CONGENITAL MALFORMATIONS

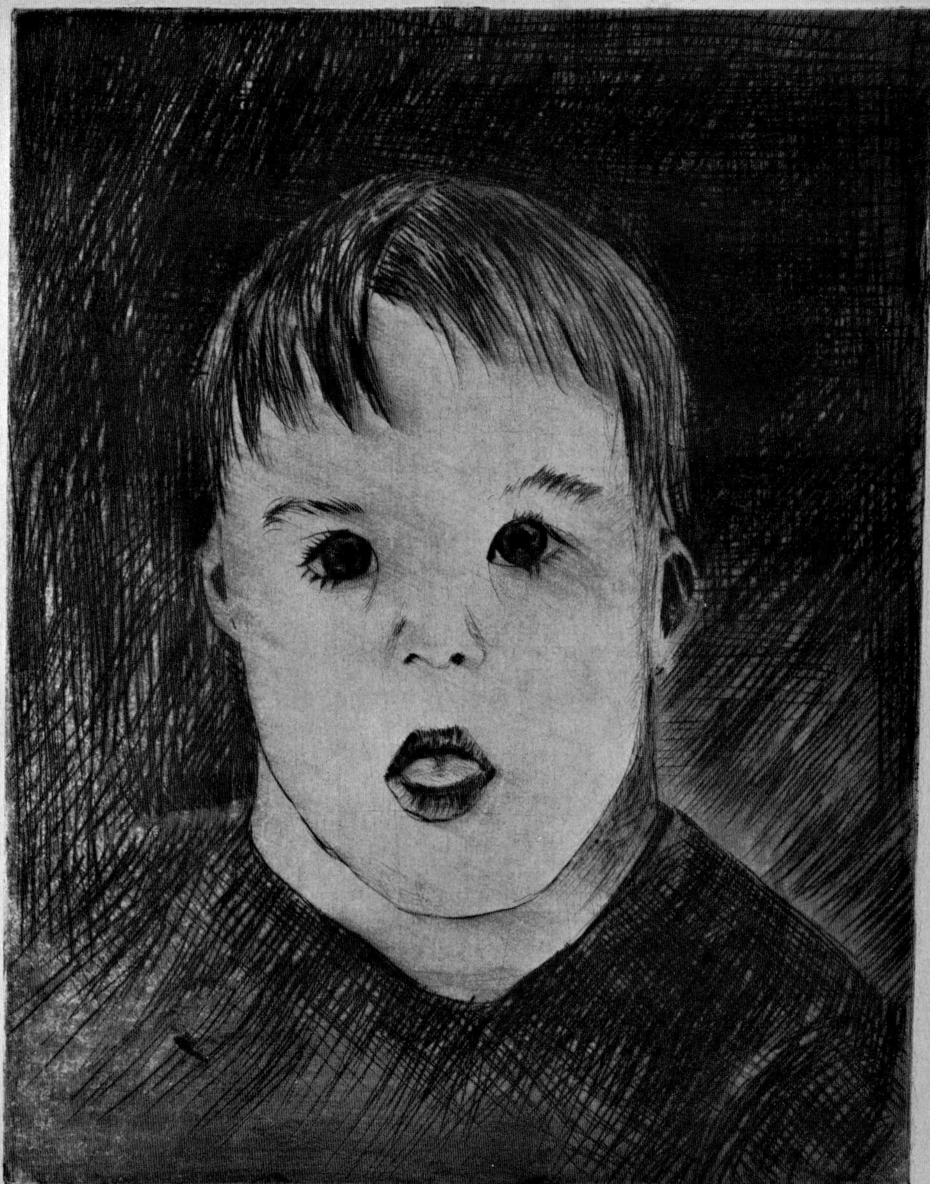

"A Child of Nondisjunction" Warkany

CONGENITAL MALFORMATIONS

Notes and Comments

JOSEF WARKANY, M.D.

Fellow of The Children's Hospital Research Foundation, Cincinnati, Ohio
Professor of Research Pediatrics, University of Cincinnati

YEAR BOOK MEDICAL PUBLISHERS · INC.
35 EAST WACKER DRIVE · CHICAGO

Library of Congress Catalog Card Number: 76-152353

International Standard Book Number: 0-8151-9098-0

Published December 1971

TO

THE CHILDREN'S HOSPITAL

RESEARCH FOUNDATION

IN

CINCINNATI, OHIO

Preface

THE NOTES AND COMMENTS published in this book are a portion of the data on congenital malformations that I have gathered over a 35-year period in which my interests have centered on this topic. During this time span, I have accumulated many books and more than 20,000 reprints concerned with congenital malformations—old and new, clinical, anatomic and experimental. It seemed timely to collect my notes and references and to make them available to others working in this field.

My interest in congenital malformations began when pediatrics was at a turning point. Following the remarkable successes in the challenges of nutritional and infectious diseases which led to prevention or quick remedy of many of the pediatric problems of the past, it became clear that there were still numerous disorders of children that needed solution. Also, it was obvious that new approaches and ways had to be found to combat and prevent the remaining disorders, which were different in origin and nature from those faced by earlier pediatricians who had concentrated on improvement of the postnatal environment of children. Congenital malformations were and are among the unsolved topics of pediatrics and it seemed worth while to focus on maladies that have their roots in prenatal life. It should be emphasized that there has been great interest and progress in diagnosis and treatment of congenital malformations during these past decades. With roentgenology, many diseases of childhood have been recognized as malformations, diseases that formerly were thought to be infectious or nutritional because postnatal complications masked the basic structural defects. The surgical specialties succeeded in repair of malformations that appeared hopeless not long ago and pediatricians learned to manage preoperative and postoperative problems of deformed children. But pediatrics has always aimed at prevention, and prevention of congenital malformations seems as necessary as prevention of contagious and alimentary disorders.

In order to avert diseases, one has to study their etiology. Like all phenomena that we observe, diseases are multifactorial in origin and the numbers of causative factors are infinite. Etiologic research must go in many directions to find factors that are not only clearly recognizable but also manageable and removable at will. Usually it cannot be predicted which approach will be rewarding and which findings will lead to preventive measures, and it seems most helpful to present all aspects of etiologic research whether they appear of practical importance today or not. This principle applies to prenatal disorders as well as to diseases of postnatal origin. In the 1930s, there was a strong belief that all congenital malformations are inherited; in fact, the terms "congenital" and "hereditary" often were equated and used interchangeably. Although there was and is no doubt that many congenital malformations are genetically determined, it seemed unwise to neglect the possibility of involvement of nongenetic factors in the etiology of congenital malformations. That environmental disturbances can lead to embryonic malformations was known from countless experiments in submammalian animals, but the mammalian embryo was thought to be so well protected by the mother that prenatal malformations were not attributed to external influences. To test this belief, it seemed desirable to develop mammalian models of congenital malformations produced by exogenous factors in the hope that such models would contribute to an understanding of malformations in children. Animal experiments had proved most successful in combating many children's diseases of the past. Attempts to provide teratologic research tools were most successful. Teratologic mammalian models are now available that can duplicate almost any type of malformation known in man. There also are animal models that exemplify spontaneous, genetically determined malformations and there are models that illustrate interaction of genetic and environmental factors. Needless to say, interpretations of animal experiments and applications to human conditions must be made with caution and prudence, since the models never simulate human circumstances completely. Fortunately, the rise of experimental mammalian teratology was paralleled by discovery of environmental causes of congenital malformations in man, discoveries that, in some instances, led to specific preventive measures. Elimination of malformations of actinic, chemical or viral origin has strengthened the belief that many aspects of experimental teratology are relevant to human disorders.

Much progress has been made in the search for genetic causes of congenital malformations. A remarkable step forward was the finding of chromosomal abnormalities as causes of certain types and combinations of congenital malformations. Although such chromosomal aberrations had been suspected for Down syndrome before, demonstration of comparable cytogenetic changes in patients with other teratologic disease pictures provided a firm basis for their explanation and led to abandonment of erroneous theories of the past.

Causes of point mutations are also under intensive study, with particular emphasis on factors created by recent changes in man's environment through modern living conditions and industrialization. To the contemporary physician dealing with congenital malformations, mutagenic factors of the past are of equal importance, and research into mutagenesis that has been with man for millennia must not be neglected because of modern threats. Many advances have been made also in classification and differentiation of gene-determined teratologic disorders, which were considered unitary entities before. Distinction of many chondrodystrophies with differing etiologic backgrounds exemplifies this point. The concept of a single chondrodystrophy (achondroplasia) as a dominantly inherited trait often led to erroneous explanations and genetic prognoses. Although many explanations of heritable disorders now appear more complicated and confused than before, they are nearer to the truth than simple and dogmatic interpretations of the past.

Despite significant progress in etiologic research on many fronts, it seems fair to say that, at present, satisfactory explanations are still wanting for the majority of congenital malformations that are seen daily in hospitals and clinics; most malformations, whether single or multiple, cannot be attributed to well-defined causes as we know them. There is understandable overemphasis of known etiologic factors—genetic or environmental—whereas the more frequent cases of unknown origin remain out of sight. Such cases may have complex causation (multifactorial or polygenic are recurrent terms) or they may be due to factors not yet discernible. Although such patients are not good subjects for teaching or publication, they are presented daily to clinicians, showing variable signs and symptoms in kaleidoscopic combinations; they need attention more than those that are easily labeled and readily explained. It must be realized that congenital malformations are manifestations of prenatal pathology, an area as large and complex as that of postnatal pathology and an area obscured by the inaccessibility of the unborn as it develops within the mother's body, concealed from direct observation and unresponsive to investigative methods traditional in postnatal research. It is not surprising that so many congenital malformations encountered by physicians remain incomprehensible and unsuitable for parental counseling. Such enigmatic cases are seldom treated in texts of medical genetics or in publications on environmental causes of malformations. But in teratologic presentations they deserve mention and description irrespective of their value to such other sciences as genetics, virology or toxicology.

Although etiologic data are most important because of their significance for preventive measures, they are treated only briefly in Part II and limited to well-established facts. Additional findings of etiologic investigations are added in chapters on specific malformations. There, observations concerning etiology often are recorded without conclusions, since the available information seemed insufficient for recognition of decisive causative factors, for parental counseling and for prevention.

It is not easy to decide how congenital malformations should be presented and arranged in a work published in a period of intensive investigation, rapid progress and change of attitudes. Aside from the general parts, most malformations are treated here according to their occurrence in organ systems. This may seem old-fashioned to those who believe that the solutions of teratologic questions are to be found in genetics, molecular biology, removal of toxic factors from the environment or protection of the mother from undue stress. Although one can hope that such beliefs and theories will contribute to elucidation of many malformations, unitary attitudes and approaches are not recommendable at a time when etiologic classifications are still in flux. Generalizations and imaginative concepts are, of course, attractive, particularly to the lay public, but one must remember that in the field of congenital malformations human imagination has ruled for millennia. There is less need for imagination than for facts—"dry" as they may be. Therefore, I have omitted explanations and theories that are unproved and controversial at this time.

There are difficulties in presenting malformations according to organ systems, since often the anomalies involve several regions and many organs. Which malformation is the most important and where should combinations of defects be dealt with? There are obvious dilemmas, and arbitrary decisions had to be made. As explained in Chapter 6 on Syndromes, different specialties have differing classifications of and attitudes toward syndromes of multiple malformations, and expositions acceptable to all teratologists—clinical and experimental—are not possible. Some types of multiple congenital malformations have established etiologic bases; they can be treated according to causation and independent of their teratologic spectra. But others are held together by signs and symptoms only and they are hard to classify. Use of the Table of Contents, of cross references and of the Index will guide the reader to areas related to but not included in the perused chapter.

Some remarks are in order to explain inclusion or omission of certain topics. The number of malformations and their combinations are infinite and most of those mentioned were selected because of common occurrence or emphasis in the medical literature. Personal experience with some of them also played a role in the selection. Since there was a lack of interest in prenatal pathology in the 1930s when I began collecting old and new data, it seemed possible to keep up with current publications, but in the following decades many fields of prenatal pathology were cultivated intensively, leading to a renaissance of teratology and of related sciences. The expansion of knowledge and information necessitated limitation of my studies, reading and notations to structural congenital malformations and to exclusion of some chapters which have assumed such proportions that they are now specialties of their own. To give an example: At first, inborn errors of metabolism were included in my studies and my notes. Now, inborn errors of metabolism are investigated and discussed so intensively that it became impossible and unnecessary to treat them in this book. Congenital malformations, i.e., structural errors present at birth, which represent the hard core of prenatally determined pathology, need more attention and research. Against the widespread belief that the problems of congenital malformations and those of inborn errors of metabolism are identical, it should be emphasized that there are striking differences in these disorders requiring different approaches. It may be true that many malformations are due to inborn errors of metabolism, but usually teratogenic metabolic errors act early in gestation and are not recognizable in postnatal life. Investigation and elucidation of their causes are much more difficult than research in inborn errors of metabolism that continue in postnatal life as biochemical anomalies accessible to chemical and enzymatic analyses. There is a danger that etiologic studies of congenital malformations will be neglected because investigators turn to fields of prenatal pathology in which harvests seem nearer and more profitable. We must not disregard structural congenital anomalies in favor of the better understood and more tractable inborn errors of metabolism recognizable in postnatal life. Other chapters considered but omitted dealt with dental malformations, twins and conjoined twins and monstrous births. Although these subjects have not been treated in special chapters, they are mentioned in places where they are relevant to the topic under discussion.

There are, on the other hand, chapters that deal with congenital defects which may not be seen in the United States by physicians trained today. The thalidomide embryopathy, endemic cretinism and the prenatal rubella syndrome were, at certain times and places, serious threats to the unborn; now they are preventable. It is worth while to recall how these disorders were investigated and how they were eliminated. In the search for prevention of existing disorders, one can learn a great deal from the successful battles of the past. Also, one could object to inclusion of some disorders which are not completely manifest at birth. Yet such conditions, although not congenital in their entire spectrum, may be foreshadowed by minor signs at or soon after birth and recognizable in early stages. The importance of their predictive signs is obvious.

Teratology reaches into many fields of medicine and into many special sciences that have accumulated huge stores of knowledge and information. There exist books, monographs and journals that deal with subjects treated in this book only briefly as chapters or as sections. My short comments often deal merely with areas of contact of such topics with teratology and my notes must be considered introductions rather than complete presentations. References to special publications can guide the reader to more detailed information and references may help the scholar who seeks answers to questions that I left unresolved. Although references to previous publications are ample, they are not exhaustive. Some publications were not available to me, and of those obtainable only a fraction could be cited. The selections made may seem arbitrary in places, but there were obvious difficulties. Should one quote the authors who opened up a subject or should one quote those who made the latest contribution with good reviews of previous work? Or should one quote important publications made in between? In many places I have cited old publications as well as new; but this could be done only to a limited extent. In teratology, much outstanding work was done decades ago. Some thoughts and studies published in books and journals long relegated to the basements of our libraries occasionally are presented as original by recent authors. Perusal of the old literature would disclose that many "new" theories and "new" syndromes are not as new as some authors believe. I have attempted to bridge some generation gaps but could do so merely to a limited extent, since I have only a modest knowledge of the treasures accumulated in the old teratologic literature.

A few words should be said about the illustrations. Most of the photographs reproduced show malformations seen in children but there also are pictures of animals with malformations produced experimentally. Since I have pointed out that extrapolations from animal experiments to human situations must be made with caution, the intermingling of pictures of human malformations with malformations induced by teratogenic procedures may seem surprising. I wish to emphasize that the illustrations derived from animal experiments should not convey the idea that corresponding human malformations have similar or identical causes. Pictures of deformed animals, particularly of histologic sections of such animals, are used because often they show malformations better than their human counterparts. It is obvious that it is difficult to obtain human specimens in proper stages of development and preservation. Sections of an entire head, chest or abdomen of a small laboratory animal are most helpful in illustrating deviations from the normal; they can serve in place of diagrams when they demonstrate features resembling those of human malformations.

Finally, I should like to acknowledge the encouragement, help and support I was given in the efforts that made this work possible. But here I find myself in a position of frustration, since there were so many men and women over these years who contributed to the collection of data, references, illustrations, writing of the manuscript, reading of proofs and so forth that even the longest list would be incomplete. The best way to acknowledge the help I received is to point out that The Children's Hospital Research Foundation of Cincinnati with its affiliated hospitals and institutions created the atmosphere of freedom of inquiry, cooperation and scholarship that enabled me to read, study, investigate and experiment in search for answers to pediatric questions. It seems appropriate to thank all those who helped me by dedicating this book to the institution with which most of those who made contributions were connected in one way or another.

JOSEF WARKANY

Table of Contents

PART I
General Considerations

1. **Definitions** 3
2. **Teratology of the Past** 6
   - Images 6
   - Malformations as Portents 7
   - Maternal Impressions 12
   - Hybridization 15
   - Devils and Witches 15
   - Infanticide 16
   - Biologic Theories of the Past 17
3. **Present Trends in Teratology** 21
4. **Beginnings of Experimental Mammalian Teratology** 29
5. **Some Problems of Statistics** 38
   - Incidence 38
   - Congenital Malformations and Morbidity 40
   - Congenital Malformations and Natural Screening 41
6. **Syndromes** 43
7. **Sensitive or Critical Periods in Teratogenesis: Uses and Abuses of Embryologic Timetables** 49

PART II
Etiologic Factors

Introduction 55

SECTION ONE

8. **Genetic and Chromosomal Factors** 57
   - Genetic Factors 57
   - Chromosomal Abnormalities 58

SECTION TWO

Environmental Factors **61**
9. Infections **62**
Rubella 62
Pathogenesis and Pathology 63
Clinical Manifestations 65
Prognosis 68
Prevention 68
Cytomegalic Inclusion Disease 71
Herpesvirus 75
Viruses as Experimental Teratogens 75
Various Infectious Diseases 76
Toxoplasmosis 78
10. Irradiation **82**
11. Drugs **84**
Thalidomide 84
Some Other Drugs 96
Aminopterin (4-aminopteroylglutamic acid) and Methotrexate . . . 96
Cyclophosphamide 97
Myleran 97
Quinine 97
Anticonvulsant Drugs 98
Antituberculosis Drugs 99
Meclizine 99
Masculinizing Progesterones and Estrogens 100
Cortisone and ACTH 100
Experimental Teratology and Drug Testing 101
12. Maternal Disorders **102**
Endemic Goiter and Cretinism 102
Etiology 106
Accessory Etiologic Factors 107
Pathogenesis 109
Symptomatology 111
Treatment 116
Prevention 116
Diabetes 124
Phenylketonuria 125
Thyroid Disease 126
Tuberculosis 127
Hypoxia 127
Vitamin A Deficiency 127

Carbon Monoxide Poisoning . . . 128
Minamata Disease . . . 128
Lead Poisoning . . . 129

PART III
General Disturbances of Growth and Development

13. Dwarfism . . . **133**
14. Intrauterine Growth Retardation . . . **134**
Children with Intrauterine Growth Retardation . . . 136
Clinical Disease Pictures Sometimes Associated with Intrauterine Growth Retardation . . . 136
Etiology . . . 143
Mothers of Children with Intrauterine Growth Retardation . . . 147
Dietary Deficiencies of Women . . . 147
Placental Insufficiency . . . 147
Hypoxia . . . 149
Exposure to X-Rays . . . 149
Other Exogenous Teratogens . . . 149
Twinning . . . 151
Pathogenesis . . . 151
Prognosis . . . 152
Treatment . . . 153
Telangiectatic Erythema and Stunted Growth (Bloom Syndrome) . . . 157
Leprechaunism . . . 159
Progeria . . . 160
15. Hemidystrophies and Hemisyndromes . . . **162**
Hemihypertrophy . . . 163
Hemidystrophies . . . 167
Hemiatrophy . . . 168
16. Visceromegaly (Beckwith-Wiedemann Syndrome) . . . **171**
17. Cerebral Gigantism . . . **173**
Congenital Generalized Lipodystrophy . . . 174
18. Diencephalic Cachexia . . . **174**
19. Laurence-Moon-Biedl Syndrome . . . **176**
Tumors and the Laurence-Moon-Biedl Syndrome . . . 180
20. Prader-Willi Syndrome . . . **182**
21. Situs Inversus . . . **183**

PART IV
Malformations of the Central Nervous System

SECTION ONE: CEREBRUM AND CEREBELLUM

22. Anencephaly **189**
Morphogenesis 191
Malformations 195
23. Cyclopia-Arhinencephaly Series **201**
Cyclopia 202
Ethmocephaly and Cebocephaly 206
Arhinencephaly with Double Proboscis 207
Arhinencephaly with Median Harelip 207
Arhinencephaly with Lateral Cleft Lips and Cleft Palate 208
Arhinencephaly with Trigonocephaly 209
Microcephaly and Olfactory Deficiency 210
24. Cephaloceles **211**
25. Hydrocephaly **217**
Incidence 217
Etiology 217
Pathogenesis 219
Symptoms 226
Diagnosis 227
Treatment 228
26. Hydranencephaly **231**
27. Iniencephaly **234**
28. Microcephaly **237**
Etiology 238
Pathology 242
Symptoms 242
29. Macrencephaly (Megalencephaly) **244**
Pseudohydrocephaly 245
30. Congenital Porencephaly and Schizencephaly **246**
31. Cerebrovascular Malformations **249**
Arteriovenous Malformations 249
Congenital Aneurysms 250
32. Agenesis and Hypoplasia of the Corpus Callosum **252**
Cavum Septi Pellucidi; Cavum Vergae; Cavum Veli Interpositi . . . 254
33. Cerebral Palsy **255**

34. Mental Retardation **262**
35. Cerebellar Malformations **267**
Pathology 268
Symptoms 269
Ataxia-Telangiectasia 270

SECTION TWO: SPINAL CORD

36. Spina Bifida **272**
Incidence 272
Etiology 273
Pathogenesis 275
Pathology 282
Symptoms 285
Prognosis 288
Genetic Prognosis 288
Treatment 288
Hydromyelia 291
Diastematomyelia 291
Myelodysplasia, Syringomyelia and Status Dysraphicus 292
Myelodysplasia 294
Syringomyelia 294
Familial Osseous Atrophy 295

SECTION THREE: SOME SYNDROMES INVOLVING MALFORMATIONS OF THE CENTRAL NERVOUS SYSTEM

37. Syndromes of Chromosomal Abnormalities **296**
Trisomy 13-15 (D_1) 296
Deficiency of the Long Arm of a Chromosome D 303
Trisomy 18 303
Clinical and Pathologic Characteristics 305
Deficiency of the Short Arm of Chromosome 18 310
Deficiency of the Long Arm of Chromosome 18 311
Ring Chromosome 18 311
Down Syndrome (Mongolism, Trisomy 21) 311
Incidence 312
Etiology 313
Translocation Down Syndrome 316
Mosaicism 319
Prevalence of Trisomy 21 in Patients with Down Syndrome 320
Down Syndrome with Normal Karyotype 320
Partial Down Syndrome 321
Offspring of Women with Down Syndrome 321
Down Syndrome in Young Mothers 322
Multiple Aneuploidies 322

Indications for Chromosome Analysis . . . 322
Some Present Etiologic Theories . . . 323
Clinical and Pathologic Characteristics . . . 324
Dermatoglyphics . . . 331
Biochemical Data . . . 331
Blood . . . 333
Differential Diagnosis . . . 333
Prevention . . . 334
Treatment . . . 334
Monosomy G (Antimongolism) . . . 339
Cat-Cry Syndrome (Syndrome du Cri du Chat: Partial Deletion of the Short Arm of Chromosome 5) . . . 340
Ring-1 Chromosome and Microcephalic Dwarfism . . . 343
Triploidy . . . 343
38. Some Syndromes of Uncertain Origin . . . 344
Cornelia de Lange Syndrome (Brachmann-de Lange Syndrome [Typus Amstelodamensis]) . . . 344
Cerebro-Hepato-Renal Syndromes . . . 347
Microcephaly and Genital Anomalies . . . 348
Microcephaly and Cleft Palate . . . 348
Puppet Syndrome . . . 349
Sturge-Weber Syndrome . . . 349

PART V
Malformations of the Eye

39. Ocular Defects . . . 355
The Lids . . . 355
The Lacrimal Apparatus . . . 355
Dyskeratosis . . . 356
Anophthalmia and Microphthalmia . . . 356
The Eye in Cyclopia and Anencephaly . . . 361
Congenital Cystic Eye . . . 361
Cryptophthalmia . . . 361
Congenital Coloboma . . . 361
Orbital Cysts . . . 365
Hydrophthalmia (Infantile Glaucoma, Buphthalmos) . . . 365
Anomalies of the Cornea . . . 367
Microcornea . . . 367
Megalocornea . . . 367
Keratoconus . . . 367
Congenital Corneal Opacities . . . 367

Systemic Disorders Involving the Cornea 368

The Iris 369

Aniridia 369

Anomalies of Iris Color 370

Heterochromia 370

Brushfield Spots 371

Cysts of the Iris 371

Mesodermal and Ectodermal Dysgenesis (Rieger Disease) 371

The Pupils 371

Persistent Pupillary Membrane 371

Congenital Anisocoria 372

Corectopia (Ectopic Pupil) 372

Slit Pupil 372

Polycoria 372

The Lens 372

Congenital Cataract 372

Cataract in Galactosemia 374

Cataract in Down Syndrome 374

Cataract with Skeletal Disorders 375

Cataract following Prenatal Rubella 375

Cataract with Skin and Dental Disorders 376

Ectopia of the Lens 376

The Retina 377

Retinal Aplasia (Congenital Amaurosis; Heredo-Retinopathia Congenitalis Monohybrida Recessiva Autosomalis) 377

Congenital Detachment of the Retina 377

Congenital Retinoschisis (Congenital Vascular Veil in the Vitreous) . 378

Choroideremia 378

Myelinated Nerve Fibers in the Retina 378

Retinitis Pigmentosa (Tapetoretinal Degenerations) 378

Hereditary Degeneration of the Macula (Macular Dystrophy) 379

Macular Dysplasia (Pseudocoloboma) 379

Coloboma of the Disc 379

Congenital Crescents of the Optic Disc 379

Aplasia and Hypoplasia of the Optic Nerve 379

Congenital Atrophy of the Optic Nerve 380

Gliomas of the Optic Nerve 380

Retinoblastoma 380

Toxoplasmosis of the Eye 381

Cytomegalic Inclusion Disease 382

Ocular Changes in Hamartoses 382

Ocular Changes in Sturge-Weber Disease 383

The Eye in the Thalidomide Embryopathy 383

40. Some Syndromes Involving Ocular Defects **388**
Oculoauriculovertebral Syndrome (Goldenhar Syndrome; Mandibulofacial Dysostosis with Epibulbar Dermoids) 388
Oculodentodigital Dysplasia 388
Oculocerebrorenal Syndrome (Lowe Syndrome) 389
Craniofacial Dysostosis with Congenital Cataract, Hypotrichosis and Dwarfism (Hallermann-Streiff Syndrome; François Syndrome; Dyscephalia Mandibulo-oculofacialis) 390
Congenital Cataract and Ataxia (Marinesco-Sjögren Syndrome) . . . 392
Rothmund-Thomson Syndrome (Poikiloderma Congenitale) 392
Marchesani Syndrome, Brachydactyly and Congenital Spherical Lens (Microphakia) 395
Waardenburg Syndrome 395
Möbius Syndrome (Nuclear Agenesis; Congenital Facial Diplegia) . . 397
Cockayne Syndrome (Mental Retardation, Dwarfism, Retinal Pigmentation and Deafness) 398
Pseudoglioma with Mental Retardation (Norrie Disease) 398

PART VI
Malformations of the Ear

41. Aural Defects **401**
Anotia 401
Cryptotia 401
Uncomplicated Hereditary Microtia 401
Microtia with Atresia of the External Meatus 401
Synotia and Melotia (Otocephaly) 402
External Meatus 402
Congenital Auricular Fistulas 403
Auricular Appendages 403
Darwinian Tubercle and Other Variations 404
Lop Ear 404
Malformations of the Middle Ear 404
Malformations of the Inner Ear 406
Deafness 407
Recessively Inherited Deafness and Deaf-Mutism 407
Dominantly Inherited Deafness and Deaf-Mutism 408
Sex-Linked Recessive Deafness 409
The Ear in Chromosomal Syndromes 409
The Ear in Anencephaly 410
The Ear in Hydrocephaly 411
The Ear in Mandibulofacial Dysostosis 411

Oculoauriculovertebral Dysplasia . . . 411
The Ear in Congenital Renal Disorders . . . 411
The Ear in the Rubella Embryopathy . . . 412
The Ear in Toxoplasmosis . . . 413
The Ear in Endemic Cretinism (Maternal Iodine Deficiency) . . . 413
Maternal Pseudohypoparathyroidism . . . 414
Deafness and Kernicterus . . . 414
Congenital Deafness due to Drugs . . . 414
Auriculo-osteodysplasia . . . 415

PART VII

Malformations of Endocrine Glands

42. The Pituitary Gland . . . 419
Congenital Absence of the Pituitary Gland . . . 419
Congenital Hypoplasia of the Pituitary Gland . . . 420
Duplication of the Pituitary . . . 420
Persistence of the Craniopharyngeal Canal . . . 420
The Pharyngeal Pituitary . . . 421
Pituitary Dystopia . . . 421
Rathke-Cleft Cysts . . . 422
Craniopharyngioma (Adamantinoma, Ameloblastoma) . . . 423
Pituitary Dwarfism . . . 423
Teratomas in the Pituitary Area . . . 424
Hyperpituitarism and Acromegaly . . . 424
Goliath Syndrome . . . 425
43. The Adrenal Gland . . . 427
Adrenal Aplasia . . . 427
Congenital Adrenal Hypoplasia . . . 428
Dystopia of the Adrenal Gland . . . 429
Accessory Adrenals . . . 429
The Adrenal in Anencephaly . . . 430
Fusion of the Adrenals . . . 431
Congenital Adrenal Cysts . . . 431
Adrenal Atrophy Occurring in Familial Aggregation with Manifestations Beginning in Postnatal Life . . . 431
Hypoadrenocorticism and Hypoparathyroidism . . . 432
Cushing Syndrome . . . 433
Adrenal Hypertrophies . . . 434
Adrenal Tumor and Hemihypertrophy . . . 434

Adrenal Tumor and Visceromegaly . . . 435
Pheochromocytoma . . . 435
44. The Thyroid Gland . . . 437
Sporadic Cretinism . . . 437
Congenital Athyrosis and Thyroid Ectopia . . . 438
Ectopic Thyroid . . . 438
Nonendemic Goitrous Cretinism ("Familial Goiter") . . . 441
Congenital Goiter or Hypothyroidism Attributed to Maternal Drug Intake . . . 442
Thiouracil and Derivatives . . . 442
Iodide . . . 443
Radioactive Iodine . . . 443
Congenital Hyperthyroidism . . . 443
45. The Parathyroids . . . 445
Absence of Parathyroids . . . 445
Hypoparathyroidism . . . 445
Pseudohypoparathyroidism . . . 446
Pseudo-pseudohypoparathyroidism (Metacarpal Dwarfism without Tetany; Albright Hereditary Osteodystrophy without Hypocalcemia) . . . 448
Congenital Hyperparathyroidism . . . 449
46. The Pineal Body . . . 450
Aplasia of the Pineal Gland . . . 450
Hypoplasia of the Pineal Gland . . . 451
Pineal Hyperplasia . . . 451
Pineal Tumors . . . 451
Cysts of the Pineal Body . . . 452
47. Endocrine-Hypothalamic Disorders . . . 453
Diabetes Insipidus . . . 453
Oliguria . . . 454
Cushing Syndrome . . . 454
Precocious Puberty . . . 454

PART VIII
Cardiovascular Malformations

SECTION ONE

48. Etiologic Factors in Congenital Heart Disease . . . 459
Congenital Heart Disease in More than One Generation . . . 460
Congenital Heart Disease in Siblings . . . 461
Congenital Heart Disease and Chromosomal Anomalies . . . 462
Environmental Factors . . . 463
49. Experimental Production of Cardiovascular Malformations in Mammals . . . 470

SECTION TWO

50. Acardia **473**
Ectopia Cordis 475
Incomplete Ectopia Cordis 475
Parchment Heart 477
51. Dextrocardia **477**
52. Atrial Septal Defects **480**
Persistent Ostium Atrioventriculare Commune 485
Cor Triloculare Biventriculare 486
Cor Triatriatum 487
Prenatal Closure of the Interatrial Foramen 488
Juxtaposition of the Atrial Appendages 489
53. Ventricular Septal Defects **489**
Tetralogy of Fallot 494
Eisenmenger Syndrome 503
Cor Triloculare Biatriatum (Single Ventricle) 503
54. Tricuspid Malformations **505**
Tricuspid Atresia 505
Tricuspid Hypoplasia 506
Congenital Tricuspid Insufficiency 506
Duplication of the Tricuspid Valve 506
Ebstein Malformation 507
55. Congenital Mitral Malformations **509**
Mitral Stenosis 509
Mitral Atresia 510
Duplication of the Mitral Valve 510

SECTION THREE

56. Persistent Truncus Arteriosus **512**
57. Transposition of the Great Vessels **515**
Corrected Transposition of the Great Vessels 523
58. Aortic Arch Anomalies **526**
Persistence of a Third Aortic Arch 528
Anomalous Innominate Artery and Anomalous Left Common Carotid Artery 529
Fourth Aortic Arch Anomalies 529
Double Aortic Arch 529
Left Aortic Arch with Right Descending Aorta 531
Right Aortic Arch 531
Interruption of the Aortic Arch ("Steidele Complex") 532
Kinking of the Aortic Arch 533
Anomalous Subclavian Artery 533
Sixth (Pulmonary) Aortic Arch Anomalies 534
Anomalies of the Ductus Arteriosus 534

Aberrant Left Pulmonary Artery . . . 535
Agenesis of a Pulmonary Artery . . . 535
59. The Aorta . . . 537
Congenital Atresia of the Aorta . . . 537
Congenital Aortic Stenosis . . . 539
Supravalvar Aortic Stenosis . . . 541
Subvalvar Aortic Stenosis and Idiopathic Cardiomegaly . . . 542
Coarctation of the Aorta . . . 542
Severe Forms . . . 546
Coarctation of the Abdominal Aorta . . . 546
Congenital Aortic Aneurysm . . . 547
Congenital Aneurysm of a Sinus of Valsalva . . . 548
60. The Pulmonary Arteries . . . 548
Classification of Congenital Malformations of the Pulmonary Arteries . 548
Congenital Absence of the Pulmonary Valve . . . 549
Etiology of Pulmonary Stenosis . . . 549
Pulmonary Atresia . . . 550
Pulmonary Stenosis with Normal Aortic Root . . . 551
61. Ductus Arteriosus . . . 553
Absence of the Ductus Arteriosus . . . 553
Physiologic Closure of the Ductus . . . 554
Persistent Patent Ductus Arteriosus . . . 555
Intrauterine Closure of the Ductus . . . 559
62. The Coronary Arteries . . . 561
Anomalies of the Coronary Arteries . . . 561
Aneurysm of the Coronary Arteries . . . 562
Single Coronary Artery . . . 562
Coronary Arteriovenous Fistula . . . 563
63. Anomalies of Venous Return . . . 564
Systemic Veins . . . 564
Pulmonary Veins . . . 565

SECTION FOUR

64. Systemic Disorders Involving Cardiovascular Malformations . . . 568
Associated Malformations . . . 568
Neurologic, Ocular and Mental Complications . . . 570
Gastrointestinal Malformations . . . 571
Skeletal Malformations . . . 571
Cleft Lip and Cleft Palate . . . 573
Urinary Tract Malformations . . . 574
Genital Tract Malformations . . . 574
Metabolic Disorders . . . 574
Chromosomal Anomalies and Congenital Heart Disease . . . 576
Down Syndrome (Mongolism) . . . 576

Palmar Dermatoglyphics and Fingerprints in Congenital Heart Disease . . . 578
Supravalvar Aortic Stenosis Complex ("Supravalvar Aortic Stenosis," Facial Anomalies and Hypercalcemia) . . . 578
Familial Syndrome of Right-Sided Aortic Arch, Mental Retardation and Facial Characteristics . . . 580
Cardiofacial Syndromes . . . 580
Cardio-Auditory Syndromes . . . 581
65. Other Congenital Disorders of the Heart . . . 582
Congenital Tumors . . . 582
Tumors Associated with Congenital Heart Disease . . . 582
Congenital Heart Block . . . 583
Obstructive Cardiomyopathy (Asymmetric Hypertrophy of the Heart in Young Adults) . . . 584

PART IX
Malformations of the Respiratory Tract

66. The Nose . . . 587
Nasal Aplasia . . . 587
The Nose In Arhinencephaly . . . 587
Proboscis Lateralis . . . 589
Bilateral Proboscis . . . 589
Median Nasal Clefts . . . 589
Lateral Nasal Clefts . . . 590
Duplication of the Nose (Polyrhinia) . . . 591
Gliomas and Encephaloceles in the Nasal Area . . . 591
Congenital Dermoid Cysts of the Nose . . . 593
Mucoids . . . 594
Congenital Saddle Nose . . . 594
Choanal Atresia . . . 594
Trisomy 13-15 (D_1) and Nasal Anomalies . . . 595
67. The Larynx . . . 596
Congenital Subglottic Hemangioma . . . 596
Papillomas . . . 596
Congenital Webs . . . 597
Congenital Cysts . . . 597
Congenital Atresia . . . 597
Laryngotracheo-esophageal Cleft . . . 597
Laryngocele (Aerocele) . . . 598

68. The Trachea and Bronchi . . . 599
Absence and Stenosis of the Trachea . . . 599
Abnormal Segmentation of the Cartilaginous Skeleton of the Trachea or Bronchi . . . 599
Tracheal Diverticula . . . 599
Congenital Fistulas of the Trachea . . . 600
Bronchial Atresia . . . 600
Tracheal Bronchi . . . 600
Left Eparterial Bronchus . . . 601
Displacement of Segmental and Subsegmental Bronchi . . . 601
Congenital Bronchiectases . . . 601
Kartagener Syndrome . . . 602
Bronchogenic Cysts of the Mediastinum . . . 603
Endobronchial Hamartomas . . . 603
Congenital Bronchomalacia . . . 603
Congenital Bronchobiliary Fistula . . . 603
69. The Lung . . . 604
Agenesis, Aplasia and Hypoplasia . . . 604
Bilateral Agenesis and Aplasia . . . 604
Unilateral Agenesis . . . 605
Hypoplasia . . . 606
Accessory or Supernumerary Lungs . . . 607
Supernumerary Fissures and Congenitally Fused Lobes . . . 608
Lobe of the Azygos Vein . . . 609
Sequestration of Lung Tissue Associated with an Abnormal Pulmonary Artery . . . 609
Congenital Pulmonary Cysts . . . 610
Congenital Emphysema . . . 612
Congenital Cystic Lymphangiectasis . . . 613
Pulmonary Arteriovenous Fistulas . . . 613
Relation of Pulmonary Tumors to Malformations . . . 615

PART X
Malformations of the Face

70. Facial Anomalies . . . 621
Agnathia . . . 621
The Face and Mouth in Otocephaly (Synotia) . . . 621
Micrognathia . . . 621
Macrognathia . . . 622
Cherubism (Familial Fibrous Dysplasia of the Jaws) . . . 622

Microstomia . . . 623
Macrostomia . . . 623
Hemifacial Hypoplasia (Hemifacial Microsomia, Unilateral Mandibulofacial Dysostosis) and Hemifacial Hyperplasia . . . 624
Median Cleft of the Upper Lip . . . 624
Oblique Facial Clefts . . . 624
Lip Anomalies . . . 625
Short and Long Upper Lip . . . 625
Double Lip . . . 626
Clefts of the Mandible and Lower Lip . . . 626
Congenital Pits and Fistulas of the Lips . . . 626
Bilateral Clefts of the Lower Lip . . . 627
Cysts of the Jaws . . . 627
Temporomandibular Joint . . . 627
Cleft Lip and Palate . . . 628
Frequency of Cleft Lip and Palate . . . 628
Etiology . . . 629
Development of the Face and Palate . . . 633
Pathogenesis and Experimental Work . . . 636
Clinical Classifications . . . 640
Associated Malformations . . . 642
71. Some Syndromes Involving the Face . . . 650
Mandibulofacial Dysostosis (Treacher Collins Syndrome; Franceschetti-Zwahlen Syndrome) . . . 650
Unilateral Mandibulofacial Dysostosis (Weyers) . . . 653
Micrognathia with Glossoptosis (Pierre Robin Syndrome) . . . 654
Cerebro-Costo-Mandibular Syndrome . . . 658

PART XI
Malformations of the Oro-gastrointestinal Tract

72. The Mouth and Pharynx . . . 661
Fusion of the Gums . . . 661
Ankyloglossia . . . 661
Aglossia and Microglossia . . . 661
Macroglossia . . . 662
Accessory Tongue . . . 663
Long Tongue . . . 663

Cleft or Bifid Tongue 663
Glossitis Rhombica Mediana 663
Lingual Thyroid 664
Developmental Anomalies of the Thyroid 664
Partial Agenesis and Hypoplasia of the Thyroid 664
Fordyce Granules 664
Leukokeratosis 665
Melanin Pigmentation Associated with Intestinal Polyposis (Peutz-Jeghers Syndrome) 665
Oral Leukoplakias 665
Torus Buccalis 665
Torus Palatinus 665
Torus Mandibularis 665
Congenital Cysts of the Mouth 666
Salivary Glands 666
Tumors 667
Teratoma of the Tonsil 668
Teratoid Parasites of the Mouth 668
Congenital Atresia of the Oropharynx 668
The Pharynx 668
Branchiogenic Fistulas and Cysts 669
Congenital Pharyngeal Pouches (Diverticula) 670

73. Some Syndromes Involving Oral and Pharyngeal Anomalies 673

Craniocarpotarsal Dystrophy (Freeman-Sheldon Syndrome) 673
Orodigitofacial Syndrome (Syndrome of Papillon-Léage and Psaume) 674
Otopalatodigital Syndrome 677

74. The Esophagus 678

Tracheo-Esophageal Fistula and Esophageal Atresia 678
Congenital Esophageal Stenoses 683
Congenital Esophageal Ulcer; Esophagitis 684
Hiatus Hernia, Partial Thoracic Stomach and Short Esophagus 684

75. The Stomach 686

Congenital Gastric Obstruction 686
Congenital Prepyloric Gastric Atresia 686
Hypertrophic Pyloric Stenosis 687
Congenital Defect of Gastric Musculature and Perforation 688
Duplication 688
Gastric Diverticula 689
Situs Inversus 689
Enterogenous Cysts 689
Teratoma 689
Polyposis 689

76. The Intestine **690**
Rotation and Malrotation of the Intestine 690
Underdevelopment of the Intestine 693
Congenital Atresias of the Intestine 694
Duplications of the Alimentary Tract 696
Intestinal Diverticula 698
Intestinal and Mediastinal Malformations Attributed to Abnormal Neurenteric Connections 700
Persistence of the Vitelline Duct and Meckel Diverticulum 701
Malformations of the Appendix 703
Congenital Mesenteric Cysts 703
Congenital Megacolon (Hirschsprung Disease) 704
Malformations of the Hindgut and Anus 709
Ano-Rectal Malformations 710
Exstrophia Splanchnica (Exstrophy of the Cloaca) 712
Polyposes 714
Gastrointestinal Polyposis with Pigmentation of the Oral Mucosa (Peutz Syndrome) 714
Hereditary Polyposis of the Colon 714
Benign Lymphoid Polyposis 715

77. The Liver **716**
Malformations 716
Anomalies of the Bile Ducts 718
Congenital Atresia of the Extrahepatic Bile Ducts 718
Congenital Atresia of the Intrahepatic Bile Ducts 720
Congenital Hepatitis 720
Congenital Choledochal Cysts 721
Congenital Malformations of the Gallbladder; Absence of the Gallbladder 722
Duplication of the Gallbladder 722
Tracheobiliary Fistula 723
Congenital Polycystic Disease; Congenital Hepatic Fibrosis 724
Arteriovenous Fistula of the Hepatic Artery and Portal Vein 726
Congenital Absence of the Terminal Portal Vein 726
Congenital Tumors 727
Chorioepithelioma 727
Hamartomas 727
Teratomas 728
Hemangiomas 728
Familial Intrahepatic Cholestasis 729

78. The Pancreas **729**
Malformations 729

Congenital Lipomatosis . . . 732
Cystic Fibrosis of the Pancreas (Mucoviscidosis) . . . 732

PART XII
Malformations Related to the Oro-gastrointestinal Tract

79. The Thymus . . . 739
Agenesis . . . 739
Hypoplasia . . . 740
Abnormal Shape and Position . . . 741
80. The Spleen . . . 745
Agenesis . . . 745
Hypoplasia . . . 748
Accessory Spleens . . . 748
Double Spleen . . . 748
Wandering Spleen . . . 748
Cysts and Hemangiomas . . . 749
Splenic-Gonadal Fusion . . . 749
81. Congenital Diaphragmatic Hernias . . . 751
Dorsolateral Hernias . . . 753
Left Dorsolateral Hernias . . . 753
Hernia of the Right Diaphragm . . . 755
Retrosternal Hernias . . . 755
Pericardo-Diaphragmatic Hernia . . . 756
Hiatus Hernias . . . 756
Eventration of the Diaphragm . . . 756
Accessory Diaphragm . . . 756
82. The Umbilicus . . . 758
Hernias . . . 758
Omphalocele (Exomphalos, Umbilical Eventration) . . . 758
Gastroschisis . . . 761
Remnants of the Vitelline Duct (Omphalo-Mesenteric Sinus; Omphalo-Enteric Duct) . . . 762
Schizosomia Reflexum (Strophosomia) . . . 762
Single Umbilical Artery . . . 763

PART XIII
Systemic Skeletal Malformations

Chondrodystrophies 767

83. Achondroplasia 768

84. Atypical Chondrodystrophies I (Transmitted Like Dominant Hereditary Traits) 782

Hypochondroplasia 783

Peripheral Chondrodysplasia 783

"Pseudoachondroplasia" (Spondylo-Epiphyseal Dysplasia) 783

Dysplasia Epiphysealis Multiplex 786

Madelung Deformity and Familial Dyschondrosteosis 790

Metaphyseal Dysostosis 791

Micromelia with Hypoplasia of Ulna and Fibula 792

Dwarfism with Medullary Stenosis of Tubular Bones and Transitory Tetany 792

Benign Achondroplasias 793

85. Atypical Chondrodystrophies II (Transmitted Like Recessive Hereditary Traits) 793

Chondroectodermal Dysplasia (Ellis-van Creveld Syndrome) 793

Asphyxiating Thoracic Dystrophy of the Newborn 795

Cartilage-Hair Hypoplasia 797

Chondrodystrophia Calcificans Congenita (Stippled Epiphyses, Dysplasia Epiphysealis Punctata, Conradi's Disease) 797

Diastrophic Dwarfism 801

Metatropic Dwarfism 803

Chondrodystrophy with Retinal Detachment and Deafness 804

"Achondrogenesis" 804

86. Atypical Chondrodystrophies III (Transmitted Like a Sex-Linked Recessive Trait or of Unknown Etiology) 805

Hereditary Osteochondrodystrophia Deformans (Jacobsen) (Dysplasia Spondylo-Epiphysealis Tarda) 805

Chondrodystrophy and Acrocephaly 805

87. Epiphyseal Dysgenesis in Cretinism; Kaschin-Beck Disease 806

Cretinism 806

Kaschin-Beck Disease (Osteochondroarthrosis Deformans, Osteoarthritis Endemica, Osteochondral Epiphyseopathy, Urow Disease) 807

88. Gargoylism and Other Mucopolysaccharidoses (Dysostosis Multiplex; Lipochondrodystrophies) 808

Hurler Syndrome 809

Hunter Syndrome . . . 816
Sanfilippo Syndrome (Polydystrophic Oligophrenia) . . . 817
Scheie Syndrome . . . 817
Polydystrophic Dwarfism . . . 817
Morquio-Ullrich Syndrome (Late Hurler Syndrome) . . . 817
Morquio Disease (Brailsford Chondro-osteodystrophy; Familial Osseous Dystrophy; Hereditary Osteochondrodystrophy) . . . 819
Lipomucopolysaccharidosis . . . 821

89. Osteogenesis Imperfecta (Osteopsathyrosis) . . . 824

90. Other Heritable Skeletal Disorders . . . 836

Cleidocranial Dysostosis . . . 836
Hereditary Multiple Exostoses (Hereditary Deforming Chondrodysplasia; Diaphyseal Aclasis) . . . 840
Osteopathia Hyperostotica Sclerotisans (Camurati-Engelmann Disease) . . . 844
Osteopoikilosis (Osteopathia Condensans Disseminata; "Spotted Bones") . . . 846
Pleonosteosis (Léri) . . . 847
Hereditary Hypertrophic Osteoarthropathy (Familial Idiopathic Osteoarthropathy; Pachydermoperiostosis) . . . 848

91. Arachnodactyly and Homocystinuria . . . 850

The Arachnodactyly Syndrome (Marfan Syndrome; Dolichostenomelia) . . . 850
Homocystinuria . . . 857

92. Hypophosphatasia and Hyperphosphatasia . . . 859

Hypophosphatasia . . . 859
Hyperphosphatasia (Familial Osteoectasia with Macrocranium) . . . 862

93. Osteopetrosis; Pyknodysostosis; Pyle Disease . . . 863

Osteopetrosis (Marble Bones; Albers-Schönberg Disease; Osteosclerosis Fragilis Generalisata) . . . 863
Pyknodysostosis (Osteopetrosis Acro-osteolytica, etc.) . . . 869
Pyle Disease (Familial Metaphyseal or Craniometaphyseal Dysplasia) . . . 870

94. Skeletal Disorders of Uncertain Etiology . . . 872

Ollier Disease (Dyschondroplasia) . . . 872
Systemic Chondromatosis (Enchondroma and Ecchondroma) . . . 874
Fibrous Dysplasia of Bone . . . 875
Fibrous Dysplasia with Areas of Pigmentation and Endocrine Dysfunction (Albright Disease) . . . 878
Maffucci Syndrome (Dyschondroplasia with Hemangiomatosis) . . . 882
Melorheostosis (Osteosis eburnisans monomelica) . . . 884
Infantile Cortical Hyperostosis (Roske-Caffey Disease) . . . 885

PART XIV
Malformations of the Axial and Appendicular Skeleton

95. The Skull **889**

Congenital Defects 889

Cranioschisis and Cranium Bifidum 889

Cranial Dysostosis 889

Craniolacunia (Lacunar Skull, Lückenschädel) 890

Persistent Metopic Fontanelle 890

Enlarged Parietal Foramina and Third Fontanelle 891

Occipital Foramina 892

Cranial Defects due to Bone Replacement by Heterologous Tissues 892

Craniostenosis (Craniosynostosis, Stenocephaly) 893

Acrocephalosyndactyly (Apert Syndrome) 899

Carpenter Syndrome 901

Craniofacial Dysostosis (Crouzon) 901

Craniofacial Dysostosis with Dental, Cardiac and Genital Anomalies 902

Sporadic Craniofacial Dysostosis 903

Craniostenosis with Vitamin D-Resistant Rickets 904

Unilateral Coronostenosis 904

Trigonocephaly 904

Cloverleaf Head (Kleeblatts chädel) 904

Bathrocephaly 905

96. Craniovertebral Anomalies **907**

Basilar Impression (Basilar Invagination, Platybasia) 907

Absence of the Odontoid Process 908

Occipitalization of the Atlas 908

Klippel-Feil Syndrome 909

Sprengel Deformity 915

97. The Spine **916**

Malformations 918

Rachischisis 919

Meningocele 920

Congenital Scoliosis 920

Block Vertebrae . . . 921
Transverse (Coronal) Vertebral Clefts . . . 921
Idiopathic Scoliosis . . . 921
Ankylosing Spondylitis . . . 922
Cleft Spinous Processes . . . 922
Intervertebral Calcifications . . . 922
Spondylolisthesis . . . 922
Malformations of the Caudal Areas of the Body . . . 922
Lumbar Anomalies . . . 923
Agenesis of the Sacrum . . . 923
Caudal Appendages (Human Tails) . . . 925
Notochord and Chordoma . . . 927
Caudal Dysplasia Syndrome (Caudal Regression) . . . 927

98. The Chest . . . 930
Rib Anomalies . . . 931
Fissure of the Sternum . . . 933
Funnel Chest (Pectus Excavatum) . . . 934
Pigeon Breast (Congenital Pectus Carinatum) . . . 936
Spondylothoracic Dysplasia . . . 937

99. The Pelvis . . . 938

100. The Extremities . . . 939
Reduction Malformations (Amputations) . . . 941
Primary Reduction Malformations (Aplasias or Hypoplasias of Limbs) . . . 941
Secondary Reduction Malformations (True Intrauterine Amputations) . . . 944
Excess Malformations . . . 947
Amelias . . . 949
Complete Amelia (Tetra-Amelia) . . . 949
Brachial Amelia . . . 950
Crural Amelia . . . 950
Sympodia . . . 950
Phocomelia . . . 951
Peromelia (Stump Formations; Terminal Transverse Hemimelia) . . . 954
Hypermelia . . . 955
Prenatal Bowing of Tubular Bones . . . 957

101. The Upper Extremities . . . 959
Hypoplasia of the Shoulder Girdle . . . 959
Congenital Hypertrophy of Upper Extremity . . . 959
Defects of the Humerus . . . 959
Congenital Defects of the Radius . . . 960
Duplication of the Radius . . . 961
Congenital Dislocation of the Radius . . . 961

Congenital Defects of the Ulna 961
Ulnar Duplication (Ulnar Dimelia) 961
Radio-Ulnar Synostosis 962
Congenital Ankylosis of the Elbow 962
The Hand 962
Split Hands and Split Feet (Lobster Claws; "True Ectrodactyly") 963
Brachydactyly 965
Symphalangy 969
Symbrachydactyly 970
Syndactyly 971
Adactyly, Oligodactyly, Ectrodactyly, Perodactyly 974
Microdactyly and Progressive Myositis Ossificans 976
Absence of the Thumb 976
Floating Thumb ("Pouce Flottant") 977
Broad Thumb 977
Potter's Thumb (Brachymegalodactyly) 977
Triphalangeal Thumb 977
Clutched Thumb (Congenital Aplasia of Extensor Tendons of the Thumb and Other Fingers) 978
Trigger Thumb 978
Polydactyly 978
Duplication of Thumb or First Toe 980
Duplication of the Fifth Digits 982
Median Duplications 983
Polydactylies of High Degree (Diplocheiria and Diplopodia) 983
Macrodactyly (Megalodactyly) 984
Camptodactyly 984
Congenital Synostoses 984

102. The Lower Extremities **992**
Congenital Dislocation of the Hip (CDH) 992
Other Anomalies Involving the Lower Extremities 997
Anomalies of the Femur 997
Absence and Hypoplasia of the Patella 998
Defects of the Tibia 998
Congenital Pseudarthrosis of the Tibia 1000
Tibia Vara (Blount Osteochondrosis Deformans Tibiae) 1001
Congenital Kyphoscoliotic Tibia 1002
Metaphyseal Dysostosis 1002
Absence of the Fibula 1002
Congenital Dislocation of the Knee 1004
Clubfoot (Talipes Equinovarus) 1004

103. Some Syndromes Involving the Extremities 1011

Arthrogryposis (Arthrogryposis Multiplex Congenita; Amyoplasia Congenita; Myodystrophia Foetalis Deformans; Multiple Congenital Articular Rigidities) 1011

Kuskokwim Disease 1015

Larsen Syndrome 1016

Osteo-Onycho Dysplasia (Nail-Patella Syndrome) 1016

Broad Thumb and Big Toe Syndrome (Rubinstein-Taybi Syndrome) 1018

Tricho-Rhino-Phalangeal Syndrome 1020

Skeletal Malformations of Patients with Fanconi Anemia 1020

PART XV
The Muscular System

104. Malformations of the Muscular System 1025

Congenital Absence of Muscles 1025

Congenital Absence of the Abdominal Muscles 1026

Congenital Muscular Torticollis 1028

Muscular Hypertrophy in Hypothyroidism (Kocher-Debré-Sémélaigne Syndrome) 1030

Congenital Muscular Hypertrophy with Extrapyramidal Motor Disturbances and Mental Deficiency 1030

Congenital Muscular Dystrophy 1032

Dystrophia Myotonica 1032

Schwartz-Jampel Syndrome 1033

PART XVI
Malformations of the Urogenital System

105. The Kidney 1037

Bilateral Renal Agenesis 1037

Unilateral Renal Agenesis (Congenital Solitary Kidney) 1039

Renal Hypoplasia and Dysplasia 1041

Renal Hypoplasia 1041

Renal Dysplasia 1041
Congenital Cystic Disease of the Kidney 1042
Type 1 1043
Type 2 1044
Type 3 1045
Type 4 (Polycystic Kidneys Due to Urethral Obstruction) 1046
Simple (Solitary) Cysts in Children 1046
Congenital Polycystic Disease of the Adult Type 1046
Multilocular Cysts or Cystadenomas 1048
Cystic Disease of the Renal Medulla 1048
Fused Kidneys (Horseshoe Kidney) 1050
Ectopia and Malrotation 1053
Supernumerary Kidney 1053
Hydronephrosis 1054
Hereditary Renal Diseases 1058
Wilms Tumor 1061
Congenital Mesoblastic Nephromas 1065
Renal Lesions in Hamartoses 1065
Malformations of Ear and Kidney 1066

106. The Ureter 1067
Duplication of the Ureter 1068
Ectopic Ureters 1068
Ureterocele 1070
Hydro-ureter and Mega-ureter 1070
Mega-ureter 1071
Mega-ureter-Megacystis Syndrome 1071
Retrocaval Ureter 1072
Obstruction of Lower Ureter by Distal Hypogastric Artery 1072

107. The Bladder 1073
Agenesis; Hypoplasia; Duplication 1073
Agenesis of the Bladder 1073
Hypoplasia of the Bladder 1073
Duplication of the Bladder 1073
Exstrophy of the Bladder and of the Cloaca; Urachal Anomalies 1074
Exstrophy of the Bladder 1074
Exstrophy of the Cloaca (Exstrophia Splanchnica) 1077
Urachal Anomalies 1077
Other Bladder Anomalies 1078
Hourglass Bladder 1078
Vesical Diverticula 1078
Congenital "Bladder Neck Obstruction" and Urethral Fibroelastosis 1078

The Urogenital Tract with Absence of the Abdominal Muscles . . . 1079
Tumors . . . 1079

108. The Urethra . . . 1080
Congenital Obliteration of the Urethra . . . 1080
Urethral Diaphragms and Strictures . . . 1080
Posterior Urethral Valves . . . 1081
Anterior Urethral Valves . . . 1081
Hypertrophy of the Verumontanum . . . 1081
Congenital Urethral Diverticula . . . 1081
Mega-urethra . . . 1081
Duplication of the Urethra . . . 1082
Epispadias . . . 1082
Hypospadias . . . 1082
Stenosis of the Urethral Meatus . . . 1083
Malformations of the Urinary Tract Associated with Anal Atresia . . . 1083

109. Female Genitalia . . . 1085
The Ovaries . . . 1085
Absence of the Ovaries . . . 1085
Ovarian Hypoplasia . . . 1085
Ovarian Deficiencies . . . 1086
Supernumerary and Accessory Ovaries . . . 1086
The Uterus . . . 1087
Aplasia and Hypoplasia . . . 1088
Absence of the Uterus . . . 1088
Uterus Arcuatus . . . 1088
Uterus Septus . . . 1088
Uterus Bicornis . . . 1088
Uterus Didelphys (Uterus Duplex Separatus with Vagina Duplex Separata) . . . 1089
Uterus Pseudodidelphys (Uterus Bicornis Bicollis; Uterus Duplex Separatus) . . . 1090
Uterus Unicornis . . . 1090
Congenital Prolapse of the Uterus . . . 1090
Tubes . . . 1091
Other Anomalies of the Female Genitalia . . . 1093
Duplication of External Genitalia . . . 1093
Vulvar Fusion . . . 1093
The Vagina . . . 1093
Congenital Absence of the Vagina . . . 1093
Transverse Vaginal Septa . . . 1095
Congenital Hydrometrocolpos . . . 1095
Hematocolpos with Imperforate Hymen . . . 1096

Double Vagina and Septate Vagina 1096
Congenital Vaginal Cysts 1096
Vaginal Fistulae 1096

110. Male Genitalia 1098
The Testes 1098
Absence of the Testes (Congenital Anorchia and Monorchia) 1098
Undescended Testes (Cryptorchidism) 1098
Testicular Intratubular Bodies 1101
Supernumerary Testes (Polyorchidism) 1101
Synorchidism 1101
Other Anomalies of the Male Genitalia 1103
Absence of External Male Genitalia 1103
Congenital Absence of the Penis 1103
Micropenis 1103
Torsion of the Penis 1103
The Prepuce 1103
Diphallus 1104
Transposition of the Penis and Scrotum (Prepenile Scrotum) 1104

111. Hermaphrodism 1105
True Hermaphrodism 1105
Female Pseudohermaphrodism 1107
Adrenal Female Pseudohermaphrodism (Virilizing Adrenal Hyperplasia) 1107
Nonadrenal Female Pseudohermaphrodism 1111
Male Pseudohermaphrodism 1113
Syndrome of Testicular Feminization 1114
Incomplete Forms of Testicular Feminization 1116
Reifenstein Syndrome 1117
Hernia Uteri Inguinalis in the Male (Internal Male Pseudohermaphrodism) 1117
Feminization of Males with Lipoid Adrenal Hyperplasia 1117
Incomplete Masculinization with 3β-Hydroxysteroid Dehydrogenase Deficiency 1117
Feminizing Adrenal Tumors 1117
Pseudohermaphrodism and Wilms Tumor 1118
Male Pseudohermaphrodism with Chromosomal Abnormalities 1118
Men with 46, XX Karyotype 1118
Pseudohermaphrodism in Syndromes of Congenital Malformations: Ullrich-Feichtiger Syndrome (Typus Rostockiensis); Smith-Lemli-Opitz and Other Syndromes 1119

112. Sex Chromosomal Anomalies . . . 1122
Turner Syndrome (Gonadal Dysgenesis) . . . 1122
XO (Turner Syndrome) . . . 1124
Turner Syndrome in the Male . . . 1131
Mixed Gonadal Dysgenesis (Asymmetric Gonadal Differentiation) . . . 1137
Pure Gonadal Dysgenesis . . . 1139
Triplo-X, Tetra-X and Penta-X . . . 1140
XXY to XXXXY (Klinefelter Syndrome) . . . 1141
XXYY . . . 1142
XYY and XYYY . . . 1144

PART XVII
Malformations of the Skin

113. Congenital Skin Defects . . . 1149
114. Epidermolysis Bullosa . . . 1151
115. Ichthyosis and Keratosis . . . 1156
Ichthyosis Simplex (Vulgaris) . . . 1156
Ichthyosis Congenita (Congenital Ichthyosiform Erythroderma) . . . 1157
Ichthyosis Fetalis (Harlequin Fetus) . . . 1159
Ichthyosis Lamellaris; Collodion Skin . . . 1160
Ichthyosis Hystrix . . . 1160
Keratosis Palmarum et Plantarum (Tylosis Palmaris et Plantaris) . . . 1161
116. Ectodermal Dysplasias . . . 1163
Mild or Hidrotic Forms . . . 1163
Anhidrotic Ectodermal Dysplasia (Hereditary Ectodermal Dysplasia; Congenital Ectodermal Defect) . . . 1165
117. Pigmented Skin Lesions . . . 1168
Pigmented Nevi . . . 1168
Nevus Pilosus (Hairy Mole) . . . 1170
Sacral Spot ("Mongolian Blue Spot") . . . 1171
Blue Nevus . . . 1171
Incontinentia Pigmenti (Bloch-Sulzberger Syndrome) . . . 1171
Acanthosis Nigricans . . . 1173
Dyskeratosis Congenita . . . 1173
Urticaria Pigmentosa . . . 1173
Xeroderma Pigmentosum . . . 1173
Nevus Unius Lateralis . . . 1175
118. Vascular Lesions . . . 1176
Blood Vessels . . . 1176

Nevus Vasculosus (Strawberry Mark and Angioma Vasculosum) 1176
Giant Hemangioma with Thrombocytopenia (Kasabach-Merritt Syndrome) 1179
Nevus Flammeus 1179
Nevus Vasculosus or Flammeus with Osteohypertrophy (Klippel-Trenaunay Syndrome) 1180
Generalized Congenital Phlebectasia (Cutis Marmorata Telangiectatica Congenita) 1180
Spider Nevi 1181
Lymph Vessels 1181
Lymphangiomas 1181
Elephantiasis Congenita Angiomatosa 1183
Lymphangiectasia and Enchondromas 1183
Milroy Disease (Nonne-Milroy-Meige Disease, Congenital Hereditary Lymphedema) 1183
Vascular Hamartoses 1185
Hereditary Hemorrhagic Telangiectasia (Rendu-Osler-Weber Syndrome) 1185
Blue Rubber-Bleb Nevus Syndrome 1185
Glomus Tumors 1185

119. Other Skin Anomalies 1186

Ehlers-Danlos Syndrome and Cutis Laxa 1186
Congenital Cutis Laxa (Dermatomegaly) 1188
Cutaneous Webs (Pterygium Syndromes) 1189
Cutis Verticis Gyrata 1192
Linear Nevus Sebaceus of the Face 1194
Lipodystrophy 1194
Focal Dermal Hypoplasia with Ocular, Dental and Digital Malformations 1195
Congenital Absence of Dermal Ridges and Congenital Milia 1196

PART XVIII

Tumors and Malformations

120. Tumors 1199

Leukemias 1207
Intracranial Tumors 1209
Congenital and Infantile Brain Tumors 1211
Gliomas 1212
Medulloblastomas 1213
Craniopharyngiomas and Rathke Pouch Tumors 1214
Intracranial Teratomas 1215

Epidermoids and Dermoids 1216
Congenital Spinal Tumors 1217
Chordomas 1218
Retinoblastoma 1218
Thyroid Tumors 1219
Cardiac Tumors 1220
Tumors of the Respiratory Tract 1221
Hepatic Tumors 1222
Neuroblastoma 1223
Adrenocortical Tumors 1226
Pheochromocytoma 1226
Renal Tumors 1228
Tumors of the Gonads 1229
Ovary 1229
Testis 1229
Congenital Malformations of the Genital Organs and Tumor Formation 1231
Soft Tissue Tumors 1235
Osteosarcoma and Other Bone Tumors 1238
Teratomas 1239

PART XIX
Hamartoses and Adenomatoses

Hamartoses and Adenomatoses **1251**
121. Recklinghausen Neurofibromatosis **1252**
122. Tuberous Sclerosis **1260**
123. Other Hamartoses **1266**
Hippel-Lindau Disease 1266
Gardner Syndrome 1268
Basal Cell Nevi Syndrome 1268
124. Adenomatoses (Multiple Endocrine Neoplasias) **1269**
Multiple Endocrine Neoplasia, Type 1 and Gastrointestinal Ulcers (MEA or MEN, Type 1) 1269
Multiple Endocrine Neoplasia, Type 2 (MEN, Type 2) 1270

PART I

General Considerations

1

Definitions

CONGENITAL MALFORMATIONS are structural defects present at birth. They may be gross or microscopic, on the surface of the body or within it, familial or sporadic, hereditary or nonhereditary, single or multiple.[1]

"Teratology" was originally the science dealing with monstrosities. It has a long history because observations, explanations and superstitions concerned with deformities of newborn infants have occupied the minds of men and women since prehistoric times. As a science, teratology flourished in the first half of the nineteenth century, when there was great interest in conjoined twins and severe malformations not compatible with life. Later, the interest changed to milder forms of "monstra," when congenital malformations were recognized to be important contributors to postnatal medical problems. There was no word available for a science of congenital malformations. To have a short name for such a science, a word that lent itself to adjectival and adverbial usage, the term "teratology" was usurped by those who wanted to promote work on congenital malformations. "Teratologic" became a useful adjective relating to the science. One speaks of "teratologic" research, observations or manifestations. "Teratogenic" implies causation or production of congenital malformations. Although the word "teratogen" is chiefly applied to environmental causes of congenital malformations such as drugs, chemicals and viruses, it is obvious that abnormal genes and chromosomes can also be teratogenic.

The use of "congenital" as meaning "present at birth" is now generally accepted.[2,3] Although other uses have been customary and other definitions are in use, it seems advisable to limit the term to indicate "present at birth."

"Malformation" is a faulty formation or structure of parts.[2] A congenital malformation is, therefore, a congenital anomaly, but not all congenital anomalies are malformations. Abnormal behavior, function and chemistry, when present at birth, are congenital anomalies but not malformations. In the large circle of congenital anomalies, malformations make up a part, a sector or a circle smaller than the whole (Fig. 1-1).

Originally, the word "malformation" signified a gross structural anomaly. Only defects on the surface of the body were recognized at first, but with the progress of pathology and practice of necropsy, internal structural defects were included in the term. One cannot contest that a horseshoe kidney, a deformed heart, an annular pancreas or an absent corpus callosum is a congenital structural defect. Yet, such malformations concealed within the body may escape recognition at birth, so that incidences are underestimated without necropsy. Many internal congenital malformations are symptomless in the neonate but become manifest with advancing age so that, even in planned investigations, incidence figures of congenital malformations may double when the search is extended beyond the first year of life.[4] Because of their location, life-threatening malformations can be overlooked in early life, whereas minor blemishes such as moles, nevi or anomalies of digits can be seen at the first inspection of an infant. A survey that combines minor and major malformations can be greatly influenced by the thoroughness of the examination. One can separate in statistical statements minor malformations from major ones by arbitrary decisions, but it is more difficult to separate the unimportant from the important. An incurved little finger can be an unimportant hereditary variation in one

Fig. 1-1.—Relationship of congenital malformations to congenital anomalies.

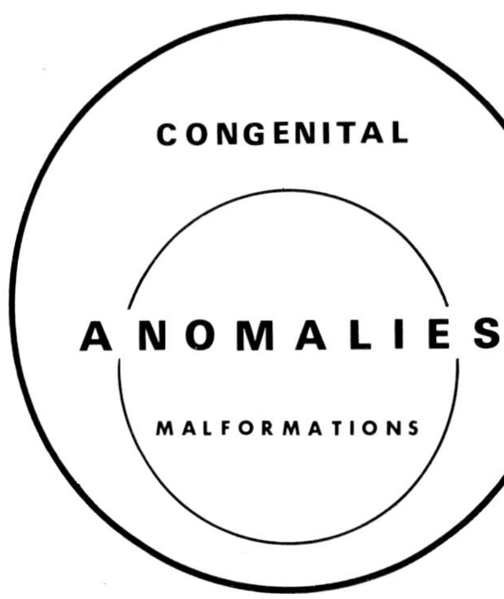

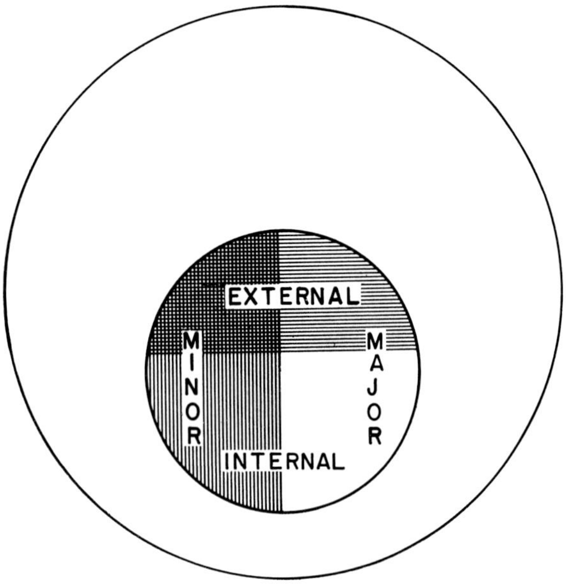

Fig. 1-2.—Interrelationship of external, internal, major and minor congenital malformations within the area of congenital anomalies.

child and a sign of Down syndrome in another. A sixth finger can be an insignificant deviation or a serious prognostic sign of the handicapping Laurence-Moon-Biedl syndrome. One café au lait spot may be a minor defect, but several café au lait spots can be indicative of Recklinghausen neurofibromatosis and all its implications. Thus, a malformation considered minor by one observer may be a sign of major trouble to another.

In addition to malformations seen on inspection, there are defects that can be recognized with the aid of the stethoscope, fluoroscope, ophthalmoscope, cystoscope, catheters or necropsy. Incidence figures depend on the methods of examination and change with progress in diagnostic measures. In general, teratologic incidence figures increase with experience of the observers and improvement of the methods of their observations. These facts illustrate some of the pitfalls of statistical evaluations and comparisons. Changes of general incidence figures from one decade to another, from one city or one country to another depend so much on the methods of ascertainment that they are almost meaningless unless the terms and the examinations used are clearly defined.

If a child appears normally formed on external inspection and at necropsy, histologic examination of tissues may still reveal structural anomalies or microscopic malformations. Changes in the arrangement of cerebral cortical layers, heterotopias, tiny cysts, malformations of nephrons, alterations of epithelia or endocrine tissues detectable with the microscope are congenital malformations according to definition. One could go further and call some ultrastructural anomalies seen with the electron microscope congenital malformations. Even inborn errors of metabolism have been considered congenital malformations because they are defects of molecular structures present at birth. But this extension of the term conflicts with its use in the past and may contribute little to progress, since not all congenital malformations are due to abnormal molecular structure. It is likely that some of the gross structural malformations of man go back to congenital molecular "malformations" caused by genetic changes or inborn errors of metabolism, but it is known that some are not, e.g., the rubella syndrome or the thalidomide embryopathy. At present, only a few gross congenital malformations have been satisfactorily shown to be due to inborn errors of metabolism. The adrenogenital syndromes belong in this category, but congenital malformations included in hypophosphatasia or in the Lowe syndrome, although closely associated with metabolic disturbances, may not be caused but merely accompanied by them. Homocystinuria may cause the malformations developing in persons with this disorder, but it remains to be seen whether they are congenital or develop after birth. Until it is demonstrated that many or most structural congenital malformations are due to molecular malformations, it is recommended that inborn errors of metabolism be separated from structural malformations and considered congenital anomalies.

Terms such as "familial," "sporadic," "hereditary" and "nonhereditary" require definition. Although in recent times these words usually have been used with care and discrimination, the confusion in medical circles with regard to them was general until lately. "Sporadic" means "scattered or of isolated occurrence." "Family" means either a group living in one house, i.e., parents, children and servants(!) or a group descended from a common ancestor. This double meaning can cause much confusion. The term "familial" is often used for attributes and disorders of siblings, although father and mother certainly are also members of a family. The word "kindred" can be applied to a group that includes the family, ascendants, descendants and collaterals. "Hereditary" was and is used for traits transmitted by direct descent from affected members of a family to their children. Today, one often considers both horizontal and vertical distribution of characteristics as hereditary and equates hereditary with "genetically determined." This should be done with caution, since the term "hereditary" had different meanings in the past. Hereditary were houses, cattle, priesthoods, kingdoms, lands, curses and contagious diseases such as syphilis and tuberculosis. Although genes entered into such transactions, the laws governing transmission of such entities were certainly different from the Mendelian. The old concepts of heredity still deserve consideration. Today, when the occurrence of almost any set of signs and symptoms in two children of healthy parents is often rashly attributed to recessive inheritance, it is good to remember that inheritance of environmental goods, deficiencies and diseases can result in traits of siblings that are not genetically determined. Familial endemic cretinism and some forms of familial mental retardation or deafness have disappeared because of measures based on the knowledge that these defects were not due to recessive inheritance but to concealed environmental factors such as deficiency of iodine or abundance of spirochetes.

Conversely, "sporadic" was and still is used synonymously for "nonhereditary" or "nongenetic." This is also incorrect, since a genetically determined trait can be sporadic in a kindred or a pedigree for various reasons: smallness of the pedigree, skipping of one or several generations, new mutation, recessive or sex-linked recessive inheritance or a chromosomal change.

As a rule, "familial" and "sporadic" should be used as descriptive and not as etiologic terms. Chromosomal changes are genetic changes, but their origin and transmission differ from those of gene changes so that often it is advisable to differentiate between gene-determined and chromosomal effects.

Malformations may be single or multiple. Abnormal genes can lead to single malformations or to syndromes, having a "pleiotropic" effect. Environmental causes such as rubella or thalidomide can also result in single or multiple abnormal traits. Chromosome changes usually bring about multiple malformations and anomalies. Occasionally, an affected child is oligosymptomatic, but single malformations probably are not attributable to chromosomal abnormalities. Multiple malformations are extremely common. They form more or less characteristic disease pictures or syndromes, which are dealt with in Chapter 6.

At times, doubts have been expressed whether malformations produced late in fetal life by diseases such as toxoplasmosis or cytomegalic inclusion disease should be considered "congenital malformations." Some investigators believe that only "developmental" malformations should be included in the term, i.e., malformations that are due to primary disturbances of organogenesis. Late teratogenic disorders can deform organs, such as the brain or eye, that were originally well developed; it is said that they resemble in their action and pathologic effects postnatal diseases that damage organs by secondary disorganization. Yet, exclusion of malformations of late prenatal origin would lead to conceptual difficulties. It may not always be possible, for instance, to distinguish clinically a genetically determined hydrocephaly from one produced by a late fetal disease. In many instances, the etiology of hydrocephaly remains obscure. Would it be reasonable to exclude one type because we know its origin and to include another whose etiology is not known? How can one distinguish clinically a patent foramen ovale that is due to arrest of development of the valvular mechanism from one that is due to excessive resorption of septum primum?[5] Genetically determined disease processes can lead to secondary destruction of organs that were originally well formed just as infectious agents do. This has been demonstrated in rabbits, which inherit a disorder leading to secondary loss of fingers or paws that had been normal before[6] and in mice with hereditary "blebs disease," which damages parts that are at first adequately developed.[7] Incidence figures could be significantly influenced and rendered arbitrary by inclusion or exclusion of cases according to their origin. It is preferable, therefore, to consider all structural anomalies present at birth as congenital malformations irrespective of cause and time of origin.

REFERENCES

1. Warkany, J.: Etiology of Congenital Malformations, in Levine, S. Z. (ed.), *Advances in Pediatrics* (New York: Interscience Publishers, Inc., 1947), Vol. II, p. 1.
2. *The Oxford Universal Dictionary on Historical Principles* (Oxford: At the Clarendon Press, 1955).
3. *Webster's Third New International Dictionary of the English Language* (Springfield, Mass.: G. & C. Merriam Company, 1961).
4. McIntosh, R., Merritt, K. K., Richards, M. R., Samuels, M. H., and Bellows, M. T.: The incidence of congenital malformations: A study of 5,964 pregnancies, Pediatrics 14:505, 1954.
5. Patten, B. M.: Varying developmental mechanisms in teratology, Pediatrics 19:734, 1957.
6. Green, H. S. N., and Saxton, J. A.: Hereditary brachydactylia and allied abnormalities in the rabbit, J. Exper. Med. 69:301, 1939.
7. Bagg, H. J., and Little, C. C.: Hereditary structural defects in descendants of mice exposed to roentgen-ray irradiation, Am. J. Anat. 33:119, 1924.

2

Teratology of the Past

FROM TIME IMMEMORIAL, men and women of all countries and continents have been fascinated by monstrous human beings and animals. Primitive man had little regard for the wonders of everyday life and never expressed any admiration for the precise and delicate reactions of embryogenesis that result in the formation of a healthy child. But when the miraculous processes of prenatal development were disturbed and a monstrosity was born, then man's emotions were aroused and he reacted to such misfortune with admiration, awe or terror. His emotions toward reproductive anomalies often have led to extreme measures; he exterminated or adored the deformed of the species—and sometimes he did both. After killing a monster, he often made an image in its likeness and set it up as an idol—god or demigod. Sculptures, carvings and drawings of abnormal births by ancient peoples antedate the arts of reading and writing; they reflect early teratologic knowledge and interest in rare and unusual human beings. That such deviants were made gods or goddesses is understandable. During times when human deities were worshiped, it was the unusual human being who assumed divine status, and rarities such as double-headed or other conjoined twins sometimes served as prototypes of divinities with magic powers.

Images

The most ancient sculpture known of a double-headed twin goddess was discovered by Mellaart[1] at the neolithic site of Catal Hüyük in southern Turkey. The marble statuette (Fig. 2-1) dates from approximately 6500 B.C. Brodsky,[2] from Sydney, Australia, compiled evidence of primitive man's knowledge as expressed in art and lore in Oceania, the islands near Australia and on the continent itself. A chalk carving from New Ireland in the South Pacific represents a double-headed human figure (Fig. 2-2, *A*) in a sitting position, a dicephalus dibrachius. A rock drawing from New South Wales shows a double-headed human male figure, 9 feet 6 inches long. There are six fingers on the right hand and four on the left (Fig. 2-2, *B*). A wooden carving from the Solomon Islands suggests conjoined twins of the pygopagus type with union of the bodies and heads (Fig. 2-3). Brodsky thought that there was a suggestion of achondroplasia, the head being relatively large and the arms and legs short. The teratologic knowledge of man living in Stone Age civilizations is expressed in such works of art, which show remarkable powers of detailed observation and description. That such sculptures represent actual teratologic specimens and not imaginary figments can be concluded from the existence of sculptures pertaining to these civilizations that show rather naturalistic deliveries of children from female figures.[1,2] The fascination of man for double-headed human beings is also expressed in pre-Columbian clay figures found in graves and tombs in Mexico and

Fig. 2-1.—White marble figurine representing double-headed twin goddess from a shrine of neolithic Anatolia (southern Turkey) dating from approximately 6500 B. C. (Courtesy of J. Mellaart and the journal *Archeology*.)

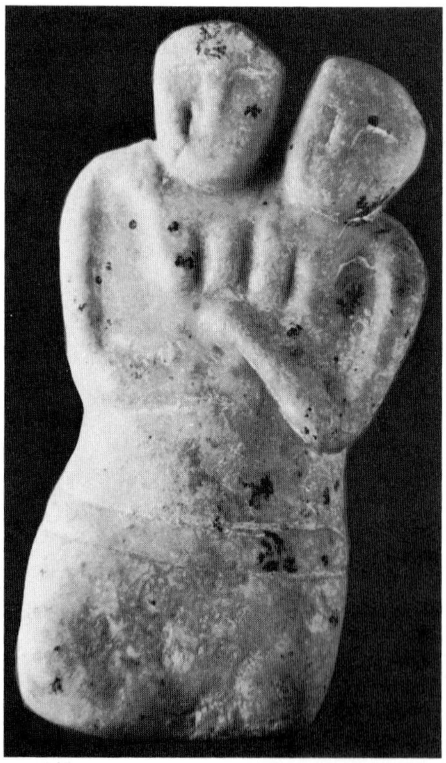

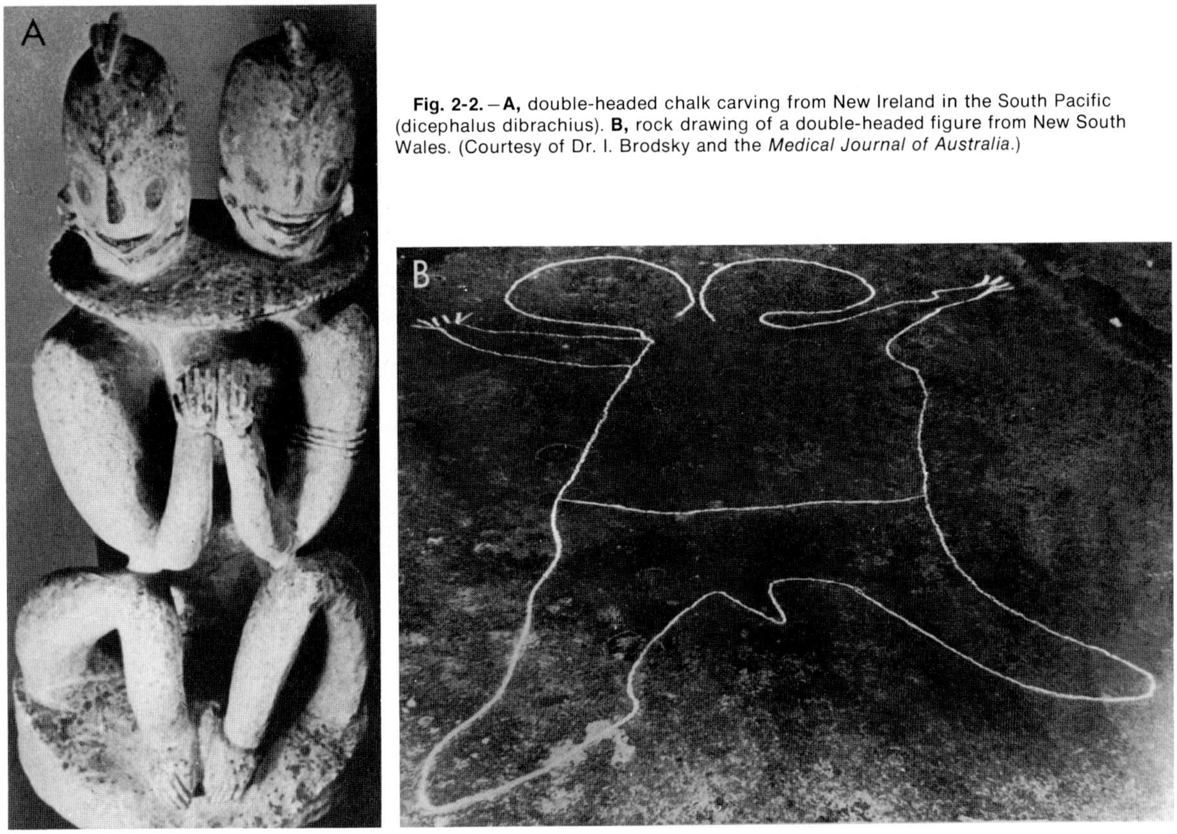

Fig. 2-2.—**A,** double-headed chalk carving from New Ireland in the South Pacific (dicephalus dibrachius). **B,** rock drawing of a double-headed figure from New South Wales. (Courtesy of Dr. I. Brodsky and the *Medical Journal of Australia*.)

Central America that probably date from 500 B.C. to A.D. 800. Some of them are contained in the Weisman Collection of Pre-Columbian Medical Sculpture[3] (Fig. 2-4). Dicephalic conjoined twins have remained favorite subjects of pictorial presentations throughout the ages. During the Middle Ages, they were recorded in pamphlets illustrated by woodcuts, and even today they are welcome subjects for articles and cartoons in popular magazines.

There are many other descriptive sculptures of antiquity that reveal teratologic knowledge of nonmonstrous, viable deformities, such as the Egyptian statuettes of dwarfs with achondroplastic proportions. Figure 2-5, *A* shows one of the dwarfs, who also has facial features characteristic of achondroplasia, whereas the one in Figure 2-5, *B*, with rather regular facial features, may be classified today as "spondyloepiphyseal dysplasia" (p. 783).

Malformations as Portents

Written records of congenital malformations and their meaning for the future have come down to us from the ancient inhabitants of Babylonia. Such records were found in the form of clay tablets covered with cuneiform characters in a mound near the Tigris River in the nineteenth century. The tablets belonged to the Royal Library of Nineveh, which was assembled under the Assyrian king, Ashurbanipal, who lived in the seventh century B.C. It is thought, however, that these records, written in Assyrian, represent copies of older Babylonian texts. The series dealing with births and congenital malformations (izbu-series) may have been recorded at the time of the first Babylonian dynasty during the period of Hammurabi.[4] Thus, the recorded divinations may be almost 4,000 years old.

Divination was a well-developed science in Babylonia. The Akkadian scholars, convinced of causal connections of natural phenomena and historical events, catalogued associated events in the belief that their observations could be used to predict the future. Divination was entrusted to a hereditary caste of priests, who studied celestial and terrestrial omens in a systematic way and established an art or science that was recognized not only in Babylonia and Assyria but subsequently also in Syria, Greece and Rome. Even in China, divinations were transmitted that closely resembled those of Babylonia, suggesting a common source.[5] The Babylonians are known as the founders of astrology—the science of foretelling the future from the stars, the sun and the moon. The fu-

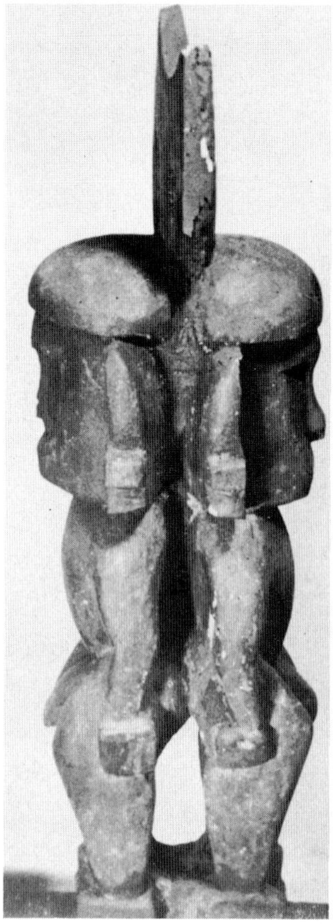

Fig. 2-3.—Wooden carving from the Solomon Islands suggesting Siamese twins of the pygopagus type and possibly achondroplasia. (Courtesy of Dr. I. Brodsky and the *Medical Journal of Australia.*)

ture was predictable not only from the course of the heavenly bodies, but also from terrestrial events. Lightning, thunder, rain and hail served as omens. The behavior of living animals and the appearance of the liver (hepatoscopy) or intestines of sacrificial animals, the flight of birds, the mixing of oil and water, and many other systems served as omens for the future. Among the events found useful for divination were the births of children with malformations. The tablets concerned with monstrous births represent merely a small part of the omen literature, which is of special interest to us because they demonstrate a remarkable knowledge of teratology.[5,6] Many of the omens enumerated can be recognized as congenital malformations as we know them today. Others seem nonsensical to us if we accept them in their literal translation. There are many repetitions on different tablets, and some of the words used remain enigmatic and ambiguous.[4]

The most interesting publication on "the teratological records of Chaldea" is that of Ballantyne[7] in 1894. It is based on the Assyriologic knowledge of his time and on sound knowledge of teratology. A series of approximately 100 tablets relating to various terrestrial occurrences had been deciphered by a number of scholars, and Ballantyne referred to one of these tablets—the sixty-fifth—which was of particular interest to the teratologist. Its first translation apparently was made by J. Oppert[8] in 1871, and modified in a few particulars by F. Lenormant[9] in 1875. The tablet contains a list of sixty-two teratologic cases in man, with the prognostic statements of the Babylonian diviners. A few of the forecasts listed by Ballantyne follow:

"When a woman gives birth to an infant
"(1) that has the ears of a lion, there will be a powerful king in the country;
"(2) that wants the right ear, the days of the master (king) will be prolonged (reach old age);
"(3) that wants both ears, there will be mourning in the country, and the country will be lessened (diminished). . . .
"(6) whose right ear is 'mudissu tehaat' (monstrous), there will be an androgyne in the house of the new born."

Eleven malformations of the ear are enumerated, and their prognostic value is specified. Other malformations are listed that may be of interest to the pediatric and plastic surgeon:

"When a woman gives birth to an infant
"(15) whose nostrils are absent, the country will be in affliction, and the house of the man will be ruined;
"(18) that has no tongue, the house of the man will be ruined;
"(20) that has no nose, affliction will seize upon the country, and the master of the house will die;
"(23) that has no lips, affliction will seize upon the land, and the house of the man will be destroyed;
"(26) that has no fingers, the town will have no births, the 'bar' shall be lost;
"(30) that has six toes on each foot, the people of the world will be injured (calamity to the troops)."

The orthodontist may be interested in an infant

"(22) whose upper lip overrides the lower, the people of the world will rejoice (or good augury for the troops)."

There are also statements of interest to the urologist and the endocrinologist:

"When a woman gives birth to an infant
"(32) that has no penis, the master of the house will be enriched by the harvest of his fields;
"(34) that has no well-marked sex, calamity and affliction will seize upon the land; the master of the house shall have no happiness. . . ."

And the cardiologist will find that

"When a woman gives birth to an infant
"(31) that has the heart open, and that has no skin, the country will suffer from calamities."

Ballantyne[7] believed that most of the deformities mentioned could be identified with anomalies known at his time, and that in the tablet cited none of the recorded anomalies could be regarded as impossible or mythical. He added examples from a tablet dealing with royal births and twins, for instance:

"If a queen give birth to—
"a male . . . royalty will be reduced to misery;
"an androgyne, royalty will be thrown down;

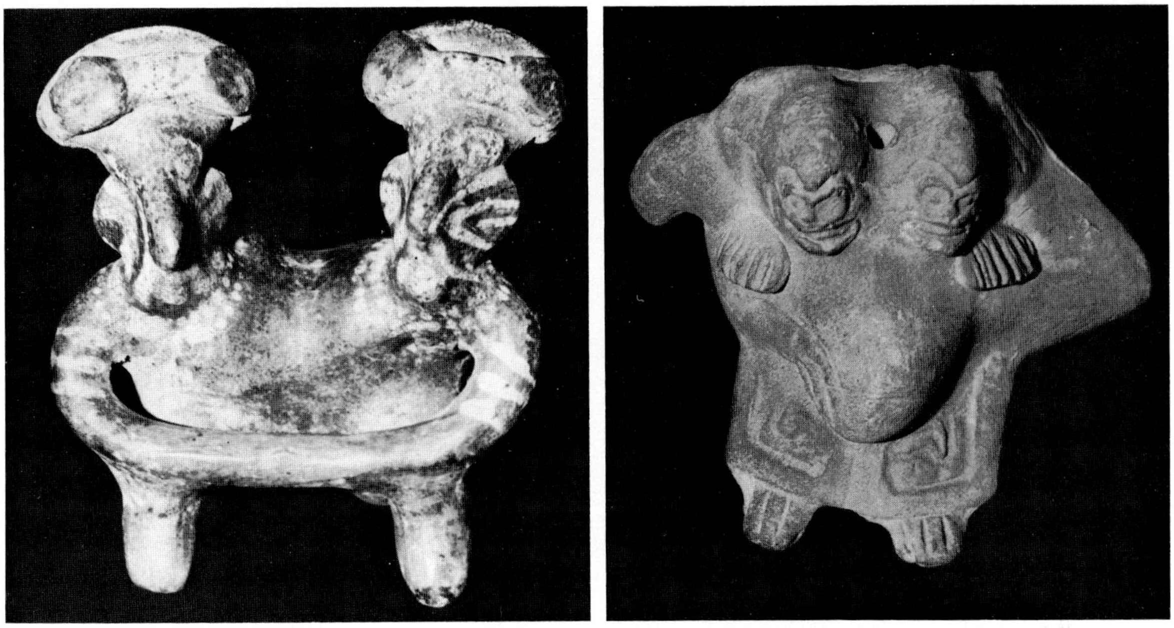

Fig. 2-4.—Dicephalic figures from Mexico—pre-Columbian sculptures. (Courtesy of Dr. Abner I. Weisman, from the Weisman Collection of Pre-Columbian Medical Sculpture.)

"an infant whose teeth are already cut, the days of the king will be prolonged." . . . etc!

But mixed in with such scientific teratologic observations one can find a statement that "if the queen give birth to a *serpent* the king will be powerful"—a statement that makes us doubt the perfection of the Assyrian writer—or that of the translator.

The fragments of birth omens were translated, edited and published in Volumes 27 and 28 of *Cuneiform Texts from Babylonian Tablets* by the British Museum, where most of the tablets still are stored. Monographs on Babylonian birth omens were published in 1914 in German by Dennefeld[4] and in French by Fossey[10] 43 years after Oppert's translation[8] appeared. According to these re-evaluations, it seems that not all teratologic records of the Babylonians were quite so clear and reliable as they appeared in the early translations. Of the existing tablets, some are originals, others copies or excerpts that can be arranged and classified in different ways. Of the tablets extant, only about one-sixth dealt with human malformations. Many of them are either senseless or not understandable to us. Thus, in tablet K258, the omens consist of births by women of lions, dogs, pigs, calves, donkeys, birds, fish, serpents, and so forth, observations that do not seem compatible with rational modern concepts. From a remark in Cicero's treatise,[11] we can assume that such fantastic births referred to dreams and not to actual occurrences. But it is also possible that the Babylonians believed that women could give birth to animals, a belief that existed in the Middle Ages in Europe (see below) and came to the surface again as late as 1726 in England, when Mary Toft of Godalming delivered some parts of a pig and later numerous rabbits.[12]

Fig. 2-5.—**A,** ancient Egyptian statuette showing achondroplastic proportions and facial features. **B,** achondroplastic proportions with "normal" facial features in an ancient Egyptian statuette. (Courtesy of the Hy-Karlsberg Glyptothek, Copenhagen.)

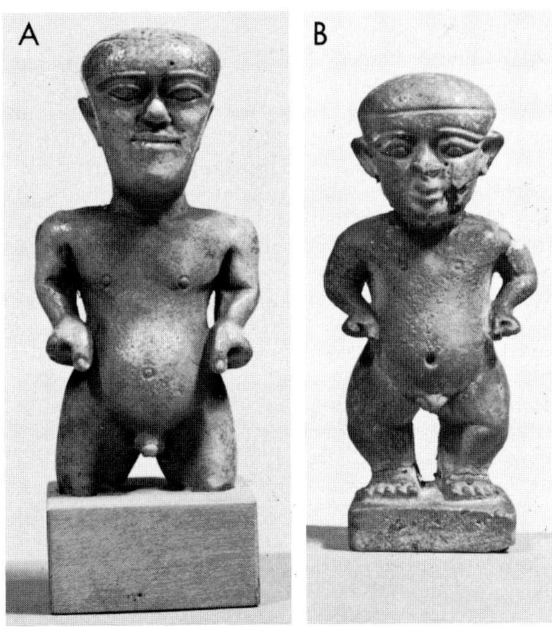

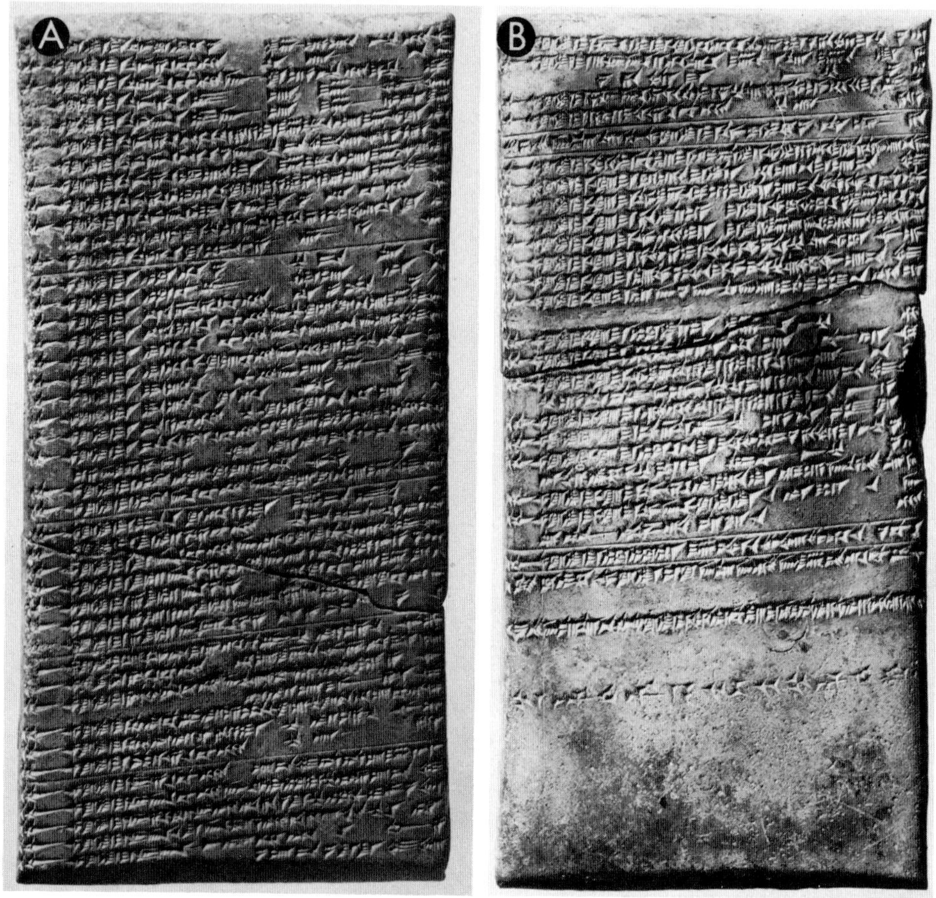

Fig. 2-6.—Clay tablet K2007. **A,** obverse side. **B,** reverse side. (Published with permission of the trustees of the British Museum, London.)

Many observations indicate remarkable knowledge of human congenital malformations. Figure 2-6 shows tablet K2007 from the British Museum in London. It apparently is the tablet translated by Oppert[8] and Lenormant[9] and cited by Ballantyne[7] in 1894. According to Dennefeld's translation,[4] the tablet contains five sections. The first deals with ears; the second with other parts of the head, namely, mouth, nose, lips and jaws; the third with arms, hands and fingers; the fourth with intestines, genitals, anus and hips; the fifth with feet and their parts. But the texts are followed by long commentaries by Dennefeld that indicate that in 1914 there was still much doubt about interpretations and translation. In general, the interpretations by Oppert and by Lenormant are recognized as basically correct by later Assyriologists, but, in some cases, newer translations are less definite. For instance, in item (6) it is prophesied, according to Ballantyne (Oppert-Lenormant), that there will be an "androgyne" in the house, whereas in Dennefeld's translation there will be a "blockhead" born in the house. Or in items (18) and (20) Ballantyne referred to absence of the "tongue" and "nose"; but Dennefeld was less certain, and left "Zag. Ga" and "Bi" untranslated, with comment that the terms are "parts of the face." Thus, the remarkable teratologic knowledge attributed to the author of tablet K2007 is in part attributable to interpretations of scientists of the nineteenth century.

There are other tablets that deal with various teratologic omens in *animals*. For instance, K3171 enumerates reduction malformations of the extremities ("amputations"), thoraco- and gastroschisis, exomphalos, anal prolapse and volvulus. Tablet K3166 deals with diaphragmatic hernia ("intestines in the chest"), volvulus and absence and prolapse of intestines. In tablets K3867 + K4065[4] there is reference to a monster who has one eye on the forehead (cyclopia), which will bring calamity to the country. There also are provisions for eyes located on the neck, back and anus (iniencephaly?) (K11889, K12001), and there is ample information concerning double monsters

(K209). Each of the anomalies had prognostic meaning for the king, the country, the cities or the house. Whatever the value of these divinations, the attention given to newborn children and animals resulted in good knowledge of congenital malformations occurring in human beings and animals. The Babylonian priests were excellent observers and diligent recorders. It is worth mentioning that their ancient teratology was not limited to the knowledge of monstrosities but encompassed also minor congenital malformations such as polydactyly, micrognathia and deformities of the external ear.

There must have been spoken traditions regarding children with congenital malformations in every community and civilization throughout the world. Legends from Oceania about conjoined twins were mentioned in the article by Brodsky.[2] But the Babylonian opinions are of outstanding importance because they were written down, copied and abstracted, and thus transmitted through centuries and millenia.

The people and the cities of Babylonia disappeared, but Babylonian belief in divination has never died. Divination from the birth of monsters and from other impressive events survived in Egypt, Persia, Syria and Asia Minor and spread from there through Greece and Rome to the countries of Europe.[13] To the minds of our educated contemporaries, Babylonian divination is merely superstition, but it is worth while to ask why such strange ideas were perpetuated until recent times.

The Babylonian soothsayers left no explanations of the basic theories of divination, but their successors, who transplanted the old methods into Europe, defended them most vigorously and in modern language. We are told that Pythagoras, Democritus, Socrates and particularly the Stoics, Zeno and Chrysippus, were firm believers in prognostication; and Cicero[11] gave us interpretations of their thoughts. In two fascinating volumes devoted to discussions of divination, he lets his brother Quintus present the arguments in favor of divination, while he himself argues vigorously against it. We learn that the Stoic philosophers were the chief defenders of the idea that the future can be foretold through careful observation and interpretation of monsters and other portents. They considered those diviners as competent "who having learned the known by observation, seek the unknown by deduction." The Stoic philosophers, and probably their Babylonian predecessors, were firm believers in Providence and Fate; by Fate, they meant "an orderly succession of causes wherein cause is linked to cause and each cause itself produces an effect. . . . If there were a man whose soul could discern the links that join each cause with every other cause, then surely he would never be mistaken in any prediction he might make. For he who knows the causes of future events, necessarily knows what every future event will be. But since such knowledge is possible only to a god, it is left to man to presage the future by means of certain signs which indicate what will follow them. . . . Auguries, and the same may be said of auspices, omens and all other signs are not the causes of what follows; they merely foretell what will occur unless precautions are taken." It is not easy to refute such wisdom and if it is combined with the claim of the Babylonian diviners that their observations cover a period of 470,000 years (considered untrue by Cicero), it is understandable that divination took a firm hold on the mind of ancient man. Our basic thinking resembles that of the old philosophers, but we employ different signs and symptoms for our prognostications. In order to predict a man's fate, we do not look at the stars but at his blood and urine, and we prefer the microscope to the telescope in our search for useful auspices.

Augury played an enormous role in Roman history: "In the first place, according to tradition, Romulus, the father of this city, not only founded it in obedience to the auspices, but was himself a most skilled augur."[11] The other Roman kings employed augurs, and, after the expulsion of the kings, no public business was transacted without first taking the auspices. Numerous examples of correct prognostications are quoted from Greek and Roman history by Quintus, Cicero's brother, but we recognize the voice of the old Babylonian diviners when he relates: "When a girl was born with two heads this foretold sedition among the people and adultery in the home"; or "when a woman dreamed that she had been delivered by a lion, this signified that the country in which she had the dream would be conquered by foreign nations." These remarks from Cicero's treatise tally with tablets K258 and K2945 of the Assyrian izbu-series, although animal malformations may have been changed to human births in the transition from Asia to Rome.

Caesar, Cicero's contemporary, was the owner of a horse having toes instead of hoofs; this indicated that the world would one day belong to his master; and shortly before Caesar's death "no heart was found in the vitals of the votive ox." On the following day, there was no head to the liver of the sacrificial animal (diaphragmatic hernia?). These portents were sent by the immortal gods to Caesar that he might foresee his death, but although Spurinna warned him to beware of the Ides of March, Caesar remained unmoved.[11] The consequences of this shocking neglect of teratologic divination are generally known and have become history.

That the Babylonian attitude toward multiple births was taken over by the Romans is attested by Pliny,[14] who stated that quadruplets and larger multiple births were considered portentous. In his time, "Fausta of Ostia was delivered of two male and two female infants, which unquestionably portended the food shortage that followed." The birth of a hermaphrodite was considered an ill omen by the early Romans, and such bisexual children were executed. The situation of hermaphrodites remained precarious because they were thought to indicate disaster, and they therefore needed special legal protection. In the Hebrew book Tosefta, detailed laws are laid down for androgynes—"whoever slays him intentionally is slain, and whoever does so unwittingly is exiled."[15]

From the Latin, such words as "portent," "monster" and "prodigy" entered the English language. They are closely related to the belief in divination, and their derivation is explained by Cicero[11] as follows: "Quia enim ostendunt, portendunt, monstrant, praedicunt, ostenta, portenta, monstra, prodigia dicuntur." Because they "make manifest," "portend," "intimate," "predict," they are called "manifestations," "portents," "monsters" and "prodigies."

During the Middle Ages, the interpretation of monsters as portents continued and played an important role during the religious controversies of the Reformation. In 1523, Luther and Melanchthon jointly published a work under the title *Der Papstesel*, interpreting the significance of a strange ass-like monster that had been found floating in the Tiber. The monster was assigned from God, indicating the doom of the papacy.[16] This prediction was balanced by the birth in 1569 of twins who were conjoined at the chest, with only one of the twins being baptized in time. The physician, Jacques Roy, who performed the necropsy interpreted this event as intimating that the Catholic faith would survive that of the Huguenots.[17]

In his great *Chyrurgery* of 1579, Ambroise Paré devoted a section to the classification and explanation of monsters. He believed that monsters could have many causes, among them "that God may either punish men's wickedness or show signs of punishment at hand."[18]

Montaigne,[19] the enlightened essayist of the sixteenth century, also showed great interest in monsters, and among his essays there is one entitled "Of a Monstrous Child." He had seen a child, 14 months old, who "under the breast was joined to another child, but without a head and which had the spine of the back without motion, the rest entire. . . . they were joined breast to breast. . . ." Montaigne was familiar with the general belief in the prognostic value of deformed children, but he, himself, thought little of it: "It is better to let it alone, for in things already past there needs no divination." He avoided following the Cretan philosopher, Epimenides, of whom it is said "that he always prophesied things past."[19]

Belief in the birth of deformed children as omens and portents can be followed through many popular pamphlets and broadsheets published for the entertainment of the public from the fifteenth to the eighteenth century.[20] Actually, the belief in monsters as portents never disappeared, but rather went underground. While enlightened and scientific explanations may appear to be generally accepted, old fears and deeply rooted prejudices persist.

It is of interest that the Babylonian beliefs crossed the Atlantic and traveled with European settlers into the New World. Although they seldom come to the surface, these beliefs are still transmitted in whispers and have not lost their grip on the human mind. In 1945, a candid autobiography by an American physician[21] appeared in which an account is given of the emotions and thoughts aroused in the author on the occasion of delivery of a monstrous child. The physician, who practiced in a German community in Pennsylvania, was undecided at the time whether to get married or not, and he relates how his decision was influenced: "During this time I delivered a monstrosity and I suppose with all the other things I inherited from my distant German ancestry was a strong streak of mysticism. The monster became a portent. . . . It was a sign, a portent that I could expect nothing good from the way things were drifting along. Silly, you say. Granted, but a doctor can't be coldly scientific all the time, and if he could, I believe that he would lack the kinship with the rest of humanity that makes for a good physician." This author's thoughts probably were not very different from those of other people of our time, but his candor and frankness were unusual and permit a glimpse into popular belief. It seems worth while to keep in mind that even in our day parents of a monstrous child may be plagued by antiquated views that must be discussed and corrected by an understanding physician.

Objective presentation of malformations and description of congenital anomalies for the purpose of divination fail to explain causation of abnormal births. Explanations of such unusual events have been forthcoming since man began asking for causes, and the answers given by different cultural groups were surprisingly similar.

Maternal Impressions

Ballantyne[13] gave a splendid exposition of the ubiquitous theory of "maternal impressions." He pointed out that the belief of psychogenic factors in the etiology of congenital malformations appears in many forms, but that essentially two subgroups can be distinguished. One belief is that parental mental impressions at the time of conception, or mental impressions of the mother during pregnancy, influence the formation of the child by producing a kind of photographic effect on the offspring. A different theory suggests that maternal frights, worries, shock or stress can produce malformations in the child in a rather nonspecific way, so that the exciting factor has no direct relationship to the morphology of the defect.

The idea that mental impressions have a formative and molding effect on the fetus apparently originated independently among peoples who were widely separated geographically as well as culturally. It existed not only among all the peoples of Europe, but also in the Near East, India, China, Japan and South America. It developed among the Eskimos and the African

Negroes.[13] It seems that this idea is inbuilt in the human brain and finds expression wherever children are observed who do not resemble their parents. This "photographic" theory was not originally used as an explanation of congenital anomalies, but was employed for eugenic purposes with the intention of changing and improving the fruit of man or animal. One of the best-known examples is found in the Bible (Genesis, Chapter 30) in the story of Jacob. Promised to be rewarded by certain sheep and goat mutants, he tried to obtain a large number of speckled offspring in Laban's flocks from which all the ring-streaked and spotted animals had been removed. To this purpose, Jacob peeled branches of various trees, thus producing white streaks on the rods, which he placed in the watering troughs of the flocks. As the flocks conceived before the troughs, they brought forth ring-streaked, speckled and spotted offspring. This method was applied chiefly to the stronger animals, which went to Jacob, while the feeble, not exposed to the visual stimulus, belonged to Laban. Needless to say, Jacob became exceedingly prosperous by this procedure.

Methods of mental "modification" were used in Greece, where expectant mothers were encouraged to look at beautiful statues and pictures so that their children would be strong and beautiful. The method was considered effective by Empedocles[22] and by the Spartans, whose law ordered pregnant women to look at statues of Castor and Pollux to make their children well formed and strong. The Romans continued the belief, and Pliny wrote that maternal and paternal thoughts at conception could shape the child.[13] It seems that expectant mothers still visit the Louvre in Paris and other museums in order to influence the looks of their children by viewing beautiful statues and pictures. That this custom is superstitious can be deduced from the fact that visits to modern art galleries, which are often full of monstrous images and sculptures, apparently have not led to an increase in monstrous births.[23]

The concept of maternal impressions was also used in reverse to explain ill-formed children. For instance, the resemblance to monkeys of microcephalic or anencephalic children gave rise to the opinion that it is dangerous for women to look at monkeys during pregnancy. The birth of a black child to white parents was attributed to a picture of a Moor. It is most interesting to trace this concept through the centuries. Ambroise Paré considered a wayward maternal imagination as one of his thirteen causes of monsters. In his writings, we see that this belief can be combined with scientific knowledge of embryology. Paré mentioned that some people believed that after 42 days in the womb, the fetus is not endangered by the mother's imagination because once it has acquired a perfect figure it cannot be altered by external impressions.[13] Thus, in the sixteenth century, it was believed by some that the organogenetic period of the embryo was passed after 6 weeks of gestation and that maternal impressions after that time could not be accused of deforming the child, which shows that knowledge of embryologic timetables is compatible with superstitious beliefs. The best minds of the sixteenth century adopted the theory of maternal impressions, including the skeptic Montaigne,[19] who, in an essay entitled "On the Power of Imagination," explained why this belief was so prevalent. Since man had observed that the mind had definite influence on such organic functions as yawning, vomiting, potency and impotence, many unexplained somatic disturbances were attributed to the mind. In the past, as well as today, psychosomatic influences are blamed for unexplained disorders. It was thought that the imagination worked not only on one's own body, but also on that of others. In the days of Montaigne, transmission of contagious diseases was attributed to visual impressions. "And as an infected body communicates its maladies to those that approach or live near it, as we see in the plague, the smallpox and sore eyes, that run through whole families and cities . . . so the imagination, being vehemently agitated, darts out infection capable of offending the foreign object." Thus, at a time when neither bacteria nor viruses were known as causative agents of contagious diseases, it was believed that communicable diseases could be transferred by visual exposure. Since imagination and fear could influence involuntary functions of the body, and since diseases could be transmitted by visual perception, it seemed likely that maternal impressions could modify the growth of the developing fetus that was considered a part of the mother's body. Therefore, Montaigne stated, "We know by experience that women impart the marks of their fancy to the bodies of the children they carry in their womb; witness her who gave birth to the Black-a-moor. And there was presented to Charles, king of Bohemia and emperor, a girl from near Pisa who was all rough and hairy, whom her mother said to be so conceived by reason of an image of Saint John the Baptist, that hung within the curtains of her bed." These thoughts of an enlightened man of the sixteenth century explain why mental factors were and are used in the explanation of disorders for which no visible causes could or can be found. Similarly, we can and must expect that maternal impressions will be employed as explanations for malformations as long as we have no satisfactory explanations for the birth of defective children.[24]

In the seventeenth and eighteenth centuries, the theory of maternal impressions continued to flourish, and we find the names of many outstanding scientists among its adherents. The French philosopher Nicolas de Malebranche (1638–1715), who was himself deformed and therefore personally interested in congenital anomalies, reported that a pregnant woman attended the execution of a criminal who had been sentenced to die on the wheel. She was greatly perturbed by this spectacle and when she gave birth to a child some time later, she noticed that the bones of the infant were broken in the places where those of the executed sinner had been broken by the wheel. Today, we occasionally see similar infants and we call their abnormal tendency to intrauterine fractures "osteogenesis imperfecta" (p. 824); we have learned that it can occur by mutation in children whose mothers did not attend executions by the wheel. It is of interest that in 1880 Ernest Martin, from whose *Histoire des Monstres*[17] I quoted the report of Malebranche, suggested a modified theory of maternal impression, that is, that the mother's excitement could have caused the fractures by sudden and forceful contractions of the uterus. He had a similar explanation for an intrauterine amputation reported by Lavater (1741–1801): A noble but curious lady attended an execution while she was pregnant. The executioner cut off one of the condemned's hands before proceeding to his main task, the separation of the head from the body. After the hand was cut off, the lady became extremely excited, began to tremble and left hastily. Several days later she gave birth to a child who had only one hand. The severed hand was born some time later. Martin believed that a sudden contraction of the uterus could sever a hand of the fetus, but he admitted that it was pure coincidence that the hand was separated in the same place where the axe of the executioner fell.

Concomitant with such beliefs in maternal impressions there were voices objecting to their validity and denying that they had any scientific foundation. Some of these objections were listed by Ballantyne.[13] It was pointed out that in consideration of the multiplicity of maternal impressions during the long 9 months of pregnancy, all children born should have marks and some should be spotted like leopards. It was observed that adverse maternal impressions were not always followed by the birth of defective children and that often abnormal children were born to mothers who did not have frightening experiences. Anatomy had progressed sufficiently to demonstrate that there were no nervous connections between mother and fetus. How could the mother's thoughts or fears be transmitted to her unborn child? It was known that the maternal and fetal circulations were separated. How could images be transmitted through the placenta? During the nineteenth century, the theory lost ground continually and German teratologists were particularly opposed to it. It was known then that most malformations are determined in the first weeks of gestation, whereas the tales of maternal impressions or frights usually referred to events late in pregnancy.

The American settlers believed in maternal impressions. In the eighteenth century, Dr. John Morgan of Philadelphia knew of a "piebald Negro girl with splotches all over her body" whose mother, while pregnant, delighted in lying out all night in the open air and contemplating the stars and planets. And there was a mulatto boy with a white aigrette on his forehead whose grandmother on his father's side had been frightened by having some milk spilled on her. Thus, it seemed that "grandmaternal impressions" could have a mutagenic effect![25] In the United States, the theory of maternal impressions survived throughout the nineteenth century. Physicians and surgeons continued to publish reports of cases in support of the imagination theory. Keating's *Cyclopaedia of the Diseases of Children*, published in 1889 in Philadelphia, contained a chapter by W. C. Dabney[26] on "Maternal Impressions" in which 90 cases recorded in reputable medical journals between 1853 and 1886 were tabulated, listing "Causes or Nature of Impression," "Nature of Defect" and "Period of Pregnancy" in which the maternal impression occurred. Only "facts connected with cases have been reported without being obscured by theories and conjectures," but the cases were screened and analyzed by the author, a Professor of Obstetrics and Practice of Medicine at the University of Virginia. Many of the cases showed "photographic" effects of the maternal impression. Thus, mothers who saw a man with a harelip or who were frightened by a rabbit had children born with a harelip, and a mother who daily saw a milkman with one finger amputated had a child with only four fingers on one hand. In another case, the mother lived next door to a man with a harelip and was apprehensive lest her child should be similarly deformed, and the child had a harelip. Another unfortunate mother was in her fourth month of pregnancy when she scuffled with a man who attempted undue liberties with her. The mother noticed that he had but one ear. When the child was born, he had but one ear. In 76% of the cases, the defect in the child was similar to the object causing the maternal impression. The author carefully considered possible embryologic periods for developmental defects such as harelip and cleft palate, but he accepted cases in which the maternal impression occurred as late as 3 or 4 months in pregnancy, although lip formation and palate closure are completed at about the end of the ninth week of gestation as calculated from onset of the last menses.[27]

Has the theory of maternal impressions been disproved? As late as the eighteenth century William Hunter, in a prospective study, asked mothers before their confinement about psychic traumas during pregnancy. The answers were recorded, but " . . . in no one instance could a coincidence be detected between the woman's answer and any abnormal structure; but when she knew the nature of the structure she frequently suggested some fresh cause" (cited by Darwin[28]).

In our own times, the theory of maternal impressions existed not only in the Ozarks[29] but it has appeared in modern scientific garb. Since fright can release adrenal hormone and since cortisone can induce cleft palate in certain strains of mice, a new mechanism has been found for those who want to believe in the ancient theory. We thought that this modern belief could be tested experimentally.[30] Mice of two strains in which cortisone injections on certain days of pregnancy induce cleft palate in the young were subjected to audiogenic "stress" on the same days. Whereas the cortisone injections resulted in a high incidence of cleft palate in the offspring, the audiogenic stress did not induce cleft palate or other congenital malformations. This limited experimental approach did not bear out the contention of some that cortisone injection can be equated with maternal "stress."

Hybridization

In the past, there might have been humanitarian reasons for enlightened and progressive minds to support the theories of maternal impressions. Such theories were rather humane and harmless if compared with some other ancient explanations of birth defects.

There was a widespread belief that members of different species might be fertile with one another and thus produce monstrous offspring. This theory, which was termed the "hybridity theory" by Ballantyne,[13] probably originated in India and Egypt, where the transmigration of souls from man to animal was taught and animals were considered as equal or superior to human beings. A cross between different species was not considered repulsive, and if a woman produced a monstrous child who resembled a particular animal, the child was paid the same respect due that animal in the official religion. For instance, at Hermopolis in Egypt, the mummy of a human anencephalus was found in a grave reserved for sacred animals. Since the monster seemed to resemble a monkey, it probably was thought to be of animal origin and was embalmed and buried with other sacred creatures. The birth of such sacred monsters, considered the result of unnatural though not sinful cohabitation, did not lead to persecution of the mother.[13] Crosses of human and terrestrial beings also are found in Greek mythology as centaurs, minotaurs, satyrs and many other more or less respectable personalities, suggesting that fertility between different species was considered possible in those days.

In contrast to these pagan ideas, the Mosaic and Christian laws condemned relations of man with animals as criminal. With the acceptance of these religious laws, the hybridity theory became extremely dangerous to the mother or the suspected father of a monstrous creature. Many examples could be cited,[31] but I shall limit discussion of this unpleasant period to two events that consign the survival of this theory and its cruel consequences to more recent times.

One of these stories is told in the *Records of the Colony and Plantation of New Haven, from 1638 to 1649*.[32] Landauer[31] discussed the pertinent events at New Haven Colony in detail. Three years after the founding of the colony, a monstrous pig was born that had "butt one eye in the midle of the face" and over the eye "a thing of flesh grew forth and hung downe, itt was hollow, and like a mans instrum' of genration." This obviously was a cyclopic pig with a proboscis, a malformation not rare in that species. However, to the good people of New Haven, cyclopia was not known as a spontaneous defect in pigs, and they attributed the birth of this monster to the "unnatureall spell and abominable filthynes" of a servant, George Spencer, who had "butt one eye for use, the other hath (as itt is called) a pearle in itt" and closely resembled the eye of the miraculous pig. The court procedures, the confessions and retractions, as well as the testimonies are recorded in great detail. This trial continued from 1641 to 1642, but finally the prisoner was executed on April 8, 1642, after the cyclopic sow had been "slaine in his sight, being run through wth a sworde.[31,32] On reading the account of this trial, one realizes that the hybridity theory of India and Egypt was, with modifications, imported to this country—but, also, the proceedings demonstrate that "brainwashing" was not invented in recent times.[24]

It is impossible to estimate how many persons became victims of the hybridity belief during the Dark Ages. That punishment probably was not rare may be gathered from the second example to be cited. The Danish anatomist Bartholin mentions in his writings that a girl who gave birth to a monster with a "cat's head" was burned alive in the public square of Copenhagen "ob lasciviorem cum fele jocum." This happened in 1683 in a civilized country, only a little more than 285 years ago. The fact is reported by Bartholin without criticism or expression of disapproval.[17] The event occurred 12 years after Niels Stensen, another Danish anatomist, had demonstrated his teratologic knowledge by an admirable description of a fetus with tetralogy of Fallot.[33]

Comparisons of malformations with structures seen in animals have been continued to our own times in many languages by the use of such expressions as harelip, bec-de-lièvre, gueule-de-loup, Hasenscharte, Wolfsrachen, phocomelia and others.

Interspecies hybridization between mammals is well recognized, the best-known case being that of the horse and donkey. Whereas the resulting mules are useful because of their hardiness, most other hybrids are inferior to their parental species and many fail to reproduce.[34] Sterility may be due to divergence of parental chromosomes, but true congenital malformations do not occur despite odd karyotypes. No hybridization of man and animal has been observed.

Devils and Witches

Related to the hybridity theory was the belief that malformations are the result of the association of human beings with demons, witches and other evil consorts. Especially in Europe during the fifteenth and sixteenth centuries it was imagined that the world was populated by demonic creatures, sorcerers, witches, incubi and succubi who plagued human beings awake or asleep. When a deformed child showed any sign that resembled the imaginary features of the devil, a demonic origin was suggested. Hairy nevi, ichthyosis, clubfeet, shortening of the upper extremities, long and deformed ears, syndactyly and similar anomalies could be interpreted as signs of satanic origin. Many pamphlets and broadsheets are extant that show such creatures of unmistakable demonic origin.[20] In these pamphlets, the devilish creature shows wings in place of arms, probably illustrating such malformations as phocomelia, syndactyly or polydactyly. Repeatedly one hears of a monster born in Kraków, Poland, in 1543, whose head was comparable to that of a cat. It had fiery eyes and near each axilla a small monkey head. On the arms and knees small dog heads were attached. The fingers and toes were webbed, and a tail and a trunk were well developed (Fig. 2-7). The description of this child and his picture were published many times in pamphlets and in books; the monstrosity was ascribed to an evil spirit by some of the learned authors. Whatever the anomalies of this child may have been, they cannot have resembled the description and the pictures reproduced. However, printing and reprinting and a wide distribution made this fabulous child an accepted fact, an example of the power of written or printed records, which, with a minimum of factual content, can create psychologic realities lasting for centuries. In those days demonology, with all its ramifications,

Fig. 2-7.—Satan's birth of Kraków (1543). (From E. Holländer.[20]) Illustration from *Wunder, Wundergeburt und Wundergestalt* used with permission of Ferdinand Enke Verlag, Stuttgart, Germany.

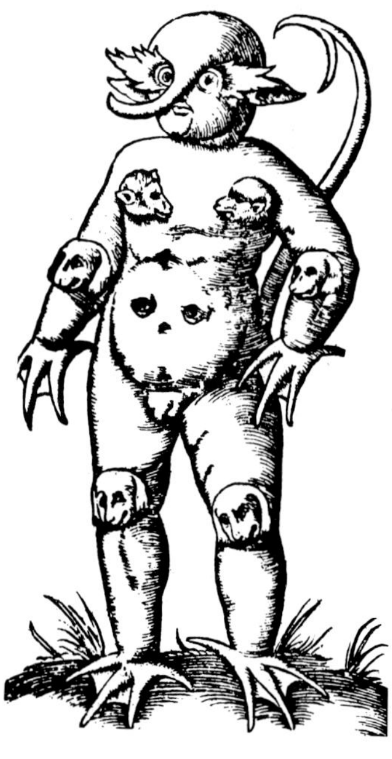

had developed into a pseudoscience incomprehensible to the modern mind and was exacting many sacrifices of human lives.[24] Sometimes it was observed that honest and pious women gave birth to monstrous children, and such mothers were not punished like the sinners who were burned at the stake. In many broadsheets still extant, such unusual births were interpreted as manifestations of the divine anger aroused by the depravity of the world. Man's haughtiness and arrogance, and particularly his innovations, obviously were going too far, as intimated by the birth of deformed children. Holländer[20] gave many examples of pamphlets that compare certain malformations with new and foreign fashions, a clear indication of divine disapproval of the prevailing trends. In Germany in the seventeenth century, the birth of a child with pterygium colli (Fig. 2-8) was attributed to the new fashion of the ruff.[20] In India, pterygium colli in a Hindu child was attributed by the mother to being frightened by a cobra during pregnancy—a maternal impression.[35]

Infanticide

Because of the alleged demonic origin of deformed children, abnormal offspring were in danger of being slain. But, in justice to the medieval world, it should be said that execution of the deformed child or of the mother did not originate in those relatively recent times. Although there are indications that primitive peoples sometimes kept deformed children, twins or conjoined twins alive and treated them well,[2] there can be little doubt that among many savage tribes deformed children were quickly disposed of. Infanticide was practiced not only on children with malformations[36] but also on normals when economic or religious considerations demanded it. In certain tribes, female infants were endangered; in others, males. Twins sometimes were killed together with their mothers.

Infanticide was widespread among the early Greeks and Romans. It was practiced, according to Aristotle,[36] when there were too many children, and Plato[37] advocated it for the inferior or deformed in his Republic. However, it was in national socialist Sparta that infanticide was incorporated in the constitution and practiced for the good of the commonwealth[38]—"Lycurgus was of a persuasion that children were not so much the property of their parents as of the whole commonwealth" and if "puny and ill shaped ordered it [the child] to be taken to what was called the Apothetae a sort of chasm under Taygetus." There the child was disposed of "if it did not, from the very outset, appear made to be healthy and vigorous." With such eugenic measures, the Spartans became a courageous, hardy and ruthless people, but to art and culture they contributed nothing. This is not surprising, since they probably threw into the chasm at Mount Taygetus the Spartan equivalents of such weak children as New-

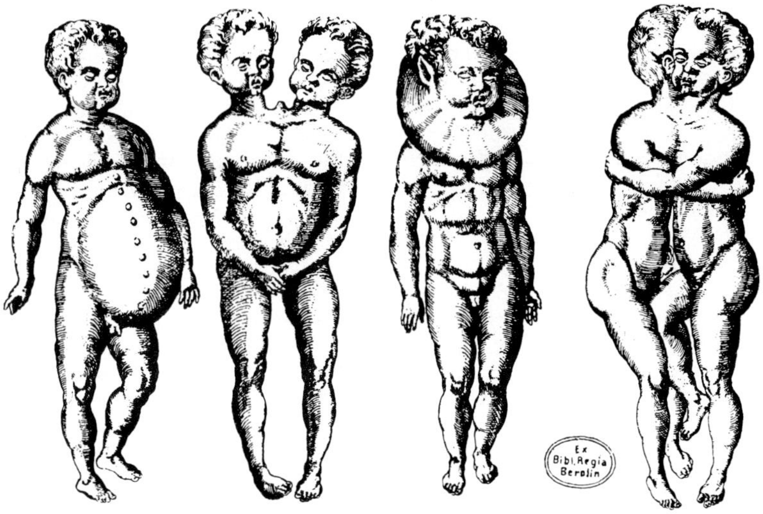

Fig. 2-8.—Malformations depicted in a German woodcut of 1693 are related to newly introduced fashions. There were objections to the new neck frills and to the ruff, as seen in the third figure from the left, which probably represents a pterygium colli. (From E. Holländer.[20]) Illustration from *Wunder, Wundergeburt und Wundergestalt* used with permission of Ferdinand Enke Verlag, Stuttgart, Germany.

ton, Kepler, Darwin, Voltaire and Rousseau, who, although puny at birth, made important contributions to later civilizations.[39] Lycurgus would have been surprised to learn that another tiny premature developed into Napoleon Bonaparte, a military commander who would have won the admiration of the most virile of Spartans.[24]

In Rome, deformed children sometimes were exposed in the Tiber, and it was particularly hermaphrodites who were chosen as victims and were executed. Other monstrous children also were sacrificed, especially in times of danger or when a catastrophe occurred. When the Roman republic was threatened, Arnus, chief of the Etruscan augurs, ordered that all monstrous children be killed and burned.[13] Thus, the treatment of deformed children often was unfavorable among savage and pagan peoples, but the hybridity theory and the demonology of the Middle Ages extended the danger to the mother, neighbors or other persons not conforming to the customs and beliefs of the land.

Biologic Theories of the Past

It would be erroneous to assume that only superstitious and primitive ideas and attitudes prevailed in the past and that the ideas we now have concerning congenital malformations originated entirely in recent times. Biologic theories and explanations of deformities that appear rational to us date back to early periods of history. Some ancient concepts are rather similar to our own, although some of the basic facts of human reproduction were then unknown and the terminology has changed. The Greek philosopher, Empedocles, who lived in the fifth century B.C., apparently was so impressed by the existence of human monstrosities that he considered them as the forerunners of man as we know him. He developed a theory of evolution that was somewhat related to the modern one. It assumed an accidental appearance of disjointed organs that formed a variety of combinations and permutations, with survival of the fittest. On the earth, "many heads sprung up without necks and arms wandered bare and bereft of shoulders. . . . Eyes strayed up and down in want of foreheads. . . . Solitary limbs wandered, seeking for union. . . . Many creatures with faces and breasts looking in different directions were born. . . . Some, offspring of oxen with faces of men, while others, again, arose as offspring of men with the heads of oxen, and creatures in whom the nature of women and men was mingled, furnished with sterile parts. . . . But as divinity was mingled still further with divinity, these things joined together as each might chance, and many other things besides them continually arose. . . ." The monstrous forms that came into being by the fortuitous union of these parts soon became extinct, but finally the fit formations survived as animals and men.[13,22,40]

Aristotle had a surprising knowledge of teratologic facts.[41] He knew of redundance and reduction of the fingers, toes, hands and feet. He knew of imperforate anus, absence of the gall bladder, spleen or one kidney; he mentioned situs inversus and cases of two spleens. He knew that milder malformations can occur in viable animals and that those that depart more severely from the normal do not live beyond the newborn period. Aristotle's description of a hermaphrodite or pseudohermaphrodite agrees perfectly with present-day observations. His knowledge of and approach to malformations represent the height of ancient teratology. The fact that his statements were uncritically repeated and passed on for centuries without verification cannot be held against him. His writings on embryology and teratology were not surpassed for many centuries.

Pliny the Elder[14] who lived in the first century A.D., mentioned many teratologic curiosities in his *Natural History*. Unfortunately, he was an uncritical writer, so that some fantastic statements are intermingled with pertinent observations and excellent descriptions. He knew that some moles and birthmarks can be transmitted through several generations. He related that in the Lepidus family three children were born with a membrane over the eye. Without knowledge of the Mendelian laws it was hard to explain "that sound parents may have deformed children and deformed parents sound children or children with the same deformity as the case may be. . . ." He knew of sex reversal and hermaphrodism. And he gave a brief description of a boy with precocious sex development and premature growth who was carried off by a sudden attack of paralysis when he reached age 3. Such cases still occur and one is tempted to make a belated differential diagnosis. But, in contrast to Aristotle, Pliny had no general concepts or explanations for the anomalies he described.

New ideas were also lacking during the following centuries, and the decline of teratology as a biologic science during the Middle Ages has been illustrated by the superstitions mentioned before that were repeated again and again in teratologic writings.

A new approach to congenital malformations was found through the growing knowledge of embryology. Among the students of embryology in the sixteenth and seventeenth centuries, Fabricius ab Aquapendente (1537–1619) probably exerted an important influence by his treatises *De Formato Foetu* and *De Formatione Ovi et Pulli*, which appeared about the time William Harvey, a student of Fabricius', received his doctor's degree in Padua.[36] There can be little doubt that Harvey was exposed to and stimulated by the embryologic teaching of the Italian master, but he went far beyond him by original observations. Harvey had opportunities to study reproductive processes by direct inspection and he acquired a good knowledge of embryology by observation of hen's eggs and by dissection of deer, which were available to him during the hunting expeditions of his patron, Charles I. Needham[42] summarized Harvey's contributions to embryology with an appreciation of the advances made by him. But it was Ballantyne[13] who pointed out that a new biologic explanation was introduced into teratology, the explanation of congenital malformations by arrest of embryonic development, when Harvey's *De Generatione Animalium* appeared in 1651. There, in the sixty-ninth exercises, are the following sentences: "In the foetuses of all animals, indeed that of man inclusive, the oral aperture without lips or cheeks is seen stretching from ear to ear; and this is the reason, unless I much mistake, why so many are born with the upper lip divided as it is in the hare and camel, whence the common name of harelip for the deformity. In the development of the human foetus, the upper lip only coalesces in the middle line at a very late period."[13] Although the comparison with the hare and camel is erroneous, it seems that here, for the first time, the idea of arrest of development during embryonic life is mentioned as a cause of congenital anomalies, and with this thought a new period of teratology began. The principle of embryonic arrest expressed by Harvey was not applied by many during the next century. It seems that von Haller and C. F. Wolff, in the second half of the eighteenth century, applied the principle of arrested development to explain ectopia cordis and exomphalos,[13] but acceptance of the principle as a general explanation of teratogenesis had to wait for the nineteenth century. By then, comparative anatomy had also been sufficiently developed so that the resemblance of certain malformations with structures occurring normally in lower animals made certain deviations from the normal understandable. Even in the twentieth century, Spitzer's phylogenic theory[43] of the transpositions of the great vessels and related anomalies found many enthusiastic adherents (p. 517). It is of interest that Ballantyne,[13] in 1904, thought that the embryologic theories of teratogenesis were not only the latest but also the last; yet he conceded that it is dangerous to speak of finality in these matters and that the way is not closed against the advance of new theories. It is clear that ontogenic and phylogenic facts can serve as illustrations of the origins of abnormal formations but they do not elucidate causation of the defects. Embryologic theories deal with pathogenesis but not with etiology of congenital malformations.

The nineteenth century represents a peak of the science of teratology. Malformations were intensively studied in man, and experiments in lower animals began to supplement morphologic investigations. It would take more than a volume to evaluate fully the contributions made to teratology between A.D. 1800 and 1900. Many books were entirely devoted to congenital malformations, and illustrations became realistic and true to life: J. F. Meckel's *Handbuch der pathologischen Anatomie*, 1812–1816[44]; Étienne Geoffroy Saint-Hilaire's *Philosophie Anatomique des Monstruosités Humaines*[45]; Isidore Geoffroy Saint-Hilaire's *Histoire Générale et Particulière des Anomalies de l'Organisation chez l'Homme et les Animaux*, 1832[46]; Otto's *Monstrorum sexcentorum descriptio anatomica*, 1841[47]; A. Förster's *Die Missbildungen des Menschen*, 1865[48]; F. Ahlfeld's *Die Missbildungen des Menschen*, 1880–1882[49]; and C. Taruffi's eight-volume *Storia della teratologia*, 1881–

1894[50]. Based on these sound foundations, there appeared at the beginning of the twentieth century J. W. Ballantyne's classic *Manual of Antenatal Pathology and Hygiene*[13] (1904) and in 1906 began the series of Schwalbe's,[51] which is still being continued and supplemented. It can be said that in systematic and taxonomic teratology the masters of the nineteenth century have not been equaled by their successors and much known to these scientists has been forgotten, as shown by some of the rediscoveries in recent times.

One of the greatest contributions to teratology during the nineteenth century was made by a man who had no interest in congenital malformations and no reputation among his contemporary scientists—a man who failed to pass his examinations for a high school teacher's position, with particular deficiencies in natural history. It was the monk, Gregor Mendel, who, working in the monastery garden of Brünn in Moravia on plant hybrids, discovered the fundamental laws of heredity, laws that apply to the transmission of many congenital malformations. His small publication of 1866[52] got little attention for almost 40 years, when it was found that some malformations in man were passed on like normal traits of the garden pea. Whereas the teratologists of the nineteenth century were generally concerned with the study of environmental modifications of embryos, Mendel's work led to genetic explanations, indicating that in many instances the origin of malformations dates back to events that occurred generations before conception of the deformed child.

The ancient history of teratology does not teach us much about the origin, prevention or treatment of congenital malformations, but it tells us a great deal about the human mind and its reactions to unexplained phenomena. If an abnormal child is born in a family or tribe, man insists on an explanation. He does not put off his question and does not wait until science gives him a satisfactory answer. Considering the millenia of observations, explanations have been relatively few, and most of the theories of the past are now considered superstitions. History reveals that primitive and superstitious explanations can coexist with naturalistic and scientific views. In our own time we have witnessed how in the Third Reich the discoveries of genetics were distorted, misinterpreted and transformed into a law that entirely failed to prevent defective offspring. To popularize insufficient knowledge does not pay. It is of interest that the various theories of defective offspring encountered in European civilizations are also found in the Āyurvedas of ancient India.[53] Knowledge of the old and deep-rooted superstitions is of some practical importance, since ancient beliefs often plague parents even today, as they interpret them as portents or punishments. Such beliefs should be brought out into the open, discussed and treated as a possible source of emotional disturbances. But let there be no mistake—as long as we cannot explain to a mother why *her* child is deformed, she will retain her own explanation and remain unconvinced by our general statements. It is not easy to define the borderline between a superstition and a theory. Superstitions generally are based on a disproportion between knowledge and belief. Since, even in our time, knowledge concerning the etiology of congenital malformations is limited, and beliefs abound, we must be aware of the possibility that we can create new superstitions in place of the old. To blame, without proof, congenital malformations on faulty DNA, RNA, mutant genes, viruses, anoxia or diet, to transfer animal experiments uncritically to human conditions, may be substituting contemporary superstitions for those of the past. Such unfounded applications usually are not made by the experimenter but by a reader whose imagination and beliefs exceed his knowledge. If such a reader is also a writer with access to medical or popular journals, his unfounded beliefs are carried to millions, whereby new superstitions are established. Considerations of the past have shown how inflexible statements become once they are written down on clay tablets, papyrus or paper. A single observation of an abnormal child born to a mother who had been in an automobile accident becomes, if reported in a popular magazine, psychologically a hundred thousand observations that seem to establish a causal relationship between the two events. The whispered word is powerful—but the written word endures.

Superstitions disappear quickly when replaced by scientific theories that lead to preventive or curative measures. When the "King's Evil," the "French disease" and childbed fever, which only yesterday also were surrounded by crude superstitions, were eliminated by scientific methods, the superstitions associated with them disappeared rapidly. Since malformations and monstrosities will be with us for some time to come, a knowledge of the beliefs about their origin, ancient or modern, ridiculous or rational, is still a necessity in dealing with parents and the public.

REFERENCES

1. Mellaart, J.: Deities and shrines of neolithic Anatolia, Archaeology 16:29, 1963.
2. Brodsky, I.: Congenital abnormalities, teratology and embryology: Some evidence of primitive man's knowledge as expressed in art and lore in Oceania, M. J. Australia 1:417, 1943.
3. Weisman, A. I.: The Weisman Collection of Pre-Columbian Medical Sculpture, National Library of Medicine, U.S. Department of Health, Education, and Welfare, Public Health Service Publication No. 1539.
4. Dennefeld, L.: *Babylonisch-Assyrische Geburts-Omina* (Leipzig: J. C. Hinrichsche Buchhandlung, 1914).
5. Meisner, B.: *Babylonien und Assyrien* (Heidelberg: C. Winter, Publisher, Vol. 1, 1920; Vol. 2, 1925).
6. Jastrow, M.: Omens from Terrestrial Phenomena. *The Religion of Babylonia and Assyria.* Chapter 20: Various Classes of Omens (Boston: Ginn & Company, Publishers, The Athenaeum Press, 1898), pp. 383–397.
7. Ballantyne, J. W.: The teratological records of Chaldea, Teratologia 1:127, 1894.

8. Oppert, J.: Tablettes Assyriennes, J. Asiatique 18:449, 1871.
9. Lenormant, F.: *La Divination et la Science des Présages chez les Chaldéens* (Paris: Maisonneuve et Cie, 1875).
10. Fossey, Ch.: Présages, tirés des naissances. *Babyloniaca.* Vol. V (Paris: Libr. P. Geuthner, 1914).
11. Cicero: *De Senectute, de Amicitia, de Divinatione.* Trans. by W. A. Falconer (Cambridge, Mass.: Harvard University Press, 1908).
12. Seligman, S. A.: Mary Toft—The Rabbit Breeder, Med. Hist. 5:349, 1961.
13. Ballantyne, J. W.: *Manual of Antenatal Pathology and Hygiene. The Embryo* (Edinburgh: William Green & Sons, 1904).
14. Pliny (The Elder): *Natural History.* Trans. by H. Rackham (Cambridge, Mass.: Harvard University Press, 1939), Vol. II, Book 7.
15. Young, H. H.: *Genital Abnormalities, Hermaphroditism and Related Adrenal Diseases* (Baltimore: The Williams & Wilkins Company, 1937).
16. White, A. D.: *A History of the Warfare of Science with Theology in Christendom* (New York: George Braziller, Inc., 1955), Vol. II.
17. Martin, E.: *Histoire des Monstres depuis l'Antiquité jusqu'a Nos Jours* (Paris: C. Reinwald et Cie, 1880).
18. Thompson, C. J. S.: *Mystery and Lore of Monsters* (London: Williams & Norgate, Ltd., 1930).
19. Montaigne, M. E.: *Essays.* Trans. by C. Cotton. Hazlitt, W. C. (ed.) (New York: A. L. Burt Company, 1892).
20. Holländer, E.: *Wunder, Wundergeburt und Wundergestalt in Einblattdrucken des fünfzehnten bis achtzehnten Jahrhunderts* (Stuttgart: F. Enke, 1922).
21. Tryon, L. R.: *Poor Man's Doctor* (New York: Prentice-Hall, Inc., 1945).
22. Burnet, J.: *Early Greek Philosophy* (4th ed.; London: A. & C. Black, 1930).
23. Warkany, J.: Birth Defects Through the Ages, in Fishbein, M. (ed.), *Birth Defects* (Philadelphia: J. B. Lippincott Company, 1963), Chap. 2, pp. 18–24.
24. Warkany, J.: Congenital malformations in the past, J. Chron. Dis. 10:84, 1959.
25. Flexner, J. T.: *Doctors on Horseback* (New York: Collier Books, 1962).
26. Dabney, W. C.: Maternal Impressions, in Keating, J. M. (ed.), *Cyclopaedia of the Diseases of Children* (Philadelphia: J. B. Lippincott Company, 1889), Vol. I.
27. Fulton, J. T.: Closure of the human palate in embryo, Am. J. Obst. & Gynec. 74:179, 1957.
28. Darwin, C. R.: *The Variation of Animals and Plants under Domestication* (New York: D. Appleton & Company, 1896), Vol. II, p. 251.
29. Randolph, V.: *Ozark Superstitions* (New York: Columbia University Press, 1947).
30. Warkany, J., and Kalter, H.: Maternal impressions and congenital malformations, Plast. & Reconstruct. Surg. 30:628, 1962.
31. Landauer, W.: Hybridization between animals and man as a cause of congenital malformations, Arch. Anat. 44: 155, 1962.
32. Hoadly, C. J. (ed.): *Records of the Colony and Plantation of New Haven, from 1638 to 1649* (Hartford, Conn.: Case, Tiffany & Company, 1857), pp. 62–63.
33. Willius, F. A.: An unusually early description of the so-called tetralogy of Fallot, Proc. Staff Meet. Mayo Clin. 23: 316, 1948.
34. Benirschke, K.: Sterility and Fertility of Interspecific Mammalian Hybrids, in Benirschke, K. (ed.), *Comparative Aspects of Reproductive Failure* (New York: Springer-Verlag, 1967), pp. 218–234.
35. Hoffman, H.: Das Pterygium colli im Rahmen multipler Abartungen, Arch. Kinderh. 110:1, 1937.
36. Encyclopedia Britannica: Infanticide, Vol. XIV; Fabricius, Vol. X (11th ed.; Cambridge, England: Cambridge University Press, 1910).
37. Plato: *Dialogues of Plato.* Trans. by B. Jowett (New York: Random House, 1937), Vol. I. The Republic, Book V.
38. Plutarch: *Lives of the Noble Grecians and Romans.* Trans. by J. Dryden (New York: Modern Library, 1934).
39. Laughlin, R. A.: Famous premature babies, A.M.A. Hygeia 17:203, 1939.
40. Osborn, H. F.: *From the Greeks to Darwin* (New York: The Macmillan Company, 1899).
41. Aristotle: *Generation of Animals.* Trans. by A. L. Peck (Cambridge, Mass.: Harvard University Press, 1943).
42. Needham, J.: *A History of Embryology* (Cambridge, England: Cambridge University Press, 1934).
43. Spitzer, A.: Über den Bauplan des normalen und missbildeten Herzens. Versuch einer philogenetischen Theorie, Virchows Arch. path. Anat. 243:81, 1923.
44. Meckel, J. F.: *Handbuch der Pathologischen Anatomie* (Leipzig: Redum, 1812–1816).
45. Geoffroy Saint-Hilaire, E.: *Philosophie Anatomique des Monstruosités Humaines* (Paris: Rignaux, 1822).
46. Geoffroy Saint-Hilaire, I.: *Histoire Générale et Particuliere des Anomalies de l'Organisation chez l'Homme et les Animaux* (Paris: J. B. Baillière et fils, 1832).
47. Otto, A. W.: *Monstrorum sexcentorum descriptio anatomica* (Vratislaviae: F. Hirt, 1841).
48. Förster, A.: *Die Missbildungen des Menschen. Systematisch Dargestellt* (Jena: Druck und Verlag von Friedrich Mauke, 1865).
49. Ahlfeld, F.: *Die Missbildungen des Menschen* (Leipzig: F. W. Grunow, 1880–1882).
50. Taruffi, C.: *Storia della Teratologia* (Bologna: Regia Typographia, 1881–1894), 8 vols.
51. Schwalbe, E.: *Die Morphologie der Missbildungen des Menschen und der Tiere* (Jena: Gustav Fischer, 1906).
52. Mendel, G.: Versuche an Pflanzen-Hybriden, Verh. Naturf. Ver. Brünn 4:3, 1866.
53. Singhal, G. D., Şingh, S., and Gaur, D. S.: The concept of hereditary and congenital anomalies in Āyurveda, J. Anat. Soc. India 12:77, 1963.

3

Present Trends in Teratology

Although the teratologists of the nineteenth century had admirable knowledge of morphology, embryology and taxonomy of congenital malformations, their ideas concerning etiology were rather limited. Ballantyne,[1] after describing notions regarding teratogenesis of the past, outlined the theories prevalent at the turn of the century, when crude superstitions had given way to scientific theories and explanations thought to have objective and factual bases. The laws of mechanics had been formulated and proved most heuristic in the understanding and conquest of the physical environment of man, and the resulting concepts were, understandably, applied to biology and teratology. Hippocrates had attributed crippling of the fetus to fall or injury of the mother or to narrowness of the womb. Aristotle considered proximity of germs and the resulting pressure among the causes of monstrosities. Ballantyne reviewed the continuation of these explanations through the centuries and brought them up to date. External pressure due to maternal traumatism and injuries as well as internal pressure – intra-abdominal, intrapelvic and intrauterine – were mechanical forces discussed as possible teratogenic factors. Mechanical explanations are still given for many malformations. They are proffered particularly by physicians dealing with orthopedic problems such as congenital positional deformities of limbs and curvatures of the spine. It is generally admitted that fetal deformities caused by an external injury to the mother are extremely rare but possible. If a child is born with a facial scar and brain damage after a serious maternal injury in the sixth month of pregnancy,[2] the case seems acceptable as an example of prenatal traumatic damage. But explanation of the Down syndrome by an automobile accident involving a mother in the seventh week of pregnancy is scientifically untenable, although it may be believed by a court of law and a jury.

Dislocation of a hip and knee combined with clubfoot in a child delivered from a bicornuate uterus[3] could be attributed to the uterine deformity, but it is not likely that many or all clubfeet and clubhands are due to malposition or increased mechanical or hydraulic pressure.[4] Uterine anomalies responsible for such defects are usually assumed but seldom proved. It was suggested, therefore, that abnormal position in utero could be indirectly demonstrated after birth by the "position of comfort" of the baby.[5] Although it is likely that some anomalies of position of postnatal life are similar to fetal position in utero, there is no proof that the faulty intrauterine position was the cause of the deformity. It is possible, for instance, that more remote factors (e.g., chromosomal or genetic) bring about anomalies in embryonic life that result in abnormal position of the fetus in utero. The abnormal intrauterine position could lead to secondary malformations that are seen and stressed by the mechanically minded observer. Thus, mechanical factors may play a contributory role, whereas more distant basic factors are at the root of the malformations. To illustrate the situation by an example from postnatal medicine: postural habits of rachitic children determined and explained the location and shape of some deformities of extremities and spine, but the important causes – lack of sunshine and vitamin D – determined the rachitic process. Investigation of these basic causes led to preventive measures that made the children's postural habits irrelevant as etiologic factors. Similarly, some orthopedic defects, although closely associated with intrauterine position, may be primarily due to abnormal genes, chromosomes or early damage by the external environment.

Extrauterine and extra-amniotic pregnancies must be considered as sources of congenital malformations.[6,7] Winckel,[8] in 1902, reported on malformations in ectopic conceptuses illustrating deformities in the products of tubal pregnancies. Torpin,[7] in 1966, stated that extramembranous pregnancies show a tendency to production of fetal pressure deformities, particularly of feet and long bones. Advanced extrauterine pregnancies have become rare in highly organized communities, but they still occur in underdeveloped areas. Dixon and Stewart[6] described 10 cases from Jamaica, dealing essentially with the obstetric problems involved. They found 6 of the fetuses macerated or stillborn, but there was no mention of malformations. Four infants were live-born; one of these "was distorted at birth from the position it had been forced to adopt during growth but it survived and developed normally." Another survivor was found to be mildly spastic at the age of 18 months. Even after abdominal pregnancies, the resulting babies may exhibit no evidence of gross deformities.[9]

Amniotic anomalies and diseases were high on the list of etiologic factors at the end of the nineteenth century. Among experimentalists, it was particularly Dareste,[10] who, using many teratogenic agents in the production of malformations in chicks, considered amniotic changes an important deforming mechanism. To Ballantyne,[1] disease, pressure and arrested growth of the amnion were possible factors of teratogenesis, but he presented also the weaknesses of "the great amniotic theory." Schwalbe,[11] in 1906, devoted the bulk of his chapter on causes of congenital malformations to amniotic anomalies. The discussions by these experts on congenital malformations reflect the general opinions of their time. Both authors warned against uncritical generalization of the amniogenic theories and recognized the difficulties of proving the role of the amnion in the origin of many malformations. They also realized the need for finding the causes of narrow and defective amnions and of amniotic constrictions and bands. But, lacking other theories, amniotic explanations were applied to malformations from anencephaly to polydactyly; and when no traces of strands or bands could be found, one could always resort to assumption of amniotic threads, which had disappeared by the time of birth. But, as new theories came to the foreground, the interest in amniotic anomalies waned. It seemed more likely that amniotic bands, oligohydramnios and polyhydramnios usually were the results rather than the causes of the malformations associated with them. While many clinical observations led to doubts concerning the importance of mechanical and amniotic factors in teratogenesis, there emerged new experimental evidence that congenital malformations can be produced in mice and rats by amniotic sac puncture. Cleft palate[13] and deformities of the limbs ranging from talipes and ring constrictions to intrauterine amputations and phocomelia have been reported as sequelae of early loss of amniotic fluid.[14] A monograph of Torpin's[53] was published in 1968 on fetal malformations caused by rupture of the amnion. These developments show that the old Hippocratic mechanical theories must not be entirely discarded. But it is certain that estimates of the relative importance of mechanical factors in teratogenesis have changed greatly since the end of the nineteenth and the beginning of the twentieth century.

The embryologic theory in teratogenesis was considered the most important by Ballantyne,[1] who believed that "if all the facts were known, they would be found to fit this theory." Although Harvey apparently was the first to compare facial clefts with the lips and cheeks as they appear in fetuses, the embryologic "explanations" of arrested development flourished chiefly during the nineteenth century. Cleft lip and palate, spina bifida, uterus bicornis, exomphalos and ectopia cordis "were so easily and evidently explicable as arrested developments that they insured for the theory a permanent place in teratogenesis."[1] But other anomalies such as excess malformations, some genital anomalies, situs inversus, exstrophy of the bladder and sympodia have no correspondents in normal embryonic life. It also was recognized that although arrested ontogenesis aids in interpreting many anomalies, it does not give any hint as to the "causa causans." Why is there an arrest at all?[1] In more recent times, arrested development has been used again to clarify teratogenesis. Following the experiments by Stockard,[12] which disclosed a certain lack of specificity of exogenous teratogens, arrest of development in human embryos could be attributed to heterogeneous—and mostly unknown or innocuous—environmental accidents at specific developmental periods and stages. This led to some correct and many incorrect statements concerning the time and type of determination of malformations, a subject discussed in Chapter 7, which deals with sensitive or critical periods in teratogenesis.

The nosologic theory was called by Ballantyne[1] the "teratogenic theory of the 19th century," a time when pathologists were greatly interested in congenital malformations. It is understandable that they considered *diseases* of the embryo and its membranes among the leading causes of structural defects present at birth. Much of the discussion dealt with the puzzling question of the origin of anencephaly, which was explained by many as a sequela of hydrocephaly. It seems that hydrocephaly was considered an understandable disease, whereas anencephaly remained an enigmatic monstrosity. Dropsy and inflammation—although of unknown origin themselves—were accepted as causes of many congenital malformations. It was particularly the disarray of the fetal membranes with their adhesions, shreds and bands that pointed to disease and secondary destruction of the fetuses to which they were attached. At a time when neither bacteria nor viruses were known as causes of inflammation, the debate centered around the question of primary faulty development versus secondary disorganization of structures that originally had been well formed. Ballantyne[1] pointed out that embryologic knowledge weakened the hypothesis of disease of the fetal membranes as a cause of deformity and monstrosity since it was recognized that formation of the embryo and its parts took place in the early weeks of antenatal life, whereas growth and functions of fetal parts progressed in the later weeks and months. "To say that a disease of the fetus is the cause of its malformation is to invert the order of events; until the part is formed it cannot become the seat of the changes which constitute a disease."[1] The argument is sometimes continued today, when definition of the term "congenital malformation" is discussed (see Chapter 1). Should only defects due to faulty development in the early organogenic periods be considered congenital malformations, or should the deformities resulting from secondary destruction by microorganisms or chemical agents be included? Although Ballantyne was not an adherent of the nosologic theory, his objective attitude is worth remembering. He pointed out that "there is no hard-and-fast line between embryonic life and foetal life; all formation is not completed in what we term the embryonic epoch (first six weeks or thereby), neither is the performance of functions limited entirely to the foetal period (last thirty-two weeks); some of the organs are capable of performing functions and therefore having diseases in the embryonic period; and there is still some formation going on in the foetal period, and, therefore, the possibility then exists of some malformations arising. I hold, therefore, that the nosological theory has not been altogether discredited by the new conception of antenatal life which has been arrived at; I maintain that diseases of formed parts of the embryo may occur and possibly interfere with the formation of the other parts, and I think that parts which have been developed monstruously in the embryonic epoch will be very liable to become the seat of disease in the foetal period." It is as if Ballantyne had foreseen the discovery of antenatal rubella, cytomegalic inclusion disease and toxoplasmosis as teratogenic agents that can act in early embryonic or late fetal periods and interfere with normal formation of parts as well as with normal function and growth. The nosologic theory has not been discredited; it is still alive and stimulates the search for teratogenic microorganisms, chemical compounds and maternal diseases that can contribute to congenital malformations. Although only a few of these pathogenic causes have been discovered, they lend themselves to preventive measures similar to those developed in postnatal medicine. We must hope, therefore, that this trend of etiologic research will be continued and further supported as a promising approach to prophylaxis of prenatal deformities.

Nutritional deficiencies as a cause of congenital malformations have been widely discussed. There is ample evidence that in animals congenital malformations of many types can be produced by various nutritional deficiencies, but there is little proof that the teratogenic conditions in animals are simulated by human living conditions. That a prenatal dietary deficiency can be deleterious in man is demonstrated by endemic cretinism. If the concept of nutritional deficiency is extended from maternal dietary deficiency to lack of nutrition of the embryo brought about by abnormal connections with the maternal organism, it may indeed be a factor in teratogenesis. The same may be true, of course, for disturbances of gas exchanges between the mother and her embryo. Disturbances of the microenvironment of embryos in mammals, including man, are not easily discovered, but observations of monozygotic twins, discordant in regard to congenital malformations, suggest that minute differences in early environmental conditions can determine normality or abnormality of the fetus.

Chemical compounds, particularly drugs, have been widely used in experimental teratology, and much attention is given at present to the possibility that they can cause congenital malformations in man. The readiness to acknowledge that changes in our chemical environment can be teratogenic contributed to the relatively rapid recognition of thalidomide, certain progesterones or antimetabolites and organic mercury compounds as sources of prenatal damage (see Chapters 11 and 12). The public is so aware of these possibilities that some chemical compounds are now outlawed and discarded, although they may be harmless in the amounts commonly used. It is to be hoped that a proper balance will be found between irresponsible promotion and use of chemicals and the reactions against them, lest oxygen, water, salt and vitamins—all dangerous in overdoses—will also be prohibited by law.

The teratogenic theories so far considered in this chapter are successors of theories proposed in the past; they are in line with the thinking of early teratologists, who considered postconceptional modification as the chief source of deformities. The teratologists of the nineteenth century were directed and supported in their beliefs by the splendid results of the experimental teratology of their times, which proved that chicks, during incubation, could be sufficiently modified by environmental manipulations to develop monstrosities and malformations of many kinds. Only a few considered malformations as inherent in the constitution of the egg itself and not dependent on external states. It is true that in antiquity alterations in quantity or quality of the male semen or menstrual disturbances were held responsible for monstrous births and that the idea of the "germ originally monstrous" continued through the Middle Ages and was much discussed during the eighteenth century.[1] But the discussions were of a purely theoretical nature and were greatly influenced by teleologic and theologic beliefs. The rationalism of the nineteenth century, combined with increasing knowledge of embryology and experimental teratology, did not readily accept the idea of monstrosities preformed in the germ. The conviction that congenital malformations arise during epigenesis by modification of the originally normal embryo prevailed. Yet, early in the nineteenth century, Meckel pointed out that hereditarily transmitted structural anomalies could not be explained by mechanical causes and Ballantyne[1] admitted that twinning is determined in the pre-embryonic stage of antenatal life and that heredity of some malformations such as polydactyly, perodactyly, polymastia and cleft palate pointed to the "existence of morbid tendencies prior to the embryonic epoch."

In Schwalbe's volume of 1906,[11] heredity was treated together with questions of comparative anatomy and Darwin's deliberations on transmission of normal and abnormal traits from one generation to another. Chromosomes as carriers of the hereditary units, continuity of germ plasm and the concept of mutation were already known and the place of teratology in the important systems and theories of biology were discussed. The causes of malformations were divided into endogenous (believed to be present in the germ cells) and exogenous (acting during postconceptional stages). There was mention of the thought that hereditary metabolic disturbances could be considered as "chemical malformations," with a reference to a publication by Garrod in 1902.[15] But there were no indications that teratologists foresaw and appreciated the importance of the basic laws discovered by Mendel,[16] published in 1866 and rediscovered simultaneously by De Vries, Ćorrens and Tschermak in 1900.[17] Although Mendel's work remained unrecognized during the last third of the nineteenth century, important contributions were made to cytology by scientists who studied cell division and fertilization. It was about 1885 that it became understood that the cell nucleus contained the physical elements of inheritance and that its chromatin carried the heritable material from parent to offspring. Between 1870 and 1890, European cytologists examined and described cell divisions in plants and animals, giving particular attention to the cell nucleus. They observed that the nucleus divided after losing its membrane, concentrating its chromatin about its middle plane. They saw the middle plane dividing subsequently and its halves migrating in opposite directions, thus forming two daughter nuclei. Details of the chromatin and the achromatic structures characteristic of cell division had been well described by 1882 and the colorable rods were named "chromosomes" by 1888.[17,18] It was known early that minute anomalies of the chromosomes, namely gene defects, were responsible for some congenital malformations, but it took more than 80 years to correlate "gross" chromosomal abnormalities and human teratologic phenomena. Few scientists believed that abnormalities of entire chromosomes could be responsible for congenital malformations. It was commonly held that absence of a chromosome or addition of a chromosome to the karyotype would be incompatible with life. Cytogenetic studies were made in plants and lower animals, but comparable observations in human cells were not possible until tissue culture methods and other technical advances made visualization of human chromosomes possible. It was not until 1956 that the correct chromosome number of man was established[19] and it was not until 1959 that some patients with congenital malformations were found to have cells with abnormal chromosome numbers.[20-22] It was then disclosed that many conceptuses with chromosomal anomalies die in utero and are aborted,[23] but it was also learned that many reach the perinatal period and some contribute to early neonatal deaths. Others survive as children and adults with mental and physical handicaps. The human karyotype has been established and sex chromosomes can be distinguished from autosomes. Simple methods permit, in the nuclei of interphase cells, the identification of the sex chromatin (Barr body) that corresponds to the physiologically inactive X chromosome.[24,25] More than one Barr body may be present in persons with various sex anomalies, indicating an abnormal number of X chromosomes. Absence or duplication of entire chromosomes, deletions and translocations of chromosomal parts and ring formations have been observed in persons with congenital malformations. It was found that chromosomal aberrations can arise before conception or in early postconceptional cell divisions. Chromosomes are studied in meiosis and mitosis and attempts are under way to map gene loci on individual chromosomes. Autoradiography is being used for identification of individual chromosomes that cannot be clearly distinguished by conventional staining from similar chromosomes of the same group; but the results often are contradictory, and definitive solutions must await methodologic improvements. After fertilization, chromosomes can be lost, displaced or altered in early cell divisions, sometimes resulting in individuals who are mosaics in regard to their chromosomal constitutions, having two or more cytogenetic cell lines in their tissues. Minor chromosomal changes from one mitotic cell division to another can be surmised. Thus, nuclear disturbances may occur before fertilization, in the zygote and in differentiating cells of embryos, causing prenatal death or malformation. In general, chromosomal abnormalities recognizable in present-day preparations result in broad spectra of malformations, but they do not consistently bring about specific anatomic malformations as they are known to the clinician and pathologist. Absence or addition of a chromosome leads to a general disturbance of the body-building plan, but in the resulting syndromes there are significant variations in the anomalies of specific organs (see Chapter 8).

Long before chromosomal abnormalities were investigated in connection with human malformations, much work was in progress associating abnormal genes with malformations. The principles of segregation and recombination of hereditary units were at first recognized by botanists and applied to plant characteristics, but soon it was shown that some human traits, including malformations, were transmitted in a similar manner. In 1905, Farabee[26] published a pedigree of brachydactyly in an American kindred that is thought to be the first demonstration of dominant Mendelian inheritance in man.[27] It is clear that similar observations had been made many times before, but there was no understanding of Mendelian ratios and of segregation of hereditary units. Systematic collection of human pedigrees containing congenital malformations began in the first decade of the twentieth century. In 1909 there appeared the first volume of *The Treasury of Human Inheritance*,[28] published by the Francis Galton Laboratory of the University of London, which contained a collection of pedigrees on split-foot, polydactyly and brachydactyly. Parenthetically, it may be mentioned that the same volume also had chapters on the inheritance of pulmonary tuberculosis and of "ability," which explains why many scientists received such early publications on human heredity with skepticism. But publication of *The Treasury of Human Inheritance* continues to the present time and many other books and journals record countless examples of inherited congenital malformations that lend themselves to genetic investigations well, often being conspicuous and relatively easily traced.

It was soon recognized that not all hereditary congenital malformations are passed on from parent to child, since recessive and sex-linked recessive modes of transmission are involved in many cases. It was also recognized that numerous anomalies, although obviously hereditary, do not always conform to Mendelian rules and that the hereditary units do not always penetrate and express themselves in persons who carry them.

In 1909, the permanent and independent units located on the chromosomes were called "genes" by the Danish botanist Johannsen,[29] who also recognized that the "genotype" of an organism is not altered by most environmental conditions that can influence the "phenotype" considerably. In regard to congenital malformations, the genotype corresponds to the concepts of older scientists concerning endogenous causes, whereas the phenotype is influenced by environmental, exogenous factors acting after conception in fetal and postnatal life. It was known that the fertilized ovum or zygote can contain a pair of identical genes on a chromosomal locus (homozygosity) or the genes of the pair can differ (heterozygosity). In the latter case, one gene may be dominant, the other recessive. A congenital malformation can be determined by only one member of a pair if the gene is dominant, or the malformation may be determined by two equal recessive genes, each contributed by a parent. As a rule, a single recessive gene, although present in the genotype, does not express itself in the phenotype.

The concept of the gene has persisted now for 60 years, but it has undergone changes and development. The gene was first a statistical concept based on the occurrence of Mendelian segregation and assortment.[17] Then the genes were assigned to a linear system of bead-like loci in the chromosomes. Now it is thought that the genetic material consists of a linear sequence of base pairs whose sequence in the deoxyribonucleic acid molecule determines the amino acid sequence in the corresponding polypeptides and proteins. Distinction has been made between the gene as a unit of function (the cistron), as a unit of mutation (the muton) and as a unit of recombination (the recon).[30]

It is assumed that it is deoxyribonucleic acid (DNA) in the cell nucleus that carries genetic information to the cytoplasm, where the proteins are synthesized. DNA is found in the chromosomes, where it is halved in meiosis and restored to diploid amounts following fertilization.[31] DNA is a polymer composed of many nucleotides, i.e., molecules containing a purine or pyrimidine base linked to a 5-carbon sugar, which is connected with a phosphate group. The 5-carbon sugar is deoxyribose, the purines are adenine and guanine and the pyrimidines are thymine and cytosine. The proportions of the four bases are constant in all the cells of a species but they vary from one species to another. According to the Watson-Crick[32] model, the DNA molecule is bipartite and has a helical configuration. The two parts of the molecule are polydeoxynucleotide strands wound around each other. The sugar-phosphates of each strand are on the outside of the helix and travel in opposite directions, whereas the bases of each strand confront each other in the internal aspects of the molecule, connected by hydrogen bonds.[31] Guanine always pairs with cytosine, and adenine with thymine. The DNA is copied in every cell division, each strand serving as a template for the production of its complement. Mutation arises by tautomeric change in a base in one of the two strands on the DNA molecule so that adenine can pair with cytosine, and thymine with guanine. It is believed that the sequence of nucleotides in a certain region of the DNA molecule determines the sequence of amino acids in a corresponding polypeptide chain, combinations of nucleotides being a code for amino acid sequence. Mutations, including those leading to hereditary congenital malformations, are thought to consist of structural changes in a DNA molecule that are responsible for subsequent developmental processes, but the biochemical changes postulated have not been identified. There is much hope and expectation that such biochemical changes will reveal the source of hereditary malformations.

The genetic information of the cell's DNA molecule must be brought from a specific area of the nucleus to the cytoplasm, where the polypeptides are determined by the alignment of their amino acids. The role of ribonucleic acid (RNA) in cellular protein synthesis had been known for 30 years when it was found that the RNA content of cells parallels their protein-synthesizing activities.[33] Since RNA is present in the nucleus as well as in the cytoplasm, it was considered likely that RNA carries information from the nucleus to the cytoplasmic constituents that manufacture proteins. Much information about RNA has been gathered since these early observations. It was found that the ribonucleotides differ from the deoxyribonucleotides in regard to their 5-carbon sugar, which is ribose instead of deoxyribose; they also differ in one of their pyrimidines, uracil, which replaces the thymine of DNA. There are different kinds of RNA. Messenger RNA is thought to carry information from the nuclear DNA to the cytoplasmic ribosomes. Its molecules vary in composition according to the nucleotide sequence of the DNA from which it is derived and sent to the ribosomes. Transfer RNA aids in transport of amino acids to the ribosomes, where the amino acids are aligned and the proteins synthesized. Ribosomal RNA is a stable component of the ribosomes that is not broken down during protein synthesis.[31]

Books dealing with molecular genetics are available,[34-38] and there is neither need nor space to deal here with these rapidly changing aspects of genetics. At present, the gaps between the biochemical concepts of mutation and the facts of congenital malformations are immense and bridged mostly by beliefs and speculations. Many writers mistakenly identify problems of congenital malformations, i.e., structural defects present at birth, with the "chemical malformations" recognized by Garrod[15] and alluded to by Schwalbe[11] at the turn of the century; but "chemical malformations" or inborn errors of metabolism are present and identifiable as chemical disorders at and after birth, whereas structural malformations are seen many months after the molecular disturbances that brought about the anomaly. There are exceptions, such as the adrenogenital syndromes, that still disclose after birth the metabolic errors that caused the genital changes, but most children with structural congenital defects do not show, after birth, the biochemical abnormalities that led to their deformities in embryonic life.

Little is known about the normal and abnormal mechanisms that are interposed between conception and birth, but the enigmas of differentiation are under investigation. What determines the differences in tissues and cells that have apparently identical sets of chromosomes? Different cytoplasmic portions of the zygote may get into the daughter cells and may account for their cytoplasmic differences. The genetic material of the cleaved nuclei may produce different reactions in cytoplasmic constituents of daughter cells that, in turn, may influence the nuclear material of differentiating cells. There is experimental evidence that nuclei lose their totipotency in embryos after the gastrula stage, proving that they differ from the nucleus of the zygote. The phenotypes of embryo, fetus and child are the result of continual interaction of nuclear and cytoplasmic functions and of intrinsic and extrinsic influences. Many geneticists attempted to elucidate the developmental processes intervening between gene and character. Morgan, in 1934,[39] considered the possibility of alterations of the nucleus and gene during embryonic development. Goldschmidt, in 1938,[40] emphasized the importance of physiologic genetics. He introduced the term "phenocopy for such forms, produced experimentally from the Wild-type form, the phenotype of which copies or duplicates the appearance of a mutant of the same form." Since there could be physiologic parallelism in the development of the phenocopy and that of the mutant, it seemed possible to obtain, through study of the imitating process, a better understanding of the ways and actions of the gene. The "new paths of genetics" were described by Haldane in 1942.[41] Whereas many attempts have been made and are being made to study differentiation from the zygote toward the embryo, other investigations deal with development in the opposite direction. Much work of this kind has been done in mammals with congenital malformations. Starting with an abnormal character present at birth, the anomaly is also observed in various fetal and embryonic stages and traced back to a period during which its abnormal development first becomes discernible.[42,43] This approach is supplemented by experimental teratology, which deals with malformations induced in embryos with normal developmental capability. It seems possible that the latter method, by producing phenocopies, can contribute to an understanding of certain gene effects. It may even lead to prevention of genetically determined anomalies by shedding light on the abnormal channels of development traveled by a mutant gene. That this approach is feasible was shown in mice with an inherited ataxia that could be rectified in the young by treatment of the mother during pregnancy with manganese.[44] The lead to this preventive measure was obtained by previous production in normal mice of a similar ataxia by a manganese-deficient diet. In other experiments, genetic differences have been demonstrated by differing teratologic reactions of inbred strains of animals to identical teratogenic procedures.[45] Studies of interaction between genetic and environmental factors in teratogenesis are of importance because combinations of such factors play a significant role in the etiology of human congenital malformations. Many of these malformations, and particularly some common ones, have a definite tendency to heredity without showing Mendelian ratios. Cleft lip and palate, spina bifida, anencephaly, hydrocephaly, dislocation of the hip and clubfoot are examples of such malformations with a complex etiology.[46] Another important point in etiologic analysis of human malformations is the fact that hereditary defects can be imitated by phenocopies, i.e., similar malformations of environmental origin. There are forms of microcephaly that are autosomal recessive traits and there are forms attributable to prenatal x-ray exposure, cytomegalic inclusion disease or toxoplasmosis. There are genetically determined cataracts and cataracts due to rubella. Hereditary cleft palate can be imitated by aminopterin-induced cleft palate and hereditary limb defects can be simulated to a certain extent by malformations produced by thalidomide. Clinical as well as experimental investigations have demonstrated the heterogeneous origin of many types of malformations that appear homogeneous on inspection.

The use of similar terms for malformations of differing etiologies and pathogenesis is sometimes an obstacle to meaningful epidemiologic studies. Epidemiology has become an important branch of teratologic research. Statisticians deserve credit for pointing out the significant role played by congenital malformations in postnatal mortality and morbidity (see Chapter 5). They have emphasized that congenital malformations represent a large public health problem that is gaining in importance as diseases of postnatal origin recede. Owing to this emphasis, public support has been made available for intensification of research in areas of prenatal development and pathology. Awe and superstition have been replaced by understanding of scientific approaches and hope for prevention by scientific methods. Many epidemiologic studies are under way that encompass national, international and interracial surveys. Congenital malformations are studied in isolated and in mixing populations. In the search of etiologic hypotheses, such factors as maternal age, birth order, seasonal and secular variations and socioeconomic status of the parents are investigated. The role of maternal diseases is explored by the recording of histories, clinical observations and laboratory research. The physical and chemical environments of parents and their kindreds are scrutinized.

The wide range of investigators from molecular biologist, geneticist, experimenter and clinician to epidemiologist and statistician results in problems of differing language, terminology and conceptions that are gradually overcome by national and international meetings[47-50, 51] and publications of many kinds.

The medical management of congenital malformations is at an all-time high. Children with cleft lip and palate; choanal atresia; tracheo-esophageal, intestinal and anal atresias; cardiovascular malformations; urinary and sex anomalies; and many skeletal malformations can be kept alive and be repaired. The brilliant surgical successes in repair sometimes result in complete or nearly complete restoration and function of the deformed organs and of the child. In other cases, the multiplicity of congenital malformations or involvement of the brain permits only partial amelioration of extensive prenatal damages. As a result, a crippled or mentally retarded child may be saved—a child who often needs permanent support by family, community and state.

There is general agreement that prevention is the final goal. To this end, etiologic factors must be found and their interactions explained. There is, understandably, no unanimity about the general directions and specific lines to be followed. Differences of opinion are justified to some extent, since many sciences are involved and different views are prevalent. There are those who believe that a molecular approach to hereditary malformations is feasible and that genetic transformation by DNA substitutions may bring success. Many ideas concerning biologic engineering on the molecular level have been put forward. The recognition of chromosomal abnormalities as a cause of malformations has stimulated investigations into the causes of chromosomal aberrations (see Chapter 8). Genetic counseling can, in selected cases, prevent malformations in a family or kindred. Prenatal cytogenetic and chemical diagnosis combined with attempts to interrupt abnormal pregnancies has become the objective of preventive endeavors. The finding of environmental teratogenic agents is of particular importance, since medicine has acquired great skills in the management of pathogenic factors of man's surroundings. Rubella, a cause of certain congenital malformations and anomalies, can be prevented by a vaccine, and there is a good chance that the rubella embryopathy will soon disappear together with the disease. When the drug thalidomide became the source of a widespread epidemic of malformations, it was quickly recognized as the causative agent; its distribution was prohibited and the epidemic stopped. Pollution of Minamata Bay in Japan by mercurial compounds was found to be the source of a small endemic of a neuropathy and of congenital brain damage. The pollution was rectified, and further brain injuries were avoided. The greatest success in prevention of a syndrome of physical and mental incapacitation was, and is, the iodine prophylaxis of endemic cretinism; it can free whole populations from a disastrous disorder prevalent for centuries in many areas of the globe (see Chapter 12). The role of environmental factors in many structural congenital malformations is less specific than in the examples cited; it may be merely contributory in cases with genetic backgrounds. Yet, removal of contributory factors can be quite effective and result in prophylaxis. As an example of a possible way of preventing chromosomal irregularities and their consequences, one could cite the theory of overripeness of ova as a cause of malformations. The dependence of some chromosomal abnormalities on advanced maternal age suggests that hormonal changes of the mother can lead to overripeness of eggs, faulty distribution of chromosomes and embryonic malformations (see Chapter 8). Overripeness of ova could become preventable by endocrine treatment of women of advanced age or by prevention of fertilization of abnormal eggs by regulation of sexual intercourse. These theoretical considerations are cited as an illustration of a medical approach to prevention of some cytogenetic disorders. In mammals, where minute cytogenetic anomalies are not accessible to direct biologic management and engineering, indirect preventive measures could be applied. To find etiologic factors and mechanisms that are manageable or avoidable is the way of preventive medicine and preventive teratology.

Although beginnings have been made in the prevention of congenital malformations, progress is slow and the goals are still distant. As pointed out before, treatment of children with congenital malformations is much more successful at present than is prophylaxis. The preservation of defective children by complicated and costly surgical and medical measures sometimes is viewed with concern by scientists conscious of the social and genetic aspects of the problem. Sometimes it is said that too much is done for the crippled and the mentally retarded and not enough for the superior who cannot get adequate attention because of lack of special facilities. It seems doubtful that it is necessary in our times to sacrifice the weak for the strong, the retarded for the advanced and to look at the management of the extremes as alternatives. There are situations in which the physician may doubt that preservation of life of a severely defective child is justified or defensible. But preservation of life is the physician's task. Our society and our laws protect and guarantee human life—perfect or imperfect—and that is fortunate. There have been other societies—savage, Spartan, Viking and national socialist—that had other rules and customs. They practiced infanticide or execution of the deformed in order to protect or improve their society and race. But somehow these civilizations did not flourish very long—and this may not be accidental. It seems that the inability to agree on what is perfect, what imperfect, what superior and what inferior in human beings destroys such "virile" societies rapidly. On the other hand, a charitable attitude toward the weak, the deformed and the mentally handicapped—irrational as it may seem sometimes to clever analysts—apparently has a beneficial effect on the society that maintains it and fosters it. We have witnessed in our lifetime fine civilizations and states go down to ruin, destroyed and disgraced not by the burden of their weak and deformed but by apparently well-formed physical specimens whose minds were considered superior by millions of their fellow citizens. During the Third Reich in Germany the Law for the Prevention of Heritable Diseases may have eliminated, by its crude and cruel methods, a number of defective genes, but the spirit that motivated this law led also to the elimination of twenty million healthy people with an inestimable treasure of sound and valuable genes.[52]

Since our society and our laws protect the life of the imperfect child, we must contribute to its care and rehabilitation. It does not seem right to leave the entire financial and emotional burden to the parents, whose misfortune is undeserved. Abnormal children teach us a great deal about the causes of physical and mental handicaps, and a great deal is learned through their treatment and training. To contribute to their care is the price to be paid by those who have normal children—the price to be paid for overcoming the barbarism and cruelty inherent in societies that eliminate the weak and dispose of the deformed.

REFERENCES

1. Ballantyne, J. W.: *Manual of Antenatal Pathology and Hygiene. The Embryo* (Edinburgh: W. Green & Sons, 1904).
2. Hinden, E.: External injury causing foetal deformity, Arch. Dis. Childhood 40:80, 1965.
3. Browne, D.: Congenital deformity, Brit. M. J. 2:1450, 1960.
4. Browne, D.: Congenital deformities of mechanical origin, Arch. Dis. Childhood 30:37, 1955.
5. Chapple, C. C., and Davidson, D. T.: Relationship between fetal position and certain congenital deformities, J. Pediat. 18:483, 1941.
6. Dixon, H. G., and Stewart, D. B.: Advanced extrauterine pregnancy, Brit. M. J. 2:1103, 1960.
7. Torpin, R.: Extramembranous pregnancy, J. M. A. Georgia, p. 174, May, 1966.
8. Winckel, F.: *Über die Missbildungen von ektopisch entwickelten Früchten und deren Ursachen* (Wiesbaden: J. F. Bergmann, 1902).
9. Henderson, D. N., and Wilson, R.: Abdominal pregnancy, Am. J. Obst. & Gynec. 88:356, 1964.
10. Dareste, M. C.: *Recherches sur la Production Artificielle des Monstruosités, ou Essais de Tératogénie Expérimentale* (2d ed.; Paris: C. Reinwald & Cie, 1891).
11. Schwalbe, E.: Allgemeine Missbildungslehre, in Schwalbe, E. (ed.) *Die Morphologie der Missbildungen des Menschen und der Tiere* (Jena: Gustav Fischer, 1906), Vol. 1, pt. 1.
12. Stockard, C. R.: *The Physical Basis of Personality* (New York: W. W. Norton & Company, Inc., 1931).
13. Walker, B. E.: Effects on palate development of mechanical interference with the foetal environment, Science 130:981, 1959.
14. Poswillo, D.: Observations of fetal posture and causal mechanisms of congenital deformity of palate, mandible, and limbs, J. D. Res. 45:584, 1966.
15. Garrod, A. E.: The incidence of alcaptonuria: A study in chemical individuality, Lancet 2:1616, 1902.
16. Mendel, G.: Versuche über Pflanzenhybriden, Verh. Naturforsch. Verein, Brünn 4:3, 1866.
17. Dunn, L. C.: *A Short History of Genetics* (New York: McGraw-Hill Book Company, Inc., 1965).
18. Nordenskiöld, E.: *The History of Biology* (New York: Tudor Publishing Company, 1942).
19. Tjio, J. H., and Levan, A.: The chromosome number of man, Hereditas 42:1, 1956.
20. Lejeune, J., Gautier, M., and Turpin, R.: Étude des chromosomes somatiques de neuf enfants mongoliens, Compt. rend. Acad. Sc. (Paris) 248:1721, 1959.
21. Ford, C. E., Jones, K. W., Miller, O. J., Mittwoch, U., Penrose, L. S., Ridler, M., and Shapiro, A.: The chromosomes in a patient showing both mongolism and the Klinefelter syndrome, Lancet 1:709, 1959.
22. Jacobs, P., and Keay, A. J.: Somatic chromosomes in a child with Bonnevie-Ullrich syndrome, Lancet 2:732, 1959.
23. Carr, D. H.: Chromosome anomalies as a cause of spontaneous abortion, Am. J. Obst. & Gynec. 97:283, 1967.
24. Barr, M. L., and Bertram, E. G.: A morphological distinction between neurones of the male and female, and the behavior of the nucleolar satellite during accelerated nucleoprotein synthesis, Nature, London 163:676, 1949.
25. Lyon, M. F.: Sex chromatin and gene action in the mammalian X-chromosome, Am. J. Human Genet. 14:135, 1962.
26. Farabee, W. C.: Inheritance of digital malformations in man. Papers, Peabody Museum, Harvard University 3:69, 1905.
27. Stern, C.: *Principles of Human Genetics* (2d ed.; San Francisco: W. H. Freeman & Company, 1960).
28. *The Treasury of Human Inheritance*. Parts I and II (London: Dulau & Company, 1909).
29. Johannsen, W. L.: *Elemente der exakten Erblichkeitslehre* (Jena: Gustav Fischer, 1909).
30. Benzer, S.: The Elementary Units of Heredity, in McElroy, W. D., and Glass, B. (eds.), *Chemical Basis of Heredity* (Baltimore: The Johns Hopkins Press, 1957).
31. Ravin, A. W.: *The Evolution of Genetics* (New York: Academic Press, Inc., 1965).

32. Watson, J. D., and Crick, F. H. C.: The structure of DNA, Cold Spring Harbor Symp. Quant. Biol. 28:123, 1953.
33. Brachet, J.: *Biochemical Cytology* (New York: Academic Press, Inc., 1957).
34. Wagner, R. P., and Mitchell, H. K.: *Genetics and Metabolism* (New York: John Wiley & Sons, Inc., 1964).
35. Watson, J. D.: *Molecular Biology of the Gene* (New York: W. A. Benjamin, Inc., 1965).
36. Hartman, P. E., and Suskind, S. R.: *Gene Action* (Englewood Cliffs, N. J.: Prentice-Hall, Inc., 1965).
37. Taylor, J. H.: *Molecular Genetics* Parts I and II (New York: Academic Press, Inc., 1963 and 1967).
38. Hsia, D. Y-Y.: *Human Developmental Genetics* (Chicago: Year Book Medical Publishers, Inc., 1968).
39. Morgan, T. H.: *Embryology and Genetics* (Princeton, N. J.: Princeton University Press, 1934).
40. Goldschmidt, R.: *Physiological Genetics* (New York: McGraw-Hill Book Company, Inc., 1938).
41. Haldane, J. B. S.: *New Paths in Genetics* (New York: Harper & Row, Publishers, 1942).
42. Grüneberg, H.: *The Genetics of the Mouse* (2d ed.; The Hague: Martin Nijhoff, 1952).
43. Gluecksohn-Waelsch, S.: Genetic Control of Mammalian Differentiation, in *Genetics Today*, Proc. XI Internat. Cong. Genetics, The Hague, 1963 (Oxford: Pergamon Press, Inc., 1964).
44. Erway, L., Hurley, L. S., and Fraser, A.: Neurological defect: Manganese in phenocopy and prevention of a genetic abnormality of inner ear, Science 152:1766, 1966.
45. Fraser, F. C., Fainstat, T. D., and Kalter, H.: The experimental production of congenital defects with particular reference to cleft palate, Etudes néo-natales 2:43, 1953.
46. Carter, C. O.: The Inheritance of Common Congenital Malformations, in Steinberg, A. G., and Bearn, A. G. (eds.), *Progress in Medical Genetics* (New York: Grune & Stratton, Inc., 1965), Vol. 4.
47. Wolstenholme, G. E. W., and O'Connor, C. M. (eds.): *A Ciba Foundation Symposium on Congenital Malformations* (London: J. & A. Churchill, Ltd., 1960).
48. Fishbein, M.: *First International Conference on Congenital Malformations* (Philadelphia: J. B. Lippincott Company, 1961).
49. Fishbein, M.: *Second International Conference on Congenital Malformations* (New York: International Medical Congress, Ltd., 1964).
50. Wilson, J. G., and Warkany, J.: *Teratology: Principles and Techniques* (Chicago and London: The University of Chicago Press, 1965).
51. Fishbein, M.: *Third International Conference on Congenital Malformations* (Amsterdam: Excerpta Medica Foundation, 1970).
52. Warkany, J.: Pediatric problems of the future: Remarks on the occasion of the Wall Memorial Lecture on Congenital Malformations, Clin. Proc. Child. Hosp. (Wash.) 20: 281, 1964.
53. Torpin, R.: *Fetal Malformations Caused by Amnion Rupture during Gestation* (Springfield, Ill.: Charles C Thomas, Publisher, 1968).

4

Beginnings of Experimental Mammalian Teratology

Experimental mammalian teratology can be best appreciated against the background of opinions prevalent among medical investigators in the 1920s and 1930s, who thought that most congenital malformations in man, except those caused by mechanical injuries, were genetically determined and hereditary. It was believed, for instance, that when malformations were symmetrical or serial (affecting hands and legs), there could be little doubt that they were hereditary. This thought was so general that during the Third Reich in Germany sterilization was advocated for persons with such defects. There existed no concepts of nongenetic mechanisms that could interfere with the regular development of the well-protected mammalian embryo and fetus and there were no animal experiments to serve as models for

Note: This chapter is an adaptation of Chapter 1, Development of Experimental Mammalian Teratology, by Josef Warkany, in Wilson, J. G., and Warkany, J. (eds.), *Teratology: Principles and Techniques* (Chicago and London: The University of Chicago Press, 1965).

environmental teratologic research in mammals.

When experimental mammalian teratology began in the 1930s, the science of experimental teratology practiced in lower classes of animals was at least 100 years old. Experiments on avian and amphibian eggs were performed most successfully during the nineteenth and twentieth centuries, and many principles and fundamental facts were already known. But it was doubted by many investigators of human congenital malformations that the results obtained on eggs of lower classes could be applied to mammalian or human situations. It was thought that mammalian embryos and fetuses were so well protected by the maternal organism that they could not be modified by methods teratogenic to embryos of lower classes. It also was thought that adverse environmental conditions would either kill a mammalian embryo or leave it unharmed. There were, of course, some observations that suggested that such gross mechanical factors as trauma, hemorrhage or amniotic anomalies could deform a fetus in utero, and there were observations, clinical and experimental, showing that large (therapeutic) doses of x-rays could result in congenital malformations of the embryo.[1,2] But such observations were considered uncommon and exceptional and completely insufficient to explain the bulk of human and mammalian congenital defects. It was known that many congenital malformations were hereditary and passed on from generation to generation. When it was realized that genetic mechanisms can be at work without clear transmission from parent to child, congenital malformations without signs of mechanical causation often were attributed to genetic factors, usually without proof. The terms "congenital" and "hereditary" often were considered to be identical.

The first experiments in mammalian teratology were done to test these assumptions. Methods more subtle than mechanical ones were sought to demonstrate environmental teratogenic effects on the mammalian embryo.

The science of nutrition furnished the early tools for this task. Interest in the effects of maternal malnutrition on the fetus had existed for some time, and, in 1925, Jackson[3] summarized the earlier nutrition experiments that resulted in either normal development of the fetuses, reduced birth weight or resorption, i.e., prenatal death. But congenital malformations were not produced by maternal inanition or general malnutrition. There was a single observation made by Zilva *et al.*[4] in 1921 during a study of the "fat-soluble factor" of four pigs with rudimentary extremities littered by a sow that was fed a deficient diet. It is clear that such a single observation could not be considered proof of teratogenicity of maternal dietary deficiency. In 1932, when Hale made his first experiments with a deficient maternal ration, the science of nutrition had progressed further and the fat-soluble factor had been divided into vitamin A and vitamin D. Between 1933 and 1937, Hale reported that sows fed a vitamin A-free diet during early pregnancy farrowed pigs "all of which were born without eyeballs." Some of the pigs also had other defects such as facial clefts, accessory ears, misplaced kidneys and, occasionally, malformed hind legs. Hale believed "the condition as illustrative of the marked effect that a deficiency may have in the disturbance of the internal factors that control the mechanism of development."[5] He also furnished good evidence that the malformations were not hereditary[6] and that normal pigs resulted from matings of a blind male to his dam or to his blind sister when the females were fed adequate rations.[7] Although we now consider the pioneer experiments by Hale as well established, doubts were then expressed about the dietary etiology of the ocular changes,[7] and it took many years before these experiments were confirmed in pigs.[8]

Although the size of such large animals sometimes could be advantageous, for instance, in experimental surgery, the expense and requirements of space preclude their use on a large scale. Further development of experimental mammalian teratology became possible when it was found that small rodents could also be used for this purpose.

When Dr. Rose Nelson and I began our experiments, we were not acquainted with the brief and scattered reports by Hale. It was our idea to induce an endocrine deficiency in female rats to damage their young in utero. That this could be possible was suggested by the existence of endemic goiter and cretinism in many areas of the world where iodine deficiency prevailed[9] (Chapter 12). It was thought that maternal goiter of a severe degree led to cretinism in the child. To produce goiter, we used the rachitogenic Steenbock and Black Diet No. 2965, which, with or without vitamin D supplementation, is goitrogenic. Animals fed this diet matured slowly, and breeding was delayed for many months. However, when the young finally were born, severe congenital malformations could be recognized in about one-third of them[10] (Fig. 4-1). We soon learned that we had failed to produce endemic cretinism; iodized salt added to the maternal diet prevented goiter in the mother and the young, but not the malformations. Yet, we had found a diet that produced skeletal malformations. When dried liver was given as a supplement, the malformations were prevented. Even before we knew what the preventive nutrient in liver was, various teratologic studies could be done. One could ascertain a definite pattern of skeletal malformations by clearing the newborn animals, one could study the histologic picture of the affected bones and follow the abnormal development back to mesenchymal stages of the skeleton, and one could demonstrate that liver was preventive up to the thirteenth day of gestation but not later. In fact, one could conclude[9] that the chronic nutritional deficiency of the mother, which began long before pregnancy and lasted throughout gestation, exercised its teratogenic effect on the young between the thirteenth and fourteenth days of gestation. Although one could

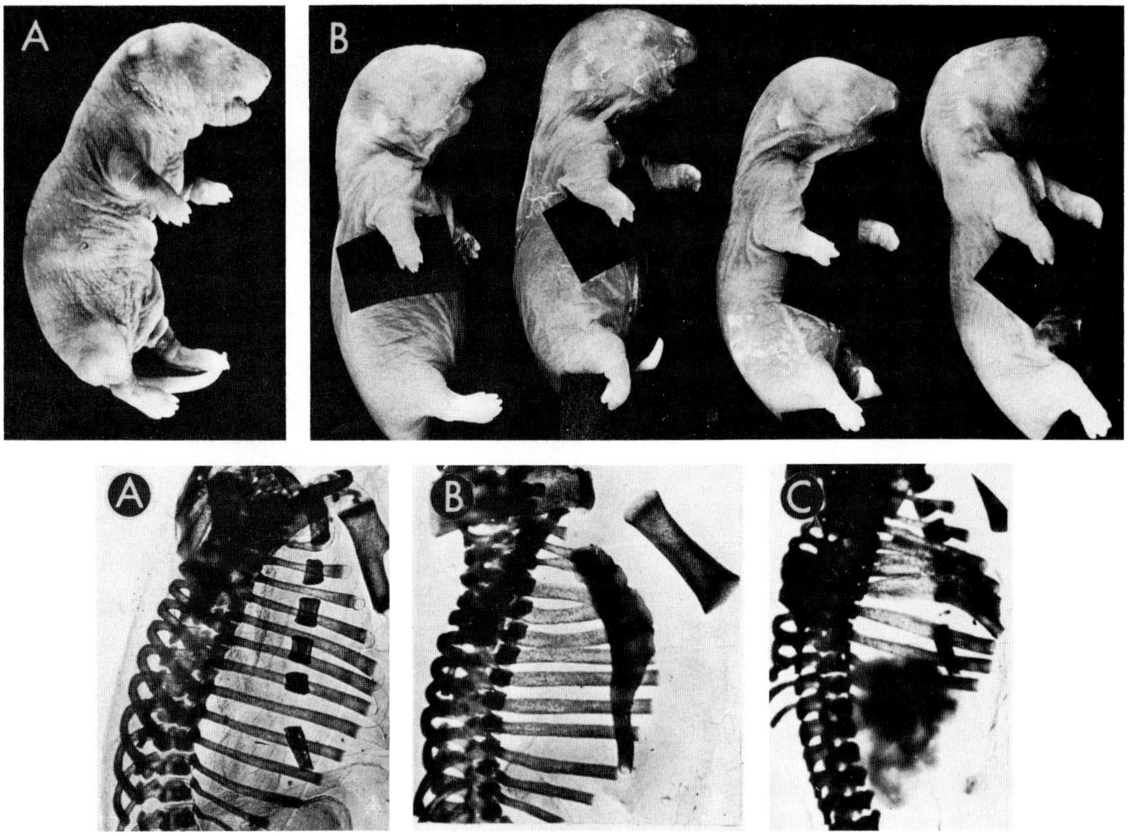

Fig. 4-1.—*Upper row:* **A,** normal newborn rat. **B,** a litter of 4 abnormal newborn rats showing brachygnathia, protruding tongue and various deformities of the extremities. *Lower row:* **A,** chest of normal cleared newborn rat showing normal ribs and sternum. **B** and **C,** chests of abnormal newborn rats showing costal and sternal abnormalities. This syndrome of skeletal malformations was produced in 1939 by a diet deficient in riboflavin. (From J. Warkany and R. C. Nelson.[10])

establish a critical period at which the abnormal environment brought on the malformations, nothing unusual happened to the mother at this critical period; the external situation was the same, weeks before and weeks after the day on which the deforming changes occurred. These findings can still serve as a warning to those who believe that they can ascertain and time environmental teratogenic events with the help of an embryologic timetable (Chapter 7). But the most important result of these experiments probably was that they showed that symmetrical, serial and "familial" (repetitive) congenital malformations could be induced in mammals by environmental manipulation.

In 1943, Warkany and Schraffenberger showed, thanks to the rapid progress of the science of nutrition, that the preventive factor in liver was riboflavin,[11,12] a rather startling finding in those days when skeletal malformations often were investigated by calcium- and phosphorus-balance studies. Subsequently, purified diets became available, and it could be shown that such a semisynthetic diet without riboflavin induced skeletal defects identical to those induced by the original "goitrogenic" diet.[11,12]

These early experiments indicated that formation of the membranous or mesenchymal skeleton, which precedes the cartilaginous as well as the osseous skeleton, is inhibited by riboflavin deficiency.[12] Since riboflavin is a constituent of several enzyme systems, it seemed likely that the riboflavin deficiency resulted in an enzyme deficiency that interfered with normal differentiation of the early skeleton at a time when the demands of the developing tissue were particularly high.[9,12] This supposition was shown to be correct many years later. Miller *et al.*,[74] in 1962, showed a lower flavin content in fetuses from riboflavin-deficient rats than in control fetuses, which suggested corresponding deficiencies in the activities of flavin-dependent enzymes such as the terminal electron transport systems. Mackler *et al.*[75,76] studied, in embryos exposed to riboflavin deficiency and galactoflavin, the terminal electron transport systems that are responsible for the generation of cellular energy from molecular oxygen and inorganic phosphate and found them markedly reduced compared to the activity of preparations from control animals during days 12–16 of gestation. It was thought that galactoflavin

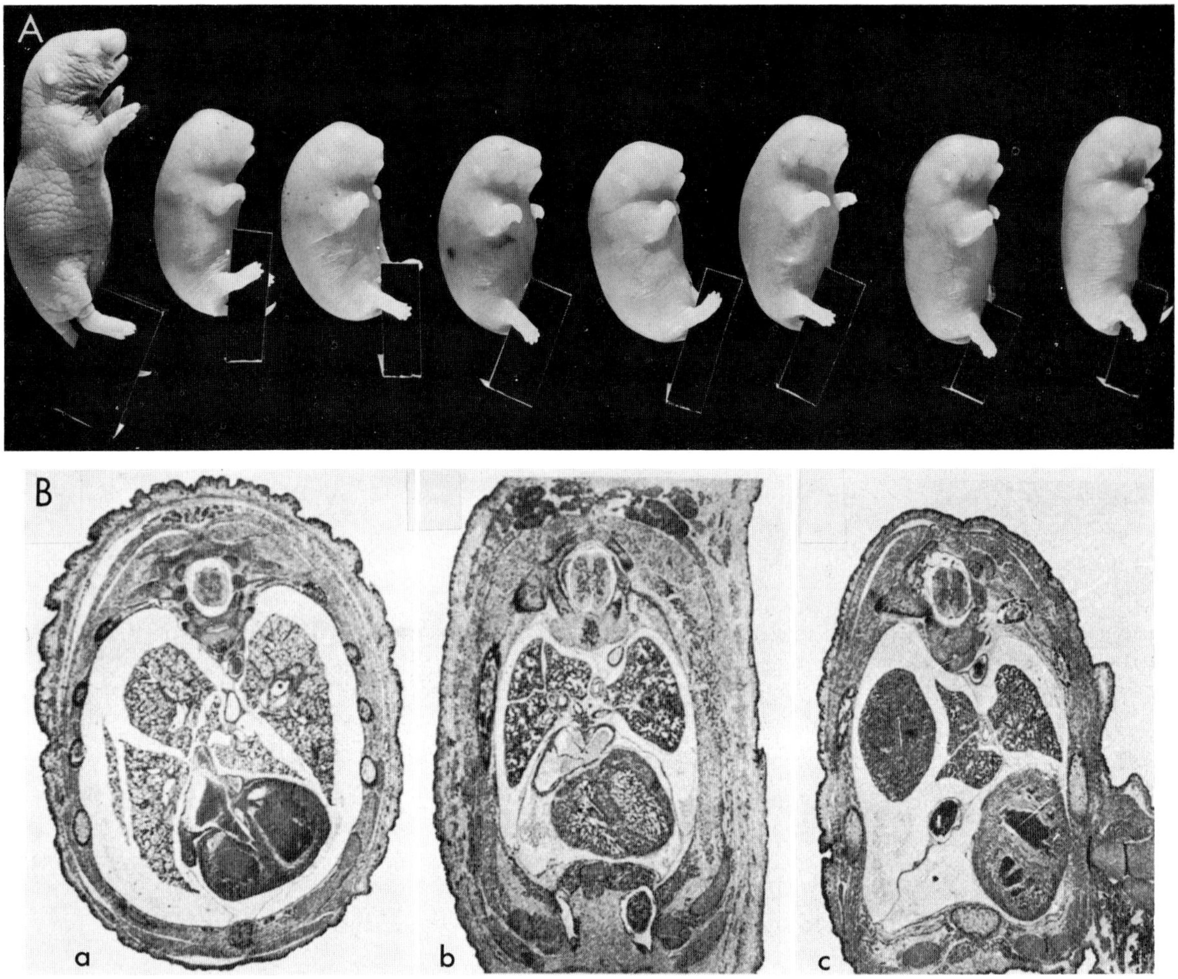

Fig. 4-2.—**A,** at the far left is a normal newborn rat. The other young, offspring of a vitamin A-deficient mother, show edema and abnormal positions of feet. "Open eye" can be seen in some specimens. **B,** sections through the chests of newborn rats. (*a*), control; (*b*) and (*c*), offspring of vitamin A-deficient mothers. In *b*, the lung, the pleura and the heart muscle show retarded development. In *c*, a lobe of the liver is seen in the right pleural cavity (diaphragmatic hernia). (From J. Warkany and C. B. Roth.[78])

produces an effect on the electron transport systems of fetal tissue by hindering the binding of the reduced amounts of flavin mononucleotide and flavin adenine dinucleotide that are present during synthesis of the enzymes. Faulty differentiation and increased mesenchymal cellular death between the twelfth and fourteenth days of gestation parallel the marked decrease in activity of the electron transport systems, which is accompanied by a decrease in the rate of formation of high-energy phosphate compounds at a time when the cellular demands for energy may be greatly increased as a result of the high rate of cellular multiplication and differentiation.[76]

With the advent of purified diets, the experiments could be varied by omission of various constituents of the diet, particularly of vitamins. There was an opportunity to induce vitamin A deficiency in pregnant rats and to conduct an experiment comparable to that performed by Hale. It was found that maternal vitamin A deficiency did indeed induce ocular anomalies in rat as in pig embryos,[13] but, in addition, there were many other soft-tissue malformations in the genitourinary and cardiovascular systems and in the diaphragm.[14] There were no malformations of the skeleton resembling those induced by riboflavin deficiency, and there was no overlapping of the two syndromes of congenital defects. The specificity of the defects produced by these dietary deficiencies is still not sufficiently appreciated, and one can still hear the opinion that all "bad maternal diets" result in malformations, or that these deficiencies probably damage the placenta and affect the embryo secondarily. I have assumed all along that these deficiencies affect the embryo directly by withholding from it important nu-

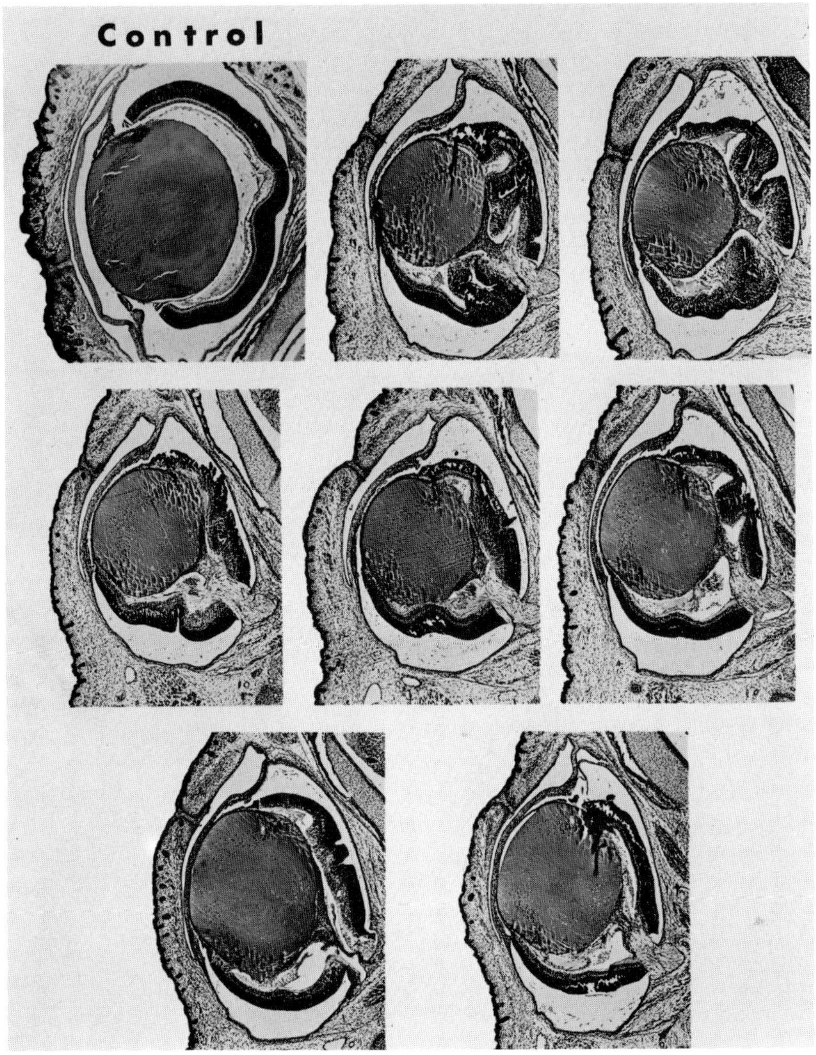

Fig. 4-3.—Sections through eyes of newborn rats. Except for the control, all eyes show the retrolenticular membrane characteristic of prenatal vitamin A deficiency. (From J. Warkany and C. B. Roth.[78])

trients, possibly enzyme constituents, and have not found any reason to change this working hypothesis; but I admit that direct proof for this assumption is still scant.

Although the mechanisms of these deficiencies are still unexplored, the results were welcome finds for the teratologist interested in abnormal morphogenesis. The development of ocular malformations (Figs. 4-2 and 4-3) produced by vitamin A deficiency (colobomas, persistence of the primary vitreous, and others) could be followed through various embryonic and fetal stages.[13] With Wilson, we could study the great variety of aortic arch anomalies and cardiac defects.[15] With vitamin A deficiency, one could also throw into disorder the development of the genital ducts and produce male and female pseudohermaphrodism, a fact that should be of interest to the endocrinologist.[16] Another experiment resulted in a change in the vitamin A deficiency syndrome by restoration of vitamin A at various times during gestation.[17] Thus, a relationship could be established between the lack of these substances and the origin of malformations of various organs.

In 1948, two "positive" teratogens, nitrogen mustard and trypan blue, were found. Haskin[18] described severe malformations in the young of rats treated with a radiomimetic and cytotoxic nitrogen mustard, and comparable results were later also obtained in mice.[19] Gillman *et al.*[20] introduced trypan blue as a teratogen that produced hydrocephaly, spina bifida and other congenital anomalies in the young of treated rats. Trypan blue has been used by many investigators and still is a favorite teratogen. Gillman and associates believed that reproductive failure among Africans was due to chronic malnutrition, which "could be complicated by the steady flooding of the circulation with particles derived from the abnormal metabolism or from the increased permeability of the gut, one of the consequences of malnutrition." They decided to use "selected particles injected into animals in different physiological states." They chose trypan blue for this purpose and succeeded in producing a wide range of gross malformations in the young born of rats treated with dye before and during pregnancy.

In 1950 and 1952, Ingalls *et al.*[21,22] reported on anoxia as a cause of fetal death and congenital defects in mice. These investigators placed female mice in a low-pressure chamber for 5 hours at 260–280 mm. Hg from the second to the eighteenth day of gestation. A significant number of young had hemivertebrae, fused ribs, cleft palate and cranioschisis. Later, Ingalls *et al.*[23] showed that hypoxia-induced congenital anomalies depended to a certain extent on the strain of mice used in the experiment. Murakami *et al.*[24] examined embryos of female mice exposed to reduced atmospheric pressures long before birth and found changes in the central nervous system and the eye. Degenhardt[25] extended this line of investigation to rabbits and found vertebral, costal and ocular defects. Some of the malformed females were mated to malformed brothers, and all the young were normal.[26]

Many hormones have been used as teratogens.[27] Only a few will be mentioned here. In 1950, Baxter and Fraser[28] announced the production of congenital defects in the offspring of female mice treated with cortisone, and in 1951 Fraser and Fainstat[29] showed that the frequency of cleft palate produced in the offspring varied with the dose administered, the time of treatment and the mouse strain used. Kalter[30] and Fraser *et al.*[31] continued this experimental system in many studies that demonstrated the inheritance of susceptibility to the teratogenic action of cortisone. Needless to say, the blending of teratologic and genetic studies was an important milestone in mammalian experimental teratology. These experiments explain, in part, why those who work with animals of variable genotype cannot expect uniform results; but they show also that, in addition to known genetic and exogenous teratogenic factors, some intangible influences may determine whether a malformation occurs or not. The uncertainties in well-controlled experiments should be made known to those who look for simple and general explanations of human congenital malformations.

The great interest in radiobiology that followed World War II led to renewed interest in x-rays as a teratogenic tool. We were curious to see whether rat embryos exposed to x-rays between the thirteenth and fourteenth days of gestation would produce malformations similar to those induced by riboflavin deficiency. The syndrome obtained (Figs. 4-4 and 4-5) was indeed superficially similar to that of the dietary deficiency, but there also were differences which have been described.[32] Since 1950, many exact and detailed studies were made by Russell,[33-35] Wilson,[36-38] Hicks[39-41] and many others who successfully used x-rays as an acute and well-defined teratogen. This line of investigation, which is still being continued in many laboratories, represents a special chapter which has been reviewed in several articles.[41-43]

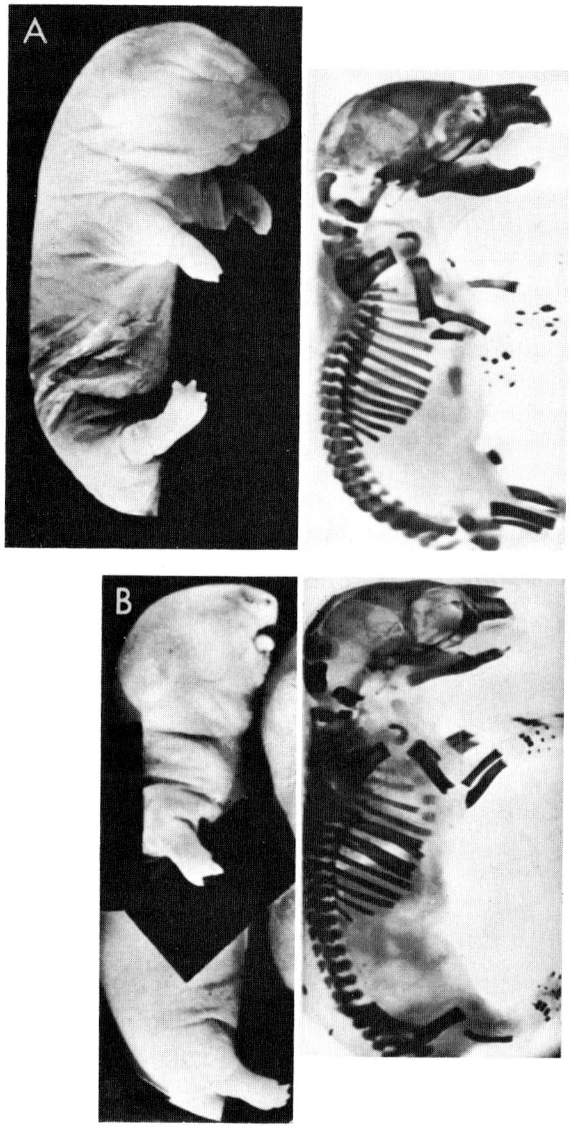

Fig. 4-4. —Comparison of patterns of congenital malformations produced in newborn rats by **A,** x-irradiation on the thirteenth day of pregnancy and **B,** maternal riboflavin deficiency. Despite external resemblance, the young had completely different patterns of skeletal malformations, as seen in cleared specimens. (From J. Warkany and E. Schraffenberger.[32])

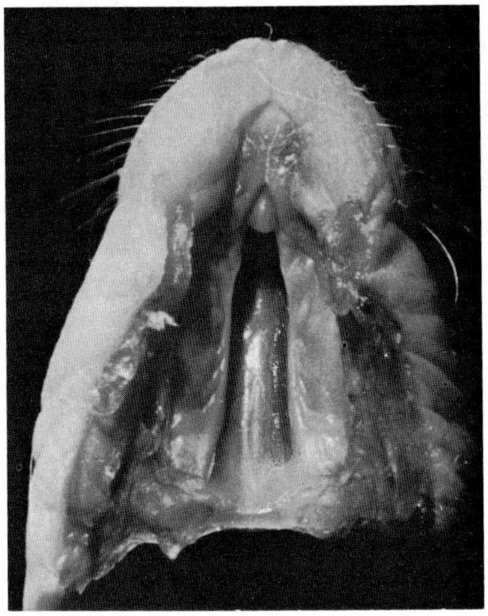

Fig. 4-5.—Cleft palate in newborn rat produced by x-irradiation on the fifteenth day of gestation. (From J. Warkany and E. Schraffenberger.[32])

It was mentioned before that the use of purified diets made possible the testing of various vitamin deficiencies for their teratogenic effects. It was found that, under certain experimental conditions, maternal deficiency of vitamin E,[44] pantothenic acid,[45-47] folic acid or nicotinic acid can result in congenital malformations of the young. To produce some of these deficiencies, special measures had to be taken to overcome the synthetic capacities of the maternal intestinal flora. To obtain folic acid (pteroylglutamic acid) deficiency in rats, an antimetabolite[48,49] or an antibiotic[50] had to be introduced in the deficient diet. With the help of x-methyl folic acid,[51] acute folic acid deficiency could be induced. This deficiency proved highly teratogenic in pregnant rats. The antimetabolites pantoyltaurine[46] and sodium omega-methyl pantothenate[47] were used to produce rapid pantothenic acid deficiency, and galactoflavin accelerated the effects of a riboflavin-deficient diet.[52] The late Dr. Marjorie M. Nelson was a leader in this important development.[53] Antimetabolites became powerful teratogenic tools that made possible conversion of long-term nutritional experiments into short-term chemical experiments. Whereas the chronic deficiency created an abnormal environmental background for the developing embryo, which led to malformations at times of increased nutritional requirements, the metabolic antagonist created a sudden deficiency at selected stages of development. It is understandable that the new methods shortened teratologic experiments greatly; but the new sharp tools also made possible the production of large numbers of certain congenital malformations that previously had seldom been obtained. To give one example: In contrast to cleft palate, cleft lip was only rarely produced in rat fetuses by teratogenic procedures. But Nelson *et al.*[54] obtained cleft lip in more than 90% of the young of rats subjected, with the help of an antimetabolite, to a transitory folic acid deficiency during days 9–11 of gestation. Being sharp tools, antagonists are often more effective and sometimes more devastating than simple deficiencies. Although galactoflavin added to a riboflavin-deficient diet induces skeletal malformations similar to those produced by the chronic dietary deficiency alone, it results also in additional cardiovascular, cerebral and urogenital anomalies.

The nicotinamide antagonist 6-aminonicotinamide can inhibit the action of the vitamin in rat and mouse embryos, even without dietary restriction of the mothers.[55,56] This brings us to the long list of teratogenic chemical compounds found during the past 10 years that permit production of congenital malformations and monstrosities in fetuses after a single dose administered to a pregnant rodent. Many of these chemicals were at first used in tumor-inhibition screening programs and subsequently tested for teratogenic effects. Murphy[57] reviewed this topic and presented comparative dosages producing toxic and teratogenic effects on the pregnant rat and its fetuses for eight tumor-inhibiting chemicals. These compounds were alkylating agents, antimetabolites and triazene. In addition to tumor-inhibiting compounds, many other drugs were found to be teratogenic in animal experiments. One of these is vitamin A, which, given in excess to rats, mice or rabbits,[58-61] has become a favorite teratogen used in many experiments dealing with abnormal morphogenesis.[61-63] It is curious that both vitamin A deficiency and hypervitaminosis A are effective in the production of congenital malformations. Whether there is a common denominator or whether the two mechanisms have nothing in common remains unknown, since the mode of action has not been elucidated for either method. Some antibiotics[27,64,65] and many hormones[27] have been found to be teratogenic in various experimental arrangements. Not all can be enumerated here; there are review articles available[27,65,66] to which the reader is referred. By 1961, it was known to the teratologist that many drugs, including salicylates,[67] are teratogenic if given at the right time, in the right dose, to the right animal. It was also known that aminopterin[68-70] and certain progesterones[71] could be teratogenic in man. The surprising feature of thalidomide[72,73] was that this drug, which appeared completely harmless when given for a limited time in postnatal life, had deleterious effects in minimal doses in prenatal life. It was also unusual that the rat embryo so extensively used in previous teratologic experiments proved extremely resistant to thalidomide (p. 86). Despite this, when the thalidomide epidemic was recognized in 1961, it was soon assumed by all investigators that there was an environmental cause for the deformities of these children. This illustrates the change of thought and attitude brought about by experimental mammalian teratology.

REFERENCES

1. Goldstein, L., and Murphy, D. P.: Etiology of ill health in children born after maternal pelvic irradiation: Defective children born after postconception pelvic irradiation, Am. J. Roentgenol. 22:322, 1929.
2. Kaven, A.: Das Auftreten von Gehirnmissbildungen nach Roentgenbestrahlung von Mäuseembryonen, Ztschr. menschl. Vererb.-u. Konstitutionslehre 22:247, 1938.
3. Jackson, C. M.: *Effects of Inanition and Malnutrition upon Growth and Structure* (Philadelphia: P. Blakiston's Son & Company, 1925).
4. Zilva, S. S., Golding, J., Drummond, J. C., and Coward, K. H.: The relation of the fat-soluble factor to rickets and growth in pigs, Biochem. J. 15:427, 1921.
5. Hale, F.: Pigs born without eyeballs, J. Hered. 24:105, 1933.
6. Hale, F.: The relation of vitamin A to anophthalmos in pigs, Am. J. Ophth. 18:1087, 1935.
7. Hale, F.: The relation of maternal vitamin A deficiency to microphthalmia in pigs, Texas J. Med. 33:228, 1937.
8. Palludan, B.: The teratogenic effect of vitamin A deficiency in pigs, Acta vet. scandinav. 2:32, 1961.
9. Warkany, J.: Congenital malformations induced by maternal dietary deficiency: Experiments and their interpretation, Harvey Lect. 18:89, 1952–1953.
10. Warkany, J., and Nelson, R. C.: Skeletal abnormalities in offspring of rats reared on deficient diets, Anat. Rec. 79:83, 1941.
11. Warkany, J., and Schraffenberger, E.: Congenital malformations induced in rats by maternal nutritional deficiency. V. Effects of a purified diet lacking riboflavin, Proc. Soc. Exper. Biol. & Med. 54:92, 1943.
12. Warkany, J., and Schraffenberger, E.: Congenital malformations induced in rats by maternal nutritional deficiency. VI. The preventive factor, J. Nutrition 27:477, 1944.
13. Warkany, J., and Schraffenberger, E.: Congenital malformations induced in rats by maternal vitamin A deficiency. I. Defects of the eye, Arch. Ophth. 35:150, 1946.
14. Warkany, J., Roth, C. B., and Wilson, J. G.: Multiple congenital malformations: A consideration of etiologic factors, Pediatrics 1:462, 1948.
15. Wilson, J. G., and Warkany, J.: Aortic arch and cardiac anomalies in the offspring of vitamin A deficient rats, Am. J. Anat. 85:113, 1949.
16. Wilson, J. G., and Warkany, J.: Malformations in the genitourinary tract induced by maternal vitamin A deficiency in the rat, Am. J. Anat. 83:357, 1948.
17. Wilson, J. G., Roth, C. B., and Warkany, J.: An analysis of the syndrome of malformations induced by maternal vitamin A deficiency. Effects of restoration of vitamin A at various times during gestation, Am. J. Anat. 92:189, 1953.
18. Haskin, D.: Some effects of nitrogen mustard on the development of external body form in the fetal rat, Anat. Rec. 102:493, 1948.
19. Danforth, C. H., and Center, E.: Nitrogen mustard as a teratogenic agent in the mouse, Proc. Soc. Exper. Biol. & Med. 86:705, 1954.
20. Gillman, J., Gilbert, C., Gillman, T., and Spence, I.: A preliminary report on hydrocephalus, spina bifida, and other congenital anomalies in the rat produced by trypan blue, South African J. M. Sc. 13:47, 1948.
21. Ingalls, T. H., Curley, F. J., and Prindle, R. A.: Anoxia as a cause of fetal death and congenital defect in the mouse, Am. J. Dis. Child. 80:34, 1950.
22. Ingalls, T. H., Curley, F. J., and Prindle, R. A.: Experimental production of congenital anomalies. Timing and degree of anoxia as factors causing fetal deaths and congenital anomalies in the mouse, New England J. Med. 247:758, 1952.
23. Ingalls, T. H., Avis, F. R., Curley, F. J., and Temin, H. M.: Genetic determination of hypoxia-induced congenital anomalies, J. Hered. 44:185, 1953.
24. Murakami, U., Kameyama, Y., and Kato, T.: Effects of maternal anoxia upon the development of embryos, Ann. Report, Res. Inst. of Environmental Med., Nagoya Univ. 76, March, 1956.
25. Degenhardt, K-H.: Durch O_2-mangel induzierte Fehlbildungen der Axialgradienten bei Kaninchen, Ztschr. Naturforsch. 96:530, 1954.
26. Degenhardt, K-H., and Kladetzky, J.: Wirbelsäulenmissbildung und Chordaanlage. Experimentelle teratogenetische und embryohistologische Untersuchungen bei Kaninchen, Ztschr. menschl. Vererb.-u. Konstitutionslehre 33:151, 1955.
27. Kalter, H., and Warkany, J.: Experimental production of congenital malformations in mammals by metabolic procedures, Physiol. Rev. 39:69, 1959.
28. Baxter, H., and Fraser, F. C.: Production of congenital defects in offspring of female mice treated with cortisone, McGill M. J. 19:245, 1950.
29. Fraser, F. C., and Fainstat, T. D.: Production of congenital defects in offspring of pregnant mice treated with cortisone, Pediatrics 8:527, 1951.
30. Kalter, H.: The genetics and physiology of susceptibility to the teratogenic effects of cortisone in mice, Ph.D. dissertation, McGill University, Montreal, 1953.
31. Fraser, F. C., Fainstat, T. D., and Kalter, H.: The experimental production of congenital defects with particular reference to cleft palate, Études néo-natales 2:43, 1953.
32. Warkany, J., and Schraffenberger, E.: Congenital malformations induced in rats by roentgen rays, Am. J. Roentgenol. 57:455, 1947.
33. Russell, L. B.: X-ray induced developmental abnormalities in the mouse and their use in the analysis of embryological patterns. I. External and gross visceral changes, J. Exper. Zool. 114:545, 1950.
34. Russell, L. B.: X-ray induced developmental abnormalities in the mouse and their use in the analysis of embryological patterns. II. Abnormalities of the vertebral column and thorax, J. Exper. Zool. 131:329, 1956.
35. Russell, L. B., and Russell, W. L.: An analysis of the changing radiation response of the developing mouse embryo, J. Cell. & Comp. Physiol. 43:103, 1954.
36. Wilson, J. G., and Karr, J. W.: Effects of irradiation on embryonic development. I. X-rays on the tenth day of gestation in the rat, Am. J. Anat. 88:1, 1951.
37. Wilson, J. G., Jordan, H. C., and Brent, R. L.: Effects of irradiation on embryonic development. II. X-rays on the ninth day of gestation in the rat, Am. J. Anat. 92:153, 1953.
38. Wilson, J. G., Brent, R. L., and Jordan, H. C.: Neoplasia induced in rat embryos by roentgen irradiation, Cancer Res. 12:222, 1952.
39. Hicks, S. P.: Some effects of ionizing radiation and metabolic inhibition on the developing mammalian nervous system, J. Pediat. 40:489, 1952.
40. Hicks, S. P.: Developmental malformations produced by radiation, Am. J. Roentgenol. 69:272, 1953.
41. Hicks, S. P., and D'Amato, C. J.: Effects of ionizing radiations on mammalian development, Adv. in Teratology 1: 195, 1966.
42. Russell, L. B.: The Effects of Radiation on Mammalian Prenatal Development, in Holländer, A. (ed.), *Radiation Biology* (New York: McGraw-Hill Book Company, Inc., 1954).
43. Wilson, J. G.: Differentiation and the reaction of rat embryos to radiation, J. Cell. & Comp. Physiol. 43:11, 1954.
44. Cheng, D. W., and Thomas, B. H.: Relationship of time of therapy to teratogeny in maternal avitaminosis E, Proc. Iowa Acad. Sc. 60:290, 1953.
45. Lefebvres-Boisselot, J.: Rôle tératogène de la déficience

en acide pantothénique chez le rat, Ann. méd. (Paris) 52: 225, 1951.

46. Zunin, C., and Barrone, C.: Embriopatie da carenza di acido pantotenico, Acta vitam. 8:263, 1954.
47. Nelson, M. M., Wright, H. V., Baird, C. D. C., and Evans, H. M.: Teratogenic effects of pantothenic acid deficiency in the rat, J. Nutrition 62:395, 1957.
48. Hogan, A. G., O'Dell, B. L., and Whitley, J. R.: Maternal nutrition and hydrocephalus in newborn rats, Proc. Soc. Exper. Biol. & Med. 74:293, 1950.
49. Evans, H. M., Nelson, M. M., and Asling, C. W.: Multiple congenital abnormalities resulting from acute folic acid deficiency during gestation, Science 114:479, 1951.
50. Giroud, A., and Lefebvres-Boisselot, J.: Influence tératogène de la carence en acide folique, Compt. rend. Soc. biol. 145:526, 1951.
51. Nelson, M. M., Asling, C. W., and Evans, H. M.: Production of multiple congenital abnormalities in young by maternal pteroylglutamic acid deficiency during gestation, J. Nutrition 48:61, 1952.
52. Nelson, M. M., Baird, C. D. C., Wright, H. V., and Evans, H. M.: Multiple congenital abnormalities in the rat resulting from riboflavin deficiency induced by the antimetabolite galactoflavin, J. Nutrition 58:125,1956.
53. Nelson, M. M.: Mammalian Fetal Development and Antimetabolites, in Rhoads, E. P. (ed.), *Antimetabolites and Cancer* (Washington, D. C.: American Association for the Advancement of Science Monograph, 1955).
54. Nelson, M. M., Wright, H. V., Asling, C. W., and Evans, H. M.: Multiple congenital abnormalities resulting from transitory deficiency of pteroylglutamic acid during gestation in the rat, J. Nutrition 56:349, 1955.
55. Murphy, M. L., Dagg, C. P., and Karnofsky, D. A.: Comparison of teratogenic chemicals in the rat and chick embryo, Pediatrics 19:701, 1957.
56. Pinsky, L., and Fraser, F. C.: Production of skeletal malformations in the offspring of pregnant mice treated with 6-aminonicotinamide, Biol. Neonat. 1:106, 1959.
57. Murphy, M. L.: Teratogenic Effects of Tumour-Inhibiting Chemicals in the Foetal Rat, in Wolstenholme, G. E. W., and O'Connor, C. M. (eds.), *A Ciba Foundation Symposium on Congenital Malformations* (London: J. & A. Churchill, Ltd., 1960).
58. Cohlan, S. Q.: Excessive intake of vitamin A as a cause of congenital anomalies in the rat, Science 117:535, 1953.
59. Cohlan, S. Q.: Congenital anomalies in the rat produced by excessive intake of vitamin A during pregnancy, Pediatrics 13:556, 1954.
60. Giroud, A., and Martinet, M.: Malformations oculaires avec fibrose du vitré chez des embryons de lapin soumis à l'hypervitaminose A, Bull. Soc. opht. Franç. No. 3, 1959.
61. Kalter, H., and Warkany, J.: Experimental production of congenital malformations in strains of inbred mice by maternal treatment with hypervitaminosis A, Am. J. Path. 38:1, 1961.
62. Giroud, A., and Martinet, M.: Morphogenèse de l'anencéphalie, Arch. Anat. Micr. 46:247, 1957.
63. Giroud, A., Martinet, M., and Roux, C.: Malformations urinaires dans l'hypervitaminose A, Compt. rend. Soc. biol. 151:1811, 1957.
64. Tuchmann-Duplessis, H., and Mercier-Parot, L.: The Teratogenic Action of the Antibiotic Actinomycin D, in Wolstenholme, G. E. W., and O'Connor, C. M. (eds.), *A Ciba Foundation Symposium on Congenital Malformations* (London: J. & A. Churchill, Ltd., 1960).
65. Wilson, J. G.: Experimental studies on congenital malformations, J. Chron. Dis. 10:111, 1959.
66. Giroud, A., and Tuchmann-Duplessis, H.: Malformations congénitales. Rôle des facteurs exogènes, Path.-biol. 10: 119, 1962.
67. Warkany, J., and Takacs, E.: Experimental production of congenital malformations in rats by salicylate poisoning, Am. J. Path. 35:315, 1959.
68. Thiersch, J. B.: Therapeutic abortions with a folic acid antagonist, Am. J. Obst. & Gynec. 63:1298, 1952.
69. Meltzer, H. J.: Congenital anomalies due to attempted abortion with 4-aminopteroglutamic acid, J.A.M.A. 161: 1253, 1956.
70. Warkany, J., Beaudry, P. H., and Hornstein, S.: Attempted abortion with 4-aminopteroglutamic acid (aminopterin); malformations of the child, Am. J. Dis. Child. 97:274, 1960.
71. Wilkins, L., Jones, H. W., Jr., Holman, G. H., and Stemfel, R. S., Jr.: Masculinization of the female fetus associated with administration of oral and intramuscular progestins during gestation: Non-adrenal female pseudohermaphrodism, J. Clin. Endocrinol. 18:559, 1958.
72. Lenz, W.: Diskussinonsbemerkung zu dem Vortrag von Pfeiffer, R. A., and Kosenow, K.: Zur Frage der exogenen Entstehung schwerer Extremitätenmissbildungen, Tagung der Rheinisch-Westfälischen Kinderärztevereinigung in Düsseldorf 19:11, 1961.
73. McBride, W. G.: Thalidomide and congenital abnormalities, Lancet 2:1358, 1961.
74. Miller, Z., Poncet, I., and Takacs, E.: Biochemical studies on experimental congenital malformations: Flavin nucleotides and folic acid in fetuses and livers from normal and riboflavin-deficient rats, J. Biol. Chem. 237:968, 1962.
75. Aksu, O., Mackler, B., Shepard, T. H., and Lemire, R. J.: Studies of the development of congenital anomalies in embryos of riboflavin-deficient, galactoflavin-fed rats. II. Role of the terminal electron transport systems, Teratology 1:93, 1968.
76. Mackler, B.: Studies of molecular basis of congenital malformations, Pediatrics 43:915, 1969.
77. Giroud, A.:*The Nutrition of the Embryo* (Springfield, Ill.: Charles C Thomas, Publisher, 1970).
78. Warkany, J., and Roth, C. B.: Congenital malformations induced in rats by maternal vitamin A deficiency. II. Effect of varying the preparatory diet upon the yield of abnormal young, J. Nutrition 35:1, 1948.

5

Some Problems of Statistics

Incidence

THE RECOGNITION OF congenital malformations as an important factor in human morbidity and mortality led to a desire for reliable incidence figures that would make possible observations of variations in time and locality under changing genetic and environmental conditions. It should be understood that "congenital malformations" is a collective term for so many heterogeneous structural anomalies present at birth that little meaning can be attached to incidence figures without definition and description of the circumstances under which the estimates were obtained. To give only one example: Ehrat,[1] in 1948, tabulated incidence figures of "malformations expressed in percentages of total birth figures" that were recorded in the world literature up to that time and found variations of from 0.03% to 3.03%! It is not difficult to understand such variations if one scans the authors' names and considers their differing interests and points of view on the subject, and it is clear that attempts to evaluate variations in incidence figures under such conditions must fail. Although present-day estimates differ less widely, there still is much room for better delineation and ascertainment when variations are to be judged. Ehrat charted malformations observed in newborn infants between 1921 and 1944 at the Zurich University Obstetrical Clinic. According to her tabulation, the number of births resulting in malformed children rose from 0.26% in 1921 to 1.48% in 1944. The more than fivefold increase was essentially due to attention paid in the latter years of the survey to "clubfoot," which accounted for 25% of the malformations, and to increased recognition of congenital heart disease. Whereas mongolism was not diagnosed once in the newborn population between 1921 and 1924, its incidence was 0.19% between 1940 and 1944. The study showed that better observation of the infants and inclusion of minor defects were chiefly responsible for the apparently continual increase in congenital malformations. The findings in Zurich, with an average incidence figure of 0.89% over the years, were similar to a figure obtained by Greenhill[2] from many clinics – 0.94%. These "obstetric incidence figures" often remained under 1%, but there were many exceptions. Malpas,[3] for instance, arrived at an incidence figure of 2.1% in Liverpool, England. Half the malformations tabulated there were gross central nervous system defects. Similar figures (between 2 and 3%) were reported from a number of German obstetric clinics, and, in Berlin, Schenk[4] came to an incidence figure of more than 3%. This estimate approaches that of 3.2% ascertained in the newborn period by McIntosh *et al.*,[5] which represents malformations detectable soon after birth by teams of pediatricians, roentgenologists and pathologists. Even prospective and intensive studies of this type can be influenced by exclusion or inclusion of abortuses, prematures, stillbirths, complicated pregnancies, twins, necropsy findings, minor or multiple defects, products of consanguineous marriages, and others. In Edinburgh, Nelson and Forfar,[46] examining 8,684 babies born in three maternity units, found congenital abnormalities in 470 (5.4%). Major abnormalities were seen in 2.1% and minor abnormalities in 3.3%. Among the infants were 172 stillborn, of whom 31.5% had congenital abnormalities. Of practical importance is that among surviving children, 4.7% had congenital malformations, of which only 1.3% were judged to be major. Stewart *et al.*,[47] in another Edinburgh survey in the years 1965–1967, found among 2,500 consecutive live-born infants in one hospital 184 (7.4%) malformed. In Sweden, Ekelund *et al.*[48] noted in a prospective study of 6,200 children that 3.3% had major and 9.6% had minor malformations. For explanation of the differences, the reader is referred to the original articles.

Since there are marked differences even in hospital observations, it is not surprising that figures derived from birth and death certificates are not uniform and not comparable to institutional estimates. Estimates from birth registration records are understandably lower than those obtained in obstetric and newborn units. In the United States, incidences from birth registration records varied from 0.74% to 1.16%. With special efforts, higher figures, between 1.37% and 1.98%, were obtained in directed studies.[6] In a follow-up study in Pennsylvania it was found that only about 60% of the malformed live-born babies were reported as malformed on their birth certificates.[7] There is a possibility that in some hospital series the incidence of congenital malformations is increased by concentration of complicated pregnancies in obstetric clinics. But it also appears increased by more reliable observation and reporting. Birth certificates may fail to reveal malformations because of neglect or because the findings are considered confidential by the physician who wishes to "protect" an affected family by withholding information concerning the tragic outcome of a pregnancy. Some certificates are made out by persons not familiar with the subject of congenital malformations. Hay[8] has listed some entries of "rare" congenital malformations on birth certificates that indicate medical illiteracy–if not ignorance–of the reporters. On the other hand, thorough examinations of infants will reveal many minor congenital malformations that have no adverse effects on the child; this can result in extremely high estimates. The importance of distinguishing between major and minor congenital anomalies can be learned from a study by Marden *et al.*,[9] which showed major defects in 2% of newborn babies and at least one minor anomaly in 14.7%.

Variations in incidence figures in different groups of conceptuses are mentioned here to show how overall estimates can be influenced by inequality of the populations observed and prevalence of one class or another in the total population. Embryos 3–10 weeks old have more malformations than fetuses at the end of pregnancy. Nishimura *et al.*[10] examined such human embryos obtained by curettage for social reasons and found that myeloschisis and polydactyly were at least ten times more frequent among them than in newborn infants. Many malformations were not yet detectable at these early stages of gestation. Stevenson[11] stated that more than half of aborted fetuses are grossly abnormal. Carr[12] found chromosomal anomalies in tissues of 22% of spontaneous abortions, an incidence 50 times that in live-born infants. It has been estimated that 17–20% of stillborn infants are deformed,[11,13] but lower incidence figures were obtained in some series.[14] Thus, inclusion or exclusion of abortuses and stillbirths will influence teratologic incidence figures. McIntosh *et al.*[5] examined products of conception over 500 Gm. and arrived at an estimate of 7% of congenital malformations for infants born alive and surviving the neonatal period. The corresponding figures were 13.6% for antepartum deaths, 23.3% for intrapartum deaths, 29.6% for neonatal deaths and 70.6% for deaths occurring between the ages of 1 and 12 months. A study in a Vermont county[15] showed that a third of early infant deaths were associated with congenital malformations, but this was less definite in late infant deaths. In the British Perinatal Mortality Survey, congenital malformations were associated with more than 21% of early neonatal deaths.[13]

It has been stated by some authors that viable infants surviving threatened abortion have an increased number of malformations,[16,17] but others thought that this increase is only slight.[18,19] In abortions during the second trimester of pregnancy, congenital malformations may play a minor role.[20] Deformities of conceptuses occur more often in cases of placenta previa than otherwise.[2]

Incidences of congenital malformations higher than those in children with adequate birth weights were reported for prematures and infants with low birth weights.[5,21-24] Children with intrauterine growth retardation have an increased incidence of congenital malformations (Chapter 14). Malformation rates among children dying in the perinatal period are much higher than those among survivors.[5,15,25] It is understandable that the number of total deaths and the number of necropsies will influence estimates of congenital malformations in the neonatal period. Approximately 18% of children dying unexpectedly in early life die of congenital malformations.[26]

In multiple births, the incidence of anomalies was found by Hendricks[27] to be three times that in the general population. Among congenitally malformed infants born in the Boston Lying-in Hospital, twinning occurred with approximately twice the expected frequency.[21] Frequency of neural tube defects and frequency of dizygous twinning show a significant positive correlation.[28] In at least one series, malformations in twins were not significantly above the number expected.[29]

The ages of the children observed are of prime importance. It is obvious that incidence figures obtained in the neonatal period can represent only a part of the actual incidence of congenital malformations. There are many malformations that do not manifest themselves and are not detectable in newborn children. McIntosh *et al.*[5] found that even expert teams detected at birth less than half of the malformations present in live-born infants. Neel[30] reported a frequency of major congenital defects found shortly after birth of 1.02%, but the estimate rose to 3.12% on re-examination at age 9 months. In McKeown and Record's series,[29] the incidence of congenital malformations estimated to be 1.7% soon after birth was revised to 2.3% at 5 years. But such figures are still underestimates of the actual incidence of congenital malformations, since many malformations are known to remain silent for years or decades until morbid processes convert the malformations into disease. In Kauai (Hawaiian island), Bierman *et al.*[49] estimated that by age 2, 10% of the surviving infants had perinatal handicaps that required special medical and educational services for physical defects, mental retardation or a combination of the two. Approximately the same number sustained minor defects requiring little or no specialized care. These high incidence figures refer not only to prenatal but also to natal damages. Furthermore, there is no certainty that minor defects recognizable at birth will remain harmless throughout life or that they are isolated and without future complications. Some café au lait spots are harmless pigment lesions, whereas others are forerunners of neurofibromatosis. Polydactyly may be an innocent variation rather common in certain ethnic groups (p. 978), but it can also presage serious consequences when it occurs as a symptom of the Ellis-van Creveld syndrome (p. 793) or of the Laurence-Moon-Biedl syndrome (p. 178). Classifications and evaluations of minor malformations without knowledge of clinical teratology may be of limited value and misleading.

Ethnic, racial or geographic factors can influence incidence figures greatly. It has been found repeatedly that in certain localities the general incidence of congenital malformations was higher in Negro infants than in Caucasian.[31-35] But it was always found that these high incidence figures in Negroes are strongly influenced by the frequent occurrence of polydactyly, an extra digit being attached to the proximal phalanx of the fifth finger. The incidence of polydactyly is approximately 1% in newborn Negroes![33,34] Other anomalies common in Negro children are umbilical hernias[35] and prehelicine fistulas.[34] If one omits such harmless malformations, one usually finds the incidence figures in Negroes lower than those in whites. In contrast, anencephaly occurs frequently in Ireland and Scotland, whereas it is rarer in other localities. In a world-wide study, there was a 40-fold difference in the frequency of anencephaly between the highest and lowest occurrences in various cities.[28] In a series reported from Ireland, the frequency of anencephaly was 1 per 175 births,[36] but it was only 1 per 2,700 in Kampala, Uganda.[34] It would be rash to attribute the difference to racial factors, since the incidence was 1 per 1,000 in Nairobi, Kenya, which is similar to that in other populations.[37] In a world-wide study, the frequency of anencephaly was extremely high in hospitals of Belfast and Alexandria (Egypt) and extremely low in Bogotá (Colombia) and Ljubljana (Yugoslavia),[28] findings that do not bear out an important role of race or ethnic origin in the etiology of this striking malformation. Observations of socioeconomic and geographic variations, together with incomplete concordance in monozygotic twins, suggest that neural tube defects, such as anencephaly and spina bifida, are predominantly "environmental" in origin.[28,38]

The harelip-cleft palate complex seems to be more dependent on racial factors; it occurs more often in Japanese than in Caucasian infants, and is least common in American Negroes.[30] Yet, among some Negroes living in Africa, the frequency resembled that of Caucasians.[34,37] Until we understand better the complex etiology of such malformations (Chapter 70), and until observations are more numerous and more detailed, it may be wise to delay explanations of localized clusters of such malformations by race or ethnic origin.

A different type of racial influence on statistical data is illustrated by the Down syndrome, which is more easily recognized in Caucasian than in Mongol or Negro infants. Experienced observers should have no difficulty in recognizing typical cases in all races.

Children born to consanguineous parents may show more major defects than those born to nonconsanguineous parents.[30]

The foregoing remarks show that incidences of congenital malformations are variable in time and dependent on many changeable factors. Such changeability makes statistical comparisons impossible without corrections for differences in ascertainment. There is little merit in comparing incidence figures of congenital malformations unless the types of malformations and the classes of population included are well defined. Much of the present confusion concerning the statistical dynamics of human congenital malformations can be attributed to attempts to compare the incomparable. Statistical studies must be planned for circumscribed entities of malformations rather than for all-inclusive and heterogeneous estimates.

Congenital Malformations and Morbidity

It would be valuable to know the role played by congenital malformations in the general morbidity of children. A quantitative estimate of this role is extremely difficult to obtain. Many congenital malformations represent merely points of reduced resistance that cause disease only when postnatal pathogenic factors intervene. A deformity of the ureter or a congenital structural anomaly of bone may be converted into disease by minor infections or trauma. In such cases, it is difficult to evaluate the importance of prenatal and postnatal factors. Another obstacle to such estimates is presented by the vague borderlines of congenital malformations and congenital microscopic or functional disturbances. Although congenital metabolic errors or microscopic malformations may be closely related etiologically to gross malformations, they usually are classified differently in medical usage.

Anybody working in an infants' ward of a children's hospital will be impressed by the number of children found there because of congenital defects. In 1956, Dr. B. B. Monroe conducted a survey of the incidence of congenital malformations and anomalies in the infants' ward population of the Children's Hospital in Cincinnati. During a period of 5 months he found that 36.5% of the children were on the ward because of structural congenital malformations.[39] McCrory[40] stated that, in 1958, 43% of all admissions to the Pediatric Service of the University of Iowa Hospitals were caused by conditions arising from congenital malformations. It is obvious that such estimates demonstrate the contribution of congenital malformations to children's morbidity, but they are of limited value because of selection of patients according to age, location, social milieu, medical services available, and so forth. As postnatal causes of children's diseases are reduced, prenatal causes emerge as important factors. Congenital malformations, which are always prenatally determined, play an increasing role in mortality and morbidity of childhood.

Congenital Malformations and Natural Screening

It deserves emphasis that congenital malformations, i.e., malformations present at birth, represent only a limited group of defective conceptuses, since some of the deformed are eliminated before birth. From a pediatric point of view, we are chiefly interested in deformed live-born infants and particularly in those who survive the neonatal period, because they require special treatment and care. But obstetricians, statisticians and demographers are interested also in conceptuses dead before or at the time of birth, i.e., in the entire field of fetal and perinatal wastage. By the time infants are born, they have undergone rigorous intrauterine screening processes that eliminate many defective embryos and fetuses. This intrauterine process of natural selection leads to prenatal death of many deformed or diseased conceptuses, resulting in miscarriage, abortion or stillbirth. Other abnormal embryos and fetuses can live through the intrauterine period and reach the end of gestation. Elimination of many defective zygotes or early embryos has been observed repeatedly. More than half of aborted ova have been shown to be pathologic.[11,41,42] Even embryos obtained by early curettage for social reasons show a much higher incidence of recognizable structural defects than fetuses at the end of gestation.[10] Spontaneously aborted conceptuses have chromosomal aberrations much more often than do live-born infants.[12] In the United Kingdom, approximately 20% of the stillborn fetuses were found to be grossly malformed.[11] In New York City, congenital malformations were present in about 16% of conceptuses dead before and during birth.[5]

Although elimination of conceptuses with congenital malformations proceeds effectively during prenatal life, there remain many deformed fetuses that grow and develop until birth. Some of the deformed infants who survive intrauterine life die after birth, contributing to perinatal and infant mortality. Anencephalic infants and children with severe and irreparable cardiovascular malformations or absent kidneys are examples of incompatibility with postnatal existence. Cleft palate, esophageal and intestinal obstructions, imperforate anus, exomphalos and large diaphragmatic hernias present problems immediately after birth. Such malformations, lethal in animals, often are correctable by surgery. Even under relatively favorable hospital conditions, the screening process continues in the newborn period. In children lost during the neonatal period at the hospitals of Columbia University, New York, the incidence of congenital malformations was approximately 30%.[5] In a necropsy series of newborn infants in Japan, the incidence of congenital malformations was 67.5%[43]; but there can be little doubt that this figure included minor defects that were not responsible for the neonatal deaths. Yet, it is certain that structural defects present at birth do contribute greatly to neonatal mortality.[44] The process of elimination of children with congenital malformations proceeds throughout infancy. Whereas in former times and in undeveloped countries, infectious and nutritional diseases overshadowed and still conceal congenital malformations as a cause of infant deaths, malformations come to the foreground when postnatal morbid factors subside. In the United States, only 5% of deaths under 1 year were attributed in 1910 to congenital malformations, whereas 29% were due to diarrhea and enteritis. As of 1964, diarrheal disorders declined to 2.5% and congenital malformations rose to about 14% as a contributing factor to infant mortality (Fig. 5-1). The same trend was observed in other countries; for instance, in Australia, where the contribution of malformations to infant mortality was 3% in 1900, 12% in 1941–1945 and 18.3% in 1956.[14]

Natural selection continues throughout postnatal life in the form of many diseases of children and adults. Severe brain, ear and eye defects, renal anomalies and reduction malformations of the extremities are handicapping disorders; they do not interfere with life directly but are lethal without the help and care of fellow men. They contribute to mental retardation, sensory and physical handicaps and delayed mortality. Stockard[45] contended: "One may go far in defense of the thesis that the human personality finally dies from some defect, weak spot, that was present at birth. In other words the individual dies of a disease (faulty construction) with which he was born." It is one of the tragedies of mammalian life that the criteria for continuation of prenatal and of postnatal life differ substantially. Some embryos and fetuses, although anatomically normal, are aborted because of maternal anomalies. One-fourth of the spontaneous abortions may belong to this group.[42] On the other hand, there are severely deformed conceptuses that do well in utero but die as soon as they are born, or soon thereafter. Much human suffering and misery is due to the differences in prenatal and postnatal viability that permit survival in utero of conceptuses that are not viable in the outer world. If anomaly of embryos is judged by chromosome analyses,[12] one finds that approximately three-fourths of spontaneously aborted conceptuses would have developed into phenotypes of little promise for adequate physical and mental development. But the most common type of chromosome anomaly encountered in spontaneous abortions (XO), which accounts for one-fourth of those with cytogenetic deviations, would lead to the Turner syndrome, a disorder that often is compatible with a long postnatal life and normal mental development (Chapter 112).

If it were possible to prevent all fetal wastage and to keep every conceptus alive and to nurse it through to the time of delivery, one would save a population of which many would have congenital malformations. Others probably would be damaged by adverse maternal conditions. Thus, preservation of all conceptuses lost before the end of the normal gestation time would keep alive many deformed and diseased fetus-

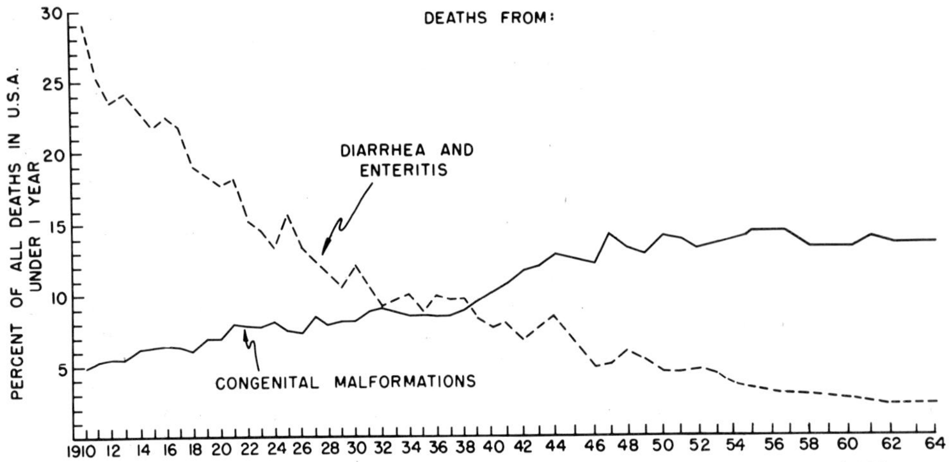

Fig. 5-1.—In 1910, 29% of all deaths of infants under 1 year in the United States were attributed to diarrhea and enteritis and only 5% to congenital malformations. In 1964, 2.5% of the deaths were due to diarrhea and enteritis and 14% to congenital malformations. (U. S. Vital Statistics, Department of Health, Education, and Welfare.)

es. This obviously cannot be considered a desirable goal. It is thinkable that methods can be found to save some of the viable and healthy conceptuses without preserving those who are irreparably damaged before birth. Such differential treatments of the unborn should be made the subject of experimental investigations in the hope that eventually they could be applied to human conditions. There is also the possibility that preventive measures and medical treatment during embryonic and fetal life can interfere with pathologic processes leading to congenital malformations.

The intrauterine prenatal screening process prevents congenital malformations to a certain extent by eliminating deformed conceptuses, but the process is not very effective. Improvement of the screening process by preservation of healthy fetuses and withdrawal of support from the malformed long before birth could be a method of reducing congenital malformations. To implement such preventive measures, a much better knowledge of prenatal physiology and pathology is needed.

REFERENCES

1. Ehrat, R.: *Die Missbildungen der Neugeborenen an der Universitätsfrauenklinik Zürich 1921–1944* (Zürich: Buchdruckerei Jak. Villiger & Cie–Wädenswil, 1948).
2. Greenhill, J. P.: Increased incidence of fetal abnormalities in cases of placenta previa, Am. J. Obst. & Gynec. 37:624, 1939.
3. Malpas, P.: The incidence of human malformations and the significance of changes in the maternal environment in their causation, J. Obst. & Gynaec. Brit. Emp. 44:434, 1937.
4. Schenk, H.: Über die Missbildungen der Jahre 1938–1941 an der Universitäts-Frauenklinik Berlin, Zentralbl. Gynäk. 66:2076, 1942.
5. McIntosh, R., Merritt, K. K., Richards, M. R., Samuels, M. H., and Bellows, M. T.: The incidence of congenital malformations: A study of 5,964 pregnancies, Pediatrics 14:505, 1954.
6. Warkany, J., and Kalter, H.: Congenital malformations, New England J. Med. 265:993 and 1046, 1961.
7. Babbott, J. G., and Ingalls, T. H.: Field studies of selected congenital malformations occurring in Pennsylvania, Am. J. Pub. Health 52:2009, 1962.
8. Hay, S.: New discoveries of rare diseases, New England J. Med. 275:1387, 1966.
9. Marden, P. M., Smith, D. W., and McDonald, M. J.: Congenital anomalies in the newborn infant, including minor variations. A study of 4,412 babies by surface examination for anomalies and buccal smear for sex chromatin, J. Pediat. 64:357, 1964.
10. Nishimura, H., Takano, K., Tanimura, T., Yasuda, M., and Uchida, T.: High incidence of several malformations in the early human embryos as compared with infants, Biol. Neonat. 10:93, 1966.
11. Stevenson, A. C.: Frequency of congenital and hereditary disease, with special reference to mutation, Brit. M. Bull. 17:254, 1961.
12. Carr, D. H.: Chromosome anomalies as a cause of spontaneous abortion, Am. J. Obst. & Gynec. 97:283, 1967.
13. Butler, N. R., and Bonham, D. G.: *Perinatal Mortality by British Perinatal Mortality Survey* (Edinburgh: E. & S. Livingstone, Ltd., 1963).
14. Green, C. R.: The incidence of human maldevelopment, Am. J. Dis. Child. 105:301, 1963.
15. Wulf, R., Gibson, T. C., and Meyer, R. J.: Congenital abnormalities in a Vermont county, New England J. Med. 274:861, 1966.
16. Kotz, J., Parker, E., and Kaufman, M. S.: Treatment of recurrent and threatened abortion: Report of 226 cases, J. Clin. Endocrinol. 1:838, 1941.
17. Turnbull, E. P. N., and Walker, J.: The outcome of pregnancy complicated by threatened abortion, J. Obst. & Gynaec. Brit. Emp. 63:553, 1956.
18. Burge, E. S.: Relationship of threatened abortion of fetal abnormalities, Am. J. Obst. & Gynec. 61:615, 1951.
19. King, A. G.: Threatened and repeated abortion. Present status of therapy, Obst. & Gynec. 1:104, 1953.
20. Stromme, W. B., and Haywa, W.: Intrauterine fetal death in the second trimester, Am. J. Obst. & Gynec. 85:223, 1963.
21. Worcester, J., Stevenson, S. S., and Rice, R. G.: 677 congenitally malformed infants and associated gestational

characteristics. II. Parental factors, Pediatrics 6:208, 1950.
22. Hendricks, C. H.: Congenital malformations. Analysis of 1953 Ohio records, Obst. & Gynec. 6:592, 1955.
23. Keuth, U., Gosztonyi-Lex, E., and Weidtman, V.: Missbildungen bei Frühgeborenen, Ztschr. Kinderh. 97:114, 1966.
24. Landtman, B., and Wallgren, E. I.: Infant mortality due to congenital malformations, Ann. paediat. Fenniae 12:47, 1966.
25. Stevenson, S. S., Worcester, J., and Rice, R. G.: 677 congenitally malformed infants and associated gestational characteristics. I. General considerations, Pediatrics 6:37, 1950.
26. Arey, J. B., and Sotos, J.: Unexpected death in early life, J. Pediat. 49:525, 1956.
27. Hendricks, C. H.: Twinning in relation to birth weight, mortality, and congenital anomalies, Obst. & Gynec. 27: 47, 1966.
28. Stevenson, A. C., Johnston, H. A., Stewart, M. I. P., and Golding, D. R.: Congenital malformations. A report of a study of series of consecutive births in 24 centres, Supp. to Vol. 34, Bull. World Health Organization, 1966, p. 1.
29. McKeown, T., and Record, R. G.: Malformations in a Population Observed for Five Years after Birth, in Wolstenholme, G. E. W., and O'Connor, C. M. (eds.), *A Ciba Foundation Symposium on Congenital Malformations* (London: J. & A. Churchill, Ltd., 1960).
30. Neel, J. V.: A study of major congenital defects in Japanese infants, Am. J. Human Genet. 10:398, 1958.
31. Shapiro, R. N., Eddy, W., Fitzgibbon, J., and O'Brien, G.: Incidence of congenital anomalies discovered in neonatal period, Am. J. Surg. 96:396, 1958.
32. Frazier, T. M.: A note on race-specific congenital malformation rates, Am. J. Obst. & Gynec. 80:184, 1960.
33. Altemus, L. A., and Ferguson, A. D.: Comparative incidence of birth defects in Negro and white children, Pediatrics 36:56, 1965.
34. Simpkiss, M., and Lowe, A.: Congenital abnormalities in the African newborn, Arch. Dis. Childhood 36:404, 1961.
35. Ingalls, T. H., and Klingberg, M. A.: Implications of epidemic embryopathy for public health, Am. J. Pub. Health 55:200, 1965.
36. Coffey, V. P., and Jessop, W. J. E.: A three-year study of anencephaly in Dublin, Irish J. M. Sc. 6:391, 1958.
37. Khan, A. A.: Congenital malformations in African neonates, J. Trop. Med. 68:272, 1965.
38. Editorial: The world's deformities, Lancet 2:1401, 1966.
39. Warkany, J.: Congenital malformations and pediatrics, Pediatrics 19:725, 1957.
40. McCrory, W. W.: Child health in the United States, Quart. Rev. Pediat. 15:94, 1960.
41. Mall, E. P.: Localized anomalies in human embryos, Am. J. Anat. 22:49, 1917.
42. Hertig, A. T.: The Overall Problem in Man, in Benirschke, K., and Jones, T. C. (eds.), *Comparative Aspects of Reproduction Failure* (New York: Springer-Verlag, 1967).
43. Shirasuna, K., Sawasaki, M., and Yonemoto, S.: On the pathological finding of the stillborn and the early neonatal corpses, Congen. Anom. (Japan) 6:15, 1966.
44. Davis, M. E., and Potter, E. L.: Congenital malformations and obstetrics, Pediatrics 19:719, 1957.
45. Stockard, C. R.: *The Physical Basis of Personality* (New York: W. W. Norton & Company, 1931).
46. Nelson, M. M., and Forfar, J. O.: Congenital abnormalities at birth: Their association in the same patient, Developmental Med. & Child Neurol. 11:3, 1969.
47. Stewart, A. L., Keay, A. J., and Smith, P. G.: Congenital malformations; a detailed study of 2500 liveborn infants, Ann. Human Genet. 32:353, 1969.
48. Ekelund, H., Kullander, S., and Källén, B.: Major and minor malformations in newborns and infants up to one year of age, Acta paediat. scandinav. 59:297, 1970.
49. Bierman, J. M., Siegel, E., French, F. E., and Simonian, K.: Analysis of the outcome of all pregnancies in a community, Am. J. Obst. & Gynec. 91:37, 1965.

6

Syndromes

IT IS WELL KNOWN that congenital malformations have a marked tendency to aggregate in persons damaged by adverse prenatal influences. Abnormal genes, chromosomes and environmental factors show little respect for the limits of organs as we know them in postnatal life. Teratogenic factors act at a time when organs and organ systems are in stages of differentiation, with a biochemistry, physiology and anatomy of their own. Disturbing factors often lead to widespread pathologic changes and multiple defects that can occur in a bewildering number of combinations and permutations. The teratologic taxonomist has an understandable desire to bring a modicum of order to this medley and to find principles of classification for the apparent chaos. To this purpose, "syndromes" of congenital malformations that show a tendency to "run together" have been suggested and established in the past and, with the renewed interest in clinical teratology, new syndromes are now being introduced with increasing frequency and in rapid succession. Unfortunately, the confusion created by the zeal of some new taxonomists is considerable.

The kaleidoscopic combinations of malformations can be classified according to different principles. One can, for instance, make anatomic anomalies the central theme of a syndrome, a method most often used in clinical medicine. It is understandable that different specialties will see syndromes from different points of view. The ophthalmologist, for instance, makes certain ocular changes the core of syndromes that include extraocular organs with variable frequency. The otologist, stomatologist, "cheilognathologist," neurologist, dermatologist, roentgenologist or pathologist tends to establish syndromes according to his chief interest. Since syndromes spread from their cores to different spheres and in different directions, patients with similar malformations may be grouped and described in dissimilar terms. It is obvious that on anatomic grounds one classification or viewpoint is as justified as another and that new aspects may appear as methods of examination are improved. Thus, the ophthalmoscope may reveal that the original description of the ocular component of a syndrome was superficial; or new cardiologic methods or roentgen examinations may require regrouping of symptoms. In general, a specialist's inclination to extend his examination beyond the organ of his main interest is meritorious, but attempts to group and classify may lead to disagreements if the outlines of syndromes are drawn too rigidly and it may be difficult to decide which classification is right and which is wrong. Even within a specialty, there can be dissension when the observations of associated symptoms of one authority differ from those of another.

The situation is further complicated by the fact that the principles of classification need not be limited to anatomic or clinical findings. Sometimes, systems of similar histologic or embryonic origin are made the basis of classification. Changes chiefly affecting connective tissue or endocrine glands may be considered together. Anomalies of organs of ectodermal, mesodermal or entodermal origin have been classified according to their embryologic past, and disorders with a tendency to early degeneration or tumor formation have been viewed together on account of their future. With progress of chemical analyses of abnormal tissues, criteria of chemical properties can be made the principle of classification so that lipidoses, mucopolysaccharidoses or an altered amino acid metabolism becomes the basis of classification. But even such classifications are sometimes short-lived when the chemical determinations shift from urine to blood or tissues or when clinical and chemical analyses are refined.

In 1937, we described the difficulties encountered in attempts to classify cases that had some but not all of the features of the Laurence-Moon-Biedl syndrome (Chapter 19) and published the results of a review of the literature then available on this subject.[1] The syndrome was thought to consist of five symptoms: obesity, hypogenitalism, retinitis pigmentosa, polydactyly and mental retardation. But, when the case reports were surveyed, we found that only about one-fourth of the patients showed the pentad of cardinal symptoms, whereas the remaining cases were incomplete. Even some of the patients reported by Laurence and Moon[2] and one of Biedl's[3] did not have all the characteristics of the syndrome. In others, there were more anomalies than those making up the pentad. We concluded that it was unjustified to designate the five cardinal symptoms as a syndrome. Since 1937, the Laurence-Moon-Biedl syndrome has been further enlarged and many variations of the cardinal symptoms have been described.[4] In addition, it has been asserted[5] that Laurence and Moon's original patients did not have the Laurence-Moon-Biedl syndrome! It would seem, therefore, that our doubts concerning the existence of an entity made up of the five cardinal constituents were warranted. Yet, I have learned that the syndrome is a valuable concept, since it represents an autosomal recessive trait. If a child with the pentad is born, there is a risk of 1 in 4 for recurrence in subsequent children, and a sixth finger in a baby born into such a family in most instances presages difficulties in later development. The value of the syndrome for genetic counselling is lessened by its variability and by the absence of most of the cardinal manifestations at birth and in infancy, but the fully developed syndrome is of definite prognostic usefulness if it is remembered that in homozygous persons the gene has a pleiotropic effect with variable expression. Affected persons do not always show the pentad but rather a symptom complex with a narrower or broader spectrum of manifestations. Knowledge of the heredity of the symptom complex is of value if it is applied with judgment and caution.

A syndrome more recently described represents another example of variability of a genetic entity. Smith *et al.*[6] reported siblings with polycystic kidneys and intrahepatic biliary dysgenesis who had eleven additional developmental defects. Although the siblings differed in regard to congenital heart defects, hepatic anomalies and other developmental deviations, it is likely that the authors observed a complex of anomalies attributable to autosomal recessive inheritance. It has been stated[7] that siblings described earlier by Bowen *et al.*[8] had the same "syndrome," although they showed also congenital glaucoma, heart disease, brain defects, genital malformations and calcifications in cartilage. Later, Passarge and McAdams[7] described 5 siblings who appeared to them sufficiently similar to the patients mentioned above[6,8] to group them together into a "cerebro-hepato-renal syndrome." Although the 5 siblings of their remarkable family in all probability had a genetic disorder and were etiologically related, they differed in important cardiovascular, ocular and hepatic changes. Many other examples of such intrafamilial variability could be cited. When pleiotropic abnormal genes produce variable clinical disease pictures in single patients, i.e., without familial recurrence, recognition of such cases as entities is difficult or impossible.

Broad spectra of signs and symptoms are also produced by chromosomal abnormalities, which can lead to variable clinical manifestations.[9] Even trisomy 13–15 (D_1), which, when fully developed, results in a characteristic and devastating syndrome of congenital malformations, can in exceptional cases express itself in few and inconspicuous signs.[10] Trisomy 18 also is variable in symptomatology and causes a spectrum of signs and symptoms.[11] Patients with trisomy 21 (Down syndrome) usually can be recognized at a glance because of characteristic external features. Yet, analysis of the constituents of the syndrome shows significant variations in regard to pathology of the affected organs.[9]

Similarly, there are great differences in the symptoms brought about by prenatal rubella and by other environmental teratogenic agents. Congenital malformations induced by rubella remained unrecognized as a syndrome and unidentified etiologically for many decades until an epidemic revealed the picture of this embryopathy. Without the experiment of nature in Australia in 1940,[12] the entity could long have remained unrecognized. The variety of anomalies appearing after the prenatal infection and the occurrence of the full syndrome in children of mothers who did not give a history of rubella in early pregnancy concealed the connection of cause and effect and confused the casual observer.[13] Mental retardation, cataracts and deafness are rather nonspecific signs that singly or in combination did not lend themselves to establishing a characteristic clinical syndrome. In contrast to the disease picture of prenatal rubella, the thalidomide embryopathy was relatively quickly recognized because it included severe limb defects, which occur only rarely without the use of the drug.[14,15] If the effects of thalidomide had been limited to variable malformations of the heart, intestine, kidney or internal genitalia, it might have taken many years to recognize the syndrome and its cause. Yet, thalidomide did not bring about the same disease picture in all cases. How much individual patients damaged by this drug can vary is best illustrated by twins affected by the drug in the same maternal environment but differing completely in symptoms (see Fig. 11-19). Many syndromes are now proposed because of the repeated "running together" of two or several anatomic anomalies but, in some instances, concurrence by chance seems possible. Even in some familial "syndromes," the variability of individual signs is such that coincidence by chance must be considered.

With the increasing interest in congenital malformations, a syndrome fever is spreading through many specialties, and it is difficult for editors of medical journals and readers to separate spurious from durable and meaningful syndromes. The confusion is due, in part, to lack of agreement concerning the use of the term "syndrome." In the strict sense of the word, any case of multiple congenital malformations represents a "syndrome," since several anomalies "run together" in the patient. But it has become customary to consider as syndromes only malformations that run together frequently. There are no rules regarding the frequency required or the role of familial recurrence or etiologic unity and there is, therefore, much room for difference of opinion and disagreement.

Many attempts have been made in the past to evaluate statistically syntropisms or synchronisms of malformations. An interesting study was made recently in Sweden by Källén and Winberg,[16] who analyzed multiple malformations ascertained by a national registry. According to probability calculations, positive and negative associations were tabulated for 120 children with multiple malformations. Positive associations, e.g., two or more malformations occurring together more often than could be explained by chance, included such well-known concurrences as esophageal and anal atresia, craniostenosis and syndactyly or renal agenesis and pulmonary hypoplasia. A more complicated syndrome, closure defects of the central nervous system, microphthalmia, facial clefts and reduction malformation of the limbs, was found particularly in children born during the first half of 1965, but its etiology was not recognized. It remains to be seen how this type of statistical syndrome research done in newborn children will compare with clinical observations based on relatively few cases seen under specific circumstances or with observations extending beyond the neonatal period. For instance, statistical analysis of malformations in the newborn may fail to find syndromes that manifest themselves gradually. To use the Laurence-Moon-Biedl syndrome as an example again: A child in whom this disease picture develops in late childhood is not born with the syndrome. Even if the entire pentad develops later, only polydactyly is present at birth. Mental retardation, obesity, retinitis pigmentosa and sexual deficiency appear later.

The difficulties of classification are further enhanced by the terminologies used for syndromes. It would be logical to define syndromes by naming the malformations that run together. It has been suggested, for instance, that we speak of "oculo-auriculo-vertebral," "oculo-dento-digital," "oro-facio-digital," "cranio-carpo-tarsal," "cerebro-hepato-renal" and many other combinations. This kind of terminology has many shortcomings, principally because there exist innumerable ocular, auricular or vertebral deviations that differ from those characteristic of the oculo-auriculo-vertebral or "Goldenhar syndrome,"[17] and the same can be said of other components of such disease pictures and of other syndromes that have different constituents. There are cases of

Laurence-Moon-Biedl syndrome with ocular, auricular and spinal anomalies differing completely from those of the Goldenhar syndrome. The same is true for many other combinations of eye, ear and spine defects. How many children have cranial, carpal and tarsal anomalies without having the cranio-carpotarsal dystrophy described by Freeman and Sheldon,[18] in which microstomia (not mentioned in the name suggested) probably is the outstanding sign? For these and other reasons, classification by organ involvement is nonspecific, colorless and not capable of evoking the *picture* to be remembered.

Assignment of proper names to syndromes has long been practiced. The eponymic nomenclature has advantages and disadvantages.[19-21] It avoids limitation to organs or anatomic structures, and the syndrome can be contracted or expanded as new cases are described and new facets are recognized. A single, short name, if properly chosen, can evoke in the listener or reader a picture of signs and symptoms without prejudgment of etiology and pathogenesis. The eponymic system can serve well as an interim terminology until causes, mechanisms and preventive measures are found. It was widely used in the nineteenth century and apparently has been successful, since it is continued to some extent in our times. In theory, the proper name to give to a syndrome should be that of the person who first described it, but this rule seldom is followed. Achondroplasia, for instance, was well "described" in antiquity by Egyptian and Roman sculptors (see Fig. 2-5) whose names are not known. In 1878, it was outlined in words by Parrot,[22] who gave it a well-sounding (though technically incorrect) Greek name. As a result, one does not speak of "Parrot's disease." In many instances, questions of priority have complicated the eponymic system when it was found that a syndrome named after one author had been described by another or others before. In some cases, more or less important data were supplied by later observers whose names were added to the original term. Occasionally, this led to accumulations of proper names such as Laurence-Moon-Biedl-Bardet-Biemond syndrome. A well-circumscribed syndrome of facial angioma, convulsions, hemiparesis and intracranial calcifications, often called the Sturge-Weber syndrome, should be termed the Luschka-Schirmer-Sturge-Kalischer-Hebold-Dimitri-Brushfield-Wyatt-Weber-Krabbe syndrome[21] to do justice to some of those who contributed to its delineation. Since this name would be longer than an account of the signs and symptoms, an abbreviation—Sturge-Weber syndrome—is in use, although F. Parkes Weber "disclaimed the honor of having his name associated to Dr. Sturge's" and suggested "Sturge-Kalischer disease."[23] Whatever the eponym chosen, it is superior to such other, more objective names as encephalotrigeminal angiomatosis, congenital neuroectodermal dysplasia, congenital ectodermosis cutaneous and similar colorless and complicated terms. The same is true for many other syndromes that are named after a person, even though the disorder had been reported before, possibly at an inopportune time, in a little-read journal, by a writer with an unmelodious name who considered a different age group with a chief interest in another aspect of the syndrome. National and ethnic preferences sometimes played a role and resulted in differing terminologies.[21] When it was suggested that the term "mongolism" be replaced by "Down syndrome," French scientists rejected the proposal, since the condition had been described by Séguin before Down's publication. Rare names are advantageous, whereas Smith and Jones are less suitable unless the term is made more distinctive by addition of other proper names or numerals. Some syndromes honor outstanding scientists and teachers who, unfortunately, occasionally established more than one disease picture and thus inadvertently caused confusion. Others are named after a casual observer who published the case because he did not know its etiology, pathogenesis, diagnosis, prognosis and treatment. In such instances, if the uncertainties concerning the disorder persist, the author may become immortal. If, on the other hand, the etiology is recognized, the eponym becomes unnecessary. Thus, Emed described a "pterygium syndrome" in 1956,[24] and in 1960 Edwards *et al.*[25] considered the same disorder "a new trisomic syndrome," which is now termed "trisomy 18" and not "Emed-Edwards syndrome." When Gregg[12] recognized maternal rubella as the cause of certain congenital cataracts and cardiac defects, there remained no need for a "Gregg syndrome." If a less astute observer had described the repeated occurrence of patent ductus arteriosus with congenital cataract without finding the cause of the malformations, his name attached to the syndrome would be familiar to students, physicians and the public who may not know of the role played by Gregg in the discovery of the syndrome and its cause.

Thus, as a rule, eponymic terminology is merely a substitute for understanding more basic concepts of complex disease pictures and usually an admission of failure to find a meaningful explanation of the phenomenon. Despite this, many authors graciously lent their names to disfiguring conditions that await further exploration and significant interpretation. Other writers seem to be unduly proud of their interim role, become possessive, write of "their" syndromes and try to expand their property beyond its original borders by absorbing syndromes described before by others. To counter such imperialistic tendencies, it has been suggested that only dead authors' names be used as eponyms. Or one could use the names of patients whose disease was so distinctive that it led to its description in the medical literature, e.g., Hartnup disease, Hagner[19] disease, Catlin mark[26] and others. Some disorders have been named after cities in which they were observed, as exemplified by Typus Rostockiensis,[27] Typus Amstelodamensis[28] and Minamata disease,[29] but the "Typus" terminology showed little durability and soon gave way to the use of authors' names.

There is no simple solution to the dilemma of syndrome terminology. When etiology and pathogenesis are elucidated, old names can be discarded or maintained according to their value. Although such meaningful terms as trisomy 18 and Minamata disease are much preferable to meaningless eponyms, the use of a proper name to designate an unexplained disease picture seems acceptable as a temporary practice as long as it is understood as an exhortation to further research. Eponyms are used in this book if they have become generally accepted or if there is no good alternative; introduction of new names would only add further confusion. In general, proper names are not apostrophized. Pierre Robin syndrome, for instance, seems preferable to Pierre Robin's syndrome, since the name-giver neither had nor owned the anomaly. At times, the apostrophic form is useful. In speaking of "Pyle disease," the speaker may evoke a picture of piles rather than the osseous dysplasia named after Pyle.

Every case of multiple congenital malformations is of interest and deserves analysis and treatment. The child's parents deserve explanations concerning prognosis, etiology and risk of recurrence. But should every case be published? Recording a single case can be justified if it poses a specific question or suggests an etiologic factor. We recorded a single case of multiple congenital malformations when we suspected that it was induced by aminopterin intake by the mother.[30] Subsequent observations confirmed the suspicion and an "aminopterin syndrome" can be considered established. Zellweger *et al.*[31] published the case of a child with unilateral fibular aplasia, asking the question: "Is lysergic-acid diethylamide a teratogen?" Time will tell whether the suspected causal relationship was real or not. Gregg[12] observed 13 cases of congenital cataract following German measles in the mother, and published when 78 cases had been ascertained. McBride[14] noticed that almost 20% of the babies delivered of women who had been given thalidomide had multiple abnormalities and sent a letter to the *Lancet* asking whether its readers had seen similar babies of women who had taken the drug. One, 2 or 20 cases can be of interest and worthy of publication if specific anatomic, physiologic or etiologic questions are raised or answered by the report. But what should be done about the flood of "new" syndromes that are now hurriedly reported and which may never be seen again in the same combination of symptoms, being variable even within the same family? Some of these "new" syndromes, probably are as old as mankind and have been described before, unknown to the new discoverer. The combinations of anomalies and malformations probably are infinite. Consider those that go with microcephaly, anencephaly, hydrocephaly, spina bifida, ocular coloboma, cataract, ear deformities, congenital heart defects, horseshoe kidney, skeletal malformations and other congenital defects. How many permutations of these malformations do actually exist? To give a specific example, there is much room for syndromes in children with imperforate anus, a striking and most serious anomaly. Gross[32] listed congenital heart disease, esophageal atresia, cleft lip and palate, vertebral malformations, spina bifida, absence of the radius, dislocated hip, clubfoot, digital deformities, kidney anomalies, exstrophy of the bladder, hypospadias, ectopic penis, bifid scrotum, vaginal malformations and many other associated defects – a total of 65 entries. Many combinations and permutations of these malformations exist. How many syndromes could be created by syndrome lovers who want their names immortalized in this area? The list of malformations associated with anal atresia shows that frequency of concurrence does not create meaningful syndromes. To give a single example: The most frequent "syndrome," congenital heart disease + anal atresia, has been observed in the Laurence-Moon-Biedl complex, in trisomy 13–15, in trisomy 21 and in the thalidomide embryopathy, i.e., in disease pictures caused by changes of genes, chromosomes or environment.

Any observation of a syndrome can be of practical or theoretical importance, particularly if it stimulates etiologic research, statistical evaluation or experimentation. But if it is named without consideration of its meaning, it can become a superficial label that inhibits rather than promotes thinking and research.

Of the thousands of syndromes existing in the field of congenital malformations only a few are mentioned in this book. Some syndromes were selected because of their special interest as representatives of etiologic or pathogenetic entities; others are mentioned because their names are familiar and in general use. No claim is made for justice of terminology, selection or allocation. When a syndrome is composed of malformations of several organ systems, its location in the book sometimes can be explained by the importance of one of its components, by its significance to a specialty or by historical factors – but sometimes location is arbitrarily assigned. For many syndromes, more than one name is mentioned and the reader can select his preferred terminology. The Index will be helpful in locating the descriptions of disease pictures in which congenital malformations "run together." The inconsistencies in handling of the syndromes are due in part to the chaotic state of the subject.

REFERENCES

1. Warkany, J., Frauenberger, G. S., and Mitchell, A. G.: Heredofamilial deviations. 1. The Laurence-Moon-Biedl syndrome, Am. J. Dis. Child. 53:455, 1937.
2. Laurence, J. Z., and Moon, R. C.: Four cases of retinitis pigmentosa occurring in the same family and accompanied by general imperfections of development, Brit. Ophth. Rev. 2:32, 1866.

3. Biedl, A.: Ein Geschwisterpaar mit adiposo-genitaler Dystrophie, Deutsche med. Wchnschr. 48:1630, 1922.
4. Bell, J.: The Laurence-Moon-Biedl Syndrome, in *Treasury of Human Inheritance*, Vol. 5 (London: Cambridge University Press, 1958).
5. Franceschetti, A., and Klein, D.: Les manifestations tapétorétiniennes et leur importance clinique et génétique, Rev. otoneuroophth. 20:109, 1948.
6. Smith, D. W., Opitz, J. M., and Inhorn, S. L.: A syndrome of multiple developmental defects, including polycystic kidneys and intrahepatic biliary dysgenesis in two siblings, J. Pediat. 67:617, 1965.
7. Passarge, E., and McAdams, A. J.: Cerebro-hepato-renal syndrome, J. Pediat. 71:691, 1967.
8. Bowen, P., Lee, C. S. N., Zellweger, H., and Lindenberg, R.: A familial syndrome of multiple congenital defects, Bull. Johns Hopkins Hosp. 114:402, 1964.
9. Warkany, J., Passarge, E., and Smith, L. B.: Congenital malformations in autosomal trisomy syndromes, Am. J. Dis. Child. 112:502, 1966.
10. Hecht, F.: Phenotypic differentiation of autosomal chromosomal abnormalities. Anomalies on the gross, radiologic, autopsy, cellular, and molecular levels in the D_1 (13–15) trisomy syndrome, Alabama J. M. Sc. 3:489, 1966.
11. Heinrichs, E. H., and Allen, S. W., Jr.: The 18-trisomy syndrome—a spectrum?, Clin. Pediat. 2:25, 1963.
12. Gregg, N. M.: Congenital cataract following German measles in mother, Tr. Ophth. Soc. Australia 3:35, 1942.
13. Beswick, R., Warner, R., and Warkany, J.: Congenital anomalies following maternal rubella, Am. J. Dis. Child. 78:334, 1949.
14. McBride, W. G.: Thalidomide and congenital abnormalities, Lancet 2:1358, 1961.
15. Lenz, W.: Diskussionsbemerkung zu dem Vortrag von R. A. Pfeiffer und K. Kosenow: Zur Frage der exogenen Entstehung schwerer Extremitätenmissbildungen, Tagung der Rheinisch-Westfälischen Kinderärztevereinigung in Düsseldorf 19:11, 1961.
16. Källén, B., and Winberg, J.: Multiple malformations studied with a national register of malformations, Pediatrics 44:410, 1969.
17. Goldenhar, M.: Associations malformatives de l'oeil et de l'oreille, en particulier le syndrome dermoide épibulbaire-appendices auriculaires-fistula auris congenita et ses relations avec la dysostose mandibulo-faciale, J. Génét. Hum. 1:243, 1952.
18. Freeman, E. A., and Sheldon, J. H.: Cranio-carpo-tarsal dystrophy—an undescribed congenital malformation, Arch. Dis. Childhood 13:277, 1938.
19. Fischer, I.: Zur Geschichte der Krankheitsnamen, Med. Klin. 25:412, 1929.
20. Schönfeld, W.: Syndromatologie, Deutsche med. Wchnschr. 79:324, 1954.
21. Leiber, B., and Olbrich, G.: *Wörterbuch der Klinischen Syndrome* (München-Berlin: Urban & Schwarzenberg, 1963).
22. Parrot, J.: Sur la malformation achondroplasique et le dieu Ptah, Bull. Soc. anthropol. (Paris) 1:296, 1878.
23. Weber, F. P.: The Sturge-Kalischer disease and the Sturge-Weber panathenaic amphora at Toronto, Brit. M. J. 1:708, 1936.
24. Emed, A.: Pterygium syndrome, J. Pediat. 48:73, 1956.
25. Edwards, J. H., Harnden, D. G., Cameron, A. H., Crosse, V. M., and Wolff, O. H.: A new trisomic syndrome, Lancet 1:787, 1960.
26. Goldsmith, W. M.: The Catlin mark: The inheritance of an unusual opening in the parietal bones, J. Hered. 13:69, 1922.
27. Hövels, O., and Müllereisert, F.: Der "Typus Rostockiensis" als charakteristisches Kombinationsbild multipler Missbildungen (Polydaktylie, Hypospadie, Kryptorchismus und Mikrognathie), Ztschr. Kinderh. 77:454, 1955.
28. de Lange, C.: Nouvelle observation du "Typus Amstelodamensis" et examen anatomo-pathologique de ce type, Arch. méd. Enf. 41:193, 1938.
29. Takeuchi, T., Kambara, T., Morikawa, N., Matsumoto, H., Shiraishi, Y., and Ito, H.: Pathologic observations of the Minamata disease, Acta Path. Jap. 9:769, 1959.
30. Warkany, J., Beaudry, P. H., and Hornstein, S.: Attempted abortion with 4-amino-pteroylglutamic acid (aminopterin); malformations of the child, Am. J. Dis. Child. 97:274, 1959.
31. Zellweger, H., McDonald, J. S., and Abbo, G.: Is lysergic-acid diethylamide a teratogen?, Lancet 2:1066, 1967.
32. Gross, R. E.: *Surgery of Infancy and Childhood* (Philadelphia: W. B. Saunders Company, 1953).
33. Gellis, S. S., and Feingold, M.: *Atlas of Mental Retardation Syndromes* (Washington, D. C.: Department of Health, Education, and Welfare, 1968).
34. Smith, D. W.: *Recognizable Patterns of Human Malformation* (Philadelphia: W. B. Saunders Company, 1970).

7

Sensitive or Critical Periods in Teratogenesis:

Uses and Abuses of Embryologic Timetables

THERE IS A COMMON BELIEF often expressed in the medical literature that one can ascertain the time of causation of congenital malformations by consideration of sensitive periods in embryologic development. It is thought that malformations are due to interference of teratogenic factors acting during critical periods of organogenesis, which leave their imprints on the child. This belief is based on numerous embryologic experiments which show that specific malformations can be produced at certain stages of development, irrespective of the nature of the teratogenic agent. Classic experiments of this type were performed by C. R. Stockard,[1] who emphasized the critical moments during early embryonic development and their importance in the outcome of teratologic experiments. He found that the same inhibiting influence, if allowed to act on the embryo during different developmental stages, will induce entirely different responses because several embryonic organs reach their most critical stages of origin at different times. He stated that a given organ must be interrupted during the early stage of its development to be completely suppressed or grossly modified. The same interruption introduced at a much earlier or a much later time will fail to influence it seriously, although at these other times some other organ, then in its critical stage of origin, will be grossly affected. It seemed that the moment of origin of an organ, its "budding stage," was the most critically susceptible time in its development. These conclusions were derived from experiments with fish embryos that showed a graded series of anomalies induced by treatment of eggs with many different chemical and physical arresting agents.[1] There can be little doubt that Stockard's observations were correct and that his conclusions were justified in the context of his experiments. But there is a wide gap between his opinions and the belief that morphologic anomalies observed in human beings indicate the time of their causation and that, with the help of embryologic timetables, one can assign a specific date of causation according to known or imagined sensitive periods of development. Since this topic is not only of theoretical interest but also of legal importance, and since correct and incorrect opinions are intermingled in this area, the uses and abuses of embryologic timetables in etiologic research on congenital malformations are worth discussing.

It is true that in human as well as in fish and amphibian embryos, sensitive periods exist that may be the time of origin of certain malformations. But it is also true that we know few examples of such causative events—if any. A single exposure of an embryo to a large dose of x-rays or a single exposure to a damaging chemical compound would correspond to the experimental setup of the embryologist. Such "acute" teratologic events may occur in man, but they seldom are recognized and are hard to prove. Most teratologic factors known at present are "chronic" in nature; they often are with the individual throughout life, as exemplified by genetic and chromosomal determinants. X-irradiation, administration of drugs and exposure to chemical compounds often occur repeatedly and differ in this respect from well-planned acute embryologic experiments.

Another source of error in assigning dates of origin to congenital malformations is the confusion of the concept of "termination period" with that of "determination period." To avoid faulty timing of teratologic events, Schwalbe[2] and others introduced at the beginning of this century the valuable concept of teratologic "termination periods." According to this concept, one can determine, with the help of embryologic facts, the *latest* possible time at which a disturbing factor could have brought about certain types of malformations. It is possible to state that a malformation must have originated before the teratologic termination period of the structure involved. Schwalbe knew that one could, at best, establish a period after which a teratogenic agent could not have deformed an organ because the structure had been shaped in principle at an earlier stage of development. No teratologic factor, whether genic, chromosomal or environmental, can bring about a cleft palate, spina bifida, a single cerebral ventricle or an ocular coloboma after the fourth month of gestation, but at no time did Schwalbe or his contemporaries assert that one could determine with the aid of embryologic knowledge or timetables the exact date at which the deformity was caused. These early embryologists knew that periods of termination are not identical with periods of determination and that the time of causation always precedes the period of termination. Teratologic determination can take place moments before the termination period or it can occur, as in cases of genetic causation, generations and centuries before the termination period. To give a simile: In the case of a derailment of a train, the timetable can be useful in the search for causes of the accident because it indicates (if the train was on time) the last moment at which the damage could have been caused. Somebody may have committed an act of sabotage immediately before the accident, but he could also have put an obstacle on the rails hours before the accident; or the derailment could have been due to neglect of the roadbed for years and decades preceding the disaster. Similar considerations should be taken into account in etiologic investigations of derailments of human prenatal development. When, in the search for the etiology of mongolism (Down syndrome), an author concluded after consideration of abnormal anatomic features of the patients that the anomalies probably originated before the third month of gestation,[3] he was on solid ground. But when he deduced from some features common in mongoloids and from their synchronous origin that anoxia and other maternal disorders operating at about 8 weeks might be an important mechanism in the causation of mongolism, he was in error.[4] The chromosomal changes responsible for mongolism date back to preconceptional or periconceptional times. The abnormal anatomic features of the child with mongolism are not determined by disease of the mother during the eighth week of pregnancy.

Embryologic developmental data can be used to test the hypothesis that an external event during pregnancy could have caused a child's malformations. This was done in a case of attempted abortion with aminopterin.[5] Considering the possibility that the drug taken by the mother from the tenth to the twelfth week of pregnancy was responsible for her child's anomalies, the authors found that cranial dysostosis, posterior palate cleft, mandibular hypoplasia and ear anomalies could be explained by arrested development at the time of the drug intake, which was not past the termination period of any of the anomalies. The hypothesis was further supported by previous observations of fetuses with malformations after aminopterin intake,[6] by animal experiments that showed folic acid antagonists to be teratogenic[7] and by the family history, which was negative for the malformations of the abnormal infant. It "seemed probable that this unusual syndrome was caused by ingestion of the drug, which interfered with normal fetal development in the third month of gestation."[5] That this cautious conclusion was correct was shown later, when similar cases were observed following maternal intake of aminopterin in early pregnancy[7,8]

It is naïve to assume that one can date from embryologic timetables the origin of malformations accurately to the day. Even Stockard[1] expressed caution by writing that interruption of organic development "at a *much* earlier or a *much* later time" will fail to influence it seriously. It should be kept in mind that a complicated structure such as a palate may be vulnerable for some time and have several critical periods of development. It can be shown in the rat that x-irradiation of fetuses on the fifteenth day of gestation results in cleft palate; but the same anomaly can be produced by irradiation on the tenth, twelfth, thirteenth and fourteenth days.[9] Similarly, it can be shown that an injection of galactoflavin given at any time between the seventh and fifteenth days of gestation can produce cleft palate in the young of mothers kept on a short-term riboflavin-deficient diet. The palate has many phases of development – phase of "budding" to phase of perfection – that are sensitive to teratogenic agents. The formation of the nasal floor, the establishment of the preincisive or anterior palate, the downward growth of the palatine shelves, their elevation and fusion with each other are stages of active and rapid cell multiplication. Each of these stages can be inhibited by teratologic factors, resulting in cleft palate. Which of these formative periods is *the* critical period for the palate? Even if a cleft palate is caused by a single environmental insult, it is impossible to single out in retrospect the exact time at which damage leading to arrest of the palatine anlage was done. The Russells,[10] after x-irradiation of pregnant mice with different doses at different days of gestation, concluded that at any one stage during major organogenesis a number of different critical periods come to their peak. This holds for cleft palate and many other malformations.

If *syndromes* of congenital malformations are considered, attempts at timing are even more hazardous. This is best illustrated by teratologic experiments with animals that carry many young at the same time. It sometimes happens that after a single administration of a teratogen a litter is obtained that contains young with quite different malformations and syndromes (Fig. 7-1). If these young were singletons, a retrospective observer using embryologic timetables would come up with quite different estimates of the time of the teratogenic insult. The same is true for human twins, who can differ in regard to congenital malformations even though they were exposed to the same drug in the same uterus, presumably at the same time. There are many reasons that could ac-

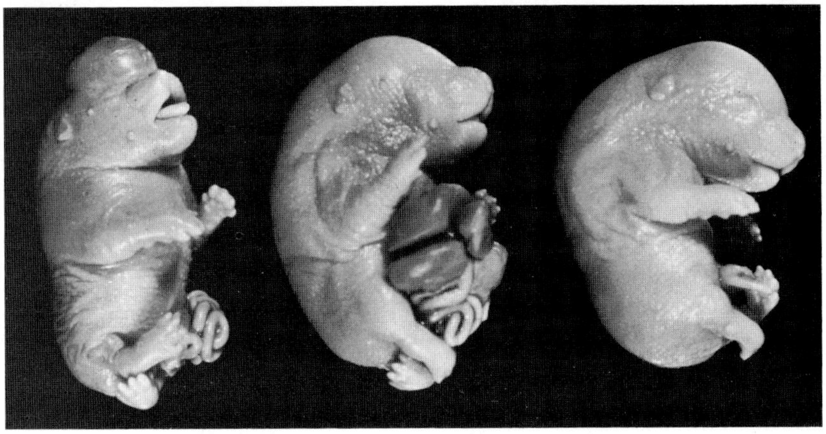

Fig. 7-1.—Three rat fetuses removed on the twentieth day of gestation. The mother had been treated by a single injection of streptonigrin on the tenth day. Note differing malformations in these litter mates.

count for discordance of litter mates after identical exposure. The young may be heterogeneous in genetic constitution; they may be of slightly but significantly differing ages; they are in different uterine positions; they may differ in blood supply, and so forth.

Many congenital malformations cannot be used for any attempts at timing because they have no teratologic termination periods. Termination periods can be found for such malformations as anencephaly, cyclopia, spina bifida, ocular colobomas, facial clefts, choanal atresia, tracheo-esophageal fistula, most aortic arch anomalies, errors of cardiac septation, some renal heterotopias, horseshoe kidney, exomphalos, exstrophy of the bladder and cloaca, imperforate anus, hemivertebrae, block vertebrae, many limb deformities and other malformations that can be recognized as arrested embryonic stages. But other congenital malformations such as microcephaly, hydrocephaly, porencephaly, microphthalmia, micrognathia, high palate, patent ductus arteriosus, anomalies of the valves of the heart and the great vessels, hydronephrosis and hydroureter, abnormal curvatures of the spine and others can be due to growth disturbances or diseases in early or in late prenatal life or to genetic and chromosomal abnormalities. There are no termination periods for abnormal size and disease effects. Structures normally formed during the organogenic period can be retarded in growth later or can undergo secondary destruction by various pathologic processes. Malformations of many kinds can be produced experimentally by necrotizing agents.[11] Secondary necrosis of previously well-formed organs can also be genetically determined, as demonstrated by certain strains of rabbits born with acheiropodia[12] or in some strains of mice with a variety of malformations.[13] Congenital gut atresia in infants can be due to lack of recanalization of the intestinal tube at the end of the second month of fetal life. But congenital atresias of the jejunum and ileum can also be due to injuries and accidents to a fetal intestine that previously had been normal.[14] It would be wrong to assign the origin of such atresias to the second month of gestation. Amputations of extremities or parts of them are, in rare cases, truly secondary severances of once normally formed parts.[15] By the time a congenital malformation is seen in a child, abnormal organogenesis, secondary destructive processes and regeneration may have influenced the disease picture. There are many critical periods before birth, and speculations concerning the time of origin of malformations should be made with caution. According to Patten,[16] too little growth, too little resorption, too much resorption, resorption in the wrong location, normal growth in an abnormal position and local overgrowth of a tissue or structure can result in prenatal malformations. To reduce these complicated mechanisms to a single concept of "arrested development," to time and to "synchronize" the origin of malformations in order to find the causative agent seems a futile exercise in speculative embryology.

In summary, it can be stated that embryologic timetables are useful and necessary in animal experiments that attempt production of certain malformations by a single environmental insult, but it is erroneous to assume that human malformations observed after birth are always due to such a single event occurring at a sensitive period. Embryologic timetables are helpful in human teratology for testing hypotheses that attempt to connect a known prenatal environmental event with congenital malformations observed in a child. The knowledge of teratologic termination periods is useful in ruling out a suspected environmental incident as causative if the event occurred after the termination period of a deformed organ or structure, but for many malformations clear-cut termination periods cannot be established. Retrospective use of embryologic timetables for ascertainment of times of origin and causes of congenital malformations is hazardous. Etiologic hypotheses derived from embryologic speculations have no validity unless they are supported by additional evidence.

REFERENCES

1. Stockard, C. R.: *The Physical Basis of Personality* (New York: W. W. Norton & Company, Inc., 1931).
2. Schwalbe, E.: Allgemeine Missbildungslehre, in Schwalbe, E. (ed.), *Die Morphologie der Missbildungen des Menschen und der Tiere* (Jena: Gustav Fischer, 1906).
3. Ingalls, T. H.: Pathogenesis of mongolism, Am. J. Dis. Child. 73:279, 1947.
4. Ingalls, T. H.: Etiology of mongolism, Am. J. Dis. Child. 74:147, 1947.
5. Warkany, J., Beaudry, P. H., and Hornstein, S.: Attempted abortion with 4-amino-pteroylglutamic acid (aminopterin); malformations of the child, Am. J. Dis. Child. 97:274, 1959.
6. Thiersch, J. B.: Therapeutic abortions with a folic acid antagonist, 4-aminopteroylglutamic acid (4-amino P.G.A.), Am. J. Obst. & Gynec. 63:1298, 1952.
7. Emerson, D. J.: Congenital malformations due to attempted abortion with aminopterin, Am. J. Obst. & Gynec. 84:356, 1962.
8. Shaw, E. B., and Steinbach, H. L.: Aminopterin-induced fetal malformation. Survival of infant after attempted abortion, Am. J. Dis. Child. 115:477, 1968.
9. Warkany, J., and Schraffenberger, E.: Congenital malformations induced in rats by roentgen rays, Am. J. Roentgenol. 57:455, 1947.
10. Russell, L. B., and Russell, W. L.: An analysis of the changing radiation response of the developing mouse embryo, J. Cell. & Comp. Physiol. 43:103, 1954.
11. Gruenwald, P.: Malformations caused by necrosis in the embryo, illustrated by the effect of selenium compounds on chick embryos, Am. J. Path. 34:77, 1958.
12. Greene, H. S. N., and Saxton, J. A., Jr.: Hereditary brachydactylia and allied abnormalities in the rabbit, J. Exper. Med. 69:301, 1939.
13. Bonnevie, K.: Embryological analysis of gene manifestations in Little and Bagg's abnormal mouse tribe, J. Exper. Zool. 67:443, 1934.
14. Santulli, T. V., and Blanc, W. A.: Congenital atresia of the intestine: Pathogenesis and treatment, Ann. Surg. 154: 939, 1961.
15. Torpin, R.: *Fetal Malformations* (Springfield, Ill.: Charles C Thomas, Publisher, 1968).
16. Patten, B. M.: Varying developmental mechanisms in teratology, Pediatrics 19:734, 1957.

PART II

Etiologic Factors

Introduction

EVERY AGE has had its explanation of congenital malformations according to its religious or philosophic concepts. Thousands of years ago, the birth of deformed children was considered a link between behavior of the stars and terrestrial events to come. Whenever a society firmly believed in a god or in multiple deities, deformities of newborn children were attributed to the wrath, or a benign warning, of the super-being that ruled the world. In times of fear of witches and sorcerers, fellow-men or fellow-women were suspected of deforming unborn children in the mother's womb. Throughout the ages, external events were thought to reach the fetus through the mother's eyes or mind. Concurrent with such "superstitious" beliefs there existed more "natural" explanations, i.e., explanations more related to our own beliefs and theories, which attributed—with little proof—unusual teratologic events to male "semen" or female "materia." It is difficult to prove, with our limited knowledge of teratogenicity, that all the ancient theories were nonsensical, i.e., outside the causal nexus. As William James put it: "Not a sparrow falls to the ground but some of the remote conditions of his fall are to be found in the milky way, in our federal constitution, or in the early history of Europe." Yet, causes that are so remote that they are useless for prediction or prevention of events should not be included in etiologic explanations aiming at practical solutions. This applies to ancient theories as well as those accepted without substantial proof by modern science. Our present concepts of teratogenicity reflect the general thinking of today and contain many beliefs which are not equally shared by all scientists and which require substantiation. They reflect present-day concepts of prenatal development whose disturbances are held responsible for prenatal malformations. There still are huge areas of human teratology that remain obscure, and there are malformations for which we have reasonable explanations but no practical ways of prevention. In such areas as the latter, modern scientific concepts of causation are *beliefs* in modern garb. There are scientists who believe that the bulk of unexplained congenital malformations are caused by genetic factors or by chromosomal changes that cannot yet be visualized. There are others who attribute them to molecular changes—without proof. Some scientists believe that diseases of the mother—viral, metabolic or nutritional—are responsible and others are convinced that drugs are the devils that turn normal embryos into monsters. There is some truth in all of these beliefs, as there was some truth in the beliefs of the ancients. As long as our unproved opinions are treated as hypotheses that stimulate research and experimentation, they are useful and necessary for progress. But if they are mistaken for facts and solutions, and if they are stifling the work of others who have different theories, they may become superstitions even when expressed in the most modern of scientific terms.

In the following pages, etiologic factors that contribute to congenital malformations will be discussed. They are numerous, but obviously not sufficient to explain all human teratologic facts. Like diseases of postnatal beginning, disorders of prenatal life are complex in origin and there often are many etiologic factors that contribute to their existence. No explanation of a disease or malformation is entirely satisfactory until it leads to successful preventive measures. There are only a few prenatal diseases and disorders that can be prevented and eradicated like their counterparts of postnatal origin. But there are hopeful signs that indicate that modern science is going in the right direction or, better, in right directions. But most of the work of etiologic research and preventive teratology remains to be done.

The child's life begins with fertilization of the ovum and formation of the zygote, in which many of the physical and mental traits of the new organism are predetermined. Development of the first cell, which weighs only 0.005 mg., into the highly differentiated organism of the newborn of more than 3,000 Gm. requires about 44 successive cell divisions that are directed by the genes contained in the zygote and influenced by the intrauterine and extrauterine environments. Abnormalities of the nuclear elements of the zygote as well as prenatal environmental disturbances may result in congenital malformations. The nucleus of the zygote contains 46 chromosomes, the carriers of the genes, derived from the sperm and ovum, which contribute 23 chromosomes each. Normal as well as abnormal genes can be passed on along the "germ track" through many generations,

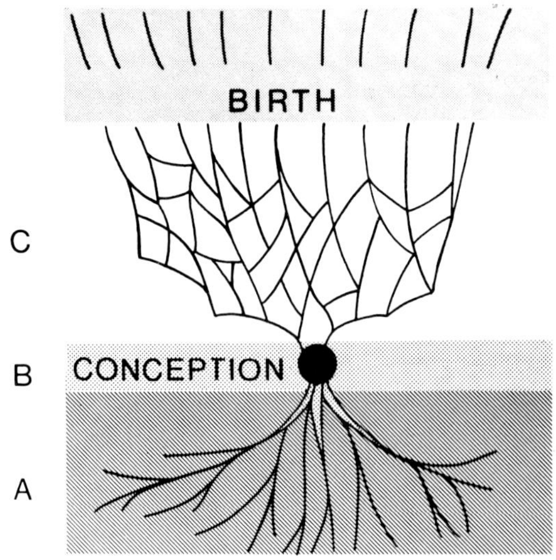

The pathways of development. The germ tracks are the roots that bring the genetic material to the zygote at the time of conception. The embryo and fetus develop from the zygote by growth and differentiation to the time of birth. Congenital malformations can be caused by **A,** genetic changes before conception, **B,** chromosomal changes before or soon after conception or **C,** environmental factors interfering with development between conception and birth.

and the origins of numerous congenital malformations date back to events, decades or centuries before conception (see *A* in the illustration above). Entire chromosomes in the zygote can be abnormal in number or structure and determine malformations in the developing organism (*B*). Chromosomal abnormalities are genetic deviations, but they differ from gene mutations in origin and mode of transmission. A healthy zygote can be damaged during its intrauterine development by various agents – infectious, actinic or chemical – and become deformed before birth (*C*). It is customary at present to divide the causes of congenital malformations into genetic, chromosomal and environmental determinants, although it often is impossible to separate clearly such causative factors, which can interact and bring about the defects encountered or prevent them.

SECTION ONE

8

Genetic and Chromosomal Factors

Genetic Factors

IT IS A REMARKABLE FACT that some congenital malformations are transmitted as hereditary characteristics like normal Mendelian traits. Some malformations can be attributed to a gene or to genes inherited from one or both parents or arising sporadically through a new mutation. Such genes may be dominant or recessive. A long list of *dominantly inherited congenital malformations* could be cited. In a catalog of human anomalies inherited like Mendelian traits, McKusick[1] enumerated more than 150 congenital malformations or teratologic syndromes transmitted as autosomal dominants. Anomalies such as short fingers, incurved little fingers, extra digits, lobster claw, certain cataracts, aniridia, ectopia of the lens, polycystic kidneys (adult type) and many others can occur in otherwise normal persons belonging to kindreds in which a mutant dominant gene is passed on from generation to generation, causing a single abnormal trait. A dominant gene can also deform an entire region of the body, as in mandibulofacial (Treacher Collins) or craniofacial (Crouzon) dysostosis; or the entire skeleton can be affected, as in achondroplasia, cleidocranial dysostosis, osteopetrosis (benign), multiple exostoses and others. Sometimes a dominant gene adversely influences several organs or body systems and brings about a syndrome of diverse anomalies. The effects of such "pleiotropic" genes are exemplified by the Waardenburg, Marfan, Ehlers-Danlos, Holt-Oram and nail-patella syndromes.

As a rule, these dominant traits are brought about by a single gene in the heterozygous state. Each patient has an affected parent and has a 50:50 risk of having affected offspring. Members of the family who are free of the trait do not carry the gene and should have normal offspring only. If the parents of a patient are normal and the dominant trait appears to be "sporadic," the disorder can be due to a new mutation, and the risk for the offspring of the affected person is 50:50. Numerous kindreds are known in which such "sporadic" patients started pedigrees typical of dominant inheritance. In general, transmission of dominant traits is regular and genetic counseling rather reliable. Unfortunately, the rules of transmission sometimes are changed by various modifications of the phenotype. The carrier of an abnormal dominant gene may fail to show the trait or have it in subclinical form yet transmit it to some of his children. Skipping of a generation is attributed to low *penetrance* (failure of the gene to manifest itself) or to low *expressivity* (mild manifestation, sometimes difficult to ascertain). Reduced penetrance and reduced expressivity often are not understood, but it is conceivable that various genes besides the one under consideration, or environmental factors, influence the expression of the abnormal gene. Achondroplasia, for instance, could be modified to a certain extent by a familial tendency to tallness or shortness or be altered by endemic cretinism, a disorder that depends on adverse environmental conditions. But, in most cases, changes of penetrance and expressivity are much more subtle and remain unexplained.

Many congenital malformations are attributed to *autosomal recessive inheritance*. Autosomal recessive genes manifest themselves only when homozygous. The parents of affected children usually are heterozygous for the abnormal gene and phenotypically normal. Each sibling in such a family has a 25% risk of being phenotypically abnormal by showing the trait. If a recessive gene is rare in a population, a homozygous affected person may appear only once ("sporadically") in a pedigree. Absence of a pathologic trait in the traceable relatives of the patient does not exclude genetic determination. Marriage between relatives increases the probability that both parents carry the same gene, so that the frequency of consanguinity is higher in parents of patients with recessive disorders than in the general population. If two persons mate who exhibit an abnormal recessive trait (and are homozygous), they risk the possibility that all their children will be abnormal. Such matings sometimes occur with deleterious effects among hereditary deaf-mutes who are handicapped by the same recessive genes.

In McKusick's catalog of Mendelian inheritance in man[1] more than 150 congenital malformations and syndromes are listed as recessive autosomal traits. Some types of limb defects, microcephaly, hydrocephaly, microphthalmia, anophthalmia, infantile polycystic kidney, Morquio disease, Ellis-van Creveld syndrome, asphyxiating thoracic dysplasia, cartilage-hair hypoplasia, chondrodystrophia calcificans, diastrophic dwarfism, Hurler gargoylism, osteopetrosis (severe form), Laurence-Moon-Biedl syndrome, adrenogenital syndromes and many others are due to autosomal recessive genes.

Some congenital malformations are caused by *sex-linked inheritance*. If an abnormal gene is located on the X chromosome of a male, it can manifest itself even if it is recessive, since it is not checked by a corresponding normal gene on the Y chromosome. In the female, manifestation of the abnormal trait is prevented by the corresponding normal dominant gene located on the second X chromosome. In this way, certain hereditary abnormal traits appear in males of a kindred without manifestation in females. The anomaly is transmitted through phenotypically normal females to approximately half of their sons. If a father is affected, all his daughters carry the abnormal recessive gene even though they are phenotypically normal; all his sons (who received their X chromosome from their genotypically normal mother) are normal. More than 30 congenital malformations or syndromes have been cataloged as sex-linked recessive traits.[1] Some forms of hydrocephaly, imperforate anus, microphthalmia, Lowe syndrome, Hunter gargoylism, anhidrotic ectodermal dysplasia, testicular feminization and others exemplify this group of inherited defects.

Sex-linked dominant traits can be transmitted in kindreds from one generation to another like autosomal dominant traits; but since affected males transmit their abnormal X chromosome to all their daughters but not to their sons, all daughters show the trait, whereas the sons are spared. Vitamin D-resistant rickets is considered a sex-linked dominant disorder. Although the basic metabolic error of this disorder is congenital, the resulting skeletal deformities usually develop after birth.[2-6]

Chromosomal Abnormalities

Many congenital malformations, particularly multiple defects and syndromes, are seen in persons who have chromosomal abnormalities. The best-known changes of this kind involve absence or duplication of an entire chromosome. As a result of nondisjunction of a pair of chromosomes during meiosis, the resulting gametes may receive an abnormal number of chromosomes – for instance, 22 or 24, instead of the normal 23. Fertilization of such an abnormal gamete by a normal one with 23 chromosomes results in zygotes with 45 or 47 chromosomes so that monosomy or trisomy ensues. In addition to the errors involving whole chromosomes, there may occur structural changes such as deletions, translocations, inversions and partial duplications. As it became possible to visualize the human chromosomes by relatively simple laboratory methods, it was soon recognized that many clinical disease pictures were associated with demonstrable cytogenetic changes. Recognition of the autosomal *trisomies* revealed new aspects of the well-known Down syndrome and of the rarer trisomy D and E syndromes. With these discoveries, cytogenetic bases were established for the numerous congenital malformations contained in these syndromes. It evolved that the trisomies caused definite patterns of malformations, yet, for each trisomy, a spectrum of malformations was discerned with a significant degree of clinical variability sometimes resulting in great dissimilarities of signs and symptoms.[2] Children with apparently equal trisomies may differ clinically by unequal involvement of organs or, if the same organs are involved, by dissimilarity of the malformations as the pathologist or clinician knows them. The trisomies create general disorders that can differ in teratologic effects. This probably is best illustrated by the variability of cardiovascular malformations caused by autosomal trisomies.[7,8] The effects on the brain by trisomy 13-15 (D_1), which include arhinencephalies and cyclopias, seem more homogeneous, but quantitative differences are considerable and may decide compatibility or incompatibility with life. Sometimes absence of an entire autosome is encountered. If, for instance, a chromosome 21 is absent, a syndrome called "antimongolism" can result, but its symptomatology apparently is not specific.[9] Duplication of an X chromosome as seen in Klinefelter syndrome causes few structural defects in the patient except those of the testis. Duplication of the Y chromosome seems to be associated with a tendency to tall stature and violence but not with malformations. Absence of an X chromosome resulting in Turner syndrome is associated in some cases with a whole spectrum of congenital malformations; in other cases, stunting of growth and lack of sexual development are the only manifestations.[10,11]

Partial *deletions* of chromosomes of the B group lead to structural phenotypic defects, mental retardation and, in the case of deletion of part of the short arm of chromosome 5, to a characteristic cat cry, which often betrays the cytogenetic abnormality. Partial deletions of chromosomes 18 and 21 and of X chromosomes have also been observed. Pieces of both ends of a chromosome may break off and the broken ends of the chromosome join with each other, forming a *ring chromosome*. Ring chromosomes derived from several autosomes have been found in children who are born small, remain small and have congenital defects. Many *translocations* in various combinations have occurred in association with mental and physical defects but, with few exceptions, the resulting disease pictures are not diagnostic and the chromosomes involved often remain unidentified. Exceptions are children with typical Down syndrome who have D/G or G/G translocation. Clinical findings are variable in patients whose karyotypes include *fragments* of usually unidentified chromosomes. A connection between anomalies of the patient and the fragment probably exists but it is seldom firmly established.

There are persons whose bodies contain two or more cell lines with different karyotypes. In the majority of cases, such persons are *mosaics* whose differing cell lines have arisen after fertilization during mitosis of early cell divisions. By nondisjunction or anaphase lag, daughter cells that have unequal numbers of chromosomes can be formed. Autosomes as well as sex chromosomes may be involved in mosaicisms that can lead to a great variety of phenotypes from normal to severe mental and physical imperfection. Malformations of many parts, including sex organs, have been observed in mosaics.

Chimeras have two or more cell lines like mosaics, but these cell lines are not derived from a single embryo but from different organisms.

In *polyploidy*, the cells contain multiples of the haploid number 23. If they contain 69 chromosomes, one speaks of triploidy; if there are 92, the cell is tetraploid. Most embryos with polyploidy probably are aborted,[12,13] but live-born infants with complete triploidy have been observed.[40,41] Children with polyploidy usually are mosaics born with signs of intrauterine growth retardation and skeletal defects.[14-16]

Several studies have been attempted to estimate the incidence of infants born with recognizable chromosomal abnormalities. Despite the great efforts involved in such investigations, the numbers of abnormalities discovered are still small and subject to corrections as experiences increase. It seems that approximately 0.5 – 1% of infants are born with recognizable chromosomal aberrations.[14,17-19,24] Sex chromosomal abnormalities account for about 0.2%.[25,26] Among live-born babies with recognizable malformations, about 4% have a chromosomal malformation detectable in mitotic cells.[26] Many embryos with chromosomal abnormalities do not reach term, as the pregnancy is terminated by spontaneous abortion. Twenty-two per cent of tissues of spontaneous abortuses were found to have numerical chromosomal anomalies, but the incidences in various studies varied between 10% and 65%.[20-22,45-47] It seems that the incidence of chromosomal anomalies in spontaneous abortions is 40 to 50 times as high as that in live-born infants. This indicates a prenatal screening process and natural elimination of a considerable portion of abnormal conceptuses. In studies by Carr,[12,13] about half the cytogenetically abnormal abortuses had one extra chromosome, resulting in trisomy. One quarter were monosomic for the X chromosome (XO), and nearly a quarter were triploid. Chromosomal anomalies occur most commonly in first-trimester abortions, particularly those with empty chorionic sacs.[21] Among induced abortuses in Japan, 7 of 140 (5%) had chromosomal abnormalities.[23] Mikamo[42] found that structural and chromosomal anomalies were particularly frequent in the younger age groups of spontaneous abortions.

Recognition of the important role played by cytogenetic abnormalities in the origin of congenital malformations was followed by inquiries into the causes of chromosomal irregularities. Many of these investigations were directed by the knowledge that the incidence of some cytogenetic disorders, e.g., Down syndrome, trisomy 18 or Klinefelter syndrome, is related to maternal age, so that this factor's role in the causation of nondisjunction has become a subject of speculation and investigation.

A rise in the incidence of Down syndrome with a power of the mother's age suggested to Penrose[27] that the error in the ovum that leads to nondisjunction depends on a succession of independent accidents. A sufficient number in a given cell causes the meiotic divisions to become inaccurate on account of degeneration of the spindle mechanism that relies on the integrity of an exact number of separate strands. After a certain number of breaks, the spindle mechanism would be unable, in the first meiotic division, to overcome the resistance of the paired chromosomes to separate, especially those supplied with nucleolus organizers like the acrocentrics.[28]

Other hypotheses associate overripeness of eggs with cytogenetic errors. In amphibians, overripeness of eggs due to intrauterine retention can lead to degeneration and to malformations. Chromosomal anomalies may be brought about in intrauterine overripe eggs by nondisjunction.[29] In mammalian eggs, delayed fertilization results in an increase in abnormalities of early zygote development and nonviability.[30] Intrafollicular overripeness of ovocytes has also been described as a cause of high mortality, malformations and abnormal behavior of meiotic chromosomes in animals. Retention of eggs in follicles may lead to a high frequency of chromosomal aberrations in rat embryos.[31] The possibility of changes in the endocrine system with advancing maternal age as a cause of intrafollicular retention and overripeness of eggs has been considered.[32] That a hormonal maternal imbalance can be responsible for an increase of triploidy in spontaneous abortuses was suggested by chromosome studies of women who conceived within 6 months of discontinuing oral contraceptives.[47] According to another hypothesis,[33] the frequency of nondisjunction is equal at all ages but the aging uterus loses the ability to reject implantation of trisomic fertilized eggs. Thus, investigations of endocrine conditions of the mother and of local changes in her reproductive organs with advancing age are likely to yield, eventually, explanations for many types of congenital malformations.

Not all factors considered in the causation of cytogenetic disturbances are associated with advancing maternal age. It has been estimated that in Down syndrome approximately 40% of the cases may be independent of the mother's age.[28] Mothers with Down syndrome or mosaics of any reproductive age can pass on an extra chromosome 21 to their offspring and bring about a trisomic zygote and embryo. This kind of trisomy could be associated with advanced grandmaternal age.[34] Inherited translocations that sometimes result in familial aggregation of chromosomal anomalies are also not dependent on maternal age. A general tendency to nondisjunction seen in some families and kindreds has been attributed to genes transmitted in such relationships.

Some observations point to environmental causes of nondisjunction. Exposure of mothers to x-irradiation has been considered an etiologic factor in Down syndrome,[35,36] but the evidence is still tenuous. The occurrence of clusters of patients with Down syndrome in time or space gave rise to various etiologic hypotheses. Such temporospatial clustering in different geographic areas was reviewed and tabulated by Lilienfeld.[37] Streptococcal infections and infectious hepatitis at the time of conception have been under suspicion in some areas, but in others there was no association of the infections with the incidence of the syndrome. A statistical analysis devised by Robinson *et al.*[38] led to the impression of nonrandom occurrence of sex chromosome anomalies. It seemed that variations occurred with intrauterine viral infections and with season of the year. These authors considered the possibility that all chromosomal irregularities, including that of no. 21, are susceptible to environmental influences. Human chromosome damage by chemical agents must be considered; the subject was reviewed by Shaw[48] in 1970.

Maternal thyroid disease, long suspected as a contributing factor in the etiology of mongolism, is again considered in a new version. Thyroid autoantibodies have been found more often in mothers of children with Down syndrome than in control mothers. A direct or indirect connection with the chromosomal anomalies is under examination, particularly with cytogenetic changes that are not dependent on maternal age.[39]

The genetic component in child morbidity and mortality is difficult to assess. As environmental causes are successfully eliminated, genetic causes come to the foreground. It was estimated in 1964 that in a pediatric unit in British Columbia approximately 50% of the beds were occupied by children whose illnesses were entirely or partially of genetic origin.[43] The genetic component in child mortality was estimated in Newcastle upon Tyne in 1970 as 42%, single gene defects accounting for 8.5% and chromosomal disorders for 2.5%. Included in the estimate were disorders of probable but complex genetic origin, contributing 31%. Malformations of the central nervous and cardiovascular systems played an important role in this complex category.[44]

REFERENCES

1. McKusick, V. A.: *Mendelian Inheritance in Man: Catalogs of Autosomal Dominants, Autosomal Recessives and X-Linked Phenotypes* (Baltimore: The Johns Hopkins Press, 1966).
2. Bartalos, M.: *Genetics in Medical Practice* (Philadelphia: J. B. Lippincott Company, 1968).
3. Hsia, D. Y-Y. (ed.): *Lectures in Medical Genetics* (Chicago: Year Book Medical Publishers, Inc., 1966).
4. Knudson, A. G.: *Genetics and Disease* (New York: The Blakiston Division, McGraw-Hill Book Company, Inc., 1965).
5. Roberts, J. A. F.: *An Introduction to Medical Genetics* (London: Oxford University Press, 1963).
6. Thompson, J. S., and Thompson, M. W.: *Genetics in Medicine* (Philadelphia: W. B. Saunders Company, 1966).
7. Warkany, J., Passarge, E., and Smith, L. B.: Congenital malformations in autosomal trisomy syndromes, Am. J. Dis. Child. 112:502, 1966.
8. Thompson, H.: Abnormalities of the autosomal chromosomes associated with human disease, Am. J. M. Sc. 250: 718, 1965; 251:706, 1966.
9. Challacombe, D. N., and Taylor, A.: Monosomy for a G autosome, Arch, Dis. Childhood 44:113, 1969.
10. Miller, O. J.: The sex chromosome anomalies, Am. J. Obst. & Gynec. 90:1078, 1964.
11. Mittwoch, U.: Sex chromatin. Review article, J. M. Genetics 1:50, 1964.
12. Carr, D. H.: Cytogenetics of Abortions, in Benirschke, K., and Jones, T. C. (eds.), *Comparative Aspects of Reproductive Failure* (New York: Springer-Verlag, 1967).
13. Carr, D. H.: Chromosome anomalies as a cause of spontaneous abortion, Am. J. Obst. & Gynec. 97:283, 1967.
14. Turpin, R., and Lejeune, J.: *Les Chromosomes Humains* (Paris: Gauthier-Villars, 1965).
15. Hamerton, J. L.: *Chromosomes in Medicine* (London: William Heinemann, Ltd., 1962).
16. Bartalos, M., and Baramski, T. A.: *Medical Cytogenetics* (Baltimore: The Williams & Wilkins Company, 1967).
17. Court Brown, W. M., Buckton, K. E., Jacobs, P. A., Tough, I. M., Kuenssberg, E. V., and Knox, J. D. E.: *Chromosome Studies on Adults* (London: Cambridge University Press, 1966).
18. Sergovich, F., Valentine, G. H., Chen, A. T. L., Kinch, R. A. H., and Smout, M. S.: Chromosome aberrations in 2159 consecutive newborn babies, New England J. Med. 280: 851, 1969.
19. Walzer, S., Breau, G., and Gerald, P. S.: A chromosome survey of 2400 normal newborn infants, J. Pediat. 74: 438, 1969.
20. Thiede, H. A., and Metcalfe, S.: Chromosomes and human pregnancy wastage, Am. J. Obst. & Gynec. 96:1132, 1966.
21. Kerr, M., and Rashad, M. N.: Chromosome studies on spontaneous abortions, Am. J. Obst. & Gynec. 94:322, 1966.
22. Waxman, S. H., Arakaki, D. T., and Smith, J. B.: Cytogenetics of fetal abortions, Pediatrics 39:425, 1967.
23. Sasaki, M., Makino, S., Muramoto, J-I., Ikeuchi, T., and Shimba, H.: A chromosome survey of induced abortuses in a Japanese population, Chromosoma 20:267, 1967.
24. Boué, J. G., Boué, A., and Lazar, P.: Les aberrations chromosomiques dans les avortements, Ann. Génét. 10:179, 1967.
25. Mikamo, K.: Sex chromosomal anomalies in newborn infants, Obst. & Gynec. 32:688, 1968.
26. Stewart, A. L., Keay, A. J., and Jacobs, P. A.: A chromo-

some survey of unselected live-born children with congenital abnormalities, J. Pediat. 74:449, 1969.
27. Penrose, L. S.: *Mongolism as a Problem in Human Biology. Symposium on the Early Conceptus, Normal and Abnormal* (Dundee, Scotland: D. C. Thomson, 1965).
28. Penrose, L. S., and Smith, G. F.: *Down's Anomaly* (Boston: Little, Brown & Company, 1966).
29. Witschi, E., and Laguens, R.: Chromosomal aberrations in embryos from overripe eggs, Develop. Biol. 7:605, 1963.
30. Blandau, R. J.: The female factor in fertility and infertility; effects of delayed fertilization in the development of the pronuclei in rat ova, Fertil. & Steril. 3:349, 1952.
31. Butcher, R. L., and Fugo, N. W.: Overripeness and the mammalian ova. II. Delayed ovulation and chromosome anomalies, Fertil. & Steril. 18:297, 1967.
32. Mikamo, K.: Intrafollicular overripeness and teratologic development, Cytogenetics 7:212, 1968.
33. Matsunaga, E.: Parental Age, Live-Birth Order and Pregnancy-Free Interval in Down's Syndrome in Japan, in Wolstenholme, G. E. W., and Porter, R. (eds.), Ciba Foundation Study Group No. 25, *Mongolism* (Boston: Little. Brown & Co., 1967).
34. Weinstein, E. D., and Warkany, J.: Maternal mosaicism and Down's syndrome, J. Pediat. 63:599, 1963.
35. Uchida, I. A., and Curtis, E. J.: A possible association between maternal radiation and mongolism, Lancet 2: 848, 1961.
36. Sigler, A. T., Lilienfeld, A. M., Cohen, B. H., and Westlake, J. E.: Radiation exposure of parents of children with mongolism (Down's syndrome), Bull. Johns Hopkins Hosp. 117:374, 1965.
37. Lilienfeld, A. M.: *Epidemiology of Mongolism* (Baltimore: The Johns Hopkins Press, 1969).
38. Robinson, A., Good, W. B., Puck, T. T., and Harris, J. S.: Studies on chromosomal nondisjunction in man, III, Am. J. Human Genet. 21:466, 1969.
39. Fialkow, P. J.: Autoimmunity and chromosomal aberrations, Am. J. Human Genet. 18:93, 1966.
40. Butler, L. J., Chantler, C., France, N. E., and Keith, C. G.: A liveborn infant with complete triploidy (69,XXX), J. M. Genetics 6:413, 1969.
41. Schindler, A-M., and Mikamo, K.: Triploidy in man, Cytogenetics 9:116, 1970.
42. Mikamo, K.: Anatomic and chromosomal anomalies in spontaneous abortion, Am. J. Obst. & Gynec. 106:243, 1970.
43. Miller, J. R.: Human Genetics in Public Health Research and Programming, in Schacht, L. E. (ed.), *Human Genetics in Public Health* (Minneapolis: Minnesota Department of Health, 1964).
44. Roberts, D. F., Chavez, J., and Court, S. D. M.: The genetic component in child mortality, Arch. Dis. Childhood 45: 33, 1970.
45. Arakaki, D. T., and Waxman, S. H.: Chromosome abnormalities in early spontaneous abortions, J. M. Genetics 7: 118, 1970.
46. Boué, J-G., and Boué, A.: Les aberrations chromosomiques dans les avortements spontanés humains, Presse méd. 78:635, 1970.
47. Carr, D. H.: Chromosome studies in selected spontaneous abortions: 1. Conception after oral contraceptives, Canad. M.A.J. 103:343, 1970.
48. Shaw, M. W.: Human chromosome damage by chemical agents, Ann. Rev. Med. 21:409, 1970.

SECTION TWO

Environmental Factors

IT IS CUSTOMARY to consider interference with normal prenatal development between conception and birth as "environmental," in contrast to genetic interference, which is predetermined by the time the sperm and ovum unite to form the zygote. Actually, genetic and chromosomal abnormalities are also attributable to environmental causes. Actinic and chemical factors are responsible for mutagenesis, and some chromosomal disturbances are influenced by the age of the mother, which points to the role of the maternal environment in the origin of cytogenetic changes. Mitotic nondisjunction after conception apparently is one of the first damages to the embryo caused by adverse situations of the inner environment that lead to defects through chromosomal imbalances. Other less subtle environmental disturbances of the embryo during the first 2 weeks of life and before organogenesis have been called "blastopathies"[1]; they often are lethal and end in abortion. In later embryonic stages, radiations or viruses penetrating the mother's protective barriers, maternal metabolic or vascular disturbances or injurious chemical compounds from the outside are considered "embryopathies"[2] that can deform the embryo during the first trimester of gestation.

Disorders of the second and third trimesters resemble, in their pathologic and clinical effects, postnatal diseases to a certain extent. Infectious and chemical or mechanical traumas during these fetal stages have been named "cyemopathies," a term derived from "cyema," which was used by Aristotle[3] for "all stages of the creature's development." There are no sharp borderlines between these periods and there is much to be learned about the pathogenic processes that disturb their normal course. Ascertainment of environmental teratologic factors acting between conception and birth is difficult, and only a few of the disturbances have been investigated thoroughly in man. Those that have been analyzed showed why they are so elusive. But experimental mammalian teratology has shown that it is relatively easy to produce congenital malformations of many types by various heterogeneous methods. These facts suggest that the small number of known environmental teratogenic agents is only a sample of the nongenetic causes of congenital malformations in man.

REFERENCES

1. Thalhammer, O.: "Missbildung," Vorschlag zu einer neuen Nomenklatur angeborener Störungen, Arch. Kinderh. 145:100, 1952.
2. Bamatter, F.: L'image pathognomique clinique et anatomopathologique des embryopathies, Rapports XIIIth Congrès de Langue Française, 1951.
3. Aristotle: *Generation of Animals* (London: William Heinemann, Ltd., 1943). English translation by Peck, A. L., Loeb Classical Library.

9

Infections

Rubella

IN 1941, IT BECAME KNOWN that German measles during early pregnancy could deform an embryo and lead to a rather typical syndrome of congenital malformations.[1] The spectrum of anomalies produced and attributed to rubella consisted of ocular, cardiovascular, aural and mental defects. It also became known that this virus infection can result in miscarriages and stillbirths. In 1961, we summarized the huge literature accumulated in the 20 years following Gregg's discovery and pointed out the many questions that remained unanswered at that time.[2] The first surveys made concerning prenatal rubella damages were retrospective and suggested that rubella contracted during the first trimester resulted in congenital defects, varying from 50% to 90% and averaging about 75%.[3-6] Since retrospective estimates started with abnormal newborns and worked back to a history of maternal rubella during pregnancy, the data were selected and the estimates were too high. Prospective studies were initiated in the 1940s and reviewed in 1966.[7] Only 15% of live-born children resulting from pregnancies complicated by rubella in the first trimester showed typical anomalies. Rubella in the first 4 weeks had a risk of anomalies of 61%, in weeks 5–8 it was 26% and in weeks 9–12 it was 8%. The chance of having a normal infant after rubella in the first 8 weeks of pregnancy seemed to be 36%. A prospective study undertaken by the British Ministry of Health regarding mothers who had had rubella during the first 16 weeks of pregnancy during 1950–1952 was summarized by Sheridan.[8] "Major" abnormalities, mainly of the eye, ear and heart, occurred in 15% of the children, 8% having more than one abnormality. "Minor" abnormalities were present in a further 16%, 4% having more than one anomaly. Other prospective investigations resulted in similar findings,[9] but prospective studies are likely to underestimate congenital defects following prenatal rubella, since deafness is not easily detected in small infants and probably is not fully appreciated in early appraisals. Mental development is also not evaluable as early as congenital malformations are. In addition, prospective investigations cannot take into consideration subclinical cases of maternal rubella, which sometimes result in the fully developed rubella syndrome[10-12] and sometimes in rather nonspecific hearing loss. With improved laboratory methods, it may become possible to diagnose subclinical rubella and to recognize some constituents of the prenatal rubella syndrome early, which will change prospective incidence figures again. But such estimates are not yet available. It has been shown that rubella before conception or after the third trimester of pregnancy can also have adverse effects on the conceptus.[13,14] All this suggests that the effects of maternal rubella have never been correctly ascertained and probably will never be known, as we hope that the disease will become preventable and be eradicated.

There were some observations in the 1940s suggesting that maternal rubella before conception could cause congenital malformations in the embryo conceived after the mother's disease had passed. Such reports were not readily compatible with the concepts of acute rubella and its subsequent immunity. Yet, similar observations were made repeatedly and it has been demonstrated now that preconceptional rubella can be followed by abortion or the birth of a child with congenital rubella.[13] These findings suggest that in adults also immunologic conditions following rubella sometimes may be more complicated than has been assumed in the past.

Fetuses exposed to maternal rubella in early pregnancy show an infection rate of approximately 80%.[15] To the malformation rates cited above, which refer to live-born children, must be added other types of fetal wastage. It has been estimated that approximately 16–18% of the pregnancies complicated by early rubella end in spontaneous abortions or stillbirths.[2,16] Approximately one-third of the live-born whose disease picture includes thrombocytopenic purpura die during the first year of life.[15]

Rubella-induced malformations do not contribute heavily to the total incidence of congenital malformations, but their impact can be appreciable in times of severe rubella epidemics. It has been estimated that in 1964 in New York City 1% of pregnancies became rubella casualties and that in the United States, despite therapeutic abortions, approximately 20,000 children developed birth defects associated with rubella.[15,17]

When, in 1962, the rubella virus became demonstrable in tissue culture,[18,19] there was rapid progress in the areas of pathogenesis, clinical definition, epidemiology and therapy. Cooper and Krugman[17] summarized the advances made possible 22 years after the basic discovery. It was found that the rubella virus acquired in utero persists throughout pregnancy, is present at birth and is shed by the rubella-infected child for many months.[20] Pharyngeal secretions, urine, cerebrospinal fluid and many tissues contain the virus. In a cataractous lens, rubella virus can be demonstrated months and years after birth.[21-23] Infants with congenital rubella have serum neutralizing antibody titers comparable to those of their mothers, particularly IgM (19S) up to 7 months and IgG (7S) by the end of the first year. Some levels of neutralizing antibody persist for many years.[17] The apparent paradox of virus excretion in the presence of continuing synthesis of antibody points to an immunologic unresponsiveness that is still under investigation.[24,25] It has been shown by virus isolation and presence of neutralizing antibody that congenital rubella infection can exist in infants who appear normal at birth and in the early months or years of life and that infants with clinical signs of congenital rubella (and sometimes without them) can be contagious and infect nurses, doctors and medical students who are exposed to the virus-shedding infants.[17,26-28]

The finding of rubella virus in infants and children who had acquired the infection in prenatal life led to the term "congenital rubella." Before 1964, one spoke of "prenatal rubella," which sometimes resulted in congenital anomalies and malformations. Now the two terms often are used alternatively, although they are somewhat different. Prenatal rubella precedes congenital rubella. Prenatal rubella can end in abortion and expulsion of fetuses that do not reach infancy and do not show the signs and symptoms of congenital rubella.

Pathogenesis and Pathology

It seems established now that the rubella virus reaches the embryo through the mother's blood stream and placenta. According to the intensity of the infection and the time of gestation, the embryo is either aborted or deformed. As mentioned before, in later fetal life and infancy the virus can cause diseases of various organs. Congenital malformations are brought about by disturbances of cell divisions or by cell destruction. Selzer,[29] who first isolated rubella virus from the fetus of a woman who had had clinical German measles 10 days previously, saw inclusion bodies in the fetal cells, whereas the chromosome pattern in cultured cells appeared normal. Normal chromosomes were also reported by Neu[30] in the tissues of a fetus of an artificially aborted infected mother and by Mellman *et al.*[31] in cultured leukocytes of infants with congenital rubella. In contrast, Nusbacher *et al.*[32] noted a higher percentage of chromosome breaks in cultured cells of 1-year-old children with congenital rubella than in normal children of the same age. When rubella virus is added to tissue cultures of human embryonic origin, chromosomal breaks occur frequently.[33] Intrauterine growth retardation of fetuses affected by rubella has been attributed to inhibition of cell multiplication[34] and a subnormal number of cells in many body organs.[35] It is established that rubella causes malformations by direct attack on embryonic cells. It is curious, however, that the virus recovery rates from conceptuses is much higher than the incidence of congenital malformations.[36] But it seems now quite likely that rubella infections occurring after the first trimester can also lead to persistent virus infestation of the fetus and cause some anomalies in the child though not malformations.

Effects of prenatal rubella have been observed in dizygotic twins. In one pair, both twins had the rubella syndrome[10]; in another pair, only one of the twins had clinical evidence of the disease, although both of them had laboratory evidence.[90]

Many fetuses and embryos whose mothers had rubella during pregnancy have been submitted to anatomic and histologic examination.[34,37-39]

Spontaneous abortuses usually are poorly preserved, and changes seen in them often are postmortem effects. It should be pointed out that from the products of induced abortion only about 50% have demonstrable rubella virus.[15] In 1944, Swan[41] reported anatomic studies of 3 infants dying from congenital defects following maternal rubella in early pregnancy. All 3 had a widely open ductus and one had a defect of the membranous septum. There was some replacement of muscle fibers by connective tissue near the margins of the septal defect. The walls of the enlarged ductus arteriosus were thin and a definite internal elastic lamina was absent or ill-defined. In one case there was unilateral cataract associated with microphthalmia. The central portion of the lens was amorphous and necrotic. There were breaks in primary and secondary lens fibers. In cortical areas, disintegrating lens fibers were replaced by vacuoles (Fig. 9-1). Baertschi[38] examined 73 conceptuses, many of them obtained after therapeutic abortion; 50 were considered abnormal and 23 normal. Histologic changes frequently were seen in the heart, where cell necrosis of the myocardium and destruction of the endocardium were noted. Early changes of the lens consisted of conversion of fibers to hyalin droplets, which became confluent under the anterior epithelium of the lens, whereas the nuclei were pyknotic and dispersed. In the inner ear, necrotic foci were noted in embryos in which the cochlear epithelium was still undifferentiated, whereas the cochlea in the newborn showed secondary destructive processes. Early dental anomalies consisted of vacuoles near the inner enamel epithelium, and in an older fetus many ameloblasts were abnormal or destroyed. The enamel and inner epithelium of the enamel were separated by droplets derived from cytoplasmic vacuoles. Töndury and Smith[39] examined fetuses obtained by therapeutic abortion following rubella during the first trimester. Histologic evidence of disease was found in two-thirds of them. It seemed that the virus entered through the chorion and spread to other fetal tissues, which showed cell damage and necrosis without inflammatory or fibrotic response. Foci of cell damage were found in the chorionic epithelium, endothelial lining of the blood vessels and heart, myocardium, skeletal muscles and particularly in cells of the developing lens, inner ear and teeth.

Several investigations dealt with the pathology of children born with the rubella syndrome at or near term. Korones *et al.*[42] emphasized myocardial necrosis, interstitial pneumonitis and swelling and vacuoli-

Fig. 9-1.—Cataractous lens of eye of a child with prenatal rubella syndrome. The nuclear portion is amorphous and stained poorly; degenerated lens fibers, comprising cortical zone, separated by vacuoles, especially in the equatorial region. (From C. Swan.[41])

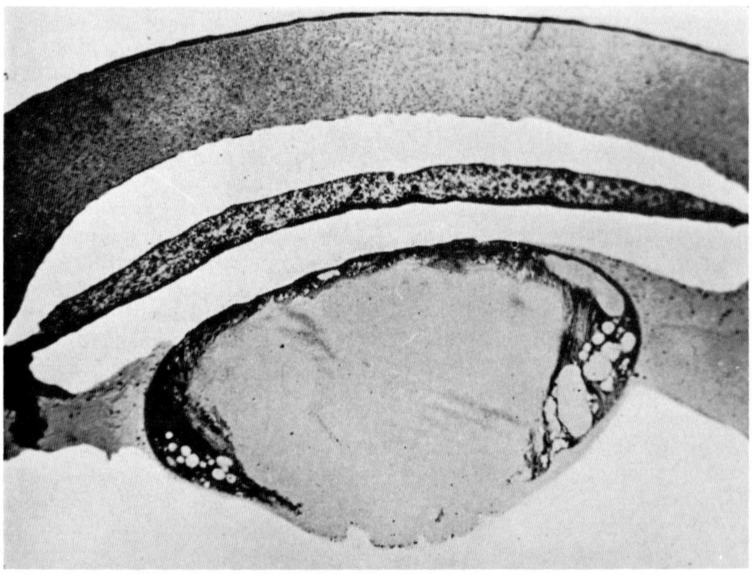

zation of liver cells. Chronic inflammation was present in the leptomeninges, lung and uveal tract of the eye in most of the cases examined by Singer *et al.*[34] but was less conspicuous in the kidney, liver, peritoneum and testes. Noninflammatory changes were noted in cardiovascular lesions, particularly patent ductus arteriosus, and there was nodular sclerosis of the cardiac valves. Cytomegaly in the adrenal cortex and precocious development of lymphoid germinal centers were noted. Atrophy of the thymus, calcifications in the kidneys and brain and nephrosclerosis were described by Thorburn and Miller.[43]

Clinical Manifestations

Not only concepts of pathogenesis and epidemiology but also the spectrum of clinical manifestations of prenatal rubella has changed since 1964. This is partly due to the new laboratory techniques and partly due to more intensive diagnostic investigations such as roentgenography, cardiac catheterization and pyelography. Intrauterine growth retardation, though noted by Gregg[1] and pointed out early by others,[3,10,44] was not generally recognized because all infants with low birth weights were considered prematures until rather recently. It is more difficult to explain why signs such as purpura, hepatosplenomegaly, adenopathy and cerebrospinal fluid pleocytosis were not recognized by pediatricians two decades ago. Whatever the reasons, there have been additions to the original disease picture described by Gregg[1] and other early students of prenatal rubella.[3]

In the neonatal period, thrombocytopenic purpura seen particularly about the face and trunk is a striking sign that carries a poor prognosis for life. Affected infants often have low birth weights and complicating diseases, so that more than one-third of them die within the first year.[15] The megakaryocytes of the bone marrow are reduced in number. In children who survive, the platelet disturbance is transitory. Sometimes hemolytic and hypoplastic anemia were noted in early infancy.[28,45] The hepatitis in the congenital rubella syndrome was studied microscopically and by electron microscopy and found to be similar to that seen in infants with neonatal hepatitis.[46,47] Hepatosplenomegaly, radiotranslucencies in the metaphyses of the long bones, bulging anterior fontanelle and cerebrospinal fluid changes are other early though transient manifestations regularly reported in recent years.[15]

Among the permanent changes, ocular defects are still common. Nuclear cataracts, microphthalmia, cloudy cornea and glaucoma can be present at birth or develop during infancy. High degrees of myopia may interfere with adequate vision.[15] The cataracts, unilateral or bilateral, often go unnoticed for several weeks or months. In the absence of cataract, chorioretinal (pepper-and-salt) changes can be seen in some instances.[48,49] Active anterior uveitis,[50] iris hypoplasia, shallow anterior chamber, strabismus and nystagmus may be additional findings.[21] Children with bilateral congenital cataract sometimes press hard with their index finger or hand on their eyes, showing the "oculo-digital syndrome of Franceschetti."[21,51] The rubella retinopathy is not progressive and does not

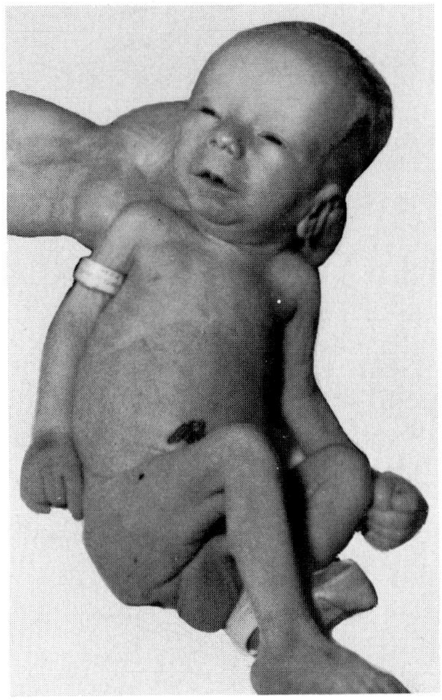

Fig. 9-2.—Prenatal rubella syndrome in a boy born after 40 weeks' gestation weighing 1,620 Gm. He had bilateral cataracts. At the age of 3 years he was deaf and could not sit or stand. The mother had had "measles" in the first month of pregnancy.

Fig. 9-3.—Child with congenital cataracts and congenital heart disease whose mother had had rubella during early pregnancy. (Courtesy of Dr. Laura Bickel, Houston, Texas.)

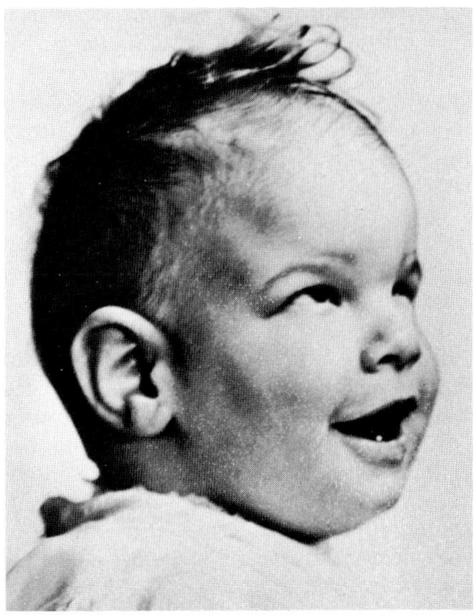

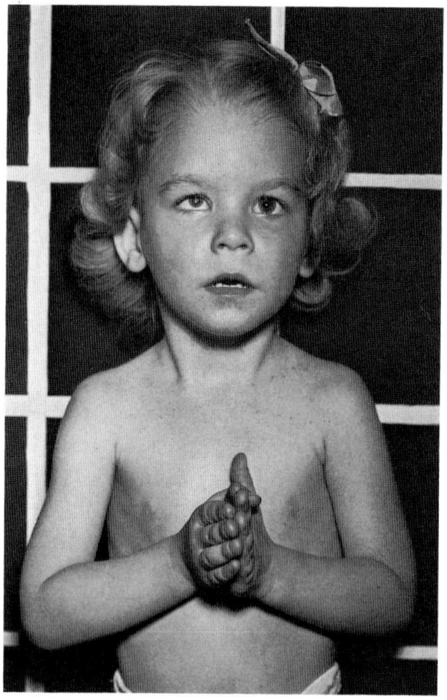

Fig. 9-4.—Prenatal rubella syndrome in a child whose mother was not aware of rubella during pregnancy. Intrauterine growth retardation, deafness, microphthalmia and cataract of the right eye and congenital heart disease. Patent ductus was corrected surgically when she was 8 years of age. Although she had scholastic difficulties, her social adjustment was good.

seriously impair visual acuity,[52] but delayed development of cataract and retinitis in the second year after birth have been reported.[53] Adverse postnatal factors may contribute to cataract formation in a lens that contains rubella virus.[54] Following the rubella epidemic of 1964 in New York City there was a fourfold increase in the number of congenital cataracts as compared with the incidence in nonepidemic years.[55]

Congenital cardiovascular malformations remain high on the list of anomalies in children with congenital rubella. Among abnormal children followed beyond infancy, congenital heart disease is noted in more than 50%.[15,27] Patent ductus arteriosus with or without stenosis of the pulmonary valve, pulmonary artery and its branches is still the leading anomaly, as it was 20 years ago. Involvement of the pulmonary artery, limited to the right or affecting both arteries, can be demonstrated by cardiac catheterization and angiography.[56-58] Coarctation of the aortic isthmus has also been described.[58] In necropsies, fibromuscular proliferation of the intima is common in pulmonary and systemic arteries (p. 464).[59] Atrial septal and ventricular septal defects occur, but they are more rare than the vascular anomalies.[58] Tricuspid atresia, transposition of the great vessels and complex cardiac anomalies seldom are seen.[58] In most cases, the cardiac defects are well tolerated, but some children develop congestive heart failure in the first months of life.[15] Pulmonary complications ranging from generalized pneumonia with hyaline membrane formation to chronic interstitial pneumonitis can be fatal.[91] Hepatosplenomegaly occurring in the neonatal period must not be interpreted as evidence of heart failure.[60] Jejunal atresia in twins with presumed congenital rubella has been reported.[61]

Renal and ureteric malformations were noted by Gregg[1] in one child when he described the results of prenatal rubella in 1941. Only a few cases with renal involvement have been reported subsequently.[62,63] Agenesis of the left kidney and nephritis were described in a child with the typical prenatal rubella syndrome and prolonged urinary virus excretion.[64] Hypospadias has been observed repeatedly in boys with congenital rubella.[3,62]

Hearing loss can be mild or severe, unilateral or bilateral. Early investigations suggested that unexplained deafness in about 10% of children was caused by maternal rubella. In a prospective study,[65] it was found that following rubella in the first 16 weeks of pregnancy, 30% of the children were deaf, but in two-thirds of them the hearing loss was not recognized until they were 4 years of age. That subclinical maternal rubella can contribute substantially to idiopathic deafness was demonstrated by serologic tests for rubella antibodies in a group of children in Trinidad.[11] Hemorrhages and inflammatory changes in the inner ear may account for the hearing loss.[66] Vestibular function also may be impaired by prenatal

Fig. 9-5.—Prenatal rubella syndrome in a child whose mother was unaware of any illness during pregnancy but nursed two of her older children who had rubella during her second month of pregnancy. The patient had bilateral cataract and congenital heart disease.

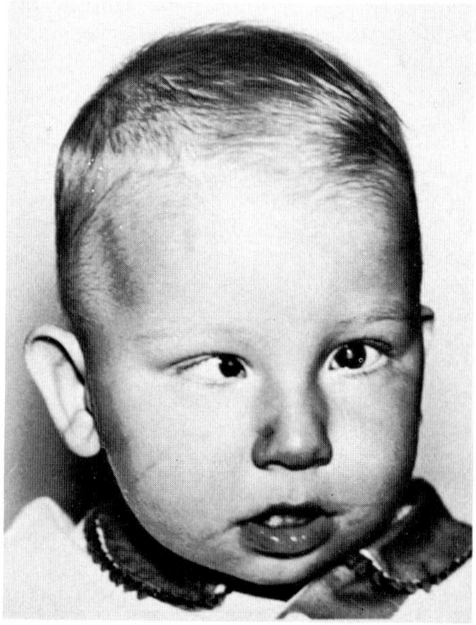

rubella, as shown by caloric tests. Vestibular defects probably are better demonstrable in early life than is hearing loss and may lead to early diagnosis of congenital rubella.[15] Audiograms are variable, but most of them suggest sensorineural impairment.[92]

Reports concerning involvement of the central nervous system are contradictory. Retardation of psychomotor activities is noted in some of the children,[62] but it is not known whether this is due to brain injury or to sensory deprivation. Desmond *et al.*[67] noted neurologic abnormalities between birth and 18 months in 81 of 100 congenital rubella patients. Lethargy, irritability, full fontanelle, increased protein in the cerebrospinal fluid and persistence of virus therein were observed. Developmental delay, motor paresis and mannerisms and restlessness were seen in 44 of 64 patients surviving to 18 months of age. Reduced head size was noted often.[62,67] Chronic infection of the central nervous system,[68] leptomeningitis, cerebral vasculitis, perivascular calcification and parenchymal necrosis have been described.[67,69] Developmental delay and central nervous system involvement, including quadriplegia, were seen in young affected children.[15] Rorke and Spiro[70] reviewed cerebral findings in such cases and described degenerative changes in arteries and foci of necrosis in the deep white matter and in gray nuclei. In apparent contrast is the 25-year follow-up of 50 original patients of Gregg's.[71] Only 1 of 50 was severely retarded, and 4 were mildly retarded. Most had made good socioeconomic adjustments and the majority had average intelligence. It seemed that because of impaired vision and hearing, the developmental potential of the patients had been underestimated during early life. This, as well as a tendency to healing of encephalitic lesions, may explain the apparent contradiction of serious central nervous system findings during infancy and the relatively favorable outcome seen in adults. Another possibility is that many children with severe involvement of the central nervous system died early and were not included in the surviving adult population. In the prospective study by the British Ministry of Health, the distribution of intelligence quotients among the children was normal.[8]

Roentgenography of the long bones of a considerable number of children with congenital rubella shows irregular mineralization at the areas of ossification and in the metaphyses, alternating radiolucent and dense metaphyseal striations and sometimes subperiosteal new bone formation.[27,69,72,73] The zones of translucency disappear spontaneously within a few weeks after birth. In a case of microcephaly and neurologic deficit, generalized cerebral atrophy was shown in a pneumoencephalogram. Cardiovascular anomalies can be demonstrated by angiography.[74]

Unusual dermatoglyphics associated with the congenital rubella syndrome were described by Achs *et al.*[75] Bilateral distal axial triradii, radial loops on other than the second digit and simian lines were found in 40 infants exposed to rubella in utero. The authors thought that these observations prove that an environmental teratogen can affect dermatoglyphics. Changes in dermatoglyphics were also noted in adults damaged by prenatal rubella. There was an increased incidence of digital whorl patterns[76] but not of simian creases. Instead, an atypical palmar line was demonstrated ("Sydney line"), which consists of an extension of the proximal transverse crease across the palm to its ulnar border.[77]

Congenital dental defects in infants with a history of maternal rubella during pregnancy have been reported by Evans[78] and others. Delayed eruption of teeth, aplasia of incisors and other teeth, malposition and malocclusion and enamel defects were observed.[79] Deciduous and permanent teeth can be missing. Susceptibility to caries and other dental changes attributed to prenatal rubella appeared somewhat doubtful in controlled studies.[62]

It seems well established that the rubella virus can interfere with normal organogenesis of the heart, and one must ask whether structural anomalies of other organs occurring following maternal rubella in the first 8 weeks of pregnancy could also be caused by the infection. Recent observations with laboratory documentation of rubella have failed to disclose such lesions as cleft palate, myelomeningocele or phocomelia[15,67] in children with congenital rubella. But there were reports in the past of posterior cleft palate,[10,62] encephalocele and spina bifida, anencephaly, renal anomalies and hypospadias[3,62] following maternal rubella that usually were considered coincidental.

When it was recognized that rubella acquired by the embryo is a chronic infection that can persist throughout fetal life and infancy,[20,29] re-examination of the concept of rubella as an acute disease that bestows immunity for life became necessary. It was found that, in the newborn, the virus can bring about thrombocytopenia, purpura, hepatitis and bone lesions. This threw doubt on the notion that the rubella virus is completely harmless after the first trimester of pregnancy. It is true that rubella infections after the fourteenth week of pregnancy do not result in malformations, but they do endanger the fetus to some extent. Hardy *et al.*[14] followed 24 women who had rubella between the fourteenth and thirty-first weeks of pregnancy. Two suffered fetal loss and 22 had live-born babies. Fifteen of the live-born children were suspected of some abnormalities of development and only 7 were considered normal. There were some hearing and speech difficulties, as well as delayed motor function and mental retardation. Most of the children were of normal birth weight but some were slow in postnatal weight gain and growth of head circumference. Over-all, manifestations were less severe and more subtle than those of infections during the first trimester.

Considering the increased exposure risk of nurses to viral infections during pregnancy, Haldane *et al.*[93] ascertained the outcome of pregnancies of nurses caring for infants with congenital defects both in hospitals and under home conditions; the incidence of congenital defects was significantly increased in the offspring of such nurses.

Prognosis

In general, the outlook for children damaged by prenatal rubella looks grave in the neonatal period and during infancy. As stated before, approximately one-third of the children die during the first 12 postnatal months. Congenital heart failure, sepsis and general debility cause many of the deaths.[15] The prognosis for the survivors who have congenital anomalies is better, as one would anticipate after observations during the early years, but intrauterine growth retardation often is followed by postnatal growth retardation.[71,80] Children infected early in utero and those with prolonged infection after birth are rather severely affected. Deafness of minor degrees, speech defects, cataract or results of its surgical treatment, hypertension and Eisenmenger syndrome were some of the sequelae found in the 25-year follow-up of the Australian survivors.[71] Of 50 patients, 45 were mentally normal and had made good social, psychologic and economic adjustments. Eleven patients were married and 7 had children. Of 8 children, 7 were normal, including the first son of a mother whose second son had bilateral congenital cataracts, microphthalmia and hypotonia; rubella virus was isolated from the urine of this child, and the mother had a high titer of rubella virus antibody.[81] This remarkable case raises the question of the mode of infection of the child. Had the mother harbored the virus since the time of her prenatal infection or was she reinfected? The high titer of antibody in the mother speaks for reinfection rather than persistence of the virus in her tissues for 26 years. Reinfection with rubella virus of a 16-year-old girl with the congenital rubella syndrome has been reported,[82] so that the occurrence of the congenital rubella syndrome in two generations is best explained by renewed susceptibility of the mother to the infection in adult life.

Prevention

The dangers of rubella to the conceptus require prophylactic measures, and various methods have been recommended to protect mother and embryo against the infection. Avoidance of exposure is to be recommended but is seldom practicable. Immunization by exposure of female children to known cases of rubella has been tried, but there is no guarantee that children who acquire the disease in this way will get through it without complications. The use of human gamma globulin for passive immunization has been a controversial issue for many years and for many reasons. One of the grounds for the controversy may be that lots of commercial gamma globulin from humans varied greatly in titers of antibody to neutralizing rubella virus.[83] In many cases, it is too late to give passive immunization by the time the mother finds out that she was exposed. Most important is the fact that a significant number of mothers in whom prophylaxis with gamma globulin had been attempted had children with congenital rubella.[15,84] Passive immunization cannot be relied on. Therapeutic abortion was and often is recommended and practiced for women who had rubella in the first trimester of pregnancy. But, aside from legal questions, there was the fact that some children were born normal even though the mothers had rubella in early pregnancy; there were problems of clinical diagnosis and there were no methods of recognizing subclinical maternal rubella. As mentioned before, rubella virus has been recovered in only 50% of the fetuses obtained by therapeutic abortions.[15,40]

The frequency of susceptibility to rubella has been estimated in females of reproductive age of different populations. Of 600 pregnant women in the United States, 17.5% did not have demonstrable antibody. Among Negro women, the absence of neutralizing antibody was significantly greater than among whites, and susceptibility decreased with increasing age. Young Indian and Eskimo women in Alaska were similar to women in the United States, with 18% without antibody.[85] Among Hawaiian pregnant women, lack of antibody amounted to 44%.[86] Other figures obtained in various countries were listed by Lundström *et al.*[87] In general, such data provide some indication of the considerable size of the population at risk for rubella infection.[84]

Mass immunization with attenuated live virus is the most probable solution for eradication of rubella. Several vaccines of this type have been produced and some are commercially available. A well-tested vaccine was produced by prolonged serial passage in monkey kidney cells and, by 1965, a 77th passage monkey kidney virus (high-passage virus-77 or HPV-77) was found to be modified so that a vaccine could be developed for clinical testing.[88] The vaccine did not cause illness in vaccinees or their contacts, but it did stimulate the production of protective antibodies. When pregnant monkeys were inoculated with the attenuated virus, maternal and fetal organs contained no virus. After vaccination of humans, antibodies could be detected by the third or fourth week. Virus was recovered from the throat 10–20 days following inoculation, but the shed virus was low in quantity and did not infect contact controls.[89] The levels of antibody induced by the vaccine were lower than those developed by natural rubella but they appeared to be sufficient for protection. Although prolonged immunity is likely, it is too early to say how long HPV-77 will protect against the disease without revaccination. It is possible that vaccines now available or some to be developed may prevent major rubella epidemics in the future.[88] In recent years, many studies have been made of rubella vaccines and their effects in mass immunizations. After an International Conference on Rubella Immunization, the U.S. Public Health Service Advisory Committee on Immunization

Practices made recommendations for the use of live rubella virus vaccines and emphasized precautions to be observed in the use of these vaccines.[94]

REFERENCES

1. Gregg, N.: Congenital cataract following German measles in mother, Tr. Ophth. Soc. Australia 3:35, 1942.
2. Warkany, J., and Kalter, H.: Congenital malformations, New England J. Med. 265:993, 1961.
3. Swan, C., Tostevin, A. L., Moore, B., Mayo, H., and Black, G. H. B.: Congenital defects in infants following infectious diseases during pregnancy, M. J. Australia 2:201, 1943.
4. Aycock, W. L., and Ingalls, T. H.: Maternal disease as principle in epidemiology of congenital anomalies: With review of rubella, Am. J. M. Sc. 212:366, 1946.
5. Wesselhoeft, C.: Rubella (German measles), New England J. Med. 236:943, 1947.
6. Swan, C.: Rubella in pregnancy as an aetiological factor in congenital malformation, stillbirth, miscarriage and abortion, J. Obst. & Gynec. Brit. Emp. 56:341, 1949.
7. Sallomi, S. J.: Rubella in pregnancy. A review of prospective studies from the literature, Obst. & Gynec. 27:252, 1966.
8. Sheridan, M. D.: Final report of a prospective study of children whose mothers had rubella in early pregnancy, Brit. M. J. 29:536, 1964.
9. Tartakow, I. J.: The teratogenicity of maternal rubella, J. Pediat. 66:380, 1965.
10. Beswick, R., Warner, R., and Warkany, J.: Congenital anomalies following maternal rubella, Am. J. Dis. Child. 78:334, 1949.
11. Karmody, C. S.: Subclinical maternal rubella and congenital deafness, New England J. Med. 278:809, 1968.
12. Sever, J. L., Nelson, K. B., and Gilkeson, M. R.: Rubella epidemic, 1964: Effect on 6,000 pregnancies. I. Preliminary clinical and laboratory findings through the neonatal period: A report from the collaborative study on cerebral palsy, Am. J. Dis. Child. 110:395, 1965.
13. Hardy, J. B., Minif, G. R. G., and Sever, J. L.: Studies in congenital rubella, Baltimore 1964–65. II. Clinical and virologic, Bull. Johns Hopkins Hosp. 118:97, 1966.
14. Hardy, J. B., McCracken, G. H., Jr., Gilkeson, M. R., and Sever, J. L.: Adverse fetal outcome following maternal rubella after the first trimester of pregnancy, J.A.M.A. 207:2414, 1969.
15. Cooper, L. Z.: Rubella: A preventable cause of birth defects, The Nat. Fdn. March of Dimes, 1968.
16. Siegel, M., Fuerst, H. T., and Peress, N. S.: Fetal mortality in maternal rubella. Results of a prospective study from 1957 to 1964, Am. J. Obst. & Gynec. 96:247, 1966.
17. Cooper, L. Z., and Krugman, S.: Diagnosis and management: Congenital rubella, Pediatrics 37:335, 1966.
18. Weller, T. H., and Neva, F. A.: Propagation in tissue culture of cytopathic agents from patients with rubella-like illness, Proc. Soc. Exper. Biol. & Med. 111:215, 1962.
19. Parkman, B. D., Buescher, E. L., and Artenstein, M. S.: Recovery of rubella virus from Army recruits, Proc. Soc. Exper. Biol. & Med. 111:225, 1962.
20. Alford, C. A., Neva, F. A., and Weller, T. H.: Virologic and serologic studies on human products of conception after maternal rubella, New England J. Med. 271:1275, 1964.
21. Roy, F. H., Hiatt, R. L., Korones, S. B., and Roane, J.: Ocular manifestations of congenital rubella syndrome. Recovery of virus from affected infants, Arch. Ophth. 75:601, 1966.
22. Cotlier, E., Fox, J., and Smith, M.: Rubella virus in the cataractous lens of congenital rubella syndrome, Am. J. Ophth. 62:233, 1966.
23. Menser, M. A., Harley, J. D., Hertzberg, R., Dorman, D. C., and Murphy, A. M.: Persistence of virus in lens for three years after prenatal rubella, Lancet 2:387, 1967.
24. Michaels, R. M.: Immunological aspects of congenital rubella, Pediatrics 43:339, 1969.
25. Medearis, D. N., Jr.: Rubella and immunologic response, Pediatrics 43:322, 1969.
26. Plotkin, S. A., Oski, F. A., Hartnett, E. M., Hervada, A. R., Friedman, S., and Gowing, J.: Some recently recognized manifestations of the rubella syndrome, J. Pediat. 67:182, 1965.
27. Rudolph, A. J., Yow, M. D., Phillips, A., Desmond, M. M., Blattner, R. J., and Melnick, J. L.: Transplacental rubella infection in newly born infants, J.A.M.A. 191:843, 1965.
28. Dudgeon, J. A.: Maternal rubella and its effect on the foetus, Arch. Dis. Childhood 42:110, 1967.
29. Selzer, G.: Virus isolation, inclusion bodies, and chromosomes in a rubella-infected human embryo, Lancet 2:336, 1963.
30. Neu, R. L., Schlegel, R. J., Leao, J. C., and Gardner, L. I.: Chromosomes of foetus following maternal rubella, Lancet 2:1185, 1964.
31. Mellman, W. J., Plotkin, S. A., Moorhead, P. S., and Hartnett, E. M.: Rubella infection of human leucocytes, Am. J. Dis. Child. 110:473, 1965.
32. Nusbacher, J., Hirschhorn, K., and Cooper, L. Z.: Chromosomal abnormalities in congenital rubella, New England J. Med. 276:1409, 1967.
33. Plotkin, S. A., and Boué, J. G.: In vitro growth of rubella virus in human embryo cells, Am. J. Epidemiol. 81:71, 1965.
34. Singer, D. B., Rudolph, A. J., Rosenberg, H. S., Rawls, W. E., and Boniuk, M.: Pathology of the congenital rubella syndrome, J. Pediat. 71:665, 1967.
35. Naeye, R. L., and Blanc, W. A.: Pathogenesis of congenital rubella, J.A.M.A. 194:1277, 1965.
36. Monif, G. R. G., and Sever, J. L.: Pathogenesis of the teratogenic effect of rubella virus, Obst. & Gynec. 27:741, 1966.
37. Töndury, G.: *Embryopathien*, Vol. XI of *Pathologie und Klinik* (Berlin: Springer-Verlag, 1962).
38. Baertschi, U.: Unsere heutigen Kenntnisse über das Rubeolenvirus und die Embryopathia rubeolica, Fortschr. Geb. Gynäk. 27:1, 1966.
39. Töndury, G., and Smith, D. W.: Fetal rubella pathology, J. Pediat. 68:867, 1966.
40. Heggie, A. D.: Intrauterine infection in maternal rubella, J. Pediat. 71:777, 1967.
41. Swan, C.: Study of 3 infants dying from congenital defects following maternal rubella in early stages of pregnancy, J. Path. & Bact. 56:289, 1944.
42. Korones, S. B., Ainger, L. E., Monif, G. R. G., Roane, J., Sever, J. L., and Fuste, F.: Congenital rubella syndrome: New clinical aspects with recovery of virus from affected infants, J. Pediat. 67:166, 1965.
43. Thorburn, M. J., and Miller, C. G.: Pathology of congenital rubella in Jamaica, Arch. Dis. Childhood 42:389, 1967.
44. Warkany, J., Monroe, B. B., and Sutherland, B. S.: Intrauterine growth retardation, Am. J. Dis. Child. 102:249, 1961.
45. Rausen, A. R., Richter, P., Tallal, L., and Cooper, L. Z.: Hematological effects of intrauterine rubella, J.A.M.A. 199:75, 1967.
46. Esterly, J. R., Slusser, R. J., and Ruebner, B. H.: Hepatic lesions in the congenital rubella syndrome, J. Pediat. 71: 676, 1967.
47. Alagille, D., Habib, E-C., Gautier, M., Boue, A., and Kocher, S.: L'hépatite de la rubéole néonatale, Arch. franç. pédiat. 25:393, 1968.
48. Murphy, A. M., Reid, R. R., Pollard, I., Gillespie, A. M., Dorman, D. C., Menser, M. A., Harley, J. D., and Hertzberg, R.: Rubella cataracts, Am. J. Ophth. 64:1109, 1967.
49. Kresky, B., and Nauheim, J. S.: Rubella retinitis, Am. J. Dis. Child. 113:305, 1967.
50. Wolter, J. R., Inset, P. A., Willey, N., and Brittain, H. P.: Eye pathology following maternal rubella. A study of four children, J. Pediat. Ophth. 3:29, 1966.

51. Franceschetti, A.: Rubéole pendant la grossesse et cataracte congénitale chez l'enfant, accompagnée du phénomène digito-oculaire, Ophthalmologia 114:332, 1947.
52. Hertzberg, R.: Twenty-five-year follow-up of ocular defects in congenital rubella, Am. J. Ophth. 66:269, 1968.
53. Hancock, M. P., Huntley, C. C., and Sever, J. L.: Congenital rubella syndrome with immunoglobulin disorder, J. Pediat. 72:636, 1968.
54. Menser, M. A., Harley, J. D., Housego, C. J., and Murphy, A. M.: Possible chemical factors in the postnatal development of rubella cataracts, Lancet 2:771, 1966.
55. Siegel, M., Fuerst, H. T., and Duggan, W.: Rubella in mother and congenital cataracts in child. Comparative data in periods with and without epidemics from 1957 to 1964, J.A.M.A. 203:632, 1968.
56. Rowe, R. D.: Maternal rubella and pulmonary artery stenoses, Pediatrics 32:180, 1963.
57. Emmanouilides, G. C., Linde, L. M., and Crittenden, I. H.: Pulmonary artery stenosis associated with ductus arteriosus following maternal rubella, Circulation 29:514, 1964.
58. Hastreiter, A. R., Joorabchi, B., Pujatti, G., van der Horse, R. L., Patacsil, G., and Sever, J. L.: Cardiovascular lesions associated with congenital rubella, J. Pediat. 71:59, 1967.
59. Esterly, J. R., and Oppenheimer, E. H.: Vascular lesions in infants with congenital rubella, Circulation 36:544, 1967.
60. Jeresaty, R. M., and Russell, W.: Hepatosplenomegaly and heart disease in the congenital rubella syndrome, Pediatrics 39:36, 1967.
61. Esterly, J. R., and Talbert, J. L.: Jejunal atresia in twins with presumed congenital rubella, Lancet 1:1028, 1969.
62. Lundström, R.: Rubella during pregnancy; a follow-up study of children born after an epidemic of rubella in Sweden, 1951, with additional investigations on prophylaxis and treatment of maternal rubella, Acta paediat., supp. 133, 1962.
63. Bellanti, J. A., Artenstein, M. S., Olson, L. C., Buescher, E. L., Luhrs, C. E., and Milstead, K. L.: Congenital rubella, Am. J. Dis. Child. 110:464, 1965.
64. Menser, M. A., Robertson, S. E. J., Dorman, D. C., Gillespie, A. M., and Murphy, A. M.: Renal lesions in congenital rubella, Pediatrics 40:901, 1967.
65. Jackson, A. D. M., and Fisch, L.: Deafness following maternal rubella. Results of a prospective investigation, Lancet 2:1241, 1958.
66. Friedmann, I., and Wright, M. I.: Histopathological changes in the foetal and infantile inner ear caused by maternal rubella, Brit. M. J. 2:20, 1966.
67. Desmond, M. M., Wilson, G. S., Melnick, J. L., Singer, D. B., Zion, T. E., Rudolph, A. J., Pineda, R. G., Ziai, M-H., and Blattner, R. J.: Congenital rubella encephalitis. Course and early sequelae, J. Pediat. 71:311, 1967.
68. Monif, G. R. G., and Sever, J. L.: Chronic infection of the central nervous system with rubella virus, Neurology 16: 111, 1966.
69. Peters, E. R., and Davis, R. L.: Congenital rubella syndrome. Cerebral mineralizations and subperiosteal new bone formation as expressions of this disorder, Clin. Pediat. 5:743, 1966.
70. Rorke, L. B., and Spiro, A. J.: Cerebral lesions in congenital rubella syndrome, J. Pediat. 70:243, 1967.
71. Menser, M. A., Dods, L., and Harley, J. D.: A twenty-five-year follow-up of congenital rubella, Lancet 1:1347, 1967.
72. Rausen, A. R., London, R. D., Mizrahi, A., and Cooper, L. Z.: Generalized bone changes and thrombocytopenic purpura in association with intrauterine rubella, Pediatrics 36:264, 1965.
73. Singleton, E. B., Rudolph, A. J., Rosenberg, H. S., and Singer, D. B.: The roentgenographic manifestations of the rubella syndrome in newborn infants, Am. J. Roentgenol. 97:82, 1966.
74. Williams, H. J., and Carey, L. S.: Rubella embryopathy. Roentgenologic features, Am. J. Roentgenol. 97:92, 1966.
75. Achs, R., Harper, R. G., and Siegel, M.: Unusual dermatoglyphic findings associated with rubella embryopathy, New England J. Med. 274:148, 1966.
76. Alter, M., and Schulenberg, R.: Dermatoglyphics in the rubella syndrome, J.A.M.A. 197:685, 1966.
77. Purvis-Smith, S. G.: Dermatoglyphics in adults with congenital rubella, Lancet 2:141, 1968.
78. Evans, M. W.: Congenital dental defects in infants subsequent to maternal rubella during pregnancy, M. J. Australia 2:225, 1944.
79. Stocker, A.: Ein Beitrag zur Kenntnis der Embryopathia rubeolosa, Inaugur. Dissert., Zurich, 1951.
80. Michaels, R. H., and Kenny, F. M.: Postnatal growth retardation in congenital rubella, Pediatrics 43:251, 1969.
81. Menser, M. A., Slinn, R. F., Dods, L., Hertzberg, R., and Harley, J. D.: Congenital rubella in a mother and son, Australian Paediat. J. 4:200, 1968.
82. Doege, T. C., and Kim, K. S. W.: Studies of rubella and its prevention with immune globulin, J.A.M.A. 200:584, 1967.
83. Schiff, G. M., Sever, J. L., and Huebner, R. J.: Rubella virus: Neutralizing antibody in commercial gamma globulin, Science 142:58, 1963.
84. McDonald, J. C., and Peckham, C. S.: Gamma globulin in prevention of rubella and congenital defect: A study of 30,000 pregnancies, Brit. M. J. 3:633, 1967.
85. Sever, J. L., Schiff, G. M., and Huebner, R. J.: Frequency of rubella antibody among pregnant women and other human and animal populations, Obst. & Gynec. 23:153, 1964.
86. Sever, J. L., Fabiyi, A., McCallin, P. F., Chu, P. T., Weiss, W., and Gilkeson, M. R.: Rubella antibody among pregnant women in Hawaii, Am. J. Obst. & Gynec. 92:1006, 1965.
87. Lundström, R., Svedmyr, A., Hagbard, L., and Kaijser, K.: Rubella immunity as related to age and history of overt disease, Acta paediat. scandinav. 56:279, 1967.
88. Parkman, P. D.: Research prospects—rubella vaccine, Ment. Retard., pp. 11–16, April, 1969.
89. Lepow, M. L., Veronelli, J. A., Hostetler, D. D., and Robbins, F. C.: A trial with live attenuated rubella vaccine, Am. J. Dis. Child. 115:639, 1968.
90. Montgomery, R. C., and Stockdell, K.: Congenital rubella in twins, J. Pediat. 76:772, 1970.
91. Phelan, P., and Campbell, P.: Pulmonary complications of rubella embryopathy, J. Pediat. 75:202, 1969.
92. Borton, T. E., and Stark, E. W.: Audiological findings in hearing loss secondary to maternal rubella, Pediatrics 45: 225, 1970.
93. Haldane, E. V., Van Rooyen, C. E., Embil, J. A., Tupper, W. C., Gordon, P. C., and Wanklin, J. M.: A search for transmissible birth defects of virologic origin in members of the nursing profession, Am. J. Obst. & Gynec. 105: 1032, 1969.
94. Krugman, S. (ed.): Proceedings of the International Conference on Rubella Immunization, Am. J. Dis. Child. 118:1, 1969.

Cytomegalic Inclusion Disease

THE LARGE CELLS characteristic of cytomegalic inclusion disease (CID) have been known to pathologists since the end of the nineteenth century, when they were seen in renal tubules, lungs, liver and salivary glands of children who died of lues and other diseases.[1,2] At first, they were mistaken for protozoan cells; later, the phenomenon was named "cytomegalia infantum"[3] and "salivary gland virus disease,"[4] a term that foresaw its viral origin. The giant cells with inclusion bodies were found in various human tissues and, by 1957, approximately 200 cases of generalized cytomegaly were on record.[5] The human virus was demonstrated in 1956 in tissue culture material obtained from submaxillary glands and kidneys of infected infants[6] and from adenoids of older children.[7] The filterable agents capable of producing typical inclusions are viruses of about 100 millimicron particle size.[8,9] The virus produces neutralizing and complement-fixing antibodies.

The inclusions are found in the salivary glands of approximately 20% of children coming to necropsy, but in only 3% are they seen in the viscera. Premature and newborn children tend to infection and dissemination of the virus, which can also be transmitted in utero.[10] The virus is disseminated widely in certain geographic areas but shows little pathogenicity in the adult population. There, it spreads throughout the body only if illnesses weaken the resistance to infections. It is assumed that only prenatal or neonatal infections with the CID virus lead to serious disease. Deaths attributable to CID occur essentially in the first 6 months of postnatal life.[11] Later, the infection rate increases, as demonstrated by serologic methods, but most of these infections take a subclinical course. In pregnant women, the primary infection can result in a symptom-free viremia and transmission of the virus to chorionic villi and various fetal tissues. There, it can cause destruction from the end of the first trimester on to the end of gestation and throughout the neonatal period.[12] It has not been established that earlier infections can lead to abortion or congenital malformations. It is assumed that fetal infectivity lasts only through the period of viremia and that there is little risk of repetition of congenital CID in a family.[11] Infection during pregnancy does not always lead to fetal CID. In Atlanta, Georgia, 3% of 185 pregnant women excreted the virus in the urine during the second trimester of gestation. The pregnancies ended in full-term normal deliveries and the children did not show neurologic deficits 6 months after delivery. One of the children had the virus in the throat and urine, and petechiae were observed on the face.[12] In a study of 59 instances of pregnancy wastage, cytomegalovirus was isolated in 5 cases.[36] It has been estimated that in Vienna, Austria, 1 case of congenital CID occurs in 1,000 live-born children.[11] In the United States, 3 of 545 newborn infants examined excreted cytomegalovirus in the urine; none of the 3 had classic cytomegalic inclusion disease.[37]

Congenital CID involves many organs, but the clinical picture depends on the severity, time and duration of the infection. Hepatosplenomegaly, jaundice, thrombocytopenic purpura, intrauterine growth retardation, anemia and cytomegalic epithelial cells in the urine aid in the early diagnosis of the disease, which

Fig. 9-6. – Markedly enlarged cells from a child with cytomegalic inclusion disease. Inclusion bodies are separated from the nuclear membranes by light halos.

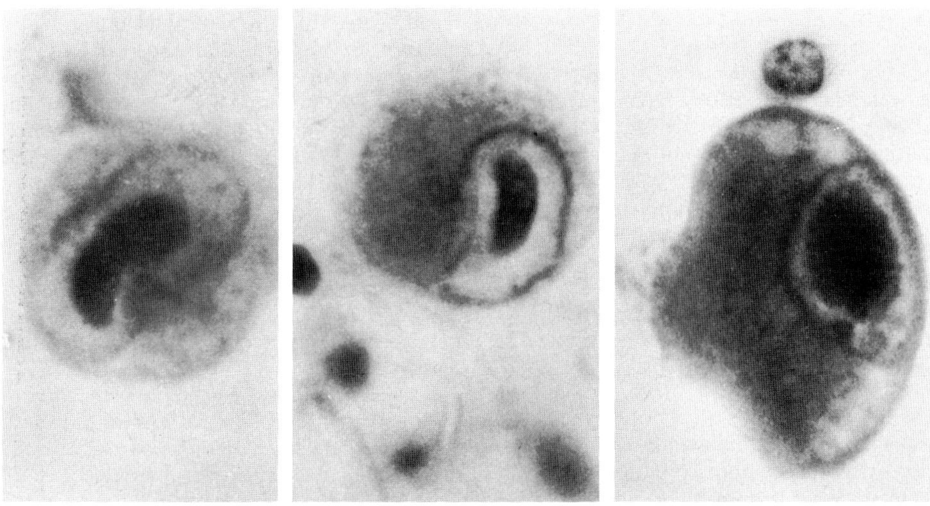

may end in neonatal death or microcephaly and mental retardation. Generalized edema, interstitial pneumonia and gastrointestinal disturbances may influence the disease picture. Ocular changes, roentgenograms of the skull and long bones, virus isolation and antibody studies confirm the diagnosis.

The CID virus that invades the unborn child can persist in the fetal and neonatal organism for many months. Pathologic-anatomic changes consist of localized, interstitial inflammatory processes with a marked tendency to necrosis, fibrosis and calcification and of destructive alterations of epithelial structures that show many characteristic CID cells but few signs of inflammation.[11] Foci of inflammation are seen in liver, lungs, pancreas, salivary glands, kidneys, myocardium, thyroid, adrenals, pituitary, brain and meninges. Diseased epithelial cells are derived particularly from ducts of excretory glands, which can be obstructed by degenerating cell masses and disturbed by accumulation of secretions. Permanent damage to the brain, eye, liver, thyroid and other organs has been observed in children who survive congenital CID. Symptoms and signs of the disease noticeable at the time of birth are not always the final manifestations, since destructive processes of CID may continue in postnatal life. Sometimes it is difficult to decide whether an infection was prenatal or postnatal.

Patients have been described who, at the time of birth, showed signs of brain damage but no visceral involvement,[13,14] as if the disease had become inactive at the time of birth. Calcifications in the brain[13] or sparse cytomegalic cells in the urine suggested the diagnosis of CID.[14] Hanshaw[15] determined cytomegalovirus complement-fixing antibody in the sera of 41 children with head circumferences 2 standard deviations below the mean. Antibody was present in 44% of these children who had no typical symptoms of extraneural CID. Such observations suggest that the role of CID in the etiology of congenital malformations of the brain and of mental retardation may be greater than demonstrable at present.

The livers of infants with congenital CID may show signs of acute or subacute hepatitis or even cirrhosis. Biopsy specimens of patients with proved CID show changes compatible with the picture of neonatal hepatitis.[16] Nuclear swelling, focal infiltration and necrosis, bile stasis, giant cell transition and disorganization of the liver architecture may be seen.[17] Jaundice is often, but not always, present.[16]

Thrombocytopenia, erythroblastemia, leukocytosis, purpura and general bleeding tendencies have been observed. Petechiae occur in approximately one-half of the infants.[16] Anemias usually develop several weeks after birth. Transitory rashes are noticed in some infants.

The kidneys are involved in many cases of disseminated congenital CID, as evidenced by secretion of virus and occurrence of cytomegalic cells in the urine.[18] Inclusion-bearing cells are located chiefly in distal convoluted and peripheral collecting tubules, whereas proximal tubules are free of inclusions.[19] Excretion of inclusion cells can last for many months[20] without manifest renal disease.

Respiratory complications are frequent. Interstitial pneumonia, bronchitis, tracheitis and cylindrical bronchiectases can be found in necropsy specimens.[21]

The most important changes occur in the brain. A disseminated meningo-encephalitis can affect many parts of the brain and cerebellum, with typical preference for subependymal layers of the ventricles. There, necrotizing inflammatory foci tend to calcifications that can be so marked that the lateral ventricles can be outlined by linear shadows in roentgenograms. Mononuclear infiltrates, perivascular gliosis and arterial changes lead to brain atrophy and malacia. Micrencephaly and microcephaly are common. Cortical lesions are variable. Whereas histologic changes of the cortex and white matter can be attributed to late fetal disease, microgyria, which has been observed repeatedly,[11,22,23] points to relatively early brain damage. It has been estimated that some of these lesions date back to the third or fourth month of gestation. Hydrocephaly can be congenital and due to early blocking of the aqueduct or develop following brain atrophy in combination with micrencephaly.[11,20,24] Weller and Hanshaw,[16] who studied 17 infants with CID, observed microcephaly in 14, which was present at birth or became noticeable during early childhood. Mental retardation was noted in 13 and motor disability in 12 of the survivors. Blindness, epileptic seizures and spastic diplegia were among the sequelae of CID.

Ocular changes have been described repeatedly, but proof of CID seldom was given.[25] Conjunctivitis, keratomalacia, uveitis, cataract, chorioretinitis and optic atrophy have been reported. The occurrence of chorioretinitis, cerebral calcifications and hepatosplenomegaly suggests toxoplasmosis as well as CID, but it seems that the retinal lesions of CID are milder and more peripheral than those of toxoplasmosis.[20,25]

Involvement of endocrine glands by generalized congenital CID may be of importance, since permanent damage to one or several of these organs could explain the etiology of some congenital endocrine disturbances. France[26] described a child with visceral manifestations of CID who developed signs of hypothyroidism when 9 weeks of age. When the child died 2 months later, there were severe changes in the structure of the thyroid, including transition of many cells to cytomegaly. Medearis[10] reported the case of a child born with an enlarged thyroid who died at the age of 2½ months. Necropsy revealed cytomegalic inclusions in many epithelial cells, but the thyroid showed merely hyperplasia and interstitial fibrosis.

Roentgenograms of the skull contribute greatly to the diagnosis, as the subependymal calcifications in the walls of the lateral ventricles are characteristic of

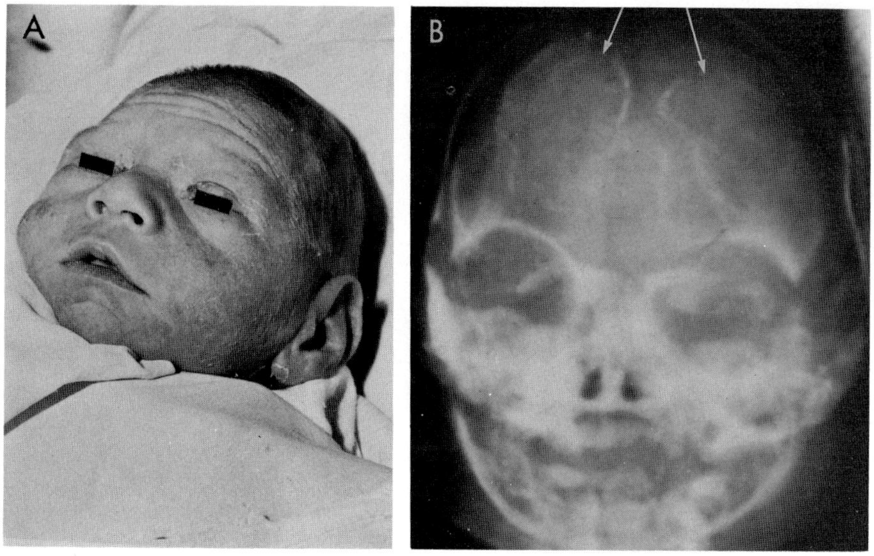

Fig. 9-7. – **A,** microcephalic child with cytomegalic inclusion disease. **B,** paraventricular calcification in the child.

CID. Diaphyseal translucencies,[5,27] osteosclerosis and double contours of the calcaneus have been reported in the appendicular skeleton.[11]

Intrauterine growth retardation is a frequent result of prenatal infection with CID. Many authors have mentioned that infants with congenital CID had subnormal weights for their gestational ages.[11,14,16,20,23,28,29] It is understandable that destruction of cells by CID results in smallness of many body organs[28] and that intrauterine growth retardation can be present in a newborn who is past the stage of active prenatal CID.[14]

There are some resemblances and some differences in the pathogenesis of congenital CID and congenital rubella. One of the differences is that abortions and congenital malformations determined in the first 2 months of pregnancy have not been demonstrated as sequelae of CID. With the conception of prenatal rubella as a chronic infection like prenatal CID, one will be inclined to look for similar manifestations. Rubella as well as CID beginning in fetal life can continue as active infections into childhood. Is there any proof that CID can affect an embryo during organogenesis and cause congenital malformations during the first 2 months of life? There are reports of children with CID who had such malformations,[11,21,30] but it is too early to decide whether the viral infection in these cases was the cause, the result or a coincidence in the teratologic process.

An exact evaluation of the prognosis of prenatal CID is not yet possible. It is not known whether infection with CID virus is possible in the first 8 weeks of pregnancy and what the fate of embryos affected early would be. The prognosis for children born with signs of CID seems extremely grave, as evidenced by the many necropsy reports and descriptions of patients with permanent central nervous system damage.[11,15,16] But it must be kept in mind that most reports so far have dealt with selected and severe cases of congenital CID and that it will take time to obtain

Fig. 9-8. – Paraventricular calcifications in a child with cytomegalic inclusion disease.

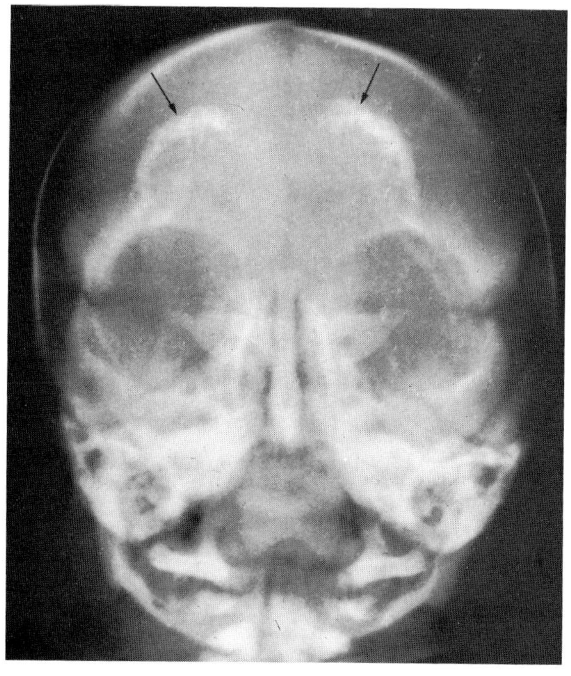

prospective data on the disease. In an Australian study of 20 children who seemed to have acquired the virus in utero, 8 recovered completely from congenital CID.[31]

Since infection with the CID virus of older children in good general health apparently is harmless, deliberate exposure of young girls has been recommended as a preventive measure to forestall infection of women during pregnancy.[32]

The uncertainty of the natural course of the disease makes it difficult to evaluate treatments. If one assumes that most cases of congenital CID are hopeless, recovery after treatment with corticosteroids[11,27,33] will seem a great success, but relatively few children have had the benefit of this therapy. As cases with spontaneous recovery become known, the value of the treatment seems less assured.[34] Administration of idoxuridine has been attempted, with some signs of improvement.[35]

REFERENCES

1. Ribbert, H.: Über protozoenartige Zellen in der Niere eines syphilitischen Neugeborenen und in der Parotis von Kindern, Zentralbl. allg. Path. 15:945, 1904.
2. Jesionek and Kiolemenoglou: Über einen Befund von protozoënartigen Gebilden in den Organen eines hereditärluetischen Fötus, München. med. Wchnschr. 51:1905, 1904.
3. Goodpasture, E. W., and Talbot, F. B.: Nature of "protozoan-like" cells in certain lesions of infancy, Am. J. Dis. Child. 21:415, 1921.
4. Farber, S., and Wolbach, S. B.: Intranuclear and cytoplasmic inclusions (protozoan-like bodies) in the salivary glands and other organs of infant, Am. J. Path. 8:123, 1932.
5. Seifert, G., and Oehme, J.: *Pathologie und Klinik der Zytomegalie* (Leipzig: Georg Thieme, 1957).
6. Smith, M. G.: Propagation in tissue cultures of a cytopathogenic virus from human salivary gland virus disease, Proc. Soc. Exper. Biol. & Med. 92:424, 1956.
7. Rowe, W. F., Hartley, J. W., Waterman, S., Turner, H. C., and Huebner, R. J.: Cytopathogenic agent resembling human salivary gland virus recovered from tissue cultures of human adenoids, Proc. Soc. Exper. Biol. & Med. 92:418, 1956.
8. Luse, S. A., and Smith, M. G.: Electron microscopy of salivary gland viruses, Am. J. Path. 32:642, 1956.
9. Weller, T. H., Macouley, J. C., Craig, J. M., and Wirth, P.: Isolation of intranuclear inclusion producing agents from infants with illnesses resembling cytomegalic inclusion disease, Proc. Soc. Exper. Biol. & Med. 94:4, 1957.
10. Medearis, D. N., Jr.: Cytomegalic inclusion disease. An analysis of the clinical features based on the literature and six additional cases, Pediatrics 19:467, 1957.
11. Thalhammer, O.: *Pränatale Erkrankungen des Menschen* (Stuttgart: Georg Thieme, 1967).
12. Feldman, R. A.: Cytomegalovirus infection during pregnancy. A prospective study and report of six cases, Am. J. Dis. Child. 117:517, 1969.
13. Thalhammer, O., and Zweymüller, E.: Angeborene Cytomegalie; nach embryonaler Infektion im Stadium des inaktiven Schadens geboren, Wien. klin. Wchnschr. 73: 762, 1961.
14. Rath, F.: Angeborene Cytomegalie; ein Kind im Stadium des inaktiven Schadens mit Mikrocephalie ohne intracerebrale Verkalkungen geboren, Monatsschr. Kinderh. 113: 565, 1965.
15. Hanshaw, J. B.: Cytomegalovirus complement-fixing antibody in microcephaly, New England J. Med. 275:476, 1966.
16. Weller, T. H., and Hanshaw, J. B.: Virologic and clinical observations on cytomegalic inclusion disease, New England J. Med. 266:1233, 1962.
17. Medearis, D. N., Jr.: Observations concerning human cytomegalovirus infection and disease, Bull. Johns Hopkins Hosp. 114:181, 1964.
18. Fetterman, G. H.: A new laboratory aid in the clinical diagnosis of inclusion disease of infancy, Am. J. Clin. Path. 22:424, 1952.
19. Fetterman, G. H., Sherman, F. E., Fabrizio, N. S., and Studnicki, F. M.: Generalized cytomegalic inclusion disease of the newborn. Localization of inclusions in the kidney, Arch. Path. 86:86, 1968.
20. Guyton, T. B., Ehrlich, F., Blanc, W. A., and Becker, M. H.: New observations in generalized cytomegalic-inclusion disease of the newborn, New England J. Med. 257: 803, 1957.
21. Ebert, W.: Zur Frage der lokalisierten und generalisierten Cytomegalie und ihre Bedeutung für die Entstehung von Fehlbildungen, Ztschr. Kinderh. 98:350, 1967.
22. Haymaker, W., Bertram, R., Girdany, R., Stephens, J., Lillie, R. D., and Fetterman, G. H.: Cerebral involvement with advanced periventricular calcification in generalized cytomegalic inclusion disease in the newborn, J. Neuropath. & Exper. Neurol. 13:562, 1954.
23. Mégevand, A.: Embryopathie cérébrale dans un case de maladie généralisée des inclusions cytomégaliques, Ann. paediat. 201:410, 1963.
24. Potter, E. L.: Placental transmission of viruses, Am. J. Obst. & Gynec. 74:505, 1957.
25. Burns, R. P.: Cytomegalic inclusion disease uveitis, A.M.A. Arch. Ophth. 61:376, 1959.
26. France, V. E.: Inclusion disease in childhood, Arch. Dis. Childhood 26:588, 1951.
27. van Gelderen, H. H.: Successfully treated case of cytomegalic disease in a newborn infant, Acta paediat. 48:169, 1959.
28. Naeye, R. L.: Cytomegalic inclusion disease, Am. J. Clin. Path. 47:738, 1967.
29. Silverman, W. A.: Clinical conference. Cytomegalic inclusion disease, Pediatrics 21:682, 1958.
30. Benyesh-Melnick, M., Rosenberg, H., and Watson, B.: Viruses in cell cultures of children with congenital heart malformations and other diseases, Proc. Soc. Exper. Biol. & Med. 3:452, 1964.
31. Jack, I., Turner, E. K., Danks, D. M., Maddison, T. G., and Colebatch, J. H.: Cytomegalovirus infection in Melbourne children, Australian Paediat. J. 3:61, 1967.
32. Elliott, G. B., and Elliott, K. A.: Cytomegalic inclusion disease of the developing fetus: A potentially preventable cause of congenital mental defect, Clin. Pediat. 1:87, 1962.
33. Margileth, A. M.: The diagnosis and treatment of generalized cytomegalic inclusion disease of the newborn, Pediatrics 15:270, 1955.
34. Hanshaw, J. B.: Congenital and acquired cytomegalovirus infection, Pediat. Clin. North America 13:279, 1966.
35. Conchie, A. F., Barton, B. W., and Tobin, J. O'H.: Congenital cytomegalovirus infection treated with idoxuridine, Brit. M. J. 4:162, 1968.
36. Kriel, R. L., Gates, G. A., Wulff, H., Powell, N., Poland, J. D., and Chin, T. D. Y.: Cytomegalovirus isolations associated with pregnancy wastage, Am. J. Obst. & Gynec. 106: 885, 1970.
37. Birnbaum, G., Lynch, J. I., Margileth, A. M., Lonergan, W. M., and Sever, J. L.: Cytomegalovirus infections in newborn infants, J. Pediat. 75:789, 1969.

Herpesvirus

RECENT CASE REPORTS[1,2] suggest that the genital herpesvirus (type 2) can result in congenital malformations similar to those produced by cytomegalic inclusion disease. Microcephaly, micrencephaly, intracranial calcifications, microphthalmia, cloudy lenses, retrolental masses and retinal dysplasia were described in children born with cutaneous lesions from which herpesvirus type 2 could be isolated. It seems likely that the virus was transmitted to the fetus transplacentally early in gestation. It is thought that the fetus can be infected when herpesvirus type 2 infection occurs at any stage of pregnancy in a mother who had no previous herpesvirus infection.

REFERENCES

1. Schaffer, A. J.: *Diseases of the Newborn* (2d ed.; Philadelphia: W. B. Saunders Company, 1965).
2. South, M. A., Tompkins, W. A. F., Morris, C. R., and Rawls, W. E.: Congenital malformations of the central nervous system associated with genital type (type 2) herpesvirus, J. Pediat. 75:13, 1969.

Viruses as Experimental Teratogens

IN CONTRAST TO the wealth of experiments that demonstrate teratogenic effects of chemical compounds or of nutritional deficiencies—for which there are few analogues in man—there are few teratogenic experiments in mammals to supplement the observations on human congenital malformations produced by viral diseases. So much attention has been given to the etiology, pathogenesis, pathology and clinical aspects of rubella and cytomegalic inclusion disease in man that the lack of experimental models for the study of viral teratogens is hard to understand. There is a possibility that many still unidentified microorganisms can invade embryos and fetuses and deform them and that they could account for congenital malformations for which we have no explanations as yet. Experimental work in mammals along these lines is needed. Even for rubella and cytomegalovirus, animal models are scanty and little used for investigative purposes.

Congenital infection of monkeys with rubella has been reported. In one study only were lesions produced in the monkey embryo following inoculation at the twenty-fifth day of gestation. Lenticular, cutaneous, osseous and chorionic lesions were reported.[1] Confirmation of this report would be of great importance. Rubella infection of newborn ferrets resulted in chronic infection and antibody production, but corneal opacities in 10% of the animals were seen only if newborns were inoculated intracerebrally. Other malformations observed in infected ferrets were not clearly related to the virus.[2] Cotlier *et al.*[3] injected rats on the sixth day of gestation and noted runting, lens opacities, malformations and neonatal deaths in the young. This report needs confirmation.

Many experiments have been done with cytomegaloviruses in mice but only the generalized type of the disease has been produced in newborn animals. Congenital infections and malformations have not been reported.[2,4]

A few viruses not known to be teratogenic in man have been reported to produce congenital malformations in animals. Attenuated hog cholera virus vaccination of sows has resulted in cerebellar hypoplasia, pitted livers and kidneys, edema and ascites in the young.[5,6] Attenuated blue tongue virus causes intrauterine death and resorption or runting, spasticity and blindness in sheep.[2,7] Congenital subcortical encephalopathies occurred only in the progeny of ewes vaccinated during early gestation.[8] Cystic cavities in subcortical tissues of the neopallium and cerebellum and dilatation of the lateral ventricles were observed.[9]

Injection of newborn hamsters with rat virus (RV) results in growth retardation, flat face, protruding eyes and tongue, abnormal teeth and bone fragility—a "mongoloid-like" disease picture.[10,11] This syndrome is postnatal in origin. Injection of RV into pregnant hamsters does not cause malformations in the young. H-1 virus injected intravenously early in gestation may be lethal to the embryos or induce exencephaly, microcephaly, facial clefts and umbilical hernias.[12] A strain of RV was reported to cause cerebellar hypoplasia in rat fetuses.[13]

Confirmation and extension of these experiments is needed. Much could be learned from animal models that can be reproduced at will and in sufficient numbers to study the role of viruses as teratogens. A comprehensive review on congenital and neonatal anomalies linked with viral infections in experimental animals was published by Elizan and Fabiyi[14] in 1970.

REFERENCES

1. Delahunt, C. S., and Rieser, N.: Rubella-induced embryopathies in monkeys, Am. J. Obst. & Gynec. 99:580, 1967.
2. Sever, J. L., and London, W. T.: Viruses and embryos, Teratology 2:39, 1969.
3. Cotlier, E., Fox, J., Bohigian, G., Beaty, C., and DuPree, A.: Pathogenic effects of rubella virus on embryos and newborn rats, Nature, London 217:38, 1968.
4. Henson, D., Smith, R. D., and Gehrke, J.: Non-fatal mouse cytomegalovirus hepatitis. Combined morphologic, virologic and immunologic observations, Am. J. Path. 49:871, 1966.
5. Young, G. A., Kitchell, R. L., Luedke, A. J., and Santter, J. H.: The effect of viral and other infections of the dam on

fetal development in swine. I. Modified live hog cholera viruses–immunological, virological, and gross pathological studies, J.A.V.M.A. 126:165, 1955.
6. Emerson, J. L., and Delez, A. L.: Cerebellar hypoplasia, hypomyelinogenesis and congenital tremors of pigs associated with prenatal hog cholera vaccination of sows, J.A.V.M.A. 147:47, 1965.
7. Shultz, G., and Delay, P. D.: Losses in newborn lambs associated with blue tongue vaccination of pregnant ewes, J.A.V.M.A. 127:224, 1955.
8. Cordy, D. R., and Shultz, G.: Congenital subcortical encephalopathies in lambs, J. Neuropath. & Exper. Neurol. 20:554, 1961.
9. Young, S., and Cordy, D. R.: An ovine fetal encephalopathy caused by bluetongue vaccine virus, J. Neuropath. & Exper. Neurol. 23:635, 1964.
10. Toolan, H. W.: Experimental production of mongoloid hamsters, Science 131:1446, 1960.
11. Kilham, L.: Rat virus (RV) infections in hamsters, Proc. Soc. Exper. Biol. & Med. 106:825, 1961.
12. Ferm, V.: Congenital anomalies induced in hamster embryos with H-1 virus, Science 145:510, 1964.
13. Kilham, L., and Margolis, G.: Spontaneous hepatitis and cerebellar "hypoplasia" in suckling rats due to congenital infections with rat virus, Am. J. Path. 49:457, 1966.
14. Elizan, T. S., and Fabiyi, A.: Congenital and neonatal anomalies linked with viral infections in experimental animals, Am. J. Obst. & Gynec. 106:147, 1970.

Various Infectious Diseases

MANY MATERNAL INFECTIOUS DISEASES are accompanied by fever, toxemia and cardiac, pulmonary or renal disturbances that can influence the outcome of a pregnancy. In addition to rubella and cytomegalic inclusion disease, smallpox, varicella, measles and influenza are some of the viral diseases that have been considered as probable teratogenic factors. It is known that these and other diseases can bring about fetal death or miscarriage, but there is no proof that they cause congenital malformations. It is possible that some of these diseases in early pregnancy destroy or damage cells in a selective manner and that such cell deficits would result in malformations if the injured embryo survived to birth. If, however, the disease is lethal during fetal life, leading to death of the embryo and miscarriage, such an illness will not be a cause of congenital malformations. This may explain why severe febrile diseases during pregnancy are not considered teratogenic, whereas mild infections such as rubella, cytomegalic inclusion disease and toxoplasmosis are. If this explanation were true, there could be a host of maternal diseases taking a mild or subclinical course that could damage a fetus and yet escape blame because the mother's illness goes unnoticed.

Smallpox has become so rare in Western countries that only a few reliable observations of pregnancy outcome have been made in recent years. It is believed that the disease can cause abortion or death of the fetus but not congenital malformations. An interesting belief has been reported by Schick.[1] Women in areas in which smallpox is or was prevalent were told to avoid contact with smallpox patients even if they had been successfully vaccinated or if they had had the disease. It seemed possible that cellular immunity of the mother protected her from smallpox by mobilization of antibodies without protection of the fetus, which could be infected transplacentally before the mother's antibodies stopped the viremia.[1] Occasionally, infants are born with a mild form of the disease or with scars, indicating residuals of prenatal variola. Infection of the fetus may be delayed after maternal disease. Dissimilarity of the expression of the disease has been reported in twins of infected mothers.[2]

Vaccination against smallpox seemed to be harmless in New York City, where 9,000,000 vaccinations were given in 1 month in 1945 without ill effects during pregnancy. There was no increase in the incidence of congenital malformations in children whose mothers had been vaccinated in the first trimester or later.[3] But in Scotland there was an increase in fetal loss after early vaccination,[4] and in one case of vaccination in the third month of gestation a stillborn fetus was delivered at 6 months with generalized vaccinia demonstrating persistence of the virus in the fetus for several months.[5]

Varicella can be transferred to the fetus, as evidenced by rashes in newborn children whose mothers acquired the disease late in pregnancy. There are many reports on congenital and neonatal varicella that deserve attention, particularly since fatal cases or stillbirths were described,[6] but there is no proof that this infection can be held responsible for congenital malformations. In some instances, intrauterine growth retardation was noted.[2]

Herpes zoster deserves attention because this disease, which is related to varicella, has been reported in association with congenital malformations. Duehr[7] described cataracts in 2 patients whose mothers had herpes zoster in early pregnancy. Microphthalmia, clubfoot and mental retardation were noted in one of the patients.

Herpes simplex can occur in a generalized form in newborn infants of infected mothers.[2,6] The disease sometimes takes a fulminating course, with widespread visceral manifestations, including hepatitis and encephalitis.[6,8] Intrauterine growth retardation has been observed repeatedly.[2] Teratogenic effects of the genital type (type 2) herpesvirus have been mentioned on page 75.

Influenza. The role of influenza in adverse sequelae of pregnancy is difficult to establish. The symptoms of the disease often are vague, and in a prospective study 39% of the cases were clinically inapparent.[9] In mild epidemics, the reporting of the disease and negative statements of the mothers are quite unreliable. During the severe epidemic of 1918, the maternal mortality was reported as 27% in uncomplicated and 50% in pneumonia-complicated cases. Abortion, stillbirth and premature delivery were similarly distributed according to severity of the disease.[10] Asian influenza seemed to exert an unfavorable influence on pregnancy outcome for the women in a prospective Baltimore study of 1957–1958. The incidence of abortion, stillbirth, low birth weight, neonatal morbidity and congenital malformations was higher in pregnancies with proved influenzal infection during the first trimester as compared with subsequent trimesters, but the outcome seemed to be independent of the severity of the disease. The numbers of cases were admittedly too small to be conclusive. Coffey and Jessop[11] found an incidence of congenital malformations among the children of women with Asian influenza 2.4 times that of a control group. Damages were chiefly to the nervous system, including anencephaly, encephalocele and spina bifida. Seventeen of the 24 malformations recorded can be attributed to nonclosure of the neural tube (which is effected by the end of the first month). Since only 4 of the 24 mothers who had children with congenital malformations had influenza during the first 2 months of pregnancy, the majority of the central nervous system malformations cannot be attributed to maternal Asian influenza, and the difference between control and influenza pregnancies becomes insignificant. Suggestive results were reported by Leck,[12] Pleydell[13] and Leck *et al.*,[28] but Campbell,[14] Wilson *et al.*,[15] Walker and McKee[16] and D'Antona[17] failed to find an increase in congenital malformations following influenza.

Poliomyelitis. Transplacental transmission of the poliomyelitis virus has been demonstrated. Congenital infection, premature delivery, stillbirth and abortion have been observed. In a number of cases of maternal infection occurring near the end of pregnancy, children were born with mild or paralytic poliomyelitis present at birth or developing soon after birth. Meningeal signs were absent. At first, the children were lethargic and floppy. Later, flaccid paralyses and atrophies developed in the children who survived. Neonatal deaths due to respiratory arrest or aspiration were not rare.[2] Mild and subclinical cases diagnosed by demonstration of the virus in the child have also been recorded.[6] There have been some reports of congenital malformations following maternal poliomyelitis, but they are not convincing.[9] In a prospective study in New York City,[18] an increase in neonatal mortality was noted following maternal poliomyelitis, but there was no increase in congenital malformations. There is no evidence to suggest that the vaccines used in the prevention of poliomyelitis have any adverse effects on the fetus.[9]

Mumps. Miscarriage following severe parotitis of the mother has been reported repeatedly.[6] A number of observations are on record of congenital defects following maternal mumps,[19] but there is no agreement on the types of defects supposedly induced by the infection.[20] In a prospective study, Manson *et al.*[21] found no significant differences in the outcome of 501 pregnancies complicated by maternal mumps as compared with controls.

Measles (morbilli, rubeola). Several cases have been reported of defective children born after maternal measles or of spontaneous abortion terminating pregnancy.[6] Packer,[22] in 1950, studied the outcome of 18 pregnancies complicated by measles at various stages of gestation. Twelve of the pregnancies were not affected by the disease and 4 ended in abortions. One child was deaf and 1 was mentally retarded. Similar complications, as well as children born with measles, have been observed in other series. In the prospective study by Manson *et al.*,[21] a number of children were recorded who were malformed after maternal measles in the first trimester, and neonatal mortality was increased. Despite suggestive reports and the assertion that the virus can cross the placental barrier,[6] teratogenic effects of rubeola have not been established. Observations are few, and no teratologic pattern associated with the disease has been recognized.

Coxsackie virus infections. Coxsackie B viruses, held responsible for pleurodynia and aseptic meningitis, can cause severe illnesses in newborn infants that can lead to death, with signs of myocarditis and meningo-encephalitis. Other organs such as the liver, pancreas and adrenals can also be involved.[6] Sometimes it is difficult to distinguish postnatal infections from late fetal ones.[23] Intrauterine infection in late pregnancy seems likely for several Coxsackie strains, and teratologic effects by early infection have been considered.[24] In one study,[25] more mothers of infants with congenital heart disease had experienced infection with Coxsackie virus than did matched controls.

ECHO virus infections. These infections occur in widespread epidemics with various clinical manifestations, including rashes, or in subclinical form. Several studies of incidences of congenital malformations have been made in different geographic areas following epidemics of ECHO 9 infections. No increase in congenital malformations was observed.[26,27]

REFERENCES

1. Schick, B.: Diaplacental infection of the foetus with the virus of German measles despite immunity of the mother, Acta paediat. 38:563, 1949.
2. Thalhammer, O.: *Pränatale Erkrankungen des Menschen* (Stuttgart: Georg Thieme, 1967).
3. Greenberg, M., Yankauer, A., Krugman, S., Osborn, J. J., Ward, R. S., and Dancis, J.: The effect of smallpox vaccination during pregnancy on the incidence of congenital malformations, Pediatrics 3:456, 1949.
4. McArthur, P.: Congenital vaccinia and vaccinia gravidarum, Lancet 2:1104, 1952.
5. MacDonald, A. M., and MacArthur, P.: Foetal vaccinia, Arch. Dis. Childhood 28:311, 1953.

6. Blattner, R. J., and Heys, F. M.: Role of viruses in the etiology of congenital malformations, Prog. Med. Virol. 3: 311, 1961.
7. Duehr, P. A.: Herpes zoster as a cause of congenital cataract, Am. J. Ophth. 39:157, 1955.
8. Zuelzer, W. W., and Stullberg, C. S.: Herpes simplex as a cause of fulminating visceral disease and hepatitis in infancy, A.M.A. Am. J. Dis. Child. 83:421, 1952.
9. Hardy, J. B.: Viral infection in pregnancy: A review, Am. J. Obst. & Gynec. 93:1052, 1965.
10. Harris, J. W.: Influenza occurring in pregnant women; a statistical study of thirteen hundred and fifty cases, J.A.M.A. 72:978, 1919.
11. Coffey, V., and Jessop, W. J. E.: Maternal influenza and congenital deformities, Lancet 2:935, 1959.
12. Leck, I.: Incidence of malformations following influenza epidemics, Brit. J. Prev. & Social Med. 17:70, 1963.
13. Pleydell, M. J.: Anencephaly and other congenital abnormalities; an epidemiological study in Northamptonshire, Brit. M. J. 1:309, 1960.
14. Campbell, W. A. B.: Influenza in early pregnancy: Effects on the foetus, Lancet 1:173, 1953.
15. Wilson, M. G., Heins, H. L., Imagawa, D. T., and Adams, J. M.: Teratogenic effects of Asian influenza, J.A.M.A. 171:638, 1959.
16. Walker, W. M., and McKee, A. P.: Asian influenza in pregnancy. Relationship to fetal anomalies, Obst. & Gynec. 13:394, 1959.
17. D'Antona, N.: Virological investigations in pregnant women with influenza caused by virus of the type Singapore A_1/57, Quad. Clin. Ostet. Ginec. 13:675, 1958.
18. Siegel, M., and Greenberg, M.: Polio in pregnancy: Effect on the fetus and the newborn infant, J. Pediat. 49:280, 1956.
19. Hallowach, J., Thurston, D. L., and Becker, B.: Congenital defects in infants following mumps during pregnancy, J. Pediat. 50:689, 1957.
20. Flamm, H.: *Die pränatalen Infektionen des Menschen* (Stuttgart: Georg Thieme, 1959).
21. Manson, M. M., Logan, W. P. D., and Loy, R. M.: Rubella and other virus infections during pregnancy, Ministry of Health Reports on Public Health and Medical Subjects, No. 101, Her Majesty's Stationery Office, London, 1960.
22. Packer, A. D.: The influence of maternal measles (morbilli) on the unborn child, M. J. Australia 1:835, 1950.
23. Kibrick, S.: The role of Coxsackie and ECHO viruses in human disease, M. Clin. North America 43:1291, 1959.
24. Makower, H., Skurska, Z., and Halazinska, L.: On transplacental infection with Coxsackie virus, Texas Rep. Biol. & Med. 16:346, 1958.
25. Brown, G. C., and Evans, T. N.: Serologic evidence of Coxsackie virus etiology of congenital heart disease, J.A.M.A. 199:183, 1967.
26. Kleinman, H., Prince, J. T., Mathey, W. E., Rosenfield, A. B., Bearman, J. E., and Syverton, J. T.: ECHO 9 virus infection and congenital abnormalities: A negative report, Pediatrics 29:261, 1962.
27. Landsman, J. B., Grist, N. R., and Ross, C. A.: ECHO 9 virus infection and congenital malformations, Brit. J. Prev. & Social Med. 18:152, 1964.
28. Leck, I., Hay, S., Witte, J. J., and Greene, J. C.: Malformations recorded on birth certificates following A2 influenza epidemics, Pub. Health Rep. 84:971, 1969.
29. Monif, G. R. G.: *Viral Infections of the Human Fetus* (London: Collier-Macmillan, Ltd., 1969).
30. Overall, J. C., Jr., and Glasgow, L. A.: Virus infections of the fetus and newborn infant, J. Pediat. 77:315, 1970.

Toxoplasmosis

PRENATAL INFECTION with the protozoan Toxoplasma gondii can lead to destructive changes in the brain and eye, to hydrocephaly and microcephaly and to a variety of functional disturbances in postnatal life. The disorder exemplifies causation of gross human congenital malformations by a protozoan.

Toxoplasma occurs in a free and in a cystic form. The free protozoan has a crescentic shape and a size of about $3 \times 6\,\mu$. Pseudocysts or cysts, composed of many parasites and seen in chronic stages of the disease, assume a size of $15-20\,\mu$ and a round or oval shape. Whereas the free organisms are extremely sensitive to heat, cold, desiccation, gastric juice, medication and antibodies, the cysts are resistant to physical and chemical external influences. The parasites can invade almost any tissue of mammals and birds and multiply in living cells. All strains of toxoplasma are serologically homogeneous.[1-3] The dangers of the protozoan to human infants were pointed out in 1939 by Wolf *et al.*,[4] who isolated the organism from children dead of congenital encephalomyelitis. Prenatal infections during the last 6 months of gestation were recognized as the beginning of the congenital form of toxoplasmosis. Acquired toxoplasmosis is widespread in man, but usually it takes its course without clinical manifestations. In rare instances, the acquired infection can result in encephalitis, pneumonitis and rash but, as a rule, the invasion of the mother's blood stream that results in prenatal toxoplasmosis is subclinical.

Since most infections with toxoplasma are subclinical and overt cases are not always accompanied by specific clinical signs, the diagnosis of toxoplasmosis often requires laboratory tests for confirmation. The Sabin-Feldman dye test,[5] complement-fixation, hemagglutination and skin tests are in use for diagnostic purposes to demonstrate antibodies.[3,6,7] An important difficulty in the diagnosis of congenital toxoplasmosis is the fact that children born of immune mothers who are free of the disease have antibody titers at birth corresponding to those of the mother. These titers usually decline during the first half of postnatal life. In children with congenital toxoplasmosis, the antibody titers remain elevated or increase during the first months of infancy. The diagnosis is made by establishing a titer curve that shows, in cases of active toxoplasmosis, titers above those transmitted through the placenta.[1] But there are questionable situations, since some infected newborns, particularly prematures, do not produce antibodies rapidly and in sufficient quantity. In older children suspected of toxoplasmosis, the titers sometimes are reduced to those of inactive disease, whereas high titers can be due to postnatal disease. Distinction of 19S from 7S gamma globulins[1] or demonstration of macroglobulin antibodies may aid in the recognition of acute congenital toxoplasmosis.[8]

For many years it has been assumed that a mother who has had a child with congenital toxoplasmosis cannot have another child with the same disease, since fetal infection is possible only through acute toxoplasmosis of the mother during pregnancy.[6,9] Against this opinion is the concept that a mother can have more than one child with congenital infection owing to a chronic maternal infection and latent foci in the uterus.[10] The subject is controversial,[11,29] and most investigators believe that chronic maternal infection has not been established as a cause of congenital toxoplasmosis, stillbirths and abortions.[1,3,6,12] It is likely that congenital toxoplasmosis in two successive sibs occurs only in exceptional cases.[13]

Incidence estimates on prenatal and congenital toxoplasmosis vary greatly. In the United States[8] and in Sweden,[14] the prevalence of clinically recognizable cases is of a magnitude of approximately 0.25 per thousand births. In France[15] and in other European areas, 2 cases of overt toxoplasmosis per 1,000 pregnancies were ascertained. Desmonts *et al.*[15] found, in a prospective study in Paris, that approximately 16% of pregnant women were lacking protective antibodies and were at risk of infection during pregnancy. The risk was greater for young females and for foreigners living in France. The frequency of maternal infections with toxoplasmosis during pregnancy was about 8 per 1,000. None of the children of mothers who had toxoplasmosis before pregnancy had clinical or latent infection. By 1966, Desmonts *et al.*[8,15] had studied 47 infants whose mothers had acquired the infection during pregnancy. Four infants died in the neonatal period with generalized toxoplasmosis, 3 were living with sequelae, 13 were infected but alive and without sequelae and 27 escaped infection. Congenital toxoplasmosis always resulted from an infection acquired by the mother during her pregnancy. There was no proof that the parasite was transmitted to the fetus by a mother with chronic toxoplasmosis.[1,3,15] About half the children born with toxoplasmosis infection remained free of the disease. Why some infected infants develop serious illness whereas others are infected without clinical signs remains unexplained. The variability of manifestations is particularly striking in twins with differing symptoms.[8,16] Some central European estimates of congenital toxoplasmosis, which were based on general epidemiologic calculations and included oligosymptomatic cases, amounted to approximately 7 per 1,000 live-born children.[1]

After primary infection of a pregnant woman with toxoplasma, the parasites reach the fetus through the placenta and spread throughout the fetal tissues, leading to generalized prenatal toxoplasmosis. This disease can be of variable severity according to the time and massiveness of the infection. The child may be born during the florid, primary stage of the disease or in various stages of healing. If the infection is generalized when the child is born, dyspnea, cyanosis, pneumonia, hepatosplenomegaly, jaundice, purpura and edema may be some of the presenting signs. Manifestations of encephalitis and chorioretinitis are absent in generalized congenital toxoplasmosis, which is the rarest type of congenital toxoplasmosis.[1] Somewhat more frequent is the subacute form, which consists of encephalitis and symptoms of nervous system disturbances; there are no signs of visceral involvement. Lethargy, feeding difficulties and progressive enlargement of the head are noted. The spinal fluid shows increased protein values without pleocytosis. Beginning chorioretinitis is recognized in some cases, and roentgenograms may reveal internal hydrocephaly and calcifications. In this stage, the disease sometimes can be diagnosed by finding parasites in the sediment of cerebrospinal fluid and by a high dye-test titer in mother and child. In the first and second stages—those of generalized and encephalitic toxoplasmosis—death may terminate the disease, or the active process can change to a chronic stage.

Another form of congenital toxoplasmosis is the postencephalitic chronic disorder.[1] The children are born after the active process has ceased and with the brain damages established. Psychomotor retardation, convulsions, microcephaly and hydrocephaly due to aqueduct stenosis or disturbances of cerebrospinal fluid exchange may be noticeable. Sometimes cerebral calcifications and chorioretinitis are present at birth or they may develop weeks or months later.

Approximately half of the clinically recognizable cases of congenital toxoplasmosis show hydrocephaly or microcephaly.[17,18] Hydrocephaly can be recognized soon after birth or become noticeable several months later. Intrauterine development of hydrocephaly has been reported. In some cases, hydrocephaly is due to cerebral atrophy and demonstrable by ventriculography only; in others, it follows aqueduct stenosis and develops rapidly to remarkable dimensions (see Fig. 25-2). Enlarged fontanelles, wide-open sutures and dilated veins are noticeable. If the brain substance is markedly reduced, transillumination may be possible. The fact that the frontal lobes are relatively less affected than other parts of the brain may aid in differentiation of severe cerebral toxoplasmosis from hydranencephaly.[18] Microcephaly is less frequent and less conspicuous than hydrocephly as a sequela of toxoplasmosis.

Intracerebral calcifications of the choroid plexus can appear in roentgenograms as linear or reticular shadows or as irregular, ill-defined spots with preference for the parieto-occipital areas. They can be distinguished from calcifications due to cytomegalic inclusion disease, which characteristically follow the outlines of the walls of the ventricles.

Chorioretinitis seldom is seen in the acute phases of toxoplasmosis but rather in its permanent stage of scar formation. The typical lesion is a pseudocoloboma, an atrophic focus of the choroid near the macula surrounded by deeply pigmented areas. Such foci can be single or multiple, unilateral or bilateral. Rupture of cysts and recurrence of chorioretinitis can occur many years after the primary infection in otherwise inactive and in latent cases.[1] Microphthalmia is not rare if the eye is affected; it can be congenital or follow birth owing to postnatal inflammatory processes such as uveitis and iridocyclitis. Cataracts and pupillary membranes have been observed repeatedly.[19] Nystagmus and strabismus are common. Blindness can result from some of the ocular changes mentioned.[18,20,21]

Deafness due to damage of the inner ear by toxoplasma seems to be rare, but some cases have been reported.[22]

Endocrine disturbances attributable to congenital toxoplasmosis, hypothyroidism,[23] precocious puberty,[24] hypogenitalism, pituitary dwarfism[25] and diabetes insipidus[1,19] have been reported in association with brain and eye damages and intracerebral calcifications.

The spectrum of manifestations is best illustrated by twins affected with this disease.[8,16] Fatal toxoplasmosis may occur in one twin whereas the other, although infected, can develop normally and remain without sequelae other than antitoxoplasma antibodies.

It has been estimated that only 15% of the children with congenital toxoplasmosis have cerebral calcifications and chorioretinitis,[1] so that the majority do not develop the full clinical picture. Epileptiform seizures and mental retardation are more common sequelae of prenatal toxoplasmosis than are microcephaly, hydrocephaly and chorioretinitis. Since these manifestations are nonspecific, estimates of the role played by toxoplasmosis in the etiology of mental retardation, cerebral palsy and epilepsy are based on serologic determinations. Antibody titer curves aid in the diagnosis, but they are influenced by transplacental maternal antibodies, the stage of the disease, postnatal infections and geographic factors. As a result, there are differences of opinion regarding the contribution of toxoplasmosis to cerebral deficits and congenital malformations of children. Whereas Feldman[17] thought that in the United States toxoplasmosis is not an important cause of prematurity, cerebral palsy, blindness and mental retardation, Thalhammer[1] stated that in Vienna, Austria, 16% of all brain damages in children that cannot be explained by postnatal factors are due to congenital toxoplasmosis and that 7.8 of 1,000 live-born infants are irreparably damaged by this disease. Whether the difference of opinion concerning the importance of toxoplasma as an agent responsible for brain damage of children is due to local differences or to differing interpretations of laboratory findings is difficult to decide. In England, Burkinshaw *et al.*[26] found positive dye and skin tests as common among institutionalized patients as in the general population, increasing in frequency with advancing age. Ocular lesions suggestive of toxoplasmosis were seen in only 0.3% of the patients and characteristic roentgenographic lesions were absent. These authors concluded that toxoplasmosis is not a common cause of mental deficiency. In an Australian study,[27] 1.4% of retarded children had positive dye tests and clinical features consistent with congenital toxoplasmosis. There is, therefore, a marked difference of opinion between those investigators who, on epidemiologic grounds, believe that congenital toxoplasmosis is a common disease that leads frequently to mental retardation and those who look for toxoplasmosis as an etiologic agent among the mentally retarded surviving to ages represented in institutions.

It seems likely that primary toxoplasmosis during the first trimester of pregnancy can result in abortion[1] and that prenatal infection with this protozoan is associated with prematurity in approximately one-third of the cases.[17] Whether such children are truly prematures or suffer from intrauterine growth retardation will have to be decided in individual cases. But there is no proof that congenital malformations arising during organogenesis in the first 2 months of gestation occur in children with congenital toxoplasmosis with greater frequency than in the general newborn population.[1]

The three stages of congenital toxoplasmosis mentioned – generalized, encephalitic and chronic – occur with unequal frequencies. Thalhammer[1] believed that their relative incidences are 1:10:100 and that most infants infected in utero and born with signs of the disease are in an irreparable postencephalitic condition. It is important, however, that in some infants with congenital toxoplasmosis signs of all three stages can be present.[19]

As mentioned before, positive serologic tests for toxoplasmosis in a mother without symptoms of disease indicate immunity. Mothers without immunity run the risk of an infection. Such an infection usually is asymptomatic, yet approximately half of the fetuses developing during such a pregnancy become infected and of these half may have overt congenital toxoplasmosis. Thalhammer[1] recommended a schedule for testing of women during pregnancy. Frenkel[3] advised treatment of newly infected pregnant women during the second and third trimesters but not during the first, when survival of an infected fetus is improbable, whereas a possibility exists of a teratologic effect of pyrimethamine, the drug prescribed for the disease. Sulfadiazine and pyrimethamine[28] supplemented by Leucovorin (folinic acid) and Baker's yeast suppress the proliferation of toxoplasma. Treatment of the mother, if initiated in time, would prevent congenital toxoplasmosis in her child.

Treatment of children with congenital toxoplasmosis is indicated as long as there are signs of active disease; it is recommended that even asymptomatic infected children be treated, since immunity in the neonate may be marginal. Delayed signs of damage have been observed repeatedly.[1] Sulfadiazine 100 mg./kg./day, pyrimethamine (Daraprim) 1 mg./kg./day, Leucovorin 1 mg./day and Baker's yeast 100 mg./day have been recommended. Leukocyte and platelet counts have to be observed. Treatment for 3 weeks has been considered adequate by Thalhammer,[1] but the prognosis is beclouded because of permanent brain damage present in many cases at the time of diagnosis.

REFERENCES

1. Thalhammer, O.: *Pränatale Erkrankungen des Menschen* (Stuttgart: Georg Thieme, 1967).
2. Jacobs, L.: Propagation, morphology and biology of toxoplasma, Ann. New York Acad. Sc. 64:154, 1956.
3. Frenkel, J. K.: Toxoplasmosis, in Benirschke, K., and Jones, T. C. (eds.), *Comparative Aspects of Reproductive Failure* (New York: Springer-Verlag, 1967).
4. Wolf, A., Cowen, D., and Paige, B. H.: Toxoplasmic encephalomyelitis; new case of granulomatous encephalomyelitis due to a protozoon, Am. J. Path. 15:657, 1939.
5. Sabin, A. B., and Feldman, H. A.: Dyes as microchemical indicators of a new immunity phenomenon affecting a protozoon parasite (toxoplasma), Science 108:660, 1948.
6. Feldman, H. A.: Toxoplasmosis, Pediatrics 22:559, 1958.
7. Desmonts, G.: Etat actuel du problème de la toxoplasmose humaine, Arch. franç. pédiat. 11:57, 1954.
8. Miller, M. J., Seaman, E., and Remington, J. S.: The clinical spectrum of congenital toxoplasmosis: Problems in recognition, J. Pediat. 70:714, 1967.
9. Eichenwald, H. F.: A Study of Congenital Toxoplasmosis with Particular Emphasis on Clinical Manifestations, Sequelae and Therapy in Siim, J. C. (ed.), *Human Toxoplasmosis* (Baltimore: The Williams & Wilkins Company, 1960).
10. Langer, H.: Repeated congenital infection with Toxoplasma gondii, Obst. & Gynec. 21:318, 1963.
11. Blattner, R. J.: Repeated congenital infection with Toxoplasma gondii, J. Pediat. 64:452, 1964.
12. Kräubig, H.: Präventive Behandlung der konnatalen Toxoplasmose, in Kirchhoff, H., and Kräubig, H. (eds.), *Toxoplasmose* (Stuttgart: Georg Thieme, 1966).
13. Garcia, A. G. P.: Congenital toxoplasmosis in two successive sibs, Arch. Dis. Childhood 43:705, 1968.
14. Holmdahl, S. C. S., and Holmdahl, K.: The frequency of congenital toxoplasmosis and some viewpoints on the diagnosis, Acta paediat. 44:322, 1955.
15. Desmonts, G., Couvreur, J., and Rachid, M-S. B.: Le toxoplasme, la mère et l'enfant, Arch. franç. pédiat. 22:1183, 1965.
16. Zuelzer, W. W.: Infantile toxoplasmosis with a report of three new cases, including two in which the patients were identical twins, Arch. Path. 38:1, 1944.
17. Feldman, H. A.: Toxoplasmosis, in Nelson, W. E. (ed.), *Textbook of Pediatrics* (8th ed.; Philadelphia: W. B. Saunders Company, 1964).
18. Couvreur, J.: *Etude de la Toxoplasmose Congénitale* (Gien: Imprimerie Jeanne-D'Arc, 1955).
19. Silver, H. K., and Dixon, M. S., Jr.: Congenital toxoplasmosis—report of case with cataract, "atypical" vasopressin-sensitive diabetes insipidus and marked eosinophilia, A.M.A. Am. J. Dis. Child. 88:84, 1954.
20. Koch, F. L. P., Wolf, A., Cowen, D., and Paige, B. H.: Toxoplasmic encephalomyelitis; significance of ocular lesions in diagnosis of infantile or congenital toxoplasmosis, Arch. Ophth. 29:1, 1943.
21. François, J.: *La Toxoplasmose et ses Manifestations Oculaires* (Paris: Masson & Cie, 1963).
22. Kelemen, G.: Toxoplasmosis and congenital deafness, A.M.A. Arch. Otolaryng. 68:547, 1958.
23. Aagaard, K., and Melchior, J.: The simultaneous occurrence of congenital toxoplasmosis and congenital myxoedema, Acta paediat. 48:164, 1959.
24. Bruhl, H. H., Bahn, R. C., and Hayles, A. B.: Sexual precocity associated with congenital toxoplasmosis, Proc. Staff Meet. Mayo Clin. 33:682, 1958.
25. Wolfe, S. M., Sawitz, W. G., and Paschkis, K. E.: Pituitary dwarfism and toxoplasmosis, J. Clin. Endocrinol. 15:745, 1955.
26. Burkinshaw, J., Kirman, B. H., and Sorsby, A.: Toxoplasmosis in relation to mental deficiency, Brit. M. J. 1:702, 1953.
27. Pitt, D., and Roboz, P.: Congenital toxoplasmosis, Australian Paediat. J. 3:238, 1967.
28. Eyles, D. E., and Coleman, N.: Synergistic effect of sulfadiazine and Daraprim against experimental toxoplasmosis in the mouse, Antibiotics & Chemother. 3:483, 1953.
29. Feldman, H. A.: Toxoplasmosis, New England J. Med. 279:1370, 1968.

10

Irradiation

FETAL X-IRRADIATION can lead to congenital malformations in man and in other mammals. The earliest findings[1,2] were summarized by Murphy[3] and Goldstein and Murphy,[4] who cited microcephaly, skull defects, spina bifida, microphthalmia, cleft palate, micromelia, clubfoot and other malformations recorded in the medical literature as effects of treatment of women during pregnancy with large doses of roentgen rays and radium. As this danger became widely known, therapeutic pelvic irradiation largely ceased being used during pregnancy, and there can be no doubt that today this particular source of radiation need be of little concern. Animal experiments,[5,6] as well as the observations made on man in the past, clearly show that fetal irradiation is teratogenic. In addition to irradiation from medical procedures, new sources of radiation, such as explosions of atomic and hydrogen bombs, have to be considered. To determine what danger there is from such sources of radioactivity, several studies were made on the offspring of Japanese women pregnant at the time they were exposed to the atomic bomb explosions in Hiroshima and Nagasaki. Two reports[7,8] noted a relatively high incidence of microcephaly and mental retardation in children whose mothers were close, at the time of the explosion, to the hypocenter—that is, the point over which the bomb exploded. In addition, a high incidence of fetal and neonatal death was found,[8] but an increased incidence of skeletal defects could not be detected.[9] The apparent lack of fetal effects, except for microcephaly sometimes associated with mental retardation, was confirmed by Miller,[10] who, in addition, established a relation between incidence of microcephaly and distance from the hypocenter and gestational age. Re-examination of the children exposed in utero to the Hiroshima bomb was made when they were 17 years of age. The results did not alter the interpretation of the observations made previously.[11,12]

The effects of actinic teratogenic agents on developing embryos and fetuses must be clearly distinguished from malformations caused by genetic changes in the germ cells through exposure to radiation. The ontogenic modification of an embryo induced by its direct irradiation is limited to its own life and generation, but irradiation of germ cells can lead to mutations producing congenital malformations that can be transmitted through many generations. It has been found that mutations in germ cells of mammals can be induced by relatively small doses of radiation.[13] And from various lines of evidence it has been inferred that an accumulated dose of radiation to the gonads of between 30 and 80 R may cause the spontaneous incidence of mutation in man to be doubled.[14,15]

The degree of the mutagenic effect of irradiation in man has not begun to be satisfactorily measured. The difficulties inherent in a study of this subject are complicated by the unsatisfactory information available concerning spontaneous mutation rates in human beings.[16] The best investigations of germ cell changes induced by irradiation in man are those by Crow[17] on the children of radiologists and Neel and Schull[18] on the Japanese populations exposed to the atomic bombs, in neither of which was clear evidence of genetic damage in the children of exposed parents found. Some positive indication that such damage did result was forthcoming from analysis of the sex ratio in the offspring.[19,20] In these studies, alterations were found in the sex ratio in the direction to be expected if exposure had resulted in the induction of sex-linked lethal mutations. The investigators cautioned, however, that such studies are subject to various errors that must be taken into consideration before judgments are made. In 1968, Miller[12] stated that the composite results thus far indicate that genetic effects were not great enough to be revealed under the conditions of the investigations conducted by the Atomic Casualty Commission. Chromosome studies of survivors of the atomic bombs showed that in approximately one-third of them there were exchange type chromosomal abnormalities in 1–4% of their peripheral leukocyte metaphases.[21]

Despite the fragmentary and hardly conclusive findings, one cannot neglect the possible dangers of the genetic effects of irradiation in man. This possibility is reinforced by the results obtained in radiation experiments with the mouse, the only mammal besides man whose sensitivity to the mutagenic action of irradiation has been investigated and been found[22] to be some fifteen times more sensitive in this regard than the fruit fly, Drosophila.

The dangers of large doses of radiation to the embryo are generally recognized, but there is less agreement concerning exposure to smaller doses. As an example of the suspicion expressed of the effects of exposure to small amounts of continued radiation, studies investigating the possible association between background radiation and incidence of congenital malformations can be cited. Gentry *et al.*[23] surveyed the incidence of congenital malformations in the townships of upstate New York and, correlating this information with geologic radioactivity, found differences in incidence between regions of low and high radioactivity that, to them, indicated "radiation as a primary etiological agent."

Another effort to correlate incidence of congenital malformations and background radiation was that by Wesley,[24] who reported this association to be worldwide and to be responsible for 96% of all deaths from congenital malformations. This author apparently believed that congenital malformations are due solely to mutations, contrary to such information as is presented in this chapter. Criticism has been experienced[25,26] of the physical facts presented by Wesley[24] and of his acceptance of estimates of incidence of congenital malformations derived from birth certificates and other documents.[25] Kratchman and Grahn[27] also found an association between mortality incidence from congenital malformations and background radiation, but cautioned that the association may have been an artifact produced by statistical biases, as, indeed, was found to be true by Henle.[28]

To explain the bulk of congenital malformations by a single cause or mechanism does not promise success. This holds for radiation as well as other environmental causes that have been suspected.[29]

Possible dangers to the fetus of diagnostic radiographic procedures are under consideration.[30-32] Whereas there is no proof that congenital malformations have been caused by exposure of pregnant women to diagnostic radiography, some authors recommend that, in order to avoid irradiation of the conceptuses of undiagnosed early pregnancies, irradiation should, as far as is possible, be performed only during the first half of the menstrual cycle and that women who are known to be pregnant should be examined roentgenologically only on strong clinical grounds.[31,33] But all writers agree that there is great need for further studies along these lines.

REFERENCES

1. Aschenheim, E.: Schädigung einer menschlichen Frucht durch Röntgenstrahlen, Arch. Kinderh. 68:131, 1920.
2. Bottaro, L. P., and DeBengoa, M. B.: El radium en las embarazadas, An. Fac. med. Montevideo 5:209, 1920.
3. Murphy, D. P.: Outcome of 625 pregnancies in women subjected to pelvic radium or roentgen irradiation, Am. J. Obst. & Gynec. 18:179, 1929.
4. Goldstein, L., and Murphy, D. P.: Microcephalic idiocy following radium therapy for uterine cancer during pregnancy, Am. J. Obst. & Gynec. 18:189, 1929.
5. Russell, L. B.: Effects of Radiation on Mammalian Prenatal Development, in Hollaender, A. (ed.), *Radiation Biology*, Vol. 1. *High Energy Radiation*, Parts 1 and 2 (New York: McGraw-Hill Book Company, Inc., 1954).
6. Hicks, S. P., and D'Amato, C. J.: Effects of Ionizing Radiations on Mammalian Development, in Woollam, D. H. M. (ed.), *Advances in Teratology* (London: Logos Press, Ltd., 1966).
7. Plummer, G.: Anomalies occurring in children exposed in utero to atomic bomb in Hiroshima, Pediatrics 10:687, 1952.
8. Yamazaki, J. N., Wright, S. W., and Wright, P. M.: Outcome of pregnancy in women exposed to atomic bomb in Nagasaki, A. M. A. Am. J. Dis. Child. 87:448, 1954.
9. Sutow, W. U., and West, E.: Studies on Nagasaki (Japan) children exposed in utero to atomic bomb: Roentgenographic survey of skeletal system, Am. J. Roentgenol. 74: 493, 1955.
10. Miller, R. W.: Delayed effects occurring within first decade after exposure of young individuals to Hiroshima atomic bomb, Pediatrics 18:1, 1956.
11. Wood J. W., Johnson, K. G., and Omori, Y.: In utero exposure to the Hiroshima atomic bomb. An evaluation of head size and mental retardation: Twenty years later, Pediatrics 39:385, 1967.
12. Miller, R. W.: Effects of ionizing radiation from the atomic bomb on Japanese children, Pediatrics 41:257, 1968.
13. Carter, T. C., Lyon, M. F., and Phillips, R. J. S.: Genetic hazard of ionizing radiations. Nature, London 182:409, 1958.
14. Great Britain, Medical Research Council: The hazards to man of nuclear and allied radiations: Presented to the Lord President of Council to Parliament by command of Her Majesty, June, 1956, London: Her Majesty's Stationery Office, 1956. (Command Paper 9780.)
15. National Academy of Sciences, National Research Council: Biological effects of atomic radiation: Summary reports from study by National Academy of Sciences, National Research Council, Washington, D. C.: Government Printing Office, 1956.
16. Penrose, L. S.: Mutation, in *Recent Advances in Human Genetics* (London: J. & A. Churchill, Ltd., 1961).
17. Crow, J. F.: Comparison of fetal and infant death rates in progeny of radiologists and pathologists, Am. J. Roentgenol. 73:467, 1955.
18. National Academy of Sciences, National Research Council. Neel, J. V., and Schull, W. J.: The effect of exposure to the atomic bombs on pregnancy termination in Hiroshima and Nagasaki, Washington, D. C.: Government Printing Office, 1956. (Pub. No. 461.)
19. Turpin, R., Lejeune, J., and Rethoré, M-O.: Étude de la descendance de sujets traités par radiothérapie pelvienne, Acta genet. 6:204, 1956.
20. Schull, W. J., and Neel, J. V.: Radiation and sex ratio in man, Science 128:343, 1958.
21. Bloom, A. D., Neriishi, S., Kamada, N., Iseki, T., and Keehn, R. J.: Cytogenetic investigation of survivors of the atomic bombings of Hiroshima and Nagasaki, Lancet 2: 672, 1966.
22. Russell, W. L.: Comparisons of x-ray-induced mutation rates in Drosophila and mice, Am. Nat. 90:69, 1956.
23. Gentry, J. T., Parkhurst, E., and Bulin, G. V., Jr.: An epidemiological study of congenital malformations in New York State, Am. J. Pub. Health 49:1, 1959.
24. Wesley, J. P.: Background radiation as cause of fatal congenital malformation, Internat. J. Rad. Biol. 2:97, 1960.
25. Spiers, F. W., Burch, P. R. J., and Reed, G. W.: Background radiation as cause of fatal congenital malformation, Internat. J. Rad. Biol. 2:235, 1960.
26. Brues, A. M.: Background radiation as cause of congenital malformation: Further comment on this subject, Internat. J. Rad. Biol. 3:99, 1961.
27. Kratchman, J., and Grahn, D.: Relationships between geologic environment and mortality from congenital malformation, U.S. Atomic Energy Commission (TID-8204), 1959.

28. Henle, R. C.: Study of mortality from congenital malformation for Benton County, Washington, Hanford Atomic Products Operation (HW-66344, Revised), 1960.
29. Warkany, J., and Kalter, H.: Congenital malformations, New England J. Med. 265:993, 1961.
30. Hammer-Jacobsen, E.: Therapeutic abortion on account of x-ray examination during pregnancy, Danish M. Bull. 6:113, 1959.
31. Hammer-Jacobsen, E.: Congenital malformations induced by radiation; a brief survey of the literature, Strahlentherapie 116:152, 1961.
32. Griem, M. L., Meier, P., and Dobben, G. D.: Analysis of the morbidity and mortality of children irradiated in fetal life, Radiology 88:347, 1967.
33. Jacobsen, L.: *Low Dose X-Irradiation and Teratogenesis* (Copenhagen: Munksgaard, 1968).

11

Drugs

Thalidomide

THALIDOMIDE was introduced as a remedy against influenza in 1956 and recommended as a sedative in the same year.[1] It proved to be an excellent sleeping medicine without acute toxic effects in high doses, and was taken against nausea and vomiting in pregnancy. The remarkable qualities of the drug rapidly made it popular, particularly in West Germany and Great Britain, where consumption rose rapidly until 1961, when its harmlessness became questionable. The year before, an increase in severe limb deformities that assumed epidemic proportions had become noticeable in a number of hospitals and clinics[2,3] of certain areas. Children were born who had amelia or various degrees of "phocomelia," sometimes affecting the upper and lower extremities; usually, both sides were involved, although to different degrees. Some of the children also had congenital heart disease, ocular, intestinal and renal anomalies and deformities of the external ears, but it was the limb defects, which were so unusual and striking, that distinguished this disease picture from other syndromes and drew attention to the infants. Once the unusual epidemic nature of these malformations had been recognized, the search was on for their causation.[4-8] Although an environmental causation of the syndrome was considered likely by several observers, it was Lenz[9] in Germany and McBride[10] in Australia who first singled out thalidomide (α-phthalimidoglutarimide) as the causative agent. Many doubts were expressed at that time concerning the correctness of this opinion, but the drug was withdrawn from the market at the end of November, 1961 in Germany and in early December, 1961 in England.[11] By August of 1962 the epidemic had subsided.[4]

McBride[10] and Lenz[9] recognized the causal connection between thalidomide and the epidemic of malformations almost intuitively.[4] Lenz[8] was guided by the suspicion concerning a physician's wife who had taken thalidomide for 6 months before conception and throughout her pregnancy. She developed severe polyneuritis and gave birth to a child with multiple congenital malformations. Although much evidence had been added to this suspicion, Lenz said in November of 1961[9]: "From a scientific point of view it seems premature to discuss it. But as a human being and as a citizen, I cannot remain silent about my observations."

At the same time, Weicker[4] initiated a broader search for the new teratogen by investigating the geographic distribution of the embryopathy and by considering many possible causes. It is of interest that many parents in Germany suspected that the malformations were due to radiation damage (atomic bomb tests) or television! These were ruled out by the fact that surrounding countries were spared and areas with better-developed television systems remained unaffected. Weicker also excluded abortives, contraceptives, x-rays, infections, antibiotics and sulfonamides. In a questionnaire, detergents, preservatives,

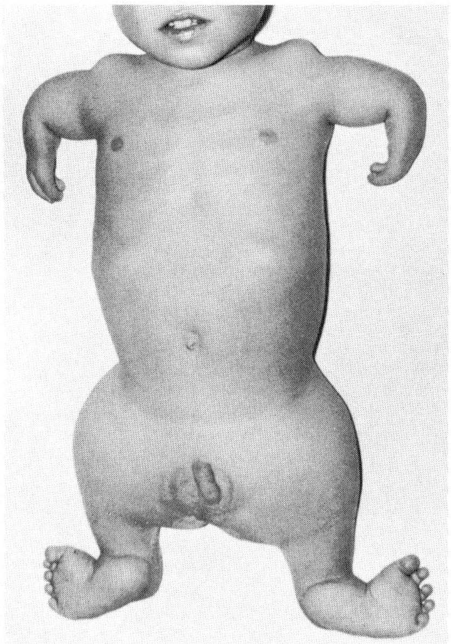

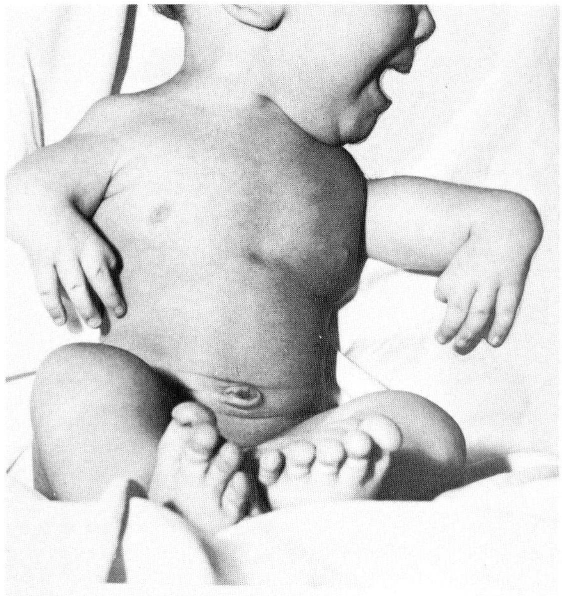

Fig. 11-1 (left).—Typical thalidomide embryopathy with reduction malformations of the limbs. (Courtesy of Prof. H. Weicker, Bonn, Germany.)

Fig. 11-2 (right).—Typical thalidomide embryopathy with reduction malformations of the limbs observed in the United States.

Fig. 11-3 (left).—Typical "clubhand" position in a rabbit fetus whose mother was treated with thalidomide.

Fig. 11-4 (right).—Anomalies of forepaws of a rabbit fetus whose mother was treated with thalidomide.

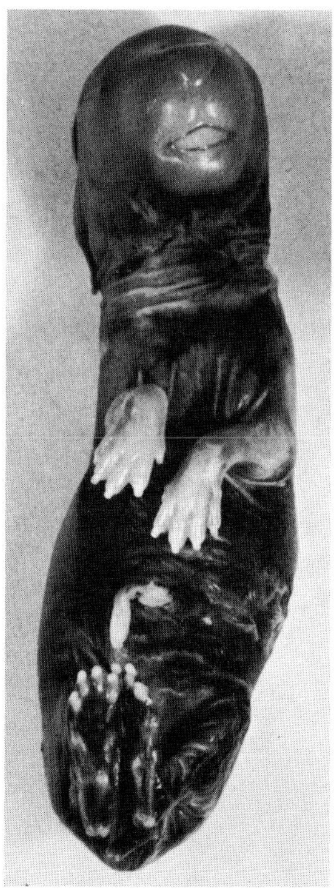

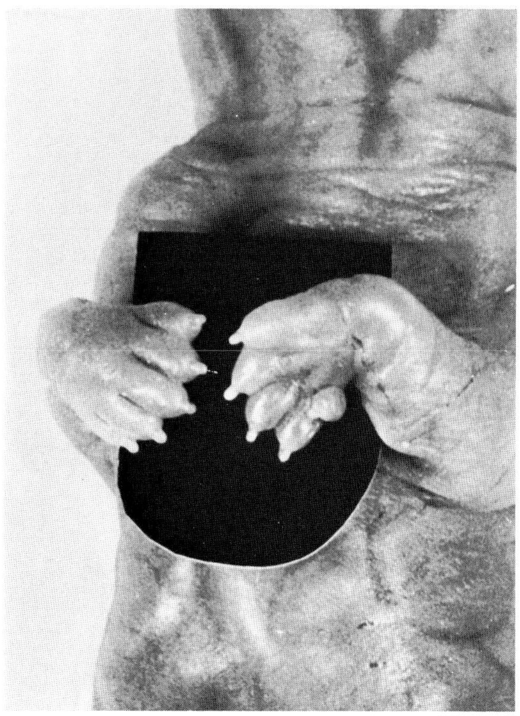

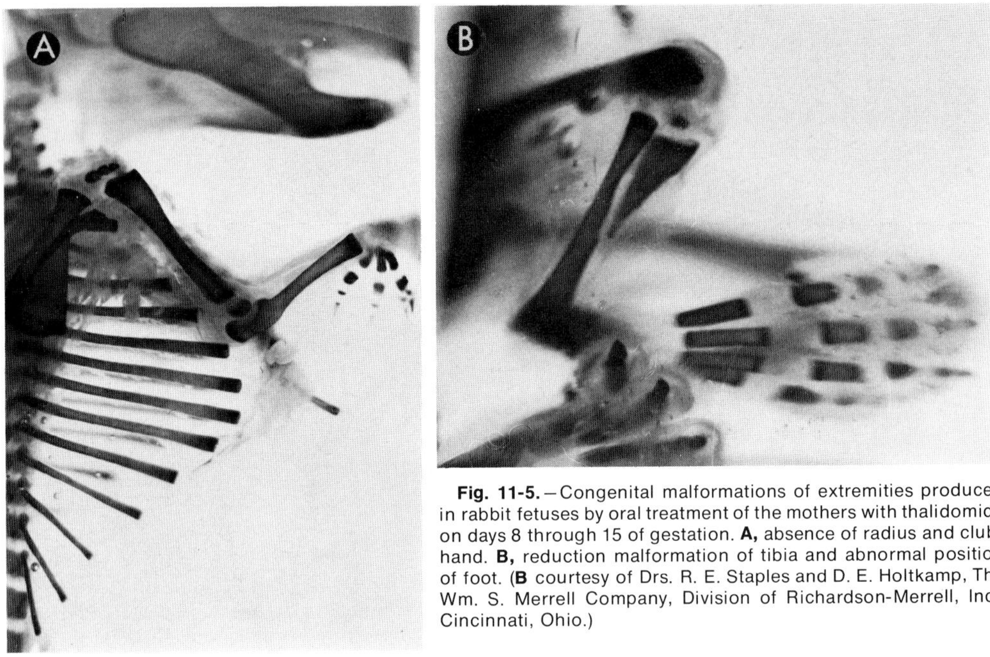

Fig. 11-5. – Congenital malformations of extremities produced in rabbit fetuses by oral treatment of the mothers with thalidomide on days 8 through 15 of gestation. **A,** absence of radius and club-hand. **B,** reduction malformation of tibia and abnormal position of foot. (**B** courtesy of Drs. R. E. Staples and D. E. Holtkamp, The Wm. S. Merrell Company, Division of Richardson-Merrell, Inc., Cincinnati, Ohio.)

insecticides, dyes, varnishes, waxes, toothpastes, hand lotions, antiemetics, hormone tests, analgesics and sedatives were considered as possible causative agents. When Lenz expressed his suspicion of thalidomide, this substance was in eighth place in Weicker's list of associated factors.[4] In the same study, only 24% of the mothers of defective children had given histories of thalidomide intake. But when asked specifically about this drug, positive answers rose to 68%. Soon thereafter it was learned[4] that 70% of the mothers of affected children had ingested thalidomide during the first 3 months of pregnancy, 14% had taken it without being able to give accurate data regarding the time of ingestion, in 8% there was a possibility of thalidomide intake and in only 8% was the history entirely negative. After expressing his suspicion,[9] Lenz established strong epidemiologic evidence that thalidomide was the cause of the malformations. His observations before and after removal of thalidomide from the market have been published.[8,11]

The association was not equally clear in other areas. Some observers of the phocomelia epidemic reported that many mothers of the affected children denied intake of the drug – or of any drug. Thus, Jones and Williamson[12] reported that they obtained a history of thalidomide ingestion in only 1 of 8 cases with typical malformations. Others who did retrospective investigations also failed to obtain "positive" histories in many instances. These retrospective studies with negative results are of great importance to the epidemiologist because they demonstrate that superficial interrogation, even if directed to a specific drug or agent, may fail to yield results unless an in-

Fig. 11-6. – Rhesus monkey fetus whose mother was treated with thalidomide on the thirtieth day after conception. Note severe malformations of lower extremities. (Courtesy of Dr. J. G. Wilson, Cincinnati, Ohio.)

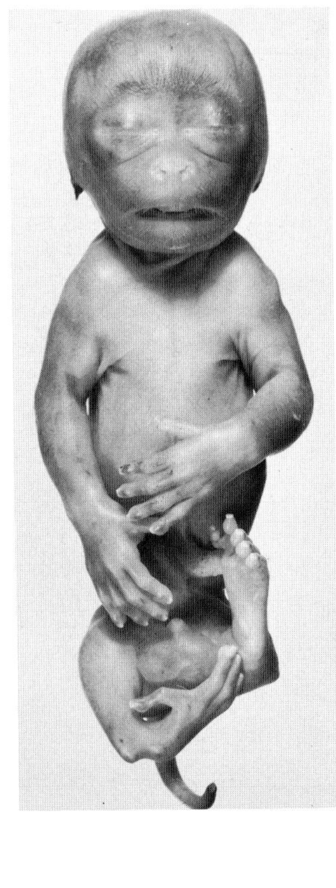

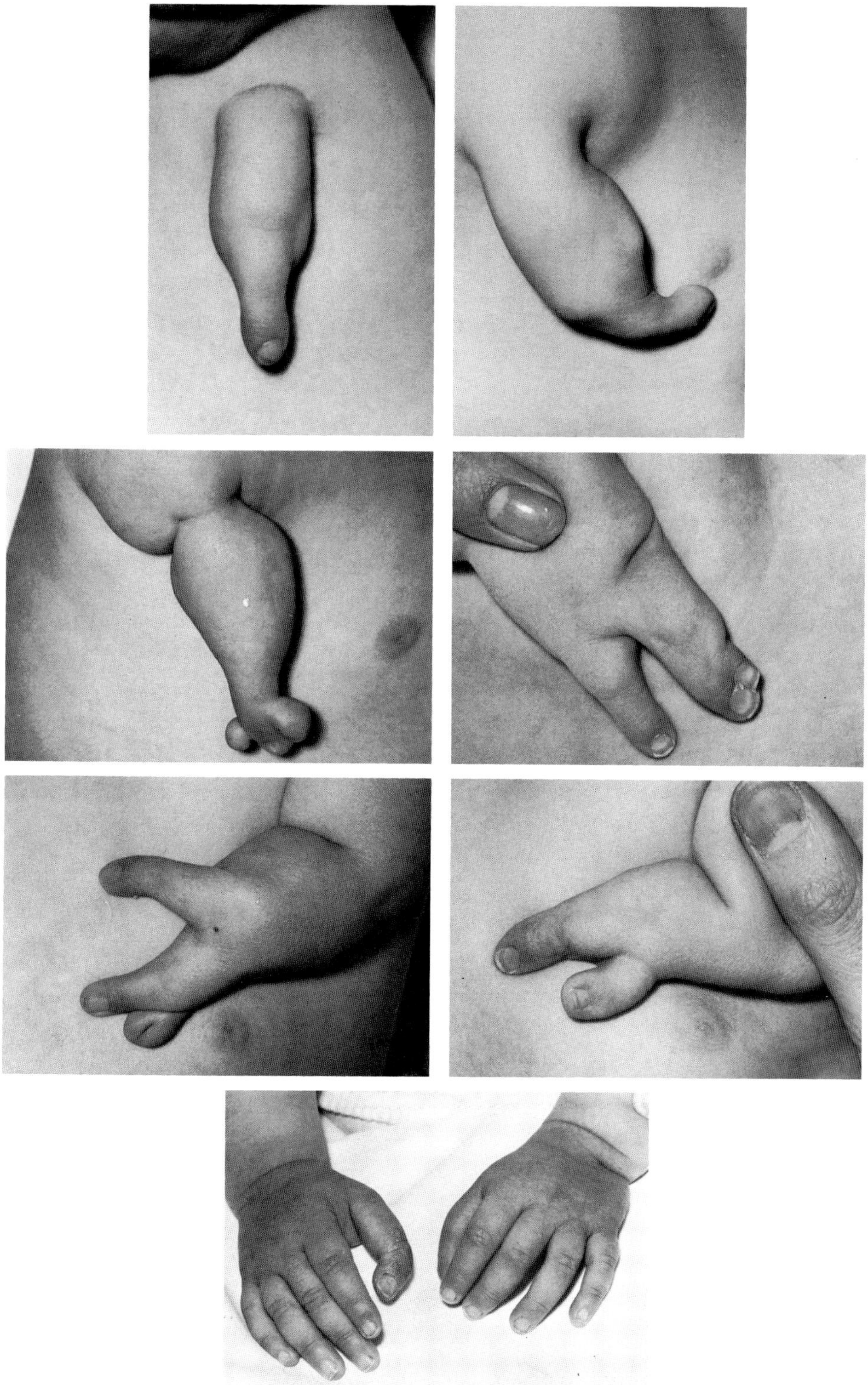

Fig. 11-7.—Various defects of upper extremities of children with thalidomide embryopathy. (Courtesy of Prof. H. Weicker, Bonn, Germany.)

tensive search is made for the suspected culprit. In some cases, the intake of thalidomide could be ascertained only after intensive and repeated investigations.[8] Prospective studies soon supplemented the initial suspicion and retrospective investigations.[8]

However, before the results of prospective affirmative studies were available, another obstacle to proof of the thalidomide embryopathy association had to be overcome. This obstacle involved reports of children born without malformations even though the mother *had* taken thalidomide. Many of the cases could be explained by the fact that the drug was taken after the first trimester, when typical malformations can no longer be induced. It is during the sixth and seventh weeks of pregnancy (thirty-fifth to fiftieth day after the last menstrual period, or twenty-third to thirty-eighth day after conception) that the embryo is most endangered by thalidomide.[13] But even during this period some embryos apparently escaped injury even though the mother had taken thalidomide. Such individual resistance to a drug cannot be used against the argument of drug-induced malformations, since individual susceptibility and resistance have been demonstrated for many other drugs. Indeed, it would be surprising to find drug injuries in 100% of the exposed cases. Unfortunately, the malformation rate was extremely high in those infants who were exposed to thalidomide during the first weeks of pregnancy. Knapp[14] stated that he knew of no case in which thalidomide had been taken during the sensitive period of gestation without some manifestation in the child. Sometimes, as in the case of hypoplasia of the thumb, the anomaly was demonstrated only after careful x-ray examination.

Another complicating factor in the search for a teratogen can be the apparent "guilt by association" of an innocent drug or agent. Thus, in one series,[4] meclizine had been taken in more than 25% of the cases involving children with phocomelia. This drug could be absolved from complicity because it had been taken with equal frequency by mothers who had healthy babies. But, in single cases, "intuition" may fail the physician confronted with a deformed child whose mother had taken two or more drugs during early pregnancy.

In early stages of the investigation of thalidomide as a teratogen, it was puzzling to find that the drug did not produce a regular syndrome in mice and rats fed thalidomide. Later, it became possible to induce in rabbits[16] and in monkeys[17,18] malformations that closely simulated the human syndrome.

Epidemiologic and experimental evidence clearly pointed to thalidomide as the cause of the syndrome of reduction malformations of the limbs and of de-

Fig. 11-8 (left).—Grossly deformed upper extremity with reduction of rays, including incomplete longitudinal separation of phalanges, incomplete segmentation of carpal bones and deformed masses representing the bones of the upper arm and/or forearm.

Fig. 11-9 (right).—Defective bones of upper extremity and defective segmentation of carpal bone, hand without thumb and osseous duplications in index finger.
(Courtesy of Prof. H. Weicker, Bonn, Germany.)

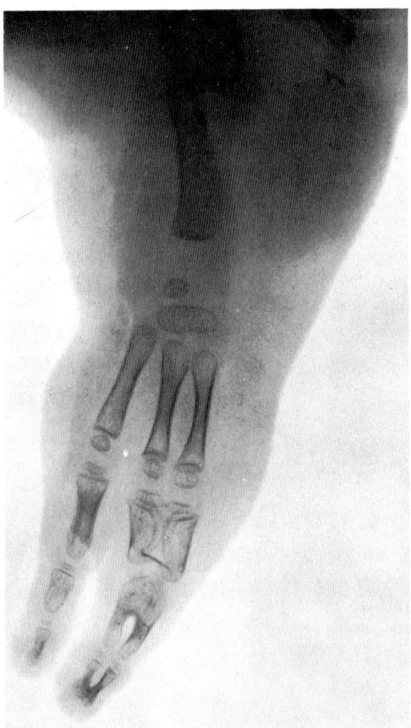

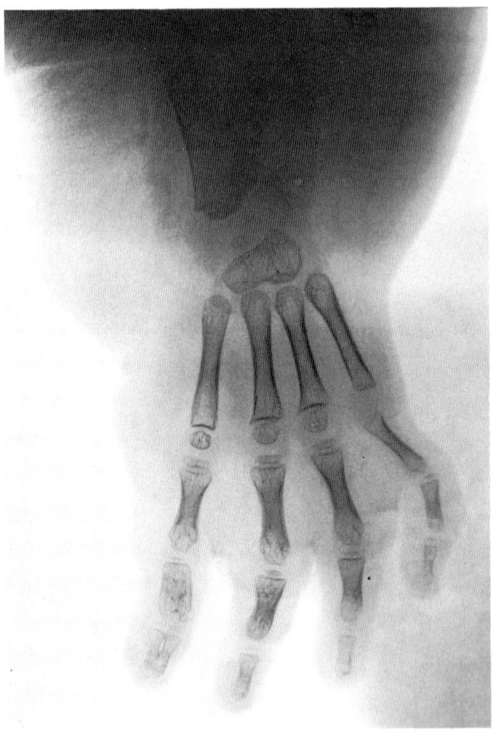

fects of the ear, eye, heart, intestine and kidney that assumed epidemic proportions in countries in which the drug was consumed in great quantities.[1] After the association of drug intake and malformations of the limbs was pointed out, confirmations soon came from many countries[15,20] in which the drug was marketed, whereas there were only a few cases reported from the United States, where its sale was delayed by Dr. Frances Kelsey of the Food and Drug Administration. In general, the incidence of phocomelic children paralleled the sale of thalidomide in various countries[1] and the epidemic of deformities declined in Germany 9 months after the sale of the drug was stopped.[4,11] It was found that thalidomide taken for short periods was harmless even in pregnancy except if taken between 35 and 50 days after the first day of the last menstrual period.[13] No familial or racial differences of susceptibility were noted. It has been estimated that approximately 7,000 children were deformed by thalidomide,[1] which is by far the largest number damaged by a known chemical but probably a small number if compared with the hundreds of thousands of endemic cretins who were mentally and physically handicapped by deficiency of a chemical, namely, iodine (Chapter 12).

The malformations produced by thalidomide in children represent a spectrum of anomalies in which certain patterns have been established. Authors describing the morphology of the thalidomide syndrome sometimes disagree in regard to details according to their personal experiences. Tabulations of the single malformations involving large numbers of affected children are few at this time. There has been a tendency to report the severely deformed and to overlook those with minor anomalies. Clinical observations differed from roentgen or necropsy reports so that quantitative data are still not satisfactory. From 1959 to 1962, more than 400 children with thalidomide embryopathy were observed at the Department of Pediatrics of the University of Bonn, Germany, but by March of 1964 about 45% of these children had died of congenital heart disease, duodenal or other intestinal atresias, malformations of the kidneys and fever of undetermined origin.[19] During the year 1964, more than 100 children were thoroughly re-examined by Weicker,[19] and their pictures, roentgenograms and analyses of individual malformations were demonstrated in 1965 at the XIth International Congress of Pediatrics in Tokyo. In approximately 60% of the surviving children, only the arms were involved and in a few only the legs; in more than 10%, both arms and legs were affected. In approximately 10%, the ears were the only deformed parts and in another 10% arms and ears were defective. In 5%, eyes and arms were involved. These findings and other combinations exemplify the difficulties in establishing well-circumscribed syndromes of the thalidomide embryopathy.

Sometimes the *extremities* were damaged so severely that their changes dominated the disease picture. Malformations generally were characterized by reduction of skeletal elements in size or number, but in a few cases duplication of digits was observed. There was a definite tendency to reduction of preaxial bones, a fact that made it possible to differentiate the thalidomide syndrome from reduction malformations of different etiology. The most impressive type was amelia – complete absence of all extremities or of the upper extremities. In some cases, the humerus was markedly reduced in size, although portions of the forearm and the hand remained (proximal phocomelia). In such cases, the radius was shortened or absent and preaxial digits – thumb and index finger – were not developed. The ulna and postaxial fingers or a monodactylous structure sometimes were the only elements preserved.[20] Three-phalangeal thumb occurring as an isolated anomaly or in combination with other defects of the arm was emphasized by Lenz *et al.*[21] When the lower extremity was damaged, the femur and the tibia were chiefly affected, whereas the fibula was maintained. In the absence of a femoral head and deformed acetabulum, the hip joint was

Fig. 11-10. – Unusual deformity of forearm in thalidomide embryopathy with radial rudiment fused with thick and short ulna. A rudimentary thumb with a tiny bone enclosed can be seen. The proximal carpal bones are not separated. (Courtesy of Prof. H. Weicker, Bonn, Germany.)

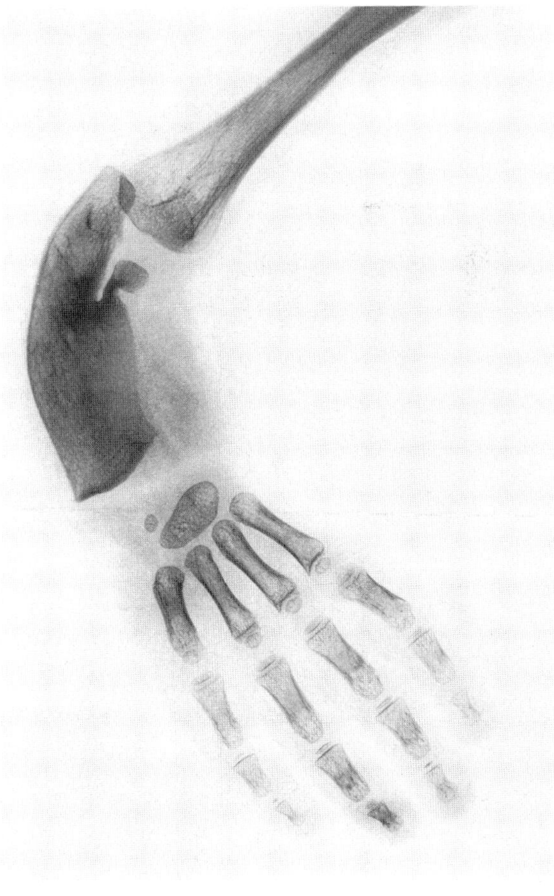

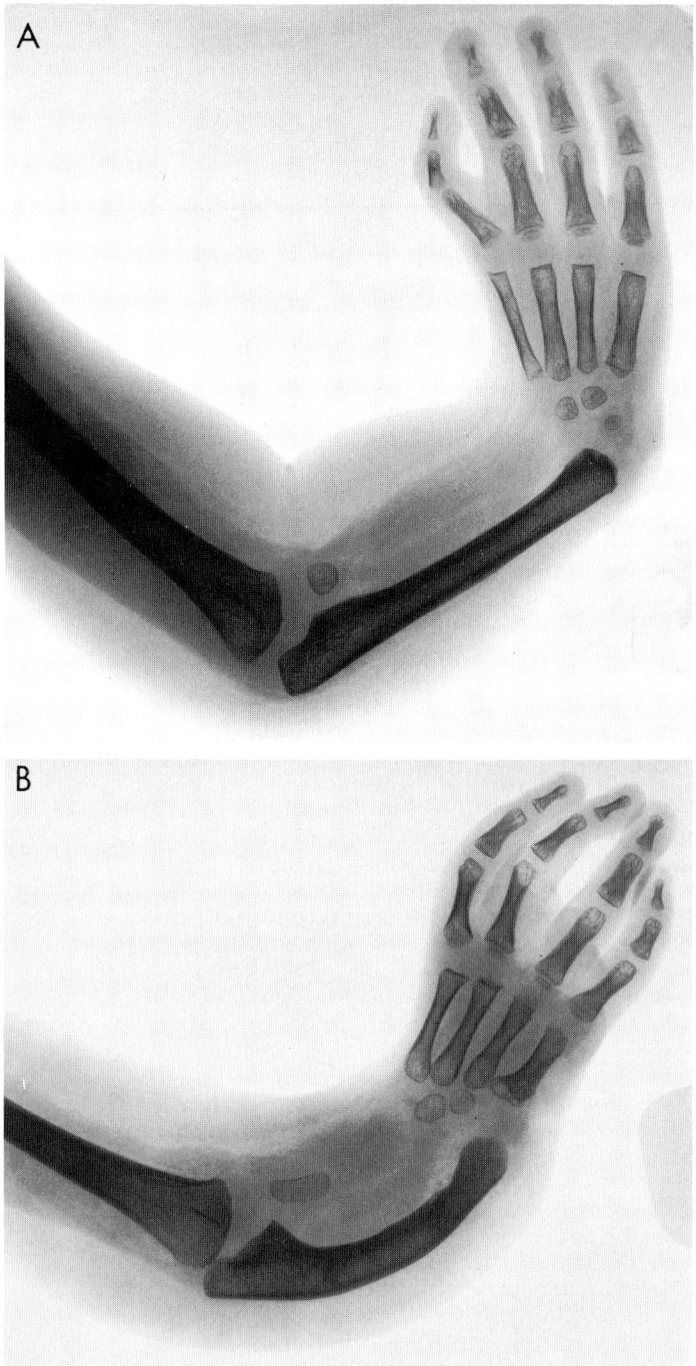

Fig. 11-11.—Typical forearms and hands in thalidomide embryopathy. **A,** rudimentary radius and thumb. **B,** rudimentary radius and absence of thumb. (Courtesy of Prof. H. Weicker, Bonn, Germany.)

severely distorted. Clubfoot with marked adduction resulted from absence or shortness of the tibia. The toes were deformed in various ways and often widely spaced; in some cases, the first toe was absent and in others there was polydactyly.

In the review of survivors by Weicker[19] in 1964, approximately 5% had total amelia, 65% total or subtotal aplasia of the humerus involving the proximal part, combined with total aplasia of the radius and of digits I–III. In 15% there was a total aplasia or partial (distal) aplasia of the radius with hypoplasia or dysplasia of the ulna and absence of digits I and III.

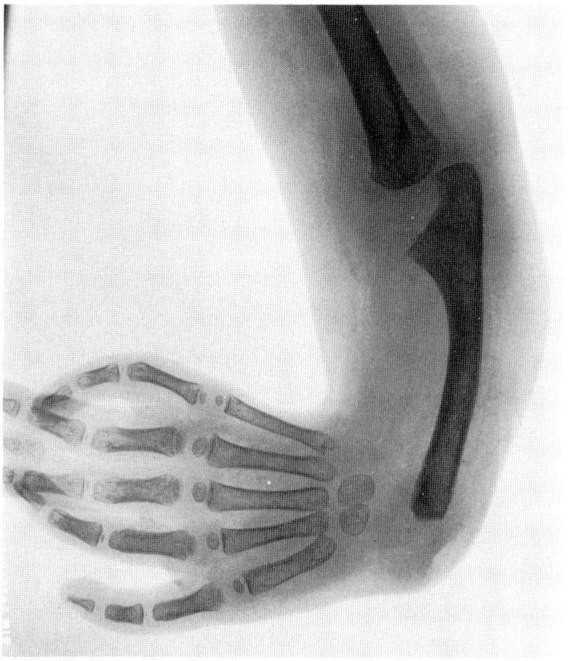

Fig. 11-12. – Typical clubhand with triphalangeal thumb, partial duplication of middle finger and absence of radius in a child with thalidomide embryopathy. (Courtesy of Prof. H. Weicker, Bonn, Germany.)

Approximately 10% of the children had only malformations of the thumb and 5% had radio-ulnar synostosis and thumb anomalies.

Malformations of the pelvic bones were quite frequent. In the lower extremities, reduction malformations of the femur and tibia were seen most often.

Cleft palate was not a sign of the thalidomide embryopathy[19] and it is doubtful that the drug induced this malformation. Smithells[20] thought that both choanal atresia and cleft palate were associated with reduction deformities of the limbs more often than would be expected by chance. Fogh-Andersen[22] reviewed suspected cases and considered the possibility of a causal connection between the drug and palate cleft. Kajii[23] recorded 4 cases of cleft lip and/or palate among 99 children with a positive thalidomide history.

Dental anomalies have been considered by Axrup *et al.*,[24] who noted higher incidences of hypodontia, deviation in crown shape and enamel hypoplasia in thalidomide children than in controls. Stahl[25] noted gray-blue discoloration but no changes of shape in the deciduous teeth. Notches in the tip of the tongue and anomalies of the frenulum linguae were seen repeatedly. Schübel and Partsch[26] examined histologically a dental primordium of a severely affected child and found no pathologic changes.

The *ears* were deformed in approximately 30% of the children; half of these had isolated malformations of the pinna and half also had other defects.[19] Hypoplasia or aplasia of the pinna, sometimes combined with atresia of the external meatus, and preauricular appendages occurred. Facialis and abducens paralysis was frequent in such cases.[27] Sometimes signs of cranial nerve damage disappeared spontaneously.[28] In some instances, the middle and inner ears were normal despite deformities of the pinna[20] but in others they were involved in the pathologic process.[19,29] Deafness was present in at least 10% of surviving children.[19]

The *eyes* were involved in some of the children, with colobomas of the iris and retina or microphthalmia of various degrees occurring (Fig. 11-18). Since the eye is derived in part from the brain, one could expect brain damages to be associated with ocular malformations. But, as a rule, children with thalidomide

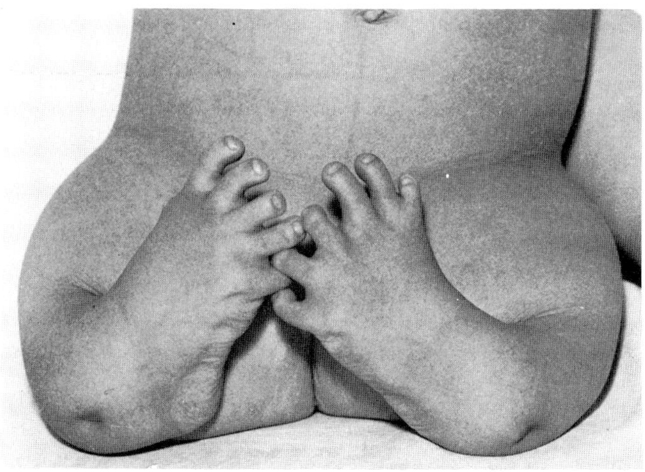

Fig. 11-13 (left). – Severe reduction malformations of lower extremities. Polydactyly on the left.

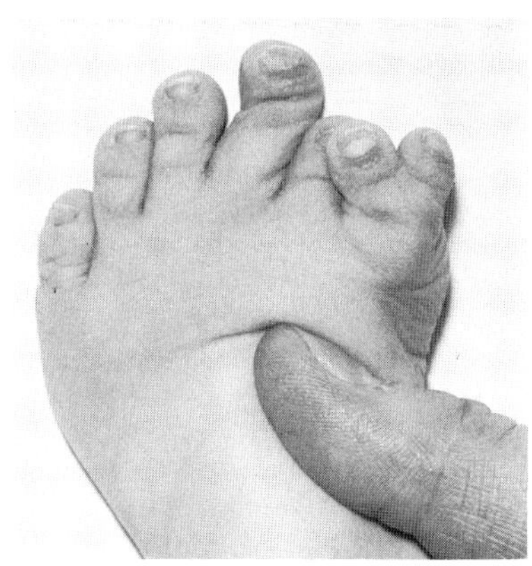

Fig. 11-14 (right). – Foot with 7 toes in a child with thalidomide embryopathy.
(Courtesy of Prof. H. Weicker, Bonn, Germany.)

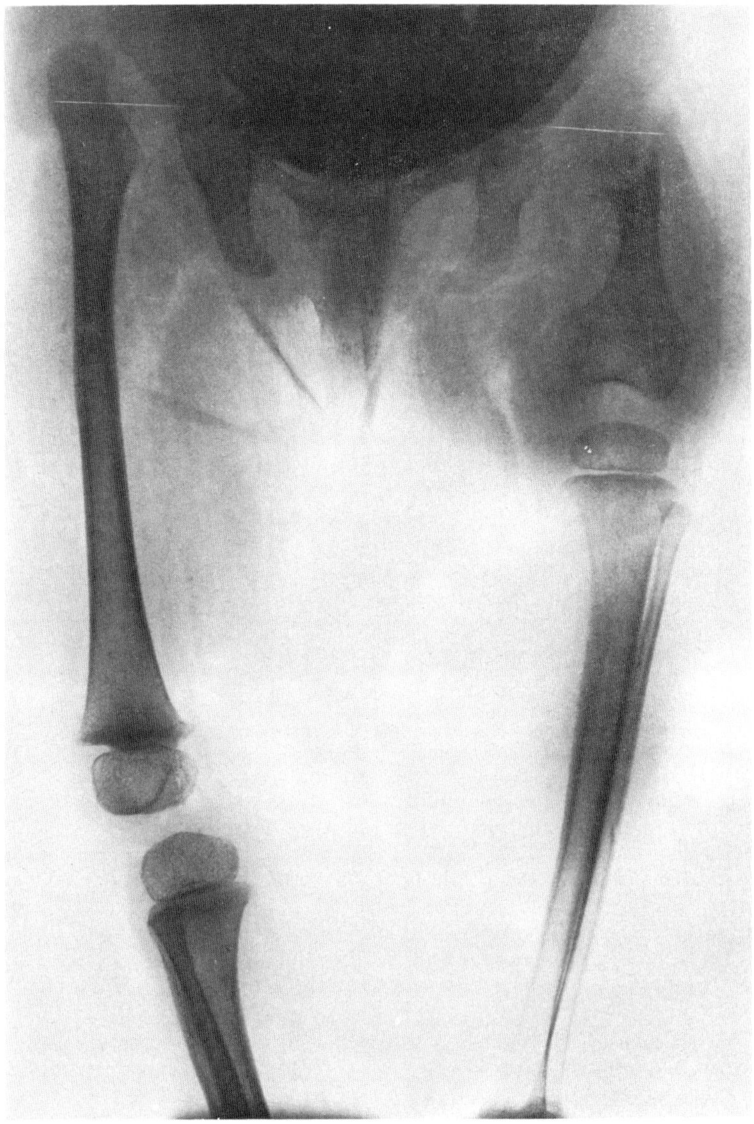

Fig. 11-15. – Congenital dislocation of hips. Severe malformation of left femur in a child with thalidomide embryopathy. (Courtesy of Prof. H. Weicker, Bonn, Germany.)

injuries were mentally alert and free of signs of cerebral involvement. Weicker[19] found good intelligence and alert facial expression in 95% of the surviving children. In exceptional cases, brain damage was observed in children with aural and ocular anomalies.[30]

The *face* often was characterized by a vascular nevus that extended from the center of the forehead down to the nose and the mouth. The nasal bridge was flat and the forehead broad.[20]

Many malformations of the *cardiovascular system* were observed, particularly in children on whom necropsy was performed. In one report,[31] 10 of 14 necropsies revealed such lesions as ventricular septal defect or tetralogy of Fallot. Weicker[19] found cardiovascular malformations in 15% of children surviving the third year. Aortic coarctation and hypoplasia, persistent ductus arteriosus, pulmonary stenosis, transposition of the great vessels,[20,32] truncus arteriosus[19,32] and anomalous pulmonary venous return[20] were recorded.

Missing lower lobe of the right lung was noted in some cases at necropsy.[19]

Urinary tract anomalies were noticed particularly in necropsies. Pliess[31] listed 10 urinary tract anomalies in 14 necropsies of "dysmelia malformations" between 1959 and 1962. Renal agenesis or hypoplasia, hydronephrosis, double kidney and horseshoe kidney have been reported.[20] Cystic kidneys were mentioned in some of the cases.[8,32] Hauke and Weicker,[33] who examined 100 children with thalidomide embryopathy, using special urologic methods, found 25 affected by renal anomalies. Single kidney, anom-

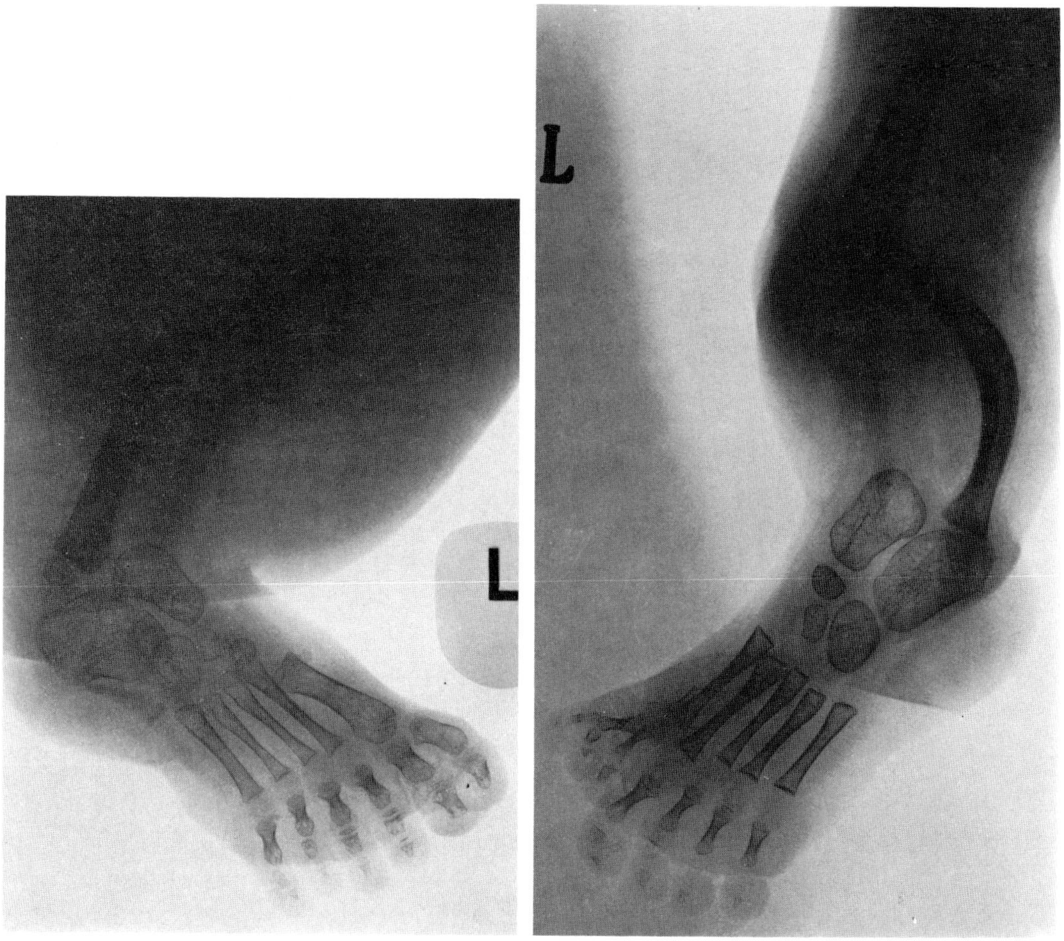

Fig. 11-16. – Typical thalidomide deformities of lower legs. Absence of tibiae, curved fibulae and polydactylies. (Courtesy of Prof. H. Weicker, Bonn, Germany.)

alies of rotation, double kidney, hydronephrosis, lump or horseshoe kidney and ectopias were ascertained with much higher frequencies than those expected in a general children's population.

The *genital tract anomalies* consisted of undescended testes and hypospadias in boys or, in girls, duplications of the uterine horns, hypoplasia of a uterine horn and agenesis or double vagina.[19,32]

The *intestinal tract* was commonly involved by esophageal atresia (sometimes associated with tracheo-espophageal fistula) or by obstruction of the small or large bowel or of the rectum. Apparently, duodenal obstruction was most often encountered.[32] These obstructions, complete or incomplete, sometimes were the cause of death. Malrotation of the intestine and hypoplasia or aplasia of the appendix or gallbladder were noted repeatedly.[20] Pyloric stenosis was recorded in a number of infants.[14,32] Anal atresia with vaginal fistula and rectal stenosis were combined with a variety of malformations of other organ systems.[32]

The teratologic findings in the thalidomide embryopathy reveal a wide spectrum of malformations. The defects of the extremities were most conspicuous because they were externally noticeable and were uncommon anomalies. Yet, malformations of the cardiovascular, intestinal and urinary systems, which were less distinctive than those of the skeleton, were more dangerous and even lethal in many cases. In general, one must agree with Lenz and Knapp[5] and Nowack[13] that thalidomide damaged the embryos between the thirty-fifth and fiftieth days after the last menstrual period, but to pinpoint the sensitive periods for specific malformations and to date their origin according to morphologic findings is a hazardous procedure. There were few mothers who could make reliable statements concerning their thalidomide consumption and fewer who took single doses at certain dates of gestation. There were observations of twins who were in the same uterus at the same time but differed greatly in phenotype (Fig. 11-19) and malformations.[7] It is true that, in monkeys, timed adminis-

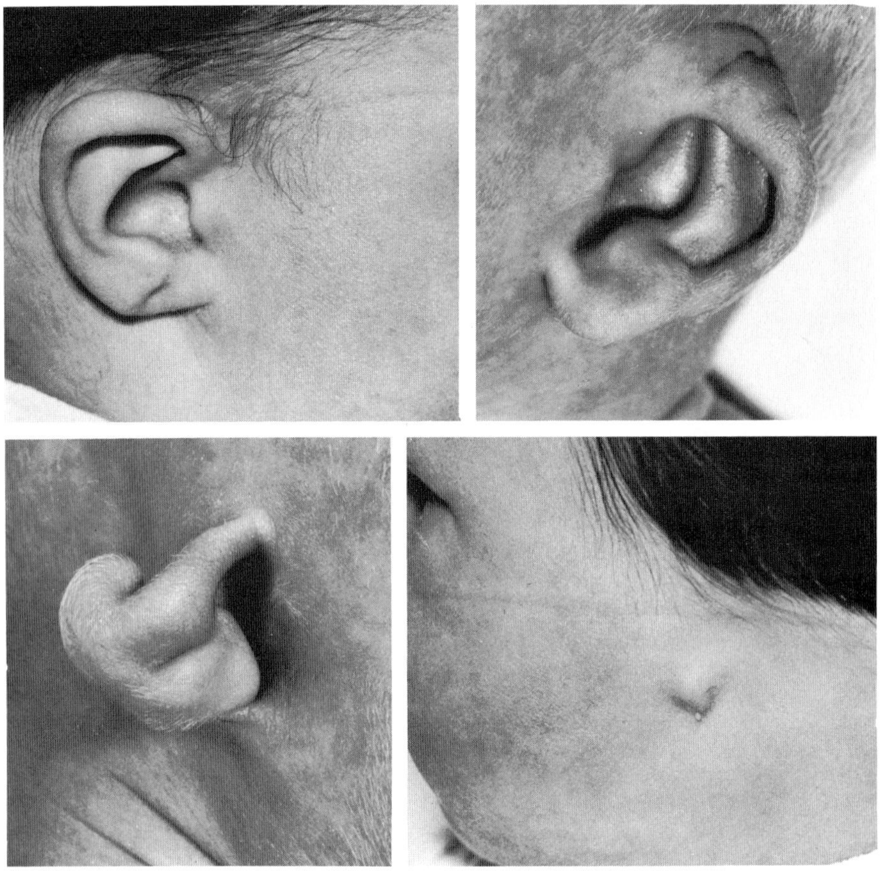

Fig. 11-17.—Abnormal external ears of children with thalidomide embryopathy. (Courtesy of Prof. H. Weicker, Bonn, Germany.)

tration of thalidomide can produce specific limb anomalies,[18] but human situations seldom simulate such experiments. In rats, which have more than one young in a litter, administration of a single dose of teratogenic drugs (not thalidomide) can produce quite different malformations in members of the same litter (see Fig. 7-1). I do not recommend calculations of the date of thalidomide intake based on morphologic

Fig. 11-18.—Microphthalmia in a child with thalidomide embryopathy. (Courtesy of Prof. H. Weicker, Bonn, Germany.)

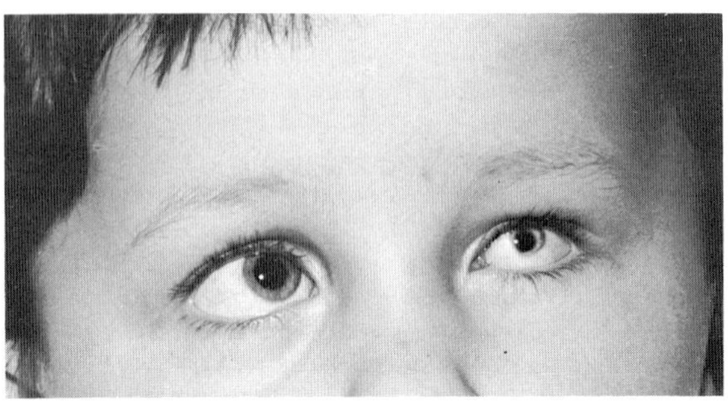

changes; all that one usually can say is that the drug was taken before the end of the organogenic period.

In the differential diagnosis, the thalidomide syndrome must be compared with other types of "phocomelia" and reduction malformations. There are reduction malformations that are genetically determined, such as the acheiropodias and defects of the upper extremities reported from Brazil (p. 955) as recessive traits. Among dominant limb defects are ectrodactyly and lobster claw, which can involve the upper and lower extremities (p. 963). Such malformations usually are limited to the skeleton. In other situations, the limb defects appear as parts of a syndrome. The Holt-Oram syndrome, a dominant trait, combines atrial and ventricular septal defects and other cardiovascular anomalies with skeletal malformations of the upper extremities involving particularly preaxial elements.[34] Similar skeletal defects occur in Fanconi pancytopenic anemia, a recessive trait. A rather characteristic phocomelia, i.e., a 5-fingered hand sitting near the shoulder, is complicated by episodes of thrombocytopenia and leukemoid reactions.[35] Similar hematologic complications have been de-

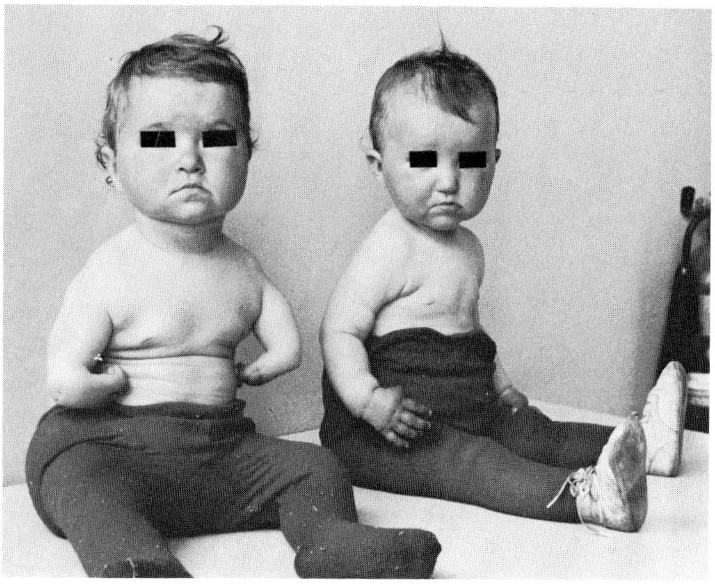

Fig. 11-19.—Dizygotic twins whose mother had taken thalidomide during the first 4 months of pregnancy. The boy had typical reduction malformations of the upper extremities. The girl had only anomalies of the thumbs but she was born with duodenal atresia and rectoperineal fistula. Note the different malformations in these twins who were exposed to the drug in the same uterus at the same time.

scribed repeatedly with radial aplasia.[36] The last two disorders have been observed in siblings. The same is true for de Lange syndrome, which sometimes includes reduction malformations of the upper extremities and regularly syndactyly of toes (Chapter 38).

In trisomy 18, "phocomelia" has been reported in exceptional cases (p. 308).

Children of diabetic mothers sometimes have reduction malformations of the lower extremities involving the femur and fibula but also the sacrum and other parts of the lower spinal column.[37] Tetraphocomelia has been described together with cleft lip and palate and hypertrophy of the clitoris.[38] A syndrome of defect of the femur and fibula and of severe reduction malformations of the upper extremities has been reported repeatedly; the etiology is obscure, but differentiation from the thalidomide embryopathy is possible since postaxial skeletal elements are affected.[39]

Thalidomide is an unusual drug that in doses harmless to the mother can cause severe malformations in embryos during their organogenic period. This embryo specificity made possible the widespread damages to children whose mothers did not realize that they were consuming a dangerous drug. For this and many other reasons, it is important to elucidate the mode of action of thalidomide, the sensitivity of the embryo to the drug and the relative resistance of adults to its harmful potentialities. It is important to understand why the oral administration of thalidomide is teratogenic in man, in macaques and to a lesser degree in rabbits, whereas rat and mice embryos are not harmed by large doses.

At first, it seemed likely that thalidomide, which contains a glutarimide ring, exerts its teratogenic action as an antimetabolite of glutamate and it was suggested by some writers that drugs containing the glutarimide ring may have comparable teratogenic effects. But Schuhmacher *et al.*[40] found that phthalimidophthalimide, an analogue that contains no glutarimide moiety, is a potent teratogen in rabbits that may be responsible for the thalidomide damages in man.

REFERENCES

1. Lenz, W.: Malformations caused by drugs in pregnancy, Am. J. Dis. Child. 112:99, 1966.
2. Wiedemann, H-R., and Aeissen, K.: Zur Frage der derzeitigen Häufung von Gliedmassen-Fehlbildungen, Med. Monatsschr. 12:816, 1961.
3. Pfeiffer, R. A., and Kosenow, W.: Thalidomide and congenital abnormalities, Lancet 1:45, 1962.
4. Weicker, H.: Klinik und Epidemiologie der Thalidomid-Embryopathie, Bull. Soc. roy. belge gynec. et obst. 33:21, 1963.
5. Lenz, W., and Knapp, K.: Die Thalidomid-Embryopathie, Deutsche med. Wchnschr. 87:1232, 1962.
6. Taussig, H. B.: A study of the German outbreak of phocomelia, J.A.M.A. 180:1106, 1962.
7. Mellin, G. W., and Katzenstein, M.: The saga of thalidomide: Neuropathy to embryopathy, with case reports of congenital anomalies, New England J. Med. 267: 1184 and 1238, 1962.
8. Lenz, W.: Das Thalidomid-Syndrom, Fortschr. Med. 81: 148, 1963.
9. Lenz, W.: Diskussionsbemerkung zu dem Vortrag von R. A. Pfeiffer und K. Kosenow: Zur Frage der exogenen Entstehung schwerer Extremitätenmissbildungen, Tagung

der Rheinisch-Westfälischen Kinderärztevereinigung in Düsseldorf 19:11, 1961.
10. McBride, W. G.: Thalidomide and congenital abnormalities, Lancet 2:1358, 1961.
11. Lenz, W.: Epidemiologie von Missbildungen, Pädiat. u. Pädol. 1:38, 1965.
12. Jones, E. E., and Williamson, D. A. J.: Thalidomide and congenital abnormalities, Lancet 1:222, 1962.
13. Nowack, E.: Die sensible Phase bei der Thalidomid-Embryopathie, Humangenetik 1:516, 1965.
14. Knapp, K.: Das Thalidomid-Syndrom, Bull. Soc. roy. belge gynec. et obst. 33:37, 1963.
15. Weicker, H., and Hungerland, H.: Thalidomid-Embryopathie. I. Vorkommen inner-und ausserhalb Deutschlands, Deutsche med. Wchnschr. 87:992, 1962.
16. Somers, G. F.: Thalidomide and congenital abnormalities, Lancet 1:912, 1962.
17. Delahunt, C. S., and Lassen, L. J.: Thalidomide syndrome in monkeys, Science 146:1300, 1964.
18. Wilson, J. G., and Gavan, J. A.: Congenital malformations in nonhuman primates: Spontaneous and experimentally induced, Anat. Rec. 158:99, 1967.
19. Weicker, H.: 100 children with thalidomide embryopathy, XIth International Congress of Pediatrics, 1965.
20. Smithells, R. W.: Drugs and Human Malformations, in Woollam, D. H. M. (ed.), *Advances in Teratology* (New York: Academic Press, 1966).
21. Lenz, W., Theopold, W., and Thomas, J.: Triphalangie des Daumens als Folge von Thalidomidschädigung, München. med. Wchnschr. 106:2033, 1964.
22. Fogh-Andersen, P.: Thalidomid und Lippen-Kiefer-Gaumen-Spalte, Deutsche Stomat. 15:343, 1965.
23. Kajii, T.: Thalidomide experience in Japan, Ann. paediat. 205:341, 1965.
24. Axrup, K., d'Avignon, M., Hellgren, K., Henrikson, C-O., Juhlin, I-M., Larsson, K. S., Persson, G. E., and Welander, E.: Children with thalidomide embryopathy: Odontologic observations and aspects, Dent. Digest 72:403, 1966.
25. Stahl, A.: Dysplasien im Bereich des Mundes, der Kiefer und der Zähne bei Dysmelie. Ein Beitrag zur Thalidomid-Embryopathie, Deutsche Zahnaerztl. Ztschr. 22:356, 1967.
26. Schübel, F., and Partsch, C. J.: Thalidomid-Embryopathien und ihre Einwirkungen auf die Zahnanlage, Deutsche Zahnaerztl. Ztschr. 20:1278, 1965.
27. Miehlke, A., and Partsch, C. J.: Ohrmissbildung, Facialis und Abducens – Lähmung als Syndrom der Thalidomidschädigung, Arch. Ohren-Nasen-u. Kehlkopfh. 181: 154, 1963.
28. d'Avignon, M., and Barr, B.: Ear abnormalities and cranial nerve palsies in thalidomide children, Arch. Otolaryng. 80:136, 1964.
29. Livingstone, G.: Congenital ear abnormalities due to thalidomide, Proc. Roy. Soc. Med. 58:493, 1965.
30. Horstmann, W.: Hinweise auf zentralnervöse Schäden im Rahmen der Thalidomid-Embryopathie. Pathologisch-anatomische, elektrencephalographische und neurologische Befunde, Ztschr. Kinderh. 96:291, 1966.
31. Pliess, G.: Thalidomide and congenital abnormalities, Lancet 1:1128, 1962.
32. Kreipe, U.: Missbildungen innerer Organe bei Thalidomid-embryopathie, Arch. Kinderh. 176:33, 1967.
33. Hauke, H., and Weicker, H.: Thalidomid-Embryopathie: V. Die Nierenfehlbildungen, Deutsche med. Wchnschr. 90:2200, 1965.
34. Pruzanski, W.: Familial congenital malformations of the heart and upper limbs; a syndrome of Holt-Oram, Cardiologia 45:21, 1964.
35. Dignan, P. St. J., Mauer, A. M., and Frantz, C.: Phocomelia with congenital hypoplastic thrombocytopenia and myeloid leukemoid reactions, J. Pediat. 70:561, 1967.
36. Schönenberg, H., and Scheidhauer, E.: Beidseitige radiale Hemimelie mit Megakaryocytopenie, Ztschr. Kinderh. 97:240, 1966.
37. Kučera, J., Lenz, W., and Maier, W.: Missbildungen der Beine und der kaudalen Wirbelsäule bei Kindern diabetischer Mütter, Deutsche med. Wchnschr. 90:901, 1965.
38. Appelt, H., Gerken, H., and Lenz, W.: Tetraphokomelie mit Lippen-Kiefer-Gaumenspalte und Clitorishypertrophie – ein Syndrom, Paediat. Path. 2:119, 1966.
39. Kühne, D., Lenz, W., Petersen, D., and Schönenberg, H.: Defekt von Femur und Fibula mit Amelie, Peromelie oder ulnaren Strahldefekten der Arme, Humangenetik 3:244, 1967.
40. Schuhmacher, H., Blake, D. A., and Gillette, J. R.: Acylation of subcellular components by phthalimidophthalimide as a possible mode of embryotoxic action, Fed. Proc. 26:739, 1967.

Some Other Drugs

Aminopterin (4-aminopteroylglutamic acid) and Methotrexate

Aminopterin

This folic acid antagonist, employed originally in the treatment of leukemia, proved to be an effective abortive. It was used to produce therapeutic and illegal abortions until it was demonstrated that in borderline situations an embryo could be deformed but survive to the end of gestation and even beyond it. It has been demonstrated that pteroylglutamic acid (PGA, folic acid) plays an important role in many biologic reactions, and that maternal PGA deficiency can lead to death of embryos or multiple congenital malformations.[1,2] Skeletal malformations and severe deformities of the ear were observed in sheep exposed to aminopterin at different times of gestation.[3]

Aminopterin was given by Thiersch[4] to tuberculous women for therapeutic abortion. Oral doses of 6–12 mg. induced fetal death in the first trimester of pregnancy, usually followed by abortion. In older fetuses, the drug failed to produce immediate death of the embryos, so they had to be removed surgically. In some fetuses, congenital malformations such as hydrocephaly, encephalomeningocele or cleft lip or palate were observed. One fetus went to term, was born with anencephaly and lived for 12 days. Meltzer[5] reported a case of attempted abortion with aminopterin in the second month of pregnancy. Bleeding was provoked but abortion failed to occur. Following a normal labor, a child was born who had a left talipes equinovarus and multiple skull anomalies such as partial craniosynostosis and "Lückenschädel."

Warkany *et al.*[6] described a well-documented case of a woman who attempted abortion with aminopterin in the second month of pregnancy. The mother developed signs of PGA deficiency, was successfully treated and the pregnancy continued. The child, born 2 weeks after term, showed marked intrauterine growth retardation (1,280 Gm.), large head, small mandible, deformed ears, long upper lip, posterior palate cleft, pterygia colli and clubhands and clubfeet (Fig. 11-20). The cranial bones were incompletely ossified (cranial dysostosis), suggesting hydrocephaly, but the brain within the cranial cavity was relatively large and the ventricular system was not expanded. The child died 29 hours after birth. The authors cautiously attributed the syndrome of congenital anomalies to aminopterin ingestion of the mother, since the disease picture was unique, the malformations were compatible with the time of administration of the drug, the family history was negative and folic acid antagonists had been proved to be teratogenic in human and other mammalian embryos. That this interpretation was correct was shown by subsequent cases. Emerson[7] reported a 24-week-old fetus aborted after intake of aminopterin by the mother. Hydrocephaly, cerebral aplasia, retardation of ossification of the skull bones, malformed ears, cleft palate and micrognathia were observed.

Fig. 11-20.—Newborn infant delivered after a gestation of 42 weeks weighing 1,280 Gm. The mother had taken aminopterin tablets in early pregnancy. (From J. Warkany, P. H. Beaudry and S. Hornstein.[6])

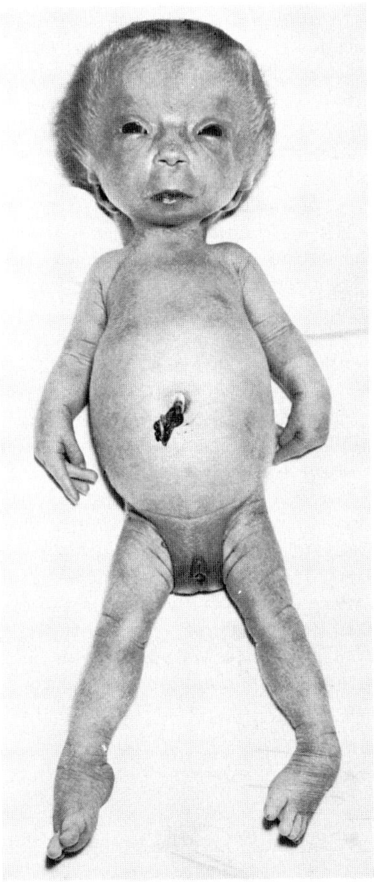

Shaw and Steinbach[8] reported the case of a girl damaged by aminopterin in early pregnancy, with survival of the child. She was born at term showing intrauterine growth retardation (1,750 Gm.), marked deficiencies of ossification of the cranial bones, micrognathia, high-arched palate and short forearms. Ossification of the skull proceeded slowly, growth and weight gain were subnormal, motor development was good and mental retardation mild. Chromosome studies revealed a normal female karyotype.

Methotrexate

Unsuccessful attempted abortion with methotrexate (a methyl derivative of aminopterin) was recorded by Milunsky *et al.*[9] Absence of the frontal bone, synostosis of the lambdoid and coronal sutures, anomalous ribs, facial peculiarities, absence of digits on the left foot and monodactyly on the right were observed at birth. The child survived birth and showed normal psychomotor development but growth was retarded.

Cyclophosphamide

A woman with Hodgkin disease was treated with cyclophosphamide, an alkylating agent of the nitrogen mustard group, throughout pregnancy.[10] Treatment was most intensive during a period corresponding approximately to the seventh or eighth week of fetal life. A male infant was born who had 4 toes on each foot, grooves on each side of the midline of the hard palate and other minor anomalies. Related compounds given to pregnant women for Hodgkin disease had no adverse effects on their fetuses.

Myleran

A girl born to a mother who received 6-mercaptopurine and x-ray therapy early in pregnancy and Myleran (busulfan) throughout most of her pregnancy had severe intrauterine growth retardation (1,077 Gm. at term), cloudy corneae, posterior palate cleft and hypoplastic ovaries. Cytomegaly was noted in many organs and tissues. There were many possibly teratogenic factors involved in this pregnancy and there is no proof that Myleran caused the anomalies of the child.[11]

Quinine

Quinine, often used in attempted abortions, has been accused of causing congenital deafness[12,13] but this has not been generally accepted.[14] Other reports of quinine as a teratogen have not described a definite pattern of malformations. Tracheo-esophageal fistula, pseudohermaphrodism, congenital heart disease, reduction malformations of the limbs and others have been observed in children born after attempted abortion with quinine.[15-17]

REFERENCES

1. Nelson, M. M., Asling, W., and Evans, H. M.: Congenital abnormalities in fetal rats resulting from pteroylglutamic (folic) acid deficiency during gestation, Anat. Rec. 106: 309, 1950.
2. Giroud, A., and Lefebvres, J.: Anomalies caused in the fetus by the absence of folic acid, Arch. franç. pédiat. 8: 648, 1951.
3. James, L. F., and Keller, R. F.: Teratogenic effects of aminopterin in sheep, Teratology 1:407, 1968.
4. Thiersch, J. B.: Therapeutic abortions with a folic acid antagonist, 4-aminopteroylglutamic acid (4-amino PGA), Am. J. Obst. & Gynec. 63:1298, 1952.
5. Meltzer, H. J.: Congenital anomalies due to attempted abortion with 4-aminopteroylglutamic acid, J.A.M.A. 161: 1253, 1956.
6. Warkany, J., Beaudry, P. H., and Hornstein, S.: Attempted abortion with 4-aminopteroylglutamic acid (aminopterin), malformations of the child, Am. J. Dis. Child. 97:274, 1960.
7. Emerson, D. J.: Congenital malformations due to attempted abortion with aminopterin, Am. J. Obst. & Gynec. 84:356, 1962.
8. Shaw, E. B., and Steinbach, H. L.: Aminopterin-induced fetal malformation. Survival of infant after attempted abortion, Am. J. Dis. Child. 115:477, 1968.
9. Milunsky, A., Graef, J. W., and Gaynor, M. F.: Methotrexate-induced congenital malformations, J. Pediat. 72:790, 1968.
10. Greenberg, L. H., Verdes, P., and Tanaka, K. R.: Congenital anomalies probably induced by cyclophosphamide, J.A.M.A. 188:423, 1964.
11. Diamond, I., Anderson, M. M., and McCreadie, S. R.: Transplacental transmission of busulfan (Myleran) in mother with leukemia (production of fetal malformation and cytomegaly), Pediatrics 25:85, 1960.
12. Taylor, H. M.: Prenatal medication and its relation to the fetal ear, Surg., Gynec. & Obst. 64:542, 1937.
13. Reed, H., Briggs, J. N., and Martin, J. K.: Congenital glaucoma, deafness, mental deficiency and cardiac anomaly following attempted abortion, J. Pediat. 46:182, 1955.
14. Winckel, C. W. F.: Quinine and congenital injuries of ear and eye of the foetus, Trop. Med. & Hyg. 51:3, 1948.
15. Uhlig, H.: Missbildungen unerwünschter Kinder, Ärztl. Wchnschr. 12:61, 1957.
16. Kup, J.: Multiple Missbildungen nach Chinin-Einnahme in der Schwangerschaft, München. med. Wchnschr. 108: 2293, 1966.
17. Fuhrmann, W.: Genetische und peristatische Ursachen angeborener Angiokardiopathien, Ergebn. inn. Med. u. Kinderh. 18:45, 1962.

Anticonvulsant Drugs

Because of progress in the treatment of epilepsy, many epileptic girls now get married and some of them go through pregnancies while under medication. Following the thalidomide incident, the question was raised whether treatment of pregnant women with antiepileptic drugs could damage the fetus. Should the general advice to avoid drugs during pregnancy be applied to epileptic women? It is clear that withdrawal of anticonvulsants could endanger pregnant women, so withholding of such drugs cannot be recommended lightly. Janz and Fuchs,[1] who made a retrospective inquiry in 1964 into this matter, found that antiepileptic medication did not increase abortions and stillbirths. Among 225 live-born infants of treated mothers there were 5 (2.2%) with congenital malformations, which was not an excessive incidence. But among the 225 infants there were 3 (1.3%) with facial clefts; this incidence is high compared with 0.15% in the general newborn population (p. 628). Since 17 anticonvulsant drugs had been used by these mothers, no specific compound could be suspected as a possible cause of the increased incidence of facial clefts. The over-all figures were too small to draw definite conclusions concerning teratogenicity of anticonvulsant treatments.

Subsequently, it was shown that diphenylhydantoin (Dilantin, phenytoin) produced cleft palate in A/Jax mice[2] and in Swiss-Webster mice.[3,4] Single injections of large amounts of this drug produced open eye, ectrodactyly, fused vertebrae, hydronephrosis and internal hydrocephaly.[4]

In 1968, Meadow[5] reported observations on 6 children with cleft lip and palate whose mothers had received regular anticonvulsant therapy; 4 of these children also had congenital heart lesions; minor skeletal abnormalities and peculiarly shaped skulls were also noted. Two years later, Meadow[6] listed 32 children with facial clefts born to treated epileptic mothers. He calculated the expected incidence and found the actual incidence excessive; the same was true for the occurrence of congenital heart disease in the children with facial clefts. Elshove[7] reported on cleft palate in the offspring of female mice treated with phenytoin and mentioned 7 babies of epileptic mothers who had congenital abnormalities, 4 of them showing facial clefts. He considered the possibility that phenytoin, like some other anticonvulsants, lowers serum folate levels and that its teratogenic action is the result of its antagonism to folic acid.

In contrast to these reports that throw suspicion on anticonvulsant drugs is a statement by Bird,[8] who, in more than 20 years, did not see a single case of congenital anomaly in a baby born to a mother on anticonvulsant therapy. Thus, the possibility of teratogenic action of anticonvulsant drugs must be considered, but there is, as yet, no evidence that these drugs are at fault in cases of congenital malformations.

REFERENCES

1. Janz, D., and Fuchs, U.: Sind antiepileptische Medikamente während der Schwangerschaft schädlich?, Deut-

sche med. Wchnschr. 89:241, 1964.
2. Massey, K. M.: Teratogenic effects of diphenylhydantoin sodium, J. Oral Therap. & Pharmacol. 2:380, 1966.
3. Gibson, J. E., and Becker, B. A.: Teratogenic effects of diphenylhydantoin in Swiss-Webster and A/J mice, Proc. Soc. Exper. Biol. & Med. 128:905, 1968.
4. Harbison, R. D., and Becker, B. A.: Relation of dosage and time of administration of diphenylhydantoin to its teratogenic effect in mice, Teratology 2:305, 1969.
5. Meadow, S. R.: Anticonvulsant drugs and congenital abnormalities, Lancet 2:1296, 1968.
6. Meadow, S. R.: Congenital abnormalities and anticonvulsant drugs, Proc. Roy. Soc. Med. 63:48, 1970.
7. Elshove, J.: Cleft palate in the offspring of female mice treated with phenytoin, Lancet 2:1074, 1969.
8. Bird, A. V.: Anticonvulsant drugs and congenital abnormalities, Lancet 1:311, 1969.

Antituberculosis Drugs

There are no indications that modern antituberculosis treatments with drugs are teratogenic,[1] but there are some reports of hearing loss in children whose mothers had been treated with streptomycin during the first 4 months of pregnancy.[2,3] Ethionamide, which has been shown to have adverse effects on the course of pregnancy and on the fetus in animal experiments, has been suspected also of damaging human fetuses. Potworowska *et al.*[4] warned against the use of this drug for treatment of pregnant women.

REFERENCES

1. Lowe, C. R.: Congenital defects among children born to women under supervision or treatment for pulmonary tuberculosis, Brit. J. Prev. & Social Med. 18:14, 1964.
2. Kern, G.: On the problem of intrauterine streptomycin damage, Schweiz. med. Wchnschr. 92:77, 1962.
3. Robinson, G. C., and Cambon, K. G.: Hearing loss in infants of tuberculous mothers treated with streptomycin during pregnancy, New England J. Med. 271:949, 1964.
4. Potworowska, M., Sianožecka, E., and Szufladowicz, R.: Ethionamide treatment and pregnancy, Polish M. J. 5: 1152, 1966.

Meclizine

Following the thalidomide crisis, an antihistaminic drug, meclizine, was accused of causing limb defects similar to those of thalidomide, but it was soon concluded that this was "guilt by association," as in some pregnancies both thalidomide and meclizine were given as sedatives to expecting women. A number of careful studies failed to detect an excess of congenital malformations in children whose mothers had taken meclizine during pregnancy.[1,2] The question was reopened when it was found that the drug, when given to pregnant rats, caused cleft palate and other oral anomalies in the young.[3] A special advisory committee was formed by the Food and Drug Administration in the United States, which considered the evidence or lack of evidence for meclizine teratogenicity. Sadusk and Palmisano[4] summarized the opinions of the committee, which considered both the efficacy and the possible teratogenic effects of the drug. The difficulties encountered in judging such drugs are brought out by this short report on lengthy meetings. There were some scientists who strongly believed that the available evidence is against adverse effects of meclizine on the fetus.[5] Yet, when Lenz[6] pooled data from 15 studies, among 3,333 infants whose mothers had been given meclizine there were 12 with cleft lip or palate or both, which is two to three times the expected number. Interpretation of these data is difficult because a selection of publications with "positive" results cannot be excluded. There also may be a selection of mothers who vomited because they carried an abnormal child and were given the drug because of their hyperemesis. Recent reports indicate that meclizine is not teratogenic in man (p. 633).

REFERENCES

1. Smithells, R. W., and Chinn, E. R.: Meclizine and foetal malformations: A prospective study, Brit. M. J. 1:217, 1964.
2. Mellin, G. W.: Drugs in the first trimester of pregnancy and the fetal life of Homo sapiens, Am. J. Obst. & Gynec. 90: 1169, 1964.
3. Kendrick, F. J., and King, C. T. G.: Oral anomalies induced in the rat by meclizine hydrochloride, Oral Surg. 18:690, 1964.
4. Sadusk, J. F., Jr., and Palmisano, P. A.: Teratogenic effect of meclizine, cyclizine, and chlorcyclizine, J.A.M.A. 194: 139, 1965.
5. Yerushalmy, J., and Milkovich, L.: The evaluation of the teratogenic effect of meclizine in man, Am. J. Obst. & Gynec. 93:553, 1965.
6. Lenz, W.: Malformations caused by drugs in pregnancy, Am. J. Dis. Child. 112:99, 1966.

Masculinizing Progesterones and Estrogens

ATTEMPTS to avert abortion by administration of synthetic progestins have led to masculinization of female fetuses. Seventy cases of masculinization of female infants associated with such treatment were reported by Wilkins[1] in 1960. Enlarged clitoris and various degrees of fusion of the labioscrotal folds were among the anomalies observed. It is of interest that as early as 1943 Van Wagenen and Hamilton[2] produced pseudohermaphrodism in rhesus monkeys by administration of androgens to mothers from day 41 to day 99 of gestation. In human fetuses, ethisterone, norethisterone and norethynodrel prescribed for pregnant women have had virilizing effects.[3] It may be added parenthetically that fetal virilization has been attributed to nonendocrine drugs such as the anticonvulsants Elipten and Mebaral.[4]

REFERENCES

1. Wilkins, L.: Masculinization of female fetus due to use of orally given progestins, J.A.M.A. 172:1028, 1960.
2. Van Wagenen, G., and Hamilton, J. B.: The Experimental Production of Pseudohermaphroditism in the Monkey, in *Essays in Biology* (Berkeley: University of California Press, 1943).
3. Venning, G. R.: The Problem of Human Foetal Abnormalities with Special Reference to Sex Hormones, in Robson, J. M., Sullivan, F. M., and Smith, R. L. (eds.), *Embryopathy Activity of Drugs* (Boston: Little, Brown & Company, 1965).
4. Iffy, L., Ansell, J. S., Bryant, J. S., and Herrmann, W. L.: Nonadrenal female pseudohermaphroditism: An unusual case of fetal masculinization, Obst. & Gynec. 26:59, 1965.

Cortisone and ACTH

CORTISONE is used in experimental teratology to produce cleft palate in mice. The experiment can be done with almost 100% success if one uses A/Jax mice, but in other inbred strains the incidence is much lower and similar experimental conditions in rats fail to produce cleft palate. These specificities illustrate the difficulty of evaluating these drugs in human heterogeneous populations. Sometimes cleft palate has been seen in babies whose mothers had been treated with cortisone.[1,2] In a review of 260 pregnancies in which the drug had been administered there were 2 cleft palates in the children born.[3] There was one series of 28 pregnancies in which such treatment had been given without any resulting malformation[4] and another series of 28 in which 1 cleft palate was observed.[5] In other publications, anomalies such as gastroschisis, hydrocephaly, tetralogy of Fallot, hypospadias or clubfoot and others were encountered – anomalies that sometimes occur in children whose mothers were not treated with any drugs.[6] We need quantitative evaluations, but even these often are biased because most of the mothers given cortisone had some complications of pregnancy that in themselves could be teratogenic. Whereas Rolf[7] stated that no catastrophes due to previous cortisone treatment have been identified in maternity departments of the Los Angeles area, Warrell and Taylor,[8] of Sheffield, England, recorded stillbirths and fetuses at risk in 18 of 34 pregnancies. In contrast, there were 30 healthy babies from 34 pregnancies of women not receiving glucocorticoids.

REFERENCES

1. Harris, J. W., and Ross, I. P.: Cortisone therapy in early pregnancy: Relation to cleft palate, Lancet 1:1045, 1956.
2. Doig, R. K., and Coltman, O. M.: Cleft palate following cortisone therapy in early pregnancy, Lancet 2:730, 1956.
3. Bongiovanni, A. M., and McPadden, A. J.: Steroids during pregnancy and possible fetal consequences, Fertil. & Steril. 2:181, 1960.
4. Margulis, R. R., and Hodgkinson, C. P.: Evaluation of safety of corticotropin (ACTH) and cortisone in pregnancy, Obst. & Gynec. 1:276, 1953.
5. Popert, A. J.: Pregnancy and adrenal cortical hormones, Brit. M. J. 1:967, 1962.
6. Smithells, R. W.: Drugs and Human Malformations, in Woollam, D. H. M. (ed.), *Advances in Teratology* (New York: Academic Press, 1966).
7. Rolf, B. B.: Corticosteroids and pregnancy, Am. J. Obst. & Gynec. 95:339, 1966.
8. Warrell, D. W., and Taylor, R.: Outcome for the foetus of mothers receiving prednisolone during pregnancy, Lancet 1:117, 1968.

Experimental Teratology and Drug Testing

THE FACT THAT thalidomide and other drugs can produce, under certain conditions, congenital malformations plus evidence resulting from the skills acquired by experimental teratologists in producing congenital malformations in mammals by administration of drugs has led to demands to test drugs in pregnant animals before admitting them for use in humans. Although such tests are to be recommended, it must be pointed out that observations in animals can be transferred to humans only with reservations. The difficulties are best illustrated by the fact that thalidomide does not produce malformations in rats and mice, whereas salicylates do.

It is important to know some of the principles of teratogenesis to understand the values and the limits of animal experiments. If one tries to produce congenital malformations, the results depend on the nature of the teratogen, the dose, the route of administration, the choice of test animal, the stage of pregnancy and many other important factors. Congenital malformations arise in borderline situations in which the embryo is damaged but not destroyed. If one uses a drug in a small dose, the embryo may go unharmed; if the dose is too large, the embryo is killed. There may be a teratogenic dose between the harmless and the lethal that can deform the embryo without killing it.

The reaction to a teratogen may vary greatly according to the route of administration. Oral administration to the mother may be harmless, whereas intravenous injection may reach the embryo and damage it. There exist differential susceptibilities to drugs at different ages. The effects of a drug differ greatly before, during and after organogenesis. A drug often adversely affects the embryo before organogenesis and leads to its death; in late pregnancy, it may cause disease or death. Even within the periods of organogenesis, different malformations are produced by administration of a drug on different days of gestation, since the effects depend to a great extent on the developmental stage of the embryo. Experiments in animals that carry more than one young demonstrate that a teratogen applied to the mother may produce different types of malformations in different members of a litter (see Fig. 7-1). The time of administration does not always determine the morphologic changes in the embryos. The young can be genetically different, unless inbred strains of animals are used, or they can be of slightly different ages and damaged in different stages of development. An organ, once formed correctly, can still be deformed by secondary destructive forces, so that malformations can arise after the organogenic periods (p. 51). Drugs harmless to the adult and to the mother may damage the embryo and deform it.

Different drugs or chemical compounds can affect specific cellular processes and, therefore, show differing results, even if applied at similar developmental stages. The reactions to a teratogen vary greatly in different species. There are teratogens, including drugs, that regularly are effective in rats but not in mice, and vice versa. Effective doses sometimes vary greatly in different species even when adjusted to the weight of the test animal. These well-established facts imply that animal experiments, which can vary from one species to another, are not necessarily applicable to human beings. Even within a species, a drug may have different teratogenic effects on the embryos of different strains. This has been shown clearly by cortisone effects on different inbred strains of mice.

Among contributory factors, season, climate, age or weight of the mother, position in the uterus and others may decide the presence or type of malformation produced. And there are intangible factors that cannot be evaluated. Thus, the production of congenital malformations depends on administration of a specific drug in a particular dosage to a genetically susceptible animal at a time when the embryos are in a susceptible stage of development. If not all of these conditions are fulfilled, no young with congenital malformations will be obtained. Yet, a minor change of the experimental conditions may result in production of young with malformations. Failure to observe offspring with congenital malformations may be due also to drug effects that are so serious that the abnormal embryos die in utero long before they are born. Since such embryos can be resorbed in some species, teratogenic effects will go undetected unless a special search is made for deformed embryos in early stages. Even in fetuses near term and in newborn animals, the finding of malformations depends on the methods of examination. Malformations can be obvious and visible on external inspection or they may be located internally and be small in size. Whether malformations are detected depends on the methods of examination used. An animal may appear normal on external examination but show severe malformations on dissection or histologic sectioning.

These are some of the facts that explain the limited value of tests performed in animals for predicting drug effects on human embryos. Teratologic animal experiments can only suggest similar effects in man but never prove them.

Animal experiments as well as clinical observations have taught us that congenital malformations of certain types can result from quite different causes. Microcephaly, hydrocephaly, congenital cataract, heart disease, limb defects and others can be genetically determined and appear after completely undisturbed pregnancies. Clinically similar malformations can be due to environmental damages to genetically normal embryos during gestation. A specific environmental teratogen, such as a drug, can cause a whole spectrum of congenital malformations that may make their appearance singly or in syndromes, on the body surface or internally, at birth or in later life. The lack of specificity of causes and the lack of specificity of effects make it difficult to establish in man causal relationships between events observed during pregnancy and malformations manifested after birth.

Although in the foregoing the insufficiencies of animal tests have been emphasized, there exist possibilities to improve them. The empirical tests now employed can be replaced by more significant investigations of drug disposition and transport in animals and man, of transplacental permeability and of intraembryonic teratogenic processes.[1,2] Good beginnings have been made in primate teratology that promise that certain tests in subhuman primates may be more meaningful than those now practiced in rodents. The simulation of human malformations caused by thalidomide in macaques is remarkable[3,4] and should stimulate more attempts along these lines. Although it seems that primate testing is very expensive, it may prove cheaper in the long run than testing in rodents, which often is not indicative of effects on human embryos.

REFERENCES

1. Report of the Commission on Drug Safety, Subcommittee on Teratology, Chicago, 1964.
2. Warkany, J.: Drugs and Teratology, in Shirkey, H. C. (ed.), *Pediatric Therapy 1968–1969* (3d ed.; St. Louis: The C. V. Mosby Company, 1968).
3. Delahunt, C. S., and Lassen, L. J.: Thalidomide syndrome in monkeys, Science 146:1300, 1964.
4. Wilson, J. G., and Gavan, J. A.: Congenital malformations in nonhuman primates: Spontaneous and experimentally induced, Anat. Rec. 158:99, 1967.

12

Maternal Disorders

Endemic Goiter and Cretinism

Endemic goiter and cretinism associated with iodine deficiency have disappeared from most civilized countries in which they once represented important health problems. There are huge areas on this planet where man can exist and subsist on the products of the land and where nutrition seemingly is adequate; yet, lack of iodine in the soil, water and vegetation results in hazards that threaten the health of the population from birth on—and even before. In such areas, good health can be maintained only by import of iodine as a chemical or in the form of foods grown on better soil or in the sea. In these regions without adequate communications and commerce, the thyroid gland lacks an element needed for synthesis of its endocrine products, reacts by hyperplasia to make up for the shortage in iodine supply and often fails to provide an adequate environment for the unborn child. Endemic cretinism is an example of a congenital anomaly caused by an environmental adversity—nutritional deficiency. Since the condition is preventable by relatively simple measures, it has become so rare that in areas open to commerce few physicians have ever seen a case of this physical and mental anomaly. Yet, endemic cretinism must never be forgotten, since it illustrates that even human embryos and fetuses can be endangered in their development by maternal nutritional deficiency. In animals, many types of congenital malformations have been produced by deficiencies of well-defined nutritional elements in the mother's diet. But few, if any, comparable situations have been found in man. Endemic cretinism shows beyond any doubt that the human fetus, like that of animals, can be damaged by absence of an essential dietary element during intrauterine development. But human conditions never simulate animal experiments completely, and adequate controls usually are not available for human populations. Secondary factors enter into the etiology and pathogenesis of goiter and cretinism in man, often beclouding the primary role of iodine deficiency as the main pathogenic cause. But, if one reviews retrospectively the huge literature on this subject, the arguments and disagreements of the past and the outcome of preventive measures, it is possible to discern primary and secondary factors in the causation of goiter and cretinism. Unfortunately, there are big gaps in our knowledge of the pathogenesis of cretinism because studies of mothers carrying future cretins were and are difficult.

Since early times, goiter and cretinoid degeneration have been thought to be interdependent. Paracelsus, in the sixteenth century, believed that goiter, mental weakness, lack of memory and deafness were connected as results of ascending "liquor mineralis" into the neck, brain and ears. Before Paracelsus, cretins were known in the Pyrenees, where they were called cagots and considered leprous and contagious. Merke[1] pointed out that Jacques de Vitry, in the thirteenth century, mentioned that in certain regions, particularly in the Alps, there were women with gigantic goiters that hung like squashes down to the belly. Many of them were dwarfed, and "from the dumb and deaf, dumb and deaf children were derived." In the thirteenth century, Haute-Savoie, Savoie and some parts of western Switzerland were within Burgundy, and Merke[2] believed that Jacques de Vitry's encounter with goiter and cretinism was in the region of the Great Saint Bernard Pass.

A study on "The Discovery of Cretinism" by Cranefield[3] related that Josias Simler, in the sixteenth century, wrote about the prevalence of goiter in the Valais, and blamed the drinking water for it. In the Valais, when a normal child was born congratulations were offered: "God be thanked, the child will not become a gouch." In German, a similar word, "gauch," was used in the Alps, and in English "gawk" and "gowk" are comparable terms for fools. As Cranefield pointed out, this passage suggests that the midwives of the Valais could diagnose cretinism at birth. This suggestion is of interest because in more recent times many physicians doubted that cretinism was present or recognizable at birth. In 1602, a Swiss physician, Felix Platter, wrote that he had seen in the Valais and in Carinthia (Austria) infants who were dumb, suffered from folly, had misshapen heads, huge tongues and goitrous throats.

The origin of the term "cretin" is obscure. It became a scientific term after it appeared in print in 1754 in the great French *Encyclopédie*, where it was stated that the name was given to a species of men born in the Valais in rather great numbers who carried goiters hanging down to the waist and were deaf, dumb, imbecile and insensitive to blows. These attributes were passed on to their children, but not all of them were born as cretins. It is noteworthy that the Valais was mentioned again as the region in which cretinism was prevalent and prototypal. Toward the end of the eighteenth century, Fodéré[4] stated that the word cretin comes from "chrétien," a good Christian – a pauvre chrétien incapable of committing any sin.[5,6] Other interpretations relate the term to "cretura" (creature), to "creta" (chalk, pale) and other origins.

From early days, most writers believed that *endemic cretinism* was somehow connected with endemic goiter. Goiter was called the "father" of, or the "first step" to, cretinism.[4,7] At the turn of the century, McCarrison[8] noticed that in the Himalayas cretinism arose among the Chitral people in families that had been affected by goiter for at least two or three generations. Taussig,[7] in Austria, and Eugster,[9] in Switzerland, stated that there is no cretinism without goiter of the mother. Authors disagreed on many aspects of cretinism, but none doubted that there was a close association of the two disorders. There are and were, of course, many goiter endemics without cretinism, but there was never an endemic of cretinism without prevalence of goiter in the adult population. Kelly and Snedden,[10] in an exhaustive review on the prevalence of goiter, mentioned cretinism as a resulting complication of regional goiter endemics in the following countries: Argentina, Brazil, Colombia, Guatemala, Dominican Republic, Peru, Norway, Sweden, Russia, Rumania, Switzerland, Czechoslovakia, Italy, Spain, England, France, French West Africa and Cameroun, Nigeria, Egypt, Congo, India, Burma, Malaya, Indonesia and China. These authors dealt with endemic goiter in Austria, but they did not mention cretinism in that country, although the condition was quite prevalent there in the past and still existed in 1954 (see below). In some Andean villages in Peru, visible goiter was found in the late 1960s in 52% of all persons.[75]

There is no way to estimate the incidence of cretinism in these countries, since the disorder usually is limited to rather inaccessible areas and remarkable changes can take place within one or two generations. Eggenberger,[11] in 1928, estimated that the number of cretins and half-cretins placed in Swiss institutions because of social incompetence amounted to approximately 6,000. It was not possible to estimate the number of those who were cared for by their relatives at home. The incidence of institutionalized cretins was thus greater than that of mongolism. But in contrast to mongolism, cretinism was concentrated in certain regions and villages, whereas other localities were completely free of the disorder. As a result, the burden of cretinism was disastrous in affected areas. Toward the end of the nineteenth century, in an Austrian village, 17% of the children of school age were mentally retarded or deaf-mute,[12] and in 1918 Diviak and Wagner-Jauregg[13] found in a Styrian town that more than 8% of the children were affected by cretinism. Even in 1954, I was told in a Tirolean hamlet that of 9 children who went to the first grade, 6 did not pass to the second! That was at a time when new cases of cretinism in children could not be found in Switzerland. In a Swiss village that once had been a spa located in a beautiful broad valley, Eugster,[9] in 1938, counted 3.5% full cretins and 1.5% borderline cases. In New Guinea, among the Dani people of the Mulia valley who are affected by severe goiter, Gajdusek,[14] in 1959, found mental defects, deafness and mutism in about 12% of the childhood population. These estimates illustrate the prevalence and importance of this disorder in many areas of the world. In 1962, Merke[2] wrote that there may still exist hundreds of thousands of endemic cretins in various continents, particularly in undeveloped countries.

Endemic goiter, the preliminary condition for endemic cretinism, was and is much more prevalent than cretinism. In 1958, Kelly and Snedden[10] thought that the number of goitrous people in the world probably was not far short of 200,000,000. The valleys of the high mountain masses—the Alps, Carpathians, Pyrenees, Himalayas and the Andes—are typical goiter regions. Since the topic to be discussed here is cretinism and not goiter, the reader is referred to reviews that deal with prevalence and geographic distribution of goiter.[10,15] In general, goiter endemics have receded as communications and commerce increased during the past century, but there are people still alive in civilized countries who remember that goiter was so common in their homeland that an enlarged neck was considered normal, whereas a goiter-free neck was unusual. I was told in the Savoie, France, that in a girl, two generations ago, thyroid hyperplasia was considered an attribute of beauty; a neck without anterior protrusion was called disparagingly "cou de chèvre," or goat's neck. Larger goiters, of course, were less attractive, some hanging down to the chest and others compressing the trachea or the blood vessels of the neck (Fig. 12-1), resulting in respiratory and cardiac difficulties.

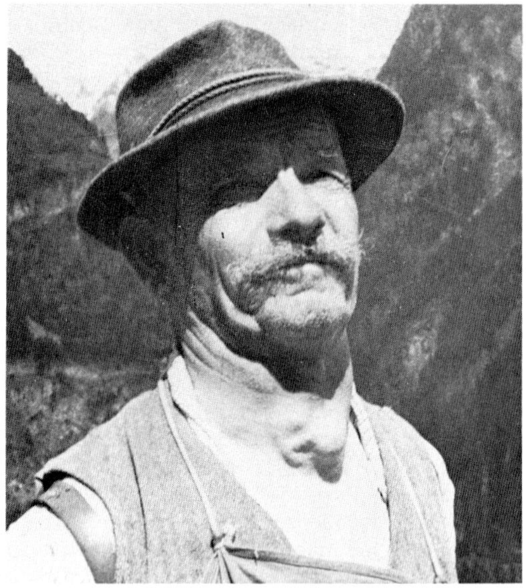

Fig. 12-1.—Dilated veins and goiter in a mentally normal Tirolean peasant who had serious respiratory difficulties.

Kelly and Snedden[10] reviewed the goiter problem of 114 countries in the Americas, Europe, Africa, Asia and Oceania in 1958 and found that endemic goiter was still prevalent in many regions. Although the endemics had receded and become localized in many instances to remote and mountainous areas, goiter remained a significant public health problem. It was found that goiter and hypothyroidism were not limited to mountainous regions. With a locally restricted diet, the danger of iodine deficiency exists right down to the seacoast. This was shown to be true for Beirut, Lebanon, where Najjar and Woodruff[16] found that 78% of children permanently residing in an orphanage were affected by goiter, whereas in a control population of similar ages 12% (boys) to 24% (girls) had goiter. The water supply was the same for the two groups, but the orphans were on a low-calorie and low-protein diet and an iodine deficiency state was demonstrated by marked avidity of the thyroids for iodine and low excretion of iodine in the urine.

Another flat region of an altitude of only 100–300 meters above sea level was investigated in 1961 by deVisscher *et al.*,[17] who studied endemic goiter in the Uele region of the Republic of Congo. There were areas in which up to 100% of the population had goiter and there were neighboring regions with milder endemics. The people affected were primitive and poor; the diet was limited, particularly in protein; salt and water were low in iodine content. Leprosy, malaria and intestinal parasites were common. All types and sizes of thyroid swellings were found. Goiter appeared at an early age and was observed occasionally in newborns and infants. Eighty per cent of the schoolchildren were goitrous, and in many cases the goiters became nodular before puberty. Hypothyroidism could be recognized in approximately 10% of the goitrous patients, who sometimes were dwarfed. "Cretinism was evident everywhere," mainly in villages far away from the centers, and all degrees of mental deficiency existed.

The endemic area found by Gajdusek[14] in 1959 in the Mulia valley (Netherlands New Guinea) is inhabited by Dani-speaking people who were still at a neolithic cultural level. About two-thirds of the females and one-fourth of the males had goiters that were either huge trilobular structures encompassing the neck or asymmetrical or nodular (Fig. 12-2). In children, there were mental defects, deafness and mutism. The entire population of the endemic area was subnormal by standards of culturally similar natives from surrounding regions. The soil of the Mulia region is extremely poor and slaty and the diet inferior to that of more fortunate neighboring tribes. Sweet potato leaves were the major staple, and Gajdusek thought that they might have a goitrogenic action. Investigations of goiter endemics in modern times are of great interest because they can answer questions raised by authors in the past when the circumstances encountered in endemic areas were more complex

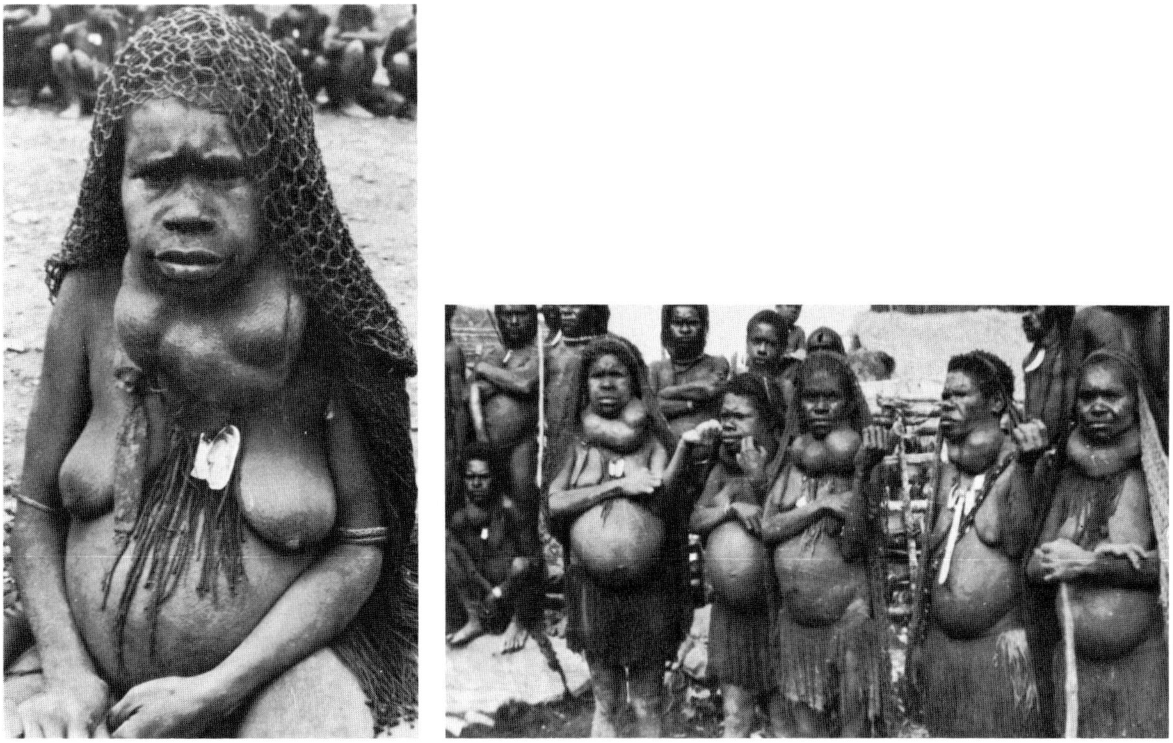

Fig. 12-2. – Goitrous neolithic people from the Mulia region, New Guinea, 1960. (Courtesy of Dr. Carleton Gajdusek, Bethesda, Md.)

and confusing than those found today. The study from Lebanon, for instance, showed that in an isolate, such as an orphanage, the goiter endemic was not due to the water supply or a local well, as asserted often in the old literature, but rather to nutritional deficiency.[16] In the Uele region of the Congo, an epidemic could be studied far from the mountains once covered by glacial ice and complicated by diseases such as leprosy, malaria and intestinal parasites.[17] The endemic in New Guinea is of interest because it affected a population that had no contact with the civilized world until 1959. This discovery speaks against Greenwald's thesis[18] that goiter is an infectious disease attributable in remote areas to the arrival of Europeans.

Endemic goiter has disappeared from the United States, but its existence in recent times should be remembered. It was still prevalent in certain areas 40 or 50 years ago. During World War I, among men drafted for service in the United States, "simple goiters" existed that were so large that military collars would not button around them.[15] In 18 states, the incidence of these huge goiters was between 5 and 27 per thousand, but these figures do not give the true picture of endemic goiter, since they do not include women and less conspicuous enlargements of the gland. Olesen,[19,20] in 1926 and 1929, published results of surveys of schoolchildren in 43 states and his figures show from 10 to 50 times as much goiter as was reported by the draft boards. One can conclude, therefore, that the 18 states heading the list of goiter incidence of drafted men were truly endemic areas.[15] Olesen's goiter map[20] shows goiter in men examined for military service most prevalent in the Pacific West and the Great Lakes Basin of the United States; it indicates that the southern states were free of the anomaly. This generally agrees (though with completely different absolute prevalence figures) with results obtained in schoolboys and schoolgirls. Only a few figures will be cited here because they may surprise the reader not yet born at the time these surveys were made. For instance, there are reports stating that in some localities of Wisconsin the percentage of goiter in boys and girls was from 90 (Ashland) to 100 (Lake Nebagamon). Girls in Terre Haute, Indiana, showed a goiter percentage figure of 82; in Torch Lake, Michigan, it was 80; in Billings, Montana, 70; in Syracuse, New York, 73; in Virgin Valley, Utah, 75; and in Charleston, West Virginia, 75. For Cincinnati, Ohio – a "borderline area" – the percentage figures in 1927 were 52 for girls and 30 for boys. Similar figures – over 50% – were cited by Marine and Kimball[21] for Akron, Ohio. In contrast, the southern states of the United States were almost free of endemic goiter although poverty was then more prevalent there than in many northern states. This is of interest because in many countries endemic goiter was attributed by some to "poverty." But there were some small endemic pockets in the South. In St. James and St. Charles parishes, Louisiana, the percentages of goiter in girls reached 72 and 68.[15]

Although endemic goiter was prevalent in many regions of the United States, there is no proof that endemic cretinism existed here. Gordon[22] stated that not a single case of true endemic cretinism has ever been reported in America. Such a general statement may be difficult to prove, and Stoddard,[23] in 1933, considered the possibility that cretinism could become endemic in Wisconsin because of the severe goiter endemic there. No doubt there were and there are goitrous cretins in the United States, but we know now that some of these are affected by inborn errors of metabolism that can result in cretinism even in regions of iodine abundance.[24]

Etiology

Since earliest times, man has searched for the causes of goiter and, long ago, travelers and writers added explanations to their descriptions of thyroid enlargement and cretinism. "Metallic and mineral waters," "fault in the waters," "waters contaminated by veins of gold, silver, lead, antimony," "coarse food," uncleanliness and excessive heat in affected valleys were named by the inhabitants or visitors. Miasmas, malaria, bacteria, intestinal parasites, toxins, domestication, filth, housing, heredity, inbreeding and many other factors were accused.[3,25] St. Lager,[26] in 1867, could enumerate 43 goiter theories.

Iodine deficiency. Iodine was discovered in 1811 by the French chemist Courtois, who found it in the waste ashes of seaweed. Soon thereafter it was recognized as an element, but it was considered to be rare. The fact that seaweed and sea sponges had been used successfully for the cure of goiter for centuries and even millenia[27] contributed, no doubt, to the introduction of iodine as a treatment for goiter by Coindet[28] as early as 1820. Although this scientist obtained some favorable results with the new element, there were also some cases that remained refractory and others that developed hyperthyroidism. For about 100 years after Coindet, iodine was given as a remedy for goiter in many forms, often in amounts 2,500–50,000 times the daily optimal dose and often with disastrous results.[11] In 1849, Prévost (cited by McClendon[15]) assumed that goiter occurred in regions in which drinking water was lacking in iodine and bromide, anticipating a deficiency theory. Chatin,[29] in 1850 and in subsequent years, systematically analyzed plants, animals, water, air, foodstuffs and soil, and he too came to the conclusion that a causal connection existed between lack of iodine in the environment and goiter; he also recognized the possibility of accessory etiologic factors[30] and arrived at a theory of the etiology of endemic goiter that seems fully valid today. Yet, his opinion and his findings were not accepted for many decades.

There was little belief in the merits of iodine until Baumann,[31] in 1895, recognized the element as an integral constituent of the thyroid gland, a discovery that gave some credence and scientific status to the "iodine superstition" of the past. In 1908, Marine and Williams[32] explained the relation of iodine to the structure of the thyroid gland and concluded that iodine deficiency was the main cause of goiter. In 1915, Kendall[33] isolated thyroxine as the active principle of the thyroid, and showed that it contained 65% iodine by weight. Other surveys followed in West Virginia and Michigan. An association could be shown between iodine deficiency of the salt used and goiter of the population.[15]

In Switzerland, Hunziker,[34] a physician in Adliswil, a town of 2,000 inhabitants, at the suggestion of a pharmacist gave "minimal doses" of iodine to some patients to reduce the size of their thyroids. He found this treatment successful and concluded that the thyroid gland requires iodine for formation of its hormone, since iodine is lost incessantly to the environment and there is a constant need for replenishment. In the absence of this necessary nutrient and in the presence of "iodine hunger," a healthy gland responds by enlargement and goiter formation. This concept, quite similar to that of Marine and Kimball,[21] was presented in a lecture in 1914 and printed at the author's expense in 1915 after rejection of the manuscript by the leading Swiss medical journal. Hunziker[34] also calculated the daily requirement of iodine (1/10th of a milligram of potassium iodide), which became the basis for artificial iodization of salt in Switzerland.

A classic and objective study of the occurrence, circulation and metabolism of iodine was made by Fellenberg.[30] Comparative examinations showed that in localities in which the inhabitants were markedly affected by goiter, the iodine content of the environment was lower than in localities spared by goiter. Differences were shown in iodine content of foodstuffs and drinking water, in minerals, soils, and so forth, for villages that were geographically closely situated. Differences in iodine availability were best demonstrated by daily iodine excretion through the urine.

In the United States, McClendon[15] showed that goiter rates were inversely correlated with the distribution of iodine. He made a comprehensive review of the occurrence of iodine in minerals, plants and animals and surveyed the prevalence of goiter and cretinism on all continents. McClendon stressed the fact that iodine is not only a drug but also an essential food constituent, and that lack of it may lead to deficiency diseases – goiter, hypothyroidism and cretinism – just as may the lack of vitamins.

Since the establishment of the iodine deficiency theory, there have always been strong opponents to it.

It is true that a beneficial effect of iodine does not prove that endemic goiter is due to lack of iodine. Greenwald[18] thought that such beneficial results obtained with the prophylactic use of iodides are due not to their rectification of a deficiency but to some pharmacodynamic action.

Although, today, few people doubt that iodine deficiency is the main factor in the etiology of goiter and cretinism, criticism of the iodine theory is useful because it points to the existence of accessory factors that may have played an important role in some endemics.

If iodine deficiency is acknowledged as the prime cause of goiter and cretinism, there remains the question of the cause of iodine deficiency itself. Geochemistry can explain the main endemics by glaciation of the affected areas during the Quaternary ice age. It is thought[35,36] that the masses of ice, melting water and fluvioglacial gravel resulted, in the course of tens of thousands of years, in iodine loss from the soil through erosion, extraction and transportation toward lowlands and the oceans, which became large iodine stores. This theory admirably fits the situations of goiter distribution in the Alps and in North America. Maps of the ice sheets that covered Canada and parts of the United States are almost identical with that of endemic goiter distribution. This fact can be used as an explanation of the existence of endemic goiter in the northern parts of the United States and its absence in southern states, which remain free of endemics despite great poverty in some segments of the population. In Switzerland, the absence of endemic goiter and cretinism in the Jura, which was not involved in the Quaternary glaciation, and their presence in other parts of the same canton (Bern) that were affected by that ice age, favor the glaciation theory also.[36] Occurrence of goiter in the Himalayas and its limitation to provinces north of the Ganges river[37] likewise can be considered in agreement with this theory.

But there are many other areas in which goiter and cretinism are or were endemic even though they were not affected by glaciation during the Quaternary ice age, Lebanon (p. 108), the Uele district of the Congo (p. 104) and numerous other goiter regions must be deficient in iodine for other reasons that are less obvious than glaciation.

The variability of iodine in air, water and foodstuffs renders it difficult to establish simple rules for the distribution of the element on earth. Even in neighboring villages, the iodine content of the soil can vary sufficiently to account for the differing incidences of goiter.[30] Changes in living conditions and habits can alter iodine intake and goiter incidence and some of these changes may go unnoticed. Although consumption of iodized salt probably is the most important factor in the decline of goiter and cretinism, administration of cod-liver oil to infants or use of Chile saltpeter as fertilizer may have contributed greatly to the same effects in many regions. The habit of eating seaweed has kept most of Japan goiter-free.

Accessory Etiologic Factors

"Water" has been blamed for goiter and its complications since early times, but there was disagreement about the reasons why some waters were goitrogenic whereas others were not. Changes of water sources often were associated with the appearance or disappearance of goiter. The water's calcium, iron, copper, fluorine, manganese or silica content was considered of importance. Others accused vitamin A deficiency, excessive intake of cabbage or related vegetables or excessive wine consumption. Infections and parasites were thought to play a role and so were fog, lack of sunshine, humidity and excessive physical effort. There were many observers who believed that the injurious agent was bound to certain houses ("cretin houses") and localities, since sometimes entire families were severely affected whereas neighbors were spared. For the same reason, heredity was considered an etiologic factor by many writers. That accessory factors play a role was shown by the fact that even in recent times goiter endemics have been described in areas in which the iodine supply was ample. There exist puzzling observations of a goiter endemic in Vietestranden, Norway,[38] where the water contained large amounts of iodine and the daily urinary iodine excretion was high. Costa[39] mentioned that in schoolchildren living in areas of endemic cretinism in northern Italy, hyperplastic thyroids occurred even though the iodine content of the drinking water and the children's daily urinary excretion of iodine were in the normal range. In Austria, a similar situation was observed in the spa Hall, where iodine supply and intake were ample, but schoolchildren living within the city showed a goiter incidence of 11% and those in surrounding localities an incidence of 50%. Although there were fewer goiters in the "iodine spa" than in the surrounding countryside, there were children in Hall who had goiter. Since water, air and food contained more iodine than average, these goiters are puzzling and one must look for a positive goitrogen[40] or other deficiencies.

The role of *calcium* as a goitrogen has a long history, which was reviewed by Taylor.[41] The question is related to the belief that hard water or "lime eating" is goitrogenic and related to the role of calcium in iodine metabolism. It has been asserted that calcium forms an insoluble compound with iodine, or that it absorbs iodine, thus preventing utilization. Other theories state that a high calcium intake leads to increased iodide excretion. It is now believed that calcium can act as an accessory goitrogenic factor if the available dietary iodine is at a critical level.

From early times, *metals* contained in water were suspected as goitrogens, and this actually is true for cobalt under certain conditions. Cobaltous chloride prescribed for correction of certain anemias occasionally has led to enlargement of the thyroid gland,[42] which subsided after cobalt treatment was stopped. In some children, cobalt can bring about goiter and even hypothyroidism, whereas in others the drug is without adverse effect. It is thought that cobalt inhibits thyroid binding of iodine[43] and that individual susceptibility is related to a defect at the enzymatic level in the conversion of inorganic iodine to thyroxine.[44]

Fluoride has been considered a goitrogen since the middle of the nineteenth century, and there have been many publications linking goiter with increased fluoride intake. But there were other observations that could not confirm such an association. Wespi[45] found that addition of sodium fluoride to iodized salt during pregnancy had no goitrogenic effect on the newborn. He admitted that a certain antagonism between fluorine and iodine is possible but that it would become manifest only in the presence of iodine deficiency or thyroid disturbances.

Many investigations dealt with *organic goitrogenic agents* occurring naturally.[46] It has been known since 1928 (Chesney *et al.*[47]) that cabbage can be goitrogenic in rabbits, and several years later it was found that seeds of cabbage, rutabaga, rape and mustards produced thyroid enlargement in rats.[48] Similarly, soybeans, soy flour and peanuts proved goitrogenic in rats.[37] Turnips fed to pregnant ewes brought about congenital goiter in lambs. Experiments showed that some of these goitrogens are species-specific and therefore do not necessarily act in man. Some studies demonstrated that yellow turnips and rutabagas have antithyroid activity, whereas cabbage has not.[46] Soybean milk has been found to be goitrogenic in infants, yet it seems that this effect is not due to a goitrogenic substance but rather to iodine deficiency.[49] A thyroid-blocking agent in the etiology of endemic goiter of children was reported from Tasmania by Clements and Wishart.[50] There, increased consumption of milk and introduction of kale as a food for cows led to ingestion by children of a substance that interfered with the uptake of ^{131}I and led to thyroid increase. Astwood *et al.*[51] demonstrated a goitrogenic compound, 5-vinyl-2-thiooxazolidone, in the rutabaga, and Greer found this "goitrin" present in relatively large amounts of kale, from where it could get into milk. It was thought that the only edible materials in which goitrin had been found in amounts sufficient to make it potentially goitrogenic for man are rutabagas and turnips.[46]

One of the accessory factors in goitrogenesis may be *vitamin A deficiency*. It has long been known that goiter epidemics and night blindness can occur together, particularly in certain military, civilian and religious residences. It is not difficult to understand such outbreaks, which have been observed repeatedly – even in recent times. Inadequate nutrition could lead to both iodine deficiency and vitamin A deficiency. A goiter wave in Bavaria in 1948 was reported by Haubold[52] affecting more than 70% of the indigenous children and sparing completely the children of the American occupation troops who lived in the same locality but who had different diets (and possibly different salt) bought in military supply stores. Horvat and Maver[53] described a goiter endemic on the island of Krk in Yugoslavia, with average incidence figures of 62% in girls and 54% in boys in certain localities, although fish was a constant item of food. It was concluded that dietary lack of iodine did not play a major role in the etiology of goiter on the island, but there was parallelism of vitamin A intake and absence of goiter. Administration of 3,000 I.U. of vitamin A daily for 3 months resulted in a decrease of goiter incidence from 66% to 37%.

Relationships of thyroid and vitamin A were examined by Eggenberger,[54] who pointed out peripheral antagonisms of thyroxine and vitamin A and synergistic effects in the thyroid. He found a certain parallelism of abnormal dark adaptation of mothers and of goiter in their newborn infants. He concluded that vitamin A deficiency contributed to goitrogenesis in endemic areas of Switzerland but that, in the presence of ample iodine supply, vitamin A-deficiency goiters do not develop.

Since endemic cretinism has a tendency to occur repeatedly in families, *heredity* often was suspected in the past. Before medical genetics was developed, such suspicions were based on superficial observations only. Today, it would appear plausible that families differ greatly in thyroid physiology, so that some have glands that can function in the presence of moderate iodine deficiency, whereas others respond by thyroid hyperplasia and failure.[77] It is known that cretinism can develop in areas with adequate and rich iodine supplies because of inborn errors of metabolism (p. 441). But there is no proof that genetic factors play an important role in the etiology of endemic cretinism. When Eugster[9] re-examined the question in 1938, he could not find proof for Mendelian inheritance. There were many examples of cretin children born to normal parents and sometimes there were normal children born to cretinoid parents, so that dominant transmission did not seem likely. Recessive inheritance was also ruled out. Although there often were several cretin siblings in the same family, sometimes there were normal children resulting from matings in which both parents were cretinoid. Cretinoid fathers had normal children if the mothers were normal. Parental consanguinity was not more frequent than in the general population. Of 9 monozygotic twins, 6 were concordant and 3 discordant. Of 15 dizygotic twins, 10 were concordant and 5 discordant.

Eugster's findings did not reveal the importance of genetic factors, but it seems that, in Lebanon, heredity played a role in some cases of endemic goiter and hypothyroidism. Najjar and Woodruff[16] examined 47 hypothyroid children in that endemic area. There was a low incidence of athyreosis, the sex ratio failed to show the predominance of females usual in athyreosis (p. 439) and the familial incidence was high. The consanguinity rate was 53%, which was higher than that of a control population. It seems likely that both iodine deficiency and inborn errors of thyroid metabolism combined in the etiology of hypothyroidism in that area.[55]

Although genetic predisposition may play a role in the etiology of endemic goiter and cretinism, it probably results in pathologic manifestations only in the presence of iodine deficiency. If iodine supply is ample, the assumed genetic weakness does not manifest itself, as demonstrated in the disappearance of the endemics in areas in which inbreeding persists (p. 119).

Eugster[9] confirmed many older observations concerning the roles of *maternal and external environments*.[8] The mothers of cretins always had goiters, usually nodular or cystic. The sibships in which cretins occurred were large, averaging 7, and about one-third of the mothers of cretins had 10 children or more. Abortions and stillbirths were frequent, and there was an increasing risk of cretinism with increasing birth order. These observations point to the importance of maternal factors in the etiology of cretinism.

Change of domicile influenced the outcome of pregnancies. Emigration from the endemic area resulted in normal children even if the parents showed cretinoid symptoms. Immigration of healthy parents into an endemic area did not lead to cretinism in the first filial generation, but there was cretinism in the second generation. Eugster's findings confirm many older statements to this effect: ". . . it has been constantly observed that when a new family moves into a goitrous district, goitre appears in the first generation, cretinism in the second" (*Encyclopaedia Britannica*, Eleventh Edition, 1911). It seems as if a woman had to be exposed to the goitrogenic environment from birth on to induce the adverse conditions that resulted in cretinism of her children. Although the abnormal maternal thyroid seems most likely to be the injurious factor that brings about cretinism in the offspring, Eugster[9] found no close correlation between the type of goiter in the mothers and the degree of cretinism in their children. Occasionally, a mother who had had one or more cretin children gave birth to a normal child subsequently. The placentas as well as abnormal thyroid hormones were considered as possible factors endangering the fetus, but there was no proof for these opinions.

The role of chronic *infections* in the endemics remains unexplained. A parallelism of infections such as malaria, leprosy, intestinal parasites, and so on, and incidence of endemic thyroid disorders has been observed repeatedly, but this could be coincidental. In the United States, malaria, leprosy and parasitic infections were more frequent in the South than in the North, but the incidences of goiter were reversed.

That acute infections may lead to loss of iodine was shown by Fellenberg,[30] who demonstrated that fever could bring about a markedly increased urinary iodine excretion. But this factor probably was of little significance in the etiology of cretinism and goiter.

Pathogenesis

The association of maternal goiter with endemic cretinism is well established, but there is no satisfactory explanation for the association.

Endemic cretinism could be a form of hypothyroidism due to postnatal iodine deficiency. If this were true, all cretins should show thyroid hyperplasia in early childhood, curable by administration of small doses of iodine. This concept is not tenable and has no adherents at present. It is true that some cretin children have hyperplastic thyroids that become smaller after iodine treatment, but this does not cure their mental deficiency or their deafness.

Are endemic cretins irreversibly damaged at the time of birth? This question may be debatable in such mild endemics as those observed in modern times in advanced countries, but in severe endemics there was and is no doubt that most cretins are hopeless creatures by the time they are born. As mentioned before (p. 103), in the Valais, 300 years ago, the women could recognize cretins immediately after birth. In 1912, Taussig[7] asserted that cretinism was congenital even though the appearance of symptoms often was delayed to the end of the first year. The parents of full cretins often reported that their child had been born both "obese" and with a large tongue, that it slept much and was apathetic from birth on. A goitrous stillborn full cretin, the child of a goitrous cretin mother, was described by Gamper[56] in 1928. Observers of cretinism, dealing with improving conditions in Europe in this century, reported diverse findings. Diviak and Wagner-Jauregg[13] examined all newborn children in Zeltweg, a village in Styria, where 8% of the children developed cretinism. In some of these children, saddle nose, large tongue, goiter, swelling of the skin, pallor, eczema and umbilical hernia permitted an early diagnosis. In others, cretinism could not be recognized during the first months of life. But absence of early symptoms does not exclude the possibility that endemic cretinism is congenital. Even athyreotic sporadic cretins appear normal at birth and develop the typical disease picture during the first months of postnatal life. The endemic cretin is never born without any thyroid tissue, as was shown in the few cases in which the glands of neonates were histologically examined. Eugster[57] described the thyroid of a 2-month-old child whose mother had had a nodular goiter. This child was small, had typical cretinoid features and retarded ossification. The thyroid was in situ but had signs of atrophy and sclerosis. In a few other cases, struma diffusa parenchymatosa was present at birth, but these hyperplastic thyroids were made up of epithelial cells with nuclei of irregular size and shape, indicating prenatal damage.

As stated before, whether there is little functioning

thyroid tissue or only remnants or thyroid hyperplasia, the glandular deficiency cannot be greater than that of athyreosis as seen in sporadic cretins. Yet, thyroid treatment of endemic cretins is less successful than that of the athyreotic cretin. These observations speak against the belief that endemic cretinism is simple hypothyroidism. There is proof that tissues other than the thyroid are congenitally damaged at birth. Lotmar[58] found in the brain and cerebellum of cretins changes that suggest developmental disturbances between the second and last third of fetal life. There are also observations that point to prenatal damage of the ear.[59,60] These changes explain the irreparability of cerebral and aural functions by iodine or thyroid treatment after birth.

If endemic cretinism commences in prenatal life, one must ask how and when the fetus is damaged. Some investigators assume that iodine deficiency renders the fetal thyroid abnormal, damaging, by some unknown mechanism, the brain and ear of the unborn child. Since such irreparable damages usually do not occur in athyreosis, this explanation does not hold. An alternative explanation is that the injuries of the fetus are due to disorders of the mother or of other ancestors. There were many observations that emphasized that endemic cretinism did not appear in the first generation of immigrants into endemic areas, and that the disorder occurred only in the second or subsequent generations. The remote possibility of gene or chromosome mutations by severe thyroid disease can be ruled out because of the disappearance of endemic cretinism soon after the introduction of goiter prophylaxis. It is much more likely that endemic cretinism, with its congenital brain damage and deafness, is due to the mother's thyroid disease, which could affect the fetus in utero.

There are now many examples of maternal disorders that can damage the unborn child. The mother's thyroid deficiency or toxic products of the gland could cause prenatal brain damage and aural injuries. There is also the possibility of maternal antithyroid immune reactions interfering with normal fetal development. There is general agreement that endemic cretinism does not arise without maternal goiter, usually cystic or nodular in type. The thyroid changes progress with age and repeated pregnancies. Eugster[9] pointed out that the risk for cretinous children increased with advancing age of the mother and for late-born children. His findings point to maternal thyroid disease as the most likely cause of the postnatally incurable symptoms of endemic cretinism.

Endemic cretinism disappears when iodized salt is distributed in an affected population. Such treatment improves thyroid hyperplasia but does not cure adenomatous and cystic goiters – the forms usually seen in mothers and cretins. Does iodine treatment of women with such goiters prevent cretinism in their children? Eggenberger[11] stated that the newborn death rate due to thyroid disease decreased promptly after introduction of iodized salt. But there are no good observations demonstrating that mothers with goiter who had given birth to cretins regularly bore normal children after receiving iodine prophylaxis. In such cases, the unborn children would receive iodine and develop normal thyroids, whereas the mothers' thyroids would remain deranged. There are no definitive statements to tell us whether cretinism can be eradicated in one generation or whether it takes two, i.e., raising of goiter-free girls who, when grown up, produce only normal children. Even Eggenberger, one of the most outspoken and optimistic advocates of iodine prophylaxis, admitted that it might take two generations to wipe out endemic cretinism. This seems to be the case. After iodized salt or other prophylactic measures are introduced and children grow up without goiter, their children are entirely free from endemic cretinism (p. 117).

The concept of maternal iodine deficiency and thyroid dysfunction as the cause of endemic cretinism resolves a controversy that has persisted for at least two generations.[9,11,39,61] Endemic cretinism cannot be simply equated with hypothyroidism nor should it be considered an ill-defined "constitutional" disease unassociated with iodine deficiency. A model from experimental teratology may exemplify our view. Vitamin A deficiency of pregnant female rats results in young with multiple congenital malformations. These malformations cannot be equated with the symptoms of postnatal vitamin A deficiency, but it would be wrong to say that they have no connection with vitamin A deficiency. Just as vitamin A deficiency manifests itself completely differently in the unborn rat from that of rats after birth, iodine deficiency manifests itself in the unborn child differently from that of persons exposed to iodine deficiency after they are born. In the case of endemic cretinism, the situation was complicated by the fact that children already damaged in utero often were also raised in an iodine-deficient milieu, acquiring thyroid hyperplasia if there was thyroid tissue present. Thyroid pathology was only a part of the syndrome of endemic cretinism – and usually not the most important one. Prenatal cerebral and aural defects were more important because they could not be removed by substitution therapy.

It would be desirable to study the pathogenesis of endemic cretinism in animal experiments, but so far it has not been possible to obtain a model that simulates the disease picture of endemic cretinism. In rats, prenatal iodine deficiency produces fetal thyroid hyperplasia but not cretinism. Even if iodine deficiency continues in postnatal life, the animals develop normally and can reproduce even though they have chronic thyroid hyperplasia. We have raised and bred such goitrous rats through several generations without inducing signs of thyroid deficiency or cretinism.

Experimental production of pathologic thyroids in the offspring of treated mothers has been achieved in mice.[62] When pregnant animals received radioactive iodine (^{131}I) after the seventeenth day of gestation –

the point at which fetal thyroids begin to develop follicles—neonatal growth was retarded in the young. But, later, their reproductive performance was normal, at least in the male offspring. It was possibly impaired in the females. The thyroids of the offspring showed pathologic changes such as fibrosis and follicular destruction, but there followed compensatory hyperplasia with adenoma formation and development of colloid goiters. Despite these changes and subsequent progression of the pathologic process, there were no demonstrable functional disturbances in the offspring. There is no proof that endemic cretinism was produced in the young.

Smith *et al.*[63] induced congenital hypothyroidism in puppies by administration of radioactive iodine to pregnant dogs 3, 9 or 10 days before delivery. The neonatal mortality was high and the surviving puppies grew slowly and were lethargic. They had short bowlegs and potbellies. The skin was coarse, dry, redundant and tough. The puppies did not play together, were not active and did not bark. Ossification was delayed and the blood chemical values indicated hypothyroidism. In puppies that were dissected there was replacement of thyroid by areolar tissue, with occasional islands of fetal thyroid tissue. These hypothyroid dogs behaved like thyroidectomized or athyreotic creatures.

Symptomatology

In most patients, physical and mental retardation is noticeable during the first 2 years. Eruption of teeth is always delayed and the anterior fontanelle remains open beyond normal closure time. Retardation of ossification centers can be demonstrated in roentgenograms. Growth in height is unsatisfactory, particularly in the second half of childhood.[13] In some cases, the thyroid is small or atrophic from birth on. Patients with atrophic thyroids remain dwarfed or small; the degree of growth retardation depends on remnants of thyroid tissue. In other infants, goiter is present at birth, and in approximately one-fourth of the endemic cretins thyroid enlargement develops during childhood. The thyroid becomes visible if it surpasses a weight of about 8 Gm. In endemic areas, goiters weighing 50 or even 100 Gm. have been observed in infants.[11] Such goiters can cause difficulties in delivery or suffocation after birth. Dyspnea, stridor and cardiac failure may lead to early death. Most goiters are hyperplastic and hyperemic without formation of follicles, but early atrophy can occur.

During the second year, it is noticed that the cretinous child does not walk or talk and the skin may become myxedematous. Subsequently, mental and physical development show further retardation and regular schooling is impossible.

The cranium usually is brachycephalic and its capacity somewhat reduced. Dentition is delayed and malocclusion not rare. Centers of ossification appear late in dwarf cretins. The hand is short and broad. There is marked brachydactyly, with particular shortness of the thumb.[64] In roentgenograms, the long bones are plump and the metaphyses show transverse growth lines. The hip joint often is abnormal. The caput femoris is characterized by delayed ossification and apparent fragmentation. It develops into a flat and dented plate sitting on a shortened femoral neck that moves in a flat and deformed acetabulum. Osteoarthritis deformans is common. The pelvis is narrow, presenting difficulties in childbirth not only in cretinous women but also in many mentally normal women living in endemic areas. Eggenberger[11] stated that more than 10% of all deliveries were pathologic in the canton of Appenzell, so that one wonders how much the narrow pelvis contributed to infant mortality, neuromuscular disease and mental retardation in such regions.

With increasing age, the symptoms become more striking. Dwarf cretins with atrophic thyroids reach heights of only 110–130 cm. (Fig. 12-3), whereas goitrous cretins can attain near normal height (Fig. 12-4). The head and trunk are relatively large, the extremities short. The myxedematous skin becomes wrinkled and yellowish brown. The hairs are coarse and turn gray late. Beards develop only rarely in male full cretins. The nails show trophic disturbances.

Cretinism in Europe was similar to that in other races, regions and continents. Bastenie *et al.*,[65] describing cretins in the flat and low-lying Uele district of the Congo, pointed out the stunted growth, large head, large, widely separated orbits, flat nose, protruding lips, underdeveloped mandible, short neck, protruding abdomen, umbilical hernia, increased lumbar lordosis, dry skin, sparse hair and delayed sexual development. Puffiness of the face, enlargement of the tongue, coldness of the skin, delayed ossification, enlarged sella turcica and speech difficulties were variably expressed. Mental retardation paralleled the physical clinical signs. In only one-fifth of the cretins examined could the thyroid be felt.

The *thyroids* of endemic cretins are quite variable. De Quervain and Wegelin[6] emphasized that goitrous and nongoitrous endemic cretinism must be distinguished; but transitional types exist. Nongoitrous cretins have thyroid glands that were reduced by early or late atrophy. Approximately two-thirds of the cretins of the canton Bern had goiters. Goitrous and nongoitrous cretins can occur in the same family.

Atrophy of cretin thyroids can be so marked that the entire organ weighs as little as 5–15 Gm. The follicles, if present, are small or replaced by solid epithelial areas. The epithelial cells vary, are sometimes small and flat, sometimes large and swollen. The cell borders are indistinct, the nuclei vary in size, shape and chromatin content. The cytoplasm often contains large amounts of lipid deposits, fat and free vacuoles. Colloid, if present, seems to be thick, mostly basophilic in the center and eosinophilic in the marginal parts, appearing old and unused. The connective tissue is much augmented. In general, the blood supply

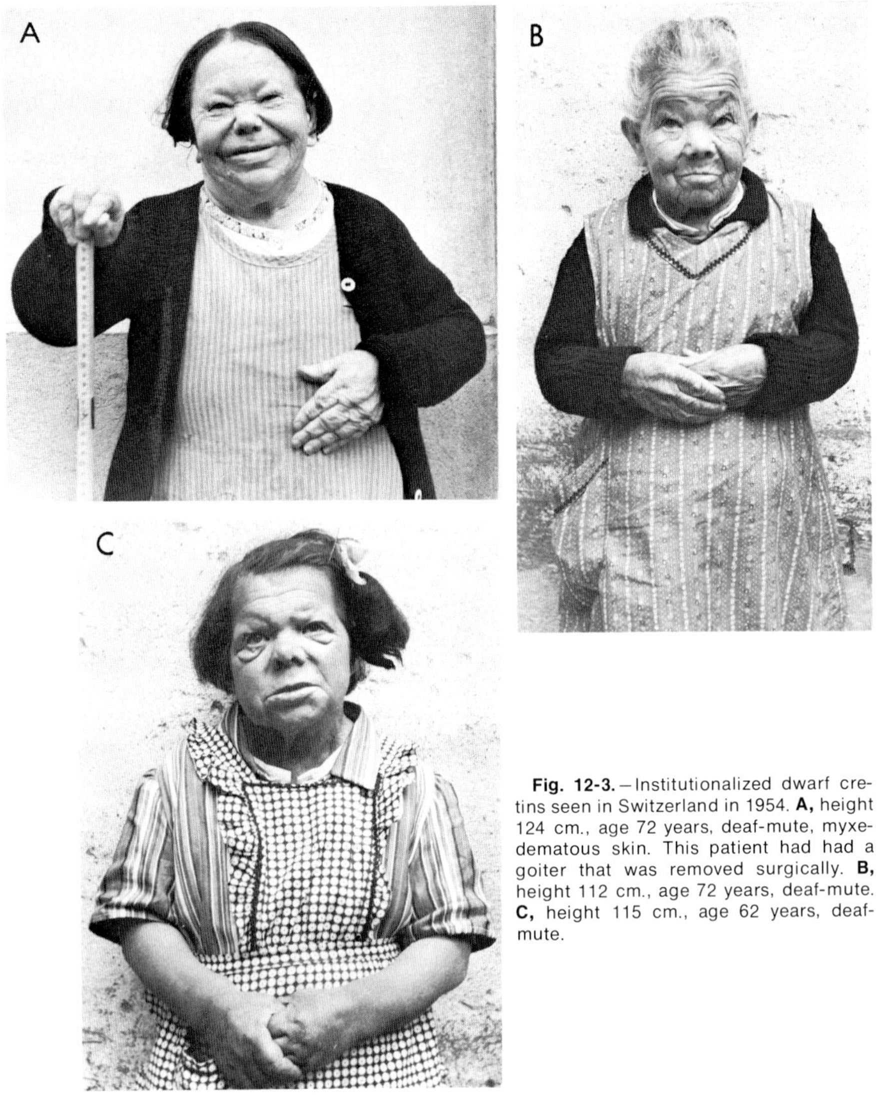

Fig. 12-3.—Institutionalized dwarf cretins seen in Switzerland in 1954. **A,** height 124 cm., age 72 years, deaf-mute, myxedematous skin. This patient had had a goiter that was removed surgically. **B,** height 112 cm., age 72 years, deaf-mute. **C,** height 115 cm., age 62 years, deaf-mute.

seems sufficient in both atrophic and goitrous glands. Even the sclerotic cretin thyroid shows regenerative epithelial foci that form small vesicles containing thin eosinophilic colloid with vacuoles and small cysts. Such foci can develop into nodular adenomas that compress the surrounding thyroid tissue.

The cretin goiter is, in most cases, an adenomatous goiter and not a diffuse hyperplastic struma. In the epithelia of the nodes, the same degenerative processes occur as in the atrophic cretin thyroid. Also, in the nodes there are regressive changes with hyalin degeneration, secondary fat deposits and calcifications, particularly around the blood vessels. Most nodes are parenchymatous and only rarely colloidal.

In young cretins, one often sees a diffuse goiter, free of adenomatous nodes. The histologic picture of such goiters corresponds to a struma diffusa parenchymatosa, rich in cells but poor in colloid. Such strumas are not necessarily functionally inferior. In fact, one could suspect that they are overactive. However, even these active thyroids have some signs of degeneration and nuclear changes. But such changes are not limited to cretinism, since they also occur in mentally normal persons with enlarged thyroids (see Figs. 12-1, 12-6 and 12-8).

These observations show that there is no typical thyroid of cretinism, although an inclination of the glandular tissue to degeneration can always be recognized. Degeneration can occur early during childhood, and sometimes there is atrophy and sclerosis in young cretins.[6]

Pathophysiologic investigations of the thyroid in endemic cretins also point to variability and yield contradictory results. Costa *et al.*[66] found in northern

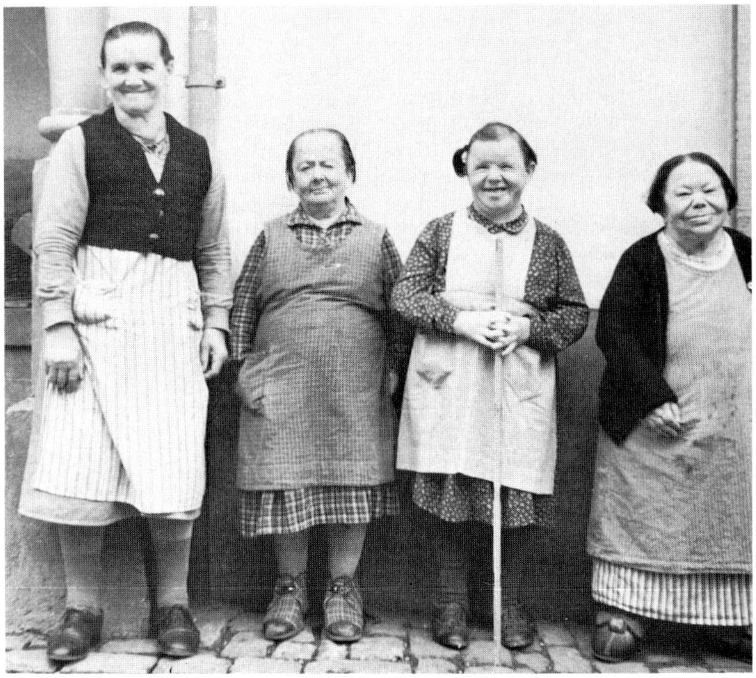

Fig. 12-4.—Four institutionalized cretins. A goitrous cretin (**left**) is of near-normal height (156 cm.). The woman holding the yardstick shows, in addition to cretinism, features of Down syndrome. (Riggisberg, Switzerland, 1954.)

Italy a normal and often an increased basal metabolism, normal or subnormal blood cholesterol values and normal serum protein-bound iodine levels (doubled after treatment with TSH). The thyroid radioiodine uptake was prompt and high, and these authors considered the endocrine metabolism of endemic cretinism as clearly distinct from that of hypothyroidism. Costa[39] objected not only to the concept of endemic cretinism as hypothyroidism but also to the theory that the disorder is caused by iodine deficiency.

In contrast to Costa *et al.*,[66] Bastenie *et al.*[65] reported from the Uele region in the Congo that the levels of plasma protein-bound ^{127}I were extremely low. There was reduced thyroidal ^{131}I uptake and a poor response to stimulation with TSH. There was a normal ratio of butanol extractable ^{131}I to protein-bound ^{131}I, a relatively high plasma level of protein-bound ^{131}I and there was thyroxine present in the plasma. These authors suggested that iodine deficiency plays a major role in the etiology of endemic cretinism.

In the majority of cases of endemic cretinism, the anterior lobe of the *pituitary* is hyperplastic and the sella turcica enlarged.[6] Histologically, one sees large cells that resemble pregnancy cells but which are, in fact, "thyroidectomy cells." The nuclei of these cells are irregular in size and shape and give way, with increasing age, to smaller eosinophilic cells. The size of the gland becomes reduced but the sella remains enlarged. The cretin pituitary resembles that of the athyreotic cretin. In contrast to these findings is the report by Costa *et al.*,[66] who considered the sella normal in size.

The *thymus* is found to be small and involuted in a number of cases. But most of the patients dissected died after protracted diseases or during adult life. The reduction in size of the organ, therefore, is not necessarily connected with the cretinism.

Neuromuscular deficiencies contribute to the cretin's abnormal posture and gait. They also play a role in the marked tendency to hernias. In the most severe cases, locomotion is completely absent, as the patients do not learn to sit or walk. But such cases have become extremely rare. Most cretins can walk, but they learn to do so late, move slowly and develop a waddling gait. Muscle tone sometimes is increased, but focal symptoms and seizures are rare. Cerebral palsy is exceptional and probably coincidental. Strabismus and hyperopia seem to be rather frequent; early opacification of the lens has been observed.

In India, McCarrison[8] observed a syndrome of "nervous cretinism." In addition to deaf-mutism, there occurred in one-third of the cretins symptoms of tetany, spasticity, cerebral diplegia, with increased patellar reflexes and loss of cutaneous sensibility; there were tremors, nystagmus and strabismus in some cases. These symptoms could be explained by prolonged and difficult labor undergone by some of the cretins. In the Alps, de Quervain and Wegelin[6] observed increased tendon reflexes in approximately one-half of the cretins, but there were no signs of tetany and the calcium level in the blood was normal. In the older literature, various brain anomalies were attributed to endemic cretinism because they were encountered in an endemic region, but the internal hydrocephaly described by early authors was not seen by de Quervain and Wegelin,[6] who found the brains of endemic cretins macroscopically normal. Microscopic changes due to developmental arrest were observed by Lotmar[58] in the cerebral cortex, which, although of normal thickness, showed alterations in the ganglion cells and in the fibers. There were ectopic cell accumulations and deformed pyramidal cells interpreted as anomalies of fetal origin. Ectopic Purkinje cells and other deviations of the cerebellar cortex were also described. In addition to developmental disturbances, Lotmar found degenerative processes that could not be attributed to advanced age or terminal disease. It is of interest that similar changes of prenatal origin were noted in the brains of some athyreotic cretins, which may explain that in some of these patients thyroid treatment does not result in normal mentality.[67]

Deaf-mutism or *deafness* is a regular symptom of endemic cretinism. Many anatomic studies have been made of the auditory apparatus, and changes were found chiefly in the middle ear. Thickening of the promontory, the roof, the ossicles, the periosteum and the mucous membranes of the middle ear reduced the tympanic spaces, and the mastoid process remained

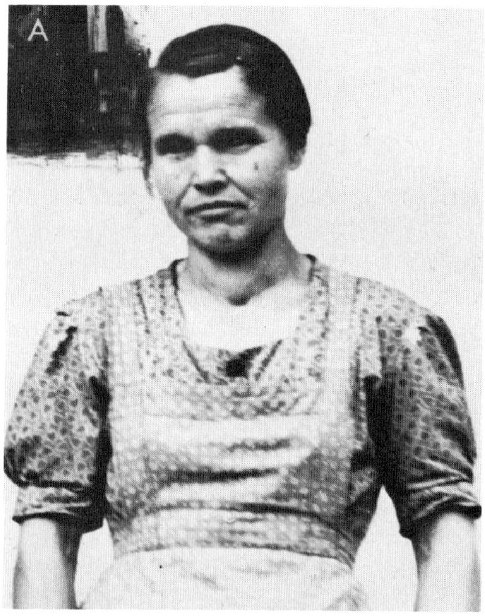

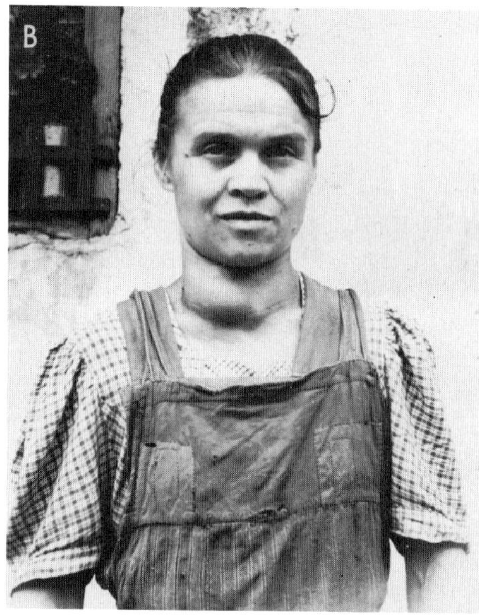

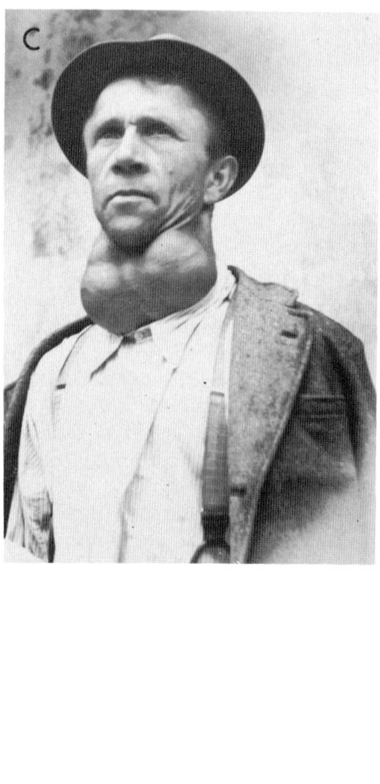

Fig. 12-5.—Three siblings, children of goitrous parents. There were 5 siblings in this family; the oldest and youngest brothers were said to be normal. **A,** 40 years of age, small stature, nodular goiter, speech defect, but lively facial expression. She had 2 children, 1 with goiter. **B,** cretin, 38 years of age, small stature, typical posture, nodular goiter, speech unintelligible, deaf. **C,** brother with huge goiter, small stature, but no signs of hypothyroidism; he was an active farm worker and could hear and talk. (Tirol, 1954.)

undeveloped and without cavitation. Changes in the inner ear were less characteristic, but some degenerative signs were seen in the cochlea. Whether the aural changes are to be considered as malformations dating back to fetal life[59,60] or as the result of secondary degeneration[11] has been debated. The important fact is that deafness is not correctable by thyroid treatment after birth, which points to a prenatal origin and speaks against its explanation by thyroid deficiency in postnatal life. Furthermore, there are many observations that show that the athyreotic, sporadic cretin's hearing is satisfactory and that these patients do not have anomalies in the middle ear like endemic cretins.[59] There exists some unexplained connection between thyroid anomalies and deafness, as manifested in their association in endemic cretinism and also in the genetically determined Pendred syndrome[78] (p. 442).

Mental development is delayed and incomplete. Cretins are described as slow in activity and reactivity. Intellectually, all degrees from mediocrity to idiocy occur. Description of "the mentality" of the cretin is, therefore, impossible. Yet, lack of imagination and initiative is a common finding. Caution, conservatism and ability to imitate make them socially good "subjects." They are generally good-natured but occasionally their wrath can be aroused. Some cretins show a tendency to collect various objects, including money, but few have a desire to work. There is a general impression that cretins have a good sense of local orientation and that they can find their way home at any time of day or night. Gratitude is another favorable trait.[6]

An interesting observation was made in the Swiss canton of Bern, where, in the endemic areas, mental retardation was almost three times as frequent as in the Jura, where goiter was rare.

As a rule, goitrous cretins learn better than those with atrophic thyroids, but their learning capacity is nonetheless limited. In endemic areas, goiter is seen in mentally normal and in some cretinous persons. In the same family, some children with goiter may be good students, whereas others are cretinous (Fig. 12-6). In such situations, it is possible that any type of mental retardation, if combined with goiter, is mistaken for cretinism, and erroneous diagnoses probably were made often in the past. But such exceptional errors should not cast doubt on the descriptions and statements of older authors, who were generally correct in their diagnosis of cretins and cretinism.

Various classifications have been attempted for mental and social achievements of endemic cretins. In endemic areas, one sees many mildly affected persons who are employed in agriculture or handicrafts, support themselves and sometimes are married. They may learn to read and write in school, but often forget these accomplishments soon after their education is terminated. Such cretinoid persons or cretins of the first degree[6] gradually blend into the normal population or into the group of cretins of the second degree, who are much more affected. These cannot do regular work and they are just barely capable of some primitive communication with their environment. The third degree of cretinism corresponds to the full-cretins who do not talk, are often deaf and remain limited to the house or institution to which they are committed. They represent the striking disease picture that usually is described as endemic cretinism and is seen only in areas of severe goiter endemics. They resemble untreated, athyreotic, sporadic cretins. Since some of

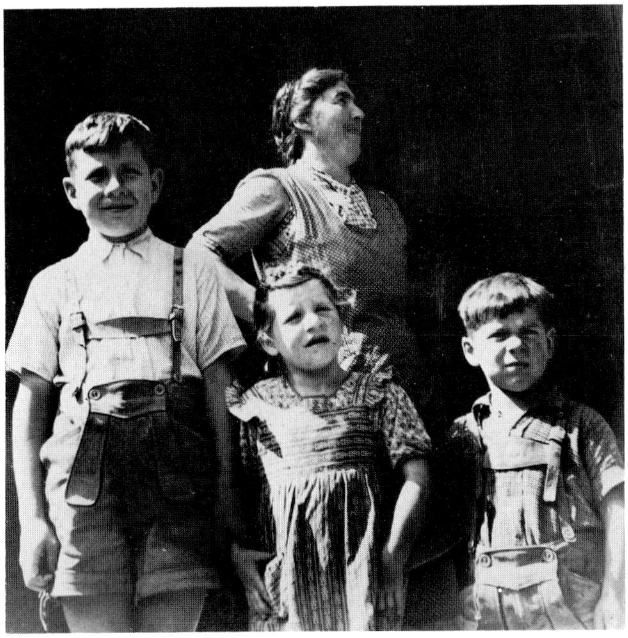

Fig. 12-6.—Goitrous mother and her children. The girl was small, mentally retarded and had no goiter. The boys, intelligent, had goiters. (Tirol, 1954.)

them have thyroid remnants of various sizes and function, a certain variability of symptoms can be expected.

The most complete descriptions of cretins are those of adults in whom the deviations from the normal are most pronounced and signs of secondary degeneration complicate the disease picture.

The *sex development* is variable. Signs of puberty usually are less expressed in cretins than in normal youths. Many cretins, particularly the nongoitrous dwarf cretins, fail to mature. Male full-cretins have no sexual drive, but male half-cretins sometimes are married and are capable of procreation (p. 122). Females who are not too severely affected can become pregnant and sometimes prove quite fertile. There are many examples of matings between normal and cretinous people and of cretinoids with each other.

Life expectancy is good for cretins who have reached the adult stage. Living in a favorable environment, they can reach old age (see Fig. 12-3).

Treatment

Iodine and thyroid treatment have been recommended. Iodine treatment can improve only those conditions that are due to lack of hormone production by an iodine-starved thyroid capable of normal function. If the gland is atrophic or made up of degenerated tissue only, iodine administration cannot be successful. There are reports that favorable effects have been observed in mild cases of cretinism. No doubt a hyperplastic thyroid can be reduced in size by intake of iodine (Fig. 12-7, *A*), but this does not render a cretin normal.

Thyroid tablets administered during childhood can improve growth, ossification and sexual development. There are reports of mental improvement but none concerning improved hearing. Evaluation of favorable reports is difficult, since the diagnosis of endemic cretinism is dubious in early childhood and one has to rely on the impressions of the writers. There is general agreement that thyroid treatment is not effective in adult full-cretins except that some symptoms of hypothyroidism, such as myxedema, can be alleviated. There are also reports of adverse effects of thyroid treatment that have been ascribed to overdosage of iodine and thyroid.[11]

Neither thyroid nor iodine treatment of endemic cretinism has resulted in spectacular successes comparable to those observed in the treatment of sporadic athyreosis with thyroid medication.

Prevention

Various methods of active prevention of endemic goiter and cretinism are available. The use of iodized salt is the method of choice. It is of interest that Boussingault, a French agricultural chemist, as early as 1831 – that is, 20 years after the discovery of iodine by Courtois – recommended to the government of Colom-

Fig. 12-7. – Siblings with moderate cretinism. The mother had "3 goiters" (trilobar goiter). **A,** the girl, 17 years of age, talked with difficulty and was hard to understand. Her goiter had been larger but became reduced in size when she took iodized salt for 6 months. **B,** her brother, 24 years of age, speech defect, moderate goiter, somewhat wrinkled skin. (Tirol, 1954.)

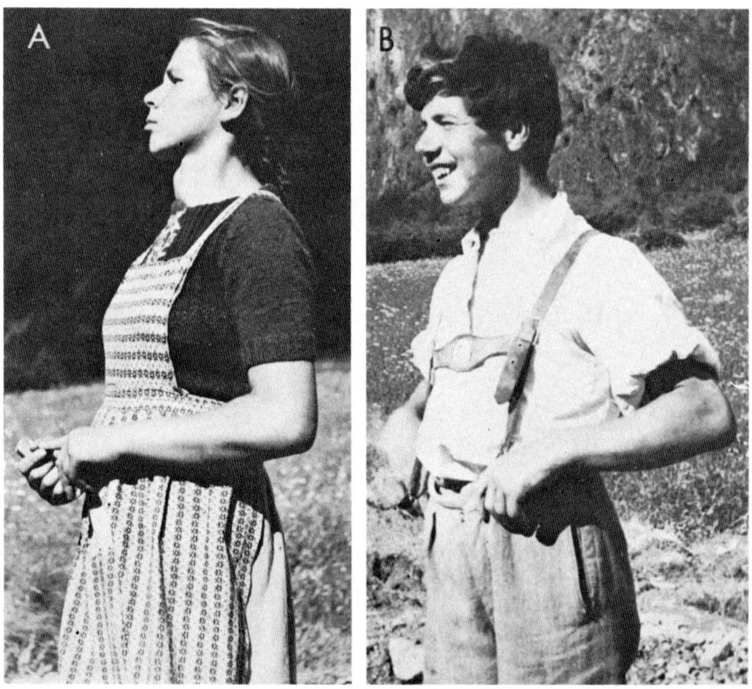

bia, South America, that iodized salt be sold by the government to prevent goiter.[10] He had found that the salt preferred by inhabitants of goitrous localities contained more iodine than salt considered ineffective. In Austria, Köstl,[68] in 1855, considered endemic cretinism a subject of public health care, and he recommended either iodine-containing sea salt or the addition of potassium iodide to rock salt as a prophylactic measure. Supplementation of salt by iodine to make up for the iodine deficiency of foodstuffs was again recommended in 1898 by Wagner-Jauregg[69] of Vienna. In the United States, it was Marine and Kimball[21] who began prophylactic experiments in Akron, Ohio, schoolchildren, not with iodized salt but with sodium iodide tablets. In Switzerland, in 1917, Bayard[70] used iodized salt in three mountain communities of the canton of Valais, and Eggenberger[11] introduced iodized salt into the canton of Appenzell in 1922. Wherever iodized salt was generally used, cretinism and simple goiter receded rapidly. There was and is a wide variation in the levels of iodization officially recommended. For instance, 1 part of iodide per 10,000 parts of salt is the level used in the United States and Canada, whereas in Switzerland the level is 1 part of potassium iodide per 100,000 parts of salt. Other countries use levels in between. To avoid the uncertainties of iodized salt intake, injections of iodized oil are now given for prophylaxis and treatment.[75,76]

This is the official and brief story of the eradication of endemic cretinism, but it is not the full story. The slow progress and the devious course of the fight against cretinism would make a worthy subject for a study of the obstacles encountered in the translation of scientific knowledge into practical measures. Thus, for instance, it was not until relatively recently that active steps were taken to stamp out by means of iodized salt the serious goiter and cretinism endemic in some valleys of Colombia, where 120 years before Boussingault had recommended a useful prophylactic method. In Austria, there was still no general goiter prophylaxis in 1954,[40,71] although there were some isolated experiments in progress. In one town of upper Austria there were still 68% of the pregnant women afflicted with goiter and 47% of the newborn children had goiter. In such areas, goiter was considered a normal attribute, and one mother, gravida XII, asked 5 days after delivery whether her child had already "goitered"; she thought that development of a goiter after birth was a sign of good health.[40] In the same year (1954), I had an opportunity to revisit regions in Europe in which goiter and cretinism had been endemic. In Switzerland and France, I could still see, examine and photograph adult cretins. However, there were no cretin children, since improved living conditions, import of foodstuffs and iodized salt had removed the basic conditions on which cretinism depends. But in Austria, in the valley of the Ötz, there were still cretin children (see Figs. 12-6, 12-7 and 12-8). I was told in the salt works of Hall in the Tirol that the salt available in this area was not iodized.

The fact that there were still goiter and cretinism in Austria in 1954 is particularly tragic, since iodized salt had been recommended there 99 years earlier for the prevention of endemic cretinism by Köstl,[68] and advocated again, in 1898, by Wagner-Jauregg.[69] Actually, iodized salt was manufactured to a certain extent in 1923 and subsequently, and there was some reduction of goiter within a few years. But iodized salt reached less than 50% of the population. There was much opposition to iodization of salt because of alleged dangers. The iodine prophylaxis terminated in Austria in 1938, when, by special order of the "Reichspräsident" (Adolf Hitler), the population was warned against iodized food, including salt.[69]

The battle of iodized salt in Switzerland, and the eradication of endemic goiter and cretinism there, is of special interest because this highly civilized coun-

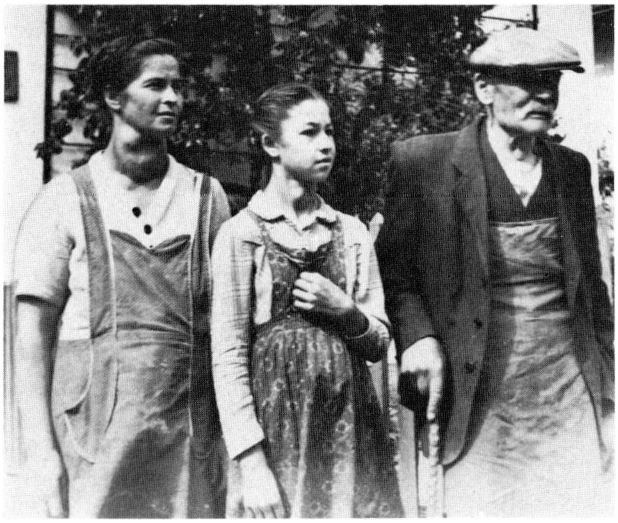

Fig. 12-8.—Goiter in three generations. The grandfather and the mother were intelligent. The girl was hard of hearing and did poorly in school. Three intelligent siblings had slight goiters. (Tirol, 1954.)

try was plagued in many areas by severe endemics. The prophylaxis was effected chiefly by three practicing physicians who had to overcome not only the resistance of the lay population but also the objections of some of their academic colleagues. It has been mentioned that in 1914 Hunziker,[34] a physician in a village near Zurich, had developed a sound theory of the need for iodine as a foodstuff, but that he had gained little recognition from his academic colleagues and the authorities. Yet, his concept was appreciated by some physicians who began preventive experiments on their own. In 1917, Bayard,[70] in St. Niklaus (population 600) in the canton of Valais – one of the worst endemic areas – gave to several goitrous children salt to which small amounts of iodine were added by the village pharmacist. Within 6 months, the goiters disappeared (Fig. 12-9). In 1954, while I was visiting St. Niklaus, Bayard kindly gave me the original photographs, since "Nobody else seemed to be interested in them." This experiment was of particular interest because the Valais was the classic land of goiter and cretinism, as mentioned by old travelers and writers (p. 103). As late as 1852, a historian of the Valais wrote, "It is known that cretinism is the most terrible plague of the Valais." This Swiss canton is surrounded by high mountains that open only toward the west. Between 1860 and 1870, a railroad opened up the Valais to commerce and traffic, which resulted in the import of foodstuffs from other cantons and other countries and led to the decrease of goiter and cretinism.[72] Yet, in 1920, more than 70% of the schoolchildren still were affected by goiter. Beginning in 1924, after Bayard's pioneer experiments had impressed the population and the authorities, iodized salt was used in increasing amounts, and after 1933 the entire salt supply was iodized. By 1934, the incidence of goiter in schoolchildren had fallen to 30%. In 1954, when I visited Evolène in the Valais, a small community that could be reached only by a one-way winding mountain road, the physician there could not show me a single case of cretinism, and there was only one case of goiter (with hyperthyroidism). The people assembling for church on Sunday – adults and children alike – appeared healthy and goiter-free (Fig. 12-10, *A*). Yet, the inhabitants of this village lived under conditions similar to those of their ancestors, cultivating small terraced fields and inhabiting old wooden houses (Fig. 12-10, *B* and *C*) without a sewer-

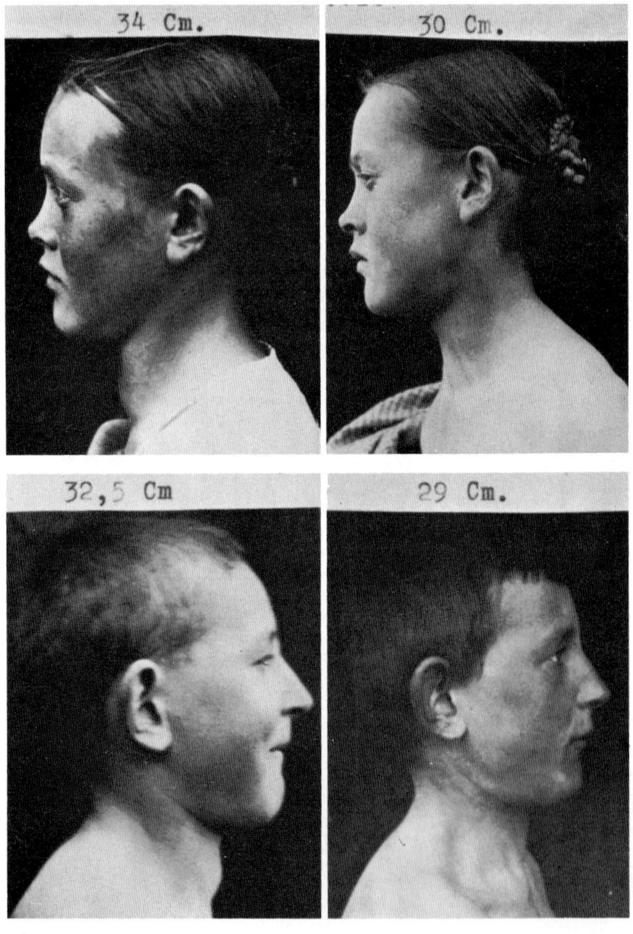

Fig. 12-9. – Effect of iodized salt (5 mg. NaI per kg. salt) prepared by the village pharmacist at the request of Doctor Bayard for the children of Graechen, where approximately 80% of the population were goitrous in 1917. After 6 months of treatment, the thyroid became visibly smaller. (Courtesy of Dr. O. Bayard, St. Niklaus, Switzerland.)

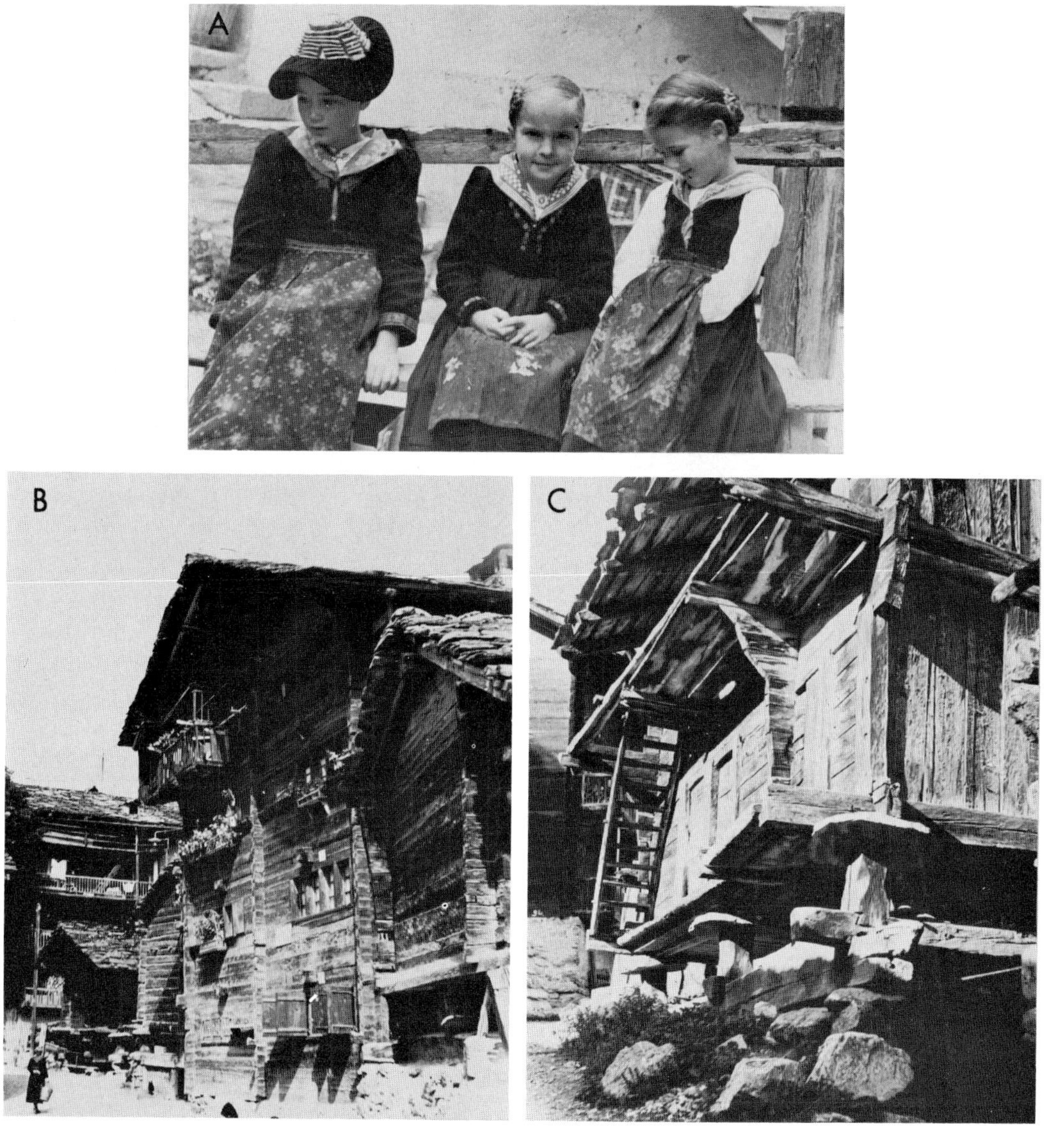

Fig. 12-10.—**A,** healthy and goiter-free children in Evolène, Switzerland, 21 years after iodized salt had become universally used in the Valais. There were no new cases of goiter and cretinism to be found in this still-remote village. **B** and **C,** houses and foundation of houses in Evolène in 1954. The people still lived in houses built by ancient methods, but goiter and cretinism had been wiped out.

age system. Consanguineous marriages were still common, the same names occurring in many families of the village. This community serves as an example of a village that continued in isolation and unchanged habits yet was freed of goiter and cretinism. Whereas one cannot give all the credit for the improvement of the situation to iodized salt, the complete eradication of goiter probably was due to this measure.

Some preventive experiments with iodized salt were begun in 1923 by Messerle in some villages in the canton of Vaud, where the entire salt supply was iodized by 1924, with excellent results. One of the most energetic proponents of iodized salt in Switzerland was a surgeon in the town of Herisau (population 12,000), H. Eggenberger,[11] who devised a method for iodization of salt and a simple practical test for demonstration of iodine in supplemented salt. He carried the message to the people, who accepted the recommended measures.[73,74]

It took approximately 100 years from the suggestion of Coindet[28] to use iodine for the treatment of goiter to the establishment of effective prophylactic measures in civilized countries, in which a more rap-

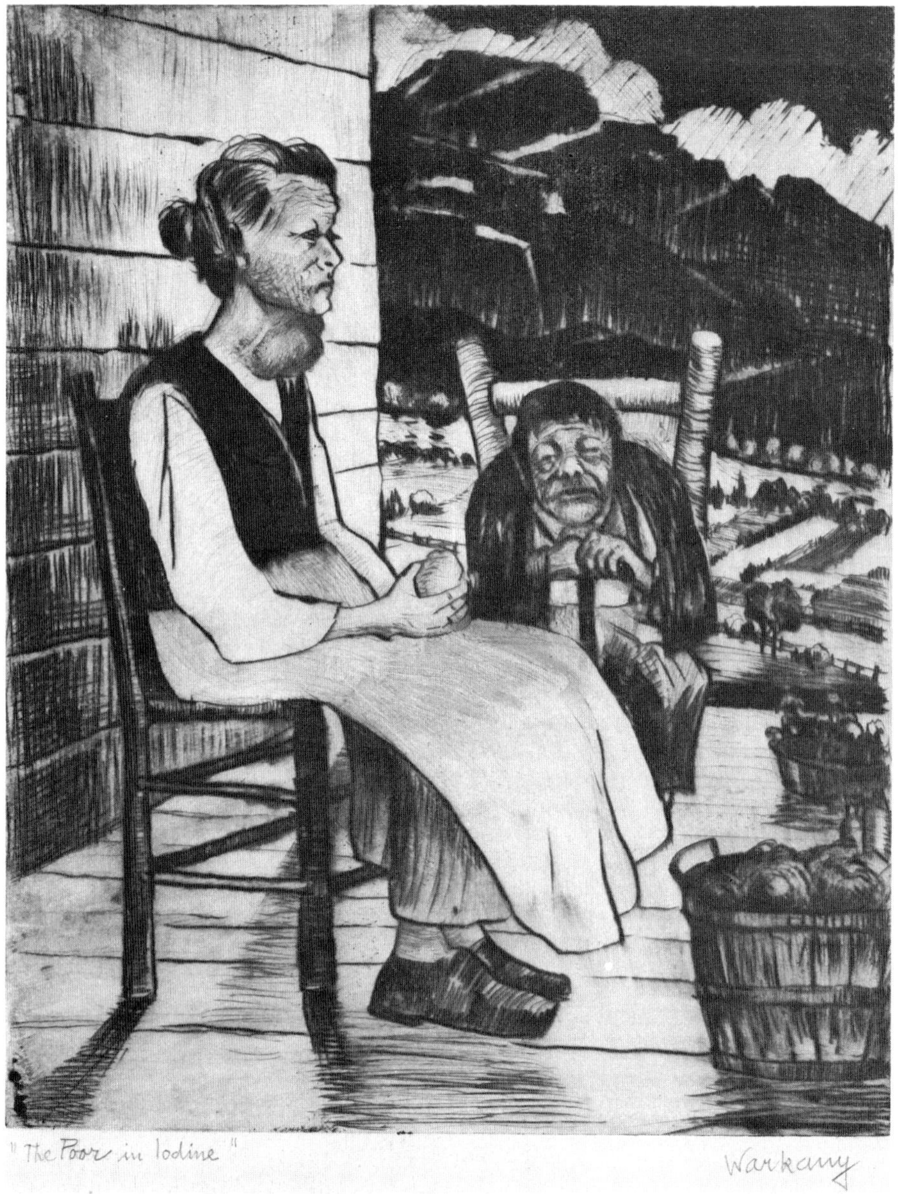

Fig. 12-11.—"The Poor in Iodine." (An etching by J. Warkany.)

id acceptance of a scientific truth should be expected. This delay in prophylactic measures is not entirely due to human torpor. At first, iodine was recommended as a remedy against goiter and cretinism; it failed in most cases because the pathologic processes in the thyroids had progressed too far to be reversible. Given in excessive doses, iodine caused adverse effects in many patients. In addition, the etiology of goiter and cretinism was obscured by many accessory factors that seemed of prime importance to some investigators. Finally, it must be realized that iodine reached isolated iodine-starved regions in many subtle ways that were not recognized. As a consequence, endemic goiter and cretinism decreased as a public health problem with increasing commerce and communication. The building of roads and railroads into endemic areas brought foodstuffs from regions and countries in which there was no lack of iodine. Cod-liver oil, if given systematically to an infant population, prevented simple goiter because of its high iodine content. But none of these silent prophylactic procedures had the general preventive effect of iodized salt.

The phenomenon of endemic cretinism and the saga of its eradication have importance beyond the narrow field of thyroid pathology. The objective description of the symptoms of endemic cretins cannot convey the impression made on the observer who saw these deformed and demented human beings in their natural environment. In contrast to mental retardation and physical handicaps due to cultural deprivation as seen in slums or desolate swamps, cretinism could be seen in lovely mountain areas and valleys where city dwellers went for recreation and recuperation. I became acquainted with the problem of endemic cretinism on hikes through Alpine valleys of Austria in about 1920. As one approached some of the farmhouses in these regions, one could see sitting on chairs or benches dwarfed, old-looking people, shivering in the warm sunshine, grimacing or grinning and mumbling unintelligible sounds. These little people usually were shy, and fled as strangers approached. On the road or in the fields, one encountered taller, often goitrous men doing some minor chores for their family or household but unable to speak clearly or to understand when they were spoken to. Goitrous deaf-mute women with little mental ability stayed in or close to the house. The abnormal posture and gait of these people betrayed their condition from a distance. Even the mentally normal people in these regions usually were burdened by goiters of variable size that sometimes interfered with their breathing and working capacity. One could not help wondering why the populations of such beautiful mountain areas were afflicted by these goiters and by relatives who obviously were physically and mentally handicapped. There were plenty of space and fresh air, but there apparently were some hidden adverse forces acting in this treacherously beautiful environment that condemned the people forced to live there permanently to mental and physical deterioration. One was told that goiter and cretinism were due to lack of iodine and that these conditions could be made to disappear by iodized salt. Although this answer probably presented the problem in an oversimplified way, it contained, if not a complete explanation of the etiology, a correct statement concerning the possibility of eradication of the disorders. The information that a nutritional deficiency could lead to congenital physical and mental disturbances became to me later a stimulus to do animal experiments that resulted in congenital malformations produced by deficient maternal diets. It remained a reminder that the unborn child can be damaged by adverse environmental factors beyond restoration in postnatal life. Endemic cretinism proved that "hereditary" transmission of congenital disorders through several generations or aggregation in families (Fig. 12-13) is not limited to genetic mechanisms but can be caused by hidden environmental agents or deficiencies that persist through more than one generation (Figs. 12-8 and 12-12). If genetic and environmental factors are intertwined in the etiology of endemic cretinism—and they probably are—it proves how widespread such genetic weakness can be and how easily it can be overcome sometimes by regulation of the environment—addition of a few micrograms of an available nutritional element to a deficient diet, in the case of cretinism.

It was indeed fortunate that endemic cretinism was associated with hyperplasia of the thyroid gland. The striking goiters seen in endemic areas suggested to ancient and modern observers a connection between the high incidence of mental retardation and the endemic of "bronchocele." If iodine deficiency had not manifested itself on an endocrine gland in the neck but in a gland concealed in the interior of the body, the connection between cretinism and glandular hyperplasia and iodine deficiency might have escaped early recognition and could have delayed eradication of the mental disorder. One can speculate about man's fate if iodine had been scarce on the entire earth; and one can speculate whether there are other limiting environmental factors to man's optimal development and how man's appearance and actions are influenced by scarcities of other elements or compounds in his environment.

The chain of events that causes endemic cretinism deserves consideration. There were cosmic events that resulted in glaciation of the Quaternary ice age

Fig. 12-12.—Goiter in three generations with cretinism in the third. There is more cretinism in the late-born children than in siblings born earlier. These pedigrees show that familial aggregation of diseases and disorders does not prove genetic determination. It exemplifies "pseudoheredity." (After J. Eugster.[9])

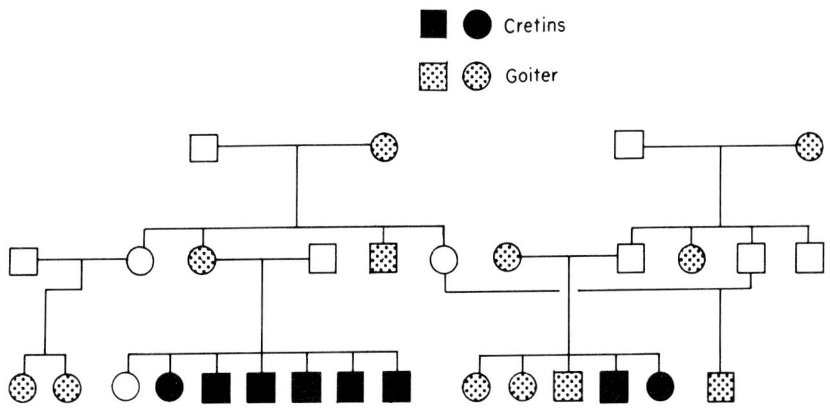

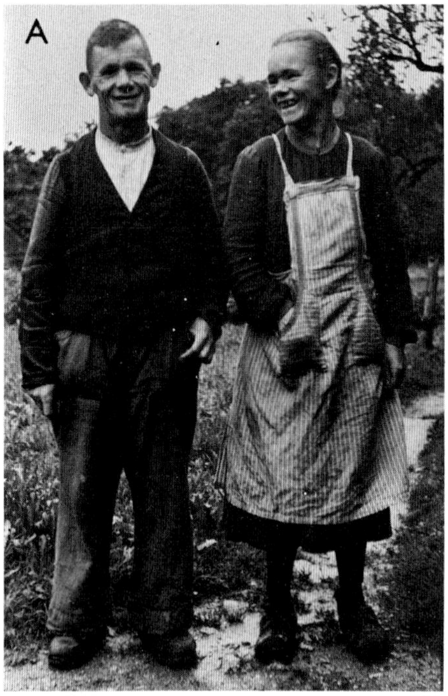

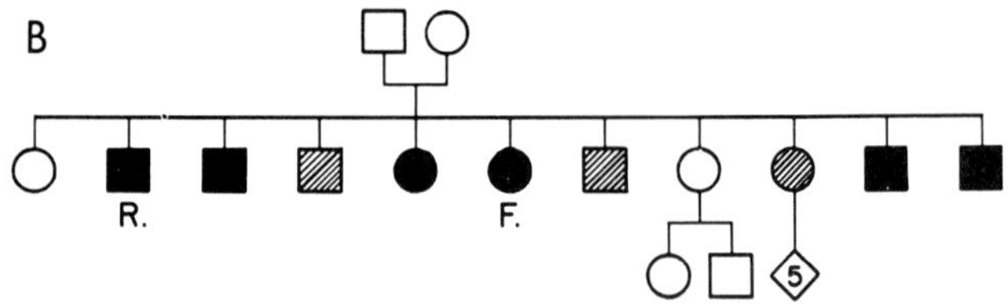

Fig. 12-13. – **A,** siblings, children of goitrous parents. The brother was 41 years of age, the sister 36. Both were mentally retarded and deaf-mute. Both had nodular goiters (Switzerland, 1954). **B,** pedigree of family in which parents were not consanguineous. Both had goiter. Of 11 living children, 6 were cretins, 3 half-cretins and 2 were normal. In the third generation, all children were normal. The siblings illustrated in **A** are those marked R and F in the pedigree (**B**). Solid squares and circles represent cretins; lined squares and circles represent half-cretins. This family was studied for many years by Prof. J. Eugster, Bern, Switzerland (see J. Eugster[9]).

that led to iodine deprivation of many areas that became endemic centers.[35,36] The iodine scarcity caused goiter in the local population, and the resulting thyroid disease in females interfered with normal brain development of their offspring. The "population explosions" of ancient times or defeat in war forced some populations into remote areas, where they lived in isolation. They could survive and feed themselves but they were deprived of an essential foodstuff. Long-lasting peace, which made possible safe conduct and communications, permitted introduction of foods that contained more iodine than the products grown in the homeland – and the incidence of goiter decreased. But war brought back the endemic with regularity. And, finally, it was man's intelligence that defined the etiology of cretinism in scientific terms and made possible complete eradication of this disabling disorder. Parenthetically, it must be added that there was resistance by extremely learned men and experts to the simple prophylactic measures that proved so successful in the elimination of the disease. The causative chain was not quite so linear as described above; accessory factors formed a complicated causative web that made the way out difficult. But endemic cretinism can be and has been eliminated in many parts of the world by simple public health measures. Unfortunately, the pathogenesis of the disorder has not yet been clearly elucidated, and its relationship to endemic goiter has remained unexplained on biochemical and embryologic levels. That such a complicated disorder as endemic cretinism could be wiped out without explanation of the intricate mechanisms involved in its pathogenesis may be disappointing to some scientific purists but consoling to those who like shortcuts in prevention of congenital disorders.

With the elimination of endemic cretinism, a portion of the mental retardation problem at least as large as that of the Down syndrome has disappeared during the past 25 years from most endemic regions of advanced countries (p. 117). This is quite an achievement, if one considers that the Down syndrome contributes approximately 10% to the mental retardation problem in goiter-free countries and that it still is not preventable. But in "hyperendemic" areas in which cretins sometimes accounted for 10% of the entire population, overshadowing all other causes of mental retardation, the eradication of this disorder meant much more – namely, a complete reorganization and recovery of the social structure of communities and countries.

REFERENCES

1. Merke, F.: Hat Paracelsus als erster über den Kretinismus berichtet und dessen Zusammenhang mit dem endemischen Kropf vermutet? Karger Gaz. Nr. 9/10, September, 1964.
2. Merke, F.: Sind die zwei Volksseuchen endemischer Kropf und Kretinismus in der Schweiz erloschen? Schweiz. Rundsch. Med., Feb.–Mar., 1962, pp. 101–117.
3. Cranefield, P.: The discovery of cretinism, Bull. Hist. Med. 36:489, 1962.
4. Fodéré: *Über den Kropf und Kretinismus. Für Ärzte und Philosophen.* Deutsche Übersetzung von Dr. Lindemann (Berlin, 1796).
5. Cranefield, P.: L'origine probable de l'introduction du mot

"Crétin" dans la langue écrite. Un manuscrit de 1750 par le Comte de Maugiron, Gesnerus 19:89, 1962.
6. De Quervain, F., and Wegelin, C.: *Der endemische Kretinismus* (Berlin and Wien: Julius Springer, 1936).
7. Taussig, S.: *Kropf und Kretinismus* (Jena: Gustav Fischer, 1912).
8. McCarrison, I. M. S.: Observations on endemic cretinism in the Chitral and Gilgit valleys, Lancet 2:1275, 1908.
9. Eugster, J.: Zur Erblichkeitsfrage des Endemischen Kretinismus – Untersuchungen an 204 Kretinen und deren Blutsverwandten, Arch. Klaus Stift. Vererbungsforsch. 13:383, 1938.
10. Kelly, F. C., and Snedden, W. W.: Prevalence and geographical distribution of endemic goitre, Bull. World Health Organ. 18:5, 1958.
11. Eggenberger, H.: In Hirsch, M. (ed.), *Kropf und Kretinismus. Handbuch der inneren Sekretion* (Leipzig: Kabitzsch, 1928).
12. Rupilius, K.: Ein Beitrag zu den verschiedenen Schwachsinnsformen mit besonderer Berücksichtigung des Kretinismus in Steiermark, Wien. klin. Wchnschr. 47:1060, 1934.
13. Diviak, R., and Wagner-Jauregg, J.: Über die Entstehung des endemischen Kretinismus nach Beobachtungen in den ersten Lebensjahren, Wien. klin. Wchnschr. 31:149, 1918.
14. Gajdusek, D. C.: Congenital defects of the central nervous system associated with hyperendemic goiter in a neolithic highland society of Netherlands New Guinea, Pediatrics 29:345, 1962.
15. McClendon, J. F.: *Iodine and the Incidence of Goiter* (Minneapolis: University of Minnesota Press, 1939).
16. Najjar, S., and Woodruff, C. W: Some observations on goiter in Lebanon, Am. J. Clin. Nutrition 13:46, 1963.
17. DeVisscher, M., Beckers, C., van den Schrieck, H-G., DeSmet, M., Ermans, A. M., Galperin, H., and Bastenie, P. A.: Endemic goiter in the Uele region (Republic of Congo). I. General aspects and functional studies, J. Clin. Endocrinol. 21:175, 1961.
18. Greenwald, I.: The history of goiter in Africa, Bull. Hist. Med. 23:155, 1949.
19. Olesen, R.: Distribution of endemic goiter in the United States as shown by thyroid surveys, Pub. Health Rep. 41: 2691, 1926.
20. Olesen, R.: Distribution of endemic goiter in the United States as shown by thyroid surveys, Pub. Health Rep. 44: 1463, 1929.
21. Marine, D., and Kimball, O. P.: Prevention of simple goiter, J. Lab. & Clin. Med. 3:40, 1917.
22. Gordon, M. B.: Childhood myxedema or so-called sporadic cretinism in North America, Endocrinology 6:235, 1922.
23. Stoddard, C. H.: Will cretinism become endemic in Wisconsin?, Wisconsin M. J. 32:389, 1933.
24. Stanbury, J. B., and Hedge, A. N.: A study of a family of goitrous cretins, J. Clin. Endocrinol. 10:1471, 1950.
25. Cranefield, P., and Federn, W.: Paracelsus on goiter and cretinism: A translation and discussion of "De struma, vulgo der Kropf," Bull. Hist. Med. 37:463, 1963.
26. St. Lager, J.: *Étude sur les causes du crétinisme et du goitre endémique* (Paris, 1867).
27. Matovinović, J., and Ramalingaswami, V.: Therapy and prophylaxis of endemic goitre, Bull. World Health Organ. 18:233, 1958.
28. Coindet: Découverte d'un nouveau remède contre le goitre, Ann. chim. et phys. 15:49, 1820.
29. Chatin, A.: Recherche de l'iode dans l'air, les eaux, le sol et les produits alimentaires des Alpes de la France et du Piémont, Gaz. d'hôp. Paris 25:14, 38, 50, 82, 86, 94, 1852.
30. Fellenberg, Th.: Das Vorkommen, der Kreislauf und der Stoffwechsel des Jods, Ergebn. Physiol. 25:176, 1926.
31. Baumann, E.: Über das normale Vorkommen von Jod im Tierkörper, Ztschr. Physiol. Chem. 21:319, 1895.
32. Marine, D., and Williams, W. W.: The relation of iodine to the structure of the thyroid gland, Arch. Int. Med. 1:349, 1908.
33. Kendall, E. C.: The isolation in crystalline form of the compound containing iodine which occurs in the thyroid; its chemical nature and physiological activity, Tr. A. Am. Physicians 30:420, 1915.
34. Hunziker-Schild, H.: *Der Kropf, eine Anpassung an jodarme Nahrung* (Bern, 1915).
35. Goldschmidt, V. M.: *Geochemistry* (Oxford: Clarendon Press, 1954).
36. Merke, F.: Die Eiszeit als primordiale Ursache des endemischen Kropfes, Schweiz. med. Wchnschr. 95:1183, 1965.
37. McCarrison, R.: The distribution of goitre in India, Indian J. M. Res. 2:778, 1914–1915.
38. Lunde, G.: *Ein Inland-Kropfgebiet ohne Jodmangel.* Internationale Kropfkonferenz, Bern, 1933; Verhandlungsbericht, Bern, 1935.
39. Costa, A.: Has endemic cretinism any relation to thyroid deficiency?, J. Clin. Endocrinol. 17:801, 1957.
40. Kopf, H.: Neuere Behandlungsergebnisse kropfbehafteter Neugeborener und Schulkinder in Oberösterreich, Wien. klin. Wchnschr. 66:96, 1954.
41. Taylor, S.: Calcium as a goitrogen, J. Clin. Endocrinol. 14:1412, 1954.
42. Gross, R. T., Kriss, J. P., and Spaet, T. H.: Hematopoietic and goitrogenic effects of cobaltous chloride in patients with sickle-cell anemia, A.M.A. Am. J. Dis. Child. 88:503, 1954.
43. Paley, K. R., Sobel, E. S., and Yalow, R. S.: Effect of oral and intravenous cobaltous chloride on thyroid functions, J. Clin. Endocrinol. 18:850, 1958.
44. Chamberlain, J. L.: Thyroid enlargement probably induced by cobalt, J. Pediat. 59:81, 1961.
45. Wespi, H. J.: Besteht ein Antagonismus zwischen Fluor und Jod?, Schweiz. Rundsch. Med. 43:616, 1954.
46. Greer, M. A.: The natural occurrence of goitrogenic agents, Recent Prog. Hormone Res. 18:187, 1962.
47. Chesney, A. M., Clawson, T. A., and Webster, B.: Endemic goitre in rabbits; incidence and characteristics, Bull. Johns Hopkins Hosp. 43:261, 1928.
48. Hercus, C. E., and Purves, H. D.: Goitre in New Zealand, New Zealand M. J. 35:83, 1936.
49. Shepard, T. H., Pyne, G. E., Kirschvink, J. F., and McLean, M.: Soybean goiter. Report of three cases, New England J. Med. 262:1099, 1960.
50. Clements, F. W., and Wishart, J. W.: A thyroid blocking agent in the etiology of endemic goiter, Metabolism 5: 623, 1956.
51. Astwood, E. B., Greer, M. A., and Ettlinger, M. G.: L-5-vinyl-2-thiooxazolidone, antithyroid compound from yellow turnip and from Brassica seeds, J. Biol. Chem. 181: 121, 1949.
52. Haubold, H.: Die Bedeutung des Karotinoidmangels für die Entstehung der neuen Kropfwelle, München. med. Wchnschr. 92:329, 1950.
53. Horvat, A., and Maver, H.: The role of vitamin A in the occurrence of goitre on the island of Krk, Yugoslavia, J. Nutrition 66:189, 1958.
54. Eggenberger, H. U.: *Vitamin A und Kropf* (Zurich: Buchdruckerei Schläpper & Co., 1954).
55. Najjar, S. S.: Hypothyroidism in children from an endemic goiter area, J. Pediat. 64:372, 1964.
56. Gamper, E.: Der endemische Kretinismus, in Bumke, O. (ed.), *Handbuch der Geisteskrankheiten* (Berlin: J. Springer, 1928–1932).
57. Eugster, J.: Wie sieht die Schilddrüse eines Kretinen aus zur Zeit der Geburt?, Beitr. path. Anat. 100:392, 1938.
58. Lotmar, F.: Entwicklungsstörungen in der Kleinhirnrinde beim endemischen Kretinismus, Ztschr. Neurol. u. Psychiat. 136:412, 1931.
59. Siebenmann, F.: Taubstummheit und Taubstummzählung in der Schweiz, Cor. Bl. F. Schweiz. Aerzte, Basel 48:1, 1918.
60. Nager, F. R., and Meyer, M.: Beiträge zur normalen und pathologischen Histologie der knöchernen Labyrinthkapsel; die Labyrinthkapsel beim endemischen Kretinismus,

Beitr. Anat. Physiol. Path. u. Therap. d. Ohres. 30:45, 1932.
61. Stanbury, J. B., and Querido, A.: On the nature of endemic cretinism, J. Clin. Endocrinol. 17:803, 1957.
62. Speert, H., Quimby, E. H., and Werner, S. C.: Radioiodine uptake by the fetal mouse thyroid and resultant effects in later life, Surg., Gynec. & Obst. 93:230, 1951.
63. Smith, C. A., Oberhelman, H. A., Jr., Storer, E. H., Woodward, E. R., and Dragstedt, L. R.: Production of experimental cretinism in dogs by the administration of radioactive iodine, Arch. Surg. 63:807, 1951.
64. Plattner, W.: Grössen- und Formverhältnisse der Kretinenhand, Ztschr. menschl. Vererb.-u. Konstitutionslehre 23:699, 1939.
65. Bastenie, P. A., Ermans, A. M., Thys, O., Beckers, C., van den Schrieck, H. G., and de Visscher, M.: Endemic goiter in the Uele region. III. Endemic cretinism, J. Clin. Endocrinol. 22:187, 1962.
66. Costa, A., Cottino, F., Ferraris, G. M., Marchis, E., Marocco, F., Mortara, M., and Pietra, R.: Nouvelles acquisitions sur l'equilibre endocrino-métabolique du cretinisme endémique, Ann. endocrinol. 14:995, 1953.
67. Lotmar, F.: Histopathologische Befunde in Gehirnen von kongenitalem Myxödem (Thyreoaplasie), Ztschr. Neurol. u. Psychiat. 119:491, 1929.
68. Köstl, F.: *Der endemische Cretinismus als Gegenstand der öffentlichen Fürsorge* (Jena, 1855).
69. Wagner-Jauregg, J.: In Schönbauer, L., and Jantsch, M. (eds.), *Lebenserinnerungen* (Wien: Springer Verlag, 1950).
70. Bayard, O.: *Beiträge zur Schilddrüsenfrage* (Basel: Benno Schwabe & Co., 1919).
71. Sallgruber, K.: Zum Problem der Säuglingsstruma, Österr. Ztschr. Kinderh. 10:312, 1954.
72. Bayard, O.: Ergebnisse der Kropfprophylaxe im Kanton Wallis, nebst Bemerkungen zur Kropffrage, Schweiz. med. Wchnschr. 67:1093, 1937.
73. Eggenberger, H.: Die Kropfprophylaxe, München. med. Wchnschr. 29:972, 1924.
74. Wespi, H. J.: 40 Jahre Kropfprophylaxe mit jodiertem Salz, Bull. des Eidg. Gesundheitsamtes, March 24, 1962.
75. Pretell, E. A., Moncloa, F., Salinas, R., Kawano, A., Guerra-Garcia, R., Gutierrez, L., Beteta, L., Pretell, J., and Wan, M.: Prophylaxis and treatment of endemic goiter in Peru with iodized oil, J. Clin. Endocrinol. 29:1586, 1969.
76. McCullagh, S. F.: The Hyon Peninsula endemic: I. The effectiveness of an intramuscular depot of iodized oil in the control of endemic goiter, M. J. Australia 1:769, 1963.
77. Podoba, J., Stukovsky, R., and Kovac, R.: Thyroid function in sibships in endemic goiter region, J. Clin. Endocrinol. 31:134, 1970.
78. Fraser, G. R.: The association of congenital deafness with goitre (Pendred's syndrome). A study of 207 families, Ann. Human Genet. 28:201, 1965.
79. Stanbury, J. B.: Research on endemic goiter in Latin America, WHO Chron. 24:537, 1970.

Diabetes

THERE IS GENERAL AGREEMENT that the perinatal mortality of children of diabetic mothers is relatively high and that many neonates have specific characteristics associated with many dangers. Most of these characteristics arise late in pregnancy. There is little agreement concerning damages in the first trimester of pregnancy and the incidence of congenital malformations in the offspring of diabetic mothers. There exist many publications that contend that the incidence is definitely increased, but some of the statements rely on impressions that are not adequately controlled and suffer from lack of clear definition of the term "congenital malformations." Some include stillbirths and necropsies; others deal with surviving children. Some conclusions are based on single examinations, others on repeated examinations. It is also probable that infants of diabetic mothers often are more thoroughly examined than the controls. Taking these factors into consideration, Rubin and Murphy,[1] in 1958, concluded that the assumed high frequency of malformations in the offspring of diabetic mothers had not been established. Subsequently, Farquhar,[2] in Edinburgh, after a small but careful study of children of diabetic and nondiabetic mothers, thought that the individual diabetic mother need have no greater fear of fetal malformation than the nondiabetic. Hagbard,[3] in Sweden, discovered (within a week of the children's births) congenital malformations in approximately 6% of those born to diabetic mothers. In a series followed for the whole first year, the rate of malformations was 7.6%. Pedersen,[4] in Denmark, found, among 843 infants, 6.4% affected by congenital malformations versus 2.1% in the control group. The difference in major malformations was 5.2 against 1.2; of lethal malformations 2.1 against 0.3; of multiple malformations 1.6 versus 0.2%. With severe diabetes of the mother, complicated by vascular nephropathy and/or proliferative retinopathy, the malformation rate of the infants was 14%. Congenital heart disease and severe limb deformity were more common in infants of mothers with vascular disease. Most important was the discovery that among these children a syndrome existed of malformations of the lower spine combined with limb defects, especially the femora. It was present in approximately 1% of the infants and in 13% of those with congenital malformations. It had been observed before that a significant number of children with sacral agenesis were born of diabetic mothers,[5] and Miller,[6] in 1946, had described a child with hypoplasia of the right humerus and femur, agenesis of the left femur and fibula, anomalies of the lower spine and cleft lip. Subsequently, Kučera *et al.*[7] added several cases and collected a total of 31 reports. Passarge[8] and Thalhammer *et al.*[9] found more than 40 reported cases. This syndrome of *caudal dysplasia* is accompanied, in many cases, by such other malformations as cleft lip and palate, Pierre Robin syndrome, congenital heart disease, renal and cerebral anomalies, syndactyly, polydactyly and others.[12] Some association with diabetes exists, but it is not known why some diabetic mothers have such deformed children, whereas the majority are not affected during the organogenic period. It seems that there is a risk for certain diabetic mothers to have children with multiple congenital malformations. These mothers are few in number, and little is known concerning their type of diabetes and treatment. Small surveys may not contain cases of this type, or if they include one, it would appear to be coincidental. On the other hand, in general surveys such as those of Rubin and Murphy,[1] such cases could be inconspicuous among the many normal offspring of average diabetic mothers whose embryos are not damaged in the organogenic period. Comess *et al.*[11] found in the offspring born after the onset of diabetes to Pima Indian mothers whose disease was diagnosed before age 25, congenital anomalies in 38%, i.e., approximately ten times more than noted in nondiabetic mothers. Anomalies were not more frequent in children of prediabetic mothers or of mothers whose disease started at or after age 25. In children whose mothers required hypoglycemic medication, anomalies were more frequent than in those whose mothers did not need medication, but there was no evidence of a teratogenic action of insulin. Although the series was small and some of the anomalies were "variations" rather than serious malformations, the study suggests that similar distinctions should be made in all types of diabetes under consideration.

Since it now seems established that maternal diabetes sometimes is associated with certain congenital malformations in children, reports of teratogenic actions of drugs used in the treatment of diabetes, such as insulin and tolbutamide,[10] will have to be re-examined in the light of recent surveys and the discovery of the caudal dysplasia syndrome.

The continued discussion of teratogenic effects of maternal diabetes illustrates the difficulties of ascertaining maternal factors in the etiology of congenital malformations. There is little doubt that infants of diabetic mothers tend to be large and that they are likely to die as the end of pregnancy approaches; they have a tendency to hypoglycemia and respiratory distress after delivery,[13] but there are marked differences in observations of congenital malformations. In many series, the incidence of congenital malformations is similar to that of control populations, and it seems that malformations contribute little to the perinatal mortality of the infants.[14] The differences in observations and opinions may be due to different sampling. There probably are several types of maternal diabetes that have differing teratogenic effects and that should be considered separately.[4,13] The classifications and evaluations of congenital malformations differ; differing treatment and reactions to treatment may influence the outcome of pregnancies. It appears that some diabetic women have a tendency to early abortions and to production of malformed fetuses, whereas the majority of diabetic women do not. In a general review, the rare cases with malformations may be overshadowed by the normal ones, which, fortunately, result from the majority of diabetic pregnancies.

REFERENCES

1. Rubin, A., and Murphy, D. P.: Studies in human reproduction. III. The frequency of congenital malformations in the offspring of nondiabetic and diabetic individuals, J. Pediat. 53:579, 1958.
2. Farquhar, J. W.: The Influence of Maternal Diabetes on Fetus and Child, in Gairdner, D. (ed.), *Recent Advances in Paediatrics* (3d ed.; Boston: Little, Brown & Company, 1965).
3. Hagbard, L.: *Pregnancy and Diabetes* (Springfield, Ill.: Charles C Thomas, Publisher, 1961).
4. Pedersen, J.: *The Pregnant Diabetic and Her Newborn* (Baltimore: The Williams & Wilkins Company, 1967).
5. Blumel, J., Butler, M. C., Evans, E. B., and Eggers, G. W. N.: Congenital anomaly of the sacrococcygeal spine, Arch. Surg. 85:982, 1962.
6. Miller, H. C.: The effect of diabetic and prediabetic pregnancies on the fetus and newborn infant, J. Pediat. 29: 455, 1946.
7. Kučera, J., Lenz, W., and Maier, W.: Missbildungen der Beine und der kaudalen Wirbelsäule bei Kindern diabetischer Mütter, Deutsche med. Wchnschr. 90:901, 1965.
8. Passarge, E.: Congenital malformations and maternal diabetes, Lancet 1:324, 1965.
9. Thalhammer, O., Lachmann, D., and Scheibenreiter, S.: "Caudale Regression" beim Kind einer 18 jährigen Frau mit Prädiabetes, Ztschr. Kinderh. 102:346, 1968.
10. Smithells, R. W.: Drugs and human malformations, Adv. in Teratology 1:251, 1966.
11. Comess, L. J., Bennett, P. H., Man, M. B., Burch, T. A., and Miller, M.: Congenital anomalies and diabetes in the Pima Indians of Arizona, Diabetes 18:471, 1969.
12. Williamson, D. A. J.: A syndrome of congenital malformations possibly due to maternal diabetes, Developmental Med. & Child Neurol. 12:145, 1970.
13. Delaney, J. J., and Ptacek, J.: Three decades of experience with diabetic pregnancies, Am. J. Obst. & Gynec. 106:550, 1970.
14. Gellis, S. S., and Hsia, D. Y-Y.: The infant of the diabetic mother, A.M.A. J. Dis. Child. 97:1, 1959.

Phenylketonuria

Because excessive phenylalanine can damage the developing brain, fetuses carried by phenylketonuric women may suffer brain damages in utero. Since most phenylketonuric women do not reproduce because of severe mental retardation, observations of intrauterine brain damage by excessive phenylalanine or its products remained scanty until recently, although Dent,[1] as early as 1956, mentioned a phenylketonuric mother who had 3 nonphenylketonuric retarded children by 3 different illegitimate matings. There also are reports of normal children born to phenylketonuric mothers, so that one must assume that differing maternal serum phenylalanine levels can result in variable intrauterine brain development or that other factors influence the outcome of such pregnancies. The situation is comparable, to a certain extent, to that of families in which cretin and normal children alter even though the mothers' goiters persist throughout their reproductive period (see Endemic Goiter and Cretinism).

In 1963, Denniston[2] reported the case of a 70-year-old phenylketonuric woman who had 5 nonphenylketonuric surviving children with severe mental retardation. Mabry *et al.*[3] described two separate kindreds with 3 phenylketonuric mothers who had 1, 5 and 8 mentally retarded but nonphenylketonuric children; 2 of the fathers had normal children through other marriages. Richards[4] observed a phenylketonuric mother who had 3 nonphenylketonuric children with mental retardation of greater severity than that of the mother. Subsequently, Fisch *et al.*[5] found that 2 children, 1 homozygous and 1 heterozygous for phenylketonuria, born of an untreated phenylketonuric mother had intrauterine growth retardation and persistent postnatal growth retardation. Of special interest was the fact that microcephaly was present in both children at birth. Stevenson and Huntley[6] reported 2 phenylketonuric females on nonrestricted diets who had 16 abortions, 6 infants who died in infancy and 4 surviving children. The live-born children had varying combinations of intrauterine growth retardation, microcephaly, cardiovascular defects, mental and physical retardation and dislocated hips. Additional cases have been published since of nonphenylketonuric children born of phenylketonuric mothers showing prenatal and postnatal growth retardation, microcephaly, mental retardation[7,8,12,13] and congenital malformations.[9,10] Menkes and Aeberhard[11] analyzed the cerebral lipids and the fatty acid pattern in a severely retarded heterozygote offspring of a phenylketonuric mother. The lipid abnormalities were similar to those in homozygote phenylketonurics, which was interpreted as evidence that exposure of the fetus to an abnormal amino acid environment produced irreversible neurochemical changes.

The importance of this discovery of prenatal damage by an abnormal maternal metabolite is enhanced by the fact that some of the phenylketonuric mothers were mentally normal or near normal,[7] so that it will be advisable to screen all mothers of mentally retarded children for metabolic defects, particularly those who have more than one retarded child.

Experimental maternal hyperphenylalaninemia in rhesus monkeys resulted in intrauterine growth retardation and reduction in learning behavior of the offspring.[14]

REFERENCES

1. Dent, G. E.: Discussion of Armstrong, M. D., in Etiologic Factors in Mental Retardation, Ross Pediatric Research Conference, November, 1956, pp. 32–33, Ross Laboratories, Columbus, Ohio. Reported in 1957.
2. Denniston, J. C.: Children of mothers with phenylketonuria, J. Pediat. 63:461, 1963.
3. Mabry, C. C., Denniston, J. C., Nelson, T. L., and Son, C. D.: Maternal phenylketonuria; a cause of mental retardation in children without the metabolic defect, New England J. Med. 269:1404, 1963.
4. Richards, B. W.: Maternal phenylketonuria, Lancet 1:829, 1964.
5. Fisch, R. O., Walker, W. A., and Anderson, J. A.: Prenatal and postnatal developmental consequences of maternal phenylketonuria, Pediatrics 37:979, 1966.
6. Stevenson, R. E., and Huntley, C. C.: Congenital malformations in offspring of phenylketonuric mothers, Pediatrics 40:33, 1967.
7. Mabry, C. C., Denniston, J. C., and Coldwell, J. G.: Mental retardation in children of phenylketonuric mothers, New England J. Med. 275:1331, 1966.
8. DeMénibus, C. H., Graic, F., Lemonnier, A., and Fleury, J.: Les enfants nés de mères phénylcétonuriques, Ann. pédiat. 43:1746, 1967.
9. Fisch, R. O., Doeden, D., Lansky, L. L., and Anderson, J. A.: Maternal phenylketonuria, Am. J. Dis. Child. 118: 847, 1969.
10. Frankenburg, W. K., Duncan, B. R., Coffelt, R. W., Koch, R., Coldwell, J. G., and Son, C. D.: Maternal phenylketonuria: Implications for growth and development, J. Pediat. 73:560, 1968.
11. Menkes, J. H., and Aeberhard, E.: Maternal phenylketonuria, J. Pediat. 74:924, 1969.
12. Yu, J. S., and O'Halloran, M. T.: Children of mothers with phenylketonuria, Lancet 1:210, 1970.
13. Hansen, H.: Epidemiological considerations on maternal hyperphenylalaninemia, J. Ment. Defic. Res. 75:22, 1970.
14. Kerr, G. R., Chamove, A. S., Harlow, H. F., and Waisman, H. A.: "Fetal PKU": The effect of maternal hyperphenylalaninemia during pregnancy in the rhesus monkey (Macaca mulatta), Pediatrics 42:27, 1968.

Thyroid Disease

HYPOTHYROID AND HYPERTHYROID women may have normal babies but, in some instances, children with various abnormalities have been reported. Cretinism and other disorders have occurred (p. 440), but it often is difficult to establish a causal connection between the disease of the mother and the child's anomaly. In modern times, analyses have been complicated by drugs used for the mother's treatment, and there are many cases of congenital goiter on record that are attributed to maternal drug intake. Drugs used for hyperthyroidism in pregnancy may depress the functions of the fetal thyroid, stimulate increased output of thyrotropic hormone and result in thyroid hyperplasia. The subject is discussed under Endemic Goiter and Cretinism and in Chapter 44.

Tuberculosis

In a study of maternal health in early pregnancy and congenital defects, McDonald[1] noted that women with a history of pulmonary tuberculosis had an excess of children with serious defects. Lowe[2] considered the possibility that some of the drugs used in the treatment of tuberculosis could be teratogenic, but a series of 74 pregnancies during which isoniazid, *p*-aminosalicylic acid and streptomycin had been administered did not reveal any teratogenic effects of the drugs. Streptomycin and dihydrostreptomycin have been suspected as causes of congenital deafness and disturbances of equilibrium,[3,4] and there is a possibility that ethionamide can interfere with normal development of the fetus.[5]

REFERENCES

1. McDonald, A. D.: Maternal health in early pregnancy and congenital defects, Brit. J. Prev. & Social Med. 15:154, 1961.
2. Lowe, C. R.: Congenital defects among children born to women under supervision or treatment for pulmonary tuberculosis, Brit. J. Prev. & Social Med. 18:14, 1964.
3. Kern, G.: On the problem of intrauterine streptomycin damage, Schweiz. med. Wchnschr. 92:77, 1962.
4. Robinson, G. C., and Cambon, K. G.: Hearing loss in infants of tuberculous mothers treated with streptomycin during pregnancy, New England J. Med. 271:949, 1964.
5. Potworowska, M., Sianožecka, E., and Szufladowica, R.: Ethionamide treatment and pregnancy, Polish M. J. 5: 1152, 1966.

Hypoxia

Because hypoxia induces congenital malformations in laboratory animals[1,2] and has been said to be implicated in the origin of human congenital malformations,[3] a study of children born at relatively high altitudes is of great importance. Although such children were found to have lighter birth weights[4] and to be smaller[5] than children born at or near sea level, an elevated incidence of congenital malformations was not found.[4] Women with cyanotic cardiovascular disorders may also give birth to infants reduced in size but without gross congenital malformations.[6,7] The often-cited report by Alzamora *et al.*[8] has not been found convincing.[9] The influence of high altitude on the incidence of patent ductus arteriosus is discussed on page 465.

REFERENCES

1. Ingalls, T. H., Curley, F. J., and Prindle, R. A.: Experimental production of congenital abnormalities: Timing and degree of anoxia as factors causing fetal deaths and congenital abnormalities in mouse, New England J. Med. 247: 758, 1952.
2. Degenhardt, K. H., and Knoche, E.: Analysis of intrauterine malformations of vertebral column induced by oxygen deficiency, Canad. M.A.J. 80:441, 1959.
3. Ingalls, T. H.: Preventive Prenatal Pediatrics, in Levine, S. Z. (ed.), *Advances in Pediatrics* (Chicago: Year Book Medical Publishers, Inc., 1953), Vol. VI, p. 33.
4. Lichty, J. A., Ting, R. Y., Bruns, P. D., and Dyar, E.: Studies of babies born at high altitude. I. Relation of altitude to birth weight, A.M.A. J. Dis. Child. 93:666, 1957.
5. Howard, R. C., Lichty, J. A., and Bruns, P. D.: Studies of babies born at high altitude. II. Measurement of birth weight, body length, and head size, A.M.A. J. Dis. Child. 93:670, 1957.
6. Black-Schaffer, B.: Fetal nanosomia and bone athrepsia in newborn of woman with severe cyanotic cardiovascular anomaly, Am. J. Obst. & Gynec. 59:656, 1950.
7. Simon, D. L., and Lustberg, A.: Case of truncus arteriosus communis compatible with full-term pregnancy, Am. Heart J. 42:617, 1951.
8. Alzamora, A., Rotta, A., Battilana, G., Abugattas, R., Rubio, C., Bouroncle, J., Zapata, C., Santa-Maria, E., Binder, T., Subiria, R., Paredes, D., Pando, B., and Graham, G. G.: On the possible influence of great altitudes on the determination of certain cardiovascular anomalies, Pediatrics 12: 259, 1953.
9. Warkany, J.: Etiologic factors of congenital heart disease. In American Association for Advancement of Science. *Congenital Heart Disease* (Washington, D. C.: The Association, 1960).

Vitamin A Deficiency

Maternal vitamin A deficiency has been proved to be teratogenic in rats, rabbits and pigs. It results in rather similar malformations in different species, and one might expect that this nutritional deficiency, which is or was common in man, could cause comparable congenital defects in children. Actually, only a few observations have been made along this line. The most suggestive case is that of a child born in India to an almost completely blind mother who had signs of severe vitamin A deficiency. The infant had microcephaly and microphthalmia or anophthalmia.[1] Another case from India was reported by Lamba and Sood,[2] who observed a blind and mentally retarded girl with bilateral microphthalmia, coloboma of the iris and choroid and retinal aplasia. The mother gave a history of night blindness during pregnancy, which was treated with tablets and injections in a hospital. Congenital xerophthalmia and bilateral cleft lip in an infant born to a mother who had suffered from multiple vitamin deficiencies was reported by Houet and Ramioul-Lecomte.[3] Vitamin A as a possible factor in human teratology was considered by Gal *et al.*,[4] who examined vitamin A levels in blood plasma collected from mothers shortly after the production of malformed and normal offspring. No abnormally low levels were found after the birth of malformed children.

REFERENCES

1. Sarma, V.: Maternal vitamin A deficiency and fetal microcephaly and anophthalmia, Obst. & Gynec. 13:299, 1959.
2. Lamba, P. A., and Sood, N. N.: Congenital microphthalmus and colobomata in maternal vitamin A deficiency, J. Pediat. Ophth. May, 1968, pp. 115–117.
3. Houet, R., and Ramioul-Lecomte, S.: Répercussions sur l'enfant des avitaminoses de la mère pendant la grossesse, Ann. paediat. 175:378, 1950.
4. Gal, I., Sharman, I. M., Pryse-Davies, J., and Moore, T.: Vitamin A as a possible factor in human teratology, Proc. Nutrition Soc. 28:9A, 1969.

Carbon Monoxide Poisoning

FETAL DEATH OR DAMAGE[1] has been reported repeatedly after accidental or suicidal maternal exposure to illuminating gas or other sources of carbon monoxide. In a girl mentioned by Ingalls and Philbrook,[2] the extremities were grossly deformed except for a normal right arm; the mother's pregnancy had been complicated by an episode of severe carbon monoxide poisoning at 5–7 weeks of gestation. No comparable malformations were reported in other cases of carbon monoxide poisoning. In a case of Crothers and Paine,[3] the mother was overcome by illuminating gas when 2 months pregnant; the child had mild athetosis, impairment of ocular movements and borderline intelligence. In general, little correlation can be found between time of exposure to carbon monoxide and symptomatology of the children born alive. Microcephaly,[4] hydrocephaly,[5,6] retarded psychomotor development,[6,7] athetosis,[8] tremors,[9] hypertonicity of limbs,[6] tetraplegia,[4] convulsions,[6] low mentality[6,10] and arthrogryposis[11] have been observed. Cortical atrophy, enlargement of the ventricles, softening and cavitation of the basal ganglia, microgyria, destruction of the white matter and other changes have been described in the central nervous systems[5,8,9] of damaged children. The subject was reviewed in 1969 by Beaudoing *et al.*[12]

REFERENCES

1. Muller, G. L., and Graham, S.: Intrauterine death of fetus due to accidental carbon monoxide poisoning, New England J. Med. 252:1075, 1955.
2. Ingalls, T. H., and Philbrook, F. R.: Monstrosities induced by hypoxia, New England J. Med. 259:558, 1958.
3. Crothers, B., and Paine, R. S.: *The Natural History of Cerebral Palsy* (Cambridge, Mass.: Harvard University Press, 1959).
4. Brander, T.: Microcephalie u. Tetraplegie bei einem Kinde nach Kohlenmonoxydvergiftung der Mutter während der Schwangerschaft, Acta paediat. 28:123, 1940.
5. Neuburger, F.: Fall einer intrauterinen Hirnschädigung nach einer Leuchtgasvergiftung der Mutter, Beitr. Gerichtl. Med. 13:85, 1935.
6. Desclaux, P., Soulairac, A., and Morlon, C.: Intoxication oxycarbonée au cours d'une gestation (cinquième mois) arriération mentale consecutive, Arch. franç. pédiat. 8: 316, 1951.
7. Zourbas, J.: Encephalopathie congénitale avec troubles du tonus neuro-musculaire vraisemblablement consécutive à une intoxication par l'oxyde de carbone, Arch. franç pédiat. 4:513, 1947.
8. Hallervorden, J.: Über eine Kohlenoxydvergiftung im Fetalleben mit Entwicklungsstörungen der Hirnrinde, Allg. Ztschr. Psychiat. 124:289, 1949.
9. Maresch, R.: Über einen Fall von Kohlenoxydgasschädigung des Kindes in der Gebärmutter, Wien. med. Wchnschr. 79:454, 1929.
10. Lombard, J.: Du role de l'intoxication oxycarbonée comme facteur de malformations, Thése médecine Nancy, 1950.
11. Pollak, K.: Kindliche Missbildungen nach Suizidversuch der Mutter während der Schwangerschaft, Zentralbl. Gynäk. 81:1830, 1959.
12. Beaudoing, A., Gachon, J., Butin, L-P., and Bost, M.: Les conséquences foetales de l'intoxication oxycarbonée de la mère, Pédiatrie 24:539, 1969.

Minamata Disease

THIS DISORDER exemplifies fetal damages caused by maternal intake of methyl mercury contained in fish and shellfish from Minamata Bay, Kumamoto prefecture, Japan. The organic mercury compounds were derived from the wastes from chemical industry, which contaminated the water of the bay, were taken up by the fish and ingested by the population of the area.[1] Between 1953 and 1965, more than 100 men and women, chiefly fishermen and their wives, developed symptoms of a general disease of the central nervous system. Ataxia, impairment of gait, tremor, constriction of visual fields and disturbances of sensation were seen most often. The disease also occurred in infants, and there were at least 22 congenital cases that presented in the form of cerebral palsy. Spastic, ataxic and athetotic forms were observed. There were diplegias and tetraplegias and all children were mentally retarded. In some villages, 6–12% of the children were affected. The disease, which occurred only between the years 1954 and 1960, illustrates that water pollution can cause an endemic fetal disease.[2,3]

REFERENCES

1. Study Group of Minamata Disease, Kumamoto University, Japan: *Minamata Disease*, 1968.
2. Matsumoto, H., Koya, G., and Takeuchi, T.: Fetal Minamata disease. A neuropathological study of two cases of intrauterine intoxication by a methyl mercury compound, J. Neuropath. & Exper. Neurol. 24:563, 1965.
3. Harada, Y.: Congenital (or Fetal) Minamata Disease, in *Minamata Disease*, Study Group of Minamata Disease, Kumamoto University, Japan, 1968.

Lead Poisoning

THERE EXIST many reports on lead poisoning in women associated with sterility, abortions and high fetal and neonatal losses, and lead has long been used as an abortifacient.[1] One would expect to find some reports on congenital malformations in children who survived attempted abortion, but such cases have not been published. There are, however, reports on infants of mothers with lead poisoning who showed small size, delayed growth, postnatal convulsions, nervous system disorders and macrocranium. In many of these cases, postnatal exposure to lead cannot be excluded.[1] In recent times, maternal lead intoxication has become rare, since women cannot be employed in industries involving a lead hazard,[2] but it has been reported in a family in which lead poisoning was due to inhalation of fumes from burning battery cases.[1] The mother, who was 8 months pregnant, was treated with calcium disodium edetate; the infant, born 4 weeks following treatment of the mother, appeared normal and remained normal to the age of 4 years. But Palmisano *et al.*,[3] in 1969, described a child born with intrauterine growth retardation who showed failure to thrive, spasticity, tremors and ankle clonus; the mother had chronic plumbism attributed to habitual ingestion of untaxed (moonshine) whiskey. Such whiskey often has a high lead concentration.[3] Since such women usually are chronic alcoholics and not available for systematic investigations, the single case reported[3] is only suggestive of prenatal lead damage of the central nervous system; yet, it should direct attention to the possibility of concealed sources of maternal metal poisoning. The possibility of lead intoxication of the infant through mother's milk must also be considered, since neuropathologic changes have been produced in suckling rats[4] and mice[5] by adding lead to the maternal diet; however, the histologic responses in the young mice differed from those of the suckling rats.

REFERENCES

1. Angle, C. R., and McIntire, M. S.: Lead poisoning during pregnancy, Am. J. Dis. Child. 108:436, 1964.
2. Hamilton, A.: *Industrial Poisons in the United States* (New York: The Macmillan Company, 1925).
3. Palmisano, P. A., Sneed, R. C., and Cassady, G.: Untaxed whiskey and fetal lead exposure, J. Pediat. 75:869, 1969.
4. Pentschew, A., and Garro, F.: Lead encephalo-myelopathy of the suckling rat and its implications on the porphyrinopathic nervous diseases, Acta neuropath. 6:266, 1966.
5. Rosenblum, W. I., and Johnson, M. G.: Neuropathologic changes produced in suckling mice by adding lead to the maternal diet, Arch. Path. 85:640, 1968.

PART III

General Disturbances of Growth and Development

13

Dwarfism

THE TERM "DWARF" originally was used to describe an adult of markedly reduced size with normal proportions or deformed by disease. As a rule, the term was applied to persons who failed to attain a height of 140 cm. Small children were seldom called dwarfs, since experience showed that many of them grew at puberty and during adolescence sufficiently to outgrow their dwarfed state.

There are dwarf races like the Pygmies, whose genetic make-up keeps them small despite rather adequate living conditions and good health. Their sex development and intelligence permit them to reproduce and maintain their race. Such racial dwarfism is not pathologic.

Other persons are small because of disease, deficient diets or adverse living conditions. Although born normally sized and with genetic endowment to normal growth, they become dwarfed by bacterial or parasitic infestation or by other acquired disorders. Protein deficiency or lack of vitamin D combined with lack of sunshine can dwarf a genetically sound child. Cardiac, pulmonary, hepatic, renal, endocrine and metabolic disorders, whether inborn or acquired, can prevent adequate postnatal growth.

In contrast to dwarfism of postnatal origin there are types that are congenital. These children, whose growth has been stunted before they are born, are a heterogeneous group. They may remain small and become dwarfs in the common sense—or they may outgrow their intrauterine dwarfism and acquire normal stature in postnatal life (Chapter 14).

Many dwarfing disorders are discussed in this book under various headings. They could be treated here in a special chapter. But such a chapter limited to congenital forms of dwarfism would be incomplete and remain a fragmentary discourse on dwarfism. The subject of dwarfing in utero or intrauterine growth retardation will be treated thoroughly in the following pages. Other types of dwarfism are dealt with in various chapters and can be looked up there. A list of such conditions leading to reduced height or dwarfism follows. Because of the confused terminology, some syndromes are mentioned more than once.

	Page
Achondroplasia	768
"Amputations" (reduction malformations)	941
Arthrogryposis	1011
Asphyxiating thoracic dystrophy	795
Bird-headed dwarfs	137
Bloom syndrome	157
Cartilage-hair hypoplasia	797
Cat-cry syndrome	340
Chondrodystrophia calcificans	797
Chondrodystrophies	767
Chondrodystrophy with detached retina and deafness	804
Chondroectodermal dysplasia (Ellis-van Creveld syndrome)	793
Cleidocranial dysostosis	836
Cockayne syndrome	398
Cretinism, endemic	102, 806
Cretinism, sporadic	437
de Lange syndrome	139, 344
Diastrophic dwarfism	801
Down syndrome	311
Dysplasia epiphysealis multiplex	786
Ellis-van Creveld syndrome	793
Engelmann disease	844
Epidermolysis bullosa dystrophica	1151
Exostoses	840
Familial dyschondrosteosis	790
Fanconi pancytopenia	1020
Fibrous dysplasia (McCune-Albright)	878
Gargoylism	808
Hallermann-Streiff-François syndrome	390
Hemidystrophy	167
Hunter syndrome	816
Hurler syndrome	809
Hyperphosphatasia	862
Hypophosphatasia	859
IUGR	134
Leprechaunism	142, 159
Lowe syndrome	389
Madelung deformity	790
Marchesani syndrome	395
Marinesco-Sjögren syndrome	392
Metaphyseal dysostosis	791
Metatropic dwarfism	803
Microcephalies	136, 237
Mitral insufficiency and deafness	409
Morquio disease	819
Morquio-Ullrich syndrome	817
Oculocerebrorenal (Lowe) syndrome	389
Osteochondrodystrophia deformans (Jacobsen)	805

Osteochondrodystrophy (Morquio) 819
Osteogenesis imperfecta 824
Osteopetrosis 863
Osteopsathyrosis 824
Ovarian dysgenesis (Turner syndrome) 1122
Pituitary dwarfism 419-424
Prenatal rubella syndrome 62
Progeria 141, 160
Pseudoachondroplasia 783
Pseudohypoparathyroidism 446
Pseudo-pseudohypoparathyroidism 448
Pyknodysostosis 869
Reduction malformations 941-957
Rothmund-Thomson syndrome 392
Russell dwarfism 140
Silver syndrome 139
Spinal malformations 909, 918-925
Spondylo-epiphyseal dysplasia 783
Stippled epiphyses 797
Turner syndrome 1122

REFERENCES

Clayton, B. E., Tanner, J. M., Newns, G. H., Whitehouse, R. H., and Renwick, A. G. L.: Differential diagnosis of children with short stature not associated with metabolic, chromosomal, or gross nervous system defects, Arch. Dis. Childhood 42:245, 1967.

Di George, A. M., and Paschkis, K. E.: Dwarfism, Pediat. Clin. North America 4:925, 1957.

Horstmann, P.: Dwarfism. With special reference to the significance of endocrine factors, Acta endocrinol. 3:1, 1949.

Langer, L. O.: Short stature. Check list of conditions associated with retarded longitudinal growth, Clin. Pediat. 8:142, 1969.

Mason, A. S., and Tanner, J. M.: Human Growth Hormone in the Treatment of Dwarfism, in *Modern Trends in Endocrinology* (New York: Appleton-Century-Crofts, 1967).

Rischbieth, H., and Barrington, A.: Dwarfism, in *Treasury of Human Inheritance* (London: University of London, Francis Galton Laboratory for National Eugenics, 1912), Memoir 15, pts. 7 and 8.

Smith, D. W.: Compendium on shortness of stature, J. Pediat. 70:463, 1967.

Weinberg, M. S.: The problems of midgets and dwarfs and organizational remedies: A study of the little people of America, J. Health & Social Behav. 9:65, 1968.

Wilkins, L.: *The Diagnosis and Treatment of Endocrine Disorders in Childhood and Adolescence* (3d ed.; Springfield, Ill.: Charles C Thomas, Publisher, 1965).

14

Intrauterine Growth Retardation

IT WAS WELL KNOWN at the beginning of this century that there were dwarfs whose growth retardation was present at birth and dwarfs whose growth retardation developed in postnatal life. Hansemann,[1] in 1902, distinguished between primordial dwarfism and infantile dwarfism, the latter corresponding to the pituitary dwarfism of today. Fetal ateleiosis[2] and fetal microsomia[3] were alternative terms used for dwarfism present at birth. Just as postnatal growth retardation may have many causes, intrauterine growth retardation can be due to many heterogeneous factors.

Although intrauterine growth retardation is a striking and long-known phenomenon, our knowledge of this abnormal growth process is still limited. There are natural and man-made reasons for this. It is natural that growth in utero cannot be studied as well as growth in postnatal life. The man-made haze over the area is pediatric in origin. It was with good intention that early pediatricians declared all children weighing less than 2,500 Gm. at birth as "premature," irrespective of their gestational age, and gave them the care and attention required by infants born too early. Ylppö,[4] who suggested the term "premature" for every child with a birth weight under 2,500 Gm., was well aware that even children with birth weights of 2,000 Gm. can result from full-term pregnancies, but he believed that such small term children – "with few exceptions" – behave like immature children. The misnomer may have benefited these small children, but it impeded etiologic research and prognostic knowledge concerning the true prematures as well as the pseudoprematures, i.e., children with intrauterine growth retardation (IUGR).

There can be no doubt that occasionally children are born with a birth weight far below that expected at their gestational age, although it must be admitted that errors are possible in the calculation of confinement and that the mother may give erroneous information concerning her last menstrual period. Despite the uncertainty of gestational estimates and age, one can safely assume that some mothers of such pseudoprematures are right when they state that they carried their small babies for 9 months and that their children were actually born at term. Time-controlled animal experiments and observations show that sometimes young are born whose growth was stunted in utero, and there is no reason to believe that intrauterine growth retardation is limited to animals. It cannot be merely coincidental that mothers who give birth to children with the de Lange syndrome or with trisomy 18 so often report full-term gestation for their children under 2,500 Gm. and that their physicians err so frequently in the calculation of the expected date of delivery.

Once the existence of infants born at term with low birth weights is admitted, a number of questions arise concerning these children who have been incorrectly called prematures. What is their fate in postnatal life, what their physical and mental development? Do they have specific somatic characteristics? Do they represent an etiologic and pathologic entity? What is their incidence in the general population? What is the cause of their stunted growth in utero? What is their behavior in utero? What is known about their fetal membranes and their placentas?

It is clear that only extensive, longitudinal, prospective studies could answer these questions. Obstetricians observe such children for a short time only. The same is true for pediatricians in charge of newborn nurseries. On the other hand, there is also bias in the point of view of the physician who sees only handicapped children and may find among them a large proportion of children with a history of IUGR. He does not see or follow systematically children who, although born at term and underweight, develop normally and do not require consultation because of physical or mental retardation. It must be expected, therefore, that he, too, cannot present a well-balanced picture of this topic.

Although the existence of such children is common knowledge, publications concerned with them were relatively few until 1960. Some obstetricians were aware of the difficulties arising from the use of the word "premature" for infants born at term. In 1947, McBurney[5] pointed out the dilemma of the obstetrician who delivers such a baby. Since the presumptive signs of pregnancy accompanying a 2-month period of amenorrhea enable the physician to predict the time of delivery, obstetricians recognized the possible discrepancy between birth weight and gestational age: "In such instances, when the patient has been delivered of her baby within 1 or 2 weeks, or even after the estimated date of parturition, it is extremely annoying to have a pediatrician insist that the baby is premature because it weighs only 4½ or 5 lb." In Los Angeles, McBurney found that the incidence of babies delivered at term weighing 5 lb. 8 oz. (2,500 Gm.) or less was approximately 1%. Colman and Rienzo,[6] at Long Island, New York, noted that 2% of the babies born at term weighed 2,500 Gm. or less, and Yerushalmy *et al.*[7] found that 3.7% of single white live births in New York City weighing under 2,500 Gm. had been carried 37 weeks or more. But the incidence of the pseudoprematures was different in New York City and in Oakland, California, in males and in females and in whites and in Negroes. Gruenwald *et al.*[8,9] estimated that for every two truly premature babies in the low birth weight group there is one pseudopremature. In areas of high altitude, the incidence may be much higher. In a county of high altitude in Colorado, Lichty *et al.*[10] found the incidence of "prematurity," as defined by birth weight, to be 30.8%, in contrast to the state average of 10.4%. A comparison of average birth weights for newborns in this county and a comparable group of newborns in Denver showed that the high-altitude babies were approximately three-quarters of a pound lighter than the Denver babies. These small babies apparently were not abnormal in any way; their neonatal mortality was not elevated, and the incidence of congenital defects was approximately the same as that reported from other areas. Therefore, it seems well established that a considerable portion of the children born weighing under 2,500 Gm. are not premature and that McBurney's[5] complaint was entirely justified. It also seems that many of these pseudoprematures develop into normal and healthy children. Not only those born at high altitudes, but also infants in various ethnic groups other than Caucasians normally often show birth weights below 2,500 Gm.

Physicians interested in handicapped children are not much concerned with infants who were only slightly underweight at the time of birth, but rather with more extreme cases whose birth weights were under 2,000 Gm. This figure lies far below the third percentile value (2,630 Gm.) for children born at term, and represents a weight deficit of over 40% of 3,400 Gm., the average or median value given for mature infants.[11,12] The number of these children is much smaller than that of those between 2,000 and 2,500 Gm. Their incidence is approximately only one-tenth of the total of the pseudopremature population – namely, 0.1%, using McBurney's figures,[5] or 0.17% according to Colman and Rienzo.[6] It is in these more marked or extreme cases that we must look for pathologic prenatal conditions that may continue after birth.

A contribution from the obstetric point of view was made along these lines by Rumbolz and McGoogan,[13] who discussed small, "undernourished full-term babies" and who, like McBurney, attributed their growth deficiency to placental insufficiency. They considered the more severe forms of IUGR. Reporting the results of pregnancies at or near term with a delivery of infants weighing 2,000 Gm. or less, they found in a series of 7,058 pregnancies 17 babies born after 36 weeks' gestation or longer with a birth weight under 2,000 Gm. This suggests an incidence of about 0.25%, which is twice that of a comparable group in McBurney's series. The difference is explained by the fact that McBurney considered only live-born children, whereas Rumbolz and McGoogan included stillborn babies in their series. Since the perinatal mortality in the latter series amounted to about 50%, the incidence figures of the two series agree fairly well: 0.1 or 0.12% of the pregnancies observed by these obstetricians ended in babies born alive at or near term weighing 2,050 Gm. or less. In a second series, Rumbolz *et al.*[14] again found an incidence of 0.25% of small full-term babies, this time with a perinatal mortality of 35%. In both series it seemed that 90% of the survivors of IUGR had no difficulty in postnatal life, and within a short period attained the accepted normal growth pattern and were living and well at the time of the reports. In a large Finnish series,[15] comparable infants were observed in only 0.05% of the pregnancies. In the prospective Fetal Life Study of the Columbia-Presbyterian Medical Center[16] there were, in a series of 5,382 live-born infants surviving 28 days, 9 who weighed 2,000 Gm. or less after a gestation of at least 37 completed weeks. This is an incidence of 0.17% live-born children with severe IUGR (2,000 Gm. or less) surviving the neonatal period. This estimate, and those of Rumbolz *et al.*[14] (0.16%) and Colman and Rienzo[6] (0.17%) tally closely. Thus, the incidence of infants weighing 2,000 Gm. or less, although born at term, equals approximately that of the Down syndrome. Of course, fetuses with IUGR and a weight deficit of 40% can also be born before term, but their number could not be ascertained easily in the past, since their weight and gestation time usually were not recorded in publications, although the growth retardation could have been ascertained by comparison with the standard weights of Streeter or Scammon and Calkins.[17] Now, percentile curves of intrauterine growth, constructed from the birth weights of infants at gestational ages ranging from 24 to 42 weeks, are available.[18-20, 158, 161, 169-176] There are differences for geographic areas and socioeconomic and ethnic groups, but these will hardly change the important results already obtained with older standards.[20] Whatever the classification and procedure used, certain facts have emerged regarding children with IUGR that are of general biologic and teratologic interest. Details will be worked out in years to come.

As pointed out before, children with IUGR were not sufficiently investigated in the past because they were submerged in the collective pool of "prematurity." This has been corrected in recent years but, again, a tendency to oversimplification can be noted. General statements are being made about "low birth weight" or "small for dates" babies, about children with "fetal malnutrition" and "dysmatures" as if they were an entity or two entities. Even with the crude evaluations available 10 years ago, one could show that intrauterine growth retardation has many causes and that it can affect many types of abnormal fetuses.[21] One must doubt that there are only two general groups—a "malnourished" group (fetal malnutrition, placental insufficiency) and a "hypoplastic" group (fetal rubella, congenital malformations, etc.),[22] and one cannot accept the generalizations made in regard to these two groups. Although only crude observations concerning intrauterine growth were available in the past, and data on both birth weight and duration of gestation are still scarce, the heterogeneity of the growth-retarded population can be demonstrated easily by naming a few types that have been recognized so far.

Children with Intrauterine Growth Retardation

Between the stillborn infant with IUGR and the children who achieve normal growth and development, a spectrum of conditions can be discerned ranging from semilethal syndromes to conditions of slight impairment of physical and mental growth. Some of these syndromes are rather well defined, others are nonspecific. Only a few of the disease pictures are understood etiologically. Despite our lack of knowledge in this area, one point is clear: intrauterine growth retardation has many causes and it results in many clinical pictures. To consider children with IUGR as an entity or as one syndrome should not be encouraged.

Clinical Disease Pictures Sometimes Associated with Intrauterine Growth Retardation

Microcephaly.—Microcephaly often has been observed in children with IUGR. It occurs in a semilethal and extreme form and in various milder types described in surviving children. Warkany *et al.*[21] reported a case (Case 1) of extreme microcephaly and posterior cleft palate, the child being born at full term weighing 1,360 Gm. (Fig. 14-1). The placenta was very small. The child died at the age of 4 weeks. Dr. S. P. Horwood[23] observed 2 children in a family in which the mother, after four normal pregnancies, delivered these 2 with severe IUGR. In both pregnancies, growth of the uterus ceased early. The fifth pregnancy terminated in the forty-first week with the delivery of a stillborn infant weighing 920 Gm! The placenta weighed 185 Gm. The fetus showed microcephaly and cleft lip and palate. The sixth pregnancy terminated at term with delivery of a female infant weighing 1,080 Gm. (Fig. 14-2). The placenta weighed 400 Gm. There was microcephaly and a

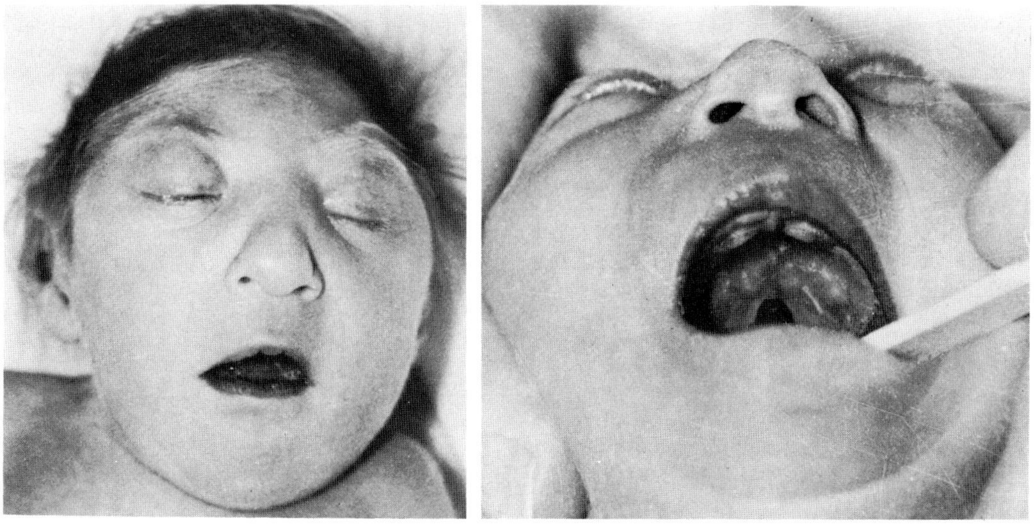

Fig. 14-1.—Microcephalic girl with cleft palate born at full term weighing 1,360 Gm.

highly arched palate. Toxoplasma skin test was negative and the chromosomal complement was normal. This child survived birth, but she appeared spastic, developed twitching and died at the age of 4 months. Stringaris[24] gave a detailed description of the brain of a male infant who was born at term weighing 2,000 Gm. The brain weighed 180 Gm. after the child's death at the age of 5½ months (the normal brain weight for this age is approximately 650 Gm.). Gruenwald[9] recorded an infant with micrencephaly (brain weight 195 Gm.) who weighed 1,320 Gm. after 37 weeks of gestation.

Among surviving microcephalics with IUGR are some of the well-known dwarfs of history and the "bird-headed dwarfs" so carefully recorded by Seckel.[25] Seckel did not include IUGR among the identifying criteria of bird-headed dwarfs, but the 2 patients studied by him were born after a gestation of 40 weeks, weighing 1,715 and 1,960 Gm., respectively, and therefore had typical IUGR. Seckel also collected 13 cases of bird-headed dwarfs from the literature published between 1746 and 1951. Of these, 10 weighed less than 2,000 Gm. when born at term. Among them were such famous dwarfs as Caroline Crachami (said to have weighed 450 Gm. at full term), who was cited as an example of "ateleiosis, Group I" or "foetal ateleiosis" by Gilford[2] in 1903; Edouard Placereau, who, after a gestation of normal duration, was small enough to be wrapped in a pocket handkerchief; Frank Flynn (General Mite) born at term weighing 900 Gm.; Pauline Muster, whose mother's "abdomen had never grown during 9 months of pregnancy," weighed 1,000 Gm. at term; Janos Dobos, who weighed, at full term, between 500 and 1,000 Gm. and had 3 brothers who were also dwarfs, born small at full term; a Dutch dwarf born at term weighing 1,250 Gm.; and 2 brothers, Carroll and James Flu,

Fig. 14-2.—Girl supposedly born at term weighing 1,080 Gm. An older stillborn sibling weighed 920 Gm. (supposedly at term). (Courtesy of Dr. S. P. Horwood, Cleveland, Ohio.)

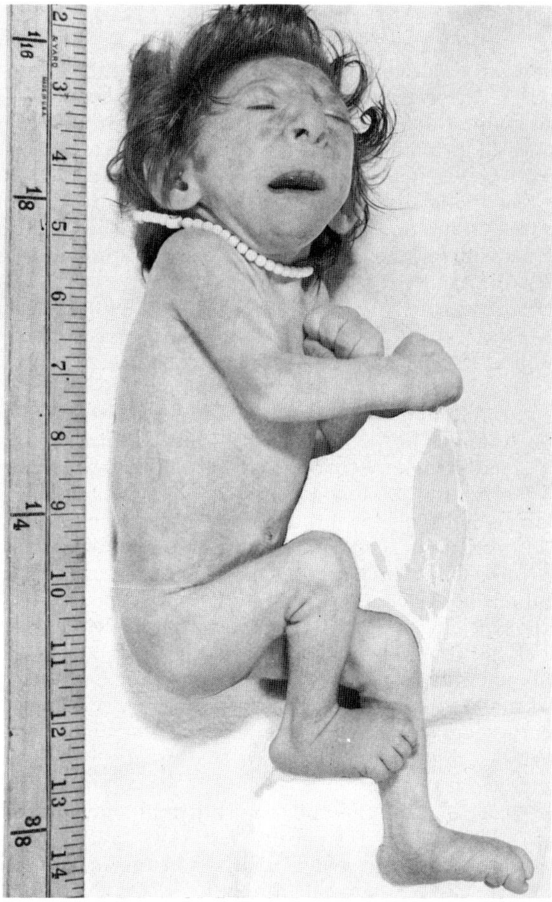

born at term weighing 1,350 and "between 1,350 and 1,500 Gm.," respectively.[25-27] The last are of special interest, since both developed anemia, granulocytopenia and thrombocytopenia and belong in the group described by Fanconi[28] as "Familiäre infantile perniziosaartige Anämie" and by Upjohn[29] as "Familial dwarfism associated with microcephaly, mental retardation and anaemia." Fanconi described this syndrome in 3 siblings, and Upjohn in 5. Fanconi mentioned "low birth weight" and one suspects that all these cases had IUGR, but this can be documented only for the brothers reported by Panos[27] and Seckel[25] who were dwarfed when born *at term.*

However, IUGR with microcephaly is much more frequent than cases conforming to Seckel's definition of bird-headed dwarfs. Menichella[177,179] pointed out that the prognosis for infants with low birth weights born at term or later is worse than that for truly premature babies. Mental retardation and dwarfism may become manifest in later life. This was also shown in some of the cases reported by Warkany *et al.*[21] Laurance[30] observed a family in which 5 children were dwarfed. Three siblings died of pneumonia. Two examined by Laurance were born at term, a boy weighing 1,960 Gm. and a girl weighing 2,268 Gm. Both were microcephalic but "alert," and both had similar old-looking faces. The "Aztecs," Maximo and Bartola, who were microcephalic idiots, were said to have been "dwarfish" at their birth.[25] A microcephalic girl, born at full term weighing only 1,165 Gm., was described by Grossman *et al.*[31] as a case of pseudosenilism with a progeroid syndrome. De Toni[32] reported the case of a child who weighed 1,300 Gm. at birth and who was a microcephalic dwarf when seen at the age of 19 months. Mann and Russell[33] studied a microcephalic midget who weighed 1,600 Gm. when born a few days after term.

Other types of microcephaly associated with IUGR have been recorded after exposure to large doses of x-ray in utero and following prenatal rubella and cytomegalic inclusion disease (Chapters 9 and 10). A peculiar familial tendency to microcephaly was reported by Warkany *et al.*[21] (Cases 4–6). In that family, some males and females were born small for their gestational ages, but the IUGR was more pronounced in males; microcephaly was not observed in females who developed normally in postnatal life. In a number of cases of microcephaly and IUGR, various chromosomal aberrations have been noted and held responsible for the pathologic development.[34-36] Some children with the cat-cry syndrome had IUGR (p. 340).

MACRENCEPHALY (MEGALENCEPHALY; PSEUDOHYDROCEPHALY).—This condition is characterized by enlargement of the head (macrocrania, megalocephaly) and enlargement of the brain. In contrast to hydrocephaly, the ventricular system is not enlarged (p. 244). Some of the children with macrencephaly have IUGR. Russell[37] pointed out that his "intrauterine dwarfs" showed a relatively large cranium and small facial bones. Closure of the anterior fontanelle was delayed but the circumference of the head was not above normal. Szalay[38] described 3 patients of this type with birth weights of 1,560, 1,730 and 2,130 Gm., respectively, although born at term. He emphasized that such children may have a normal cranium sitting on a dwarfed body. Knowledge of this syndrome will aid in the differentiation from hydrocephaly and make unnecessary repeated air ventriculograms. Sudden death occurred in one of Szalay's cases. The brain at age 41 months weighed 1,320 Gm. and was, therefore, above the average of 1,170 Gm. for that age. One patient had an I.Q. between 75 and 80. Chromosomes appeared normal in one case.

An infant described by us[39] with IUGR due to aminopterin poisoning can be considered as a nonviable case of macrencephaly. Another patient, a boy (Fig. 14-3), seen in the Cincinnati Children's Hospital, was born after a pregnancy of 42 weeks weighing 1,990 Gm. Failure to thrive led to several hospital admissions. The marked craniofacial dysostosis, the low-set ears and the enlarged anterior fontanelle suggested hydrocephaly but air encephalograms showed a normal ventricular system. His physical and mental development appeared slow and at the age of 6 years his height was only 87.5 cm. and his weight 12 kg. But his I.Q. was within normal limits. A chromosome analysis showed a normal karyotype. A similar patient, reported by Ammann,[40] was born 10 days after term with a birth weight of only 1,660 Gm. The cranium was large, suggesting hydrocephaly, and the facial bones were hypoplastic. The child had microphthalmia and the setting-sun sign but there was no enlargement of the ventricular system. Physical development was extremely slow but the mental development appeared normal. Figure 14-4 illustrates another pseudohydrocephalic child.

CEREBRAL PALSY.—Cerebral palsy is a clinical diagnosis of admittedly heterogeneous origin. Since the time of William J. Little, premature labor has been blamed for some of the cases (Chapter 33), and it is well established that low birth weight is associated with the condition carrying this name. McDonald[41] found that 6.5% of the children weighing not more than 1,800 Gm. at birth developed cerebral palsy. Alberman[42] considered both birth weight and length of gestation in cerebral palsy and found evidence that some patients with cerebral palsy had shown a tendency to growth retardation before birth, suggesting prenatal factors acting in the development of certain types of cerebral palsy. It was among the diplegics that, with a gestation of 39 weeks and over, a mean birth weight significantly lower than that of the corresponding controls was found. Among the patients with IUGR described by Warkany *et al.*[21] there were several who could be considered to have "cerebral palsy."

MARINESCO-SJÖGREN SYNDROME.—In siblings with this syndrome of congenital cataract, mental and

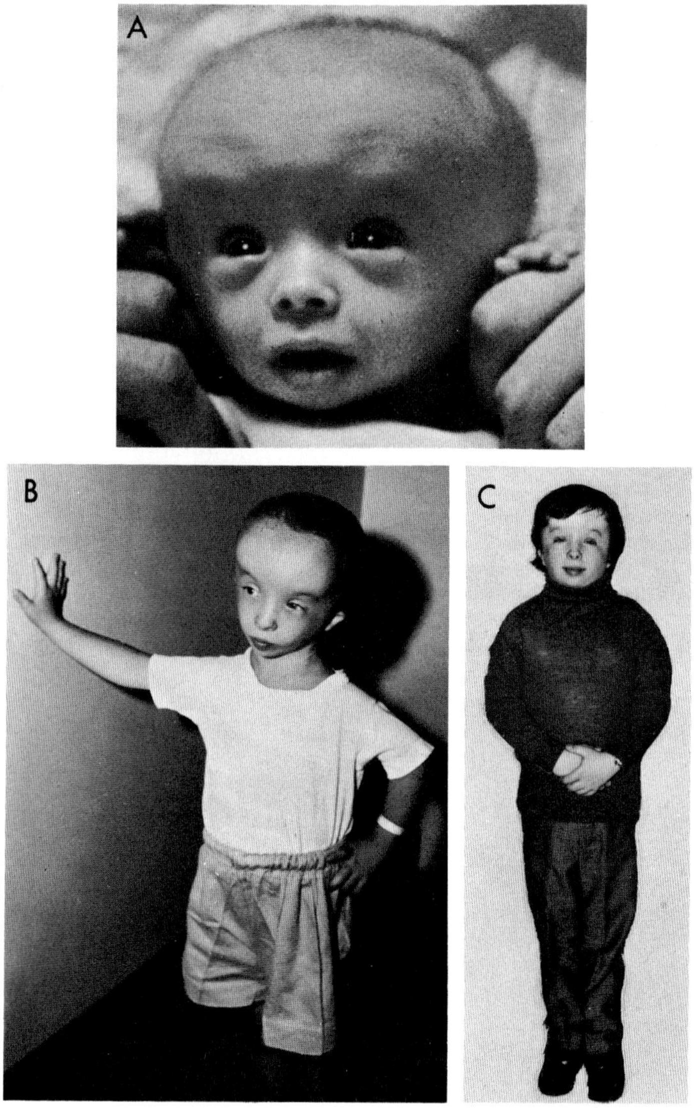

Fig. 14-3. – **A,** infant with pseudohydrocephaly who was born after a gestation of 42 weeks weighing 1,990 Gm. Air encephalograms showed a normal ventricular system. **B,** the boy at the age of 6 years. His I.Q. was normal. **C,** at the age of 11½ years he had a height of 121 cm., which is far below the 3d percentile, but he was well adjusted and good in school. His I.Q. was about 100.

physical retardation and ataxia, Norwood[43] noted IUGR and thus established onset of the disorder before birth.

DE LANGE SYNDROME. – This syndrome, as described by Cornelia de Lange[44] in 1933, consisted of brachycephaly, low-set ears, heavy eyebrows and lashes, small hands and feet, proximal position of thumb and syndactyly of the toes. Intrauterine growth retardation was marked in these children. As the syndrome became better known, new symptoms had to be included and then it was discovered that a patient showing this disease picture had been described by Brachmann[45] 17 years before de Lange. Although the symptoms described by the two authors differed greatly, IUGR was present in all. Brachmann stated that birth occurred at term and that the birth weight was 1,600 Gm. According to Jervis and Stimson,[46] intrauterine growth retardation seems to be the rule (p. 344) in de Lange syndrome, but some of the reported patients[47] had normal birth weights.

SILVER SYNDROME. – A syndrome of congenital "hemihypertrophy," shortness of stature and elevated urinary gonadotropins was described by Silver *et al.*[48] in 1953. Two patients, a girl and a boy, born at term and weighing 1,818 and 1,730 Gm., respectively, were reported. These children, who had marked IUGR,

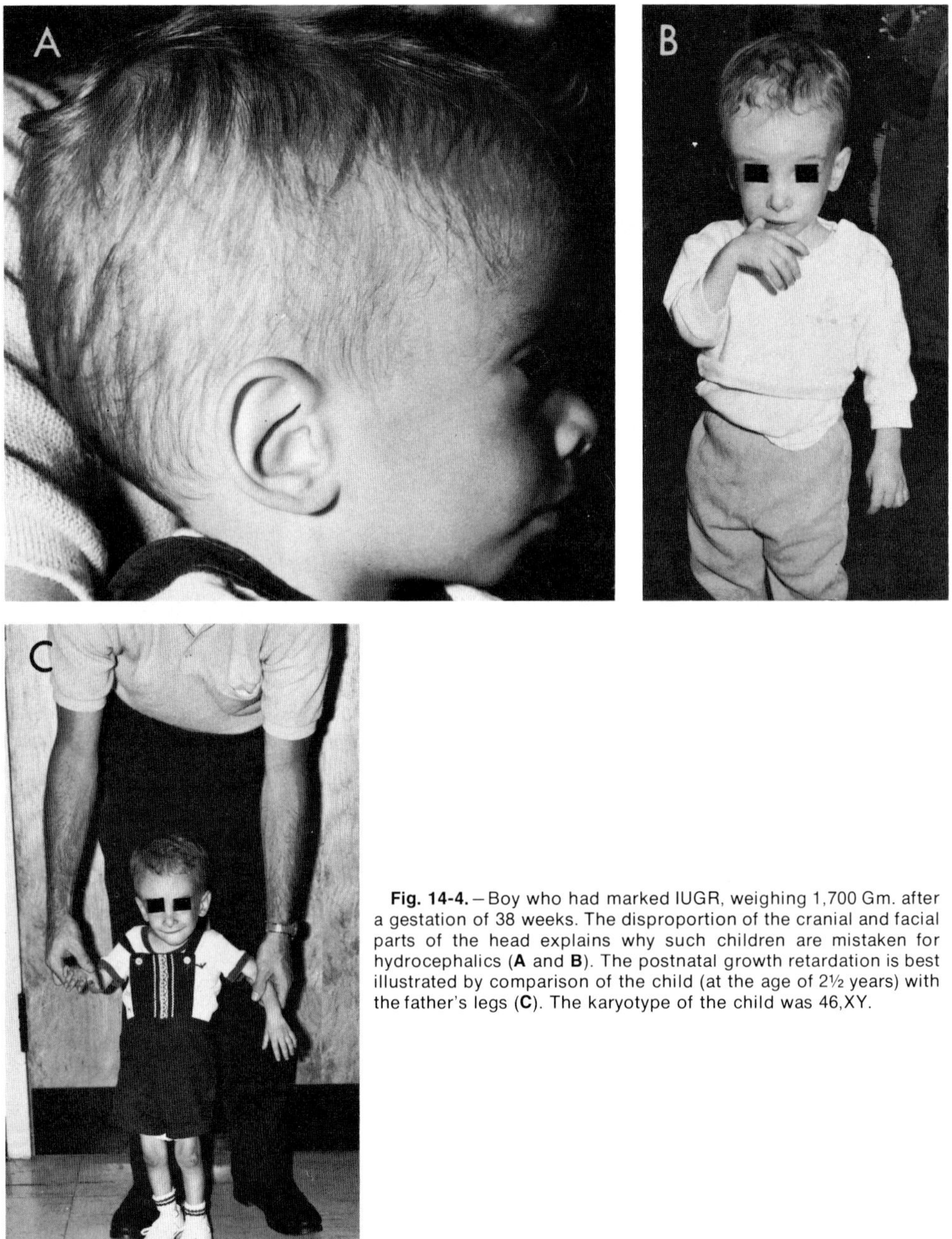

Fig. 14-4.—Boy who had marked IUGR, weighing 1,700 Gm. after a gestation of 38 weeks. The disproportion of the cranial and facial parts of the head explains why such children are mistaken for hydrocephalics (**A** and **B**). The postnatal growth retardation is best illustrated by comparison of the child (at the age of 2½ years) with the father's legs (**C**). The karyotype of the child was 46,XY.

were still small at the time of examination. In the girl, the entire right side of the body was *smaller* than the left, and in the boy the left side was *smaller* than the right. As pointed out on page 163, the term "hemihypertrophy" does not seem fitting for such children with bilateral growth retardation and growth more retarded on one side than on the other. Children with true hemihypertrophy born at term have normal birth weights.

Russell intrauterine dwarfism.—In 1954, Russell[37] demonstrated in London 5 examples of "intrauterine dwarfism" recognizable at birth, with craniofacial dysostosis, disproportionately short arms and other anomalies. These children obviously had IUGR, as they weighed between 1,360 and 1,810 Gm. at birth, and prematurity was denied by the mothers. There was threatened abortion in 3, and a small placenta in 4 of the cases. The faces of these children were small in comparison with the skull, closure of the anterior fontanelle was delayed, the upper extremities were short, the fifth fingers incurved and a slight degree of hemiatrophy was present. The children were hyperactive and alert and showed normal mental development. The final outcome of these cases was not known at the time of publication, since none of the children had reached adulthood.

Russell failed to find in the families of his patients abnormal growth patterns or other abnormal traits, and believed that a case could be made of acquired intrauterine growth failure because of the history of threatened abortions of the mothers and placental pathology. His concept approached that of obstetricians such as McBurney[5] and Rumbolz and McGoogan[13,14] but, in contrast to them, he did not consider the survivors entirely normal physically. He pointed out that the smallness of the face relative to the skull often conveys an impression of hydrocephaly in infancy, although the head circumference seldom exceeded the appropriate value. He described the sharply updrawn philtrum and the downdrawn angles of the mouth resulting in an inverted 'V" or "shark mouth." The skeleton was characterized by shortening of the upper limbs, slight lordosis, tubular chest and incurved little finger. Thus, one can recognize in Russell's cases certain features described by de Lange[44] in 1933, but, in contrast to her patients, those of Russell were mentally normal. Hemiatrophy in two cases is comparable to the "hemihypertrophy" stressed by Silver[48] in 1953. The "impression of hydrocephalus in infancy" was mentioned before him by Thomson[49] in a patient with poikiloderma congenitale (p. 393) and later described by Szalay[38] as "pseudohydrocephalus" with IUGR. The importance of Russell's contribution lies in his emphasis on "intrauterine dwarfism" in contrast to prematurity and in his description of threatened abortion and smallness of the uterus of some of the mothers and of their small placentas.

Warkany *et al.*,[21] who reported 27 cases of IUGR, saw only one child who conformed to the syndromes of Silver[48] and Russell.[37] Obviously, only a small portion of the children with IUGR have the characteristics described by these authors. We suggested that the term "intrauterine dwarfism" be avoided. Since children with IUGR may eventually attain normal or near-normal height, they should not be spoken of as "dwarfs" until one can be certain that growth has stopped and the final height attained. The term "intrauterine growth retardation" is less euphonic and harder to pronounce than "intrauterine dwarfism," but it appears preferable, since it will avoid unnecessary anxiety in the parents.

Bloom syndrome.—In some children with IUGR, telangiectatic erythema develops after exposure to sunlight. Bloom[50] described several children of this type and reviewed the literature. Szalay[51] reported three cases, two in a brother and his sister. Although the gestation times were 40 weeks or more, the birth

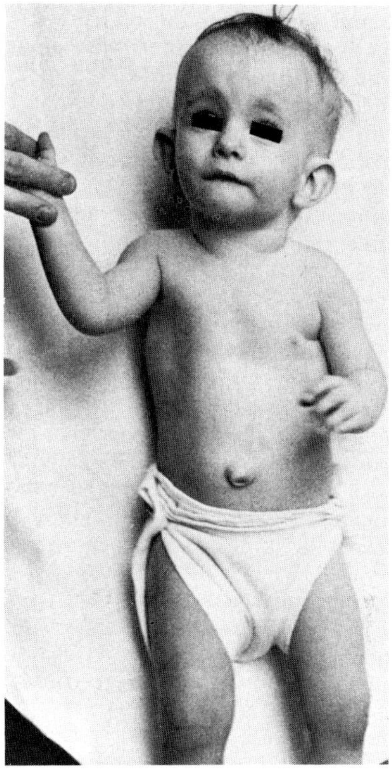

Fig. 14-5.—Girl with "Russell" or "Silver" type of intrauterine growth retardation at age 11 months. The birth weight was 1,650 Gm. at full term. The left eye is somewhat smaller than the right. Normal intelligence but slow growth. (From J. Warkany, B. B. Monroe and B. S. Sutherland.[21])

weights were 2,013, 2,098 and 2,041 Gm., respectively. Congenital malformations and anomalies often are associated with the skin disease (p. 157). A similar, though not identical, condition of familial low birth weight, unusual facies and a skin eruption was recorded by Dubowitz.[52]

Progeria and progeroid syndromes.—Among children with progeria or progeroid syndromes, a birth weight low for the gestational age has been observed repeatedly. Wiedemann[53] listed some of these cases and added one of his own, a child weighing 1,850 Gm. at term. A case of progeria in a child born at term with an estimated birth weight of 2,000 Gm. was described in great detail by Zeder.[54] This patient also had scleroderma, but probably not "hypophyseal dwarfism," as suggested in the title of the paper, since patients with pituitary dwarfism usually have normal weight at birth. Schondel[55] described a girl with progeria and microphthalmia who weighed 1,750 Gm. although born at term. Grossman *et al.*[31] reported an atypical patient classified by them as having a progeroid syndrome who, born at full term, weighed only 1,165 Gm. Her growth retardation persisted, and by the age of 6 years she attained a weight of only 3,640 Gm. and a length of 66 cm.

LEPRECHAUNISM.—The syndrome described by Donohue and Uchida[56] is associated with IUGR (p. 159). In both of their cases there was apparent cessation of fetal growth about the seventh month of pregnancy, and the mother reported cessation of abdominal growth at the same time of gestation. Intrauterine fetal movements were barely detectable from this time on in the first pregnancy, which ended at term with the birth of an infant weighing 1,780 Gm. The second child, the result of the mother's seventh pregnancy, was delivered prematurely after a pregnancy of 7½ months, weighing 1,600 Gm. Although the IUGR appeared less marked in this case, one can assume that it would have been more conspicuous at a later date, since growth probably had stopped by the time of the premature delivery. In some cases published subsequently as "leprechauns," IUGR was absent, but they had little resemblance to the patients reported by Donohue and Uchida. In two sisters entirely comparable with those of Donohue and Uchida and reported by Kálló *et al.*,[57] there was marked IUGR.

ROTHMUND-THOMSON SYNDROME.—In some instances, IUGR could be established for children with this syndrome[58,59] but, unfortunately, both birth weight and gestation time were recorded in only a few case reports (Chapter 40).

CONGENITAL CARDIOVASCULAR MALFORMATIONS.—Prenatal growth of children with cardiac malformations has not yet been examined adequately. There are some data that suggest IUGR in some of the fetuses with abnormal hearts. Engle,[60] writing about infants with ventricular septal defect, found it remarkable that 7 of 9 babies with this anomaly had birth weights in the "premature" range although, with one exception, the pregnancies were full term. Naeye[61] noted that most infants with congenital heart disease considered premature because of low birth weights are rather dysmature, since their birth measurements are subnormal for gestational age. Although all infants with CHD combined had 91% of normal birth weights, there were some whose weights were 40–50% of the expected weight for their gestational age. In contrast, an elevated birth weight seemed to be characteristic for infants with transposition of the great vessels. There is a tendency to low birth weight for gestational age in children with supravalvar aortic stenosis.

VARIOUS CONGENITAL MALFORMATIONS.—It is well known to experimental teratologists that abnormal young born of mothers exposed to various teratogens during pregnancy are often small and underweight for their gestational ages. An extreme case is shown in Figure 14-8, where rats exposed to heavy x-irradiation during pregnancy and removed from the uterus just before term are compared with a normal control young of the same gestational age. Smaller doses of x-rays and other teratogens result in less IUGR. Riboflavin deficiency results in young with a pattern of skeletal defects; in general, their IUGR parallels the severity of the skeletal abnormalities.

IUGR is not uncommon in children with severe and multiple malformations,[178] although it seldom can be documented because the recorders often fail to state both birth weight and gestational age. Sometimes low birth weight and full-term delivery are mentioned. A monstrous full-term child, weighing 1,200 Gm. was described by Crelin.[62] The child, born to a mother 40 years of age, showed eventration of the abdominal viscera, intestinal malrotation and imperforate anus. There also were renal anomalies, an atrial septal defect and a single umbilical artery. Newbill[63] described a sirenomelic monster born at full term that weighed 1,565 Gm. and was 39 cm. long. Agenesis of both kidneys often is associated with IUGR. Potter,[64] in a review of 50 of these cases, found that of 20 infants with this anomaly delivered after 37 weeks of pregnancy, only 3 weighed more than 2,500 Gm. Of 17 infants of more than 37 weeks' gestation, 11 weighed less than 2,000 Gm. and 6 from 2,000 to 2,500 Gm. In those of younger gestational age the weight was less than the average for the period of gestation. This was true for a large share of fetuses with renal agenesis and multiple malformations. Necropsy of a "male infant with a uterus" born at term weighing 1,580 Gm. was done by Richard and Benirschke.[65] The placenta, which weighed 660 Gm., had but one umbilical artery. Associated malformations such as omphalocele, intestinal malrotation, ventricular septal defect and others were present. Landau *et al.*[66] reported an infant with arhinencephaly that weighed 1,390 Gm. when born at term. Nitowsky *et al.*[67] and Sedano and Gorlin[68] described cases of cyclopia with IUGR.

Schutt[20] found retarded weight gain in utero of children with osteogenesis imperfecta. Infants with arthrogryposis sometimes have IUGR. Their mothers state that they did not gain weight adequately during pregnancy and that the activity of the fetus was weak (p. 147). The related Möbius syndrome can also be associated with IUGR.[69] Such examples of IUGR in deformed children can be found accidentally in the literature when birth weight and gestational age are contained in case reports. In a statistical study, Yerushalmy *et al.*[7] compared two groups of infants weighing between 1,588 and 2,500 Gm. who differed in length of gestation. It was found that the frequency of severe congenital malformations was greater for the group with longer gestation (i.e., those with IUGR), whereas the neonatal mortality was greater for the group with shorter gestation (i.e, prematures). Gruenwald[8,9] stated that 38% of malformed children of a necropsy series had a low birth weight index.

INFANTS WITH CONGENITAL TUMORS.—Congenital tumors can be present in children with IUGR. Wells[70] described an infant with congenital neuroblastoma. The child, who had a persistent omphalomesenteric duct, a cyst in the thymus and vascular anomalies of the brain, weighed 1,815 Gm. at full term. Batchelor and Mann[71] reported a full-term female infant weighing 2,119 Gm. with congenital rhabdomyoma.

SYNDROMES OF CHROMOSOMAL ORIGIN.—The effect of chromosomal abnormalities on prenatal growth is discussed on page 145.

ETIOLOGY

During the description of various syndromes on the foregoing pages it has evolved that heterogeneous etiologic factors can result in IUGR. Although the etiology of IUGR is known in a minority of cases only, it is possible to discern abnormal genes, chromosomes and certain environmental agents as responsible for some cases.

GENETIC FACTORS.—That genetic factors can lead to retarded growth in utero was suggested to us by some of our observations[21] and from the literature. In rare instances, primordial dwarfism has been transmitted from a parent to one or more of his children. The older literature was reviewed by Ballantyne[3] in his chapter on fetal microsomia and by Rischbieth and Barrington[26] in their monograph on dwarfism. Since gestational age and size at birth are mentioned in only a few of the older publications, IUGR sometimes is hard to prove. But in the kinship reported by Gilford,[2,26] in which dwarfism occurred in three generations, one dwarf is said to have been "a small child, like a doll at birth."[26] In the Magro family described by Levy, II_5, born at term, his son (III_1) and daughter (III_2) were "extremely small at birth." In another kinship reported by this author, dwarfism was observed in three generations. In the fourth generation, the child (IV_1) of a dwarf woman (III_1) weighed 1,930 Gm. at birth and measured 44 cm. In Dubois' case, dwarfism was inherited through two and, possibly, three generations. Of one dwarf it is said that "she was very small at birth" and that one of her children weighed 1,360 Gm. when labor was induced in the eighth month.[26] In more recent times, Selle[72] described a kinship in which primordial dwarfism was transmitted through three generations, 10 persons being affected. De Toni[32] observed a dwarfed girl, 11½ years of age, who weighed 1,980 Gm. when born at term to a dwarfed mother who had not weighed more than 2,000 Gm. when she was born at term. The maternal grandmother of the patient also was a dwarf. These rare cases illustrate that dominantly inherited primordial dwarfism can be manifest during prenatal development, so that IUGR may be recognized at birth. DeRudder and Kipper[73] described several patients considered primordial dwarfs, whose growth retardation was not attributed to primordial dwarfism of a parent but to an additive effect of nonpathologic "smallness-factors" that accumulated through several generations by marriages of small persons.

In our series[21] published in 1961 there were several instances of IUGR extending through more than one generation. In Case 4, the child's mother had been born after IUGR but had reached normal measurements in postnatal life, matured and had children. A sister of the patient also had IUGR. The mother and sister of another patient (Case 12) were quite small at birth. The gestation time was not known for the mother; the sister was a premature, too small for her gestational age. The family history in our Cases 5 and 6 deserves particular attention (Fig. 14-6). There, a sibship of 3 showed marked growth retardation at birth. These children were born of one mother (II_2) in two marriages. Patients III_2 and III_3 remained abnormal in postnatal life, whereas their sister (III_1) showed normal mental and physical development. Three of her sons are mentally retarded. The mother (II_2) of the patients and her mother (I_1) were both small at birth, and one of the patient's maternal uncles (II_5) apparently was a lethal case of IUGR. Although this family shows a hereditary tendency to IUGR, the genetic mechanisms involved are not clear. The mother of patient 23 had been an extremely small "premature" twin, and his sister born at term weighed only 1,360 Gm. These cases illustrate that IUGR may occur in subsequent generations. Some children thus affected may outgrow their prenatal dwarfism, whereas others remain stunted in postnatal life. Ounsted and Ounsted[74] noted that the birth weights of mothers who bore growth-retarded offspring were reduced as compared with those of control mothers; the smaller the proband infant, the smaller the mother at birth.

Intrauterine growth retardation has been observed repeatedly in more than one member of a sibship whose parents were normal. Such sibships can be found in Rischbieth's and Barrington's[26] review. Other cases were published by Verschuer and Conradi,[75] who wrote of recessive inheritance of primordial dwarfism, and by Grebe,[76] who pointed out that primordial dwarfism can be inherited according to different modes of transmission. Kirchhoff *et al.*,[77] who described 7 patients with primordial dwarfism, included one sibship that contained 2 sisters at term weighing 1,500 Gm. Among the cases of nanocephalic dwarfs with IUGR cited by Seckel,[25] there were three sibships containing more than 1 patient. His cases 3 and 4 were brothers. The dwarf Janos Dobos had 3 dwarfed brothers born small at full term, and Barbara Schreier (Case 14) had a sibling who was said to be "rather small at full term." Case 15 in our series[21] had 7 siblings, of whom 3 were said to be undersized, 2 of them mentally retarded.

Repeated births of infants with IUGR in one family do not prove genetic determination of the anomaly. If 2 or more children of phenotypically normal parents are affected, one can consider that a recessive gene is at work, but it is also possible that the external environment or the mother as environment exerts a repeated inhibitory effect on the developing fetus. The mother's genotype or maternal disease could result repeatedly in IUGR. But for several disease pictures

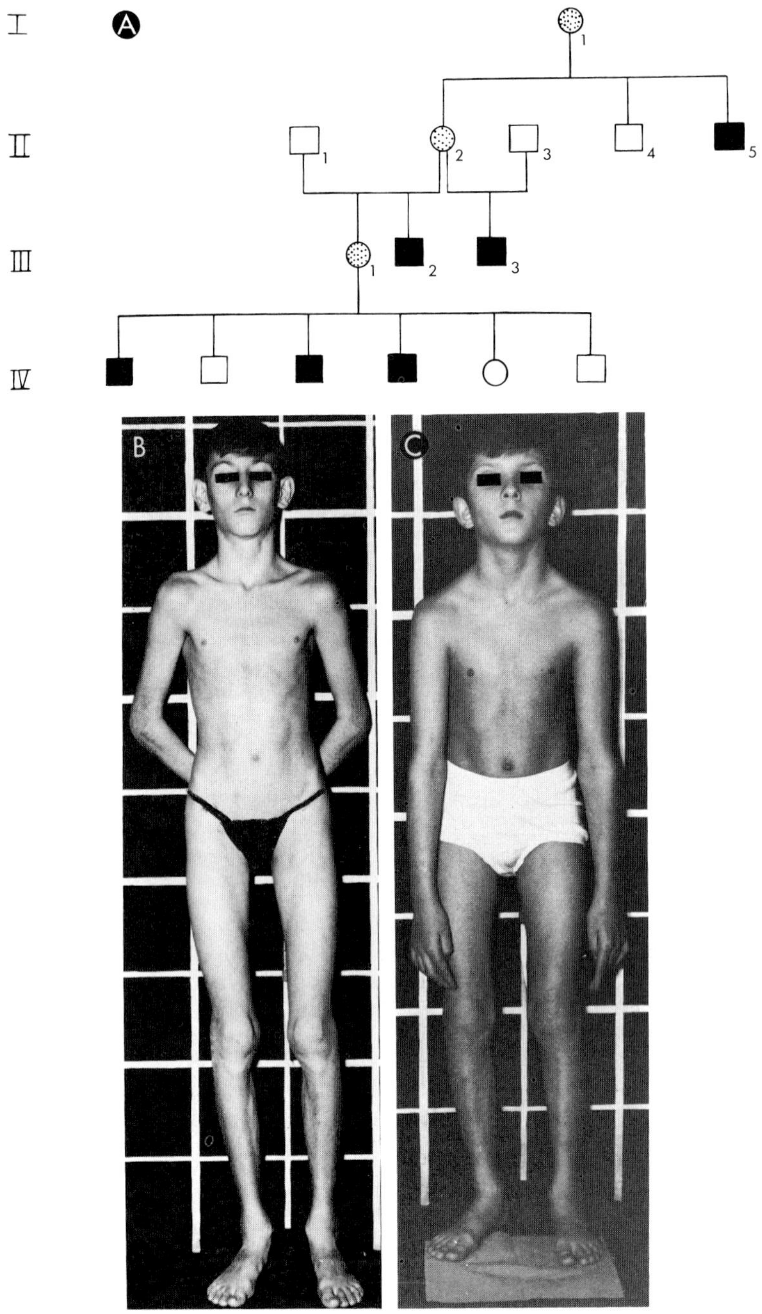

Fig. 14-6. – **A,** pedigree of a kindred with several cases of IUGR. **B,** III_2 weighed 1,610 Gm. after a gestation of 38 weeks. At the age of 14 years he was 136 cm. tall and weighed 23 kg. His head circumference was only 44 cm. and his I.Q. was about 50. **C,** III_3 weighed 2,270 Gm. after a gestation of 38 weeks. At the age of 12 years he was 131 cm. tall and weighed 25 kg. His I.Q. was about 50. III_1, the sister of these boys, was born after a gestation of 38 weeks weighing 1,590 Gm. She outgrew her IUGR and became a normal, intelligent woman who has 3 mentally retarded children.

such as Bloom syndrome,[50] leprechaunism (p. 159) and Fanconi anemia[78] recessive inheritance seems established. Intrauterine growth retardation occurred in brothers with congenital hypoplastic thrombocytopenia and micrencephaly.[168] It would be difficult to understand how maternal disease or placental insufficiency could lead repeatedly to similar specific disease pictures in the same family. General nutritional deficiency or hypoxia in man can result in IUGR but not in specific congenital malformations.[10,79] Yet, the possibility of environmental causation of repeated cases of IUGR in one family should always be kept in mind before recessive genes are invoked as culprits.

CHROMOSOMAL ABERRATIONS.—Chromosomal determination of IUGR has come to light in many cases in recent years. Böök and Santesson[80] reported a patient born at full term weighing 2,190 Gm. and showing micrognathia, syndactyly and localized lipomatosis. Chromosome analyses showed mosaic patterns with triploid, diploid and other aneuploid cells derived from fascia lata. Another case of diploid-triploid mosaicism was reported by Ferrier *et al.*[81] The patient was born near term weighing 1,850 Gm. The right side was smaller than the left, there was syndactyly, and on the right half of the trunk large serrated pigmented spots were seen. Although this child showed some signs of the syndrome of Silver *et al.*,[48] there also were some differences, as the urinary gonadotropins were low and mental retardation marked. Kohn *et al.*[82] found tetraploid-diploid mosaicism in an infant weighing 1,700 Gm. at birth after a 42-week gestation.

IUGR has been recorded in some of the abnormal phenotypes associated with ring chromosomes. Bain and Gauld[83] described a fetus delivered after a gestation of 42 weeks weighing 1,347 Gm. The brain was abnormal, resembling the cyclopean series and showing arhinencephaly. Ventricular septal defect, hypoplastic kidneys, uterus bicornis, digital anomalies, simian creases and clubfeet were also present. Some of these findings, together with bilateral microphthalmia, were reminiscent of the trisomy 13-15 syndrome. Interestingly, the ring chromosome seemed to represent an abnormal chromosome of the 13-15 group, since that group was represented by only five large acrocentrics. A ring D chromosome was present in a child with multiple congenital abnormalities who weighed 2,160 Gm. after 44 weeks of gestation.[84] In a dwarfed microcephalic female,[85] a ring chromosome replacing a no. 1 chromosome was found. The child, born at term, weighed 1,644 Gm. She remained small, underweight and mentally retarded. Except for microcephaly, there were no congenital malformations. Wolf *et al.*,[86] reporting on ring 1 chromosome and dwarfism, described a girl born at term weighing 1,080 Gm. Unfortunately, birth weight and gestation time were not always recorded in cases with ring chromosomes.

IUGR may occur in the cat-cry syndrome, which is associated with partial deletion of the short arm of one of the chromosomes 5. The patient in Case 1 of Lejeune *et al.*[87] weighed only 1,700 Gm. at term. Their Cases 5 and 6 showed patients with mild IUGR (2,400 and 2,500 Gm.). The patient in Case 3 had a normal birth weight. A patient reported by Dumars *et al.*[88] weighed 1,928 Gm. after a 36-week gestation. The twins recorded by Hijmans and Shearin[89] are of interest because the one with the cat-cry syndrome weighed 2,160 Gm. and the normal one 2,610 Gm.

A translocation of two chromosomes 13-15 was found in the father of a child with multiple congenital malformations and IUGR.[90] Two anencephalic siblings of this child were born at term but birth weights were not recorded.

The average birth weight of infants with trisomy 21 (Down syndrome, mongolism) is significantly lower than that of controls. The low birth weight is not entirely explained by the early onset of labor, but is believed to be attributable in part to a low rate of prenatal growth. The prenatal growth retardation usually is not extreme in mongoloids (2,900 Gm., with a mean duration of gestation of 269 days). Schachter[91] found that in 100 mongoloid infants 12.6% weighed under 1,500 Gm. at birth (in contrast to 2.3% of normal controls), but in his series premature infants were not separated from term children, so that the contribution of the latter group to the total is not discernible, and the role of IUGR cannot be evaluated.

We saw one mongoloid child who weighed only 1,500 Gm. although born at term. She was a dizygotic twin whose twin brother weighed 2,580 Gm. at birth, indicating marked IUGR in the mongoloid. But twinning probably was an additional growth-retarding factor. Another child with typical Down syndrome and a karyotype of trisomy 21 weighed 1,360 Gm. after 36 weeks' gestation. There was one mongoloid child in the series of Rumbolz and McGoogan[13] who weighed 1,705 Gm. after a gestation of 39 weeks. Thus, trisomy 21 inhibits normal prenatal growth, but IUGR is striking in exceptional cases only.

With trisomy 18, IUGR is more pronounced. The first patient recorded[92] weighed 2,296 Gm. at term, thus showing mild retardation. Among the cases reported by Smith *et al.*,[93,94] uterine and intrauterine growth retardation was clearly described. In one case, the birth weight was 2,098 Gm. at term. The mother "did not feel pregnant." Fetal movements were delayed and feeble. In another case, the maternal history was similar and the placenta was small but the birth weight was 2,950 Gm. In their report of 1962, Smith *et al.*[94] listed 2 children with trisomy 18 with a gestation of 40 and 44 weeks, respectively. One of these weighed 2,098 and the other 2,211 Gm. The placenta was noted to be small in 5 cases and polyhydramnios was present in 4 of these. According to Hecht *et al.*,[95] the average birth weight of babies with trisomy 18 is 2,325 Gm. Twenty cases of trisomy 18 examined in our laboratory were charted on a graph of the University of Colorado Medical Center. The low birth weights for gestational age are obvious (Fig. 14-7). Similar findings were recorded by Schutt.[20]

The association of trisomy 13-15 (D_1) with IUGR is not as well established as that of trisomy 18. Some of the infants with trisomy 13-15 weighing under 2,000 Gm. were born prematurely, whereas others born at term weighed between 2,000 and 2,500 Gm. The majority of the cases reported showed rather adequate intrauterine growth. The first patient reported by Patau *et al.*[96] weighed 2,860 Gm. at term.

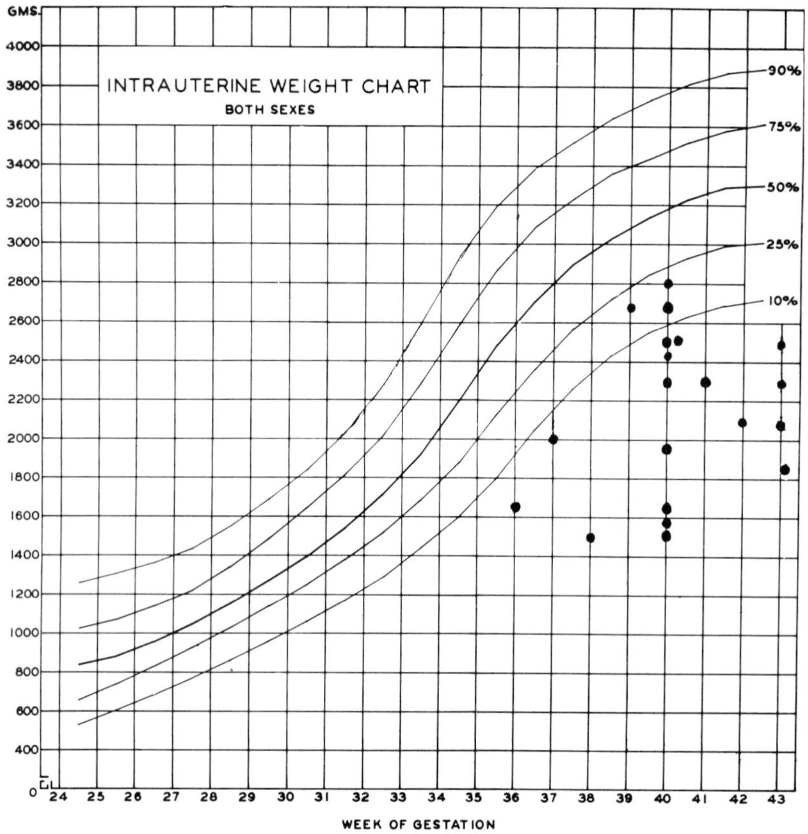

Fig. 14-7.—Trisomy 18—distribution of birth weights shown on a Lubchenco chart.

Most children who have signs of Turner syndrome have normal birth weights, but a few patients have been described who showed IUGR. In Turner's original article,[97] Case 7 was that of a twin who weighed 1,135 Gm. at birth and presented "a rather typical picture of infantilism with congenital webbed neck and cubitus valgus." Her twin sister and "control," who had weighed 2,270 Gm. at birth, showed normal growth and normal physical and sexual development, but in such a case twinning could account for the IUGR of the child with Turner syndrome. Grumbach *et al.*,[98] listing 22 cases of gonadal dysgenesis, recorded birth weights between 1,270 Gm. and 2,180 Gm. in 5 patients. Since the gestation time was not listed, prematurity cannot be ruled out in these patients. But in their Case 1, the birth weight was 2,040 Gm. at full term, so that IUGR can be diagnosed. Spence and Havard[99] observed an unusual case of gonadal dysgenesis and remarked "Her birth weight was only 4 lb. (1,800 Gm.) though the pregnancy had run to full term." Richard and Benirschke[65] reported a case of gonadal dysgenesis in a newborn infant who, after a gestation of 37½ weeks, weighed only 1,700 Gm. Thus, prenatal growth retardation may not be too rare in children with Turner syndrome, particularly in those who do not survive birth (p. 1122).

In a child with the XXXXY syndrome, the gestation time was recorded as 43 weeks but the weight was only 2,360 Gm. and the length 45 cm.[100]

There is a close association of monosomy G with IUGR.[157]

Exogenous factors.—In addition to abnormalities of genes and chromosomes, some environmental or exogenous factors are known to result in IUGR. Physiologic and pathologic factors must be considered as prenatal growth regulators.

Control of prenatal growth in mammals depends to a certain extent on the intrauterine environment.[101] Maternal effects on weight at birth have been clearly demonstrated in crosses of Shire mares to Shetland stallions that yielded foals that were almost as large as pure Shire newborns, whereas the offspring of the reciprocal cross were as small as newborn Shetlands.[102] Comparable effects of the maternal environment on prenatal growth have been demonstrated by egg transfers in rabbits, sheep and mice. Maternal age plays a role. Young ewes that are themselves still growing usually produce smaller young at birth than do adult mothers. This can be explained on the theory that in a young mother the competition of the maternal tissues for nutrients would be more severe than in adult mothers.[103] It was shown in mice that litter size has a definite influence on the weights of the term fetuses and that fetal growth depends on uterine blood flow. At the ends of the uterine horns, which are supplied by offshoots of the uterine arteries with relatively high blood pressure, the fetuses are larger than those situated in the middle portions of the uterine horns, where the pressure is lower. The placental sizes parallel the sizes of the fetuses.[101] Similar observations were made in guinea pigs.[104] Fetal and placental weights are inversely related to the number of fetuses in the same horn of the uterus and to the number of fetuses in the other horn, but the variation in placental weight does not wholly account for the variation of fetal weight. Fetuses with placentas of the same weight reflect both a general effect due to litter size and a local effect determined by contiguity of fetuses within the same horn. Such observations in animals suggest that – genetic factors being equal – fetal size is not entirely dependent on placental size but that both fetal and placental sizes parallel each other to a great extent and are influenced by rather complex circumstances of the uterine and maternal environment.

In sheep,[105] restriction of maternal diet resulted in the birth of lambs reduced in size and weight, but this was the case only if the dietary restriction was enforced during the last 8 weeks of gestation. Maternal undernutrition during early pregnancy did not reduce the birth weight of the lambs significantly. In lambs underweight because of maternal undernutrition, the mass of nerve tissue, skeleton and heart was less reduced than the body generally, whereas skin, spleen, thymus and liver were more affected than the entire body. Chow and Lee[106] found that dietary restriction of female rats during gestation resulted in young born with reduced weights. When the mothers received unrestricted diets after delivery, the young's weight remained below that of controls and growth retardation persisted for many months even though the young's food intake was not restricted.

Mothers of Children with Intrauterine Growth Retardation

Mothers of children with marked IUGR often relate that they believed that their pregnancy was not normal. They did not "grow" sufficiently and did not gain much weight. The fetus seemed less active than their previous unborn children and fetal activity was delayed. The maternal statements are supplemented by obstetric observations. In none of the patients studied by Rumbolz and McGoogan[13] did the growth of the fundus approach normal. The average growth curve of the fundus paralleled the normal until about the thirty-first week, when the curve leveled off to an almost horizontal line. Approximately one-third of the mothers had toxemia of pregnancy. Similar observations were made by McDonald,[107] who found that more than a third of the "small for date" children's mothers had toxemia. But there is no agreement on this point. Other investigators who made controlled studies found no increased rates of toxemia or ill health in the mothers of children with IUGR.[108,109,162] Beaudry and Sutherland[110] saw no growth reduction of infants of toxemic mothers. Brent and Jensh[111] listed additional studies on this subject and thought that reduction of birth weight is related to the severity of the toxemia.

Dietary Deficiencies of Women

There can be little doubt that malnutrition of women can reduce the weight of their fetuses, but in many human situations various adverse environmental factors usually are so intertwined that the role of undernutrition is not always well defined. A careful study in Holland after World War II by Smith[79] showed a decline of fetal growth following maternal starvation, but the amount of decline was less than 10% of the weights in normal times; the maternal dietary deficiency reduced the weight of the fetus, particularly during the last trimester of gestation. Malnutrition before and during pregnancy may cause complications that result in IUGR.[162] In Holland and in Greece, starvation of women led rather rapidly to amenorrhea and sterility, so that the marked IUGR discussed in this chapter was not attained by dietary limitations of women. There are, of course, other types of malnutrition that could interfere with fetal growth.

Placental Insufficiency

The role of the placenta in fetal nutrition is so prominent that explanations of IUGR by placental defects are understandable. But to accept axiomatically placental insufficiency as the cause of IUGR cannot be recommended.

Obstetricians who observe an association of placental anomalies with IUGR tend to relate the poor development of the infant to poor prenatal nutrition. Thus, McBurney[5] spoke of the "undernourished full-term infant" when he described IUGR. Rumbolz and McGoogan[13] believed that either a small placenta or a placenta reduced in surface area by multiple infarcts or necrosis could be responsible for the small, undernourished, full-term infant. They considered the possibility that hypertension or toxemia of the mother leads to poor placental development but conceded that in the majority of their cases there was no evidence obtainable from the history that a pre-existing local or generalized abnormal condition affected the proper development of the endometrium and of the placenta.

There can be little doubt that placental anomalies sometimes are associated with IUGR.[163] In our series[21] of 27 cases, occurrence of an extremely small placenta could be established in 5 and it may have been more frequent, as most mothers did not know anything concerning the appearance of the afterbirth. It is possible that some cases of IUGR are due to the placental condition observed in such instances. But the coexistence of a small or abnormal placenta with IUGR does not prove that the retarded growth of the fetus is due chiefly to "placental insufficiency." It could be, for instance, that both the placental anomaly and the fetal growth retardation are parallel phenomena caused by a common and more remote factor. Thus, it is likely that an abnormal gene or chromosome or an exogenous teratogenic factor results in smallness of the placenta and smallness of the fetus. One could argue that in such cases the growth retardation of the fetus is brought about by the small size or insufficiency of the placenta, but this theory does not explain the persistence for years of the small stature of many children with IUGR. Why do so many of these children fail to resume normal growth after birth when they are offered food of good quality and sufficient quantity? In many children, growth retardation begun in prenatal life continues after birth even though the nutritional conditions are significantly altered. Other children born small at term grow well in postnatal life, soon catching up with their fellows with normal birth weights. Prenatal undernutrition cannot be the only cause of failure to thrive in all children with IUGR. Some of the failures to respond to adequate postnatal feeding remain unexplained despite thorough clinical and laboratory examinations.

The parallelism of fetal and placental growth retardation is not consistent. Thus, in the cases observed by Horwood,[23] the fetuses born at term of the same mother weighed 920 Gm. and 1,080 Gm., respectively. But, in one case, the placenta weighed 185 Gm. and in the second 400 Gm. Is the first fetus to be classified as a "malnourished" and the second as a "hypoplastic" child? In many cases of trisomy 18, both IUGR and smallness of the placenta have been noted, but a small placenta can also be associated with a more adequate birth weight and size, as shown in a boy with this syndrome who weighed nearly 3,000 Gm. at term even though the placenta was small.[94] In such an instance, the child's growth is satisfactory in utero but postnatal growth is not. Failure to thrive is one of the constant features of trisomy 18 that is understandable because of the congenital malformations so characteristic of this disease picture and the disturbances resulting from the chromosomal anomaly. Could a small or abnormal placenta produce in one case the disease picture of trisomy 18 and in others leprechaunism, de Lange, Bloom or Russell syndrome? In such cases, it is obvious that genetic or chromosomal mechanisms are responsible for IUGR and placental anomalies and that placental insufficiency can be merely a contributory factor for the reduced growth rate before birth. The same probably is true for cases of IUGR caused by such exogenous factors as x-rays, rubella or cytomegalic inclusion disease.

That in some cases of IUGR maternal and placental disorders may play an important role is not to be denied, but this role is not too clear and must not be taken for granted. Neither size nor structure of the placenta is necessarily changed in pregnancies resulting in children with IUGR. Vascular changes in the mother's body[162,164] during pregnancy could influence the placental blood supply. The role of placental infarction in fetal mortality, morbidity and growth is a controversial subject. As Little[113] has pointed out, the term "placental infarction" is ill-defined and means different things to different authors. It is not surprising, therefore, that estimates of the general incidence of placental infarction vary between 2 and 100%. Most authors have believed that the placenta usually has sufficient reserve to overcome extensive infarction without damage to the fetus. But Little, after definition and classification of five types of placental infarction, concluded that necrosis of chorionic villi due to vascular obstruction is associated with pre-eclampsia, bleeding disorders of pregnancy, abruptio placentae and adverse fetal effects, as expressed in placental coefficients, fetal distress and fetal mortality. In placentas that were more than 30% infarcted there was a progressive decrease in the weight of term infants with increasing amounts of placental infarction. There are compensatory adjustments that may maintain adequate placental metabolic activity and fetal oxygenation up to a point, but beyond this point compensatory changes may be inadequate to maintain gaseous exchange, so that fetal hypoxia and IUGR result.[114] Gruenwald[115] discussed abnormalities of placental vascularity in relation to intrauterine "deprivation" and retardation of fetal growth, with emphasis on avascular chorionic villi. In another study,[74] the placentas were found to have a relatively small quantity of villous tissue, but what there was of this usually appeared histologically normal. Naeye,[116] discussing the general growth retardation of twins, considered it possibly related to inadequate placental function but not to inadequacy of placental tissue per se, since in most of such twins normal or increased placental coefficients were ascertained. A deficient uteroplacental blood flow in twin pregnancies, especially when combined with pre-eclampsia, could be responsible for growth retardation of twins. But in such cases the causes of twinning – whatever they may be – would be the primary factors of IUGR, with pre-eclampsia, reduced blood flow and hypoxia as mediators. Morris *et al.*[117] found effective circulation in the uterine wall in late pregnancy about half the normal in mild and only one-fourth the normal in severe cases of pre-eclampsia.

It is understandable that, in the past, placental pathology and placental insufficiency were satisfactory explanations for IUGR, particularly to obstetricians who frequently saw the association of placental or maternal pathology with children too small for their gestational ages. But considerations of family histories, pregnancy histories, chromosomal karyotypes, virus studies and variability of disease pictures associated with IUGR indicate that placental insufficiency can be only a preliminary and partial explanation

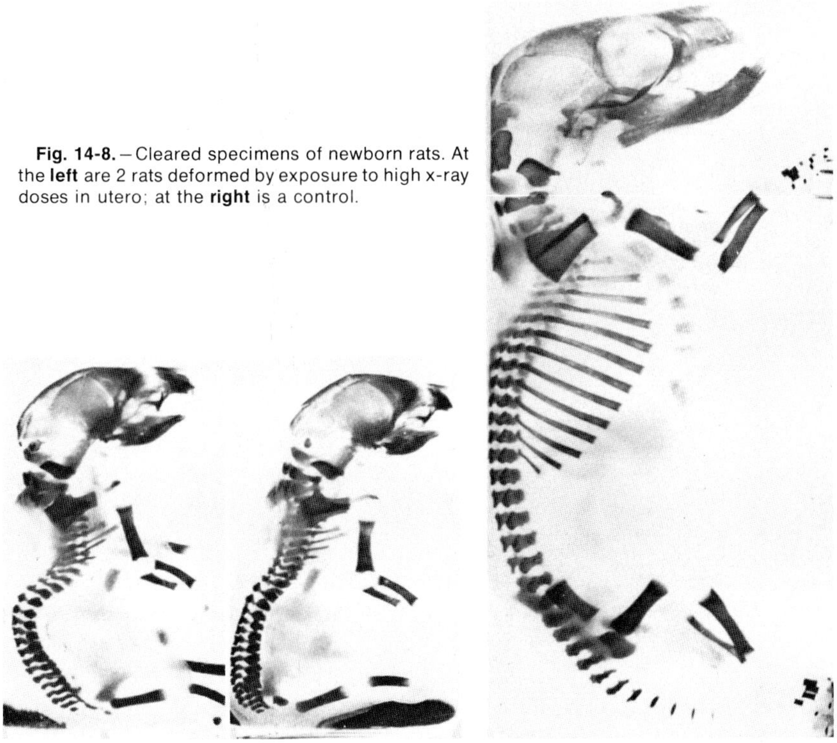

Fig. 14-8. – Cleared specimens of newborn rats. At the **left** are 2 rats deformed by exposure to high x-ray doses in utero; at the **right** is a control.

of IUGR. Time will tell what the various causes and mechanisms are that lead to prenatal retardation of growth. At this time, it should be emphasized that a general explanation of IUGR by "placental insufficiency" is an oversimplification that again may obstruct investigation of the complex area of "pseudo-prematurity."

Hypoxia

That hypoxia may lead to moderate IUGR has been shown by the relatively low birth weights of children carried and born in areas of high altitude.[10, 118, 119] Even marked IUGR may be caused by maternal hypoxia. Black-Schaffer[120] reported as "fetal nanosomia" the case of a newborn child born to a woman with a severe cyanotic cardiovascular anomaly, and Simon and Lustberg[121] described a child born at full term weighing 1,814 Gm. whose mother had a truncus arteriosus communis and cyanosis.

Exposure to X-Rays

Pathologic environmental factors acting between conception and birth can reduce intrauterine growth to a great extent. This has been shown with almost experimental precision in children born to mothers who were exposed to massive x-irradiation during pregnancy. One child observed by us[21] weighed 2,070 Gm. when born at term. The mother had received many x-ray treatments during early pregnancy after removal of a kidney that contained malignant tissue. Before that time, the medical literature contained numerous similar reports on prenatal exposure to x-rays resulting in IUGR. Unfortunately, in many of these reports, the birth weight and duration of pregnancy were not stated, but in some[21] a birth weight low for the gestational period was mentioned and IUGR documented. Intrauterine growth retardation produced experimentally in rats is shown in Figure 14-8.

Other Exogenous Teratogens

A variety of experimental teratogenic experiments have resulted in IUGR.

Vitamin A deficiency of the mother often leads to marked growth retardation of the newborn rat.[122] In this case, the retardation is much more marked than the size and weight of the young indicate, since a large amount of subcutaneous edema makes the extremely small body appear larger and heavier than it actually is. Other teratogenic factors resulting in IUGR can be found in the literature dealing with experimental production of congenital malformations, but often little attention was paid to the stunting of the young, whereas the more spectacular malformations are described in detail.[111] Lee *et al.*,[123] in 1955,

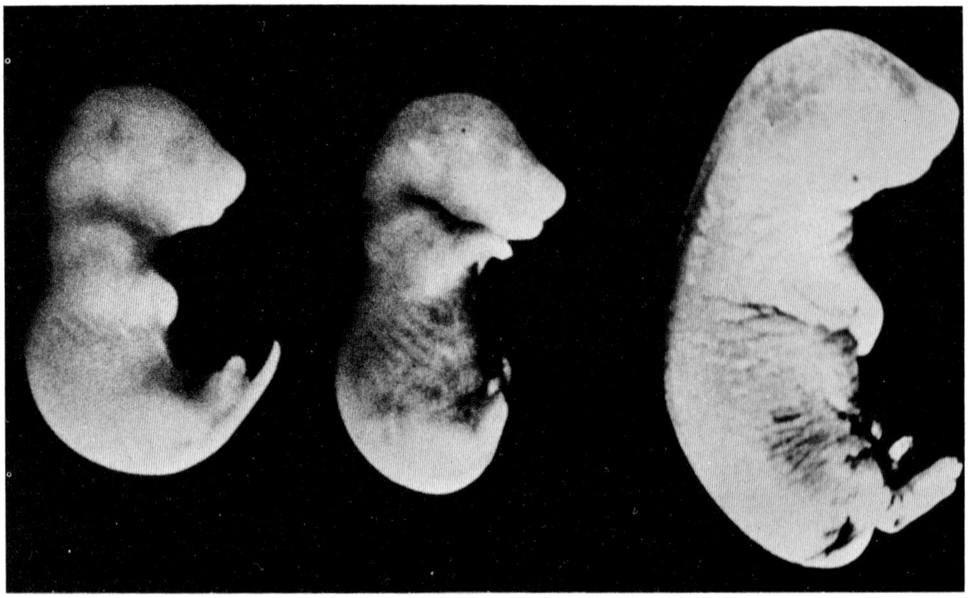

Fig. 14-9.—At the **left** are 2 newborn rats stunted by treatment of the mother with ethionine. At the **right** is a control for comparison. (From C. M. Lee, J. T. Wiseman, S. A. Kaplan and J. Warkany.[123])

produced marked IUGR in the young of rats whose mothers received injections of ethionine. Whereas the pancreas of the mothers were severely damaged, those of the young appeared normal; there were no congenital malformations. In recent years, growth studies have been included in teratogenic experiments. Before that, the work of Nelson *et al.*[124] demonstrated in animals that maternal pteroylglutamic (folic) acid deficiency during gestation results in multiple congenital anomalies and in marked reduced birth weights of the young. Maternal folic acid deficiency in humans has similar results. Warkany *et al.*[39] described a child born to a mother who had attempted abortion with sodium aminopterin (4-aminopteroylglutamic acid) in early pregnancy. This nonviable infant, born 2 weeks after term, weighed only 1,280 Gm. A similar case recorded by Shaw and Steinbach[125] also showed IUGR, the child weighing

Fig. 14-10.—Three near-term rat fetuses. At the **left** is a control. The other young are dwarfed (IUGR) and have congenital malformations. These anomalies were produced by treatment of the mother with a teratogenic dose of streptonigrin on the tenth day of gestation.

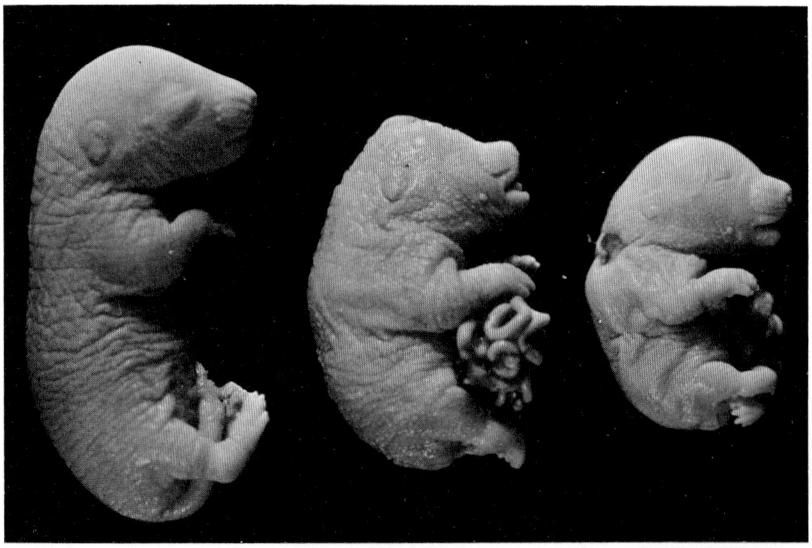

1,750 Gm. at term. Another patient with intrauterine stunting of growth by a chemical was reported by Diamond *et al.*,[126] who described the case of a mother with leukemia, treated with busulfan (Myleran) through most of her pregnancy. The child weighed only 1,336 Gm. after a 40-week gestation. These cases suggest that antimetabolites or alkylating agents can result in IUGR. The relationship of IUGR and teratogenicity was discussed by Brent and Jensh,[111] who emphasized the need for investigation of this casually treated area.

Viral infections such as rubella and cytomegalic inclusion disease can deform the fetus and retard its growth. Gregg[127] mentioned that most of the babies with congenital cataract following German measles were of small size and ill-nourished, and Swan *et al.*[128] found that after maternal rubella ". . . even when born at or near full time, the congenitally defective babies were sometimes subnormal in weight . . ." and they listed two cases with marked IUGR. Töndury[129] stated that 15% of the children with defects attributable to rubella have subnormal weights even when born at term. Warkany *et al.*[21] cited some cases of severe IUGR due to prenatal rubella (see Fig. 9-2) but it was not until the rubella epidemic of 1964 that the growth deficit of children affected by maternal rubella was clearly recognized. There was no change in the manifestations of rubella during this epidemic but there was a change in the terminology of the pediatricians who had learned to distinguish between prematurity and IUGR. Cooper *et al.*[130] showed in a scattergram that 40% of the children affected by rubella had birth weights below the tenth percentile of normal infants.

Cytomegalic inclusion disease can also interfere with intrauterine growth, as shown by an infant with this disease who weighed only 1,070 Gm. when born during the thirty-sixth week of pregnancy.[131] Other cases of this type were described by Weller and Hanshaw,[132] who reported on 17 infants with this disease. Of 12 whose gestation time was known, 4 had marked IUGR. Quantitative data on the effects of cytomegalic inclusion disease and other infectious diseases on prenatal growth will become available in the future and make possible evaluation of the scattered data now obtainable. Maternal phenylketonuria[159] and maternal lead poisoning[160] can result in growth retardation of the fetus.

Twinning

Prenatal growth and growth retardation of twins represent a special chapter that deserves monographic treatment. Only a few pertinent points can be made here. McKeown and Record[133] showed that the incidence of low-birth-weight infants increases with the number of offspring per pregnancy but that there was also an increase of true prematurity. Growth retardation sets in earlier in quadruplets and triplets than in twins. The combined birth weights of 9 symmetrical conjoined twins born at or near term averaged 3,700 Gm.[156] All this gives the impression that it is the struggle for nutrients that retards the growth of multiple-birth infants. Again, one must warn against uniform concepts of IUGR of twin fetuses. Monozygotic twins are more affected than dizygotic; they show intra-pair discordance when associated with hydramnios and possibly the cross-placental transfusion syndrome. Although it has been stated that the growth retardation of twins evident at birth disappears by the end of the first postnatal year,[116] this does not hold for all twins.[134] It is clear that there will be permanent growth differences in twins discordant for Turner syndrome or mongolism[21]; but even apparently normal twins can retain their growth differences for many years (Fig. 14-11). Such cases demonstrate that there was more than prenatal malnutrition to the IUGR of the smaller twin, who could not attain the height and weight of her co-twin in many years.

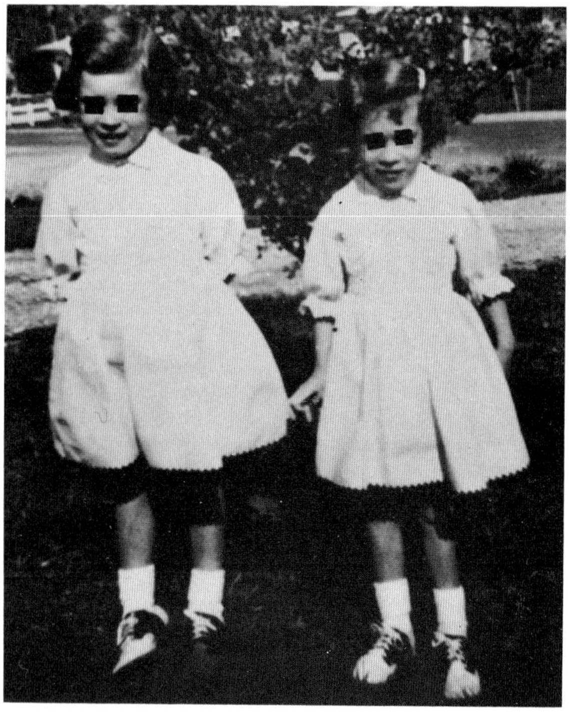

Fig. 14-11.—Identical twin girls of different birth weights. The larger twin weighed 2,900 Gm. and the smaller 1,650 Gm. at birth. At the age of 7 years their weights still differed greatly, being 21 and 13.5 kg., respectively. Both were healthy and mentally normal.

Pathogenesis

The fact that some of the children who suffer IUGR remain small and "undernourished" after they are born, despite adequate food offered them, raises the question of why they fail to thrive in postnatal life. There are animal experiments that demonstrate that fetuses damaged by severe dietary restriction of their mothers remain small in extrauterine life.[106,112] But this obviously cannot apply to all children with IUGR, since some of them gain weight rapidly and grow even though they start out with low weights for their gestational ages. Some children with IUGR have organic defects—cardiac, intestinal, renal or cerebral—but in others no explanation can be found for their failure to thrive. Long hospital stays often result in a mass of laboratory data and huge charts that contain little that explains the failure to thrive, and the children remain small. Sometimes, after many years, such children begin to grow, again without explanation, so that one has the impression that their organs or cells had to be rebuilt before normal growth and development could take place.

It would be of great interest to know the cellular basis of intrauterine growth retardation. Are affected infants small because they have a reduced number of cells or are they small because their cells are reduced in size? Naeye[135] examined the organs of 11 infants with marked intrauterine growth retardation (whose birth weights were 2 or more standard deviations below the mean values for their gestational ages) and found that cells in many organs had a *subnormal amount of cytoplasm*—but there was also a subnormal number of cells in several organs. Since similar findings were obtained in control infants with postnatal alimentary malnutrition, Naeye concluded that the similarity of cellular abnormalities in the two groups suggests *malnutrition* as a common cause for their growth retardation. Placental abnormalities in the prenatally retarded infants accounted for their malnourished state. The results were different in a study made in infants with trisomy 21, 18 and 13-15. The basis of their growth retardation was a *subnormal number of cells* in many body organs.[136] A comparable search for the basis of dysmaturity of infants with congenital cardiac anomalies also showed a subnormal number of cells in many body organs. Naeye[137] thought that the reduction of cell number together with the growth pattern of individual organs distinguishes these types of dysmaturity from those of prenatal malnutrition. No common denominator was found on the cellular level for all forms of intrauterine growth retardation, but it seems that there is now a tendency to distinguish two kinds of dysmaturity—a "malnourished" type resulting from multiple or prolonged pregnancy, maternal toxemia, uterine abnormalities, and so on, and a "hypoplastic" group represented by infants with congenital malformations, prenatal rubella and possibly other infections.[22] It seems that we are headed again for an oversimplification of the situation. But this dichotomy cannot be upheld. Infants retarded in growth who have chromosomal abnormalities often have small and defective placentas, and children with various congenital malformations, teratologic syndromes and prenatal growth retardation often have mothers with toxemia and other complications of pregnancy that would place them in the "malnourished" group. Distinction of two types will not do. Already many differing etiologic entities—genetic, chromosomal and environmental—are known to result in IUGR, and it seems doubtful that their pathogenesis, morphology, physiology, clinical course, prognosis and treatment can be presented in simple dualistic schemes.

Some valuable physiologic and pathologic data have been collected in infants with intrauterine growth retardation, but they were obtained in small numbers of children of differing ages and states of health. Useful as the findings are, they should not be generalized and considered applicable to all infants with IUGR. Sinclair and Silverman,[22] dealing mostly with nonspecific cases of the "malnutrition" type, found that the oxygen consumption per kilogram body weight of those undergrown in utero is increased compared to normally grown babies of similar birth weight. Cassady[138] noted an elevated average plasma volume of infants with intrauterine growth retardation immediately after birth and a more persisting average blood volume. Studies of immunoglobulins may aid in differential treatment of premature and pseudopremature children.[139] Inability to achieve normal adult pH values and bicarbonate levels after the first week of life with a tendency to acidosis was noted in low-birth-weight infants by Schain and O'Brien,[140] and a lack of clinical storm signs in such acidotic infants was emphasized. A finding of importance is the occurrence of idiopathic hypoglycemia in some infants with dysmaturity[141,142] and the relatively large number of infants with IUGR among neonates with hypoglycemia.[143] Low levels of glucose were found particularly in the smaller of twins and in children of mothers who had had toxemia of pregnancy. Symptomatic hypoglycemia occurred predominantly in male infants of low birth weight for their gestational age. It was thought that the prenatal malnutrition of such children could result in reduced stores of glycogen at birth associated with an abnormally sensitive insulin-release mechanism leading to hypoglycemia. Intravenous glucose and ACTH or steroids were recommended for treatment.[143,144] The role of the adrenal medulla in the hypoglycemia of these children was considered by Stern *et al.*[145]

Although one will agree that there is need for treatment of hypoglycemia and for other symptomatic treatments, it must be emphasized that hypoglycemia can occur in the neonatal period in infants with IUGR and prenatal brain damage that cannot be repaired by glucose and steroids. If this is kept in mind, one will not lightly blame cerebral deficiencies seen in later life on insufficient treatment of hypoglycemia. It is also possible that children with IUGR are prone to postnatal infections, meningitis and encephalitis,[146] which can be responsible for subsequent inadequate mental development.

Prognosis

The optimistic outlook for the survivors of severe IUGR expressed by the obstetricians and cited above was shared by some pediatricians, who believed that pseudopresmatures or infants suffering from "placental malnutrition," when properly fed after birth, gain rapidly and develop into normal children. In fact, Pick[147] stated that they differed from premature children in that they regained their weight more rapidly and doubled their weight in less than 10 weeks. Hepner and Bowen[148] also found that infants with IUGR adjusted rapidly to extrauterine life and began to grow immediately without the prolonged and severe adjustment period characteristic of the usual premature infant. Yerushalmy *et al.*[7] reported that, in their series, the neonatal mortality of the pseudopremmatures was much lower than that of the truly prematures. Thus, it appears that IUGR results in stillbirth or perinatal death in almost half the cases but that the survivors of the neonatal period do quite well in postnatal life. There are, however, reports which indicate that the prognosis of these children is not always as favorable as it appears to observers during the neonatal period. It seems that after an early return to birth weight, the pseudopremature gains much below the standard for full-term infants and, when plotted on weight and height standards for truly premature infants, it falls off continuously after the early spurt in growth.[8,9,148]

Yerushalmy *et al.*,[7] after pointing out the high neonatal mortality of the truly prematures, stressed the greater frequency of severe congenital malformations among the pseudoprematures. Baird,[149] in a discussion of physical and mental handicaps of premature babies, stated that the intelligence tested at the age of 9 years in all low-birth-weight babies born with weights between 4 and 5½ lb. was much lower in those born at or near term than in those born at 36 weeks or less. "A foetal weight of 5 pounds at 36 weeks' gestation suggests a normal rate of growth, whereas at 40 weeks it may represent a serious disturbance of intrauterine nutrition and growth." Wiener *et al.*,[150,151] correlating low birth weight and psychologic status at 6–10 years of age, likewise noted that babies of less than 2,500 Gm. who had a gestational period of 40 weeks or more showed a greater degree of impairment than did babies of like weight with shortened gestational period. Hockey and Hawks[146] compared birth weight and gestational period in a mentally retarded population and in a control population. Children with marked intrauterine growth retardation (weighing 2,000 Gm. after a gestation of 36 weeks or more) were found thirteen times more often in the retarded group than in the control group. Truly prematures weighing 2,000 Gm. or less were seen six times more often in the retarded group than in the control group. Horn *et al.*,[165] comparing truly premature with small-for-dates children aged 8–11 years, found the latter group less talented and often lower in intelligence; those with birth weights under 2,000 Gm. showed particularly poor performance. The situation was less clear in children examined by Eaves *et al.*,[166] who noted alternating performances with increasing age. Bazsó *et al.*,[167] examining twins 6–16 years of age, found in monozygotic and like-sexed dizygotic twins that the level of intelligence of the smaller member of the pair was lower than that of its co-twin of normal birth weight.

These observations are in accord with my experience in taking histories with mothers of handicapped children who had had IUGR. Many of these infants do well in the newborn nursery but, after discharge from the hospital, feeding difficulties arise and there is a lack of weight gain and of growth and development. There have been other reports on the physical and mental handicaps in school-age children of extremely low birth weights,[152,153] but since in the past a clear distinction of the truly prematures from the pseudoprematures was not made, children with IUGR could not be evaluated. Increasing attention is now given to the differences of the premature and the infants with low birth weights for their gestational period. There are monographs that deal with the relationship of gestational age, size and maturity,[154] with children of extremely low birth weight[107] and with IUGR.[21,111] But there are still many publications that treat children of low birth weight as an entity. It is understandable that in retrospective studies of this type the relation of birth weight to gestational period cannot be established. This will be corrected in future follow-up studies. One point still needs emphasis: All generalizations concerning the dysmature, "small for dates" and low-birth-weight child and the infant with IUGR should be accepted with skepticism. This small group of small babies is so heterogeneous in origin and outlook that they require individual consideration. Not only the many handicapped children in this group should be considered but also the important sector of those who do well soon after birth and disappear from the view of the hospital personnel and the worried physician. And there are those who, despite poor beginnings in early childhood, attain normal or near-normal mental and physical characteristics. Some of them outgrow their "dwarfism" at puberty and become normal adults. It is for this reason that we discourage the use of the term "intrauterine *dwarfism*" during the period of childhood until one can be certain that growth has stopped and the final height is reached. The word "dwarf" implies to most people a permanent characteristic, and to apply it to a child must have a shocking effect on parents. It is not justified to give such a severe prognosis as long as there is hope for growth into the normal range. It is better to say that a child had "intrauterine growth retardation," which may be overcome or not, in postnatal life.

Treatment

What has been said about prognosis can be repeated about treatment of children with IUGR. Whether their treatment as prematures, as in the past, was good or bad, I cannot judge. Some of the pseudoprematures outgrow their prenatal retardation without any special care and treatment; others will need specific therapy, protection and supervision throughout life. How many belong to the first group, how many to the second and how many are in between will be known when longitudinal studies are available for the various types of children with IUGR. There is a need for distinction of children retarded in utero in weight and those retarded in linear growth; there is a need for quantitative evaluation of IUGR of children with specific diagnoses; and there is a need for constant vigilance against the idea that "low-birth-weight" infants are an entity that can be treated as one group.

No specific treatment has been found. Attempts to promote growth of some of these children with human growth hormone have been discouraging,[155] but when this hormone is in ample supply it may be found that some types respond to it. Some children with IUGR may be small because of inadequate pituitary function even if the majority are not.

REFERENCES

1. Hansemann, D.: Echte Nanosomie, mit Demonstration eines Falles, Berl. Klin. Wchnschr. 39:1209, 1902.
2. Gilford, H.: Ateleiosis: A form of dwarfism, Practitioner 70:797, 1903.
3. Ballantyne, J. W.: *Manual of Antenatal Pathology and Hygiene. The Embryo* (Edinburgh: W. Green & Sons, 1904).
4. Ylppö, A.: Zur Physiologie, Klinik und zum Schicksal der Frühgeborenen, Ztschr. Kinderh. 24:1, 1920.
5. McBurney, R. D.: The undernourished full term infant. A case report, West. J. Surg. 55:363, 1947.
6. Colman, H. I., and Rienzo, J.: The small term baby, Obst. & Gynec. 19:87, 1962.
7. Yerushalmy, J., van den Berg, B. J., Erhardt, C. L., and Jacobziner, H.: Birth weight and gestation as indices of "immaturity," Am. J. Dis. Child. 109:43, 1965.
8. Gruenwald, P., Dawkins, M., and Hepner, R.: Chronic deprivation of the fetus, Sinai Hosp. J. 11:51, 1963.
9. Gruenwald, P.: Chronic fetal distress and placental insufficiency, Biol. Neonat. 5:215, 1963.
10. Lichty, J. A., Ting, R. Y., Bruns, P. D., and Dyar, E.: Studies of babies born at high altitude. 1. Relation of altitude to birth weight, A.M.A. J. Dis. Child. 93:666, 1957.
11. Streeter, G. L.: Weight, sitting height, head size, foot length, and menstrual age of the human embryo, Contrib. Embryol. 9:143, 1920.
12. Stuart, H. C., and Stevenson, S. S.: Physical Growth and Development, in Nelson, W. E. (ed.), *Textbook of Pediatrics* (7th ed.; Philadelphia: W. B. Saunders Company, 1959).
13. Rumbolz, W. L., and McGoogan, L. S.: Placental insufficiency and the small undernourished full-term infant, Obst. & Gynec. 1:294, 1953.
14. Rumbolz, W. L., Edwards, M. C., and McGoogan, L. S.: The small full-term infant and placental insufficiency, West. J. Surg. 69:53, 1961.
15. Jarvinen, P. A., Pankamao, P., and Kinunen, O.: The full-term, underdeveloped live-born infant, Études néonatales 6:3, 1957.
16. Mellin, G. W.: Personal communication.
17. Scammon, R. E., and Calkins, L. A.: *The Development and Growth of the External Dimensions of the Human Body in the Fetal Period* (Minneapolis: University of Minnesota Press, 1929).
18. Lubchenco, L. O., Hansman, C., Dressler, M., and Boyd, E.: Intrauterine growth as estimated from liveborn birth-weight data at 24 to 42 weeks of gestation, Pediatrics 32:793, 1963.
19. Yerushalmy, J.: The low-birthweight baby, Hosp. Practice 3:62, 1968.
20. Schutt, W.: Foetal factors in intrauterine growth retardation, Spastics Soc. Med. Ed. and Information Unit, 1965.
21. Warkany, J., Monroe, B. B., and Sutherland, B. S.: Intrauterine growth retardation, Am. J. Dis. Child. 102: 249, 1961.
22. Sinclair, J. C., and Silverman, W. A.: Intrauterine growth in active tissue mass of human fetus, with particular reference to the undergrown baby, Pediatrics 38: 48, 1966.
23. Horwood, S. P.: Personal communication.
24. Stringaris, M. G.: Mikrenkephalia. Ein Beitrag zur Lehre und Kasuistik der Missbildungen, Frankfurt Ztschr. Path. 37:396, 1929.
25. Seckel, H. P.: *Bird-headed Dwarfs* (Springfield, Ill.: Charles C Thomas, Publisher, 1960).
26. Rischbieth, H., and Barrington, A.: Dwarfism, in *Treasury of Human Inheritance* (London: Dulau & Company, 1912).
27. Panos, T. C.: Observations on siblings with primordial dwarfism associated with hypersplenism, Soc. Pediat. Res., 1951.
28. Fanconi, G.: Familiäre infantile perniziosaartige Anämie (perniziöses Blutbild und Konstitution), Jahrb. Kinderh. 117:257, 1927.
29. Upjohn, C.: Familial dwarfism associated with microcephaly, mental retardation and anaemia, Proc. Roy. Soc. Med. 48:334, 1955.
30. Laurance, B.: Familial dwarfism, Proc. Roy. Soc. Med. 44:735, 1951.
31. Grossman, H. J., Pruzansky, S., and Rosenthal, I. M.: Progeroid syndrome. Report of a case of pseudo-senilism, Pediatrics 15:413, 1955.
32. de Toni, G.: Importanza dell 'eraditarieta,' dell 'ambiente'e dell 'alimentazione nell' eziopatogenesi dei nanismi, Ereditarieta-Ambiente-Alimentazione, Ferrara – 7 – 8 Giugno, 1958.
33. Mann, T. P., and Russell, A.: Study of a microcephalic midget of extreme type, Proc. Roy. Soc. Med. 52:1024, 1959.
34. Atkins, L., and Feingold, M.: Enlarged B-group chromosome (4-5). Association with the cri du chat syndrome, Am. J. Dis. Child. 113:277, 1967.
35. de Grouchy, J., Brissaud, H. E., Repessé, G., and Lamy, M.: Anencéphalie familiale et remaniement de deux chromosomes 13-15, Compt. rend Acad. Sc. (Paris) 258: 691, 1964.
36. de Grouchy, J., Thieffry, S., Aicardi, J., Chevrie, J-J., and Zucker, G.: Trisomie partielle C par translocation t(Cq−;Dp+) et remaniement d'un C(p−q+), Arch. franç. pédiat. 24:859, 1967.
37. Russell, A.: A syndrome of "intra-uterine" dwarfism recognizable at birth with cranio-facial dysostosis, disproportionately short arms, and other anomalies (5 examples), Proc. Roy. Soc. Med. 47:1040, 1954.
38. Szalay, G. C.: Pseudohydrocephalus in dwarfs: The Russell dwarf, J. Pediat. 63:622, 1963.
39. Warkany, J., Beaudry, P. H., and Hornstein, S.: Attempted abortion with aminopterin (4-aminopteroylglutamic acid); malformations of the child, A.M.A. J. Dis. Child. 97:274, 1959.
40. Ammann, P.: Beitrag zum Syndrom des "low birth weight dwarfism," Helvet. paediat. acta 18:438, 1963.
41. McDonald, A. D.: Cerebral palsy in children of very low birth weight, Arch. Dis. Childhood 38:579, 1963.
42. Alberman, E.: Birth weight and length of gestation in cerebral palsy, Developmental Med. & Child Neurol. 5: 388, 1963.
43. Norwood, W. F., Jr.: The Marinesco-Sjögren syndrome, J. Pediat. 65:431, 1964.

44. de Lange, C.: Sur un type nouveau de dégenération (Typus Amstelodamensis), Arch. méd. Enf. 36:713, 1933.
45. Brachmann, W.: Ein Fall von symmetrischer Monodactylie durch Ulnadefekt und symmetrischer Flughautbildung in den Ellenbeugen, sowie anderen Abnormitäten, Jahrb. Kinderh. 84:225, 1916.
46. Jervis, G. A., and Stimson, C. W.: De Lange syndrome; the "Amsterdam type" of mental defect with congenital malformation, J. Pediat. 63:634, 1963.
47. Dodge, J. A.: De Lange's Amsterdam dwarfs syndrome, Developmental Med. & Child Neurol. 7:31, 1965.
48. Silver, H. K., Kiyasw, W., George, J., and Deamer, W. C.: Syndrome of congenital hemihypertrophy, shortness of stature, and elevated urinary gonadotropins, Pediatrics 12:368, 1953.
49. Thomson, M. S.: Poikiloderma congenitale, Brit. J. Dermat. 48:221, 1936.
50. Bloom, D.: The syndrome of congenital telangiectatic erythema and stunted growth, J. Pediat. 68:103, 1966.
51. Szalay, G. C.: Dwarfism with skin manifestations, J. Pediat. 62:686, 1963.
52. Dubowitz, V.: Familial low birthweight dwarfism with an unusual facies and a skin eruption, J. M. Genetics 2:12, 1965.
53. Wiedemann, H-R.: Progerie, Arch. Kinderh. 135:169, 1948.
54. Zeder, E.: Über Progerie, eine seltene Form des hypophysären Zwergwuchses mit diffuser Sklerodermie, Monatsschr. Kinderh. 81:167, 1940.
55. Schondel, A.: Two cases of progeria complicated by microphthalmos, Acta paediat. 30:286, 1943.
56. Donohue, W. L., and Uchida, I.: Leprechaunism: A euphemism for a rare familial disorder, J. Pediat. 45:505, 1954.
57. Kálló, A., Lakatos, I., and Szijártó, L.: Leprechaunism (Donohue's syndrome), J. Pediat. 66:372, 1965.
58. Habermann, P., and Fleck, M.: Über das Rothmund-Syndrom, Ztschr. Kinderh. 77:306, 1955.
59. Silver, H. K.: Rothmund-Thomson syndrome: An oculocutaneous disorder, Am. J. Dis. Child. 111:182, 1966.
60. Engle, M. A.: Ventricular septal defect in infancy, Pediatrics 14:16, 1954.
61. Naeye, R. L.: Unsuspected organ abnormalities associated with congenital heart disease, Am. J. Path. 47:905, 1965.
62. Crelin, E. S.: Eventration of the abdominal viscera and other uncommon anomalies in a newborn infant, Anat. Rec. 115:485, 1953.
63. Newbill, H. P.: Sirenomelian monster (sympus), Am. J. Dis. Child. 62:1233, 1941.
64. Potter, E. L.: Bilateral absence of ureters and kidneys. A report of 50 cases, Obst. & Gynec. 25:3, 1965.
65. Richard, R., and Benirschke, K.: Gonadal dysgenesis in a newborn infant, New England J. Med. 258:974, 1958.
66. Landau, J. W., Barry, J. M., and Koch, R.: Arhinencephaly, J. Pediat. 62:895, 1963.
67. Nitowsky, H. M., Sindhvananda, N., Konigsberg, U. R., and Weinberg, T.: Partial 18 monosomy in the cyclops malformation, Pediatrics 37:260, 1966.
68. Sedano, H. O., and Gorlin, R. J.: The oral manifestation of cyclopia. Review of the literature and report of two cases, Oral Surg. 16:823, 1963.
69. Dalloz, J. C., and Nocton, F.: Le syndrome de Moebius, Arch. franç. pédiat. 21:1025, 1964.
70. Wells, H. G.: Occurrence and significance of congenital malignant neoplasms, Arch. Path. 30:535, 1940.
71. Batchelor, T. M., and Mann, M. E.: Congenital glycogenic tumors of the heart, Arch. Path. 39:67, 1945.
72. Selle, G.: Über Vererbung des echten Zwergwuchses, (University of Jena: Inaugural Dissertation, 1920).
73. DeRudder, B., and Kipper, E.: Zur Phaenogenese primordialen Zwergwuchses, Ztschr. Kinderh. 68:567, 1950.
74. Ounsted, M., and Ounsted, C.: Maternal regulation of intra-uterine growth, Nature, London 212:995, 1966.
75. Verschuer, O., and Conradi, L.: Eine Sippe mit rezessiv erblichem primordialem Zwergwuchs, Ztschr. menschl. Vererb.-u. Konstitutionslehre 22:261, 1938.
76. Grebe, H.: Über Differentialdiagnose und Erbverhältnisse beim primordialen Zwergwuchs, Der Erbarzt 10:195, 1942.
77. Kirchhoff, H. W., Lehmann, W., and Schaefer, U.: Klinische, erbbiologische und körperbauliche Untersuchungen bei primordialen Zwergen, Ztschr. Kinderh. 75:243, 1954.
78. Nilsson, L. R.: Chronic pancytopenia with multiple congenital abnormalities (Fanconi's anaemia), Acta paediat. 49:518, 1960.
79. Smith, C. A.: The effect of wartime starvation in Holland upon pregnancy and its product, Am. J. Obst. & Gynec. 53:599, 1947.
80. Böök, J. A., and Santesson, B.: Malformation syndrome in man associated with triploidy (69 chromosomes), Lancet 1:858, 1960.
81. Ferrier, P., Stalder, G., Bamatter, F., Ferrier, S., Bühler, E., and Klein, D.: Congenital asymmetry associated with diploid-triploid mosaicism and large satellites, Lancet 1:80, 1964.
82. Kohn, G., Mayall, B. H., Miller, M. E., and Mellman, W. J.: Tetraploid-diploid mosaicism in a surviving infant, Pediat. Res. 1:461, 1967.
83. Bain, A. D., and Gauld, I. K.: Multiple congenital abnormalities associated with ring chromosome, Lancet 2:304, 1963.
84. Teplitz, R. L., Miller, D., Hansson, K. M., and Rundall, T. S.: A human ring D chromosome associated with multiple congenital abnormalities, J. Pediat. 70:936, 1967.
85. Gordon, R. R., and Cooke, P.: Ring-1 chromosome and microcephalic dwarfism, Lancet 2:1212, 1964.
86. Wolf, C. G., Peterson, J. A., LoGrippo, G. A., and Weiss, L.: Ring 1 chromosome and dwarfism—a possible syndrome, J. Pediat. 71:5, 1967.
87. Lejeune, J., Lafourcade, J., Grouchy, J., Berger, R., Gautier, M., Salmon, C., and Turpin, R.: Délétion partielle du bras court du chromosome 5. Individualisation d'un nouvel état morbide, Semaine hôp. Paris 40:1069, 1964.
88. Dumars, K. W., Gaskill, C., and Kitzmiller, N.: Le cri du chat (crying cat) syndrome, Am. J. Dis. Child. 108:533, 1964.
89. Hijmans, J. C., and Shearin, D. B.: Partial deletion of short arms of chromosome no. 5, Am. J. Dis. Child. 109: 85, 1965.
90. de Grouchy, J., Brissaud, H. E. Repessé, G., and Lamy, M.: Anencéphalie familiale et remaniement de deux chromosomes 13-15, Compt. rend. Acad. Sc. (Paris) 258: 691, 1964.
91. Schachter, M.: Contribution à l'étude étiologique de l'-arriération mongolienne, J. Génét. Hum. 1:201, 1952.
92. Edwards, J. H., Harnden, D. G., Cameron, A. H., Crosse, V. M., and Wolff, O. H.: A new trisomic syndrome, Lancet 1:787, 1960.
93. Smith, D. W., Patau, K., Therman, E., and Inhorn, S. L.: A new autosomal trisomy syndrome: Multiple congenital anomalies caused by an extra chromosome, J. Pediat. 57:338, 1960.
94. Smith, D. W., Patau, K., Therman, E., and Inhorn, S. L.: The no. 18 trisomy syndrome, J. Pediat. 60:513, 1962.
95. Hecht, F., Bryant, J. S., Motulsky, A. G., and Giblett, E. R.: The no. 17-18 (E) trisomy syndrome; studies on cytogenetics, dermatoglyphics, paternal age, and linkage, J. Pediat. 63:605, 1963.
96. Patau, K., Smith, D. W., Therman, E., Inhorn, S. L., and Wagner, H. P.: Multiple congenital anomaly caused by an extra autosome, Lancet 1:790, 1960.
97. Turner, H. H.: A syndrome of infantilism, congenital webbed neck and cubitus valgus, Endocrinology 23:566, 1938.
98. Grumbach, M. M., Van Wyk, J. J., and Wilkins, L.: Chro-

mosomal sex in gonadal dysgenesis (ovarian agenesis): Relationship to male pseudohermaphrodism and theories of human sex differentiation, J. Clin. Endocrinol. 15:1161, 1955.
99. Spence, A. W., and Havard, C. W. H.: Unusual case of gonadal dysgenesis (Turner's syndrome), Brit. M. J. 2: 1288, 1959.
100. Scherz, R. G., and Roeckel, I. E.: The XXXXY syndrome, J. Pediat. 63:1093, 1963.
101. McLaren, A., and Michie, D.: Control of pre-natal growth in mammals, Nature, London 187:363, 1960.
102. Walton, A., and Hammond, J.: The maternal effects on growth and conformation in Shire horse-Shetland pony crosses, Proc. Roy. Soc. 125:311, 1938.
103. Hammond, J.: Physiological factors affecting birth weight, Proc. Nutrition Soc. 2:8, 1944.
104. Eckstein, P., McKeown, T., and Record, R. G.: Variations in placental weight according to litter size in the guinea pig, J. Endocrinol. 12:108, 1955.
105. Barcroft, J.: *Researches on Prenatal Life* (Springfield, Ill.: Charles C Thomas, Publisher, 1947).
106. Chow, B. F., and Lee, C-J.: Effect of dietary restriction of pregnant rats on body weight gain of the offspring, J. Nutrition 82:10, 1964.
107. McDonald, A.: Children of very low birth weight. A survey of 1128 children with a birth weight of 4 lb. (1800 g.) or less, Res. Monograph No. 1, Spastics Soc. Med. Ed. and Information Unit, 1967.
108. Scott, K., and Usher, R.: Fetal malnutrition, its incidence, causes, and effects, Am. J. Obst. & Gynec. 94: 951, 1966.
109. Ounsted, M.: Maternal constraint of foetal growth in man, Developmental Med. & Child Neurol. 7:479, 1965.
110. Beaudry, P. H., and Sutherland, J. M.: Birth weights of infants of toxemic mothers, J. Pediat. 56:505, 1960.
111. Brent, R. L., and Jensh, R. P.: Intra-uterine growth retardation, Adv. in Teratology 2:139, 1967.
112. McCance, R. A.: Food, growth, and time, Lancet 2:671, 1962.
113. Little, W. A.: The significance of placental/fetal weight ratios, Am. J. Obst. & Gynec. 79:134, 1960.
114. Little, W. A.: Placental infarction, Obst. & Gynec. 15: 109, 1960.
115. Gruenwald, P.: Abnormalities of placental vascularity in relation to intrauterine deprivation and retardation of fetal growth, New York J. Med. 61:1508, 1961.
116. Naeye, R. L.: The fetal and neonatal development of twins, Pediatrics 33:546, 1964.
117. Morris, N., Osborn, S. B., and Wright, N. P.: Effective circulation of the uterine wall in late pregnancy measured with[24] NaCl, Lancet 1:323, 1955.
118. Mazees, R. B.: Neonatal mortality and altitude in Peru, Am. J. Phys. Anthropol. 23:209, 1965.
119. Grahn, D., and Kratchman, J.: Variation in neonatal death rate and birth weight in the United States and possible relations to environmental radiation, serology and altitude, Am. J. Human Genet. 15:329, 1963.
120. Black-Schaffer, B.: Fetal nanosomia and bone athrepsia in the newborn of a woman with a severe cyanotic cardiovascular anomaly, Am. J. Obst. & Gynec. 59:656, 1950.
121. Simon, D. L., and Lustberg, A.: A case of truncus arteriosus communis compatible with full-term pregnancy, Am. Heart J. 42:617, 1951.
122. Warkany, J., and Roth, C. B.: Congenital malformations induced in rats by maternal vitamin A deficiency, J. Nutrition 35:1, 1948.
123. Lee, C. M., Wiseman, J. T., Kaplan, S. A., and Warkany, J.: Effect of ethionine injections on pregnant rats and their offspring, Arch. Path. 59:232, 1955.
124. Nelson, M. M., Asling, C. W., and Evans, H. M.: Production of multiple congenital abnormalities in young by maternal pteroylglutamic acid deficiency during gestation, J. Nutrition 48:61, 1952.
125. Shaw, E. B., and Steinbach, H. L.: Aminopterin-induced fetal malformation. Survival of infant after attempted abortion, Am. J. Dis. Child. 115:477, 1968.
126. Diamond, I., Anderson, M. M., and McCreadie, S. R.: Transplacental transmission of busulfan (Myleran) in a mother with leukemia. Production of fetal malformation and cytomegaly, Pediatrics 25:85, 1960.
127. Gregg, N.: Congenital cataract following German measles in mother, Tr. Ophth. Soc. Australia 3:35, 1942.
128. Swan, C., Tostevin, A. L., Moore, B., Mayo, H., and Barham Black, G. H.: Congenital defects in infants following infectious diseases during pregnancy, M. J. Australia 2:201, 1943.
129. Töndury, G.: *Embryopathien* (Berlin: Springer-Verlag, 1962).
130. Cooper, L. Z., Green, R. H., Krugman, S., Giles, J. P., and Mirick, G. S.: Neonatal thrombocytopenic purpura and other manifestations of rubella contracted in utero, Am. J. Dis. Child. 110:416, 1965.
131. Silverman, W. A.: Clinical conference. Cytomegalic inclusion disease, Pediatrics 21:682, 1958.
132. Weller, T. H., and Hanshaw, J. B.: Virologic and clinical observations on cytomegalic inclusion disease, New England J. Med. 266:1233, 1962.
133. McKeown, T., and Record, R. G.: The influence of placental size on fetal growth in man, with special reference to multiple pregnancy, J. Endocrinol. 9:418, 1953.
134. Babson, S. G., Kangas, J., Young, N., and Bramhall, J. L.: Growth and development of twins of dissimilar size at birth, Pediatrics 33:327, 1964.
135. Naeye, R. L.: Malnutrition, Arch. Path. 79:284, 1965.
136. Naeye, R. L.: Prenatal organ and cellular growth with various chromosomal disorders, Biol. Neonat. 11:248, 1967.
137. Naeye, R. L.: Anatomic features of growth failure in congenital heart disease, Pediatrics 39:433, 1967.
138. Cassady, G.: Plasma volume studies in low birth weight infants, Pediatrics 38:1020, 1966.
139. Berg, T.: Immunoglobulin levels in infants with low birth weights, Acta paediat. scandinav. 57:369, 1968.
140. Schain, R. J., and O'Brien, K.: Longitudinal studies of acid-base status in infants with low birth weight, J. Pediat. 70:885, 1967.
141. Neligan, G. A., Robson, E., and Watson, J.: Hypoglycaemia in the newborn. A sequel of intrauterine malnutrition, Lancet 1:1282, 1963.
142. Cox, M., and Dunn, H. G.: Idiopathic hypoglycaemia and children of low birth-weight, Developmental Med. & Child Neurol. 9:430, 1967.
143. Cornblath, M., Wybregt, S. H., Baems, G. S., and Klein, R. I.: Symptomatic neonatal hypoglycemia: Studies of carbohydrate metabolism in newborn infant, Pediatrics 33:388, 1964.
144. Cornblath, M., Joassin, G., Weisskopf, B., and Swiatek, K.: Hypoglycemia in the newborn, Pediat. Clin. North America 13:905, 1966.
145. Stern, L., Sourkes, T. L., and Raiha, N.: The role of the adrenal medulla in the hypoglycemia of foetal malnutrition, Biol. Neonat. 11:129, 1967.
146. Hockey, K. A., and Hawks, D. V.: An analysis of birth weight and period of gestation in relation to mental deficiency with particular reference to "small for dates" babies, J. Ment. Defic. Res. 11:185, 1967.
147. Pick, W.: Malnutrition of the newborn secondary to placental abnormalities, New England J. Med. 250:905, 1954.
148. Hepner, R., and Bowen, M.: The placenta and the fetus, J.A.M.A. 172:427, 1960.
149. Baird, D.: Contribution of obstetrical factors to serious physical and mental handicap in children, J. Obst. & Gynaec. Brit. Emp. 66:743, 1959.
150. Wiener, G., Rider, R. V., Oppel, W. C., Fischer, L. K., and Harper, P. A.: Correlates of low birth weight: Psychological status at six to seven years of age, Pediatrics 35: 434, 1965.
151. Wiener, G., Rider, R. V., Oppel, W. C., and Harper, P. A.:

Correlates of low birth weight. Psychological status at eight to ten years of age, Pediat. Res. 2:110, 1968.
152. Drillien, C. M.: Growth and development in a group of children of very low birth weight, Arch. Dis. Childhood 33:10, 1958.
153. Lubchenco, L. O., Horner, F. A., Reed, L. H., Hix, I. E., Jr., Metcalf, D., Cohig, R., Elliott, H. C., and Bourg, M.: Sequelae of premature birth. Am. J. Dis. Child. 106:101, 1963.
154. Dawkins, M., and MacGregor, W. G.: *Gestational Age, Size and Maturity* (London: Spastics Society Medical Education and Information Unit in association with William Heinemann Medical Books, Ltd., 1965).
155. Mason, A. S., and Tanner, J. M.: *Human Growth Hormone in the Treatment of Dwarfism* (New York: Appleton-Century-Crofts, 1967).
156. Milham, S., Jr.: Symmetrical conjoined twins: An analysis of the birth records of twenty-two sets, J. Pediat. 69: 643, 1966.
157. Challacombe, D. N., and Taylor, A.: Monosomy for a G autosome, Arch. Dis. Childhood 44:113, 1969.
158. Usher, R., and McLean, F.: Intrauterine growth of liveborn Caucasian infants at sea level: Standards obtained from measurements in 7 dimensions of infants born between 25 and 44 weeks of gestation, J. Pediat. 74:901, 1969.
159. Fisch, R. O., Walker, W. A., and Anderson, J. A.: Prenatal and postnatal developmental consequences of maternal phenylketonuria, Pediatrics 37:979, 1966.
160. Palmisano, P. A., Sneed, R. C., and Cassady, G.: Untaxed whiskey and fetal lead exposure, J. Pediat. 75:869, 1969.
161. Bazsó, J., Vachter, J., and Lányi, I.: Die Schätzung der fetalen Gewichtszunahme und ihrer Variationen aus dem Geburtsgewicht bei ungarischen Neugeborenen, Geburtsh. u. Frauenh. 29:845, 1969.
162. Bazsó, J., Gaál, J., and Boros, A.: Untergewichtige Neugeborene auf Termin, Zentralbl. Gynäk. 86:364, 1964.
163. Bazsó, J., and Abonyi, D.: Untersuchung der auf das Geburtsgewicht wirkenden Faktoren bei Zurückgebliebenheit im fetalen Wachstum, Zentralbl. Gynäk. 90: 384, 1968.
164. Caldeyro-Barcia, R.: Fetal malnutrition: The role of maternal blood flow, Hosp. Practice 5:33, 1970.
165. Horn, R., Grävinghoff, C., and Wolf, H.: Ergebnisse psychologischer Nachuntersuchungen von ehemals frühgeborenen und ehemals hypotrophen Neugeborenen, Monatsschr. Kinderh. 117:442, 1969.
166. Eaves, L. C., Nuttall, J. C., Klonoff, H., and Dunn, H. G.: Developmental and psychological test scores in children of low birth weight, Pediatrics 45:9, 1970.
167. Bazsó, J., Lipák, J., Soós, A., Malán, M., and Zsadányi, O.: The later effects of prenatal malnutrition on the physical and mental development of twins, Proc. First Congress of the International Association for the Scientific Study of Mental Deficiency, Montpellier, France, 1967.
168. Høyeraal, H. M., Lamvik, J., and Moe, P. J.: Congenital hypoplastic thrombocytopenia and cerebral malformations in two brothers, Acta paediat. scandinav. 59:185, 1970.
169. Babson, S. G., Behrman, E., and Lessel, R.: Liveborn birth weights for gestational age of white middle class infants, Pediatrics 45:937, 1970.
170. Neligan, G.: A Community Study of the Relationship between Birth Weight and Gestational Age, in Dawkins, M., and McGregor, B. (eds.), *Gestational Age, Size and Maturity*, Clinics in Develop. Med. No. 19 (London: Spastics Society Medical Education and Information Unit, William Heinemann Medical Books, Ltd., 1965), p. 28.
171. Gruenwald, P.: Growth of the human fetus. 1. Normal growth and its variations, Am. J. Obst. & Gynec. 94: 1112, 1966.
172. Battaglia, F. C., Frazier, T. M., and Hellegers, A. E.: Birth weight, gestational age, and pregnancy outcome with special reference to high birth weight-low gestational age infant, Pediatrics 37:417, 1966.
173. Pusey, W. A., and Haworth, J. C.: The relationship between birth weight and gestational age for a Winnipeg hospital population, Canad. M.A.J. 100:842, 1969.
174. Rantakallio, P.: Groups at risk in low birth weight infants and perinatal mortality, Acta paediat. scandinav., No. 193, 1969.
175. Betheras, F. R., White, J. G., and Betheras, G. W.: Intrauterine growth in an Australian population, Australian & New Zealand J. Obst. & Gynaec. 9:153, 1969.
176. Freeman, M. G., Graves, W. L., and Thompson, R. L.: Indigent Negro and Caucasian birth weight-gestational age tables, Pediatrics 46:9, 1970.
177. Menichella, V.: Rapporti tra oligofrenie ed iposomie neonatali in feti nati da gravidanze a termine e prolungate, Proc. VIII Congresso Nazionale di Nipiologia e delle IV Giornate Internazionali Nipiologiche, Napoli, 1955.
178. Lugo, G., and Cassady, G.: Intrauterine growth retardation, Am. J. Obst. & Gynec. 109:615, 1971.
179. Menichella, V.: Le iposomie del neonato, Matern. e Infanz. 11:1013, 1967.

Telangiectatic Erythema and Stunted Growth (Bloom Syndrome)

In 1954, Bloom[1] described a syndrome of congenital telangiectatic erythema "resembling lupus erythematosus in dwarfs." There were three cardinal features – congenital telangiectatic erythema of the face, sun sensitivity and stunted growth. Bloom's report was based on the observation of 3 cases. He has since added 2 cases and reviewed 12 additional reports in the literature.[2]

The patients show telangiectatic erythema of the face, but the lesions are only rarely present at birth. The erythema, which is due to dilatation of blood vessels in the upper dermis, is combined with nonspecific inflammatory infiltration. The diagnosis of lupus erythematosus made in the early cases was erroneous. Following exposure to sunlight, there is marked exacerbation of the erythema of the face. The light reaction usually consists of bullae on the lips, with bleeding, crusting and exfoliation. Only telangiectatic areas react adversely to light exposure. The inflammatory episodes caused by sunlight result in atrophy of the skin of the face and formation of milia. Uroporphyrin and protoporphyrin are not found in the urine and blood of such patients.

Stunted growth, an important component of this syndrome, usually is present at birth. The patients show intrauterine growth retardation, i.e., low birth

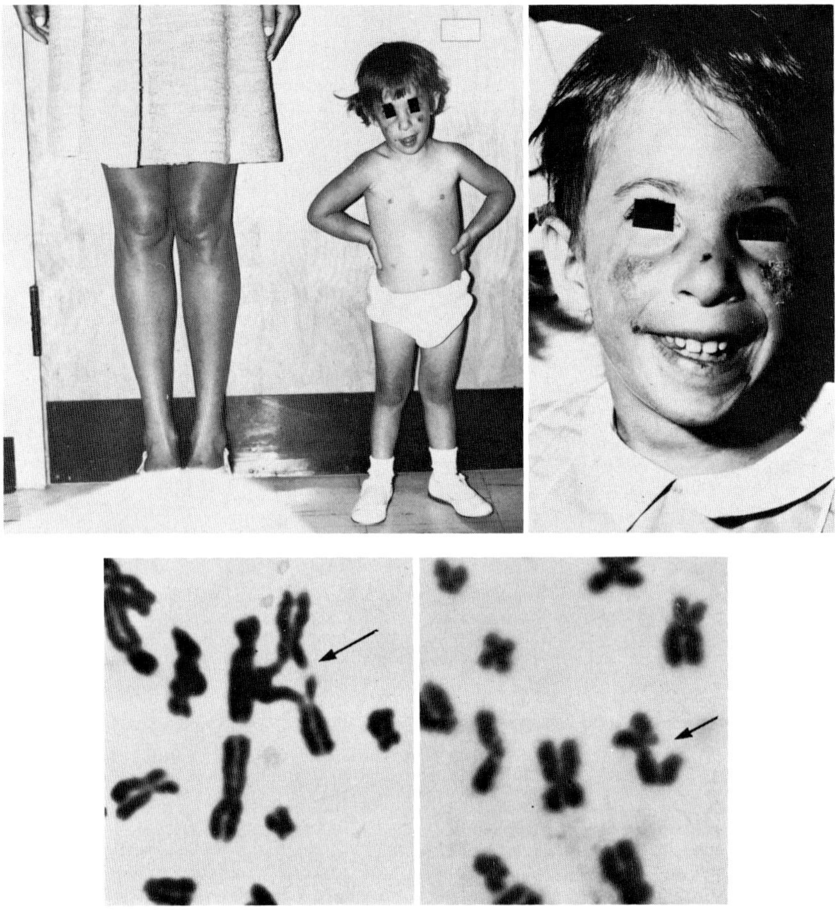

Fig. 14-12.—**Above,** girl 2½ years of age with Bloom syndrome showing growth retardation and facial lesions. **Below,** chromosomes with breaks and exchanges.

weights, although born at term[3,4] (p. 141). In postnatal life, growth continues to be slow but epiphyseal development is normal. The patients are characterized by their slender build, narrow, fine-featured face, with erythematous lesions and a dolichocephalic head. Despite slow growth, the patients' final height is above that of dwarfs, and they become undersized adults.

The cardinal symptoms may be associated with ichthyosis, lichen pilaris, café au lait spots, acanthosis nigricans, pilonidal cysts, supernumerary digits, absence of digits, clinodactyly, short lower extremity, pes equinus, absence of upper lateral incisors, prominent ears, hypospadias or cryptorchidism.

The syndrome has been seen twice in siblings, and parental consanguinity has been recorded. Males and females are affected. Recessive autosomal inheritance seems to be responsible for this syndrome. It is likely that this gene is relatively more frequent among Jewish parents than among other ethnic groups.

Hypogammaglobulinemia has been reported repeatedly.[5-8,11]

Chromosomal irregularities have been observed in increased numbers in leukocytes and fibroblast cultures of patients with this syndrome; breaks, exchanges and dicentrics have been seen.[2,8,9,11] By 1966, 3 of 23 recognized patients with Bloom syndrome had died of leukemia and a male patient 31 years of age developed a squamous cell carcinoma.[10]

REFERENCES

1. Bloom, D.: Congenital telangiectatic erythema resembling lupus erythematosus in dwarfs, A.M.A. Am. J. Dis. Child. 88:754, 1954.
2. Bloom, D.: The syndrome of congenital telangiectatic erythema and stunted growth, J. Pediat. 68:103, 1966.
3. Warkany, J., Monroe, B. B., and Sutherland, B. S.: Intrauterine growth retardation, Am. J. Dis. Child. 102:249, 1961.
4. Szalay, G. C.: Dwarfism with skin manifestations, J. Pediat. 62:686, 1963.
5. Landau, J., Sasaki, M., Newcomer, V., and Norman, A.: Bloom's syndrome, Arch. Dermat. 94:687, 1966.
6. Schoen, E., and Shearn, M.: Immunoglobulin deficiency in Bloom's syndrome, Am. J. Dis. Child. 113:594, 1967.
7. Keutel, J., Marghescu, S., and Teller, W.: Bloom-Syndrom: Bericht über einen Fall mit dermatohistologischen,

endokrinologischen, immunologischen und cytogenetischen Untersuchungen, Ztschr. Kinderh. 101:165, 1967.
8. Rauh, J. L., and Soukup, S. W.: Bloom's syndrome, Am. J. Dis. Child. 116:409, 1968.
9. German, J., and Grippa, L.: Chromosome breakage in diploid cell lines from Bloom's syndrome and Fanconi's anemia, Ann. Génét. 9:143, 1966.
10. Sawitsky, A., Bloom, D., and German, J.: Chromosomal breakage and acute leukemia in congenital telangiectatic erythema and stunted growth, Ann. Int. Med. 65:487, 1966.
11. Keutel, J.: Cytogenetische, immunologische und cytologische Familienuntersuchungen bei Bloom-Syndrom, Humangenetik 8:142, 1969.

Leprechaunism

IN 1954, Donohue and Uchida[1] recorded a family in which the first and the seventh pregnancies ended in the delivery of infants with a rare and distinctive disease picture. There were 2 normal siblings in this family, and 3 pregnancies had ended in abortion. The parents were first cousins once removed. The pregnancies resulting in the delivery of the patients were characteristic in that the uterus of the mother ceased to grow after the seventh month. The first patient, although born at term, weighed only 1,760 Gm. Intrauterine movements were barely detectable from the seventh month on. The younger patient, who was delivered after 7½ months' gestation, weighed 1,590 Gm. Both children were unviable, one dying at age 46 days and the other at 69 days. Failure to thrive and marked emaciation were outstanding symptoms. The siblings resembled each other externally as well as in necropsy findings. The facial features were coarse, the eyes large, protruding and far apart, and there were epicanthic folds. The forehead was hairy, the cranial sutures were wide and the external ears large and low-set. The nose was broad, the mouth large and the lips were thick. The skin of the thin neck was in folds. The breasts and nipples were enlarged, the abdomen was protruding and the clitoris prominent. Necropsies performed on these children yielded similar findings. The inner organs appeared grossly rather normal with the exception of the kidneys, which were large, and the liver, which in one child contained numerous small, pale, grayish yellow nodules. The ovaries were markedly enlarged, each measuring approximately 3 cm. in the long axis. The head and brain, including the pituitary, appeared normal.

Microscopic examination of the livers revealed within the nodules swollen cells with indistinct boundaries and clumping of nuclei. The cytoplasm of the liver cells had many vacuoles and there were large deposits of glycogen in the abnormal areas. The pancreas showed a marked prominence of the islets of Langerhans. Beta cells predominated and in one case the insulin content of the pancreas was six times the upper limit of normal for the age. In the ovaries of both infants, marked follicular maturation and cyst development were noted and in the breasts there was duct hypoplasia with early cyst formation. In the pituitary, there was an increase in the number of basophilic cells and in the thymus prominence and distention of Hassall's corpuscles. Many of the distended corpuscles had coalesced, whereas the lymphoid tissue was atrophic. The adrenals, the thyroid and parathyroid appeared normal. The kidneys exhibited diffuse dilatation of the collecting tubules, which contained conglomerate masses of calcareous, granular material.

Donohue and Uchida believed that the syndrome probably was a rare recessive trait. The case of the older sibling, published previously as "dysendocrinism," had found little attention under this modest name. When the authors coined the term "leprechaunism" for the same disorder, the condition became popular at once. But only a few cases of leprechaunism have been published since 1954, and for some of these the diagnosis is doubtful. In 1955, Evans[2] reported 2 cases as possible examples of leprechaunism, but the birth weights of both patients were normal and there were no signs of intrauterine growth retardation. The first of Evans' cases had definite external resemblance to the patients of Donohue and Uchida.[1] This girl had, like the original leprechauns, enlargement of the nipples and clitoris, defective growth and cystic changes of the ovaries, but the ears were not particularly large. There was no facial hairiness, and no histologic changes were found in the liver or pancreas. Evans' second case, also a girl, had large ears, congenital mammary enlargement, increased liver glycogen, large cystic ovaries and retarded bone age. Pregnancy, birth weight and feeding history were normal. The facial appearance was not characteristic and the clitoris was not enlarged. Patterson and Watkins[3] recorded leprechaunism in a male infant. The child's birth weight was 4,250 Gm., the pregnancy had been normal and weight gain was poor, but the physical features were not typical and the child was mentally retarded. Other cases, possibly resembling leprechaunism and blending into generalized lipodystrophy (p. 174), were reported by Bamatter.[4] Whether such cases are really related to those described by Donohue and Uchida[1] remains to be seen. But the case of 2 sisters reported in 1965 from Hungary by Kálló *et al.*[5] demonstrates that the syndrome exists in the form originally described and suggests that its explanation by homozygosity of a recessive gene may be correct. These sisters had marked intrauterine growth retardation, the facial and body features shown by the 2 original cases, hypertrichosis, hyperplasia of the islets of Langerhans and large cystic ovaries with premature follicular maturation. Furuncles and other skin infections apparently are also characteristic of the disease picture, which includes cystic enlargement of Hassall's bodies and deficiency of the lymphoid system of the thymus. Rogers[6] reported a male child with features of leprechaunism and basophilic hyperplasia of the pituitary gland. It seemed that excess gonadotropin resulted in Leydig cell hyperplasia with precocious development of secondary sex characteristics.

In another case, necropsy revealed, in addition to suggestive features of leprechaunism, absence of the corpus callosum, hydromelia, vascular anomalies, eventration of the diaphragm and abnormalities of the thymolymphatic system.[7]

REFERENCES

1. Donohue, W. L., and Uchida, I.: Leprechaunism: A euphemism for a rare familial disorder, J. Pediat. 45:505, 1954.
2. Evans, P. R.: Leprechaunism, Arch. Dis. Childhood 30:479, 1955.
3. Patterson, J. H., and Watkins, W. L.: Leprechaunism in a male infant, J. Pediat. 60:730, 1962.
4. Bamatter, F.: Leprechaunisme, Rev. méd. Suisse Rom. 84: 494, 1964.
5. Kálló, A., Lakatos, I., and Szijártó, L.: Leprechaunism (Donohue's syndrome), J. Pediat. 66:372, 1965.
6. Rogers, D. R.: Leprechaunism (Donohue's syndrome), Am. J. Clin. Path. 45:614, 1966.
7. Summitt, R. L., and Favara, B. E.: Leprechaunism (Donohue's syndrome): A case report, J. Pediat. 74:601, 1969.

Progeria

PROGERIA is a term used by Gilford[1] for a form of dwarfism combined with "senilism" or "premature senility in which death takes place from old age long before it is due." Only about 40 cases were described in the 80 years[2,3] following Hutchinson's[4] report of the first case in 1886.

One may doubt that progeria, or senile dwarfism, is a congenital disease since, in many instances, the patient is described as normal at birth. But Hutchinson reported his patient because of "congenital absence of hair and mammary glands." The child was born at full term and was a small and fretful infant; his birth weight is not known. There are signs of prenatal onset of the disorder in some cases. Although the average birth weight is only moderately reduced to 2,650 Gm.,[5] intrauterine growth retardation is marked in some cases. In addition, some patients show congenital defects which suggest that the disorder began in prenatal life. Zeder[6] reported a case in which the patient was born at term with an estimated birth weight of 2,000 Gm. Schondel[7] recorded 2 patients; one of them weighed 1,750 Gm. at term; the second, who was premature, weighed 2,250 Gm. Only the first of these patients had definite intrauterine growth retardation, but both had congenital microphthalmia. In the first case there was also a double row of incisors and a rudimentary uvula. Wiedemann[8] mentioned that his patient weighed 1,800 Gm. at term. She had hypoplastic terminal phalanges, anonychia, blue sclerae and hypoplastic ears. One of Cooke's[9] patients weighed 2,270 Gm. at full term. Beginning scleroderma was noticed in several patients shortly after birth, and Moynahan[10] believed that such early scleroderma presages conversion to progeria by the age of 2 years. Micrognathia and faulty anlage of the teeth point to prenatal onset of the disorder. The same can be said of anomalies of the external ears, particularly of aplasia of the lobules, which often is emphasized. It is less certain that malformations of the chest, clavicles and femora are always congenital. In fact, in one instance, clavicles appeared normal during the first year but seemed to be absent in roentgenograms at the age of 5½ years, when they were thought to be fibrotic[11]; but such behavior is not typical of the disease. It seems, from the recorded observations, that some patients have their first manifestations in utero, whereas others appear normal at birth and develop their changes in postnatal life.[21]

As a rule, the outstanding anomaly—marked retardation in growth and weight—becomes evident in the second year and more marked subsequently, so that all patients are dwarfed as they get older. From the

Fig. 14-13.—Gilford's patient at the age of 17 years. (From H. Gilford,[1] with permission of *The Practitioner*.)

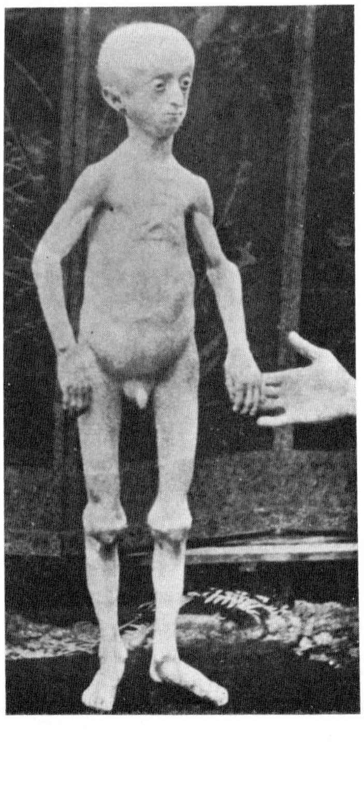

second year on, height and weight curves remain far below the third percentiles.[12] Cooke[9] stated that after an almost normal growth during the first year, the weight of the typical patient becomes stabilized, and thereafter remains in the zone of a normal child in the second year with a maximum at the normal 3-year level. Similarly, the height increases slowly but regularly during the first decade, to reach, eventually, the normal 4–5-year range, which seems to be the maximum obtainable. Height and weight curves for progeria patients were published by Thomson and Forfar[5] and by Cooke.[9]

Typical patients can be recognized at a glance, since they resemble one another greatly. If the disease picture is fully developed, the patients look like "plucked birds"—an unkind but fitting description. The face is small but the cranium, although also reduced in size, is relatively large, so that the patients appear hydrocephalic. The anterior fontanelle remains open beyond the second year and, in some cases, to the time of adolescence.[1-3] The veins of the scalp are large, irregular and quite conspicuous. The eyes are prominent, but the palpebral fissures may be small.[1] The orbits usually are shallow. The mouth cannot be opened completely because of stiffness of the temporomandibular joints. The tongue is small and smooth, the palate high. The neck is thin and long, and the voice is high pitched. The shoulders are narrow and the upper aperture of the chest is small. The clavicles are short. In about one-half of the patients, cardiac murmurs are reported but they rarely are present soon after birth. More often, they develop after the patient is 5 years of age, and become more conspicuous in subsequent years, when atherosclerosis of the cusps of mitral and aortic valves progresses. Elevation of blood pressure is noted after the patients become 5 or 6 years of age. At the same time, signs of angina pectoris become manifest in many cases.[13] The abdomen usually is protuberant and the liver enlarged. The umbilicus is a "mere indentation in the skin without folds."[1] The genitalia appear normal until the age of adolescence, when there is little evidence of sexual maturation. The muscles are poorly developed and the extremities are thin. The joints appear enlarged and show limitation of extension. The posture has been described as a "horse-riding stance," as the knees and hips are flexed, the trunk and head held forward, the arms adducted and the fingers flexed.[5] Arthritis sets in early and becomes a prominent feature in older patients. There are no characteristic changes in the central nervous system, and most of the patients have been described as mentally normal or precocious.

An outstanding symptom is the lack of subcutaneous fat in the skin and the absence of hair of the scalp. Eyebrows and eyelashes also are underdeveloped. There usually is some subcutaneous fat around the pubic region. The skin shows some brownish pigmentation sprinkled with nonpigmented spots. The nails are described as atrophic, short and furrowed. Scleroderma has been observed in several patients.

In roentgenograms of the skull, the craniofacial disproportion is outstanding.[14] Bones of the skull are thin and an open anterior fontanelle may be noticed. The sella turcica can be normal or enlarged. The vertebral bodies often show ventral notches in the lateral view. The clavicles are short and sometimes rudimentary. The distal phalanges are hypoplastic and subject to acrolysis. The appearance of the femora usually is striking, as the neck and the shaft form almost a straight line, and coxa valga is marked. There is a marked contrast in the long delay of closure of the anterior fontanelle and the normal ossification in the long bones.

Arteriosclerotic changes can occur as early as the fifth year and be well marked in older patients. Most patients with progeria die at an early age, 16 years being the average age at death. Arteriosclerotic changes, coronary occlusion or stroke have been reported as terminal events.

Differentiation from dyscephalia mandibulo-oculofacialis (Hallermann-Streiff syndrome, p. 390) is not always easy, since the two disorders have many symptoms in common. Atrophy of subcutaneous fat and muscles, arthritis, early arteriosclerotic changes and absence of cataracts speak for progeria. But there exist borderline cases[7,22] in which the differential diagnosis is difficult.

Pathogenesis and etiology of progeria are still obscure. Deficiency of eosinophilic cells of the anterior pituitary gland has been considered the underlying lesion, but such pituitary changes are seen in many other diseases with different symptoms.[15]

Talbot *et al.*,[16] after thorough study, concluded that their patient with progeria was suffering from a metabolic disturbance, characterized chiefly by excessive utilization of calories for energy metabolism, that apparently was not due to hyperthyroidism. Owing to the hypermetabolism, there were only a few calories available for growth even when the patient was assimilating a good diet. Rosenthal *et al.*[12] found lipoproteins in the serum abnormally high and thought that a metabolic error caused the atherosclerosis, but lipoproteins were not raised in patients of Ghosh and Varma.[3] Blood cholesterol values have varied, with a definite tendency to increased blood levels. Relative insulin resistance and lack of response to growth hormone were found by Villee *et al.*[20]

Only one instance of familial occurrence has been reported[11]; the parents of the 2 affected sisters were consanguineous. Parental consanguinity was also mentioned by Broc *et al.*[17] and Bhakoo *et al.*[2] Some of the cases with suggestive family history[11,18] are not entirely typical of the progeria described by Gilford. In Hutchinson's case, the mother had been almost wholly bald from alopecia areata from the age of 6, and the sister of the patient had similar signs of a temporary nature. Normal chromosomes in bone marrow cells have been reported.[19]

REFERENCES

1. Gilford, H.: Progeria, a form of senilism, Practitioner 73: 188, 1904.
2. Bhakoo, O. N., Garg, S. K., and Sehgal, V. N.: Progeria with unusual ocular manifestations: Report of a case with a review of the literature, Indian Pediat. 2:164, 1965.
3. Ghosh, S., and Varma, K. P. S.: Progeria: Report of a case with review of the literature, Indian Pediat. 1:146, 1964.
4. Hutchinson, J.: Congenital absence of hair and mammary glands, Med. Chir. Tr. 69:473, 1886.
5. Thomson, J., and Forfar, J. O.: Progeria (Hutchinson-Gilford syndrome). Report of a case and review of the literature, Arch. Dis. Childhood 25:224, 1950.
6. Zeder, E.: Über Progerie, eine seltene Form des hypophysären Zwergwuchses mit diffuser Sklerodermie, Monatsschr. Kinderh. 81:167, 1940.
7. Schondel, A.: Two cases of progeria complicated by microphthalmus, Acta paediat. 30:286, 1943.
8. Wiedeman, H.-R.: Über Greisenhaftigkeit im Kindesalter, insbesondere die Gilfordsche Progerie, Ztschr. Kinderh. 65:670, 1948
9. Cooke, J. V.: The rate of growth in progeria, J. Pediat. 42: 26, 1953.
10. Moynahan, E.: Progeria (Hastings Gilford) presenting as scleroderma in early infancy, Proc. Roy. Soc. Med. 55: 232, 1962.
11. Gabr, M., Hashem, N., Hashem, M., Fahmi, A., and Safouh, M.: Progeria, a pathologic study, J. Pediat. 57:70, 1960.
12. Rosenthal, I. M., Bronstein, I. P., Dallenbach, F. D., Pruzansky, S., and Rosenwald, A. K.: Progeria, Pediatrics 18: 565, 1956.
13. Makous, N., Friedman, S., Yakovac, W., and Maris, E. P.: Cardiovascular manifestations in progeria, Am. Heart J. 64:334, 1962.
14. Margolin, F. R., and Steinbach, H. L.: Progeria. Hutchinson-Gilford syndrome, Am. J. Roentgenol. 103: 173, 1968.
15. Atkins, L.: Progeria, report of a case with post-mortem findings, New England J. Med. 250:1065, 1954.
16. Talbot, N. B., Butler, A. M., Pratt, E. L., MacLachlan, E. A., and Tannheimer, J.: Progeria, Am. J. Dis. Child. 69: 267, 1945.
17. Broc, R., Nicolle, M., and Jaubert de Beaujen, A.: Progeria. Études des lésions du système osseux, Presse méd. 43: 786, 1935.
18. Bamatter, F., Franceschetti, A., Klein, D., and Sierro, A.: Gérodermie ostéodysplastique héréditaire, Ann. paediat. 174:126, 1950.
19. Djupesland, T.: Progeria, Acta paediat. 51:438, 1962.
20. Villee, D. B., Nichols, G., and Talbot, N. B.: Metabolic studies in two boys with classical progeria, Pediatrics 43: 207, 1969.
21. Kaiman, H., Lambie, R. W., and Metzl, K.: Progeria, Clin. Pediat. 8:411, 1969.
22. Wiedemann, H-R: Über einige progeroide Krankheitsbilder und deren diagnostische Einordnung, Ztschr. Kinderh. 107:91, 1969.

15

Hemidystrophies and Hemisyndromes

ALTHOUGH the external appearance of the human body usually is considered a bilaterally symmetrical structure, internal asymmetry is normal and dates back to early embryonic stages. The external apparent symmetry of the body is also imperfect when tested by exact measurements. As early as 1822, Meckel[1] wrote about lateral asymmetry of the body. Cox, in 1875,[2] wrote "On the want of symmetry in the length of opposite sides of persons who have never been the subjects of disease or injury to their lower extremities." He demonstrated differences in the lengths of the limbs of normal persons by simple measurements. Liebreich, in 1908,[3] pointed out that asymmetry of the skull and face is a constant and characteristic feature of the human species and that Negroes showed less asymmetry than white persons. Halperin[4] stated that "it is now common knowledge that the left cerebral hemisphere, the left half of the skull and the left side of the face are larger than those on the right." But it is said that the right halves of the vertebral bodies and of the sternum and the right upper extremities and the right ribs are larger than their left counterparts, and that the left lower extremities are stronger than the right. The ears, the eyes and the nipples usually are seen on different levels. These asymmetries have been known to artists since ancient times, inasmuch as no likeness can be achieved by the sculptor or painter who repeats the observations made on one side on the contralateral side. In trick photographs, the picture of one half of a face can be joined to a reversed print of the same half with the result of an image quite dissimilar to the complete photograph, which generally consists of two asymmetrical halves. Yet, there are people with striking asymmetry of the face, of extremities or of the entire body that are considered abnormal and of medical interest. Since, however, measurable asymmetries are a normal feature, asymmetry in itself cannot be considered a pathologic symptom without quantitative evaluation. "The real marvel is not the occurrence of hypertrophy but the fact that hemihypertrophy is such an extreme rarity."[5] Obvious and marked asymmetry has been reported often in the medical literature. Some patients show definite hemiatrophy of the face or of a limb, and others present definite hemihypertrophy that cannot be disputed. Minor asymmetries are difficult to define and to separate from normal variations. It is also difficult in many cases to distinguish between hemiatrophy and hemihypertrophy. Thus, general statements made in the literature concerning patients with hemihypertrophy of parts or an entire half of the body often refer to observations of heterogeneous entities.

There are cases of obvious "hemihypertrophy" in which overgrowth is demonstrated by unusual size or number of parts (teeth, centers of ossification, etc.) or of an entire half of the body for a child's age or by monstrous enlargement beyond normal variation. But it does not make sense to talk of hemihypertrophy in cases of asymmetry of children who are generally retarded in growth and dwarfed,[9] since in such patients the "hypertrophic" half is nearer to normal proportions than the smaller half. It is doubtful that the so-called hemihypertrophy (or asymmetry) associated with intrauterine growth retardation is biologically and etiologically identical with that seen in children of normal birth weight and normal size in postnatal life. Chromosome analyses and recording of tendency to tumor formation and of association with other malformations may permit, in the future, a biologic classification not definitely possible at present. In the meantime, discussion of hemidystrophies and hemisyndromes must be considered tentative and subject to reconsideration. Johnston and Penrose,[10] in speaking of congenital asymmetry, pointed out that there is no indication that these conditions have a uniform etiology. They applied dermatoglyphic methods to the problem and found that varying times of onset are likely for different types of hemidystrophies. In only 2 of 9 patients were dermatoglyphic patterns sufficiently different to suggest early onset (before the eighth week of gestation) of the growth anomaly. In other cases, the pattern was normal but distorted by overgrowth of the underlying tissues after the dermal ridges had been formed.

"Hemiatrophy" should signify reduction of a half that was once well developed. It should refer to a usually postnatal, progressive process that may have its roots in prenatal life. These conditions can be variable in etiology; they clearly show a deficit of one half in comparison to the other and normal half.[6-8] Ward and Lerner[11] suggested the following classification, which distinguishes chiefly the congenital and acquired hypertrophies:

Congenital
- I. Total hypertrophy (involving all systems)
  - A. Segmental
  - B. Crossed
  - C. Hemihypertrophy
- II. Limited hypertrophy (in which one or more, but not all, systems are involved)
  - A. Muscular
  - B. Vascular
  - C. Skeletal
  - D. Neurologic

Acquired
- I. Total hypertrophy
  - A. Gigantism–hyperpituitarism
  - B. Neurofibromatosis
- II. Limited hypertrophy
  - A. Milroy's disease
  - B. Elephantiasis
  - C. Lipomatosis
  - D. Neurofibromatosis
  - E. Vascular anomalies
  - F. Multiple A-V aneurysms

A number of objections can be made to such a classification, but since some recent contributions to this subject promise a better insight into fundamental mechanisms associated with some hemihypertrophies it may be best to refrain at this time from establishing a new classification that may require revision in the near future.

Hemihypertrophy

Hemihypertrophy can be partial, involving merely the face, the tongue, a breast, one or both extremities of one side, etc., or it can be total, affecting an entire half of the body. In total hemihypertrophy, corresponding parts of the right and left side differ in size, but the structures of the same sides are rather well proportioned. The condition is congenital but it may become more noticeable after birth or with puberty and again less pronounced with increasing age. It can occur on either side but it is more frequent on the right than on the left.[5,12] Males seemed to be more often affected than females when Ward and Lerner[11] reviewed the subject but the ratio was reversed in the review by Ringrose *et al.*[13]

The birth weight of children with true hypertrophy usually is normal for their gestational age.[14-18]

The hypertrophied parts often appear swollen or edematous but the skin actually may be thickened and the hair darker, coarser and overgrown on the larger side. There may be differences of temperature and perspiration[19,20] on the two sides. Skin lesions are present in approximately 50% of the patients.[15] Pigmented nevi of many shapes and types such as nevus pilosus,[21] nevus unius lateralis,[22] telangiectases, prominent veins, varices and ichthyosis[23-25] may be seen on the affected side, but sometimes such cuta-

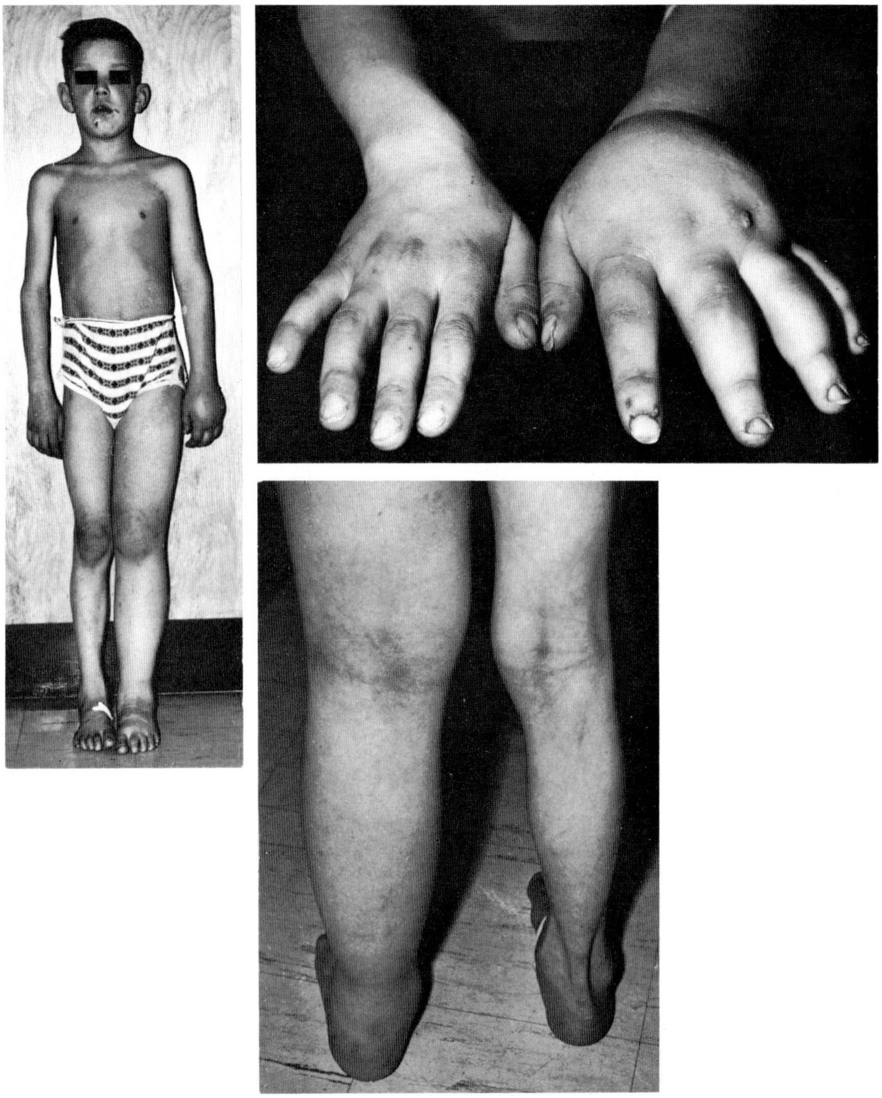

Fig. 15-1.—Hypertrophy of the left side affecting particularly the leg, arm and hand. Fibroblast culture from skin of hypertrophic site showed cells with 46,XY chromosomes.

neous anomalies are contralateral.[5] Supernumerary nipples or enlargement of one breast may be present on the hypertrophic[5,18,19,26] or on the smaller side.[4] The nails may be dry or dystrophic.[27]

Asymmetry of the face can be the only manifestation[28] or it can be a part of total hemihypertrophy. Usually, a bulging cheek is noticeable and the lips of the involved side are enlarged, with lowering of the angle of the mouth on the same side. Asymmetry of the nasal halves is not rare. The palpebral fissure and the pupils sometimes are larger on the hypertrophic side.[16,19,27] Heterochromia iridis and eccentric pupil have been observed.[29] The enlargement of one auricle is sometimes striking.[19] The tongue may show hypertrophy of the affected side, with sharp demarcation at the midline and enlargement of the fungiform papillae on the larger half.[16,19,27,29] The palate can be correspondingly enlarged and the alveolar ridges markedly thickened on the hypertrophic side. Uvula fissa has been observed.[5] Enlargement of the maxilla and mandible contributes to the unilaterally swollen appearance of the face. Dentition is precocious on the larger side in some of the patients. There may be marked enlargement of the teeth ("giant teeth"[19]) in one half of the jaw, a feature particularly characteristic of the permanent set.[5,29] Asymmetry of the jaws and teeth may result in malocclusion.[30] Rowe[28] pointed out that hemifacial hypertrophy is congenital and that after birth the enlarged portion of the face grows at a rate proportional to the normal

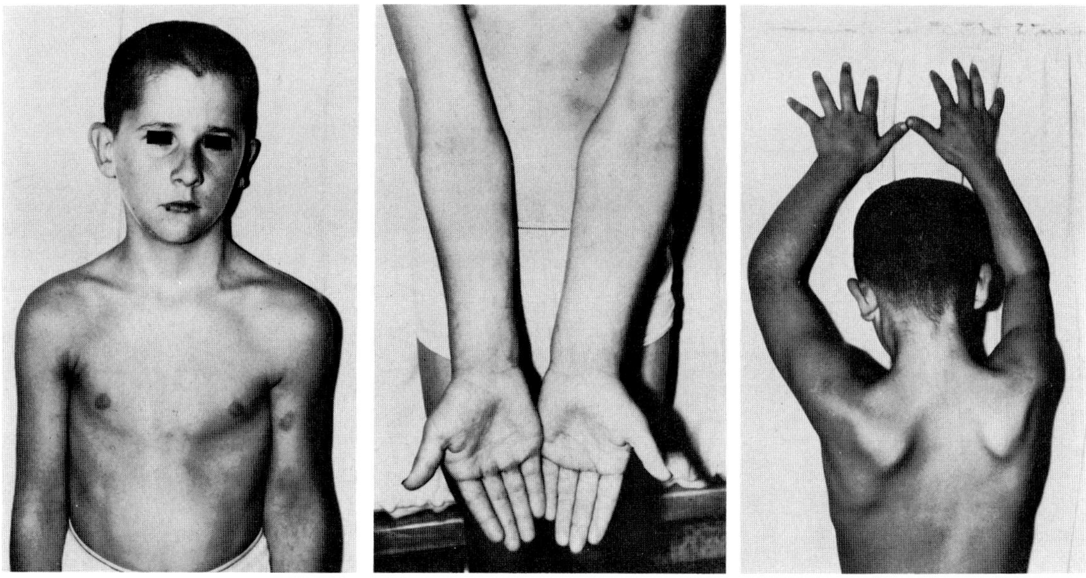

Fig. 15-2. – Crossed hemihypertrophy in a healthy 9-year-old boy. The right half of the face is larger than the left and the left arm and the left shoulder are larger than their right fellows.

side; growth of the larger side ceases at the time of skeletal maturation and the subsequent course of the disorder may be relatively benign. Bone, soft tissues and teeth are enlarged and the abnormality seems to be a quantitive one rather than qualitative. The enlargement results from an increased number of cells and not an increase in cell size. Enlargement of the long bones on one side can be demonstrated by roentgenography and necropsy. In children, the ossification centers may appear several years ahead of schedule on the hypertrophic side. Precocious ossification and dentition clearly indicate that the hypertrophic side is the abnormal one. Scoliosis, asymmetry of the chest and pelvis and limping are frequent symptoms.[5,14] Polydactyly,[11,18] syndactyly[19,29] and other skeletal malformations[18] point to early embryonic errors of mesenchymal differentiation. Macrodactyly limited to one or two digits occurs in neurofibromatosis and in macrodystrophia lipomatosa progressiva, entities that probably differ in etiology from true hemihypertrophy.

Enlargement of one kidney, adrenal, testis or ovary has been observed.[21,31-34] Congenital bronchiectasis[21] and congenital heart disease have been reported.[14,18] Not only superficial veins but also arteries may be involved in the process of overgrowth, with thickening of the media and enlargement of the lumen.[24] Hypogenitalism,[35] hypospadias and cryptorchidism[18] were mentioned in some of the reports.

It has been estimated that approximately 25% of the patients with hemihypertrophy have mental retardation.[13,16,23,36] Psychotic manifestations[23,27] are rare. Hemihypertrophy of the brain has been seen on the larger side of the body,[5,23,37] but it is not always present in hemihypertrophy. Roget *et al.*[38] reported a case with abnormal cerebral cysternae. Convulsions complicated some of the cases.[19,29,33] Unilateral enlargement of peripheral nerves has been described,[21,24] as well as sciatica and intermittent attacks of pain and swelling.

One of the most interesting and disturbing features of hemihypertrophy is a significant association with development of tumors. Wilms tumor developed in at least 21 reported patients, adrenal neoplasm in 6 and hepatoblastoma in 4.[39] Miller *et al.*,[26] reviewing the records of 440 children with Wilms tumor, found hemihypertrophy recorded in 3. In 7 of the 21 reported patients with Wilms tumor, the hypertrophy was contralateral, which suggests that there probably is no "normal" side in patients with hemihypertrophy. It seems worth emphasis that the tendency to development of Wilms tumor exists not only in patients with total hemihypertrophy but also in those with hemihypertrophy limited to the face and in cases of crossed hemihypertrophy.[26] Children with hemihypertrophy who developed tumors apparently did not show intrauterine growth retardation at birth.[41] According to Reister and Scherz,[17] the birth weights of children with hemihypertrophy and Wilms tumor ranged from 3,000 to 5,000 Gm. Association of hemihypertrophy, abdominal tumors and visceromegaly has been reported (Chapter 16).

The etiology of hemihypertrophy is still obscure. Many of the older theories on this subject were reviewed by Gesell,[5] who thought that the disorder might be related to atypical or imperfect twinning: "It is not as monstrous as the double monster, but it may have a related morphogenesis." Yet, twinning

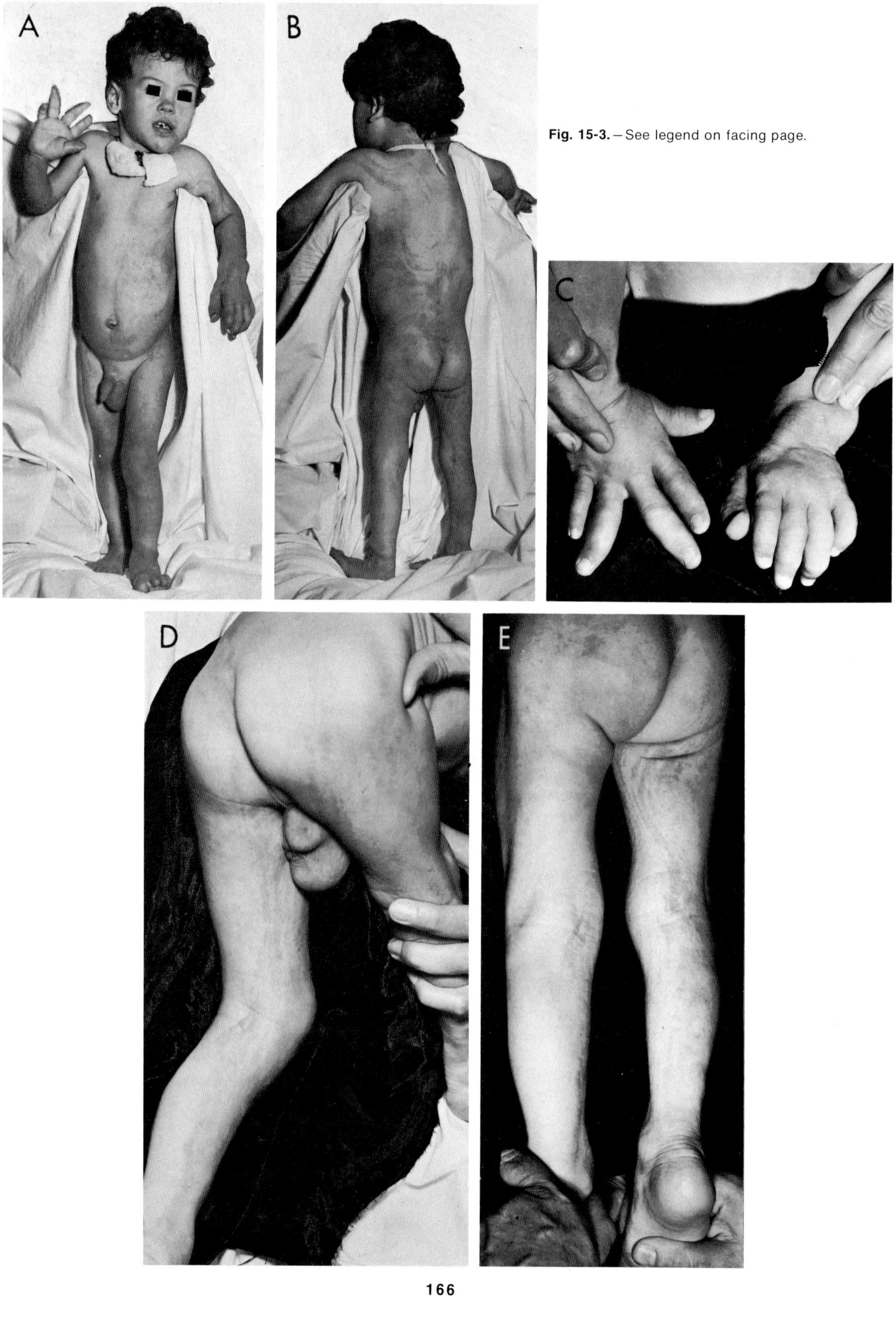

Fig. 15-3. — See legend on facing page.

has been mentioned only rarely[23,42,43] in the families of patients with hemihypertrophy.

In several families, the disorder was seen in a parent of an affected child.[14,23,44] In one case of partial hemihypertrophy, the patient's mother and grandmother had limited signs of the disorder, and in at least two instances[23,45] siblings were affected. Hemifacial hypertrophy has been observed in a mother and daughter,[30] but the cases were not adequately documented.[28] Signs of hemihypertrophy were occasionally mentioned in more distant relatives.[44] But most cases on record were sporadic.

Experimental work has been cited to explain hemihypertrophy. Speeman (cited by Gesell[5]) obtained a large number of twins in Triton by constricting the eggs in segmentation or in early blastula stages. In many of these cases, one individual—usually the right one—developed complete situs inversus viscerum. It is of interest in this respect that situs inversus viscerum apparently has not been observed in association with hemihypertrophy.

Gesell[5] mentioned that, in gynandromorphism of a wasp, the male half of the body was black and winged like the normal male, whereas the female half was red and wingless. In Drosophila, gynandromorphism was attributed by Morgan and Bridges[46] to elimination of one X chromosome in an early cell division, and Gesell[5] stated: "It is tempting . . . to relate true hemihypertrophy and certain not infrequent forms of cranial asymmetry to some quantitative abnormality in the chromosomal mechanism." This suggestion, made in 1921, is still worth considering. There are observations and experiments on asymmetries in animals resulting from heteroploidy,[47] but they probably are not relevant to the hemihypertrophy discussed in this section. The karyotypes of children with hemihypertrophy repeatedly have been found to be normal.[48-50] But chromosomal abnormalities have been reported in children with hemidystrophies, which will be discussed in the next section.

Hemidystrophies

Partial or total underdevelopment of one side of the body may occur for various reasons. It has been observed repeatedly in children with intrauterine growth retardation. It should be emphasized that such hemidystrophies do not occur in all children with intrauterine growth retardation and that hemidystrophy is only one form of irregular growth in such children. While it was stressed by Silver *et al.*[9] (and called "hemihypertrophy"), Russell[51] directed attention to disproportionate shortening of the upper limbs and to reduction of span relative to height. Yet, in 2 of the 5 patients described by him, a slight degree of "hemiatrophy" was noticeable.

To my knowledge, "hemihypertrophy," i.e., overgrowth beyond normal size, has not occurred in any of the children affected by intrauterine growth retardation. Conversely, no child with obvious hemihypertrophy was born with a weight far below the average for his gestational age. Silver *et al.*[9] described 2 children with a syndrome of "congenital hypertrophy, shortness of stature, and elevated urinary gonadotropins" who were born small and remained small to the time of the report. In Case 1, the entire right side of the body was *smaller* than the (small) left and, in Case 2, the entire left side of the body of an extremely small boy was *smaller* than the right. Dentition was delayed in both children. Bone age was normal in Case 1 and somewhat retarded on the smaller side in Case 2. Thus, these children had neither hemihypertrophy nor precocious development on the larger side. Similarly, the children described by Silver in 1959[52] had neither hemihypertrophy nor precocious development of one side, and the author adopted the term "congenital asymmetry" instead of "congenital hypertrophy." Patients with intrauterine growth retardation described by Russell,[51] Warkany *et al.*,[53] Reister and Scherz[17] and Ferrier *et al.*[54] also showed more retarded growth and development on one side than on the other. The patient with congenital asymmetry associated with diploid-triploid mosaicism described by Ferrier *et al.*[54] weighed only 1,850 Gm., although born near term.[55] He had intrauterine growth retardation and conformed to the Silver syndrome of 1953.[9] The authors stated clearly that one could not speak of "hemihypertrophy" in this case, since there was no excessive growth anywhere and even the taller side was below average height for age. In another patient born with intrauterine growth retardation and asymmetry, Ferrier and Ferrier[56] pointed out that ossification was retarded on both sides, more so on the smaller side. Neither side was hypertrophic. It would be justified to speak of "hemiatrophy" in these asymmetric patients with intrauterine growth retardation. This expression was used by Russell[51] to describe 2 of his patients, but the term "hemiatrophy" has been pre-empted for other conditions (p. 168). It is suggested, therefore, that the term "hemidystrophy" be used to signify unequal growth of the two halves of the body occurring in some children with intrauterine

Fig. 15-3.—Hemihypertrophy of the left in a boy 16 months of age. Breathing difficulties from birth on were due to a mucous membrane fold across the larynx. Finger deformities were also congenital. The birth weight was 3,000 Gm. Overgrowth of the left side was noticed in the second year. **A,** front view showing hypertrophy of the left side of face and left leg. **B** shows distribution of linear nevi with predominance on the left. **C,** hands with deformities of fingers and marked enlargement of veins on the left forearm. **D,** legs seen from the right. Enlargement of the left scrotum is shown. Linear nevus streaks are noticeable on the left. **E** shows that the right leg also has linear nevi.

In roentgenograms, hypertrophy of the left half of the skull and hyperostoses were noted. The long bones of the left arm and left leg were larger than the corresponding bones on the right. No enchondromas were seen, so that the diagnosis of Maffucci syndrome could not be made.

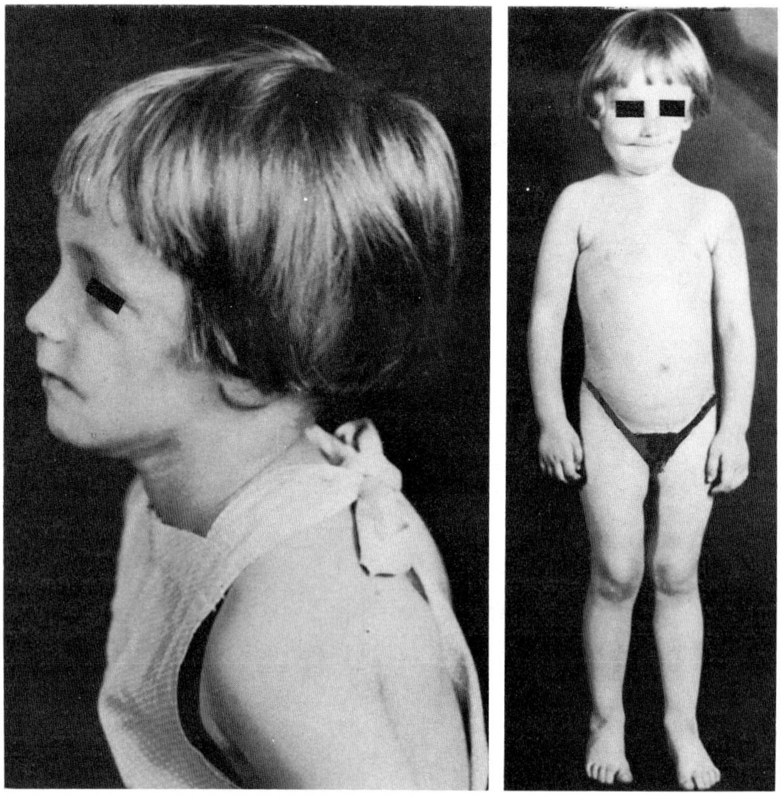

Fig. 15-4. – Hemiatrophy of the left half of the face in a 3-year-old girl. She had fallen at age 16 months, striking the left malar region. After formation of a hematoma, progressive atrophy of the left side of the face was noted at age 18 months. In front of the left ear the skin is atrophic, free of hair and there is no sweating.

growth retardation. Parenthetically, it may be added that a boy described by Silver and Gruskay[57] in 1957 probably had true hemihypertrophy. Born at term weighing 3,100 Gm., he did not have intrauterine growth retardation. His stature was not short and there was diffuse *enlargement* of the left buttock, leg and foot, and roentgenograms showed diffuse enlargement of bones and soft tissues on the left. Except for elevated urinary gonadotropins, he had little in common with the children described by Silver *et al.*[9] in 1953.

It may seem of little importance to distinguish true hemihypertrophy from the dystrophies occurring in children with intrauterine growth retardation, but it seems likely that the two growth disturbances are biologically quite different. As stated before, an association has been found of hemihypertrophy with a tendency to tumor formation, but no such tendency has been noted in children born with intrauterine growth retardation and hemidystrophy. On the other hand, a chromosomal abnormality, diploid-triploid or tetraploid mosaicism, has been noted in some children with intrauterine growth retardation.[54,58,59] Although oncologic and chromosomal studies of hemisyndromes are still in the early stages, it is recommended, at least for the present, that the term "hemihypertrophy" be reserved for cases of true overdevelopment and precocity of one side and that "hemidystrophy" be spoken of in cases of asymmetry of generally underdeveloped children.

The asymmetries seen in some children with intrauterine growth retardation are, of course, not the only hemidystrophies known. Facial asymmetry in the newborn may be due to juxtaposition of shoulder and jaw in utero showing a predilection for infants with craniotabes and for offspring of primiparas.[6] A much more severe facial hemidystrophy has been described as unilateral mandibulofacial dysostosis[7] and as hemifacial microsomia.[8] Hemidystrophies often are seen in patients with cerebral palsy. There is also a possibility that children with various chromosomal abnormalites might show some form of asymmetry whether they are small at birth or not.[60,61]

Hemiatrophy

Progressive hemiatrophy occurs chiefly in adults, with onset in preadolescence in 75% of the cases. It is therefore not a congenital disorder but rather a postnatal process; yet, in some of the patients, congenital anomalies are present, suggesting a prenatal disposition to the disease process, which manifests itself in later years. Congenital palsies of ocular and facial muscles, torticollis, defect of a pectoral muscle, supernumerary nipples, heterochromia iridis, nevi and pseudohermaphrodism have been observed as associated anomalies. Genetic transmission is noticeable in some of the cases,[62] and recessive inheritance has been suggested.[63]

Hemiatrophy most often affects the face, but extension to the neck, shoulder, trunk and extremities can occur. Internal organs such as the kidney, adrenal and ovary may be affected. The brain also may show hemiatrophy or be diffusely involved. Homolateral migraine and heterolateral epilepsy have been observed repeatedly. The cardinal symptom is hemiatrophy of fat and subcutaneous tissue. Sometimes the skin is not involved in the early stage of the disease, but scleroderma, particularly morphea or scleroderma "en coup de sabre," may develop. Alopecia and blanching of the hair can occur early, often being located in a paramedian area, i.e., about two fingerbreadths lateral and parallel to the midline of the forehead and face. Moles, nevus flammeus, white eyelashes and gray hair are also often noticeable in paramedial locations, whereas the central part of the face remains unaffected.

Wartenberg[62] emphasized that hemiatrophy, in contrast to congenital facial asymmetry and hypotrophy due to cerebral palsy or poliomyelitis, is the result of a progressive and destructive process. It has been thought that the sympathetic nervous system is primarily at fault, as suggested by phenomena of sympathetic irritation, which are often present. But irritation of cranial and spinal nerves, hyperesthesias and neuralgias are also frequent symptoms.

After a progressive and irritative stage, hemiatrophy may become stationary and remain unchanged for many years. Arrest of the process may occur early, resulting in abortive or borderline forms.

REFERENCES

1. Meckel, J. F.: *Über die seitliche Asymmetrie im tierischen Körper. Anatomisch physiologische Beobachtungen und Untersuchungen* (Halle: Renger, 1822).
2. Cox, W. C.: On the want of symmetry in the length of opposite sides of persons who have never been the subject of disease or injury to their lower extremities, Am. J. M. Sc. 69:438, 1875.
3. Liebreich, R.: *Die Asymmetrie des Gesichtes und ihre Entstehung* (Munich: J. F. Bergmann, 1908).
4. Halperin, G.: Normal asymmetry and unilateral hypertrophy, Arch. Int. Med. 48:676, 1931.
5. Gesell, A.: Hemihypertrophy and twinning: Further study of the nature of hemihypertrophy with report of a new case, Arch. Neurol. & Psychiat. 6:400, 1921.
6. Boder, E.: A common form of facial asymmetry in the newborn infant: Its etiology and orthodontic significance, Am. J. Orthodont. 39:895, 1953.
7. Franceschetti, A., and Klein, D.: Mandibulofacial dysostosis; new hereditary syndrome, Acta ophth. 27:143, 1949.
8. Gorlin, R. J., and Pindborg, J. J.: *Syndromes of the Head and Neck* (New York: McGraw-Hill Book Company, 1964).
9. Silver, H. K., Kigasu, W., George, J., and Deamer, W. C.: Syndrome of congenital hemihypertrophy, shortness of stature, and elevated urinary gonadotropins, Pediatrics 12:368, 1953.
10. Johnston, A. W., and Penrose, L. S.: Congenital asymmetry, J. M. Genetics 3:77, 1966.
11. Ward, J., and Lerner, H. H.: A review of the subject of congenital hemihypertrophy and a complete case report, J. Pediat. 31:413, 1947.
12. Landauer, W.: Supernumerary nipples, congenital hemihypertrophy and congenital hemiatrophy, Human Biol. 2: 447, 1939.
13. Ringrose, R. E., Jabbour, J. T., and Keele, D. K.: Hemihypertrophy, Pediatrics 36:434, 1965.
14. Scott, A. J.: Hemihypertrophy. Report of four cases, J. Pediat. 6:650, 1935.
15. Gesell, A.: Hemihypertrophy and twinning. A further study of the nature of hemihypertrophy with report of a new case, Am. J. M. Sc. 173:542, 1927.
16. Schwartzman, J., Grossman, L., and Dragutsky, D.: True total hemihypertrophy, Arch. Pediat. 59:637, 1942.
17. Reister, H. C., and Scherz, R. B.: Silver syndrome, Am. J. Dis. Child. 107:410, 1964.
18. Wakefield, E. G., and Hines, E. A., Jr.: Congenital hemihypertrophy. A report of eight cases, Am. J. M. Sc. 185:493, 1933.
19. Wiseberg, M.: An unusual case of hemigigantism, Canad. M.A.J. 25:591, 1931.
20. Mayers, L. H.: Hemihypertrophy, Surg., Gynec. & Obst. 43:746, 1926.
21. Arnheim, G.: Über einen Fall von congenitaler halbseitiger Hypertrophie mit angeborenen Bronchiektasien, Virchows Arch. path. Anat. 154:300, 1898.
22. Lenson, N.: Nevus unius lateralis, New England J. Med. 248:757, 1953.
23. Morris, J. V., and MacGillivray, R. C.: Mental defect and hemihypertrophy, Am. J. Ment. Deficiency 59:645, 1955.
24. Cagiati, L.: Klinischer und pathologischer Beitrag zum Studium der halbseitigen Hypertrophie, Deutsche Ztschr. Nervenh. 32:282, 1907.
25. Carter, C. H., Howard, F. H., and Connolly, J.: Unilateral ichthyosiform erythroderma, Clin. Pediat. 7:605, 1968.
26. Miller, R. W., Fraumeni, J. F., and Manning, M. D.: Association of Wilms' tumor with aniridia, hemihypertrophy and other congenital malformations, New England J. Med. 270:922, 1964.
27. Lisser, H.: Congenital total hemihypertrophy, J.A.M.A. 82:1046, 1924.
28. Rowe, N. H.: Hemifacial hypertrophy. Review of the literature and addition of four cases, Oral Surg. 15:572, 1962.
29. Gorlin, R. J., and Meskin, L. H.: Congenital hemihypertrophy, J. Pediat. 61:870, 1962.
30. Rudolph, C. E., and Norvold, R. W.: Congenital partial hemihypertrophy involving marked malocclusion, J. Dent. Res. 23:133, 1944.
31. Harwood, J., and O'Flynn, E.: Specimens from a case of right-sided hemihypertrophy associated with pubertas praecox, Proc. Roy. Soc. Med. 25:951, 1932.
32. Hutchinson, R.: A case of hemihypertrophy in which the internal organs were affected, Brit. J. Child. Dis. 1:258, 1904.
33. Lenstrup, E.: Eight cases of hemihypertrophy, Acta paediat. 6:205, 1926.
34. Carter, F. S., and Dockeray, G. C.: A case of congenital hemihypertrophy showing variations in bone age and development, Arch. Dis. Childhood 28:321, 1953.
35. Curtius, F.: Kongenitaler partieller Riesenwuchs mit endokrinen Störungen, Deutsche Arch. klin. Med. 147: 310, 1925.
36. Davies, P. A.: Congenital hemihypertrophy, Developmental Med. & Child Neurol. 8:213, 1966.
37. Steffen, W.: Angeborene Hypertrophie der einen Körperhälfte, Jahrb. Kinderh. 38:379, 1894.
38. Roget, J., Beudoing, A., and Guilhot, J.: Un cas d'-

hémihypertrophie congénitale avec aspect anormal des cisternes de la base du crâne, Pédiatrie 10:195, 1955.
39. Fraumeni, J. F., Jr., and Miller, R. W.: Adrenocortical neoplasms with hemihypertrophy, brain tumors, and other disorders, J. Pediat. 70:129, 1967.
40. Fraumeni, J. F., Jr., Geiser, C. F., and Manning, M. D.: Wilms' tumor and congenital hemihypertrophy: Report of five new cases and review of literature, Pediatrics 40:886, 1967.
41. Benson, P. F., Vulliamy, D. G., and Taubman, J. O.: Congenital hemihypertrophy and malignancy, Lancet 1:468, 1963.
42. Simpson, B. S.: A case of unilateral hypertrophy, Edinburgh M. J. 33:623, 1926.
43. Schaeffer, E.: Halbseitenriesenwuchs und Wilms' Tumor, Monatsschr. Kinderh. 11:504, 1960.
44. Gruber, G. B., and Kuss, O. D.: Der angeborene örtliche Riesenwuchs, in Schwalbe, E., and Gruber, G. B. (eds.), *Die Morphologie der Missbildungen des Menschen und der Tiere* (Jena: Gustav Fischer, 1909–1937), Vol. III, pt. 1, Chap. 7, p. 423.
45. Reed, E. A.: Congenital total hypertrophy, Arch. Neurol. & Psychiat. 14:824, 1925.
46. Morgan, T. H., and Bridges, C. B.: *Contributions to the Genetics of Drosophila Melanogaster* (Washington, D. C.: Carnegie Institution, 1919).
47. Fankhauser, G., and Humphrey, R. R.: The origin of spontaneous heteroploids in the progeny of diploid, triploid, and tetraploid axolotl females, J. Exper. Zool. 142: 379, 1959.
48. Wiedemann, H.-R., Tolksdorf, M., and Hansen, H-G.: Congenital asymmetry with diploid-triploid mosaicism, Lancet 1:1166, 1964.
49. The Human Chromosome Letter Nos. 14, 18, 19.
50. Cincinnati Children's Hospital.
51. Russell, A.: A syndrome of "intra-uterine" dwarfism recognizable at birth with cranio-facial dysostosis, disproportionately short arms, and other anomalies (5 examples), Proc. Roy. Soc. Med. 47:1040, 1954.
52. Silver, H. K.: Syndrome of congenital asymmetry (hemihypertrophy), shortness of stature, and elevated gonadotropins, Abst. American Pediatric Society 69th Annual Meeting, p. 66, 1959.
53. Warkany, J., Monroe, B. B., and Sutherland, B. S.: Intrauterine growth retardation, Am. J. Dis. Child. 102:249, 1961.
54. Ferrier, P., Ferrier, S., Stalder, G., Bühler, E., Bamatter, F., and Klein, D.: Congenital asymmetry associated with diploid-triploid mosaicism and large satellites, Lancet 1: 80, 1964.
55. Bamatter, F.: Personal communication.
56. Ferrier, P. E., and Ferrier, S. A.: Silver's syndrome: Report of a case with chromosomal and dermatoglyphic study, J. Pediat. 70:438, 1967.
57. Silver, H. K., and Gruskay, F. L.: Syndrome of congenital hemihypertrophy and elevated urinary gonadotropins, A.M.A. J. Dis. Child. 93:559, 1957.
58. Böök, J. A., and Santesson, B.: Malformation syndrome in man associated with triploidy (69 chromosomes), Lancet 1:858, 1960.
59. Kohn, G., Mayall, B. H., Miller, M. E., and Mellman, W. J.: Tetraploid-diploid mosaicism in a surviving infant, Pediat. Res. 1:461, 1967.
60. Hook, E. B., and Yunis, J. J.: Congenital asymmetry associated with trisomy 18 mosaicism, Am. J. Dis. Child. 110: 551, 1965.
61. Brøgger, A., von der Hagen, C. B., and Støren, A.: Mosaicism involving two karyotypes with 45 chromosomes and a new autosomal translocation in girl with mental defect, asymmetry, congenital heart disease and other malformations, Acta paediat. Supp. 159:44, 1965.
62. Wartenberg, R.: Progressive facial hemiatrophy, Arch. Neurol. & Psychiat. 54:75, 1945.
63. Bramley, P., and Forbes, A.: A case of progressive hemiatrophy presenting with spontaneous fractures of the lower jaw, Brit. M. J. 1:1476, 1960.

16

Visceromegaly
(Beckwith-Wiedemann Syndrome)

A SYNDROME OF fetal visceromegaly, macroglossia, omphalocele and overgrowth of the kidneys and pancreas was described by Beckwith *et al.*[1] Cytomegaly in the fetal adrenal cortex and Leydig cell hyperplasia without masculinization were added characteristics noted in several premature or newborn children. Life expectancy for such children generally is limited, but survival is possible. Hypoglycemia due to hyperplasia of the pancreatic islets may occur during the first months of postnatal life.[9,15] There is also postnatal somatic gigantism and possibly a tendency to cortical carcinoma of the adrenal gland occurring in infancy.[2] A combination of macroglossia, omphalocele, intestinal malrotation and anomalies of the diaphragm was reported by Wiedemann[3] in 3 siblings whose parents probably were consanguineous. Hydramnios was associated with the pregnancies resulting in 2 of the male infants whose omphaloceles contained liver and intestines. The boys died soon after birth, but a sister with similar signs survived operation of the umbilical hernia. When seen at the age of 6 years she still had macroglossia and was unusually tall for her age. Her clitoris was enlarged and bone development was precocious. The mandible was protruding and there was some webbing of the neck. The joints were hyperextensible. Mental development was normal. A wedge of the enlarged tongue was excised and hyperplasia of the lingual muscles was found in histologic sections. The chromosomal pattern was normal 46,XX.

The syndrome of visceromegaly is now well established and additional cases are being published. It is also recognized that cases were recorded before 1964. Among patients with macroglossia there were some who had exomphalos or umbilical hernia.[4,5] Pannullo[6] observed an enormous protruding tongue in an overweight fetus. The newborn girl had generalized muscular hypertrophy, misshapen bones of the extremities and a markedly enlarged liver. Hydramnios complicated the pregnancy, which terminated 30 weeks after the last menstrual period when the child weighed 3,572 Gm. Visceromegaly may be the basis of cases described in the past because of muscular hypertrophy (p. 1031) and macroglossia.[7]

Recurrence in siblings[3,8] and in a second cousin of

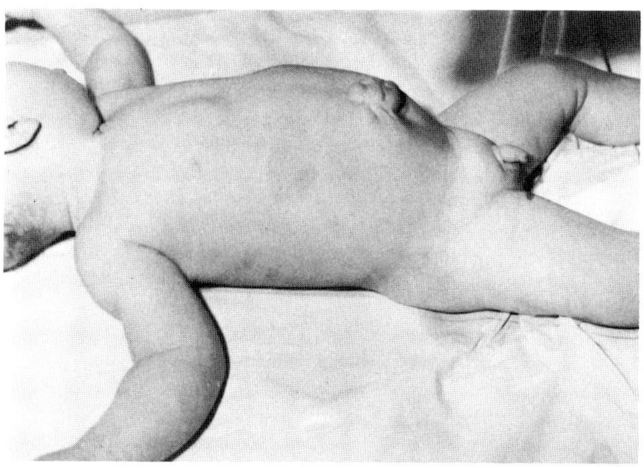

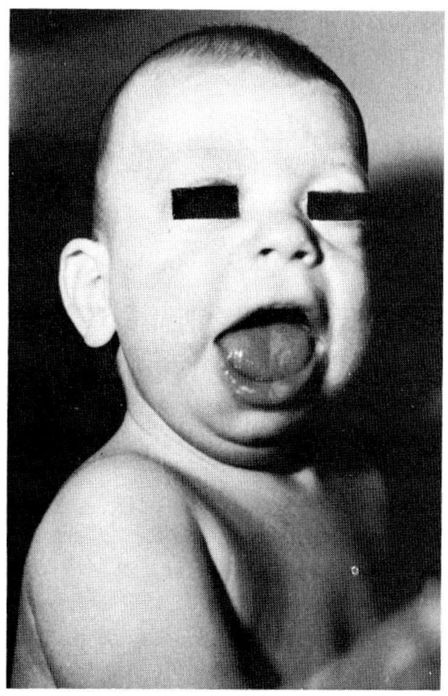

Fig. 16-1.—Boy born with omphalocele and macroglossia. He was tall for his age and had advanced bone age.

patients[8] has been reported and maternal diabetes has been suspected, but the etiology of the disorder is still obscure.

The birth weight is high, usually at or above the 90th percentile. A large protruding tongue, nevus flammeus and umbilical hernia or exomphalos constitute the typical disease picture in the neonate. A peculiar ear anomaly was emphasized by Irving,[8] namely a transverse linear indentation on the lobule; protruding occiput was conspicuous in some instances. The umbilical hernia may be of moderate size or consist of a large sac tending to rupture. Enlargement of the kidneys and hepatosplenomegaly have been observed repeatedly in the neonatal period. Immaturity of the renal tubules in the presence of mature glomeruli was described in some cases.[1,9] Pancreatic hyperplasia[1] and hypoglycemia[9,15] were emphasized by some authors. The fetal cortex of the adrenals shows cytomegaly.[4,8] Hypoglycemia at birth may be followed by prediabetes and hyperlipemia.[10,11]

Prognosis is uncertain. Sudden death may occur in the newborn period. Hypoglycemia may lead to convulsions and cerebral damage. A clinical picture simulating myxedema, gigantism, genital hypertrophy or latent diabetes with hyperlipidemia can develop.[13]

If the children survive, they may attain good health and intelligence. The large tongue can become accommodated as the oral cavity and its constituents grow. In some cases, partial glossectomy results in improved function and appearance,[8,12] but malocclusion may persist. The middle third of the face remains underdeveloped, leading to shortness of the orbital floor and exophthalmos. Mandibular prognathism and a midline frontal ridge add to a typical physiognomy. Advanced physical development, including accelerated bone age, remains characteristic of the condition.[8,10] Association with hemihypertrophy, adrenal carcinoma and nephroblastoma has been observed in some instances.[16]

REFERENCES

1. Beckwith, J. B., Wang, C-I., Donnell, G. N., and Gwinn, J. L.: Hyperplastic fetal visceromegaly with macroglossia, omphalocele, cytomegaly of the adrenal fetal cortex, postnatal somatic gigantism, and other abnormalities: A newly recognized syndrome, Abst. American Pediatric Society 74th Annual Meeting, p. 56, 1964.
2. Sherman, F. E., Bass, L. W., and Fetterman, G. H.: Congenital metastasizing adrenal cortical carcinoma associated with cytomegaly of the fetal adrenal cortex, Am. J. Clin. Path. 30:439, 1958.
3. Wiedemann, H-R.: Complexe malformatif familial avec hernie ombilicale et macroglossie – un "syndrome nouveau?", J. Génét. Hum. 13:223, 1964.
4. Stones, H. H.: *Oral and Dental Diseases* (Edinburgh: E. & S. Livingstone, Ltd., 1948).
5. Bell, H. G., and Millar, R. G.: Congenital macroglossia, Surgery 24:125, 1948.
6. Pannullo, J. N.: Congenital macroglossia, Obst. & Gynec. 7:97, 1956.
7. Goldstein, R.: Congenitale Muskelhypertrophie, Ann. paediat. 189:51, 1957.
8. Irving, I. M.: Exomphalos with macroglossia: A study of eleven cases, J. Pediat. Surg. 2:499, 1967.
9. Combs, J. T., Grunt, J. A., and Brandt, I. K.: New syndrome of neonatal hypoglycemia. Association with visceromegaly, macroglossia, microcephaly and abnormal umbilicus, New England J. Med. 275:236, 1966.
10. Hooft, C., Boedts, F., and Van Acker, K.: Le syndrome de Wiedemann et Beckwith (omphalocèle-macroglossie-gigantisme), Ann. Pédiat. (Paris) 16:49, 1969.
11. Wiedemann, H-R., Spranger, J., Mogharei, M., Kübler, W., Tolksdorf, M., Bontemps, M., Drescher, J., and Gunschera, H.: Über das Syndrom Exomphalos-Makroglossie-Gigantismus, über generalisierte Muskelhypertrophie, progressive Lipodystrophie und Miescher-Syndrom im Sinne diencephaler Syndrome, Ztschr. Kinderh. 102:1, 1968.
12. Shafer, A. D.: Primary macroglossia, Clin. Pediat. 7:357, 1968.
13. Wiedemann, H-R.: Das EMG-Syndrom: Exomphalos, Makroglossie, Gigantismus und Kohlenhydratstoffwechsel-Störung, Ztschr. Kinderh. 106:171, 1969.
14. Filippi, G., and McKusick, V. A.: The Beckwith-Wiedemann syndrome. (The exomphalos-macroglossia-gigantism syndrome), Medicine 49:279, 1970.
15. Sotelo-Avila, C., and Singer, D. B.: Syndrome of hyperplastic fetal visceromegaly and neonatal hypoglycemia (Beckwith's syndrome): A report of seven cases, Pediatrics 46:240, 1970.
16. Beckwith, J. B.: Macroglossia, omphalocele, adrenal cytomegaly, gigantism and hyperplastic visceromegaly, Birth Defects: Original Article Series, The National Foundation 2:188, 1969.

17

Cerebral Gigantism

GIGANTISM IN CHILDREN with mental retardation, macrocrania, dilated ventricular system, dolichocephaly, flat face with frontal bossing, hypertelorism, high arched palate and prognathism are manifestations of a syndrome termed "cerebral gigantism."[1] Clumsy, awkward gait or ataxia, seizures, large hands and feet and many other signs have been noted in such children.[2] Normal (fasting) plasma growth hormone levels have been reported. The levels failed to rise following marked hypoglycemia, which was interpreted as impaired function of the hypothalamic-pituitary axis. Oral glucose tolerance curves were of the diabetic type.[2] Serum growth hormone and insulin assays during glucose tolerance tests were normal in most patients, so that the pathogenesis could not be defined by laboratory methods.[3-5]

Intrauterine onset of accelerated growth is shown by increased birth weight and length in most of the cases[2,6] and by congenital gigantism in 1 patient.[4] Occasionally, the growth rate becomes excessive several years after birth. Dentition is precocious and ossification is advanced. Some patients who have manifestations of the syndrome are mentally normal. Hook and Reynolds[4] emphasized the wide spectrum of the symptomatology and considered the possibility of a "pseudosyndrome." There is also a resemblance of these children to patients with gigantism, lipodystrophy and endocrine manifestations as described by Seip[7] or to those with the diencephalic emaciation syndrome of Russell,[8] in which early advance in stature and lipodystrophy occur.

Familial recurrence has been reported by Hooft *et al.*[9] The chromosomes appear normal.[5] Prolonged gestation, pre-eclampsia of the mother and neonatal problems of the children have been noted.[6]

Roentgenograms show a large skull with a normal sella turcica, increased interorbital distance and advanced bone age. Pneumoencephalograms reveal ventricular dilatation and cavum septi pellucidi in some cases.[5,6,10]

In 1969, Abraham and Snodgrass[11] reviewed 43 published cases and recorded 2 of their own. They found that the patients had the following characteristics in common: (1) high birth weight for gestational age, (2) macrocrania, dolichocephaly, hypertelorism, high arched palate, prognathism and facial plethora, (3) accelerated growth and skeletal maturation from early infancy, with some features of acromegaly and (4) clumsiness without neurologic deficit. Endocrine functions and dermatoglyphics were not abnormal,[11] but Bejar *et al.*[12] considered the dermatoglyphics of their patients abnormal. These authors noted elevation of essential amino acids and deviation in the glycine-valine ratio in the plasma.

REFERENCES

1. Sotos, J. F., Dodge, P. R., Murhead, D., Crawford, J. D., and Talbot, N. B.: Cerebral gigantism in childhood, New England J. Med. 271:109, 1964.
2. Milunsky, A., Cowie, V. A., and Donoghue, E. C.: Cerebral gigantism in childhood, Pediatrics 40:395, 1967.
3. Sizonenko, P-C., Job, J-C., Sebouk, S., and Rossier, A.: Gigantisme cérébral de l'enfant; dosage de l'hormone de croissance dans le plasma, Arch. franç. pédiat. 25:151, 1968.
4. Hook, E. B., and Reynolds, J. W.: Cerebral gigantism: Endocrinological and clinical observations of six patients including a congenital giant, concordant monozygotic twins, and a child who achieved adult gigantic size, J. Pediat. 70:900, 1967.
5. Stephenson, J. N., Mellinger, R. C., and Manson, G.: Cerebral gigantism, Pediatrics 41:130, 1968.
6. Ott, J. E., and Robinson, A.: Cerebral gigantism, Am. J. Dis. Child. 117:357, 1969.
7. Seip, M.: Lipodystrophy and gigantism with associated endocrine manifestations; a new diencephalic syndrome?, Acta paediat. 48:555, 1959.
8. Russell, A.: A diencephalic syndrome of emaciation in infancy and childhood, Arch. Dis. Childhood 26:274, 1951.
9. Hooft, C., Schotte, H., and Van Hooren, G.: Gigantisme cérébral familial, Acta paediat. belg. 22:173, 1968.
10. Poznanski, A. K., and Stephenson, J. M.: Radiographic findings in hypothalamic acceleration of growth associated with cerebral atrophy and mental retardation, Radiology 88:446, 1967.
11. Abraham, J. M., and Snodgrass, G. J. A. I.: Sotos' syndrome of cerebral gigantism, Arch. Dis. Childhood 44: 203, 1969.
12. Bejar, R. L., Smith, G. F., Park, S., Spellacy, W. N., Wolfson, S. L., and Nyhan, W. L.: Cerebral gigantism: Concentrations of amino acids in plasma and muscle, J. Pediat. 76:105, 1970.

Congenital Generalized Lipodystrophy

IT IS POSSIBLE that the "undiagnosed endocrinometabolic syndrome" of Berardinelli[1] described by Seip[2] as lipodystrophy and gigantism and reviewed by Senior and Gellis[3] is related in pathogenesis, though not in etiology, to the syndrome of diencephalic cachexia. In the latter condition, lipodystrophy, despite good appetite, early enhanced growth rate and external appearance, is reminiscent of the hypophysiodiencephalic syndrome,[1,2] which is characterized by increased growth rate, advanced bone age, muscular hypertrophy, emaciation, hyperlipemia, hepatosplenomegaly, moderate precocious puberty, hyperpigmentation, hypertrichosis and dilatation of cerebral ventricles. This disorder seems to be an autosomal recessive trait, or it can be associated with brain atrophy of unknown origin.[2] Astrocytomas have not been observed, in contrast to the children with diencephalic cachexia. Seip[2] pointed out that idiopathic familial hyperlipemia with infantilism and growth retardation[4] could be a primary hypothalamic disorder that results in secondary hyperlipemia.

A hypothalamic disturbance has also been considered in the etiology of progressive lipodystrophy,[5] which is characterized by fat depletion in the upper parts of the body with adiposity in the lower parts. Changes in the cerebral ventricular system have been demonstrated in affected children, but "constitutionally determined deficiency of adipose tissue" has also been postulated as an additional factor. A genetic factor seems to play a role in many cases.[5] (See also Chapter 119.)

REFERENCES

1. Berardinelli, W.: An undiagnosed endocrinometabolic syndrome: Report of 2 cases, J. Clin. Endocrinol. 14:193, 1954.
2. Seip, M.: Lipodystrophy and gigantism with associated endocrine manifestations; a new diencephalic syndrome?, Acta paediat. 48:555, 1959.
3. Senior, B., and Gellis, S. S.: The syndromes of total lipodystrophy and of partial lipodystrophy, Pediatrics 33:593, 1964.
4. Harslöf, E.: Idiopathic familial hyperlipemia attended with hepatosplenomegaly, Acta med. scandinav. 130:140, 1948.
5. Schönenberg, H., and Theil, H.: Zur Pathogenese der Lipodystrophia Progressiva, Ann. paediat. 187:425, 1956.

18

Diencephalic Cachexia

IN 1951, Russell[1] briefly announced observations on a diencephalic syndrome of emaciation in infancy and childhood. In 5 children, the cardinal feature was profound emaciation linked with initial growth acceleration, often with locomotor overactivity and euphoria. All cases had a common pathologic basis in the form of a neoplastic process involving the anterior hypothalamus and, indirectly, the hypophysis. In 4 of these cases, craniotomy confirmed the location, and biopsy revealed astrocytoma in each. Subsequently, Dods[2] reported 4 cases of this syndrome in 2 males and 2 females. The syndrome, which had its onset within the first few months of life, was described as follows: Apparently well infants began to suffer from irregular vomiting, failed to thrive and rapidly became emaciated and pallid but not anemic. The infants remained exceptionally alert, vigorous, hyperkinetic, happy and even euphoric. Excessive sweating could be noted, and nystagmoid movements of the eyes and signs suggesting optic atrophy were evident during the later months of life. Death occurred within the first or second year, and postmortem examinations disclosed oligodendroglioma, astrocytoma or spongioblastoma near or in the third ventricle. Optic glioma[3] and ependymoma have been added to the list of tumors observed.[4] The early onset of symptoms suggests that these tumors are congenital.

Braun and Forney[6] reported a case of diencephalic

syndrome in a fraternal twin girl who began to lose weight at the age of 3 months and developed the rather typical disease picture thereafter. When she died at the age of 1 year, a massive multiloculated cystic mass was found at the base of the brain arising just anterior to the infundibulum. The tumor, which merged with the wall of the 3d ventricle, was a cystic glioma that could be called a small-cell astrocytoma or multipolar spongioblastoma. Another finding was a perforated duodenal ulcer. It is worth mentioning that a congenital hypothalamic neoplasm has also been observed by Mossberger[7] as the probable cause of a fatal perforated duodenal ulcer in a newborn child. In this case, a globular nodule was found projecting from the undersurface of the hypothalamus and lying in a shallow midline depression of the tuber eminence, in front of the mamillary bodies attached to the depression by an eccentric pedicle. The lesion was considered a hamartoma of the tuberal region of the hypothalamus. This child did not live long enough to develop other hypothalamic symptoms.

In a case of anorexia and severe inanition from birth on, Kagan[8] observed a tumor involving the hypothalamus. Despite normal birth weight, the appetite was so poor immediately after birth that the child never gained weight. At the age of 4 months, nystagmus, signs of brain tumor and hydrocephaly developed rather suddenly. Pneumoencephalograms showed both ventricles markedly enlarged. When the girl died 2 months later, necropsy revealed an astrocytoma originating in the hypothalamus and extending into and blocking the 3d ventricle. It seems that this child was the youngest patient with an astrocytoma on record and that the astrocytoma was congenital.

In a boy reported by Aas,[9] vomiting leading to emaciation began at the age of 2 months. Ventriculography demonstrated a probable tumor in the 3d ventricle.

The "syndrome of diencephalic emaciation in infancy" represents a rather uniform disease picture attributable to congenital brain tumors. It seems quite likely that such brain tumors are the result of developmental errors during prenatal life.

Bain *et al.*[10] described 3 cases of "diencephalic syndrome due to silent brain tumor." They also brought up to date the literature to the year 1966, adding some French and German publications antedating that of Russell.[1] It appeared that radiation treatment resulted in remission in several patients and that therapy with beam-directed cobalt irradiation was partly successful. According to these authors, it is likely that with increasing knowledge the clinical spectrum of this syndrome will be broadened and that one might sometimes expect to find anorexia rather than increased appetite, lassitude rather than hyperactivity, irritability rather than euphoria and obesity rather than emaciation.[3] Combination with diabetes insipidus has been reported.[11] Dods[12] reviewed 30 cases, and by 1966 Vassella and Rossi[4] found 40 cases on record.[5]

REFERENCES

1. Russell, A.: A diencephalic syndrome of emaciation in infancy and childhood, Arch. Dis. Childhood 26:274, 1951.
2. Dods, L.: A diencephalic syndrome of early infancy, M. J. Australia 44:689, 1957.
3. Gamstorp, I., Kjellman, B., and Palmgren, B.: Diencephalic syndromes of infancy. Report of 3 children with emaciation syndrome and disproportionately large hands and feet, J. Pediat. 70:383, 1967.
4. Vassella, F., and Rossi, E.: Diencephales Abmagerungssyndrom des Säuglings und Kleinkindes (Russell-Syndrom), Helvet. paediat. acta 21:548, 1966.
5. Hamilton, W.: Diencephalic syndromes of infancy and childhood, Developmental Med. & Child. Neurol. 9:497, 1967.
6. Braun, F. C., Jr., and Forney, W. R.: Diencephalic syndrome of early infancy associated with brain tumor: Report of a case and review of the literature, Pediatrics 24: 609, 1959.
7. Mossberger, J. I.: Perforated duodenal ulcer and neoplasm of tuber cinereum in newborn, J. Neuropath. & Exper. Neurol. 6:391, 1947.
8. Kagan, H.: Anorexia and severe inanition associated with a tumour involving the hypothalamus, Arch. Dis. Childhood 33:257, 1958.
9. Aas, K.: Diencephalic syndrome of emaciation. Report of a case, Acta paediat. 52:161, 1963.
10. Bain, H. W., Darte, J. M. M., Keith, W. S., and Kruyff, E.: The diencephalic syndrome of early infancy due to silent brain tumor: With special reference to treatment, Pediatrics 28:473, 1966.
11. Stanescu, V., Bona, C., Ionescu, V., Florea, I., Arseni, C., and Horvath, L.: Cachexia and diabetes insipidus due to a tumour of the hypothalamus in a girl presenting an intense chromaffin reaction in the subcutaneous tissue, Helvet. paediat. acta 21:659, 1966.
12. Dods, L.: Diencephalic syndrome of early infancy, M. J. Australia 1:222, 1967.

19

Laurence-Moon-Biedl Syndrome

THIS SYNDROME is a rare disorder. In Switzerland, where the incidence probably is high because of inclusion of isolates in ascertainments, the disorder was seen at a rate of 1 in 175,000 inhabitants.[1] Yet, the syndrome has assumed importance in the medical literature because of its varied and puzzling manifestations, which reach into many specialties. The signs and symptoms are associated in some patients and dissociated in others, although a common origin often is demonstrated by family connections of persons with different phenotypes. The manifestations can be congenital malformations or functional disorders without gross signs of pathology. The hypothalamic area, which betrays anomaly by malfunction but not by anatomic or microscopic disorder, can become the site of tumors that reveal that the region was unsound. The syndrome – or the genes responsible for it – includes teratologic, oncologic and endocrine phenomena that can be lethal at birth or in later life, handicapping or rather harmless in "formes frustes." The Laurence-Moon-Biedl syndrome[2,3] exemplifies a genetically determined disease picture in which obesity is combined with retinitis pigmentosa, hypogenitalism, mental retardation and polydactyly. It is likely that it is due to homozygosity in regard to a pleiotropic autosomal recessive gene, although alternative explanations have been given. Actually, the disease picture is not always clear-cut. Mental retardation, obesity and hypogenitalism often are difficult to assess and polydactyly, a well-defined sign, is the least constant manifestation. Ocular symptoms are rarely absent and are the main constituents of the syndrome, but they appear relatively late and are variable. In 1937, when we[4] reviewed 87 cases of the Laurence-Moon-Biedl syndrome reported in the literature and analyzed the symptoms in these cases, we found that only 24 (about 28%) had the five cardinal signs; the remaining 63 (72%) were "incomplete." This did not look like a stable syndrome useful for clinical purposes. One could object to the inclusion of incomplete cases in considerations of the syndrome, but 3 of the 4 patients of Laurence and Moon[2] did not have polydactyly and 1 of the 2 patients of Biedl[3] did not have mental retardation. It does not seem fair to exclude cases of Laurence and Moon and of Biedl from the syndrome named after them. Some writers call the disorder the Bardet-Biedl[3,5] syndrome because the five cardinal symptoms – the "pentad" – were emphasized by these authors; since the patients of Laurence and Moon[2] had paraplegic disturbances, Franceschetti and Klein[6,7] believed that they represented heredo-ataxias associated with tapeto-retinal degeneration and hypogenitalism. When we included in our tabulation[4] patients reported in the literature who had additional, "accidental" findings such as dwarfism, optic atrophy without retinitis pigmentosa, nystagmus, strabismus, deafness, congenital heart disease and deformities of the skull, we found 102 patients, of whom only 24 conformed to the "pentad." But 14 of these 24 patients had additional symptoms and were "supercomplete"; 78 cases were "incomplete." This left 10 in which the five, and only the five, symptoms said to constitute the Laurence-Moon-Biedl syndrome were present. It is true that the combination of the five cardinal symptoms appeared more often in our tabulation than any other. But this is not surprising, since the cases had been selected and published to confirm the syndrome. We concluded that "from the evidence presented, the designation as a syndrome of the five hereditary symptoms – retinitis pigmentosa, obesity, hypogenitalism, mental retardation and polydactyly – has been shown to be unjustified." Thirty years later, the limits of the syndrome were still uncertain.[8] In a nationwide study in Switzerland, Klein and Ammann[49,50] classified 26 of 57 cases as complete, 11 incomplete, 6 abortive, 5 atypical and 9 undetermined. Despite the variability of the syndrome, it is recommended that the term "Laurence-Moon-Biedl" syndrome be continued, whatever the historical justification of that name, because it is so well established in the literature and because it can be used in certain cases for genetic counseling. But it should be realized that the name as used in the literature does not correspond to the syndrome described by Laurence and Moon or to that of Bardet and Biedl. The term is used as a name for an ill-defined and changeable *syndrome complex* appearing in almost kaleidoscopic variations. When used with caution and experienced judgment, knowledge of the complex can be of definite value to the clinician and geneticist. Within the ill-defined syndrome complex, the five-symptom disease picture (retinitis pigmentosa, obesity, hypogenitalism, mental retardation and polydactyly) can be spoken of as "the pentad."

In 1958, Bell[9] collected a series of 273 patients, 160

males and 113 females, for analyses of symptoms and inheritance. The pentad was observed in 47.5% of the males and in only 37% of the females, indicating again the variability of the syndrome. Bell thought that deafness and retinitis pigmentosa, a recessively inherited association, represent a syndrome not related to that of Laurence-Moon-Biedl. But this combination is encountered in patients who also have hypogenitalism and finger deformities[10] or adiposogenital dystrophy, dwarfism and mental retardation, so that it will be difficult to exclude some of these related cases.[11] Many combinations recorded are incomplete, but others include such malformations as congenital heart disease, tower skull, microcephaly, microglossia, facial asymmetry, anomaly of the external ear, dental defects, spina bifida, atresia ani, renal disease and many others, enlarging the spectrum of the syndrome complex.[9] The pathologic findings in cases that came to necropsy are also varied,[12,13] so that there is room for many subsyndromes that could be decorated by euphonious eponyms and made illustrious. Such a syndrome complex is also ideally suited for establishment, defense and criticism of pathogenetic hypotheses, since one can, at will, exclude or include incomplete cases in support of one's opinions.

Ocular findings can vary from normality to anophthalmia.[9,49,50] Although retinitis pigmentosa is the typical anomaly in the syndrome, atypical retinal changes and retinitis without pigmentation have been observed. Optic atrophy has also been cited repeatedly as the ocular component.[4] In the "Biemond syndrome,"[14,15] coloboma of the iris appears as a variant, and even bilateral aniridia has been described.[16] Microphthalmia has been seen in combination with adiposogenital dystrophy[17] and with the complete syndrome.[18] Anophthalmia, adiposogenital dystrophy and mental retardation were observed in a patient, the offspring of a consanguineous marriage, who belonged to a kindred affected in four generations by various eye anomalies from iris coloboma to bilateral anophthalmia.[19] It seemed as if consanguinity had an additive effect in this kindred with ocular anomalies. Cataract has been observed repeatedly in affected eyes, and myopia and external ophthalmoplegia have been reported.[9] Retinitis pigmentosa, the typical eye anomaly of the Laurence-Moon-Biedl syndrome, is characterized histologically by a reduced number of cone, rod and ganglion cells and diminution of the outer nuclear layer. In the ganglion cell layer, pigment is accumulated around the retinal vessels.[13]

Obesity, although a leading symptom, is seldom recognized at birth but usually is well expressed by the age of 4 years even though, at that time, the fat accumulation rarely is excessive. Earlier appearance of obesity has been recorded,[9] and a few affected children were fat at birth. The important point is that obesity under the age of 8 years is rare in children who develop the benign adiposity of adolescence. If distinct obesity is seen before the age of 8 years, one should not rule out more serious disorders. Visual disturbances or polydactyly can lead to an early diagnosis of the Laurence-Moon-Biedl syndrome. The obesity is most marked on the trunk, abdomen, thighs and in the pelvic region, but the face also can be affected. Overweight becomes more pronounced as the children grow older and it often is excessive after puberty. In contrast to the benign adiposity of puberty, obesity of the Laurence-Moon-Biedl syndrome usually is combined with a deficit in height[9] that amounts, in some cases, to dwarfism.[4] But, in rare instances, overgrowth in height has occurred[20] (Fig. 19-1).

It is believed by many investigators that failure in development of the hypothalamus results in secondary effects extending to the pituitary that, in turn, can lead to hypogonadism.[9] But, in many instances of the Laurence-Moon-Biedl syndrome, genital dystrophy and hypopituitarism have been assumed uncritically. Keifer *et al.*[34] wrote that females with the characteristics of the syndrome and aplasia or hypoplasia of the ovaries or deficient pituitary stimulation are rare. There are several instances on record of women exhibiting three or more of the main symptoms of the disease who have borne children.[9]

There is also great variation in the development of the male sex characteristics. Normal testes with spermatogenesis have been observed in some of the patients.[21] In others, spermatogenesis was lacking even though the germinal epithelium appeared normal.[12] Congenital germinal aplasia was diagnosed by Oettlé *et al.*[22] in a 19-year-old male with the full syndrome. Pituitary function was normal, as shown by the presence of adult Leydig and Sertoli cells and normal urinary excretion of follicle-stimulating hormone and 17-ketosteroids. The authors thought that the evidence for hypopituitarism as the cause of hypogonadism in the Laurence-Moon-Biedl syndrome was not sufficient. They considered germinal aplasia as a primary defect and not secondary to pituitary deficiency. The frequent occurrence of undescended and atrophic scrotal testes was explained by them as hormonal unresponsiveness rather than as sequelae of pituitary or hypothalamic defects. The penis often is small, the scrotum bifid and there may be hypospadias or malformation of the prostatic urethra combined with renal disease.[9,12] Such malformations of the urinary tract support the view that hypogenitalism may be considered an associated anomaly like malformations of the anus, the heart or the uterus and vagina[13] and independent of the pituitary-hypothalamic apparatus.

Necropsy reports concerning the hypophysis and the hypothalamus are contradictory. Marked preponderance of basophilic cells in the anterior pituitary has been observed repeatedly,[12,23] but it has been said that the basophilia may not be the cause of the genital changes but rather the result of renal disturbances of some of these patients. Yet, even in a patient dead of uremia, the basophilic component of the anterior lobe can be within normal limits. No consistent correlation seems to exist between the Laurence-Moon-Biedl syndrome and histologic pituitary changes,[13] and there are cases in which normal

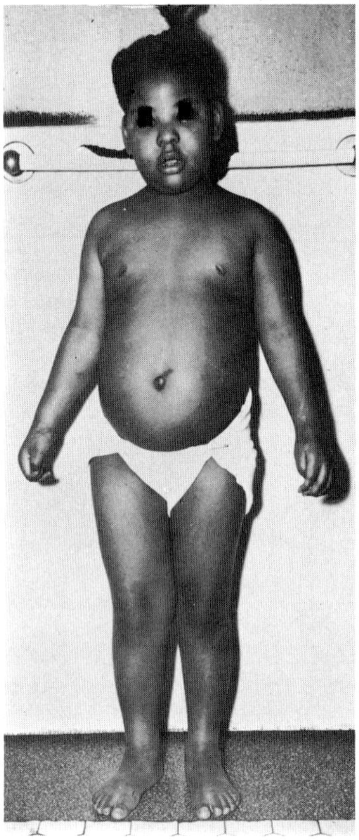

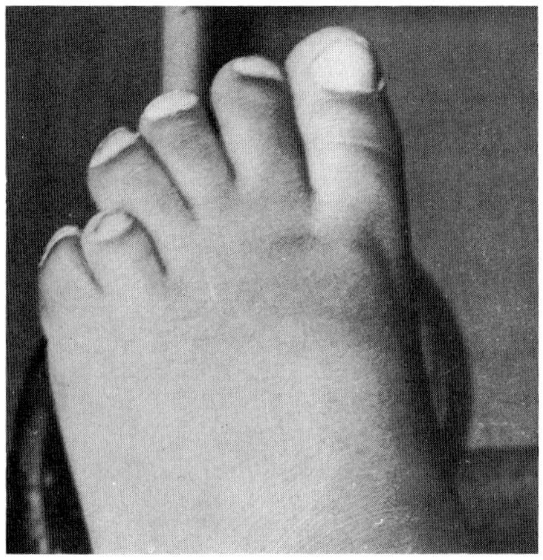

Fig. 19-1.—A 5-year-old girl with Laurence-Moon-Biedl syndrome. When first seen at the age of 3 years she weighed 29 kg., her height was 109 cm. and her bone age was much advanced. She had hexadactyly on the right hand and left foot, failing vision and mental dullness. Her unusual pedigree is shown in Figure 19-2.

function of the pituitary was demonstrated intra vitam.[22]

The role of hypothalamic anomalies in the syndrome has been stressed by some writers[9,24] and denied by others. It is obvious that mental retardation in many patients points to a cerebral defect that could include the hypothalamus. A hypothalamic lesion could be the common cause of obesity, diabetes insipidus and gonadal hypofunction occurring in the syndrome. But, as stated before, hypogonadism could be an anomaly independent of pituitary and hypothalamic conditions, and polyuria and polydipsia—mentioned in some reports—could be due to renal disease in some of the patients.[22] Yet, diabetes insipidus was observed in some patients with the syndrome. The patient of Massobrio and Boccuzzi[25] excreted 3-4 liters of urine with a specific gravity of 1.002-1.006, and the polyuria of Moussio-Fournier and Saralegni's [26] patient responded to Pitressin. Another patient had polydipsia from earliest childhood on.[27] Anatomic proof of hypothalamic defects is scanty. A slight diminution in the number of cells in hypothalamic nuclei with reduction of glial cells throughout the hypothalamus[12] as well as scarcity of large cells in the tuberal nuclei, in the subthalamic nucleus and in the nuclei of the mamillary bodies[13] has been reported. But in various severe forms of obesity the hypothalamus was found normal.[28]

Gross brain defects probably are rare in patients with the syndrome. Shrinkage of the frontal poles[23] and reduction of brain weight with widening of the sulci[13] have been seen in necropsy specimens. Extrapyramidal disturbances (hyperkinesias, choreiform and Parkinson-like movements) have been observed occasionally.[7]

Mental retardation, a symptom of the fully developed disease picture, was present in 87% of the cases compiled by Bell.[9] Most of the patients were dull, showing mental inferiority, particularly after entering school, where the situation is aggravated by ocular changes. Severe mental defects have also been observed and occasionally a psychosis is superimposed on the mental defect.[29] Yet, one sometimes finds that members of an affected kindred who have some symptoms of the pentad are mentally normal.[49,50]

Polydactyly is a relatively rare but important symptom of the Laurence-Moon-Biedl syndrome. In Bell's[9] series, digital anomalies were the least constant symptom of the disease picture, although syndactyly, brachydactyly and more serious hand defects were accepted in place of polydactyly. Seven toes on each foot occurred in a girl reported by Raab[30] and in a relative of the patients of Best and Münch.[32] In hexadactyly, the extra finger usually is postaxial, but there are exceptions, as the thumb and other fingers sometimes are duplicated. If not all extremities are affected, there is a predilection for polydactyly of the feet.

Polydactyly is important because it is – if present – a clearly discernible malformation at birth; this is in contrast to other symptoms of the disease picture that often are recognizable only years after birth. In a family in which repetition of the syndrome is feared, a child with polydactyly arouses concern immediately after birth. Polydactyly and other congenital malformations appearing within the circle of the Laurence-Moon-Biedl complex prove that some of the symptoms, if not all, are determined in early prenatal life, although some, like hypogenitalism or obesity, make their appearance years after birth. Polydactyly and other signs illustrate that the effects of a pleiotropic gene can become manifest at different times and in regions separated from one another. The common denominator that brings about such heterogeneous anomalies as polydactyly, obesity and retinitis pigmentosa is not known and is not likely to be understood through investigations undertaken in postnatal life. Although congenital malformation of fingers and toes is the only cardinal skeletal symptom of the pentad, other parts of the skeleton can be involved. Deformities of the skull include microcephaly and acrocephaly. A syndrome standing between acrocephalosyndactyly (p. 899) and the Laurence-Moon-Biedl syndrome that includes craniosynostosis has been named "Carpenter syndrome" (p. 901). It seems pertinent to emphasize that in one necropsied patient, often cited as typical of the Laurence-Moon-Biedl syndrome, a tower skull was present.[12] Legg-Perthes disease has occurred as a complication.[26,35] Genu valgum and foot deformities were reported occasionally. Dental anomalies were mentioned in some of the cases.

In our review in 1937,[4] congenital heart disease was listed in 3 cases only, and there was then little justification to include such malformations in the symptom complex. But, in 1964, McLoughlin *et al.*[36] culled from the literature 9 cases in which congenital heart disease was associated with other symptoms of the Laurence-Moon-Biedl syndrome. They also described 3 siblings with the syndrome, 2 of whom had cyanotic congenital heart disease. A patient of Landau *et al.*[33] can be added to the tabulation of McLoughlin *et al.* The diversity of the cardiovascular defects observed is worth emphasis. Atrial and ventricular septal defects, patent ductus arteriosus, pulmonary stenosis, hypoplastic aorta, transposition of the great vessels, single ventricle, dextrocardia and many other anomalies have been reported.

Congenital malformations of the urinary tract have attracted increasing attention as part of the syndrome. Malformation of the penis may be an indication of urethral anomaly leading to renal disorder.[12] Urethral stenosis and hydronephrosis were reported by Blumel and Kniker.[45] Landau *et al.*[33] diagnosed malformations of the urinary tract in a patient by pyelograms. In a number of cases, uremia and chronic nephritis were recognized as terminal diseases. Persistence of the urogenital sinus was reported in a girl who had vesicoureteral reflux and vesicovaginal fistula. Urinary tract involvement has been established in more than two-thirds of necropsies.[47]

Congenital malformations of the intestinal tract are rarely mentioned, yet anal atresia is a striking congenital symptom in some of the cases.[3,26,37,38] It sometimes has been observed as an isolated anomaly in children dead in infancy whose sibling or siblings had Laurence-Moon-Biedl syndrome. In some of these cases, atresia ani was combined with polydactyly. This association in a newborn child may foreshadow the birth of children with the full syndrome.[26,37] In the Cincinnati Children's Hospital,[35] the syndrome was seen associated with Hirschsprung disease in a boy. There were 3 children born with Laurence-Moon-Biedl syndrome in this family.

The Laurence-Moon-Biedl syndrome generally is attributed to homozygosity in a single autosomal recessive gene with pleiotropic effects. There is a high parental consanguinity rate, and affected parents are uncommon. In Switzerland, parental consanguinity was established in 52.6% of the affected sibships.[49] There are exceptions that speak for irregular dominance in some pedigrees.[39,40] Whatever their causes, such exceptions suggest caution in genetic prognosis and counseling. The genetic relationships of the pentad to its variants within the Laurence-Moon-Biedl complex cannot be considered established at this time. We pointed out in 1937[4] that the designation as a syndrome of the five symptoms (retinitis pigmentosa, obesity, hypogenitalism, mental retardation and polydactyly) was not justified. Since then, it has been pointed out that the Laurence and Moon syndrome differs significantly from that of Bardet and Biedl (p. 46). Ocular manifestations vary greatly, so that a number of new syndromes have been established in which retinitis pigmentosa is replaced by other eye defects. We had mentioned optic atrophy without retinitis pigmentosa,[4] and now iris coloboma,[14] retinal coloboma,[41] aniridia,[16] microphthalmia,[17,18]

Fig. 19-2. – Pedigree of girl shown in Figure 19-1. Propositus has Laurence-Moon-Biedl syndrome. II_3 had 6 fingers on each hand, had extremely poor vision, went to 7th grade in school and was "thin." I_7 had 6 fingers on one hand, obesity and failing vision. Never learned to read and write.

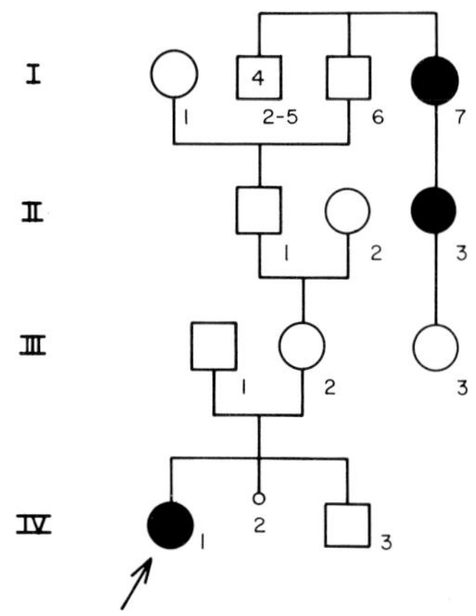

anophthalmia[19] and ophthalmoplegia externa[9] also appear as ocular substitutes within the complex. Similar variations occur in mental, skeletal, genital and metabolic symptoms.[49,50] Congenital cardiac, intestinal and renal malformations, labyrinthine deafness and diabetes mellitus[42] enter the picture. It is not surprising that the syndrome of Laurence, Moon and Biedl has been called "confused."[34]

Despite seemingly hopeless confusion, I believe now that the designation of the pentad as a syndrome is justified. It is, however, an exceptional combination of symptoms in a much wider syndrome complex and not a monolithic syndrome of unusual importance. Recording of such combinations of symptoms has its uses. Although rigid classifications and discussions about inclusion or exclusion of cases make little sense, the pentad can be used as a starting point for analysis of the numerous variants that can be grouped around it for comparison. The pentad and related symptom complexes generally are genetically determined by autosomal recessive genes, which carries significant implications for genetic prognosis and counseling. A few examples will be given to illustrate the usefulness of these symptom complexes. In an obesity clinic, a patient with polydactyly and any of the ocular defects mentioned above will be judged differently from the obese patient who has none of the associated symptoms. In an eye clinic, an obese patient with polydactyly should alert the ophthalmologist to the possibility of hypogonadism or renal complications. A newborn child with anal atresia and polydactyly requires surgical intervention. But the physician should also know that this combination of symptoms may forebode ocular, endocrine and mental disturbances for the patient and possibly also for some of his siblings. The parents of one of our patients with the pentad had another child who was born with polydactyly, a rather harmless congenital malformation, which, however, under the circumstances, predicted mental and ocular difficulties for his future. In this sense, the variants of the Laurence-Moon-Biedl syndrome are also of value for clinical and genetic prognosis. But even in an affected family, one cannot be absolutely sure that a congenital symptom like polydactyly predicts development of other and more serious manifestations. A review of the pedigrees listed in Bell's monograph[9] shows in some kinships persons who had polydactyly but who apparently were normal otherwise. Special caution is recommended if the kinship belongs to an ethnic group in which polydactyly commonly occurs as a harmless variant (p. 40).

A monograph on the syndrome was published by Stiggelbout[48] in 1969. An extensive bibliography can be found there.

Tumors and the Laurence-Moon-Biedl Syndrome

Of great interest are cases in which tumors appeared in patients with the Laurence-Moon-Biedl complex. In 1913, Rozabal Tarnés[43] reported hypophyseal tumors in two brothers with hexadactyly and adiposogenital dystrophy. Bertolotti[44] described a woman with obesity, microcephaly, retinitis pigmentosa and polydactyly who developed clinical and roentgenologic symptoms of a supra- and retrosellar tumor. In a case recorded by Loepp,[46] in which an incomplete syndrome was present, enlargement of the sella was caused by a cyst that contained epithelial rests within its walls. In the patient described by Biemond,[14] mention is made of the patient's sister, who had died of a brain tumor of undetermined nature; she had shown signs of "pituitary infantilism and polydactyly." The patient of Massobrio and Boccuzzi[25] who had polydactyly, obesity, mental retardation, diabetes insipidus and possibly precocious sex development had a disorder related to the Laurence-Moon-Biedl complex. Brain tumor symptoms developed and were fully expressed when she was 17 years of age. The tumor was localized in the pineal area. A sibling who died in infancy also had had polydactyly.

REFERENCES

1. Ammann, F., Klein, D., and Franceschetti, A.: Genetic and epidemiological investigations on pigmentary degeneration of the retina and allied disorders in Switzerland, J. Neurol. Sc. 2:183, 1965.
2. Laurence, J. Z., and Moon, R. C.: Four cases of "retinitis pigmentosa," occurring in the same family, and accompanied by general imperfections of development, Ophthalmic Rev. (London) 2:32, 1866.
3. Biedl, A.: Ein Geschwisterpaar mit adiposo-genitaler Dystrophie, Deutsche med. Wchnschr. 48:1630, 1922.
4. Warkany, J., Frauenberger, G. S., and Mitchell, A. G.: Heredofamilial deviations. 1. The Laurence-Moon-Biedl syndrome, Am. J. Dis. Child. 53:455, 1937.
5. Bardet, G.: Sur un syndrome d'obésité congénitale avec polydactylie et rétinite pigmentaire. (Contribution à l'étude des formes cliniques de l'obésité hypophysaire. Thesis, University of Paris, 1920.)
6. Franceschetti, A., and Klein, D.: Les manifestations tapéto-rétiniennes et leur importance clinique et génétique, Rév. Otoneuroophtal. 20:109, 1948.
7. Klein, D., and Franceschetti, A.: Malformations and Diseases of the Eye, in Becker, P. E. (ed.), *Humangenetik*, Vol. IV (Stuttgart: Georg Thieme, 1964).
8. Caldera, R., and Combourieux, M.: Les limites du syndrome de Laurence-Moon-Biedl-Bardet, Semaine hôp. Paris 54:2424, 1967.
9. Bell, J.: The Laurence-Moon-Biedl Syndrome, in *The Treasury of Human Inheritance*, Vol. 5 (London: Cambridge University Press, 1958).
10. Boenheim, F.: Zur Kenntnis der Laurence-Biedlschen Krankheit, Endokrinologie 4:263, 1929.
11. Weiss, E.: Cerebral adiposity with nerve deafness, mental deficiency and genital dystrophy: Variant of Laurence-Biedl syndrome, Am. J. M. Sc. 183:268, 1932.
12. Anderson, N. L.: The Laurence-Moon-Biedl syndrome; case report with complete autopsy, J. Clin. Endocrinol. 1: 905, 1941.
13. Brattgard, S. O.: The pathology of Laurence-Moon-Biedl syndrome, Acta path. et microbiol. scandinav. 26:525, 1949.
14. Biemond, A.: Het syndroom van Laurence-Biedl en een aanverwant nieuw syndroom (Laurence-Biedl syndrome and a new related syndrome), Nederl. tijdschr. geneesk. 78:1801, 1934.
15. Van Bogaert, L., and Delhaye, A.: Observations d'un syn-

drome familiel nouveau (Biemond) proche de la maladie de Laurence-Moon-Bardet, Bull. Soc. méd. hôp. Paris 52: 683, 1936.
16. Bornstein, M. B.: Aniridie bilatérale avec polydactylie. Relations des anomalies oculaires de type colobomateux associées a des malformations squelettiques avec les formes atypiques du syndrome de Bardet-Biedl, J. Génét. Hum. 1:211, 1952.
17. Warkany, J., and Weaver, T.: Heredofamilial deviations. II. Enlarged parietal foramens combined with obesity, hypogenitalism, microphthalmus and mental retardation, Am. J. Dis. Child. 60:1147, 1940.
18. Cavalacci, G.: Sindrome di Laurence Biedl con microftalmo bilaterale congenito di lieve grado; consideracioni patogenetiche, Arch. ottal. 46:111, 1939.
19. François, J.: A propos d'une famille présentant des anomalies oculaires du type colobomateux depuis le colobome unilateral de l'iris jusqu'a l'anophthalmie bilatérale associée au syndrome de Bardet-Biedl, J. Génét. Hum. 2:203, 1953.
20. Straub, W., and Heberling, V.: Beitrag zur Symptomatologie und Klinik des Laurence-Moon-Bardet-Biedlschen syndromes, Klin. Monatsbl. Augenh. 120:289, 1952.
21. McCullagh, E. P., and Leiser, A. E.: Turner's syndrome and Laurence-Moon-Biedl syndrome in siblings, J. Clin. Endocrinol. 17:985, 1957.
22. Oettlé, A. G., Rabinowitz, D., and Seftel, H. C.: The Laurence-Moon syndrome with germinal aplasia of the testis: Report of a case and review, J. Clin. Endocrinol. 20:683, 1960.
23. Griffiths, G. M.: The Laurence-Moon-Biedl syndrome. A pathological report, J. Neurol. & Psychiat. 1:1, 1938.
24. Grislain, J. R.: Les syndromes de Laurence-Moon-Biedl, Semaine hôp. Paris 31:2347, 1955.
25. Massobrio, E., and Boccuzzi, G.: Tumore (teratoma?) della pineale associato a malformazioni scheletriche come causa di pubertà precoce e sindrome iperpituitarica tipo Cushing, Endocrinologia 14:86, 1939.
26. Moussio-Fournier, J. C., and Saralegni, J. P.: Syndrome de Laurence-Moon-Biedl avec diabète insipide maladie de Legg-Perthes et doigt de Telford-Smith, Bull et mém. Soc. méd. hôp. Paris 64:34, 1948.
27. Bernhardt, H.: Ein Beitrag zur Laurence-Biedlschen Krankheit, Ztschr. klin. Med. 107:488, 1928.
28. Ritter, W.: Histologische Untersuchung des Hypothalamus bei gewöhnlicher Fettsucht, Morgagnischem und Güntherschem Syndrom sowie bei Morbus Cushing, Frankfurt. Ztschr. Path. 52:149, 1938.
29. Todd, J.: A case of the Laurence-Moon-Biedl syndrome with paranoid psychosis, Am. J. Ment. Deficiency 60:331, 1955.
30. Raab, W.: Klinische und röntgenologische Beiträge zur hypophysären und zerebralen Fettsucht und Genitalatrophie, Wien. Arch. Med. 7:443, 1924.
31. Cockayne, E. A., Krestin, D., and Sorsby, A.: Obesity, hypogenitalism, mental retardation, polydactylism, and retinal pigmentation: The Laurence-Moon-Biedl syndrome, Quart. J. Med. 4:93, 1935.
32. Best, F., and Münch, H.: Über diencephaloretinale degeneration (Laurence-Moon-Biedl syndrome), Nervenarzt 23: 292, 1952.
33. Landau, J., Bromberg, Y. M., and Schorr, J.: Laurence-Moon-Biedl syndrome with multiple congenital malformations of the urinary tract, Acta med. orient. (Jerusalem) (Israel M. J.) 8:205, 1949.
34. Keifer, W. S., Wartham, J. T., Zanartu, J., and Hamblen, E. C.: The Laurence-Moon-Biedl syndrome: A confused symptom complex, Am. J. Obst. & Gynec. 60:721, 1950.
35. Observation, Cincinnati Children's Hospital Chart #86454 (Dr. F. Silverman).
36. McLoughlin, T. G., Korvetz, L. J., and Schiebler, G. L.: Heart disease in the Laurence-Moon-Biedl-Bardet syndrome, J. Pediat. 65:388, 1964.
37. Radner, S.: On Laurence-Moon-Biedl's syndrome, Acta med. scandinav. 105:141, 1940.
38. Ricaldoni, A., and Isola, A.: Maladie congénitale et familiale caracterisée par une dystrophie adiposogénitale, associée à une rétinite pigmentaire et une polydactylie, Bull. et mém. Soc. méd. hôp. Paris 52:1131, 1928.
39. Hanhart, E.: Unregelmässige Dominanz des Syndromes von Laurence-Moon-Bardet-Biedl in Oberwaldner Sippe mit 6 Fällen, Arch. Klaus. Stift. 22:326, 1947.
40. Van Bogaert, L.: Ein Stammbaum einer Familie mit Laurence-Moon-Biedl-Bardetscher Krankheit, Ztschr. menschl. Vererb.-u. Konstitutionslehre 21:314, 1938.
41. Sorsby, A.: Familial occurrence of macular coloboma associated with apical dystrophy of hands and feet, Proc. Roy. Soc. Med. 27:694, 1934.
42. Alström, C. H., Hallgren, B., Nilsson, L. B., and Asander, H.: Retinal degeneration combined with obesity, diabetes mellitus and neurogenic deafness, Acta psychiat. scandinav. 34:1, 1959.
43. Rozabal Tarnés, F.: Tumor hypofisario con sindroms adiposogenital an dos hermanos, Rev. clin. Madrid 90:401, 1913.
44. Bertolotti, M.: Polidattilia, arresto di sviluppo nell'acrometagenesi e distrofia ipofisaria concomitante, Gior. Accad. med. Torino 20:6, 1914.
45. Blumel, J., and Kniker, W. T.: Laurence-Moon-Bardet-Biedl syndrome; review of the literature and a report of 5 cases including a family group with 3 affected males, Texas Rep. Biol. & Med. 17:391, 1959.
46. Loepp, W. H.: Gegenseitige Auswertung der Augen- und Röntgensymptome bei der Tumordiagnostik im Sellabereich, Ztschr. Augenh., Supp. 23, 1936.
47. Nadjmi, B., Flanagan, M. J., and Christian, J. R.: Laurence-Moon-Biedl syndrome, Am. J. Dis. Child. 117: 352, 1969.
48. Stiggelbout, W.: *The (Laurence-Moon)-Bardet-Biedl Syndrome* (Assen, The Netherlands: Van Gorcum & Company, 1969).
49. Klein, D., and Ammann, F.: The syndrome of Laurence-Moon-Bardet-Biedl and allied diseases in Switzerland, J. Neurol. Sc. 9:479, 1969.
50. Ammann, F.: Investigations cliniques et génétiques sur le syndrome de Bardet-Biedl en Suisse (Genève: Editions Médecine et Hygiène, 1968), Thèse No. 3045.

20

Prader-Willi Syndrome

Prader *et al.*[1] described a syndrome of obesity, small stature, cryptorchidism and mental retardation in children and adults who, in the newborn period, had had marked muscular hypotonia. In boys, who seemed to be affected more often than girls, there was delayed pubertal development followed by infertility in adult life. In girls, puberty was also delayed, but menstruation began eventually.

In 1946, we observed a 6-year-old girl (Children's Hospital Chart No. 51649) who had been born postmaturely, weighing 2,400 Gm. She did not cry, did not take food well and was flaccid. In her third year, she started to gain and weighed 35 kg. at age 4, 51 kg. at age 6 (Fig. 20-1) and 67 kg. at age 8. Developmental milestones were delayed. When she was 4 years of age, an ovarian teratoma was removed from her right side. Dental caries developed; her bone age was reported to be advanced. There was increasing lethargy and sleepiness. In her tenth year, she developed noisy respiration, cyanosis and pitting edema of the lower legs. Treatment was unsuccessful and she died of cardiac failure. Necropsy revealed microgyria in the right parietal area and slight meningeal fibrosis. The remaining ovary was approximately 2½ times normal size; it contained several small cysts but no recognizable ovarian tissue. The obesity remained unexplained. No abnormalities of the endocrine glands were revealed and the hypothalamus (examined repeatedly by various pathologists) showed no pathologic changes.

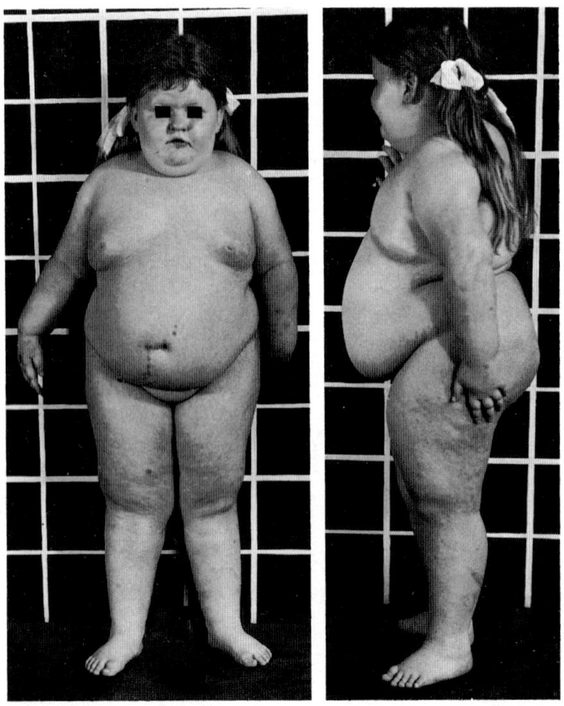

Fig. 20-1. – A 6-year-old girl who became obese after a period of malnutrition and muscular hypotonia.

Many cases have been described in recent years,[2-5] and a certain disease picture has evolved. In 1968, Dunn[8] reviewed 70 reported cases.

Gestation usually is normal except that fetal movements are weak. The gestation time may be prolonged. In the neonatal period there is marked muscular hypotonia, weakness and inability to suck. Undernutrition is followed within a year or two by obesity, which can precede the polyphagia so characteristic in later years. Mental and physical development are delayed but the muscle tone gradually is improved. The palate is highly arched and the mouth dry and there is a marked tendency to dental decay. Hands and feet are small (acromicria), as is true in most cases of children's obesity. Bone age is retarded and stature is subnormal. Convulsive seizures, if present, subside after infancy. There is a tendency to early development of diabetes mellitus, which generally is benign.[6]

Etiology and pathogenesis of the syndrome are not known. Necropsy fails to reveal gross hypothalamic changes and laboratory tests are essentially noncontributory. Prenatal onset of the disorder is suggested by reduction of fetal movements, cryptorchidism and scrotal hypoplasia. Chromosomes were normal in most cases. In some instances, cytogenetic changes have been reported but the pattern was not consistent.[8] The syndrome was seen once in a brother and sister and, in one case, the parents were first cousins.[7]

REFERENCES

1. Prader, A., Labhart, A., and Willi, H.: Ein Syndrom von Adipositas, Kleinwuchs, Kryptorchismus und Oligophrenie nach myatonieartigem Zustand im Neugeborenenalter, Schweiz. med. Wchnschr. 86:1260, 1956.
2. Laurance, B. M.: Hypotonia, mental retardation, obesity, and cryptorchidism associated with dwarfism and diabetes in children, Arch. Dis. Childhood 42:126, 1967.

3. Hoefnagel, D., Costello, P. J., and Hatoum, K.: Prader-Willi syndrome, J. Ment. Defic. Res. 2:1, 1967.
4. Juul, J., and Dupont, A.: Prader-Willi syndrome, J. Ment. Defic. Res. 11:12, 1967.
5. Evans, P. R.: Hypogenital dystrophy with diabetic tendency, Guy's Hosp. Rep. 113:207, 1964.
6. Hooft, C., Delire, C., and Thevelin, P.: Syndrome de Prader avec diabète sucré, Acta paediat. belg. 21:193, 1967.
7. Gabilan, J-C., and Royer, P.: Le syndrome de Prader, Labhardt et Willi (étude de onze observations), Arch. franç. pédiat. 25:121, 1968.
8. Dunn, H. G.: The Prader-Labhart-Willi syndrome: Review of the literature and report of nine cases, Acta paediat. scandinav., Supp. 186, 1968.

21

Situs Inversus

In complete situs inversus, both the thoracic and the abdominal viscera are in reverse position, as in a mirror image. The heart apex is in the right mamillary line and the aortic arch turns toward the right. The right lung has two lobes, the left lung three, and the main mass of the liver is in the left hypochondrium. The gallbladder and the pylorus are on the left side, the fundus of the stomach, the descending colon and the sigmoid on the right side. This arrangement of the viscera may go without functional disturbance and remain undetected during life. Total situs inversus probably is etiologically and pathogenetically different from some forms of partial situs inversus. Cockayne[1] distinguished three types of partial transposition of the viscera: (1) partial transposition involving thoracic and abdominal organs, (2) partial or complete transposition of the abdominal viscera without transposition of the thoracic viscera and (3) dextrocardia, with the chambers of the heart forming the mirror image of the normal.

The frequency of situs inversus has been estimated in adults as 1 in 10,000 or 1 in 8,400,[2,3] but its incidence among newborns may be much higher, since those with situs inversus combined with multiple congenital malformations usually do not reach adulthood. The occurrence may be 1 in 5,000 or even higher in a newborn population.[4]

Although it often is stated that a sharp distinction must be made between situs inversus totalis and partialis, this is not done in the medical literature. If one limits the term "situs inversus totalis" to the mirror image anomaly, most cases complicated by congenital malformations are excluded, since they do not represent mirror images of the normal. If, for instance, a child with situs inversus has a left-sided aortic arch and a left descending aorta,[5] one cannot speak of total situs inversus.

It seems that more males than females are affected. Cockayne[1] assembled evidence that complete transposition of the viscera is inherited as a recessive trait and determined by a single autosomal gene. As proof of this, he cited familial incidence, the ratio of affected to normal siblings in fraternities, occurrence

Fig. 21-1.—Roentgenogram of a 10-year-old girl with situs inversus.

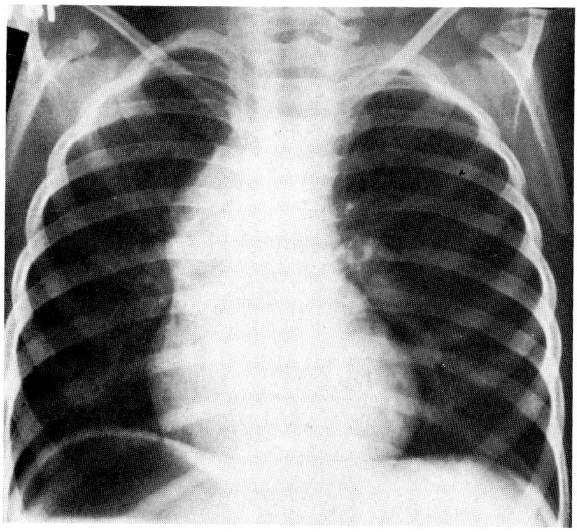

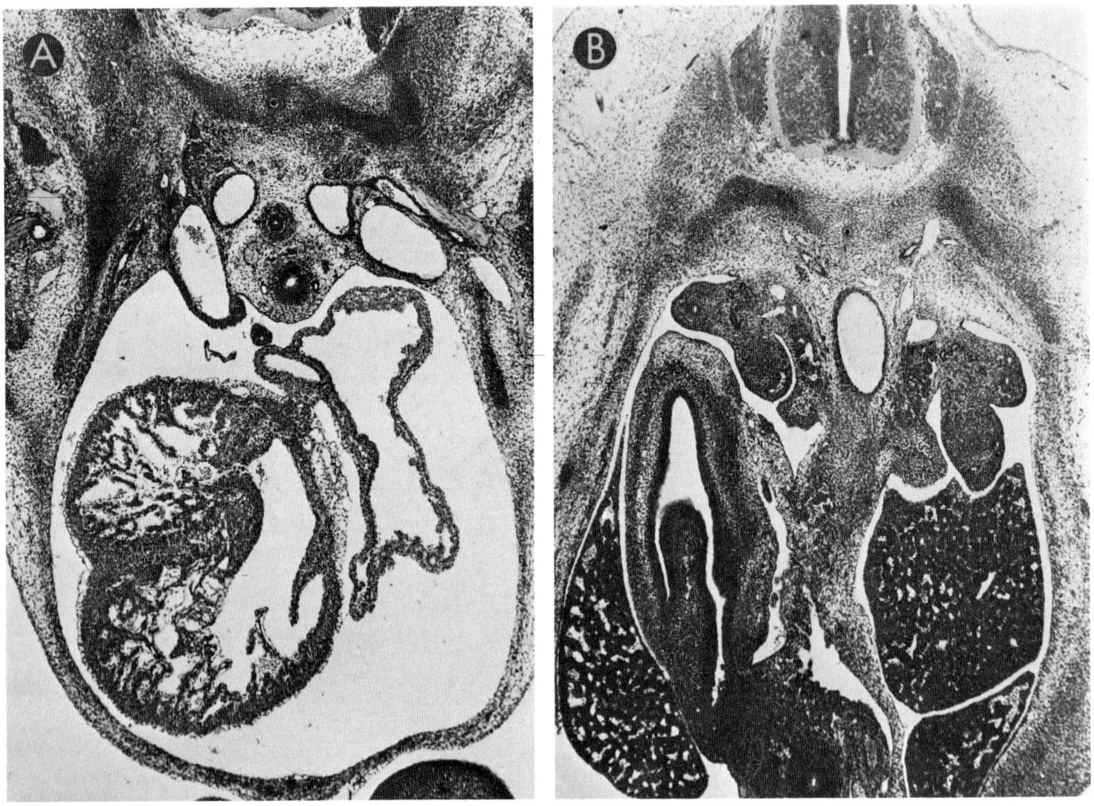

Fig. 21-2.—Situs inversus in rat fetus (fifteenth day) whose mother had been treated with trypan blue. The heart (**A**) and the stomach (**B**) are seen on the right side of the body.

in both members of a pair of monozygotic twins and the high percentage of first cousin marriages of the parents. Campbell[6] also concluded that recessive inheritance plays an important part in the etiology of situs inversus totalis, isolated dextrocardia and isolated levocardia.

Torgersen[2] collected from the literature reports of 12 pairs of probably monozygotic twins with situs inversus; 6 of these were concordant and 6 discordant. In 3 pairs of dizygotic twins, concordance was observed once and discordance twice. These observations do not elucidate the etiology of the anomaly. Torgersen,[2] like others, believed that evidence of genetic determination of situs inversus was furnished by observations of families and by the frequency of first cousin marriages among the parents of patients with situs inversus. But he stated that the hereditary mechanism was still far from being cleared up and that the relative influence of genetic and prenatal environmental factors in the causation of situs inversus could not yet be evaluated. Twinning or left-handedness apparently were not related to situs inversus. Lowe and McKeown[7] concluded that the inheritance of situs inversus cannot be attributed to a single recessive gene. They found that the incidence of affected siblings born after propositi was 1 in 31 and not the expected 1 in 4. They, as well as Brandt and Revaz[8] and Schippan *et al.*,[9] observed additional cases of monozygotic twin pairs, discordant for situs inversus. There also are reports of situs inversus totalis occurring in two and even in four generations.[10] Normal chromosomes have been demonstrated in a case of Kartagener syndrome.[11] In our cytogenetics laboratory, trisomy 18 was established in a child with multiple congenital malformations, including phocomelia and situs inversus. These findings demonstrate the etiologic heterogeneity of situs inversus.

Cockayne[1] suggested that the three types of partial transposition are not sharply separated and that there is a gradation leading up to complete situs inversus. This concept appears questionable, since most cases of the asplenia syndrome (with partial situs inversus) are sporadic and parental consanguinity is rare (p. 746). However, in at least one family with parental consanguinity, both a child with situs inversus totalis and one with situs inversus abdominalis were observed.[12]

Experiments and observations in animals point to heterogeneous causes of situs inversus. Situs inversus inherited as a recessive trait has been described in mice. Affected animals have left-right transposition of thoracic and abdominal viscera, anomalous

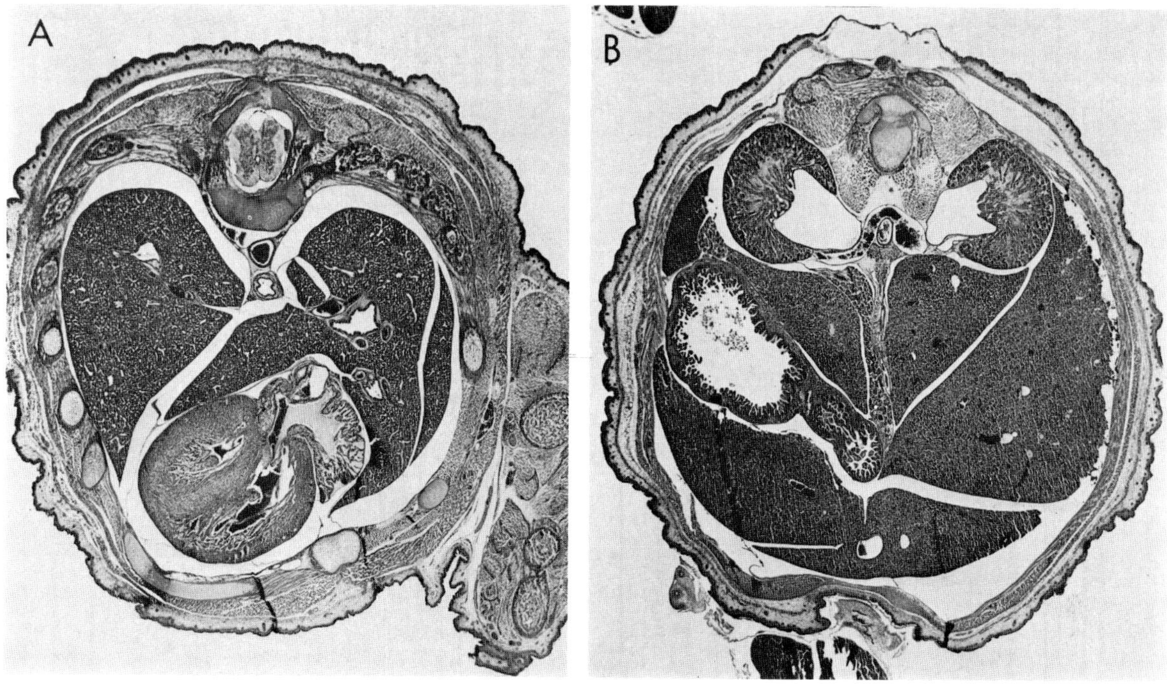

Fig. 21-3. – Situs inversus of heart (**A**) and stomach (**B**) of rat fetus (twenty-first day) whose mother had been treated with trypan blue injections from the eighth to the tenth day of gestation. Note hydronephrosis and spina bifida in **B**.

relationship of postcaval and azygos veins, anomaly of the hepatic portal vein, irregularities in spleen position and shape, and in liver and lung lobation.[13] There are no cardiac malformations in these mice. Situs inversus can also be produced experimentally in amphibia and in mammals by postconceptional manipulations. In amphibian embryos, it has been shown that the normal asymmetry of the intestine and heart is dependent on a factor situated in the roof of the gut. When the neural folds are still open, a square piece of presumptive neural tube material and the underlying gut roof can be removed, rotated through 180 degrees and grafted back into place so that the anteroposterior axis of the piece is reversed. Subsequently, the embryo develops situs inversus of the asymmetric organs, i.e., the stomach is on the right and the intestine and heart are twisted in the direction opposite to the normal. It is necessary to rotate the underlying gut roof with the piece of neural tube, or normal asymmetry develops. It is believed that symmetry and asymmetry are regulated by some factor distributed across the gut roof. Removal of the square piece without reversed back-grafting does not produce any change in the normal situs. Situs inversus of conjoined twins has been imitated by experiments in which a blastula of a newt is partially constricted by tying a fine hair around it in the plane of bilateral symmetry, which results in the production of a double-headed monster. In such conjoined twins, the left-hand member of the pair always shows the normal asymmetry, the right-hand member nearly always situs inversus. After complete separation of halves of a blastula of a newt by a hair in the plane of bilateral symmetry, the right halves develop into organisms that show situs inversus in approximately 50% of the cases. But the decisive factor apparently is not yet present in earlier stages of development because, if the separation is made at the two-cell stage, the right-hand blastomeres do not have any greater tendency to production of reversed asymmetry than do normal newts' eggs.[14]

Situs inversus has been produced experimentally in mammals. It has been observed occasionally in the young of mother rats treated with trypan blue injections (Figs. 21-2 and 21-3). X-irradiation of pregnant rats on the ninth day of gestation resulted in situs inversus in some of the young.[15] Such experiments support the view of Torgersen[2,16] that not only genetic but also environmental factors may be responsible for situs inversus in man. Spontaneous situs inversus totalis with cardiac malformations in a puppy was described by Ferencz,[17] who pointed out the similarity of the case to that of a child.

Despite complete situs inversus, human beings can live a normal life and attain a normal life span. This remarkable fact is often emphasized, but there are numerous cases that are complicated by congenital malformations that are life-threatening or life-shortening. Many infants with situs inversus are eliminated early because of the severe defects of the central nervous or cardiovascular system, hypoplastic lungs, esophageal or duodenal obstruction, diaphragmatic hernia, omphalocele, polycystic kidneys, single kidney, hydronephrosis, urethral anomaly, imperforate anus or other malformations.[1,4]

Among those who survive, bronchiectasis is found in 25% and cardiovascular malformations in 8%.[5] Kartagener syndrome–i.e., situs inversus, bronchiectasis, nasal polyposis and sinusitis (p. 602)–occurs in approximately 10% of persons with situs inversus.[18] Bronchiectasis, sometimes present in infancy,[19] probably is congenital in such cases.[20] Bronchogenic carcinoma complicating situs inversus totalis has been reported.[21] Situs inversus and cardiac malformations as observed in hospitals were analyzed by Merklin and Varano.[22] Ventricular septal defect was the most frequent anomaly, but it occurred in many heterogeneous clinical entities. Absence of the spleen or multiple spleens frequently associated with partial situs inversus (Chapter 80) occurs only rarely in cases of total situs inversus.

Situs inversus has been observed in combination with vertebral defects and even with agenesis of the spine below the first lumbar vertebra.[23] Association with Recklinghausen neurofibromatosis,[1] tuberous sclerosis,[24,25] Albright syndrome[26] and Down syndrome[27] has been reported. Observations by Everett[28] suggest an increased frequency of mental retardation in patients with situs inversus. Reduced fertility in men was noted in a kindred in which 4 cases of situs inversus occurred.[29]

The recognition of situs inversus is important when affected persons require surgical intervention. Symptoms of appendicitis or gallbladder disease can be misinterpreted in cases of visceral transposition and lead to erroneous preoperative diagnosis.[30] It is advantageous for persons with situs inversus to have early knowledge of their anomaly. According to Cleveland,[31] detection of the anomaly is possible at birth by inspection of the umbilical cord. In case of inversion, the cord, as it leaves the placenta, is wound spirally to the right instead of the left. In males with situs inversus, the right testis usually is lower than the left.

REFERENCES

1. Cockayne, E. A.: The genetics of transposition of the viscera, Quart. J. Med. 7:479, 1938.
2. Torgersen, J.: Situs inversus, asymmetry and twinning, Am. J. Human Genet. 2:361, 1950.
3. Caplan, S. M.: Visceral transposition with dextrocardia; report of eight cases with review of literature of dextrocardia, U.S. Navy M. Bull. 46:1011, 1946.
4. Varano, N. R., and Merklin, R. J.: Situs inversus; review of the literature, report of four cases and analysis of the clinical implications, J. Internat. Coll. Surgeons 33:131, 1960.
5. Schmutzer, K. J., and Linde, L. M.: Situs inversus totalis associated with complex cardiovascular anomalies, Am. Heart J. 56:761, 1958.
6. Campbell, M.: The mode of inheritance in isolated laevocardia and dextrocardia and situs inversus, Brit. Heart J. 25:803, 1963.
7. Lowe, C. R., and McKeown, T.: An investigation of dextrocardia with and without transposition of abdominal viscera, with a report of a case in one monozygotic twin, Ann. Eugenics 18:267, 1954.
8. Brandt, H., and Revaz, C.: Jumelles univitellines et situs inversus, J. Génét. Hum. 7:33, 1958.
9. Schippan, R., Hunger, H., and Hammer, H-J.: Situs inversus totalis bei einem eineiigen Zwilling, Arch. Kinderh. 175:80, 1966.
10. Grebe, H.: Beitrag zur Ätiologie des Situs Inversus, Ztschr. menschl. Vererb.-u. Konstitutionslehre 28:262, 1944.
11. Siebner, H., and Flach, A.: Chromosome findings in Kartagener triad, Monatsschr. Kinderh. 112:465, 1964.
12. Schönfeld, E. A., and Frischman, B.: Syndrome of spleen agenesis, defects of the heart and vessels and situs inversus; report of a case suggesting heredity as an etiological factor, Helvet. paediat. acta 13:636, 1958.
13. Hummel, K. P., and Chapman, D. B.: Visceral inversion and associated anomalies in the mouse, J. Hered. 50:9, 1959.
14. Huxley, J. S., and DeBeer, G. R.: *The Elements of Experimental Embryology* (London: Cambridge University Press, 1934).
15. Wilson, J. G., Jordan, H. C., and Brent, R. L.: Effects of irradiation on embryonic development. II. X-rays on the ninth day of gestation in the rat, Am. J. Anat. 92:153, 1953.
16. Torgersen, J.: The triad of Kartagener; a contribution to its hereditary and developmental basis, Schweiz. med. Wchnschr. 82:770, 1952.
17. Ferencz, C.: Visceral heterotaxy with malformed heart. Similar findings in a child and a puppy, Anat. Rec. 149: 299, 1964.
18. Torgersen, J.: Transposition of viscera–bronchiectasis and nasal polyps; a genetical analysis and a contribution to the problem of constitution, Acta radiol. 28:17, 1947.
19. Bergstrom, W. H., Cook, C. C., Scannell, J. G., and Berenberg, W.: Situs inversus, bronchiectasis and sinusitis; report of a family with two cases of Kartagener's triad and two cases of bronchiectasis among six siblings, Pediatrics 6:573, 1950.
20. Kartagener, M., and Stucki, P.: Bronchiectasis with situs inversus, Arch. Pediat. 79:193, 1962.
21. Thompson, J. R.: Bronchogenic carcinoma complicating situs inversus totalis. Report of a case, Dis. Chest 44:317, 1963.
22. Merklin, R. J., and Varano, N. R.: Situs inversus and cardiac defects, J. Thoracic & Cardiovas. Surg. 45:334, 1963.
23. Balocco, A.: Agenesis of the lumbo-sacral segment of the vertebral column with situs viscerum inversus, Minerva pediat. 15:1482, 1963.
24. Ody, R., and Berger, H.: Bourneville-Pringle phakomatosis with situs inversus, bilateral double kidney and recurrent pneumothorax, Deutsche med. Wchnschr. 91:488, 1966.
25. Arenillas, L.: Tuberous sclerosis with situs inversus, J. Ment. Defic. Res. 12:108, 1968.
26. Verghese, A.: Albright's syndrome in the male with situs inversus, Proc. Roy. Soc. Med. 55:357, 1962.
27. De Pra, M.: Description of a case of mongolism with total situs viscerum inversus without congenital heart disease, Minerva pediat. 15:526, 1963.
28. Everett, H. C.: Situs inversus totalis: A survey of laterality and some observations on the frequency of mental disorder, Am. J. Psychiat. 119:884, 1963.
29. Arge, E.: Transposition of the viscera and sterility in men, Lancet 1:412, 1960.
30. Blegan, H. M.: Surgery in situs inversus, Ann. Surg. 129: 244, 1949.
31. Cleveland, M.: Situs inversus viscerum: An anatomic study, Arch. Surg. 13:342, 1926.

PART IV

Malformations of the Central Nervous System

SECTION ONE: Cerebrum and Cerebellum

22

Anencephaly

ANENCEPHALY is one of the most striking congenital malformations recognizable at birth. Although the condition is lethal before or soon after birth and does not contribute greatly to children's morbidity, it has always aroused great interest because of its obvious manifestations, the puzzles of pathogenesis, the questions of etiology and the geographic variability of incidence. As a congenital malformation that cannot be overlooked, it exemplifies the problems and difficulties of teratologic research in man. The terminology is confusing. I use the terms "anencephaly" for partial or total absence of the brain, "exencephaly" for exposure of the brain—a congenital defect of the calvarium—and "pseudencephaly" for massive "area cerebrovasculosa" imitating the shape of the brain that it replaces.

The incidence is approximately 1 per 1,000 deliveries in hospital wards, but remarkable variations have been reported from different areas. The highest incidence figures come from Ireland. In Belfast, 6.7 and 4.6 anencephalic births have been reported per 1,000 births,[1,2] in Dublin 5.0,[3] in Liverpool 3.2, in Birmingham 2.3 and in London 1.6. (In Birmingham, about 9% of the anencephalics also had spina bifida,[4] in France 17%.[5]) In Europe, incidence rates were averaging 1 per 1,000 births; in France, the over-all incidence was 0.5, with low values of 0.2 and 0.12 per 1,000 for Lyon.[1,5] In the province of Quebec in Canada, the rate was 1.45, but in the Jewish population it was only 0.3.[6] The hypothesis of a decreasing incidence from north to south was tested by Alter,[7] who ascertained rates of 1.5 in Halifax County, Nova Scotia, and 0.6 per 1,000 live births in Charleston County, South Carolina. There were many more Negroes in the Charleston population than in the Halifax population. But, even for the white populations, the incidence of anencephalic births was significantly higher in Halifax (1.6) than in Charleston (0.9). The incidence among the Negroes in Charleston was only 0.3 per 1,000 live births. Simpkiss and Lowe[8] did not encounter anencephaly in over 2,000 African newborn infants, but in Negroes of Nairobi, Kenya, the incidence was 1 per 1,000 births,[9] so that one cannot assume a low incidence in all Negro populations. In the state of Victoria, Australia, the incidence of all anencephalic births (live and still) was only 0.72 per 1,000 total births.[90] Penrose[1] computed a table derived from many countries showing variations that are completely unexplained at present. In a comparative study in 24 cities of 16 countries, Stevenson *et al.*[10] found a 40-fold difference in the frequency of anencephaly between the highest in Belfast and the lowest in Bogotá and Ljubljana (p. 40). Extensive frequency tables were published by Hamersma.[11] Neither geographic nor ethnic factors furnish satisfactory explanations for the rather constant local variations.

It has been found repeatedly that anencephalic births occurred more often in the autumn and winter than in the spring and summer. This was shown to be true for Birmingham, England, and Scotland by McKeown and Record[12] until 1958.[12a] More recent

Fig. 22-1.—Stillborn fetus with anencephaly. Delivered in thirtieth week of gestation, weighing 1,100 Gm. The area cerebrovasculosa is well developed (pseudencephaly). External ears are deformed. A distant relative had meningocele. (Cincinnati General Hospital No. 245725.)

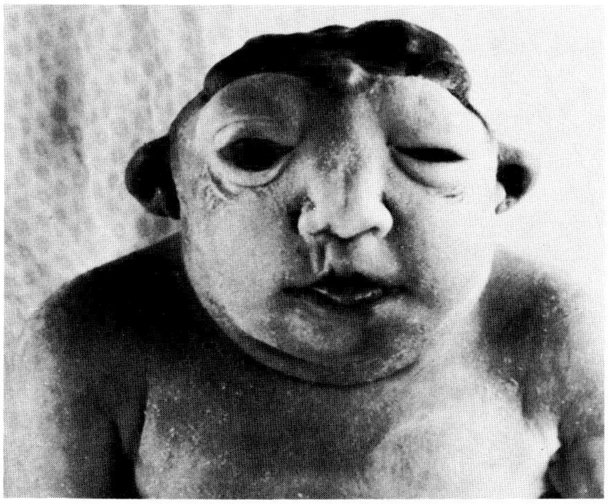

studies in England and in other countries failed to confirm these findings.[5,13]

Changes of incidences in certain years in Dublin were reported by Leck and Rogers.[91] There were peaks in 1940–1941 and 1960–1961, with 4 or 7 per 1,000 births affected. Unknown environmental changes were held responsible for the fluctuations.

Edwards[14] noted for Scotland a social class gradient in the incidence of stillbirths with anencephaly. Socioeconomic influences on development of anencephaly and spina bifida were also noted in Rotterdam by Hamersma.[11]

In some studies, maternal age and parity were found to be influential; it seemed that anencephalics were born more often to young primiparous women and to women over 40 years of age. It was difficult to separate age and parity factors.[14,15] In other investigations, there was no evidence of maternal age or parity.[11] A maternal factor was demonstrated in an unusual instance of anencephaly in 4 consecutive pregnancies.[16] The first 3 anencephalics were the offspring of a woman and her husband. After artificial insemination from a donor, who previously and subsequently had several normal children, the woman gave birth to a fourth anencephalic child.

The frequency of lethal outcome in previous or subsequent pregnancies of mothers who have given birth to children with anencephaly has been found to be increased over that in control groups.[15] But there have been exceptions to this rule.[11] Fetuses with anencephaly and related malformations can contribute to the raised abortion rate,[2] which could be due, therefore, to paternal as well as maternal influences.

A marked tendency to prematurity in anencephalic deliveries is well established, and hydramnios is observed in 30–50% of the cases.[10,17] The increased amount of amniotic fluid in such pregnancies has been explained by secretion of cerebrospinal fluid into the amniotic cavity, by lack of normal deglutition, by lack of absorption of amniotic fluid through the hypoplastic lungs and by excess urine production caused by a lack of antidiuretic hormone.[18] Hamersma[11] believed that anencephalic fetuses do not "drink" when there is a closure defect in the myelencephalon, but it seems that failure to swallow cannot explain all cases of polyhydramnios.[19] Observations in rats[20] revealed marked hydramnios in fetuses with exencephaly. Such animals often have an intact neurohypophysis and myelencephalon but show abundant choroid plexus floating in amniotic fluid. This supports the view that the hydramnios in such fetuses is due to cerebrospinal fluid excretion into the amniotic cavity.

Association of anencephaly with postmaturity has also been stressed.[11,21] Postmaturity may be connected with disturbed estrogen metabolism and normal progesterone production; it occurs often in patients without hydramnios.[11,84]

Women pregnant with anencephalics have low urinary estriol but normal pregnanediol excretion.[22,23] The reduced urinary values have been attributed to absence of the intermediary zone in the fetal adrenals. The placentas of anencephalics show changes of the epithelium of the villi and anomalies in the stroma.[22]

Some observations point to paternal influences. In a family recorded by Brooks Popham,[24] the father was married twice. With his first wife, he had one child with hydrocephaly and one with spina bifida; with a second wife, he had one child with hydrocephaly and one with anencephaly. There is a report of a family with repeated anencephaly in which a chromosomal anomaly was found in the father.[25]

It has long been known that there is a marked prevalence of females among anencephalic infants. The ratios reported vary.[11] In the world-wide study by Stevenson *et al.*,[10] two-thirds of the anencephalics (with and without spina bifida) were females. The "nuclear sex" (sex chromatin) of cells of female and male anencephalics was found concordant with the observed external sexual characteristics in each case.[26,27]

There is an increased incidence of anencephaly (and spina bifida) in siblings of anencephalics. Penrose[1] estimated the incidence in siblings to be 3% as opposed to 0.1% in the general population. Polman[28] and Milham[29] arrived at similar estimates. Masterson[15] combined published data and thought that after the birth of a child with anencephaly or spina bifida the risk of a malformation of the central nervous system in further pregnancies was about 4%; it may be 13% after the birth of two defective sibs. Similar figures were obtained in a study in South Wales.[86,87]

Recurrence of anencephaly and related malformations of the central nervous system in families or kinships can be attributed to genetic or to persistent environmental constellations. Dunn and Salter[30] recorded a pedigree in which a mother with spina bifida occulta had 2 sisters with spina bifida aperta; she gave birth to 2 anencephalic infants with spina bifida. These authors cited instances of 2, 3 and even 6 anencephalics occurring in the same sibship. In certain families or kinships, anencephaly, spina bifida, exencephaly and hydrocephaly may occur vicariously.[24,28,31-34] Polman[28] recorded findings in 30 families from 2 provinces of Holland in which anencephaly, exencephaly, hydrocephaly and spina bifida occurred with unusual frequency. Some of the families contained 3 or 4 affected children. Twenty-four of the 30 families were related. A genetic mechanism seemed to be responsible for these anomalies, but the mode of transmission could not be elucidated.

Chromosomal mechanisms have been considered in some instances. In a family,[25] there were 2 anencephalic births followed by a girl with marked intrauterine growth retardation, microcephaly, facial anomalies and spina bifida. The father showed a translocation manifested by one short and one extra-long chromosome of the 13-15 (D) group. Ellis and Penrose[35] described a pedigree in which anencephaly, spina

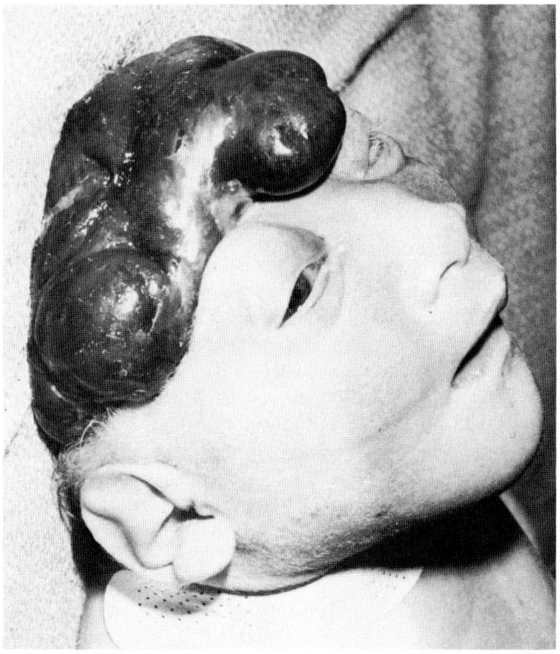

Fig. 22-2.—Female anencephalic infant with a normal 46,XX karyotype.

bifida, meningocele and other malformations occurred in two generations. In 3 unaffected surviving members (mother, son and grandson), an enlarged satellite on one of the large acrocentric chromosomes was detected in cell cultures. An anencephalic "male" with XX sex chromosome complement has been reported.[88]

Examination of chromosomes of anencephalic fetuses failed to reveal gross abnormalities.[5,15,27] We examined the chromosomes of a couple that had 2 anencephalic children and found their karyotypes to be normal. The blood groups of anencephalics and control series did not show significant differences in regard to rhesus or ABO blood groups.[36]

Observations in twins with anencephaly often are reported in the hope that they may contribute to the understanding of the etiology of the malformation. In dizygotic twins, one twin may be affected and the other spared[37]; or one male twin with hydrocephaly may be found in the same uterus with a female anencephalic[38]; or both twins—although dizygotic—may be anencephalic.

Monozygotic twins can be concordant[40-43] or discordant.[31,44-47] There also are reports of discordant twins who were monochorionic but diamniotic.[34,48] A large survey of 108 twin pairs showed that concordance is quite rare.[89]

Concordant anencephaly in conjoined twins has been recorded,[46] but Stevenson *et al.*[10] mentioned a pair of conjoined twins of whom only one had anencephaly. Observations in twins prove neither genetic nor environment hypotheses. In some cases, unfavorable local conditions, such as those associated with twinning, may be at fault. The exencephalic embryo described by Hunter[49] (p. 192) was the result of a tubal pregnancy.

Epidemiologic studies failed to provide a better understanding of the anomaly. They allow the blame to be placed on a "genotypic factor"[17] or on environmental factors.[10,50] Pleydell[51] found higher incidences of anencephaly in urban and industrial than in rural districts of Northamptonshire and suspected infectious causation. Toxoplasmosis[52] and rickettsia[53] have been considered as possible infective agents. Infectious factors were not considered of importance for anencephaly or spina bifida occurring twice in sibships.[54] One instance is on record of a young woman with tetralogy of Fallot who gave birth to 2 anencephalic premature children; after a Blalock operation, she delivered a normal child.[55] This case has been cited as proof that hypoxia was responsible for the anencephalics delivered before operation. But such a single case is not too convincing if one remembers that the risk for recurrence of anencephaly or spina bifida in pregnancies following the birth of two affected sibs is only 13%.[15] There is a single case of anencephaly on record in which the mother had taken aminopterin for therapeutic abortion.[92]

Penrose[1] summarized the facts and discussed the relative merits of the explanations available without arriving at definite conclusions. Although anencephalic infants seem similar to the observer, there is a definite possibility that a variety of etiologic factors lead to interference with the closure of the anterior neuropore and subsequently to anencephaly. Observations in animals[56] and experimental work (see below) demonstrate that exencephaly, the forerunner of anencephaly, can be caused by heterogeneous factors—genetic or environmental. If we are dealing with a symptom, the end result of various pathologic processes, general and simple explanations of the etiology often are deceptive.

Morphogenesis

The morphogenesis of anencephaly was difficult to understand, since the condition observed at birth is derived from an early malformation that is subjected to regressive changes in utero. It seemed futile to speculate about the shape and appearance of the forebrain structures that had long been destroyed by the time the child was born. But it is now generally recognized that some early *exencephalic* embryos that have been observed and described represent the forerunners of anencephalic monsters and that most anencephalics develop from the state of encephaloschisis. In anencephaly, the vault of the skull is always missing and it seems established that the forebrain anlage was abnormal and the anterior end of the neural tube not properly closed. Owing to the abnormal structure and vascularization of an exencephaly and possibly to the lack of protection by skull and skin, the neural tissue undergoes secondary degeneration until most of it is replaced by the spongy and vascular mass called the "area cerebrovasculosa." It is not rare to find remnants of an open medullary plate in the posterior cranial fossa while the anterior brain structures are absent. That such anterior structures were formed originally is indicated by the usual presence of normal eyes and optic nerves, which, by the time of birth, end blindly at the base of the skull. Formation of the eye requires the presence of a forebrain but it does not require the presence of a *normal* forebrain. This is proved by some human exencephalic embryos and also by experimental animals that show exencephaly and normal eyes (see Fig. 22-4, *A* and *C*). Hunter[49] described a human embryo of 35 mm. crown rump length, the product of a tubal pregnancy. This embryo had much-enlarged hemispheres that lay on top of a vaultless skull overhanging the eyes. Actually, the exposed brain was turned inside out, the visible surface representing the inner or ventricular wall, with the outer wall turned toward the face and joining the skin at the base of the skull. In the midline, the brain formed a deep trough and on each side there were prominences – the thalami. Although the margins of the anterior portion of the medullary plate apparently had rolled outward instead of inward at an early stage of development and the neural tube had remained unclosed, the optic cups and nerves were well developed. It is understandable that such an exposed brain undergoes degeneration and regression and that in its place connective tissue and blood vessels grow abundantly. In such everted brains, the choroid plexuses found on the surface of the open brain structures may secrete their product into the amniotic cavity and thus be responsible for the hydramnios in pregnancies resulting in anencephaly.[57] As will be described for spina bifida (p. 285), there also may be regenerative changes going hand in hand with the regressive changes in the neural tissues. From the border of skin and neural ectoderm, epithelium can extend over the remnants of the brain and the connective and vascular tissues, thus forming a sac that eventually encloses the area cerebrovasculosa (see Figs. 22-1 and 22-2). Vogel and McClenahan[58] pointed out that the destroyed parts of the brain are those normally supplied by the internal carotids, whereas the well-formed parts (eyes, brain stem and cervical cord) are supplied by the ophthalmic and vertebral arteries. It seemed possible to these authors that anencephaly might result from some alteration in the blood vessels. "Vascular starvation" was also considered but not accepted as the cause of anencephaly by Frazer,[59] who examined and reported an anencephalic embryo. In this embryo, the internal carotids abruptly came to an end with open mouths. It seemed that they had been torn, but they did not appear hypoplastic or aplastic. Frazer stated that "If we can judge from the remains of the carotid and vertebral systems, there was nothing wrong with these to account for the primary failure in development, but they have been secondarily affected as a result of the primary failure." It appears, therefore, that the anomalies of the internal carotids are the result but not the cause of the destruction that ends in anencephaly. Congenital anomalies in cephalobrachial vessels do occur in anencephalics, but this is not always the case.[42] They are to be considered associated malformations but not causative. Since the early reports of human embryos with exencephaly or encephaloschisis, many additional cases have been recorded. Politzer,[60] Wrete[61] and Dekaban[62] reviewed

Fig. 22-3. – Small exencephaly in rat produced by x-irradiation on the twelfth day of gestation. **A**, external appearance. **B**, frontal section through pituitary region.

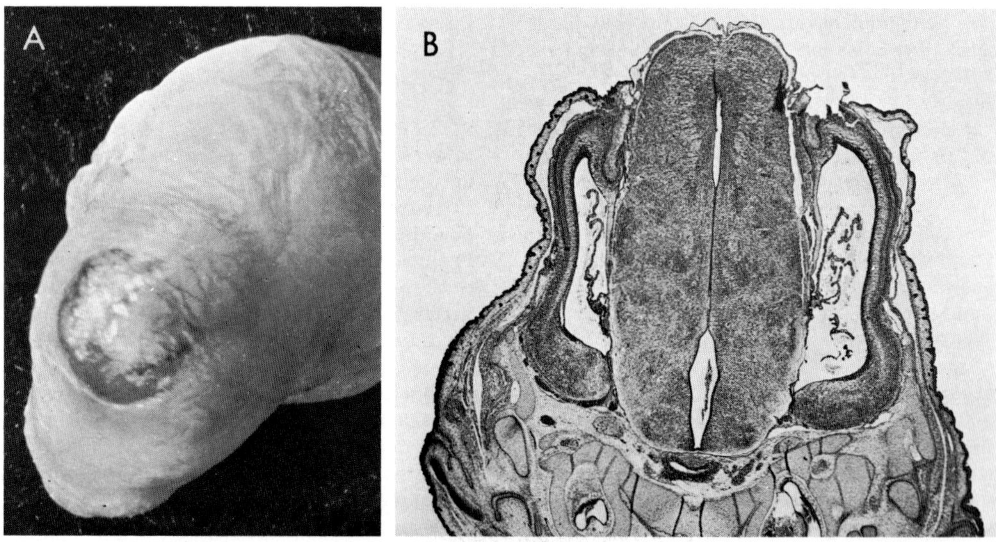

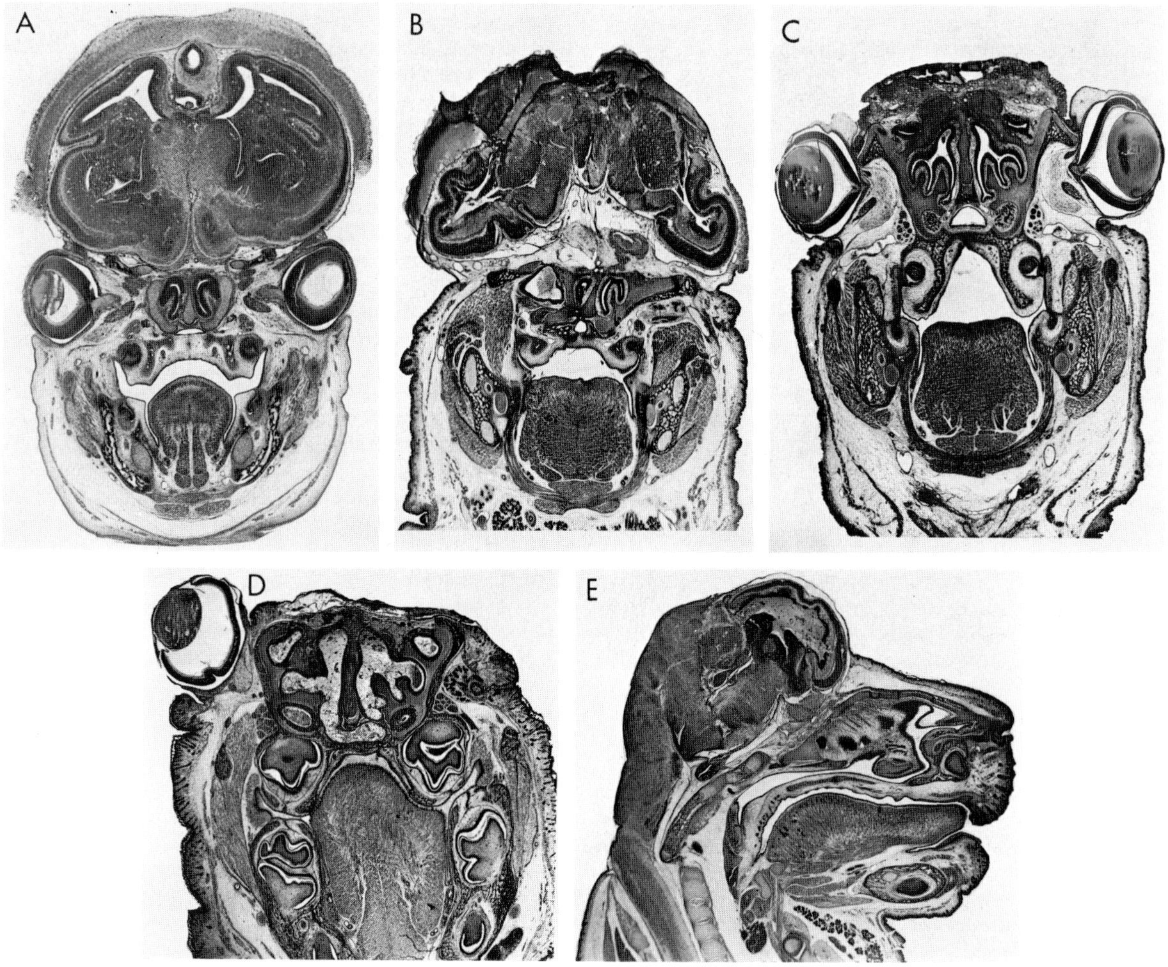

Fig. 22-4. – **A,** exencephaly in rat fetus. Section through eyes and optic nerves. The large exposed brain consists of hemispheres with abnormal ventricular system and structural anomalies. The uppermost layer consists of extroverted diencephalon. (Trypan blue injections from eighth to tenth day.) **B,** exencephaly with beginning destruction and removal of brain from skull base. (Hypervitaminosis A.) **C,** the brain has become reduced to a few remnants and angiomatous tissue but the eyes are well preserved. (Sodium salicylate on ninth day.) **D,** exencephaly has been converted into anencephaly. Right eye is still preserved, left eye microphthalmic. (Hypervitaminosis A.) **E,** sagittal section through exencephalic head. The abnormal brain and brain stem are exposed but spinal cord lies in spinal canal. (Trypan blue on eighth day.)

the literature that indicates that most anencephalics are the result of nonclosure of the neural tube. Overgrowth of brain tissue often is present in exencephalic embryos,[63] but this also is the result and not the cause of nonclosure. That disturbance in the axial cephalic mesoderm occurring before the closure of the anterior neuropore is the primary cause of anencephaly has been suggested often and is still maintained,[64] but evidence points to primary disturbance of the neural epithelium.[62] As in some other embryologic problems, ectoderm-mesoderm disputations are scholarly and enduring – but not fruitful.

Pathologic morphogenesis of exencephaly and anencephaly can be studied in rodents, which furnish genetically determined or experimentally produced models. Bonnevie[65] found exencephalic embryos in a stock of inbred mice and attributed the anomaly to a simple recessive gene. The description of the everted brain resting on a cranium without a bony roof and of the choroid plexuses on the surface of the brain closely resembles that of the Hunter[49] embryo. Similar exencephalies, but attributed to chromosomal translocations, occur in stocks originally derived from mice subjected to x-ray treatment.[66] Grüneberg[67] reviewed the work on hereditary exencephalies, which are by no means homogeneous genetically. In addition to hereditary forms, exencephalies can be produced experimentally in rodents as phenocopies by a variety of experimental procedures such as exposure of the mother during pregnancy to x-rays[68] (Fig. 22-3), trypan blue injections,[69] anoxia,[70] hypervitaminosis A,[20,71,94] salicylates[72] and many other teratogens. In

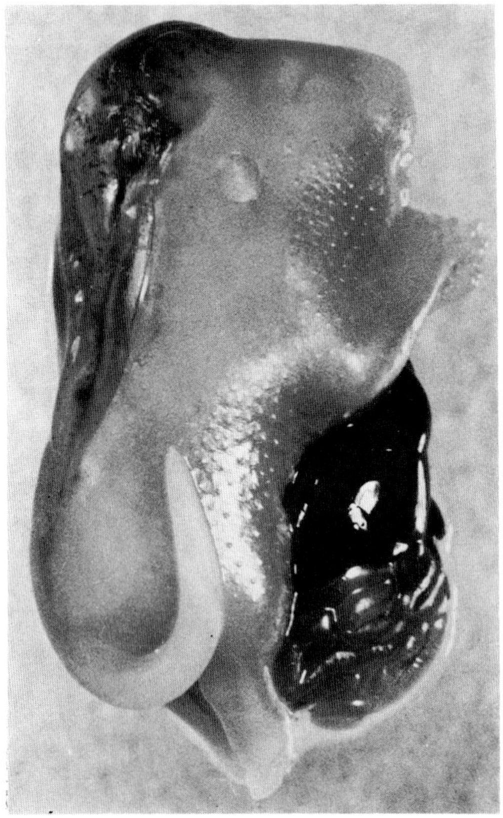

Fig. 22-5.—Craniorachischisis and exomphalos in rat fetus. (Treated with methyl salicylate on the tenth day of gestation.)

rodents, well-preserved exencephalic brains can be obtained because, in contrast to human fetuses, the embryos remain in utero for only a relatively short time after organogenesis is completed. Figure 22-4 illustrates various stages of near-term rat fetuses from exencephaly to anencephaly. In *A*, an overgrown exencephaly is in a good state of preservation. Although the brain is anatomically abnormal in many respects, the eyes appear normal. In *B*, the outline of an abnormal brain is still well preserved, but hemorrhagic areas are seen, and lifting of the brain from the base of the skull has begun. In *C*, few remnants of the brain are left, but the eyes have remained in good condition although they are not covered by lids. In *D*, the anencephalic state is almost complete. There is one protruding eye; the other eye is extremely microphthalmic. *E* shows, in a sagittal section, how the exposed brain lies on the base of the skull and continues into the spinal cord in the cervical region.

Development of exencephaly during embryogenesis has been described in great detail by Giroud and coworkers[20,73] in rats treated with hypervitaminosis A. Complete failure of the neural plate to close results in exencephaly combined with myeloschisis, a condition called "craniorachischisis." This monstrous malformation sometimes can be produced experimentally in rat embryos exposed to various teratogens. We have been most successful using salicylates.[72] Figure 22-5 shows the combination of craniorachischisis with exomphalos, a combination sometimes observed in human anencephalic fetuses. Figure 22-6 shows a series of embryos and fetuses with nonclosure of the neural tube.

Specimens obtained experimentally can also illustrate the effect of exencephaly of organs outside the central nervous system. Although the eye can be normal in exencephalic brains, it also may be damaged concomitantly by the teratogen. The anterior lobe of the pituitary may be rather normally formed in the presence of an exencephaly but, as the exposed brain is removed from the skull base and deteriorates, the pituitary stalk is stretched and torn, resulting in separation of the gland from the diencephalon (Fig. 22-7). The adrenals of such fetuses are somewhat reduced in size but differentiated into zona glomerulosa, fasciculata and reticularis. The thyroids and the gonads attain good differentiation also. It is only in rare exencephalic specimens that the anterior hypophysis is absent. Then the adrenals are markedly reduced in size and without zonation.[74]

Retention of the adenohypophysis in a persistent craniopharyngeal canal can also be illustrated by specimens obtained experimentally (Fig. 22-7, *C*). As in human fetuses, this anomaly is also seen in some rat fetuses with exencephaly.

The conditions of such experimental animals may not be identical to those of human exencephalic or anencephalic monsters, but they suggest certain possibilities for the pathogenesis of these malformations in man. It is likely that in infants, as in rodents, the malformations leading to anencephaly or exencephaly are not of a unitary origin. There may be cases that are genetically determined and cases that are due to nongenetic accidents. Ernst[75] believed that some cases of anencephaly could be derived from brains with closed neuropores, and there are some observations in animals that seem to support this view.[20] For human anencephalics, it is not advisable to assign a certain time or critical period to a supposed catastrophe or "cataclysm" that turns a developed brain into a disorganized area cerebrovasculosa. Such catastrophes have been assumed because the presence of eyes and optic nerves in the absence of hemispheres indicates clearly that the forebrain must have existed in early embryonic life before it underwent destruction. Thomas[76] assumed that the brain that results in anencephaly must develop normally, or nearly so, to the fifth or sixth week of gestation, since the ocular structures, offshoots of the anterior brain vesicle, are present and well formed in most anencephalics. Such reasoning is not justified, since observations of human and rodent brains show that extremely abnormal exencephalic brains destined to prenatal destruction can form eyes and optic nerves that can remain rather normal to the time of birth (see Fig. 22-1). The "de-

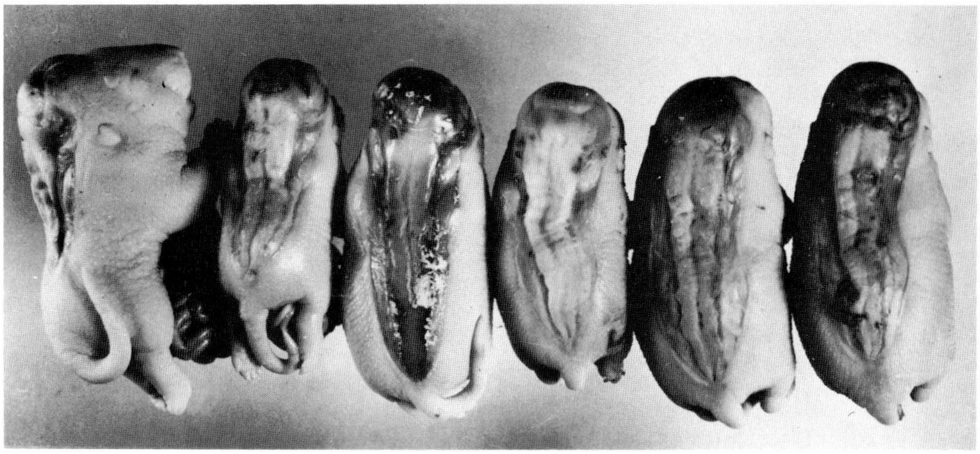

Fig. 22-6.—Craniorachischisis in 6 rat fetuses treated with methyl salicylate on the tenth day of gestation.

structive cataclysm" in the second month of gestation is actually relatively late and shows sequelae of the earlier failure of closure of the neural plate. It is possible that environmental events within the first month can prevent closure of the anterior end of the neural plate, but in the case of genetic causation, such arrest of development of the neural plate can occur without any environmental disturbance during teratogenesis. In most cases, if not in all, anencephaly is determined before the time of closure of the anterior neuropore, which takes place in age group XI of Streeter,[77] in embryos of about 24 days to 26 days of gestation. A possible causal connection with anencephaly of teratogenic events occurring in later gestational stages should be examined critically and with skepticism.

The Malformations

The extreme forms of cranioschisis are accompanied by complete or partial absence of the brain—anencephaly. When the brain is completely absent, one speaks of *holo-anencephaly* (see Fig. 22-10, *A*); when the cranium and the brain are present in rudimentary form, the term *mero-anencephaly* (Fig. 22-8) may be used.[75] Holo-anencephaly frequently is combined with spinal clefts (craniorachischisis) (Fig. 22-9). In a case of complete anencephaly, the cranial vault is entirely absent (Fig. 22-10). The frontal bone and the parietal and occipital squamae are rudimentary. The occipital foramen is open posteriorly. The base of the skull is reduced in all dimensions, the anterior and middle fossae being absent or small. The pyramides of the temporal bones are short and placed transversely. The corpus of the sphenoid bone is short and reduced in the transverse diameter,[64] the alae rudimentary, the sella turcica shallow or absent and the craniopharyngeal canal may be open. Those bones that are present are thick and compact. The foramina of the cranial nerves are relatively well formed. The orbital apertures, set far apart, are turned outward and the orbital fossae are shallow, resulting in the typical protrusion of the eyeballs. The eyes show relatively normal structure, but in the retinas the arrangements of the nerve cells may be irregular. The eyelids and orbital muscles usually are well developed. The nose is plump and the tongue large. Cleft palate often is present.[78] In some instances, the formation of the palate is irregular, showing deep grooves on both sides of the raphe without communication of the nasal and oral cavities (see Fig. 22-10, *B*).

The spine shows abnormal curvatures and often cleft formations (Fig. 22-11). The lordosis of the cervical spine may be so marked that its upper part runs parallel to the base of the skull. As a result, the neck is short and the face turned upward (see Iniencephaly, Chapter 27). The vertebral bodies often are irregular in shape, resulting in abnormal lordosis, kyphosis and scoliosis.[79] In craniorachischisis, not only the cranium but also the vertebrae are dorsally open.

In complete anencephaly, the base of the skull is covered by a spongy and vascular mass—the area cerebrovasculosa. This area may be represented by a thin membrane or by a large pseudencephalic mass that sometimes simulates the shape of the brain, showing imitations of irregular gyri and sulci (Fig. 22-2). It consists of connective tissue, abundant collagen, blood channels, blood-filled cavities, cysts, nodes of glia, irregular choroid plexuses and many hemorrhages. Its cover is a thin and transparent layer of partly keratinized cuboidal epithelium that merges with the normal skin on the margins of the area. However, in some of the cases, remnants of flattened, open medullary plates are found in the posterior fossa. The cranial nerves often are present, but they are rudimentary and end blindly in the area cerebrovasculosa. The peripheral nervous system can be well developed.

The spinal cord usually is thin and underdeveloped

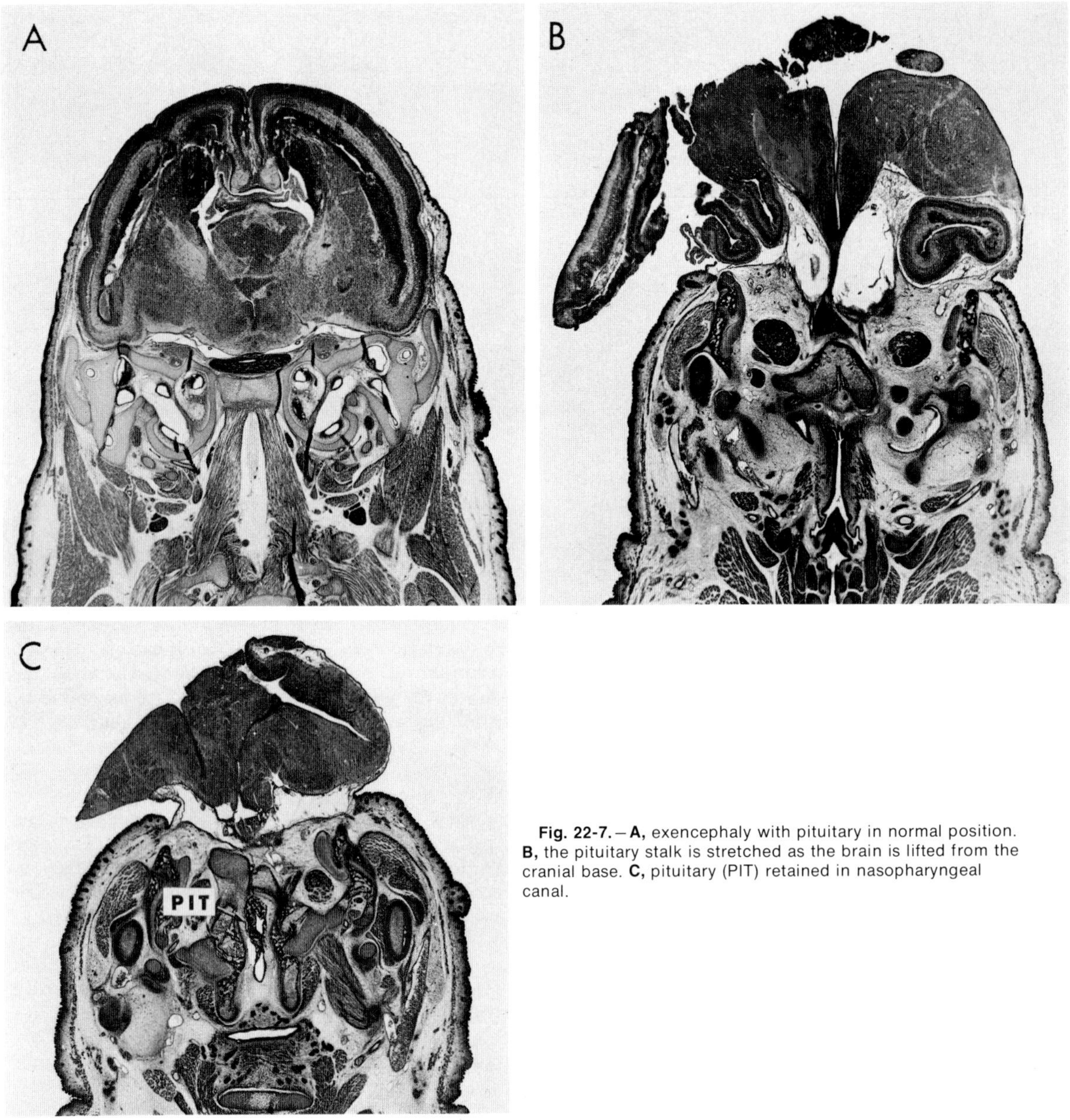

Fig. 22-7. – **A,** exencephaly with pituitary in normal position. **B,** the pituitary stalk is stretched as the brain is lifted from the cranial base. **C,** pituitary (PIT) retained in nasopharyngeal canal.

(micromyelia). The white substance is more reduced than the gray and the lateral fascicles are more affected than the anterior and posterior columns. The central canal may be irregularly shaped, showing syringomyelia or duplications of the canal. The gray matter is characterized by defects of the nerve cells and increased glia formation. The dura is markedly thickened and the pia highly vascularized.

The pituitary often is abnormal, but it seems that the anterior lobe can always be found. Shape and size of the adenohypophysis are variable, particularly when the gland is retained at the roof of the pharynx or in an open craniopharyngeal canal. The vascular channels often are greatly distended and the parenchymal cells appear compressed.[46,80] Absence or reduction in size of the neurohypophysis is common. In human anencephalics, one sees the end results of a complicated process of faulty anlage and of secondary destruction, whereas in experimental specimens the process can be observed in early stages[74] (see Fig. 22-7). Ultrastructural changes in the pars intermedia[93] have been attributed to lack of inhibitory stimuli from

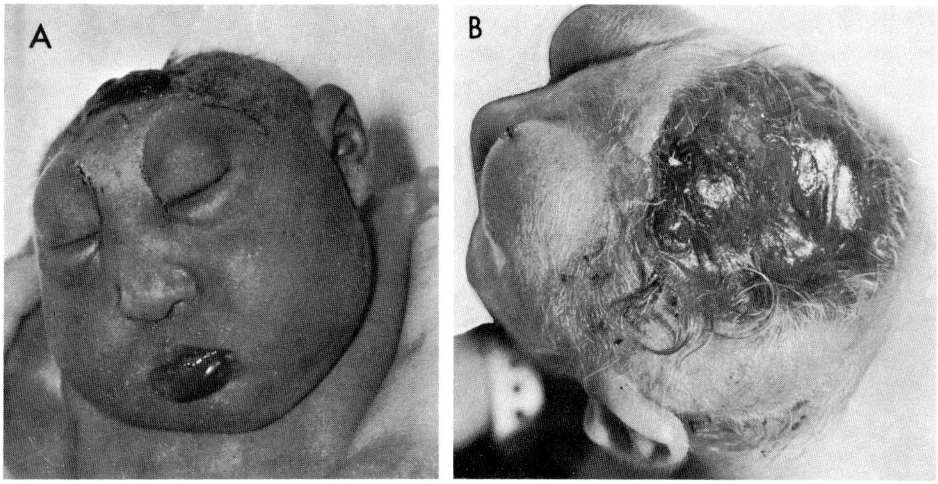

Fig. 22-8.—Mero-anencephaly. The skull and brain are rudimentary.

Fig. 22-9.—**A,** craniorachischisis in a child. (From E. L. Potter, *Pathology of the Fetus and Infant* [2d ed.; Chicago: Year Book Medical Publishers, Inc., 1961].) **B,** craniorachischisis in a 21-day rat fetus (mother treated with methyl salicylate). (From J. Warkany and E. Takacs.[72])

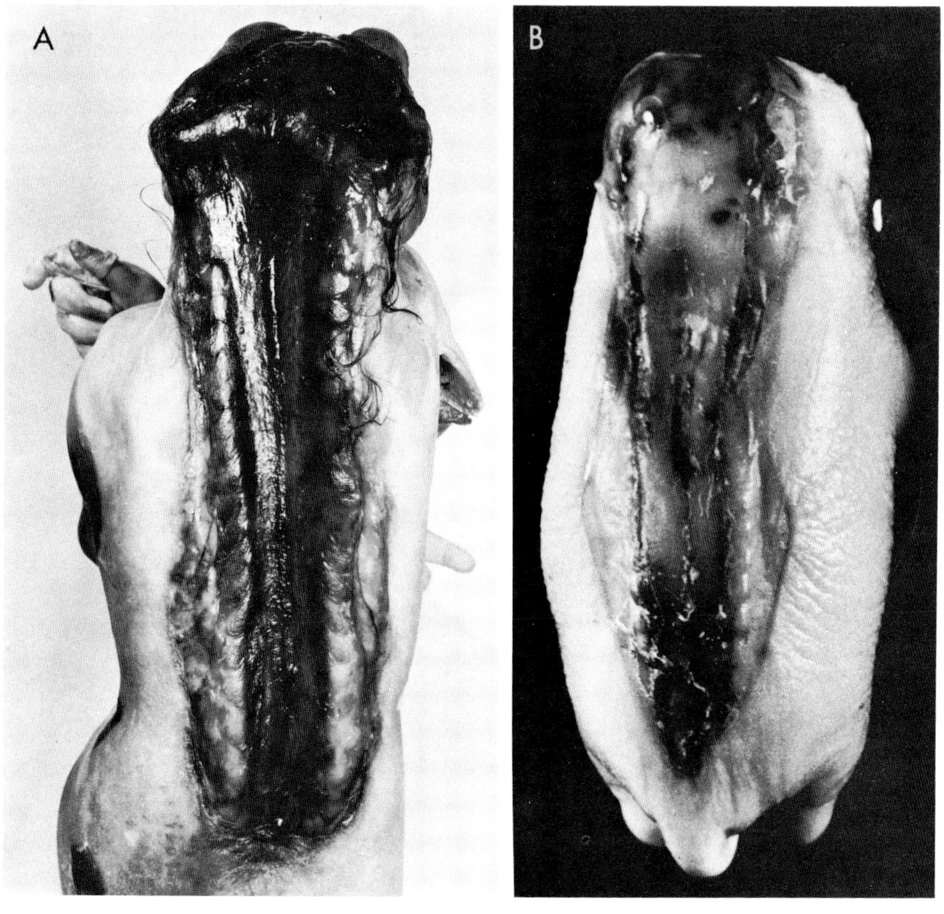

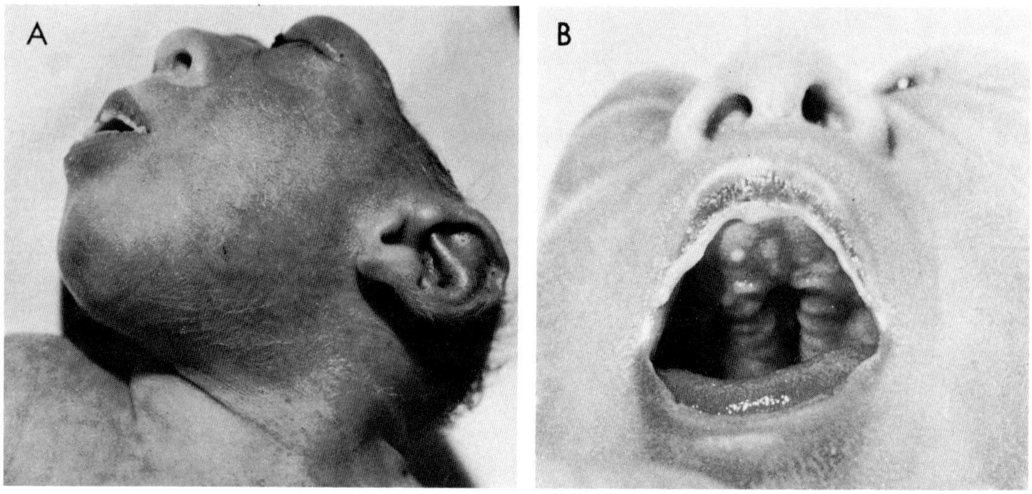

Fig. 22-10.—**A,** anencephaly with complete absence of calvarium and brain. There was only disorganized glial tissue with foci of neurons over the base of the skull. The spinal cord was hypoplastic. **B,** the palate is rather characteristic of anencephaly. Although it looks cleft, there was no communication between oral and nasal cavities. No associated congenital malformations. (Cincinnati Children's Hospital No. 159251.)

the hypothalamus. The thyroid glands show normal size and structure[81] but the adrenals are much reduced in size and resemble miniature adult glands since they lack the fetal zone. They often weigh less than 1 Gm. combined at the time of birth and sometimes they are hard to find. Study of human and rodent fetuses with exencephaly indicate that the adrenal anlage is normal[46,57] but that the glands deteriorate when the hypophysis loses contact with the diencephalon as the exencephalic brain is lifted from the cranial base and converted into area cerebrovasculosa. It is thought that secretion of corticotropic hormone ceases when the neurohypophysis fails to receive neurosecretory material from the diencephalon. But stimulation of the thyroid continues, since athyrotropic hormone production is independent of hypothalamic stimulation or releasing factor.[81]

In the milder *mero-anencephaly*, the skull is partly formed, but there is a median defect through which the area cerebrovasculosa protrudes. The occipital foramen is formed completely and rudiments of the rhombencephalon and mesencephalon can be found.

In the severest forms, *craniorachischisis*, the area cerebrovasculosa and the area medullovasculosa fill the skeletal defects of the cranium and of the spinal column (see Fig. 22-9). The neck is short, the face turned upward and the ears may touch the shoulders.

The viscera and the extremities may be well developed but the lungs often are hypoplastic. Occasionally, brain tissue has been found growing in the lungs. It is thought that brain cells from deteriorating brain are aspirated into the lungs together with amniotic fluid. Hyperplasia of the thymus has been reported.[46] Associated malformations are cleft lip and palate, cyclopia, syndactyly, absence of radius and thumb, clubfoot, exomphalos, imperforate anus, her-

Fig. 22-11.—Mero-anencephaly and thoracolumbar myeloschisis. The protruding area cerebrovasculosa was relatively small and contained glia, few neurons and vascular tissues. The adrenals weighed 0.9 Gm. together and the zones were poorly defined. (Cincinnati Children's Hospital No. 129400.)

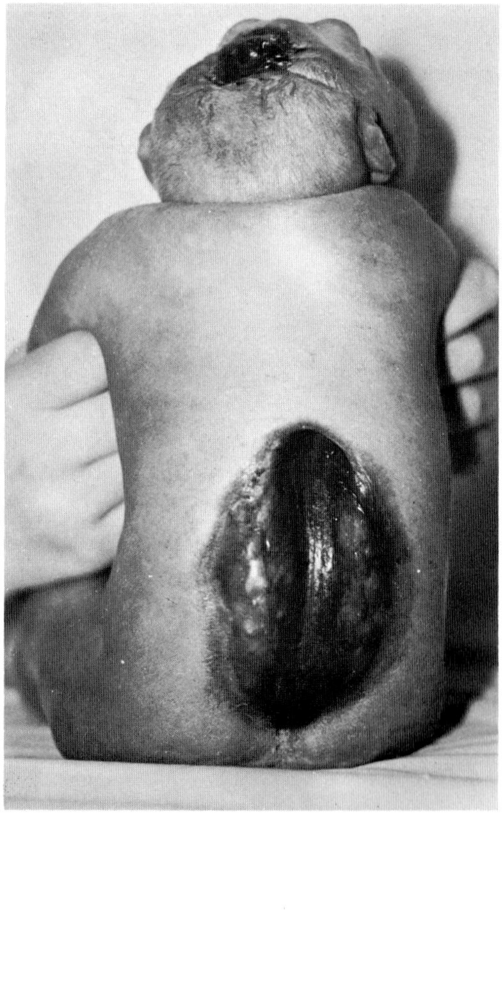

nias or renal and cardiac anomalies, but no definite pattern of the associated defects can be established.[84] Spina bifidas are closely related anomalies that often are combined with anencephaly. Dermatoglyphics have been examined by Hilman.[83] Most anencephalics are stillborn or they live only a few hours or days. Survival for 4 and even 16 days has been reported in exceptional cases.[84]

Monnier and Willi[85] made neurophysiologic studies in infants with partial anencephaly who survived birth. In infants lacking telencephalon, diencephalon, mesencephalon and the rostral portion of the rhombencephalon, the caudal rhombencephalon, medulla oblongata and spinal cord represent the central nervous system. Such infants are limited to primitive functions necessary to life, such as respiration and deglutition. Defense reactions are present, and the threshold of stimulation is reduced. The performances of these rhombencephalic or myelencephalic infants are immature and comparable in their motor actions to human fetuses of 3 or 4 months' gestation. Partial anencephalics do not have the rigidity and hypertonia of decerebrated organisms.

REFERENCES

1. Penrose, L. S.: Genetics of anencephaly, J. Ment. Defic. Res. 1:4, 1957.
2. Stevenson, A. C., and Warnock, H. A.: Observations on the results of pregnancies in women resident in Belfast. 1. Data relating to all pregnancies ending in 1957, Ann. Human Genet. 23:382, 1959.
3. Coffey, V. P., and Jessop, W. J. E.: Congenital abnormalities, Irish J. M. Sc. 344:30, 1955.
4. Record, R. G., and McKeown, T.: Congenital malformations of the central nervous system. 1. A survey of 930 cases, Brit. J. Social Med. 3:183, 1949.
5. Frézal, J., Kelley, J., Guillemot, M. L., and Lamy, M.: Anencephaly in France, Am. J. Human Genet. 16:336, 1964.
6. McDonald, A. D.: Anencephaly and spina bifida in Quebec, Seventh Annual Meeting, The Teratology Society, 1967.
7. Alter, M.: Anencephalic births in a northern and a southern community, Am. J. Dis. Child. 106:536, 1963.
8. Simpkiss, M., and Lowe, A.: Congenital abnormalities in the African newborn, Arch. Dis. Childhood 36:404, 1961.
9. Khan, A. A.: Congenital malformations in African neonates, J. Trop. Med. 68:272, 1965.
10. Stevenson, A. C., Johnston, H. A., Stewart, M. I. P., and Golding, D. R.: Congenital malformations. A report of a study of series of consecutive births in 24 centres, Bull. World Health Organ., supp. to vol. 34, p. 1, 1966.
11. Hamersma, K.: *Anencephalie en spina bifida* (Apeldoorn, The Netherlands: Drukkerij Romijn, 1966).
12. McKeown, T., and Record, R. G.: Seasonal incidence of congenital malformations of the central nervous system, Lancet 1:192, 1951.

12a. Record, R. G.: Anencephalus in Scotland, Brit. J. Prev. & Social Med. 15:93, 1961.

13. Leck, I., and Record, R. G.: Seasonal incidence of anencephalus, Brit. J. Prev. & Social Med. 20:67, 1966.
14. Edwards, J. H.: Congenital malformations of the central nervous system in Scotland, Brit. J. Prev. & Social Med. 12:115, 1958.
15. Masterson, J. G.: Empiric risk, genetic counseling and preventive measures in anencephaly, Acta Genet. 12:219, 1962.
16. Horne, H. W.: Anencephaly in four consecutive pregnancies, Fertil. & Steril. 9:67, 1958.
17. Böök, J. A., and Rayner, S.: A clinical and genetical study of anencephaly, Am. J. Human Genet. 2:61, 1950.
18. Benirschke, K., and McKay, D. G.: The antidiuretic hormone in fetus and infant, Obst. & Gynec. 1:638, 1953.
19. Nichols, J., and Schrepfer, R.: Polyhydramnios in anencephaly, J.A.M.A. 197:549, 1966.
20. Giroud, A., and Martinet, M.: Production d'un excès de liquide amniotique dans l'anencéphalie, Compt. rend. Soc. biol. 149:452, 1955.
21. Sarma, V.: Anencephalus of the fetus in obstetric practice, Clin. Obst. & Gynec. 6:429, 1963.
22. ten Berge, B. S.: The placenta in anencephali, Gynaecologia 159:359, 1965.
23. Frandsen, V. A., and Stakemann, G.: The side of production of oestrogenic hormones in human pregnancy. III, Acta endocrinol. 47:265, 1964.
24. Brooks Popham, R.: Two cases of anencephaly, Lancet 1: 1829, 1906.
25. de Grouchy, J., Brissaud, H. E., Repessé, G., and Lamy, M.: Anencéphalie familiale et remaniement de deux chromosomes 13-15, Compt. rend. Acad. Sc. (Paris) 258: 691, 1964.
26. Perrin, E. V., and Benirschke, K.: Somatic sex of anencephalic infants, J. Clin. Endocrinol. 18:327, 1958.
27. Harnden, D. G., Briggs, J. H., and Stewart, J. S. S.: Nuclear chromatin of anencephalic foetuses, Lancet 2:126, 1959.
28. Polman, A.: Anencephaly, spina bifida, and hydrocephaly, Genetica 25:29, 1950.
29. Milham, S., Jr.: Increased incidence of anencephalus and spina bifida in siblings of affected cases, Science 138: 593, 1962.
30. Dunn, H. G., and Salter, J. G.: Recurrent anencephaly; case report with note on etiology of anencephaly and allied malformations, J. Obst. & Gynaec. Brit. Emp. 51:529, 1944.
31. Grebe, H.: Eineiige Zwillinge mit diskordanter Anenzephalie, Virchows Arch. path. Anat. 316:116, 1949.
32. Murphy, D. P.: *Congenital Malformations. A Study of Parental Characteristics with Special Reference to the Reproductive Process* (2d ed.; Philadelphia: J. B. Lippincott Company, 1947).
33. Spreng, D. S.: Fetal maldevelopment recurring in mother and four daughters, Ohio M. J. 34:520, 1937.
34. Dumoulin, J. G., and Gordon, M. E.: Anencephaly in twins, J. Obst. & Gynaec. Brit. Emp. 66:964, 1959.
35. Ellis, J. R., and Penrose, L. S.: Enlarged satellites and multiple malformations in the same pedigree, Ann. Human Genet. 25:159, 1961.
36. Smithells, R. W., Chinn, E. R., and Franklin, D.: Anencephaly in Liverpool, Developmental Med. & Child Neurol. 6:231, 1964.
37. Gedda, L., and Gentili, F.: Anencefalia di un gemello dizigotico diagnosticata in utero, Analecta Genetica Monograph 6, pp. 163–172, in Genetica della Tubercolosi e dei Tumori, Simposio Internazionale, Turin, 1957.
38. Symonds, E. M.: Anencephaly and hydrocephaly in a twin pregnancy, Obst. & Gynec. 26:414, 1965.
39. Lewis, L.: A case of twin anencephalic pregnancy, Brit. M. J. 1:1500, 1960.
40. Josephson, J. E., and Waller, K. B.: Anencephaly in identical twins, Canad. M.A.J. 29:34, 1933.
41. Lin, R-K., and Plenk, H. P.: Anencephaly in twins – diagnosed ante partum by roentgen examination, Am. J. Roentgenol. 73:219, 1955.
42. Epstein, B. S., and Kolker, P.: Congenital variations in cephalobrachial vessels in anencephaly, Am. J. Roentgenol. 93:339, 1965.
43. DeHaan, Q. C.: Monozygotic anencephalic twins, Obst. & Gynec. 28:559, 1966.
44. Litt, S., and Strauss, H. A.: Monoamniotic twins, one normal, the other anencephalic; multiple true knots in

the cords, Am. J. Obst. 30:728, 1935.
45. Wilson, J. K.: Mono-amniotic multiple pregnancy; a report of 5 new cases, J. Obst. & Gynaec. Brit. Emp. 62:605, 1955.
46. Potter, E. L.: *Pathology of the Fetus and Infant* (2d ed.; Chicago: Year Book Medical Publishers, Inc., 1961).
47. Pedlow, P. R. B.: Anencephaly in a mono-amniotic twin, Brit. M. J. 2:997, 1961.
48. deSa', D. J., Strong, S. J., and Corney, G.: Anencephaly in one of monozygous twins, Biol. Neonat. 7:328, 1964.
49. Hunter, R. H.: Extroversion of the cerebral hemispheres in a human embryo, J. Anat. 69:82, 1934.
50. Ingalls, T. H., Pugh, T. F., and MacMahon, B.: Incidence of anencephalus, spina bifida, and hydrocephalus related to birth rank and maternal age, Brit. J. Prev. & Social Med. 8:17, 1954.
51. Pleydell, M. J.: Anencephaly and other congenital abnormalities; an epidemiological study in Northamptonshire, Brit. M. J. 1:309, 1960.
52. de Morsier, G., and Bammater, F.: Études sur les dysraphies cranio-cérébrales, Rev. neurol. 103:513, 1960.
53. Giroud, P., and Giroud, A.: Anencéphalie et rickettsioses maladies inapparentes, Bull. Acad. nat. méd. 148:621, 1964.
54. Milham, S.: Random distribution of affected birth ranks in anencephalic and spina bifida sibships with two affected cases, Nature, London 200:480, 1963.
55. Olim, C. B., and Turner, H. B.: Anencephaly in fetuses of mother with tetralogy of Fallot, J.A.M.A. 149:932, 1952.
56. Kalter, H.: *Teratology of the Central Nervous System in Laboratory and Domestic Mammals* (Chicago: The University of Chicago Press, 1968).
57. Angevine, D. M.: Pathologic anatomy of hypophysis and adrenals in anencephaly, Arch. Path. 26:507, 1938.
58. Vogel, F. S., and McClenahan, J.: Anomalies of major cerebral arteries associated with congenital malformations of the brain, Am. J. Path. 28:701, 1952.
59. Frazer, J. E.: Report on an anencephalic embryo, J. Anat. 56:12, 1921.
60. Politzer, G.: Über frühembryonale Encephalomyeloschisis beim Menschen, Wien. Ztschr. Nervenh. 5:1, 1952.
61. Wrete, M.: Über die Kenntnis des abnormen Offenstehens des Neuralrohres bei menschlichen Embryonen und jungen Feten, Beitr. path. Anat. 121:329, 1959.
62. Dekaban, A. S.: Anencephaly in early human embryos, J. Neuropath. & Exper. Neurol. 22:533, 1963.
63. Patten, B. M.: Overgrowth of the neural tube in young human embryos, Anat. Rec. 113:381, 1952.
64. Marin-Padilla, M.: Study of the sphenoid bone in human cranioschisis and craniorachischisis, Virchows Arch. path. Anat. 339:245, 1965.
65. Bonnevie, K.: Pseudencephalie als spontane recessive (?) Mutation bei der Hausmaus, Skr. Norske Vidensk.-Akad. Kl. 1, No. 9, pp. 39, 1936.
66. Snell, G. D.: Induction by roentgen rays of hereditary changes in mice, Radiology 36:189, 1941.
67. Grüneberg, H.: *The Genetics of the Mouse* (The Hague: Martinus Nijhoff, 1952).
68. Kaven, A.: Das Auftreten von Gehirnmissbildungen nach Roentgenbestrahlung von Mäuseembryonen, Ztschr. menschl. Vererb.-u. Konstitutionslehre 22:247, 1938.
69. Gillman, J., Gilbert, C., and Gillman, T.: A preliminary report on hydrocephalus, spina bifida and other congenital anomalies in the rat produced by trypan blue, South African J. M. Sc. 13:47, 1948.
70. Ingalls, T. H., Curley, F. J., and Prindle, R. A.: Experimental production of congenital anomalies, New England J. Med. 247:758, 1952.
71. Cohlan, S. Q.: Congenital anomalies in the rat produced by excessive intake of vitamin A during pregnancy, Pediatrics 13:556, 1954.
72. Warkany, J., and Takacs, E.: Experimental production of congenital malformations in rats by salicylate poisoning, Am. J. Path. 35:315, 1959.
73. Giroud, A., Delmas, A., and Martinet, M.: Étude morphogénétique sur des embryons anencéphales, Arch. Anat. (Strasb.) 42:203, 1959.
74. Warkany, J., and Takacs, E.: Changes of endocrine glands produced by teratogenic methods. The pituitary gland, Arch. Path. 85:101, 1968.
75. Ernst, P.: Missbildungen des Nervensystems, in Schwalbe, E. (ed.), *Die Morphologie der Missbildungen des Menschen und der Tiere* (Jena: Gustav Fischer, 1909), Vol. 3, pt. 2, pp. 67–252.
76. Thomas, A.: L'anencéphalie est-elle primitive ou secondaire?, Presse méd. 58 (Pt. 2): 1425, 1950.
77. Streeter, G.: *Developmental Horizons in Human Embryos* (Washington, D. C.: Carnegie Institution, 1951).
78. Roches, P.: Zur Frage der Anenkephalie; Präparation von 9 Fällen des Pathologischen Institutes, Inaugural Dissertation (Basel: Birkhauser, 1951).
79. Dziallas, P.: Ein Fetus von 18 mm Sitzhöhe mit Anencephalie und Amyelie, Gegenbaur. Morph. Jahrb. 103:662, 1962.
80. Kohn, A.: Anencephalie und Nebenniere, Arch. mikr. Anat. u. Entwicklungsmechanik 102:113, 1924.
81. Tuchmann-Duplessis, H.: Thyroïde et corrélations hypophysothyroïdiennes chez l'anencéphale humain, Ann. endocrinol. 20:569, 1959.
82. Jost, A.: Anterior Pituitary Function in Foetal Life, in Harris, G. W., and Donovan, B. T. (eds.), *The Pituitary Gland* (London: Butterworth & Co., Ltd., 1966), pp. 299–323.
83. Hilman, B. C.: Dermatoglyphics of anencephalic monsters, Anat. Rec. 116:295, 1953.
84. Ballantyne, J. W.: *Manual of Antenatal Pathology and Hygiene. The Embryo* (Edinburgh: William Green & Sons, 1904).
85. Monnier, M., and Willi, H.: Die integrative Tätigkeit des Nervensystems beim normalen Säugling und beim bulbospinalen Anencephalen (Rautenhirnwesen), Ann. paediat. 169:289, 1947.
86. Laurence, K. M., Carter, C. O., and David, P. A.: Major central nervous system malformations in South Wales. 1. Incidence, local variations and geographical factors, Brit. J. Prev. & Social Med. 22:146, 1968.
87. Carter, C. O., David, P. A., and Laurence, K. M.: A family study of major central nervous system malformations in South Wales, J. M. Genetics 5:81, 1968.
88. Arias-Bernal, L., and Jones, H. W., Jr.: An anencephalic male with XX sex chromosome complement, Am. J. Obst. & Gynec. 99:877, 1967.
89. Yen, S., and McMahon, B.: Genetics of anencephaly and spina bifida, Lancet 2:623, 1968.
90. Collmann, R. D., and Stoller, A.: The occurrence of anencephalus in the state of Victoria, Australia, J. Ment. Defic. Res. 12:22, 1968.
91. Leck, I., and Rogers, S. C.: Changes in the incidence of anencephalus, Brit. J. Prev. & Social Med. 21:177, 1967.
92. Thiersch, J. B.: The control of reproduction in rats with the aid of antimetabolites, and, Early experiences with antimetabolites as abortifacient agents in man, Acta endocrinol. (supp.) 28:37, 1956.
93. Salazar, H., MacAulay, M. A., and Pardo, M.: The human hypophysis in anencephaly, Arch. Path. 88:377, 1969.
94. Marin-Padilla, M.: Morphogenesis of anencephaly and related malformations, Curr. Top. Path. 51:145, 1970.

23

Cyclopia-Arhinencephaly Series

THERE EXISTS a group of malformations of the brain and face that is characterized by defects of midline structures of the head ranging from cyclopia through arhinencephaly and trigonocephaly to near-normal states. Cyclopia is a monstrosity that combines lack of separation of the eyes with lack of cleavage of the prosencephalon. The arhinencephalies were defined and classified by Kundrat[1] in 1882. They can occur as isolated anomalies or be associated with other developmental defects. The term "arhinencephaly," implying agenesis of the rhinencephalon, has been criticized by Yakovlev[2] because the praepiriform and hippocampal formations of the rhinic lobe of the telencephalon, although hypoplastic and dystopic, are always present. In addition to absence of the olfactory bulbs and tracts, there may be failure of cleavage of the cerebral hemispheres. The resulting undivided telencephalon with a single ventricular cavity was called a "holosphere"[2] in contrast to the normal hemispheres with symmetrical lateral ventricles. The terms "holotelencephaly"[2] and "holoprosencephaly"[3] are less fortunate, since "holo" signifies not only "whole" or "entire" but also "perfect" (as in "holosymmetry"), a meaning certainly not applicable to the brains with an undivided telencephalon. To replace the name "arhinencephaly" with the cumbersome "alobar holoprosencephaly" or "semilobar holoprosencephaly"[3] cannot be recommended. "Arhinencephaly," like "achondroplasia," may not be an entirely correct term but it is an expression widely accepted and useful if the variability of the rhinencephalic lesions is kept in mind.

The arhinencephalies always involve the nervous system, whereas defects of the nasal apparatus may not be present.[4] Accordingly, arhinencephaly comprises not only the cyclencephalies (cyclopia, ethmocephaly and cebocephaly) but also milder forms without external malformations. Ernst[4] believed the establishment of this group to be of great importance because it represented an excellent example of a morphologic series of malformations. To us, the series is equally important because it demonstrates that morphologically related malformations may be quite heterogeneous etiologically (p. 45). The finding of frequent association of trisomy 13-15 (D_1) with arhinencephaly[5] seemed to supply a cytogenetic basis for these midline defects, but the association is not constant. There are examples of severe arhinencephalies with normal karyotype[6-9] (see Fig. 23-6) and there are examples of trisomy 13-15 without arhinencephaly.[10-12] It is true that a case of cebocephaly reported as karyotypically normal[13] was subsequently found to have deletion of the short arms of a chromosome 18 and that a similar deficiency involving the short arm of a chromosome 18 has been seen in children with cyclopia or with arhinencephaly,[21] but it would be unwise to assume that hidden chromosomal anomalies are responsible for all arhinencephalies. Even in cyclopia, cytogenetic findings are not uniform (p. 203) and the possibility of nongenetic phenocopies must be considered (p. 205). In 32 necropsies of infants with trisomy 13-15, arhinencephaly was noted 25 times.[14] The extent of the anomalies of the olfactory system and of other brain defects varied greatly.[15] It has been suggested[8] that arhinencephalies without extracephalic malformations have normal karyotypes, whereas those combined with polydactyly or cardiac, intestinal and other extracephalic manifestations are associated with trisomy 13-15. This concept probably is an oversimplification. The patient reported by Landau *et al.*[9] who had an apparently normal karyotype had such extracephalic anomalies as ventricular septal defect, coarctation of the aorta, diaphragmatic hernia and cryptorchidism. Ferrier *et al.*[7] described a patient with 46,XY karyotype who had had, in addition to arhinencephaly, polydactyly, common mesentery, ambiguous external genitalia and testes in place of the ovaries. In the infant recorded by Marshall *et al.*,[16] the brain had a single ventricle without corpus callosum, septum pellucidum, olfactory nerves and pituitary. Cephalic and extracephalic characteristics of the trisomy 13-15 syndrome were present but the karyotype was normal. These cases do not conform to the rule proposed by DeMyer.[8]

Familial cases that have probably similar or identical causation may differ greatly in phenotype (see below). This fact should caution against the assumption that a karyotype can be safely deduced from clinical manifestations.

At present, one can state that some cases of the cyclopia-arhinencephaly series can be attributed to trisomy 13-15. Others may also be due to chromosome changes even though a normal count of 46 is found. Conen *et al.*[17] described a child with a severe brain defect and extracephalic anomalies characteristic of trisomy 13-15 who had 46 chromosomes and a D/D translocation, a karyotype equivalent to trisomy 13-15. Others have more subtle changes such as deletion of a short arm of a chromosome 18[13,18] or other chromosomal anomalies.[19] Familial arhinencephaly (holoprosencephaly) has been reported repeatedly. In one family there were 3 cases, and a fourth, presenting with congenital hydrocephaly, possibly had the same anomaly. Two of the affected children were dizygotic twins of different sex.[22] We know little of "environmental" factors that can induce arhinencephaly in man. Dekaban[20] reported two arhinencephalics born to diabetic mothers, and animal experiments and observations point to the possibility of toxic factors as causes of arhinencephaly (p. 205). As in many other malformations, the anomalies of the cyclopia-arhinencephaly series can be heterogeneous in origin.

REFERENCES

1. Kundrat, H.: *Arhinencephalie als typische Art von Missbildung* (Graz, 1882).
2. Yakovlev, P. I.: Pathoarchitectonic studies of cerebral malformations. III. Arrhinencephalies (holotelencephalies), J. Neuropath. & Exper. Neurol. 18:22, 1959.
3. DeMyer, W., and Zeman, W.: Alobar holoprosencephaly (arhinencephaly) with median cleft lip and palate: Clinical, electroencephalographic and nosologic considerations, Confinia neurol. 23:1, 1963.
4. Ernst, P.: Missbildungen des Nervensystems, in Schwalbe, E. (ed.), *Die Morphologie der Missbildungen des Menschen und der Tiere* (Jena: Gustav Fischer, 1909).
5. Miller, J. Q., Picard, E. H., Alkan, M. K., Warner, S., and Gerald, P. S.: A specific congenital brain defect (arhinencephaly) in 13-15 trisomy, New England J. Med. 268:120, 1963.
6. Bishop, K., Connolly, J. M., Carter, C. H., and Carpenter, D. G.: Holoprosencephaly, J. Pediat. 65:406, 1964.
7. Ferrier, P., Widgren, S., and Ferrier, S.: Nonspecific pseudohermaphroditism, Helvet. paediat. Acta 19:1, 1964.
8. DeMyer, W.: A 46 chromosome cebocephaly, with remarks on the relation of 13-15 trisomy to holoprosencephaly (arhinencephaly), Ann. paediat. 203:169, 1964.
9. Landau, J. W., Barry, J. M., and Koch, R.: Arhinencephaly, J. Pediat. 62:895, 1963.
10. Schade, H., Schöller, L., and Schultze, K. W.: D-trisomy (Pätau-Syndrome) mit kongenitaler myeloischer Leukämie, Med. Welt 50:2690, 1962.
11. Sergovich, F., Madronich, J. S., Barr, M. L., Carr, D. H., and Langdon, W. A.: The D trisomy syndrome, Canad. M.A.J. 89:151, 1963.
12. Blanck, C., Jalling, B., Lindsten, J., and Zetterquist, P.: Trisomy 13-15, Acta path. et. microbiol. scandinav. 60:36, 1964.
13. Uchida, I. A., McRae, K. N., Wang, H. C., and Ray, M.: Familial short arm deficiency of chromosome 18 concomitant with arhinencephaly and alopecia congenita, Am. J. Human Genet. 17:410, 1965.
14. Warkany, J., Passarge, E., and Smith, L. B.: Congenital malformations in autosomal trisomy syndromes, Am. J. Dis. Child. 112:502, 1966.
15. Neuhäuser, G., and Usener, M.: Hirnmissbildung und autosomale Trisomie, Ztschr. Kinderh. 95:244, 1966.
16. Marshall, R., Newnham, R. E., Rawstron, J. R., Ellis, J. R., and Stevens, L. J.: Features of 13-15 trisomy syndrome with normal karyotype, Lancet 1:556, 1964.
17. Conen, P. E., Erkman, B., and Metaxotou, C.: The "D" syndrome, Am. J. Dis. Child. 111:236, 1966.
18. Nitowsky, H. M., Sindhvananda, N., Konigsberg, U. R., and Weinberg, T.: Partial 18 monosomy in the cyclops formation, Pediatrics 37:260, 1966.
19. Cohen, M. M.: Chromosomal mosaicism associated with a case of cyclopia, J. Pediat. 69:793, 1966.
20. Dekaban, A. S.: Arhinencephaly in an infant born to a diabetic mother, J. Neuropath. & Exper. Neurol. 18:620, 1959.
21. McDermott, A., Insley, J., Barton, M. E., Rowe, P., Edwards, J. H., and Cameron, A. H.: Case reports. Arhinencephaly associated with a deficiency involving chromosome 18, J. M. Genetics 5:60, 1968.
22. Kahn, M., Rozdilsky, B., and Gerrard, J. W.: Familial holoprosencephaly, Developmental Med. & Child Neurol. 12:71, 1970.

Cyclopia

Cyclopia is a monstrosity characterized by a median eye. There are various degrees of ocular approximation and there are intermediate forms leading to arhinencephaly and trigonocephaly.

The true incidence of cyclopia in man is not known. In one hospital it was about 1 in 40,000 births.[1] In Japan, cyclopia was found 6 times in 3,400 embryos, but was not recorded once among 63,800 Japanese infants,[2] which suggests prenatal screening of fetuses with this severe anomaly. Sixty per cent of the patients are female.[3]

Cyclopia can occur twice in a family, and in several sibships other congenital malformations such as hydrocephaly, cebocephaly, harelip, cleft palate or imperforate anus occurred in addition to cyclopia. In an interesting family reported by Klopstock,[4] the father and mother were first cousins. There were 5 pregnancies, the third ending in miscarriage, the fourth in the birth of a cyclops and the fifth in the birth of a cebocephalus. Dominok and Kirchmair[5] described 3 cases of arhinencephaly in a family: The first, a girl, was a cyclops with situs inversus and duplication of the vagina and uterus; the second, also a girl, had cleft palate; the third, a boy, had median harelip. All had undivided prosencephalon. Chromosomes were not reported. Cyclopic dichorionic twins were reported by Ellis in 1866. There were two separate placentas. One twin was a female with a nasal proboscis and palpebral fissures and the other, who was of doubtful sex, had a nasal proboscis without a trace of eyes. The mother previously had given birth to a female infant with cleft palate and imperforate anus (cited by Ballantyne[6]). Jackson[7] described fraternal twins, one normal and the other with cyclopia. Recently, some cases of cyclopia have been found to be associated with chromosomal anomalies. Faint and Lewis[8] and

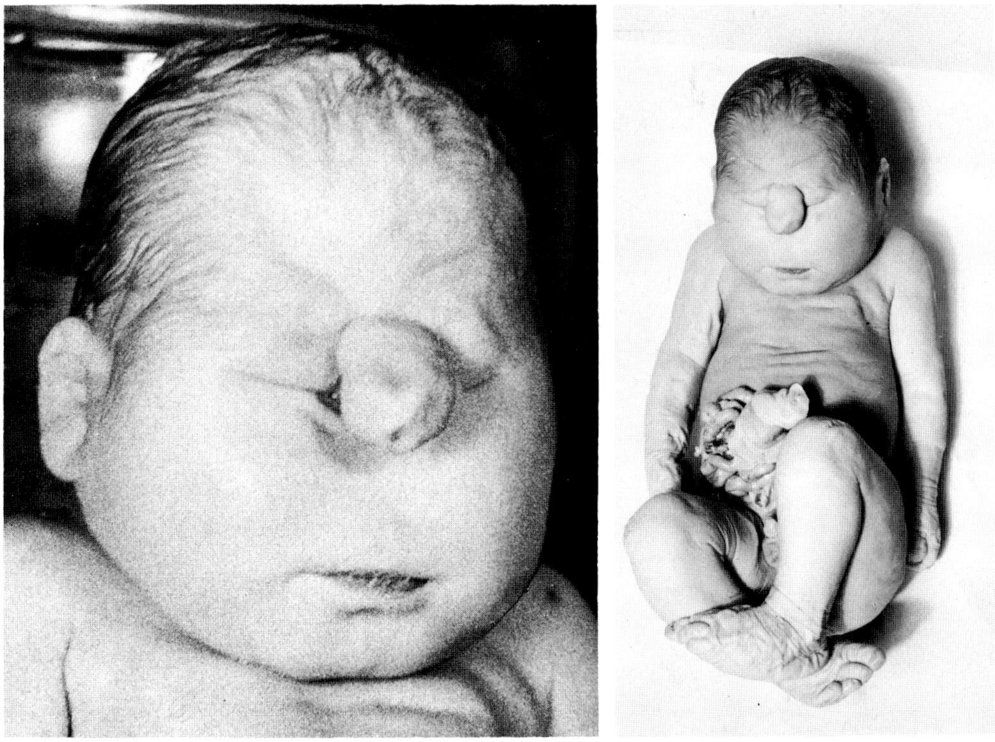

Fig. 23-1.—Cyclops with proboscis and exomphalos.

Nitowsky *et al.*[9] reported deletion of the short arms of one of the E chromosomes, probably chromosome 18, in cyclopic children. Cohen[10] noted mosaicism for monosomy of a group G chromosome in such a child. Lejeune and Juberg (cited by Cohen[10]) found normal chromosome complements in patients with cyclopia. Arakaki and Waxman[34] reported trisomy D in a cyclops and noted that in 7 other cases normal karyotype, mosaicism and deletion of the short arm of chromosome 18 had been seen.

In perfect cyclopia, the eye has a single cornea, pupil and lens without evidence of doubling. In other cases, two eyes may be found in a single orbit, or the eyes may be approximated but lie in different orbits. Occasionally, an eye with double iris, choroidea and retina can be observed within a single scleral and corneal cover. Colobomas of the iris, of the retina and of the optic nerve occur.[11,12] A single eye usually is framed by four eyelids that form a rhomboid or oval opening. The optic nerve may be single or show various degrees of duplication. The optic chiasma may be absent or imperfectly developed. The single median eye is but one component of a complex of abnormalities affecting the entire prechordal region of the head. The external nose is either lacking or situated above the eye in the form of a proboscis that is a cylindrical structure about 2 cm. in length with a central depression on its free end. It either projects forward or it hangs over the eye covering the palpebral fissure (see Fig. 23-1). If the proboscis is absent, the eye may also be lacking. When cyclopia is combined with hypognathia or synotia, absence of the proboscis has been observed repeatedly. There may be a single nasal chamber that fails to communicate with the pharynx. The lamina cribrosa and crista galli, the nasal bones, vomer, turbinates, premaxilla and other facial bones are missing. Failure of fusion of palatine processes of the maxilla due to absence of the median nasal process results in cleft palate.[3] The mouth is small and the philtrum absent. In the upper jaw, the incisors may be replaced by a single conical tooth located in the midline. This tooth may be erupted at birth.[3] Krafka[13] distinguished six types of cyclopia, depending on the variation of the nose and upper lip. Roentgenologically, the single orbit, single optic foramen, absence of nasal cavity or maxillary sinuses, lack of fusion of facial bones and abnormal dentition can be ascertained.[3,14]

The head is small and round, with a high cephalic index.[11] The forebrain is not divided into hemispheres but consists of a single sac enclosing an undivided ventricle (holosphere).[15] Usually, there are no longitudinal sulci and the corpus callosum, septum pellucidum and falx are absent. The olfactory nerve and the rhinencephalon may be a single median structure or be entirely absent. The diencephalon and the thalami can be fused in varying degrees and often the hypophysis is absent.[16] The caudal portions of the central

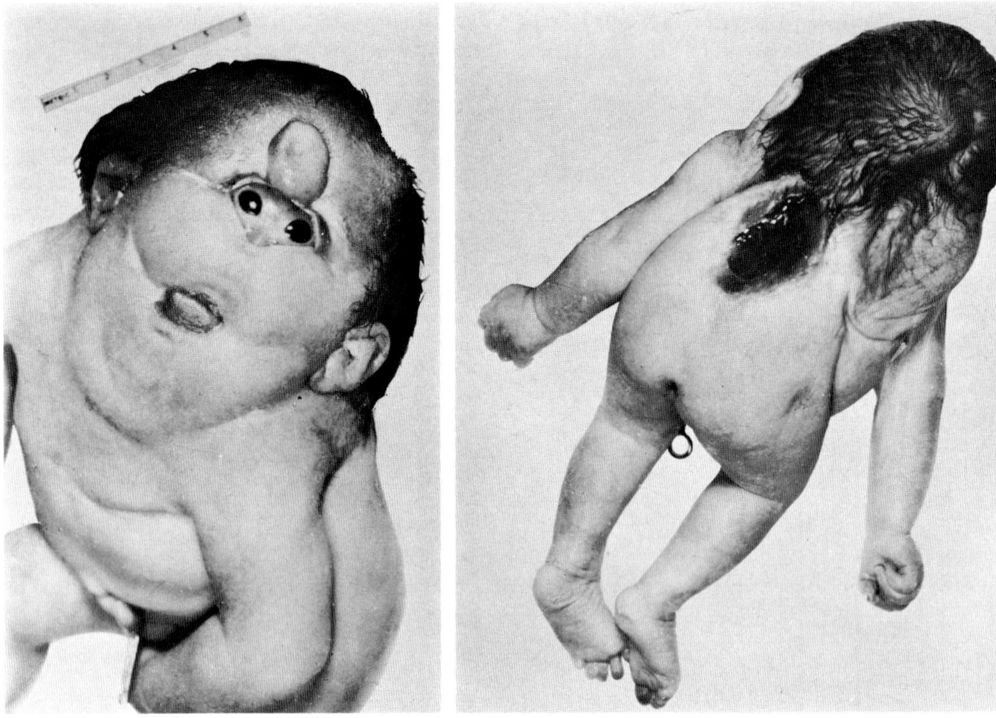

Fig. 23-2.—Incomplete cyclopia with proboscis in an infant with iniencephaly and myelomeningocele. (Courtesy of Dr. J. B. Hamblet, Cincinnati, Ohio.)

nervous system can be unaffected. For interpretation of the origins of the undivided forebrain, the single ventricle and the dorsal cyst, special publications are recommended.[15,17,18]

Cyclopia often is associated with other anomalies of the face or other organ systems. Absence or smallness of the mouth (astomia or microstomia) or absence of the lower jaw with approximation or fusion of the ears (otocephaly, synotia) may be combined with cyclopia. Anencephaly, hydrocephaly, harelip, cleft palate, spina bifida, omphalocele, situs inversus, diaphragmatic hernia, absence of the adrenal glands or renal agenesis have been observed as associated malformations.[3,6] Two children with calcareous chondrodystrophy, one a cyclopic monster, were described in the same family by Haynes and Wanger.[19]

Pregnancies ending in the birth of cyclopic infants are often but not always accompanied by hydramnios. Many cyclopic fetuses are born at term. Intrauterine growth retardation probably is frequent but seldom recorded.[3,9,20]

Cyclopia has been observed in many animals. In lambs, pigs, calves, dogs, cats and foals the malformation probably is not rare. Cyclopia can be produced experimentally. Stockard[21] obtained the malformation in Fundulus eggs treated with magnesium salts, alcohol and other chemical substances when he exposed the embryos in the 8–32-cell stage, but not later than 15 hours after fertilization. Cyclopian embryos have been produced by treating amphibian eggs in early stages of gastrulation with a variety of chemicals.[22,22a,23] The anomaly can be produced also by removal of the anterior portion of the roof of the primitive gut. Early investigators attributed cyclopia to fusion of two originally separated eyes or head structures, but there is no doubt that the cyclopian eye is single from its first appearance. It is quite likely that the eye anlagen are influenced by mesodermal organizer tissue that lies under the medullary plate in the roof of the primitive gut.[24] Early experimenters with chicken eggs produced a variety of malformations, among which they included cyclopia. Rogers[22] reviewed these reports and newer observations and came to the conclusion that production of cyclopia in chicks by chemicals was by no means established. He succeeded in inducing cyclopia in explanted chick embryos by addition of lithium chloride to the culture. In 1964, he[25] produced cyclopia in chicks at the time of beginning bilateralization of the optic vesicles by microsurgical removal of the telencephalon. Similar experiments were reported by Schowing.[26] Giroud and co-workers[27] produced cyclopia in mice whose mothers were given 100 I.U. of vitamin A from the eighth to the tenth day of gestation. The anomalies were limited to the prosencephalon, which was not subdivided into hemispheres and lacked olfactory bulbs. The third ventricle communicated with a single anterior ventricle and there was medial fusion of the eyes.

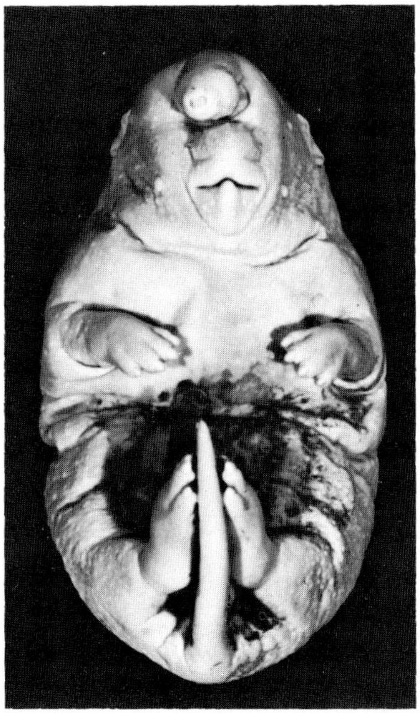

Fig. 23-3.—Cyclopia produced in rat fetus by AY 9944 (inhibitor of cholesterol synthesis). (Courtesy of Prof. Ch. Roux, Paris, France.)

The pituitary was absent. Roux[28] produced a variety of malformations in rats by triparanol. a substance that inhibits cholesterol synthesis. Occasionally, cyclopia was observed among the malformations (Fig. 23-3). Production of cyclopia by x-rays had been effected by Wolf[29] in 1936. Murakami *et al.*[30] exposed mice to a single whole-body x-irradiation of 200 R on the ninth day of pregnancy. They obtained many malformations belonging to the cyclopia-arhinencephaly series, but there were no typical cyclopias. Binns *et al.*[31] noticed an epidemic of cyclopian-type malformation in certain stocks of range sheep (Fig. 23-4). The malformations could be produced under controlled experimental conditions by feeding *Veratrum californicum* in fresh and dry green forms, but the plants varied widely in teratogenicity among different range areas. Malformations occurred in ewes fed *Veratrum californicum* on gestation day 14. Reports of experimental production of cyclopia can be found in reviews by Rogers[22] and Kalter.[32] That genetic factors may be at work in the production of head defects of the cyclopia series was demonstrated in guinea pigs by Wright and Wagner.[33]

Fig. 23-4.—Cyclopian-type malformation in a lamb with a centrally located single eye, a proboscis-like protuberance above and to the left of the eye and absence of the premaxilla bone. The anomaly is induced by maternal ingestion of a range plant, *Veratrum californicum*. (From W. Binns, L. F. James, J. R. Shupe and G. Everett.[31])

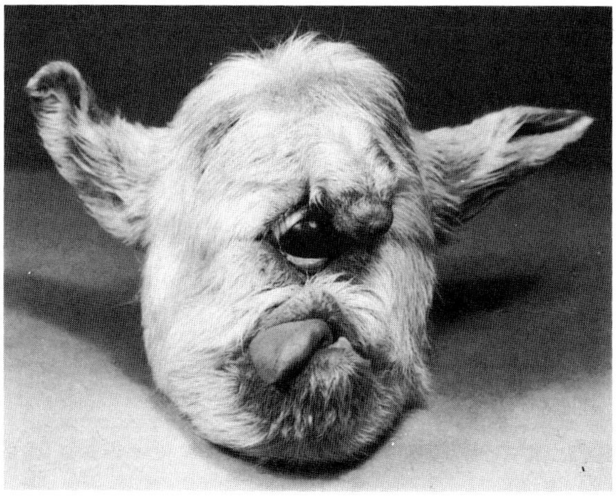

REFERENCES

1. Barber, A., and Muelling, R. J.: Cyclopia with complete separation of the neural and mesodermal elements of the eye, Arch. Ophth. 43:989, 1950.
2. Nishimura, H., Takano, K., Tanimura, T., Yasuda, M., and Uchida, T.: High incidence of several malformations in the early human embryos as compared with infants, Biol. Neonat. 10:93, 1966.
3. Sedano, H. O., and Gorlin, R. J.: The oral manifestations of cyclopia. Review of the literature and report of two cases, Oral Surg. 16:823, 1963.
4. Klopstock, A.: Familiäres Vorkommen von Cyklopie und Arrhinencephalie, Monatsschr. Geb. Gynäk. 56:59, 1921.
5. Dominok, G. W., and Kirchmair, H.: Familiäre Häufung von Fehlbildungen der Arhinencephaliegruppe, Ztschr. Kinderh. 85:19, 1961.
6. Ballantyne, J. W.: *Manual of Antenatal Pathology and Hygiene. The Embryo* (Edinburgh: William Green & Sons, 1904).
7. Jackson, H.: Cyclopian monsters; some general observations with report of a case, J.A.M.A. 53:1483, 1909.
8. Faint, S., and Lewis, F. J. W.: Presumptive deletion of the short arm of chromosome 18 in a cyclops, Human Chromosome Newsletter No. 14:5, 1964 (personal communication).
9. Nitowsky, H. M., Sindhvananda, N., Konigsberg, U. R., and Weinberg, T.: Partial 18 monosomy in the cyclops malformation, Pediatrics 37:260, 1966.
10. Cohen, M. M.: Chromosomal mosaicism associated with a case of cyclopia, J. Pediat. 69:793, 1966.
11. Shehata, R.: Human cyclops. Report of a case, Alexandria M. J. 10:210, 1964.
12. Wolter, J. R., and Schmidt, D. W.: Cyclopia with cystic coloboma of the optic nerve, J. Pediat. Ophth. 3:18, 1966.
13. Krafka, J.: Cyclopia and arhinia; new concept, Arch. Ophth. 33:128, 1945.
14. Melian, J. M.: Cyclopia, Am. J. Ophth. 57:134, 1964.
15. Yakovlev, P. I.: Pathoarchitectonic studies of cerebral malformations. III. Arhinencephalies (holotelencephalies), J. Neuropath. & Exper. Neurol. 18:22, 1959.
16. Rogers, K. T.: Presence of the pituitary in perfect cyclopia, Anat. Rec. 128:213, 1957.
17. Marburg, O., and Warner, F. J.: The brain in a case of human cyclopia, J. Nerv. & Ment. Dis. 103:319, 1946.
18. DeMyer, W., and Zeman, W.: Alobar holoprosencephaly (arhinencephaly) with median cleft lip and palate: Clinical, electroencephalographic and nosologic considerations, Confinia Neurol. 23:1, 1963.
19. Haynes, E. R., and Wanger, W. F.: Chondroangiopachia calcarea seu punctata: Review and case report, Radiology 57:547, 1951.
20. Sarma, V.: Ocular abnormalities of the foetus with spe-

cial reference to cyclopia, Brit. J. Ophth. 47:193, 1963.
21. Stockard, C. R.: Developmental rate and structural expression, Am. J. Anat. 28:115, 1921.
22. Rogers, K. T.: Experimental production of perfect cyclopia in the chick by means of LiCl with a survey of the literature on cyclopia produced experimentally by various means, Develop. Biol. 8:129, 1963.
22a. Lehmann, F. E.: Die Augen- und Linsen-Bildungen von Amphibienembryonen unter dem Einfluss chemischer Mittel, Rev. Suisse Zool. 40:251, 1933.
23. Evans, H. E., Ingalls, T. H., and Binns, W.: Teratogenesis of craniofacial malformations in animals. III. Natural and experimental cephalic deformities in sheep, Arch. Environ. Health 13:706, 1966.
24. Adelmann, H. B.: The problem of cyclopia, Quart. Rev. Biol. 11:161; 284, 1936.
25. Rogers, K. T.: Experimental production of perfect cyclopia by removal of the telencephalon and reversal of bilateralization in somite-stage chicks, Am. J. Anat. 115:487, 1964.
26. Schowing, J.: Obtention expérimentale de cyclopes parfaits par microchirurgie chez l'embryon de Poulet. Étude histologique, J. Embryol. & Exper. Morphol. 14:(pt. 3)255, 1965.
27. Giroud, A., Delmas, A., and Martinet, M.: Cyclocéphalie: Morphogénèse et mécanisme de sa production, Arch. Anat. 47:295, 1963.
28. Roux, C.: Action tératogène du triparanol chex l'animal, Arch franç. pédiat. 21:451, 1964.
29. Wolf, E.: Les bases de la tératogenèse expérimentale chez les vertébrés amniotes d'après les résultats des méthodes directes, Arch. Anat. 22:1, 1936.
30. Murakami, U., Jameyama, Y., Majima, A., and Sakurai, T.: Radiation malformations belonging to the cyclopia-arhinenocephalia-otocephalia group in the mouse foetus, J. Embryol. & Exper. Morphol. 10:64, 1962.
31. Binns, W., James, L. F., Shupe, J. R., and Everett, G.: A congenital cyclopian-type malformation in lambs induced by maternal ingestion of a range plant, *Veratrum californicum*, Am. J. Vet. Res. 24:1164, 1963.
32. Kalter, H.: *Teratology of the Central Nervous System in Laboratory and Domestic Mammals* (Chicago: The University of Chicago Press, 1968).
33. Wright, S., and Wagner, K.: Types of subnormal development of the head from inbred strains of guinea pigs and their bearing on the classification and interpretation of vertebrate monsters, Am. J. Anat. 54:383, 1934.
34. Arakaki, D. T., and Waxman, S. H.: Trisomy D in a cyclops, J. Pediat. 74:620, 1969.

Ethmocephaly and Cebocephaly

ALTHOUGH SOME AUTHORS[1,2] described these anomalies separately, the term "cebocephaly" often is used for either condition in modern clinical writing.

Ethmocephaly is morphologically closely related to cyclopia, but neither the eyes nor the orbits are fused. The nose is absent or represented by a proboscis. The forehead is narrow and there is no metopic suture. The nasal bones, maxillae, nasal septum and turbinates are missing; the lacrimal and palatine bones are united. The olfactory nerves and the olfactory lobes are not developed, but rudiments may be found. The optic nerve originates singly but may be forked at the dura. The forebrain is represented by an elongated thin vesicle that leaves the mesencephalon uncovered.[2]

Cebocephaly derives its name from a supposed resemblance to a platyrrhinic monkey face characterized by a flat and rather rudimentary nose. The forehead is keel-shaped and the anterior cranial fossa narrow. Sphenoid and ethmoid are defective. There is hypotelorism and the foramina optica are approximated; they may be contained in a common bony canal although separated by fibrous tissue. The nasal septum and premaxilla are absent, nasal bones and turbinates defective and the maxillae fused. The forebrain is incompletely cleaved and simplified; it lacks falx, corpus callosum, septum pellucidum and anterior fornix. A thin-walled vesicle occupies the free space between the forebrain, diencephalon and mesencephalon. The thalami may be fused and the corpora striata absent. In addition to agenesis of the olfactory nerves, there may be absence of the pineal gland, infundibulum, corpora mammillaria and lamina perforata. The cerebellum sometimes is defective and leaves the 4th ventricle partly exposed. Ernst[2] mentioned that microphthalmia and anophthalmia, defects of the external ears, jaws, heart, diaphragm and uterus may be associated with ethmocephaly. Bühler *et al.*[3] described fusion of the frontal, parietal and occipital lobes in a case of this type in which trisomy 13-15 was proved. There were ocular anomalies, ventricular septal defect, patent ductus arteriosus, intestinal malrotation, uterus subseptus and polydactyly. A cebocephalus with similar anomalies associated with trisomy 13-15 was reported by Conen *et al.*[4] The patient reported by Haworth *et al.*[5] resembled externally those just mentioned. The brain consisted of a central mass with a crescentic dorsal opening, as seen in cyclopia. There was no pituitary and the adrenals were hypoplastic. A brother of the cebocephalic infant was mentally and physically retarded and the mother showed mental deficiency and alopecia totalis. A deficiency of the short arms of a chromosome 18 was found in the 3 affected members of this family.[6] Short-arm deletion of chromosome 18 in cebocephaly was also reported by Gorlin *et al.*[23] In a female infant with fusion of the hemispheres and arhinencephaly combined with microphthalmia, ventricular septal defect, hypoplastic kidney and uterus bicornis, analysis showed one of the D-group chromosomes replaced by a ring chromosome.[21] The cebocephalic girl shown in Figure 23-6 had 46 chromosomes and an apparently normal karyotype. Grebe,[7] in 1944, reported an unviable cebocephalus with microphthalmia and cleft

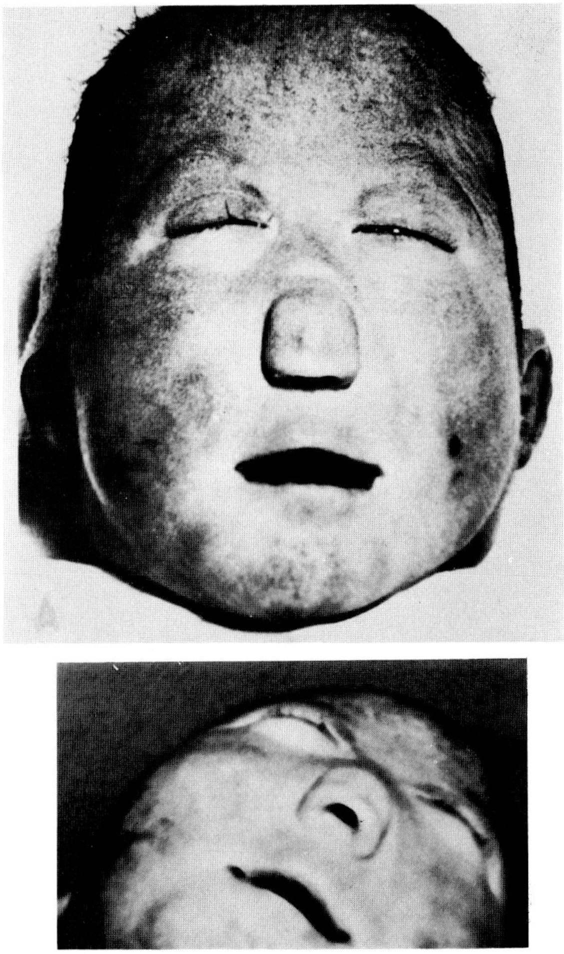

Fig. 23-5.—Cebocephaly with single nostril.

palate. There was absence of the olfactory bulb and tract, undivided forebrain, hypogyria and other cerebral anomalies. The family history was of unusual interest. A brother of the cebocephalus had a cleft lip and palate, mental deficiency and anosmia. A second brother was mentally deficient but showed no anomalies of the lip and palate. A paternal uncle had been born with wide median clefts of the upper lip and palate, absence of the nasal septum and hypoplastic nasal bones. He was mentally deficient and anosmic. The father had had another brother who lived only 3 hours and who resembled the nonviable child with arhinencephaly. This kindred shows not only heritability of these anomalies but also the variable expression in different members. It was, of course, not possible in 1944 to make chromosome studies in these patients and it was thought that the arhinencephalic anomalies were inherited as an irregular dominant trait with great variation of expressivity. Now it seems possible that a chromosomal anomaly was responsible for the various malformations in this kindred. Cebocephaly and cyclopia in a family in which the parents were consanguineous have been mentioned before.[8]

Arhinencephaly with Double Proboscis

An unusual partial arhinencephaly was present in an infant with bilateral proboscis combined with unilateral anophthalmos (Fig. 23-8, *A*). In this case, described in detail by Gitlin and Behar,[9] the frontal lobes were divided by a large midline structure that proved to be a hamartoma consisting of areas of astrocytoma, oligodendroglioma and ependymoma. This hamartoma interfered with the normal growth of the midline tissues that form the rhinencephalon and the nose (Fig. 23-8, *B*).

Arhinencephaly with Median Harelip

This form of arhinencephaly is relatively common and clinically well known because affected infants can survive birth. The philtrum is absent. The nose is flat, and cleft palate exists in most of the cases; the premaxilla, nasal septum and horizontal ethmoid with crista galli are absent (Fig. 23-9). There is a single nasal cavity with imperforate choanae. Externally and radiologically, hypotelorism is noted and the optic foramina are approximated. The metopic suture seems obliterated and the forehead is keel-shaped. The falx is reduced and the mesencephalon small and simplified. As in cebocephaly, the thalami may be fused, the corpora striata and the diencephalon defective. Olfactory nerves and bulbs are absent. Caudal to the mesencephalon, the central nervous system may be normally formed. It has long been known that polydactyly, septal defects of the heart, persistent truncus arteriosus, pulmonic stenosis, microphthalmia, malformations of the external and inner ears, umbilical and diaphragmatic hernia and spina bifida may complicate this type of arhinencephaly.[2] This syndrome with median or lateral facial clefts was obviously known to Bartholin and described by him in 1657 and it was mentioned 100 years earlier by Lycosthenes.[10] Two sisters with arhinencephaly and median cleft lip and palate were reported by DeMyer *et al.*,[11] and Hintz *et al.*[20] observed two sisters, one with median cleft lip and another with median cleft lip and palate. The mother of these children had polydactyly. A case of arhinencephaly with a ring chromosome showed multiple malformations but no cleft palate.[21] Arhinencephaly and median cleft lip and palate with deletion of the short arms of a chromosome 18 have been reported.[22,24] The chromosome count and karyotype of the sisters reported by DeMyer *et al.*[11] were normal. In many other cases, trisomy 13-15 was established.[12,13] In one instance, this type of arhinencephaly with median facial clefts was associated with a 46,XX D/D translocation[4] and in another with a ring E chromosome.[25] A thorough description

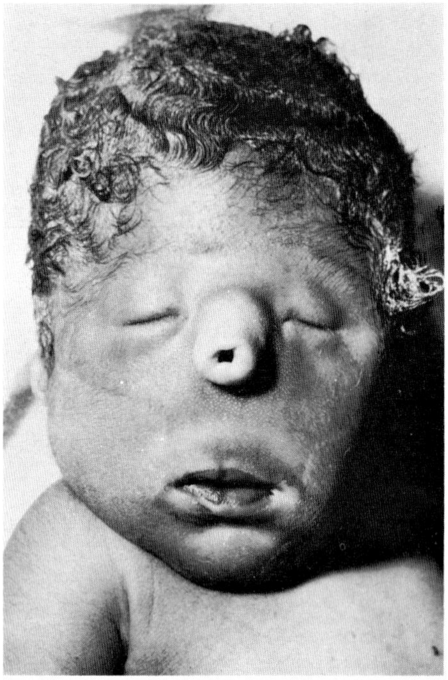

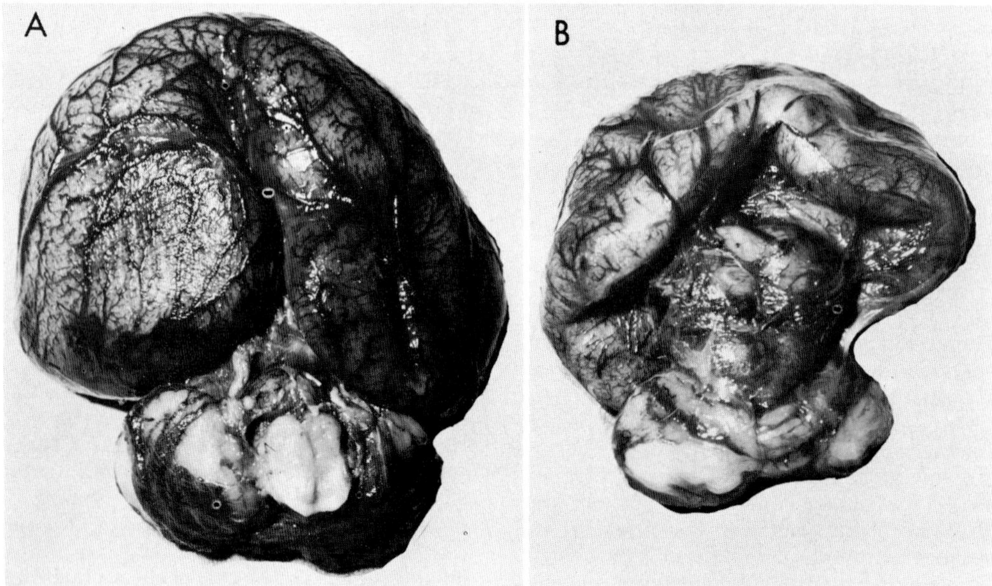

Fig. 23-6 (above).—Cebocephalic premature girl with incompletely divided telencephalon and arhinencephaly. Chromosomes (46,XX) apparently were normal. (Cincinnati General Hospital No. 447094.)

Fig. 23-7 (below).—Brain of cebocephalic girl shown in Figure 23-6. **A,** ventral view. The division of hemispheres is incomplete. **B,** dorsal view. Fused frontal lobes and fluid-filled posterior cyst.

of arhinencephaly combined with median cleft lip and palate was given by DeMyer and Zeman.[14]

Arhinencephaly with Lateral Cleft Lips and Cleft Palate

This type of arhinencephaly may be associated with and betrayed by trigonocephaly. The frontal bone originates from a single center of ossification and appears fused, the forehead is narrow and keel-shaped, the frontal lobe narrow, the rhinencephalon absent, but the occipital lobes broad. The falx may subdivide the forebrain more or less so that various degrees of communication exist between hemispheres. Defects

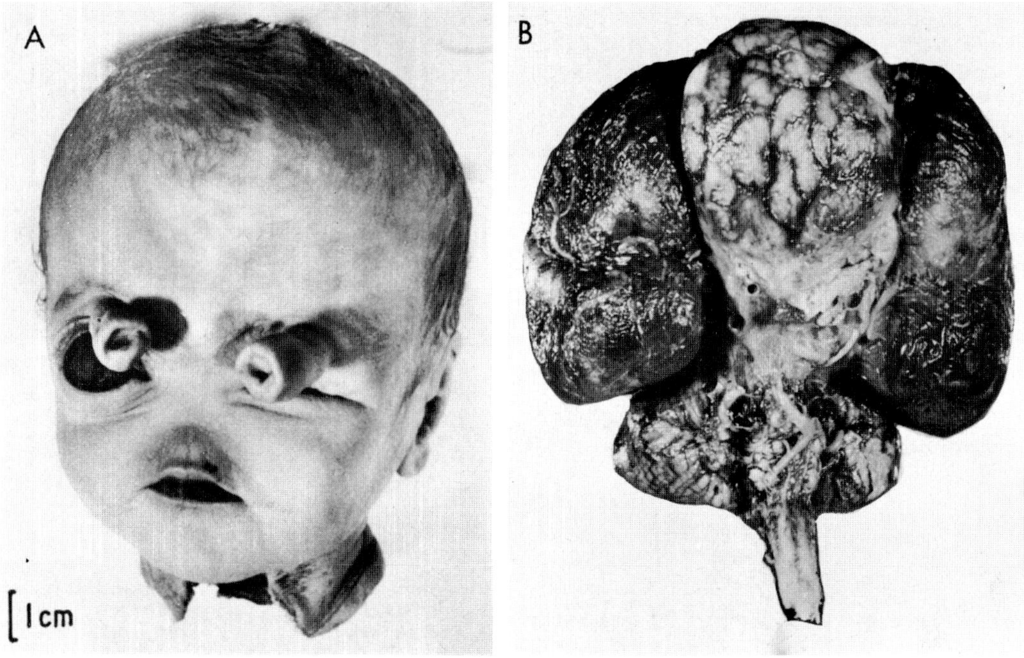

Fig. 23-8. – **A,** infant with bilateral proboscis. **B,** base of brain of the child. Between the hemispheres a large "central lobe" is seen; this is actually a hamartomatous tumor. This malformation of the brain interfered with normal formation of the nose. (From G. Gitlin and A. J. Behar.[9])

of the diencephalon may resemble those of the more serious types of arhinencephaly. In this condition, there is no fusion of the maxilla and palatine bones, giving rise to cleft palate (see Fig. 23-9). Microphthalmia, polydactyly, abnormal external ears, umbilical hernia and cardiovascular malformations were known as associated malformations many decades ago.[2] This type of arhinencephaly frequently is associated with trisomy 13-15[13, 15] but is rare in trisomy 18.[16] The trisomy 13-15 syndrome with bilateral harelip and cleft palate can be seen without brain anomalies.[17] In one of our cases of trisomy 13-15, the olfactory nerves and bulbs were absent, nerves II–VIII hypoplastic but cleavage of the cerebrum and cerebellum was normal.

Arhinencephaly with Trigonocephaly

This arhinencephaly is characterized by a narrow and keel-shaped forehead and relatively minor anomalies of the eyes. There may be microphthalmia or mongoloid slanting of the palpebral fissures. The external nose can be normal but the olfactory nerves are absent. There may be some other defects of the basal parts of the prosencephalon and diencephalon. This type is compatible with life and therefore of interest to the clinician.

The relationship of arhinencephaly, trigonocephaly and orbital hypotelorism was thoroughly discussed by Currarino and Silverman.[18] It seems that orbital hypotelorism often is more obvious radiographically than by external inspection. In trigonocephaly, the metopic suture is either prematurely obliterated or not formed at all. It is of importance that trigonocephaly can occur in association with arhinencephaly or as an isolated anomaly; it probably is found with increased

Fig. 23-9. – Median cleft of lip, flat nose, protruding eyes. Probably arhinencephaly.

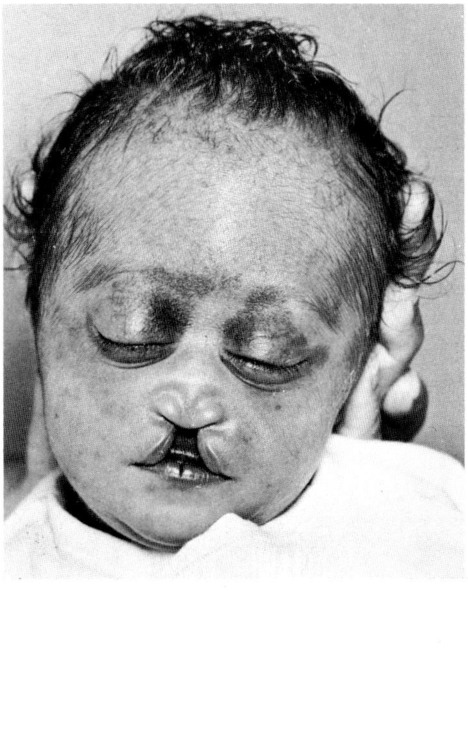

frequency in some types of mental retardation, but it can be seen in otherwise normal persons.

Arhinencephaly may be combined with another type of craniosynostosis, acrocephalosyndactyly (p. 899) and with encephalocele.[19]

Microcephaly and Olfactory Deficiency

Ernst[2] listed an additional form of arhinencephaly that manifests itself by microcephaly associated with defects of the forebrain and deficiency of the olfactory nerves. There may be absence of the corpus callosum.

REFERENCES

1. Kundrat, H.: *Arhinencephalie als typische Art von Missbildung* (Graz, 1882).
2. Ernst, P.: Missbildungen des Nervensystems, in Schwalbe, E. (ed.), *Die Morphologie der Missbildungen des Menschen und der Tiere* (Jena: Gustav Fischer, 1909).
3. Bühler, E., Bodis, I., Rossier, R., and Stalder, G.: Trisomie 13-15 mit Cebocephalie, Ann. paediat. 199:198, 1962.
4. Conen, P. E., Erkman, B., and Metaxotou, C.: The "D" syndrome, Am. J. Dis. Child. 111:236, 1966.
5. Haworth, J. C., Medovy, H., and Lewis, A. J.: Cebocephaly with endocrine dysgenesis; report of 3 cases, J. Pediat. 59:726, 1961.
6. Uchida, I. A., McRae, K. N., Wang, H. C., and Ray, M.: Familial short arm deficiency of chromosome 18 concomitant with arhinencephaly and alopecia congenita, Am. J. Human Genet. 17:410, 1965.
7. Grebe, H.: Zur Aetiologie der Arhinencephalie, Der Erbarzt 12:138, 1944.
8. Klopstock, A.: Familiäres Vorkommen von Cyklopie und Arhinencephalie, Monatsschr. Geb. Gynäk. 56:59, 1921.
9. Gitlin, G., and Behar, A. J.: Meningeal angiomatosis, arhinencephaly, agenesis of the corpus callosum and large hamartoma of the brain, with neoplasia, in an infant having bilateral nasal proboscis, Acta anat. 41:56, 1960.
10. Warburg, M.: Anophthalmos complicated by mental retardation and cleft palate, Acta ophth. 38:394, 1960.
11. DeMyer, W., Zeman, W., and Palmer, C. G.: Familial alobar holoprosencephaly (arhinencephaly) with median cleft lip and palate, Neurology 13:913, 1963.
12. Conen, P. E., Phillips, K. G., and Maunter, L. S.: Multiple developmental anomalies and trisomy of a 13-15 group chromosome ("D" syndrome), Canad. M.A.J. 87:709, 1962.
13. Neuhäuser, G., and Usener, M.: Hirnmissbildung und autosomale Trisomie, Ztschr. Kinderh. 95:244, 1966.
14. DeMyer, W., and Zeman, W.: Alobar holoprosencephaly (arhinencephaly) with median cleft lip and palate: Clinical, electroencephalographic and nosologic considerations, Confinia Neurol. 23:1, 1963.
15. Warkany, J., Passarge, E., and Smith, L. B.: Congenital malformations in autosomal trisomy syndromes, Am. J. Dis. Child. 112:502, 1966.
16. Butler, L. J., Snodgrass, G. J., France, N. E., Sinclair, L., and Russell, A.: E (16-18) trisomy syndrome: Analysis of 13 cases, Arch. Dis. Childhood 40:600, 1965.
17. Blanck, C., Jalling, B., Lindsten, J., and Zetterquist, P.: Trisomy 13-15, Acta path. et microbiol. scandinav. 60:36, 1964.
18. Currarino, G., and Silverman, F. N.: Orbital hypotelorism, arhinencephaly, and trigonocephaly, Radiology 74:206, 1960.
19. Gruber, G. B.: Beiträge zur Frage "gekoppelter" Missbildungen (Acrocephalo-Syndactylie und Dysencephalia splanchnocystica), Beitr. path. Anat. 93:459, 1934.
20. Hintz, R. L., Menking, M., and Sotos, J. F.: Familial holoprosencephaly with endocrine dysgenesis, J. Pediat. 72: 81, 1968.
21. Bain, A. D., and Gauld, I. K.: Multiple congenital abnormalities associated with ring chromosome, Lancet 2:304, 1963.
22. Pfeiffer, R. A.: Deletion der kurzen Arme des Chromosoms Nr. 18, Humangenetik 2:178, 1966.
23. Gorlin, R. J., Yunis, J., and Anderson, V. E.: Short arm deletion of chromosome 18 in cebocephaly, Am. J. Dis. Child. 115:473, 1968.
24. McDermott, A., Insley, J., Barton, M. E., Rowe, P., Edwards, J. H., and Cameron, A. H.: Arhinencephaly associated with a deficiency involving chromosome 18, J. M. Genetics 5:60, 1968.
25. Dumars, K. W., Carnahan, L. G., and Barrett, R. V.: Median facial cleft associated with ring E chromosome, J. M. Genetics 7:86, 1970.

24

Cephaloceles

ENCEPHALOCELES (encephalomeningoceles) are hernias of the brain protruding through a congenital opening of the skull, a cranium fissum. Cranial *meningoceles* are protrusions that do not contain brain. These malformations, both of which can be subsumed under the term "cephalocele," are, to a certain degree, analogous to spinal myelomeningocele and meningocele. Encephaloceles are closely related to exencephaly and anencephaly. If the protruding brain of an exencephaly deteriorates, anencephaly results. If it is covered by skin or epithelium, and persists, encephaloceles are formed.

Cranium bifidum and encephaloceles are less common anomalies than spina bifidas. In the material of Record and McKeown,[1] which dealt with fatal congenital malformations of the central nervous system, spina bifida was present in 45% of the cases, whereas encephalocele occurred in only 1.7%. In the

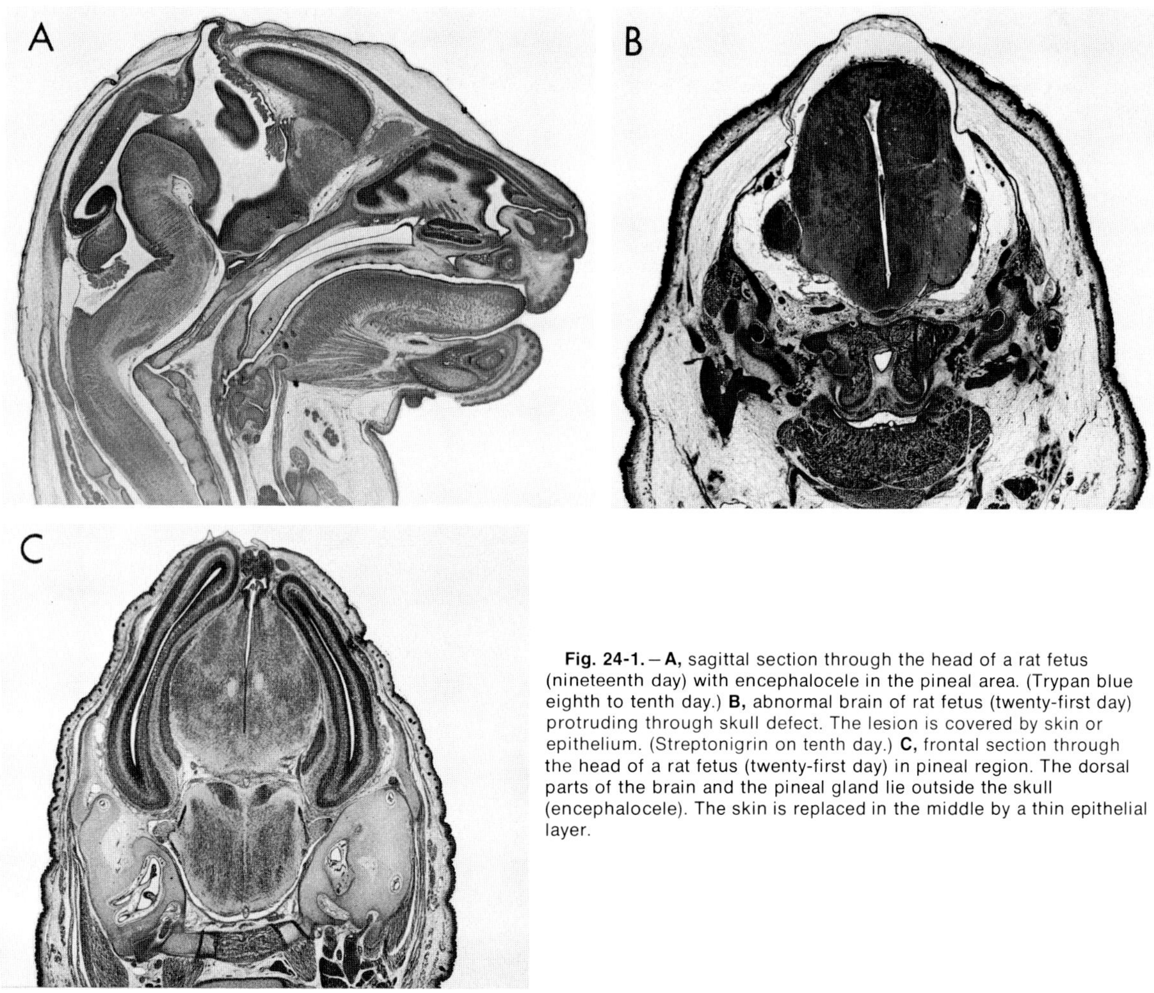

Fig. 24-1. – **A,** sagittal section through the head of a rat fetus (nineteenth day) with encephalocele in the pineal area. (Trypan blue eighth to tenth day.) **B,** abnormal brain of rat fetus (twenty-first day) protruding through skull defect. The lesion is covered by skin or epithelium. (Streptonigrin on tenth day.) **C,** frontal section through the head of a rat fetus (twenty-first day) in pineal region. The dorsal parts of the brain and the pineal gland lie outside the skull (encephalocele). The skin is replaced in the middle by a thin epithelial layer.

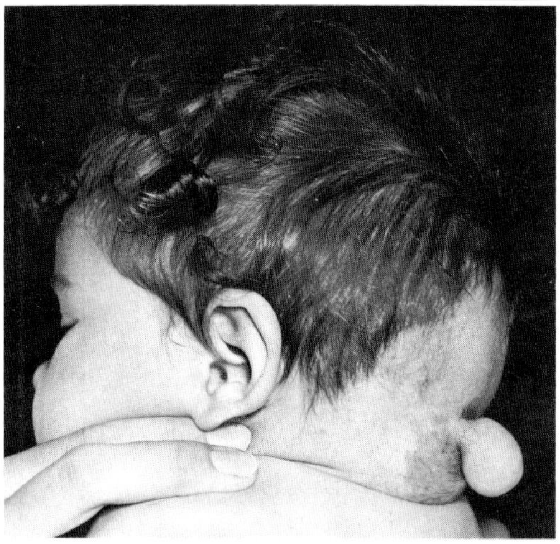

Fig. 24-2.—Pedunculated meningocele and hemangioma in occipital region. There was no osseous defect detectable in roentgenogram, but when the mass was excised the dura extruded through the pedicle, establishing a fistula.

clinical material of Ingraham and Matson,[2] which did not contain anencephalics or other nonviable infants with central nervous system lesions, spinal lesions were approximately six times more frequent than encephaloceles.

The etiology of encephaloceles occurring in children is not clear. In some cases, genetic determination is quite likely, since anencephaly, spina bifida or hydrocephaly occurring in families or kinships can alternate with encephalocele (p. 273). In most cases, the lesion is sporadic. Kappers[3] described an embryo 46 days old with exencephaly whose mother had had German measles 33 days after the beginning of pregnancy. Carr[4] observed an embryo with XO karyotype with an occipital protrusion that resembled an encephalocele; however, there was no connection with the brain, and the tumor was considered a lymphangioma. In experimental teratology, exencephalies are encountered frequently. Sometimes they are covered by skin or thin epithelium (Fig. 24-1) corresponding to encephaloceles in man. Giroud *et al.*[5] produced intranasal meningoceles and encephaloceles in mice by x-irradiation.

Cranial meningoceles usually are located over a small, well-defined bone defect and contain a hydropic arachnoidea covered by thin, hairless skin. The dura is absent. Sometimes cerebral elements can be discovered by histologic examination in a lesion that looks like a meningocele on superficial examination (Fig. 24-2). Cranium bifidum frontale in the area of the bregma sometimes is the point of exit for a meningocele. Meningoceles in the occipital area can assume large proportions.

Encephaloceles occur occasionally in the parietal, frontal, nasal or nasopharyngeal region, but the majority—about 70%—are found in the occipital area.[2] Occipital encephaloceles (Fig. 24-3) protrude through either an enlarged foramen magnum or the squama of the occipital bone. As a rule, the osseous opening is relatively small compared with the large protrusion of the sac. A sac, small at birth, can increase in size during the first months of life. Some encephaloceles are pedunculated, others are sessile on a broad base. Occipital lesions that sometimes have the size of a child's head may involve the neck region and be combined with cervical spina bifida. Some encephaloceles are covered by normal skin, others by a thin epithelium or by a parchment-like membrane that often shows necrotic areas. The contents of the sac are also variable and the size of the protrusion is not always indicative of the seriousness of the underlying malformation. Large cephaloceles may contain only fluid,

Fig. 24-3.—Occipital encephaloceles. (Courtesy of Dr. R. L. McLaurin, Cincinnati, Ohio.)

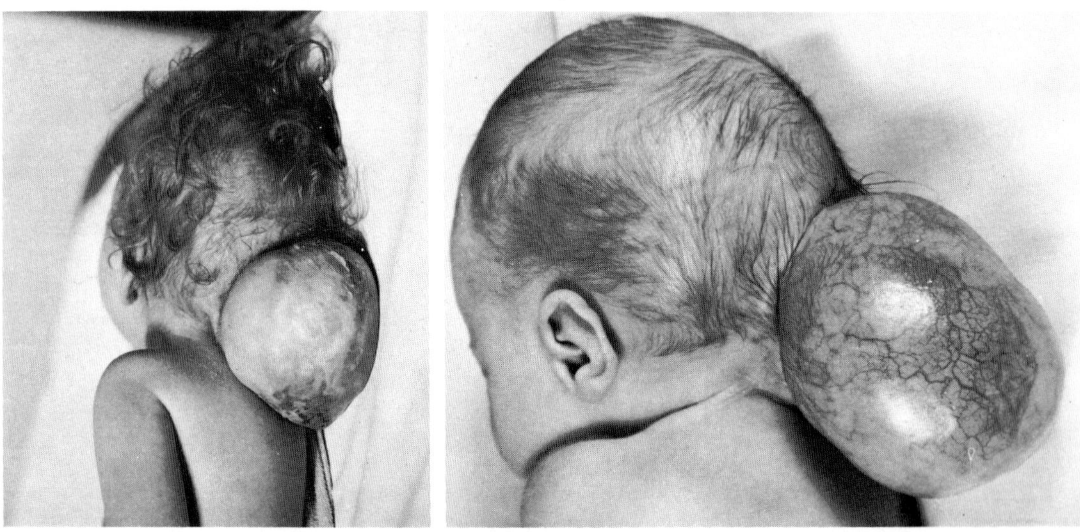

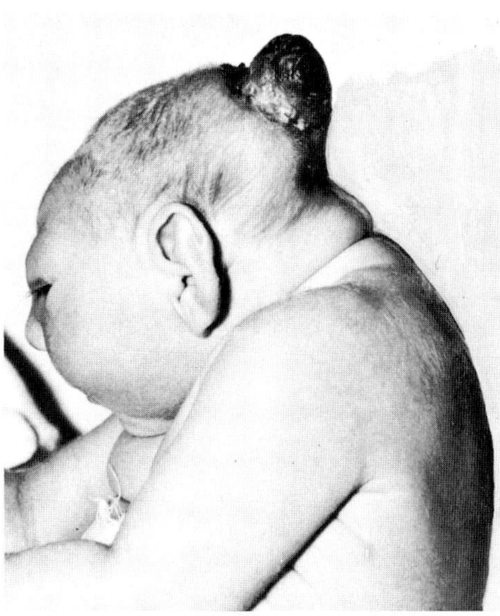

Fig. 24-4.—Child with microcephaly and encephalocele.

whereas small lesions can harbor a portion of the brain. Occipital encephaloceles sometimes are associated with hydrocephaly, since the anomaly can interfere with the circulation of the spinal fluid.

Lorber[6] reviewed the outlook of patients with occipital cephaloceles and concluded that the most important prognostic factor is the presence or absence of brain matter in the sac. He found hydrocephaly a common complication of occipital meningocele and encephalocele. Microcephaly and mental retardation are also common (Fig. 24-4). Most cases of occipital meningocele may be expected to survive without sequelae, but occipital encephalocele carries a high mortality risk, and survivors often are mentally and physically affected. Guthkelch[19] reported a follow-up of 74 patients operated on in a 17-year period. When no hydrocephaly developed, 86% of the cases of cranial meningocele showed normal mental development. With encephaloceles, however, only 40% had normal mental development.

A lethal syndrome of "coupled malformations" consisting of occipital encephalocele, ocular defects, arhinencephaly and polycystic liver and kidney was described by Gruber[7] in 1934. A case reported more recently by Marshall *et al.*[8] because of normal karyotype, despite its resemblance to the trisomy 13-15 syndrome, probably belonged in this group of "coupled" malformations. This child had—in addition to posterior encephalocele—microcephaly, unilateral microphthalmia, median cleft lip and bilateral cleft palate and polydactyly. Necropsy revealed a single ventricle of the forebrain, absence of the corpus callosum, cerebellum, pituitary and olfactory nerves, atrial septal defect and only one adrenal. Tierney[9] observed a child with occipital encephalocele, hydrocephaly and polycystic kidneys. The mother had delivered a hydrocephalic stillborn child before. Exencephaly combined with absence of the left lung was reported by Minne and Gernez.[10]

Cranial dermal sinus tracts are attributed to in-

Fig. 24-5.—Sagittal section through a newborn rat with meningocele (*M*) over pineal (*P*) area. Note thinning of skin over the small protuberance and sinus tract connecting the lesion with the subarachnoid space. (Trypan blue.)

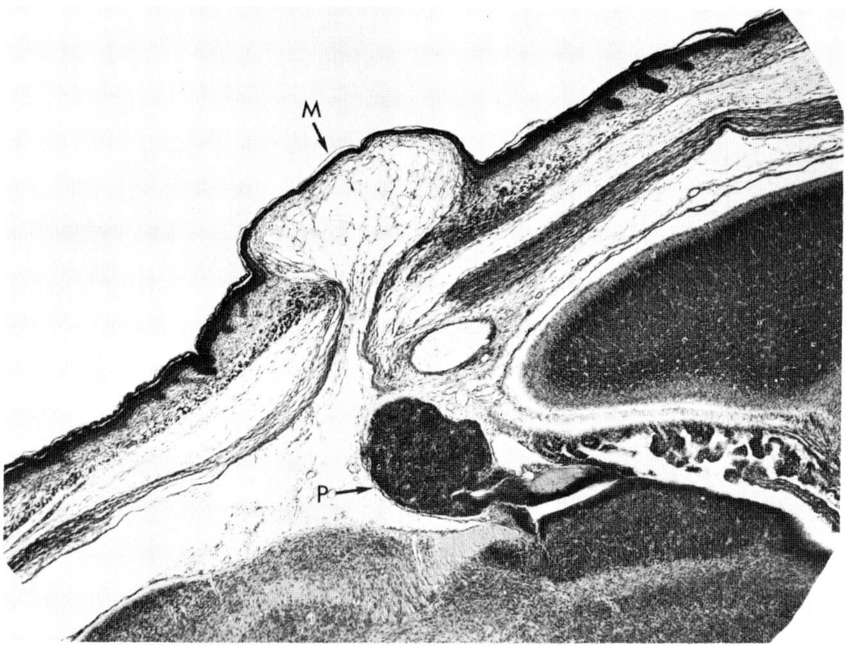

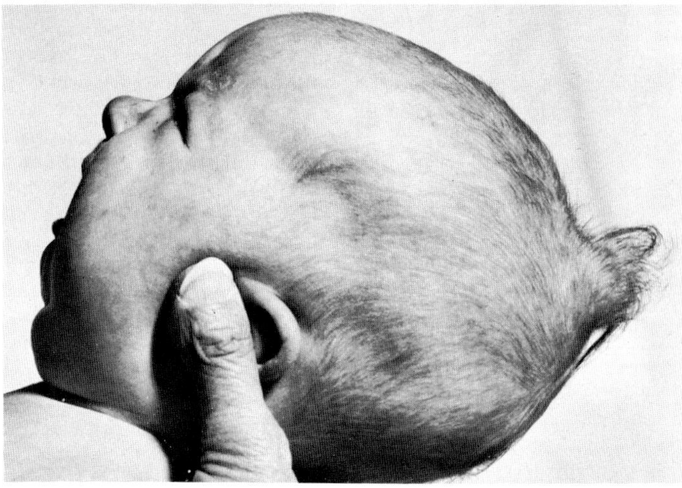

Fig. 24-6.—Parietal cephalocele covered by hair and skin. Compare with Figure 24-7.

complete separation of the neural ectoderm from the epithelial ectoderm. The tracts persist as ducts or channels lined with stratified squamous epithelium. Along the dermal sinuses, especially at their intracranial end, cystic enlargements occur that are epidermoids or dermoids. They may be palpated as subcutaneous masses or be located within the cranium. The tracts open externally on the skin near the midline and most frequently in the occipital region. The openings may be hidden by hair and be discovered only by careful examination. Sometimes the anomaly is betrayed by a vascular nevus, thickening of the scalp or by secretion of a thin fluid. The connection between the skin and the intracranial tissues represents a port of entry for microorganisms. Meningitis or an intracranial abscess can result from infection of such an abnormal communication.[2] The recognition of dermal sinus tracts often is difficult, since the external opening may be hidden or the subcutaneous swelling connected with it be mistaken for a simple dermoid or epidermoid cyst. Cranial dermal sinus tracts can be interpreted as mild forms of cranial cephaloceles. Like an occipital encephalocele,[7] the lesion can be associated with polydactyly. A boy observed in the Cincinnati Children's Hospital, born with postaxial supernumerary toes, an extra finger on the left hand and a small dermal lesion on the occipital scalp, developed meningitis after the scalp lesion was removed. He recovered after antibiotic treatment and closure of a dural defect in the posterior fossa (Children's Hospital Chart No. 122681).

Parietal cephaloceles usually protrude in the posterior parietal region but anterior to the lambda (Fig. 24-6). If the cephalocele appears more rostral (Fig. 24-7), it has graver implications than one at the more common site. These parietal lesions vary in size, are sessile or pedunculated, cystic and covered by modified skin. They may be meningoceles or encephaloceles.[11] In general, the prognosis is good in cases of parietal meningocele, but if they are combined with absence of the corpus callosum, mental retardation impairs the outlook. With parietal encephalocele, the prognosis is poor, particularly if the ventricular system is abnormal and brain participates in the hernia.

Fig. 24-7.—Huge encephalocele in parietal area. The child, a twin, died of intracranial hemorrhage.

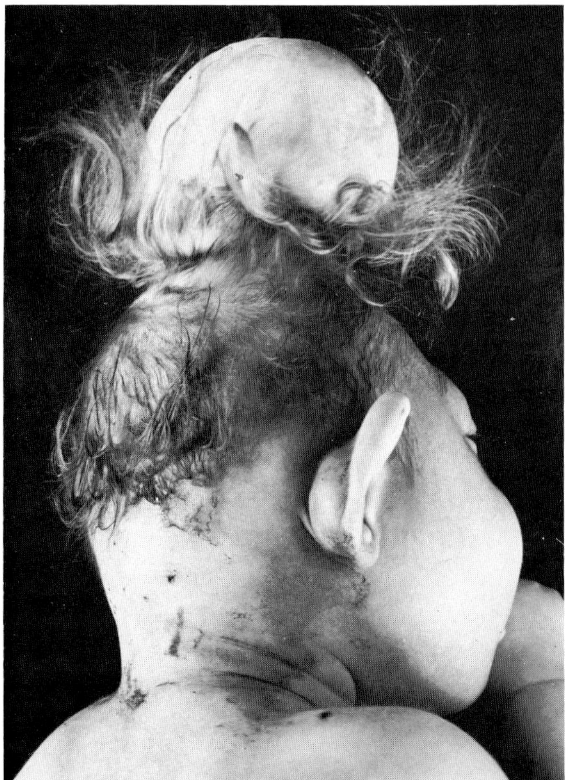

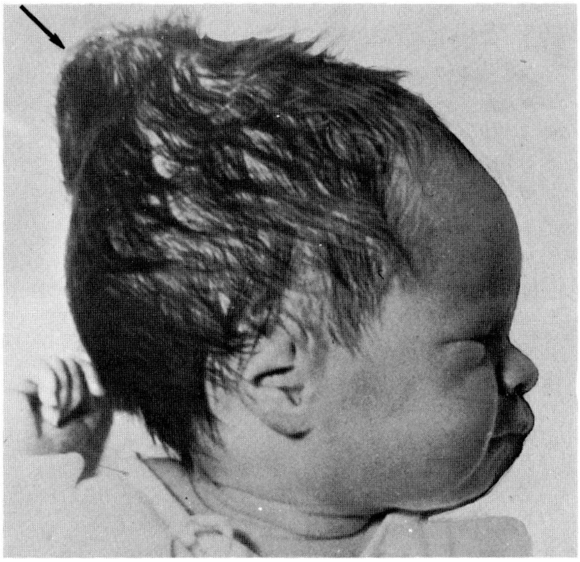

Fig. 24-8.—This lesion, which presented as an encephalocele (**arrow**), proved to be connected with a severe brain defect (absence of corpus callosum and septum pellucidum and porencephaly). (See Fig. 32:3, p. 254.)

Combination with hydrocephaly, Dandy-Walker malformation or agenesis of the corpus callosum has been observed (Fig. 24-8). If the cerebral participation consists merely of heterotopic glial rests, the outlook may be better. Management of these lesions was discussed by McLaurin.[11] Heterotopic brain tissue can be found under a flat circular midline lesion covered by modified skin in the parietal area.[12] Such brain tissue corresponds to nasal "gliomas" associated with nasal encephaloceles (Chapter 66).

A parietal encephalocele developing after birth in a boy born with a cranial defect on the right parietal bone, an umbilical hernia and loose skin was described by Dodge and Shillito.[13] By the time the boy was 14 months old, a large protrusion had developed over the skull defect, the mass communicating with the ventricular system. Although there were features of Ehlers-Danlos syndrome (p. 1186), the skin biopsy was not typical of this disorder. The patient died at the age of 2 years, 4 months with abdominal distention due to a large diverticulum of the bladder.

Encephaloceles can pass through defects of the cribriform plate into the nasopharynx. Such *nasal encephaloceles* sometimes manifest themselves in the newborn child by difficult respiration, nasal discharge and a soft gray mass in a nostril. The mass often is mistaken for a nasal polyp, but such polyps do not occur in the neonate. The obstruction of the nostril may not be noticeable until several months or years after birth when the tumor has enlarged to considera-

Fig. 24-9.—Nasofrontal encephalocele removed at age 4 months, metal plated at age 4 years. Speech delayed, but general development was normal. (Cincinnati Children's Hospital No. 32463.)

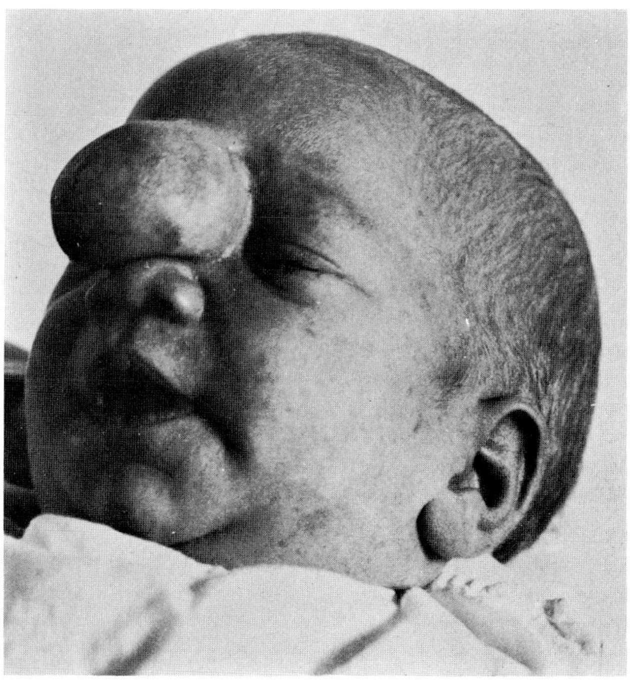

Fig. 24-10.—Nasofrontal encephalocele associated with microcephaly and hydrocephaly.

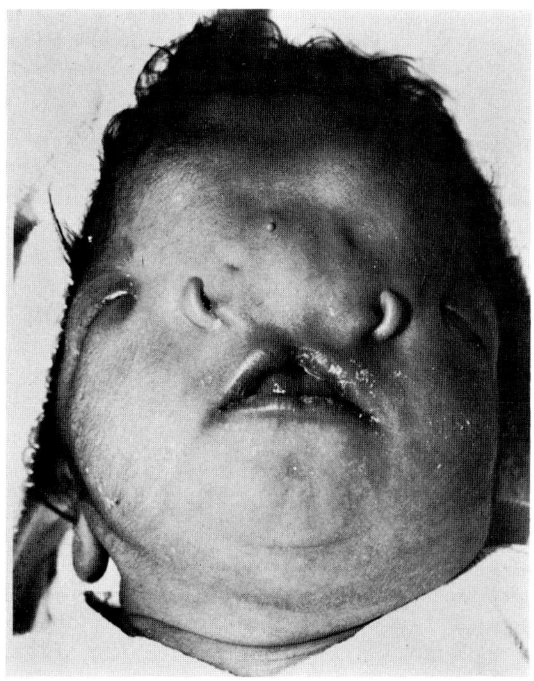

ble size. Rhinorrhea yielding cerebrospinal fluid can be a presenting symptom.[14] A nasopharyngeal encephalocele protruding through a cleft palate into the mouth was described by Ingraham and Matson.[2] A comparable lesion associated with posterior cleft palate and encroaching on the base of the tongue proved to be an encephalocele containing infundibulum, optic tracts and hypophysis.[15] Roentgenograms reveal a defect of the ethmoid bone in such cases. In other cases, the hernia passes through the orbital fissures into the orbit or into the pterygopalatine fossa. In older children and in adults, nasal encephaloceles can be distinguished from polyps by their fluctuation and by pulsation. As a rule, patients with nasal encephaloceles show marked hypertelorism. Unilateral nasal encephalocele may occur.[14]

Frontal encephaloceles manifest themselves by protrusion in the bregma, deformity of the nose, displacement of the eyes and hypertelorism (Fig. 24-10). They are closely related to nasal encephaloceles. Roentgenograms show skull defects of variable sizes involving the frontal, sphenoid and nasal bones.[2] Whereas frontal encephaloceles are rare in Europe and America, there seems to be a high incidence in Thailand. In Bangkok, Suwanwela and Hongsaprabhas[16] saw 25 cases in 3 years. The site of the cranial opening was at the junction between the frontal and ethmoid bones. Although all the lesions were congenital, some of the patients were not seen before puberty. Six of the lesions were associated with microcephaly and two with hydrocephaly. In two cases, the brain was exposed, resembling an area cerebrovasculosa. One of these microcephalic patients had a cerebral hemisphere with a single ventricle. Facial deformities and ocular anomalies were associated with the encephaloceles. Some of the patients were mentally retarded, others had normal mental development. No familial occurrence was observed.

Hereditary cranium bifidum occultum in the frontal area has been described by Terrafranca and Zellis[17] in three generations of a Negro family. In one case, the anomaly was associated with enlarged parietal foramina and spina bifida occulta in the cervical and lumbosacral regions. The frontal defects that corresponded to metopic fontanelles ossified with advancing age. It is doubtful, therefore, that this form of "cranium bifidum" is actually related to skull defects associated with lesions of the central nervous system.

As a rule, operation and removal of all types of encephaloceles is indicated. Ingraham and Matson[2] particularly recommended early removal of the pedunculated lesions to avoid infection and to make possible reasonable nursing and feeding procedures. In occipital lesions, malformations of the hindbrain may be present, causing hydrocephaly by interference with the circulation of the cerebrospinal fluid. In such cases, hydrocephaly and its relationship to the encephalocele can be demonstrated by ventriculograms, and attempts should be made to re-establish normal flow of the fluid. Neurosurgeons recommend removal of nasopharyngeal encephaloceles through a cranial approach although, occasionally, such a tumor has been successfully attacked through the nasal cavity.[18] Dermal sinus tracts and the cystic enlargements connected with them should be excised whenever they are recognized and, if possible, before infection has occurred. Extirpation of intracranial cysts connected with dermal sinus tracts requires craniectomy and exposure of the posterior fossa. It is obvious that tracts and cysts are difficult to treat after meningitis or abscess formation has set in.

REFERENCES

1. Record, R. G., and McKeown, T.: Congenital malformations of the central nervous system. 1. A survey of 930 cases, Brit. J. Social Med. 3:183, 1949.
2. Ingraham, F. D., and Matson, D. D.: *Neurosurgery of Infancy and Childhood* (Springfield, Ill.: Charles C Thomas, Publisher, 1954).
3. Kappers, J. A.: Developmental disturbance of the brain induced by German measles in an embryo of the 7th week, Acta anat. 31:1, 1957.
4. Carr, D. H.: Chromosome abnormalities and their influence on the development of the nervous system, International Copenhagen Cong. Sc. Study of Mental Retardation, 132–138, 1964.
5. Giroud, A., Martinet, M., and Deluchat, C.: Au sujets des méningocèles intra-nasaux, Bull. A. Anat. 449–452, 1966.
6. Lorber, J.: The prognosis of occipital encephalocele, Developmental Med. & Child Neurol., supp. 13, 75 pp., 1967.
7. Gruber, G. B.: Beiträge zur Frage "gekoppelter" Missbildungen (Akrocephalo-Syndactylie und Dysencephalia splanchnocystica), Beitr. path. Anat. 93:459, 1934.
8. Marshall, R., Newnham, R. E., Rawstron, J. R., Ellis, J. R., and Stevens, L. J.: Features of 13-15 trisomy syndrome with normal karyotype, Lancet 1:556, 1964.
9. Tierney, R.: Personal communication.
10. Minne, J., and Gernez, L.: Agénésie complète du poumon gauche chez un nouveau-nè exencéphale, Ann. anat. path. 10:503, 1933.
11. McLaurin, R. L.: Parietal cephaloceles, Neurology 14: 764, 1964.
12. Lee, C. M., Jr., and McLaurin, R. L.: Heterotopic brain tissue as an isolated embryonic rest, J. Neurosurg. 12:190, 1955.
13. Dodge, J. A., and Shillito, J., Jr.: Ehlers-Danlos syndrome associated with acquired encephalocele, J. Pediat. 66: 1061, 1965.
14. Mounier-Kuhn, P., Allegre, G., Charachon, R., and Tassin, M.: Méningo-encéphalocèle nasale, Confinia neurol. 25: 262, 1965.
15. Lau, B. P., and Newton, T. H.: Sphenopharyngeal encephalomeningocele, Radiol. clin. 34:386, 1965.
16. Suwanwela, C., and Hongsaprabhas, C.: Fronto-ethmoidal encephalomeningocele, J. Neurosurg. 25:172, 1966.
17. Terrafranca, R. J., and Zellis, A.: Congenital hereditary cranium bifidum occultum frontalis, with review of anatomical variations in lower midsagittal region of frontal bones, Radiology 61:60, 1953.
18. Finerman, W. B., and Pick, E. I.: Intranasal encephalomeningocele, Ann. Otol. 62:114, 1953.
19. Guthkelch, A. N.: Occipital cranium bifidum, Arch. Dis. Childhood 45:104, 1970.

25

Hydrocephaly

HYDROCEPHALY is characterized by an increase of free fluid in the cranial cavity. Accumulation of excessive fluid within the ventricular system gives rise to internal hydrocephaly, and fluid outside the brain to external hydrocephaly.

Incidence

Incidence figures vary greatly, which can be explained by inclusion or exclusion of stillbirths, of home deliveries, of patients with spina bifida and of cases developing in postnatal life. Alter[1] listed findings from different cities of Europe, Asia and North America, with variations from 0.3 to 4.2 per thousand births. Figures from Great Britain and the United States varied between 0.9 and 1.5 per thousand, but when hydrocephaly with spina bifida was included, incidence rates were between 1.3 and 2.9. In these reports, the highest rates came from Belfast, Ireland, where there is also a high rate of anencephalic births. If hydrocephaly with spina bifida is excluded, there is an excess of male hydrocephalics; if cases with spina bifida are included, there is an excess of female hydrocephalics. In some studies, a higher incidence of hydrocephaly was found among Negroes than among whites. Among Jewish children, anencephaly, spina bifida and hydrocephaly seemed to be less frequent than in non-Jewish populations.[2] In 69 necropsies of hydrocephalic patients, Malamud[3] found 31 instances of Arnold-Chiari malformation associated with spina bifida, 14 of aqueduct stenosis, 6 of atresia of the foramina of Magendie and Luschka and 18 of undetermined origin. External hydrocephaly is quite uncommon.

Etiology

Hydrocephaly is a symptom of many diverse disorders. Only those of prenatal origin will be considered here.

It is well known that hydrocephaly may occur in more than one child of a family. Schockaert and Janssens[4] reported the case of a woman who gave birth to 4 hydrocephalic children of both sexes. These investigators reviewed the literature in which even 6 and 7 cases in the same family are mentioned. In other sibships, hydrocephaly, anencephaly, encephalocele and spina bifida may alternate, thus suggesting a common causation of these anomalies. In some of these families there is also a tendency to spontaneous abortions and stillbirths. Polman[5] found that congenital malformations of the central nervous system as the cause of death were much more frequent in some provinces of Holland than in others. The incidence was particularly high in circumscribed areas characterized by inbreeding of the population. In some families, 2 to 4 children were affected either by the same

Fig. 25-1.—**A,** congenital hydrocephaly in a boy 1 month of age. The clinical diagnosis was "communicating hydrocephaly." Roentgenograms showed, in addition to ventricular enlargement, dilated cisternae and hypoplasia of the cerebellum. Necropsy revealed aqueduct stenosis. There was moderate atrophy of the cerebral cortex, microgyria and cerebellar and medullary hypoplasia. **B,** pedigree of the family of the patient shown in **A** (**arrow**). The parents were first cousins. Three boys and one girl had had hydrocephaly.

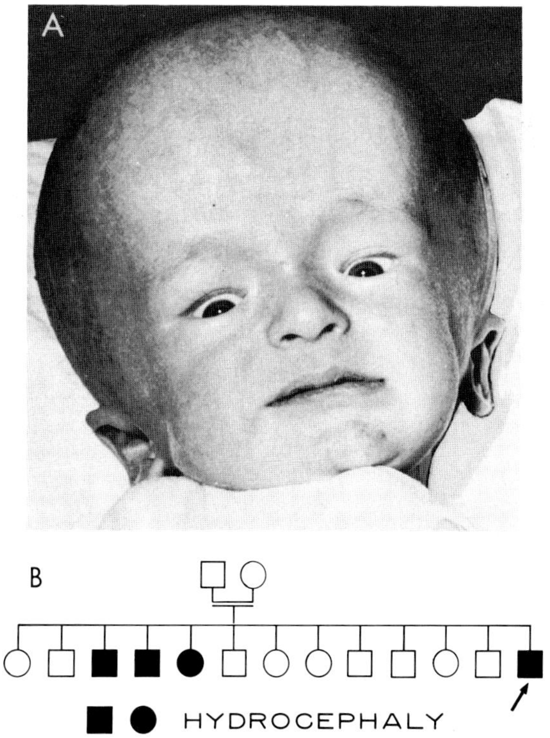

malformation of the central nervous system or by various forms alternately. Similar malformations occurred also in relatives of the parents or in their children. Polman concluded that in these districts inbreeding favored the appearence of such malformations, which could be attributed to recessive inheritance. The fact that a man might have children with such malformations with different wives[6] also suggests genetic determination. Borle[7] reviewed reports of familial hydrocephaly. The hereditary forms can be due to different genetic mechanisms, and they must not be considered an etiologic entity. As mentioned before, there are observations that suggest that, in some families, hydrocephaly is a recessively inherited trait.[5,8] Such cases can be due to aqueduct stenosis[9] (Fig. 25-1) or be associated with spina bifida.[10] In other families, hydrocephaly occurs as a sex-linked recessive trait that is also manifested by aqueduct stenosis.[11-15] Irregular dominant inheritance of hydrocephaly and incomplete fusion of fetal clefts (cleft palate, exstrophy of the bladder, spina bifida and encephalocele) was reported by Larson.[16] The Dandy-Walker malformation has been observed in siblings.[17,18]

Hydrocephaly may occur in such differing hereditary syndromes as osteopetrosis, achondroplasia,[19,20] platybasia,[21] the Klippel-Feil anomaly, Hurler syndrome, Tay-Sachs disease, tuberous sclerosis,[22] neurofibromatosis[23] and other hamartoses.[24]

Observations of twins with hydrocephaly support the view that the malformation is varied in origin. There are a few examples of monozygotic twins who were concordant in regard to hydrocephaly, but such cases are rare.[7,25,26] It is more common to find discordance in twins, but zygosity is rarely established in such cases.[2] Achondroplastic hydrocephalic monozygous twins have been reported.[19] The twins' hydrocephaly was associated with narrowing of the spaces around the base of the skull. In the same family there was another sibling whose hydrocephaly was due to aqueduct stenosis. Anencephaly in one twin and hydrocephaly with myelomeningocele in the other were observed by Symonds.[27]

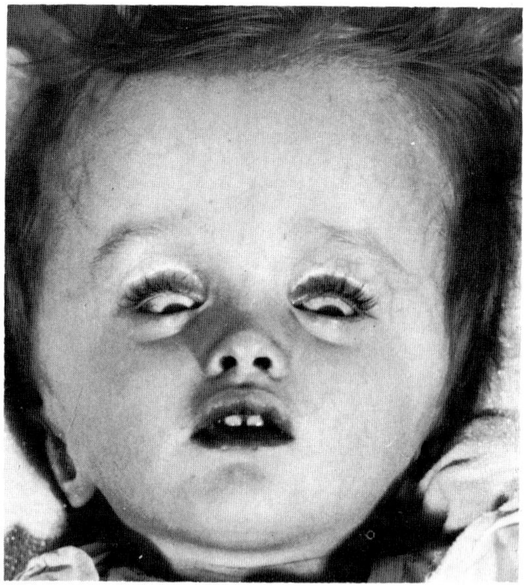

Fig. 25-2.—Hydrocephaly caused by prenatal toxoplasmosis.

Association of hydrocephaly with chromosomal anomalies has been observed, but the association is not close. In 32 necropsies of infants with trisomy 13-15, hydrocephaly was noted 4 times, and there were 4 hydrocephalics among 84 necropsies of children with trisomy 18.[28] Hydrocephaly was present in a child with B/G translocation.[29]

Not all cases of hydrocephaly are genetically determined. Congenital syphilis can result in hydrocephaly, but enlargement of the head usually develops after birth. It is well established that fetal toxoplasmosis or cytomegalic inclusion disease can result in hydrocephaly (Fig. 25-2) (p. 78).[30,31] Hydrocephaly has been observed in a newborn infant whose mother had had epidemic hepatitis in the first trimester of preg-

Fig. 25-3.—Obstructive congenital hydrocephaly in a boy 4 months of age. Necropsy showed almost complete atrophy of brain tissue. The head was reported to be of normal size at birth but measured 61 cm. at 4 months.

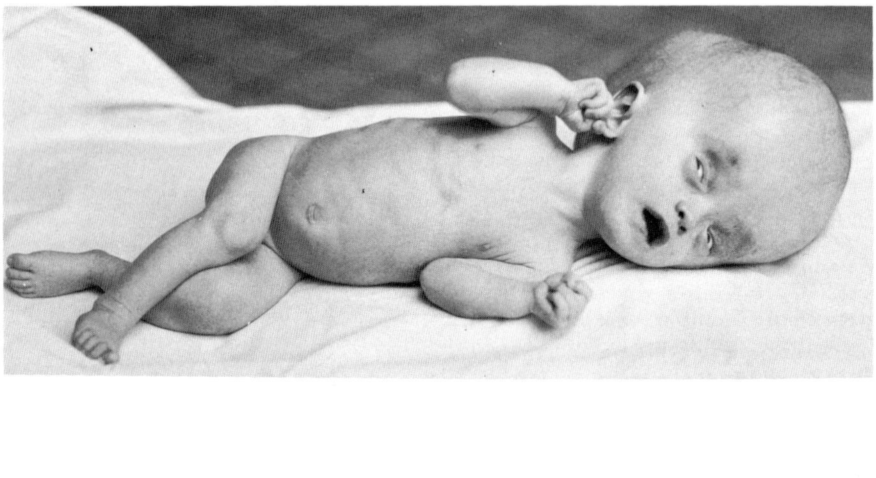

nancy[32]; it has been reported as a consequence of intrauterine meningitis[33] and of intrauterine fungal infection.[34,35] Prenatal or perinatal hemorrhage can result in hydrocephaly appearing soon after birth.[23,36] Epidemics of congenital hydrocephaly have been reported.[37] An association between births of hydrocephalic children and increasing maternal age has been found in several studies.[2]

Congenital papilloma of the choroid plexus, which accounts for 5% of intracranial tumors in childhood,[38] has been recognized repeatedly as a cause of hydrocephaly.[39] In most cases of hydrocephaly, the cause remains obscure. Association with prematurity and postmaturity has been reported. Hydramnios is present in approximately 10% of the cases. Larson and Banner[40] reported that of 62 hydrocephalic infants 27 were stillborn. Breech presentation occurred in about 30% of the cases.

Pathogenesis

Various mechanisms have been suggested to explain the formation of hydrocephaly—which is justified, since etiologies of the malformation differ. A block in the normal circulation of the cerebrospinal fluid (CSF) is considered the most frequent cause of the anomaly, but overproduction of fluid has been established in some cases. There are many gaps in the knowledge of the CSF circulation and in the explanation of many forms of hydrocephaly.

Conventional descriptions assign the formation of the CSF to the choroid plexuses and its absorption to the arachnoid spaces and villi. The fluid formed in the lateral ventricles flows through the foramina of Monro into the third ventricle and from there through the sylvian aqueduct into the fourth ventricle. It leaves the ventricular system through the foramina of Luschka and Magendie and reaches the cisterna magna. From there, the fluid is distributed through the basal cisterna, the cisterna ambiens and other subarachnoid spaces to the pia-arachnoid covers of the cerebral and cerebellar hemispheres. Caudally, the cisterna magna is in broad communication with the subarachnoid spaces of the spinal cord. The fluid is returned to the circulating blood through arachnoid villi or through the capillaries of the subarachnoid spaces. It leaves also, to a lesser extent, through perineural spaces of the cranial and spinal nerves to reach lymphatic pathways.

This concept represents, at best, a simplification of the CSF physiology. Hassin[41] insisted that the CSF represents the tissue fluids of the brain and that the absorption of the CSF is effected by the perineural spaces of the cranial nerves and spinal roots. The function of the choroid plexus is excretion and elimination of noxious substances but not secretion of fluid. Bering[42] found that CSF of unchanged composition can be formed after the choroid plexus has been removed and that in hydrocephaly fluid can originate elsewhere. It seems that the ventricular system produces only 60% of the fluid, whereas 40% is formed in the subarachnoid space. The arachnoid villi absorb only a small portion of the fluid. The sinuses, veins, brain substance and the dural venous sinuses participate in the absorption. Although the CSF generally flows from the ventricles to the surface of the brain, the flow sometimes is reversed, as shown by tracers that, when placed into the subarachnoid space, appear occasionally in the ventricle. The fluid in the aqueduct moves backward and forward with each heart beat. The intraventricular pressure can be influenced by venous obstructions, by the osmotic pressure of the blood serum, by metabolic disturbances and by other factors.[42]

The circulation of the CSF can be blocked in several places. If one foramen of Monro is closed, unilateral accumulation of fluid occurs.[43] Obstruction of the aqueduct results in dilatation of the third and lateral ventricles. Occlusion of Magendie's and Luschka's foramina leads to enlargement of all four ventricles. These forms of hydrocephaly are considered obstructive. Hydrocephaly may develop also in the presence of free communication between the ventricular system and the spinal subarachnoid space. It is thought that in communicating forms a block exists in the cerebral subarachnoid spaces that normally take up the bulk of the spinal fluid leaving the ventricles. If dye is introduced into a lateral ventricle, it appears in the lumbar space within a few minutes. If the dye does not appear within 20 minutes in the lumbar spinal fluid, obstructive hydrocephaly is diagnosed.[44]

Noncommunicating hydrocephaly of the third and lateral ventricles is attributed to obliteration or stenosis of the aqueduct. Different shapes of the aqueduct may be seen in cross section, or, more often, several narrow channels are present that are lined with normal ependyma and situated in the area in which the aqueduct is normally located. Separated by nerve tissue, they may end blindly or connect the third and fourth ventricles. Forking is considered a congenital malformation since it usually is associated with other structural changes of the central nervous system and no signs of inflammation are found (see Fig. 25-9, *D*). Gliosis of the aqueduct also causes stenosis of the cerebrospinal pathways, but it was doubted by Russell[45] that this anomaly is congenital. Occasionally, a neuroglial septum or a vascular anomaly causes an obstacle to the circulation of the spinal fluid, resulting in hydrocephaly. Alvord[46] believed that the aqueduct normally is just sufficient to allow adequate amounts of CSF to pass under pressure of approximately 100 mm. of water. It can permit moderate variations in rate of production of CSF without undue increase in third ventricular pressure, but a stenotic aqueduct cannot. In addition to anatomic stenosis there are physiologic variations in CSF production and tissue resistance, factors that contribute to fluid accumulation rostral to the aqueduct.

Cysts at the level of the incisura tentorii are rare obstacles to CSF flow. They were considered cerebellar meningoencephaloceles by Alvord.[46] Congenital atresia of the foramina of Magendie and Luschka or maldevelopment of the cerebellum results in dilatation of the lateral, third and fourth ventricles and of the aqueduct. A large cyst-like structure is formed in the posterior fossa that displaces the cerebellar hemispheres and interferes with growth of the vermis. Elevation of the tentorium, torcular and transverse sinuses accompanies this noncommunicating hydrocephaly. Such Dandy-Walker cysts are rare.[18] Diffuse melanosis[24,47,48] and other congenital neoplasms may also result in abnormal accumulation of fluid in the ventricular system.[45] Association with vascular malformations has been observed in newborn infants[49] and in adults.[50] Progress of hydrocephaly is most rapid with a blocked aqueduct of Sylvius; it is somewhat lessened with a blockage of the outlets of the fourth ventricle and decreases as the block to flow gets more and more caudal.[42]

Obstruction of the spinal fluid pathways and hydrocephaly can be caused by skeletal malformations of the base of the skull (p. 907). In platybasia, the basi-occipital bone is foreshortened, the atlas is fused to the occiput and the occipital foramen is narrow. Congenital hydrocephaly has been observed repeatedly under such conditions. In achondroplastic infants, the posterior fossa and the occipital foramen are small, and obstruction in the area of the hindbrain results in hydrocephaly. In some cases of this type, the relationship of bone and central nervous system is capable of readjustment in postnatal life, thus leading to arrested hydrocephaly.[45] Enlargement of the head in achondroplasia does not always indicate hydrocephaly; it may be due to megalencephaly.[20] Hydrocephaly in osteopetrosis is attributed to general thickening of the bones of the cranial base, which causes narrowing of the occipital foramen and of the foramina of the cranial nerves, with obstruction of circulation of CSF.

Hydrocephaly occurring in congenital toxoplasmosis may be present before or develop soon after birth. In such cases, the encephalomyelitic process destroys the ependymal lining of the ventricular system, and occlusion of the aqueduct or of the foramina of Monro results.[30]

The relationship of hydrocephaly to spina bifida and the Arnold-Chiari malformation represents an interesting but puzzling problem. Alvord[46] reviewed this controversial subject and listed 14 explanations offered by various authors. A critical analysis shows that many of the theories are compatible with one another and not contradictory. Myelomeningoceles are commonly associated with caudal displacement of the medulla oblongata and of a cerebellar process into the spinal canal. In fact, the entire spinal cord seems to be displaced caudad, since the upper cervical nerve roots descend from their intervertebral foramina toward the spinal cord, the caudal end of which is fixed in the sacral canal. In some cases, the foramina of Luschka and Magendie are located below the foramen magnum and permit communication of the ventricular fluid with the spinal subarachnoid space, but return of the fluid to the cerebral surface is not possible, since the foramen magnum is obstructed by the cerebellar process and the medulla (communicating hydrocephaly).[45] In other cases, the Arnold-Chiari malformation is associated with a noncommunicating hydrocephaly, with obstruction at the level of the fourth ventricle and foramen magnum[51] or at the level of the aqueduct. It is believed that the communicating and obstructive types are about equally common.[46]

Lichtenstein[52] attributed hydrocephaly with myelomeningocele to traction on the mesencephalon (and resulting aqueduct stenosis) owing to fixation of the spinal cord in the lumbosacral area, at the site of the vertebral defect. Such traction downward would also be the cause of the Arnold-Chiari malformation. The traction theory is suggested by the caudad course of the cervical spinal nerves from the intervertebral foramina toward the spinal cord, the reverse of the normal direction. But careful examination of angulation of all spinal nerves by Barry *et al.*[53] revealed that in thoracic and some lower levels the course of the nerves is essentially normal and does not indicate a caudad pull. There are other objections to the traction theory. Hydrocephaly is comparatively rare in pure sacral spina bifida.[54,55] The Arnold-Chiari malformation has been observed in a fetus with myelomeningocele of only 10 weeks' gestational age, i.e., long before ascent of the spinal cord occurs.[56] The Arnold-Chiari complex has been seen in the absence of spina bifida or combined with spina bifida in the cervical or thoracic region.[45] Experimental tethering of the spinal cord in newborn rats and in opossum fetuses did not result in Arnold-Chiari malformation.[57]

Attempts to explain spina bifida as the result of hydrocephaly[58,59] have also failed. It appears likely that a common denominator for myelomeningocele, Arnold-Chiari malformation and hydrocephaly exists in embryonic life[53,56] and not in conditions present at birth.[60]

Many cerebral anomalies accompany spina bifida and the Arnold-Chiari malformation.[51,61] The massa intermedia is enlarged, the falx cerebri underdeveloped and the great longitudinal cerebral fissure partially obliterated as the hemispheres are pressed together in the midline. The thalami appear fused together and the corpora quadrigemina are represented by a single mass. There is generalized microgyria and projecting heterotopic gray matter in the walls of the lateral ventricles. There also are malformations of the cerebellum, the posterior fossa is reduced in size and the tentorium attached nearer the foramen magnum than normal. In contrast to Lichtenstein,[52] who attributed the caudal displacement of the brain stem and cerebellum to pull from below, Cameron[61] believed that leakage of cerebrospinal fluid through the myeloschisis into the amniotic cavity results in reduced intraventricular and increased amniotic pressure. As a result, the cranial contents are forced through the foramen magnum into the vertebral canal "as toothpaste is squeezed out of a tube." The original "oligohydrocephaly" is converted into hydrocephaly by the Arnold-Chiari malformation, and aqueduct stenosis results from the external squeeze. One does not have to agree with this simple mechanical explanation, but the overcrowding within the cranial cavity probably is an important contribution to the formation of hydrocephaly associated with spina bifida. The intracranial contents are too large for the cranium, and they extend into the cervical vertebral canal, establishing a vicious circle by interfering with the proper exit of the CSF. Subsequently, the relatively large brain is further enlarged by increase of its ventricular fluid and development of hydrocephaly. The situation is made worse if aqueduct stenosis or obliteration occurs. There is an absolute as well as a relative decrease in the size of the aqueduct from the second fetal month to the time of birth[62] (Fig. 25-4). In postnatal life there is again an increase in size. Bickers and Adams[11] pointed out that narrowing may be excessive in prenatal life or growth retarded in postnatal life, both processes leading to stenosis. The maintenance of a proper lumen with progressive growth of the brain and changing production of cerebrospinal fluid apparently is a precarious developmental process that is likely to be disturbed under abnormal growth conditions of the brain. Such growth disturbances can affect chiefly the midbrain or, in association with spina bifida, the contents of the posterior fossa. It appears that, in the latter case, the malformations of the brain, the cord and the skeleton have a common origin in early prenatal life without being caused by one another. Mechanical conditions present at birth cannot account for the association of all the anomalies found in children with spina bifida. Some of the malformations of the brain may not be more dependent on the spina bifida than malformations of the kidney or the heart that occur occasionally in association with spina bifida. This point sometimes is illustrated by animal experiments when, after administration of a teratogen, one young is born with spina bifida and in the same litter others are born with hydrocephaly without spina bifida (p. 225). But the probability of cerebral anomalies predisposing to hydrocephaly is high when myelomeningocele is present.

One should expect that increased accumulation of fluid and increased pressure within the ventricular system existing in cases of communicating hydrocephaly should keep the communications open and even enlarge them. But this is not always the case, and communicating hydrocephaly can be converted in postnatal life into the obstructive form, particularly by closure of the aqueduct. Hemorrhage into the ventricular or cisternal system or infections ascending from a spina bifida can result in reactions of glia or connective tissue sufficient to occlude the aqueduct or the foramina of Monro.[23,36] An interesting observation was made by Foltz and Shurtleff,[63] who described such conversion in children with ventricular shunt. It seemed that overstretching of the aqueductal walls by the expanding hydrocephaly at first caused separation of ependymal cells and scarring of the lining. When the pressure was relieved by the shunt, the aqueduct collapsed, the walls came in contact and grew together. Similar effects may result from pressure changes without surgical shunt.

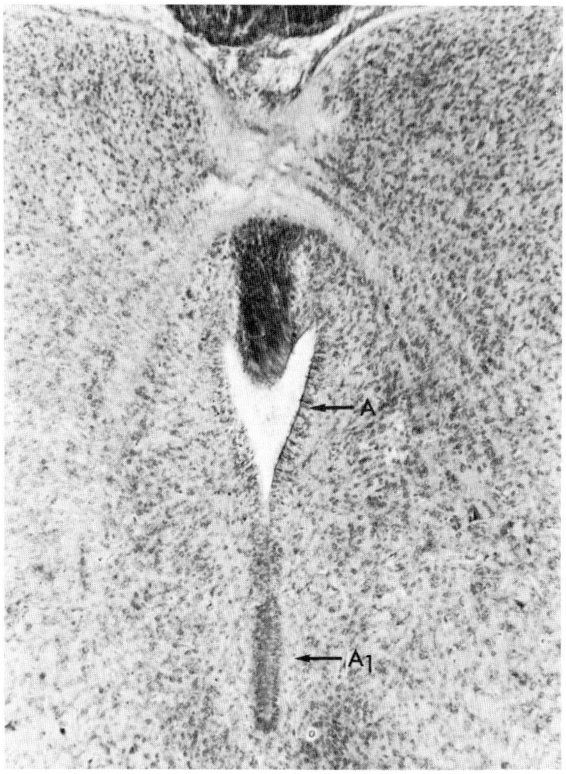

Fig. 25-4.—Frontal section through the head of a control rat fetus (twenty-first day) in pineal region. Even normally, the aqueduct (*A*) appears closed in its lower (ventral) aspects (A_1) about the time of birth.

Most of the explanations of hydrocephaly associated with myelomeningocele are offered by clinicians and pathologists whose experience is derived from children after birth and from observations far removed in time from the early stages of development. A better picture is obtained from descriptions of human fetuses and experimental animals that show early stages of spina bifida, the brain and cerebellum without secondary changes caused by birth trauma and infection. The observations by Barry *et al.*[53] dealing with three embryos of 49 mm. (10 weeks' estimated fertilization age), 141 mm. (17 weeks) and 160 mm. (18 weeks) revealed early overgrowth of the central nervous system involving different areas to different degrees. There was overgrowth of the spinal cord at the level of the myeloschisis, and the length of the spinal cord segments immediately cephalic to the defect was greater than normal in the two older fetuses. But the excessive length was less noticeable in higher levels, and within four or five segments the spinal cord appeared normal so that the tension exerted by the anchoring of the myeloschisis seemed dissipated within five segments. Angulation of the spinal nerves in the thoracic and lower cervical segments did not indicate any caudad pull exerted by the spina bifida even though an Arnold-Chiari malformation was present in the older fetuses. Of prime importance was the finding of enlargement of the brain and reduction in size of the posterior fossa. Furthermore, hydrocephaly was present in the oldest fetus even though the aqueduct was patent. Well-preserved human fetuses with spina bifida are only rarely obtained. It is, therefore, useful to supplement observations gained in human specimens with findings in animal fetuses that have similar malformations (p. 29). Brocklehurst[97] made a quantitative study of a 95-mm. (16-week) fetus with spina bifida. He concluded that this fetus did not contain an over-all excess of neural tissue, but rather less than normal. The appearance of crowding in the posterior fossa was due to a disturbance in volume relation between structures of mesodermal and neurectodermal origin.

There is a natural tendency to explain pathogenesis of hydrocephalies by mechanical changes. But there are observations that indicate that more subtle factors may be at work. Drugs, poisons and vitamins can change the fluid content of the ventricular system.[42] Children with vitamin A deficiency sometimes develop increased CSF pressure that disappears rapidly after administration of vitamin A,[64] and hypervitaminosis A can also cause acute hydrocephaly (Marie-Sée[65] syndrome).[66]

The pathogenesis of hydrocephaly can be studied in animals. Hydrocephaly occurs spontaneously in swine, cattle,[67] dogs, rabbits and mice. In the mouse, several hereditary types have been observed and analyzed.[68-70] A congenital hydrocephaly lethal at birth (Ch) has been described in mice as a recessive trait. Shortening of the basicranium is held responsible for this type of hydrocephaly. The telencephalon is forced upward and the caudal parts of the brain are telescoped and wedged against the osteogenic membrane.[68] The crowding of the cerebellum and medulla oblongata results in a situation comparable to the Arnold-Chiari complex and subsequently in hydrocephaly. Another type of hydrocephaly (hy-1), also recessively inherited, permits survival of the mice to the age of 3–6 weeks. Although obstruction of the aqueduct occurs, embryologic studies showed that the entire ventricular system, including the fourth ventricle, is dilated from the twelfth day of prenatal life on. Increased production of CSF caused by early disturbance of the embryo's fluid balance was considered responsible for the early general hydrocephaly, whereas the obstruction of the aqueduct seemed to be a secondary and late complication.[68] Another hydrocephaly (hy-3) is caused by a block due to degeneration of the meninges, which begins around the time of birth.[70] In the "Dreher" mouse (dr), the origin of hydrocephaly could be traced to thickening of the roof of the fourth ventricle present in embryos of 11 days. The foramen of Magendie is not formed, CSF accumulates in the entire ventricular system and malformations of the cerebellum develop. The aqueduct remains open or is slightly narrowed by pressure of the growing cerebral hemispheres.[69] The importance of these observations in embryonic mice lies in the fact that the origins of hydrocephaly can be traced to very early embryonic deviations that have little resemblance to the observations at the time of birth.

Hydrocephaly and related conditions can be produced experimentally in various mammals by interference with development during the organogenic period of gestation. Trypan blue injections into the mother[71] (Fig. 25-5, *A*), maternal vitamin A deficiency,[72,73] folic acid and vitamin B_{12} deficiencies,[74,75] riboflavin deficiency combined with galactoflavin administration,[76] hypervitaminosis A,[77] administration of salicylates,[78] x-irradiation and many other teratogenic methods have resulted in hydrocephaly. Despite the availability of hydrocephalic fetuses, the mechanisms leading to enlargement of the ventricular system have not been fully elucidated. In many of the young made hydrocephalic by trypan blue treatment, aqueduct stenosis or obliteration is found (Fig. 25-5, *A*). This offers a seemingly satisfactory explanation for the enlargement of the lateral and third ventricles. But some of the young have hydrocephaly even though the aqueduct is patent.[71,79,80] (See Fig. 25-9, *B*.) Such exceptions deserve attention, since they may indicate that—as in hy-1 mice—the aqueduct stenosis is the result of CSF accumulation caused by a preceding unknown mechanism. If the aqueduct closes, a vicious circle is initiated by further increase of CSF in the ventricles rostral to the obstruction. That increased secretion of CSF may precede aqueduct stenosis was also shown in newborn rabbits made hydrocephalic by vitamin A deficiency. Millen *et al.*[72] thought that the determining factor might be overproduction of CSF, a belief supported by observations of children with vitamin A deficiency who developed increased CSF pressure.[64] Hydrocephaly resulting from vitamin B_{12} deficiency is also unexplained. Although it is associated with partial or complete closure of the aqueduct, it is not clear whether the stenosis is the cause of the hydrocephaly or the result of a more primary defect.[75] Occlusion of the cerebral aq-

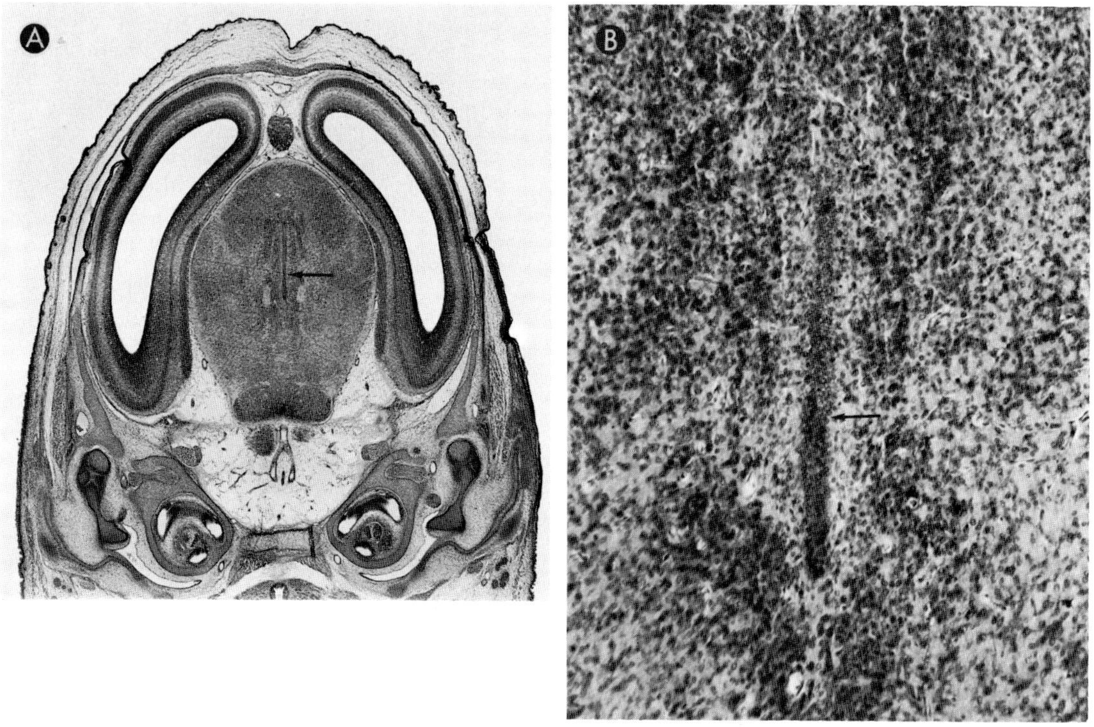

Fig. 25-5.—**A,** frontal section through the head of a rat fetus (twentieth day) showing hydrocephaly and closed aqueduct (**arrow**). The ependymal lining is still clearly seen. (Trypan blue eighth to tenth day.) **B,** frontal section through the head of a rat fetus (twenty-first day) with hydrocephaly. The aqueduct (**arrow**) is closed but ependyma is still visible in ventral portion with modification in dorsal part. (Methyl salicylate ninth day.) (Compare with Fig. 25-4.)

Fig. 25-6.—Sagittal section through the head of a mouse fetus (nineteenth day) showing communicating hydrocephaly involving all ventricles and deficiency all nerve tissue. Cerebellum is absent and the mesencephalic tectum thin (riboflavin deficiency plus galactoflavin). (From H. Kalter and J. Warkany.[76])

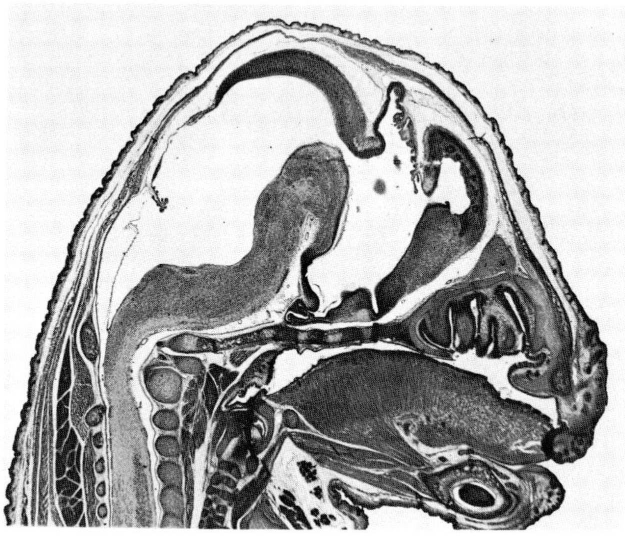

ueduct—if present—was also attributed to absence of specialized columnar ependymal cells in the roof of the aqueduct and posterior part of the roof of the third ventricle that were thought to secrete fluid into the embryonic ventricular system before the choroid plexus is fully developed.[81]

Hydrocephaly produced in mice by a riboflavin-deficient diet combined with galactoflavin administration[76] is characterized by cystic enlargement of all ventricles, including the fourth, and an enlarged aqueduct (Fig. 25-6). The enlargement of the ventricular system can be seen in embryos as soon as the treatment is finished (13 days), and it remains combined with a persisting area membranacea anterior, reduction in size of the cerebellum and reduction in thickness of the cerebral cortex.[82]

Since trypan blue or salicylate administration can produce hydrocephaly, spina bifida and the Arnold-Chiari malformation in rats,[78,83-85] one can examine the relationship of these anomalies to one another. It is commonly assumed that a myelomeningocele causes the Arnold-Chiari complex, which, in turn, results in hydrocephaly. It is of interest, therefore, that we observed in some litters of treated rats that these malformations can occur independently of one another.

The crowding seen in the midbrain and hindbrain of near-term fetuses (Fig. 25-7, *B* and *C*) with spina

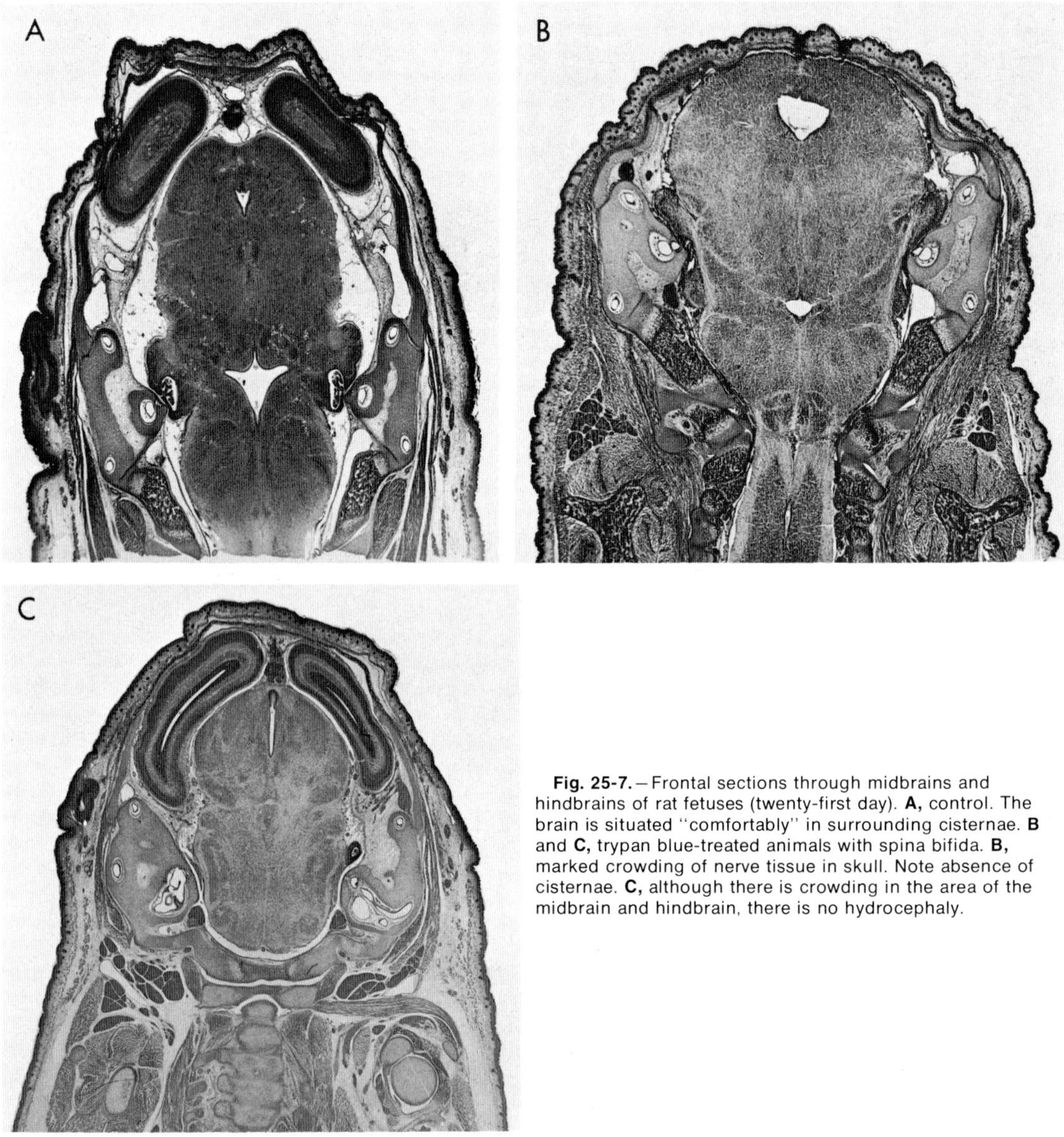

Fig. 25-7.—Frontal sections through midbrains and hindbrains of rat fetuses (twenty-first day). **A,** control. The brain is situated "comfortably" in surrounding cisternae. **B** and **C,** trypan blue-treated animals with spina bifida. **B,** marked crowding of nerve tissue in skull. Note absence of cisternae. **C,** although there is crowding in the area of the midbrain and hindbrain, there is no hydrocephaly.

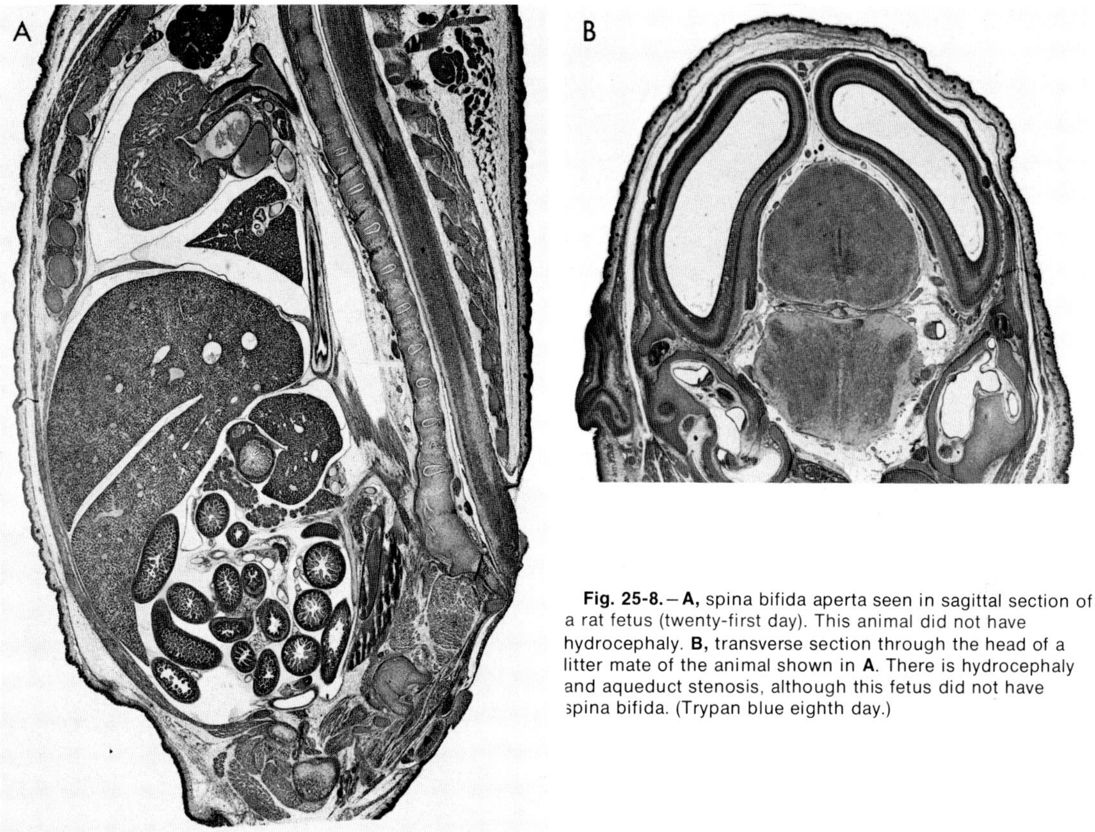

Fig. 25-8.—**A,** spina bifida aperta seen in sagittal section of a rat fetus (twenty-first day). This animal did not have hydrocephaly. **B,** transverse section through the head of a litter mate of the animal shown in **A**. There is hydrocephaly and aqueduct stenosis, although this fetus did not have spina bifida. (Trypan blue eighth day.)

bifida is associated with spina bifida but not with hydrocephaly. It is not possible to state whether or not hydrocephaly would develop after birth in such animals. More important is the fact that, in some of the young, a spina bifida aperta may be associated with no or only slight enlargement of the third and lateral ventricles, whereas in litter mates without spina bifida marked hydrocephaly with aqueduct stenosis is present. Figure 25-8, *A* shows in sagittal section a spina bifida aperta in a rat fetus that had no hydrocephaly. But its litter mate that had no spina bifida had hydrocephaly with aqueduct stenosis, as shown in Figure 25-8, *B*. The hydrocephaly illustrated in the frontal section in Figure 25-5, *A* is from an animal that did not have spina bifida. A litter mate with spina bifida had no hydrocephaly. Such dissociation of spina bifida and hydrocephaly in litter mates suggests that these malformations sometimes are parallel phenomena rather than cause and effect. Some observations in man support this view. In a large kindred reported by Polman[5] with an unusually high incidence of malformations of the central nervous system, there were children who had spina bifida and hydrocephaly; but there also were children who had only spina bifida and children with only hydrocephaly.

Another observation made in hydrocephalic near-term rat fetuses was that the enlargement of the ventricles may be present in brains with closing (Fig. 25-9, *B*) but not closed aqueducts that still have their ependymal lining (see Fig. 25-5). In other specimens, forking can be seen as described in human cases[45] (Fig. 25-9, *D*). The relationship of the malformations to one another has not been sufficiently investigated to permit definite conclusions concerning the pathogenesis of hydrocephaly induced by teratogenic methods. In general, one has the impression that the size of the brain is too large for the size of the cranial cavity and that crowding exists. Growth of the central nervous system and that of its surrounding tissues are not well coordinated. Such disorganization can be brought about by abnormal genes or by environmental teratogenic factors acting early in embryogenesis.

It seems that hydrocephaly is a tragedy limited to mammals. The subarachnoid spaces, which are important for CSF resorption, are not present in phylogenesis until the birds appear.[42] There exists in mammals a normal and physiologic narrowness of the aqueduct of Sylvius at the time of birth (see Fig. 25-4). The perinatal stresses, with their tendency to hemorrhage and infection, contribute to the danger of CSF obstruction. It is understandable that at or soon after

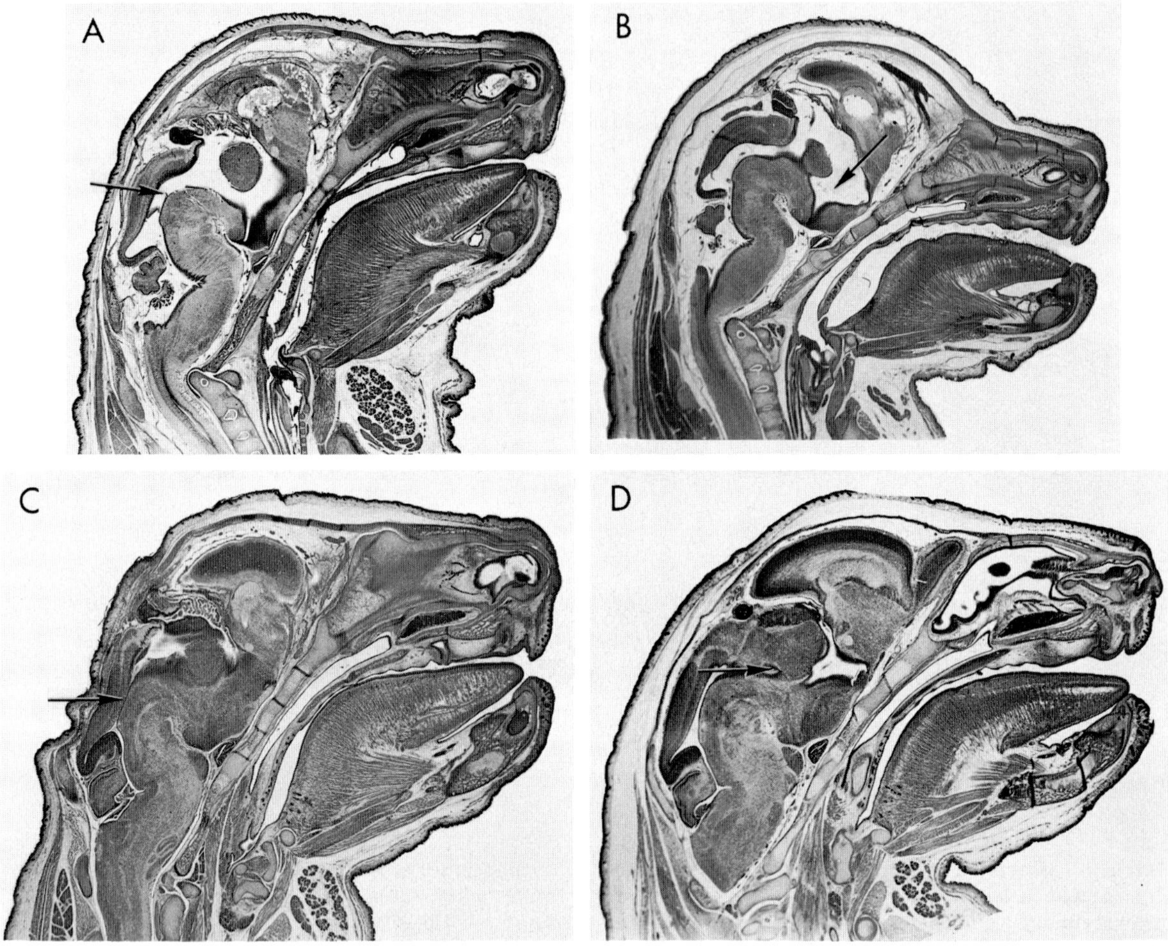

Fig. 25-9.—Sagittal sections through rat fetuses (twenty-first day). **A,** control with wide (aqueduct) communication (**arrow**). **B–D,** trypan blue-treated animals. **B,** although the aqueduct is still open, enlargement of the third ventricle (**arrow**) is seen on this section and enlargement of the lateral ventricles on parasagittal sections. Ependymal reaction in rostral part of aqueduct foreshadows closure. **C** and **D,** there is crowding in the area of the fourth ventricle with closing aqueduct (**arrow**) in **C** and forking of aqueduct (**arrow**) in **D**. Neither **C** nor **D** had hydrocephaly.

birth many heterogeneous pathologic factors can upset the balance of CSF production and resorption, with formation of hydrocephaly.

Symptoms

True congenital hydrocephaly, i.e., marked enlargement of the head present at birth, is seldom compatible with delivery and postnatal life. About half of the cases of clinical importance, although due to congenital malformations, show increase in the size of the head only after birth.[23] This increase usually is noticeable by inspection alone, but repeated measurements of the occipitobregmatic circumference, if compared with standard values (p. 237) and with measurements of the chest, are preferable, since they give objective proof of unusual cranial growth. The normal child's head should not grow more than 1 inch in each of the first 2 months, and much less subsequently.[38] The disproportion of the size of the face to that of the vault can be recognized by external inspection and in lateral roentgenograms. Bulging of the forehead, protrusion of the parietal areas and extension of the occipital region are characteristic changes. The distance between the anterior fontanelle and the external ears is markedly increased. The fontanelles are tense and enlarged. The sutures are wide and show, like the fontanelles, no tendency to close. The skin of the scalp is thin and stretched and its veins are dilated. The eyes are directed downward and the scleras are visible above the corneas ("setting sun sign"). Strabismus, nystagmus and optic atrophy may be present. Appearance of the fundi in hydrocephalic infants can be deceptive. Pallor of the disc does not always indicate optic atrophy, as proved by subsequent visual development. Papilledema is rare; if present, an intracranial tumor should be suspected.[38] Papilledema does not develop despite a high ventricular pressure if the subarachnoid space is blocked.[86] Percussion of the head results in a hollow, "cracked-pot" sound (Macewen sign). The head cannot be held up, and walking and talking are delayed. The legs are spastic, the tendon reflexes increased and convulsions may occur. Anorexia, vomiting and emaciation complicate severe cases. As a rule, hydrocephalic children are dull and lethargic. Blindness can develop, but hearing and the auditory memory may be good. Physical and mental development depend on several factors, such as rapidity of onset, intracranial pressure, compensatory growth of the head, nature of the basic malformations and progress or arrest of the process. Such variability makes the prognosis and evaluation of therapeutic measures difficult. Pressure on the hypothalamic area can cause obesity or precocious puberty in exceptional cases.

Associated malformations are not rare. Spina bifida, vertebral anomalies, microgyria, absence of the corpus callosum, cerebellar anomalies, syringomyelia and diplomyelia, harelip and cleft palate, cardiac defects, horseshoe or cystic kidneys, urethral strictures, cryptorchidism, clubfoot and micromelia have been observed repeatedly.[31,40,61] In Denmark, the incidence of hydrocephaly was 3% in babies with harelip and cleft palate.[87] Edwards[13] pointed out that boys with sex-linked hydrocephaly develop a syndrome of mental deficiency, slightly enlarged irregular head, spasticity with wasting and contractures and peculiar facies. A syndrome of polycystic kidneys, polydactyly and internal hydrocephaly has been described in siblings.[88] Special attention should be paid to the occipitocervical area, where skeletal malformations that can be causative anomalies may be found. There, bony defects may initiate or aggravate the obstruction to free CSF circulation, and surgical intervention can alleviate the hydrocephaly. D'Agostino *et al.*,[18] of the Mayo Clinic, found only 10 cases of Dandy-Walker cysts in the necropsy files of 1917–1961. This rare anomaly occurred once in two siblings who had polycystic kidneys, and a third sib of this family had polycystic kidneys without Dandy-Walker malformation.

Diagnosis

Advanced forms of hydrocephaly can be recognized at a glance, but beginning or mild cases can be overlooked or confounded with other conditions. Enlargement of the head is present in older infants with rickets, but other signs of that disorder will suggest the correct diagnosis. Subdural hematoma often is mistaken for hydrocephaly. It occurs after birth traumas or after bleeding in early infancy. It may be complicated by hydrocephaly if blood obliterates the subarachnoid spaces. The hematoma can be diagnosed by subdural puncture, which yields bloody or xanthochromic fluid with crenated cells. Congenital tumors can give rise to hydrocephaly by obstructing the aque-

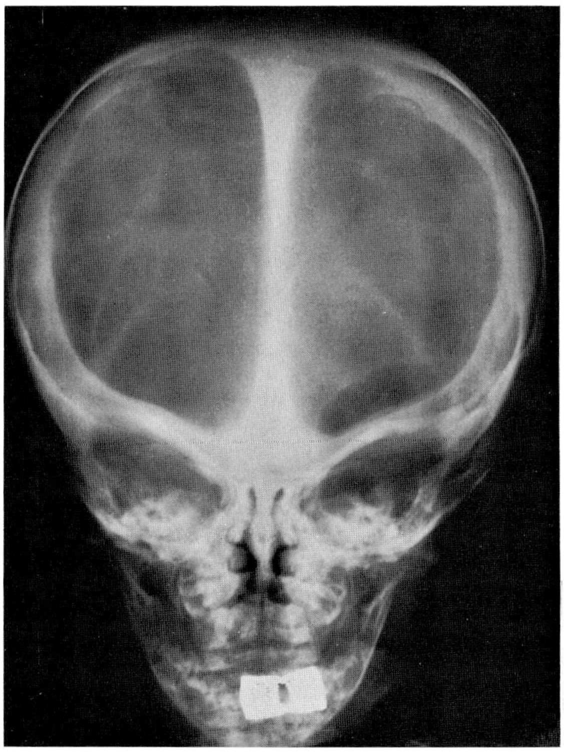

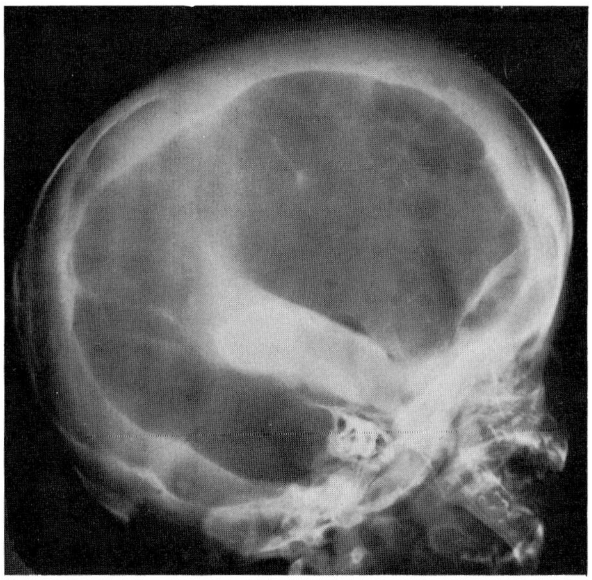

Fig. 25-10.—Air encephalogram of extreme noncommunicating hydrocephaly (aqueduct stenosis) in a boy 5 months of age. Air failed to reach the fourth ventricle and dye introduced into the lateral ventricle did not appear in lumbar spinal fluid.

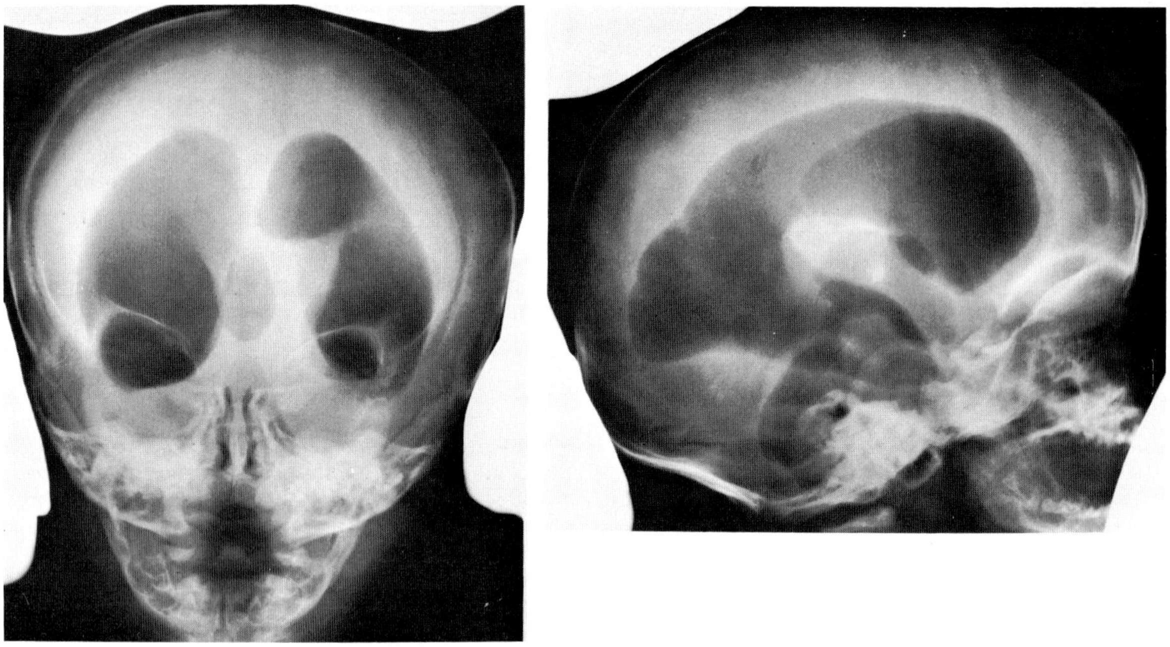

Fig. 25-11.—Air encephalograms of a boy 4 months of age showing enlargement of all ventricles. Although there seems to be a large communication between the third and fourth ventricles, necropsy at age 9 months showed aqueduct stenosis.

duct or the outlets from the fourth ventricle. They may be visualized by ventriculography or recognized at operation. Macrencephaly simulates hydrocephaly externally as well as on plain x-ray films, but ventriculograms permit differentiation of the two conditions. In achondroplasia, macrencephaly as well as hydrocephaly can occur.[20] A pseudohydrocephaly sometimes occurs in children with intrauterine growth retardation (Chapter 14).

Lumbar puncture may be dangerous in cases of obstructive hydrocephaly, since herniation of the brain stem into the occipital foramen may be brought about by withdrawal of spinal fluid. Foltz and Shurtleff[63] described the adverse effects of release of lumbar spinal fluid in a case that had converted from communicating to obstructive hydrocephaly. Neurosurgeons perform lumbar and spinal punctures simultaneously and compare the pressures as well as the properties of the fluids removed from both compartments. Dyes introduced into a lateral ventricle appear in the spinal fluid, in cases of communicating hydrocephaly, in from 2 to 12 minutes. If the dye cannot be found after 20 minutes, obstruction must be assumed. Ventriculography permits visualization of the enlarged ventricular and subarachnoid spaces and may demonstrate the site of obstruction (Figs. 25-10 and 25-11). Films of the head should be made in various positions, the most informative results being obtained by inversion, whereby air can be demonstrated in the fourth ventricle and in the cisterna magna.

In *parental counseling*, the etiology of hydrocephaly in the propositus should be ascertained, if possible. If counseling cannot be based on an established cause, an empirical risk figure of 3–5% can be given for subsequent siblings of an affected propositus.[2] It is of importance that in some families hydrocephaly is transmitted as a recessive trait and in others as a sex-linked recessive trait (p. 218), so that the genetic prognosis has to be made accordingly. Familial recurrence of hydrocephaly due to toxoplasmosis has not been reported.

Treatment

It is not possible to do justice here to the many attempts to arrest or cure hydrocephaly. There are reviews available that deal with the subject,[89-91] but even experts actively engaged in the field differ greatly in evaluation of therapeutic results.[92] Evaluation is made difficult by the variability of the types of hydrocephaly treated and by ignorance of the natural course of the individual cases. There are some who believe that spontaneous arrest is so common that cures by surgery often are doubtful. Others consider surgical intervention a necessity as soon as the diagnosis of progressive hydrocephaly is established.

The natural history of hydrocephaly was studied by Laurence[93] by a follow-up of a large unselected series of hydrocephalic patients who had not been treated surgically. After many years, of 179 patients, 81 were found to be alive with the hydrocephaly arrested spontaneously, 89 had died and in 9—all under the age of 5 years—the condition was still progressing. Of the 81 survivors, 33 had an I.Q. of 85 or above. A further 26 patients were below normal intelligence but educable, and the remaining 22 were ineducable. Laurence considered the natural course of hydrocephaly much more hopeful than expected, with survival of 46%, educability of 73% and a 57% chance of being taught in a school for normal children. It is clear that evaluation of any treatment must be made against this background of untreated cases. Pudenz[91] distinguished three main procedures: (1) reduction of cerebrospinal fluid formation at its source, (2) diversion of the fluid into some area of absorption and (3) bypassing the obstruction in the ventricular system. There are many subgroups in these main procedures, so that in 1961 a total of 24 surgical methods could be enumerated! Scarff[89] gave a historical and critical review of methods and results of treatment of hydrocephaly. He found that the operative mortality and the initial success were essentially the same with all types of operations. But the incidence of severe late complications was many times greater after most shunt operations than after third-ventriculostomy or after cauterization of the choroid plexuses. Against effectiveness of the last procedure one may cite the view that cerebrospinal fluid is not only produced by the choroid plexuses of the lateral ventricle, but also by those of the third and fourth ventricles, by the lining and vessels of the subarachnoid space, by ependymal cells and by cerebral perivascular spaces (p. 219). Ventriculoatrial shunting has become the preferred operation by many neurosurgeons for obstructive and communicating hydrocephaly.[91] It is obvious that arrest of hydrocephaly does not assure normal physical and mental development of the patients, since some of them have suffered irreversible brain damage and others are born with associated cerebral defects that cannot be removed by operation.[96] Yet, most neurosurgeons and their teams believe that surgical therapy can improve the outlook for most hydrocephalics by achieving maximal intellectual and cosmetic results.[63, 90, 94, 95]

Medical treatment of hydrocephaly is not often used. If a drug causes sufficient dehydration, it also often causes metabolic disturbances that endanger the child.

Nursing care is always of prime importance and decisive for the outcome. Follow-up examinations, training, education and many other factors influence the children's development.[98] As a rule, surgically treated children receive greater attention than children who have not been operated on. This difference in attention makes comparison of treated and untreated children difficult.

REFERENCES

1. Alter, M.: Anencephalus, hydrocephalus, and spina bifida, Arch. Neurol. 7:411, 1962.
2. Myrianthopoulos, N. C., and Kurland, L. T.: Present Concepts of the Epidemiology and Genetics of Hydrocephalus, in Fields, W. S., and Desmond, M. M. (eds.), *Disorders of the Developing Nervous System* (Springfield, Ill.: Charles C Thomas, Publisher, 1961), pp. 187–202.
3. Malamud, N.: Neuropathology, in Stevens, H. A., and Heber, R. (eds.), *Mental Retardation* (Chicago: The University of Chicago Press, 1964), pp. 429–502.
4. Schockaert, R., and Janssens, J.: Hydrocéphalies congénitales répétées, Bull. Féd. soc. gynéc. et obst. 3:560, 1951.
5. Polman, A.: Anencephaly, spina bifida and hydrocephaly; a contribution to our knowledge of the causal genesis of congenital malformations, Genetica 25:29, 1950.
6. Popham, R. B.: Two cases of anencephaly, Lancet 1:1829, 1906.
7. Borle, A.: Sur l'étiologie de l'hydrocéphalie congénitale à propos d'un cas d'hydrocéphalie concordant chez de jumeaux univitellins, J. Génét. Hum. 2:157, 1953.
8. Macklin, M. T.: Cases of hydrocephalus in one family, J.A.M.A. 101:1663, 1933.
9. Mehne, R. G.: Three hydrocephalic newborns – each of a successive pregnancy of a white female, Arch. Pediat. 78:67, 1961.
10. Chapman, J. C. F.: Occurrence of spina bifida and hydrocephalus in siblings; review of literature and case report, Am. J. Obst. & Gynec. 57:761, 1949.
11. Bickers, D. S., and Adams, R. D.: Hereditary stenosis of aqueduct of Sylvius as cause of congenital hydrocephalus, Brain 72:246, 1949.
12. Edwards, J. H., Norman, R. M., and Roberts, J. M.: Sex-linked hydrocephalus; report of a family with 15 affected members, Arch. Dis. Childhood 36:481, 1961.
13. Edwards, J. H.: The syndrome of sex-linked hydrocephalus, Arch. Dis. Childhood 36:486, 1961.
14. Needleman, H. L., and Root, A. W.: Sex-linked hydrocephalus. Report of two families, with chromosomal study of two cases, Pediatrics 31:396, 1963.
15. Warren, M. C., Lu, A. T., and Ziering, W. H.: Sex-linked hydrocephalus with aqueductal stenosis, J. Pediat. 63: 1104, 1963.
16. Larson, C. A.: Hydrocephalus and incomplete fusion of fetal clefts. Report on a kindred, Am. J. Human Genet. 6: 16, 1954.
17. Benda, C. E.: Dandy-Walker syndrome or so-called atresia of the foramen Magendie, J. Neuropath. & Exper. Neurol. 13:14, 1954.
18. D'Agostino, A. N., Kernohan, J. W., and Brown, J. R.: The Dandy-Walker syndrome, J. Neuropath. & Exper. Neurol. 22:450, 1963.
19. Cohn, S., Weinberg, A., and Rockaway, F.: Identical hydrocephalic achondroplastic twins; subsequent delivery of single sibling with same abnormalities, Am. J. Obst. & Gynec. 72:1346, 1956.
20. Dennis, J. P., Rosenberg, H. S., and Alvord, E. C., Jr.: Megalencephaly, internal hydrocephalus and other neurological aspects of achondroplasia, Brain 84:427, 1961.
21. List, C. F.: Neurologic syndromes accompanying developmental anomalies of occipital bone, atlas and axis, Arch. Neurol. & Psychiat. 45:577, 1941.
22. Krabbe, K. H.: Tuberous sclerosis of brain and hydrocephalus in relation to early puberty, Encéphale 17:281, 1922.
23. Laurence, K. M.: The pathology of hydrocephalus, Ann. Roy. Coll. Surgeons England 24:388, 1959.
24. Berblinger, W.: Ein Beitrag zur epithelialen Genese des Melanins, Virchows Arch. path. Anat. 219:328, 1915.
25. Gellman, W.: Congenital hydrocephalus in monovular twins, Arch. Dis. Childhood 34:274, 1959.
26. Record, R. G., and McKeown, T.: Congenital malformations of the central nervous system. Data on sixty-nine pairs of twins, Ann. Eugenics 15:285, 1951.
27. Symonds, E. M.: Anencephaly and hydrocephaly in a twin pregnancy, Obst. & Gynec. 26:414, 1965.
28. Warkany, J., Passarge, E., and Smith, L. B.: Congenital malformations in autosomal trisomy syndromes, Am. J. Dis. Child. 112:502, 1966.
29. Gustavson, K-H., Finley, S. C., Finley, W. H., and Jalling, B.: A 4-5/21-22 chromosomal translocation associated

with multiple congenital anomalies, Acta paediat. 53: 172, 1964.
30. Paige, B. H., Cowen, D., and Wolf, A.: Toxoplasmic encephalomyelitis; further observations of infantile toxoplasmosis; intrauterine inception of the disease; visceral manifestations, Am. J. Dis. Child. 63:474, 1942.
31. Potter, E. L.: *Pathology of the Fetus and Infant* (2d ed.; Chicago: Year Book Medical Publishers, Inc., 1961).
32. Kass, A.: Congenital hydrocephalus in newborn infant—epidemic hepatitis in mother in second-third month of pregnancy, Acta paediat. 40:239, 1951.
33. Crosby, R. M. N., Mosberg, W. H., Jr., and Smith, G. W.: Intrauterine meningitis as a cause of hydrocephalus, J. Pediat. 39:94, 1951.
34. Burry, A. F.: Hydrocephalus after intra-uterine fungal infection, Arch. Dis. Childhood 32:161, 1957.
35. Liss, L., Knoblich, R. R., and Wolter, J. R.: Cerebral mucormycosis with hydrencephaly and primary optic atrophy: In a 4-month-old child, J. Pediat. Ophth. 4:36, 1967.
36. Lourie, H., and Berne, A. S.: A contribution on the etiology and pathogenesis of congenital communicating hydrocephalus. The syndrome of delayed hemorrhage into the cisterns of the transverse cerebral fissure of infants, Neurology 15:815, 1965.
37. Carter, M. P.: A probable epidemic of congenital hydrocephalus in 1940–1941, Developmental Med. & Child Neurol. 7:61, 1965.
38. Laurence, K. M.: Infantile hydrocephalus: Its diagnosis and natural history, Quart. Rev. Pediat. 15:5, 1960.
39. Matson, D. D.: Hydrocephalus in a premature infant caused by papilloma of the choroid plexus, with report of surgical treatment, J. Neurosurg. 10:416, 1953.
40. Larson, S. L., and Banner, E. A.: Hydrocephalus: A 30-year survey, Obst. & Gynec. 28:571, 1966.
41. Hassin, G. B.: Cerebrospinal fluid; its origin, nature and function, J. Neuropath. & Exper. Neurol. 7:172, 1948.
42. Bering, E. A., Jr.: Pathophysiology of Hydrocephalus, in Shulman, K. (ed.), *Workshop in Hydrocephalus, Children's Hospital of Philadelphia, 1965* (Philadelphia: University of Pennsylvania School of Medicine, 1966), pp. 9–19.
43. Dott, N. M.: A case of unilateral hydrocephalus in an infant; operation—cure, Brain 50:548, 1927.
44. Ingraham, F. D., and Matson, D. D.: *Neurosurgery of Infancy and Childhood* (Springfield, Ill.: Charles C Thomas, Publisher, 1954).
45. Russell, D. S.: Observations on the pathology of hydrocephalus, Brit. Med. Research Council, Special Report Series, #265, 138 pp., 1949.
46. Alvord, E. C., Jr.: The Pathology of Hydrocephalus, in Fields, W. S., and Desmond, M. M. (eds.), *Disorders of the Developing Nervous System* (Springfield, Ill.: Charles C Thomas, Publisher, 1961).
47. Farnell, F. J., and Globus, J. H.: Primary melanoblastosis of leptomeninges and brain, Arch. Neurol. & Psychiat. 25:803, 1931.
48. Fanconi, A.: Neurocutane Melanoblastose mit Hydrocephalus communicans bei zwei Säuglingen, Helvet. paediat. acta 11:376, 1956.
49. Bernard, R., Carcassonne, M., Vigouroux, R., Berard-Badier, R., Mariani, R., and Passeron, P.: Hydrocéphalie du nouveau-né par angiome crânien temporal, Pédiatrie 21: 709, 1966.
50. Askenasy, H. M., Herzberger, E. E., and Wijsenbeek, H. S.: Hydrocephalus with vascular malformations of the brain, Neurology 3:213, 1953.
51. Ingraham, F. D., and Scott, H. W., Jr.: Spina bifida and cranium bifidum. Arnold-Chiari malformation; study of 20 cases, New England J. Med. 229:108, 1943.
52. Lichtenstein, B. W.: Distant neuroanatomic complications of spina bifida (spinal dysraphism); hydrocephalus, Arnold-Chiari deformity, stenosis of aqueduct of Sylvius, etc.; pathogenesis and pathology, Arch. Neurol. & Psychiat. 47:195, 1942.
53. Barry, A., Patten, B. M., and Stewart, B. H.: Possible factors in the development of the Arnold-Chiari malformation, J. Neurosurg. 14:285, 1957.
54. Laurence, K. M.: The natural history of spina bifida cystica, Arch. Dis. Childhood 39:41, 1964.
55. Smith, E. D.: *Spina Bifida and the Total Care of Spinal Myelomeningocele* (Springfield, Ill.: Charles C Thomas, Publisher, 1965).
56. Duckett, S.: Foetal Arnold-Chiari malformation, Acta neuropath. 7:175, 1966.
57. Goldstein, F., and Kepes, J. J.: The role of traction in the development of the Arnold-Chiari malformation, J. Neuropath. & Exper. Neurol. 25:654, 1966.
58. Morgagni, J. B.: *The Seats and Causes of Diseases Investigated by Anatomy* (trans. by Benjamin Alexander), Vol. 3 (London: A. Miller and T. Cadell, 1769).
59. Dandy, W. E., and Blackfan, K. D.: Internal hydrocephalus, an experimental, clinical and pathological study, Am. J. Dis. Child. 8:406, 1914.
60. Schwalbe, E., and Gredig, M.: Über Entwicklungsstörungen des Kleinhirns, Hirnstamms und Halsmarks bei Spina bifida, Beitr. path. Anat. 40:132, 1906.
61. Cameron, A. H.: The Arnold-Chiari and other neuro-anatomical malformations associated with spina bifida, J. Path. & Bact. 73:195, 1957.
62. Turkewitsch, N.: Die Entwicklung des Aquaeductus cerebri des Menschen, Morphol. Jahrb. 76:421, 1935.
63. Foltz, E. L., and Shurtleff, D. B.: Conversion of communicating hydrocephalus to stenosis or occlusion of the aqueduct during ventricular shunt, J. Neurosurg. 24:520, 1966.
64. Bass, M. H.: The relation of vitamin A intake to cerebrospinal fluid pressure: A review, J. Mt. Sinai Hosp. 24:713, 1957.
65. Marie, J., and Sée, G.: Acute vitaminosis A of the infant, A.M.A. Am. J. Dis. Child. 87:731, 1954.
66. Ehrengut, W.: Akuter benigner Hydrocephalus durch Hypervitaminosis-A (Syndrom Marie-Sée) bei Keratomalacie, Ztschr. Kinderh. 77:468, 1955.
67. Gilman, J. P. W.: Congenital hydrocephalus in domestic animals, Cornell Vet. 46:487, 1956.
68. Grüneberg, H.: *The Genetics of the Mouse* (The Hague: Martinus Nijhoff, 1952).
69. Bierwolf, D.: Die Embryogenese des Hydrocephalus und der Kleinhirnmissbildungen beim Dreherstamm der Hausmaus, Morphol. Jahrb. 99:542, 1958.
70. Berry, R. J.: The inheritance and pathogenesis of hydrocephalus-3 in the mouse, J. Path. & Bact. 81:157, 1961.
71. Gillman, J. C., Gilbert, C., and Gillman, T.: A preliminary report on hydrocephalus, spina bifida and other congenital anomalies in the rat produced by trypan blue, South African J. M. Sc. 13:47, 1948.
72. Millen, J. W., Woollam, D. H., and Lamming, G. E.: Congenital hydrocephalus due to experimental hypovitaminosis A, Lancet 2:679, 1954.
73. Carton, C. A., Pascal, R. R., and Tennyson, V. M.: Hydrocephalus and Vitamin A Deficiency in the Rabbit: General Considerations, in Fields, W. S., and Desmond, M. M. (eds.), *Disorders of the Developing Nervous System* (Springfield, Ill.: Charles C Thomas, Publisher, 1961), pp. 214–266.
74. O'Dell, B. L., Whitley, J. R., and Hogan, A. G.: Relation of folic acid and vitamin A to incidence of hydrocephalus in infant rats, Proc. Soc. Exper. Biol. & Med. 69:272, 1948.
75. Newberne, P. M., and O'Dell, B. L.: Vitamin B_{12} Deficiency and Hydrocephalus, in Fields, W. S., and Desmond, M. M. (eds.), *Disorders of the Developing Nervous System* (Springfield, Ill.: Charles C Thomas, Publisher, 1961), pp. 123–140.
76. Kalter, H., and Warkany, J.: Congenital malformations in inbred strains of mice induced by riboflavin-deficient, galactoflavin-containing diets, J. Exper. Zool. 136:531, 1957.

77. Cohlan, S. Q.: Congenital anomalies in the rat produced by excessive intake of vitamin A during pregnancy, Pediatrics 13:556, 1954.
78. Warkany, J., and Takacs, E.: Experimental production of congenital malformations in rats by salicylate poisoning, Am. J. Path. 35:315, 1959.
79. Vickers, T. H.: Concerning the mechanism of hydrocephalus in the progeny of trypan blue treated rats, Arch. mikr. Anat. u. Entwicklungsmechanik 153:255, 1961.
80. Stempak, J. G.: Etiology of trypan blue induced antenatal hydrocephalus in the albino rat, Anat. Rec. 148:561, 1964.
81. Overholser, M. D., Whitley, J. R., O'Dell, B. L., and Hogan, A. G.: The ventricular system in hydrocephalic rat brains produced by a deficiency of vitamin B_{12} or of folic acid in the maternal diet, Anat. Rec. 120:917, 1954.
82. Kalter, H.: Experimental mammalian teratogenesis, a study of galactoflavin-induced hydrocephalus in mice, J. Morphol. 112:303, 1963.
83. Gunberg, D. L.: Spina bifida and the Arnold-Chiari malformation in the progeny of trypan blue injected rats, Anat. Rec. 126:343, 1956.
84. Warkany, J., Wilson, J. G., and Geiger, J. F.: Myeloschisis and myelomeningocele produced experimentally in the rat, J. Comp. Neurol. 109:35, 1958.
85. Warkany, J.: Experimental Production of Congenital Malformations of the Central Nervous System, in Bowman, P. W., and Mautner, H. V. (eds.), *Mental Retardation, Proceedings First International Conference on Mental Retardation* (New York: Grune & Stratton, Inc., 1960).
86. Macnab, G. H.: The development of the knowledge and treatment of hydrocephalus, Developmental Med. & Child Neurol. Supp. 11:1, 1966.
87. Fogh-Andersen, P.: *Inheritance of Harelip and Cleft Palate* (Copenhagen: Arnold Busck, 1942).
88. Simopoulos, A. P., Brennan, G. G., Alwan, A., and Fidis, N.: Polycystic kidneys, internal hydrocephalus and polydactylism in newborn siblings, Pediatrics 39:931, 1967.
89. Scarff, J. E.: Treatment of hydrocephalus: An historical and critical review of methods and results, J. Neurol., Neurosurg. & Psychiat. 26:1, 1963.
90. Ransohoff, J., Shulman, K., and Fishman, R. A.: Hydrocephalus; a review of etiology and treatment, J. Pediat. 56:399, 1960.
91. Pudenz, R. H.: The Surgical Treatment of Infantile Hydrocephalus, in Fields, W. S., and Desmond, M. M. (eds.), *Disorders of the Developing Nervous System* (Springfield, Ill.: Charles C Thomas, Publisher, 1961), pp. 468–483.
92. Shulman, K. (ed.): *Workshop in Hydrocephalus, Children's Hospital of Philadelphia, 1965* (Philadelphia: University of Pennsylvania School of Medicine, 1966).
93. Laurence, K. M.: The natural history of hydrocephalus, Postgrad. M. J. 36:662, 1960.
94. Yashon, D.: Prognosis in infantile hydrocephalus, J. Neurosurg. 20:105, 1963.
95. Badell-Ribera, A., Shulman, K., and Paddock, N.: The relationship of non-progressive hydrocephalus to intellectual functioning in children with spina bifida cystica, Pediatrics 37:787, 1966.
96. Guthkelch, A. N., and Riley, N. A.: Influence of aetiology on prognosis in surgically treated infantile hydrocephalus, Arch. Dis. Childhood 44:29, 1969.
97. Brocklehurst, G.: A quantitative study of a spina bifida foetus, J. Path. 99:205, 1970.
98. Studies in Hydrocephalus and Spina Bifida, Proc. Freiburg Meeting of the Society for Research into Hydrocephalus and Spina Bifida, Developmental Med. & Child Neurol., Supp. 22, Vol. 12, No. 6, 1970.

26

Hydranencephaly

In contrast to an anencephalus, a hydranencephalus is covered by skin, bones, dura and leptomeninges, and in contrast to a hydrocephalus, the cerebral hemispheres are almost completely absent. Only basal ganglia and remnants of the mesencephalon are found at the base of the skull and above the cerebellar tentorium; from these remnants a thin membranous sac extends forward and upward, enclosing ventricular spinal fluid. The sac consists of glia and pia-arachnoid. Lateral and third ventricles cannot be distinguished; choroid plexuses, if present, are floating behind the basal ganglia. The falx cerebri, subtentorial structures and cranial nerves usually are found. Microphthalmia is common in children with hydranencephaly.[1] The fact that the cranial nerves are present indicates that a brain had been formed originally. In this respect, hydranencephaly resembles anencephaly; but, in the latter, the brain consist-

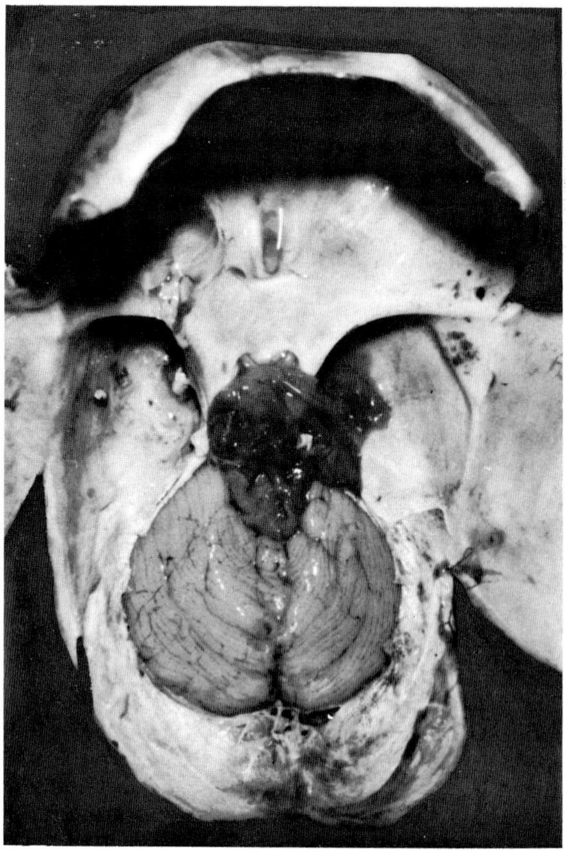

Fig. 26-1.—Hydranencephaly. Only cerebellum and cerebral rudiments are seen in opened cranium. The child lived 4½ months.

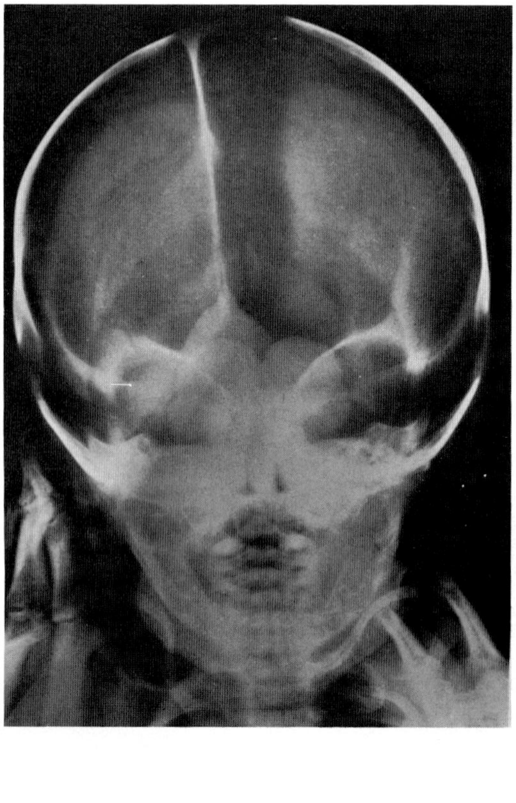

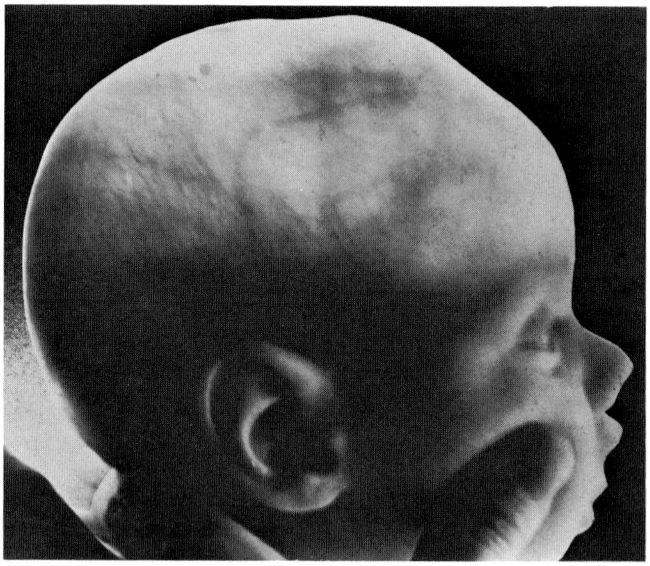

Fig. 26-2 (left).—Hydranencephaly. Falx and basal ganglia are clearly outlined in roentgenogram.

Fig. 26-3 (right).—Transillumination of a child with hydranencephaly.

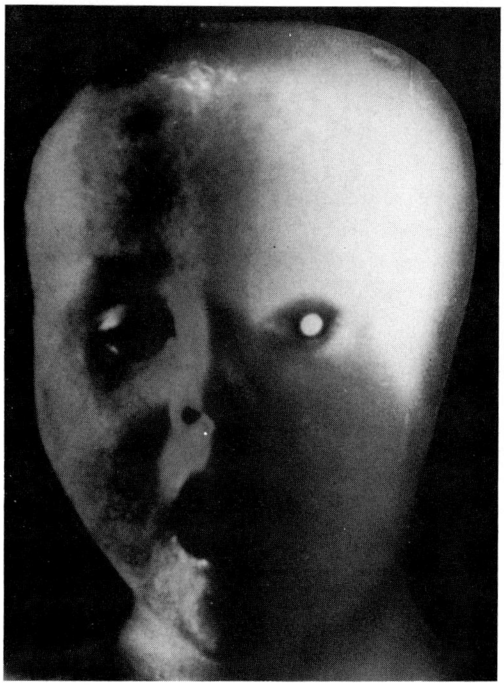

Fig. 26-4. – Hemi-hydranencephaly in a girl 3½ years of age. Transillumination shows unilateral involvement. (Courtesy of Dr. Ralph N. Hayden, Seattle, Washington.)

ed of an "araphic" or unclosed neural plate that was not covered by bones and skin. We may safely assume that hydranencephaly was preceded by a brain, with hemispheres separated by a falx and connected with cranial nerves, that was destroyed by an unknown secondary event. Convolution-like indentations on the pia-arachnoid and on the skull bones are also signs left behind by a once-existing brain in some cases.[1] Whereas in anencephaly the anterior neuropore fails to close, it does close in hydranencephaly. Hydranencephaly has been considered an extreme form of porencephaly.[2]

There have been many speculations concerning the cause of secondary destruction of the brain leading to hydranencephaly. Spielmeyer,[2] who, in 1905, apparently introduced the term "hydranencephaly" for the lesion described 70 years before by Cruveilhier,[3] saw the anomaly concordant in female twins who had two amnions and two chorions. In both, there were signs of destruction of nerve tissues, with hemorrhages and blood pigments in cerebral remnants. The hemorrhagic process was attributed by Spielmeyer to vascular anomalies. The blood vessels had extremely thin walls and showed a tendency to form cavernous spaces. Thrombosis, embolism and inflammation were excluded by Spielmeyer as causes of the hemorrhages. Hydranencephaly in such dichorionic twins and identical vascular anomalies in both are remarkable findings, but their interpretation is difficult, and they leave us without a satisfactory explanation of the cerebral malformation. What could cause such thorough destruction of the hemispheres? Attempted abortion has been considered. The mother of the twins described by Spielmeyer was unmarried and there are reports of attempted abortion in two cases.[4,5] In some instances, toxoplasmosis, syphilis, hepatitis, exposure to x-rays and venous thrombosis have been considered etiologic or pathogenic factors,[1] but in most cases the pregnancy apparently was normal. It is worth mentioning that in a number of patients for whom duration of pregnancy and birth weight were recorded, there was no indication of intrauterine growth retardation. It seems, therefore, that the destruction of the brain is due to a local process. The portions of the brain most affected are those supplied by the anterior and middle cerebral arteries. The arteries of the carotid system are hypoplastic in hydranencephaly but without obvious disease process. Muir[1] believed that the arterial hypoplasia is secondary to the loss of cerebral substance. Associated malformations are rare and the children may be so well formed that some have been adopted before the cerebral defect was recognized.[1,6]

The head seldom is enlarged at birth, but there is an increase in size after a few weeks or months. Cyanosis and jaundice are noted frequently in the neonatal period, but such symptoms are not distinctive. Irritability and whining is a common manifestation and incoordinated eye movements and nystagmus may betray the disorder. Microphthalmia and optic atrophy confirm the impression of anomaly and, in some cases, there are convulsions.[1] Transillumination and absence of electrical activity in electroencephalograms confirm the suspicion of hydranencephaly. The prognosis for life is poor, but occasionally such children can live for several years.

REFERENCES

1. Muir, C. S.: Hydranencephaly and allied disorders; a study of cerebral defect in Chinese children, Arch. Dis. Childhood 34:231, 1959.
2. Spielmeyer, W.: Ein hydranencephales Zwillingspaar, Arch. Psychiat. Nervenkr. 39:807, 1905.
3. Cruveilhier, J.: *Anatomie pathologique du corps humain* (Paris: J. B. Baillière, 1835).
4. Picaza, J. A., Cardelle, G., and Jimenez, R. M: Hydroencephalodysplasia, J. Neurosurg. 12:535, 1955.
5. Yakovlev, P. I., and Wadsworth, R. C.: Schizencephalies; study of congenital clefts in cerebral mantle; clefts with hydrocephalus and lips separated, J. Neuropath. & Exper. Neurol. 5:169, 1946.
6. Hamby, W. B., Krauss, R. F., and Beswick, W. F.: Hydranencephaly: Clinical diagnosis. Presentation of seven cases, Pediatrics 6:371, 1950.

27

Iniencephaly

THE TERM INIENCEPHALY suggests that the brain and the neck (inion) show the principal anomalies. The impressive malformation has attracted early attention, as seen in a woodcut of 1640 (Fig. 27-1), which shows the marked retroflexion of the head and the low position of the ears characteristic of iniencephaly. The child is depicted as a female, which corresponds to the fact that most iniencephalics are girls. The braids must be considered erroneous interpretations of area cerebrovasculosa, which is present when iniencephaly is combined with anencephaly (see Fig. 22-1). The text of the book in which this woodcut appears attributes the headgear to divine punishment for the then new fashion of braids that were arranged in the shape of a nest and held together by ribbons.[1]

Iniencephaly is a rare malformation. Only about 70 cases had been reported in the literature by 1962,[2] but at certain localities and times there seems to be an increased incidence. Howkins and Lawrie[3] observed 3 cases in 30 months, and Paterson[4] reported an incidence in an Edinburgh hospital of 1 in 896 births. In Winnipeg, Canada, Osborne[5] recorded 1 in 1,730 births. It appears that iniencephaly is relatively common in areas in which anencephaly is frequent. This may explain why Ballantyne[6] in Edinburgh observed 7 cases and considered the malformation not a great rarity. Little is known concerning etiologic factors. The prevalence of females seems to be even more pronounced than in anencephaly. It seems that only about 10% of iniencephalics are male.[4,7] A male iniencephalic born to a Bantu woman was described in detail by Muller.[8] Some iniencephalics were monozygotic or dizygotic twins,[7] and in one of Ballantyne's[6] cases twinning had occurred repeatedly in the families of both parents. In the same instance, a sibling of the iniencephalic had had spina bifida. Oakley and Grimshaw[14] reported a case of iniencephaly associated with cyclopia. They also cited several similar cases previously reported in the literature. In their specimen, there was a single diamond-shaped palpebral fissure in the midline, which contained a globe with two pupils and a single conjunctiva. Behind the eye, which looked upward and backward, there was a well-developed proboscis. In addition to iniencephaly, an occipital encephalocele, spina bifida aperta, umbilical hernia and bilateral clubfoot were present in the specimen. The fact that iniencephaly can be produced experimentally by treatment of the mother with a drug (p. 236) points to the possibility of environmental causation.

Pregnancy often goes to term and frequently is complicated by hydramnios,[7] although – in contrast to anencephaly – the choroid plexuses are within the cranial cavity and not secreting into the amniotic space. Because of the distortion of the fetal body form, abnormal presentation (such as breech, footling, face or chin) is frequent and sometimes endangering to the mother's life. Most iniencephalics are dwarfed at birth. The extent of intrauterine growth retardation is difficult to evaluate, since in only a few cases gestation time and birth weight are recorded. In one of Ballantyne's[6] cases, delivery was at the eighth month, the fetus weighing only 1,470 Gm.

The severely deformed fetuses show, in addition to retroflexion of the head, severe defects of the spine that always include an exaggerated cervicothoracic lordosis and often anterior or posterior spina bifida. The head is large in relation to the shortened body, the face looks upward and the neck is absent. The skin of the face is continuous with the skin of the chest, and the scalp – if present – is directly connected with the skin of the back. Lack of hair in the parietal area and abundance over the neck and back contribute to the grotesque appearance of some of these fetuses. The defective and retroflexed occiput may be joined to vertebrae of the lower spine. Rachischisis exists in most cases, but the defective spinal cord and column usually are covered dorsally by brain, cerebellum and skin (see Fig. 27-2) so that the open neural plate and vertebral trough are not seen on the surface (iniencephaly clausus). Marked retroflexion of the head also occurs sometimes in anencephalics or fetuses with open rachischisis (iniencephaly apertus). The anomalies of the occiput vary; they may involve the squama only or include all parts. In closed iniencephaly, the cranial contents remain within the cranial cavity, but in the open form they protrude into an encephalocele or present as exencephaly or anencephaly. The foramen magnum is enlarged, and through the opening, parts of the brain and cerebellum establish contact with dorsal aspects of the spine. The cervical spine is always severely deformed and shortened by formation of block vertebrae or by vertebral deficiencies. Since such anomalies of the

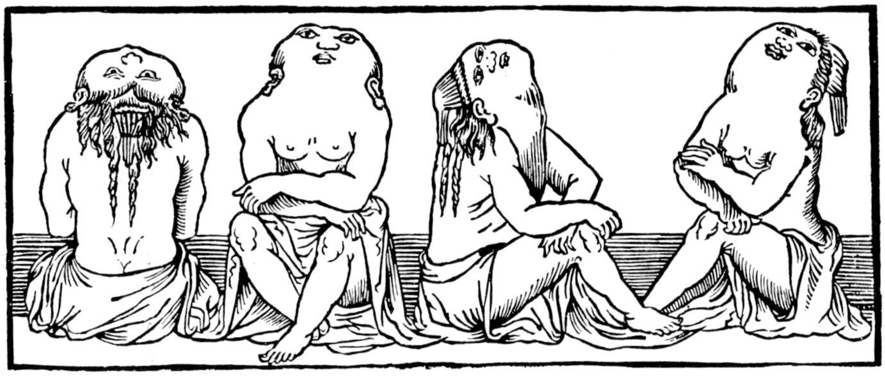

Fig. 27-1.—Four views of an iniencephalic female in a woodcut of 1640. (From E. Holländer.[1] Reproduced with permission of Ferdinand Enke, Stuttgart, Germany.)

cervical spine also occur in the Klippel-Feil syndrome (p. 909), this syndrome, which is compatible with postnatal life and is encountered in clinical medicine, has been considered a mild iniencephaly.[9] But little is gained by this identification, since the Klippel-Feil syndrome is neither a morphologic nor an etiologic entity (p. 910). In iniencephaly, vertebral anomalies are not limited to the cervical spine but also occur in other parts of the axis. Ballantyne[6] thought that the principal anomaly was an arrest of the embryo in physiologic retroflexion in the third week of gestation, but the existence of such an early retroflexion has been doubted.[10] Whatever the explanation, the normal forward bending seen in embryos from the fourth week on is not attained in iniencephaly.

Among the many associated malformations described are anencephaly, encephalocele, hydrocephaly, cyclopia, cleft lip and palate, bifid uvula, deformed ears, rachischisis, fusion or deficiency of ribs, abnormal lobation of the lungs, diaphragmatic hernia, single umbilical artery, omphalocele, situs inversus, horseshoe or polycystic kidneys, imperforate anus and

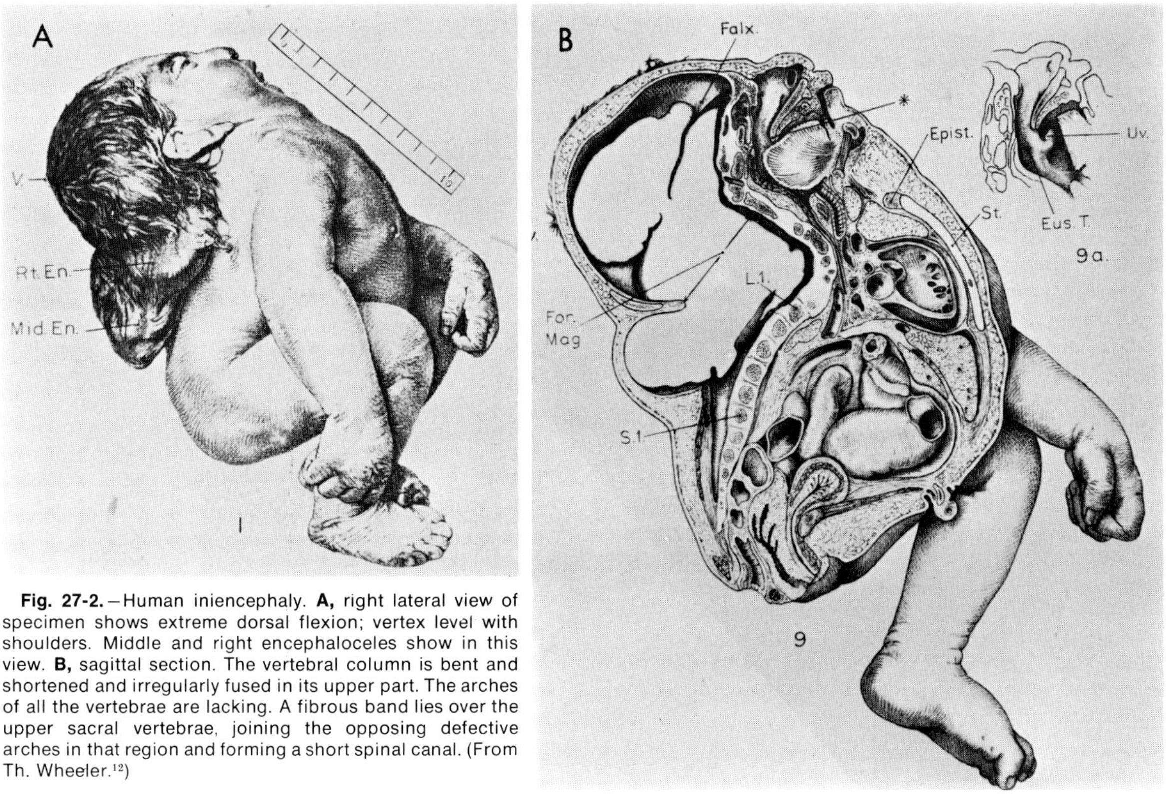

Fig. 27-2.—Human iniencephaly. **A,** right lateral view of specimen shows extreme dorsal flexion; vertex level with shoulders. Middle and right encephaloceles show in this view. **B,** sagittal section. The vertebral column is bent and shortened and irregularly fused in its upper part. The arches of all the vertebrae are lacking. A fibrous band lies over the upper sacral vertebrae, joining the opposing defective arches in that region and forming a short spinal canal. (From Th. Wheeler.[12])

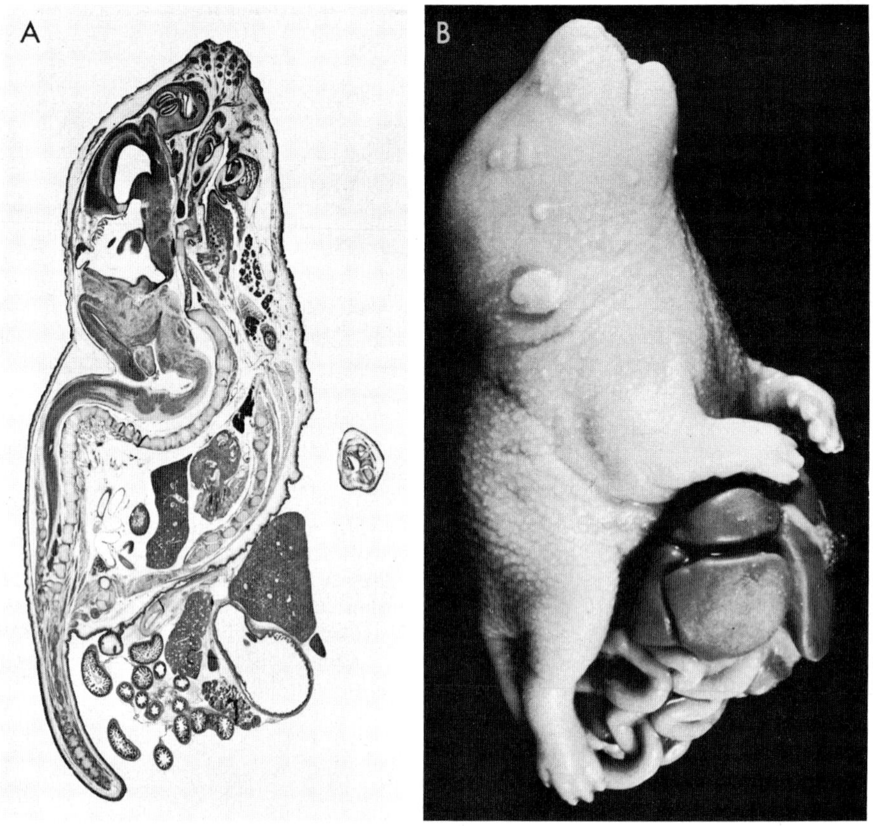

Fig. 27-3.—**A,** sagittal, near-midline section of an iniencephaly in a rat fetus (mother treated with streptonigrin). **B,** external appearance of rat shown in **A**. (From J. Warkany and E. Takacs.[13])

clubfeet.[6,7,11] The heart may be found under the chin without complete septation and connected with an abnormal aortic arch system.[8]

Iniencephaly sometimes is imitated by specimens obtained in teratologic experiments. Figure 27-3 represents a rat fetus exposed to streptonigrin on the ninth day of gestation, which is comparable to the human iniencephalic reported by Wheeler[12] (Fig. 27-2). The rat fetus had marked lordosis of the cervical and thoracic portions of the vertebral column, the concavity filled with brain and upper spinal cord, severe exomphalos, with pulmonary, intestinal, hepatic and pancreatic tissues located outside the body cavities. In both specimens the spinal cords were mere appendages of the relatively large brains. In the rat fetus, all vertebrae were open dorsally with the exception of the sacral and caudal ones, but, as in human cases, the rachischisis did not open onto the surface, since it was covered by skin and subcutaneous tissue throughout.[13] Thus, the iniencephaly produced experimentally resembles in many respects its human counterpart.

REFERENCES

1. Holländer, E.: Wunder, Wundergeburt und Wundergestalt, in *Einblattdrucken des funfzehnten bis achtzehnten Jahrhunderts* (Stuttgart: Ferdinand Enke, 1922).
2. Cimmino, Ch. V., and Painter, J. W.: Iniencephaly, Radiology 79:942, 1962.
3. Howkins, J., and Lawrie, R. S.: Iniencephaly, J. Obst. & Gynaec. Brit. Emp. 46:25, 1939.
4. Paterson, S. J.: Iniencephalus, J. Obst. & Gynaec. Brit. Emp. 51:330, 1944.
5. Osborne, D. F.: Iniencephalus, Canad. M.A.J. 59:474, 1948.
6. Ballantyne, J. W.: *Manual of Antenatal Pathology and Hygiene. The Embryo* (Edinburgh: W. Green & Sons, 1904).
7. Brodsky, I.: Four examples of iniencephalus, with a statistical review of the literature, M. J. Australia 2:795, 1939.
8. Muller, T.: An unusual anomaly of the neck, Medical Proceedings, Mediese Bydraes 11:537, 1965.
9. Gilmour, J. R.: Essential identity of Klippel-Feil syndrome and iniencephaly, J. Path. & Bact. 53:117, 1941.
10. Patten, B. M.: *Human Embryology* (2d ed.; New York: McGraw-Hill Book Company, Inc., 1953).
11. Potter, E. L.: *Pathology of the Fetus and Infant* (2d ed.; Chicago: Year Book Medical Publishers, Inc., 1961).
12. Wheeler, Th.: Study of a human spina bifida monster with encephaloceles and other abnormalities, Contrib. Embryol. 7:87 (No. 22), 1918.
13. Warkany, J., and Takacs, E.: Congenital malformations in rats from streptonigrin, Arch. Path. 79:65, 1965.
14. Oakley, N. W., and Grimshaw, J. S.: A case of iniencephaly associated with cyclopia, Brit. J. Clin. Pract. 15:845, 1961.

28

Microcephaly

A BRAIN reduced in size and enclosed in a small skull usually is termed "microcephaly." Since the disturbance is primarily a cerebral affection that involves the skull secondarily, the term "micrencephaly" actually is preferable, although it is not commonly used. As a rule, the forebrain is chiefly affected and the occipital lobes do not cover entirely the cerebellum, which is of normal size. Adults or children over 10 years with a brain weight under 900 Gm. and a head circumference under 46 cm. (18 in.) usually are classified as microcephalics. Sometimes the brain weighs not more than 300 or 400 Gm. in adults and may amount to only one-hundredth of the body weight in contrast to the normal, where the relationship is 1 to 30.[1] In children, a head circumference of about 5 cm. below average for the age is considered significant, but since small, intelligent children or pituitary dwarfs also have small heads, such measurements are of doubtful diagnostic value. Most authors now use the term "microcephaly" if the cranial circumference is 3 standard deviations below the mean. Westropp and Barber[2] published a table of head circumferences for boys and girls during the first 7 years of life, recording the mean and standard deviation for each age (Table 28-1). Some microcephalic heads are diminished in height and width but are relatively long. It was thought that patients who have cephalic indices below 73[3] are "genetic microcephalics" but, actually, attempts to correlate measurements with etiology have not been successful.[4] Since the cranial deficit is above the cranial base, it is clear that the circumference of the head is not always a satisfactory criterion for the diagnosis, but the measurement together with the head shape usually makes recognition of microcephaly easy. The narrow and receding forehead, the small cranium and the flat occiput give the head a conoidal shape that, together with the relatively large face and large ears, combine into a striking malformation described popularly as "pinhead," and recognizable by inspection alone (Figs. 28-1 and 28-2).

Description of microcephaly dates back to early times. An interesting review of the literature before 1929 was published by Stringaris.[5] Microcephaly was known to Thomas Willis in the seventeenth century; early writers often attributed it to premature closure of the cranial sutures, which, however, is not a characteristic of microcephaly. With the popularization of Darwin's theory of evolution, many malformations were considered "atavisms" or relapse to early stages of phylogenic development, and microcephaly was identified with simian brains. But it was found that the brains of microcephalics are much more human than ape-like,[3] and recognized that they resembled

TABLE 28-1.—HEAD CIRCUMFERENCE FOR BOYS AND GIRLS DURING THE FIRST SEVEN YEARS OF LIFE*

AGE	Boys			Girls		
	Number	Mean (cm.)	S.D.	Number	Mean (cm.)	S.D.
1 month	295	37.3	±1.54	282	36.5	±1.41
3 months	229	40.7	±1.43	230	39.8	±1.39
6 months	275	43.6	±1.45	262	42.5	±1.42
9 months	247	45.7	±1.40	259	44.6	±1.41
1 year	289	46.8	±1.40	275	45.6	±1.22
1½ years	255	47.9	±1.40	255	47.0	±1.30
2 years	264	49.1	±1.47	260	48.0	±1.32
2½ years	219	49.8	±1.39	221	48.8	±1.35
3 years	216	50.4	±1.35	227	49.5	±1.35
3½ years	226	51.0	±1.40	222	50.1	±1.45
4 years	233	51.2	±1.41	229	50.7	±1.46
4½ years	220	51.6	±1.45	217	51.0	±1.48
5 years	224	51.8	±1.47	225	51.2	±1.50
7 years	187	52.7	±1.48	194	52.2	±1.37

*From Westropp and Barber.[2] Reprinted with permission of the authors, editor and publishers, B. M. A. House, Tavistock Square, London, W.C. 1, England.

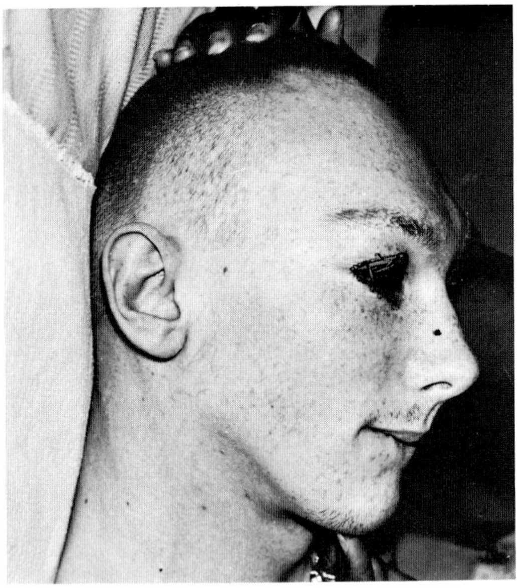

Fig. 28-1. – Microcephaly in a young man with "cerebral palsy," contractures and petit mal attacks. He was the result of a twin pregnancy. The other twin was stillborn and macerated.

rather those of human fetuses. The anomaly then usually was attributed to arrested development by fetal disease at early embryonic stages. The genetic approach of the first decades of the twentieth century and the finding of multiple cases in certain families led to the concept of hereditary or genetic microcephaly. It has been estimated that the incidence of microcephaly is 0.6–1.6 per 10,000 births.[9] The rate probably varies in different areas and populations. It has been stated that the frequency of genetic microcephaly is of the magnitude of 1 in 25,000 to 1 in 50,000 in the general population. Among institutionalized mental defectives, Böök *et al.*[9] found only one-half of 1% belonging to this group. But in institutions in which most of the patients are of idiot or imbecile level, 20% might be classed as microcephalic.[4]

Etiology

Today, we consider microcephaly a symptom of differing etiologic disturbances. Microcephaly illustrates that a congenital malformation can have various causes (Fig. 28-3) and that it is fallacious to consider a morphologic concept as an etiologic entity. Whatever the cause – known or unknown – microcephaly is always due to reduced growth of the brain

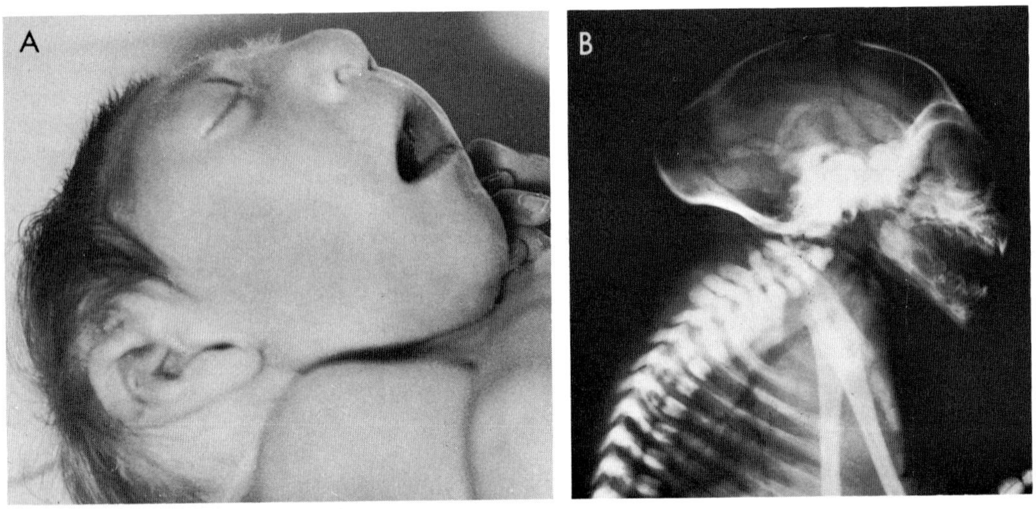

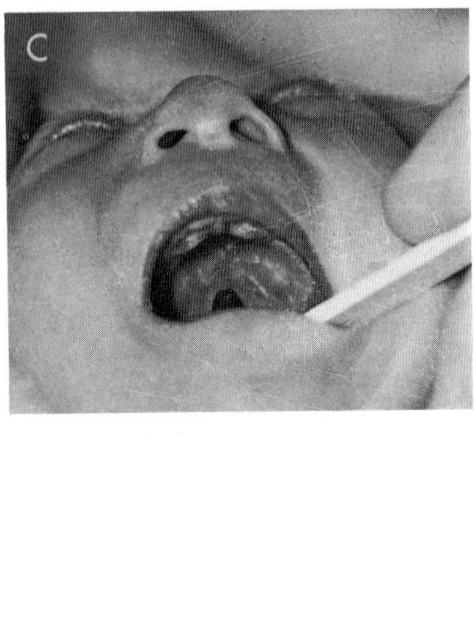

Fig. 28-2. – **A,** extreme microcephaly in a newborn child. Birth weight at term 1,360 Gm. **B,** roentgenogram showing reduced cranial capacity. **C,** posterior palate cleft, repeatedly seen in such microcephalic children. (From J. Warkany, B. B. Monroe and B. S. Sutherland.[12])

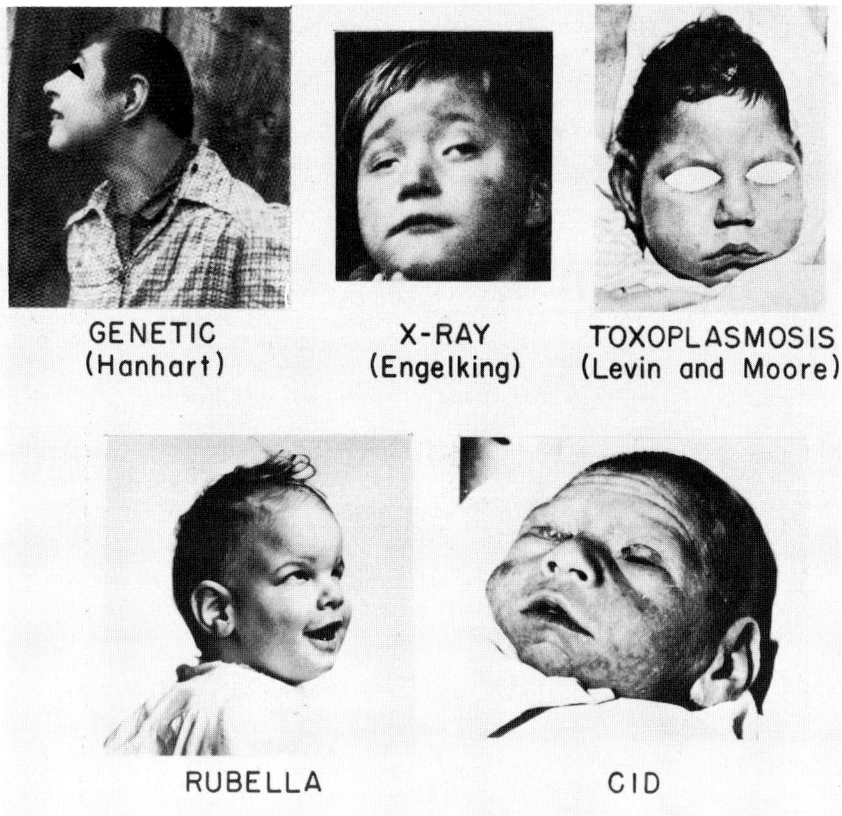

Fig. 28-3. – Microcephaly of differing etiology.

and not to smallness of the skull or premature obliteration of the cranial sutures. It is possible that some cases of microcephaly are caused by postnatal disturbances of cerebral growth.[1] During the first year, the head circumference increases from about 35 cm. (13.5 in.) to 47 cm. (18.5 in.). If the brain of an infant is affected by meningitis, retardation of brain growth may occur and microcephaly ensue,[6] but most cases probably are due to prenatal damage.

There have been many families recorded with repeated microcephaly,[5,7,8] and there is good proof that the disorder can be attributed to an autosomal recessive gene.[3,7-11] In some areas, parental consanguinity was marked,[7,8,10] but in others it was associated with only a few of the cases.[4,11] In some series, males predominated to such an extent that in order to uphold the hypothesis of autosomal recessive inheritance, one had to assume that female microcephalics were not included because they were kept at home and remained concealed.[7] But in other series the sex ratio was near 1:1.[8,11] It should also be emphasized that not all genetically determined microcephalies need be due to the same mutant gene.[4] We published a pedigree in which intrauterine growth retardation was associated with microcephaly in males but not in females[12] (Chapter 14). Smith *et al.*[13] described 3 boys with a syndrome of microcephaly, hypertonicity, growth retardation, unusual facies and incomplete development of the external genitalia. It is possible that the prevalence of males in some series is real and not due to biased ascertainment. Bird-headed dwarfs are microcephalics with intrauterine and postnatal growth retardation.[14,15] Girls and boys are affected, and autosomal recessive inheritance seems likely. The same is true for the microcephaly associated with various congenital malformations and Fanconi[16] aplastic anemia (Chapter 103).

The pedigrees published by Hanhart[8] of microcephaly in Swiss isolates are of great interest because they show that in some of the cases the anomaly, although genetically determined, can appear sporadically; only careful study of a kindred over many generations shows the common origin of familial and of sporadic cases. One can only guess how many cases of microcephaly are genetically determined and how many are of "environmental" origin. Some authors assumed that microcephaly generally is due to a recessive autosomal gene,[7] whereas others believed that only a third of the cases[11] or a minority[4] are genetically determined. Such disagreement is understandable, since sampling methods differed greatly.

There are differences of opinion concerning the

state of heterozygotes in affected families. Intellectual impairment, small stature and reduced head circumference have been found in relatives of microcephalics (Fig. 28-4). Alternate microcephaly, spastic diplegia or mental deficiency has been observed in some families.[4,11] There also are families on record in which both hydrocephaly and microcephaly occurred, but microcephaly does not alternate with anencephaly and spina bifida.[8] Concordant microcephaly in monozygotic twins has been recorded,[8,9,17,18] but there also are reports of microcephaly in only one of monozygotic twins.[19,20] These cases are of great interest because the microcephalic twins weighed much less than the normal twins at birth; in one instance,[20] the mother asserted that the microcephalic's cord came from the side of the placenta, whereas that of his brother was centrally attached. Koch[11] reported monozygotic twins, one of whom – a microcephalic idiot – died at 5 years, whereas his "normal" brother died of a cerebral tumor at the age of 6 years. Monozygotic twin boys recorded by Brenner[21] differed in that one of them was microcephalic and the other hydrocephalic.

An indirect result of a genetically determined metabolic error can be microcephaly in the child of a phenylketonuric mother.[44]

A review of congenital malformations of the central nervous system attributable to autosomal trisomies[22] did not list microcephaly as a frequent defect. Yet, a small brain is present in many cases of Down, trisomy 18 and trisomy 13-15 syndromes. The microcephaly often is overshadowed by more spectacular lesions such as arhinencephaly, fusion of hemispheres, convolutional anomalies, and so forth. As cytogenetic investigations proceed and various unusual chromosomal aberrations are described in children, microcephaly is found in many unusual cytogenetic situations.

Fig. 28-4. – Microcephalic child with cleft palate. In this family, 7 of 8 children were retarded, had speech defect and/or small heads. All had low birth weights (approximately 1,800 Gm.). Only 1 child had cleft palate.

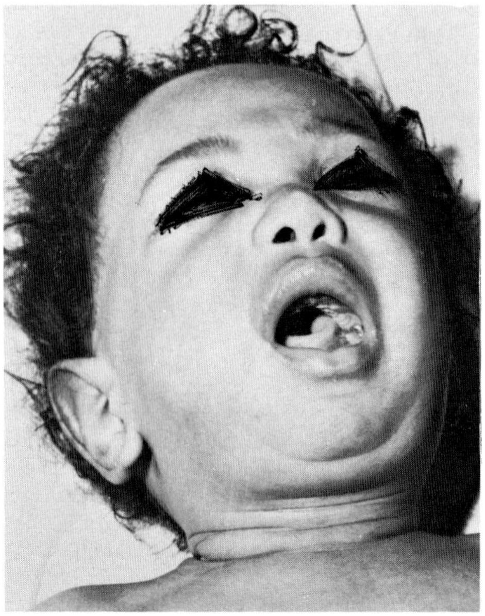

Microcephaly has been reported in patients with 47 chromosomes with a supernumerary small metacentric[45,46] or with a small submetacentric.[47,48] Extra sex chromosomes have been found associated with microcephaly.[23,49-52] Deletion of chromosomal material has been recorded repeatedly in microcephalic patients. The cat-cry syndrome with deletion of a short arm of chromosome no. 5 is rather regularly characterized by microcephaly (p. 340). The cat-cry syndrome complicated by midline clefts has been attributed to a deletion of the short arm of chromosome no. 4 (p. 342). An enlarged long arm of a B chromosome has also been found to be associated with microcephaly and cat-cry syndrome.[24] Small head or brain with deletion in an 18 chromosome, short arm[53,54] or long arm[55,56] with a ring 1 chromosome,[57] ring C chromosome[25] or ring D chromosome[26,58] has been described. A syndrome of microcephaly and absent thumbs has been attributed to a D_2 ring chromosome.[59] Ring 18 chromosomes have been found repeatedly in children with mental retardation who, in some cases, had microcephaly.[60,61] Translocations, familial or de novo, can give rise to microcephaly in various teratologic syndromes. Translocations 2/3,[62,63] 4/5,[64] 2/5,[65] D/E[66-68] and others have been recorded in association with microcephaly. It seems premature to make a systematic review of microcephaly attributable to recognizable chromosomal abnormalities, since many statements now made in the literature probably will be revised in the future. Although many cases of microcephaly are now published because of chromosomal changes, one must not assume that cytogenetic abnormalities are a frequent cause of microcephaly. In our laboratory, only 1 case with a ring D chromosome was discovered among 23 patients with microcephaly examined cytogenetically because of suggestive associated malformations.

Since sporadic microcephaly can be genetically determined, some authors in the past assumed that all or most of the cases are hereditary. But now there are several environmental causes known that lead to microcephaly, so that this concept cannot be upheld. It has long been known[27,28] that x-irradiation of the mother during pregnancy can result in microcephaly of the fetus. Such children often also have microphthalmia and mental retardation, and there may be deformities of the extremities. A variety of congenital malformations of the brain can be produced experimentally in rats and other animals by x-ray exposure during gestation,[29,30] and microcephaly is among these (Fig. 28-5). Microcephaly has also been observed in children of women exposed during pregnancy to the atomic bomb in Hiroshima.[31,32]

Small heads are noticed in children damaged

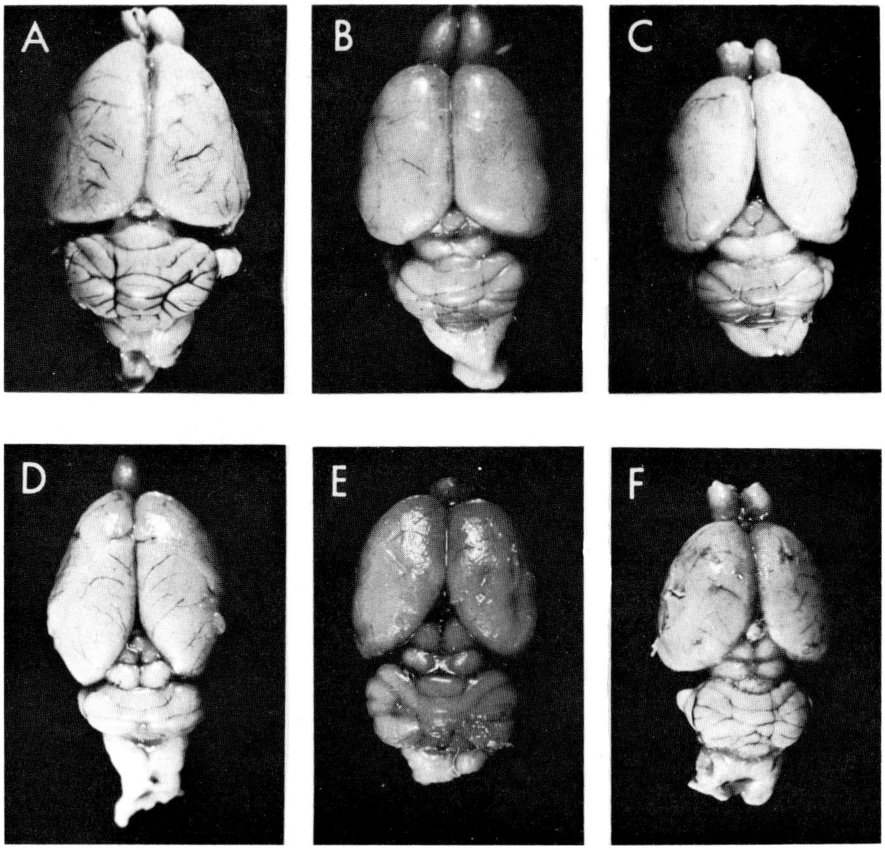

Fig. 28-5. – **A,** control rat brain. **B – F,** various degrees of microcephaly produced by x-irradiation (150 – 200 R) on fourteenth, fifteenth, sixteenth or eighteenth day of gestation.

by rubella in early intrauterine life,[33] but only a few of them have a circumference of 3 standard deviations below the normal average.[4] Prenatal toxoplasmosis[34,35] (Fig. 28-6) and cytomegalic inclusion disease[36,37] (Fig. 9-7) can result in microcephaly. Inapparent infection with cytomegalovirus may cause microcephaly in a small number of cases.[71] A certain degree of microcephaly was observed in fetal Minamata disease[38] attributed to prenatal methylmercury poisoning. After carbon monoxide poisoning of the mother, her fetus may show microcephaly and tetraplegia.[39] Microcephaly has been observed repeatedly in children of phenylketonuric mothers.[69,70] Such children may be free of phenylketonuria but damaged in utero by the mother's metabolic disturbance. Several children of such a woman may be affected and simulate recessive inheritance. Although the mother's disease is genetically determined in such cases, the children, if heterozygous, are damaged in utero by the maternal environment, i.e., excessive phenylalanine or its products. Discordance in regard to microcephaly of identical twins points to causation by abnormal intrauterine environmental factors that are still poorly understood. Intrauterine growth retarda-

Fig. 28-6. – Microcephaly and microphthalmia in a newborn child with posterior palate cleft. Toxoplasma antibody titers were high in mother and child, but there were no intracerebral calcifications seen roentgenologically.

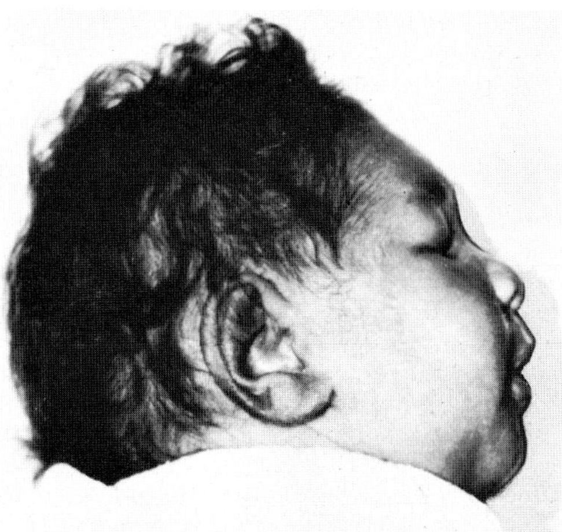

tion is associated with microcephaly in a significant number of cases. The prenatal growth retardation has been explained by many authors as the result of fetal malnutrition or maternal disease. But such a unitary explanation is not acceptable, since intrauterine growth retardation with microcephaly sometimes is obviously due to genetic or chromosomal anomalies[12] (p. 145).

In summary, it can be stated that microcephaly can result from various and heterogeneous causes. If the etiology is unknown, parental counseling is difficult and only empirical risk figures can be given. It has been estimated that the empirical risk of another mentally defective child being born to a mother who has already had one microcephalic offspring is 6%.[4]

Pathology

The capacity of the cranial cavity is diminished, chiefly by a marked reduction in the size of the anterior cranial fossa. In typical microcephaly, the frontal bone recedes and the occipital bone ascends steeply. The cerebral hemispheres are reduced in size, the convolutional pattern is simple and microgyria or macrogyria as well as marked asymmetries are observed. The frontal lobes are reduced in size and sometimes partly fused. The anterior central gyrus usually is present, the central sulcus short and the sulci of the temporal, parietal and occipital lobes are shallow. The sulcus parieto-occipitalis may be enlarged to a "simian fissure" and the island of Reil remain uncovered owing to imperfect development of the opercula. The cortex is poor in large nerve cells and contains many undifferentiated cells, neuroblasts and abnormal spindle-shaped cells.[40] Cystic degeneration of the white matter and enlargement of the ventricles and of the subdural spaces occur in some cases.[1] Porencephaly, lissencephaly, absence of the corpus callosum, heterotopias and defects of tracts and fascicles can be found in microcephalics. But the brains of some of these patients are merely small without showing any definite histopathologic changes. Cerebral atrophy in microcephalic cousins has been reported.[41] It is clear that, to the pathologist, microcephaly is not an entity.[42]

Symptoms

The clinical picture varies as the diagnosis of microcephaly applies to disorders of different origin and different severity. Some microcephalic children die soon after birth and represent a population that investigators in institutions do not see. Survivors are characterized by the cranial shape and size described before. Premature closure of the anterior fontanelle is the rule, and x-ray films reveal narrow but not obliterated sutures (see Fig. 28-2, *B*). As the child grows older, the smallness of the skull becomes more obvious, but the entire body also often is underweight and dwarfed. Development of motor functions and speech is delayed and some microcephalics never learn to talk. In contrast to children with the Down syndrome, microcephalics often show hypertonicity, increased reflex activity and, in more than one-third of the cases, convulsive disorders.[4] Most microcephalics remain sexually immature, but in some females menstruation occurs regularly. The mentality may be too low to be measured in some patients, but reach imbecile levels in others. The mental development is not always proportionate to the size of the head. Some microcephalics are slow, apathetic and immobile but others are lively, imitative, capable of acrobatic stunts and of performing simple household chores. Such patients are good-natured and socially adaptable; others are destructive, irritable and restless. In 1893 Korsakov[43] gave an excellent description of a probably genetically determined microcephalic, of her behavior and her psychologic status, an account still worth reading today.

In some cases, the etiology can be ascertained by associated symptoms. For instance, microcephaly due to maternal rubella in the first trimester of pregnancy often is combined with cataract, congenital heart disease and deafness. Microcephaly due to intrauterine irradiation of the embryo is accompanied by microphthalmia and, rarely, by malformations of the extremities. In microcephaly caused by toxoplasmosis, the diagnosis is aided if chorioretinitis, cerebral calcifications seen in roentgenograms, and convulsions are present. Calcifications are also seen in cases attributed to cytomegalic inclusion disease (see Fig. 9-8). In so-called intrauterine dwarfs with microcephaly, the low birth weight at term points to a general growth impairment (p. 136). In the differential diagnosis, it is of prime importance to distinguish microcephaly from craniosynostosis (p. 893), since in the latter condition surgical intervention may prevent mental and physical deterioration. In children with premature obliteration of the coronal suture, the anterior fontanelle usually is wide open, the forehead ascends steeply and the vertex of the cranium is in the area of the anterior fontanelle. In contrast, microcephalics have a small anterior fontanelle from birth on, the forehead recedes and the vertex is in the area of the occiput. Pituitary dwarfs who also have small heads show no disproportion in the development of the skull and the face. Closure of the fontanelle usually is delayed.

Although most microcephalics are idiots or imbeciles, some children with small heads are able to attend special schools and to learn to read and write. Some can perform simple household chores, but only a few can earn a living. In general, the life expectancy of microcephalics is low. Many die in infancy and others succumb to infectious diseases, particularly tuberculosis, but some have been known to attain ages of over 60 years.

Craniotomy is of no avail. Decades ago there was disagreement on this question as some distinguished pediatricians reported success of operative procedures. Failure to distinguish between microcephaly and craniosynostosis may have caused the controversy.

REFERENCES

1. Benda, C. C.: *Developmental Disorders of Mentation and Cerebral Palsies* (New York: Grune & Stratton, Inc., 1952).
2. Westropp, C. K., and Barber, C. R.: Growth of the skull in young children. Part 1. Standards of head circumference, J. Neurol., Neurosurg. & Psychiat. 19:52, 1956.
3. Penrose, L. S.: Microcephaly, Folia hered. path. 5:79, 1956.
4. Brandon, M. W. G., Kirman, B. H., and Williams, C. E.: Microcephaly, J. Ment. Sc. 105:721, 1959.
5. Stringaris, M. G.: Mikrokephalia. Ein Beitrag zur Lehre und Kasuistik der Missbildungen, Frankfurt. Ztschr. Path. 37:396, 1929.
6. Thelander, H. E., and Goebel, G.: Microcephalia as a complication of pneumococcic meningitis, Am. J. Dis. Child. 77:642, 1949.
7. Komai, T., Kishimoto, K., and Ozaki, Y.: Genetic study of microcephaly based on Japanese material, Am. J. Human Genet. 7:51, 1955.
8. Hanhart, E.: Über einfache Rezessivität bei Mikrocephalia vera, spuria et combinata und das herdweise Vorkommen der Mikrocephalia vera in Schweizer Isolaten, Acta genet. med. et gemel. 7:445, 1958.
9. Böök, J. A., Schut, J. W., and Reed, S.: A clinical and genetical study of microcephaly, Am. J. Ment. Deficiency 57:637, 1953.
10. Van den Bosch, J.: Microcephaly in the Netherlands, Acta Genet. 7:398, 1957.
11. Koch, G.: Genetics of microcephaly in man, Acta genet. med. et gemel. 8:75, 1959.
12. Warkany, J., Monroe, B. B., and Sutherland, B. S.: Intrauterine growth retardation, Am. J. Dis. Child. 102:249, 1961.
13. Smith, D. W., Lemli, L., and Optiz, J. M.: A newly recognized syndrome of multiple congenital anomalies, J. Pediat. 64:210, 1964.
14. Seckel, H. P. G.: *Bird-Headed Dwarfs. Studies in Developmental Anthropology Including Human Proportions* (Springfield, Ill.: Charles C Thomas, Publisher, 1960).
15. Harper, R. G., Orti, E., and Baker, R. K.: Bird-headed dwarfs (Seckel's syndrome), J. Pediat. 70:799, 1967.
16. Fanconi, G.: Familiäre infantile perniziosaartige Anaemie (perniziöses Blutbild und Konstitution), Jahrb. Kinderh. 117:257, 1927.
17. Whitney, E. A.: A microcephalic family, Eugenics 3:104, 1930.
18. Jacob, H.: Eine Gruppe familiärer Mikro- und Mikrencephalie, Ztschr. Neurol. u. Psychiat. 156:633, 1936.
19. Hinden, E.: Idiocy in one of monozygotic twins, Brit. M. J. 1:333, 1956.
20. Brandon, M. G. W., Kirman, B. H., and Williams, C. E.: Microcephaly in one of monozygous twins, Arch. Dis. Childhood 34:56, 1959.
21. Brenner, W.: Zur Frage der Erblichkeit von Mikrocephalie und Hydrocephalie, Ztschr. menschl. Vererb.-u. Konstitutionslehre 30:375, 1951.
22. Warkany, J., Passarge, E., and Smith, L. B.: Congenital malformations in autosomal trisomy syndromes, Am. J. Dis. Child. 112:502, 1966.
23. Ferguson-Smith, M. A., Johnston, A. W., and Handmaker, S. D.: Primary amentia and micro-orchidism associated with an XXXY sex-chromosome constitution, Lancet 2: 184, 1960.
24. Atkins, L., and Feingold, M: Enlarged B-group chromosome (4-5). Association with the cri du chat syndrome, Am. J. Dis. Child. 113:277, 1967.
25. Atkins, L., Pant, S. S., Hazard, G. W., and Ouellette, E. M.: Two cases with a C-group ring autosome, Ann. Human Genet. 30:1, 1966.
26. Gerald, P. S., Warner, S., Singer, J. D., Corcoran, P. A., and Umansky, I.: A ring D chromosome and anomalous inheritance of haptoglobin type, J. Pediat. 70:172, 1967.
27. Zappert, J.: Über röntgenogene fötale Mikrozephalie, Arch. Kinderh. 80:34, 1927.
28. Goldstein, L., and Murphy, D. P.: Etiology of ill-health in children born after maternal pelvic irradiation; defective children born after post-conception pelvic irradiation, Am. J. Roentgenol. 22:322, 1929.
29. Kaven, A: Das Auftreten von Gehirnmissbildungen nach Roentgenbestrahlung von Mäuseembryonen, Ztschr. menschl. Vererb.-u. Konstitutionslehre 22:247, 1938.
30. Hicks, S. P.: Some effects of ionizing radiation and metabolic inhibition on the developing mammalian nervous system, J. Pediat. 40:489, 1952.
31. Plummer, G.: Anomalies occurring in children exposed in utero to the atomic bomb in Hiroshima, Pediatrics 10: 687, 1952.
32. Miller, R. W.: Delayed effects occurring within the first decade after exposure of young individuals to the Hiroshima atomic bomb, Pediatrics 18:1, 1956.
33. Swan, C., Tostevin, A. L., Mayo, H., and Black, G. H. B.: Further observations on congenital defects in infants following infectious diseases during pregnancy, with special reference to rubella, M. J. Australia 1:409, 1944.
34. Levin, P. M., and Moore, H.: Fetal toxoplasmic encephalitis—a type of congenital cerebral disease, J. Pediat. 21: 673, 1942.
35. Couvreur, J.: *Étude de la Toxoplasmose Congénitale* (Gien: Impr. Jeanne-d'Arc, 1955).
36. Weller, T. H., and Hanshaw, J. B.: Virologic and clinical observations on cytomegalic inclusion disease, New England J. Med. 266:1233, 1962.
37. Megevand, A.: Embryopathie cérébrale dans un cas de maladie généralisée des inclusions cytomégaliques, Thèse, présentée à la Faculté de médecine, Univ. Genève, 1963 (Bâle: Editions S. Karger). Also: Ann. paediat. 201:410, 1963.
38. Takeuchi, T., Matsumoto, H., and Koya, G.: A pathological study on the fetal Minamata disease diagnosed clinically so-called infantile cerebral palsy, Shinkei-kenkyo no Shinpo (Prog. Neurol. Res.) 8:145, 1964.
39. Brander, T.: Microcephalie und Tetraplegie bei einem Kinde nach Kohlenmonoxydvergiftung während der Schwangerschaft der Mutter, Acta paediat. 28:123, 1940, Supp. 1.
40. Ernst, P.: Missbildungen des Nervensystems, in Schwalbe, E. (ed.), *Die Morphologie der Missbildungen des Menschen und der Tiere* (Jena: Gustav Fischer, 1909).
41. Sylvester, P. E.: Cerebral atrophy in microcephalic cousins, Arch. Dis. Childhood 34:325, 1959.
42. Bailey, O. T., and Woodard, J. S.: Some problems in the pathology of mental deficiency with microcephaly, Neurology 6:761, 1956.
43. Korsakov, S. S.: On the psychology of microcephalics (translated and republished by N. Raskin), Am. J. Ment. Deficiency 62:108, 1957.
44. de Ménibus, C. H., Graic, F., Lemonier, A., and Fleury, J.: Les enfants nés de mères phénylcétonuriques, Ann. Pédiat. 43:1746, 1967.
45. Frøland, A., Holst, G., and Terslev, E.: Multiple anomalies associated with an extra small autosome, Cytogenetics 2: 99, 1963.
46. Taft, P. D., Dodge, P. R., and Atkins, L.: Mental retardation and multiple congenital anomalies, Am. J. Dis. Child. 109:554, 1965.
47. Gustavson, K-H., Hagberg, B., Finley, S. C., and Finley, W. H.: An apparently identical extra autosome in two severely retarded sisters with multiple malformations, Cytogenetics 1:32, 1962.
48. Smith, G. F., Berg, J. M., Ridler, M. A. C., Faunch, J. A.,

Farnham, F. N., and Pendrey, M. J.: Familial transmission of an aberrant submetacentric chromosome, J. Ment. Defic. Res. 11:58, 1967.
49. Barr, M. L., Carr, D. H., Pozsonyi, J., Wilson, R. A., Dunn, H. G., Jacobson, T. S., and Miller, J. R.: The XXXXY sex chromosome abnormality, Canad. M.A.J. 87:891, 1962.
50. Carr, D. H., Barr, M. L., and Plunkett, E. R.: A probable XXYY sex determining mechanism in a mentally defective male with Klinefelter's syndrome, Canad. M.A.J. 84: 873, 1961.
51. Scherz, R. G., and Roeckel, I. E.: The XXXXY syndrome, J. Pediat. 63:1093, 1963.
52. Anders, G., Prader, A., Hauschteck, E., Schärer, K., Siebenmann, R. E., and Heller, R.: Multiples sex-chromatin und komplexes chromosomales Mosaik bei einem Knaben mit Idiotie und multiplen Missbildungen, Helvet. paediat. acta 15:515, 1960.
53. Pfeiffer, R. A.: Deletion der kurzen Arme des Chromosoms Nr. 18, Humangenetik 2:178, 1966.
54. Migeon, B. R.: Short arm deletions in group E and chromosomal "deletion" syndromes, J. Pediat. 69:432, 1966.
55. de Grouchy, J.: Chromosome 18: A topologic approach, J. Pediat. 66:414, 1965.
56. Insley, J.: Syndrome associated with a deficiency of part of the long arm of chromosome no. 18, Arch. Dis. Childhood 42:140, 1967.
57. Gordon, R. R., and Cooke, P.: Ring-1 chromosome and microcephalic dwarfism, Lancet 2:1212, 1964.
58. Teplitz, R. L., Miller, D., Hansson, K. M., and Rundall, T. S.: A human ring D chromosome associated with multiple congenital abnormalities, J. Pediat. 70:936, 1967.
59. Sparkes, R. S., Carrel, R. E., and Wright, S. W.: Absent thumbs with a ring D_2 chromosome: A new deletion syndrome, Am. J. Human Genet. 19:644, 1967.
60. Bernard, R., Stahl, A., Giraud, F., Hartung, M., and Brusquet, Y.: Encéphalopathie avec dysmorphie complexe et chromosome 17-18 en anneau, Ann. Pédiat. 42:2129, 1966.
61. Palmer, C. G., Fareed, N., and Merritt, A. D.: Ring chromosome 18 in a patient with multiple anomalies, J. M. Genetics 4:117, 1967.
62. Summitt, R. L.: Familial 2/3 translocation, Am. J. Human Genet. 18:172, 1966.
63. Lee, C. S. N., Bowen, P., Rosenblum, H., and Linsao, L.: Familial chromosome-2, 3 translocation ascertained through an infant with multiple malformations, New England J. Med. 271:12, 1964.
64. Shaw, M. W., Cohen, M. M., and Hildebrandt, H. M.: A familial 4/5 reciprocal translocation resulting in partial trisomy B, Am. J. Human Genet. 17:54, 1965.
65. de Grouchy, J.: A complex familial chromosome translocation, Am. J. Human Genet. 17:501, 1965.
66. Migeon, B. R., and Young, W. J.: Reciprocal (D;E) translocation: Euploid transmission in three generations, Bull. Johns Hopkins Hosp. 115:379, 1964.
67. Cohen, M. M., and Lockwood, M. A.: Familial transmission of a presumptive D/E (13-15/17-18) short arm translocation, Pediat. Res. 1:104, 1967.
68. Breibart, S., Mellman, W. J., and Eberlein, W. R.: Developmental retardation associated with an unbalanced 13-15/18 translocation, Cytogenetics 3:252, 1964.
69. Fisch, R. O., Walker, W. A., and Anderson, J. A.: Prenatal and postnatal developmental consequences of maternal phenylketonuria, Pediatrics 37:979, 1966.
70. Stevenson, R. E., and Huntley, C. C.: Congenital malformations in offspring of phenylketonuric mothers, Pediatrics 40:33, 1967.
71. Baron, J., Youngblood, L., Siewers, C. M. F., and Medearis, D., Jr.: The incidence of cytomegalovirus, herpes simplex, rubella, and toxoplasma antibodies in microcephalic, mentally retarded, and normocephalic children, Pediatrics 44:932, 1969.

29

Macrencephaly (Megalencephaly)

This is a rare condition of cerebral hypertrophy that can occur in mentally normal or in retarded persons. Normal brains of adults usually weigh less than 1,500 Gm.; weights above this are considered abnormal and macrencephalic. At birth, the normal brain weighs approximately 370 Gm. The brain weight in contrast to other tissues increases only about fourfold until adulthood is reached.[1]

Macrencephaly is not a clinical or an etiologic entity. Relatively few cases have been described in detail and they show little resemblance to one another. The thickness of the cranial bones varies, some being described as thin, others as thickened. The brain is always large and heavy, but in some cases the gray and the white substances are enlarged, whereas in others only the cortex is broad. The convolutions appear

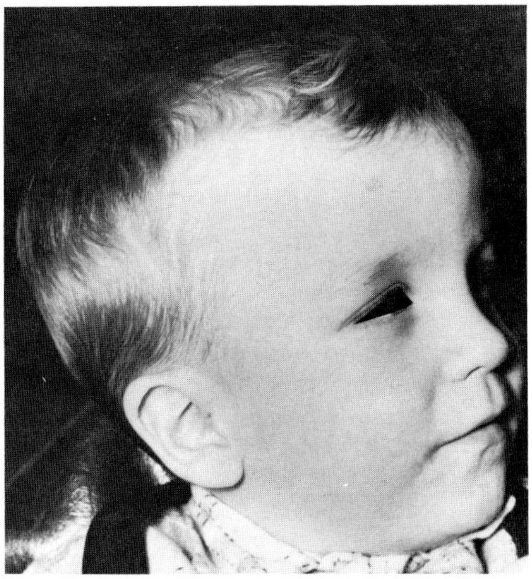

Fig. 29-1. – Mild macrencephaly in a boy with normal mentality. At the age of 2 years his head circumference was 54 cm. (mean for normal boys, 49 cm.).

wide and densely packed. The size of the cerebellum varies, but the spinal cord usually is enlarged. In the cortex, the stratification of the layers is not well defined. The nerve cells are large, but the distance between them is enhanced so that their density is reduced. Occasionally, giant cells are seen and structural abnormalities can be demonstrated by silver stains. The glia is normal in some cases, hypertrophic in others. Anomalies of the pituitary gland have been described and adrenal atrophy has been observed.[2]

Norman[3] distinguished three varieties. In the first, there is diffuse overgrowth of macroglia (interstitial macrencephaly) and the astrocytes may undergo malignant transformation. Weil[4] described a macrencephalic child who developed normally to his seventh year, when he became ataxic and paralyzed. When he died at the age of 7, hypertrophy of the hemispheres combined with diffuse glioblastomatosis of the brain stem and cerebellum were found at necropsy. In a second form, the brain generally is increased in size without neuroglial preponderance. The third type consists of macrencephalies associated with such other malformations or disorders as abnormal gyration, heterotopias, tuberous sclerosis, amaurotic idiocy and others. Macrencephaly has been found associated with achondroplasia.[5]

Children with macrencephaly may be born with large heads, or the enlargement becomes noticeable in postnatal life. When the head grows rapidly soon after birth and the fontanelles remain widely open, hydrocephaly usually is suspected. As a rule, macrencephaly results in a circumference of only 4.5–7.5 cm. above average. The forehead is high and the temporal bones fail to show the lateral bulging characteristic of hydrocephaly. There may be disproportion between cranial and facial bones as in hydrocephaly, but the eyes are not directed downward. The spinal fluid pressure is not increased and air encephalograms show ventricles of normal size. In some cases, physical and mental development is retarded. The head is not held up, speech is delayed and the children talk and walk late. Spastic diplegia or hypotonicity may be present. There often are visual disturbances, and anomalies of the macula or the optic discs are seen. Convulsions occur in about half the cases. The mental development varies; some macrencephalics are mentally normal, others are idiots or imbeciles; some can learn to read and to help in housework or simple occupations. Macrencephaly occurs more often in males than in females. Occasionally, more than one case has been observed in a family.[6] Hemimacrencephaly has been described in association with macrodystrophia lipomatosa of the face,[7] nevus, epilepsy and mental deficiency.[8]

In the differential diagnosis, hydrocephaly has to be considered. It has been pointed out that the shape of the head and the appearance of the eyes sometimes differ in the two conditions, but usually the correct diagnosis cannot be established without air encephalography. Intracranial tumors must be ruled out by the absence of signs of increased intracranial pressure. Various conditions of "pseudohydrocephaly" may be distinguished from macrencephaly only with difficulty. In these cases, the brain is normal and the cranium is enlarged or a disproportion of facial and cranial skeleton is present. Sometimes pseudohydrocephaly occurs in children who had suffered intrauterine growth retardation.[9]

The life expectancy is reduced in patients with mental and physical retardation. Macrencephalic children sometimes die suddenly, sometimes in convulsions or with infections, but other patients have lived into the seventh decade.

Pseudohydrocephaly

Enlargement of the head without enlargement of the ventricular system must be distinguished from hydrocephaly. Many pathologic conditions result in absolute or relative enlargement of the head, sometimes simulating hydrocephaly and giving cause for anxiety of parents and physicians. Generalized hyperostosis of the cranium and facial bones occurs in leontiasis ossea. A disproportionately large head often is striking in achondroplasia, a disorder in which hydrocephaly or macrencephaly can occur. In cleidocranial dysostosis (p. 836), the head may appear unduly large. Cephalhematomas and rickets can leave residuals suggesting hydrocephaly. Macrocephaly sometimes is a family trait without serious implications. It has been transmitted as a dominant autosomal characteristic in association with pseudopapilledema and hemangiomas.[10] Enlargement of the head may be a sign of intracranial tumor or of obstruction of the superior caval vein.[11]

A disproportion of facial and cranial bones has been observed repeatedly in children with intrauterine growth retardation (p. 138) who may appear so "hydrocephalic" that they are subjected repeatedly to air encephalography (Chapter 14). Russell[12] discussed this condition and Szalay[9] described several cases of pseudohydrocephaly in dwarfs. In one of his cases, the brain inside the apparently large skull was found to be normal at necropsy. Mental development may be retarded, but in some cases the abnormal physical appearance is deceptive. Ammann[13] reported such a child who had normal intelligence, and I have seen several such cases. One of these surprised all early observers by good mental development at school age (Fig. 14-3). A case of pseudohydrocephaly and intrauterine growth retardation was due to aminopterin intake of the mother during pregnancy[14] (Fig. 11-20).

REFERENCES

1. Brock, J.: *Biologische Daten für den Kinderarzt* (Berlin: Springer-Verlag, 1954).
2. Benda, C. E.: *Developmental Disorders of Mentation and Cerebration* (New York: Grune & Stratton, Inc., 1952).
3. Norman, R. M.: Malformations of the Nervous System, Birth Injury and Diseases of Early Life, in Greenfield, J. G. (ed.), *Neuropathology* (London: Edward Arnold & Company, 1960).
4. Weil, A.: Megalencephaly with diffuse glioblastomatosis of the brain stem and the cerebellum, Arch. Neurol. 30: 795, 1933.
5. Dennis, J. P., Rosenberg, H. S., and Alvard, E. C.: Megalencephaly, internal hydrocephalus and other neurological aspects of achondroplasia, Brain 84:427, 1961.
6. Ford, F. R.: *Diseases of the Nervous System in Infancy, Childhood and Adolescence* (3d ed.; Springfield, Ill.: Charles C Thomas, Publisher, 1952).
7. Feriz, H.: Makrodystrophia lipomatosa progressiva, Virchows Arch. path. Anat. 260:308, 1926.
8. Gross, H., and Uiberrak, B.: Klinisch-anatomische Befunde bei Hemimegalencephalie, Virchows Arch. 327: 577, 1955.
9. Szalay, G. C.: Pseudohydrocephalus in dwarfs: The Russell dwarf, J. Pediat. 63:622, 1963.
10. Riley, H. D., Jr., and Smith, W. R.: Macrocephaly, pseudopapilledema and multiple hemangiomata. A previously undescribed heredofamilial syndrome, Pediatrics 26:293, 1960.
11. Andersen, A. H., Hansen, A. T., Husfeldt, E., Pedersen, A., and Thomsen, G.: Superior caval vein syndrome, Acta med. scandinav. 150:81, 1954.
12. Russell, A.: A syndrome of "intra-uterine" dwarfism recognizable at birth with cranio-facial dysostosis, disproportionately short arms, and other anomalies (5 examples), Proc. Roy. Soc. Med. 47:1040, 1954.
13. Ammann, P.: Beitrag zum Syndrom des "low birth weight dwarfism," Helvet. paediat. acta 18:438, 1963.
14. Warkany, J., Beaudry, P. H., and Hornstein, S.: Attempted abortion with 4-amino-pteroylglutamic acid (aminopterin); malformations of the child, A.M.A. J. Dis. Child. 97:274, 1959.

30

Congenital Porencephaly and Schizencephaly

PORENCEPHALY is a collective term for a variety of large cerebral defects involving cortical tissue and penetrating, as a rule, through the white matter into the ventricular system. There can be no doubt that such defects may be of postnatal origin or be caused by birth trauma, but Heschl,[1] who, in 1859, coined the name "porencephaly," considered it a congenital anomaly. A typical porencephaly consists of a funnel-shaped cortical defect that communicates through a small hole with a ventricle.[2] The cavity usually is lined by connective tissue and a glial membrane, but the dura covers the opening externally, taking a normal course over the surface of the brain. Sometimes the cortical defect is filled out by cystic spaces derived from vascular elements or it is covered up by surrounding gyri. Porencephaly can be unilateral, but bilateral and symmetrical lesions have been observed in two-thirds of the cases.[3] The central gyri and the island of Reil are most often affected, but the defects can occur in any lobe. The cerebellum and the basal ganglia also may be sites of porencephalic lesions.

The origin of these defects has been discussed ever since first described,[1] when it was attributed to disease of the brain occurring during its prenatal development. Some thought that hydrocephaly, with its increased fluid pressure, causes interference with normal blood flow and brings about softening of the brain substance by ischemia. Kundrat[4] attributed porencephaly to cerebral malacia following circulatory disturbances. He pointed out that the defects occur most frequently in areas supplied by the middle cerebral artery, and that the cerebral wall can be destroyed by ischemia before and also after birth. Marburg *et al.*[5] also adhered to the vascular theory and considered porencephaly the result of hemorrhages or thrombosis of the vein of Galen or of cortical veins. They believed that such vascular changes are caused by birth injuries or other traumas that may occur before or after birth.

There are other brain defects that fall under the definition of porencephaly as usually employed that are of different origin. Yakovlev and Wadsworth[6] described clefts with fused lips occurring in the cerebral mantle and named these forms of arrested development "schizencephaly." In contrast to the porencephaly attributed to secondary destruction of a brain that at first had been formed normally (encephaloclastic porencephaly), schizencephalies are considered defects of primary formation—or "true malformations." A region reduced in thickness would later be overgrown by well-developed parts of the brain. The area of arrested growth would form a funnel-shaped groove that might remain separated from the ventricle by a thin membrane. If the area of thin cortical tissue is large, it can be pushed out as a hydrocephalic dilatation of the ventricle (Fig. 30-1). Developmental schizencephalies usually are bilateral and symmetrical. They show a departure from the fundamental structural organization of the normal brain. The entire system of the neopallium may fail to develop, whereas other systems such as the rhinencephalon and striatum show compensatory hyperplasia. Accidents of circulation such as thrombosis or phlebostasis cannot explain such radical departure in the organization of the brain, since the embryonal cerebral wall does not possess blood vessels in the terms of arteries and veins at the early stages of development, when schizencephaly is determined. There are two types of schizencephaly.[6] Schizencephaly without hydrocephaly shows clefts covered by fused lips and schizencephaly with hydrocephaly has separated lips. If necrosis, hemorrhages, thromboses, venous stasis or hydrocephaly occurs in schizencephaly, it is not the cause but, rather, the result of the developmental anomaly. Gross and Kaltenbäck[7] attributed the lesions to circumscribed, early disturbances of cell migration, formation of microgyri and subsequent difficulties of vascularization and necrosis. A rare instance of familial porencephaly was observed in the Children's Hospital and the Neuromuscular Clinic in Cincinnati. Three of 11 children had pneumoencephalograms that indicated porencephaly. As pointed out by Heschl,[1] associated malformations may occur with the developmental form of porencephaly or schizencephaly. Association of polymicrogyria and porencephaly was described by Dekaban.[11] It is of interest that porencephaly was diagnosed roentgenologically in a boy with a chromosomal anomaly, namely partial triploidy.[12]

Fig. 30-1.—Air encephalogram of a child with porencephaly, hydrocephaly and absence of corpus callosum.

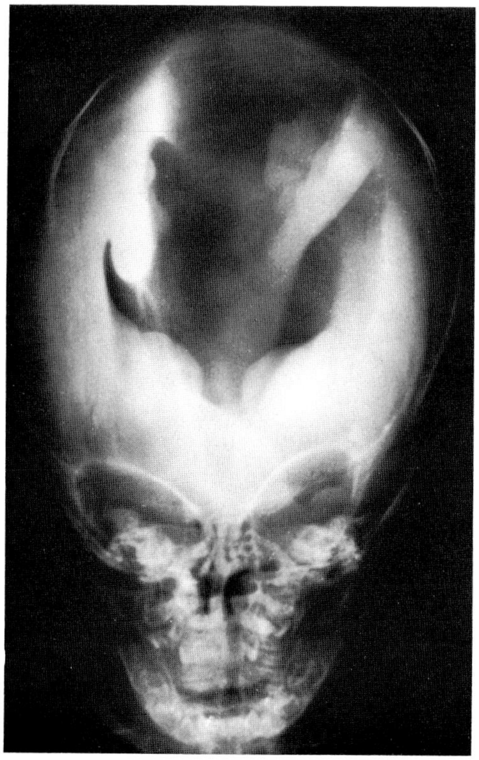

Porencephaly is found among mentally retarded persons, but not all patients with porencephaly are mentally retarded. Patten *et al.*[8] described a group of porencephalic patients who had presented abnormal neurologic signs from early childhood but survived to the second or third decade. Although these patients showed a substantial lack of brain substance at operation or necropsy, some of them suffered relatively mild functional disturbances. Patten and his colleagues suggested that porencephaly can be diagnosed clinically by a rather characteristic group of symptoms. Among these, lack of development in one half of the body is the most striking. Many have Jack-

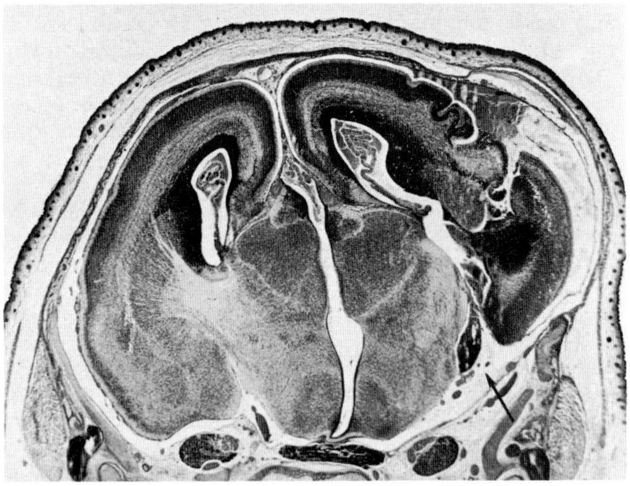

Fig. 30-2. – Cortical defect (**arrow**) in an abnormal rat brain connecting left brain surface and ventricular system. (Mother treated with trypan blue.)

sonian epilepsy but some have generalized convulsions, usually beginning in early life. Frequently there are motor weakness, hemiparesis and unilateral disturbance of reflexes. There also may be sensory disturbances such as hemianesthesia or hemianopia. Sensory anomalies are of significance because they distinguish porencephaly from spastic diplegia and related conditions with paralysis from early life in which the motor system only is involved and the neurologic findings are bilateral. In roentgenograms, it is found that one side of the skull is smaller than the other and the calvarium on the affected side is thickened. In the patients of Patten *et al.*,[8] air studies usually revealed a single cavity located in the parietal or occipital region and communicating with one of the lateral ventricles. Freeman and Gold[9] pointed out that porencephaly can simulate subdural hematoma in childhood. There is congenital hemiplegia, macrocephaly with contralateral parietal bulging, unilateral transillumination of the skull and unilateral voltage depression on EEG. The lesion was attributed to arterial occlusion, probably prenatal in origin. Naef[10] noted that the clinical picture is mild early in the course of some cases, so that studies are not made until adolescence or early adulthood.

In treatment, anticonvulsive drugs may result in improvement of seizures, but sometimes such drugs are ineffective.[10] Surgical procedures have been attempted and, in some cases, relief from convulsions has been reported. Occasionally, porencephalic brains are found at necropsy in persons who lived to old age without clinical manifestations of their cerebral defect.

REFERENCES

1. Heschl, R.: Gehirndefekt und Hydrocephalus, Vierteljschr. prakt. Heilk. Prag, 61:59, 1859; 72:102, 1861; 100:40, 1868.
2. Ernst, P.: Missbildungen des Nervensystems, in Schwalbe, E., *Die Morphologie der Missbildungen des Menschen und der Tiere* (Jena: Gustav Fischer, 1909), Vol. 3, pt. 2, pp. 67–252.
3. Hallervorden, J., and Meyer, J. E.: Cerebrale Kinderlähmung, in Lubarsch, O., Henke, F., and Rössle, R. (eds.), *Handbuch der Speziellen Pathologischen Anatomie und Histologie* (Berlin: Springer, 1956), Vol. 13, pt. 4, p. 214.
4. Kundrat, H.: *Die Porencephalie, eine anatomische Studie* (Graz: Leuschner and Lubensky, 1882).
5. Marburg, O., Rezek, P. R., and Marks, M. B.: Porencephaly. II. Studies in phlebothrombosis and phlebostasis, J. Neuropath. & Exper. Neurol. 4:43, 1945.
6. Yakovlev, P. I., and Wadsworth, R. C.: Schizencephalies. A study of congenital clefts in the cerebral mantle; clefts with fused lips, J. Neuropath. & Exper. Neurol. 5:116, 169, 1946.
7. Gross, H., and Kaltenbäck, E.: Neue Erkenntnisse über die Formalgenese der echten Porencephalie, Morphol. Jahrb. 100:517, 1960.
8. Patten, C. A., Grant, F. C., and Yaskin, J. C.: Porencephaly; diagnosis and treatment, Arch. Neurol. & Psychiat. 37:108, 1937.
9. Freeman, J. M., and Gold, A. P.: Porencephaly simulating subdural hematoma in childhood, Am. J. Dis. Child. 107: 327, 1964.
10. Naef, R. W.: Clinical features of porencephaly. A review of thirty-two cases, A.M.A. Arch. Neurol. & Psychiat. 80: 133, 1958.
11. Dekaban, A.: Large defects in cerebral hemispheres associated with cortical dysgenesis, J. Neuropath. & Exper. Neurol. 24:512, 1965.
12. Böök, J. A., and Santesson, B.: Malformation syndrome in man associated with triploidy (69 chromosomes), Lancet 1:858, 1960.

Cerebrovascular Malformations

Arteriovenous Malformations

ARTERIOVENOUS MALFORMATIONS may be seen on the surface of the brain as a tangle of abnormal blood vessels, diffusely distributed over the cortex, or as discrete masses within interlobar fissures embedded in the pia-arachnoid; sometimes they lie within a cerebral hemisphere. In children, communication of one or both posterior cerebral arteries with the vein of Galen or straight sinus may result in hydrocephaly as the presenting sign.[1]

Distinction of angiomatous malformations and of angiomatous tumors is not always easy. Cushing and Bailey[2] considered lesions consisting of vessels that are separated by brain tissue as malformations and distinguished them from vascular lesions, which they considered true neoplasms originating from angioblasts. Such neoplasms consist not only of blood vessels but also of a fine network of reticulin, but no nerve tissue is found between the vessels. Dandy[3] emphasized the congenital nature of the lesions and separated them from angiomas, and Bergstrand *et al.*[4] looked on all angiomas as malformations—even those that present as tumors. Lindau tumors, for instance, often are associated with other malformations that are manifestations of a general hamartosis (p. 1251). Scott *et al.*[5] stated that congenital arteriovenous malformations are almost always associated with angiomas capable of alteration in size and that they are composed of arteries, veins and capillaries with glial tissue between the vessels. The arterial blood may flow directly from an artery into a venous channel; more often, connection is established by a tangle of abnormal, undifferentiated vessels that forms the bulk of the malformation, provoking irritation and pressure symptoms like neoplasms. The arteries feeding the malformation and the emptying veins are distended to large channels.[5] Classification and nomenclature of angiomatous malformations and tumors are still confusing. Bergstrand *et al.*[4] distinguished:

1. Angioma cavernosum
2. Angioma racemosum
   a. Telangiectases
   b. Sturge-Weber syndrome
   c. Angioma racemosum arteriale
   d. Angioma racemosum venosum
   e. Aneurysma arteriovenosum
3. Angioreticuloma (angioblastoma of Cushing and Bailey or Lindau tumors)
4. Angioglioma

The delineations of these terms are rather indefinite, and some patients have angiomatous malforma-

Fig. 31-1.—Arteriovenous malformation (*A*) in occipital lobe with hemorrhage (*H*) into the ventricular system.

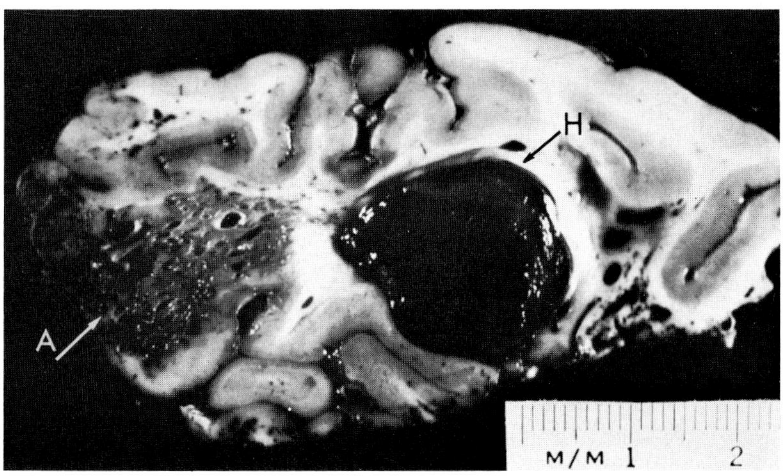

tions of different types.[6] Coexistence of arteriovenous malformations and saccular aneurysm, of persistent carotid-basilar anastomoses with saccular aneurysm and of arteriovenous angioma with carotid-basilar anastomosis (primitive trigeminal artery) has been described.[7]

The vascular malformations are the result of incomplete differentiation of the primordial vascular cerebral plexus into arteries, veins and capillaries and of failure of separation of the dural and pial circulations.[5] Although the anomalies date back to early developmental stages, their growth in postnatal life can lead to delayed manifestations during the fifth or sixth decade. As a rule, carotid-cavernous sinus or ophthalmic vein fistulas become symptomatic in adults, but arteriovenous malformations can manifest themselves in infancy and childhood.[5] Congestive heart failure in the newborn caused by cerebral arteriovenous fistulas has become a well-known complication. If the arteriovenous connections are large and the peripheral vascular resistance is lowered, the cardiac output is increased, the cardiac chambers are dilated and heart failure with cardiomegaly and cyanosis may follow. The heart can be structurally normal in such cases[8] or be affected by congenital malformations.[9,10] Arteriovenous malformations involving the vein of Galen are among the anomalies that can result in cardiac complications during infancy and childhood.[11,12] In the latter case, enlargement of the head, distention of scalp veins, discoloration of the eyelids, a bruit over the cranium and seizures may point to an intracranial lesion. Arteriovenous connections involving the vein of Galen were emphasized by Gold *et al.*,[13] who noted that neonates with this malformation present with cyanosis and respiratory distress and die with cardiovascular decompensation. Convulsions with or without hypoglycemia can occur. The cranial vascular malformations sometimes are a component of a general disturbance of cardiovascular development that may include transposition of the great vessels, patent ductus arteriosus or patent foramen ovale. Cervical cystic hygroma or polydactyly was observed in some of these patients. Congenital hydrocephaly was rare, but postnatal enlargement of the head developed in 18 of 19 infants seen after the neonatal period. In older children and adults, malformations of the vein of Galen presented with headaches and signs of subarachnoid hemorrhage.

Convulsions, aphasia, cranial nerve palsies, pareses, ataxia and mental retardation were noted in some of the cases.

Ingraham and Matson,[1] describing cerebral arteriovenous malformations of children, mentioned headaches, facial neurologic abnormalities, convulsions, spontaneous subarachnoid or intracortical hemorrhages and subjective or objective detection of intracranial bruits among the signs and symptoms. Gillingham[14] pointed out that, in contrast to the catastrophic bleeding from saccular aneurysms of the circle of Willis, the hemorrhages associated with arteriovenous malformations often are minor and intraventricular rather than subarachnoid. Askenasy[15] demonstrated that vascular malformations of the brain sometimes lead to hydrocephaly in adults, and Bailey and Woodard[16] directed attention to the fact that even small vascular malformations of the brain sometimes are associated with hydrocephaly and mental deficiency. Recognition of such a small vascular anomaly by arteriography and ventriculography is of importance, because the lesions, after production of intracerebral hematomas, can be treated by evacuation of the blood clot and removal of the small anomaly.[17] Small arteriovenous malformations usually are not associated with roentgenographic changes of the skull, but major lesions cause signs recognizable in cranial roentgenograms.[18]

Vascular intracranial malformations can be a part of generalized disorders such as Hippel-Lindau disease (p. 1266), Sturge-Weber syndrome (p. 349), hereditary hemorrhagic telangiectasia (p. 1185), multiple hemangiomas (p. 1178), ataxia-telangiectasia (p. 270) and others. In some of these diseases, the vascular anomalies are clearly congenital; in others, they become noticeable in postnatal life, although prenatal origins seem well established. Cavernous hemangiomatosis involving the brain, spinal cord, heart, skin and kidney was reported by Wood *et al.*,[19] who described a woman with multiple lesions compatible with life to the ninth decade. Multiple hemangiomas of the pons that have been observed in children and young adults can be symptomless or cause nuclear paralyses, tract disturbances and signs of diffuse brain lesions.[20]

Follow-up studies of intracranial arteriovenous malformations show growth of the lesion and increase in the caliber of afferent and efferent vessels in the majority of cases observed over many years, particularly if the vascular anomaly is situated around the sylvian fissure. In other cases, the size of the lesion remains unchanged. If the shunt through the arteriovenous aneurysm increases with advancing age and the circulation through the vessels of adjacent regions decreases, mental deterioration can occur,[21] so that for many patients the outlook is serious unless they are treated.

In recent decades, cerebral angiography has made possible visualization of the location, size and connections of the malformations,[5] and many patients can be helped by various neurosurgical procedures,[1,22] particularly dissection and excision of all the abnormal vessels and ligating and dividing of the feeding arteries and draining veins.[23]

Congenital Aneurysms

Congenital intracranial aneurysms are found in necropsies with a frequency of 0.6%. In about one-tenth of these cases, the aneurysms are multiple and sometimes associated with arteriovenous angiomas.[24]

Although the underlying anomaly is congenital and manifestation can occur in children,[25,26] most patients develop symptoms in the fifth decade of life.[27] Rupture of an aneurysm of the circle of Willis has been reported in a newborn twin.[28] Males and females are affected equally. Familial occurrence of aneurysms of cerebral arteries has been reported. A man and his son suffered rupture of cerebral vessels; in the son, an abnormal vessel was demonstrated by arteriography, pointing to a developmental error as the basis of the cerebral accident.[29] The aneurysms are seen at points of division of arteries, such as the first branching points of the middle cerebral artery in the sylvian fissure or at the junction of an anterior cerebral and an anterior communicating artery. They commonly are of pea size, but smaller and larger aneurysms have been found. They are of saccular type and lie initially in the subarachnoid space, but extension into the brain substance or the subdural space can occur. The wall is thin and made up of fibrous tissue as the muscles of the arterial media and the internal elastic membrane of the feeding vessel terminate at the neck of the aneurysm. The defect is attributed to congenital aplasia or hypoplasia of the muscle coat at the point of branching or junction of the arteries.[24] Association of intracranial aneurysms with polycystic kidneys or coarctation of the aorta has been observed repeatedly.[30] It seems that many normal persons have "weak spots" in cerebral arteries, particularly at points of bifurcation in the circle of Willis, but only a few develop aneurysms and are damaged by hemorrhages due to rupture of the sac. Blood from a ruptured sac may pass into the subarachnoid space, into the brain and ventricles or into the subdural space. Seizures, paralyses, mental symptoms or death can result from such hemorrhages, but recovery has been observed in a third of the cases.[24] Demonstration by arteriography can lead to successful surgical treatment.[1,22]

REFERENCES

1. Ingraham, F. D., and Matson, D. D.: *Neurosurgery of Infancy and Childhood* (Springfield, Ill.: Charles C Thomas, Publisher, 1954).
2. Cushing, H., and Bailey, P.: *Tumors Arising from Blood Vessels of the Brain. Angiomatous Malformations and Hemangioblastomas* (Springfield, Ill.: Charles C Thomas, Publisher, 1928).
3. Dandy, W. E.: Venous abnormalities and angiomas of brain, Arch. Surg. 17:715, 1928.
4. Bergstrand, H., Olivecrona, H., and Tonnis, W.: *Gefässmissbildungen und Gefässgeschwülste des Gehirns* (Leipzig: Georg Thieme, 1936).
5. Scott, W. G., Simril, W. A., and Seaman, W. B.: Intracerebral arteriovenous malformations: Their diagnosis and angiographic demonstration, Am. J. Roentgenol. 71:762, 1954.
6. Foroughi, E.: Coexistence of two types of congenital cerebral vascular disease, Arch. Neurol. 3:732, 1960.
7. Frugoni, P., Mingrino, S., and Giammusso, V.: Association of cerebral vascular malformations. Coexistence of arteriovenous angioma and persistent carotid-basilar anastomosis (primitive trigeminal artery), Neurochirurgia 6:74, 1963.
8. Silverman, B. K., Breckx, T., Craig, J., and Nadas, A. S.: Congestive failure in the newborn caused by cerebral A-V fistula, A.M.A. Am. J. Dis. Child. 89:539, 1955.
9. Devic, M., Girard, P. F., and Masson, R.: Malformations vasculaires dans les cardiopathies congénitales et les anomalies de la charnière occipito-vertébrale, Acta neurol. et psychiat. belg. 51:457, 1951.
10. Hernandez, A., Jr., Schwartz, H. G., and Goldring, D.: Cerebral arteriovenous fistulas and congenital heart disease, J. Pediat. 66:722, 1965.
11. Levine, O. R., Jameson, G., Nellhaus, G., and Gold, A. P.: Cardiac complications of cerebral arteriovenous fistula in infancy, Pediatrics 30:563, 1963.
12. Lehman, J. S., Jr., Chynn, K-Y., Hagstrom, J. W. C., and Steinberg, I.: Heart failure in infancy due to arteriovenous malformation of the vein of Galen, Am. J. Roentgenol. 98:653, 1966.
13. Gold, A. P., Ransohoff, J., and Carter, S.: Vein of Galen malformation, Acta neurol. scandinav. 40:1, 1964.
14. Gillingham, J.: Arteriovenous malformations of the head, Edinburgh M. J. 60:305, 1953.
15. Askenasy, H. M.: Hydrocephalus with vascular malformations of the brain, Neurology 3:213, 1953.
16. Bailey, O. T., and Woodard, J. S.: Small vascular malformations of the brain: Their relationship to unexpected death, hydrocephalus and mental deficiency, J. Neuropath. & Exper. Neurol. 18:98, 1959.
17. Papatheodorou, C. A., Gross, S. W., and Hollin, S.: Small arteriovenous malformations of the brain, Arch. Neurol. 5:666, 1961.
18. Rumbaugh, C. L., and Potts, D. G.: Skull changes associated with intracranial arteriovenous malformations, Am. J. Roentgenol. 98:525, 1966.
19. Wood, M. W., White, R. J., and Kernohan, J. W.: Cavernous hemangiomatosis involving the brain, spinal cord, heart, skin and kidney, Proc. Staff Meet. Mayo Clin. 32: 249, 1957.
20. Teilman, K.: Hemangiomas of the pons, Arch. Neurol. & Psychiat. 69:208, 1953.
21. Höök, O., and Johanson, C.: Intracranial arteriovenous aneurysms. A follow-up study with particular attention to their growth, A.M.A. Arch. Neurol. & Psychiat. 80:39, 1958.
22. Hamby, W. B.: *Intracranial Aneurysms* (Springfield, Ill.: Charles C Thomas, Publisher, 1952).
23. Norlén, G.: Arteriovenous aneurysms of the brain. Report of ten cases of total removal of the lesion, J. Neurosurg. 6:475, 1949.
24. Blackwood, W., McMenemey, W. H., Meyer, A., Norman, R. M., and Russell, D. S.: *Greenfield's Neuropathology* (2d ed.; Baltimore: The Williams & Wilkins Company, 1963).
25. Akerren, Y.: Über intrakranielle Aneurysmen als Ursache von subarachnoidal Blutungen im Kindesalter, Acta paediat. 31:109, 1943.
26. Richardson, J. C., and Hyland, H. H.: Intracranial aneurysms; clinical and pathological study of subarachnoid and intracerebral hemorrhage caused by berry aneurysms, Medicine 20:1, 1941.
27. Carmichael, R.: Pathogenesis of non-inflammatory cerebral aneurysms, J. Path. & Bact. 62:1, 1950.
28. Newcomb, A. L., and Munns, G. F.: Rupture of aneurysm of the circle of Willis in the newborn, Pediatrics 3:769, 1949.
29. Chambers, W. R., Harper, B. F., Jr., and Simpson, J. R.: Familial incidence of congenital aneurysms of cerebral arteries: Report of cases of ruptured aneurysms in father and son, J.A.M.A. 155:358, 1954.
30. Bigelow, N. H.: The association of polycystic kidneys with intracranial aneurysms and other related disorders, Am. J. M. Sc. 225:485, 1953.

32

Agenesis and Hypoplasia of the Corpus Callosum

Agenesis of the corpus callosum has long been known, but early descriptions usually referred to severe malformations of the brain, and only later did it become known that the anomaly may exist in persons who are intellectually and physically normal. The corpus callosum is phylogenically and ontogenically a relatively new structure. It develops in man in the lamina terminalis but remains small and limited to the rostral part of the brain to the fourth fetal month. After that, and particularly from the fifth month on, it grows rapidly caudad until it reaches the extent known in the adult brain. Agenesis of the corpus callosum may be complete or partial. In the latter case, the rostrum and the genu are present, whereas the posterior portions are missing. In some instances, the anterior commissure, fornix and the septum pellucidum are also defective but the longitudinal callosal bundle is clearly distinguishable. Among the severe cerebral malformations that are associated with agenesis of the corpus callosum are those of the cyclopia-arhinencephaly series (Chapter 23).

The etiology of callosal agenesis is diverse. As a rule, the anomaly occurs sporadically, but some hereditary patterns have been reported. Zellweger[1] observed it in brothers, and Naiman and Fraser[2] in sisters. Ziegler[3] continued observations in the family first reported by Zellweger and mapped the pedigree of the kindred involved. In 3 brothers, the disorder manifested itself within the first 3 weeks after birth by epileptiform convulsions leading to status epilepticus and early death. The mother of these boys had signs of latent epilepsy shown by electroencephalography. Menkes *et al.*[4] described less fulminant epilepsy associated with hypoplasia of the corpus callosum. Severe mental retardation was noted in the children, who died during the second year. Only males related through apparently normal mothers were affected. The observations were consistent with the assumption that the disorder was transmitted by a sex-linked recessive gene. Necropsy of one patient revealed abnormal convolutional pattern and heterotopias in addition to lack of development of the caudal parts of the corpus callosum. Chemical examination of the brain showed a decrease in lipid content, particularly in the cholesterol and cerebroside fractions, the latter being poor in normal fatty acids. Since the patient examined died at 19 months of age, it is not known whether the chemical changes were congenital or whether they resulted from the protracted convulsive disorder. An interesting association of complete agenesis of the corpus callosum with tuberous sclerosis has been reported.[5] In this case, the defect could be attributed to a hamartosis that is due to a dominant gene. Identical twins, both of whom had corpus callosum defects, have been observed.[2] Agenesis of the structure has been reported as a possible sequel to maternal rubella during the second month of pregnancy.[6]

Arhinencephaly due to trisomy 13-15 often is combined with hypoplasia or absence of the corpus callosum, and, in some instances of trisomy 13-15, callosal hypoplasia occurs without other serious malformations of the brain. Corpus callosum defects were also noted in rare cases of trisomy 18.[7,8] Agenesis of the corpus callosum, mental deficiency and convulsions were present in a child with a translocation involving chromosome 2 and a chromosome of the B group.[22] Some heterogeneous malformations such as hydrocephaly, microcephaly, porencephaly or absence of a hemisphere have been combined with agenesis of the corpus callosum. According to Marburg,[9] one must distinguish between primary agenesis of the corpus callosum, which is due to an early embryonic defect of the lamina terminalis, and secondary absence of the corpus callosum, which originates in a later month of fetal life by inflammation, porencephalic or hydrocephalic processes.

Defects of the corpus callosum with presence of the longitudinal callosal bundle similar to those in man have been described as a hereditary condition in mice,[10] but defect of this structure can also be produced experimentally in rats and mice by x-irradiation,[11] by maternal riboflavin deficiency[12] and by trypan blue injections in early gestation (Figs. 32-1 and 32-2).

There is no typical clinical syndrome that can be attributed to this anomaly. Some observations in man and some experimental evidence seem to indicate that absence of the corpus callosum in itself does not cause any neurologic disturbances. The clinical

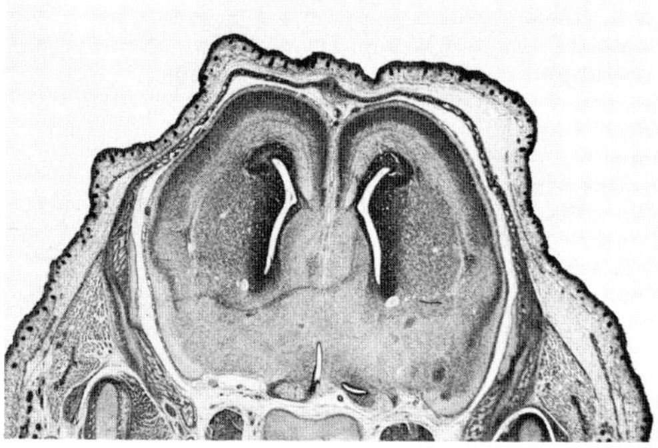

Fig. 32-1. – Absence of corpus callosum in newborn rat. (Mother treated with trypan blue injections.)

symptoms known to occur in cases of agenesis of the corpus callosum apparently are attributable to associated anomalies of the brain. Several publications indicate that some persons with this defect remained symptomless and in good mental condition throughout life.[13] In others, manifestations may exist from birth on or begin within the first 2 years of life. But cases are known in which the first symptoms appeared in the third decade only. Convulsive disorders, grand mal and petit mal attacks, Jacksonian epilepsy, athetoid movements and tremor may occur. Mental retardation is frequent. Patients with this anomaly may be diagnosed as microcephalic or as affected with cerebral palsy, but a large head may also be an early sign.[14,21] There may be neurologic findings such as hemiparesis, abnormal muscular spasticity or flaccidity, hyperactive reflexes, impaired coordination, and so forth. Hypertelorism, strabismus, corneal opacities, cataract, coloboma of the iris and the optic nerve, chorioretinitis, optic atrophy, cleft palate and lip, macroglossia and pilonidal sinus have been noted as associated findings. Defects of the corpus callosum have been found in patients with basal cell nevi and dental cysts[19] (p. 1269) and in children with the broad thumb syndrome.[20]

The electroencephalogram often is abnormal but not characteristic of the malformation. Typical x-ray findings have been established by Davidoff and Dyke.[15] The most common encephalographic findings are dorsal extension and dilatation of the third ventricle, wide separation of the lateral ventricles, dilatation of the posterior horns of the lateral ventricles, angular dorsal margins of the lateral ventricles and concave mesial borders of the lateral ventricles. These findings have made possible diagnosis of callosal agenesis during life. Angiographic studies can contribute to the diagnosis of agenesis of the corpus callosum during life.[16] In the differential diagnosis, cysts of the cavum septi pellucidi (p. 254), lipoma of the corpus callosum and neoplasm have to be considered. Lipoma can be recognized by direct radiography of the skull by radiolucency and characteristic calcifications of the fatty tissue that replaces the corpus callosum.[17,18] There is only symptomatic treatment available for agenesis or lipoma of the corpus callo-

Fig. 32-2. – Frontal section through the brain of a newborn rat in the area of the foramina of Monro (*M*). There is absence of corpus callosum and fornix. In their place, vascular and neural tissues (VN) are seen. (Mother treated with trypan blue.)

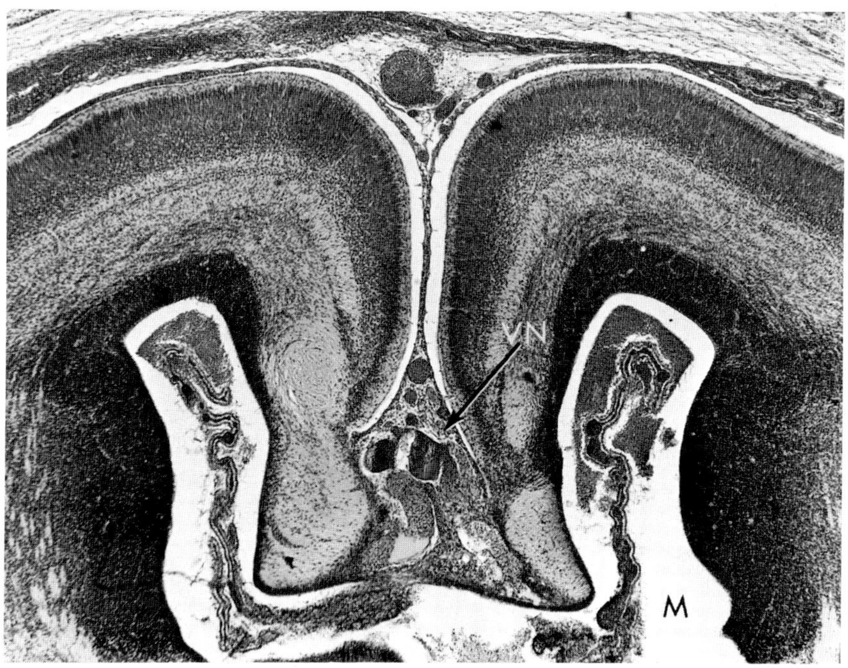

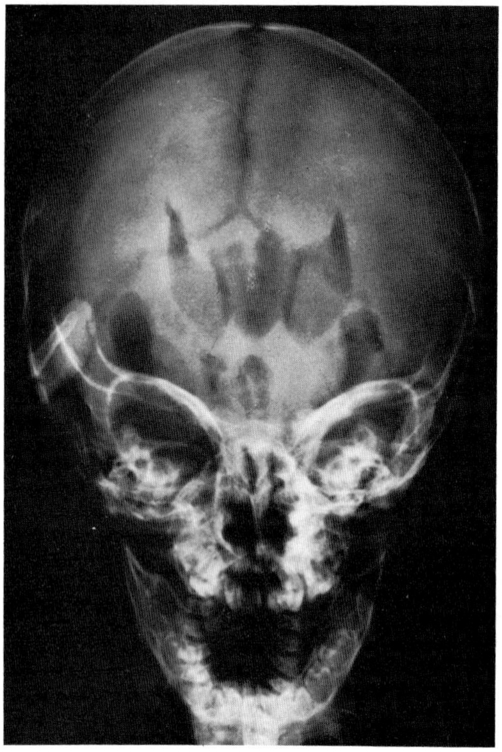

Fig. 32-3. – Pneumoencephalogram showing absence of corpus callosum. The lateral ventricles are widely separated and their dorsal angles elongated and drawn out like horns. The third ventricle is enlarged.

sum. The prognosis depends on associated anomalies of the central nervous system.

REFERENCES

1. Zellweger, H.: Agenesia corporis callosi, Helvet. paediat. acta 7:136, 1952.
2. Naiman, J., and Fraser, F. C.: Agenesis of the corpus callosum. A report of two cases in siblings, A.M.A. Arch. Neurol. & Psychiat. 74:182, 1955.
3. Ziegler, E.: Bösartige, familiäre, frühinfantile Krampfkrankheit, teilweise verbunden mit familiärer Balkenaplasie, Helvet. paediat. acta 13:169, 1958.
4. Menkes, J. H., Philippart, M., and Clark, D. B.: Hereditary partial agenesis of corpus callosum, Arch. Neurol. 11: 198, 1964.
5. Elliott, G. B., and Wollin, D. W.: Defect of the corpus callosum and congenital occlusion of fourth ventricle with tuberous sclerosis, Am. J. Roentgenol. 85:701, 1961.
6. Friedman, M., and Cohen, P.: Agenesis of corpus callosum as a possible sequel to maternal rubella during pregnancy, Am. J. Dis. Child. 73:178, 1947.
7. Warkany, J., Passarge, E., and Smith, L. B.: Congenital malformations in autosomal trisomy syndromes, Am. J. Dis. Child. 112:502, 1966.
8. Passarge, E., True, C. W., Sueoka, W. R., Baumgartner, N. R., and Keer, K. R.: Malformations of the central nervous system in trisomy 18 syndrome, J. Pediat. 69:771, 1966.
9. Marburg, O.: So-called agenesia of the corpus callosum (callosal defect): Anterior cerebral dysraphism, Arch. Neurol. & Psychiat. 61:297, 1949.
10. King, L. S.: Hereditary defects of the corpus callosum in the mouse, mus musculus, J. Comp. Neurol. 64:337, 1936.
11. Hicks, S. P.: Developmental malformations produced by radiation, Am. J. Roentgenol. 69:272, 1953.
12. Kalter, H., and Warkany, J.: Congenital malformations in inbred strains of mice induced by riboflavin-deficient, galactoflavin-containing diets, J. Exper. Zool. 136:531, 1957.
13. Ostertag, B.: Missbildungen, in Lubarsch, O., Henke, F., and Rössle, R. (eds.), *Handbuch der Speziellen Pathologischen Anatomie und Histologie* (Berlin: Springer, 1956), Vol. 13, pt. 4.
14. Koch, F. P., and Doyle, P. J.: Agenesis of the corpus callosum. Report of eight cases in infancy, J. Pediat. 50:345, 1957.
15. Davidoff, L. M., and Dyke, G. A.: Agenesis of the corpus callosum: Diagnosis by encephalography; report of 3 cases, Am. J. Roentgenol. 32:1, 1934.
16. Larsen, J. L.: Angiographic findings in agenesis of the corpus callosum, Am. J. Roentgenol. 98:579, 1966.
17. Sheinmel, A., and Lawrence, L. R.: Agenesis of the corpus callosum, Radiology 57:15, 1951.
18. Cant, W. H. P., and Astley, R.: Lipoma of corpus callosum, Arch. Dis. Childhood 27:478, 1952.
19. Binkley, G. W., and Johnson, H. H.: Epithelioma adenoides cysticum: Basal cell nevi, agenesis of the corpus callosum and dental cysts, Arch. Dermat. & Syph. 63:73, 1951.
20. Rubinstein, J. H., and Taybi, H.: Broad thumbs and toes and facial abnormalities, Am. J. Dis. Child. 105:588, 1963.
21. Butler, I. J., Beal, S., and Simpson, D. A.: Agenesis of the corpus callosum in infancy, South Australia Clin. 3:137, 1968.
22. Mantle, D. J., Mitchell, P., Kucheria, K., and Wilson, J.: A mentally retarded child with convulsions, agenesis of the corpus callosum, and a translocation involving chromosomes 2 and the B group, J. M. Genetics 6:435, 1969.

Cavum Septi Pellucidi; Cavum Vergae; Cavum Veli Interpositi

THE SEPTUM PELLUCIDUM represents a partition between the two lateral ventricles. It extends between the anterior portions of the corpus callosum and the body of the fornix. It consists of two thin laminae with a space between them. This space, or cavum, of the septum pellucidum usually is a narrow cleft that can be widened appreciably after trauma, or it is formed in the case of complete or partial agenesis of the septum. The finding of a cavum is not rare in pneumoencephalograms, but estimates of its occurrence vary, probably owing to selection of cases. In more than 1,000 formalin-fixed brains, Schwidde[1] noted a cavum septi pellucidi in 20% of the cases. Clinical features of cysts or caves of the septum include mental changes, motor defects, seizures, visual and hearing disorders and others. Hydrocephaly, agenesis of the corpus callosum or of olfactory tracts, craniolacunia and other defects may be associated.[2]

Cavum vergae, the caudal extension of a cavum septi pellucidi, is more rare and was found in only 2.3% of formalin-fixed brains.[1] It sometimes occurs in patients with mental and neurologic symptoms, but the cavum probably is not responsible for the clinical manifestations.[3] Differentiation of the cavum vergae from cavum veli interpositi was discussed by Zellweger and Van Epps.[4] The latter space is a part of the subarachnoid system that lies above and posterior to the third ventricle. It is not rare in mentally retarded children, but it is not the cause of the retardation.

REFERENCES

1. Schwidde, J. T.: Incidence of cavum septi pellucidi and cavum vergae in 1,032 human brains, A.M.A. Arch. Neurol. & Psychiat. 67:625, 1952.
2. Madonick, M. J., and Stern, W. Z.: Partial agenesis of septum pellucidum with cave of septum pellucidum, Arch. Neurol. 11:324, 1964.
3. Schönenberg, H.: Klinische und encephalographische Befunde bei Verdacht auf Cavum Vergae, Ztschr. Kinderh. 68:512, 1950.
4. Zellweger, H., and Van Epps, E. F.: The cavum veli interpositi and its differentiation from cavum vergae, Am. J. Roentgenol. 82:793, 1959.

33

Cerebral Palsy

CEREBRAL PALSY (CP) is a term for a group of motor disturbances present since early childhood that are due to nonprogressive abnormalities of the brain. It is generally admitted that this group does not represent an etiologic or clinical entity, but rather a practical problem posed by patients handicapped by motor difficulties. As Crothers and Paine[1] stated, the original lesion must occur early in life, but abnormalities of prenatal development, birth injuries and postinfectious states of early childhood are included in the term. Cerebral palsy thus defined is a frequent cause of crippling and accounts for approximately 8% of the handicapped children on State Registers.[2] The incidence of infants with CP born annually is estimated as 3.5–5.9 per 1,000 births,[3] the prevalence among school children or persons under 20 years of age, 1–2 per 1,000[4-6] and the prevalence of patients with CP in the population of the United States at about 350,000.[3] There are great variations in such estimates for various reasons, one being the lack of uniformity of definitions of CP.[4,5] The area of cerebral palsy overlaps, in part, that of mental retardation, and both areas are related to congenital malformations. Estimates of the percentage of cerebral palsied children said to be mentally deficient vary between 25% and 75%.[4,7] It is obvious that tests using verbal and motor skills are not fair to children with CP. In general, CP frequently is associated with mental retardation, but normal and even superior intelligence is found in a minority of patients who have motor disturbances classifiable as CP. In this chapter, some facts and deliberations will be cited which indicate that prenatal factors and congenital malformations are the basis of some cases of CP.

There is general agreement that prenatal factors play an etiologic and pathogenic role, but there is wide disagreement concerning the quantitative importance of these factors. This disagreement is explained in part by the differences in the patients seen by various specialists. Orthopedic surgeons examine a different group of patients with CP than observers in mental institutions. Pediatricians, neurologists, physiotherapists and pathologists deal with different samples of the entity. In addition, there often is an intermingling of adverse factors that resists analysis of etiology. There are differences of definition in clinical and neuropathologic studies, and the terminology is confusing in both. Some children suffer damage more than once. A child injured in prenatal life may undergo abnormal delivery and suffer damage from postnatal infection or trauma. It is easily understood that such a case could be attributed to prenatal, perinatal or postnatal factors.

Prenatal origin of some of the lesions sometimes is suggested by family histories or demonstrated by the presence of congenital cerebral malformations in the patients. It is not possible to give a quantitative estimate of the role played by early developmental defects and congenital malformations, but neuropathologic studies indicate that many disorders of prenatal origin result in the symptoms of cerebral palsy. Microcephaly, arrested hydrocephaly, microgyria, pachygyria, cerebellar atrophy, agenesis of the corpus callosum, various forms of sclerosis, Sturge-Weber syndrome, congenital encephalomalacia with cavity formations, agenesis of white matter and many other pathologic changes of the brain of prenatal origin may be at the root of some of the clinical syndromes often attributed to birth injury. Knowledge of the prenatal segment of CP is important, since it cannot be eliminated by improved obstetric care but must be considered together with the problem of congenital anomalies.

The conceptions on etiology and pathogenesis of infantile cerebral palsies have varied since the beginning of the nineteenth century, when scientific approaches to this problem began. Freud[8] relates that Cazauvielh, in 1827, had already distinguished between primary and secondary agenesis of the brain in cases of infantile hemiplegia. "Primary agenesis" as seen in brain dissections was his term for a reduction in size of one hemisphere, an anomaly of fetal development. His "secondary agenesis," represented by cysts or malacia, was considered the result of pathologic processes that could exert their damaging influences during fetal life or after birth. This concept probably can still be upheld today, but it seems that Cazauvielh had no etiologic explanation for these forms of cerebral agenesis. Unitary but contradictory explanations followed soon when Breschet, in 1831, attributed all cerebral atrophies to developmental disturbances, whereas Lallemand declared them all to be the result of early encephalic diseases.[8] In 1862, William John Little[9] directed attention to the role of obstetric factors in the etiology of infantile spastic diplegias in a paper "On the Influence of Abnormal Parturition, Difficult Labours, Premature Birth, and Asphyxia Neonatorum, on the Mental and Physical Condition of the Child, Especially in Relation to Deformities." In this classic paper, which has not lost its validity to the present day, Little pointed out that "the foetus in utero is subject to similar diseases to those which afflict the economy at later periods of existence." But during the period of birth "any untoward influences . . . would affect the economy in a manner different to the influence at work during the periods ordinarily characterised as those before birth and after birth." Thus, the conditions of the perinatal period were recognized as important for the spastic rigidity of the limbs of infants who survived the difficulties of parturition. Little concluded, from the histories of approximately 200 cases of spastic rigidity encountered in orthopedic practice, that they had one fact in common, namely some abnormal circumstance during parturition. Doctor Little's paper, presented to the Obstetrical Society of London, was well received. Doctor Barnes found it difficult to discuss because of "the entire novelty and originality of the subject" but mentioned the case of Samuel Johnson, who "was born almost dead, and did not cry for some time. The name of Samuel Johnson was almost synonymous with intellectual grandeur, but he was well known to be affected with certain nervous disorders which Dr. Little could better interpret than the speaker." Prematurity present in at least 26 of 47 children with spastic rigidity was also referred to by Little when he quoted Shakespeare's description of Richard III as an individual afflicted with a deformity originating at birth:

> "I, that am curtail'd of this fair proportion,
> Cheated of feature by dissembling nature,
> Deform'd, unfinish'd, sent before my time
> Into this breathing world scarce half made up,
> And that so lamely and unfashionable
> That dogs bark at me as I halt by them."

Little's paper became well known, and the spastic rigidity he described was named "Little's disease" and recognized as a substantial portion of the cerebral palsies. One hundred years after Little, Eastman *et al.*,[10] after a review of the obstetric and neonatal background of 753 children with CP, stressed again the importance of prematurity, mechanical birth trauma or intrauterine hypoxia and the poor condition at birth in the histories of these children.

Although these associations are well established, there remains the question of the prenatal state of children with perinatal difficulties. Thus, the interpretation of pathologic findings by McNutt,[11] who described a case of double infantile spastic hemiplegia in a child born after tedious labor, was severely criticized 39 years later by Collier,[12] who pointed out that McNutt's illustrations demonstrated that the pathologic process in this brain had begun long before birth. That there could be a discussion of a single case, over such a time, illustrates the importance of the question of prenatal versus perinatal origin of the cerebral palsies and also the difficulties of interpreting pathologic findings years after birth. The literature of the nineteenth century was surveyed by Freud in an extensive monograph entitled *Die Infantile Cerebrallähmung*.[8] He divided the cerebral palsies into congenital, birth and acquired paralyses, and pointed out that histories can be misleading, since congenitally abnormal children may not show obvious nervous manifestations before the second half of the first year of postnatal life. Freud quoted the case of a child considered normal for 9 months who developed rigidity, choreatic movements and intellectual impairment following an attack of enteritis and convulsions. Necropsy at the age of 3½ years showed porencephaly, microgyria and abnormal convolutions that dated back to developmental disturbances in prenatal life. It seemed that, in some cases, the obstetric difficulties might not be the true cause of the nervous disorders but rather the result of prenatal etiologic factors, and that such prenatal disturbances could also cause both prematurity and brain defect. Combination of prenatal and perinatal factors could cooperate in the pathogenesis of cerebral palsies. Familial and hereditary forms mentioned by Freud deserve attention, but some of the disorders considered by him have since been separated from the cerebral palsies because they are progressive. Collier[12] believed that cerebral diplegia was due to arrest in neuronal development caused by noxious influences of unknown origin. But Schwartz[13] maintained that malformations such as porencephaly and lobar atrophies can be attributed to difficult labor, resulting in circulatory disturbances of the areas served by branches of the vena magna Galeni, vena terminalis and vena lateralis ventriculi. Similarly, Courville[14] thought that congenital malformations of the brain are not a common cause of cerebral palsy, since any severe anomalous lesion of the brain precludes prolonged survival. In a series of 127 brains of CP patients, only 6 were classified as gross congenital defects and 6 as porencephaly, "still classed by some as congenital lesions." Cystic degeneration of the white matter, although attributed in some cases to intrauterine disease during the third trimester of pregnancy, and hydranencephaly were not considered congenital malformations by Courville because they are due to secondary destruction of the brain and not to failure of development. If congenital malformations are defined as structural defects present at birth, Courville's figures for this category would be much higher than 4.7%. Other necropsies revealed congenital malformations as the basic pathology.[15-17] Stewart,[18] who noticed that a large proportion of patients with CP had been delivered normally at term, found microcephaly, hydrocephaly, abnormal convolutional patterns, cerebellar atrophy, small pyramids and other malformations in such patients. Norman *et al.*,[19] Towbin[20] and Malamud *et al.*,[21] who studied brains of mentally retarded children with CP, considered about one-third attributable to malformations. Most of these were thought to be prenatal in origin, but in older children developmental defects masked by encephaloclastic secondary changes could not always be identified.

Neuropathology can be of only limited value in differentiation of prenatal and postnatal etiology. Even if the clinical picture is correlated with neuropathologic findings,[22] interpretation of the origin of the disorder often is uncertain. If a child is born with uncomplicated delivery but does not cry and has respiratory difficulties with cyanosis, it may show pathologic changes considered perinatal by the pathologist. But postnatal asphyxia or anoxia can occur in children damaged long before birth, and the postnatal changes of the brain can dominate the neuropathologic picture. If, for instance, polyporencephaly is accepted as a sign of perinatal damage,[22] its presence does not rule out prenatal damage.

Clinical distinction between prenatal and perinatal causes in patients with CP is also difficult. In 1924, Collier[12] acknowledged the importance of difficult birth for "Little's disease," and recognized cases of postnatal diplegias due to polioencephalitis, but he thought primary degeneration of the cerebral neurons from unknown causes to be the essential cause of diplegia. Ford[23] came to similar conclusions when he stated that the congenital diplegias, the largest group of infantile spastic palsies, cannot be attributed to meningeal hemorrhage at birth, but result from various pathologic intrauterine processes, as the neuropathology of true congenital diplegia cannot be reconciled with the theory of birth injury. Yannet,[24] who investigated the etiology of congenital CP in a population with marked mental retardation, came to the conclusion that developmental cerebral disturbances, possibly genetic in origin, are of greater importance in the causation of CP than perinatal events. Keith *et al.*,[25] reviewing 57 children with lesions of the nervous system, found that only 5 had had difficult births. They concluded that, in most of these children, difficulties during delivery had little to do with the persisting neurologic abnormalities. Approaching the problem from another side, Campbell *et al.*[26] followed the course of 89 children born with asphyxia and 178 controls. There were no significant differences in the outcome of the two groups. But Craig,[27] who examined the development of 593 children who survived symptoms of intracranial irritation following birth, noted physical or mental disability 1 or more years after birth in 8.8% and CP-like disease pictures in 6.6%.

In 1958, Illingworth[6] and Bailey[7] reviewed the literature on the etiology of CP and found opinions still divided. The role of asphyxia neonatorum, considered the leading cause of CP by many, did not seem established and proved to others. Crothers and Paine,[1] attempting an evaluation of "plausible etiologic factors" in 235 of their CP patients, attributed 20 to prenatal, 10 to prenatal plus birth factors and 205 to abnormal birth. Skatvedt[28] believed that perinatal injuries are the most frequent cause of CP. Perlstein[29] stated that the more common prenatal damages often end in stillbirths or miscarriages and that among the surviving CP patients, prenatal causes can be established in about 30%.

Eastman *et al.*[10] compared the obstetric and neonatal backgrounds of 753 children with CP with those of 759 presumably normal control children. In 8.5% of the CP children, the disease was of postneonatal origin. Prematurity was encountered in 31% of the CP series in contrast to 8.2% of the controls. Outstanding was the fact that 8.8% in the CP series weighed 1,500 Gm. or less at birth, whereas only 0.4% in the control series fell into this low-weight category. The pronounced tendency of very small prematures to develop CP was attributed to neonatal hypoxia, dehydration with hypernatremia and/or incomplete development of the pyramidal tracts. The incidence of twins was five times greater in the CP series than in the controls. Obstetric factors proved of great importance in this well-controlled study, but the incidence of gross congenital malformations, especially those of the central nervous system, was higher in the CP group than in the controls. Microcephaly and hydrocephaly were present in 4.5% of the CP series.

Attempts have been made to separate prenatal from perinatal and postnatal factors in subgroups of CP that could be of differing origin. Mitchell[30] considered etiologic factors in four separate types of cerebral palsy, namely, cerebral diplegia, hemiplegia, tetraplegia and athetoid cerebral palsy. There was also a group of mixed types. Prenatal causes accounted for all the cases of tetraplegia, about half the mixed cases and less than half the hemiplegic cases. The remaining cases were associated with birth injury and prematurity. Ingram[31] attempted an analysis of the role of developmental malformations in the various types of CP. He found strong evidence that developmental malformations were responsible for a significant proportion of patients with bilateral hemiplegia and ataxic diplegia. All the patients with bilateral hemiplegia had small heads and some of the patients with ataxic diplegia had relatives with CP or other neurologic disorders. Ten per cent of the children with congenital hemiplegia had a family history of CP.

That "prematurity" is of etiologic importance in CP was stressed by Little more than a hundred years ago; this has been confirmed in every study of perinatal factors in CP. In recent years, it has been established that 6–12% of children of very low birth weight develop CP,[32,33] and it has been shown that some children with low birth weight and CP were not prematures but had intrauterine growth retardation.[34] It will be of great importance to find out how many of these infants who are born small and develop CP are real prematures and how many are underweight because of intrauterine growth retardation (p. 134). If the two groups are equally affected by CP, perinatal or postnatal factors dangerous to small babies should be held responsible for the complications. If the children with intrauterine growth retardation are more often affected by CP than the truly premature, then prenatal factors, probably the same ones that are responsible for intrauterine growth retardation, could be incriminated for that group. X-irradiation, prenatal rubella and cytomegalic inclusion disease are examples of such prenatal factors already established for some of the cases.

In a study of cerebral palsy in children of very low birth weight (1,800 Gm. or less), McDonald[35] noted that, in single births, diplegia developed in 12% resulting from pregnancies lasting less than 31 weeks and in only 3% following pregnancies lasting 35 or more weeks. The fact that the truly prematures were more often affected rendered a perinatal origin more likely. But for twins born at or near term, Alberman[36] suspected a defect in the uterine environment associated with multiple pregnancy as the cause of the CP. Cerebral palsy was studied in twins by Griffiths.[77] It was not possible to separate monozygotic from dizygotic twins. There was a marked excess of first-born twins suffering from cerebral palsy as compared with the second twins, but there were more neonatal deaths in the second twins. The first twins were smaller and they showed a high incidence of spastic diplegia, whereas the higher-weight second twins had a tendency to tetraplegia. McDonald's finding of a lower incidence of diplegia in twins than in singletons of equally low birth weight could be related to the fact that in twins only the first acts as the dilator whereby the second twin is benefited.

Associated congenital malformations can suggest prenatal damage in some cases. Estimates of such association vary greatly. Skatvedt[28] found 1.1%, Asher and Schonell[37] 2.6%, Illingworth[38] 6.8%, Eastman and DeLeon[3] 14.6%, Ingram[31] 23.8%, Roboz[39] 34.8% and Barclay[40] 43.3% congenital anomalies in patients with CP. Such differences can be explained by differing definitions of "congenital anomaly" (minor and major) and of "cerebral palsy"; also by differing methods of search for congenital anomalies. The findings of Illingworth[38] are of interest because they were compared with the incidence of associated congenital malformations in children with mental retardation, the latter being about four times that of children with CP. If one accepts the occurrence of associated congenital anomalies as an indicator of the presence of congenital malformations in the central nervous system, it would seem that congenital malformations play a lesser role in the etiology of cerebral palsy than in that of mental retardation (p. 263). Since the athetoid group in CP is attributed to idiopathic and physiologic jaundice, Rh and ABO incompatibility and prematurity,[41] one would not expect an increased incidence of congenital malformations in this sector. Actually, congenital deformities are not more frequent, with the exception of a high, narrow arched palate noted by Koven and Lamm[42] in two-thirds of their athetoid patients. This interesting observation casts doubt on the congenital nature of high arched palate.

There is a general rule[22] that after perinatal damage the symptoms start at birth and continue throughout life, whereas patients with prenatal maldevelopment present only transient neonatal signs, develop rather normally during the first months of life and become spastic later. There is a great deal of truth in this view, but there is a possibility that a child with prenatal damage is also injured perinatally and acts accordingly soon after birth.

One way to investigate the role of prenatal determinants of CP is to search for specific causative factors acting before birth. Among prenatal infectious agents, rubella is known to cause microcephaly, sometimes associated with spastic diplegia[43,44] or athetoid movements.[44] Microcephaly with diplegia or paraplegia may follow cytomegalic inclusion disease.[45] Infection in utero with Toxoplasma can result in hydrocephaly or microcephaly with spasticity of the extremities.[46] Syphilis, now of little etiologic importance, did contribute to infantile cerebral palsy in the past.[8] Radium or x-irradiation in utero resulting in microcephaly and microphthalmia was sometimes associated with muscular rigidity and palsy.[47] Carbon monoxide poisoning in utero can result in microcephaly, tetraplegia[48] or athetosis.[1] In such cases, the basal ganglia and the thalamus may be found destroyed and replaced by cavities and the cortex atrophied and distorted by microgyria.[49] A case of cerebral palsy, mental retardation and ectrodactyly was attributed to prenatal hypoxia because the mother had mitral stenosis and rheumatic fever.[76] Endemic cretinism, generally attributed to environmental iodine deficiency, usually is characterized by hyperactive reflexes and occasionally associated with spasticity.[50] "Nervous cretinism"[51] was said to be associated with nervous disorders resembling spastic diplegia. This condition was described in India in areas in which goiter and cretinism were endemic. About one-third of the cretins showed all degrees from spastic paralysis of the lower limbs to general rigidity. Andersen[52] observed a boy with tetraplegia whose mother had suffered from night blindness during pregnancy because of an extremely deficient diet. Fetal Minamata disease caused by intrauterine intoxication by a methyl mercury compound (p. 128) manifested itself as infantile CP.[53]

Heredity repeatedly has been considered a factor in the etiology of CP, but in most general surveys the search for multiple cases in families yielded rather meager results.[24,37] It should be emphasized that the occurrence of CP in more than one child of a family could be due to genetic factors, but also to nongenetic causes such as parental syphilis or pelvic anomalies or endemic goiter of the mother. There exist, however, pedigrees that show spastic conditions transmitted through several generations or reveal genetic determination by parental consanguinity. Some of these conditions represent systemic neurologic syndromes, often of a progressive nature, and are therefore excluded by definition from the realm of CP. But, when seen in an early stage or only once, they may resemble cerebral palsy. Familial spastic paraplegias, familial athetoses, familial tremors and familial ataxias are cases in point.

Penrose[54] stated that there are many instances of cerebral diplegia in which the condition has the characteristics of recessive gene determination, since parental consanguinity and affected sibs are reported. In an institutional population, Yannet[55] found that 5 of 7 children with paraplegia and 2 of 65 with tetraplegia had affected siblings or relatives. Greenspan and Deaver,[56] in a series of 100 children with CP, ascertained that 2 patients had brothers with mild forms of spasticity and 7 had cousins with CP. Fuldner[57] ascertained 7 affected siblings or relatives in 204 cases of CP with paraplegia, hemiplegia and athetosis alternating in some family members. Illingworth[6] mentioned several families with multiple cases of CP differing in form—hemiplegia, paraplegia, quadriplegia and athetosis occurring in different members. Hanhart[58] described 7 cases of spastic diplegia in 4 related sibships in which all 8 parents had a common ancestor. Adler[59] found, in a series of 120 patients with CP, 16 children in 8 families with near relatives affected; in 5 of the families, parental consanguinity could be established. Ingram[31] mentioned that in 3 of 10 patients suffering from congenital ataxic diplegia there was a family history of CP. In 2 of these cases, the mothers also suffered from ataxic diplegia. In a study of familial cerebral palsy throughout Sweden, Gustavson *et al.*[79] ascertained 43 families in 30 of which the patients were siblings. Cerebral palsy and juvenile glaucoma have been observed in siblings.[80]

Sex-linked recessive inheritance of CP was suggested by a pedigree published by Blumel *et al.*,[60] in which 4 males were affected in two generations. Sex-linked spastic paraplegia with severe mental retardation occurred in a kinship with 13 males affected.[61]

A syndrome of cerebral palsy, mental retardation self-mutilation and hyperuricemia is inherited as a sex-linked recessive trait.[62-65] Choreoathetosis (double athetosis) present from early infancy[64] and spastic paralysis[66] justify classification of the disorder as cerebral palsy, but progressiveness of the process could be cited against inclusion in this category. A clinical observer of affected children would certainly diagnose cerebral palsy, and this was the term applied to such children in the past. The picture simulates cerebral palsy of children with double athetosis who have a definite history of neonatal asphyxia but do not show self-mutilation or hyperuricemia.[64]

Spastic disorders combined with mental retardation and ichthyosis attributed to an autosomal recessive gene was reported by Sjögren and Larsson.[67] The syndrome has also been observed outside Sweden.[68,69]

The fact that in some families with genetically determined CP[6,57,59] intrafamilial variation of clinical syndromes occurred makes it unlikely that clinical types correspond to etiologic entities.

In recent years, a few cases of CP have been found associated with chromosomal anomalies. Blumel *et al.*[70] described a chromosomal anomaly in a brother and sister with CP. Dobson and Ohnuki[71] reported a cytogenetic deviation in a boy with a convulsive disorder who had appeared normal up to the age of 3 years. Then convulsions began, craniotomy was performed and, subsequently, spasticity and rigidity of all limbs developed. Frøland *et al.*[72] found 47 chromosomes in the cells of a child with multiple anomalies.

There had been a slight degree of asphyxia in the neonatal period. At the age of 8 months, he was found to have cerebral palsy of the hypertonic tetraplegic type. The extra chromosome was a very small metacentric. Porencephaly was present in a boy with partial triploidy.[73] Hamerton *et al.*,[74] searching for sex chromosome abnormalities in a population of mentally defective children, encountered one idiotic girl with spastic tetraplegia who had two sex chromatin masses in buccal cell nuclei. Chromosome analysis revealed a triple-X chromosome pattern. This case is of specal interest, since this girl was thought to be normal until she was 2 years of age, and her deterioration was attributed to an accident. On the basis of her history, she could have been classified as a case of CP of postnatal origin. Thus, genetic and therefore prenatal causation can be proved in a relatively small number of patients with CP, but, even in such cases, birth histories and postnatal histories may confuse the situation. It should also be emphasized that familial repetition of CP does not necessarily signify genetic causation, since environmental hazards—prenatal or perinatal—can be repetitive.

Rh incompatibility, which once accounted for 10% of the cerebral palsies, represents a combination of genetic and nongenetic factors leading to kernicterus and central nervous system damage. It is now held responsible for only 1–2% of CP cases.[31] Other forms of kernicterus caused by different blood incompatibilities, hemolytic anemias, drugs, and so forth still play an important role in the etiology of CP.

Although there is good evidence that prenatal damage to the brain occurs in many children who develop CP, it is not clear which sector of the area is prenatal in origin and what its size is. Children with congenital malformations or other brain anomalies of prenatal origin can be asphyctic at birth or be born in difficult labors and/or prematurely. For instance, a child described by Insley[78] was severely mentally retarded after a difficult birth. The cord was tight around the neck and the baby was slow to breathe. In all probability, the brain damage and physical anomalies were due to a deficiency of the long arm of chromosome 18 and not to the difficult birth. The observer perceiving the last link in the chain of events accepts it as the cause of the disorder. But observations beginning at the time of birth or thereafter often fail to take into account preceding events and the fact that they deal with sequelae and complications of disturbances dating back to prenatal life.

But it is most likely that a normal fetus damaged at birth can also develop the signs and symptoms of CP. Asphyxia produced in fetal primates causes motor disturbances comparable to neurologic manifestations in children with CP.[75] Little's[9] observation of the association of cerebral palsy with abnormal parturition, difficult labors, premature birth and asphyxia neonatorum is still valid. He directed the attention of physicians to the perinatal period as the time of origin of certain types of physical and mental retardation. It is possible that Little's publication has contributed to the reduction of that portion of cerebral palsy caused by obstetric factors, which may explain why in some more recent studies[25,26] his findings could not be confirmed. As the obstetric factors lose some of their relative importance, prenatal factors come to the foreground and assume a more prominent part among the causes of CP.

REFERENCES

1. Crothers, B., and Paine, R. S.: *The Natural History of Cerebral Palsy* (Cambridge, Mass.: Harvard University Press, 1959).
2. Saffian, S.: Program trends in crippling conditions, 1950–1960, U.S. Dept. Health, Education and Welfare, Statistical Series No. 67, Children's Bureau, 1962, 40 pp.
3. Eastman, N., and DeLeon, M.: Etiology of cerebral palsy, Am. J. Obst. & Gynec. 69:950, 1955.
4. Herlitz, G., and Redin, B.: The prevalence of cerebral palsy, Acta paediat. 44:146, 1955.
5. Kurland, L. T.: Definitions of cerebral palsy and their role in epidemiologic research, Neurology 7:641, 1957.
6. Illingworth, R. S.: *Recent Advances in Cerebral Palsy* (London: J. & A. Churchill, Ltd., 1958).
7. Bailey, C. J.: Interrelationship of Asphyxia Neonatorum, Cerebral Palsy and Mental Retardation, in Windle, W. F., Hinman, E. H., and Bailey, P. (eds.), *Neurological and Psychological Deficits of Asphyxia Neonatorum* (Springfield, Ill.: Charles C Thomas, Publisher, 1958), pp. 5–30.
8. Freud, S.: *Die Infantile Cerebrallähmung* (Vienna: A. Hoelder, 1897).
9. Little, W. J.: On the influence of abnormal parturition, difficult labours, premature birth, and asphyxia neonatorum, on the mental and physical condition of the child, especially in relation to deformities. Tr. Obst. Soc. London 3:293, 1862.
10. Eastman, N. J., Kohl, S. G., Maisel, J. E., and Kavaler, F.: The obstetrical background of 753 cases of cerebral palsy, Obst. & Gynec. Surv. 17:459, 1962.
11. McNutt, S. J.: Double infantile spastic hemiplegia with the report of a case, Am. J. M. Sc. 89:58, 1885.
12. Collier, J. S.: The pathogenesis of cerebral diplegia, Brain 47:1, 1924.
13. Schwartz, P.: Die traumatischen Schädigungen des Zentralnervensystems durch die Geburt, Ergebn. inn. Med. u. Kinderh. 31:165, 1927.
14. Courville, C. B.: Structural Changes in the Brain in Cerebral Palsy, in Illingworth, R. S. (ed.), *Recent Advances in Cerebral Palsy* (London: J. & A. Churchill, Ltd., 1958).
15. Mackay, R. P.: Congenital demyelinating encephalopathy, Arch. Neurol. & Psychiat. 43:111, 1940.
16. Winkelman, N. W., and Moore, M. T.: Progressive degenerative encephalopathy; occurrence in infancy, with antenatal onset simulating "swayback" of lambs; report of a case, Arch. Neurol. & Psychiat. 48:54, 1942.
17. Yakovlev, P. J., and Wadsworth, R. C.: Schizencephalies. A study of the congenital clefts in the cerebral mantle. II. Clefts with hydrocephalus and lips separated, J. Neuropath. & Exper. Neurol. 5:169, 1946.
18. Stewart, R. M.: Observations on the pathology of cerebral diplegia, Proc. Roy. Soc. Med. 36:25, 1942.
19. Norman, R. M., Sandifer, P. H., Evans, E. S., and Tizard, J. P. M.: Discussion on infantile cerebral palsies, Proc. Roy. Soc. Med. 46:627, 1953.
20. Towbin, A.: *The Pathology of Cerebral Palsy* (Springfield, Ill.: Charles C Thomas, Publisher, 1960).
21. Malamud, N., Itabashi, H. H., Castor, J., and Messinger, H. B.: An etiologic and diagnostic study of cerebral palsy, J. Pediat. 65:270, 1964.
22. Christensen, E., and Melchior, J. C.: *Cerebral Palsy—A*

Clinical and Neuropathological Study. Clinics in Developmental Medicine No. 25 (London: Spastics Society Medical Education and Information Unit in association with William Heinemann Medical Books, Ltd., 1967).
23. Ford, F. R.: Cerebral birth injuries and their results, Medicine 5:121, 1926.
24. Yannet, H.: The etiology of congenital cerebral palsy. A statistical and clinical study, J. Pediat. 24:38, 1944.
25. Keith, H. M., Norval, M. A., and Hunt, A. B.: Neurologic lesions in relation to the sequelae of birth injury, Neurology 3:139, 1953.
26. Campbell, W. A. B., Cheeseman, E. A., and Kilpatrick, A. W.: The effects of neonatal asphyxia on physical and mental development, Arch. Dis. Childhood 25:351, 1950.
27. Craig, W. S.: Intracranial irritation in the newborn: Immediate and long-term prognosis, Arch. Dis. Childhood 25:325, 1950.
28. Skatvedt, M.: Cerebral palsy. A clinical study of 370 cases, Acta paediat. 46:1, 1958. Supp. 111.
29. Perlstein, M. A.: Cerebral palsy, incidence, etiology, pathogenesis, Arch. Pediat. 79:289, 1962.
30. Mitchell, R. G.: Some Aetiological Considerations, in Henderson, J. L. (ed.), *Cerebral Palsy in Childhood and Adolescence* (Edinburgh & London: E. & S. Livingstone, Ltd., 1961).
31. Ingram, T. T. S.: *Paediatric Aspects of Cerebral Palsy* (Baltimore: The Williams & Wilkins Company, 1964).
32. Drillien, C. M.: The incidence of mental and physical handicaps in school age children of very low birth weight, Pediatrics 27:452, 1961.
33. McDonald A.: Neurological and ophthalmic disorders in children of very low birth weight; a survey with the Society of Medical Officers of Health, Brit. M. J. 1:895, 1962.
34. Warkany, J., Monroe, B. B., and Sutherland, B. S.: Intrauterine growth retardation, Am. J. Dis. Child. 102:249, 1961.
35. McDonald, A. D.: Cerebral palsy in children of very low birth weight, Arch. Dis. Childhood 38:579, 1963.
36. Alberman, E.: Birth weight and length of gestation in cerebral palsy, Developmental Med. & Child Neurol. 5: 388, 1963.
37. Asher, P., and Schonell, F. E.: Survey of 400 cases of cerebral palsy in childhood, Arch. Dis. Childhood 25:360, 1950.
38. Illingworth, R. S.: Congenital anomalies associated with cerebral palsy and mental retardation, Arch. Dis. Childhood 34:228, 1959.
39. Roboz, P.: Etiology of congenital cerebral palsy, Arch. Pediat. 79:233, 1962.
40. Barclay, J.: Survey of cerebral palsy in Otago, New Zealand M. J. 55:199, 1956.
41. Plum, P.: Aetiology of athetosis with special reference to neonatal asphyxia, idiopathic icterus and ABO-incompatibility, Arch. Dis. Childhood 40:376, 1965.
42. Koven, L. J., and Lamm, S. S.: The athetoid syndrome in cerebral palsy. Part II. Clinical aspects, Pediatrics 14: 181, 1954.
43. Swan, C., and Tostevin, A. L.: Congenital abnormalities in infants following infectious diseases during pregnancy, with special reference to rubella: A third series of cases, M. J. Australia 1:645, 1946.
44. Beswick, R. C., Warner, R., and Warkany, J.: Congenital anomalies following maternal rubella, Am. J. Dis. Child. 78:334, 1949.
45. Weller, T. H., and Hanshaw, J. B.: Virologic and clinical observations on cytomegalic inclusion disease, New England J. Med. 266:1233, 1962.
46. Sabin, A. B.: Toxoplasmosis, in De Sanctis, A. G. (ed.), *Advances in Pediatrics* (New York: Interscience Publishers, Inc., 1942), Vol. I, p. 1.
47. Goldstein, L., and Murphy, D. P.: Microcephalic idiocy following radium therapy for uterine cancer during pregnancy, Am. J. Obst. & Gynec. 18:189, 1929.
48. Brander, T.: Microcephalus und Tetraplegie bei einem Kinde nach Kohlenmonoxydvergiftung der Mutter während der Schwangerschaft, Acta paediat. 28:123, 1940. Supp. 1.
49. Hallervorden, J., and Meyer, J. E.: Cerebrale Kinderlähmung, in Lubarsch, O., Henke, F., and Rössle, R. (eds.), *Handbuch der Speziellen Pathologischen Anatomie und Histologie* (Berlin: Springer, 1956), Vol. 13, pt. 4, pp. 194–282.
50. deQuervain, F. J., and Wegelin, K.: *Der endemische Kretinismus* (Berlin: J. Springer, 1936).
51. McCarrison, R.: Observations on endemic cretinism in the Chitral and Gilgit valleys, Lancet 2:1275, 1908.
52. Andersen, B.: Infantile cerebral palsy, Acta paediat. 46: (Supp. 109) 3, 1957.
53. Matsumoto, H., Koya, G., and Takeuichi, T.: Fetal Minamata disease. A neuropathological study of two cases of intrauterine intoxication by a methyl mercury compound, J. Neuropath. & Exper. Neurol. 24:563, 1967.
54. Penrose, L. S.: *The Biology of Mental Defect* (2d ed.; London: Sidgwick & Jackson, Ltd., 1954).
55. Yannet, H.: Infantile cerebral palsy cases with severe mental deficiency, Pediatrics 3:820, 1949.
56. Greenspan, L., and Deaver, G. G.: Clinical approach to the etiology of cerebral palsy, Arch. Phys. Med. 34:478, 1953.
57. Fuldner, R. V.: Cerebral palsy: Where next? A.M.A. Arch. Neurol. & Psychiat. 74:267, 1955.
58. Hanhart, E.: Eine Sippe mit einfach-rezessiver Diplegia Spastica Infantilis (Little'scher Krankheit) aus einem Schweizer Inzuchtsgebiet, Der Erbarzt 3:165, 1936.
59. Adler, E.: Familial cerebral palsy, J. Chron. Dis. 13:207, 1961.
60. Blumel, J., Evans, E. B., and Eggers, G. W. N.: Hereditary cerebral palsy, J. Pediat. 50:454, 1957.
61. Baar, H. S., and Gabriel, A. M.: Sex-linked spastic paraplegia, Am. J. Ment. Deficiency 71:13, 1966.
62. Riley, J. D.: Gout and cerebral palsy in a three-year-old boy, Arch. Dis. Childhood 35:293, 1960.
63. Lesch, M., and Nyhan, W. L.: A familial disorder of uric acid metabolism and central nervous system function, Am. J. Med. 36:561, 1964.
64. Hoefnagel, D., Andrew, E. D., Mireault, N. G., and Berndt, W. O.: Hereditary choreoathetosis, self-mutilation and hyperuricemia in young males, New England J. Med. 273:130, 1965.
65. Manzke, H.: Hyperuricämie mit Cerebralparese. Syndrom eines hereditären Purinstoffwechselleidens, Helvet. paediat. acta 22:258, 1967.
66. Nyhan, W. L., Pesek, J., Sweetman, L., Carpenter, D. G., and Carter, C. H.: Genetics of an X-linked disorder of uric acid metabolism and cerebral function, Pediat. Res. 1:5, 1967.
67. Sjögren, T., and Larsson, T.: Oligophrenia in combination with congenital ichthyosis and spastic disorders, Acta psychiat. et neurol. scandinav. 32:1, 1957. Supp. 113.
68. Link, J. K., and Roldan, E. C.: Mental deficiency, spasticity, and congenital ichthyosis, J. Pediat. 52:712, 1958.
69. Timpany, M. M.: Congenital ichthyosis, spastic diplegia, and mental deficiency, Lancet 1:1132, 1962.
70. Blumel, J., Ohnuki, Y., and Awa, A.: Chromosome anomaly in two cases of cerebral palsy, a brother and a sister, Nature, London 189:154, 1961.
71. Dobson, R., and Ohnuki, Y.: Chromosomal abnormalities in a child with a convulsive disorder, Lancet 2:627, 1961.
72. Frøland, A., Holst, G., and Terslev, E.: Multiple anomalies associated with an extra small autosome, Cytogenetics 2: 99, 1963.
73. Böök, J. A., and Santesson, B.: Malformation syndrome in man associated with triploidy (69 chromosomes), Lancet 1:858, 1960.
74. Hamerton, J. L., Jagiello, G. M., and Kirman, B. H.: Sex-chromosome abnormalities in a population of mentally defective children, Brit. M. J. 1:220, 1962.
75. Windle, W. F.: Anoxia and Asphyxia: Experiments in Fetal and Neonatal Monkeys, in Fields, W. S., and Desmond,

M. M. (eds.), *Disorders of the Developing Nervous System* (Springfield, Ill.: Charles C Thomas, Publisher, 1961), pp. 144–155.
76. Jancar, J.: Ectrodactyly, spastic paraplegia and mental retardation, J. Ment. Defic. Res. 11:207, 1967.
77. Griffiths, M.: Cerebral palsy in multiple pregnancy, Developmental Med. & Child Neurol. 9:713, 1967.
78. Insley, J.: Syndrome associated with a deficiency of part of the long arm of chromosome no. 18, Arch. Dis. Childhood 42:140, 1967.
79. Gustavson, K-H., Hagberg, B., and Sanner, G.: Identical syndromes of cerebral palsy in the same family, Acta paediat. scandinav. 58:330, 1969.
80. Hyams, S. W., and Jaffe, M.: Cerebral palsy and juvenile glaucoma in siblings, Developmental Med. & Child Neurol. 12:467, 1970.

34

Mental Retardation

MANY, IF NOT MOST, cases of mental retardation show physical features that betray the patient's mental condition. Posture, gait, facial expression or movements that suggest subnormal mentality develop in postnatal life. Other characteristics such as congenital malformations and abnormal dermatoglyphics point to prenatal damage. It is not only of theoretical but also of practical importance to know whether a case of mental retardation is of prenatal or postnatal origin. Histories often are unreliable and confusing; they seldom permit valid conclusions concerning the origin of mental defects. One often hears about perinatal or postnatal difficulties of a child whose disturbances date back to embryonic or fetal life. A cord around the neck, failure to breathe, cyanosis, jaundice or hypoglycemia after birth often are blamed for a child's subnormality even though the infant had been damaged before birth.[30] Such erroneous concepts of causation may place the blame on innocuous events or innocent persons. They may direct etiologic research into false channels or result in embarrassing legal situations. For these reasons, the nature of brain defects – whether congenital or postnatal in origin – should be established whenever possible. Not only investigators but also parents, siblings and other relatives may profit from knowledge of the origin of the mental impairment of a patient. If a mentally retarded child shows malformations that point to prenatal disturbance of development, perinatal and postnatal factors suspected as the cause of mental impairment will be recognized as secondary and sometimes innocent complications rather than as primary causes.

Necropsy sometimes reveals the congenital nature of a brain defect, but, at times, the interpretation of cerebral malformations seen years after confinement and illness may be uncertain. There are not many serial necropsy examinations available of mentally defective persons, and those that have been published deal with severely affected and institutionalized patients. Malamud[1] analyzed 1,410 consecutive necropsies performed in three hospitals for the mentally retarded in California. He attributed 61% of the cases to malformations. Hydrocephaly, micropolygyria, agyria, porencephaly, hydranencephaly, encephalocele and arhinencephaly were encountered. In addition, there were many kinds of multiple and nonspecific malformations. Microcephaly was not listed separately in this study, although there were many microcephalic children included who were listed in such categories as agyria, pachygyria and nonspecific types. Agenesis of the corpus callosum was common and was associated with a variety of other cerebral malformations. Down syndrome accounted for 17% of the retarded on whom necropsies were performed and for 29% of those in whom cerebral malformations were recognized. Crome,[2] studying 282 brains of institutionalized mental defectives, found established syndromes in 32% and unclassified anomalies in 68%. Only 8 brains showed no abnormalities. Such necropsy series give us valuable information concerning the pathology of institutionalized patients, but even they cannot always distinguish between malformations of prenatal and postnatal origin. Whereas agyria, microgyria, absence of the corpus callosum, hydranencephaly and arhinencephaly are clearly of prenatal origin, hydrocephaly and microcephaly are not; they can arise before or after birth. These studies show the difficulties encountered in etiologic and pathogenic classification of the various types of mental retardation; even combinations of clinical and neuropathologic analyses often fail in such retrospective studies. In the living, classification of mental deficiencies is even more difficult unless somatic characteristics help in their distinction. It has long been known that there exist associations of some forms of mental retardation with congenital malformations outside the central nervous system, and physicians have studied somatic "stigmas" in the retarded with varying success. Some external signs noted in such patients are of great significance and have led, for instance, to the recognition of a cytogenetic entity, Down syndrome, about 100 years before the chromosomes of such persons could be visualized. Other signs are of doubtful significance because they occur rather frequently in the general population; their occurrence among the retarded could be fortuitous. Yet, minor "stigmas" such as simian creases, incurved little fingers, syndactyly, polydactyly, auricular appendages, slanting eyes, retrognathia and others that occur occasionally in mentally normal persons are seen with increased frequency in many types of mental retardation. Some structural anomalies prove quite useful in the diagnosis and prognosis of mental defects, as exemplified by the Laurence-Moon-Biedl, Apert, de Lange or Rubinstein-Taybi syndrome and by many disease pictures resulting from chromosomal aberrations and the rubella embryopathy. Some of the malformations seen in such patients with regularity point to prenatal onset of the disorder. Illingworth[3] (after exclusion of cases of known postnatal origin) noted congenital malformations in 40% of mentally deficient patients. In a comparable group of children with cerebral palsy, the percentage of congenital malformations was only 6.8. Smith and Bostian,[4] in a series of children with idiopathic mental retardation, noted three or more congenital defects in 42% and assumed that in these patients the idiopathic mental defect could be attributed to abnormal embryonic differentiation.

Although associated malformations point to prenatal damage, they do not reveal the nature of etiologic factors. Before 1940, it was commonly asserted in the medical literature that multiple malformations in man, particularly internal and symmetric anomalies, must be due to genetic factors and be hereditary.[5] Since that time, numerous experiments in mammals have demonstrated that multiple congenital malformations, including deformities of the brain, can be produced by environmental agents, actinic, nutritional and toxic.

Rubella and other infectious agents were shown to be teratogenic in man and to be responsible for some cases of mental retardation. The identification of this form of mental retardation was made possible by Gregg's finding of the etiology of congenital cataracts,[6] which accompany the brain damage. It seems that all children with mental impairment attributable to rubella have characteristic somatic congenital defects.[7] Thus, the rubella syndrome illustrates the role played by malformations in the classification and recognition of subgroups of mental deficiency. Cytomegalic inclusion disease also can result in mental retardation accompanied by microcephaly and ocular anomalies, and prenatal toxoplasmosis sometimes produces a syndrome of hydrocephaly or microcephaly, chorioretinitis and cerebral calcifications in which the malformations are the basis of identification of the disease picture. Although the prenatal rubella syndrome accounts for less than 1% of institutionalized children,[8] its recognition and that of other disease pictures caused by prenatal infections made it necessary to consider nongenetic factors in the etiology of mental retardation associated with systemic structural anomalies, disorders that are not hereditary. Although familial recurrence has been reported for toxoplasmosis[9] and rubella,[10] such incidents are exceptional. This is not true for prenatal or congenital syphilis, which has a tendency to recur in families of an infected mother. Owing to involvement of the central nervous system, children with congenital syphilis can be mentally defective. No reliable prevalence and incidence figures are available for the times when the disease was endemic, but by 1940 there were still approximately 4% of the children institutionalized for mental retardation because of syphilis of the central nervous system.[11,12] By 1959, the corresponding figure had been reduced to about 0.2%[13]

An important syndrome of physical and mental subnormality can be caused by maternal iodine deficiency. Endemic cretinism, once prevalent in many countries of the world (p. 102), is now rapidly declining. Incidences varied from one locality to another and statistical reports usually were of limited reliability. Endemic cretinism did not lend itself to scientific investigation, since the disorder flourished chiefly in inaccessible and remote areas. It was (and still is in certain places) an important contributor to mental retardation of environmental origin. Endemic cretinism can occur repeatedly in children of a mother goitrous because of iodine deficiency (p. 121). Anomalies of the patient's thyroid and their consequences pointed to the root of the anomaly and aided in the recognition and eradication of the disorder in many areas.

Since 1959, many syndromes that include multiple malformations and mental retardation have been found to be associated with chromosomal abnormalities. Such syndromes can appear as a sporadic phenomenon in a family or carry a risk of recurrence. Both autosomal and gonosomal abnormalities can result in mental retardation.

Autosomal abnormalities occasionally are discovered among normal persons, but some deviant karyotypes are regularly associated with characteristic mental and physical defects. In 1865, Down singled out a type of mental deficiency because of the patient's characteristic somatic anomalies.[14] For 94 years this type was recognized as a syndrome, mongolism (p. 311), until it was found to be associated with trisomy 21.[15] The condition, which occurs with a frequency of about 0.15% in the newborn population, can be recognized, as a rule, by physical examination because of its characteristic features. It represents an important medical and social problem, since it is always associated with mental retardation. Although the mortality of patients with trisomy 21 is 40–50% during the first year of life, survival to puberty has become frequent, and now many of the patients reach adulthood because of effective treatment of diseases that formerly caused early death. The prevalence rate of children with Down syndrome reaching an age of 10 years was 1 in 4,000 in 1929; it doubled to 1 in 2,000 by 1949 and doubled again to 1 in 1,000 by 1958.[16] These patients made up approximately 10% of the institutionalized population in the past, but their number is rising and approaching 20% in some institutions[17,18] as other forms of serious mental retardation decline.[19] Trisomies 18 and 13-15 are associated with congenital mental and serious physical abnormalities. Their incidences at birth have been estimated as 0.02 and 0.007%.[20] Life expectancy is poor, and only exceptional patients live long enough to reach institutions for the mentally retarded. Malformations of the central nervous system are nearly always present in trisomy 13-15; they are less frequent in trisomy 18.[21,22] Associated malformations are sufficiently characteristic to permit, in most cases, a diagnosis by inspection alone. Monosomy G has been described as a syndrome (p. 339). Deletion of the short arm of one of the chromosomes, no. 5, results in the "cat-cry syndrome," which is associated with microcephaly and mental retardation. There are many other chromosomal anomalies, such as translocations and ring formations, that result in mental and physical defects. Although individually rare, these disorders may account for a significant percentage of the retarded population, but their incidence and prevalence cannot yet be estimated. Of 50 mentally defective children with three or more congenital anomalies not specific for a recognized disease picture, 4 had abnormal karyotypes containing ring chromosomes, deletions or translocations.[23]

Abnormalities of the sex chromosomes leading to mental retardation may or may not manifest themselves in associated congenital malformations. Patients with complex karyotypes such as XXXY or XXXXY have both mental and physical defects; they have been found in institutions with a frequency of about 0.15%. The XXY or Klinefelter syndrome is much more frequent, with an incidence of 0.27% in the general male population, but many persons with this anomaly are mentally normal and free from gross congenital malformations. It has been estimated that about one-fourth of them have mental impairment[24] and that they contribute 0.8% to institutionalized populations.[25] Persons with XXXX karyotype have been observed who are mentally retarded without showing other abnormalities.[26] Women with XXX constitution can be phenotypically normal or be mentally retarded and handicapped by congenital malformations. The anomaly has been found in institutions with a frequency of 0.4%.[25,26]

The XO condition (Turner syndrome) is rare in the neonatal population (0.03%); for unknown reasons, it is not well tolerated in prenatal life, as it accounts for 5% of spontaneous abortuses. Carr[27] estimated that an XO zygote has only a 1 in 40 chance of producing a live-born infant. Most of these children are recognizable at birth by congenital malformations and anomalies, but many are mentally normal. XO patients are only rarely found in institutions, where they contribute 0.04% to the retarded population.[25]

One can assume at this time that approximately 0.25–0.3% of all children born have brain defects attributable to chromosomal abnormalities recognizable with present methods. If this estimate is correct, such chromosomal errors would account for 10% of the children born with mental retardation. The proportion of the chromosome-determined retarded to institutionalized populations probably is more than 10% but less than that to the milder noninstitutionalized groups.

A long list of gene-determined congenital malformations associated with mental retardation could be given, and some of these syndromes are listed below. It must be emphasized that mental retardation is not obligatory and present in all patients who have the characteristic deformities. Brain malformations resulting in mental retardation, such as microcephaly, hydrocephaly and agenesis of the corpus callosum are genetically determined in some cases. Genetic factors play a role in certain syndromes of skeletal and mental defects: acrocephalosyndactyly and other craniosynostoses, Klippel-Feil syndrome, mandibulofacial dysostosis, Ellis-van Creveld syndrome, orodigitofacial syndrome and Laurence-Moon-Biedl syndrome exemplify this group. In others, skin changes are leading signs: Poikiloderma, Sjögren-Larsson syndrome, incontinentia pigmenti and others have been described in association with mental retardation.[28] The hamartoses – tuberous sclerosis, the basal cell nevi syndrome and neurofibromatosis – sometimes have congenital manifestations. In all these hereditary conditions there is an increased incidence of mental retardation, but mentally normal persons often have some signs of these disorders. If mental retardation is present in such cases, its prenatal determination is obvious.

It is assumed by many that all genetically determined forms of mental retardation are due to inborn errors of metabolism and that all congenital malformations of genetic origin are determined through biochemical mechanisms. Although these assumptions may be correct, it would be erroneous to think that the work dealing with mental retardation due to inborn errors of development that is now in progress is at the same time solving questions of etiology of congenital malformations. It is worth emphasis that most of the known inborn errors of metabolism leading to mental retardation are not associated with structural defects present at birth. If they were, patients with such inborn metabolic errors would be recognizable at birth by inspection, and there would be little need for screening the entire newborn population for chemical anomalies of blood and urine.

Much progress has been made in the classification and explanation of cases of mental retardation, but most patients are still awaiting etiologic analysis. Interaction of genetic and prenatal or postnatal environmental factors results in the disease pictures presented in hospitals and clinics. In some of these cases, the presence of congenital malformations aids in the ascertainment of causes to a certain extent.

In the following list, there are a number of congenital malformations and syndromes that are always—or with significant frequency—associated with mental retardation. "Significant frequency" is a term that requires explanation. Clubfoot, for instance, occurs in many mentally normal persons, but its incidence in institutionalized mental defectives is about ten times that of the general population (p. 1004). Conversely, about one-fourth of the patients with hemihypertrophy have mental retardation (p. 165), which is ten times the frequency of mental retardation in the general population. There exist constant associations of certain malformations and syndromes with mental retardation, and there are facultative associations, which are shown in parentheses. Because of the unsettled and changing terminology, some conditions are listed more than once. Since many syndromes and combinations have not been delineated as yet, the list is incomplete.

	Page
(Acrocephaly)	895
(Acromegaloid syndromes)	424
(Agenesis of corpus callosum)	252
Agyria	242, 262
(Aniridia)	369
(Anophthalmia)	356
Antimongolism	339
Apert syndrome	899
(Arachnodactyly)	850
(Arhinencephaly)	202, 206
(Arthrogryposis)	1011
(Ataxia-telangiectasia)	270
(Basal cell nevi syndrome)	1268
Bird-headed dwarfs	137
Broad-thumb syndrome	1018
(Brushfield spots)	326, 371
Camptodactyly	984
Cat-cry syndrome	340
(Cavum septi pellucidi)	254
Cebocephaly	206
(Cerebellar aplasia)	268
(Cerebral gigantism)	173
(Cerebral palsies)	138, 255
Cerebro-hepato-renal syndrome	347
Chondrodystrophia calcificans	797
Chondrodystrophy with retinal detachment	804
(Chondroectodermal dysplasia)	793
Chromosomal abnormalities: deletions, monosomies, translocations, trisomies and other aneuploidies	296-344
(Cleft lip and palate)	628-646
(Cleidocranial dysostosis)	836
Cloverleaf skull	904
(Clubfoot)	1004
Cockayne syndrome	398
(Colobomas of the eye)	361
(Congenital cataract)	372-377, 389
(Congenital corneal opacities)	367
(Congenital heart disease, cyanotic)	499
(Corpus callosum, agenesis or hypoplasia)	252
(Craniosynostoses)	893
Cretinism (sporadic, metabolic, endemic)	102
Cri du chat syndrome	340
(Cutis laxa)	1186
(Cutis verticis gyrata)	1192
Cyclopias	202
(Cytomegalic inclusion disease)	71
de Lange syndrome	139, 344
Down syndrome	311
(Ectodermal dysplasia anhidrotica)	1165
(Ellis-van Creveld syndrome)	793
(Epidermolysis dystrophica)	1151
(Erythroderma ichthyosiform)	1157
(Exencephalies)	211
(Fanconi pancytopenia)	1020
Gargoylism	808
(Goldenhar syndrome)	388
(Hallermann-Strieff-François syndrome)	390
(Hemihypertrophy)	165
Hunter syndrome	816
Hurler syndrome	809
Hydranencephaly	231
(Hydrocephaly)	217
(Hydrophthalmos)	365
Hypercalcemia-supravalvar aortic stenosis syndrome	578
(Hypertelorism)	326
(Hypoparathyroidism)	445
Hypothyroidism (congenital)	438
(Ichthyosiform erythroderma)	1157
(Incontinentia pigmenti)	1171
(Intrauterine growth retardation)	134
(Keratosis palmaris et plantaris)	1161
Kleeblattschädel	904
(Klinefelter syndrome)	1141
(Klippel-Feil syndrome)	909
Laurence-Moon-Biedl syndrome	176
(Lipodystrophia totalis)	174
Lissencephaly (agyria)	242
Lowe syndrome	389
(Macroencephaly)	138, 244
(Macroglossia)	171
Macrogyria (pachygyria)	262
(Mandibulofacial dysostosis)	650

(Marfan syndrome) 850
Marinesco-Sjögren syndrome 392
(Median facial clefts) 207
Microcephalies 136, 237
(Micrognathia) 621
Microgyria 262
(Microphthalmia) 356
(Möbius syndrome) 397
Mongolism 311
(Morquio disease) 819
(Mucopolysaccharidoses) 808
Myotonic dystrophy 1032
(Neurofibromatosis) 1252
Oculocerebrorenal syndrome 389
(Optic nerve, aplasia or atrophy) 380
Orodigitofacial syndrome 674
(Osteopetrosis) 863
Otocephaly 402
(Otopalatodigital syndrome) 677
(Oxycephaly) 893
(Parietal foramina, enlarged) 891
(Phocomelia) 951
(Polydactyly) 176, 978
Polymicrogyria 262
Porencephaly 246
Prader-Willi syndrome 182
Prosencephaly 201, 206
(Pseudoglioma) 398
Pseudohypoparathyroidism 446
Pseudo-pseudohypoparathyroidism 448
Puppet syndrome 349
(Pyknodysostosis) 869
(Radial hypoplasia) 960
(Radio-ulnar synostosis) 962
(Recklinghausen neurofibromatosis) 1252
(Retinal aplasia) 377
(Retinal dysplasia) 377
(Retinal pigmentation) 378
(Right aortic arch syndrome) 531, 580
Rubella syndrome 62
Rubinstein-Taybi syndrome 1018
(Rud syndrome) 1159
Sanfilippo syndrome 817
(Simian creases) 330, 341
(Situs inversus) 183
Sjögren-Larsson syndrome 1159
Smith-Lemli-Opitz syndrome 348
(Sturge-Weber syndrome) 349
Supravalvar aortic stenosis complicata 578
(Syndactyly) 971
(Synotia) 402
(Tetraphocomelia) 951
(Third fontanelle) 324
(Thumb, hypoplasia or aplasia) 976
(Toxoplasmosis (congenital) 78
(Translocation syndromes) 316
(Treacher Collins syndrome) 650
Trisomies 296-339
Tuberous sclerosis 1260
(Turner syndrome) 1122
(Tylosis palmaris et plantaris) 1161
Vascular cerebral malformations 249
(Xeroderma pigmentosum) 1173
(XXX), XXXX, XXXXX syndromes 1140
(XXY), XXXY, XXXXY, XXXYY syndromes 1141
(XXY) syndromes 1144

REFERENCES

1. Malamud, N.: Neuropathology, in Stevens, H. A., and Heber, R. (eds.), *Mental Retardation* (Chicago and London: The University of Chicago Press, 1964).
2. Crome, L.: The brain and mental retardation, Brit. M. J. 1:897, 1960.
3. Illingworth, R. S.: Congenital anomalies associated with cerebral palsy and mental retardation, Arch. Dis. Childhood 34:228, 1959.
4. Smith, D. W., and Bostian, K. E.: Congenital anomalies associated with idiopathic mental retardation, J. Pediat. 65:189, 1964.
5. Lenz, F.: Morbific Hereditary Factors, in Baur, E., Fischer, E., and Lenz, F. (eds.), *Human Heredity* (New York: The Macmillan Company, 1931).
6. Gregg, N. McA.: Congenital cataract following German measles in the mother, Tr. Ophth. Soc. Australia 3:35, 1941.
7. MacMahon, B., and Sowa, J. M.: Physical damage to the fetus, Milbank Mem. Fund Quart. 39:14, 1961.
8. Kirman, B. H.: Rubella as a cause of mental deficiency, Lancet 2:1113, 1955.
9. Garcia, A. G. P.: Congenital toxoplasmosis in two successive sibs, Arch. Dis. Childhood 43:705, 1968.
10. Menser, M. A., Slinn, R. F., Dods, L., Hertzberg, R., and Harley, J. D.: Congenital rubella in a mother and son, Australian Paediat. J. 4:200, 1968.
11. Penrose, L. S.: A clinical and genetic study of 1280 cases of mental defect, Med. Res. Counc. Spec. Rep. No. 229, London, His Maj. Stat. Off., 1938.
12. Benda, C. E.: Congenital syphilis in mental deficiency, Am. J. Ment. Deficiency 47:40, 1942.
13. Berg, J. M., and Kirman, B. H.: Syphilis as a cause of mental deficiency, Brit. M. J. 2:400, 1959.
14. Down, J. L. H.: Observations on an ethnic classification of idiots, Clin. Lect. & Rep. London Hosp. 3:259, 1866.
15. Lejeune, J., Gautier, M., and Turpin, R.: Étude des chromosomes somatiques de neuf enfants mongoliens, Compt. rend. Acad. Sc. (Paris) 248:1721, 1959.
16. Carter, C. O.: A life-table for mongols with the causes of death, J. Ment. Defic. Res. 2:64, 1958.
17. Berg, J. M., and Kirman, B. H.: Some aetiological problems in mental deficiency, Brit. M. J. 2:848, 1959.
18. Hamerton, J. L., Jagiello, G. M., and Kirman, B. H.: Sex-chromosome abnormalities in a population of mentally defective children, Brit. M. J. 1:220, 1962.
19. Goodman, N., and Tizard, J.: Prevalence of imbecility and idiocy among children, Brit. M. J. 1:216, 1962.
20. Conen, P. E., and Erkman, B.: Frequency and occurrence of chromosomal syndromes, Am. J. Human Genet. 18: 374, 387, 1966.
21. Warkany, J., Passarge, E., and Smith, L. B.: Congenital malformations in autosomal trisomy syndromes, Am. J. Dis. Child. 112:502, 1966.
22. Passarge, E., True, C. W., Sueoka, W. T., Baumgartner, N. R., and Keer, K. R.: Malformations of the central nervous system in trisomy 18 syndrome, J. Pediat. 69:771, 1966.
23. Summitt, R. L.: Cytogenetics in mentally defective children with anomalies: A controlled study, J. Pediat. 74:58, 1969.
24. Raboch, J., and Sipova, I.: The mental level in 47 cases of "True Klinefelter's syndrome," Acta endocrinol. 36:404, 1961.

25. Wright, S. W., and Tarjan, G.: Mental retardation, Am. J. Dis. Child. 105:511, 1963.
26. Carr, D. H.: Chromosome abnormalities and their influence on the development of the nervous system, International Copenhagen Congress on the Scientific Study of Mental Retardation, Denmark, 1964, pp. 132–138.
27. Carr, D. H.: Chromosome anomalies as a cause of spontaneous abortion, Am. J. Obst. & Gynec. 97:283, 1967.
28. Ewing, J. A.: The association of oligophrenia and dyskeratosis. A clinical investigation and an inquiry into its implications, Am. J. Ment. Deficiency 60:98, 1955.
29. Farrell, G.: *Congenital Mental Retardation*, Vol. 1, in the Advances in Mental Science Series (Austin: University of Texas Press, 1969).
30. Roboz, P., and Pitt, D.: Studies on 782 cases of mental deficiency, Part I, Australian Paediat. J. 4:79, 1968; Part II, *ibid.*, 4:260, 1968; Part III, *ibid.*, 5:38, 1969; Part IV, *ibid.*, 5:137, 1969.

35

Cerebellar Malformations

Malformations of the cerebellum are not rare. They have been known to anatomists and pathologists for many years, but their clinical diagnosis and evaluation have become possible only as their clinical picture became better known and pneumoencephalograms were used in the establishment of their diagnosis intra vitam. Differentiation of congenital malformations of the cerebellum and of degenerative disorders presents an old problem for which no definite solution has been found.[1] Cerebellar hypoplasia combined with Werdnig-Hoffmann disease[2] exemplifies the difficulty encountered in the differential diagnosis. *Cerebellar aplasia* or *hypoplasia* sometimes is found among the mentally retarded or among children with spastic diplegia, cerebral palsy and other motor disorders. Malformations of the cerebellum are also associated with many cases of hydrocephaly and spina bifida. In such severe malformations of the central nervous system as anencephaly or cyclopia, the cerebellum often is involved. On the other hand, unilateral or bilateral cerebellar aplasia has been found occasionally at necropsy in normal persons who had only minimal motor disturbances during life. From the normal to the severely defective, a great variety of clinical pictures have been observed and described, and some symptoms recorded probably are not due to the cerebellar disturbance but to other anomalies of the brain associated with it.[1]

Various etiologic factors can result in cerebellar malformations. Occasionally, more than one child with cerebellar hypoplasia is affected in one family.[3,4] In some cases, consanguinity of the parents can be established,[5] and recessive inheritance has been considered. Total and partial agenesis of the vermis of the cerebellum has been reviewed by de Haene,[6] who reported the anomaly in 3 brothers who showed tremor and hypotonia and died when 4–8 years of age. A relationship of cerebellar hypoplasia with systemic degeneration in early postnatal life has been found by Norman and Urich.[7] Such association of a congenital malformation of the cerebellum with a degenerative disease suggests that the onset of the abiotrophic process in prenatal life can result in congenital morphologic changes. Chromosomal anomalies can result in cerebellar malformations. In 9 of 32 necropsies of children with trisomy 13-15 and in 5 of 83 necropsies of children with trisomy 18, cerebellar anomalies were noted.[8-10] Norman[11] compared brains from children with trisomy 13-15 with those from patients with trisomy 18, paying special attention to the cerebellum. There were massive accumulations of heterotopic nerve cells in the cerebellar white matter in trisomy 13-15. Although there also were similar heterotopias in trisomy 18, they were less conspicuous than those in trisomy 13-15. Another thorough study of structural anomalies of the cerebellum in trisomies was made by Terplan *et al.*[12] Cerebellar changes are present in many cases of chromosomal anomaly, but it is doubtful that they are specific for specific cytogenetic patterns. The cerebellum was absent in a child with many features of the 13-15 trisomy syndrome whose karyotype was normal.[13] Several authors noted hypoplasia of the cerebellum in patients with Down syndrome.[9] Villaverde[14] paid special attention to the cerebellum of mongoloid patients and reviewed the literature on this subject. It is generally agreed that the cerebellum is hypoplastic in patients with Down syndrome, but the findings are not uniform.[1,9] Sometimes an association may exist between Klinefelter syndrome (XXY constitution) and familial cerebellar ataxia.[15] Some investigators believe that syphilis, toxoplasmosis[4] or transplacental virus infections may be responsible for certain cerebellar anomalies.[1] Kuru, a progressive and fatal cerebellar ataxia, is, according to Burnet,[16] transmitted from mother to offspring and is thought to be an infectious disease. Cerebellar changes due to maternal iodine deficiency are suggested by the findings of Lotmar,[17] who studied patients with endemic cretinism. He noted that the Purkinje cells were hypoplastic and displaced to the surface of the cerebellum. In one instance, intrauterine x-irradiation may have been the cause of marked cerebellar hypoplasia.[18] The mother had been irradiated in the third month of pregnancy because of genital neoplasm. The infant showed microcephaly and an ulceration on the occiput that had "signs of a Roentgen ulcer."

Pathology

Many abnormalities of the cerebellum have been described in great detail in the neuropathologic literature.[19,20] Agenesis can be limited to the vermis or to one hemisphere. Hypoplasia can be bilateral or unilateral. Malformations of individual folia have been observed.[1] Complete absence of the cerebellum may be found combined with hydrocephaly and spina bifida, as in a case described by Priestley.[21] In a 4-month-old child, the fourth ventricle was covered only by a thin sheet and the pons, peduncles and the tentorium were absent. In another case, the cerebellum showed the development of that of an embryo in the third month.[22] In cases of cerebellar hypoplasia, the vermis and the flocculi (paleocerebellum) may be present and the hemispheres absent, but in other cases the phylogenically older parts of the cerebellum may also be underdeveloped.[23] Unilateral aplasia of the cerebellum, involving the left half of the vermis, the left hemisphere and nuclei and the left choroid plexus of the fourth ventricle, was found at necropsy in a woman 60 years of age. Clinical symptoms were mild compared to the large cerebellar defect.[24]

Cleft formations of the cerebellum (dysraphism) affect the inferior vermis and the velum medullare posterius in most cases. Closure of the cerebellar area proceeds in rostro-caudal direction, and for some time a remnant of the fissura mediana may persist normally. In this area, incomplete or defective closure of the neural tube can lead to malformations. In severe cases, clefts of the cerebellum are combined with incomplete development of the occipital bone and the cervical spine, so that a cerebellomeningocele is formed. The extent of cerebellar cleft formation is variable. Some cases are combined with cerebellar cysts, some with syringobulbia and syringomyelia[23] and others with hydrocephaly.[25] In addition to the gross malformations of the cerebellum, more generalized anomalies may be found. Microgyria, macrogyria, polygyria, agyria and dystopias of the gray matter have been observed repeatedly.[23,24]

Hyperplasia of the cerebellum occurs, usually associated with megalencephaly. In one instance, unilateral hyperplasia was combined with leontiasis ossea.[26] Some hyperplastic cases have been considered diffuse hamartomas (ganglioneuromas) of the cerebellum. They show severe disturbance of the cytoarchitecture and many heterotopias. It is of interest that polydactyly may be found in persons with such

Fig. 35-1.—Brain of an infant with trisomy 18. There is agenesis of the cerebellum.

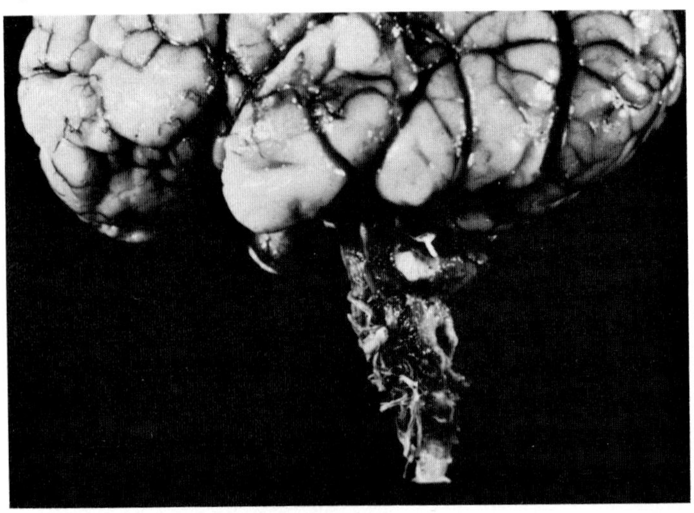

ganglioneuromas.[23] Malformations of the skull can affect the cerebellum. Basilar impressions (p. 907) may be associated with an anomaly of the hindbrain, either an Arnold-Chiari malformation or a disturbance of the closure of the neural plate.[1] Congenital vascular malformations of the cerebellum may remain symptomless for many years, yet result in sudden death when the lesion ruptures.[27] The cerebellar anomalies that occur in Hippel-Lindau disease are discussed on page 1267.

Symptoms

In recent years, congenital malformations of the cerebellum have become of clinical interest, since they are now recognized in the living. Most of these cases probably are cerebellar hypoplasias, which may cause symptoms noticeable in the first few months of life. Affected infants cannot hold up their heads and show awkwardness or tremor when reaching for objects. Even in infancy, it may be noticed that the inability to hold up the head and the flaccidity of the neck muscles contrast with an increased muscle tone in other parts of the body. For instance, the muscles of the back may be rigid and the children lie in opisthotonos. There may be hypertonicity in the muscles of the lower extremities. It is possible that such signs of increased muscle tone are due to associated cerebral damage and not to the cerebellar anomaly. The inability to swallow solid foods was pointed out by Batten,[28] and Brenner and Hagedorn[4] re-emphasized dysphagia, difficulties in feeding and anorexia as symptoms of cerebellar hypoplasia. There may be hyperkinetic manifestations – jerky movements of the arms, uncoordinated choreiform or athetoid movements and general restlessness. Strabismus is frequent, nystagmus rare. Uncoordinated movements of the head and eyes sometimes are noticeable, and convulsive disorders are present in some cases. As the children get older, it is noticed that they have difficulty in sitting and in walking. They do not find equilibrium when placed in the upright position, they cannot stand, and fall easily. When they make attempts to walk, they show a swaying gait and lack of balance, although the muscle strength may be good. Speech usually is considerably delayed and remains indistinct. The mental development may be normal, but many affected children are mentally retarded.

In contrast to the progressive degenerative ataxias, children with congenital hypoplasia of the cerebellum show a tendency to improvement. Their muscle coordination and strength and their speech may get better as they get older. A great deal depends on the development of their higher brain centers and their mental capacities. If they are intelligent, they learn to compensate for their cerebellar weakness by the use of other parts of the brain. Complete recovery is possible in mild cases.

In the differential diagnosis, atonic diplegias and progressive degenerative ataxias must be excluded. Ataxias following acute infectious diseases, tumors, tuberculomas, and so forth, usually can be distinguished from the congenital form by their relatively late and acute onset. In the diagnosis of cerebellar aplasia or hypoplasia, air encephalograms may show a marked increase in the size of the cisterna magna and sometimes an increase in the fourth ventricle. Between these two areas of decreased density, the shadow of the small cerebellum sometimes can be visualized. At the same time, one finds in some of the cases a flattening of the posterior cranial fossa and thickening of the occipital squama. Air encephalograms may reveal, as accidental findings, associated anomalies of the ventricular system or of the brain.

The treatment of cerebellar hypoplasia is limited to physiotherapy. Systematic exercises in the use of the affected extremities and in coordination may advance the progress of improvement, which in many cases also occurs spontaneously. Malformations associated with basilar impressions and vertebral anomalies can be approached surgically (p. 908).

REFERENCES

1. Dow, R. S., and Moruzzi, G.: *Physiology and Pathology of the Cerebellum* (Minneapolis: University of Minnesota Press, 1958).
2. Norman, R. M.: Cerebellar hypoplasia in Werdnig-Hoffmann disease, Arch. Dis. Childhood 36:96, 1961.
3. Sarrouy, C., Raffi, A., and Boineau, N.: À propos de deux cas d'hypoplasie cérébelleuse dans une même fratrie, Arch. franç. pédiat. 14:449, 1957.
4. Brenner, W., and Hagedorn, M.: Zur Diagnose des konnatalen Kleinhirnsyndroms beim Säugling, Ztschr. Kinderh. 74:209, 1954.
5. Fanconi, G., and Türler, U.: Kongenitale Kleinhirnatrophie mit supranucleären Störungen der Motilität der Augenmuskeln, Helvet. paediat. acta 6:475, 1951.
6. de Haene, A.: Agénésie partielle du vermis du cervelet à caractère familial, Acta neurol. belg. 55:622, 1955.
7. Norman, R. M., and Urich, H.: Cerebellar hypoplasia associated with systemic degeneration in early life, J. Neurol., Neurosurg. & Psychiat. 21:159, 1958.
8. Carr, D. H.: Chromosome abnormalities and their influence on the development of the nervous system, International Copenhagen Congress on the Scientific Study of Mental Retardation, Denmark, 1964, pp. 132–138.
9. Warkany, J., Passarge, E., and Smith, L. B.: Congenital malformations in autosomal trisomy syndromes, Am. J. Dis. Child. 112:502, 1966.
10. Passarge, E., True, C. W., Sueoka, W. T., Baumgartner, N. R., and Keer, K. R.: Malformations of the central nervous system in trisomy 18 syndrome, J. Pediat. 69:771, 1966.
11. Norman, R. M.: Neuropathological findings in trisomies 13-15 and 17-18 with special reference to the cerebellum, Developmental Med. & Child Neurol. 8:170, 1966.
12. Terplan, K. L., Sandberg, A. A., and Aceto, T., Jr.: Structural anomalies in the cerebellum in association with trisomy, J.A.M.A. 197:129, 1966.
13. Marshall, R., Newnham, R. E., Rawstron, J. R., Ellis, J. R., and Stevens, L. J.: Features of 13-15 trisomy syndrome with normal karyotype, Lancet 1:556, 1964.
14. Villaverde, J. M.: Les lésions cérébelleuses dans l'idiotie mongoloide et quelques considérations sur la pathologie du cervelle, Trav. Lab. recherches biol. Univ. Madrid 27:111, 1931.
15. Hecht, A., and Ruskin, H.: Seminiferous tubule dysgenesis

(Klinefelter's syndrome) associated with familial cerebellar ataxia, J. Clin. Endocrinol. 20:1184, 1960.
16. Burnet, F. M.: The changing face of kuru, Lancet 1:1138, 1965.
17. Lotmar, F.: Entwicklungsstörungen in der Kleinhirnrinde beim endemischen Kretinismus, Ztschr. Neurol. u. Psychiat. 136:412, 1931.
18. Miskolczy, D.: Ein Fall von Kleinhirnmissbildung, Arch. Psychiat. 93:596, 1931.
19. Brun, R.: Zur Kenntnis der Bildungsfehler des Kleinhirns, Schweiz. Arch. Neurol. u. Psychiat. 1:61, 1917.
20. Lichtenstein, B. W.: Cerebellar atrophy, analysis of various forms and analytical scheme for their study (review), J. Neuropath. 4:379, 1945.
21. Priestley, D. B.: Complete absence of the cerebellum, Lancet 2:1302, 1317, 1920.
22. Baker, R. C., and Graves, G. O.: Cerebellar agenesis, Arch. Neurol. & Psychiat. 25:548, 1931.
23. Ostertag, B.: Missbildungen, in Lubarsch, O., Henke, F., and Rössle, R. (eds.), *Handbuch der Speziellen Pathologischen Anatomie und Histologie* (Berlin: Springer, 1956), Vol. 13, pt. 4, p. 540.
24. Minkowski, M.: Prenatal neuropathologic changes leading to neurologic or mental disorders, Proceedings, International Congress of Neuropathology, Rome, September 8-13, 1952.
25. Benda, C. E.: *Developmental Disorders of Mentation and Cerebral Palsies* (New York: Grune & Stratton, Inc., 1952).
26. Spiegel, E.: Hyperplasie des Kleinhirns, Beitr. path. Anat. 67:539, 1920.
27. Thrash, A. M.: Vascular malformations of the cerebellum, Arch. Path. 75:65, 1963.
28. Batten, F. E.: Ataxia in childhood, Brain 28:484, 1905.

Ataxia-Telangiectasia

In 1941, Louis-Bar[1] reported a case of cutaneous and conjunctival telangiectases and cerebellar disturbances.* Boder and Sedgwick[2] named the syndrome "ataxia-telangiectasia" and described 7 cases. In the same year, Wells and Shy[3] reported on progressive familial choreoathetosis with cutaneous telangiectasia. By now, more than 100 cases have been recorded. Boder and Sedgwick[4] extended the syndrome to include, in addition to ataxia and telangiectasia, susceptibility to sinopulmonary infection, bronchiectases and peculiar eye movements. In several families, more than one sibling was affected, and there was no predilection for either sex.

Ataxia usually is the first symptom noted at the time the child begins to walk. Mild athetoid movements are also noticeable early. The ataxia first manifested by swaying of the head and trunk on standing and as ataxia of gait are progressive. Intention tremor follows. Initial hypertonia is succeeded by hypotonia and diminished tendon reflexes. After the age of 10 years, the children often become confined to a wheelchair. Telangiectasia usually develops later than ataxia. It begins on the conjunctiva bulbi, sometimes leaving the area near the cornea free. Cutaneous telangiectases involve the face, the palate, the neck and certain parts of the extremities. "Pink-eye" combined with ataxia suggests the diagnosis of this syndrome. Not included in the name of the disorder is the tendency to rhinitis, sinusitis, bronchitis, bronchiectases and pneumonia. Chronic pulmonary disease may dominate the disease picture and lead to early death. Clubbing of fingers and toes becomes noticeable. Roentgenograms show peribronchial infiltration suggestive of cystic fibrosis of the pancreas. Hypogammaglobulinemia is associated with the disorder in many cases and may play an etiologic role in the infectious processes that affect the patients,[5] but studies of immunoglobulins resulted in contradictory findings.[6,7] Peterson *et al.*[8] established in patients with this syndrome a thymic abnormality, immunologic deficiency and tendency to malignancy. Generalized reticulum cell sarcoma, Hodgkin disease, undifferentiated round-cell sarcoma and "malignant tumors of lymphoid tissue" have occurred in patients with ataxia-telangiectasia.[7] Other malignancies such as a cerebellar medulloblastoma,[14] glioma in a frontal lobe[15] and dysgerminomas[16] have been reported. An intracranial angioma led to subarachnoid hemorrhage in one case.[17] In lymphocyte cultures there is a high incidence of chromosome breakage.[9,10] On testing the eyes, slowly initiated and interrupted movements are noticed on lateral and upward gaze, followed by rapid blinking and completion of the movement. The facies appears relaxed, dull and emaciated in later stages. The smile is slow-spreading, and drooling is a conspicuous symptom. The children sit bent forward, the shoulders drooped and the head sunk forward. The facial expression and the stooped posture suggest mental retardation, but the intelligence quotients are within normal limits. The disposition and adjustment are good. Statural growth is retarded in most cases.

Necropsy in an 11-year-old girl revealed chronic, progressive cerebellar degeneration involving Purkinje cells, granule cells and basket cells. The Purkinje cells underwent the most marked alterations accompanied by secondary shrinkage of the cerebellar white matter. The small veins of the cerebellar

Fig. 35-2.—Telangiectases in a 16-year-old girl with ataxia-telangiectasia.

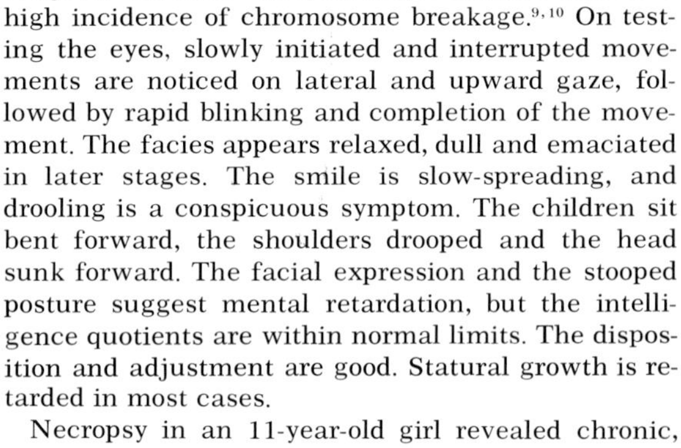

leptomeninges were thin-walled, enlarged and engorged. The lungs showed bronchiectases and severe fibrosis, the fingers and toes hypertrophic osteoarthropathy. Congenital absence of the ovaries, infantile uterus and tubes and absence of the thymus were recorded.[4] Absence or abnormality of the thymus was also noted in two necropsies reported by Peterson *et al.*[8] Ovarian changes, particularly paucity of ovarian follicles, were emphasized by Miller and Chatten.[11] Association with megalencephaly and mesenteric lymphangiectasia was noted at necropsy of an 8-month-old child.[12]

An adverse response to radiation therapy for a lymphosarcoma was reported by Gotoff *et al.*[7]

Ataxia-telangiectasia is considered an immunologic deficiency disease characterized by a defect of the thymic system and the lymphoid system. Most, but not all, patients have low or absent serum IgA levels. Skin homografts persist for prolonged periods.[12] Lymphocytes show impaired blastogenesis in vitro after stimulation with phytohemagglutinin.[13]

REFERENCES

1. Louis-Bar, D.: Sur un syndrome progressif comprenant des télangiectasies capillaires cutanées et conjonctivale symétriques, à disposition naevoide et des troubles cerebelleux, Confinia Neurol. 4:32, 1941.
2. Boder, E., and Sedgwick, R. P.: Ataxia-telangiectasia. A familial syndrome of progressive cerebellar ataxia, oculocutaneous telangiectasia and frequent pulmonary infection, Univ. Southern California M. Bull. 9:15, 1957.
3. Wells, C. E., and Shy, G. M.: Progressive familial choreoathetosis with cutaneous telangiectasia, J. Neurol., Neurosurg. & Psychiat. 20:98, 1957.
4. Boder, E., and Sedgwick, R. P.: Ataxia-telangiectasia. A familial syndrome of progressive cerebellar ataxia, oculocutaneous telangiectasia and frequent pulmonary infection, Pediatrics 21:526, 1958.
5. Gutmann, L., and Lemli, L.: Ataxia-telangiectasia associated with hypogammaglobulinemia, Arch. Neurol. 8:318, 1963.
6. Fireman, P., Boesman, M., and Gitlin, D.: Ataxia telangiectasia, Lancet 1:1193, 1964.
7. Gotoff, S. P., Amirmokri, E., and Liebner, E. J.: Ataxia telangiectasia; neoplasia, untoward response to x-irradiation, and tuberous sclerosis, Am. J. Dis. Child. 114: 617, 1967.
8. Peterson, R. D. A., Cooper, M. C., and Good, R. A.: Lymphoid tissue abnormalities associated with ataxia-telangiectasia, Am. J. Med. 41:342, 1966.
9. Hecht, F., Koler, R. D., Rigas, D. A., Dahnke, G. S., Case, M. P., Tisdale, V., and Miller, R. W.: Leukaemia and lymphocytes in ataxia-telangiectasia, Lancet 2:1193, 1966.
10. Gropp, A., and Flatz, G.: Chromosome breakage and blastic transformation of lymphocytes in ataxia-telangiectasia, Humangenetik 5:77, 1967.
11. Miller, M. E., and Chatten, J.: Ovarian changes in ataxia telangiectasia, Acta paediat. scandinav. 56:559, 1967.
12. Scott, R. E.: Ataxia-telangiectasia, Arch. Path. 88:78, 1969.
13. Hayakawa, H., Matsui, I., Yoshino, K., Hayakawa, S., and Kobayashi, N.: Immunopathological aspects of ataxia telangiectasia, Paediat. Univ. Tokyo, No. 16, 1, 1968.
14. Shuster, J., Hart, Z., Stimson, C. W., Brough, A. J., and Poulik, M. D.: Ataxia telangiectasia with cerebellar tumor, Pediatrics 37:776, 1966.
15. Young, R. R., Austen, K. F., and Moser, H. W.: Ataxia-telangiectasia and the thymus, Tr. Am. Neurol. A. 89:28, 1964.
16. Dunn, H. G., Menwissen, H., Livingstone, C. S., and Pump, K. K.: Ataxia-telangiectasia, Canad. M.A.J. 91: 1106, 1964.
17. Terheggen, H. G., Kramer, S., and Heimann, K.: Ataxia telangiectasia (Louis-Bar-Syndrom), Ztschr. Kinderh. 107:324, 1970.

SECTION TWO: **Spinal Cord**

36

Spina Bifida

MIDLINE DEFECTS of the osseous spine are called spina bifida. Most patients have the defect in the posterior aspects of the vertebral canal. If the anomaly is not visible externally, one speaks of *spina bifida occulta*. In such cases, the defect is limited to the posterior neural arches, laminae and the spines (Fig. 36-1, *A*). If there is an external saccular protrusion, one speaks of *spina bifida cystica*. Saccular enlargements protruding through osseous defects of the vertebral column that contain anomalous meninges and spinal fluid but do not have neural elements affixed to their wall[1] are called meningoceles (Fig. 36-1, *B*). If the spinal cord or nerves are included in the formation of the wall, the anomaly is called myelomeningocele (Fig. 36-1, *C*). Sometimes the open neural plate that failed to form a tube lies "like an open book" on the surface without cover by skin, meninges or vertebral arches, a condition called myeloschisis. The relationship of myeloschisis to myelomeningocele will be discussed later (p. 286). A rare cystic form of spina bifida called *myelocystocele* or *syringomyelocele* is due to dilatation of the central canal (hydromyelia) and to protrusion over the surface of the posterior aspects of the much-expanded spinal cord, which may be covered by meninges and skin (Fig. 36-2). The cavities of myelomeningoceles are traversed by nerves; those of myelocystoceles are not. Strictly speaking, the terms spina bifida and rachischisis refer to defects of the vertebral column and not to those of the spinal cord, but, clinically, the term spina bifida is used collectively and includes malformations with cord involvement.

Incidence

Estimates of *spina bifida occulta* vary widely. Ford[2] considers 2–3%, Sutherland[3] 5% and Giles[4] 24% as representative figures. Sutow and Pryde[5] made a study of spina bifida occulta in Japan and found that the differences in previous estimates could be explained by varying definitions of spina bifida occulta and by differences in age and sex. They established, for instance, that according to roentgenograms the incidence of spina bifida occulta at the 5th lumbar vertebra was 16.1% in the age group 7–8 years, whereas it was only 2.2% in the adult group. In the 1st sacral vertebra, the anomaly was found in 51.6% of the 7–8-year group and in 26.4% of the adult group. There also was a marked sex difference for the defect in the 1st lumbar vertebra, males being more affected than females. Spina bifida occulta diagnosed in x-ray film reviews usually is of no clinical significance, but there are exceptions to this rule. *Spina bifida cystica* with an externally visible sac occurs in approximately 1 of 1,000 births. The crude estimate has been made in many obstetric hospitals, but it is clear that there are variations according to definition, location, inclusion of stillbirths, geography, and so forth. In a world-wide review, the rate per thousand births was only 0.5.[6] In a prospective study in New York City it was 1.5 (including stillbirths).[7] In Charleston County, South Carolina, the rate was 1.5 per 1,000 births (including spina bifida with hydrocephaly). In that study, the incidence was 2.5 times higher in whites than in Negroes.[8] For England, the rate is 2.5,[9] but it was found to be 4.1 in South Wales.[10] Low rates (0.2) are consistently recorded in Japan. Alter,[8] summarizing hospital figures for Europe, Asia and North America, cited a variation in rates of from 0.2 to 3.2. Some of these differences are real, others are due to differing ascertainment. There also are unexplained temporary variations in certain localities. In Atlanta, Georgia, the incidence of spina bifida was 1 per 1,000 up to August of 1962 when, in a 3-month period, an "epidemic" rise to 4.4 was noticed.[11] In the same year, Lucey *et al.*[12] observed in Vermont a less impressive rise to 2.3, with a cluster of 4 children in one block of one city. Thus, great variations have been noted, and reports of alteration in incidence are acceptable only if they deal with comparable observations. Contribution of spina bifida to infant mortality is considerable.[13,14] Losses probably are high in intrauterine life. In Japan, the incidence of myeloschisis was about 13 times higher in embryos

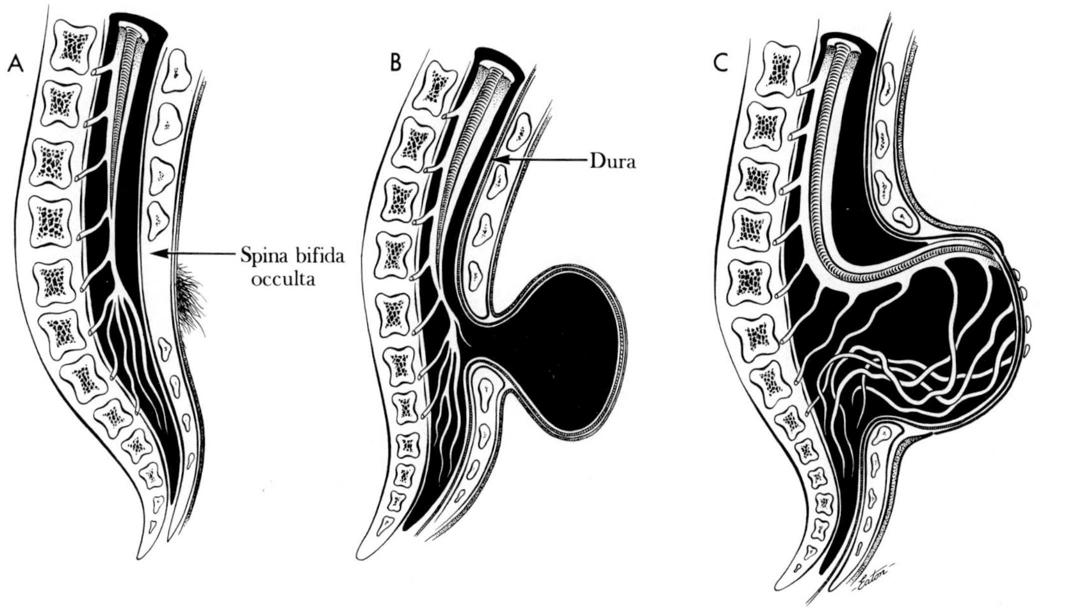

Fig. 36-1. – **A,** spina bifida occulta. **B,** meningocele. **C,** myelomeningocele.

than in infants.[14a] About 90% of the cases of spina bifida cystica seen in hospitals are lumbosacral, 7% purely lumbar and the remainder thoracic or cervical.

Etiology

In man, spina bifida usually occurs sporadically, but cases have been observed with 2, 3 or 4 siblings affected.[15-18] Sometimes an accumulation of cases has been observed not only in sibships but also in kinships.[16,18,19] Demeler[15] reported a family in which the first child had anencephaly and thoracic spina bifida, the second hydrocephaly, thoracic spina bifida and cleft lip and palate and the third anencephaly and thoracic spina bifida. All were females and stillborn. A fourth child was a normal girl. Two miscarriages followed and then a viable child with lumbosacral spina bifida was born, followed again by a miscarriage. The mother had a cervical rib and a rudimentary twelfth rib. One of her 10 sisters was born with occipital meningoencephalocele. There is a report by Wilner[20] of a woman born with meningocele or myelomeningocele who gave birth to a girl with myelomeningocele. Such observations are most unusual, but they point to genetic factors in the etiology of some cases of spina bifida, although the mode of transmission usually is irregular. There are some cases of spina bifida that are related in etiology to anencephaly, hydrocephaly and encephalocele; they occur alternately with these conditions in some families.[15-19] Sometimes there also is an increased incidence of malformations of other body systems in the family. Occasionally, spina bifida has been observed concordantly in twins[21] and in twins and in a sib.[22,23] Taking into consideration spina bifida and related malformations of the central nervous system, abortions and spina bifida occulta in affected families, Lorber[24] considered the possibility that spina bifida might be a

Fig. 36-2. – Myelocystocele (syringomyelocele) or hydromyelia.

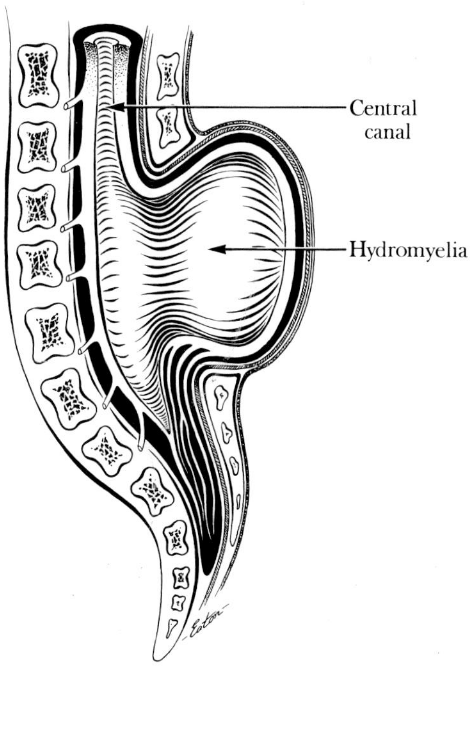

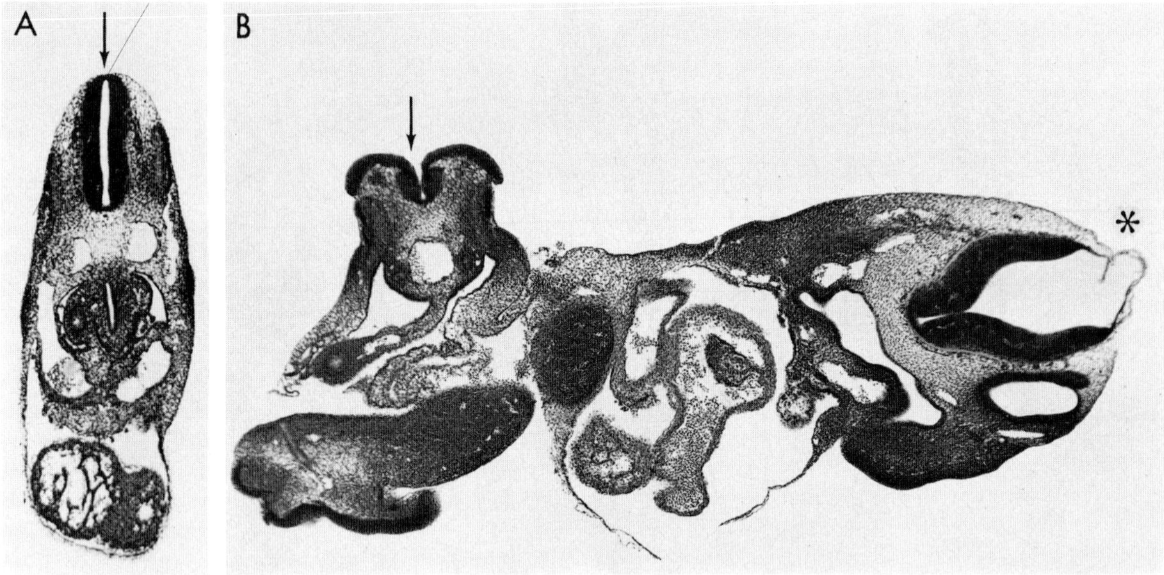

Fig. 36-3.—**A,** transverse section through control rat embryo (twelfth day). The spinal cord is closed (**arrow**). **B,** section through rat embryo (twelfth day). The neural tube is closing in cerebral area (**asterisk**) but is wide open in caudal area (**arrow**). One can distinguish between the original (thicker) folds of neural plate that failed to close and the thinner and everted overgrowths that spread laterad from the dorsal lips of the original neural plate. (Mother was treated with trypan blue on eighth to tenth day.)

recessively inherited trait. Miller *et al.*[25] found no increased frequency of vertebral and rib anomalies in the parents of children with spina bifida and meningocele, but Lorber and Levick[25a] stated that the incidence of spina bifida occulta was 20.4% among parents of children with spina bifida cystica and only 5% in a control group.

Hewitt[25b] noted that the mortality of white infants attributed to spina bifida and meningocele is not equally distributed in the United States. Of 24 states with rates below the national median, 20 lie west of the Mississippi, whereas higher rates are found in eastern states. A possible explanation is that the incidence of spina bifida is influenced by the average degree of homozygosity and that a downward time trend of recent years and a downward geographic east-west trend are due to greater outbreeding. This would be in agreement with the hypothesis of recessive inheritance.[25b]

To avoid premature generalization, it should be emphasized that in some patients anterior spina bifida can be a manifestation of neurofibromatosis that is dominantly inherited (p. 1252) and, in rare cases, spina bifida appears as a malformation in children with the trisomy 18 syndrome.[26,27] Spina bifida in trisomy 18 was also reported by Scorta *et al.*[27a] and observed in trisomy 21 by Hindse-Nielsen.[16] Among 55 patients with Turner syndrome, Haddad and Wilkins[28] listed 2 patients with cervical spina bifida and 3 patients with "mild degrees" of lumbosacral spina bifida.

Animal observations and experiments have shown that spina bifida is genetically determined in certain strains of mice.[29] In rabbits, a recessive lethal gene causes rachischisis from the calvarium to the tail. In this case, there are many malformations of the skeleton, heart and urogenital system associated with the spina bifida.[30]

There also are observations that indicate that some cases of spina bifida are due to environmental influences. Among his patients, Hindse-Nielsen[16] found 8 pairs of twins with only 1 member affected, but zygosity was not certain in all cases. Morison[31] reported a pair of identical twins; one was normal and the other was affected with spina bifida, Arnold-Chiari malformation, encephalocele and other malformations. The possibility that spina bifida can be of environmental origin is suggested by numerous animal experiments that show that in mammals, as well as in lower classes, the malformation can be induced by treatment of the mother with trypan blue,[32-34] x-rays,[35] hypervitaminosis A,[36] salicylates[37] and other teratogens. In such experiments, exencephaly, anencephaly, hydrocephaly and other malformations of the central nervous system (and of other organs) may appear together or vicariously with spina bifida in animals of the same litter. Although these experiments do not prove that spina bifida is ever caused by comparable exogenous factors in man, they should keep us from glib acceptance of heredity as the only etiologic factor possible. A belief in variable causation will help to maintain an open mind and an interest in etiologic research.

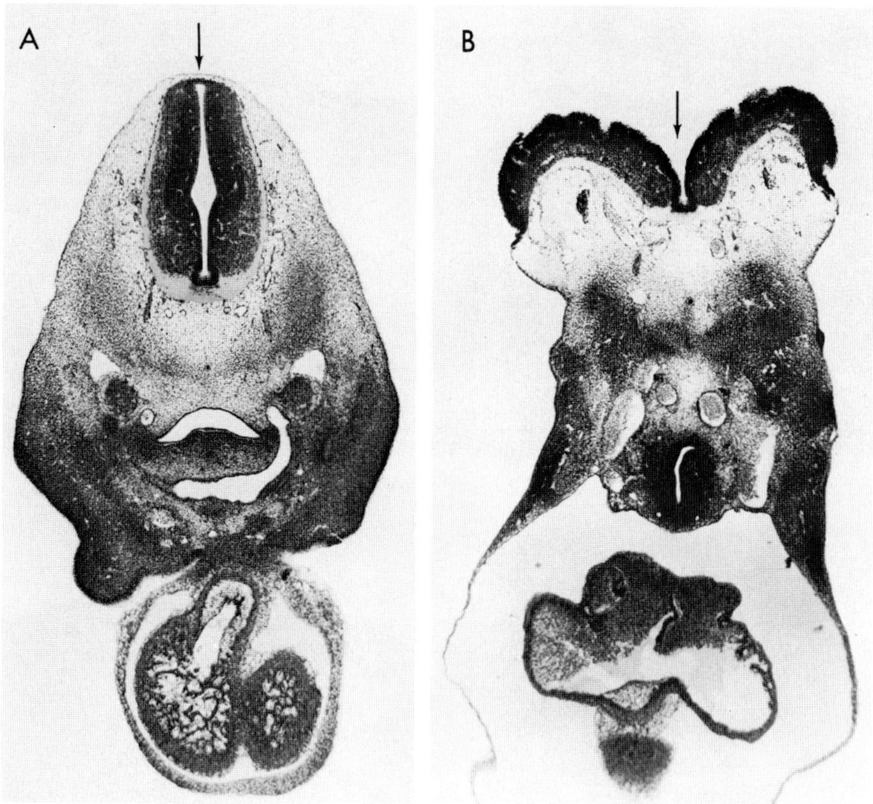

Fig. 36-4.—**A,** transverse section through control rat embryo (fourteenth day). Note closed spinal cord (**arrow**). **B,** section through rat embryo (fourteenth day) treated with trypan blue on eighth and ninth days. The neural plate is open (**arrow**), everted and overgrown. (From J. Warkany, J. G. Wilson and J. F. Geiger.[33])

The sex distribution is about equal,[1] but in some series there was a slight preponderance of females.[8]

Pathogenesis

The embryology of the central nervous system indicates that spina bifida dates back to very early life. The nervous system is derived from a thickened area of the integument located along the mid-dorsal line of the embryo, the neural plate. As the lateral parts of this plate grow dorsad and become elevated, they form a central groove that can be recognized in embryos 17–18 days of age. The elevated lateral folds approach one another dorsally in the midline, forming the neural tube. Closure begins at the cervical border of the spinal cord and brain and progresses both cephalad and caudad. In normal human embryos, closure is completed rostrally at fertilization age of about 23 days (18–20 somite-stage) and caudally somewhat later in the fourth week in embryos of 25 days of age (25 somite-stage)[38] or Streeter's horizon XII.[39] With the caudal closure of the neural tube, the primitive central nervous system is established. Spina bifida or cranium bifidum, which are due to incomplete closure of the neural tube, are thus determined before the end of the fourth week of embryonic life.

Developmental stages of spina bifida have been observed in experimental animals as well as in human embryos. In chick embryos, spina bifida can be produced by different teratogenic agents applied before 48 hours of incubation. According to Ancel,[40] the sensitive anlage is not the nerve tissue but the underlying mesoderm, the most sensitive area being situated at the Hensen knot. The sensitivity to teratogenic agents is less pronounced in early stages, when the knot is located in anterior regions of the spinal cord, than when the knot is on the level of the posterior extremities. The survival of chick embryos with spina bifida depends on the situation of the defect and is, in general, most likely if spina bifida is present in caudal regions.[40] Spina bifida produced experimentally in rats can be studied during early developmental stages. Gunberg[34] distinguished five types of spina bifida aperta produced by trypan blue. We have studied the development of experimentally induced spina bifida in rats[33,37] from the thirteenth day of gestation to the time of delivery. Myeloschisis could be recognized in an embryo removed on the twelfth day

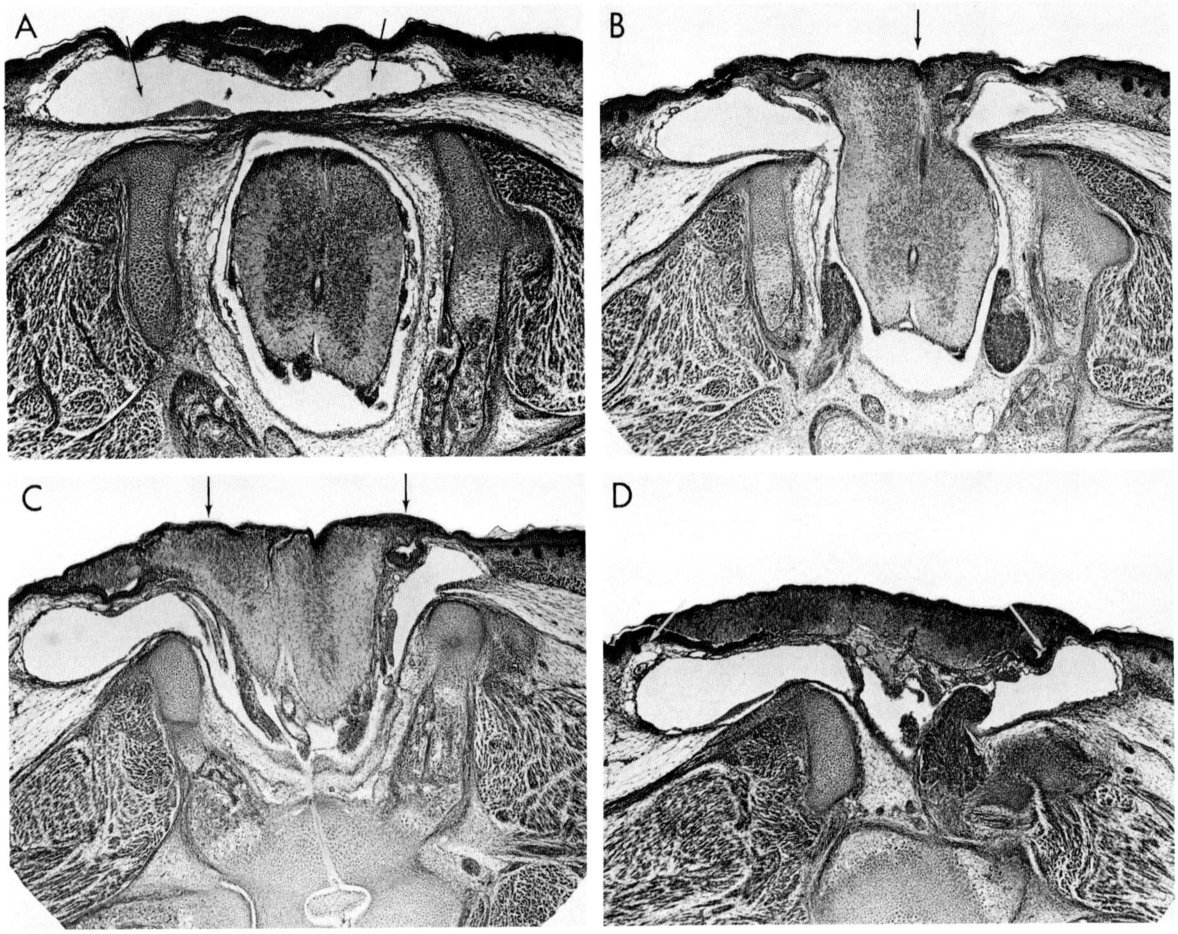

Fig. 36-5.—Transverse sections through spine of a newborn rat with spina bifida aperta. **A,** the spinal cord is shown cranial to its exit onto the surface. Dorsal to the cord is seen a compartment that represents an arachnoid space (**arrows**) lying dorsal to the cord. Note that the central canal is not dilated cranial to the spina bifida. **B** (section caudal to that of **A**), the cord reaches the body surface, opening up into a neural plate (**arrow**). **C** (section caudal to **B**), the central canal has reached the surface but it is covered by an epithelial layer (**arrows**). **D** (section caudal to **C**), neural plate bridges the fluid-filled (ventral) subarachnoid space. Note that epithelium (**white arrows**) originating from lateral edges of skin undermines the plate and separates it from underlying vascular bed. The medial portion of the neural plate is still connected with nerves and blood vessels, which course ventrad. An irregular spinal ganglion is seen between the pedicles of the abnormal vertebra. (From J. Warkany, J. G. Wilson and J. F. Geiger.[33])

of gestation. This embryo showed not only an open neural (medullary) plate but also substantial overgrowth of neural tissue lateral to the area where the neural folds should have united (Fig. 36-3). Thus, overgrowth of nerve tissue as stressed by Patten[41] could be recognized in early stages. There was no sign that the failure of the neural tube to close was attributable to an early "embryonic hydrocephaly," since this embryo had neither a choroid plexus nor hydrocephaly. The changes in myeloschisis from this early embryonic stage to the time of birth could be followed by observations of intermediate stages (Fig. 36-4). It could be seen how the open medullary plate was moved dorsad by enlargement of the ventral subarachnoid space, which became fluid-filled toward the end of gestation. The nerve tissue of the unclosed plate remained dorsally devoid of meningeal and cutaneous covers (Fig. 36-5). Degenerative changes set in, showing destruction of the exposed neural plate and proliferation of vascular elements of the pia that covered the plate ventrally. Epithelization of the degenerating neural plate progressed from the surrounding skin (Figs. 36-5, *D* and 36-6, *B* and *C*). At the end of pregnancy, a small fluid-filled sac was formed consisting chiefly of the remnants of the pia-arachnoid enforced by vascular tissue and epithelium and containing only a few elements of the original neural plate (Fig. 36-7). The conversion of the myeloschisis into a cystic spina bifida is shown diagrammatically in Figure 36-8. This type of experimental spina bifida

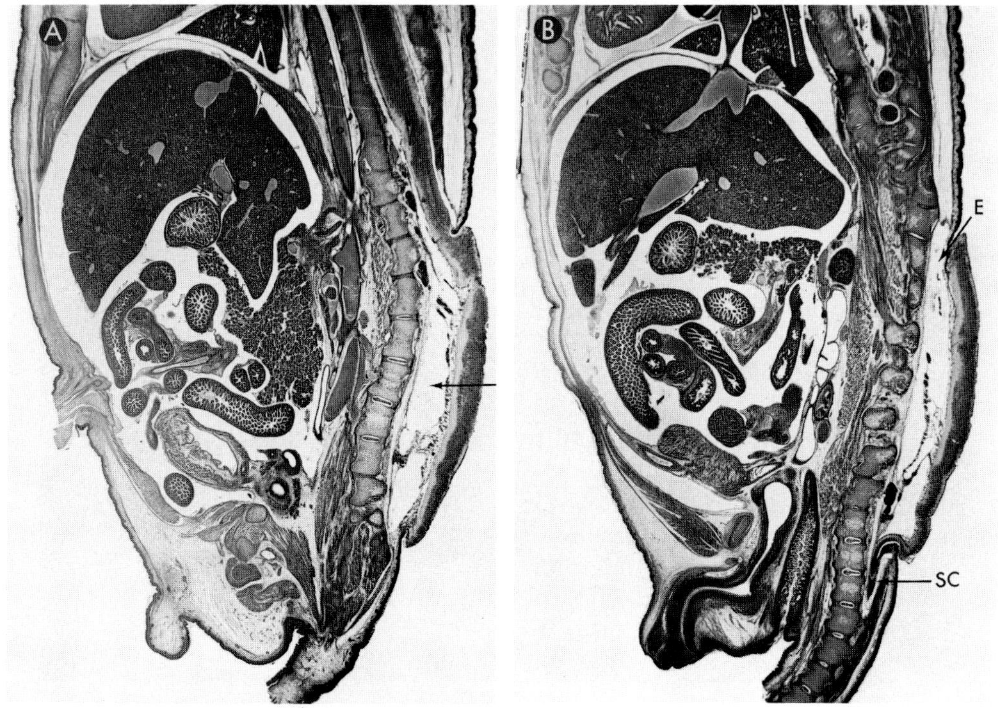

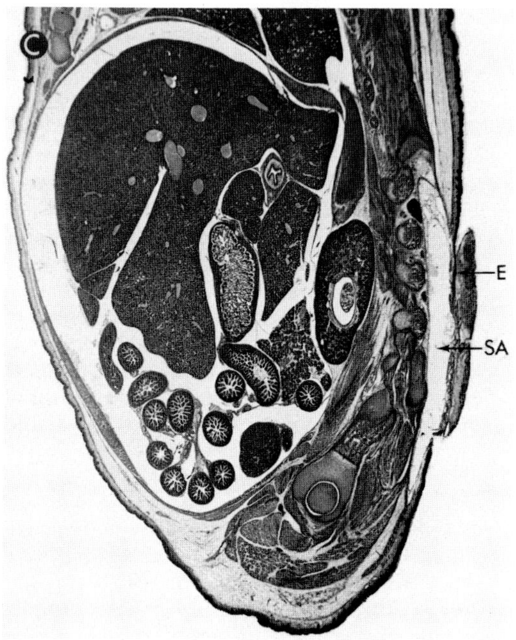

Fig. 36-6. — **A,** sagittal section of a rat fetus (twenty-first day) with lumbosacral spina bifida. The spinal cord penetrates the dorsal muscle and skin layers and joins the neural plate, which lies on the surface of the animal. Ventral to the neural plate is seen an enlarged (ventral) subarachnoid space (**arrow**) that is traversed by nerves and blood vessels. (Trypan blue eighth to tenth day of gestation.) **B,** sagittal section through same rat fetus showing re-forming of caudal spinal cord (*SC*) and central canal at caudal end of the neural plate. Note how epithelium (*E*) undermines the cranial end of the neural plate. **C,** a more lateral section shows the peripheral portion of the neural plate undermined by epithelium (*E*) in a stage of separation from the cystic subarachnoid space (*SA*). (From J. Warkany, J. G. Wilson and J. F. Geiger.[33])

closely resembles those occurring spontaneously in fetuses of man and rabbit.[42] Myeloschisis observed in young human embryos shows an open and overgrown neural plate prior to the time of formation of the vertebral bodies and neural arches. Lemire *et al.*[43] described a lumbosacral myeloschisis in a 5.5-mm. (horizon XIV) human embryo. The lesion extended from the twenty-fifth somite caudally for 1 mm. and showed findings indicating that the lesion originated before closure of the neural tube. Wrete[44] reported findings in a human embryo 18.8 mm. in length in which the entire neural plate, with the exception of some thoracic segments, remained open. He cited many other descriptions of embryos with unclosed neural tubes.

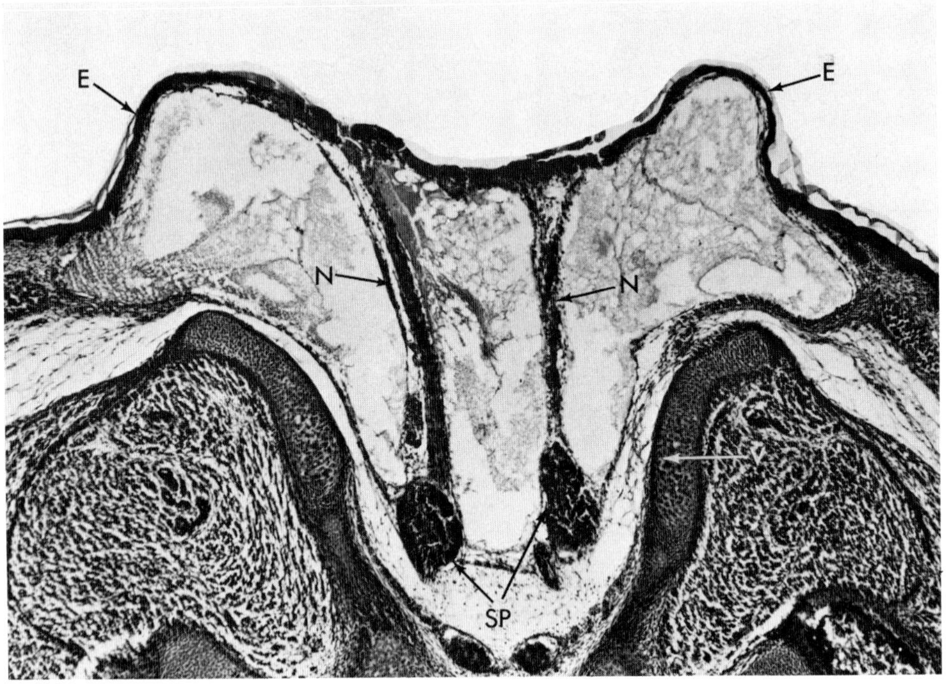

Fig. 36-7. — From a transverse section of a rat fetus (twenty-first day) with spina bifida. Note open vertebra (*V*) and fluid-filled space dorsal to it. The cystic space is bordered dorsally by a thin epithelial layer (*E*) and a few remnants of the neural plate. These remnants are connected by degenerating nerve roots (*N*) and blood vessels with the spinal ganglia (*SP*) seen in the ventral part of the vertebral trough. (Trypan blue eighth to tenth day.)

In some embryos, duplication of the spinal cord was seen in regions adjacent to the myeloschisis.[42,45] In older embryos, the open cord underwent degenerative changes. Ventral to the neural tissue, large fluid-filled subarachnoid spaces could be seen surrounded by zones of extreme vascularity. Secondary hemorrhages occurred in the defective areas, thus changing the original embryonic picture. Patten[42] described in detail 3 well-preserved human fetuses with myeloschisis that were 8, 49 and 160 mm. long and 5, 10 and 18 weeks of age. The progressive changes observed are closely simulated by the rat fetuses with myeloschisis described by us.[33] In the oldest human fetus, "externally the general configuration of the defective area was a miniature of conditions seen all too frequently in newborn infants."[42] As the fetuses with myeloschisis grew older, their lesions became more similar to myelomeningocele of the newborn period. It seems that the transformation of a myeloschisis into a myelomeningocele is achieved by degeneration of neural plate tissue and vascularization and thickening of the leptomeninges underlying the neural plate, followed by centripetal epithelization of the degenerating nerve tissue. With increasing accumulation of fluid in the subarachnoid space ventral to the pia of the neural plate, the transformed plate is pushed dorsad and a sac is formed. In human fetuses there remains little nerve tissue in the wall of the sac by the time the child is born, but nerves originating from the dorsal wall of the cyst and traversing the fluid-filled space indicate the previous site of the neural plate (Fig. 36-8). The dome of the sac often is formed by a red, velvety "area medullovasculosa" in which remnants of nerve tissue, blood vessels and pia mater are recognizable. This area is surrounded by a thin "area epithelio-serosa," which in turn is enclosed by an "area cutanea" (Figs. 36-8, *C* and 36-11, *A* and *C*). This concept of the pathogenesis of myelomeningocele goes back to Recklinghausen[46] and was accepted by Ernst.[47] Cameron[48] also found that in most of his cases of spina bifida cystica an open neural plate was the basic malformation and that in older children this exposed neural plate became covered by scar tissue and squamous epithelium.

With the cephalic portion of the sac, a flat but closed spinal cord often is seen leaving the spinal canal, running caudad and dorsad and attaching itself to the posterior wall of the sac (Figs. 36-8, *C* and 36-10). In rats, we found in the most cephalic region of the spina bifida a short segment of closed cord (containing a central canal) that was located within defective vertebrae so that it appeared that the osseous spina bifida was more extensive than the myeloschisis. Dorsal to the spinal cord, an enlargement of the subarachnoid space could be observed (Fig. 36-5, *A*). More caudally, the spinal cord became attached to the dorsal wall of the sac (Fig. 36-5, *B*) and the central canal opened onto the surface of the neural plate a short distance below the exit of the cord from the spinal canal (Fig. 36-5, *C*). In children, the segment of the cord immediately above the myeloschisis may be stretched in fetal life[49] and the dorsal arachnoid space distended by spinal fluid so that the spinal cord can be seen traversing the cranial portion of the sac. The diagrams of Figure 36-8 illustrate the conversion of the myeloschisis into a myelomeningocele of the type often seen in infants at the time of birth. Since the stages of myelomeningocele in later fetal months have not been systematically investigated, this explanation of the conversion of myeloschisis into the typical myelomeningocele must be considered hypothetical for man. But this hypothetical concept would explain why some investigators of myelomeningocele found a closed, flattened spinal cord containing a central canal in the wall of the sac,[50] whereas others described an open neural plate as the basic anomaly of myelomeningocele.[46] Sections cranial to the upper pole of the sac (the termination of the central canal) and sections caudal to the lower pole will contain a cord with central canal; sections between the poles will not (Fig. 36-5, *B* and *C*).

It has been mentioned that experimentally produced spina bifida may vary in morphology.[34] Similarly, not all cases of spina bifida seen in infants conform to the most common type of myelomeningocele described above. If the space ventral to the neural plate is not enlarged and filled by fluid, the neural plate remains near the vertebral trough (myeloschisis) (Fig. 36-8, *A*); such lesions resemble early embryonic stages. In some human cases, duplications of the spinal cord near a myelomeningocele change the picture to a certain extent.[42,45,48]

In some instances, the fluid-filled space actually is an enlargement of the central canal (hydromyelia) and the lesion represents an enormously expanded spinal cord (*myelocystocele* or *syringomyelocele*) (Fig. 36-2). In such cases, the cavity is cranially and caudally directly connected with the central canal and lined by cylindrical epithelium probably derived from ependyma. The spinal nerves do not traverse the cavity (as they do in the common myelomeningocele) but course around it. There is a defect in the posterior portions of the dura and the vertebrae, but the sac is covered dorsally by leptomeninges and skin. Myelocystocele is not rarely associated with exstrophy of the cloaca (Fig. 36-17, *A*). It seems possible that some skin-covered spina bifida lesions arise from neural tube formed, after closure of the posterior neuropore, from the differentiating caudal cell mass.[98]

Anterior spina bifida occulta associated with mediastinal neurenteric cyst and dorsal spina bifida connected with an intestinal fistula are lesions attributed to persistence of a neurenteric canal, a structure normally present only in very early embryos. These anomalies have a pathogenesis and manifestations of their own (p. 286). Intrathoracic and lumbar meningoceles may be a complication of neurofibromatosis.[51-53]

Fig. 36-8. – Conversion of myeloschisis (**A**) into myelomeningocele (**C**). In **A**, the neural plate is still near the vertebral bodies, but it is pushed dorsad by fluid that accumulates in the ventral aspects of the subarachnoid space (**B**). The nerves are stretched and deterioration of the neural plate sets in (**C**). Epithelization progresses from the margins of the lesion toward its center, undermining the remnants of the neural plate.

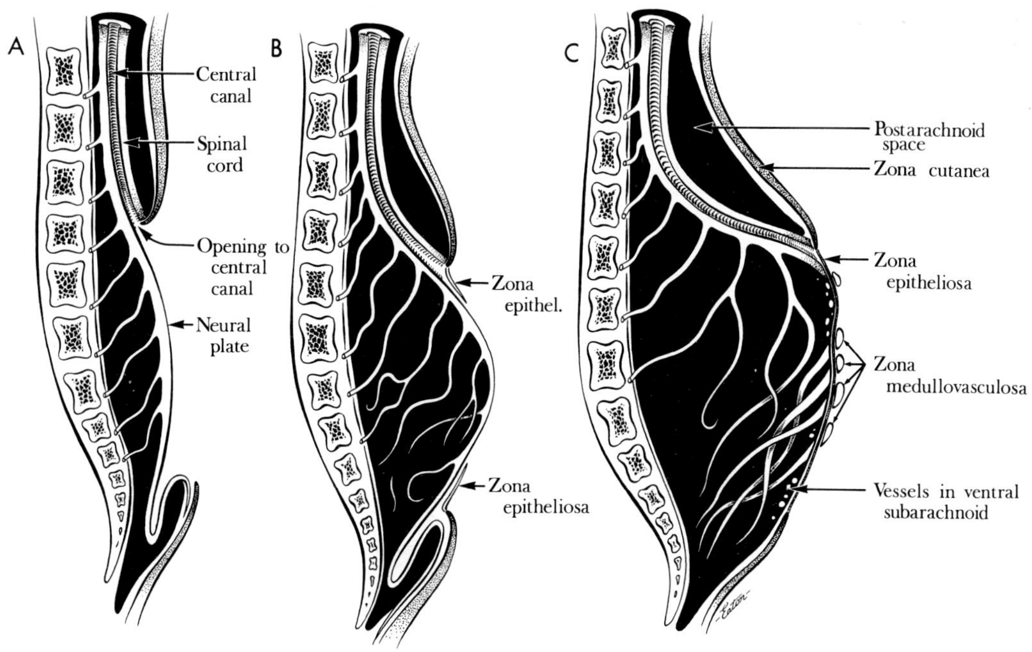

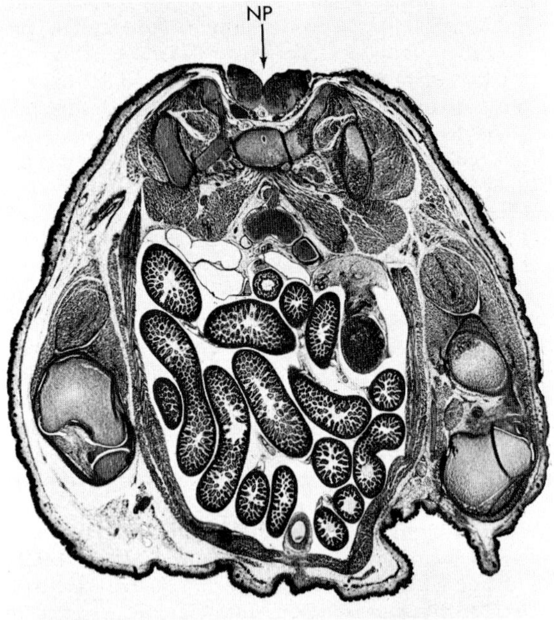

Fig. 36-9. —Transverse section through rat fetus (twenty-second day) with myeloschisis. The neural plate (*NP*) is open; there is no central canal; the ependyma lies on the dorsal surface of the animal. In this case the neural plate rests in the trough formed by open vertebra. There is no subarachnoid space and fluid pushing neural plate dorsad. (Hypervitaminosis A on tenth day.)

Morgagni,[54] in 1769, explained spina bifida, "the watery tumors of the vertebrae," as a disruption resulting from the pressure of fluid descending in the tube of the spine from the hydrocephalic head. This naïve concept of Morgagni has been generally abandoned, but it is still valiantly defended by Gardner,[55] who considers myelomeningocele the result of rupture of the embryonic neural tube and not as failure of the plate to close. Neither human embryos[42,43,56] with spina bifida nor experimentally produced specimens of animals with this lesion show distention of the central canal cranial to the spina bifida or signs of rupture in early stages. Myelomeningocele has its beginning in myeloschisis, a neural plate that has failed to close, an anatomic structure that cannot persist because of its abnormal make-up and location on the surface of the body. It can be shown in animal fetuses that degenerative and regenerative processes convert the open neural plate (myeloschisis) into the dorsal wall of the cavity represented by the space between the neural plate and the trough formed by unclosed vertebral arches. The central canal cephalad to the myelomeningocele is not dilated but irregular and even closed at some levels. The everted and open neural plate is present in the youngest embryos observed in man and animals (Fig. 36-3, *B*). There is no reason to assume that in such early stages a hydrocephalus caused rupture of a previously closed neural tube. The explanation of myelomeningocele as an altered myeloschisis does not apply to the rare myelocystocele[46] and some formations seen in monstrous specimens. Padget[99] attributed the anomalies of the spinal cord associated with spina bifida to clefts that may appear before or after closure of the neural plate.

One can compare the morphogenesis of myelomeningocele with that of anencephaly (p. 191). Both lesions are attributable to nonclosure of the neural plate; the one is due to persistence of an unclosed rostral area, the other to persistence of an unclosed caudal area. Rostral interference with normal closure leads to faulty folding and overgrowth of brain tissue (p. 192), to failure of development of dorsal meninges and cranial bones and to exposure of the abnormal brain to unnatural surroundings, which results in deterioration of brain substance and its replacement by vascular and fibrous tissues (area cerebrovasculosa). Before destruction of the brain, cranial nerves

Fig. 36-10. —Sagittal section through a myelomeningocele of a child showing spinal cord (*SC*) curving dorsad, joining the posterior wall of the cystic sac. The nerve roots (*NR*) emanating caudal to the attachment of the cord are connected with remnants of the neural plate.

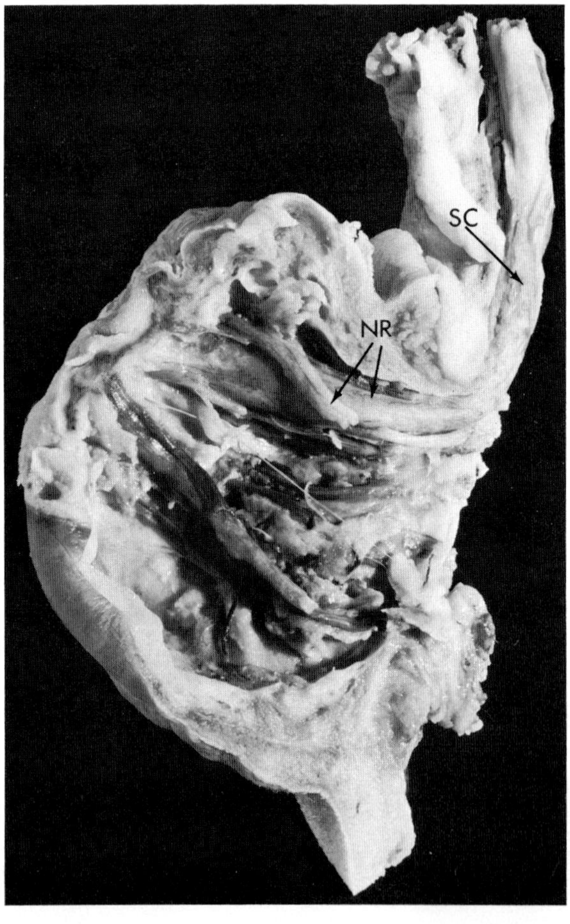

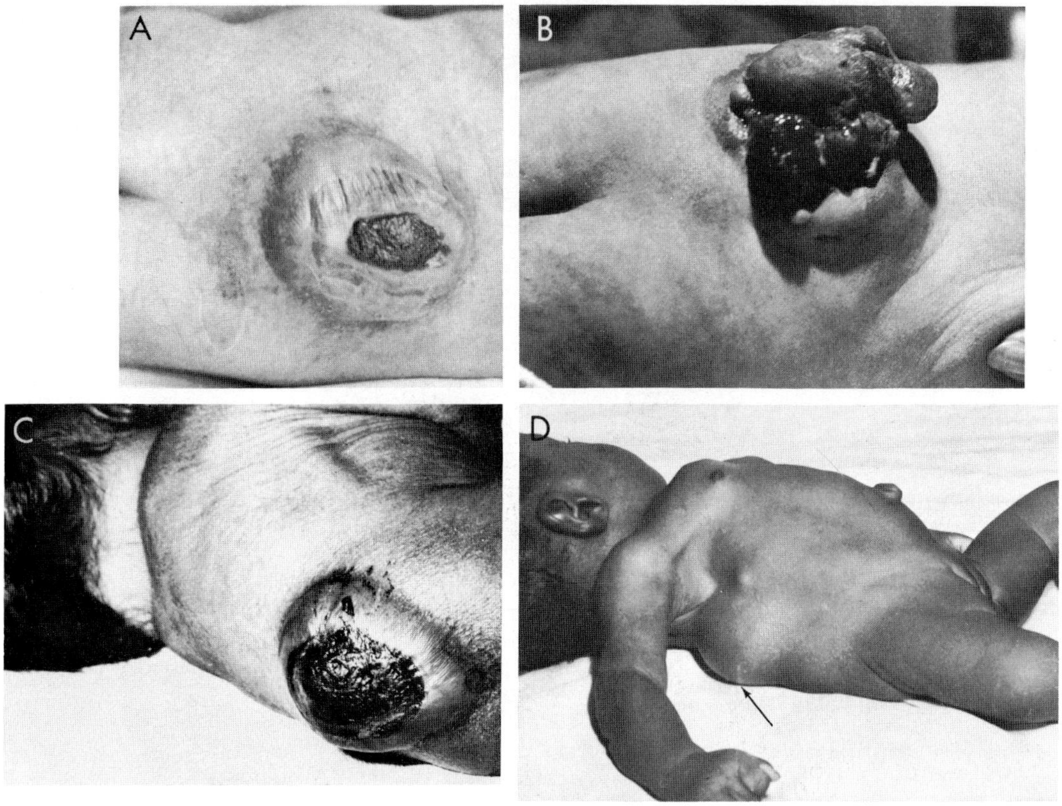

Fig. 36-11.—**A,** myelomeningocele of infant showing central area medullovasculosa surrounded by thin area epitheliosa and peripheral area cutanea. **B,** myelocystocele with dilated central canal (hydromyelia) in a child with neurenteric canal remnant (lined with gastric mucosa) and exstrophy of the bladder, hydrocephaly, microgyria and clubfeet. **C,** myelomeningocele in a child with trisomy 18. Large central area medullovasculosa surrounded by zona epitheliosa. **D,** infant with laterodorsal myelomeningocele (**arrow**) associated with gross defect of the rib cage. There was agenesis of ribs VI–XI on the right and marked scoliosis. Two soft cystic masses were seen over the right thorax and back. These masses were meningoceles beginning at the level of T7 and extending down to the coccyx. In the lower segments of the cord the central canal was much dilated, terminating dorsally at a point where the dorsal fissure was obliterated by a zone of glia that separated the central canal from the pia. There also was renal and ovarian hypoplasia. This patient was seen in the Cincinnati Children's Hospital (65–670; C-49-6).

develop at the base of the brain. The nerves course to their end organs through the foramina of the skull base. After destruction of the brain, the cranial nerves usually can be identified at the skull base of the anencephalus, where they may be seen either ending blindly or still connected with cerebral remnants. The area cerebrovasculosa may be overgrown in parts by epithelium that grows from the skin that encircles the skull base toward the overlying exposed brain remnants.

The situation is similar when the caudal end of the neural plate remains open but there is no excessive folding, as seen at the rostral end. There is overgrowth of neural tissue, failure of development of dorsal meninges and of neural arches and exposure to an abnormal extra-embryonic environment. Nerves originate from the anterior horns of the neural plate and others enter the posterior horns, which are displaced laterad. The neural plate is pushed dorsad by accumulation of fluid in its ventral meningeal spaces. The motor nerves are stretched by this dorsad movement of the plate; they may be torn or remain connected with the remnants of the neural plate that are contained in the area medullovasculosa of the posterior wall of the sac. As nerve tissue is destroyed there, epithelization progresses from the encircling skin of the lesion toward and over the area medullovasculosa in the center.

Anencephaly is not produced by a "cataclysm" that befalls a once normal brain and myelomeningocele is not produced by rupture of a once normal spinal cord. Differences of opinion concerning the pathogenesis of these lesions are not merely of theoretical interest. Since the neural tube normally is closed by the end of the first month of embryonic life, nonclosure (and anencephaly and myelomeningocele) cannot be due to events after the first month of gestation. If, however, these lesions were due to rupture or cataclysms of once well-formed organs, they could originate at any fetal period and be caused by events in the sec-

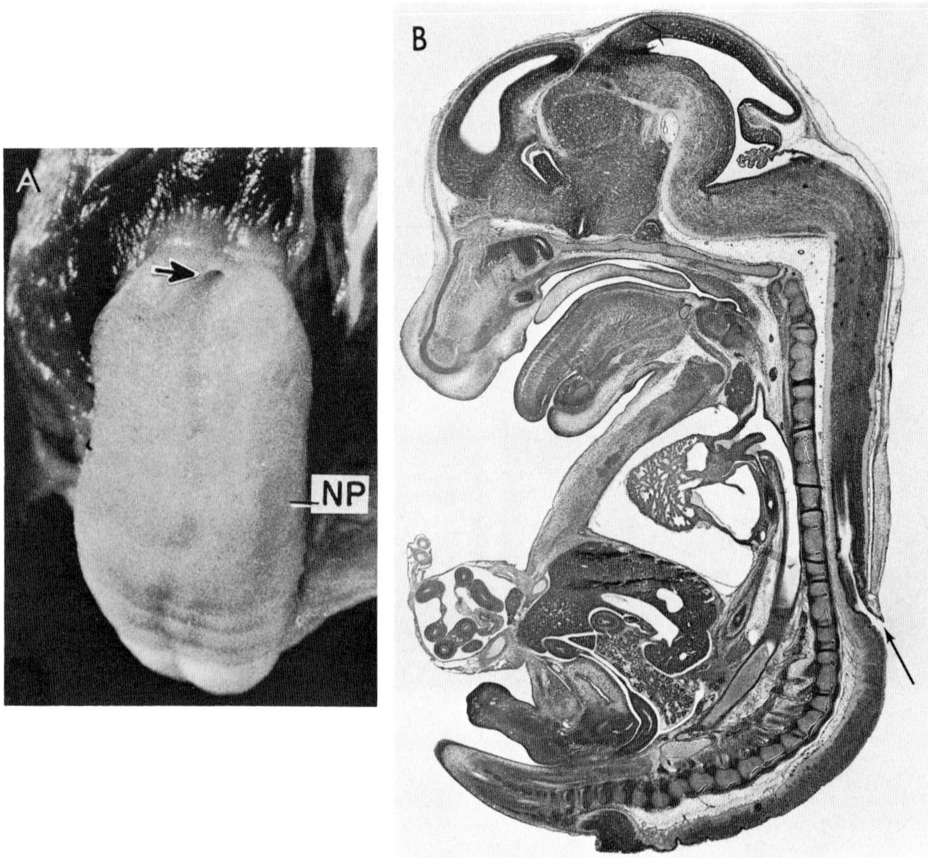

Fig. 36-12. – **A,** external appearance of a neural plate (*NP*) in a rat fetus (seventeenth day) showing opening of a central canal onto the surface at upper pole (**arrow**) of lesion. (Trypan blue eighth to tenth day.) **B,** sagittal section through rat fetus (seventeenth day) with spina bifida. The spinal cord breaks through the dorsal epidermal cover opening up into a neural plate. The central canal terminates at the upper pole (**arrow**) of the neural plate. There is no hydromyelia cranial to spina bifida. At the caudal end, the plate is again converted into a cord that is covered by epidermis. (Trypan blue.) (From J. Warkany, J. G. Wilson and J. F. Geiger.[33])

ond, third and later fetal months. It is clear that these differing theories could have differing legal consequences. It is my belief that neither anencephaly nor myelomeningocele can be caused by events after the embryo is 1 month of (fertilization) age.

Pathology

In spina bifida, the neural arches of the vertebrae fail to unite and the spinal foramina remain open dorsally. Such defects may occur in several segments and in any area of the spinal column, but the lumbosacral spine is affected most often. Minor anomalies of the lumbar and sacral spine (*spina bifida occulta*) can be found in roentgenograms of many children. The vertebral arches remain unclosed, but the defects vary greatly in degree. In the majority of these children, normal muscles and skin cover the open spinal canal, but sometimes cutaneous changes betray the lesion (p. 000). The spinal cord and the nerves usually are normal in the affected area but, rarely, underlying nerve tissue is malformed (myelodysplasia) or compressed and distorted by lipomatous, osseous or fibrous tissue lying between the skin and the nerve elements. In some instances, the caudal end of the spinal cord is attached to the dural sac in the sacral area, so that its ascent to the lumbar area is inhibited. Changes underlying a spina bifida occulta may exert traction or pressure on the spinal cord and lead to clinical symptoms[57] (p. 000). The cord may be distended by hydromyelia[58] or teratomas, or congenital dermal sinuses may be associated with spina bifida occulta.[59] Anterior spina bifida occulta may be associated with a neurenteric cyst in the mediastinum. Such cysts are connected with the meninges or spinal cord by a stalk through a defect in the vertebral bodies. The cysts are lined by esophageal, gastric or intestinal epithelium and are considered remnants of a neurenteric canal.[60,61] a structure normally existing only in very early embryos. The triad of mediastinal cyst,

intramesenteric duplication and vertebral anomaly has been pointed out by Fallon *et al.*,[62] who regarded the cysts as the result of an extension of the lumen of the foregut produced on its posterior aspects by incomplete separation of the notochord leading to interference with the anterior fusion of the vertebrae.

If the dorsal subarachnoid space under a skeletal spina bifida is distended by spinal fluid, the meninges protrude through the defect over the affected area, forming a meningocele (Fig. 36-1, *B*). Meningoceles are rarer than myelomeningoceles, accounting for only one-tenth of the cases of spina bifida cystica.[1,63] As a rule, the cord remains within the spinal canal in its normal position and the course of the spinal nerves is not disturbed (Fig. 36-1, *B*), but sometimes the terminal portion of the cord is displaced into a lumbosacral meningocele and spinal roots may traverse the sac.[1] In exceptional cases, the underlying nerve tissue is defective.[64] A meningocele usually is covered by normal skin, but a vascular malformation or a thin, transparent membrane may make the sac vulnerable. The covering sometimes is ulcerated or torn, thus permitting leakage of spinal fluid. The sac may be pedunculated or sessile on a broad base. Often, overgrowth of lipomatous tissue, adherent to the sac of the meningocele, is observed. *Anterior meningoceles* are found occasionally within the pelvis. They may form large tumors that are filled with fluid and communicate with the spinal canal through anterior defects of the sacrum[65] (p. 000). Sometimes they are associated with imperforate rectum.[1] *Intrathoracic meningocele* is a protrusion of the meninges through an intervertebral foramen or defect of the vertebrae that displaces the pleura and intercostal vessels forward. The anomaly is commonly a manifestation of neurofibromatosis (p. 000), but it can also occur without signs of that disorder.[51] *Lumbar meningocele* also has been observed in association with neurofibromatosis.[53]

In the most frequent forms of spina bifida presenting protruding sacs (the *myelomeningoceles*), a flattened "cord" usually is present in the cephalic portion of the sac, leaving the spinal canal through a defect of the spinal column and coursing dorsad to the posterior wall of the sac (Fig. 36-10), where it becomes attached to the dome of the protrusion at a point at which, in the embryo, the spinal cord opened up to join the unclosed neural plate. This area medullovasculosa appears in the center of the sac as a red, raw and often bleeding lesion that often is mistaken for an "ulcer" of the sac. But this central area (Fig. 36-11) contains the remnants of the neural plate that usually are continuous with the more or less normal spinal cord, located in the cranial portion of the sac. In the common form, the central canal is not dilated but found cephalad enclosed in the cord substance

Fig. 36-13.—**A,** myelomeningocele in a newborn child with area medullovasculosa in center of lesion. The spinal cord could be seen on upper and lower ends of lesion, and probes passed through dilated central canal emerged on the surface at the upper and lower poles of the "ulcer." **B,** there was no apparent continuity between the upper and lower spinal segments, except via the roof of the sac. The area between the upper and lower poles is represented by degenerated neural plate and vascular tissues.

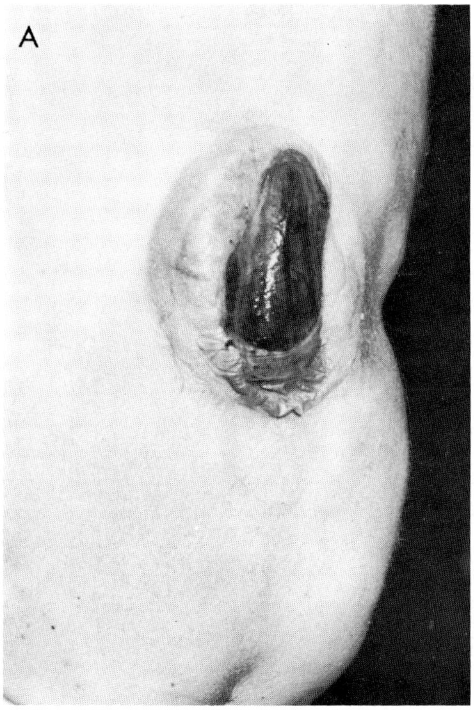

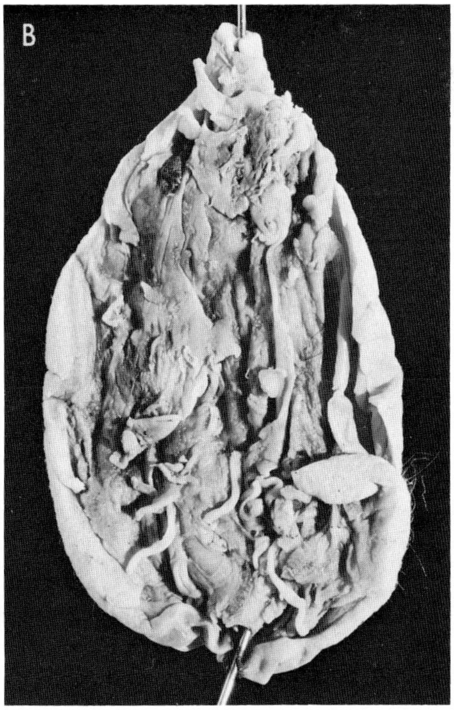

until it opens onto the surface at the point of attachment of the cord to the posterior wall of the sac. The opening of the central canal onto the surface is called the upper pole of the myelomeningocele (Fig. 36-12), from which fluid sometimes escapes. Below this upper pole is the area of myeloschisis where the neural plate has remained unclosed.[46,47] In the most caudal parts of the spina bifida sometimes one can see that the neural plate is closed again and a terminal cord is formed (Fig. 36-6, *B*). Nerves originating from or terminating at the area cerebrovasculosa (which contains the remnants of the neural plate) course through the sac of the myelomeningocele.

Myelocystoceles (hydromyelia), in which the sac is formed by expansion of the central canal, often are associated with severe malformations of the spine, exomphalos or exstrophy of the bladder and cloaca.[46,47] The sac of a myelocystocele is lined by derivatives of the ependyma. It is not traversed by nerves (Fig. 36-17).

Myelocystocele may be combined with anterior spina bifida and an intestinal fistula (p. 281) (Fig. 36-11, *B*). Dorsal intestinal fistulas, which can result in various clinical manifestations, have been described in detail by Bremer.[60] The dorsal opening may be found in the sacral, lumbar or thoracic region. These lesions represent a combination of anterior and posterior spina bifida or they may be limited to defects in the anterior aspects of the spine. Postvertebral entodermal cysts associated with axial deformities have been considered an "entodermal-ectodermal adhesion syndrome."[66] A review of spinal fissure with involvement of the alimentary canal was made by Willis.[67]

Myeloschisis with an open neural plate lying flat on the surface of the defect and without marked protrusion (Fig. 36-8) has been observed in embryos and is seen occasionally in older fetuses or infants. It may occur in the lumbosacral, the thoracic or cervical region. The entire neural plate and spine may remain open (craniorachischisis) (p. 198). The dorsal surface layer is ependyma; the mantle and marginal layers are found ventrally underneath. The neural processes of the vertebrae flare out laterally. Such early and well-preserved stages are seen commonly in young embryos; in older fetuses, the original condition is distorted by degenerative changes and hemorrhage. Sometimes the neural plate and all of its remnants have been eroded and have disappeared when a human fetus with myeloschisis or craniorachischisis is born. Only the osseous bed formed by wide-open

Fig. 36-14 (above). – Spina bifida cystica from lower thoracic to lumbar area in a child with hydrocephaly. The sac is overgrown by epithelium but there are some necrotic areas.

Fig. 36-15 (below). – Hair over spina bifida occulta. The child also had a diaphragmatic hernia.

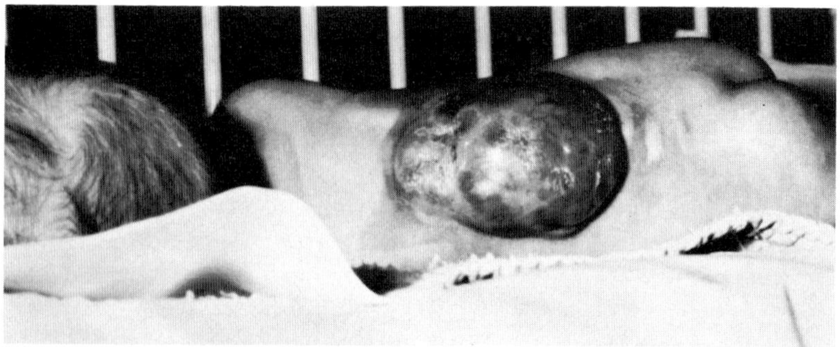

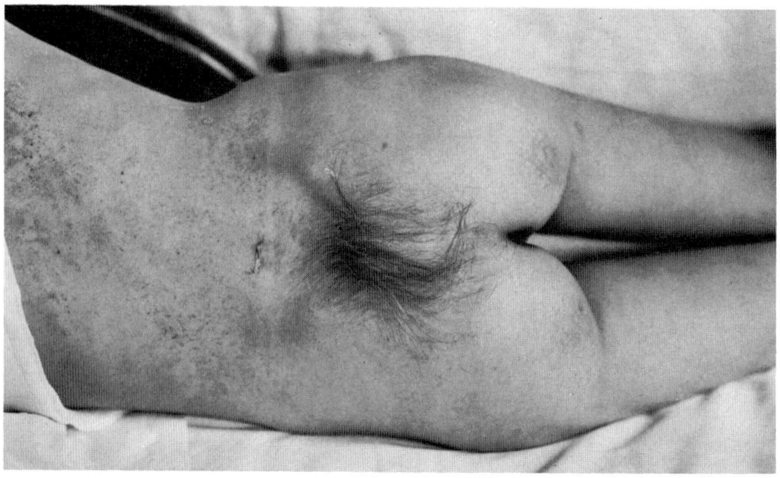

vertebral arches is seen at the back of the child. Degeneration and destruction of the neural plate progress in both myeloschisis or the more complicated myelomeningocele. At the same time, regenerative processes take place, with attempts to "heal the wounds" brought on by the destruction of the neural plate. Berndorfer[68] has emphasized and illustrated intrauterine regenerative processes in various forms of spina bifida. In rare instances, a myelomeningocele is covered completely by skin by the time the child is born, as a result of spontaneous surface repair during intrauterine life[69] (Fig. 36-14). It can be demonstrated in histologic sections that the spontaneous *epithelization* does not grow over the exposed neural plate but under it, thus unfortunately undermining the remnants of neural tissue and contributing to its deterioration (Fig. 36-6, *C*) (see also Cameron,[48] Fig. 2). Epithelization may save the infant's life by protecting it from postnatal infection, but covering of the lesion exacts a price: it undermines the neural plate, separates it from its blood supply and nerves and contributes to its destruction (Figs. 36-5 and 36-6).

Whether nerve tissue can be found in the sac or not, the existence of nerve roots and peripheral nerves demonstrates that a neural plate had once existed at the point of their origin. Smith[1] noted normal sciatic, popliteal and sural nerves in a fetus without a cord below the midthoracic region. He found normal peripheral nerve roots in every myelomeningocele. Stimulation of peripheral nerves at operation shows that these nerves conduct and produce a response in the muscle groups that they supply.

Many anomalies of the central nervous system accompany myelomeningoceles. Hydrocephaly, the most important complication, is present in about 80% of children with myelomeningocele,[1,70] and in most of these it can be demonstrated within the first month after birth.[1] But it can still develop in some children later, i.e., during the first 2 years of life. In necropsies of cases of myelomeningocele, hydrocephaly is almost always present and is accompanied by the Arnold-Chiari malformation. Aqueduct stenosis is found in about one-third of the necropsies, whereas forking is rarer.[1] In addition, overgrowth of the brain, microgyria, heterotopias of gray matter, cerebellar defects and other anomalies may be associated with the spinal lesion. Several of these anomalies can contribute to the formation of hydrocephaly, and their respective roles in its pathogenesis have been debated. The origin of the Arnold-Chiari malformation in cases of spina bifida has been discussed (p. 220). It may be mentioned that the incidence of hydrocephaly is comparatively low in pure sacral spina bifida,[1,71] a fact that does not support the theory that the Arnold-Chiari malformation is due to impaired ascent of the spinal cord and its traction on the brain stem (p. 220). Combination with a Dandy-Walker malformation is exceptional. Anencephaly is related to spina bifida etiologically and by association. Rachischisis may occur as a continuation of the cranial defect of anencephalics (Fig. 22-9). Cervical spina bifida has been observed together with cerebellar anomalies. Cameron,[72] in a series of 26 necropsies of children with spina bifida and hydrocephaly, found 12 cases of diastematomyelia (longitudinal division of the spinal cord) (p. 292). Each half of the cord contained one anterior and one posterior horn. Malformations of the vertebral column were frequent.

Spina bifida sometimes is associated with malformations of organs outside the nervous system. This is particularly true for stillborn fetuses and those who succumb early. In the survivors, there is a high association with such defects of the skeleton as unclosed vertebrae, block vertebrae or hemivertebrae, diastematomyelia, lumbar kyphosis and sacral anomalies. Barson[97] examined the roentgenograms of 510 infants with spina bifida and listed the incidences of the bony defects according to spinal levels. The skull often shows craniolacuna and craniofenestra.[73] Foot deformities and dislocation of the hip can be associated congenital malformations (Fig. 36-16) or be the result of muscle paralysis during postnatal life. Congenital heart disease, umbilical hernia, intestinal malformations (particularly imperforate rectum), harelip and cleft palate sometimes are present, but the incidence of such associations is below 5%.[1] In necropsies, associated malformations are encountered more often. Cameron[48] noted such anomalies of the urogenital tract as horseshoe kidney, cystic kidneys, bilateral double renal arteries and cryptorchidism in 8 of 26 necropsies. Fusion of the adrenals across the midline was noted in one case. A teratoid cystic tumor occurred in one instance and jejunal cyst in another. Pathologic changes in the urinary tract are of prime importance, but congenital and postnatal defects cannot always be distinguished. Hydronephrosis has been demonstrated in 10% of the patients in the neonatal period. It developed in another 15% within 3 years after birth.[74] Spina bifida has been encountered repeatedly in the asplenia syndrome combined with cardiac anomalies and partial situs inversus (p. 745). In rare instances, spina bifida has been observed in children with the trisomy 18 syndrome[26,27] (Fig. 36-11, *C*). A great variety of spina bifidas can be found in children with multiple congenital malformations. In such cases, the spinal cord may be quite different from that of the "standard" type of myelomeningocele (Fig. 36-11, *B*).

Symptoms

Children with *spina bifida occulta* usually appear normal externally and their neuromuscular functions are undisturbed. Their defect often is discovered incidentally in roentgenograms. In young children, incomplete ossification of the vertebral laminae may be mistaken for spina bifida, so that comparison with films of normal children of the same age is indicated. In older children and in adults, fusion defects seen in roentgenograms are more significant, but they, too,

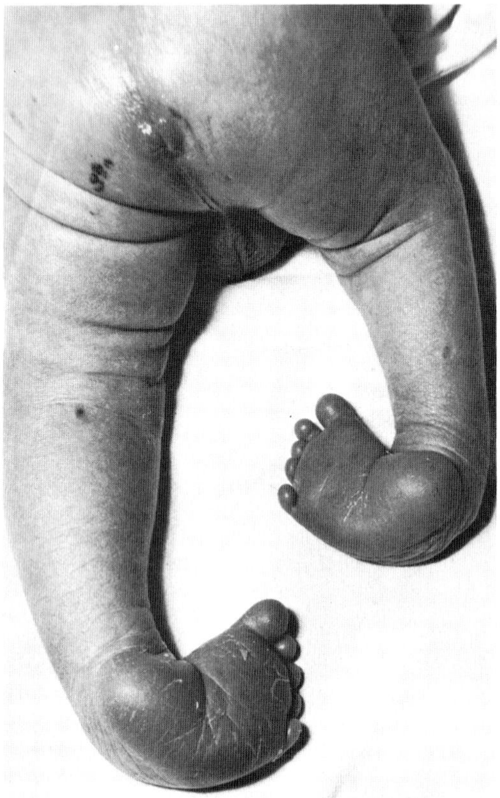

Fig. 36-16.—Bilateral talipes equinovarus in an infant with myelomeningocele, Arnold-Chiari malformation and hydrocephaly.

can be free of neurologic disturbances. Externally, hypertrichosis (Fig. 36-15), telangiectases, abnormal pigmentations, lipomas or dimples sometimes suggest an underlying skeletal defect. Neuromuscular disorders caused by spina bifida occulta with myelodysplasia ("spinal dysraphism"[57,75]) usually are discovered at the beginning of the second year, when it is noticed that the child does not learn to walk at the proper time and weakness is discovered in the lower extremities. Changes are attributed to adhesions between the spinal cord, the dura and the abnormal vertebrae. Myelograms with Pantopaque are helpful in demonstrating widening of the canal as well as abnormal contents. Spina bifida occulta is not complicated by the Arnold-Chiari malformation and hydrocephaly.

Anterior thoracic spina bifida occulta associated with a neurenteric cyst located in the mediastinum and connected with the meninges or spinal cord by a stalk through a defect in the vertebral bodies can cause respiratory infections, cough, failure to thrive or thoracic malformations.[60,61] The triad of mediastinal cyst, intramesenteric duplication and vertebral anomaly has been described by Fallon *et al.*[62] Intrathoracic meningoceles have been observed repeatedly in patients with neurofibromatosis.[52] They may be found on routine roentgenograms or manifest themselves by pain, pressure symptoms, dyspnea or generalized neurofibromatosis.

Meningoceles and myelomeningoceles are characterized by a visible sac along the spinal column. *Meningoceles* appear over the vertebral defect as protrusions covered by normal or atrophic skin. The sac shows fluctuation on palpation and sometimes translucency to light. The osseous defect and the channel connecting the intraspinal spaces with the sac usually are small and narrow, thus resulting in a pedunculated tumor. Usually, hydrocephaly does not develop, but increased cerebrospinal fluid pressure has been observed.[76] Meningoceles in the sacral area must be differentiated from sacrococcygeal teratomas. Plain roentgenograms or myelograms are helpful in the diagnosis, but the two lesions may occur together.[63]

Anterior sacral meningocele often remains unrecognized before puberty; diagnosis is assisted by roentgenograms, since the sacrum and coccyx are characteristically deformed.[65] Sometimes pyelography performed for urinary complaints reveals the sacral defect coincidentally. Pain at the lower end of the spine, constipation, urinary frequency, pyelitis or fever may be symptoms leading to the diagnosis. A pelvic mass may be found on rectal examination. Such lesions can complicate labor. The subject was reviewed by Thierry *et al.*,[95] who recommended and discussed operative procedures.

Myelomeningoceles are, as a rule, not pedunculated but form round, sessile tumors. The underlying osseous defect often is large and the cyst is not translucent, since neural tissue is closely attached to the external cover of the sac (Fig. 36-10). In the presence of lumbosacral lesions, weakness or flaccid paralysis is noticed in the muscles of the lower extremities, particularly those below the knee. There may be contracture at the hip and extension at the knee. The patellar reflexes are present in many cases, but the ankle reflexes cannot be elicited. Occurrence of upper motor neuron lesions was stressed by Stark and Baker.[91] The feet often are deformed (Fig. 36-16) and appear cold and cyanotic. In such cases there exists lack of sphincter control, and rectal prolapse may be seen. Incontinence of the vesical sphincters can be recognized by constant dribbling or by urination on abdominal pressure. Sensory disturbances are discovered by lack of response to painful or thermal stimuli, but in infants demonstration of such defects may be difficult. Ability to move can be established by tickling or a pinprick. Flaccid paralysis is the rule. Smith[1] distinguished four types of muscular disability in children according to the spinal segments involved. If the lesion is above L3 there is total paraplegia and the child needs total support to the lower limbs. If L4 and segments below are involved and the hip extensors and knee flexors are paralyzed, there are "flail feet" and vesical and rectal incontinence. Lesions of

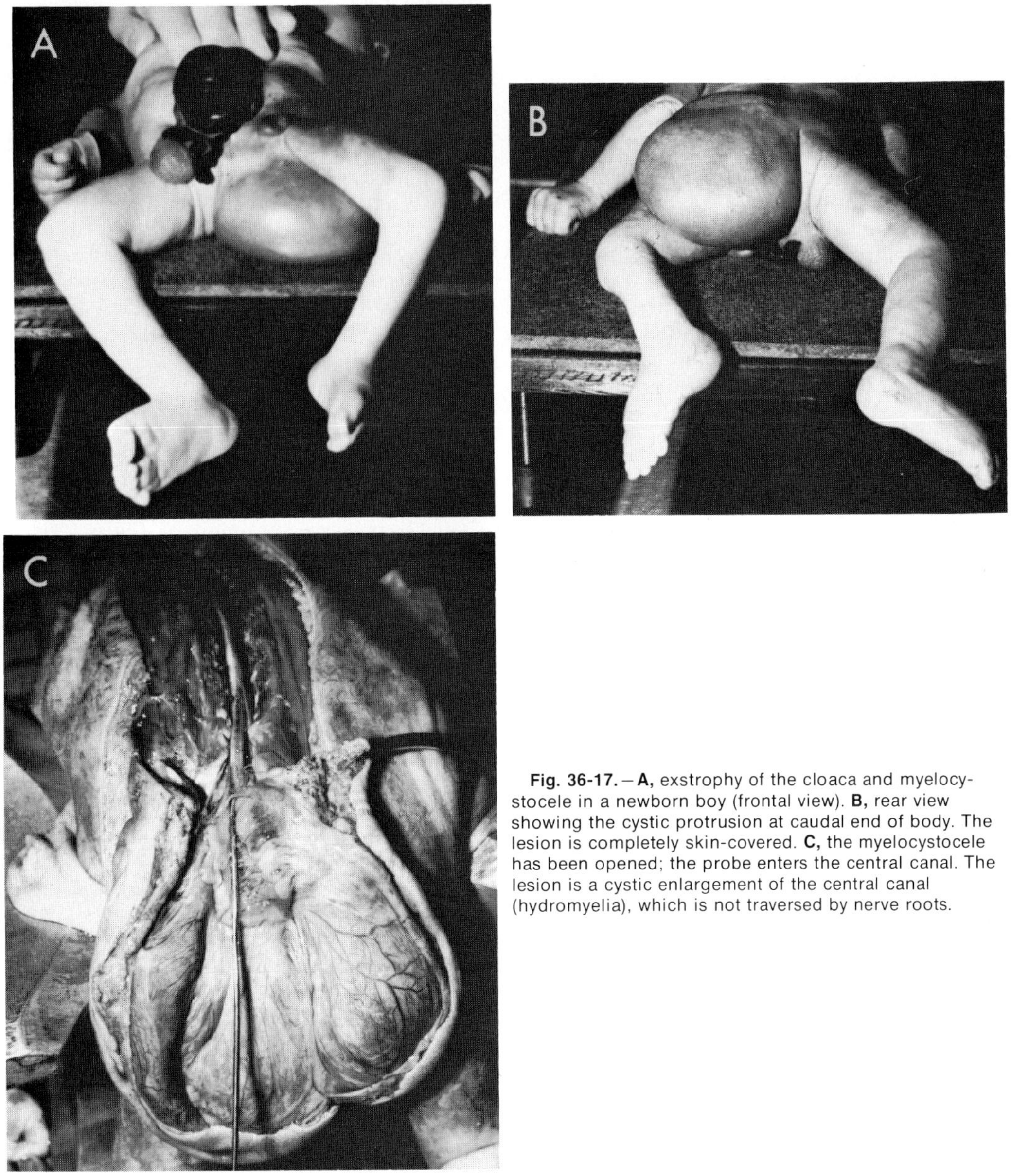

Fig. 36-17. – **A,** exstrophy of the cloaca and myelocystocele in a newborn boy (frontal view). **B,** rear view showing the cystic protrusion at caudal end of body. The lesion is completely skin-covered. **C,** the myelocystocele has been opened; the probe enters the central canal. The lesion is a cystic enlargement of the central canal (hydromyelia), which is not traversed by nerve roots.

S1 and below result in weakness of hip extensors and knee flexors and of inversion and eversion of feet; the plantar flexors of the feet are paralyzed and there is incontinence of the bladder and rectum. A spinal lesion of S3 and below leaves the lower limbs normal but the bladder and rectum are incontinent. Sensory and autonomic deficiencies cause trophic ulcerations of the perineum, buttocks, heels, vulva or prepuce and vasomotor changes. Smith[1] stated that perineal anesthesia over the third, fourth and fifth sacral dermatomes indicates some bladder disturbance. Bowel disturbances consist of constipation, rectal prolapse and lack of control. The urinary tract is seriously involved in most patients and its anomalies are life-threatening to children who survive the early dangers presented by the lesion. Bladder insufficiency is due to relaxed sphincters or to sphincter resistance, the latter being associated with sacral lesions.[1] For detailed discussions of urinary tract deficiency, which is of greatest importance to older children, I refer the reader to special publications.[1,77,78,92] Fractures of the long bones of the leg and periosteal reactions result from minor traumas in approximately 20% of the children with myelomeningocele.[79]

Cervical myelomeningoceles may result in spastic paralysis and hyperactive tendon reflexes in the lower extremities. Owing to cerebellar involvement, ataxia may be present.

Observation of the size of the head is of great importance in infants and young children. Since myelomeningoceles usually are associated with the Arnold-Chiari malformation and with anomalies of the brain, hydrocephaly develops in the majority of children with spina bifida (p. 220). Regular examination of the anterior fontanelle, of the skin of the scalp and measurements of the head circumference must be made in all children with spina bifida. Ventriculography reveals the extent of the ventricular enlargement and cortical thinning (p. 228).[70] Laryngeal stridor has been discussed in association with the Arnold-Chiari malformation.[96]

Prognosis

The prognosis for *spina bifida occulta* is favorable, as most of the patients remain symptomless throughout life. There are exceptions to this rule, because some affected persons develop neurologic manifestations. If symptoms are present at birth, surgical treatment promises little success, but if they develop later and are due to disproportion of growth between the spinal cord and the spinal column and if fixation of the spinal cord interferes with normal growth processes, surgical mobilization may be helpful.[57] Since the advent of antibiotics and advances in surgical treatment, the prognosis for *myelomeningocele* has improved considerably. In 1938, Hindse-Nielsen[16] found that 85–90% of infants born with myelomeningocele succumbed to meningitis, hydrocephaly and bladder paralysis. Laurence,[10] who studied the natural histories of more than 400 unselected cases occurring in the population of South Wales, arrived at similar figures. Twenty-five per cent of the infants with such lesions were stillborn and 14% died during the first week after birth. This heavy loss may take place even today if those born alive cannot be hospitalized quickly. Only 16% survived without surgery and intensive supportive treatment. At present, nothing can be done for the stillborn and little for those endangered immediately after birth. Including these hopeless patients, a survival rate of about 36% can be achieved by timely operation and proper management.[80] The survival rate of live-born children who receive proper treatment and care in hospitals is now 60–70%.[1,81,82]

It has been stated that the outlook is better for boys than for girls with myelomeningocele.[76] Urinary tract infection and upper urinary tract dilatation are more common in girls than in boys. But urinary tract infection does not seem to be a major cause of death in the first 5 years of life.[92]

Genetic Prognosis

If spina bifida occurs in a family, frequently the question arises as to what the chances for the outcome of future pregnancies are. The risk for a sibling born after an index case to have spina bifida or a related disorder of the central nervous system (p. 190) has been estimated to be from 3 to 4.6%.[83,94] After 2 children with spina bifida, an empirical risk figure of 10% has been cited for subsequent pregnancies.[84] But in Sheffield, England, Lorber[24] arrived at a risk figure of 8% after 1 child with spina bifida. With increasing family size there was a progressive increase in multiple cases. In sibships of 5 or more, multiple cases occurred in 24% of the families. General risk figures are, of course, not applicable to families and kindreds that repeatedly have shown a tendency to produce children with malformations of the central nervous system.[15,18,19,24]

Treatment

Treatment of myelomeningocele can be discussed here in general terms only. Infection and hydrocephaly should be prevented or treated. The patient's potentials for mental activities and physical functions should be preserved or improved. Future care, psychologic adjustment and social integration and adaptation should be initiated. These are formidable tasks that require the cooperation of many professional experts with the family. One finds greatly differing opinions in the areas of treatment and care, and no attempt will be made here to judge their respective merits. All teams working with these patients report marked improvement of survival rates and all agree on the serious problems left in the treatment of the survivors. Since the use of valves has made possible ventriculoatrial shunts for relief of cerebrospinal fluid hypertension,[85,86] and antibiotic prophylaxis and treatment have reduced the dangers of infection, differing methods of treatment have become possible. There are recommendations to close the spinal defect within 48 hours of birth and claims that muscle paralysis, sepsis, meningitis and mortality can be reduced by such early treatment.[80,81] Others believe that control of hydrocephaly before repair of the spinal lesion offers definite advantages. In fact, repair of the spinal defect may be unnecessary in 40% of the cases treated first by control of hydrocephaly.[87] An intermediate position was taken by Smith,[1] who believed that decisions concerning surgical approach are best made between the third and fifth weeks after birth. Intervention will then be directed commonly to arrest of advancing hydrocephaly, followed a week or two later by repair of the back. If no hydrocephaly is apparent, the back may be repaired first.

A great deal can be achieved for children with spina bifida by proper nursing care given while the children are waiting for operation or after the operation has been performed. It is not possible to discuss the details of nursing here, and the reader is referred to the publications by Ingraham and Matson,[63] West,[88] Shurtleff[89] and Smith.[1] Habilitation procedures have been developed successfully. By prevention of decubitus, deformities and urinary infections, the lives of many of these children can be prolonged.[1,77,78] By the proper use of wheelchairs, braces and crutches, children with neurologic deficits can be made ambulatory and adjusted to a rather normal life.[1,77,82,89,90]

Uncomplicated meningocele does not cause neurologic signs or hydrocephaly. The lesion is operated on for skin defects or cosmetic reasons. The proper time can be selected according to the situation of the individual patient. In spina bifida occulta, surgical treatment is indicated only if progressive neurologic or sphincter disturbances become noticeable. Operation consists of removal of lipomatous, fibrous, cartilaginous or osseous masses that adhere to the neural tissue.[57,93] But most persons with spina bifida occulta do not require treatment.

REFERENCES

1. Smith, E. D.: *Spina Bifida and the Total Care of Spinal Myelomeningocele* (Springfield, Ill.: Charles C Thomas, Publisher, 1965).
2. Ford, F. R.: *Diseases of the Nervous System in Infancy, Childhood and Adolescence* (3d ed.; Springfield, Ill.: Charles C Thomas, Publisher, 1952).
3. Sutherland, C. G.: Roentgenographic study of developmental anomalies of the spine, J. Radiol. 3:357, 1922.
4. Giles, R. G.: Vertebral anomalies, Radiology 17:1262, 1931.
5. Sutow, W. W., and Pryde, A. W.: Incidence of spina bifida occulta, A.M.A. Am. J. Dis. Child. 91:211, 1956.
6. Stevenson, A. C., Johnston, H. A., Stewart, M. I. P., and Golding, D. R.: Congenital malformations. A report of a study of series of consecutive births in 24 centres, Bull. WHO 34 (supp.):127, 1966.
7. McIntosh, R., Merritt, K. K., Richards, M. R., Samuels, M. H., and Bellows, M. T.: The incidence of congenital malformations: A study of 5,964 pregnancies, Pediatrics 14:505, 1954.
8. Alter, M.: Anencephalus, hydrocephalus and spina bifida, Arch. Neurol. & Psychiat. 7:411, 1962.
9. Nash, D. F. E.: Meningomyelocele, Proc. Roy. Soc. Med. 56:506, 1963.
10. Laurence, K. M.: The survival of untreated spina bifida cystica, Developmental Med. & Child Neurol., supp. 11, p. 10, 1966.
11. Boris, M., Blumberg, R., Feldman, D. B., and Sellers, T. F., Jr.: Increased incidence of meningomyeloceles, J.A.M.A. 184:768, 1963.
12. Lucey, J. F., Mann, R. W., Simmons, G. M., and Friedman, E.: An increased incidence of spina bifida in Vermont in 1962, Pediatrics 33:981, 1964.
13. Bucy, P. C.: Spina Bifida and Associated Malformations, in Brennemann, J. (ed.), *Practice of Pediatrics* (Hagerstown, Md.: W. F. Prior Company, Inc., 1948), Vol. 4, Chap. 15, pp. 1–31.
14. Record, R. G., and McKeown, T.: Congenital malformations of the central nervous system; survey of 930 cases, Brit. J. Social Med. 3:183, 1949.

14a. Nishimura, H., Takano, K., Tanimura, T., Yasuda, M., and Uchida, T.: High incidence of several malformations in the early human embryos as compared with infants, Biol. Neonat. 10:93, 1966.

15. Demeler, W.: Über familiäre Missbildungen der Wirbelsäule, Münster, 1933, 47 pp. (Inaugural Dissertation, Universität Münster.)
16. Hindse-Nielsen, S.: Spina bifida—prognosis and heredity; clinical study, Acta chir. scandinav. 80:525, 1938.
17. Murphy, D. P.: *Congenital Malformations. A Study of Parental Characteristics with Special Reference to the Reproductive Process* (2d ed.; Philadelphia: J. B. Lippincott Company, 1947), p. 127.
18. Grebe, H.: Familienbefunde bei letalen Anomalien der Körperform, (1) Acta genet. med. (Roma) 2:447, 1953; (11) Acta genet. med. (Roma) 3:93, 1954.
19. Polman, A.: Anencephaly, spina bifida and hydrocephaly; a contribution to our knowledge of the causal genesis of congenital malformations, Genetica 25:29, 1950.
20. Wilner, I. A.: Familial repetition of myelomeningocele, J. Michigan M. Soc. 48:727, 1949.
21. Newman, H. H., and Quisenberry, W. B.: One-egg twins with spina bifida and polydactyly, J. Hered. 35:309, 1944.
22. Myers, B.: Spina bifida (two other cases in same family), Proc. Roy. Soc. Med. 23:603, 1930.
23. Weidenmüller, K.: Beitrag zur Frage der Erbbedingtheit der Spina bifida. Ein Fall von familiärer Spina bifida aperta, Ztschr. menschl. Vererb.-u. Konstitutionslehre 20:42, 1936.
24. Lorber, J.: The family history of spina bifida cystica, Pediatrics 35:589, 1965.
25. Miller, J. R., Fraser, F. C., and MacEwan, D. W.: The frequency of spina bifida occulta and rib anomalies in the parents of children with spina bifida aperta and meningocele, Am. J. Human Genet. 14:245, 1962.

25a. Lorber, J., and Levick, K.: Spina bifida cystica. Incidence of spina bifida occulta in parents and in controls, Arch. Dis. Childhood 42:171, 1967.

25b. Hewitt, D.: Regional Variation in the Incidence of Spina Bifida, in *Genetics and Epidemiology of Chronic Diseases* (Washington, D.C.: U.S. Dept. of Health, Education and Welfare, 1965).

26. Warkany, J., Passarge, E., and Smith, L. B.: Congenital malformations in autosomal trisomy syndromes, Am. J. Dis. Child. 112:502, 1966.
27. Passarge, E., True, C. W., Sueoka, W. T., Baumgartner, N. R., and Keer, K. R.: Malformations of the central nervous system in trisomy 18 syndrome, J. Pediat. 69:771, 1966.

27a. Scorta, A., Franceschini, P., and Pilotti, G.: Su un caso di trisomia 18 con spina bifida e meningocele, Minerva ginec. 18:31, 1966.

28. Haddad, H. M., and Wilkins, L.: Congenital anomalies associated with gonadal aplasia. Review of 55 cases, Pediatrics 23:885, 1959.
29. Dunn, L. C., and Gluecksohn-Schoenheimer, S.: A specific abnormality associated with a variety of genotypes, Proc. Nat. Acad. Sc. 30:173, 1944.
30. Crary, D. D., Fox, R. R., and Sawin, P. B.: Spina bifida in the rabbit, J. Hered. 57:236, 1966.
31. Morison, J. E.: Congenital malformations in one of monozygotic twins, Arch. Dis. Childhood 24:214, 1949.
32. Gillman, J., Gilbert, C., and Gillman, T.: A preliminary report on hydrocephalus, spina bifida and other congenital anomalies in the rat produced by trypan blue, South African J. M. Sc. 13:47, 1948.
33. Warkany, J., Wilson, J. G., and Geiger, J. F.: Myeloschisis and myelomeningocele produced experimentally in the rat, J. Comp. Neurol. 109:35, 1958.
34. Gunberg, D. L.: Spina bifida and the Arnold-Chiari malformation in the progeny of trypan blue injected rats, Anat. Rec. 126:343, 1956.
35. Russell, L. B.: X-ray induced developmental abnormalities in the mouse and their use in the analysis of embryological patterns. I. External and gross visceral changes, J. Exper. Zool. 114:545, 1950.
36. Cohlan, S. Q.: Congenital anomalies in the rat produced by excessive intake of vitamin A during pregnancy, Pediatrics 13:556, 1954.
37. Warkany, J., and Takacs, E.: Experimental production of congenital malformations in rats by salicylate poisoning, J. Path. 35:315, 1959.
38. Arey, L. B.: *Developmental Anatomy. A Textbook and Laboratory Manual of Embryology* (6th ed.; Philadelphia: W. B. Saunders Company, 1954).
39. Streeter, G. L.: *Developmental Horizons in Human Embryos.* Embryology Reprint Vol. II (Washington, D.C.: Carnegie Institution of Washington, 1951).
40. Ancel, P.: Recherche expérimentale sur le spina bifida,

Arch. Anat. Micr. 36:45, 1946–47.
41. Patten, B. M.: Overgrowth of the neural tube in young human embryos, Anat. Rec. 113:381, 1952.
42. Patten, B. M.: Embryological stages in the establishing of myeloschisis with spina bifida, Am. J. Anat. 93:365, 1953.
43. Lemire, R. J., Shepard, T. H., and Alvord, E. C., Jr.: Caudal myeloschisis (lumbo-sacral spina bifida cystica) in a five millimeter (horizon XIV) human embryo, Anat. Rec. 152:9, 1965.
44. Wrete, M.: Über die Kenntnis des abnormen Offenstehens des Neuralrohres bei menschlichen Embryonen und jungen Feten, Beitr. path. Anat. 121:329, 1959.
45. Gruenwald, P.: Tissue anomalies of probable neural crest origin in a twenty millimeter human embryo with myeloschisis, Arch. Path. 31:489, 1941.
46. von Recklinghausen, F.: Untersuchungen über die Spina bifida, Virchows Arch. path. Anat. 105:243, 1886.
47. Ernst, P.: Missbildungen des Nervensystems, in Schwalbe, E. (ed.), *Die Morphologie der Missbildungen des Menschen und der Tiere* (Jena: Gustav Fischer, 1909), Vol. 3, pp. 67–252.
48. Cameron, A. H.: The spinal cord lesion in spina bifida cystica, Lancet 2:171, 1956.
49. Barry, A., Patten, B. M., and Stewart, B. H.: Possible factors in the development of the Arnold-Chiari malformation, J. Neurosurg. 14:285, 1957.
50. Report of the committee appointed to inquire into the anatomy of spina bifida and its treatment by the injection of Dr. Morton's iodo-glycerine solution, Tr. Clin. Soc. London 18:339, 1885.
51. YaDeau, R. E., Clagett, O. T., and Divertie, M. D.: Intrathoracic meningocele, J. Thoracic & Cardiovas. Surg. 49: 202, 1965.
52. LaVielle, C. J., and Campbell, D. A.: Neurofibromatosis and intrathoracic meningocele, Radiology 70:62, 1958.
53. Sammons, B. P., and Thomas, D. F.: Extensive lumbar meningocele associated with neurofibromatosis, Am. J. Roentgenol. 81:1021, 1959.
54. Morgagni, J. B.: *The Seats and Causes of Diseases Investigated by Anatomy.* Trans. by Benjamin Alexander. Vol. 3 (London: A. Miller and T. Cadell, 1769).
55. Gardner, W. J.: Myelomeningocele, the result of rupture of the embryonic neural tube, Cleveland Clin. Quart. 27: 88, 1960.
56. Dekaban, A. S., and Bartelmez, G. W.: Complete dysraphism in 14 somite human embryos. A contribution to normal and abnormal morphogenesis, Am. J. Anat. 115:27, 1964.
57. James, C. C. M., and Lassman, L. P.: Spinal dysraphism. An orthopaedic syndrome in children accompanying occult forms, Arch. Dis. Childhood 35:315, 1960.
58. Brickner, W. M.: Spina bifida occulta, Am. J. M. Sc. 155: 473, 1918.
59. Bucy, P. C., and Haymond, H. E.: Lumbosacral teratoma associated with spina bifida occulta; report of case with review of literature, Am. J. Path. 8:339, 1932.
60. Bremer, J. L.: *Congenital Anomalies of the Viscera. Their Embryological Basis* (Cambridge, Mass.: Harvard University Press, 1957).
61. Neuhauser, E. B. D., Harris, G. B. C., and Berrett, A.: Roentgenographic features of neurenteric cysts, Am. J. Roentgenol. 79:235, 1958.
62. Fallon, M., Gordon, A. R. G., and Lendrum, A. C.: Mediastinal cysts of fore-gut origin associated with vertebral abnormalities, Brit. J. Surg. 41:520, 1954.
63. Ingraham, F. D., and Matson, D. D.: *Neurosurgery of Infancy and Childhood* (Springfield, Ill.: Charles C Thomas, Publisher, 1954).
64. Turnbull, F. A.: Syringomyelic complications of spina bifida, Brain 56:304, 1933.
65. Leigh, T. F., and Rogers, J. V., Jr.: Anterior sacral meningocele, Am. J. Roentgenol. 71:808, 1954.
66. Prop, N., Frensdorf, E. L., and van de Stadt, F. R.: A postvertebral entodermal cyst associated with axial deformities: A case showing the "entodermal-ectodermal adhesion syndrome," Pediatrics 39:555, 1967.
67. Willis, R. A.: *The Borderland of Embryology and Pathology* (2d ed.; Washington, D.C.: Butterworth, Inc., 1962).
68. Berndorfer, A.: Die Variationstypen der Meningozelen und ihre biologischembryologische Bedeutung, Zentralbl. Chir. 88:357, 1963.
69. Bonsmann, M. R.: Über nachträgliche Überhäutung von Myelomeningozelen, Virchows Arch. path. Anat. 213:131, 1913.
70. Lorber, J.: Systematic ventriculographic studies in infants born with meningomyelocele and encephalocele. The incidence and development of hydrocephalus, Arch. Dis. Childhood 36:381, 1961.
71. Laurence, K. M.: The natural history of spina bifida cystica, Arch. Dis. Childhood 39:41, 1964.
72. Cameron, A. H.: The Arnold-Chiari and other neuro-anatomical malformations associated with spina bifida, J. Path. & Bact. 73:195–211, 213–221, 1957.
73. Barson, A. J.: Radiological studies of spina bifida cystica; the phenomenon of congenital lumbar kyphosis, Brit. J. Radiol. 38:294, 1965.
74. Rose, R. S., and Smith, J. P.: Hydronephrosis in infants with meningomyelocele: Its early recognition, J. Urol. 90: 129, 1963.
75. Lichtenstein, B. W.: "Spinal dysraphism"; spina bifida and myelodysplasia, Arch. Neurol. 44:792, 1940.
76. Doran, P. A., and Guthkelch, A. N.: Studies in spina bifida cystica. I. General survey and reassessment of problem, J. Neurol., Neurosurg. & Psychiat. 24:331, 1961.
77. Morales, P. A., Deaver, G. G., and Hotchkiss, R. S.: Urological complications of spina bifida in children, J. Urol. 75:537, 1956.
78. Nash, D. F. E.: Ileal loop bladder in congenital spinal palsy, Brit. J. Urol. 28:387, 1956.
79. Waltenspühl, J.: Traumatisch bedingte Knochenläsionen bei Meningomyelocelen, Ann. paediat. 200:280, 1963.
80. Rickham, P. P., and Mawdsley, T.: The effect of early operation on the survival of spina bifida cystica, Developmental Med. & Child Neurol., supp. 11, p. 20, 1966.
81. Sharrard, W. J. W., Zachary, R. B., Lorber, J., and Bruce, A. M.: A controlled trial of immediate and delayed closure of spina bifida cystica, Arch. Dis. Childhood 38:18, 1963.
82. Shurtleff, D. B., Gordon, L., Foltz, E. L., and Ansell, J.: Hydrocephalus and meningomyelocele: Practical considerations, Gen. Pract. 32:101, 1965.
83. Fraser, F. C.: Recent advances in genetics in relation to pediatrics, J. Pediat. 52:734, 1958.
84. Fraser, F. C.: Genetics and Congenital Malformations, in Steinberg, A. G. (ed.), *Progress in Medical Genetics* (New York: Grune & Stratton, Inc., 1961), Chap. 3.
85. Nulsen, F. E., and Spitz, E. B.: Treatment of hydrocephalus by direct shunt from ventricle to jugular vein, S. Forum 2:399, 1951.
86. Pudenz, R. H., Russell, F. E., Hurd, A. H., and Shelden, C. H.: Ventriculo-auriculostomy; a technique for shunting cerebrospinal fluid into the right auricle, J. Neurosurg. 14:171, 1957.
87. Shurtleff, D. B., and Foltz, E. L.: A comparative study of meningomyelocele repair or cerebrospinal fluid shunt as primary treatment in 90 children, Developmental Med. & Child Neurol., supp. 13, p. 57, 1967.
88. West, J. St.: *Congenital Malformations and Birth Injuries* (New York: Association for the Aid of Crippled Children, 1954).
89. Shurtleff, D. B.: Timing of learning in the meningomyelocele patient, J. Am. Phys. Ther. A. 46:136, 1966.
90. Deaver, G. G., Buck, D., and McCarthy, J.: Spina Bifida, in the *1951 Year Book of Physical Medicine and Rehabilitation* (Chicago: Year Book Publishers, 1952), pp. 9–24.
91. Stark, G. D., and Baker, G. C. W.: The neurological involvement of the lower limbs in myelomeningocele, Developmental Med. & Child Neurol. 9:732, 1967.
92. Cooper, D. G. W.: Urinary tract infection in children with myelomeningocele, Arch. Dis. Childhood 42:521, 1967.
93. James, C. C. M., and Lassman, L. P.: Results of treatment

of progressive lesions in spina bifida occulta five to ten years after laminectomy, Lancet 2:1277, 1967.
94. Yen, S., and MacMahon, B.: Genetics of anencephaly and spina bifida?, Lancet 2:623, 1968.
95. Thierry, A., Archimbaud, J-P., Fischer, G., Freidel, M., and Mansuy, L.: La méningocèle sacrée antérieure, Neuro-chir. 15:389, 1969.
96. Morley, A. R.: Laryngeal stridor, Arnold-Chiari malformation and medullary haemorrhages, Developmental Med. & Child Neurol. 11:471, 1969.
97. Barson, A. J.: Spina bifida: The significance of the level and extent of the defect to the morphogenesis, Developmental Med. & Child Neurol. 12:129, 1970.
98. Lemire, R. J.: Variations in development of the caudal neural tube in human embryos (horizons XIV–XXI), Teratology 2:361, 1969.
99. Padget, D. H.: Neuroschisis and human embryonic maldevelopment, J. Neuropath. & Exper. Neurol. 29:192, 1970.

Hydromyelia

Dilatations of the central canal may be congenital anomalies or secondary to postnatal mechanical obstructions. The dilatations vary greatly in size and extent; they can be symptomless or be associated with such severe congenital malformations (myelocystocele, syringomyelocele) as exstrophy of the cloaca (p. 713), spina bifida cystica or the Arnold-Chiari malformation. They also can be present in patients with myelodysplasia or diastematomyelia, where they are found cranial to the level of the cord division![1] In patients with syringomyelia, a congenital anomaly of the hindbrain may be present and the syrinx be in communication with the ventricular system. Failure of formation of the foramina in prenatal life may account for this form of hydromyelia.[2]

Symptoms vary greatly. In some patients, abnormal gait, muscular weakness, anesthesia and reflex changes can be manifestations. In other cases, the anomaly may remain symptomless.[1]

In some cases diagnosed as syringomyelia, surgical treatment can be of considerable benefit.[1]

REFERENCES

1. Lassman, L. P., Michael James, C. C., and Foster, J. B.: Hydromyelia, J. Neurol. Sc. 7:149, 1968.
2. Gardner, W. J.: Hydrodynamic mechanism of syringomyelia: Its relationship to myelocele, J. Neurol., Neurosurg. & Psychiat. 28:247, 1965.

Diastematomyelia

Complete or incomplete sagittal division of the neural axis into halves was recognized and described by Cruveilhier as early as 1853. At first, interest in this anomaly was limited to pathologists and teratologists,[1] but now it has been recognized that diastematomyelia can occur in living persons, causing crippling and disability. Since surgical intervention may arrest progress of adverse manifestations, recognition of the anomaly by clinical and roentgenographic measures is of practical importance. The sagittal division of a segment of the spinal cord or cauda equina usually is associated with anomalous development of the vertebrae. The two portions of the cord are separated by an osseous or fibrocartilaginous septum that is attached anteriorly to one or more vertebral bodies, posteriorly to the dura and occasionally to the deformed vertebral arches.[2]

The osseous or fibrocartilaginous septum passing through the cord fixes the cord in a low anatomic position, so that its normal ascent during growth is impaired. This septum and the arachnoid adhesions that frequently accompany it produce traction on the cord or cauda equina, which results in neurologic disturbances.

The anomaly is most frequently observed in the lumbar region and usually is associated with skeletal irregularities such as hemivertebrae, double vertebrae or incomplete arches. Ballantyne[1] described a spur from the third lumbar vertebra into the spinal canal in a case of spina bifida and hydrocephaly. In such cases, an Arnold-Chiari malformation usually is present.[2,3] Milder cases may resemble spina bifida occulta with myelodysplasia (p. 286). At birth, there may be visible manifestations such as lipoma, excessive hair, a skin dimple or a nevus. Sometimes, kyphosis, scoliosis, spina bifida cystica or clubfoot is associated with diastematomyelia but, usually, neurologic symptoms are not observed until later, when the patient fails to walk properly at the expected time or when a limp develops during the first years of life after the child has learned to walk correctly. An abnormal gait is the most frequent initial complaint. Atrophy of the lower extremities is frequent and foot deformities develop. The deep reflexes of the lower extremities vary according to the location of the lesion. Disturbances of the vesical or rectal sphincters may occur.

The anomaly has been explained by persistence and partial obliteration of a neurenteric canal.[4] It is of interest that in one observation[3] a parasitic twin was attached to the patient in the midthoracic region. The lesion occurs more often in females than in males.[5]

Roentgenograms of the spine show, at the level of diastematomyelia, spina bifida with widening of the neural canal and of the interpedicular spaces extending over several adjacent spinal segments. When the

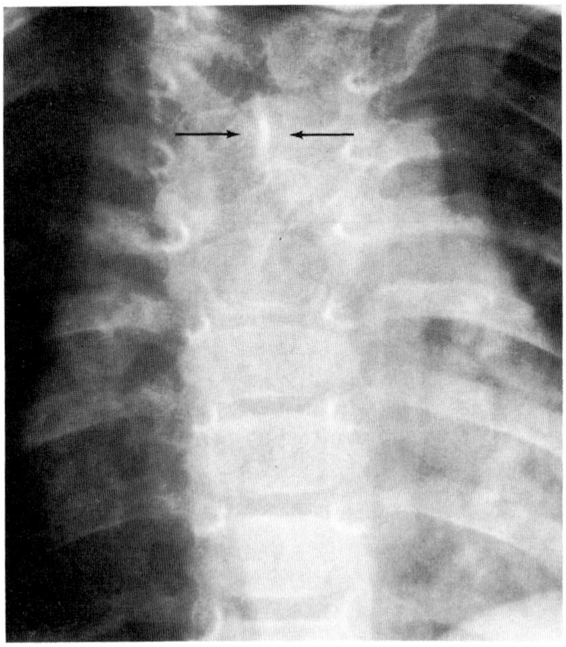

Fig. 36-18.—Density (**arrows**) is caused by bony spur of diastematomyelia.

septum that divides the cord is osseous, it can be seen in anteroposterior projection and recognized as a small linear or irregular fragment of bone lying in the midline of the neural canal (Fig. 36-18). Diminution of the anteroposterior diameter of the vertebral bodies is frequent and gross anomalies such as hemivertebrae or block vertebrae can be demonstrated. On myelography, one finds that, in addition to the osseous spicule, nonopaque tissues further widen the dividing septum and that the contrast substance is split. As the patients grow older, deformities of the spine develop that mask the typical roentgenologic picture.[2] Expanding intraspinal tumors or lipomas must be considered in the differential diagnosis, but in these conditions no dividing septum will be found.

Treatment consists of removal of the bony spur and mobilization of the spinal cord. Neurologic disorders seldom are improved by operation, but it is thought that their progress can be prevented[6] if the condition is recognized early.

In a series of 60 consecutive cases of spina bifida occulta submitted to laminectomy because of abnormality of the spinal cord or cauda equina, diastematomyelia was found in 24. Accompanying extrinsic anomalies such as angulated bands seem to be responsible for clinical symptoms rather than the diastematomyelia.[7]

REFERENCES

1. Ballantyne, J. W.: *Manual of Antenatal Pathology and Hygiene* (Chicago: Chicago Medical Book Company, 1904).
2. Neuhauser, E. B. D., Wittenborg, M. H., and Dehlinger, K.: Diastematomyelia; transfixation of the cord or cauda equina with congenital anomalies of the spine, Radiology 54:659, 1950.
3. Moes, C. A. F., and Hendrick, E. B.: Diastematomyelia, J. Pediat. 63:238, 1963.
4. Bremer, J. L.: Dorsal intestinal fistula; accessory neurenteric canal; diastematomyelia, Arch. Path. 54:132, 1952.
5. Sheptak, P. E., and Susen, A. F.: Diastematomyelia, Am. J. Dis. Child. 113:210, 1967.
6. Ingraham, F. D., and Matson, D. D.: *Neurosurgery of Infancy and Childhood* (Springfield, Ill.: Charles C Thomas, Publisher, 1954).
7. James, C. C. M., and Lassman, L. P.: Diastematomyelia, Arch. Dis. Childhood 39:125, 1964.

Myelodysplasia, Syringomyelia and Status Dysraphicus

In experimental teratology, one finds that certain teratologic conditions result not only in gross malformations of the central nervous system, such as exencephaly, anencephaly and spina bifida, but also in minor malformations of the spinal cord that are seen in histologic sections as deformities of the gray or white matter (Figs. 36-19 and 36-20). Such histologic malformations can properly be called myelodysplasias. They frequently are found in animals with gross malformations at cord levels above or below the major lesions, and they sometimes are seen in apparently normal young that had been subjected to teratogenic manipulations; they are the mild forms of the teratologic series experimentally produced. A congenital myelodysplasia changing postnatally to syringomyelia has been described in purebred Weimaraner dogs. It seems likely that the anomaly is genetically determined. The spinal lesions consist of anomalies of the central canal, anterior horns and the ventral median fissure.[1] These myelodysplasias, which show great morphologic variations, often are associated with anomalies of the vertebrae surrounding them. Such myelodysplasias occur in man also. They vary in location, morphology and extent. Their recognition is complicated by the fact that they are of differing etiology and can be imitated by postnatal disease processes and trauma. It is understandable that such minor malformations of the spinal cord that vary greatly in symptomatology are not always recognized as such and that the literature concerned with them is confusing.

The term *myelodysplasia* seems most appropriate for congenital anomalies of the cord derived from maldevelopment of the neural tube. The dysplasia may be due to imperfect closure of the neural plate

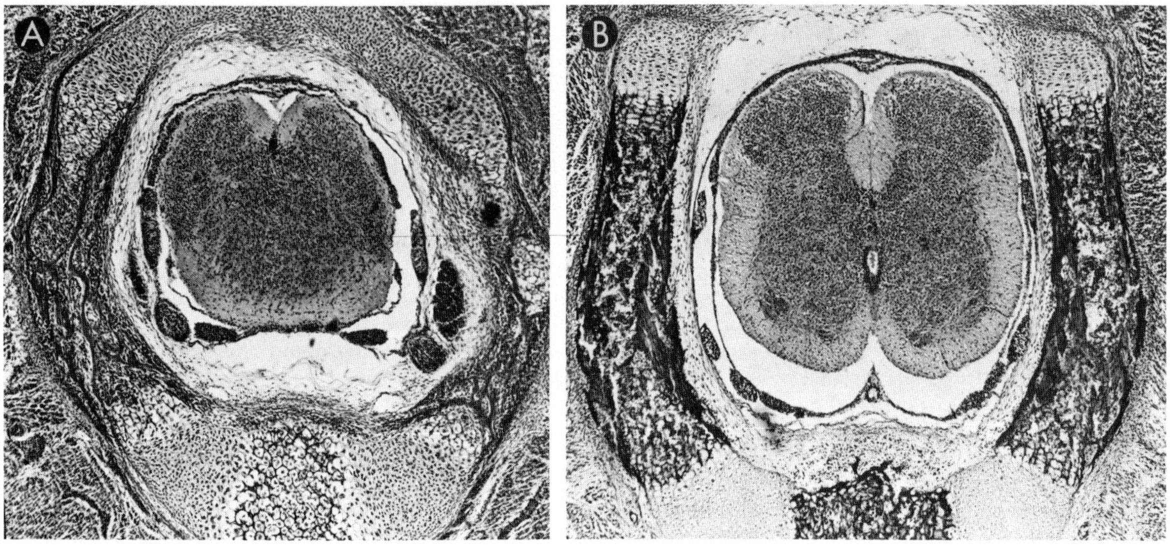

Fig. 36-19. – **A,** transverse section through spinal cord of a rat fetus (twenty-second day) showing myelodysplasia. The horns of the gray matter and the tracts of the white matter are in disorder. (Trypan blue eighth to tenth day.) **B,** section through control animal (twenty-second day).

but it can also be present in a closed spinal cord.

"Myelodysplasia" was described by Fuchs[2] as a congenital defect of the lower spinal cord, which he assumed as the basis of mild clinical symptoms that were then often attributed to "neuroses." In a number of patients, Fuchs found persistent enuresis, mild sensory disturbances in the lower portions of the body and inconspicuous reflex anomalies. He thought that, in these patients, spina bifida occulta, deformities of the feet and syndactyly pointed to an organic rather than a neurotic origin of the manifestations. Later, histologic examinations of the spinal cord revealed that a variety of anomalies could be found in the area of the central canal and in the white and gray matters, although more or less complete closure of the neural plate had taken place. In 1918, Brickner[3] discussed many clinical symptoms attributable to myelodysplasia associated with spina bifida occulta, including sensory and trophic changes. The symptoms of some of these patients resemble those of syringomyelia, and there are cases in which a clear differentiation between these disorders cannot be made.

Syringomyelia indicates cavity formation in the spinal cord. The clinical picture is well defined though variable and it is believed that the typical symptom complex can be caused by differing etiologic factors, namely infectious, vascular or neoplastic processes. There are other forms that can be attributed to congenital anomalies of the spinal cord, e.g., the myelodysplasias mentioned above. It is thought that embryonic cell rests, particularly ependymal spongioblasts, can undergo proliferation and cavitation, resulting in syringomyelia. Scott *et al.*[4] considered syringomyelia a congenital disease of glial tissue resulting from fetal malformations in the closure of the neural canal. This opinion, expressed by some authors in the nineteenth century, is still held by many today. The prenatal origin of syringomyelia, a disorder that manifests itself, as a rule, in the second or third decade of life, is further supported by findings of associated congenital malformations in some of the patients. Platybasia, Klippel-Feil syndrome, Sprengel deformity or rib anomalies[5,6] point to a malformation of the spinal cord in the cervicothoracic area.[7] In rare instances, manifestations occur during childhood[8]

Fig. 36-20. – Transverse section through rat fetus (twenty-first day) with spina bifida occulta and myelodysplasia. The shape of the cord is quite irregular, and gray and white matters are in disarray. (Streptonigrin tenth day.)

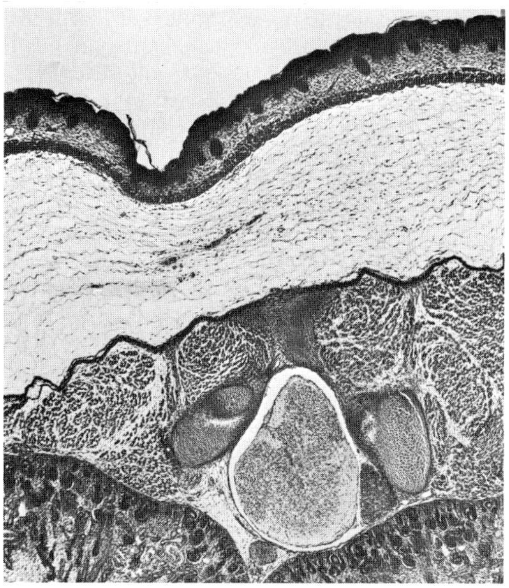

(p. 295), but early diagnosis is difficult. Familial occurrence pointing to genetic determination has been observed repeatedly.[9,10] Lumbosacral syringomyelia may be transmitted through several generations.[11] "Familial osseous atrophy" (p. 295) probably is closely related to myelodysplasia. Congenital tumors of the spinal canal and hemangioblastomas occurring in Hippel-Lindau disease[12] (p. 1267) can be associated with cavity formation in the cord.[13] In rare instances, the deficit of nerve tissue may be due to tumors such as medulloblastomas, neuroblastomas or ependymomas.[14] From the extensive and confusing literature on the subject of myelodysplasia-syringomyelia,[4,7,10,15-17] one can conclude that some cases of syringomyelia are closely related to myelodysplasia and, therefore, are prenatal in origin. Postnatal events may precipitate the appearance of the disease.

Nonclosure of the neural plate has been called "araphia," and faulty closure "dysraphia," terms that are acceptable and can be recommended. Araphia would be a collective term for exencephalies or myeloschises (p. 284). The term "spinal dysraphia" would include anomalies of the posterior septum with or without penetration of the posterior aspect of the cord by mesenchymal tissue, irregularities of the ependyma, enlargement of the central canal and also malformations of the gray or white matter and asymmetries that affect the raphe of the cord. Such cord anomalies, dysraphias, usually can be found above, but sometimes below, an open spina bifida or myeloschisis; but similar irregularities can be discovered in persons who have neither an open nor an occult spina bifida. Benda[18] pointed out that this is particularly true in mentally deficient persons. The pathology of spinal dysraphism has been studied by Ostertag,[14] Lichtenstein[15] and Benda.[18] Spinal dysraphism is a myelodysplasia, but not all myelodysplasias are dysraphic. Clinical manifestations may range from those described by Fuchs[2] to those of syringomyelia.[4] Unfortunately, the term "status dysraphicus" has been extended not only to patients with syringomyelia-like symptoms but also to their relatives and other persons who have merely minor and nonspecific congenital malformations or dysfunctions. Sternal anomalies, kyphoscoliosis, difference in the size of the breasts, long arms with spider fingers, cyanotic and cold hands, curving of fingers (particularly digit V), sensory disturbances, enuresis, high palate and aural anomalies have been considered signs of "status dysraphicus."[19] It is obvious that such frequent and nonspecific anomalies cannot be considered indicative of faulty closure of the neural tube. If "status dysraphicus" were familial and related to true "araphia," one should sometimes find myelomeningocele, meningocele or anencephaly among relatives. But this, to my knowledge, is not the case. Because of the indiscriminate use of the term "status dysraphicus" and its applicability to a host of nonspecific "stigmata of degeneration," I avoid the term. Cavitation of the spinal cord is better called "syringomyelia," and congenital malformation of the cord without cavitation should be termed "myelodysplasia."

Myelodysplasia

In contrast to typical syringomyelia, the manifestations of myelodysplasia are not progressive. In the disease picture described by Fuchs[2] and Mattauschek,[20] there is weakness of the sphincters, with enuresis persisting into adult life; disturbances in sensation of the legs, with marked thermanesthesia; trophic and vasomotor disorders; and abnormal skin and tendon reflexes of the abdomen and lower extremities. These functional disturbances often are accompanied by clefts of vertebral arches, clubfoot, syndactyly of the second and third toes and skin changes such as hypertrichosis, nevus or fovea coccygea. These anomalies are not present in every patient with myelodysplasia, but there is a tendency to the association. The extension of this symptom complex to syringomyelias and status dysraphicus was well presented by Mulvey and Riely.[10]

Syringomyelia

Syringomyelia affects the cervical region most often; in typical cases, the cord appears enlarged and flattened. Other areas also may be affected. If the medulla oblongata is involved, one speaks of "syringobulbia"; lumbosacral cavitation defects of the cord may be found also. On section, the cord shows cavities of variable size, limited to a few segments or extended over a large portion of the cord. The cavities can be single or multiple, limited to the area behind the central canal or extending into the gray matter. There usually is fibrous gliosis around the cavity, but ependyma and connective tissue may occur around it. Nerve cells and fibers near the cavity are destroyed by edema, fluid pressure or glial overgrowth. Hemorrhage or tumors originating in the defect can aggravate the symptoms. Occasionally, extensive syringomyelia is found at necropsy in persons who had no clinical symptoms of the disease.[21]

The principal symptoms of syringomyelia consist of muscular atrophy, dissociated anesthesia, trophic disturbances, arthropathies and, sometimes, spastic paraplegia.[17] If the cervical cord is chiefly affected, the fingers, hands and arms are involved, but the shoulders and the upper trunk may also show signs of disease. Manifestations sometimes are unilateral. Muscular changes are variable. As a rule, the small muscles of the hands show atrophy and contractures so that a clawhand is formed. There also may be wasting of the muscles of the arms and of the neck, spine and chest; muscular fibrillations sometimes are noticeable. The limbs may be partly atrophic, partly hypertrophic, partly flaccid and partly spastic. The patient is insensitive to painful and thermal stimuli but remains sensitive to touch. If the pyramidal tracts are involved, spastic paraplegia is present in the lower extremities. Horner syndrome and heterochromia iridis may develop. If syringomyelia affects the lumbosacral area, the patient develops atrophy and weakness of the lower limbs, loss of deep reflexes and sometimes loss of sphincter control. The syringobulbar syndrome shows great diversity. The onset can be acute or insidious. Ocular symptoms, nystagmus, strabismus, crossed analgesia, disturbance of taste, respiration, circulation and digestion, dysphagia or dysphonia, facial hemiatrophy or hemihypertrophy and many other symptoms may occur.[21,22] Deformities of the hands and fingers develop and scoliosis is quite frequent. Serious arthropathies with destruction of cartilage and relaxation of the capsule occur more often in the upper than in the lower extremities. Trophic disturbances affect the skin, which may appear rough and thickened or atrophic and paper thin. Sores and abscesses, dystrophies of the nails and absorption of the terminal phalanges develop. Various rashes can make their appearance and differences in the size of the breasts may become noticeable. Roentgenograms of the bones show porotic as well as sclerotic changes, and fractures can occur after minor traumas. Although the disease is rare in children, the onset of symptoms sometimes can be traced back to childhood. Bermann[8] described a child who developed multiple abscesses on his fingers at the age of 2 years and seemed to have lost sensitivity to pain and heat in early life. When the boy was 11 years old, he had muscular atrophy, dissociated anesthesia, scoliosis, Horner syndrome and unilaterally hyperactive patellar reflexes. Infantile syringobulbia may manifest itself as neurogenic stridor, recurrent apnea and bradycardia. A case including a necropsy report was published by Duffy and Ziter.[23] In most instances, syringomyelia does not become disabling before the second or third decade. Usually, it progresses slowly, with remissions and exacerbations, but sometimes the onset is sudden and leads to early death. The prognosis as to life is not unfavorable except in the case of the syringobulbar syndrome or septicemia, which in former times often was fatal to patients with syringomyelia.

In selected cases, improvement of symptoms has been achieved by reducing pressure on the nerve tissue by roentgen or radium therapy, or by surgical drainage of fluid from the cavity. The indications for surgical intervention were discussed by McIlroy and Richardson.[24]

Familial Osseous Atrophy

This condition of "postnatal amputations" probably is due to a circumscript myelodysplasia. The disorder is not congenital in its manifestations but the underlying anomaly (probably a defect of the nervous system) is hereditary. The disease manifests itself at first as blisters and ulcers on the soles, developing under the heads of the metacarpal bones. The ulcers, surrounded by heavy calluses, show little tendency to heal. With the secretions from the ulcers there also occurs extrusion of necrotic bone until whole phalanges and metacarpals are destroyed. In some cases, only stumps of the feet are left. Areas of anesthesia can be demonstrated around the ulcers, with a loss of sensation of pain, touch and temperature. The anesthesia probably is not congenital but it precedes the necrotic processes. It remains limited to the feet in most cases.

The disorder can be transmitted through several generations. In some pedigrees, only males are affected,[25,26] but in others, females are not spared.[27] Onset of manifestations occurs in the second or third decade of life. Although the disease can disable the patients, it is not fatal and is compatible with life for many decades.

Associated malformations such as spina bifida occulta and harelip and cleft palate have been listed in a pedigree,[27,28] but they seem to be rare and accidental occurrences not related to the disease process.

A dominantly inherited myelodysplasia seems to be at the root of this disorder. In two families, the manifestations were limited to the feet.[25,26] In one pedigree, affected members showed changes involving not only the feet but also the lower legs and the hands.[27] In the same family, males and females were affected.

The prognosis is good as to life, but crippling by loss of the ends of the extremities may occur. Temporary healing of ulcers can be achieved by protracted bed rest. Surgical amputations were required in some of the cases, and sometimes such amputations could be performed without anesthetic.

REFERENCES

1. McGrath, J. T.: Spinal dysraphism in the dog. With comments on syringomyelia, Path. Vet. (supp.) 2:1, 1965.
2. Fuchs, A.: Über den klinischen Nachweis kongenitaler Defektbildungen in den unteren Rückenmarksabschnitten (Myelodysplasia), Wien. med. Wchnschr. 59:2141, 1909.
3. Brickner, W. M.: Spina bifida occulta, Am. J. M. Sc. 155: 473, 1918.
4. Scott, E., LeFever, H., and Oliver, M.: Syringomyelia and syringobulbia, Ohio M. J. 30:213, 1934.
5. Critchley, M.: Sprengel's deformity with paraplegia, Brit. J. Surg. 14:243, 1926.
6. du Toit, F. S.: A case of congenital elevation of the scapula (Sprengel's deformity) with defect of the cervical spine associated with syringomyelia, Brain 54:421, 1931.
7. Kramer, P. W.: The pathogenesis of syringomyelia, J. Indiana M. A. 55:1635, 1962.
8. Bermann, E. J.: Syringomyelie im Kindesalter, Monatsschr. Kinderh. 37:1, 1927.
9. Kino, F.: Über heredo-familiäre Syringomyelie, Ztschr. Neurol. u. Psychiat. 107:1, 1927.
10. Mulvey, B. E., and Riely, L. A.: Familial syringomyelia and status dysraphicus, Ann. Int. Med. 16:966, 1942.
11. Van Epps, C., and Kerr, H. D.: Familial lumbosacral syringomyelia, Radiology 35:160, 1940.
12. Kinney, T. D., and Fitzgerald, P. J.: Lindau-von Hippel disease with hemangioblastoma of spinal cord and syringomyelia, Arch. Path. 43:439, 1947.
13. Kernohan, J. W., Woltman, H. W., and Adson, A.: Intramedullary tumors of spinal cord; review of 51 cases with attempt at biologic classification, Arch. Neurol. & Psychiat. 25:679, 1931.

14. Ostertag, B.: Missbildungen, in Henke, F., Lubarsch, O., and Rössle, R.(eds.), *Handbuch der speziellen pathologischen Anatomie und Histologie* (Berlin: Springer-Verlag, 1956), Vol. 13, part 4, p.283.
15. Lichtenstein, B. W.: Spinal dysraphism, spina bifida and myelodysplasia, Arch. Neurol. & Psychiat. 44:792, 1940.
16. Riley, H. A.: Syringomyelia or myelodysplasia, J. Nerv. & Ment. Dis. 72:1, 1930.
17. Schlesinger, H.: *Die Syringomyelie* (Leipzig & Wien: F. Deuticke, 1895).
18. Benda, C. E.: *Developmental Disorders of Mentation and Cerebral Palsies* (New York: Grune & Stratton, Inc., 1952).
19. Bremer, F. W.: Klinische Untersuchungen zur Aetiologie der Syringomyelie, des "Status dysraphicus," Deutsche Ztschr. Nervenh. 95:1, 1926.
20. Mattauschek, E.: Über Enuresis, Wien. med. Wchnschr. 9:2154, 1909.
21. Wilson, S. A. K.: *Neurology*, Bruce, A. N.(ed.) (2d ed.; Baltimore: The Williams & Wilkins Company, 1955).
22. Ford, F. R.: *Diseases of the Nervous System in Infancy, Childhood and Adolescence* (Springfield, Ill.: Charles C Thomas, Publisher, 1966).
23. Duffy, P. E., and Ziter, F. A.: Infantile syringobulbia. A study of its pathology and a proposed relationship to neurogenic stridor in infancy, Neurology 14:500, 1964.
24. McIlroy, W. J., and Richardson, J. C.: Syringomyelia: A clinical review of 75 cases, Canad. M.A.J. 93:731, 1965.
25. Smith, E. M.: Familial neurotrophic osseous atrophy; familial neurotrophic condition of feet with anesthesia and loss of bone, J.A.M.A. 102:593, 1934.
26. Cooper, G., Jr., Adair, N., and Patterson, W. M.: Familial osseous atrophy, Radiology 48:509, 1947.
27. Tocantins, L. M., and Reimann, H. A.: Perforating ulcers of feet, with osseous atrophy in family with other evidences of dysgenesis (harelip, cleft palate): Instance of probable myelodysplasia, J.A.M.A. 112:2251, 1939.
28. Reimann, H. A., McKechnie, W. G., and Stanisavljevic, S.: Hereditary sensory radicular neuropathy and other defects in a large family, Am. J. Med. 25:573, 1958.

SECTION THREE: **Some Syndromes Involving Malformations of the Central Nervous System**

37

Syndromes of Chromosomal Abnormalities

Trisomy 13-15 (D_1)

A STRIKING SYNDROME of congenital malformations was described by Thomas Bartholin of Copenhagen in 1657.[1] He reported a monster without eyes, with open and reddish "bregma," a nasal protrusion, absence of nostrils combined with a large and deformed mouth, a single maxillary bone and polydactyly on both hands and on the left foot (Fig. 37-1). This rare but striking combination of congenital defects has been observed many times since; some of the cases may have been included among the arhinencephalies of Kundrat (1882) and the "coupled malformations" of Gruber (1934) (p. 206).

In 1960, Patau *et al.*[2] found an association of this syndrome with trisomy of a large acrocentric chromosome of the D or 13-15 group. In modern language, the syndrome was described as consisting of anophthalmia (or microphthalmia), cleft lip and palate, capillary hemangiomas, cerebral malformations, congenital heart defect, polydactyly, trigger thumbs and simian creases (Fig. 37-2). This disease picture has become

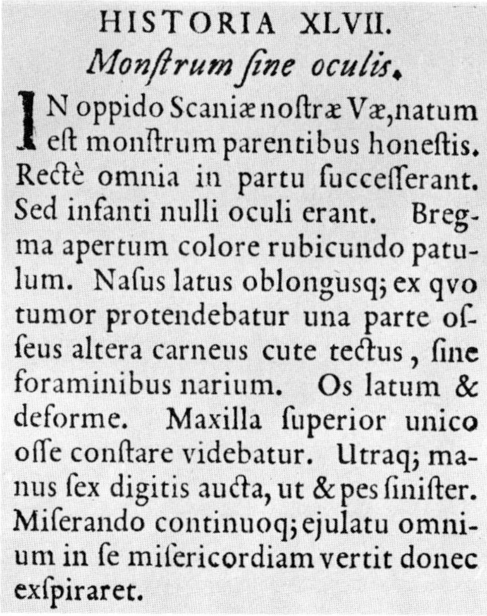
HISTORIA XLVII.
Monſtrum ſine oculis.

IN oppido Scaniæ noſtræ Væ,natum eſt monſtrum parentibus honeſtis. Rectè omnia in partu ſucceſſerant. Sed infanti nulli oculi erant. Bregma apertum colore rubicundo patulum. Naſus latus oblongusq; ex qvo tumor protendebatur una parte oſſeus altera carneus cute tectus, ſine foraminibus narium. Os latum & deforme. Maxilla ſuperior unico oſſe conſtare videbatur. Utraq; manus ſex digitis aucta, ut & pes ſiniſter. Miſerando continuoq; ejulatu omnium in ſe miſericordiam vertit donec exſpiraret.

Fig. 37-1.—Thomas Bartholin's description of a monster without eyes. (From M. Warburg.[1]) Translation:

HISTORY XLVII
Monster without eyes.

In our town Vä in Scania a monster was born of honest parentage. In the parturition everything passed off well. But the child had no eyes. There was a wide, open void of red colour. The nose broad and oblong, from which a tumour protruded, one part bony, the other part fleshy, without nostrils. The mouth wide and deformed. The upper maxilla seemed to consist of one bone. Either hand had six fingers, as had the left foot. By pitiable and continual howling it attracted everybody's compassion until it breathed its last.

firmly established as an entity, but there exist variations in clinical manifestations and cytogenetic findings. The full syndrome and similar but incomplete forms can occur with apparently normal karyotype (p. 298). Conversely, the manifestations of trisomy 13-15 can be limited to microcephaly, iris coloboma, axillary webs and a cleft in the tip of the fifth finger.[3] An incidence of 1 in 14,500 live births has been calculated for the syndrome of trisomy D_1.[4] The incidence of trisomy 21 is approximately 20 times greater and its prevalence much higher than that, since the mortality of trisomy 13-15 is nearly 100% during the first few months of infancy. The maternal age at the birth of children with trisomy D was calculated as 32 years, that of D/D translocation as 24.[4] Magenis *et al.*[45] found a bimodal distribution of maternal ages consistent with age-independent and age-dependent subgroups, the peak of the first being at about 25, that of the second at about 38 years. There seems to be no abnormal sex ratio for the disorder. The birth weight usually corresponds to the gestational age, but intrauterine growth retardation occurred in some cases.[5,6]

In the standard type of trisomy 13-15, the cells contain 47 chromosomes with a supernumerary large, acrocentric (47,XY [or XX], D+) (Fig. 37-3). Cytogenetic variations exist that can result in the standard disease picture. When a D/D translocation occurs with a supernumerary large acrocentric fused to another chromosome of the D group, the cells show in metaphase only 46 chromosomes with absence of one D and a supernumerary large mediocentric in the A group that resembles a chromosome no. 3. The karyotype is thus 46,XY,D−,t(DqDq)+. This translocation type can be sporadic[7,8] or heritable through a father[9] or a mother.[10] A pair of identical twins with trisomy D_1 syndrome and D/D translocation (46,XY,D−,t[DqDq]+) has been reported[46]; the mother and one of her daughters were translocation carriers. In a number of patients, clinical and cytogenetic variants of trisomy 13-15 were encountered. A boy with a partial clinical picture of trisomy 13-15 and 47 chromosomes showed instead of an extra D a smaller acrocentric, interpreted as a deleted chromosome of the D group. The mother, maternal grandfather and a sister were carriers of a balanced reciprocal translocation between two different chromosomes in the D group.[11] A small acrocentric, probably a deleted D chromosome similar to that found in the proband of the family cited above, was seen in a girl with cleft lip and palate, aural and ocular ear anomalies, congenital heart disease, anal atresia and other malformations.[12] In another case of multiple congenital malformations, some of them similar to those of trisomy D_1, there were 46 chromosomes, but one of the D group was enlarged and interpreted as a translocation of a supernumerary chromosomal (D?) fragment to a D chromosome.[12] A girl with iris coloboma on the right, cleft lip and palate, nevus flammeus on the forehead, umbilical hernia and diastasis recti proved to be a chromosomal mosaic. All cells had 46 chromosomes, but in 55% of the mitoses one of the 6 D chromosomes was replaced by a chromosome resembling no. 3 and interpreted as an iso-D. The remainder of the cells appeared to be normal, except for one D chromosome that had no short arms and seemed to be telocentric. It was thought that there was a telocentric D_1 in one cell type and a D_1 isochromosome in the other.[13] In a boy with absence of the patella, various malformations and mental retardation, a mosaicism was found that was interpreted at first as normal/trisomy D. In many cells the presumed D appeared telocentric.[14] But cytogenetic re-examination by autoradiography indicated that the supernumerary chromosome was not a D but rather a portion of an unidentified autosome.[15] A large translocation chromosome interpreted as a translocation D/B was noted in a woman with anophthalmia, bilateral harelip, syndactyly, simian creases and mental retardation.[16] A child with clinical signs of trisomy D had only 46 chromosomes. Two cell lines were found, one normal 46,XY and the other had one chromosome 18 and an extra chromosome believed to be a translocation between an 18 and the terminal portions of the long arms of a D chromosome.[17] In an infant with hypoplastic male external genitalia and malformations resembling those

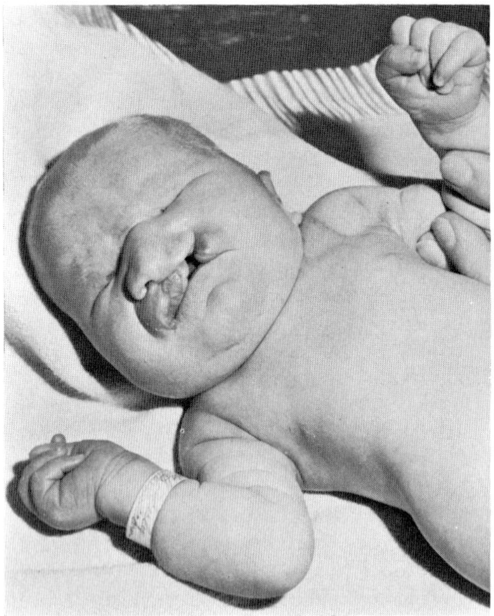
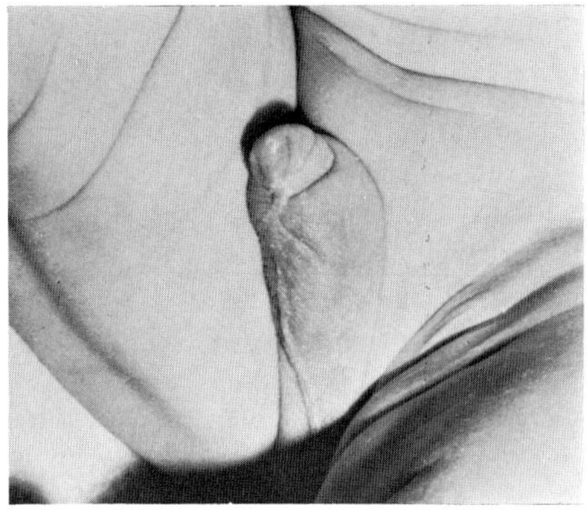

Fig. 37-2. – Child with harelip, cleft palate, microphthalmia, flexed fingers, short scrotum and rocker bottom feet. There also were ear anomalies, a healed scalp defect, abnormal thumbs (but no polydactyly), ventricular and atrial septal defects, with both aorta and pulmonary artery leaving the right ventricle, and malrotation of the bowel.

of trisomy D complicated by a sacral meningocele, rudimentary uterus and absence of gonads, cells with 46 and 47 chromosomes were found. All cells were trisomic for 13-15 but there was XO/XY mosaicism.[18] A puzzling case was reported by Bain and Gauld.[19] A term fetus with marked intrauterine growth retardation had some signs of the trisomy D_1 syndrome such as microphthalmia, arhinencephaly, ventricular septal defect and hypoplastic kidneys. There were reduction malformations of the digits instead of polydactyly. The chromosomal material was reduced and not increased as in trisomy D_1. One chromosome of the 13-15 group was missing and apparently replaced by a ring chromosome.

Double aneuploidy involving a D chromosome was reported by Becker *et al.*[20] in a child with the Down syndrome who had 48 chromosomes. She was considered trisomic for chromosome 21 and for a chromosome of the D group. The D trisomy syndrome was noted in an infant girl who had a sister with XO Turner syndrome.[21]

The central nervous system is severely defective in most of the cases. Warkany *et al.*[22] reviewed reports of 32 necropsies. Table 37-1 shows the most frequent malformations noted. This list gives merely the general type of malformation associated with trisomy 13-15. There are, in some cases, combinations and degrees of various defects that defy classification. The "arhinencephalies" mentioned varied greatly in extent. Some patients showed fused frontal lobes and single ventricles suggestive of the cyclopia series, whereas in others only deficiencies of the olfactory nerves and lobes[29] were mentioned. Cyclopia is the severest malformation characterized by absence of the rhinencephalon, approximation of the cerebral hemispheres, union of ventricles and midline structures (thalami) and defects of the corpus callosum, falx and commissures. The cerebellar anomalies (p. 267) mentioned included abnormal convolutional patterns, dysplasias and hypoplasias, heterotopias of nerve cells into the white matter and other microscopic defects. In 1966, Norman[23] and Terplan *et al.*[24] gave detailed descriptions of the cerebellum in this trisomy (p. 267).

In three cases the brain was considered normal at necropsy[25-27] and in one it was small but otherwise grossly and histologically unremarkable.[28] It is of interest that in these cases the brain appeared normal in the presence of severe malformations of other organs, including the eye.

Although arhinencephaly and related malformations are now considered typical of trisomy 13-15 (D_1), they have been found in children with an apparently normal karyotype (p. 203). A review dealing with central nervous system changes in trisomy 13-15 was published by Neuhäuser and Usener.[29]

A trisomy 13-15 with cebocephaly was reported by Bühler *et al.*[5] The mother was 41 years of age when the child was born with a weight of 2,320 Gm. 2 weeks before term. The frontal, parietal and occipital

TABLE 37-1. – CENTRAL NERVOUS SYSTEM MALFORMATIONS, TRISOMY 13–15 (D_1) (32 NECROPSIES)

Arhinencephalies	25
Cerebellar anomalies	9
Corpus callosum defect	7
Hydrocephaly	4

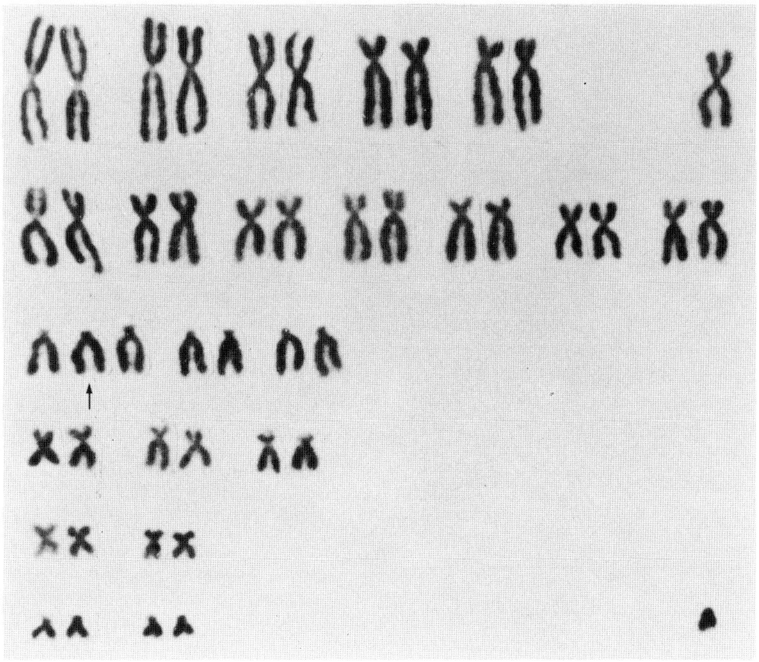

Fig. 37-3.—Karyotype of a child showing 47 chromosomes, of which 7 are large acrocentrics (**arrow**).

lobes appeared fused, the palpebral fissures were narrow, and the right eye was situated near the midline. There was choanal atresia and arhinencephaly with other findings characteristic of trisomy 13-15. Cebocephaly with this trisomy was also described by Conen *et al.*[31]

Ocular defects usually are recognized at birth. Anophthalmia or microphthalmia of variable degree often is combined with coloboma of the iris, cloudy cornea, cataract, retrolental fibroplasia (persistent hyperplastic primary vitreous) and retinal dysplasia. Such anomalies have also been observed in eyes of normal size in children with trisomy 13-15. Histologic examination of microphthalmic eyes shows rudimentary irides, detached retinas with rosettes and disorganization and absence of the retinal ganglion cell layer. The optic nerves are devoid of myelin and nerve fibers. Masses of cartilage surrounded by dense fibrous tissue is a characteristic finding. They are situated behind the lens adjacent to dysplastic retinal tissue and extend through the ciliary body.[32] Intraocular cartilage occurs in microphthalmic eyes of patients with this syndrome but not in eyes of normal size. Detailed analyses of ocular changes have been published.[6,28,33,34] Among 37 cases of trisomy 13-15 reported, Warkany *et al.*[22] found mention of microphthalmia in 13, and in 5 instances anophthalmia was recorded in one eye and microphthalmia in the other. Colobomata were noticed in 17 eyes and cataracts in 8. In a few cases there were no gross malformations of the eyeballs.

Ossification of the cranial bones often is markedly retarded. Cranial defects may be associated with skin defects in the parieto-occipital area. Harelip and cleft palate are rather regular constituents of the syndrome (see Fig. 37-2). Sometimes median clefts with absence of the premaxillary area, the nasal septum and nasal bones[31] cause severe facial malformations, but normal lip and palate sometimes are seen.[32] Among 40 cases of trisomy 13-15 reported by 1966, facial cleft formation was noted in 30. In 10 cases, this manifestation was absent. In 25 cases, there was cleft lip (with or without cleft palate) and in 5 there was isolated cleft palate.[32]

The external ears usually are low set, deformed in various ways (Fig. 37-4) and carry auricular appendages. The external auricular canal may be occluded.[35] Deafness usually is noticeable. Kos *et al.*[36] reported detailed studies of the inner ear in 2 cases.

Congenital heart disease is an integral part of the syndrome, but a normal heart does not exclude trisomy 13-15. A review of 32 necropsy reports[22] showed a variety of cardiovascular malformations (Table 37-2). In 21 cases, combinations of anomalies were listed, most often ventricular septal defect with patent ductus arteriosus, which occurred 10 times (with or without other lesions). There were 2 cases of dextrocardia, 1 of dextroversion and 4 of dextroposition. One dextrocardia was combined with tetralogy of Fallot. Many anomalies were listed only once, and in 6 hearts only a single lesion was encountered. Five hearts appeared anatomically normal.[22]

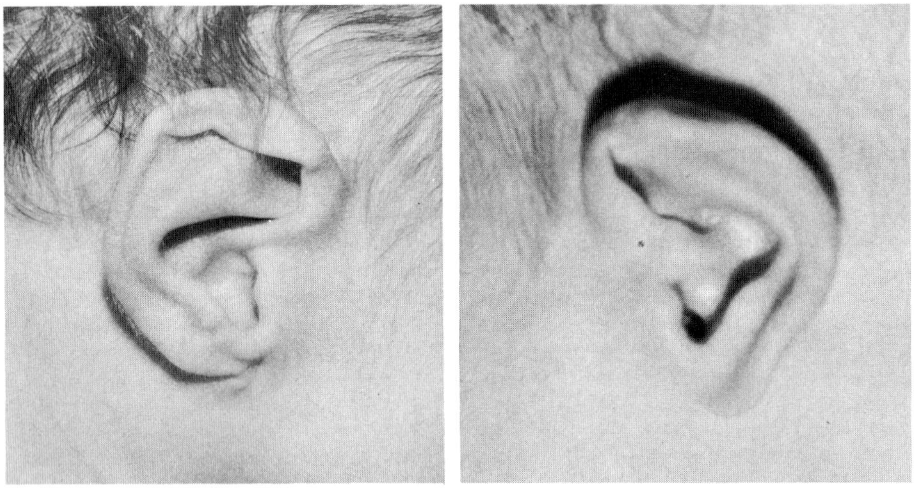

Fig. 37-4.—Aural deformities in 13-15 trisomy.

TABLE 37-2.—CARDIOVASCULAR MALFORMATIONS, TRISOMY 13–15 (D_1) (32 NECROPSIES)

Ventricular septal defect	15	Bicuspid aortic valve	3
Patent ductus arteriosus	12	Transposition of the great vessels	2
Atrial septal defect	8	Truncus arteriosus	2
Dextrocardia/dextroposition	7	Pulmonary atresia	2
Patent foramen ovale	4	Aortic coarctation	2
Pulmonary stenosis	4	Left superior vena cava	2

Reports concerning anomalies of the respiratory system are scanty. A single nostril combined with choanal atresia was reported in a case of cebocephaly with trisomy 13-15. Situs inversus of the lungs with anomalous pulmonary venous return and abnormal lobation of the lungs has been reported.[22] Small foci of cartilage were observed in the lungs by Marin-Padilla *et al.*[37]

Malformations of the intestinal tract are not rare but they are not as conspicuous as other defects that are visible by inspection or audible by auscultation. In a group of 32 necropsies, malformations of the alimentary tract were present in 21. There was malrotation of the colon in 8 cases and unattached mesentery in 5. A mesenteric cyst was present in 1 patient and Meckel diverticulum in 3. There was a high incidence of abnormalities of the spleen; an accessory spleen was present in 9 cases and ectopic splenic tissue within the pancreas in 2. Other anomalies observed only once included hypoplastic bile ducts, abnormal lobation of the liver and true diverticula of the appendix. Umbilical defects, consisting of omphalocele or umbilical hernia, were recorded in 13 of 32 cases. No anomalies of the gastrointestinal tract were found in 10 of 32 necropsies.[22]

Malformations of the urogenital system are found in necropsies in the majority of cases (Table 37-3). Cystic kidneys, including microcysts, are common. Osathanondh and Potter[38] described polycystic kidneys of their type 3 (p. 1045) in a case of trisomy 13-15. Unilateral renal agenesis and stenosis of the prostatic urethra were recorded in 1 infant. A persistent urachus was present in the first case of trisomy 13-15 published by Patau *et al.*[2] in 1960. Interestingly, no horseshoe kidney has been reported, although this is the leading renal malformation in trisomy 18 (p. 307). Cryptorchidism was present in 9 of 16 boys and uterus bicornis in 9 of 16 girls. Uterus duplex and abnormal fallopian tubes were also observed. Partially duplicated labia minora, hypoplastic ovaries and slight abnormalities of the penis and clitoris were mentioned in some cases.

Flexion contractures of the fingers are an outstanding symptom, as in trisomy 18, but polydactyly is characteristic of trisomy 13-15 (Fig. 37-5). Among 40 recorded cases, polydactyly occurred in 28. It is present on both hands and feet or is limited to one extremity or it can be entirely absent. In most of the cases, one or several postaxial extra digits were described. The thumbs often are abnormal, as retroflexion is not possible. All fingers may be in permanent flexion. Syndactyly is observed occasionally. Transverse simian creases on one or both hands are common. Convexity of the soles and protrusion of the heels (rocker bottom feet) are not mentioned as often as in trisomy 18. Fused vertebrae are seen occasionally in roentgenograms.

TABLE 37-3.—UROGENITAL MALFORMATIONS, TRISOMY 13–15 (D_1) (32 NECROPSIES—16 BOYS, 16 GIRLS)

Cystic kidney	10	Double kidney	3
Cryptorchidism	9	Double ureter	3
Uterus bicornis	9	Abnormal fallopian tubes	3

Uchida *et al.*[39] described characteristic dermal ridge patterns. Distal axial triradius, a trait also typical for the Down syndrome, has been observed in most cases of trisomy 13-15. If the mean of the distance of the axial triradius from the wrist crease in per cent of the vertical distance from the wrist crease to the base of the middle finger is 35 or more, one speaks of a "distal mean axial triradius." In the hallucal area, a pattern—an S-shaped modification of a simple arch fibular (A^f)—is considered typical of the syndrome (A^f-S). In one case,[31] all fingers had arch patterns (as in trisomy 18) and there were hallucal whorls.

In 17 of 40 cases of trisomy 13-15 there were hemangiomas on the forehead, upper eyelids, nasal bridge, nape of the neck or lower back. Congenital defects of the scalp (see Fig. 37-5), often involving skull bones, are not rare. Hypoplastic nails have been observed in many cases.

In the peripheral blood of patients with trisomy 13-15 neutrophils with multiple nuclear projections ranging from small sessile nodules to long pedunculated excrescences can be seen[40,41] (Fig. 37-6). Congenital leukemia in an infant was reported by Schade *et al.*[27]

Huehns *et al.*[42] found that trisomy 13-15 affects hemoglobin synthesis in several ways. Both increased Hb F and Hb Gower-2 could be demonstrated in neonates with trisomy 13-15. Older children still had slightly elevated amounts of Hb F. But the Hb A_2 concentration was found to be decreased. The hemoglobin and leukocyte changes have been explained as a maturational retardation in trisomy 13-15.[43,44]

Histopathologic studies were made of several cases of trisomy 13-15 by Marin-Padilla *et al.*[37] and by Mottet and Jensen.[26]

Soon after birth, attacks of apnea and cyanosis occur; resuscitation may revive the child, but the at-

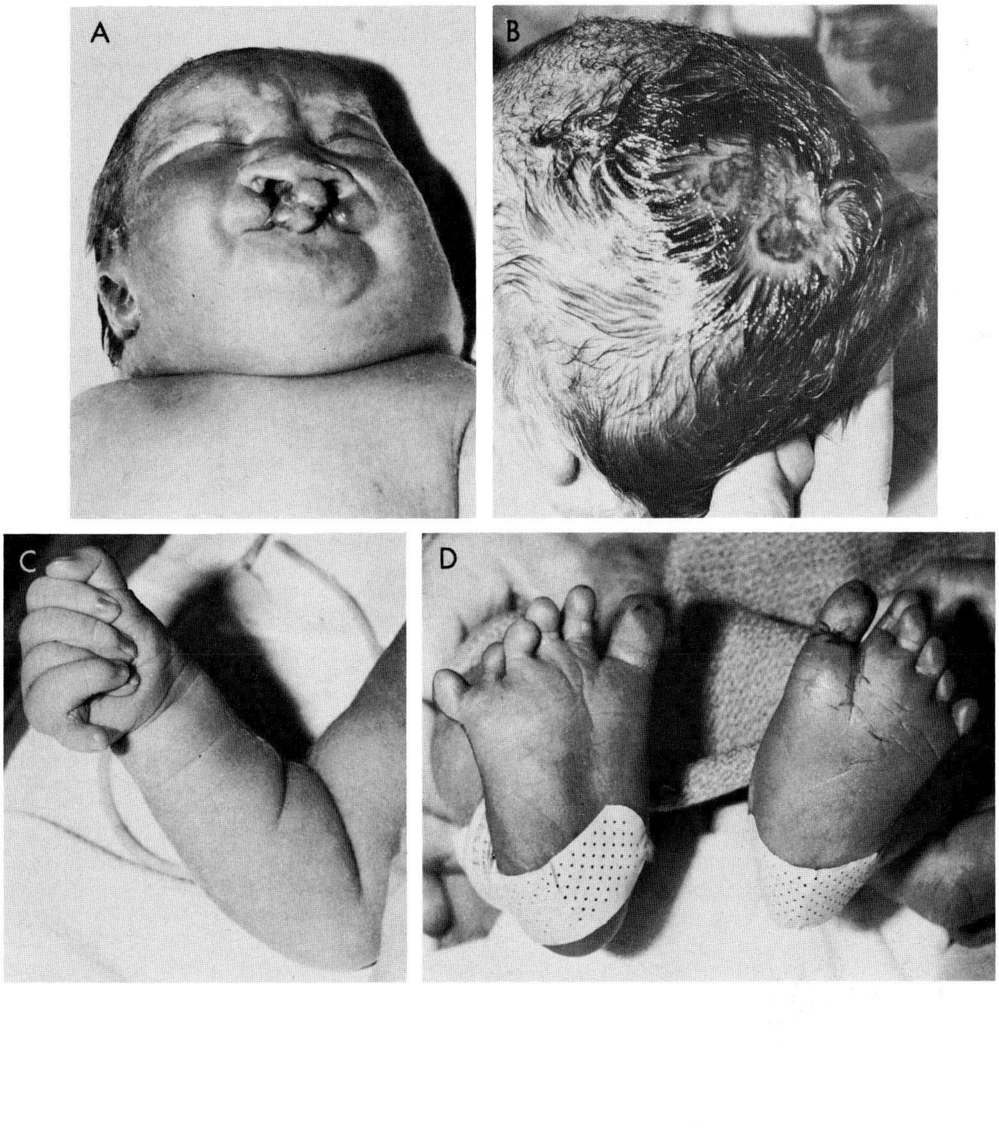

Fig. 37-5.—**A,** double harelip and cleft palate, microphthalmia. **B,** scalp defects. **C,** typical hand with flexion of fingers, polydactyly and hypoplastic nails. **D,** feet showing polydactyly.

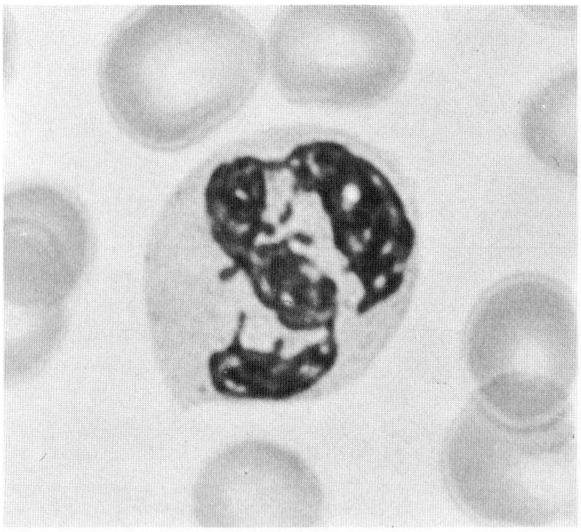

Fig. 37-6.—Leukocyte with multiple nuclear projections.

tacks recur. Convulsions are common. Life expectancy of children with the trisomy 13-15 syndrome is short. Most of the patients die within hours, weeks or months after birth, but Therman *et al.*[21] reported a patient 2 years of age. In a group of more than 200 patients with trisomy 13-15, 44% were dead by 1 month of age, 73% by 4 months and 86% by 1 year.[45]

REFERENCES

1. Warburg, M.: Anophthalmos complicated by mental retardation and cleft palate, Acta ophth. 38:394, 1960.
2. Patau, K., Smith, D. W., Therman, E., Inhorn, S. L., and Wagner, H. P.: Multiple congenital anomaly caused by an extra autosome, Lancet 1:790, 1960.
3. Hecht, F.: Phenotypic differentiation of autosomal chromosomal abnormalities. Anomalies on the gross, radiologic, autopsy, cellular, and molecular levels in the D_1 (13-15) trisomy syndrome, Alabama J. M. Sc. 3:489, 1966.
4. Conen, P. E., and Erkman, B.: Frequency and occurrence of chromosomal syndromes. I. D-trisomy, Am. J. Human Genet. 18:374, 1966.
5. Bühler, E., Bodis, I., Rossier, R., and Stalder, G.: Trisomie 13-15 mit Cebocephalie, Ann. paediat. 199:198, 1962.
6. Cogan, D. G., and Kuwabara, T.: Ocular pathology of the 13-15 trisomy syndrome, Arch. Ophth. 72:246, 1964.
7. Jongbloet, P., van Winckel, H., Adriaenssens, K., and Hooft, C.: Sporadic trisomy D_1 with translocation D/D, Helvet. paediat. acta 19:121, 1964.
8. Tolksdorf, M., Wiedemann, H-R., Hansen, H-G., and Lehmann, W.: Pätau-Syndrom mit Trisomie D_1 und D/D-Translokation, Med. Welt 41:2304, 1965.
9. Dill, F. J., and Miller, J. R.: D trisomy with a translocation, Human Chromosome Newsletter No. 9:10, 1963.
10. Oikawa, K., Gromults, J. M., Hirschhorn, K., and Novins, J.: 13-15 trisomy with translocation, Human Chromosome Newsletter No. 7:11, 1962. (References 9 and 10 cited by Turpin, R., and Lejeune, J.: Les chromosomes humains, 1965.)
11. Jacobsen, P., Dupont, A., and Mikkelsen, M.: Translocation in the 13-15 group as a cause of partial trisomy and spontaneous abortion in the same family, Lancet 2:584, 1963.
12. Zellweger, H., Mikamo, K., and Abbo, G.: Two cases of multiple malformations with an autosomal chromosomal aberration—partial trisomy D?, Helvet. paediat. acta 17:290, 1962.
13. Therman, E., Patau, K., DeMars, R. I., Smith, D. W., and Inhorn, S. L.: Iso/telo-D mosaicism in a child with an incomplete D_1 trisomy syndrome, Portugal acta biol. 7:211, 1963.
14. Warkany, J., Rubinstein, J. H., Soukup, S. W., and Curless, M. C.: Mental retardation, absence of patellae and other malformations with chromosomal mosaicism, J. Pediat. 61:803, 1962.
15. Nakagome, Y., Warkany, J., and Rubinstein, J. H.: Mental retardation, absence of patellae, and other malformations with chromosomal mosaicism, J. Pediat. 72:695, 1968.
16. Wallace, C., and Anderson, I. F.: A large translocation chromosome in a mentally defective female patient with multiple congenital abnormalities, Human Chromosome Newsletter No. 10:16, 1963.
17. Craig, A. P., and Luzzatti, L.: Translocation in trisomy D syndrome. A case of a probable D/18 translocation, J. Pediat. 70:264, 1967.
18. France, N. E., Evison, P. G. H., Butler, L. J., Snodgrass, G. J. A. I., Crome, L., and Keith, C. G.: Trisomy D_1 (13-15) associated with XO/XY mosaicism, J. M. Genetics 4:134, 1967.
19. Bain, A. D., and Gauld, I. K.: Multiple congenital abnormalities associated with ring chromosome, Lancet 2:304, 1963.
20. Becker, K. L., Burke, E. C., and Albert, A.: Double autosomal trisomy (D trisomy plus mongolism), Proc. Staff Meet. Mayo Clin. 38:242, 1963.
21. Therman, E., Patau, K., Smith, D. W., and DeMars, R. I.: The D trisomy syndrome and XO gonadal dysgenesis in two sisters, Am. J. Human Genet. 13:193, 1961.
22. Warkany, J., Passarge, E., and Smith, L. B.: Congenital malformations in autosomal trisomy syndromes, Am. J. Dis. Child. 112:502, 1966.
23. Norman, R. M.: Neuropathological findings in trisomies 13-15 and 17-18 with special reference to the cerebellum, Developmental Med. & Child Neurol. 8:170, 1966.
24. Terplan, K. L., Sandberg, A. A., and Aceto, T., Jr.: Structural anomalies in the cerebellum in association with trisomy, J.A.M.A. 197:557, 1966.
25. Blanck, C., Jalling, B., Lindsten, J., and Zetterqvist, P.: Trisomy 13-15, Acta path. et microbiol. scandinav. 60:36, 1964.
26. Mottet, N. K., and Jensen, H.: The anomalous embryonic development associated with trisomy 13-15, Am. J. Clin. Path. 43:334, 1965.
27. Schade, H., Schoeller, L., and Schultze, K. W.: D-Trisomie (Pätau-syndrom) mit kongenitaler myeloischer Leukämie, Med. Welt 50:2690, 1962.
28. Sergovich, F., Madronich, J. S., Barr, M. L., Carr, D. H., and Langdon, W. A.: The D trisomy syndrome: A case report with a description of ocular pathology, Canad. M.A.J. 89:151, 1963.
29. Neuhäuser, G., and Usener, M.: Hirnmissbildung und autosomale Trisomie, Ztschr. Kinderh. 95:244, 1966.
30. Passarge, E., True, C. W., Sueoka, W. T., Baumgartner, N. R., and Keer, K. R.: Malformations of the central nervous system in trisomy 18 syndrome, J. Pediat. 69:771, 1966.
31. Conen, P. E., Erkman, B., and Metaxotou, C.: The "D" syndrome. Report of four trisomic and one D/D translocation case, Am. J. Dis. Child. 111:236, 1966.
32. Atkins, L., and Rosenthal, M. K.: Multiple congenital abnormalities associated with chromosomal trisomy, New England J. Med. 265:314, 1961.
33. Ginsberg, J., and Perrin, E. V. D.: Ocular manifestations of 13-15 trisomy, Arch. Ophth. 74:487, 1965.
34. Roch, L. M., II, Petrucci, J. V., and Barber, A. N.: Studies on the development of the eye in the 13-15 trisomy syndrome, Am. J. Ophth. 60:1067, 1965.
35. Conen, P. E., Phillips, K. G., and Mauntner, L. S.: Multiple developmental anomalies and trisomy of a 13-15 group chromosome ('D' syndrome), Canad. M.A.J. 87:709, 1962.

36. Kos, A. O., Schuknecht, H. F., and Singer, J. D.: Temporal bone studies in 13-15 and 18 trisomy syndromes, Arch. Otolaryng. 83:439, 1966.
37. Marin-Padilla, M., Hoefnagel, D., and Benirschke, K.: Anatomic and histopathologic study of two cases of D_1 (13-15) trisomy, Cytogenetics 3:258, 1964.
38. Osathanondh, V., and Potter, E. L.: Pathogenesis of polycystic kidneys; historical survey, Arch. Path. 77:459, 1964.
39. Uchida, I. A., Patau, K., and Smith, D. W.: The dermal patterns of the new autosomal trisomy syndromes, Am. J. Dis. Child. 102:588, 1961.
40. Powars, D., Rohde, R., and Graves, D.: Foetal haemoglobins and neutrophil anomaly in the D_1 trisomy syndrome, Lancet 1:1363, 1964.
41. Hecht, F., Huehns, E. R., and Lutzner, M.: Nuclear abnormalities of neutrophils in D_1 trisomy syndrome, J. Pediat. 65:1089, 1964.
42. Huehns, E. R., Hecht, F., Keil, J. V., and Motulsky, A. G.: Developmental hemoglobin anomalies in a chromosomal triplication: D_1 trisomy syndrome, Proc. Nat. Acad. Sc. 51:89, 1964.
43. Walzer, S., Park, S. G., Breau, G., O'Neill, D., and Diamond, L. K.: Hematologic changes in the D_1 trisomy syndrome, Pediatrics 38:419, 1966.
44. Lee, C. S. N., Boyer, S. H., Bowen, P., Weatherall, D. J., Rosenblum, H., Clark, D. B., Duke, J. R., Liboro, C., Bias, W., and Borgaonkar, D. S.: The D_1 trisomy syndrome: Three subjects with unequally advancing development, Bull. Johns Hopkins Hosp. 118:374, 1966.
45. Magenis, R. E., Hecht, F., and Milham, S., Jr.: Trisomy 13 (D_1) syndrome: Studies on parental age, sex ratio, and survival, J. Pediat. 73:222, 1968.
46. Yu, F-C., Gutman, L. T., Huang, S-W., Fresh, J. W., and Emanuel, I.: Trisomy 13 syndrome in Chinese infants, J. M. Genetics 7:132, 1970.

Deficiency of the Long Arm of a Chromosome D

In 1969, twenty-three cases with the karyotype 46,Dq− or 46,Dr were available for clinical analysis. Allderdice *et al.*[1] described a chromosome deletion syndrome caused by partial monosomy for a distal segment of the long arm of chromosome 13. Mental retardation, microcephaly, trigonocephaly, micrognathia, large malformed ears, hypertelorism, prominent nasal bridge, microphthalmia and ptosis were observed repeatedly. Facial asymmetry was noticeable in several patients. Protruding teeth and lateral neck folds were described in some of the cases. Variations of ocular and genital changes occur. Retinoblastoma was observed in 4 cases; it was attributed to deletion of chromosome 14.[2] In one of these cases there were no associated malformations,[3] and in another the child had an attractive appearance but cleft palate and transverse palmar creases.[2] Aplasia or hypoplasia of the thumb has been emphasized.[4] Congenital heart disease and imperforate anus were present in several cases.[1] Monosomy for a distal segment of a D chromosome, whether seen as Dq− or as a ring, was held responsible for the syndrome,[1] but it remains to be seen whether chromosome 13 or 14 is affected.[1,2]

REFERENCES

1. Allderdice, P. W., Davis, J. G., Miller, O. J., Klinger, H. P., Warburton, D., Miller, D. A., Allen, F. H., Jr., Abrams, C. A. L., and McGilvray, E.: The 13− deletion syndrome, Am. J. Human Genet. 21:499, 1969.
2. Wilson, M. G., Melnyk, J., and Towner, J. W.: Retinoblastoma and deletion D (14) syndrome, J. M. Genetics 6:322, 1969.
3. Lele, K. P., Penrose, L. S., and Stallard, H. B.: Chromosome deletion in a case of retinoblastoma, Ann. Human Genet. 27:174, 1963.
4. Sparkes, R. S., Carrel, R. E., and Wright, S. W.: Absent thumbs with a ring D_2 chromosome. A new deletion syndrome, Am. J. Human Genet. 19:644, 1967.

Trisomy 18

In 1960, Edwards *et al.*[1] described a trisomy syndrome, identifying the extra chromosome as a no. 17; it is now generally believed that the extra chromosome corresponds to no. 18 (Denver classification) (Fig. 37-7). The child's head was long and narrow, the metopic suture open and the ears low-set, with their long axis running downward and forward. There was an abnormally great distance between the crus anthelicis and the helix margin, giving the ear "a pixie look." The mouth was small and the chin receding. The chest was shield-like, with nipples almost in the anterior axillary line. The fingers were tightly clenched but could be straightened. Mental development was retarded.

The association of this syndrome with trisomy 18 was soon confirmed by Smith *et al.*[2] By 1964, more than 100 cases could be evaluated in an incomplete review.[3] In the Cincinnati Children's Hospital alone, 10 cases had been observed by 1964, all of them diagnosed clinically and confirmed cytogenetically. It is remarkable that this syndrome apparently was not recognized as a clinical syndrome until it was identified as a cytogenetic entity, except for a single case described in 1956 by Emed[4] as a "pterygium syndrome." Conen and Erkman[5] calculated for trisomy 18 an incidence of 1 in 4,500 live births.

Life expectancy is short. The survival period for females seems to be, on the average, 7 months, whereas that of males is only 2 months.[5] The chance of survival to 1 month is 70%, to 1 year, 10% and to 10 years, 1%. Weber[6] studied survival rates and found that males have a greater fatality rate than females,

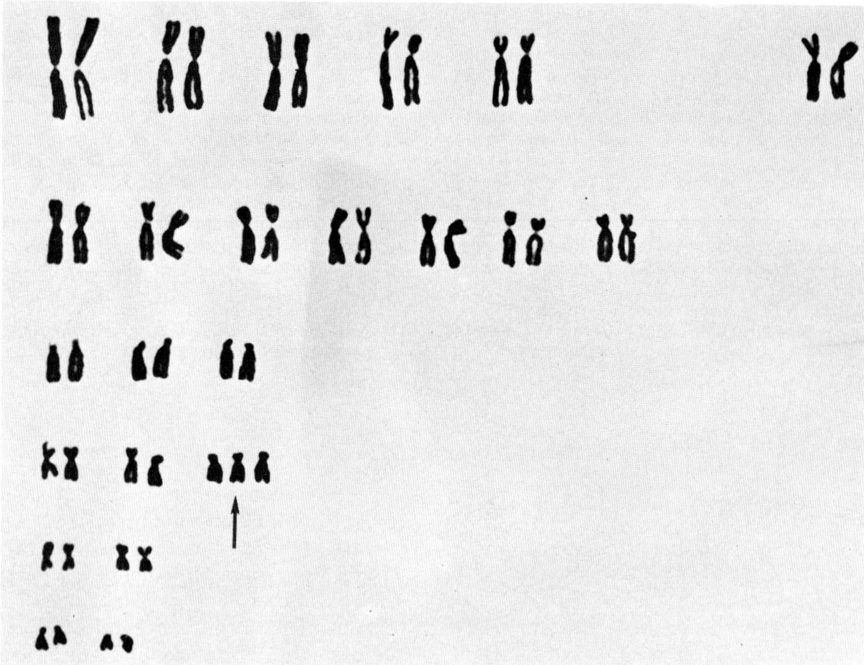

Fig. 37-7.—Karyotype showing trisomy 18 (**arrow**) (cell from skin tissue culture begun post mortem).

especially during the first few weeks of life. The sex ratio decreases from a value of 0.55 at 14 days to 0.35 at 3 months after birth, without changing much afterward. The difference in mortality may account for the excess of published cases of females with trisomy 18. Weber *et al.*[3] and Ozonoff *et al.*[7] reported girls more than 10 years of age with this disorder. We observed a girl with normal/trisomy 18 mosaicism who died at age 12 years.[8]

Soon after the discovery of trisomy 18, it was recognized that the malformations associated with it show a wide spectrum; it was also recognized that cytogenetic pictures involving chromosome 18 can vary. A fragment of chromosome 18 can be translocated to a chromosome of the 13-15 group, resulting in a rather typical disease picture of trisomy 18 even though the modal count is 46. Such a translocation can be sporadic, arising de novo,[9] or be transmitted by a parent.[10] In sisters with mental retardation and some signs of the trisomy 18 syndrome, a supernumerary chromosome was interpreted as a no. 18 with partial deletion of the long arms.[11] A possible partial trisomy 18 was also assumed for a brother and sister with mental retardation, epicanthus, low-set ears and marked hypotonia.[12] In this case, the mother had a possible D/E translocation. Partial trisomy 18 by insertion or translocation B/E was considered for a girl with signs of the trisomy 18 syndrome.[13] Miller *et al.*[14] observed an infant with many signs of trisomy 18 who had a modal count of 47 with an additional unidentified chromosome that could be considered a long arm isochromosome.

Deficiencies of parts of trisomy 18 result in mental retardation and in a variety of somatic anomalies.[15,20]

There has been at least one case report of a trisomy 18 syndrome in a female infant who showed no abnormalities of the karyotype in cells from blood, bone marrow and skin.[21]

Normal/trisomy 18 mosaicism has been observed repeatedly. Weiss *et al.*,[22] Wolf *et al.*[23] and Koulischer *et al.*[24] described disease pictures rather typical of trisomy 18. The girl reported by us[8] with such mosaicism had only a few of the typical signs but was severely retarded in motor and mental development. A familial normal/trisomy 18 mosaicism was reported by Huggert.[25] Corneal opacity, cardiac defects and skeletal anomalies were present in 3 patients, but the disease picture varied in some respects from typical trisomy 18. Trisomy 18/trisomy 21 mosaicism was recorded by Marks *et al.*[26] Since the patient had typical Down syndrome without any signs of trisomy 18, it is doubtful that the medium-sized acrocentric was an 18 chromosome. It is more likely that a large Y chromosome was present in some of the cells, as in a case with mongolism reported by us.[8]

Multiple aneuploidy involving chromosome 18 has been observed repeatedly. Trisomy 18 with triple X in infants with 48 chromosomes resembles, phenotypically, the trisomy 18 syndrome.[27-29] Trisomy 18 with Klinefelter syndrome[30] and Down syndrome with trisomy 18[31] have been recorded. In at least two families the birth of a child with Down syndrome was followed by one with trisomy 18.[32,33]

Preconceptional parental irradiation as a possible etiologic factor in trisomy 18 was considered by Townes *et al.*[34]

Clinical and Pathologic Characteristics

Infants with the trisomy 18 syndrome usually suffer growth retardation in utero. At birth, most of them are small and underweight for their gestational age. The placenta is small and a single umbilical artery may be present. In some pregnancies, the mothers did not show increased girth, in others hydramnios was present.[34-37] Although intrauterine growth retardation occurs occasionally in trisomy 21 and in trisomy 13-15, it is most characteristic for trisomy 18.[8] The average birth weight of 90 cases analyzed was 2,180 Gm., although 70% of the infants were born at or after 38 weeks' gestation. The mean maternal age is advanced. In 36 cases of trisomy 18 it was 34.3 years as compared with 26.4 years for the general population. Advanced maternal age can be responsible for recurrence of differing chromosomal disturbances in the same family.[32,33] In one instance, a young mother had two children with possible trisomy 18 but only one of these was definitely identified cytogenetically.[38]

Immediately after birth, infants with trisomy 18 appear "undernourished" because of their low weight and loose skin (Fig. 37-8). At first, they are limp, but soon become hypertonic. The face often appears triangular because of a relatively large cranium and a small, receding chin. The skull, which is long and narrow, regularly shows an occipital prominence. The sutures are wide.

Gross malformations of the central nervous system are less common in trisomy 18 than in trisomy 13-15, but the brain cannot be considered normal. The few children with the trisomy 18 syndrome who survived the first year were mentally retarded. In 84 necropsies, abnormal gyri, cerebellar anomalies and myelomeningoceles were noted 5 times, hydrocephaly 4 times, corpus callosum defect 3 times and occipital lobe defect twice. In addition, there were single cases of encephalocele, arhinencephaly and cyst of the cisterna magna. Smallness of the brain was mentioned in many reports. In more than 50 necropsies, the central nervous system showed no major malformations or was not mentioned. Microscopic anomalies consisted mainly of heterotopic ganglion cells in the cerebrum and abnormal stratification of the cerebellum. The situation is comparable to a certain extent with that in Down syndrome, in which gross malformations of the central nervous system are rare, yet alterations of the brain are always revealed by mental retardation of the patients who survive infancy. Reviews of the central nervous system changes in trisomy 18 are available.[39-41]

Ocular changes are less spectacular in trisomy 18 than in trisomy 13-15. Occasionally, colobomas, cloudy corneas or microphthalmia are recorded. Minor anomalies were mentioned in 30 of 84 necropsies.[41]

The external ears are low-set and their malformations are manifold. The helix often is rolled out or pointed in its upper posterior portion ("pixie-like"). In general, the ears can be distinguished from those of trisomy 21 but not from those of trisomy 13-15 (see Fig. 37-4). The auditory canal was occluded in several patients[35,40,42]; aplasia of the inner ear was mentioned by Wolf *et al.*[23] and studied in detail by Kos *et al.*[43] Atresia of the middle ear was noted in some patients with an 18 ring chromosome.

The mouth is small and the upper lip short. A high palate is the rule; cleft palate (Fig. 37-9) or cleft lip occur in about 15% of the cases. The cleft lip/cleft palate complex is more common than cleft palate alone.[41] Micrognathia is noted regularly (Fig. 37-10).

The neck is thin and its skin loose, sometimes giving it a webbed appearance. The chest is shield-like and short; the nipples are far apart and located near the anterior axillary line. A short sternum, characteristic for trisomy 18, contains a reduced number of ossification centers; the ribs are thin. Deformities of

Fig. 37-8.—Trisomy 18. Note loose skin, short thorax, flexed fingers and rocker bottom feet.

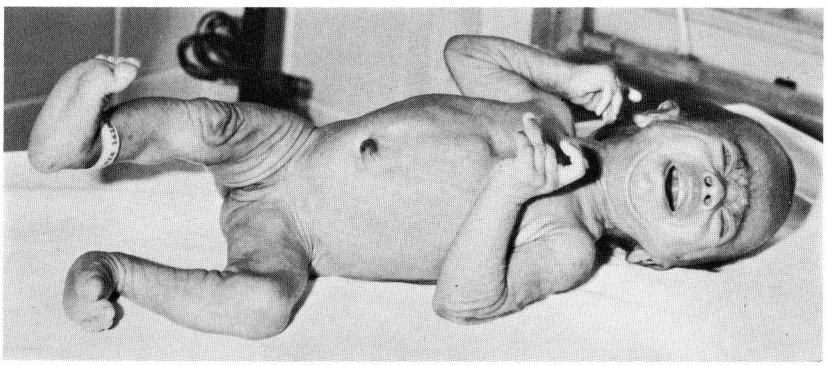

Fig. 37-9.—Trisomy 18 in a girl 5 years of age. There is a posterior palate cleft and the ears are characteristically pointed.

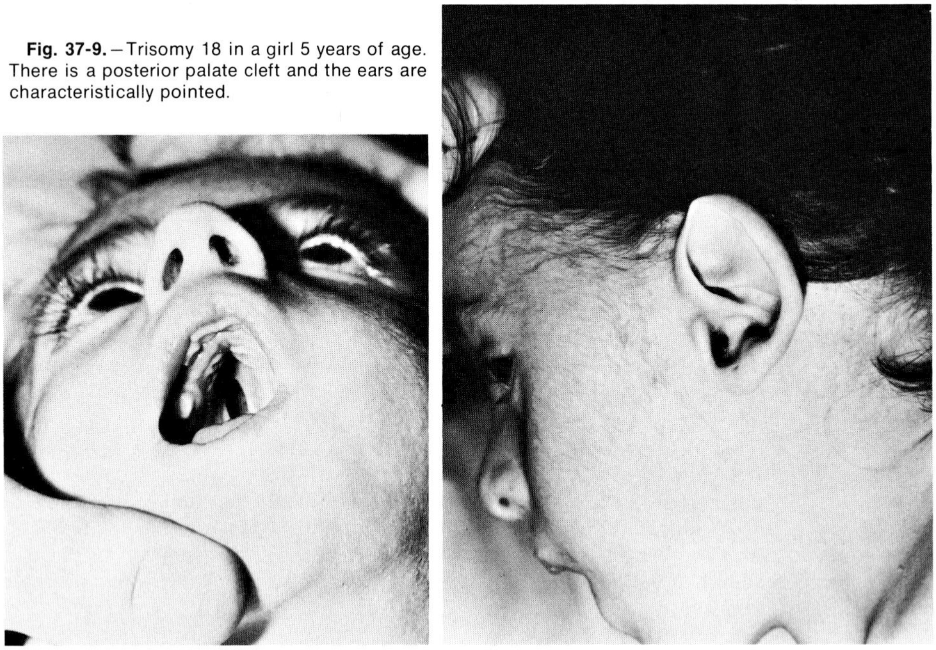

the spinal column occur. Smallness of the thymus was mentioned repeatedly. Short trachea,[44] tracheo-esophageal fistula[38] and cystic lungs[45] have been observed occasionally, but congenital heart disease is the rule. A review of 84 necropsies of children with trisomy 18 revealed that 83 had some type of congenital heart disease. Table 37-4 lists the defects noted more than once.

Ventricular septal defect and patent ductus arteriosus were leading malformations, as in trisomy 13-15 (D_1), but atrial septal defect was comparatively rare. Truncus arteriosus, right-sided aortic arch and abnormal origin of the left carotid artery were mentioned only once. In 15 hearts, a single lesion only was found; 10 of these were ventricular septal defects, whereas patent ductus arteriosus, bicuspid pulmonary valve, small left heart, hypertrophy of the interventricular septum and subendocardial fibroelastosis appeared once. In 68 cases, combined anomalies were described—ventricular septal defect with patent ductus arteriosus 12 times and ventricular septal defect and patent ductus arteriosus combined with various other lesions 28 times. Rogers *et al.*[46] stressed origin of both great vessels from the right ventricle as a characteristic lesion of the trisomy 18 syndrome.

TABLE 37-4.—Cardiovascular Malformations, Trisomy 18 (84 Necropsies)*

Ventricular septal defect	62	Coarctation of aorta	6
Patent ductus arteriosus	47	Aorta from right ventricle	5
Patent foramen ovale	19	Hypoplastic left ventricle	4
Pulmonic stenosis/ bicuspid valve	18	Abnormal coronary artery	3
Bicuspid aortic valve	15	Left superior vena cava	3
Overriding aorta	11	Transposition of great vessels	2
Atrial septal defect	9	Dextrocardia	2
Abnormal mitral valve	8	Hypoplastic left atrium	2

*From Warkany, J., *et al.*[41]

Fig. 37-10.—Trisomy 18. Note low-set ears and elongated occiput. The auricles are standing off and the helix is flattened. Micrognathia and flexed fingers are shown.

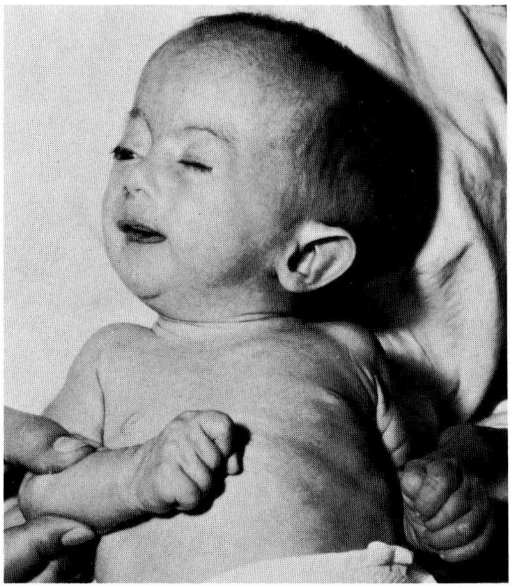

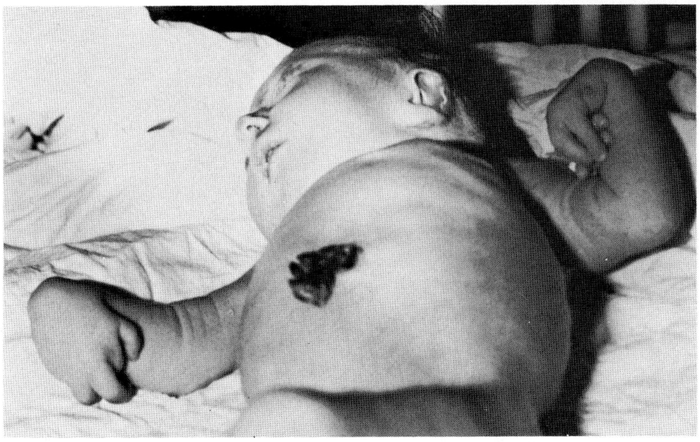

Fig. 37-11.—Clubhands in a child with trisomy 18.

TABLE 37-5.—Gastrointestinal Malformations, Trisomy 18 (84 Necropsies)*

Meckel diverticulum	19	Tracheo-esophageal fistula with or without esophageal atresia	3
Malrotation	13	Biliary atresia	2
Accessory spleen	6	Imperforate anus	2
Abnormal lobation of liver	5	Bile duct stenosis	2
Ectopic pancreas	4	Pyloric stenosis	2
Hypoplastic gallbladder	3		

*From Warkany, J., *et al.*[41]

The respiratory tract can be impaired by choanal stenosis or atresia,[34,37] shortness of the trachea[44] or tracheo-esophageal fistula.[23,38,47,48] Agenesis of one lung was noted once[49] and abnormal lobation several times. Muscular defects of the diaphragm with eventration of the diaphragm were present in approximately 20% of the cases.

The gastrointestinal system is affected by various anomalies in approximately 75% of the cases. The most common ones are listed in Table 37-5.

Supra-umbilical diastasis recti and inguinal hernias occur. Omphaloceles were present in some of the cases.[50,51] Malrotation should be thought of when intestinal symptoms appear.

Urogenital anomalies recorded in 84 necropsies are listed in Table 37-6.

The high incidence of horseshoe kidney is noteworthy (Fig. 37-12). Bladder diverticula[38] and urethral anomalies occur. Enlargement of the clitoris and urethrovaginal fistula have been recorded.[35] The general frequency of urogenital malformations in the syndrome is approximately 70%. Severe renal deformities are more often found in trisomy 18 than in the other autosomal trisomies. In patients with trisomy 18 and XXX aneuploidy (p. 1140), the external genitalia are normal female but the ovaries are histologically abnormal. A tendency to Wilms tumor has been suggested, and survival in a boy to 11½ years after removal of a tumor at 2 years of age has been reported.[56]

Variations in the size and position of the pituitary

TABLE 37-6.—Urogenital Malformations, Trisomy 18 (84 Necropsies)*

Horseshoe kidney	18	Unilateral absence or hypoplastic kidney	6
Double ureter	14	Ectopic kidney	3
Cystic kidney	9	Uterus bicornis	3
Double kidney	8	Uterus bicollis	2
Hypoplastic ovaries	7	Cryptorchidism	2

*From Warkany, J., *et al.*[41]

Fig. 37-12.—Horseshoe kidney in trisomy 18.

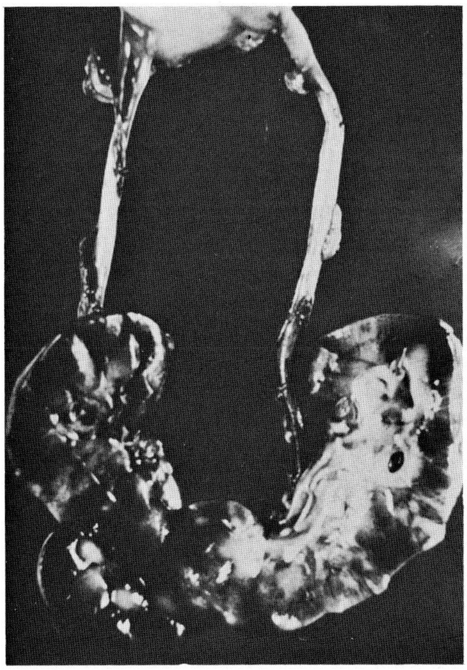

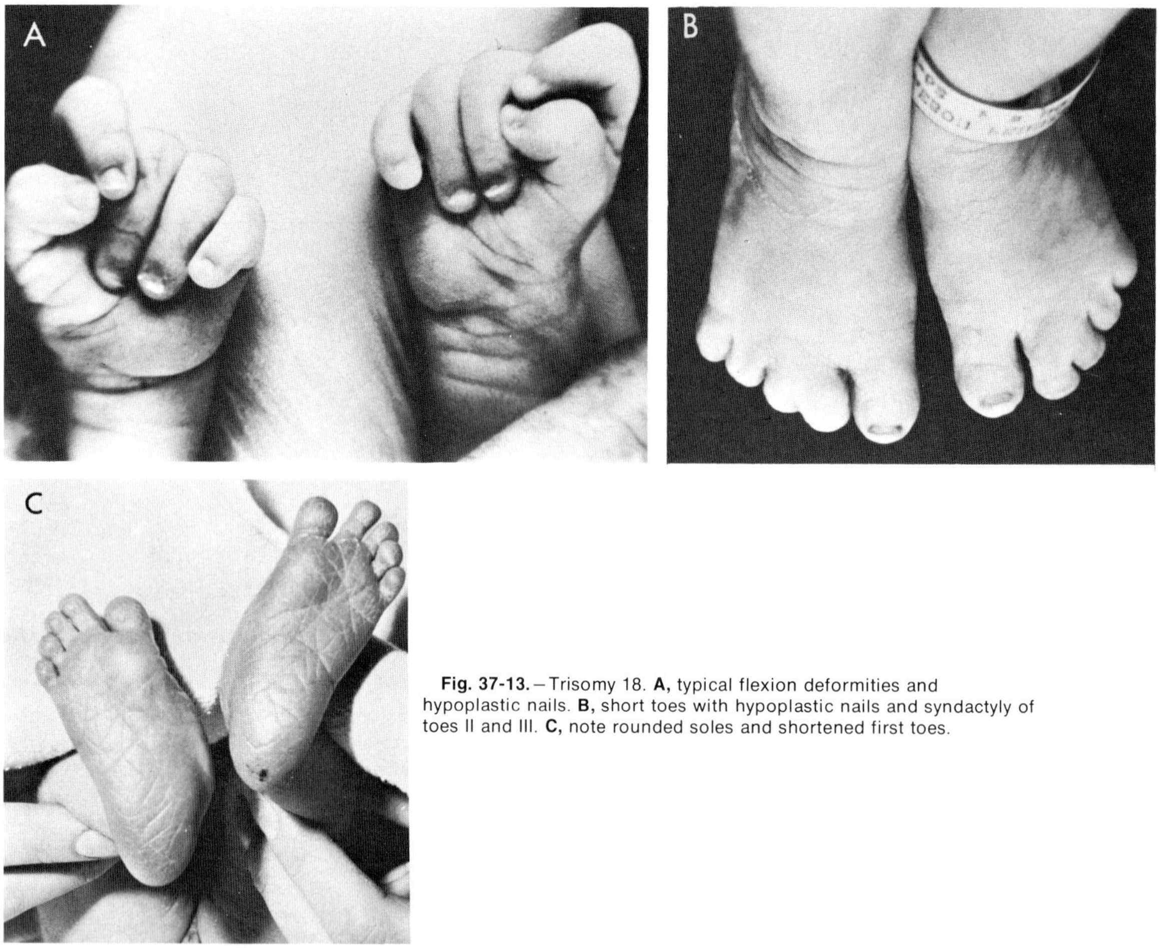

Fig. 37-13.—Trisomy 18. **A,** typical flexion deformities and hypoplastic nails. **B,** short toes with hypoplastic nails and syndactyly of toes II and III. **C,** note rounded soles and shortened first toes.

sometimes were mentioned and in one case absence of the parathyroids was noted.[3]

The appearance of the hands is characteristic for the D and E trisomies. There often is radial or ulnar deviation, but flexion of the fingers is a more typical feature (see Figs. 37-5, *C* and 37-10). The index finger often overlaps the third, and the fifth finger overlaps the fourth. The nails are hypoplastic (see Fig. 37-5). A single palmar crease and a single crease on the fifth finger are typical signs. The pelvis is small and abduction is limited in the hip joints. The feet are characterized by protruding heels and rounded soles (rocker bottom feet) (see Fig. 37-8). Clubfeet have been seen in several cases. Shortness of the dorsiflexed first toe and syndactyly of toes II and III—or IV and V—are seen frequently (Fig. 37-13, *B*). Ossification of the bones usually is retarded and joint movements are limited. Muscular hypertonicity develops and the tendon reflexes appear increased.

The large array of skeletal malformations noted in 115 recorded cases is shown in Table 37-7.

TABLE 37-7.—Skeletal Malformations, Trisomy 18 (115 Cases)*

Flexion contractions	89	Talipes equinovarus	18
Short or abnormal sternum	52	Abnormal nails	15
Limited hip abduction	30	Ulnar deviation	14
Rocker bottom feet	29	Hyperextensible joints	13
Syndactyly	25	Hypoplastic thumbs	5
Hammer toe	22	Hypoplastic clavicles	3
Hypoplastic toes	22	Phocomelia	2
Small pelvis	20		

*From Warkany, J., *et al.*[41]

The malformations vary from minor deviations to severe reduction malformations recorded as phocomelia[52] or amputation.[53] Trisomy 18 with a disease picture of malformed radii, esophageal atresia and congenital hypoplastic thrombocytopenia was reported by Rabinowitz *et al.*[48] Median cleft of the feet, resembling lobster claws, can occur.[42] Klippel-Feil syndrome[7] and changes of the clavicle have been observed. Roentgen signs of the syndrome were summarized by Moseley *et al.*[54] Congenital asymmetry associated with trisomy 18 mosaicism has been reported.[57]

The dermal pattern of trisomy 18 was described by Uchida *et al.*[55] and Penrose.[58] Presence of arches on all or nearly all of the digits is characteristic of trisomy 18. Patients with this syndrome often have short fingers with only one crease. They resemble mongoloids in this respect but differentiation of the patterns is not difficult, since trisomics 18 have mostly arches and mongoloids mostly ulnar loops on the fingers.

Soon after birth, infants show episodes of dyspnea, apnea and cyanosis. Food intake and weight gain are poor, and death ensues a few months after birth. Few children live longer than 1 year, but unusual cases have been described involving patients 10 years of age.[7] Severe mental and physical retardation, flexion deformities and hypertonia of the lower extremities were present. A similar severe disease picture was reported by us[8] in a girl with normal/trisomy 18 mosaicism.

REFERENCES

1. Edwards, J. H., Harnden, D. G., Cameron, A. H., Crosse, V. M., and Wolff, O. H.: A new trisomic syndrome, Lancet 1:787, 1960.
2. Smith, D. W., Patau, K., Therman, E., and Inhorn, S. L.: A new autosomal trisomy syndrome: Multiple congenital anomalies caused by an extra chromosome, J. Pediat. 57: 338, 1960.
3. Weber, W. W., Manunes, P., Day, R., and Miller, P.: Trisomy 17-18 (E): Studies in long-term survival with report of two autopsied cases, Pediatrics 34:533, 1964.
4. Emed, A.: Pterygium syndrome, J. Pediat. 48:73, 1956.
5. Conen, P. E., and Erkman, B.: Frequency and occurrence of chromosomal syndromes. II. E-trisomy, Am. J. Human Genet. 18:387, 1966.
6. Weber, W. W.: Survival and the sex ratio in trisomy 17-18, Am. J. Human Genet. 19:369, 1967.
7. Ozonoff, M. B., Steinbach, H. L., and Mamunes, P.: The trisomy 18 syndrome, Am. J. Roentgenol. 91:618, 1964.
8. Warkany, J., Weinstein, E. D., Soukup, S. W., Rubinstein, J. H., and Curless, M. C.: Chromosome analyses in a children's hospital: Selection of patients and results of studies, Pediatrics 33:290 and 454, 1964.
9. Hecht, F., Bryant, J., Arakaki, D., Kaplan, E., and Gentile, G.: Trisomy-18 syndrome due to de-novo translocation, Lancet 1:114, 1963.
10. Brodie, H. R., and Dallaire, L.: The E syndrome (trisomy 17-18) resulting from a maternal chromosomal translocation, Canad. M.A.J. 87:559, 1962.
11. Gustavson, K-H., Hagberg, B., Finley, S. C., and Finley, W. H.: An apparently identical extra-autosome in two severely retarded sisters with multiple malformations, Cytogenetics 1:32, 1962.
12. Vislie, H., Wehn, M., Brogger, A., and Mohr, J.: Chromosome abnormalities in a mother and two mentally retarded children, Lancet 2:76, 1962.
13. Gagnon, J., Archambault, L., Laberge, E., and Katyk-Longtin, N.: Trisomie partielle 18 par insertion ou translocation 4/18, Union méd. Canada 92:311, 1963.
14. Miller, J. Q., Rostafinski, M. J., and Hyde, M. S.: A defective extra chromosome associated with clinical 17-18 trisomy syndrome, Pediatrics 36:135, 1965.
15. de Grouchy, J.: Chromosome 18: A topologic approach, J. Pediat. 66:414, 1965.
16. Pfeiffer, R. A.: Deletion der kurzen Arme des Chromosoms Nr. 18, Humangenetik 2:178, 1966.
17. Uchida, I. A., McRae, K. N., Wang, H. C., and Ray, M.: Familial short arm deficiency of chromosome 18 concomitant with arhinencephaly and alopecia congenita, Am. J. Human Genet. 17:410, 1965.
18. Lejeune, J., Berger, R., Lafourcade, J., and Réthoré, M-O.: La délétion partielle du bras long du chromosome 18. Individualisation d'un nouvel état morbide, Ann. Génét. 9: 32, 1966.
19. Insley, J.: Syndrome associated with a deficiency of part of the long arm of chromosome no. 18, Arch. Dis. Childhood 42:140, 1967.
20. Bernard, R., Stahl, A., Giraud, F., Hartung, M., and Brusquet, Y.: Encéphalopathie avec dysmorphie complexe et chromosome 17-18 en anneau, Ann. pédiat. 13:2129, 1966.
21. Hook, E. B., and Yunis, J. J.: Trisomy-18 syndrome in a patient with normal karyotype, J.A.M.A. 193:184, 1965.
22. Weiss, L., DiGeorge, A. M., and Baird, H. W.: Four infants with trisomy 18 syndrome and one with trisomy 18 mosaicism, Am. J. Dis. Child. 104:533, 1962.
23. Wolf, U., Reinwein, H., and Schröter, R.: Bericht über vier Trisomien 18 und ein Trisomie-18-Mosaik, Humangenetik 1:232, 1965.
24. Koulischer, L., Pelc, S., and Périer, O.: A case of trisomy-18 mosaicism, Lancet 2:945, 1963.
25. Huggert, A.: The trisomy 18 syndrome; a report of three cases in the same family, Acta ophth. 44:186, 1966.
26. Marks, J. F., Wiggins, K. M., and Spector, B. J.: Trisomy 21-trisomy 18 mosaicism in a boy with clinical Down's syndrome, J. Pediat. 71:126, 1967.
27. Uchida, I. A., Bowman, J. M., and Wang, H. C.: The 18-trisomy syndrome, New England J. Med. 266:1198, 1962.
28. Ricci, N., Castoldi, G. L., Borgatti, L., and Alberti, R.: Malformazioni congenite multiple associate ad une doppia Anomalia cromosomica: Triplo-X e trisomia 17-18, Acta genet. med. 13:253, 1964.
29. Haas, L., and Lewis, F. J. W.: Double trisomy: Trisomy 17-18 with triple X in a female infant, J. Pediat. 69:660, 1966.
30. Cohen, M. M., and Bumbalo, T. S.: Double aneuploidy; trisomy-18 and Klinefelter's syndrome, Am. J. Dis. Child. 113:483, 1967.
31. Gagnon, J., Katyk-Longtin, N., deGroot, J. A., and Barbeau, A.: Double trisomie autosomique à 48 chromosomes (21 + 18), Union méd. Canada 90:1220, 1961.
32. Turner, B., den Dulk, G. M., and Watkins, G.: The 17-18 trisomy and 21 trisomy syndromes in siblings, J. Pediat. 64:601, 1964.
33. Hecht, F., Bryant, J. S., Motulsky, A. G., and Giblett, E. R.: The no. 17-18 (E) trisomy syndrome; studies on cytogenetics, dermatoglyphics, paternal age, and linkage, J. Pediat. 63:605, 1963.
34. Townes, P. L., DeHart, G. K., Jr., and Ziegler, N. A.: Trisomy 17-18 – an evaluation of preconceptional parental irradiation as a possible etiologic factor, J. Pediat. 65:870, 1964.
35. Smith, D. W., Patau, K., Therman, E., and Inhorn, S. L.: The no. 18 trisomy syndrome, J. Pediat. 60:513, 1962.
36. Hecht, F.: The placenta in trisomy 18 syndrome, Obst. & Gynec. 22:147, 1963.
37. Heinrichs, E. H., and Allen, S. W., Jr.: The 18-trisomy syndrome – a spectrum?, Clin. Pediat. 2:25, 1963.
38. Holman, G. H., Erkman, B., Zacharias, D. L., and Koch, H. F.: The 18-trisomy syndrome – two new clinical variants; one with associated tracheoesophageal fistula and the other with probable familial occurrence, New England J. Med. 268:982, 1963.
39. Neuhäuser, G., and Usener, M.: Hirnmissbildung und autosomale Trisomie, Ztschr. Kinderh. 95:244, 1966.
40. Passarge, E., True, C. W., Sueoka, W. R., Baumgartner, N. R., and Keer, K. R.: Malformations of the central nervous system in trisomy 18 syndrome, J. Pediat. 69:771, 1966.

41. Warkany, J., Passarge, E., and Smith, L. B.: Congenital malformations in autosomal trisomy syndromes, Am. J. Dis. Child. 112:502, 1966.
42. Butler, L. J., Snodgrass, G. J. A. I., France, N. E., Sinclair, L., and Russell, A.: E (16-18) trisomy syndrome: Analysis of 13 cases, Arch. Dis. Childhood 40:600, 1965.
43. Kos, A. O., Schuknecht, H. F., and Singer, J. D.: Temporal bone studies in 13-15 and 18 trisomy syndromes, Arch. Otolaryng. 83:439, 1966.
44. Gibson, D. A., Uchida, I. A., and Lewis, A. J.: A review of the 18 trisomy syndrome, Med. & Biol. Illus. 13:80, 1963.
45. Levkoff, A. H., Mather, G. B., and Eisenstein, R. P.: A case of trisomy 16-18 syndrome, Am. J. Dis. Child. 107:300, 1964.
46. Rogers, T. R., Hagstrom, J. W. C., and Engle, M. A.: Origin of both great vessels from the right ventricle associated with the trisomy-18 syndrome, Circulation 32:802, 1965.
47. Hustinx, T. W. J., *et al.*: Het syndrom met drie chromosomen 17-18 (17-18 of E_1 trisomie), Maandschr. kindergeneesk. 32:655, 1964.
48. Rabinowitz, J. G., Moseley, J. E., Mitty, H. A., and Hirschhorn, K.: Trisomy 18, esophageal atresia, anomalies of the radius, and congenital hypoplastic thrombocytopenia, Radiology 89:488, 1967.
49. Voorhees, M. L., Vaharu, T., and Gardner, L. I.: Trisomy 16-18 syndrome, Lancet 2:992, 1962.
50. Kajii, T., Oikawa, K., Itakura, K., and Ohsawa, T.: A probable 17-18 trisomy syndrome with phocomelia, exomphalos, and agenesis of hemidiaphragm, Arch. Dis. Childhood 39:519, 1964.
51. Scorta, A., Franceschini, P., and Pilotti, G.: Su un caso di trisomia 18 con spina bifida e meningocele, Minerva ginec. 18:31, 1966.
52. Zellweger, H., Huff, D. S., and Abbo, G.: Phocomelia and trisomy E, Acta genet. med. 14:164, 1965.
53. Weichsel, M. E., Jr., and Luzzatti, L.: Trisomy 17-18 syndrome with congenital extrahepatic biliary atresia and congenital amputation of the left foot, J. Pediat. 67:324, 1965.
54. Moseley, J. E., Wolf, B. S., and Gottlieb, M. I.: The trisomy 17-18 syndrome; roentgen features, Am. J. Roentgenol. 89:905, 1963.
55. Uchida, I. A., Patau, K., and Smith, D. W.: Dermal patterns of 18 and D_1 trisomics, Am. J. Human Genet. 14:345, 1962.
56. Geiser, C. F., and Schindler, A. M.: Long survival in a male with 18-trisomy syndrome and Wilms' tumor, Pediatrics 44:111, 1969.
57. Hook, E. B., and Yunis, J. J.: Congenital asymmetry associated with trisomy 18 mosaicism, Am. J. Dis. Child. 110:551, 1965.
58. Penrose, L. S.: Dermatoglyphics in trisomy 17 or 18, J. Ment. Defic. Res. 13:44, 1969.

Deficiency of the Short Arm of Chromosome 18

By 1968, more than 25 cases had been reported with karyotypes suggesting deletion of the short arm of one of the chromosomes 18.[1] In general, the clinical findings were not sufficiently characteristic to permit a diagnosis without cytogenetic examination. Mental retardation, failure to thrive, short stature, epicanthic folds, ptosis, floppy ears, saddle nose, dental caries and fish mouth are among the more frequent features.[2-5] Rare but striking anomalies include cyclopia, cebocephaly,[6] pterygium colli and facial clefts.[7,8] Minor anomalies of fingers and toes have been recorded often. Hypotonia, speech defects and delayed verbal development have been noted in some cases. More females with deletion of the short arm of chromosome 18 (46,XX,18p−) than males have been reported. Survival to adult life and reproduction are possible. In a case published by Uchida *et al.*,[6] an affected woman had two children, both of whom showed the same cytogenetic anomaly. The children, one a boy and one a girl, had different fathers and different phenotypes. Whereas the girl had cebocephaly, a single nostril and choanal atresia, the boy had rather uncharacteristic signs of mental and physical retardation.

REFERENCES

1. Reinwein, H., Struwe, F. E., Bettecken, F., and Wolf, U.: Defizienz am kurzen Arm eines Chromosoms Nr. 18 (46,XX,18p−) Ein einheitliches Missbildungssyndrom, Monatsschr. Kinderh. 116:511, 1968.
2. De Grouchy, J., Lamy, M., Thieffry, S., Arthuis, M., and Salmon, C.: Dysmorphie complexe avec oligophrénie: Délétion des bras courts d'un chromosome 17-18, Compt. rend. Acad. Sc. (Paris) 256:1028, 1963.
3. De Grouchy, J., Bonnette, J., and Salmon, C.: Délétion du bras court du chromosome 18, Ann. Génét. 9:19, 1966.
4. Migeon, B. R.: Short arm deletions in group E and chromosomal "deletion" syndromes, J. Pediat. 69:432, 1966.
5. Weiss, L., and Mayeda, K.: Case reports: A patient with a short arm deletion of chromosome 18 (46,XY,18p−), J. M. Genetics 6:216, 1969.
6. Uchida, I. A., McRae, K. N., Wang, H. C., and Ray, M.: Familial short arm deficiency of chromosome 18 concomitant with arhinencephaly and alopecia congenita, Am. J. Human Genet. 17:410, 1965.
7. Pfeiffer, R. A.: Deletion der kurzen Arme des Chromosoms Nr. 18, Humangenetik 2:178, 1966.
8. McDermott, A., Insley, J., Barton, M. E., Rowe, P., Edwards, J. H., and Cameron, A. H.: Arhinencephaly associated with a deficiency involving chromosome 18, J. M. Genetics 5:60, 1968.

Deficiency of the Long Arm of Chromosome 18

MENTAL RETARDATION, microcephaly, short stature, impaired hearing with malformations of the auricles and external auditory canals, retinal changes, facial peculiarities and a high count of whorls on the fingers are signs observed in patients with partial deletion of the long arm of chromosome 18. Congenital heart disease, horseshoe kidney, cryptorchidism, spinal defects and foot anomalies were described in some of the patients.[1-6] The disorder is compatible with life and has been seen in children beyond infancy.

REFERENCES

1. De Grouchy, J., Royer, P., Salmon, C., and Lamy, M.: Délétion partielle des bras longs du chromosome 18, Path.-biol. 12:579, 1964.
2. Lejeune, J., Berger, J. R., Lafourcade, J., and Réthoré, M-O.: La délétion partielle du bras long du chromosome 18, Ann. Génét. 9:32, 1966.
3. Insley, J.: Syndrome associated with a deficiency of part of the long arm of chromosome no. 18, Arch. Dis. Childhood 42:140, 1967.
4. Kushnick, T., and Matsushita, G.: Partial deletion of long arms of chromosome 18, Pediatrics 42:194, 1968.
5. Reinwein, H., Gorman, L. Z., and Wolf, U.: Defizienz am langen Arm eines Chromosoms Nr. 18 (46,XX,18q−), Ztschr. Kinderh. 101:152, 1967.
6. Wertelecki, W., and Gerald, P. S.: Clinical and chromosomal studies of the 18q− syndrome, J. Pediat. 78:44, 1971.

Ring Chromosome 18

NUMBER 18 RING CHROMOSOMES have been reported repeatedly.[1,2] As with other deletions of no. 18, the clinical manifestations vary. Mental retardation is present in all cases and microcephaly in some.[3,5] Intrauterine growth retardation[1,4] seems to be the exception rather than the rule.[2,5-7] Short stature in postnatal life is present more often.[6] Round face, flat occiput, hypertelorism, epicanthic folds, ear anomalies and deafness, clubfoot and syndactyly have been reported, but there is no definite clinical picture that betrays the cytogenetic anomaly.[5,6] Variable losses of chromosome 18 probably account for the variance in manifestations. The mothers of the children with ring chromosome 18 show no tendency to advanced age at the time of conception.[6]

REFERENCES

1. De Grouchy, J., Léveque, B., Debauchez, C., Salmon, C., Lamy, M., and Marie, J.: Chromosome 17-18 en anneau et malformations congénitales chez une fille, Ann. Génét. 7: 17, 1964.
2. Bernard, R., Stahl, A., Giraud, F., Hartung, M., and Brusquet, Y.: Encéphalopathie avec dysmorphie complexe et chromosome 17-18 en anneau, Ann. paediat. 42:2129, 1966.
3. Lucas, M., Kemp, N. N., Ellis, J. R., and Marshall, R.: A small autosomal ring chromosome in a female infant with congenital malformations, Ann. Human Genet. 27:189, 1963.
4. Lejeune, J., Réthoré, M-O., Berger, R., Baheux, G., and Chabrun, J.: Sur un cas de chromosome 18 en anneau, Ann. Génét. 9:173, 1967.
5. Palmer, C. G., Fareed, N., and Merritt, A. D.: Ring chromosome 18 in a patient with multiple anomalies, J. M. Genetics 4:117, 1967.
6. Hooft, C., Haentjens, P., Orye, E., Kluyskens, P., and D'Hont, G.: Chromosome 18 en anneau, Acta paediat. 22: 69, 1968.
7. Leisti, J., Gripenberg, U., Kivalo, E., Palo, J., von Schoultz, B., and Suomalainen, E.: Two patients with a 46,XX,Er chromosome constitution, Acta paediat. scandinav. 57: 441, 1968.

Down Syndrome

(Mongolism, Trisomy 21)

AMONG the congenital anomalies that result in mental retardation, Down syndrome plays an outstanding role. It is recognizable at birth by some nonspecific and elusive characteristics. Although no one symptom is pathognomonic, a correct diagnosis usually can be made by an experienced physician or nurse at the time of the child's birth. The suspicion aroused by some facial features makes possible prediction of the mental retardation of the child in years to come.

As early as 1846, Séguin[1] gave a good description of mongoloid children, whom he considered a special type of cretin. In 1866, John Langdon Haydon Down,[2] a London physician, described in a publication of 3½ pages a disease picture that is still recognized as an entity today. This author, who obviously had a large experience with mentally retarded children, attempted to classify his patients according to their external resemblance to racial stocks. He believed that many of the feeble-minded "can be referred to one of the great divisions of the human family other than the class from which they have sprung." He saw among his patients resemblances to Caucasians, Ethiopians, Malayans or originals of the American continent, and he believed that the great Mongolian family had numerous representatives among his mentally defective. He saw the likeness of these so-called Mongols to one another, and stated that it was difficult to believe that the specimens compared were not children of the same parents. Then Langdon Down proceeded to describe one defective member of the "mongolian racial division," as he called it, selected from the large number that had come under his observation.

There followed a superb description of this patient that included the facial features, the abnormal coordination, the speech difficulties, the feeble circulation, the power of imitation and the sense of humor. He stated that ". . . the improvement which training effects in them is greatly in excess of what would be predicated, if one did not know the characteristics of the type." But, he added, "The life expectancy . . . is far below the average. . . ." His estimate of the incidence of this mongoloid type as "more than ten per cent of the cases which are presented to me" is not far off the figures obtained in large institutions today. It is not surprising that this excellent 1866 description of the syndrome is still retained today.

There are statements in Down's brief paper to which one cannot subscribe today. Langdon Down believed that tuberculosis in the parents "is able to break down the barrier . . . of racial differences. . .," a phenomenon that, in a way, seemed to prove "the unity of the human species." This ingenious explanation—given 7 years after the publication of Darwin's *Origin of Species*—reflects the knowledge and thinking of the times, which is not in line with our ideas. But for 93 years there were no great improvements over the explanation given by Langdon Down for the origin of "mongolism" among Caucasians. Although the syndrome has been known to physicians since 1866, its etiology remained obscure until 1959, when it was recognized that the cells of these patients contained 47 instead of 46 chromosomes.[3a,3b] Numerous theories and hypotheses concerning its etiology had been advanced previously, but no explanation found general acceptance. Several monographs have been written on the subject.[4-12] Since only a short review of some questions about Down syndrome can be given here, the reader is referred to the more extensive publications, which present the topic in detail and supply extensive bibliographies.

Langdon Down's concept of a racial relationship of the disorder has been abandoned, but the term "mongolism" has remained a household word in medical practice. There are important objections to the use of the term "mongolism" for these defective children, and many suggestions have been made to replace it, but it is unlikely that it will be abandoned completely. The term "Down syndrome" is now widely accepted and used, but it is not a complete substitute for "mongolism." No adjective can be formed, and in place of "mongoloid" one has to say "patient with Down syndrome." Although I am in favor of the latter term, I still use "mongoloid" at times as an adjective and a noun. The term cannot be eliminated from quotations of past publications on the subject.

Incidence

Down syndrome occurs once in approximately 700 births and can be expected to have an incidence of 0.14% in the neonatal population. All recent estimates resulted in similar figures, but incidence rates quoted in the literature vary from 1 in 292 (0.34%) to 1 in 1,935 (0.05%).[13] Surprisingly, such differing estimates can come from the same hospital service. There are many explanations for such variations. Most studies were made in hospitals, a fact that could influence the results. Collmann and Stoller[14] made a complete survey in Victoria, Australia, and Renwick *et al.*[15] one in British Columbia. They found very similar incidence rates (0.145 and 0.146 per hundred live births). There may be changes over time, and ethnic groups may differ. Groups with different average maternal ages included in the samples could greatly influence incidence figures, since advanced maternal age increases the risk significantly.

Several studies are available showing incidence figures for various maternal age groups.[8,14,16] Collmann and Stoller[14] noted the following incidences according to maternal age distribution in quinquenniums: In mothers between 15 and 19 years there occurred 1 patient with Down syndrome in 2,300 births (0.043%); between 20 and 24, 1 in 1,600 (0.062%); between 25 and 29, 1 in 1,200 (0.083%); between 30 and 34, 1 in 870 (0.115%); between 35 and 39, 1 in 300 (0.33%); between 40 and 44, 1 in 100 (1.0%); and at 45 and over, 1 in 45 (2.2%). These figures show the increasing risk with advancing maternal age. In 1954, Penrose[17] found that the paternal age and birth order of the child are of no significance in the etiology of the disorder. Incidence figures could be changed by changing reproductive patterns. Fewer children in the maternal age groups over 35 years could reduce the incidence significantly. It is doubtful, however, that the variable estimates of birth rates of mongoloid children[13] can be explained by differences in the maternal age factor in the various localities and hospitals.

There is no proof that incidences have changed greatly over the years, but there can be no doubt that the prevalence of Down syndrome has increased because of improved medical facilities. It was estimated in Germany in 1938 that there was 1 mongoloid in 7,000 persons, or that the prevalence was 0.14 per 1,000.[18] Carter[19] pointed out a remarkable increase of prevalence in England. In 1929, it was 0.24 per 1,000 at age 10 years. In 1949, it was 0.46 per 1,000 and in 1958, 1.06 per 1,000. These figures suggest that the prevalence of the disorder at age 10 doubled in England between 1929 and 1949 and doubled again between 1949 and 1958. The rate of Down syndrome in institutions is definitely increasing. It doubled during the years between 1905 and 1915[20]; it was estimated at about 10% in recent years,[20-22] but may be much higher in some institutions at present.[23] Increasing prevalence in institutions is not only due to survival of patients with Down syndrome but also to the decline in the over-all prevalence of serious forms of mental retardation during the past 30–40 years.[24] In institutions, adults with Down syndrome are not rare. In Swedish institutions (about 10 years ago), 37% of the patients with Down syndrome were over 20 years of age, and 2.6% were over 50.[20]

In 1958, Carter[19] prepared a life table for nearly 700 mongoloid children seen at the Hospital for Sick Children in London between 1944 and 1955. He found that of live-born patients, 30% were dead at the age of 1 month, 53% by 1 year and 60% by the age of 10 years. The ratio of males to females increased with age. Analysis of deaths of 136 children with Down syndrome showed that 39% died of pneumonia, 35% of congenital heart disease, 8% of other congenital anomalies such as esophageal atresia, diaphragmatic hernia, duodenal stenosis, Hirschsprung disease, imperforate anus or exstrophy of the bladder, 2% of leukemia and the rest of various infections. There is good agreement concerning causes of death between the London study and one made in Denmark by Øster *et al.*[25]

A preponderance of male patients over females has been claimed,[26] but this seems to apply to institutional populations only. When all cases are considered, the sexes seem to be affected equally.[27]

There are reports of ethnic differences in the incidence of Down syndrome. It was thought to be quite low among Negroes, but this may be due to underestimates because of lack of proper examination and recognition of the condition in Negroes in the past. Parker[28] found similar incidences for Caucasians and Negroes in Washington, D. C.

Etiology

In 1958, before aneuploidy of patients with Down syndrome had been recognized, a review of explanations of the disorder revealed approximately 40 theories (approximately, because some popular explanations were not recorded and there was overlapping of others). Numerous hypotheses existed that were opposed to one another but were, according to their authors, compatible with the facts then known. Some of these hypotheses were well circumscribed and many could be refuted easily. Others were so broad and ill-defined that it was difficult to prove or disprove them. Now we know that many of the theories were wrong, that some are compatible with the cytogenetic discoveries made since and that some were correct, as the authors held chromosomal changes responsible for the condition. It may seem unnecessary to recall the situation in 1958, but much can be learned by past approaches, by past correct conjectures and by past mistakes, after the puzzle is solved—or partly solved. In an unpublished manuscript that I prepared in 1958, I cited the following explanations: (1) Reversion to a primitive racial type.[2,29] (2) Reversion to the orangutan.[29] (3) Heredodegeneration with strong psychopathic family background.[30] (4) Combination of microsymptoms demonstrable in sibs and other relatives.[18,31] (5) A dominant factor with greatly reduced penetrance or a chromosomal aberration.[32] (6) Hereditary "bleb disease" due to one main recessive and other modifying genes.[33] (7) Presence in the germ cells of 5 pairs of recessive factors, or 2 dominant and 4 pairs of recessive factors, carried in as many different chromosomes.[34] (8) "Germinal changes."[35] (9) Germinal mutation with consideration of chromosomal changes.[36-38]

The theories mentioned so far can be considered genetic explanations of mongolism. The following hypotheses consider change in the embryo after fertilization of the ovum or a combination of genetic and environmental factors: (10) Injury to germ cell or zygote.[31,39-41] (11) Hereditary factors combined with insufficiency of maternal organism.[42] (12) Maternal and fetal genetic predisposition and precipitating environmental factors.[43]

The following theories must be considered nongenetic. They incriminate environmental factors from cytoplasmic changes in the ovum to growth disturbances in the embryonic or fetal period: (13) "Dysplasmatic" or cytoplasmic changes.[6,44] (14) Overaged or immature ova.[45,46] (15) Maternal exhaustion by many pregnancies, advanced age or toxic influences.[47] (16) Abnormal nidation of ovum.[8,48] (17) Diseased uterine mucosa.[4,8,49]

There are many "subcauses" to this explanation: contraceptives, abortives, curettage,[50] shock, fall, collapse of uterus and operations preceding the pregnancy resulting in mongolism have been incriminated for mucosal changes. Contraceptives and x-ray exposures could be considered causes of modification or causes of mutation. In the latter case, they should be listed with the "genetic" theories. (18) Threshold conditions of sterility[7] or reduced reproductive faculty.[27] (19) Maternal infantilism.[49] (20) Maternal worries.[51] (21) Parental alcoholism. (22) Tuberculosis.[2] (23) Syphilis.[52,53] (24) Maternal hypothyroidism.[7,54] (25) Maternal uterine retroflexion or descent.[55] (26) Maternal hyperthyroidism.[56] (27) Maternal x-ray treatment.[57] (28) A host of maternal diseases and disorders acting in early months of pregnancy,[51,58] bleeding,[55] influenza, mumps, rubella, typhus, grippe or pleurisy,[58] vomiting, toxemia, rheumatism, streptococcal infections,[59] sinusitis and nephritis. (29) Increased amniotic pressure acting between the sixth and eighth weeks of gestation.[4]

The following explanations refer to the mongoloid organism itself: (30) Imperfection of fetal development.[47] (31) Fetal retardation[60] or deceleration of developmental rate[7] during early weeks of gestation. (32) Polyglandular deficiency.[61] (33) Thyroid deficiency.[62] (34) Fetal hyperthyroidism.[63] (35) Pituitary deficiency.[7] (36) Adrenal deficiency.[64] (37) Gonadal deficiency.[65] (38) Thymus deficiency.[66] (39) Deficiency of an undiscovered endocrine gland.[67] (40) Blockage of an enzyme system by an inhibitor such as fluorine at an early stage of fetal development.[68]

By 1958, some of the explanations listed above had long been discarded, whereas others were still flourishing and accepted by students of the disease. To a certain extent, these theories reflected the biologic thinking of their times. Often, when a new discovery was made in biology or medicine it was used to explain mongolism in some way or another, but it seemed clear that the biologic principles involved in the abnormal mechanisms of this disorder remained unknown.

A satisfactory theory had to be in agreement with a few well-established facts and these facts could not be integrated easily into a lucid and acceptable concept.

Shuttleworth,[47] in 1909, apparently was the first to point out the advanced age of many mothers at the time of birth of their mongoloid children. This observation was confirmed by many careful statistical studies. In 1938, Bleyer[69] computed the maternal age at birth of 2,822 mongoloid children and compared it with that of the mothers of 2,000,000 normal children. This comparison showed clearly the tendency of the mongoloid to be born of an older mother. The peak maternal age in the general population was found to be 24 years, but in the group producing mongoloid children it was 41 years (Fig. 37-14).

These findings were confirmed by Penrose,[17] whose careful analysis showed that the paternal age and birth order of the child probably were not significant. In Denmark, Øster[9] demonstrated the abnormal age distribution of mothers of more than 500 mongoloid children. Approximately 28% of all children with mongolism are born to mothers under 30 and 72% to older women.[70] It is of interest that Macklin,[34] who proposed a complicated genetic etiology, considered advanced maternal age as unimportant in the etiology of mongolism because many mothers of these patients were young.

Another fact that had to be considered in an acceptable theory of mongolism was the concordance of monozygotic twins and the overwhelming discordance of dizygotic twins. It is true that it often was difficult to establish the zygosity of sex-like twins. In one instance,[71] a case of discordant twins was considered uniovular, but there was not sufficient proof of monozygosity. In rare cases, both members of probably dizygotic pairs were affected,[72] and in one instance a definitely dizygotic pair (a boy and a girl) were both mongoloid,[73] but, despite the few exceptions, the rule mentioned above seemed well established. The importance of this behavior of twins for the theory of Down syndrome was first pointed out by

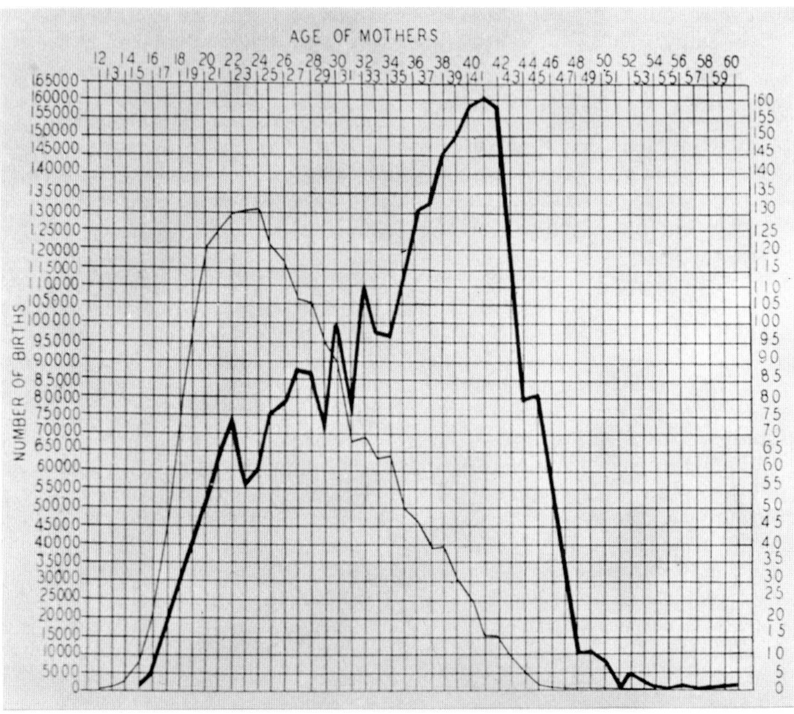

Fig. 37-14. – Maternal age at the birth of 2,822 mongoloids compared with maternal age at the birth of approximately 2,000,000 children in the United States in the year 1934 (exclusive of Massachusetts and New Hampshire). This shows the tendency of the mongoloid imbecile to be born of an old mother. The peak maternal age in the general population is 24 years; in the group producing mongoloid imbeciles it is 41 years. (From A. Bleyer.[69])

McLean[74] in 1922, and later re-emphasized by others.[34,35,41,75,76] These observations generally supported the genetic explanations, but Penrose[17] noted that the genotype of mongolism apparently was dependent on more than one pair of genes. If it depended on one gene pair only, at least a fourth of the dizygotic partners should be affected.

The idea that an external event or a maternal disease in the early weeks of pregnancy can be the cause of mongolism is an old one. In 1913, Thompson (cited by Halbertsma[35]) concluded from the nature of the cardiac defects that a disturbance in the second month of gestation might be responsible for mongolism. There were observations of children exposed to x-irradiation in utero during the second month of pregnancy who had some resemblance to mongoloids.[57,77] Although such children had epicanthic folds, broad nose, and so forth, the resemblance was superficial. Microphthalmia and microcephaly were more characteristic of radiation damage than was mongolism. With the discovery of German measles as a teratogen acting in early pregnancy, it seemed plausible to some writers that mongolism might have a similar origin. The symptoms of mongolism were explained by various events coinciding with the "timetable" of embryologic development. It was not difficult to find a few mongoloid children whose mothers had had influenza, rubella, mumps or other infections in early pregnancy. In other instances, the mothers had undergone an operation or been in an automobile accident between the sixth and ninth weeks of fetal life.[58,78]

Against the theory of accidents during the second month of gestation as causes of mongolism there were observations in multiple pregnancies. Twins, whether monozygotic or dizygotic, should, in general, be equally affected by disturbances of the external environment or maternal disorders. It was thought that such events occurring in the organogenic period should change both twins; there should be no persistent difference between monozygotic and dizygotic twins in cases of viremia, bacteremia, x-irradiation or maternal endocrinopathies.

Ascertainment of the etiology of congenital malformations by timetables is a doubtful principle (Chapter 7). Although some of the malformations occurring in Down syndrome make their appearance in the second month of pregnancy, that does not mean that they are determined at that time. In addition, there occur malformations in mongoloids that date back to earlier periods of organogenesis. Down syndrome has been found combined with situs inversus[79] or with spina bifida,[80] anomalies that are determined before the end of the second month. Despite all the evidence against it, the belief in modification during the second month of pregnancy as the cause of mongolism

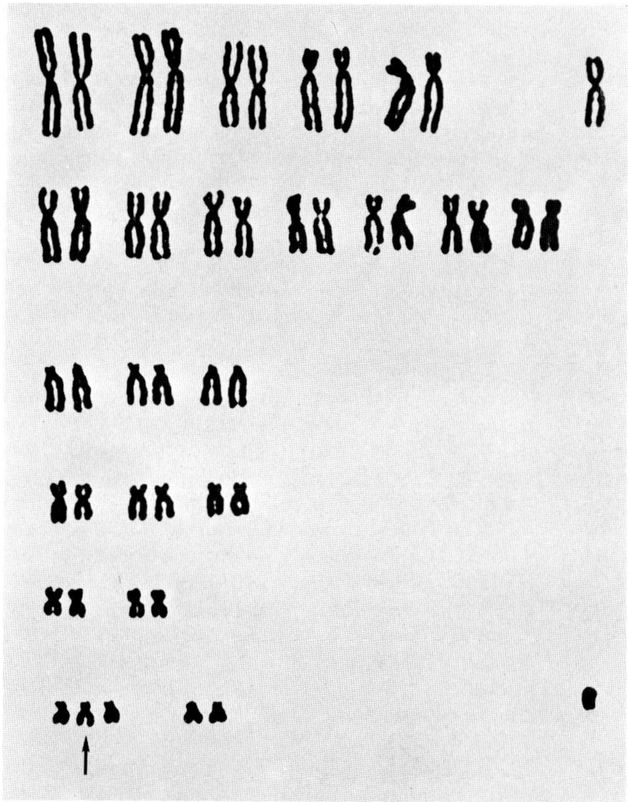

Fig. 37-15.—Karyotype of an 18-year-old patient with Down syndrome, showing 47 chromosomes and trisomy 21 (**arrow**).

became so popular that it was expressed in leading textbooks of pediatrics and accepted by some courts, which held accidents in early pregnancy responsible for mongolism.[81]

The theory of pathologic nidation suggested by the reproductive histories of some mothers of mongoloid children moved the origin further back in embryogenesis. A period of apparent sterility may precede the birth of a mongoloid, and a history of miscarriage, curettage or gynecologic disturbances before conception is obtained in some cases. The theory of faulty nidation was consistent with the observations on maternal age, with multiple cases of Down syndrome in one family and, to a certain extent, with twin observations. It was not consistent with observations made in children resulting from extrauterine pregnancies. In such cases, nidation is extremely pathologic, but mongolism does not result. This argument[6] also spoke against theories that considered other uterine anomalies (uterine retroflexion, etc.) as a cause of mongolism.

These notes illustrate the thinking of most medical writers before 1959.

Among the many essayists who wrote about the etiology of mongolism there were some who astutely deduced that a chromosomal abnormality could account for the syndrome. In 1932, the ophthalmologist Waardenburg[36] suggested to cytologists that they search for a chromosomal aberration in mongolism. He thought of a chromosomal deficiency by nondisjunction, a chromosome duplication, partial deficiency, translocation or partial duplication. At about the same time, the pediatrician Bleyer[37] made some deductions that are worth recounting. He remarked that looking at "mongoloid imbeciles" is like looking at the stars—the more one looks, the more one sees. He thought that sometime it might be known that no part of the entire body is spared by this disease, a conjecture confirmed 27 years later by cytogenetic findings that demonstrated that every cell in the body is abnormal in trisomy 21. Bleyer believed that mongolism might be due to a deviation present at the time of fertilization or even before, and foresaw that the problem of mongolism might belong to the cytologist rather than to the common-clay clinician. In 1934, he considered that an unequal migration of the chromosomes to the poles of the germ cell during the reduction period "may result in a cell progeny having a number of chromosomes unlike the number present in the parent." Bleyer thought that the origin of mongolism may be due to an alteration in the normal number of chromosomes, a very early alteration in the germ cell or a true gametic alteration that would repeat itself in every cell derived therefrom throughout the entire body. To appreciate the following, it must be remembered that in 1934 it was taught that the cells of man have 48 chromosomes. "Whether in the mongoloid imbecile one is dealing with forty-nine or forty-seven, with fifty or forty-six or with some other number of chromosomes must be left to the cytologist, in whose field the richest prizes in genetics now seem to lie." In 1937, Turpin *et al.*[82] and in 1939, Penrose[83] and Fanconi[38] considered a chromosomal aberration as a possible cause of mongolism.

The theory of a chromosomal change was substantiated when, in January of 1959, Lejeune, Gautier and Turpin[3a] announced that they had found in fibroblasts of 3 mongoloid boys a chromosomal number of 47, the supplementary chromosome being a small acrocentric. This discovery soon was confirmed in several other laboratories,[84-86] and now it is well established that mongolism in the majority of cases is associated with a chromosomal pattern considered at present as a "trisomy 21." It is assumed that trisomy 21 is brought about by a faulty chromosomal separation or nondisjunction occurring during formation of an ovum. Although there are statements that the supernumerary chromosome is number 22 of the set,[87] there is no definite proof of this. To avoid confusion, it seems reasonable to uphold the terminology introduced by Lejeune *et al.*[3a]

The discovery of trisomy 21 represents a milestone in the search for the origin of mongolism, since the hypothesis that this chromosomal aberration is responsible for the clinical disease picture is in good agreement with many of the known facts and observations.

The experiences with twins (p. 315) can be explained by the derivation of monozygotic pairs from one zygote with trisomy 21 and of dizygotic pairs from one normal and one trisomic zygote. The fact that women with Down syndrome can bear normal or mongoloid children[88-90] with about equal chance is due to their ability to form ova with 23 or 24 chromosomes, which, when fertilized by sperm containing 23 chromosomes, results in normal or trisomic zygotes (Fig. 37-16, *C*).

Translocation Down Syndrome

Not all patients with Down syndrome have 47 chromosomes and trisomy 21. Deviations from the standard type are rare, comprising only about 6–10% of the population with Down syndrome.[91-93]

Some mongoloid patients have 46 chromosomes even though they have a supernumerary chromosome 21. The small supernumerary acrocentric chromosome appears fused by translocation with a large or a small acrocentric. In 1960, Polani *et al.*[94] reported a girl with typical Down syndrome who had 46 chromosomes . There were only 5 chromosomes in the 13-15 (D) and 4 chromosomes in the 21-22 (G) group, but there was a supernumerary submetacentric chromosome in group 6-12. Such a translocation of a 21 to a 13, 14 or 15 chromosome can be written as 13-15/21 or D/G (Fig. 37-17) translocation or, according to the new, clumsy and precise standardization, 46,XX,D−,t(DqGq)+. Many cases of this type (Fig. 37-17, *A*) have been described since. Another form of translocation mongolism is characterized by 46 chro-

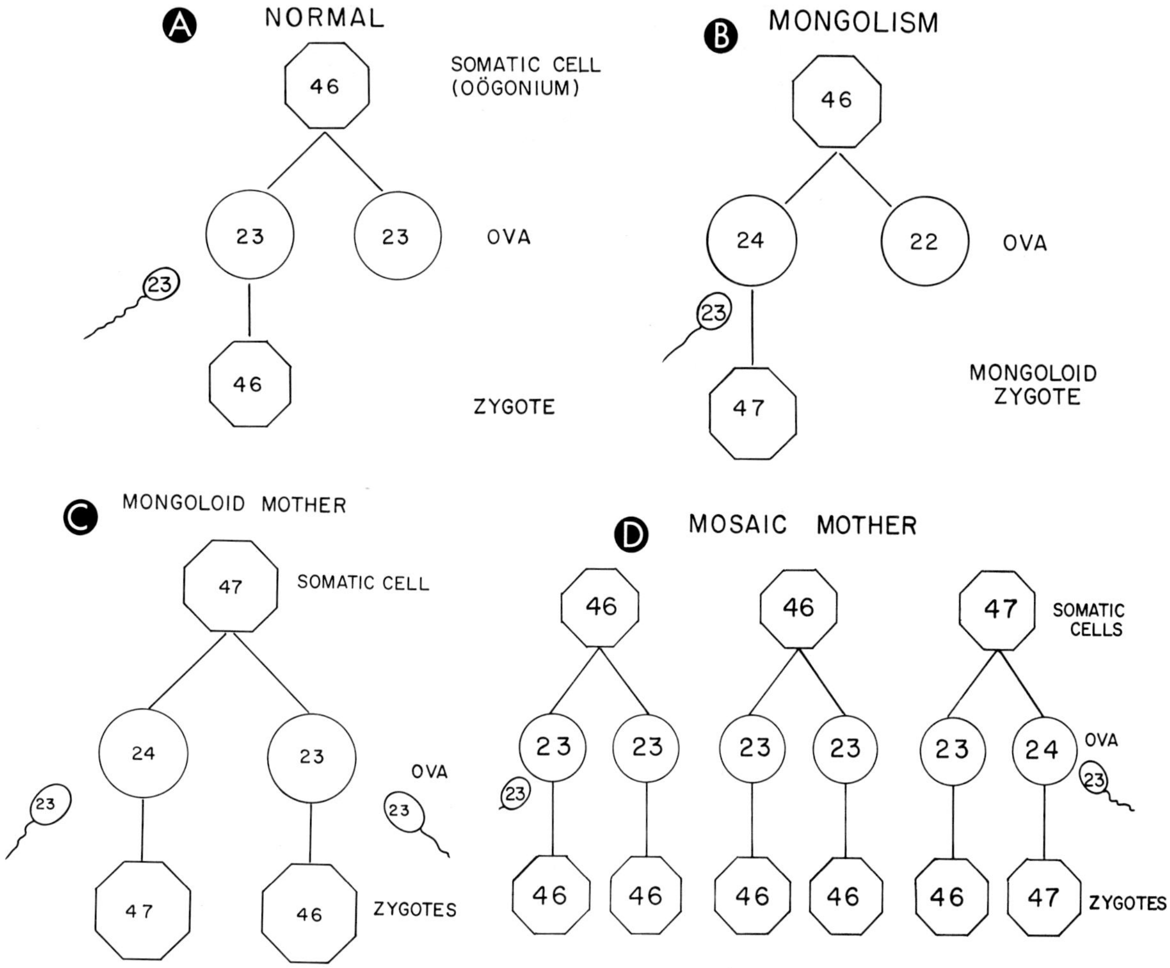

Fig. 37-16. – Diagrams showing formation of zygotes from germ cells with normal or abnormal chromosome number. **A,** normal germ cells (**circles**) with 23 chromosomes are formed from a somatic cell (**octagonal**) with 46 chromosomes. By union of two germ cells, a zygote with 46 chromosomes is formed. **B,** by nondisjunction, an ovum receives 24 chromosomes. Fertilization results in a zygote with 47 chromosomes. **C,** a woman with Down syndrome produces ova with 23 or 24 chromosomes. Zygotes with 46 or 47 chromosomes result from fertilization. **D,** a mother, mosaic of normal and trisomic somatic cells, produces ova with 23 or 24 chromosomes. Normal or 47 chromosome-zygotes can be formed by fertilization.

mosomes and an extra chromosomal mass equivalent to a supernumerary 21 attached to a small chromosome 21 or 22 (Fig. 37-18). Such a G/G translocation can be a 21/22 or 21/21 type, both now written 46,XY,G–,t(GqGq)+. There is no evidence that translocation mongolism differs clinically from the standard type, although slight differences have been reported.[95] The parents of children with translocation mongolism may have normal karyotypes. There is little danger of recurrence of Down syndrome in such families. But in other families the risk of translocation mongolism is greatly enhanced. Penrose *et al.*[96] investigated a family in which two translocation mongoloids of the (13-15)/21 type had been born. There were two normal children and a history of two abortions. The mother had only 45 chromosomes, with absence of one large (13-15) and one small (21) acrocentric chromosome and presence of an extra chromosome in the (6-12) group, considered a fusion product of a 21 chromosome with one of the 13-15 group (45,XX,D–,G–,t(DqGq)+). The mother, having normal chromosomal material despite the translocation, was phenotypically normal. The mother's mother and a sister of the children with mongolism were also translocation carriers with 45 chromosomes.

We[97] have observed a similar family and many comparable cases have been recorded from other centers.[12] Recognition of translocation mongolism with a parental translocation carrier is of importance because of the great increase in risk of recurrence in such families. In the translocation carrier, many germ cell types can be formed; some of them, being monosomic, are unviable and others are very rare. One type of germ cell containing normal acro-

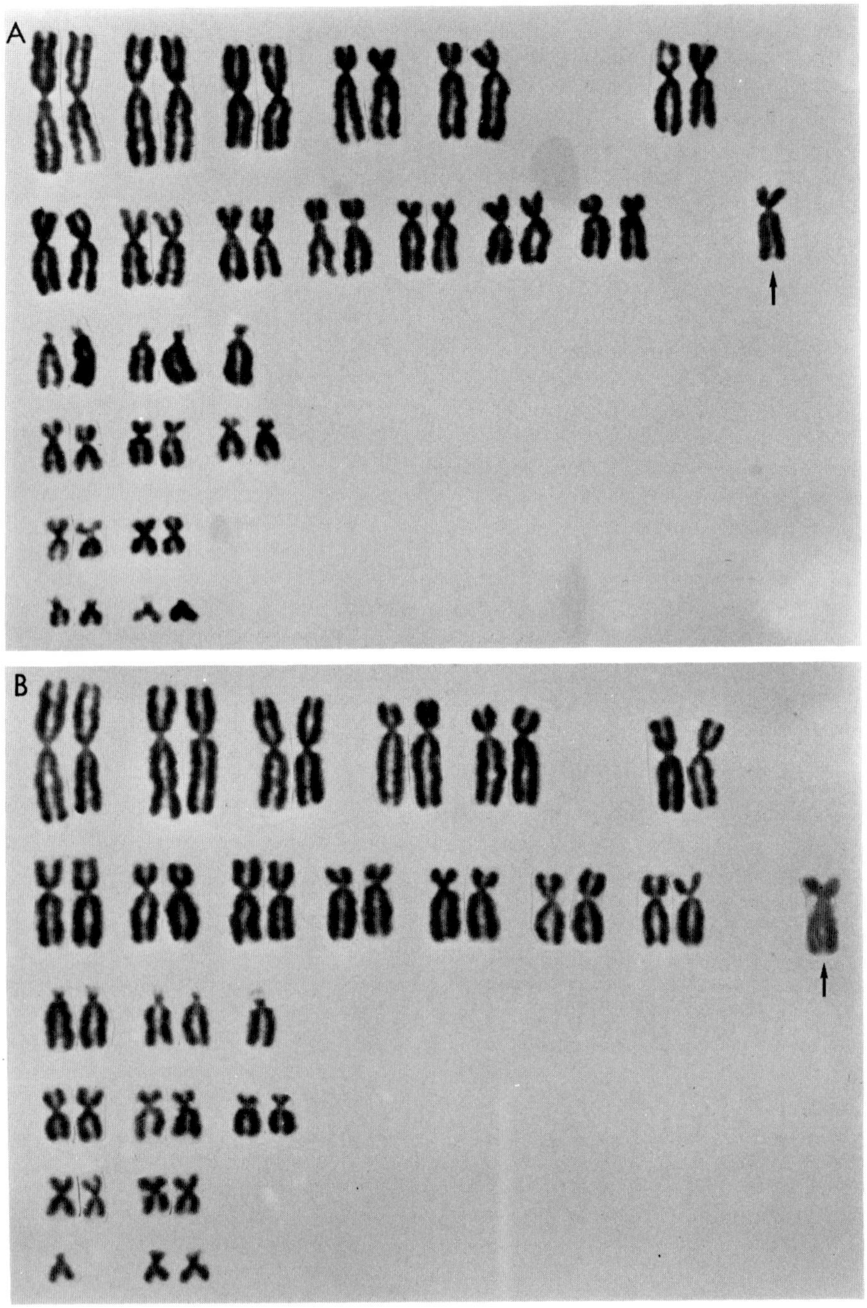

Fig. 37-17. – **A,** D/G translocation Down syndrome. There are 46 chromosomes. One chromosome of the D group is replaced by a chromosome (**arrow**) that shows fusion of a D chromosome with a supernumerary small acrocentric (46,XX,D–t(DqGq)+). **B,** karyotype of the mother of the patient in **A.** There are only 45 chromosomes. In place of one D and one G chromosome a translocation chromosome (**arrow**) is seen (45,XX,D–,G–,t(DqGq)+).

centrics of groups 13-15 and 21 is normal and capable of forming a normal zygote with a normal mate. A second type, containing a (13-15)/21 translocation chromosome, can form a phenotypically normal translocation carrier resembling the cytogenetically abnormal parent. The third type, a germ cell with a translocation chromosome and a 21, will result in a zygote with two "free" and one translocated chromosome 21 and in translocation mongolism.[12] The outlook for such a family appears dim, since for one normal

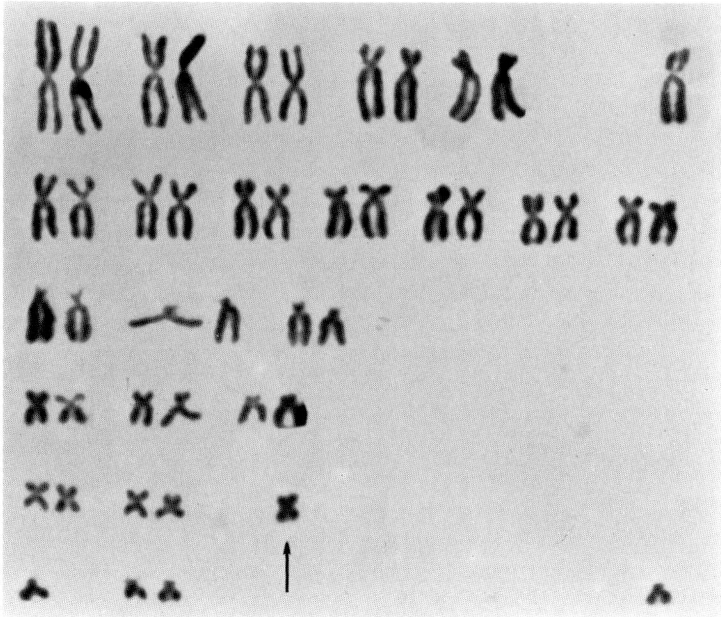

Fig. 37-18.—Karyotype of translocation (G/G) Down syndrome. The translocation chromosome (**arrow**) replaces one G chromosome: 46,XY,G−,t(GqGq)+.

child, one translocation carrier and one mongoloid might be expected.[98]

But there are exceptions to these expectations. Male translocation carriers rarely produce mongoloid children, most of their offspring being normal or translocation carriers.[12] However, in some instances, male translocation carriers have fathered children with translocation mongolism.[99,100] In other families, carriers produced an excess of phenotypically normal children, many being male and female carriers.[101]

The situation is similar for G/G or 21/22 fusion (see Fig. 37-18). Mongoloids of this type, written 46,XY,G−,t(GqGq)+, cannot be distinguished clinically from cytogenetically differing types. The parents can be normal or one of them may show a cytogenetic deviation. It seems that this kind of translocation mongolism, if transmitted through a parent, is more often passed on through the father than the mother.[102] Penrose[103] noted advanced paternal age in cases of 21/22 translocation mongolism. In the majority of cases of this type the parents are cytogenetically normal but in a number of them paternal mosaicism has been noted.[96,101,104] Rarely, translocation of chromosomes not involving 21 occurring in a parent can contribute to nondisjunction and thus result in mongolism of a child.[105,106] If a parent has 45 chromosomes and a 21/21 translocation (45,XX,G−,G−,t[GqGq]+), all children will have Down syndrome (46,XX,G−,t[GqGq]+).[216-218]

Translocation "in tandem" involves translocation of the long arm of one chromosome 21 onto the long arm of another with loss of centromere and short arms of one of them.[226-228] It seems that this translocation is associated with a higher level of intelligence than the regular trisomy 21 karyotype (Fig. 37-19).

Mosaicism

Trisomy 21 cells can coexist in human beings with cell types of other chromosomal constitution. Many cases have been reported of persons who have mosaicism of trisomy 21 and normal cells. Clarke *et al.*[107] described a girl who had some physical features of mongolism and an intelligence somewhat above average for this disorder. Leukocyte and fibroblast cultures showed normal and trisomy 21 karyotypes, the latter being in the minority and more frequent in fibroblasts than in leukocytes. Mosaicism can vary from patient to patient and from tissue to tissue and more than two stem lines can coexist.[108] The subject was reviewed by Richards.[224] In one of our cases[97] that was clinically dubious, the rare trisomy 21 cells were at first missed in leukocyte culture but found in 23% of fibroblasts (Fig. 37-20). In a clinically typical mongoloid,[109] skin cultures showed predominantly trisomic cells, but leukocyte cultures consistently yielded cells with normal karyotype. Many other cases of normal/trisomy 21 mosaicism have been reported, but the resulting phenotypes do not necessarily parallel the quantitative composition of the cellular mosaicism.[229] Some mosaics are mentally normal, others are intermediate in intelligence between average mongoloids and normal persons, and others are severely retarded. In a mongoloid adult with very low mentality, Fitzgerald and Lycette[110] found normal karyotype in 42 and trisomy 21 in 53% of cells derived from leukocyte culture. The proportion of trisomic cells may change in the course of years.[230] Phenotypically normal or near-normal persons with normal/trisomy 21 mosaicism can reproduce and run an increased risk of having mongoloid offspring.[111-114] If

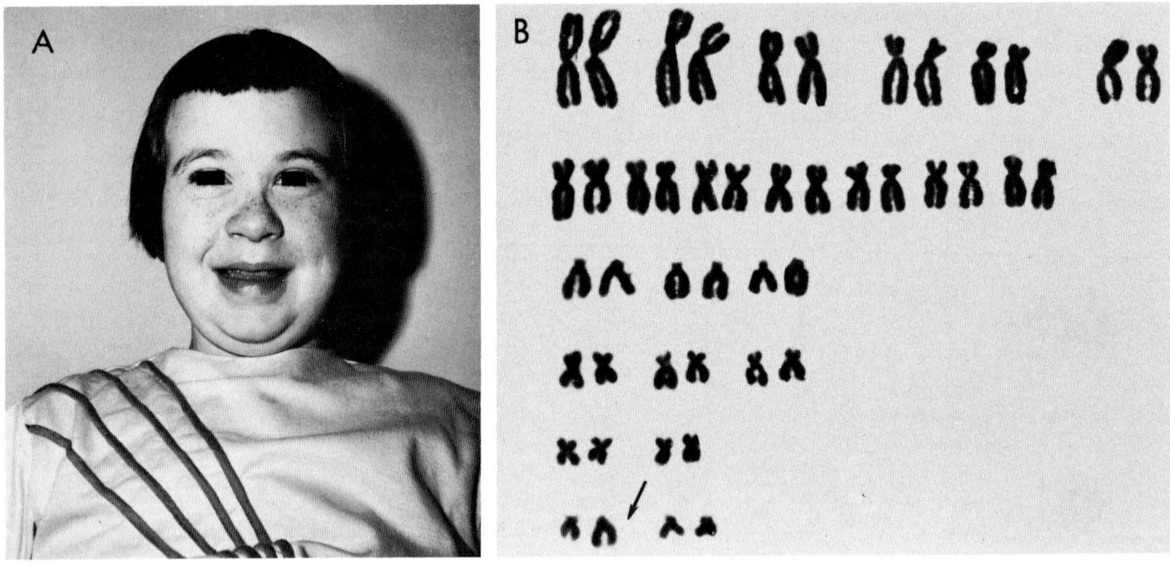

Fig. 37-19.—Translocation 21 "in tandem." **A,** girl with atypical and mild Down syndrome at the age of 10 years. **B,** the karyotype shows the enlarged chromosome 21 (**arrow**). (From J. Warkany and S. Soukup.[226])

such mosaics have normal and trisomy 21 cells in their gonads, they may form gametes with 23 and 24 chromosomes. The latter, when fertilized by a normal mate, will result in a trisomy 21 zygote and a mongoloid child (see Fig. 37-16, *D*).

The age of a mosaic mother probably is irrelevant in such cases, but advanced age of the grandmother at the time of the birth of the mosaic mother may play an etiologic role.[111-113] It is recommended that in taking a history of a child with Down syndrome not only the age of the mother but also the age of the grandmother be recorded. If the mother was young at the birth of her mongoloid child, and the maternal grandmother of advanced age at the birth of her daughter, cytogenetic investigation of the family may be rewarding. But in a general review of grandmaternal ages at birth of mothers of mongoloid children there was no indication that a young maternal age is associated with a high grandmaternal age.[225] It is believed that normal/trisomy 21 mosaicism may arise from a trisomy 21 zygote by loss of a chromosome at mitotic division; or it may arise from a normal zygote with 46 chromosomes after the first cell division by nondisjunction in one of the daughter's cells.

Prevalence of Trisomy 21 in Patients with Down Syndrome

In serial examinations of patients with Down syndrome, trisomy 21 is always the most frequent type encountered. Hayashi[91] analyzed 79 mongoloids and found trisomy 21 in 74 (93.7%), mosaics in 2 (2.5%) and (13-15)/21 translocation in 3 (3.8%). Hamerton *et al.*,[92] studying a series of 157 mongoloids, found 144 (90%) with trisomy 21, 6 with mosaicism, 4 with G/G and 2 with D/G translocation; 1 had a trisomy 21 and XXY karyotype. In an analysis of compiled data, Wright *et al.*[93] attributed 1,304 of 1,382 (94.3%) to trisomy 21 or mosaics of normal/trisomy 21-type and 78 (5.7%) to D/G and G/G translocation.

Down Syndrome with Normal Karyotype

Three years after the discovery of trisomy 21, Hall[115] described a 2½-year-old boy with typical Down syndrome and a normal karyotype in cells from skin and blood. The author considered the possibility of an undiscovered mosaicism or a concealed translocation, but expressed the belief that the correlation between Down syndrome and trisomy 21, and possibly the etiology, might not be an absolute one. Sergovich *et al.*[116] observed a boy, diagnosed as a mongoloid by a majority of pediatricians, who had a normal karyotype in cells from peripheral blood, skin, esophagus and duodenum. We have seen a girl suspected by all observers to have Down syndrome who consistently had a karyotype not distinguishable from the normal in cells from blood and skin. It is likely that similar cases have been seen in other centers without being published. In some cases, mosaicism could be demonstrated (p. 319), in others, extra chromosomal material was found attached to another chromosome. The phenotype of such patients is variable and the outcome not predictable. In a family described by Day and Miles,[117] mongolism was associated with a normal karyotype in one sibling and trisomy, with the long arm of a presumed chromosome 21 deleted, in another sibling. The fact remains that Down syndrome can be associated with a karyotype in which the extra chromosome cannot be detected with methods now available. Such exceptions should be emphasized and not explained away. A discrepancy

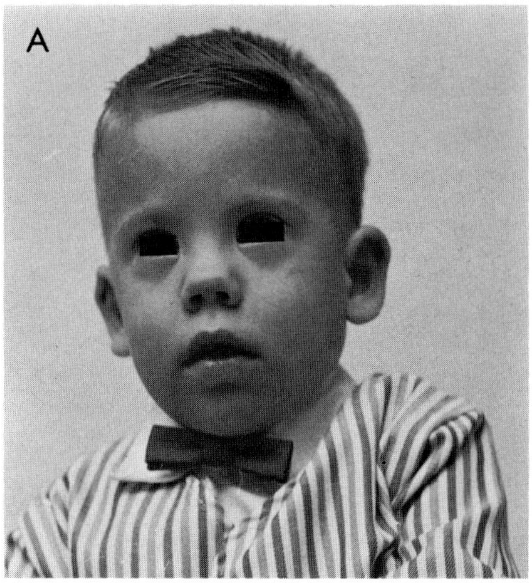

Fig. 37-20. – **A,** patient with mosaicism (46,XY/47,XY,21+) at the age of 3 years. He has two cell types with: **B,** normal 46,XY karyotype and **C,** karyotype showing trisomy 21.

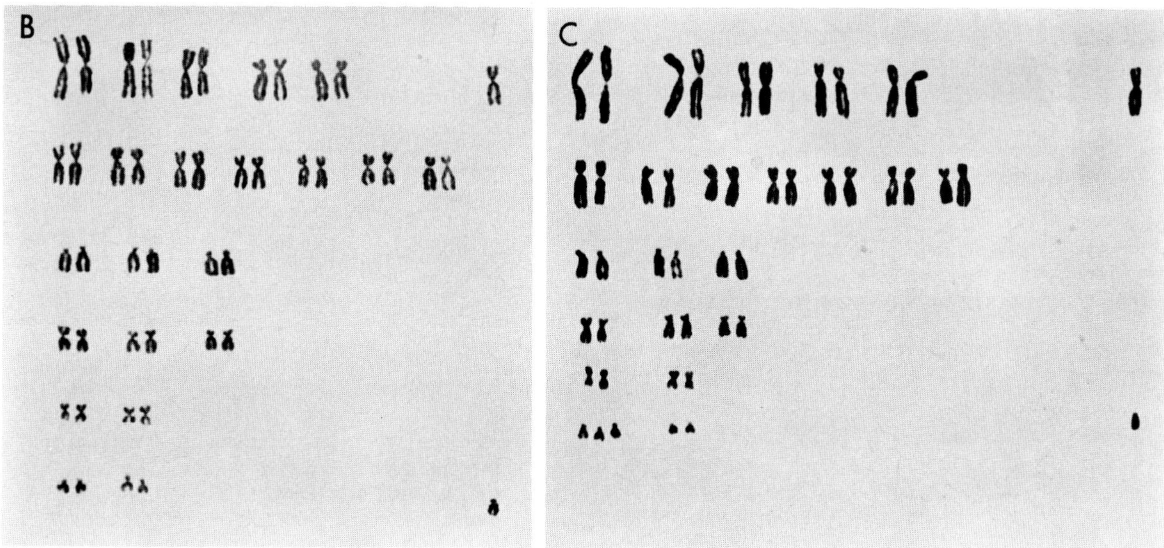

between clinical and cytogenetic findings could become of legal importance. There are other examples of such discrepancy in cases of trisomy 13-15 (p. 297) and in various syndromes of sex anomalies. In the latter case, it can be proved that some deviations are not due to chromosomal changes but rather to environmental injuries during embryonic or fetal life or to gene anomalies.

Partial Down Syndrome

In some patients, the disease picture is not fully expressed, although sufficient signs are present to suggest Down syndrome. In some of these cases, mosaicism (p. 319) accounts for the reduced expression. In others, the extra chromosomal material may be reduced in quantity. Dent *et al.*[118] reported such a case with 47 chromosomes. One of the G chromosomes was smaller than the rest of the group. In other cases, some of the cells contained a fragment rather than a supernumerary chromosome.[119,120] The extra chromosomal material may be so small that, when attached to a chromosome of the 13-15(D) group; it cannot be easily recognized as a D/G translocation.[116,121] The importance of these patients with partial Down syndrome is that they – like persons with normal/trisomy 21 mosaicism – can produce mongoloid offspring.[121]

Offspring of Women with Down Syndrome

Women with Down syndrome form ova with 24 chromosomes, containing 2 chromosomes no. 21, and ova with 23 chromosomes, containing a normal haploid set (see Fig. 37-16, *C*). If fertilized by a normal sperm with 23 chromosomes, zygotes with 47 and zygotes with 46 chromosomes are formed with a chance of equal numbers of mongoloid and nonmongoloid children. By 1966, 14 females with Down syndrome who had produced offspring were on record. The offspring consisted of 5 mongoloids and 9 nonmongoloids.[12,90]

The offspring of women with normal/trisomy 21 mosaicism will vary according to their ovarian mosaicism (p. 320).

Down Syndrome in Young Mothers

In general, Down syndrome is associated with advanced maternal age, but there are cases that arise independently of the maternal age factor. In some of these cases, the risk of recurrence is increased because of maternal mosaicism or translocation. This renders cytogenetic examinations desirable in families in which Down syndrome occurs at a young maternal age. Day and Wright[122] analyzed 41 patients with Down syndrome whose mothers were under 20 years of age when the affected child was born. Thirty-five had trisomy 21, 3 were G/G mosaics and 3 showed translocations (21/22, 13-15/21, 21/22 and mosaicism). In all 41 families, the index case was the only one with Down syndrome. Combining their results with comparable preceding publications on mothers under 30 years of age led to similar results. Young mothers had children with mosaic Down syndrome in 8%, and with translocation Down syndrome in 8% of the cases. In mothers under 30 years of age, translocation mosaicism was noted in 11% of the children, but in only 3% was the translocation inherited from the carrier parent. Day and Wright concluded that when the maternal age is less than 30 years and no cytogenetic studies are performed, the maximum empirical risk that a second child may be affected by a maternally transmitted D/G or (13-15)/21 translocation is approximately 1%; if chromosomal analysis shows that the child has trisomy 21, the risk of recurrence is less than 1%; if the child has a D/G translocation inherited from a carrier mother, the risk is 1 in 3. Giannelli *et al.*[106] examined 96 consecutive families in which mongoloids had been born at a maternal age of less than 30 years. There were 7 translocation cases (7.3%) and 89 with trisomy 21 (92.7%). Petersen and Luzzatti[123] arrived at similar figures. Mikkelsen,[124] compiling data of several series, found that 8.4% of mothers under 30 years of age who had given birth to mongoloid children had translocation mongoloids; in only 2.1% was the translocation inherited from the parent. Mothers over 30 years of age had only 1.3% translocation mongoloids. The condition was transmitted by a parent in only 0.3%. Wright *et al.*,[93] in a similar survey, arrived at comparable conclusions. Mothers under 30 years of age have 8.9% translocation mongoloids. One-fourth of these are inherited. Mothers over 30 years of age have 2.1% translocation mongoloids.

Fig. 37-21. – Phenotypically normal mosaic mother with her son who has trisomy 21 Down syndrome.

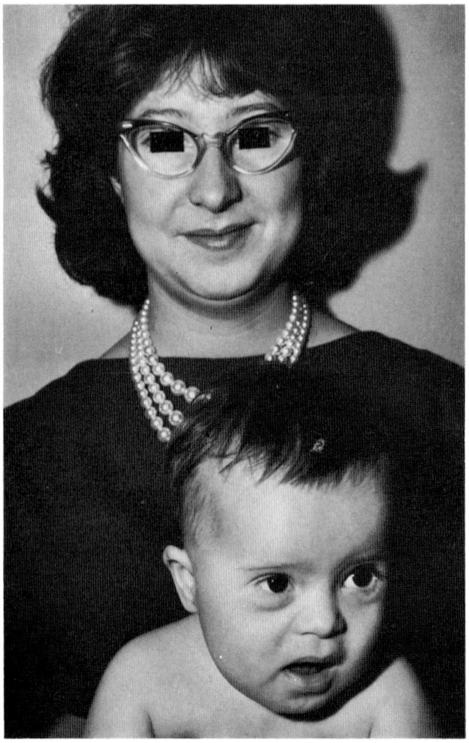

Multiple Aneuploidies

Down and Klinefelter syndromes in the same person result from double aneuploidy. Ford *et al.*[84] described a mongoloid male with symptoms of Klinefelter syndrome with 48 chromosomes, 2 X chromosomes and a supernumerary G. Hustinx *et al.*[125] reported mongoloid twins with 48 chromosomes and karyotypes of the kind described by Ford *et al.*[84] and by others.[12]

Down syndrome can be associated with Turner syndrome,[126,127] with triple X syndrome,[117] with XYY complement,[128] with trisomy 18[129] and with trisomy 13-15.[130] There can be different cell lines (mosaicism) in such cases, with variable admixture of aneuploidy.

Indications for Chromosome Analysis

Diagnosis of patient. – In most instances, Down syndrome can be diagnosed by clinical examination without any difficulty. In the newborn, the diagnosis may have grave consequences, and a careful analysis of signs and manifestations is indicated (p. 324). Roentgenographic examination of the pelvis and other skeletal parts or, in some cases, of the heart and intestinal tract can aid in the diagnosis. Cytogenetic confirmation of the diagnosis is most useful but not always possible. The amounts of blood available are small and leukocytes may fail to grow. In questionable cases, the cytogenetic findings may be ambiguous. Experienced physicians and nurses seldom err in the early diagnosis of Down syndrome.

EUGENIC PROGNOSIS.—The risk of a mother having a mongoloid child is approximately 1 in 650, but the risk varies greatly for different age groups (p. 312) from 1 in 2,300 for mothers between 15 and 19 to 1 in 45 for mothers over 45 years of age. But there are great deviations from the general risk in mothers of certain chromosomal constitutions. Women carriers of (13-15)/21 or 21/22 translocation have a risk of almost 1 in 3,[106] mongoloid women with trisomy 21 have a risk of 1 in 2 and women carriers of a 21/21 translocation have a risk of 1 in 1 (or 100% certainty) of having a mongoloid child. The last group cannot be distinguished cytogenetically from a 21/22 translocation carrier, which reduces the usefulness of the cytogenetic analysis to a certain extent. If the father carries a translocation 13-15/21, the risk of having a mongoloid child apparently is smaller than for a mother with this translocation, but he occasionally fathers children who are translocation carriers.[131]

Approximately 90–95% of all patients with Down syndrome have trisomy 21. It has been stated that such patients have parents with normal chromosomes.[132] This is not necessarily correct. In a number of cases of this type, a phenotypically normal parent was found to have normal/trisomy 21 mosaicism (p. 322). Since such parents have an increased risk for mongoloid children, establishment of trisomy 21 does not render unnecessary examination of the parental karyotypes. We recommend cytologic analysis when the mother is young and the maternal grandmother was of advanced age at the mother's birth.

Translocation mongolism is rare. Only about 5% of the patients with Down syndrome have such forms, and of these only a minority inherited it from a parent. The chance of detecting such a heritable translocation in serial examinations is 1 in 50 mothers under 30 years of age, and only 1 in 330 in mothers over 30 years.[93] This is a small yield for costly and time-consuming cytogenetic mass analyses. But if a young mother of a child with Down syndrome gives a history of Down syndrome or other chromosomal abnormalities or of many miscarriages in the family, then a cytogenetic examination of the child, the parents and other relatives is indicated.

Often, parents are not interested in a genetic prognosis and fail to promise cooperation. Analyses usually remain incomplete in such cases. A risk of 1 in 3 may be accepted by some parents. On the other hand, anxious parents who desire a promise that there will be no recurrence of mongolism in the family can never be reassured completely, even if their karyotype appears normal. There may be an unexplained genetic tendency to nondisjunction, or a parent may have mosaicism not manifest in the tissues examined, or a parent may have an unrecognized translocation. At best, one can state that the chromosome analysis did not prove that the parents run an increased risk of recurrence.

Some Present Etiologic Theories

Discovery of the cytogenetic basis of mongolism was of outstanding importance because it showed that many of the old theories were incorrect and misleading and that research must concentrate on the mechanisms that lead to normal and abnormal distribution of chromosomes during gametogenesis and during the earliest cell divisions of the young embryo. But we are still far from a true understanding of the causes of nondisjunction and translocation, and prevention of Down syndrome—the true test of understanding etiology—is not yet in sight. In place of the many etiologic theories of the past, we must expect a similar abundance of theories concerned with causation of abnormal cytogenetic behavior. Possible causes have been separated into those independent of the mother's age (Class A) and those influenced by the mother's age (Class B).[12] In Class A belong secondary nondisjunction in mothers with fully developed Down syndrome or with standard trisomy mosaicism, translocations, genes tending to produce nondisjunction and environmental influences such as exposure to infection[133-135] or to irradiation.[136] In Class B belong nondisjunction during oogenesis and possibly unknown factors present in very young mothers of mongoloids.[12]

A relationship between the presence of maternal thyroid antibodies and the birth of aneuploid children has been considered. It was found in some studies that mothers of mongoloid children had thyroid autoantibodies more often than mothers of controls. The increase of antibodies was noted particularly in mothers who were under 35 years of age and in those who had mongoloids of the nontrisomic type.[213] There has been a suggestion that an association exists between epidemics of infectious hepatitis and the birth of children with Down syndrome. The serum of patients who had infectious hepatitis was studied by Dallaire *et al.*[214] It was found that thyroid antibodies are present in a large number of patients with hepatitis shortly after the onset of the disease. These authors believed that an immunologic mechanism may be involved in meiotic nondisjunction, leading to Down syndrome. Interpretations of these findings are still at variance and investigations proceed along these lines.[231]

If one looks back at the reasoning concerning the etiology of mongolism before 1959, one finds that the investigators who proffered genetic explanations and timed the origin of the disturbance at or before the time of conception based their opinion on twin observations that showed that monozygotic twins were concordant, whereas dizygotic twins usually were discordant (p. 315). Curiously, subsequent cytogenetic experience showed that the reasoning that led to correct hypotheses was not quite correct. It was learned that occasionally monozygotic twins can be discordant for mongolism[189,210] as the result of faulty mitosis of a zygote. Turpin and Lejeune[189] spoke of "monozygotisme heterocaryote" in such cases.

Much of the recent work concerned with the etiology of mongolism deals with epidemiologic findings. A review of these investigations was published by Lilienfeld in 1969.[215]

Clinical and Pathologic Characteristics

Although Down syndrome is a well-established disease picture in which nearly every organ differs more or less from the normal, the picture is not easily described, since every anomaly found in these patients can be seen occasionally in normal people or in persons with other mental or physical defects.

As a rule, mongoloids are lighter and smaller at birth than normal babies,[137] but many have normal birth weight and length. Their postnatal growth is retarded. According to Benda,[7] the retardation is most conspicuous during the first 3 years. After a period of better growth during the following years, the retardation becomes increasingly apparent during adolescence, and at the end of that period few of the patients exceed 150 cm.

HEAD.—The head is small and round and the occipital area flat. At birth, the cranial sutures are wide, the anterior fontanelle is large and the posterior fontanelle open. A third fontanelle along the sagittal suture is not rare. The fontanelles are late in closing. This distinguishes Down syndrome from microcephaly. The cephalic index, which is obtained by dividing the breadth of the skull by its length and multiplying the result by 100, is increased because of the shortness of the skull. Although it normally is between 75 and 79, it is 80 or over in mongolism.

Many studies have been made of the cranium and its growth. A critical review was published by Roche,[138] who presented an extensive bibliography. At birth, cranial size and brain weight are about the same in mongoloid as in normal children, but their growth is slow during the first years of life. Cranial growth is fair between 3 and 6 years but there is no corresponding increase in brain weight. Ossification of the fibrous cranial capsule is slow, as manifested by slow closing of fontanelles and sutures and by slow thickening of the bones. The cranial base is short because of depressed growth at the spheno-occipital synchondrosis.[138]

BRAIN.—Although the brain of children with Down syndrome has long been the subject of anatomic and histologic research, no specific neuropathologic picture has emerged as characteristic of the condition. The reports available are varied and they appear contradictory in many respects. This situation, once baffling and difficult to understand, can now be accepted in the light of observations of variability in other trisomy syndromes which show that an extra chromosome may result in a clinically recognizable disease picture that can vary in regard to malformations of single organs such as the heart, the kidney, the brain and others. Such variability is also present in children with Down syndrome, and it is not surprising that no distinctive neuropathologic picture has been found regularly associated with trisomy 21. It is also understandable that certain anomalies of the central nervous system reported by some investigators could not be confirmed by others.

Fraser,[139] in 1876, described the brain of an adult with Down syndrome as small, asymmetrical and characterized by flat convolutions and simple gyri. Hill[140] found the cortex thinned and myelin fibers and nerve cells scarce. Many studies were made by French investigators early in this century. They were summarized by Apert,[141] who stated that in necropsies no well-marked lesions visible to the naked eye are discernible but that the brain is small and globular, like the skull. The anterior parts of the brain are comparatively less developed than the posterior and lateral parts. The brain is simplified, resembling that of an animal. The most striking microscopic feature is paucity of cells in the cerebral cortex. The processes of the nerve cells are few in number and short, with scanty ramifications. Not infrequently, pyramidal cells are heterotopic and situated far from the cortex in the midst of the white matter. Although agenesis of the cellular elements of the cortex is the main lesion, it is difficult to say whether it is primary and followed by secondary vascular and meningeal reactions or whether the cellular deficiency is secondary to meningovascular changes.

In 1928, Brousseau[5] and Davidoff[142] reviewed the literature. Davidoff, reporting 10 cases, found few constant morphologic changes, with the exception of a small cerebellum and brain stem, an embryonic convolutional pattern and a small content of ganglion cells of the third cortical layer. In one case there was porencephaly, a tuber flocculi and misplaced large ganglion cells. Benda[143] stressed the need for separation of findings in infants and young children from those of older patients who have confusing degenerative and secondary changes. In contrast to many other authors, he believed that the neuropathology of mongolism is quite uniform and characteristic despite the variations in degree of the changes. There is hypoplasia of the frontal poles with retroflexion and "compression" of the temporal and occipital poles. The brain stem, medulla and cerebellum are hypoplastic, appearing pushed forward and originating almost anteriorly to the center of the brain. Benda found the loss of nerve cells not restricted to one layer but dependent on the vascular conditions. The nuclei are swollen and surrounded by bright halos of watery cytoplasm showing confluence in areas where nerve cells have more or less disappeared. "This picture is typical for almost every section from infants below the age of 9 months." The white matter appears moth-eaten, the fibers being interrupted by numerous small patches of necrosis. Degenerative processes in the white matter can be observed early. Benda also described changes in the spinal cord identical with those seen in myelodysplasia. He thought that the spinal cord is never normal but that the degree of pathology varies. In addition, there are changes in the central canal and fetal configuration of gray matter with lack of separation of Clarke's columns. Various degrees of hydromyelia, shaft ependymopathy and true syringomyelia are not rare. Some of the illustrations show asymmetry of the anterior horns and partly or completely missing posterior horns. But such changes obviously are not found in all children with Down syndrome, since, for instance, the most conspicuous malformation of the spinal cord observed by Benda was in a mongoloid with congential clubfeet, an anomaly not typical for this disorder. Jacob[144] described reduction of the angle between the brain stem and the brain as 80–100 degrees instead of 110–120 degrees, as in the normal. Hypoplasia of the hypothalamus or the mamillary bodies sometimes is noticeable. The ganglion cells in the cerebral cortex may be reduced in number and appear immature and fetal in type. The cell deficiencies differ in different lobes, but there is no agreement concerning the areas most affected. Hilliard and Kirman[145] stated that the neuropathologic changes in Down syndrome usually are diffuse and rather nonspecific. The brain often is round when viewed from above, and the frontal lobes, brain stem and cerebellum are small. The ratio of the weight of the cerebrum to that of the cerebellum plus brain stem is increased. This finding confirms the statement of older investigators, who found the brain stem and cerebellum particularly reduced in size. Hilliard and Kirman considered the evidence for simplification of gyral patterns insufficient. Some authors reported sparseness and others excessive density of cortical cells. Patients with Down syndrome may be more likely than other persons to develop incidental secondary lesions because of frequent congenital heart disease, embolism and cerebral abscess. Solitare and Lamarch[146] described in 5 adults with Down syndrome neuropathologic changes consistent with the diagnosis of Alzheimer disease (presenile dementia).

From the numerous reports available, one can conclude that the abnormalities of the central nervous system of patients with Down syndrome are varied and inconstant. It has been said[144] that there probably are no two mongoloid brains that are alike. It is futile to look for a description of "the mongoloid brain." It seems more fruitful to register the many neuropathologic aberrations and malformations resulting from trisomy 21, to classify them and to establish their variability.

Neurologic signs in mongoloids are not distinctive. The reflexes are variable. Diseases of the central nervous system rarely are associated with mongolism. Epilepsy is not more frequent than in the general population. The gait and posture of adult patients with Down syndrome are characteristic. They walk with a stoop and unsteadily. Movements are slow and

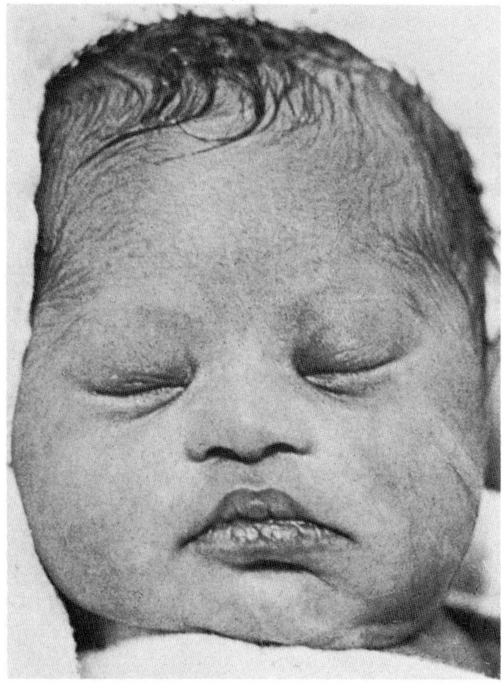

Fig. 37-22.—Newborn child with Down syndrome.

coordination is poor. Pathologic neurologic signs and symptoms can be observed in the majority of patients with Down syndrome, increasing in frequency and intensity with increasing age. Hypotonia decreases as the patients grow older. In general, pathologic reactions parallel the mental impairment and are most pronounced in patients with the lowest intelligence.[211]

Mental development.—There are variations in mental development,[147] but a general description characteristic of the type can be given. In infancy, the mongoloid child is quiet and placid (Fig. 37-22). Movements of the tongue and grimacing must not be mistaken for early facial expressions. Most mongoloids sleep a great deal and do not take or demand food as normal children do. They sit up and walk late. Talking may be delayed for years, and when they learn to speak they pronounce either simple words or short sentences but are not able to converse. Their attention span and power of concentration are low and memory generally is poor, although exceptions occur. Ability to learn is limited, but they often are observant, curious and able to imitate. Generally, mongoloids are cheerful, love music, dance and are well liked because they are good-natured, affectionate and responsive to love. There are some unfortunate exceptions of mongoloids who are restless, aggressive and destructive. Psychoses are rare. The degree of the mental defect varies to some extent and prognosis of mentality is difficult. In general, mongoloids with severe physical defects also show more marked mental deficiency. The mental development is influenced to a certain degree by the environment.

Usually, mongoloids living at home and in the community are superior to those in institutions. Some of them learn to read and to write, but they are poor in arithmetic. Although they love music, they do not learn to play an instrument. Many are capable of performing household chores and errands. As a rule, they are reliable and show no tendency to lie, steal or be violent.

Many studies have been made to evaluate the mentality of patients with Down syndrome by intelligence tests.[5,9,12,148-150] Such studies are difficult and results vary greatly. In mongoloids in hospitals, mean I.Q. values of 23 were reported,[12] wheras in those living in the community the mean I.Q. may be 44.[150] Whereas in Brousseau's[5] study 38% were classified as idiots (I.Q. below 25), only 10% tested as low in Øster's[9] study. Of mongoloids living in the community, only 5% were classified as idiots.[150] It is not clear whether the difference between institutionalized and clinic patients is due to removal of the severe forms to institutions or whether living in the community can improve the performance of the patient significantly. In institutions, only about 2% rated above imbecile level (I.Q. 50),[5,8] whereas in the community more than 20% reached higher levels.[150] For a recent review of this difficult subject, the reader is referred to the book by Penrose and Smith.[12]

FACE.—The appearance of the eyes contributes greatly to the character of the mongoloid facies. Much has been said and written about the epicanthic fold of patients with Down syndrome since Down had noticed it and considered it an attribute of the Mongolian race. Now it is stated that the epicanthic fold of Mongolian peoples is continuous with the pars orbitalis as it sweeps down over the inner angle of the eye and covers the pars tarsalis, whereas in mongoloids—patients with Down syndrome—the fold arises within the pars orbitalis and courses downward without covering the pars tarsalis. But the difference in epicanthic folds cannot be recommended for the differentiation of a Mongolian from a "mongoloid." There are millions of Mongolian people and their epicanthic folds vary greatly, there are older patients with Down syndrome who have no epicanthic folds (Fig. 37-23) and Oriental children with Down syndrome may have epicanthic folds resembling those of normal Oriental children.[12,151,152] Many normal children of toddler age have apparent hypertelorism and epicanthic folds like patients with Down syndrome, a fact that often confuses and worries the young pediatrician. The palpebral fissures of mongoloids run upward and outward. They often are narrow with drooping eyelids, which gives the face a somewhat tired expression. Under the lower eyelid, one or two horizontal skin creases often are present that run from the inner angle of the eye laterad, a peculiarity that contributes to the appearance of the mongoloid newborn.

Gifford[151] devoted an interesting article to the Mongolian eye. Slanting eyes are not frequent among Mongolian peoples (except possibly in the Kyoto district of Japan), but there is narrowness of the fissure combined with fullness and width of the space below the eyebrow and the margin of the fissure. For some reason, Japanese artists have selected persons with eyes of exaggerated obliqueness and upward and outward extended eyebrows for their woodcuts and theatrical masks.[151] Personally, I was quite happy to observe that there are only a very few ladies in Japan who have the formidable slant of the eyes that prevails in Japanese art.

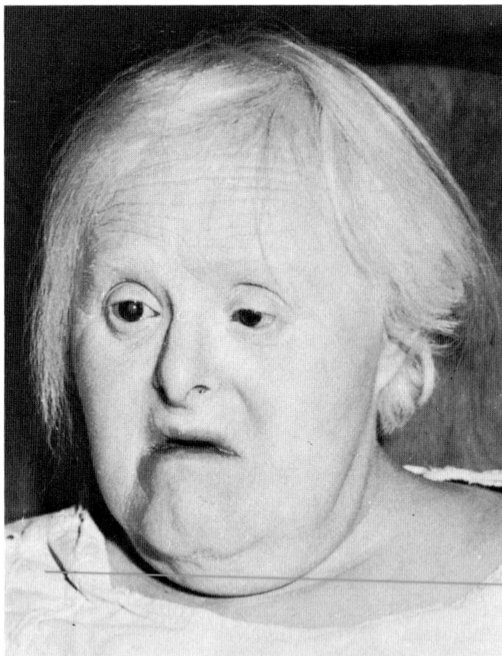

Fig. 37-23.—Down syndrome in a woman 63 years of age. Cataract visible in right eye.

Because of the epicanthic folds, which make the nasal root appear broad, the eyes seem widely separated, and "hypertelorism" often is described clinically. Actually, hypotelorism exists in most cases, as is shown in roentgenograms that reveal reduction of the interorbital distance in Down syndrome.[153]

Convergent strabismus is frequent in Down syndrome, divergent strabismus rare. It has been estimated to occur in one-third of the patients.[154] Nystagmus, which is present in about 15% of the patients,[155] is attributed to ocular or cerebral defects. It is seen more often in severe than in mild cases of Down syndrome. Refractive errors are common. If the irides are light, one often sees white nodules of pinpoint size placed at regular intervals in a ring near the outer margin. These so-called Brushfield spots are said to be present in all mongoloid children with blue eyes and to disappear when the color changes to brown. They also can be seen in normal infants, and their diagnostic value is not great. Congenital lamellar cataract is rare and occurs in not more than 3% of

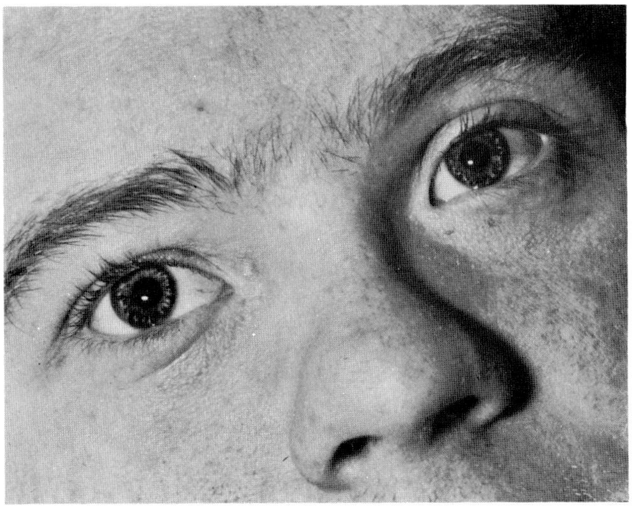

Fig. 37-24. – Brushfield spots of the iris in a 25-year-old patient with Down syndrome.

mongoloids but, in patients over 8 years of age, flake-like and punctate opacities develop frequently.[4,156] There is a marked tendency to conjunctivitis, blepharitis and ectropion. In many patients with Down syndrome, epicanthic folds and slanting of the eyes disappear with advancing age. Blindness is found in approximately 5% of institutionalized patients.[157] It occurs more often in older mongoloids owing to development of cataracts and to keratoconus. Detailed descriptions of ocular changes in patients with Down syndrome can be found on page 374.

The nose is short and button-shaped, the bridge depressed and the nostrils face forward. The mucous membranes often are infected and a purulent discharge erodes the skin of the upper lip. The nasopharynx is narrow and the tonsils and adenoids usually are enlarged. The nasal sinuses are underdeveloped.[158] The palatal vaults appear of normal height but they are narrow; the palatal length is greatly reduced.[159]

The behavior of the tongue aids in the diagnosis, particularly in the newborn period, when the tongue is constantly pushed forward and then withdrawn. This, combined with the characteristic grimacing that often is mistaken by lay persons for smiles or early facial expression, leads the experienced observer to early recognition of the disorder. Later, the tongue becomes large and fissured. In older mongoloids, the lips are thick, everted and cracked. Dentition usually is delayed and teeth are irregular in size, shape and position, with a tendency to early decay and early loss. Gingivitis and pyorrhea are frequent and salivation is marked. Occlusal anomalies and periodontal disorders are common.[160]

The external ears are situated low and appear "round" rather than oblong. The helix often is broad and folded over the anthelix and the lobule is missing. Sometimes the right and left ear differ greatly in shape. The external canal, which usually is narrow, should always be tested for patency. Betlejewski *et al.*[161] compared the external ears of 100 mongoloids with those of 200 controls and made quantitative studies. The ear in Down syndrome is further discussed on page 409. The voice usually is harsh and hoarse.

NECK, TRUNK AND ABDOMEN.—The neck is broad and flat. In newborn mongoloids, the skin around the

Fig. 37-25. – Boy with Down syndrome showing epicanthic folds and protruding tongue.

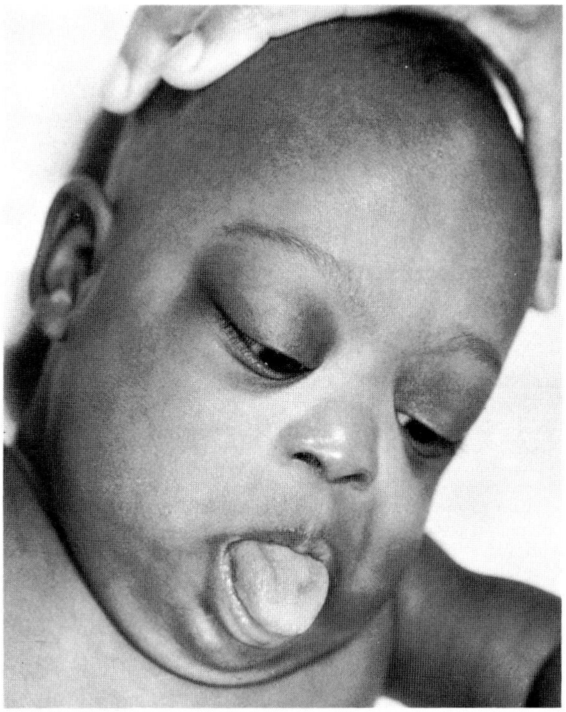

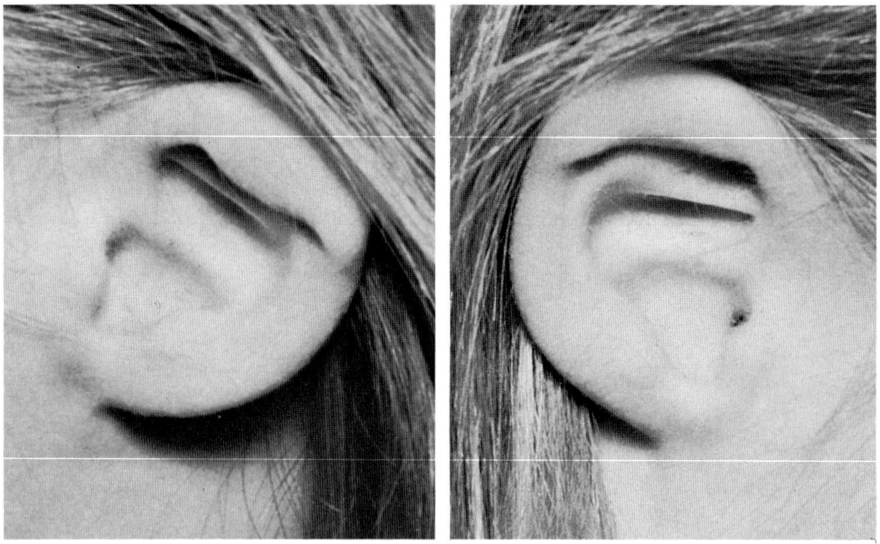

Fig. 37-26. – A frequent form of auricles in Down syndrome: "round ear" with overhanging upper helix.

neck often is loose and forms folds. Occiput, neck and back lie in one plane, a very characteristic and almost diagnostic feature in older patients. The curvatures of the spine often are not well pronounced. In many mongoloids, the vertebral arches are not closed.[162] Dislocation of the atlas was observed by Martel and Tishler[163] in 20% of these patients of various ages. "Scheuermann-like" lesions may be present in young adult mongoloids. Two or three ossification centers sometimes are seen in the manubrium sterni within the first few years. The multiple centers revealed in lateral chest roentgenograms show no significant relationship to congenital heart disease.[164, 165] Absence of one pair of ribs has been observed repeatedly.[166]

Congenital heart disease is an important feature of Down syndrome, but reliable estimates of its frequency in mongoloids are hard to find, since they vary according to age of the patient and with diagnostic methods. The most serious cardiovascular anomalies result in early death and are, therefore, not encountered in older, institutionalized patients. Necropsies (Table 37-8) cannot be considered representative of the entire population with mongolism, since they include too many patients with congenital heart disease who entered hospitals because of cardiac failure and related diseases. Even in necropsy series there are marked variations according to the age composition. Ostium atrioventriculare commune (p. 485) was thought to be typical for Down syndrome. Although this anomaly is found in mongoloids more often than in other children with cardiac defects, it is not the leading heart lesion in mongolism. Ventricular and atrial septal defects and patent ductus arteriosus are more common than atrioventricularis communis. Details concerning the cardiovascular system in Down syndrome are given on page 576.

TABLE 37-8. – Cardiovascular Malformations, Trisomy 21 (272 Necropsies)

Ventricular septal defect	68	Transposition of the great vessels	6
Atrial septal defect	61	Truncus arteriosus	3
Patent ductus arteriosus	35	Coarctation of the aorta	3
Atrioventricularis communis	27	Abnormal aortic valve	3
Ostium primum	24	Eisenmenger complex	3
Abnormal mitral valve	19	Cor triloculare	3
Abnormal tricuspid valve	17	Pulmonic stenosis	2
Abnormal pulmonary valve	11	Endocardial fibroelastosis	2
Foramen ovale	7	Left superior vena cava	1
Tetralogy of Fallot	7	Aberrant right subclavian artery	1

A number of congenital malformations occur more often in children with Down syndrome than in the general population. Esophageal atresia, annular pancreas and exomphalos belong in this category.[232–234]

Intestinal anomalies are not rare, and many cases of duodenal occlusion have been reported (p. 694)[167]; imperforate anus and megacolon can also occur. It seems that about 2% of all children with Hirschsprung disease have Down syndrome, but few patients with Down syndrome have Hirschsprung disease (approximately 0.5%).[168]

Genitalia and endocrine glands. – The genitalia usually are underdeveloped. In boys, the testes remain undescended in many cases. Maturation is slow in both sexes. In girls, the genitalia often remain infantile and the breasts develop late. Menstruation begins late and ceases early. Precocious puberty occurs in rare instances. Female patients with Down syndrome reproduce only in exceptional cases, but at least 14 completed pregnancies have been reported

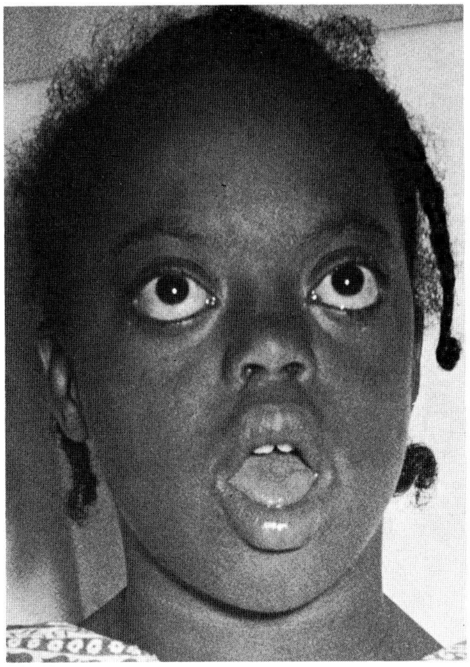

Fig. 37-27. – Girl with Down syndrome and hyperthyroidism.

(p. 321). An extensive literature exists on the pathology of the endocrine glands, particularly of the thyroid and the pituitary. Although the reports are contradictory,[7,8] it can safely be assumed that these glands are in some ways pathologic, just as other organs of the body frequently are abnormal in mongoloids.[219,220] In the past, such endocrine anomalies were considered the cause of Down syndrome by some (p. 313), but it is not justified to attribute the syndrome to disturbances of the endocrine glands that constitute only a symptom but not the cause of the disorder. Hypothyroidism as well as hyperthyroidism can occur (Fig. 37-27). Hypothyroidism and precocious puberty have been described in an 8-year-old girl with Down syndrome.[221] In the newborn period, the skin is soft but later it becomes rough and dry. There is a lack of normal secretion, and dermatitis and eczema develop. The hair, which is at first normal, later becomes dry and stiff. Mongoloid patients turn gray early.

THE PELVIS. – In young mongoloid infants, Caffey and Ross[169] observed flattening of the acetabular roofs and widening of the iliac wings and bodies. The acetabular angles (formed by a line connecting the two ends of the caudal edge of the ilium and by the Y-Y line drawn through the two Y cartilages) and the iliac angles (formed by a line connecting the lateral end of the lower edge of the ilium with the outermost point of the lateral edge of the ilium and by the Y-Y line) are greatly reduced in mongoloid children throughout the first year. The mongoloid pelvis generally is smaller than the normal. The iliac wings are shortened cephalocaudally and there are coxa valga deformities in the femurs. The ischial rami lag in growth during the first 6 months. They appear slender and tapering in contrast to the heavy normal ischia.[170] Kaufmann[171] made a statistical and anatomic study of mongoloid pelves and emphasized the diagnostic value of roentgenograms in the newborn period, particularly in prematures. He stated that in 4 out of 5 cases Down syndrome can be diagnosed from roentgenograms of the pelvis. After 3–6 months of age, hypoplasia of the ischia with valgus postion of the femora becomes noticeable, and abnormal features of the mongoloid pelvis persist throughout life. The diagnostic value of the pelvic findings in the newborn period is considerable, but before the diagnosis of

Fig. 37-28. – **A,** diagram of pelvis showing acetabular (*a*) and iliac (*i*) angles. **B,** pelvis of newborn with Down syndrome. The ilium is short in craniocaudal and wide in transverse diameter. The acetabular roof is flat and nearly horizontal.

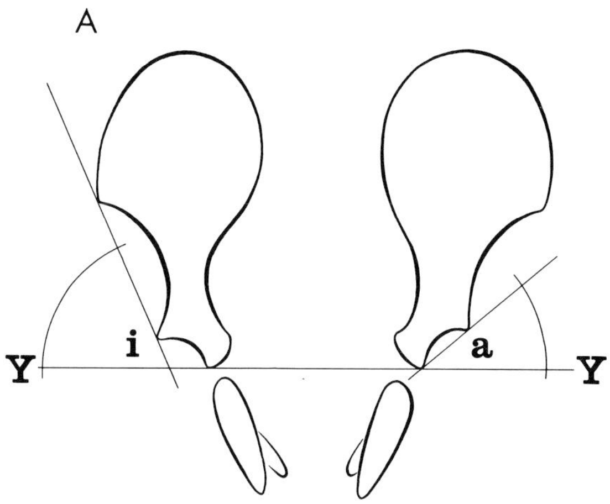

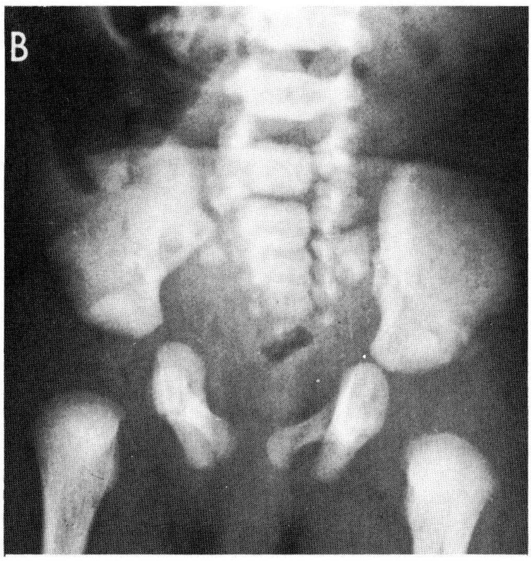

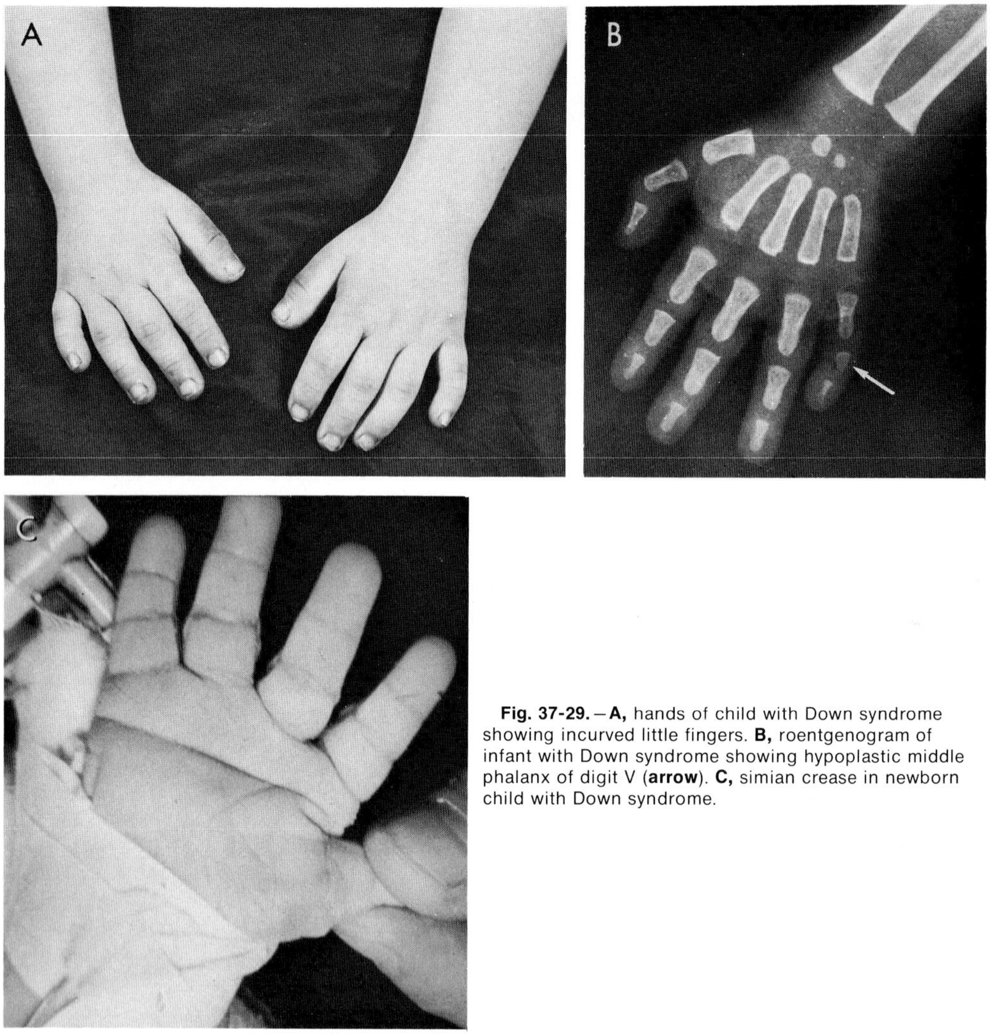

Fig. 37-29. – **A,** hands of child with Down syndrome showing incurved little fingers. **B,** roentgenogram of infant with Down syndrome showing hypoplastic middle phalanx of digit V (**arrow**). **C,** simian crease in newborn child with Down syndrome.

Down syndrome can be based on the roentgenographic findings alone, the latter must be compared not only with those of normal children but also with deviations seen in abnormal children of various kinds.

EXTREMITIES. – The hands are plump, the fingers stubby and the thumbs and fifth fingers short. Incurving of the little fingers is present in about half of the older mongoloids, but it seldom is recognizable at birth; it is also found in about 5% of normal children. The middle phalanx of the little finger is small and the digit may have one instead of two flexion creases. The so-called simian line (or 4-finger crease) is present in about 50% of mongoloids and in 2% of normal individuals and various types of feeble-minded people.[8] The distal palmar crease, which normally runs from the ulnar margin of the hand to the base of the index finger, is absent and the middle crease takes a transverse course (Fig. 37-29, *C*). The simian crease is unilateral in many mongoloids. Absence of the entire hand occurs in exceptional cases (Fig. 37-30). Cummins *et al.*,[172] in 1950, found that the dermal ridges, which, in the normal palm, take a generally diagonal course from the base of the index finger to the proximal portion of the hypothenar, show a marked tendency to transversality in the mongoloid. These ridges contribute to formation of a central (distal) triradius that is rather characteristic of Down syndrome (see Fig. 37-32).

The toes often terminate distally in a straight line and there is a cleft between the first and second toes (Fig. 37-31). But this anomaly, characteristic of older patients, is not specific in infancy, since many normal babies show a more or less pronounced distance between the first two toes. Syndactyly is not rare. Lax ligaments and hypertonicity of the muscles result in the overextensibility of joints so characteristic of Down syndrome. After children with Down syndrome learn to sit up, they often bend forward and place

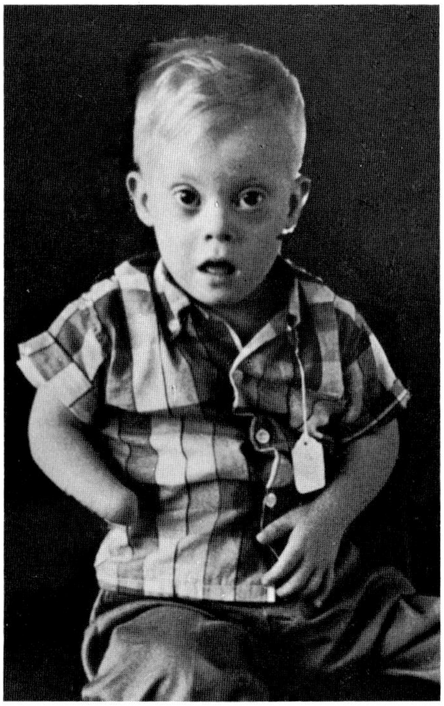

Fig. 37-30.—Absence of the right hand in a boy with Down syndrome.

their head and trunk between their abducted legs. Knock-knees and flat feet develop. Reduction in height is due chiefly to shortness of the lower extremities. Growth of long bones was studied by Rarick *et al.*[173] The tibiae at age 7 were about 4 years behind the standard, but the annual increments were within normal limits. Epiphyseal closure usually is delayed, paralleling pubertal development. The shortness of the legs cannot be attributed to premature epiphyseal closure.

Fig. 37-31.—Feet of patient with Down syndrome showing space between toes I and II.

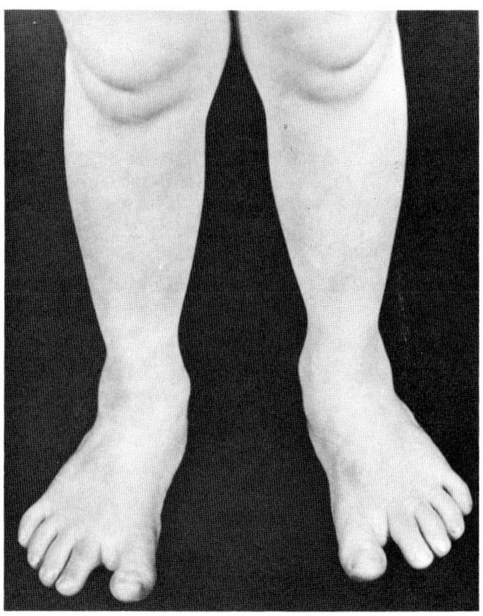

Dermatoglyphics

With other morphologic changes of the extremities there are alterations of the dermal ridge patterns on the digits, palms and soles of patients with Down syndrome. As with other signs, the alterations of the dermatoglyphics are variable and therefore of diagnostic value only as a part of the whole disease picture. In doubtful cases they may be dubious too. There is no definitive dermatoglyphic pattern of Down syndrome. Variations exist in males and females, on the right and on the left side and in individual cases. For statistical variations and formulas useful in the diagnosis of Down syndrome the reader is referred to detailed articles on the subject.[12, 174-177]

The frequencies of the dermal ridge patterns on the fingers of mongoloids differ from those in the general population. Patients with Down syndrome have few whorls, few arches and a reduced number of radial loops. There is an increased frequency of ulnar loops,[174] which are seen in more than 80% of the fingers of mongoloids. In fact, between 30% and 40% of the patients have ulnar loops on all 10 fingers. Normally, a palmar triradius is formed by dermal ridges between the thenar and hypothenar near the flexion creases of the wrist. Mongoloids often have a more distal triradius located in the central area of the palm (t' or t''). The angle formed by the most distal palmar triradius and the triradiuses at the bases of digits II and V (*atd*) angle is much larger in mongoloids than in normal persons. The sum of the maximal *atd* angles has been used by Penrose for quantitative comparisons of palmar ridge patterns in mongoloids and controls. It was noted that, if this measurement were the sole means of diagnosis, only 12% of patients with Down syndrome would be wrongly classified.[177] More than 90% of the patients have a pattern in the third interdigital area between the bases of the middle and ring fingers.

On the soles, tibial arches occur in nearly half the patients, a characteristic seen in less than 1% of controls. A distal loop in the fourth interdigital area is two to three times more common in mongoloids than in controls.[12, 176] In mosaic mongoloids, dermatoglyphic patterns are intermediate between fully affected patients and controls.[12]

Biochemical Data

After the discovery of extra chromosomal material contained in every cell of mongoloids, it was hoped to find specific metabolic changes that would correspond to the cytologic alterations. It was hoped partic-

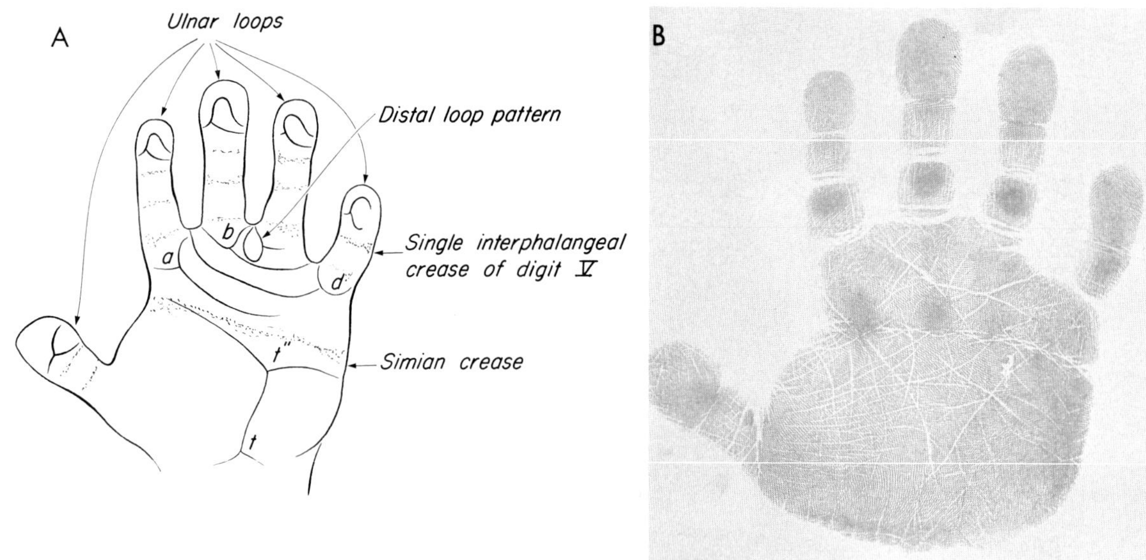

Fig. 37-32.—Dermatoglyphics of a 2-year-old boy with Down syndrome.

ularly that "triple enzyme doses" might be discovered that could be attributed to the extra chromosome 21. There have been claims along these lines but it is too early to accept them as proved, since they have not always been confirmed or found to be specific for Down syndrome. Gershoff *et al.*[178] reported that following an oral tryptophan load children with mongolism excreted in the urine less of the tryptophan metabolite xanthurenic acid than nonmongoloid controls. Jérôme *et al.*[179] noted in mongoloids decreased excretion of xanthurenic, indoleacetic and 5-hydroxyindoleacetic acid following a tryptophan load. Based on these findings, several theories were developed to coordinate the chemical deviations with theories of triple enzyme doses. Unfortunately, some of the basic observations could not be duplicated.[180] When a pyridoxine antagonist was administered, tryptophan load caused the mongoloid children to excrete greater amounts of xanthurenic acid and 3-HO-kynurenine than the controls, which suggested that the mongoloid is more sensitive to pyridoxine deficiency than the normal child.[180] Blood serotonin values of trisomic mongoloid children were found to be as low as those of normal infants.[181,182] Signs of depressed tryptophan metabolism in the normal newborn and the mongoloid child still need clarification, and effects on cerebral metabolism are still hypothetical. It is curious that whole blood serotonin was diminished in trisomic mongolism but normal in translocation cases.[183] The mean value of galactose-1-phosphate-uridyl transferase was found to be about 50% higher in mongoloid patients than in normals.[184] For this enzyme, similar elevations were noted in trisomy 21 and in translocation mongoloids but also in nonmongoloid oligophrenics. Hsia *et al.*[185] reported that the transferase activity was increased in leukocytes but not in red cells of mongoloids. Baikie *et al.*[186] found an increase of erythrocyte-phosphohexokinase in mongolism, but other erythrocyte enzymes showed normal activity. Leukocyte alkaline phosphatase was elevated in mongoloids over that of controls,[187] but there was overlap in the distributions in the two groups and elevation proved to be nonspecific for Down syndrome. In fact, elevated leukocyte alkaline phosphatase has also been observed in so-called antimongolism.[188] Hyperuricemia in Down syndrome was reported by Pant *et al.*[235] Interpretation of increased leukocyte phosphatase activity as a marker for chromosome 21 seems to be premature. The same is true for galactose transferase and other enzyme changes reported in Down syndrome. It must be admitted that such determinations are still of very limited value in the diagnosis of the disorder.[184] Many other chemical data have been gathered from patients with Down syndrome and normal values have been recorded for many constituents of blood and urine. For other elements and compounds contradictory results were obtained or abnormal values were noted not only in mongoloid but also in other oligophrenic patients. There have been findings of abnormal glucose tolerance, vitamin A resorption and cerebral oxygen consumption in patients with Down syndrome but they cannot be considered as specific or diagnostic. Some biochemical deviations noted were due to institutionalization or to dietary habits of the mentally defective. Before chemical changes can be accepted as specific they have to be compared with values of mentally normal and of nonmongoloid defective controls. Reviews of biochemical data in Down syndrome are available.[12,189,190]

Blood

Routine blood examination results are normal as a rule, but anemia is not rare. The blood group distribution is not different from that of the normal population. Attempts to locate the ABO locus on chromosome 21 were not successful.[12] The total leukocyte count is within normal limits. The lymphocyte count is low in the age group 3–6 years and the neutrophil count is elevated correspondingly.[143] The mean lobe count of circulating polymorphonuclear cells is lower in mongoloids than in normal males.[191,192] There is also a reduced incidence of drumsticks in female mongoloids.

LEUKEMIA.—In 1930, Brewster and Cannon[193] reported a case of Down syndrome associated with acute lymphatic leukemia, and 17 years later Ingalls[194] mentioned, as a curiosity, that 2 of 50 necropsied children with that syndrome died of leukemia. Subsequently it was found that the occurrence of the combined disorders was many times higher than that which might be expected to result from chance association. Krivit and Good,[195] after a survey in the United States, thought that the actual occurrence of simultaneous leukemia and Down syndrome was approximately three times higher than that to be expected from chance association. Stewart *et al.*[196] noted, in a survey of childhood malignancies, that 17 of 677 children with leukemia had Down syndrome, which was about twelve to fifteen times that of the prevalence of Down syndrome for the age group involved. In an analysis of deaths of 136 children with Down syndrome by Carter,[19] 3 were attributed to leukemia. Occurrence of leukemia in institutionalized patients with Down syndrome is many times above that in the general population, but variations of leukemia risks have been observed in different places.[222,223] The hematologic picture of the leukemias in mongolism is variable. When we reviewed the subject,[197] in 31 cases the leukemia was thought to be acute lymphogenous and in 18 myelogenous; 4 were diagnosed as stem-cell leukemia, 2 as monocytic, 1 as aleukemia and 1 as atypical acute. Thus, the type of leukemia associated with Down syndrome is not specific. In a number of cases, aneuploid karyotypes have been seen before clinical leukemia developed.[198-200] It is of interest that in some mongoloid children leukemoid reactions occur that imitate acute myeloblastic leukemia but result in hematologic recovery.[201,202] In a number of cases, leukemia was congenital in patients with Down syndrome.[197]

Down syndrome and leukemia have alternated in the same family.[203] Miller,[204] surveying 1,000 sibs of leukemic children, found that 5 had Down syndrome; one of the patients with Down syndrome also had leukemia. In some families, a tendency to leukemia, Down syndrome and other conditions characterized by chromosomal anomalies has been reported.[205]

Advanced age of the mother at the birth of the patient was recorded in some cases of leukemia in Down syndrome, which suggests that advanced maternal age, known as an etiologic factor in Down syndrome, may also be a factor in the etiology of some leukemias. MacMahon and Newill,[206] studying birth characteristics of children dying of malignant neoplasms, found the risk of death from leukemia to be greater with increasing maternal age.

In most cases of Down syndrome complicated by leukemia the karyotype is trisomy 21, but the combined disorders have also been observed in patients who have 46 chromosomes with D/G or G/G translocation Down syndrome.[203,207,208] The karyotypes of cells derived from skin or other tissues, with the exception of blood, correspond to the karyotypes mentioned. But, in leukocytes derived from peripheral blood, cell lines with 48, 49, 51 and 54 chromosomes have been described.[17,197] In some of these cases, the chromosome count returned to 47 or 46 after treatment.[197] It is possible that some of these variations in chromosome count are due to variations of techniques and depend on the duration of the leukocyte culture.

Differential Diagnosis

Considering the great variability of the syndrome, it is surprising how seldom an incorrect diagnosis of mongolism is made by experienced physicians or nurses. Even in the newborn period, the round head, the appearance of the eyes, the movements of the tongue and the flaccidity of the joints usually are sufficient for an early diagnosis. It is rather rare that a child diagnosed as a mongoloid by a trained observer develops normal mentality, but exceptional cases do occur.[209] I saw one girl of high school age who had been diagnosed in infancy by a competent pediatrician as a definite mongoloid. She still had marked mongoloid features, but she was a good student. These observations were made before cytogenetic examinations could be done, but even now children are seen occasionally who have features of Down syndrome—including mental retardation—without having chromosomal anomalies. In some of these children, mosaicism explains the dilemma but in others no cells with trisomy 21 can be detected (p. 320). Although pronounced mongoloid features are rare in normal children, they occur more often under pathologic conditions. Children with congenital heart disease sometimes have hypertelorism, epicanthic folds and other mongoloid characteristics. Slanting of the eyes can be marked in trigonocephaly. A superficial resemblance occurs also in congenital syphilis or after intrauterine x-ray damage (p. 82). Many normal children have widely spaced eyes and epicanthic folds at toddler age. The difficulty in differentiating between cretinism and mongolism has been emphasized by many authors. Cretinism is rarely recognizable at birth. In contrast to the mongoloid with his lively facial movements, the cretin is immobile and dull.

His tongue is large but not in constant motion. He does not show the characteristic palmar creases, the incurved little finger and the hyperextensibility of the joints. Hair and skin are dry and the temperature is low. The cretin responds to thyroid treatment well, whereas the mongoloid shows little improvement; in case of doubt, however, thyroid treatment is always indicated. Roentgenograms help in the diagnosis and differential diagnosis.

The responsibility for diagnosing Down syndrome in the newborn period is great, since an error could have grave consequences. It is often thought that the diagnosis in the newborn period is particularly difficult. This, however, is not the case, as pointed out by Hall,[11] who made a valuable study of mongolism in newborns. In this study, 38 mongoloid newborn children were compared, symptom by symptom, with 40 controls. Of special control value was the analysis of 5 children suspected of Down syndrome but found to be cytogenetically normal. Hall chose the following ten signs as cardinal in the newborn period: (1) lack of Moro reflex, (2) muscle hypotonia, (3) flat facial profile, (4) oblique palpebral fissures, (5) abnormal ears, (6) abundant neck skin, (7) typical or atypical simian crease, (8) hyperflexibility, (9) abnormal pelvis, (10) abnormal middle phalanx of the fifth finger. The last two signs are ascertained roentgenologically. Hall believed that the iliac index is not a suitable diagnostic sign in newborn patients. Some signs usually described in children with Down syndrome were not chosen as cardinal in the neonate. Epicanthic folds are only slightly pronounced in the newborn mongoloid. The newborn patients do not have the flat occiput typical of older mongoloids, but the head is rounder than that of normal newborn children. Also, the head circumference is smaller than that of normals with corresponding birth weight. The pregnancy period is shorter for mongoloids than for normal infants and the birth weight lower than can be explained by the curtailed pregnancy period (intrauterine growth retardation). But when mongoloids are full term, the birth weight is not reduced. Hall thought that a chromosome study is not necessary for diagnosis when six or more of the cardinal signs are positive. Of great interest were suspected cases sent for study that proved to be cytogenetically normal. None of these children had six of the cardinal signs but 3 children had four. Two of these proved to be mentally retarded at age 1 year. Consideration of such "pseudomongoloid" patients shows that there is little danger of mistaking a normal child for a mongoloid; however, there are children with other physical and mental anomalies who can be mistakenly considered to have Down syndrome in the neonatal period.

Prevention

Despite great progress in etiologic research, no successful preventive measures have been developed as yet. Since the mechanisms leading to the chromosomal anomalies of mongolism are still not known (p. 323), rational prophylaxis is not yet possible. Genetic advice will be sought particularly by young mothers who have given birth to a child with Down syndrome or by young persons who have a relative with the disorder. Cytogenetic examinations sometimes may reveal the great risk for mongoloid offspring of some of these people. Others may be happy to learn that they are free of detectable cytogenetic abnormalities. The results of chromosome studies can be beneficial to some of these families, but the general incidence of Down syndrome will not be influenced greatly by measures taken after chromosome analysis. As pointed out before, most mongoloids have trisomy 21 and most of their mothers have normal karyotypes. But such normal parental karyotypes are not entirely reassuring (p. 323), since the recurrence risk is increased somewhat in such cases. Penrose and Smith[12] concluded from dermatoglyphic studies of mothers of mongoloids and from grandmaternal age studies that about 10% of all mothers of patients with Down syndrome could be mosaics. Recognition of trisomy 21 mosaicism with its increased risk for offspring would represent a dilemma for such women but provide no clear answer to their request for genetic prognosis.

The most important factor, advanced maternal age, cannot be eliminated easily. If no conception occurred after maternal age of 37 years, about one-third of all cases of mongolism would be prevented.[12] In Victoria, Australia, a shift of childbirth to younger mothers between 1939 and 1964 resulted in decreasing mean percentage incidences of mongoloid births.[212] But this is not the solution to the problem. Even mothers between 40 and 44 years have a chance of 99 to 1 of having a nonmongoloid child. With the prevention of each mongoloid, too many normal children would be deprived of existence. Until more accurate genetic predictions can be made than those now available, prophylaxis by genetic advice and birth control remains limited to a few exceptional cases.

Treatment

Although many suggestions have been made concerning treatment, no specific therapy has been found. In the successes claimed, deception and self-deception played a major role. A great deal can be achieved by symptomatic treatment. Correction of refractive errors, of strabismus, of orthopedic handicaps or of cardiac defects will improve the outlook for the child. Antibiotic treatment given in respiratory diseases overcomes crises that were fatal in years past. Thyroid treatment is indicated for those mongoloids who have symptoms of thyroid deficiency. Pituitary preparations given by mouth or injection have not resulted in improvement of these patients' handicaps. Much can be done for the child by teaching and by developing his capacities. Although he will not reach a normal mental level, he may become a useful and often beloved member of his family. Special education combined with living in the family and community results in significant improvement of the average patient. Many mongoloids can be taught some productive occupation; work in sheltered workshops or similar institutions is the best treatment for adults with Down syndrome. The parents deserve sound advice from their physician and help from their relatives and neighbors. Every affected family presents a different situation and there is no simple formula for their guidance. Much could be said about this part of the treatment, but this is not the place to do it.

REFERENCES

1. Séguin, E.: Traitement moral, Hygiène et Education des Idiots, Paris & London, 1846.
2. Down, J. L. H.: Observations on an ethnic classification of idiots, Clin. Lect. & Rep. London Hosp. 3:259, 1866.

3a. Lejeune, J., Gautier, M., and Turpin, R.: Les chromosomes humains en culture de tissus, Compt. rend. Acad. Sc. (Paris) 248:602, 1959.

3b. Lejeune, J., Gautier, M., and Turpin, R.: Étude des chromosomes somatiques de neuf enfants mongoliens, Compt. rend. Acad. Sc. (Paris) 248:1721, 1959.

4. Van der Scheer, W. M.: Beiträge zur Kenntnis der mongoloiden Missbildung, Neurol., Psychiat., Psychol. 41 (Berlin: S. Karger, 1927).
5. Brousseau, K.: *Mongolism* (Baltimore: The Williams & Wilkins Company, 1928).
6. Geyer, H.: *Zur Aetiologie der Mongoloiden Idiotie* (Leipzig: Georg Thieme, 1939).
7. Benda, C. E.: *Mongolism and Cretinism* (2d ed.; New York: Grune & Stratton, Inc., 1949).
8. Engler, M.: *Mongolism (Peristatic Amentia)* (Bristol, England: John Wright & Sons, Ltd., 1949).
9. Øster, J.: *Mongolism* (Opera ex domo biologiae hereditariae humanae Universitatis Hafniensis, vol. 32) (Copenhagen: Danish Science Press, Ltd., 1953).
10. Gustavson, K-H.: *Down's Syndrome. A Clinical and Cytogenetical Investigation* (Uppsala, Sweden: Almqvist & Wiksells, 1964).
11. Hall, B.: Mongolism in newborns, Acta paediat. scandinav., supp. 154, pp. 1–95, 1964.
12. Penrose, L. S., and Smith, G. F.: *Down's Anomaly* (Boston: Little, Brown & Company, 1966).
13. Cohen, B. H., Lilienfeld, A. M., and Sigler, A. T.: Some epidemiological aspects of mongolism: A review, Am. J. Pub. Health 53:223, 1963.
14. Collmann, R. D., and Stoller, A.: A survey of mongoloid births in Victoria, Australia, 1942–1957, Am. J. Pub. Health 52:813, 1962.
15. Renwick, D. H. G., Miller, J. R., and Paterson, D.: Estimates of incidence and prevalence of mongolism and of congenital heart disease in British Columbia, Canad. M. A. J. 91:365, 1964.
16. Carter, C., and MacCarthy, D.: Incidence of mongolism and its diagnosis in the newborn, Brit. J. Social Med. 5: 83, 1951.
17. Penrose, L. S.: Observations on the etiology of mongolism, Lancet 2:505, 1954.
18. Doxiades, L., and Portius, W.: Zur Ätiologie des Mongolismus unter besonderer Berücksichtigung der Sippenbefunde, Ztschr. menschl. Vererb.-u. Konstitutionslehre 21:384, 1938.
19. Carter, C. O.: A life-table for mongols with the causes of death, J. Ment. Defic. Res. 2:64, 1958.
20. Forssman, H.: Mongolism among inmates of Swedish institutions for mentally deficient–rate and age distribution, Am. J. Ment. Deficiency 65:32, 1960.
21. Allen, G., and Kallman, F. J.: Frequency and types of mental retardation in twins, Am. J. Human Genet. 7:15, 1955.
22. Tarjan, G., Wright, S. W., Kramer, M., Person, P. H., and Morgan, R.: The natural history of mental deficiency in a state hospital, A.M.A. J. Dis. Child. 96:64, 1958.
23. Berg, J. M., and Kirman, B. H.: Some aetiological problems in mental deficiency, Brit. M. J. 2:848, 1959.
24. Goodman, N., and Tizard, J.: Prevalence of imbecility and idiocy among children, Brit. M. J. 1:216, 1962.
25. Øster, J., Mikkelsen, M., and Nielsen, A.: The mortality and causes of death in patients with Down's syndrome (mongolism), Internat. Copenhagen Cong. Ment. Retard., pp. 231–235, 1964.
26. Hug, E.: Das Geschlechtsverhältnis beim Mongolismus, Ann. paediat. 177:31, 1951.
27. Øster, J.: The causes of mongolism, Danish M. Bull. 3: 158, 1956.
28. Parker, G. F.: The incidence of mongoloid imbecility in the newborn infant, J. Pediat. 36:493, 1950.
29. Crookshank, F. G.: *The Mongol in our Midst* (3d ed.; London: Kegan Paul, 1931).
30. Lahdensuu, S.: Über Vorkommen und Ätiologie der Idiotia mongoloidea im Lichte des in Finnland gesammelten Materials, Acta paediat. 21:256, 1937.
31. Orel, H.: Zur Aetiologie des Mongolismus, Ztschr. Kinderh. 42:440, 1926.
32. Snyder, L. H.: *Medical Genetics* (Durham, N. C.: Duke University Press, 1941).
33. Engel, D.: Etiology of multiple deformities, Am. J. Dis. Child. 60:562, 1940.
34. Macklin, M. T.: Mongolian idiocy. The manner of its inheritance, Am. J. M. Sc. 178:315, 1929.
35. Halbertsma, T.: Mongolism in one of twins and the etiology of mongolism, Am. J. Dis. Child. 25:350, 1923.
36. Waardenburg, P. J.: *Das Menschliche Auge und seine Erbanlagen* (The Hague: Martinus Nijhoff, 1932).
37. Bleyer, A.: Indications that mongoloid imbecility is a gametic mutation of degressive type, Am. J. Dis. Child. 47:342, 1934.
38. Fanconi, G.: Die Mutationstheorie des Mongolismus, Schweiz. med. Wchnschr. 69:81, 1939.
39. Rasonoff, A. J., and Handy, L. M.: Etiology of mongolism with special reference to its occurrence in twins, Am. J. Dis. Child. 48:764, 1934.
40. MacKaye, L.: Mongolism in nonidentical twins, Am. J. Dis. Child. 52:141, 1936.
41. Allen, G., and Baroff, G. S.: Mongoloid twins and their siblings, Acta Genet. 5:294, 1956.
42. Illing, J.: Beiträge zum Krankheitsbild der mongoloiden Idiotie, Monatsschr. Kinderh. 78:353, 1939.
43. Penrose, L. S.: Mongolian idiocy (mongolism) and maternal age, Ann. New York Acad. Sc. 57:494, 1954.
44. Gérard-Lefebvre, M., Mollet, F., Lefebvre, R., and Bernard, F.: Enquête sur le mongolisme dans le nord de la France: essai d'étude étio-pathogénique, Arch. franç. pédiat. 10:834, 1953.
45. Blandau, R. J.: The female factor in fertility and infertility; effects of delayed fertilization on the development of the pronuclei in rat ova, Fertil. & Steril. 3:349, 1952.
46. Witschi, E.: Overripeness of the egg as a cause of twinning and teratogenesis; review, Cancer Res. 12:763, 1952.
47. Shuttleworth, G. E.: Mongolian imbecility, Brit. M. J. 2: 661, 1909.
48. Bennholdt-Thomsen, C.: Über den Mongolismus und andere angeborene Abartungen in ihrer Beziehung zu hohem Alter der Mütter, Ztschr. Kinderh. 53:427, 1932.
49. Still, G. F.: Place-in-family as a factor in disease, Lancet 2:795 and 853, 1927.
50. Mayerhofer, E.: Die mongoloide Idiotie in ihrer ursächlichen Beziehung zum Curettage-Abortus, Ann. paediat. 154:57, 1939.
51. Comby, J.: Nouvelles observations de mongolisme, Arch. méd. Enf. 30:86, 1927.

52. Sutherland, G. A.: Mongolian imbecility in infants, Practitioner 63:632, 1899.
53. Pollet, L.: Étude étiologique du mongolisme. Rôle de la syphilis héréditaire, Thèse de Paris, 1922.
54. Stöltzner, W.: Zur Aetiologie des Mongolismus, München. med. Wchnschr. 66:1943, 1919.
55. Schröder, H.: Haben gynäkologische Erkrankungen eine Bedeutung für die Genese des Mongolismus?, Ztschr. Neurol. u. Psychiat. 163:390, 1938.
56. Dollinger, A.: Zur Aetiologie des Mongolismus, Ztschr. Kinderh. 27:337, 1921.
57. Zappert, J.: Hat eine Strahlenbehandlung der graviden Mutter einen schädlichen Einfluss auf das Kind?, Wien. klin. Wchnschr. 38:669, 1925.
58. Ingalls, T. H.: Etiology of mongolism. Epidemiologic and teratologic implications, Am. J. Dis. Child. 74:147, 1947.
59. Pleydell, M. J.: Mongolism and other congenital abnormalities; an epidemiological study in Northamptonshire, Lancet 1:1314, 1957.
60. Greig, D. M.: Skull of mongolian imbecile, Edinburgh M. J. 34:253, 1927.
61. Verga, P.: Ricerche anatomo-pathologiche sull'encefalo e le ghiandole a secrezione interna in un caso di idiozia mongoloide, Pediatria 36:1261, 1928.
62. Bourneville: Du traitement tyréoidien chez les idiots mongoliens, Cong. Aliénistes Neurol., 1903.
63. Clark, R. M.: The mongol, a new explanation, J. Ment. Sc. 75:261, 1929.
64. Vas, J.: Beiträge zur Pathogenese und Therapie der Idiotia Mongoliana, Jahrb. Kinderh. 111:51, 1925.
65. Goldstein, K.: Zwei Geschwister mit Myxidiotie und vorhandener, sicher nicht grob veränderter Schilddrüse, Deutsche Ztschr. Nervenh. 49:103, 1913.
66. Barnes, N. P.: Mongolism. Importance of early recognition and treatment, Ann. Clin. Med. 1:302, 1923.
67. Rachid, K.: Quelques considérations sur la pathogénie du mongolisme, Arch. méd. Enf. 36:31, 1933.
68. Rapaport, I.: Contribution à l'étude du mongolisme; rôle pathogénique du fluor, Bull. Acad. nat. méd. 140:529, 1956.
69. Bleyer, A. S.: Role of advancing maternal age in causing mongolism; study of 2822 cases, Am. J. Dis. Child. 55: 79, 1938.
70. Polani, P. E., Hamerton, J. L., Giannelli, F., and Carter, C. O.: Cytogenetics of Down's syndrome (mongolism). III. Frequency of interchange trisomics and mutation rate of chromosome interchanges, Cytogenetics 4:193, 1965.
71. van Beukering, J. A., and Vervoorn, J. D.: A case of uniovular twins of which one child was normal and the other had the syndrome of mongolism, Acta genet. med. 5:113, 1956.
72. Jervis, G. A.: Mongolism in twins, Am. J. Ment. Deficiency 47:364, 1943.
73. Nicholson, D. N., and Keay, A. J.: Mongolism in both of twins of opposite sex, Arch. Dis. Childhood 32:325, 1957.
74. McLean, S.: Mongolian idiocy in one of twins, J.A.M.A. 78:13, 1922.
75. Warner, R.: Mongolism in one of twins and in another sibling, Am. J. Dis. Child. 78:573, 1949.
76. Friedman, A.: Mongolism in twins, A.M.A. Am. J. Dis. Child. 90:43, 1955.
77. Engelking, E.: Augenärztlich wichtige Röntgenschädigungen der Frucht nach Bestrahlung Schwangerer, Klin. Monatsbl. Augenh. 94:151, 1935.
78. Brown, E. E.: Pathogenesis of mongolism following maternal illness: Role of adrenals, Arch. Pediat. 71:47, 1954.
79. Cockayne, E. A.: The genetics of transposition of the viscera, Quart. J. Med. 7:479, 1938.
80. Hindse-Nielsen, S.: Spina bifida – prognosis and heredity; clinical study, Acta chir. scandinav. 80:525, 1938.
81. Pediatric Herald 2: Pediatric Herald Publishing Company, New York, February, 1961.
82. Turpin, R., Caratzali, A., and Rogier, H.: Étude étiologique de cent quatre cas de mongolisme et considérations sur la pathogénie de cette maladie, Prem. Cong. Féd. Internat. Latine des Stés Eug. (Paris: Masson, 1937), pp. 154–164.
83. Penrose, L. S.: Maternal age, order of birth and developmental abnormalities, J. Ment. Sc. 85:1141, 1939.
84. Ford, C. E., Jones, K. W., Miller, O. J., Mittwoch, U., Penrose, L. S., Ridler, M., and Shapiro, A.: The chromosomes in a patient showing both mongolism and the Klinefelter syndrome, Lancet 1:709, 1959.
85. Jacobs, P. A., Baikie, A. G., Court-Brown, W. M., and Strong, J. A.: The somatic chromosomes in mongolism, Lancet 1:710, 1959.
86. Böök, J. A., Fraccaro, M., and Lindsten, J.: Cytogenetical observations in mongolism, Acta paediat. 48:453, 1959.
87. Yunis, J. J., Hook, E. B., and Mayer, M.: Identification of the mongolism chromosome by DNA replication analysis, Am. J. Human Genet. 17:191, 1965.
88. LeLong, M., Borniche, P., Kreisler, and Baudy, Mongolien issue de mère mongolienne, Arch. franç. pédiat. 6: 231, 1949.
89. Hanhart, E.: Mongoloide Idiotie bei Mutter und zwei Kindern aus Inzesten, Acta genet. med. 9:112, 1960.
90. Tagher, P., and Reisman, L. E.: Reproduction in Down's syndrome (mongolism): Chromosomal study of mother and normal child, Obst. & Gynec. 27:182, 1966.
91. Hayashi, T.: Karyotypic analysis of 83 cases of Down's syndrome in Harris County, Texas, Texas Rep. Biol. & Med. 21:28, 1963.
92. Hamerton, J. L., Giannelli, F., and Polani, P. E.: Cytogenetics of Down's syndrome (mongolism). I. Data on a consecutive series of patients referred for genetic counselling and diagnosis, Cytogenetics 4:171, 1965.
93. Wright, S. W., Day, R. W., Muller, H., and Weinhouse, R.: The frequency of trisomy and translocation in Down's syndrome, J. Pediat. 70:420, 1967.
94. Polani, P. E., Briggs, J. H., Ford, C. E., Clarke, C. M., and Berg, J. M.: A mongol girl with 46 chromosomes, Lancet 1:721, 1960.
95. Gibson, D., and Pozsoni, J.: Morphological and behavioral consequences of chromosome subtype in mongolism, Am. J. Ment. Deficiency 69:801, 1965.
96. Penrose, L. S., Ellis, J. R., and Delhanty, J. D. A.: Chromosomal translocations in mongolism and in normal relatives, Lancet 2:409, 1960.
97. Warkany, J., Weinstein, E. D., Soukup, S. W., Rubinstein, J. H., and Curless, M. C.: Chromosome analysis in a Children's Hospital, Pediatrics 33:290 and 454, 1964.
98. Hamerton, J. L., and Steinberg, A. G.: Progeny of D/G translocation heterozygotes in familial Down's syndrome, Lancet 1:1408, 1962.
99. Sergovich, F. R., Soltan, H. C., and Carr, D. H.: A 13-15/21 translocation chromosome in carrier father and mongol son, Canad. M.A.J. 87:852, 1962.
100. Tips, R. L., Smith, G. S., and Meyer, D. L.: Paternal transmission of a 15/21 translocation, Am. J. Dis. Child. 106:630, 1963.
101. Hamerton, J. L., Briggs, S. M., Giannelli, F., and Carter, C. O.: Chromosome studies in detection of parents with high risk of second child with Down's syndrome, Lancet 2:788, 1961.
102. Forssman, H., and Lehmann, O.: Translocation-carrying phenotypically normal males and the Down syndrome, Lancet 1:1286, 1961.
103. Penrose, L. S.: Paternal age in mongolism, Lancet 1: 1101, 1962.
104. Fraccaro, M., Kaijser, K., and Lindsten, J.: Chromosomal abnormalities in father and mongol child, Lancet 1: 724, 1960.
105. Lejeune, J.: Autosomal disorders, Pediatrics 32:326, 1963.
106. Giannelli, F., Hamerton, J. L., and Carter, C. O.: Cytogenetics of Down's syndrome (mongolism). II. The frequency of interchange trisomy in patients born at a

maternal age of less than 30 years, Cytogenetics 4:186, 1965.
107. Clarke, C. M., Edwards, J. H., and Smallpeice, V.: 21-trisomy/normal mosaicism in an intelligent child with some mongoloid characters, Lancet 1:1028, 1961.
108. Gustavson, K-H., and Ek, J. I.: Triple stem-line mosaicism in mongolism, Lancet 2:319, 1961.
109. Ridler, M. A. C., Shapiro, A., Delhanty, J. D. A., and Smith, G. F.: A mosaic mongol with normal leucocyte chromosomes, Brit. J. Psychiat. 111:183, 1965.
110. Fitzgerald, P. H., and Lycette, R. R.: Mosaicism involving the autosome associated with mongolism, Lancet 2: 212, 1961.
111. Blank, C. E., Gemmell, E., Casey, M. D., and Lord, M.: Mosaicism in a mother with a mongol child, Brit. M. J. 2:387, 1962.
112. Smith, D. W., Therman, E. M., Patau, K. A., and Inhorn, S. L.: Mosaicism in mother of two mongoloids, Am. J. Dis. Child. 104:534, 1962.
113. Weinstein, E. D., and Warkany, J.: Maternal mosaicism and Down's syndrome (mongolism), J. Pediat. 63:599, 1963.
114. Ferrier, S.: Enfant mongolien-parent mosaique. Étude de deux familles, J. Génét. Hum. 13:315, 1964.
115. Hall, B.: Down's syndrome (mongolism) with normal chromosomes, Lancet 2:1026, 1962.
116. Sergovich, F. R., Valentine, H., Carr, D. H., and Soltan, H. C.: Mongolism (Down's syndrome) with atypical clinical and cytogenetic features, J. Pediat. 65:197, 1964.
117. Day, R. W., and Miles, C. P.: Familial Down's syndrome with undetected translocation, J. Pediat. 67:399, 1965.
118. Dent, T., Edwards, J. H., and Delhanty, J. D. A.: A partial mongol, Lancet 2:484, 1963.
119. Ilbery, P. L. T., Lee, C. W. G., and Winn, S. M.: Incomplete trisomy in a mongoloid child exhibiting minimal stigmata, M. J. Australia 2:182, 1961.
120. Migeon, B. R., Kaufmann, B. N., and Young, W. J.: A chromosome abnormality with centric fragment in a paramongoloid child, Am. J. Dis. Child. 104:533, 1962.
121. Shaw, M. W.: Familial mongolism, Cytogenetics 1:141, 1962.
122. Day, R. W., and Wright, S. W.: Down's syndrome at young maternal ages: Chromosomal and family studies, J. Pediat. 66:764, 1965.
123. Petersen, C. D., and Luzzatti, L.: The role of chromosome translocation in the recurrence risk of Down's syndrome, Pediatrics 35:463, 1965.
124. Mikkelsen, M.: DNA replication analysis of six 13-15/21 translocation families, Ann. Human Genet. 30:325, 1967.
125. Hustinx, T. W. J., Eberle, P., and Geerts, S. J.: Mongoloid twins with 48 chromosomes ($AA+A_{21}XXY$), Ann. Human Genet. 25:111, 1961.
126. Root, A. W., Bongiovanni, A. M., Breibart, S., and Mellman, W. J.: Double aneuploidy: Trisomy 21 and XO/XX sex chromosome mosaicism, J. Pediat. 65:937, 1964.
127. van Wijck, J. A. M., Blankenborg, G. J., and Stolte, L. A. M.: XO/XX mosaicism and mongolism in the same person, Lancet 1:171, 1964.
128. Uchida, I. A., Ray, M., and Duncan, B. P.: 21 trisomy with an XYY sex chromosome complement, J. Pediat. 69:295, 1966.
129. Gagnon, J., Katyk-Longtin, N., de Groot, J. A., and Barbeau, A.: Double trisomie autosomique à 48 chromosomes (21 + 18), Union méd. Canada 90:1220, 1961.
130. Becker, K. L., Burke, E. C., and Albert, A.: Double autosomal trisomy (D trisomy plus mongolism), Proc. Staff Meet. Mayo Clin. 38:242, 1963.
131. MacIntyre, M. N., Staples, W. I., Steinberg, A. G., and Hempel, J. M.: Familial mongolism (trisomy-21 syndrome) resulting from a "15/21" chromosome translocation in more than three generations of a large kindred, Am. J. Human Genet. 14:335, 1962.
132. McKay, R. J., Jr.: Whose chromosomes to count in mongolism?, Pediatrics 36:620, 1965.
133. El-Alfi, O. S., Smith, P. M., and Biesele, J. J.: Chromosomal breaks in human leucocyte cultures induced by an agent in the plasma of infectious hepatitis patients, Hereditas 52:285, 1964.
134. Stoller, A., and Collmann, R. D.: Virus aetiology for Down's syndrome (mongolism), Nature, London 208: 903, 1965.
135. Robinson, A., and Puck, T. T.: Sex chromatin in newborns: Presumptive evidence for external factors in human nondisjunction, Science 148:83, 1965.
136. Uchida, I. A., and Curtis, E. J.: A possible association between maternal radiation and mongolism, Lancet 2: 848, 1961.
137. Smith, A., and McKeown, T.: Pre-natal growth of mongoloid defectives, Arch. Dis. Childhood 30:257, 1955.
138. Roche, A. F.: The cranium in mongolism; a critical review, Acta neurol. Scandinav. 42:62, 1966.
139. Fraser, J.: Kalmuc idiocy: Report of a case with autopsy. With notes on sixty-two cases (by Mitchell, A.), J. Ment. Sc. 22:169, 1876.
140. Hill, W. B.: Mongolism and its pathology: An analysis of eight cases, Quart. J. Med. 2:49, 1908.
141. Apert, E.: Mongolism (mongoloid idiocy; mongoloid backwardness), Le Monde Médical 24:201, 1914.
142. Davidoff, L. M.: The brain in mongolian idiocy, Arch. Neurol. & Psychiat. 20:1229, 1928.
143. Benda, C. E.: *The Child with Mongolism* (New York: Grune & Stratton, Inc., 1960).
144. Jacob, H.: Mongolismus, in Lubarsch, O., Henke, F., and Rössle, R. (eds.), *Handbuch der Speziellen Pathologischen Anatomie und Histologie* (Berlin: Springer-Verlag, 1956), Vol. 13, Part 4, pp. 82–98.
145. Hilliard, L. T., and Kirman, B. H.: *Mental Deficiency* (2d ed.; Boston: Little, Brown & Company, 1965).
146. Solitare, G. B., and Lamarche, J. B.: Alzheimer's disease and senile dementia as seen in mongoloids: Neuropathological observations, Am. J. Ment. Deficiency 70: 840, 1966.
147. Levinson, A., Friedman, A., and Stamps, F.: Variability of mongolism, Pediatrics 16:43, 1955.
148. Malzberg, B.: Some statistical aspects of mongolism, Am. J. Ment. Deficiency 54:266, 1950.
149. Penrose, L. S.: A clinical and genetic study of 1280 cases of mental defect, Med. Res. Counc. Spec. Rep. No. 229, London, His Maj. Stat. Off., 1938.
150. Quaytman, W.: The psychological capacities of mongoloid children in a community clinic, Quart. Rev. Pediat. 8:255, 1953.
151. Gifford, H.: The "Mongolian eye," Am. J. Ophth. 11:887, 1928.
152. Wagner, H. R.: Mongolism in Orientals, Am. J. Dis. Child. 103:706, 1962.
153. Gerald, B. E., and Silverman, F. N.: Normal and abnormal interorbital distances, with special reference to mongolism, Am. J. Roentgenol. 95:154, 1965.
154. Lowe, R. F.: The eyes in mongolism, Brit. J. Ophth. 33: 131, 1949.
155. Eissler, R., and Longenecker, L. P.: The common eye findings in mongolism, Am. J. Ophth. 54:398, 1962.
156. Igersheimer, J., and Mautner, H.: About changes of the crystalline lens in mongoloids, Am. J. Ment. Deficiency 55:370, 1951.
157. Cullen, J. F.: Blindness in mongolism (Down's syndrome), Brit. J. Ophth. 47:331, 1963.
158. Betlejewski, S., Klajman, S., and Walczyński, Z.: Radiologische Untersuchungen der Entwicklung der Nasennebenhöhlen im Down-Syndrom, Ann. paediat. 203: 355, 1964.
159. Shapiro, B. L., Gorlin, R. J., Redman, R. S., and Bruhl, H. H.: The palate and Down's syndrome, New England J. Med. 276:1460, 1967.
160. Cohen, M. M., and Winer, R. A.: Dental and facial characteristics in Down's syndrome (mongolism), J. Dent. Res. 44:197, (supp.), January–February, 1965.
161. Betlejewski, S., Jordan, J., and Walczyński, Z.: Le pavil-

lon de l'oreille chez les enfants atteints du syndrome de Down, Ann. paediat. 207:247, 1966.
162. Mautner, H.: Abnormal findings on the spine in mongoloids, Am. J. Ment. Deficiency 55:105, 1950.
163. Martel, W., and Tishler, J. M.: Observations on the spine in mongoloidism, Am. J. Roentgenol. 97:630, 1966.
164. Currarino, G., and Swanson, G. E.: Developmental variant in ossification of the manubrium sterni in mongolism, Radiology 82:916, 1964.
165. Horns, J. W., and O'Loughlin, B. J.: Multiple manubrial ossification centers in mongolism, Am. J. Roentgenol. 93:395, 1965.
166. Beber, B. A.: Absence of a rib in Down's syndrome, Lancet 2:289, 1965.
167. Bodian, M., White, L. L. R., Carter, C. O., and Louw, J. H.: Congenital duodenal obstruction and mongolism, Brit. M. J. 1:77, 1952.
168. Passarge, E.: The genetics of Hirschsprung's disease. Evidence of heterogeneous etiology and a study of sixty-three families, New England J. Med. 276:138, 1967.
169. Caffey, J., and Ross, S.: Mongolism (mongoloid deficiency) during early infancy–some newly recognized diagnostic changes in pelvic bones, Pediatrics 17:642, 1956.
170. Caffey, J., and Ross, S.: Pelvic bones in infantile mongoloidism; roentgenographic features, Am. J. Roentgenol. 80:458, 1958.
171. Kaufmann, H. J.: Das Mongoloidenbecken, Fortschr. Geb. Röntgenstrahlen 94:57, 1961.
172. Cummins, H., Talley, C., and Platou, R. V.: Palmar dermatoglyphics in mongolism, Pediatrics 5:241, 1950.
173. Rarick, G. L., Rapaport, I. F., and Seefeldt, V.: Long bone growth in Down's syndrome, Am. J. Dis. Child. 112:566, 1966.
174. Cummins, H.: Dermatoglyphic stigmata in mongoloid imbeciles, Anat. Rec. 74:407, 1939.
175. Holt, S. B.: Finger-print patterns in mongolism, Ann. Human Genet. 27:279, 1964.
176. Ford-Walker, N.: The use of dermal configurations in the diagnosis of mongolism, Pediat. Clin. North America, May, 1958, p. 531.
177. Penrose, L. S.: The distal triradius *t* on the hands of parents and sibs of mongol imbeciles, Ann. Human Genet. 19:10, 1954.
178. Gershoff, S. N., Hegsted, D. M., and Trulson, M. F.: Metabolic studies of mongoloids, Am. J. Clin. Nutrition 6:526, 1958.
179. Jérôme, H., Lejeune, J., and Turpin, R.: Étude de l'excrétion urinaire de certains métabolites du tryptophane chez les enfants mongoliens, Compt. rend. Acad. Sc. (Paris) 251:474, 1960.
180. McCoy, E. E., and Chung, S. I.: The excretion of tryptophan metabolites following deoxypyridoxine adminstration in mongoloid and nonmongoloid patients, J. Pediat. 64:227, 1964.
181. Bazelon, M.: Serotonin metabolism in Down's syndrome, Clin. Proc. Child. Hosp. (Wash.) 23:58, 1967.
182. Tu, J., and Zellweger, H.: Blood-serotonin deficiency in Down's syndrome, Lancet 2:715, 1965.
183. Rosner, F., Ong, B. H., Paine, R. S., and Mahanand, D.: Blood-serotonin activity in trisomic and translocation Down's syndrome, Lancet 1:1191, 1965.
184. Brandt, N. J., Frøland, A., Mikkelsen, M., Nielsen, A., and Tolstrup, N.: Galactosemia locus and the Down's syndrome chromosome, Lancet 2:700, 1963.
185. Hsia, D. Y-Y., Inouye, T., Wong, P., and South, A.: Studies on galactose oxidation in Down's syndrome, New England J. Med. 270:1085, 1964.
186. Baikie, A. G., Loder, P. B., de Gruchy, G. C., and Pitt, D. B.: Phosphohexokinase activity of erythrocytes in mongolism; another possible marker for chromosome 21, Lancet 1:412, 1965.
187. Alter, A. A., Lee, S. L., Pourfar, M., and Dobkin, G: Studies of leukocyte alkaline phosphatase in mongolism: A possible chromosome marker, Blood 22:165, 1963.
188. Lejeune, J., Berger, R., Réthoré, M-O., Archambault, L., Jérôme, H., Thieffry, S., Aicardi, J., Broyer, M., Lafourcade, J., Cruveiller, J., and Turpin, R.: Monosomie partielle pour un petit acrocentrique, Compt. rend. Acad. Sc. (Paris) 259:4187, 1964.
189. Turpin, R., and Lejeune, J.: *Les Chromosomes Humains* (Paris: Gauthier-Villars, 1965).
190. Rosner, F., Ong, B. H., Paine, R. S., and Mahanand, D.: Biochemical differentiation of trisomic Down's syndrome (mongolism) from that due to translocation, New England J. Med. 273:1356, 1965.
191. Turpin, R., and Bernyer, G.: De l'influence de l'hérédité sur la formule d'Arneth (cas particulier du mongolisme) Rev. hémat. 2:189, 1947.
192. Kiossoglou, K. A., Garrison, M., Jr., Walker, A., and Wolman, I. J.: The leukocyte, differential and polymorphonuclear lobe counts in mongols and in "organic" mental retardation, J. Ment. Defic. Res. 7:69, 1963.
193. Brewster, H. F., and Cannon, H. E.: Acute lymphatic leukemia: Report of a case in eleventh month mongolian idiot, New Orleans M. & S. J. 83:872, 1930.
194. Ingalls, T. H.: Pathogenesis of mongolism, Am. J. Dis. Child. 73:279, 1947.
195. Krivit, W., and Good, R. A.: Simultaneous occurrence of mongolism and leukemia; report of a nationwide survey, A.M.A. J. Dis. Child. 94:289, 1957.
196. Stewart, A., Webb, J., and Hewitt, D.: A survey of childhood malignancies, Brit. M. J. 1:1495, 1958.
197. Warkany, J., Schubert, W. K., and Thompson, J.: Chromosome analyses in mongolism (Langdon Down syndrome) associated with leukemia, New England J. Med. 268:1, 1963.
198. Honda, F., Punnett, H. H., Charney, E., Miller, G., and Thiede, H. A.: Serial cytogenetic and hematologic studies on a mongol with trisomy-21 and acute congenital leukemia, J. Pediat. 65:880, 1964.
199. Freireich, E. J., Whang, J., Tijio, J. H., Levin, R. H., Brittin, G. M., and Frei, E., III: Refractory anemia, granulocytic hyperplasia of bone marrow and a missing chromosome in marrow cells. A new clinical syndrome?, Clin. Res. 12:284, 1964 (abstract).
200. DeMayo, A. P., Kiossoglou, K. A., Erlandson, M. E., Notterman, R. F., and German, J.: A marrow chromosomal abnormality preceding clinical leukemia in Down's syndrome, Blood 29:233, 1967.
201. Ross, J. D., Moloney, W. C., and Desforges, J. F.: Ineffective regulation of granulopoiesis masquerading as congenital leukemia in a mongoloid child, J. Pediat. 63:1, 1963.
202. Lahey, M. E., Beier, F. R., and Wilson, J. F.: Leukemia in Down's syndrome, J. Pediat. 63:189, 1963.
203. Buckton, K. E., Harnden, D. G., Baikie, A. G., and Woods, G. E.: Mongolism and leukemia in the same sibship, Lancet 1:171, 1961.
204. Miller, R. W.: Down's syndrome (mongolism), other congenital malformations and cancers among the sibs of leukemic children, New England J. Med. 268:393, 1963.
205. Miller, O. J., Breg, W. R., Schmickel, R. D., and Tretter, W.: A family with an XXXXY male, a leukaemic male and two 21-trisomic mongoloid females, Lancet 2:78, 1961.
206. MacMahon, B., and Newill, V. A.: Birth characteristics of children dying of malignant neoplasms, J. Nat. Cancer Inst. 28:231, 1962.
207. German, J. L., deMayo, A. P., and Bearn, A. G.: Inheritance of an abnormal chromosome in Down's syndrome (mongolism) with leukemia, Am. J. Human Genet. 14: 31, 1962.
208. Cooper, H. L., and Hirschhorn, K.: Enlarged satellites as a familial chromosome marker, Am. J. Human Genet. 14:107, 1962.
209. Cant, W. H. P., Gerrard, J. W., and Richards, B. W.: A girl of mongoloid appearance and normal intelligence, J. Ment. Sc. 99:560, 1963.
210. Dekaban, A.: Twins, probably monozygotic: One mongo-

loid with 48 chromosomes, the other normal, Cytogenetics 4:227, 1965.
211. Loesch-Mdzewska, D.: Some aspects of the neurology of Down's syndrome, J. Ment. Defic. Res. 12:237, 1968.
212. Collmann, R. D., and Stoller, A.: Shift of childbirth to younger mothers and its effect on the incidence of mongolism in Victoria, Australia, 1939–1964, J. Ment. Defic. Res. 13:13, 1969.
213. Fialkow, J.: Thyroid antibodies, Down's syndrome and maternal age, Nature, London 214:1253, 1967.
214. Dallaire, L., Flynn, D. K., and Leboeuf, G.: Thyroid antibodies in relation to infectious hepatitis and Down's syndrome, J. Ment. Defic. Res. 12:93, 1968.
215. Lilienfeld, A. M.: *Epidemiology of Mongolism* (Baltimore: The Johns Hopkins Press, 1969).
216. Dallaire, L., and Fraser, F. C.: Two unusual cases of familial mongolism, Canad. J. Genet. & Cytol. 6:540, 1964.
217. de Capoa, A., Miller, O. J., Mukherjee, B. B., and Warburton, D.: Autoradiographic studies on a mother and aborted fetus from a family with four mongoloid children and a presumptive 21/21 translocation, Ann. Human Genet. 31:243, 1967.
218. Lawton, S. B., Stoddard, G. R., and Seely, J. R.: Familial 21/21 translocation, J. Pediat. 74:305, 1969.
219. Ruvalcaba, R. H. A., Ferrier, P. E., and Thuline, H. C.: Incidence of goiter in patients with Down's syndrome, Am. J. Dis. Child. 118:451, 1969.
220. Aarskog, D.: Autoimmune thyroid disease in children with mongolism, Arch. Dis. Childhood 44:454, 1969.
221. Pabst, H. F., Pueschel, S., and Hillman, D. A.: Etiologic interrelationship in Down's syndrome, hypothyroidism, and precocious sexual development, Pediatrics 40:590, 1967.
222. Turner, J. H.: *The Mongoloid Phenotype; Its Incidence, Etiology and Association with Leukemia and other Neoplastic Disease* (Ann Arbor, Mich.: Univ. Microfilm, Inc. No. 63-7539, 1962).
223. Jackson, E. W., Turner, J. H., Klauber, M. R., and Norris, F. D.: Down's syndrome: Variation of leukemia occurrence in institutionalized populations, J. Chron. Dis. 21: 247, 1968.
224. Richards, B. W.: Mosaic mongolism, J. Ment. Defic. Res. 13:66, 1969.
225. Stoller, A., and Collmann, R. D.: Grandmaternal age at birth of mothers of children with Down's syndrome (mongolism), J. Ment. Defic. Res. 13:201, 1969.
226. Warkany, J., and Soukup, S.: A chromosomal abnormality in a girl with some features of Down's syndrome (mongolism), J. Pediat. 62:890, 1963.
227. Lejeune, J., Berger, R., Vidal, O. R., and Réthoré, M-O.: Un cas de translocation G/G en tandem, Ann. Génét. 8: 60, 1965.
228. Garson, O. M., Baikie, A. G., Pitt, D. B., and Newman, N. M.: Down's syndrome with translocation-en-tandem: A report of two unrelated cases, Australian Paediat. J. 6: 53, 1970.
229. Kohn, G., Taysi, K., Atkins, T. E., and Mellman, W. J.: Mosaic mongolism. I. Clinical correlations, J. Pediat. 76: 874, 1970.
230. Taysi, K., Kohn, G., and Mellman, W. J.: Mosaic mongolism. II. Cytogenetic studies, J. Pediat. 76:880, 1970.
231. Vanhaelst, L., Hayez, F., Bonnyns, M., and Bastenie, P. A.: Thyroid auto-immune disease and thyroid function in families of subjects with Down's syndrome, J. Clin. Endocrinol. 30:792, 1970.
232. Gross, R. E.: *The Surgery of Infancy and Childhood* (Philadelphia: W. B. Saunders Company, 1953).
233. Shapiro, D. J., Dzurick, F. J., and Gerrish, E. W.: Obstruction of duodenum in the newborn infant due to annular pancreas, Pediatrics 9:764, 1952.
234. McKeown, T., MacMahon, B., and Record, R. G.: An investigation of 69 cases of exomphalos, Am. J. Human Genet. 5:169, 1953.
235. Pant, S. S., Moser, H. W., and Krane, S. M.: Hyperuricemia in Down's syndrome, J. Clin. Endocrinol. 28: 472, 1968.

A Reference Bibliography on Down syndrome (mongolism) was compiled by R. F. Vollman and published by the U.S. Department of Health, Education and Welfare, 1969.

Monosomy G
(Antimongolism)

COMPLETE OR PARTIAL monosomy for a G autosome has been observed repeatedly. Intrauterine growth retardation apparently is a regular sign and postnatal growth is impaired also. Hypertonia is a constant finding and mental and physical development are retarded. Pyloric stenosis with typical vomiting was reported in some of the cases. The palpebral fissures slope down and outward in antimongoloid fashion and congenital cataracts or corneal opacities may occur. The auricles are large and low-set. The nasal bridge is described as prominent. Micrognathia is a regular feature and posterior palate cleft may be present.[1] Systolic murmurs were noticed in some cases, but the nature of the heart anomaly has not been established. Hypospadias and cryptorchidism were seen in the male infants. The thumbs are low-set and held in flexion. The dermatoglyphics showed absence of the C triradius on one or both palms in several children. Thrombocytopenia was recorded in several cases and the leukocyte alkaline phosphatase was normal. Most of the patients were mosaics with one cell line with 45 chromosomes (G−) and the other with 46, including a small ring or centric fragment. Death occurs in most cases within the first year but survival beyond infancy has been reported.[2-5]

REFERENCES

1. Challacombe, D. N., and Taylor, A.: Monosomy for a G autosome, Arch. Dis. Childhood 44:113, 1969.
2. Lejeune, J., Berger, R., Réthoré, M-O., Archambault, L., Jérôme, H., Thieffry, S., Aicardi, J., Broyer, M., Lafourcade, J., Cruveiller, J., and Turpin, R.: Monosomie partielle pour un petit acrocentrique, Compt. rend. Acad. Sc. (Paris) 259: 4187, 1964.
3. Reisman, L., Kasahara, S., Chin-Young Chung, Darnell, A., and Hall, B.: Anti-mongolism. Studies in an infant with a partial monosomy of the 21 chromosome, Lancet 1:394, 1966.
4. Thorburn, M. J., and Johnson, B. E.: Apparent monosomy of a G autosome in a Jamaican infant, J. M. Genetics 3: 290, 1966.
5. Böhm, R., and Fuhrmann, W.: Lebensfähigkeit bei Monosomie G, Monatsschr. Kinderh. 117:184, 1969.

Cat-Cry Syndrome

(Syndrome du Cri du Chat: Partial Deletion of the Short Arm of Chromosome 5)

IN 1963, Lejeune *et al.*[1] described, in 3 cases of mental and physical retardation, deletion of the short arm of a B chromosome, and by 1964 they[2] had collected 6 similar cases with craniofacial anomalies and a phonetic characteristic resembling a cat's cry. By now, about 60 cases have been observed,[3,4] so that the syndrome seems well established. It is possible that a deficiency of the short arm of a no. 4 chromosome results in a disease picture that differs from the cat-cry syndrome (p. 342).[5]

In most cases, the cat-cry syndrome seems to originate de novo by loss of a segment of the short arm of one chromosome no. 5. The parents of such patients are cytogenetically normal. In other cases, a balanced translocation can exist in antecedents who can have offspring with deficient arms of chromosome 5. Koulischer and Quersin[6] reported a patient with cat-cry syndrome whose father was a balanced carrier of a translocation of a short arm of a chromosome 5 to a 13-15. In a patient of de Grouchy and Gabilan,[7] the mother carried a translocation of the short arm of a chromosome 5 to a chromosome of the 21-22 group, but in this case the mechanism of transmission was complex. The possibility of a trisomy of the short arm of chromosome 5 must be considered. Carriers of a balanced translocation of a short arm may have normal children, translocation carriers, children with cat-cry syndrome and children with trisomy for the short arm of a chromosome 5. The last type, which represents the "counterpart" of the cat-cry syndrome, shows severe mental retardation and small stature without other external characteristics.[8] Another case of such a trisomy resulted from a maternal balanced translocation of a short arm of a B group to a G group chromosome.[9] Cat-cry syndrome with mosaicism of normal cells and of cells with deletion of a short arm of chromosome 5 has been reported.[3] Another mosaicism consisted of cells with a deleted short arm of chromosome 5 and some cells with a translocation of a fragment to the long arms of a no. 4. The clinical picture was that of the cat-cry syndrome complicated by congenital heart disease, hypospadias, cryptorchidism, skeletal malformations and increased amino acid levels of the serum.[10] In a severely retarded girl with ocular and cardiac malformations, partial deletion of the short arm of a B group chromosome was combined with deletion of most of the material of a G group member.[11] The disorder was considered as a cat-cry and antimongolism syndrome. A case showing the clinical signs of the cat-cry syndrome with an apparently normal karyotype was presented by McGavin *et al.*[12] These authors tabulated 50 cases of the syndrome reported in the literature.

More female than male children with cat-cry syndrome have been reported. Parental age, position in the family and consanguinity probably are not of etiologic importance. Intrauterine growth retardation is common. More than half the patients reported had birth weights of 2,500 Gm. or less, although the gestation time was normal in most of them.[13] Failure to thrive and to grow continues after birth. Feeding difficulties prevail. They may be due to muscular deficiencies or to laryngeal stridor. The feeble, high-pitched and plaintive cry contributes to the extremely weak appearance. Yet, many of these children survive infancy and childhood despite severe mental and physical handicaps.[36]

As other syndromes due to chromosomal abnormalities, the cat-cry syndrome shows variations that could be explained by differing losses of genetic material from the short arm of chromosome 5. Mental retardation and microcephaly are the leading signs in addition to the cat cry. The microcephaly is associated with brachycephaly and a "moon face." The cranial deficiency can be more pronounced in the occipital than in the frontal region,[14] where bossing may mask the microcephaly. In one case, the anterior fontanelle was wide open at 5 months but closed at 1 year.[15] The pathology of the brain is but little known. In one instance, necropsy revealed a quite small left cerebellar hemisphere. Since this was seen in a child with the asplenia syndrome (p. 745) combined with cat-cry syndrome,[2] the finding probably is not typical. In another instance, the brain of a 19-year-old female with cat-cry syndrome was found to be uniformly small and considered a primary micrencephaly.[29] Pneumoencephalograms revealed, in some cases, cortical cerebral atrophy and dilatation of the ventricular system.[2] The mental retardation usually is severe and can amount to idiocy. The cat cry is so typical that it often aids in the differentiation from other forms of retardation. Malacia of the cartilages and smallness and subglottic malformations of the larynx have been observed,[2,16] but laryngoscopic findings can be normal despite a high-pitched voice.[17] After careful acoustic analyses, Schroeder *et al.*[30] concluded that the cat cry is caused by an organic or functional cerebral lesion and not by a malformation of the voice-forming organs. Micheau and Schlumberger[31] found minimal changes in the vestibule of the larynx as the only anomaly and concluded that a malformation of the nerve centers or pathways controlling phonation must be responsible for the characteristic cry. The round face, hypertelorism, strabismus and low-set ears contribute to the disease picture. Antimongoloid slant of the palpebral fissures and epicanthic folds are less constant. Eyeground changes have been observed.[2,18] Auricular appendages are seen in some cases.[19,20] The bridge of the nose is broad, micrognathia is common. Cleft palate and high palate have been observed,[28] but cleft lip and palate or uvula fissa was seen in exceptional cases only.[16,20,21] It remains to be seen whether patients with facial clefts have the cat-cry syndrome or a cytogenetically similar condition.

There are cases that involve congenital heart defects[2,10,21-23]; some of these may represent deviant syndromes (p. 342). Usually, muscular hypotonia is noted but hypertonicity has been observed also.[17] Scoliosis, dislocation of the hip, hyperextensibility of fingers and toes, incurved little fingers and clubfoot occur.[14,17] Simian creases or transverse but interrupted palmar creases are the rule. The dermatoglyphics are abnormal, but some of the findings are contradictory.[24,27] Cutaneous hemangiomas were noticeable in some cases.[14]

The phenotypes of some of the patients reported deviate so much from the standard cat-cry syndrome that some authors believe that the deviant disease

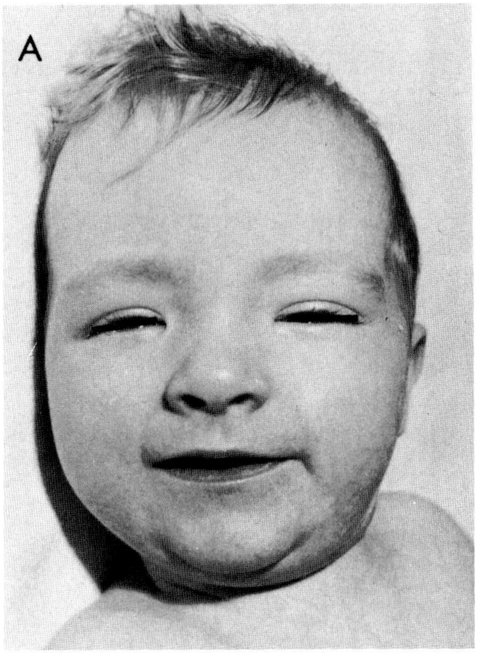

Fig. 37-33.—**A,** girl with cat-cry syndrome. Peculiar cry was noted from birth. Microcephaly (−4 cm.), moon face and, **B,** transverse but interrupted palmar creases. **C,** karyotype of a child with cat-cry syndrome showing deletion of short arms of a no. 5 chromosome (**arrow**).

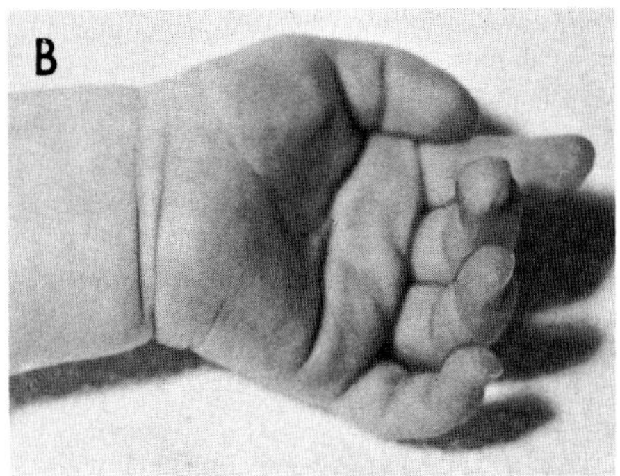

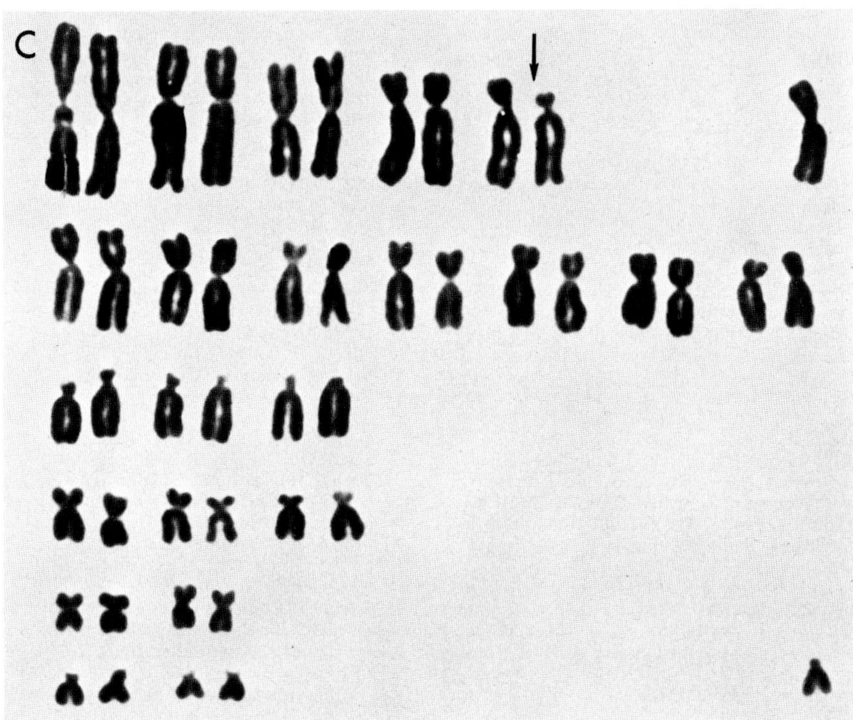

pictures are not due to deletion of the short arm of chromosome 5. Hirschhorn *et al.*[25] reported deletion of short arms of chromosome 4–5 in a child with defects of midline fusion. Wolf and Reinwein[5] considered patients who resemble those with cat-cry syndrome to a certain extent but who have facial clefts, iris colobomas, congenital heart disease, hypospadias and convulsions as a separate entity. They are said to have a deletion of a short arm of chromosome 4. Other cases with similar karyotypes have been reported.[32-35]

The patient reported by Hijmans and Shearin,[20] whose malformations were attributed to partial deletion of short arms of a chromosome 5, represented a disease picture of severest mental and somatic retardation. With a developmental quotient of 20, a height of 97 cm. and weight of 9 kg. at 13 years of age, the child differed from the standard type. Cleft lip and palate, scoliosis and the inability to stand or walk were outstanding signs. The face was asymmetrical. The antimongoloid position of the palpebral fissures, macrostomia and skin tags on the left cheek and ear are reminiscent of mandibulofacial dysostosis (p. 650). But one of the B chromosomes did show partial deletion of the short arms, which is not an attribute of mandibulofacial dysostosis, a dominantly inherited trait.

Wolf *et al.*[26] described a 13-year-old girl with many features of the cat-cry syndrome but with some deviations. Moon face, epicanthus, low-set ears and hypotonicity were absent. Growth was enhanced and brachymetacarpy, kyphoscoliosis and analgesia were present. Only 45 chromosomes were found and there was a translocation of chromosome 5 to a D_2 chromosome with partial deletions of the short arms of the fused chromosomes.

REFERENCES

1. Lejeune, J., Lafourcade, J., Berger, R., Vialatte, J., Boeswillwald, M., Seringe, P., and Turpin, R.: Trois cas de délétion partielle du bras court d'un chromosome 5, Compt. rend. Acad. Sc. (Paris) 257:3098, 1963.
2. Lejeune, J., Lafourcade, J., de Grouchy, J., Berger, R., Gautier, M., Salmon, C., and Turpin, R.: Délétion partielle du bras court du chromosome 5. Individualisation d'un nouvel état morbide, Semaine hôp. Paris 40:1069, 1964.
3. Zellweger, H.: Cri-du-chat with chromosomal mosaicism, Lancet 2:57, 1966.
4. German, J., Lejeune, J., Macintyre, M. N., and de Grouchy, J.: Chromosomal autoradiography in the cri du chat syndrome, Cytogenetics 3:347, 1964.
5. Wolf, U., and Reinwein, H.: Klinische und cytogenetische Differentialdiagnose der Defizienzen an den kurzen Armen der B-Chromosomen, Ztschr. Kinderh. 98:235, 1967.
6. Koulischer, L., and Quersin, C.: La délétion des bras courts d'un chromosome du groupe 4-5, Acta paediat. belg. 19:167, 1965.
7. de Grouchy, J., and Gabilan, J. C.: Translocation 5/21-22 et syndrome du cri du chat, Ann. Génét. 8:31, 1965.
8. Lejeune, J., Lafourcade, J., Berger, R., and Turpin, R.: Ségrégation familiale d'une translocation 5-13 déterminant une monosomie et une trisomie partielle du bras court du chromosome 5: Maladie du "cri du chat" et sa "reciproque," Compt. rend. Acad. Sc. (Paris) 258:5767, 1964.
9. Böök, J. A., Atkins, L., and Santesson, B.: Some new data on autosomal aberrations in man, Path.-biol. 11:1159, 1964.
10. Genest, P., Tremblay, M., and Mortezai, M.: Le syndrome du "cri du chat." Étude d'un cas de délétion partielle du bras court du chromosome 5 et translocation au chromosome 4, Laval méd. 36:319, 1965.
11. Engel, E., Hastings, C. P., Merrill, R. E., McFarland, B. S., and Nance, W. E.: Apparent cri-du-chat and "antimongolism" in one patient, Lancet 1:1130, 1966.
12. McGavin, D. D. M., Cant, J. S., Ferguson-Smith, M. A., and Ellis, P. M.: The cri-du-chat syndrome with an apparently normal karyotype, Lancet 2:326, 1967.
13. Silber, D. L., Engel, E., and Merrill, R. E.: So-called "cri du chat syndrome," Am. J. Ment. Deficiency 71:486, 1966.
14. Schmid, W., and Vischer, D.: Cri-du-chat syndrome. Case report, Helvet. paediat. acta 22:22, 1967.
15. Lichtenberger, M., and Morineaud, J-P.: Un cas de délétion du bras court du chromosome 5 au Vietnam (syndrome du cri du chat), Ann. pédiat. 43:234, 1967.
16. Macintyre, M. N., Staples, W. I., LaPolla, J. J., and Hempel, J. M.: The "cat cry" syndrome, Am. J. Dis. Child. 108:538, 1964.
17. Schneegans, E., Rohmer, A., Levy-Silagy, J., Rumpler, Y., Ruch, J-V., and Gerlinger, P.: Un cas de maladie du cri du chat. Délétion partielle du bras court du chromosome 5, Pédiatrie 21:823, 1966.
18. Hustinx, T. W. J., and Wijffels, J. C. H. M.: "Cri du chat" syndrome, Lancet 2:135, 1965.
19. Dyggve, H. V., and Mikkelsen, M.: Partial deletion of the short arms of a chromosome of the 4-5 group (Denver), Arch. Dis. Childhood 40:82, 1965.
20. Hijmans, J. C., and Shearin, D. B.: Partial deletion of short arms of chromosome no. 5, Am. J. Dis. Child. 109:85, 1965.
21. Giorgi, P. L., Ceccarelli, M., and Paci, A.: Su un caso di sindrome del "cri du chat" con peculiari anomalie fenotipiche, Minerva pediat. 17:1972, 1965.
22. Cavalieri, S., Mastella, G., and Tiepolo, L.: La sindrome della voce da gatto, Fracastoro 57:369, 1964.
23. MacCracken, J. S., and Gordon, R. R.: "Cri du chat" syndrome, Lancet 1:23, 1965.
24. Pfeiffer, R. A., and Simon, H. A.: "Cri du chat," ein neues Missbildungssyndrom als Folge einer Chromosomenaberration, München. med. Wchnschr. 107:2669, 1965.
25. Hirschhorn, K., Cooper, H. L., and Firschein, I. L.: Deletion of short arms of chromosome 4-5 in a child with defects of midline fusion, Humangenetik 1:479, 1965.
26. Wolf, U., Reinwein, H., Gey, W., and Klose, J.: Cri-du-chat-Syndrome mit Translokation 5/D_2, Humangenetik 2:63, 1966.
27. Warburton, D., and Miller, O. J.: Dermatoglyphic features of patients with a partial short arm deletion of a B-group chromosome, Ann. Human Genet. 31:189, 1967.
28. Olive, D., Gilgenkrantz, S., Cabrol, C., and Wolkowicz, M. W.: Maladie du Cri du Chat (5p−) avec gueule de loup, Pediatrie 23:795, 1968.
29. Solitare, G. B.: The cri du chat syndrome: Neuropathologic observations, J. Ment. Defic. Res. 11:268, 1967.
30. Schroeder, H. H., Schleiermacher, E., Schroeder, T. M., Bauer, H., Richter, C., and Schwenk, J.: Zur klinischen Differentialdiagnose des Cri du Chat-Syndroms, Humangenetik 4:294, 1967.
31. Micheau, C., and Schlumberger, J. R.: Étude anatomopathologique du larynx dans la maladie du cri du chat, Ann. pédiat. 15:748, 1968.
32. Šubrt, I., Blehová, B., and Sedlácková, E.: Mewing cry in a child with the partial deletion of the short arm of chromosome no. 4, Humangenetik 8:242, 1969.
33. Arias, D., Passarge, E., Engle, M. A., and German, J.: Human chromosomal deletion: Two patients with the

4p− syndrome, J. Pediat. 76:82, 1970.
34. Wilcock, A. R., Adams, F. G., Cooke, P., and Gordon, R. R.: Deletion of short arm of no. 4 (4p−)—A detailed case report, J. M. Genetics 7:171, 1970.
35. Wilson, M. G., Towner, J. W., and Negus, L. D.: Wolf-Hirschhorn syndrome associated with an unusual abnormality of chromosome no. 4, J. M. Genetics 7:164, 1970.
36. Breg, W. R., Steele, M. W., Miller, O. J., Warburton, D., de Capoa, A., and Allerdice, P. W.: The cri du chat syndrome in adolescents and adults: Clinical findings in 13 older patients with partial deletion of the short arm of chromosome no. 5 (5p−), J. Pediat. 77:782, 1970.

Ring-1 Chromosome and Microcephalic Dwarfism

IN A GIRL born with marked intrauterine growth retardation, the head circumference was 28 cm. and the anterior fontanelle was small. Her height and weight remained subnormal but she had no congenital malformations other than microcephaly. The chromosome number was 46, but in place of one chromosome many cells had a ring chromosome. Some cells had a supernumerary chromosome of the C group in place of a missing no. 1.[1]

REFERENCE

1. Gordon, R. R., and Cooke, P.: Ring-1 chromosome and microcephalic dwarfism, Lancet 2:1212, 1964.

Triploidy

THREE SETS OF chromosomes (triploidy) instead of the normal two (diploidy), frequently seen in aborted products of conception, are extremely rare in children. Chromosomal abnormalities have been recognized in approximately 20% of abortuses examined and one-fifth of them had a triploid karyotype. The three sex chromosomes present in a triploid karyotype vary. The XXY type has been found twice as often as the XXX, and XYY was quite exceptional.[1] Triploid karyotypes have been noted repeatedly in hydatidiform moles and in hydatidiform areas in the placenta of triploid infants.[2-4] The origin of triploid zygotes has been explained by fertilization of the egg by two spermatozoa (diandry), by incorporation of a polar body (digyny) or by a mitotic error of a germ cell precursor, leading to a diploid gamete (aneugamy).[1]

In children surviving to term or near term, diploid/triploid mosaicism was established in 7 of 11 cases,[5-11] and in only 4 a single triploid cell line was found.[1,12-14] Intrauterine growth retardation of fetuses with triploidy is the rule. Underdevelopment of one half of the body (hemidystrophy) has been noticed in 2 instances of diploid/triploid mosaicism[6,7] but this partial growth retardation was not present in others. Syndactyly of the third and fourth fingers has been seen repeatedly in patients with triploidy and diploid/triploid mosaicism.[1] Colobomas involving ocular structures in varying degrees have been observed in 3 cases.[1,10,13] One child with homogeneous triploidy was described in detail by Schindler and Mikamo.[1] The boy, born in the thirty-ninth week of gestation weighing 1,450 Gm., lived only 6 hours after delivery. The karyotype was 69,XXY. Hypotonia and marked respiratory distress were present. Hypertelorism, prominent upper jaws, deviation of the nose, large posterior fontanelle, microphthalmia and bilateral coloboma, macroglossia, low-set small ears, syndactyly of the third and fourth fingers, bilateral simian creases, low insertion of the umbilical cord on the abdomen, cryptorchidism and a small penis with hypospadias were seen on inspection. Necropsy revealed unilateral hydronephrosis and testes with well-developed seminiferous tubules that were decreased in number and lined by many germ cells and Sertoli cells. The coloboma involved the optic nerve, choroid, ciliary body and the iris. Despite the 69,XXY karyotype, only a few sex-chromatin-positive cells were found in buccal smears and cultured fibroblasts. Although in most instances of intrauterine growth retardation the placenta is small, a large placenta, nearly twice normal size and weighing 880 Gm. was present in this case; it was histologically immature and showed hydatidiform-like changes in the stroma of the stem villi.[1]

Some cases of diploid/triploid mosaicism were discussed in Chapter 14, Intrauterine Growth Retardation.

REFERENCES

1. Schindler, A-M., and Mikamo, K.: Triploidy in man, Cytogenetics 9:116, 1970.
2. Atkin, N. B., and Klinger, H. P.: The superfemale mole, Lancet 2:727, 1962.
3. Makimo, S., Sasaki, M. S., and Fukushima, T.: Triploid chromosome constitution in human chorionic lesions, Lancet 2:1273, 1964.
4. Carr, D. H.: Cytogenetics and the pathology of hydatidiform degeneration, Obst. & Gynec. 33:333, 1969.
5. Böök, J. A., Masterson, J. G., and Santesson, B.: Malformation syndrome associated with triploidy. Further chromosome studies of the patient and his family, Acta Genet. 12:193, 1962.
6. Ellis, J. R., Marshall, R., Normand, I. C. S., and Penrose,

L. S.: A girl with triploid cells, Nature, London 198:411, 1963.
7. Ferrier, P., Stalder, G., Bamatter, F., Ferrier, S., Buehler, E., and Klein, D.: Congenital asymmetry associated with diploid-triploid mosaicism and large satellites, Lancet 1: 8082, 1964.
8. Gropp, A., Jussen, A., and Odunjo, F.: Near-triploid chromosome constitution in epithelial cell cultures of palatal mucosa from a case of cleft palate, Lancet 1:1167, 1964.
9. Sacrez, R., Clavert, J., Willard, D., Rumpler, Y., M'Bede, J., Meyer, R., and Korn, R.: La triploidie chez l'enfant, Pédiatrie 22:267, 1967.
10. Schmid, W., and Vischer, D.: A malformed boy with double aneuploidy and diploid-triploid mosaicism 48,XXYY/71,XXXYY, Cytogenetics 6:145, 1967.
11. Lejeune, J., Salmon, C., Berger, R., Réthoré, M-O., Rossier, A., and Job, J. C.: Chimère 46,XX/69,XXY, Ann. Génét. 10:188, 1967.
12. Bernard, R., Stahl, A., Colgnet, J., Giraud, F., Hartung, M., Brusquet, Y., and Passeron, P.: Triploidie chromosomique chez un nouveau-né polymalformé, Ann. Génét. 10:70, 1965.
13. Edwards, J. H., Yuncken, C., Rushton, D. I., Richards, S., and Mittwoch, U.: Three cases of triploidy in man, Cytogenetics 6:81, 1967.
14. Papiernik-Berkhauer, E.: Enfant triploide à terme et thérapeutique hormonale, Bull. Féd. soc. gynéc. et obst. 20: 248, 1968.

38

Some Syndromes of Uncertain Origin

Cornelia de Lange Syndrome

(Brachmann-de Lange Syndrome [Typus Amstelodamensis])

In 1933, Cornelia de Lange[1] described two cases of congenital malformations that she considered "a new type of degeneration (Typus Amstelodamensis)." These cases were sporadic, showing no familial disorder. The children had severe intrauterine growth retardation, weighing at term 1,250 and 2,000 Gm. The growth retardation and weight deficit continued after birth and developmental milestones were delayed. There was hirsutism over the forehead, the eyelashes were long and the eyebrows well developed, meeting in the midline (synophrys). A bluish tint of the skin was noticeable about the face and the temporal region. The ears were low set, the nostrils directed forward. Mandible and chin were hypoplastic. The mouth was small, the angles turned downward (fish mouth). The palate was arched and dentition delayed. The skull was brachycephalic and the occiput flat. The arms were short, the hands and feet small and plump, the digits short and the fifth fingers incurved. The thumb and thenar were situated more proximally than normal. There was cutaneous syndactyly between some of the toes. Roentgenograms revealed hypoplasia of the second and third phalanges of the little fingers. De Lange considered mental retardation, undersize at birth (weight below one-half of the normal at term), brachycephaly, heavy eyebrows and lashes, small hands and feet, proximal position of the thumb and thenar, low-set ears and syndactyly of the toes as essential signs of the typus Amstelodamensis. A third case reported in 1938[2] closely resembled those observed before and, in addition, showed simian palmar creases, contractures of the elbows and a "heavy" appearance of the diaphyses of the forearm bones. These traits were considered accidental, since they were absent in the first 2 cases. One of the children described was studied post mortem. Incomplete fixation of the intestine was noticed. The brain was smaller than normal, the convolutions were gross and the cortex underdeveloped.

The condition is not too rare, and many cases have been described since de Lange's original report. In 1961, Richter[3] added 3 new cases to 13 collected from the literature, and additional characteristics were established. Antimongoloid slanting, elongation of the upper lip, ocular fundus changes, congenital heart disease, inguinal hernias, small genitalia, hypospadias,[3] phocomelia[4] and muscular hypertrophy were found in patients with the syndrome. In several cases there was a tendency to infections of the skin and of the respiratory tract. Jervis and Stimson[5] described 5 cases and pointed out that the etiology remained obscure. They observed the presence of fragments in some cells of 4 of their patients subjected to chromosome analysis. Intrauterine growth retardation seemed to be the rule, with an average birth weight of 2,150 Gm. for males and 1,842 Gm. for females who were born at term.

By 1967, more than 100 cases had been recorded,[6-8] including patients from various ethnic groups.[9,10] More than 250 cases could be analyzed in a monograph by Berg *et al.*,[26] which appeared in 1970. Necropsy findings were reviewed by France *et al.*[24]

With publication of additional cases, the spectrum of manifestations broadened. Some of the somatic defects described were more serious than those mentioned by de Lange.[2] Cleft palate,[11,12] microcornea and other ocular anomalies,[13] pyloric stenosis, duodenal obstruction, volvulus, ventricular and auricular septal defect, hypoplasia of the aorta, small left ventricle and persistent left superior vena cava[13] were observed. One patient had adrenals conjoined in front of the aorta and polycystic kidneys.[12] Hypoplasia of the left heart, mitral and aortic stenosis, coarctation of the aorta and patent ductus arteriosus were seen at necropsy in a patient with severe deformities of the upper extremities observed in the Cincinnati Children's Hospital (Fig. 38-1).

In some of these cases, severe reduction deformities of the upper extremities were the most striking symptoms.[3,12,14] Shortening of the forearms, contractures of the elbow joints, deformities of the hands and monodactyly were seen repeatedly in children with facial features typical of the de Lange syndrome. It was also recognized[15] that a case conforming to the expanded syndrome had been published by Brachmann[16] 17 years before de Lange had published her cases. But it must be emphasized that Brachmann's case of symmetrical monodactyly, ulnar defects, pterygia of the elbows, dwarfism, cervical ribs and hirsutism presented a disease picture greatly differing from that described by de Lange.[1] Whereas the descriptions by Brachmann and de Lange had little in common, the connecting links reported much later by other authors suggested that the cases belonged to the same syndrome.

In one study,[17] thyroid function was found to be abnormal, but growth hormone was detectable in the plasma of all the patients examined. Simulation of de Lange syndrome by hypothyroidism was reported by Beer *et al.*[23] in a child of a kindred in which synophrys was a dominant hereditary trait. Roentgen findings are most characteristic in the upper extremities. They range from those of phocomelia to minor changes such as short first metacarpals and small middle phalanges of digits V (incurved little fingers). Anomalies and dislocation of the radial heads have been observed repeatedly.[7,8]

Fig. 38-1 (left). – Infant boy with de Lange syndrome. Note forward-facing nostrils, fish mouth, micrognathia and webbing of neck. Monodactyly flexion deformity of elbow. Bilateral absence of radius. The child had mitral and aortic stenosis, coarctation of the aorta and malrotation of the intestines. He did not have intrauterine growth retardation. (Courtesy of Cincinnati Children's Neuromuscular Diagnostic Clinic.)

Fig. 38-2 (right). – De Lange syndrome in a 4-year-old girl. Note heavy eyebrows, forward-facing nostrils and fish mouth.

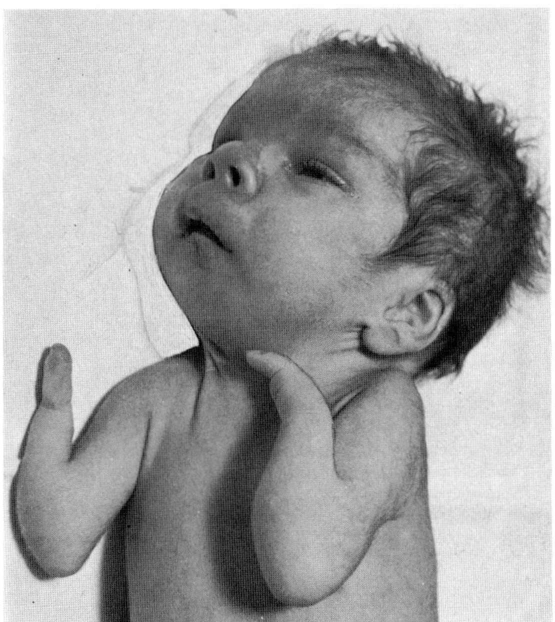

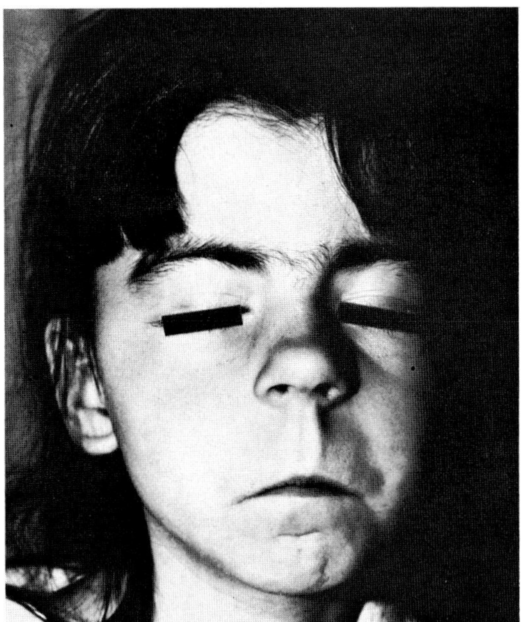

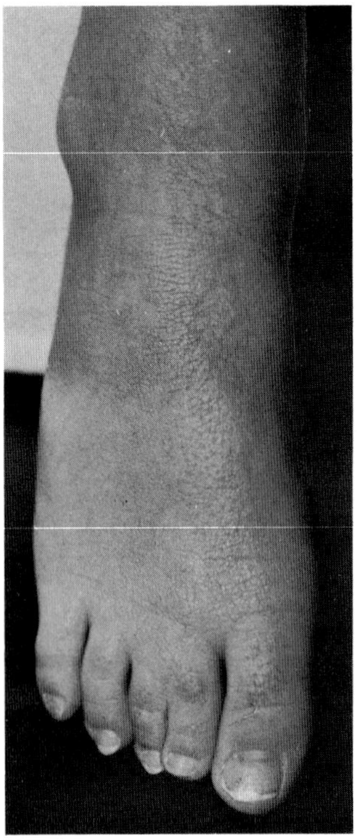

Fig. 38-3.—Syndactyly of toes II and III of girl with de Lange syndrome.

Most cases of de Lange syndrome are sporadic, but recurrence in some families has been reported.[15] In some patients, seemingly heterogeneous chromosomal abnormalities have been seen.[5,18-21] In one kindred,[22] the syndrome appeared in 4 members, with 3 siblings and a maternal first cousin being affected. Three of the patients had an abnormal metacentric chromosome in the absence of a small acrocentric of the G group. Some of the relatives were carriers of a deletion of one of the A-3 chromosomes. Interestingly, none of the patients in this kindred had intrauterine growth retardation. In most cases, however, the karyotype appeared normal.[6] Concordance has been observed in monozygotic twins.[15] Pashayan *et al.*[25] rejected the hypothesis of simple autosomal recessive inheritance and suggested that the empirical risk of recurrence in siblings of an affected child is between 2% and 5%. The etiology remains obscure and the possibility of the existence of several forms of the de Lange syndrome has been considered.[26]

REFERENCES

1. de Lange, C.: Sur un type nouveau de dégénération (Typus Amstelodamensis), Arch. méd. Enf. 36:713, 1933.
2. de Lange, C.: Nouvelle observation du "Typus Amstelodamensis" et examen anatomo-pathologique de ce type, Arch. méd. Enf. 41:193, 1938.
3. Richter, H.: Drei neue Beobachtungen des Cornelia de Lange syndroms, Arch. Kinderh. 164:249, 1961.
4. Arnaud-Battandier, R., and Gillot, F.: Un nouveau cas de typus Amstelodamensis (Maladie de Cornelia de Lange), Pédiatrie 8:100, 1953.
5. Jervis, G. A., and Stimson, C. W.: De Lange syndrome; the "Amsterdam type" of mental defect with congenital malformation, J. Pediat. 63:634, 1963.
6. McArthur, R. G., and Edwards, J. H.: De Lange syndrome: Report of 20 cases, Canad. M.A.J. 96:1185, 1967.
7. Kurlander, G. J., and DeMyer, W.: Roentgenology of the Brachmann-de Lange syndrome, Radiology 88:101, 1967.
8. Lee, F. A., and Kenny, F. M.: Skeletal changes in the Cornelia de Lange syndrome, Am. J. Roentgenol. 100:27, 1967.
9. Familant, J. W.: Cornelia de Lange syndrome; a second case is reported in the Negro, Clin. Pediat. 7:411, 1968.
10. Noé, O., and Hammond, J.: De Lange's Amsterdam dwarfism: Case report and etiological considerations, Am. J. Ment. Deficiency 71:994, 1967.
11. Laurence, K. M., and Ishmael, J.: Chromosomes in typus degenerativus Amstelodamensis (Cornelia de Lange syndrome), Lancet 1:1426, 1963.
12. Gans, B., and Thurston, J. G. B.: De Lange's Amsterdam dwarfs syndrome, Developmental Med. & Child Neurol. 7:42, 1965.
13. Aberfeld, D. C., and Pourfar, M.: De Lange's Amsterdam dwarfs syndrome, Developmental Med. & Child Neurol. 7:35, 1965.
14. Smithells, R. W.: De Lange's Amsterdam dwarfs syndrome, Developmental Med. & Child Neurol. 7:27, 1965.
15. Opitz, J. M., Segal, A. T., Lehrke, R. L., and Nadler, H. L.: The etiology of the Brachmann-de Lange syndrome, Birth Defects Reprint Series, National Foundation, New York, 1965.
16. Brachmann, W.: Ein Fall von symmetrischer Monodactylie durch Ulnadefekt und symmetrischer Flughautbildung in den Ellenbeugen, sowie anderen Abnormitäten (Zwerghaftigkeit, Halsrippen, Behaarung), Jahrb. Kinderh. 84:225, 1916.
17. Hillman, J. C., Hammond, J., Noé, O., and Reiss, M.: Endocrine investigations in de Lange's and Seckel's syndromes, Am. J. Ment. Deficiency 73:30, 1968.
18. Geudeke, M., Bijlsma, J. B., and De Bruijne, J. I.: Chromosomenonderzaek bij typus degenerativus Amstelodamensis, Maandschr. kindergeneesk. 31:248, 1963.
19. Dodge, J. A.: De Lange's Amsterdam dwarfs syndrome, Developmental Med. & Child Neurol. 7:31, 1965.
20. Berg, J. M., Smith, G. F., Ridler, M. A. C., McCreary, B. D., Faunch, J. A., Farnham, F. N., and Allen, M. L.: De Lange syndrome: Report of a case with an unusual karyotype, J. M. Genetics 4:184, 1967.
21. Craig, A., and Luzzatti, L.: Translocation in de Lange's syndrome, Lancet 2:445, 1965.
22. Falek, A., Schmidt, R., and Jervis, G. A.: Familial de Lange syndrome with chromosome abnormalities, Pediatrics 37:92, 1966.
23. Beer, S., Wallis, K., and Czerniak, P.: Two cases of de Lange's syndrome (typus degenerativus Amstelodamensis), J. Ment. Defic. Res. 12:128, 1968.
24. France, N. E., Crome, L., and Abraham, J. M.: Pathological features in the de Lange syndrome, Acta paediat. scandinav. 58:470, 1969.
25. Pashayan, H., Whelan, D., Guttman, S., and Fraser, F. C.: Variability of the de Lange syndrome: Report of 3 cases and genetic analysis of 54 families, J. Pediat. 75:853, 1969.
26. Berg, J. M., McCreary, B. D., Ridler, M. A. C., and Smith, G. F.: *The De Lange Syndrome* (Oxford: Pergamon Press, 1970).

Cerebro-Hepato-Renal Syndromes

UNDER THIS TERM may be cited some familial syndromes attributed to autosomal recessive genes with strongly pleiotropic effects. Affected children fail to develop physically and mentally, have some facial resemblance and are hypotonic in infancy. Outlook for survival and improvement is poor.

Bowen *et al.*[1] recorded a familial syndrome of multiple congenital defects with hypotonia, congenital cataracts or glaucoma and minor skeletal anomalies, including calcification of the patella. One of the children had hepatomegaly, gastrointestinal bleeding, cardiovascular defects and renal cysts. Punnett and Kirkpatrick[2] observed a similar patient with marked micrencephaly, eyeground changes and elevated intraocular tension. Hepatomegaly and diffuse interstitial fibrosis were noted. The kidneys were small and had minimal renal dysplasia. As in the cases observed by Bowen and associates,[1] calcifications were seen in roentgenograms of the patella. The facial features, epicanthic folds, low-set ears and simian creases suggested Down syndrome but the karyotype appeared normal.

Intrahepatic biliary dysgenesis combined with polycystic kidneys, various minor developmental defects and a characteristic facies was observed in a brother and sister by Smith *et al.*[3] and reported as a syndrome. A high forehead, flat supraorbital ridges, epicanthic folds, a narrow palatal arch, camptodactyly, flexion at the knees, incomplete descent of gonads and hypotonia were constituents of the syndrome. The infants failed to thrive, developed jaundice and died at the age of 10 weeks. The authors considered autosomal recessive inheritance the most likely etiology. The histologic pictures of the liver were not identical in these two cases. Whereas in the boy the lobular architecture was preserved and the bile canaliculi were dilated and terminal cholangioles absent, the liver architecture was radically distorted in his sister, as liver intrahepatic bile ducts were not seen and identification of bile canaliculi was difficult. There was generalized fibrosis pervading her liver.

A cerebro-hepato-renal syndrome probably comparable to that described above was reported by Passarge and McAdams.[4] Five sisters of a family of 13 children were affected; 8 children and the parents apparently were normal. Hypotonia and craniofacial characteristics were noticeable at birth. Hepatomegaly and cortical renal cysts were present in all children; morphologic anomalies of the brain were noted in 2 but cardiovascular defects in only 1. Broad gyri and deficient development and sclerosis of white matter were seen in 2 of the infants.

Since these syndromes occur repeatedly in families, a genetic etiology has been assumed and the manifestations were considered "syndromes." But, on careful analyses, these syndromes show great interfamilial and intrafamilial variation. Except for craniofacial resemblance, hypotonia, failure to thrive, variable degrees of hepatomegaly and renal cysts—rather uncharacteristic signs—the variability of the changes seen in different organs is considerable. If such syndromes occurred sporadically, their differing constituents often would fail to suggest a similar origin. To give some examples: Patient 4 of Passarge and McAdams[4] had bilateral cataracts and a histologically normal liver, whereas patient 5 had no cataracts but cirrhosis of the liver and gastrointestinal bleeding. Patient 2 had a large anterior fontanelle that extended anteriorly almost to the nasal bridge, a large posterior fontanelle, dextroposed and stenotic pulmonary artery, atrial and ventricular septal defects and patent ductus arteriosus, but the liver was histologically normal. Patient 3 had normal fontanelles, no septal or pulmonary anomalies but she had hepatitis and a subcapsular cavernous hemangioma. Thus, the genes—or whatever the cause of these anomalies—have variable, pleiotropic effects that would be quite nonspecific and unclassifiable when seen in a sporadic case.

REFERENCES

1. Bowen, P., Lee, C. S. N., Zellweger, H., and Lindenberg, R.: A familial syndrome of multiple congenital defects, Bull. Johns Hopkins Hosp. 114:402, 1964.
2. Punnett, H. H., and Kirkpatrick, J. A., Jr.: A syndrome of ocular abnormalities, calcification of cartilage and failure to thrive, J. Pediat. 73:602, 1968.
3. Smith, D. W., Opitz, J. M., and Inhorn, S. L.: A syndrome of multiple developmental defects including polycystic kidneys and intrahepatic biliary dysgenesis in two siblings, J. Pediat. 67:617, 1965.
4. Passarge, E., and McAdams, A. J.: Cerebro-hepato-renal syndrome, J. Pediat. 71:691, 1967.
5. Poznanski, A. K., Nosanchuk, J. S., Baublis, J., and Holt, J. F.: The cerebro-hepato-renal syndrome, Am. J. Roentgenol. 109:313, 1970.

Microcephaly and Genital Anomalies

SMITH, LEMLI AND OPITZ[1] described a syndrome of microcephaly, mental retardation, failure to thrive, short nose with anteverted nostrils, broad maxillary alveolar ridges, hypospadias, cleft scrotum, horizontal upper palmar creases and syndactyly between the second and third toes. In two cases, the dermal pattern showed 10 whorls. Pinsky and DiGeorge[2] pointed out that there were genital abnormalities in males and normal genitals in females with this syndrome. Gibson[3] found the syndrome associated with dysplasia epiphysealis punctata. Blair and Martin[4] reported 2 siblings with this syndrome and pointed out that cleft uvula and unusual dermal pattern may be of diagnostic help. The dermatoglyphics of 6 patients examined revealed 10 whorls in 3 patients and 1 had 9 whorls, a finding that confirmed those of Smith *et al.*[1] In some patients, an arch tibial hallucal pattern was found. Dallaire and Fraser[5] observed 2 male patients with the same syndrome. The patients also had simian creases and high palmar triradii. Chromosomal studies have been normal. Autosomal recessive mode of inheritance is suspected.

REFERENCES

1. Smith, D. W., Lemli, L., and Opitz, J. M.: A newly recognized syndrome of multiple congenital anomalies, J. Pediat. 64:210, 1964.
2. Pinsky, L., and DiGeorge, A. M.: A familial syndrome of facial and skeletal anomalies associated with genital abnormality in the male and normal genitals in the female, J. Pediat. 66:1049, 1965.
3. Gibson, R.: A case of the Smith-Lemli-Opitz syndrome of multiple congenital anomalies in association with dysplasia epiphysialis punctata, Canad. M.A.J. 92:574, 1965.
4. Blair, H. R., and Martin, J. K.: A syndrome characterized by mental retardation, short stature, craniofacial dysplasia, and genital anomalies occurring in siblings, J. Pediat. 69:457, 1966.
5. Dallaire, L., and Fraser, F. C.: The syndrome of retardation with urogenital and skeletal anomalies in siblings, J. Pediat. 69:459, 1966.

Microcephaly and Cleft Palate

CLEFT PALATE with and without cleft lip sometimes is associated with microcephaly. It has been estimated that in Sweden 1.6 microcephalics occur in 10,000 unselected births.[1] In contrast, 3 microcephalics were noted among 105 cases of cleft lip and palate during a study in Birmingham, England.[2] The association of microcephaly and posterior palate cleft is also frequent, so that one could speak of a "syndrome." But this association probably is of heterogeneous etiology. We have seen a family in which at least 7 of 9 children were microcephalic and mentally retarded. The ninth child, a boy with microcephaly, also had cleft palate (Cincinnati Children's Hospital Chart No. 145705). It was mentioned in Chapter 14 that microcephaly and cleft palate occur in some children with intrauterine growth retardation. In addition to the cases mentioned there, a girl weighing 1,700 Gm. (after a pregnancy of 36 weeks) who had microcephaly, posterior palate cleft, iris coloboma and clubfoot on the right was seen in the Cincinnati Children's Hospital (Chart No. 166813). She developed convulsions and weighed 5,000 Gm. at the age of 2½ years. The karyotype was 46,XX. The birth weight can be normal, as noted in a girl who combined microcephaly with micrognathia and posterior palate cleft (Pierre Robin syndrome) (Cincinnati Children's Hospital Chart No. 164144). In the severest form of microcephaly (pinhead), which occurs as an autosomal recessive trait, associated malformations, including cleft palate, are rare.[3] Microcephaly with cleft palate (with or without lip) occurs in trisomy 13-15, cat-cry syndrome,[4-6] deficiency of the short arm of chromosome no. 4[7] and other chromosomal abnormalities.

REFERENCES

1. Böök, J. A., Schut, J. W., and Reed, S. C.: A clinical and genetical study of microcephaly, Am. J. Ment. Deficiency 57:637, 1953.
2. MacMahon, B., and McKeown, T.: The incidence of harelip and cleft palate related to birth rank and maternal age, Am. J. Human Genet. 5:176, 1953.
3. Hanhart, E.: Über einfache Rezessivität bei Mikrocephalia vera, spuria et combinata und das herdweise Vorkommen der Mikrocephalia vera in Schweizer Isolaten, Acta genet. med. 7:445, 1958.
4. Olive, D., Gilgenkrantz, S., Cabrol, C., and Wolkowica, M. W.: Maladie du cri du chat (5p−) avec gueule de loup, Pédiatrie 23:795, 1968.
5. Giorgi, P. L., Ceccarelli, M., and Paci, A.: Su un caso di sindrome del (cri du chat) con peculiari anomalie fenotipiche, Minerva pediat. 17:1972, 1965.
6. Hijmans, J. C., and Shearin, D. B.: Partial deletion of short arms of chromosome no. 5, Am. J. Dis. Child. 109:85, 1965.
7. Wolf, U., and Reinwein, H.: Klinische und cytogenetische Differentialdiagnose der Defizienzen an den kurzen Armen der B-Chromosomen, Ztschr. Kinderh. 98:235, 1967.

Puppet Syndrome

AFFECTED CHILDREN are severely retarded from the first months. They have convulsions and spasms at an early age combined with paroxysms of laughter, ataxic jerky movements resembling those of puppets and ability to protrude the tongue to an unusual degree.[1] The head is brachycephalic, the face round, the ears large and the chin protruding. There is a horizontal occipital depression and roentgenograms of the skull reveal a vertical inclination of the base and microcephaly. The EEG shows slow wave and spike activity and absence of hypsarrhythmia.[2] The etiology is not known.

REFERENCES

1. Angelman, H.: "Puppet" children. A report on 3 cases, Developmental Med. & Child Neurol. 7:681, 1965.
2. Bower, B. D., and Jeavons, P. M.: The "happy puppet" syndrome, Arch. Dis. Childhood 42:298, 1967.

Sturge-Weber Syndrome

STURGE-WEBER SYNDROME, which consists of a facial port-wine nevus, convulsions and other neurologic manifestations, has appeared in the literature under a wide variety of names, including "encephalofacial," "cerebrocutaneous," "encephalo-trigeminal" and "meningeal angiomatosis." Other names are "calcified pseudoangiomas of the brain," "benign subcortical calcifications" and "nevoid amentia." Although the names of Sturge,[1] Weber,[2] Dimitri,[3] Kalischer[4] and Krabbe[5] have been linked eponymically with the syndrome, some of its features were first recorded by Schirmer[6] in 1860.

The syndrome in its complete form includes: (1) cutaneous angioma, (2) seizures, (3) hemiparesis, (4) characteristic intracranial calcifications, (5) mental retardation and (6) glaucoma. Many of the cases reported are incomplete and show only some of the above characteristics. Several reviews on the subject are available.[7-12]

The syndrome in its complete form is rare. In institutions for mental patients it is found in 1 of 1,000 patients. The incidence of trigeminal port-wine nevus as an isolated anomaly is more frequent and is said to occur once in 5,000 persons of the general population. Estimates of the sex ratio vary widely.[13]

In the majority of cases, Sturge-Weber syndrome occurs sporadically. The triad consisting of cutaneous, ocular and cerebral manifestations has not been found in familial aggregation. In only 19 of approximately 500 published cases could Koch[13] ascertain some suggestion of heredity. Even in these patients, the syndrome usually was incomplete. Some of the cases with suggestive familial symptomatology were cited by Warkany and Rubinstein.[12] In these families, the relatives of the patients afflicted with Sturge-Weber syndrome had incomplete manifestations. The fact that the syndrome itself is variable and that many cases are incomplete, or "formes frustes," makes family studies difficult. According to Blum and Mutrux,[14] 85% of the cases have only one or two of the cardinal signs said to be sufficiently characteristic to ensure specificity. Furthermore, the complete picture may not be present at birth, yet develop with increasing age.[13] Therefore, an affected member of the family may die before the entire syndrome has developed and thus escape recognition. Such variability may cause the lack of pedigrees showing transmission of the disorder through several generations. In addition, even in cases of determination by a dominant gene, a syndrome or symptom may not be transmitted if the first person to manifest the new mutation is not capable of reproducing. Thus, sporadic cases could be genetically determined. If the pedigrees of patients with Sturge-Weber syndrome showed such incomplete manifestations consistently, one could assume that a dominant gene with low expressivity was responsible for the symptoms or the entire syndrome. But, on the basis of isolated pedigrees containing such nonspecific symptoms as seizures, migraine, mental retardation, angiomas, and so forth, one cannot draw definite conclusions, since it is possible that in such families pathologic manifestations of differing etiology accumulated by chance. The pedigrees that have been referred to are selected and not convincing examples of determination by an incompletely dominant gene. It is somewhat unusual in a disease with dominant inheritance that no case of the complete syndrome is transmitted through more than one generation or that it is not observed in more than one sibling. The only case of transmission of the syndrome, the case of Sorsby,[15] was not described in detail.

The patients of Geyelin and Penfield,[16] reported as "cerebral calcification epilepsy" in a father and 4 of his children, were not cases of Sturge-Weber syndrome, although they are cited at times as an example of the familial occurrence of the disorder. The same can be said of a report by Touraine *et al.*,[17] in which they described a pair of twins who had epileptic attacks and "voluminous varicose formation inscribed into the internal table of the parietal bones" but apparently no port-wine nevi. Since no illustrations of the patients or their roentgenograms were given, it is not possible to make a definite diagnosis or draw impartial conclusions from the report. In the older literature, reports of dominantly inherited

Sturge-Weber syndrome probably were cases of Hippel-Lindau disease (Chapter 123).

Yakovlev and Guthrie[18] gave an interesting example of "a combined heredity" transmitted to a patient with Sturge-Weber syndrome from both paternal and maternal sides. There were congenital cutaneous malformations (considered to be abortive forms of neurofibromatosis) in the patient, in her mother and in several brothers and sisters, a vascular nevus in a brother, fainting spells and convulsions in the mother and in several brothers and sisters. On the father's side there were nervous disorders, migraine and psychopathic disposition. In this family there apparently was a partial overlapping of Sturge-Weber syndrome with neurofibromatosis. The same was true in the case of Kissel and Arnould,[19] in which the mother had neurofibromatosis and the daughter signs of Sturge-Weber syndrome. Possible transitions from Osler's hereditary hemorrhagic telangiectasis to Sturge-Weber syndrome were discussed by Chao.[8] Recessive inheritance is also doubtful. A few case reports recorded parental consanguinity[13]; many others did not. It is to be hoped that in future publications attention will be paid to this part of the family history. Possible explanations suggested by Penrose[20] were "fresh mutations of a gene presumably dominant," "intrauterine environmental accidents at a very early stage of development," "somatic mutation of an unstable gene" and "infective disease of the fetus." Spiller[21] reported a case of Sturge-Weber syndrome in which a history was obtained of the mother having been exposed to roentgen rays of unstated dosage when she was 3½ months pregnant; the significance of this association cannot be evaluated.

With lack of adequate genetic evidence to explain the etiology of the syndrome, the chromosomal study by Hayward and Bower[22] was encouraging in suggesting a possible cause. They reported trisomy of one of the five smallest acrocentric chromosomes, which they identified as probably chromosome 22. But, following their publication, Lehmann and Forssman[23] reported normal idiograms in two cases of Sturge-Weber syndrome. Many subsequent reports also failed to discover a chromosomal abnormality,[12] but Patau *et al.*[24] found a possible "partial trisomy" in one of their cases.

The first clinical finding usually is a cutaneous angioma in the form of a "port-wine" nevus in the distribution area of one or more of the major sensory trigeminal divisions, most often the ophthalmic branch. In almost two-thirds of the cases the nevus is present at birth. It usually is flat, but occasionally covered with rough nodules. Most often it is unilateral, tending to stop at the midline. Occasionally, the entire face is involved and more rarely the nevus extends to the trunk. The mucous membranes may be affected by cavernous nevi of the lips and the tongue.

Convulsions occur in more than two-thirds of the

Fig. 38-4 (left). – Girl with vascular nevus on the left in the area of the ophthalmic branch of the trigeminal nerve. Normal 46,XX karyotype. (From J. Warkany and J. Rubinstein.[12])

Fig. 38-5 (right). – Roentgenogram of a 10-year-old girl with nevus flammeus on the left side showing left hemicranium smaller than the right and intracranial calcifications arranged in parallel lines and following the convolutions – a pattern typical of Sturge-Weber syndrome.

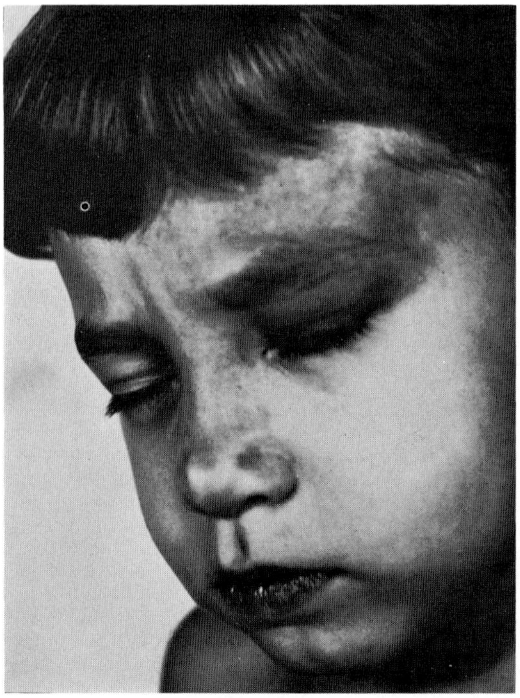

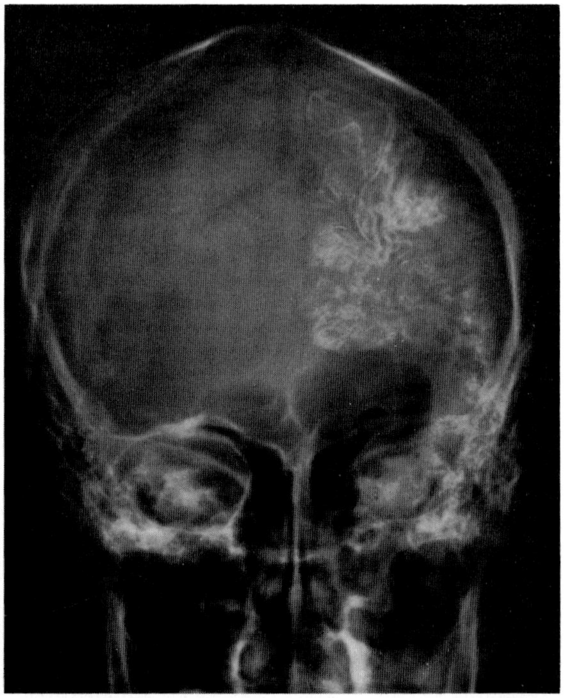

cases, with onset from infancy to adulthood. They may be generalized or, more often, focal and contralateral to the facial lesion. Contralateral transient or permanent hemiplegia or hemiparesis usually is noted in about half the cases after the onset of seizures, but sometimes they precede the convulsive disorder. The neurologic evidence for weakness and spasticity may be rather inconspicuous.

Mental retardation of variable severity is found in about half the cases and the eye is involved (on the side of the nevus) in about one-third, the lesions varying from dilated vessels in the sclera and conjunctiva to glaucoma that may be secondary to angiomatous malformation in the choroid or uvea. Engorgement of retinal veins or actual retinal angiomas have been reported. Heterochromia of the iris has been observed repeatedly.[25]

Roentgenographic examination of the skull may reveal characteristic sinuous calcifications arranged in double lines 1–2 mm. apart. Their parallel arrangement is comparable to that of railroad tracks. Such calcifications are most often unilateral and on the side of the facial nevus. They are most prominent in the occipital area and can be associated with cranial asymmetry. Pneumoencephalograms sometimes show atrophy of the affected side of the cortex with ventricular dilatation. The calcifications are not in the angioma of the meninges but rather in the substance of the cortex below. Calcification has been reported as early as 4 months, but it can take a number of years before it becomes visible in roentgenograms. Angiograms occasionally demonstrate angiomatous malformations of the meninges. Associated angiomas of viscera have also been observed.[9] Hemiatrophy or hemihypertrophy on the side of the cutaneous nevus has been noted in some instances.

For some time, a group of syndromes involving the skin and the central nervous system have been collectively named "phakomatoses,"[26] "congenital ectodermoses,"[18] "neurocutaneous syndromes"[8] and so forth. Conditions such as tuberous sclerosis, Recklinghausen neurofibromatosis, Hippel-Lindau disease and, recently, ataxia telangiectasia have been covered by these terms. There have been suggestions to include Sturge-Weber syndrome in this group of disorders, which are admittedly genetically determined, although their modes of transmission differ. Unlike the other conditions named, the etiology of Sturge-Weber syndrome is still obscure. It has not been shown to have a simple hereditary or even familial pattern, although some authors believe in a more subtle mode of hereditary transmission.

Patients with the triad of symptoms are handicapped by convulsions, pareses, ocular changes and often mental retardation. A survey by Greenwald and Koota[27] showed that the majority of patients died in the second or third decade of life, but a number of them lived on into middle age.

Successful treatment with radium or x-rays has been reported. In some cases, surgery and radiotherapy were combined.[27]

REFERENCES

1. Sturge, W. A.: A case of partial epilepsy, apparently due to a lesion of one of the vasomotor centres of the brain, Tr. Clin. Soc. London 12:162, 1879.
2. Weber, F. P.: Notes on association of extensive haemangiomatous naevus of skin with cerebral (meningeal) haemangioma, especially cases of facial vascular naevus with contralateral hemiplegia, Proc. Roy. Soc. Med. (Sect. Neurol.) 22:25,1929.
3. Dimitri, V.: Congenital cavernous angioma, Rev. Asoc. méd. argent. 36:1029, 1923.
4. Kalischer, S.: Demonstration des Gehirns eines Kindes mit Teleangiectasie der links-seitigen Gesichts-Kopfhaut und Hirnoberfläche, Klin. Wchnschr. 34:1059, 1897.
5. Krabbe, K. H.: Facial and meningeal angiomatosis associated with calcifications of brain cortex; clinical and anatomopathologic contribution, Arch. Neurol. & Psychiat. 32:737, 1934.
6. Schirmer, R.: Ein Fall von Teleangiektase, von Graefes Arch. Ophth. 7:119, 1860.
7. Peterman, A. F., Hayles, A. B., Dockerty, M. B., and Love, J. G.: Encephalotrigeminal angiomatosis (Sturge-Weber disease); clinical study of thirty-five cases, J.A.M.A. 167: 2169, 1958.
8. Chao, D. H-C.: Congenital neurocutaneous syndromes of childhood. III. Sturge-Weber disease, J. Pediat. 55:635, 1959.
9. Wohlwill, F. J., and Yakovlev, P. I.: Histopathology of meningofacial angiomatosis (Sturge-Weber's disease); report of four cases, J. Neuropath. & Exper. Neurol. 16: 341, 1957.
10. King, G., and Schwarz, G. A.: Sturge-Weber syndrome (encephalo-trigeminal angiomatosis), A.M.A. Arch. Int. Med. 94:743, 1954.
11. Brushfield, T., and Wyatt, W.: Hemiplegia associated with extensive naevus and mental defect (pathological changes), Brit. J. Child. Dis. 25:96, 1928.
12. Warkany, J., and Rubinstein, J. H.: Etiology of the Sturge-Weber syndrome with chromosome analysis of a case, J. Maine M. A. 53:76, 1962.
13. Koch, G.: Neuere Betrachtungen über die Erblichkeit der Sturge-Weberschen und von Hippel-Lindauschen Krankheit, Med. Welt 38:1955, 1960.
14. Blum, J. D., and Mutrux, S.: La maladie de Sturge-Weber-Krabbe (angiomatose encéphalo-trigeminée); considérations sur ses formes complètes et incomplètes, à propos de deux cas, Ophthalmologica 118:781, 1949.
15. Sorsby, A.: *Clinical Genetics* (St. Louis: The C. V. Mosby Company, 1953).
16. Geyelin, H. R., and Penfield, W.: Cerebral calcification epilepsy; endarteritis calcificans cerebri, Arch. Neurol. & Psychiat. 21:1020, 1929.
17. Touraine, A., Golé, L., and Sambron, J.: Epilepsie et angiomatose intra-cranienne chez deux jumeaux, Bull. Soc. franç. dermat. et syph. 43:618, 1936.
18. Yakovlev, P. I., and Guthrie, R. H.: Congenital ectodermoses (neurocutaneous syndromes) in epileptic patients, Arch. Neurol. & Psychiat. 26:1145, 1931.
19. Kissel, P., and Arnould, G.: Neuro-ectodermose familiale à type de maladie de Recklinghausen chez la mère, de maladie de Sturge-Weber chez la fille, Rev. neurol. 91: 381, 1954.
20. Penrose, L. S.: *The Biology of Mental Defect* (London: Sidgwick and Jackson, Ltd., 1954).
21. Spiller, W. G.: Congenital tumor of brain (telangiectasis) and associated cerebral movements, Arch. Neurol. & Psychiat. 2:50, 1919.
22. Hayward, M. D., and Bower, B. D.: Chromosomal trisomy associated with the Sturge-Weber syndrome, Lancet 2: 844, 1960.

23. Lehmann, O., and Forssman, H.: Chromosomes in the Sturge-Weber syndrome, Lancet 2:1450, 1960.
24. Patau, K., Therman, E., Inhorn, S. L., and Picken, B. F.: The cytogenetics of the Sturge-Weber syndrome, Proc. Am. Soc. Human Genetics, Atlantic City, 1961.
25. Walsh, F. B.: *Clinical Neuro-Ophthalmology* (Baltimore: The Williams & Wilkins Company, 1947).
26. van der Hoeve, J.: Doyne Memorial Lecture: Eye symptoms in phakomatoses, Tr. Ophth. Soc. U. Kingdom 52: 380, 1932.
27. Greenwald, H. M., and Koota, J.: Associated facial and intracranial hemangiomas, Am. J. Dis. Child. 51:868, 1936.

PART V

Malformations of the Eye

39

Ocular Defects

The Lids

PALPEBRAL COLOBOMAS are triangular gaps in the lid margins. According to Mann,[2] colobomas of the upper lid usually are located at the junction of the inner and middle thirds of the lids, colobomas of the lower lid at the junction of the outer and middle thirds. The gaps can be unilateral or bilateral. Amniotic bands have been seen attached to colobomas of the lids, but this does not signify that they are the cause of the gap.[1] Palpebral colobomas often are combined with ocular anomalies such as iris coloboma, corneal opacities, microphthalmia and others. There also may be dermal or hairy connections of the coloboma with the cornea or hair of the scalp, indicating a more comprehensive linear defect in which the eyelids are involved. Hereditary transmission of colobomas of the upper lid is rare but some instances have been reported. Coloboma of the lower lid is a constituent of the Treacher Collins syndrome (mandibulofacial dysostosis) (p. 650). This syndrome has been observed repeatedly as an autosomal dominant trait with irregular expression. In some mildly affected persons there may be no coloboma but the palpebral fissure appears widened as an alternative manifestation, so that the lid opening looks "square." Coloboma of the upper lid is a constituent of the Goldenhar syndrome (p. 388), in which it is associated with epibulbar dermoids, malformed auricles and defective segmentation of the spine.

Epicanthic folds. When the skin of the nasal bridge extends laterad over the inner canthus and covers the inner angle of the orbital fissure, one speaks of epicanthic folds. The upper end of the fold can begin at the eyebrow, at the skin of the upper lid or at the tarsal fold.[2] This variability makes differentiation of the pathologic epicanthus from the true mongol fold difficult. Epicanthus is normal in the Mongolian race and in the fetuses of Europeans.[2] It also is frequent in infants and toddlers. It has been estimated that approximately 30% of Europeans have epicanthic folds up to 6 months but only 3% at ages 12–25 years.[1] Whatever the figures are in various populations, it generally is observed that the epicanthus disappears with increasing age. Since pediatricians are trained to observe epicanthic folds in various disease pictures, particularly Down syndrome, they may worry unnecessarily when they see these folds in otherwise normal infants who lose this trait later and attain normal intelligence.

In some families, epicanthus is transmitted as a dominant hereditary trait. In such cases, congenital ptosis of the upper lids with absence of the levator palpebrae superioris occurs frequently as an associated symptom.

Epicanthus is a frequent symptom of Down syndrome (p. 326). Although it persists in these patients longer than normally, there is a tendency to disappearance of the epicanthic folds in mongoloid patients too. They often are present in such heterogeneous conditions as trisomy 18, Turner syndrome, craniosynostosis, renal agenesis and Ehlers-Danlos syndrome.

Blepharophimosis is a small or short palpebral fissure. This anomaly can occur in otherwise normal persons as a hereditary dominant trait, but it also can be associated with severe malformations of the eye such as anophthalmia or microphthalmia. It occurs in Down syndrome (p. 326), Waardenburg syndrome (p. 395), hemiatrophy of the face and with congenital ptosis of the upper eyelid.[1] I have seen it repeatedly in infants with arthrogryposis (p. 1014).

Distichiasis is the term for double rows of eyelashes, one row in the normal position, the other behind it and located at the site of the openings of the Meibomian glands. These glands are hypoplastic or absent in such cases. All four lids can be affected. This rare condition is hereditary and is transmitted as an autosomal dominant trait. Falls and Kertesz[3] described a syndrome in which distichiasis is combined with pterygium colli and Milroy's disease. The disorder can be transmitted as a dominant hereditary trait. Lymphedema of the lower extremities is not congenital but appears at the time of puberty.

The Lacrimal Apparatus

The lacrimal glands develop as outgrowths from the conjunctival epithelium, at first as solid cords, later forming lumina; they are located over the external angle of the eye and consist of a larger orbital and a smaller palpebral portion. Congenital absence of tear secretion in 3 sisters was described as early as 1900; neurologic complications appeared later. Alacrimia is a symptom of familial autonomic dysfunction (Riley-Day syndrome). It may also occur in anhidrotic ectodermal dysplasia (p. 1165).

The nasolacrimal sac and duct exist at first, in 12-mm. embryos, as an epithelial thickening of the nasolacrimal groove, which connects the inner angle of the eye with the primitive olfactory sac, separating the maxillary and lateral nasal processes. The epithelial thickening is later covered up by mesenchymal tissue and becomes the solid forerunner of the lacrimal sac and nasolacrimal duct. From its upper end secondary branches extend to the eyelids (lacrimal canaliculi), and its lower end establishes a communication with the nasal cavity. The lacrimal puncta, the opening of the canaliculi into the conjunctival sac and the other lacrimal passages canalize just before birth. The nasal opening of the lacrimal duct can still be closed at birth. The lacrimal passages may fail to develop, fail to canalize or take an abnormal course.

Delay until after birth of perforation of the membrane at the nasal end of the lacrimal duct is not rare. As long as tear secretion is absent in the newborn the anomaly remains symptomless, but when stagnation of tears and debris leads to infection, purulent discharge occurs into the conjunctival sac (dacryocystitis). Probing through the lower canaliculus is performed to dilate the nasal opening of the duct.

Absence of the puncta and canaliculi occurs if the branches from the lacrimal duct fail to grow in the direction of the lids. More often, the puncta fail to open, although they and the canaliculi are present. Laterad dislocation of the lacrimal puncta and elongation of the canaliculi is a symptom of the Waardenburg syndrome (p. 395).

Dyskeratosis

Involvement of the ocular tissues in cases of ichthyosis of the skin is rare.[4] In mild cases there may be no symptoms, but sometimes photophobia, blepharospasm, epiphora and diminution of vision do occur. The conjunctiva may be swollen, thickened and glazed. In rare instances, the disorder involves the cornea, which may be irritated by the hyperplastic conjunctiva or be primarily affected by keratosis. Infiltration and pannus formation can result in diminution of vision.

Witkop *et al.*[5] described a congenital and hereditary bulbar conjunctivitis that is accompanied by oral lesions of intra-epithelial dyskeratosis. There are raised gelatinous plaques that overlie intensely injected conjunctiva. The plaques are triangular in shape, having their base on the limbus. In the spring, the lesions sometimes extend over the cornea, causing temporary blindness, but these corneal membranes sometimes are shed in late summer. Affected children have corneal vascularization and marked photophobia. Corneal opacities may become permanent, but carcinoma does not develop. The syndrome of oral and ocular dyskeratotic lesions is transmitted as a dominant autosomal trait. Witkop *et al.* found it widely distributed in a large kindred in North Carolina that constitutes part of a triracial isolate in that area.

Anophthalmia and Microphthalmia

The clinical distinction between anophthalmia and microphthalmia is difficult, since, without microscopic examination, severe microphthalmia can be mistaken for anophthalmia. Traces of an eyeball or remnants of an optic nerve often are found when histologic sections are made. True anophthalmia is due to failure of formation of the optic pit and of optic outgrowths from the forebrain.[1] The lens, which normally is induced by the optic outgrowth, the optic nerves, the chiasma and the foramen opticum are absent, but the eyelids, the conjunctival sac, the extrinsic ocular muscles and the lacrimal apparatus are present. It follows that anophthalmia cannot be diagnosed with certainty by clinical observation alone and that clinical reports of this condition often probably are cases of microphthalmia. In necropsy reports, the diagnosis of anophthalmia should be based not only on the absence of ocular rudiments in serial section but also on absence of the optic nerves, chiasma and tracts. In discussing clinical cases, I shall use the term microphthalmia rather than anophthalmia, but sometimes it will be necessary to use the terms vicariously because of the terminology used by other writers. Anophthalmia and microphthalmia can both occur in the same individual.[6] Primary bilateral anophthalmia was proved by necropsy in a boy whose family history was negative for the condition; there was a teratoma at the base of the brain between the mamillary bodies. In this case,[7] in which the optic vesicle had failed to grow out, there were no optic tracts, no chiasma and no geniculate bodies.

Congenital anophthalmia may be unilateral or bilateral. It usually is sporadic but sometimes it occurs in kinships or sibships. It sometimes alternates with colobomatous conditions and there are pedigrees in which such ocular defects are transmitted as dominant traits with variable expression. In other families, anophthalmia recurs in sibs; in several such cases, parental consanguinity could be established. Autosomal recessive inheritance is assumed in such cases.[1,8] In one member of a family group in which several patients with anophthalmia occurred, chromosome analysis showed a normal pattern[9] but in many sporadic cases to be mentioned later abnormal chromosomal patterns have been established (p. 358). To this group in which anophthalmia or microphthalmia usually is combined with facial clefts and polydactyly possibly belonged the case recorded in 1657 by Thomas Bartholin of Copenhagen, who described a "monstrum sine oculis" with a mouth wide and deformed that had 6 digits on either hand and on the left foot (see Fig. 37-1)—a condition since described

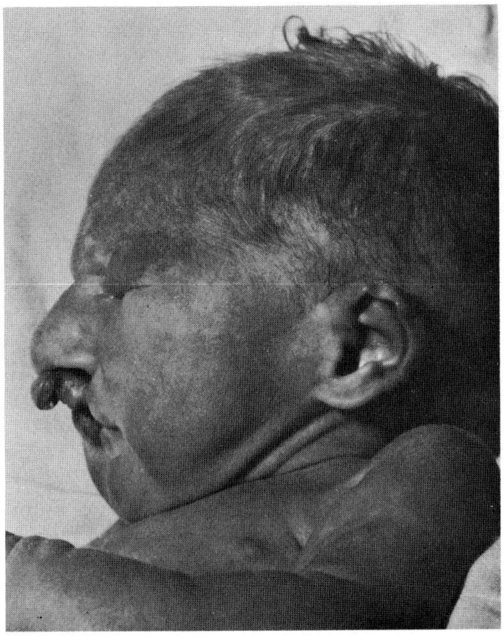

Fig. 39-1. – Microphthalmia in an infant with trisomy 13–15.

as trisomy D_1 (13-15) by Patau *et al.*[10] There also are pedigrees in which sex-linked inheritance of microphthalmia seems likely.[8]

The incidence of microphthalmia in the general population has been estimated at 0.1%. In Sweden, Sjögren and Larsson[11] found that the defect accounted for 8% of children admitted to schools for the blind. About half of these children were mentally retarded.

Microphthalmia and anophthalmia are neither clinical nor genetic entities, and many classifications have been attempted. Mann[2] spoke of primary anophthalmia when the optic outgrowth failed to develop and of secondary anophthalmia when there was suppression of the forebrain with consequent failure of eye development. In the third type, an optic vesicle is formed that subsequently is destroyed completely so that no trace of an eye is found in postnatal life. Other classifications distinguish between true anophthalmia and microphthalmia as variants of colobomatous malformations, microphthalmia associated with other ocular malformations – particularly orbital cysts – microphthalmia associated with syndromes involving other parts of the body and nanophthalmia (pure microphthalmia).[1] Although most reports deal with hereditary cases, sporadic instances of microphthalmia probably are the most frequent ones. Zeiter,[12] who reviewed hospital records of 44 cases of microphthalmia, encountered only 1 with a history of the same malformation in the family. There was no predilection of sex or race in these cases. Only 36 of the patients survived the neonatal period, as cerebral and cardiovascular anomalies associated with the eye defect were fatal. Mental retardation, brain atrophy, hydrocephaly, microcephaly, congenital heart disease, omphalocele, urogenital malformations, cleft lip and palate, polydactyly or syndactyly and other anomalies were recorded in about half the microphthalmic patients. Toxoplasmosis accounted for only 2 of the cases. Congenital cataract, corneal scarring, muscle imbalance, colobomas of the iris and choroid and pupillary obstruction were the most frequent ocular anomalies associated with microphthalmia. Sjögren and Larsson[11] divided their patients into those with and without mental retardation. Of the oligophrenic patients, more than 70% had skeletal anomalies such as clubfoot or scoliosis, 28% had epilepsy and more than 8% had spastic diplegia. Toxoplasmosis and syphilis could not be established in any of the cases and rubella was not considered an important etiologic factor. In certain families, definite hereditary patterns are likely but it seems premature to give general rules about the mode of inheritance of microphthalmia, because clinical entities recognized are not always etiologic entities. Thus, Sjögren and Larsson thought that in cases with oligophrenia a partially sex-linked recessive mode of inheritance was responsible, whereas, in cases with normal mentality, dominant inheritance prevailed. But it is not justified to assume that microphthalmia with and microphthalmia without mental retardation are definite and separate genetic entities. This was shown in a family recorded by Kallmann *et al.*,[13] in which recessive autosomal inheritance was likely. There, of 4 children with microphthalmia, 2 were mentally normal and 2 (monozygotic twins) were retarded. Roberts[14] reported a pedigree with probably sex-linked recessive inheritance of microphthalmia. Some of the patients with microphthalmia were mentally normal, whereas others had various degrees of mental deficiency. Zeiter[12] published a pedigree showing bilateral microphthalmia in three generations. Males and females had the anomaly. One affected mother had 4 normal and 4 affected children. Microphthalmia was associated with congenital cataract in all the microphthalmic children but mental retardation was present in only 2.

To assume that genetic entities can be recognized by ocular anomalies that accompany microphthalmia also seems precarious. For instance, the assumption by Waardenburg *et al.*[1] that microphthalmia as a variant of colobomatous malformations shows autosomal dominance (with variable penetrance) cannot be generally correct, since, in some pedigrees, recessive or sex-linked recessive transmission seemed probable. In the pedigree reported by Roberts,[14] associated ocular malformations differed not only among affected persons but also between the eyes of the same patient. The variability of ocular manifestations in the trisomy 13-15 syndrome (p. 299) shows that the manifestations of a well-defined etiologic entity are not uniform. The pedigrees available[1,8] demonstrate that various modes of transmission are likely for microphthalmia complicated by cataract, opacity of the cornea, aniridia, dystrophia retinae pigmentosa or glaucoma.

Both anophthalmia and microphthalmia often occur in combination with extraocular anomalies or malformations that permit an etiologic classification. For other syndromes the etiology remains obscure.

In an anencephalic fetus, Timm[6] found failure of eye development with no ocular remnants on the left and rudiments of the eyeball on the right. There was no optic chiasma but the anterior pituitary was present. Association with arhinencephaly and prosencephaly is now emphasized in syndromes with or without chromosomal anomalies. Microphthalmia with absence of occipital lobes[16] or with absence of the corpus callosum has been recorded.[15] Combinations with encephalocele have been seen repeatedly.[8] Microphthalmia associated with spastic diplegia has been described as a syndrome.[11] Skeletal malformations, particularly syndactyly and polydactyly, have been observed often, sometimes combined with obesity and hypogenitalism, resulting in syndromes related to the Laurence-Moon-Biedl complex[8,17,18] (p. 176). Associated genital anomalies can be minor or present as pseudohermaphrodism[19] or true hermaphrodism.[20] The Ullrich-Feichtiger syndrome sometimes includes microphthalmia and other ocular anomalies, polydactyly, micrognathia, cryptorchidism or uterine malformations, congenital heart disease and others (p. 1120). The chromosomes are normal in these patients, although they are now often suspected of trisomy 13-15.

Lenz[21] presented a pedigree of sex-linked recessive microphthalmia in three generations. The proband had congenital microphthalmia and cataract associated with congenital heart disease, agenesis of the left kidney, unilateral cryptorchidism, cleidal dysostosis, highly arched palate and crooked fingers. One maternal uncle had microphthalmia and a double thumb on the right; another had crooked fingers like the propositus and his mother. Microphthalmia, coloboma of the optic papilla and hexadactyly were present in 1 of 2 brothers with atypical orodigitofacial syndrome.[22]

Weyers and Thier[23] separated an "oculovertebral" syndrome from that of mandibulofacial dysostosis. They believed that unilateral cases of so-called mandibulofacial dysostosis showing malformations of the eyeballs and of the vertebral column represent a special entity. Microphthalmia was among the ocular manifestations. We have seen repeatedly in the Cincinnati Children's Hospital patients who had unilateral microphthalmia and vertebral malformations, but the syndromes included other skeletal defects as well as cardiac and renal malformations. A syndrome of ocular anomalies such as microphthalmia, corneal dysplasia and blindness, cutaneous hypopigmentation resembling albinism, spastic diplegia and mental retardation has been described as an autosomal recessive trait. Four siblings out of 10 were affected in a highly inbred Amish family.[24] Microphthalmia occurs frequently in the Hallermann-Streiff-François syndrome (p. 390).

Dental anomalies in patients with microphthalmia have been described as familial traits since the middle of the nineteenth century.[8] An "oculodentodigital" syndrome of microphthalmia with iris anomalies, thin nose without alar flare, enamel defects, syndactyly and finger contractures has been observed repeatedly.[25] Heredity was not proved in these cases.

In children who develop Fanconi pancytopenia, skeletal anomalies often are present at birth. Occasionally, microphthalmia is among the congenital malformations.[8,26] Parental consanguinity and recessive inheritance has been established in these cases. Another autosomal recessive trait, Goltz syndrome,[27] includes focal dermal hypoplasia, skeletal anomalies, microphthalmia and colobomas.[28] Microphthalmia is present in some patients with Rothmund-Thomson disease (p. 392).

The combination of microphthalmia or other ocular anomalies with cardiac and skeletal malformations was known before chromosome analyses could be done, but the interest in these eye anomalies grew when their association with trisomy D_1 (13-15) became known.[10] Although anophthalmia and microphthalmia are the most striking ocular manifestations of trisomy 13-15, such other eye defects as coloboma iridis, cataract, cloudy cornea or persistent hyperplastic vitreous can represent the developmental errors of the eye.[32,33] Normal eyes have also been observed in children with trisomy 13-15.[34] This spectrum from normality to anophthalmia illustrates the futility of overemphasis of clinical signs in place of etiologic knowledge. A microphthalmic eye of the 13-15 trisomy syndrome was examined histologically by Sergovich *et al.*,[32] who found persistence of the fetal type of irido-corneal angle, anomalous sphincter pupillae, absence of the dilator pupillae and abnormal ciliary body. The retina was dysplastic, showing folds, tubes and rosettes about the hyaloid canal. The hyaloid artery could be traced from the optic disc to the retrolental area, where the vessels ramified in hyperplastic primary vitreous, which was extremely vascular and covered the posterior surface of the lens. There was cataract formation and the optic nerve was hypoplastic. The olfactory bulb and lobe were present in that case and the cerebral and cerebellar cortex appeared normal. It is quite likely that the case of Yudkin[35] in 1928 was one of trisomy 13-15, since the histologic ocular findings were similar to those of Sergovich *et al.* In 1965, Ginsberg and Perrin[33] reviewed reports on ocular manifestations of trisomy 13-15 and gave a detailed description of the eyes of a typical case. Bilateral microphthalmia, uveal tract colobomas, cataracts, retinal dysplasia and ectopic cartilage formation were among the significant findings. Anophthalmia was present in a case of B/D translocation.[36]

As pointed out before, hereditary anophthalmia and microphthalmia have been emphasized in the medical literature, but surveys of affected persons have shown that sporadic cases outnumber by far those for whom genetic determination can be demonstrated. Some of the sporadic cases probably are new mutations or due to cytogenetic abnormalities; others can be attributed to damage during the embryonic period and be considered nonhereditary. A wealth of experimental material shows that the eye is extremely sensitive to teratogenic factors and there is some evidence that exogenous factors can also cause microphthalmia in human beings.

One of the best examples of this type is microphthalmia induced by maternal exposure to x-rays. As early as 1920, Aschenheim[37] published a case of microphthalmia, microcephaly, cloudy lens, chorioretinitis and abnormal optic nerves in a child whose mother had been irradiated with roentgen rays during the first 4 months of pregnancy. The same author reviewed the then existing literature on experimental production of malformations by irradiation in which much attention had been paid to ocular damages. This report was followed by many others that showed a significant association of microphthalmia with x-ray-induced microcephaly.[38,39] Other teratogenic agents

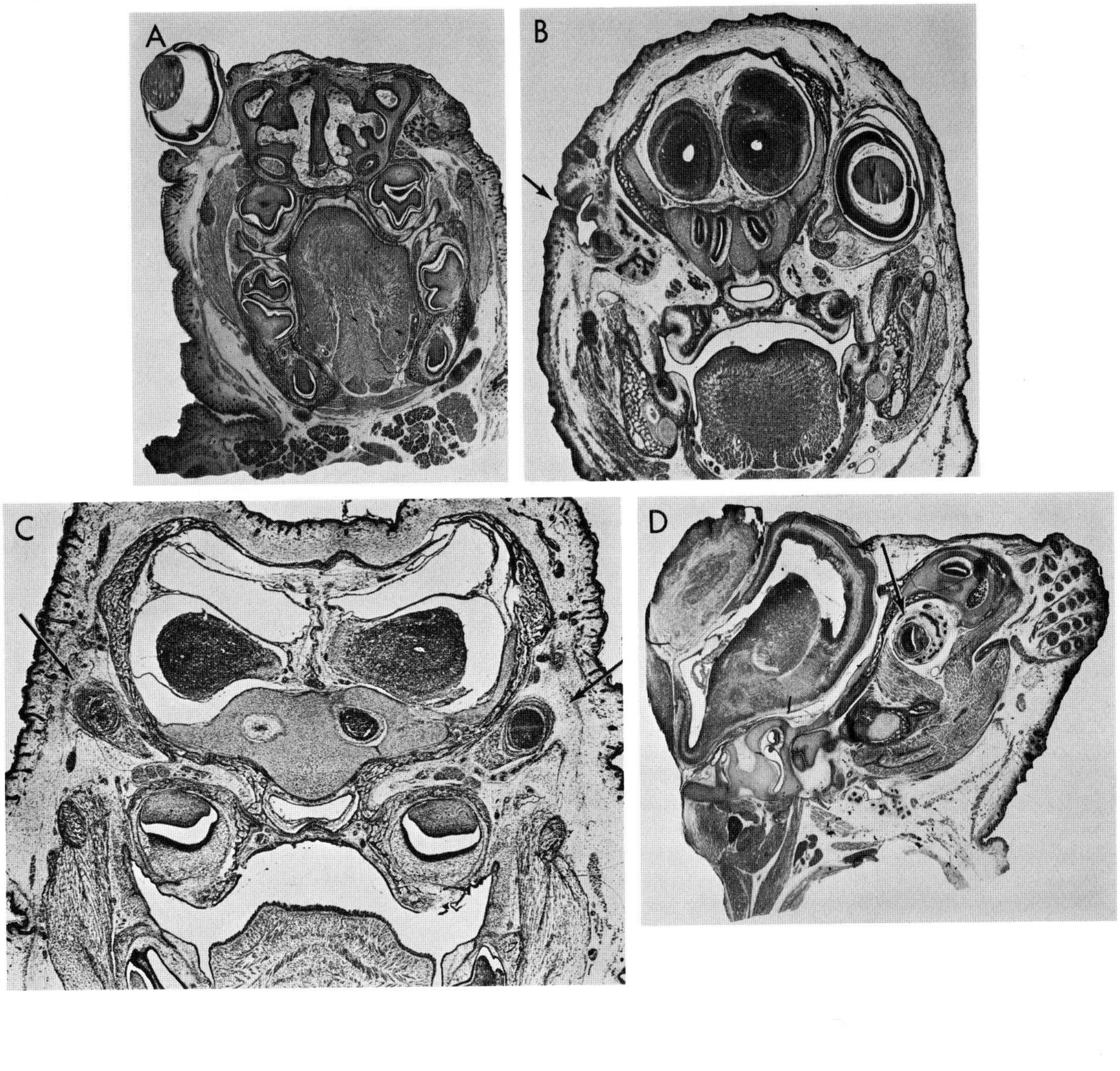

Fig. 39-2. – **A–C,** frontal sections through the head of a newborn rat. **A,** anencephaly produced by hypervitaminosis A (100,000 units by mouth on the ninth day). On the animal's right is a large protruding eye; microphthalmia on the left. **B,** microphthalmia of animal's right eye produced by treatment of mother with methyl salicylate on the tenth day of gestation. **C,** bilateral microphthalmia and cryptophthalmia produced by x-irradiation (250 R) on the twelfth day of gestation. **D,** sagittal section through the head of a newborn rat showing exencephaly and microphthalmia produced by injection of mother with methyl salicylate on the ninth day of gestation.

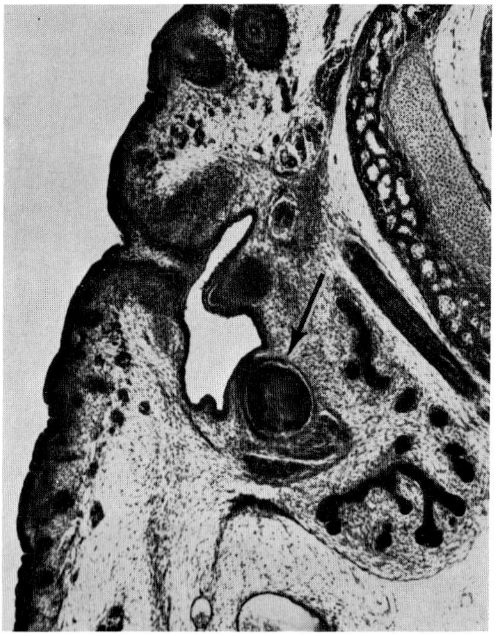

Fig. 39-3.—Apparent anophthalmia on the right of a newborn rat whose mother had been treated with an injection of 0.15 ml. of methyl salicylate on the ninth day of pregnancy. The frontal section shows a tiny lens (**arrow**) inside the lower part of the conjunctival sac.

capable of producing congenital microphthalmia in human beings are the rubella virus[40] and toxoplasmosis.[41]

Spontaneous microphthalmia in animals has been observed often and many reports dealing with hereditary forms have been made.[42] Thorough investigations of hereditary anophthalmia and microphthalmia have been made in mice. Anophthalmia occurs in mice, with 91% eyelessness and 9% intermediate eye reductions in strain B, which is said to be homozygous for two pairs of recessive genes.[43,44] In completely eyeless animals of this strain no eye remnants are present at birth. In embryos of 10 days, the growth of the optic vesicle is inhibited and by the age of 13 days nothing is left of the eye anlage. A strain called microphthalmia is characterized by a semidominant gene (mi) that is lethal in the homozygous condition. The gene is pleiotropic and results in ocular and skeletal changes. Hair color and spotting are also dependent on the action of this gene.[44] In mice homozygous for the gene "ocular retardation," the eyes appear normal up to age 11 days but they fail to grow after this because of failure of the central artery and vein to establish a pathway along the choroid fissure. In the adult, the lens is distorted in shape, the retina contains no sensory cells and there are no optic nerves or optic chiasma.[45] An association between anophthalmia and polydactyly of the hind foot has been detected in crosses of certain inbred strains of mice.[46] Eye defects occur spontaneously in C57 Black strains of mice, but incidence as well as phenotypic expression vary in different sublines. Russell[47] found that in some sublines more than 20% of the females exhibit eye anomalies ranging from slight cataract to an eyeless condition. Inbred strains in the Jackson Laboratory in Bar Harbor, Maine, showed more variation in eye development than that recorded from random-bred stocks.

Many reports of hereditary microphthalmia in laboratory rats have appeared, but in most of these observations the mode of inheritance was not established. By brother-sister matings of microphthalmic rats, Browman and Ramsey[48] obtained an incidence of 85% of microphthalmic young, which enabled them to study the embryology of the anomaly. They could trace the deviation from the normal to about 12½ days of gestation and attributed it to failure of formation of the embryonic blood supply to the eye and particularly to failure of development of the hyaloid artery.

Anophthalmia and microphthalmia frequently are produced in teratologic experiments. Of the many teratogenic agents employed in experiments with mammals, x-rays were used very early, producing ocular defects.[37] Anophthalmia, microphthalmia and other ocular anomalies have resulted from prenatal exposure to x-rays (Fig. 39-2,C). Special attention has been paid to ocular changes by Hicks.[49] Majima[50,51] produced anophthalmia and microphthalmia by exposure on various days of gestation and correlated the results with types described in clinical classifications.

Fig. 39-4.—Microphthalmia with coloboma (on animal's right side) and anophthalmia (on left side) of rat fetus. Induced by injection of streptonigrin on the tenth day of gestation.

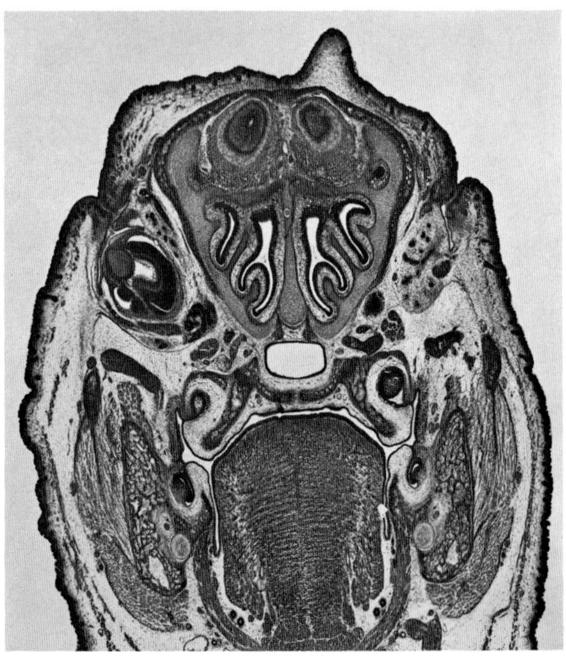

Figure 39-2, *A* shows anencephaly produced by hypervitaminosis A, with a large eye on the right and microphthalmia on the left side of the animal. In Figure 39-4, a frontal section through a rat fetus near term is shown with a coloboma and microphthalmia on the right and apparent anophthalmia on the left side of the animal. Figure 39-2, *B* and *D* show microphthalmia induced by methyl salicylate.

Pantothenic acid deficiency[52] results in microphthalmia in rats, and a hypoglycemia-inducing compound (aminophenurobutane [carbutamide]) in anophthalmia or microphthalmia.[53] Hypoxia can cause microphthalmia in mice[54] and in rabbits.[55]

The Eye in Cyclopia and Anencephaly

In cyclopia, there is either a single median eye or the eyes are in various stages of fusion or approximation. If the nasal septum and the ethmoids are absent, there is only a single median orbital opening located under a proboscis. In extreme cyclopia, a single median eye may be contained in a median orbit. Sometimes a double lens is found in such a median eye or there may be duplication of the retina, whereas the cornea and sclera are single. A further step of separation leads to duplication of all ectodermal derivatives of the eye, enclosed in a common sclera. Two completely separated eyes can be encompassed by united sclerae. Sometimes a diamond-shaped opening leads into a single orbit containing two eyes lying side by side. Less pronounced cases are cebocephaly and arhinencephaly with approximated but not fused eyes.[2] Concordance has been found in probably monozygotic twins with different degrees of cyclopia in the members of the pair.[1]

In anencephaly, the eye usually is well developed, since in this malformation the brain is at first well formed – although not closed at its rostral end – so that the optic stalk and vesicle can take their normal course from the brain toward the orbital region. Although the uncovered and exposed brain (exencephaly) degenerates more or less completely during intrauterine life, the eyes often persist and contribute to the peculiar appearance of the anencephalus. The eyes and lids appear normal but there is proptosis because of shallowness of the orbits. Microscopically, the nerve-fiber layer of the retina is absent and the ganglion cell layer often imperfect. The optic nerve consists of glial and connective tissues but the fibers are absent. The nerves can be followed toward the optic foramina, where they end in the remnants of the brain. The eye muscles usually are preserved, although their nerves are degenerated because of separation from their cerebral origins.[2]

Congenital Cystic Eye

This is a rare anomaly dating back to early differentiation of the eye. It represents an optic vesicle that failed to invaginate and appears as a cyst without any trace of a microphthalmic eye. There is an outer wall composed of fibrous (scleral) tissue and an inner membrane of abnormal retinal tissue. Such cysts expanding the lower lids can be a sign of anophthalmia.[8] A congenital cyst may be microscopically small or reach a size sufficiently large to make the lids bulge. A small lens may be found outside the cyst and attached to its border.[2]

Cryptophthalmia

In cryptophthalmia, the skin of the forehead continues over the eye to the cheek. The lids are not formed, the cornea is absent and it is believed that the cornea has been transformed into skin by metaplasia. A conjunctival sac may never have been formed or may have been occluded secondarily, resulting in fusion of skin and cornea. In some cases, a scar-like line suggests an attempt at lid formation, but failure of differentiation of a conjunctival sac rather than its secondary obliteration seems likely. Under the skin, the eyeball may be visible in the form of a protrusion or it may be palpable, but the bulbus is small and defective. The eyebrows are not developed. Bilateral cryptophthalmia has been observed repeatedly.[56] Experimental production of such a situation is illustrated in Figure 39-2, *C*. According to Mann,[2] "hereditary" cases are rare, but Waardenburg *et al.*[1] cited observations that suggest recessive inheritance in some cases. Transmission from a mother to two of her children has also been reported.[57]

Associated anomalies often are found in the affected as well as in the contralateral eye. Some of the patients had no extraocular anomalies besides cryptophthalmia. Others were severely deformed by cyclopia, facial clefts, syndactyly of hands and feet, atresia of the larynx, aplasia of the kidneys or genital anomalies, including hermaphrodism.[1,2,56]

Congenital Coloboma

Coloboma is a fissure, notch or hole in the iris, the choroid or the retina. A typical coloboma is situated in the area of the fetal ocular cleft and runs downward and slightly inward from the optic disc toward the periphery of the affected structure. The typical iris coloboma often is associated with colobomas of the choroid and retina. Isolated iris coloboma may be seen in atypical positions not corresponding to the fetal fissure. Approximately 45% of the clefts are directed downward and/or inward.[2] According to the literature, iris colobomas outnumber by far colobomas in other parts of the eye, but such reports may give a false picture, since iris colobomas are more obvious than those of the fundus. In 26 eyes, Hird[58] saw the iris affected in 22, the choroid in 20, the optic nerve in 10, the lens in 8 and the macula in 1. No predilection seems to exist for males or females. Estimates of prevalence vary between 0.02% and 0.04%.[1,8]

Typical iris colobomas are triangular, becoming narrower toward the periphery, but sometimes they

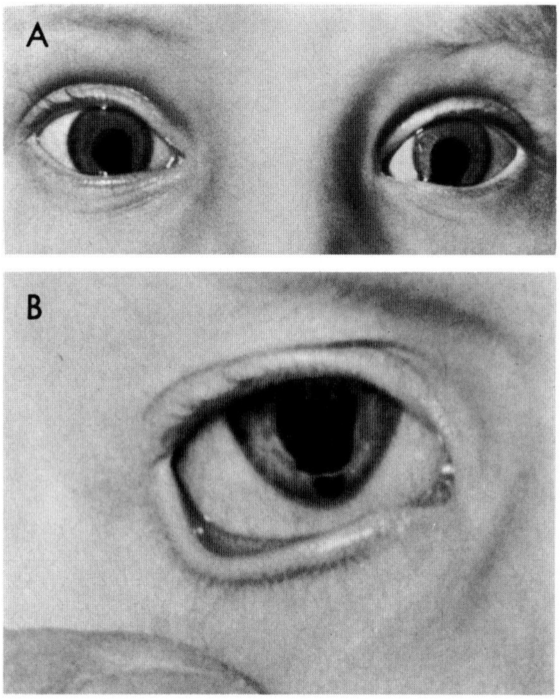

Fig. 39-5.—**A,** bilateral colobomas in typical position in a 13-month-old girl. There also were colobomas of the choroid and retina. **B,** right eye of same patient with lower lid pulled down: bridge coloboma. This girl's twin brother had normal eyes. An older sibling had similar colobomas.

are separated from the ciliary area by a bridge of iris tissue (bridge coloboma). Remnants of pupillary membrane are commonly seen on the edges of the defect.

Failure of closure of the choroid fissure can be genetically determined or be due to environmental factors.

Of the various forms of coloboma, that of the iris is recognized most easily. Hereditary cases of this type were observed and described centuries ago. In 1673, Bartholin mentioned a unilateral coloboma in a boy whose father had a similar bilateral condition. This case and other early reports of apparently dominantly transmitted cases were cited by Waardenburg *et al.*,[1] who added numerous more recent publications of pedigrees in which one or more generations were skipped and expressivity varied in affected members. There are pedigrees that include three or five generations.[8] Modern reports include iridochoroidal colobomas, which also may be transmitted as regular or irregular dominant traits. In such a kinship, colobomas were associated in some members with heterochromia of the iris and signs of the arachnodactyly syndrome[59] (p. 850). In a kinship described by Grebe,[60] atypical colobomas, mental retardation, epilepsy and dislocation of the hip occurred in many members. Irregular dominance of the gene responsible for the ocular anomalies seemed likely. It is probable that recessively inherited forms exist. Waardenburg[61] observed patients with colobomas whose parents were first cousins. Other cases of coloboma that apparently are recessively inherited have been found combined with obesity, sexual infantilism, mental retardation and polydactyly. It is obvious that this syndrome[62] blends into the Laurence-Moon-Biedl syndrome (p. 176), which is attributable to a recessive pleiotropic gene showing great variation of expressivity.[63] Sometimes coloboma of the iris has been noted in the Ellis-van Creveld syndrome (p. 793), an autosomal recessive trait. In a disorder that includes focal dermal hypoplasia, syndactyly and other malformations, coloboma of the iris, retina and choroid can complicate the syndrome.[25]

Atypical iris coloboma and partial aniridia may be indistinguishable. For both traits, dominant inheritance has been demonstrated occasionally. Aniridia and iris coloboma, in both its typical and atypical forms, may alternate in the eyes of one patient or in different members of the same family.[1] Iris coloboma can be associated with the D_1 (13-15) syndrome[64-66] and with partial trisomy due to translocation in the 13-15 group.[67] Lele *et al.*[68] studied the chromosomes of 5 patients with coloboma of the iris and other congenital anomalies. Two of the patients had a pericentric inversion of the no. 1 chromosome, which was also present in the normal mother of one of them. Iris colobomas were present in an infant who had some signs of trisomy 13-15. In 60% of the cells there was an extra, small metacentric chromosome that was interpreted as a part of an additional chromosome of the D group.[69] We examined 3 other children cytogenetically because of coloboma. Two had normal chromosomes; one of these was mentally retarded and had an older sibling with colobomas and mental retardation. A third child, who had a coloboma of the iris on the right side only, bilateral lenticular cataracts, high palate, pectus excavatum, horseshoe kidney and slight eventration of the left leaf of the diaphragm, had 47 chromosomes in cells derived from blood; it could not be decided with certainty whether the extra chromosome belonged to the D or E group.

Multiple congenital malformations may be associated with colobomas in syndromes of unknown etiology. Angelman[70] described 4 unrelated children with typical colobomas, 3 of them affected also by fissures of the retina and choroid. All 4 had cerebral defects and 3 had congenital heart disease. Hydrocephaly, occipital encephalocele, pulmonary stenosis, patent ductus and hydronephrosis were some of the malformations listed.

Development of colobomas can be observed and induced in animals. In rabbits and in many other animals, hereditary colobomas associated with microphthalmia and orbital cysts have been examined.[2] The occurrence of such anomalies makes possible embryologic studies of the deviations from the normal.[71-73] The colobomas are inherited as a recessive trait in rabbits. The defect seems to be primarily in the optic cup, which fails to close its fetal fissure properly. Persistence of mesoderm separating the lips of the fissure is not seen in every case and may be a secondary defect. In affected animals, colobomas of the iris, retina, optic nerve, choroid and orbital cysts can occur together or interchangeably. Cyclopia and anophthalmia do not belong in this series of congenital defects.[2] In the coloboma series, one can observe that the cleft that, in the rabbit, closes normally on the thirteenth day remains open and that the physiologic eversion of the inner retinal layer becomes more pronounced. If there is no intervening mesoderm between the margins of the fetal cleft, the space between the proximal portion of the inner layer and its everted part may become distended, thus preparing the development of an orbital cyst. Aberrant nerve fibers emanate from the abnormal retina, sometimes forming abnormal optic nerves. The choriocapillaris does not develop over the retinal defect. The formation of cysts and the appearance of degenerative and reparative processes result in ocular anomalies similar to those that occur in man.

In the rabbits studied, the defects were genetically determined. Many imitations of these hereditary anomalies have been produced experimentally in the rat. Warkany and Schraffenberger[74] analyzed the abnormal eyes of the young of female rats subjected to severe vitamin A deficiency. Among many other ocular anomalies, colobomas of the retina were observed frequently. Figure 39-6, *B* shows a beautiful example with a cleft on the lower and posterior aspect of the eye, transgressed by a thin mesodermal strand that is connected with a thick retrolenticular

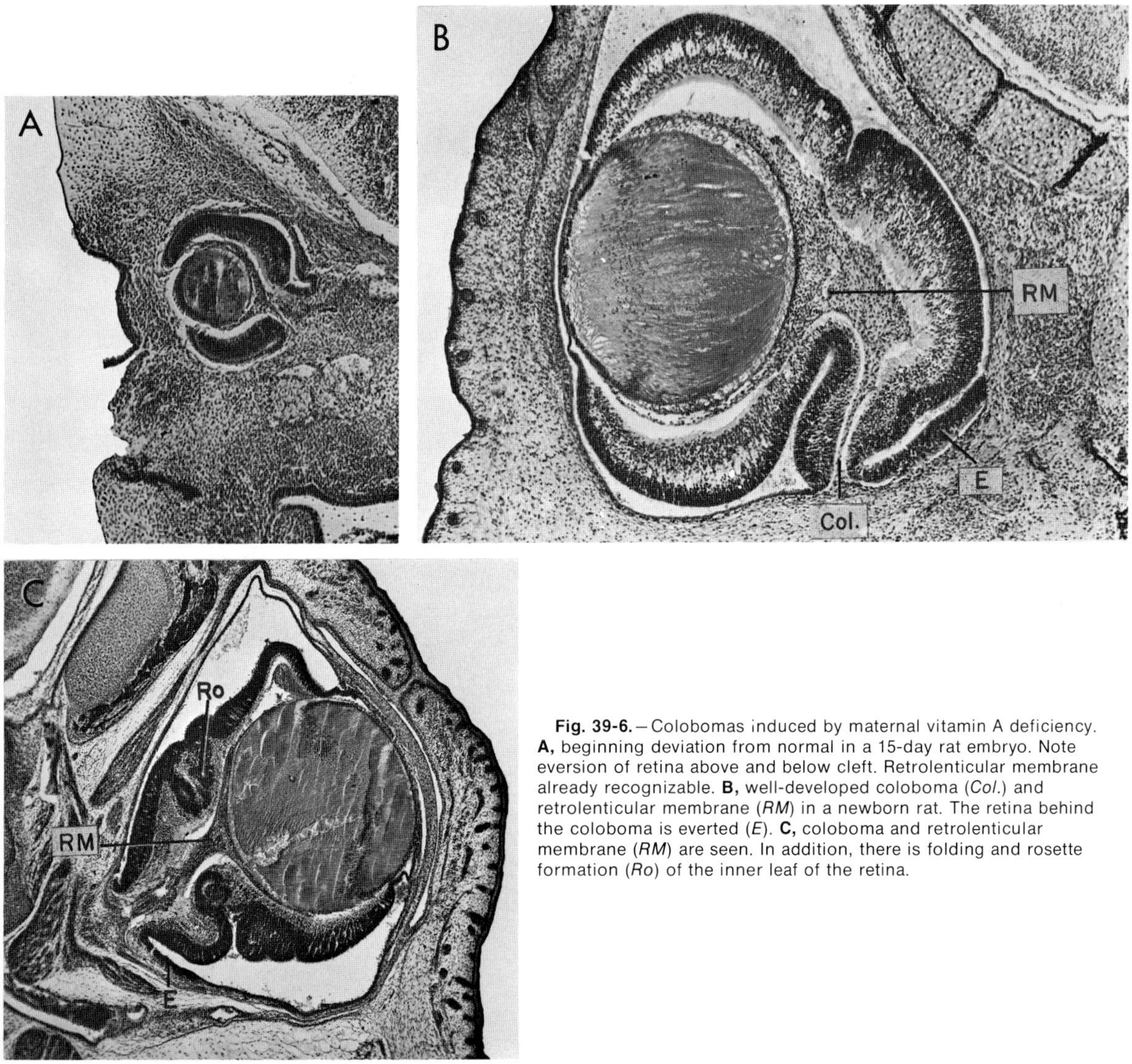

Fig. 39-6.—Colobomas induced by maternal vitamin A deficiency. **A,** beginning deviation from normal in a 15-day rat embryo. Note eversion of retina above and below cleft. Retrolenticular membrane already recognizable. **B,** well-developed coloboma (*Col.*) and retrolenticular membrane (*RM*) in a newborn rat. The retina behind the coloboma is everted (*E*). **C,** coloboma and retrolenticular membrane (*RM*) are seen. In addition, there is folding and rosette formation (*Ro*) of the inner leaf of the retina.

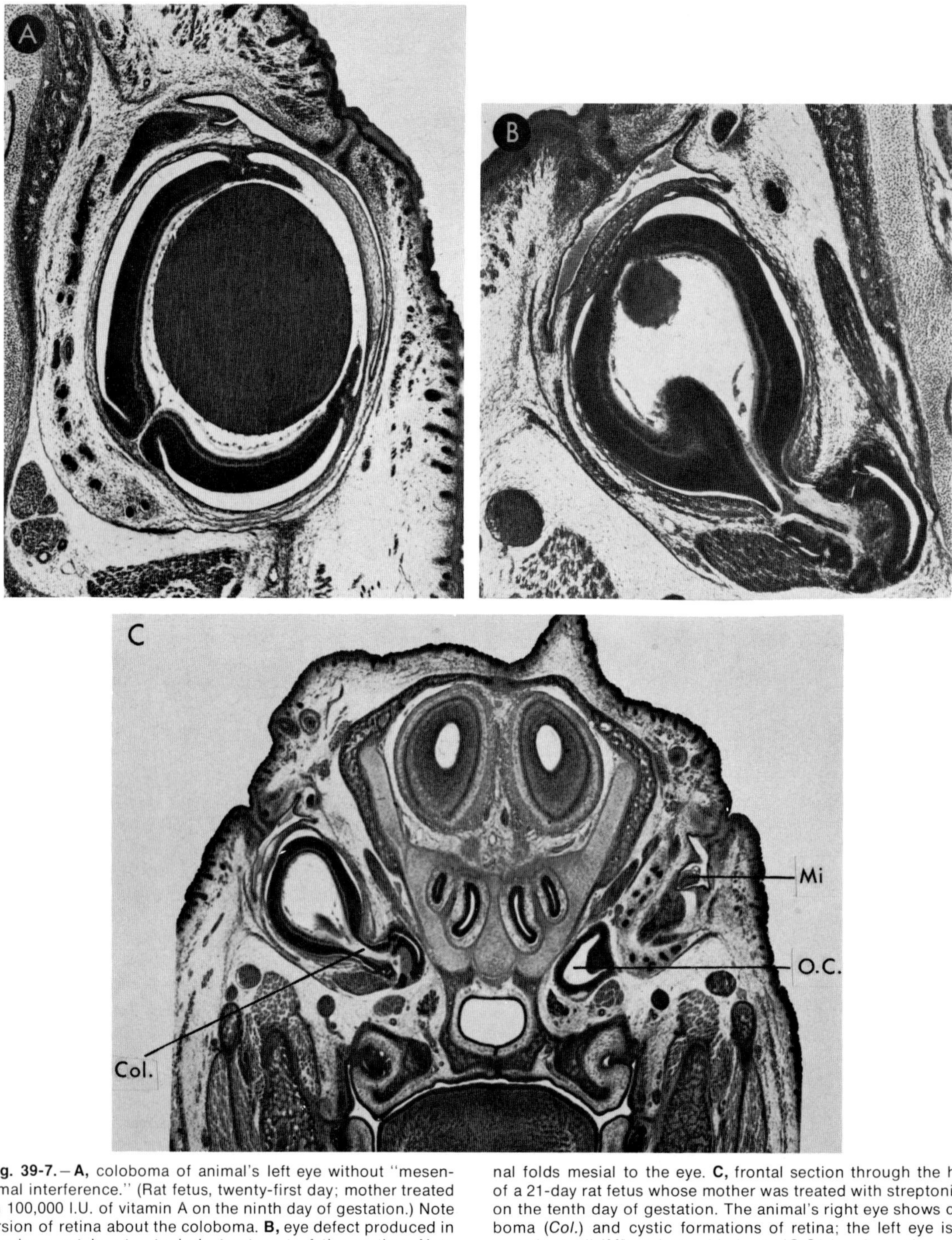

Fig. 39-7.—**A,** coloboma of animal's left eye without "mesenchymal interference." (Rat fetus, twenty-first day; mother treated with 100,000 I.U. of vitamin A on the ninth day of gestation.) Note eversion of retina about the coloboma. **B,** eye defect produced in a newborn rat by streptonigrin treatment of the mother. Note absence of retrolenticular tissue in colobomatous eye and retinal folds mesial to the eye. **C,** frontal section through the head of a 21-day rat fetus whose mother was treated with streptonigrin on the tenth day of gestation. The animal's right eye shows coloboma (*Col.*) and cystic formations of retina; the left eye is extremely small (*Mi*) and an orbital cyst (*O.C.*) has formed.

membrane. There is considerable eversion of the inner leaf of the retina, with abnormal inversion of the cell layers of the everted portion. The everted retina terminates abruptly on both sides of the cleft and joins the external leaf of the retina. The space between the two leaves is clearly visible but not cystically distended. Other abnormalities of the eyes occurring in this experimental series have been described in detail by Warkany and Schraffenberger,[74] who also illustrated the deviation of these eyes from the normal development in fetuses. In vitamin A deficiency experiments, retention and overdevelopment of retrolenticular connective tissue is the rule. The retrolenticular tissue is found in all abnormal eyes even if coloboma is absent and the retinal lips have closed. Fibrosis of the vitreous was also seen associated with colobomas induced in rabbits by hypervitaminosis A.[75] Thus, these experimentally produced colobomas could be cited in favor of the oldest theory of coloboma formation, which attributed the retinal cleft to persistence of mesoderm interposed between the margins of the retinal fissure.[2]

Ocular malformations, including coloboma, have been produced by teratogenic methods other than vitamin A deficiency. Figure 39-7, *A* illustrates a coloboma of the eye of a 21-day-old rat fetus that differs from that described above since it is not associated with overdeveloped retrolenticular connective tissue. Figure 39-7, *B* shows retinal folds, probably forerunners of orbital cysts mesial to the eye. In Figure 39-7, *C*, the connection of the retinal folds with the colobomatous retina of the eye is demonstrated. Interestingly, the left side of the same specimen shows marked microphthalmia and a well-developed "orbital cyst" that greatly exceeds in size the microphthalmic eye. This specimen is one of a series of abnormal fetuses whose mothers were treated with streptonigrin. Figure 39-7, *A* could be cited as an example of coloboma without mesenchymal interference and as supporting the theories that attribute colobomas to primary ectodermal failure of development.[2]

Orbital Cysts

Orbital cysts are outgrowths from the cleft of a colobomatous eye. The space between a portion of the retina near the cleft and the everted retina becomes distended by fluid and may enlarge considerably, often growing to a size many times that of the abnormal eye. The cyst may be connected with a colobomatous eye or be separated from it by the time the fetus is born. Figure 39-7, *C* illustrates well the variability observable in two eyes of the same rat fetus. On the right (of the animal), retinal folds are seen proximal to a colobomatous eye, but no distention has yet taken place. On the left, only remnants of the eye can be seen microscopically, but below and mesiad a cystic space enclosed by retinal tissue has formed. Another orbital cyst is shown in Figure 39-8. These experimentally induced ocular anomalies are similar to those

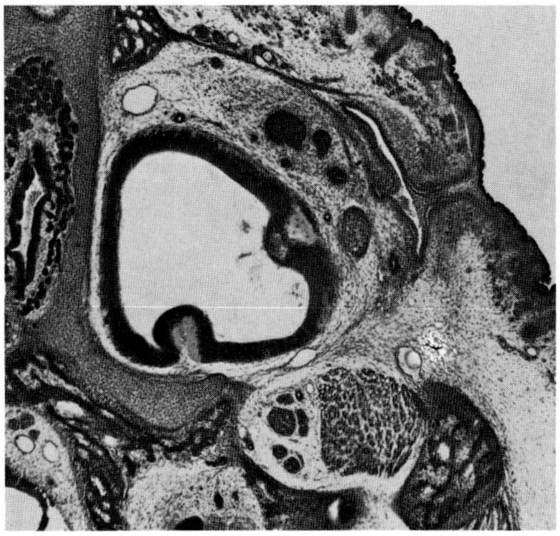

Fig. 39-8. – Frontal section through the orbital region of a newborn rat whose mother was treated with 100,000 I.U. of vitamin A. In place of the left eye, an orbital cyst has formed from retinal tissue.

that occurred in colobomatous stocks in rabbits that were studied in great detail by Szily.[73]

In children, the origin of orbital cysts may not be recognizable at the time of birth. The eye can be extremely small and the cyst so distended that it causes bulging of the eyelids. Cysts can be multiple or loculated. Owing to its origin, a cyst usually is attached to the lower portion of the eye, which is microphthalmic and colobomatous. The lining of the cyst, which may show rosette formation, consists of neuroglia and malformed retina.[2]

In man, heredity of orbital cysts can seldom be established, but, in rabbits, such cysts are found as variations of colobomas that occur as a recessive trait.

Hydrophthalmia (Infantile Glaucoma, Buphthalmos)

This anomaly is caused by developmental errors of the anterior segment of the eyeball but it involves the whole eye. The enlargement of the eye, the flattened lens, iris atrophy, optic atrophy and associated anomalies are due to increased intraocular tension within an eye that cannot yet resist internal pressure. The increased tension is brought about by a faulty drainage mechanism attributed to absence of the canal of Schlemm or to its incomplete development. Persistence of the fetal ligamentum pectinatum or a rudimentary scleral spur can also inhibit normal drainage.[2] Maumenee[76] suggested that the raised intraocular pressure is due to abnormal insertion of the bundles of the ciliary muscle into the trabecular fibers, which tends to compress the scleral spur forward and outward, thus narrowing the Schlemm canal. Anomalies in the iris such as atrophy or absence of crypts usually are considered secondary changes, but a forward displacement of the root of the iris or developmental anomalies of the iris may be responsible for or connected with changes of the angle of the anterior chamber and thus cause inhibition of free circulation of fluid. Sometimes the angle is blocked by products of more general disorders such as neurofibroma or facial nevus flammeus.[77] Some investigators differentiate between primary and secondary hydrophthalmia,[2] others distinguish between genetic types and their phenocopies.[1] Primary hydrophthalmia is due to blockage at the filtration angle, whereas the secondary intrauterine type is thought to be due to adhesions between the iris and the lens and to fetal iritis.[2] In the latter case, the iris is pushed forward by increased pressure (iris bombé) and the anterior chamber is rendered shallow. The classic type, on the other hand, is characterized by faulty development of the angle of the anterior chamber and by a deep anterior chamber.

The cornea of a hydrophthalmic eye is cloudy and enlarged. The anterior chamber is deep and the peripheral portion of the iris is in close contact with the cornea, obliterating the filtration angle. The lens may become subluxated by damage to the zonular fibers. As the eye enlarges, vision is diminished. Approximately 80% of the cases are bilateral. In Denmark, the prevalence in the population was estimated at 0.0008%.[78]

Many familial cases have been published, and autosomal recessive inheritance has been demonstrated in some of them. But there is predominance of males, who account for about 70% of the patients. There are instances that suggest dominant or sex-linked recessive inheritance. In the majority of cases, single gene inheritance seems unlikely.[79] In 1961,[1] 6 pairs of concordant monozygotic twins and 3 pairs of discordant dizygotic twins had been recorded. It has been estimated that only 12% of the patients showed familial recurrence.[80] Development of juvenile glaucoma has been reported in association with ectodermal dysplasia[205] and with familial cerebral palsy.[206] Occasionally, the condition has been observed in more than one generation, which suggests a somewhat guarded prognosis for the offspring. A peculiar case is presented in Figure 39-10. There, hydrophthalmia, cataract, myopia and cleft palate occurred combined or vicariously in members of one kindred. The patient, seen in the Cincinnati Children's Hospital (Chart no. 23812), had hydrophthalmia associated with posterior palate cleft. His father also had been born with hydrophthalmia but he did not have cleft palate. An irregular dominant gene affecting the eye and palate led to these apparently unrelated malformations.

Fig. 39-9.—Bilateral congenital hydrophthalmia with opacification of the corneae.

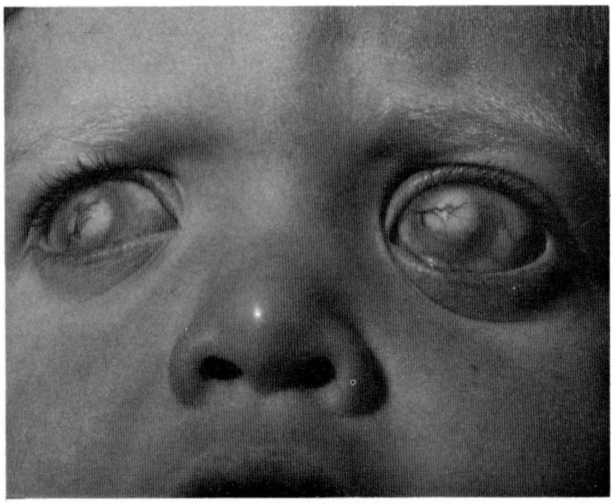

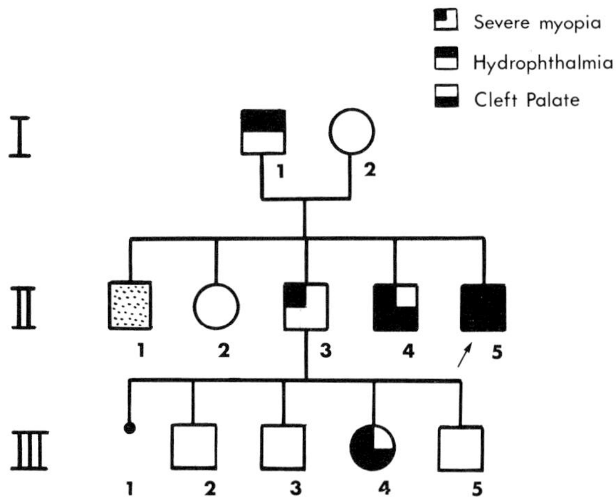

Fig. 39-10.—Pedigree of a kindred in which ocular anomalies and cleft palate recurred. I_1, congenital hydrophthalmia; II_1, congenital heart disease, died when 24 hours of age; II_3, severe myopia; II_4, severe myopia and cleft palate; II_5, propositus. Congenital hydrophthalmia, posterior palate cleft and "spider fingers"; III_4, severe myopia and cleft palate, hearing defect.

Bowen *et al.*[81] reported a familial syndrome of multiple congenital malformations in which glaucoma plays a leading role. These children also have a high, arched palate, joint contractures, congenital heart disease, agenesis of the corpus callosum and of the olfactory bulbs and other (variable) anomalies. Although there was some suggestion of trisomy 13-15, the karyotypes were normal in these patients. Neurofibromatosis, the basal cell nevi syndrome (p. 1268) and Sturge-Weber disease can lead to hydrophthalmia.[207]

Congenital cataract, hydrophthalmia, organic aciduria, decreased renal ammonia production and mental retardation are known as a clinical entity (Lowe syndrome, p. 389). This syndrome is genetically determined. It occurs in males only and seems to be a sex-linked recessive trait. An association of glaucoma with homocystinuria has been shown.[82]

Some cases are not genetic in origin. Prenatal rubella can result in hydrophthalmia,[40,83] and obstetric or perinatal difficulties have been considered as possible causes.[79] Congenital glaucoma, deafness, cardiac anomaly and mental retardation have been observed following attempted abortion with quinine and slippery elm.[84]

Hydrophthalmia occurs in rabbits as an autosomal recessive trait. It can be unilateral or bilateral in young of the same litter of albino New Zealand stock. Buphthalmic rabbits have more extraocular associated malformations than their normal litter mates.[85] Sometimes large, bulging eyes with corneal opacities are seen in the offspring of female rats treated during pregnancy with extremely large doses of vitamin A.[86] Deuschle *et al.*[87] examined histologic sections of such animals and found a rather normal appearance of the globes despite their protrusion and absence of lids. The orbital floor was defective and there was no support for the bulging eye. There is no proof that these large eyes were hydrophthalmic.

A long list of associated ocular anomalies was given by Kwitko,[82] who also presented theories on the pathogenesis of congenital glaucoma.

Anomalies of the Cornea

Absence of the cornea occurs in cryptophthalmia when the lid and conjunctival sac fail to form and the outer skin covers the globe, which has fibrous tissue in place of a transparent cornea (p. 361).

Microcornea

Microcornea consists of a reduction in the size of the cornea to a diameter of 10 mm. or less (in normal children over 5 years of age the horizontal diameter of the cornea varies between 10.5 and 13 mm.).[88] In the case of microcornea, the entire anterior part of the eye shows growth failure and incomplete development of the angle. Approximately 20% of the patients develop glaucoma in later life.[2] If the posterior part of the eye is also small, one speaks of microphthalmia. Several pedigrees showing dominant autosomal inheritance of microcornea have been recorded. In one kindred,[89] the affected members through five generations had microcornea and cataract in eyes that were not microphthalmic. A syndrome of microcornea, glaucoma, platyspondyly, generalized osteoporosis and geroderma was reported by Bamatter *et al.*[90]

Megalocornea

Megalocornea can be a symptom of hydrophthalmia (p. 366) or it occurs as an isolated malformation. The diameter may be 13–18 mm. even without ocular hypertension. If the anomaly is limited to the anterior portion of the globe, visual acuity can be normal, but frequently subluxation of the lens and cataract complicate the disease picture. The ciliary ring is also enlarged and iridodonesis is noticeable. There is a predilection for males, and X-linked recessive inheritance is likely for some kinships. However, autosomal recessive transmission of megalocornea combined with ectopia of the lens and pupil and late glaucoma has been reported.[91] Autosomal dominant inheritance has also been observed for Marfan syndrome, in which megalocornea has been observed repeatedly.[1]

Keratoconus

If this anomaly is congenital, it occurs together with microcornea, anterior polar cataract, optic atrophy and particularly retinitis pigmentosa.[92] Typical keratoconus, although inherited, has a delayed onset at puberty. Dominant and recessive inheritance can occur. Females are affected more often than males.

The cornea has the shape of an obtuse conus whose vertex is in or near the corneal center. The anomaly can be demonstrated by distortion of the rings of Placido's keratoscope. Refraction is rendered abnormal by the irregular curving of the cornea.

Keratoconus has been concordant in several pairs of monozygotic twins.[1] It occurs in the simple form or it develops acutely in a relatively high percentage of patients with Down syndrome. Acute keratoconus begins in mongoloids of higher age groups with sudden cloudiness and ectasia of the cornea associated with pain, redness and lacrimation. It seems that a rupture of Descemet's membrane occurs, which allows a sudden influx of aqueous into the cornea, leading to deformation. In serial examinations, about 6% of patients with Down syndrome were found to have keratoconus.[93,94] Association of keratoconus with retinitis pigmentosa has been seen in many cases.[8]

Congenital Corneal Opacities

Among the many hereditary corneal dystrophies only a limited number are congenital. Such opacities, which are not accompanied by inflammation or vascularization, may be stationary or progressive. They can be localized in the parenchyma or in the limiting membranes or involve the entire cornea. Congenital parenchymatous dystrophies of the cornea must be distinguished from syphilitic parenchymatous keratosis, which is seldom congenital. In the absence of signs of syphilis and vitamin A deficiency, one has to consider hereditary congenital dystrophy as the basis of congenital corneal opacities.[1,88] Franceschetti and Klein (in Waardenburg *et al.*[1]) distinguished between a degenerative and a "malformative" type of congenital corneal opacity. The degenerative type generally is not associated with other anomalies of the eye and consists of diffuse cloudiness of the cornea. Recessive and dominant inheritance has been observed. In the malformative type, other parts of the eye are affected also. Two groups can be distinguished. In one, the border of the cornea is more or less effaced and the limit between the opacified cornea and the sclera is difficult to find. Microcornea, microphthalmia, staphyloma, glaucoma and malformations of the brain[95] and ear can be associated anomalies. Various diffuse peripheral opacities and dermoids of the cornea belong in this group. A second group, which shows distinct corneal borders, includes anterior embryotoxon (arcus juvenilis), posterior embryotoxon (marginal dysplasia of Descemet's membrane) and central discoid opacities.

For the diffuse corneal opacities with indistinct corneal borders, recessive and dominant inheritance has been observed.[96] In the dominant type, cataract and dental anomalies have been reported as associated malformations.[1]

Dermoids of the cornea are tumors consisting chiefly of fibrous and fatty tissue and an ectodermal cover with hair follicles, sebaceous glands and sweat glands. A minor form is limited to the limbus, whereas the cornea and the rest of the eye remain normal. In more severe forms, the entire cornea can be replaced by fibro-fatty tissue and be covered by skin, or the dermoid can replace all the tissues between the pigment epithelium of the iris and the surface ectoderm, so that there is no anterior chamber or iris stroma. Mann[2] described and illustrated such a case in detail. Dermoids of the cornea often accompany other congenital anomalies such as auricular appendages, auricular fistulas, colobomas of the upper lid, iris or retina, microphthalmia, micrognathia, macrostomia[97] and mandibulofacial dysostosis.[88] Multiple corneal dermoids associated with miliary aneurysms of the retina were reported by Lichter.[98] Anterior embryotoxon (arcus juvenilis) is a ring-shaped opacity near the limbus of the cornea, usually separated from it by a transparent ring. It resembles the arcus senilis, but the infantile form involves deeper corneal layers than that of advanced age. Embryotoxon can occur as an isolated anomaly or in association with blue sclerae or megalocornea.[2] Dominant and recessive inheritance have been reported.[88] Posterior embryotoxon is a ring-shaped opacity of the posterior layers of the cornea located near the limbus. This annular opacity may be associated with iris anomalies and be inherited like a dominant trait.[2]

Systemic Disorders Involving the Cornea

Gargoylism (Hurler syndrome). Cloudy corneae are seen in 75% of patients with gargoylism (p. 809). Boys show the corneal symptoms less often than girls, since there are two genetic types. In the recessive form, males and females are affected equally and corneal dystrophy is frequent. In the X-linked recessive forms, the male patients have no corneal dystrophy. In Morquio disease, ocular anomalies generally are absent, but cases have been described that have corneal involvement (Morquio-Ullrich disease, p. 817).

The gray spots within the cornea are not visible at first without the slit lamp. They can be present at birth or they appear soon after. They are said to be more numerous in the anterior layers and in Bowman's membrane and more pronounced at the center than at the periphery of the cornea,[88] but the deposition of mucopolysaccharides within the stroma cells of the cornea probably is irregular and variable. With advancing age, the cloudiness of the cornea usually increases, so that it becomes clearly visible and interferes with the vision of the patients. Histologically, one finds that the basal cells of the epithelium are vacuolated, but more marked changes are seen in the stroma. The interlamellar spaces are enlarged and they contain a granular material. Bowman's membrane may be missing and be replaced by large vacuolated cells containing the same granular material found in the interlamellar spaces. In addition to corneal changes, patients with gargoylism may have megalocornea, infantile glaucoma or pigmentary chorioretinal changes.[88] In *Hand-Schüller-Christian disease*, a lipoid impregnation of the cornea or of the limbus may take place; the lids and the palpebral conjunctivae probably are more often the seat of lipoid deposits, and exophthalmos is one of the common symptoms of the disease. *Cystinosis* leads to cystine crystal deposits in many organs, the cornea among them. The cornea becomes cloudy as punctate opacities appear in its anterior layers. Vision is somewhat impaired and photophobia may become disturbing. The irides and conjunctivae may contain similar cystine deposits.[1]

A syndrome of corneal opacities, ankylosis of the temporomandibular joints and multiple anomalies of the appendicular skeleton was described by Pillay[99] as "ophthalmo-mandibulo-melic dysplasia." There are striking deformities of the forearm bones, with marked shortening of the ulna, ulnar-deviated clubhands and flexion deformities of the fingers. The syndrome can be inherited as an autosomal dominant trait.

In rare instances, *neurofibromatosis* may cause corneal tumors.[100] A syndrome of *cutis verticis gyrata*, acromegaly and corneal leukoma has been described.[101] The corneal lesions begin in the first decade of life in the epithelium as gray areas. Then the lesions thicken and opacify and develop into raised leukomas that can, over many years, involve the entire cornea. The syndrome has been inherited as an autosomal dominant trait. Corneal opacities are involved in a recessively inherited syndrome[102] that includes growth failure, contractures of the elbows and mental retardation. In one family 4 children were affected.[102] An association of epibulbar dermoid, coloboma of the upper lid, iris coloboma, microtia, auricular appendages, micrognathia and macrostomia with dental anomalies has been reported[97] (Oculoauriculovertebral [Goldenhar] syndrome, Chapter 40).

The epithelium of the cornea is of ectodermal origin and represents a modified epidermis.[103] The parenchyma of mesodermal origin is a transparent continuation of the fibrous sclera. The cornea can become involved in various disorders of the skin. In *ichthyosis*, opacities of the cornea occur, primarily as an ichthyosis of the ectodermal epithelium with secondary changes in the parenchyma, but opacities have also been observed in the posterior corneal stroma. *Keratosis palmaris et plantaris* may be complicated by corneal opacities located chiefly in the epithelium. Mental retardation accompanies some of these findings. In *ectodermal dysplasia* and in *epidermolysis bullosa dystrophica*, the cornea can be affected. In the latter disorder, blebs may form between epithelium and Bowman's membrane. This process can result in corneal scars and even in ulceration and perforation of the cornea.[1] Cloudy corneae can complicate trisomy 18[104] and normal/trisomy 18 mosaicism.[105,106]

Keratomalacia has been described in cytomegalic inclusion disease.[107,108]

The Iris

The iris is formed from mesoderm and neural ectoderm. The stroma and the pupillary membrane are derived from mesoderm, the sphincter and dilator of the pupil and the pigment epithelium from ectoderm. Mann[2] pointed out the phylogenic stability of the sphincter and the rarity of its malformations. In contrast, the stroma varies greatly in different phylogenic classes and tends to anomalies and malformations. The stroma of the iris develops early in embryonic life, whereas the uveal pigment formed by the forward extension of the rim of the optic cup is late in developing. The iris consists of a large outer ring (annulus major or pars ciliaris) and a smaller inner ring (annulus minor or pars pupillaris), the two rings being separated by the iris frill. There is a radial striation or reticular design of great variability and, between the strands, pits or crypts are seen. In the anteroposterior direction, there is first an indefinite and incomplete endothelial layer that is a continuation of the posterior endothelium of the cornea; this anterior limiting membrane is followed by the anterior iris leaf containing connective tissue, chromatophores, blood vessels and nerves. Behind this layer one finds the posterior iris leaf (myovascular layer) in which radial blood vessels, connective tissue, the sphincter muscle, nerve plexuses and chromatophores are seen. The sphincter muscle is of ectodermal origin. The layers that follow are derived from the pars iridica of the retina. There are radial contractile fibers that make up the dilator pupillae; they are covered posteriorly by the pigment layer (inner leaf of the secondary optic vesicle). This pigment layer, which forms the posterior free surface of the iris, consists of cells that are so heavily pigmented that one can hardly distinguish cell membranes or nuclei. Toward the pupillary margin, this pigment layer, turning forward toward the anterior leaf of the iris, can be seen as a dark seam around the pupil.[1]

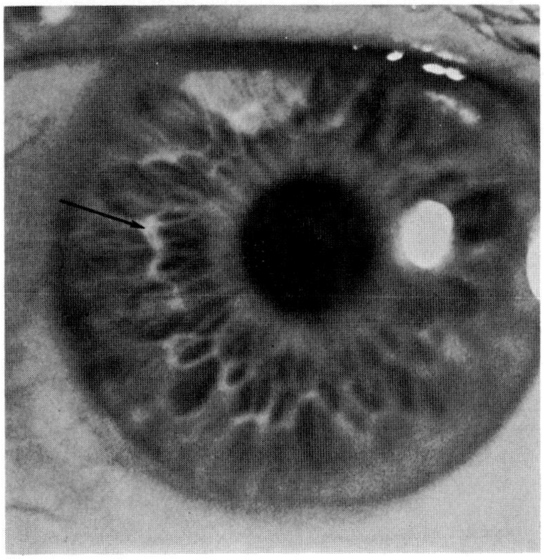

Fig. 39-11.—The normal iris is divided by (white) irregular iris frill (**arrow**) into a central (pupillary) and a peripheral (ciliary) portion. The radial as well as the arcuate elevations correspond to blood vessels in the stroma. Between them, the iris crypts or lacunae are clearly seen.

Aniridia

Absence of the iris usually is incomplete, since iris remnants can be found in most instances of so-called aniridia. The anomaly often is bilateral. Males and females are affected equally.[1] The incidence was 1 in 100,000 in the Danish population.[109] Aniridia is related to coloboma of the iris, as evidenced by patients showing aniridia in one eye and coloboma in the other and by alternating of the two conditions in pedigrees. Aplasia of the macula is almost always associated with aniridia but not with iris coloboma.[1] Nystagmus and photophobia frequently are associated anomalies.[110] In some cases only the stroma is absent, in others the posterior layer only—or both. Whether aniridia is due to mesodermal or to ectodermal failure of development remains undecided.[2]

Aniridia is, in many cases, attributable to a dominant autosomal gene. An Amsterdam family had 22 cases in four generations.[1] Møllenbach,[109] in Denmark, reviewed 48 cases of aniridia and calculated an incidence of 1 in 95,000. Heredity could be demonstrated in 31 cases. In some cases in which heredity could not be proved, new mutations were considered possible. Two persons who were thought to be sporadic cases later had children with the same anomaly. Dominant autosomal inheritance appeared to be responsible for the condition. Many affected persons were of low intelligence. About one-third of the children with aniridia could do regular school work, but all adults needed public financial support. Reed and Falls[110] studied a Michigan kindred consisting of 23 aniridic and 99 apparently normal persons distributed over four generations. The gene behaved as a dominant of high penetrance. Only one case showed incomplete expression. The first occurrence of aniridia was in a sibship of 4 affected and 6 normal individuals, the parents apparently being normal. It was considered possible that one of the parents had the gene for aniridia with nonpenetrance, but an alternative explanation was that a parental gonad consisted of normal and mutant tissue (gonadal mosaicism), so that several children received the abnormal gene and transmitted the trait as a dominant. In other families in which iris defects, including aniridia, are transmitted as a dominant trait, there is great variability of the ocular defects.[112] In some instances, recessive inheritance has been considered.

Many associated ocular defects have been described, such as cataract, ectopia lentis, coloboma lentis and choroidea, microphthalmia and others.[111] The iris stump present in so-called aniridia often is adherent to the posterior surface of the cornea, which can lead to interference with the function of the Schlemm canal and to glaucoma.[2]

Extraocular anomalies include mental retardation, craniofacial dysostosis, cleft palate and Wilms tumor.[1, 113] One form of aniridia shows an association with hemihypertrophy, Wilms tumor and other neoplasms,[113] genital abnormalities and mental retardation.[114] These cases usually are sporadic.[115] A relationship to the Laurence-Moon-Biedl syndrome was suggested by an association of aniridia with hexadactyly.[116] There was aniridia in a case of congenital lipomatosis of the central nervous system.[117]

Anomalies of Iris Color

Iris color depends on mesodermal or stromal pigment. There is good evidence that the stromal pigment develops from mesoderm and not from the ectodermal pigment layer of the iris. The chromatophores of the iris stroma are stellate cells with branching processes and amorphous pigment in contrast to the sharply defined epithelial cells with crystalline granules. The epithelial cells derived from the optic cup show pigment in embryos of 5 weeks, whereas the stromal pigment does not appear until shortly before birth in pigmented races or several months after birth in Europeans.[2]

In albinism, which probably occurs in all racial groups, there is absence of mesodermal pigment in the iris and all other parts of the body and a partial absence of ectodermal pigment. The iris stroma appears white and hypoplastic and usually the sphincter can be seen. There also are anomalies of the retina. The fovea, which normally is completed about 6 months after birth, remains underdeveloped in albinism, a fact held responsible for the reduced visual acuity of affected persons. Nystagmus usually is present.

Generalized albinism often is used as a textbook example of a recessively inherited trait. Parental consanguinity is estimated to be 25–50% and albinism has been observed repeatedly in the offspring of incestuous matings. A child, the result of a brother-sister mating, who was albinotic and mentally and physically retarded was seen in the Cincinnati Children's Hospital. There are examples of matings of two albinotic parents that resulted in albinism of all their children. But there also are reports of such matings that resulted in pigmented children. This suggests that phenotypically similar types of albinism may differ genetically. As a rule, monozygotic twins are concordant in regard to albinism, whereas dizygotic twins are discordant.

Ocular albinism is a localized pigment deficiency seen in persons with pigmented hair and skin. The iris is translucent and the fovea underdeveloped. Ocular albinism is linked to the X chromosome and is seen fully developed in males. But female transmitters of the X-linked trait may have translucent irides and pigment anomalies in the fundus periphery. Waardenburg[1] mentioned X-linked intermediate inheritance of ocular albinism.

Heterochromia

Unilateral hypopigmentation can occur without complications in hypoplastic irides (*heterochromia simplex*). Dominant inheritance has been observed in several families of various races. The anomaly has also been seen in monozygotic twins who, in some cases, showed mirror imaging. In *heterochromia with sympathetic paralysis*, the lighter eye has a smaller pupil and is enophthalmic (Horner syndrome), suggesting that disturbances of the sympathetic nervous system can influence mesodermal pigment. Such changes can result from birth injury or they are prenatally determined, as demonstrated by heredity of the condition in some cases. Dominant inheritance with irregular penetrance has been claimed for some cases.[1] Heterochromia iridis, Horner syndrome and "status dysraphicus" have been considered a complex of congenital anomalies by Passow.[118] In some kinships, these anomalies occur interchangeably in persons who may have such defects as funnel chest, scoliosis, scapula alata or asymmetry of the breasts and nipples. Syringomyelia seems to be responsible for the ocular symptoms. DiGeorge *et al.*[119] mentioned that the case of Anastasius, a Byzantine emperor in the fifth century A.D., may have been the first case of heterochromia on record. Anastasius was called "Dicorus," which probably indicates a man with differently colored eyes. In modern ophthalmology, however, dicoria means "double pupil."

Heterochromia complicata (Fuchs syndrome) includes cataract, corneal opacities in the vitreous body and sometimes secondary glaucoma developing in the lighter eye. A congenital basis of this anomaly can be assumed, although the fully developed disease picture develops slowly, progressing in postnatal life. The posterior part of the eye remains normal.[2] In some families, irregularly dominant transmission seems likely. Occasionally, heterochromia simplex and complicata alternate in a kinship.[1] In monozygotic twin sisters with Fuchs syndrome, the disorder led to serious visual disturbances in the fifth decade of life.[120] In one twin, the right eye, showing the syndrome, appeared lighter than the left. In the other, the color difference was slight but other symptoms of

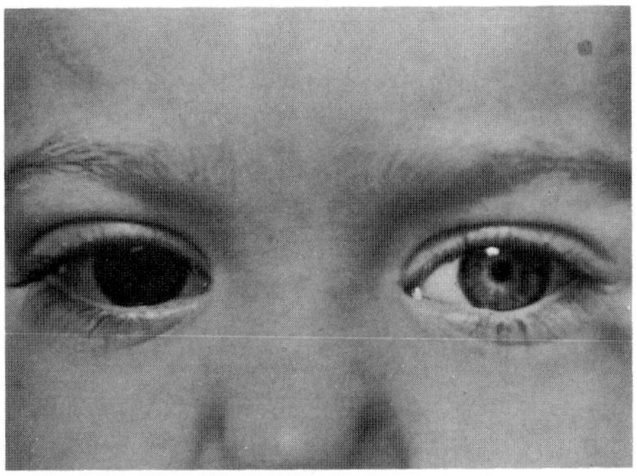

Fig. 39-12.—Congenital anisocoria and heterochromia in a girl with Waardenburg syndrome.

the syndrome developed. The oldest daughter of this patient showed a suggestion of color difference of the irides. It was not certain that the mutation had occurred in the twins, since their maternal grandfather had had some ocular anomaly. The Fuchs syndrome sometimes is associated with a syndrome of facial hemiatrophy and alopecia.[121] This combination has been observed in females only.

Heterochromia iridis, partial or total, is one of the constituents of the Waardenburg syndrome (p. 395) that is a dominant trait, but the penetrance of heterochromia is estimated to be only 25%[119] in that syndrome, in which hypoplasia of the iris is more often observable than heterochromia. Such hypoplastic irides appear pale blue; they may occur in both eyes, so that isochromic blue eyes can represent the faulty development of the irides in the Waardenburg syndrome.

Heterochromia of the irides has been observed repeatedly in patients with arachnodactyly or Marfan syndrome (p. 850). In some of these patients, depigmentation may be partial or iris atrophy may be present. This syndrome is a dominant trait, in which dislocation of the lens is the leading ocular symptom, whereas the iris anomalies are present only occasionally.[122] François and Verriest[123] observed heterochromia iridis in 2 children whose mothers had had rubella during pregnancy.[1] These observations are of interest because they show that iris color, often considered a purely genetically determined trait, is not independent of prenatal environmental factors. Heterochromia iridis combined with Horner syndrome, vertebral anomalies and duplication of the foregut was described by Robinson *et al.*[124]

Brushfield Spots

A description of the peculiarities of the irides of infants with Down syndrome was given by Brushfield,[125] who referred to white or light yellow, "clearly defined pin-points near the outer margin, generally placed at regular intervals in a ring and appearing to be placed on the iris." He did not find these spots in brown irides. Wallis[126] examined 7 newborn mongoloids and found that all had blue irides with white spots which he named "Brushfield's spots." The spots disappeared when the color of the iris changed to brown as the child grew older. Since the spots can be seen in normal children also, their diagnostic value was not thought to be great "except in the negative sense." Lowe[127] studied the irides of mongoloids in detail and believed that thinning was a more prominent feature than the spots. Donaldson[128] found the spots in 85% of mongoloids and somewhat similar spots in 24% of normal persons. In mongoloids, the spots were located nearer to the pupillary margin and were also more numerous and more distinct than in the normals. There was no correlation of spotting with age or I.Q. of the mongoloids.

Cysts of the Iris

Congenital cysts of the iris can be located in the stroma or in the neuroepithelium. In the latter case, the cyst develops between the two leaves contributed to the iris by the anterior portion of the optic cup. Such cysts, which can be located near the periphery or near the pupillary portion of the iris, can be associated with lenticular opacities or colobomas. Stromal cysts may be lined with stratified epithelium or with flat endothelial cells. They are thought to be derived from misplaced surface ectoderm or from ectoderm of the anterior leaf of the optic cup.[129]

Mesodermal and Ectodermal Dysgenesis (Rieger Disease)

A triad of ocular disease (malformation of the anterior chamber angle, iris atrophy, glaucoma), of malformation of the upper jaw with partial anodontia and of myopathy occurs occasionally as a hereditary disorder that may behave like a dominant trait.[130,131] Iris atrophy with failure of complete separation of the cornea and iris, cloudy cornea, obstruction of the angle, ectopia pupillae, perforation of the iris and glaucoma slowly become recognizable during the first and second decades, so that the visual disturbance is not congenital. But occlusion of the angle, occasional colobomas, hypoplasia of the maxilla and partial anodontia point to a congenital basis of the syndrome, which has been observed repeatedly as a familial disorder. Short stature has been reported in a member of a kindred in which Rieger syndrome occurred in three generations.[204] Myopathies combined with iris atrophy occurring in families have been described.[132]

The Pupils

Persistent Pupillary Membrane

The pupil is covered in fetal life by a thin membrane consisting of vascular arcades that have their convexity turned toward the center of the pupil and of mesodermal cells between the blood vessels. As the eye grows in the second half of gestation, the vascular arcades normally fail to reach the pupillary area and, at the same time, the centrally located blood vessels begin to atrophy. Normally, the membrane begins to disappear after the fifth month of gestation, so that the pupil is almost freed of it by the time of birth. Postnatal atrophy of remnants is possible during the first year. Mann[2] believed that genetic factors play no role in persistence of the membrane, but Waardenburg *et al.*[1] pointed out that there is great similarity of remnants in monozygotic but discordance in dizygotic twins. There also are reports of pupillary membranes in a parent and some of the children and transmission of the anomaly through more than two generations. Usually, other ocular defects such as coloboma, cataract or glaucoma are associated with such hereditary cases.[1] Associated anomalies (aniridia, coloboma or polycoria) have also been reported in sporadic cases.[2] Persistent pupillary membrane occurs occasionally in eyes affected by toxoplasmosis.[133,134]

Congenital Anisocoria

Inequality in diameter of the pupils has long been a sign of pathologic conditions following trauma, infection, intoxication and so forth. There exists also a congenital and hereditary anisocoria that occurs in eyes free of functional disturbances. The frequency of this "innocent" anisocoria depends on the degree considered. If only anisocorias of more than 20% difference in pupillary diameters are included, 1–2% of the general population show the anomaly. To diagnose this innocent form of anisocoria, neurologic, ocular and pleuropulmonary disorders have to be excluded. Irregular dominant transmission has been observed in some families.[135]

Corectopia (Ectopic Pupil)

Corectopia signifies an out-of-place pupil. Normally, the pupil is in a slightly inferior-mesial position from the iris center, but displacement in almost any direction is possible. Such pupils can be functionally normal, or the displacement, when due to strands attached to the pupillary margin or when associated with dislocation of the lens, can be seen in an eye with impaired vision. Uncomplicated corectopia occurred in a kindred through five generations, 25 members being affected, and there are other kindreds with this dominant trait.[1] The same mode of inheritance was seen in a pedigree in which heart disease was associated with corectopia.[135,136] In association with ectopia lentis, the anomaly of the pupil has occurred repeatedly as a recessively inherited trait.[137] Ectopic pupils have also been seen in 3 siblings with a variant of the Laurence-Moon-Biedl syndrome, which suggests a recessive mode of inheritance.[138]

Slit Pupil

A slit-like pupil replacing a round one can run in any direction; sometimes it is connected with strands of aberrant zonular fibers.[2]

Polycoria

True polycoria, i.e., presence of more than one pupil in an eye, is extremely rare. In such cases, the accessory pupil is surrounded by a sphincter, as is the main pupil. In contrast, iris dehiscence (splitting) is attributed to defective development of mesoderm, resulting in one or several holes in the iris. Such holes are not surrounded by sphincters and represent false polycoria. Some cases on record suggest dominant inheritance.[1]

The Lens

Absence of the lens (aphakia) may be due to a failure of development of the lens placode or due to secondary degeneration or absorption of a lens originally formed. True aphakia is very rare and probably recognizable only by microscopic examination, especially in early embryos. Mann[2] illustrated such a case of a 13-mm. embryo in which a fairly normal eye cup was found without a lens within its cavity. Secondary aphakia is more common than its primary counterpart. There, the lens is present in a rudimentary form as a wrinkled capsule invaded by mesoderm and forming a white membrane in the pupil. Spontaneous rupture of the lens capsule has been assumed in such cases, an opinion supported by observations in some rodents in which rupture of the lens occurs as a hereditary trait.[2]

Congenital Cataract

There are many forms of congenital cataract and many more forms that are prenatally determined, although they become manifest at various times in postnatal life. François,[139] in 1963, wrote a monograph on congenital cataracts and in a lecture discussed syndromes in which congenital cataracts occur. Cataracts assume various shapes and forms that cannot always be classified according to etiology.

Total (diffuse) congenital cataracts have been observed repeatedly as genetically determined traits. Dominant recessive and sex-linked recessive transmissions have been described.[1] Meissner[140] reported a pedigree of 22 affected members out of 48, distributed over six generations. All layers of the lens may be present and opaque or only a capsular sac may be left from which fluid has been resorbed (membranous cataract). Membranous cataract and congenital aphakia have been seen interchangeably in families.[1]

Total nuclear cataracts are limited to the embryonic nucleus. They consist of dense and chalky opacities impairing vision to a considerable extent. François[88] collected 14 pedigrees showing irregular autosomal dominance; one of these pedigrees comprised six generations. X-linked cataract was recorded by Fraccaro *et al.*[141] The cataract described by Gregg[40] in children with the prenatal rubella syndrome was essentially central nuclear but other shapes and positions were also observed. Swan *et al.*[142] stated that most of these cataracts were of the central nuclear type.

Capsular cataracts are found on the anterior or posterior pole of the lens. *Anterior polar cataracts* consist of small opacities of the lens attached to its anterior pole and sometimes connected with strands of persistent pupillary membrane. Such small opacities do not interfere seriously with vision, but if the anterior pole extends forward into the anterior chamber as a pyramidal prominence almost touching the cornea, vision can be impaired. The same is true for anterior polar cataracts associated with other ocular malformations such as corneal anomalies, colobomas, hydrophthalmia and so forth. The anomaly has been attributed to imperfect separation of the lens from the surface ectoderm. This partial persistence of the lens stalk probably is a rare cause of anterior polar cataract, which is more often due to secondary changes of the epithelial cells of the lens capsule. In this way, an abnormal mass is formed that lies over the anterior pole separated from the main mass by a rather normal epithelial layer. New lens fibers may grow over the abnormal cells, thus placing the cataract behind the lens surface.[2] In this case, the cataract can be connected with the surface by strands attached to the surface (capsulolenticular cataract). Another origin of anterior polar cataracts could be incomplete resorption of blood vessels and mesoderm present in front of the lens of embryos.[2] This would explain the association of these cataracts with remnants of the pupillary membrane. In some families, anterior polar cataract has been inherited as a regular or irregular dominant trait[1,88]; occasionally, recessive inheritance seems likely.[1]

Posterior polar cataracts usually are associated with persistence of the hyaloid artery or parts of it. They consist of circular opacities limited to the posterior capsule or extending forward to the interior of the lens. Vision usually is not affected. Dominant inheritance has been observed in several pedigrees. In one kindred, the anomaly has been traced through seven generations, with 37 of 117 members being affected. In this pedigree, congenital cataracts and cataracts of postnatal development occurred interchangeably.

Suture cataracts consist of abnormal deposits along the lines of the anterior or posterior Y sutures of the fetal nucleus.[2] These deposits usually remain static and cause no visual disturbances. If both the anterior and posterior Y sutures are involved, a stellate cataract may be formed. Sometimes there occur many irregular opacities between the sutures, yet they are arranged in a stellate pattern. This type has been described in Down syndrome, but suture cataracts have also been reported repeatedly as a dominant hereditary trait.[1]

Lamellar (zonular) cataracts consist of fine white dots limited to one layer of the lens. It seems that the primary lens fibers are not involved, but secondary fibers are affected, so that a clear center is surrounded by an opaque sphere. The area outside the opaque lamella also remains clear. These opacities usually are bilateral; they can be formed before or soon after birth; it is believed that this type represents the most frequent congenital cataract. A gray area is seen in the center of the lens surrounded by a translucent area in which radially arranged opaque "riders" may be seen. The opacities vary in density and vision is variably affected.

This type of cataract often is associated with metabolic disturbances and hypoplasia of dental enamel. Parathyroid disturbances, rickets, tetany and hypocalcemia have been held responsible for its appearance. There are many prematures among the children with such cataracts. But zonular cataract can also be inherited through many generations without demonstrable metabolic disorders. Marner[143] published a pedigree of eight generations with 542 members, 132 affected by cataract. Although many of these had the zonular form, there were others who had nuclear, polar or stellate cataracts. In some patients, the cataracts were congenital; in others, they developed in postnatal life. Several observations in monozygotic twins showed discordance in regard to zonular cataract, which suggests an environmental causation in such cases.[1,88] Thus, it is likely that genetic as well as environmental injurious factors can bring about lamellar cataracts.

Congenital cataract often is present in microphthalmic eyes. The combination of this condition can occur sporadically or in familial aggregations. In the prenatal rubella syndrome, microphthalmia and cataract often are combined. In some families, the combination occurring repeatedly can be attributed to a recessive gene, but in other kindreds dominant inheritance seems likely. Microcornea and cataract (without microphthalmia) appears to be an autosomally dominant trait.[1] Microphthalmia and cataract occur in patients with trisomy 13–15, sometimes combined with iris coloboma.[65]

François,[88] in 217 cases of large lens opacities, established the etiology in about one-third. In 45 cases, a hereditary factor played a role and in 12 the mother had had rubella. Toxoplasmosis was held responsible for 6 cases, syphilis for 1, maternal influenza for 1 and sulfonamide poisoning for 1. Two cases of galactosemia accounted for the rest. Wilson[144] found etiologic factors in two-thirds of 72 cases, assigning heredity (including galactosemia and Lowe syndrome) to 30, rubella to 9 and mongolism and tuberous sclerosis to 1 each. McDonald[145] analyzed 68 children with congenital cataract. There were 15 cases that were genetically determined, 9 were attributable to early prenatal rubella, 5 were associated with Down syndrome and 5–10 with low birth weight; the last group had a tendency to epilepsy and often a prenatal history of toxemia.

Cataract in Galactosemia

In this metabolic disorder, cataract usually is not congenital but develops in the neonatal period. Owing to an inborn deficiency in uridyl-transferase, affected infants are incapable of converting ingested galactose into glucose. Galactosemia, galactosuria, aminoaciduria, hepatosplenomegaly, jaundice and mental retardation ensue.

In 1953, Johnson[146] reviewed the cases with cataract then reported. All children with cataract had been 6 weeks of age or older when examined. But, in one of his own cases, the lenses showed nuclear opacities when the infant was 3 weeks of age. The opacities disappeared when milk was withdrawn. In another infant, the cataracts were cortical and in a third they were nuclear, with spoke-shaped peripheral opacities. In previous publications, the cataracts had been termed nuclear, lamellar (zonular), cortical or central anterior. There was no correlation between the type of lenticular change and the age of the patient. Removal of milk from the diet before the third month was considered imperative for the prevention of irreversible lens changes. Wilson and Donnell[147] followed 12 cases of galactosemia for 6 months to 9 years. Four children did not develop cataract, because of early diagnosis and immediate inception of dietary treatment. In 8 patients with cataract (diagnosed between 6 weeks and 13 months of age), no regression of cataract was found, although the children developed well otherwise. The lens in galactosemia is lacking in galactose-1-phosphate-uridyl-transferase.[148]

Congenital cataract can be produced experimentally in the young of rats by feeding large amounts of galactose to the pregnant mother.[149]

Cataract in Down Syndrome

It has long been known that mongoloid patients surviving the first decade of life have a strong predilection to pathologic changes of the lens. Ormond,[208] in 1912, found such changes in 25 of 42 mongoloids. Congenital cataract is rare, but it has been reported occasionally,[1,150] and I have seen some cases with obvious prenatal onset (Fig. 39-13). It is believed by some authors that such congenital cataracts are not characteristic of the disorder and that their appearance in mongoloids is fortuitous. However, congenital cataract is much more frequent in children with Down syndrome than in the general newborn population,[93,151] so that a tendency to prenatal damage to the lens must be assumed.

Van der Scheer[152] examined 60 mongoloid patients with oblique illumination. He found no lenticular opacities in 10 of those aged 8 years or younger. Of 36 patients between 8 and 17 years, 22 had cataracts. In all 14 patients over 17 years bilateral opacities were present. The author concluded that cataracts in mongolism are not congenital and that the opacities progress slowly with advancing age. He considered the Y-figure opacities in the central portion of the lens, stellate opacities in the anterior and posterior portions of the cortex and generally distributed flaky and punctate opacities as characteristic of cataracts in mongolism. It seemed that the cataracts originated from the lens sutures and from borderlines of the various fiber systems.

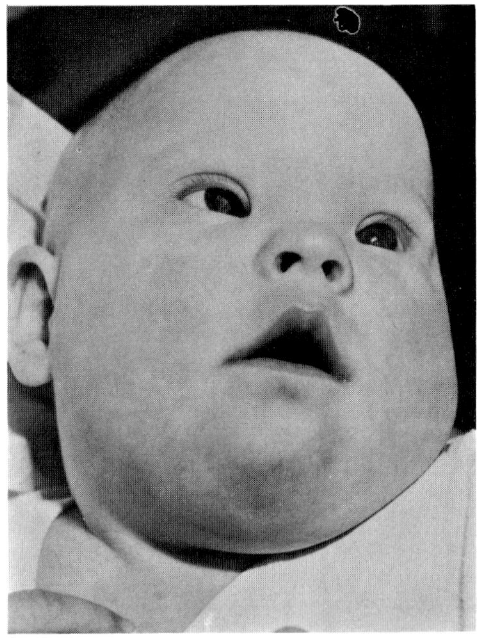

Fig. 39-13.—Down syndrome in a girl who shows a small cranium, hypertelorism, epicanthic folds and congenital cataract.

Lowe[127] examined 52 patients with Down syndrome and found four types of cataracts: arcuate opacities, thought to commence during the formation of the fetal nucleus; sutural opacities mainly affecting the anterior Y of the fetal nucleus, but occasionally also showing in later sutures; and flake opacities within the infantile and adult nuclei. In 3 patients, there were congenital cataracts (disk-shaped, lamellar or posterior polar). Lowe thought that the arcuate opacities seen in one-sixth of the patients were the most distinctive of mongolism. He believed that they developed during fetal life owing to the presence of abnormal vessels. This belief probably was based on the faulty concept of dating the onset of the cataracts by their location in areas of different developmental ages. That the method of dating malformations by embryologic timetables is fraught with danger has been pointed out before (Chapter 7).

Igersheimer and Mautner[151] examined 165 mongoloid patients with the slit lamp. The most frequent findings were punctate and flake-like opacities (cataracta cerulea). In addition, the sutures often were grayish and occasionally cataractous. These typical lenticular opacities were so fine that they could not be seen by external inspection or ophthalmoscope but only by slit lamp. There was no tendency to rapid progression, and vision was not seriously impaired. With the exception of 8% of the patients who had coarse congenital cataracts, the lenses were clear in all children in the first 6 years of life. From then on, the lenticular changes appeared with increasing frequency until age 17, when most patients showed opacities, but the nuclear part was always free. The authors emphasized that arcuate opacities are quite rare and not characteristic of mongolism, as stated by Lowe.[127] Igersheimer and Mautner believed that cataracts in Down syndrome usually do not commence in fetal life but result from early aging and that they resemble the opacities developing in patients with myotonia dystrophica or those of early senile cataract.

The occurrence of coarse congenital cataracts in 8% of Igersheimer and Mautner's patients was not considered characteristic of mongolism, yet this incidence is too high to be regarded as fortuitous. It seems likely that two different mechanisms, a prenatal and a postnatal one, can adversely affect the lens of patients with Down syndrome.

Cataract with Skeletal Disorders

In *chondrodystrophia calcarea* (p. 797), cataract usually is present at birth, but in some cases it develops postnatally. It occurs bilaterally and is total or nuclear with radial opacities. Illustrations of such a cataract can be seen in François'[88] excellent article on syndromes with congenital cataract. There was diffuse degeneration of the lens fibers, globules derived from the fibers were between the lens and the capsule and a homogenized area was seen on the anterior pole. Optic atrophy and retinal changes have been observed occasionally.[88] The syndrome, which often includes other skeletal anomalies, congenital heart disease and malformations of the skin, is inherited as a recessive trait. The "minor" form of stippled epiphyses and the "regular" forms of achondroplasia are not associated with congenital cataract. Cataract has also been observed in patients with the Ellis-van Creveld syndrome (p. 793).

Oxycephaly (acrocephaly). The involvement of the ectodermal lens in this deformity, which is brought about by premature ossification of the mesoderm between flat bones of the skull (p. 893), is worth emphasis. The connection between these anomalies is not clear, but it has been described repeatedly.[88,153] Other ocular anomalies in patients with this cranial malformation, such as exophthalmos and optic atrophy, are explained by the orbital shallowness, which in some cases may lead to nutritional disturbances of the lens. An association between oxycephaly, congenital hemolytic icterus and cataract has also been reported.[154]

Malformations of digits. Cataract in patients with polydactyly and syndactyly has been reported repeatedly. The association is considered significant by some[88] and fortuitous by others.[1] Reduction malformation of a leg, progressive scoliosis and congenital cataract were found as a syndrome in an Amish group by McKusick *et al.*[155] The disorder is inherited as an autosomal recessive trait.

Cataract following Prenatal Rubella

In the first half of the year 1941, Gregg[40] observed in Sydney, Australia, an unusual number of cases of congenital cataract that he correctly attributed to an epidemic of rubella occurring in Australia in 1940. From the involvement of central nuclear fibers, he concluded that the noxious factor had acted during the early months of gestation. Two types were observed. In one, there was a marked contrast between a dense white central zone and a smaller, cloudy and peripheral one. In the other type, the density was uniform. Gregg thought that the appearance of these cataracts did not exactly correspond to any of the lenticular congenital opacities described before. Sometimes the cataracts were unilateral. In such cases, pigmentary degeneration of the retina could be seen in the other eye. Despite the opacities, response to light was good; nystagmus developed if treatment was delayed. Cloudy corneae and microphthalmia were also noted. Swan *et al.*[142] described additional cases from Australia, confirming that early maternal rubella resulted in central nuclear cataract appearing as a flattened, dense white disk in which six radiating lines, presumably the superimposed two Y sutures of the lens, could be discerned. The whole lens was very small, but, after good mydriasis, a clear zone was seen peripheral to the opacity. Swan[156] published pictures of sections through eyes damaged by prenatal rubella. The lens was reduced in size and the central portion amorphous and necrotic. Primary and secondary lens fibers showed breaks, and disintegrated lens fibers of the cortical area were replaced by vacuoles. A number of reports dealing with the histopathology of such eyes appeared subsequently. They were summarized by Töndury,[157] who added his own description of eyes found in rubella embryopathies. When the damage occurred early, the primary fibers of the embryonic nucleus appeared swollen and, near the anterior pole, filled with vacuoles. There, under the epithelium, a vesicle interpreted as a product of disintegrated fibers could be seen. In older fetuses (50 mm.), the embryonal nucleus of the lens was hyaline without well-defined fibers, whereas the middle zone around it consisted of swollen fibers whose contours were darkly stained. A third and outer layer showed fibers terminating at the equator and containing many hyaline droplets. Although the central embryonal portion of the lens was in dissolution, new secondary fibers were formed on the periphery, but these were also included in the degenerative process. In still older fetuses (64 mm.), three zones could be recognized: an inner homogeneous zone in which the embryonal fibers had been dissolved but on the periphery of which darkly stained droplets formed a well-defined border against the middle zone, which was made up of darkly outlined, swollen fibers. The outer zone was composed of fibers of variable caliber. In abnormal eyes examined after birth, small and flattened lenses were found with complete disintegration of the embryonal nucleus and some degeneration of the outer secondary fibers of the lens. Frequently, the iris also was damaged by the prenatal rubella process.

As pointed out by Gregg,[158] the pupils react sluggishly to light in such cases and mydriasis is difficult to obtain. Iris atrophy has been observed clinically as well as histologically. Damage to the sphincter and dilator of the pupil may be responsible for the sluggish reaction of the pupil, but adhesions between iris and lens can also interfere with iris movements. Iris atrophy, thickening and abnormal curvature of the cornea and folding of the retina coexist in microphthalmic eyes of children damaged by prenatal rubella.[157]

Cytomegalic inclusion disease has been seen in association with congenital cataract.[159]

Cataract with Skin and Dental Disorders

Cole *et al.*[160] described sisters who had ectodermal dysplasia of the anhidrotic type in whom congenital cataract occurred. The cataract was lamellar and associated with marked internal strabismus. Hypoplastic teeth and nails, alopecia and atrophy of the skin and of the nasal mucosa were additional symptoms. Marshall[161] reported on ectodermal dysplasia associated with ocular anomalies and hearing defects. The trait occurred in 7 individuals of a kindred through three generations. There were congenital and juvenile cataracts, some of which showed spontaneous maturation and absorption, whereas others showed spontaneous luxation with complications. In addition, there was myopia, fluid vitreous and one instance of retinal detachment in the presence of a lens luxated into the vitreous. The nose was saddle shaped. The nasal bones were small and appeared absent clinically. Hearing was reduced approximately 50%. Congenital cataracts associated with congenital ichthyosiform erythroderma has been described in siblings whose father had psoriasis. The parents were not consanguineous.[162] Skin and eye symptoms are combined in the Rothmund-Thomson syndrome (p. 392).

A relationship between tooth anomalies and congenital cataract was known to Hutchinson, who, in 1875, wrote about imperfect teeth and zonular cataract. An association between dental anomalies and cataract has been seen occasionally in children with incontinentia pigmenti,[163] but cataracts are not congenital in this condition.[88] Congenital cataract may accompany congenital ichthyosis (harlequin fetus) and congenital atrophy of the skin (Siemens syndrome). Both anomalies apparently are recessively inherited traits. Palmoplantar keratosis combined with cicatricial alopecia, pachyonychia, microcephaly, nanism and congenital cataract has been named Schäfer[164] syndrome.

Ectopia of the Lens

Simple congenital ectopia of the lens usually is associated with anomalies of the zonula fibers and tremulous iris (iridodonesis). Since the dislocation often is upward and laterad, the aphakic part is found in the inferior and internal portion of the pupil. Lens coloboma may be present. Dominant inheritance through as many as five generations has been reported.

Fig. 39-14.—Pedigree of an Ohio kindred with dislocation of the lens dominantly inherited.

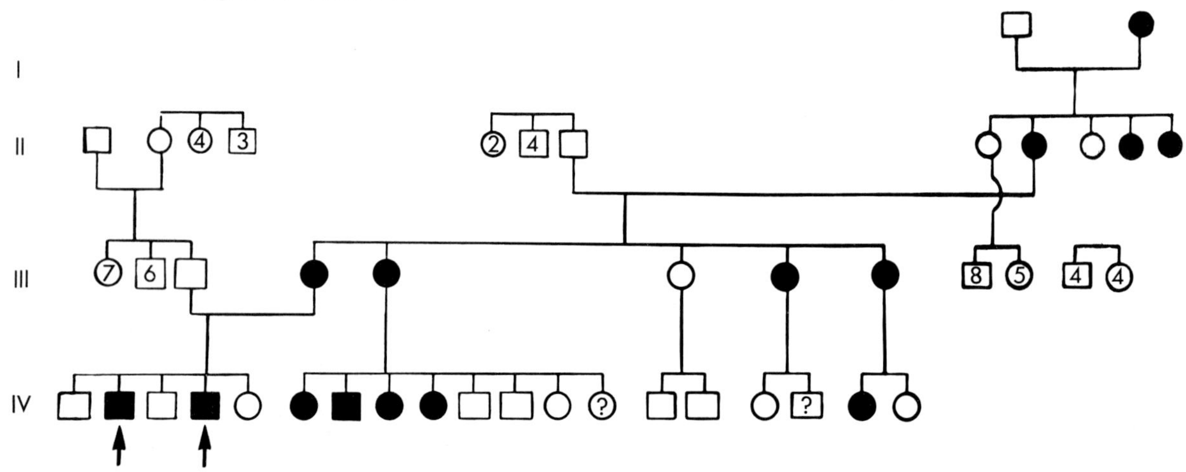

In *ectopia lentis and pupillae* there is not only displacement of the lens but also abnormal position and shape of the pupil, both anomalies being bilateral and symmetrical. Recessive inheritance seems to be responsible for these defects. In some of these families, ectopia of the lens and pupil may alternate with simple ectopia.[1]

Ectopia of the lens is, together with arachnodactyly, cited as an essential constituent of Marfan syndrome. Approximately 70% of these patients are said to have ectopic lenses (p. 850). If the lens is displaced into the anterior chamber, glaucoma can result; if it is displaced into the vitreous, the retina can become detached. The dislocated lens in Marfan syndrome is small and spherical and sometimes colobomatous. Iridodonesis and miosis are often present. Aplasia of the dilator muscle and iris hypoplasia have been observed. Other ocular anomalies mentioned repeatedly are megalocornea, hydrophthalmia, microcornea, microphthalmia, coloboma of the iris and lens, aniridia, heterochromia iridis, eccentric pupils, coloboma of the macula and optic nerve, choroidal atrophy and retinal pigmentary dystrophy.[1,122] The fact that the lens and the zonula fibers are of ectodermal origin does not fit too well into the concept of Marfan syndrome as a mesodermal dystrophy.

The Retina

Congenital anomalies of the fundus oculi, of the retina and choroidea are so numerous and intricate that they cannot possibly be dealt with here satisfactorily. Ida Mann, in her book *Developmental Abnormalities of the Eye*,[2] devoted 124 pages to this topic. The ophthalmoscope permits such detailed studies of this small area of the body that innumerable congenital anomalies have been observed and studied. Only some of these anomalies can be mentioned here. Special attention will be paid to those deviations that are associated with other congenital malformations of the body. They sometimes make possible the diagnosis of a prenatal disease or syndrome and sometimes permit us to make a eugenic prognosis.

Retinal Aplasia (Congenital Amaurosis; Heredoretinopathia Congenitalis Monohybrida Recessiva Autosomalis)

This disorder is of outstanding importance to the pediatrician and the ophthalmologist dealing with blind infants. Between 10% and 20% of congenitally blind children belong in this group.[8] As early as 1869, Leber[165] dealt with retinitis pigmentosa and congenital blindness. In the first months of life there were no definite alterations in the fundus in his cases. Later, pigmentary changes appeared accompanied by narrowing of the blood vessels and optic atrophy. Cataracts followed in some patients with advancing age. A high consanguinity rate of the apparently normal parents and occurrence in sibs were also stressed by Leber. In Sweden, Alström and Olson[166] emphasized that this disorder was congenital, hereditary and attributable to an autosomal recessive gene. Cataract and keratoconus occurred in some of the patients. The importance of this form of congenital blindness can be gathered from the fact that these authors held it responsible for 10% of all cases of blindness in Sweden. In Holland, Schappert-Kimmijser *et al.*[167] found among 600 blind children 109 (18%) affected by this amaurosis congenita, which at first shows no definite fundus changes but leads to retinochoroidal changes with advancing age. The trait was particularly prevalent on isolated islands, where consanguineous marriages were common. There is markedly reduced electric activity of the retina. Nystagmus is present in the majority of cases and photophobia in some. Cataract and keratoglobus or keratoconus are facultative symptoms.[167] Sorsby and Williams[168] reported two family groups in which cases of retinal aplasia occurred repeatedly. The eyes were normally formed and the media were clear. Ophthalmoscopically, either a normal fundus or some mottling with pallor of the disc was found initially, but retinal changes developed progressively as the patients grew older. In one family, the trait was dominant and there were 2 mentally defective children in the third generation. On necropsy, one of these children showed a completely disorganized retina but the brain was free of macroscopic anomalies. The authors believed that there is a failure of the retina to develop into a functional tissue and that this undeveloped retina subsequently undergoes secondary degeneration. They compared the condition with retinal dystrophy in the mouse, in the Irish setter and in the rat, where the affection is due to failure in the final differentiation of the rod layer.

Whereas in typical cases the funduscopic findings are minimal, there are peripheral changes in some and extensive macular atrophic lesions in others.[79] In about one-fourth of the children, the ocular findings are associated with deafness, spastic paralysis and mental deficiency.[8]

Although recessive inheritance is assumed in most of these cases, the genes responsible for the disorders may be heterogeneous. Mating of two affected parents can result in normal children.[79] In rare instances, children with retinal aplasia have polydactyly and develop mental retardation, obesity and hypogonadism,[79] i.e., the Laurence-Moon-Biedl syndrome (Chapter 19).

Congenital Detachment of the Retina

Mann[2] has emphasized the discrepancies of growth of the outer and inner layers of the optic cup in normal development. The two layers are separated up to the third month but later they appear in apposition in normal eyes. Congenital detachment, however, is common in microphthalmia, in which the detached area is tightly stretched between its points of attachments, as if it were too small for the outer layer of the cup. Persistent hyaloid vessels also occur in such eyes. Mann stated that a relationship has been noted occasionally between congenital cystic disease of the retina and congenital cystic disease of the lung and possibly other congenital cystic states. Congenital detachment of the retina is rare in otherwise normal eyes, but it may occur as a hereditary congenital retinoschisis.

Congenital Retinoschisis (Congenital Vascular Veil in the Vitreous)

Retinal detachment due to cystic degeneration of the retinal periphery was described by Sorsby *et al.*,[169] who observed the condition in a kindred in which 8 men belonging to three generations were affected. It is possible that the retina had split, with detachment following, but other explanations of the disorder, which results in slow retinal atrophy, have also been proferred. In 1938, Mann and McRae[170] described the condition as congenital vascular veil in the vitreous. Unilateral and bilateral involvement can occur in the same kindred. Gieser and Falls[171] observed the disorder in five generations with evidence of sex-linked transmission. Great variation in expressivity was demonstrated in the pedigree, in which a female carrier showed a macular cyst in one eye.

Choroideremia

This anomaly is characterized by night blindness from earliest childhood and by reduced central vision. Ophthalmoscopically, the fundus appears glistening white, with the exception of the macular region, which has normal color and a plexus of choroidal vessels. The optic disc usually is normal. There seems to be absence of the choroid and retina in certain parts of the eye, which has been attributed to failure of prenatal development. The condition occurs only in males and seems to be an X-linked recessive trait. In female carriers, who have no visual disturbances, changes in pigmentation can be seen with the ophthalmoscope.[172]

Myelinated Nerve Fibers in the Retina

Since myelin sheaths normally do not pass the lamina cribrosa, the nerve fibers of the retina usually are not myelinated. Myelinization beyond the lamina into the retina can occur as a harmless variation that produces a rather impressive ophthalmoscopic picture. Myelinated fibers may appear as silk-like opacities irregularly distributed about the disc, covering blood vessels at the margin of the disc and beyond its periphery. Sometimes they look like arcuate isolated patches at some distance from the disc. A hereditary tendency to myelinated retinal nerve fibers has been reported. As a rule, vision is not disturbed but scotomas in affected areas can be demonstrated in some cases.[172]

Retinitis Pigmentosa (Tapetoretinal Degenerations)

This group of ocular disorders has been classified according to various characteristics. In hereditary cases, it can be shown that the same genotypic form can have various phenotypic manifestations, so that classifications have found no general acceptance and applicability. All forms have in common the fact that the retinal and pigmentary epithelia undergo partial or total destruction because of an innate weakness of the tissues, which deteriorate earlier than the rest of the body. Such processes of degeneration, called "abiotrophies," lead to tapetoretinal changes without inflammation or trauma, but they can be imitated by such infections as rubella, toxoplasmosis or cytomegalic inclusion disease. The typical form is the generalized pigmentary retinopathy with "osteoblast-like" pigmentary clusters, optic atrophy, shrinking retinal blood vessels and sclerosis of the choroid. Other characteristics are hemeralopia, narrowing of visual fields, diminution of central vision and absence of electroretinographic response.[88] Most of the tapetoretinal degenerations progress and lead to blindness in adult life, but onset of visual disturbances dates back to early infancy in the majority of cases. There also is a congenital form (amaurosis congenita or retinal aplasia) that is of great practical importance, since it is the cause of a considerable portion of congenital blindness (p. 377).

The typical tapetoretinal degenerations are genetically determined and attributed to autosomal recessive inheritance in most cases. It has long been known that parental consanguinity is quite high, and recurrence in sibs, children of phenotypically normal parents, has been recorded many times. However, there also are pedigrees showing transmission of the disorder through many generations as an apparently dominant trait.[88,173] In some of these cases, pseudodominance seems likely as in a case of Klein and Franceschetti's,[8] in which triple consanguinity resulted in pigmentary retinopathy in two generations, with direct transmission in one instance. There exist pedigrees that are best interpreted on the basis of X-linked recessive inheritance.[88,174] Among these kinships are some with intermediate X-linked inheritance that are of special practical and theoretical interest. Weiner and Falls[175] recorded a family in which male members had retinitis pigmentosa, and there were female carriers who, although they had no evidence of abnormal retinal function, had abnormal opthalmoscopic findings. In this and other pedigrees of this type, a tapetoretinal silvery reflex is obtained, sometimes covering the entire surface of the retina in female carriers of the gene.[88] It is obvious that this finding makes possible distinction of carrier and normal daughters of affected males, thus improving genetic counseling. The most frequent complication of pigmentary retinopathy is cataract, particularly in the region of the posterior pole. Myopia is frequent, but macular involvement and glaucoma are rare complications.[88, 172]

Association with extraocular disorders is of great biologic and diagnostic interest. It is especially in the recessive type that such complications are observed. Labyrinthine deafness has been reported in 20–30% of patients with pigmentary retinopathy. In about 6% of deaf-mutes, pigmentary retinal changes have been found. The deafness can be congenital or it develops in postnatal life. The association of the ocular and aural defects is considered by some investigators as coincidental, by others as etiologically related. François[88] believed that the evidence points to association of pigmentary retinopathy and deafness as manifestations of a single gene with pleiotropic effects. Mental retardation has been recorded repeatedly in patients with these retinopathies, but estimates of its frequency vary between 4% and 18%. It is likely that families with a high incidence of mental impairment represent special entities. The Laurence-Moon-Biedl syndrome (Chapter 19) is an example of this.

Hereditary Degeneration of the Macula (Macular Dystrophy)

There are many forms of this disorder, which can appear at various periods of life. Among them there is a congenital or infantile type. Best[176] described a kindred of 59 that had 8 affected members (Best disease). Irregular dominant inheritance has been reported.[88] Pigmentation and stippling of the macula is present at an early age and it seems possible that degeneration of the retinal layers sets in before the macula is fully formed.[2] As a rule, the lesion is stationary, but slow progression has also been reported. Cystic macular degeneration may also be transmitted as a dominant trait.[88]

Barkman[177] published a large pedigree from a limited area in Sweden in which 39 men and 30 women were affected by central retinal degeneration. The patients belonged to six frequently intermarrying kindreds, but the author believed that irregular autosomal dominant inheritance was responsible for the trait. The great variability of funduscopic pictures of central degeneration is of interest. The variability of age at onset—from 1 week to 40 years—is also worth emphasis. Such observations demonstrate that the gene does not always conform to rigid clinical classification.

Macular Dysplasia (Pseudocoloboma)

Macular dysplasias are extensive oval defects of the retina in the area of the macula. They have some superficial resemblance to colobomas but they are not related in origin or position to the fetal fissure. They can be pigmented or not pigmented; the retinal vessels may pass over them undisturbed or they stop at their borders. The atrophic area can be excavated. In rare cases, abnormal blood vessels may be connected with a dysplastic macula. The retina, the pigment epithelium and the choriocapillaris are involved in the defect. Some of the cases are due to developmental errors, others are the result of disease. It has been learned that ocular toxoplasmosis can result in the classic picture of (pseudo-) coloboma of the macula. The white zones are due to chorioretinal destruction with persistence of some choroidal vessels. The pigmented areas are fragments of pigment epithelium on the border of the destroyed area.[41] There were 47 patients with "coloboma of the macula" in Møllenbach's Danish series,[109] the defect being bilateral in about half of them. There was no connection between this anomaly and the iris colobomas, and no hereditary background could be ascertained for them.

Although typical macular dysplasia has been shown to be due to toxoplasmosis in some cases, the anomaly also can be of different origin. Hereditary macular dystrophy has been described in some families, occurring in at least two generations. Sorsby[178] reported the case of a mother and 5 of her 7 children affected by bilateral pigmented "macular colobomas." These patients also had apical skeletal and nail defects of the hands and feet. Genetic determination of macular dysplasia was further suggested by identical appearance of the lesions in monozygotic twin girls.[179]

Coloboma of the Disc

As with other ocular structures, the disc may show a coloboma with or without connection with coloboma of the choroid below. The disc appears deeply cupped and the blood vessels show abnormal arrangement. If limited to the disc, the coloboma presents one end of the fetal fissure, which has remained open to a minimal degree.

Congenital Crescents of the Optic Disc

Congenital crescents of the disc are very frequent anomalies that do not interfere with vision and do not progress. They are seen most often below the disc, whereas acquired (myopic) crescents have a predilection for the temporal side. Mann[2] believed that the fetal fissure is the determining factor in the inferior type, in which the pigmented outer layer of the optic cup does not reach up to the insertion of the optic stalk.

Aplasia and Hypoplasia of the Optic Nerve

Congenital absence or rudimentary development of the optic nerve occurs in anophthalmia, microphthalmia, cyclopia or orbital encephalocele; it can also be seen in otherwise normal eyes. In the case of absence, excavations may be seen with the ophthalmoscope in place of the disc; in the case of hypoplasia, the disc is reduced in size and altered in shape. Sometimes these anomalies alternate with microphthalmia or anophthalmia in members of the same kindred. Congenital aplasia of the optic nerve probably is more common than true congenital optic atrophy.[153]

Congenital Atrophy of the Optic Nerve

Optic atrophy is a frequent cause of blindness in childhood. Approximately 20% of the children in schools for the blind are handicapped by optic atrophy. Although only a few of these probably had optic atrophy at birth, many of them became blind because of a congenital disorder. In the past, congenital syphilis was a rather frequent cause of optic atrophy, but this form, which usually did not manifest itself before the third year,[180] has lost its importance in recent years. Hydrocephaly, congenital or developing soon after birth, is a leading cause of optic atrophy in infants. Atrophy can develop without preceding papillary edema. Stretching of the nerve may be responsible for its atrophy.[153] Spina bifida complicated by hydrocephaly or other malformations of the brain can be associated with optic atrophy. Secondary optic atrophy may follow chorioretinitis or toxoplasmosis. In craniostenoses, such as oxycephaly (acrocephaly) and Crouzon craniofacial dysostosis, optic atrophy is attributed to increased intracranial pressure and also to stretching of the nerve. In microcephaly, optic atrophy may occur among other ocular symptoms. Optic atrophy was seen with microcephaly caused by intrauterine exposure to radiation.[181] Retinal and optic nerve atrophy was observed by Ford[182] in siblings with macrencephaly. In osteopetrosis (p. 863), blindness can be one of the early symptoms that is thought to be due to narrowing of the optic foramina. Occasionally, optic atrophy has been reported in achondroplastic dwarfs.[153] Primary optic atrophy can develop in Recklinghausen neurofibromatosis.[183]

Hereditary congenital or infantile optic atrophy occurs as an uncomplicated anomaly that is not associated with general and nervous disorders or it can be complicated by manifestations of central nervous system disease. In the uncomplicated form, optic atrophy is present at birth or in early infancy and is recognizable by a pale and excavated disc. Severe cases with early loss of vision generally are seen in sibships with parental consanguinity, recessive inheritance being responsible for the trait. A milder dominant form that develops gradually without leading to complete blindness can be passed on through many generations.[88] Complicated infantile hereditary optic atrophy usually is limited to the temporal side and remains incomplete, but the patients are handicapped by a spastic gait, muscular hypertonia and poor coordination. Nystagmus, increased tendon reflexes and a positive Babinski sign are noted. Both sexes are affected, and recessive inheritance is likely. The condition has been seen concordant in monozygotic twins.[88] Irregular dominant inheritance with various ocular manifestations has also been observed.[8]

Gliomas of the Optic Nerve

This term has been applied to tumors of the optic nerves, chiasma and optic tracts. Gliomas contribute significantly to tumors of the orbit. Dodge *et al.*[184] believed that many of these tumors were congenital, and Davis[185] considered them "a phenomenon of Recklinghausen's disease." Dodge *et al.* distinguished two groups – glioma of the optic nerve and glioma of the chiasma or optic tract. The first group generally is found unilaterally and in younger children than is the second. Proptosis, loss of vision, strabismus, papilledema and optic atrophy are signs of glioma of the optic nerve. Females are affected much more often than males. The symptoms are similar in the second group but loss of vision is the leading symptom in these cases. They may cause early endocrine signs because of their intracranial situation. Both groups are identified as astrocytomas microscopically. They resemble in this and other respects pontine and cerebellar tumors occurring in children. Ganglion cells found in some of these tumors suggest that they may be derived from heterotopic brain tissue.[184] Gliomas of the optic nerve occur about four times more often than meningiomas of the optic nerve that are derived from the nerve sheath. They are seen in older age groups than the gliomas, but occasionally children are affected.

Retinoblastoma

It has been estimated that retinoblastoma occurs once in 20,000–30,000 births. It makes its appearance most often around the age of 2 years[88] but it probably is determined prenatally in the majority of cases. Gradual appearance of bilateral retinoblastoma in a premature infant has been observed[186] but late formation in the sixth or even seventh decade of life has also been reported.[153] There are striking observations in kinships and sibships that indicate genetic determination. Pedigrees showing retinoblastoma in three or four generations and concordance in 4 monozygotic twin pairs[8] (as compared with discordance in 8 dizygotic pairs) support this point of view. Autosomal dominant inheritance has been assumed. Observation of sibships with more than one sibling affected, although both parents were free of the disorder, have been explained by reduced penetrance of the gene in one of the parents. The mother of several children with retinoblastoma seen in the Cincinnati Children's Hospital had one microphthalmic eye. She attributed the anomaly to an injury, but it is more likely that she had had a retinoblastoma that was spontaneously arrested and retrogressed, an event observed occasionally. In this family, 6 of 9 children developed retinoblastoma.[187,188] Estimates of penetrance of the gene vary considerably and it is possible that it is different in different families. Although genetic determination has been demonstrated many times, sporad-

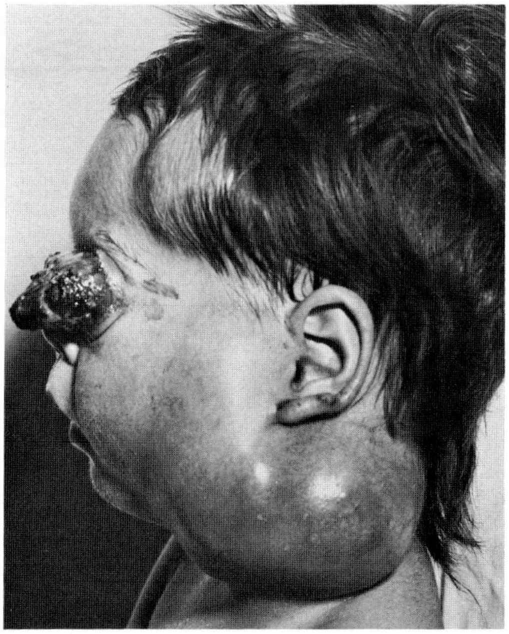

Fig. 39-15.—Retinoblastoma with metastases to cervical lymph glands.

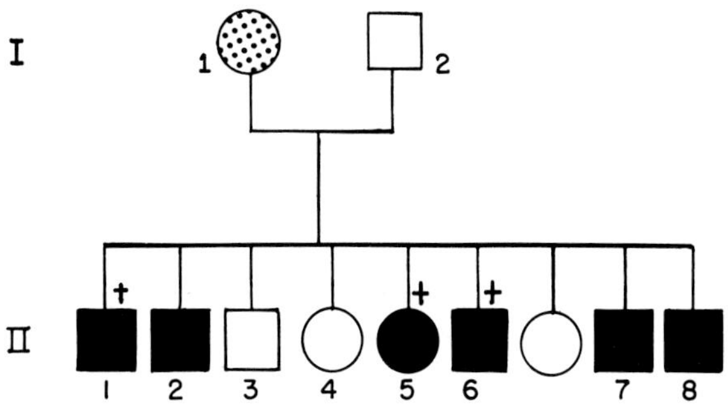

Fig. 39-16.—Pedigree of a family with retinoblastomas. Figure 39-15 shows II_5 with metastases. *I*, the mother, had unilateral microphthalmia, which she attributed to an injury. But this eye probably was small because of shrinking due to spontaneous retrogression of a retinoblastoma. This family was seen for many years in the Cincinnati General and Children's Hospitals and was recorded by W.E. Sovik.[187]

ic occurrence is much more common. Opinions concerning such sporadic cases differ. Some investigators believe that they all represent germinal mutations that are not passed on because of early death of their bearers. However, there are many survivors who had had normal children only, a fact that allows differing interpretations. Vogel[189] believed that only 25% of the sporadic cases are new mutants, whereas 75% are nonhereditary phenocopies. Retinoblastoma has been described in a child with XXX,21-trisomy.[190] Deletion of the long arm of a chromosome D has been observed repeatedly[209-211] (Chapter 37). Thus, the etiology of retinoblastoma is heterogeneous and obscure in many cases, so that eugenic prognosis is difficult. For normal parents with 1 affected child, the empirical risk for a future child seems to be only 4%, but if 2 children are affected, the risk is 50%. The risk is high for a cured patient's children, but reliable risk figures are not available.[88,191]

Clinically, the tumor may be recognized by a white reflex (cat's eye) or by lack of fixation or by enlargement of the pupil. Ophthalmoscopically, the tumor begins as a circumscribed gray lesion with dilatation and tortuosity of blood vessels. Sometimes two tumors may be seen in one eye. A tumor may grow forward into the vitreous (endophytum) or toward the choroid (exophytum). In the latter type, the retina becomes detached, which accentuates the white reflex from the pupil.[172] The glioma endophytum fills the vitreous with a white mass that is friable and furnishes movable vitreous opacities. Increased intraocular tension, protrusion of the globe and ulceration of the cornea occur. In some cases, retrogression of the tumor and shrinking of the globe become noticeable. This process may be temporary or, rarely, lead to phthisis bulbi or microphthalmia, with arrest of malignant growth. Such spontaneously cured persons can transmit the condition to some of their offspring.[187,192] This course, however, is the exception. More often, the tumor progresses beyond the eye, perforating the cornea and sclera, or grows into the optic nerve or metastasizes through the blood stream. From the optic nerve, the tumor spreads into the orbit, the skull, the chiasma, the optic nerve of the other side, the meninges or the lymph nodes of the neck. Metastases have been observed in many organs.[172]

In retinoblastomas, the nuclear layers are involved and there is typical rosette formation in the tumor. Mann[2] believed that the malignant change in the inner layer of the optic cup must occur late in intrauterine life or in infancy after vascularization of the retina and before its final differentiation. The tumor cells are small and polygonal, with a relatively large nucleus. They show perivascular aggregation and early tendency to degeneration. Numerous mitotic figures can be observed.

Early recognition and treatment of the tumor can save the patient's life. When found in only one eye, enucleation often cures the disease. In complicated and widespread disease, radium and roentgen treatment, cobalt applicators and triethylenemelamine (TEM) have been used with differing results.[191]

Toxoplasmosis of the Eye

Lavat[41] reviewed the reports on ocular toxoplasmosis and came to the following conclusions. Microphthalmia is a frequent manifestation. It can be unilateral or bilateral; it can be congenital or be due to atrophy following uveitis. Searching nystagmus is noted frequently, accompanied by internal strabismus or other pareses of the eye muscles. Iridocyclitis is not rare, but the lens is seldom involved. Occasionally, the vitreous is affected, as retrolental masses, infiltrates, hemorrhages or a hyaloid artery may interfere with examination of the retina, but chorioretinitis is the principal sign. Macular dysplasia (pseudocoloboma of the macula) is the result of severe chorioretinitis of the posterior pole of the globe. The white areas are remnants of necrosis of the retina and choroidea, with persistence of some large choroidal vessels. The black areas are hypertrophied fragments of the pigment epithelium around the destroyed regions. The macular lesions usually are large and bilateral. Similar lesions may be seen in areas outside the macula. In addition, active foci can be visible, showing edema and hemorrhages. The lesions can also be limited in extent or have the appearance of a detached retina, pseudoglioma or cysts surrounded by chorioretinitis. Histologic studies showed that the choroid usually is less affected than the retina, which is involved in most of the cases. The optic nerves often are affected by inflammatory reactions.

Cytomegalic Inclusion Disease

In cytomegalic inclusion disease (CID), the eye may be affected by prenatal, perinatal or postnatal infection. Involvement of the lacrimal glands and keratomalacia have been reported.[107,108] Necrotic membranous conjunctivitis with involvement of the sclera and ciliary body has been observed in a baby 1 month of age.[193] Cataract, retinal autolysis, hemorrhage and gliosis were found in another infant with the disease.[159] Burns[194] observed and described CID uveitis in an infant who developed chorioretinitis with perivascular and macular exudates. The areas of chorioretinitis were seen chiefly in the periphery and consisted of white and pigmented foci. The optic nerves appeared white and atrophic. These findings are different from those of toxoplasmosis, in which typically distinct macular or posterior polar lesions are seen and which leave, on healing, punched-out areas of white sclera surrounded by pigment[194] (Chapter 9).

Ocular Changes in Hamartoses

Diseases tending to formation of multiple tumors or tumor-like lesions have been termed in this book "hamartoses" (Chapters 121–123). Recklinghausen neurofibromatosis, tuberous sclerosis and Hippel-Lindau disease are inherited as dominant traits with polymorphic expression. Other authors have summarized them under the name of "phakomatoses."[195] They show "marks" or birthmarks, according to this rather nonspecific term. Sturge-Weber disease, which is essentially limited to one side of the body and is etiologically more obscure than the three mentioned hamartoses, often is incorrectly included in this group. Other authors prefer the term "neuroectodermal dysplasias," a rather misleading term, since mesodermal tissues are often affected.

The eye often is involved in these general disorders, which can manifest themselves in so many tissues. In patients with *tuberous sclerosis* (Chapter 122), tumors may be detectable in the retina. Ophthalmoscopically, round or oval grayish spots are seen in some of the patients near the papilla, more or less elevated and covering the retinal vasculature. Other ocular manifestations are corneal or lens opacities, glaucoma and hemorrhages.[88] A rare anomaly is coloboma of the choroid[196]; it is one of the manifestations that point to an early prenatal onset of the disease. In *neurofibromatosis*, the eye may be affected by many lesions. Neurofibromas can be located on the eyelids, in the conjunctiva, ciliary body, iris, retina, optic nerve and orbit. Exophthalmos can occur and congenital hydrophthalmia can result from involvement of the ciliary nerves and blocking of the angle. It is unilateral and sometimes associated with facial hemihypertrophy.[197] Ocular anomalies are also caused by intracranial tumors occurring in central neurofibromatosis[88] (Chapter 121).

In 1904, Hippel[198] described a rare anomaly of the retina observed in 2 patients. There was a yellowish tumor in the periphery of the fundus that was entered by a pair of enlarged retinal vessels originating from the optic disc. There had been reports of similar cases before and the angiomatous nature of the disorder was recognized, but the lesion was named "von Hippel disease" and became the first symptom of a much larger symptom complex or hamartosis, now termed *Hippel-Lindau disease*. The ocular findings are enlargement of pairs of retinal vessels and nodular tumors accompanied by secondary exudative changes.[172] The vessels are tortuous and their enlargement increases toward the peripheral tumor. The lesions may be multiple, each tumor being supplied by a pair of vessels. With advancing of the disease, exudates and detachment of the retina appear as secondary changes. With development of cerebellar tumors (Lindau disease), papilledema caused by increased intracranial pressure may develop. In the early stage, before a tumor can be seen ophthalmoscopically, a capillary angioma consisting chiefly of endothelial capillaries filled with blood and replacing some of the retinal layers may be found on histologic examination.[199] Later, the endothelial cells may fill the capillary tubes completely, converting them into cords. Connective tissue intervenes between the capillaries and cords. Vacuoles appear in some of the cells, which results in formation of a "pseudoxanthoma." Glial cells may form a reticulum within the tumor (angioreticuloma) and cystic cavities appear. Glial and connective tissue reactions progress as the disease advances, and occasionally the angioma breaks into the vitreous. Angiomatosis of the retina is rare. It usually is recognized in young adults but it has been observed in children. It is a component of a general disorder that is characterized by cerebellar cysts or tumors, angiomas in the medulla oblongata or spinal cord, cysts in the pancreas or kidneys or hypernephroma. Hippel-Lindau disease is a dominant hereditary trait with great variability in expression. Its manifestations can appear alternately in the various members of an affected kinship.

Ocular Changes in Sturge-Weber Disease

This disorder is characterized by a facial nevus flammeus, intracranial calcifications, convulsions and glaucoma (Chapter 38). The facial hemangioma is always congenital; glaucoma may be present at birth. Unilateral glaucoma is the rule, but bilateral cases have been observed. In these patients, glaucoma is attributed to angiomas of the choroid, which impede outflow of blood from the eye and increase intraocular pressure. In some cases, tortuosity of retinal veins has been noted ophthalmoscopically. The facial vascular nevus usually involves the lid of the glaucomatous eye. Tortuosity and dilatation of conjunctival vessels have been observed and heterochromia of the irides may be present in patients with this syndrome.[153, 172]

The Eye in the Thalidomide Embryopathy

Ocular involvement in the thalidomide syndrome has been reported in approximately one-fourth of the children damaged by the drug in early gestation. Gilkes and Strode[200] found visual defects in 7 of 20 children with congenital limb deformities, and 5 of the 7 had colobomatous defects. Cullen[201] saw eye defects in 3 of 12 "thalidomide babies." Colobomas of the iris, lens, choroid, optic disc and retina have been described in various combinations and degrees. Microphthalmia was present in some of the cases but, in others, the eye defects were less obvious. Pigmentary retinopathy, high refractive error and reduced visual acuity are among less noticeable anomalies.[202] One child with phocomelia of the upper extremities had microphthalmia on one side and "clinical anophthalmia" on the other. Despite a high suspicion of thalidomide damage, the mother denied taking any drug during pregnancy.[203]

REFERENCES

1. Waardenburg, P. J., Franceschetti, A., and Klein, D.: *Genetics and Ophthalmology* (Springfield, Ill.: Charles C Thomas, Publisher, 1961).
2. Mann, I.: *Developmental Abnormalities of the Eye* (2d ed.; Philadelphia: J. B. Lippincott Company, 1957).
3. Falls, H. F., and Kertesz, E. D.: A new syndrome combining pterygium colli with developmental anomalies of the eyelids and lymphatics of the lower extremities, Tr. Am. Ophth. Soc. 62:248, 1964.
4. Cordes, F. C., and Hogan, M. J.: Ocular ichthyosis, Arch. Ophth. 22:590, 1939.
5. Witkop, C. J., Jr., Shankle, C. H., Graham, J. B., Murray, M. R., Rucknagel, D. L., and Byerly, B. H.: Hereditary benign intraepithelial dyskeratosis. II. Oral manifestations and hereditary transmission, Arch. Path. 70:696, 1960.
6. Timm, G.: Über Anophthalmie und Mikrophthalmie bei Anenzephalie, Klin. Monatsbl. Augenh. 137:430, 1960.
7. Recordon, E., and Griffiths, G. M.: A case of primary bilateral anophthalmia, Brit. J. Ophth. 22:353, 1938.
8. Klein, D., and Franceschetti, A.: Missbildungen und Krankheiten des Auges, in Becker, P. E.: *Humangenetik*, Vol. 4 (Stuttgart: Georg Thieme, 1964).
9. Hoefnagel, D., Keenan, M. E., and Allen, F. H., Jr.: Heredofamilial bilateral anophthalmia, Arch. Ophth. 69:760, 1963.
10. Patau, K., Smith, D. W., Therman, E., Inhorn, S. L., and Wagner, H. P.: Multiple congenital anomaly caused by an extra autosome, Lancet 1:790, 1960.
11. Sjögren, T., and Larsson, T.: Microphthalmos and anophthalmos with or without coincident oligophrenia. A clinical and genetic-statistical study, Acta psychiat. et neurol., Supp. 56, 1949.
12. Zeiter, H. J.: Congenital microphthalmos: A pedigree of four affected siblings and an additional report of forty-four sporadic cases, Am. J. Ophth. 55:910, 1963.
13. Kallmann, F. J., Barrera, S. E., and Metzger, H.: The association of hereditary microphthalmia with mental deficiency, Am. J. Ment. Deficiency 45:25, 1940.
14. Roberts, J. A. F.: Sex-linked microphthalmia sometimes associated with mental deficiency, Brit. M. J. 2:1213, 1937.
15. Pospiech, K. H.: Encephalographische und anatomische Befunde bei angeborenem Balkenmangel und bei Erweiterung des Cavum Septi Pellucidum, Ztschr. Neurol. u. Psychiat. 74:249, 1942.
16. Monthus, A., and Opin,: Étude histologique et pathogénique d'un cas de microphthalmie, Arch. opht. 23: 32, 1903.
17. François, J.: À propos d'une famille présentant des anomalies oculaires du type colobomateux depuis le colobome unilateral de l'iris jusqu'à l'anophthalmie bilatérale associée au syndrome de Bardet-Biedl, J. Génét. Hum. 2:203, 1953.
18. Warkany, J., and Weaver, T.: Heredofamilial deviations. II. Enlarged parietal foramens combined with obesity, hypogenitalism, microphthalmos and mental retardation, Am. J. Dis. Child. 60:1147, 1940.
19. Ferrier, P., Widgren, S., and Ferrier, S.: Nonspecific pseudohermaphroditism. Report of two cases with cytogenetic investigations, Helvet. paediat. acta 19:1, 1964.
20. Root, A. W., Eberlein, W. R., Briebart, S., Moorhead, P. S., and Mellman, W. J.: Chromosomal analysis of multiple tissues from a true hermaphrodite, J. Clin. Endocrinol. 24:467, 1964.
21. Lenz, W.: Recessive geschlechtsgebundene Mikrophthalmie mit multiplen Missbildungen, Ztschr. Kinderh. 77:384, 1955.
22. Hooft, C., and Jongbloet, J.: Syndrome oro-digito-facial chez deux frères, Arch. franç. pédiat. 21:729, 1964.
23. Weyers, H., and Thier, C. J.: Malformations mandibulo-faciales et délimitation d'un syndrome oculo-vertebral, J. Génét. Hum. 7:143, 1958.
24. Cross, H. E., McKusick, V. A., and Breen, W.: A new oculocerebral syndrome with hypopigmentation, J. Pediat. 70:398, 1967.
25. Gorlin, R. J., Meskin, L. H., and St. Geme, J. W.: Oculodento-digital dysplasia, J. Pediat. 63:69, 1963.
26. Silver, H. K., Blair, W. C., and Kempe, C. H.: Fanconi syndrome. Multiple congenital anomalies with hypoplastic anemia, A.M.A. Am. J. Dis. Child. 83:14, 1952.
27. Goltz, R. W., Peterson, W. C., Gorlin, R. J., and Ravits, H. G.: Focal dermal hypoplasia, Arch. Dermat. 86:708, 1962.
28. Holden, J. D., and Akers, W. A.: Goltz's syndrome: Focal dermal hypoplasia. A combined mesoectodermal dysplasia, Am. J. Dis. Child. 114:292, 1967.
29. Harris, H. A., and Thompson, G. C.: Persistent truncus arteriosus communis with microphthalmos, orbital cyst and polydactyly, Arch. Dis. Childhood 12:59, 1937.
30. Apfelbaum, M. A., and Marmelstein, M.: Congenital bi-

lateral anophthalmos vera with unilateral polydactyly and cleft palate, Arch. Ophth. 29:258, 1943.
31. Warburg, M.: Anophthalmos complicated by mental retardation and cleft palate, Acta ophth. 38:394, 1960.
32. Sergovich, F., Madronich, J. S., Barr, M. L., Carr, D. H., and Langdon, W. A.: The D trisomy syndrome: A case report with a description of ocular pathology, Canad. M.A.J. 89:151, 1963.
33. Ginsberg, J., and Perrin, E. V. D.: Ocular manifestations of 13-15 trisomy, Arch. Ophth. 74:487, 1965.
34. Lubs, H. A., Jr., Koenig, E. U., and Brandt, I. K.: Trisomy 13-15: A clinical syndrome, Lancet 2:1001, 1961.
35. Yudkin, A. M.: Congenital bilateral microphthalmos accompanied by other malformations of the body, Am. J. Ophth. 11:128, 1928.
36. Wallace, C., and Anderson, I. F.: Group B/D translocation chromosome in a case with stigmata of the D trisomy, South African M. J. 38:352, 1964.
37. Aschenheim, E.: Schädigung einer menschlichen Frucht durch Röntgenstrahlen, Arch. Kinderh. 68:131, 1920.
38. Murphy, D. B.: Outcome of 625 pregnancies in women subjected to pelvic radium or roentgen irradiation, Am. J. Obst. & Gynec. 18:179, 1929.
39. Engelking, E.: Augenärztlich wichtige Röntgenschädigungen der Frucht nach Bestrahlung Schwangerer, Klin. Monatsbl. Augenh. 94:151, 1935.
40. Gregg, N. M.: Congenital cataract following German measles in mother, Tr. Ophth. Soc. Australia 3:35, 1942.
41. Lavat, J.: Toxoplasmose oculaire, Arch. opht. 13:252, 1953.
42. Schultz, G. A.: Postnatal developmental anatomy of a heritable rat microphthalmia, J. Morphol. 113:49, 1963.
43. Chase, H. B.: Studies on an anophthalmic strain of mice. IV. A second major gene for anophthalmia, Genetics 29:264, 1944.
44. Grüneberg, H.: *The Genetics of the Mouse* (The Hague: Martinus Nijhoff, 1952).
45. Truslove, G. M.: A gene causing ocular retardation in the mouse, J. Embryol. & Exper. Morphol. 10:652, 1962.
46. Beck, S. L.: Response to a teratogen of mice heterozygous for anophthalmia, Proc. XI Internat. Cong. Genet. 1:183, 1963.
47. Russell, W. L.: *Inbred and Hybrid Animals and Their Value in Research in Biology of the Laboratory Mouse* (Philadelphia: Blakiston Company, 1941).
48. Browman, L. G., and Ramsey, F.: Embryology of microphthalmos in Rattus Norvegicus, Arch. Ophth. 30:338, 1943.
49. Hicks, S. P.: Mechanism of radiation anencephaly, anophthalmia, and pituitary anomalies, Arch. Path. 57:363, 1954.
50. Majima, A.: Eye-abnormalities in mouse embryos caused by x-radiation of mothers. On changes in the initial stage of development by irradiation on the 8th day of pregnancy, Nagoya J. M. Sc. 24:85, 1961.
51. Majima, A.: Eye-abnormalities in mouse embryos and fetuses caused by x-radiation of mothers. Processes of production in case of exposure with 200r on the 8th day of pregnancy, Nagoya J. M. Sc. 24:171, 1962.
52. Boisselot, J.: Malformations foetales par insuffisance en acide pantothénique, Arch. franç. pédiat. 6:225, 1949.
53. Tuchmann-Duplessis, H., and Mercier-Parot, L.: Sur l'action tératogène d'un sulfamide hypoglycémiant. Étude expérimentale chez la ratte, J. Physiol. 51:65, 1959.
54. Ingalls, T. H., Tedeschi, C. G., and Helpern, M. M.: Congenital malformations of eye induced in mice by maternal anoxia, Am. J. Ophth. 35:311, 1952.
55. Degenhardt, K-H.: Cranio-facial dysplasia induced by oxygen-deficiency in rabbits, Biol. Neonat. 2:93, 1960.
56. Avizonis, P.: Über Kryptophthalmus congenitus, Ztschr. Augenh. 64:240, 1928.
57. Coover, D. H.: Cryptophthalmia, Ophthalmoscope 13: 586, 1915.
58. Hird, R. B.: An exhaustive treatise on the various colobomata, Ophth. Rev. 31:162, 1912.
59. Ammann, F., Klein, D., and Jöhr, P.: Une famille atteinte de colobomes iridochoroidiens, d'hétérochromie irienne et de syndrome de Marfan abortif, Ophthalmologica 147:118, 1964.
60. Grebe, H.: Biemond syndrom in einer Sippe mit Iriskolobomen, Hüftgelenks-dysplasie und Epilepsie, Acta genet. med. 9:197, 1960.
61. Waardenburg, P. J.: *Das menschliche Auge und seine Erbanlagen* (The Hague: Martinus Nijhoff, 1932).
62. Biemond, A.: Het syndroom van Laurence-Biedl en een aanverwant nieuw syndroom, Nederl. tijdschr. geneesk. 78:1801, 1934.
63. Warkany, J., Frauenberger, G. S., and Mitchell, A. G.: Heredofamilial deviations. 1. The Laurence-Moon-Biedl syndrome, Am. J. Dis. Child. 53:455, 1937.
64. Therman, E., Patau, K., DeMars, R. I., Smith, D. W., and Inhorn, S. L.: Iso/telo-D_1 mosaicism in a child with an incomplete D_1 trisomy syndrome, Portugal acta biol. 7: 211, 1963.
65. Conen, P. E., Phillips, K. G., and Mauntner, L. S.: Multiple developmental anomalies and trisomy of a 13-15 group chromosome (D_1 syndrome), Canad. M.A.J. 87: 709, 1962.
66. Ellis, J. R., and Marwood, J. C.: Autosomal trisomy syndromes, Lancet 2:263, 1961.
67. Jacobsen, P., Dupont, A., and Mikkelsen, M.: Translocation in the 13-15 group as a cause of partial trisomy and spontaneous abortion in the same family, Lancet 2:584, 1963.
68. Lele, K. P., Dent, T., and Delhanty, J. D. A.: Chromosome studies in five cases of coloboma of the iris, Lancet 1:576, 1965.
69. Ginsberg, J., Dignan, P., and Soukup, S.: Ocular abnormality associated with extra small autosome, Am. J. Ophth. 65:740, 1968.
70. Angelman, H.: Syndrome of coloboma with multiple congenital abnormalities in infancy, Brit. M. J. 2:1212, 1961.
71. Hippel, von, E.: Embryologische Untersuchungen über die Entstehungsweise der typischen angeborenen Spaltbildungen, von Graefes Arch. Ophth. 45:313, 1903.
72. Koyanagi, Y.: Embryologische Untersuchungen über die Genese der Augenkolobome und des Mikrophthalmus mit Orbitalcyste, von Graefes Arch. Ophth. 104:1, 1921.
73. Szily, von, A.: Die Ontogenese der idiotypischen (erblichen) Spaltbildungen des Auges des Mikrophthalmus und' der Orbitalcysten, Arch. mikr. Anat. u. Entwicklungsmechanik 74:1, 1924.
74. Warkany, J., and Schraffenberger, E.: Congenital malformations induced in rats by maternal vitamin A deficiency. I. Defects of the eye, Arch. Ophth. 35:150, 1946.
75. Giroud, A., and Martinet, M.: Malformations oculaires avec fibrose du vitré chez des embryons de lapin soumis à l'hypervitaminose A, Bull. Soc. opht. France No. 3, 1, 1959.
76. Maumenee, A. E.: The pathogenesis of congenital glaucoma, Am. J. Ophth. 47:827, 1959.
77. Dunphy, E. G.: Glaucoma accompanying nevus flammeus, Am. J. Ophth. 18:709, 1935.
78. Westerlund, E.: *Clinical and Genetic Studies of the Primary Glaucoma Diseases* (Copenhagen: Munksgaard, 1947).
79. Franceschetti, A.: Heredity of hydrophthalmia, J. Pediat. Ophth. 2:35, 1965.
80. Delmarcelle, Y.: Considérations sur l'hérédite du glaucome infantile, J. Génét. Hum. 6:33, 1956.
81. Bowen, P., Lee, C. S. N., Zellweger, H., and Lindenberg, R.: A familial syndrome of multiple congenital defects, Bull. Johns Hopkins Hosp. 114:402, 1964.

82. Kwitko, M. L.: Congenital glaucoma. A clinical study, Canad. J. Ophth. 2:91, 1967.
83. Alfano, J. E.: Ocular aspects of the maternal rubella syndrome, Tr. Am. Acad. Ophth. 70:235, 1966.
84. Reed, H., Briggs, J. N., and Martin, J. K.: Congenital glaucoma, deafness, mental deficiency, and cardiac anomaly following attempted abortion, J. Pediat. 46: 182, 1955.
85. Hanna, B. L., Sawin, P. B., and Sheppard, L. B.: Recessive buphthalmos in the rabbit, Genetics 47:519, 1962.
86. Cohlan, S. Q.: Congenital anomalies in the rat produced by excessive intake of vitamin A during pregnancy, Pediatrics 13:556, 1954.
87. Deuschle, F. M., Geiger, J. F., and Warkany, J.: Analysis of an anomalous oculodentofacial pattern in newborn rats produced by maternal hypervitaminosis A, J. Dent. Res. 38:149, 1959.
88. François, J.: *Heredity in Ophthalmology* (St. Louis: The C. V. Mosby Company, 1961).
89. Friedman, M. W., and Wright, E. S.: Hereditary microcornea and cataract in five generations, Am. J. Ophth. 35:1017, 1952.
90. Bamatter, F., Franceschetti, A., Klein, D., and Sierro, A.: Gérodermie ostéodysplasique héréditaire, Ann. paediat. 174:126, 1950.
91. Franceschetti, A., Dieterle, P., and Forni, S.: Megalocornea, ectopia lentis et pupilla é glaucoma tardivo: Sindrome ereditaria recessiva, Atti 42 Cong. Soc. Oftal. ital, Napoli 16:357, 1956.
92. Römer, A.: Untersuchung über die Erblichkeit d. Spiesskatarakt, Arch. Klaus Stift. Vererbungsforsch. 2:207, 1926.
93. Skeller, E., and Øster, J.: Eye symptoms in mongolism, Acta ophth. 29:149, 1951.
94. Cullen, J. F., and Butler, H. G.: Mongolism (Down's syndrome) and keratoconus, Brit. J. Ophth. 47:321, 1963.
95. Speakman, J. S., and Crawford, J. S.: Congenital opacities of the cornea, Brit. J. Ophth. 50:68, 1966.
96. Ioannides, T., Charemis, C., and Economou-Mavrou, C.: Congenital familial diffuse corneal dystrophy with dominant heredity, J. Pediat. Ophth. 3:9, 1966.
97. Goldenhar, M.: Associations malformatives de l'oeil et de l'oreille, en particulier le syndrome dermoide épibulbaire-appendices auriculaires-fistula auris congenita et ses relations avec la dysostose mandibulo-faciale, J. Génét. Hum. 1:243, 1952.
98. Lichter, P. R.: Multiple corneal dermoids associated with miliary aneurysms of the retina, J. Pediat. Ophth. 4:31, 1967.
99. Pillay, V. K.: Ophthalmo-mandibulo-melic dysplasia, J. Bone & Joint Surg. 46-A:858, 1964.
100. Gasteiger,: Über seltene Augenveränderungen bei Neurofibromatose, Klin. Monatsbl. Augenh. 100:768, 1938.
101. Rosenthal, J. W., and Kloepfer, H. W.: An acromegaloid, cutis verticis gyrata, corneal leukoma syndrome, Arch. Ophth. 68:722, 1962.
102. Mietens, C., and Weber, H.: A syndrome characterized by corneal opacity, nystagmus, flexion contracture of the elbows, growth failure, and mental retardation, J. Pediat. 69:624, 1966.
103. Arey, L. B.: *Developmental Anatomy* (Philadelphia: W. B. Saunders Company, 1965).
104. Weber, W. W., Manunes, P., Day, R., and Miller, P.: Trisomy 17-18(E): Studies in long-term survival with report of two autopsied cases, Pediatrics 34:533, 1964.
105. Huggert, A.: The trisomy 18 syndrome. A report of three cases in the same family, Acta ophth. 44:186, 1966.
106. Warkany, J., Weinstein, E. D., Soukup, S. W., Rubinstein, J. H., and Curless, M. C.: Chromosome analysis in a children's hospital, Pediatrics 33:290 and 454, 1964.
107. Wilson, J. R., and DuBois, R. O.: Report of a fatal case of keratomalacia in an infant with postmortem examination, Am. J. Dis. Child. 26:431, 1923.
108. Farber, S., and Wolbach, S. B.: Intranuclear and cytoplasmic inclusions in salivary glands and other organs of infants, Am. J. Path. 8:123, 1932.
109. Møllenbach, C. J.: *Congenital Defects in the Internal Membranes of the Eye* (Copenhagen: Munksgaard, 1947).
110. Reed, T. E., and Falls, H. F.: A pedigree of aniridia with a discussion of germinal mosaicism in man, Am. J. Human Genet. 7:28, 1955.
111. Bachmann, K. D., Nover, A., and Kwa, S. D.: Über das angeborene Fehlen der Regenbogenhaut des Auges (Aniridie), Ztschr. Kinderh. 99:119, 1967.
112. Drenckhahn, F. O., and Behnke, H.: Die Variabilität der klinischen Ausprägung des Irisdefektes in zwei Familien mit erblicher Aniridie, Klin. Monatsbl. Augenh. 138: 545, 1961.
113. Miller, R. W., Fraumeni, J. F., and Manning, M. D.: Association of Wilms' tumor with aniridia, hemihypertrophy and other congenital malformations, New England J. Med. 270:922, 1964.
114. DiGeorge, A. M., and Harley, R. D.: The association of aniridia, Wilms' tumor, and genital abnormalities, Arch. Ophth. 75:796, 1966.
115. Fraumeni, J. F., Jr., and Glass, A. G.: Wilms' tumor and congenital aniridia, J.A.M.A. 206:825, 1968.
116. Bornstein, M. B.: Aniridie bilatérale avec polydactylie. Relations des anomalies oculaires du type colobomateux associées à des malformations squelettiques avec les formes atypiques du syndrome de Bardet-Biedl, J. Génét. Hum. 1:211, 1952.
117. Baker, A. B., and Adams, J. M.: Lipomatosis of central nervous system, Am. J. Cancer 34:214, 1938.
118. Passow, A.: Horner syndrom, Heterochromie und Status dysraphicus, ein Symptomen Komplex, Arch. Augenh. 107:1, 1933.
119. DiGeorge, A. M., Olmsted, R. W., and Harley, R. D.: Waardenburg's syndrome; a syndrome of heterochromia of the irides, lateral displacement of the medial canthi and lacrimal puncta, congenital deafness, and other characteristic associated defects, J. Pediat. 57:649, 1960.
120. Makley, T. A.: Heterochromic cyclitis in identical twins, Am. J. Ophth. 41:768, 1956.
121. Franceschetti, A., and Maeder, G.: Hémiatrophie faciale avec alopécie (syndrome de Romberg) associée à une cyclite hétérochromique (syndrome de Fuchs), J. Génét. Hum. 7:116, 1958.
122. Ross, L. J.: Arachnodactyly. Review of recent literature and report of a case with cleft palate, Am. J. Dis. Child. 78:417, 1949.
123. François, J., and Verriest, G.: Les effets malformatifs chez l'enfant des infections virales de la mère, Ann. ocul. 189:269, 1956.
124. Robinson, G. C., Kidrainian, D. A., and Roseborough, G. F.: Congenital Horner's syndrome and heterochromia iridum, Pediatrics 35:103, 1965.
125. Brushfield, T.: Mongolism, Brit. J. Child. Dis. 21:241, 1924.
126. Wallis, H. R. E.: The significance of Brushfield's spots in the diagnosis of mongolism in infancy, Arch. Dis. Childhood 26:495, 1951.
127. Lowe, R.: The eyes in mongolism, Brit. J. Ophth. 33:131, 1949.
128. Donaldson, D. D.: The significance of spotting of the iris in mongoloids, Arch. Ophth. 65:26, 1961.
129. Klein, B. A., and Tanner, G. S.: Congenital epithelial cyst of the iris stroma, Am. J. Ophth. 55:291, 1963.
130. Rieger, H.: Erbfragen in der Augenheilkunde, Arch. opht. 143:277, 1941.
131. Busch, G., Weiskopf, J., and Busch, K-T.: Dysgenesis mesodermalis et ectodermalis Rieger oder Rieger'sche Krankheit, Klin. Monatsbl, Augenh. 136:512, 1960.

132. Löhlein, H.: Zur Kenntniss der essentiellen fortschreitenden Iris Atrophie mit Lochbildung und Glaukom, Klin. Monatsbl. Augenh. 118:379, 1951.
133. Couvreur, J.: *Étude de la Toxoplasmose Congénitale* (Gien: Impr. Jeanne d'Arc, 1955).
134. Silver, H. K., and Dixon, M. S., Jr.: Congenital toxoplasmosis—Report of case with cataract, "atypical" vasopressin-sensitive diabetes insipidus and marked eosinophilia, A.M.A. Am. J. Dis. Child. 88:84, 1954.
135. Berryman, M. L.: L'anisocorie congénitale familiale, Dissertation, Geneva, 1953.
136. Strebel, J., and Steiger, O.: Korrelation der Vererbung von Augenleiden (Ectopia lentium cong., Ectopia pupillae, Myopie) und sog. nicht angeborenen Herzfehlern, Arch. Augenh. 78:208, 1915.
137. Franceschetti, A.: Ectopia lentis et pupillae congenita als recessives Erbleiden und ihre Manifestierung durch Konsanguinität, Klin. Monatsbl. Augenh. 78:351, 1927.
138. Straub, W., and Heberling, V.: Beitrag zur Symptomatologie und Klinik des Laurence-Moon-Bardet-Biedlschen Syndroms, Klin. Monatsbl. Augenh. 120:289, 1952.
139. François, J.: *Congenital Cataract* (Assen, The Netherlands: Royal Van Gorcum, 1963).
140. Meissner, M.: Augenärztliches aus dem Blindeninstitut, Ztschr. Augenh. 80:49, 1933.
141. Fraccaro, M., Morone, G., Manfredini, U., and Sanger, R.: X-linked cataract, Ann. Human Genet. 31:45, 1967.
142. Swan, C., Tostevin, A. L., Moore, B., Mayo, H., and Black, G. H. B.: Congenital defects in infants following infectious diseases during pregnancy, M. J. Australia 2: 201, 1943.
143. Marner, E.: A family with generations of hereditary cataract, Acta ophth. 27:538, 1949.
144. Wilson, W. A.: Congenital cataracts, Arch. Ophth. 67: 143, 1962.
145. McDonald, A. D.: Congenital cataract, Developmental Med. & Child Neurol. 8:301, 1966.
146. Johnson, J.: Cataracts in galactosemia, Am. J. Ophth. 36:1380, 1953.
147. Wilson, W. A., and Donnell, H. N.: Cataracts in galactosemia, Arch, Ophth. 60:215, 1958.
148. Lerman, S.: The lens in congenital galactosemia, Arch. Ophth. 61:88, 1959.
149. Bannon, S. L., Higginbottom, R. M., McConnell, J. M., and Kaan, H. W.: Development of galactose cataract in albino rat embryo, Arch. Ophth. 33:224, 1945.
150. Rhode, J., and Grom, E.: Un cas de mongolisme avec cataracte congénitale totale, J. Génét. Hum. 8:275, 1959.
151. Igersheimer, J., and Mautner, H.: About changes of the crystalline lens in mongoloids, Am. J. Ment. Deficiency 55:370, 1951.
152. Van der Scheer, W.: Cataracta lentis bei mongoloider Idiotie, Klin. Monatsbl. Augenh. 62:155, 1919.
153. Walsh, F. B.: *Clinical Neuro-Ophthalmology* (Baltimore: The Williams & Wilkins Company, 1957).
154. Gänsslen, M., Lambrecht, K., and Werner, M.: Erbbiologie und Erbpathologie des Kreislaufapparates, in Bauer, K. H., Hanhart, E., and Lange, J. (eds), *Handbuch der Erbbiologie des Menschen* (Berlin: Julius Springer, 1940).
155. McKusick, V. A., Weilbaecher, R. G., and Gragg, G. W.: Recessive inheritance of a congenital malformation syndrome, J.A.M.A. 204:113, 1968.
156. Swan, C.: Study of 3 infants dying from congenital defects following maternal rubella in early stages of pregnancy, J. Path. & Bact. 56:289, 1944.
157. Töndury, G.: Embryopathien, Vol. XI of *Pathologie und Klinik in Einzeldarstellungen* (Berlin: Springer-Verlag, 1962).
158. Gregg, N. M.: Congenital cataract following German measles in the mother, Tr. Ophth. Soc. Australia 3:35, 1941.
159. Christensen, L., Beeman, H. W., and Allen, A.: Cytomegalic inclusion disease, Arch. Ophth. 57:90, 1957.
160. Cole, H. N., Giffen, H. K., Simmons, J. T., and Stroud, G. M.: Congenital cataracts in sisters with congenital ectodermal dysplasia, J.A.M.A. 129:723, 1945.
161. Marshall, D.: Ectodermal dysplasia. Report of a kindred with ocular abnormalities and hearing defect, Am. J. Ophth. 45:143, 1958.
162. Rubenstein, R. A., and Eggleston, T. F.: Congenital cataracts associated with congenital ichthyosiform erythroderma, J. Pediat. Ophth. 2:53, 1965.
163. Gorlin, R. J., and Anderson, J. A.: The characteristic dentition of incontinentia pigmenti, J. Pediat. 57:78, 1960.
164. Schäfer, E.: Zur Lehre von den kongenitalen Dyskeratosen, Arch. Dermat. u. Syph. 148:425, 1925.
165. Leber, T.: Über Retinitis pigmentosa und angeborene Amaurose, Arch. opht. 15:1, 1869.
166. Alström, C. H., and Olson, O.: Heredo-retinopathia congenitalis monohybrida recessiva autosomalis, Hereditas 43:1, 1957.
167. Schappert-Kimmijser, J., Henkes, H. E., and van den Bosch, J.: Amaurosis congenita, Arch. Ophth. 61:211, 1959.
168. Sorsby, A., and Williams, C. E.: Retinal aplasia as a clinical entity, Brit. M. J. 1:293, 1960.
169. Sorsby, A., Klein, M., Gann, J. H., and Siggins, C.: Unusual retinal detachment, possibly sex-linked, Brit. J. Ophth. 35:1, 1951.
170. Mann, I., and MacRae, A.: Congenital vascular veil in the vitreous, Brit. J. Ophth. 22:1, 1938.
171. Gieser, E. P., and Falls, H. F.: Hereditary retinoschisis, Am. J. Ophth. 51:1193, 1961.
172. Elwyn, H.: *Diseases of the Retina* (Philadelphia: Blakiston Company, 1946).
173. Bell, J.: Retinitis Pigmentosa and Allied Diseases, in *Treasury of Human Inheritance*, Vol. 21 (London: Cambridge University Press, 1922).
174. Usher, C. H.: On a few hereditary eye affections, The Bowman Lecture, Tr. Ophth. Soc. U. Kingdom 55:164, 1935.
175. Weiner, R. L., and Falls, H. F.: Intermediate sex-linked retinitis pigmentosa, Arch. Ophth. 53:530, 1955.
176. Best, F.: Über eine hereditäre Makulaffektion, Ztschr. Augenh. 13:199, 1905.
177. Barkman, Y.: A clinical study of a central tapetoretinal degeneration, Acta ophth. 39:663, 1961.
178. Sorsby, A.: Ocular lesions in bony dystrophies, Tr. Ophth. Soc. U. Kingdom 55:499, 1935.
179. Gesell, A., and Blake, M.: Twinning and ocular pathology, with a report of bilateral macular coloboma in monozygotic twins, Arch. Ophth. 15:1050, 1936.
180. Cordes, F. C.: Optic atrophy in infancy, childhood, and adolescence, Am. J. Ophth. 35:1272, 1952.
181. Goldstein, L.: Radiogenic microcephaly: A survey of nineteen recorded cases with special reference to ophthalmic defects, Arch. Neurol. & Psychiat. 24:102, 1930.
182. Ford, F. R.: *Diseases of the Nervous System in Infancy, Childhood and Adolescence* (3d ed.; Springfield, Ill.: Charles C Thomas, Publisher, 1952).
183. Dresner, E., and Montgomery, D. A. D.: Primary optic atrophy in von Recklinghausen's disease, Quart. J. Med. 18:93, 1949.
184. Dodge, H. W., Jr., Love, J. G., Craig, W. M. K., Dockerty, M. B., Kearns, T. P., Holman, C. B., and Hayles, A. B.: Gliomas of the optic nerves, A.M.A. Arch. Neurol. & Psychiat. 79:607, 1958.
185. Davis, F. A.: Primary tumors of the optic nerve (a phenomenon of Recklinghausen's disease), Arch. Ophth. 23:735, 1940.
186. Hix, I. E., Jr., and Danielson, R. W.: Bilateral retinoblastoma in a premature infant, Am. J. Ophth. 35:1647, 1952.
187. Sovik, W. E.: Bilateral retinoblastomas in six siblings,

Am. J. Ophth. 35:1611, 1952.
188. Macklin, M. T.: A study of retinoblastoma in Ohio, Am. J. Human Genet. 12:1, 1960.
189. Vogel, F.: Über Genetik und Mutationsrate des Retinoblastoms (Glioma retinae), Ztschr. menschl. Vererb.-u. Konstitutionslehre 32:308, 1954.
190. Day, R. W., Wright, S. W., Koons, A., and Quigley, M.: XXX,21-trisomy and retinoblastoma, Lancet 2:154, 1963.
191. Birge, H. L.: Congenital cataracts; strabismus; congenital obstruction of the lacrimal canal; adolescent myopia and glasses; infantile retinoblastoma, Am. J. M. Sc. 245: 244, 1963.
192. Hine, M.: Spontaneous cure of retinal glioma, Tr. Ophth. Soc. U. Kingdom 57:173, 1937.
193. Kalfayan, B.: Inclusion disease of infancy, Arch. Path. 44:467, 1947.
194. Burns, R. P.: Cytomegalic inclusion disease uveitis, A.M.A. Arch. Ophth. 61:376, 1959.
195. Van der Hoeve, J.: Eye symptoms in phakomatoses, Doyle Memorial Lecture, Tr. Ophth. Soc. U. Kingdom 52:380, 1932.
196. François, J., and Deweer, J. P.: Sclérose tubéreuse cérébrale de Bourneville, Ophthalmologica 124:321, 1952.
197. Turpin, R., Saraux, H., Defranoux, A., Cruveiller, J., Bocquet, H., and Lecoq, F.: L'hémihypertrophie faciale neurofibromateuse avec buphtalmie; à propos d'une nouvelle observation, Ann. pédiat. 36:1921, 1960.
198. Hippel, von E.: Über eine sehr seltene Erkrankung der Netzhaut, Arch. opht. 59:83, 1904.
199. Lindau, A.: Zur Frage der Angiomatosis Retinae und ihrer Hirnkomplikationen, Acta ophth. 4:193, 1927.
200. Gilkes, M. J., and Strode, M.: Ocular anomalies in association with developmental limb abnormalities of drug origin, Lancet 1:1026, 1963.
201. Cullen, J. F.: Ocular defects in thalidomide babies, Brit. J. Ophth. 48:151, 1964.
202. Cant, J. S.: Minor ocular abnormalities associated with thalidomide, Lancet 1:1134, 1966.
203. Cullen, J. F.: Clinical anophthalmos in a ?thalidomide child, J. Pediat. Ophth. 3:10, 1966.
204. Feingold, M., Shiere, F., Fogels, H. R., and Donaldson, D.: Rieger's syndrome, Pediatrics 44:564, 1969.
205. Samuelson, G.: Hereditary ectodermal dysplasia, Acta paediat. scandinav. 59:94, 1970.
206. Hyams, S. W., and Jaffe, M.: Cerebral palsy and juvenile glaucoma in siblings, Developmental Med. & Child Neurol. 12:467, 1970.
207. Petri, H.: Körperliche Missbildungen und Syndromerkrankungen bei angeborenem Glaukom, Monatsschr. Kinderh. 114:327, 1966.
208. Ormond, A.: Notes on the ophthalmic condition of 42 mongolian imbeciles, Tr. Ophth. Soc. U. Kingdom 32:69, 1912.
209. Lele, K. P., Penrose, L. S., and Stallard, H. B.: Chromosome deletion in a case of retinoblastoma, Ann. Human Genet. 27:171, 1963.
210. Wilson, M. G., Melnyk, J., and Towner, J. W.: Retinoblastoma and deletion D (14) syndrome, J. M. Genetics 6:322, 1969.
211. Allerdice, P. W., Davis, J. G., Miller, O. J., Klinger, H. P., Warburton, D., Miller, D. A., Allen, F. H., Jr., Abrams, C. A. L., and McGilvray, E.: The 13q− deletion syndrome, Am. J. Human Genet. 21:499, 1969.

40

Some Syndromes Involving Ocular Defects

Oculoauriculovertebral Syndrome

(Goldenhar Syndrome; Mandibulofacial Dysostosis with Epibulbar Dermoids)

CHILDREN WITH THIS SYNDROME have many features of mandibulofacial dysostosis, but in some of them the facial features are unilateral. In addition, there are epibulbar dermoids, vertebral anomalies and sometimes hypoplastic bones of digit I.

The skull and the face may be unilaterally underdeveloped, with mandibular and molar hypoplasia and macrostomia. There are various ocular anomalies, epibulbar dermoids being the most common.[1] Such dermoids are located on the lower outer margin of the cornea and extend onto the conjunctiva bulbi. Coloboma of the iris or of the upper eyelid, microphthalmia,[2] microcornea and cataract have also been observed. There may be microtia, with or without occlusion of the external auditory canal, and deafness. Preauricular fistulas and appendages are the rule. The palate may be high or cleft and can be combined with cleft lip and palate, cleft tongue or uvula fissa. Micrognathia, malocclusion and dental anomalies often are present. In the vertebral column, block vertebrae and hemivertebrae occur, particularly in the cervical spine,[3] sometimes combined with occipitalization of the atlas. There also may be irregularities in the thoracic, lumbar and sacral spine. Goldenhar[1] emphasized the association of epibulbar dermoids and auricular appendages and fistulas. Unilateral mandibulofacial dysostosis with vertebral anomalies was stressed as a syndrome by Weyers and Thier.[4] Hypoplasia of the thumb has been observed.[5] In contrast to mandibulofacial dysostosis, dominant inheritance has not been recorded in Goldenhar syndrome.[1,5]

REFERENCES

1. Goldenhar, M.: Associations malformatives de l'oeil et de l'oreille, en particulier le syndrome dermoide épibulbaire-appendices auriculaires-fistula auris congenita et ses relations avec la dysostose mandibulo-faciale, J. Génét. Hum. 1:243, 1952.
2. Christiaens, L., Walbaum, R., Farriaux, J. P., and Fontaine, G.: À propos de deux cas de dysplasie oculo-auriculo-vertébrale, Pédiatrie 21:935, 1966.
3. Sugar, H. S.: An unusual example of the oculoauriculovertebral dysplasia syndrome of Goldenhar, J. Pediat. Ophth. 4:9, 1967.
4. Weyers, H., and Thier, C. J.: Malformations mandibulo-faciales et délimitation d'un "syndrome oculo-vertébral," J. Génét. Hum. 7:143, 1958.
5. Gorlin, R. J., and Pindborg, J. J.: *Syndromes of the Head and Neck* (New York: McGraw-Hill Book Company, Inc., 1964).
6. Pashayan, H., Pinsky, L., and Fraser, F. C.: Hemifacial microsomia: Oculo-auriculo-vertebral dysplasia. A patient with overlapping features, J. M. Genetics 7:185, 1970.

Oculodentodigital Dysplasia

MICROPHTHALMIA of moderate degree is included in a syndrome called by Gorlin *et al.*[1] "oculodentodigital dysplasia." One finds hypotelorism, reduced size of the palpebral fissures, reduced distance of the inner canthi and pupils, changes in iris structure and remnants of the pupillary membrane. Glaucoma may be present. The teeth, which have marked enamel hypoplasia, appear yellow because of exposure of the dentin. The osseous width of the mandible is increased, the nose thin, the alae are hypoplastic and the nostrils anteverted. Incurved little finger due to hypoplasia of its middle phalanx, syndactyly between digits IV and V and abduction deformities of fingers may occur. The 6 patients reviewed by Gorlin *et al.* showed no familial aggregation or parental consanguinity. In 1 patient, the chromosomal pattern was ascertained and found to be normal. Mental development may be normal.

REFERENCE

1. Gorlin, R. J., Meskin, L. H., and St. Geme, J. W.: Oculodentodigital dysplasia, J. Pediat. 63:69, 1963.

Oculocerebrorenal Syndrome
(Lowe Syndrome)

THIS DISEASE PICTURE is characterized by congenital cataract, hypotonia, metabolic acidosis, hyperaminoaciduria, proteinuria, growth retardation, rickets and mental retardation. The syndrome was described by Lowe *et al.*[1] in 1952 and, by 1968, Abbassi *et al.*[2] had collected 70 cases for comparison of its signs and its course. Reviews were written also by Hooft *et al.*,[3] Richards *et al.*[4] and others. The external appearance of these children is said to be characteristic, but few of the typical features are present at birth.[3] When the disease picture is developed, the children are blind, have cataracts and often glaucoma, large and cloudy corneae, increased intraocular pressure, nystagmus and hand movements characteristic of infantile blindness. They show failure to thrive and loss of fat, pallor, frontal bossing, hypotonia, hyporeflexia, overextensibility of joints, inattentiveness, hyperexcitability, high-pitched cry, repetitive movements and mental deficiency. Osteoporosis develops in all patients and rickets with fractures in some. Irregular thickening of the bones of the calvarium has been described. Intravenous pyelograms may be normal[4] but, in some cases, roentgenograms reveal marked nephrolithiasis.[3] Biochemical deviations are metabolic acidosis, proteinuria, aminoaciduria, decreased renal ammonia production and decreased ability to excrete hydrogen ions, which results in urinary bicarbonate wastage.[2]

It seems that all patients are male. In one report, 2 females were described. Although the disorder could theoretically occur in homozygous females,[4] this is extremely unlikely, since male patients do not reach reproductive age and cannot transmit the trait to their offspring. A certain resemblance because of oculocerebrorenal involvement with other syndromes may explain reports of occurrence in girls. Crome *et al.*[5] described a syndrome of congenital cataracts, renal tubular necrosis and encephalopathy in 2 sisters. Limitation to males, recurrence in sibships, relationship of affected individuals (outside the sibship) to maternal kins and apparent normality of parents are characteristic of the Lowe oculocerebrorenal syndrome. In some cases, ocular symptoms such as opacification of the lens in mothers and other female family members[2,4] suggested manifestation of the disorder in heterozygous females. But, occasionally, punctate lenticular lesions were also seen in fathers of patients, so that interpretation of these findings is difficult. Although X-linkage of the mutant gene is likely, final proof is not yet available.

Pathologic changes in the kidneys are variable, nonspecific and age-dependent. Patients in the early stages of the disease show no renal pathology. Later, tubular changes develop without glomerular involvement. Finally, fibrotic and hyalinized glomeruli embedded in scar tissue are found. Cerebral changes seem to be age-specific also. In some patients, no characteristic findings were obtained at dissection of the brain.[2] The eyes show cataracts and anomalies in the cornea, ciliary body, macula and ora serrata.[6]

It is of interest that the metabolic disturbances characteristic of Lowe syndrome are not present at birth although the eye changes are.[2,3] By the time the children are 6 months of age, metabolic acidosis and aminoaciduria with their clinical consequences set

Fig. 40-1.—Boy with Lowe syndrome. Cloudy corneae and cataracts were noticed at birth.

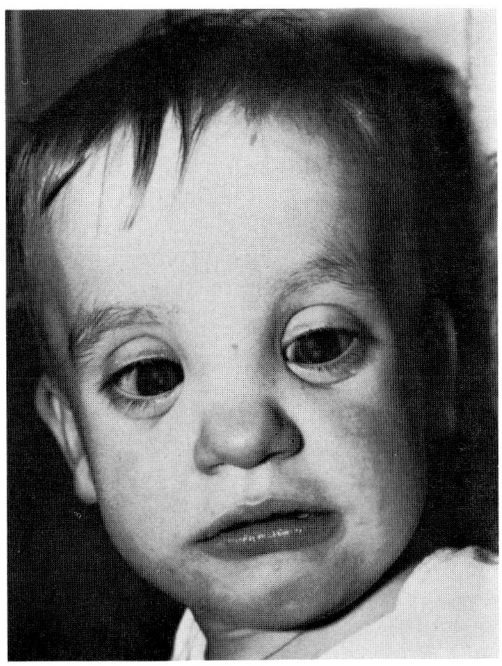

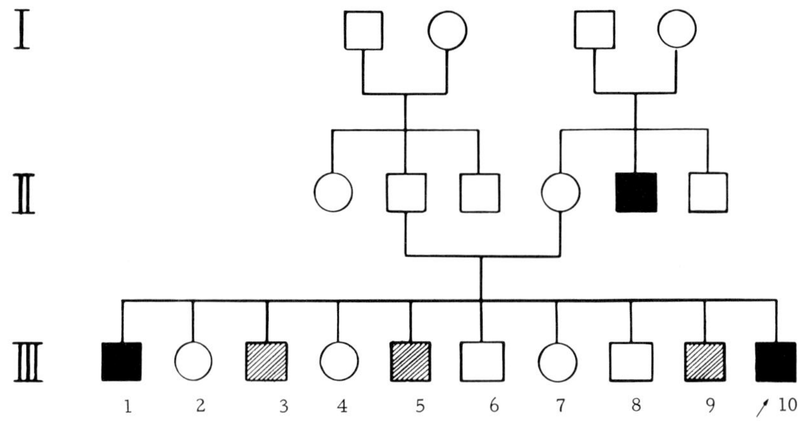

Fig. 40-2.—Pedigree of a kindred with multiple cases of oculocerebrorenal (Lowe) syndrome. *II₅*, at 6 months of age, boy had photophobia, cloudy corneae, cataracts and strabismus. The abdomen was large and development slow. III_1, born with glaucoma and cataracts. Did not develop physically or mentally. Had rickets and convulsions. Died at 3½ years of age. III_3, born after 6½ months' pregnancy. Lived several hours only. III_5, born after 7 months' pregnancy. Lived 30 hours. III_9, delivered by cesarean section after 7 months' pregnancy. Died on third day. III_{10}, delivered by cesarean section 2 weeks before term. Atonia and cataracts were noticed at birth. He did not develop physically or mentally. He had rickets and osteoporosis that responded to treatment. (Cincinnati Children's Hospital Chart No. 166672.)

in. Several years later, the metabolic abnormalities may subside and the patients can live on without intensive therapy.

REFERENCES

1. Lowe, C. U., Terrey, M., and MacLachlan, E. A.: Organic-aciduria, decreased renal ammonia production, hydrophthalmos, and mental retardation, A.M.A. Am. J. Dis. Child. 83:164, 1952.
2. Abbassi, V., Lowe, C. U., and Calcagno, P. L: Oculo-cerebro-renal syndrome. A review, Am. J. Dis. Child. 115: 145, 1968.
3. Hooft, C., Valcke, R., and Herpol, J: Étude clinique du syndrome de Lowe, Acta paediat. belg. 18:197, 1964.
4. Richards, W., Donnell, G. N., Wilson, W. A., Stowens, D., and Perry, T.: The oculo-cerebro-renal syndrome of Lowe, Am. J. Dis. Child. 109:185, 1965.
5. Crome, L., Duckett, S., and Franklin, A. W.: Congenital cataracts, renal tubular necrosis and encephalopathy in two sisters, Arch. Dis. Childhood 38:505, 1963.
6. François, J., and Hanssens, M.: Syndrome oculo-cerebro-rénale de Lowe: Examen histopathologique oculaire, Bull. Soc. belg. ophth. 35:412, 1963.

Craniofacial Dysostosis with Congenital Cataract, Hypotrichosis and Dwarfism

(Hallermann-Streiff Syndrome; François Syndrome; Dyscephalia Mandibulo-oculofacialis)

A PECULIAR AND RARE SYNDROME of dwarfism and multiple congenital anomalies affecting chiefly the head and face has been reported under a variety of names,[1-3] most cases being published in ophthalmologic journals. It seems that the first record on this disorder was made by Aubry[4] in 1893. By 1968, 63 cases had been published.[5] The facial appearance is so similar to that of progeria that a number of authors considered their cases "progeria with congenital cataract." The face has been described as "bird-like" because of a beak-shaped nose, small eyes and mandibular hypoplasia. Although the birth weight is normal or only moderately reduced,[13] there develops during childhood a proportionate dwarfism, with retarded bone age. In contrast to Seckel's bird-headed dwarfs, these patients do not have microcephaly but scaphocephaly or brachycephaly are mentioned often. The sutures and fontanelles remain wide open during infancy. Eyelashes and eyebrows often are absent and hypotrichosis of the anterior portion of the head or alopecia areata is present. Bilateral microphthalmia, microcornea and congenital cataract are characteristic findings. Antimongoloid inclination of the palpebral fissures, bluish sclerae, pupillary membrane, nystagmus, strabismus, retinal anomalies and other ocular defects have been described. Atrophy of the skin often is noted in the face. The mouth and the

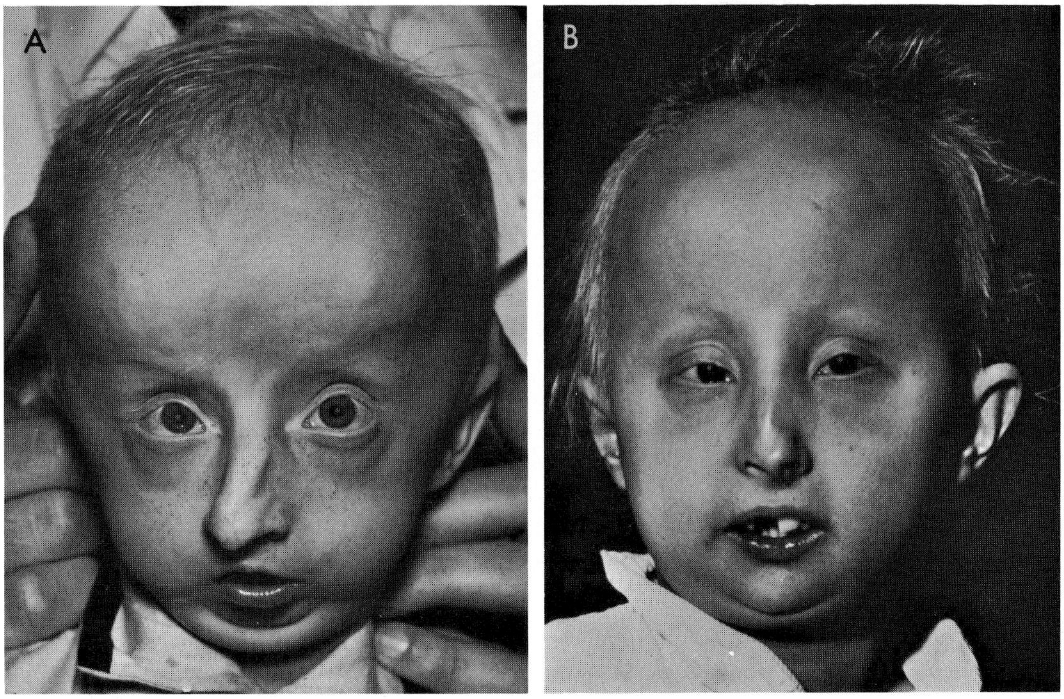

Fig. 40-3. – Hallermann-Streiff-François syndrome in a boy (**A**) and in a girl (**B**). (Courtesy of Dr. D. Hoefnagel, Hanover, N.H.)

tongue are small and the palate is high. Micrognathia and glossoptosis occur, as in the Pierre-Robin syndrome. The alveolar processes are hypoplastic and some teeth may be erupted at birth; others are never formed. Malocclusion is the rule. Anterior displacement of the temporomandibular joint occurs.[5] The external ears are low set but otherwise normal. The beak-shaped nose may have a deviating septum and be asymmetric.[6,7] A typical patient can be recognized at a glance. One must agree with Ravin and Hodge,[8] who believed that "La Niña," painted by Raphael Coronel, had this syndrome. Roentgenograms show reduced interorbital distance, small orbits and underdeveloped paranasal sinuses. The ascending ramus of the mandible appears underdeveloped or is absent. The temporomandibular joint may be undeveloped. The hypoplastic facial portion of the head contrasts with the relatively large cranial part. Muscular weakness, hyperextensible joints and winged scapulae are present in some patients.

Other anomalies mentioned are scoliosis, osteoporosis, syndactyly, double ureter, cryptorchidism or absent testes, speech defects and mental retardation, but these findings are not always present. Despite their handicaps, several of these patients have been encountered as adults living a rather normal life.[3,7] Good intelligence[9] and normal height[5,9] are achieved by some patients. In some patients, respiratory difficulties lead to early death. Parental consanguinity was present in two instances.[10,11] Familial occurrence has been reported[11] and concordance has been seen in male twins.[12] In several instances,[6,9,11] the karyotype was found to be normal, but deletion of the short arm of chromosome no. 4 or no. 5 has been asserted by Jalbert *et al.*[10]

REFERENCES

1. Hallermann, W.: Vogelgesicht und Cataracta congenita, Klin. Monatsbl. Augenh. 113:315, 1948.
2. Streiff, E. B.: Dysmorphie mandibulo-faciale (tête d'oiseau) et altérations oculaire, Ophthalmologica 120:79, 1950.
3. François, J.: A new syndrome: Dyscephalia with bird face and dental anomalies, nanism, hypotrichosis, cutaneous atrophy, microphthalmia, and congenital cataract, A.M.A. Arch. Ophth. 60:842, 1958.
4. Aubry, M.: Variété singulière d'alopecie congénitale, alopécie suturale, Ann. dermat. et syph. 4:899, 1893.
5. Caspersen, I., and Warburg, M.: Hallermann-Streiff syndrome, Acta ophth. 46:385, 1968.
6. Hoefnagel, D., and Benirschke, K.: Dyscephalia mandibulo-oculo-facialis, Arch. Dis. Childhood 40:57, 1965.
7. Falls, H. F., and Schull, W. J.: Hallermann-Streiff syndrome, A.M.A. Arch. Ophth. 63:409, 1960.
8. Ravin, J. G., and Hodge, G. P.: Hallermann-Streiff syndrome diagnosed from a painting, J. Pediat. Ophth. 5:124, 1968.
9. Walbaum, R., Woillez, M., François, P., and Mayolle, P.: Le syndrome de Hallermann-Streiff-François, Pédiatrie 23:787, 1968.
10. Jalbert, P., Gilbert, Y., Léopold, P., Mouriquand, C., and Beaudoing, A.: Syndrome d'Hallermann-Streiff-François.

À propos d'une nouvelle observation associée à une anomalie, Pédiatrie 23:703, 1968.
11. Sánchez, M. B.: Sindrome de Hallermann-Streiff-François a propósito de una presentación familiar, Bol. S. Vasco-Nav. Ped. 1:21, 1966.
12. Van Balen, A. T.: Dyscephaly with microphthalmos, cataract and hypoplasia of the mandible, Ophthalmologica 141:53, 1961.
13. Suzuki, Y., Fujii, T., and Fukuyama, Y.: Hallermann-Streiff syndrome, Developmental Med. & Child. Neurol. 12:496, 1970.

Congenital Cataract and Ataxia

(Marinesco-Sjögren Syndrome)

CONGENITAL or rapidly progressive infantile cataract, ataxia, mental retardation, sexual infantilism in females, dwarfism, hypotrichosis, lack of ossification of the distal phalanges of the fingers and hypocalcemia have been described as a syndrome sometimes occurring in siblings.[1] Similar cases collected in Sweden[2] showed an increased incidence of consanguinity among the phenotypically normal parents. By 1964,[3] approximately 40 cases had been recorded. Of 20 families reported, parental consanguinity was noted in 12. Norwood[3] described the condition in siblings. Both showed growth retardation at birth and remained below the third percentiles in height and weight. Postnatal development was slow, sitting, standing, walking and talking being delayed. Cataract, strabismus and nystagmus were noted in infancy. Walking with assistance was on a wide base and ataxic. Scalp hair was sparse, fine and without pigment and medulla. Outlook for life is good but physical and mental development remain retarded. The chromosomes appear normal.

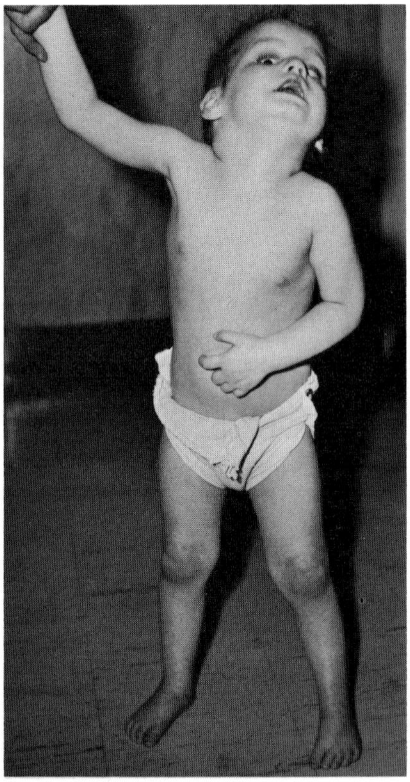

Fig. 40-4.—Girl with Marinesco-Sjögren syndrome. Her brother had the same disease.

REFERENCES

1. Marinesco, G., Draganesco, S., and Vasiliu, D.: Nouvelle maladie familiale, caractérisée par une cataracte congénitale et un arrêt du developpement somato-neuropsychique, Encéphale 26:97, 1931.
2. Sjögren, T.: Hereditary congenital spinocerebellar ataxia accompanied by congenital cataract and oligophrenia, Confinia neurol. 10:293, 1950.
3. Norwood, W. F., Jr.: The Marinesco-Sjögren syndrome, J. Pediat. 65:431, 1964.

Rothmund-Thomson Syndrome

(Poikiloderma Congenitale)

IN 1868, ROTHMUND[1] described a disease picture of "cataracts associated with peculiar skin degeneration." At first, he saw a 5-year-old boy who apparently had just developed a cataract in one eye. The boy also showed a cutis marmorata. Several weeks later, Rothmund saw two other children with the same symptoms from the same small valley of Vorarlberg in Austria. Their parents asserted that there were several blind children with similar "rashes" in the vicinity. In that valley there were three villages with a total of 1,500 inhabitants, and in every village there was a family with several children with cataract and skin lesions. Parents and unaffected children had neither general nor local symptoms; only one grandmother was said to have been partly affected.

Rothmund examined 8 children with the cutaneous symptoms. The skin of the patients was normal during the first half year after birth but then some red spots appeared on the cheeks and the skin became mottled. A network of fine red lines enclosing patches of healthy skin made up the initial lesion. Subsequently, the lines became wider and the enclosed healthy areas smaller. The rash spread to the ears and to the extremities. As a rule, the lesions reached their full extent by the end of the first year. With time, the red lines became yellow and finally they were converted into scars. The unaffected skin was soft, velvety and transparent. Perspiration was most noticeable on the scalp. Lanugo hair was not visible, scalp hair was blond and copious. There were no hairs on the red lines, which were reminiscent of striae gravidarum. The nails were well formed. The extensor surfaces of the extremities were more affected than the flexor sides. Only the palms and cubital fossae remained free. The lower extremities were similarly involved. The red lines changed color with the outside temperature. Except for desquamation, there were no further changes of the affected skin. Rothmund thought that the disease process was an inflammatory one ending in fatty degeneration and scar formation without purulence. He stated that heredity played a definite role in the disorder and that consanguinity of the parents was of importance.

Cataracts appeared rapidly between the fourth and sixth years of life, i.e., much later than the skin lesions. They began as radial, triangular densities that involved the entire lens within a few days. The lesions resembled cataracts with "cortical onset." Rothmund then described in detail the families, the patients and the operations that were successful, with one exception. His detailed description makes good reading now, more than 100 years after its publication.

In 1936, M. Sidney Thomson[2] recorded "poikiloderma congenitale," a disorder resembling the skin lesions described by Rothmund 68 years earlier. Two of the cases had been recorded in 1923 as "An Hitherto Undescribed Familial Disease" and were followed until one of the patients was 14 years of age. In the first of these cases, a girl, there were telangiectatic networks enclosing white patches as in Rothmund's patients, but onset was on the buttocks and swelling and cyanosis of the hands were disturbing symptoms. The condition resembled "erythema ab igne" but, when the acute symptoms subsided, the outcome of the lesions was similar to that described by Rothmund. On the limbs, the dilated vessels had disappeared and were replaced by pigmentations at age 14 years. The hair was normal except for thinness of the eyebrows and sparsity of the lashes. The teeth, nails and skeleton were normal and the eyes apparently were in no way affected. The facies appeared triangular. Hyperkeratosis, slight edema, irregular acanthosis, loss of papillae, confusion of the epidermo-dermal boundary and hyperpigmentation among the basal cells and the adjacent spinous cells were noticed on microscopic examination. Case 2, the sister of this patient, developed lesions on the face and buttocks when 3½ months of age. The exanthema spread rapidly and terminated in a skin condition resembling that of the first patient. But the younger sister was not well developed otherwise. She had been "small and puny from birth." The membrane bones of the skull were large in proportion to the cartilage bones so that the child looked hydrocephalic, but at necropsy, a year later, no hydrocephaly was noticed. The metacarpals and phalanges of the thumbs were absent and ulnae and radii were rudimentary. In a third girl, 6 years of age, Thomson recorded sudden loss of hair of the scalp, eyebrows and lashes as outstanding symptoms, but there were also the well-developed symptoms of poikiloderma that had begun in infancy.

Fig. 40-5.—One of the children seen by Rothmund in 1868. (From A. Rothmund.[1])

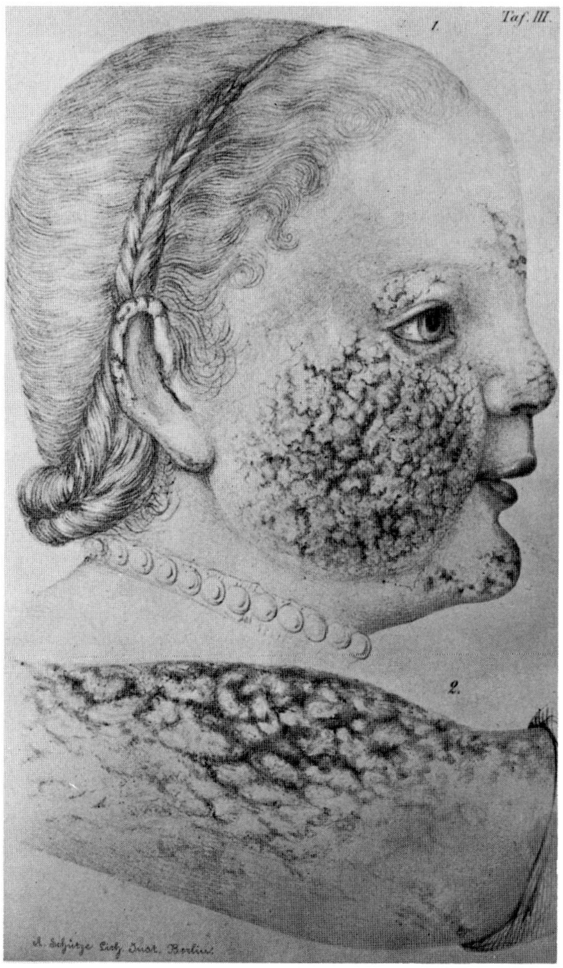

Nails and teeth were normal, the face was triangular, and there was "microcephaly" and microphthalmia, high myopia and partial optic atrophy. Cataract was not mentioned and mentality was normal. Thomson cited some patients with similar skin lesions described before and in one of them there had been cataracts,[3] as in some of Rothmund's patients. Thomson apparently was not aware of Rothmund's publication, which is not surprising, since the two physicians were separated by barriers of language and specialization. Furthermore, the syndromes were not identical, since Thomson's patients did not show cataracts. Taylor[4] suggested the term "Rothmund-Thomson syndrome," since the name of Rothmund had priority, but Thomson's poikiloderma congenitale had become established in the literature. Time will tell whether these are good reasons to create a syndrome. But neither the framework established by Rothmund nor that by Thomson encompasses all the symptoms occurring with poikiloderma congenitale. It may be noted, by the way, that the poikiloderma seen in these cases probably is never congenital but rather dependent on postnatal factors such as exposure to light and sunshine. In rare instances,[5,6] red spots were noticed immediately after birth. Unfortunately, birth weight and/or gestation time seldom are recorded. Thomson mentioned that his second patient was small and puny from birth. Some patients were said to have been prematures,[7] weighing 2,170 Gm.[8] or 1,814 Gm.[5] Since gestation time was not mentioned in these cases and low birth weight term children usually were called "prematures" in the past, it is possible that some of these children suffered intrauterine growth retardation. Two patients reported by Habermann and Fleck[9] weighed under 2,400 Gm., one of them 2,300 Gm. at term. Case 2 of Silver[10] weighed 1,430 Gm. after 37 weeks' gestation, thus showing marked prenatal growth retardation; his brother, who also was affected, weighed 1,750 Gm. after 33 weeks' gestation. The patient of Koch *et al.*[11] had definite intrauterine growth retardation. Thus, there are signs of prenatal onset of the syndrome and we can expect more information on this point in the future.

Postnatally, shortness of stature was present in 54% of the cases reviewed by Taylor.[4] General symptoms of abnormal growth and reproduction were not mentioned by Rothmund, but Bloch and Stauffer[7] stressed endocrine deficiencies of their patients and believed that the skin manifestations were of endocrine origin. Subsequently, hypogonadism, cryptorchidism and amenorrhea were emphasized by some observers,[12-14] but there is no proof that the cutaneous manifestations are the result of endocrine disturbances. Re-examination of Rothmund's patients after 67 years by Seefelder[14] revealed infertility and small stature in some cases. But one woman who had the skin anomaly without cataracts had had 13 children. In addition to the poikiloderma, cutaneous appendages often are involved. Sparseness of hair has been mentioned and complete alopecia was added in some cases. Dystrophic nails—not present in Rothmund's cases—were described in about one-fourth of subsequent reports.[4] Carcinomas of the skin developed in some of the adult patients.[12,15] There is evidence that some of the skin manifestations are brought out by sunlight, and sensitivity to sunlight was definite in some of the patients. Transitional forms to epidermolysis bullosa[6] and to ectodermal dysplasia[16] occur. A transitional case of late Rothmund or early Werner syndrome was described by Engleson and Widell[17] in a girl 9 years of age. Werner syndrome usually has its onset in the third or fourth decade, with graying of hair, sclero-poikiloderma,[13] cataract formation, hypogonadism and speech difficulties.[18] Microdontia, delayed dentition[5] and dental decay have been observed in patients with Rothmund-Thomson syndrome.

Among the ocular symptoms, juvenile cataract is mentioned in about half the cases. Other ocular symptoms include microphthalmia, myopia and partial optic atrophy.[2,19]

Skeletal defects were noted in Thomson's Case 2, which probably had pseudohydrocephaly (p. 138) and, in addition, rudimentary forearm bones and absence of the thumbs. Taylor[4] found skeletal defects mentioned in 39% of the cases on record. Frontal bossing, lacunar skull,[9] saddling of the nose, reduction of fingers,[5] bowing of long bones[4,8,9] and cystic rarefactions in metaphyseal and epiphyseal portions of the long or pelvic bones[4,5,9] have been reported. Hemidystrophy has been observed.[5]

Familial occurrence and parental consanguinity have been recognized since Rothmund's report. Seefelder[14] clarified some of the interrelationships of these kindreds and added another affected family to the literature. There is general agreement that the disorder is recessively inherited. Concordance in probably monozygotic twins has been reported by Feldreich.[19] There is a single observation of "congenital" poikiloderma in a mother and her newborn son.[20] In one instance,[11] the patient had remarkable cytogenetic changes, namely a 48 chromosome complement with trisomies D and G. His mother had mosaicism in which cells with trisomy D prevailed, sometimes combined with defect of an X chromosome.

REFERENCES

1. Rothmund, A.: Über Cataracten in Verbindung mit einer eigenthümlichen Hautdegeneration, von Graefes Arch. Ophth. 14:159, 1868.
2. Thomson, M. S.: Poikiloderma congenitale, Brit. J. Dermat. 48:221, 1936.
3. Lutz, W.: Poikiloderma atrophicans, Schweiz. med. Wchnschr. 58:1118, 1928.
4. Taylor, W. B.: Rothmund's syndrome-Thomson's syndrome; congenital poikiloderma with or without juvenile cataracts. A review of the literature, report of a case, and discussion of the relationship of the two syndromes, A.M.A. Arch. Dermat. 75:236, 1957.
5. Hailey, H., Hailey, H., and Clemens, H.: Poikiloderma congenitale: Report of a case in America, Arch. Dermat. u. Syph. 44:345, 1941.

6. Kindler, T.: Congenital poikiloderma with traumatic bulla formation and progressive cutaneous atrophy, Brit. J. Dermat. 66:104, 1954.
7. Bloch, B., and Stauffer, H.: Skin diseases of endocrine origin (dyshormonal dermatoses): Poikiloderma-like changes in connection with underdevelopment of the sexual glands and dystrophia adiposogenitalis, Arch. Dermat. u. Syph. 19:22, 1929.
8. Jäckli, W.: Ein Fall von Infantiler Poikilodermie (Atrophodermia reticularis cum incontinentia pigmenti) kombiniert mit Alopecie, Mikrodontie und frühzeitiger Cataracta complicata, Monatsschr. Kinderh. 78:73, 1939.
9. Habermann, P., and Fleck, M.: Über das Rothmund-Syndrom, Ztschr. Kinderh. 77:306, 1955.
10. Silver, H. K.: Rothmund-Thomson syndrome: An oculocutaneous disorder, Am. J. Dis. Child. 111:182, 1966.
11. Koch, F., Santamouris, C., and Ulbrich, F.: D + G Trisomie bei einem Patienten mit Rothmund-Syndrom, Ztschr. Kinderh. 99:1, 1967.
12. Rook, A., and Whimster, I.: Congenital cutaneous dystrophy (Thomson's type), Brit. J. Dermat. 61:197, 1949.
13. Franceschetti, A.: Les dysplasies ectodermiques et les syndromes héréditaires apparantes, Dermatologica 106: 145, 1953.
14. Seefelder, R.: Über familiäres Auftreten von Katarakt und Poikilodermie (Poikilodermia vascularis atrophicans Jakobi), Ztschr. Augenh. 86:81, 1935.
15. Sexton, G. B.: Thomson's syndrome (poikiloderma congenitale), Canad. M.A.J. 70:662, 1954.
16. Cole, H. N., Giffen, H. K., Simmons, J. T., and Stroud, G., III: Congenital cataracts in sisters with congenital ectodermal dysplasia, J.A.M.A. 129:723, 1945.
17. Engleson, G., and Widell, S.: Rothmund-Werner's disease, Acta dermat.-venereol. 34:353, 1954.
18. Werner, C. W. O.: Über Katarakt in Verbindung mit Sklerodermie, Thesis, Schmidt and Klauning, Kiel, 1904.
19. Feldreich, H.: Poikiloderma congenitale in twins, Acta dermat.-venereol. 35:86, 1955.
20. Hallman, N., and Patiala, R.: Congenital poikiloderma atrophicans vasculare in mother and her son, Acta dermat.-venereol. 31:401, 1951.

Marchesani Syndrome, Brachydactyly and Congenital Spherical Lens (Microphakia)

IN 1939, MARCHESANI[1] described a syndrome of brachydactyly, spherophakia and glaucoma. The patients are of short stature, heavyset, severely myopic because of spherophakia and microphakia and often mentally retarded. Ectopia lentis and glaucoma occur in some of the patients. The fingers are short and stubby and the *atd* angles markedly increased.[2] In one family of French descent, 4 of 12 siblings had the full syndrome. In another family observed in the United States, the patients were of Italian descent. In this case, 1 of 7 siblings was affected. In the first family, the parents were related. An autosomal recessive mode of inheritance seems likely for most of the cases. Heterozygous carriers may be of short stature and have *atd* angles intermediate between those of patients with the fully developed syndrome and those of normals.[3] Families have been described in which the syndrome, or certain parts of it, are transmitted through several generations. It is possible that heterozygotes have short stature and short fingers, whereas homozygotes have spherophakia and marked growth retardation.[4] In 1958, Zabriskie and Reisman[5] reviewed 14 published cases and reported 2 brothers with the disorder.

REFERENCES

1. Marchesani, O.: Brachydaktylie und angeborene Kugellinse als Systemarkrankung, Klin. Monatsbl. Augenh. 103:392, 1939.
2. Rosenthal, J. W., and Kloepfer, H. W.: The spherophakia-brachymorphia syndrome, Am. J. Ophth. 55:28, 1956.
3. Kloepfer, H. W., and Rosenthal, J. W.: Possible genetic carriers in the spherophakia-brachymorphia syndrome, Am. J. Human Genet. 7:398, 1955.
4. Waardenburg, P. J., Franceschetti, A., and Klein, D.: *Genetics and Ophthalmology* (Springfield, Ill.: Charles C Thomas, Publisher, 1961).
5. Zabriskie, J., and Reisman, M.: Marchesani syndrome, J. Pediat. 52:158, 1958.

Waardenburg Syndrome

WAARDENBURG[1] described a syndrome of lateral displacement of the medial canthi (dystopia canthi medialis lateroversa), prominent broad root of the nose, growing together of the eyebrows with hypertrichosis of their medial portion (hyperplasia supercilii medialis), white forelock as a form of partial albinism, partial or total heterochromia iridis and deaf-mutism or incomplete congenital deafness. It seemed that dystopia canthi was the most frequent manifestation of the syndrome, whereas deaf-mutism, the most serious feature, was the least frequent. In contrast to hypertelorism, dystopia canthi shows laterad displacement of the lacrimal points, reduced visibility of the nasal portion of the sclera, shortening of the palpebral fissures and increased distance between the pupils and outer canthi. The lacrimal points are situated in front of (and below) the corneae. Waardenburg believed the trait to be inherited as an autosomal dominant characteristic. The syndrome, which occurs in both sexes, showed variable expressivity, the various symptoms having differing penetrance. With dystopia canthi as the leading manifestation, prominent nasal root, overgrowth of medial eyebrows, heterochromia iridis, deaf-mutism and partial albinism seemed to follow, with the penetrance of symptoms varying in different families. Most of the component anomalies of the syndrome had been recognized as separate hereditary traits before. Waardenburg estimated that the frequency of the syndrome in the Dutch population was 1 per 42,000. Among 1,050 patients in Dutch institutions for the deaf, there were 13 with the eye anomaly. In Canada, Partington[2] found in an institution for the deaf 1 case of Waardenburg syndrome among 343 congenitally deaf children and Ahrendts[9] in Germany ascertained 5 cases among 176 deaf pupils.

Of course, the syndrome had been reported before 1951[3] and other cases have been published since. McKenzie[4] described a pedigree with affected members in three generations and considered the condition "the first arch syndrome"; but many patients have pigmentary changes outside the facial area and show that the anomaly is not limited to the first visceral arch and its blood vessels. Partington[2] observed an English family with the syndrome in which only the propositus was severely affected, whereas her ancestors had rather harmless variations of pigmentation and of facial features. DiGeorge *et al.*[5] added 11 probands to the literature, including Negro patients, investigated their families and analyzed the individual symptoms. They recognized additional manifestations among their patients such as premature graying of the hair of the scalp and of the medial portions of the eyebrows, depigmentation of the skin and pigmentary changes of the fundi and estimated that 2% of congenital deafness in the United States may result from this disorder. The inner canthal distances, which vary in normal children under 10 years between 22 and 30 mm., were increased to 32–45 mm. Thorkilgaard[6] reported a Danish family in which 12 of 73 members through five generations had the syndrome. He believed that hypoplasia of the iris is of primary importance and heterochromia of secondary importance in the definition of the syndrome. In the same year, Aasved[7] described a kindred from Norway, and Rugel and Keates[8] one from America with four and six generations affected, respectively. Additional contributions came from Germany[9] and France.[10] Chromosome analyses resulted in normal findings.[2,8,10]

Fisch[11] made histologic studies of the inner ear and noted absence of the organ of Corti and of the greater part of the ganglion cells of the spiral ganglion, whereas the basilar membrane and the bony cochlea were normal. He described a pedigree in which early graying, deafness and heterochromia iridis occurred without anomalies of the eyelids and spoke of the "early graying" syndrome. An observation by Feingold *et al.*[12] was of interest because it showed that a white forelock present at birth can disappear by age 6 weeks and that heterochromia iridis appeared at age 3 months. The entire facial skeleton can be involved, with cleft lip and palate[13] or abnormalities of the jaws with malocclusion.[9]

REFERENCES

1. Waardenburg, P. J.: A new syndrome combining developmental anomalies of the eyelids, eyebrows and nose root with pigmentary defects of the iris and head hair and with congenital deafness, Am. J. Human Genet. 3:195, 1951.
2. Partington, M. W.: Waardenburg's syndrome and heterochromia iridum in a deaf school population, Canad. M.A.J. 90:1008, 1964.
3. Wilbrandt, H. R., and Ammann, F.: Nouvelle observation de la forme grave du syndrome de Klein-Waardenburg, Arch. Klaus Stift. Vererbungsforsch. 39:80, 1964.
4. McKenzie, J.: The first arch syndrome, Arch. Dis. Childhood 73:477, 1958.
5. DiGeorge, A. M., Olmsted, R. W., and Harley, R. D.: Waardenburg's syndrome; a syndrome of heterochromia of the irides, lateral displacement of the medial canthi and lacrimal puncta, congenital deafness, and other characteristic associated defects, J. Pediat. 57:649, 1960.
6. Thorkilgaard, O.: Waardenburg's syndrome in father and daughter, Acta ophth. 40:590, 1962.
7. Aasved, H.: Waardenburg's syndrome, Acta ophth. 40: 622, 1962.
8. Rugel, S. J., and Keates, E. U.: Waardenburg's syndrome in six generations of one family, Am. J. Dis. Child. 109: 579, 1965.
9. Ahrendts, H.: Das Waardenburg-Syndrom, dargestellt an fünf Familien, Ztschr. Kinderh. 93:295, 1965.
10. Boniface, L., and Fontaine, G.: Le syndrome de Waardenburg (à propos de 5 observations), Ann. pédiat. 42:788, 1966.
11. Fisch, L.: Deafness as part of an hereditary syndrome, J. Laryng. & Otol. 73:355, 1959.
12. Feingold, M., Robinson, M. J., and Gellis, S.: Waardenburg's syndrome during the first year of life, J. Pediat. 71: 874, 1967.
13. Giacoia, J. P., and Klein, S. W.: Waardenburg's syndrome with bilateral cleft lip, Am. J. Dis. Child. 117:344, 1969.

Möbius Syndrome
(Nuclear Agenesis; Congenital Facial Diplegia)

IT SEEMS THAT the first description of congenital facial diplegia was given by von Graefe[1] in 1880, but Möbius in 1888 and 1892[2] added to the subject considerably and directed attention to nuclear aplasia. Reviews on the subject were written by Henderson[3] in 1939, by Danis[4] in 1945 and by Gorlin and Pindborg[5] and Dalloz and Nocton[6] in 1964.

Möbius expressed the belief that the anomaly was due to degeneration of the nuclei of the sixth and seventh cranial nerves. In 1900, Huebner[7] demonstrated in a necropsy of a 2-year-old child complete absence of the nucleus of the abducens and diminished number of cells of that of the facialis. Pathologic findings were summarized by Henderson[3] and by Dalloz and Nocton.[6] More recently, it has been said that the syndrome is due primarily to a mesodermal defect because there is complete absence of muscles in the involved areas and there are associated musculoskeletal anomalies of the extremities in many affected children. The situation is similar to that of arthrogryposis, in which anterior horn cells as well as muscles and joints are defective (p. 1014) and, as in arthrogryposis, it will remain difficult to decide where the primary anomaly is located. The fact that Möbius syndrome includes associated malformations of different body systems, including Klippel-Feil syndrome,[8] points to early general disturbances of development. Arthrogryposis and Möbius syndrome can occur together[9] and may be closely related in some cases.

Facial diplegia usually is noticed soon after birth and is manifested by difficulties in sucking and inability to close the eyes. Later, it is noted that the child does not smile or move its facial muscles on crying. Bilateral facial palsy results in a mask-like facies. Paralysis of the sixth cranial nerve with inability to abduct the eyes is a frequently associated anomaly. The oculomotor and trigeminal nerves sometimes are involved and strabismus is not rare. The hypoglossal nerve is affected in about one-fourth of the cases, resulting in palsy and atrophy of the tongue.[10] Movement of the palate and speech sometimes are impaired and laryngeal stridor causes early difficulties.[8] It is understandable that the mask-like face, drooling and inability to follow subjects arouse suspicion of mental retardation. In the majority of cases, intelligence is normal but in approximately 10% there is mental retardation.[10] Because of the presence of epicanthic folds, hypertelorism and the habit of keeping the mouth open, an erroneous diagnosis of mongolism may be made.[11] Among associated malformations, clubfoot, occurring in about one-third of the cases, is most frequent. Other important anomalies are epicanthic folds, hypertelorism, ear deformities, micrognathia, bifid uvula, palatal palsy, Klippel-Feil syndrome,[8] absence of the sternal head of the pectoralis major, rib defects, brachial muscle defects, perodactyly, syndactyly and brachydactyly.[10,12] Intrauterine growth retardation has been recognized in some of the cases.[6]

Most cases are sporadic; others are clearly hereditary.[13-17] Some of the latter suggest dominant, others recessive inheritance.[5,16,17] It is likely that different etiologic factors can result in congenital facial diplegia.

REFERENCES

1. von Graefe, A.: In von Graefe, A., and Saemisch, T. (eds.), *Handbuch der gesammten Augenheilkunde* (Leipzig: W. Engelmann, 1880), Vol. 6.
2. Möbius, P. J.: Über infantilen Kernschwund, München. med. Wchnschr. 39:17, 41 and 55, 1892.
3. Henderson, J. L.: The congenital facial diplegia syndrome, Brain 62:381, 1939.
4. Danis, P.: Les paralysies oculo-faciales congénitales, Ophthalmologica 110:113, 1945.
5. Gorlin, R. J., and Pindborg, J. J.: *Syndromes of the Head and Neck* (New York: McGraw-Hill Book Company, Inc., 1964).
6. Dalloz, J. C., and Nocton, F.: Le syndrome de Moebius, Arch. franç pédiat. 21:1025, 1964.
7. Huebner, O.: Über angeborenen Kernmangel (infantiler Kernschwund, Moebius), Charité-Ann. 25:211, 1900.
8. Evans, P. R.: Nuclear agenesis. Moebius' syndrome, Arch. Dis. Childhood 30:237, 1955.
9. Sprofkin, B. E., and Hillman, J. W.: Moebius syndrome; congenital oculofacial paralysis, Neurology 6:50, 1956.

Fig. 40-6. – Möbius syndrome in a 1-year-old boy who also had bilateral clubfoot. The sixth, seventh and twelfth nerves were involved. Family history was negative.

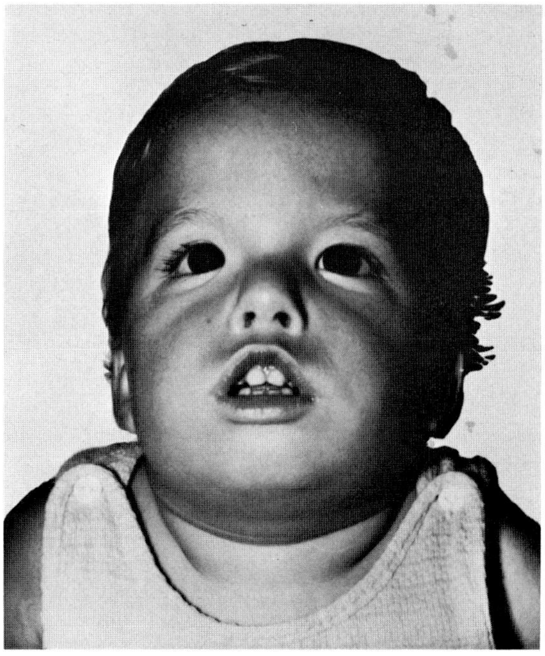

10. Hellström, B.: Congenital facial diplegia, Acta paediat. 37:464, 1949.
11. Nisenson, A.: Masklike facies with associated congenital anomalies, J. Pediat. 46:255, 1955.
12. Richards, R. N.: The Moebius syndrome, J. Bone & Joint Surg. 35-A:437, 1953.
13. Van der Weil, H. J.: Hereditary congenital facial paralysis, Acta Genet. 7:348, 1957.
14. Fortanier, A. H., and Speijer, N.: Eine Erblichkeitsforschung bei einer Familie mit angeborenen Beweglichkeits Störungen der Hirnnerven, Genetica 17:471. 1935.
15. Hicks, A. M.: Congenital paralysis of lateral rotators of eyes with paralysis of muscles of face, Arch. Ophth. 30: 38, 1943.
16. Cadwalader, W. R.: A clinical report of two cases of agenesis (congenital paralysis) of the cranial nerves, Am. J. M. Sc. 163:744, 1922.
17. Harrison, M., and Parker, N.: Congenital facial diplegia, M. J. Australia 1:650, 1960.

Cockayne Syndrome

(Mental Retardation, Dwarfism, Retinal Pigmentation and Deafness)

Cockayne[1] described a syndrome of dwarfism with retinal atrophy and deafness in 2 siblings who apparently had had a normal infancy. Growth retardation was noticed in the second year, with kyphosis and ankylosis; the extremities were long and the hands and feet large. The children had an old appearance, because of lack of subcutaneous fat of the face, and sunken eyes. The skin was sensitive to sunlight and there was retinal degeneration, with pigmentation and optic atrophy. Cataract, partial deafness, thickening of the skull bones and mental retardation developed.[2] Neill and Dingwall[3] saw 2 brothers with similar symptoms who showed, in addition, coarse tremor, hepatosplenomegaly, arteriosclerosis and intracranial calcifications. They compared the syndrome with progeria. Macdonald *et al.*[4] reported 3 siblings affected in a family of 5 children. Lack of facial fat, scarred and pigmented skin in areas exposed to the sun, sunken eyes, carious teeth and an unsteady gait gave a wizened and cachetic appearance. The elbow and knee joints were semiflexed, the posture was stooped, the limbs were long and the hands and feet large. Roentgenograms showed shortened metacarpals and ivory density of some epiphyses of the terminal phalanges. The vertebral bodies were flattened and biconvex and the skull bones thickened. The fundi were characterized by speckled pigmentation of the retina, optic atrophy and extremely narrow vessels.

The syndrome has a superficial resemblance to progeria, but familial incidence, mental retardation, skin sensitivity to sunlight and retinal pigmentation are quite distinctive features. Cockayne syndrome is thought to be inherited as a recessive trait. Absence of ocular findings has been reported.[5]

REFERENCES

1. Cockayne, E. A.: Dwarfism with retinal atrophy and deafness, Arch. Dis. Childhood 11:1, 1936.
2. Cockayne, E. A.: Case reports: Dwarfism with retinal atrophy and deafness, Arch. Dis. Childhood 21:52, 1946.
3. Neill, C. A., and Dingwall, M. M.: A syndrome resembling progeria; a review of two cases, Arch. Dis. Childhood 25: 213, 1950.
4. Macdonald, W. B., Fitch, K. D., and Lewis, I. C.: Cockayne's syndrome. An heredofamilial disorder of growth and development, Pediatrics 25:997, 1960.
5. Tympner, K. D., Eichin, F., and Fendel, H.: Cockayne's syndrome, Ztschr. Kinderh. 104:298, 1968.

Pseudoglioma with Mental Retardation

(Norrie Disease)

Congenital pseudoglioma combined with mental deficiency has been described as an X-linked recessive hereditary trait. At birth, vascular proliferating tissue behind the lens or pseudogliomatous tumor masses may be observed in male infants. Cataract and iris atrophy can be congenital or develop after birth. Severe progressive mental retardation has been described in brothers and one of their maternal uncles.[1] In other instances of pseudoglioma of this type, the mental retardation can be mild or mental development can be normal.[2] The congenital blindness is due to a malformation of the retina, which lacks rods, cones and ganglion cells. Persistence of the primary vitreous, cataract and elongation of the ciliary bodies have been seen in histologic sections. Necropsy of the brain of a blind and severely retarded boy showed scarce myelinated nerve fibers in the visual pathways and abnormal stratification of the cortex.[2]

REFERENCES

1. Forssman, H.: Mental deficiency and pseudoglioma, a syndrome inherited as an X-linked recessive, Am. J. Ment. Deficiency 64:984, 1960.
2. Warburg, M.: Norrie's disease, J. Ment. Defic. Res. 12:247, 1968.

PART VI

Malformations of the Ear

Aural Defects

Anotia

COMPLETE ABSENCE of the auricle is extremely rare. It must be distinguished from microtia, in which vestiges of the external ear are present. In 1948, Ruzic[1] published the "seventh case" of complete anotia and re-examined the cases previously recorded. In contrast to microtia, the anomaly usually was unilateral and sporadic. In addition, the middle ear always – and the inner ear sometimes – seemed included in the pathologic process. Externally, the skin of the cheek passes smoothly over the aural area without definite elevation or depression. The malformation may be associated with congenital facial paralysis or with absence of the tonsil on the abnormal side. Ellwood *et al.*[2] reported bilateral anotia with meatal atresia in a brother and sister, children of consanguineous parents.

Cryptotia

Abnormal adherence of the upper part of the auricle to the head is a rare anomaly. As the skin of the postauricular region directly joins the skin of the upper portion of the auricle, the ear seems to be pushed upward into a pocket of skin. The upper part of the auricle becomes detached from the head in the fourth month of gestation.[3] Cryptotia is attributed to persistence of fetal attachment of the auricle to the underlying skin.

Fig. 41-1 – Anotia. (From J. Ruzic.[1])

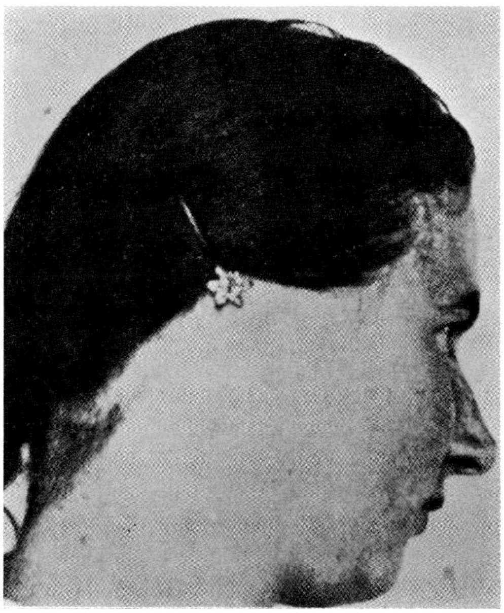

Uncomplicated Hereditary Microtia

Microtia combined with cup shape, infolding and other anomalies of the auricle can be transmitted as a dominant and rather harmless trait. Potter[4] reported this malformation in five generations of a kinship. The gene was regular in expression. Normal members of the kinship did not transmit the trait and affected members passed it on to approximately half their children. Hanhart[5] published two large pedigrees from Switzerland. In one of these, microtia could be traced through seven generations, in the other through five. Although in some cases the external ears were reminiscent of those seen in mandibulofacial dysostosis (p. 650), the external meatuses were patent and there were no complications such as middle ear infections, otosclerosis or deafness. Congenital cup-shaped ears can also be transmitted through several generations. A relationship to the Pierre Robin syndrome was suggested by a kindred recorded by Peterson and Schimke.[6]

Microtia with Atresia of the External Meatus

This more serious form of microtia usually is unilateral. Of 31 cases reported by Hanhart,[5] only 6 were bilateral. Auricular fistulas (or appendages), cleft or high palate and middle ear disease complicated the disorder. The auditory canal was either absent or rudimentary. Males seemed to be more often affected than females. Ellwood *et al.*[2] observed unilateral microtia with meatal atresia in 2 siblings whose parents did not show the trait. The inner ear may be intact in such cases. Improvement of hearing has been achieved surgically by fenestration and construction of an external canal.[7]

Bilateral microtia or anotia with atresia of the external meatus was observed in approximately 15% of children with thalidomide embryopathies.[8]

Synotia and Melotia (Otocephaly)

If the mandible is absent or markedly hypoplastic, the temporal bones are in close proximity. The external ears assume a horizontal position, with the lobules located near the midline. The external meatuses and the tympanic cavities are also close together at the undersurface of the head. The tubes are quite short or absent, so that the tympanic cavities open directly into the pharynx. The bases of the petrous bones are located quite low over the neck, whereas their tips are situated higher and are in contact with the body of the sphenoid bone. In such cases, the ascent of the auricles did not take place and their embryonic position is maintained. A more severe degree of synotia is found in the cyclopia series. If the eyes are close together and the nasal cavities are fused, the tympanic spaces may form, together with the pharynx, a saccular enlargement that hangs like a big goiter over the anterior aspects of the neck.[9] In cyclopia, the eyes are in a common orbit or they are fused completely and a proboscis is formed over the midline eye. In such cases, the temporal bones are moved forward and downward, approaching each other in the midline. But complete fusion of both ears to a single organ with a single external meatus has been observed only in animals with the highest degrees of central facial defects (aprosopia [absence of the face]).

Synotia occurs in certain types of conjoined twins. In monosymmetric cephalothoracopagi, approachment or union of the auricles and middle ear chambers occurs. If the duplication is limited to the cranial portion of the body (diprosopus or dicephalus), various degrees of synotia occur, according to the location and degree of fusion. The aural anomalies that occur in such cases have been described and reviewed by Marx.[9]

Milder degrees of synotia can occur in various types of micrognathia. The "low-set" ears described in many syndromes represent a lack of aural ascent due to underdevelopment of the mandibular area. If the ear is located on the cheek, one speaks of "melotia." In such cases, the lobule of the auricle is located near the angle of the mouth. In rare cases, the auricle is represented by several hillocks that may be distributed between the normal site of the auricle and the angle of the mouth.

Synotia can be produced experimentally. Giroud *et al.*[10] achieved this in mice by x-irradiation in utero. We have seen the anomaly in rats whose mothers were treated with streptonigrin. Synotia is understandably associated with agnathia.

External Meatus

The external meatus opens at the level of the upper margin of the ala nasi if the head is held in an erect position. It consists of an outer cartilaginous part and an inner membranous part derived from the meatal plate. The osseous canal develops in postnatal life when it replaces the membranous part. The width of the external meatus varies widely in individuals and in races. Hyperostosis and exostoses were discussed by Altmann.[3]

Atresia of the external meatus may be osseous or membranous. In osseous atresia, the os tympanicum is replaced by a solid bony wall. A membranous atresia may be located on the external opening of the canal or at the blind end of a short canal. Duplication of the external meatus is a rare anomaly. In such a case, the accessory canal, which ends blindly, can be located above or below the canal, which leads to the drum. Auricular appendages accompany such malformations.[9] Various types of septa dividing the external meatus have been described. A rare anomaly consists

Fig. 41-2.—Agnathus or synotus. The mandible is missing, the oral cavity rudimentary. The petrous bones and ears approach each other. Note the typical embryonic position of the external ears. From Förster, A.: *Missbildungen des Menschen* (Jena: Friedrich Mauke, 1865.)

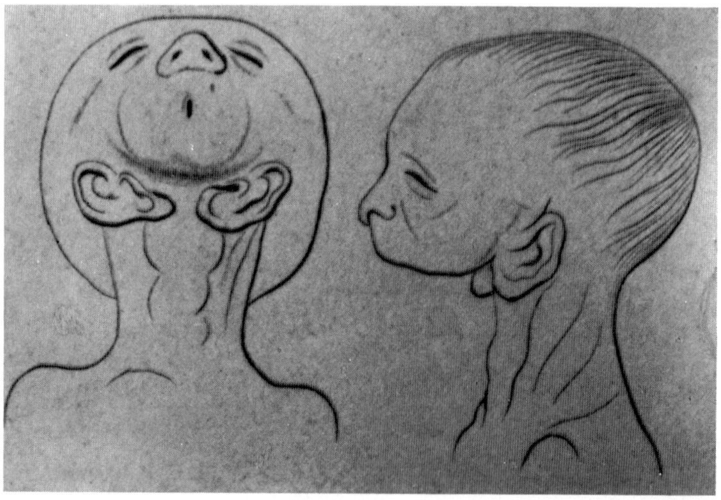

in absence of the external part of the canal in the presence of the inner part.[3]

Atresia of the meatus is present in severe cases of mandibulofacial dysostosis. In a case of bilateral atresia, Altmann[11] found the obstruction effected mainly by the tympanic bones. The external canals ended blindly approximately 5 mm. from the well-developed external meatuses.

Congenital Auricular Fistulas

Thorough reviews of this subject were made by Selkirk[12] and Altmann.[3] Auricular fistulas are blindly ending narrow tubes or pits, most often located at the anterior margin of the ascending limb of the helix. Other sites are along a curve passing from the temple to the anterior margin of the crus helicis and from there through the interspace between the crus helicis and the upper part of the tragus to the concha, the external auditory meatus, the interspace between the tragus and antitragus and to the skin at the junction of the concha and the cheek,[13] but other locations can be seen. A rare one is in the center of the lobule, which, when perforating, has been called a "natural earring hole." Another rare type is the colloaural fistula that extends from the floor of the external meatus down to the angle of the mandible. Connection of a fistula with the middle ear or a tonsillar pillar has also been observed. Aural fistulas often are overlooked and incidence figures vary. In Oriental races, estimates ranged from 4% to 6%; in some African Negroes the fistulas occurred in 5.2% of the females and in 3.6% of the males. Selkirk[12] found them in the United States in 0.9% of Caucasian and in 5.2% of Negro school children. An incidence of about 0.9% was found in European populations.[14] Most auricular fistulas are harmless and uncomplicated anomalies. Occasionally, they become infected, form retention cysts and cause a chronic discharge. Some fistulas occur in conjunction with more severe deformities of the ear and the face, such as microtia, auricular appendages, branchiogenic fistulas, facial clefts, microphthalmia or others. In mandibulofacial dysostosis, a typical location of the fistulas is between the ear and the angle of the mouth.

In most cases, auricular fistulas occur sporadically,[12] but many selected pedigrees show that irregular dominant inheritance can play an etiologic role, with great variability of penetrance and expressivity. The anomaly sometimes can be traced through many generations. The rare "natural earring holes" have also been observed as a hereditary trait.[12]

Hereditary deafness in a family with hereditary aural fistulas was reported by Fourman and Fourman.[14] Some members of this kinship had branchial fistulas also. The authors believed that the three defects may be the effects of one dominant gene.

Fig. 41-3.—Normal external ear. *AH*, anthelix; *AT*, antitragus, *CH*, crus helicis, *H*, helix; *L*, lobule; *T*, tragus.

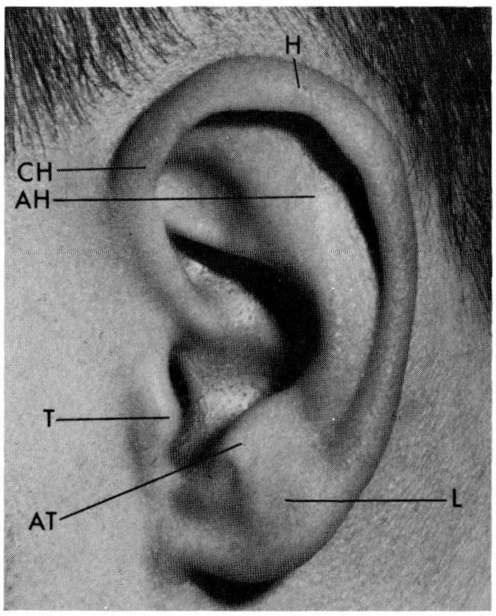

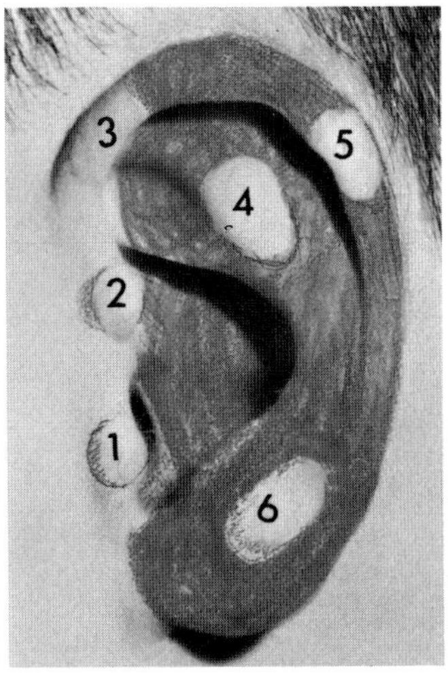

Fig. 41-4.—Auricle of adult male. The shaded areas are derived from the hyoid bar and the light areas from the mandibular bar. The numbers *1-6* correspond to the branchial hillocks as seen in embryos of approximately 14 mm. in length. (After Streeter, G. L.: Development of the auricle in the human embryo, Contrib. Embryol. 14:111, 1922.)

Auricular Appendages

Auricular appendages are rather common malformations found, in most cases, in front of the auricle and occasionally within or behind the ear or on the lobule. It is estimated that they occur in approximately 1.5% of the population, more often unilaterally than bilaterally. Appendages vary greatly in size and may be sessile or pedunculated. They are made up of skin, but they also contain a cartilaginous base that can be anchored deeply in the underlying tissues.[3]

The most frequent location of auricular appendages is the line of junction of the mandibular and hyoid

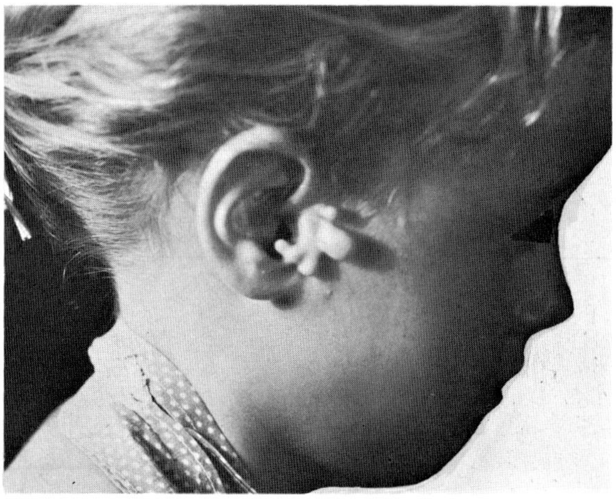

Fig. 41-5.—Multiple auricular appendages in an otherwise normal girl.

arches, where they often are attached to otherwise normal ears. Less frequently, they occur in the line of junction of the mandibular and maxillary processes, i.e., on the cheek between the auricle and the angle of the mouth. Appendages in this area are more often associated with microtia, melotia or oblique facial fissures. They may, if well developed, simulate an extra ear, but true polyotia seems to be extremely rare. A case of proved polyotia has been reported by Bol and deKleyn[15] in a newborn boy with cleft lip and palate. On the left side, two auricles were grown together by their conchae, which enclosed a narrow external canal.

Darwinian Tubercle and Other Variations

Much has been written about a small projection from the descending part of the helix since Darwin regarded this variation as a remnant of the erect pointed ears of some anthropoids. Actually, many variations in shape can be observed in this area that have been compared with the ears of macaques (pointed and directed backward), of cercopithecidae (sharp angle on tip of auricle, satyr ear) and of cats (upper and posterior portion of helix is enlarged and bent forward). Both Darwin's point and satyr point are normal features in human fetal stages. Cat ears may be associated with ptosis of the upper eyelid.[9]

Fig. 41-6—Darwinian tubercle (**arrow**).

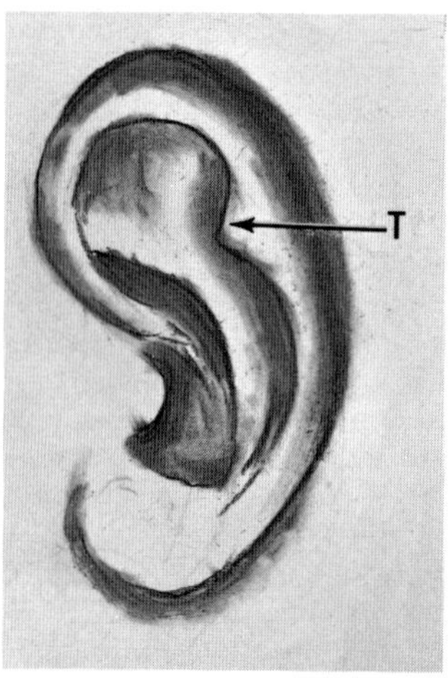

Adherent lobules are a frequent variation that occurs less often in men than in women. Complete absence of the lobule is rare. Split lobule (coloboma) may result in equal anterior and posterior portions or in predominance of either part. "Wildermuth ear" is a rare but striking anomaly. It consists in relative overdevelopment of the anthelix, which protrudes laterad over the plane of the helix and tragus.[9] Cup-shaped ears are small auricles that grow forward over the meatus.

Lop Ear

The angle of the auricle to the median plane averages 25 degrees in boys and 18 degrees in girls. If the external ear stands away from the head at a greater angle, one speaks of "lop ears" or "bat ears." The angle between the attached medial concha and the free lateral scapha is increased in such flaring ears. Lop ears often are larger than normal ears (macrotia) and have a less marked relief.[3]

Malformations of the Middle Ear

In former decades, studies of the middle ear and its malformations were limited to anatomic examinations. Abnormal specimens could be obtained only

Fig. 41-7.—Low-set lop ears.

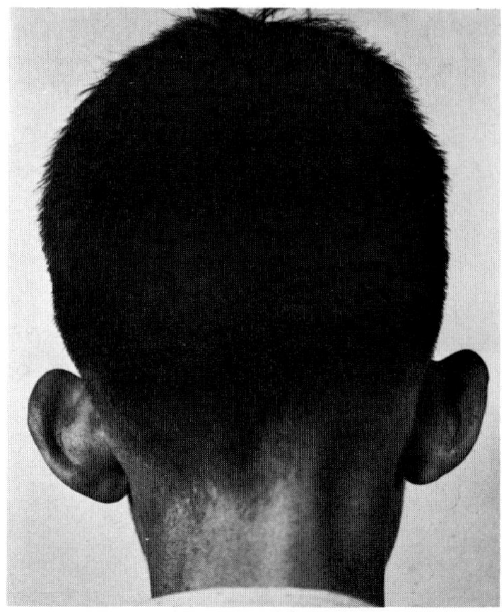

rarely. Marx,[9] in 1911, could evaluate only 40 anatomic analyses of malformations of the middle ear, and in 1955 Altmann[11] stated that the total number of usable histologic observations of the temporal bones was 63. With the advent of modern middle ear surgery in conjunction with mobilization operations and with microscopic surgical approaches, the variety of middle ear anomalies has become appreciated. Only a superficial survey of malformations as recognized at present can be given here.

Marx[9] distinguished four types of middle ear malformations. In type I, there is an abnormal drum with minor anomalies of the ossicles. The annulus tympanicus is abnormally thick, the drum is undifferentiated and the malleus lacks the manubrium and short process. Malleus and drum are not connected. Type II is characterized by a bony plate in place of the drum. Otherwise, the middle ear can be normal or be diminished in size, with its contents deformed in varying degrees. These changes blend into those of type III, which show narrowing of the tympanic cavity by osseous tissue and anomalies or absence of ossicles. In type IV, the tympanic cavity is entirely absent and replaced by spongy bone. There are no ossicles and the pyramid of the temporal bone can be absent.

The ossicles often are deformed in abnormal tympanic cavities. The *stapes* can be altered in many respects. Some parts, such as the head or base, may be overdeveloped, a crus may be abnormally bent, the crura can be connected by a bony plate, there may be exostoses on a crus or on the footplate or both crura can be united to a compact bony pillar. Complete absence of the crura or of the footplate has also been observed.[9]

Hough[16] stated that "from the bone most neglected before 1952 in human anatomy, the stapes has now become the most investigated bone in our skeleton." He also stressed that the stapes is not formed exclusively by the second pharyngeal arch (or Reichert cartilage) as previously taught, but from this arch and the labyrinthine capsule as well. During differentiation, the otic capsular area around the footplate of the stapes begins to thin out and the cells develop into fibrous tissue (instead of precartilage) and into the annular ligament. The stapes originally is continuous with the vestibular window, but by the thinning out of the periphery the annular ligament is formed, which makes the stapes a bone capable of vibratory motion. Failure of differentiation of the annular ligament results in chondrification and ossification and finally in stapedial fixation. Without differentiation of the annular ligament, the stapes remains a part of the labyrinthine capsular bone, as the footplate fails to develop as a separate part. Children affected with this malformation sometimes are considered mentally retarded, but their hearing and mentation can be improved by surgical correction of the stapedial malformation.[16] Shambaugh[17] operated on patients with patent meatus and intact tympanic membrane but affected by congenital stapes fixation. Patients with this disorder have deafness from birth, nonprogressive hearing loss and a family history negative for otosclerosis. Malformations are found at operation of the stapes and other tympanic structures. Associated malformations such as meatal atresia, micrognathia, mandibulofacial dysostosis and others have been observed. Two cases of congenital absence of the fenestra ovalis were reported by Pou,[18] who stated that this anomaly should be considered in all patients with a history of conductive, nonprogressive deafness since birth or early childhood. In such cases, the facial nerve is in an abnormal, inferior position. Rudiments of the superstructure of the stapes such as the neck or parts of the crura are present but they are not connected with a footplate. In one of these cases, the patient had situs inversus and dextrocardia. At least 13 cases of absent oval window have now been recorded[19] and in some of these there was also absence of the round window.[20]

Persistent stapedial artery was considered rare in man until recently, but it is now, according to Hough,[16] considered a common variation that must be expected at operations on the middle ear. Early case reports were reviewed by Marx.[9] Originating from the internal carotid, such a stapedial artery can enter the tympanic cavity through its floor, run across the promontory and through the stapes and from there reach through an opening in the cranial cavity. A large stapedial artery was encountered at operation and described by Hough.[16] This vessel disappeared into the bone of the promontory on one side and into the facial canal on the other.

Malformations of the *incus* and *malleus* had long been known to anatomists, but a better knowledge has been acquired more recently by aural surgeons. Marx[9] mentioned enlargement and exostoses of the body and changes in the crura of the incus. He was also acquainted with rudimentary manubrium and processes of the malleus. There also existed descriptions of bony union of the malleus head and incus body or union of all ossicles. Supernumerary ossicles had been reported.

Hough[16] emphasized that the anomalies of the malleus and incus can be better understood by a revised concept of their development. It seems that the ancestral cells of these ossicles are not entirely derived from the mandibular arch but also from the hyoid arch. It is now believed that the long process of the incus and the manubrium of the malleus are differentiated from primordial mesenchyme of the second arch, whereas the body of the incus and the head of the malleus are formed from that of the first arch. Thus, the lower parts of the ossicular chain and the stapes are closely related as products of the second arch. One finds, therefore, frequent associations of malformations of the stapes with those of the long process of the incus and of the handle of the malleus. Hough[16] described a case in which bony union of these lower tympanic parts was present from birth, manifested by congenital bilateral conductive deafness. The handle of the malleus was not attached to the tympanic membrane but was directed dorsad to join the head of the stapes. In other cases, the incudostapedial joint was not developed and the handle of the malleus was missing. Sometimes congenital anomalies of all three ossicles were found and it was assumed that both branchial arches and the labyrinthine capsule had failed to develop properly.

The *tendon of the stapedius muscle* is not rarely involved in congenital anomalies of the middle ear. The stapedius muscle, its tendon and the pyramidal eminence that houses the muscle are derived from histologically different ancestor cells of the second arch but they finally fuse and form the smallest muscular unit in the body.[16] The stapedius tendon varies greatly in position. It may be absent, together with the pyramidal eminence and the stapedial muscle. This developmental defect is thought to be present in approximately 1% of human ears without obvious hearing loss.[16]

Malformations of the eustachian tube are not frequent, according to Marx.[9] The tube can be normal in the presence of severe middle ear defects. But there are reports of absence of the tube, atresia of the ostium pharyngeum, abnormal course with angular bends and of abnormal lumen. Enlargements at the ostium pharyngeum or diverticula may be acquired anomalies. Shortened tubes occur in anencephaly and absence of the tube has been observed in cyclopia.[9]

Malformations of the Inner Ear

Congenital deafness can be due to inherited anomalies of the ear but also to infection or other exogenous factors during intrauterine life. Inherited deafness can be congenital or its onset can be delayed, so that it becomes manifest many years and decades after birth. Although in late-appearing inherited deafness congenital anomalies may be present, they are not easily detectable since, by the time of anatomic or histologic examination, hereditary and environmental factors often have combined in the production of the final disease picture. Deaf-mutism may be due to early postnatal disease, such as infections in infancy or erythroblastosis fetalis. Thus, it is generally admitted that etiologic explanations of seemingly congenital deafness are difficult and that in man the knowledge of the anatomic basis is limited. In animals, particularly in mice, hereditary disorders of the inner ear have been studied intensively, and from these studies it is obvious that many differing mutations and disease processes can lead to similar disease pictures.[21]

Marx[9] attempted a classification of congenital malformations of the inner ear by establishing three groups. In the first group were cases of minor changes in the osseous capsule of the labyrinth, particularly those of its lateral wall. It also included cases of narrowing or absence of the fenestra cochleae or vestibuli and similar anomalies usually described with malformations of the middle ear. The second group included epithelial metaplasia, particularly in the cochlea. Absence or hypoplasia of the organ of Corti, hypoplasia of the ganglion spirale, of the membrana tectoria or of the stria vascularis and ectasia or collapse of the membranous labyrinth were among changes found repeatedly in cases of congenital deaf-mutism. The third group was composed of the most severe forms, with complete aplasia of the entire labyrinth. Such defects can occur in the presence of a normal external and middle ear or they can be combined with anomalies of the middle ear. The entire pyramid may be absent in such cases.

Altmann,[22] in a critical review of the literature on the histologic findings in inherited nerve deafness, distinguished between cases of regressive change in the end organs and the truly developmental anomalies of the cochlear duct or of the saccule. The developmental group includes the congenital malformations of the "typus Mondini," named after an observer in the eighteenth century. These cases are bilateral. The osseous capsule of the cochlea is flattened, and in the upper part of the cochlea the septa are absent and a scala communis is formed. The turns of the cochlear duct are reduced in number and altered in width. There also are changes in the utricle and saccule but the semicircular canals usually are normal. The organ of Corti is absent or abnormal, particularly in the upper portion of the duct. The spiral ganglion is reduced in regard to the number of cells and nerve fibers or it is in atypical positions. This "typus Mondini" obviously belongs in group two of the classification of Marx.[9] Malformations of the Mondini type may show clinically complete deafness or only a partial hearing loss, with hearing of the low notes more affected than that of the high.[22] The malformations may result in congenital deafness and deaf-mutism or in slowly progressive loss of hearing. Simple dominant inheritance was found in a number of kinships. Concordance in monozygotic twins has been reported.[23]

Ormerod[24] gave a good review of the pathology of congenital deafness. He listed six types of congenital deafness, the classification depending on the completeness of their agenesis: (1) Michel type—complete lack of development of the internal ear, (2) Mondini-Alexander type—development only of a single curved tube representing the cochlea and similar immaturity of the vestibule and canals, (3) Bing-Siebenmann type—bony labyrinth well formed but the membranous part, particularly the sense organ, underdeveloped, (4) Scheibe type or cochlear-saccular type—vestibular part of the ear developed and functioning; malformation restricted to membranous cochlea and saccule, (5) Siebenmann type—changes mainly in the middle ear and often due to hormone deficiency and (6) microtia and atresia of meatus—abnormalities mainly in the external ear.

Older classifications of hereditary deafness often distinguished between the common "sporadic" type attributed to a recessive gene and a rarer dominant variety. The term "sporadic," although widely used for the recessive trait, was never justified, since such genes can occur in the homozygous state in several members of a kindred,[25] thus leading to "familial" deafness. On the other hand, it is now known that sporadic congenital deaf-mutism can be due to nongenetic factors such as prenatal rubella, toxoplasmosis, syphilis and others. An article by Ormerod[24] presents good illustrations of the histopathology of various types of congenital deafness. Ward *et al.*[26] described the pathology of the inner ear in a 17-year-old male with probable congenital deafness. The findings corresponded to those of the so-called cochlear-saccular degeneration of Scheibe. Partial absence of the organ of Corti, aplasia or atrophy of the stria vascularis, deformity of the tectorial membrane and partial collapse of the Reissner membrane and of the saccule were noted. The patient had interesting associated anomalies, such as hypoplasia of the aorta, Milroy disease (Chapter 118), cryptorchidism and signs of past inflammatory diseases.

Deafness

In many cases of profound deafness in children, causes can be ascertained only with difficulty. Fraser,[27] studying more than 2,000 children in special schools, analyzed 1,500 children's deafness according to etiology. Aproximately 60% of the causes were considered prenatal and/or genetic, about 10% perinatal and 30% postnatal. Among genetic causes, recessive inheritance was considered of greatest importance and rubella accounted for the majority of patients damaged by intrauterine postconceptional factors. An excellent review of the present knowledge of the causes of profound deafness in childhood was published by Fraser in 1964.[28] Konigsmark[93] discussed associations of hereditary deafness with external-ear abnormalities.

Recessively Inherited Deafness and Deaf-Mutism

This group is by no means uniform, as different genes are involved in different families and in different ethnic groups. Parental consanguinity is high in such cases and can amount to from 7% to 11%[29,30] The anatomic basis consists of atrophy of the sensory elements in the acoustic labyrinth and the sacculus, whereas the vestibular labyrinth usually is intact. Although most investigators believe that the pathologic changes are chiefly in the peripheral aural organs, there are some who localize them in the central nervous system. The organ of Corti is rudimentary and the nervus cochlearis and its ganglion cells are defective. Although in these cases hearing defects or remnants usually are symmetric, symmetry cannot be accepted as proof of heredity. Bilateral deafness can occur following prenatal rubella (p. 66), and unilateral deafness can be hereditary.

That different recessive genes exist which, in the homozygous condition, cause deaf-mutism can be deduced from observations of matings of deaf-mutes that result in normal children even though both parents have recessively inherited deafness as suggested by consanguinity of their parents or deafness of their siblings.[31] If both parents were homozygous for the same genes, all their children should be deaf-mutes. If this is not the case, different genes must be responsible for the disorders in the parents. Associated hereditary anomalies often suggest that recessively inherited deafness is diverse in origin.[32]

The association of deafness with retinitis pigmentosa has long been known as a hereditary entity (Usher syndrome). Bell,[33] in her review of retinitis pigmentosa, found deaf-mutism or deafness in 10% of her cases. But in selected pedigrees in which deafness occurred as a complication in at least one case of retinitis pigmentosa, approximately 75% of the retinitis pigmentosa cases were complicated by deafness and in some pedigrees the association was 100%. The parents of the patients with both defects usually were phenotypically normal, but consanguinity was high among them. Similar observations were made by Lindenov[23] in Sweden, where it appeared that the gene for deafness and retinitis pigmentosa was a pleiotropic one and different from the more common gene responsible for uncomplicated deafness. This opinion was based on observation of a pedigree showing a normal child born to parents, one of whom had uncomplicated deaf-mutism and the other deaf-mutism with retinitis pigmentosa.

Another syndrome sometimes combines deafness with retinitis pigmentosa, polydactyly, obesity, hypogenitalism and mental retardation. The gene for this disorder, the Laurence-Moon-Biedl syndrome (Chapter 19), is also considered a recessive one with pleiotropic effect in the homozygous condition. A variant of this syndrome was described by Alström *et al.*[34] and attributed to a single recessive gene. This disease picture includes nerve deafness, retinal degeneration, obesity and diabetes mellitus.

Congenital deafness associated with goiter (Pendred syndrome[35]) has been observed repeatedly in familial aggregation.[39] Most authors believe that the trait is inherited as a recessive, but there are suggestions of dominant transmission.[36] It has been suggested that the patient's deafness is due to hypothyroidism in utero and that the sporadic form can be linked to the form found in endemic areas.[37] Elman[38] described a family in which 4 of 7 female siblings had congenital or infantile nerve deafness associated with nodular goiter. In 2 of the 4 patients, invasive carcinoma was found on histologic examination of the glands. An inborn enzymatic defect of thyroid cellular metabolism was suspected. The patients showed good intelligence and health with the exception of the aural and thyroid defects.

Congenital deaf-mutism combined with a peculiar heart disease was described by Jervell and Lange-Nielsen[40] in 4 of 6 children of a Norwegian family. The parents and 2 children appeared entirely healthy. The deaf-mute children suffered attacks of fainting, probably caused by standstill of the heart, and 3 of them died suddenly at the ages of 4, 5 and 9 years, respectively. Electrocardiograms showed marked prolongation of the Q-T interval. Necropsy performed in 1 of the children showed no anatomic or microscopic changes in the heart.

Deafness develops in a number of congenital and/or recessively inherited disorders such as gargoylism (p. 808), Morquio disease (p. 819), Morquio-Ullrich disease (p. 817), osteopetrosis (p. 863), Klippel-Feil syndrome (p. 909) and others. It seems that in the sex-linked form of gargoylism deafness is particularly frequent (p. 816). Perceptive deafness associated with split-hand and split-foot was observed in 2 brothers and considered a syndrome due to a rare recessive gene.[41] Winter *et al.*[91] described a family in which 4 female siblings showed a syndrome of middle ear deafness (due to malformation of the ossicles), renal malformations and genital anomalies, particularly vaginal atresia. One unviable sibling had bilateral renal agenesis, pulmonary hypoplasia, atrial septal defect, undescended ovaries and vaginal atresia. The auricles were low set and the external canals stenotic.

Dominantly Inherited Deafness and Deaf-Mutism

It has been estimated that approximately 25% of the cases of deaf-mutism are dominantly inherited.[42] There are various types of dominantly inherited deafness. As pointed out before, the developmental anomalies described as the "Mondini type" have been considered the basis of a dominantly transmitted form of deafness (p. 406). Although this deafness sometimes is congenital and results in deaf-mutism, most cases develop later in life. A large pedigree showing transmission through generations was published by Stephens and Dolowitz.[43] In this large kindred, nerve deafness appeared late in life but some of the younger members had high tone loss without conscious deafness. The trait was dominant with complete penetrance.

Congenital deaf-mutism is a constituent of the Waardenburg syndrome, a combination of traits attributed to an irregular autosomal dominant gene with pleiotropic effects (p. 395). In Holland, more than 1% of all congenitally deaf persons have this type of hearing loss. From the ophthalmologist's point of view, lateral displacement of the medial canthi and of the inferior lacrimal puncta is the leading symptom, whereas deafness occurs in only 20% of the patients. The syndrome was described from the otologist's point of view by Fisch,[44] who stated that it was rather common within the group of congenital deafness disorders. Deafness is either very severe, with almost total hearing loss, or it is moderate and unilateral, with hearing for high frequencies better than for the lower ones. In a case in which a complete histologic study was done, the organ of Corti was absent in all coils and the basilar membrane was thickened and smooth. The vascular stria was atrophic, the spiral ganglion poor in cells and the nerve fibers were sparse.

In the Waardenburg syndrome, abnormal pigmentation of irides and hair is associated with the ocular and aural symptoms. Since there is some evidence that both the otic vesicle and pigment cells are derivatives of the neural crest, Fisch[44] believed that this common origin may explain the frequent association of aural and pigmentary disturbances. He also described a kindred in which deafness and early graying was transmitted through four generations. A syndrome of deaf-mutism associated with partial albinism was recorded by Tietz.[45] There is generalized albinism but there are no ocular symptoms and melanin is present in the irides. There is underdevelopment of the eyebrows. In this kindred, deaf-mutism and albinism, constantly associated, were dominantly inherited through six generations. Deafness combined with cataracts, myopia and ectodermal dysplasia of the anhidrotic type was observed by Marshall[46] in 7 members of a kindred through three generations. In a family in which pulmonary stenosis seemed to be transmitted from the mother to 3 of her children – 1 boy and 2 girls – congenital deaf-mutism was noticed in 2 of the children with the heart anomaly.[47]

There are other dominantly inherited disorders in which auditory disturbances occur. Mandibulofacial dysostosis and ear defects are discussed on page 650. Deafness in neurofibromatosis, a disorder attributable to a dominant gene, can be caused by acoustic neuromas. Such neuromas are rare in children. Most patients develop symptoms of this form of neurofibromatosis in adult life. Thus, they can reproduce and transmit the disorder, as shown in a number of pedigrees by Gardner and Turner.[48] Deafness and tinnitus usually precede vertigo. Twitching of the face and unsteady gait, reduction of the corneal reflex and facial weakness are early symptoms. Deafness in osteogenesis imperfecta, a dominant trait of brittle bones and blue sclerae, usually develops in or after the third decade. Because of its variable onset, different incidence figures of deafness will be ascertained in patients with osteogenesis imperfecta (Chapter 89). Approximately one-fourth of the patients are deaf, usually bilaterally and progressively. Although the deafness in this disorder is commonly attributed to otosclerosis, there may be a labyrinthine component. Laxity of the tympanic membrane and of the ligaments of the ossicles may also contribute to the hearing difficulties. Impaired hearing was found by Mørch[49] in 22% of the achondroplastic dwarfs examined in Denmark. Many of these had had otitis media, but it is likely that they were predisposed to this by the skeletal anomalies of the skull characteristic of this disorder. Nager and Meyer[50] studied the osseous labyrinth in stillborn or newborn children with severe achondroplasia and found that the changes were essentially the same in the labyrinth capsule as those in other parts of the skeleton, namely a failure in longitudinal growth. There were disturbances of enchondral ossification with irregular invasion of cartilage by marrow spaces and premature formation of compact bone. In lethal cases, the cartilage canals were much increased in number and were permeated by connective tissue strands that became the basis of fibrous ossification replacing normal enchondral ossification. Deafness has been observed repeatedly in persons with hereditary symphalangism.[51] It seems that ankylosis of the finger joints is paralleled in such cases by ankylosis of the joints of the ossicles.

Hereditary deafness, hematuria and nephropathy have been described as a syndrome that can be transmitted through several generations. The deafness is attributed to defects in the auditory nerve or the organ of Corti. The males of the kindred are more seriously affected than the females, who are able to survive to adult age and transmit the disorder. Ocular lesions such as spherophakia and cataracts sometimes are associated with the nephro-aural syndrome (p. 1059). A syndrome of deafness, mitral insufficiency, skeletal malformations and short stature has been described as a dominantly inherited trait.[52] Conductive deafness combined with deformities of the external ears was recognized as an autosomal recessive trait in a genetic isolate by Mengel *et al.*[90] Malformations of the middle ear bones, mental retardation and hypogonadism were established in some of the patients.

Unilateral deafness, once considered an acquired condition, is now considered hereditary in 25–30% of the cases and attributed to an irregular dominant gene. There was an early report by Smith[54] of a kindred in which 9 persons of four generations had congenital unilateral deafness. In affected families, deafness can be congenital or there is an inherent weakness that leads to deafness following febrile diseases.

Sex-Linked Recessive Deafness

A congenital form of nerve deafness was described by Sataloff *et al.*[55] as a sex-linked recessive trait. There were 7 male members with deaf-mutism in this kindred. Parker[56] constructed a pedigree in Australia with 15 male members affected. The audiograms were similar in both families. Other pedigrees are mentioned by McRae *et al.*[87] Sex-linked deaf-mutism associated with total albinism was reported by Margolis.[57] This syndrome was present in 14 males of a pedigree that was composed of more than 100 persons of six generations. Hearing impairment may be found in female carriers.[88] Since there is evidence that both the auditory nerve and pigment cells arise from neural crest cells, syndromes involving hearing and pigment disturbances are now sometimes attributed to "faults of the neural crest." But such theories do not explain why the auditory organ is affected even though most of the cranial and all of the spinal sensory ganglion cells that are derived from neural crest cells remain intact.

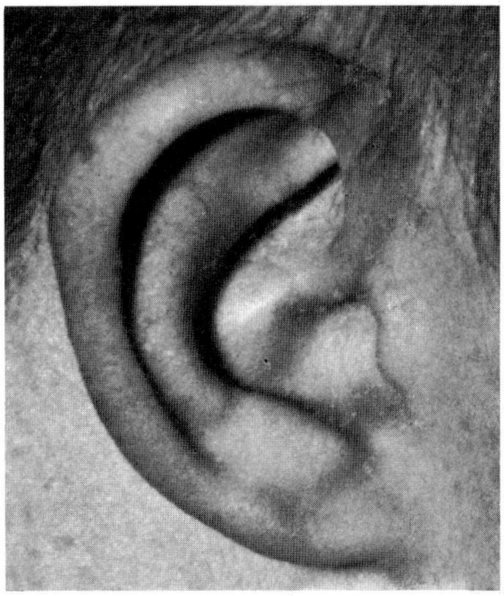

Fig. 41-8.—Ear of an adolescent with Down syndrome. The ear is round, the fold between the helix and the anthelix continues down to the lobular area, which is underdeveloped.

The Ear in Chromosomal Syndromes

The external ears often are abnormal in trisomy 21 or mongolism. There frequently are differences between the right and left ear. In most cases, the auricle is shortened in its vertical diameter, so that a

Fig. 41-9.—Deformed external ear of a child with trisomy 18.

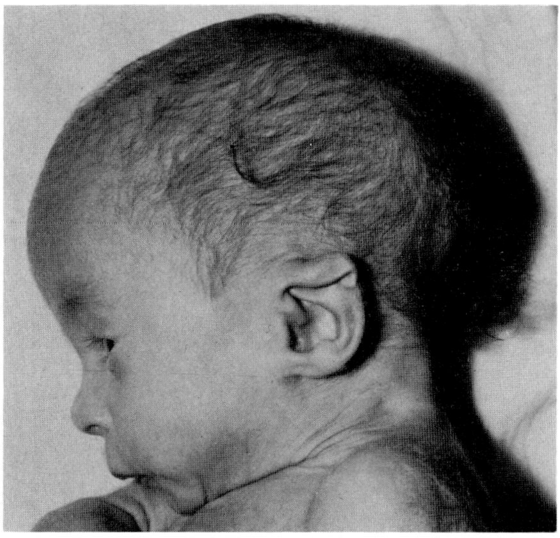

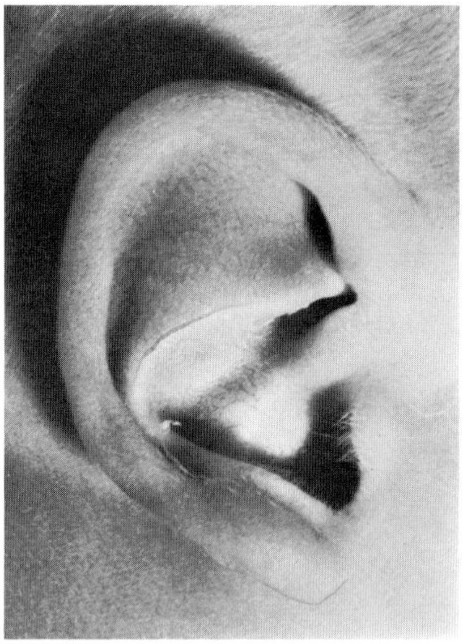

Fig. 41-10.—Ear of a child with trisomy 13-15. Note the sharp angulation of the crus helicis, the fold paralleling the lower end of the helix, and hypoplasia of the anthelix and lobule.

"round" ear is formed. In addition, there are variations such as folding over of the superior portion of the helix, prolongation of the crus helicis through the concha, flaring of the auricle, underdevelopment of the lobule and others. The external canal often is narrow but only rarely completely occluded.

In trisomy 18, the ears are low set and often deformed by folding and appendages.

The auricles show various anomalies in trisomy 13-15, and deafness is a frequent characteristic. Underdevelopment of the tragus and lobule, skin tags in front of the ear, Darwinian tubercle, atresia of an external meatus and other anomalies have been observed.

Auricular deformities occur in the cat-cry syndrome, in patients with ring chromosomes and in cases of translocation.

Ears with a long vertical axis are seen in patients with 45,XO karyotype and boys with the male Turner syndrome (Chapter 112). Such elongated ears have long been known to occur in "eunuchoid" men.

The Ear in Anencephaly

The skeletal aural anomalies of anencephaly have been thoroughly studied. There are variations according to the severity of the cranial defect.[9] The squamous portion of the temporal bone usually is rudimentary. The petrous bones assume an abnormal transverse position, forming an obtuse angle or an angle of 180 degrees. The bases of the pyramides are situated lower than their tips, as the cranial base slants on both sides like a roof toward the periphery. The pyramides are plump and their eminentiae arcuatae lie close to their obtuse tips. The canal of the facial nerve may be defective so that the nerve runs in an open groove. The tympanic rings are turned forward and the temporomandibular joints are situated anterior to them.

The auricles usually appear large and fleshy. Sometimes the ear is folded so that the cranial portion of the helix lies near the lobulus or it is represented by a deformed rudiment. The tympanic cavity may be enlarged or obliterated by bony excrescences, the tympanic membrane assumes a perpendicular position and the stapes has a small footplate. The eustachian tubes are short. The inner ears show various deformi-

Fig. 41-11.—Ears of an infant with cat-cry syndrome.

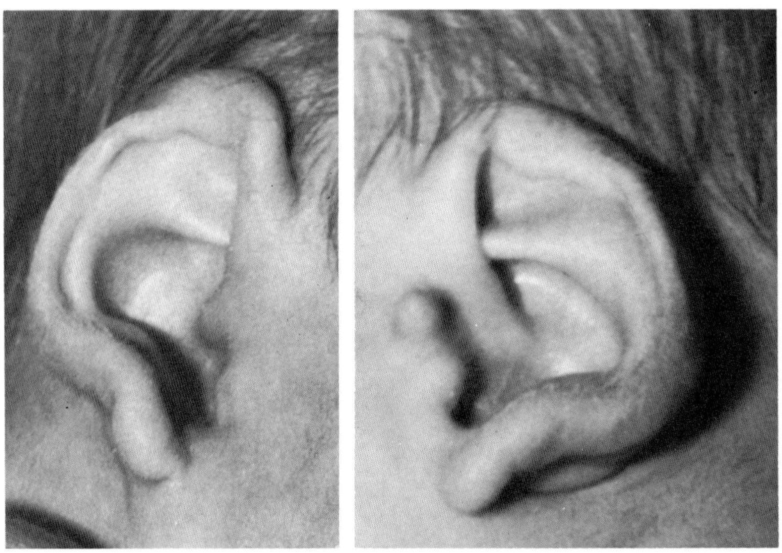

ties. The cochleae are nearer to each other than in normal skulls and the vestibular ducts appear compressed. The fenestrae often are narrow or completely closed. Changes in the membranous labyrinth are not pronounced.[9] The ears of 3 anencephalic fetuses have been described in detail by Altmann.[58]

The Ear in Hydrocephaly

Congenital hydrocephaly affects the labyrinth by hydrops. An interdependence between the increase in cerebrospinal liquor pressure and endoperilymphatic hypertension can be explained by the connections between the cerebrospinal and labyrinthine circulations.[59]

The Ear in Mandibulofacial Dysostosis

In mandibulofacial dysostosis (p. 650), microtia is a frequent symptom. In a typical case, the ear is represented by a skin fold that is only poorly supported by cartilaginous vestiges. Atresia of the external auditory meatus and middle ear deafness usually are found. In milder cases, the ears are small and the parts usually seen in a normal ear are hypoplastic. Sometimes the small auricle is bent forward and shaped like a shell. Such a "crumpled" ear has no helix or anthelix (Fig. 41-12) and the external canal and the drum are reduced in size. The aural changes are a part of the syndrome, which is transmitted as a dominant trait. Some members of an affected kinship may have no external deformity but manifest an inherent weakness of the auditory organ by repeated and tenacious infections resulting in hearing loss. Herberts[60] described the ears of 3 patients with mandibulofacial dysostosis. In one case, normal external ears and external canals were combined with marked malformation of the middle and inner ears. A second case had pronounced malformations of the external ears, lack of external meatuses and malformed middle ears, but conditions were normal from the stapes inward to the labyrinths. In a third case, the external structures were also severely deformed but there was some residual hearing, especially in the lower frequencies, and roentgenograms showed normal ossicles and bony labyrinth bilaterally. It was concluded that such cases should be examined early otologically, since surgical improvement is possible in some cases.

Oculoauriculovertebral Dysplasia

Microtia, auricular fistulae and appendages combined with epibulbar dermoids have been described as a syndrome possibly related to unilateral mandibulofacial dysostosis (Goldenhar syndrome, p. 388). There are anomalies of the spine in such patients such as hemivertebrae and block vertebrae, spina bifida and others. In contrast to mandibulofacial dysostosis, heredity of this syndrome has not been demonstrated. The resemblance between this syndrome and mandibulofacial dysostosis seems to be superficial and without etiologic connection.

The Ear in Congenital Renal Disorders

In renal agenesis (p. 1066), the ears are large, low set and flabby, having little cartilaginous support. Mal-

Fig. 41-12.—Ears of children with mandibulofacial dysostosis.

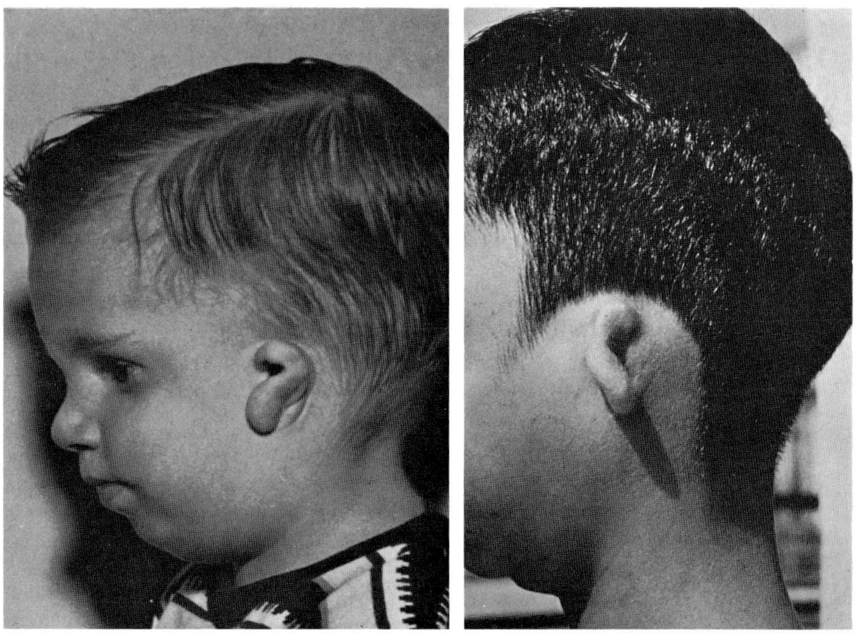

formation of the ears has also been described with less severe anomalies of the genitourinary tract. Hilson[61] pointed out that not all infants who die with renal agenesis have the large flabby ears described with renal agenesis and that other patterns, such as small folded ears, can occur in this lethal anomaly. He found that in malformations of the genitourinary tract compatible with life, deformed ears may also be large and flabby or they may be folded over, with the helix squared across its upper margin; they may be "elfin-shaped" or "bat-ears"; or they may be small and cockleshell-shaped. Asymmetry of the ears is also said to be a sign of urinary tract deformity. The association between aural and renal anomalies is said to be high but not absolute.[61]

The Ear in the Rubella Embryopathy

Soon after the discovery of prenatal rubella as a teratogenic disease, it was found that some of the affected children were deaf-mute. In general, the patients were not totally deaf, since ability to hear high-pitched sounds persisted. Bone conduction seemed to be better than air conduction for high tones but low tones seemed not to be appreciated. The external canal and the tympanic membrane were normal.

Hopkins,[62] in a school for the deaf in Massachusetts, inquired how many mothers of the pupils had had German measles during the early months of pregnancy. After exclusion of mothers of children deaf of known causation, 10 of 116 mothers (8.6%) remembered that they had had the disease but there probably were some mothers of older deaf children who had forgotten that they had had rubella during pregnancy. Similarly, in England, Clayton-Jones[63] reported that in two schools for the deaf 19 of 141 children (13.5%) were born to mothers who had had rubella during the first 4 months of pregnancy. The children with a prenatal rubella history had bilateral, incomplete inner-ear deafness, usually fairly uniform throughout the frequency range. There was no obvious relation between the severity of the mother's rubella and the degree of the child's defect. It is clear that the percentage contribution of maternal rubella to deafness in a population changes with the trends of rubella epidemiology. Goodhill[64] found maternal rubella in the first 3 months of pregnancy to be the potential cause of deafness in 186 (20.5%) of 904 cases of deafness studied in questionnaires.

To ascertain how many children exposed to rubella during early gestation have hearing losses, several prospective studies were undertaken. Jackson and Fisch,[65] in such a prospective study, detected congenital deafness following maternal rubella in the first 16 weeks of pregnancy in 30% of the children examined. One-third of these children had unilateral deafness. The deafness was detected before the age of 4 years in only one-third of them; or—in other words—deafness remained undetected during the first years in two-thirds. Half of the children with hearing defects had speech defects. The audiograms in the cases of congenital deafness were "flat," with a similar degree of hearing loss in all frequencies.

Barr and Lundström[66] made retrospective and prospective studies along these lines in Sweden. In a series of 752 children with severe hearing defect, histories of maternal rubella were obtained in 92 (12%). In 91 cases with a rubella history, the maternal infection occurred within the first 4 months of gestation; in one case, the illness was in the fifth month. There was a tendency to more severe hearing loss with histories of the disease in the second month. The vestibular function was normal. In schools and special classes for the deaf, 25% of the pupils born shortly after an epidemic of rubella had histories of maternal rubella in early gestation. These results are similar to those obtained by Goodhill.[64] In a prospective study, Barr and Lundström[66] found that 22% of the children exposed to maternal rubella during the first 4 months of pregnancy had hearing losses. Among 1,509 deaf children, maternal rubella was the apparent cause in 133, i.e., approximately 9%, according to Fraser,[27] who examined children in residential schools in 1959–1961. But such estimates may be too low, since among cases of idiopathic deafness a significant number may be due to subclinical maternal rubella.[67]

Histologic examinations of the ears in rubella embryopathies did not yield uniform results. This is understandable, since time of infection and the intervals between infection and examination varied; some ears were those of fetuses, others were of children of differing ages. Some negative findings could correspond to cases that escaped rubella injuries. Some of the positive results may be attributable to agonal or postmortem changes. Carruthers[68] examined the ears of a 6-month-old child with the signs of rubella embryopathy. The middle ears, eighth nerve, spiral ganglion and osseous labyrinth were normal, but differentiation of the cells forming the organ of Corti was lacking. The tectorial membrane and Reissner membrane were not present. This severe defect probably represents the end result of the disease process; other observations made by later investigators may show earlier effects of the virus.

Töndury[69] summarized published cases and added excellent illustrations. He also gave descriptions of the ears of 2 fetuses injured by rubella, showing interruption of the ductus cochlearis with destruction of basal epithelial cells. Gray[70] examined the ears of a 53-mm. fetus whose mother had had rubella 51 days after her last menstrual period. Fixation of the fetus was a half hour after hysterotomy. The cochlear ducts were abnormal bilaterally, and in the basal and middle coils the cytoplasm of the epithelium of the organ of Corti was in lysis, with disappearance of the cells. The vestibular apparatus was normal. This case was considered by the author as an earlier stage of cochlear lesion than that described by Carruthers.[68] The changes were thought to be the result of cell destruction following invasion by the rubella virus.

Friedmann and Wright[71] thought that inflammatory

changes in the vascular stria found in infants were the primary lesion caused by the rubella virus, which, followed by secondary degenerative changes in the cochlear duct and organ of Corti, could lead to profound childhood deafness.

The Ear in Toxoplasmosis

There are a few reports on congenital aural changes in toxoplasmosis. Callahan *et al.*[72] and Koch *et al.*[73] found mastoiditis in infants with proved toxoplasmosis. Kelemen[74] gave good accounts of aural toxoplasmosis in an infant and in a stillborn child. Changes were demonstrable in the soft tissues, mesenchyme and mucoperiosteum. In one case, calcification was present in the spiral ligament, predominantly in the stria vascularis. The changes were most marked in the niche of the oval window. The picture was that of an otitis media with extensive organization. The skeleton and the sensory elements were not involved in the process.

The Ear in Endemic Cretinism (Maternal Iodine Deficiency)

Deafness and endemic cretinism (p. 114) are closely associated. Since endemic cretinism is determined by environmental factors, the deafness in this disorder can also be attributed to exogenous causes. The external ear usually is normal but the middle ear shows changes. The mastoid process is small and often without pneumatization. Enchondral bone of the labyrinth capsule is normal, but the periosteal layer of the capsule that borders the middle ear is thickened over the promontorium and the tympanic roof. The fenestrae are narrowed.[75] The periosteal part of the stapes is thick and the ossicles are plump and immobilized. The mucous membrane of the tympanic cavity is also increased in thickness by abnormal amounts of subepithelial connective tissue. The inner ear often shows an anomaly of the cochlea, namely hyaline columellae in the organ of Corti and swelling of the Corti membrane. It is possible that the deaf-

Fig. 41-13.—External ears of 4 children with thalidomide embryopathy. (Courtesy of Prof. H. Weicker, Bonn, Germany.)

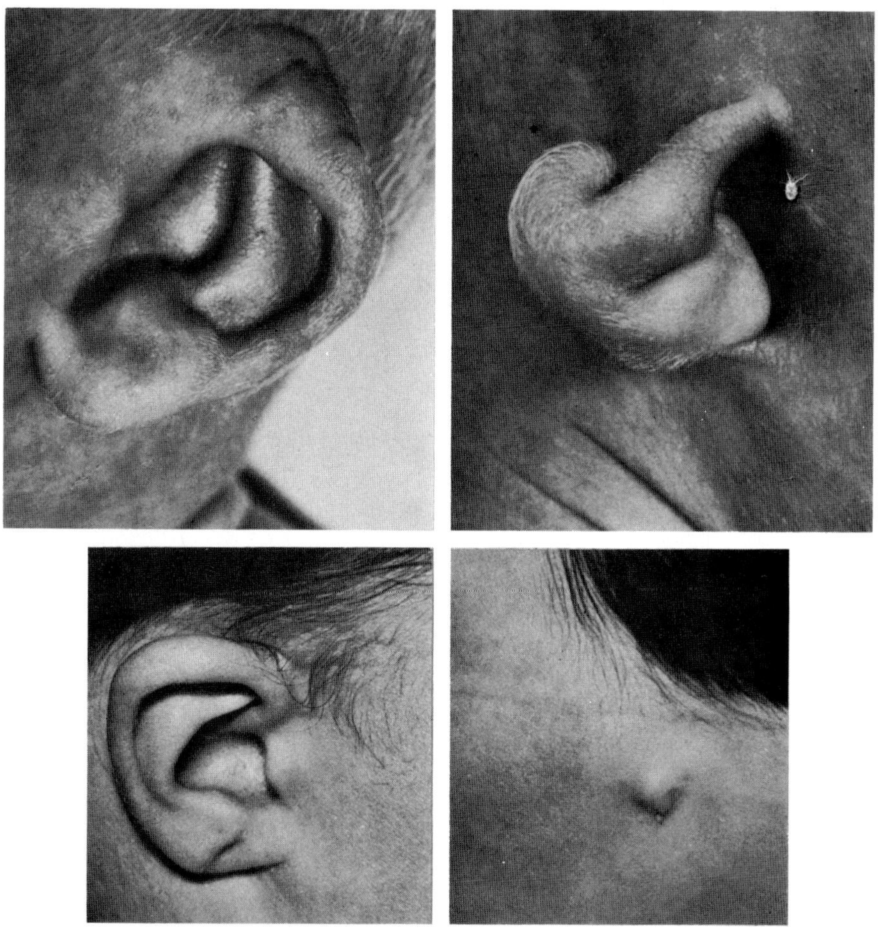

ness of endemic cretins is partly due to changes in the acoustic centers.

Maternal Pseudohypoparathyroidism

There is a report of a child born to a mother with pseudohypoparathyroidism.[76] In the ear of the newborn, calcifications were found in the spiral ligament and there were corpora amylacea in the meatus internus. The center of the stapedial plate was found in reabsorption by a granulating focus.

Deafness and Kernicterus

Deafness as a sequela of kernicterus has been known for some time but it still is difficult to ascertain the contribution made to congenital deafness by blood incompatibilities. Goodhill[64] pointed out an association of moderate perceptive deafness, athetoid cerebral palsy and history of erythroblastosis. Since kernicterus can cause athetosis in such patients, it also seemed related to the deafness. Among perceptibly deaf children, the incidence of erythroblastosis was significantly higher than would be expected in the general population. The deafness seemed to be localized in the nuclear masses of the brain and brain stem. Cavanagh[77] found 3 cases of rhesus sensitization among 118 deaf children and among 124 "rhesus babies" 6 cases of deafness. Byers *et al.*[78] followed 23 patients with extrapyramidal cerebral palsy due to erythroblastosis and believed that hearing loss was demonstrable but not obvious in the majority of them. The hearing loss was partial, most marked in high frequencies and serious enough to interfere with speech development. Severe forms of deafness are only rarely attributable to kernicterus. Barton *et al.*[79] found only 2 cases with known hemolytic disease of the newborn among 270 severely deaf children, but there was a history of neonatal jaundice in 16.

A follow-up study by Keaster *et al.*[89] of 405 patients who had hemolytic disease of the newborn or hyperbilirubinemia as neonates showed that 17 (4.2%) had sensorineural hearing loss that varied from mild to profound.

Congenital Deafness due to Drugs

Taylor[80] pointed out that certain drugs such as quinine and salicylates have a selective injurious effect on the auditory apparatus and are known to cause degenerative changes in the ear. Since they pass the placenta and reach the fetal circulation, they could be toxic to the fetus. Quinine frequently used during pregnancy and in labor could be an etiologic factor in deafness in the newborn. Taylor cited a number of cases of hearing loss of children whose mothers had taken quinine before the child's birth. Winkel[81] did not accept this etiologic factor as proved, since only a few cases of deafness attributable to quinine have been reported despite the extremely large consumption of the drug all over the world. There was no higher rate of deaf-mutism in countries with endemic malaria than in countries without malaria and there was no dose effect.

Streptomycin and dihydrostreptomycin treatment of tuberculosis sometimes results in disturbances of equilibrium and hearing. Kern[82] reported the case of a deaf child whose mother had had dihydrostreptomycin treatment during the first 4 months of gestation. He also mentioned 3 cases in the literature of deafness following similar treatment. It has been shown that these drugs pass the placenta and reach the fetal circulation and cerebrospinal fluid. There are many observations of normal children born to mothers treated with these antibiotics, but there is the possibility of cochlear damage to children with exceptional susceptibility.

Robinson and Cambon[83] reported 2 cases of congenital hearing loss that probably were due to prenatal streptomycin treatment and quoted a few comparable cases from the literature.

The ear often was deformed in children damaged by thalidomide in prenatal life. Knapp and Lenz[84] recognized malformations of the external and inner ear in 39 of 117 children with thalidomide embryopathy. In 15 cases, there was agenesis of the external ear and in 5 agenesis of the inner ear. Malformations

Fig. 41-14. – Defective helix in a newborn child damaged prenatally by aminopterin.[86] Note the low position of the auricle.

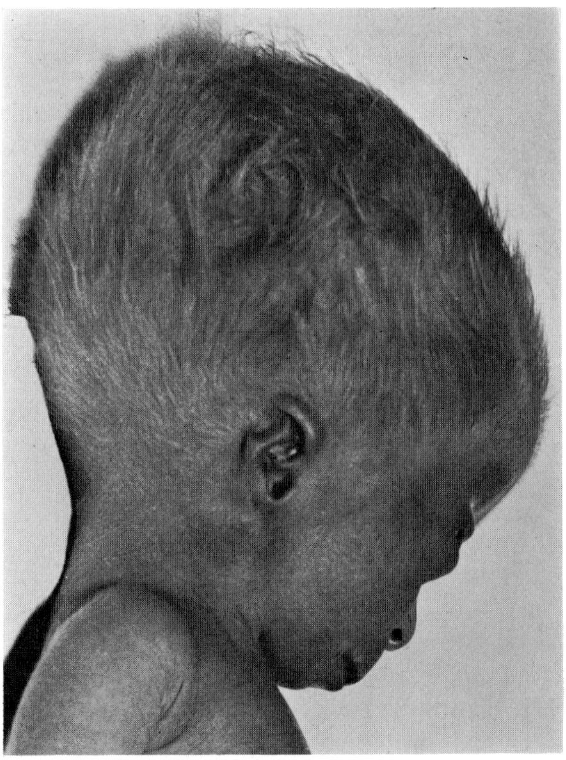

were present in 19. Anotia usually was bilateral, microtia unilateral. Differentiation of helix and lobule often was subnormal. In some cases, pedunculated appendages were seen in front of the tragus. Other reports concerning aural damage by thalidomide were cited by Rosendal,[85] who described aplasia and hypoplasia of the otic labyrinth in a girl exposed to the drug in utero.

In a case of prenatal exposure to aminopterin,[86] the ears were asymmetric and very low set (Fig. 41-14). On the right side, the helix was interrupted, terminating near the tip of the ear. The anthelix continued as a bar to the posterior aspect of the ear, where the helix was missing. On the left side, the ear was small and round, with abnormal molding.

Auriculo-osteodysplasia

Beals[92] described a syndrome of elbow dysplasia or dislocation, broad shoulders and an auricular anomaly. The external ear is characterized by a divided lobule, a failure of the helix and anthelix to unite inferiorly. The shape of the ear permits identification of the syndrome in neonates of affected kindreds. Dislocation of the hip in females, ulnarward sloping of the distal part of the radius and short stature are additional characteristics. The trait is inherited as an autosomal dominant characteristic.

REFERENCES

1. Ruzic, J.: Der siebente Fall kompletter Anotie, Acta oto-laryng. 36:186, 1948.
2. Ellwood, L. C., Winter, S. T., and Dar, H.: Familial microtia with meatal atresia in two sibships, J. M. Genetics 5:289, 1968.
3. Altmann, F.: Malformations of the auricle and the external auditory meatus, A.M.A. Arch. Otolaryng. 54:115, 1951.
4. Potter, E. L.: A hereditary ear malformation transmitted through 5 generations, J. Hered. 28:255, 1937.
5. Hanhart, E.: Nachweis einer einfach-dominanten, unkomplizierten sowie einer unregelmässig-dominanten, mit Atresia auris, Palatoschisis und anderen Deformationen verbundenen Anlage zu Ohrmuschelverkümmerung (Mikrotie), Arch. Klaus Stift. Vererbungsforsch. 24:374, 1949.
6. Peterson, D. M., and Schimke, R. N.: Hereditary cup-shaped ears and the Pierre Robin syndrome, J. M. Genetics 5:52, 1968.
7. Sharp, H. S.: Improvement of hearing in malformation of the external auditory meatus and middle ear, Brit. M. J. 2:758, 1952.
8. Livingstone, G.: Congenital ear abnormalities due to thalidomide, Proc. Roy. Soc. Med. 58:493, 1965.
9. Marx, H.: Die Missbildungen des Ohres, in Schwalbe, E. (ed.), *Die Morphologie der Missbildungen des Menschen und der Tiere* (Jena: Verlag-Fischer, 1911), Vol. III.
10. Giroud, A., Martinet, M., and Deluchat, C.: Otocéphalie, Compt. rend. Soc. franç. oto-rhino-laryngol. Cong. Paris, 1965.
11. Altmann, F.: Congenital atresia of the ear in man and animals, Ann. Otol. 64:824, 1955.
12. Selkirk, T. K.: Fistula auris congenita, Am. J. Dis. Child. 49:431, 1935.
13. Jones, F. W., and Wen, I. C.: The development of the external ear, J. Anat. 68:525, 1934.
14. Fourman, P., and Fourman, J.: Hereditary deafness in family with ear-pits, Brit. M. J. 2:1354, 1955.
15. Bol, G., and deKleyn, A.: Über einen Fall von Polyotie, Acta oto-laryng. 1:187, 1918.
16. Hough, J. V. D.: Congenital malformations of the middle ear, Arch. Otolaryng. 78:335, 1963.
17. Shambaugh, G. E., Jr.: Developmental anomalies of the sound conduction apparatus and their surgical correction, Ann. Otol. 61:873, 1952.
18. Pou, J. W.: Congenital absence of the oval window, Laryngoscope 73:384, 1963.
19. Bernstein, L.: Congenital absence of the oval window, Arch. Otolaryng. 83:535, 1966.
20. Nakamura, S., and Sando, I.: Congenital absence of the oval window, Arch. Otolaryng. 84:35, 1966.
21. Deol, M. S.: Inherited diseases of the inner ear in man in the light of studies on the mouse, J. M. Genetics 5:137, 1968.
22. Altmann, F.: Histologic picture of inherited nerve deafness in man and animals, Arch. Otolaryng. 51:852, 1950.
23. Lindenov, H.: The Ear, in Sorsby, A. (ed.), *Clinical Genetics* (St. Louis: The C. V. Mosby Company, 1953).
24. Ormerod, F. C.: The pathology of congenital deafness, J. Laryng. & Otol. 74:919, 1960.
25. Gedda, L., Maltarello, A., and Rédeky, M.: Les jumeaux sourds-muets – analyse génétique et clinique de sept couples de jumeaux atteints de surdi-mutité, J. Génét. Hum. 2:1, 1953.
26. Ward, P. H., Kinney, C. E., and Lindsay, J. R.: Inner ear pathology in congenital deafness, Laryngoscope 72:435, 1962.
27. Fraser, G. R.: A Study of Causes of Deafness Amongst 2,355 Children in Special Schools, in Fisch, L. (ed.), *Research in Deafness in Children* (Oxford: Blackwell Scientific Publications, 1964).
28. Fraser, G. R.: Profound childhood deafness, J. M. Genetics 1:118, 1964.
29. Van Egmond, A. A. J.: Congenital deafness, J. Laryng. & Otol. 68:429, 1954.
30. Fisch, L. (ed.): *Research in Deafness in Children* (Oxford: Blackwell Scientific Publications, 1964).
31. Mühlmann, W. E.: Ein ungewöhnlicher Stammbaum über Taubstummheit, Arch. Ross. ges. Biol. 22:181, 1929.
32. Danish, J. M., Tillson, J. K., and Levitan, M.: Multiple anomalies in congenitally deaf children, Eugenics Quart. 10:12, 1963.
33. Bell, J.: Retinitis Pigmentosa and Allied Diseases, in *Treasury of Human Inheritance*, Vol. III (London: Cambridge University Press, 1922).
34. Alström, C. H., Hallgren, B., Nilsson, L. B., and Asander, H.: Retinal degeneration combined with obesity, diabetes mellitus and neurogenous deafness, Acta psychiat. et neurol. scandinav., Supp. 129, 1, 1959.
35. Pendred, V.: Deaf-mutism and goiter, Lancet 2:532, 1896.
36. Sacrez, R., Juif J-G., Mandry, J., Kellershohn, C., Rivière, R., and Comar, D.: Le syndrome de Pendred. I. Étude critique, clinique et génétique, Ann. pédiat. 43:5, 1967.
37. Thould, A. K., and Scowen, E. F.: The syndrome of congenital deafness and simple goitre, J. Endocrinol. 30:69, 1964.
38. Elman, D. S.: Familial association of nerve deafness with nodular goiter and thyroid carcinoma, New England J. Med. 259:219, 1958.
39. Fraser, G. R.: Deafness with goitre (syndrome of Pendred) and some related aspects of thyroid disease, Thesis, University of London, 1960.
40. Jervell, A., and Lange-Nielsen, F.: Congenital deaf-mutism, functional heart disease with prolongation of the Q-T interval and sudden death, Am. Heart J. 54:59, 1957.
41. Wildervanck, L. S.: Perceptive deafness associated with split-hand and -foot, a new syndrome?, Acta Génét. Basel 13:161, 1963.
42. Sank, D.: The Genetic and Adjustive Aspects of Early Total Deafness, in Kallmann, F. J. (ed.), *Expanding*

Goals of Genetics in Psychiatry (New York: Grune & Stratton, Inc., 1962).
43. Stephens, F. E., and Dolowitz, D. A.: Hereditary nerve deafness, Am. J. Human Genet. 1:37, 1949.
44. Fisch, L.: Deafness as part of an hereditary syndrome, J. Laryng & Otol. 73:355, 1959.
45. Tietz, W.: A syndrome of deaf-mutism associated with albinism showing dominant autosomal inheritance, Am. J. Human Genet. 15:259, 1963.
46. Marshall, D.: Ectodermal dysplasia, Am. J. Ophth. 45: 143, 1958.
47. Lewis, S. M., Sonnenblick, B. P., Gilbert, L., and Biber, D.: Familial pulmonary stenosis and deaf-mutism: Clinical and genetic considerations, Am. Heart J. 55:458, 1958.
48. Gardner, W. J., and Turner, O.: Bilateral acoustic neurofibromas. Further clinical and pathologic data on hereditary deafness and Recklinghausen's disease, Arch. Neurol. & Psychiat. 44:76, 1940.
49. Mørch, E. T.: *Chondrodystrophic Dwarfs in Denmark* (Copenhagen: Munksgaard, 1941).
50. Nager, F. R., and Meyer, M.: Beiträge zur normalen und pathologischen Histologie der knöchernen Labyrinthkapsel; die Labyrinthkapsel beim endemischen Kretinismus, Beitr. Anat. Physiol. Path. Therap. Ohres. 30:45, 1932.
51. Strassburger, A. K., Hawkins, M. R., Eldridge, R., Hargrave, R. L., and McKusick, V. A.: Symphalangism: Genetic and clinical aspects, Bull. Johns Hopkins Hosp. 117: 108, 1965.
52. Forney, W. R., Robinson, S. J., and Pascoe, D. J.: Congenital heart disease, deafness, and skeletal malformations: A new syndrome?, J. Pediat. 68:14, 1966.
53. Everberg, G.: Further studies on hereditary unilateral deafness, Acta oto-laryng. 51:615, 1960.
54. Smith, A.: Unilateral hereditary deafness, Lancet 2:1172, 1939.
55. Sataloff, J., Pastore, P. M., and Bloom, E.: Sex-linked hereditary deafness, Am. J. Human Genet. 7:201, 1955.
56. Parker, N.: Congenital deafness due to a sex-linked recessive gene, Am. J. Human Genet. 10:196, 1958.
57. Margolis, E.: A new hereditary syndrome—sex-linked deaf-mutism associated with total albinism, Acta. Génét. Basel 12:12, 1962.
58. Altmann, F.: The ear in severe malformations of the head, Arch. Otolaryng. 66:7, 1957.
59. Vallesi, R. N.: L'orecchio nell'idrocefalo congenito, Boll. Mal. Orecch. 76:465, 1958.
60. Herberts, G.: Otological observations on the "Treacher Collins" syndrome, Acta oto-laryng. 54:457, 1962.
61. Hilson, D.: Malformation of ears as sign of malformation of genito-urinary tract, Brit. M. J. 2:785, 1957.
62. Hopkins, L. A.: Rubella-deafened infants, Am. J. Dis. Child. 78:182, 1949.
63. Clayton-Jones, E.: Rubella as a cause of congenital deafness in England, Lancet 1:56, 1947.
64. Goodhill, V.: The nerve-deaf child: Significance of Rh, maternal rubella and other etiologic factors, Ann. Otol. 59:1123, 1950.
65. Jackson, A. D. M., and Fisch, L.: Deafness following maternal rubella. Results of a prospective investigation, Lancet 2:1241, 1958.
66. Barr, B., and Lundström, R.: Deafness following maternal rubella. Retrospective and prospective studies, Acta oto-laryng. 53: 413, 1961.
67. Karmody, C. S.: Subclinical maternal rubella and congenital deafness, New England J. Med. 278:809, 1968.
68. Carruthers, D. G.: Congenital deaf-mutism as sequela of rubella-like maternal infection during pregnancy, M. J. Australia 1:315, 1945.
69. Töndury, G.: *Embryopathien*, Vol. XI of *Pathologie und Klinik in Einzeldarstellungen* (Berlin: Springer-Verlag, 1962).
70. Gray, J. E.: Rubella in pregnancy. Fetal pathology in the internal ear, Ann. Otol. 68:170, 1959.
71. Friedmann, I., and Wright, M. I.: Histopathological changes in the foetal and infantile inner ear caused by maternal rubella, Brit. M. J. 2:20, 1966.
72. Callahan, W. J., Russel, W. O., and Smith, M. G.: Human toxoplasmosis, Medicine 25:343, 1946.
73. Koch, F., Schorn, J., and Ule, G.: Über Toxoplasmose, Deutsch. Ztschr. Nervenh. 166:315, 1951.
74. Kelemen, G.: Toxoplasmosis and congenital deafness, A.M.A. Arch. Otolaryng. 68:547, 1958.
75. Kelemen, G., and Gotlib, B. N.: Pathohistology of fetal ears after maternal rubella, Laryngoscope 69:385, 1959.
76. Hinojosa, R.: Pathohistological aural changes in the progeny of a mother with pseudohypoparathyroidism, Ann. Otol. 67:964, 1958.
77. Cavanagh, F.: The rhesus factor in deafness, J. Laryng. & Otol. 68:444, 1954.
78. Byers, R. K., Paine, R. S., and Crothers, B.: Extrapyramidal cerebral palsy with hearing loss following erythroblastosis, Pediatrics 15:248, 1955.
79. Barton, M. E., Court, S. D., and Walker, W.: Causes of severe deafness in school children in Northumberland and Durham, Brit. M. J. 1:351, 1962.
80. Taylor, M.: Prenatal medication and its relation to the fetal ear, Surg., Gynec. & Obst. 64:542, 1937.
81. Winkel, C. W. F.: Quinine and congenital injuries of ear and eye of the foetus, J. Trop. Med. 51:2, 1948.
82. Kern, G.: On the problem of intrauterine streptomycin damage, Schweiz. med. Wchnschr. 92:77, 1962.
83. Robinson, G. C., and Cambon, K. G.: Hearing loss in infants of tuberculous mothers treated with streptomycin during pregnancy, New England J. Med. 271:949, 1964.
84. Knapp, K., and Lenz, W.: Die Formen der Thalidomid-Embryopathie, Roentgen, Europ. No. 5, 105, 1963.
85. Rosendal, T.: Thalidomide and aplasia-hypoplasia of the otic labyrinth, Lancet 1:724, 1963.
86. Warkany, J., Beaudry, P. H., and Hornstein, S.: Attempted abortion with 4-amino-pteroylglutamic acid (aminopterin); malformations of the child, A.M.A. J. Dis. Child. 97:274, 1959.
87. McRae, K. N., Uchida, I. A., and Lewis, M.: Sex-linked congenital deafness, Am. J. Human Genet. 21:415, 1969.
88. Fried, K., Feinmesser, M., and Tsitsianov, J.: Hearing impairment in female carriers of the sex-linked syndrome of deafness with albinism, J. M. Genetics 6:132, 1969.
89. Keaster, J., Human, C. B., and Harris, I.: Hearing problems subsequent to neonatal hemolytic disease or hyperbilirubinemia, Am. J. Dis. Child. 117:406, 1969.
90. Mengel, M. C., Konigsmark, B. W., Berlin, C. I. , and McKusick, V. A.: Conductive hearing loss and malformed low-set ears, as a possible recessive syndrome, J. M. Genetics 6:14, 1969.
91. Winter, J. S. D., Kohn, G., Mellman, W. J., and Wagner, S.: A familial syndrome of renal, genital, and middle ear anomalies, J. Pediat. 72:88, 1968.
92. Beals, R. K.: Auriculo-osteodysplasia. A syndrome of multiple osseous dysplasia, ear anomaly, and short stature, J. Bone & Joint Surg. 49-A:1541, 1967.
93. Konigsmark, B. W.: Hereditary deafness with external-ear abnormalities: A review, Johns Hopkins M. J. 127: 228, 1970.

PART VII

Malformations of Endocrine Glands

42

The Pituitary Gland

THE PITUITARY GLAND is derived from two ectodermal primordia that unite to form a composite structure situated at the base of the brain (hypophysis). In the fourth week, when the neural and digestive tubes are still in close proximity and not separated by prechordal mesoderm, two diverticula of these tubes come into contact with each other, constituting the pituitary primordium. The buccal evagination (Rathke pocket) arises external to the oropharyngeal membrane, extends upward and toward the brain, contacting with its blind end a diverticulum that comes down from the neural tube as the infundibular process. The communication of the Rathke pocket with the stomodeum is soon narrowed and converted into a cylindrical stalk that remains inserted into the roof of the pharynx. The Rathke pocket subsequently is divided into an upper cranial and a lower pharyngeal portion by the primordium of the sphenoid. The lower remnant persists in man as the pharyngeal pituitary, whereas the upper portion assumes the shape of a vesicle or cup into which the neural lobe of the infundibular process is implanted from above and behind. The rostral portion of the vesicle thickens greatly, assumes glandular appearance and becomes the pars anterior or distalis of the pituitary (adenohypophysis). The posterior layers of the vesicle remain in close contact with the infundibular process, constituting the pars intermedia of the pituitary. The lumen of the former pouch, surrounded by pars anterior and intermedia, persists as the residual lumen. Lateral lobes of the pars anterior, consisting of thin epithelial shelves, grow forward and backward and surround the infundibular process like a collar, forming the pars tuberalis.[1] In 3–4-month-old embryos, the pituitary gland has assumed its permanent shape and location.

Congenital Absence of the Pituitary Gland

Blizzard and Alberts[2] described a well-developed newborn boy who had a small penis and scrotum without palpable gonads. At necropsy, no hypophysis or infundibulum was found. The adrenal glands were small, the testes undescended, undersized and devoid of interstitial cells. Brewer[3] reported the case of a premature girl with bilateral harelip and anterior palate cleft who died after an attack of cyanosis. At necropsy, the sella was found empty; there was merely a small round knob in place of the pituitary stalk that histologically resembled normal posterior lobe tissue. The anterior lobe was completely absent. The adrenal cortices were thin and there was increased interstitial fibrous tissue in the thyroid; otherwise, the endocrine glands appeared normal. Reid[4] observed a full-term boy with erythroblastosis fetalis who died at the age of 19 hours in a period of apnea. Necropsy revealed a normal brain that had in the position of the pituitary stalk a small nodule that did not contain pituitary cells. The sella turcica was normally formed and covered by a fibrous diaphragm but did not contain a hypophysis. The thyroid and testes were hypoplastic. There was no adrenal gland on the right side but there were two disorganized adrenals on the left.

Congenital absence of the pituitary gland is extremely rare in infants who are free of serious congenital malformations. In anencephalic monsters, anomalies of the pituitary gland are frequent but it seems that the anterior lobe is always present.[5-7] The shape of the adenohypophysis sometimes is abnormal, particularly if it is retained at the roof of the pharynx or in an open craniopharyngeal canal

Fig. 42-1.—Transverse section through a near-term rat fetus with exencephaly and absence of pituitary gland produced by treatment of the mother with sodium salicylate on the ninth day of gestation. (From J. Warkany and E. Takacs.[52])

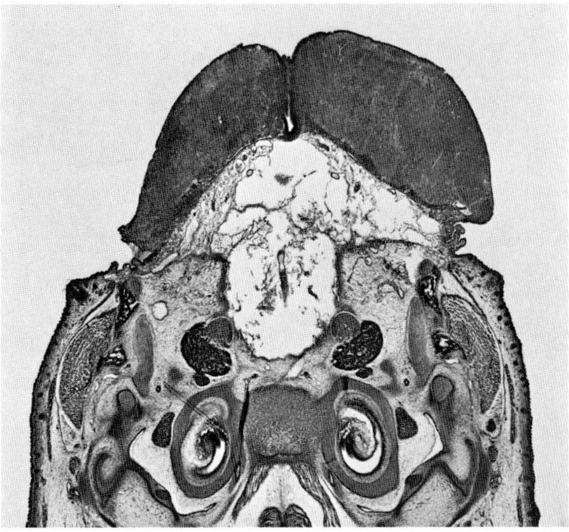

("Kanalhypophyse").[8] Absence or reduction in size of the neurohypophysis is common. If present, the pars neuralis may have no connection with the adenohypophysis or it may be separated from the cerebral remnants. Despite the presence of the adenohypophysis, the adrenal glands commonly are hypoplastic in anencephalic infants. It seems likely that separation from the hypothalamus results in abnormal function of the gland and in failure of adrenal stimulation.

In cyclopic infants, the pituitary gland may be absent as a manifestation of the median regional deficit characteristic of this anomaly. In such cases, the sella likewise is absent. Edmonds[9] examined 5 cyclopic fetuses; the pituitary was absent in 3 and present in 2. Fetuses without pituitary had small adrenal cortices and thyroids. In ethmocephaly, the pituitary can be absent and the adrenals small.[10]

Congenital Hypoplasia of the Pituitary Gland

Hypoplasia of the pituitary gland was reported by Mosier.[11] The patient was a normally formed twin girl who died 4 days after birth with symptoms of adrenal insufficiency. In the adenohypophysis, there was absence of acidophils, a decrease in PAS-positive material and a relative increase in basophils. The adrenals were minute.

Duplication of the Pituitary

Two pituitary glands lying on either side of the midline, posteromedial to the ends of the internal carotid arteries, were found at the base of the skull of an infant with multiple oral malformations.[12] Each pituitary consisted of a neurohypophysis and an adenohypophysis. There were large pharyngeal pituitaries that were composed of cells similar to those of the intracranial adenohypophysis. There also were two infundibula separated by a median elevation that contained nerve cells. The olfactory tracts were absent. Associated malformations were duplication of the lower lip, duplication of the mandible, frenula connecting the upper lip to the gum, a bar connecting the floor to the roof of the mouth and separating two tongues that were united to a single lingual mass behind the vertical bar, bilateral cleft palate and polyps.

Fig. 42-2.—Duplication of pituitary (*P–P*) in a cephalothoracopagus.

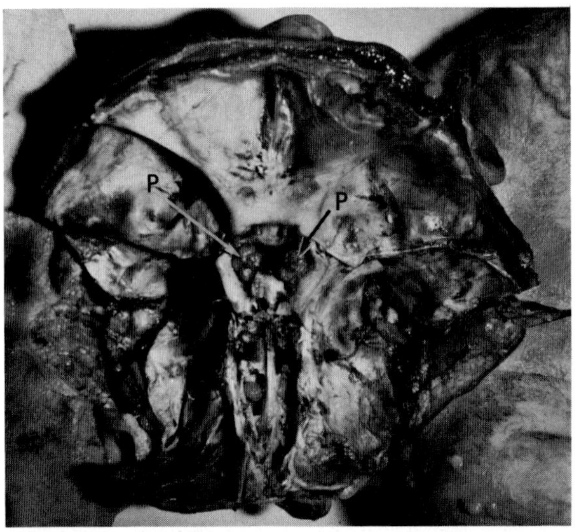

Persistence of the Craniopharyngeal Canal

As the Rathke pocket is divided by mesodermal tissue into a cranial and an oral portion, it is surrounded in part by the primordium of the sphenoid. The craniopharyngeal connection through the sphenoid regularly disappears as chondrification and ossification progress. Older statements in the literature that made it appear that persistence of a craniopharyngeal canal is common were refuted by Haberfeld,[13] who never found it in 256 normal skulls. But patent canals have been described repeatedly in association with congenital malformations. The skull anomalies occurring in anencephalic infants sometimes—but not always—are accompanied by a persistent craniopharyngeal canal that is situated in the midline, taking a course from the posterior cranial aspect of the sella to the anterior lower surface of the sphenoid body. Such canals vary in width and often contain pituitary tissue and blood vessels. Encephaloceles, which often are related in origin to anencephaly, can also be associated with craniopharyngeal communications. Haberfeld[13] described a canal in a child with harelip, cleft palate and hydrocephaly. In hydrocephalic individuals, pituitary tissue or encephalomeningoceles may be found in open canals. In cases of teratomas of the pituitary region, widely open craniopharyngeal canals are the rule.

In rare instances, a craniopharyngeal canal containing pituitary tissue can occur in otherwise well-formed persons and cause endocrine disturbances. Nichols and Delp[14] described a young man who had signs of Fröhlich syndrome, namely, small stature, obesity, hypogenitalism and symptoms of brain tumor. At operation, a calcified suprasellar cystic meningioma was found and removed. The patient lived 24 years after the operation with signs of panhypopituitarism. After death, pituitary tissue was found encased in the sphenoid bone but not in the sella. The thyroid gland and the gonads showed atrophy and the adrenal cortices were only partly maintained. Nichols and Delp concluded that in this case anterior lobe tissue failed to migrate to the sella and that the embryologic defect in the craniopharyngeal canal led subsequently to development of the cystic meningioma.

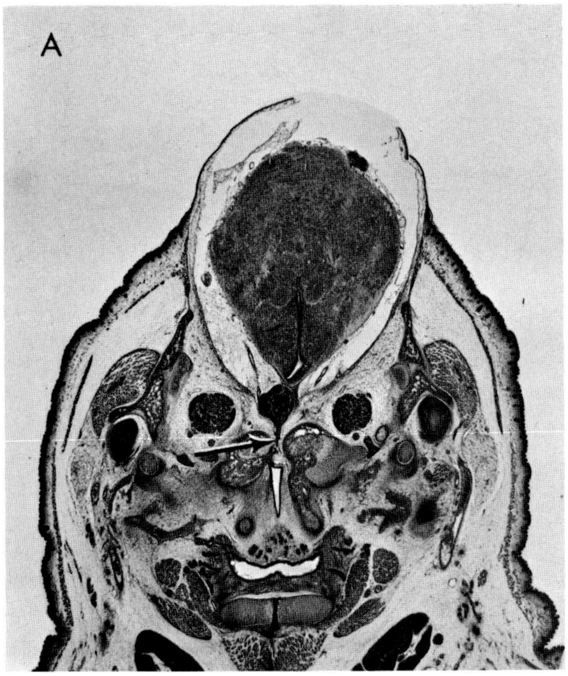

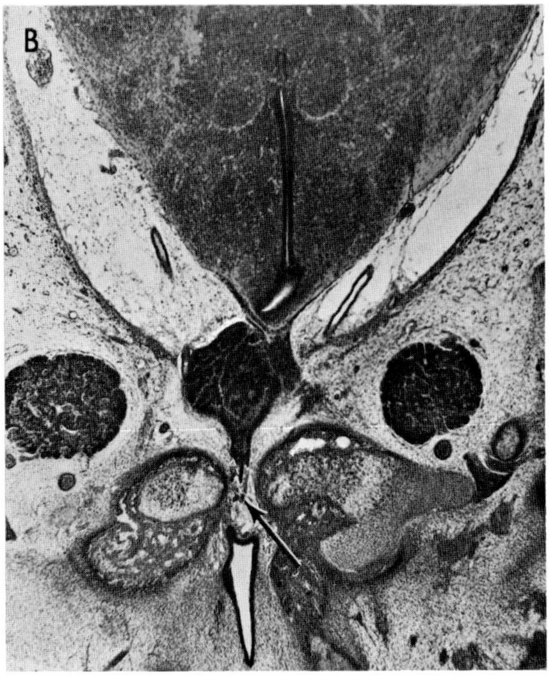

Fig. 42-3. – Frontal section through the head of a near-term rat fetus whose mother had been treated with large doses of streptonigrin on the tenth day of gestation. **A**, a craniopharyngeal canal connects the cranial and pharyngeal spaces (**arrow**). There are epithelial rests in the canal (**B**). Note the abnormal connection of the adenohypophysis with the infundibulum.

The Pharyngeal Pituitary

The Rathke pouch, from its origin in the stomodeum, migrates upward through mesenchymal tissue that later becomes the body of the sphenoid bone and comes to rest in the anlage of the sella turcica. There always remains a small piece of pituitary tissue in the pharyngeal mucosa at the place of the original oral end of the pouch. Melchionna and Moore,[15] in histologic studies, found a pharyngeal pituitary gland in 51 of 54 human bodies examined. Located in the midline, deep in the mucosa or in the periosteum beneath or near the vomerosphenoid articulation, it appeared most frequently as a single well-circumscribed and encapsulated structure.

The pharyngeal pituitary cells are chiefly chromophobes but there also are some eosinophilic cells. It seems that the cells of the pharyngeal pituitary can undergo differentiation even though they are away from vascular and nerve association with the hypothalamus.[16] Under normal conditions, it is unlikely that the pharyngeal pituitary gland has any significant physiologic function, but in some cases of altered activity of the cranial pituitary it is possible that the pharyngeal pituitary may undergo structural alterations and serve as an endocrine organ. After pregnancy, large cells of transitional epithelium have been seen in the pharyngeal pituitary, and in a patient with teratoma of the testes there were abundant acidophilic cells in it.[15] Although a pharyngeal pituitary is always present in man, it does not regularly occur in other mammals except the dog.

Pituitary Dystopia

Failure of proper union of the adenohypophysis with the neurohypophysis results in pituitary dystopia.[17] This term has been applied chiefly to malformations that show the posterior lobe outside and above the sella. The neurohypophysis can be located on the tuber cinereum (dystopia tuberalis), in the stalk (dystopia infundibularis) or above the adenohypophysis and solidly connected with it (dystopia opercularis). In dystopia tuberalis, the posterior lobe sits like a small tumor on the base of the brain. It can be connected with the anterior lobe in the sella by a short stalk. The adenohypophysis can also be deformed in such cases and be retained in the craniopharyngeal canal. In dystopia infundibularis, the posterior lobe is in a somewhat lower position and separated from the tuber cinereum by a portion of the infundibulum. Dystopia opercularis resembles the normal pituitary more than the other forms, since the neural lobe is embedded in the upper layers of the adenohypophysis, sometimes above and in front of its cranial surface. The neural lobe usually is not altered in its cytologic structure and the pituitary functions can be normal, but in some of the cases pituitary dwarfism,[17,18] adipo-

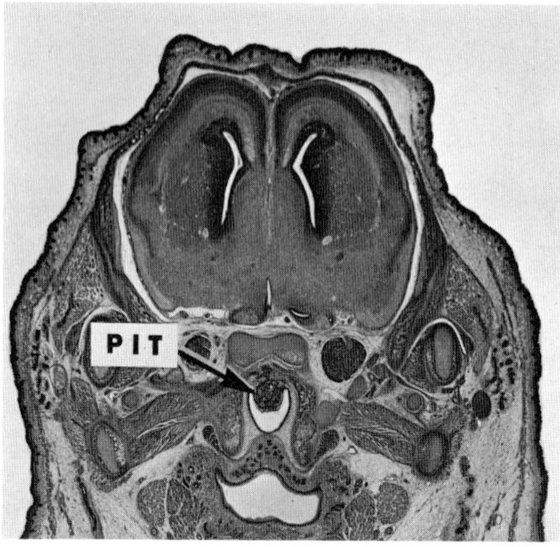

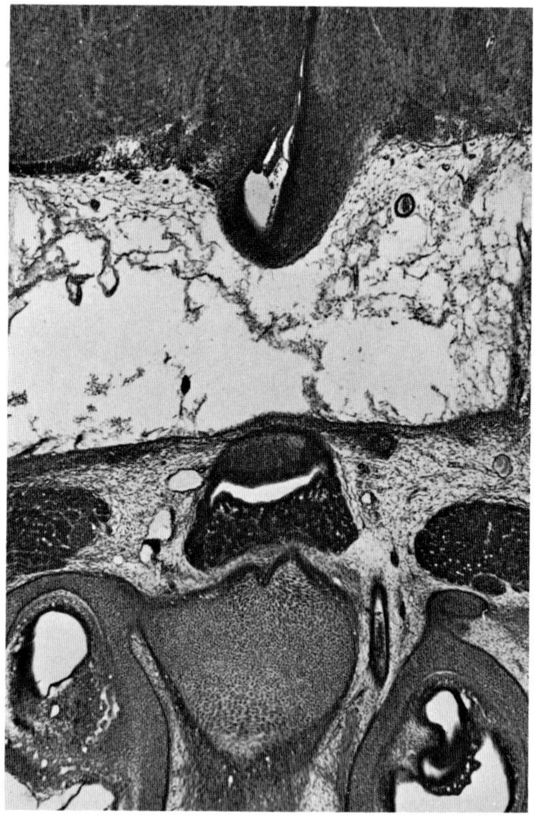

Fig. 42-4 (left). – Transverse section through the head of a newborn rat whose mother had been treated with trypan blue on the eighth to tenth day of gestation. Note the pituitary tissue hanging down into the pharynx and craniopharyngeal canal (**arrow**).

Fig. 42-5 (right). – Transverse section through the head of a near-term rat fetus whose mother had been treated with methyl salicylate on the ninth day of gestation. The pituitary gland and the infundibulum are separated by a wide space.

sogenital dystrophy[19] or diabetes mellitus[20] has been observed. Pituitary dystopia can be associated with craniopharyngioma.[21]

A different type of pituitary dystopia with hypoplasia of the gland was found in a 15-year-old girl who died in status epilepticus.[18] There were two separate nodules between the optic chiasm and the pedunculi that consisted of anterior and posterior pituitary tissues but in abnormal situation to each other and outside the sella turcica. Pharyngeal pituitary tissue was without signs of activity or hypertrophy. The suprasellar, small pituitary was deficient in eosinophilic cells. The child's birth weight had been within normal limits but she was very small and underweight at the time of death and thought to be a pituitary dwarf. Faulty alignment of the pituitary lobes can occur in persons who are mentally normal or sometimes it can account for dwarfism of mentally retarded patients. Joseph and Yannet[21a] described two cases of congenital idiocy, sexual infantilism and dwarfism. Necropsy of the brain of one of these patients showed widely disseminated focal ganglion cell loss, gliosis and ventricular malformation. The changes observed in the endocrine glands were compatible with a primary pituitary deficiency. The authors interpreted the clinical picture as the result of widespread cerebral maldevelopment, including failure of hypothalamic neural connections with the pituitary gland, leading to pituitary dysfunction and gonadotropic and growth hormone deficiency.

Rathke-Cleft Cysts

Tumors in the pituitary area can arise from the cleft of the Rathke pouch, which normally disappears in postnatal life, leaving only a residual cystic space between pars anterior and intermedia. Shanklin[22] observed 22 small cysts in 100 human pituitaries. Ciliated epithelium often was found lining the cysts, which suggested that they are derived from the Rathke cleft. It seems that tubules bearing ciliated epithelium grow from the cleft into the adjacent lobes, usually the anterior lobe. Although small cysts are frequent, they seldom grow sufficiently large to cause clinical symptoms. Cysts filled with mucus or colloid can expand within the sella or they can extend beyond it. Pituitary cachexia, dwarfism, infantilism and diabetes insipidus have been observed as clinical manifestations. Sometimes Rathke-cleft cysts are seen as incidental necropsy findings in persons who had no clinical disturbances.

Baar[23] observed pituitary cachexia in childhood brought about by large colloidal cysts of the Rathke cleft that caused pressure atrophy of the anterior lobe. The cysts can be associated with changes in the adrenal and parathyroid glands as well as in the gonads. Sandison[24] described a 15-year-old girl who died of malignant astrocytoma. She had been a proportionate dwarf from birth. There also was retarded mental development and poor sexual maturation. Dwarfism was due to hypoplasia of the pituitary gland, which was damaged by a Rathke-cleft cyst lined by cuboidal and columnar ciliated epithelium, and there was a chromophobic adenoma in the pars anterior of the pituitary. The combination of astrocytoma, adenoma and Rathke-cleft cyst suggests that developmental disturbances were responsible for these dissimilar tumors.

Craniopharyngioma (Adamantinoma, Ameloblastoma)

These tumors are thought to arise from nests of squamous epithelial cells in the pars tuberalis of the pituitary gland, which is derived in part from remnants of the craniopharyngeal duct. Atwell[1] believed that the epithelial layer on the anterior surface of the infundibular stalk, which can give rise to tumors in the hypophyseal region, is the pars tuberalis of the gland. The oral end of the craniopharyngeal duct is carried upward by "rotation" of the developing pituitary to the anterior infundibular surfaces of the adenohypophysis. This high location of the duct can explain the presence of displaced squamous epithelium on the anterior surface of the pituitary, on the stalk or on the infundibulum. The cells of the pars infundibularis are arranged in acini that in the adult consist mostly of chromophobic cells.

Erdheim[25] attributed certain tumors in the pituitary region to remnants of the craniopharyngeal duct. The pars tuberalis shows enlargements containing small groups of squamous cells derived from buccal epithelium that could be the source of squamous cell carcinomas or craniopharyngiomas. The embryologic origin of these tumors has been doubted by some authors[26] because squamous cell nests have been found rarely in pituitary glands of young persons, but Goldberg and Eshbaugh,[27] examining more than 100 pituitary glands of newborn infants, found nests of squamous cells in the pituitaries of 4 of them, 1 a premature. This finding supports the theory of the origin of craniopharyngiomas from embryonic squamous cell nests. The theory is further supported by the fact that craniopharyngiomas can occur in young children. A congenital adamantinoma was observed by Iyer[28] in the interpeduncular fossa encroaching on the third ventricle and producing hydrocephaly. It seems that 50% of adamantinomas occur in the first two decades of life and 14% in the first. Approximately 5% of all intracranial tumors in children are adamantinomas.[26,29] But craniopharyngiomas can manifest themselves as late as the seventh decade. Tiberin *et al.*[30] called attention to the fact that this congenital tumor may remain silent until old age.

Tumors derived from the hypophyseal duct do not elaborate hormones but they can bring about endocrine symptoms by pressure on neighboring organs. Craniopharyngiomas can be solid or present as cysts lined by smooth epithelium or by papillary excrescences. They can be malignant or benign. Some of these tumors grow slowly and some can regress. There is a strong tendency to calcification, which can be seen in roentgenograms. Localization of craniopharyngiomas varies. Intrasellar tumors occur but they are rare. If they begin in early childhood, they can destroy the anterior lobe and produce pituitary dwarfism. Children with such tumors are born normal in size but show growth failure 1 or several years after birth, remaining subnormal in progress of ossification and immature in sexual development.

Craniopharyngiomas arise more often in the pituitary stalk or in the infundibulum than within the sella. In such cases, the gland is only indirectly affected while the tumor exerts pressure on the brain. The results can be those of Fröhlich syndrome with pituitary dwarfism, obesity and sexual impairment. Cysts lined with squamous epithelium and lying over the sella turcica have been found repeatedly in patients presenting with these signs. Infundibular epiphyseal duct tumors compressing the third ventricle and assuming its place can cause pituitary as well as hypothalamic signs.[31] Combination of craniopharyngioma with pituitary dystopia (p. 421) has been observed. Apitz[21] described it in a man 46 years of age who had pituitary dwarfism and infantilism. At necropsy, complete separation of the pars anterior and pars nervosa of the pituitary was found. The neurohypophysis was suprasellar and separated from the adenohypophysis by a small craniopharyngioma. The case is of interest because it shows that separation of the two lobes (pituitary dystopia) can result in dysfunction of the pars anterior. Furthermore, it seems noteworthy that the malformation of the hypophysis was combined with a tumor derived from the hypophyseal duct, betraying the teratologic nature of this craniopharyngioma. But the congenital malformation of the pituitary failed to manifest itself before the patient was 10 years of age.

Pituitary Dwarfism

The causes of pituitary dwarfism are only partially known but it is established that they are varied and heterogeneous. Martin and Wilkins[32] analyzed 26 cases of pituitary dwarfism past the age of puberty. Seven patients had neoplasms in the region of the sella turcica, whereas 19 had so-called idiopathic pituitary insufficiency. The tumors were not specified and it is not clear how many of them could be attributed to congenital defects. All cases took a chronic course. Tumor symptoms occurred between the ages of 4 and 12 years. In 19 patients with idiopathic pituitary insufficiency, growth retardation commenced at an early age. The sex distribution in the two groups is of interest because in the tumor group there were 5 females and 2 males, whereas in the idiopathic group there was only 1 female and 19 males. It is possible that many idiopathic cases are determined by genetic factors. A great deal can be learned about this type by the fact that genetically determined pituitary dwarfism has been identified in various strains of mice as an autosomal recessive characteristic.[33,34] Like human pituitary dwarfs, mice destined to become dwarfed appear normal at birth and cannot be distinguished easily from their normal litter mates, but in the third week they are recognizable by their smaller size, shorter snout and shorter tail. In some strains, the dwarfs become emaciated, in others they develop obesity. Both sexes are sterile. Histologically, the posterior lobe looks normal, whereas the anterior lobe is much reduced in size. Interestingly, at birth, the anterior lobe appears normal, whereas at the age of 12 days abnormal size and structure become noticeable. The changes in the adenohypophysis, the thyroid, the adrenals and the gonads have been studied thoroughly in pituitary dwarf mice.[34]

It can be assumed that in human beings some cases of pituitary dwarfism are comparable to those observed in mice. Rischbieth and Barrington[35] collected examples of pituitary dwarfs and their pedigrees. Many of the cases listed are compatible with the hypothesis of autosomal recessive inheritance. It is true that the diagnosis of pituitary dwarfism cannot be considered established in all the patients because laboratory data or roentgenograms are not available, but the description of the dwarfs and their pictures are in some cases most suggestive of pituitary dwarfism.

A rather impressive sibship was reported by Schmolck[36] from the Samnaun Valley in the Alps, where, among 356 inhabitants of an isolated village, 7 dwarfs were found who, according to their photographs, were pituitary dwarfs. There was a great deal of intermarriage in that area, as the same names recurred repeatedly. Hanhart[37] discovered recessively inherited dwarfism with adiposogenital dystrophy of variable degree in Swiss isolates in whom inbreeding had existed for centuries. Kirchhoff and Schaefer[38] mentioned 3 dwarfed siblings in a family with 4 children. Among 14 pituitary dwarfs, they established minor malformations of the extremities in 7.

Trygstad and Seip[39] published cases of hereditary pituitary dwarfism that were analyzed with modern methods and treated successfully with human growth hormone. These dwarfs were found in a family in which 8 members – 4 males and 4 females – through five generations had been abnormally short. Three of the dwarfs, a brother and a sister among them, were studied in detail. They were normal in size and weight at birth but showed growth retardation either during the first year of life or in early childhood. Some of the small members of this kinship were married and proved to be fertile. These were thought to have isolated growth hormone deficiency without concomitant lack of gonadotropic hormone. The disorder was considered to be hereditary with an autosomal recessive mode of transmission.

It is possible that some of the sporadic or "idiopathic" pituitary dwarfs seen in endocrine clinics are also affected because of recessive inheritance, but the genetic origin of their anomaly cannot be proved because of lack of familial repetition and parental consanguinity. But sporadic cases also can be due to tumors in the sellar region or due to postnatal pathologic processes. One may find dwarfism (associated with diabetes insipidus) subsequent to scarlet fever, pertussis or in the course of xanthomatosis.[40] That anterior hypopituitarism can be determined by nongenetic factors is shown in instances of discordance of this trait in monozygotic twins.[41,42]

Wolfe *et al.*[43] described a case of pituitary dwarfism associated with signs of congenital toxoplasmosis. The patient showed retarded growth and sexual immaturity at the age of 19 years. The authors considered the possibility that toxoplasma infection of the pituitary or hypothalamus may have been the cause of the pituitary hypofunction.

Teratomas in the Pituitary Area

Dislocation of cells and faulty differentiation that has a rather complicated origin can occur in the area of the pituitary. The normal pituitary results from coordinated growth of the oral cavity, the Rathke pouch, neural tube, notochord and intermediate mesoderm. Faulty development in the pituitary angle can result in teratomas of the epignathus type that protrude from the mouth and may be connected above with the cranial cavity. Such teratomas go through the craniopharyngeal canal, where they are constricted, mushrooming into the cranial and oral cavities.[19] Or a teratoma can originate at the cranial end of an open canal and grow toward the brain and penetrate it. Association with malformations such as dextroposition of the aorta, malrotation of the intestine, and so forth, indicates that such tumors are closely related to general developmental errors.[44] Less serious malformations in this area can be compatible with postnatal life. A teratoma-like tumor containing bone, teeth and other tissues was described by Beck[45] in a 74-year-old woman who died of old age. The tumor, situated in an enlarged sella, compressed the chiasma opticum and was covered on its upper surface by remnants of adenohypophyses and neurohypophyses. The complicated embryology of the pituitary angle probably is responsible for other tumors in that area as well as for malformations that can elicit endocrine and general disturbances.

Hyperpituitarism and Acromegaly

Congenital infantile hyperpituitarism is rare. Behrens and Barr[46] reported a case of hyperpituitarism beginning soon after birth. They described a boy who weighed 4,050 Gm. at birth and began almost immediately to grow at an abnormal rate. When he was 9 years of age, he measured 185 cm. and weighed 76 kg.; he was able to pick his father up and carry him about. His lips were thick and the chin somewhat protruding, but his hands and feet were normally shaped. His appearance was not typical of acromegaly. The sella turcica was very large in its anteroposterior diameter and roentgenograms suggested a persistent craniopharyngeal canal. The boy was shy and reticent but his progress in school was good. At the age of 13, he was more than 210 cm. tall, towered over his father and brother, who were of normal size, and weighed 125 kg. His growth from birth on apparently was continuous, without spurts or notable periods of quiescence. Except for the large size of the sella turcica, there were no local signs of pituitary involvement or brain tumor. Another case of pituitary gigantism was observed by Hurxthal[47] in a child 5 years of age whose symptoms had begun at age 3 years. The sella was large and overgrowth was attributed to an eosinophilic adenoma of the pituitary, which responded to x-ray treatment. Todd[48] reported a case of acromegaly in a girl of 8 years whose symptoms—enlarged hands and abnormal facial appearance—were present when she was 5½ years of age. There was rapid growth of the skeleton without acceleration of skeletal maturation; the sella turcica was enlarged but there were no destructive changes and no intracranial calcifications. At the age of 9 years, bilateral papilledema appeared and a ventriculogram revealed a large suprasellar lesion that was blocking the spinal fluid. Chromophobe adenomas of the pituitary in a father and son were reported by Koch and Tiwisina.[49] In both patients, the pituitary tumors were removed surgically and histologic examination proved adenoma of the pituitary in both, but the clinical syndrome of acromegaly was present only in the son.

Since acromegaly usually begins during late childhood or in adult life, one does not consider this anomaly in the context of congenital malformations. But, in some cases, the pituitary anomaly that causes acromegaly is part of a developmental disturbance that goes back to early prenatal life. Persistence of the craniopharyngeal canal was described by Levi[50] in two skeletons with obvious signs of acromegaly. He quoted Cunningham, who found in an acromegalic giant not only an enormous dilatation of the sella turcica, but also a communication between the pituitary fossa and the nasal cavity. Behrens and Barr,[46] describing the Alton giant who had gigantism beginning soon after birth (see above), stated that roentgenograms showed in the floor of the sella turcica a tubular structure that extended downward and forward from the sella and reached almost to the posterior wall of the pharynx, where there was an indefinite soft tissue shadow encroaching on the lumen of the pharynx.

Goliath Syndrome

According to the Bible (I Samuel, 17), a Philistine giant named Goliath challenged the Israelites to select a representative to fight him. Young David, who was supposed to supply his brothers with victuals sent by their father, volunteered to fight the heavily armed Goliath with a stick and five smooth stones. When the Philistine giant arose and went to meet David, the young lad took a stone from his pouch, slung it and struck the Philistine on his forehead. The stone sank into his forehead and Goliath fell to the ground on his face. David ran and stood by the Philistine, took his sword and cut off his head. When the Philistines saw that their champion was dead, they fled. This victory started David on his career and his complicated relationship to Saul, the king.

There is a possibility that the Philistine champion actually was less formidable than he appeared. It seems that another member of the giant family, possibly a brother of Goliath—but in any case a man of great stature—was slain in a battle in Gath. This Philistine giant "had on every hand six fingers, and on every foot six toes, in all, four and twenty in number" (II Samuel, 21:20). Since polydactyly can be associated with pituitary-hypothalamic anomalies, one could suspect that the family of giants may have had some handicaps resembling those of persons with the Laurence-Moon-Biedl syndrome, although stature usually is subnormal in patients with that syndrome. But there is a report by de Cyon[51] that deals with juvenile acromegaly and polydactyly, a syndrome that may correspond to the condition of Goliath and his brother, the sons of Raphah. De Cyon described a boy, 12 years of age, who from early infancy showed excessive skeletal development and adiposity, intellectual apathy, intense headaches, narrowing of the pupils, nystagmus, drooping of the eyelids and small, frequent and irregular pulse. He had 2 brothers, 7½ and 5½ years of age, who had the same disorder, although in differing degrees. All 3 had 6 toes bilaterally. If Goliath and his brother were acromegalics suffering from headaches, eye trouble and intellectual apathy, their defeat appears understandable. One can only speculate what a stone thrown at the forehead of an acromegalic could do to a person with such a pituitary anomaly.

REFERENCES

1. Atwell, W. J.: Development of hypophysis cerebri in man with special reference to pars tuberalis, Am. J. Anat. 37: 159, 1926.
2. Blizzard, R. M., and Alberts, M.: Hypopituitarism, hypoadrenalism and hypogonadism in the newborn infant, J. Pediat. 48:782, 1956.
3. Brewer, D. B.: Congenital absence of the pituitary gland and its consequences, J. Path. & Bact. 73:59, 1957.
4. Reid, J. D.: Congenital absence of the pituitary gland, J. Pediat. 56:658, 1960.
5. Covell, W. P.: A quantitative study of the hypophysis of the human anencephalic monster, Am. J. Path. 3:17, 1927.

6. Kraus, E. J.: Die Entwicklungsstörungen der Hypophyse, in Schwalbe, E., and Gruber, G. B. (eds.), *Die Morphologie der Missbildungen des Menschen und der Tiere* (Jena: Gustav Fischer, 1929), Vol. 3.
7. Angevine, D. M.: Pathologic anatomy of hypophysis and adrenals in anencephaly, Arch. Path. 26:507, 1938.
8. Kohn, A.: Anencephalie und Nebenniere, Arch. mikr. Anat. u. Entwicklungsmechanik 102:113, 1924.
9. Edmonds, H. W.: Pituitary, adrenal and thyroid in cyclopia, Arch. Path. 50:727, 1950.
10. Haworth, J. C., Medovy, H., and Lewis, A. J.: Cebocephaly with endocrine dysgenesis; report of 3 cases, J. Pediat. 59:726, 1961.
11. Mosier, H. D.: Hypoplasia of the pituitary and adrenal cortex, J. Pediat. 48:633, 1956.
12. Morton, W. R. M.: Duplication of the pituitary and stomatodaeal structures in a 38-week male infant, Arch. Dis. Childhood 32:135, 1957.
13. Haberfeld, W.: Zur Pathologie des Canalis craniopharyngeus, Frankfurt. Ztschr. Path. 4:96, 1910.
14. Nichols, J., and Delp, M.: Craniopharyngeal pituitary gland, J.A.M.A. 185:643, 1963.
15. Melchionna, R. H., and Moore, R. A.: The pharyngeal pituitary gland, Am. J. Path. 14:763, 1938.
16. Boyd, J. D.: Observations on the human pharyngeal hypophysis, J. Endocrinol. 14:66, 1956.
17. Priesel, A.: Über die Dystopie der Neurohypophyse, Virchows Arch. path. Anat. 266:407, 1927.
18. Ehrlich, R. M.: Ectopic and hypoplastic pituitary with adrenal hypoplasia, J. Pediat. 51:377, 1957.
19. Kraus, E. J.: Über ein epignathisches Teratom der Hypophysengegend, Virchows Arch. path. Anat. 271:546, 1929.
20. Lennox, B., and Russel, D. S.: Dystopia of the neurohypophysis, J. Path. & Bact. 63:485, 1951.
21. Apitz, K.: Zur Pathogenese des hypophysären Kleinwuchses, Virchows Arch path. Anat. 302:555, 1938.
21a. Joseph, C., and Yannet, H.: Congenital idiocy, sexual infantilism, and dwarfism, Yale J. Biol. & Med. 24:257, 1952.
22. Shanklin, W. H.: Incidence and distribution of cilia in the human pituitary with a description of micro-follicular cysts derived from Rathke's cleft, Acta anat. 11:361, 1951.
23. Baar, H. S.: Dysontogenic pituitary cysts: Pituitary cachexia in childhood, Arch. Dis. Childhood 22:118, 1947.
24. Sandison, A. T.: Autopsy findings in a case of pituitary dwarfism, Arch. Dis. Childhood 33:469, 1958.
25. Erdheim, J.: Über einen Hypophysentumor von ungewöhnlichem Sitz, Beitr. path. Anat. 46:233, 1909.
26. Kernohan, J. W., and Sayre, G. P.: Tumors of the Pituitary Gland and Infundibulum, in *Atlas of Tumor Pathology*, Sec. X, Fasc. 36 (Washington, D. C.: Armed Forces Institute of Pathology, 1956).
27. Goldberg, G. M., and Eshbaugh, D. E.: Squamous cell nests of the pituitary gland as related to the origin of craniopharyngiomas; a study of their presence in the newborn and infants up to age four, Arch. Path. 70:293, 1960.
28. Iyer, C. G. S.: Case report of an adamantinoma present at birth, J. Neurosurg. 9:221, 1952.
29. Ingraham, F. D., and Scott, H. W., Jr.: Craniopharyngiomas in children, J. Pediat. 29:95, 1946.
30. Tiberin, P., Goldberg, G. M., and Schwartz, A.: Craniopharyngioma in the aged, Neurology 8:51, 1958.
31. Erdheim, J.: Die pathologisch-anatomischen Grundlagen der hypophysären Skelettveränderungen (Zwergwuchs, Typus Fröhlich, Akromegalie, Riesenwuchs), Fortschr. Geb. Röntgenstrahlen 52:234, 1935.
32. Martin, M. M., and Wilkins, L: Pituitary dwarfism: Diagnosis and treatment, J. Clin. Endocrinol. 18:679, 1958.
33. Snell, G. D.: Dwarf, a new Mendelian recessive character in the house mouse, Proc. Nat. Acad. Sc. 15:733, 1929.
34. Grüneberg, H.: *The Genetics of the Mouse* (2d ed.; The Hague: Martin Nijhoff, 1952).
35. Rischbieth, H., and Barrington, A.: Dwarfism, in *Treasury of Human Inheritance* (London: Dulau & Company, Ltd., 1912), Vol. 1, pts VII and VIII.
36. Schmolck: Mehrfacher Zwergwuchs in verwandten Familien eines Hochgebirgstales, Virchows Arch. path. Anat. 187:105, 1907.
37. Hanhart, E.: Über die Bedeutung der Erforschung von Inzuchtsgebieten an Hand von Ergebnissen bei Sippen mit hereditärer Ataxie, heredodegenerativem Zwergwuchs und sporadischer Taubheit, Schweiz. med. Wchnschr. 54:1143, 1924.
38. Kirchhoff, H. W., and Schaefer, U.: Hypophysärer Zwergwuchs im Kindesalter. Eine klinische und anthropologische Studie, Ztschr. Kinderh. 75:267, 1954.
39. Trygstad, O., and Seip, M.: Hereditary pituitary dwarfism treated with human growth hormone, Acta paediat. 53: 527, 1964.
40. Warkany, J., and Mitchell, A. G.: Diabetes insipidus in children, Am. J. Dis. Child. 57:603, 1939.
41. Rosenbloom, A. L., and Smith, D. W.: Idiopathic anterior hypopituitarism in one of identical twins, J. Pediat. 67:84, 1965.
42. Rosenfield, R. L., Root, A. W., Bongiovanni, A. M., and Eberlein, W. R.: Idiopathic anterior hypopituitarism in one of monozygous twins, J. Pediat. 70:114, 1967.
43. Wolfe, S. M., Sawitz, W. G., and Paschkis, K. E.: Pituitary dwarfism and toxoplasmosis, J. Clin. Endocrinol. 15:745, 1955.
44. Gautier, R.: Zur Kenntnis der Mischgeschwülste der Hypophysengegend, Frankfurt. Ztschr. Path. 19:247, 1916.
45. Beck, H.: Über ein Teratom der Hypophysis cerebri, Ztschr. Heilkunde. 4:393, 1883.
46. Behrens, L. H., and Barr, D. P.: Hyperpituitarism beginning in infancy. The Alton giant, Endocrinology 16:120, 1932.
47. Hurxthal, L. M.: Pituitary gigantism in a child five years of age: Effect of x-radiation, estrogen therapy and self-imposed starvation diet during an eleven-year period, J. Clin. Endocrinol. 21:343, 1961.
48. Todd, R. M.: Acromegaly in a girl of 8 years, Arch. Dis. Childhood 33:49, 1958.
49. Koch, G., and Tiwisina, T.: Beitrag zur Erblichkeit der Akromegalie und der Hyperostosis generalisata mit Pachydermie, Ärztliche Forschung 13:489, 1959.
50. Levi, E.: Persistenza del canale cranio-faringèo in due cranii di acromegalici: Significata ed importanza di questo nuovo reperto in rapporto alla patogenesi dell'acromegalia e delle sindromi ipofisarie in genere, Riv. crit. clin. med. 10:361, 1909.
51. de Cyon, E.: Traitement de l'acromégalie par hypophysine, Acad. méd. Paris, 1898.
52. Warkany, J., and Takacs, E.: Changes of endocrine glands by teratogenic methods, Arch. Path. 85:101, 1968.

43

The Adrenal Gland

THE ADRENAL GLAND of mammals, including man, is a composite structure formed by cortex and medulla. The latter is made up of cells derived from the neural crest but transformed into glandular cells after temporary contact with the sympathetic ganglia. The medulla is surrounded by the adrenal cortex, which is derived from splanchnic mesoderm located on both sides of the root of the mesentery mesial to the urogenital folds.

Crowder[1] described in great detail the development of the human adrenal, with special reference to origin and ultimate location of cell types. The earliest evidence of the adrenal primordium is found in the fifth week, when cells derived from the celomic epithelium enter the mesenchyme between the aorta and the mesonephros on the level of the sixth to the twelfth thoracic segments. Soon thereafter, similar cells enter the ventral surface of the primordium from the capsule of the mesonephric glomeruli. These cells migrate into the adrenal periphery during the sixth week to become the capsule. The dorsal portion of the whole cortical primordium is invaded by medullary elements, sympathetic nerves and paraganglion cells.

Development of the adrenal medulla begins during week five, when nerve fibers appear ventrally and laterally from the sympathetic ganglia accompanied by paraganglion cells. The most important part of this system is located above the developing kidneys. It is this part that is destined to form the adrenal medulla, whereas other paraganglion cells are situated at various levels along the aorta, constituting, in places, sizable cell aggregations on both sides of the aorta or joining in front of it (aortic chromaffin body of Zuckerkandl). During the eighth week, there is rapid multiplication of paraganglion elements scattered along the nerve tracts, a process that continues into the neonatal period. The neural tissue invades the cortical portions in such quantity that the volume of the adrenal primordium is greatly increased.

The adrenal cortex is well developed and clearly recognizable in embryos of the seventh and eighth weeks, and in the third month a differentiation into permanent and provisional cortex can be recognized. At first, only the inner part of the cortex (the provisional cortex) consists of mature cell cords separated by sinusoids, whereas the outer part is less differentiated and destined to become the permanent cortex. The glomerular zone is formed as arterial capillaries penetrate the capsule, packing the glomeruli between them. From the end of week seven to week ten, the adrenal gland is shaped like a pyramid with an overhanging lip on its medioanterior border. The position of the adrenal glands over the kidneys is established by cephalic migration of the latter, whereby the large fetal adrenals become situated over the cranial renal poles, equaling in size the kidneys from the third fetal month to the time of birth. After the twelfth week, the growth of the gland is extremely rapid in a limited space and the cords assume a reticular appearance. In the central reticulofascicular portion (the provisional zone), cell destruction sets in toward the end of gestation.

The adrenal of the human fetus is ten to twenty times larger than the adult gland relative to body weight, but not all portions of the gland are equally involved in the enlargement.[2] Four-fifths of the fetal gland are made up of fetal zone, a centrally located structure composed of large cells with pale-staining nuclei and abundant, eosinophilic cytoplasm. The remaining fifth of the gland consists of a thin fascicular zone and a poorly differentiated glomerular zone, both containing small cells with small, dense nuclei and scanty cytoplasm. Within a few hours or days after birth, the fetal zone rapidly undergoes involution, often with hemorrhage and necrosis and with the appearance of abundant fat-staining material. Simultaneously, the fascicular zone lengthens, the glomerular zone assumes the adult architecture and the cells of both permanent zones acquire more abundant cytoplasm. As these changes take place, there is a loss of approximately 50% in the total weight of the gland within 2 or 3 weeks.

Tähkä[3] made a study of the weight and structure of the adrenal glands in children from birth to 2 years of age. The absolute weight of the adrenals decreases from birth to the age of 3 months from 6.5 to 3.5 Gm. Then the weight rises slowly without attaining the weight of the newborn by the age of 2 years. The relative weight of the adrenals decreases continually from birth to 2 years. The reduction of the adrenals in the earliest months of life is due largely to the involution of the fetal cortex.

Adrenal Aplasia

Absence of both adrenals has been reported repeatedly in children as well as in adults. It is obvious that postnatal life without adrenals is impossible, and most pertinent reports should be considered with skepticism. Even with anencephaly and other severe cerebral anomalies, adrenals are found in rudimentary form if a thorough search is made.[4] But there are numerous reliable reports of unilateral absence of an adrenal gland. Pagel[5] listed several examples from the older literature. Absence of one adrenal has been observed in cases of fusion of the extremities. Absence of the right adrenal can be associated with aplasia or malformation of the kidney, ureter and colon, but, in general, the adrenals are normal in cases of malformed kidneys. It is of interest that in most instances unilateral adrenal aplasia occurs on the right side, which generally is more subject to adrenal variations than the left. The adrenal of the opposite side may be so affected by various pathologic processes that Addison disease results. In other instances, hypertrophy of the contralateral adrenal has been observed.[5] Absence of both adrenals and the anterior pituitary in a live-born normocephalic child has been reported.[20]

Congenital Adrenal Hypoplasia

When Jaudon,[6] in 1946, made a critical review of Addison disease in children, he could find only 4 proved cases under 5 years of age. The youngest case presented by him probably was not congenital but resulted from acquired tuberculosis. Two years later, in 1948, Sikl[7] reported briefly a case of Addison disease due to congenital hypoplasia of the adrenals in a boy 33 days of age. The child had appeared normal at birth but failed to thrive, and from 3 weeks on the skin became increasingly darker. After the child died, the adrenals were found to be extremely hypoplastic, the volume being about 1/100th that of the normal. Histologically, the cortex and medulla could not be distinguished. The pituitary appeared grossly and microscopically normal. Deamer and Silver[8] reported the case of a boy who failed to gain weight because of vomiting that began shortly after birth and suggested pyloric stenosis. On laparotomy, no pyloric hypertrophy was demonstrated. The patient died at the age of 10 months, and at necropsy the adrenals showed only small islands of a markedly hypoplastic cortex on one side and complete absence of cortical elements on the other. Other cases were described by Williams and Robinson,[9] but Mosier's[10] patients were of special interest because there was hypoplasia of the adrenal cortex in twin girls. Necropsy performed in one infant, dead at 4 days, revealed adrenals that, together, weighed only 0.35 Gm. (normal weight at birth for both adrenals is approximately 6.5 Gm.). The cortex was yellow on cut sections and its lipids histologically appeared normal or increased in amount. Glomerulosa, fasciculata and reticularis were developed but there were only traces of fetal cortex. The small pituitary showed an absence of acidophils, a decrease in PAS-positive material and a relative increase in basophils. In the twin sister, who had died before, the adrenals together had weighed less than 1 Gm. The adrenal hypoplasia observed by Ehrlich[11] was associated with a congenital malformation of the pituitary gland. At necropsy, performed at age 15 months, there were two extrasellar nodules near the optic chiasma that proved to be ectopic pituitary tissue. The adrenals had a combined weight of only 1.2 Gm. but microscopically the three layers of the cortex were evident and they were present in their usual proportions. The medulla also was normal. But such miniature adrenals, similar in structure to the normal adult gland, are not always found in adrenal insufficiency. There are cases of adrenal failure in infancy in which the cortex is composed of one type of cells only that look like those of fetal adrenal.[12,13] The entire cortical area is occupied by eosinophilic cells, many of which are several times larger than normal. There is no division of the cortex into zones and no peripheral permanent cortex made up of small basophilic cells arranged in compact orderly rows, as is normally seen at this age. These glands are different from the miniature adrenals commonly associated with the anencephalic condition and those described above.[10,11] The cells also differ from those seen in the adrenals of children suffering from Addison disease associated with the adrenogenital syndrome. It was assumed that the absence of the zona glomerulosa explained the disease picture, which consisted of failure of electrolyte control. The same kind of congenital adrenal hypoplasia with large cells resembling those found in the fetal cortex has been observed in a boy whose brother, who apparently had the same disorder, survived with the aid of treatment of his electrolyte disturbance.[14] Kerenyi[15] tabulated 9 cases of congenital adrenal hypoplasia and divided them into two classes: The "miniature adult" type, which occurs in anencephalics and sometimes in infants without associated congenital malformations,[10,11] is commonly associated with a lesion of the pituitary, either hypoplasia, absence (p. 419) or marked decrease of acidophilic cells. A second type of adrenal hypoplasia has a cortex composed mostly of large cells without any distinct arrangement and resembling cells of the fetal adrenal zone.[7,8,12-14] The characteristic layers of the cortex cannot be identified and there is no marginal permanent cortex. The medulla usually is present but arranged irregularly in eccentric islets.[15] Roselli and Barbosa[16] reviewed 23 cases of congenital adrenal hypoplasia in which necropsy had been performed. These included 15 males and 8 females and one pair of identical twins.[10] They also reported the cases of two sisters with extreme bilateral adrenal hypoplasia verified at necropsy. Two other siblings who had died in infancy with symptoms compatible with the diagnosis of congenital adrenal hypoplasia may also have died of the same disorder. Necropsy revealed in two of these infants both pituitary and extreme adrenal hypoplasia, which probably can be classified as miniature adult type. Thus, familial occurrence has been observed in the large cell type[14] and in the miniature adult type. Other cases of familial congenital adrenal hypoplasia have been reported.[68,69] An X-linked form characterized by lack of organization of the adult cortex into cords and the presence of clumps of large, pale-staining cells has been seen in males only.[70]

Some of the symptoms of congenital adrenal hypoplasia, such as vomiting, dehydration and electrolyte disturbances, may suggest pyloric stenosis.[8] But pyloric stenosis and adrenal hypoplasia can occur together,[17,18] and volvulus of the large bowel can be associated.[19] Cecum mobile was also found in the patient of MacMahon *et al.*[13] which was combined with coarctation of the aorta and a widely patent foramen ovale.

Dystopia of the Adrenal Gland

Displacement of the adrenal is most frequent into the kidney or the liver. Adrenal rudiments found under the capsule of the kidney may be disk shaped or divided into small irregular nodules. The normal relationship of cortex and marrow usually is disturbed in such cases. Malformations of the brain seem to be associated frequently with such adrenal dystopias.[5] Miloslavich[23] described disk-like, flat adrenals fused with the upper pole of the kidney in patients who lack adrenals in their normal location. The adrenal anomalies were associated with "hypertrophy of the brain" and, in one case, with glioma of the brain stem. Subcapsular position and malformations of the adrenals have also been found together with horseshoe kidney, cystic kidneys, ectopic kidneys, cystic liver, small testis and epididymis, epispadias or abnormal ovaries.[5] Adrenohepatic union probably is not rare. Dystopic adrenals have been observed combined with diaphragmatic and abdominal hernias. In such cases, hyperplasia and hypoplasia of the adrenal have been described.[5] Dystopias of the adrenals seem to be characteristic for craniorachischisis. In such cases, the adrenals may be found ventral to the kidney or behind the great vessels. As in accessory adrenals (p. 430), tumors may develop in ectopic adrenals. Dystopic adrenocortical tissue, located in the right lobe of the liver, was found in a boy with virilism and Cushing syndrome. The right adrenal was absent in this case.[25]

Dahl and Bahn[26] examined microscopically the testes and immediate adjacent structures from 100 infants less than 1 year of age for the presence of adrenal cortex. Fifteen of the 200 testes contained adrenocortical nodules. It was estimated that the incidence of adrenocortical tissue near the testes in human infants is between 7% and 15%. The histologic structure of the aberrant adrenals was closely comparable to that of the cortex of the adrenal glands in the same patients in respect to degeneration of the provisional cortex and to cortical differentiation. No medullary tissue was found in any of the aberrant adrenal nodules.

Heterotopic adrenocortical tissue may modify the symptoms of adrenal hormonal insufficiency. Certain neoplasms within and near the male gonads have been attributed to adrenocortical rests. In both pseudohermaphrodism and macrogenitosomia praecox, proliferation of tissue morphologically similar to adrenocortical tissue within and near the testes has been observed.

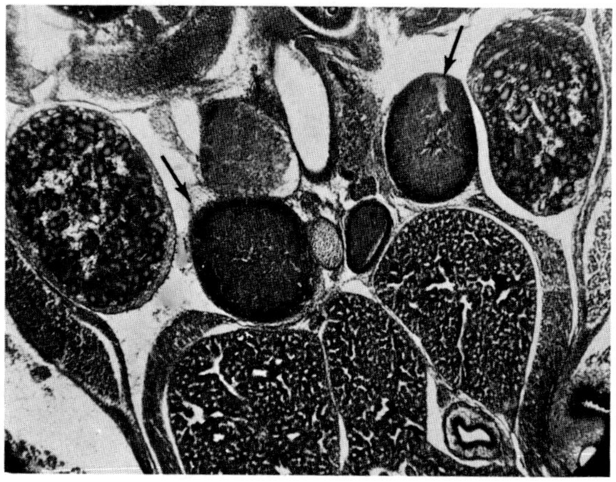

Fig. 43-1.—Ectopic adrenals. Transverse section through a near-term rat fetus showing the adrenals (**arrows**) beside the undescended testes. The anomalies were produced by toxic doses of streptonigrin. (From J. Warkany and E. Takacs.[71])

A strange location of heterotopic adrenal tissue was reported by Wiener and Dallgaard.[27] An adrenal gland measuring about 5 × 3 × 2 cm. was found attached to the pia mater of the inferior surface of the left frontal lobe. The patient was a man 49 years of age who died with signs of cerebral thrombosis or brain tumor. The intracranial adrenal contained both cortical and medullary tissue. There were no adrenal glands at the normal retroperitoneal sites.

Accessory Adrenals

Accessory adrenal tissue can be found near the adrenals and also at some distance from them. In infants, more or less isolated nodules of accessory adrenal cortex located in an adrenal gland are by no means rare, but after the second year they decrease in frequency and size. Such nodules may be located in the capsule or appear as adenomas of the cortex or as nodes within the marrow substance. Other nodules of adrenal cortex are found in the environment of the main adrenals, particularly in the kidneys. There they may form complicated formations made up of adrenal and renal tissue. Adrenal nodules can occur along blood vessels in the plexus solaris or renalis, between colon transversum and spleen, in the right lobe of the liver or in the pancreas. Accessory adrenals may also be located retroperitoneally below the lower pole of the kidney on the sacroiliac joint, along the spermatic veins and on the iliopsoas muscle. Accessory adrenal tissue sometimes is seen along the seminal ducts or, rarely, within a testis or in a paradidymis. A common location of nodules is between testis and epididymis. In some boys with virilizing adrenal hyperplasia, the testes are enlarged by masses of cells that resemble cells of the adrenal reticular zone. They probably are hyperplastic aberrant adrenocortical cells that shrink after treatment with cortisone.[28] In females, adrenal tissue is rather common in the ligamentum latum, where it occurs in nodules 2–5 mm. in diameter, but much larger disk-shaped formations have been observed occasionally. Other accessory adrenals have been seen in the mesosalpinx, ligamentum suspensorium of the ovary or in the ovary itself.[5]

The fate of accessory adrenal tissue varies. It seems that accessory nodules usually disppear as a child gets older, but sometimes compensatory enlargement is possible if the main adrenal's function is reduced. They also can be the origin of tumors in the kidney, ligamentum latum, ovary, testes, liver, solar plexus or between the spleen and transverse colon.[5]

The Adrenal in Anencephaly

Since early times, pathologists have known that the adrenals are small in anencephalics and it was stated that the glands are absent in such infants. The defect often was found associated with absence or anomaly of the pituitary gland. But it seems that both adenohypophysis and adrenals can be found in every case of anencephaly if an intensive search is made. Angevine,[4] in 1938, confirmed this in 18 anencephalics, but in a few instances the adrenals were located with considerable difficulty. It has long been known that the adrenals of anencephalics resemble "in miniature" the well-differentiated adrenal of the adult, and Angevine noted that smaller and younger anencephalic fetuses had larger amounts of adrenal tissue than larger and older fetuses. This suggested that the adrenals had increased in size for a time before they atrophied to the small size usually seen in anencephalic fetuses in the second half of gestation. These findings and conclusions agree with those of earlier investigators,[32] who had stated that the adrenal growth retardation in human anencephalic fetuses becomes noticeable only from the fifth month of gestation. It seems logical to conclude that the changes in the adrenals are secondary to those of the hypophysis, which follow destruction of the brain as intrauterine life progresses. But the relationship of these glandular systems may be rather complex, since some large hypophyses can be associated with extremely small adrenal glands and marked adrenocortical atrophy, and vice versa.[4] It must be assumed that it is not the *size* of the pituitary gland but its *function* that determines the condition of the fetal adrenals. Even large anterior lobes present in anencephalic fetuses

Fig. 43-2. – **A,** adrenal gland (**arrow**) of a near-term rat that had a dystopic pituitary. The adrenal is of near-normal size. **B,** the adrenal gland (**arrow**) of a litter mate that had no pituitary. The adrenal is much reduced in size. The anomalies were produced by treatment of the mother with sodium salicylate. (From J. Warkany and E. Takacs.[72])

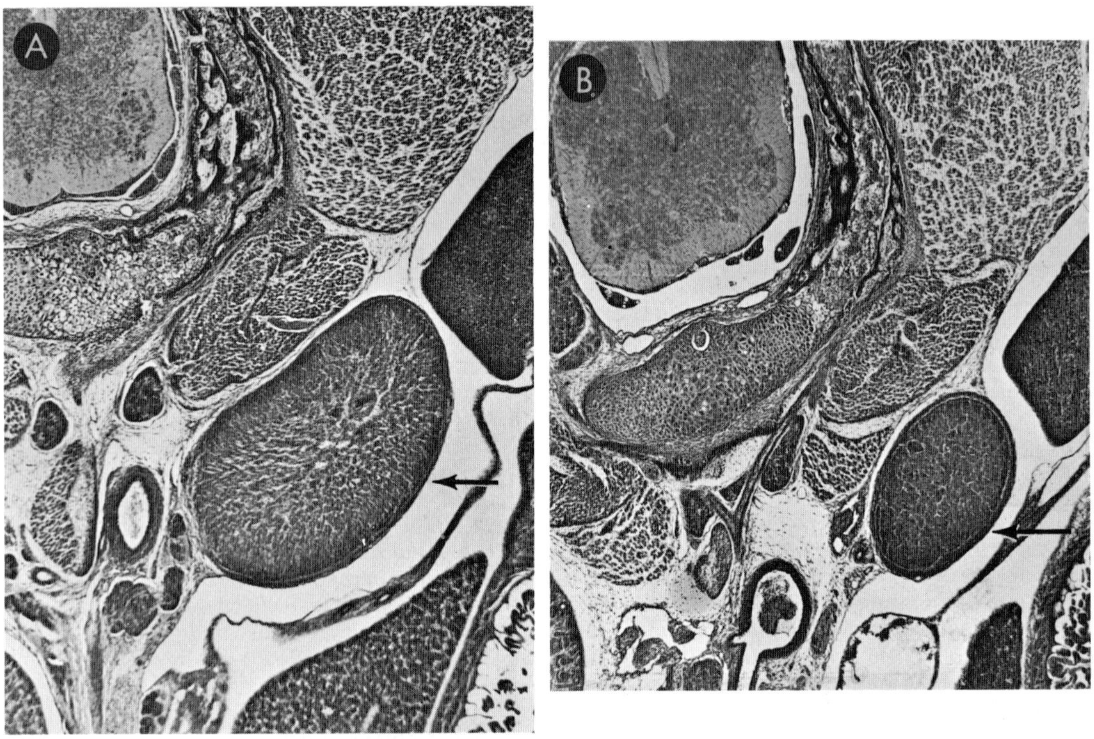

may fail to stimulate adrenocortical tissue because of their separation from the influences of the diencephalon. There exists experimental evidence that adrenocortical atrophy in anencephalic rat fetuses is dependent on deficiency in hypothalamic releasing factors.[29] It seems likely that separation of the connections between the pituitary and the hypothalamus results in deficiency of adrenocorticotropic hormone.[30,31] This belief is supported by numerous teratologic experiments that result in exencephaly of rat fetuses, which is the forerunner of anencephaly. But brain destruction is only partially effected in rat fetuses near term, because of the relative and absolute shortness of intrauterine growth after termination of organogenesis. In such rat fetuses, the destruction of the brain and its separation from the diencephalon begin near term and, consequently, the adrenals still show adequate size and differentiation; there has not been time for atrophy of the adrenal cortex in such fetuses. In contrast are adrenals of rat fetuses without any adenohypophysis. Such adrenals are small and undifferentiated near term. Thus, observations in human anencephalics and experimental evidence suggest that development and growth of the fetal adrenal cortex depend on stimulation by the adenohypophysis, which, in turn, functions through stimulation by the diencephalon. Anencephaly results in deficiency of cerebral influences on the adenohypophysis and consequently in failure of production of adrenocorticotropins and adrenal atrophy. The adrenal medulla of human anencephalic fetuses is normal.[32]

Fig. 43-3. – Fusion of the adrenals in the midline (**arrow**) in a case of spina bifida and renal aplasia. (From W. Helmreich.[33])

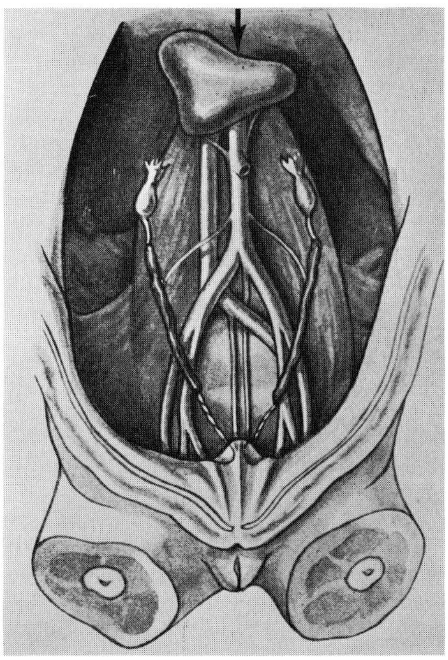

In cebocephaly, the pituitary can be absent and the adrenals reduced in size (p. 206).

Fusion of the Adrenals

When adrenal tissue appears fused in the midline, "horseshoe" or "butterfly" adrenals result. Such anomalies are not rare in conjoined twins. They sometimes are associated with malformations of the lower half of the body, such as renal and vesical anomalies, ovarian defects, uterus unicornis, myeloschisis and others. Encephalocele and other malformations of the brain have also been combined with fused adrenals.[5,33] Fused adrenals were observed in a child with de Lange syndrome.[34] Fused adrenals have been produced experimentally (Fig. 43-4).

Congenital Adrenal Cysts

Congenital adrenal cysts are quite rare but have to be considered in the diagnosis of cystic abdominal masses. They are pseudocysts that may show a curvilinear calcification in roentgenograms. Intestinal obstruction can result if the cysts are not resected.[35]

Adrenal Atrophy Occurring in Familial Aggregation with Manifestations Beginning in Postnatal Life

The familial occurrence observed in several instances of congenital adrenal hypoplasia suggests

Fig. 43-4. – Adrenal approximation (**arrow**) in a near-term rat with multiple congenital malformations produced by a large dose of streptonigrin administered on the tenth day of gestation.

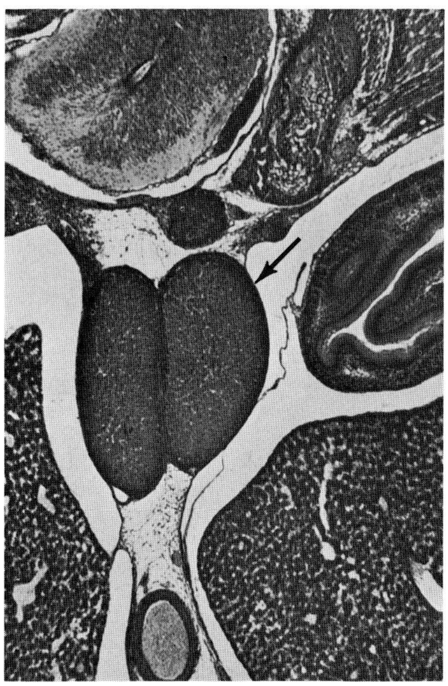

genetic mechanisms in their etiology (p. 428). Similar mechanisms may be responsible for cases of "idiopathic" or familial adrenal atrophy beginning at various ages in postnatal life. Although such cases are not congenital, prenatal determination justifies mentioning some of these conditions that sometimes are associated with other hereditary disorders of great medical interest.

Shepard *et al.*[36] reported 2 sisters with hyperpigmentation, weakness and convulsions, symptoms beginning with the second year and attributed to absence of corticoid production in the presence of normal aldosterone production. In one case, histologic sections showed marked atrophy of cortical tissue. There were occasional clumps of cortical cells in the zona glomerulosa but all cells of the zona fasciculata and reticularis were absent. Chromaffin cells of the medulla were abundant. It was thought that the anterior pituitary had a specific inability to secrete corticotropins.

Meakin *et al.*[37] described Addison disease in 2 brothers. The patients were 10 and 6 years of age, respectively, when examinations began, but it was thought that the onset of the disease had been at the age of 3 or 4 years. It seemed likely that atrophy or degeneration of the adrenals was present in both cases. Urinary steroid excretion showed no activity of adrenocortical function. These authors cited 15 publications on familial Addison disease, but emphasized that not in all the cases was the diagnosis substantiated by steroid studies or necropsy findings. A strange accumulation of Addison disease in two related families was reported by Nöthiger.[44] He mentioned the occurrence of Addison disease in more than one generation of some families.

Moehlig[38] described a male patient followed for 9 years who died in an Addisonian crisis. At necropsy, no adrenal tissue was found. A maternal aunt had died of Addison disease and a niece was developing pigmentation. Brøchner-Mortensen[39] reported 4 cases of Addison disease in two generations of a family in which 2 brothers and 2 of their maternal uncles were affected. Although tuberculosis could not be ruled out in the first generation, one can assume that the illness was due to atrophy of the adrenal cortex.

Harris-Jones and Nixon[40] described 2 brothers with Addison disease and spastic paraplegia. These patients were 32 and 40 years of age, respectively, when Addison disease was diagnosed. In one brother, paraplegia developed 12 years after onset of Addison disease, but in the second brother the spastic gait with increased muscle tone and diminished power in the legs began simultaneously with the adrenal insufficiency. Adrenal cortical atrophy was assumed in both cases because there were no signs of tuberculosis. The authors found in the literature nine families in which Addison disease occurred in more than one member. In a number of these cases, postmortem records showed atrophy of the adrenal cortex. Spastic paraplegia often behaves like a dominant hereditary trait. Although there were no signs of this disorder in the parents and in preceding generations, the authors believed that spastic paraplegia was the correct diagnosis for the brothers.

Some familial disorders of the central nervous system are associated with adrenocortical atrophy. Hoefnagel *et al.*[41] described a young boy who died of a diffuse demyelinating disease of the central nervous system. When he was about 5½ years of age, there were changes in behavior followed by incontinence of feces and urine, breathing difficulties, slurring of speech and ataxia of gait. At necropsy, the patient had histologic abnormalities in several endocrine glands, such as absence of basophilic cells in the pituitary, marked atrophy of the adrenal cortices and an interstitial cell tumor of one testis. Similar abnormalities of the pituitary and adrenal glands had been present in a brother of the patient who had died at an earlier age after a brief illness. Interestingly, clinical evidence of endocrinologic disease, including hypoadrenocorticism, was absent in both patients. These authors reviewed the literature of similar cases. In none of these was adrenal insufficiency congenital, but familial occurrence may be due to genetic determination of the disorder.

Fanconi *et al.*[42] observed Addison disease with cerebral sclerosis in a boy who had the first signs of adrenal insufficiency in his fifteenth year, followed soon thereafter by ataxia, spastic paralysis and mental deterioration. Death occurred in his eighteenth year. Necropsy showed primary atrophy of the adrenal cortex and a spotty demyelinization of the brain, with destruction of neurons. The authors mentioned 9 other cases with the syndrome. All patients were male, and it is believed that the disorder is genetically determined and a sex-linked recessive trait.

Gordon and Marsden[43] reviewed the subject of diffuse cerebral sclerosis and adrenal atrophy and reported the case of a boy of 7 years who showed this association. The onset of both diseases was rather sudden and the patient died within 6 months. The adrenals were small and, on microscopic examination, they contained swollen glandular cortical cells with little lipoid. In some places, the cortex was absent.

Hypoadrenocorticism and Hypoparathyroidism

Association of hypoadrenocorticism and hypoparathyroidism has been observed repeatedly. Hiekkala[66] found 20 published cases. There can be more than one child with both conditions in the same family (p. 445). Sweetnam[45] described 2 sisters, one 7 years of age, the other 4½. In the older sister, hypoadrenocorticism was diagnosed clinically and confirmed by endocrine studies. Later, hypoparathyroidism was diagnosed clinically and low serum calcium and high serum phosphorus values were found. In the second sister, there were clinical and chemical signs of hypoparathyroidism, and endocrine biochemical

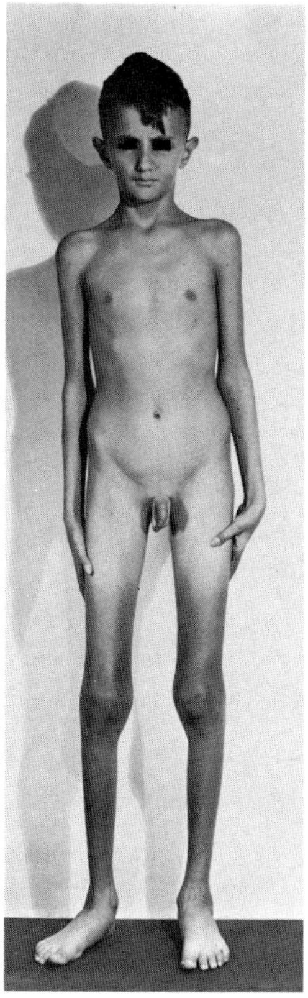

Fig. 43-5. – Boy with Addison disease whose sister had idiopathic hypoparathyroidism. The picture shows general emaciation and abnormal pigmentations.

tests showed a gradual failure of adrenocortical function. Both patients were free from moniliasis. Complement-fixing antiadrenal antibodies were not found in these cases.

Cushing Syndrome

Fully developed congenital Cushing syndrome apparently has not yet been observed, but in a girl reported by Bernheim *et al.*[46] hirsutism and pubic hair were present at birth. There also was some enlargement of the clitoris. Weight gain was rapid and at the age of 17 months she presented both Cushing and adrenogenital syndromes. A malignant tumor of the right adrenal gland was found at operation. In other cases, symptoms made their appearance within a few weeks after birth, suggesting that a prenatal disturbance must be considered. Greenblatt *et al.*[47] recorded such a case in which adrenal calcification was present at the age of 5 months in a girl with fully developed Cushing disease. She showed extreme obesity, moon face with acne, slight hair growth on pubis and vulva and some enlargement of the clitoris. Polyphagia, polydipsia and polyuria had been present for several months. The weight was 9,400 Gm. and the blood pressure only 30/30 mm. Hg. A calcification above the right kidney was demonstrated in roentgenograms. A tumor mass that weighed 11 Gm. and replaced the right adrenal was removed transperitoneally; the left adrenal appeared normal. The yellow adrenal tumor was an adenoma consisting of cells arranged in cords like zona fasciculata. The child was cured by the removal of the adenoma. In a case of Guin and Gilbert,[48] obesity began at the age of 6 weeks, and at 3 months the girl weighed 5,500 Gm. The face was round and there was hirsutism on the upper lip but no pubic hair. A mass could be palpated to the right of the umbilicus. Systolic blood pressure varied between 115 and 210 mm. Hg. A tumor replacing the right adrenal was removed surgically but the infant died on the fourth day after the operation. The tumor, which weighed 105 Gm., was partly hemorrhagic-necrotic. It was diagnosed as cortical carcinoma, and many metastatic foci were found. This case is of interest because of its early onset and the fact that the infant's mother had suffered from diabetes since the age of 4 years. Overstimulation of the adrenal by maternal hormones was considered a possible cause of the child's adrenal changes. Marks *et al.*[49] described a girl who was born apparently normal but developed a ravenous appetite at the age of 3 months. She began to gain weight rapidly and red cheeks and a harsh voice became noticeable. In her eleventh month, she had the grotesque appearance seen in Figure 43-6, *A*. Hirsutism was present on the forehead, cheeks, back and pubis but the external genitalia were normal. The systolic blood pressure rose to 245 mm. Hg. Ossification was normal for her age. She died because of cardiac failure, and at necropsy a tumor, 3 cm. in diameter, was found in the region of the right adrenal gland, which was identified along one border of the tumor mass. The pituitary was normal. The well-encapsulated neoplasm was considered to be an adenoma of adrenal cortex tissue with strands of nests of large, foamy, well-differentiated cells. It seems likely that in this case aberrant and abnormal adrenal cortex adjacent to the right adrenal gland was responsible for the bizarre clinical picture. With similar disease pictures,[28,50] malignant tumors of the right adrenal gland have been found. In the case of Goldstein,[50] the tumor had developed in the presence of an adrenal gland on the same side. Although Cushing syndrome has been observed repeatedly in infancy,[48,49] the etiology of such cases is still puzzling. Causation by developmental error is suggested by the findings in the case of Wilkins and Ravitch,[25] in which an adrenocortical tumor leading to virilism and Cushing syndrome was found and removed from the right lobe of the liver. The right adrenal gland was absent and there was no indication that the displaced tissue had originated from an adrenal in its proper place. It seemed that the neoplasm arose from aberrant adrenal cells within the liver. In the early embryo, the root of the mesogastrium lies along the adrenogenital ridge, and cells from the

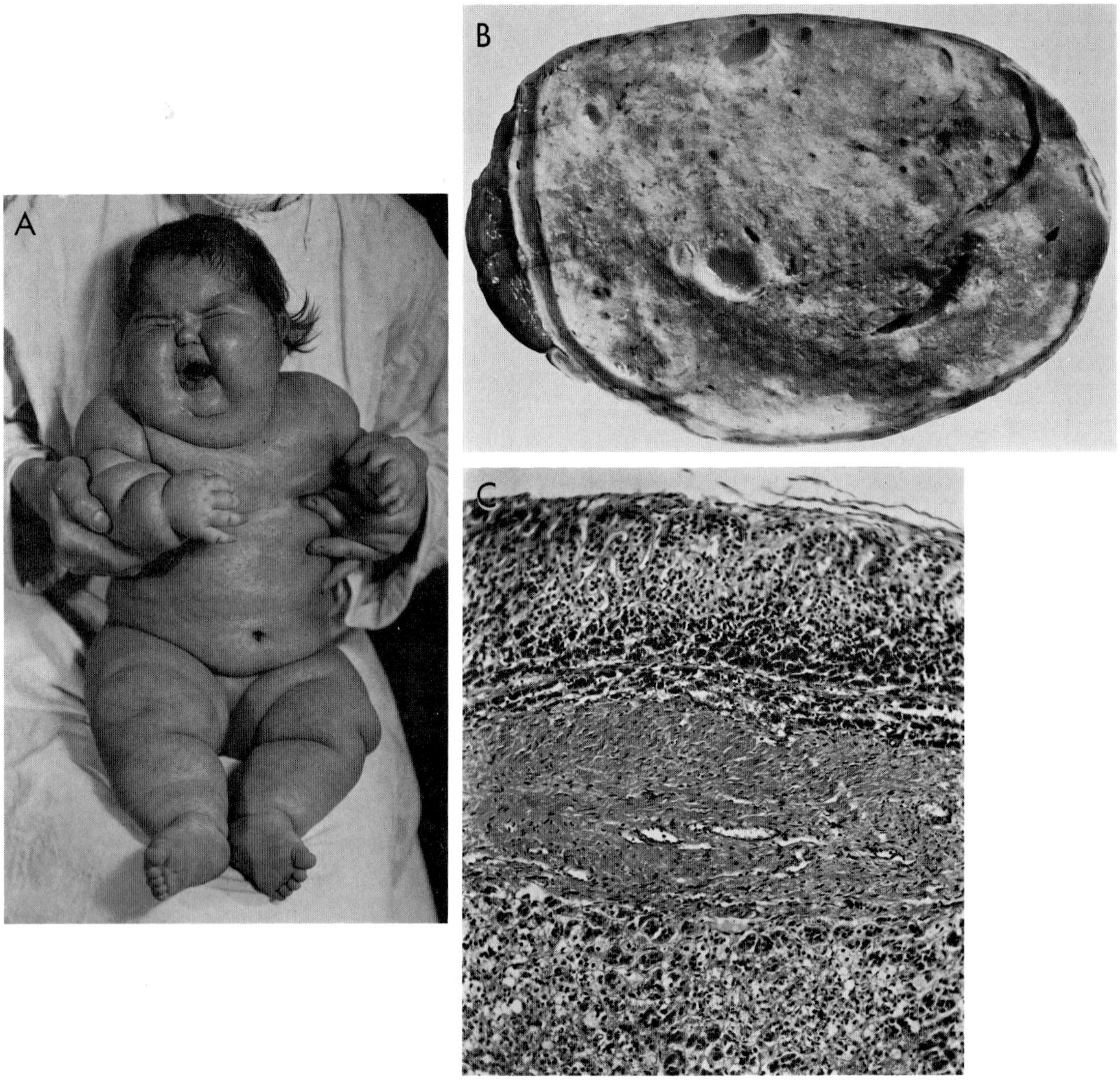

Fig. 43-6.—**A**, Cushing syndrome in a girl 10 months of age. Onset of symptoms at 3 months. Obesity, hirsutism, elevated blood pressure. **B**, tumor connected with the right adrenal gland was found at necropsy. **C**, adrenal tissue is seen on top of the section, separated by a capsule from adenoma consisting of well-differentiated epithelial cells that resemble in appearance and arrangement normal adrenocortical tissue. (From T. M. Marks, J. M. Thomas and J. Warkany.[49])

ridge could migrate along the mesogastrium toward the gut and be included in the hepatic anlage. Despite the congenital presence of this developmental error, the boy with the anomaly had appeared entirely normal until he was $2\frac{1}{2}$ years of age. An unusual finding in an infant with Cushing syndrome was reported by Kogut and Donnell.[67] Onset of polydipsia and obesity was noticed when the child was 9 months of age and this was followed by hypertrichosis and typical signs of Cushing disease. The adrenal glands were normal but a ganglioneuroblastoma was found that had originated in the lower pole of the left kidney. After removal of the tumor, the abnormal clinical symptoms subsided. The authors thought that catecholamines secreted by the tumor stimulated the adrenals or pituitary to hyperactivity.

Adrenal Hypertrophies

Virilizing adrenal hyperplasia and macrogenitosomia praecox are discussed in Chapter 111.

Adrenal Tumor and Hemihypertrophy

In a few instances, adrenocortical hyperplasia or tumor was associated with hemihypertrophy (p. 165), pointing to prenatal determination of the adrenal pathology. Hutchison[51] found left-sided hemihypertrophy associated with marked enlargement of the left adrenal gland, and Harwood and O'Flynn[52] observed right-sided hemihypertrophy in a boy who had a tumor of the right adrenal. But Riedel[53] reported contralateral pathology – an adenoma of the right adrenal in a boy with left-sided hemihypertrophy. In this case, the tumor caused signs of precocious puberty beginning at the age of 5 months. Although the tumor was removed toward the end of the first year, a mass that proved to be an adenosarcoma of the right kidney developed 5 years later in the right abdomen. Other adrenocortical tumors associated with hemihypertrophy were recorded by Lewis and Geschickter[54] and Benson *et al.*[55] The relationship of oncogenesis to hemihypertrophy seems well established[56] but remains unexplained. Fraumeni and Miller[56] found records of hemihypertrophy in two hospital charts of 62 children with adrenocortical neoplasm. Children with adrenal or Wilms tumor should be examined for asymmetric body development. It seems possible that other adrenal tumors reported in children may belong in the group associated with asymmetry.

Adrenal Tumor and Visceromegaly

Congenital adrenal cortical carcinoma was observed in a girl born with macroglossia[57] and enlarged kidneys and pancreas. Both adrenals presented cytomegalic changes in the fetal cortex, and in one adrenal an intracapsular and a large extracapsular adenoma were found. There were metastatic cytomegalic nodules in the choroid plexus, lungs and pancreas (Chapter 16).

Pheochromocytoma

There have been no reports on congenital pheochromocytoma. In one case that manifested itself in high blood pressure, hirsutism and obesity, onset was at age 8 months and the disease picture was fully developed at 16 months.[58] That prenatal factors play an important role in the etiology of pheochromocytomas is evidenced by the fact that heredity can be demonstrated in some families. Carman and Brashear[59] analyzed ten kindreds in which pheochromocytoma appeared in more than one member. They concluded that the trait probably is due to a dominant gene. The diagnosis in these hereditary cases had been made at various ages from 4 to 57 years. In many of the patients, the tumors appeared at multiple sites and individual lesions sometimes developed at various ages, so that recurrence of the disease must be anticipated. By 1968, familial pheochromocytoma had been described in at least twenty-nine families involving 85 individuals.[60]

The association of pheochromocytomas with Recklinghausen neurofibromatosis is of great interest,[61] since it points to an etiologic entity known to be a dominantly inherited trait. This hamartosis (Chapter 121) has many manifestations that, when present, can help in the diagnosis and classification of pheochromocytomas. Cutaneous lesions, pigmentation, deformities of the vertebral column and other symptoms of neurofibromatosis can occur in patients with pheochromocytomas.[61] Multiple neoplasia must be considered possible in combination with pheochromocytoma: sarcoma, neurinoma, ependymoma, meningioma, astrocytoma[62] and granulosa cell tumor[63] can accompany the adrenal tumors. Aganglionic megacolon (Hirschsprung disease), megaloureter and neurofibroma may be associated anomalies.[64] There also is the possibility that pheochromocytoma can be a manifestation of another dominantly heritable hamartosis, namely Hippel-Lindau disease (p. 1266). Angiomatosis retinae has been observed in patients with pheochromocytoma.[61] These ocular lesions must be distinguished from those caused by hypertension.

Pheochromocytoma is a leading manifestation in an "endocrine tumor diathesis" described by Steiner *et al.*,[60] which also includes medullary thyroid carcinoma, parathyroid hyperplasia and Cushing disease. The disorder of multiple endocrine neoplasia is transmitted as an autosomal dominant trait. The adrenal medullary tumors frequently are bilateral and multicentric. Manifestations of the tumor begin in adult life (Chapter 124).

Discordant pheochromocytoma with renal artery compression has been reported in a monozygotic twin.[65]

REFERENCES

1. Crowder, R. E.: The development of the adrenal gland in man, with special reference to origin and ultimate location of cell types and evidence in favor of the "cell migration" theory, Contrib. Embryol. 36:193, 1957.
2. Lanman, J. T.: The adrenal gland in the human fetus; an interpretation of its physiology and unusual developmental pattern, Pediatrics 27:140, 1961.
3. Tähkä, H.: On the weight and structure of the adrenal glands and the factors affecting them in children of 0–2 years, Acta paediat. 40:1, 1951.
4. Angevine, D. M.: Pathologic anatomy of hypophysis and adrenals in anencephaly, Arch. Path. 26:507, 1938.
5. Pagel, W.: Missbildungen der Nebennieren, in Schwalbe, E., and Gruber, G. B. (eds.), *Die Morphologie der Missbildungen des Menschen und der Tiere* (Jena: Gustav Fischer, 1929), Vol. 3, p. 525.
6. Jaudon, J. J.: Hypofunction of the adrenals in early life, J. Pediat. 29:696, 1946.
7. Sikl, H.: Addison's disease due to congenital hypoplasia of the adrenals in an infant aged 33 days, J. Path. & Bact. 60:323, 1948.
8. Deamer, W. C., and Silver, H. K.: Abnormalities in the secretion of the adrenal cortex during early life, J. Pediat. 37:490, 1950.
9. Williams, A., and Robinson, M. J.: Addison's disease in infancy, Arch. Dis. Childhood 31:158, 1956.
10. Mosier, H. D.: Hypoplasia of the pituitary and adrenal cortex, J. Pediat. 48:633, 1956.
11. Ehrlich, R. M.: Ectopic and hypoplastic pituitary with adrenal hypoplasia, J. Pediat. 51:377, 1957.
12. Harlem, O. K., and Myhre, E.: Congenital adrenal hypoplasia, A.M.A. J. Dis. Child. 94:696, 1957.
13. MacMahon, H. E., Wagner, R., and Weiner, D. B.: Acute adrenal insufficiency due to congenital defect, A.M.A. J. Dis. Child. 94:282, 1957.

14. Mitchell, R. G., and Rhaney, K.: Congenital adrenal hypoplasia in siblings, Lancet 1:488, 1959.
15. Kerenyi, N.: Congenital adrenal hypoplasia; report of a case with extreme adrenal hypoplasia and neurohypophyseal aplasia, drawing attention to certain aspects of etiology and classification, Arch. Path. 71:336, 1961.
16. Roselli, A., and Barbosa, L. T.: Congenital hypoplasia of the adrenal glands, Pediatrics 35:70, 1965.
17. Morec, G. J.: Hypertrophic pyloric stenosis associated with adrenal insufficiency, J. Pediat. 42:359, 1953.
18. Rosenberg, P.: Temporary adrenal insufficiency with associated pyloric stenosis, J. Pediat. 48:63, 1956.
19. Boyd, J. F., and MacDonald, A. M.: Adrenocortical hypoplasia in siblings, Arch. Dis. Childhood 35:561, 1960.
20. Dunn, J. M.: Anterior pituitary and adrenal absence in a live-born normocephalic infant, Am. J. Obst. & Gynec. 96: 893, 1966.
21. O'Donohoe, N. V., and Holland, P. D.: Familial congenital adrenal hypoplasia, Arch. Dis. Childhood 43:717, 1968.
22. Uttley, W. S.: Familial congenital adrenal hypoplasia, Arch. Dis. Childhood 43:724, 1968.
23. Miloslavich, E.: Über Bildungsanomalien der Nebennieren, Virchows Arch. path. Anat. 218:131, 1914.
24. Dolan, M. F., and Janovski, N. A.: Adreno-hepatic union. Adrenal dystopia, Arch. Path. 86:22, 1968.
25. Wilkins, L., and Ravitch, M.: Adrenal cortical tumor arising in the liver of a three year old boy with signs of virilism and Cushing's syndrome, Pediatrics 9:671, 1952.
26. Dahl, E. V., and Bahn, R. C.: Aberrant adrenal cortical tissue near the testis in human infants, Am. J. Path. 40: 587, 1962.
27. Wiener, M. F., and Dallgaard, S. A.: Intracranial adrenal gland. A case report, A.M.A. Arch. Path. 67:228, 1959.
28. Wilkins, L.: *The Diagnosis and Treatment of Endocrine Disorders in Childhood and Adolescence* (3d ed.; Springfield, Ill.: Charles C Thomas, Publisher, 1965).
29. Jost, A.: Problems of Fetal Endocrinology: The Adrenal Glands, in *Recent Progress in Hormone Research* (New York: Academic Press, Inc., 1966).
30. Benirschke, K.: Adrenals in anencephaly and hydrocephaly, Obst. & Gynec. 8:412, 1956.
31. Tuchmann-Duplessis, H.: Etude des glandes endocrines des anencéphales. Déduction sur les corrélations hypophysonerveuses du foetus humain, Biol. Neonat. 1:8, 1959.
32. Meyer, R.: Nebennieren bei Anenzephalie, Virchows Arch. path. Anat. 210:158, 1912.
33. Helmreich, W.: Über eine Beobachtung von Nebennierenverschmelzung bei Spina bifida und Aplasie der Nieren, Beitr. path. Anat. 109:511, 1947.
34. Huang, C. C., Emanuel, I., Huang, S. W., and Chen, T. Y.: Two cases of the de Lange syndrome in Chinese infants, J. Pediat. 71:251, 1967.
35. Van de Water, J. M., and Fonkalsrud, E. W.: Adrenal cysts in infancy, Surgery 60:1267, 1966.
36. Shepard, T. H., Landing, B. H., and Mason, D. G.: Familial Addison's disease. Case reports of two sisters with corticoid deficiency unassociated with hypoaldosteronism, A.M.A. J. Dis. Child. 97:154, 1959.
37. Meakin, J. W., Nelson, D. H., and Thorn, G. W.: Addison's disease in two brothers, J. Clin. Endocrinol. 19:726, 1959.
38. Moehlig, R.: Addison's disease followed for nine years: Case report with autopsy, J. Clin. Endocrinol. 7:134, 1947.
39. Brøchner-Mortensen, K.: Familial occurrence of Addison's disease, Acta med. scandinav. 156:205, 1956.
40. Harris-Jones, J. N., and Nixon, P. G. F.: Familial Addison's disease with spastic paraplegia, J. Clin. Endocrinol. 15:739, 1955.
41. Hoefnagel, D., Van den Noort, S., and Ingbar, S. H.: Diffuse cerebral sclerosis with endocrine abnormalities in young males, Brain 85:553, 1962.
42. Fanconi, A., Prader, A., Isler, W., Lüthy, F., and Siebenmann, R.: Morbus Addison mit Hirnsklerose im Kindesalter. Ein hereditäres Syndrom mit X-chromosomaler Vererbung?, Helvet. paediat. acta 18:480, 1963.
43. Gordon, N., and Marsden, H. B.: Diffuse cerebral sclerosis and adrenal atrophy, Developmental Med. & Child Neurol. 8:719, 1966.
44. Nöthiger, F.: Familiärer Morbus Addison, Ztschr. Kinderh. 99:14, 1967.
45. Sweetnam, W. P: Juvenile familial endocrinopathy, Lancet 1:463, 1966.
46. Bernheim, M., Wertheimer, P., Guinet, P., François, R., and Sutet, J.: Les syndromes d'hyperfonctionnement cortico-surrénal d'origine tumorale chez l'enfant, Semaine hôp. Paris 41:1, 1954.
47. Greenblatt, R. B., Manautou, J. M., Zimmerman, A. M., and Lucas, W. T.: Cushing's syndrome in infancy, A.M.A. J. Dis. Child. 94:691, 1957.
48. Guin, G. H., and Gilbert, E. F.: Cushing's syndrome in children associated with adrenal cortical carcinoma, A.M.A. Am. J. Dis. Child. 92:297, 1956.
49. Marks, T. M., Thomas, J. M., and Warkany, J.: Adrenocortical obesity in children, Am. J. Dis. Child. 60:1147, 1940.
50. Goldstein, H. M.: Cushing's syndrome due to tumor of the adrenal cortex, Am. J. Dis. Child. 78:260, 1949.
51. Hutchison, R.: Case of hemihypertrophy in which internal organs were affected, Brit. J. Child. Dis. 1:258, 1904.
52. Harwood, J., and O'Flynn, E.: Specimens from case of right-sided hemihypertrophy associated with pubertas precox, Proc. Roy. Soc. Med. 28:837, 1935.
53. Riedel, H. A.: Adrenogenital syndrome in a male child due to adrenocortical tumor, Pediatrics 10:19, 1952.
54. Lewis, D., and Geschickter, C. F.: Tumors of sympathetic nervous system: Neuroblastoma, paraganglionoma, ganglioneuroma, Arch. Surg. 28:16, 1934.
55. Benson, P. F., Vulliamy, D. G., and Taubman, J. O.: Congenital hemihypertrophy and malignancy, Lancet 1:468, 1963.
56. Fraumeni, J. F., Jr., and Miller, R. W.: Adrenocortical neoplasms with hemihypertrophy, brain tumors, and other disorders, J. Pediat. 70:129, 1967.
57. Sherman, F. E., Bass, L. W., and Fetterman, G. H.: Congenital metastasizing adrenal cortical carcinoma associated with cytomegaly of the fetal adrenal cortex, Am. J. Clin. Path. 30:439, 1958.
58. Neff, F. C., Tice, G., Walker, G. A., and Ockerblad, N.: Adrenal tumor in female infant. With hypertrichosis, hypertension, overdevelopment of external genitalia, obesity, but absence of breast enlargement, J. Clin. Endocrinol. 2:125, 1942.
59. Carman, C. T., and Brashear, R. E.: Pheochromocytoma as an inherited abnormality; report of the tenth affected kindred and review of the literature, New England J. Med. 263:419, 1960.
60. Steiner, A. L., Goodman, A. D., and Powers, S. R.: Study of a kindred with pheochromocytoma, medullary thyroid carcinoma, hyperparathyroidism and Cushing's disease: Multiple endocrine neoplasia, type 2, Medicine 47:371, 1968.
61. Glushien, A. S., Mansuy, M. M., and Littman, D. S.: Pheochromocytoma. Its relationship to neurocutaneous syndromes, Am. J. Med. 14:318, 1953.
62. Lichtenstein, B. W.: Neurofibromatosis (von Recklinghausen's disease of the nervous system), Arch. Neurol. & Psychiat. 62:822, 1949.
63. Lopez, J. F.: Pheochromocytoma of the adrenal gland with granulosa cell tumor and neurofibromatosis, Ann. Int. Med. 48:187, 1958.
64. Shocket, E., and Teloh, H. A.: Aganglionic megacolon, pheochromocytoma, megaloureter and neurofibroma, A.M.A. J. Dis. Child. 94:185, 1957.
65. Kerzner, M. S., Reeves, J. A., DeNyse, D., and Claunch, B. C.: Pheochromocytoma with renal artery compression in an identical twin, Arch. Int. Med. 121:91, 1968.
66. Hiekkala, H.: Idiopathic hypoparathyroidism, adrenal

insufficiency and moniliasis in children, Ann. paediat. Fenniae 10:213, 1964.
67. Kogut, M. D., and Donnell, G. N.: Cushing's syndrome in association with renal ganglioneuroblastoma, Pediatrics 28:566, 1961.
68. Uttley, W. S.: Familial congenital adrenal hypoplasia, Arch. Dis. Childhood 43:724, 1968.
69. O'Donohoe, N. V., and Holland, P. D. J.: Familial congenital adrenal hypoplasia, Arch. Dis. Childhood 43:717, 1968.
70. Weiss, L., and Mellinger, R. C.: Congenital adrenal hypoplasia—an X-linked disease, J. M. Genetics 7:27, 1970.
71. Warkany, J., and Takacs, E.: Congenital malformations in rats from streptonigrin, Arch. Path. 79:65, 1965.
72. Warkany, J., and Takacs, E.: Changes of endocrine glands by teratogenic methods, Arch. Path. 85:101, 1968.

44

The Thyroid Gland

THE PRIMORDIUM of the thyroid can be recognized quite early in embryonic life. In a 2–4-mm. human embryo (22–26 days), the median and lateral thyroid components can be seen as evaginations from the foregut. Between the first and second pharyngeal arches a midline diverticulum develops, marked by the foramen cecum. It extends caudally at first as a solid primordium that shows communicating cavities in the 6-mm. stage. Soon, two lobes can be recognized in the median component, and in embryos 8 mm. in length, the lobes are connected with each other by an isthmus and with the ventral epithelium of the pharynx by a thin pedicle. In 16-mm. embryos, there is active cell proliferation and formation of anastomosing cellular plates but there is no follicle formation up to the third month. The thyroid lobes extend caudally along the ventral aspects of the pharynx and later along the larynx and trachea, at first being connected with the area of the foramen cecum by a ductus thyroglossus. This duct disappears as a continuous structure, but not rarely remnants can be found even in adults anywhere between the foramen cecum and the thyroid isthmus. Of special importance are remnants of thyroid tissue in the area of the foramen cecum and in the lingual muscle masses. Accessory thyroid glands can also be located ventral to the larynx or behind the sternum. Such accessory thyroid glands can become hypertrophic and develop into dystopic goiters.

All functioning thyroid tissue is derived from the median component of the thyroid gland. The lateral components (ultimobranchial bodies) contribute no active tissue. They degenerate and sometimes form cysts. In cases of lingual thyroid there is no ^{131}I accumulation in the lower regions of the neck, and removal of a lingual thyroid results in hypothyroidism.[1] Intracellular colloid appears at about 70 days (60 mm. length) and follicles a few days later. Studies with radioactive material have shown iodine concentration in the thyroid between 70 and 84 days' gestation and thyroxine production begins approximately 5 weeks later.[1,2]

Sporadic Cretinism

Sporadic cretinism due to "athyrosis" or "hypothyrosis," once thought to be a simple congenital malformation, is now recognized as a complex anomaly. It can be caused by agenesis or dysgenesis of the thyroid gland, by an inborn enzymatic defect or by maternal ingestion of antithyroid drugs. Although it formerly was thought that sporadic cretinism was always of the athyrotic type, it is now established that it can occur in the presence of a thyroid gland and goiter. Goitrous sporadic cretinism is interpreted as a response to faulty hormonogenesis.

The frequency of sporadic cretinism is not well established. In contrast to endemic cretinism occurring in certain areas (Chapter 12), the sporadic form is rare. But, according to Wilkins,[3] in the United States sporadic hypothyroidism is more common than any other thyroid disturbance of childhood and is one of the most frequent of all endocrine disorders during that period of life. Yet, only 141 cases of congenital agenesis or dysgenesis of the thyroid were diagnosed in the Endocrine Clinic of the Harriet Lane Home in Baltimore during a period of 20 years and there were only 26 cases of defective hormonogenesis. In Michigan, Carr *et al.*[1] found 94 sporadic cretins in State Homes and at the University Hospital. After critical evaluation with modern diagnostic methods, it was estimated that of these sporadic cretins 32% were goitrous and probably 68% athyrotic.

Congenital Athyrosis and Thyroid Ectopia

Absence of the thyroid gland has long been noticed in necropsies of sporadic cretins. The first cases of athyrosis verified by necropsy apparently were those of Curling[5] in 1850. As early as 1871, Fagge[6] distinguished sporadic from endemic cretinism in England. In Austria, Pineles[7] wrote about "thyreoaplasia" and cited 12 cases in which necropsy had failed to demonstrate any thyroid tissue and 6 similar cases in which no thyroid rests could be found histologically. He distinguished clearly athyrotic sporadic cretinism from endemic goitrous cretinism. There was a marked prevalence of girls with thyroaplasia. In 1904, Erdheim[8] demonstrated, in serial sections from the base of the tongue through the neck, complete aplasia of the thyroid gland in 3 cases of sporadic cretinism. The thymus was very small. Breast feeding did not prevent the clinical symptoms of cretinism.

Fig. 44-1.—Infant with sporadic cretinism.

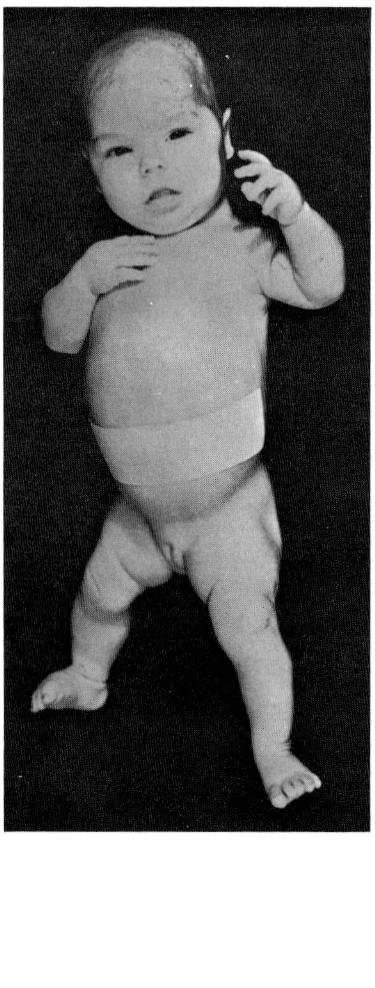

Whether in sporadic cretinism thyroid tissues present in fetal life underwent atrophy after birth remains uncertain. The presence of parathyroids in athyrotic patients suggested primary aplasia to Pineles,[7] but other authors emphasized that in some cases remnants of thyroid tissue or fat and connective tissue in the neck indicated former existence of the gland. More recently, Hubble[8a] demonstrated, in the thyroid area of a cretin dead at 3 months of age, residual thyroid tissue 2 mm. in diameter. The thyroid remnant showed degenerated tissue without colloid formation and cysts containing serous fluid. Failure of thyroid-stimulating hormone was considered the cause of the thyroid atrophy. In other cases of hypothyroidism, the thyroid gland was arrested in its descent ventral to the pharynx.

Ectopic Thyroid

Lingual thyroid is a well-known disease picture characterized by glandular tissue behind the foramen cecum in the midline of the tongue. Local and systemic effects vary. In 1897, Boucourt[9] described a dwarfed cretin woman who developed a thyroid tumor at the root of the tongue. In the same year, myxedema following removal of a lingual thyroid was observed. In recent years, thyroid remnants have been demonstrated in many sporadic cretins by scanning with radioactive iodine. McGirr and Hutchison,[10] examining 4 hypothyroid children with radioactive iodine, showed absence of ^{131}I accumulation in the neck in all cases, but in 2 of them there was marked accumulation above the hyoid bone, indicative of functioning thyroid tissue in the sublingual region. In the third case, hypothyroidism had followed surgical removal of a midline swelling under the chin that contained active thyroid tissue. These authors believed that in the fetus destined to cretinism, small foci of functioning thyroid tissue may satisfy the needs in utero but prove inadequate in postnatal life when the metabolic needs increase. Neimann *et al.*[11] found a similar high incidence of lingual thyroid tissue in 20 of 28 myxedematous patients by scintiscanning, but Gabr[12] ascertained sublingual thyroid remnants in only 8 of 35 patients with sporadic cretinism, and no thyroid tissue could be demonstrated in 18. In 9 cases, tissue remnants were noted in prelaryngeal sites. Andersen,[13] in 38 nongoitrous hypothyroid children, noted no uptake of ^{131}I over the thyroid gland in 24 and sublingual uptake in 14. These isotope studies confirmed numerous older anatomic observations[14,15] that showed that maldescent of the thyroid can bring about sporadic cretinism. Since the descent of the thyroid begins in 6-mm. embryos (fifth week), the origin of this form of cretinism must begin in early embryonic life. It should be emphasized that ectopic thyroid glands, lingual or sublingual, can occur in euthyroid children. Hung *et al.*[16] described 5 children with midline lingual or sublingual masses that were composed of thyroid tissue. Such patients present various problems in diagnosis and management. The presence or absence of normally located thyroid gland should be ascertained by physical examination and by scintiscan with ^{131}I. According to these authors, all children with ectopic thyroid glands should have a trial of full-replacement thyroid therapy before excision is contemplated. Thyroid therapy prevents further hypertrophy and hyperplasia. Surgical intervention should be reserved for those children in whom there is dysphagia, dysphonia, ulceration or hemorrhage from a lingual thyroid gland or if ectopic thyroid gland fails to decrease in size following a course of treatment with thyroid hormones.

Genetic factors in the etiology of sporadic athyroid cretinism have been considered repeatedly. Among 50 propositi, Bernheim *et al.*[17] found only 2 sisters affected, but among ancestors simple and exophthalmic goiter were more frequent than in those of controls. Clinically normal parents showed a high uptake of radioactive iodine, a finding not confirmed by Neel *et al.*[18] In the latter series, there was no recurrence of athyrotic cretinism in 34 families in which a cretin "with no evidence of thyroid tissue" (type I) had occurred. Childs and Gardner[19] recorded 2 affected siblings in a series of 88 athyrotic propositi and Wilkins[3] a pair of siblings in 152 cases. Federman *et al.*[20] described 2 and Ainger and Kelley[21] 3 cretin siblings in whom radioiodine studies revealed no thyroid tissue. There was no thyroid disease in the parents of the 3 cretins, but the histories of more distant relatives were "strikingly suggestive of cretinism." Thus, repetition of athyrotic cretinism in a family is quite rare but the possibility of recurrence must be considered.

There is a marked excess of females among cretins without goiter. The ratio was 1 male to 3.3 females in one series[18] and 1 to 3.6 in another.[17] Consanguinity of the parents of athyrotic cretins is slightly increased, although it is less marked than that of parents of goitrous cretins.[19] The parents of the 3 athyrotic cretin siblings described by Ainger and Kelley[21] were first cousins.

Associated congenital malformations are rare in cretins. If incomplete descent or failure of formation of the thyroid were a teratologic phenomenon comparable to other developmental defects, one would expect a significant incidence of associated oral or cervical malformations in athyrotic cretins. Some authors mention that these patients are normal except for the symptoms of thyroid deficiency, but most publications fail to consider this aspect. Mental retardation, spasticity, strabismus and deafness sometimes occurring despite early treatment have been considered independent anomalies by some authors. But it is possible that thyroid deficiency is responsible for such nerve defects. Among 34 athyrotic cretins, Neel *et al.*[18] observed 1 case of absence of a cervical vertebra, 1 case

Fig. 44-2. – Sporadic cretinism in a boy 2½ years of age. He began to walk at 17 months but had not learned to talk. He was 67 cm. tall. At the age of 9 years, after inadequate treatment, he was 87 cm. tall.

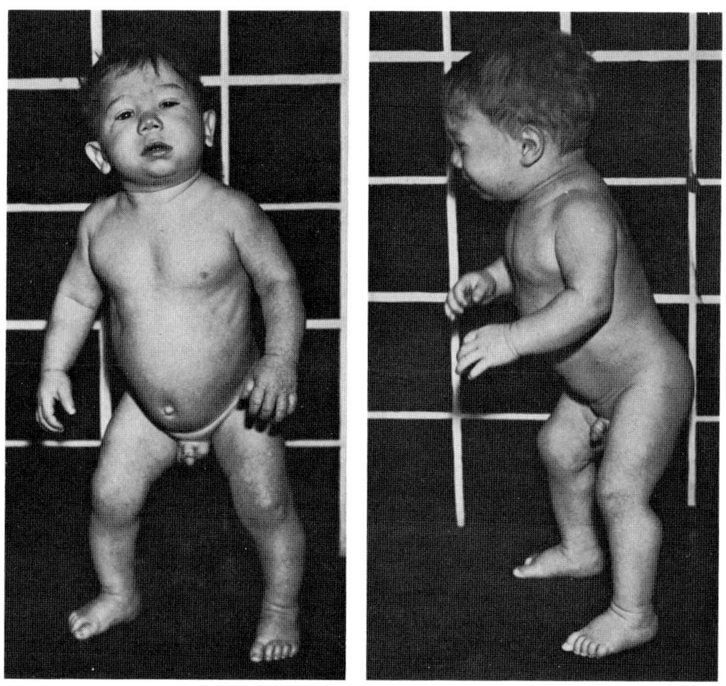

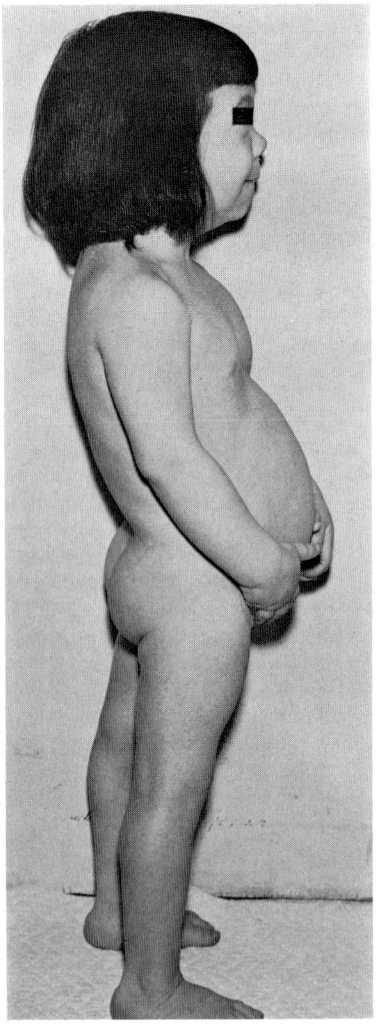

Fig. 44-3. – Hypothyroidism in a girl 14 years of age. She was the thirteenth of 17 children of a mother who had an "internal goiter." She did not walk until age 7 and did not talk until age 10. Her height was 94 cm. at 14 years.

of a large hemangioma of the right face combined with a large pilose nevus of the left scapular region and 1 case of cavernous hemangioma on the back. Recording of associated malformations in all cases of athyrotic cretinism may aid in evaluation of the developmental disturbance leading to the thyroid anomalies. At present, it seems that inhibition of thyroid development in athyrotic cretinism differs from other more generalized teratologic processes, so that search for thyroid-specific injurious factors appears justified.

Blizzard and Chandler[22] suggested that autoimmune disease of the mother transmitted to the fetus could lead to the destruction of the fetal thyroid and thus cause some cases of cretinism. Sutherland *et al.*[23] reported 2 and perhaps 3 siblings, infants of a hypothyroid mother, and considered them "athyrotic." Antithyroid antibodies were present in the serum of the mother and her serum could damage fetal thyroid tissue in vitro, which was considered an explanation of the familial nongoitrous cretinism in this family. It seems questionable that these children can be called athyrotic, since in one of them "the thyroid gland was abnormally firm, pale and yellow-white and was thought to be slightly enlarged." Microscopically, the thyroid was atrophic and fibrotic. In the second child, the thyroid and liver were relatively small, but microscopically the thyroid was within normal limits. The third child survived, treated with desiccated thyroid from the sixth day. These children cannot be considered representative of the common form of athyrosis, in which maldescent or maldevelopment of the thyroid leads to cretinism.

There are reports of hyperthyroid and of hypothyroid mothers who gave birth to cretin children.[24] The fact that overfunction and underfunction of the gland occurs in mothers is difficult to explain by maternal-fetal hormone exchanges. If any type of thyroid disease of the mother could damage the thyroid of the child by transfer of thyroid antibodies, such apparently contradictory findings could be reconciled. But antithyroid antibodies were present in only 29% of mothers who had cretin children and in other instances, when both mother and child had antibodies, the infant had no evidence of disease.[22] The occurrence of monozygotic twins, discordant in regard to hypothyroidism,[25] born to mothers who had thyroid disease, makes it difficult to explain the hypothyroid-

Fig. 44-4. – Sporadic cretinism in a 16-year-old girl. Note myxedema, protruding tongue and umbilical hernia.

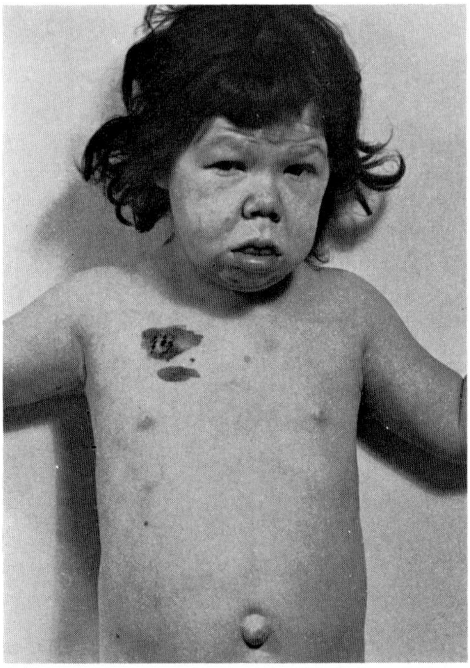

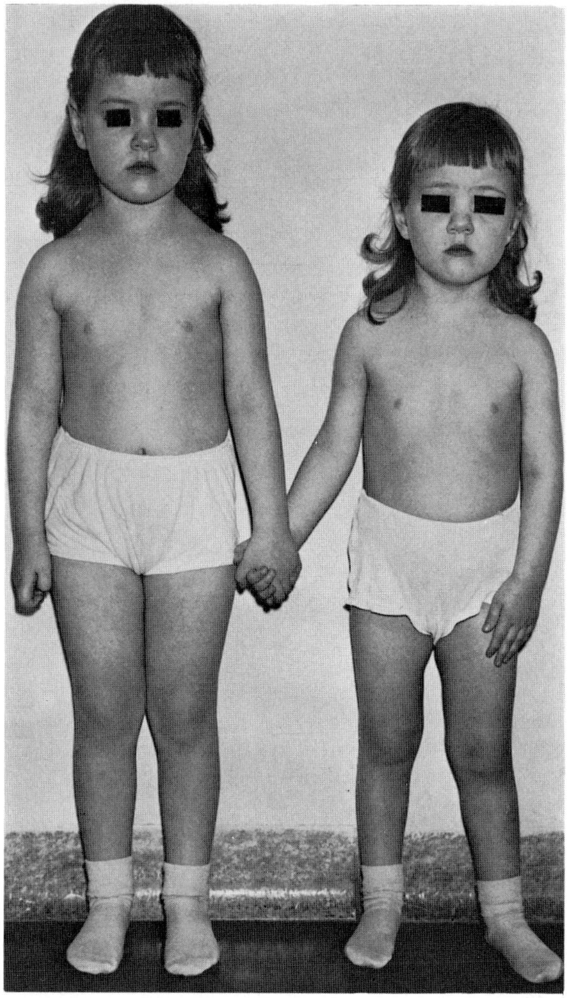

Fig. 44-5. – Discordant hypothyroidism in monozygotic twins. The child at the reader's left was normal; the one at the right was recognized as hypothyroid at age 3 months. Treatment subsequently was irregular. The twins' mother had been treated for hypothyroidism for many years, including the entire time of the pregnancy that resulted in the birth of the twins. (From J. Warkany and T. K. Selkirk.[27])

ism of one twin by placental transfer of thyroid antibodies. In one of the twin cases reported, the mother was hyperthyroid,[26] in the other the mother was hypothyroid.[27] In a third case of such discordant twins, the mother was thought to be in good health.[28] Thus, it appears that there exists a connection between maternal thyroid disease and some cases of athyrotic cretinism, but the reasons for this association are still not known. Some of the most severe forms of thyroid disease occur in endemic areas, and one should expect development of thyroid antibodies in women with such goiters and abundance of athyroidism in their offspring. Yet, the children of mothers with large endemic goiters usually are born goitrous and not athyrotic.

Nonendemic Goitrous Cretinism ("Familial Goiter")

In this type of cretinism, goiter can be present at birth or it develops during childhood. Retardation of development becomes noticeable soon after birth. Cases of this type sometimes recur in families, even in regions in which iodine is plentiful in food and water. Familial goitrous cretinism is due to inborn errors of metabolism that are genetically determined. The disorders are caused by inadequate synthesis or delivery of thyroid hormone.[29] Osler,[30] in 1897, suggested that goitrous cretinism in nonendemic areas might be due to an inborn inability to synthesize thyroid hormone.

Impaired hormone synthesis and hypothyroidism can be present in newborn infants and children who do not yet have enlarged thyroid glands. Goiter often develops later in these children as a compensatory mechanism by increase of thyroid-stimulating pituitary hormone. The degree of cretinism varies and may be absent in the case of sufficient hyperplasia and compensation for the deficient hormonogenesis.[3] Differing degrees of thyroid hormone deficiency may occur in the same family, and sibships have been observed with two types of hypothyroidism – the athyrotic form and the goitrous form with deficiency in hormone synthesis.[18] Such findings suggest that the distinction between athyrotic and goitrous cretinism may not be as clear-cut as previously thought.

It is not possible to discuss thoroughly here the inborn errors of metabolism leading to hypothyroidism. Review articles are available.[29,31] The thyroid glands resulting in "hypothyroidism" or cretinism may be hyperactive and accumulate iodine more rapidly and in greater concentration than in normal persons.

A number of families have been reported with goiter from failure to *form organic iodine compounds* (organification defect). In one study, such a defect was found only once in 50 sibships containing one or more patients with hypothyroidism.[18] The clinical findings in persons with this defect are not uniform. They may show severe cretinism or even be euthyroid. They are not deaf. The metabolic defect seems to be inherited as an autosomal recessive trait.[29]

Cretinism with *failure of coupling iodotyrosines* has been reported in a number of cases of familial goiter with euthyroidism or hypothyroidism. The fault in the thyroid gland is an inability to couple monoiodotyrosine and diiodotyrosine into triiodothyronine (T_3) and thyroxine (T_4). All patients with this defect have been female, and the genetic defect has not yet been elucidated.[29]

Cretinism from *failure of deiodination of iodotyrosine* was reported by McGirr and Hutchison[10] in 12 patients, 4 of whom were siblings and another a relative. They all had goiters that had a high avidity for iodide. Uptake of ^{131}I was completed rapidly but the accumulated iodine left the gland within 24 hours. The sera of the patients then contained monoiodotyrosine and diiodotyrosine but little thyroxine and triiodothyronine. Analysis of the thyroid and of the patients' urines indicated that the principal product of the glands was monoiodotyrosine. Intravenous injection of labeled diiodotyrosine showed that such patients were unable to remove iodine from the benzene ring, and the injected diiodotyrosine appeared in the urine. There was no mechanism to remove iodine from iodotyrosines and an iodine-want was established, resulting in a hyperplastic thyroid devoted to the production and secretion of hormone precursors. This biochemical anomaly may be fairly common among nonendemic goitrous cretins.[29]

Cretinism with *abnormal iodinated polypeptides in the serum* is characterized by iodinated amino acids that are in peptide linkage and which are not extractable into acid butanol. The PBI may be normal or elevated. The gland apparently excretes an ineffective product thought to be an iodoprotein. Untreated patients develop mental retardation and goiter.[29] Observations, although few, suggest recessive autosomal inheritance.

Familial goiter from *failure to transport iodide*, an extremely rare defect, is attributed to an autosomal recessive genetic mechanism.[29]

Familial goiter and deaf-mutism (Pendred syndrome) (p. 407) was described by Pendred in 1896 and recognized as a familial syndrome by Brain.[32] Goiter can be present at birth or appear within the first two decades of life. Nerve deafness is congenital or develops during childhood. Intelligence and growth usually, but not always, are normal. The patients may appear euthyroid but the PBI values tend to be low. The thyroids are moderately enlarged and there is a tendency to malignant degeneration of the gland. The sex distribution is equal. The pattern of inheritance is not entirely clear and the reason for the constant association of thyroid enlargement and deafness is not known. The metabolic error probably is an organification defect but it may be milder or different from that leading to familial goitrous cretinism.[29]

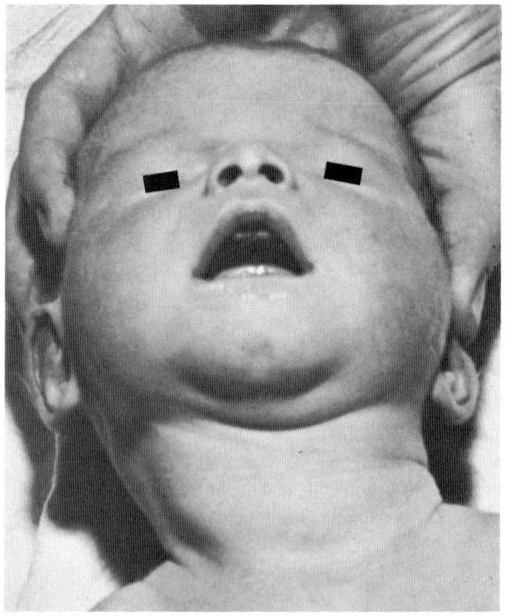

Fig. 44-6. – Congenital goiter in a girl whose mother had been treated for "goiter" with methimazole during pregnancy.

Congenital Goiter or Hypothyroidism Attributed to Maternal Drug Intake

Thiouracil and Derivatives

Most women treated during pregnancy with thiouracil received the drug for treatment of thyrotoxicosis. Some of the children resulting from such pregnancies were normal but a significant number were born with goiter and thyroid hyperplasia.[33,34] Other offspring were aborted, stillborn or died soon after birth. Survivors with goiter sometimes showed spontaneous recovery. Of interest is a case of twin girls[35] born with congenital thyroid hyperplasia following treatment of the mother during pregnancy for thyrotoxicosis with propylthiouracil and iodine. One twin was stillborn, with a conspicuous tumor at the middle of the neck. The surviving twin had an enlarged thyroid but was otherwise normal. In another instance, a woman with mild thyrotoxicosis treated with thiouracil died during the sixth month of pregnancy. The thyroid of the fetus was enlarged and hyperplastic.[36] The case reported by Hone and Magarey[37] is of interest because the child had cretinism at birth and death ensued rapidly. The mother had been treated for hyperthyroidism with thiouracil. Interpretation of such cases is difficult, since maternal disease and thiouracil and iodine treatment often were so intertwined that the antithyroid drug cannot be considered the sole and certain cause of the children's difficulties. More convincing are cases of goiter in the newborn when the mother was treated with thiouracil for vague symptoms without having proved thyroid disease. Such a child was seen in the Cincinnati Children's Hospital for many years (Chart No. 57012). The mother had been treated for "supposed hyperthyroidism" with iodide and thiouracil even though her BMR was +6. The child, a girl, was born with a goiter. At first, she appeared euthyroid but was considered hypothyroid when 1 year of age. Treatment with thyroid was instituted. At the age of 4 years, hyperthyroidism was diagnosed and she was treated with Lugol solution and propylthiouracil. At the age of 5 years, thyroidectomy was done and mild mental retardation (I.Q. 86) was established at the age of 10 years. Hepner,[33] in reviewing the literature, found that of 30 infants born of mothers with hyperthyroidism treated with thiourea derivatives during pregnancy, 25 were normal and 2 had transient enlargement of the thyroid. One pregnancy produced a cretin, two pregnancies ended in abortion, one of the fetuses had a goiter and one pregnancy resulted in an anencephalic with a normal thyroid. Another review of this subject was made by Bongiovanni *et al.*[34]

Iodide

It seems well established that protracted treatment with iodides can lead to thyroid enlargement and goiter in adults[38] and in children.[39] There have been a number of reports of congenital goiter with a history of protracted iodide intake by the mother.[50] Potassium iodide for asthma[40,41] or Lugol solution for tachycardia[40] taken during pregnancy resulted in fetal hyperplasia. If there are no symptoms of choking, the goiter may disappear spontaneously after birth. But in several cases such goiters were fatal. A child recorded by Bernhard *et al.*[42] had a huge goiter (75 Gm.) encircling the trachea. The baby died 1 hour after birth and diffuse epithelial hyperplasia of the thyroid was found at necropsy. In another child dead 30 minutes after delivery, the follicles of the thyroid (42 Gm.) were filled with colloid. The mother had taken saturated solution of potassium iodide freely during pregnancy for the treatment of asthma.[43] Concordant iodine goiter in dizygotic twins has been reported.[49]

Radioactive Iodine

Russell *et al.*[44] reported the case of a woman operated on for carcinoma of the thyroid and treated with radioactive iodine at the thirteenth week of pregnancy. Her child was born with an umbilical hernia and at 2 months of age clinical signs of hypothyroidism developed. In another case of ^{131}I treatment following surgical removal of a thyroid cancer, the drug was given at approximately 13 weeks' gestation and the child was born with slightly dry skin and a small umbilical hernia. At 9 days of age, the PBI was 1.4 μg./100 ml. and at 17 days the external appearance was suggestive of hypothyroidism. Despite thyroxine treatment, the child expired during the third month of life and at necropsy no thyroid tissue was found. Hamill *et al.*[45] recorded the case of a woman treated for thyroid metastases with ^{131}I when 3 months pregnant. A boy was born after 38 weeks' pregnancy weighing 2,050 Gm. At 8 days of age, the PBI was 9.6 μg./100 ml. but it fcll to 3.9 μg./100 ml. at age 4 weeks. At approximately 3 months of age, a large tongue, an umbilical hernia and retardation of ossification indicated hypothyroidism. Thyroid treatment was begun and seemed to be successful. Later, the child developed convulsions and mental retardation. Since he had suffered head trauma, these manifestations cannot be attributed to prenatal ^{131}I treatment with certainty. Fischer[46] described hypothyroidism in a boy 18 months of age whose mother had been treated for thyrotoxicosis with therapeutic doses of ^{131}I at the end of the first trimester of pregnancy.

Congenital Hyperthyroidism

This rare condition was reviewed by Sclare[47] in 1960. The babies with congenital hyperthyroidism are thin, develop diarrhea and are hungry and restless. The pulse rate is very high. If they survive, they recover by about 3 months of age. Treatment with potassium iodide may lead to rapid weight increase and euthyroidism. The disease has been attributed to stimulation of the infant's thyroid by long-acting thyroid stimulator, which can cross from the maternal to the fetal circulation.[48]

REFERENCES

1. Shepard, T. H.: Onset of function in the human fetal thyroid: Biochemical and radioautographic studies from organ culture, J. Clin. Endocrinol. 27:945, 1967.
2. Yamazaki, E., Noguchi, A., and Slingerland, D. W.: The development of hormonal biosynthesis in human fetal thyroids, J. Clin. Endocrinol. 19:1437, 1959.
3. Wilkins, L.: *The Diagnosis and Treatment of Endocrine Disorders in Childhood and Adolescence* (3d ed.; Springfield, Ill.: Charles C Thomas, Publisher, 1965).
4. Carr, E. A., Jr., Beierwaltes, W. H., Neel, J. V., Davidson, R., Lowrey, G. H., Dodson, V. N., and Tanton, J. H.: The various types of thyroid malfunction in cretinism and their relative frequency, Pediatrics 28:1, 1961.
5. Curling: Sporadic cretinism, Med. Chir. Tr. 33:303, 1850.
6. Fagge, C. H.: On sporadic cretinism occurring in England, Brit. M. J. 1:279, 1871.
7. Pineles, F.: Über Thyreoaplasie (kongenitales Myxoedem) und infantiles Myxoedem, Wien. klin. Wchnschr. 15:1129, 1902.
8. Erdheim, J.: Über Schilddrüsenaplasie, Beitr. path. Anat. 35:366, 1904.

8a. Hubble, D.: Thyroid disorders in childhood, Brit. M. J. 1:875, 1956.

9. Boucourt, A. C.: Struma der Zungenwurzel, Beitr. klin. Chir. 19:281, 1897.
10. McGirr, E. M., and Hutchison, J. H.: Dysgenesis of the thyroid gland as a cause of cretinism and juvenile myxedema, J. Clin. Endocrinol. 15:668, 1955.
11. Neimann, N., Kellershohn, C., Pierson, M., and Martin, J.: Le role de l'ectopie thyroidienne dans la génèse du myxoedème, Arch. franç. pédiat. 15:315, 1958.
12. Gabr, M.: The role of thyroid dysgenesis and maldescent in the etiology of sporadic cretinism, J. Pediat. 60:830, 1962.
13. Andersen, H. J.: Studies on hypothyroidism in children, Acta paediat. 50:50, 1961.
14. Montgomery, M. L.: Lingual thyroid, West. J. Surg. 43: 661, 1935.
15. Montgomery, M. L.: Lingual thyroid, West. J. Surg. 44: 303, 1936.
16. Hung, W., Randolph, J. G., Sabatini, D., and Winship, T.: Lingual and sublingual thyroid glands in euthyroid children, Pediatrics 38:647, 1966.
17. Bernheim, M., Berger, M., and Uzan, R.: Le role des facteurs génétiques dans le development du myxoedème congénital, Conf. Internat. sur l'utilisation de l'energie atomique a des fins pacifiques, France, July 7, 1955.
18. Neel, J. V., Carr, E. A., Beierwaltes, W. H., and Davidson, R. T.: Genetic studies on the congenitally hypothyroid, Pediatrics 27:269, 1961.
19. Childs, B., and Gardner, L.: Etiologic factors in sporadic cretinism: An analysis of ninety cases, Ann. Human Genet. 19:90, 1954.
20. Federman, D., Robbins, J., and Rall, J. E.: Some observa-

tions on cretinism and its treatment, New England J. Med. 259:610, 1958.
21. Ainger, L. E., and Kelley, V. C.: Familial athyreotic cretinism: Report of 3 cases, J. Clin. Endocrinol. 15:469, 1955.
22. Blizzard, R. M., and Chandler, R. W.: The history and present concepts of autoimmunization in thyroid disease, J. Pediat. 57:399, 1960.
23. Sutherland, J. M., Esselborn, V. M., Burket, R. L., Skillman, T. B., and Benson, J. T.: Familial nongoitrous cretinism apparently due to maternal antithyroid antibody, New England J. Med. 263:336, 1960.
24. Mayer, J. B., and Hemmer, A.: Die Embryopathia Thyreotica, Arch. Kinderh. 153:123, 1956.
25. Moncrieff, M. W., and McArthur, R. G.: Hypothyroidism in one of monozygotic twins, Postgrad. M. J. 44:423, 1968.
26. Harnack, G. A.: Eineiige Zwillinge mit diskordanter Hypothyreose, Arch. Kinderh. 146:60, 1953.
27. Warkany, J., and Selkirk, T. K.: Discordant monozygotic twins. Hypothyroidism, A.M.A. Am. J. Dis. Child. 89:144, 1955.
28. Pickering, D. E., and Koulischer, N.: Discordance of cretinism in monozygotic twins, A.M.A. Am. J. Dis. Child. 92:63, 1956.
29. Stanbury, J. B.: Familial Goiter, in Stanbury, J. B., Wyngaarden, J. B., and Fredrickson, D. S. (eds.), *The Metabolic Basis of Inherited Disease* (2d ed.; New York: McGraw-Hill Book Company, 1966).
30. Osler, W.: Sporadic cretinism in America, Tr. Cong. Am. Physicians & Surgeons 4:169, 1897.
31. Hutchison, J. H.: Hypothyroidism, in Gairdner, D. (ed.), *Recent Advances in Pediatrics* (2d ed.; Boston: Little, Brown & Company, 1958).
32. Brain, W. R.: Heredity in simple goiter, Quart. J. Med. 20: 303, 1927.
33. Hepner, W. R.: Thiourea derivatives and the fetus. Review and report of a case, Am. J. Obst. & Gynec. 63:869, 1952.
34. Bongiovanni, A. M., Eberlein, W. R., Thomas, P. Z., and Anderson, W. B.: Sporadic goiter of the newborn, J. Clin. Endocrinol. 16:146, 1956.
35. Saye, E. B., Watt, C. H., Foushee, J. C., and Palmer, J. I.: Congenital thyroid hyperplasia in twins, J.A.M.A. 149: 1399, 1952.
36. Davis, L. J., and Forbes, W.: Thiouracil in pregnancy; effect on foetal thyroid, Lancet 2:740, 1945.
37. Hone, G. M., and Magarey, I.: Cretinism associated with methyl thiouracil therapy, M. J. Australia 2:524, 1948.
38. Paris, J., McConahey, W. M., Owen, C. A., Jr., Woolner, L. B., and Bahn, R. C.: Iodide goiter, J. Clin. Endocrinol. 20:57, 1960.
39. Turner, H. H., and Howard, R. B.: Goiter from prolonged ingestion of iodide, J. Clin. Endocrinol. 16:141, 1956.
40. Parmelee, A. H., Allen, E., Stein, I. F., and Buxbaum, H.: Three cases of congenital goiter, Am. J. Obst. & Gynec. 40:145, 1940.
41. Talbot, N. B., Sobel, E. H., McArthur, J. W., and Crawford, J. D.: *Functional Endocrinology* (Cambridge, Mass.: Harvard University Press, 1952).
42. Bernhard, W. G., Grubin, H., and Scheller, C. A.: Congenital goiter; report of fatal case with postmortem findings, A.M.A. Arch. Path. 60:635, 1955.
43. Petty, C. S., and DiBenedetto, R. L.: Goiter of the newborn. Report of an unusual case, New England J. Med. 256:1103, 1957.
44. Russell, K. P., Rose, H., and Starr, P.: The effects of radioactive iodine on maternal and fetal thyroid function during pregnancy, Surg., Gynec. & Obst. 104:560, 1957.
45. Hamill, G. C., Jarman, J. A., and Wynne, M. D.: Fetal effects of radioactive iodine therapy in a pregnant woman with thyroid cancer, Am. J. Obst. & Gynec. 81:1018, 1961.
46. Fischer, P. M. S.: Hyperthyroidism in the first year of life; report of a case occurring in the neonatal period, South African M. J. 25:217, 1951.
47. Sclare, G.: Congenital hyperthyroidism, Biol. Neonat. 2: 132, 1960.
48. Adams, D. D., Lord, J. M., and Stevely, H. A. A.: Congenital thyrotoxicosis, Lancet 2:497, 1964.
49. Anderson, G. S., and Bird, T.: Congenital iodide goitre in twins, Lancet 2:742, 1961.
50. Carswell, F., Kerr, M. M., and Hutchison, J. H.: Congenital goitre and hypothyroidism produced by maternal ingestion of iodides, Lancet 1:1241, 1970.

45

The Parathyroids

THE PARATHYROID GLANDS originate from the third and fourth pharyngeal pouches in the form of solid epithelial strands that contact the dorsal surfaces of the lateral lobes of the thyroid. The parathyroids of the third pharyngeal pouches at first lie near the main anlage of the thymus, with which they migrate caudad, becoming the inferior parathyroids located below the parathyroids originating from the fourth pharyngeal pouches, which become the superior parathyroids. Thus, there is a craniocaudad inversion of the parathyroids in position as development progresses.

The primordia of the parathyroids appear in the sixth week, and they join the thyroid lobes during the seventh week. The superior parathyroids (parathyroids IV) usually are found on the posterior or medial surfaces of the thyroid, above their lower thirds. The inferior parathyroids (parathyroids III) usually are located near the inferior poles of the thyroid. As they are derived from the third pharyngeal pouches, they are associated with the thymus, and occasionally situated in the mediastinum several centimeters below the inferior pole of the thyroid. If one of the parathyroid primordia fails to separate from the pharynx, the gland can develop within the pharyngeal wall; in such a case, an aberrant parathyroid is embedded in the pharyngeal submucosa.[1]

Abnormal location of parathyroid glands is of importance in cases of adenoma and surgical intervention. In approximately 10% of the cases, adenomas are located within the mediastinum, more often in the anterior than in the posterior mediastinum.[2]

Absence of Parathyroids

Congenital absence of the parathyroid glands is rare. Lobdell,[3] in 1959, stated that there were only 5 reported cases. He described a full-term infant boy born with neuromuscular hyperirritability noted at birth who had a serum calcium level of 4.9 mg./100ml. 12 hours after birth. There was a positive Chvostek sign but no carpopedal spasms. The child emitted a high-pitched "cerebral cry." The serum calcium could be raised by parathormone, vitamin D and calcium administration. At 1 month of age, signs of tetany were diminished, but pneumonia and enteritis developed and the child died when 55 days of age. At necropsy, no thymus tissue and no thyroid isthmus were found. Serial sections showed absence of parathyroid tissue. Derivatives of branchial pouches I and II, namely, the middle ears, eustachian tubes and tonsillar fossae were intact. There also was a double aortic arch with predominance of the right arch. Other cases of congenital absence of parathyroid glands reviewed by Lobdell[3] were accompanied by such malformations as acrania, microcephaly with external hydrocephaly, aniridia, absent macula lutea, malformed ears, branchiogenic cyst, agenesis of a thyroid lobe, cleft uvula, reduplication of a renal pelvis and ureter, or heterotopic pancreas.

Hypoparathyroidism

Infants born without parathyroid glands represent a form of congenital hypoparathyroidism, but it is doubtful that such cases are etiologically related to the forms of hypoparathyroidism that develop postnatally during childhood or in adult life.[4] The average age of onset of symptoms is 17 years in patients with idiopathic hypoparathyroidism, which therefore cannot be considered a congenital disease in most of the cases. But it is possible that the glandular deficiency may exist for many years prior to the appearance of overt symptoms, so that a congenital hypoparathyroid tendency cannot be ruled out in all cases. The overt signs are tetany, convulsions, lenticular opacities, trophic ectodermal lesions, basal ganglia calcifications, and low serum calcium and high serum phosphorus levels. Mental development can range from deficiency to superiority.[5]

Hypoparathyroidism has occurred repeatedly in siblings. Familial aggregation may be due to genetic or adverse environmental factors. Peden[6] recorded neonatal idiopathic hypoparathyroidism in 2 male siblings and assumed sex-linked inheritance in this family. A case of neonatal idiopathic hypoparathyroidism was also reported by Smith and Zike,[7] who pointed out the importance of early diagnosis for successful treatment. Congenital familial hypoparathyroidism also has been reported in a female and a male sibling.[51] Sutphin *et al.*[8] described a family in which there were 3 cases of idiopathic hypoparathyroidism and thalassemia. Two or possibly 3 of the patients had chronic moniliasis. By 1968, seven families with more than one member affected by idiopathic hypoparathyroidism had been reported. The disorder developed during adolescence or thereafter. The trait seemed to be transmitted as an autosomal recessive.[9] Neuhaus *et al.*[10] believed that hypocalcemia and tetany can be the result of cerebral disorders that, in some cases, are present in the neonatal period. They reported a case of congenital microcephaly associated with neonatal tetany and severe hypocalcemia. Nichols *et al.*[11] recorded a kindred in which 9 of 13 members had abnormal intracranial calcifications. The disorder was transmitted through three generations like an autosomal dominant hereditary trait. In 2 members, calcification of basal ganglia was demonstrated, although there were no abnormalities of serum calcium, serum phosphorus or neuromuscular irritability. A kindred in which 6 members had calcification of the basal ganglia but no other symptoms of idiopathic hypoparathyroidism or pseudohypoparathyroidism has been reported. In only 2 of these persons latent abnormalities of phosphorus balance and a subnormal response to parathormone administration could be shown.[12] Lachmann[13] reported a family of 5 siblings, of whom 3 and possibly 4 had idiopathic hypoparathyroidism. Interestingly, the 3 affected children had associated abnormalities of the hands and feet, 2 of them showing partial syndactyly. There are a number of observations of patients with hypoparathyroidism combined with hypoadrenocorticism[14,15] and there are families in which siblings developed hypoparathyroidism and other siblings developed adrenal insufficiency. We have seen a family in which a girl suffered from idiopathic hypoparathyroidism, chronic tetany and hypocalcemia. Many years later, her brother developed symptoms of Addison disease (see Fig. 43-5). Other cases were discussed by Sweetnam,[16] who pointed out the occurrence of the two conditions separately or together in siblings in several families. He thought that genetic factors might be important in the etiology of these disorders. No doubt the association of such familial endocrine disorders is not understood. One theory has considered an inborn inferiority of the organs. Familial hypoparathyroidism with pernicious anemia, steatorrhea and adrenocortical insufficiency was reported as a variant of mucoviscidosis by Morse *et al.*[17] and idiopathic hypoparathyroidism and adrenocortical insufficiency occurring with cystic fibrosis by McMahon *et al.*[18] A case of hypoparathyroidism associated with megaloblastic anemia has been described.[19] A familial autoimmune reaction was considered by Blizzard *et al.*[20] as the basis of parathyroid and adrenocortical damages. But the possibility that idiopathic hypoparathyroidism is an acquired disease cannot be excluded from consideration, since, in some of the familial cases, the patients have monilial infections. Growth of monilia could be the result of the metabolic disturbance, yet moniliasis does not occur in parathyroid deficiency following thyroidectomy or in pseudohypoparathyroidism. In some instances, the moniliasis preceded the appearance of symptoms of hypoparathyroidism.[21] A case report of cytomegalic inclusion disease associated with hypoparathyroidism also deserves attention in this connection.[22] It seems probable that idiopathic hypoparathyroidism is not an etiologic entity.

Hypoparathyroidism as a reaction to maternal hyperparathyroidism points to a different mechanism. There is one report of chronic hypoparathyroidism (associated with a multicystic kidney) that probably can be blamed on the mother's hyperparathyroidism.[23] It was thought[24] that the development of the child's parathyroid glands in utero was suppressed by the excess of diffusible calcium in the mother's serum and that the glands failed to recover when the repressive stimulus was withdrawn. The child's symptoms did not begin until he was 1 year of age. The delay in onset of the symptoms was thought to be due to the lower phosphate content of breast milk, since the first manifestations of tetany did not appear until shortly after breast feeding was stopped. Permanent damage to the parathyroid of the fetus by maternal hyperparathyroidism probably is rare. Temporary hypoparathyroidism in the newborn period due to hyperparathyroidism of the mother has been observed repeatedly. It is believed that neonatal tetany may, at times, be the only clinical lead to the diagnosis of hyperparathyroidism in the mother.[25,26] If more than one child develops tetany in infancy, the parathyroid function of a mother, even if free of symptoms, should be investigated. There seems to be an increased incidence of stillbirths, miscarriages and premature births in mothers with primary hyperparathyroidism.[25] But idiopathic hypoparathyroidism can also occur in newborn children of diabetic mothers.[27]

The incidence of primary hypoparathyroidism in the first year of life seems to be low, as by 1966 only 20 cases had been reported. An infant with congenital absence of both the parathyroid and thymus glands has been described by Taitz *et al.*[4] and Huber *et al.*[28] The patient developed renal tubular acidosis and nephrocalcinosis. The disease picture was named by these authors the "three and four pharyngeal pouch syndrome." It is believed that this syndrome, which should be differentiated from the nonlethal sex-linked form[6] of hypoparathyroidism, has a high mortality because of absence of the thymus and immunologic incompetence[4] (Chapter 79).

Geertinger[29] examined the parathyroid sites at the thyroid capsule in 82 infants between 2 and 11 months of age who had died suddenly and unexpectedly of unknown cause. In 28 cases, the parathyroid could not be found and in 54 thymus tissue occurred within the parathyroid capsule. The sudden deaths were attributed to embryologic maldevelopment of the branchial apparatus and a disorder of calcium metabolism.

PSEUDOHYPOPARATHYROIDISM

Pseudohypoparathyroidism was described in 1942 by Albright *et al.*[30] as a disorder resembling idiopathic hypoparathyroidism in patients who do not respond to parathyroid hormone. Biopsy shows that such persons have functioning parathyroid glands and it seems that their symptoms are due to an inability of the end organs to respond to parathyroid hormone.[31,32] In fact, exploration of the neck revealed hyperplastic parathyroid glands in some cases.

The condition has been observed repeatedly in siblings[34] and in two successive generations.[32] Concordance has been reported in at least three pairs of twins.[35] Some of the physical features of the disorder are at times seen in relatives who have no signs of hypoparathyroidism. Females are affected about twice as often as males.

The average age at onset of symptoms is 8½ years,[36] but in many instances congenital or early signs have been observed.[37] Talbot *et al.*[38] noted calcification in soft tissues in newborn twins. Slow development from birth was reported by Oberst and Tompkins,[39] Cohen and Donnell[35] and others. One patient had always been small for his age and was unable to run and play from earliest childhood because of cramps and discomfort in the extremities.[40] Early obesity was seen in some instances.[35]

Tetany, convulsions, twitching and muscle cramps are alarming manifestations. Low serum calcium and high serum phosphorus levels are found. Urinary excretion of calcium and phosphorus is decreased. Response to parathormone injection is insignificant. Round face, obesity and short stature are external characteristics. Dentition may be delayed and incomplete. The neck is short and the hands are broad, small and stubby. The digits of the hands and feet are short and irregular in length, the index finger usually being longer than the middle finger. Shortening of the metacarpals and metatarsals is quite characteristic but not all are equally affected. As a rule, the first, fourth and fifth metacarpal bones are reduced in length more than their neighbors. This anomaly can be demonstrated by clenching of the patient's fist, which brings out a (distally) concave arching of a line connecting the metacarpophalangeal joint. Roentgenograms show, in addition to shortened metacarpal and metatarsal bones, short and wide digital phalanges. Often there are soft tissue and cerebral calcifications, the calvarium is thickened and the diploic space wide. Ossification is irregular and sometimes accelerated. Osteoporosis and osteosclerosis have been described. Modeling of the long bones often is disturbed, and curving of the forearm bones is seen occasionally.[35] The outstanding skeletal symptom, brachydactyly, has been explained by early closure of the epiphyses, but the cause of this is not clear.

Mental retardation is common. In some cases, mental deterioration follows attacks of tetany or seizures, and it seems likely that early treatment can prevent such oligophrenia. But in other cases development is slow from infancy on, long before tetany or convulsions appear. Association with hypothyroidism may be responsible for mental retardation in such cases.[35] Cretinoid appearance has been pointed out repeatedly in some of the patients, and hypothyroidism has been suspected often. Hypogenitalism was reported in some patients,[41] but one woman with self-limited pseudohypoparathyroidism went through a normal pregnancy and gave birth to a normal child.[42] The disorder can be passed on by a patient to her children.[32]

Treatment with dihydrotachysterol (AT-10) sometimes has been used successfully but has failed in other cases. Vitamin D in large doses – initially 100,000 – 400,000 I.U. – has been successful. Supplemental oral calcium therapy has been given to hasten the initial rise in serum calcium and to stop tetany and convulsions. If hypothyroidism is present, administra-

Fig. 45-1. – Roentgenogram of a child with pseudohypoparathyroidism, showing marked shortening of metacarpals IV and V.

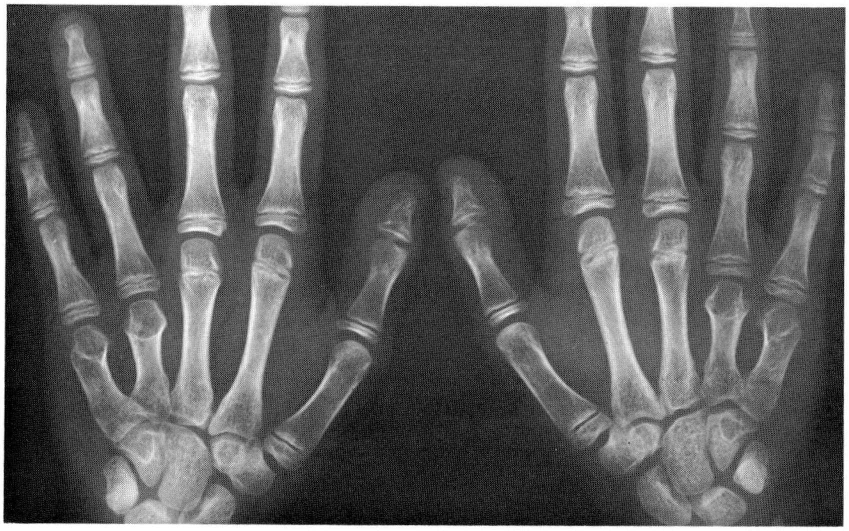

tion of thyroid should be added to the treatment. Mental improvement has been observed in some treated cases but it was questionable in others.

Pseudo-pseudohypoparathyroidism

(Metacarpal Dwarfism without Tetany; Albright Hereditary Osteodystrophy without Hypocalcemia)

The term pseudo-pseudohypoparathyroidism (PPH) was first used in 1952 by Albright *et al.*[43] for a woman with signs of pseudohypoparathyroidism (PH) (p. 446) but without tetany or hypocalcemia. Since it was found out subsequently that this condition is only loosely connected with hypoparathyroidism, many attempts have been made to find a better term. Jancar,[44] in 1965, enumerated seven names suggested for this disease and contributed a new one: cerebro-metacarpo-metatarsal dystrophy. A review of the terms suggested leads one to the impression that Albright "pseudo-pseudohypoparathyroidism," inadequate as it is, is not inferior to those proposed by others, and it at least has the merit of being fairly well established.

Pseudo-pseudohypoparathyroidism cannot be distinguished from pseudohypoparathyroidism by external inspection or roentgenographically and there are reasons to believe that the two disorders are etiologically related.[45] Early convulsions in infancy have been reported.[44,46] Since, in these cases, calcium determinations were not done during the early convulsive state, it is possible that the seizures were due to hypocalcemia and that the disorder actually began as PH, developing into PPH with cessation of tetanic manifestations. This explanation would be in accord with the finding of lenticular opacities in some of the patients.[47] That PH and PPH are variants of the same disorder is also suggested by the fact that the two diseases have been seen in members of the same family.[46]

Short stature, obesity, round face, mental retardation, short metacarpal or metatarsal bones and soft tissue calcifications are symptoms common to both disorders. It has been said that exostoses occur more often in the form without tetany and cerebral calcifications more often in PH with hypocalcemia.[46]

Hypoparathyroidism is only one of the endocrine symptoms complicating the varied disease picture of PPH. Disturbances of sexual functions (Turner syndrome) were observed by Engel *et al.*[48] and emphasized by van der Werff.[33] Diabetes mellitus was mentioned by Engel *et al.*[48] and by Tanz.[50] In PH, diabetes insipidus and hypothyroidism have been observed as complicating symptoms. The common denominator for the vicarious endocrine disturbances is still not known.

Mental retardation occurs in many patients with PPH. Sometimes not only the patients with the entire syndrome are affected but also relatives may have neurologic, intellectual and psychiatric difficulties.[49]

PPH in all probability is genetically determined but the mode of inheritance is not established. Familial incidence has been reported in approximately one-third of the cases. Repetitive cases occurred in siblings, but the condition has also been transmitted from mothers to their children; in no instance was a male-to-male transmission observed.[46] Schwarz and Bahner,[45] who considered PH and PPH as one entity, found in the medical literature 56 familial cases that belonged to twenty-two different families. In fourteen families, the disorder was transmitted from parents to children, which suggests some form of dominant inheritance. There was no transmission from a father to a son. Females were affected twice as often as males. One-fifth of the cases of PPH reported were associated with chromatin-negative gonadal dysgenesis (Turner syndrome). From these facts, Schwarz and Bahner concluded that PH and PPH probably are inherited as an irregular dominant trait attributable to a gene located on an X chromosome. In one case, one large acrocentric chromosome showed elongated short arms with prominent satellites.[44]

The treatment of PPH is symptomatic.

REFERENCES

1. Herrold, K. M., Rabson, A. S., and Ketcham, A. S.: Aberrant parathyroid gland in pharyngeal submucosa, Arch. Path. 71:60, 1961.
2. Black, B. M.: Surgical aspects of hyperparathyroidism, Am. Surgeon 20:1044, 1954.
3. Lobdell, D. H.: Congenital absence of the parathyroid glands, A.M.A. Arch. Path. 67:412, 1959.
4. Taitz, L. S., Zarate-Salvador, C., and Schwartz, E.: Congenital absence of the parathyroid and thymus glands in an infant (III and IV pharyngeal pouch syndrome), Pediatrics 38:412, 1966.
5. Money, J., and Ehrhardt, A. A.: Preservation of IQ in hypoparathyroidism of childhood, Am. J. Ment. Deficiency 71:237, 1966.
6. Peden, V. H.: True idiopathic hypoparathyroidism as a sex-linked recessive trait, Am. J. Human Genet. 12:323, 1960.
7. Smith, F. G., Jr., and Zike, K.: Idiopathic hypoparathyroidism in neonatal period, Am. J. Dis. Child. 105:182, 1963.
8. Sutphin, A., Albright, F., and McCune, D.: Five cases (three in siblings) of idiopathic hypoparathyroidism associated with moniliasis, J. Clin. Endocrinol. 3:625, 1943.
9. Bronsky, D., Kiamko, R. T., and Waldstein, S. S.: Familial idiopathic hypoparathyroidism, J. Clin. Endocrinol. 28:61, 1968.
10. Neuhaus, T., Zellweger, H., and Fanconi, G.: Cerebral bedingte chronische Hypocalcämie und Tetanie, Helvet. paediat. acta 8:237, 1953.
11. Nichols, F. L., Holdsworth, D. E., and Reinfrank, R. F.: Familial hypocalcemia, latent tetany and calcification of the basal ganglia, Am. J. Med. 30:518, 1961.
12. Palubinskas, A. J., and Davies, J.: Calcification of the basal ganglia of the brain, Am. J. Roentgenol. 82:806, 1959.
13. Lachmann, A.: Hypoparathyroidism in Denmark; clinical study, Acta med. scandinav. 121:1, 1941.
14. Leifer, E., and Hollander, W., Jr.: Idiopathic hypoparathyroidism and chronic adrenal insufficiency: A case report, J. Clin. Endocrinol. 13:1264, 1953.
15. Hiekkala, H.: Idiopathic hypoparathyroidism, adrenal

insufficiency and moniliasis in children, Ann. paediat. Fenniae 10:213, 1964.
16. Sweetnam, W. P.: Juvenile familial endocrinopathy, Lancet 1:463, 1966.
17. Morse, W. I., Cochrane, W. A., and Landrigan, P. L.: Familial hypoparathyroidism with pernicious anemia, steatorrhea and adrenocortical insufficiency, New England J. Med. 264:1021, 1961.
18. McMahon, F. G., Cookson, D. U., Kabler, J. D., and Inhorn, S. L.: Idiopathic hypoparathyroidism and idiopathic adrenal cortical insufficiency occurring with cystic fibrosis of the pancreas, Ann. Int. Med. 51:371, 1959.
19. Hurwitz, L. J.: Spontaneous hypoparathyroidism with megaloblastic anaemia, Lancet 1:234, 1956.
20. Blizzard, R. M., Chee, D., and Davis, W.: The incidence of parathyroid and other antibodies in the serums of patients with idiopathic hypoparathyroidism, Clin. & Exper. Immunol. 1:119, 1966.
21. McLean, M. M.: Chronic idiopathic hypoparathyroidism associated with moniliasis, Arch. Dis. Childhood 29:419, 1954.
22. Curtis, J. C., Dodge, W. F., and Daeschner, C. W.: Cytomegalic inclusion disease associated with hypoparathyroidism, Pediatrics 29:52, 1962.
23. Mitchell, R. G.: Chronic hypoparathyroidism associated with a multicystic kidney, Arch. Dis. Childhood 29:349, 1954.
24. Bruce, J., and Strong, J. A.: Maternal hyperparathyroidism and parathyroid deficiency in the child, Quart. J. Med. 24:307, 1955.
25. Walton, R. L.: Neonatal tetany in two siblings: Effect of maternal hyperparathyroidism, Pediatrics 13:227, 1954.
26. Hutchin, P., and Kessner, D. M.: Neonatal tetany. Diagnostic lead to hyperparathyroidism in the mother, Ann. Int. Med. 61:1109, 1964.
27. Kunstadt, R. H., Oh, W., Tanman, F., and Cornblath, M.: Idiopathic hypoparathyroidism in the newborn, Am. J. Dis. Child. 105:499, 1963.
28. Huber, J., Cholnoky, P., and Zoethout, H. E.: Congenital aplasia of parathyroid glands and thymus, Arch. Dis. Childhood 42:190, 1967.
29. Geertinger, P.: Sudden, unexpected death in infancy, Pediatrics 39:43, 1967.
30. Albright, F., Burnett, C. H., Smith, P. H., and Parson, W.: Pseudohypoparathyroidism—an example of "Seabright-Bantam syndrome"; report of 3 cases, Endocrinology 30: 922, 1942.
31. Mautalen, C. A., Dymling, J-F., and Horwith, M.: Pseudohypoparathyroidism 1942–1966. A negative progress report, Am. J. Med. 42:977, 1967.
32. Lee, J. B., Tashjian, A. H., Jr., Streeto, J. M., and Frantz, A. G.: Familial pseudohypoparathyroidism. Role of parathyroid hormone and thyrocalcitonin, New England J. Med. 279:1179, 1968.
33. van der Werff ten Bosch, J. J.: The syndrome of brachymetacarpal dwarfism ("pseudo-pseudohypoparathyroidism") with and without gonadal dysgenesis, Lancet 1:69, 1959.
34. Christiaens, L., Fontaine, G., Farriaux, J. P., and Biserte, G.: Le pseudohypoparathyroidisme chronique. A propos de trois cas familiaux, Acta paediat. belg. 21:5, 1967.
35. Cohen, M. L., and Donnell, G. N.: Pseudohypoparathyroidism with hypothyroidism; a case report and review of literature, J. Pediat. 56:369, 1960.
36. Bronsky, D., Kushner, D. S., Dubin, A., and Snapper, I.: Idiopathic hypoparathyroidism and pseudohypoparathyroidism: Case reports and review of the literature, Medicine 37:317, 1958.
37. Taitz, L. S.: Pseudohypoparathyroidism in infancy, Arch. Dis. Childhood 35:506, 1960.
38. Talbot, N. B., Sobel, E. H., McArthur, J. W., and Crawford, J. D.: *Functional Endocrinology from Birth Through Adolescence* (Cambridge, Mass.: Harvard University Press, 1952).
39. Oberst, B. B., and Tompkins, C. A.: Pseudohypoparathyroidism, A.M.A. Am. J. Dis. Child. 90:205, 1955.
40. Butterworth, C. E., Hamilton, L. C., and Zheutlin, N.: Pseudohypoparathyroidism, Am. J. Med. 21:644, 1956.
41. MacGregor, M. E., and Whitehead, T. P.: Pseudo-hypoparathyroidism, Arch. Dis. Childhood 29:398, 1954.
42. Gershberg, H., and Weseley, A. C.: Pseudohypoparathyroidism and pregnancy. Is pseudo-pseudohypoparathyroidism a mild form of pseudohypoparathyroidism?, J. Pediat. 56:383, 1960.
43. Albright, F., Forbes, A. P., and Hermeman, P. H.: Pseudo-pseudohypoparathyroidism, Tr. A. Am. Physicians 65: 337, 1952.
44. Jancar, J.: Cerebro-metacarpo-metatarsal dystrophy (pseudo-pseudohypoparathyroidism) with chromosomal anomaly, J. M. Genetics 2:32, 1965.
45. Schwarz, G., and Bahner, F.: Die Genetik des Pseudohypoparathyreoidismus und des Pseudo-Pseudohypoparathyreoidismus, Deutsche med. Wchnschr. 88:240, 1963.
46. Papaioannou, A. C., and Matsas, B. E.: Albright's hereditary osteodystrophy (without hypocalcemia). (Brachymetacarpal dwarfism without tetany, or pseudo-pseudohypoparathyroidism.) Report of a case and review of the literature, Pediatrics 31:599, 1963.
47. Casey, T. R., Fast, B. B., and Cherniack, R. M.: Pseudo-pseudohypoparathyroidism. Report of a case with associated cardiopulmonary syndrome of obesity, J.A.M.A. 169: 1988, 1959.
48. Engel, E., Haenni, A., and Ducommun, P.: Agénésie ovarienne et pseudohypoparathyroidisme sans hypocalcémie, Schweiz. med. Wchnschr. 86:1260, 1956.
49. Cruz, C. E., and Barnett, N.: Mental retardation on pseudo-pseudohypoparathyroidism. Case reports of siblings and review of the literature, Am. J. Ment. Deficiency 67:381, 1962.
50. Tanz, S. S.: Pseudo-pseudohypoparathyroidism; three cases in one family, Am. J. M. Sc. 239:453, 1960.
51. Gorodischer, R., Aceto, T., Jr., and Terplan, K.: Congenital familial hypoparathyroidism, Am. J. Dis. Child. 119:74, 1970.

Congenital Hyperparathyroidism

HYPERPARATHYROIDISM is rare in children and only 8 cases have been observed in infants. Parental consanguinity[1,2] and familial recurrence[3] suggest that recessive inheritance may play a role in the etiology. Congenital hyperparathyroidism secondary to the mother's hypoparathyroidism has been reported.[5] Failure to thrive, marked hypotonia, dehydration, constipation, craniotabes and bulging fontanelle are some of the signs of the disorder. Rarefactions of the long bones are seen in radiograms. Hypercalcemia and hypophosphatemia are marked.[2,4] The condition is extremely serious; with one exception, all the children died in infancy. Subtotal parathyroidectomy at an early age seems to be the only hope for survival.[3]

REFERENCES

1. Philips, R. N.: Primary diffuse parathyroid hyperplasia in an infant of four months, Pediatrics 2:428, 1948.
2. Corbeel, L., Casaer, P., Malvaux, P., Lormans, J., and Bourgeois, N.: Hyperparathyroidie congénitale, Arch. franc. pédiat. 25:879, 1968.
3. Hillman, D. A., Schriver, C. R., Pedvis, S., and Shragovitch, I.: Neonatal familial primary hyperparathyroidism, New England J. Med. 270:483, 1964.
4. Pratt, E. L., Geren, B. B., and Neuhauser, E. B. D.: Hypercalcemia and idiopathic hyperplasia of the parathyroid glands in an infant, J. Pediat. 30:388, 1947.
5. Landing, B. H., and Kamoshita, S.: Congenital hyperparathyroidism secondary to maternal hypoparathyroidism, J. Pediat. 77:842, 1970.

46

The Pineal Body

IN HUMAN EMBRYOS of 5 weeks (or 8 mm.), a diverticulum develops from the posterior portion of the roof of the diencephalon that represents the first pineal anlage. The rostral wall of the diverticulum thickens rapidly by development of cell masses (anterior pineal lobe), whereas the caudal wall at first remains limited to a single cell layer. In embryos of 2 months, the anterior cell masses show formation of tubules that appear in sections as rosettes with small lumina. This tubular arrangement is of short duration, as the parenchymal cells are condensed to cords and clusters that are separated by mesodermal tissue and vascular channels. In the third month, proliferation of cells in the posterior wall of the diverticulum progresses whereby the pineal ventricle is narrowed and finally obliterated. Although the anterior lobe develops before the posterior, the two components consist of similar cells, all derived from ependyma of the pineal diverticulum.

The pineal gland is situated in the roof of the diencephalon between the habenular and posterior commissures and its body lies between the anterior colliculi of the corpora quadrigemina. An evagination of the third ventricle – the recessus pinealis – extends into the base of the pineal gland. The dorsal surface of the pineal is in contact with the lamina tectoria of the third ventricle, which encloses the recessus suprapinealis. Size and weight of the gland vary with age.[1] The neuroepithelial or parenchymal cells of the pineal body are arranged in lobules that are separated by a meshwork of connective tissue, capillaries and glia fibers. Lobules or follicles are more visible in old than in young persons and more often present in the central than in the peripheral parts of the pineal body. The parenchymal chief cells (pineocytes) are characterized by a large nucleus and nucleolus and multiple cytoplasmic processes.[2]

Aplasia of the Pineal Gland

Only a few instances of aplasia of the pineal gland have been recorded. Zandrén[3] described absence of the pineal body in a 16-year-old boy with infantilism, retarded growth and hypoplastic testes. The boy's retardation had begun when he was 9 years of age. The pituitary gland appeared normal. Zandrén concluded that the pineal normally initiates puberty and stimulates the sex glands. Kitay and Altschule[4] listed 6 cases of pineal aplasia; in 3 of these, hypogonadism was reported. This does not support the view that the pineal inhibits sex development and is in contrast with reports of hypergonadism associated with pineal hypoplasia. In children with hydrocephaly, absence of the pineal may be due to pressure atrophy. A case of male pseudohermaphrodism associated with adrenal hyperplasia and absence of the pineal was reported by Healey and Guy.[5]

Hypoplasia of the Pineal Gland

Kitay and Altschule[4] listed 9 cases of pineal hypoplasia. Eight of the patients had genital precocity, but in 5 of these there were associated pituitary changes such as eosinophilic hyperplasia or adenoma. Askanazy and Brack[6] reported hypoplasia of the pineal in a girl 23 years of age who had microcephaly, microgyria, porencephaly, chorioretinitis, goiter, bronchiectasis, cecum mobile and precocious isosexual development with onset before the age of 10 years. There was no hydrocephaly that could explain pineal atrophy. Dietrich[7] found hypoplasia of the pineal with microscopic cysts in glial tissue in a woman of 25 years with hirsutism of the masculine type and undeveloped breasts. There were small aggregates of pineal cells in the stalk of the gland (accessory pineal). Thus, of 2 females with pineal hypoplasia, 1 showed somewhat precocious isosexual development, whereas the other had hirsutism of the heterosexual type. Testicular hypertrophy associated with pineal hypoplasia and eosinophilic adenoma of the anterior pituitary was observed by Kup.[8] The same author[9] reported macrogenitosomia praecox in a boy who died of tuberculosis. There was a reduction of pineal parenchyma and weight increase of the pituitary. In another case,[9] there was an association of macrogenitosomia praecox with adenocarcinoma of the adrenal cortex, enlargement of the pituitary and pineal hypoplasia.

Pineal Hyperplasia

Rabson and Mendenhall[10] reported a family in which 3 children, 2 sisters and a brother, presented a syndrome of precocious dentition and precocious isosexual development, insulin-resistant diabetes, hirsutism, old and "heavy" features, protuberant abdomen, thick and pigmented skin, thickened nails and mental precocity. The children died at ages 7½, 8 and 9 years. Necropsy in one girl showed a hyperplastic pineal body measuring 30 × 20 × 10 mm. "The brain proper was grossly not unusual." The pituitary was not enlarged but it contained a relatively large cyst. The adrenals reached adult weight. The pancreas was remarkably enlarged but showed hyalinizing fibrosis of both the islets and acini. The authors assumed that the sister and brother, who had shown similar disease pictures, also had pineal hypertrophy and adrenal hyperplasia. A fourth child in the family had the same abnormal anatomic features but died of intestinal intussusception when 5 months of age.

Pineal Tumors

Although the incidence of pineal tumors is low, these neoplasms have aroused a great deal of interest because of their peculiarities and the physiologic implications of their symptoms. The incidence is three times as frequent in males as in females and a third of the reported cases were in children under 15 years of age. According to Kitay and Altschule,[4] mixed tumors have occurred almost exclusively in males, whereas cysts were observed more often in females. The terminology is varied, but the names given to many of the tumors suggest that the authors considered them the result of developmental errors: teratomas, dermoids, chorioepitheliomas, pinealomas, angiomas and others. A striking effect of some pineal tumors in boys is macrogenitosomia praecox, an effect that has been used for elucidation of questions of pineal function. There are two main theories concerning this function. Marburg[11] collected evidence to prove that sexual precocity associated with pineal tumors is due to deficiency of a hormone that normally inhibits gonadal development. Destruction by neoplasms of pineal parenchyma would account for hormonal deficiency. An alternative explanation attributed precocity to a pineal hormone that stimulates the gonads or to an indirect effect of expanding tumors on hypothalamic-pituitary mechanisms that result in increased secretion of gonadotropins and precocious testicular development.[12] This widely accepted theory is based on the fact that intracranial lesions that are not pineal in origin are capable of producing precocious puberty (p. 454) and that the nature of the pineal tumors causing precocity is variable. Lists of pineal tumors causing sexual precocity can be found in reviews.[4,13] Kitay and Altschule[4] compared effects on sexual development of parenchymal and glial tumors and found that sexual precocity was associated with more than three times as many nonparenchymal as parenchymal tumors. They thought that the "hypothalamus pressure" theory cannot explain the fact that 78% of nonparenchymal tumors were associated with precocious puberty although their general incidence was only 49% and that this finding would agree better with Marburg's theory, which attributed precocity to pineal destruction. There also are records of pineal tumors associated with hypogonadism in males. The majority of such tumors were parenchymal, an observation that also could be used against the "hypothalamus pressure" theory, which assumes that the pineal body has no function. In addition, there is increasing evidence that the pineocytes secrete potent physiologic substances, and a theory of a control over sexual maturation through melatonin has been suggested.[14] The pendulum is swinging back and it is now believed that gonadal abnormalities in patients with pineal tumors are not caused exclusively by pressure on the hypothalamus[4] and that either suppression of pineal secretion or secretion from teratomatous tumors is responsible for some forms of precocious puberty.[13]

Evidence from tumors is difficult to obtain for either theory, since these neoplasms can destroy the pineal tissue, can include it within its structure or can give rise to pineal tissue as new growth material.[15]

A review published by Puschett and Goldberg[27] includes data on endocrine determinations performed in patients with pineal tumors.

Teratomas of the pineal body, although rare, constitute the leading type of embryonal pineal tumor. Epidermoids of the pineal apparently are unknown and dermoids are extremely rare.[15] Teratomas are derived from a primitive cell or a cell group that has become separated from the main organizational pattern of the organism during embryonic life and which has retained pluripotential powers of differentiation. Teratomas derived from all three primitive germ layers have been diagnosed in a number of pineal tumors. The complexity of pineal teratomas suggests departure of the aberrant cell group very early in embryonic development. The location of displaced cells in the roof of the posterior diencephalon has not been explained. Krabbe[16] suggested that the superficial position of the pineal in intrauterine life may expose it to penetration of foreign tissue elements. Russell[17] pointed out that the more common pinealomas may be atypical teratomas and that there is a similarity of pinealomas to spheroidal-cell carcinomas of the testis, which are also widely regarded as atypical teratomas. Numerous similarities seem to exist between the pineal and the testis in regard to cell structure and neoplasia.[15] Harris and Cairns[18] stressed the marked resemblance of the cell type of the pineal adenoma or pinealoma to that of the testicular seminoma (with spheroidal cells). Epithelioid cells that have the characteristics of interstitial cells of testis have been found in pineal teratomas. "The pineal body ranks second to the testis as a source of multipotential neoplastic material, and together they form the principal locations of teratomas in the male."[15] There must be some connections and relations between the pituitary and the male gonads that are not understood at present. Although most teratomas of the pineal occurred in boys, a congenital pineal teratoma has been observed in a girl who developed hydrocephaly.[19] Two additional cases of congenital teratoma, probably pineal, causing congenital hydrocephaly have been reported.[20,21]

Associated congenital malformations apparently are rare in cases of pineal teratoma. Most reports emphasize that the patients were normal until manifestations of the tumor began. A probable tumor of the pineal associated with precocious puberty and skeletal malformations was reported by Massobrio and Boccuzzi.[22]

Chorioepithelial elements in pineal tumors have been noted[23] and association of pineal chorioepithelioma with precocious puberty has been reported. Zondek *et al.*[24] observed a boy with precocious puberty suffering from recurrent cerebral accidents; there was increased excretion of urinary gonadotropins. At operation, a tumor involving the pineal region was found that proved to be a chorioepithelioma. David *et al.*[13] also described a boy with macrogenitosomia praecox who had a pineal chorioepithelioma.

Cysts of the Pineal Body

Small cysts frequently are found in human pineals and are considered normal by some authors. In infants, one can see cysts lined by parenchymal cells but, with increasing age, the inner walls of such cysts become covered by glia fibers. Lining by ependyma cells has also been described. Sometimes such cysts are large enough to expand the pineal body and to cause tumor symptoms. The contents of the cysts are made up of a thin liquor (hydrops cysticus). The age of patients with pineal cysts usually is beyond that of adolescence. A congenital cyst of the pineal was reported by Joukovsky[25]; it caused hydrocephaly by compression of the aqueduct.[26]

REFERENCES

1. Bargmann, W.: Die Epiphysis Cerebri, in Möllendorff, W. (ed.), *Handbuch der Mikroskopischen Anatomie des Menschen, Vol. VI* (Berlin: Springer-Verlag, 1943).
2. Quay, W. B.: Histologic Structure and Cytology of Pineal Organ in Birds and Mammals, in Dappers, J. A., and Schadé, J. P. (eds.), *Structure and Function of the Epiphysis Cerebri,* Progress in Brain Research, Vol. 10 (Amsterdam: Elsevier Publishing Company, 1965).
3. Zandrén, S.: Function of pineal gland, Acta med. scandinav. 54:323, 1921.
4. Kitay, J. I., and Altschule, M. D.: *The Pineal Gland: A Review of the Physiologic Literature* (Cambridge, Mass.: Harvard University Press, 1954).
5. Healey, C. E., and Guy, C. C.: Pseudohermaphroditism masculinus externus associated with suprarenal hyperplasia and vascular hypertension, Arch. Path. 12:543, 1931.
6. Askanazy, M., and Brack, W.: Sexuelle Frühreife bei einer Idiotin mit Hypoplasie der Zirbel, Virchows Arch. path. Anat. 234:1, 1921.
7. Dietrich, A.: Mangel der Zirbeldrüse mit Hirsutism, Zentralbl. allg. Path. 48:209, 1930.
8. Kup, J.: Zusammenhang zwischen Makroorchie und Zirbeldrüsenhypoplasie, Beitr. path. Anat. 97:385, 1936.
9. Kup, J.: Zur Frage der Funktion der Zirbel (Beobachtungen bei einem Fall von Makrogenitosomia praecox), Frankfurt. Ztschr. Path. 51:12, 1938.
10. Rabson, S. M., and Mendenhall, E. N.: Familial hypertrophy of pineal body, hyperplasia of adrenal cortex and diabetes mellitus, Am. J. Clin. Path. 26:283, 1956.
11. Marburg, O.: Die Klinik der Zirbeldrüsenerkrankungen, Ergebn. inn. Med. 10:146, 1913.
12. Bing, J. F., Globus, H. H., and Simon, H.: Pubertas praecox: A survey of the reported cases and verified anatomical findings, with particular reference to tumors of the pineal body, J. Mount Sinai Hosp. New York 4:935, 1938.
13. David, M., de Ajuriaguerra, J., and Bonis, A.: Les pubertés précoces des tumeurs cérébrales, Semaine hôp. Paris 33:3935, 1957.
14. Relkin, R.: The pineal gland, New England J. Med. 274: 944, 1966.
15. Bochner, S. J., and Scarff, J. E.: Teratoma of the pineal body, classification of the embryonal tumors of the pineal body. Report of a case of teratoma of the pineal body presenting formed teeth, Arch. Surg. 36:303, 1938.
16. Krabbe, K. H.: The pineal gland, especially in relation to the problem of its supposed significance in sexual development, Endocrinology 7:379, 1923.
17. Russell, D. S.: The pinealoma: Its relationship to teratoma, J. Path. & Bact. 56:145, 1944.
18. Harris, W., and Cairns, H.: Diagnosis and treatment of pineal tumors, Lancet 1:3, 1932.

19. Lichtenstein, B. W.: Teratoma of the pineal body, Arch. Neurol. & Psychiat. 44:153, 1940.
20. Hulst, J. P. L.: Ein Teratom in der Schädelhöhle als Ursache eines kongenitalen Hydrocephalus, Beitr. Geb. Gynäk. 8:168, 1904.
21. Schuster, H.: Ein das Hirn ersetzendes Teratom in der Schädelhöhle eines Neugeborenen, Zentralbl. allg. Path. 59:163, 1933.
22. Massobrio, E., and Boccuzzi, G.: Tumore (teratoma?) della pineale associato a malformazioni scheletriche come causa di puberta precoce e cindrome iperpituitarica tipo Cushing, Endocrinologia 14:86, 1939.
23. Askanazy, M.: Teratom und Chorionepitheliom der Zirbel, Verhandl. deutsch. Gesellsch. Path., p. 58, 1906.
24. Zondek, H., Kaatz, A., and Unger, H.: Precocious puberty and chorioepithelioma of the pineal gland, with report of a case, J. Endocrinol. 10:12, 1953.
25. Joukovsky, V.: Hydrocéphalie et tumeur congénitale de la glande pinéale chez un nouveau-né, Rev. Mens. Mal. Enf. 19:197, 1901.
26. Wurm, H.: Die Missbildungen der Epiphyse des Gehirns, in Schwalbe, E. (ed.), *Die Morphologie der Missbildungen des Menschen und der Tiere* (Jena: Gustav Fischer, 1929), Vol. 3.
27. Puschett, J. B., and Goldberg, M.: Endocrinopathy associated with pineal tumor, Ann. Int. Med. 69:203, 1968.

47

Endocrine-Hypothalamic Disorders

Diabetes Insipidus

DIABETES INSIPIDUS is determined before birth in many cases. There are hereditary forms that are transmitted from generation to generation like a dominant trait.[1-3] Polyuria and polydipsia probably are present at birth in most of these hereditary cases. There are reports that the patient "always" drank a great deal or that the disorder began in infancy. But there are variations in intensity with age, febrile diseases and other circumstances. The pathologic basis of genetically determined cases has not been well established, but there are reports which indicate that hypoplasia of the nucleus supraopticus and the nucleus paraventricularis with a reduced number of ganglion cells and a decrease in the volume of the posterior pituitary lobe occurs in patients with hereditary diabetes insipidus.[4] "Idiopathic" cases, therefore, may be due to a microscopic congenital malformation of the hypothalamus. According to another concept, the primary defect in familial diabetes insipidus may be in the osmoreceptor mechanism rather than at the site of production of antidiuretic hormone. The osmoreceptors are thought to be situated on the branches of the carotid arteries.[5] The teratologic nature of diabetes insipidus is more manifest in rare cases in which the disorder is included in a syndrome of congenital malformations such as the Laurence-Moon-Biedl syndrome.[6-8] In other familial cases, diabetes insipidus is associated with mental retardation. In such families and in those with the Laurence-Moon-Biedl syndrome, diabetes insipidus is inherited as a recessive trait.

Diabetes insipidus due to brain tumors sometimes can be attributed to developmental errors. In fact, polyuria and polydipsia are, in some instances, early manifestations that can precede pressure symptoms caused by the expanding lesion by many years. Such early onset suggests that the lesion that terminates as a glioma, carcinoma or sarcoma of the hypothalamus possibly was present as a minor anomaly or malformation from birth on, or before.[8]

Sometimes the nature of a tumor betrays its prenatal origin. For instance, diabetes insipidus has been known as a manifestation of teratomas. Cushing[9] described a girl 16 years of age who had polyuria and polydipsia because of a teratoma at the base of the diencephalon. Globus[10] reported diabetes insipidus in a girl 6 years of age with brain tumor symptoms due to a teratoid cyst. A Rathke-cleft cyst was the cause of diabetes insipidus in a girl 3 years of age[11] and in at least 2 children diabetes insipidus was a symptom of ganglioneuroma of the hypothalamus.[12,13] Carcinoma in the region of the infundibulum[14] or in the posterior pituitary lobe[15] causing diabetes insipidus in young children could be derived from hypophyseal duct remnants or other developmental abnormalities in the hypothalamic region.

Hereditary hypothalamic diabetes insipidus that can be used as an experimental model of the disorder has been observed in a strain of rats. The trait is transmitted as an autosomal recessive.[16]

Vasopressin-resistant diabetes insipidus is a congenital and hereditary renal failure to respond to antidiuretic hormone.[40]

Oliguria

A case of pituitary dwarfism with oliguria and oligodipsia was described by Debré *et al.*[17] The authors believed that this patient suffered from pure and isolated insufficiency of the anterior lobe of the pituitary, which is opposed, in regard to water metabolism, to the function of the posterior lobe. But oliguria was also present in a girl who had precocious puberty owing to a hamartoma of the floor of the third ventricle.[12]

Cushing Syndrome

Visscher-Jolles and Cornelia de Lange[18] described Cushing syndrome in a 3-year-old boy with congenital malformation of the hypothalamus and without adenoma of the pituitary gland. This boy appeared normal at birth but toward the end of the second year he developed marked obesity showing particularly on the face, breasts and abdomen. His weight was about 50% over the norm for his age. During the course of his illness he had, at times, sugar in his urine but he did not have diabetes insipidus. He developed dark violet striae typical of Cushing syndrome. Also, the red cell count was increased and the blood pressure was high. He died at the age of 3 years. The brain appeared externally normal but when microscopic sections were made through the area of the tuber cinereum and the infundibulum, a malformation was found. There were large clefts in the infundibulum lined by ependyma. In the tuber cinereum, there were no ganglion cells and the glia was markedly increased. The shape and position of the paraventricular nuclei were abnormal. The authors believed that the malformation was a congenital hypoplasia of the hypothalamus. It is noteworthy that this malformation was not recognizable macroscopically but was revealed in serial histologic sections.

Precocious Puberty

Precocious puberty has been caused repeatedly by tumors of prenatal origin. One of these cases was attributed to a teratoma,[19] and a teratoma in the area of the third ventricle was reported as a cause of precocious puberty by Bruton *et al.*[20] A boy in his seventh year showed rapid weight increase and signs of precocious puberty. After adrenal dysfunction, testicular tumor and abdominal teratoma were ruled out as the cause of these signs, a tumor of the third ventricle was found that proved to be a teratoma containing a secreting chorioepithelioma. The teratoma, which was responsible for the precocity of the boy, contained many different tissues such as sarcoma, leiomyosarcoma, epithelial structures resembling glands of the gastrointestinal and respiratory tracts and sebaceous glands. There also were tissues resembling embryonal carcinoma or seminoma of the testis. Most significant were large areas of unmistakable choriocarcinoma with malignant syncytial trophoblasts interposed between blood-filled sinuses and seats of malignant cytotrophoblasts. Other cases of sexual precocity were brought about by hamartomas in the hypothalamic region. LeMarquand and Russell[21] reported such a case, and Driggs and Spatz[22] recognized the basic lesion as a hyperplastic malformation of the tuber cinereum in a boy whose precocious sex development began at the age of 4 months. A hamartoma of hazelnut size was found at operation behind the infundibulum and covering the corpora mamillaria. Gross[12] described the difficulties in finding the cause of precocious puberty in a girl who suddenly developed signs of puberty at the age of 19 months. Laparotomy failed to show the origin of the disorder but ventriculograms revealed enlargement of the third and fourth ventricles. Masses projecting into the posterior portion of the third ventricle were attributed to a pineal neoplasm but, after death, the cause of precocious puberty was recognized as a mass that arose from the floor of the third ventricle and extended from the chiasma opticum to the pons. The lesion, which consisted chiefly of glial elements and had no invasive tendencies, was classified as a hamartoma. A boy reported by Weinberger and Grant[23] rapidly developed signs of precocious puberty and brain tumor at the age of 7 years. Ventriculograms showed changes that indicated blocking of the aqueduct. Operation revealed a large tumor filling the third ventricle and originating from its walls. It was thought to be "a malformation rather than true neoplasm." A lesion described by Hooft *et al.*[24] in a girl 2 years of age was just a small node sitting on the left corpus mamillare without involvement of the tuber cinereum or the stalk of the pituitary. Microscopically, the growth consisted of mature brain tissue with ganglion cells, neuroglia and nerve fibers. In other words, it was not a tumor but rather a malformation. Bronstein *et al.*[25] studied a 22-month-old girl who had enlarged breasts and signs of precocity since birth. Necropsy revealed ectopic brain tissue between infundibulum and mamillary bodies. This tumor-like structure contained ganglion cells, axis cylinders and a few myelinated fibers in a glial stroma. The hyperplastic malformation at the base of the brain was considered a hamartoma. Pubertas praecox due to a "hyperplastic malformation" was recorded by Meyer.[26] Signs of precocious puberty often appear late in childhood even though the underlying lesion is a congenital malformation. A girl who developed signs of puberty in her third year was observed by Richter.[27] At the age of 7 years she had the appearance of a 16-year-old adolescent girl. She died during laparotomy and at necropsy a hamartoma was found overlying the mamillary bodies and bridging the interpeduncular and pontine cisterns. A girl reported by Ernould *et al.*[28] developed menstrual bleeding at the age of 5 months and enlargement of the breasts and uterus were present at the age of 3 years. Ventriculograms suggested a paramamillary hyperplasia. In this case, the hypothalamic lesion was associated with a cyst of the septum pellucidum. Treatment with x-rays and an inhibitor of gonadotropins led to temporary improvement. There was a café au lait spot on the hip that disappeared after treatment.

The nature of these hamartomas that result in precocious puberty remains to be elucidated. Are they possibly early malformations of generalized hamartoses (Chapters 121–123)? The single café au lait spot mentioned in the case of Ernould *et al.*[28] does not prove a relationship to neurofibromatosis, but in another case[29] precocious puberty in a 9-year-old boy was attributed to a neurofibroma of the floor of the third ventricle. Barta[30] and Levin[31] mentioned precocious puberty caused by neurofibromatosis. Tuberous sclerosis was the basis of an egg-sized nodule between the infundibulum and mamillary bodies in a mentally retarded boy who had genital enlargement quite early. It seems advisable, therefore, to search for manifestations of general hamartoses in cases of precocious puberty with signs of hypothalamic involvement.

There also are reports of precocious puberty caused by craniopharyngiomas, i.e., tumors attributable to developmental errors.[32] Other tumors such as astrocytoma or ependymoma causing precocious puberty will not generally be recognized as teratologic. However, there are observations that show precocious puberty preceded by several years of tumor symptoms,[23] so that one must consider the possibility that a benign and possibly congenital anomaly of the hypothalamus that produced the endocrine disturbances was later transformed into a more or less malignant tumor. Thus, in the case of Vickers and Tidswell,[33] a walnut-sized astrocytoma was found in a boy 8 years of age in the floor of the third ventricle, destroying the mamillary bodies and tuber cinereum; but rapid enlargement of the genitals occurred from birth on, which is proof that a congenital lesion had been in the hypothalamus long before a "tumor" developed. The teratoma described by Frazier[19] did not cause precocious maturation before the age of 10 years, showing again the discrepancy between the time of origin of a tumor and that of its clinical manifestation. In a review by Bauer[34] of 60 lesions in the hypothalamus with endocrine or other clinical manifestations, there were 51 neoplasms, of which 22 (43%) can be attributed to disturbances of prenatal origin (5 hyperplastic malformations, 14 craniopharyngiomas, 1 angioma, 1 neurofibroma and 1 lesion of tuberous sclerosis). Hydrocephaly can be added to the organic cerebral lesions that can cause precocious puberty[35,36] (Fig. 47-1).

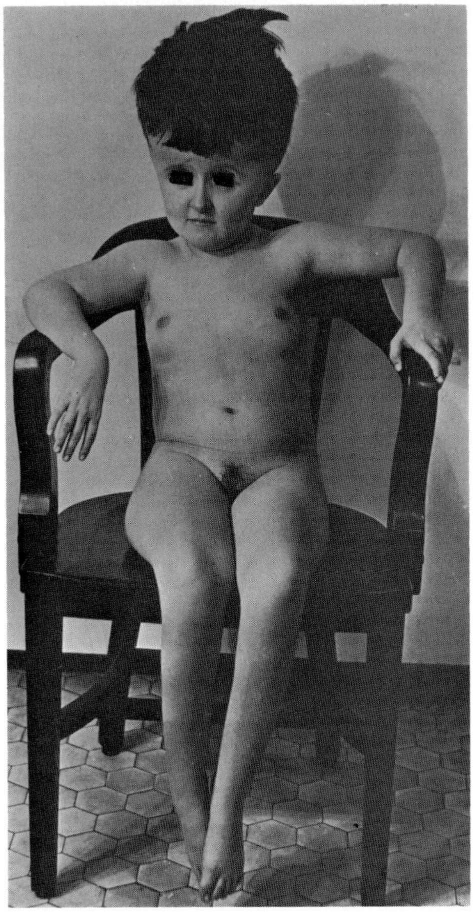

Fig. 47-1.—Isosexual precocity in a girl with hydrocephaly.

Precocious puberty owing to tumors or hamartomas in the hypothalamic area is relatively rare. In most cases of isosexual precocity, no abnormality is found in the nervous system or in the endocrine glands. Such cases are considered "idiopathic" or "constitutional" forms of sexual precocity that take a physiologic course, with spermatogenesis or ovulation at early ages. The mechanisms leading to precocious onset of sexual maturation are not known, but, in some instances, genetic determination can be demonstrated. Hereditary sexual precocity in a kindred with 27 affected members in four generations has been reported by Jacobsen and Macklin.[37] The trait was dependent on a sex-limited autosomal gene with almost complete penetrance that was transmitted by affected males and carrier females to approximately half their offspring.

Walker[38] reported a family in which male true sexual precocity occurred like a dominant hereditary trait. Signs of maturation appeared in the first few years of childhood. Precocity was manifested by pubic hair, enlargement of penis and testicles, strong muscular development and premature ossification. There also were signs of early spermatogenesis. True sexual precocity was transmitted in 7 male members of this family, with sexual precocity appearing prior to the age of 5 years. There were no signs of neurologic or mental disturbance.

De Lange[39] and Bierich *et al.*[36] believed that precocious puberty without an anatomic substrate is unlikely and that the constitutional form is diencephalic in origin, with a small hamartoma concealed and containing a surplus of tumor tissue. But there is no anatomic confirmation of these beliefs.

Isosexual precocious puberty was seen in a girl with hydrocephaly (Fig. 47-1). The child died at home and the nature of the hydrocephaly was not explained.

REFERENCES

1. Weil, A., Jr.: Über die hereditäre Form des Diabetes insipidus, Deutsche Arch. klin. Med. 93:180, 1908.
2. Pender, C. B., and Fraser, F. C.: Dominant inheritance of diabetes insipidus, Pediatrics 11:246, 1953.
3. Forssman, H.: On hereditary diabetes insipidus, Acta med. scandinav. 159:1, 1945.
4. Gaupp, R., Jr.: Über den Diabetes insipidus, Ztschr. Neurol. u. Psychiat. 171:514, 1942.
5. Martin, F. I. R.: Familial diabetes insipidus, Quart. J. Med. 28:573, 1959.
6. Bernhardt, H.: Ein Beitrag zur Laurence-Biedlschen Krankheit, Ztschr. klin. Med. 107:488, 1928.
7. Reilly, W. A., and Lisser, H.: Laurence-Moon-Biedl syndrome, Endocrinology 16:337, 1932.
8. Warkany, J., and Mitchell, A. G.: Diabetes insipidus in children: A critical review of etiology, diagnosis and treatment with report of 4 cases, Am. J. Dis. Child. 57: 603, 1939.
9. Cushing, H.: *Pituitary Body and Its Disorders* (Philadelphia: J. B. Lippincott Company, 1912).
10. Globus, J. H.: Teratoid cyst of the hypophysis, Arch. Neurol. & Psychiat. 9:417, 1923.
11. Moffett, R. D.: Craniopharyngeal pouch cyst arising from pituitary body, Am. J. Dis. Child. 32:89, 1926.
12. Gross, R. E.: Neoplasms producing endocrine disturbances in childhood, Am. J. Dis. Child. 59:579, 1940.
13. Horrax, G., and Bailey, P.: Pineal pathology; further studies, Arch. Neurol. & Psychiat. 19:394, 1928.
14. Wieland, E.: Macrogenitosomia praecox bei 4½ jährigem Knaben mit Carcinom des dritten Hirnventrikels und intakter Zirbeldrüse, Praxis 17:9, 1928.
15. Wentzler, E.: Ein Fall von Carcinom der Hypophyse bei 9 jährigem Knaben, Monatsschr. Kinderh. 69:86, 1937.
16. Valtin, H.: Hereditary hypothalamic diabetes insipidus in rats (Brattleboro strain). A useful experimental model, Am. J. Med. 42:814, 1967.
17. Debré, R., Royer, R., Alloiteau, J. J., and Spahr, A.: Nanisme hypophysaire avec oligurie et oligodipsie, Arch. franç. pédiat. 11:1, 1954.
18. Visscher-Jolles, J. M. C., and de Lange, C.: Cushing's Syndrom bei einem 3½ jährigen Knaben bei angeborener Missbildung des Hypothalamus und Fehlen eines Hypophysenadenoms, Ann. paediat. 163:57, 1944.
19. Frazier, C. H.: Lesions in and adjacent to the sella turcica (Case 8), Am. J. Surg. 16:199, 1932.
20. Bruton, O. C., Martz, D. C., and Gerard, E. S.: Precocious puberty due to secreting chorionepithelioma (teratoma) of the brain, J. Pediat. 59:719, 1961.
21. LeMarquand, H. S., and Russell, D. S.: A case of pubertas praecox (macrogenitosomia praecox) in a boy associated with a tumor in the floor of the third ventricle, Roy. Berkshire Hosp. Rep., p. 31, 1934.
22. Driggs, M., and Spatz, H.: Pubertas praecox bei einer hyperplastischen Missbildung des Tuber cinereum, Virchows Arch. path. Anat. 305:567, 1939.
23. Weinberger, L. M., and Grant, F. C.: Precocious puberty and tumors of the hypothalamus. Report of case and review of the literature with pathophysiologic explanation of precocious sexual syndrome, Arch. Int. Med. 67:762, 1941.
24. Hooft, C., Dierickx, K., and Cieters, P.: Pubertas praecox bij een Meisje van 2 Jaar met een Tumor van het linker Corpus mammillare, Maandschr. kindergeneesk. 12:87, 1943.
25. Bronstein, L. P., Luhan, J., and Mavrelis, W. B.: Sexual precocity associated with hyperplastic abnormality of the tuber cinereum, Am. J. Dis. Child. 64:211, 1942.
26. Meyer, J.: Pubertas praecox bei einer hyperplastischen Missbildung des Hypothalamus, Arch. Psychiat. 119:378, 1948.
27. Richter, R. B.: True hamartoma of the hypothalamus associated with pubertas praecox, J. Neuropath. & Exper. Neurol. 10:368, 1951.
28. Ernould, H. J., Thibaut, A., and Decamps, G.: Puberté précoce avec néoformation développée dans la région des corps mamillaires. Traitement par radiothérapie interstitielle de Talairach, Ann. endocrinol. 26:181, 1965.
29. Schmalz, A.: Über einen Fall von Hirntumor mit Pubertas praecox, Beitr. path. Anat. 73:168, 1925.
30. Barta, L.: Pubertas praecox bedingt durch Neurofibromatosis generalisata (Recklinghausensche Krankheit), Ann. paediat. 170:15, 1948.
31. Levin, B.: Neurofibromatosis: Clinical and roentgen manifestations, Radiology 71:48, 1958.
32. Bailey, P., Buchanan, D. N., and Bucy, P. C.: *Intracranial Tumors of Infancy and Childhood* (Chicago: University of Chicago Press, 1939).
33. Vickers, W., and Tidswell, F.: A tumor of the hypothalamus, M. J. Australia 2:116, 1932.
34. Bauer, H. G.: Endocrine and metabolic conditions related to pathology in the hypothalamus: A review, J. Nerv. & Ment. Dis. 28:323, 1959.
35. Lowrey, G. H., and Brown, T. G.: Precocious sexual development; study of 30 cases, J. Pediat. 38:325, 1951.
36. Bierich, J. R., Blunck, W., and Schönberg, D.: Über Frühreife. II. Mitteilung. Frühreife bei cerebral-organischen Erkrankungen, Monatsschr. Kinderh. 115:509, 1967.
37. Jacobsen, A. W., and Macklin, M. T.: Hereditary sexual precocity: Report of a family with twenty-seven affected members, Pediatrics 9:682, 1952.
38. Walker, S.: Constitutional true sexual precocity, J. Pediat. 41:251, 1952.
39. de Lange, C.: Zur Klinik und pathologischen Anatomie der hypothalamischen Form von Pubertas praecox, Ann. paediat. 161:113, 1943.
40. Orloff, J., and Burg, M. B.: Vasopressin-Resistant Diabetes Insipidus, in Stanbury, J. B., Wyngaarden, J. B., and Fredrickson, D. S. (eds.), *The Metabolic Basis of Inherited Disease* (2d ed.; New York: McGraw-Hill Book Company, Inc., 1966), Chap. 55.

PART VIII

Cardiovascular Malformations

SECTION ONE

48

Etiologic Factors in Congenital Heart Disease

UNTIL ABOUT 30 years ago, fairly good agreement existed concerning the etiology of congenital heart disease (CHD). On anatomic grounds, two types of cardiac anomalies were then distinguished. There were the malformations attributed to developmental errors and those thought to be due to fetal endocarditis. Fetal endocarditis, in turn, was ascribed to infectious or toxic agents that damaged the heart, particularly its valves, endocardium or myocardium in the fetal period after normal development of the basic cardiac structures and after closure of the septa. Herxheimer,[1] for instance, distinguished between the "vitia primae formationis" and cardiac anomalies due to "congenital fetal inflammation." Maude Abbott believed that most cardiac defects were due to a primary arrest of development of unknown origin but that "in cases of stenosis of the pulmonary and tricuspid valves in which the interventricular septum is closed and the lesion is limited only to the thickened and fused valve leaflets, the cause is certainly a fetal endocarditis beginning in late embryonic life after the heart is fully formed. The cause of this fetal valvulitis might be an intercurrent infection including rheumatic fever, though the latter so rarely attacks the mother during her pregnancy that it must be regarded as an infrequent cause" (cited by Gross[2]).

The concept of arrested development in cardiac defects can be traced to Meckel,[3] who, in 1802, compared such anomalies with the hearts of lower classes of animals, thus initiating the *phylogenic* explanations that continued to flourish in our century. But Rokitansky,[4] in 1875, at a time when the knowledge of human embryology already afforded a better understanding of *ontogenic* processes, related most malformations to phases of arrested development of the human embryo. The concept of fetal endocarditis apparently was introduced by Kreysig,[5] who, early in the nineteenth century, suggested that cases of pulmonary stenosis could be due to disease of the pulmonary artery and its valves, a concept subsequently accepted by many outstanding pathologists. Maternal rheumatic fever, bronchitis and influenza thus were held responsible for certain forms of CHD.[1,6]

Not all investigators accepted the concept of fetal endocarditis. In 1941, Paul Gross[2] reviewed the literature on this subject and pointed out that the criteria for the diagnosis of fetal endocarditis often were quite loose, entirely macroscopic and based on a superficial resemblance of certain cardiac defects to postnatal rheumatic valvulitis. He pointed out that the acute form of this so-called inflammation had never been observed, that scar tissue is absent in the deformed valves, that the assumed etiologic pathogens in the reported cases have been either anamnestically absent or variable in identity, and he came to the conclusion that the occurrence of fetal endocarditis has not been established. Gross considered valvular and parietal endocardial changes previously attributed to fetal endocarditis as developmental defects, since they showed no inflammatory residua.

By a strange coincidence, it became known in the same year (1941) that infection of the mother with the rubella virus can cause CHD in her child. This discovery by the ophthalmologist Gregg[7] changed the concepts of the relationship of infection to cardiac pathology. It showed that the results of this infection usually did not resemble anatomically those attributed to fetal endocarditis by the older pathologists, that the virus acting in the first months of gestation often led to cardiac malformations previously ascribed to arrested development and that infection and arrested development are not antithetic concepts. As will be shown later, congenital cardiovascular malformations attributed to arrested development, such as atrial or ventricular septal defects and others, can be induced by prenatal rubella infection and other environmental factors. At present, one can look at CHD as gene-determined, chromosome-determined or as resulting from injurious exogenous factors. Examples of all three teratogenic categories can be cited but it should be emphasized that the majority of congenital cardiovascular defects still remain unexplained. A monograph on genetic and environmental causes of angiocardiopathies was published in 1962 by Fuhrmann.[10]

Congenital Heart Disease in More than One Generation

Genetic mechanisms are suggested by familial aggregation of cases[8-10] or by inclusion of CHD in syndromes known to be gene-determined. Many instances of transmission of CHD from a parent to one or several children have been recorded. In some cases, more than two generations were affected.

Walker and Ellis[11] reported a father with patent ductus arteriosus who had 8 children, 4 of them affected with the same anomaly. Taussig[12] reported patent ductus arteriosus in three generations. G. C. Walker and Ellis[11] and W. G. Walker[13] mentioned the case of a father and son with coarctation of the aorta, and, more recently, heredity of supravalvar aortic stenosis has been stressed.[14,15] Jörgensen and Beuren[16] reviewed the literature and suggested that the uncomplicated form of supravalvar aortic stenosis is due to an irregular dominant gene, whereas the congenital aortic stenosis complicated by disturbed calcium metabolism, mental retardation and typical facial features (p. 578) is of different origin, since, until now, only sporadic cases have been recorded. But the fact that there are no pedigrees available showing transmission of the complicated form may be due to reduced marriageability of these patients. Pulmonary stenosis was transmitted from a mother to 3 of her children[17]; 2 of these children were also deaf-mutes. In another family, the mother and 4 of her 6 children had pulmonary stenosis.[18] Two of the 4 affected children were deaf-mutes. Malformations of the chest, digits and ears as well as scoliosis were also observed. Ventricular septal defect in parent and child has been seen repeatedly.[19-22] Apert and Cambessédès[23] observed an acyanotic mother with probable ventricular septal defects who had, in each of two marriages, a child with the same defect. Atrial septal defect was established by necropsy in a woman who had transmitted the same defect to her daughter and granddaughter.[24] Another woman transmitted the anomaly to her son[25] and still another to her daughter.[8]

Weil and Allenstein[26] reviewed familial incidence of atrial septal defect. There were then five families with 2 affected members and four families with 4 affected members. A pedigree reported by these authors showed a father who had 4 children with proved atrial septal defect, 2 children with the defect suspected and 5 normal children. Three of the affected children also had pulmonic stenosis and 2 had ventricular septal defects. Zetterquist[27] recorded the pedigree of a family with 4 certain and 4 probable cases of atrial septal defect. Ehlers and Engle[28] listed a family in which atrial septal defect possibly occurred in three generations. Nora *et al.*[29] analyzed the overall data available on hereditary cases of atrial septal defect and concluded that multifactorial inheritance is the explanation most consistent with the reports, but Bizarro *et al.*[181] pointed out that, while the majority of atrial septal defects are sporadic with little likelihood of recurrence in siblings or children, the atrial septal defect of the fossa ovalis type with prolonged A-V conduction is due to an autosomal dominant gene involving a risk of almost 50% of recurrence in subsequent siblings or children of affected persons. Endocardial fibroelastosis in a mother and son was reported by Moller *et al.*[30] Hypoplasia of the right ventricle and of the tricuspid valve has been diagnosed in a father and his daughter.[171] A unique observation of a father and son with dextrocardia was made by Doolittle.[31] Both father and son had normal twin sisters. Situs inversus transmitted through four generations apparently was observed by Lancisi (cited by Gänsslen *et al.*[32]).

In the cases mentioned so far, the same anomaly was transmitted through two or more generations. Sometimes, clinically differing anomalies occur in a pedigree. A mother with coarctation of the aorta had 2 children with patent ductus,[33] or a mother with patent ductus had a daughter with aortic coarctation. A father with Wolff-Parkinson-White syndrome had 2 sons with congenital complete A-V heart block.[176] Of 3 sisters with atrial septal defect, 1 had a daughter with ventricular septal defect and pulmonary stenosis.[8] More impressive pedigrees of this type were published in the older literature,[32,34] but the diagnosis was understandably doubtful in some of these early publications. Thus, the "morbus coeruleus" in four generations reported by Burwinkel[35] probably was not due to CHD but to hereditary noncardiac cyanosis as described by Thysell[36] more recently. Additional families with parents and 1 or 2 children affected can be found in a publication by Ehlers and Engle.[28] Other instances of inherited anomalies of the conduction system are mentioned in Chapter 65. These reports suggest that dominantly inherited CHD exists but it must be rather rare, since in some extensive surveys of unselected cardiac patients no index cases have been found with parents affected by CHD,[37] or the incidence in parents was not higher than that in the general population.[38,39]

The fact that dominant genes can be responsible for congenital cardiovascular anomalies is better demonstrated by dominantly inherited syndromes that include CHD. In recent years, the Holt-Oram[40] syndrome (p. 481), consisting of upper limb and cardiovascular defects, has been emphasized. Cardiac septal defects and thumb abnormalities are the rule. Holmes[41] reviewed the literature and added a report of two families. In addition to the atrial defects reported previously, there were observations of ventricular septal and endocardial cushion defects, coarctation of the aorta and patent ductus arteriosus. The abnormal thumbs were either triphalangeal or vestigial or absent. Lewis *et al.*[42] recorded a family with the "upper limb-cardiovascular syndrome" transmitted through three generations. In addition to the cardiac defects enumerated before, there were anomalies of the coronaries, retro-esophageal right subclavian artery and transposition of the great vessels. Pruzanski[43] described severe malformations of the extremities through four generations and in several of the 11 affected persons acyanotic CHD was established. Phocomelia, deformities of the humerus, radius and ulna, absence of carpal and metacarpal bones and other malformations were noted. Thus, the pleiotropic gene exerts its influence not only over differentiation of the heart but also over that of the upper limbs.

An extensive pedigree containing 28 persons with Holt-Oram syndrome in four successive generations was published by Gall *et al.*[44] Of 13 affected members who underwent cardiac catheterization, 9 showed evidence of anatomic malformation of the great vessels or of the heart. Ventricular and atrial septal defects, persistent left superior vena cava, patent ductus arteriosus and an anomalous left coronary were diagnosed. Short clavicles and hypoplasia of other bones of the shoulder girdle and upper extremity were observed. The hand deformities were variable. The palmar dermatoglyphics were studied.

An interesting syndrome of mitral insufficiency, deafness, short stature and skeletal malformations was described in a woman and 2 of her daughters.[45]

Patients with arachnodactyly and congenital dislocation of the lens typically develop cystic media necrosis of the aorta and aortic aneurysm after childhood. But the dominant gene responsible for these changes also causes *congenital* cardiovascular defects in some of the patients. Ventricular and atrial septal defects, tetralogy of Fallot, aortic and pulmonic stenosis, patent ductus arteriosus, pseudotruncus arteriosus, persistent left superior vena cava and abnormal pulmonary venous return have been described in patients with Marfan syndrome (p. 850). Pulmonary stenosis, café au lait spots and dull intelligence have been reported in three pedigrees. The skin pigmentations were inherited as an autosomal dominant, as in Recklinghausen disease[46] (Chapter 121).

Idiopathic cardiomegaly has been recognized in recent years as a hereditary entity that can be transmitted through several generations. Evans,[47] in 1949, recorded "familial cardiomegaly" and Paré *et al.*[48] reported "hereditary cardiovascular dysplasia, a form of familial cardiomyopathy" in a large kinship in which 30 members were affected in five generations. Necropsies have shown hypertrophy and fibrosis of the myocardium, hypoplasia of the aorta and hypertrophy of the ventricular septum leading to subaortic stenosis. Death occurs in affected members of such families in adult life but dyspnea may be present in childhood and some yet unknown changes probably are present at birth. A dominant gene is held responsible for this cardiopathy,[49] but sex-linked transmission has also been considered.[50]

CHD in several generations suggests, but does not prove, genetic determination. On the other hand, it is likely that sporadic cases of CHD sometimes are genetically determined. If some of the children with CHD who die in infancy or before reaching the reproductive period represent dominant lethal or semilethal mutations, these cannot be transmitted to subsequent generations. They would appear as sporadic cases in the pedigree and their genetic determination would escape us. How often this occurs is not known. Some information concerning this type of sporadic CHD will be obtained by analyses of the offspring of persons who, although born with disabling forms of CHD, were restored to normal function and reproductivity by cardiac surgery. In the meantime, it is well to remember that the conventional criteria for heredity or nonheredity (familial vs. sporadic occurrence) cannot be accepted in the search for etiologic factors.

Congenital Heart Disease in Siblings

Repeated occurrence of CHD in siblings probably is more frequent than transmission through several generations. However, such familial cases in the same generation are not convincing proof of genetic etiology, since repetitive or persistent environmental or maternal factors could be responsible for cardiac defects in several children born to the same mother. The same holds true for findings indicating that approximately 2% of the siblings of patients with CHD have a cardiovascular defect. This incidence is higher than that of the general population, but consanguinity rates among parents of patients were only slightly elevated in some of these studies.[42]

To give some examples of cardiac defects in siblings, Joyce and O'Toole[51] reported 3 children with patent ductus and 1 with cyanotic CHD, and others (Ehlers and Engle,[28] Kjaergaard[52] and Ekström[53]) observed 3 siblings with patent ductus. Two siblings with this anomaly have been seen in many families.[38,53-57] Ventricular septal defect has been reported in 3[57] or in 2 siblings.[28,37,38,57-59] Interatrial septal defect,[28,60] interatrial septal defect with mitral stenosis,[61] patent foramen ovale,[37] congenital aortic stenosis,[62] aortic coarctation,[37] tetralogy of Fallot,[28,37,57] pulmonary valvar stenosis,[28,37,46,63] Eisenmenger complex,[37] transposition of the great vessels[38] and endocardial fibroelastosis[64-67] have been observed in siblings. Familial (fraternal) incidence of dextrocardia with situs inversus is a well-recognized phenomenon. There are reports of at least ten sibships with 3 affected and twenty-nine with 2 affected by this anomaly.[68] Cockayne[69] believed that this anomaly is due to a single recessive autosomal gene, but other investigators assert that more complicated genetic mechanisms are at work.[68,70] Campbell[71] recorded another case of situs inversus in a member of a sibship, with situs inversus also occurring in more distant relatives. Hypoplasia of the right ventricle and of the tricuspid valve, although a rare condition, has been observed several times in siblings.[170,171] Ebstein anomaly was reported in siblings by Gueron *et al.*[172] Congenital heart block has been described in 2 sisters[173] of one family and in 3 brothers of another.[174] Although recurrence in siblings suggests genetic determination, alternative explanations must be kept in mind. Latta and Crittenden[175] reported the case of a woman who had 8 children, 4 of whom had congenital heart block. Two came to necropsy, which showed absence of the A-V node and of adjacent atrial muscle fibers associated with calcification and fibrosis that seemed to be the result of fetal myocarditis.

There are many observations of siblings affected by differing types of congenital cardiac anomalies.[24,37,38,69] A special study was made by Davison[178] on concordance and discordance of congenital heart disease. Such isolated records of families with more than one affected member are paralleled by broader statistical studies on the familial incidence of congenital malformations of the heart. The data of McKeown *et al.*[38] indicate that the incidence of congenital cardiac malformations is raised in siblings but is not raised in parents and in cousins of affected individuals. Lamy *et al.*[37] also found an elevated familial incidence with a high rate of consanguineous marriages in their series of patients with CHD, suggesting that genetic factors are operative in the etiology of these disorders. In both studies, it was found that the consanguinity rate varied in different clinical types, being high in situs inversus[69] and in pulmonary stenosis.[37] This is of interest, since pulmonary stenosis in the past was considered the prototype of a cardiac malformation produced by "fetal endocarditis" (p. 459).

A few general disorders known to be recessively inherited include CHD. The Ellis-van Creveld syndrome (Chapter 85) is one of these syndromes that may show, among other congenital malformations,[177] ventricular and atrial septal defects. The Laurence-Moon-Biedl syndrome (Chapter 19), attributed to a recessive pleiotropic gene, can include a variety of congenital cardiovascular defects. Dextrocardia, ventricular and atrial septal defects, single ventricle, complete and corrected transposition of the great vessels, patent ductus arteriosus, right-sided aortic arch, aortic hypoplasia, pulmonary stenosis, defects of the aortic and pulmonary cusps, anomalies of the coronary arteries and anomalous pulmonary venous return have been observed in this syndrome.[72] A combination of deaf-mutism, functional heart disease with prolonged Q-T interval and sudden death has been described in 4 children of a family of 6.[73] Although the parents were not related, recessive inheritance can be suspected. Gargoylism (Hurler syndrome) (Chapter 88) is attributed to an autosomal or, in some cases, to a sex-linked recessive gene that leads to a storage disease. Although cardiac symptoms may appear early in life, the lesions observed seldom are congenital. Cardiomegaly, valvular lesions, shortening of the chordae tendineae, narrowing of the ostia and lumina of the coronary vessels and endocardial and myocardial changes result from storage of abnormal mucopolysaccharides in diseased cells. Glycogen-storage disease of the heart with early failure and death in infancy has occurred repeatedly in siblings. The basic metabolic error is considered a recessively inherited trait.[74]

The magnitude of familial incidence of congenital heart disease is illustrated by a study conducted by Christiaens *et al.*,[75] who encountered 25 familial cases among 920 cardiopathies (2.7%).

Twins were included in this estimate. Nora and Meyer[76] investigated 517 families selected through a proband having a congenital heart disease and ascertained 3.4% affected siblings and 1.8% affected parents. The findings suggest a higher frequency of familial congenital heart disease than has been reported before.

Congenital Heart Disease and Chromosomal Anomalies

Associations of CHD and chromosomal abnormalities are now well established. CHD frequently is a constituent of the syndromes characteristic of trisomy 21, 18 and 13-15 (D_1); there is also a rather high association of congenital cardiovascular disease with Turner syndrome. In other instances, the association is less regular, so that the findings of CHD and of chromosomal changes sometimes could be coincidental.

Most cases of trisomy 13-15 and trisomy 18 are lethal within a few months after birth. Sufficient necropsies have been done in such cases to demonstrate the high incidence of CHD and the great variability of the clinical and pathologic findings in these syndromes.[77] The types of CHD occurring in the patients have been listed on page 300.

The situation is different from these trisomies in trisomy 21 (Down syndrome, mongolism), which often permits survival of affected persons and therefore contributes to clinical cardiology. It is for this reason that a special section is devoted to cardiovascular anomalies in Down syndrome (p. 328).

Chromosome analyses of many children with multiple congenital malformations including cardiovascular defects revealed a variety of cytogenetic abnormalities that probably are responsible for the anomalies of the heart. But no regular relationship between the chromosomal and cardiac anomalies has yet been established, and it would be unrewarding to survey the situation at this time. Many of the cytogenetic anomalies are not classifiable with present-day methods, so that it seems too early to correlate the cardiac defects found with the cytogenetic interpretations. Only a few examples will be cited, therefore, to illustrate some of the associations recorded.

Additional chromosomal material in the karyotype has been demonstrated in many children with congenital cardiovascular defects, the outstanding examples being trisomies 21, 18 and 13-15. A small supernumerary submetacentric chromosome, considered a deleted 18, was noted in a girl with multiple malformations, including atrial septal defect, by Gustavson *et al.*,[78] but in the sister, who had an apparently identical extra autosome and many similar malformations, the heart was not involved. Böök *et al.*[79] reported atrial septal defect in a mother and son who had 47 chromosomes with a supernumerary autosome of the 19-20 group. Koulischer *et al.*[80] observed CHD associated with trisomy considered as 22, and Atkins and Feingold[81] reported CHD in a patient with an enlarged B-group chromosome.

Congenital cardiovascular anomalies were mentioned in descriptions of patients with 2/3 translocation,[82,83] D/E translocation,[84,85] C/D translocation,[86] and with more complex rearrangements.[87]

In the cat-cry syndrome with deletion of the short arm of chromosome 5,[88-91] CHD has been observed occasionally; it seems to occur more regularly with deletion of the short arm of chromosome 4.[92] Ring chromosome 18 combined with CHD has been reported.[93]

Serial cytogenetic examinations of patients with congenital heart disease revealed aberrations in a small percentage of patients. Sasaki *et al.*[94] noted reduction in size of one chromosome 16 in a number of patients with CHD, but Anders *et al.*[95] could not confirm this finding; chromosome 16 is recognized as a polymorphic structure, and anomalies observed must be interpreted with caution. Moores *et al.*[96] studied 6 examples of marker chromosomes encountered in an investigation of 250 cases of CHD. The presence of similar marker chromosomes in many normal relatives of the patients proved that there was no correlation between these chromosomes and CHD. German *et al.*[97] analyzed the chromosomes of 35 patients with CHD selected because of multiple instances of cardiac anomalies in their families. Although in four families various cytogenetic aberrations were discovered, the biologic significance of the variants and their relation to the etiology of CHD remained unexplained.

Absence of an X chromosome leading to Turner syndrome and cardiovascular anomalies is a well-known phenomenon, but it is difficult to give quantitative data of the incidence of cardiac defects in the 45,X anomaly. Few of the patients were examined by necropsy and reliable clinical diagnoses were supplied in recent years only. Rainier-Pope *et al.*[98] cited 15 publications from the literature that named coarctation of the aorta in patients with Turner syndrome without exact analysis of associated cardiovascular malformations. They examined 36 of their patients with this syndrome and found cardiovascular disease in 16 (44%). Pulmonic stenosis was as frequent as the more commonly reported coarctation of the aorta (7 cases each). Atrial and ventricular septal defects, endocardial cushion defect, patent ductus arteriosus and aortic stenosis were also diagnosed. In other series, additional forms of CHD such as dextrocardia, aortic stenoses and atresias and endocardial fibroelastosis were observed occasionally.[99,100]

Congenital heart disease sometimes is mentioned in patients with various abnormalities of the sex chromosomes. Atkins and Connelly,[101] Fraccaro *et al.*[102] and Joseph *et al.*[103] reported such patients with XXXXY karyotype. Day *et al.*[104] described a patient with XXX constitution and an atrial septal defect. A girl with presumed XXXXX karyotype had a rough grade 3 systolic murmur without "evidence of cardiac failure."[105] In her and in another girl[180] with penta-X karyotype, ligation of a ductus arteriosus was performed at the end of the first year.

Since sex is chromosome-determined, its influence on certain types of CHD shown in large-scale inquiries can be discussed here. CHD as a whole seems to be equally distributed in males and females.[37] However, definite sex preponderance exists in certain anatomic and clinical entities. Of patients with patent ductus, only about 30% are male and 70% female.[106-108] Record and McKeown[108] pointed out that the proportion of affected males is related to the age of the patients at the time of observation, as there is a higher early mortality of males with this anomaly. This differential mortality could, to a certain extent, account for the excess of female survivors. There seems to be general agreement also that atrial septal defects affect females and males in a proportion of 65 to 35%.[61, 109-111]

The sex ratio is reversed in other cardiovascular anomalies. Of necropsy cases with aortic coarctation, 75% are males and 25% are females.[1,106,112] In clinical studies of this malformation, the differences of the sexes is not so marked, but there is still an incidence of more than 60% males.[37,39] The prevalence of males in aortic stenosis also seems well established.[113,114] Transposition of the great vessels is another defect prevalent in males. In reported series of transposition, the patients were males in 59%,[39] 72%[115] and 75%[116] of the cases. In the Cincinnati Children's Hospital 74% were males. More males than females seem to have tetralogy of Fallot[1,37,39] and congenital mitral stenosis.[117,118] A list of sex ratios in CHD found in a Cincinnati Children's Hospital necropsy series was published by Landing *et al.*[119] These sex ratios must have some meaning, but their interpretation is still dubious. Although one could blame early male mortality for prevalence of females with ductus arteriosus in clinical populations, differential mortality does not account for excess of males with aortic defects or transposition of the great vessels.

Environmental Factors

There are many observations that indicate that nongenetic, postconceptional or environmental factors can induce CHD. Experimental work has shown that many adverse situations during pregnancy can result in CHD in mammals. Vitamin A deficiency,[120] hypervitaminosis A,[121] folic acid deficiency,[122] hypoxia,[123] administration of trypan blue,[124] salicylates[125] and many other experimental devices can be used to interfere with the normal development of the heart in experimental animals (p. 470).

In man, observations of maternal rubella, of thalidomide damage and of discordant monozygotic twins point to the importance of nongenetic factors in the etiology of CHD.

Rubella as a cause of CHD was discovered in Australia in 1941.[7] Maternal rubella infection during the first trimester of pregnancy can lead to a variety of congenital malformations, cardiovascular anomalies being among them. The risks of having children with congenital malformations have been discussed on page 62. From a prospective study by the British Ministry of Health,[126] it appears that CHD occurred in 7% of the children whose mothers had rubella in early pregnancy; this was fourteen times as common as among controls. Re-examination of surviving children at ages 8–11 arrived at a definite diagnosis of CHD in 6% but murmurs were heard in an additional 8%.[127] Comparable figures were reported from New York State,[128] where, in a prospective study, 2 children with CHD were found among those born of 36 mothers (5.5%) who had rubella during the first trimester of pregnancy. But it is important to remember that subclinical rubella can cause CHD[129,130] and that its effect could go unnoticed in a prospective study. According to a report from the collaborative study on cerebral palsy in the United States, of 54 mothers who had clinical rubella during the first trimester, 8 had therapeutic abortion, 1 a stillbirth and 1 an infant dead in the neonatal period. Five children had a congenital rubella syndrome and all of these had CHD. Of the mothers exposed to rubella without clinical manifestations of the disease, 4 had children with the congenital rubella syndrome, including CHD. These observations suggest a higher incidence of CHD in children following maternal rubella than those cited above. But, even in times of epidemics, prospective studies deal with small samples of mothers affected during the first trimester and variations in incidence figures are to be expected. There also is uncertainty concerning the role played by maternal rubella as a contributor to CHD in general. Estimates vary between 1% and 8%, but such estimates are of little value, since they differ according to the places in which the patients were examined (referral, etc.) and to the time the observations were made (relation to rubella epidemics). Campbell[131] concluded that rubella is not one of the major causes of CHD and that it is responsible for only 2–4% of all cases of CHD. In Toronto, Canada, in 100 cases of simple ductus arteriosus, a history of rubella in the first trimester was obtained in 8 cases and denied in 92. But, in the 3 years immediately following the peak of a New Zealand rubella epidemic, 17 of 50 babies under 2 years of age with patent ductus had a definite rubella background.[132] These observations exemplify differing estimates according to time, location and relation to rubella epidemics.

From the beginning, Gregg[7] and Swan *et al.*[133] thought that patent ductus arteriosus was the leading malformation in the maternal rubella syndrome. When Rutstein *et al.*[134] reviewed the reported cases in which specific heart lesions were mentioned, they found that in 77 cases patent ductus arteriosus was diagnosed 42 times and septal defects 36 times. Rare diagnoses of tetralogy of Fallot, of coarctation of the aorta and of patent foramen ovale had also been made. In the series of Gibson and Lewis,[135] of 16 cases of CHD attributable to maternal rubella in early pregnancy, 14 had patent ductus, 1 a tetralogy of Fallot and 1 an interatrial septal defect. Ten of the 14 patients with patent ductus were operated on and 4 of them were found to have complications caused by such other lesions as pulmonary stenosis, coarctation of the aorta or ventricular septal defect. Jackson[136] reported 7 cases, all confirmed by operation or postmortem examination, showing patent ductus, 1 of them complicated by pulmonary stenosis and ventricular septal defect. In a prospective rubella study, Pitt[137] found 1 patient with patent ductus and 1 with tricuspid atresia, ventricular septal defect and abnormal ductus. Campbell,[131] combining three samples with well-established diagnoses, considered 136 patients with 153 cardiac malformations. Persistent ductus arteriosus was the most common malformation, being present in 58% of the cases. Ventricular septal defect was the malformation next in frequency (18%), followed by atrial septal defect (7%), tetralogy of Fallot (7%) and pulmonary valvular stenosis (6%). There also were several instances of aortic coarctation and single cases of aortic stenosis, transposition and tricuspid atresia. Campbell found it worth emphasis that the combination of persistent ductus and ventricular septal defect occurred in 6% of the cases, as, generally, this combination is not a frequent one.

With the improvement in diagnostic methods and with necropsy experience, the knowledge of cardiovascular lesions following prenatal rubella was augmented. It was found that sometimes patent ductus arteriosus may dominate the disease picture and conceal associated cardiac anomalies.[138] Stenosis of the main pulmonary artery or its branches has become increasingly recognized[139-141]; in fact, in one series,[142] anatomic lesions of the pulmonary arterial system were noted in all cases with cardiovascular involvement, whereas patent ductus arteriosus was present in 75% and hypoplasia of the aortic isthmus in 16% of the patients. Insufficiency of the pulmonary valves has been shown by the use of contrast medium in the presence of a patent ductus arteriosus.[143] Examination of the blood vessels in necropsies of infants with congenital defects due to rubella revealed not only lesions in the pulmonary artery but also fibromuscular proliferation of the intima of systemic arteries and ostial stenosis of a renal artery.[144] The possibility of postnatal cardiovascular damage must be considered in the presence of a persistent active rubella infection in infancy.[145]

Although maternal rubella accounts for only a small percentage of the cases of CHD, the discovery of this infection as an etiologic factor is of great theoretical importance. A possibility exists that other viral infections may play a similar role, but it is difficult to indict them. The experience with rubella has shown that the maternal infection causes malformations in some children, whereas others are spared. Sometimes women who are exposed to rubella without getting sick have children with the fully developed rubella syndrome.[129] And, in rare cases, the syndrome is seen in children of mothers who are not aware of either exposure or illness during pregnancy.[133,146]

These lessons learned from rubella demonstrate how difficult it is to discover a causal connection between a prenatal virus infection and a congenital cardiac malformation without an experiment of nature like the Australian epidemic. One can suspect that other maternal viral or bacterial diseases during pregnancy are responsible for CHD in children,[37,147,148] but convincing proof is lacking in most of the cases. Placental transmission of a number of viruses is well established[149] and may lead, in the case of Coxsackie group B virus infection, to myocarditis in the late fetal or neonatal period,[150-151] but it has not been shown that this virus interferes with the development of the heart in its early formative periods. The role of intrauterine mumps virus infection in the etiology of endocardial fibroelastosis has been discussed in recent years. Some of the patients with the primary form of this disorder have cutaneous delayed hypersensitivity to the mumps virus antigen and, in a number of cases, the patients' mothers had parotitis or exposure to mumps during pregnancy, yet virus neutralizing antibodies are uncommon in the patients and the virus has not been recovered from them after birth.[152,153]

In the search for other environmental etiologic factors, *hypoxia* has been considered repeatedly. Reports exist indicating that ductus arteriosus is more common in populations living at high altitudes than in those living near sea level. Alzamora *et al.*[154] reported from Lima, Peru, that in their clinical material of 42 cases of patent ductus, 26 (62%) were born at an altitude of more than 3,000 meters (9,843 feet), although, if equally distributed, only 15% of the patient population should have been born in these elevated areas. Dexter[155] stated that in Lima, Peru, only 0.8 per 100,000 population have patent ductus, whereas in Junín, an area of high altitude, 3 per 100,000, i.e., four times more, have patent ductus. However, this incidence of 3 per 100,000 is not impressive, since in the United States, according to Anderson,[107] 25 cases of patent ductus can be expected per 100,000 births. Much more convincing are the observations made by Penaloza *et al.*,[156] who reported from Peru that patent ductus arteriosus is more frequent among school children at high altitudes than at sea level and that the incidence increases gradually as altitude above sea level increases. The frequency of patent ductus was more than 1% at altitudes over 4,500 meters, i.e., thirty times greater than at sea level. These authors believed that, at high altitude, hypoxia and pulmonary hypertension remaining as chronic conditions after birth are factors related to the patency of ductus arteriosus. There also is experimental work that indicates that hypoxia after birth tends to keep the ductus open. If this is correct, patent ductus due to hypoxia is a postnatal and not a congenital cardiovascular anomaly.

Concerning other cardiac malformations caused by hypoxia, one may cite that a few infants with CHD have been born of mothers with cyanotic CHD.[22,157] Before such observations are accepted as proof of maternal hypoxia as a cause of CHD, a few other facts must be taken into consideration. A number of reports exist of normal though sometimes small children born to mothers with cyanotic CHD.[158-160,179] Then there also are reports of mothers with noncyanotic CHD who transmitted CHD to their children.[19,20,23] And there are observations of fathers with CHD who had children with CHD.[12,24,53,56] These factors point to the possibility of involvement of genetic factors in the transmission of CHD from cyanotic or noncyanotic mothers to their children. It appears that the role of hypoxia is difficult to prove by consideration of mothers with *congenital* heart disease. It would be much more convincing if *acquired* cyanotic heart disease would often result in cardiac or other congenital defects in the child. This, however, does not seem to be the case. There is no evidence that women with acquired heart disease have children with an excess of congenital malformations.[158] Thus, the evidence for hypoxia as an etiologic factor in CHD often has been overestimated.

Thalidomide is best known as a teratogen that causes congenital malformations of the limbs. But it was learned from early reports that cardiac malformations may be included in the thalidomide syndrome, and there was an early report of a case of cor triloculare with truncus arteriosus following maternal thalidomide intake from conception to the thirty-fifth day of pregnancy.[161] Interestingly, there was no evidence of other malformations. In 1965, Weicker[162] stated at the XIth International Congress of Pediatrics in Tokyo that by March of 1964 approximately 45% of the children damaged by thalidomide had died because of their cardiac, gastrointestinal or renal malformations. Truncus arteriosus communis, Fallot tetralogy and pentalogy were found often in such children. Among the survivors, 15% had CHD, most frequently tetralogy of Fallot and rarely pseudotruncus arteriosus. In the noncyanotic group, large patent ductus arteriosus was common but septal defects were rare.

Kajii[163] reported 41 necropsies of children damaged by thalidomide who had malformations of the limbs and ears. Of these, 16 (39%) had malformations of the heart. Ventricular septal defects (7), patent ductus arteriosus (5), atrial septal defect and transposition of the great vessels (2), truncus arteriosus (1) and aortic isthmus stenosis (1) were encountered. Kreipe[164] listed 17 cases of cardiovascular malformations, expressing the belief that thalidomide intake from the thirty-sixth to the forty-fifth postmenstrual day of pregnancy was responsible for the CHD. In 10 cases, specific diagnoses were available. Ventricular and atrial septal defects, cor biloculare, tetralogy of Fallot, aortic hypoplasia and coarctation, truncus arteriosus, transposition of the great vessels, patent ductus arteriosus and absent ductus arteriosus were present in various combinations.

The association of hypercalcemia with supravalvar pulmonic stenosis and other cardiovascular malformations (p. 578) led to the hypothesis that maternal hypervitaminosis D may in some way be responsible for the syndrome in children.[165] But critical evaluation of this hypothesis failed to disclose excessive intakes of vitamin D in either the mothers or infants. No evidence was found for increased responsiveness to the hypercalcemic effect of vitamin D or for prolonged retention of the vitamin in the patients or their mothers.[166]

Studies of *twins* showing that discordance is more frequently observed than concordance[167,168] suggest that postconceptional factors play an important role in the determination of normality or abnormality of their hearts. Such twin studies afford interesting glimpses into the etiology of CHD, but interpretation of the observations is not always easy. The fact is that in pairs of identical twins (monozygotic twins) occasionally both members of the pair have congenital heart disease (concordance), but more often only one twin is affected (discordance). Nonidentical (dizygotic) twins usually are discordant in regard to CHD. Monozygotic discordant twins, i.e., identical twins who differ in regard to cardiac defects, demonstrate that postconceptional factors play a role in the etiology of CHD. Such twins also grow and develop in the same maternal environment. If their genetic endowment or their extrauterine maternal environment were at fault, both twins should be affected equally by adverse factors. Since this is not the case, it must be their intrauterine or their "microenvironment" that differs and decides that the heart of one twin develops normally and that of the other abnormally. About such microenvironmental factors we know little, if anything, at present.

Maternal age plays an etiologic role, since it is somehow responsible for Down syndrome, trisomy 18 and trisomy 13-15 and for CHD associated with these disorders. It also appears that mothers over 39 years of age are at a greater risk than younger mothers of having children with congenital heart disease who are otherwise normal.[169] An epidemiologic perspective on the etiology of congenital heart disease as seen in 1969 was outlined by Miller.[182] Genetics of congenital heart disease was discussed in 1970 by Emanuel.[183]

REFERENCES

1. Herxheimer, G.: Missbildungen des Herzens und der grossen Gefässe, in Schwalbe, E. (ed.), *Die Morphologie der Missbildungen des Menschen und der Tiere* (Jena: Gustav Fischer, 1909).
2. Gross, P.: Concept of fetal endocarditis: General review with report of illustrative case, Arch. Path. 31:163, 1941.
3. Meckel, J. F.: De cordis conditionibus abnormibus. Halae typ. Batheanis. 1802 (cited by Herxheimer[1]).
4. Rokitansky, C.: *Die Defecte der Scheidewände des Herzens. Pathologisch-anatomische Abhandlung* (Vienna: W. Braumüller, 1875).
5. Kreysig, F. L.: Krankheiten des Herzens systematisch bearbeitet. Berlin, 1814–17 (cited by Herxheimer[1]).
6. Fischer, B.: Über fötale Infektionskrankheiten und fötale Endokarditis, nebst Bemerkungen über Herzmuskelverkalkung, Frankfurt. Ztschr. Path. 7:83, 1911.
7. Gregg, N. M.: Congenital cataract following German measles in mother, Tr. Ophth. Soc. Australia 3:35, 1942.
8. Carleton, R. A., Abelmann, W. A., and Hancock, E. W.: Familial occurrence of congenital heart disease, New England J. Med. 259:1237, 1958.
9. Warkany, J.: Etiologic Factors of Congenital Heart Disease, in Bass, A. D., and Moe, G. K. (eds.), *Congenital Heart Disease* (Washington, D. C.: Pub. No. 63, American Association for the Advancement of Science, 1960).
10. Fuhrmann, W.: Genetische und Peristatische Ursachen Angeborener Angiokardiopathien, Ergebn. inn. Med. u. Kinderh. 18:47, 1962.
11. Walker, G. C., and Ellis, L. B.: The familial occurrence of congenital cardiac anomalies, Proc. New England Heart A. 1940–1941, p. 26.
12. Taussig, H. B.: *Congenital Malformations of the Heart* (London: Commonwealth Fund, 1947).
13. Walker, W. G.: Coarctation of the aorta in father and son, New England J. Med. 211:1192, 1934.
14. Eisenberg, R., Young, D., Jacobson, B., and Bioto, A.: Familial supravalvular aortic stenosis, Am. J. Dis. Child. 108:341, 1964.
15. Zoethout, H. E., Carter, R. E. B., and Carter, C. O.: A family study of aortic stenosis, J. M. Genetics 1:2, 1964.
16. Jörgensen, G., and Beuren, A. J.: Genetische Untersuchungen bei supravalvulären Aortenstenosen, Humangenetik 1:497, 1965.
17. Lewis, S. M., Sonnenblick, B. P., Gilbert, L., and Biber, D.: Familial pulmonary stenosis and deaf-mutism: Clinical and genetic considerations, Am. Heart J. 55:458, 1958.
18. Koroxenidis, G. T., Webb, N. C., Jr., Moschos, C. B., and Lehan, P. H.: Congenital heart disease, deaf-mutism and associated somatic malformations occurring in several members of one family, Am. J. Med. 40:149, 1966.
19. Debré, R., Cordey, F., and Olivier: Une mère et son enfant atteints de maladie de Roger. Hérédité similaire d'une cardiopathie congénitale, Bull. Soc. méd. hôp. Paris 47:1742, 1923.
20. Lund, C. J.: Maternal congenital heart disease as obstetric problem, Am. J. Obst. & Gynec. 55:244, 1948.
21. Seitz, R., and Baumann, H.: Familiäres Vorkommen von angeborenen Herzfehlern, Ztschr. Kreislaufforsch. 27: 13, 1935.
22. Tucker, A. W., and Kinney, T. D.: Interventricular septal defect (Roger's disease) occurring in a mother and her six-month fetus, Am. Heart J. 30:54, 1945.
23. Apert, E., and Cambessédès: Malformations cardiaques (maladie de Roger) chez une mère et deux de ses enfants, Bull. Soc. pédiat. Paris 28:340, 1930.
24. Campbell, M.: Genetic and environmental factors in congenital heart disease, Quart, J. Med. 18:379, 1949.
25. Weinstein, A.: Congenital heart disease in successive

generations. Interatrial septal defect in a 63-year-old woman and her 31-year-old son, J. Chron. Dis. 8:669, 1958.
26. Weil, M. H., and Allenstein, B. J.: A report of congenital heart disease in five members of one family, New England J. Med. 265:661, 1961.
27. Zetterquist, P.: Multiple occurrence of atrial septal defect in a family, Acta paediat. scandinav. 49:741, 1960.
28. Ehlers, K. H., and Engle, M. A.: Familial congenital heart disease, I. Genetic and environmental factors, Circulation 34:503, 1966.
29. Nora, J. J., McNamara, D. G., and Fraser, F. C.: Hereditary factors in atrial septal defect, Circulation 35:448, 1967.
30. Moller, J. H., Fisch, R. O., From, A. H. L., and Edwards, J. E.: Endocardial fibroelastosis occurring in a mother and son, Pediatrics 38:918, 1966.
31. Doolittle, W. F.: Congenital dextrocardia, Boston M. & S. J. 157:662, 1907.
32. Gänsslen, M., Lambrecht, K., and Werner, M.: Die kongenitalen Missbildungen des Herzens, in *Handbuch der Erbiologie des Menschen* (Berlin: Springer, 1940), Vol. 4, pt. 2, pp. 198–217.
33. Stein, I., and Barber, D. J.: Congenital heart disease. Case reports on 3 members of a family, Am. Heart J. 30: 118, 1945.
34. Tedesco, P. A.: Su due casi di cardiopatia congenita familiare, Cuore e circolaz. 17:76, 1933.
35. Burwinkel, O.: Morbus coeruleus bei vier Generationen, Berl. Klin. Wchnschr. 47:968, 1910.
36. Thysell, T.: Non-cardiac familiar cyanosis, Acta paediat. scandinav. 30:212, 1942.
37. Lamy, M., DeGrouchy, J., and Schweisguth, O.: Genetic and non-genetic factors in the etiology of congenital heart disease: A study of 1188 cases, Am. J. Human Genet. 9:17, 1957.
38. McKeown, T., MacMahon, B., and Parsons, C. G.: The familial incidence of congenital malformations of the heart, Brit. Heart J. 15:273, 1953.
39. Polani, P. E., and Campbell, M.: An aetiological study of congenital heart disease, Ann. Human Genet. 19:209, 1955.
40. Holt, M., and Oram, I.: Familial heart disease with skeletal malformations, Brit. Heart J. 22:236, 1960.
41. Holmes, L. B.: Congenital heart disease and upper-extremity deformities; a report of two families, New England J. Med. 272:437, 1965.
42. Lewis, K. B., Bruce, R. A., Baum, D., and Motulsky, A. G.: The upper limb-cardiovascular syndrome. An autosomal dominant genetic effect on embryogenesis, J.A.M.A. 193:1080, 1965.
43. Pruzanski, W.: Familial congenital malformations of the heart and upper limbs; a syndrome of Holt-Oram, Cardiologia 45:21, 1964.
44. Gall, J. C., Jr., Stern, A. M., Cohen, M. M., Adams, M. S., and Davidson, R. T.: Holt-Oram syndrome: Clinical and genetic study of a large family, Am. J. Human Genet. 18:187, 1966.
45. Forney, W. R., Robinson, S. J., and Pascoe, D. J.: Congenital heart disease, deafness, and skeletal malformations: A new syndrome?, J. Pediat. 68:14, 1966.
46. Watson, G. H.: Pulmonary stenosis, café-au-lait spots, and dull intelligence, Arch. Dis. Childhood 42:303, 1967.
47. Evans, W.: Familial cardiomegaly, Brit. Heart J. 11:68, 1949.
48. Paré, J. A. P., Fraser, R. G., Pirozynski, W. J., Shanks, J. A., and Stubington, D.: Hereditary cardiovascular dysplasia. A form of familial cardiomyopathy, Am. J. Med. 31:37, 1961.
49. Kariv, I., Szeinberg, A., Fabian, I., Sherf, L., Kreisler, B., and Zeltzer, M.: A family with cardiomyopathy, Am. J. Med. 40:140, 1966.
50. Walther, R. J., Madoff, I. M., and Zinner, K.: Cardiomegaly of unknown cause occurring in a family; report of three siblings and review of the literature, New England J. Med. 263:1104, 1960.
51. Joyce, J. C., and O'Toole, S. P.: Congenital heart disease. Report of an unusually high incidence in one family, Brit. M. J. 1:1241, 1954.
52. Kjaergaard, H.: Patent ductus Botalli in three sisters, Acta med. scandinav. 125:339, 1946.
53. Ekström, G.: The surgical treatment of patent ductus arteriosus; a clinical study of 290 cases, Acta chir. scandinav., supp. 169, 1952.
54. Jewesbury, R. C.: Two similar but somewhat unusual heart conditions in sisters, Proc. Roy. Soc. Med. 6:100, 1912–1913.
55. Nadas, A. S.: *Pediatric Cardiology* (Philadelphia: W. B. Saunders Company, 1957).
56. Starer, F.: Analysis of 50 cases of persistent ductus arteriosus, Brit. M. J. 1:971, 1953.
57. Uchida, I.: Familial Occurrence of Congenital Heart Disease, in Keith, J. D., Rowe, R. D., and Vlad, P. (eds.), *Heart Disease in Infancy and Childhood* (New York: The Macmillan Company, 1958), Chap. 9.
58. Ellis, R. W. B.: Congenital morbus cordis in two sisters, Brit. J. Child. Dis. 33:286, 1936.
59. Snelling, D. B.: Familial congenital heart disease: Patent ductus arteriosus in sisters, J.A.M.A. 108:1502, 1937.
60. Dexter, L.: Atrial septal defects, Brit. Heart J. 18:209, 1956.
61. Courter, S. R., Felson, B., and McGuire, J.: Familial interauricular septal defect with mitral stenosis (Lutembacher's syndrome), Am. J. M. Sc. 216:501, 1948.
62. Schöne, G.: Congenital defects, their diagnosis and familial occurrence, Deutsche Arch. klin. Med. 184:129, 1939.
63. Coblentz, B., and Mathivat, A.: Sténose pulmonaire congénitale chez deux soeurs, Arch. mal. coeur 45:490, 1952.
64. Dordick, J. R.: Diffuse endocardial fibrosis and cardiac hypertrophy in infancy, Am. J. Clin. Path. 21:743, 1951.
65. Kelly, J., and Andersen, D. H.: Congenital endocardial fibroelastosis. II. A clinical and pathologic investigation of those cases without associated cardiac malformations including report of two familial instances, Pediatrics 18:539, 1956.
66. Rosahn, P. D.: Endocardial fibroelastosis: Old and new concepts, Bull. New York Acad. Med. 31:453, 1955.
67. Weinberg, T., and Himmelfarb, A. J.: Endocardial fibroelastosis (so-called fetal endocarditis); report of 2 cases occurring in siblings, Bull. Johns Hopkins Hosp. 72:299, 1943.
68. Lowe, C. R., and McKeown, T.: Investigation of dextrocardia with and without transposition of abdominal viscera with report of case in one monozygotic twin, Ann. Eugenics 18:267, 1954.
69. Cockayne, E. A.: The genetics of transposition of the viscera, Quart. J. Med. 7:479, 1938.
70. Torgersen, J.: Concordant situs inversus in dizygotic twins, J. Hered. 39:293, 1948.
71. Campbell, M.: The genetics of congenital heart disease and situs inversus in sibs, Brit. Heart J. 21:65, 1959.
72. McLoughlin, T. G., Krovetz, L. J., and Schiebler, G. L.: Heart disease in the Laurence-Moon-Biedl-Bardet syndrome, J. Pediat. 65:388, 1964.
73. Jervell, A., and Lange-Nielsen, F.: Congenital deafmutism, functional heart disease with prolongation of the Q-T interval and sudden death, Am. Heart J. 54:59, 1957.
74. Childs, A. W., Crose, R. F., and Henderson, P. H.: Glycogen disease of heart; report of 2 cases occurring in siblings, Pediatrics 10:208, 1952.
75. Christiaens, L., Dupuis, C., Poingt, O., Belbenoit, C., and Fovet, A.: Les cardiopathies congénitales familiales,

Arch. franç. pédiat. 21:921, 1964.
76. Nora, J. J., and Meyer, T. C.: Familial nature of congenital heart diseases, Pediatrics 37:329, 1966.
77. Warkany, J. Passarge, E., and Smith, L. B.: Congenital malformations in autosomal trisomy syndromes, Am. J. Dis. Child. 112:502, 1966.
78. Gustavson, K-H., Hagberg, B., Finley, S. C., and Finley, W. H.: An apparently identical extra autosome in two severely retarded sisters with multiple malformations, Cytogenetics 1:32, 1962.
79. Böök, J. A., Santesson, B., and Zetterquist, P.: Association between congenital heart malformation and chromosomal variations, Acta paediat. scandinav. 50:217, 1961.
80. Koulischer, L., Kulakowski, S., and Malherbe, A.: Trisomie 22 possible chez un enfant polymalforme, Arch. franç. pédiat. 23:839, 1966.
81. Atkins, L., and Feingold, M.: Enlarged B-group chromosome (4-5). Associated with cri du chat syndrome, Am. J. Dis. Child. 113:277, 1967.
82. Summitt, R. L.: Familial 2/3 translocation, Am. J. Human Genet. 18:172, 1966.
83. Lee, C. S. N., Bowen, P., Rosenblum, H., and Linsao, L.: Familial chromosome-2, 3 translocation ascertained through an infant with multiple malformations, New England J. Med. 271:12, 1964.
84. Migeon, B. R., and Young, W. J.: Reciprocal (D/E) translocation: Euploid transmission in three generations, Bull. Johns Hopkins Hosp. 115:379, 1964.
85. Cohen, M. M., and Lockwood, M. A.: Familial transmission of a presumptive D/E (13-15/17-18) short arm translocation, Pediat. Res. 1:104, 1967.
86. Jensen, M. K., and Melchior, J. C.: Possible partial trisomy of a chromosome of group 6-X-12 and familial translocation heterozygosity in a child with congenital abnormalities, Developmental Med. & Child Neurol. 9:313, 1967.
87. de Grouchy, J., Aussannaire, M., Brissaud, H. E., and Lamy, M.: Aneusomie de recombinaison: Three further examples, Am. J. Human Genet. 18:467, 1966.
88. Lejeune, J., Lafourcade, J., de Grouchy, J., Berger, R., Gautier, M., Salmon, C., and Turpin, R.: Délétion partielle du bras court du chromosome 5. Individualisation d'un nouvel état morbide, Semaine hôp. Paris 40:1069, 1964.
89. Pfeiffer, R. A., and Simon, H. A.: "Cri du Chat," ein neues Missbildungssyndrom als Folge einer Chromosomenaberration, München med. Wchnschr. 107:2669, 1965.
90. Genest, P., Tremblay, M., and Mortezai, M.: Le syndrome du "cri du chat." Etude d'un cas de délétion partielle du bras court du chromosome 5 avec translocation au chromosome 4, Laval méd. 36:319, 1965.
91. Cavalieri, S., Mastella, G., and Tiepolo, L.: The crying cat syndrome, Fracastoro 57:369, 1964.
92. Wolf, U., and Reinwein, H.: Klinische und cytogenetische Differentialdiagnose der Defizienzen an den kurzen Armen der B-Chromosomen, Ztschr. Kinderh. 98: 235, 1967.
93. Palmer, C. G., Fareed, N., and Merritt, A. D.: Ring chromosome 18 in a patient with multiple anomalies, J. M. Genetics 4:117, 1967.
94. Sasaki, M. S., Makino, S., and Kajii, T.: Chromosomal aberrations in congenital vascular disorders of man, Proc. Jap. Acad. 39:394, 1963.
95. Anders, J. M., Moores, E. C., and Emanuel, R.: Chromosome studies in 156 patients with congenital heart disease, Brit. Heart J. 27:756, 1965.
96. Moores, E. C., Anders, J. M., and Emanuel, R.: Inheritance of marker chromosomes from a cytogenetic survey of congenital heart disease, Ann. Human Genet. 30:77, 1966.
97. German, J., Ehlers, K. H., and Engle, M. A.: Familial congenital heart disease. II. Chromosomal studies, Circulation 34:517, 1966.
98. Rainier-Pope, C. R., Cunningham, R. D., Nadas, A. S., and Crigler, J. F., Jr.: Cardiovascular malformations in Turner's syndrome, Pediatrics 33:919, 1964.
99. Haddad, H. M., and Wilkins, L.: Congenital anomalies associated with gonadal aplasia. Review of 55 cases, Pediatrics 23:885, 1959.
100. Conen, P. E., and Glass, I. H.: 45/XO Turner's syndrome in the newborn: Report of two cases, J. Clin. Endocrinol. 23:1, 1963.
101. Atkins, L., and Connelly, J. P.: XXXXY sex-chromosome abnormality, Am. J. Dis. Child. 106:514, 1963.
102. Fraccaro, M., Kaijser, K., and Lindsten, J.: A child with 49 chromosomes, Lancet 2:899, 1960.
103. Joseph, M. C., Anders, J. M., and Taylor, A. I.: A boy with XXXXY sex chromosomes, J. M. Genetics 1:95, 1964.
104. Day, R. W., Larson, W., and Wright, S. W.: Clinical and cytogenetic studies on a group of females with XXX sex chromosome complements, J. Pediat. 64:24, 1964.
105. Kesaree, N., and Woolley, P. V., Jr.: A phenotypic female with 49 chromosomes, presumably XXXXX, J. Pediat. 63:1099, 1963.
106. Abbott, M. E.: *Atlas of Congenital Cardiac Disease* (New York: American Heart Association, Inc., 1936).
107. Anderson, R. C.: Causative factors underlying congenital heart malformation. I. Patent ductus arteriosus, Pediatrics 14:143, 1954.
108. Record, R. G., and McKeown, T.: Observations relating to aetiology of patent ductus arteriosus, Brit. Heart J. 15:376, 1953.
109. Bailey, C. P., Downing, D. F., Geckeler, G. D., Likoff, W., Goldberg, H., Scott, J. C., Janton, O., and Redondo-Ramirez, H. P.: Congenital interatrial communications: Clinical and surgical considerations with description of new surgical technic; atrio-septo-pexy, Ann. Int. Med. 37:888,1952.
110. Keith, J. D., Rowe, R. D., and Vlad, P. (eds): *Heart Disease in Infancy and Childhood* (New York: The Macmillan Company, 1958).
111. Roesler, H.: Interatrial septal defect, Arch, Int. Med. 54: 339, 1934.
112. Pritchard, J. A.: Coarctation of the aorta and pregnancy, Obst. & Gynec. Surv. 8:775, 1953.
113. Campbell, M., and Kauntze, R.: Congenital aortic valvular stenosis, Brit. Heart J. 15:179, 1953.
114. Ongley, P. A., Nadas, A. S., Paul, M. H., Rudolph, A. M., and Starkey, G. W. B.: Aortic stenosis in infants and children, Pediatrics 21:207, 1958.
115. MacMahon, B., McKeown, T., and Record, R. G.: Incidence and life expectation of children with congenital heart disease, Brit. Heart J. 15:121, 1953.
116. Edwards, J. E.: Congenital Malformations of the Heart and Great Vessels, in Gould, S. E. (ed.), *Pathology of the Heart* (Springfield, Ill.: Charles C Thomas, Publisher, 1953).
117. Ferencz, C., Johnson, A. L., and Wiglesworth, F. W.: Congenital mitral stenosis, Circulation 9:161, 1954.
118. Field, C. E.: Congenital mitral stenosis, Arch. Dis. Childhood 13:371, 1938.
119. Landing, B. H., Nakai, H., Margaretten, W., Kobayashi, N., and Beaudry, P. H.: Some genetic and biochemical implications of congenital heart disease, Quart. Rev. Pediat. 16:160, 1961.
120. Wilson, J. G., and Warkany, J.: Aortic arch and cardiac anomalies in the offspring of vitamin A deficient rats, Am. J. Anat. 85:113, 1949.
121. Kalter, H., and Warkany, J.: Experimental production of congenital malformations in strains of inbred mice by maternal treatment with hypervitaminosis A, Am. J. Path. 38:1, 1961.
122. Baird, C. D., Nelson, M. M., Monie, I. W., and Evans, H. M.: Congenital cardiovascular anomalies induced by pteroylglutamic acid deficiency during gestation in the rat, Circulation Res. 2:544, 1954.

123. Ingalls, T. H., Curley, F. J., and Prindle, R.: Medical progress: Experimental production of congenital anomalies, New England J. Med. 247:758, 1952.
124. Gillman, J., Gilbert, C., and Gillman, T.: A preliminary report on hydrocephalus, spina bifida and other congenital anomalies in the rat produced by trypan blue, South African J. M. Sc. 13:47, 1948.
125. Warkany, J., and Takacs, E.: Experimental production of congenital malformations in rats by salicylate poisoning, Am. J. Path. 35:315, 1959.
126. Manson, M. M., Logan, W. P. D., and Loy, R. M.: Rubella and other virus infections during pregnancy, Pub. Health Rep. Med. Sub. No. 101, 1960.
127. Sheridan, M. D.: Final report of a prospective study of children whose mothers had rubella in early pregnancy, Brit. M. J. 2:536, 1964.
128. Tartakow, I. J.: The teratogenicity of maternal rubella, J. Pediat. 66:380, 1965.
129. Warkany, J.: Etiology of Congenital Malformations, in Levine S. Z. (ed.), *Advances in Pediatrics* (New York: Interscience Publishers, Inc., 1947), Vol. II, p. 1.
130. Malmberg, N., Sterner, G., and Lundmark, C.: Asymptomatic maternal rubella as a probable cause of embryopathy, Ann. paediat. Fenniae 3:437, 1957.
131. Campbell, M.: Place of maternal rubella in the aetiology of congenital heart disease, Brit. M. J. 1:691, 1961.
132. Keith, J. D., Rowe, R. D., and Vlad, P. (eds.): *Heart Disease in Infancy and Childhood* (2d ed.; New York: The Macmillan Company, 1966).
133. Swan, C., Tostevin, A. L., Moore, B., Mayo, H., and Black, G. H. B.: Congenital defects in infants following infectious diseases during pregnancy, with special reference to relationship between German measles and cataract, deaf-mutism, heart disease, and microcephaly and to period of pregnancy in which occurrence of rubella is followed by congenital abnormalities, M. J. Australia 2:201, 1943.
134. Rutstein, D. D., Nickerson, R. J., and Herald, F. P.: Seasonal incidence of patent ductus arteriosus and maternal rubella, A.M.A. Am. J. Dis. Child. 84:199, 1952.
135. Gibson, S., and Lewis, K.: Congenital heart disease following maternal rubella during pregnancy, A.M.A. Am. J. Dis. Child. 83:317, 1952.
136. Jackson, A. V.: In King, E. S. J., Lowe, T. E., and Cox, L. B. (eds.), *Studies in Pathology*. Presented to Peter MacCallum (Melbourne: Melbourne University Press, 1950).
137. Pitt, D. B.: Congenital malformations and maternal rubella, M. J. Australia 1:233, 1957.
138. Heiner, D. C., and Nadas, A. S.: Patent ductus arteriosus in association with pulmonic stenosis, Circulation 17: 232, 1958.
139. Rowe, R. D.: Maternal rubella and pulmonary artery stenoses. Report of 11 cases, Pediatrics 32:180, 1963.
140. Venables, A. W.: The syndrome of pulmonary stenosis complicating maternal rubella, Brit. Heart J. 27:49, 1965.
141. Emmanouilides, G. C., Linde, L. M., and Crittenden, I. H.: Pulmonary artery stenosis associated with ductus arteriosus following maternal rubella, Circulation 29: 514, 1964.
142. Hastreiter, A. R., Joorabchi, B., Pujatti, G., van der Horse, R. L., Patacsil, G., and Sever, J. L.: Cardiovascular lesions associated with congenital rubella, J. Pediat. 71:59, 1967.
143. Williams, H. J., and Carey, L. S.: Rubella embryopathy. Roentgenologic features, Am. J. Roentgenol. 47:92, 1966.
144. Esterly, J. R., and Oppenheimer, E. H.: Vascular lesions in infants with congenital rubella, Circulation 36:544, 1967.
145. Jeresaty, R. M., and Russell, W.: Hepatosplenomegaly and heart disease in the congenital rubella syndrome: Report of eight cases, Pediatrics 39:36, 1967.
146. Beswick, R. C., Warner, R., and Warkany, J.: Congenital anomalies following maternal rubella, Am. J. Dis. Child. 78:334, 1949.
147. Bass, M. H.: Diseases of the Pregnant Woman Affecting the Offspring, in Dock, W., and Snapper, I. (eds.), *Advances in Internal Medicine* (Chicago: Year Book Medical Publishers, Inc., 1952), Vol. V, p. 15.
148. Dogramaci, I., and Green, H.: Factors in the etiology of congenital heart anomalies, J. Pediat. 30:295, 1947.
149. Potter, E. L.: Placental transmission of viruses, with special reference to the intrauterine origin of cytomegalic inclusion body disease, Am. J. Obst. & Gynec. 74: 505, 1957.
150. Benirschke, K., and Pendleton, M. E.: Coxsackie virus infection, an important complication of pregnancy, Obst. & Gynec. Surv. 12:305, 1958.
151. Javett, S. N., Heymann, S., Mundel, B., Pepler, W. J., Lurie, H. I., Gear, J., Measroch, V., and Kirsch, Z.: Myocarditis in the newborn infant, J. Pediat. 48:1, 1956.
152. Noren, G. R., Adams, P., and Anderson, R. C.: Positive skin reactivity to mumps virus antigen in endocardial fibroelastosis, J. Pediat. 62:604, 1963.
153. St. Geme, J. W., Jr., Noren, G. R., and Adams, P., Jr.: Proposed embryopathic relation between mumps virus and primary endocardial fibroelastosis, New England J. Med. 275:339, 1966.
154. Alzamora, V., Rotta, A., Battilana, G., Abugattas, R., Rubio, C., Bouroncle, J., Zapata, C., Santa-Maria, E., Binder, T., Subira, R., Paredes, D., Pando, B., and Graham, G. G.: On the possible influence of great altitudes on the determination of certain cardiovascular anomalies, Pediatrics 12:259, 1953.
155. Dexter, L.: Congenital defects of the heart in high altitudes, New England J. Med. 247:851, 1952.
156. Penaloza, D., Arias-Stella, J., Sime, F., Recavarren, S., and Marticorena, E.: The heart and pulmonary circulation in children at high altitudes; physiological, anatomical, and clinical observations, Pediatrics 34:568, 1964.
157. Selzer, A., and Laquer, G. L.: Eisenmenger complex and its relation to uncomplicated defect of ventricular septum; review of 35 cases of Eisenmenger's complex including 2 new cases, A.M.A. Arch. Int. Med. 87:218, 1951.
158. Burwell, C. S., and Metcalfe, J.: *Heart Disease and Pregnancy* (Boston: Little, Brown & Company, 1958).
159. Scherlis, S., and Soloway, L. R.: Pregnancy and labor in patient with cardiac anomaly, probable tetralogy of Fallot, Am. J. Obst. & Gynec. 44:697, 1942.
160. Simon, D. L., and Lustberg, A.: Case of truncus arteriosus communis compatible with full term pregnancy, Am. Heart J. 42:617, 1951.
161. Owen, R., and Smith, A.: Cor triloculare and thalidomide, Lancet 2:836, 1962.
162. Weicker, H.: 100 children with thalidomide embryopathy, XIth International Congress of Pediatrics, 1965.
163. Kajii, T.: Thalidomide experience in Japan, Ann. paediat. 205:341, 1965.
164. Kreipe, U.: Missbildungen innerer Organe bei Thalidomid-Embryopathie, Arch. Kinderh. 176:33, 1967.
165. Taussig, H. B.: Possible injury to the cardiovascular system from vitamin D, Ann. Int. Med. 65:1195, 1966.
166. Anita, A. U., Wiltse, H. E., Rose, R. D., Pitt, E. L., Levin, S., Ottesen, O. E., and Cooke, R. E.: Pathogenesis of the supravalvular aortic stenosis syndrome, J. Pediat. 71: 431, 1967.
167. Uchida, I. A., and Rowe, R. D.: Discordant heart anomalies in twins, Am. J. Human Genet. 9:133, 1957.
168. Ross, L. J.: Congenital cardiovascular anomalies in twins, Circulation 20:327, 1959.
169. Renwick, D. H., Miller, J. R., and Paterson, D.: Estimates of incidence and prevalence of mongolism and of congenital heart disease in British Columbia, Canad. M.A.J. 91:365, 1964.
170. Davachi, F., McLean, R. H., Moller, J. H., and Edwards,

J. E.: Hypoplasia of the right ventricle and tricuspid valve in siblings, J. Pediat. 71:869, 1967.
171. Sackner, M. A., Robinson, M. J., Jamison, W. L., and Lewis, D. H.: Isolated right ventricular hypoplasia with atrial septal defect or patent foramen ovale, Circulation 24:1388, 1961.
172. Gueron, M., Hirsch, M., Stern, J., Cohen, W., and Levy, M. J.: Familial Ebstein's anomaly with emphasis on the surgical treatment, Am. J. Cardiol. 18:105, 1966.
173. Aylward, R. D.: Congenital heart block, Brit. M. J. 1:943, 1928.
174. Wallgren, G., and Agorio, E.: Congenital complete A-V block in three siblings, Acta paediat. 49:49, 1960.
175. Latta, H., and Crittenden, I. H.: Acquired lesions of the conduction system in familial congenital heart block, Lab. Invest. 13:214, 1964.
176. Wendkow, M. H., and Study, R. S.: Familial congenital complete A-V heart block, Am. Heart J. 34:138, 1947.
177. Lynch, J. I., Perry, L. W., Takakuwa, T., and Scott, L. P.: Congenital heart disease and chondroectodermal dysplasia, Am. J. Dis. Child. 115:80, 1968.
178. Davison, B. C. C.: Concordance and discordance of congenital heart disease in 20 families, J. M. Genetics 4: 245, 1967.
179. Barnes, A. C., and Vernon, C. P.: Discussion of Cannell, D. E., and Vernon, C. P.: Congenital heart disease and pregnancy, Am. J. Obst. & Gynec. 85:744, 1963.
180. Brody, J., Fitzgerald, M. G., and Spiers, A. S. D.: A female with five X chromosomes, J. Pediat. 70:105, 1967.
181. Bizarro, R. O., Callahan, J. A., Feldt, R. H., Kurland, L. T., Gordon, H., and Brandenburg, R. O.: Familial atrial septal defect with prolonged atrioventricular conduction, Circulation 41:677, 1970.
182. Miller, R. W.: Origins of congenital heart disease: An epidemiologic perspective, Teratology 2:77, 1969.
183. Emanuel, R.: Genetics and congenital heart disease, Brit. Heart J. 32:281, 1970.
184. Passarge, E.: Genetische Faktoren in der Ätiologie angeborener Fehlbildungen des Herzens, in Keck, E. W. (ed.), *Herzkrankheiten des Säuglings- und Kindesalters* (Berlin: Urban & Schwarzenberg, 1970).

49

Experimental Production of Cardiovascular Malformations in Mammals

About 30 years ago, it became possible to produce congenital malformations in mammals by maternal dietary deficiencies. Among the malformations produced by vitamin A deficiency,[1] there were malformations such as ventricular septal defects and various anomalies of the aortic arches.[2] Malformations could be produced in rats with regularity and in sufficient numbers to establish a pattern that, despite individual variations, proved rather characteristic of prenatal vitamin A deficiency. Wilson and Warkany[3] analyzed the cardiovascular anomalies of the syndrome and found that an astounding variation of arch pattern occurred in the young under the conditions of maternal vitamin A deficiency (Chapter 58) together with ventricular septal defect and general retardation of myocardial development. Some of the malformations were compatible with intrauterine life, others were not, as shown by the fact that the cardiovascular defects were more common in younger fetuses than in term animals. Another significant observation was that fetuses of the same litter were rarely affected by the same malformations. Such discordance in litter mates illustrates by analogy the fallacy of the belief that dizygotic twins are regularly concordant if their malformations are due to an environmental cause. Another point of interest was that the cardiovascular malformations were associated with marked intrauterine growth retardation of the affected fetuses,[4] thus demonstrating a relationship recognized in clinical cardiology many years later.[5] The first teratologic experiments of vitamin A deficiency consisted of maternal depletion throughout pregnancy, which resulted in a high rate of infertility and resorptions. When the vitamin A deficiency was interrupted by supplements of vitamin A between the tenth and fifteenth days of gestation, the patterns of congenital malformations were altered, as some malformations and fetal deaths were prevented, whereas others still appeared. When, for instance, supplements were given on the twelfth or thirteenth day of pregnancy, the incidence of cardiovascular defects was increased, whereas ocular malformations became rare.[6]

Palludan[7] produced cardiac malformations in pigs by maternal vitamin A deficiency. Septal defects, aortic arch anomalies and myocardial hypoplasia were noted in 15% of the pigs when the deficiency lasted throughout pregnancy. As in rats, the incidence of cardiac malformations was raised when the vitamin A deficiency was arrested during pregnancy. This may be explained by salvage of fetuses with cardiovascular defects by vitamin A supplied in later stages of gestation. The similar outcome of these experiments in rats and pigs is worth emphasis, since other teratogens, although effective in one species, often fail to produce similar malformations in others.

Vitamin A deficiency experiments are difficult and prolonged. It was of great importance that a much simpler method became available when Gillman *et al.*[8] demonstrated that injections of trypan blue into pregnant rats produced congenital malformations in the offspring. This easy procedure became an excellent instrument of cardiovascular teratology. Interestingly, the pattern of cardiac malformations produced by trypan blue differs in many respects from that of vitamin A deficiency. Among the aortic arch anomalies produced by trypan blue, transposition of the great vessels was frequent[9] and there was a high incidence of atrioventricular valve malformations. The transposition complexes produced resembled human malformations of this type in many respects.[10] Abnormal rotation and position of the atria were observed[11,12] and combination with situs inversus totalis occurred in some animals.[12] Postnatal survival of offspring with ventricular septal defect has been reported.[13] The method was employed in prenatal studies to observe the development of the malformations during embryogenesis.[11,14-16] Deviations from normal development could be recognized from the twelfth or thirteenth day of gestation on. Inversion of the atria, narrowness of the atrioventricular canal, abnormal looping of the heart tube resulting in inversion of the ventricles and absence (or stenosis) of the tricuspid or mitral valves could be observed in embryos. Atrioventricular cushions appeared enlarged and tricuspid or mitral ostia were stenotic or absent, resulting in reduction in size or absence of the corresponding ventricle. Retarded development of the truncus leading to prolongation of its sinuous stage and to reduction of its length plays an important role in the sinistral location of the truncus. As spiraling of the trunco-bulbar cushions is minimal, the dorsally placed pulmonary trunk communicates directly with the left ventricle and the ventrally located aorta retains its connection with the right ventricle. Thus, the problem of transposition of the great vessels (Chapter 57) could be reduced to alterations of growth of the cardiac structures, but the cellular basis of the growth changes is still not known.[15]

Growth inhibition of the developing heart can be achieved experimentally by many other procedures. X-irradiation of pregnant rats on the ninth day of gestation results in a variety of malformations in the young.[6] Transposition of the great vessels and other aortic arch anomalies result. Atrial, ventricular and atrioventricular septal defects and atresia of the interatrial foramen secundum with hypoplasia of the left-sided chambers were observed. Ventricular septal defect has been observed in the young of mice whose mothers were exposed to hypoxia[17] and in the offspring of rats whose mothers were exposed to carbon dioxide during pregnancy.[18] In the latter case, partial transposition, narrowing of the pulmonic or aortic outflow tracts and mitral or tricuspid atresia have been reported.

Production of congenital malformations by vitamin deficiencies was greatly facilitated when antimetabolites became available. Cardiovascular anomalies were induced in rats by folic acid deficiency,[19] with the highest percentage obtained when the deficiency was maintained from day 9 to day 11 of gestation. The malformations were similar to those brought about by vitamin A deficiency and pantothenic acid deficiency.[20] Riboflavin deficiency produced by diet alone results in skeletal malformations,[21] but when the antimetabolite galactoflavin is incorporated in the deficient diet, other organ systems are affected also.[22] Cardiovascular malformations are particularly prevalent when the deficiency period lasts from day 7 to day 11.

Not only hypovitaminoses but also hypervitaminosis A can induce cardiovascular malformations. In certain strains of inbred mice, with a single dose of 10,000 I.U. of vitamin A given by mouth, many malformations are produced in the young of females treated at 8 days after conception.[23] Narrow ductus arteriosus, transposition of the great vessels, double outlet of the right ventricle, ventricular septal defect and coronary aneurysm can be observed. Among the effects of thalidomide on rabbit fetuses, such cardiovascular malformations as ventricular septal defect, truncus arteriosus, transposition and other anomalies of the great vessels may appear.[24] The antibiotic and antitumor compound streptonigrin is an effective teratogen that can induce transposition of the great vessels, among many other malformations.[25] Dextroamphetamine sulfate given intraperitoneally to pregnant A/Jax mice induced cardiac malformations in 12% of the offspring.[26] There probably are numerous other compounds that can derange the development of the circulatory system of mammals. Even the widely used salicylates, including aspirin, are teratogenic in rats and, when given in toxic doses, they produce varying degrees of transposition of the aorta, particularly double outlet of the right ventricle. Defects of septation are also effected.[27] A review of experimentally produced cardiovascular malformations was published by Le Douarin.[28]

Thus, experimental teratology has made possible production of congenital cardiovascular malformations in mammals and provided opportunities to study abnormal morphogenetic processes in early embryonic stages. In the past, anatomists and pathologists were greatly interested in the formal genesis of the various malformations of the heart and great vessels; they had to substitute speculations for observations in abnormal embryos, which were not available in sufficient numbers. It is regrettable that at this time, when innumerable animal models are available to test the theories, only a few anatomists and pathologists show an interest in this subject. It is for this reason that the studies of the pathogenesis of cardiac malformations have not been developed in depth. Old ideas of torsion and detorsion of the cardiac primordia could now be replaced by exact observations of local cell growth and differentiation. It is possible that the lack of interest in this subject is due to the fact that teratologic experiments in mammals have shown that the development of pathologic entities that are of interest to the clinician apparently are due to "chance" once the normal course of development is disturbed by a teratogen. Whether a certain embryo of a litter develops transposition of the great vessels or a simple ventricular septal defect is beyond the power of the experimenter and a rather disappointing fact. But it is a fact worth knowing, because it exemplifies the "chance" element in the pathogenesis of cardiac malformations also expressed in discordance of twins and diversity of heart defects caused by thalidomide. It points to the need for exploration of the so-called chance factors of the microenvironment that decide the morphology of clinical entities.

REFERENCES

1. Hale, F.: The relation of vitamin A to anophthalmos in pigs, Am. J. Ophth. 18:1087, 1935.
2. Warkany, J., Roth, C. B., and Wilson, J. G.: Multiple congenital malformations: A consideration of etiologic factors, Pediatrics 1:462, 1948.
3. Wilson, J. G., and Warkany, J.: Aortic-arch and cardiac anomalies in the offspring of vitamin A deficient rats, Am. J. Anat. 85:113, 1949.
4. Warkany, J., and Roth, C. B.: Congenital malformations induced in rats by maternal vitamin A deficiency. II. Effect of varying the preparatory diet upon the yield of abnormal young, J. Nutrition 35:1, 1948.
5. Engle, M. A., Holswade, G. R., Goldberg, H. P., and Glenn, F.: Present problems pertaining to patency of the ductus arteriosus. I. Persistence of growth retardation after successful surgery, Pediatrics 21:70, 1958.
6. Wilson, J. G., Jordan, H. C., and Brent, R. L.: Effects of irradiation on embryonic development. II. X-rays on the 9th day of gestation in the rat, Am. J. Anat. 92:153, 1953.
7. Palludan, B.: *A-Avitaminosis in Swine* (Copenhagen: Munksgaard, 1966).
8. Gillman, J., Gilbert, C., and Gillman, T.: A preliminary report on hydrocephalus, spina bifida and other congenital anomalies in the rat produced by trypan blue, South African J. M. Sc. 13:47, 1948.
9. Wilson, J. G.: Teratogenic activity of several azo dyes chemically related to trypan blue, Anat. Rec. 123:313, 1955.
10. Fox, M. H., and Goss, C. M.: Experimentally produced malformations of the heart and great vessels in rat fetuses. Transposition complexes and aortic arch abnormalities, Am. J. Anat. 102:65, 1958.
11. Fox, M. H., and Goss, C. M.: Experimentally produced malformations of the heart and great vessels in rat fetuses. Atrial and caval abnormalities, Anat. Rec. 129:309, 1957.
12. Wegener, K.: Über die experimentelle Erzeugung von Herzmissbildungen durch Trypanblau, Arch. Kreislaufforsch. 34:99, 1961.
13. Richman, S. M., Thomas, W. A., and Konikov, N.: Survival of rats with induced congenital cardiovascular anomalies, A.M.A. Arch. Path. 63:43, 1957.
14. Christie, G. A.: An embryological analysis of certain cardiac abnormalities produced in rats by the injection of trypan blue, Scottish M. J. 6:465, 1961.
15. Monie, I. W., Takacs, E., and Warkany, J.: Transposition of the great vessels and other cardiovascular abnormalities in rat fetuses induced by trypan blue, Anat. Rec. 156:175, 1966.
16. Smith, W. N. A.: The site of action of trypan blue in cardiac teratogenesis, Anat. Rec. 147:507, 1963.
17. Ingalls, T. H., Curley, F. J., and Prindle, R.: Medical progress: Experimental production of congenital anomalies, New England J. Med. 247:758, 1952.
18. Haring, O. M.: Cardiac malformations in rats induced by exposure of the mother to carbon dioxide during pregnancy, Circulation Res. 18:1218, 1960.
19. Baird, C. D. C., Nelson, M. M., Monie, I. W., and Evans, H. M.: Congenital cardiovascular anomalies induced by pteroylglutamic acid deficiency during gestation in the rat, Circulation Res. 11:544, 1954.
20. Nelson, M. M., Wright, H. V., Baird, C. D. C., and Evans, H. M.: Teratogenic effects of pantothenic acid deficiency in the rat, J. Nutrition 62:395, 1957.
21. Warkany, J., and Nelson, R. C.: Appearance of skeletal abnormalities in the offspring of rats reared on a deficient diet, Science 92:383, 1940.
22. Nelson, M. M., Baird, C. D. C., Wright, H. V., and Evans, H. M.: Multiple congenital abnormalities in the rat resulting from riboflavin deficiency induced by the antimetabolite galactoflavin, J. Nutrition 58:125, 1956.
23. Kalter, H., and Warkany, J.: Experimental production of congenital malformations in strains of inbred mice by maternal treatment with hypervitaminosis A, Am. J. Path. 38:1, 1961.
24. Roux, C., Cahen, R., and Dupuis, R.: Malformations viscérales provoquées par le thalidomide chez le lapin, Compt. rend. Soc. biol. 159:1059, 1965.
25. Warkany, J., and Takacs, E.: Congenital malformations in rats from streptonigrin, Arch. Path. 79:65, 1965.
26. Nora, J. J., Trasler, D. G., and Fraser, F. C.: Malformations in mice induced by dexamphetamine sulphate, Lancet 2:1021, 1965.
27. Takacs, E., and Warkany, J.: Experimental production of congenital cardiovascular malformations in rats, Teratology 1:109, 1968.
28. Le Douarin, G.: Les malformations cardiaques expérimentales, Rev. Anat. et Morphol. Expér. 37:168, 1964.

SECTION TWO

50

Acardia

Absence of the heart occurs only in monsters that are members of a pair of monozygotic twins and are associated with twin fetuses who have a functioning heart. It has been estimated that an acardius occurs once in approximately 35,000 deliveries and that somewhat less than 1% of identical twin pregnancies contain an acardius. Acardiac monsters were described in the sixteenth century[1] and many times thereafter, but Hempel,[2] in 1850, made probably the most important contribution to an understanding of the anomaly by pointing out vascular placental anastomoses between the acardius and his twin and reversal of the circulation in the acardius. Large artery-to-artery and vein-to-vein anastomoses exist that make possible nutrition of the acardiac fetus through his umbilical artery or arteries, which are supplied by the heart of the twin. Acardii can also occur in triplet pregnancies. Hydramnios quite often is associated with pregnancies that yield an acardius. There is always a monochorial placenta but there can be double amnion. In human cases, the sex of the acardius and his twin has always been the same; sex chromatin and chromosomes support the belief that the twins are monozygotic.[3] There has never been recurrence of the condition in a family.[1]

Two pathogenetic theories have long been discussed.[4] According to one opinion, the acardius never developed a heart and was kept alive by his twin's heart from early embryonic times. The second theory asserts that the acardius originally was a normal twin whose heart degenerated later during fetal life. An obstacle to the venous return of the acardius could have caused the reversal of circulation.[5]

Acardii show various defects in addition to absence of the heart. The most highly developed type is the *hemiacardius* or *acardius anceps* who has a partly developed head, deformed face, trunk and extremities. This relatively "mild" form is rare. Holoacardii

Fig. 50-1. – Acardius acephalus. **A,** external appearance. **B,** sagittal section. **C,** roentgenogram of acardius.

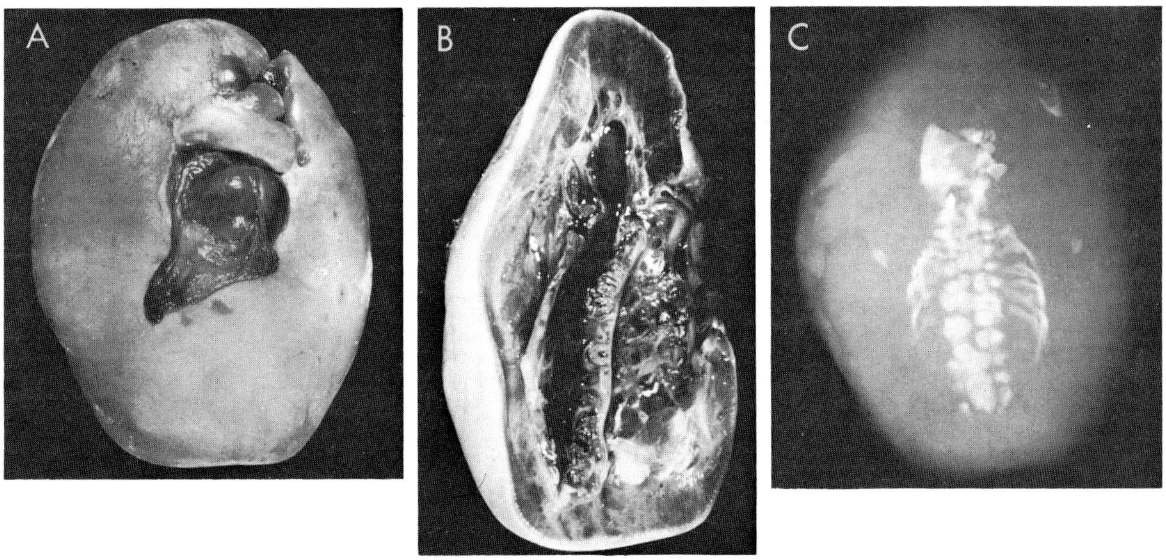

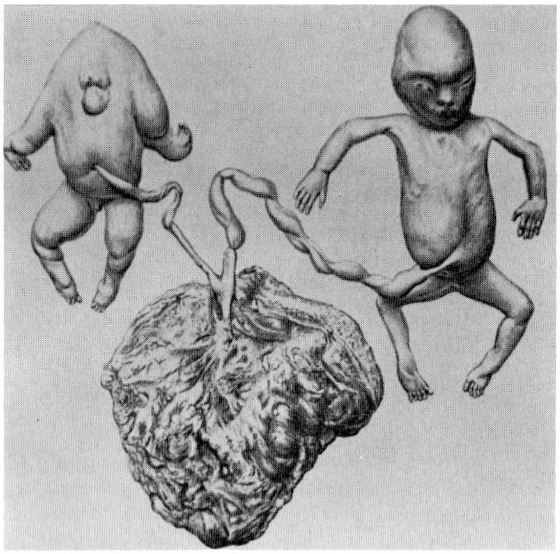

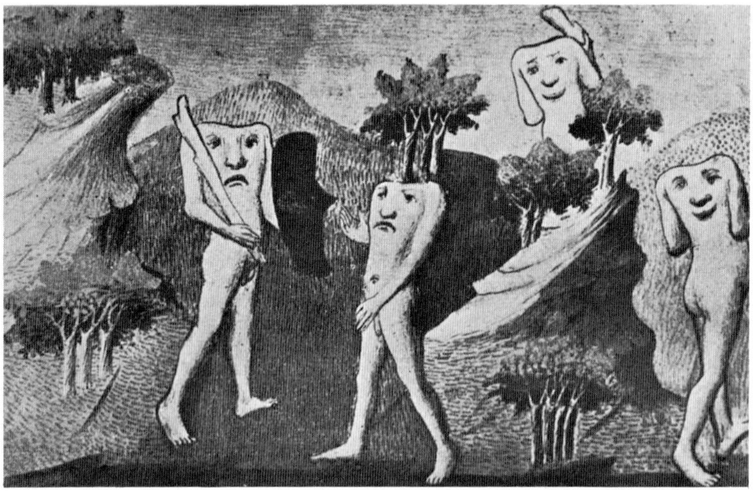

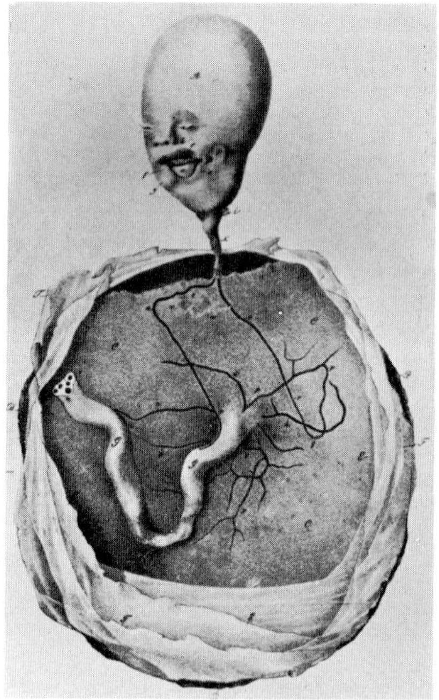

Fig. 50-2 (top). – Monochorionic, monoamniotic twins. Acardius acephalus on the left. Such acardii may have served as prototypes for imaginary headless men (Fig. 50-3). (From F. Schatz.[5])

Fig. 50-3 (bottom left). – Men without heads depicted in the *Livre de merveilles* (thirteenth century) are imaginary creatures that resemble, to a certain extent, the acardii acephali. (From E. Holländer, *Wunder, Wundergeburt und Wundergestalt* [Stuttgart: Ferdinand Enke, 1922].)

Fig. 50-4 (bottom right). – Acardius acormus. (From F. Schatz.[5])

occur more often; they vary greatly in regard to differentiation. The most common form is the *acardius acephalus*, of which more than 90 cases are on record. They are headless and lack thoracic organs but ribs or vertebrae may be present; upper extremities are either absent or defective. The abdominal organs are rudimentary and the genitalia sometimes are developed. Lower vertebrae, pelvis and lower extremities are clearly recognizable. These monstrous formations, which still show some resemblance to human beings, stimulated the imagination of observers in the past and served as prototypes for men of unexplored countries and of beings from outer space.

The *acardius acormus* is the oddest form. A head without a body is attached to the placenta by an umbilical cord that terminates in the cervical region. Some parts of the trunk or the extremities may be developed as rudimentary appendages. The *acardius amorphus* is a shapeless mass covered by skin and some hair and containing undifferentiated cartilage, bone, muscle and fibrous tissue. The mass is connected to the placenta by an umbilical cord that often is dark and edematous. Rudimentary organs sometimes are recognizable and transitional forms to acardius acephalus exist.[1,4]

REFERENCES

1. Napolitani, F. D., and Schreiber, I.: The acardiac monster; a review of the world literature and presentation of two cases, Am. J. Obst. & Gynec. 80:582, 1960.

2. Hempel: De monstris acephalis, Dissert. Hafniae, 1850. Cited by Schwalbe, E. (ed.), in *Die Morphologie der Missbildungen des Menschen und der Tiere* (Jena: Gustav Fischer, 1907), Vol. 2, chap. X.
3. Richart, R., and Benirschke, K.: Holoacardius amorphus. Report of a case with chromosome analysis, Am. J. Obst. & Gynec. 86:329, 1963.
4. Schwalbe, E.: Acardii und Verwandte. Die Doppelbildungen, Part II of *Die Morphologie der Missbildungen des Menschen und der Tiere* (Jena: Gustav Fischer, 1907).
5. Schatz, F.: Die Gefässverbindungen der Placentarkreisläufe eineiiger Zwillinge, ihre Entwickelung und ihre Folgen. *Die Acardii und ihre Verwandten* III. Gruppe. Arch. Gynäk. 58:1, 1899.

Ectopia Cordis

THE HEART can be displaced outward through a sternal fissure, upward into the neck or downward by a diaphragmatic hernia into the sac of an exomphalos. Accordingly, one speaks of thoracic, cervical or abdominal ectopia cordis. It is asserted that the first case report was by Haller (cited by Blatt and Zeldes[1]) in 1706, but it seems that the monstrous infant described by Stensen in 1671 (p. 495) (cited by Willius[2]) had not only tetralogy of Fallot but also a thoraco-omphalocele with ectopia cordis. In 1942, there appeared a review by Blatt and Zeldes,[1] who tabulated 52 cases from the literature, and in 1948 Byron[3] listed 142 cases of thoracic, abdominal and cervical ectopia. The most frequent type is the extrathoracic ectopia, which shows the heart outside the chest and protruding through a sternal fissure. Millhouse and Joos[4] found 45 cases of extrathoracic ectopias of the heart in the literature and added 5 cases by personal communication. Some of the cases involved stillbirths and many prematures. A pair of discordant twins was reported by Rolland.[5] Only rarely was the heart found to be normal. Ventricular septal defect was the most frequent associated cardiac anomaly. Left superior vena cava, aortic and pulmonary stenosis, transposition of the aorta, cor triloculare or biloculare, atrioventricularis communis, atrial septal defects, tetralogy, tricuspid atresia and other malformations have been described.[1,4,6] Associated malformations frequently are present, with harelip and cleft palate in the lead.[4]

Fig. 50-5.—Ectopia cordis (**arrow**) in a newborn rat produced by streptonigrin given to the mother on the tenth day of gestation. Note bilateral harelip and protrusion of intestinal loops through defect in the abdominal wall.

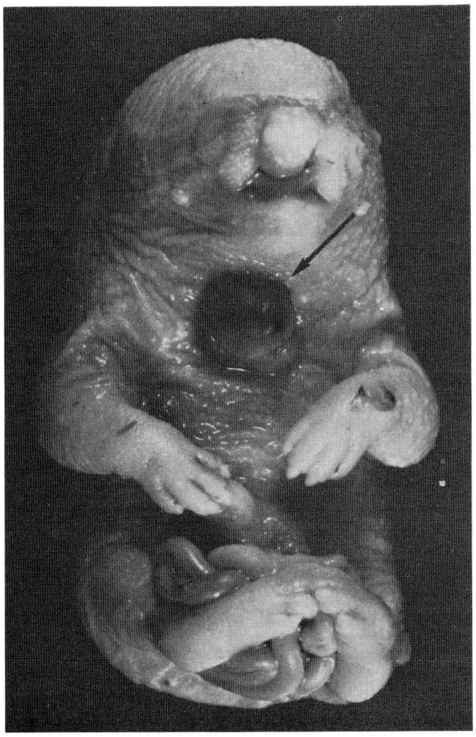

Life expectancy is limited for extrathoracic ectopia. Most of the premature babies die soon after birth and some of the term infants live only several days. However, if all types of ectopia cordis are included, the outlook is better. Blatt and Zeldes[1] found reports of 12 infants who survived the neonatal period. The best prognosis involves those with abdominal ectopia; these can survive for years and decades. Some women with this type underwent repeated pregnancies.[1]

Surgical correction of extrathoracic ectopia has been attempted repeatedly but no success has been reported. There is not sufficient space in the thorax, and embarrassment of the cardiac action follows manipulation as the great vessels assume altered angulation.[4]

According to Patten,[7] the defect of ectopia cordis must be established about the third week of development, when the demarcation between intra-embryonic and extra-embryonic coelom is perfected by the folding off of the body. This early termination period is of importance because, in some cases, attempted abortion has been reported[8] or suspected. In a case of incomplete ectopia cordis, the mother had ingested quinine in early pregnancy.[9]

Incomplete Ectopia Cordis

A syndrome of congenital defects involving the abdominal wall, sternum, diaphragm, pericardium and heart was described by Cantrell *et al.*[10] in 1958. The defect of the abdominal wall is in the midline and above the umbilicus. The lower portion of the sternum is defective and there are deficiencies of the anterior diaphragm and of the diaphragmatic pericardium, and congenital intracardiac anomalies. Such patients sometimes show a large omphalocele immediately after birth and the cardiac pulsations are

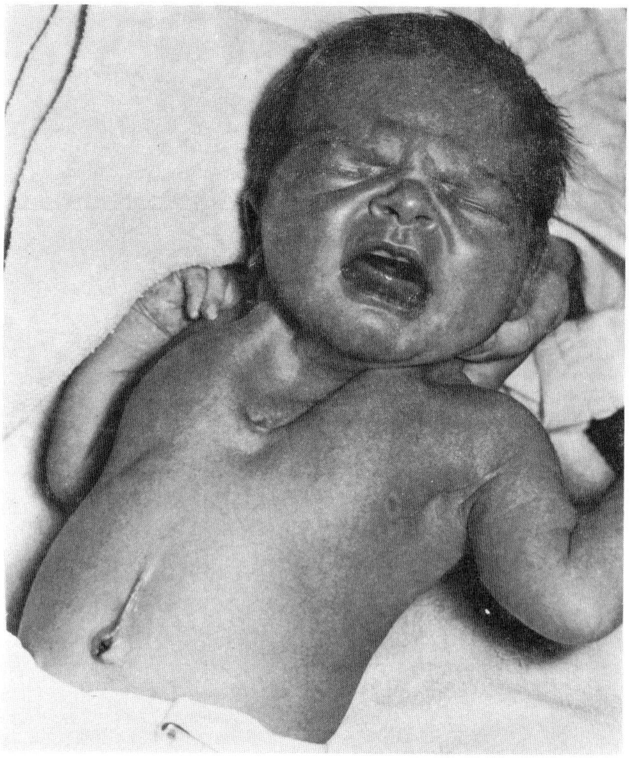

Fig. 50-6. – Incomplete ectopia cordis in an infant. There was a large sternal defect through which pulsations of the heart could be felt. The lower ribs joined in the midline in the area of the xiphoid process. Pericardium was found under the thinned cutis that bridged the defect. The child died at the age of 4 weeks. There was a large ventricular septal defect, patent ductus arteriosus and dextroposition of the aorta. The scar running upward from the umbilicus was a remnant of the abnormally attached umbilical cord. (Cincinnati Children's Hospital Chart No. 42209.)

prominent under the shortened sternum. The contour of the heart is visible beneath the skin of the unusually high epigastrium. The medial edges of the rectus muscles are widely separated and inserted on the costal margins at the midclavicular line. Such defects of the anterior body wall combined with diaphragmatic and pericardial defects apparently are always associated with ventricular septal defects and, in more than half the cases, with atrial septal defects. Pulmonary stenosis and tetralogy of Fallot are rarer. An interesting anomaly, a diverticulum extending subcutaneously from the apex of the left ventricle downward through the diaphragmatic defect, was observed in 3 patients with this body wall anomaly. Patent ductus arteriosus, anomalous venous return, tricuspid atresia or truncus arteriosus have also been associated in some instances.

Cantrell *et al.*[10] believed that this syndrome is caused by an alteration of the development of the mesoderm at a very early period in embryonic life. The deviations must occur prior to or immediately after the differentiation of the primitive intraembryonic mesoderm into its splanchnic and somatic layers, since derivatives of both these layers are involved. The termination period for this process is estimated to be at about 14–18 days of embryonic life. The etiologic factors leading to this anomaly are obscure. There were no disturbances during pregnancy that could account for the anomaly nor were there suggestions in the family histories that would indicate a hereditary origin. Related to the disease picture described by Cantrell *et al.*[10] is the syndrome of sternal and diaphragmatic defects combined with deficiency of the anterior abdominal wall and congenital heart disease reviewed by Crittenden *et al.*[9]

REFERENCES

1. Blatt, M. L., and Zeldes, M.: Ectopia cordis: Report of a case and review of the literature, Am. J. Dis. Child. 63: 515, 1942.
2. Willius, F. A.: An unusually early description of so-called tetralogy of Fallot, Proc. Staff Meet. Mayo Clin. 23:316, 1948. (Stensen, cited by Willius.)
3. Byron, F. X.: Ectopia cordis – case with attempted operative correction, J. Thoracic Surg. 7:717, 1948.
4. Millhouse, R. F., and Joos, H. A.: Extrathoracic ectopia cordis: Report of cases and review of literature, Am. Heart J. 57:470, 1959.
5. Rolland, W.: A case of ectopia cordia, Brit. M. J. 2:121, 1913.
6. Repciuc, E., Simionescu, N., and Cernaianou, G.: Ectopie cardiaque associée à des malformations multiples, Rev. roumaine embryol. & cytol. 2:101, 1965.
7. Patten, B. M.: *Human Embryology* (2d ed.; Philadelphia: Blakiston Company, 1953).
8. Lintgen, C.: Case of ectopia cordis, Am. J. Obst. & Gynec. 25:449, 1933.
9. Crittenden, I. H., Adams, F. H., and Mulder, D. G.: A syndrome featuring defects of the heart, sternum, diaphragm, and anterior abdominal wall, Circulation 20: 396, 1959.
10. Cantrell, J. R., Haller, J. A., and Ravitch, M. M.: A syndrome of congenital defects involving the abdominal wall, sternum, diaphragm, pericardium, and heart, Surgery 107:602, 1958.

Parchment Heart

PARTIAL ABSENCE of the right ventricular musculature as a congenital defect was reported by Gould *et al.*[1] in a patient who died at the age of 66 years of chronic myelogenous leukemia. At necropsy, a "parchment"-like right ventricle was found; 6 previously described cases were reviewed. In these cases, the walls of all the chambers were reduced in myocardial substance or the thinning was limited to the right ventricle. The anomaly has been observed in infancy.[2]

REFERENCES

1. Gould, L., Guttman, A. B., Carrasco, J., and Lyon, A. F.: Partial absence of the right ventricular musculature. A congenital lesion, Am. J. Med. 42:636, 1967.
2. Uhl, H. S. M.: A previously undescribed congenital malformation of the heart. Almost total absence of the myocardium of the right ventricle, Bull. Johns Hopkins Hosp. 91: 197, 1952.

51

Dextrocardia

IF THE HEART is found in the right hemithorax, one speaks of dextrocardia. Dextrocardia may follow disease or be the result of thoracic or abdominal malformations. In such cases, one speaks of secondary dextrocardia, a condition that will not be considered here. Primary dextrocardia is a developmental disorder that either is associated with complete situs inversus or occurs as an isolated anomaly. In itself, dextrocardia may be a harmless congenital malformation compatible with a long life. It is the associated cardiac or extracardiac anomalies that make it a pathologic disorder.

Aristotle had observed dextrocardia in animals, and the first description of dextrocardia in man was given by Fabricius in 1600.[1] It is said that Marie de Medici, the wife of Henry IV of France, had dextrocardia with situs inversus.[2] This, in itself, is not of great interest but may be a fact of some value to genealogists interested in the background of this lady, since dextrocardia often has been found in the offspring of consanguineous matings.

There is general agreement that isolated dextrocardia is more often combined with severe forms of congenital heart disease than dextrocardia with complete situs inversus, in which the heart, the great vessels and other thoraco-abdominal organs may present a mirror image of the normal. Such hearts, if not associated with cardiac or vascular anomalies, can function perfectly normally. In isolated dextrocardia, however, afferent and efferent vessels must somehow connect with the normally situated organs of the chest and abdomen and it is understandable that anomalous connections can easily come about.

Dextrocardia with situs inversus and dextrocardia as an isolated anomaly are etiologically and pathologically different entities and will, therefore, be discussed separately. Van Praagh *et al.*[3] distinguished 8 anatomic types of congenital dextrocardia, creating subgroups of situs solitus, situs inversus and asplenia. No doubt many other classifications are possible according to associated defects. A classification illustrated by roentgenographic and angiographic data was offered by Ellis *et al.*[24] Experimental work[4] has shown how closely related dextrocardia, transposition of the great vessels, tricuspid atresia and mitral atresia are, and how a well-defined teratogenic procedure can bring about a variety of combinations that fail to follow existing classifications.

DEXTROCARDIA WITH SITUS INVERSUS TOTALIS OR PARTIALIS.—All persons with total situs inversus have dextrocardia. The prevalence of dextrocardia with situs inversus is approximately 1:10,000 in an adult population,[5] but it probably is higher in a newborn population since, even in this group, some individuals are born with severe congenital defects and may die in infancy. It is estimated that not more than 3%[6] to 9%[7] of persons with dextrocardia and situs inversus are affected by congenital heart disease. In the series of Lowe and McKeown,[8] only 1 of 20 propositi with situs inversus had a defective ventricular septum and a patent foramen ovale.

Of 51 patients with dextrocardia, one-third were classified as mirror image cases by Van Praagh and Vlad.[9]

A great deal of thought has been given to the etiology of situs inversus and thus indirectly to dextrocardia associated with it. It seems that a few families are on record who show transmission of situs inversus through more than one generation. Doolittle[10] reported a man, himself a (dizygotic) twin, who had a pair of dizygotic twins, a boy and a girl. The father had dextrocardia and the son had transposition of the viscera. Gänsslen *et al.*[11] stated in 1940 that situs inversus occurring in more than one generation had been reported in four families. In a family described by Lancisi, situs inversus is said to have occurred in four generations.[11] This would indicate that in rare instances situs inversus and dextrocardia can be transmitted like a dominant trait. More often, situs inversus is inherited as a recessive trait. Occurrence in sibships has been observed repeatedly. There are ten sibships on record in which 3 members were affected and twenty-eight with 2 affected.[6,8,12] In siblings of propositi with situs inversus, the same anomaly was reported in 1 in 20[7] or 1 in 50[8] or 1 in 90.[5] In addition, there can be no doubt that cousin marriages are relatively frequent among the parents of patients with situs inversus.[5,7,8] Cockayne[7] came to the conclusion that situs inversus is a genetically determined anomaly and that homozygosity for a simple recessive gene is responsible for it. But the incidence of the anomaly in siblings found by other investigators and quoted above is not compatible with an explanation of simple recessive inheritance. Torgersen[5] and Lowe and McKeown[8] are of the opinion that situs inversus is genetically determined but they recognize that a complicated genetic mechanism must be at work. Dextrocardia and dextroposition have been observed in trisomy 13-15 and in trisomy 18.[13]

It seems that 12 pairs of monozygotic twins have been reported, 6 of which were concordant in regard to situs inversus and 6 discordant. In addition, 3 dizygotic pairs of twins 1 of which was concordant were reported. Although such twin data are not easily interpreted, it seems that the existence of so many monozygotic twins discordant for situs inversus points definitely to the possibility that the anomaly is not genetically determined in all cases, or that nongenetic factors play an important role in its expression. Gänsslen[11] stated that 2 cases of conjoined twins discordant in regard to dextrocardia have been observed.

Many authors have expressed the opinion that a high incidence of twinning exists in families in which dextrocardia has been observed.[10] Torgersen,[5] who made an extensive study of situs inversus and twinning in Norway, did not believe that this is true, since he found that among 100 selected cases of situs inversus and their siblings and parents, neither twinning nor left-handedness was observed with greater frequency than that to be expected by chance. Despite such statistical findings, it is possible that in certain cases of situs inversus and dextrocardia, twinning is of decisive importance. One should not assume that dextrocardia and situs inversus have a unitary etiology. Although genetic determination can be assumed to be proved for some cases, one should consider the possibility that environmental factors may result in similar disorders in others. This is suggested by monozygotic twins discordant in regard to situs inversus as mentioned before and also by experimental work. It has long been shown that dextrocardia can be produced experimentally in chicks[14] and in amphibia.[15] In recent years, situs inversus has been produced experimentally in mammals also. Wilson obtained situs inversus by x-irradiation on the ninth day of gestation in the rat,[16] and situs inversus totalis can be produced occasionally by trypan blue injections (see Figs. 21-2 and 21-3). Monie *et al.*[4] produced dextrocardia together with the transposition complex in rats by trypan blue injections. In this embryologic study, dextrocardia was combined with a variety of anomalies such as tricuspid or mitral atresia, transposition of the great vessels, inversion of the ventricles, left or double aorta and total or partial situs inversus.

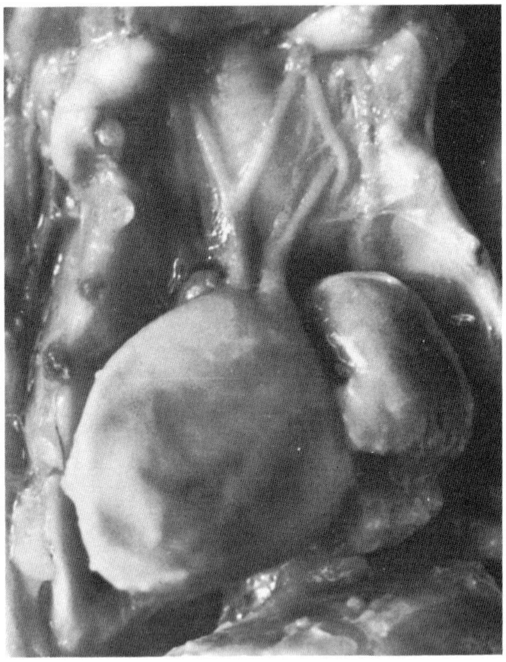

Fig. 51-1.—Dextrocardia and auricular shift in a newborn rat produced by trypan blue treatment on the eighth day of gestation. There is no spiraling of great vessels.

PATHOLOGY.—As a rule, situs inversus totalis is

combined with uncomplicated mirror-image dextrocardia. In such cases, the venae cavae are found on the left entering the pulmonic atrium on the left. Venous blood thus reaches the pulmonic ventricle, also located on the left, leaving through the pulmonary artery. The pulmonary veins return oxygenated blood to a systemic atrium located on the right and this blood reaches the aorta through a systemic ventricle located on the right. Such a situation is not pathologic, and affected persons may go through life without any difficulties derived from the anomaly. In less than 10% of the cases,[5,7] dextrocardia combined with situs inversus is complicated by congenital anomalies of the heart. Keith *et al.*[1] analyzed the cardiac anomalies of 20 anatomically proved cases of complicated dextrocardia with situs inversus. Approximately one-fifth of these cases were combined with noncyanotic anomalies such as ventricular septal defect, atrial septal defect or partial anomaly of the pulmonary veins. Among the cyanotic anomalies, which accounted for four-fifths of the cases, single ventricle, common atrium, transposition of the great vessels, truncus arteriosus, atrioventricularis communis and total anomalous venous return were recorded but there was no tetralogy of Fallot.

Among patients with situs inversus and dextrocardia, noncardiac abnormalities also are common. The Kartagener syndrome, consisting of situs inversus, bronchiectasis and paranasal sinusitis, is a well-known combination (p. 602). Other anomalies reported were duodenal and other intestinal atresias, common mesentery, agenesis of the spleen, multiple spleens, thyroglossal cyst, congenital absence of the left breast, spina bifida[1,8,17] and anomalies of the spine and the mandible.[6]

Mirror-image dextrocardia may remain completely asymptomatic throughout life. Only the position of the apical thrust and the intensity of the heart sounds on the right side betray the anomaly. X-ray films show the heart in the right hemithorax and demonstrate the situs inversus by gastrointestinal examination, which reveals that not only is the stomach on the right side but that the ileocecal region is abnormally located. The prognosis is less favorable in those patients who have associated malformations. Bronchiectasis may cause protracted illness, and the congenital cardiac defects mentioned above can interfere with health according to the abnormal anatomy and physiology of the specific malformation. The treatment depends entirely on the complications of the dextrocardia.

Isolated dextrocardia.—This condition is much more rare than dextrocardia combined with situs inversus. It is estimated that 1 case occurs in 30,000 live births[8] and 1 in 900,000 adults.[5] The difference between the incidence in live births and adults reflects the high mortality resulting from this anomaly. It is not surprising that in necropsied cases isolated dextrocardia accounted for 51% and proved to be the most common type of dextrocardia.[3]

There is general agreement that congenital heart disease is very frequent in isolated dextrocardia, estimates varying between 70% and 98%.[1,8,18] Little is known about the etiology and pathogenesis of this disorder. Lowe and McKeown[8] found neither familial incidence nor parental consanguinity in their cases. Ostertag and Spaich[19] reported monozygotic twins discordant in regard to isolated dextrocardia, which indicates that the anomaly may be, in some cases, of nongenetic origin. Some authors believed that isolated dextrocardia may show normal or mirror-image arrangement of the chambers,[8] but Keith *et al.*[1] doubted that isolated dextrocardia with inversion of the chambers exists and suggested that some of the cases reported as such were associated with partial situs inversus.

Isolated dextrocardia without chamber inversion is combined with congenital heart disease in most instances, although rare cases have been reported with normal cardiac function. Keith *et al.*[1] analyzed the cases anatomically proved and found that 85% were cyanotic. Transposition of the great vessels was present in approximately 70% of the cases. Tricuspid atresia or stenosis, right ventricular hypoplasia, single ventricle, pulmonary stenosis, tetralogy of Fallot and atrioventricularis communis were observed in this group. Among the noncyanotic complications were ventricular septal defect, corrected transposition, stenosis and coarctation of the aorta.[20]

Noncardiac associated malformations were agenesis of the spleen, tracheo-esophageal fistula, pulmonary hypoplasia, imperforate anus, polydactyly,[8] spina bifida,[18] pelvic kidney, hydrocephaly, horseshoe kidney, absence of the radius, craniostenosis[1] and hemivertebrae.[9] The prognosis is poor and most patients die of their serious cardiac complications within the first year. Lowe and McKeown[8] found that some of their patients considered as isolated dextrocardias survived to adolescence. An exceptional patient may survive to adulthood despite pulmonary stenosis, functionally single ventricle and transposition of the great vessels.[21]

The treatment depends on the cardiac malformation and associated anomalies. Repair of ventricular septal defect, atrial septal defect and tetralogy of Fallot in patients with mirror-image dextrocardia has been reported.[22]

Levocardia with situs inversus.—In 1958, Keith *et al.*[1] discussed this condition in detail, but in 1966 they[23] abandoned their concept as a definite entity and pointed out that most of these cases belong to the asplenia or polysplenia syndrome (Chapter 80).

REFERENCES

1. Keith, J. D., Rowe, R. D., and Vlad, P. (eds.): *Heart Disease in Infancy and Childhood* (New York: The Macmillan Company, 1958).
2. Ballantyne, J. W.: *Manual of Antenatal Pathology and Hygiene* (Chicago: Chicago Medical Book Company, 1904).
3. Van Praagh, R., Van Praagh, S., Vlad, P., and Keith, J. D.: Anatomic types of congenital dextrocardia. Diagnostic

and embryologic implications, Am. J. Cardiol. 13:510, 1964.
4. Monie, I. W., Takacs, E., and Warkany, J.: Transposition of the great vessels and other cardiovascular abnormalities induced by trypan blue, Anat. Rec. 156:175, 1966.
5. Torgersen, J.: Situs inversus, asymmetry and twinning, Am. J. Human Genet. 2:361, 1950.
6. Torgersen, J.: Genic factors in asymmetry and in the development and pathological changes of lungs, heart and abdominal organs, Arch. Path. 47:566, 1949.
7. Cockayne, E. A.: The genetics of transposition of the viscera, Quart. J. Med. 7:479, 1938.
8. Lowe, C. R., and McKeown, T.: An investigation of dextrocardia, Ann. Eugenics 18:267, 1954.
9. Van Praagh, R., and Vlad, P.: Dextrocardia, Mesocardia, and Levocardia, in Keith, J. D., Rowe, R. D., and Vlad, P. (eds.), *Heart Disease in Infancy and Childhood* (2d ed.; New York: The Macmillan Company, 1966).
10. Doolittle, W. F.: Congenital dextrocardia, Boston, M. & S. J. 157:662, 1907.
11. Gänsslen, M., Lambrecht, K., and Werner, M.: Die kongenitalen Missbildungen des Herzens, *Handbuch der Erbiologie des Menschen* (Berlin: Springer, 1940).
12. Leininger, C. R., and Gibson, S.: Transposition of viscera in siblings, J. Pediat. 37:195, 1950.
13. Warkany, J., Passarge, E., and Smith, L. B.: Congenital malformations in autosomal trisomy syndromes, Am. J. Dis. Child. 112:502, 1966.
14. Dareste, C.: *Recherches sur La Production Artificielle des Monstruosités ou Essais de Tétratogénie Expérimentale* (2d ed.; Paris: C. Reinwald et Cie, 1891).
15. Pressler, K.: Beobachtungen und Versuche über den normalen und inversen Situs viscerum et cordis bei Anurenlarven, Arch. Entwicklungsmechanik d. Organ. 22:1, 1911.
16. Wilson, J. G., Jordan, H. C., and Brent, R. L.: Effects of irradiation on embryonic development. II. X-rays on the ninth day of gestation, Am. J. Anat. 92:153, 1953.
17. Moller, J. H., Nakib, A., Anderson, R. C., and Edwards, J. E.: Congenital cardiac disease associated with polysplenia, a developmental complex of bilateral "left-sideness," Circulation 36:789, 1967.
18. Lichtman, S. S.: Isolated congenital dextrocardia. Report of 2 cases with unusual findings, Arch. Int. Med. 48:683, 1931.
19. Ostertag, M., and Spaich, D.: Diskordantes Auftreten einer isolierten Dextrokardie bei einem eineigen Zwillingspaar, Ztschr. menschl. Vererb.-u. Konstitutionslehre 19: 577, 1935.
20. Gilbert, E. F., Nishimura, K., and Wedum, B. G.: Congenital malformations of the heart associated with splenic agenesis, Circulation 17:72, 1958.
21. Fisher, J., and Suh, S. K.: Dextrocardia with pulmonary stenosis and functionally single right ventricle, Circulation 17:266, 1958.
22. Cooley, D. A., and Billig, D. M.: Surgical repair of congenital cardiac lesions in mirror-image dextrocardia with situs inversus totalis, Am. J. Cardiol. 11:518, 1963.
23. Keith, J. D., Rowe, R. D., and Vlad, P. (eds.): *Heart Disease in Infancy and Childhood* (2d ed.; New York: The Macmillan Company, 1966).
24. Ellis, K., Fleming, F. J., Griffiths, S. P., and Jameson, A. G.: New concepts in dextrocardia. Angiocardiographic considerations, Am. J. Roentgenol. 97:295, 1966.

52

Atrial Septal Defects

COMMUNICATIONS between the atria can assume quite different forms, from a small patent foramen ovale to complete absence of the interatrial septum. Such communications may be combined with a variety of other cardiac anomalies, and it is clear that general statements about etiology, incidence or clinical data are difficult to make and that marked differences exist in the opinions of various authors in regard to some of the basic facts.

INCIDENCE.—Atrial septal defect (ASD) was diagnosed once in 6,000 children examined in a prospective study[1] and occurrence among a general children's population was estimated at 1 in 13,500.[2] Prevalence figures vary according to age of the group examined. Atrial septal defect accounts for approximately 17% of the total population with congenital heart disease,[3] but in children's series it is less conspicuous, being fourth in frequency and making up 7% of the total. The relatively low prevalence of ASD in children is due to frequency of other forms of congenital heart disease that are eliminated by death in infancy or early childhood. Atrial septal defect, which may be well tolerated into adult life, thus emerges as an important lesion in older age groups. It has been estimated that in approximately half the cases ASD remains undetected before the age of 18 years.

Among newborn children who die of congenital heart disease, ASD seldom is seen as an isolated lesion. Disenhouse *et al.*,[4] reviewing 202 necropsied cases of congenital heart disease in children, found only 6 in which ASD was considered the cause of death. In Abbott's[5] series, ASD amounted to 3.3% and patent foramen ovale to 4% of necropsied cases.

The subgroups in a children's population with ASD were estimated to be 68% ostium secundum, 12% ostium primum and 20% atrioventricularis communis defects.[2]

Etiology.—Genetic determination of some cases of ASD can be accepted as proved. Familial occurrence has been known for some time. It has been observed in three generations by Campbell.[6] Zetterquist[7] recorded a pedigree in which four generations contained 8 certain and 5 probable cases of ASD and listed other reports of repetition of the defect in more than one generation. Lamy *et al.*[8] had 2 patients with this anomaly who had siblings with congenital heart disease. One of the siblings had an open foramen ovale and another had tetralogy of Fallot. These authors observed a high consanguinity rate in the parents of patients with ASD but they believed that nongenetic factors also may be at work relatively often in the etiology. Campbell and Polani[9] investigated the families of 170 patients with ASD. Sixteen per cent of these had other cardiac malformations that, however, were of minor importance. Congenital heart disease, most often ASD, was found more often in siblings and their parents than would be expected by chance. The parents of patients were first cousins more often than could be expected (1.9%), which suggests that some of the cases were due to recessive Mendelian inheritance; but in other families dominant inheritance with incomplete penetrance seemed to be responsible. In such cases, ASD may be combined with pulmonary stenosis.[10] Dominant transmission is now well established for patients with ASD and associated skeletal anomalies.

Holt and Oram[11] described a kindred in which ASD was transmitted through four generations. Affected members also had abnormal thumbs. But the Holt-Oram syndrome is not limited to ASD and the skeletal defects are not limited to abnormal thumbs, so that the name "upper limb-cardiovascular syndrome" has been suggested (p. 461). Another dominantly inherited trait, Marfan syndrome, occasionally is combined with ASD (p. 850). Nora *et al.*[12] found pedigrees with hereditary ASD that could be interpreted as dominant and others that seemed to indicate recessive inheritance. They concluded that multifactorial inheritance was the best explanation consistent with available observations and thought that environmental hazards played an important role in the production of ASD, an opinion also expressed by Campbell and Polani.[9] Forsyth and Uchida[13] studied a pair of identical twins, of whom only 1 was affected by ASD.

It is now well known that ASD can occur in autosomal trisomy syndromes.[33] It was mentioned in 25% of necropsy reports involving trisomy 13-15 and in 10% of trisomy 18 cases. Atrial septal defects are particularly prominent in trisomy 21 (Down syndrome); they were encountered in 41% of necropsied cases. ASD was noted in 22%, atrioventricularis communis in 10% and ostium primum defect in 9% of the necropsies. Considering that only 52% of the necropsy cases had congenital heart disease, the various septal defects were found in 77% of the cases of Down syndrome with congenital heart disease.

A few cases of ASD following early maternal rubella have been reported.[14,15] Dogramaci and Green[16] found a probable ASD in a child whose mother had had poliomyelitis during the second month of pregnancy, but they recommended caution in claiming a causal relationship. ASD occurred as a rare complication in the thalidomide embryopathy (Chapter 11).

It is estimated that slightly over 60% of the patients are female.[2,9]

Congenital ASD can be produced experimentally in the young of rats injected with trypan blue 7 or 8 days after conception. Defects of septum primum, septum secundum and auricular displacement have been reported in the young examined.[17]

There are various types of atrial septal defects that usually are classified as patent foramen ovale, ostium secundum, ostium primum, ostium atrioventricularis communis, cor triloculare biventriculare and cor biloculare.

Foramen ovale. Although the function of the foramen ovale terminates at the time of birth, anatomic closure usually is not achieved until several months after birth.[18] Probe-patency of the foramen ovale persists in approximately 25% of all persons and is not

Fig. 52-1.—Foramen ovale with fenestrae.

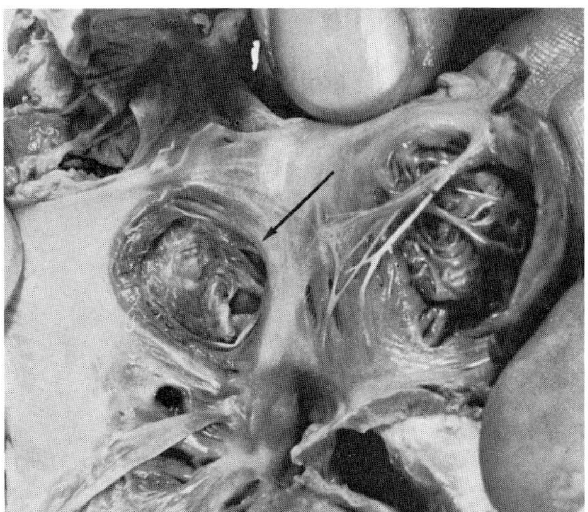

considered an anomaly, since all the atrial structures can be normal even though the opening is not sealed. If the pressure in the left atrium is larger than in the right, the valve of the foramen remains closed; there are no shunts and circulation is normal. If, however, for any reason the pressure on the right side becomes larger than that on the left, the foramen ovale can be functionally opened. As a rule, the right-to-left shunt does not suffice to cause cyanosis, but the defect of the septum may manifest itself by paradoxic emboli.

Ostium secundum is a defect in the area of the foramen ovale, ostium primum a defect in the lowest portion of the septum, located near the atrioventricular valves. In Figure 52-2, the formation of the interatrial septum is presented diagrammatically as seen from the right atrium. In Figure 52-2, *A*, a stage is illustrated that corresponds approximately to the sixth embryonic week. The sickle-shaped septum primum is developed, but there is still in its lower portion a communication between the right and the left auricle – the foramen or ostium primum. Figure 52-2, *B* shows the septum reaching the atrioventricular canal at the beginning of the seventh week. At this time, a new opening is being formed between the two auricles – the foramen secundum. This communication is narrowed by another sickle-shaped septum that descends like a curtain over the septum primum and the foramen secundum, partially covering these structures on the right side (Fig. 52-2, *C*). The two septa fuse in the lower portion of the atrium with each other and with the endothelial cushion masses of the atrioventricular canal. In the normal heart, the foramen primum disappears. The foramen secundum persists during fetal life, guarded on the left by the valve of the foramen ovale, which is derived from the septum primum.

An opening in the area of the foramen ovale representing an interatrial communication larger than 2 or 3 millimeters in diameter is classified as an ostium secundum. This anomaly is the most frequent pathologic communication between the atria. It is estimated that almost 70% of the ASD belong in this subgroup.[19] Such openings, however, may be of differing origin embryologically. The foramen secundum may be larger than normal so that the valve of the foramen ovale is not sufficient to cover the opening; or the remnant of the septum primum may be markedly reduced by overresorption, thus forming an incompetent valve flap (Fig. 52-3, *A*). Instead of a single opening in the septum primum, several fenestrations may be formed (Fig. 52-3, *B*), producing a defective valve. Another defect may originate by insufficient development of the septum secundum, resulting in a defect of the cranial portion of the septum (Fig. 52-3,*C*).[20] Sometimes the interatrial defect is even higher and near the entrance of the superior vena cava. In such cases, abnormal pulmonary veins may enter the right atrium. Finally, there may be combinations of the defects described. In children, the openings created by these deficiencies vary in size and range from about 2 millimeters to 2 centimeters. When the opening becomes 2 × 2 cm. or larger, one considers the result a common atrium. In adults, the communications may be larger. With ostium secundum, the heart is enlarged, the right atrium and the great veins are distended and the right ventricular chamber usually is more spacious than the hypoplastic left. The pulmonary artery is larger than the aorta and may become huge in case of added mitral stenosis.

As a rule, the pressure is higher in the left atrium than in the right and some oxygenated blood enters the right atrium, from where it reaches the lungs. The deficiency of blood in the left heart leads to reduction in size of the left ventricle and the aorta. If the right ventricle becomes overburdened, heart failure may ensue. If there is stenosis of the pulmonary artery, a right-to-left shunt occurs. Stenosis of the mitral valve (Lutembacher syndrome) enhances the left-to-right shunt.

Ostium secundum is a congenital defect that usually goes undetected in early life. Occasionally, a systolic murmur or arrhythmia may betray the defect and, in rare instances, such an ASD can cause early cardiac failure and death in infancy. Transitory cyanosis, feeding difficulties, recurrent respiratory infections and retardation of growth are the principal symptoms. There are no pathognomonic cardiac signs.[4] Many cases are discovered in schoolchildren when the symptoms become more pronounced. Such children usually are of normal height but some are thin and underweight; they may show a bulge of the left chest over the cardiac area and scoliosis. Their exercise tolerance usually is good but they have a tendency to respiratory infections. In former years, rheumatic fever frequently was a complicating factor. Cyanosis usually is absent in children except for short periods during illness or in heart failure. Adults more than 20 years of age may develop "cyanosis tardive,"

Fig. 52-2. – Diagrams showing closure of atrial septum. Septum primum (black), foramen primum (F_1) and foramen secundum (F_2). The septum secundum (S_2) is seen in **C**.

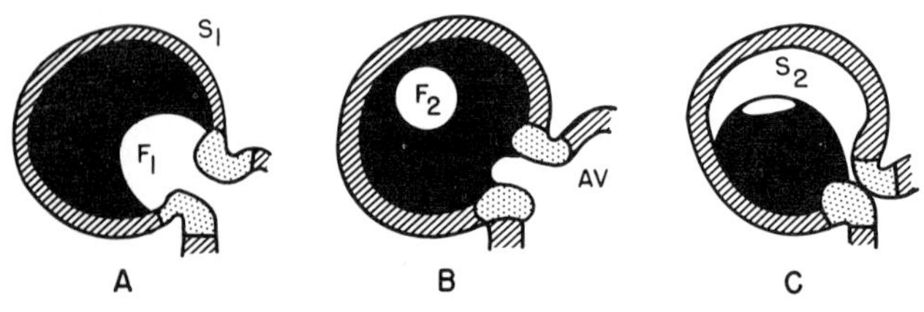

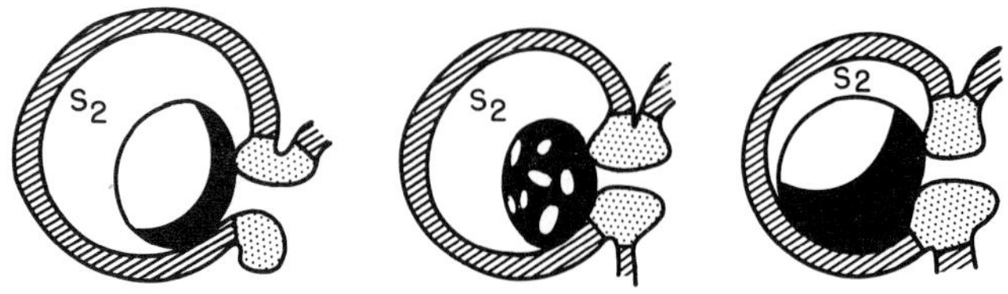

Fig. 52-3.—Diagrams showing defects of atrial septum. (See text, p. 482.)

the oxygen unsaturation increasing with increasing age.[21] There is no clubbing. The heart beat usually is forceful and a systolic murmur is heard in the first and second interspace on the left sternal border. With a large defect there may also be a mid-diastolic murmur. In roentgenograms, the heart is moderately enlarged, chiefly by expansion of the right atrium and right ventricle. The pulmonary artery and its branches are also prominent and there are large pulsating hilar shadows. Rheumatic fever, cardiac arrhythmias, respiratory infections and pulmonary hypertension and pulmonary artery thrombosis are complications.[22]

Death is uncommon in infancy unless infections endanger the child's life. The outlook for older children is good and longevity is the rule. In 1934, Roesler[23] estimated the average life expectancy at 36 years but now it has risen to about 50 years.[24] A number of persons with interatrial defects have reached old age.[22] The prognosis is less favorable if ASD is combined with other cardiac lesions or if pulmonary vascular disease develops.[25] Death, if caused by the cardiac defect, is attributable to heart failure in most, to emboli or to thromboses in rare cases. Pregnancy usually is well tolerated by patients with ASD,[23,26,27] and some women have undergone repeated pregnancies without serious difficulty. Repair of an ASD during pregnancy has been reported.[28]

Ostium primum is rare as an isolated defect, but combined with cleft mitral valve it accounts for 10% of the ASD group.[2] The opening is low in the atrial septum just above the atrioventricular valve tissue. A separate tricuspid and mitral valve can be recognized but, as stated before, the aortic leaf of the mitral valve often is cleft. Such cases should be distinguished from atrioventricularis communis but the differentiation sometimes is difficult because both conditions have a low atrial septal defect.[29] The separation of the atrioventricular valves may be imperfect, particularly in cases that are combined with ventricular and tricuspid anomalies. In ostium primum, the foramen ovale may be normal, or an additional high septal defect may be present. The valvar anomalies mentioned change the clinical picture and are responsible for the severity of symptoms. If the valves are not involved, the clinical findings are like those of ostium secundum defects, although, as a rule, the course is more serious. Affected children have normal birth weights but they fail to thrive, remain thin and underweight and have a tendency to respiratory infection, dyspnea and fatigability. The precordial bulge to the left of the sternum is pronounced and a systolic murmur can be heard at the apex and along the left sternal border. Usually a diastolic murmur and a split second heart sound are present.

Roentgenograms show an enlarged heart with raised apex, bulging pulmonary artery and pulsating prominent hilar shadows. In addition to the increased size of the right ventricle there may also be hypertrophy of the left. In general, the prognosis of ostium primum is not as good as that of ostium secundum.

Associated malformations.—Many cardiac anomalies can be combined with atrial septal defects. Some of the combinations result in cyanotic and others in noncyanotic congenital heart disease. ASD

Fig. 52-4.—Ostium primum (**single arrow**) and secundum (**double arrow**) defects.

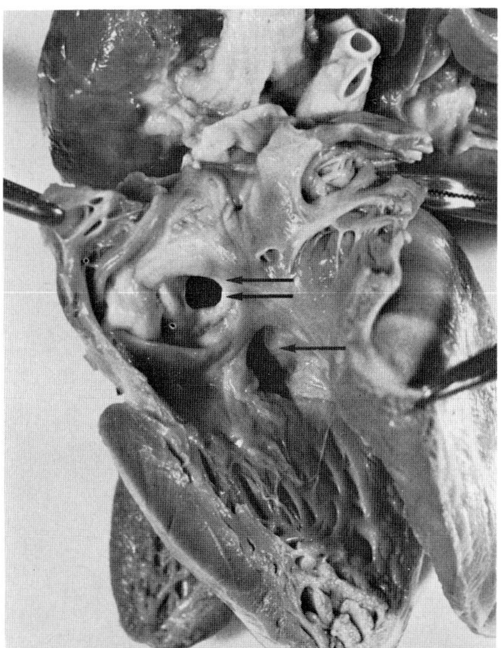

with open ductus arteriosus, coarctation of the aorta, ventricular septal defect or mitral valve anomalies usually remain noncyanotic. Tricuspid atresia, common ventricle, tetralogy of Fallot, pulmonary stenosis or atresia, or transposition of the great vessels leads to cyanotic congenital heart disease.[2] It is estimated that 15–20% of patients with atrial defect have some abnormal pulmonary veins terminating in the right atrium.[30] Extracardiac malformations were found by Lamy *et al.*[8] in more than 25% of the cases. Of 97 patients, 5 (5.1%) were mongoloids. Large atrial defects were present in 40% of mongoloid children dying of heart disease in early life.[31,32] Scoliosis, chest deformities, skeletal malformations of the extremities and spina bifida may also accompany atrial defects. Patent foramen ovale and large ASD occasionally have occurred in children with Marfan syndrome (p. 853). Atrial septal defects are quite common in the asplenia and polysplenia (Chapter 80) syndromes.

TREATMENT.—If there is a significant left-to-right shunt in an ostium secundum defect, surgical repair usually is recommended, since the mortality is low in operations of this kind. Dalen *et al.*[25] suggested that because of danger of pulmonary vascular disease, all atrial septal defects without pulmonary vascular disease should be corrected surgically. Direct-vision, open heart surgery utilizing cardiopulmonary bypass apparently is the method of choice. With ostium primum defect, the mitral and tricuspid clefts are repaired before the ASD is closed by a prosthesis.

REFERENCES

1. Richards, M. R., Merritt, K. K., Samuels, M. H., and Langman, A. G.: Congenital malformations of the cardiovascular system in a series of 6,053 infants, Pediatrics 15:12, 1955.
2. Keith, J. D., Rowe, R. D., and Vlad, P. (eds.): *Heart Disease in Infancy and Childhood* (2d ed.; New York: The Macmillan Company, 1966).
3. Wood, P., Magidson, O., and Wilson, P. A. O.: Ventricular septal defect with note on acyanotic Fallot's tetralogy, Brit. Heart J. 16:387, 1954.
4. Disenhouse, R. B., Anderson, R. C., Adams, P., Jr., Novick, R., Jorgens, J., and Levin, B.: Atrial septal defect in infants and children, J. Pediat. 44:269, 1954.
5. Abbott, M. E.: *Atlas of Congenital Heart Disease* (New York: American Heart Association, 1936).
6. Campbell, M.: Genetic and environmental factors in congenital heart disease, Quart. J. Med. 18:379, 1949.
7. Zetterquist, P.: Multiple occurrence of atrial septal defect in a family, Acta paediat. scandinav. 49:741, 1960.
8. Lamy, M., De Grouchy, J., and Schweisguth, O.: Genetic and non-genetic factors in the etiology of congenital heart disease: A study of 1188 cases, Am. J. Human Genet. 9:17, 1957.
9. Campbell, M., and Polani, P. E.: Factors in the aetiology of atrial septal defect, Brit. Heart J. 23:477, 1961.
10. Weil, M. H., and Allenstein, B. J.: A report of congenital heart disease in five members of one family, New England J. Med. 265:661, 1961.
11. Holt, M., and Oram, S.: Familial heart disease with skeletal malformations, Brit. Heart J. 22:236, 1960.
12. Nora, J. J., McNamara, D. G., and Fraser, F. C.: Hereditary factors in atrial septal defect, Circulation 35:448, 1967.
13. Forsyth, C., and Uchida, I.: Auricular septal defect in one of monozygotic twins, Arch. Dis. Childhood 26:582, 1951.
14. Stuckey, D.: Congenital heart defects following maternal rubella during pregnancy, Brit. Heart J. 18:519, 1956.
15. Gibson, S., and Lewis, K. C.: Congenital heart disease following maternal rubella during pregnancy, A.M.A. Am. J. Dis. Child. 83:317, 1952.
16. Dogramaci, I., and Green, H.: Factors in etiology of congenital heart anomalies, J. Pediat. 30:295, 1947.
17. Fox, M. H., and Goss, C. M.: Experimentally produced malformations of the heart and great vessels in rat fetuses; atrial and caval abnormalities, Anat. Rec. 129:309, 1957.
18. Christie, A.: Normal closing time of the foramen ovale and the ductus arteriosus, Am. J. Dis. Child. 40:323, 1930.
19. Keith, J. D., Rowe, R. D., and Vlad, P. (eds): *Heart Disease in Infancy and Childhood* (New York: The Macmillan Company, 1958).
20. Patten, B. M.: Developmental defects at the foramen ovale, Am. J. Path. 14:135, 1938.
21. Dexter, L.: Atrial septal defects, Brit. Heart J. 18:209, 1956.
22. Kelly, J. J., Jr., and Lyons, H. A.: Atrial septal defect in the aged, Ann. Int. Med. 48:267, 1958.
23. Roesler, H.: Interatrial septal defect, Arch. Int. Med. 54:339, 1934.
24. Cosby, R. S., and Griffith, G. C.: Interatrial septal defect, Am. Heart J. 38:80, 1949.
25. Dalen, J. E., Haynes, F. W., and Dexter, L.: Life expectancy with atrial septal defect, J.A.M.A. 200:442, 1967.
26. Lund, C. J.: Maternal congenital heart disease as obstetric problem, Am. J. Obst. & Gynec. 55:244, 1948.
27. Burwell, C. S., and Metcalfe, J.: *Heart Disease and Pregnancy. Physiology and Management* (Boston: Little, Brown & Company, 1958).
28. Kirklin, J. W., Weidman, W. H., Burroughs, J. T., Burchell, H. B., and Wood, E. H.: The hemodynamic results of surgical correction of atrial septal defects: A report of thirty-three cases, Circulation 13:825, 1956.
29. Kiely, B., Adams, P., Jr., Anderson, R. C., and Lester, R. G.: The ostium primum syndrome, A.M.A. J. Dis. Child. 96:381, 1958.
30. Gilman, R. A., Skowron, C. A., Musser, B. G., and Bailey, C. P.: Partial anomalous venous drainage, Am. J. Surg. 94:688, 1957.
31. Hambach, R.: Ein Beitrag zur Frage der Kombination von Habitus mongoloides mit angeborenen Herzmissbildungen, Ann. paediat. 183:77, 1954.
32. Evans, P. R.: Cardiac anomalies in mongolism, Brit. Heart J. 12:258, 1950.
33. Warkany, J., Passarge, E., and Smith, L. B.: Congenital malformations in autosomal trisomy syndromes, Am. J. Dis. Child. 112:502, 1966.

Persistent Ostium Atrioventriculare Commune

THIS ANOMALY represents a severe defect of cardiac septation. The atrioventricular canal, which should be subdivided into a right and a left portion in the sixth week of embryonic life, persists as a single opening and the mitral and tricuspid valves are not formed. Combined with the persistent separation of the dorsal and ventral atrioventricular cushions are defects of the atrial and ventricular septa.

Atrioventricularis accounts for 20% of atrial septal defects. Chromosomal anomalies are relatively frequent, since atrioventricularis communis is found in approximately one-fourth of patients with Down syndrome who have congenital heart disease (p. 328). Both sexes seem to be affected equally.[1] Morison[2] described the anomaly in one of identical twins.

PATHOLOGY.—The characteristic lesion is an H-shaped common outlet from the atrial cavities into the ventricular cavities (Fig. 52-5). This common outlet is reminiscent of the connection that exists between the atrium and the ventricle in embryos before the 11-mm. stage, before fusion of the anterior and posterior atrioventricular cushions. From this connecting opening originate valvar leaflets that can be more or less identified with the leaflets of the mitral and tricuspid valves.[1] As a rule, the anomaly is combined with a large defect in the lower portion of the atrial septum and with a ventricular septal defect of variable size. The foramen ovale may be normal or in its place there may be a defect due to absence of the valve. The ventricular septal defect may appear closed by a meshwork of trabeculae,[3] but, as a rule, there are sickle-shaped defects of the septa above and below the common atrioventricular canal. If the atrial and ventricular septa are rudimentary or absent, a cor biloculare may exist. The weight of the heart as found at necropsy usually is twice the normal.[1] The right atrium, the right ventricle and its infundibulum are markedly enlarged and the pulmonary artery usually is larger than the aorta. If ostium primum is combined with an imperfection of the mitral valve, the delineation from atrioventricularis communis may become difficult. Atrioventricularis communis often is combined with other cardiovascular defects.

SYMPTOMS.—Children with atrioventricularis communis usually are poorly developed, showing dyspnea, tachycardia and a tendency to respiratory infections and heart failure. Cyanosis may be present at birth or may remain inconspicuous if a left-to-right shunt prevails. The heart is enlarged on physical examination and in roentgenograms. A systolic and an apical diastolic murmur often are heard. X-ray examination shows marked enlargement of the right atrium and ventricle, but the left cardiac border and the shadow of the pulmonary artery also may be prominent. The hilar shadows are increased.

Most of these children die in the first year of life, but occasionally survival has been reported for several years. Patients who reach adult life[1] and are said to have atrioventricularis communis probably are patients with an ostium primum and a split mitral valve, a cardiac anomaly related to but not identical with that of a common atrioventricular canal. The infants who die early succumb to respiratory infections or heart failure.

Extracardiac malformations frequently are present. It is well known that atrioventricularis communis and mongolism often are associated. However, this association has been overemphasized when it was stated that acyanotic mongoloid children with congenital heart disease usually have a common atrioventricular canal. Ventricular septal defect is the most common congenital heart disease in patients with Down syndrome; it accounts for 68% of congenital heart disease in necropsied mongoloids, and atrioventricularis communis for 27%.[4]

Another syndrome with high incidence of a common atrioventricular canal is asplenia (p. 745). It seems that approximately 60% of the published cases of agenesis of the spleen are combined with atrioventricularis communis.[5,6] In these cases, atrial septal defect, ventricular septal defect, transposition of the

Fig. 52-5.—Atrioventricularis communis seen from right side. Atrial septal defect of secundum type is seen. Cleft of the tricuspid valve is present.

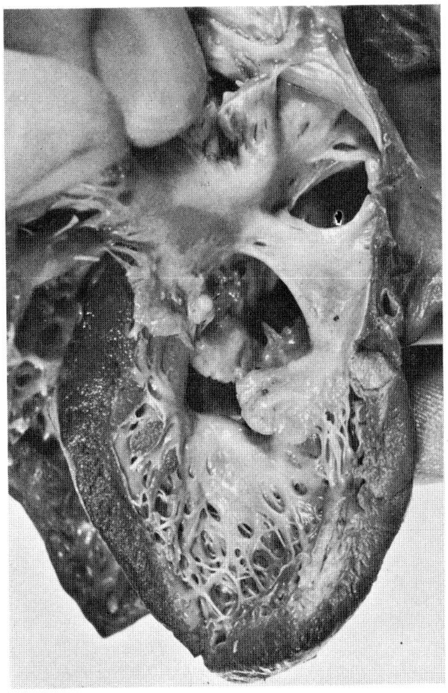

great vessels and other anomalies characteristic of the asplenia syndrome often are present, and signs of partial situs inversus and accessory lobes of the lungs usually are found. A sibling of a patient with the asplenia syndrome had atrioventricularis communis.[6] In the asplenia syndrome, mongolism does not seem to occur frequently and there is little overlapping between these two syndromes that include atrioventricularis communis so frequently. However, in Hambach's[7] series, a mongoloid with persistent atrioventricular canal and transposition of the great vessels had an abnormal spleen and another had asplenia. Atrioventricularis communis occurs also with polysplenia (p. 748).

TREATMENT.—Surgical repair has been attempted successfully, but the anomaly and concomitant malformations represent difficult problems. Operative mortality is said to be about 70%, which is a relative success since, without operation, more than 90% of the patients die in the first few years after birth.[3]

REFERENCES

1. Rogers, H., and Edwards, J.: Incomplete division of the atrioventricular canal with patent interatrial foramen primum (persistent common atrioventricular ostium), Am. Heart J. 36:28, 1948.
2. Morison, J. E.: Congenital malformations in one of identical twins, Arch. Dis. Childhood 24:214, 1949.
3. Keith, J. D., Rowe, R. D., and Vlad, P. (eds.), *Heart Disease in Infancy and Childhood* (2d ed.; New York: The Macmillan Company, 1966).
4. Warkany, J., Passarge, E., and Smith, L. B.: Congenital malformations in autosomal trisomy syndromes, Am. J. Dis. Child. 112:502, 1966.
5. Gilbert, E. F., Nishimura, K., and Wedum, B. G.: Congenital malformations of the heart associated with splenic agenesis; with a report of five cases, Circulation 17:72, 1958.
6. Polhemus, D. W., and Schafer, W. B.: Congenital absence of the spleen. Syndrome with atrioventricularis and situs inversus, Pediatrics 9:696, 1952.
7. Hambach, R.: Ein Beitrag zur Frage der Kombination von Habitus mongoloides mit angeborenen Herzmissbildungen, Ann. paediat. 183:77, 1954.

Cor Triloculare Biventriculare

THIS IS a rare malformation of the heart. Only 5 cases were included in Abbott's[1] tabulation. In the complete form of "common atrium" there is absence of the atrial septum in the presence of a ventricular septum, two ventricles and two auricular appendages. Both mitral and tricuspid valve leaflets may be cleft. The anomaly can be combined with ostium atrioventriculare commune. The blood is mixed in the atrium, but differential pressure is maintained so that the right heart receives most of the blood.[2] The life expectancy is short, but occasionally survival to adulthood is possible. An unusual case was reported by Cunningham,[3] the case of a man who died at the age of 51 years. In his youth he could walk 20–30 miles per day but later he was disturbed by attacks of palpitation, dyspnea and cyanosis. By the time he was 46 years of age, marked cyanosis, dyspnea and polycythemia were present. Finally, auricular fibrillations and hemoptysis occurred and he died of congestive heart failure. Necropsy showed his heart markedly enlarged and the pulmonary artery twice the size of the aorta. There was only a single atrial cavity; this was dilated. In addition, atrioventricularis communis and a defect of the membranous portion of the ventricular septum were present. Giknis[4] reported a typical case of Ellis-van Creveld syndrome in a girl who had no atrial septum as revealed in an exploratory operation. He pointed out that in 7 of 36 case reports of the Ellis-van Creveld syndrome absence of the atrial septum was mentioned.

Surgical repair in 5 cases was reported by Ellis *et al.*[5]

REFERENCES

1. Abbott, M. E.: *Atlas of Congenital Heart Disease* (New York: American Heart Association, 1936).
2. Edwards, J. E.: Congenital Malformations of the Heart and Great Vessels, in Gould, S. E. (ed.), *Pathology of the Heart* (Springfield, Ill.: Charles C Thomas, Publisher, 1953), pp. 266–503.
3. Cunningham, G. J.: Trilocular heart with bilateral aneurysmal dilatation of the pulmonary arteries, J. Path. & Bact. 60:379, 1948.
4. Giknis, F. L.: Single atrium and the Ellis-van Creveld syndrome, J. Pediat. 62:558, 1963.
5. Ellis, F. H., Jr., Kirklin, J. W., Swan, H. J., Dushane, J. W., and Edwards, J. E.: Diagnosis and surgical treatment of common atrium (cor triloculare biventriculare), Surgery 45:160, 1959.

Cor Triatriatum

THIS IS a rare malformation produced by a diaphragm stretching across the left atrium subdividing it into a distal, funnel-shaped chamber that receives all the pulmonary veins and a lower, proximal chamber connected with the mitral orifice and the auricular appendage. Abbott[1] included in her 1,000 cases 10 with this anomaly, and by 1966 there had been approximately 50 cases reported.[2]

The thickness of the septum is variable and the opening that connects the two left atrial chambers (cor triatriatum sinistrum) may be from 2 to 10 mm. in diameter. The border of the perforation often is thickened, rigid and calcified. The pulmonary veins entering the distal chamber vary in number and abnormal connections between them and a left superior vena cava and left innominate veins occur occasionally. Atrial septal defects commonly are associated with this anomaly but the mitral valve usually is normal. Only rarely is the diaphragm complete without any opening into the proximal chamber. In such cases, circulation is possible only if there is an atrial septal defect. Tetralogy of Fallot, dextrocardia or patent ductus arteriosus[3] may be associated anomalies.

The stenosis in the diaphragm results in pulmonary congestion, hypertrophy of the right atrium and ventricle and in enlargement of the pulmonary artery. A related but less serious anomaly consists in fibrous bands or cords within the left atrium that do not form a diaphragm and are not of any clinical significance. A divided right atrium (cor triatriatum dextrum) has also been described wherein the coronary sinus opens into the intermediate chamber that opens into the tricuspid.[4]

The anomaly probably is due to incomplete incorporation of the early single pulmonary vein into the left atrium. In young embryos of about 5 weeks' gestational age, a single pulmonary vein enters the area to the left of the septum primum. As the heart grows and the atria develop, this vessel is incorporated into the wall of the left atrium so that in the seventh week its four branches enter the left atrium separately. The abnormal distal chamber of the left atrium can be considered a persistent common pulmonary vein that is stenotic at the entrance into the true atrium and dilated distal to it.[5-7] Other pathogenetic explanations were cited by Niwayama.[8] An accessory median atrial chamber was described by Patten and Taggart[9] and considered a space located between the septum primum and septum secundum, which were not normally fused.

The symptoms depend on the opening between the two left atrial chambers. If there is a wide opening there are no clinical symptoms. If the opening is small, symptoms appear in early infancy. The anomaly causes pulmonary congestion and hypertension and eventually right heart failure. Approximately 50% of patients with this anomaly die within the first year. These infants have early dyspnea and signs of congestive heart failure. They appear malnourished and are difficult to feed. Patients with openings of more than 5 mm. in diameter show a delay of symptoms such as exertional dyspnea and moderate cyanosis. Recurrent infections complicate the case. The heart may be of normal size or enlarged. There may be systolic and diastolic murmurs. The second heart sound is accentuated.[2] On x-ray examination, the heart often appears enlarged, the pulmonary arch prominent, the pulmonary fields mottled and the vasculature increased.

Kyphoscoliosis and absence of the middle lobe of the right lung have been reported as associated extracardiac anomalies.[3]

If the opening between the two left atrial chambers is larger than 5 mm., survival to adulthood or even old age is possible. The diaphragm in Loeffler's[5] case was found accidentally at the necropsy of a woman 70 years of age. Pedersen and Therkelsen[3] described a woman with this anomaly who had lived an active life to the age of 24, when she underwent a pregnancy without complications. After delivery, her health deteriorated and she finally succumbed following a surgical attempt to alleviate her symptoms. Mitral stenosis had been suspected but on necropsy two left atria were found divided by a septum that had a foramen 5–7 mm. in diameter.

In patients who show early symptoms and in whom an early diagnosis is made, surgical repair is indicated.[8,10]

REFERENCES

1. Abbott, M. E.: *Atlas of Congenital Heart Disease* (New York: American Heart Association, 1936).
2. Keith, J. D., Rowe, R. D., and Vlad, P. (eds): *Heart Disease in Infancy and Childhood* (2d ed.; New York: The Macmillan Company, 1966).
3. Pedersen, A., and Therkelsen, F.: Cor triatriatum: A rare malformation of the heart, probably amenable to surgery, Am. Heart J. 47:676, 1954.
4. Kjellberg, S. R., Mannheimer, E., Rudhe, U., and Jonsson, B.: *Diagnosis of Congenital Heart Disease* (2d ed.; Chicago: Year Book Medical Publishers, Inc., 1959).
5. Loeffler, E.: Unusual malformation of the left atrium pulmonary sinus, Arch. Path. 48:371, 1949.
6. Edwards, J. E., du Shane, J. W., Alcott, D. L., and Burchell, H. E.: Thoracic venous anomalies, Arch. Path. 51: 446, 1951.
7. Parsons, C. G.: Cor triatriatum: Concerning the nature of an anomalous septum in the left auricle, Brit. Heart J. 12:327, 1950.
8. Niwayama, G.: Cor triatriatum, Am. Heart J. 59:291, 1960.
9. Patten, B. M., and Taggart, W. B.: Unusual type of triatrial heart, Arch. Path. 8:894, 1929.
10. Jegier, W., Gibbons, J. E., and Wiglesworth, F. W.: Cor triatriatum: Clinical, hemodynamic and pathological studies: Surgical correction in early life, Pediatrics 31: 255, 1963.

Prenatal Closure of the Interatrial Foramen

PRENATAL CLOSURE of the interatrial foramen causes developmental defects of the heart that are not compatible with postnatal life more than a few hours or days. The absence of an interatrial communication during fetal life deprives the left atrium and left ventricle of all blood except the small amount brought by the pulmonary veins. It has been estimated that the foramen ovale normally transmits at least half of the blood that enters the left side of the fetal heart.[1] Since the pulmonary circulation in fetal life is limited, the pulmonary veins bring extremely small amounts of blood to the left atrium, so that normal expansion of the left chambers does not take place. As a result, the left side is hypoplastic, whereas the right chambers become hypertrophic and distended. Although this condition is tolerated in intrauterine life, it is incompatible with postnatal life, since the increased blood volume delivered from the lungs after birth to the left side of the heart cannot be accommodated by the underdeveloped left atrium and ventricle. Venous congestion of the lungs, cyanosis, dyspnea and death result soon after birth. Wilson *et al.*[2] described 2 cases of this type, an extreme form with diminutive left atrium and ventricle, and a milder form with a relatively well-developed left-sided heart. They also stated that at that time (1953) 20 cases of prenatal closure of the interatrial foramen had been reported in the literature. In the same year, Brody[3] reported 2 cases.

If the left side of the heart is extremely underdeveloped, it may seem that only a single atrium and a single ventricle are present. The left atrium and the left ventricle may be enclosed in the posterior wall of such a heart, appearing as a slit-like cleft containing a diminutive mitral valve. From such a rudimentary left ventricle, the aorta originates as a small blood vessel that seems to join a larger innominate artery. The left atrium has the appearance of an accessory auricular appendage that is entered by a small, single pulmonary vein. The fossa ovalis and the foramen ovale are absent. The right ventricle is well developed, and from its left superior aspect a large pulmonary trunk turns backward, giving off two pulmonary arteries. It continues in the form of a large ductus arteriosus that joins the descending aorta. At the junction of the ductus and the descending aorta, a vessel arises that gives off, from left to right, the left subclavian, the left carotid and, finally, the innominate arteries. This vessel is joined by the tiny ascending aorta. In other cases, one can recognize in the interatrial septum that the foramen ovale had been formed and that it obliterated prematurely. Under these conditions, the left atrium and ventricle are better developed, since the left side of the heart apparently was supplied with blood through a foramen ovale for some time during intrauterine life. In these milder cases, the closure of the foramen ovale is not always complete, but the slit-like opening found between the atria does not permit normal interatrial communication. Wilson *et al.*[2] pointed out that premature closure of the interatrial foramen may result from three different developmental errors. The normal perforation of septum primum that should occur in the sixth week of prenatal life may not take place, thus interrupting interatrial communication at a very early age. A second possibility is the overgrowth of septum secundum, which results in formation of a complete interatrial partition in the third month of intrauterine life, thus precluding formation of the foramen ovale. The third form of prenatal closure of interatrial communication consists in prenatal obliteration of the foramen ovale, which should not occur in intrauterine life.

Owing to the scarcity of reported cases, nothing is known about the etiology of this disorder, but in a case described by Wilson *et al.*[2] there were clinical signs of congenital heart disease in 5 siblings of the patient.

Premature intrauterine interruption of interatrial communication has been produced experimentally by early roentgen irradiation of pregnant rats by Wilson *et al.*[4] In these animals, interatrial communication was interrupted because of failure of normal perforation of the septum primum.

Associated cardiac defects are mitral atresia or stenosis, aortic atresia, anomalies of the aortic valve, absence of the left ventricle, ventricular septal defect and absence of the ductus arteriosus. Among the noncardiac malformations, diaphragmatic hernia has been observed.[2] A truncus communis was present in one of Brody's[3] cases.

Children with this anomaly are either stillborn or they die soon after birth. Maximum life expectancy is 5 weeks.

REFERENCES

1. Patten, B. M.: Developmental defects at the foramen ovale, Am. J. Path. 14:135, 1938.
2. Wilson, J. G., Lyon, R. A., and Terry, R.: Prenatal closure of the interatrial foramen, A.M.A. Am. J. Dis. Child. 85:285, 1953.
3. Brody, H.: Antenatal occlusion of foramen ovale, Am. J. Clin. Path. 23:37, 1953.
4. Wilson, J. G., Jordon, H. C., and Brent, R. L.: Effects of irradiation on embryonic development. II. X-rays on the ninth day of gestation in the rat, Am. J. Anat. 92:153, 1953.

Juxtaposition of the Atrial Appendages

DIXON,[1] in 1954, described two hearts that showed the atrial appendages lying side by side instead of enclosing the great vessels. In one case, the two appendages lay to the right of the great vessels and the right side of the heart was hypoplastic, so that a functional cor biloculare was formed. In addition, there was an atrial septal defect, a common pulmonary vein, right-sided venae cavae emptying into the left atrium, tricuspid hypoplasia, partial transposition of the great vessels, coarctation of the arch of the aorta, patent ductus arteriosus and malrotation of the intestines. Death due to cardiac failure occurred when the child was 3 weeks of age. This form of dextrojuxtaposition seems to be extremely rare and the case observed apparently is the first of its kind on record.

Juxtaposition with both atrial appendages situated on the left of the great vessels has been observed repeatedly. Dixon's second case was that of a girl of 8 years in whom cyanosis was first noticed at 1 year of age. She was undersized, intensely cyanotic and had marked clubbing of fingers and toes. In addition to juxtaposition, there was an atrial septal defect, a common pulmonary vein, accessory septa in the right ventricle, partial transposition of the great vessels and stenosis of the pulmonary artery. Reviews of similar cases were made by Dixon[1] and Smyth.[2] In this type of juxtaposition, atrial septal defects, ventricular septal defects, stenosis of the pulmonary trunk and partial transposition of the great vessels are found regularly.

Fox and Goss[3] produced similar syndromes by injecting trypan blue into rats 8½ days after insemination. Displacement of major portions of both auricles to either the right or left of the arterial trunks, ventricular septal defects, dextroposition of the aorta and subpulmonary stenosis were recognized in the young. The heart appeared elongated and the ventricles rotated in counterclockwise fashion.

REFERENCES

1. Dixon, A. S. J.: Juxtaposition of the atrial appendages: 2 cases of unusual congenital cardiac deformity, Brit. Heart J. 16:153, 1954.
2. Smyth, N. P. D.: Lateroposition of the atrial appendage, Arch. Path. 60:259, 1955.
3. Fox, M. H., and Goss, C. M.: Experimental production of a syndrome of congenital cardiovascular defects in rats, Anat. Rec. 124:189, 1956.

53

Ventricular Septal Defects

IT IS ESTIMATED that half of all cases of congenital heart disease show a ventricular septal defect (VSD) and that approximately half of these are complicated by other cardiovascular malformations, which may dominate the disease picture.[1] The uncomplicated form of VSD ("maladie de Roger"), originally considered a rather harmless anomaly, is characterized by a harsh systolic murmur and absence of cyanosis. In the past, all cases with these characteristics often were diagnosed as VSD, but modern diagnostic methods have demonstrated that other cardiac malformations may show the same signs and symptoms.

INCIDENCE.—Estimates of incidence and prevalence of VSD are influenced by the ages of the patients in the group considered, by the diagnostic methods used and by complication of the septal defect by other cardiovascular anomalies. In necropsy material of patients with congenital heart disease, uncomplicated ventricular septal defect is not adequately represented because the lesion is relatively benign and compatible with a long life. In Abbott's[2] material, 6.2% of the cases were classified as ventricular septal defect. Wood *et al.*,[3] reviewing the literature on postmortem studies, found an average incidence of 15%, but this figure included some complicated cases. In infants dying in the neonatal period of congenital heart disease, Ober and Moore[4] classified 18% of the cases as ventricular septal defect. In general necropsy material, the rate of VSD is about 6 per 10,000.[5]

The rate per 10,000 live births is thought to be 20.[6] If approximately 10% of children with VSD died during childhood, one would expect 18 VSDs per 10,000 schoolchildren, but surveys yield only one-half[6] or one-third of that rate.[1] It is thought, therefore, that in a large percentage of children born with VSD the clinical signs disappear or spontaneous closure of the defect occurs within several years after birth.

In children born with a weight of 2,500 Gm. or less, the incidence of VSD is much higher than in the general newborn population, and the same is true of stillbirths.[6] Thus, the incidence of VSD varies according to the composition of the population examined.

In children's clinics and hospitals dealing with cardiac patients, VSD accounts for 12%[7,8] to 22%[1] of the cases.

Etiology.—The final closure of the ventricular septum is a complicated process, so that many different circumstances can interfere with the final perfection of cardiac septation. One must expect, therefore, that various pathogenic factors can result in this common anomaly. Yet, there are only a few cases of known origin. Occasionally, ventricular septal defects are observed in a mother and her child.[9-11] In one instance, a father and 4 of his children had this cardiac malformation.[12] VSD occurs in some patients with the Holt-Oram syndrome, which is attributed to a pleiotropic dominant gene (p. 481). Recurrence in sibships has been recorded several times.[13-15] In the same sibship, one child may have VSD and another tetralogy of Fallot.[13] In the study by Lamy *et al.*[8] there were no indications that genetic factors played a prominent role in the etiology of VSD. The parental consanguinity rate was low and there was a relatively high incidence of nongenetic factors mentioned in pregnancy histories.

In autosomal trisomy syndromes, VSD is the most frequent cardiac anomaly seen in necropsied patients. It was found in 47% of patients with trisomy 13-15, in 74% of those with trisomy 18 and in 25% of those with trisomy 21. Many of these VSDs were complicated by other cardiac malformations[16]; in two series,[17,18] uncomplicated VSD was noted in 18–25% of the patients with Down syndrome and CHD. There are other chromosomal anomalies that lead to VSD (Chapter 48), but in most of the patients exact diagnoses were not established.

Although VSD can be produced experimentally by numerous teratogenic procedures (Chapter 49), there is little known regarding environmental causes of the defect in man. Stecher[19] reported a pair of identical twins discordant for ventricular septal defect. MacMahon[20] came to the conclusion that older mothers have a greater tendency to bear children with "septal defects" than younger mothers. It seems possible that rubella in the first trimester can result in uncomplicated ventricular septal defect.[21-23] Uncomplicated VSD was rare in children with the thalidomide embryopathy but was quite frequent as a constituent of tetralogy and pentalogy of Fallot caused by this drug (Chapter 11). A cor triloculare biatriatum with truncus arteriosus following thalidomide intake was reported by Owen and Smith.[24]

Pathogenesis.—Until recently, it was generally assumed that defects of the membranous septum are due to incomplete fusion of the atrioventricular endocardial cushions with the ventricular muscular septum and the conus ridges. If proper union is disturbed by any process, the final closure of the interventricular septum cannot be effected. The termination period for perfection of the closure and formation of the membranous interventricular septum was thought to be between 22 and 35 days after conception (Horizons X to XVII),[25] a concept that still holds for the majority of cases. But it seems very likely that in some children final closure of the septum can occur at any time in pregnancy or even after birth. It has been suggested that the bulbar ridges, the endocardial cushions and possibly the muscular portions of the ventricular septum can still grow in later stages of pregnancy and during the first few years after birth.[26] That postnatal closure is possible had long been suspected[27] and has been demonstrated by repeat cardiac catheterization by Evans *et al.*[28] in 1960 and by many other investigators subsequently. Although in some cases of late closure the defects probably were small, spontaneous closure of defects large enough to cause cardiac failure in infancy can also occur.[1,29] It seems possible that approximately 10–25% of VSDs present in infants undergo spontaneous closure.[1,30] Anatomic evidence points to fibrous obliteration of the defects, which can occur in adults as well as in children.[31] Closure can be effected by adherence of the medial leaflet of the tricuspid valve to the edge of the defect, by formation of a fibrous membrane or by muscular hypertrophy, which can eliminate low defects. Signs of late closure of VSD were found by Simmons *et al.*[32] in 1 of 225 necropsies.

Defects of the muscular septum probably differ in origin from the junctional defects. Wimsatt and Lewis[33] pointed out that the muscular septum originally is trabeculated and that open, tortuous communications exist between the ventricles in early embryonic life. Enlargement and persistence of early sinusoidal communications result in the rare perforation foramina found at various levels of the ventricular septum.

The morphogenesis of ventricular septal defects can be studied experimentally, since various methods are available to produce this anomaly in mammals. In the rat, the ventricular septum is closed on the seventeenth day of gestation. Wilson and Warkany[34] studied the offspring of vitamin A-deficient rats.

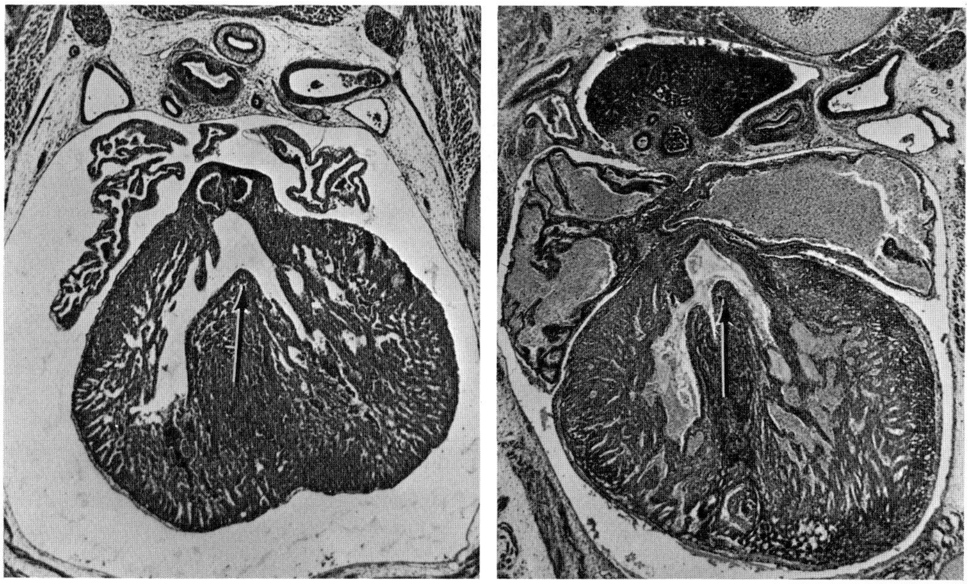

Fig. 53-1.—Sections showing VSD produced experimentally in rat fetuses by maternal vitamin A deficiency. Arrows point to communications of ventricles.

Among 64 fetuses older than 17 days, they found 22 (34%) with VSD. Most of these interventricular foramina were found in the membranous portion, but in some fetuses the muscular septum was defective also. In one young, a cor triloculare biatriatum was found. Most, but not all, of the affected offspring had aortic arch anomalies in addition to the septal defects. In animals with absent fourth and/or sixth arches and in all patterns containing only one functional arch there was always a septal defect that apparently made possible adequate blood circulation. Baird *et al.*[35] produced a variety of cardiovascular anomalies by folic acid deficiency. Of 130 fetuses with such anomalies, 92 (70%) had VSD but only 25% were uncomplicated. Cardiovascular malformations can be produced by trypan blue injections into pregnant rats.[36,37] In the young with such cardiovascular anomalies, approximately one-third have isolated VSD. Richman *et al.*,[38] after using the same teratogenic method, examined young rats surviving 30 days of postnatal life. Of 50 young dissected, 38% had VSD; 24% of these were uncomplicated. Conn and Hardy[39] attempted to produce congenital cardiovascular malformations in dogs by injections of trypan blue. Of 160 puppies, only 7 had significant cardiovascular defects, 2 being ductus arteriosus, 2 ventricular septal defect, 2 atrial septal defect and 1 a single coronary ostium. VSD is among the cardiovascular malformations induced in rats by salicylates[40] and is a manifestation of many other teratogens.

Pathology.—Interventricular defects are most common in the membranous septum, but in 10% of the cases defects are located in the muscular portion. The size of the openings varies from a few millimeters to 2 cm. in diameter. Approximately half the defects are 6–10 mm. in diameter, one-fourth less than 6 mm. and one-fourth more than 10 mm.[1] The shape may be oval, round or triangular. Most defects are located immediately below the aortic valve to the left of the septal leaf of the tricuspid and behind the crista supraventricularis. These lesions in the region of the membranous septum (junctional defects) account for 70% of the VSDs. Bulbar septal defects (uncomplicated, truncus arteriosus or Taussig-Bing malformation), atrioventricular septal defects and muscular defects in the ventricular sinus septum each accounts for approximately 10% of the cases of VSD.[1]

With overriding and dextraposed aortae, the openings usually are large and associated with increased pulmonary blood flow. There is increased pressure in the pulmonary artery, persistence of the normal hypertrophy of the small muscular arteries into childhood and development of intima changes. Progressive histologic changes in the pulmonary arteries and arterioles associated with VSD were classified by Heath and Edwards,[41] who distinguished six grades of structural alterations. It was thought that defects of the muscular septum are functionally unimportant because they can be occluded in systole,[42] but multiple muscular defects can cause growth retardation and cardiac failure.[43] As a rule, the pulmonary artery is larger than the aorta and the left ventricular wall thicker than the right. Abnormal blood currents can produce endocardial thickening in the area below the defect on the septal leaflet of the tricuspid valve or on the wall of the right ventricle and form places of predilection for bacterial endocarditis. The changes below the septal opening may involve the bundle of His

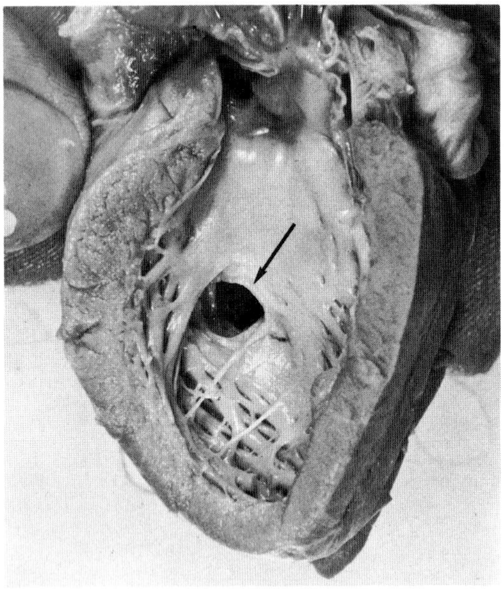

Fig. 53-2. – Muscular ventricular septal defect (**arrow**) seen from left ventricle.

and lead to heart block.[44] The course of the bundle is of importance in surgical repair of VSD, and special studies have been made to localize its path.[45,46]

SYMPTOMS. – The symptoms of ventricular septal defect vary greatly. The anomaly probably does not cause strain in fetal life, at which time the lungs are not unfolded. In postnatal life, the higher pressure in the left ventricle effects shunting of blood through the defect into the right ventricle and through the pulmonary artery to the lungs, from where shunted oxygenated blood returns via the pulmonary veins to the left atrium. This puts an extra load on the heart, but the symptoms depend on the size of the defect, on the resistance of the pulmonary vasculature and possibly on the extent of overriding of the aorta. It has been stated that a defect of more than 1 – 1.5 cm. in diameter – a defect larger than the diameter of the aortic orifice – leads to serious disturbance of the circulation unless flow is regulated by increased pulmonary resistance.[42]

It is thought that approximately two-thirds of the patients with uncomplicated VSD are asymptomatic and discovered on routine examination by auscultation. There is no cyanosis and no clubbing of the fingers and toes. Cyanosis is noticed if pulmonary vascular resistance is marked or in the case of congestive heart failure. Growth and development of children with simple VSD usually are normal, except in infants with large defects who show poor growth. A loud, harsh systolic murmur is audible in the third and fourth interspaces near the left sternal border. This murmur radiates, and may be heard clearly over the back. If the pressure in the right ventricle is smaller than in the left, there is a marked thrill felt over the precordium and if the pulmonary blood flow is large, a diastolic murmur can be heard.

Congestive heart failure occurs in approximately 10% of the patients with VSD, particularly in infants and children in the first year of life. Death is not necessarily due to the VSD, and in recent years the mortality of these infants has decreased.[1] An interesting fact was noted by Engle,[47] namely that 7 of 9 infants with early failure due to uncomplicated VSD had intrauterine growth retardation as if their growth had been disturbed in utero by the altered systemic blood supply. Necropsy revealed that the interventricular defects were high and variable in size, ranging from 2 to 18 mm., so that the size of the defect could not explain the early failure of circulation. It is possible that some of these infants had suffered some general prenatal damages, as indicated by their intrauterine growth retardation (Chapter 14).

Fig. 53-3. – High ventricular septal defect (**arrow**) seen from right ventricle.

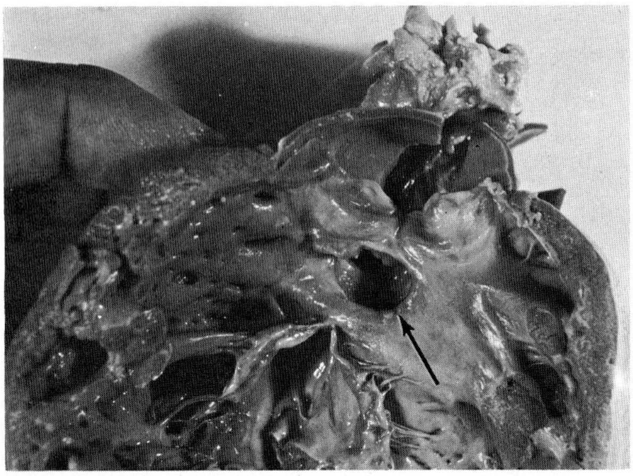

Fig. 53-4. – Right ventricle with ventricular septal defect (**arrow**). Pulmonary artery and valves are visible.

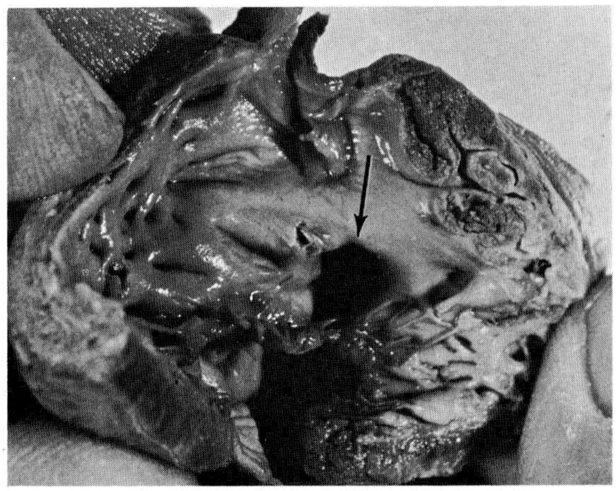

Beyond the period of infancy, VSD can be complicated by bacterial endocarditis or by emboli thrown into the pulmonary circulation, causing infarcts and pneumonic consolidation.[48] Cerebral abscess is a rare complication.[44]

In roentgenograms, the heart is enlarged in the majority of cases during the first 2 years of life but the cardiothoracic ratio falls in later childhood. The pulmonary artery is enlarged and the hilar shadows vary with the degree of blood flow and the pressure in the pulmonary artery.[1]

Extracardiac associated malformations are found occasionally. There may be chest deformities, scoliosis, syndactyly and malformations of the alimentary tract.[8] In one series, 3.5% of patients with VSD had Down syndrome.[8] Of 45 mongoloids who died early of congestive heart disease and were necropsied,[17,18] between 10% and 22% had simple defects in the ventricular septum. Association of VSD with congenital malformations of the urinary tract was discussed by Vince and Vanandel[49] and by Mehrizi.[50] Turner syndrome, trisomy 18, trisomy 13-15 and the thalidomide embryopathy represent some specific examples of conditions in which VSD and urogenital anomalies can be associated.

PROGNOSIS.—Many factors enter into prognostic evaluation of VSD. The natural history of VSD in infancy and childhood has been described in several publications[5,51-53] that point out the great variability of the course of this malformation. There is a large group of patients who remain asymptomatic without increase in heart size, pulmonary artery pressure or resistance. Some infants repeatedly develop respiratory infections and congestive heart failure and some develop pulmonary hypertension. Marked pulmonary hypertension with reversed shunt through a VSD represents a form of Eisenmenger syndrome, with its serious implications. Development of pulmonary stenosis that serves as a protection to the pulmonary circulation may mask the VSD.[54] Bacterial endocarditis is rare in children. Spontaneous closure of the VSD occurs in a significant number of patients (p. 490).

Lund[10] considered VSD a serious complication of pregnancy, since he noted 1 case of heart failure in 8 women observed during gestation, but the milder types of this malformation are compatible with normal pregnancy, normal delivery and birth of a normal child. Roger,[55] in 1879, mentioned a woman with this disease who was in good health when she was more than 50 years of age and the mother of 4 children. In some patients, complications develop after delivery.[56] In several instances, a mother with this defect gave birth to a child with the same anomaly (p. 490).

TREATMENT.—Many patients do not require special treatment and get along with moderate restriction of activity. Pulmonary infections and bacterial endocarditis are treated by antibiotics and heart failure by digitalization. Treatment by open heart surgery and patch closure is practiced for some of the patients. Those more than 2 years of age with large left-to-right shunts and moderate pulmonary hypertension are the best candidates for surgical treatment. Others are less favored by operation, and with significant right-to-left shunt surgical treatment is contraindicated. Infants developing serious symptoms usually are treated medically and some refractory cases are treated by banding of the pulmonary artery, which may prevent congestive heart failure and reduce pulmonary infections.[1,54]

REFERENCES

1. Keith, J. D., Rowe, R. D., and Vlad, P. (eds.): *Heart Disease in Infancy and Childhood* (2d ed.; New York: The Macmillan Company, 1966).
2. Abbott, M. E.: *Atlas of Congenital Heart Disease* (New York: American Heart Association, 1936).
3. Wood, P., Magidson, O., and Wilson, P. A. O.: Ventricular septal defect with note on acyanotic Fallot's tetralogy, Brit. Heart J. 16:387, 1954.
4. Ober, W. B., and Moore, T. E., Jr.: Congenital cardiac malformations in neonatal period; autopsy study, New England J. Med. 253:271, 1955.
5. Kaplan, S., Daoud, G. I., Benzing, G., III, Devine, F. J., Glass, I. H., and McGuire, J.: Natural history of ventricular septal defect, Am. J. Dis. Child. 105:581, 1963.
6. Hoffman, J. I. E.: Natural history of congenital heart disease. Problems in its assessment with special reference to ventricular septal defects, Circulation 37:97, 1968.
7. Nadas, A. S.: *Pediatric Cardiology* (Philadelphia: W. B. Saunders Company, 1957).
8. Lamy, M., De Grouchy, J., and Schweisguth, O.: Genetic and non-genetic factors in the etiology of congenital heart disease: A study of 1188 cases, Am. J. Human Genet. 9:17, 1957.
9. Debré, R., Cordey, F., and Olivier: Une mère et son enfant atteints de maladie de Roger: Hérédité similaire d'une cardiopathie congénitale, Bull. Soc. méd. hôp. Paris 47: 1742, 1923.
10. Lund, C. J.: Maternal congenital heart disease as obstetric problem, Am. J. Obst. & Gynec. 55:244, 1948.
11. Tucker, A. W., and Kinney, T. C.: Interventricular septal defect (Roger's disease) occurring in a mother and her six-month fetus, Am. Heart J. 30:54, 1945.
12. Seitz, R., and Baumann, H.: Familiäres Vorkommen von angeborenen Herzfehlern, Ztschr. Kreislaufforsch. 27: 13, 1935.
13. McKeown, T., MacMahon, B., and Parsons, C. G.: Familial incidence of congenital malformation of heart, Brit. Heart J. 15:273, 1953.
14. Tedesco, P. A.: Su due casi di cardiopatia congenita familiare, Cuore e circolaz. 17:76, 1933.
15. Fuhrmann, W.: Genetische und peristatische Ursachen angeborener Angiokardiopathien, in Heilmeyer, L., Schoen, R., and De Rudder, B. (eds.), *Ergebnisse der Inneren Medizin und Kinderkeilkunde* (Berlin: Springer, 1962).
16. Warkany, J., Passarge, E., and Smith, L. B.: Congenital malformations in autosomal trisomy syndromes, Am. J. Dis. Child. 112:502, 1966.
17. Evans, P. R.: Cardiac anomalies in mongolism, Brit. Heart J. 12:258, 1950.
18. Hambach, R.: Ein Beitrag zur Frage der Kombination von Habitus mongoloides mit angeborenen Herzmissbildungen, Ann. paediat. 183:77, 1954.
19. Stecher, R. M.: Identical twins discordant for interventricular septal defect and absent radius and thumb, Am. J. Human Genet. 9:218, 1957.
20. MacMahon, B.: Association of congenital malformation of heart with birth rank and maternal age, Brit. J. Social Med. 6:178, 1952.

21. Stuckey, D.: Congenital heart defects following maternal rubella during pregnancy, Brit. Heart J. 18:519, 1956.
22. Gibson, S., and Lewis, K. C.: Congenital heart disease following maternal rubella during pregnancy, A.M.A. Am. J. Dis. Child. 83:317, 1952.
23. Dogramaci, I., and Green, H.: Factors in etiology of congenital heart anomalies, J. Pediat. 30:295, 1947.
24. Owen, R., and Smith, A.: Cor triloculare and thalidomide, Lancet 2:836, 1962.
25. Streeter, G. L.: *Developmental Horizons in Human Embryos*. X–XVII (Washington, D. C.: Carnegie Institution of Washington, 1951 and 1957).
26. Mitchell, S. C., Berendes, H. W., and Clark, W. M., Jr.: The normal closure of the ventricular septum, Am. Heart J. 73:334, 1967.
27. Parkes-Weber, F.: Can the clinical manifestation of congenital heart disease disappear with the general growth and development of the patient?, Brit. J. Child. Dis. 15: 113, 1918.
28. Evans, J. R., Rowe, R. D., and Keith, J. D.: Spontaneous closure of ventricular septal defects, Circulation 22:1044, 1960.
29. Moore, D., Vlad, P., and Lambert, E. C.: Spontaneous closure of ventricular septal defect following cardiac failure in infancy, J. Pediat. 66:712, 1965.
30. Bloomfield, D. K.: The natural history of ventricular septal defect in patients surviving infancy, Circulation 29: 914, 1964.
31. Suzuki, H., and Lucas, R. V., Jr.: Spontaneous closure of ventricular septal defects. Anatomical evidence in three patients, Arch. Path. 84:31, 1967.
32. Simmons, R. L., Moller, J. H., and Edwards, J. E.: Anatomic evidence of spontaneous closure of ventricular septal defect, Circulation 34:38, 1966.
33. Wimsatt, W. A., and Lewis, F. T.: Duplication of the mitral valve and a rare apical interventricular foramen in the heart of a yak calf, Am. J. Anat. 83:67, 1948.
34. Wilson, J. G., and Warkany, J.: Aortic-arch and cardiac anomalies in the offspring of vitamin A deficient rats, Am. J. Anat. 85:113, 1949.
35. Baird, C. D. C., Nelson, M. M., Monie, I. W., and Evans, H. M.: Congenital cardiovascular anomalies induced by pteroylglutamic acid deficiency during gestation in rats, Circulation Res. 2:544, 1954.
36. Wilson, J. G.: Teratogenic activity of several azo dyes chemically related to trypan blue, Anat. Rec. 123:313, 1955.
37. Fox, M. H., and Goss, C. M.: Experimental production of a syndrome of congenital cardiovascular defects in rats, Anat. Rec. 124:189, 1956.
38. Richman, S. M., Thomas, W. A., and Konikov, N.: Survival of rats with induced congenital cardiovascular anomalies, A.M.A. Arch. Path. 63:43, 1957.
39. Conn, J. H., and Hardy, J. D.: Experimental production of cardiovascular anomalies in dogs using trypan blue, S. Forum 9:294, 1958.
40. Takacs, E., and Warkany, J.: Experimental production of congenital cardiovascular malformations in rats by salicylate poisoning, Teratology 1:109, 1968.
41. Heath, D., and Edwards, J. E.: The pathology of hypertensive pulmonary vascular disease. A description of six grades of structural changes in the pulmonary arteries with special reference to congenital cardiac septal defects, Circulation 18:533, 1958.
42. Selzer, A.: Defects of the cardiac septums, J.A.M.A. 154: 129, 1954.
43. Friedman, W. F., Mehrizi, A., and Pusch, A. L.: Multiple muscular ventricular septal defects, Circulation 32:35, 1965.
44. Edwards, J. E.: Congenital Malformations of the Heart and Great Vessels, in Gould, S. E. (ed.), *Pathology of the Heart* (Springfield, Ill.: Charles C Thomas, Publisher, 1953).
45. Lev, M.: The architecture of the conduction system in congenital heart disease. III. Ventricular septal defect, A.M.A. Arch. Path. 70:529, 1960.
46. Titus, J. L., Daugherty, G. W., and Edwards, J. E.: Anatomy of the atrioventricular conduction system in ventricular septal defect, Circulation 28:72, 1963.
47. Engle, M. A.: Ventricular septal defect in infancy, Pediatrics 14:16, 1954.
48. Taussig, H. B.: *Congenital Malformations of the Heart* (New York: Commonwealth Fund, 1947).
49. Vince, D. J., and Vanandel, M.: Ventricular septal defect and congenital malformations of the urinary tract. Clinical indications for intravenous urography, Clin. Pediat. 6: 16, 1967.
50. Mehrizi, A.: Congenital malformations of the heart associated with congenital anomalies of the urinary tract, J. Pediat. 61:582, 1962.
51. Fyler, D. C., Rudolph, A. M., Wittenborg, M. H., and Nadas, A. S.: Ventricular septal defect in infants and children. A correlation of clinical, physiologic, and autopsy data, Circulation 18:833, 1958.
52. Lynfield, J., Gasul, B. M., Arcilla, R., and Luan, L. L.: The natural history of ventricular septal defects in infancy and childhood; based on serial cardiac catheterization studies, Am. J. Med. 30:357, 1961.
53. Ash, R.: Natural history of ventricular septal defects in childhood lesions with predominant arteriovenous shunts, J. Pediat. 64:45, 1964.
54. Kaplan, S.: Congenital Heart Disease, in Nelson, W. E. (ed.), *Textbook of Pediatrics* (8th ed.; Philadelphia: W. B. Saunders Company, 1964).
55. Roger, H.: Recherches cliniques sur la communication congénitale des deux coeurs, par inocclusion du septum interventriculaire, Bull. Acad. méd. Paris 8:1074, 1879.
56. Burwell, C. S., and Metcalfe, J.: *Heart Disease and Pregnancy; Physiology and Management* (Boston: Little, Brown & Company, 1958).

Tetralogy of Fallot

In 1888, Fallot[1] described a pathologic syndrome encountered in cyanotic heart disease that has become an established entity in cardiology. This syndrome consists of pulmonary stenosis, ventricular septal defect, overriding of the aorta and right ventricular hypertrophy. After establishment of a syndrome named for an author, it usually is soon discovered that the syndrome is variable and that the author whose name it bears was not the first to describe it. This is true for the tetralogy of Fallot. It is understandable that the combination of anomalies mentioned, which occurs in approximately half of all cyanotic patients, had been known to anatomists before the end of the nineteenth century. In 1948, Willius[2a] reviewed the history of tetralogy and stated that in 1777 Sandifort, of Leyden, Holland, had given a comprehensive description of all the cardinal factors that Fallot enumerated 111 years later. In 1784, William Hunter, of Glasgow and London (cited by Willius[2a]), also gave a complete description of the combination of anomalies. As soon as the article by Willius was published, he learned that Sandifort's publication was antedated more than a hundred years by a remarkable description of the tetralogy of Fallot by the Danish scientist Niels Stensen (or Nicholas Steno), who saw the tetralogy in a monstrous embryo in 1671 and wrote: "The unusual form of the arteries arising from the heart attracted the chief attention and called for admiration. In particular, the pulmonary artery, which was much narrower than the aorta, seemed to be suggestive of something new, and hence I opened this vessel from the right ventricle to the hilus pulmonum, and then I could plainly see that the communication between the pulmonary artery and the aorta which usually is quite distinct in any fetus, was completely absent. When I opened the right ventricle, however, the probe that was passed forward and upward along the interventricular septum entered directly into the aorta just as readily as the probe passed from the left ventricle into the aorta. Thus, no less than three openings led into the right ventricle: one from the right atrium, the other two being connected with the arteries. The same aortic canal that was common to both ventricles, found, together with the interventricular septum, a double opening. The auricles were normal."[2b] This description not only contains the basic anomalies of the tetrad but demonstrates a good understanding of the normal and fetal circulation. It is now known that approximately 7% of patients with the tetralogy of Fallot have absence of the ductus arteriosus.[3b] The fact that this anomaly was observed in an embryo is still of great interest today. The associated malformations are also of interest, as the embryo apparently had a midline cleft that can be called a thoraco-omphalocele. On the left hand, all the fingers—with the exception of the thumb—were united by a common skin fold, and the third finger was short. There also was a cleft palate and harelip on the right side, which anomaly the mother attributed to the fact that she was fond of rabbit stew. This was a rather harmless explanation if one considers that in 1683, 12 years after this first careful anatomic description of the tetrad of Fallot, in the same city (Copenhagen, Denmark), a woman was burned alive because she had given birth to a monster whose head resembled that of a cat (p. 15). The tetrad may be combined with other cardiovascular anomalies, and one of these, the right-sided aortic arch, which occurs in approximately 25% of the patients, sometimes is termed "Corvisart disease."[4] *Triad* of Fallot is characterized by pulmonary stenosis and auricular septal defect, whereas an auricular septal defect added to the tetralogy leads to a *pentalogy* of anomalies. Several cases, beautifully illustrated, were recorded by Peacock[5] in 1866 (Fig. 53-5).

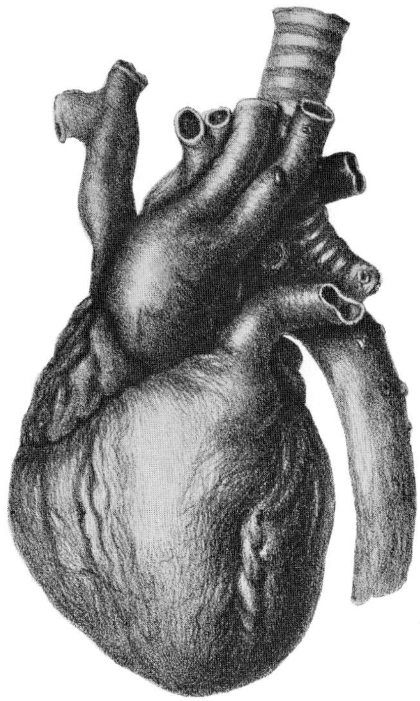

Fig. 53-5.—Tetralogy of Fallot seen and described by Peacock in 1866 (22 years before Fallot's description) in a boy 11½ months of age. The pulmonary artery was of small size, the aorta arose in part from the right ventricle, crossed over the right bronchus and then behind the trachea and gave off four vessels—the right and left carotid and the right and left subclavian artery. There was a ventricular septal defect and a right aortic arch. (From T. B. Peacock.[5])

INCIDENCE.—It has been estimated that tetralogy of Fallot occurs once in approximately 8,500 children,[3a] but in the prospective study conducted in the Babies Hospital in New York[6] there were 5 (and possibly 8) cases of tetrad of Fallot in approximately 6,000 births, i.e., possibly 1 in about 1,000. It remains to be seen which estimate is correct. Among children with cardiovascular disease, 20% were thought to have tetralogy until, in the past decade, a more accurate differentiation became possible between this anomaly and pulmonary stenosis with normal aortic root. Since then, estimates of the incidence of tetralogy have come down and now it is thought that approximately 10% of children with congential heart disease have tetralogy of Fallot. Similarly, the contribution of this syndrome to cyanotic congenital heart disease has also undergone some change. Although Fallot, in 1888, thought that 70% of all children with cyanotic congenital heart disease have the tetrad, it is now believed that the actual figure is 30%.[3b] Age does not seem to influence the prevalence of this anomaly as much as that of other congenital cardiovascular diseases. Stuckey[7] found that the tetrad accounts for 15% of children with cardiovascular anomalies below 2 years of age and also of those between 2 and 13 years.

In necropsy material of patients dying of congenital heart disease, the tetrad makes up 11% of the cases. In the neonatal period, it is found in only 4% of those who suffer cardiac deaths,[8] but if the entire first year is considered, the tetrad exacts many more deaths.[3a]

ETIOLOGY.—In only a few cases can leads be obtained concerning etiology of this common anomaly. Hereditary factors can be suspected only in exceptional cases. In the older literature,[9] several pedigrees were recorded indicating that cyanotic heart disease occasionally can be transmitted from one generation to another. It is clear that, in the past, the tetralogy of Fallot, with an average life expectancy of approximately 12 years, was not passed on directly from patients to their children. The offspring of women operated on will be observed with interest, but so far no direct transmission has been reported. There are a number of families recorded in which more than one child was affected with cyanotic heart disease, but in most of these the diagnosis was only assumed. In more recent times, Pitt[10] reported a large kindred in which 11 members had congenital heart disease, 8 of whom were cyanotic. Three members had proved tetralogy of Fallot. Lynch *et al.*[11] described tetralogy in a brother and sister. The brother had additional facial and neurologic anomalies and was mentally retarded, whereas the sister was normal except for congenital heart disease. The brother's malformations resembled those seen in patients with the "male Turner syndrome" (Chapter 112). A few cases have been reported that indicate that in siblings one child was affected with the tetrad of Fallot while another child had another form of congenital heart disease. Campbell,[12] in 1949, mentioned 3 patients with the tetralogy of Fallot who had siblings with different forms of congenital heart disease. In the material of McKeown *et al.*,[13] a boy with the tetralogy had had a sister who had died at the age of 3 weeks of an unspecified cardiac defect. Genetic factors occasionally do enter into the etiology of the tetrad when they contribute to situs inversus,[14] a condition commonly associated with congenital heart disease, particularly with tetralogy of Fallot. But Lamy *et al.*[15] stated that in Fallot tetralogy, genetic factors appear less important than nongenetic factors, since consanguinity and familial incidence are both low, and irregularities of pregnancy are common occurrences. This is in contrast to pulmonary stenosis, in which genetic factors appear more important (Chapter 48). A nongenetic determination must also be assumed in the affected members of two pairs of discordant identical twins who had tetralogy and pentalogy respectively, reported by Yuceoglu and Dresdale.[16] Tetralogy of Fallot is seldom diagnosed in autosomal trisomies. There is one patient on record with dextrocardia combined with tetralogy in a case of trisomy 13-15. In necropsies of patients with Down syndrome, tetralogy was diagnosed in 2.5% of the cases.[17] And Down syndrome was present in 3% of patients with tetralogy.[15]

Although rubella in early gestation does not often result in the tetrad of Fallot, a number of cases have been reported in which this virus probably had caused this complicated cardiac anomaly. In Campbell's[12] series there were only 4 children with congenital heart disease attributable to prenatal rubella, and all 4 had the tetrad of Fallot. This is an unusual observation, since this syndrome is absent in other reports on postrubella malformations. But there can be little doubt that the tetrad can be caused, in exceptional cases, by rubella in the first trimester of gestation.[18-22] Tetralogy of Fallot and some variations of it were seen in children with the thalidomide syndrome[23] (Chapter 11).

It seems that more males are affected than females, although the sex difference is not as striking as in some other forms of congenital heart disease. Polani and Campbell,[24] finding 58% of their 380 patients with the tetrad to be male, thought that this anomaly belongs to the group of the "aortic defects," headed by aortic stenosis, that show a definite male preponderance. Other authors had less impressive sex differences, but in the series of Lamy *et al.*[15] there were 55% and in the necropsy material of Abbott[25] and Herxheimer[26] 54–55% males. Tetralogy of Fallot has been observed in dogs, cattle, horses and pigs.[11] Some of its features can be produced in rats by maternal treatment with trypan blue.[27]

PATHOGENESIS.—In contrast to pure pulmonary stenosis, the tetralogy of Fallot represents a complete disturbance of the central vascular system. This is suggested by the fact that not only are the pulmonary artery and the aorta abnormal but there exists also, in a high percentage of cases, a derangement of the aortic arch derivatives.

The frequent combination of pulmonary stenosis and septal defect with dextroposition of the aorta has aroused speculation since early times and many attempts have been made to explain it. It was often discussed whether the ventricular septal defect or the pulmonary stenosis is the primary defect. Old theories concerning the pathogenesis of the tetralogy of Fallot were reviewed and discussed by Herxheimer.[26]

In Spitzer's[28] concept, tetralogy represents the type I transposition (Chapter 57). The human heart, like that of reptiles, has the potential of developing a right and left aorta. In the tetralogy, the large overriding aorta covers the location of the normal left ventricular aorta as well as the conus of the right ventricular aorta. It represents a fusion of the two aortae, which did not become separated by the septum aorticum. As this large aorta is connected with both ventricles, there exists necessarily a subaortic communication—a small septal defect—between the ventricles. The septum aorticopulmonale, which corresponds in such cases to that of the reptiles, should divide the outflow tract in such a manner that the pulmonary artery has only two cusps. This actually was the case in one of Mautner's[29] patients with tetralogy, who was one of the first to be analyzed by Spitzer with regard to his theory of the development of the heart,[28] a fact that is of some historical interest. The heart was shown to Spitzer with the large vessels unopened. Spitzer examined the septal defect and the large overriding aorta, and thought that this malformation could be the result of fusion of the two conuses of the right ventricular and the left ventricular aorta. He added, as Mautner[29] relates it: "If my theory is correct, then the arteria pulmonalis must have two cusps only." The artery was cut and there were the two cusps. Mautner adds: "This prophecy was such a surprise to me that I definitely believed in his theory and tried to make it as widely known as I could." It is a fact that the pulmonary valve may be bicuspid in cases of tetralogy,[25,30] but this seems to be true in only 25% of the cases.[3b] Thus, Spitzer's chance to make a correct "prophecy" was only 1 in 4, and one wonders what would have happened to his theory if this first heart had had a pulmonary artery with three cusps. The concept of aortic transposition has been challenged and underdevelopment of the subpulmonary conus has been considered the primary defect of tetralogy in a more recent concept.[31] Subpulmonary stenosis, ventricular defect, overriding aorta and right ventricular hypertrophy are consequences of the primary conus anomaly.

It is of interest that some of the features of the tetrad that have been "explained" by phylogenic theories have been produced experimentally in animals by environmental interference with early embryonic development. Fox and Goss,[27] by injecting trypan blue into rats 8½ days after insemination, observed in many of the young a ventricular septal defect and, in addition, a syndrome that included displacement of major portions of both auricles to either the right or the left of the arterial trunks, elongation and craniocaudal orientation of the heart, counterclockwise rotation of the ventricles, dextroposition of the aorta usually accompanied by a subpulmonary stenosis or some degree of pulmonary transposition. This syndrome was also combined with aortic arch anomalies and malformations of the atrioventricular valve.

Pathology.—The leading anomaly in the tetrad is stenosis or atresia of the pulmonary artery, stenosis being more frequent than complete atresia. In 1909, Herxheimer[26] reviewed 700 cases then published and found that 550–580 patients had stenosis and only 100–120 had atresia, which suggests a relation of 5 or 6 stenoses to 1 atresia. In the case of pulmonary atresia, patent right and left pulmonary arteries are present. If the pulmonary valve or the pulmonary trunk is completely obliterated, blood cannot reach the lungs directly from the heart. In fetal life or in early infancy, the blood leaving the aorta and reaching the ductus arteriosus may flow to the lungs through the branches of the pulmonary artery. If such a ductus undergoes normal obliteration after birth, before adequate collateral anastomoses are established, the lungs are not supplied with blood, and death results. This may be an explanation for the relative high mortality of patients with the tetralogy of Fallot during the first year of life. Survival is possible if bronchial or esophageal arteries arising from the aorta establish anastomoses with the pulmonary vasculature. In the absence of a ductus arteriosus, such collaterals may be established in fetal life, and the patients can survive the neonatal period better than those who are affected by the closure of a once-patent ductus.

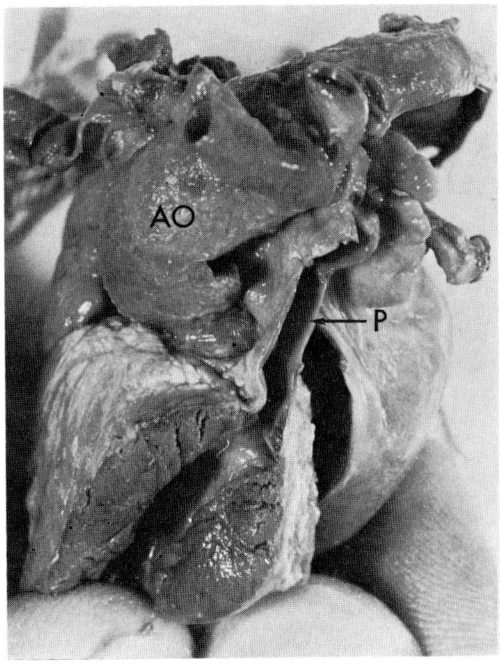

Fig. 53-6.—Tetralogy of Fallot. Narrow pulmonary artery (*P*) leaving hypertrophic right ventricle. The aorta (*AO*) is much enlarged.

Pulmonary stenosis is found most often in the subvalvar or valvar region and rarely in the trunk of the pulmonary artery, but the trunk is hypoplastic and narrow in most patients; it is normal in some and wider than normal in exceptional cases. Stenosis of the subpulmonary outflow tract probably is the most common cause of resistance to normal pulmonary circulation. Infundibular stenosis can be located immediately under the valves or more proximal near the main chamber of the right ventricle. The outflow tract may be straight or tortuous. It may be contracted by muscle, particularly a hypertrophic crista supraventricularis, or by fibrous tissue that may form a transverse diaphragm. In addition, the infundibulum is narrowed by thickened endocardial tissue and by deposits of fibrin and other blood elements. In valvar stenosis, the pulmonary cusps are fused, leaving an opening of variable size. There is no agreement concerning the frequency of infundibular versus valvar stenosis. In general, it is thought that the majority of cases with tetralogy have chiefly an infundibular narrowing and that valvar stenosis occurs in a minority of cases. But combinations of the two types exist and it is understandable that a strict classification is impossible.

The aorta usually is of normal size and arises from both ventricles sitting over the septal defect. As a rule, the aortic valves are normal. The origin of the coronary arteries may be irregular or one of them may be absent.[30] The ventricular septal defect is located in the membranous portion. The wall of the right ventricle that forms the apex is thickened, its chamber being normal or large. Anatomic variations of the tetralogy of Fallot are numerous. Baffes *et al.*[32] and Brinton and Campbell[20] described in detail the conditions in pulmonary valvar and in infundibular stenosis associated with tetralogy of Fallot. Baffes *et al.* found that stenosis of the pulmonary valve, when present, was in all instances associated with some degree of infundibular deformity. After study of 30 hearts with patent pulmonary artery associated with stenosis of the infundibulum, they stated that in their series no two hearts were alike. Most of the hearts showed either a narrow tubular or a band stenosis constricting the ostium of the infundibulum. In some cases, a subvalvar or intermediate stenosis was encountered. Brinton and Campbell[20] found the level of infundibular stenosis variable and detected a functional defect in the atrial septum in 10 of 25 patients.

Aortic arch anomalies are frequent. Right aortic arch occurs in 20–30% of the patients with the tetrad. As a rule, in such cases, the aorta descends on the right side and crosses to the left at the level of the seventh or eighth thoracic vertebra.[30] The origin of the vessels arising from the aortic arch is reversed, the innominate artery being on the left, followed by the right common carotid and by the right subclavian artery. Sometimes there are four branches and no innominate artery. In some cases of right aortic arch, the aorta crosses to the left behind the esophagus on a high level to form a left descending aorta. Double aortic arch is rare but retroesophageal subclavian artery is common; there were 26 cases in Blalock's[33] series of 610 cyanotic patients. In the same series there were 9 cases of single pulmonary artery. When the aorta descends on the left, the ductus arteriosus usually is on the left. If the aorta is on the right, the ductus may join the left innominate or left subclavian artery. In approximately 30% of necropsied patients with tetrad of Fallot, patent ductus arteriosus is seen, and in about 7% the ductus is absent on both sides. In the remaining cases the ductus normally is closed.[3b]

In the case of pulmonary atresia, blood reaches the lungs through collateral channels (p. 550). In pulmonary stenosis, some blood reaches the lungs through the pulmonary artery, but a great deal of the pulmonary vasculature is supplied by collateral circulation, which increases with age. The collaterals are derived from the posterior bronchial, esophageal, inferior phrenic, pericardiophrenic, subclavian and even the inferior thyroid arteries. These arteries pass to the lungs with the bronchi or through the pulmonary ligaments directly, anastomosing not only with the pulmonary vessels but also with the lung tissue directly. Collister *et al.*[34] emphasized the great irregularities of these anastomoses. Arteries may cross from one side of the mediastinum to the other and from the anterior to the posterior aspects of the lungs. These anomalous vessels are not normal arteries that increase in size but newly formed blood channels chosen almost accidentally from a widespread vascular network. Absence of the pulmonary valve in the tetralogy of Fallot results in peculiar features of the complex, which were described by Ruttenberg *et al.*[35] Congenital pericardial defect associated with the tetralogy can result in herniation of normal lung into the pericardial cavity.[36] In necropsies, intrapulmonary thromboses frequently are found. The lesions vary with severity of the stenosis and they often are absent in patients who have undergone shunt operations.[37] Alterations of the conduction system associated with the tetralogy complex were described by Lev.[38]

Symptoms.—Cyanosis is an outstanding symptom that usually is noticed in the first 6 months of life. Its delay in appearance may be related to the closure of the ductus arteriosus or, in rare cases, to increasing obstruction of the pulmonary outflow tract.[39] Paroxysmal dyspnea on exertion is the rule. It is particularly frequent in the first 3 years of life and may become less serious after the second year, after collateral channels are established. Attacks of dyspnea and cyanosis may lead to states of unconsciousness and paralysis. Exercise causes fall of oxygen content and saturation of the arterial blood, resulting in the paroxysms.[40] The children can breathe more easily in a squatting position and sleep better with the knees drawn up. Clubbing of the fingers and toes is typical of the tetrad. General physical development usually is retarded, growth and weight gain being slow. The children are thin and the onset of puberty often is delayed.[40] Polycythemia amounting to 6 million to 10 million red cells per cubic millimeter develops and the hemoglobin increases to more than 20 Gm./100 ml. Typically, there is a systolic murmur on the left border of the sternum. The heart is small but the right ventricle may be enlarged and cause chest deformity. Roentgenograms show a small heart with the apex elevated above the diaphragm. Owing to absence of the pulmonary shadow, a concavity is seen on the left outline of the heart shadow. In the case of a right aortic arch, the aortic knob may be seen on the right side of the sternum. The hilar areas and the lung fields usually are clear, indicating poor vascularization of the lungs. In recent years, however, it has been learned that this typical picture of the tetralogy of Fallot is not seen in all cases. If the infundibular chamber is large, a bulge may be visible on the left outline of the heart shadow. In the case of a right aortic arch, the heart usually appears long and narrow. In older children, the pulmonary vascular markings may be pronounced owing to a well-established collateral circulation to the lungs. Absence of one pulmonary artery may cause an increase in the vascular markings in the opposite lung. Barium swallows re-

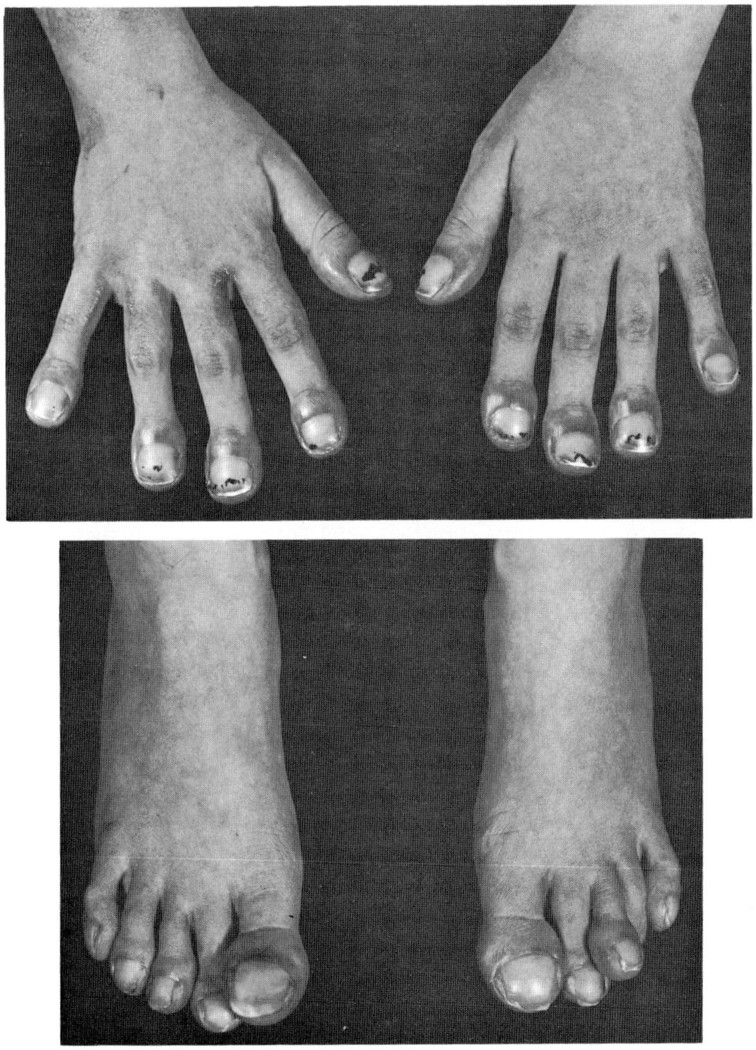

Fig. 53-7. —Clubbing of fingers and toes in a 7-year-old girl with tetralogy of Fallot. A twin brother was normal.

veal retro-esophageal vessels, which are not rare in patients with the tetralogy. Selective angiocardiography reveals the pulmonary stenosis, VSD, immediate filling of the aorta and simultaneous filling of the pulmonary artery.

ASSOCIATED MALFORMATIONS.—Many children with the tetralogy of Fallot are mentally normal and are free of associated congenital defects. Yet, the group as a whole is affected by a relatively high incidence of associated congenital malformations of the heart, the blood vessels and other organs. Cardiovascular variations have been discussed by Nagao *et al.*[61] Estimates of associated malformations outside the cardiovascular system vary. In necropsies, 20% of the patients with the tetralogy have noncardiac associated malformations.[3b] In the series of Lamy *et al.*,[15] 15% were affected by a variety of associated anomalies. It is of interest that mongolism was present in 3% of the patients with tetralogy and another 2.5% were mentally retarded. Thus, in this series, more than 5% of the patients with tetrad were mentally defective. In contrast to these high estimates of associated anomalies, Polani and Campbell[24] found only 2.2% affected with noncardiac congenital defects in a series of 181 patients. Associated malformations vary greatly. Those that are mentioned repeatedly in different series are harelip and cleft palate, diaphragmatic hernia, various types of renal anomalies and many variations of skeletal anomalies.[6,15,26] Wood *et al.*[41] found an association of tetralogy with polydactyly. It has been said that situs inversus and dextrocardia are not rarely associated with the tetralogy of Fallot,[14] but Keith *et al.*[3a] stated that this association has not been proved.

COURSE AND PROGNOSIS.—The most frequent compli-

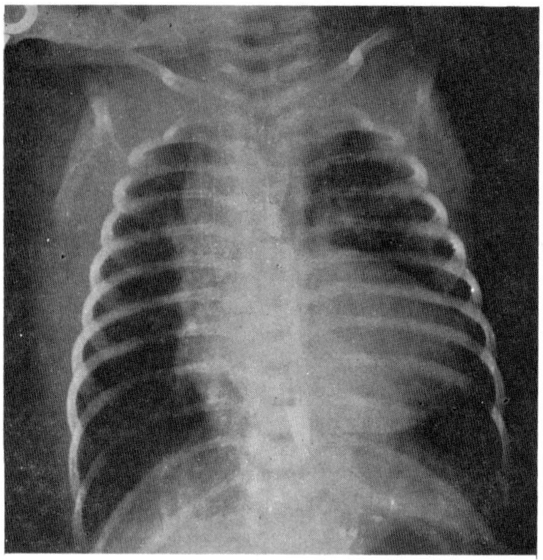

Fig. 53-8.—Roentgenogram of a child with tetralogy of Fallot. The apex is elevated and there is a defect on the left border at the cardiac base because of smallness of the pulmonary artery. The wide shadow above the heart on the right suggests right aortic arch. Pulmonary vascular markings are reduced.

cations related to anoxia are cerebral thrombosis, cerebral abscess and pneumonia. Patients with the most severe form of the tetrad may die in the neonatal period[41] or during the first year of life. Other children tolerate the transition from intrauterine to extrauterine life well and develop such symptoms as cyanosis and dyspnea several months after birth. Many reach childhood without serious difficulties and adapt themselves well to their impaired circulation after the first 2 years by reduction of activity and postural preferences. However, with adolescence, cyanosis and dyspnea increase and often lead to death in the second decade. This course makes the tetralogy of Fallot the typical cyanotic congenital heart disease of childhood. But there are exceptions, as some patients have mild forms and show little cyanosis and dyspnea, and there apparently are infants who, at first, merely have ventricular septal defects and develop infundibular pulmonary stenosis later.[39] Exceptional cases are known with survival to middle or old age. The noted musician who lived until his sixtieth year, reported by White and Sprague,[42] is such a well-known exception. Longevity in tetralogy and trilogy of Fallot was discussed by Bowie,[43] who reported 2 women 69 and 71 years of age with these conditions. There were 20 cases of tetralogy on record with survival beyond the age of 40 years and 4 over 60 years. A number of patients with the trilogy survived the fourth decade and one man reached 75 years of age. Such exceptions without surgical treatment are possible, but the average age of patients with tetralogy and pulmonary stenosis was about 12 years and that of patients with pulmonary atresia about 6 years.

PREGNANCY.—It is understandable that the incidence of pregnancy in patients with the tetralogy of Fallot is low, since the life expectancy averaged only 12 years. Pregnancy and delivery are more dangerous for women with tetralogy than for normal women, but this fact did not lead to general prohibition of pregnancy. Careful and individual treatment of each patient was recommended.[44] Black-Schaffer[45] described the pregnancy of a woman with severe cyanotic cardiovascular disease, in whom the diagnosis of tetralogy of Fallot, Eisenmenger syndrome or tricuspid atresia had been considered, who gave birth to an infant who, at term, weighed only 1,400 Gm., with a length of 38 cm. This child with intrauterine growth retardation showed osseous anomalies on histologic examination. The retardation of growth in utero was attributed by the author to fetal hypoxemia. Olim and Turner[46] described a woman who, at the age of 16 and again at the age of 18 years, was delivered prematurely of anencephalic fetuses. She was extremely cyanotic, with clubbing of fingers and toes, and gave a history of dyspnea. A Blalock procedure was carried out and 7 months later the patient became pregnant again. After a pregnancy of 39 weeks, she gave birth to a baby weighing 2,693 Gm. who had no congenital abnormalities. The authors surmised that "the low arterial oxygen saturation of the mother's blood interfered with fetal nutrition during the cephalic phase of development" and that repair of the cardiac lesion resulted in the normal outcome of pregnancy. This is a suggestive case report, but before any definite conclusions concerning the etiology of the anencephalic children can be drawn, it will be necessary to find similar cases. It has happened that a woman without congenital heart disease and without cyanosis gave birth to 2 consecutive anencephalics and later to a normal child without the benefit of a Blalock operation.[47] It must also be taken into consideration that a number of women with tetralogy of Fallot and persistent cyanosis have given birth to normal children.[44,48]

Russell *et al.*[49] reported the case of a woman with tetralogy of Fallot with right-sided aortic arch who, $1\frac{1}{2}$ years after a Blalock operation, gave birth to a girl weighing 2,282 Gm. During the fifth month there was an episode suggesting incipient cardiac failure. Busky *et al.*[50] observed a similar case of pregnancy 6 years after a Blalock operation. An apparently normal girl weighing 2,610 Gm. was born after a good pregnancy that was disturbed only once by signs of beginning heart failure in the sixth month. Kaufman *et al.*[51] described a woman who had been operated on twice for tetralogy of Fallot who underwent a pregnancy of 36 weeks with delivery of a normal boy. Pregnancy, delivery and postpartum course were uneventful.

TREATMENT.—Until 1945, medical treatment was the only therapy offered to patients with the tetralogy of Fallot. Even now, this treatment is of great importance because the ideal time for operation is late in childhood and it is necessary to carry the patient through the difficulties of infancy and early childhood. Taussig[52] described the measures necessary for the care of the cyanotic infant and child.

Now, a number of surgical procedures are available that are recommended for improvement of the tetralogy of Fallot. The Blalock-Taussig[53] operation, consisting of anastomosis of a subclavian artery with a main branch of the pulmonary artery, represents a milestone in medical history. Through this operation many thousands of cyanotic patients with the tetrad have been enabled to lead a normal life. By creation of an artificial anastomosis, the circulation is approximated to conditions that existed prior to the closure of the ductus arteriosus. In many children, the color of the lips becomes normal and clubbing of fingers and toes gradually subsides. The child who had been unable to walk and run can play like a normal child. The oxygen saturation of the arterial blood rises rapidly and usually reaches 80–88%. With an oxygen saturation of over 80% combined with adequate circulation to the lungs, the stimulus for the development of polycythemia is removed. Over a period of time there is a marked fall in the blood count and the hemoglobin. In the majority of cases, the child is able to live a relatively normal life. In 1953, Taussig and Bauersfeld[54] reported follow-up studies on the first 1,000 patients operated on for pulmonary stenosis or atresia. Of 857 patients with the tetralogy of Fallot, 78% had good results, 4% fair results, 3% remained unimproved and 15% died immediately after operation. The mortality in patients between the ages of 2 and 12 years has now been reduced to 2%.[55] Complications of shunt operations were discussed by Keith *et al.*[3b] In general, those patients who were operated on late in childhood had the best results, whereas those operated on early, usually because of the severity of their illness, had a less favorable outcome. In 1946, Potts *et al.*[56] performed an anastomosis of the aorta to a pulmonary artery, thus conducting the blood directly from the aorta to the circulation of the lung. This operation has also been successful in tetralogy of Fallot and may be more satisfactory than the subclavian anastomosis for infants.[3a] The Waterston operation (side-to-side anastomosis of the ascending aorta and right pulmonary artery) was advised in patients under the age of 2 years because palliation is prolonged and during later corrective surgery the shunt can be closed with greater ease than after a Potts anastomosis.[62] A different approach was made by Sellors[57] and Brock,[58] who attacked the pulmonary stenosis and the infundibular stenosis through an incision into the right ventricle outflow tract, which has the advantage that some of the anomalies prohibiting the free flow of blood to the lungs actually are removed. These operations are now more and more replaced by direct-vision intracardiac surgery performed with the help of heart-lung machines, procedures that permit adjustment to the individual anomalies of the patient as seen by direct inspection of the heart at the operating table. Closure of the ventricular defect, resection of the infundibular stenosis, valvotomy and relief of pulmonary artery stenosis are now practiced.[59] The mortality of this approach is now approximately 15%. Complications have been discussed by Keith *et al.*[3b] Patients successfully operated on have a normal arterial oxygen saturation, normal exercise tolerance and hemoglobin and hematocrit levels. Mental development and learning capacity are improved. Keith *et al.*[3b] believed that the reported relatively high incidence of mental retardation in tetralogy of Fallot may be, in part, a consequence of hypoxia, which may constitute a reversible situation. Individual surgical treatment is strongly recommended by Taussig.[60]

REFERENCES

1. Fallot, E. A.: Contribution à l'anatomie pathologique de la maladie bleu (cyanose cardiaque), Marseille-méd. 25:77, 138, 207, 270, 341, 403, 1888.

2a. Willius, F. A.: Cardiac clinics; comments on historical aspects of certain congenital anomalies of heart and great vessels, Proc. Staff Meet. Mayo Clin. 23:99, 1948.

2b. Willius, F. A.: An unusually early description of the so-called tetralogy of Fallot, Proc. Staff Meet. Mayo Clin. 23: 316, 1948.

3a. Keith, J. D., Rowe, R. D., and Vlad, P. (eds.): *Heart Disease in Infancy and Childhood* (New York: The Macmillan Company, 1958).

3b. Keith, J. D., Rowe, R. D., and Vlad, P. (eds.): *Heart Disease in Infancy and Childhood* (2d ed.; New York: The Macmillan Company, 1966).

4. Soulié, P.: *Les Cardiopathies Congénitales* (Paris: L'Expansion Scientifique Française, 1952).

5. Peacock, T. B.: *On Malformations of the Human Heart* (2d ed.; London: J. Churchill & Sons, 1866).

6. Richards, M. R., Merritt, K. K., Samuels, M. H., and Langmann, A. G.: Congenital malformations of the cardiovascular system in a series of 6,053 infants, Pediatrics 15:12, 1955.

7. Stuckey, D.: Pattern of congenital heart disease in infancy and childhood, M. J. Australia 2:433, 1954.

8. Ober, W. B., and Moore, T. E., Jr.: Congenital cardiac malformations in neonatal period; autopsy study, New England J. Med. 253:271, 1955.

9. Tedesco, P. A.: Su due casi di cardiopatia congenital familiare, Cuoree circolaz. 17:76, 1933.

10. Pitt, D. B.: A family study of Fallot's tetrad, Australasian Ann. Med. 11:179, 1962.

11. Lynch, H. T., Tips, R. L., and Krush, A. J.: Tetralogy of Fallot in two siblings, Am. J. Dis. Child. 111:304, 1966.

12. Campbell, M.: Genetic and environmental factors in congenital heart disease, Quart. J. Med. 18:379, 1949.

13. McKeown, T., MacMahon, B., and Parsons, C. G.: Familial incidence of congenital malformation of heart, Brit. Heart J. 15:273, 1953.

14. Cockayne, E. A.: Genetics of transposition of viscera, Quart. J. Med. 7:479, 1938.

15. Lamy, M., DeGrouchy, J., and Schweisguth, O.: Genetic and non-genetic factors in the etiology of congenital heart disease: A study of 1,188 cases, Am. J. Human Genet. 9:17, 1957.

16. Yuceoglu, Y. Z., and Dresdale, D. T.: Cyanotic congenital heart disease in one of identical twins: Report of two cases, Am. Heart J. 55:255, 1958.

17. Warkany, J., Passarge, E., and Smith, L. B.: Congenital malformations in autosomal trisomy syndromes, Am. J. Dis. Child. 112:502, 1966.

18. Dogramaci, I., and Green, H.: Factors in etiology of congenital heart anomalies, J. Pediat. 30:295, 1947.

19. Gibson, S., and Lewis, K. C.: Congenital heart disease

following maternal rubella during pregnancy, A.M.A. Am. J. Dis. Child. 83:317, 1952.
20. Brinton, W. D., and Campbell, M.: Necropsies in some congenital disease of the heart, mainly Fallot's tetralogy, Brit. Heart J. 15:335, 1953.
21. Jackson, A. V.: In King, E. S. J., Lowe, T. E., and Cox, L. B. (eds.), *Studies in Pathology*. Presented to Peter MacCallum (Melbourne: Melbourne University Press, 1950).
22. Stuckey, D.: Congenital heart defects following maternal rubella during pregnancy, Brit. Heart J. 18:519, 1956.
23. Weicker, H.: 100 children with thalidomide embryopathy, XIth International Congress of Pediatrics, 1956.
24. Polani, P. E., and Campbell, M.: Aetiological study of congenital heart disease, Ann. Human Genet. 19:209, 1955.
25. Abbott, M. E.: *Atlas of Congenital Heart Disease* (New York: American Heart Association, 1936).
26. Herxheimer, G.: Missbildungen des Herzens und der grossen Gefässe, in Schwalbe, E. (ed.), *Die Morphologie der Missbildungen des Menschen und der Tiere* (Jena: Gustav Fischer, 1909), Vol. 3, pt. 3.
27. Fox, M. H., and Goss, C. M.: Experimental production of a syndrome of congenital cardiovascular defects in rats, Anat. Rec. 124:189, 1956.
28. Spitzer, A.: Über den Bauplan des normalen und missbildeten Herzens. Versuch einer philogenetischen Theorie, Virchows Arch. path. Anat. 243:81, 1923.
29. Mautner, H.: The developmental mechanics of heart malformations, Arch. Pediat. 73:47, 1956.
30. Edwards, J. E.: Congenital Malformations of the Heart and Great Vessels, in Gould, S. E. (ed.), *Pathology of the Heart* (Springfield, Ill.: Charles C Thomas, Publisher, 1953).
31. Van Praagh, R., and Van Praagh, S.: The anatomy of common aorticopulmonary trunk (truncus arteriosus communis) and its embryological implications; a study of 57 necropsy cases, Am. J. Cardiol. 16:406, 1965.
32. Baffes, T. G., Johnson, F. R., Potts, W. J., and Gibson, S.: Anatomic variations in the tetralogy of Fallot, Am. Heart J. 46:657, 1953.
33. Blalock, A.: Surgical procedures employed and anatomical variations encountered in the treatment of congenital pulmonic stenosis, Surg., Gynec. & Obst. 87:385, 1948.
34. Collister, R. M., Dankmeijer, J., and Snellen, H. A.: Les vaisseaux collatéraux dans l'atrésie de l'artère pulmonaire, Compt. rend. A. anatomistes 39 (6):734, 1953.
35. Ruttenberg, H. D., Carey, L. S., Adams, P., Jr., and Edwards, J. E.: Absence of the pulmonary valve in the tetralogy of Fallot, Am. J. Roentgenol. 91:500, 1964.
36. Hipona, F. A., and Crummy, A. B., Jr.: Congenital pericardial defect associated with tetralogy of Fallot; herniation of normal lung into the pericardial cavity, Circulation 29:132, 1964.
37. Ferencz, C.: The pulmonary vascular bed in tetralogy of Fallot. I. Changes associated with pulmonic stenosis, Bull. Johns Hopkins Hosp. 106:81, 1960.
38. Lev, M.: The architecture of the conduction system in congenital heart disease. II. Tetralogy of Fallot, A.M.A. Arch. Path. 67:572, 1959.
39. Gasul, B. M., Dillon, R. F., Vrla, V., and Hait, G.: Ventricular septal defects: Their natural transformation into those with infundibular stenosis or into the cyanotic or noncyanotic type of tetralogy of Fallot, J.A.M.A. 164:847, 1957.
40. Taussig, H. B.: *Congenital Malformations of the Heart* (New York: The Commonwealth Fund, 1947).
41. Wood, P., McDonald, L., and Emanuel, R.: The clinical picture correlated with physiological observations in the diagnosis of congenital heart disease, Pediat. Clin. North America 5:981, 1958.
42. White, P. D., and Sprague, H. B.: The tetralogy of Fallot: Report of a case in a noted musician who lived to his sixtieth year, J.A.M.A. 92:787, 1929.
43. Bowie, E. A.: Longevity in tetralogy and trilogy of Fallot. Discussion of cases in patients surviving 40 years and presentation of two further cases, Am. Heart J. 62:125, 1961.
44. Burwell, C. S., and Metcalfe, J.: *Heart Disease and Pregnancy* (Boston: Little, Brown & Company, 1958).
45. Black-Schaffer, B.: Fetal nanosomia and bone athrepsia in the newborn of a woman with a severe cyanotic cardiovascular anomaly, Am. J. Obst. & Gynec. 59:656, 1950.
46. Olim, C. B., and Turner, H. B.: Anencephaly in fetuses of mothers with tetralogy of Fallot, J.A.M.A. 149:932, 1952.
47. Polman, A.: Anencephaly, spina bifida and hydrocephaly; a contribution to our knowledge of the causal genesis of congenital malformations, Genetica 25:29, 1950.
48. Scherlis, S., and Soloway, L. R.: Pregnancy and labor in a patient with cardiac anomaly, probably tetralogy of Fallot, Am. J. Obst. & Gynec. 44:697, 1942.
49. Russell, K. P., Dallke, W. E., and Buell, J. I.: Pregnancy following Blalock operation for tetralogy of Fallot, J.A.M.A. 149:266, 1952.
50. Busky, A. H., Grusetz, M. W., Wagman, W., and Grossman, F. E.: Pregnancy and delivery following operation for tetralogy of Fallot, Am. J. Obst. & Gynec. 70:1143, 1955.
51. Kaufman, J. M., Campeau, L. A., Ruble, P. E., Monahan, J., and Dodrill, F. D.: Pregnancy and successful delivery in a case of tetralogy of Fallot, Arch. Int. Med. 99:487, 1957.
52. Taussig, H. B.: Tetralogy of Fallot, especially the care of the cyanotic infant and child, Pediatrics 1:307, 1948.
53. Blalock, A., and Taussig, H. B.: The surgical treatment of malformations of the heart in which there is pulmonary stenosis or pulmonary atresia, J.A.M.A. 128:189, 1945.
54. Taussig, H. B., and Bauersfeld, S. R.: Follow-up studies on the first 1000 patients operated on for pulmonary stenosis or atresia (results up to March 1952), Ann. Int. Med. 38:1, 1953.
55. Taussig, H. B., Crawford, H., Pelargonio, S., and Zacharioudakis, S.: Ten to thirteen year follow-up on patients after a Blalock-Taussig operation, Circulation 25:630, 1962.
56. Potts, W. J., Smith, S., and Gibson, S.: Anastomosis of the aorta to a pulmonary artery, J.A.M.A. 132:627, 1946.
57. Sellors, T. H.: Surgery of pulmonary stenosis: A case in which the pulmonary valve was successfully divided, Lancet 1:988, 1948.
58. Brock, R. C.: Pulmonary valvulotomy for the relief of congenital pulmonary stenosis: Report of three cases, Brit. M. J. 1:1121, 1948.
59. Lillehei, C. W., Cohen, M., Warden, H. E., Read, R. C., Aust, J. B., DeWall, R. A., and Varco, R. L.: Direct vision intracardiac surgical correction of the tetralogy of Fallot, pentalogy of Fallot and pulmonary atresia defects, Ann. Surg. 142:418, 1955.
60. Taussig, H. B.: Tetralogy of Fallot—indications for operation, Am. J. Cardiol. 12:90, 1963.
61. Nagao, G. I., Daoud, G. I., McAdams, A. J., Schwartz, D. C., and Kaplan, S.: Cardiovascular anomalies associated with tetralogy of Fallot, Am. J. Cardiol. 20:206, 1967.
62. Kaplan, S., Helmsworth, J. A., Ahearn, E. N., Benzing, G., III, Daoud, G., and Schwartz, D. C.: Results of palliative procedures for tetralogy of Fallot in infants and young children, Ann. Thoracic Surg. 5:489, 1968.

Eisenmenger Syndrome

THIS SYNDROME is not associated with any specific morphologic entity. The condition is characterized by pulmonary hypertension at systemic level due to a high pulmonary vascular resistance with reversed or bidirectional shunt through a large ventricular septal defect[1] or through an atrial septal defect or a patent ductus arteriosus.[2] The normal fall of the pulmonary vascular resistance fails to occur in infancy in some patients with VSD who develop dyspnea, feeding difficulties and respiratory infections. Cyanosis becomes increasingly noticeable and, by the time of puberty, polycythemia, clubbing, angina pectoris and hemoptysis may be present. The fully developed Eisenmenger syndrome is rare in early childhood. Approximately 10% of the patients with VSD over the age of 2 years have the pulmonary hypertension and pulmonary vascular resistance characteristic of the syndrome, which actually is more prevalent during the second and third decades of life than during the first. In most patients, the increased resistance becomes noticeable during later childhood and adolescence and by the age of 30 or 40 years about 30% of the patients with VSD have developed Eisenmenger syndrome. Because of progressive changes in the pulmonary vasculature, the disease picture becomes more pronounced, with cyanosis, hemoptysis and heart failure,[3] so that the average length of life of these patients has been estimated at 35 years.[1] Surgical closure of the ventricular defect is not successful if there is a right-to-left shunt.

REFERENCES

1. Wood, P.: The Eisenmenger syndrome, or pulmonary hypertension with reversed central shunt, Brit. M. J. 2:701 and 755, 1958.
2. Kaplan, S.: Congenital Heart Disease, in Nelson, W. E. (ed.), *Textbook of Pediatrics* (8th ed.; Philadelphia: W. B. Saunders Company, 1964).
3. Keith, J. D., Rowe, R. D., and Vlad, P. (eds.): *Heart Disease in Infancy and Childhood* (2d ed.; New York: The Macmillan Company, 1966).

Cor Triloculare Biatriatum
(Single Ventricle)

IF THE interventricular septum does not develop, or if it remains rudimentary, a single ventricle results. In cor triloculare biatriatum there are two atria, but in many cases the interatrial septum is not perfectly developed. If the atrial septum is completely absent, a cor biloculare exists. In both conditions there is a single ventricle, and some reports on this subject include both conditions. The true single ventricle should be distinguished from apparent single ventricles with mitral or tricuspid atresia resulting in marked hypoplasia of the corresponding ventricle.

Cor triloculare biatriatum is a rare malformation. Abbott[1] listed an incidence of 1.3% in necropsy material, and single ventricle contributes approximately 2% to clinical cardiac cases.[2] Ober and Moore,[3] combining cor triloculare and biloculare in their analysis of patients dying of congenital heart disease in the newborn period, found them in 12% of these early cardiac deaths. Little is known concerning the etiology of the anomaly but it probably is related to those malformations that result from disturbed asymmetry of the body. Single ventricle may be associated with dextrocardia or with mongolism.[4] Of the patients reported because of agenesis of the spleen, 40% have a single ventricle.[5] Chauss[6] reported a necropsied patient with Ellis-van Creveld syndrome and cor triloculare biatriatum. It seems that 60% of the patients with single ventricle are male.[7]

PATHOLOGY.—The septum seems to be absent or rudimentary. Actually, absence of the septum is rare. Normal walls of the right and left ventricular sinuses seldom are found. Most of the cases are due to failure of development of one of the sinuses. The appearance of the myocardium indicates whether a left, a right, an undivided or an infundibular ventricle is present. Arrangement of the great vessels can be normal or the aorta is in dextro- or levoposition. In approximately 80% of the cases, the single ventricle has the characteristics of a left chamber. Dextro- and levotransposition of the aorta are present in 85% of the cases. with normal arrangement of the great vessels accounting for the remainder. Aortic or pulmonary stenoses frequently are present. Their type and degree are of decisive prognostic importance. With dextrotransposition, the aortic outflow tract is always obstructed; with levotransposition, only one-third of the patients have a narrow outflow tract.[7] The ventricular walls are hypertrophic. The inflow portion of the ventricle is connected with the atria by separate mitral and tricuspid valves or by a common atrioventricularis. The outflow portion often is subdivided by a muscular band that corresponds to the embryonic conoventricular flange.[8,9] There often is a rudimentary chamber from which one or both large vessels originate. If the pulmonary artery arises from this rudimentary chamber and the aorta from the large ventricle, the pulmonary trunk usually is small. If the aorta arises from the rudimentary chamber, it is reduced in size.[8] The normal spiraling of the great vessels is absent in approximately 80% of the cases.

The single ventricle with its rudimentary outflow chamber is reminiscent of the condition of the heart in embryos 5–10 mm. in length, and single ventricle

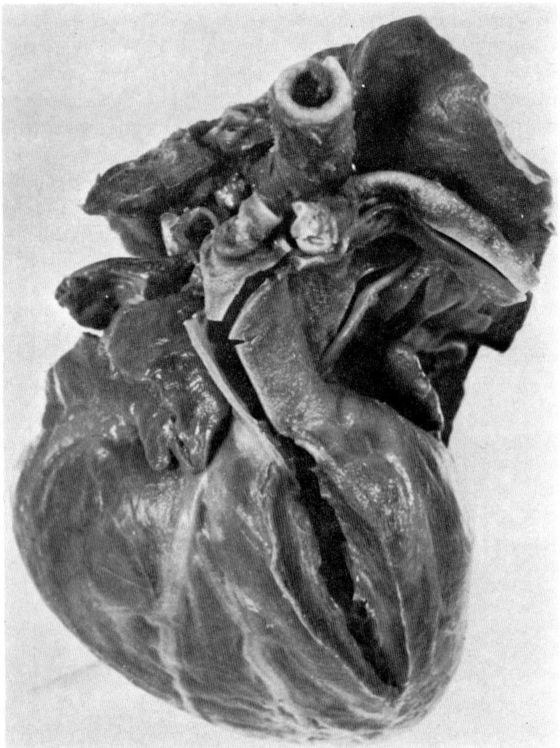

Fig. 53-9.—Anterior view of a heart with single ventricle and transposition. The rudimentary chamber, which has been opened, gives rise to the anteriorly placed aorta.

has been attributed to arrest of development in such early stages. However, with the arrest in this stage, malformations frequently occur in the great vessels and other cardiac structures that do not correspond to normal embryonic stages. The well-developed muscle ledge that separates the ventricle from the rudimentary outflow tract and corresponds to the conoventricular flange often causes obstruction to the free flow of blood to the smaller chamber.

SYMPTOMS.—With the exception of the patients who have a large pulmonary artery arising from the common ventricle, most children with this anomaly show early cyanosis and dyspnea. Patients with pulmonary stenosis have marked cyanosis. If the aorta is connected with the large ventricle and the pulmonary artery with the rudimentary chamber, a small amount of blood reaches the lung and the patients are intensely cyanotic. If, on the other hand, the pulmonary artery arises from the large ventricle and the aorta from the rudimentary outflow tract, the lungs are well supplied with blood and little cyanosis should be seen. But this situation is rare and mixed blood is always present in the single chamber. Physical development is poor and respiratory infections are frequent.

The heart size and murmurs are variable. In roentgenograms, the heart can be normal but, with increasing age, enlargement usually is seen. The shape of the heart often is determined by cardiac anomalies associated with the single ventricle. Roentgenograms usually show an enlarged heart shadow, with the rudimentary outflow chamber sometimes visible on the left cardiac border. The hilar shadows vary with the size of the pulmonary artery. Angiocardiography demonstrates the single ventricle and associated malformations.

PROGNOSIS.—More than half the patients reported because of single ventricle died below the age of 1 year, but 18 of 85 patients reviewed by Campbell *et al.*[10] reached the age of 20 and the oldest was 56 years. The average age at death of those with a bilocular heart was under 3 years and of those with a closed atrial septum 17 years. The prognosis depends on the state of the outflow tracts. Severe aortic or pulmonary stenosis (or atresia) leads to early death. Moderate pulmonary stenosis may prevent severe pulmonary vascular changes and permit survival to adult life.[7]

TREATMENT.—Patients with single ventricle, large aorta and pulmonary stenosis often are benefited by a Blalock-Taussig operation. Cyanosis and exercise tolerance can be improved. In cases of excessive pulmonary flow, banding of the pulmonary artery can be helpful.

REFERENCES

1. Abbott, M. E.: *Atlas of Congenital Heart Disease* (New York: American Heart Association, 1936).
2. Keith, J. D., Rowe, R. D., and Vlad, P. (eds.): *Heart Disease in Infancy and Childhood* (New York: The Macmillan Company, 1958).
3. Ober, W. B., and Moore, T. E., Jr.: Congenital cardiac malformations in neonatal period; autopsy study, New England J. Med. 253:271, 1955.
4. Hambach, R.: Ein Beitrag zur Frage der Kombination von Habitus mongoloides mit angeborenen Herzmissbildungen, Ann. paediat. 183:77, 1954.
5. Gilbert, E. F., Nishimura, K., and Wedum, B. G.: Congenital malformations of the heart associated with splenic agenesis; report of five cases, Circulation 17:72, 1958.
6. Chauss, J. M.: Chondroectodermal dysplasia (Ellis-van Creveld disease); case report, Radiology 65:213, 1955.
7. Van Praagh, R.: Single (Common) Ventricle, in Keith, J. D., Rowe, R. D., and Vlad, P. (eds.), *Heart Disease in Infancy and Childhood* (2d ed.; New York: The Macmillan Company, 1966), pp. 745–769.
8. Taussig, H. B.: *Congenital Malformations of the Heart* (New York: Commonwealth Fund, 1947).
9. Edwards, J. E.: Congenital Malformations of the Heart and Great Vessels, in Gould, S. E. (ed.), *Pathology of the Heart* (Springfield, Ill.: Charles C Thomas, Publisher, 1953), pp. 266–503.
10. Campbell, M., Reynolds, G., and Trounce, J. R.: Six cases of single ventricle with pulmonary stenosis, Guy's Hosp. Rep. 102:99, 1953.

54

Tricuspid Malformations

Tricuspid Atresia

TRICUSPID ATRESIA combined with defective development of the right ventricle, interatrial defect and hypertrophy of the left ventricle is a well-established cardiac entity that accounts for 2–3% of cardiac necropsy or clinical material.[1,2] It has been estimated that the incidence is 1 case in 5,000 births.[2] The etiology is obscure. Association with other serious cardiac malformations in many cases points to an early and profound disturbance of development. In one instance,[3] a case of tricuspid atresia and ventricular septal defect was found at necropsy in a child whose mother had had rubella 7 weeks after the time of (probable) ovulation.

The right ventricle may be reduced to a small slit-like space in the wall of the left ventricle, separated from it by a complete ventricular septum, or it may be connected with the left ventricle through a ventricular septal defect. If the septum is complete, the right ventricle is a blind sac that does not communicate with the circulation. Blood from the right atrium enters the left atrium by an interatrial defect or by a foramen ovale that is held open by the high pressure in the right atrium. The tricuspid valve, which is atretic or markedly hypoplastic, sometimes is difficult to identify, but occasionally the fused cusps are recognizable. The pulmonary artery may be atretic, hypoplastic or large. In the case of pulmonary atresia, the blood reaches the lungs through a patent ductus arteriosus. The foramen ovale is wide open in two-thirds of the patients and there is a gross defect in the atrial septum in one-third. In the absence of separate atria and of a distinct right ventricle, a bilocular heart is simulated and it may seem that both venae cavae enter the left atrium. The left ventricle is hypertrophic and the mitral valve usually competent. Tricuspid atresia is compatible with intrauterine life, since blood reaching the right atrium can be distributed throughout the body through the aorta and via the ductus arteriosus into the branches of the pulmonary artery. The heart is of normal size at birth.[4] After birth, circulation to the lungs is established through an open ductus arteriosus or through a transposed pulmonary artery. There are many variations, according to the origin of the great vessels, the size of the pulmonary artery and other criteria. Herxheimer[5] enumerated many cases reported in the older literature and pointed out that ventricular and atrial defects and transposition of the great vessels often are combined with tricuspid atresia. He cited Valleix,[6] who, in 1834, described a case associated with anomalous venous return, situs inversus, absence of the spleen and cleft lip and palate.

Tricuspid atresia is subdivided into two or even three main groups. Type I includes the forms without and type II the forms with transposition of the great vessels.[2,7,8,20] Type I accounts for approximately 70% and type II for 30% of the cases. Each type is subdivided into three groups, according to the size of the pulmonary artery. Type I (a) is characterized by pulmonary atresia, a closed ventricular septum and a slit-like right ventricular chamber. The pulmonary artery may be occluded at the valve or, more rarely, the entire trunk is cord-like. The right ventricle looks like an endocardial fold that can easily be overlooked so that it seems that one is dealing with a single ventricle. This form accounts for less than 10% of the cases of tricuspid atresia. Type I (b) shows a hypoplastic pulmonary artery, subpulmonary stenosis and a small interventricular defect. The small right ventricle consists of a tubular infundibulum and a thick-walled inflow chamber. A small ventricular septal defect or even multiple septal defects may be present. Some blood can reach the lungs through the ventricular septal defects. This type accounts for half of all cases of tricuspid atresia. Type I (c) has a large pulmonary artery that is supplied with blood by way of a large ventricular defect. Such an arrangement permits rather adequate pulmonary blood flow and a pulmonary-systemic balance. Less than 10% of the patients belong in this category.[2]

In type II, the great vessels are either completely or partially transposed. In these cases, the right ventricle appears larger than in the cases without transposition, but the ventricular compartments are not divided, since there always are ventricular septal defects of considerable size or the septum is completely absent. Type II (a) is associated with complete pulmonary atresia. The overriding aorta arises from the right ventricle and the lungs are supplied by a wide ductus arteriosus. This type, which accounts for only 2% of the cases,[2] may be associated with dextrocardia, situs inversus or right aortic arch. Ivemark[9] listed

3 cases of tricuspid atresia among those recorded for agenesis of the spleen, and Levy[10] added another case to this group. Type II (b) shows pulmonary stenosis and an overriding aorta originating from the right ventricle, with the narrow left pulmonary artery leaving the left ventricle. The stenosis may be valvar, subpulmonary or a combined form. In this type, juxtaposition of the atrial appendages to the left of the great vessels has been observed (p. 489). Type II (b) occurs in only 8% of the cases of tricuspid atresia. Type II (c) is more frequent. There is a large pulmonary artery that arises to the left of a hypoplastic aorta. Coarctation of the aorta may occur in this type, which accounts for less than 20% of the cases.[2] Keith *et al.*[2] added a rare third type to this classification, which is characterized by levotransposition of the great vessels. There can be subpulmonary or subaortic stenosis. Only 3% of the cases show these features.

In experiments, atresia of the tricuspid orifice has been observed in combination with transposition of the great vessels in the offspring of rats treated with trypan blue 8 days after insemination[11] and after treatment with carbon dioxide.[12] Monie *et al.*[13] studied the development of these anomalies in rat embryos. Tricuspid atresia or stenosis was found in 12% of the treated young. The anomalies could be recognized as early as day 12 of gestation. The right atrium was already enlarged in many of these young embryos. It seemed that inadequate expansion of the atrioventricular ring and deformation of the dorsal and ventral atrioventricular cushions were responsible for absence or stenosis of the tricuspid orifice.

Symptoms.—Because of admixture of venous and arterial blood in the left atrium, there is persistent cyanosis. In most patients, cyanosis is present at birth or appears very early in life, but in exceptional cases the cyanosis appears later. Clubbing of the fingers is observed in older patients. Signs of venous congestion and heart failure may be encountered in cases of transposition with large pulmonary blood flow. The heart may be enlarged on physical examination. Frequently, murmurs are heard but they seldom are diagnostic.

Roentgenograms show, in the anteroposterior view, a heart of normal or slightly increased size without a prominent shadow of the pulmonary conus. The area of the right ventricle appears flat and the dilated superior vena cava may be seen. The shadow of the great vessels is narrow but, in the left anterior oblique view, the cardiac shadow does not project forward to the anterior chest walls. The left ventricle is enlarged.[4] In some instances, the roentgenogram is quite similar to that of the tetralogy of Fallot. In other cases it resembles that of transposition of the great vessels. The pulmonary vasculature appears reduced in the majority of cases. A right aortic arch is present in 10% of the patients. Angiocardiography shows, after entry of the dye into the right atrium, immediate filling of the left atrium, left ventricle and the great vessels. The right ventricle does not opacify. The origin of the great vessels is seen in lateral views.

Prognosis.—The average life expectancy is approximately 15 months.[4] Half the patients die before they are 6 months of age, two-thirds are dead at 1 year and 90% at 10 years.[2] There is no agreement as to life expectancy in the different types, but Keith *et al.*[14] estimate the life expectancy of patients with types I (a) and II (a), who have pulmonary atresia, as only 2–3 months. The patient with common type I (b), characterized by pulmonary stenosis and a small ventricular defect, has an average life expectancy of 1 year. Those with type I (c), in which the pulmonary and systemic blood flow are well balanced, have a relatively good outlook and an average life expectancy of 8 years. Pulmonary stenosis combined with transposition (II [b]) is relatively favorable, with an average life expectancy of several years.[2] In general, the prognosis is poor if cyanosis appears during the first days or months of life.

Treatment consists in shunt procedures for improvement of pulmonary blood flow, if this is deficient.[15] Cavopulmonary artery anastomosis is one of the techniques now applied. If the interatrial communication is insufficient, the atrial septum is removed. In cases of excessive pulmonary blood flow, the pulmonary artery can be banded.

Tricuspid Hypoplasia

Tricuspid hypoplasia combined with hypoplasia of the right ventricle probably is rare, since only a few cases have been reported. Apparently this combination occurs as an entity without complicating cardiovascular anomalies. Familial recurrence has been observed in 7 of 10 reported cases.[16] In one family, two generations were affected. Two brothers had hypoplasia of the right ventricle and one of them transmitted the anomaly to his daughter.[17] In one patient examined, the chromosomal pattern was normal.[16]

The onset of symptoms and the course vary greatly, according to the degree of the malformations. Cyanosis can be present soon after birth and present a differential diagnostic problem. Early death occurs in some of the patients, but one of the patients reported died when 39 years of age.

Congenital Tricuspid Insufficiency

This rare anomaly is of interest because it can present at birth with cyanosis, marked cardiomegaly and congestive heart failure. Ventricular angiocardiography shows regurgitation of contrast material into the right atrium. The tricuspid valve is normally inserted, has a dilated orifice and short, thickened chordae tendineae.[18]

Duplication of the Tricuspid Valve

Only a few cases of this anomaly, which is rarer than duplication of the mitral valve, have been reported.[19] Cyanosis from birth and a large globular heart with hypertrophy of the right atrium and ventricle are among the manifestations. Combination with Ebstein anomaly has been observed, with survival into adolescence.

REFERENCES

1. Lamy, M., De Grouchy, J., and Schweisguth, O.: Genetic and non-genetic factors in the etiology of congenital heart disease: A study of 1,188 cases, Am. J. Human Genet. 9:17, 1957.
2. Keith, J. D., Rowe, R. D., and Vlad, P. (eds): *Heart Disease in Infancy and Childhood* (2d ed.; New York: The Macmillan Company, 1966).
3. Pitt, D. B.: Congenital malformations and maternal rubella, M. J. Australia 1:233, 1957.
4. Taussig, H. B.: *Congenital Malformations of the Heart* (New York: Commonwealth Fund, 1947).
5. Herxheimer, G.: Missbildungen des Herzens und der grossen Gefässe, in Schwalbe, E. (ed.), *Die Morphologie der Missbildungen des Menschen und der Tiere* (Jena: Gustav Fischer, 1909).
6. Valleix, M.: Transposition irrégulière des organes, Soc. anat. Paris 9:264, 1834.
7. Kühne, M.: Über zwei Fälle kongenitaler Atresie des ostium venosum dextrum, Jahrb. Kinderh. 63:235, 1906.
8. Edwards, J. E.: In Gould, S. E. (ed.), *Pathology of the Heart* (Springfield, Ill.: Charles C Thomas, Publisher, 1950).
9. Ivemark, B. I.: Implications of agenesis of the spleen on the pathogenesis of conotruncus anomalies in childhood, Acta paediat. scandinav. 44:(supp.)104, 1955.
10. Levy, D.: Congenital malformations of the heart and the great vessels associated with congenital absence of the spleen, Arch. Dis. Childhood 32:131, 1957.
11. Fox, M. H., and Goss, C. M.: Experimentally produced malformations of the heart and great vessels in rat fetuses. Transposition complexes and aortic arch abnormalities, Am. J. Anat. 102:65, 1958.
12. Haring, O. M.: Cardiac malformations in rats induced by exposure of the mother to carbon dioxide during pregnancy, Circulation Res. 8:1218, 1960.
13. Monie, I. W., Takacs, E., and Warkany, J.: Transposition of the great vessels and other cardiovascular abnormalities in rat fetuses induced by trypan blue, Anat. Rec. 156: 175, 1966.
14. Keith, J. D., Rowe, R. D., and Vlad, P. (eds.): *Heart Disease in Infancy and Childhood* (New York: The Macmillan Company, 1958).
15. Riker, W. L., Potts, W. J., Grana, L., Miller, R. A., and Lev, M.: Tricuspid atresia or stenosis complexes. A surgical and pathologic analysis, J. Thoracic & Cardiovas. Surg. 45:423, 1963.
16. Davachi, F., McLean, R. H., Moller, J. H., and Edwards, J. E.: Hypoplasia of the right ventricle and tricuspid valve in siblings, J. Pediat. 71:869, 1967.
17. Sackner, M. A., Robinson, M. J., Jamison, W. L., and Lewis, D. H.: Isolated right ventricular hypoplasia with atrial septal defect or patent foramen ovale, Circulation 24: 1388, 1961.
18. Reisman, M., Hipona, F. A., Bloor, C. M., and Talner, N. S.: Congenital tricuspid insufficiency, J. Pediat. 66:869, 1965.
19. Cascos, A. S., Rábago, P., and Sokolowski, M.: Case reports. Duplication of the tricuspid valve, Brit. Heart J. 29: 943, 1967.
20. Folger, G. M., Witham, A. C., and Ellison, R. G.: Tricuspid atresia with transposition of the great vessels, J. Pediat. 74:946, 1969.

Ebstein Malformation

This is a malformation of the tricuspid valve, which seems displaced downward into the right ventricle so that space normally occupied by this ventricle is incorporated into the right atrium. The malformation is rare, occurring in less than 1% of clinical cardiac cases.[1] Since the anomaly was first described by Ebstein[2] in 1866, approximately 300 cases have been recorded in the literature.[3]

Little is known concerning the etiology. One instance of recurrence in siblings has been reported[4] and in 2 cases siblings had some form of congenital heart disease.[3,5] Ebstein anomaly was also reported in a boy and his maternal uncle.[17] Of 2 patients with Ebstein anomaly, each had a nonidentical twin who did not have the malformation.[3,4] Males and females are affected equally.

The septal and posterior valves of the tricuspid originate low from the wall of the ventricle and not from the annulus fibrosus. The anterior leaflet may be normally formed and placed. The papillary muscles and chordae tendineae also are deformed. The low origin of the leaflets of the tricuspid valve results in a cone-shaped extension of the right atrium into the right ventricular space, which is thus markedly reduced in size. The tricuspid opening is always narrow but the valve not always insufficient. There usually is a defect in the area of the foramen ovale, either an open foramen, or fenestration of its valve or a gross interatrial defect. The wall of the right ventricle is always thin.[5,6]

The clinical symptoms are variable.[14] Ebstein anomaly has been seen in stillborn and premature children but it can be compatible with a long life. The spectrum of manifestations has been described by Genton and Blount.[3] Cyanosis may be present from birth on and be intermittent or it may begin in early infancy[7]; in other cases, onset is delayed. Some neonates with Ebstein anomaly who manifest symptoms and signs may improve if helped during their early difficulties. They can make up for their early failure to thrive by gains in subsequent months.[8] The malformation exists in adults,[9] in whom it can be mistaken for acquired heart disease.[10] Dyspnea, palpitation, cough and respiratory infections may be among the symptoms. The patients are said to be of the asthenic type,[6] but athletic body build has also been observed.[10] Systolic and diastolic murmurs usually are heard but they are not diagnostic. Cardiac arrhythmias are common. In roentgenograms, the heart usually is enlarged. The left border is prominent because of dilatation of the outflow tract of the right ventricle, and the right border because of enlargement of the right atrium.[11] Pulmonary vasculature is normal or decreased. Angiocardiographically, the immediate filling of the right ventricular area is characteristic, since it seems as though a large atrium occupying more than half of the cardiac shadow would be filled by the entering dye.[12] Owing to interatrial communication, the left atrium may be filled before the pulmonary artery. Difficulty in entering the right ventricle and delay in emptying of the right atrium and right ventricle contribute to the diagnosis.

Associated cardiovascular anomalies were listed by Rebolledo,[13] who reported a case combined with a right aortic arch.

The prognosis is variable. Infants with this anomaly may die early. The average life expectancy is approximately 30 years, but one-fourth of the patients die in the first 10 years of life. Ebstein's case was that of a man of 19 years, and the oldest patient died at the age of 70 years.[12] Patients with tricuspid insufficiency and a large right-left shunt apparently are endangered and die in early infancy. Association with double tricuspid valve has been reported.[13] Sudden death attributed to cardiac arrhythmias has occurred repeatedly.

Yamauchi and Cayler[8] succeeded in keeping alive neonates with Ebstein anomaly by medical treatment. Older patients with this anomaly are told to avoid excessive exercise and fatigue, yet a 60-year-old man with proved Ebstein anomaly was employed as a message runner for Western Union.[9] By surgical closure of the atrial septal defect, cyanosis and other symptoms may be reduced.[15] Anastomosis of the superior vena cava with the right pulmonary artery relieves the right heart of part of its load.[16] Surgical replacement of the tricuspid valve has also been accomplished successfully.[18] The steps to be considered in surgical correction of Ebstein anomaly were outlined by Ross and Somerville in 1970.[19]

REFERENCES

1. Nadas, A. S.: *Pediatric Cardiology* (Philadelphia: W. B. Saunders Company, 1957).
2. Ebstein, W.: Über einen sehr seltenen Fall von Insuffizienz der Valvula Tricuspidalis bedingt durch eine angeborene hochgradige Missbildung derselben, Arch. Anat., Physiol. u. Wissensch, Med., Leipsig, pp. 238–254, 1866.
3. Genton, E., and Blount, S. G., Jr.: The spectrum of Ebstein's anomaly, Am. Heart J. 73:395, 1967.
4. Gueron, M., Hirsch, M., Stern, J., Cohen, W., and Levy, M. J.: Familial Ebstein's anomaly with emphasis on the surgical treatment, Am. J. Cardiol. 18:105, 1966.
5. Taussig, H. B.: *Congenital Malformations of the Heart* (New York: Commonwealth Fund, 1947).
6. Keith, J. D., Rowe, R. D., and Vlad, P. (eds.): *Heart Disease in Infancy and Childhood* (New York: The Macmillan Company, 1958).
7. Broadbent, J. C., Wood, E. H., Burchell, H. B., and Parker, R. L.: Ebstein's malformation of the tricuspid valve, Proc. Staff Meet. Mayo Clin. 28:79, 1953.
8. Yamauchi, T., and Cayler, G. G.: Ebstein's anomaly in the neonate; a clinical study of three cases observed from birth through infancy, Am. J. Dis. Child. 107:165, 1964.
9. Oldenburg, F. A., and Nichol, A. D.: Ebstein's anomaly in the adult, Ann. Int. Med. 52:710, 1960.
10. Blount, S. G., McCord, M. C., and Gelb, I. J.: Ebstein's anomaly, Circulation 15:210, 1957.
11. Schiebler, G. L., Adams, P., Jr., Anderson, R. C., Amplatz, K., and Lester, R. G.: Clinical study of twenty-three cases of Ebstein's anomaly of the tricuspid valve, Circulation 19:165, 1959.
12. Keith, J. D., Rowe, R. D., and Vlad, P. (eds.): *Heart Disease in Infancy and Childhood* (2d ed.; New York: The Macmillan Company, 1966).
13. Rebolledo, J. R.: Ebstein's anomaly with right aortic arch. Review of the cardiovascular defects associated with Ebstein's malformation of the tricuspid valve, J. Pediat. 71:66, 1967.
14. Cascos, A. S., Rábago, P., and Sokolowski, M.: Case reports. Duplication of the tricuspid valve, Brit. Heart J. 29: 943, 1967.
15. Wright, J. L., Burchell, H. B., Kirklin, J. W., and Wood, E. H.: Congenital displacement of the tricuspid valve (Ebstein's anomaly), Proc. Staff Meet. Mayo Clin. 29:278, 1954.
16. Weinberg, M., Jr., Bicoff, J. P., Agustsson, M. H., Steiger, Z., Gasul, B. M., Fell, E. H., and Laun, L. L.: Surgical palliation in patients with Ebstein's anomaly and congenital hypoplasia of the right ventricle, J. Thoracic & Cardiovas. Surg. 40:310, 1960.
17. Donegan, C. C., Jr., Moore, M. M., Wiley, T. M., Jr., Hernandez, F. A., Green, J. R., Jr., and Schiebler, G. L.: Familial Ebstein's anomaly of the tricuspid valve, Am. Heart J. 75:375, 1968.
18. Barnard, C. N., and Schrire, V.: Surgical correction of Ebstein's malformation with prosthetic tricuspid valve, Surgery 54:302, 1963.
19. Ross, D., and Somerville, J.: Surgical correction of Ebstein's anomaly, Lancet 1:280, 1970.

55

Congenital Mitral Malformations

Mitral Stenosis

CONGENITAL MITRAL STENOSIS is considered a rare malformation but it accounts for approximately 4% of the cardiac cases seen in children's hospitals.[1,2] In necropsies of patients with congenital malformations of the heart, mitral stenosis or atresia was found in 7.5% of the cases by Bower *et al.*[3] Ferencz *et al.*[1] reviewed 43 cases and included 9 of their own. Most of the patients with congenital mitral stenosis have associated cardiac anomalies, but 6 of 7 cases reported by Daoud *et al.*[4] were isolated, only 1 being complicated by aortic coarctation. These authors found 30 case reports of isolated mitral stenosis in the literature.

ETIOLOGY.—The older opinion that fetal endocarditis is responsible for this type of mitral stenosis has been abandoned. Histologic examinations show no evidence of inflammation or scarring, but the pattern of stratification is confused in the leaflets.[1] Since congenital mitral stenosis usually is combined with aortic anomalies and patent ductus arteriosus, it may somehow be related to the etiology of these disorders. In one case,[3] a patient with this anomaly had a sibling with patent ductus arteriosus. Mitral stenosis may develop in patients with Hurler syndrome and other mucopolysaccharidoses,[5] and mitral insufficiency in patients with Marfan syndrome (Chapter 91). Although such cases occur in syndromes of congenital anomalies, it is unlikely that the cardiac lesions themselves are congenital. Mitral atresia has been observed repeatedly together with the asplenia syndrome[6] (Chapter 80). Since mitral atresia and mitral stenosis cannot always be sharply differentiated, it is possible that some cases of mitral stenosis are also present in patients with agenesis of the spleen. More males than females seem to have congenital mitral stenosis,[1,7] but this is not found in all series.[4] In one instance, the mother had had rubella during the third month of gestation.[4]

PATHOLOGY.—The heart size is variable, but enlargement is found in most of the cases. Hypertrophy of the right ventricle usually is responsible for the size of the heart, but the left ventricle may be involved also if stenotic malformations of the aorta are present. The mitral leaflets and chordae tendineae are thickened, fused and hard, forming a small narrow funnel with a small opening into the left ventricle. Hypertrophy and dilatation of the left atrium correspond to the severity of the stenosis. The endocardium of the left atrium is thickened in most of the cases, the thickening usually paralleling the age of the patient and the severity of the disease. Ferencz *et al.*[1] considered the thickening of the endocardium not as congenital but as a reaction to stenosis of the mitral valve and the aorta. Endocardial thickening may be present in the ventricle also, if blood flow is impaired by aortic stenosis. The lungs show marked changes of the arteries due to pulmonary hypertension. Hypertrophy of the medial muscular layers and reduction in the size of the lumina have been observed.

SYMPTOMS.—The birth weight usually is normal but, later, most children with this anomaly are underweight. They may be ill from birth, but more often they appear well until they suddenly are taken ill when several months old. Marked dyspnea is the most common symptom but cyanosis is seen in less than half the cases. Pulmonary congestion and infections are responsible for the distress of most patients. With increased pulmonary pressure, reversal of flow may

Fig. 55-1.—Mitral stenosis (**arrow**) seen from left atrium.

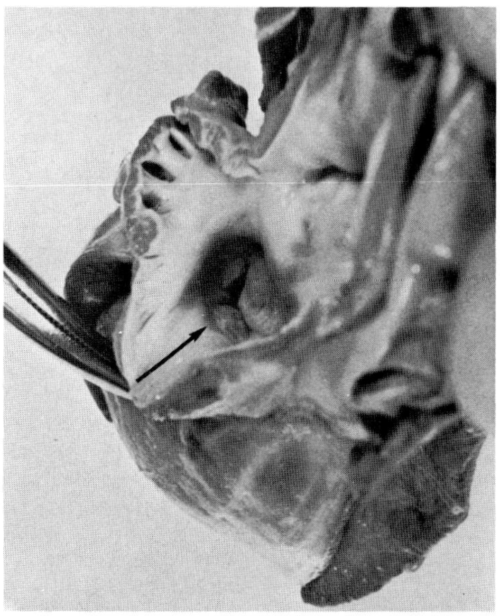

occur through an open ductus, so that venous blood is directed from the pulmonary artery into the aorta, and differential cyanosis may develop in the lower extremities. Heart murmurs are variable. There are apical, diastolic and systolic murmurs but associated anomalies influence these findings.

ASSOCIATED MALFORMATIONS.—Associated malformations were present in 35 of 43 cases reviewed by Ferencz *et al.*[1] Patent ductus arteriosus, aortic stenosis, hypoplasia and coarctation, aortic, tricuspid and pulmonary valve anomalies, patent foramen ovale, ventricular septal defect and double aortic arch have been observed. Endocardial fibroelastosis was present in more than half the cases.

PROGNOSIS.—More than 50% of the reported patients die within the first year, but it remains to be seen whether this serious picture applies to all cases of mitral stenosis of congenital origin. Some survivors with congenital mitral stenosis are thought to have the acquired form. In a case reported by Swan *et al.*,[8] the patient, who also had patent ductus arteriosus and coarctation of the aorta, survived 18 years. A woman 32 years of age underwent commissurotomy for mitral stenosis and had no history or signs of rheumatic fever. Since she had situs inversus, it is possible that her lesion was congenital.[9]

TREATMENT.—Bower *et al.*[3] reported successful valvotomy in a case of congenital mitral stenosis combined with patent ductus arteriosus with reversal of flow. Successful operation was performed when the patient, a girl, was 5½ years of age. The patient of Berkowitz and Likoff[9] also was successfully operated on. In the isolated form, operation seldom is successful.[4]

Mitral Atresia

Isolated mitral atresia is a rare anomaly but combinations with pulmonary and aortic atresia probably are not too rare.[10] Abbott[11] listed 5 cases of mitral atresia among 1,000 cardiac postmortem cases. Only 2 of these patients had a normal aortic valve. Brockman[12] reviewed 48 cases and added 1 of his own. Teller[13] listed 17 cases of isolated mitral atresia and Watson *et al.*[14] reported 11 patients with normal aortic valve. The etiology is obscure. Mitral atresia has been observed at least five times combined with other cardiac malformations in the asplenia syndrome.[6] Males account for 60% of the patients.[12]

PATHOLOGY.—The heart is large, the right atrium and right ventricle accounting for its size. The left side of the heart always is poorly developed. The ductus arteriosus, the foramen ovale and the ventricular septum may be open. If the foramen ovale is closed, a levoatrio-cardinal vein, connecting the left atrium through a systemic vein with the right atrium, may represent the only channel for oxygenated blood to the circulation.[15] Approximately half the patients have transposition of the great vessels.[12] There may be a single ventricle (cor triloculare biatriatum). In Brockman's case, the left atrium entered by one pulmonary vein was small. There was no mitral orifice and atrioventricular leaflets could not be identified on the left side. There was a truncus arteriosus that terminated distally in a right aorta and a left pulmonary artery. The pulmonary artery continued through a large ductus arteriosus into a narrowed aortic arch. The morphogenesis of this case was explained by Brockman as lack of fixation of the bulbus to the atrial canal. Consequently, the atrial canal moved far to the right and the septum primum inserted over the mitral orifice, fusing with the lateral, dorsal and ventral endocardial cushions and obliterating the mitral orifice.

As mentioned before, mitral atresia occurs in combination with many other cardiovascular anomalies, such as pulmonary, tricuspid and aortic stenosis, ventricular septal defect, transposition of the great vessels, patent ductus arteriosus and atrial septal defects. It is of interest that transposition of the great vessels and mitral atresia were found associated in rat fetuses whose mothers had been treated with trypan blue during early pregnancy.[16] Of noncardiac malformations, harelip and cleft palate, horseshoe kidney[10] and partial atresia of one ureter[12] have been reported. In mitral atresia with normal aortic valve, the left atrium is small, the right atrium large. Usually, a communication exists between the atria; anomalies of the venous return are frequent, especially with asplenia. The right ventricle is large but the left ventricle is rudimentary unless there is a septal defect. Pulmonary atresia or stenosis may be present. Dextroposition of the aorta or transposition of both great vessels is found in many, and the ductus is open in most cases.

The prognosis is poor. Neither medical nor surgical treatment has been successful.

Duplication of the Mitral Valve

This rare condition has been reviewed by Schraft and Lisa.[17] Only 14 cases had been reported in man up to 1948, when Wimsatt and Lewis[18] studied this subject; in 1958, Soloff *et al.*[19] brought the number up to 18. Although duplication of the mitral ostium is rare, it has been described more often than duplication of the tricuspid orifice.

Duplication of the mitral ostium may occur in a competent and otherwise normal valve. Consequently, the anomaly is compatible with a long life and it may be discovered accidentally at necropsy. Prior[20] found such a double mitral valve in a man 72 years of age, and the patient of Soloff *et al.*,[19] whose case was complicated by aortic coarctation and aortic stenosis, died postoperatively at the age of 57 years.

In most of the cases, the accessory orifice lies in the anterior mitral leaflet. It has a normal valvar structure and is connected with an anterior papillary muscle. Although in former years an inflammatory origin of the anomaly was considered possible, it is now generally assumed that the duplication is the result of a developmental error. A thorough discussion of the morphogenesis of duplication of the mitral valve was given by Wimsatt and Lewis.[18] These authors described the anomaly combined with an apical interventricular foramen in the heart of a yak calf that died at the age of 3 months. They pointed out that the medial and lateral cusps of the mitral valve differ in their origin. The medial arises from fusion of the anterior and posterior cushions, whereas the lateral cusp is derived from the single lateral cushion. The medial cushion is large and redundant and the accessory ostium seems to arise within its limits. On the left, fusion of the anterior and posterior cushion is somewhat delayed, so that in a normal 9-mm. embryo a crevice may be found medial to the definitive mitral ostium. Persistence of this crevice could account for duplication of the mitral orifice.

Schraft and Lisa[17] described in detail 12 reported cases and a patient of their own. The anomaly may be complicated by associated cardiac anomalies. Persistent ostium primum, coarctation or stenosis of the aorta and patent ductus arteriosus have been described.[17] The patient of Soloff *et al.*[19] had a horseshoe kidney.

REFERENCES

1. Ferencz, C., Johnson, A. L., and Wiglesworth, F. W.: Congenital mitral stenosis, Circulation 9:161, 1954.
2. Keith, J. D., Rowe, R. D., and Vlad, P. (eds.): *Heart Disease in Infancy and Childhood* (2d ed.; New York: The Macmillan Company, 1966).
3. Bower, B. D., Gerrard, J. W., D'Abreu, A. L., and Parsons, C. G.: Two cases of congenital mitral stenosis treated by valvotomy, Arch. Dis. Childhood 28:91, 1953.
4. Daoud, G., Kaplan, S., Perrin, E. V., Dorst, J. P., and Edwards, F. K.: Congenital mitral stenosis, Circulation 27: 185, 1963.
5. Vanace, P. W., Friedman, S., and Wagner, B. M.: Mitral stenosis in an atypical case of gargoylism; a case report with pathologic and histochemical studies of the cardiac tissues, Circulation 21:80, 1960.
6. Ivemark, B.: Implications of agenesis of the spleen on the pathogenesis of cono-truncus anomalies in childhood, Acta paediat. 44:(supp.)104, 1955.
7. Field, C. E.: Congenital mitral stenosis, Arch. Dis. Childhood 13:371, 1938.
8. Swan, H., Trapnell, J. M., and Denst, J.: Congenital mitral stenosis and systemic right ventricle with associated pulmonary vascular changes frustrating surgical repair of patent ductus arteriosus and coarctation of the aorta, Am. Heart J. 38:914, 1949.
9. Berkowitz, D., and Likoff, W.: Mitral stenosis complicating situs inversus: A case successfully treated by commissurotomy, Ann. Int. Med. 40:784, 1954.
10. Herxheimer, G.: Missbildungen des Herzens und der grossen Gefässe, in Schwalbe, E. (ed.), *Die Morphologie der Missbildungen des Menschen und der Tiere* (Jena: Gustav Fischer, 1909), Vol. 3, pt. 3.
11. Abbott, M. E.: *Atlas of Congenital Heart Disease* (New York: American Heart Association, 1936).
12. Brockman, H. L.: Congenital mitral atresia, transposition of the great vessels and congenital aortic coarctation, Am. Heart J. 40:301, 1950.
13. Teller, W. M.: Congenital mitral atresia, Am. Heart J. 56: 304, 1958.
14. Watson, D. G., Rowe, R. D., Conen, P. E., and Duckworth, J. W. A.: Mitral atresia with normal aortic valve; report of 11 cases and review of the literature, Pediatrics 25:450, 1960.
15. Edwards, J. E.: Congenital Malformations of the Heart and Great Vessels, in Gould, S. E. (ed.), *Pathology of the Heart* (Springfield, Ill.: Charles C Thomas, Publisher, 1953).
16. Monie, I. W., Takacs, E., and Warkany, J.: Transposition of the great vessels and other cardiovascular abnormalities in rat fetuses induced by trypan blue, Anat. Rec. 156: 175, 1966.
17. Schraft, W. C., and Lisa, J. R.: Duplication of the mitral valve, Am. Heart J. 39:136, 1950.
18. Wimsatt, W. A., and Lewis, F. T.: Duplication of the mitral valve and a rare apical interventricular foramen in the heart of a yak calf, Am. J. Anat. 83:67, 1948.
19. Soloff, L. A., Zatuchni, J., and Licata, R.: Double mitral valve, A.M.A. Arch. Int. Med. 101:103, 1958.
20. Prior, J. T.: Congenital anomalies of the mitral valve, Am. Heart J. 46:649, 1953.

SECTION THREE

56

Persistent Truncus Arteriosus

A TRUNCUS ARTERIOSUS is a single large vessel that carries blood from the heart. It represents the persisting original truncus arteriosus, which has remained undivided by an aortopulmonary septum. Such a single arterial vessel is rare. It was observed by Benešova and Sikl[1] only seven times in 20,000 necropsies. In Abbott's[2] series of 1,000 cases of congenital heart disease, there were 21 with persistent truncus. Incomplete separation of the great vessels, with a communication of the aorta and pulmonary artery distal to the semilunar valves, was listed in 10 of Abbott's 1,000 cases, but Evans[3] found 4 cases in 50 necropsies of children with congenital heart disease. Keith *et al.*[4] estimated that less than 1% of children with congenital heart disease have persistent truncus arteriosus.

Male preponderance has been reported for truncus arteriosus, but this was not the case in the series of MacMahon *et al.*[5]

Among the many forms of congenital heart disease occurring with trisomy 21, truncus arteriosus is relatively rare. It was noted in only 3 of 272 necropsies but was listed twice among 32 necropsies of trisomy 13-15 and once among 84 necropsies of trisomy 18.[6] Persistent truncus arteriosus was present in a number of infants with thalidomide embryopathy who died soon after birth.[7,8] In most cases, no cause can be ascertained. It is of interest that concordance in regard to persistent truncus has been observed twice in identical male twins. In the cases of Benešova and Sikl,[1] the twins were monochorionic and biamniotic. Both twins had truncus arteriosus communis, with three cusps of the semilunar valve and a septal defect. Both also had a right aortic arch and no ductus arteriosus. In a case of Giustra and Tosti,[9] it is somewhat doubtful that the twins were identical, since there were two placentas; yet, both twins had persistent truncus. Thoracopagus with double truncus arteriosus was observed by Kreutner *et al.*[10]

Persistent truncus arteriosus can be subdivided into various types, according to the origin of the vessels that supply the lungs.[11] The most frequent type shows an aorta and pulmonary artery originating from a common trunk. This form represents an incomplete division of the truncus, which appears partitioned in its distal portion but not in the proximal conal area. A second type is characterized by a single aortic trunk with two pulmonary arteries arising from its ascending portion. In the third type, no pulmonary arteries can be found and the lungs are supplied by bronchial arteries that originate in the descending aorta. This third type obviously results from absence of both sixth aortic arches and is always combined with absence of a ductus arteriosus. The persistent truncus usually is a large vessel that arises either from both ventricles, from the right ventricle or from a single ventricle. Hypertrophy of the right ventricle is always present. A truncus communis usually has three cusps of the semilunar valves, but there may also be two, four or six.[11] The coronary arteries arise from the base of the truncus but they may vary in number or course. Ductus arteriosus is absent in more than half the cases and always absent in the third type mentioned—the truncus without pulmonary arteries. Right aortic arch is quite frequent, estimates varying from 14%[11] to 60%.[4] There is always a ventricular septal defect. Truncus arteriosus with interrupted aortic arch is a rare combination.[12]

Related to truncus arteriosus embryologically but not clinically is the congenital defect of the aortopulmonary septum, which is located between the ascending aorta and the pulmonary artery and distal to the semilunar valves. It effects an arteriovenous shunt comparable to that of a patent ductus arteriosus.

If partition of the aortic trunk has taken place but the pulmonary artery remains rudimentary, a clinical situation arises that simulates persistent truncus but actually represents a "pseudotruncus."[13] This condition is not related anatomically or embryologically to true persistent truncus arteriosus.

In truncus arteriosus, an embryonic condition persists, since the septation of the truncoconal outflow tract, which normally takes place at the end of the sixth and the beginning of the seventh embryonic week, is not accomplished. The ridges that lead to septation of the common arterial trunk at birth can be noticed during the sixth week of embryonic life. The septation begins between the roots of the fourth and sixth aortic arches. Two ridges, a dextro-dorsal and a sinistro-ventral ridge, take their origin distally from the sixth aortic arches spiraling downward 225 degrees in a clockwise direction. The right dorsal ridge terminates on the ventral wall of the heart where the conus joins the left ventricle. The left ventral ridge ends on the dorsal wall of the conoventricular juncture. These ridges grow toward each other and unite early in the seventh week, thus forming the aortopulmonary septum. The caudal ends of these ridges fuse with the atrioventricular endocardial cushion tissue, forming the pars membranacea of the ventricular septum and completing this septum eventually. The spiral course of the truncus ridges and of the resulting septum explain the twisting of the aorta and pulmonary artery around each other.

Failure of the truncal ridges to develop at the end of the sixth or early seventh week leads to persistent truncus arteriosus. In one type of this anomaly that shows a distal separation of the aorta from the pulmonary artery, the cephalic portion of the truncus septum has developed but it did not continue downward to the conus area. If the distal and proximal portions of the septum develop but the middle portion above the semilunar valves remains defective, then an aortopulmonary fistula results.

Incomplete septation of the truncus arteriosus has been produced experimentally in rats. Wilson and Warkany[14] observed incomplete or irregular partitioning of the truncus arteriosus in rat fetuses rendered abnormal by maternal vitamin A deficiency (Fig. 56-1). The specimens obtained also had such aortic arch anomalies as absent ductus arteriosus, right-sided or double aortic arch, and there always were ventricular septal defects. Truncus arteriosus also has been observed occasionally in the offspring of female rats injected with trypan blue in early pregnancy.[15-17] Baird *et al.*[17] found truncus arteriosus in 16% of the young with cardiovascular anomalies produced by folic acid deficiency. The pulmonary arteries originated from the truncus and the abnormal specimens showed double aortic arch, right aortic arch, anomalous origin of the left subclavian artery and ventricular septal defect. Large doses of aspirin given to pregnant rats have resulted in persistent truncus arteriosus in some of the young.[25]

The symptomatology of truncus arteriosus varies according to presence or absence of pulmonary arteries. If a pulmonary artery arises from the trunk, some oxygenated blood goes to the lungs and venous blood reaches the systemic circulation. But since a large volume of oxygenated blood is mixed with this blood, cyanosis may be minimal or absent. If, however, the pulmonary arteries are absent and the lungs are supplied by bronchial arteries only, then the pulmonary blood supply is insufficient and cyanosis usually is intense.[13] In other cases, cyanosis is absent at birth but appears later, or it may be intermittent.[4] There often is dyspnea, clubbing and polycythemia paralleling the intensity of cyanosis.

Fig. 56-1 (left). – Transverse section through a rat fetus showing incomplete partitioning of trunco-conal segment of ventral aorta (**arrow**) produced by maternal vitamin A deficiency. (From J. G. Wilson and J. Warkany.[14])

Fig. 56-2 (right). – Persistent truncus arteriosus in a rat fetus whose mother had been treated with large doses of aspirin. (From E. Takacs and J. Warkany.[25])

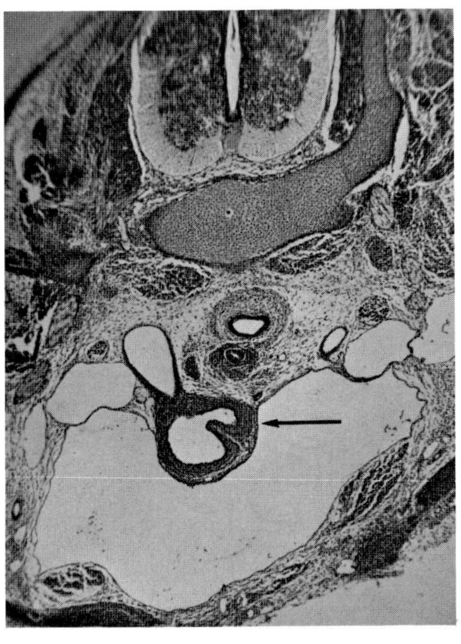

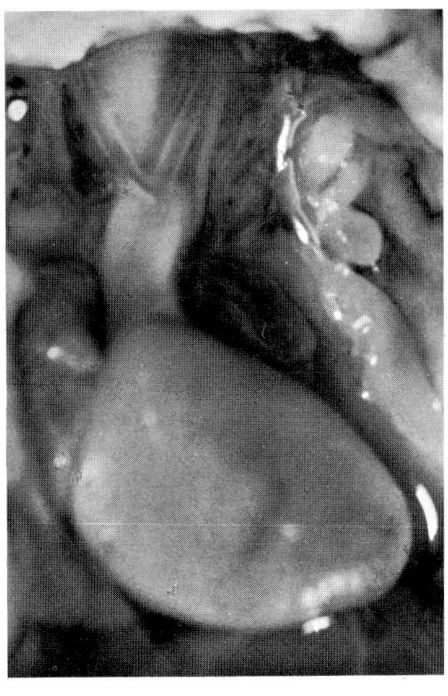

The heart, and especially the right ventricle, is always enlarged. In most cases, a harsh systolic murmur is audible over the entire cardiac area and a thrill over the sternum at the base of the heart.[13] Roentgenograms reveal a greatly enlarged heart shadow with a concavity at the upper left margin that is due to absence of the shadow of the pulmonary artery. The truncal shadow is large and may indent the esophagus.[13]

A partial defect in the aortopulmonary septum can simulate clinically ductus arteriosus or ventricular septal defect. This anomaly, which represents a window between the aorta and the pulmonary artery above the semilunar valves, can be demonstrated in aortograms, which show filling of the pulmonary arteries from the aorta.

ASSOCIATED MALFORMATIONS.—Persistent truncus arteriosus is always combined with other septal anomalies. The ventricular septum is defective in its cephalic portion, since its closure cannot be established owing to absence of the proximal portion of the conotruncal septum. Mitral atresia may be associated with persistent truncus.[18] Truncus arteriosus is also found combined with more extensive defects of the ventricular septum and with atrial septal defects. It is not rare in cor biloculare or triloculare. In fact, a single ventricle is found in approximately one-fourth of the cases of persistent truncus.[4] Right aortic arch, absence of the ductus arteriosus, interruption of the aortic arch or coarctation of the aorta are also often combined with truncus arteriosus. Gilbert *et al.*,[19] reviewing 85 cases of agenesis of the spleen, listed persistent truncus arteriosus in 12 of these cases. The same association had been noted by Ivemark.[20] Aplasia of the left kidney and ureter, accessory pancreas in the duodenum and ileum, accessory spleen in the tail of the pancreas[21] and abnormal lobation of the lungs[1] are among the associated extracardiac malformations.

The prognosis is poor, as about 60–70% of children born with persistent truncus arteriosus die within the first 6 months of life. Approximately 10% of the patients may live longer than 10 years. In rare instances, patients with persistent truncus may reach the third or fourth decade of life. A case of truncus arteriosus compatible with a full-term pregnancy was reported by Simon and Lustberg.[22] The mother died after delivery of an infant who weighed only 4 lb. at term but was otherwise mentally and physically normal.

No effective treatment was available until recently, when surgical separation of the systemic and pulmonary circulation became possible. Partial defect of the aortopulmonary septum is accessible to surgical treatment and several patients have been operated on successfully by closure of the communication.[23] Wallace *et al.*[24] repaired the ventricular septal defect and constructed a pulmonary trunk from the right ventricle to the arteries supplying the lungs with a homograft of the ascending aorta and aortic valve.

REFERENCES

1. Benešova, D., and Sikl, H.: Rare concordant malformation in monochoriate twins: Persistent common arterial trunk, J. Path. & Bact. 67:367, 1954.
2. Abbott, M. E.: *Atlas of Congenital Heart Disease* (New York: American Heart Association, 1936).
3. Evans, P. R.: Cardiac anomalies in mongolism, Brit. Heart J. 12:258, 1950.
4. Keith, J. D., Rowe, R. D., and Vlad, P. (eds.): *Heart Disease in Infancy and Childhood* (New York: The Macmillan Company, 1958).
5. MacMahon, B., McKeown, T., and Record, R. G.: The incidence and life expectation of children with congenital heart disease, Brit. Heart J. 15:121, 1953.
6. Warkany, J., Passarge, E., and Smith, L. B.: Congenital malformations in autosomal trisomy syndromes, Am. J. Dis. Child. 112:502, 1966.
7. Weicker, H.: 100 children with thalidomide embryopathy, XIth International Congress of Pediatrics, 1965.
8. Kreipe, U.: Missbildungen inner Organe bei Thalidomidembryopathie, Arch. Kinderh. 176:33, 1967.
9. Giustra, F. X., and Tosti, V. G.: True cor biloculare in identical twins, Am. Heart J. 17:249, 1939.
10. Kreutner, A. K., Levine, J., and Thiede, H.: A double truncus arteriosus in thoracopagus twins, New England J. Med. 268:1388, 1963.
11. Edwards, J. E.: Congenital Malformations of the Heart and Great Vessels, in Gould, S. E. (ed.), *Pathology of the Heart* (Springfield, Ill.: Charles C Thomas, Publisher, 1953).
12. Morgan, A. D., Brinsfield, D., and Edwards, F. K.: Persistent truncus arteriosus, Am. J. Dis. Child. 109:74, 1965.
13. Taussig, H. B.: *Congenital Malformations of the Heart* (New York: Commonwealth Fund, 1947).
14. Wilson, J. G., and Warkany, J.: Aortic-arch and cardiac anomalies in the offspring of vitamin A deficient rats, Am. J. Anat. 85:113, 1949.
15. Wilson, J. G.: Teratogenic activity of several azo dyes chemically related to trypan blue, Anat. Rec. 123:313, 1955.
16. Fox, M. H., and Goss, C. M.: Experimentally produced malformations of the heart and great vessels in rat fetuses. Atrial and caval abnormalities, Anat. Rec. 129:309, 1957.
17. Baird, C. D. C., Nelson, M. M., Monie, I. W., and Evans, H. M.: Congenital cardiovascular anomalies induced by pteroylglutamic acid deficiency during gestation in rat, Circulation Res. 2:544, 1954.
18. Brockman, H. L.: Congenital mitral atresia, transposition of great vessels, and congenital aortic coarctation. Case report and interpretation of anomaly, Am. Heart J. 40: 301, 1950.
19. Gilbert, E. F., Nishimura, K., and Wedum, B. G.: Congenital malformations of the heart associated with splenic agenesis; with a report of five cases, Circulation 17:72, 1958.
20. Ivemark, B. I.: Implications of agenesis of the spleen on the pathogenesis of cono-truncus anomalies in childhood, Acta paediat. 44:(supp. 104), 1955.
21. Beaver, D. C.: Persistent truncus arteriosus and congenital absence of one kidney with other developmental defects, Arch. Path. 15:51, 1933.
22. Simon, D. L., and Lustberg, A.: Case of truncus arteriosus communis compatible with full-term pregnancy, Am. Heart J. 42:617, 1951.
23. Gross, R. E.: Surgical closure of aortic septal defect, Circulation 5:858, 1952.
24. Wallace, R. B., Rastelli, G. C., Ongley, P. A., Titus, J. L., and McGoon, D. C.: Complete repair of truncus arteriosus defects, J. Thoracic & Cardiovas. Surg. 57:95, 1969.
25. Takacs, E., and Warkany, J.: Experimental production of congenital cardiovascular malformations in rats by salicylate poisoning, Teratology 1:109, 1968.

Transposition of the Great Vessels

If the aorta arises from the right ventricle and the pulmonary artery from the left, one speaks of transposition of the great vessels. There are many variations of this anomaly, such as complete, incomplete and corrected transposition. The great vessels may be of normal size or one may be hypoplastic or oversized. Association with other cardiovascular defects influences the course and symptoms of the disease to a great extent. In fact, complete transposition of the aorta and pulmonary artery without associated anomalies making possible interchange of blood of the two circulations is not compatible with life, since by such an arrangement only venous blood returning through the vena cava would be pumped into the systemic circulation and only oxygenated blood returning through the pulmonary veins would reach the pulmonary circulation. Either patency of a ductus arteriosus or foramen ovale, or auricular or ventricular septal defects (VSD), make survival possible.

The definitions and classifications of the various types of transposition become increasingly confused as embryologists, anatomists, pathologists, pediatricians and surgeons devise their own schemes. From the distinction of complete and corrected transposition of Rokitansky[1] in 1874 to Spitzer's[2] four types and Harris and Farber's[3] eight possible combinations, classifications have been extended to numerous anatomic and physiologic uncorrected and corrected transpositions complicated not only by capricious variations of anatomic parts but by many semantic disagreements. Whereas Spitzer[2] called overriding and dextroposed aortae transposition type I and type II, Van Mierop and Wiglesworth[4] excluded these anomalies from the transpositions on embryologic grounds. Van Praagh *et al.* (in Keith *et al.*[5]) presented a "basic" classification of normal and abnormal relationships of great arteries, ventricles and atria consisting of twelve combinations. But they emphasized that many more permutations exist if one includes the various types of double-outlet right ventricle, the various types of single ventricle, combinations with morphologically unidentified atria and/or ventricles and the various overridings of each great artery. Van Praagh *et al.* recommended the terms dextrotransposition and levotransposition to indicate the right-sided or left-sided location of the transposed aortic valve relative to the transposed pulmonary valve. Fortunately, some of the errors of transposition cancel one another out functionally, so that more than one "transposition" can result in physiologic correction. It may become difficult eventually to find two hearts with transposition that can be considered alike by conscientious pathologists. The only hope for a workable classification rests with the surgeons, who will need some grouping of the deviations for a reasonable approach to repair.

In necropsied patients with congenital heart disease, approximately 12% are affected by transposition, but in some series the incidence may be as high as 18% or 21%.[5] Since many children born with transposition die soon after birth, the contribution of this anomaly to cardiac infant mortality is high. Ober and Moore[6] attributed 27% of their cardiac patients necropsied in the newborn period to transposition of the great vessels. Approximately half of these had no intracardiac shunts. In clinical material of congenital cardiovascular disorders passing through children's clinics or hospitals, about 5% are transpositions. To congenital heart disease of children under 2 years, transpositions contribute 10%, of those over 2 years, only 0.5%.[7] In the cyanotic group, approximately 8% are affected by transposition of the great vessels.

As will be seen, tremendous efforts have been made to elucidate the pathogenesis of transpositions but little thought has been given to their etiology. Mönckeberg, in 1912 (cited by Bremer[8]), saw in the frequent occurrence of this anomaly in families and kindreds, and in its frequent association with other bodily anomalies, a sign of involvement of the "germ plasma." Actually, there are only a few reports that indicate repetition of this anomaly or of related anomalies in families. In 1871, Kelly (cited by Gänsslen *et al.*[9]) observed in one family 2 cases of transposition confirmed by necropsy. Transposition is, in rare instances, a manifestation of the Holt-Oram syndrome,[10] a dominantly inherited disease entity. There are a number of children on record who had siblings with other congenital heart defects. Transposition of the great vessels in one sibling has been recorded in families in which another sibling had septal defect (Broemser in 1898, cited by Gänsslen *et al.*[9]), patent ductus arteriosus,[11] tetralogy of Fallot,[12,13] dextrocardia[14] or an uncertain congenital heart disease (Lucksch and Stohr, cited by Gänsslen *et al.*[9] and

Noonan *et al.*[15]). In one instance, a patient with corrected transposition and dextrocardia proved by necropsy had 2 siblings with congenital heart disease (Hellmer, cited by Gänsslen *et al.*[9]). The frequency of familial recurrence of congenital heart disease in cases of transposition can be estimated from two series[13,15] in which in 2 of 89 cases a sibling with cyanotic congenital heart disease could be ascertained. Complete and corrected transposition of the great vessels associated with agenesis of the spleen and situs inversus has been stressed repeatedly in recent years.[16-18] In one instance of the asplenia syndrome (Chapter 80), a child with transposition had a sibling with cyanotic congenital heart disease. Necropsy of the sibling revealed persistent atrioventricularis communis, partial transposition of the abdominal viscera and multiple accessory spleens.[19] Since situs inversus is genetically determined in some of the cases, if not in most of them, one may assume a hereditary basis for some of these patients with transposition.

Chromosome changes causing transposition must be considered among the etiologic factors, but complete transposition of the great vessels is relatively rare in autosomal trisomy syndromes. It was found in 6% of necropsied children with trisomy 13-15 and in 2% of those with trisomy 18. It is quite rare in Down syndrome, although it was listed in 2% of necropsied patients with mongolism.[20] The cases of Down syndrome with transposition were all from one series,[21] which consisted chiefly of stillborn and infant mongoloids. Early death of such children explains the absence of transposition in other series that include chiefly older mongoloids. But transposition cannot be ruled out in patients with Down syndrome,[22] and Bar and Ledererova (cited by Hambach[21]) found 2 mongoloids among 26 cases of transposition. Uchida *et al.*[23] reported a mongoloid patient with an XYY sex chromosome complement who showed, at necropsy, transposition of the great vessels with atrial and ventricular septal defects. Minor degrees of transposition, such as overriding aorta or double-outlet right ventricle with pulmonary stenosis, are more frequent in autosomal trisomy syndromes. Overriding aorta was mentioned in 12% and aorta from the right ventricle in 6% of necropsies of trisomy 18 cases. Rogers *et al.*[24] believed that origin of both great vessels from the right ventricle is a common lesion of the trisomy 18 syndrome.

The male sex is affected more often than the female; in the series of Keith *et al.*,[5] 66%, and in other series 75%, were male.[25,26] It is curious that of 6 cases of transposition in mongoloids, 5 were female.[21]

Rubella is certainly a rare cause of transposition. Campbell[27] mentioned 1 case among 136 cardiovascular anomalies due to rubella. Stuckey[28] attributed 1 transposition to this infection, but it seems that the mother had rubella too late to account for this profound disturbance of cardiac development. Transposition of the great vessels was found in rare cases of the thalidomide embryopathy (p. 92).

The average birth weights of infants with transposition of the great vessels often are somewhat greater than expected for gestational age. Naeye[29] noted a moderately increased cytoplasmic mass in parenchymal cells, hyperplasia in pancreatic islet cells and a relative enlargement of the fetal zone of the adrenal cortex. These cellular abnormalities resemble, to a certain extent, changes found in children of diabetic mothers, but transpositions have not been obvious in children of diabetic mothers.[29] The relationship of transposition to diabetes in grandparents[15,26] needs further investigation.

Explanation of transposition of the great vessels and of related anomalies of the trunco-conal complex has been of special interest to pathologists, embryologists and clinicians since early times. In contrast to other malformations of the heart or the great vessels that can be "explained" by arrest of development, transpositions of the great vessels represent profound disturbances of the basic architecture of the heart. Tremendous efforts have been made to find a unitary concept for the great variety of malformations connected with this complex according to various principles. Unfortunately, no explanation of pathogenesis has been generally accepted and it would take a book of its own to do justice to the differing theories. To get a clear picture of the authors' opinions and presentations, the reader is referred to the original publications or to abbreviated interpretations that have appeared in the medical literature.[1-5,30-33]

Early anatomists explained transposition as a lack of the spiral twisting of the large vessels around each other or as abnormal division of the truncus arteriosus. Rokitansky,[1] in 1874, developed a theory of transposition based on the embryologic knowledge of his time. He assumed that the truncus septum originates posteriorly on the left and grows toward the right anterior wall of the truncus in a curved line, with the convexity directed forward. The normal aorta was thought to be on the concave side of this septum, i.e., in the right posterior position and the pulmonary artery in the left anterior position. A faulty origin or a faulty direction of the septum would result in positional changes of the vessels. The ventricular septum was thought to grow backward from the left anterior aspect of the aorta around its right circumference, forming the pars membranacea on the right posterior wall of the aorta. By abnormal origin and course of the truncus septum, by change of its convexity and by abnormal course of the ventricular septum, the relative positions of the aorta and pulmonary artery could be altered and each vessel planted in either ventricle. There are many permutations possible in this scheme and many corrected and uncorrected forms of transposition can be explained in this way. Detailed presentations of Rokitansky's theory can be found in the publications of Herxheimer[30] and Harris and Farber.[3] This theory had to be revised when it was recognized that at the distal end of the truncus the aorta is in the anterior position and the pulmonary artery in the posterior position. To achieve this change of position, the truncus septum, formed from two truncus ridges, had to descend in a clockwise spiral of 225 degrees from the origin of the sixth aortic arches toward the heart. If the spiraling were limited to 45 degrees or less, the aorta would be in the right anterior position and the pulmonary artery in the left posterior position, i.e., the great vessels would be transposed. This again "explained" transposition of the great vessels. Subsequently, various modifications were developed, but the most elaborate theory of transposition and related malformations of the heart was established by Spitzer[2] in 1923. This theory was the outgrowth of Spitzer's original concept of the development of the normal heart in terrestrial vertebrates. His publication entitled "Über den Bauplan des normalen und missbildeten Herzens. Versuch einer philogenetischen Theorie" represents a monograph of 191 pages. A translation into English of the essential passages was made by Lev and Vass.[34] According to Spitzer, the partition of the vertebrate heart into a left arterial and a right venous half commences with the replacement of the gills by the lungs. The fishes have a simple, purely venous heart without longitudinal septation. The septum appears first in the lung fishes, develops further in the amphibia and reptiles, until in the crocodiles two completely separated atria and chambers are formed. There, from each of the two chambers, a special aorta originates and through their communication the blood is still partially mixed. Only in the warm-blooded birds and mammals is the separation of both circulations perfected. Some transpositions of the great vessels would appear like atavistic reversions to the reptilian condition in which two aortic trunks normally are present, one arising from the left ventricle, the other from the right. The pulmonary artery also originates from the right ventricle but in a more ventral position than the right aorta and separated from it by a ridge, identified as the crista supraventricularis. Normally, the lost right aorta is represented in the human heart by a niche in the wall of the right ventricle, located between the crista and the base of the left (anterior) cusp of the tricuspid valve. To achieve separation of the pulmonary and systemic circulations, the heart tube must undergo, according to Spitzer,[2] a torsion of 180 degrees at its arterial end and the septum, when formed, would be similarly rotated. This would produce the desired direction of blood flow, but since the heart is fixed on both ends, a rotation on one end would lead to a counter-rotation at the other end. To prevent the nullification of the effects of torsion on the arterial end by the countertorsion at the venous end, one must assume that the countertorsion occurs at a point peripheral to the point of division between pulmonary and systemic veins, so that this torsion would affect only the systemic veins. The hypothesis further assumes connection of the atria first in series, then in parallel; initial position of the pulmonary venous ostium proximal to that of the cava; formation of an acutely kinked ventricular bow; establishment of a transverse ventricular septum in the plane of the kink; and secondary transformation of the transverse into a longitudinal septum by torsion of the septal plane in the longitudinal axis of both limbs.[34] Originally, Spitzer's theory was concerned only with the development of the normal heart, but subsequently he found that it was applicable to congenital malformations. He considered four types of transposition (Fig. 57-1). Type I is the anomaly commonly called tetralogy of Fallot (p. 494), characterized by a small defect of the ventricular septum with a

Fig. 57-1.—Diagrams showing four types of transpositions of the great vessels described by A. Spitzer.[2]

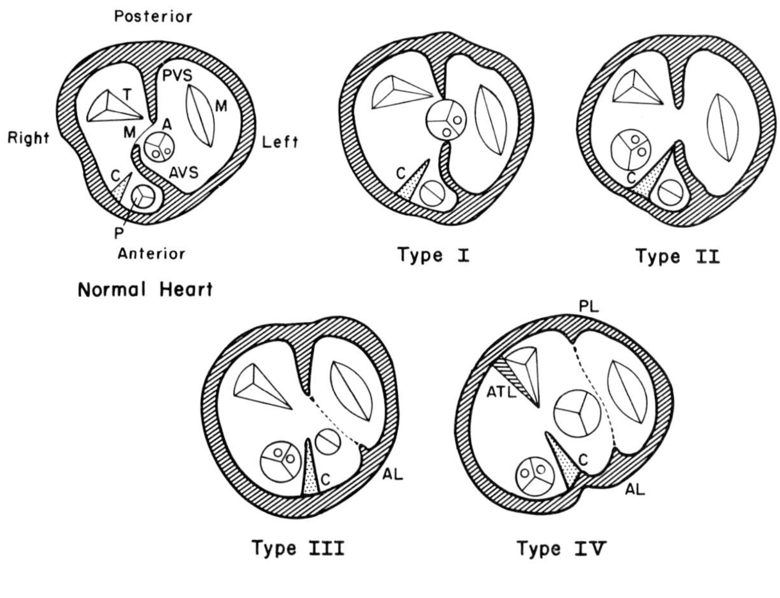

dextroposed overriding aorta that communicates with both ventricles. The aortic ostium lies behind that of the pulmonary artery, which is narrow and often bicuspid. The pulmonary conus of the right ventricle is separated posteriorly from the aortic ostium by a protruding ridge, the crista supraventricularis. In type II, both arteries arise from the right ventricle, the aorta lying to the right of a narrow pulmonary artery. The septal defect is larger. This anomaly is called simple transposition of the aorta into the right ventricle. Type III represents the common type of "crossed" or complete transposition where the aorta arises from the right and the pulmonary artery from the left. The aorta is at the right of and anterior to the pulmonary artery. The septal defect is large. There are two subgroups. In group IIIA, the VSD is so large that a cor biatriatum univentricularis exists, whereas in group IIIB "the septum-forming force" is so increased that no VSD results. The ostium of the pulmonary artery may be narrow or wide. Type IV, called mixed transposition, shows the pulmonary and tricuspid ostia moved into the left ventricle, whereas the aortic ostium is located in a small right ventricle, anterior to and to the right of the pulmonary ostium. The VSD appears relatively small, but no complete septum has developed. The pulmonary ostium is large.

Spitzer[2] assumed a phylogenic "cause" for transposition, an arrest in development at a lower phylogenic level, related to but not identical with that of the reptiles. The basic anomalies in transposition are a lesser torsion (or detorsion) of the heart tube and incomplete migration and fusion of both primary septa. The anomalies represent a return, further development and fixation of certain tendencies common to the ancestral type of both reptiles and mammals. In malformations, a combination of specifically mammalian features with those more characteristic of other branches of the common ancestral tree is possible. Ontogenic forces may initiate and complete normal or pathologic phenomena that are phylogenically "preordained."[34]

This short exposition does not do justice to Spitzer's theory, which includes many detailed facts and observations of comparative and pathologic anatomy not mentioned here. If one can accept Spitzer's[2] basic tenets, his theory represents a logical system that can interpret many, though not all, forms of transposition. It also furnishes a basis for an understanding of such related cardiovascular malformations as the tetralogy of Fallot, double aortic ostium, corrected transposition and others.

Although Spitzer's theory was accepted by many investigators, there also were many dissenters. The value of phylogenic explanations in the field of congenital malformations has been questioned. Pernkopf and Wirtinger[35] insisted that the ontogeny of a human malformation can be understood only by comparison of the anomaly with the known ontogenic facts. They asserted that the heart tube is rotated around its axis in two phases, each with its own countertorsion, one in the region of the atrial canal and one in the region of the semilunar valves. The two are independent of each other and in transposition the semilunar torsion fails to take place. Doerr[36] could not accept the theory of Pernkopf and Wirtinger. He believed that transposition can be brought about by abnormal junction of the bulbo-truncal septum with the ventricular septum. The wall and septum of the bulbo-truncus form an entity. Incomplete bulbo-truncus rotation is the essential feature of transposition.

According to Bremer,[37] the lower part of the bulbus cordis is transformed into the right ventricle by the outgrowth of sinusoids sprouting from the convex surface of the heart tube, which points caudad, laterad and ventrad in the normal embryo of the fifth week. The deep sinusoidal invasion causes the corresponding walls of the bulb to bulge and assume the shape of the right ventricle. If the sharpest curve points downward and backward, continued growth in this dorsal direction would meet the opposition of the right atrium and septum transversum, and the right ventricle would be forced ventrad. Since the left wall of the embryonic right ventricle is attached to the ventricular canal, such ventral displacement can be accomplished only by a rotary counter-clockwise motion that, when transmitted to the distal bulb, would counteract the normal dextrotorsion and result in transposition.[8]

De la Cruz and da Rocha[33] proposed an ontogenic theory to explain congenital trunco-conal malformations. Their theory is based on investigations of human embryos and the study of pathologic specimens. They considered trunco-conal congenital malformations a result of developmental alterations of the conoventricular flange, the trunco-conal ridges and the primordia of the aortic and pulmonary cusps. They proposed some revisions of the older theories and emphasized that only an arbitrary limit exists between the truncus arteriosus and the conus. There is no clockwise or counterclockwise rotation of the truncus-conus. The trunco-conal ridges appear from the beginning with a clockwise rotation of 180 degrees. No portion of the conus is absorbed into the ventricle. The conus goes into the formation of the cephalic portion of the outflow tracts of both ventricles and the trabecular zone of the right ventricle. The authors stated that these facts are not in agreement with Pernkopf and Wirtinger's[35] findings and discussed application of their theory to the interpretation of the most frequent congenital trunco-conal malformatións such as common truncus, Eisenmenger complex, tetralogy of Fallot, the Taussig-Bing complex and others. Transposition of the great vessels was attributed to complete lack of rotation of the trunco-conal septum.

Van Mierop and Wiglesworth[4] assumed that in transposition of the great vessels without inversion of ventricles the bulboventricular loop develops normally, since the morphology of ventricles and atrioventricular valves is normal. The error seems to lie in the truncus region. Normally, the truncus swellings appear earlier and grow faster than the intercalated valve swellings, but in true transposition there is a reversal of this sequence. If the intercalated valve swellings appear earlier than the truncus swellings and become the major structures in the truncus, they execute the division of the truncus. In contrast, transposition of the great vessels with inversion of the ventricles (corrected transposition) is attributed to inverted formation of the cardiac loop. If subsequently the truncus swellings develop normally relative to the bulboventricular loop, and the trunco-aortic sac divides normally, transposition of the great vessels results, since the position of the truncus swellings in relation to the trunco-aortic sac is identical with that occurring in transposition without ventricular inversion. This theory[4] reduces inversion of the ventricles associated with transposition of the great vessels to a single embryologic error.

The diversity of theories of transposition is bewildering. It must be realized that most of these interpretations are attempts to reconcile known facts of phylogeny or ontogeny with pathologic findings obtained in postnatal life. It is obvious that there exists a tremendous gap between the beginnings of abnormal morphology in the embryo and end results that has been bridged chiefly by speculation. One must admire the learning and sagacity of the investigators, their knowledge of human and comparative anatomy and their ability to think, but it is not easy to follow their speculations, in which fact and theory are so closely intermingled. As Bremer[37] wrote frankly after such a hypothetical explanation: "However, with all these theories, it may still be said that the ultimate cause of the transposition of the great vessels of the heart is as yet unknown. All types seem to be derived from chance variations in the shape of the growing heart tube in a constricted space." Owing to the rarity of transposition in human hearts, there are no prospects of systematic studies of this anomaly in human embryos.

It is possible, however, to do embryologic studies in animals. A beginning in this direction was made by Shaner,[38] who examined 20,000 pig embryos and recovered 48 distinctly abnormal hearts. Among these were some in early stages of transposition. He found complete transposition in an 18-mm. pig embryo, and believed that the "master defect" was not in the heart but outside it, above the semilunar valves and in the truncus arteriosus, as assumed by Doerr[36] after study of human hearts. It appeared that the anomaly was brought about by a delayed descent of the aortopulmonary septum in an otherwise normal heart. Owing to this delay, the tips of the descending aortopulmonary septum do not meet the proper conus cushions, which have undergone their normal rotation before they joined these tips. Another type of transposition may originate at an earlier embryonic stage when the ventricles are reversed by a twist of the early ventricular loop to the left instead of the usual twist to the right. When normal septation occurs later, the atria retain their normal position, whereas the ventricles are reversed. The right atrium will discharge into the left ventricle and through it into the aorta. In another form of transposition, both the aorta and pulmonary artery arise from the right ventricle. Shaner found two early stages of this form in pig embryos and established that this anomaly begins early when the aorta still arises from the right ventricle. There was an early "breakdown" of the ventricular muscular septum, with enlargement of the foramen and subsequent hypertrophy of the crista and the moderator band. A pseudoseptum was formed. The larger part of the right ventricle to the right of this pseudoseptum emptied into the aorta, the smaller portion of the right ventricle and the entire left ventricle into the pulmonary artery. This would resemble a transposition with overriding pulmonary artery.

Examination of large numbers of mammalian embryonic hearts may thus occasionally yield hearts with developing malformations. The process of collecting abnormal hearts can now be speeded up by modern teratologic methods. It has become possible to produce transposition of the great vessels in rats by trypan blue injections.[39,40] When efforts comparable to those made by investigators of the past are made along experimental lines in the future, a better understanding of these baffling problems can be expected. Concepts such as torsion, countertorsion, detorsion, rotation, absorption, fixation of some parts and movability of others represent, at best, symbolic and auxiliary terms for the end effect of cell growth and differentiation in certain areas of the heart occurring at times when direct observation in man is not possible. Animal experiments could teach us a great deal about the factual growth changes during development that appear to the observer of human material obtained after birth as faulty "movements" of tubes and septa.

Monie *et al.*[41] made an embryologic study of transposition of the great vessels and other cardiovascular abnormalities induced by trypan blue in rats. The injections of trypan blue were given on either the eighth or ninth day of pregnancy and fetuses were removed from the eleventh to the twenty-second day of pregnancy. Histologic sections and wax plate reconstructions were made from 40 experimental fetuses. With the method used, 30% of 226 embryos examined showed abnormalities of the heart and great vessels. In addition to transposition, anomalies of the tricuspid and mitral valves as well as dextrocardia were encountered often. The hearts of embryos removed on the eleventh day, i.e., 2 or 3 days after the teratogenic insult, resembled those of controls. The same generally was true for embryos of the twelfth day, but in some cases the atrioventricular canal appeared narrow or the common pulmonary vein terminated in the right horn of the sinus venosus, indicating possible inversion of the atria. In several embryos the appearance of the branchial arch arteries was delayed. These were the first anomalies detectable in damaged embryos. More deviations from the normal were seen in embryos of the thirteenth, fourteenth and fifteenth days, i.e., 5–7 days after injection of trypan blue. There were some embryos whose truncus still followed a sinuous path and in others the region of the trunco-bulbar junction was so sinistrally placed that it communicated with both the left and right ventricles. Separation of the aortic and pulmonary trunks was delayed and minimal spiraling of the trunco-bulbar cushions was noted in some embryos. The tricuspid was not developed in several of these embryos and the mitral was absent in some. In such cases, the atrioventricular cushions usually were large and misshapen and the corresponding atria were distended. Dextrocardia was recognized in several specimens, accompanied by inversion of the ventricles or by absence of the mitral or tricuspid valve in some cases. Occasionally, isolated dextrocardia, complete situs inversus and partial situs inversus occurred. In sixteenth and seventeenth day fetuses, delayed separation of the aorta and pulmonary trunk accompanied by patency of the interventricular foramen was recognized and in eighteenth to twenty-second day embryos transposition of the great vessels, VSD, dextrocardia and absence of the tricuspid were the most frequent anomalies noted.

Monie *et al.*[41] described many other details of "clinical importance" in these fetuses and summarized their findings as follows: "Hearts with transposition of the great vessels were usually characterized by shortness of the aorta and pulmonary trunk, cranial location of the aortic valve, displacement of the coronary arteries and a channel or 'track' extending from the cranial portion of the right ventricle to the commencement of the transposed pulmonary trunk. Inadequate expansion of the atrioventricular ring about the 12th or 13th day of gestation possibly leads to deformity of the atrioventricular cushions and to absence or stenosis of the tricuspid or mitral valves. Sinuosity of the truncus arteriosus seen in many 13th day and older embryos of the trypan blue series is considered a significant factor in the development of transposition of the great vessels." Owing to sinistral location of the truncus whose lumen lay over the cranial edge of the ventricular septum and to minimal spiraling of the trunco-bulbar cushions, the dorsally placed pulmonary trunk communicated directly with the left ventricle, whereas the ventrally located aorta retained its connection with the right ventricle. Thus, on the fourteenth or fifteenth day (or about 6 days after injection of trypan blue and 7 or 8 days before birth) the essential elements for complete transposition were present and recognizable. Aside from detailed morphologic observations, it was of interest that embryos from treated mothers usually were smaller than controls, cardiovascular abnormalities observed in litter mates were commonly dissimilar and males predominated (57%) over female fetuses with transposition.

The early changes actually observed in embryos and fetuses exposed to a single teratogenic insult il-

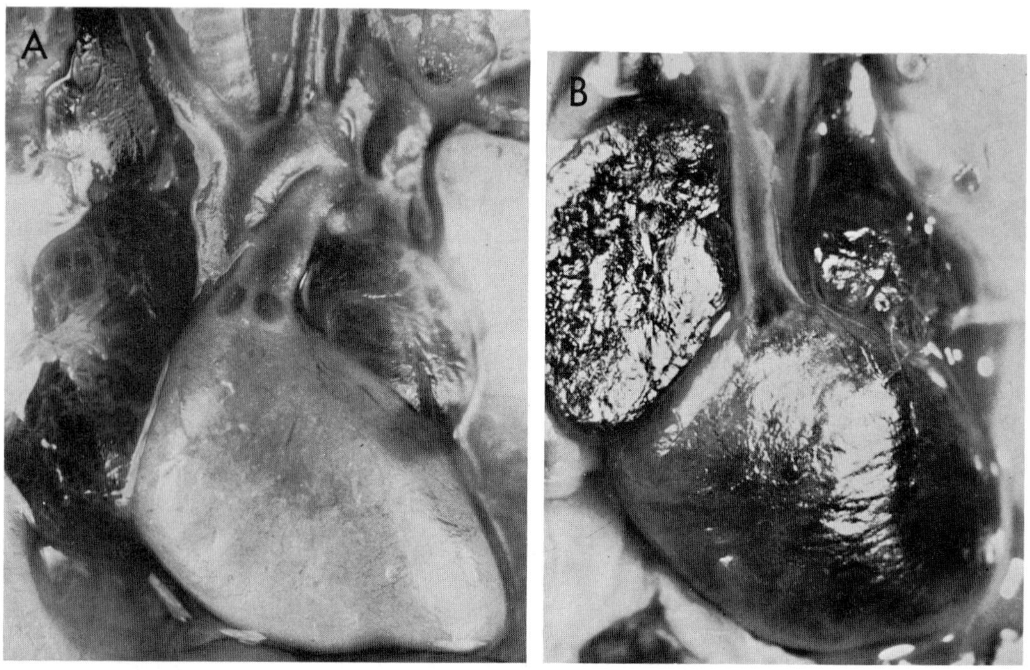

Fig. 57-2. – **A,** heart of a newborn control rat fetus showing the pulmonary artery leaving the heart ventral to the aorta and spiraling of the great vessels. **B,** transposition of the great vessels in a newborn rat produced by trypan blue injection on the ninth day of gestation. The aorta is anterior to the pulmonary artery and there is no spiraling of the great vessels.

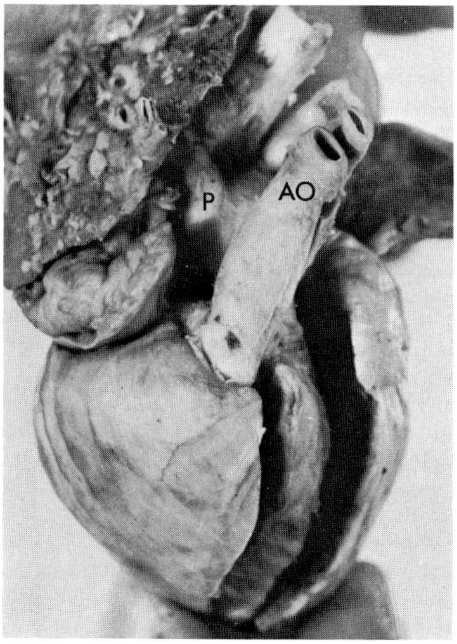

Fig. 57-3.—Human heart. Transposition of the great vessels, with aorta (*AO*) leaving the right ventricle ventral to the pulmonary artery (*P*).

lustrate the beginnings of the malformations of the transposition series, but even in rat experiments the first deviations are not recognized until about 4 days after the teratogenic injection. There could be less obvious changes on the cellular level before the twelfth day that have not been discovered yet, but an approach has been made by the experiments by Monie *et al.*[41] toward an understanding of early—though not the earliest—morphogenetic changes leading to transposition. These experiments showed that rather-well-defined external interference can throw the normal growth processes of the developing heart into disorder and that transposition of the great vessels can occur under such conditions as well as anomalies of the aortic arch system or of the ventricles and atria. At present, we consider these differences as "chance variations," but only a beginning has been made in mammalian experimental teratology. In the future, it may become possible to find teratogenic agents that lead to transposition with great regularity. Then it will be possible also to observe directly in mammalian embryos the abnormal cellular processes of growth and differentiations that result in transposition of the great vessels.

From a practical point of view, a simplified classification by Keith *et al.*[5] seems useful. In necropsies they found a closed ventricular septum in 57%, ventricular septal defect (VSD) in 32%, VSD and pulmonary stenosis in 7% and intact ventricular septum with pulmonary stenosis in 4% of their patients with transposition. Lev *et al.*[42] distinguished transpositions with normal and those with abnormal atrioventricular (A-V) orifices. In the first group, 35% of a total of 147 hearts examined had intact ventricular septa, 37% had VSD and 5% had pulmonary stenosis. Cor biatriatum triloculare accounted for 3% and single ventricle with small outlet chamber for 5% of the cases. A total of 16% had abnormal A-V orifices, such as tricuspid stenosis or atresia, mitral stenosis or atresia and common A-V orifice. Complete transposition with mitral stenosis or with common A-V orifice was found associated with pulmonary stenosis, whereas transposition with tricuspid stenosis or atresia, or with common ventricle, or single ventricle and small outlet chamber was associated with increased pulmonary flow. It is of interest in this context that in the experimental work of Monie *et al.*[41] more A-V malformations were found in embryos than transposition of the great vessels. It is possible that some embryos and fetuses with A-V anomalies are eliminated before birth. Elliott *et al.*[43] analyzed 60 cases of complete transposition of the great vessels, but they excluded from their survey cases of transposition with single ventricle, with atretic A-V valves and with straddling pulmonary trunk. Interatrial communications were present in all patients with a valvar competent patent foramen in one half and a small atrial defect in the other half. The ductus arteriosus was patent in 57% of the cases and a VSD in 37%. In 3 instances, a left ventricular-right atrial communication was found. The aorta was only exceptionally located anterior to the pulmonary trunk (3% of the cases). The relationship of the great vessels usually was oblique (65%) and less often side-to-side (32%). With one exception, the right coronary artery arose above the posterior aortic sinus and the left coronary artery above the left aortic sinus. If the aorta is transposed and the pulmonary artery overrides the ventricular septum (Taussig-Bing complex), the clinical picture is domi-

Fig. 57-4.—Transposition of the great vessels with aorta (*AO*) anteriorly placed. A coronary artery leaving the root of the aorta (**arrow**) indicates the place of the ventricular septum.

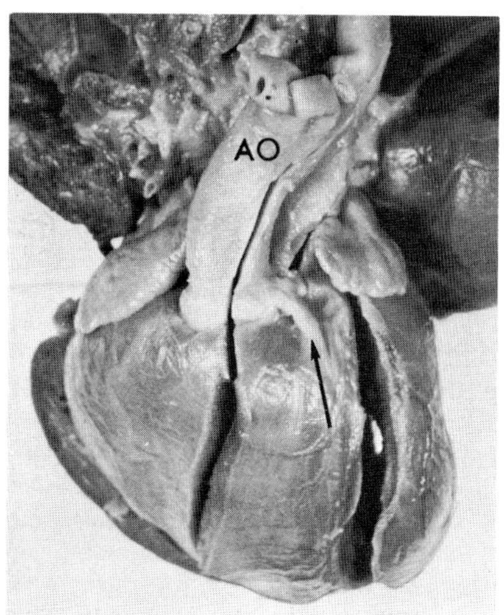

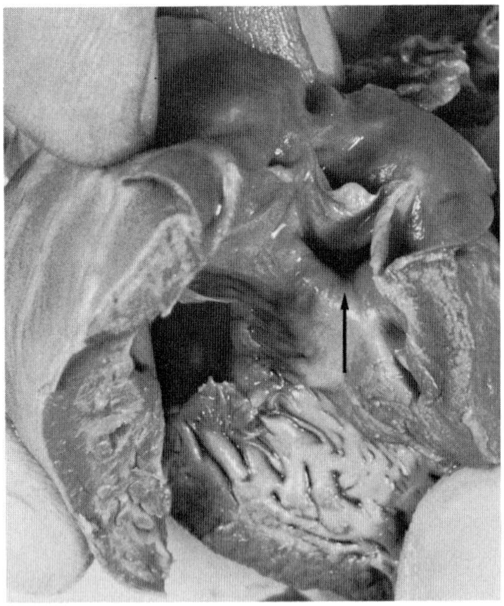

Fig. 57-5. – Supracristal ventricular septal defect of the Taussig-Bing type (**arrow**) seen from the right ventricle and below a pulmonary valve.

nated by pulmonary hypertension. There always is a VSD. The semilunar valves usually are side by side.[5] The pulmonary trunk receives blood from both ventricles and the oxygen saturation of its blood is greater than that of the aorta or the peripheral arteries. The aorta is supplied by venous blood from the right ventricle and in part by oxygenated blood entering the right side through the ventricular septal defect. The pulmonary arterioles show narrowing of the lumina, resulting in increased resistance to pulmonary blood flow, which may be responsible for a reasonable balance of flow to the two circulations and for maintenance of life for some years.[25]

Associated malformations. – Right and double aortic arch, coarctation of the aorta, interruption of the aortic arch, pulmonary stenosis, abnormal A-V orifices, juxtaposition of the atrial appendages, endocardial fibroelastosis and abnormal venous return occur in some cases.[15,42,43] The combination of agenesis of the spleen with congenital malformations of the heart and transposition of the great vessels has been known since Breschet, in 1826 (cited by Ivemark[16]), described a case. This syndrome has attracted great interest in recent times (Chapter 80). Ivemark[16] found transposition in 27 of 69 cases of splenic agenesis reported in the literature or observed by himself. Gilbert *et al.*[44] listed 52 cases of transposition in 85 cases of splenic agenesis, so that a high correlation of these anomalies exists. That this syndrome is related to situs inversus (Chapter 21) has been mentioned before. Cases of asplenia and transposition may be combined with atrial and ventricular septal defects, cor biloculare or triloculare, common atrioventricular valve, abnormal venous return, transposition of the stomach or liver, abnormal lobation of the lungs and so forth. Mongolism and transposition is a rare combination[21,22] (p. 516). A mongoloid child with transposition who had no spleen has been observed, linking the asplenia syndrome with that of mongolism, and in others atrioventricularis communis and large septal defects were combined with transposition.[21] That transposition can occur among the malformations characteristic of trisomies 13-15 and 18 has been mentioned before (p. 516). But, in general, children with transposition seen in cardiac clinics do not have congenital malformations in other systems. Occasionally, craniorachischisis, meningocele,[45] porencephaly,[15] diaphragmatic hernia, harelip, cleft palate and anomalies of the urogenital tract have been observed.[21]

Symptoms. – Most infants with transposition have normal birth weights and some are even overweight,[29] which suggests that the abnormal arterial arrangement need not interfere with normal intrauterine growth. But patients surviving infancy show marked stunting of growth.[46]

Cyanosis is present at birth in most, and at the age of 3 months in all children with complete transposition. If, in the newborn period, a large patent ductus permits flow of oxygenated blood from the left ventricle through the pulmonary artery to the descending aorta, the lower extremities will be less cyanotic than the upper parts of the body.[47] A similar situation may be due to preductal coarctation or interrupted aortic arch,[48] resulting in "cyanose en pèlerine," i.e., cyanosis above the legs. In infants with transposition, cardiac failure occurs between 1 and 4 months in approximately two-thirds of the cases. Dyspnea, cough, enlargement of the heart and liver, edema, gallop rhythm, etc., appear within the first few weeks in most of the cases. Keith *et al.*[5] pointed out that cardiac failure begins, as a rule, in transposition later than in congenital aortic atresia. Since it takes some time to develop clubbing of the fingers and toes, this symptom is absent in those who die in early infancy, but patients surviving the first half year do develop clubbing. Such children show retarded growth and generalized weakness. Auscultation does not result in typical findings. The murmurs are inconstant and in only one-third of the cases a loud and harsh murmur is heard that is attributable to a VSD or pulmonary stenosis. If the septum is closed, there may be no or only faint murmurs.[5,13] Apical diastolic murmurs are common.[5] Roentgenograms of typical patients are characterized in the anteroposterior view by a narrow vascular shadow, since the pulmonary artery runs behind the aorta,[49] but the vascular shadow is wide in oblique views. The heart is described as large and egg-shaped, with the long axis oblique to the left downward. The pulmonary vasculature is increased in the majority of cases, but if the ventricular septum is intact and the ductus arteriosus closed, it is normal.[13,50] Within a few weeks, all cardiac chambers become enlarged. Angiocardiography can demonstrate dextrotransposition or levotransposition of the aorta, communications between the two circulations, single or common ventricle and pulmonary artery obstruction.[51]

Clinically, transposition with pulmonary stenosis and VSD resembles tetralogy of Fallot, but cyanotic spells and loss of consciousness are rare, squatting is unusual, the heart is enlarged radiologically and pulmonary vascularity is slightly increased.[52]

It is obvious that survival depends on associated defects that permit interchange of blood between the two circulations. Thus, transposition represents a paradoxic situation, since, to a certain extent, additional cardiovascular defects improve the prospect for life. Keith *et al.*[5] quoted an equal average life expectancy of 3.5 months for patients with transposition with closed ventricular septum and those with VSD. But if VSD is combined with pulmonary stenosis, the life expectancy is 17.6 months and with intact ventricular septum and pulmonary stenosis it is 46 months. A large VSD resembling cor biatriatum triloculare is compatible with survival for several decades, particularly if the transposed pulmonary artery assumes a certain dextroposition. Intact ventricular septum with a large atrial septal defect is favorable; intact ventricular and intact atrial septa result in the least tolerated situation. But with transposition and ventricular septal defect,[13] presence of an atrial septal defect reduces the life expectancy.[53] VSD or single ventricle with high pulmonary resistance or pulmonary stenosis may permit survival for several decades. Patent ductus usually is an unfavorable adjunct.[5] Cardiac failure, anoxia and cerebral complications are the most frequent causes of death.

Oxygen and digitalis represent the medical therapeutic measures but, in most cases, the outlook is so unfavorable that surgical corrections are attempted. Keith *et al.*[5] enumerated eight types of operations devised for transposition. It seems that the most satisfactory results have been obtained in young children with creation of an atrial septal defect leading to a common atrium and mixing of venous and arterialized blood. Operation particularly helps children with intact ventricular septum.[13,54,63] Baffes'[55] procedure directs the right pulmonary vein blood into the right atrium and shunts inferior vena caval blood into the left atrium. In children over 2 years, an intra-atrial baffle operation[56] has been successful. A pericardial segment is sewed into the left and right atrium, which directs blood of the superior and inferior venae cavae into the left ventricle and blood of the pulmonary veins into the right ventricle and from there to the aorta. This operation is best suited for the most common situation, namely transposition with intact ventricular septum.[5] If there is a VSD, creation of an atrial septal defect is not recommended.[53]

Corrected Transposition of the Great Vessels

In corrected transposition, the aorta lies anterior to the pulmonary artery but arises from a ventricle that receives oxygenated blood. The pulmonary artery located behind the aorta originates from a ventricle containing venous blood. Both vessels ascend in a parallel fashion without the normal twist around each other.

Corrected transposition is said to be a very rare anomaly, but Anderson *et al.*[57] reported 17 cases, Schiebler *et al.*[58] and Ellis *et al.*[59] 30 cases observed in individual hospital units. Several patients are on record who had a sibling with congenital heart disease. In one of these cases, the parents were consanguineous.[58] Whereas in some previous series the sexes were equally represented,[62] summarization of subsequent reports[57-59] showed that 55 of 80 cases (69%) were male. Various concepts of the pathogenesis of corrected transpositions have been developed. De la Cruz *et al.*[60] explained inversion of the ventricles as changes limited to the bulboventricular loop. The position of the ventricles does not correspond with the viscero-atrial situs. Grant[61] believed that deviations in the timing or distribution of growth potentials could result in coilings of the primary heart tube, with abnormal positioning of the otherwise normal cardiac components.

There are several possibilities of correction of the derangement of the great vessels but in all corrected cases the pulmonary veins enter the heart on the side on which the aorta leaves. The relatively common form, called "bulboventricular inversion," shows the aorta arising from the left side (levotransposition) from a ventricle that has anatomic characteristics of a right ventricle, namely a tricuspid valve, extensive trabeculation and a crista supraventricularis. Thus, of the four heart chambers, only the ventricles are inverted, the atria receiving the usual blood return. Since the aorta and the pulmonary veins both lie on the left side, the transposition is corrected. The pulmonary artery lies behind the aorta. In another form, which probably is the next in frequency, all chambers are properly located, the only abnormality being that the aorta originates anterior to the pulmonary artery and the vessels ascend without the normal twist. This type is called corrected transposition with "bulbus inversion." In other rare forms in which the aorta arises from the right side and the pulmonary artery from the left, the situation is corrected by "atrial inversion" when the atrium receiving the pulmonary veins lies on the right side or by "atrioventricular inversion" when both the atrium receiving the pulmonary veins and the ventricle containing the mitral valve are also located on the right. But, as mentioned before, there are other positional variations that can be considered corrected transpositions,[5] and the variability of defects is further increased by associated malformations, which are the rule. Pure corrected transposition of the "bulboventricular inversion" type without ventricular septal and other associated defects is rare but some cases have been reported. Schiebler *et al.*[58] observed such a patient who had no symptoms of his anomaly before death at age 60 years. This patient was 1 of 33 necropsied patients, but this ratio may not be representative of the true incidence of pure corrected transposition, since such patients could go through life undiagnosed. Another patient of this type diagnosed on the basis of chest films was reported by Ellis *et al.*[59]

The most common associated lesions are ventricular septal defect, anomalies of the left atrioventricular valve usually causing incompetence, pulmonary valvar stenosis and disturbances of atrioventricular conduction. Atrial septal defects are less common. Patent ductus arteriosus, abnormal coronaries, coarctation of the aorta and other cardiovascular anomalies occur. Corrected transposition with situs inversus is compatible with a prolonged life.[58,62] Extracardiac associated malformations are rare in patients with corrected transposition.[57,58]

Symptoms are not specific. They may be absent in uncomplicated corrected transposition and depend on associated cardiovascular anomalies in complicated cases. Ellis *et al.*[59] suspect corrected transposition in cases of congenital heart block, mesocardia or dextrocardia without visceral situs inversus and congenital insufficiency of the left atrioventricular valve. Anteroposterior roentgenograms show a narrow waist at the base of the heart, absence of a pulmonary-artery knob and an enlarged left atrium.[58] Electrocardiograms[5,58] aid in the diagnosis and angiocardiography is diagnostic.[59]

Life expectancy is better than that of complete (noncorrected) transposition and has been estimated to average 14 years,[62] with some patients known to have reached the fifth and sixth decades.[58]

Treatment depends on symptoms, which, in turn, depend on associated cardiovascular malformations. Many associated lesions now can be corrected surgically, but anomalous coronary arteries, defects of the atrioventricular valves and a tendency to develop complete heart block represent high risks.[5,58]

REFERENCES

1. Rokitansky, C. F.: *Die Defecte der Scheidewände des Herzens* (Vienna: W. Braumüller, 1874).
2. Spitzer, A.: Über den Bauplan des normalen und missbildeten Herzens. Versuch einer philogenetischen Theorie, Virchows Arch. path. Anat. 243:81, 1923.
3. Harris, J. S., and Farber, S.: Transposition of the great cardiac vessels, Arch. Path. 28:428, 1939.
4. Van Mierop, L. H. S., and Wiglesworth, F. W.: Pathogenesis of transposition complexes. II. Anomalies due to faulty transfer of the posterior great artery. III. True transposition of the great vessels, Am. J. Cardiol. 12:226, 1963.
5. Keith, J. D., Rowe, R. D., and Vlad, P. (eds.): *Heart Disease in Infancy and Childhood* (2d ed.; New York: The Macmillan Company, 1966).
6. Ober, W. B., and Moore, T. E., Jr.: Congenital cardiac malformations in the neonatal period; an autopsy study, New England J. Med. 253:271, 1955.
7. Stuckey, D.: Pattern of congenital heart disease in infancy and childhood, M. J. Australia 2:433, 1954.
8. Bremer, J. L.: Transposition of the aorta and the pulmonary artery; embryologic study of its causes, Arch. Path. 34:1016, 1942.
9. Gänsslen, M., Lambrecht, K., and Werner, M.: Die kongenitalen Missbildungen des Herzens, in *Handbuch der Erbbiologie des Menschen* (Berlin: Springer, 1940), Vol. 4, pt. 2, pp. 198–217.
10. Lewis, K. B., Bruce, R. A., Baum, D., and Motulsky, A. G.: The upper limb-cardiovascular syndrome. An autosomal dominant genetic effect on embryogenesis, J.A.M.A. 193: 1080, 1955.
11. McKeown, T., MacMahon, B., and Parsons, C. G.: Familial incidence of congenital malformation of heart, Brit. Heart J. 15:273, 1953.
12. Polani, P. E., and Campbell, M.: Aetiological study of congenital heart disease, Ann. Human Genet. 19:209, 1955.
13. Gallaher, M. E., Fyler, D. C., and Lindesmith, G. G.: Transposition with intact ventricular septum, Am. J. Dis. Child. 111:248, 1966.
14. Cockayne, E. A.: Genetics of transposition of viscera, Quart. J. Med. 7:479, 1938.
15. Noonan, J. A., Nadas, A. S., Rudolph, A. M., and Harris, G. B. C.: Transposition of the great arteries; a correlation of clinical, physiologic and autopsy data, New England J. Med. 263:592, 637, 684, 739, 1960.
16. Ivemark, B. I.: Implications of agenesis of the spleen on the pathogenesis of cono-truncus anomalies in childhood, an analysis of the heart malformations in the splenic agenesis syndrome, with fourteen new cases, Acta paediat. 44(supp.):104, 1944.
17. Putschar, W. G. J., and Manion, W. C.: Congenital absence of the spleen and associated anomalies, Am. J. Clin. Path. 26:429, 1956.
18. Terslev, E.: A case of agenesis of the spleen, congenital heart disease and complete situs inversus, Acta paediat. 47:297, 1958.
19. Polhemus, D. W., and Schafer, W. B.: Congenital absence of the spleen; syndrome with atrioventricularis and situs inversus, Pediatrics 9:696, 1952.
20. Warkany, J., Passarge, E., and Smith, L. B.: Congenital malformations in autosomal trisomy syndromes, Am. J. Dis. Child. 112:502, 1966.
21. Hambach, R.: Ein Beitrag zur Frage der Kombination von Habitus mongoloides mit angeborenen Herzmissbildungen, Ann. paediat. 183:77, 1954.
22. Mannheimer, E.: *Morbus Caeruleus* (Basel-New York: S. Karger, 1949).
23. Uchida, I. A., Ray, M., and Duncan, B. P.: 21 trisomy with an XYY sex chromosome complement, J. Pediat. 69:295, 1966.
24. Rogers, T. R., Hagstrom, J. W. C., and Engle, M. A.: Origin of both great vessels from the right ventricle associated with the trisomy-18 syndrome, Circulation 32:802, 1965.
25. Edwards, J. E.: Congenital Malformations of the Heart and Great Vessels, in Gould, S. E. (ed.), *Pathology of the Heart* (Springfield, Ill.: Charles C Thomas, Publisher, 1953), pp. 266–503.
26. Landing, B. H., Nakai, H., Margaretten, W., Kobayashi, N., and Beaudry, P. H.: Some genetic and biochemical implications of congenital heart disease, Quart. Rev. Pediat. 16:160, 1961.
27. Campbell, M.: Place of maternal rubella in the aetiology of congenital heart disease, Brit. M. J. 1:691, 1961.
28. Stuckey, D.: Congenital heart defects following maternal rubella during pregnancy, Brit. Heart J. 18:519, 1956.
29. Naeye, R. L.: Transposition of the great arteries and prenatal growth, Arch. Path. 82:412, 1966.
30. Herxheimer, G.: Missbildungen des Herzens und der grossen Gefässe, in Schwalbe, E. (ed.), *Die Morphologie der Missbildungen des Menschen und der Tiere* (Jena: Gustav Fischer, 1909), Vol. 3, pt. 3.
31. Lev, M., and Saphir, O.: A theory of transposition of arterial trunks based on the phylogenetic and ontogenetic development of the heart, Arch. Path. 39:172, 1945.
32. Mautner, H.: The developmental mechanics of heart malformations, Arch. Pediat. 73:47, 1956.
33. De la Cruz, M. V., and da Rocha, J. P.: An ontogenetic theory for the explanation of congenital malformations involving the truncus and conus, Am. Heart J. 51:782, 1956.
34. Lev, M., and Vass, A.: *The Architecture of Normal and*

Malformed Hearts. A Phylogenetic Theory of Their Development (Springfield, Ill.: Charles C Thomas, Publisher, 1951).
35. Pernkopf, E., and Wirtinger, W.: Das Wesen der Transposition im Gebiete des Herzens; ein Versuch der Erklärung auf entwicklungsgeschichtlicher Grundlage, Virchows Arch. path. Anat. 295:143, 1935.
36. Doerr, W.: Zur Transposition der Herzschlagadern, Virchows Arch. path. Anat. 303:168, 1938.
37. Bremer, J. L.: *Congenital Anomalies of the Viscera. Their Embryological Basis* (Cambridge, Mass.: Harvard University Press, 1957).
38. Shaner, R. B.: Complete and corrected transposition of the aorta, pulmonary artery and the ventricles in pig embryos, and a case of corrected transposition in a child, Am. J. Anat. 88:35, 1951.
39. Wilson, J. G.: Teratogenic activity of several azo dyes chemically related to trypan blue, Anat. Rec. 123:313, 1955.
40. Fox, M. H., and Goss, C. M.: Experimentally produced malformations of the heart and great vessels in rat fetuses. Transposition complexes and aortic arch abnormalities, Am. J. Anat. 102:65, 1958.
41. Monie, I. W., Takacs, E., and Warkany, J.: Transposition of the great vessels and other cardiovascular abnormalities in rat fetuses induced by trypan blue, Anat. Rec. 156: 175, 1966.
42. Lev, M., Alcalde, W. M., and Baffes, T. G.: Pathologic anatomy of complete transposition of the arterial trunks, Pediatrics 28:293, 1961.
43. Elliott, L. P., Anderson, R. C., Tuna, N., Adams, P., Jr., and Neufeld, H. N.: Complete transposition of the great vessels. II. An electrocardiographic analysis, Circulation 27:1118, 1963.
44. Gilbert, E. F., Nishimura, K., and Wedum, B. G.: Congenital malformations of the heart associated with splenic agenesis, Circulation 17:72, 1958.
45. Miskall, E. W., and Fraser, J. A.: Complete transposition of the great cardiac vessels, Ohio M. J. 44:709, 1948.
46. Pung, S., Gottstein, W. K., and Kirsch, E. F.: Complete transposition of great vessels in male aged 18 years, Am. J. Med. 18:155, 1955.
47. Taussig, H. B.: *Congenital Malformations of the Heart* (New York: The Commonwealth Fund, 1947).
48. Peacock, T. B.: *On Malformations of the Human Heart* (2d ed.; London: J. Churchill & Sons, 1866).
49. Fanconi, G.: Die Transposition der Grossen Gefässe, Arch. Kinderh. 95:202, 1932.
50. Carey, L. S., and Elliott, L. P.: Complete transposition of the great vessels, Am. J. Roentgenol. 91:529, 1964.
51. Barcia, A., Kincaid, O. W., Davis, G. D., Kirklin, J. W., and Ongley, P. A.: Transposition of the great arteries. An angiocardiographic study, Am. J. Roentgenol. 100:249, 1967.
52. Mehrizi, A., Rowe, R. D., Hutchins, G. M., and Folger, G. M., Jr.: Transposition of the great vessels with pulmonary stenosis and ventricular septal defect, Bull. Johns Hopkins Hosp. 119:200, 1966.
53. Shaher, R. M.: Prognosis of transposition of the great vessels with and without atrial septal defect, Brit. Heart J. 25:211, 1963.
54. Blalock, A., and Hanlon, C. R.: The surgical treatment of complete transposition of the aorta and the pulmonary artery, Surg., Gynec. & Obst. 90:1, 1950.
55. Baffes, T. G.: A new method for surgical correction of transposition of the aorta and pulmonary artery, Surg., Gynec. & Obst. 102:227, 1956.
56. Mustard, W. T.: Successful two-stage correction of transposition of the great vessels, Surgery 55:469, 1964.
57. Anderson, R. C., Lillehei, C. W., and Lester, R. G.: Corrected transposition of the great vessels of the heart. A review of 17 cases, Pediatrics 20:626, 1957.
58. Schiebler, G. L., Edwards, J. E., Burchell, H. B., DuShane, J. W., Ongley, P. A., and Wood, E. H.: Congenital corrected transposition of the great vessels: A study of 33 cases, Pediatrics 27 (supp.):851–888, 1961, No. 5, Pt II.
59. Ellis, K., Morgan, B. C., Blumenthal, S., and Anderson, D. H.: Congenitally corrected transposition of the great vessels, Radiology 79:35, 1962.
60. De la Cruz, M. V., Espino-Vela, J., Attie, F., and Munoz, L.: An embryologic theory for ventricular inversions and their classification, Am. Heart J. 73:777, 1967.
61. Grant, R. P.: The morphogenesis of corrected transposition and other anomalies of cardiac polarity, Circulation 29:71, 1964.
62. Cardell, B. S.: Corrected transposition of the great vessels, Brit. Heart J. 18:186, 1956.
63. Newfeld, E. A., Eisenberg, R. N., and Young, D.: Transposition of the great arteries. The changing prognosis, Am. J. Dis. Child. 120:320, 1970.

58

Aortic Arch Anomalies

The aortic arches and the vessels derived from them occur in many variations that have attracted the attention of anatomists and pathologists since early times. Since few of these variations cause pathologic manifestations, clinicians have paid little attention to them until relatively recent times. It is true that dysphagia lusoria has long been attributed to an aberrant subclavian artery pressing on the esophagus,[1] but many other types had escaped clinical description until they became recognizable by x-ray methods and amenable subsequently to surgery. In 1964, Stewart *et al.*[2] published an atlas of vascular rings and related malformations of the aortic arch system, with detailed descriptions of the pathologic and roentgenologic aspects of the anomalies.

The incidence of nonpathogenic anomalies of the aortic arch system is high. For instance, aberrant right subclavia is found in 0.5–1% of cadavers observed in dissecting rooms,[3] and other harmless vascular variations also are not too rare. But, quantitatively, pathogenic aortic arch anomalies do not play an important role in cardiovascular diseases of children or adults. Usually, they do not appear as separate entities in hospital or mortality statistics. Abbott[4] listed, in 1,000 necropsies of cardiovascular anomalies, only 30 aortic arch anomalies as primary defects, but there were others that accompanied more serious malformations and are not listed separately. There were 14 right aortic arches (but 21 associated with other defects), 5 double aortic arches, 5 anomalies of the right subclavian, 1 anomaly of the left subclavian, 3 cases of absent aortic arch and 2 cases of common brachiocephalic trunk. Poynter,[3] analyzing a variety of vascular anomalies, found an abnormal right subclavian in 31%, right aortic arch in 9% and double aortic arch in 2% of dissected subjects. This author reviewed the literature of aortic arch anomalies up to 1916, and the references cited occupy 53 pages.

Although an abnormal right subclavian artery, right aortic arch or double aortic arch may be entirely harmless in childhood and in early adulthood, such variations from the normal may become troublesome when arteriosclerosis sets in and the vessels become rigid, causing compression of adjacent organs.

With the advent of cardiac surgery, aortic arch anomalies associated with other cardiovascular malformations have assumed increased importance, since surgical procedures may be greatly influenced by the variations of the vessels originating from the aortic arches.[5] In a series of surgically evaluated arch anomalies, Mahoney and Manning[6] encountered ten varieties. They found that the true vascular rings usually cause severe symptoms that require surgical intervention. Other arch anomalies may cause tracheal or esophageal compression, or both.

To understand the great variety of aortic arch variations, some knowledge of the normal development of the permanent aortic arch system is necessary. Poynter[3] made an excellent review of this subject, and Congdon[7] gave the definitive description of the transformation of the aortic arch system during the development of the human embryo. Edwards[8] established a system of existing and hypothetically possible aortic arch anomalies, explaining them from a common basic pattern.

The aortic arches and some of their anomalies were known to anatomists in the eighteenth century, but it was in the early nineteenth century that the basic pattern of aortic arch development was established by von Baer[9] in 1828 and Rathke in 1832, although some corrections had to be made in later years.[10]

Figure 58-1, *A* shows a hypothetic embryonic pattern of aortic arches, but at no time during mammalian development are all the arches present simultaneously; the fifth pair, which remains rudimentary, is omitted in the diagram. The truncus arteriosus and the ventral aortae are seen near the midline, whereas the dorsal aortae are projected to both sides, uniting caudally in the midline to form the descending aorta. Of the six pairs of aortic arches connecting the ventral with the dorsal aortae in embryonic life, only a limited number of blood channels persist to form the definitive pattern. In Figure 58-1, *B* the first and second aortic arches have disappeared, but both third arches are being used by the internal carotid arteries. The left fourth arch forms an important part of the permanent aortic arch and connects the ascending with the descending aorta. On the right side, the fourth aortic arch is transformed into the proximal portion of the right subclavian artery. The last pair of arches, the pulmonary or sixth, is connected with the pulmonary arteries, but only the left one persists to the time of birth as ductus arteriosus. Figure 58-1, *B*

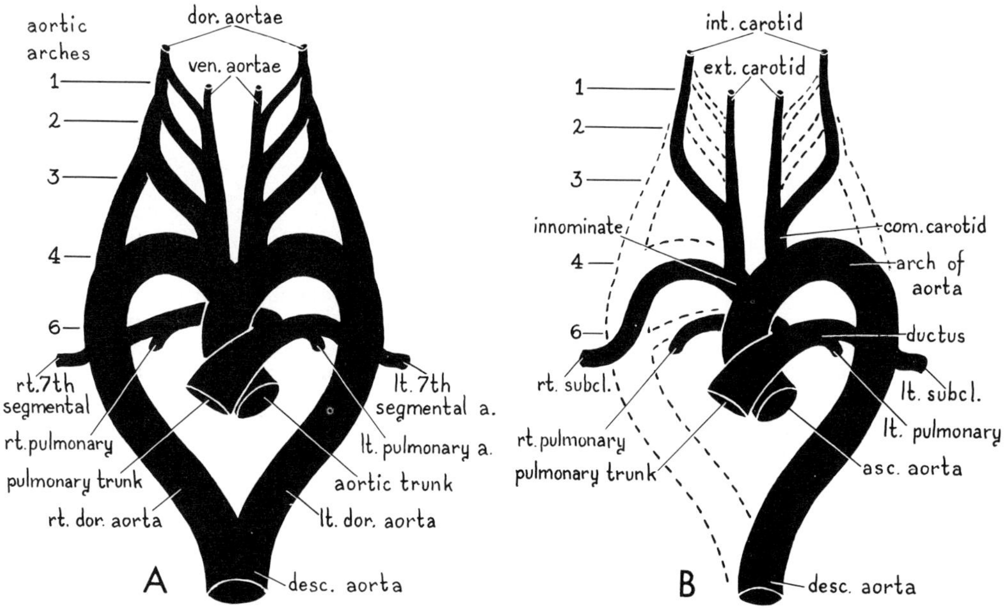

Fig. 58-1. – Diagram of hypothetic embryonic pattern of aortic arches (**A**) and definitive pattern of arteries derived from embryonic aortic arch system (**B**). Parts of embryonic system that underwent complete or partial regression are indicated by broken lines. (From J. G. Wilson and J. Warkany.[14])

shows that large portions of the dorsal aortae are destined for obliteration. On both sides the sections between the third and fourth arches, and on the right side the section between the right subclavian and the descending aorta, disappear. The pulmonary arch distal to the right pulmonary artery normally degenerates also. The first pairs of aortic arches are formed in the fourth week and the definitive pattern (present at birth) is established by the eighth week of intrauterine life.

The forces that determine the obliteration of some channels and the maintenance of others are not known. Some of the changes can be explained by the growth of the cephalic end of the embryo and by the apparent caudad migration of the heart. Hemodynamic forces can be used to interpret alterations of the original basic pattern but such explanations are not convincing. Even less understood are the anomalies of the aortic arch pattern as encountered in man or animals. Heredity plays a role in dextrocardia and the mirror-image right aortic arch associated with it. That heredity also plays a role in some variations of the arteries arising from the aortic arch was shown by Sawin and Edmonds[11] in rabbits. Although there was little indication found in breeding experiments of the segregation characteristic of Mendelian inheritance, there seemed to be evidence that some vascular anomalies are determined by their relation to hereditary regional growth patterns. Some of the variations observed by Sawin and Edmonds, such as anomalous innominate or anomalous left common carotid arteries can cause pathologic manifestations in man. Chromosomal anomalies occasionally result in aortic arch anomalies. Right-sided aortic arch has been observed in trisomies 13-15 and 18, and aberrant right subclavian artery in trisomy 21.[12]

That environmental factors may disturb the development of the aortic arch system was demonstrated experimentally by Wilson and Warkany,[13,14] and several investigators subsequently (Chapter 49). Among the experimental malformations were many variations of the aortic arch system, some of which had been described in human pathology, whereas others had been postulated on theoretic grounds. Such environmental disturbances acting at the time of organogenesis were capable of disorganizing the normal development of embryonic arches and their derivatives. The experiments also showed that teratogenic agents are not specific for any type of arch anomaly. Different methods resulted in similar types of aortic arch anomaly, whereas a specific environmental disturbance such as vitamin A deficiency resulted in a variety of unpredictable aortic arch irregularities. Differing aortic arch anomalies sometimes occurred in the young of the same litter. It appears that once the basic disturbance is produced, the resulting morphologic variation is due to factors that are difficult to ascertain. The position of the embryo in utero may have some influence by determining hemodynamic factors, or its age or the genetic constitution may play a role. An important factor in the morphologic end results is the viability of the injured embryos. For instance, some aortic arch anomalies, such as bilateral absence of the fourth and pulmonary arches, would result in interruption of the blood flow to the lower half of the body and in death of the embryo. Other combinations that do not interfere with intrauterine life may be incompatible with postnatal life. Most of the experimental animals with induced aortic arch anomalies also have associated malformations in other organs and may be eliminated because of them before birth. Thus, a combination of factors probably is responsible for the aortic arch anomalies encountered in man and in animals.

There is little evidence of environmental factors causing aortic arch anomalies in man, but in children damaged by thalidomide, truncus arteriosus, pseudotruncus and patent ductus arteriosus were encountered (p. 92). Foley[15] reported a child with interrupted aortic arch and septal defects whose mother had had a febrile illness when the embryo was 4 weeks old, but no conclusions as to etiology can be drawn from such an isolated case.

In the following pages, some arch anomalies that are of medical interest will be described. Third arch anomalies will be discussed first, to be followed by variations of the fourth and sixth (pulmonary) arches.

Persistence of a Third Aortic Arch

In the absence of both fourth aortic arches, the ascending aorta may pass high into the neck to the level of the larynx, give off the carotid arteries and then turn caudally to form the descending aorta. In such rare cases, the arch of the aorta represents a persisting third embryonic arch. The recurrent laryngeal nerve arising from the vagus in the neck goes directly to the larynx by passing under the third arch (Fig. 58-2). The vessels originating from the aortic arch vary, but the important point is that the apex of the arch may appear in the supraclavicular region of the neck as a pulsating mass that can be mistaken for an aneurysm of the common carotid artery. Only a few cases of this anomaly have been described in the literature, but other instances probably have been observed or gone unrecognized. It is of interest that persistent third arch has been experimentally produced in rats by vitamin A deficiency (Fig. 58-2, *A*).[13,14] Ductus arteriosus on the contralateral side has been noted in such animals as well as in one child.[16]

Beavan and Fatti[16] described the case of a girl 9 years of age with a pulsating swelling of the neck that was clinically diagnosed as an aneurysm of the right common carotid. This swelling grew slowly and reached the size of a pigeon's egg when the child was about 10 years of age. The trachea was pushed to the left and there was shortness of breath on exertion and slight dysphagia on extending the neck. At operation, it was found that the recurrent laryngeal nerve curved around the exposed dilated vessel. The large

Fig. 58-2. – **A,** diagram of persistent left third aortic arch, which ascends into the neck to the level of the larynx and gives off separate external and internal carotid arteries. No fourth arch persists on either side. Pulmonary trunk and enlarged right-sided ductus arteriosus constitute additional communication between the heart and the descending aorta. **B,** drawing of postmortem specimen of the heart and great vessels of a child diagnosed during life as having aneurysm of the common carotid artery. This arterial pattern represents mirror image of that shown in **A**; that is, the right instead of the left third embryonic arch has been retained as the arch of the aorta. (Courtesy of T. E. D. Beavan and L. Fatti[16] and J. G. Wilson and J. Warkany.[14])

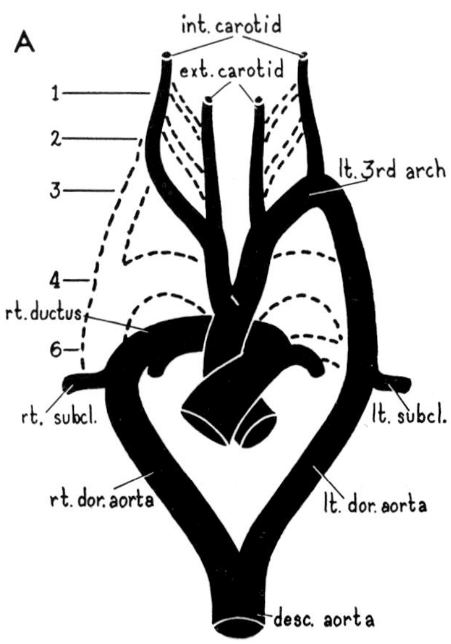

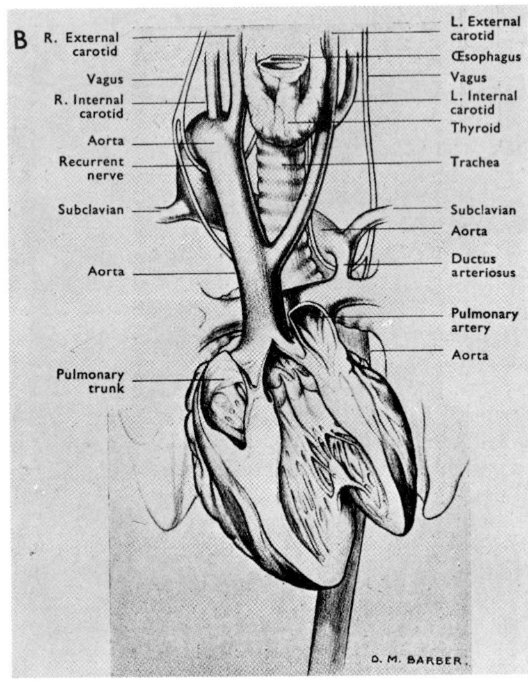

vessel was ligated and the child died suddenly about 15 minutes after application of the ligature. Necropsy showed the aorta passing upward and to the right into the neck, up to the level of the thyroid, then backward and downward, and to the left behind the esophagus. The subclavian arteries arose on each side from the descending portion of the arch. On the left side, the subclavian was joined by a ductus arteriosus that was patent only to a slight degree. Another case was reported by Lewis and Rogers,[17] who noticed in a 5-year-old boy a pulsating swelling in the lower part of the right side of the neck that had been expanding since the age of 2. The boy often was tired, short of breath and his lips occasionally became cyanotic. An oval tumor was present in the region of the right common carotid artery. No pulsations were felt in the left arm but the radial pulse was normal and equal pulses were palpable in both femoral arteries. At operation, a grossly enlarged arterial trunk was found in the position of the common carotid artery but there was no arteriovenous communication. The arterial trunk extended to the hyoid bone, where it formed an anteroposterior arch, with its afferent loop lying slightly internal to its efferent loop. The internal and external carotid arteries originated from the apex of the arch and a nerve descending from high in the neck was related to the arch. In a second operation, it was noted that compression of the vessel stopped the femoral pulses. After further investigation with angiography and radiography, it was concluded that the large cervical vessel represented a right-sided aortic arch derived from the third arch, with a descending aorta passing behind the esophagus in the region of the tracheal bifurcation. Knowledge of this rare arch anomaly is of practical importance, since, when mistaken for an aneurysm, ligation may lead to death. Removal of the first rib has been recommended for alleviation of the symptoms.[17] In 1967, Lipchik and Young[18] stated that only 4 cases of the cervical aorta syndrome have been reported in the English literature. They added 1 case with radiologic findings.

Anomalous Innominate Artery and Anomalous Left Common Carotid Artery

Figure 58-1, *A* shows the junction of the ventral aortae with the fourth aortic arches. If the division of the ventral aortae does not reach down completely to the aortic arch, the innominate artery and the left common carotid artery may arise from one common stem, or the innominate artery may arise more to the left, or vice versa, the left common carotid originating more to the right than normal. In such cases, the displaced vessel must cross the trachea to reach the side for which it is destined, or the innominate and the left common carotid artery may form a fork that compresses the trachea anteriorly. Such slight deviations from the normal can cause respiratory distress in infants, groaning respiration, retractions or a tendency to infection. Visualization with contrast medium shows the anterior surface of the trachea indented. Vascular indentation remains fixed during the entire respiratory cycle in contrast to respiratory difficulties caused by softness of the tracheal cartilages. The trachea can be freed of the oppressing vessel by dislocating the offending artery anteriorly and stitching it to the sternum.[19] But a common origin of the left common carotid or the innominate does not often cause trouble; the variation has been noted in 10–20% of adults while symptoms are rare. Even when symptoms are present in infancy they may disappear spontaneously.[18]

Fourth Aortic Arch Anomalies

Double Aortic Arch

Double aortic arch is a striking but relatively rare anomaly. It was described by Hommel[20] as early as 1737, but when Griswold and Young[21] reviewed the subject in 1949, they could find only 47 cases reported in the literature and, by 1966, 82 cases were on record.[22] Some persons with this anomaly probably are asymptomatic, but there exists a syndrome of stridor and dysphagia that occurs during the first few months of life that is produced by constriction of the esophagus and trachea by a double aortic arch.[23] In 1936, Arkin[24] demonstrated that the anomaly can be diagnosed by x-ray examination, and Neuhauser[25] elaborated more specifically the roentgenologic criteria for the diagnosis. In 1945, Gross[26] obtained surgical relief for tracheal obstruction from a double aortic arch. Although rare, double aortic arch anomalies show great variability. In the majority of cases, the right aortic arch is larger than the left, with the smaller left arch being stenotic or atretic. The ascending aorta divides into two arches. The left anterior arch, as a rule, follows the course of the normal aortic arch and passes in front of the trachea over the left major bronchus, joining a descending aorta situated on the left side of the vertebral column. The right posterior arch passes over the right major bronchus and then turns to the left behind the esophagus and in front of the vertebral column, joining the left arch either behind the esophagus or farther to the left at the point at which the latter arch joins the descending aorta (Figs. 58-3 and 58-4).[8] Mahoney and Manning[6] encountered a major right aortic arch with a right descending aorta more often than other types. In rare cases, the aortic arches may be of equal size or the left larger than the right. This type is of importance to the surgeon because, on inspection, a left aortic arch of normal size taking a normal course is seen and the smaller right aortic arch, which is concealed behind the trachea and esophagus, may be overlooked (Gordon[27]). Such a larger left aortic arch may also be combined with an aorta descending on the right, taking a retro-esophageal course.

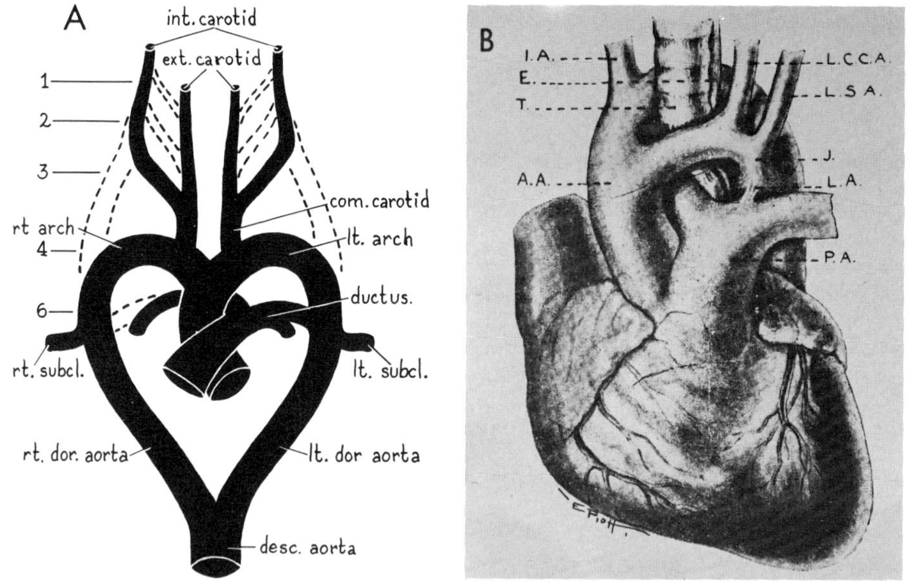

Fig. 58-3. – **A,** diagram of double aortic arch with left-sided ductus arteriosus. **B,** double aortic arch in a child operated on by R. E. Gross.[26] The ascending aorta (A.A.) bifurcates into two branches, one passing behind the esophagus, the other in front of the trachea. The two branches join to form the descending aorta. (From J. G. Wilson and J. Warkany.[14])

One of the arches, usually the left one, may show complete or partial atresia and be replaced by a fibrous band. The ductus arteriosus usually is on the left.[2] Right-sided ductus combined with a double aortic arch and other forms of double aortic arch have been produced experimentally in rats[13,14,28] (Fig. 58-3, *A*). Griswold and Young[21] emphasized that double aortic arch causes symptoms chiefly in children under 2 years of age. Beyond that age, double aortic arch can be tolerated well,[6] and occasions symptoms only when the vessels become rigid by arteriosclerosis in later life. As a rule, double aortic arch is an isolated anomaly, but it has been observed associated with tetrad of Fallot,[5,21] with nonfunctioning left ventricle and with transposition of the great vessels.[21] Double aortic arch with open ductus was reported by Dalton and Jones.[29] An interesting, but so far unique, observation was a double aortic arch in a child with a cerebellar angioreticuloma of the Lindau type.[30]

The symptoms most frequently observed in infants with double aortic arch are respiratory stridor, chronic cough, head retraction, dysphagia, malnutrition

Fig. 58-4. – Double aortic arch (*AO*) surrounding the trachea. The white arrow points to the anterior component of the double arch. The posterior arch encircles the trachea posteriorly, completing the ring. The dark arrow points to the first branch given off from the right arch.

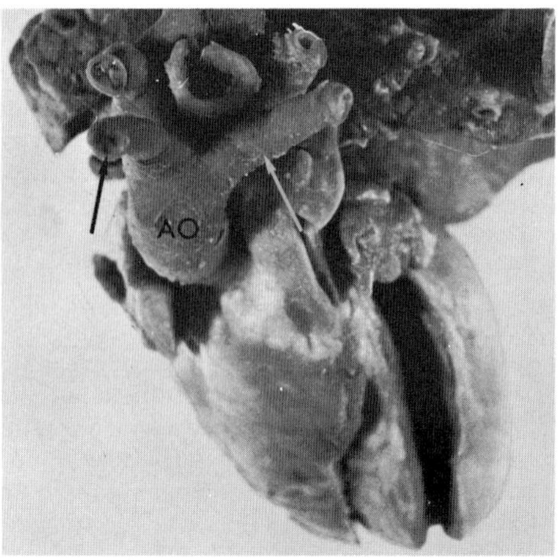

Fig. 58-5. – Esophagogram of a child with double aortic arch showing constriction of the esophagus by right and left arches.

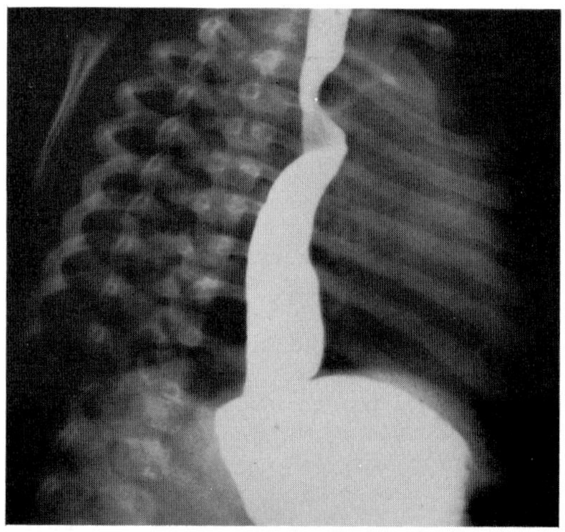

and susceptibility to respiratory infections. Double aortic arch impressions on the esophagus as seen in a roentgenogram are shown in Figure 58-5.

Surgical treatment consists in division of the smaller arch. If the posterior arch is the smaller of the two, it can be exposed in the posterior mediastinum and divided, which relieves esophageal and tracheal constriction.[19] If the anterior arch is smaller, it is divided between the origins of the left common carotid and the left subclavian arteries. In the case of arterial anomalies, the surgical procedure must be adapted to the existing conditions.[5]

Left Aortic Arch with Right Descending Aorta

Paul[31] described 2 patients with this anomaly at first considered to have tetralogy of Fallot because of cyanosis, dyspnea, clubbing, fatigability and squatting. Administration of barium showed the esophagus coursing to the left of the descending aorta instead of its normal position to the right of this structure. It also showed the aorta crossing retro-esophageally.

Right Aortic Arch

A right aortic arch probably is not rare. In Poynter's[3] postmortem material of vascular abnormalities it accounted for 9% of the cases. It seems to occur relatively often in patients with cyanotic heart disease, particularly tetralogy of Fallot. At operation, Blalock[5] found right aortic arch in 24% of cyanotic patients, and Keith *et al.*[22] estimated that it occurs in nearly 50% of cases of truncus arteriosus; it is not rare to find it associated with agenesis of the left pulmonary artery.[2] It is always present in patients with double arch. A right aortic arch may be a harmless variation, or it may even be a favorable anomaly in patients undergoing shunt operations, since a left subclavian artery arising from a left innominate usually is a long vessel that can be approximated easily to the left pulmonary artery. In other cases, the right aortic arch may be involved in a taut ring formation and cause obstructive symptoms.

The mirror image of the normal aorta is a right-sided aortic arch that passes over the right major bronchus and joins a right descending aorta. A left innominate artery arises as the first branch of the aortic arch and divides into a left common carotid and a left subclavian artery. A right common carotid and a right subclavian follow. There is no ring formation caused by this mirror-image right aortic arch, which occurs in approximately 25% of patients with tetralogy of Fallot[5,32] (Fig. 58-6). In some of these cases, the left subclavian does not arise from the left innominate artery but from the descending aorta on the right. In this case, it crosses to the left behind the esophagus and represents the mirror image of the aberrant right subclavian artery discussed on page 533. This configuration may cause symptoms by compression of the esophagus. If a left ductus arteriosus is present, a vascular ring is formed that usually is loose and asymptomatic, except in children with a tendency to respiratory infections. This vascular anomaly occurs often in persons who have no cardiac malformation.[2] If a left ductus connects the left pulmonary artery with the upper descending aorta through a partially persistent left aortic root, a constricting ring is formed, but this is not the case if there is a right duc-

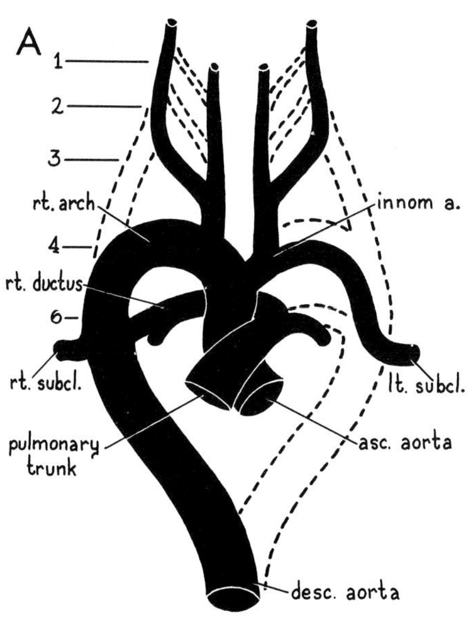

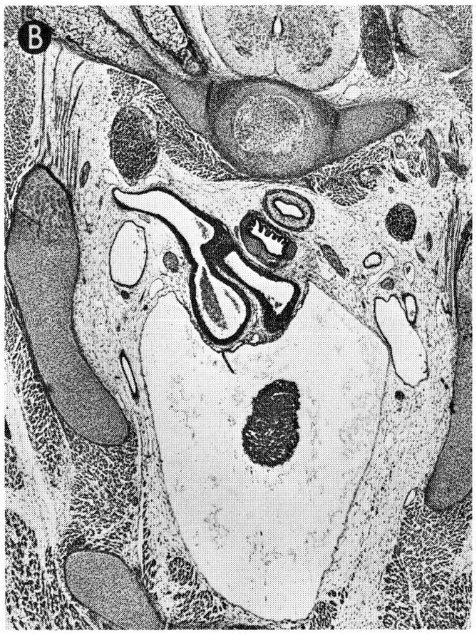

Fig. 58-6. — **A,** diagram of right aortic arch with right-sided ductus arteriosus. **B,** section through a newborn rat (vitamin A deficiency) showing similar malformation. (From J. G. Wilson and J. Warkany.[14])

tus. If the left subclavian artery is completely disconnected from the right aortic arch, no ring is formed in the presence of a left or bilateral ductus.[2]

Neuhauser[33] and Gross[19] described the clinical and x-ray findings of right aortic arch anomalies with left ligamentum arteriosum, which can have results similar to those produced by a double aortic arch. An alleviating operation consists of division of the ligamentum arteriosum, which breaks the constricting ring. If a left subclavian artery is found behind the esophagus, it is divided also. Respiratory distress and dysphagia improve following surgical intervention.[19] Felson and Palayew[34] distinguished two main types of right aortic arch. With cyanotic heart disease, especially the tetralogy of Fallot, the right arch is almost invariably the mirror image of the normal left arch and lies anterior and to the right of the trachea and esophagus. But when the right arch exists as an isolated anomaly, it extends posteriorly behind the esophagus.

Recognition of a right aortic arch is of importance in patients scheduled for shunt operations, since the side of the arch determines the place of incision. In most of these cases, a ductus arteriosus is found that connects the first part of the left subclavian branch of the innominate to the pulmonary artery. A right ductus apparently is the exception in such cases even if the aorta descends on the right side. In patients with dextrocardia who often have a left aortic arch,[32] the aorta may descend on the right or the left. It is of surgical importance that the innominate artery usually arises on the right when the aorta descends on the left, and on the left when the aorta descends on the right.[5] Ebstein anomaly with right aortic arch has been reported by Rebolledo.[35]

Right-sided aortic arch has been produced experimentally and many vascular variations with it.[13,14,28] Mirror image of the normal with a left innominate artery (Fig. 58-6) or with an aberrant left subclavian artery has been observed. The left subclavian artery in one animal arose from the left pulmonary artery and in another there was a right and a left ductus arteriosus.

Interruption of the Aortic Arch ("Steidele Complex")

This malformation is rare. In 1967, Lie[36] collected 88 cases from the literature, added 2 cases of his own and suggested the term "Steidele complex" for the anomaly, which apparently was first described by a Viennese obstetrician in the late eighteenth century.[37] The left aortic arch may be interrupted distal to the origin of the left subclavian,[38] distal to the origin of the left common carotid[39] or distal to the origin of the innominate artery (types A, B and C of Celoria and Patton[40]). There are other variants, such as that shown diagrammatically in Figure 58-7, which illustrates an ascending aorta terminating in two common carotid arteries, whereas both subclavian arteries arise from a descending left aorta. Such cases have been seen in children,[41,42] and the same anomaly has been produced experimentally in rats.[13,14] In all these cases, the lower half of the body receives its blood via a large ductus that connects the left pulmonary artery with the descending aorta. A case with patent

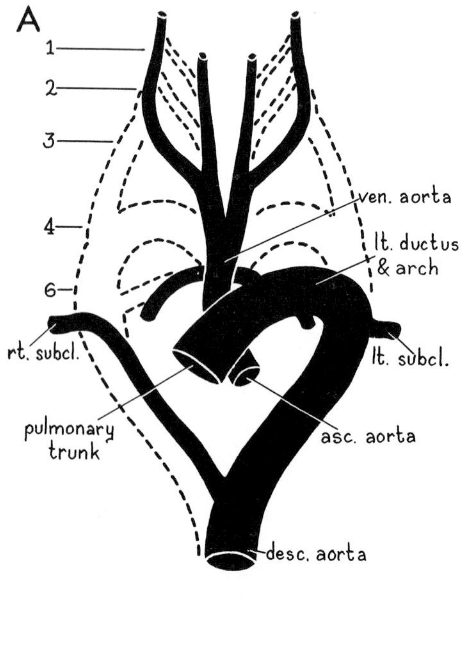

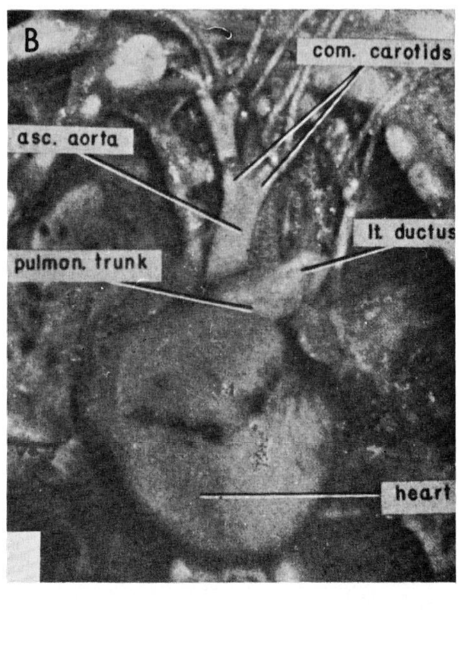

Fig. 58-7. – **A,** diagram of arterial pattern in one variety of absence of the fourth aortic arch. Pulmonary trunk and ductus arteriosus serve as connection between the heart and the descending aorta. Small ascending aorta terminates by dividing into two common carotids but does not communicate with the descending aorta. **B,** heart and large vessels of a newborn child with similar malformation. (From J. G. Wilson and J. Warkany.[14])

right ductus arteriosus shunting blood to a right-sided descending aorta has been observed.[41] Evans[42] described 3 infants ages 2, 3 and 11 days, respectively, with interrupted aortic arch, and in each case the arterial branches arising from the aortic arch were different in origin. In all patients, the left ventricle supplied blood for the head and neck and in some for the arms, but the lower half of the body was always supplied with blood from the right ventricle. One should expect, therefore, cyanosis of the lower half of the body (differential cyanosis), but this theoretic postulate was not always fulfilled, since septal defects usually permitted communications between the two circulations.[15] In 1876, Barlow[43] recorded a case of an aortic arch interrupted between the left subclavian and the (patent) ductus arteriosus in a boy 3 months of age with a septal defect and overriding aorta (Eisenmenger complex).[8] Persistent truncus arteriosus with interruption of the arch was reported by Morgan *et al.*[44] Neufeld *et al.*[45] observed interruption of the aortic arch in siblings with biventricular origin of the pulmonary trunk and subaortic stenosis above the ventricular septal defect. Interrupted aortic arch with tetralogy of Fallot was described by Altshuler.[74]

Although interrupted aortic arch is rare, Kleinerman *et al.*[41] reported 6 cases from one hospital and Lie[36] 2 cases seen within 5 weeks in an obstetric service. The mortality rate is approximately 75% in the first year of life. Only 4 patients diagnosed during life had successful corrections by surgery. Tyson *et al.*[72] reported successful repair of a type A aortic arch interruption in a neonate. The anomaly was associated with a large ventricular septal defect and incomplete closure of a patent ductus arteriosus. A palliative operation in a case of aortic arch atresia with transposition of the great vessels and ventricular septal defect was described by Norton *et al.*[73]

Respiratory distress is the most common symptom and cyanosis, as a rule, appears a few days after birth. The ascending aorta is hypoplastic and there usually is a bicuspid aortic valve. Ventricular septal defect and patent foramen ovale are seen in most cases, permitting a shunt of oxygenated blood to the descending aorta. Kleinerman *et al.*[41] believed that faulty partition of the truncus arteriosus, resulting in a small aorta and a large pulmonary artery, represents the primary lesion that leads to disuse of the fourth aortic arch and its eventual disappearance. Cleft palate, anencephaly, renal agenesis or hypoplasia, double vagina and absence of the spleen have been observed as associated malformations.

Kinking of the Aortic Arch

Kinking or buckling of the aortic arch represents a "pseudocoarctation" that does not cause hemodynamic disturbances and is compatible with normal arm and leg pressures. Roentgenograms show a double rounded shadow in the left superior mediastinum that may lead to a mistaken diagnosis of tumor.[46]

Anomalous Subclavian Artery

A right subclavian artery arising distally to the left subclavian and passing behind the esophagus is not a rare anomaly. It is seen in approximately 1% of necropsies,[22] and many hundreds of cases have been reported in the literature. The embryologic derivation of

Fig. 58-8. – **A,** diagram of right subclavian artery arising distally and passing dorsally behind the esophagus. **B,** section through the upper thoracic region of an abnormal newborn rat (produced by vitamin A deficiency) showing distally arising right subclavian artery as it leaves the descending aorta to cross midline behind the esophagus. (From J. G. Wilson and J. Warkany.[14])

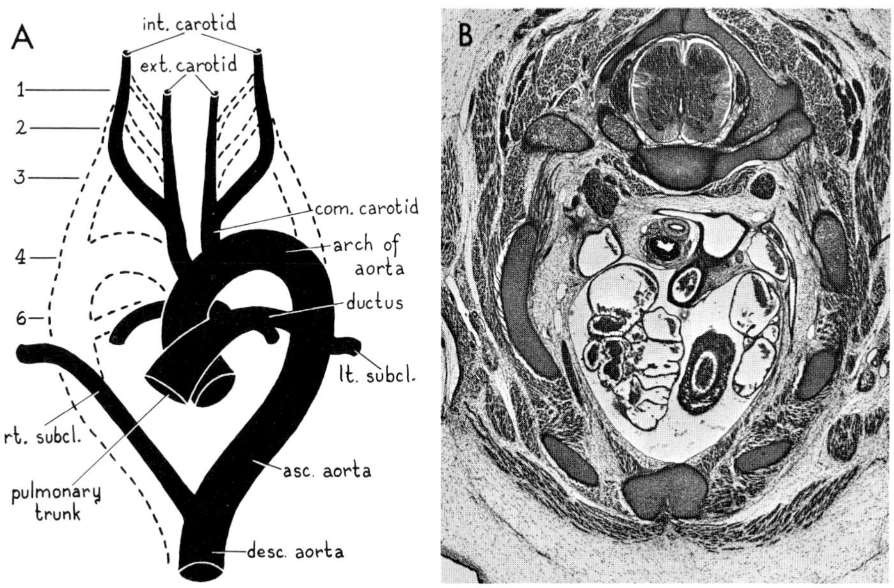

this anomaly can be gathered from Figure 58-8, *A*, which shows the right subclavian arising from the aorta descending on the left, utilizing the most distal part of the right dorsal aorta and the right seventh segmental artery. It must be realized, however, that both the left and the right subclavian arteries migrate cephalad and take their origin at the time of birth immediately distal to the left common carotid. To reach the right side, the anomalous right subclavian must cross the midline. It usually runs behind the esophagus, but in exceptional cases it crosses between the esophagus and the trachea or even in front of the trachea. These exceptional cases are difficult to explain embryologically, since normally the esophagus and the trachea are situated anterior to the point of union of the dorsal aortae. It most likely is that such ventral position of the vessel is best explained by the assumption that the subclavian trunk behind the esophagus becomes connected with the capillary plexus encircling and supplying the esophagus or the trachea, whereby a new channel is formed that runs ventral to the esophagus or trachea.[47] As a rule, however, the right subclavian artery arising from the aortic arch on the left crosses in a right and upward direction behind the esophagus to reach the right apex of the chest. In the case of a right aortic arch, a left subclavian may have a low origin and cross behind the esophagus to the left side. These traversing subclavian arteries were known in the eighteenth century, and as early as 1794 Bayford[1] recognized one as a cause of "dysphagia lusoria." He described the case of a woman who had lifelong difficulty in deglutition. She was confined to a hospital for 20 years and died of extreme emaciation at 62 years of age. After thorough examination of the body, Bayford finally found the source of her difficulties: ". . . At length, by mere accident I discovered an extraordinary lusus naturae in the disposition of the right subclavian artery which will easily be understood by reference to the annexed figure." This illustration, reprinted in 1952 in an article by Asherson,[48] shows the right subclavian originating distally to the left subclavian, turning to the right between the trachea and the esophagus. The compression of the esophagus between this artery and the vertebral column behind it may have had something to do with the severity of the patient's symptoms. Actually, the anomaly rarely causes pathologic manifestations but, in rare cases, it can cause difficulties in swallowing even in infants. Some of the children have more difficulty with liquids and others more with solid food retained in the pharynx. An interesting point is that persons who tolerate the anomaly well in childhood and early adulthood may experience their first symptoms when the situation is aggravated by hypertension or arteriosclerosis of the vessel. Palmer[49] emphasized that such older patients may also suffer from fear of having cancer or from accusations of being hypochondriacs. Roentgen examination with a barium swallow shows a small defect of the esophagus at the height of the third or fourth thoracic vertebra, the defect coursing obliquely upward and to the right.

Children experiencing difficulty because of this anomaly can obtain relief by ligation and division of the abnormal subclavian near its origin. Collateral blood flow is soon established and the right arm remains well supplied with blood. Aberrant subclavian arteries are also important in association with cardiac defects amenable to surgery. Bahnson and Blalock[50] encountered 18 instances of aberrant right and 18 instances of aberrant left subclavian arteries in 841 patients operated on for pulmonary stenosis. Pattinson[51] also found aberrant right subclavian artery in 4.4% of patients with congenital heart disease. Blalock[5] pointed out that retro-esophageal location of a subclavian artery is not a deterrent to the performance of a satisfactory anastomosis and that the wall of such an aberrant subclavian is thinner than that of a normally located artery. Other congenital anomalies related to the subclavian arteries may be mentioned briefly. Perry and Massey[52] described a case of bilateral subclavian and axillary aneurysms believed to be congenital. Vascular anomalies of the upper limbs associated with cervical ribs were reviewed by Hill.[53] Subclavian origin of bronchial arteries was discussed by O'Rahilly *et al.*[54] Beabout *et al.*[55] expressed doubt concerning the role of aberrant right subclavian artery in the production of dysphagia.

Variations and anomalies of the subclavian arteries are of importance to the surgeon in many operations. Daseler and Anson[56] discussed the clinical significance of the various patterns that must be known to avoid hazards in surgery of the neck and in the upper thorax. An interesting variation is congenital atresia of a subclavian artery, which can result in the "subclavian steal syndrome." In such cases, the affected extremity is supplied by collateral vessels. If blood is derived from the ipsilateral vertebral artery, a shortage may occur in the basilar system, leading to symptoms of cerebral ischemia. Mental retardation may be associated with this anomaly.[57]

Sixth (Pulmonary) Aortic Arch Anomalies

Anomalies of the Ductus Arteriosus

Absence of a functional ductus arteriosus connecting the pulmonary and systemic circulations during fetal life is not compatible with normal development of the heart. Survival of the fetus is possible only if an open ventricular septum permits a shunt between the pulmonary and systemic circulations. Failure to find the ligamentum arteriosum connecting a pulmonary artery with the aorta may be indicative of a septal defect in the ventricles or of an aortopulmonary fistula. In rats treated by prenatal vitamin A deficiency, bilateral absence of a ductus arteriosus was found occasionally, and in all cases ventricular septal defects were associated with this anomaly.[13]

In a patient operated on for pulmonary stenosis, Blalock[5] noted a right ductus arteriosus connecting the innominate artery with the area of the pulmonary artery. Since the pulmonary end of this vessel was narrow or obliterated, anastomosis between its open section and the right pulmonary artery was surgically established and the patient showed striking improvement following the operation.

Blalock[5] observed several patients at operation in whom the pulmonary artery did not connect with the heart or the aorta. The circulation to the lungs was by way of collateral vessels, usually bronchial arteries. There was a functional truncus arteriosus with a blind pulmonary artery and there was no ductus arteriosus on either side. Absence of a ductus arteriosus combined with tetralogy of Fallot probably is not too rare. It was described in an embryo by Stensen in 1671 (cited by Willius[58]) and illustrated by Peacock[59] in 1866.

An unusual congenital anomaly causing tracheoesophageal obstruction associated with tetralogy of Fallot was reported by Wagner and Price.[60] A retroesophageal vascular anomaly, probably representing a right ductus arteriosus connecting the pulmonary artery with the right subclavian artery, passed behind the esophagus and caused dysphagia lusoria.

Aberrant Left Pulmonary Artery

Several cases have been described of infants born with respiratory obstruction because of an anomalous course of the left pulmonary artery. In such cases, the left pulmonary artery passed between the trachea and the esophagus and indentations can be seen on these structures by x-ray examination. The patients have noisy respiration, head retraction, cyanotic spells and they fail to gain weight. Pulmonary emphysema may be present. This anomaly often is accompanied by cardiovascular and other malformations. Coarctation of the aorta, dextroposition of the aorta, aberrant right subclavian artery, persistent left superior vena cava, patent foramen ovale, ventricular septal defect, absence of one kidney, malrotation of the intestine and fusion of vertebrae have been found. The obstruction may affect the distal end of the trachea or the right main bronchus. Embryologically, the anomaly can be explained by abnormal union of the left pulmonary artery with the esophago-tracheal plexus.[61,62] Surgical relief has been attempted by Potts *et al.*[63]

Agenesis of a Pulmonary Artery

Agenesis of a pulmonary artery, long known as an anatomic curiosity, has become a clinical topic in recent years. Many cases diagnosed in vivo have been published, and Steinberg[64] reviewed the subject. Congenital absence of a main branch of the pulmonary artery may be classified in two categories: the isolated form and that associated with septal defects. Isolated absence of a pulmonary artery usually is on the right side. There are no septal defects, but right-sided aortic arch, coarctation of the aorta or patent ductus arteriosus has been observed in such patients.[65] As a rule, the patients are asymptomatic but, in some cases, bronchiectases are present, dominating the disease picture. Diagnosis of congenital absence of a pulmonary artery can be made by inspection of the conventional roentgenogram, which shows a hypoplastic, poorly vascularized lung on one side with a fully vascularized, distended opposite lung that causes mediastinal herniation.

Patients with an absent pulmonary artery combined with a septal defect present a quite different clinical picture. Absence of the left pulmonary artery has been described repeatedly in combination with tetralogy of Fallot and more rarely with the Eisenmenger complex. In such cases, a right aortic arch frequently is present. The patients often are ill with recurrent infections, dyspnea and cyanosis. Diagnosis from conventional roentgenograms is difficult, but angiocardiography is helpful and provides information regarding the circulation in the lung with the absent pulmonary artery. Indirect evidence of bronchial anastomoses can be obtained or direct visualization of aortic branches supplying the lungs can be achieved.

Blalock[5] encountered a single pulmonary artery in 9 of 610 cyanotic patients with a preoperative diagnosis of pulmonic stenosis. During operation, the heart action becomes impaired in such cases by temporary occlusion of the single pulmonary artery, but collateral circulation may permit occlusion for a sufficiently long time to allow for the anastomosis. Congenital absence of the right pulmonary artery in a newborn infant, with resulting necrosis of the lung and spontaneous pneumothorax, was reported by Miller.[66]

Douglass[67] described 4 instances in which pulmonary arteries arose from the descending aorta. He also reviewed 23 additional cases of anomalous origin of pulmonary arteries from various sources, including subclavian and innominate arteries.

Schneiderman[68] believed that the defect is not due to failure of development of the right sixth aortic arch but due to misplaced attachment. It is possible that during the migration of the right sixth arch and the simultaneous division of the truncus, the former is retarded sufficiently so that when the truncus divides, the right sixth arch is retained on the wrong side. It then appears as an anomalous artery arising from the aorta proximal to the innominate artery.

Wilson and Warkany[13,14] found agenesis of the left pulmonary artery in several young of vitamin A-deficient rats. In most of these cases, the absence of the pulmonary artery was associated with agenesis of the left lung. This situation may be considered a somewhat exaggerated form of the hypoplasia of the lung seen in clinical cases on the side of the absent pulmonary artery. In some rat fetuses, the left lung was well developed and the blood supply derived from large bronchial arteries.

An abnormal course of the left pulmonary artery may lead to tracheobronchial obstruction. Contro *et al.*[69] described 3 patients in whom the left pulmonary artery coursed abnormally anterior to the right bronchus and behind the trachea, with consequent compression of these structures. Tetralogy combined with aneurysm of the pulmonary artery and bronchial obstruction was observed in 2 infants by Contro *et al.*[70] Congenital malformations of the lung and associated anomalies of the pulmonary arteries were discussed by Ferencz.[71]

REFERENCES

1. Bayford, D.: An account of a singular case of obstructed deglutition, Mem. M. Soc. London 2:271, 1794.
2. Stewart, J. R., Kincaid, O. W., and Edwards, J. E.: *An Atlas of Vascular Rings and Related Malformations of the Aortic Arch System* (Springfield, Ill.: Charles C Thomas, Publisher, 1964).
3. Poynter, C. W. M.: Arterial anomalies pertaining to the aortic arches and the branches arising from them, Univ. Studies, Lincoln, Nebr. 16:229, 1916.
4. Abbott, M. E.: *Atlas of Congenital Heart Disease* (New York: American Heart Association, 1936).
5. Blalock, A.: Surgical procedures employed and anatomical variations encountered in the treatment of congenital pulmonic stenosis, Surg., Gynec. & Obst. 87:385, 1948.
6. Mahoney, E. B., and Manning, J. A.: Congenital abnormalities of the aortic arch, Surgery 55:1, 1964.
7. Congdon, E. D.: Transformation of the aortic arch system during development of the human embryo, Contrib. Embryol. 14:47, 1922.
8. Edwards, J. E.: Anomalies of derivatives of aortic arch system, M. Clin. North America 32:925, 1948.
9. von Baer, K. E.: Des branches et des vaisseaux branchiaux dans les embryonales animaux vértébralés, Ann. Sc. Nat., vol. 15, 1828.
10. Rathke, M. H.: Untersuchungen über die Aortenwurzeln und die von ihnen ausgehenden Arterien der Saurier, Denkschr. Akad. Wissen., Wien 13:51, 1857.
11. Sawin, P. B., and Edmonds, H. W.: Morphogenetic studies of rabbit; aortic arch variations in relation to regionally specific growth differences, Anat. Rec. 105:377, 1949.
12. Warkany, J., Passarge, E., and Smith, L. B.: Congenital malformations in autosomal trisomy syndromes, Am. J. Dis. Child. 112:502, 1966.
13. Wilson, J. G., and Warkany, J.: Aortic-arch and cardiac anomalies in the offspring of vitamin A deficient rats, Am. J. Anat. 85:113, 1949.
14. Wilson, J. G., and Warkany, J.: Cardiac and aortic arch anomalies in the offspring of vitamin A deficient rats correlated with similar human anomalies, Pediatrics 5:708, 1950.
15. Foley, B. V.: Congenital interruption of the aortic arch, Arch. Dis. Childhood 33:131, 1958.
16. Beavan, T.E.D., and Fatti, L.: Ligature of the aortic arch in the neck, Brit. J. Surg. 34:414, 1947.
17. Lewis, C., and Rogers, L.: The cervical aortic knuckle which resembles an aneurysm, Lancet 1:825, 1953.
18. Lipchik, E. O., and Young, L. W.: Unusual symptomatic aortic arch anomalies, Radiology 89:85, 1967.
19. Gross, R. E.: *The Surgery of Infancy and Childhood* (Philadelphia: W. B. Saunders Company, 1953).
20. Hommel: Commercium litterarium, Norimbergae, p. 162, 1737.
21. Griswold, H. E., Jr., and Young, M. D.: Double aortic arch; report of 2 cases and review of the literature, Pediatrics 4:751, 1949.
22. Keith, J. D., Rowe, R. D., and Vlad, P. (eds.): *Heart Disease in Infancy and Childhood* (2d ed.; New York: The Macmillan Company, 1966).
23. Wolman, I. J.: Syndrome of constricting double aortic arch in infancy, J. Pediat. 14:527, 1939.
24. Arkin, A.: Double aortic arch with total persistence of right and isthmus stenosis of left arch; new clinical and x-ray picture: Report of 6 cases in adults, Am. Heart J. 11:444, 1936.
25. Neuhauser, E. B. D.: Roentgen diagnosis of double aortic arch and other anomalies of great vessels, Am. J. Roentgenol. 56:1, 1946.
26. Gross, R. E.: Surgical relief for tracheal obstruction from a vascular ring, New England J. Med. 233:586, 1945.
27. Gordon, L.: Double aortic arch, J. Pediat. 30:428, 1947.
28. Baird, C. D. C., Nelson, M. M., Monie, I. W., and Evans, H. M.: Congenital cardiovascular anomalies induced by pteroylglutamic acid deficiency during gestation in rat, Circulation Res. 2:544, 1954.
29. Dalton, E. G., and Jones, H. E.: Congenital anomalies of the aortic arch, Lancet 1:537, 1952.
30. Krepler, P.: Zur Klinik des angeborenen Stridors bei doppeltem Aortenbogen, Oesterreich. Ztschr. Kinderh. 9:225, 1954.
31. Paul, R. N.: New anomaly of aorta; left aortic arch with right descending aorta, J. Pediat. 32:19, 1948.
32. Taussig, H. B.: *Congenital Malformations of the Heart* (New York: Commonwealth Fund, 1947).
33. Neuhauser, E. B. D.: Tracheo-esophageal constriction produced by right aortic arch and left ligamentum arteriosum, Am. J. Roentgenol. 62:493, 1949.
34. Felson, B., and Palayew, M. J.: The two types of right aortic arch, Radiology 81:745, 1963.
35. Rebolledo, J. R.: Ebstein's anomaly with right aortic arch. Review of the cardiovascular defects associated with Ebstein's malformation of the tricuspid valve, J. Pediat. 71:66, 1967.
36. Lie, J. T.: The malformation complex of the absence of the arch of the aorta – Steidele's complex, Am. Heart J. 73: 615, 1967.
37. Roberts, W. C., Morrow, A. G., and Braunwald, E.: Complete interruption of the aortic arch, Circulation 26:39, 1962.
38. Sewart, M.: Congenital interruption of the aortic arch, Arch. Dis. Childhood 23:63, 1948.
39. Herzog, W.: Über eine seltene Herz-Gefässmissbildung. Fehlen des Aortenbogens, Frankfurt. Ztschr. Path. 59: 454, 1948.
40. Celoria, G. C., and Patton, R. B.: Congenital absence of the aortic arch, Am. Heart J. 58:407, 1959.
41. Kleinerman, J., Yang, W. M., Hackel, D. B., and Kaufman, N.: Absence of the transverse aortic arch, A.M.A. Arch. Path. 65:490, 1958.
42. Evans, W.: Congenital stenosis (coarctation), atresia, and interruption of aortic arch; study of 28 cases, Quart. J. Med. 2:1, 1933.
43. Barlow, T.: Congenital heart disease, two cases, Tr. Path. Soc. London 27:140, 1875–1876.
44. Morgan, A. D., Brinsfield, D., and Edwards, F. K.: Persistent truncus arteriosus, Am. J. Dis. Child. 109:74, 1965.
45. Neufeld, H. N., Ongley, P. A., Swan, H. J. C., Purgert, E. O., and Edwards, J. E.: Biventricular origin of the pulmonary trunk with subaortic stenosis above the ventricular septal defect, Am. Heart J. 61:189, 1961.
46. Steinberg, I.: Anomalies (pseudocoarctation) of the arch of the aorta; report of 8 new and review of 8 previously published cases, Am. J. Roentgenol. 88:73, 1962.
47. Bremer, J. L.: *Congenital Anomalies of the Viscera, Their Embryological Basis* (Cambridge, Mass.: Harvard

University Press, 1957).
48. Asherson, N.: Dysphagia lusoria with a record of 3 cases, J. Laryng. & Otol. 66:111, 1952.
49. Palmer, E. D.: Dysphagia lusoria: Clinical aspects in adult, Ann. Int. Med. 42:1173, 1955.
50. Bahnson, H. T., and Blalock, A.: Aortic vascular rings encountered in surgical treatment of congenital pulmonic stenosis, Ann. Surg. 131:356, 1950.
51. Pattinson, J. N.: Anomalous right subclavian artery, Brit. Heart J. 15:150, 1953.
52. Perry, S. P., and Massey, C. W.: Bilateral aneurysms of the subclavian and axillary arteries, report of case, Radiology 61:53, 1953.
53. Hill, R. M.: Vascular anomalies of upper limbs associated with cervical ribs: Report of case and review of literature, Brit. J. Surg. 27:100, 1939.
54. O'Rahilly, R., Debson, H., and King, T. S.: Subclavian origin of bronchial arteries, Anat. Rec. 108:227, 1950.
55. Beabout, J. W., Stewart, J. R., and Kincaid, O. W.: Aberrant right subclavian artery, Am. J. Roentgenol. 92:855, 1964.
56. Daseler, E. H., and Anson, B. J.: Surgical anatomy of the subclavian artery and its branches, Surg., Gynec. & Obst. 108:149, 1959.
57. Gerber, N.: Congenital atresia of the subclavian artery, producing a "subclavian steal syndrome," Am. J. Dis. Child. 113:709, 1967.
58. Willius, F. A.: Comments on the historical aspects of certain congenital anomalies of the heart and great vessels, Proc. Staff Meet. Mayo Clin. 23:99, 1948.
59. Peacock, T. B.: *On Malformations of the Human Heart* (2d ed.; London: J. Churchill & Sons, 1866).
60. Wagner, B. M., and Price, W. S.: Dysphagia lusoria: An unusual case, Am. Heart J. 44:452, 1952.
61. Wittenberg, M. H., Tantivongse, T., and Rosenberg, B. F.: Anomalous course of the left pulmonary artery, Radiology 67:345, 1956.
62. Welsh, T. M., and Munro, I. B.: Congenital stridor caused by an aberrant pulmonary artery, Arch. Dis. Childhood 29: 101, 1954.
63. Potts, W. J., Holinger, P. H., and Rosenblum, A. H.: Anomalous left pulmonary artery causing obstruction to right main bronchus; report of case, J.A.M.A. 155:1409, 1954.
64. Steinberg, I.: Congenital absence of a main branch of the pulmonary artery, Am. J. Med. 24:559, 1958.
65. Emanuel, R. W., and Pattinson, J. N.: Absence of the left pulmonary artery in Fallot's tetralogy, Brit. Heart J. 18: 289, 1956.
66. Miller, J. F.: Congenital absence of right pulmonary artery in new-born infant with resulting necrosis of lung and spontaneous pneumothorax, Am. J. Dis. Child. 53: 1268, 1937.
67. Douglass, R.: Anomalous pulmonary vessels, J. Thoracic Surg. 17:712, 1948.
68. Schneiderman, L. J.: Isolated congenital absence of the right pulmonary artery: A caution as to its diagnosis and a proposal for its embryogenesis; report of a case with review, Am. Heart J. 55:772, 1958.
69. Contro, S., Miller, R. A., White, H., and Potts, W. J.: Bronchial obstruction due to pulmonary artery anomalies. I. Vascular sling, Circulation 17:418, 1959.
70. Contro, S., Miller, R. A., White, H., and Potts, W. J.: Bronchial obstruction due to pulmonary artery anomalies. II. Pulmonary artery aneurysm, Circulation 17:424, 1958.
71. Ferencz, C.: Congenital abnormalities of pulmonary vessels and their relation to malformations of the lung, Pediatrics 28:993, 1961.
72. Tyson, K. R. T., Harris, L. C., and Nghiem, Q. X.: Repair of aortic arch interruption in the neonate, Surgery 67: 1006, 1970.
73. Norton, J. B., Jr., Ullyot, D. J., Stewart, E. T., Rudolph, A. M., and Edmunds, L. H., Jr.: Aortic arch atresia with transposition of the great vessels: Physiologic considerations and surgical management, Surgery 67:1011, 1970.
74. Altshuler, G.: The ventricular septal defect, Am. J. Dis. Child. 119:407, 1970.

59

The Aorta

Congenital Atresia of the Aorta

In congenital atresia, the hypoplastic aorta ends blindly and is separated from the hypoplastic (or absent) left ventricle. In approximately one-fourth of the cases, the mitral valve is also completely closed, whereas in the majority of cases the valve is small but open. The left ventricle is markedly reduced in size in 90% of the cases. As a rule, there is progressive narrowing of the aorta toward the left ventricle and, in the area of stenosis, rudiments of the semilunar valves can be recognized. The ascending aorta is hypoplastic to the point of entrance of the ductus arteriosus. The right side of the heart is markedly enlarged and the pulmonary artery carries blood through a widely patent ductus arteriosus into the descending aorta. There always is an opening between the right and left atrium, or the left atrium is connected with the superior vena cava through an anomalous channel whereby an anastomosis is established between the atria. Ventricular septal defects are present only rarely.[1]

Aortic atresia probably is a rare congenital malformation. Abbott[2] noted it only twelve times in 1,000 necropsied patients with cardiovascular anomalies. Aortic atresia is thought to occur once in 39,000 births,[3] but it probably is not rare in newborn pathology. It is thought that it is a common cause of heart failure in the newborn period and that 25% of patients dying of congenital heart disease in the first month of life have this anomaly.[3] The etiology of aortic atresia has always been a controversial subject. It has been attributed to fetal intrauterine infection,[4] but in some cases examined histologically no evidence of inflammation could be found.[5] In 1909, Herxheimer[6] distinguished two types: atresia on a developmental basis and atresia on an inflammatory basis; it is, of course, possible that both types occur. Unequal partitioning of the truncus arteriosus is not an accepted explanation of this anomaly, which is almost always associated with a normal ventricular septum.[1] Brekke[7] reported a case of atresia and a case of hypoplasia of the aortic orifice in 2 brothers. Aortic valvar atresia in 2 brothers was described by Rao *et al.*[9] There is a definite predominance of males among patients with this disease.

Fig. 59-1.—Aortic valve atresia with hypoplasia of the ascending aorta (*AO*). The pulmonary artery (*P*) is much enlarged.

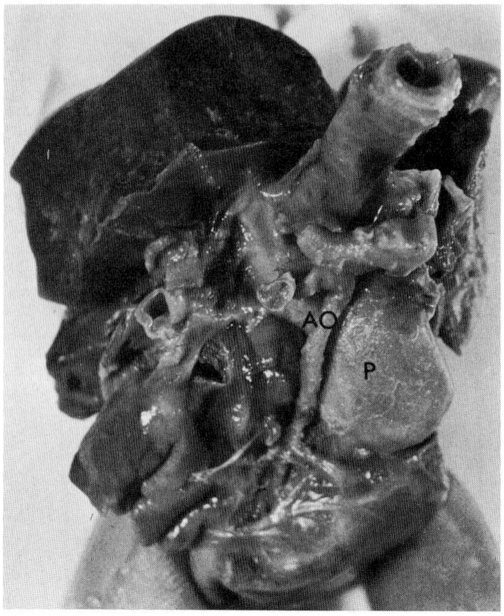

The blood leaving the right ventricle through the pulmonary artery reaches the lungs and oxygenated blood returns to the left atrium. There may be no inlet to the left ventricle because of mitral atresia and if blood can enter a small left ventricle there is no outflow through the aorta. The only outlet for the blood from the left atrium is through an interatrial defect that permits admixture of oxygenated with venous blood of the right atrium. The right heart, which in such cases propels the blood not only through the lungs but also through the rest of the body, is markedly enlarged and the pulmonary artery and ductus arteriosus are dilated. Taussig[8] pointed out that in the majority of other malformations cyanosis is due to the shunting of venous blood into the systemic circulation, whereas in aortic atresia the body is primarily supplied with venous blood.

It is quite likely that many fetuses with aortic atresia die early in utero. Those born alive show early signs of heart failure. Dyspnea, tachycardia and enlargement of the liver usually appear in the first week of postnatal life and cyanosis becomes apparent within a few days. A murmur may be audible but it is not characteristic. The heart is always enlarged and electrocardiograms show right ventricular hypertrophy. Venous angiograms or aortography are helpful in the diagnosis.[3]

Mitral atresia and absence or marked hypoplasia of the left ventricle can be a part of the syndrome, but ventricular septal defect is only rarely associated with it. Endocardial fibroelastosis is found in the left atrium, but the left ventricle is affected only in those cases in which the mitral valve is open.[3]

The prognosis is extremely poor. Most infants with aortic atresia die within the first 2 weeks, but occasionally some survive for several months. No appropriate surgical treatment has been devised.

REFERENCES

1. Edwards, J. E.: Congenital Malformations of the Heart and Great Vessels, in Gould, S. E. (ed.), *Pathology of the Heart* (Springfield, Ill.: Charles C Thomas, Publisher, 1953), pp. 266–503.
2. Abbott, M. E.: *Atlas of Congenital Heart Disease* (New York: American Heart Association, 1936).
3. Keith, J. D., Rowe, R. D., and Vlad, P. (eds.): *Heart Disease in Infancy and Childhood* (New York: The Macmillan Company, 1958).
4. Farber, S., and Hubbard, J.: Fetal endomyocarditis: Intrauterine infection as a cause of congenital cardiac anomalies, Am. J. M. Sc. 186:705, 1933.
5. Rossman, J. I.: Congenital atresia and stenosis of great cardiac vessels, Am. J. Dis. Child. 64:872, 1942.
6. Herxheimer, G.: Missbildungen des Herzens und der grossen Gefässe, in Schwalbe, E. (ed.), *Die Morphologie der Missbildungen des Menschen und der Tiere* (Jena: Gustav Fischer, 1909), Vol. 3, pt. 3.
7. Brekke, V. G.: Congenital aortic atresia and hypoplasia of the aortic orifice, Am. Heart J. 45:925, 1953.
8. Taussig, H. B.: *Congenital Malformations of the Heart* (New York: The Commonwealth Fund, 1947).
9. Rao, S. S., Gootman, N., and Platt, N.: Familial aortic atresia. Report of a case of aortic atresia in siblings, Am. J. Dis. Child. 118:919, 1969.

Congenital Aortic Stenosis

IT WAS CUSTOMARY in the past to distinguish merely between valvar and subvalvar aortic stenosis, but in recent years the classification of the aortic stenoses has become more complex. The story of aortic stenoses in adults is somewhat confused by the fact that it is not always possible to separate acquired from congenital forms; for children, however, one can safely assume that aortic stenoses generally are congenital. Some of the congenital forms seen in adults and children are rather benign but there is an infantile type that is rapidly fatal and contributes to neonatal and infant mortality. Only about 5% of the congenital aortic stenoses are encountered in children under 1 year of age, 65% between 1 and 15 years and approximately 30% beyond the age of 15 years.[1]

Aortic valvar, subvalvar (fibrous ring) and supravalvar stenoses are the important subgroups, but Keith *et al.*[2] in their classification also considered aortic stenosis with underdevelopment of the left chamber, hypoplastic aortic ring, aortic stenoses combined with other cardiovascular defects and endocardial fibroelastosis with aortic valve involvement.

Valvar aortic stenosis is characterized by fusion and thickening of the valvar cusps, which are variable in number in such cases. The commissures usually are recognizable but in some cases there is only a single flap, resulting in a "unicommissural" valvar stenosis.[3] The fused cusps form a dome-shaped diaphragm with an opening of variable size that protrudes distally into the aorta. Distal to the stenosis, the aorta usually is dilated. Valvar stenosis can be complicated by aortic insufficiency, endocardial fibroelastosis and left ventricular hypertrophy. The valvar stenoses account for 60–80% of the congenital aortic stenoses.[1,3]

Fig. 59-2. – Left ventricle with anterior mitral leaflet reflected upward, exposing rudimentary aortic outflow tract with marked valvar stenosis. Endocardial sclerosis can be seen.

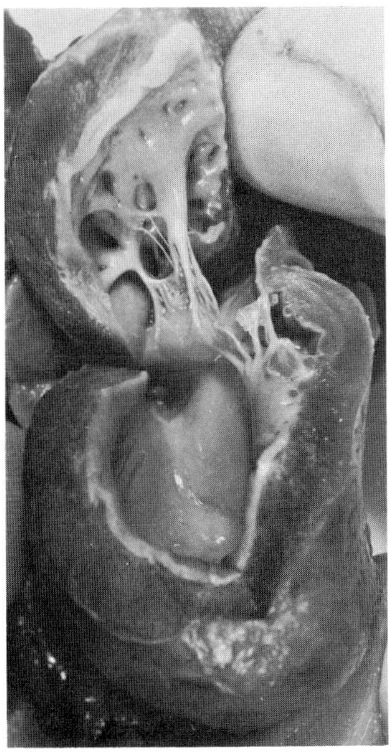

Subaortic (subvalvar) stenosis consists in a fibrous ring that is located in the left ventricular outflow tract, several millimeters below the aortic valve. Sometimes subvalvar stenosis is combined with valvar stenosis. Subaortic stenosis may be a harmless accidental finding at necropsy or cause obstruction and symptoms comparable to the valvar form. This type is encountered in 10–20% of the cases of congenital aortic stenosis.[1,3]

Supravalvar stenosis is relatively rare, accounting for approximately 5% of the cases, but the literature concerning this form has become quite voluminous because of the syndrome associated with the aortic anomaly (p. 578). The narrowing of the aorta may be localized above the sinuses of Valsalva or be diffuse and include the entire ascending aorta.

ETIOLOGY. – In the old literature, fetal endocarditis was considered the cause of some cases of congenital aortic stenosis, but this opinion is not prevalent at present. That an infectious agent can be the cause of such anomalies has been shown by rare cases of aortic stenosis following early maternal rubella.[4,5] In many instances, associated cardiovascular malformations suggest that the aortic stenosis originated in embryonic life and not in late fetal life, as assumed by early writers. Occasionally, aortic stenosis has been observed in the thalidomide syndrome.[6]

Genetic determination of congenital aortic stenosis sometimes can be assumed because of familial aggregation. Schöne[7] reported 2 brothers with congenital aortic stenosis, 1 confirmed by necropsy, and Landtman and Wallgren[4] 2 cases in one family. Polani and Campbell[8] saw 1 sibling affected by aortic stenosis and another by the tetrad of Fallot. A rare kind of aortic stenosis can be attributed to xanthoma tuberosum, an (incomplete) dominantly inherited disorder that is due to hypercholesterolemia.[9] An interesting family of this kind was described by Bloom *et al.*[10] Apparently normal parents had at least 5 children with xanthoma tuberosum, and the most serious effect of this disease was cardiovascular involvement with sudden death in some of the children. In some of these cases, clinical signs pointed to aortic valve involvement.[2] Subaortic stenosis due to hypertrophy of the ventricular septum has been observed in cases of familial cardiomegaly.[11] Congenital organic subvalvar aortic stenosis shows familial recurrence less frequently. In the families of 45 propositi Jörgensen[18] found 11 relatives affected with similar or – rarely – dissimilar congenital heart disease. He advanced the hypothesis of a "multifactorial genetic" background as the mode of inheritance.

Aortic stenosis is rare in autosomal trisomy syndromes. Abnormal aortic valve was mentioned only three times in necropsies of 272 cases of Down syndrome.[12]

The prevalence of males among the patients with aortic stenosis is a well-established but unexplained fact. In most series, approximately 80% of the patients were males.[1,13,14] But there are some types of aortic stenosis with less definite male prevalence. The sex ratio probably is less elevated for subvalvar than for valvar stenosis[2] and for aortic stenosis symptomatic in the first year of life, which may affect more females than males.

Symptoms.—The majority of children with aortic stenosis remain symptom-free for a long time. They also show good physical development, except for those who have associated malformations interfering with growth.[4,16] As a rule, aortic stenosis is discovered in routine examinations when a harsh systolic murmur is noticed in the right second intercostal space. Some children have a diastolic murmur, which is pronounced if a concomitant aortic insufficiency is present. During childhood, angina pectoris, syncope or left ventricular failure is rare. The pulse usually is normal and the blood pressure variable. The electrocardiogram is normal, but in severe cases there are signs of left ventricular hypertrophy. Roentgenograms are within normal limits, but sometimes the heart appears enlarged and the ascending aorta dilated. Calcifications may be seen in the valvar area. Cardiac catheterization reveals the systolic gradient between the left ventricle and the aorta, which may be an important guide in the treatment of the case. Left ventriculography can demonstrate the site of the obstruction.[2]

Aortic stenosis, symptomatic in the first year of life, is a serious cardiovascular anomaly that may lead to congestive heart failure at an early age. It occurs in approximately 5% of children with aortic stenosis.[1,14] The majority of cases of aortic stenosis resulting in congestive heart failure in the first year of life[1,2] is made up of infants who often have a combination of aortic stenosis and endocardial fibroelastosis.[2] Intermittent cyanosis and respiratory difficulties commonly precede the final heart failure. Necropsy usually shows a unicommissural aortic valve.[15] Subaortic ring stenosis does not endanger the life of infants.[2]

Associated malformations.—These occur in the cardiovascular system or in other systems. Some may be found in the aorta. Aortic insufficiency may be combined with aortic stenosis, and bicuspid valves are not rare. Association of valvar and subaortic stenosis occurs. Patent ductus arteriosus, coarctation of the aorta, atrial or ventricular septal defect,[4,5] pulmonary stenosis[17] and dextrocardia[13] may be present in patients with aortic stenosis. Aortic hypoplasia, although rare in these cases, has been observed.[17] Bonham Carter *et al.*[5] found aortic stenosis and incompetence in more than 4% of their patients operated on for patent ductus arteriosus. Some of the patients observed who had this combination of anomalies also had coarctation or aneurysm of the aorta, arachnodactyly, eye defects or deafness. Extracardiac associated malformations occur in only 6% of the cases and they are rather nonspecific except for those occurring with supravalvar aortic stenosis (p. 541).[1]

Prognosis.—The prognosis is poor for infants with valvar aortic stenosis combined with endocardial fibroelastosis who show early signs of congestive heart failure. After the first year, many children seen with aortic stenosis are symptom-free and not endangered by heart failure. The prognosis is less favorable for adults with this anomaly. Severe valvar or subvalvar stenosis may lead to sudden death in 1–2% of the patients with aortic stenosis. Aortic regurgitation develops in approximately one-third of the patients[1] with valvar or subvalvar stenosis. Bacterial endocarditis is rare. Syncope becomes more frequent with increasing age. Angina pectoris is rare in children.[2] Some patients with aortic stenosis survive to old age without serious illness. Persons with subaortic stenosis can also remain symptom-free, but ventricular hypertrophy, heart failure or sudden death can occur.[2]

Treatment.—In a disorder with widely varying prognosis, treatment must be individual. Congestive heart failure in infants represents an emergency that requires intensive medical treatment, generally followed by surgical intervention. The same is true for aortic stenoses beyond the first year of age, which sometimes are subjected to open heart surgery. Surgical mortality is between 5% and 10% and the survivors may need a second operation. The majority of children with aortic stenosis do not require surgery. The degree of exercise permissible varies greatly for individual patients.[2] Overexercise and competitive sports should be avoided in all cases.

REFERENCES

1. Hohn, A. R., Van Praagh, S., Moore, D., Vlad, P., and Lambert, E. C.: Aortic stenosis, Circulation 32 (supp. 3): 4, 1965.
2. Keith, J. D., Rowe, R. D., and Vlad, P. (eds.): *Heart Disease in Infancy and Childhood* (2d ed.; New York: The Macmillan Company, 1966).
3. Takekawa, S. D., Owings, W. K., Titus, J. L., and DuShane, J. W.: Congenital aortic stenosis, Am. J. Roentgenol. 98:800, 1966.
4. Landtman, B., and Wallgren, E. I.: Congenital aortic stenosis in children; a study of twenty-four cases, Ann. paediat. Fenniae 2:259, 1956.
5. Bonham Carter, R. E., Walker, C. H. M., Daley, R., Matthews, M. B., and Medd, W. E.: Patent ductus arteriosus with abnormal aortic valve, Brit. Heart J. 17:255, 1955.
6. Kajii, T.: Thalidomide experience in Japan, Ann. paediat. 205:341, 1965.
7. Schöne, G.: Über angeborene Herzfehler. Ein Beitrag zu ihrer Diagnostik, Zirkulationsgrösse und ihrem familiären Vorkommen, Deutsche Arch. klin. Med. 184:129, 1939.
8. Polani, P. E., and Campbell, M.: Aetiological study of congenital heart disease, Ann. Human Genet. 19:209, 1955.
9. Cook, C. D., Smith, H. L., Giesen, C. W., and Berdez, G. L.: Xanthoma tuberosum aortic stenosis, coronary sclerosis and angina pectoris; report of case in boy 13 years of age, Am. J. Dis. Child. 73:326, 1947.
10. Bloom, D., Kaufman, S. R., and Stevens, R. A.: Hereditary xanthomatosis; familial incidence of xanthoma tubero-

sum associated with hypercholesteremia and cardiovascular involvement with report of several cases of sudden death, Arch. Dermat. & Syph. 45:1, 1942.
11. Paré, J. A. P., Fraser, R. G., Pirozynski, W. J., Shanks, J. A., and Stubington, D.: Hereditary cardiovascular dysplasia; a form of familial cardiomyopathy, Am. J. Med. 31: 37, 1961.
12. Warkany, J., Passarge, E., and Smith, L. B.: Congenital malformations in autosomal trisomy syndromes, Am. J. Dis. Child. 112:502, 1966.
13. Campbell, M., and Kauntze, R.: Congenital aortic valvular stenosis, Brit. Heart J. 15:179, 1953.
14. Ongley, P. A., Nadas, A. S., Paul, M. H., Rudolph, A. M., and Starkey, G. W. B.: Aortic stenosis in infants and children, Pediatrics 21:207, 1958.
15. Moller, J. H., Nakib, A., Eliot, R. S., and Edwards, J. E.: Symptomatic congenital aortic stenosis in the first year of life, J. Pediat. 69:728, 1966.
16. Kjellberg, S. R., Mannheimer, E., Rudhe, U., and Jonsson, B.: *Diagnosis of Congenital Heart Disease* (Chicago: Year Book Medical Publishers, Inc., 1955).
17. Downing, D. F.: Congenital aortic stenosis; clinical aspects and surgical treatment, Circulation 14:188, 1956.
18. Jörgensen, G.: Genetische Untersuchungen bei angeborener organischer subvalvulärer Aortenstenose, Humangenetik 7:51, 1969.

Supravalvar Aortic Stenosis

ALTHOUGH A RARE FORM of aortic stenosis, the supravalvar type has attracted much attention in recent years. The incidence may be only 1 in 300,000,[1] but there are three anatomic types and possibly three clinical types. The relationship of these subgroups is not clear. Anatomically, a localized zone of obstruction may appear as a band just distal to the sinuses of Valsalva, a localized narrowing of the ascending aorta may be present or there may be diffuse narrowing of the ascending aorta.[2] The clinical subgroups consist of the syndrome of cardiovascular, facial, dental and mental abnormalities (p. 578), the familial form and the sporadic form. These three clinical forms may show localized obstruction above the sinuses of Valsalva, or more distally in the ascending aorta or diffuse narrowing of the ascending aorta.

The "supravalvar aortic stenosis complex" is discussed on pages 578–580. In addition to the aortic changes, many cardiovascular anomalies have been recognized in patients with a rather typical facies, hypercalcemia, dental changes and mental retardation. This complex associated with supravalvar aortic stenosis obviously represents a severe general disorder. Most cases reported so far have been sporadic, but familial repetition cannot be excluded.[3,4] There are familial cases of "simple" supravalvar aortic stenosis that do not have the syndrome of associated anomalies. McCue *et al.*[8] described the anomaly in a mother and 4 of her 5 children. A pair of concordant identical twins was included in the sibship. Jörgensen and Beuren[5] reviewed the simple supravalvar aortic stenoses and presented pedigrees showing repetition of the disorder not only in families but also in kindreds through several generations. But it seems that in such families of simple stenosis sometimes one affected member shows the entire syndrome of supravalvar aortic stenosis.[6] Add to this the finding that the "supravalvar aortic stenosis complex" occasionally can go with a normal supravalvar region,[4] and the confusion concerning these vascular anomalies will become obvious.

The diagnosis of supravalvar aortic stenosis is based on auscultation, catheterization and angiography. Surgical correction is possible. The aorta can be widened by insertion of a patch or by excision of the aortic narrowing.[1,7]

REFERENCES

1. Keith, J. D., Rowe, R. D., and Vlad, P. (eds.): *Heart Disease in Infancy and Childhood* (2d ed.; New York: The Macmillan Company, 1966).
2. Neufeld, H. N., Wagenvoort, C. A., Ongley, P. A., and Edwards, J. E.: Hypoplasia of ascending aorta. An unusual form of supravalvular aortic stenosis with special reference to localized coronary arterial hypertension, Am. J. Cardiol. 10:746, 1962.
3. Hebedank, M., and Bücheler, E.: Kardiovasculäre Fehlbildungen mit konstitutionellen Charakteristika und Debilität, Ztschr. Kinderh. 98:268, 1967.
4. Wiltse, H. E., Goldbloom, R. B., Antia, A. U., Ottesen, O. E., Rowe, R. D., and Cooke, R. E.: Infantile hypercalcemia syndrome in twins, New England J. Med. 275:1157, 1966.
5. Jörgensen, G., and Beuren, A. J.: Genetische Untersuchungen bei supravalvulären Aortenstenosen, Humangenetik 1:497, 1965.
6. Antia, A. U., Wiltse, H. E., Rowe, R. D., Pitt, E. L., Levin, S., Ottesen, O. E., and Cooke, R. E.: Pathogenesis of the supravalvar aortic stenosis syndrome, J. Pediat. 71:431, 1967.
7. De Bakey, M. E., and Beall, A. C., Jr.: Successful surgical correction of supravalvular aortic stenosis, Circulation 27: 858, 1963.
8. McCue, C. M., Spicuzza, T. J., Robertson, L. W., and Mauck, H. P., Jr.: Familial supravalvular aortic stenosis, J. Pediat. 73:889, 1968.

Subvalvar Aortic Stenosis and Idiopathic Cardiomegaly

THIS DISORDER (p. 584) has been recognized in patients who die suddenly or following an episode of heart failure and show, at necropsy, hypertrophy and fibrosis of the myocardium without evidence of valvar disease.[1] There exists, however, a functional-obstructive subvalvar aortic stenosis that is not recognizable on dissection or operation and is thought to be due to functional muscular conus stenosis effected by hypertrophy of the interventricular septum and anterior walls of the ventricles.[2] The condition is familial and has been observed in several generations. In a genetic study, Jörgensen[2] found familial recurrence in about half the cases. Autosomal dominant inheritance seems likely, but penetrance and expression of the disease vary. The risk of siblings being affected was calculated as approximately 0.3%.

REFERENCES

1. Paré, A. P., Fraser, R. G., Pirozynski, W. J., Shanks, J. A., and Stubington, D.: Hereditary cardiovascular dysplasia, Am. J. Med. 31:37, 1961.
2. Jörgensen, G.: Genetische Untersuchungen bei funktionell-obstruktiver subvalvulärer Aortenstenose, Humangenetik 6:13, 1968.

Coarctation of the Aorta

THERE IS A MARKED DISCREPANCY between estimates of the frequency of coarctation of the aorta in clinical material and in necropsy findings. In necropsies, this malformation of the aorta is not rare, and reviews indicate that 1 case can be found in 1,500 necropsies. In series that include a large infant material, the incidence may be much higher. Sloan and Cooley,[1] for instance, found 24 cases of coarctation of the aorta in 13,000 necropsies, which corresponds to 1 in 540 cases. Twenty-one of the 24 cases occurred in stillborn or young infants with additional cardiovascular anomalies. Ober and Moore[2] observed coarctation of the aorta in 11% of the infants dying of congenital cardiovascular malformations in the first month. Abbott[3] found the anomaly in 8.5% of necropsied patients with cardiovascular anomalies, coarctation of the aorta being the third most frequent anomaly.

In clinical material, the disorder is much more rare. Keith *et al.*[4] stated that it occurred only once in every 12,000 children between the ages of birth and 15 years in the Toronto Cardiac Registry and that it was seventh in order of frequency among congenital heart defects. Perlman[5] found it once in 10,000 army recruits. In general hospital and clinic material, coarctation of the aorta accounts for from 4% to 11% of cardiac patients.[4,6] This marked discrepancy between necropsy and clinical findings indicates a high early mortality of some patients and freedom from symptoms in many others who do not appear as patients in children's hospitals or clinics. They either develop clinical manifestations later or not at all.

Coarctation can occur in many locations in the aorta, but the most important areas are those distal to the left subclavian artery. Ever since Morgagni (cited by Keith *et al.*[4]), in 1760, observed and described an extreme stenosis of the aorta, anatomists have been greatly interested in the different types and forms of coarctation, and many cases were reported in the literature of the nineteenth century. It was soon noticed that some patients with this anomaly died in early infancy, whereas others survived to adulthood or sometimes to old age. In 1903, Bonnet[7] divided the various forms of coarctation into two main groups. The infantile type is characterized by stenosis proximal to the ductus arteriosus and usually distal to the left subclavian artery. This coarctation lies in the area of the isthmus aortae, which is a physiologic constriction in prenatal life. In this form, which is also called the preductal type, the ductus arteriosus often remains patent in early life. The second main form established by Bonnet is the adult type, which usually is located near the aortic termination of the ductus arteriosus or below it. The coarctation of the adult type, as a rule, is a rather abrupt constriction with a lumen of variable size. Bonnet's classification was quite useful as long as coarctation was chiefly of interest to the anatomists, who commonly found in necropsies preductal stenosis in infants, whereas the postductal form occurred in adults. The value of this classification was reduced when exact clinical methods became available for investigation of coarctation, and especially when surgery made repair feasible. Nadas[6] pointed out that a classification of coarctation into adult and infantile types based on the location and length of the constricted segment is meaningless in view of present-day physiologic and therapeutic concepts, since the so-called adult type, a localized constriction near the insertion of the ductus arteriosus, may cause death in congestive failure in infancy. On the other hand, the so-called infantile type, the long, narrow coarctation between the left subclavian artery and the ligamentum arteriosum, may occur in adults and be associated with relative longevity. Ober and Moore[2] reported 11 cases of coarctation of the aorta seen in necropsies of neonates and 3 of them were of the "adult" type.

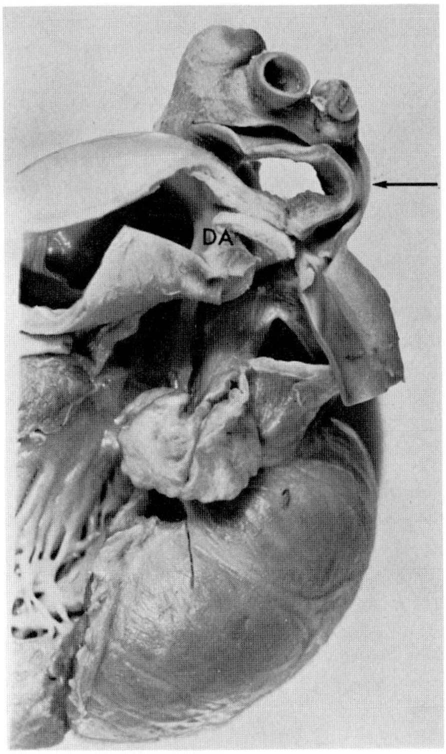

Fig. 59-3.—Aortic coarctation (**arrow**) with hypoplasia of the aortic isthmus and thickened ductus (*DA*).

Most clinicians agree that the old classification must be abandoned, but there is no unanimity on a new one. Nadas recommended a general division into coarctations in which the left ventricle directly, or by means of collaterals, supplies the entire systemic circuit with blood, and those in which the left ventricle supplies only the upper half of the body, whereas the parts below the coarctation are supplied from the right ventricle through a ductus arteriosus. A classification of a postductal-adult type and a preductal-infantile type was recommended by Keith *et al.*,[4] who, however, found it necessary to subdivide the postductal type in cases encountered in children under or over 1 year of age; the same subdivision is necessary for the preductal type.

Coarctation of the aorta with a closed ductus usually shows an area of marked constriction opposite the aortic insertion of the ligamentum arteriosum or somewhat distal to it. The lumen of the constricted area often is much more narrow than the external appearance of the constricted area indicates, since it may be occluded by a diaphragm with a very small opening. In approximately half the cases, the lumen is less than 5 mm. in diameter and in some cases no opening can be found. The basis for the aortic narrowing is, according to Edwards *et al.*,[8] a deformity of the aortic media, which shows a characteristic thickening and projects into the lumen, making it narrow and eccentric. The medial thickening is seen in cases of coarctation of all ages, including infancy. In adolescents and adults, there often is an additional change, namely, intimal thickening that develops progressively in postnatal life. The aorta proximal to the coarctation is normal in size or dilated and thick walled. Distal to the coarctation, the aortic lumen may also be enlarged, but the wall is thin. In this distal area of the aorta, Edwards *et al.* described a corrugated patch rising above the intimal surface, a lesion explained as the result of a jet of blood that strikes the wall after passing through the zone of aortic narrowing. This jet lesion develops into a point of minor resistance and an area susceptible to bacterial infection. Congenital bicuspid aortic valve is associated with coarctation of the aorta in one-fourth to one-half the cases. Generally, the heart is enlarged in coarctation, with hypertrophy of the left ventricle.

Collateral circulation is present in most cases, a fact known since the end of the eighteenth century. A detailed description of the collateral circulation in coarctation was given by Edwards *et al.*[8] Stenosis of the aorta is compensated for by branches originating in the subclavian arteries, which join blood vessels connected with the lower part of the aorta. The intercostal arteries, with the exception of the first two pairs, are most important anastomotic bridges, particularly the fourth through the seventh pairs. They connect the aorta below the level of the coarctation with the internal mammary, musculophrenic, superior epigastric, anterior spinal and lateral thoracic arteries. In addition, collateral circulation is established by the vessels around the scapula. The intercostal arteries are markedly enlarged and tortuous.

Edwards[9] stated that the collateral circulation in aortic coarctation begins during intrauterine life. In cases of coarctation distal to the ductus arteriosus, fetal life would be impossible without collateral circulation, since the ductus would have no outlet to the descending aorta. In cases of coarctation proximal to the ductus, a collateral circulation need not develop during fetal life, since blood can pass from the right ventricle through the open ductus and reach directly the lower part of the body, whereas the upper part can be supplied by the left ventricle. However, in such cases, if the ductus obliterates in postnatal life, the blood flow becomes insufficient for the lower half of the body and life is endangered. Infants with this type of anomaly often are also carriers of associated malformations that may contribute to early death.

Etiology.—Little is known of etiologic factors in coarctation. The prevalence of males among necropsy cases with coarctation of the aorta was noted by early observers. Herxheimer[10] reviewed 100 cases described anatomically and found that 75 patients were male and 25 female. A similar sex distribution was noted by Pritchard[11] and by Abbott.[3]

In the clinical material, which usually includes cases diagnosed by clinical methods, operation or necropsy, the difference in the sexes is not so marked. For instance, Campbell and Polani[12] found 63% and Lamy *et al.*[13] 64% males, whereas MacMahon *et al.*[14] observed a female prevalence of 56%.

It is well known that coarctation of the aorta occurs with some frequency in Turner syndrome (Chapter 111). This association seemed curious as long at it was thought that these patients were females characterized by ovarian agenesis, but now it has been established that most of them are sex-chromatin negative. In 1954, Polani *et al.*[15] demonstrated, in 3 patients with Turner syndrome and coarctation, a sex chromatin pattern normally seen in males. It has been shown since that patients with phenotypic Turner syndrome tend to other cardiovascular anomalies, particularly pulmonic stenosis; they may differ in etiology from the XO Turner syndrome (Chapter 111). Ikeda[16] studied the sex chromatin in fetal coarctation of the aorta. Only 2% of a series of patients investigated by Campbell and Polani[12] had Turner syndrome.

Coarctation of the aorta occurs with increased frequency in trisomy syndromes. In necropsies of patients with Down syndrome, coarctation was noted in 1.1% of the cases, which is approximately five times the frequency reported in a general infant population. In trisomy 18 the frequency was 7% and in trisomy 13-15 it was 6%.[17] Freundlich *et al.*[18] saw 1 child with Down syndrome among 33 infants with coarctation.

Genetic determination may play a role in some of the cases. Walker[19] reported coarctation in a father and son, and Taylor and Pollock[20] observed it in a mother, her daughter and her son. In the son, who died at the age of 16 years while playing basketball, necropsy revealed an abrupt coarctation of the aorta immediately above the aortic cusps and extending past the origin of the left subclavian artery. Klemola[21] observed two families with 2 brothers each showing signs of coarctation, and Moss[22] reported a brother and a sister in whom the diagnosis was confirmed by surgery. In Marfan syndrome (Chapter 91), coarctation has been observed in at least one instance.[23] Many other etiologic factors were considered by Campbell and Polani.[12] They observed a case in which the mother had rubella in early pregnancy.

Pathogenesis.—The pathogenesis of coarctation has never been explained satisfactorily, and there may be no unitary explanation for the many forms of the anomaly. In the nineteenth century, it was believed that coarctation of the aorta, which so frequently is located near the aortic opening of the ductus arteriosus, is closely related to the closure of the ductus. It was thought that the obliterating process of the ductus may extend to the aorta and constrict that vessel, but microscopic examination of the aorta adjacent to the ligamentum arteriosum did not show overgrowth of the closing tissue into the constricted area of the aorta. Other objections to this theory, which dates the origin of coarctation after birth, have been summarized by Evans.[24] In some cases, the constriction lies at some distance from the site of insertion of the ductus. Coarctation near the ductus may occur in patients with patency of the ductus arteriosus. At the time of birth, the pressure within the ductus is lowered and that within the aorta is raised, which should help to produce dilatation rather than constriction of the aortic lumen. A marked degree of periductal constriction of the aorta sometimes is present in infants less than 1 week old and in fetuses.[16,25]

The alternative explanation of coarctation also goes back to the early nineteenth century, when Reynaud,[26] in 1828, suggested that the anomaly was the result of faulty development during embryonic life. This theory is now more generally accepted, although, according to Evans, no early embryos have been found showing congenital coarctation of the aorta. The theory of disturbed prenatal development is supported by the finding of associated congenital malformations that often are present in patients with coarctation of the aorta.

The portion of the aorta that is the most frequent site of coarctations undergoes many changes in prenatal life and represents, therefore, a sensitive point of development. The permanent arch of the aorta develops from the fourth left aortic arch; the fifth aortic arch is rudimentary and disappears early in embryonic life. The portion of the dorsal aorta that connects the left third and fourth aortic arches disappears also and the subclavian artery "migrates" cephalad along the aortic wall until it approaches the origin of the common carotid. Such changes can be a source of growth disturbances and could account for stenotic areas of the aorta. The amount of blood in the fetus that passes through the portion of the aorta located between the left subclavian and the ductus arteriosus is relatively small, since it is bypassed by the blood stream, which reaches the lower half of the body through the ductus arteriosus. Normally, this portion of the aorta forms an isthmus, but this isthmus is capable of rapid expansion if its walls have normal structure. The degenerative processes that obliterate aortic arches and branches normally in fetal life may extend, according to Bremer,[27] to the aorta itself. The disappearance of the segment of the dorsal aorta connecting the third and fourth aortic arches may be responsible for the fetal type of coarctation. Bremer pointed out that the aortic isthmus is matched embryologically by the less well-known right subclavian isthmus situated a short distance along that artery beyond its origin from the innominate trunk. At about 6 or 7 weeks of fetal life, the section of the dorsal aorta between the third and fourth arches degenerates on both sides (Fig. 58-1). The obliterative processes of these two sections of the dorsal aortae may extend to the caudal ends of the two fourth arches in the form of a slight local endothelial thickening and a more noticeable increase of constricting musculature, with consequent narrowing of the lumen. In the right subclavian, the constrictive processes soon yield to the counterpressure of the increasingly more powerful force of the blood stream until, at birth, the subclavian isthmus is rarely noticeable. On the left, the aortic isthmus lying in the "stagnant section" of the descending aorta, which, in fetal life, carries relatively little blood, may remain undistended[27] if its wall has been affected by the obliterating process extended from adjacent transitory blood channels.

SYMPTOMS.—From a clinical point of view, it probably is best to distinguish those patients who have no manifestations or symptoms in infancy from those who present signs early in the first year of life.

The "simple form" of coarctation usually is located in the area of the ductus or distal to it (postductal coarctation, adult type). Most children with this anomaly have no signs or symptoms until they reach school age. Then a heart murmur may be found on routine examination and a suprasternal pulsation may be noticed. Examination of the blood pressure reveals a discrepancy between the arms and the legs, and the femoral arteries may not be palpable at all. These children, usually boys, are well developed, but the lower half of the body may be relatively underdeveloped. In older children, pulsations of dilated collateral vessels occasionally are palpable in the scapular or interscapular region. There is no cyanosis or clubbing. The heart murmur is systolic, but in the presence of an abnormal aortic valve a diastolic murmur may be present also. Electrocardiography can be normal or show left ventricular hypertrophy. In roentgenograms, left ventricular enlargement is seen and sometimes an indentation of the barium-filled esophagus at the site of the coarctation.

As a rule, these children have few complaints during childhood, but occasionally they may have dyspnea, muscle pains in the legs or suffer complications such as bacterial endocarditis, rheumatic fever or cerebrovascular accidents. However, most complications occur in the years after adolescence, and the mean life expectancy of these patients is not more than 35 years. Only one-fourth of the patients with clinical manifestations live through the fourth decade unless an operation is performed. The most common fatal complications are left ventricular failure, bacterial endocarditis or aortitis, dissecting aneurysm of the aorta or rupture of an aneurysm of the circle of Willis. Bacterial endocarditis usually develops on a bicuspid aortic valve but, in some cases, the infection may be located in the ascending or descending aorta. Ruptured aneurysm may be found in the aorta proximal or distal to the coarctation. Many patients have been described who were in apparently good health and capable of strenuous physical exercise who died suddenly of a ruptured aneurysm or sudden heart failure.

Although most patients with this form of coarctation are males, many females with this anomaly have reached adult life and some went through successful pregnancies. Pritchard[11] reviewed 77 cases of coarctation and pregnancy and added 2 cases of his own. Approximately 10% of the patients died during pregnancy or during the postpartum period. Three women with this malformation were pregnant more than ten times. However, in general, one-fourth of the patients showed some cardiac embarrassment and 2 deaths resulted from heart failure during pregnancy. Therapeutic abortion probably is not often indicated and cesarean section should be done only for the usual obstetric indications. The second stage of labor should be limited to a short period if possible. The condition of the children born of successful pregnancies of these mothers usually was not described, but in some of the cases it was stated that the children were normal and that their birth weight was normal. Resection of the constricted segment of the aorta has been performed during pregnancy.[28] In 1958, Goodwin[29] reviewed the outcome of 136 pregnancies complicated by coarctation. The mortality was 9.5 per 100 patients and 3.7 per 100 pregnancies (many of the patients had multiple pregnancies). Goodwin stated that pregnancy is not necessarily an added hazard to the patient with coarctation. It should be allowed to continue in uncomplicated cases but be interrupted if heart disease complicates the situation. Toxemia of pregnancy is rare in these patients and fetal mortality low.[30]

ASSOCIATED MALFORMATIONS.—Among 151 patients with aortic coarctation, Campbell and Polani[12] recognized aortic stenosis, aortic regurgitation, persistent ductus and berry aneurysm of the cerebral vessels as complications. Twelve (8%) had malformations of the heart. Noncardiac malformations were observed in 13% (including 2% with Turner syndrome). Most of the patients in this series were adolescents or adults with coarctation who usually were well and of good physique. Associated cardiac lesions are much more frequent among infants with aortic coarctation; they amounted to 70% in the series of Freundlich *et al.*[18] and to 87% in the series of Becker *et al.*[38]

TREATMENT.—To avoid the complications mentioned and to ensure normal life expectancy, surgical treatment of coarctation is now recommended.[39] Operations have been performed on hundreds of patients successfully. The optimal age is between 10 and 15 years, the operative risk in this age group being less than 5%. Operation consists of excision of the constricted segment and end-to-end anastomosis if possible. If the gap between the aortic ends is too large, a graft can be inserted. Aneurysms found either in the aorta beyond the constriction or in the terminal portion of an intercostal artery joining the aorta are also accessible to surgical treatment.[31] In 1962, Schuster and Gross[32] had performed nearly 500 surgical repairs (chiefly on patients between 8 and 20 years), with a mortality of 4% and a morbidity rate of 4% in the survivors. In general, the blood pressure becomes normal after the operation, and the anastomosis grows with the child. If coarctation is associated with an open ductus with pulmonary hypertension, the prognosis should be guarded because of the greater risk of operation.[33]

Severe Forms

For unknown reasons, some patients with this type of coarctation develop congestive heart failure in infancy. Such children may lack a collateral circulation or the degree of coarctation may be unusually severe at the time of birth. The infants have general signs of congestive heart failure, but some can be recognized by the weak and late femoral pulse. At first, treatment should be medical,[18] operation being delayed to an age more favorable for surgical treatment.[6] However, some prefer early surgical intervention when immediate response to medical treatment is inadequate.[4]

There are other forms of coarctation that cause severe symptoms in infancy. Among these is coarctation with left-to-right shunt through an open ductus or a ventricular defect. In this situation, the ductus usually opens above the coarctation but it may be at or even below the site of the constriction. The left-to-right shunt is understandable in the first case and can be explained by good collateral anastomoses in the second case. These infants frequently are poorly developed but they have neither cyanosis nor clubbing. Hypertension of the upper extremities is present. If the patent ductus is large, a typical machinery murmur may be heard, but if the ductus is small there is only a systolic murmur. In the case of ventricular septal defect, a murmur characteristic for this anomaly may be noted.[6] Medical treatment is indicated in such cases.

The most serious form of coarctation, which is a frequent cause of death in early infancy, consists of a constriction located proximal to a large patent ductus that, in this case, supplies the descending aorta with blood from the pulmonary artery. In these patients, the coarctation usually is located between the origin of the left subclavian and the ductus. This form, which is the prototype of "infantile coarctation," frequently is associated with such other cardiovascular anomalies as transposition of the great vessels, aortic or mitral valvar disease, ventricular septal defect or endocardial fibroelastosis. The associated defects may determine the clinical picture. If the anomaly is limited to coarctation and open ductus, the latter supplies unoxygenated blood to the lower half of the body, and there is right ventricular hypertension.[6] The children develop congestive heart failure in early infancy, with dyspnea, cyanosis and feeding difficulties. The cyanosis may be limited to the lower extremities. Auscultation is not characteristic, there may be no differences in blood pressure of the upper and lower extremities and the femoral pulse may be palpable. The diagnosis is difficult in such cases because neither the roentgen aspects nor the electrocardiogram betray the coarctation. The prognosis is poor and surgery only rarely successful. There exists an aortic arch anomaly that is functionally related to the "infantile" form of coarctation. In this anomaly, the aortic arch is completely interrupted between the left subclavian (or carotid) and the ductus so that only the vessels to the upper part of the body are derived from the ascending aorta, whereas the descending aorta receives blood from the ductus only (p. 532).

Freundlich *et al.*[18] reported their experience with medical treatment of aortic coarctation in infancy. Of 30 infants with cardiac symptoms, 15 died during infancy; all had intracardiac defects that often masked the coarctation. There were no deaths among 8 patients with uncomplicated coarctation. In another series of infantile coarctation, 15 of 17 patients were operated on, with survival of 10.[34]

Coarctation of the Abdominal Aorta

Coarctation of the abdominal aorta is rare but, according to Gerbasi *et al.*,[35] more cases have been reported in the past few years than in the 100 years following the first case described in 1847. The subject was reviewed by Inmon and Pollock,[36] and the possible relationship of this anomaly to renal hypertension was discussed by Fisher and Corcoran.[37] A coarctation of the abdominal aorta limited to the area of the celiac axis was treated successfully by Gerbasi *et al.*, who used an aortic homograft as a shunt around the constricted area.

REFERENCES

1. Sloan, R. D., and Cooley, R. N.: Coarctation of the aorta; the roentgenologic aspects of 125 surgically confirmed cases, Radiology 61:701, 1953.
2. Ober, W. B., and Moore, T. E., Jr.: Congenital cardiac malformations in neonatal period; autopsy study, New England J. Med. 253:271, 1955.
3. Abbott, M. E.: *Atlas of Congenital Heart Disease* (New York: American Heart Association, 1936).
4. Keith, J. D., Rowe, R. D., and Vlad, P. (eds.): *Heart Disease in Infancy and Childhood* (2d ed.; New York: The Macmillan Company, 1966).
5. Perlman, L.: Coarctation of aorta; clinical and roentgenologic analysis of 13 cases, Am. Heart J. 28:24, 1944.
6. Nadas, A. S.: *Pediatric Cardiology* (Philadelphia: W. B. Saunders Company, 1957).
7. Bonnet, L. M.: Sur la lésion dite sténose congénitale de l'aorte dans la région de l'isthme, Rev. méd. Paris 23:108, 255, 335, 418, 481, 1903.
8. Edwards, J. E., Clagett, O. T., Drake, R. L., and Christensen, N. A.: Collateral circulation in coarctation of aorta, Proc. Staff Meet. Mayo Clin. 23:333, 1948.
9. Edwards, J. E.: Congenital Malformations of the Heart and Great Vessels, in Gould, S. E. (ed.), *Pathology of the Heart* (Springfield, Ill.: Charles C Thomas, Publisher, 1953).
10. Herxheimer, G.: Missbildungen des Herzens und der grossen Gefässe, in Schwalbe, E. (ed.), *Die Morphologie der Missbildungen des Menschen und der Tiere* (Jena: Gustav Fischer, 1909).
11. Pritchard, J. A.: Coarctation of the aorta and pregnancy, Obst. & Gynec. Surv. 8:775, 1953.
12. Campbell, M., and Polani, P. E.: Aetiology of coarctation of the aorta, Lancet 1:473, 1961.
13. Lamy, M., de Grouchy, J., and Schweisguth, O.: Genetic and non-genetic factors in the etiology of congenital heart disease: Study of 1188 cases, Am. J. Human Genet. 9:17, 1957.
14. MacMahon, B., McKeown, T., and Record, R. G.: Incidence and life expectation of children with congenital

heart disease, Brit. Heart J. 15:121, 1953.
15. Polani, P. E., Hunter, W. F., and Lennox, B.: Chromosomal sex in Turner's syndrome with coarctation of aorta; preliminary communication, Lancet 2:120, 1954.
16. Ikeda, T.: On the sex chromatin in fetal coarctation of the aorta, Jap. J. Human Genet. 8:241, 1963.
17. Warkany, J., Passarge, E., and Smith, L. B.: Congenital malformations in autosomal trisomy syndromes, Am. J. Dis. Child. 112:502, 1966.
18. Freundlich, E., Engle, M. A., and Goldberg, H. P.: Coarctation of aorta in infancy; analysis of a 10-year experience with medical management, Pediatrics 27:427, 1961.
19. Walker, W. G.: Coarctation of the aorta in father and son, New England J. Med. 211:1192, 1934.
20. Taylor, R. R., and Pollock, B. E.: Coarctation of aorta in 3 members of family, Am. Heart J. 45:470, 1953.
21. Klemola, E.: Über familiäres Auftreten von Isthmusstenose der Aorta, Acta med. scandinav. 98:355, 1939.
22. Moss, A. J.: Coarctation of aorta in siblings, J. Pediat. 46:707, 1955.
23. Fischl, A. A., and Ruthberg, J.: Clinical implications of Marfan's syndrome, J.A.M.A. 146:704, 1951.
24. Evans, W.: Congenital stenosis (coarctation), atresia, and interruption of aortic arch; study of 28 cases, Quart. J. Med. 2:1, 1933.
25. Marks, D. N., Shapiro, R. S., and Joseph, L. G.: Roentgenographic diagnosis of coarctation of aorta in two-day-old infant, J. Pediat. 43:453, 1953.
26. Reynaud, A.: Observation d'une oblitération presque complète de l'aorte, J. hebd. méd. 1:161, 1828.
27. Bremer, J. L.: *Congenital Anomalies of the Viscera, Their Embryological Basis* (Cambridge, Mass.: Harvard University Press, 1957).
28. Peterson, L. T., Paul, O., and Fell, E.: Surgical correction of coarctation of aorta in pregnancy, Am. J. Obst. & Gynec. 65:199, 1953.
29. Goodwin, J. F.: Pregnancy and coarctation of the aorta, Lancet 1:16, 1958.
30. Shanahan, W. R., Romney, S. L., and Currens, J. H.: Coarctation of the aorta and pregnancy; report of ten cases with twenty-four pregnancies, J.A.M.A. 167:275, 1958.
31. Gross, R. E.: Coarctation of aorta, Circulation 7:757, 1953.
32. Schuster, S. R., and Gross, R. E.: Surgery for coarctation of the aorta; a review of 500 cases, J. Thoracic & Cardiovas. Surg. 43:54, 1962.
33. Cooley, J. C., Kirklin, J. W., Clagett, O. T., DuShane, J. D., Burchell, H. B., and Wood, E. H.: Coarctation of aorta associated with patent ductus arteriosus, Circulation 13:843, 1956.
34. Hartmann, A. F., Jr., Goldring, D., and Staple, T. W.: Coarctation of the aorta in infancy; hemodynamic studies, J. Pediat. 70:95, 1967.
35. Gerbasi, F. S., Kibler, R. S., and Margileth, A. M.: Coarctation of the abdominal aorta; a case successfully treated surgically, J. Pediat. 52:191, 1958.
36. Inmon, T. W., and Pollock, B. A.: Coarctation of the abdominal aorta: Review of the literature, Am. Heart J. 52:314, 1956.
37. Fisher, E. R., and Corcoran, A. C.: Congenital coarctation of abdominal aorta with resultant renal hypertension, A.M.A. Arch. Int. Med. 89:943, 1952.
38. Becker, A. E., Becker, M. J., and Edwards, J. E.: Anomalies associated with coarctation of aorta, Circulation 41:1067, 1970.
39. Shearer, W. T., Rutman, J. Y., Weinberg, W. A., and Goldring, D.: Coarctation of the aorta and cerebrovascular accident: A proposal for early corrective surgery, J. Pediat. 77:1004, 1970.

Congenital Aortic Aneurysm

A CONGENITAL AORTIC ANEURYSM involving the first part of the descending aorta and located just inferior to the origin of the left subclavian artery was described and repaired by Woods and Kenney.[1] An abnormal shadow extending outward from the left upper mediastinum was seen in a chest roentgenogram. Because mediastinal tumor or cyst was considered a possibility, thoracotomy was performed and a thin-walled, egg-shaped aneurysm was found. Since rupture threatened, the sac was infolded, tamponaded against the approximated edges of the defect and repaired.

An aneurysm of the thoracic aorta in an infant was treated by resection and arterial homograft by Cooley and Taylor.[2]

A large congenital aneurysm of the abdominal aorta was described by Howorth[3] in an infant born with a large abdominal mass measuring 11 cm. in diameter. At operation, the patient died when the aneurysm was entered to dissect the "tumor." In another case,[4] the child survived until the aneurysm ruptured at age 16 months.

REFERENCES

1. Woods, F. M., and Kenney, L. J.: Congenital aortic aneurysm; report of a case, J.A.M.A. 148:1216, 1952.
2. Cooley, D. A., and Taylor, F. M.: Aneurysm of thoracic aorta in infant treated by resection and arterial homograft, J. Pediat. 49:185, 1956.
3. Howorth, M. B., Jr.: Aneurysm of abdominal aorta in the newborn infant, New England J. Med. 276:1133, 1967.
4. Gibson, T. A.: Aneurysm of lower aorta with rupture in 16 month old infant, Am. J. Dis. Child. 71:654, 1946.

Congenital Aneurysm of a Sinus of Valsalva

AN ANEURYSM of a sinus of Valsalva may rupture into the right or left ventricle, right auricle or into the pulmonary artery. Such aneurysms have been attributed to abnormal fusion of the aortopulmonary septum with the bulbar septum or to congenital defects in the elastic tissue of the sinuses. The latter assumption is more plausible, since aneurysms can develop in all three sinuses.[1] The anomaly may be associated with ventricular septal defect, coarctation of the aorta, mitral stenosis, bicuspid aortic valve and aortic insufficiency. Jones and Langley[2] reviewed 25 cases in 1949. Nineteen of the patients were male. In most of the published cases, the aneurysm originated from the right sinus and penetrated into the right ventricle. There are no symptoms before the rupture unless associated anomalies are present. Rupture of the aneurysm produces a critical situation, with precordial pain, shortness of breath and collapse. A systolic-diastolic murmur develops, with its maximum intensity in the third and fourth left intercostal space. The time of survival after rupture of the aneurysm into the right side of the heart may vary from a few seconds to many years; the oldest patient reported was 64 years of age. Bacterial endocarditis, heart block or heart failure may be the cause of death. Falholt and Thomsen[3] diagnosed a congenital aneurysm of the right sinus by aortography. In recent years, a number of unperforated aortic sinus aneurysms have been described, and associated coarctation of the aorta, congenital aortic and mitral stenosis and arachnodactyly have been mentioned as associated symptoms. Steinberg and Geller[4] demonstrated, by angiocardiography in 3 consecutive patients with arachnodactyly, aneurysmal dilatation of the aortic sinuses. Two of these patients were asymptomatic. Sakakibara and Konno[5] estimated the average age of rupture to be approximately 32 years. The sex ratio was about 4 males to 1 female. These authors discussed diagnosis of the malformation and its surgical treatment.

REFERENCES

1. Micks, R. H.: Congenital aneurysms of all three sinuses of Valsalva, Brit. Heart J. 2:63, 1940.
2. Jones, A. M., and Langley, F. A.: Aortic sinus aneurysms, Brit. Heart J. 11:325, 1949.
3. Falholt, W., and Thomsen, G.: Congenital aneurysm of the right sinus of Valsalva, diagnosed by aortography, Circulation 8:549, 1953.
4. Steinberg, I., and Geller, W.: Aneurysmal dilatation of aortic sinuses in arachnodactyly: Diagnosed during life in 3 cases, Ann. Int. Med. 43:120, 1955.
5. Sakakibara, S., and Konno, S.: Congenital aneurysm of the sinus of Valsalva, Am. J. Cardiol. 12:100, 1963.

60

The Pulmonary Arteries

Classification of Congenital Malformations of the Pulmonary Arteries

SINGLETON *et al.*[1] classified the congenital abnormalities of the pulmonary arteries encountered in a children's hospital. Some of the defects were of clinical significance, others merely of anatomic interest. The authors mentioned as abnormalities of the undivided pulmonary artery: valvar stenosis, supravalvar stenosis, idiopathic dilatation, valvar insufficiency and coronary artery arising from the pulmonary artery. The following abnormalities of the pulmonary arteries were considered: atresias and hypoplasias, branch stenoses, retrotracheal left pulmonary artery and anomalous origin. Abnormalities of the pulmonary vascular bed mentioned were: arteriovenous fistula, arterial sclerosis and telangiectasias. Embryology and clinical and roentgenographic findings of these conditions were discussed and illustrated.

Congenital Absence of the Pulmonary Valve

Absence of the pulmonary valve cusps is a rare congenital defect that usually is associated with tetralogy of Fallot and occasionally with ventricular septal and other defects. Osman *et al.*[2] reviewed the literature on this subject and added clinical and roentgenographic findings of 8 observations of their own. They credited the first description to Chevers,[3] who noted the anomaly at necropsy of an 8-year-old child. Repeated respiratory infections with wheezing, to-and-fro murmurs, absent diminished second pulmonary sounds, enlarged pulmonary arteries and right ventricular hypertrophy are said to be characteristic of absent pulmonary valve cusps associated with other congenital cardiac malformations.[2]

REFERENCES

1. Singleton, E. B., Leachman, R. D., and Rosenberg, H. S.: Congenital abnormalities of the pulmonary arteries, Am. J. Roentgenol. 91:487, 1964.
2. Osman, M. Z., Meng, C. C. L., and Girdany, B. R.: Congenital absence of the pulmonary valve: Report of eight cases with review of the literature, Am. J. Roentgenol. 106:58, 1969.
3. Chevers, N.: Recherches sur les maladies de l'artère pulmonaire, Arch. gen. méd. 15:488, 1847.

Etiology of Pulmonary Stenosis

MANY PUBLICATIONS containing information about etiology of pulmonary stenosis appeared before modern terminology and classifications were introduced, so that the various types often were lumped together. There is no proof that the different clinical and anatomic forms have specific etiologies. The few etiologic data known for "pulmonary stenosis" therefore will be treated as if the anomaly were an entity, unless a publication specifies the type in modern terms.

Several cases are on record in which more than one member of a family was affected. In 1844, Friedberg (cited by Gänsslen *et al.*[1]) reported a man who had 2 boys with pulmonary stenosis by his first wife and a pair of nonidentical twins by his second wife, one of whom had pulmonary stenosis confirmed by necropsy. Coblentz and Mathivat[2] observed 2 sisters with pulmonary stenosis. Lamy *et al.*[3] found that in pulmonary valvar stenosis siblings were affected with cardiac malformations in 3.7% of the cases, which was about seven times the incidence of cardiac malformations in the general population. There also was a high consanguinity rate of the parents. Lamy and co-workers believed that in pulmonary valvar stenosis genetic factors appear more important than in other cardiac malformations, since there was a high consanguinity rate and a high familial incidence. A recessive genetic mechanism may therefore be responsible for some of the cases. A number of authors reported pulmonary valvar stenosis in siblings (p. 461), and pulmonary stenosis has been diagnosed as one of the many cardiovascular anomalies occurring in some patients with Laurence-Moon-Biedl syndrome,[4] which is a recessive trait (Chapter 19).

Transmission of pulmonary stenosis from mothers to some of their children has been reported. Deaf-mutism and congenital malformations may be associated anomalies in such cases.[5,6] Supravalvar aortic stenosis of the hereditary type (p. 541) sometimes is associated with pulmonary stenosis.[7] In families in which atrial septal defect occurs as a dominant hereditary trait, pulmonary stenosis also has been diagnosed in some members of the affected families.[8] The anomaly was observed occasionally in patients with Marfan syndrome (Chapter 91) and in a dominantly inherited syndrome of café au lait spots and dull intelligence.[9] Pulmonary stenosis is not rare in patients with phenotypic Turner syndrome,[10] particularly in male patients with anomalies usually seen in Turner syndrome.[11]

Some chromosomal abnormalities lead to pulmonary stenosis. In postmortems of children with trisomy 13-15, the anomaly was mentioned in approximately 13% of the cases, and with trisomy 18 in 20%.[12] Evans[13] found pulmonary stenosis four times in 28 patients with Down syndrome, but in a large necropsy series of patients with trisomy 21 this anomaly was mentioned in less than 1% of the cases.[12]

Rubella can result in pulmonary stenosis, although the diagnosis was only rarely mentioned in early reports. But during operations for patent ductus arteriosus it was encountered occasionally as an associated malformation,[14] and later it was recognized with increasing frequency.[15] Stenosis of the main pulmonary artery or of its branches has found much attention in analyses of the prenatal rubella syndrome in recent years. Involvement of the pulmonary arteries is now considered an important cardiovascular sequela of infection with the rubella virus in utero[16] (p. 66). In a series of 69 cases of pulmonary stenosis with normal aortic root, 2 could be attributed to rubella.[17]

REFERENCES

1. Gänsslen, M., Lambrecht, K., and Werner, M.: Die kongenitalen Missbildungen des Herzens, in *Handbuch der*

Erbiologie des Menschen (Berlin: Springer, 1940), Vol. 4, pt. 2, pp. 198–217.
2. Coblentz, B., and Mathivat, A.: Sténose pulmonaire congénital chez deux Soeurs, Arch. mal. coeur 45:490, 1952.
3. Lamy, M., DeGrouchy, J., and Schweisguth, O.: Genetic and non-genetic factors in the etiology of congenital heart disease: A study of 1188 cases, Am. J. Human Genet. 9:17, 1957.
4. McLoughlin, T. G., Krovetz, L. J., and Schiebler, G. L.: Heart disease in the Laurence-Biedl-Bardet syndrome, J. Pediat. 65:388, 1964.
5. Lewis, S. M., Sonnenblick, B. P., Gilbert, L., and Biber, D.: Familial pulmonary stenosis and deaf-mutism: Clinical and genetic considerations, Am. Heart J. 55:458, 1958.
6. Koroxenides, G., Webb, N. C., Jr., Moschos, C. B., and Lehan, P. H.: Congenital heart disease, deaf-mutism and associated somatic malformations occurring in several members of one family, Am. J. Med. 40:149, 1966.
7. Antia, A. U., Wiltse, H. E., Rowe, R. D., Pitt, E. L., Levin, S., Ottesen, O. E., and Cooke, R. E.: Pathogenesis of the supravalvular aortic stenosis syndrome, J. Pediat. 71:431, 1967.
8. Weil, M. H., and Allenstein, B. J.: A report of congenital heart disease in five members of one family, New England J. Med. 265:661, 1961.
9. Watson, G. H.: Pulmonary stenosis, café-au-lait spots, and dull intelligence, Arch. Dis. Childhood 42:303, 1967.
10. Rainier-Pope, C. R., Cunningham, R. D., Nadas, A. S., and Crigler, J. R., Jr.: Cardiovascular malformations in Turner's syndrome, Pediatrics 33:919, 1964.
11. Summitt, R. L., Opitz, J. M., and Smith, D. W.: Noonan's syndrome in the male, Abstracts, Annual Meeting, Society for Pediatric Research, p. 19, May, 1965.
12. Warkany, J., Passarge, E., and Smith, L. B.: Congenital malformations in autosomal trisomy syndromes, Am. J. Dis. Child. 112:502, 1966.
13. Evans, P. R.: Cardiac anomalies in mongolism, Brit. Heart J. 12:258, 1950.
14. Gibson, S., and Lewis, K. C.: Congenital heart disease following maternal rubella during pregnancy, A.M.A. Am. J. Dis. Child. 83:317, 1952.
15. Campbell, M.: Place of maternal rubella in the aetiology of congenital heart disease, Brit. M. J. 1:691, 1961.
16. Hastreiter, A. R., Joorabachi, B., Pujatti, G., van der Horst, R. L., Patacsil, G., and Sever, J. L.: Cardiovascular lesions associated with congenital rubella, J. Pediat. 71: 59, 1967.
17. Abrahams, D. G., and Wood, P.: Pulmonary stenosis with normal aortic root, Brit. Heart J. 13:519, 1951.

Pulmonary Atresia

THIS ANOMALY can occur with intact ventricular septum or with VSD. Cases with intact ventricular septum and normal aortic root are rare. Keith *et al.*[1] estimated that it occurs once in 70,000 children and that it accounts for 1% of the total group of congenital cardiac malformations. In the majority of cases, the pulmonary valve is replaced by an imperforate diaphragm formed by completely fused leaflets.

Owing to the rarity of the condition, little is known in regard to its etiology. Campbell[2] mentioned a family in which 3 siblings had cyanotic CHD. In a girl there were signs of pulmonary atresia. In another family, a boy had severe Fallot tetralogy, "perhaps with pulmonary atresia"; his brother had severe pulmonary valvar stenosis with a closed ventricular septum. A sister was thought to have pulmonic stenosis. The possibility of rubella as a cause of pulmonary atresia is shown by a case (Case 36) mentioned by Hastreiter *et al.*[3] that was associated with a VSD and a small patent ductus arteriosus.

If the ventricular septum is closed, the thick-walled right ventricle and the tricuspid valve are small. The right atrium and the interatrial communication are large. The ductus arteriosus can be large or just probe-patent with a tendency to early closure. The tricuspid valve usually is small but well formed. Anomalous coronary vessels connect the right ventricular myocardial vessels with the coronary arterial system.[4] In some cases, the right ventricle is of normal size or enlarged and the tricuspid valve grossly deformed as in Ebstein malformation.

Cyanosis is present on the first day or develops within a few days. Tachypnea is marked and cardiac failure is common. The prognosis is very poor, as approximately 50% of the patients die within the first 2 weeks; occasionally there is survival to puberty.[1]

Pulmonary valvotomy can improve the situation if the infundibulum is not atretic and the right ventricle is large.[4] If the right ventricle is small and the infundibulum atretic, caval-pulmonary artery shunt or pulmonary-to-systemic artery anastomosis has been attempted without great success.[1]

Obliteration of the main pulmonary artery with VSD usually is combined with dextroposition of the aorta. The hemodynamics and the clinical manifestations are similar to those of Fallot tetrad, but cyanosis appears earlier in cases of pulmonary atresia. Although the main pulmonary artery is atretic, its two

Fig. 60-1. – Clamps holding pulmonary artery (*P*) with pulmonary valve atresia. Commissures and sinuses (**arrow**) are well formed.

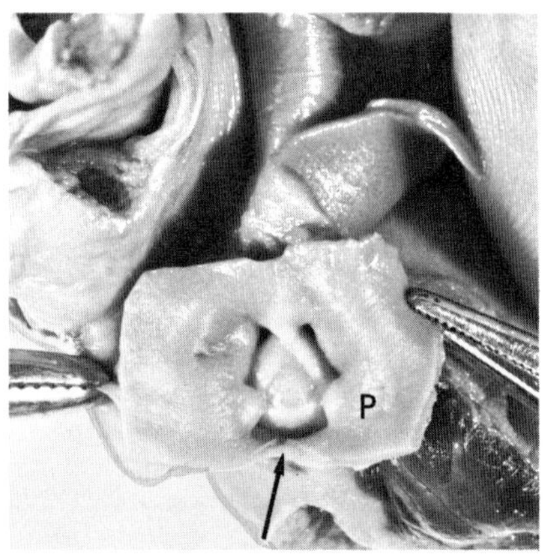

primary branches may be of sufficient size to permit an anastomotic procedure.[5]

REFERENCES

1. Keith, J. D., Rowe, R. D., and Vlad, P. (eds.): *Heart Disease in Infancy and Childhood* (2d ed.; New York: The Macmillan Company, 1966).
2. Campbell, M.: The genetics of congenital heart disease and situs inversus in sibs, Brit. Heart J. 21:65, 1959.
3. Hastreiter, A. R., Joorabachi, B., Pujatti, G., van der Horst, R. L., Patacsil, G., and Sever, J. L.: Cardiovascular lesions associated with congenital rubella, J. Pediat. 71:59, 1967.
4. Davignon, A. L., Greenwold, W. E., DuShane, J. W., and Edwards, J. E.: Congenital pulmonary atresia with intact ventricular septum. Clinicopathologic correlation of two anatomic types, Am. Heart J. 62:591, 1961.
5. Kaplan, S.: Congenital Heart Disease, in Nelson, W. E. (ed.), *Textbook of Pediatrics* (8th ed.; Philadelphia: W. B. Saunders Company, 1964).

Pulmonary Stenosis with Normal Aortic Root

THE MALFORMATION now called pulmonary stenosis with normal aortic root has an interesting history. It has long been known to pathologists but was thought to be extremely rare. Herxheimer,[1] for instance, stated that in cases of pulmonary stenosis the aorta is almost always involved and displaced, and Abbott[2] found only 25 cases in 1,000 necropsies with cardiovascular anomalies that could be considered as belonging to this group. Abrahams and Wood[3] in compiling several series of necropsies, found that only 3.1% of cardiovascular anomalies were congenital pulmonary stenosis with normal aortic root. The condition also was little known to clinicians, and Taussig,[4] in 1947, believed it to be rare, stating that she had had no opportunity to study a proved case of pure pulmonary stenosis. Since then, the diagnosis has been made with increasing frequency and now about 10% of cardiovascular anomalies are thought to belong in this category.[5] The diagnosis has become of great importance because the lesion is operable and the treatment differs from that for the tetralogy of Fallot. It is not easy to understand why this diagnosis has now come to the foreground. It must be assumed that, in the past, pathologists considered cases of congenital pulmonary stenosis in adults as acquired conditions and that the diagnosis could not be made clinically in children before modern diagnostic methods were available.

PATHOGENESIS.—Little is known concerning the pathogenesis of valvar pulmonary stenosis, but Edwards[6] believed that the lesion, like pulmonary atresia, is congenital even though it may develop relatively late in embryonic life or at least after the membranous portion of the ventricular septum has formed. If the stenosis or atresia developed earlier, one would expect that the interventricular foramen would fail to close. This anomaly is an example of a congenital malformation that cannot be explained by arrest of development, since it does not correspond to any normal embryonic stage. Yet, that the narrowing dates back to an early stage of the valve is suggested by the fact that in many cases the number of cusps is abnormal, two or four fusing to form the stenosis. In the past, it was thought that the fusion of cusps, as well as their thickening, was due to fetal endocarditis, but in postnatal life histologic studies showed no evidence of inflammation.[7] Thus, the mechanisms leading to fusion and thickening of the valvar cusps are still poorly understood but it seems now that they are governed by genetic, infectious (rubella) and possibly other factors.

PATHOLOGY.—Pulmonary valvar stenosis is characterized by fusion of the valvar cusps, which results in the formation of a dome-shaped diaphragm with a central opening of variable size. The size of the aperture determines the severity of clinical symptoms. Two, three or four cusps may participate in the formation of the diaphragm, as indicated by persisting raphae that run from the diaphragm to the wall of the pulmonary artery. Distal to the pulmonary stenosis, the trunk of the pulmonary artery usually is dilated in older children and adults but not in infants.[5] This indicates that the dilatation of the pulmonary artery is not congenital but develops in postnatal life.

Although in patients with normal aortic root the stenosis usually is valvar, in about 10% of the patients it is located in the infundibulum approximately

Fig. 60-2.—Dome-shaped pulmonary stenosis (**arrow**) seen from pulmonary artery.

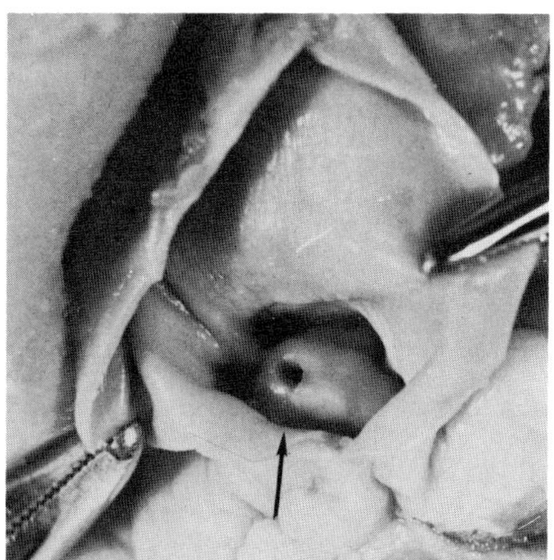

1 cm. below the valve and is formed by a fibrous or muscular ring. In some patients, valvar and infundibular stenoses are combined. An infundibular chamber of variable size may be found lined by endothelium of ground-glass appearance considered as endocardial fibroelastosis.[5] Patients with infundibular pulmonary stenosis sometimes have a hypoplastic pulmonary artery. It is of interest that pulmonary stenosis with normal aortic root usually is not combined with right aortic arch or other arch anomalies so frequently found in tetralogy of Fallot, but ventricular septal defects may be present. The foramen ovale may be well formed but unsealed or the valve guarding the foramen may be small or missing. Sometimes large atrial defects are present that are attributable to lack of development of the septum secundum. The weight of the heart usually is much increased. There always is marked hypertrophy of the right ventricle but the right ventricular cavity may be small. The right atrium is large. The tricuspid valve usually is normally formed but the leaves of the valve are thickened. A patent ductus arteriosus is present only rarely. Pulmonary stenosis associated with an underdeveloped right ventricle and hypoplasia of the tricuspid valve ring may result in cyanotic CHD with characteristic clinical signs. The abnormal filling resistance of the small right ventricle results in a right-to-left shunt at the atrial level.[8] Pulmonary atresia with intact ventricular septum can be associated with a tiny right ventricle (type 1) or with a right ventricle of normal size. In type 2, the tricuspid valve is deformed as in Ebstein malformation. In the presence of a well-developed right ventricle, surgical improvement is possible.[9]

SYMPTOMS. – The symptomatology of pulmonary stenosis varies greatly according to the size of the aperture in the pulmonary diaphragm and the condition of the atrial septum. In all cases there is a systolic pressure gradient between the right ventricle and the pulmonary artery, but this gradient varies according to the severity of the lesion. In mild cases in which there is a sizable blood flow through the pulmonary ostium, the patients are always free of cyanosis and have dyspnea only rarely. The jugular venous pulse is normal and the general physical development satisfactory. In valvar stenosis, there is always a systolic murmur and a thrill in the second left intercostal space; in infundibular stenosis, the murmur may be heard better in the fourth left intercostal space.

In the severe form, cyanosis is present if there is a right-to-left shunt through an atrial defect, and there may be clubbing of the fingers. There always is dyspnea on exertion. The onset of these symptoms varies; they may be present in infancy or develop in childhood or after adolescence. Manifestations of valvar pulmonary stenosis in infancy were described by Luke,[10] who pointed out the need for surgery in severely affected infants. In older children, fainting spells and precordial pain are not uncommon but squatting is reported only rarely. An interesting but unexplained symptom is the "moon face"[3] that can be observed in approximately half the patients with severe pulmonary stenosis. Catheterization shows a marked difference of pressure in the pulmonary artery and the right ventricle. In infundibular stenosis, a pressure difference is also found between the infundibulum and the ventricle. X-ray examination reveals enlargement of the right atrium, usually bulging in the area of the pulmonary artery, and decreased pulmonary vascularity. The entire heart is enlarged in severe and advanced cases. The stenosis, the jet through the opening and the dilated pulmonary artery, can be visualized by angiocardiography.

Congestive heart failure, anoxic spells and subacute bacterial endocarditis are complications of severe pulmonary stenosis causing sudden death in some cases. Another complication always mentioned in older texts was tuberculosis, which has now become rare as a complicating factor. In the presence of patent foramen ovale, cerebral abscess may develop.[6] The prognosis is good for mild cases of pulmonary stenosis, and several patients have been described who lived beyond the sixth decade.[11] Lund[12] mentioned a woman with pulmonary stenosis who tolerated pregnancy without serious difficulty. Severe cases may be fatal in infancy or patients may survive (without therapy) to the second or third decade, when complications may endanger the patient's life.

TREATMENT. – Mild cases can be treated medically but severe cases with a right ventricular pressure over 100 mm. in systole require surgical relief. Direct valvotomy has been practiced since 1948. Although this operation has been successful in the hands of many surgeons, it is being replaced in recent years by an approach through the pulmonary artery under direct vision.[13] It is now thought that death of those with severe lesions is due to delay of surgical treatment, and that recurrence of severe stenosis after operation is not likely.[5]

REFERENCES

1. Herxheimer, G.: Missbildungen des Herzens und der grossen Gefässe, in Schwalbe, E. (ed.), *Die Morphologie der Missbildungen des Menschen und der Tiere* (Jena: Gustav Fischer, 1909), Vol. 3, pt. 3.
2. Abbott, M. E.: *Atlas of Congenital Heart Disease* (New York: American Heart Association, 1936).
3. Abrahams, D. G., and Wood, P.: Pulmonary stenosis with normal aortic root, Brit. Heart J. 13:519, 1951.
4. Taussig, H. B.: *Congenital Malformations of the Heart* (New York: Commonwealth Fund, 1947).
5. Keith, J. D., Rowe, R. D., and Vlad, P. (eds.): *Heart Disease in Infancy and Childhood* (2d ed.; New York: The Macmillan Company, 1966).
6. Edwards, J. E.: Congenital Malformations of the Heart and Great Vessels, in Gould, S. E. (ed.), *Pathology of the Heart* (Springfield, Ill.: Charles C Thomas, Publisher, 1953).
7. Rossman, J. I.: Congenital atresia and stenosis of great cardiac vessels, aortic atresia, pulmonary stenosis, Am. J. Dis. Child. 64:872, 1942.

8. Williams, J. C. P., Barratt-Boyes, B. G., and Lowe, J. B.: Underdeveloped right ventricle and pulmonary stenosis, Am. J. Cardiol. 11:458, 1963.
9. Davignon, A. L., Greenwold, W. E., DuShane, J. W., and Edwards, J. E.: Congenital pulmonary atresia with intact ventricular septum. Clinicopathologic correlation of two anatomic types, Am. Heart J. 62:591, 1961.
10. Luke, M. J.: Valvular pulmonic stenosis in infancy, J. Pediat. 68:90, 1966.
11. Geraci, J. E., Burchell, H. R., and Edwards, J. E.: Congenital pulmonary stenosis with intact ventricular septum in persons more than 50 years of age, Proc. Staff Meet. Mayo Clin. 28:346, 1953.
12. Lund, C. J.: Maternal congenital heart disease as obstetric problem, Am. J. Obst. & Gynec. 55:244, 1948.
13. Blount, S. G., Jr., McCord, M. C., Mueller, H., and Swan, H.: Isolated valvular pulmonic stenosis. Clinical and physiologic response to open valvuloplasty, Circulation 10:161, 1954.

61

Ductus Arteriosus

AMONG the congenital cardiovascular anomalies, persistent patent ductus arteriosus represents a malformation of a special type. In the strict sense, it is not a *congenital* malformation, since an open ductus is a normal structure at the time of birth. However, it is likely that in many—if not in most—cases patency of the ductus is determined long before birth and it is justified, therefore, to consider the tissue changes in the wall of the ductus that determine postnatal patency as congenital anomalies even though they become manifest only after birth. Thus, the patent ductus is a good example of a malformation that often is determined long before it is recognizable as an anomaly. The period of determination is separated from the period of termination by many months (Chapter 7).

The ductus arteriosus connects the pulmonary artery with the aorta inserting distal to the left subclavian artery. It is a relatively large structure in fetal life but its lumen is narrowed considerably soon after birth. The ductus is embryologically derived from the sixth left aortic arch. A right-sided ductus is uncommon in man, but in animal experiments leading to cardiovascular anomalies right ductus has been observed repeatedly.[1] It was found associated with right aortic arch or connecting the heart with the right dorsal aorta in the absence of both fourth arches. Even both right and left ductus may occur in such experimental animals. Double ductus, always associated with other cardiovascular anomalies, has been observed only rarely in children.[2,3]

In man, patent ductus usually assumes a cylindrical shape; occasionally it assumes a funnel shape. In the less common window type of patent ductus, the aorta and the left pulmonary artery are in communication by means of a large opening without formation of a ductus canal. The cylindrical and funnel types may have a length of between 1 and 2 cm., the width varying considerably. In the normally closing ductus, the intima is thick but in the persistent patent ductus it remains thin. According to Edwards,[4] the entire wall of the patent ductus is thin and does not show the cord-like texture of the closing ductus of the newborn. In adults, the media of a patent ductus contains much collagen that is intermingled with muscular tissue.

Absence of the Ductus Arteriosus

This may occur in conjunction with such malformations of the heart as a common ventricle, ventricular septal defect or communication between the pulmonary artery with the aorta. It is absent in approximately half of the patients with persistent truncus arteriosus. The left-sided ductus acts in the normal fetus as an overflow valve that permits blood leaving the right ventricle to reach the descending aorta through the ductus. If other overflow mechanisms exist, the amount of blood that flows through the

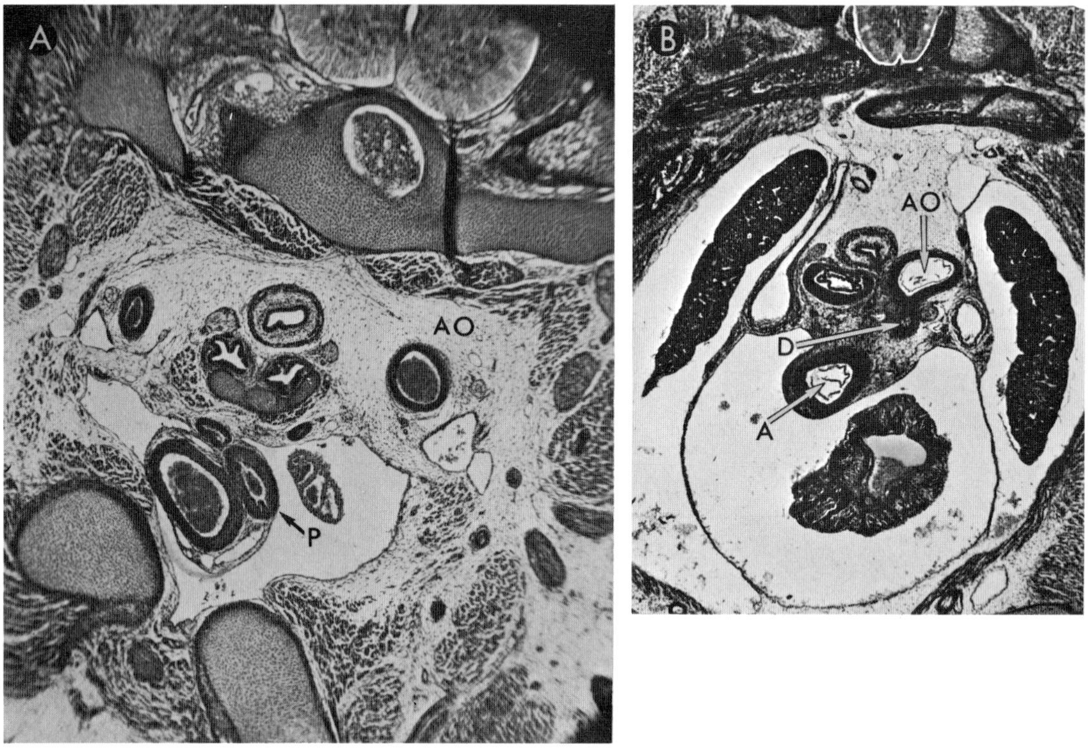

Fig. 61-1.—Transverse sections through the upper thorax of near-term rat fetuses. **A,** absence of ductus arteriosus; there is a small pulmonary trunk (*P*) without any connection with the descending aorta (*AO*) (produced by maternal vitamin A deficiency). **B,** extreme stenosis of ductus arteriosus (*D*). Ascending aorta (*A*) and descending aorta (*AO*) are shown. The pulmonary artery is not seen in this section. (Mother was treated with sodium salicylate.)

ductus during fetal life can be minimal and the ductus may disappear.[4] It is of interest in this connection that Wilson and Warkany,[1] analyzing the cardiovascular malformations induced in rat fetuses by maternal vitamin A deficiency, found ventricular septal defect in every animal without ductus arteriosus, so that the interventricular foramen compensated to some extent for the deficiency of normal outlet by conveying blood directly into the left ventricle. If at least one fourth and one sixth arch were functional, ventricular septal defects were present in only half the animals. When the number of functional arches exceeded two, provided one sixth arch was included, the ventricular septum usually was closed. From these findings it appeared that the number of functional arches available for delivering blood from the heart to the aorta was a factor in determining whether or not the ventricular septum closed. Whereas Edwards[4] explained the absence of the ductus by the existence of other overflow mechanisms, Wilson and Warkany[1] explained the open ventricular septum by absence of a ductus. A third possibility is that the two anomalies develop independently of each other and that all embryos without any overflow mechanism die early, whereas those with an overflow mechanism can survive through fetal life and be observed at or near term. It is worth pointing out that absence of the ductus arteriosus occurred in the thalidomide syndrome. Kreipe[5] mentioned two cases of tetralogy of Fallot combined with agenesis of the ductus.

Physiologic Closure of the Ductus

In discussing closure of the ductus, it is necessary to distinguish between functional closure, which normally takes place soon after birth, and anatomic obliteration, which usually is delayed several weeks after birth. In most infants, the ductus is closed as an effective channel by the end of the second week after birth.[4,6] Normally, the process leading to the closure of the ductus starts in fetal life when, during the last trimester, intimal ridges are being formed that later, at the time of birth, proliferate together with medial tissue.[4] After birth, obliteration progresses gradually. According to Christie,[7] the ductus is anatomically patent in two-thirds of infants 2 weeks old, in 12% at 8 weeks, and in 1% at 1 year.

Barclay *et al.*,[8] observing the lamb fetus by cineradiography, thought that interruption of the placental circulation was followed by closure of the foramen ovale and by closure of the ductus within a few minutes, but Dawes *et al.*[9] found the ductus arteriosus patent in newborn lambs for many hours after birth. Within a few minutes of birth, blood begins to flow through the ductus from the aorta to the lungs, but the lungs are still inefficient and the arterial oxygen saturation rises only slowly after birth. Thus, it appeared that the continued patency of the ductus for some hours after birth served a useful function so long as the lungs were not fully expanded. Working with guinea pigs, Kennedy and Clark[10] found the ductus different from other great arteries in structure and in physiologic reactivity. During fetal life, it was able to close in response to certain stimuli – electrical, mechanical or respiratory. Normally, closure took place within a few minutes following birth and the ductus remained closed. Breathing seemed to be the most important stimulus for its closure, and oxygen proved to be a necessary component of the gas mixture breathed, since inflation of the lungs with pure nitrogen did not cause closure. But, a few hours after birth, changes occurred in the ductus that made it no longer sensitive to changes of the oxygen tension of its environment. Record and McKeown,[11] studying the anatomic closure of the ductus in guinea pigs, saw the lumen obliterated by 24 hours after birth. The mechanism of closure was disturbed in some animals by induction of labor, separation of the young from the mother at birth and by oxygen deficiency. Barron[12] did not accept the chemical explanation of the mechanism of closure, pointing out that the ductus remains open during fetal life even though the percentage of oxygen saturation in the blood may be high and that it does close in lambs before the oxygen content of their blood returns to the intrauterine level. Thus, the role of oxygenation of the blood in closure of the ductus was not entirely elucidated by animal experiments. Hörnblad[78] studied closure of the ductus with the help of whole-body freezing. Pigs, guinea pigs, rats, rabbits and mice were used. There were definite species differences in the ductal closure rate.

Although such experiments are of great interest for explanation of the mechanism of closure of the normal ductus arteriosus, they do not necessarily contribute to an understanding of the etiology of permanently persistent patent ductus. The experiments usually are terminated soon after birth and, to my knowledge, permanent patent ductus has not been produced in this way. In human infants, increased oxygen tended to constrict the ductus arteriosus and hypoxia tended to cause dilatation.[13] But, in premature infants, closure of the ductus may be delayed for weeks and spontaneous closure can still take place several months after birth.[14] The cause of the delay is not known.[15] The fact that spontaneous closure can occur in the presence of severe congestive heart failure[16] and in children with cyanotic heart disease and significant hypoxemia[15] speaks against a dominating role of hypoxemia in delay of closure.

Persistent Patent Ductus Arteriosus

Wilkins[79] estimated that 1 case of persistent patent ductus occurs in 2,000 births; Anderson[17] 1 in 2,500–5,000; Stuckey[18] 1 in 3,000; Gardiner and Keith[19] 1 in 3,850. In 1943, Keys and Shapiro[20] thought that there were then approximately 20,000 persons with a patent ductus in the United States, i.e., 1 case per 6,800 persons. Joyce and O'Toole[21] found an unusual number of cases in Roscommon County, Ireland, among schoolchildren. There were 15 cases among 9,250 of these schoolchildren, which would correspond to a rate of 1 in 616. In Peru, the frequency of patent ductus increases with altitude.[22] It is 1 in 2,500 for schoolchildren at sea level and rises to 1 in 300 at 9,000 feet, 1 in 170 at 12,000 feet and 1 in 90 at 15,000 feet elevation.

Patent ductus plays an important role in cardiac clinics and hospitals, in which it accounts for 10–18% of cardiovascular malformations.[23-25] Stuckey,[18] in Sydney, Australia, found among children with congenital heart disease up to the age of 2 years only 5% with patent ductus, but 30% among those from 2 to 13 years, which illustrates the shift in the percentage contribution of patent ductus to congenital heart disease with progressing age.

In the necropsy material of Abbott,[26] patent ductus accounted for 10.5%, but it played a minor, if any, role in the infants dying in the first month of life reported by Ober and Moore.[27]

Etiology. – The malformation called patent ductus arteriosus is heterogeneous in origin. In some cases, it probably is genetically determined, as suggested by kinships showing more than one generation affected by the anomaly. An affected father may transmit the disorder to one or more of his children. Walker and Ellis[28] reported a man with this anomaly who had 8 children, 4 of whom were affected with patent ductus. Transmission through three generations was observed by Taussig,[29] who saw a man with patent ductus who had 2 children and 1 grandchild with the same anomaly. In some instances, patent ductus occurred in a mother and her child,[30] in others, in a daughter[23,31] or a son.[32,33] Such reports suggest that patent ductus can be transmitted in some families like a dominant hereditary trait. In other families, two generations were affected by different cardiovascular anomalies. Campbell[34] mentioned a mother who had a patent ductus whereas her daughter had coarctation of the aorta. Stein and Barber[35] observed a mother with coarctation of the aorta who had a boy and a girl both affected with patent ductus arteriosus. Hereditary transmission of patent ductus arteriosus has been reported in dogs.[36]

Since patent ductus arteriosus has become correctable by surgery, many treated patients have reached reproductive age. In a group of 86 patients with patent ductus, Wilkins[79] found that 1 in 60 of their offspring had congenital heart disease and 1 in 90 had patent ductus arteriosus.

Multiple cases of ductus arteriosus have been observed repeatedly in one generation of a family. Two sisters, both affected with patent ductus arteriosus, have been reported.[37-39] In Ekström's[32] series of 150 cases of patent ductus there was an unusually high incidence of familial cases. In four families, 2 cases of patent ductus were observed in sisters, and in one family a brother and a sister had the anomaly. Kjaergaard[40] noted 3 sisters affected in a sibship, the parents being well and not consanguineous, and 3 sisters were affected in a family in Ekström's series. There were 2 affected brothers in a family observed by Wade.[41] Joyce and O'Toole[21] reported a sibship of 9 children, 3 boys of which had patent ductus arteriosus; a fourth was a blue baby who died at the age of 7 weeks. Lamy *et al.*[42] mentioned patent ductus in a patient whose cousin also was affected with the same anomaly. In several instances, a patient with patent ductus had a sibling with a different type of congenital heart disease. McKeown *et al.*[43] mentioned a family in which 1 sibling had patent ductus and the other transposition of the great vessels. In some families, 1 child was affected with patent ductus, whereas another sibling showed signs of unspecified congenital heart disease.[30,42]

Such observations of familial incidence are of great interest, but it is difficult to interpret them from an etiologic point of view. Several such siblings occurring in a family with healthy parents could be attributed to an autosomal recessive gene, but consanguinity of the parents is not prevalent.[17] On the other hand, it would appear possible that a reproductive anomaly of the mother results in repeated interference with the normal closure of the ductus arteriosus.

There are reports of monozygous twins, both of whom were affected with this anomaly,[44,45] but other pairs of identical twins were discordant. Anderson[17] reported 4 sets of monozygous twins, 3 female and 1 male, in whom only 1 member had patent ductus. Discordant pairs of monozygous twins were also observed by others.[30,41,46,47]

Patent ductus arteriosus is a frequent anomaly in patients with autosomal trisomies. In fact, in necropsies of patients with trisomies 13-15 and 18, patent ductus together with ventricular septal defect appears as a leading form of congenital heart disease, whereas it is less prominent in trisomy 21.[48] It is also occasionally mentioned in patients with other chromosomal anomalies such as translocations and deletions, but such cases are rare and atypical. Two girls with XXXXX karyotype have been described and both had patent ductus arteriosus that required surgical treatment toward the end of the first year (see Chapter 112).

Of many possible environmental factors, maternal rubella has been generally accepted as a cause of persistent patent ductus. In the rubella epidemic of 1941 in Australia,[49] approximately half the children affected by malformations had cardiac defects of the acyanotic type (p. 66). Necropsy in 3 cases revealed a wide patency of the ductus arteriosus. Swan and coworkers[50] confirmed the relationship of maternal rubella to congenital heart disease, particularly patency of the ductus arteriosus, but septal defects were also observed occasionally. Swan and Tostevin[51] noticed, on microscopic examination of 3 patients with patent ductus arteriosus following maternal rubella, absence of a well-defined elastic lamina and of intimal mounds, which normally are present in the ductus. At the margins of the ventricular septal defect there was occasional replacement of muscle fibers by connective tissue. Since then, many other forms of congenital heart disease have been observed to follow maternal rubella,[34,42,52] but patent ductus probably is still considered the most frequent lesion among them.[53-55] Recently, changes in the pulmonary vasculature have been emphasized as sequelae of maternal rubella.[56]

Although there can be no doubt that rubella can be a cause of patent ductus arteriosus, it probably is not a frequent – and certainly not a leading – cause of this anomaly. Rutstein *et al.*[54] obtained a history of maternal rubella in 6.7% of children in whom patent ductus had been diagnosed. Seasonal variation of the cases was noticed, as the first gestational trimester of the children with patent ductus fell in the late winter and early spring months, coinciding with a rubella epidemic in Massachusetts. Record and McKeown,[33] in Birmingham, England, found a different seasonal distribution and came to the conclusion that rubella caused only 2% of the cases of patent ductus. Lynxweiler and Wells[57] obtained a history of rubella in 5.0% and Anderson[17] in 3.4% of patients with ductus, whereas Starer[30] got no history of rubella in his series. In 100 cases of simple ductus arteriosus seen in Montreal, a history of maternal rubella in the first trimester was obtained in 8 cases. But during 3 years following a rubella epidemic in New Zealand, 17 of 50 infants with patent ductus had a rubella history.[58] Thus, according to proximity to a rubella epidemic, the percentage contribution of that infection to patent ductus can vary between 0% and 34%.

There are only a few examples of drug-induced cases in man. Patent ductus has been reported by Weicker[59] in patients damaged by thalidomide. In another series there were 3 patent ductus among 17 cases of congenital heart disease attributed to thalidomide.[5]

Anderson[17] observed no birth order effect in a series of patent ductus, but MacMahon[60] and Record and McKeown[33] noted some influence of birth rank. Polani and Campbell[61] could not show any difference between observed and expected values in regard to either maternal or paternal age or birth rank.

Record and McKeown[33] thought that a history of fetal distress at birth could be obtained in a higher proportion of children with ductus than would be expected among normal births. There is some experimental evidence that defective oxygenation of the blood during birth delays closure of the ductus, but Polani and Campbell[61] pointed out that asphyxia also may cause the ductus to close. They believed that both failure of the ductus to close and neonatal cyanosis may at times be due to a common factor that could be the primary event.

There are reports that indicate that ductus arteriosus is more often found in populations living in high altitudes than in those living at or near sea level.[62,63] This question is discussed on page 465.

There can be no doubt that a marked preponderance of females exists among children with patent ductus. In general, there are only 30 males in 100 children with this anomaly as compared with 70 females. Ekström,[32] reviewing earlier reports of more than 500 cases, found that 69% were female. Adding the figures of Anderson[17] and Record and McKeown,[33] one finds 71% females in a total of 350 children, a ratio also observed in many other reports. No satisfactory explanation exists for the female preponderance. An interesting change in the sex ratio with increasing age was detected by Record and McKeown,[33] who found in their series 62% males in those patients with ductus who died in the neonatal period, 44% in those dying between 1 and 12 months and 29% in those alive at 1 year. A similar change in the sex ratio with age of the patients was noted by these authors in 244 cases reported in the literature. They considered it possible, therefore, that the proportion of males among all children affected may be higher than most estimates suggest, since the incidence of the two sexes may be nearly equal at birth. The high proportion of surviving females would thus be "explained" by high mortality rates of males in early life.

Associated malformations may throw some light on the etiology of certain cases of patent ductus. The presence of cataract, deafness, and so forth, would point to an early infection with rubella. Association with cardiac or other defects dating back to embryonic life suggests an early determination of the anomalous ductus. Anderson[17] found in his series an incidence of associated cardiac defects in 8% and of noncardiac abnormalities in 14% of the patients with ductus. Some of these associated defects pointed to early fetal damage, but others could be attributed to late fetal or to perinatal injurious agents.

It was mentioned before that reports of twins discordant in regard to patent ductus do not indicate that genetic factors were responsible for the persistent patency of the ductus in one twin. But it is possible that the process of twinning itself may somehow contribute to the etiology of the anomaly or that after faulty mitosis of the zygote one twin is rendered abnormal whereas the other develops normally. The incidence of twinning among the patients of Anderson[17] was high (4 in 105), but the sample was too small to draw definite conclusions concerning its role in the etiology of patent ductus.

Symptoms.—Owing to the higher aortic pressure, the blood flows through the persistent patent ductus from the aorta to the pulmonary artery. The amount of blood shunted depends on the size of the ductus and the pressure gradient between the aorta and the pulmonary artery. In extreme cases, one-half to two-thirds of the left ventricular output may be shunted through the ductus and the oxygenated blood recirculated through the pulmonary circulation.

Although heart failure may occur occasionally in early life,[64] many children with patent ductus arteriosus have no symptoms and their anomaly is discovered during routine physical examination. A systolic thrill is present frequently in the second left interspace and a typical machinery murmur is heard best in the second left intercostal space. But many variations of the murmur are noted; sometimes it is only systolic and sometimes only diastolic in time.[58] The heart size is normal in many cases but there may be moderate enlargement. The pulse pressure is large. The electrocardiogram is normal in the majority of patients. In typical cases, roentgenograms show a prominent and pulsating pulmonary artery and pulmonary vascular markings are increased, showing pulsation or hilar dance. In atypical cases, the diagnosis is aided by catheterization and angiocardiography.

As a rule, children with patent ductus are described as underdeveloped and small,[65] but Shapiro[66] stated that approximately half the children in his series were developed normally and some of them were even obese. Ekström[32] found that the heights and weights of his patients with patent ductus were similar to those of healthy Swedish boys and girls. Porter[47] reported identical twin boys, of whom only 1 had a patent ductus. At the age of 11, the affected twin was smaller and weighed less than his co-twin, but after operation the affected twin grew better than his normal brother. Starer[30] observed a pair of identical twin sisters, of whom only 1 had a patent ductus. The patient showed rapid progress in general development after ligation of the ductus. But children with patent ductus do not represent an etiologic entity that explains their differing behavior in regard to physical growth and response to operation. Review of a large series of these patients by Umansky and Hauck[67] showed a tendency to reduced height and weight. After operation, a marked acceleration occurred in only 20% for height and 28% for weight. The lack of response of the majority was interpreted as a sign that growth retardation was not due to the abnormal hemodynamic pattern of the patent ductus but to prenatal factors. In cases of patent ductus due to rubella, intrauterine growth retardation is present at birth in many cases (p. 65) and a rapid response to repair of the vascular anomaly cannot be expected to repair the general growth retardation imposed by the rubella virus. Occasionally, the lack of growth and development is the presenting symptom and the cardiac findings are obtained in examinations for physical underdevelopment. In other patients, repeated respiratory infections and fatigability dominate the picture.

The typical murmur often is not recognizable at

birth and the diagnosis may be missed within the first few months of life, but it is important to diagnose uncomplicated patent ductus arteriosus early because surgical treatment can bring relief from symptoms and prevent secondary late effects. Lyon and Kaplan[64] pointed out that symptoms produced by patent ductus in infancy vary widely. The anomaly may cause congestive heart failure, atypical murmurs, respiratory infections, normal systolic blood pressure combined with a lowered diastolic pressure or retarded physical growth. Cardiac catheterization, aortography or angiocardiography assist in an early diagnosis and may thus make possible early surgical treatment. Although many patients with this anomaly remain asymptomatic for many years, the condition is not harmless. In 1943, Shapiro and Keys[68] estimated that a person with a patent ductus arteriosus has, at the age of 17 years, only half the average life expectancy if the defect is not corrected by operation. These patients are endangered by congestive heart failure, subacute bacterial endocarditis, acquired rheumatic heart disease or aneurysm of the ductus. Despite these dangers, many persons with open ductus arteriosus have reached old age without serious illness. The anomaly is of interest because it is one of the congenital malformations that may not cause disease until late in life.

Patency of the ductus arteriosus in adults was reviewed by Keys and Shapiro.[20] Final analysis was applied to 60 patients, of whom 77% were women. The average age at death of the 14 men was 38.9 years, that of the 46 women 35.5 years. The oldest man died at 58 and the oldest woman at 66. The authors believed that patent ductus reduces the life expectancy by approximately 20 years in men and 28 years in women. In approximately 40% of the cases the cause of death was subacute bacterial endocarditis and in 28% it was congestive heart failure. Rupture of a pulmonary or aortic aneurysm accounted for 7% of the deaths. Aneurysms of the pulmonary artery were found in 10 of the 60 patients. In general, the ductus is short in adults and it may be reduced to a mere fistula-like opening between the aorta and pulmonary artery. In some adults with this anomaly, no murmur is heard, particularly in cases of congestive heart failure. Uncomplicated patent ductus probably prevails in adults because complicated cases are eliminated in infancy or childhood. If complications are present in adults, they occur more often in males than in females. Many of the patients with patent ductus lived a normal life, went to school and could earn a living. None of them was a cardiac cripple.[20] Usually, they maintained good compensation until either subacute bacterial endocarditis or cardiac failure intervened. The natural history of patency of the ductus in the adult indicates a prognosis that is good to the extent that the patient can expect to live a considerable number of years with relatively slight disability, but then he is faced with the threat of subacute bacterial endocarditis and a shortened life expectancy. From this analysis, Keys and Shapiro[20] concluded that operation is justifiable despite the absence of signs of decreasing adjustment to the defect, but it must be expected that in adults difficulties frequently are encountered in surgery.

Associated malformations.—Although many cases of patent ductus are isolated lesions, some are complicated by associated cardiovascular or noncardiac malformations. How many cases are combined with other cardiac malformations is not known. In reports of serious cardiac lesions, patent ductus often is dealt with as an accidental finding. In series of patients operated on for patency of the ductus, other cardiac malformations are noted in 5–15% of the cases.[17,32,69,70] Keith *et al.*[58] stated that ventricular septal defect, coarctation of the aorta, aortic stenosis, pulmonary stenosis and mitral regurgitation are frequent complicating lesions. Bonham Carter *et al.*[71] reported on patients with a patent ductus and aortic valve lesion and reviewed related case reports. With a right descending aorta a retro-esophageal ductus may cause dysphagia lusoria in infancy.[72] Patent ductus combined with ventricular septal defect occurred in 30% of trisomy 13-15 patients and in approximately 50% of trisomy 18 patients who were necropsied.[48]

Noncardiac abnormalities were found to be associated with patent ductus in 14% of the patients of Anderson.[17] Scoliosis, sternal deformities, clubfoot, eye defects and mental retardation were observed repeatedly. Polani and Campbell[61] noted noncardiac malformations in only 6% of their patients.

The association of patent ductus with congenital cataract, deafness and physical and mental retardation is seen following prenatal rubella and occasionally in children whose mothers deny any infection during pregnancy.[73] The malformations of children damaged by thalidomide are described in Chapter 11.

Prognosis.—No uniform prognosis is possible in cases taking their natural course without operation. In the presence of pulmonary stenosis or atresia with tetrad of Fallot, a patent ductus may be a beneficial malformation. In some persons, the uncomplicated persistent ductus is a harmless anomaly and its bearer may live a long and active life, but in most of those reaching adulthood, the life expectancy is reduced markedly.[20] Some patients with patent ductus die in infancy of congestive heart failure or intercurrent infections. Since such children do not show typical symptoms of the anomaly, the patent ductus may go unrecognized and, therefore, their number cannot be assessed.

It is obvious that the prognosis given by authors who refer to necropsy reports appears more unfavorable than that of observers who take into account the living. Some recent series are complicated by the fact that operated on and unoperated on survivors have to be considered. Cosh[74] recorded 34 persons of an average age of 26 years whose ductus had not been ligated and who did not suffer serious restriction of activity. Whereas Lund[75] considered patent ductus a serious complication of pregnancy, Cosh[74] thought that pregnancy is well tolerated in the presence of a patent ductus of small or moderate size.

TREATMENT.—The prognosis is greatly improved in the majority of cases by surgical closure of the ductus. Since Gross,[76] in 1938, performed the first successful operation for patent ductus arteriosus, the surgical technique has been modified to some extent, but ligation or division of the ductus is now a well-established treatment for the anomaly. Children who are stunted in physical growth and development or handicapped by cardiac fatigue or failure are candidates for surgical treatment. Patients with superimposed infections should be operated on after antibiotic treatment. There remains a large number of children who have no disturbing symptoms and do not require immediate help. Gross[69] recommended surgical closure for all children and young adults, even those who are symptom-free at the moment. It is clear that such advice depends on the availability of good surgical and medical facilities. Operation is more difficult in infants than in older children, and in adults the vessels may be rigid or affected by degenerative changes. In young prematures, delay of operation has been recommended because of the possibility of spontaneous closure[14] (p. 555). The age most suitable for operation varies and depends on the urgency of the situation. For elective cases, optimal ages range between 3 and 20 years, the best chances being claimed for the ages of 6–12[69] or 3–7,[32] according to different authors. In most cases, division of the ductus is technically more difficult than ligation but preferable because it precludes recanalization. Waterman *et al.*,[77] in 1956, calculated the over-all mortality in 2,929 operations in children under 14 years as 2.3%. In uncomplicated cases, the heart diminishes in size after closure, the pulse pressure becomes normal and the machinery murmur is replaced by normal heart sounds. If pulmonary hypertension was present in patients with left-to-right shunts, the pressure returns to normal after operation in many cases. The general physical development of most patients improves, but a gain in height and weight is achieved in only one-third of the cases.[67,74] Continued failure to grow may be due to extracardiac defects. Patients who had intrauterine growth retardation may continue their slow growth pattern even after operation.

Ventricular or atrial septal defect or isolated pulmonary stenosis is not a contraindication to surgical closure. In patients with cyanosis, the ductus should not be closed surgically. Surgical complications and mortality occur chiefly in atypical cases. Variations in postoperative behavior have been discussed by Keith *et al.*[58]

Intrauterine Closure of the Ductus

Ductal closure during fetal life can lead to congestive heart failure at birth, with spontaneous subsequent recovery. A child with this anomaly was born to a mother who developed polyarthritis and fever 10 days before delivery and was treated with salicylates and penicillin.[80]

REFERENCES

1. Wilson, J. G., and Warkany, J.: Aortic-arch and cardiac anomalies in the offspring of vitamin A deficient rats, Am. J. Anat. 85:113, 1949.
2. Kelsey, J. R., Jr., Gilmore, C. E., and Edwards, J. E.: Bilateral ductus arteriosus representing persistence of each sixth aortic arch; report of case in which there were associated isolated dextrocardia and ventricular septal defects, A.M.A. Arch. Path. 55:154, 1953.
3. Stewart, J. R., Kincaid, O. W., and Edwards, J. E.: *An Atlas of Vascular Rings and Related Malformations of the Aortic Arch System* (Springfield, Ill.: Charles C Thomas, Publisher, 1964).
4. Edwards, J. E.: Congenital Malformations of the Heart and Great Vessels, in Gould, S. E. (ed.), *Pathology of the Heart* (Springfield, Ill.: Charles C Thomas, Publisher, 1953).
5. Kreipe, U.: Missbildungen innerer Organe bei Thalidomid-embryopathie, Arch. Kinderh. 176:33, 1967.
6. Adams, F. H., and Lind, J.: Physiological studies on the cardiovascular status of the normal newborn infant (with special reference to the ductus arteriosus), A.M.A. J. Dis. Child. 93:12, 1957.
7. Christie, A.: Normal closing time of the foramen ovale and the ductus arteriosus, Am. J. Dis. Child. 40:323, 1930.
8. Barclay, A. E., Barcroft, J., Barron, D. H., and Franklin, K. J.: Radiographic demonstration of circulation through the heart in adult and in fetus and identification of ductus arteriosus, Am. J. Roentgenol. 47:687, 1942.
9. Dawes, G. S., Mott, J. C., and Widdicombe, J. G.: The patency of the ductus arteriosus in newborn lambs and its physiological consequences, J. Physiol. 128:36, 1955.
10. Kennedy, J. A., and Clark, S. L.: Observations on the ductus arteriosus of the guinea pig in relation to its method of closure, Anat. Rec. 79:349, 1941.
11. Record, R. G., and McKeown, T.: Anatomical closure of the ductus arteriosus in the guinea pig, Clin. Sc. 14:213, 1955.
12. Barron, D. H.: The changes in the fetal circulation at birth, Physiol. Rev. 24:277, 1944.
13. Moss, A. J., Emmanouilides, G. C., Adams, F. H., and Chuang, K.: Response of ductus arteriosus and pulmonary and systemic arterial pressure to changes in oxygen environment in newborn infants, Pediatrics 33:937, 1964.
14. Powell, M. L.: Patent ductus arteriosus in premature infants, M. J. Australia 2:58, 1963.
15. Danilowicz, D., Rudolph, A. M., and Hoffman, J. I. E.: Delayed closure of the ductus arteriosus in premature infants, Pediatrics 37:74, 1966.
16. Auld, P. A. M.: Delayed closure of the ductus arteriosus, J. Pediat. 69:61, 1966.
17. Anderson, R. C.: Causative factors underlying congenital heart malformations; patent ductus arteriosus, Pediatrics 14:143, 1954.
18. Stuckey, D.: Congenital heart defects following maternal rubella during pregnancy, Brit. Heart J. 18:519, 1956.
19. Gardiner, J. H., and Keith, J. D.: Prevalence of heart disease in Toronto children: 1948–1949. Cardiac registry, Pediatrics 7:713, 1951.
20. Keys, A., and Shapiro, M. J.: Patency of the ductus arteriosus in adults, Am. Heart J. 25:158, 1943.
21. Joyce, J. C., and O'Toole, S. P.: Congenital heart disease; report on unusually high incidence in one family, Brit. M. J. 1:1241, 1954.
22. Penaloza, D., Arias-Stella, J., Sime, F., Recavarren, S., and Marticorena, E.: The heart and pulmonary circulation in children at high altitudes; physiological, anatomical, and clinical observations, Pediatrics 34:568, 1964.

23. Nadas, A. S.: *Pediatric Cardiology* (Philadelphia: W. B. Saunders Company, 1957).
24. Wood, P.: *Diseases of the Heart and Circulation* (2d ed.; London: Eyre and Spottiswoode, 1956).
25. Richards, M. R., Merritt, K. K., Samuels, M. H., and Langmann, A. G.: Congenital malformations of cardiovascular system in series of 6,053 infants, Pediatrics 15:12, 1955.
26. Abbott, M. E.: *Atlas of Congenital Heart Disease* (New York: American Heart Association, 1936).
27. Ober, W. B., and Moore, T. E., Jr.: Congenital cardiac malformations in neonatal period; autopsy study, New England J. Med. 253:271, 1955.
28. Walker, G. C., and Ellis, L. B.: The familial occurrence of congenital cardiac anomalies, Proc. New England Heart A. p. 26, 1940-41.
29. Taussig, H. B.: *Congenital Malformations of the Heart* (New York: The Commonwealth Fund, 1947).
30. Starer, F.: Analysis of 50 cases of persistent ductus arteriosus, Brit. M. J. 1:971, 1953.
31. Lamy, M., and Schweisguth, O.: Étiologie des malformations du coeur, Ann. paediat. 171:245, 1948.
32. Ekström, G.: The surgical treatment of patent ductus arteriosus, Acta chir. scandinav. 169 (supp.):1, 1952.
33. Record, R. G. and McKeown, T.: Observations relating to the etiology of patent ductus arteriosus, Brit. Heart J. 15: 376, 1953.
34. Campbell, M.: Genetic and environmental factors in congenital heart disease, Quart. J. Med. 18:379, 1949.
35. Stein, I., and Barber, D. J.: Congenital heart disease: Case reports on 3 members of family, Am. Heart J. 30: 118, 1945.
36. Patterson, D. F., and Detweiler, D. K.: Hereditary transmission of patent ductus arteriosus in the dog, Am. Heart J. 74:289, 1967.
37. Jewesbury, R. C.: Two similar but somewhat unusual heart conditions in sisters, Proc. Roy. Soc. Med. 6:100, 1912-1913.
38. Ellis, R. W. B.: Congenital morbus cordis in two sisters, Brit. J. Child. Dis. 33:286, 1936.
39. Snelling, D. B.: Familial congenital heart disease, J.A.M.A. 108:1502, 1937.
40. Kjaergaard, H.: Patent ductus Botalli in 3 sisters, Acta med. scandinav. 125:339, 1946.
41. Wade, G.: Congenital heart disease in one of uniovular twins, Brit. Heart J. 14:475, 1952.
42. Lamy, M., DeGrouchy, J., and Schweisguth, O.: Genetic and non-genetic factors in the etiology of congenital heart disease: A study of 1,188 cases, Am. J. Human Genet. 9:17, 1957.
43. McKeown, T., MacMahon, B., and Parsons, C. G.: Familial incidence of congenital malformations of the heart, Brit. Heart J. 15:273, 1953.
44. McAleese, J. J.: A survey of congenital heart disease in a children's hospital, Am. J. Surg. 83:755, 1952.
45. Smith, K. S.: Congenital heart disease in identical twins, Arch. Dis. Childhood 4:330, 1929.
46. McClintock, K.: Congenital malformation of the heart in one of identical twins, Arch. Dis. Childhood 20:47, 1945.
47. Porter, W. B.: The effect of patent ductus arteriosus on body growth, Am. J. M. Sc. 213:178, 1947.
48. Warkany, J., Passarge, E., and Smith, L. B.: Congenital malformations in autosomal trisomy syndromes, Am. J. Dis. Child. 112:502, 1966.
49. Gregg, N. M.: Congenital cataract following German measles in mother, Tr. Ophth. Soc. Australia 3:35, 1942.
50. Swan, C., Tostevin, A. L., Moore, B., Mayo, H., and Black, G. H. B.: Congenital defects in infants following infectious diseases during pregnancy, with special reference to relationship between German measles and cataract, deaf-mutism, heart disease, and microcephaly, and to period of pregnancy in which occurrence of rubella is followed by congenital abnormalities, M. J. Australia 2:201, 1943.
51. Swan, C., and Tostevin, A. L.: Congenital malformations in infants following infectious diseases during pregnancy, with special reference to rubella. A third series of cases, M. J. Australia 1:645, 1946.
52. Dogramaci, I., and Green, H.: Factors in etiology of congenital heart anomalies, J. Pediat. 30:295, 1947.
53. Jackson, A. V.: In King, E. S. J., Lowe, T. E., and Cox, L. B. (eds.), *Studies in Pathology*. Presented to Peter MacCallum (Melbourne: Melbourne University Press, 1950).
54. Rutstein, D. D., Nickerson, R. J., and Heald, F. P.: Seasonal incidence of patent ductus arteriosus and maternal rubella, A.M.A. Am. J. Dis. Child. 84:199, 1952.
55. Gibson, S., and Lewis, K. C.: Congenital heart disease following maternal rubella during pregnancy, A.M.A. Am. J. Dis. Child. 83:317, 1952.
56. Hastreiter, A. R., Joorabachi, B., Pujatti, G., van der Horst, R. L., Patacsil, G., and Sever, J. L.: Cardiovascular lesions associated with congenital rubella, J. Pediat. 71: 59, 1967.
57. Lynxweiler, C., and Wells, C.: Patent ductus arteriosus: A report of 180 operations, South. M. J. 43:61, 1950.
58. Keith, J. D., Rowe, R. D., and Vlad, P. (eds.): *Heart Disease in Infancy and Childhood* (2d ed.; New York: The Macmillan Company, 1966).
59. Weicker, H.: 100 children with thalidomide embryopathy, XIth International Congress of Pediatrics, 1965.
60. MacMahon, B.: Association of congenital malformations of the heart with birth rank and maternal age, Brit. J. Social Med. 6:178, 1952.
61. Polani, P. E., and Campbell, M.: Factors in the causation of persistent ductus arteriosus, Ann. Human Genet. 24: 343, 1960.
62. Alzamora, V., Rotta, A., Battalani, G., Abugattas, R., Rubio, C., Bouroncle, J., Zapata, C., Santa Maria, E., Binder, T., Subiria, R., Paredes, D., Panto, B., and Graham, G. G.: On the possible influence of great altitudes on the determination of certain cardiovascular anomalies, Pediatrics 12:259, 1953.
63. Dexter, L.: Congenital defects of the heart in high altitudes, New England J. Med. 247:851, 1952.
64. Lyon, R. A., and Kaplan, S.: Patent ductus arteriosus in infancy, Pediatrics 13:357, 1954.
65. Adams, F. H., and Forsyth, W. B.: The effect of surgery on the growth of patients with patent ductus arteriosus, J. Pediat. 39:330, 1951.
66. Shapiro, M. J.: Preoperative diagnosis of patent ductus arteriosus, J.A.M.A. 126:934, 1944.
67. Umansky, R., and Hauck, A. J.: Factors in the growth of children with patent ductus arteriosus, Pediatrics 30:540, 1962.
68. Shapiro, M. J., and Keys, A.: The prognosis of untreated patent ductus arteriosus and the results of surgical intervention: A clinical series of 50 cases and an analysis of 139 operations, Am. J. M. Sc. 206:174, 1943.
69. Gross, R. E.: The patent ductus arteriosus. Observations on diagnosis and therapy in 525 surgically treated cases, Am. J. Med. 12:472, 1952.
70. Krovetz, L. J., and Warden, H. E.: Patent ductus arteriosus. An analysis of 515 surgically proved cases, Dis. Chest 42:46, 1962.
71. Bonham Carter, R. E., Walker, C. H. M., Daley, R., Mathews, M. B., and Medd, W. E.: Patent ductus arteriosus with abnormal aortic valve, Brit. Heart J. 17:255, 1955.
72. Wagner, B. M., and Price, W. S.: Dysphagia lusoria: Unusual case, Am. Heart J. 44:452, 1952.
73. Beswick, R., Warner, R., and Warkany, J.: Congenital anomalies following maternal rubella, Am. J. Dis. Child. 78:334, 1949.
74. Cosh, J. A.: Patent ductus arteriosus; a follow-up study of 73 cases, Brit. Heart J. 19:13, 1957.
75. Lund, C. J.: Maternal congenital heart disease as an obstetric problem, Am. J. Obst. & Gynec. 55:244, 1948.
76. Gross, R. E.: A surgical approach for ligation of a patent ductus arteriosus, New England J. Med. 220:510, 1939.
77. Waterman, D. H., Samson, P. C., and Bailey, C. P.: The

surgery of patent ductus arteriosus; a report of the section on cardiovascular surgery, Dis. Chest 29:102, 1956.
78. Hörnblad, P. Y.: Experimental studies on closure of the ductus arteriosus utilizing whole-body freezing, Acta paediat., Supp. 190, 1969.
79. Wilkins, J. L.: Risks to offspring of patients with patent ductus arteriosus, J. M. Genetics 6:1, 1969.
80. Arcilla, R. A., Thilenius, O. G., and Ranninger, K.: Congestive heart failure from suspected ductal closure in utero, J. Pediat. 75:74, 1969.
81. Desligneres, S., and Larroche, J. C.: Ductus arteriosus, Biol. Neonat. 16:278, 1970.

62

The Coronary Arteries

Anomalies of the Coronary Arteries

THE RIGHT OR THE LEFT OR BOTH coronary arteries may arise from the pulmonary trunk. Such anomalies have assumed additional clinical significance since surgical correction has become possible for many patients with congenital heart disease. The condition is rare and only about 80 cases have been recorded.[1] It amounted to only one-quarter of 1% of cardiovascular cases seen in a hospital[2] and the incidence is 1 in 300,000 births. The sexes seem to be affected equally.[2] Approximately 80% of the reported cases are of the infantile type,[1] which differs from that seen in adults. Most observations concern anomalous left coronary arteries.

Since before birth the oxygen content of the blood of both ventricles is nearly the same, the anomaly is well tolerated in prenatal life. After birth, difficulties arise as the pressure in the pulmonary artery falls and the abnormal coronary artery receives venous blood under low pressure. Within a few weeks or months, pathologic changes occur in the wall of the left ventricle. As subendocardial and myocardial fibrosis set in, the left ventricle becomes greatly enlarged. In its thin and expanded wall, an increase of fibrous and elastic tissue becomes noticeable, calcareous deposits are formed and endocardial fibrosis develops, particularly on the posterior aspects.

In embryos of 42–45 days,[3] the coronary arteries develop as solid endothelial buds in the not completely divided truncus arteriosus from that portion that later forms the aorta. It seems that, in development, the left coronary artery somewhat precedes the right. In the case of a left heterotopic coronary artery, this vessel takes its origin from the portion that later develops into the pulmonary artery. An alternative explanation, that abnormal division of the truncus arteriosus results in displacement of the left coronary artery, has not been accepted since, in most cases, there are no signs of such abnormal division and the cusps of both semilunar valves are normal. In most of the reported cases there are no serious cardiac malformations associated with heterotopic left coronary artery.[4]

Patients seen by pediatricians are children with serious manifestations in early infancy. They usually are of normal birth weight and appear normal in the first few weeks of life. In the second and third months, however, the first symptoms appear in the form of irritability, restlessness, crying in pain, feeding difficulties and respiratory infections. Dyspnea, tachycardia, retractions and enlargement of the liver are observed and there may be intermittent cyanosis. Enlargement of the heart becomes noticeable but usually there are no murmurs. Within a few months the children succumb to heart failure. In these infantile cases, a rather typical x-ray picture is observed. The heart is markedly enlarged, the apex reaching almost to the axillary line. The lung fields are congested and in the left anterior oblique view the enlargement of the left ventricle can be seen clearly by extension of the heart shadow backward. Angiography shows the continuity between the pulmonary artery and the left coronary artery and the marked disproportion between the small right and the large left ventricle.[1,5]

This rather typical clinical and pathologic picture of infants is quite different from that of persons who, despite this anomaly, reach adult life.[5] Such persons can be entirely symptom-free for many years and do strenuous work as well as healthy people. A continuous murmur may betray the condition.[6] Adult patients with heterotopic coronaries who reach middle or old age report no symptoms during childhood. Their fate may be sudden death or heart failure. At necropsy, a large right coronary artery usually is found that supplies blood to the left ventricle by anastomoses. The left coronary artery seems anatomically and functionally transformed into a vein and carries venous blood to the pulmonary artery. Although most patients with the infantile form die within the first 6 months, those with the adult form usually reach middle age. In recent years, it has been recognized that manifestations can occur throughout childhood.[7]

Surgical treatments have been suggested and attempted, the most promising theoretically being anastomosis of the abnormal left coronary with a systemic artery.[8] If the anomalous artery functions as a vein with blood flowing from it into the pulmonary artery, ligation of the left coronary may be helpful.[2]

Heterotopic right coronary artery arising from the pulmonary artery apparently is not of functional significance if the left coronary artery originates normally from the aorta. It is not clear why this anomaly is so well tolerated. The few cases described have been found as accidental anomalies at necropsy of adults. One patient reported by Cronk *et al.*[9] was 90 years of age at the time of death.

Origin of both coronary arteries from the pulmonary artery is a very rare anomaly that has been reported only five times.[10] Three infants with heterotopic origin of both coronaries had complicating serious cardiovascular malformations such as tetralogy of Fallot, atresia of the tricuspid valve or ventricular septal defect. In two cases,[10,11] only patent ductus arteriosus was found, which could not be considered a malformation, since the children were under 2 weeks of age. Four of the 5 infants with heterotopic origin of both coronary arteries died within the first 2 weeks.

Single Coronary Artery

Single coronary artery may follow the course of either the right or left coronary artery and supply blood to the entire myocardium by extension of its subdivisions; or it may branch shortly after its origin from the aorta and follow the courses of the normal right and left coronaries; or it may be so abnormal that it cannot be compared with either the right or left coronary.[12] Such anomalies can occur in children with complex cardiovascular malformations that require surgery and may present serious hazards to successful operation.[13]

REFERENCES

1. Bookstein, J. J.: Aberrant left coronary artery, Am. J. Roentgenol. 91:515, 1964.
2. Keith, J. D., Rowe, R. D., and Vlad, P. (eds.): *Heart Disease in Infancy and Childhood* (2d ed,; New York: The Macmillan Company, 1966).
3. Wilson, J. G.: Unpublished data, 1959.
4. Wüthrich, R.: Über den Abgang der Arteria coronaria sinistra aus der Arteria pulmonalis. Zugleich ein Beitrag zum Problem des plötzlichen Todes, Cardiologia 18:193, 1951.
5. Kaunitz, P. E.: Origin of left coronary artery from pulmonary artery; review of the literature and report of two cases, Am. Heart J. 33:182, 1947.
6. Lampe, C. F. J., and Verheugt, A. P. M.: Anomalous left coronary artery. Adult type, Am. Heart J. 59:769, 1960.
7. Nadas, A. S., Gamboa, R., and Hugenholitz, P. G.: Anomalous left coronary artery originating from the pulmonary artery. Report of two surgically treated cases with a proposal of hemodynamic and therapeutic classification, Circulation 29:167, 1964.
8. Keith, J. D., Rowe, R. D., and Vlad, P. (eds.): *Heart Disease in Infancy and Childhood* (New York: The Macmillan Company, 1958).
9. Cronk, E. S., Sinclair, J. G., and Rigdon, R. H.: An anomalous coronary arising from the pulmonary artery, Am. Heart J. 42:906, 1951.
10. Tedeschi, C. G., and Helpern, M. M.: Heterotopic origin of both coronary arteries from the pulmonary artery. Review of literature and report of a case not complicated by associated defects, Pediatrics 14:53, 1954.
11. Limbourg: Über den Ursprung der Kranzarterien des Herzens aus der Arteria pulmonalis, Beitr. path. Anat. 100:191, 1937.
12. Smith, J. C.: Review of single coronary artery, with report of two cases, Circulation 1:1168, 1950.
13. Friedman, S., Ash, R., Klein, D., and Johnson, J.: Anomalous single coronary artery complicating ventriculotomy in a child with cyanotic congenital heart disease, Am. Heart J. 59:140, 1960.

Aneurysm of the Coronary Arteries

THE SUBJECT OF ANEURYSM of the coronary arteries was reviewed by Scott[1] in 1948. It is now believed that many of these aneurysms are of congenital origin, although arteriosclerosis and infections are also causative in some of the cases. Approximately one-third of the reported cases are thought to be congenital and among these many more males are found than females. The left coronary artery is more often involved than the right. In some instances, these aneurysms are well tolerated, whereas in others rupture or occlusion may become fatal. In the congenital form, the ages of the patients observed varied between 5 and 84 years. Valdivia *et al.*[2] reported a patient who was well to the age of 21 years when, during her first pregnancy, she developed heart palpitations. At the age of 25 years, a huge shadow was found on x-ray examination of the chest, and exploration revealed a tumor that was vascular and yielded blood on aspiration. Four years later, the patient died of heart failure and, at necropsy, a large globular tumor arising from the posterior wall of the left ventricle was found that occupied almost completely the left pleural cavity, pushing the collapsed left lung upward. The heart together with the mass weighed 1,800 Gm. The left coronary artery was normal but the right coronary was enlarged and its dilated and tortuous descending branch communicated with the large aneurysmal mass and the right atrium. Gore *et al.*[3] presented a case in a 26-year-old man.

REFERENCES

1. Scott, D. H.: Aneurysm of the coronary arteries, Am. Heart J. 36:403, 1948.
2. Valdivia, E., Rowe, G. G., and Angevine, D. M.: Large congenital aneurysm of the right coronary artery, A.M.A. Arch. Path. 63:168, 1957.
3. Gore, I., Smith, J., and Clancy, R.: Congenital aneurysms of the coronary arteries with report of a case, Circulation 19:221, 1959.

Coronary Arteriovenous Fistula

ABNORMAL COMMUNICATIONS between coronary arteries and the coronary venous system constitute arteriovenous lesions in which blood is shunted into vascular channels without first passing through capillaries.[1] Since coronary arteriovenous fistulas are potentially serious lesions that can be treated surgically, their diagnosis is of importance and many studies have been devoted to them in recent years. In 1962, Upshaw[2] analyzed 73 reported cases. Such fistulae probably are due to defective differentiation of coronary capillaries and continuation of primitive sinusoidal spaces of the coronary system resulting in communications between the coronary arteries and veins. Another origin of intercoronary communication is found in cases of heterotopic coronary arteries (p. 562). Approximately 90% of the fistulae empty into the right side of the heart and 10% into the left side.[2] Diagnosis can be made intra vitam by a continuous murmur resembling that of patent ductus arteriosus but atypical in location. Catheterization of the heart reveals the presence and volume of a left-to-right shunt and angiocardiography may reveal the anomaly clearly by demonstrating the site of the fistula.

The prognosis varies widely. In some instances there has been long life with freedom from symptoms. In others, heart failure has caused death of the patients. In approximately one-third of the patients, associated cardiovascular malformations are present. Surgical closure of the fistula has been performed with success.[2-5]

REFERENCES

1. Steinberg, I., Baldwin, J. S., and Dotter, C. T.: Coronary arteriovenous fistula, Circulation 17:372, 1958.
2. Upshaw, C. B., Jr.: Congenital coronary arteriovenous fistula; report of a case with an analysis of seventy-three reported cases, Am. Heart J. 63:399, 1962.
3. Björck, G., and Crafoord, G.: Arteriovenous aneurysm of the pulmonary artery simulating patent ductus arteriosus botalli, Thorax 2:65, 1947.
4. Keith, J. D., Rowe, R. D., and Vlad, P. (eds.): *Heart Disease in Infancy and Childhood* (2d ed.; New York: The Macmillan Company, 1966).
5. McNamara, J. J., and Gross, R. E.: Congenital coronary artery fistula, Surgery 65:59, 1969.

63

Anomalies of Venous Return

Systemic Veins

PERSISTENT LEFT SUPERIOR VENA CAVA.—If the left innominate vein fails to cross to the right to join the right innominate vein, but descends vertically to join the coronary sinus, a persistent left superior vena cava is formed. In such cases, the coronary sinus is enlarged but it empties normally into the right atrium. In rare instances, the right innominate vein crosses to the left to join a left superior vena cava, which empties into the coronary sinus. In such cases, the coronary sinus delivers the entire blood from the upper portion of the body to the right atrium and there are no functional disturbances. But persistent left superior vena cava often is associated with such serious cardiovascular anomalies as atrial septal defects, partial anomalies of pulmonary venous return and many others. More than 50% of patients with splenic agenesis have anomalous systemic venous return.[1]

Persistent left superior vena cava sometimes can be recognized in roentgenograms by a vertical shadow in the left mediastinum.

No treatment is needed for persistent left superior vena cava.

In the rat, a left superior vena cava terminating in the right atrium is a normal structure. Transposition of this left superior vena cava can be produced experimentally by trypan blue injections during early organogenesis.[2] The abnormal vessel may enter the left atrium, both atria or the inferior vena cava. Rarely, all three venae cavae may terminate in a common sinus venosus communicating with the right atrium. These anomalies of the left superior vena cava usually are accompanied by auricular shift, but they are independent of defects of the auricular septum.

ABSENCE OF INFERIOR VENA CAVA.—In the presence of this anomaly, the blood from the lower extremities reaches the lower portion of the vena azygos, which empties into the superior vena cava. This is in itself a benign anomaly, but frequently it is associated with such severe cardiac malformations as dextrocardia, levocardia, cor biloculare, pulmonary atresia, septal defects and anomalies of the pulmonary veins. The hepatic veins may enter the right or left atrium directly.[3] Venous angiograms from the leg show the contrast medium entering the right atrium through the superior vena cava.[4] Stackelberg *et al.*[5] reported 2 cases of absent inferior vena cava. The vein, demonstrated in its place by angiocardiography, was considered by these authors to be a right posterior cardinal vein. In one of their cases, the venous anomaly was not combined with other malformations. In the second case, a persistent left superior vena cava emptying into the left auricle and an auricular septal defect were present. Anderson *et al.*[6] described a case of absent inferior vena cava or "anomalous inferior vena cava with azygous drainage" associated with a dextroposed bilocular heart, pulmonary atresia and patent ductus arteriosus, and reviewed 7 additional cases from the literature. In several instances, the anomaly was combined with partial or complete situs inversus. In roentgenograms, the dilated, forward-coursing azygos vein may be recognized as a rounded density in the superior mediastinum.[3]

Atresia of the postrenal segment of the inferior vena cava, the common iliac veins and the left innominate vein was described by Swaiman *et al.*[7] Extensive superficial collateral circulation was present in a newborn boy with this rare vascular malformation.

VENAE CAVAE ENTERING THE LEFT AURICLE.—Taussig[8] described anomalous entrance of both venae cavae into the left auricle. In such cases, the right auricle is a small chamber that receives blood from the left auricle through a defect in the interatrial septum. The clinical syndrome and the cardiac findings are identical to those of a defective development of the right ventricle. An inferior vena cava entering the left atrium is a rare malformation. Gardner and Cole[9] described such a patient who survived to an age of 32 years even though cyanosis had existed from birth, and Meadows *et al.*[10] reported a 37-year-old man with this anomaly who had clubbing, cyanosis and polycythemia. There were reports of heart trouble in many members of this patient's family.

LEVOATRIO-CARDINAL VEIN.—This represents a communication of a systemic vein with the left atrium without the aid of a left superior vena cava or coronary sinus. The systemic vein may be the right superior vena cava, a right internal jugular or left innominate vein. The connection was considered by Edwards[11] to be a residual of communications of early pulmonary venous primordia with cardinal veins. In the case of mitral atresia and closed foramen ovale, such a vein may be the only outlet for oxygenated blood to the right atrium. This anomaly may also be combined with transposition of the great vessels and provide a communication between the two circulations.[11]

Pulmonary Veins

TOTAL ANOMALOUS PULMONARY VENOUS RETURN.—If all pulmonary veins drain into the right auricle and the left auricle has no direct connection with the lungs, the left heart can receive blood only through a patent foramen ovale or an atrial septal defect. Both the left atrium and the left ventricle are small, whereas the right atrium, ventricle and the pulmonary artery are considerably enlarged. The anomaly is found in 1–2% of necropsied cases of congenital heart disease.[12]

Total anomalous venous return sometimes is associated with such cardiac malformations as ventricular septal defects, cor biloculare, single ventricle, transposition of the great vessels, pulmonary stenosis, truncus arteriosus and others.[12,13] Such cases can be combined with partial or complete situs inversus and agenesis of the spleen. Of 85 cases with agenesis of the spleen reviewed by Gilbert *et al.*,[1] 45 had anomalous pulmonary venous return. In patients with these anomalies, the pulmonary veins empty directly into the right atrium or they are connected with it by subdiaphragmatic channels, a superior vena cava or an innominate vein. Occasionally, anomalous pulmonary venous return can partially correct complicated forms of congenital heart disease and prove life-prolonging.[12]

Anomalous pulmonary venous return sometimes is combined with anomalies of the lungs, particularly hypoplasia. Malformations of the spine also may be present.[14,15] The pulmonary hypoplasia usually is located on the right side, but anomalous venous drainage of the left hypoplastic lung into the inferior vena cava also has been reported.[16]

Failure of connection between the venous outgrowth from the atrium with the early pulmonary network derived from the foregut plexus is held responsible for the lack of pulmonary venous drainage into the left atrium and drainage through systemic veins into the right. In the case of direct return of pulmonary veins into the right atrium, abnormal deviation of the atrial septum to the left has been postulated as a pathogenic factor.[13]

The more common form is the isolated type, which is not associated with severe cardiac malformations; it is compatible with life only if the foramen ovale is patent or an atrial septal defect exists. Thus, the isolated form actually is not so isolated but is combined with an interatrial defect. As long as the ductus arteriosus is open, the high pressure in the pulmonary artery can drive some oxygenated blood from the right through the ductus into the aorta. With the obliteration of the ductus, more blood flows through the lungs, but oxygenated blood can still reach the left heart through an open foramen ovale. The ductus remains open in approximately 25% of the cases. The pulmonary veins may have supracardiac, cardiac, infracardiac or mixed connections with the right atrium. The supracardiac connection through the superior vena cava probably is the most frequent form, the pulmonary veins draining into the right superior vena cava or into the left innominate vein through a remnant of the left superior vena cava. A second way of anomalous drainage is represented by direct connections of the pulmonary veins with the right atrium or the coronary sinus. In the third type of total anomalous venous drainage, the pulmonary veins are connected with the inferior vena cava through the portal system subdiaphragmatically. Finally, there may be connections at different levels.[13] Subdiaphragmatic anomalous pulmonary venous return has been reported in siblings.[26]

In infants with such anomalous pulmonary venous return, symptoms frequently appear early. Those with infradiaphragmatic connections usually die before 3 months of life.[13] They commonly have pulmonary venous obstruction. Children who survive the neonatal period show poor weight gain and feeding difficulties, tachypnea and often—though not always—cyanosis. Cardiac arrhythmias are common, murmurs variable. The heart shows progressive enlargement to the right and pulmonary congestion is common. As a rule, cardiac failure develops within the first year, presumably because of closure of compensatory shunts.[13]

Roentgenograms show the progressive cardiac enlargement and sometimes a supracardiac shadow formed by the right and the remnant of the left superior vena cava and the enlarged innominate veins ("figure of 8"). Return below the diaphragm is suggested by a heart within normal limits in size and configuration in a patient with cyanosis and evidence of congestive heart failure.[17] A characteristic reticulated appearance of the lungs in chest films suggests the diagnosis.[18]

The prognosis is poor. Without surgical treatment, 80% of these children die in infancy.[12,13] A small group of patients survive to adult life. It is possible that associated atrial defects or some other mechanism that permits mixing of pulmonary and systemic blood make such survival possible.[4]

Successful surgical treatment has been reported in older children by establishment of an anastomosis of the pulmonary veins with the left atrium. In infants, surgical procedures are difficult, but successful open-heart correction has been reported in children under 1 year of age,[19] including some with infradiaphragmatic return.[20] The best results are achieved in patients with low pulmonary artery pressure.[12]

PARTIAL ANOMALOUS PULMONARY VENOUS RETURN.—If one or two of the pulmonary veins enter the right atrium while others open into the left, a portion of the

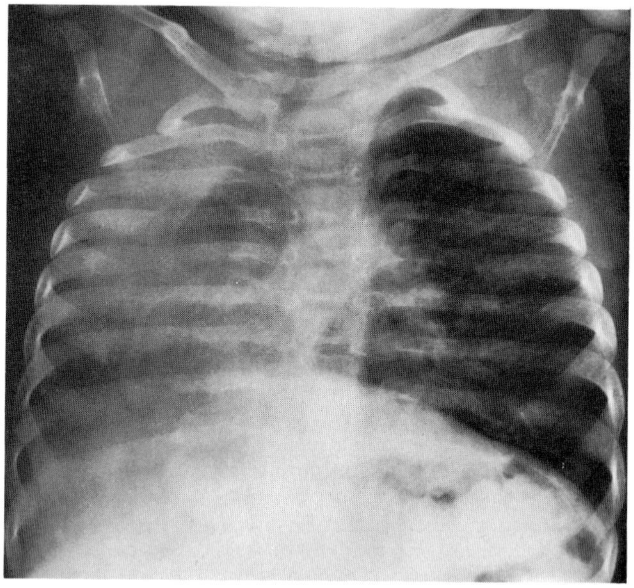

Fig. 63-1.—Roentgenogram of a boy 1 year of age with hypoplasia of the right lung and scimitar syndrome.

Fig. 63-2.—Angiogram showing connection of right pulmonary vein with inferior vena cava.

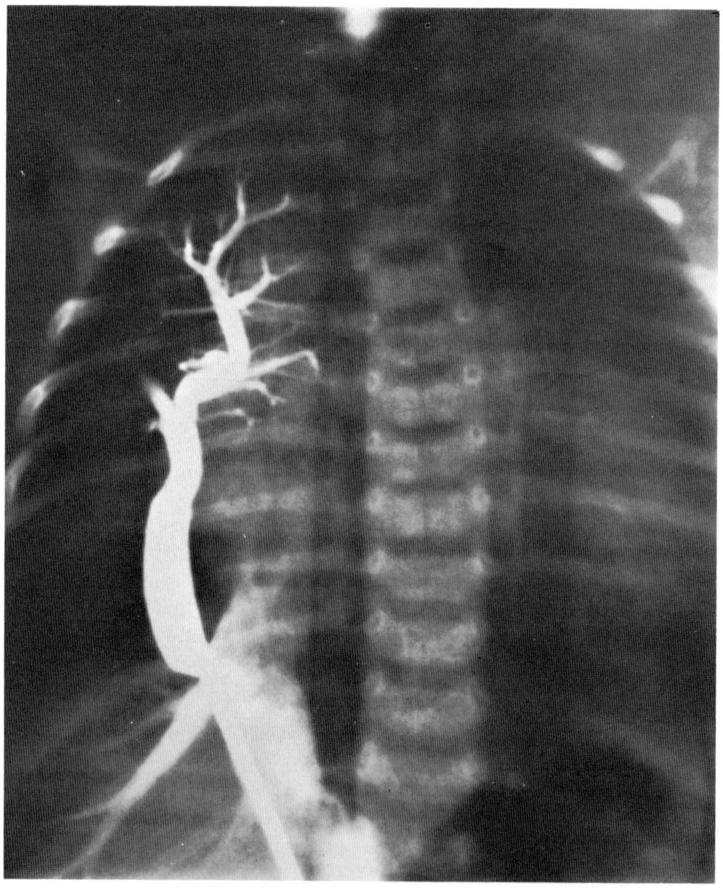

oxygenated blood is shunted into the pulmonary circulation and the remainder reaches the systemic circulation. Thus, the right atrium and ventricle receive more than their normal share of blood and are subjected to unusual strain.[8] It is estimated that such partial anomalies of the pulmonary veins are not rare and occur once in 140 necropsies.[21] The right lung is involved twice as often as the left.[13] Familial occurrence has been recorded.[14,22] Anomalous pulmonary venous return may occur as an isolated anatomic variation or be combined with congenital defects of the heart.

In the isolated form, one usually sees one or two right pulmonary veins joining either one of the venae cavae or the right auricle. If the left pulmonary veins are also involved, they are connected, as a rule, with the left innominate vein or the coronary sinus.

Such limited pulmonary venous anomalies usually cause no symptoms in children. One abnormal pulmonary vein may remain asymptomatic throughout life. If more than one vein is involved, the right side of the heart may become hypertrophic, the chambers dilated and the pulmonary artery enlarged. If less than 50% of the pulmonary venous blood is shunted to the right, early symptoms usually are absent. If more than 50% is returned to the wrong chamber, signs of fatigue, exertional dyspnea and eventually congestive heart failure may develop.[23] But the anatomic findings do not always parallel the clinical manifestations. Such differential response is explained by different reactions of the pulmonary vasculature to the extra blood flow.[12] In roentgenograms, an anomalous pulmonary vein may be visible as it enters the inferior vena cava. Its crescentic shape has been compared to a scimitar. The *scimitar syndrome* consists of hypoplasia of the right lung, bronchial anomalies, hypoplasia of the right pulmonary artery, dextroposition of the heart and anomalous right pulmonary veins.[24] This syndrome has been observed in a father and one of his daughters.[24]

Partial anomalous pulmonary venous return commonly is combined with other cardiac anomalies. Atrial septal defect is the most important associated anomaly. It is estimated that 15–20% of patients with atrial defect have abnormal pulmonary veins entering the right atrium.[12,25] Tetralogy of Fallot, single ventricle, tricuspid atresia and other malformations also may show abnormal return of pulmonary veins. In such cases, it usually is the right pulmonary veins that enter the right atrium directly or contact the superior vena cava or the coronary sinus.[12] It is believed that the combination of atrial septal defect with abnormal pulmonary venous return aggravates the symptoms of atrial defects, leading to signs of fatigue, dyspnea and even heart failure in children or young adults. If infants with partial anomalous drainage die early, it is because of the large amount of oxygenated blood that reaches the right atrium or because of severe associated cardiac malformations.[13]

Asymptomatic patients require no treatment. If there are symptoms, the aberrant veins can be connected surgically to the left atrium. An atrial defect, if present, can be closed simultaneously.

REFERENCES

1. Gilbert, E. F., Nishimura, K., and Wedum, B. G.: Congenital malformations of the heart associated with splenic agenesis; report of five cases, Circulation 17:72, 1958.
2. Fox, M. H., and Goss, C. M.: Experimentally produced malformations of the heart and great vessels in rat fetuses; atrial and caval abnormalities, Anat. Rec. 129:309, 1957.
3. Downing, D. F.: Absence of inferior vena cava, Pediatrics 12:675, 1953.
4. Keith, J. D., Rowe, R. D., and Vlad, P. (eds.): *Heart Disease in Infancy and Childhood* (New York: The Macmillan Company, 1958).
5. Stackelberg, B., Lind, J., and Wegelius, C.: Absence of the inferior vena cava diagnosed by angiocardiography, Cardiologia 21:583, 1952.
6. Anderson, R. C., Heilig, W., Novick, R., and Jarvis, C.: Anomalous inferior vena cava with azygous drainage: So-called absence of inferior vena cava, Am. Heart J. 49: 318, 1955.
7. Swaiman, K. F., Austrian, S., and Raile, R. B.: Congenital atresia of the inferior vena cava, common iliac veins, and left innominate vein, A.M.A. J. Dis. Child. 96:81, 1958.
8. Taussig, H. B.: *Congenital Malformations of the Heart* (New York: Commonwealth Fund, 1947).
9. Gardner, D. L., and Cole, L.: Long survival with inferior vena cava draining into left atrium, Brit. Heart J. 17:93, 1955.
10. Meadows, W. R., Bergstrand, I., and Sharp, J. T.: Isolated anomalous connection of a great vein to the left atrium; the syndrome of cyanosis and clubbing, "normal" heart, and left ventricular hypertrophy on electrocardiogram, Circulation 24:669, 1961.
11. Edwards, J. E.: Congenital Malformations of the Heart and Great Vessels, in Gould, S. E. (ed.), *Pathology of the Heart* (Springfield, Ill.: Charles C Thomas, Publisher, 1953).
12. Keith, J. D., Rowe, R. D., and Vlad, P. (eds.): *Heart Disease in Infancy and Childhood* (2d ed.; New York: The Macmillan Company, 1966).
13. Darling, R. C., Rothney, W. B., and Craig, J. M.: Total pulmonary venous drainage into the right side of the heart; report of 17 autopsied cases, not associated with other major cardiovascular anomalies, Lab. Invest. 6:44, 1957.
14. Ferencz, C.: Congenital abnormalities of pulmonary vessels and their relation to malformations of the lung, Pediatrics 28:993, 1961.
15. Jue, K. L., Amplatz, K., Adams, P., Jr. and Anderson, R. C.: Anomalies of great vessels associated with lung hypoplasia. The scimitar syndrome, Am. J. Dis. Child. 111: 35, 1966.
16. D'Cruz, I. A., and Arcilla, R. A.: Anomalous venous drainage of the left lung into the inferior vena cava; a case report, Am. Heart J. 67:539, 1964.
17. Harris, G. B. C., Neuhauser, E. B. D., and Giedion, A.: Total anomalous pulmonary venous return below the diaphragm; the roentgen appearance in three patients diagnosed during life, Am. J. Roentgenol. 84:436, 1960.
18. Levin, B., and White, H.: Total anomalous pulmonary venous drainage into the portal system, Radiology 76:894, 1961.
19. Ryan, N. J., Williams, G. R., Cayler, G. G., Snyder, D. S., Taybi, H., Richardson, W. R., and Campbell, G. S.: Total anomalous pulmonary venous drainage; results of open-heart correction in four infants, Am. J. Dis. Child. 105:42, 1963.
20. Cooley, D. A., and Balas, P. E.: Total anomalous pulmonary venous drainage into inferior vena cava; report of a successful surgical correction, Surgery 51:798, 1962.

21. Hughes, C. W., and Rumore, P. C.: Anomalous pulmonary veins, Arch. Path. 37:364, 1944.
22. Kittle, C. F., and Crockett, J. E.: Vena cava bronchovascular syndrome – a triad of anomalies involving the right lung: Anomalous pulmonary vein, abnormal bronchi and systemic pulmonary arteries, Ann. Surg. 156:222, 1962.
23. Brody, H.: Drainage of the pulmonary veins into the right side of the heart, Arch. Path. 33:221, 1942.
24. Neill, C. A., Ferencz, C., Sabiston, D. C., and Sheldon, H.: The familial occurrence of hypoplastic right lung with systemic arterial supply and venous drainage: "Scimitar syndrome," Bull. Johns Hopkins Hosp. 107:1, 1960.
25. Gilman, R. A., Skowron, C. S. R., Musser, B. G., and Bailey, C. P.: Partial anomalous venous drainage, Am. J. Surg. 94:688, 1957.
26. Vinh, L. T., Van Duc, T., Alcardi, J., and Thieffry, St.: Retour veineux pulmonaire anormal total infra-diaphragmatique familial, Arch. franç. pédiat. 25:1141, 1968.

SECTION FOUR

64

Systemic Disorders Involving Cardiovascular Malformations

Associated Malformations

EXTRACARDIAC MALFORMATIONS occur more often in children with congenital heart disease than in the general population. Associated malformations in children with congenital heart disease are enumerated in many places in this book but quantitative correlations vary in different studies. Estimates of malformations associated with congenital cardiopathies range between 18% and 36%.[1] Boesen *et al.*[2] examined 615 children with congenital heart disease for extracardiac malformations; they found such malformations in 70 patients (11.4%). Mongolism per se was not included in this estimate but obvious extracardiac malformations in mongoloids were counted. When mongolism was counted as a malformation, the incidence rose to 15.6%. In necropsy material, extracardiac malformations were found in 13.4% of children under 4 years of age with congenital heart disease or in 22.8% when mongolism was included. The fact that no extracardiac malformations were noted clinically in patients with transposition of the great vessels or with tricuspid atresia is noteworthy. In the necropsy material of Boesen *et al.*,[2] extracardiac malformations associated with transposition were also rare, but some anomalies of the asplenia syndrome (p. 745) were discovered that were missed in clinical observations. Extracardiac malformations do occur occasionally in infants with transposition (p. 522), but such patients probably are not viable and do not reach clinical cardiac services. In experimental studies in rats, the transposition complex (which includes tricuspid atresia) produced by trypan blue is also only seldom associated with extracardiac malformations, with the exception of ocular anomalies, which occur commonly in abnormal fetuses.[3]

In the series of Boesen *et al.*,[2] harelip and/or cleft palate were present in 1.8% of the patients with congenital heart disease. This is not a striking association, but it is more than ten times the incidence in the general population in Denmark (p. 628). The association of harelip and/or cleft palate with atrial septal defects was more marked than with other types of congenital heart disease. Ventricular septal defects were relatively often combined with malformations of bones, joints and lungs. Clinical and necropsy observations of extracardiac malformations generally were in agreement; only the number of malformations within the gastrointestinal tract and the lungs was higher in the necropsy than in the clinical material.

MacMahon *et al.*,[4] whose sampling differed from that of Boesen *et al.*,[2] included stillborn and neonatal children as well as mongoloids in their series. They estimated associated malformations to be 21%; of these, 6% referred to mongolism and 4% to the alimentary tract. Malformations of the central nervous system, the skeleton and the genitourinary tract each accounted for 2–3%.

Emerit *et al.*[1] examined associated malformations in 1,000 patients with cardiovascular anomalies evaluated by modern clinical methods. Extracardiac anomalies were noted in 41.7% of the patients, the majority being minor deviations. After exclusion of patients who had only a single minor malformation, the percentage was reduced to 20 if only serious anomalies and syndromes were included or 30 if patients with multiple minor defects were added. Control patients had fewer malformations in all categories. Tetralogy of Fallot and ventricular septal defect (VSD) more often were complicated by extracardiac malformations than coarctations, patent ductus arteriosus, aortic stenosis and atrial septal defect. Severe kyphoscolioses were outstanding in frequency, particularly among patients with cyanotic CHD. Mental retardation was also a frequent anomaly, especially with tetralogy, VSD, coarctation and atrioventricularis communis. Limb defects were not clearly associated with subgroups of CHD, but severe deformities more often were combined with tetralogy, pulmonary stenosis and atrial septal defect than with anomalies of the great vessels. Eight per cent of the patients in this series had well-defined syndromes such as Turner, Down, Marfan or postrubella signs. In 92%, the etiology remained unexplained even though in 7% of them some familial aggregation pointed to heredity as a factor; no regular transmission was noted. In 10–15% of the cases there were reports of incidents during pregnancy. The resulting disease pictures more often were complicated syndromes than isolated cardiovascular anomalies.

A detailed study of extracardiac malformations associated with CHD was made by Okada *et al.*[5] in the Chicago area. These authors tabulated the anomalies of the cardiovascular system of 1,287 necropsied cases and the anomalies noted in other organ systems. The diagnoses of the heart and vessels were carefully established and 54 types were listed. In contrast, the malformations of other systems were lumped into rather meaningless classes such as "anomalies of cephalic end," "genetic system," "musculoskeletal system" and others. The lack of specificity of the associated malformation classes reduced the value of the tabulation. The over-all incidence of extracardiac malformations was 37.1%, i.e., higher than that of Boesen *et al.*[2] and MacMahon *et al.*[4] Since it is not clear whether minor associated malformations were included, comparisons are not possible. Extracardiac defects were more frequent than the over-all incidence with VSD, atrioventricularis communis, combined shunts and dextrocardia; they were less frequent with complete transposition of the great vessels, hypoplasia of the aortic tract complex and idiopathic hypertrophy. The incidence was higher with complicated lesions than with simple lesions of the same type. Associations with gastrointestinal and musculoskeletal defects were leading. Abnormalities of the spleen were particularly frequent in combination with positional abnormalities of the heart, transposition of the great vessels and atrioventricularis communis. With fetal coarctation there was polydactyly, arachnodactyly, deformed digits, dislocation of the hip, cleft palate or micrognathia; with adult coarctation there were chiefly anomaliies of the urinary system. Other combinations were listed in general terms. A valuable list of references on the subject of cardiac and extracardiac malformations was included.

Naeye,[6] working with necropsy material that included stillborn and newborn infants, pointed out an association of intrauterine growth retardation with congenital heart disease (p. 142) and considered a subnormal number of cells in many body organs as the basis of the prenatal and postnatal growth retardation of some infants with congenital heart disease.

The results of over-all studies of CHD and their associated defects give general figures of complications, but attempts to assign specific malformations to specific types of CHD end in failure. No etiologic relations emerge from such general studies, except those that had been known before the investigation was begun. These conclusions are disappointing but not unexpected. From the few etiologically defined entities (Down, Turner, Laurence-Moon-Biedl, Oram-Holt syndromes, rubella embryopathy and others), one learns that the effect of the mutant gene or the exogenous teratogen usually leads to a variety of types of CHD as they are known to the clinician and the pathologist. These etiologic factors do not recognize clinical or pathologic cardiology and behave accordingly. To establish syndromes of associated defects will remain, as in the past, the task of individual observers who can use their memory, the results of experiments of nature, meaningful epidemiologic methods, useful laboratory techniques and serendipity.

REFERENCES

1. Emerit, I., Vernant, P., Corone, P., and de Grouchy, J.: Malformations extracardiaques associées à des cardiopathies congénitales (étude statistique portant sur 1000 cas), Acta genet. med. et gemel. 16:27, 1967.
2. Boesen, I., Melchior, J. C., Terslev, E., and Vendel, S.: Extracardiac congenital malformations in children with congenital heart disease, Acta paediat. (supp.) 146:28, 1963.
3. Monie, I. W., Takacs, E., and Warkany, J.: Transposition of the great vessels and other cardiovascular abnormalities induced by trypan blue, Anat. Rec. 156:175, 1966.

4. MacMahon, B., McKeown, T., and Record, R. B.: The incidence and life expectation of children with congenital heart disease, Brit. Heart J. 15:121, 1953.
5. Okada, R., Johnson, D., and Lev, M.: Extracardial malformations associated with congenital heart disease, Arch. Path. 85:649, 1968.
6. Naeye, R. L.: Unsuspected organ abnormalities associated with congenital heart disease, Am. J. Path. 47:905, 1965.

Neurologic, Ocular and Mental Complications

TYLER AND CLARK[1] found that one-fourth of the patients in the cardiac clinic at the Harriet Lane Home of the Johns Hopkins Hospital had signs or symptoms of neurologic disorders. Loss of consciousness or convulsions occurred in approximately 20% of patients with cyanotic heart disease who had anatomic and physiologic potentiality for a rapid variation in the amount of venous blood reaching the systemic circulation. In other forms of congenital heart disease, the incidence of these complications was only 3%. The frequency of cerebrovascular accidents was highest in transposition of the great vessels and tricuspid atresia. Cerebral abscess occurred rather constantly (1.6%) in all types in which it was anatomically possible for venous blood to reach the systemic circulation without passing through the lungs. The incidence of mental retardation was higher in patients with cyanotic CHD than in the acyanotic, but this difference cannot be attributed to hypoxia, since, in some cases (mongoloids, microcephalics), the mental deficiency was associated with and not caused by the cardiac defect. Linde *et al.*,[2] who evaluated mental development in CHD, excluded children in whom the heart anomaly was part of a general syndrome. They reported that cyanotic children scored lowest in developmental and intelligence tests (mean I.Q. 96) and acyanotic children higher (I.Q. 104), but children without CHD scored significantly above those in both cardiac groups. Emerit *et al.*[3] listed mental retardation as a major complication (3.9% of the patients) of congenital heart disease, although they excluded established syndromes from this count.

Association of cerebral arteriovenous fistulas with CHD was reported by Hernandez *et al.*[4] This finding is of clinical importance, since cardiomegaly or congestive heart failure may be attributed to the arteriovenous fistula, whereas the associated cardiovascular malformations may be overlooked. Patent ductus arteriosus, ASD and anomalous venous connections have been found in such cases.

CHD often is found together with severe defects of the cyclopia series and the arhinencephalies. This includes trisomy 13-15 (p. 300), in which cardiovascular malformations occur in 85% of the cases. The brain anomalies of Down syndrome are associated with CHD in approximately 50% of the patients (p. 328).

Gardiner and Joseph[5] studied the eyes of 85 children with congenital heart disease between the ages of 6 and 15 years. In general, more eye defects were found in children with cyanotic heart disease than in those with left-to-right shunts or those with pulmonary or aortic stenosis. In the cyanotic group, 1 child had choroid coloboma and 2 had cataracts, but amblyopia was present in 50% of the children with tetralogy of Fallot. There also was a relatively high incidence of myopia and astigmatism in these children.

Combination of ocular colobomas with congenital heart disease and brain anomalies was emphasized by Angelman.[6] In 3 cases, colobomas were associated with severe types of congenital heart disease, particularly pulmonary stenosis. We have seen, without special search, several children of this type; the heart disease was either cyanotic or acyanotic. In one patient, cyanotic congenital heart disease, left iris coloboma, simian creases and bifid first toe on the right were present. In such a case, trisomy 13-15 would now be considered. This is particularly true when the coloboma occurs in microphthalmia.

It is of interest that ocular colobomas quite often are associated with congenital heart disease in fetuses made abnormal by vitamin A deficiency.[7] Microphthalmia and CHD are combined in many cases of trisomy 13-15 (p. 296).

REFERENCES

1. Tyler, H. R., and Clark, D. B.: Incidence of neurological complications in congenital heart disease, Arch. Neurol. & Psychiat. 77:17, 1957.
2. Linde, L. M., Rasof, B., and Dunn, O. J.: Mental development in congenital heart disease, J. Pediat. 71:198, 1967.
3. Emerit, I., Vernant, P., Corone, P., and de Grouchy, J.: Malformations extracardiaques associées à des cardiopathies congénitales (étude statistique portant sur 1000 cas), Acta genet. med. et gemel. 16:27, 1967.
4. Hernandez, A., Jr., Schwartz, H. G., and Goldring, D.: Cerebral arteriovenous fistulas and congenital heart disease, J. Pediat. 66:722, 1965.
5. Gardiner, P. A., and Joseph, M.: Eye defects in children with congenital heart lesions: A preliminary study, Developmental Med. & Child Neurol. 10:42, 1968.
6. Angelman, H.: Syndrome of coloboma with multiple congenital abnormalities in infancy, Brit. M. J. 1:1212, 1961.
7. Wilson, J. G., and Warkany, J.: Aortic-arch and cardiac anomalies in the offspring of vitamin A deficient rats, Am. J. Anat. 85:113, 1949.

Gastrointestinal Malformations

In reviews of large groups of patients with CHD, gastrointestinal malformations were frequent in one study[1] but rare in another.[2] They appear more frequently in necropsy series of children with CHD than in clinical material.[3] If one considers cardiovascular malformations associated with stenoses and atresias of the gastrointestinal tract, associations appear stronger. Of 111 children with such anomalies of the alimentary tract, Buchs[4] noted that 16 (14.4%) had cardiovascular anomalies that affected chiefly the distal part of the cardiac tube. Developmental errors of the primitive left ventricle, the bulbus, truncus and the primitive branchial arteries apparently were predominant. Mellins and Blumenthal,[5] limiting their study to esophageal atresia, ascertained CHD in 26% of the cases. Patent ductus arteriosus, VSD, coarctation of the aorta, tetralogy, atrioventricularis communis, transposition of the great vessels and Ebstein anomaly were noted. Many of these children had low birth weights. Mehrizi *et al.*[6] reviewed the records of 39 infants who died of tracheo-esophageal atresia or fistula and found that 16 of them had associated cardiovascular malformations. The most common anomaly was coarctation of the aorta, but patent ductus arteriosus, VSD, ASD, tetralogy and other defects were seen also. The mortality rate of patients with esophageal atresia and CHD is high.

REFERENCES

1. Okada, R., Johnson, D., and Lev, M.: Extracardiac malformations associated with congenital heart disease, Arch. Path. 85:649, 1968.
2. Emerit, I., Vernant, P., Corone, P., and de Grouchy, J.: Malformations extracardiaques associées à des cardiopathies, congénitales (étude statistique portant sur 1000 cas), Acta genet. med. et gemel. 16:27, 1967.
3. Boesen, I., Melchior, J. C., Terslev, E., and Vendel, S.: Extracardiac congenital malformations in children with congenital heart diseases, Acta paediat. (supp.) 146:28, 1963.
4. Buchs, S.: Über die Missbildung des Herzens und der Gefässe bei den Stenosen und Atresien des Verdauungstraktes, Ann. paediat. 203:256, 1964.
5. Mellins, R. B., and Blumenthal, S.: Cardiovascular anomalies and esophageal atresia, Am. J. Dis. Child. 107:160, 1964.
6. Mehrizi, A., Folger, G. M., Jr., and Rowe, R. D.: Tracheoesophageal fistula associated with congenital cardiovascular malformations, Bull. Johns Hopkins Hosp. 118:246, 1966.

Skeletal Malformations

Anomalies of the skeleton are relatively important complications of CHD. In the series of Emerit *et al.*,[1] they were leading as associated malformations, with particular prominence of kyphoscoliosis. Okada *et al.*[2] listed them second in frequency as associated malformations. There is a constant association of CHD and malformation of the upper extremities in the Holt-Oram syndrome (p. 481), and the limb defects of the thalidomide embryopathy often were complicated by CHD (p. 92). Congenital heart disease sometimes occurs in acrocephalosyndactyly (p. 899), arthrogryposis (p. 1014), broad-thumb syndrome (p. 1019), hemihypertrophy (p. 163), Laurence-Moon-Biedl syndrome (p. 179), Pierre Robin syndrome (p. 654) and others. Some of these disorders are discussed in the following pages.

Arachnodactyly (Marfan syndrome).—The cardiovascular lesions associated with arachnodactyly are of interest because they can be suspected and predicted, to a certain extent, by external inspection of the patient or sometimes of a relative. They also are interesting as manifestations of a dominant pleiotropic gene, thus representing one of the few cases in which inheritance of cardiovascular lesions can be proved by association with recognized hereditary features.

Arachnodactyly (Marfan syndrome) is described in Chapter 91. It is estimated that 30–60% of the patients with this syndrome have cardiovascular lesions,[3] but the incidence may be higher. Aortic and pulmonary arterial aneurysms, valvar lesions and septal defects occur in some affected persons.

The pathologic defect underlying the aortic and pulmonary arterial lesions consists of degenerative changes of the elastic and muscle fibers of the media, resulting in cystic medial necrosis,[4] a term considered inaccurate by Macleod and Williams,[5] since there are neither true cysts nor definite necrosis. Such microscopic lesions are found in the aortic wall in 80% of the patients with or without aortic dilatation. Aneurysmal dilatation of the aorta or of the aortic sinuses occurs in two-thirds of necropsied patients and dissecting aneurysm in one-third. Aortic valvar deformities and aortic insufficiency are not rare.[6,7] Steinberg and Geller[8] reported 3 cases of aneurysmal dilatation of aortic sinuses in adult patients, diagnosed by angiocardiography. In the pulmonary artery, the changes may remain microscopic or lead to aneurysmal dilatation with dissection. The mitral valve sometimes shows thickening of the cusps and chordae tendineae, resulting in valvar insufficiency.

One of the most interesting but controversial questions is the significance and frequency of truly congenital malformations of the heart in patients with arachnodactyly. In the older literature on this subject, it was generally assumed that atrial septal defects are common, but necropsies have not confirmed this assumption. Goyette and Palmer[3] listed only 1 case of auricular septal defect in 34 postmortem cases. There was 1 incidence of patent ductus and 7 of patent foramen ovale. But now there are many cases of structural congenital cardiovascular anomalies on record, so that one must assume that in some cases the abnormal gene acts during organogenic periods.

BRACHYDACTYLY.—Brachydactyly and stenotic lesions of the outflow tract of the heart were reported by Cascos.[10] The situation is similar in Ehlers-Danlos syndrome, in which a hereditary connective tissue disorder causes general vascular weaknesses; but some patients also have atrial septal defects, atrioventricularis communis or tetralogy of Fallot, lesions that date back to embryologic times.[11]

Skeletal and cardiovascular malformations are associated in gargoylism, which is discussed on pages 574 and 810.

LAURENCE-MOON-BIEDL SYNDROME.—Congenital heart disease may appear in the Laurence-Moon-Biedl syndrome as a "supernumerary" constituent.[12] McLoughlin *et al.*[13] observed a sibship in which at least 2 brothers with the Laurence-Moon-Biedl syndrome had congenital heart disease, established by clinical examination and necropsy. One brother had tetralogy of Fallot and the other had complete transposition of the great vessels, a single ventricle, ventricular septal defects and anomalous drainage of the inferior vena cava and of the pulmonary veins. In other cases of the Laurence-Moon-Biedl syndrome in which congenital heart disease was documented, a variety of malformations such as patent ductus arteriosus, hypoplasia of the aorta, defective development of aortic cusps, abnormal coronary arteries, ventricular septal defect, atrial septal defect, dextrocardia and corrected transposition of the great vessels have been reported.[13] Thus, the Laurence-Moon-Biedl syndrome (Chapter 19) represents an example of a gene-determined disorder that begins in embryonic life (polydactyly, cardiovascular malformations) and continues as a "degenerative disease" in postnatal life.

ELLIS-VAN CREVELD SYNDROME.—Congenital heart disease is a frequent constituent of the Ellis-van Creveld syndrome.[14] It has been diagnosed in 11 of 15 reported cases,[15] ventricular septal defect usually being suspected. But subsequent studies revealed a surprising variety of congenital cardiovascular defects in this disorder, in which probably half the patients have CHD. Lynch *et al.*[16] reviewed 18 cases studied by catheterization or necropsy. In 16 patients there was a defect of the atrial septum and in 10 of these a single atrium seemed to exist. In at least 13 patients the defect was of the endocardial cushion type. Ventricular septal defect was present in 9 patients, persistent left superior vena cava in 4 and total anomalous venous return in 2. The usual causes of death are CHD and pulmonary hypoplasia. It seems that the cardiovascular malformations of this recessively inherited syndrome resemble those of the chromosome-determined Down syndrome (Chapter 37).

KLIPPEL-FEIL SYNDROME.—Nora *et al.*[17] discussed the association of CHD with Klippel-Feil syndrome (p. 909). Review of the world literature uncovered only 4 instances of CHD in approximately 200 patients with Klippel-Feil syndrome, but the authors noted 5 cases of CHD among 8 patients with this skeletal anomaly in Madison, Wisconsin. These patients had either VSD alone or VSD combined with other heart lesions. Five of their 8 patients had cyanotic CHD. Congenital heart disease and scoliosis proved to be associated in a significant number of children examined by Luke and McDonnell.[18] Vertebral anomalies were present in a minority of these patients.

PIERRE ROBIN SYNDROME.—In the Pierre Robin syndrome (p. 654), congenital heart disease has been observed repeatedly. Necropsies revealed patent ductus arteriosus, auricular septal defects, cor triloculare, dextrocardia and coarctation of the aorta.[19]

CHOANAL ATRESIA.—Choanal atresia and congenital heart disease in newborn children was pointed out to be a likely combination by Stool and Kemper.[20]

HOLT-ORAM SYNDROME.—This disease picture has been cited and described as an example of a dominantly inherited syndrome that involves congenital heart disease (p. 481). Holt and Oram,[21] in 1960, recorded a kindred in which 9 members in four generations were affected by cardiac malformations and skeletal abnormalities of the upper extremities. Shortened, displaced or absent thumbs, shortened forearms and carpal defects were observed; the most common cardiac malformation was atrial septal defect combined with arrhythmias. As additional cases were described, the spectrum of anomalies enlarged to include ventricular septal defects, anomalous coronary and subclavian arteries, transposition of the great vessels, coarctation of the aorta, patent ductus arteriosus and congenital myocardial disease[22-24] and skeletal defects such as phocomelia, deformed humerus, radio-ulnar synostosis,[25] shortened clavicles and deformed scapulae.[23] Muscular and neurologic anomalies were also noted.[24]

BONY FUSION.—Bony fusion of vertebrae and carpal and tarsal bones, short stature and conductive deafness combined with mitral insufficiency was reported as a syndrome inherited like a dominant trait.[26]

REFERENCES

1. Emerit, I., Vernant, P., Corone, P., and de Grouchy, J.: Malformations extracardiaques associées à des cardiopathies congénitales (étude statistique portant sur 1000 cas), Acta genet. med. et gemel. 16:27, 1967.
2. Okada, R., Johnson, D., and Lev, M.: Extracardial malformations associated with congenital heart disease, Arch. Path. 85:649, 1968.
3. Goyette, E. M., and Palmer, P. W.: Cardiovascular lesions in arachnodactyly, Circulation 7:373, 1953.
4. Baer, R. W., Taussig, H. B., and Oppenheimer, E. H.: Congenital aneurysmal dilatation of aorta associated with arachnodactyly, Bull. Johns Hopkins Hosp. 72:309, 1943.
5. Macleod, M., and Williams, A. W.: Cardiovascular lesions in Marfan's syndrome, A.M.A. Arch. Path. 61:143, 1956.
6. Griffin, J. F., and Koman, G. M.: Severe aortic insufficiency in Marfan's syndrome, Ann. Int. Med. 48:174, 1958.

7. McKusick, V. A.: Cardiovascular aspects of Marfan's syndrome: Heritable disorder of connective tissue, Circulation 11:321, 1955.
8. Steinberg, I., and Geller, W.: Aneurysmal dilatation of aortic sinuses in arachnodactyly: Diagnosis during life in 3 cases, Ann. Int. Med. 43:120, 1955.
9. Piper, R. K., and Irvine-Jones, E.: Arachnodactylia and its association with congenital heart disease; report of a case and review of literature, Am. J. Dis. Child. 31:832, 1926.
10. Cascos, A. S.: Brachydactyly and outflow heart tract obstruction. Report of two cases, Cardiologia 50:330, 1967.
11. McKusick, V. A.: *Heritable Disorders of Connective Tissue* (3d ed.; S. Louis: The C. V. Mosby Company, 1966).
12. Warkany, J., Frauenberger, G. S., and Mitchell, A. G.: Heredofamilial deviations. I. The Laurence-Moon-Biedl syndrome, Am. J. Dis. Child. 53:455, 1937.
13. McLoughlin, T. G., Krovetz, L. J., and Schiebler, G. L.: Heart disease in the Laurence-Moon-Biedl-Bardet syndrome, J. Pediat. 65:388, 1964.
14. Ellis, R. W. B., and van Creveld, B.: A syndrome characterized by ectodermal dysplasia, polydactyly, chondrodysplasia and congenital morbus cordis; report of three cases, Arch. Dis. Childhood 15:65, 1940.
15. Mitchell, F. N, and Waddell, W. W., Jr.: Ellis-van Creveld syndrome. Report of two cases in siblings, Acta paediat. 47:142, 1958.
16. Lynch, J. I., Perry, L. W., Takakuwa, T., and Scott, L. P.: Congenital heart disease and chrondro-ectodermal dysplasia. Report of two cases, one in a Negro, Am. J. Dis. Child. 115:80, 1968.
17. Nora, J. J., Cohen, M., and Maxwell, G. M.: Klippel-Feil syndrome with congenital heart disease, Am. J. Dis. Child. 102:858, 1961.
18. Luke, M. J., and McDonnell, E. J.: Congenital heart disease and scoliosis, J. Pediat. 73:725, 1968.
19. Smith, J. L., and Stowe, F. R.: The Pierre Robin syndrome. A review of 39 cases with emphasis on associated ocular lesions, Pediatrics 27:128, 1961.
20. Stool, S. E., and Kemper, B. I.: Choanal atresia and/or cardiac disease, Pediatrics 42:525, 1968.
21. Holt, M., and Oram, S.: Familial heart disease with skeletal malformations, Brit. Heart J. 22:236, 1960.
22. Holmes, L. B.: Congenital heart disease and upper-extremity deformities. A report of two families, New England J. Med. 272:437, 1965.
23. Lewis, K. B., Bruce, R. A., Baum, D., and Motulsky, A. G.: The upper limb-cardiovascular syndrome, J.A.M.A. 193: 1080, 1965.
24. Ashby, D. W., Chadha, J. S., and Henderson, C. B.: Associated skeletal and cardiac abnormalities: The Holt-Oram syndrome, Quart. J. Med. 38:267, 1969.
25. Pruzanski, W.: Familial congenital malformations of the heart and upper limbs, Cardiologia 45:21, 1964.

Cleft Lip and Cleft Palate

In clinics and hospital services dealing with congenital heart disease (CHD), cleft lip (CL) and cleft palate (CP) are not prevalent. Yet, such facial clefts do occur among these patients more often than in the general population. The association of CHD and facial clefts is rather pronounced in infants who die early because of multiple congenital anomalies. An example of a lethal syndrome that combines CHD and CL and/or CP is trisomy 13-15. That the association of cardiac and facial malformations is not too obvious is evidenced by a necropsy series of 100 neonates with CHD in which facial clefts were not encountered.[1] But Okada *et al.*,[2] reporting on extracardiac malformations in 1,287 necropsied patients with CHD, mentioned that cleft palate and abnormal extremities "often" were seen associated with tetralogy of Fallot, tricuspid stenosis and atresia without transposition, hypoplasia of the aortic tract and premature closure of the foramen ovale. The Pierre Robin syndrome was associated with coarctation of the aorta and tetralogy of Fallot. In a series of 39 cases of Pierre Robin syndrome, Smith and Stowe[3] encountered 6 with probable CHD. Among 574 live-born children with cleft palate, Knox and Braithwaite[4] mentioned 4 and among those with cleft lip and cleft palate 3 who had CHD.

The subject of cardiac malformations and facial clefts was dealt with by Shah *et al.*,[5] who reported from Chicago. In 32 children with cleft lip or cleft palate who had died, heart disease was present in 21 (66%). Of these 21 patients, 18 died during infancy, 17 had cleft palate (2 with Pierre Robin syndrome), 3 had cleft lip and palate and only 1 – a patient with trisomy 18 – had cleft lip without palate involvement. In 16 patients, multiple cardiac lesions were recognized. Tetralogy of Fallot, coarctation of the aorta, atrial septal defect, patent ductus arteriosus, VSD and tricuspid stenosis were seen in more than one patient.

Shah and co-workers listed 10 living children who were known to have both facial clefts and CHD; only 3 of these had cleft lip and palate, whereas 7 had cleft palate only. In 150 consecutive patients with cleft lip and/or palate (average age 9½ years), only 2 had CHD. The rate of 13 per 1,000 is more than eight times that found among a general population of schoolchildren.[6] Among the types of CHD diagnosed in patients with facial clefts, transposition of the great vessels and single ventricle were not encountered.

REFERENCES

1. Ober, W. B., and Moore, T. E.: Congenital cardiac malformations in the neonatal period. An autopsy study, New England J. Med. 253:271, 1955.
2. Okada, R., Johnson, D., and Lev, M.: Extracardial malformations associated with congenital heart disease, Arch. Path. 85:649, 1968.
3. Smith, J. L., and Stowe, F. R.: The Pierre Robin syndrome (glossoptosis, micrognathia, cleft palate). A review of 39 cases with emphasis on associated ocular lesions, Pediatrics 27:128, 1961.
4. Knox, G., and Braithwaite, F.: Cleft lips and palates in Northumberland and Durham, Arch. Dis. Childhood 38:66, 1963.
5. Shah, C. V., Pruzansky, S., and Harris, W. S.: Cardiac malformations with facial clefts, Am. J. Dis. Child. 119:238, 1970.
6. Miller, R. A., *et al.*: The detection of heart disease in children, Circulation 25:85, 1962.

Urinary Tract Malformations

EXAMINATION of the urinary tract following angiocardiography[1,2] reveals urinary tract anomalies in a relatively high percentage of cases.[4] In many instances, there are no signs or symptoms pointing to urinary tract involvement. Lawlah *et al.*[1] found some type of urinary tract anomaly in 10% of their patients examined for various congenital or acquired diseases. Bruns[3] examined 453 children with congenital heart disease and found such complicating features in 67 (15.4%). In 28 (6.5%), the urinary tract anomalies were serious, some of them requiring surgical intervention. Estimates of renal anomalies in patients with CHD vary between 3% and 16% after clinical evaluation. Such associations were found in 4–18% in necropsies and in approximately 2–17% in roentgenograms following angiocardiography (Bruns[3]).

REFERENCES

1. Lawlah, J. W., Johnson, J. B., and Failey, A. I.: Genitourinary tract screening as a routine procedure in angiocardiography, J.A.M.A. 158:921, 1955.
2. Hipona, F. A., and Melnick, G. S.: The value of postangiographic pyelograms, Am. J. Roentgenol. 95:413, 1965.
3. Bruns, H. A.: Überraschende Befunde im Bereich des Harntraktes bei Kindern mit angeborenen Herzfehlern, Monatsschr. Kinderh. 116:564, 1968.
4. Vince, D. J., and Vanandel, M.: Ventricular septal defect and congenital malformations of the urinary tract, Clin. Pediat. 6:16, 1967.

Genital Tract Malformations

MALFORMATIONS of the genital tract that are included in the Ullrich-Feichtiger (typus rostockiensis) or Smith-Lemli-Opitz syndrome (Chapter 111) may be combined with cardiovascular anomalies. In cases considered Ullrich-Feichtiger syndrome, atrial and ventricular septal defects, valvar lesions, patent ductus arteriosus with aortic atresia[1] and truncus arteriosus[2] have been observed. In similar cases called Smith-Lemli-Opitz syndrome, patent ductus arteriosus, tetralogy of Fallot and ventricular septal defect have been recorded.[3,4]

REFERENCES

1. Hövels, O., and Müllereisert, F.: Der Typus Rostockiensis als charakteristisches Kombinationsbild multipler Missbildungen (Polydaktylie, Hypospadie, Kryptorchismus und Mikrognathie), Ztschr. Kinderh. 77:454, 1955.
2. Kunze, J.: Das Ullrich-Feichtiger-syndrom, Arch. Kinderh. 179:182, 1969.
3. Dallaire, L.: Syndrome of retardation with urogenital and skeletal anomalies (Smith-Lemli-Opitz syndrome): Clinical features and mode of inheritance, J. M. Genetics 6:113, 1969.
4. Park, S. C., Needles, C. F., Dimich, I., and Sussman, L.: Congenital heart disease in an infant with the Smith-Lemli-Opitz syndrome, J. Pediat. 73:896, 1968.

Metabolic Disorders

CARDIOVASCULAR CHANGES occur in several hereditary metabolic disorders, particularly in storage diseases. Manifestations of heart disease sometimes are present in early infancy and delayed in other instances. Little is known regarding manifestations of the abnormal genes in prenatal life and often it is doubtful whether one is dealing with a congenital disorder or with a disease that is brought out by postnatal factors.

GARGOYLISM.—Although cardiovascular manifestations in gargoylism may not be congenital, the underlying condition is. Gargoylism is a heritable metabolic disorder that affects many organs, the cardiovascular system among them (p. 810). Necropsy reports indicate that most children affected with this disorder have cardiac involvement, although in some reports this fact was overlooked. Approximately half the deaths can be attributed to heart failure.[1,2] Krovetz *et al.*[2] found the median age of death for males to be 7 years and that of females 6 years. No girl survived after the age of 11, but 13 of 49 males lived past that age. These survivors probably belonged to the milder "Hunter type" of gargoylism. A case reported by Lindsay[3] shows that infants can die of heart failure due to gargoylism before other symptoms of the disorder become manifest, and in the Cincinnati Children's Hospital characteristic histologic changes were found in the heart of an infant with gargoylism who was 2½ months of age.

Cardiac hypertrophy, thickening of the epicardium, endocardium and valves, stenosis of the coronary orifices and lumina, thickening of the aortic intima and that of other vessels have been observed.[3]

Hypertrophy of the left ventricle usually is present; the right ventricle may be affected also.[4] The mitral valve is, as a rule, most severely involved by the disease process, which may cause marked thickening of the valve and formation of nodules on the mitral cusps. The aortic and pulmonary cusps are also thickened and they form rounded, heavy edges. The changes in the tricuspid valve resemble those of the mitral valve but usually are less pronounced. Cardiovascular findings in necropsy reports were tabulated by Krovetz *et al.*[2]

The affected tissues show similar histologic alterations. The fibroblastic cells are swollen and enlarged and their cytoplasm is clear, vacuolated or granular. Several investigators have pointed out an increase in the amount of intercellular collagenous stroma, which lacks the normal fibrillary characteristics and shows edema of the fibers. The cellular swelling and the alteration of the intercellular collagen often produce a picture reminiscent of cartilage. Occasionally, myocardial alterations have been described. Fibrous thickening and cellular alterations were marked in the endocardium and accounted for the nodular deformities of the valves and the widening of the chordae tendineae. Similar thickening of the intima and media of the coronary arteries has been described,[3,5] alterations that may lead to narrowing of the arterial lumina. The abnormal storage reaction also involves the intima and the media of the aorta. Lagunoff *et al.*,[6] using histochemical and electron microscopic techniques, distinguished two types of gargoyle cells—a clear cell containing pure mucopolysaccharide and a small cell containing glycolipid. The conduction system may be involved by increased fibrous tissue in and around the bundle and bundle branches.[7] In addition to the changes in the heart, extracardiac factors may contribute to cardiac embarrassment. The deformities of the chest, elevation of the diaphragm by the enlarged liver and spleen, chronic interstitial pneumonitis and anemia contribute to the difficulties of the heart.[3]

Approximately half the patients affected by gargoylism show clinical evidence of cardiac involvement. Usually, there is a definite heart murmur present, which may increase with increasing age of the child. Cardiac enlargement and congestive heart failure may be the presenting features of cardiac involvement but, in some cases, sudden death may be the first sign of heart disease.[1] In the early literature on this anomaly, the cardiac murmurs usually were interpreted as signs of congenital malformations of the heart, but this interpretation is not correct. Cardiac changes characteristic of gargoylism develop either in late fetal life or in postnatal life, but there are no signs of disturbed embryologic organogenesis; persistent patent ductus arteriosus has been observed.[7]

Glycogen storage disease (Pompe disease).—This storage disease is a specific metabolic disturbance that can lead to enlargement of the heart in infants and to early death.[8-10] The metabolic disturbance is attributed to homozygosity for a recessive gene; the cardiac lesion has been observed repeatedly in siblings. Absence of lysosomal acid alpha-glucosidase has been ascertained in all tissues, including heart muscle.[11] Whether pathologic manifestations are present before birth is now under investigation. After birth, the cardiac ventricles become thick-walled, resulting in marked enlargement of the heart. The muscle cells appear large and vacuolated with glycogen deposits in the clear spaces. The atria and valves are not altered by the disorder but they become involved by ventricular failure. The tongue, the diaphragm and other muscle groups are variously affected. Clinical manifestations begin in infancy with failure to thrive, dyspnea and muscular weakness. Enlargement of the heart can be demonstrated and heart failure results early. Death occurs, with few exceptions, within the first year.[1] Special hemodynamic and angiographic studies were made by Ruttenberg *et al.*,[12] who also reported positive skeletal muscle biopsies for glycogen storage disease in affected infants.

Pseudoxanthoma elasticum.—It is known that pseudoxanthoma elasticum affects the skin, the eyes and the blood vessels. Signs and symptoms of heart disease are quite common.[13] Valvar heart disease was emphasized by Coffman and Sommers,[14] who described a family with pseudoxanthoma elasticum suggesting dominant inheritance of the basic disorder.

Hereditary xanthomatosis.—In 1942, Bloom *et al.*[15] discussed hereditary xanthomatosis, familial incidence of xanthoma tuberosum associated with hypercholesterolemia and cardiovascular involvement, and reported several cases of sudden death.

The tendency of xanthoma tuberosum to occur in several members of a family has long been known and it is assumed that the disorder is inherited as a dominant trait or incomplete dominant trait. It is likely that the disturbance of cholesterol metabolism is inherited as a dominant trait, although cutaneous lesions are not always present in those affected by hypercholesterolemia.

The heart, the aorta, pulmonary arteries and other blood vessels and the mitral and aortic valves may be affected by xanthomatosis.

Bloom *et al.*[15] described a consanguineous couple with 7 affected children. Four of these had the full syndrome of xanthomatosis and died suddenly. One daughter died suddenly at the age of 23 and necropsy showed myocardial degeneration with coronary sclerosis throughout the aorta; her lipoid deposits gave the appearance of advanced arteriosclerosis. Similar lipoid deposits were found in all the arteries of the body.

REFERENCES

1. Keith, J. D., Rowe, R. D., and Vlad, P. (eds.): *Heart Disease in Infancy and Childhood* (2d ed.; New York: The Macmillan Company, 1966).
2. Krovetz, L. J., Lorincz, A. E., and Schiebler, G. L.: Cardiovascular manifestations of the Hurler syndrome, Circulation 31:132, 1965.
3. Lindsay, S.: Cardiovascular system in gargoylism, Brit. Heart J. 12:17, 1950.
4. Emanuel, R. W.: Gargoylism with cardiovascular involvement in two brothers, Brit. Heart J. 16:417, 1954.
5. Strauss, T.: Pathology of gargoylism; report of a case and review of the literature, Am. J. Path. 24:855, 1948.
6. Lagunoff, D., Ross, R., and Benditt, E. P.: Histochemical

and electron microscopic study in a case of Hurler's disease, Am. J. Path. 41:273, 1962.
7. Okada, R., Rosenthal, I. M., Scaravelli, G., and Lev, M.: A histopathologic study of the heart in gargoylism, Arch. Path. 84:20, 1967.
8. Pompe, J. D.: Over idiopatische hypertrophy van het hart, Nederl. tijdschr. geneesk. 76:304, 1932.
9. Putschar, W.: Über angeborene Glykogenspeicherkrankheit des Herzens, Beitr. path. Anat. 90:222, 1932.
10. Di Sant'Agnese, P. A.: Diseases of glycogen storage with special reference to cardiac type of generalized glycogenosis, Ann. New York Acad. Sc. 72:439, 1959.
11. Hers, H. G.: α-Glucosidase deficiency in generalized glycogen storage disease (Pompe's disease), Biochem. J. 86: 11, 1963.
12. Ruttenberg, H. D., Steidl, R. M., Carey, L. S., and Edwards, J. E.: Glycogen-storage disease of the heart, Am. Heart J. 67:469, 1964.
13. Szymanski, F. J., and Caro, M. R.: Pseudoxanthoma elasticum: Review of its relationship to internal diseases and report of an unusual case, A.M.A. Arch. Dermat. 71:184, 1955.
14. Coffman, J. D., and Sommers, S. C.: Familial pseudoxanthoma elasticum and valvular heart disease, Circulation 19:242, 1959.
15. Bloom, D., Kaufman, S. R., and Stevens, R. A.: Hereditary xanthomatosis. Familial incidence of xanthoma tuberosum associated with hypercholesteremia and cardiovascular involvement, with report of several cases of sudden death, Arch. Dermat. & Syph. 45:1, 1942.

Chromosomal Anomalies and Congenital Heart Disease

SINCE CHROMOSOME ANALYSES in man became possible, association of cytogenetic anomalies with congenital cardiovascular malformations has been reported frequently. The subject has been discussed on page 462, and the cardiac malformations in trisomy syndromes and Turner syndrome are treated on pages 463 and 1127. Congenital heart anomalies in Down syndrome represent a special chapter in the area of congenital heart disease that will be dealt with here.

Down Syndrome (Mongolism)

It has long been known that many mongoloid children have congenital heart disease and it has been surmised that they show a predilection for certain types. Langdon Down,[1] in 1866, mentioned the feeble circulation of these patients, and, ever since, their cardiac status has been under scrutiny. Despite this continued interest, estimates vary in regard to incidence and prevalence of and predilection to specific congenital cardiac defects of mongoloid patients. Berg *et al.*[2] reviewed the literature and compiled estimates of earlier authors. The percentage of cardiac malformations found in mongoloids varied between 7.1 and 70.8, with an average percentage of 18.9 for all the publications reviewed. This remarkable variation is understandable if one considers that various authors dealt with different age groups and based their diagnosis on widely different criteria. The diagnostic methods used varied from auscultation to necropsy. Some series were based on hospital patients, others on institutional populations. In recent years, attempts have been made to evaluate unselected cases and to apply, in the living, modern diagnostic methods that included, in addition to physical examination, roentgenograms, fluoroscopy, electrocardiograms, cardiac catheterization and angiocardiography. Before more recent findings based on clinical studies are discussed, some necropsy surveys deserve to be mentioned.

Evans[3] found cardiac anomalies in 28 of 63 mongoloid children necropsied at The Hospital for Sick Children, Great Ormond Street, London. The incidence of 44.4% of cardiac malformations in mongoloids, ascertained between 1911 and 1949, and the individual classifications of defects may not be quite correct, since, according to the author, the descriptions of some of the cardiac lesions must be viewed critically. The author stated that atrioventricularis communis, which occurred in only 4 of 28 cases (14.3%), should not be regarded as the typical cardiac lesion of mongolism, although it occurred within this syndrome more often than in a group of nonmongoloid children with congenital heart disease. No particular combination of anomalies was characteristic of the abnormal heart in mongolism. Atrial and ventricular septal defects each accounted for more than one-third of the cases and patent ductus arteriosus for one-sixth. Most of the remaining lesions were pulmonary stenoses. Defect of the pars membranacea of the ventricular septum was the most common anomaly. In contrast to the control series of nonmongoloid children with cardiovascular defect, there were no malformations due to malrotation of the bulbus cordis in the mongoloids. Transposition of the great vessels, truncus arteriosus and aortic coarctation did not occur in this rather small series. Nine (32%) of the mongoloids with heart disease showed other congenital anomalies such as Meckel diverticulum, esophageal and duodenal atresia, intestinal malrotation and skeletal malformations. There was one case of spina bifida with meningocele. This is of special interest, since it proves that abnormal development in mongoloid children dates back to earlier embryonic periods than those stressed by some authors (Chapter 7).

Berg *et al.*[2] gathered data on 141 necropsy cases from several hospitals in England. These cases covered the whole age range of childhood, but did not include adult patients. They also used as controls nonmongoloid patients with congenital heart disease necropsied in these hospitals. Of 141 patients, 79 (56%) had cardiovascular malformations. Such malformations were, of course, much more frequent among mongoloids dying in the first 3 years of life (66%) than in those dying from the fourth to the tenth year (19%). Only about 70% of the cardiac defects were diagnosed during life. As in Evans'[3] series, ventricular and atrial septal defects were the leading anomalies, persistent atrioventricularis communis was present in 20% and ostium primum in 28% of the cases. Patent ductus arteriosus and anomalies of the valves were found in approximately one-fifth of the cases. Many other anomalies occurred with low frequency, but there was no example of transposition of the great vessels. Yet, in contrast to Evans' series, there were 3 cases of truncus arteriosus and 2 with coarctation of the aorta. Of 141 children with mongolism, 34 (24%) had noncardiac malformations of various types, with duodenal anomalies in the lead.

These necropsy reports show that the abnormal hearts of mongoloid children display as wide a variety of malformations as those of subjects without mongolism.[2] There is no typical "mongol heart." However, it is correct that atrioventricularis communis and ostium primum occur relatively more often in mongoloid children than in nonmongoloid children with congenital heart disease. Ventricular and auricular septal defects are the most frequent cardiac anomalies in both groups. Although transposition of the great vessels was not encountered in the two series mentioned, it can occur in mongoloid children. A surprisingly high incidence was reported by Hambach,[4] who found 6 instances of it in 17 necropsies. Three of these cases also showed atrioventricularis communis. Transposition was also reported by Mannheimer[5] in a case of mongolism. It is worth emphasis that transposition of the great vessels was found in a boy with Down syndrome who had 48 chromosomes with trisomy 21 and XYY sex chromosomes.[8] It is clear that various types of cardiac malformations occur often in the same mongoloid child, so that classifications listing the main anomaly often are incomplete and subjective. Thus, overemphasis of atrioventricularis communis and ostium primum may be due to the fact that some authorities singled out this malformation as typical for mongolism.

Liu and Corlett[6] studied congenital heart defects in 173 mongoloid patients admitted to the Fountain Hospital in London. Of these, 51 patients died and necropsies were performed in 44. Congenital heart defects were found in 16 (36%). Again, ventricular and atrial septal defects were the most common anomalies. Of 122 patients who were living, having a mean age of 10 years, only 9% had demonstrable congenital heart defects.

Rowe and Uchida[7] examined the entire mongoloid population of The Hospital for Sick Children in Toronto, Canada. Most of the 184 patients included in their study were referred for medical or genetic counseling. Although selection was excluded in this series to a certain extent, the group was heavily weighted by very young patients, whereas only 17 were between 5 and 15 years of age. Only 6 patients were first seen at necropsy, whereas all others received clinical evaluation by modern cardiodiagnostic methods. Of 184 patients, 70 (38%) had cardiac malformations, with 10 (5.4%) being uncertain. Thus, 56.6% had normal hearts. Atrioventricular canal defects (atrioventricularis communis and ostium primum) were diagnosed in 25 (36%), ventricular septal defect in 23 (33%), patent ductus arteriosus in 7 (10%), secundum atrial septal defect in 6 (9%), aberrant subclavian artery in 5 (7%), with other malformations occurring only rarely.

Table 64-1, which summarizes four necropsy series,[2-4,6] gives a general picture of the findings obtained in necropsies.

In summary, it can be said that, despite great efforts, truly representative figures of incidence and type of congenital cardiac malformations in mongoloids are still not available. It seems that well over 50% of the mongoloid population have normal hearts. Ventricular and atrial septal defects probably are the most common cardiac malformations in mongoloid patients. Atrioventricularis communis and ostium primum occur more often in mongoloids than in nonmongoloid patients with congenital heart disease. There is no cardiac malformation that is typical for mongolism.

TABLE 64-1.—CARDIOVASCULAR MALFORMATIONS: TRISOMY 21 (272 NECROPSIES)[9]

Ventricular septal defect	68	Tetralogy of Fallot	7
Atrial septal defect	61	Transposition of great vessels	6
Patent ductus arteriosus	35	Truncus arteriosus	3
Atrioventricularis communis	27	Coarctation of aorta	3
Ostium primum	24	Abnormal aortic valve	3
Abnormal mitral valve	19	Eisenmenger complex	3
Abnormal tricuspid valve	17	Cor triloculare	3
Abnormal pulmonary valve	11	Pulmonic stenosis	2
Foramen ovale	7	Endocardial fibroelastosis	2
		Left superior vena cava	1
		Aberrant right subclavian artery	1

REFERENCES

1. Down, J. L. H.: Observations on an ethnic classification of idiots, Clin. Lect. & Rep. London Hosp. 3:259, 1866.
2. Berg, J. M., Crome, L., and France, N. E.: Congenital cardiac malformations in mongolism, Brit. Heart J. 22:331, 1960.
3. Evans, P. R.: Cardiac anomalies in mongolism, Brit. Heart J. 12:258, 1950.

4. Hambach, R.: Ein Beitrag zur Frage der Kombination von Habitus mongoloides mit angeborenen Herzmissbildungen, Ann. paediat. 183:77, 1954.
5. Mannheimer, E.: *Morbus caeruleus* (Basel: S. Karger, 1949).
6. Liu, M. C., and Corlett, K.: A study of congenital heart defects in mongolism, Arch. Dis. Childhood 34:410, 1959.
7. Rowe, R. D., and Uchida, I. A.: Cardiac malformation in mongolism: A prospective study of 184 mongoloid children, Am. J. Med. 31:726, 1961.
8. Uchida, I. A., Ray, M., and Duncan, B. P.: 21 trisomy with an XYY sex chromosome complement, J. Pediat. 69:295, 1966.
9. Warkany, J., Passarge, E., and Smith, L. B.: Congenital malformations in autosomal trisomy syndromes, Am. J. Dis. Child. 112:502, 1966.

Palmar Dermatoglyphics and Fingerprints in Congenital Heart Disease

Takashina and Yorifuji[1] compared palmar dermatoglyphic patterns of patients with CHD with patterns of patients with acquired heart disease. Distal displacement of the palmar axial triradii occurred with greater frequency in the first group (64%) than in the second (17%). Fingerprint patterns were examined by Cascos.[2] Arches were quite frequent in pulmonary stenosis and rare in aortic coarctation. Ulnar loops were the most frequent type in all groups. Radial loops were quite rare except in atrial septal defect. Whorls were frequent in aortic stenosis, aortic coarctation and tetralogy of Fallot.

REFERENCES

1. Takashina, T., and Yorifuji, S.: Palmar dermatoglyphics in heart disease. Differential studies in Japanese and American populations with congenital and acquired heart disease, J.A.M.A. 197:689, 1966.
2. Cascos, A. S.: Fingerprint patterns in congenital heart disease, Brit. Heart J. 26:524, 1964.
3. Alter, M., and Schulenberg, R.: Dermatoglyphics in congenital heart disease, Circulation 41:49, 1970.

Supravalvar Aortic Stenosis Complex

("Supravalvar Aortic Stenosis," Facial Anomalies and Hypercalcemia)

In 1952, Fanconi *et al.*[1] described 2 children with chronic hypercalcemia, osteosclerosis, hyperazotemia, congenital cardiac malformation, premature closure of cranial sutures, microcephaly, mental retardation and dwarfism. These children had a peculiar facial appearance that since has become recognized as typical of supravalvar aortic stenosis and related vascular disorders. One of the children described in 1952 died at the age of 16 years from hypertension and renal failure, showing supravalvar aortic stenosis at necropsy.[2] Although the disease picture varies and the association of the heterogeneous symptoms remains unexplained, physicians have learned to recognize some children with supravalvar aortic stenosis by their facial features. It must be emphasized, however, that there exists a simple or uncomplicated form of supravalvar aortic stenosis (Chapter 59) and a benign form of infantile hypercalcemia that must be distinguished from the syndrome discussed here, which has more serious implications.

The face is described as full, the forehead broad, the eyes set far apart, the nasal bridge depressed, the cheeks heavy and dependent, the mouth wide, the lips thick and pouting and the chin receding or pointed. Strabismus, irregularities of dentition, malocclusion, high palate, open mouth, macroglossia and abnormal external ears contribute to the facial expression. The facial peculiarities can best be illustrated in family pictures, which show the dissimilarity between the patient and his siblings.[3] The voice is hoarse. There often is a history of vomiting and failure to thrive beginning in infancy. Small stature and retarded psychomotor development are the rule. Hypercalcemia in infancy has been demonstrated in some cases and assumed in many others.[4] Resemblance to myxedema was pointed out occasionally.[1,5,6]

Supravalvar aortic stenosis can vary in degree and extent. A short ascending portion with narrowing, stenosis of the proximal segment of an aorta of normal length, localized narrowing above shallow sinuses of Valsalva with distal dilatation of the aorta and membranous or fibrous diaphragm at the upper margins of the sinuses of Valsalva can be distinguished.[7] In the syndrome of complicated supravalvar aortic stenosis, narrowing of the proximal segment or of the entire ascending aorta has been observed. In addition to aortic stenosis, there may exist postvalvar pulmonary artery stenosis of various degrees and types and single or multiple peripheral stenoses of the branches of the pulmonary artery. In the arterial system, coarctation, stenosis or hypoplasia have also been found in the descending or abdominal aorta and in the coronary, celiac mesenteric or renal arteries.[7,8] Stenosis of the origins of the brachiocephalic vessels may be

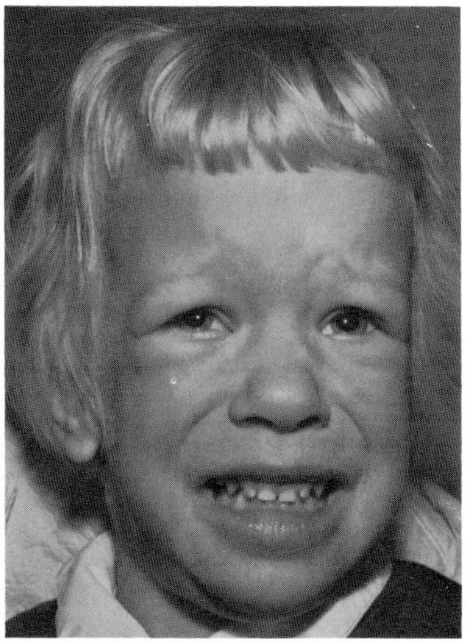

Fig. 64-1. – Child with proved supravalvar aortic stenosis. (Courtesy of Hamilton County, Ohio, Diagnostic Clinic for the Mentally Retarded.)

found in some patients with asymmetric pulses or blood pressures in the upper extremities.[9] Tortuosity of retinal and cerebral arteries has been observed in some cases.[3,10] It seems that the disorder can express itself by vascular changes with differing localization[11,25] and that some forms are "sine supravalvar stenosis."[8]

Mental retardation varies in degree, with I.Q. values between 40 and 80.[6] As a rule, the children are good-natured and appear happy. Sometimes the retardation is more severe and associated with microcephaly and premature obliteration of the sagittal sutures. Osteopetrosis of the skull and other skeletal structures, so marked in the cases of Fanconi *et al.*,[1] were absent in most of the cases reported. Craniosynostosis, block vertebrae and kyphoscoliosis were observed occasionally.[6,12,25]

The relationship of the complicated form of supravalvar aortic stenosis to hypercalcemia is under discussion. In some instances, hypercalcemia has been demonstrated, in others it has been surmised because of anorexia and irritability in infancy or because of the presence of facial features "typical of hypercalcemia." Even if vague symptoms in early infancy were due to idiopathic hypercalcemia, there is doubt that such transitory hypercalcemia always has serious consequences. Mitchell[13] reviewed 13 cases of idiopathic hypercalcemia of infancy 3–6 years after the metabolic disturbance. He found 12 of the children in good health and mentally normal.

There are many observations that speak against a causal relationship between vitamin D intake, hypercalcemia and the syndrome of complicated supravalvar aortic stenosis.[4] Some mothers state that they did not take any vitamin supplements during pregnancy[6] and others assert that they, as well as their affected children, took only conventional doses of vitamin D.[8,10,12,14] The mother of a boy with osteosclerosis, hypercalcemia and renal failure had taken "the usual supplements" during her pregnancy and the child had "a very occasional teaspoonful of cod-liver oil." At necropsy, cellular mucoid thickening of the valve cusps and calcification of the valve ring were found. There also was diffuse mucoid edema of the myocardium, but aortic stenosis was not mentioned and intelligence apparently was good.[15] Schlesinger *et al.*[16] were unable to find that infants with the severe type of infantile hypercalcemia or their mothers had had an abnormally high intake of vitamin D. To uphold the role of vitamin D in the etiology of the syndrome, hypersensitivity to vitamin D or a disturbance of vitamin D metabolism has been assumed by many authors,[17] but proof of hypersensitivity to vitamin D in mothers and affected children could not be obtained.[4,26] A case report by Hjelt *et al.*[18] dealt with the effects of huge doses of vitamin D on the cardiovascular and other systems of children. The results differed greatly from the findings in most children with complicated supravalvar pulmonary stenosis. There were calcifications of the cardiac valves, of arteries and of other tissues. A mother who had had a child with the supravalvar aortic stenosis complex received 10,000 units of vitamin D from the thirteenth to the thirty-first day of a subsequent pregnancy; the child apparently was normal.[26] Changes found in rabbits whose mothers were treated with huge doses of vitamin D during pregnancy[19,24] are of interest but not comparable to those of children and mothers who received only moderate doses of vitamin D or no supplements at all.

An etiologic role of postnatal hypercalcemia or vitamin D intake seems doubtful, since many children with the complicated syndrome have signs that point to prenatal onset of the disorder. Intrauterine growth retardation is marked in some patients[5,6,8,16] and moderate in others.[3,10,12,17,20] Although the weight at birth is within normal limits in some cases, a general tendency to prenatal growth retardation exists. In a number of patients, a heart lesion was diagnosed at or soon after birth,[10,12,17,20] or anorexia[5,20] or peculiar facial features[6,10] were noted in early infancy.

Males and females are affected. Concordance has been reported in monozygotic twins in regard to typical facies, arterial stenoses (without supravalvar aortic and pulmonary stenosis), mental retardation, craniosynostosis and abnormal dentition.[8]

Whereas in simple supravalvar stenosis an autosomal dominant mode of inheritance is likely,[21] the etiology of the complicated form is not established. Familial repetition of complicated cases is rare but it has been observed.[6,8] If one assumes that the complicated form of supravalvar aortic stenosis is due to a new mutation of a dominant gene, one can explain the absence of pedigrees with the complicated form by the inability of the first patient to reproduce. It is possible that in some kinships the simple and the complicated forms can alternate. Chromosome studies reveal normal karyotypes.[21-23]

REFERENCES

1. Fanconi, G., Gircudet, P., Schlesinger, B., Butler, N., and Black, J.: Chronic hypercalcemia, combined with osteosclerosis, hyperazotemia, dwarfism and congenital malformations, Helvet. paediat. acta 7:314, 1952.
2. Black, J. A., Butler, N. R., and Schlesinger, B. E.: Aortic stenosis and hypercalcemia, Lancet 2:546, 1965.
3. Williams, J. C. P., Barratt-Boyes, B. G., and Lowe, J. B.: Supravalvular aortic stenosis, Circulation 24:1311, 1961.
4. Antia, A. U., Wiltse, H. E., Rowe, R. D., Pitt, E. L., Levin, S., Ottesen, O. E., and Cooke, R. E.: Pathogenesis of the supravalvular aortic stenosis syndrome, J. Pediat. 71:431, 1967.
5. Hooft, C., Vermassen, A., and Blancquaert, A.: Observations concerning the evolution of the chronic form of idiopathic hypercalcaemia in children, Helvet. paediat. acta 18:138, 1963.
6. Habedank, M., and Bücheler, E.: Kardiovasculäre Fehlbildungen mit konstitutionellen Charakteristika und Debilität, Ztschr. Kinderh. 98:268, 1967.
7. Kurlander, G. J., Petry, E. L., Taybi, H., Lurie, P. R., and Campbell, J. A.: Supravalvar aortic stenosis: Roentgen analysis of twenty-seven cases, Am. J. Roentgenol. 98: 782, 1966.
8. Wiltse, H. E., Goldbloom, R. B., Antia, A. U., Ottesen, O. E., Rowe, R. D., and Cooke, R. E.: Infantile hypercalcemia syndrome in twins, New England J. Med. 275:1157, 1966.
9. Kupic, E. A., and Abrams, H. L.: Supravalvular aortic stenosis, Am. J. Roentgenol. 98:822, 1966.
10. Fay, J. E., Lynn, R. B., and Partington, M. W.: Supravalvular aortic stenosis, mental retardation and a characteristic facies, Canad. M.A.J. 94:295, 1966.
11. Ottesen, O., Antia, A. U., and Rowe, R. D.: The peripheral vascular anomalies associated with the supravalvular stenosis syndrome, Radiology 86:430, 1966.
12. Black, J. A., and Bonham Carter, R. C.: Association between aortic stenosis and facies of severe infantile hypercalcaemia, Lancet 2:745, 1963.
13. Mitchell, R. G.: The prognosis in idiopathic hypercalcaemia of infants, Arch. Dis. Childhood 35:383, 1960.
14. Farrehi, C., Dotter, C. T., and Griswold, H. E.: Supravalvular aortic stenosis. Underdevelopment and characteristic facies, Am. J. Dis. Child. 108:335, 1964.
15. Fletcher, R. F.: A case of osteosclerosis with hypercalcaemia and renal failure, Arch. Dis. Childhood 32:245, 1957.
16. Schlesinger, B. E., Butler, N. R., and Black, J. A.: Severe type of infantile hypercalcaemia, Brit. M. J. 1:127, 1956.
17. Beuren, A. J., Apitz, J., and Harmjanz, D.: Supravalvular aortic stenosis in association with mental retardation and a certain facial appearance, Circulation 26:1235, 1962.
18. Hjelt, L., Tähkä, H., and Hallman, N.: Chronic hypercalcemia and vitamin D in early childhood, Ann. paediat. Fenniae 2:75, 1956.
19. Friedman, W. F., and Roberts, W. C.: Vitamin D and the supravalvar aortic stenosis syndrome. The transplacental effects of vitamin D on the aorta of the rabbit, Circulation 34:77, 1966.
20. Rashkind, W. J., Golinko, R., and Arcasoy, M.: Cardiac findings in idiopathic hypercalcemia of infancy, J. Pediat. 58:464, 1961.
21. Jörgensen, G., and Beuren, A. J.: Genetische Untersuchungen bei supravalvulären Aortenstenosen, Humangenetik 1:497, 1965.
22. Joseph, M. C., Polani, P. E., and Gold, R. G.: Chromosome studies in patients with supravalvular aortic stenosis, Lancet 2:788, 1963.
23. de Grouchy, J., and Emerit, J.: Chromosome studies in patients with supravalvular aortic stenosis, Lancet 2:789, 1963.
24. Friedman, W. F., and Mills, L. F.: The relationship between vitamin D and the craniofacial and dental anomalies of the supravalvular aortic stenosis syndrome, Pediatrics 43:12, 1969.
25. Ebeling, J., Bette, L., and Schiefer, I.: Ein weiterer Beitrag zu den kardiovaskulären Veränderungen und der Klinik defektgeheilter infantiler Hyperkalzämien, Arch. Kinderh. 180:1, 1969.
26. Forbes, G. B., Cafarelli, C., and Manning, J.: Vitamin D and infantile hypercalcemia, Pediatrics 42:203, 1968.

Familial Syndrome of Right-Sided Aortic Arch, Mental Retardation and Facial Characteristics

A SYNDROME of right-sided aortic arch, mental retardation, prominent nose with septal deviation, underdevelopment of the left side of the face and small mouth with downturned corners was described in a mother, 2 of her daughters and 1 son. The mother had given birth to a girl with anal atresia and ventricular and atrial septal defects; another female infant was a stillborn anencephalic.[1]

REFERENCE

1. Strong, W. B.: Familial syndrome of right-sided aortic arch, mental deficiency, and facial dysmorphism, J. Pediat. 73:882, 1968.

Cardiofacial Syndromes

ASSOCIATION OF ventricular septal defect with unilateral facial paralysis involving only the mentalis and the quadratus labii inferioris muscles was reported by Cayler,[1,2] who observed 14 patients with this syndrome. In addition to ventricular septal defect, tetralogy, pulmonary stenosis, atrioventricularis communis, aortic coarctation, single ventricle and atrial septal defect were diagnosed. The facial paralysis, which was noted only when the children cried, was limited to the right side in 12 of the 14 cases.

Mental retardation, microcephaly, lop ear, aplasia of the radius or distal phalanges, renal aplasia, fusion of the labia minora, anal stenosis or imperforation and arthrogryposis of the knees complicated some of the cases. Although viral studies were essentially negative, Cayler thought that the syndrome might be due to a subclinical viral infection occurring in the mother during the fifth week of pregnancy. The karyotypes of 3 children were normal, but breaks seen in the long arms of some chromosomes were considered excessive.

A syndrome of acyanotic congenital heart disease, dwarfism and bilateral ptosis in 2 boys was described by Schönenberg.[3] Both children were born at term and had low birth weights. Associated "facultative" anomalies were vertebral defects in one of the boys and hypospadias and mental retardation in the other. In the latter case, swelling of the dorsa pedis was present in early childhood, suggesting that the patient had the "male Turner syndrome." In that disease picture, ptosis, epicanthic folds and cardiovascular anomalies often are combined[4] (Chapter 112).

REFERENCES

1. Cayler, G. G.: An "epidemic" of congenital facial paresis and heart disease, Pediatrics 40:666, 1967.
2. Cayler, G. G.: Cardiofacial syndrome, Arch. Dis. Childhood 44:69, 1969.
3. Schönenberg, H.: Über ein neues Kombinationsbild multipler Abartungen, Ann. paediat. 182:229, 1954.
4. Heller, R. H.: The Turner phenotype in the male, J. Pediat. 66:48, 1965.

Cardio-Auditory Syndromes

CONGENITAL deaf-mutism, functional heart disease with prolongation of the Q-T interval and sudden death were described by Jervell and Lange-Nielsen[1] in 1957 as a familial anomaly that is now attributed to autosomal recessive inheritance.[2,3] A syndrome of deaf-mutism with cardiac and dermatoglyphic anomalies was suggested by Cascos *et al.*[3]

A syndrome that involves familial pulmonary stenosis and deaf-mutism was reported by Lewis *et al.*[4] The mother and 4 of her 8 children had pulmonary stenosis and 2 of the 4 were deaf-mutes. The affected children showed hypertelorism, broad nasal root, low-set ears with hypoplastic auricular helices, spine and chest deformities and hypoplastic fifth digits.[5]

Deafness, bony fusions and mitral insufficiency were reported as a syndrome inherited like a dominant trait.[6]

REFERENCES

1. Jervell, A., and Lange-Nielsen, F.: Congenital deaf-mutism, functional heart disease with prolongation of the Q-T interval and sudden death, Am. Heart J. 54:59, 1957.
2. Fraser, G. R., Froggatt, P., and Murphy, T.: Genetical aspects of the cardio-auditory syndrome of Jervell and Lange-Nielsen (congenital deafness and electrocardiographic abnormalities), Ann. Human Genet. 28:133, 1964.
3. Cascos, A., Sánchez-Harguindey, L., and de Rábago, P.: Cardio-auditory syndromes, Brit. Heart J. 31:26, 1969.
4. Lewis, S. M., Sonnenblick, B. P., Gilbert, L., and Biber, D.: Familial pulmonary stenosis and deaf-mutism: Clinical and genetic considerations, Am. Heart J. 55:458, 1958.
5. Koroxenidis, G. T., Webb, N. C., Moschos, C. B., and Lehan, P. H.: Congenital heart disease, deaf-mutism and associated malformations occurring in several members of one family, Am. J. Med. 40:149, 1966.
6. Forney, W. R., Robinson, S. J., and Pascoe, D. J.: Congenital heart disease, deafness and skeletal malformations: A new syndrome?, J. Pediat. 68:14, 1968.

65

Other Congenital Disorders of the Heart

Congenital Tumors

PRIMARY TUMORS of the heart are rare. Although "polyps of the heart" had been described since the seventeenth century, it was generally thought that the heart is an organ "too noble to be attacked by a primary tumor."[1] In necropsies, the frequency of primary heart tumors amounts to only 0.001%.[2] Primary tumors of the heart in infancy and early childhood were discussed by Bigelow *et al.*[3] Congenital primary cardiac tumors are even greater rarities. Rhabdomyoma is the best-known tumor of the heart in children. In approximately half the cases, such tumors are associated with manifestations of tuberous sclerosis.[4] Rhabdomyoma of the heart can cause the first symptoms of tuberous sclerosis in the neonatal period.[4,5] The tumors can be 1–2 cm. in diameter and extend into the cavity of the heart. They contain large vacuolated cells that show striations of their peripheral cytoplasm and contain glycogen.[6,7] A case of special interest was that of a girl whose rhabdomyoma was located in a heart with tetralogy of Fallot.[4] Seizures in the patient and her brother suggested tuberous sclerosis as the basic disorder.

Myxomas, intramural fibromas, angiomas and pericardial tumors can occur in small infants.[7,8] Basora-Defilló and Lichtenberg[9] cited 8 cases of intrapericardial teratoma and added a case of their own, which occurred in an infant 3 months of age. The tumor was attached to the aorta and proved to be a polycystic teratoma composed of many well-differentiated tissues.

Primary cardiac malignancies in children were reviewed by Arshadi *et al.*,[10] who described the case of a teratocarcinoma of the heart in a girl 4 years of age. Vascular hamartoma of the right atrium with successful resection was reported by May *et al.*[11] Although their patient was 10 years of age, the cardiac lesion was considered a malformation rather than a neoplasm.

Tumors Associated with Congenital Heart Disease

Among the many malformations known to occur in patients with Wilms tumor, cardiovascular anomalies have been observed occasionally.[12] In a 4½-year-old boy whose mother had had four primary malignant neoplasms, a Wilms tumor developed that led to the patient's death at the age of 6 years. Necropsy revealed corrected transposition of the great vessels and Ebstein malformation.[13]

In situ neuroblastomas have been reported in infants with various congenital cardiovascular malformations.[14,15] A small adrenal tumor was found in a patient with complete transposition of the great vessels who survived to adulthood by Roberts *et al.*,[16] who believed that the association of endocrine tumors with heart disease of the cyanotic variety may be more than coincidental.

Pheochromocytoma associated with congenital heart disease has been observed in several instances.[17]

REFERENCES

1. Coe, G. C.: Tumors of the heart. A review of the literature, Chicago M. School Quart. 19:158, 1958.
2. Straus, R., and Merliss, R.: Primary tumor of the heart, Arch. Path. 39:74, 1945.
3. Bigelow, N. H., Klinger, S., and Wright, A. W.: Primary tumors of the heart in infancy and early childhood, Cancer 7:549, 1954.
4. Golding, R., and Reed, G.: Rhabdomyoma of the heart, New England J. Med. 276:957, 1967.
5. Debré, R., Thieffry, S., Mozziconacci, P., Bargeton, E., and Ramade, J.: La sclérose tubéreuse de Bourneville chez le nourrisson et le petit enfant, Arch. franç. pédiat. 9:342, 1952.
6. Farber, S.: Congenital rhabdomyoma of the heart, Am. J. Path. 7:105, 1931.
7. Potter, E. L.: *Pathology of the Fetus and Infant* (2d ed.; Chicago: Year Book Medical Publishers, Inc., 1961).
8. Keith, J. D., Rowe, R. D., and Vlad, P. (eds.): *Heart Disease in Infancy and Childhood* (2d ed.; New York: The Macmillan Company, 1966).
9. Basora-Defilló, J., and Lichtenberg, F.: Intrapericardial teratoma, J. Pediat. 48:77, 1956.
10. Arshadi, S., and Watson, D. G.: Teratocarcinoma of the heart, Am. J. Dis. Child. 112:87, 1966.
11. May, I. A., Hardy, K. L., Char, F., and McAdams, J.: Vascular hamartoma of the right atrium with successful resection, Ann. Thoracic Surg. 1:64, 1965.
12. Miller, R. W., Fraumeni, J. F., Jr., and Manning, M. D.: Association of Wilms's tumor with aniridia, hemihypertrophy and other congenital malformations, New England J. Med. 270:922, 1964.
13. Lynch, H. T., and Green, G. S.: Wilms' tumor and congenital heart disease, Am. J. Dis. Child. 115:723, 1968.

14. Beckwith, J. B., and Perrin, E. V.: In situ neuroblastomas: A contribution to the natural history of neural crest tumors, Am. J. Path. 43:1089, 1963.
15. Reisman, M., Goldenberg, E. D., and Gordon, J.: Congenital heart disease and neuroblastoma, Am. J. Dis. Child. 111:308, 1966.
16. Roberts, W. C., Mason, D. T., and Braunwald, E.: Survival to adulthood in a patient with complete transposition of the great vessels, including a note on the association of endocrine tumors with heart disease, Ann. Int. Med. 57: 834, 1962.
17. Reynolds, J. L., and Gilchrist, T. F.: Congenital heart disease and pheochromocytoma, Am. J. Dis. Child. 112:251, 1966.

Congenital Heart Block

CONGENITAL HEART BLOCK generally is attributed to malformations of the conduction system. Although such infections as syphilis, German measles, and so forth have been considered as possible causative factors, no case has been observed that definitely could be explained in this way. But Latta and Crittenden[1] reported acquired lesions of the conduction system by demonstration of scarring and calcification in the bundle of His and surrounding myocardium, with round cell infiltration. In other cases, the conduction system was found to be interrupted by noninflammatory fibrous tissue.[2] There are many instances of congenital heart block associated with congenital cardiac malformations that support the concept of heart block as a developmental anomaly. Familial cases have been known since Morquio,[3] in 1901, described a sibship of 8 children in which 5 boys had very slow and irregular pulse rates. Aylward[4] reported 2 sisters affected and Wendkos and Study[5] recorded a family in which the father had signs of the Wolff-Parkinson-White syndrome and his 2 children had complete heart block. In a family observed by Wallgren and Winblad,[6] a brother and sister affected with complete congenital heart block transmitted this condition as well as other forms of congenital heart disease to some of their children. Later, Wallgren and Agorio[7] reported 3 boys in one family whose heart block was diagnosed in utero. Gazes *et al.*[8] observed 35 patients with congenital arrhythmias occurring over three or four generations. Such familial cases probably are due to inherited congenital malformations of the conduction system. Other patients with congenital heart block have associated cardiovascular malformations that probably are heterogeneous in origin. Ventricular and atrial septal defects, atrioventricularis communis, inversion of the atria or ventricles, transposition or corrected transposition of the great vessels, single ventricle, hypoplasia or coarctation of the aorta, atresia of the pulmonary artery, patent ductus arteriosus, endocardial fibroelastosis and other anomalies may be combined with congenital heart block.[9]

The incidences of complicated versus isolated cases of heart block in different series vary. Keith *et al.*[10] stated that among 50 children with heart block 40 had no obvious evidence of heart involvement other than the block, whereas Donoso *et al.*,[11] in reviewing 17 necropsies, found only 4 isolated cases. Malformations of the conductive system are compatible with a long and active life, and patients with complete congenital heart block have reached the third or fourth decade without serious complications except occasional syncope. Some of them transmitted the anomaly to some of their offspring. Campbell[12] observed 7 adult patients with congenital heart block for 9 years who had no cardiac symptoms, and Turner[13] reported asymptomatic congenital heart block in an Army Air Force pilot. In other patients, sudden death occurred with Stokes-Adams attacks. Two brothers of the family reported by Wallgren and Agorio[7] died on the fourth and tenth days of life, whereas the third brother survived. In patients with associated cardiovascular malformations, the prognosis is influenced by the nature of the basic defect. Despite the presence of complicated forms of congenital heart disease, survival to adulthood is possible,[14] as exemplified by a man with congenital heart block who died at the age of 20 years. Necropsy revealed transposition of the great vessels, juxtaposition of the left atrium, double mitral ostium, cor biatriatum triloculare, right conus stenosis and pulmonary arteriovenous aneurysm.[15]

REFERENCES

1. Latta, H., and Crittenden, I. H.: Acquired lesions of the conduction system in familial congenital heart block, Lab. Invest. 13:214, 1964.
2. Monnet, P., and Perrin, A.: Bloc auriculo-ventriculaire congénital sous la dépendance d'une interruption du système Hisien vérifiée par coupes sériées et sans anomalie macroscopique cardiaque, Arch. franç. pédiat. 15: 1337, 1958.
3. Morquio, L.: Sur une maladie infantile et familiale caractérisée par des modifications permanentes du pouls, des attaques syncopales et épileptiformes et la morte subite, Arch. méd. Enf. 4:467, 1901.
4. Aylward, R. D.: Congenital heart block, Brit. M. J. 1:943, 1928.
5. Wendkos, M. H., and Study, R. S.: Familial congenital complete A-V heart block, Am. Heart J. 34:138, 1947.
6. Wallgren, A., and Winblad, S.: Congenital heart block, Acta paediat. 20:175, 1937.
7. Wallgren, G., and Agorio, E.: Congenital complete A-V block in three siblings, Acta paediat. scandinav. 49:49, 1960.
8. Gazes, P. C., Culler, R. M., Taber, E., and Kelly, T. E.: Congenital familial cardiac conduction defects, Circulation 32:32, 1965.
9. Lev, M.: The normal anatomy of the conduction system in man and its pathology in atrioventricular block, Ann. New York Acad. Sc. 111:817, 1964.
10. Keith, J. D., Rowe, R. D., and Vlad, P. (eds.): *Heart Disease in Infancy and Childhood* (2d ed.; New York: The Macmillan Company, 1966).

11. Donoso, E., Braunwald, E., Jick, S., and Grishman, A.: Congenital heart block, Am. J. Med. 20:869, 1956.
12. Campbell, M.: Congenital complete block, Brit. Heart J. 5:15, 1943.
13. Turner, L. B.: Asymptomatic congenital complete heart block in Army Air Force pilot, Am. Heart J. 34:426, 1947.
14. Aitchison, J. D., Duthie, R. J., and Young, J. S.: Palpable venous pulsations in a case of transposition of both arterial trunks and complete heart block, Brit. Heart J. 17:63, 1955.
15. Abbott, M. E., and Moffatt, D.: Congenital Heart Disease, in *Nelson Loose Leaf Medicine* (New York: Thomas Nelson & Sons, 1932).
16. Mitchell, S. C. (ed.): Proceedings of the Conduction Development Conference, U.S. Government Printing Office, 1970.

Obstructive Cardiomyopathy

(Asymmetric Hypertrophy of the Heart in Young Adults)

IT MAY NOT BE JUSTIFIED to list this anomaly as a congenital malformation, since it has not yet been observed in infancy. But since a congenital origin has been considered and since the lesion has been called a hamartoma[1] that can be transmitted like a dominant hereditary trait,[2] it must be mentioned, if only briefly. Teare[1] described asymmetric hypertrophy of the heart as a benign tumor of striped muscle in 8 of 16,000 necropsies; it obviously is a rare cardiac condition, which Schrader *et al.*[3] considered a congenital myocardial anomaly. This fact emphasizes the importance of the occurrence of 3 certain and 6 probable cases of this type in one kinship of 23 persons examined by Hollman *et al.*[2] Men and women were affected equally.

Hypertrophy of the interventricular septum and of the anterior wall of the heart is the striking feature at necropsy. The muscular hypertrophy may impinge on the mitral valve or the aortic valve or obstruct the right ventricular inflow tract, leading to symptoms of valvar stenosis. Histologically, one finds bizarre arrangements of muscle bundles associated with hypertrophy of muscle fibers and their nuclei. Teare[1] considered the anomaly as possibly congenital but not identical with glycogenic tumors and not associated with renal cysts or tuberous sclerosis.

Clinical manifestations are palpitations, blackouts, auricular fibrillations, systolic and diastolic murmurs and enlargement of the cardiac silhouette in roentgenograms. Sudden death may occur in adolescence or in adult life. Manifestations may resemble those of Ebstein disease[2] or those of mitral or aortic stenosis.[4]

REFERENCES

1. Teare, D.: Asymmetrical hypertrophy of the heart in young adults, Brit. Heart J. 20:1, 1958.
2. Hollman, A., Goodwin, J. F., Teare, D., and Renwick, J. W.: A family with obstructive cardiomyopathy (asymmetrical hypertrophy), Brit. Heart J. 22:449, 1960.
3. Schrader, W. H., Pankey, G. A., Davis, R. B., and Theologides, A.: Familial idiopathic cardiomegaly, Circulation 24:599, 1961.
4. Goodwin, J. F., Hollman, A., Cleland, W. P., and Teare, D.: Obstructive cardiomyopathy simulating aortic stenosis, Brit. Heart J. 22:403, 1960.

PART IX

Malformations of the Respiratory Tract

The Nose

Nasal Aplasia

COMPLETE NASAL APLASIA can occur in otherwise normal persons, but the anomaly is very rare. A concavity is seen in place of the nose between the forehead and the upper lip[1] or there may be a small button representing a nasal tip without nares over an apertura piriformis closed by bone.[2] In a case of Berndorfer[3] there was a small hole in place of a normal nostril but the nasal cavities were absent. Regression of a nasal anlage once present was considered by the author. The same author reported a case of arhinia in a patient with mandibulofacial dysostosis (Fig. 66-1).

Unilateral nasal aplasia can also occur in otherwise normal persons. The undeveloped half is indicated by a small pit in place of a nostril. The nasal bone, vomer, septum, choana and nasolacrimal duct are absent on the affected side (unilateral arhinia). The absent half of the nose may be represented by a unilateral proboscis. Despite unilateral absence of the external nose, there may be a nasal cavity on the abnormal side.[1] Unilateral underdevelopment of the nose associated with various malformations is illustrated in Figures 66-2 and 66-3.

Fig. 66-1.—Failure of nasal development in a child with signs of mandibulofacial dysostosis (antimongoloid slanting of eyes, microtia). (From A. Berndorfer.[3])

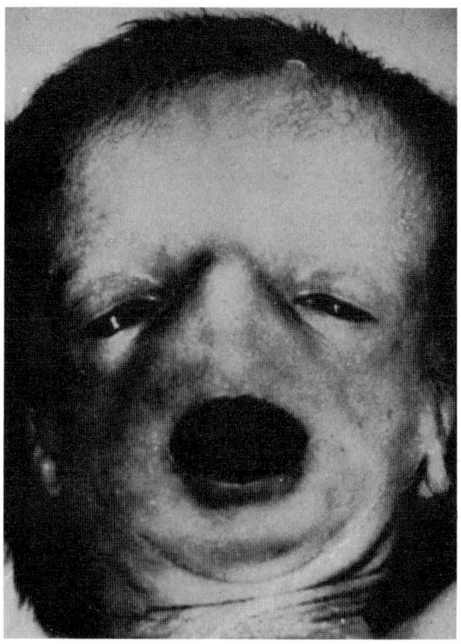

The Nose in Arhinencephaly

The arhinencephalies[4] include a series of malformations from cyclopia through ethmocephaly and cebocephaly to milder and sometimes viable defects of midline structures. They all have in common deficiencies of the olfactory lobes and nerves, but the peripheral olfactory organ can vary greatly from formation of a proboscis and union of the nasal sacs to simple hypoplasia of some of the nasal components.

In *ethmocephaly*, two orbits and bulbi sit close together without being united as in cyclopia. The nose is absent and a proboscis arises in the area of the nasal root. The proboscis, situated between the eyes, may have one or two nares but always lacks choanal openings. The ethmoid, the nasal conchae, the nasal and lacrimal bones and the premaxilla are absent. The prosencephalon represents a single cavity that does

Fig. 66-2.—Absence of left nostril in a child with cleft lip and palate (cleft repaired) and rudimentary left ear.

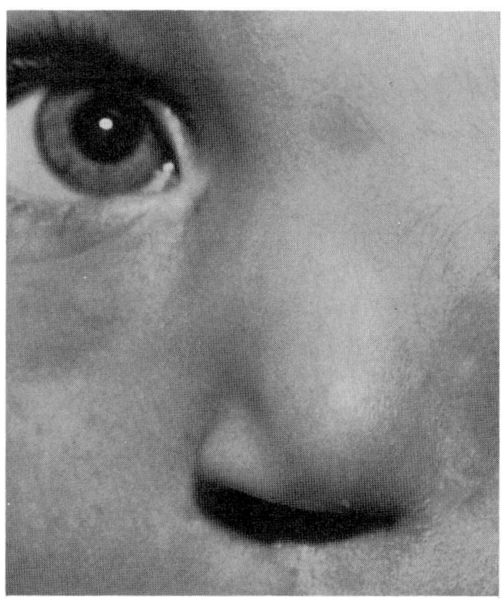

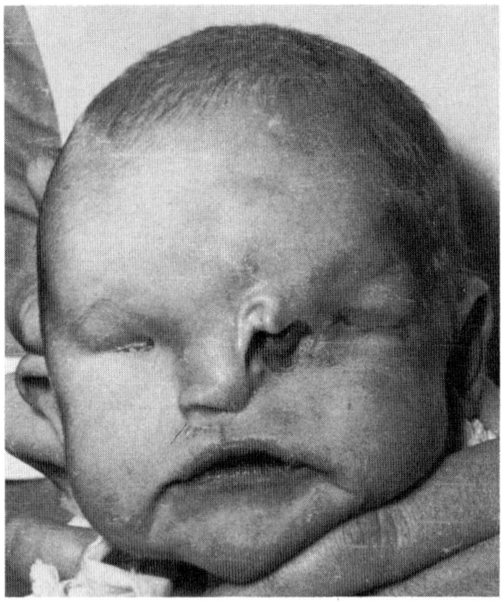

Fig. 66-3.—Faulty development of the left nasal half in a child with bilateral microphthalmia. Bilateral choanal atresia. Scar on right side of upper lip ("spontaneous healing" of cleft lip). The etiology is obscure. The mother had severe heart disease, decompensation and bleeding during pregnancy treated with many drugs. Chromosome analysis was not made. (From A. Berndorfer.[3])

not cover the midbrain. There are transitional forms between cyclopia and ethmocephaly. Tracheo-esophageal fistula and duplication of the central canal have been observed as associated malformations.[2]

Unilateral arhinencephaly with one proboscis and one "normal" nasal half has been described in an anencephalic female fetus.[5] Such unilateral arhinencephaly can be compatible with life. It was described by Selenkoff[6] in a man 34 years of age. The right half of the nose was replaced by a proboscis (proboscis lateralis) that had only a small opening at its distal end leading into a canal with a blind proximal end. The left half of the nose was "well formed" but had only one nostril connected with a nasal cavity and a single choanal opening. The olfactory apparatus, the ethmoid and nasal bones, the sinuses, the vomer and the premaxilla were absent on the right side. With the exception of the rudimentary right olfactory bulbus, which was underdeveloped, the brain was normal. Ethmocephaly is an extremely rare malformation in man.

In *cebocephaly* ("monkey head"), a rudimentary nose is seen in its normal position between the eyes. The orbits and the bulbi are approximated and hypotelorism exists. Usually, there is one nasal opening and one nasal cavity with underdeveloped conchae. The nasal bones and the septum are absent and the premaxilla is underdeveloped. The maxillae are approximated and the palate is long and narrow. Rudimentary or occluded choanae have been observed. The brain weight is markedly reduced in such cases, since portions of the frontal, parietal and occipital lobes are absent. Behind the fused rostral portions of the brain there is a crescent-shaped opening through which the lateral and third ventricles can be seen united to a single cavity. The pituitary gland is absent and the adrenals are hypoplastic in some of these cases.[7] In some instances of cebocephaly, hydrocephaly, encephalocele, microphthalmia, cardiac and genital malformations and polydactyly have been recorded as associated defects.[2] Although this condition is rare, Haworth *et al.*[7] observed 2 cases within 6 months. In one of these patients, a short arm deficiency of chromosome 18 was found.[8] Bühler *et al.*[9] reported a trisomy 13-15 with cebocephaly.

Median cleft of the lip with arhinencephaly occurs more often than the forms mentioned before, and children with this anomaly can live for some time. The philtrum, the premaxilla and the nasal bones and septum are absent and the nose is flat. Usually, there is a concomitant median palatine cleft but this is not so in all cases. If the palatine processes are developed and united with each other, there exists only one choanal connection between the nasal cavity and the pharynx. There is a single nasal cavity with hypoplastic conchae. Olfactory nerves, bulbi and tracts often are absent, but rudiments of these structures have been observed. Choanal atresia can occur in such cases. Polydactyly, ocular, aural, cardiac and other anomalies were reported as associated malformations[2,10] long before some of these cases were identi-

Fig. 66-4.—Cebocephaly showing single median nostril. (From J. C. Haworth *et al.*[7])

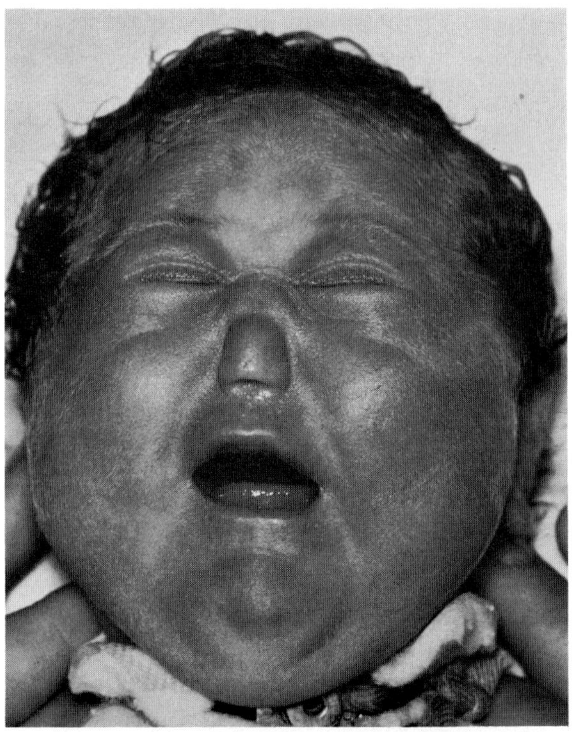

fied as trisomy 13-15 (D_1) (Chapter 37). However, not all patients with median cleft of the lip show this chromosomal pattern. There also are patients with unilateral or double harelip and cleft palate and patients with normal facies who have arhinencephaly and trigonocephaly.

Proboscis Lateralis

Proboscis lateralis is a rare trunk-like malformation that hangs down from the inner canthus, resembling—except for its location—the median proboscis well known in cyclopia (p. 202). At its lower end, this skin covered formation shows a dimple that may be connected with a central canal lined by cylindrical epithelium. Usually, it is combined with absence of the isolateral half of the nose. On the side of the proboscis, the bulbus olfactorius may be rudimentary, the ethmoid and nasal bones absent and the choana as well as the nasal cavity missing. Bremer[11] explained this strange formation by absence of the nasal and globular processes of one side and by meeting of the remaining median and nasal and globular processes with the contralateral maxillary process at its normal place. There may be anomalies of the maxilla, colobomas of the eyelids and of the iris and choroidea or anophthalmia.[6,12]

Bilateral Proboscis

Bilateral proboscis associated with unilateral anophthalmia and anomalies of the skull and brain and hydramnios were reported by Rosen and Gitlin.[13] There was no external nose and no nostrils, and the proboscises were attached symmetrically to the supraorbital margins. There was an accessory bone within the metopic suture. In this case,[14] there was concomitant partial arhinencephaly, lissencephaly, agenesis of the corpus callosum and meningeal angiomatosis. A hamartoma ("central lobe") was found between the two hemispheres (see Fig. 23-8). This midline malformation of the brain apparently interfered with the normal mediad movement and descent of the olfactory sacs, resulting in conditions resembling those seen in a 10-mm. embryo. Double proboscis in a male infant with cerebral defect is shown in Figure 66-5.

Median Nasal Clefts

In this anomaly, the septum narium is split anteriorly in two diverging halves so that a skin-covered median furrow is formed on the dorsum nasi. The extent of the dividing furrow varies.[52] It may split the nose completely so that two separate halves are formed, both having their own median wall. In such cases of bifid nose there usually is hypertelorism and often association with other malformations such as facial clefts, colobomas of the lower eyelids, encephalocele, choanal atresia and others (Figs. 66-6 and 66-7). Nasal fistulas, dermoids or teratomas have been observed between the halves. The two nasal halves may be symmetric or one half be underdeveloped. In milder cases, only the lower part of the nose appears divided as the cartilaginous septum narium is split and the nasal openings and the two nasal tips are separated by a furrow variable in extent. In most cases, the median cleft is wider on the lower end than

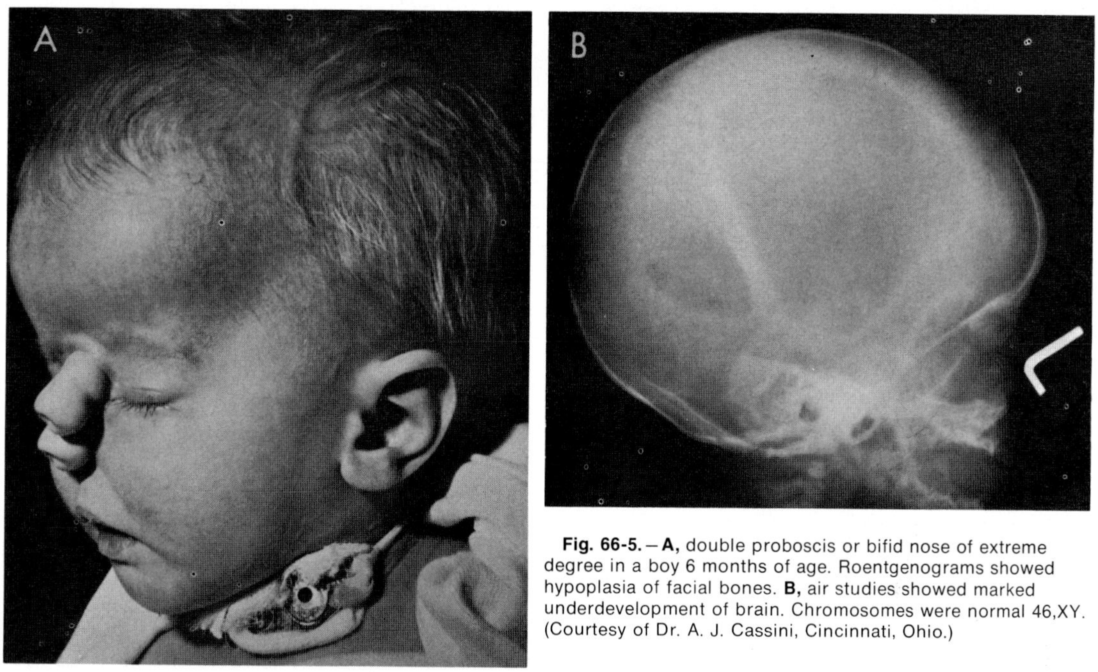

Fig. 66-5.—**A,** double proboscis or bifid nose of extreme degree in a boy 6 months of age. Roentgenograms showed hypoplasia of facial bones. **B,** air studies showed marked underdevelopment of brain. Chromosomes were normal 46,XY. (Courtesy of Dr. A. J. Cassini, Cincinnati, Ohio.)

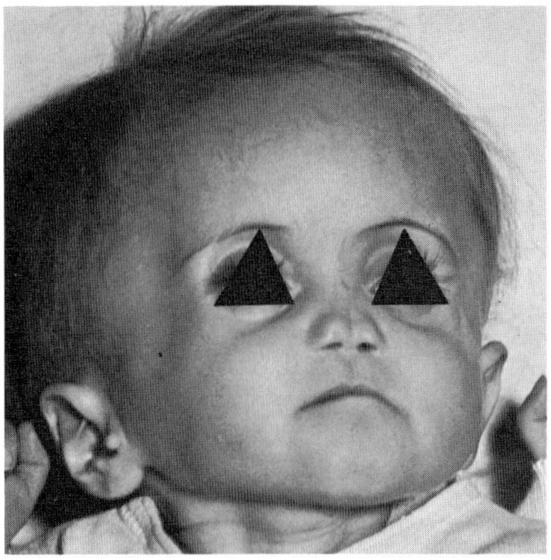

Fig. 66-6. – Median nasal cleft of mild degree. Necropsy showed cerebral dysplasia and marked internal hydrocephaly, fusion of frontal lobes, absence of parietal, temporal and occipital lobes, corpus callosum and falx. (Cincinnati Children's Hospital Chart No. 63280.)

on the upper end of the nose and hypertelorism is absent. A median "scar" on the nasal dorsum probably represents the mildest form of this anomaly.

In some cases, amniotic bands have been found connected to the skin of the scalp or the nasal furrow, which led to explanations of bifid nose as a result of amniotic concrescences.[2] But there may be more subtle mechanisms involved. In young embryos (10 mm.), the nasal pits are relatively widely separated from each other by the central portion of the frontal process, and median nasal furrows are present on the tip of the nose in many human embryos. These depressions are filled out later by connective tissue, and the olfactory sacs approach each other. Failure of this normal process of development would result in median clefts. Complete failure of mediad migration of the nasal sacs would lead to bilateral proboscises and a partial approach to a split nose broader at the root than at the split lower end.[13] Displacement of surface ectoderm into the prenasal space, resulting in midline dermoids or fistulas, may account for those median clefts that are associated with such anomalies.

Fig. 66-7. – Incomplete midline clefts of nose and upper lip in a child whose twin had craniostenosis, small brain, dextrocardia and clubfeet.

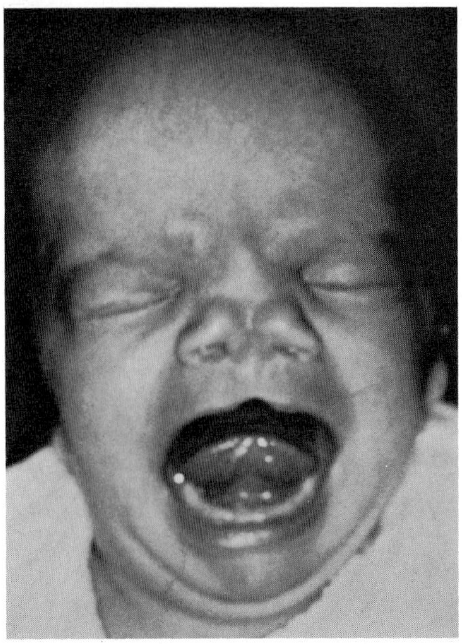

Lateral Nasal Clefts

These are rare triangular defects that divide an ala nasi or the lateral nasal wall more or less completely (Fig. 66-8). In all probability, the clefts are secondary tears in a primarily normal area. The tear may go through the ala nasi and reach into the nasal cavity, or the nasal cleft may run upward and terminate median to the inner epicanthus. The mildest form is a scar-like line in the same area. More severe types are seen in association with such other malformations as choanal atresia, facial clefts or coloboma of the lower lid, teratomas, fibromas and others. Morphogenetic explanation of these clefts encountered difficulties, since they do not correspond to any of the known facial furrows seen during embryonic life. The anomaly has been explained, therefore, as a failure of formation of a complete mesenchymal wall around the olfactory pits. In embryos of approximately 10 mm., one sees that the medial and lateral nasal processes are clearly elevated around the olfactory pits with the exception of the anterolateral portion of the circular ring, which is not well set off from the surrounding nasofrontal process. If this area does not participate

Fig. 66-8. – Lateral nasal cleft in a child 18 months of age. A nasal meningocele had been removed soon after birth. (From A. Berndorfer.[3])

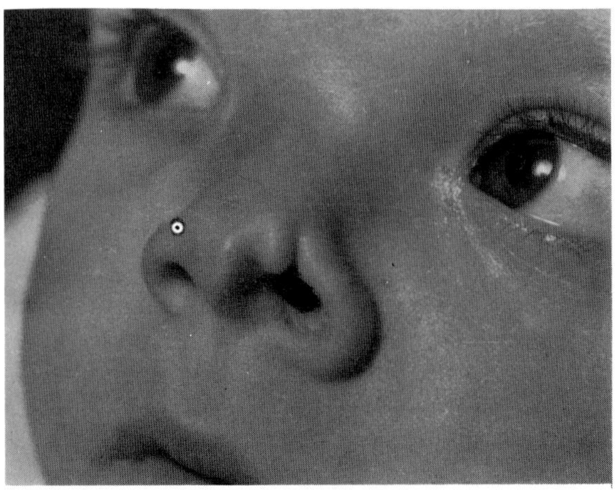

in the molding of the ala by its underlying mesenchyme, a defect in the characteristic lateral cleft position can be expected.[2] Another concept was advanced by Berndorfer,[3] who believed that lateral nasal clefts occur as anomalies secondary to changes of the brain or of the cranial capsule. In every one of his cases he found some kind of "tumor" or remnants of tumors regressed in utero. In one case, a typical lateral nasal cleft was associated with a frontal meningocele (see Fig. 66-8).

Duplication of the Nose (Polyrhinia)

There are many nasal malformations in conjoined twins of different types; these have been discussed thoroughly by Wilder.[15] Duplication of the nose in an otherwise normal body (rhinodymia) occurs in various forms. In a case reported by Muecke and Souttar,[16] two complete noses with four nostrils were present in the face of an otherwise normal girl. Each nose had its own septum, two nares and two alae. There are less complete forms with one normal and one underdeveloped half that may have only one nostril and one choana. An extra nostril may be situated over one of the normal nostrils.[2]

Gliomas and Encephaloceles in the Nasal Area

Encephaloceles can occur extranasally and intranasally (p. 215). Among the extranasal ones, one distinguishes nasofrontal, naso-ethmoidal, spheno-ethmoidal and naso-orbital lesions, which usually prolapse through "areas of weakness." There exists, for instance, in newborn children a membranous region between the upper end of the nasal bones and the frontal bone that has been called "fonticulus nasofrontalis." Between the nasofrontal bony skeleton and the cartilaginous capsule behind it a "prenasal space" exists that extends downward to the tip of the nose.[17] In postnatal life, the area of the fonticulus nasofrontalis becomes ossified, thus sealing off the approximation of the dura from the skin of the nasal bridge. If some surface ectoderm remains in contact with the dura in this area, a dermoid cyst may be formed that can be connected with the skin by a sinus. These dermoid sinuses have been considered homologous to pilonidal sinuses at the coccyx. Another point of possible prolapse of nerve tissue exists at the foramen caecum of the frontal bone's contact with the ethmoid, where a projection of the dura reaches down into the prenasal space. This gap is closed later during normal development, but it represents another possible pathway for cerebral tissue into the nasal area. Extranasal gliomas may be connected with the brain by fibrous or glial tissue passing through this gap[18] and encephaloceles penetrate through a skeletal defect in the same area.

Fig. 66-9. – Nasal glioma in a boy 5 months of age.

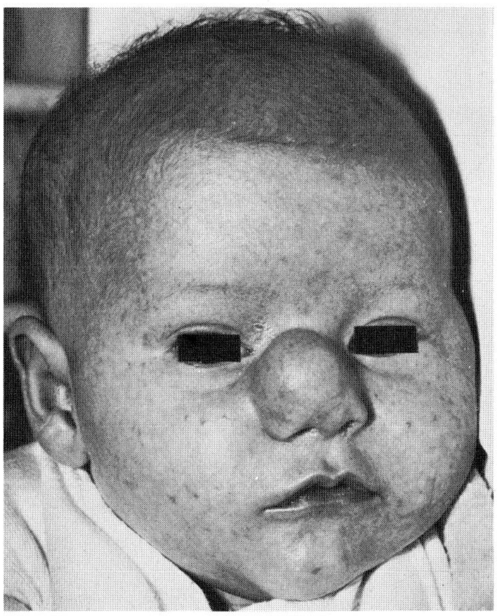

Gliomas of the nose are rare congenital tumors usually seen over or below the bridge of the nose (Fig. 66-9) and associated with hypertelorism. They do not pulsate and do not change in size when the patient cries. Usually, no defect of the skull is seen roentgenographically. Intranasal gliomas arise from the lateral wall of the nasal cavity or from a turbinate. Coexisting extranasal and intranasal tumors connected through a nasal bone have been observed. They can be mistaken for polyps. Nasal gliomas are considered benign tumors with little growth tendency, but sometimes they increase in size rapidly and recur after excision.[17] In general, nasal gliomas are similar in origin to nasal encephaloceles. Transitional forms have been observed that were directly connected by a stalk with the subarachnoidal space and represent surgical risks like encephaloceles. Microscopically, they consist of nests of glia cells intermingled with vascular fibrous tissue septa. The cells are astrocytes with pale-staining nuclei (Fig. 66-10). Mitoses are rare. Intranasal tumors are covered by respiratory epithelium, extranasal tumors by skin.

Nasal gliomas must be distinguished from encephaloceles and nasal neurofibromata; from dermoid, sebaceous, ethmoid and lacrimal duct cysts; and from lipomas and hemangiomas.[17]

Reviews[18,19] showed that excessive growth or recurrence was exceptional. Associated congenital malformations have not been reported and there is no evidence of heredity.[19]

A different neurogenic tumor (neuroepithelioblastoma, esthesioneuroblastoma) of the nose is thought to be of peripheral origin. It is attributed to displaced cells of the olfactory placodes, to sensory olfactory cells or to glial supporting tissue of the olfactory mucosa. These tumors are radiosensitive. In contrast to gliomas, the majority of them have been reported in adults.[20]

Encephaloceles in the nasal area are rare. In a se-

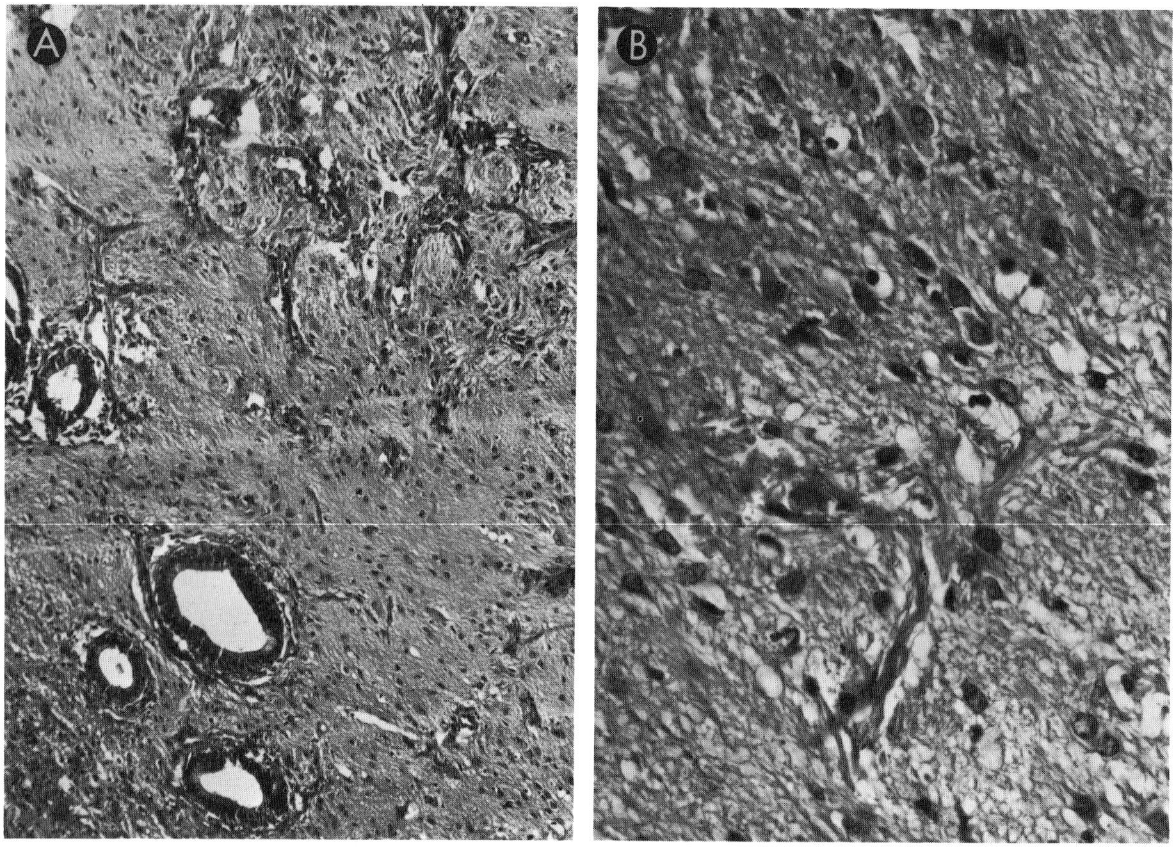

Fig. 66-10.—Sections of nasal tumor shown in Figure 66-9. **A,** glioma and ependymal channels. **B,** glioma cells. This case showing spaces lined by ependyma represents a transitional form between glioma nasi and encephalocele. (Cincinnati Children's Hospital Chart No. 102-597.)

ries of 187 encephaloceles,[21] nasal encephaloceles accounted for 4.8% of the cases. But, in Thailand and Indonesia, such lesions seem to be much more frequent than in Western countries (p. 216).

Nasofrontal encephaloceles pass through the nasofrontal fonticulus and have no relation to the nasal cavities. They can attain various sizes,[22] extending over the forehead and nose. A nasofrontal encephalocele in an infant was described by Browder and de Veer[23] and interpreted as an anomaly of the rhinencephalon. A resemblance to nasal glioma was stressed. Ventricular septal defect was an associated malformation. A defect of bone at the bregma may be the site of a pedunculated meningocele without any brain tissue. A child with nasofrontal encephaloceles and various cerebral malformations is shown in Figure 66-11.

Naso-ethmoidal or prenasal encephaloceles pass through the foramen caecum into the prenasal space. They appear below the nasal bones and are also unrelated to the nasal cavities.

Naso-orbital encephaloceles break through the anterior portion of the lamina cribrosa into the medial portion of the orbita. The lacrimal bone and other skeletal elements may be absent and the bulbus oculi be displaced laterad. Bilateral and multiple encephaloceles have been described.[2] Encephaloceles of the orbita, of the external auditory meatus and of the temporal squama have been observed simultaneously in an adult patient.[24]

Transethmoidal encephaloceles usually reach a nasal cavity through an opening in the lamina cribrosa. These protrusions of the brain often are mistaken for polyps. But, since polyps are quite rare in infancy, such tumors should always be suspected to be connected with the brain. Intranasal encephaloceles sometimes are compressible and they may show pulsation. Sometimes they grow after birth and cause respiratory and feeding difficulties. The tumor is located on the roof of a nasal cavity or in front of the middle concha. The nasal septum is bent toward the normal side and the conchae of the affected side are compressed or underdeveloped. The tumor may appear within a nostril or, if associated with facial and palatine clefts, reach the oral cavity or even pass through the mouth onto the body surface.[2] Successful operation of a transethmoidal encephalocele protruding into the left nostril and through a cleft palate was

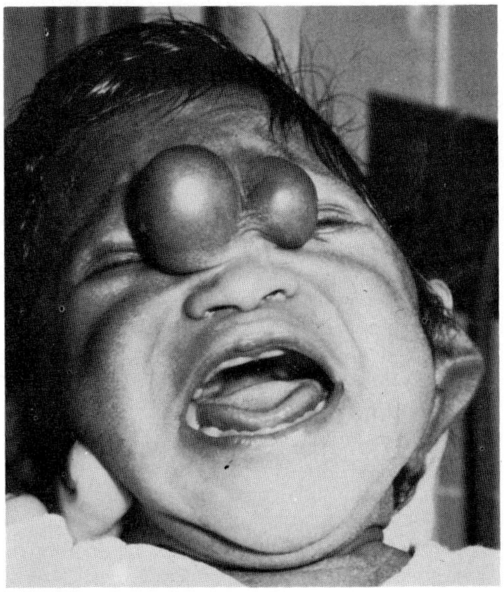

Fig. 66-11.—Nasofrontal encephalocele. The child also had internal hydrocephaly, absence of the anterior horn of the left lateral ventricle, microgyria and cerebellar malformations with cerebellar tongues projecting downward on the dorsal aspect of the brain stem. The child died of meningitis at 1 year of age. (Cincinnati Children's Hospital Chart No. 130-148.)

reported and well illustrated by Ingraham and Matson.[21]

Spheno-ethmoidal encephaloceles pass through a defect between the sphenoid and ethmoidal bones and reach the oral cavity. Both the external nose and the nasal cavities are deformed in such cases. The posterior part of the palate and the uvula may be cleft. In a case described by Exner,[25] a boy, the ninth child in an otherwise normal family, showed median cleft through the upper lip and the soft palate. A nonpulsating cyst seen over the tongue burst 5 days after birth and meningitis resulted in death of the child. The cyst represented an encephalocele that passed through an opening bordered by sphenoid and ethmoid.

The differential diagnosis between nasal encephaloceles and gliomas may be difficult. Encephaloceles, if well developed, contain a lumen lined by ependyma and filled with cerebrospinal fluid. A communication exists between the lumen and the cerebral ventricular system. Often there is a defect in the base of the skull, pulsation of the tumor and enlargement when the child cries. In contrast, the glioma is a solid tumor consisting of glia cells separated by fibrous septa. The glioma is not connected directly with the brain. But transitional forms exist[26] that make the clinical differential diagnosis difficult; sometimes, even the pathologic findings are ambiguous.[17] In Figure 66-9, a nasal glioma is shown that histologically showed ependymal channels, proving its cerebral origin.

In cases of sacrolumbar myelomeningocele, hydrocephaly develops in many cases with and without removal of the tumor. The association between the two anomalies often is the subject of discussion, since it is not clear whether the myelocele causes hydrocephaly by leading to an Arnold-Chiari malformation or whether operation and removal of a fluid-resorbing sac results in accumulation of fluid in the ventricular system. It is of interest in this respect that temporary enlargement of the head followed removal of a nasal encephalocele.[17] This observation could be used in support of the explanation of hydrocephaly by removal of a fluid-resorbing surface. Development of an Arnold-Chiari malformation in a case of nasal encephalocele shows that the malformations around the foramen magnum are not always associated with fixation of the spinal cord (p. 220), but rather are a part of a complex of cerebral malformations.

Congenital Dermoid Cysts of the Nose

Among all congenital dermoids, those of the nose make up less than 1%.[27] In most instances, these cysts are present at birth, but in rare cases first manifestations occur in early childhood or even later. The location of the cysts may range from the frontal area to the tip of the nose, but the majority occupy the upper nasal dorsum.

There is no complete agreement on the embryologic origin of these cysts. Some authors attribute them to developmental errors in early intrauterine life, such as abnormal epidermal sequestration during fusion of the nasal segments, whereas others explain them by displacement of ectoderm by the ingrowing membranous bone.[28] During formation of the nasal bones, displaced parts of ectoderm may be situated in the prenasal space between the cartilaginous nasal wall and nasal bone. The displaced parts of ectoderm eventually form dermoids that may or may not remain in connection with the skin.[28]

As a rule, dermoid cysts of the nose occur sporadically, but in one instance the anomaly was found in both mother and daughter, and in another it occurred in twin brothers.[27]

Most of these cysts present as small, rather firm tumors in the region of the mid-frontal suture, but some lie lateral to the midline. Sinus openings to the surface are crater-like, vary in size from almost complete occlusion to 1 mm. in diameter and have small tufts of fine hair growing from the orifice. Most cysts are unilocular; they can be filled with lipiodol through the sinus tract and be demonstrated in x-ray films.

Dermoid cysts must be differentiated from sebaceous cysts, gliomas, meningoceles and lipomas. Meningoceles, like dermoid cysts, occur at closure lines in embryonic development. They often become more tense with crying and straining. They readily transmit light. Lipomas move more freely than dermoid cysts.

Congenital malformations rarely are associated with cysts of the nose, but bifid nose, harelip and cleft palate and multiple malformations have been observed in affected persons. Complete surgical removal and plastic reconstruction represent the treatment of these congenital anomalies.[27,29]

Mucoids

The site of these cystic tumors is on the dorsal wall of the nostril between the insertions of the ala and the septum nasi. This corresponds to a point at which the lateral and median nasal processes unite with the maxillary process. The cysts, which are covered by cylindrical epithelium, are filled with a yellow mucin-containing fluid. Usually, they are of pea to hazelnut size and may compress the premaxilla. In contrast to dental root cysts, their walls are not osseous but fibrous. Interestingly, they occur more often in females than in males. Transmission from a father to his daughter has been described.[30] Although they are of prenatal origin, they make their appearance after puberty.[2] A rare form of mucoids sometimes occurs on the upper end of the nasolacrimal canal. Such cysts, which occur in the naso-ethmoidal area, sometimes are considered serous orbital cysts.

Congenital Saddle Nose

In several syndromes of multiple congenital anomalies, saddle nose has been mentioned as a symptom. Marshall[31] observed saddle nose in members of a kinship who had ectodermal dysplasia, hearing defects and cataract. Dominant inheritance was suggested. Saddle nose is also mentioned among the symptoms of the Rothmund-Thomson syndrome (p. 392).

Choanal Atresia

Bilateral choanal atresia is a rare condition that usually causes severe symptoms in infants. Unilateral choanal atresia, although more common than the bilateral form, may go unrecognized in many cases. It is said that this condition was first described in 1829 by Otto, who found choanal atresia in a child at necropsy (cited by Beinfield[32]). According to Wilson,[33] approximately 500 cases had been reported by 1955. Unilateral cases are said to occur more often on the right side; females are affected more often than males.[33] Reviews on this subject are available.[32,34-36]

Choanal atresia probably is due to persistence of the nasobuccal membrane, which, in young embryos, separates the nasal pits from the primitive mouth. Normally, this membrane ruptures early in the sixth week of fetal life, but if rupture does not take place, mesodermal tissue migrates between the epithelial layers, which later leads to a membranous or a bony separation between the nasal cavity and the nasopharynx.

Most cases are sporadic, but a hereditary tendency has been observed in some families, particularly those with unilateral involvement. Thus, Lang,[37] in 1912, described a mother and her daughter and son, all with choanal atresia, and Stewart,[38] in 1931, reported 2 sisters with the anomaly. There was concordance of congenital choanal atresia in twin girls reported by Dickson.[39] Choanal atresia may be associated with trisomy 13-15[8,9,40] and with trisomy 18.[40,46,47] Choanal atresia can be bilateral or unilateral, complete or incomplete, osseous or membranous. Lemoyne[41] pointed out that the choanae are almost horizontal in newborn infants.

Bilateral complete choanal atresia may represent an emergency situation in newborn children who, as a rule, have not learned to breathe through their mouths and develop dyspnea and cyanosis in case of complete obstruction of the nasal air passages. Such infants present a picture of asphyxia neonatorum that is not alleviated by oxygen medication. The cardiac rate may be very high, so that congenital heart disease sometimes is suspected in children with complete choanal atresia. It is believed that the anomaly, if it goes unrecognized and untreated, may be a cause of death in many newborn infants,[42] but not all children with choanal atresia die in infancy. Cases have been reported of survival of bilaterally affected patients for months and even years. Such children have chronic prenasal secretion without postnasal discharge. They are mouth breathers; they cannot blow their noses and they are completely anosmic. The palate is high and the children appear underweight, pale and listless. Their sleep is disturbed by respiratory difficulties. Enlargement of the adenoids and tonsils is suspected, but the symptoms are not relieved by removal of these structures. Ersner[43] described a girl operated on at the age of 8 years and the improvement of her condition after operation. She had to re-educate herself and learn "that her nose was not there as an ornament but was for breathing purposes." Smelling and tasting food increased her appetite to such an extent that she gained 25 pounds within the year following the operation.

Unilateral cases may cause few symptoms and be overlooked for many years. A tenacious mucous discharge from the affected nostril is noticed and the obstruction can be demonstrated by a catheter that does not pass from the nose into the nasopharynx, or by roentgenograms that show that iodized oil does not reach the nasopharynx.

Associated malformations have been observed repeatedly in children with choanal atresia. Asymmetry of the face, high arched palate, irregularities of the upper incisors, double tragus, cleft palate, coloboma of the lower lids, coloboma of the iris, congenital absence of the puncta and canaliculi of the lower lids, atresia of the external auditory canal and hydrocephaly have been observed.[35] The combination of choanal atresia and congenital heart disease[44] is of practical importance, since either condition can result in cyanosis, increased heart rate and other symptoms that could be explained by one or the other anomaly. Cleft palate may mitigate the manifestations of choanal atresia.[45] In a patient of Hanckel's,[34] polydactyly was present, and choanal atresia has been observed in monstrous infants.[10] Hydramnios may accompany the nasal anomaly,[35] which suggests that swallowing may be impaired in the prenatal period.

Treatment of complete bilateral choanal atresia consists in surgical establishment of an air passage from the nose into the nasopharynx, the operation being preceded in severe cases by tracheostomy. Many operative procedures have been described since a first surgical attempt was made in 1853 by Emmert (cited by Hanckel[34]). Direct transnasal removal of the osseous or membranous obstruction of the choanae is difficult because of the small size of the nasal cavity. Transpalatal and transseptal attacks can be made.[32-34,41] But conservative treatment and delay of operation have also been recommended. Insertion of an oropharyngeal airway and teaching of the infants to breathe by mouth has been successful in some cases.[48]

Trisomy 13-15 (D_1) and Nasal Anomalies

Abnormalities of the nose occur frequently in children with trisomy 13-15. With harelip and cleft palate, one or both nostrils may be incompletely formed. In cases of median clefts, the nose is flat and depressed and the premaxilla, the nasal septum[49] and the nasal bones[50] are absent. Absence of the olfactory bulbs and tracts has been described[49,51] (p. 298). Cebocephaly associated with trisomy 13-15 was reported by Bühler *et al.*[9] As was mentioned before, choanal atresia may be associated with trisomy 13-15.[8,9,40]

REFERENCES

1. Blair, V. P.: Congenital atresia or obstruction of nasal air passages, Ann. Otol. 40:1021, 1931.
2. Stupka, W.: *Die Missbildungen und Anomalien der Nase und des Nasenrachenraumes* (Vienna: Springer, 1938).
3. Berndorfer, A.: Über die seitliche Nasenspalte, Acta otolaryng. 55:163, 1962.
4. Kundrat, H.: Arhinencephalie als typische Art von Missbildungen, Wien. M. Bull. 5:1395, 1882.
5. Lang, B.: Über seltene Nasenmissbildungen, Virchows Arch. path. Anat. 285:93, 1932.
6. Selenkoff, A.: Ein Fall von Arhinencephalia unilateralis bei einem erwachsenen Manne, Virchows Arch. path. Anat. 95:95, 1884.
7. Haworth, J. C., Medovy, H., and Lewis, A. J.: Cebocephaly with endocrine dysgenesis, J. Pediat. 59:726, 1961.
8. Uchida, I. A., McRae, K. N., Wang, H. C., and Ray, M.: Familial short arm deficiency of chromosome 18 concomitant with arhinencephaly and alopecia congenita, Am. J. Human Genet. 17:410, 1965.
9. Bühler, E., Bodis, I., Rossier, R., and Stalder, G.: Trisomie 13-15 mit Cebocephalie, Ann. paediat. 119:198, 1962.
10. Gruber, G. B.: Beiträge sur Frage "gekoppelter" Missbildungen (Akrocephalo-Syndactylie und Dysencephalia splanchnocystica), Beitr. path. Anat. 93:459, 1934.
11. Bremer, J. L.: *Congenital Anomalies of the Viscera* (Cambridge, Mass.: Harvard University Press, 1957).
12. Grünberg, K.: Die Gesichtsspalten und die zu ihnen in genetischer Beziehung stehenden anderweitigen Missbildungen des Gesichtes, in Schwalbe, E. (ed.), *Die Morphologie der Missbildungen des Menschen und der Tiere* (Jena: Gustav Fischer, 1909), Vol. 3.
13. Rosen, Z., and Gitlin, G.: Bilateral nasal proboscis associated with unilateral anophthalmia, unilateral diffuse pigmentation of the conjunctiva and anomalies of the skull and brain, A.M.A. Arch. Otolaryng. 70:545, 1959.
14. Gitlin, G., and Behar, A. J.: Meningeal angiomatosis, arhinencephaly, agenesis of the corpus callosum and large hamartoma of the brain, with neoplasia, in an infant having bilateral nasal proboscis, Acta anat. 41:56, 1960.
15. Wilder, H. H.: The morphology of Cosmobia; speculations concerning the significance of certain types of monsters, Am. J. Anat. 8:355, 1908.
16. Muecke, F. F., and Souttar, H. S.: Case of double nose, Proc. Roy. Soc. Med. (Sect. Laryngol.) 17:8, 1924.
17. Macomber, W. B., and Wang, M. K.: Congenital neoplasms of the nose, Plast. & Reconstruct. Surg. 11:215, 1953.
18. Black, B. K., and Smith, P. E.: Nasal glioma: Two cases with recurrence, Arch. Neurol. & Psychiat. 64:614, 1950.
19. Walker, E. A., Jr., and Resler, D. R.: Nasal glioma, Laryngoscope 73:93, 1963.
20. Riemenschneider, P. A., and Prior, J. T.: Neuroblastoma originating from olfactory epithelium (esthesioneuroblastoma), Am. J. Roentgenol. 80:759, 1958.
21. Ingraham, F. D., and Matson, D. D.: Spina bifida and cranium bifidum. IV. An unusual nasopharyngeal encephalocele, New England J. Med. 228:815, 1943.
22. Ernst, P.: Missbildungen des Nervensystems, in Schwalbe, E. (ed.), *Die Morphologie der Missbildungen des Menschen und der Tiere* (Jena: Gustav Fischer, 1909), Vol. 3, pt. 2.
23. Browder, J., and deVeer, J. A.: Rhino-encephalocele, Arch. Path. 18:646, 1934.
24. Schreyer, W., and Sprenger, W.: Über basale Cephalocelen, Ztschr. Hals-, Nasen- u. Ohrenh. 17:252, 1927.
25. Exner, A.: Über basale Cephalocelen, Deutsche Ztschr. Chir., Leipzig 90:23, 1907.
26. Jamieson, K. G.: Nasal glioma, Pediatrics 35:342, 1965.
27. Crawford, J. K., and Webster, J. P.: Congenital dermoid cysts of the nose, Plast. & Reconstruct. Surg. 9:235, 1952.
28. Brunner, H., and Donnelly, W. A.: Nasal and auricular fistulae, Plast. & Reconstruct. Surg. 2:497, 1947.
29. Taylor, B. W., and Erich, J. B.: Dermoid cysts of the nose, Mayo Clinic Proc. 42:488, 1967.
30. Kasche, F.: Klinische und pathologische Beiträge zu den Erkrankungen der oberen Luftwege und des Ohres: Vorkommen von Gesichtsspaltencysten bei Vater und Tochter, Ztschr. Laryng. Rhin. Otol. 16:113, 1927.
31. Marshall, D.: Ectodermal dysplasia. Report of a kindred with ocular abnormalities and hearing defect, Am. J. Ophth. 45:143, 1958.
32. Beinfield, H. H.: Treatment of complete unilateral bony atresia of posterior nares; new technique and brief reference to asphyxia neonatorum, A.M.A. Arch. Otolaryng. 53:530, 1951.
33. Wilson, T. G.: *Diseases of the Ear, Nose and Throat in Children* (New York: Grune & Stratton, Inc., 1955).
34. Hanckel, R. W.: Bilateral choanal atresia: Report of case in infant and review of literature, Ann. Otol. 58:852, 1949.
35. Beinfield, H. H.: Congenital bilateral bony atresia of the posterior nares in a one-month premature infant who survived. Experiences with a case, J. Pediat. 45:679, 1954.
36. Campbell, W., Stokes, D. E., and Jennings, R. E.: Choanal atresia—report of five cases and a review of recent literature, J. M. Soc. New Jersey 58:468, 1961.
37. Lang, J.: Über Choanenatresie (Heredität derselben), Monatsschr. Ohrenh. 46:970, 1912.
38. Stewart, J. P.: Congenital atresia of the posterior nares, Arch. Otolaryng. 13:570, 1931.
39. Dickson, J. C.: Congenital atresia of the posterior nares, Texas J. Med. 46:115, 1950.
40. Warkany, J., Passarge, E., and Smith, L. B.: Congenital malformations in autosomal trisomy syndromes, Am. J. Dis. Child. 112:502, 1966.

41. Lemoyne, J.: Traitement de l'imperforation chonale du nourrisson, Arch. franç. pédiat. 11:354, 1954.
42. Beinfield, H. H.: Ways and means to reduce infant mortality due to suffocation: Importance of choanal atresia, J.A.M.A. 170:647, 1959.
43. Ersner, M. S.: Operative and postoperative management of bilateral bony atresia of the choana, A.M.A. Arch. Otolaryng. 58:96, 1953.
44. McGovern, F. H.: The association of congenital choanal atresia and congenital heart disease, Ann. Otol. 62:894, 1953.
45. Kiel, F. W.: Mitigation of posterior choanal atresia by cleft palate, J. Pediat. 56:516, 1960.
46. Heinrichs, E. H.: The 18-trisomy syndrome—a spectrum?, Clin. Pediat. 2:25, 1963.
47. Erickson, D. J., Lodge, J. L., and Tomsovic, E. J.: Medical management of bilateral choanal atresia; report of 4 cases, J. Pediat. 63:561, 1963.
48. Townes, P. L., DeHart, G. K., and Ziegler, N. A.: Trisomy 17-18. An evaluation of preconceptional parental irradiation as a possible etiologic factor, J. Pediat. 65:870, 1964.
49. Smith, D. W., Patau, K., Therman, E., Inhorn, S. L., and DeMars, R. I.: The D_1 trisomy syndrome, J. Pediat. 62: 326, 1963.
50. Conen, P. E., Phillips, K. G., and Mauntner, L. S.: Multiple developmental anomalies and trisomy of a 13-15 group chromosome ("D" syndrome), Canad. M.A.J. 87: 709, 1962.
51. Miller, J. Q., Picard, E. H., Alkan, M. K., Warner, S., and Gerald, P. S.: A specific congenital brain defect (arhinencephaly) in 13-15 trisomy, New England J. Med. 268:120, 1963.
52. Sedano, H. O., Cohen, M. M., Jr., Jirasek, J., and Gorlin, R. J.: Frontonasal dysplasia, J. Pediat. 76:906, 1970.

67

The Larynx

Congenital Subglottic Hemangioma

JUDGING FROM THE LITERATURE, this anomaly was thought to be rare, since only 14 cases had been reported up to 1958, when Campbell *et al.*[1] summarized these cases and added 5 of their own. But, in 1961, the number of published cases had risen to 24 and Ferguson and Flake[16] stated that 17 infants with the anomaly had been seen and treated in 9 years at the Children's Hospital Medical Center in Boston. Tefft[17] reported 28 cases from the same Center, with emphasis on radiotherapeutic management in children. Maier[18] discussed hemangiomas of the subglottic region together with similar hemangiomas of the trachea and mediastinum. Subglottic hemangioma occurs more often in females than in males.[16] It may manifest itself as asphyxia neonatorum or, later, by feeding difficulties or attacks of cyanosis. The cry usually is vigorous but hoarse; there may be inspiratory stridor and retractions. Serious respiratory difficulty or sudden death can occur because of the location of the tumor, but the attacks of respiratory impairment may change from hour to hour, according to the filling of the hemangioma.

The anomaly may be suggested by hemangiomas in other parts of the body[2] or, as in one case of Campbell *et al.*,[1] by a port-wine nevus of the head and neck. Otherwise, the lesion is difficult to visualize and diagnose. Roentgenograms sometimes show a subglottic constriction of the trachea. The laryngoscope may show a bluish red bulge in the region of the subglottis distal to the vocal cord. Bronchoscopy, if not preceded by tracheostomy, may be dangerous because it can produce hemorrhage.

These hemangiomas usually are small, sessile and variable in size, as the capillaries and large cavities may be filled with blood or be empty at times. The tumors can be overlooked even at necropsy, since they may collapse after death. Histologically, they consist of capillaries and large cavities filled with blood.

Treatment consists of tracheostomy followed by radium or roentgen therapy. Satisfactory results have been reported.[16,17]

Papillomas

Papillomas can be present at birth but in the majority of cases they are formed after birth. A hereditary tendency has been demonstrated in some of the cases.[3]

Congenital Webs

As a rule, this anomaly consists of thin bands across the anterior margins of the vocal cords. The webs usually are wedge-shaped, with the thin concave border posteriorly extending between the anterior portions of the true vocal cords. Only a few webs are supraglottic or extend to the posterior portions of the larynx. Some of the cases are discovered in infancy but others are diagnosed much later. In infants, the common symptoms are aphonia, inspiratory and expiratory stridor, difficulty in feeding, dyspnea and cyanosis and sometimes suffocation with retraction and convulsions.[4] A rare supraglottic type was described by Hudson.[5] The morphogenesis probably is explained by the embryology of the larynx as seen in 9-mm. embryos (fifth week), when there exists in the area of the fifth branchial arches a slit (the primitive glottis) that is bordered laterally by two arytenoid swellings. In the seventh week, the laryngeal cavity is temporarily obliterated owing to fusion of the epithelium in the upper larynx, which persists to the tenth week.[6] Only in the second half of the third month, as connection is established with the trachea, does the laryngeal entrance become more oval in contour and the laryngeal ventricles become formed. These are bounded cranially and caudally by projecting lateral shelves; the caudal pair lying at the same level as the primitive laryngeal slit represents the vocal folds.[6] Disturbance of the dissolution of the separating epithelium between the primitive glottis and the trachea results in formation of congenital webs of the larynx.

Congenital Cysts

Laryngeal cysts have been found on the epiglottis, on the aryepiglottic folds and on the lateral walls of the larynx. They may block the entrance to the larynx so that extrauterine life becomes impossible, leading to death of the child in the first weeks of life. The lining of the cysts consists of stratified or ciliated epithelium, which distinguishes them from retention cysts of the mucous glands. The origin of such cysts is not always clear, but sometimes they result from constriction of the mouth of a laryngeal sacculus.[3]

Congenital Atresia

In 1965, Smith and Bain[7] stated that only about 27 cases of larynx atresia had been described in the literature up to that time. But they observed 9 examples at necropsy within one decade. This lethal anomaly probably is related to congenital webbing of the larynx, a malformation compatible with life.

Complete occlusion of the larynx by muscle, cartilage and connective tissue from the epiglottis to the trachea represents the most extensive form of the anomaly. Occlusion from the vocal cords down to the trachea, fusion of the arytenoid cartilages, obliteration by the cricoid and occlusion by a membrane have been described as less extensive atresias. Sayre and Hall[8] reported a case of laryngeal atresia in which the vestibule ended blindly above the level of the cricoid and a case of laryngeal stenosis below the glottis, where the opening of the cricoid cartilage was only 2 mm. in diameter. Smith and Bain[7] described a type in which the supraglottic and infraglottic parts are atretic as well as an infraglottic and a glottic form.

A temporary epithelial occlusion of the infraglottic space exists normally in human embryos from the seventh week to the tenth week. Failure of dissolution of this occlusion leads to ingrowth of mesenchyme into the occluding membrane, which is later replaced by muscle, cartilage and connective tissue. During the normal epithelial occlusion of the arytenoid bulges, a capillary communication persists in the dorsal aspects of the larynx connecting the pharynx with the trachea. A ductus pharyngotrachealis has been observed repeatedly in cases of laryngeal atresia,[7-9] suggesting persistence of early embryonic conditions in such cases. But it has been pointed out that atresias of the glottis or of the supraglottic space require differing explanation, and arrest of development can occur at different stages.[7]

Associated malformations frequently are found in infants with atresia of the larynx. Tracheo-esophageal fistula and esophageal atresia have been observed repeatedly, so that Sayre and Hall[8] emphasized that children with such anomalies who have signs of respiratory obstruction should be examined for laryngeal stenosis or atresia and that, vice versa, the presence of a tracheo-esophageal fistula should be borne in mind when a laryngeal atresia or stenosis has been diagnosed in a newborn infant. Many other malformations have been found associated with laryngeal atresia: hydrocephaly, symblepharon and concrescence of the lids and cornea, occlusion of the lacrimal ducts, harelip and cleft palate, vertebral and radial anomalies, absence of the trachea, duodenal atresia, imperforate anus, urethral and vaginal atresia, ventricular septal defect and renal agenesis have been recorded. The lungs often are large and distended. Hydramnios may complicate the pregnancy preceding the birth of these children.[8,9] It has been pointed out correctly[9] that the teratologic termination periods of these malformations differ significantly, so that it is not justified to attribute these anomalies to short environmental stresses. It is more likely, at least in some of these cases, that genetic mechanisms are at work. This is suggested by a case of a girl with laryngeal atresia whose sister had atresia ani, hypoplasia of the uterus, aplasia of the vagina, syndactyly and other congenital malformations.[10]

Laryngotracheo-esophageal Cleft

This anomaly consists of a failure of fusion of the two bilateral centers of the cricoid cartilage and of an arrest of the rostral advancement of the tracheo-esophageal septum. A communication between the trachea and esophagus extending cephalad through the entire length of the larynx results. The signs and symptoms, including roentgenographic findings, can simulate those of tracheo-esophageal fistulas. Only 12 cases had been recorded by 1965, although as early as 1792 an infant with this anomaly had been described in a doctor's thesis.[11] Stridor, choking, cyanosis and regurgitation are manifestations of the anomaly. The cleft can extend caudally as far as the tracheal bifurcation. Combination with cleft lip and palate, esophageal atresia, tracheo-esophageal fistula, cyst of the brain, vertebral and costal anomalies, atrial and ventricular septal defects, coarctation of the aorta and hypoplasia of the penis and testes has been observed. Hydramnios complicated 5 of the cases. Successful surgical repair has been reported.

Laryngocele (Aerocele)

This is a rare abnormality in man, with fewer than 90 cases reported in the literature by 1959. The anomaly consists of a cystic dilatation of the ventricular appendix or sacculus of the larynx, which may remain confined within the borders of the larynx (internal laryngocele) or may herniate through the thyrohyoid membrane into the soft tissues of the neck, presenting as a cervical mass (external laryngocele).[12] The internal laryngocele is an abnormal distention of the ventricle and the sacculus above the cords that may displace the mucous membranes deep to the false cords and encroach on the intralaryngeal airway. The external laryngocele is formed when the sacculus of the ventricle perforates the thyrohyoid membrane at a point of weakness; it may be found in the neck as a small cyst the size of a pea or it may be as large as an orange. Laryngoceles usually are described in adults but some have been observed in children. Kan[13] reported suffocation of a 16-day-old baby by a laryngocele and Freedman[14] observed a unilateral laryngocele in a 9-week-old infant. Although the symptoms and the tumor may not appear before adulthood, then being provoked by such postnatal stresses as coughing or straining and activities such as blowing wind instruments, continuous use of the voice or lifting heavy weights, the tendency to laryngocele probably is congenital. In fact, laryngoceles are phylogenically normal structures in apes, in which they may reach large proportions, extending down to the base of the neck and even to the axilla. In man, they are abnormally enlarged ventricular laryngeal sacculi. The normal sacculus is an upward elongation of the anterior third of the laryngeal ventricle that forms a vertical blind pouch reaching the upper border of the thyroid cartilage. The sacculi are more prominent in newborn than in older children, since regression sets in at approximately 6 years.[15]

Laryngoceles appear as unilateral or bilateral tumors of variable size located anterior to the sternomastoid muscle. The tumor may be fluctuant and compressible or hard. It may increase on speaking, coughing or straining, and sometimes be emptied by external pressure. Large laryngoceles sound tympanitic on percussion and they are transilluminable if not infected. They can influence the voice, cause hoarseness, dyspnea, obstruction, cough or dysphagia. Following colds and other upper respiratory infections, they may become infected, forming pyoceles that can be emptied internally on coughing. In roentgenograms, laryngoceles can be recognized as air-containing tumors connected with the larynx and opening into the piriform sinus. Laryngoceles can be excised, but spontaneous regression and fibrosis have been observed.[15]

REFERENCES

1. Campbell, J. S., Wiglesworth, F. W., Latarroca, R., and Wilde, H.: Congenital subglottic hemangiomas of the larynx and trachea in infants, Pediatrics 22:727, 1958.
2. Dargeon, H. W., and Daly, J. F.: Hemangioma of the larynx in an infant, J. Pediat. 39:738, 1951.
3. Schneider, P.: Die Missbildungen der Atmungsorgane, in Schwalbe, E. (ed.), *Die Morphologie der Missbildungen des Menschen und der Tiere* (Jena: Gustav Fischer, 1911), Vol. 3, pts. 8–11.
4. McHugh, H. E., and Loch, W. E.: Congenital webs of the larynx, Laryngoscope 52:43, 1942.
5. Hudson, P.: Congenital web of the larynx, A.M.A. Am. J. Dis. Child. 81:545, 1951.
6. Arey, L. B.: *Developmental Anatomy* (7th ed.; Philadelphia: W. B. Saunders Company, 1965).
7. Smith, I. I., and Bain, A. D.: Congenital atresia of the larynx, Ann. Otol. 74:338, 1965.
8. Sayre, J. W., and Hall, E. G.: Anomalies of the larynx associated with tracheoesophageal fistula, Pediatrics 13: 150, 1954.
9. Heineken, H.: Beitrag zur angeborenen Kehlkopfatresie, Frankfurt. Ztschr. Path. 63:30, 1952.
10. Kovacs, E.: Angeborene Atresie des Kehlkopfes mit beiderseitiger Lungenhyperplasie und Hydrops fetus universalis, Virchows Arch. path. Anat. 288:243, 1933.
11. Blumberg, J. B., Stevenson, J. K., Lemire, R. J., and Boyden, E. A.: Laryngotracheoesophageal cleft, the embryologic implications: Review of the literature, Surgery 57: 559, 1965.
12. Forrester, H. C., Morrow, R. C., and Soule, A. B., Jr.: Laryngocele: A case report, Am. J. Roentgenol. 81:322, 1959.
13. Kan, P. T. L.: Über einen Fall von kongenitalen Larynxluftsäcken bei einem Kinde von sechzehn Tagen, Ztschr. Laryng. Rhin. Otol. 1:51, 1908.
14. Freedman, A. O.: Diseases of the ventricle of Morgagni with special reference to pyocele of a congenital air sac of the ventricle, Arch. Otolaryng. 28:329, 1938.
15. Horowitz, S.: Laryngoceles, J. Laryng. & Otol. 65:724, 1951.
16. Ferguson, C. F., and Flake, C. G.: Subglottic hemangioma as cause of respiratory obstruction in infant, Ann. Otol. 70:1095, 1961.
17. Tefft, M.: The radiotherapeutic management of subglottic hemangioma in children, Radiology 86:207, 1966.
18. Maier, H. C.: Hemangiomas of the subglottic region, trachea, and mediastinum in infancy and childhood, Ann. Thoracic Surg. 3:514, 1967.

68

The Trachea and Bronchi

Absence and Stenosis of the Trachea

COMPLETE ABSENCE of the trachea sometimes is seen in monstrous cyclopic, acephalic or acardiac fetuses but not in viable infants. It is of interest that in such cases the lungs may be formed and be connected directly with the larynx, or both the larynx and the trachea may be absent despite formation of lungs. The bifurcation of the trachea may originate in the esophagus.[1] Joshi,[36] in 1969, found 16 cases in the literature and added the description of a newborn girl who also had ureteric atresia and tetralogy of Fallot. Communication between bronchi and esophagus is the rule.

Congenital constrictions or stenoses of the trachea are compatible with life and therefore are of clinical importance. They may be congenital fibrous strictures consisting of webs or fibrous stenoses of tracheal segments. A different type of stenosis is due to cartilaginous deformity and a third type is caused by vascular compression.

Fibrous constrictions or webs may be located in the upper or lower trachea. If a central opening is present and visible with the bronchoscope, dilatation of the opening may lead to relief of the tracheal obstruction.[2] Fibrous strictures have been observed postoperatively in the tracheas of infants with tracheo-esophageal fistula, the stenosis being located at the point from which the lower esophageal segment had been removed from the trachea. It is not certain that in such cases the tracheal obstruction was congenital or rather the result of the operation,[2] but anomalies of the respiratory tract do accompany tracheo-esophageal fistulas.

Congenital stenosis of the trachea in its entire length may be combined with dwarfing of the larynx.[1] If due to absence or deformity of tracheal cartilages, it may be located in the upper, the middle, or the lower trachea.[1] In infants with tracheomalacia, the tracheal wall is extremely flaccid because of retarded development. Symptoms of severe stridor with dyspnea and cyanosis disappear with the passage of a bronchoscope, and eventually subside entirely with increasing age.[2]

Hemangiomas of the trachea in infants causing airway obstruction are rare. Although such hemangiomas are congenital, symptoms may be delayed until several months after birth. Stridor, dyspnea, wheezing, cough and cyanosis can alternate with periods of well-being. Sometimes the symptoms are attributed to an infection or foreign body. Hemangiomas on other parts of the body may suggest a similar lesion in the trachea. It has been said that females are affected more often than males. Roentgenograms may show a mass projecting into the trachea. Treatment by irradiation, surgical excision or cautery has been successful.[3]

Congenital anomalies of the cardiovascular system may produce tracheal and esophageal stenosis. Stridor and dysphagia can be caused in infants by a right aortic arch, right descending thoracic aorta and a ligamentum arteriosum producing a constrictive ring. These vascular anomalies are well known (p. 530), and division of the ligamentum arteriosum leads to relief of stridor and dysphagia. Holinger *et al.*,[2] who observed similar symptoms in patients with tracheal stenosis due to vascular constriction, always found deformity or absence of tracheal cartilage at the site of the vascular anomaly.

Abnormal Segmentation of the Cartilaginous Skeleton of the Trachea or Bronchi

Segmentation of the cartilaginous skeleton may be very irregular. Rarely, the trachea forms an almost completely cartilaginous tube with quite defective formation of the pars membranacea. In milder cases, some of the cartilaginous rings are completely or partially connected by cartilaginous bridges with one another. Such connected cartilaginous rings are particularly developed in the upper part of the trachea, where union of the first tracheal ring with the cricoid is common. Another variation consists of posterior continuation of the rings, so that they extend into the membranous part of the trachea. Intercalary cartilages are flat, irregular, small cartilages in the posterior wall of the trachea.[1] Deficient cartilage in a bronchus can result in bronchomalacia and repeated attacks of pneumonia.[4]

Tracheal Diverticula

True tracheal diverticula represent rudimentary tracheal bronchi. Such diverticula usually occur in males and on the right side of the trachea, originating from the lateral wall at its transition to the membranous portion. They appear as short, cylindrical projections that have the composition of the tracheal wall and are directed obliquely downward, like bronchi.[1]

Acquired diverticula, which also have a predilection for the right posterolateral border of the trachea and usually are situated below the lower pole of the thyroid gland, have been distinguished from true congenital diverticula. According to MacKinnon,[5] their structure indicates that they arise by cystic distention of the ducts of mucous glands. They are always associated with chronic respiratory disease and are found in approximately 1 of 100 necropsies of adults. Ettman and Keel[6] described roentgenographic features of tracheal diverticulosis in adults and found it associated with bronchiectasis. They thought that weakness of the tracheal and bronchial walls must be present and coupled with chronic lung disease to produce this condition.

Congenital Fistulas of the Trachea

The most common tracheal fistulas are associated with esophageal anomalies. Usually, they originate near the carina and lead into the lower half of the esophagus. The openings vary greatly in size. Other types of tracheo-esophageal fistulas are discussed in Chapter 74.

Bronchial Atresia

Sante[7] believed that congenital bronchial atresia follows failure of a bronchial bud's growth. If the failure is complete, the bronchiole is represented only by a cord. If growth is resumed after a time, tubularity is established distal to an area of atresia and a cyst may develop. A congenital bronchial atresia can be represented in later life by a smooth, thin septum that separates a patent bronchus from a fluid-filled intrapulmonary bronchogenic cyst.[8]

Tracheal Bronchi

An abnormal partition of the trachea occurs occasionally, showing, in addition to the main bronchi, a smaller branch of variable size that usually originates over the right and exceptionally over the left main bronchus.[1] The anomalous tracheal branch runs obliquely downward into the upper lobe, which it supplies in part.

In many mammals, such as swine, cattle, sheep, goats, camels and giraffes, the bronchus supplying the right upper lobe arises regularly from the trachea. In man, normally the bronchus to the right upper lobe divides into an apical, a posterolateral and an anterolateral bronchus (Fig. 68-1, *A*). If, in addition to this normal segmental bronchial pattern, a bronchus arises above the point of origin of the right main bronchus, one speaks of a supernumerary apical bronchus (Fig. 68-1, *B*). If, however, the bronchus to the right upper lobe divides only into the posterolateral and anterolateral branches, the tracheal bronchus is considered a displaced apical bronchus (Fig. 68-1, *C*) called "pre-eparterial bronchus" by Boyden.[9]

The abnormal bronchus may vary greatly in size and may arise anywhere from the point above the right main-stem bronchus to as high as 5 cm. above the carina, the majority being located 2 cm. or less above the bifurcation. Sometimes the supernumerary bronchus may give rise to a supernumerary apical lobe separated from the remainder of the upper lobe by a fissure. Neuhauser *et al.*[10] described a congenital communication between the biliary system and the respiratory tract, an anomaly caused by an accessory bronchus that penetrated the diaphragm and, below it, joined an aberrant hepatic duct. Holinger *et al.*[2] reported a case in which the bronchus leading to the right lung was found to originate on the medial aspect of the left main bronchus. This observation was made bronchoscopically and confirmed on exploratory thoracotomy, which had been performed to relieve dyspnea from tracheal compression. These authors also observed right and left upper lobe bronchi originating from the trachea. The trachea continued downward to give rise to both the right and left main bronchi, from each of which originated a distinct middle and lower lobe and bronchus. Such an abnormal bifurcation was seen in a female infant who also had dextrocardia, mild rotation of the intestine, single accessory digits, deformities of the pelvis and right foot and congenital absence of the spleen. There were three lobes of both the right and left lungs. Abnormal branching of the trachea and bronchi has been observed in other cases with the asplenia syndrome.[11] Bremer[12] found, in 80 embryos examined, 4 with abnormal bronchial buds from the right side of the trachea. He explained the relatively frequent occurrence of such accessory tracheal buds by their ready spread in the mass of loose mesenchyme that surrounds the respiratory anlage in embryos of 5–6 weeks and believed that some of these abnormal buds are absorbed into the growing walls of the parent stem and disappear before the child is born. If they persist, they may develop into an accessory lung, a diverticulum or a cyst within the lung or within the pleural cavity.[13] Such accessory bronchi and cysts have a wide distribution, since, at the time of their first appearance in embryos of 5 or 6 weeks, the trachea and esophagus lie in a mass of loose mesenchyme through which the new buds can penetrate readily. The tissue into which they grow becomes mediastinum, which is continuous with the base of the neck, the dorsal wall of the chest and the septum transversum. The accessory bronchi may, therefore, grow into any of these regions, where they can be found as cysts or as masses of atelectatic lung, free or attached by tube or pedicle. Bronchial cysts have been reported behind the manubrium, near the suprarenal gland, in the diaphragm or coronary ligament or in the septa within the liver. A common location for small cysts is at the bifurcation of the trachea.[13]

Often, the finding of a supernumerary tracheal

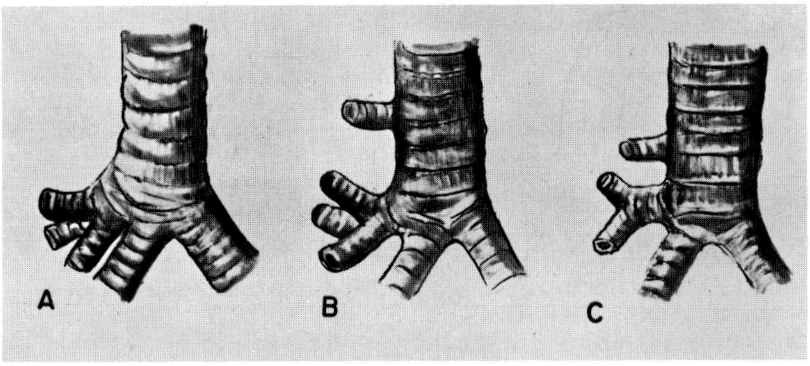

Fig. 68-1. – **A,** normal bronchial division. **B,** supernumerary apical bronchus. **C,** pre-eparterial bronchus.

bronchus is accidental in bronchoscopy or bronchography without causing symptoms,[14] but occasionally patients have complaints due to pathologic conditions involving the abnormal bronchus. A chronic productive cough with copious sputum, repeated episodes of pneumonia and pain in the right hemithorax can be symptoms of this anatomic anomaly.

Left Eparterial Bronchus

On the right side, the superior lobe bronchus normally comes off above the pulmonary artery and is called, therefore, the eparterial bronchus. A left eparterial bronchus occurs, according to Boyden,[9] in not more than 1% of necropsy cases. In such specimens, the left pulmonary artery enters the left lung between two bronchial stems that arise separately from the left primary bronchus. Boyden believed that in embryos of 7–8 mm. length, or on the thirtieth to thirty-second day, two left upper lobe buds instead of one must have arisen from the left primary lung sac to explain a left eparterial bronchus. One case of such a bronchus was found in a twin girl who also had agenesis of the right lung. These anomalies were absent in the identical twin sister of the affected child.[9] Bilateral eparterial bronchi seem to occur rather frequently in the asplenia syndrome (Chapter 80) together with symmetric lobation of the lungs.[15]

Displacement of Segmental and Subsegmental Bronchi

These changes of the smaller bronchi represent variations rather than malformations of the bronchial tree. However, in recent years it has become likely that such anomalous bronchi may occasionally predispose to disease and become of practical importance in cases of surgical resection. Boyden[9] stated that the displacement occurs at the time when the segmental and subsegmental buds appear, namely, in embryos 8–11 mm. long, 34–40 days after ovulation. Ando[16] has shown that even in monozygotic twins the respective right and left lungs have slightly different patterns. Boyden[9] mentioned some of these variants. On the right side, a bronchus that supplies all or part of the apical segment may branch off the trachea or from the lateral wall of the right primary bronchus before the lobar bronchus is given off. Such a pre-eparterial bronchus, as mentioned before, should not be considered a supernumerary bronchus but merely a displaced apical ramus or apical bronchus. Conversely, one of the upper lobe bronchi may originate at a lower level. For instance, the right anterior bronchus may arise from the middle lobe stem – a variation termed "post-eparterial bronchus" by Boyden.[9] Although normally the left medial basal bronchus and left anterior basal bronchus arise from a common stem, Boyden[9] found in 7% of his specimens that the left medial basal bronchus arose alone at a level higher on the tree. Another anomaly on the left side may be absence of the posterior ramus of the anterior segment.

Congenital Bronchiectases

The existence and frequency of congenital bronchiectases has been a controversial subject ever since Grawitz,[17] in 1880, published 4 cases of cystic bronchiectasis found in a 5-month-old fetus, in a newborn infant, in a child 1 year of age and in a man 25 years of age. In these cases, a main bronchus and its branches were dilated, so that a central cyst existed into which many secondary cysts opened. In one instance, the cysts were separated from the bronchial tree but in three cases there were open communications. The lining of the cyst walls by ciliated columnar epithelium suggested that the anomalies were bronchiectases. Despite these and similar findings before and after Grawitz, there is still no agreement concerning this subject. Although some experienced clinicians and pathologists believe that congenital bronchiectases are rare curiosities or nonexistent, others assert that, in children, 80% of the bronchiectases of the lower lobes are congenital.[18] Such differing opinions are due partly to different observations and experiences and partly to semantic confusion. Generally, it is admitted that many congential cysts of the lung are lined by bronchial mucosa and have walls containing smooth muscle and cartilage, thus resembling greatly dilated bronchi (p. 610). Since the existence of such congenital bronchogenic cysts cannot be denied, the existence of congenital bronchiectases – dilated bronchi – must be admitted. Another source of misunderstanding is the erroneous use of the word "congenital" for "hereditary." By showing that a tendency to bronchiectases can be hereditary, one has not proved that such bronchiectases are congenital, i.e., present at birth. It is likely that most bronchiectases for which hereditary tendency can be demonstrated are not present at birth and should, therefore, not be called "congenital."

The history of the controversy on congenital bronchiectases was told in detail by Kartagener.[19] Bronchiectases, as first recognized by Laënnec in 1819 (cited by Kartagener[19]), were acquired and attributable to infections, trauma, and so forth. When Bard,[20] in 1899, stressed the activities of endogenous pathogenetic factors in the enlargement of hollow organs such as the bronchi, he referred to a congenital *disposition* for these changes. Peiser,[21] writing on congenital bronchiectases in 1910, considered them not a rarity; he enumerated many cases from the literature and added a few of his own. His cases were either lung cysts of bronchial origin or the congenital nature of the pulmonary lesions was deduced from the presence of associated congenital defects of the lung or of similar lesions in a relative. Hueter,[22] who, in 1914, discussed congenital bronchiectases and congenital honeycomb lung, believed that the number and size of congenital cavities depends on the time of bronchial development in which the arrest occurs. If the arrest occurs in an early stage, few, but large, cavities are formed, whereas, in later stages, arrest results in more numerous but smaller cavities. In the latter case, the afferent bronchi usually are open. Sauerbruch's[18] belief in the prevalence of congenital bronchiectases in children represents a surgeon's point of view. He found no pleural adhesions associated with the bronchial dilatations but noticed thickening of the bronchial tree within normal lung tissue. Bronchiectases often were combined with pulmonary cysts and symptoms dated from early childhood. Kartagener,[19] reporting on 142 cases of bronchiectases in children and adults, stressed the predilection of certain lobes, particularly accessory lobes, for bronchial dilatations and the presence of so-called acquired bronchiectases in bronchial walls without signs of inflammation. In addition, bronchiectases frequently are associated with other malformations of the lung, of the respiratory tract or of other organs. Their association with situs inversus and sinus disease has been established as the Kartagener syndrome. Congenital bronchiectases in a case of Turner syndrome were reported by Koch and Rossipal.[23] Turpin and Cany[24] described a syndrome of bronchiectases, tracheo-esophageal fistula, diverticulum of the trachea, costovertebral anomalies, heterotopic thoracic duct and mega-esophagus. Kartagener[19] believed that the occurrence of bronchiectases in certain families and in pairs of twins points to a congenital origin, but he realized that such an observation actually proved only a congenital predisposition to the disorder. To this may be added that in cases of cystic fibrosis of the pancreas, a genetically determined disease, bronchiectases occur occasionally in late stages of the disease. They are attributable to hereditary factors but are not congenital and appear only after exposure to injurious environmental agents.

Kartagener Syndrome

There exists a relatively frequent association between bronchiectases, situs inversus and nasal disorders such as polyposis, chronic sinusitis or rhinitis,[19,25] but the interdependence of these pathologic manifestations is not clear. Attempts to find a common denominator for these anomalies have failed, but it is assumed that for unknown reasons persons with certain types of situs inversus also have underdevelopment of the paranasal sinuses and a tendency to develop bronchiectases in early life. Apparently there exists a hereditary constitutional disposition to develop these anomalies, but a specific basis for this is not known. That the combination of situs inversus and bronchiectases is not coincidental was shown by Adams and Churchill,[26] who found the incidence of bronchiectases in cases of situs inversus to be 21.7% in the Massachusetts General Hospital population, whereas the incidence of bronchiectases in the hospital population in general was 0.3%. The Kartagener syndrome has been observed repeatedly in siblings. Gorham and Merselis[27] stated that of 125 reported cases, 23 occurred among siblings, but it seems that inheritance through several generations has not been observed. The triad described by Kartagener may be found dissociated in a family. Thus, Bergstrom *et al.*[28] described 2 brothers with the fully developed Kartagener syndrome and in the same family a sister and a brother with bronchiectases and chronic sinusitis but without situs inversus. This family report, as well as others,[29] demonstrates that dissociation of the symptoms is possible and that explanations of bronchiectases and sinusitis as secondary complications of situs inversus are not convincing.

Torgersen[30] reported a 25% incidence of bronchiectases and nasal polyposis among 77 siblings of persons with Kartagener syndrome, whereas among 496 siblings of persons with situs inversus alone he found only 3 with nasal polyps.

Patients with this syndrome show nasal discharge, frequent colds and chronic bronchitis or pneumonia from early infancy on. As the disease progresses, chronic productive cough, foul smelling sputum, hemoptysis, asthma, emphysema, bronchiectases, pulmonary osteoarthropathy and cor pulmonale may develop. Often there is absence of the frontal sinuses and hypoplasia of the paranasal sinuses. Nasal polyposis and tubular bilateral bronchiectases are common, but it is likely that the bronchiectases are not congenital, since they develop during childhood or even later. Stillborn or newborn infants with dextrocardia have not been found to have bronchiectases.[28]

Associated malformations are relatively rare in complete situs inversus, and it seems that they are not frequent in cases of Kartagener syndrome. However, in the family reported by Bergstrom *et al.*,[28] one brother with situs inversus also had hypospadias and the other had cyanotic congenital heart disease. Ocular anomalies in Kartagener syndrome were reported by Collier,[31] who observed myopia, iris coloboma, pseudopapilledema and other changes. Segal *et al.*[32] reported pigmentary degeneration of the retina and congenital cataract in a case of Kartagener syndrome. There were similar eye changes in the mother and 2 siblings of the patient.

Bronchogenic Cysts of the Mediastinum

The respiratory tract has a common origin with the esophagus from the primitive foregut, which leads to a close association of developmental anomalies of these two systems. Bronchogenic cysts result from an abnormal budding of the tracheobronchial tree. If the continuity of the bronchial tree is maintained, the cyst is intrapulmonary, but if the mass of cells becomes separated from the tracheobronchial tree, there may be no continuity with the bronchial lumen. Separated cysts gradually increase in size because of the distention produced by the secretion within the cavity. The majority of bronchogenic cysts are found in relationship to the trachea or main bronchi, but occasionally the cyst may be in close association with the esophagus or the vertebral bodies.[33]

Endobronchial Hamartomas

These benign tumors can cause bronchial obstruction, with cough, bloody sputum, atelectasis, pneumonia and pleurisy. Males are affected more often than females. Bronchus carcinoma is erroneously suggested by signs and symptoms. The hamartomas are made up of masses of cartilage, bone, smooth muscle, adipose and fibrous tissue and are covered by respiratory epithelium. Although they are developmental errors, they do not seem to be related to the systemic hamartoses (Chapters 121–123). Manifestations occur in adult life.[34]

Congenital Bronchomalacia

A case of isolated left bronchomalacia was described by Gupta *et al.*[4] Recurrent episodes of pneumonia resulted from the anomaly, which was treated by left pneumonectomy. Congenital segmental bronchomalacia[37] can lead to collapse of the bronchus on expiration, with trapping of air resulting in regional emphysema, recurrent pneumonia and death.

Congenital Bronchobiliary Fistula

This rare malformation manifests itself as aspiration pneumonia with bile-stained sputum. It can be diagnosed by bronchoscopy and treated by surgical excision of the intrathoracic portion of the fistula.[35]

REFERENCES

1. Schneider, P.: Die Missbildungen der Atmungsorgane, in Schwalbe, E. (ed.), *Die Morphologie der Missbildungen des Menschen und der Tiere* (Jena: Gustav Fischer, 1911), Vol. 3, pts. 8–11.
2. Holinger, P. H., Johnston, K. C., Parchet, V. N., and Zimmerman, A.: Congenital malformations of the trachea, bronchi and lung, Ann. Otol. 61:1159, 1952.
3. Hudson, H. L., and McAlister, W. H.: Obstructing tracheal hemangioma in infancy, Am. J. Roentgenol. 93:428, 1965.
4. Gupta, T. G. C. M., Goldberg, S. J., Lewis, E., and Fonkalsrud, E. W.: Congenital bronchomalacia, Am. J. Dis. Child. 115:88, 1968.
5. MacKinnon, D.: Tracheal diverticula, J. Path. & Bact. 65: 513, 1953.
6. Ettman, I. K., and Keel, D. T., Jr.: Tracheal diverticulosis, Radiology 78:187, 1962.
7. Sante, L. R.: Cystic disease of the lung, Radiology 33:152, 1939.
8. Ramsay, B. H., and Byron, F. X.: Mucocele, congenital bronchiectasis and bronchiogenic cyst, J. Thoracic Surg. 26:21, 1953.
9. Boyden, E. A.: Developmental anomalies of the lungs, Am. J. Surg. 89:79, 1955.
10. Neuhauser, E. B. D., Elkin, M., and Landing, B. H.: Congenital direct communication between biliary system and respiratory tract, Am. J. Dis. Child. 83:654, 1952.
11. Ivemark, B. F.: Implications of agenesis of the spleen on the pathogenesis of conotruncus anomalies in childhood, Acta paediat. scandinav. 44 (supp.) 104:1, 1955.
12. Bremer, J. L.: Accessory bronchi in embryos; their occurrence and probable fate, Anat. Rec. 54:361, 1932.
13. Bremer, J. L.: *Congenital Anomalies of the Viscera. Their Embryological Basis* (Cambridge, Mass.: Harvard University Press, 1957).
14. Harris, J. H., Jr.: The clinical significance of the tracheal bronchus, Am. J. Roentgenol. 79:228, 1958.
15. Hjelt, L., and Hakosalo, J.: Congenital asplenia. Case reports and a review of the literature, Ann. paediat. Fenniae 5 (supp.) 12:3, 1959.
16. Ando, T.: Über die bronchiale Ramifikation bei den Japanischen Zwillingsfeten, Folia anat. jap. 23:167, 1951.
17. Grawitz, P.: Über angeborene Bronchiektasie, Virchows Arch. path. Anat. 82:217, 1880.
18. Sauerbruch, F.: Die operative Behandlung der kongenitalen Bronchiektasen, Arch. klin. Chir. 180:312, 1934.
19. Kartagener, M.: Das Problem der Kongenitalität und Heredität der Bronchiektasien, Ergebn. inn. Med. u. Kinderh. 49:378, 1935.
20. Bard, L.: *Précis d'Anatomie Pathologique* (2d ed.; Paris: Masson & Cie, 1899).
21. Peiser, J.: Über angeborene Bronchiektasie, Monatsschr. Kinderh. 8:602, 1910.
22. Hueter, C.: Über angeborene Bronchiektasien und angeborene Wabenlunge, Beitr. path. Anat. 59:520, 1914.
23. Koch, J., and Rossipal, E.: Turnersyndrom mit angeborenen Bronchiektasien und passagerem Auftreten eines ungewöhnlichen Globulins, Arch, Kinderh, 174:342, 1966.

24. Turpin, R., and Cany, J.: Bronchectasies et malformations congénitales. Syndrome d'ectasies broncho-oesophagiennes avec fistule oesophago-trachéale et malformations vertébrocostales, Arch. franç. pédiat. 13:797, 1956.
25. Kartagener, M.: Zur Pathogenese der Bronchiektasen; Bronchiektasien bei Situs viscerum inversus, Beitr. Klin. Erforsch. Tuberk. 83:489, 1933.
26. Adams, R., and Churchill, E. D.: Situs inversus, sinusitis, bronchiectasis; report of 5 cases, including frequency statistics, J. Thoracic Surg. 7:206, 1937.
27. Gorham, G. W., and Merselis, J. G., Jr.: Kartagener's triad: A family study, Bull. Johns Hopkins Hosp. 104:11, 1959.
28. Bergstrom, W. H., Cook, C. D., Scannell, J. G., and Berenberg, W.: Situs inversus, bronchiectasis and sinusitis, Pediatrics 6:573, 1950.
29. Overholt, E. L., and Bauman, D. F.: Variants of Kartagener's syndrome in the same family, Ann. Int. Med. 48: 574, 1958.
30. Torgersen, J.: Transposition of viscera, bronchiectasis and nasal polyps; a genetical analysis and a contribution to the problem of constitution, Acta radiol. 28:17, 1947.
31. Collier, M. M.: Constatations ophtalmologiques dans le syndrome de Kartagener, Bull. Socopht. France 74:429, 1961.
32. Segal, P., Kikiela, M., Mrzyglod, S., and Zeromska-zbierska, I.: Kartagener's syndrome with familial eye changes, Am. J. Ophth. 55:1043, 1963.
33. Meier, H. C.: Bronchiogenic cysts of mediastinum, Ann. Surg. 127:476, 1948.
34. Dovenbarger, W. V., and Elstun, W.: Endobronchial hamartoma, Am. J. Med. 30:965, 1961.
35. Weitzman, J. J., Cohen, S. R., Woods, L. O., Jr., and Chadwick, D. L.: Congenital bronchobiliary fistula, J. Pediat. 73:329, 1968.
36. Joshi, V. V.: Tracheal agenesis, Am. J. Dis. Child. 117: 341, 1969.
37. MacMahon, H. E., and Ruggieri, J.: Congenital segmental bronchomalacia, Am. J. Dis. Child. 118:923, 1969.

69

The Lung

BOYDEN[1] and Breton and Dubois[2] reviewed the subject of congenital malformations of the lung and the pertinent bibliography then available. Other monographs on pulmonary diseases and anomalies[3,4] include chapters dealing with congenital defects. A symposium on the development of the lung was held in 1965. In the publication of this symposium, phylogeny, ontogeny and physiology of the lung during fetal and neonatal life are discussed thoroughly.[5] Vascular anomalies of the lungs as seen in roentgenograms were reviewed by Good.[6]

Agenesis, Aplasia and Hypoplasia

Under *agenesis* of the lung, one understands malformations with complete absence of the lungs, the bronchi and the vascular structures. In *aplasia*, the trachea shows small rudimentary bronchi but absence of pulmonary and vascular structures. In pulmonary *hypoplasia*, the bronchial tree is poorly developed and pulmonary tissue shows an abnormal histologic picture. Hypoplasia can be partial or total.[7] According to Boyden,[1] the factors that prevent the formation of the lungs must become effective not later than 26 days after ovulation, that is, early in the second month of menstrual age.

BILATERAL AGENESIS AND APLASIA

By 1958, only 4 cases of bilateral absence of the lung had been described in children carried near or to term.[8-11] These 4 cases can be discussed together irrespective of classification as agenesis or aplasia. The 4 children – 2 males, 1 female and 1 of unknown sex – were born normal in size and length for their gestational ages. They appeared externally normal and the chest size was not diminished. The trachea ended blindly or primitive bronchial buds were present. In the case of Schmit,[8] the trachea and the esophagus communicated by means of a wide opening. In all cases, the pericardial sac was present and the heart was four-chambered, but cardiac malformations were present that differed slightly. The pulmonary trunk joined the aorta at the point at which the aorta and ductus arteriosus normally meet.[11] The left auricle did not receive any pulmonary veins in the 4 infants described, but in the case of Tuynman and Gardner[10] the inferior vena cava drained into it, and in that of Claireaux and Ferreira[11] a left superior vena cava entered this chamber. The foramen ovale may be closed or an interatrial septum may be present.[11] The aorta may be normal or have a right-sided arch[10] or a coarctation.[11] The diaphragm is in a high position. In one case, half of the thorax was filled by a thymus[11] and in another case a portion of the liver extended into the right chest. Osseous abnormalities of the neck were present in Schmit's[8] case, and an accessory spleen in that of Tuynman and Gardner.[10] Respiratory movements have been observed and survival to 15 or 45 minutes has been reported.[11] Total tracheopulmonary agenesis associated with asplenia (Chapter 80), agenesis of the umbilical artery, cardiovascular anomalies and other malformations were recorded by Devi and More[12] in a girl born alive at term weighing 2,050 Gm. The authors tabulated 4 cases of bilateral pulmonary agenesis recorded previously. In addition to these children, Oyamada *et al.*[13] tabulated the cases of 2 fetuses with congenital absence of both lungs. In 1754, Roderer[14] apparently described a fetus in whom only the heart and the thymus were found in the thoracic cavity, the larynx ending blindly. The second case of Saito,[15] published in 1902, concerned a fetus in which only the heart was found in the thoracic cavity, both lungs being absent. The larynx ended blindly and the isthmus of the thyroid was lacking.

In the embryologic development of the lung, the primary bronchi appear at the 4-mm. stage, and the situation described in children with bilateral absence of the lung corresponds approximately to the 5-mm. stage of human embryos (the fourth and fifth week of fetal life).[10]

Unilateral Agenesis

Although a distinction has been made between agenesis and aplasia of the lung, the difference is not always clear-cut and the two conditions can be described together. In contrast to bilateral agenesis of the lung, unilateral absence is compatible with life, but the mortality of children with this anomaly is high, which probably is due to the great susceptibility of the single lung to infections or to the presence of other malformations. In many instances, survival to adult age is possible, as shown in the case of Heerup,[16] who found absence of the left lung at necropsy of a woman who was more than 70 years of age. But it is believed that approximately half the children with unilateral pulmonary agenesis die under 1 year of age. In reported cases, the left side was found affected somewhat more often than the right and females predominated over males.[17-19]

Unilateral agenesis of the lung has been described in identical twins, both twins showing the anomaly. In the cases of Finkelstein,[20] the left lung was rudimentary in one twin and the right in the other. In the twins reported by Yount,[21] the right lung was absent in each identical twin but 4 twin pairs were discordant in regard to unilateral pulmonary agenesis.[22-24,98] It seems possible that, in some instances, twinning may be causally related to this anomaly. Agenesis of one lung has been observed in trisomy 18[25] and in trisomy of a C-group chromosome.[26] Field,[22] taking histories of mothers of children with pulmonary agenesis, obtained, in some of the cases, reports of trauma or infection during pregnancy. Warkany *et al.*[27] induced congenital absence of one lung by maternal vitamin A deficiency in rats that had, in addition, ocular, cardiovascular and urogenital defects. Of 50 abnormal young, 5 had agenesis of the left lung associated with absence of the left pulmonary artery.

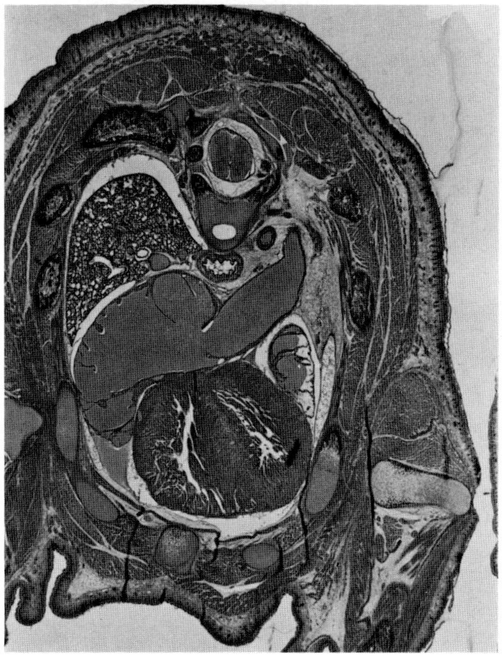

Fig. 69-1.—Transverse section through the thorax of young of a female rat that was vitamin A deficient to the twelfth day of pregnancy. Agenesis of left lung (and left pulmonary artery).

In the pathogenesis of absence of one lung, a number of associated anomalies have been considered as causative, i.e., anomalous blood vessels, a hypertrophic thymus and others, but it is unlikely that such associated anomalies can cause pulmonary agenesis, which must arise very early in embryos 5 mm. long, whereas the pulmonary vessels develop somewhat later.[2,22]

Children with unilateral agenesis of the lung may appear externally normal or show asymmetry of the thorax, with underdevelopment of the affected side, scoliosis and general deficit in weight and height. Sometimes dyspnea and cyanosis are present. On x-ray examination, a mediastinal shift to the affected side of the thorax is found, with tracheal, esophageal and skeletal scoliosis. Bronchoscopy shows the absence of the carina and a single bronchial lumen. Angiocardiography demonstrates the absence of one pulmonary artery. The single lung of the patients is always increased in volume and herniates into the empty hemithorax. Striking anomalies in the bronchovascular pattern have been reported by Thomas and Boyden.[24] In 3 cases of agenesis of the right lung observed by Boyden,[1] the left lung exhibited variants from the usual pattern. Two had lobes with variations of the segments and an eparterial bronchus. In the third case there were such vascular anomalies as coarctation of the aorta, persistent ductus arteriosus or a left postbronchial pulmonary artery. Although the histologic structure of these lungs appeared abnormal in some of the cases, the finding of enlarged alveolae and emphysema was the exception rather than the rule.

Diagnosis before death is possible by means of x-rays and bronchoscopy. In the differential diagnosis, pleurisy, empyema, diaphragmatic hernia, dextrocardia, tumors, atelectasis and foreign bodies must be considered.

Approximately half the cases are said to be complicated by associated malformations.[2,13,98] Skeletal anomalies such as scoliosis, vertebral defects, Sprengel deformity, absence of the radius[28] or ulna or clubfoot are not rare. Caffey[29] was impressed with the frequency of vertebral anomalies, especially hemivertebrae, in cases of pulmonary aplasia and believed that the two anomalies represent a syndrome. Anencephaly, hydrocephaly, microcephaly, cleft palate, facial asymmetry, micrognathia, cardiovascular anomalies, tracheo-esophageal fistula, diaphragmatic hernia, anal atresia, anomalies of the spleen, horseshoe kidney, agenesis of a kidney and others have been observed. Schultze-Jena and Kosenow[30] reviewed the cases of unilateral pulmonary agenesis associated with esophageal atresia. In 5 of 11 cases, ventricular septal defect, coarctation of the aorta, diaphragmatic hernia, renal agenesis or horseshoe kidney, or absence of the genitalia or atresia ani were found together with the anomalies mentioned. It is obvious that some of the associated anomalies can cause the deaths of the patients with unilateral pulmonary agenesis. In the case of Maier and Gould,[23] the anomalous course of the pulmonary artery and the aorta, causing tracheal narrowing, was considered the cause of death.

The prognosis is variable. Although the condition is compatible with a long life, many children die early of pulmonary infections or of complications by associated malformations. The majority of the recognized patients are dead within the first decade.[19] The prognosis is more serious in cases of absence of the right lung than that of the left.[28]

Treatment was discussed by Warner *et al.*,[31] who recommended vigorous antibiotic therapy of respiratory infections. They considered thoracoplasty or plastic fillers in the anomalous pleural space for patients with pathologic manifestations, but concluded that such treatment remains controversial.

Hypoplasia

Oyamada *et al.*[13] reviewed 38 cases of pulmonary hypoplasia reported in the literature. Of these, 13 had been diagnosed during life. The majority of published cases referred to neonates and children, but the anomaly has been described occasionally in stillborn infants and survival to adult life is also possible. Males and females are affected equally. The left lung is involved slightly more often than the right and the hypoplasia may be bilateral. The size of the underdeveloped lung can vary from that of a pea to that of a sphere several inches in diameter. The corresponding bronchi either end blindly or are markedly hypoplastic or constricted. The hypoplastic lung tissue resembles fetal lung tissue or assumes, in rare cases, more mature aspects. The pulmonary vessels leading to the hypoplastic lung usually are vestigial or absent, and sometimes the rudiment of the lung is supplied by an artery from the thoracic aorta. The hypoplastic lung may be found near the chest wall, near the vertebral column or in the diaphragmatic gutter. The pleural cavity of the underdeveloped lung is filled either by connective tissue, fluid or the emphysematous contralateral lung. The heart and the mediastinal structures are shifted toward the side of the underdeveloped lung. The affected as well as the contralateral lung may show abnormal lobation. Ferencz[32] reviewed hypoplasia and other anomalies of the lung in relation to their vascular connections and analyzed hemodynamic data available in some of the cases.

Associated malformations have been observed repeatedly. The thorax often is asymmetric and deformed. Fusion of ribs and of vertebral bodies may be present. Cleft palate, abnormalities of the digits and clubfeet have been observed in affected patients. Enlargement of the thymus has been described repeatedly. Tracheo-esophageal fistula, communications between the lower esophagus and the bronchi, intestinal atresias and imperforate anus may accompany the pulmonary anomalies. A hypoplastic lung separated from the bronchial tree may be connected with the esophagus.[33] Small liver and accessory spleens have been described. The heart usually is large and shifted to the affected side, but true dextrocardia may occur also. Ventricular and atrial septal defects are not rare. Coarctation of the pulmonary artery and persistent left superior vena cava have been found. Association of pulmonary hypoplasia with anomalous pulmonary venous return, dextroposition of the heart, hypoplasia of the right pulmonary artery, subdiaphragmatic systemic arterial supply to the lower lobe of the right lung and cardiac malformations has been emphasized by Jue *et al.*[34] (Chapter 63). Horseshoe kidney, polycystic kidney and anomalies of the ureters have been observed occasionally. In renal agenesis, pulmonary hypoplasia is the rule.[35] Microcephaly, meningoceles and spina bifida are rare com-

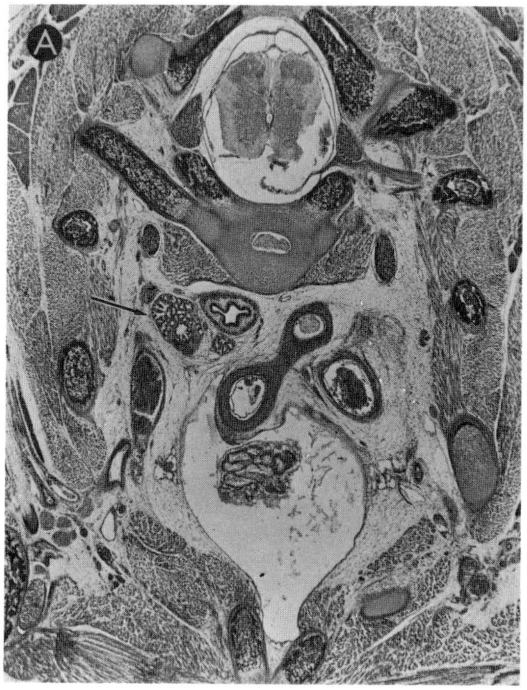

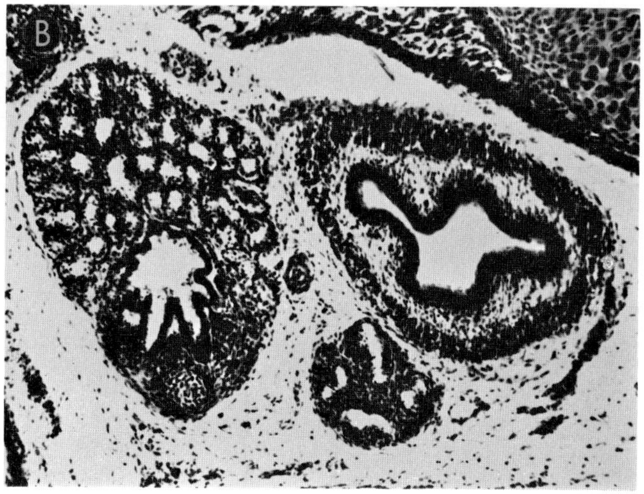

Fig. 69-2.—**A,** transverse section through a newborn rat fetus (treated with vitamin A deficiency until the fifteenth day of gestation) showing rudimentary lung tissue (**arrow**) to the right of the esophagus. There was agenesis of the left lung. **B,** high magnification of rudiments of the right lung and esophagus of the same animal.

plications. Hypoplasia of the lung is found often in cases of reduction of the thoracic space by intrathoracic cysts or diaphragmatic hernias. In the hypoplastic lungs, the bronchial branchings are reduced but size and number of the alveoli appear normal. After repair of the diaphragmatic hernia, growth within the acini can provide the lung with its normal complement of alveoli.[36] Pulmonary hypoplasia is also seen in achondroplastic infants; often it is combined with renal agenesis.[37]

Hypoplastic lungs have been produced experimentally in vitamin A-deficient rats.[27] Figures 69-2 and 69-3 show such hypoplastic lungs in rats, together with associated malformations.

In addition to hypoplasia of a whole lung, there may be hypoplasia of just one lobe. Foster-Carter[38] found, in a case of left-sided diaphragmatic hernia, a left bronchus that led into a tiny lung about the size of a hazelnut. Bronchography revealed a branching bronchial system in the hyperplastic left lung. In a case of Hepburn's,[39] the right lung appeared to have only two lobes, but in the oblique fissure a flattened piece of tissue that adhered to the right upper lobe was found. This was supplied by a small bronchus that originated at the expected site of the middle lobe bronchus.

Accessory or Supernumerary Lungs

Rudiments of lung tissue in ectopic positions are rare anomalies. According to Boyden,[1] the most common site of origin is the trachea. Small third lungs may arise from a tracheal bronchus or the posterior wall of the trachea. Such accessory lungs may be located above the lung or behind the manubrium of the sternum.

Another type of supernumerary lungs are the so-called Rokitansky lobes, which usually are found in the lower thorax, most often on the left side above the

Fig. 69-3.—Transverse section through a newborn rat treated during gestation with vitamin A deficiency. There is a ventricular septal defect. Dorsal to the atria, a rudimentary right lung is visible (**arrow**). There was no left lung.

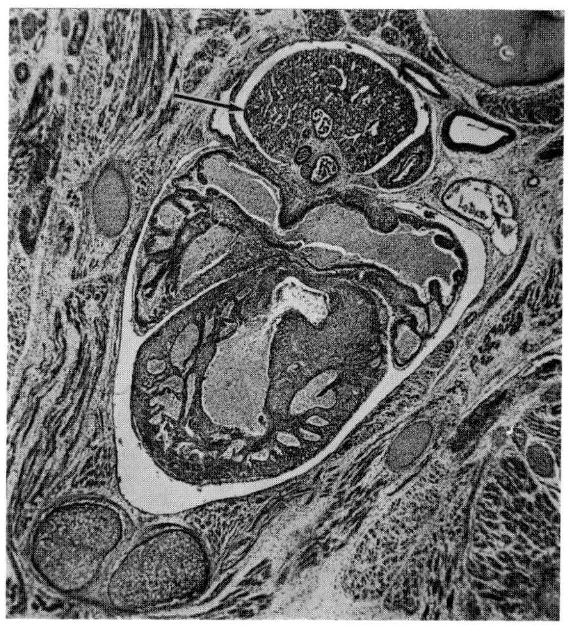

diaphragm and separated from the tracheobronchial tree and pulmonary vascular system. They may have connections with the esophagus, the diaphragm or the stomach and be associated with diaphragmatic defects. Such lungs seem to grow out of the esophagus or the stomach, and the connecting pedicle may have gastric epithelium. They, like tracheo-esophageal fistulas, are evidence of the close early connection and common origin of the intestinal and respiratory tracts. Boyden *et al.*[40] described a left lower accessory lung removed from a 10-day-old infant because of respiratory distress. The accessory lobe was attached by a short pedicle to the lower mediastinum just above the esophageal hiatus. Pulmonary ectopias have been explained as an excessive downward growth of the laryngotracheal groove to the diaphragm or as adhesions between the growing lung bud and the celomic epithelium, with separation of the normal respiratory tissue from the accessory lobe. In embryos approximately 6–10 mm. in length, the lungs project below the pleuroperitoneal membrane into the peritoneal cavity, contacting the liver and the stomach. Abnormal adhesions could hold a portion of the lung in contact with the abdominal organs.[1,41]

Supernumerary Fissures and Congenitally Fused Lobes

Supernumerary fissures are among the most frequent anomalies of the lungs. One of the more common sites for a supernumerary fissure is the line between the medial basal and anterior basal segments of the right lower lobe, which partially separates a "cardiac" or "infracardiac lobe" (Fig. 69-4, *A*). Dévé[42] and Boyden[1] found such fissures in more than one-third of human lungs examined, but they are rare on the left side. Another common abnormal fissure is a dorsal cleft that creates the so-called dorsal lobe of Nelson, which isolates the superior segment of the right or left lower lobe (Fig. 69-4, *B*). Dévé,[42] before Nelson, had found such a fissure in the right lower lobe approximately three times more often than in the left. The anomaly also can be bilateral.

Another common abnormal fissure is a left horizontal fissure that subdivides the left upper lobe into two more or less equal portions, the lower of which is called the left middle lobe even though this lobe is not always comparable to a right middle lobe (Fig. 69-4, *C*). Boyden[1] distinguished four types of left middle lobes. Abnormal supernumerary fissures were discussed in detail by Boyden[1] and by Breton and Dubois.[2]

Supernumerary lobation of the lung frequently is found in children with the asplenia syndrome (Chapter 80). Usually, both lungs have three lobes, thus being symmetrically subdivided; the bronchial bifurcation also is symmetric. Bilateral eparterial bronchi may be present.[43] In the review of the asplenia syndrome by Gilbert *et al.*,[44] supernumerary lobation was recorded in 55% of the cases. Abnormal lobation was reported in the lungs of some children damaged by thalidomide (p. 92).

Fissures, normal or supernumerary, develop during the period in which the segmental and subsegmental buds first appear and can be seen in 17–20-mm. embryos. Boyden[1] pointed out that the early appearance of fissures suggests that the infolding of visceral pleura around the bronchial buds depends partly on the prominence of certain buds at the time of their formation, a precociously appearing bronchus favoring the development of an accessory fissure. But subsequent growth may modify the early embryonic appearance, as seen in congenital fusions of lobes that are peripherally obliterated, whereas the deeper portions remain open and lined with the pleural investment.

Fig. 69-4. – **A,** diaphragmatic view of lungs and heart. The basis of the right lower lobe (*L.L.*) is divided by a supernumerary fissure that separates the medial basal and the anterior basal segments of the right lower lobe. **B,** lateral view of right lung with lower lobe divided by abnormal fissure separating the dorsal lobe of Nelson. **C,** lateral view of left lung with abnormal middle lobe. *U.L.* – upper lobe. *M.L.* – middle lobe. *L.L.* – lower lobe.

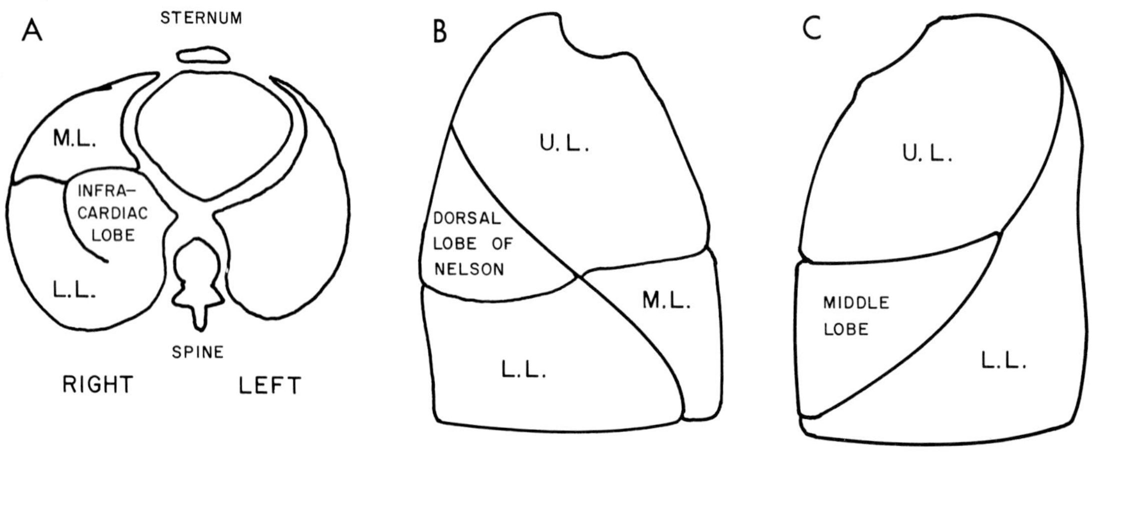

Congenital fusions of lobes are not rare. Kent and Blades[45] found the horizontal fissure absent in 21% of the lungs examined and incomplete in 67%. The oblique fissures were incomplete in 30% of both right and left lungs.

Lobe of the Azygos Vein

This malformation of the apex of the lungs has been known since the eighteenth century. Usually, it is found on the right side only, but in exceptional cases azygos lobes have been observed on the left also. In x-rayed lungs, the condition is recognized in approximately 0.3%,[1] but estimates vary from 0.1% to 4%.[46] In early fetal life, the azygos vein lies on the apex of the right upper lobe lateral to the mediastinum. As the heart descends during development and the apex ascends, the vein may become embedded in the pulmonary apex. The parietal and the visceral layers of the pleura are drawn into the fissure created by the vein, which results in a covering of the cleft by four layers. In roentgenograms, the azygos lobe is separated from the rest of the anterior lobe by a distinct pleural shadow that is convex laterally and descends downward and inward toward the hilus. At the lower extremity of the fissure, the azygos vein casts a small circular or oval shadow. The combined shadow of the pleura along the fissure and the vein (Fig. 69-5) resembles the shape of an inverted comma. The angle at which the vein descends determines the size of the wedge. The clinical importance of the shadow of the mesoazygos and its vein lies in the fact that it may be confused with pathologic markings in the apex. In the case of surgical intervention on the upper lobe, its presence or absence should be known before the operation.

Fig. 69-5.—Roentgenogram showing sign of azygos lobe (**arrow**) ("inverted comma").

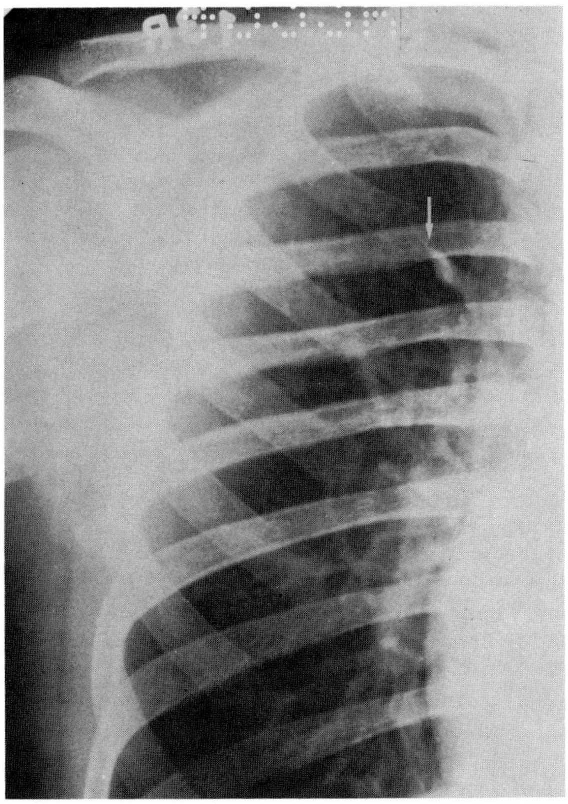

A dilated azygos vein may simulate a mediastinal tumor,[47] if in the case of faulty development of the inferior vena cava the azygos vein becomes a principal channel of venous return from the lower parts of the body to the heart. Dilatation of the azygos vein should be taken into consideration in the diagnosis of mediastinal shadows, especially when they extend to the right.

Genetic factors play a role in the development of the azygos lobe in some of the cases. It seems that this variation does not occur in Mexican Indians, although it is present in some Mexicans of European descent.[48] Pipkin *et al.*[46] found azygos lobes of the right lung in a father and 3 of his 4 children.

Sequestration of Lung Tissue Associated with an Abnormal Pulmonary Artery

The importance of this anomaly to the thoracic surgeon was stressed by Pryce *et al.*[49] The abnormal artery represents a hazard in lower lobectomy, since it is of considerable size and occurs in an inaccessible angle. Such an abnormal pulmonary artery may supply normal lung tissue, sequestered tissue or both sequestered and normal tissue. The pulmonary lesions may assume various forms and be complicated by postnatal processes that mask the congenital nature of the anomaly; the finding of an anomalous artery arising from the aorta betrays the prenatal origin of the pulmonary lesion. The bronchial abnormality may affect either lower lobe; usually it consists of bronchiectases and cysts of bronchial origin surrounded by nonfunctioning lung tissue.[50] In some cases, there is a failure of development of branches of the pulmonary artery to the affected part of the lobe. Instead of venous blood, the bronchopulmonary mass is supplied with arterial blood through the anomalous artery derived from the lower thoracic aorta or from the abdominal aorta. According to Pryce *et al.*,[49] the oxygenated blood from the anomalous artery drains in intralobar sequestration into the pulmonary vein, but Bruwer *et al.*[51] stated that the vascular connection is with the pulmonary artery. If the branches of the anomalous artery connect directly with the pulmonary vein, an unusual type of vascular shunt is established and the rate and volume of blood flow through this shunt may be considerable, whereby added work is imposed on the left ventricle.[50] Concerning the embryology of this malformation, Pryce *et al.*[49] pointed out that both normal and abnormal pulmonary arteries develop in the primitive splanchnic plexus induced by the developing lung, which lies in the neighborhood of the ventral aorta and the two dorsal aortae. The competition between these vessels usually is decided in favor of the ventral aorta, but occasionally one of the dorsal aortae "captures" a bulbous tip of the developing bronchial tree and the lung tissue derived from this tip remains connected with a branch of the dorsal aorta. If the abnormal tissue remains within the lung, intralobar ectopia or sequestration results. If the separation is more complete, the abnormal lung mass forms a lower accessory lung (extralobar sequestration). Atrophy of the affected bronchial tip leads to agenesis of part of the affected lung. Bruwer *et al.*,[51] accepting the concept of Pryce *et al.*, believed that most congenital cysts of the lung can be regarded as "sequestrations" and that an anomalous artery, after sequestration of a portion of the lower lobe, could become separated from the aorta, so that the vascular origin of the cyst is concealed. Boyden[52] did not accept this view and thought that lung cysts and systemic pulmonary arteries may occur as associated anomalies rather than as the result of one sequestration by aberrant masses. Whatever the causal relationship, the possibility of the presence of a large anomalous artery from the thoracic or abdominal aorta to the lower lobe should be borne in mind whenever cystic disease of a lower lobe is suspected.

Intralobar sequestration clinically may take the form of a cyst or a polycystic disease, anomalies that in themselves do not cause symptoms unless the abnormal parts become infected. Then, cough, fever, pain or chills may direct attention to the abnormal mass. The onset of symptoms usually occurs within the first two decades of life but it may be delayed to the sixth decade.[51] The symptoms often lead to erroneous diagnoses, such as pneumonia, empyema or bronchiectases. If sequestrations become infected, antibiotic substances or drugs can temporarily improve the acute febrile condition of the patient, but only surgical extirpation of the diseased lobe can cure intralobar sequestration and its complications. The anomalous arteries are an operative hazard.[51] Approximately 90% of the extralobar sequestrations occur on the left side, above or below the diaphragm, often associated with diaphragmatic hernia or pulmonary arteriovenous fistula. There is no communication with the respiratory tract and no function of the sequestered lung tissue.[4]

Congenital Pulmonary Cysts

The subject of cystic disease of the lungs is confusing. Many synonyms are used for various types of pulmonary cystic disease, which makes it difficult to establish a reasonable classification and to correlate pathologic and clinical pictures. For the same reason, the incidence of cystic disease of the lungs is not known.[53] Bronchial cysts accounted for 2.6% of solitary circumscribed lesions of the lung resected at the Mayo Clinic.[54] Schenck,[55] in 1936, found 232 cases of congenital cystic disease of the lungs in the world literature. Of 228 cases that could be analyzed, 82 (36%) were solitary or single cysts and 146 (64%) were multiple. The right lung alone was involved in 40% of the cases, the left in 37% and the lesions were bilateral in 23%. Lichtenstein[56] reviewed 92 cases of congenital lobar multicystic disease; two-thirds were in males and one-third in females. The right and left lungs were involved equally. In 75 cases, only one lobe was involved, in 16 cases two lobes and in 1 case three lobes. Of the 75 unilobar cases, the disease affected 30 upper, 18 middle and 27 lower lobes.

Distinction of solitary cysts, multiple cysts and ballooning cysts has been recommended.[57] Cooke and Blades[53] distinguished cysts with bronchogenic cell types that may be solitary or multiple, those with alveolar cell types that may be solitary (pneumatocele) or multiple and those with bronchogenic and alveolar types combined. Columnar, cuboidal or squamous epithelium can be found, but the shape of the epithelium may be modified by the increase in size or ballooning of the cyst, or by infection. It is of importance whether or not the cysts communicate with the neighboring bronchus. If a communication exists, the contents of the cysts are evacuated and replaced by air. Such communicating cysts are more likely to be infected than cysts without a bronchial opening.[55]

Solitary cysts rarely are found in the newborn but they may be seen within a few weeks of birth. Most of the solitary cysts contain mucous glands, smooth muscle and cartilage in the wall and resemble greatly dilated bronchi. If they communicate with the bronchus, they may become distended with air and reach considerable size or they become filled with thick mucoid fluid and compress the remaining pulmonary tissue.[35] Other solitary cysts are lined with alveolar-type cells, have a single bronchial communication and contain air. Adjacent pulmonary segments appear anatomically normal except for compression and atelectasis due to the enlarging balloon cysts.

The typical congenital lesions are seen in fetuses dead at birth or in infants who live but a short time.[100] In older children, such formations often are altered by infection and fibrosis. Diffuse cystic changes may involve a single lobe or all lobes of both lungs. The latter extreme condition was seen by Potter[35] in an iniencephalic fetus that also had complete tracheal atresia. Such cysts, not visible to the naked eye, are composed of many small cavities lined by epithelium similar to that of the bronchi. Only a few scattered areas have alveolar structure. Since it seems that a great overgrowth of bronchi is present at the expense of lung tissue, some authors looked on this form of pulmonary cystic disease as congenital bronchiectasis. In contrast to acquired bronchiectasis, which, as a rule, occurs in the basal segments of the lower lobes, congenital cystic disease or bronchiectasis is seen particularly in the upper lobes. In the congenital form

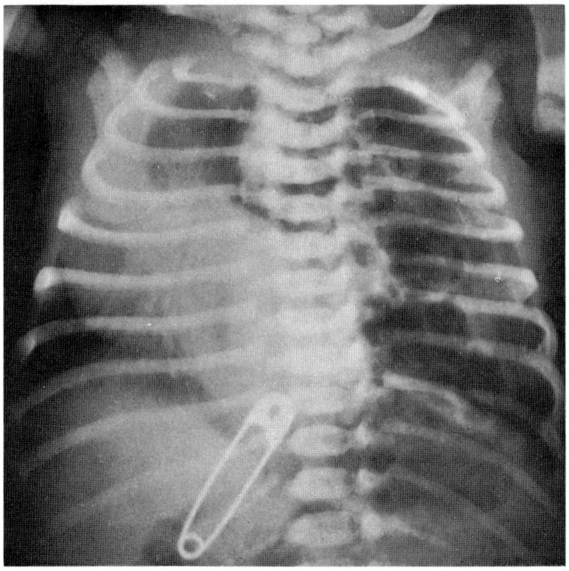

Fig. 69-6.—Congenital cystic disease of the lung in a newborn boy. He was dyspneic from birth on and was thought to have diaphragmatic hernia. However, the diaphragm was intact. The appearance of the left hemithorax was due to pulmonary cysts.

of bronchiectasis, the cysts usually are small and uniform in size, whereas in the acquired form, tubular and saccular dilatations occur.

There is general agreement that cystic disease of the lung is not an etiologic entity. In the general pool of reported cases, the male sex predominates. The age at which symptoms are first noted varies considerably. Symptoms may begin at birth or be delayed to puberty. In some cases, there are no symptoms referable to the chest, and cystic pulmonary disease is an accidental observation in necropsies of patients of advanced age.

Genetic factors seem to be involved in some of the cases. Neisser[58] described congenital bronchiectasis in a father and his son and MacRae[59] reported congenital cystic disease of the lung in 4 males of one family. Sandoz[60] observed "fetal bronchiectasis" or congenital pulmonary cysts in probably identical twin sisters. Genetic determination is evidenced by the occurrence of congenital cystic disease of the lung in patients with disorders known to be hereditary. Honeycomb lung in childhood can be a manifestation of tuberous sclerosis, a dominantly inherited trait. Familial interstitial fibrosis of the lung with multiple small cystic changes may be related to Recklinghausen neurofibromatosis.[61] Microcysts of the lung were described by Levkoff *et al.*[62] in a case of trisomy 18 syndrome in which many areas of the lung showed a spongy quality and multiple cysts lined by columnar epithelium.

Numerous theories have been proposed to explain the pathogenesis of congenital cystic disease of the lung. Schenck[55] reviewed these theories, of which many are now obsolete. Fetal inflammation, syphilis or dilatation of the lymphatics (p. 613) are inadequate explanations. Arrested development of alveoli with compensation by widening of neighboring bronchi was another interpretation. Ch'in and Tang[63] considered one form of congenital cysts as an adenomatoid malformation. They collected from the literature 10 cases observed in stillborn fetuses that were associated with general anasarca of the infant and hydramnios of the mother. The essential feature was overgrowth of the bronchioles, causing marked enlargement of one lobe and suppression of the alveolae of the area. Placental edema may accompany the anasarca in such cases, which have been attributed to obstruction of the venous return to the heart.[64] Diffuse hyperplasia of this type limited to only a portion of one lobe is compatible with life and usually is discovered only when infected or greatly distended by air. Ramsay and Byron[65] thought that pulmonary cystic changes may be due to an obstruction by a proximal bronchial septum, which could be a common cause of bronchogenic cysts.

It is known that the process of developmental growth of new bronchopulmonary elements continues in postnatal life until the seventh or eighth year and, in some instances, to as late as the fourteenth year. If at any time during such late periods, anomalies of development occur that lead to cystic disease in the

Fig. 69-7.—Congenital cystic lung disease in upper lobe of left lung of a girl 12 years of age.

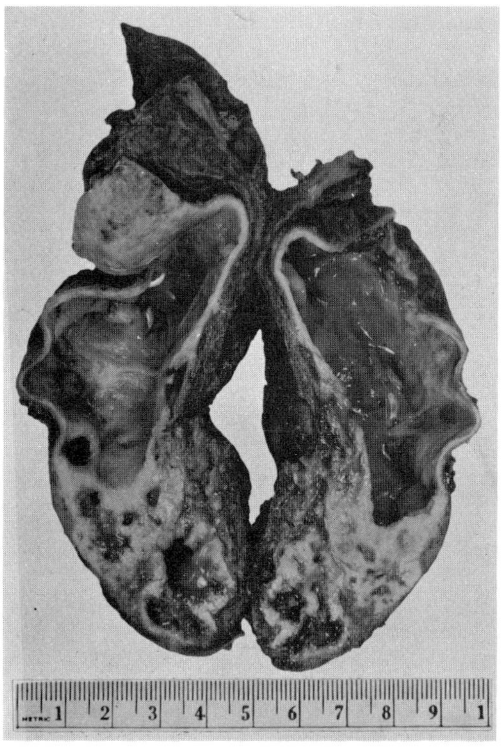

bronchopulmonary tree, it is better to speak of developmental than of congenital cysts.[66,67] Some forms of genetically determined cysts of the lung are hereditary but not congenital.

The symptomatology of solitary cystic disease depends not on the histologic make-up of the lesions but on their size, location, capsular strength and the presence or absence of infection. Many cases go unrecognized for years without symptoms, whereas, in others, symptoms are evident at birth or soon thereafter.

Infants and young children may show some embarrassment in respiration and paroxysms of dyspnea. This becomes particularly serious with balloon cysts when the air becomes trapped and the cysts enlarge, compressing the lung, flattening the diaphragm and displacing the mediastinal structures. A cyst can rupture into the pleural space, resulting in pneumothorax. Wheezing associated with a cough may suggest a diagnosis of asthma. Varying degrees of cyanosis are present. If a bronchial connection exists, a cough may be notable, especially in infected cysts when expectoration becomes marked. Elevation of temperature depends on the presence or absence of infection. In older children and adults, the balloon type of cyst seldom is seen. Beyond childhood, solitary air cysts and diffuse multiple cysts predominate. Of the patients with congenital lobar multicystic disease reviewed by Lichtenstein,[56] approximately one-third had no symptoms but more than 40% had cough with sputum. Fever, weakness or hemoptysis was rare. If hemoptysis or profuse hemorrhage occurs, tuberculosis may be suspected. There are no physical signs characteristic of congenital cystic disease, but a history of long-continued cough and expectoration dating from childhood, with signs of chronic bronchial suppuration, should arouse suspicion of congenital cystic disease.

Roentgenographic findings in solitary fluid cysts consist of an ovoid opaque area within the parenchyma of the lung that can remain unchanged over a long period. If rupture into a neighboring bronchus takes place, a horizontal fluid level with a pocket of air above it will appear. A balloon cyst may occupy the entire half of the chest and even overlap the mediastinum and heart. Such a cyst can simulate a pneumothorax. Patients with multiple cysts containing air or fluid show smaller lesions.

Potter[35] mentioned polycystic disease of the kidney and iniencephaly as associated anomalies. Accessory lobes,[55] abnormal segmentation and malformations of the small bronchi have been observed.[68] If congenital cystic disease of the lung appears as a symptom of Marfan syndrome or of tuberous sclerosis, associated anomalies are characteristic of the general disorder. McKusick and Fisher[69] found an association of a hereditary form of pulmonary cystic disease with progressive pulmonary fibrosis and carcinomatosis. Gillot[70] described 2 patients with polycystic lung disease who were retarded in growth; in regard to these, he wrote of "pulmonary infantilism."

Complications consist in infection or rupture of the cyst into the pleural cavity, resulting in pneumothorax. In patients with delayed symptoms, the condition is compatible with a long life. There is no agreement concerning the prognosis in infants and children. Some authors believed that the prognosis is grave in infants who show early symptoms, but Caffey[71] pointed out that spontaneous regression is the rule for pulmonary cysts even when they are demonstrated during the first weeks and months of life. He believed that if an excision is postponed, most early pulmonary cysts disappear spontaneously after several weeks or months and that even with a persisting cyst the patient may thrive. But Caffey admitted that acute respiratory obstruction due to sudden and marked expansion of cysts does occur and that in such cases surgical excision is urgent and life-saving. If one considers the heterogeneous character of these cysts, it is understandable that there is no agreement concerning treatment. Swan and Aragon[72] discussed surgical treatment of pulmonary cysts in infancy. Small symptomless cysts discovered on incidental chest roentgenograms should be treated expectantly, but this is not advisable in patients with such early manifestations as dyspnea or cyanosis on crying or coughing. These authors thought that persistence of the cystic condition endangers healthy lung tissue and that surgical treatment could prevent spread of pulmonary disease. The operative procedure consists in extirpation of the infected or expanding cyst, with conservation of normal pulmonary tissue.

Congenital Emphysema

Emphysema of the lung involving a segment of a lobe or a whole lobe is a rare congenital anomaly that has been attributed to a check-valve mechanism in the bronchus. The valve effect may be due to redundant folds of mucosa or a congenital weakness of the bronchial wall that causes occlusion of the lumen during expiration. Affected infants show attacks of dyspnea and cyanosis. Roentgenograms of the chest at first suggest congenital heart disease, dextrocardia, atelectasis, agenesis of a lung, congenital cysts, foreign body, diaphragmatic hernia or other disorders. But congenital heart disease can be excluded by the finding of displacement of the mediastinum and by absence of cardiac murmurs. In pulmonary atelectasis or in agenesis, the diaphragm is elevated rather than depressed as in emphysema. Foreign body is excluded by history and bronchoscopy. Robertson and James[73] pointed out that recognition of the condition is more difficult than treatment. Medical measures do not improve the ventilation of the involved segments, but surgical removal of the affected segment or lobe apparently is well tolerated by infants.[73,74] Congenital emphysema associated with cutis laxa (Chapter 119) was described by Christiaens *et al.*[75] Cystic emphysema in premature infants can be postnatal in origin and due to a type 19 ECHO virus.[76]

Congenital Cystic Lymphangiectasis

Only 32 cases of this disorder, which was known 100 years ago, had been reported by 1967.[77] Congenital cystic lymphangiectasis of the lungs may be confused with cystic pulmonary malformations.[78] The cysts predominate in positions in which the lymphatic plexuses are known to occur, namely in the subpleural connective tissue, in the interlobular septa and in close relationship to the blood vessels and bronchi. They can be so small that they cannot be seen with the naked eye or they may be 1–3 cm. in diameter.[77,79] The position of the cysts, the flat endothelial lining and the structure of the delicate walls containing elastic, muscle and collagen fibers similar to those seen in the larger lymphatics suggest a diagnosis of congenital pulmonary lymphangiectasis. Laurence[78] reviewed 5 cases from the literature and added 3 of his own. The condition was observed in fetuses or in children who died soon after birth. In 2 of the 3 cases reported by Laurence, and in a case of Javett *et al.*,[79] hydramnios complicated the pregnancy. Associated anomalies apparently are frequent; congenital heart disease, cretinism, arachnodactyly and hydronephrosis were present in some of the affected children. According to Laurence,[78] the condition dates back to the third month of intrauterine life, when the lymphatics invade the lung tissue rapidly and become large in comparison with the size of the whole organ. Normally, by the fourth month, the large lymphatics within the connective tissue divide the parenchyma into distinct lobules but by the fifth month the lobulations become less prominent as the connective tissue and the lymphatics are reduced in amount. If this reversal of the proportions does not take place and the tissue elements maintain their early condition, the anomaly described results as a continuation of the embryologic situation. Lymphangiectases may be present in organs other than the lung; for example, the heart, kidney and lymph nodes.[80]

As a rule, fetuses with this disorder are either stillborn or, if live-born, suffer dyspnea and cyanosis in the neonatal period and die within a few hours. The thorax is held as in extreme inspiration. Roentgenograms show lungs with a network of shadows surrounding round, transparent foci.[80] Survival for 9 months has been reported in a case confirmed by biopsy.[79] Associated malformations were noted in half the cases reported. Cardiovascular anomalies, particularly hypoplasia of the left heart, were frequent. Anomalous pulmonary venous return[99] and renal malformations were found in some of the cases.[80]

Pulmonary Arteriovenous Fistulas

These anomalies are congenital hemangiomatous malformations of the pulmonary vascular bed that are related to, and often associated with, telangiectasis in other parts of the body. Reviews on the subject by Stringer *et al.*[81] LeRoux[82] and Moyer *et al.*[83] are available. In many cases, the pulmonary lesions are a manifestation of hereditary hemorrhagic telangiectasia (Rendu-Osler-Weber disease) (Chapter 118), and cutaneous or mucosal manifestations are seen in approximately 40% of patients with pulmonary arteriovenous fistula (PAF). Other terms used for the pulmonary anomaly are pulmonary arteriovenous aneurysm, multiple pulmonary hemangiomas, cavernous hemangioma and others.

According to LeRoux,[82] it was Churton[84] who, in 1897, first reported a necropsy finding of multiple hemangiomatous lesions in the lungs. Other necropsy reports followed, but the first antemortem diagnosis on clinical and radiographic evidence apparently was made by Smith and Horton.[85] In 1942, Hepburn and Dauphinee[86] diagnosed such a lesion clinically and treated it surgically by pneumonectomy. Other historical details can be found in Stringer *et al.*[81]

The condition seems to be rare, and Steinberg and McClenahan[87] found only 9 pulmonary arteriovenous fistulas in 2,000 consecutive angiograms. There are numerous reports of PAF in more than one member of the same family or kinship. Thus, the lesion has been seen in sisters, in brothers and in parent and children.[88] Genetic aspects of the disease are further suggested by its frequent association with mucosal or cutaneous telangiectasis, a condition known to be hereditary.[83] A family history of hereditary hemorrhagic telangiectasia is obtained in approximately 15% of patients with PAF.[82] Thus, in many cases, PAF is a manifestation of generalized hereditary hemorrhagic telangiectasia, which may manifest itself in many parts of the body, the lung among others. Since this disorder is inherited as a dominant trait, PAF in such cases is due to a dominant gene with variable expressivity.

The developmental defect leading to such fistulas is attributed by some authors to failure of fusion of septa that normally separate the pulmonary arterial and venous channels. In addition, there is hypoplasia of both veins and arteries, which may rupture, leading to formation of arteriovenous fistulas and cavities. The resulting lesions consist of vascular channels lined with endothelium and supporting connective stroma. Muscular and elastic layers of the vessel walls are absent. The vascular channels range in size from connections of capillary diameter to large saccular cavities with walls of varying thickness. The arterial supply usually is derived from branches of the pulmonary artery, but arterial blood may also come from bronchial or intercostal arteries or directly from the aorta. The veins usually drain into the left atrium through pulmonary veins. The adjacent pulmonary tissue, as a rule, is normal.[82] Although a congenital anomaly or tendency to vascular enlargement can be assumed in all cases, the cavities leading to symptoms may be formed in postnatal life by such accessory factors as coughing, increase in pulmonary pressure or mitral stenosis.[82] In rare instances, PAF has been found in the newborn. Bowers[89] described a small

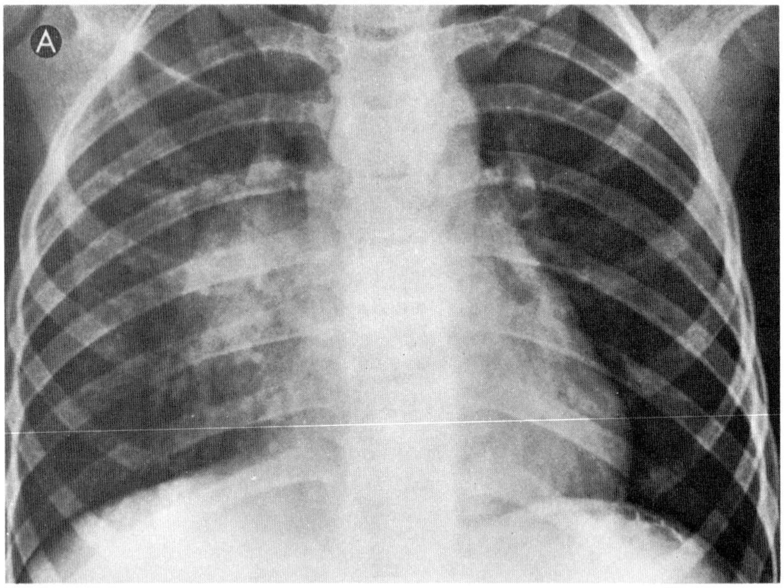

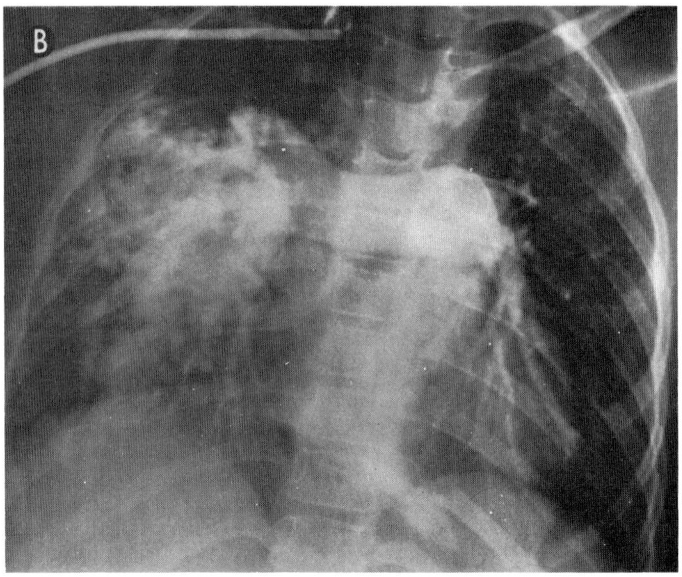

Fig. 69-8. – **A,** roentgenogram of an 8-year-old girl with congenital arteriovenous fistula in the right middle and upper lobes. She had been cyanotic since birth; clubbing of fingers and toes developed at 2 years of age. **B,** angiogram revealed the fistula. Lobectomy was performed when she was 8 years old. Right upper and middle lobes were resected.

infant, a "blue baby," who died on the second day of life. PAFs were found in both lower lobes and there was massive pulmonary hemorrhage into the left pleural cavity. Husson[90] reported the case of a 2½-year-old boy with PAF successfully treated by lobectomy.

Arteriovenous fistulas of the lung – in contrast to those in other regions of the body – can cause severe symptoms because they establish communications between afferent and efferent pulmonary vessels, which creates a shunt and bypass of the pulmonary capillary bed and permits the return of unoxygenated blood to the heart. The size of the right-to-left shunt is variable and may range from 18% to 89% of the right ventricular output. The heart usually is normal in size but it may become enlarged during the course of the disease. Maldevelopment of the pulmonary veins and pulmonary arteriovenous aneurysms were reported by Anabtawi and Ellison.[91]

The typical manifestations in well-developed cases

are cyanosis, clubbing of the fingers, polycythemia, dyspnea and an extracardiac murmur. Cutaneous and mucosal hemangiomas are frequent. The fully developed disease picture is relatively rare, as most patients are discovered in radiographic surveys. Well-developed cases can be confused with cyanotic heart disease or with polycythemia vera. Cyanosis is a consequence of the shunting of unoxygenated blood past the pulmonary capillary bed. Polycythemia results from the stimulation of erythropoiesis by anoxia. Clubbing of the fingers and toes is related to cyanosis and peripheral vasodilatation. Rarer manifestations of these lesions are osteoarthropathy, pain in the chest, epistaxis or hemoptysis. Usually, the diagnosis is made in adults when symptoms become prominent, but lesions may be discovered earlier. The right and the left lower lobe usually are the sites of PAF, but the lesions often are multiple and bilateral. All five lobes may be affected, a fact of great importance in the treatment of the disorder. A continuous murmur is commonly heard over the lesion.[83] Roentgenography shows a pulmonary opacity within the lung parenchyma with well-defined outlines and connected with the hilum by the shadows of dilated blood vessels. Pulsation of the opacity can be seen on fluoroscopy. Angiocardiography is an auxiliary method useful before surgical treatment, since it demonstrates all the fistulas present in the lung; however, the method is not without danger.[82] Hemorrhages, infections and cerebral lesions can complicate PAF. Hemoptysis may be the presenting symptom and even a fatal manifestation of the disease. Fatal pleural hemorrhage is possible but rare.[89] Headache, vertigo, dizziness, convulsions, visual and auditory disturbances and brain abscess occur as nerve complications.[82]

Treatment is surgical, and the operation of choice, according to LeRoux,[82] is "the most limited resection compatible with complete removal of the fistula." Surgical removal is clearly indicated in a patient who has only one fistula that produces definite symptoms. However, if the fistulas are small and asymptomatic, or if they are extensive and multiple, the usefulness of surgical treatment is doubtful. Removal of an entire lung is dangerous, since additional fistulas may develop subsequently in the remaining lung, reducing the patient's lung volume.

Relation of Pulmonary Tumors to Malformations

Association of lung tumors and malformations of the lung was emphasized by Schwyter.[92] He thought that pulmonary tumors in young persons develop on the basis of fetal bronchiectases; adenomas, lipomas, rhabdomyomas, chondromas and others have been considered related to malformation. In some of these cases, sometimes it is difficult to decide whether one deals with a tumor or a malformation and it is likely that such patients have hamartomas or hamartoses. Schwyter added cases of pulmonary carcinoma to these tumors thought to originate from developmental errors in the lungs. In adults of advanced ages he found pulmonary tumors associated with congenital cysts, bronchiectases and immature lung tissue and believed that the tumors had originated within malformed sectors of the lung areas not connected with the bronchial tree.

Hamartomas of the lung.—According to Taiana and Zorraquin,[93] hamartomas account for 1.65% of primary pulmonary new growths and 55% of pulmonary benign tumors. These tumors may cause no symptoms at all or result in cough, bloody sputum or pain. They usually are detected by routine radiographic examination. Hamartomas predominate in the right lung and usually are situated peripherally in roentgenograms. They appear nodular or lobulated and they tend to calcification or ossification. Increase in size is slow. They usually are discovered in adults, but Jones[94] reported a case in a newborn child. Pulmonary hamartomas consist chiefly of cartilage, but osseous, glandular, adipose, connective, lymphoid and muscular tissues are also present. The tumors are thought to be derived from aberrant bronchial buds, since they contain tissues that normally occur in bronchi. Malignant tumors such as bronchial carcinomas can simulate hamartomas and some hamartomas have undergone malignant degeneration. For these reasons, surgical exploration of pulmonary hamartomas has been recommended, but the outcome of such operations is not always favorable.[93] Cystic lesions of the lung as manifestations of tuberous sclerosis or neurofibromatosis have been mentioned (p. 611).

Tissue of extrapulmonary origin.—Potter[35] described in a fetal lung a hemangiorhabdomyoma showing a great increase in the size and number of blood vessels and large masses of striated muscle cells. Occasionally, small masses of brain tissue are found in the lungs of anencephalic monsters. Potter pointed out that such changes are limited to anencephalic monsters and believed that destruction of the brain and presence of its nerve element in the amniotic fluid may be aspirated into the lungs and be implanted there. But, in other lungs, small masses of tissue resembling the cortex of the fetal adrenal gland may be found.[35]

Tumor-like angiomas of the lung.—These have been described repeatedly in infants. De Lange and de Vries Robles[95] reported the case of an infant with symptoms thought to be due to cerebral lesions. At necropsy, multiple angiomas were found in the lungs. In the kidneys, convolutes of renal tubules were seen and the ovaries consisted of multiple cysts. Wollstein[96] described a case of malignant hemangioma of the lung with multiple visceral foci in a child 4 months of age and reviewed the literature on this subject available at the time of publication. It is doubtful that these angiomas of the lung are etiologically and pathogenetically related to pulmonary arteriovenous fistulas.

HEMANGIOMA OF THE MEDIASTINUM.—These tumors usually occur in the anterior mediastinum and cause symptoms by compression and invasion of mediastinal structures. Histologically, the lesions appear benign.[97]

REFERENCES

1. Boyden, E. A.: Developmental anomalies of the lung, Am. J. Surg. 89:79, 1955.
2. Breton, A., and Dubois, A.: *Les Malformations Congénitales du Poumon* (Paris: G. Doin & Cie, 1957).
3. Spencer, H.: *Pathology of the Lung* (New York: The Macmillan Company, 1962).
4. Levine, M. I., and Mascia, A. V.: *Pulmonary Diseases and Anomalies of Infancy and Childhood* (New York: Hoeber Medical Division, Harper & Row, Publishers, 1966).
5. de Reuck, A. V. S., and Porter, R. (eds.): *Development of the Lung* (Boston: Little, Brown & Company, 1967).
6. Good, C. A.: Certain vascular abnormalities of the lungs, Am. J. Roentgenol. 85:1009, 1961.
7. Schneider, P.: Dis Missbildungen der Atmungsorgane, in Schwalbe, E. (ed.), *Die Morphologie der Missbildungen des Menschen und der Tiere* (Jena: Gustav Fischer, 1911), Vol. 3, pts. 8–11.
8. Schmit, H.: Ein Fall von vollständiger Agenesie beider Lungen, Virchows Arch. path. Anat. 134:25, 1893.
9. Allen, and Affelbach,: Congenital absence of both lungs, Surg., Gynec. & Obst. 41:375, 1925.
10. Tuynman, P. E., and Gardner, L. W.: Bilateral aplasia of the lung, A.M.A. Arch. Path. 54:306, 1952.
11. Claireaux, A. E., and Ferreira, H. P.: Bilateral pulmonary agenesis, Arch. Dis. Childhood 33:364, 1958.
12. Devi, B., and More, J. R. S.: Total tracheopulmonary agenesis; associated with asplenia, agenesis of umbilical artery and other anomalies, Acta paediat. scandinav. 55:107, 1966.
13. Ôyamada, A., Gasul, B. M., and Holinger, P. H.: Agenesis of the lung. Report of a case with a review of all previously reported cases, A.M.A. Am. J. Dis. Child. 85:182, 1953.
14. Roderer, G. J. (cited by Schuchardt, K.): Hochgradige Atrophie (inveterierte Atelektase) der linken Lunge mit kompensatorischer Hypertrophie der rechten, Virchows Arch. path. Anat. 101:71, 1885.
15. Saito, J.: Ein Foetus ohne Trachea und Lunge, Verhandl. Aertzkong. Tokyo, 4:2, 1902.
16. Heerup, L.: Case of absence of left lung, Hospitalstid. 70: 1165, 1927.
17. Smart, J.: Complete congenital agenesis of a lung, Quart. J. Med. 15:125, 1946.
18. Lukas, D. S., Dotter, C. T., and Steinberg, I.: Agenesis of the lung and patent ductus arteriosus with reversal of flow, New England J. Med. 249:107, 1953.
19. Valle, A. R.: Agenesis of the lung, Am. J. Surg. 89:90, 1955.
20. Finkelstein, H.: *Lehrbuch der Säuglingskrankheiten* (4th ed.; Amsterdam: Elsevier, 1938).
21. Yount, F.: Agenesis of right lung in each of identical twins, Arizona Med. 5:48, 1948.
22. Field, C. E.: Pulmonary agenesis and hypoplasia, Arch. Dis. Childhood 21:61, 1946.
23. Maier, H. C., and Gould, W. J.: Agenesis of the lung with vascular compression of the tracheobronchial tree, J. Pediat. 43:38, 1953.
24. Thomas, L. B., and Boyden, E. A.: Agenesis of the right lung; report of three cases, Surgery 31:429, 1952.
25. Voorhess, M. L., Vahard, T., and Gardner, L. I.: Trisomy 16-18 syndrome, Lancet 2:992, 1962.
26. Butler, L. J., France, N. E., Russell, A., and Sinclair, L.: A chromosomal aberration associated with multiple congenital anomalies, Lancet 1:1242, 1962.
27. Warkany, J., Roth, C. B., and Wilson, J. G.: Multiple congenital malformations: A consideration of etiologic factors, Pediatrics 1:462, 1948.
28. Smith, R. A., and Bech, A. O.: Agenesis of lung, Thorax 13:28, 1958.
29. Caffey, J.: *Pediatric X-Ray Diagnosis* (4th ed.; Chicago: Year Book Medical Publishers, Inc., 1961).
30. Schultze-Jena, B. S., and Kosenow, W.: Einseitige Lungenagenesie mit Oesophagusatresie. Zugleich ein Beitrag zur Differentialdiagnose des angeborenen Lungenmangels, Ztschr. Kinderh. 81:50, 1958.
31. Warner, A. L., Palladino, N. M., Schwartz, W., and Schuster, A.: The relationship of agenesis of the lung to emphysema and cor pulmonale, J. Pediat. 46:200, 1955.
32. Ferencz, C.: Congenital abnormalities of pulmonary vessels and their relation to malformations of the lung, Pediatrics 28:993, 1961.
33. Warner, F. S., McGraw, C. T., Peterson, H. G., Jr., Cleland, R. S., and Meyer, B. W.: Lung ectopia and agenesis with heart dextrorotation, Am. J. Dis. Child. 101:514, 1961.
34. Jue, K. L., Amplatz, K., Adams, P., Jr., and Anderson, R. C.: Anomalies of great vessels associated with lung hypoplasia. The scimitar syndrome, Am. J. Dis. Child. 111:35, 1966.
35. Potter, E. L.: *Pathology of the Fetus and Infant* (2d ed.; Chicago: Year Book Medical Publishers, Inc., 1961).
36. Areechon, W., and Reid, L.: Hypoplasia of lung with congenital diaphragmatic hernia, Brit. M. J. 1:230, 1963.
37. Potter, E. L.: Bilateral renal agenesis, J. Pediat. 29:68, 1946.
38. Foster-Carter, A. F.: Bronchopulmonary abnormalities, Brit. J. Tuberc. 40:111, 1946.
39. Hepburn, D.: Note on a right lung which resembled a left lung in presenting only apical and basal lobes, J. Anat. 59:326, 1924–1925.
40. Boyden, E. A., Bill, A. H., Jr., and Creighton, S. A.: Presumptive origin of a left lower accessory lung from an esophageal diverticulum, Surgery 52:323, 1962.
41. Davies, D. V., and Gunz, F. W.: Two cases of lower accessory lung in the human subject, J. Path. & Bact. 56:417, 1944.
42. Dévé, M. F.: Les lobes surnuméraires du poumon. Le lobe cardiaque. Valeur du lobe supérieur du poumon gauche, Bull. Soc. anat. Paris 75:341, 1900.
43. Hjelt, L., and Hakosalo, J.: Congenital asplenia. Case report and a review of the literature, Ann. paediat. Fenniae 5 (supp.) 12:3, 1959.
44. Gilbert, E. F., Nishimura, K., and Wedum, B. G.: Congenital malformations of the heart associated with splenic agenesis; with a report of five cases, Circulation 17:72, 1958.
45. Kent, E. M., and Blades, B.: The surgical anatomy of the pulmonary lobes, J. Thoracic Surg. 12:18, 1942.
46. Pipkin, S. B., Kegel, R., and Pipkin, A. C.: Inheritance of the accessory lobe of the azygos vein, J. Hered. 43:260, 1952.
47. Magbitang, M. H., Hayford, F. C., and Blake, J. M.: Dilated azygos vein simulating a mediastinal tumor. Report of a case, New England J. Med. 263:598, 1960.
48. Alarcón, D. G.: Lóbulo azigos, Rev. Mex. Tuberc. 5:139, 1943.
49. Pryce, D. M., Sellors, T. H., and Blair, L. G.: Intralobar sequestration of lung associated with an abnormal pulmonary artery, Brit. J. Surg. 35:18, 1947.
50. Kergin, F. G.: Congenital cystic disease of lung associated with anomalous arteries, J. Thoracic Surg. 23:55, 1952.
51. Bruwer, A., Clagett, O. T., and McDonald, J. R.: Anomalous arteries to the lung associated with congenital pulmonary abnormality, J. Thoracic Surg. 19:957, 1950.
52. Boyden, E. A.: Bronchogenic cysts and the theory of intralobar sequestration: New embryologic data, J. Thoracic Surg. 35:604, 1958.
53. Cooke, F. N., and Blades, B.: Cystic disease of lungs, J. Thoracic Surg. 23:546, 1952.
54. Hood, R. T., Jr., Good, C. A., Clagett, O. T., and McDonald,

J. R.: Solitary circumscribed lesions of the lung. Study of 156 cases in which resection was performed, J.A.M.A. 152:1185, 1953.
55. Schenck, S. G.: Congenital cystic disease of the lungs, Am. J. Roentgenol. 35:604, 1936.
56. Lichtenstein, H.: Congenital multiple cysts of the lung, Dis. Chest 24:646, 1953.
57. Wier, J. A.: Congenital anomalies of the lung, Ann. Int. Med. 52:330, 1960.
58. Neisser, E.: Über einseitige Lungenatrophie und über angeborene Bronchiektasie, Ztschr. klin. Med. 42:88, 1900.
59. McRae, D. F.: Congenital cystic disease of the lung. A familial incidence of four males in one family, Canad. M.A.J. 57:545, 1947.
60. Sandoz, E.: Über zwei Fälle von "fötaler Bronchiektasie," Beitr. path. Anat. 41:495, 1907.
61. McKusick, V. A., and Mutalik, G. S.: Genetics and Pulmonary Disease, in Liebow, A. A., and Smith, D. E. (eds.), *The Lung* (Baltimore: The Williams & Wilkins Company, 1968).
62. Levkoff, A. H., Mather, G. B., and Eisenstein, R. P.: A case of trisomy 16–18 syndrome, Am. J. Dis. Child. 107:300, 1964.
63. Ch'in, K. Y., and Tang, M. Y.: Congenital adenomatoid malformation of one lobe of a lung with general anasarca, Arch. Path. 48, 221, 1949.
64. Gottschalk, W., and Abramson, D.: Placental edema and fetal hydrops; a case of congenital cystic and adenomatoid malformation of the lung, Obst. & Gynec. 10:626, 1957.
65. Ramsay, B. H., and Byron, F. X.: Mucocele, congenital bronchiectasis, and bronchiogenic cyst, J. Thoracic Surg. 26:21, 1953.
66. Peirce, C. B.: "Cystic" disease of the lung, Am. J. Roentgenol. 44:848, 1940.
67. Mayer, E., and Rappaport, I.: Developmental origin of cystic, bronchiectatic and emphysematous changes in the lungs. A new concept, Dis. Chest 21:146, 1952.
68. Marie, J., and Sée, G.: Les kystoïdes pulmonaires congénitaux du nourrisson. Formations aériennes circonscrites d'origine malformative et de determinisme mécanique, Arch. franç. pédiat. 13:820, 1956.
69. McKusick, V. A., and Fisher, A. M.: Congenital cystic disease of the lung with progressive pulmonary fibrosis and carcinomatosis, Ann. Int. Med. 48:774, 1958.
70. Gillot, F.: Maladie polykystique du poumon et retard de croissance à propos de deux observations, Arch. franç. pédiat. 8:888, 1951.
71. Caffey, J.: On the natural regression of pulmonary cysts during early infancy, Pediatrics 11:48, 1953.
72. Swan, H., and Aragon, G. E.: Surgical treatment of pulmonary cysts in infancy—report of three cases, Pediatrics 14:651, 1954.
73. Robertson, R., and James, E. S.: Congenital lobar emphysema, Pediatrics 8:795, 1951.
74. Shaw, R. R.: Localized hypertrophic emphysema, Pediatrics 9:220, 1952.
75. Christiaens, L., Marchand-Alphant, A., and Fovet, A.: Emphysème congénital et cutix laxa, Presse méd. 62: 1799, 1954.
76. Butterfield, J., Moscovici, C., Berry, C., and Kempe, C. H.: Cystic emphysema in premature infants; report of an outbreak with the isolation of type 19 ECHO virus in one case, New England J. Med. 268:18, 1963.
77. Fronstin, M. H., Hooper, G. S., Besse, B. E., and Ferreri, S.: Congenital pulmonary cystic lymphangiectasis; case report and a review of 32 cases, Am. J. Dis. Child. 114:330, 1967.
78. Laurence, K. M.: Congenital pulmonary cystic lymphangiectasia, J. Path. & Bact. 70:325, 1955.
79. Javett, S. N., Webster, I., and Braudo, J. L.: Congenital dilatation of the pulmonary lymphatics, Pediatrics 31: 416, 1963.
80. Giedion, A., Müller, W. A., and Molz, G.: Angeborene Lymphangiektasie der Lungen. Eine radiologisch erkennbare Ursache des Atemnotsyndroms beim Neugeborenen, Helvet. paediat. acta 22:170, 1967.
81. Stringer, C. J., Stanley, A. L., Bates, R. C., and Summers, J. E.: Pulmonary arteriovenous fistula, Am. J. Surg. 89: 1054, 1955.
82. LeRoux, B. T.: Pulmonary arteriovenous fistulae, Quart. J. Med. 28:1, 1959.
83. Moyer, J. H., Glantz, G., and Brest, A. N.: Pulmonary arteriovenous fistulas. Physiologic and clinical considerations, Am. J. Med. 32:417, 1962.
84. Churton, T.: Multiple aneurysms of pulmonary artery, Brit. M. J. 1:1223, 1897.
85. Smith, H. L., and Horton, B. T.: Arteriovenous fistula of the lung associated with polycythemia vera, Am. Heart J. 18:589, 1939.
86. Hepburn, J., and Dauphinee, J. A.: Successful removal of hemangioma of the lung followed by the disappearance of polycythemia, Am. J. M. Sc. 204:681, 1942.
87. Steinberg, I., and McClenahan, J.: Pulmonary arteriovenous fistula: Angiocardiographic observations in nine cases, Am. J. Med. 19:549, 1955.
88. Tobin, J. R., Jr., and Wilder, T. C.: Pulmonary arteriovenous fistula associated with hereditary hemorrhagic telangiectasis. A report of their occurrence in a father and son, Ann. Int. Med. 38:868, 1953.
89. Bowers, W. F.: Rupture of visceral hemangioma as a cause of death, Nebraska M. J. 21:55, 1936.
90. Husson, G. S.: Pulmonary arteriovenous aneurysm in childhood, Pediatrics 18:871, 1956.
91. Anabtawi, I. N., and Ellison, R. G.: Maldevelopment of the pulmonary veins and pulmonary arteriovenous aneurysm, Am. Surgeon 30:770, 1964.
92. Schwyter, M.: Über das Zusammentreffen von Tumoren und Missbildungen der Lungen, Frankfurt. Ztschr. Path. 36:146, 1928.
93. Taiana, J. A., and Zorraquin, V. A.: Pulmonary hamartomas. Ten cases treated surgically, West. J. Surg. 70:267, 1962.
94. Jones, C. J.: Unusual hamartoma of lung in new-born infant, Arch. Path. 48:150, 1949.
95. de Lange, C., and de Vries Robles, S. B.: Über Lungenangiome bei einem Säugling, Ztschr. Kinderh. 34:304, 1922.
96. Wollstein, M.: Malignant hemangioma of the lung with multiple visceral foci, Arch. Path. 12:562, 1931.
97. Attar, S., and Cowley, R. A.: Hemangioma of the mediastinum; collective review and case report, Am. Surgeon 30:141, 1964.
98. Booth, J. B., and Berry, C. L.: Unilateral pulmonary agenesis, Arch. Dis. Childhood 42:361, 1967.
99. Noonan, J. A., Walters, L. R., and Reeves, J. T.: Congenital pulmonary lymphangiectasis, Am. J. Dis. Child. 120: 314, 1970.
100. Benatre, A., Laugier, J., Rolland, J-C., Delvert, B., Vandooren, M., and Desbuquois, G.: Malformation pulmonaire kystique asphyxiante du nouveau-né, Arch. franç. pédiat. 27:821, 1970.

PART X

Malformations of the Face

70

Facial Anomalies

Agnathia

AGNATHIA (absence of the maxilla or mandible) is an extremely rare condition. Unilateral maxillary agnathia is due to failure of development of one maxillary process. Absence of the premaxillary area is found in cyclopia when the frontonasal process does not form. Strictly speaking, man has no premaxilla, i.e., an independent bone, but the portions of the upper jaw that lie in front of the anterior palatine foramen usually are referred to as the "premaxilla." Two skulls with absence of the premaxilla have been described by Derry,[1] one of them a skull found in an Egyptian grave dating back to 700 B.C. In this case, the hard palate was markedly reduced in size due to absence of the premaxilla and the horizontal parts of the palatine bones. There were no incisor teeth and only one canine. Since the mandible was normal, it protruded markedly over the retracted maxilla.

Fig. 70-1.—Human newborn agnathus with exencephaly and synophthalmia. The left ear joins the right ear under the frontomaxillary process (synotia). (Courtesy of Prof. Kl. Goerttler, Pathology Institute, University of Kiel.)

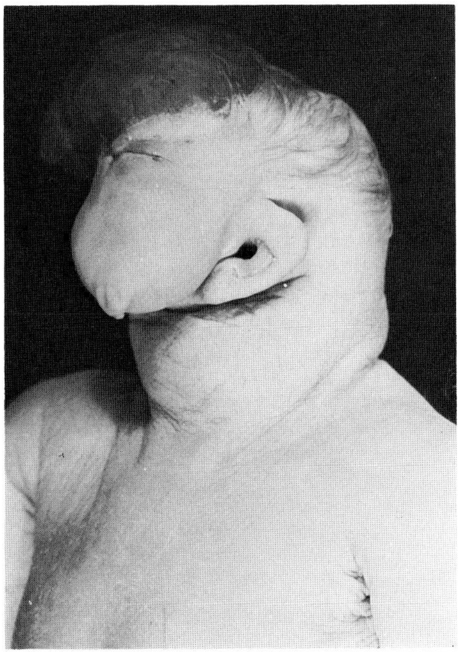

Mandibular agnathia sometimes is combined with cyclopia or synotia (p. 202). The mandible may be missing on one side only (hemignathia), a condition sometimes associated with microtia or absence of the external and internal ear[2] or with unilateral congenital fissure of the mouth (macrostomia). Kazanjian[3] reported 5 cases of this rare combination, 1 of them showing both microtia and unilateral macrostomia. Some of these cases seem to be morphologically related to mandibulofacial dysostosis (p. 650) but the etiology probably is different. Although the anomaly is primarily a developmental defect of the first branchial arch, it need not be limited to it, as the temporal area also may be involved.

The Face and Mouth in Otocephaly (Synotia)

The mouth is rudimentary, as the mandible is markedly underdeveloped (p. 402) and the tongue is incompletely developed and situated near the pharynx. The small oral cavity is connected with the pharynx by a narrow opening and sometimes there is no communication at all between these cavities. In contrast to the mouth, the pharynx may be large and dilated. Larynx, epiglottis and thyroid are rather normal. It seems that a rudiment of the mandible can be found in all human cases. There are many types of otocephaly[4]; human cases apparently belong to the ageniocephalic (chinless) group.[5] Some forms resemble cyclopia but, in contrast to this deformity, the brain is not involved in uncomplicated otocephaly; others represent true combinations of otocephaly and cyclopia.[5]

Otocephaly has been produced experimentally in mice by x-irradiation[6] and in rats by streptonigrin treatment.[7]

Micrognathia

Micrognathia occurs in some systemic anomalies such as mandibulofacial dysostosis (p. 650), the Pierre Robin syndrome (p. 654) and others. A decreased width of the dental arch is an important symptom of an undeveloped, narrow maxilla. It is spoken of as a contraction—also as a V-shaped arch or "rat bite"—and generally is associated with maxillary protrusion.[8] Maxillary micrognathia frequently is

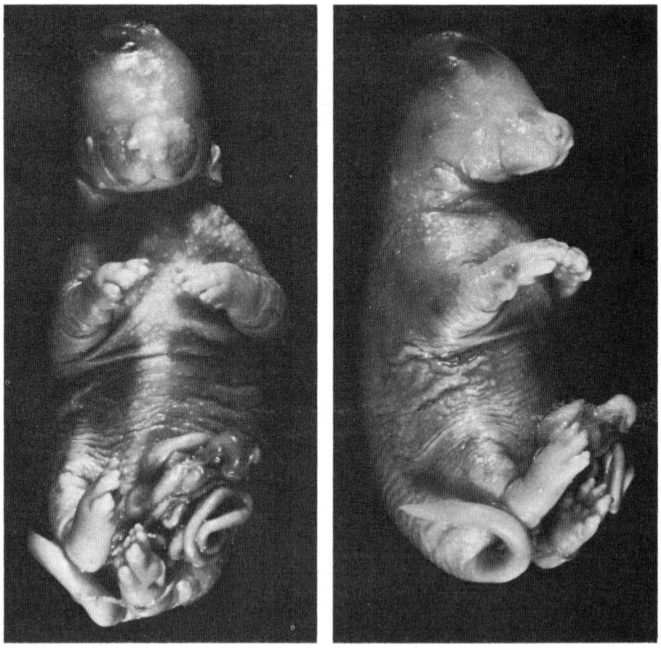

Fig. 70-2.—Agnathus with synotia in a newborn rat produced by treatment of the mother with streptonigrin. (From J. Warkany and E. Takacs.[7])

due to a deficiency of the premaxillary area, and patients with this deformity appear to have the middle third of the face retracted.[2]

Sometimes mandibular micrognathia is a hereditary characteristic.[9] It occurs in a variety of syndromes, as associated congenital malformations are not rare. A combination of peromelia (congenital stump formation of the extremities) and micrognathia was described by Hanhart,[10] who believed that simple recessive inheritance is responsible for some of these cases. If combined with posterior cleft and glossoptosis, attacks of cyanosis occur and there are difficulties in breathing and feeding (see Pierre Robin syndrome, p. 654). Micrognathia combined with microcephaly and microphthalmia occurred in children whose mothers had received x-ray treatment during pregnancy.[11]

Micrognathia can be produced experimentally in rodents by various methods.[12,13] In rats, maternal riboflavin deficiency results in a syndrome of skeletal malformations in which micrognathia is an outstanding feature[14] (Fig. 70-3). The dentofacial changes in this syndrome have been examined and described.[15]

Much has been written about the treatment of micrognathia, particularly that of the Pierre Robin syndrome. Opinions concerning the need for and type of treatment differ, as the cases differ in degree and etiology.[16]

Macrognathia

Mandibular macrognathia combined with prognathism is known to occur as a hereditary characteristic. In the Hapsburgs, the condition occurred apparently as a dominantly inherited trait through several centuries. Dental occlusion is disturbed in mandibular macrognathia.

Cherubism
(Familial Fibrous Dysplasia of the Jaws)

In 1933, Jones[17] described a familial multilocular cystic disease of the jaws that has become known as "cherubism." In the cases reported by him, 3 members (2 boys and a girl) of a Jewish family from Russia were affected by this strange deformity of both jaws that, although not present at birth, developed within the first few years of life. The parents of these children were normal and no similar deformity had been observed in the ancestry. The name "cherubism" is due to a marked fullness of the cheeks and jaws, resulting in a chubbiness of the features. Both the upper and the lower jaw can be felt as hard masses bulging outward to form bilateral, painless swelling of the face. Some teeth are irregularly placed and others are missing. The alveolar ridges are very wide in the upper jaw, which results in formation of a narrow V-shaped palate. The submandibular lymph nodes often are enlarged. The eyes are characteristically turned upward, so that white lines of sclera are visible beneath the irides. Roentgenograms reveal multilocular cysts in the jaws but other skeletal parts show no abnormality. Histologically, the lesions consist chiefly of fibrous tissue with numerous multinucleated giant cells. Several cases of this rare fibrous dysplasia have been reported, and Jones *et al.*[18] published a follow-up of the original cases in 1950. Aiken[19] reviewed the literature and added a sporadic case.

It is likely that this symmetric fibrous dysplasia is

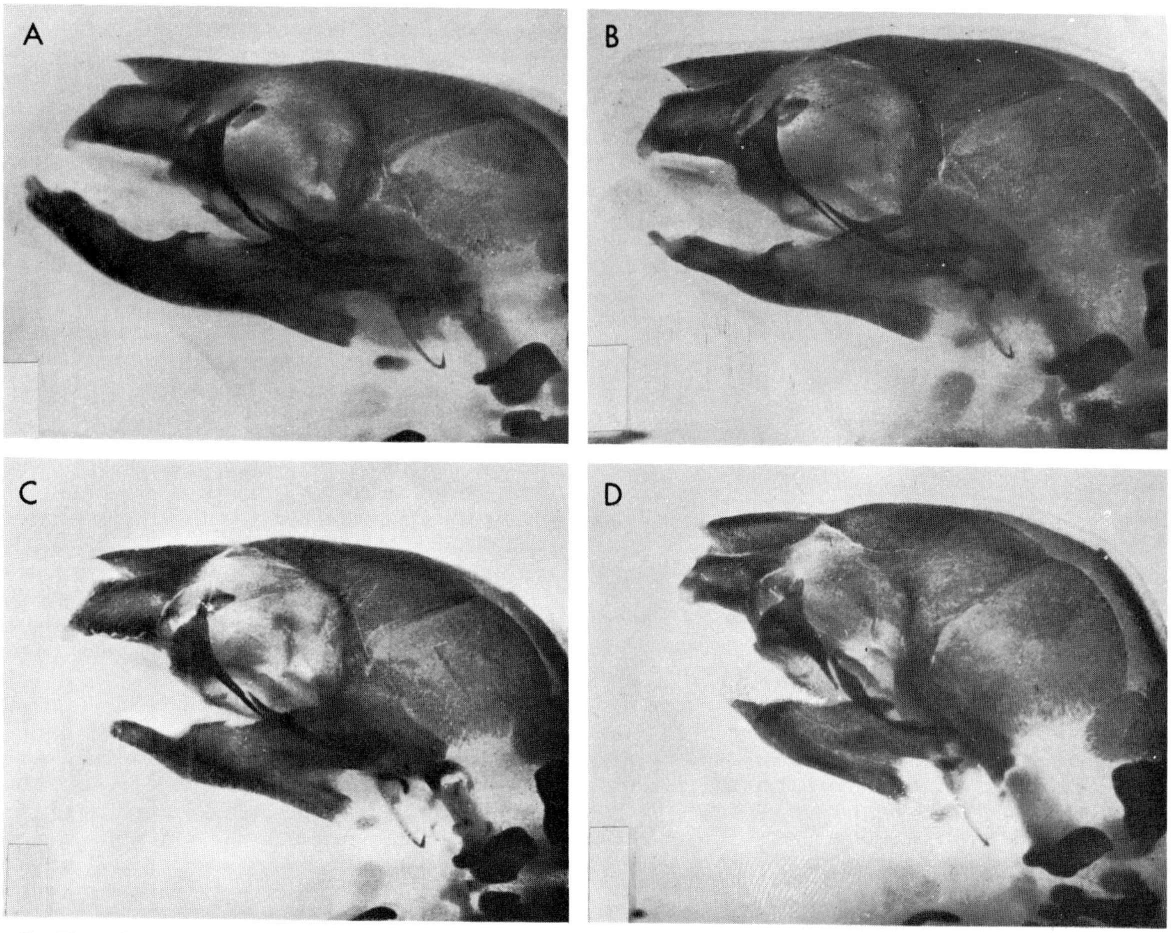

Fig. 70-3. – **A,** head of cleared specimen of a normal newborn rat. **B–D,** heads of newborn rats affected by maternal riboflavin deficiency, showing various degrees of shortening of lower and upper jaws (micrognathia).

genetically determined, but the mode of transmission is not known. As mentioned, in Jones's cases, the parents were normal and 3 children were affected. In other families, dominant transmission from parent to children seemed to occur.[19] Exogenous pathogenic factors must also be considered.

The disorder usually progresses within the first few years up to the time of puberty, when arrest or regression may occur. However, the appearance of these children may become so grotesque that plastic surgery is required.[18] The diagnosis can be made by the characteristic facies and the early bilateral mandibular swelling without x-ray evidence of a generalized skeletal disorder. The blood chemical values are normal and biopsy shows giant cells and fibrous tissue. The diagnosis is facilitated if more than one member of a family is affected.[19]

Microstomia

Agnathia and micrognathia frequently are associated with microstomia. In agnathia, the oral opening may be minute. A small mouth is seen often in children with trisomy 18, and the same is true for infants of the cyclopia series. A syndrome named "typus Rostockiensis"[20] was characterized by micrognathia, ocular and genital anomalies, congenital heart disease and polydactyly. Since these cases were described before chromosome analyses were possible, it seems likely that the patients, or at least some of them, had trisomy 13-15 (D_1) (p. 296). Microstomia sometimes is present in patients with the Hallermann-Streiff syndrome (p. 391). Microstomia, elongated philtrum, hypoplastic facial bones, ulnar deviations of the hands and clubfeet have been described as a syndrome by Freeman and Sheldon[21] (p. 673).

Microstomia can be produced experimentally in mice by maternal hypervitaminosis A.[22]

Macrostomia

Oblique facial clefts (p. 624) result in macrostomia. Such clefts may occur as isolated anomalies or be associated with such other malformations as super-

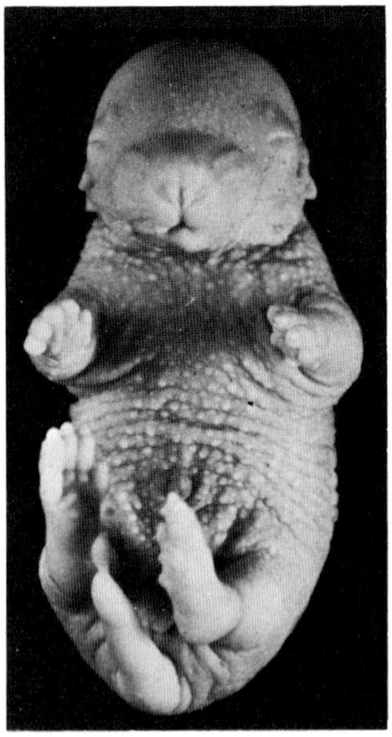

Fig. 70-4.—A mouse with microstomia produced by hypervitaminosis A. (From H. Kalter and J. Warkany.[47])

numerary teeth, congenital heart disease, costovertebral anomalies and defects of the extremities.[23] Macrostomia is a characteristic constituent of mandibulofacial dysostosis (p. 650), and is present in many cases of the Goldenhar syndrome (p. 388).

Hemifacial Hypoplasia (Hemifacial Microsomia, Unilateral Mandibulofacial Dysostosis) and Hemifacial Hyperplasia

Gorlin and Pindborg[23] considered unilateral cases of mandibulofacial dysostosis unrelated to the bilateral form (p. 650). This point of view seems justified, since dominant inheritance cannot be demonstrated in unilateral cases. On the affected side, the ear frequently is deformed and the eye may be small, colobomatous or cystic. Hemifacial hypoplasia can be combined with features of the Goldenhar syndrome (p. 388). There is aplasia or hypoplasia of the mandibular ramus accompanied by microtia of the same side.[3] There may be ipsilateral absence of the parotid gland and pulmonary agenesis. Underdevelopment of facial muscles on the affected side is common.

Congenital asymmetry of the face and jaws may be of a mechanical nature. Parmelee[24] described facial asymmetry due to intrauterine pressure of the shoulder against the jaw. There may be a marked depression on the side of the mandible or a convex deformity in the region of the angle of the jaw in the mastoid area. Facial paralysis may occur in such cases. The deformities often disappear gradually by adaptive growth of the affected side.

Unilateral hyperplasia of the mandible and of the maxilla have been reported as cases of unilateral gigantism or partial hemihypertrophy.[25] In such cases, unilateral enlargement of the maxilla, mandible, teeth, chin, cheek, lip, tongue and tonsil have been observed. The condition is noticeable at birth and becomes more pronounced with growth of the face. As a rule, there is no familial repetition of such cases. The hemihypertrophy may be limited to the face or involve other parts of the body.

Median Cleft of the Upper Lip

A median cleft of the upper lip is normal in many animals, especially in rodents. Its occurrence in humans represents the true imitation of a "harelip," whereas this term applied to lateral clefts of the lip is incorrect. Median cleft of the upper lip is seen only rarely in children. Mild cases consist of a slight notch of the vermilion border of the upper lip or, in more severe cases, in a triangular cleft that points to the nasal septum. There also may be a notch in the alveolar process, and the median incisor teeth can be more distant than normal. Sometimes, such clefts are combined with clefts of the maxilla and the posterior palate or with cleft of the nose or median cleft of the lower lip.

The most severe forms of median clefts of the upper lip represent bilateral paramedian cleft formations in which the middle portion also is missing. These median clefts, sometimes termed "false median clefts of the upper lip," often are combined with absence of the premaxillary area and of the nasal septum. The upper lip is completely split and the cleft continues through the alveolar process and the entire hard and soft palates. There is one nasal opening and the oral and nasal cavities are not separated. The external nose is flat, since it lacks a cartilaginous and osseous skeleton. The nasal root is narrow and the orbits lie close together. This condition often is combined with absence of the rhinencephalon, the olfactory tracts and nerves and belongs to the cyclopia series (Chapter 23). Other portions of the brain may be normal, or exencephaly or anencephaly may be present.[26,27] In a series of 1,000 cases of facial clefts and facial deformities, Davis[28] listed 4 cases of median cleft lip.

Median pseudocleft of the upper lip may be a manifestation of the orodigitofacial syndrome (Chapter 73).

Oblique Facial Clefts

This malformation is relatively rare. In 1887, Morian[29] collected a number of cases and established three types of the anomaly. In type 1, the cleft begins lateral to the philtrum as a typical harelip, continues into the nose and runs between the nose and cheek upward to the inner canthus or to the lower lid. The depth of the cleft varies and may be limited to the skin, or the bones are included. These cases usually

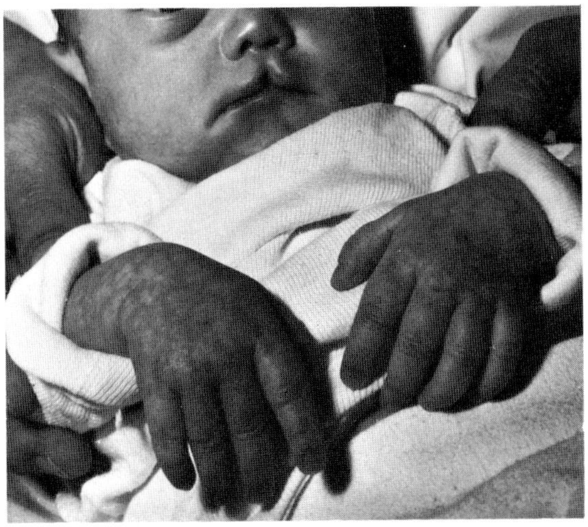

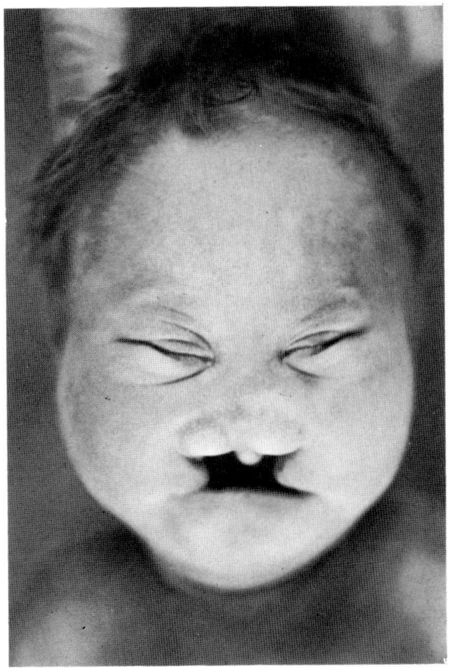

Fig. 70-5 (above).—Incomplete median cleft of lip in an infant who had bilateral colobomas.

Fig. 70-6 (right).—Median harelip and cleft palate in an infant who had fusion of the telencephalic hemispheres, absence of anterior parts of the corpus callosum and absence of olfactory nerves.

are combined with complete cleft lip and cleft palate. Morian's type 2 begins on the upper lip, continues lateral to the nose and runs obliquely through the cheek to the internal canthus or the lower lid. Type 1 and type 2 have been considered primary facial clefts that generally follow the naso-optic groove. Type 3 was recognized as a secondary facial cleft, since its course does not correspond to any of the known embryologic grooves. This type of oblique facial cleft begins in the soft parts of the angle of the mouth and runs upward in an irregular course. In these cases, the palate usually is intact. Politzer[30] doubted that any of the oblique facial clefts could be attributed to primary arrest of development and thought that they all were the result of tears of the embryonic face.

Oblique facial clefts have been induced experimentally in rats, although not with regularity. In some offspring of folic acid-deficient rats, complete clefts of the lip, palate and maxillary area have been observed by Nelson *et al.*[31] and Giroud.[32] In our laboratory, maternal hypervitaminosis A and salicylate intoxication[33] have led to oblique facial clefts. Figure 70-7 shows a unilateral oblique facial cleft produced by hypervitaminosis A in a rat that also has cleft palate and exencephaly. Histologic sections showed that the edges of the cleft were completely covered by skin and surface epithelium consisting of many layers. There is no indication of a tear, and it appears very likely that this cleft represents a primary oblique facial fissure. In a specimen induced by salicylate poisoning, the situation is less clear, as the lower portion of the cleft is covered by normal skin and the upper portion is covered by an epithelium that appears eroded and not intact. Examination of these specimens suggests that at least some cases of oblique facial fissures can be primary and attributable to insufficient growth of the maxillary and frontal processes.

Lip Anomalies

Short and Long Upper Lip

Short upper lip has been described as a symptom in the popliteal pterygium syndrome (p. 643) and the Ellis-van Creveld syndrome (p. 793), and an elongat-

Fig. 70-7.—Harelip and oblique facial cleft on the animal's right side in a rat with exencephaly (produced by hypervitaminosis A).

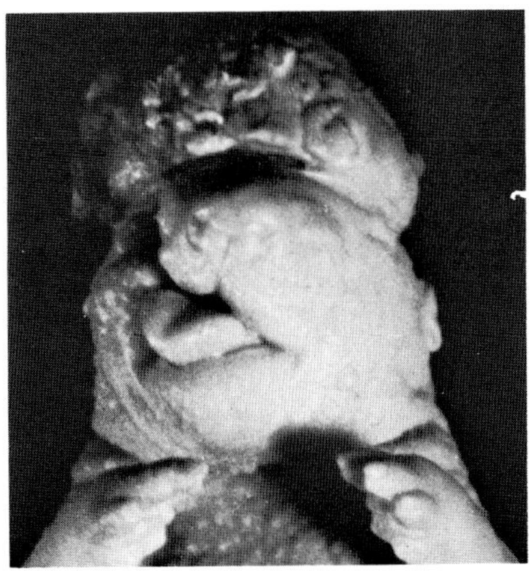

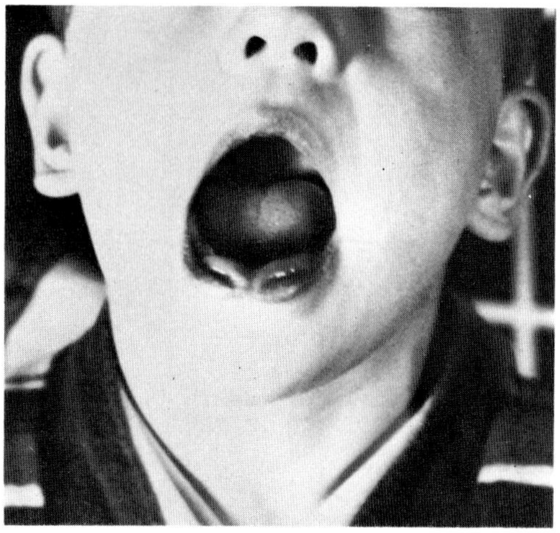

Fig. 70-8.—Congenital "double lower lip" in a 3-year-old boy whose mother had the same anomaly.

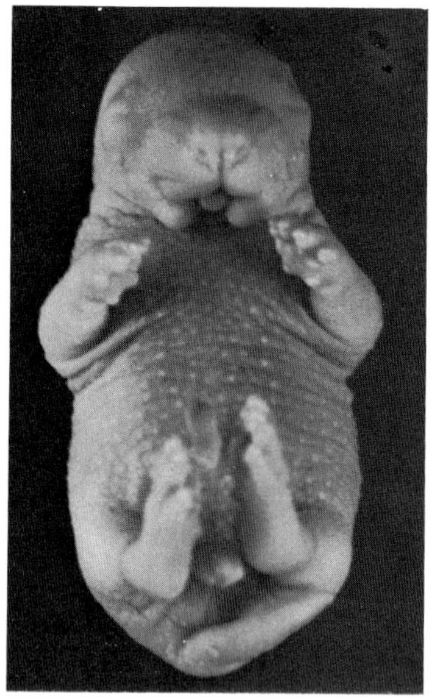

Fig. 70-9.—A mouse with median cleft mandible produced by hypervitaminosis A. (From H. Kalter and J. Warkany.[47])

ed upper lip in the de Lange syndrome (p. 344) and in craniocarpotarsal dystrophy.[21]

Double Lip

Double lip is a deformity that consists of redundant tissue in the mucosal portion of the lip just inside its vermilion border. The anomaly, which can occur in the upper or in the lower lip (Fig. 70-8), has been observed in men and women. It is more conspicuous in the upper lip, since the mucosal duplication, which shows a median notch, hangs down and partly covers the incisors. The "inner lip" becomes especially noticeable when the patient smiles. The excess fold, which is composed of mucous membrane and submucosal tissue, contains mucous glands. The deformity is, according to Dingman,[34] truly congenital, although usually it is not noticed until after eruption of the teeth. Although the deformity causes no functional difficulty, it is embarrassing to the patient and is a psychologic handicap. The condition lends itself readily to surgical treatment. Double lip may be associated with relaxation of the supratarsal fold (blepharochalasis) and with thyroid enlargement.[23,35] A "double lower lip" occurred in the mother and the child shown in Figure 70-8.

Clefts of the Mandible and Lower Lip

Clefts of the lower lip and mandible are extremely rare. The lip may be cleft merely superficially or, in severe cases, be split down to the chin, involving the mandible. In cases of mandibular cleft, the two portions are connected by bridges of connective tissue that vary in length. The two halves of the mandible, although movable against each other, can be normal otherwise and contain the normal number of teeth. In rare instances, the cleft formation continues into the mouth and includes the tongue. A symptom complex of mandibular cleft, oligodontia and polydactyly has been described by Weyers[36] as "dysostosis acrofacialis." In some cases of this type, the cleft of the mandible and of the tongue is occupied by tumors.[26] A complicated bilateral cleft of the lower lip was described by Abramson.[37] A "parasitic monster" was attached to the hard palate and a mass of tissue separated the cleft elements of the lower lip. There also was an anterior ankyloglossia. Clefts of the mandible sometimes are associated with cleft lip, cleft palate or oblique facial cleft. The anomaly has been observed in animals and has been induced experimentally in mice, rats and guinea pigs by hypervitaminosis A[13,22] (Fig. 70-9).

Congenital Pits and Fistulas of the Lips

Congenital pits or recesses usually occur in the lower lips, where they may be bilateral or unilateral, showing a well-defined circular depression on the vermilion border. In the upper lip, where they are rare, they are found lateral to the philtrum. They represent the orifice of mucous tracts that extend into the substance of the lip (Fig. 70-10). Mucus is secreted from the openings of the tracts, which diverge laterally and vary in length from 5 mm. to 25 mm. Histologically, the tracts are lined by stratified squamous epithelium that extends downward to the orbicularis oris muscles. Cleft lip and palate or isolated cleft palate is present in 70–80% of the patients with labial pits.[38] Clubfoot, syndactyly and popliteal pterygia have been observed occasionally.[23] The condition is hereditary and is considered an irregularly dominant

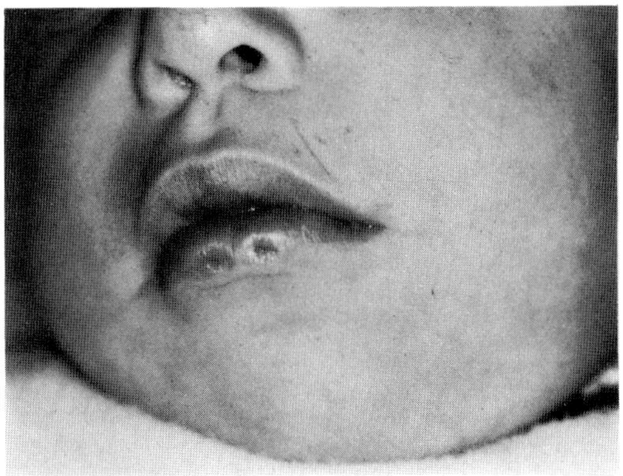

Fig. 70-10.—Congenital pits in the lower lip combined with a high palate. (Courtesy of Hamilton County, Ohio, Diagnostic Clinic for the Mentally Retarded.)

trait. The penetrance is high but the expressivity varies, as the condition can be unilateral, bilateral and combined with other facial anomalies[9,38,39] (p. 643).

Bilateral Clefts of the Lower Lip

This rare anomaly was seen in an infant with a parasitic "monster" arising from the hard palate and with ankyloglossia.[37]

Cysts of the Jaws

Multiple cysts within the jaws may be a manifestation of a hamartous syndrome that includes basal cell nevi, costovertebral anomalies and changes of the central nervous system (p. 1268). The cysts, which are scattered through the jaws, vary in size[40] and epithelial lining. They originate near the teeth, which can be disturbed in growth and development.[23] Multiple epithelial cysts of the jaws have been described in association with trichoepitheliomas, tumors originating from squamous epithelium or hair follicles.[41] These disorders can be transmitted as a dominant trait with variable expressivity and penetrance.

Temporomandibular Joint

The early development of the temporomandibular joint was studied by Furstman,[42] who noted that important histodifferentiation of the embryonic mesenchyme takes place in that area from the eighth to the tenth week of intrauterine life. At the same time, the mandibular condyle assumes its mature pattern, but formation of the articular disk follows approximately 4 weeks later. Meckel cartilage does not participate in the development of the joint.

Epithelial syngnathia in human embryos was described by Hochstetter,[43] and Mathis[44] recorded a case of fibro-epithelial concretion of upper and lower jaws in an infant girl who could not open her mouth and could not be fed normally. Prompt relief could be achieved by surgery. Partial fusion of the mandible and maxilla combined with micrognathia and microstomia was observed by Salleh[45] in an 8-year-old girl who survived by sucking her food through the small opening between her teeth.

Experimental production of syngnathia in mice has been reported by Kalter and Deuschle.[46]

REFERENCES

1. Derry, D. E.: Two skulls with absence of the premaxilla, J. Anat. 72:295, 1938.
2. Shafer, W. G., Hine, M. K., and Levy, B. M.: *A Textbook of Oral Pathology* (Philadelphia: W. B. Saunders Company, 1958).
3. Kazanjian, V. H.: Congenital absence of the ramus of the mandible, J. Bone & Joint Surg. 21-B:761, 1939.
4. Ballantyne, J. W.: *Manual of Antenatal Pathology and Hygiene. The Embryo* (Chicago: Chicago Medical Book Company, 1904).
5. Josephy, H.: Missbildungen des Halses. Otocephalie, in Schwalbe, E. (ed.), *Die Morphologie der Missbildungen des Menschen und der Tiere* (Jena: Gustav Fischer, 1913), Vol. 3, pt. 11, Chap. 6.
6. Giroud, A., Martinet, M., and Deluchat, C.: Otocéphalie, Compt. rend. Soc. oto-rhin-laryng. Oct., 1965.
7. Warkany, J., and Takacs, E.: Congenital malformations in rats from streptonigrin. Arch. Path. 79:65, 1965.
8. Thoma, K. H.: *Oral Pathology* (3d ed.; St. Louis: The C. V. Mosby Company, 1950).
9. Thoma, K. H.: *Oral Pathology* (4th ed.; St. Louis: The C. V. Mosby Company, 1954).
10. Hanhart, E.: Über die Kombination von Peromelie mit Mikrognathie, ein neues Syndrom beim Menschen, entsprechend der Akroteriasis congenita von Wriedt und Mohr beim Rinde, Arch. Klaus Stift, Vererbungsforsch. 25: 531, 1950.
11. Leist, M.: Odontologischer Befund bei sechs Kindern von intra graviditatum mit Röntgenstrahlen, beziehungsweise Radium bestrahlten Müttern, Ztschr. Stomatol. 24:448, 1926.
12. Kalter, H., and Warkany, J.: Experimental production of congenital malformations in mammals by metabolic procedures, Physiol. Rev. 39:69, 1959.
13. Giroud, A., and Martinet, M.: Fissures médianes de la machoire inférieure, Rev. stomatol. 65:796, 1964–1965.
14. Warkany, J., and Nelson, R. C.: Appearance of skeletal abnormalities in the offspring of rats reared on a deficient diet, Science 92:383, 1940.
15. Warkany, J., and Deuschle, F. M.: Congenital malformations induced in rats by maternal riboflavin deficiency: Dentofacial changes, J.A.D.A. 51:139, 1955.
16. Jolleys, A.: Micrognathos: A review of 38 cases treated in the newborn period, J. Pediat. Surg. 1:460, 1966.
17. Jones, W. A.: Familial multilocular cystic disease of the jaws, Am. J. Cancer 17:946, 1933.
18. Jones, W. A., Gerrie, J., and Pritchard, J.: Cherubism—a familial fibrous dysplasia of the jaws, J. Bone & Joint Surg. 32-B:334, 1950.
19. Aiken, H. E.: Cherubism, Am. J. Dis. Child. 103:679, 1962.
20. Hövels, O., and Müllereisert, F.: Der "Typus Rostockiensis" als charakteristisches Kombinationsbild multipler Missbildungen (Polydaktylie, Hypospadie, Kryptorchismus und Mikrognathie), Ztschr. Kinderh. 77:454, 1955.
21. Freeman, E. A., and Sheldon, J. H.: Cranio-carpo-tarsal dystrophy—an undescribed congenital malformation, Arch. Dis. Childhood 13:277, 1938.
22. Kalter, H., and Warkany, J.: Experimental production of congenital malformations in strains of inbred mice by maternal treatment with hypervitaminosis A, Am. J. Path. 38:1, 1961.

23. Gorlin, R. J., and Pindborg, J. J.: *Syndromes of the Head and Neck* (New York: McGraw-Hill Book Company, Inc., 1964).
24. Parmelee, A. H.: Molding due to intrauterine pressure, Am. J. Dis. Child. 42:1155, 1931.
25. Rushton, M. A.: A dental abnormality of size and rate, Proc. Roy. Soc. Med. 41:490, 1948.
26. Grünberg, K.: Die Missbildungen des Kopfes. I. Die Gesichtsspalten und die zu ihnen in genetischer Beziehung stehenden anderweitigen Missbildungen des Gesichts, in Schwalbe, E. (ed.), *Die Morphologie der Missbildungen des Menschen und der Tiere* (Jena: Gustav Fischer, 1913), Vol. 3, pt. 1, Chap. 4, pp. 113-204.
27. Gruber, G. B.: Über einen akrocephalen Reliefschädel. Ein Beitrag zur Frage der partiellen Chondrodystrophie, Beitr. path. Anat. 97:9, 1936.
28. Davis, W. B.: Congenital deformities of face; types found in series of 1,000 cases, Surg., Gynec. & Obst. 61:201, 1935.
29. Morian, R.: Über die schräge Gesichtsspalte, Arch. klin. Chir. 35:245, 1887.
30. Politzer, G.: Die Projektion der embryonalen Gesichtsfurchen auf das Gesicht des Erwachsenen und die Entstehung der schrägen Gesichtsspalte, Beitr. path. Anat. 97:557, 1936.
31. Nelson, M. M., Wright, H. V., Asling, C. W., and Evans, H. M.: Multiple congenital abnormalities resulting from transitory deficiency of pteroylglutamic acid during gestation in the rat, J. Nutrition 56:349, 1955.
32. Giroud, A.: Les malformations congénitales et leurs causes, Biol. méd. 44:1, 1955.
33. Warkany, J., and Takacs, E.: Experimental production of congenital malformations in rats by salicylate poisoning, Am. J. Path. 35:315, 1959.
34. Dingman, R. O.: Double lip, J. Oral Surg. 5:146, 1947.
35. Ascher, K. W.: Blepharochalasis mit Struma und Doppellippe, Klin. Monatsbl. Augenh. 65:86, 1920.
36. Weyers, H.: Hexadactylie, Unterkieferspalt und Oligodontie, ein neuer Symptomenkomplex: Dysostosis acro-facialis, Ann. paediat. 181:45, 1953.
37. Abramson, P. D.: Bilateral congenital clefts of the lower lip, Surgery 31:761, 1952.
38. Müller, D.: Über den Erbgang und die Genese der "angeborenen Unterlippenfistel," Deutsche Zahnarztl. Ztschr. 4:299, 1949.
39. Ludy, J. B., and Shirazy, E.: Concerning congenital fistulas of the lips, Internat. Clin. 3:75, 1938.
40. Nichamin, S. J., and Kaufman, M.: Gingival microcysts in infancy, Pediatrics 31:412, 1963.
41. McKelvey, L. E., Albright, C. R., and Prazak, G.: Multiple hereditary familial epithelial cysts of the jaws with the associated anomaly of trichoepithelioma; report of a case, Oral Surg. 13:111, 1960.
42. Furstman, L.: The early development of the human temporomandibular joint, Am. J. Orthodont. 49:672, 1963.
43. Hochstetter, F.: Über zwei Falle epithelialer Syngnathie bei menschlichen Keimlingen, cited by Mathis.[44]
44. Mathis, H.: Über einen Fall von Ernährungsschwierigkeit bei connataler Syngnathie, Deutsche Zahnaerztl. Ztschr. 17:1167, 1962.
45. Salleh, N. B. M.: Congenital partial fusion of the mandible and maxilla, Oral Surg. 20:74, 1965.
46. Kalter, H., and Deuschle, F. M.: Congenital malformations experimentally induced by hypervitaminosis A, in Kreshover, S. J., and McClure, F. J. (eds.), *Environmental Variables in Oral Disease* (Washington, D. C.: American Association for the Advancement of Science, 1966).
47. Kalter, H., and Warkany, J.: Experimental production of congenital malformations in strains of inbred mice by maternal treatment with hypervitaminosis A, Am. J. Path. 38:1, 1961.
48. Pashayan, H., Pinsky, L., and Fraser, F. C.: Hemifacial microsomia: Oculo-auriculo-vertebral dysplasia. A patient with overlapping features, J. M. Genetics 7:185, 1970.

Cleft Lip and Palate

Frequency of Cleft Lip and Palate

MANY ESTIMATES of the frequency of facial clefts were made in the fourth decade of this century in obstetric hospitals, and it was found that 1 case occurred in approximately 900-1,000 births. In northern Germany and in Denmark, the incidence at birth was higher, namely 1 in 600-700 (1.5 per 1,000).[1] Some of the differences may be real, since racial variations are well established. In 1924, J. S. Davis[2] found an incidence of 1 in 1,170 births in the obstetric ward at Johns Hopkins Hospital in Baltimore, Maryland, but there was a marked difference between white and Negro children. Among the white, the incidence was 1 in 915 (1.1 per 1,000) and among the Negroes 1 in 1,788 (0.56 per 1,000). Racial differences were similar 35 years later in New York City.[3] W. B. Davis[4] stated that facial clefts are rare among Hebrews. Other incidence figures in different racial groups are cited on page 631. Thus, care must be taken not to generalize the Danish figures obtained by Fogh-Andersen,[1] which, although collected with great care, were obtained from a population of northern Europeans only. In New York City, McIntosh *et al.*[5] found 8 children with facial clefts in 6,000 births, an incidence of 1 in 750 births (1.33 per 1,000). This incidence, observed in a prospective fetal life study and derived from small figures, agrees fairly well with figures obtained by other methods. It is estimated that approximately 9% of infants born with harelip and cleft palate are stillborn and about 12% die within the first 10 days. In Denmark, it was estimated that the number of patients with harelip and cleft palate living, i.e., the prevalence, was about 4,000—or somewhat higher than 1 per 1,000.

Fogh-Andersen[1] found that in Denmark 25% of the patients with clefts have harelip only, 50% have harelip and cleft palate and 25% have cleft palate alone. It is generally and correctly stated that facial clefts occur more frequently in males than in females. In Fogh-Andersen's[1] series, there were approximately 63% males and 37% females. But isolated cleft palate (CP) actually occurred more often in females than in males (66% as opposed to 34%), whereas harelip with or without cleft palate (CL/CP) was seen in 70% males as opposed to 30% females. Fogh-Andersen assumed, therefore, that harelip (with or without cleft palate) and isolated cleft palate are genetically differing malformations. It is known that cleft formations affect the left side more often than the right; simple harelip, unilateral or bilateral, is rarer than the harelip-cleft palate complex (cheilognathopalatoschisis); unilateral cleft lip is more frequent than bilateral; and simple unilateral harelip occurs more than twice as often on the left side as on the right. Double harelip without cleft palate is even rarer than right harelip. In the harelip-cleft palate complex, the left side is affected more than twice as often as the right, and double harelip and cleft palate is more frequent than the right-sided complex. It is possible that in Denmark the incidence of clefts increased from 1.5 per 1,000 in 1939 to 1.8 per 1,000 in 1960.[6] Frequency figures cited in the literature vary greatly. In a study of consecutive births in 24 centers undertaken by the World Health Organization,[7] the mean frequency of CL/CP was 0.98 per 1,000 and that of CP 0.23 per 1,000. The highest frequencies for CL/CP were in Johannesburg, Kuala Lumpur, Santiago, Hong Kong and Singapore; for CP in Melbourne, Czechoslovakia and Belfast. Tabulations show variations of from 0.5 per 1,000 to 2 per 1,000.[8,9] Some authors report incidence figures, others prevalence figures; some report large samples, others small samples; some reports come from hospitals or surgical clinics, others from birth certificates. None of these estimates comprises the total population affected. There are definitely ethnic group differences (p. 631) and there may be secular changes.[6] Differences in size of the clefts may influence frequency figures, as small posterior clefts often are overlooked or not reported. With increasing interest in facial clefts, the classes proposed by Fogh-Andersen[1] are further broken down as new syndromes and entities are described. Drillien *et al.*,[10] in a sample of 169 children in Scotland, classified 16.6% as cleft lip, 37.8% as cleft lip and cleft palate (54.4% CL/CP), 36.7% as cleft palate, 7.1% as cleft palate with micrognathia (p. 655) and 1.8% as cleft palate and lip pits (p. 626). The literature is replete with atypical facial clefts[11–13] that are relatively rare. Among 4,000 consecutive admissions for facial clefts at a Copenhagen hospital during 30 years, 48 cases (1.2%) were considered atypical by Fogh-Andersen.[11]

Etiology

Interest in the causation of cleft lip can be traced back to the seventeenth century, when William Harvey[14] gave an embryologic explanation of harelip by stating that "in fetuses the oral aperture without lips or cheeks stretches from ear to ear which was the reason why so many are born with the upper lip divided" (p. 18). This concept of arrested development was a formal but not a causal explanation of facial clefts. Some etiologic explanations are ancient but mostly superstitious. That encounter of a pregnant woman with a rabbit or a gaping fish can cause cleft palate is an old theory. Encounters with itinerant foreigners, especially gypsies, were considered definitely teratogenic.[15] Sudden fright and emotional shock served as explanations for harelip and cleft palate that were acceptable to scientists and common people alike until the beginning of this century, and well into this century,[16] when old beliefs were revived as it became known that cortisone can produce cleft palate in certain strains of mice. But it was shown experimentally in susceptible mice that cortisone injections cannot be equated with (audiogenic) stresses,[17] and there was no association of emotional stress during pregnancy to cleft lip or palate in man.[18]

Heredity has been another explanation of facial clefts, since Trew,[19] in 1757, described a family in which several members were affected in more than one generation. By 1910, Rischbieth[15] could chart 175 cases of familial harelip or cleft palate, so that heredity seemed well established by then. But few of the pedigrees conformed to Mendelian rules and many more cases were sporadic than familial.

During the 1920s and the 1930s, numerous complicated theories were offered to uphold the tenet that all facial clefts were hereditary, but these theories could not be translated into intelligible language useful in genetic counseling. In 1943, we[20] reviewed some of the older publications on this subject; we also demonstrated that cleft palate can be produced in rats with great regularity by prenatal dietary deficiency. It was pointed out that the experiments indicated that it is not justifiable to assume a priori that all cleft palates in human beings are hereditary, and we expressed the belief that the clinical material encountered was a conglomeration of hereditary malformations and their phenocopies. Many early investigators studied the family backgrounds of patients with cleft lip and palate as encountered in hospitals and clinics. The familial occurrence found by different authors ranged between 6% and 45%, but most found more than one afflicted member in the families of approximately 20% of their patients.[20] More recent studies resulted in reports showing from 30% to 40%[10,21] familial involvement. Of course, one cannot equate familial incidence with heredity, since genetically determined cases can be sporadic and recurrence in a family could be due to different etiologic factors—genetic or environmental. Consequently, different interpreters assigned the nonfamilial 80% to either genetic or nongenetic factors, according to their preference.

In 1942, Fogh-Andersen[1] published his scholarly survey of harelip and cleft palate in Denmark, a study that was superior to previous attempts not only in scope and numbers but also in its approach to the problem, which was unimpeded by theoretical prejudices. He grouped the clefts into (1) harelip, (2) harelip and cleft palate and (3) isolated cleft palate. He concluded that cleft lip with or without associated cleft palate (CL/CP) and isolated cleft palate (CP) are two different entities. Whereas the CL/CP complex occurred most frequently in males, isolated CP was more common in females. The two groups seemed genetically different and risk figures for genetic prognosis had to be separated. In the isolated cleft palate group, a considerable admixture of nonhereditary cases seemed probable. It followed that the clefts were heterogeneous in origin, a finding that was and is essential for successful etiologic research. Instead of forcing the heterogeneous results into a semblance of Mendelian rules, Fogh-Andersen established empirical risk figures for genetic prognosis. In general, these risk figures have been confirmed and are still of value[22]:

A. *Cleft lip* with or without cleft palate (CL/CP).
   1. Parents unaffected, 1 child with CL/CP: The average risk for each child of such parents lies between 4% and 7%.
   2. One parent with CL/CP, no affected children: For a person with harelip married to a normal person, the risk for affected children is 2%.
   3. One parent and 1 child with CL/CP: The average risk for other children of such parents being affected is between 11% and 14%.
   4. Parents unaffected, 2 children with CL/CP: From the combined data available, it seems that the risk for CL/CP for subsequent pregnancies is approximately 10%.

B. *Cleft palate* without cleft lip (CP).
   1. Parents unaffected, 1 child with CP: The risk of having a cleft palate is between 2% and 5% for each child of such parents.
   2. One parent with CP, no affected children: Based on small numbers, the probability that a person with cleft palate will have a child with the same anomaly was estimated as 7%.[1]
   3. One parent and 1 child with CP: Based on small figures, Fogh-Andersen found that in this case 14–17% of the siblings of the affected child also had cleft palate.[22]

These empirical figures found in families in which one or several cases of clefts occur exceed by far the frequency figures for the general population, which suggested to Fogh-Andersen[1] that for both conditions, CL/CP and CP, heredity has been proved as an etiologic factor. Although it is clear from this and other studies that genetic factors play a role in many cases of facial clefts, the risk figures are much lower than would be expected if simple dominant or recessive inheritance were apparent. The figures do not rule out that some cases of facial clefts may be strongly influenced by nongenetic factors.

Although Fogh-Andersen[1] distinguished between CL/CP and CP as different entities, this division is only a beginning in etiologic classification. It is clear that the malformations called harelip (CL/CP) or cleft palate (CP) can be subdivided into many other etiologic entities. These malformations are merely symptoms of various prenatal disturbances that may be due to genetic or nongenetic factors or combinations of them. That CL/CP and CP cannot be considered etiologic entities can be illustrated by examples of syndromes that include facial clefts (p. 650).

The examples of clefts due to various etiologic mechanisms show that empirical risk figures for CL/CP and CP must be considered merely as provisional in parental counseling, to be replaced by a better knowledge of the determining factors in individual families. Although the value of empirical risk figures is limited for eugenic prognosis and parental counseling, these figures have been extremely valuable in demonstrating that eugenic measures proposed in the past have been greatly unwarranted and unjustified. In the past, particularly during the years of the Third Reich in Germany, some authors suggested sterilization for all persons with harelip or cleft palate. One will agree with Fogh-Andersen[1] that sterilization of a patient with harelip of unknown origin would be absurd if his chances for normal children are 98%.

As stated before, one has to look at facial clefts as symptoms of disturbed development. *The disturbances can be gene-determined, chromosome-determined or they can be due to adverse environmental conditions.* In many cases, a combination of factors probably is at fault.

To find a simple mode of inheritance for genetically determined cases cannot be expected. Even the division into CL/CP and CP did not result in Mendelian ratios. There is occasional overlapping of the two groups (p. 643). Several heritable but distinct syndromes that may include cleft formations are now recognized (p. 650), and chromosome-determined clefts conform to their own rules (p. 632).

In the common CL/CP type, heredity often is recognizable, but skipping of a generation or of collaterals prohibits establishment of simple rules of inheritance. One must take recourse to such modifiers as reduced penetrance or variable expressivity to explain most of the pedigrees.

The capricious behavior of cleft formation in monozygotic twins illustrates the dilemma; whereas concordance of clefts in such twins (see Fig. 70-21) can be used as an argument in favor of genetic determination, discordance points up the power of nongenetic factors. Even conjoined twins can differ in regard to harelip. Figure 70-11 illustrates a thoracopagus tetrabrachius tripus published in 1620 showing one member affected by a cleft lip whereas the other is spared. The skeptic who doubts the accuracy of this old drawing can find a similar situation in the reports of modern authors.[23-25] If discordance in regard to cleft lip is possible in conjoined twins, it is not surprising to find it in monozygotic twins. Fogh-Andersen's[1] series contained 2 pairs of monozygotic twins; 1 pair was concordant and one discordant in regard to facial clefts. In a review of the literature, including his own cases, Fogh-Andersen found among 25 monozygotic pairs 8 concordant and 17 discordant. Of 71 dizygotic twin pairs, there were only 5 concordant and 66 discordant. Similar ratios have been ascertained by other authors. It seems that concordance occurs in approximately 30% of monozygotic twins and in only 7% of dizygotic twins.[21] These findings point to an important role of genetic factors, but also to modification by nongenetic factors in many of the cases. Of special interest is the fact that identical twins who have a

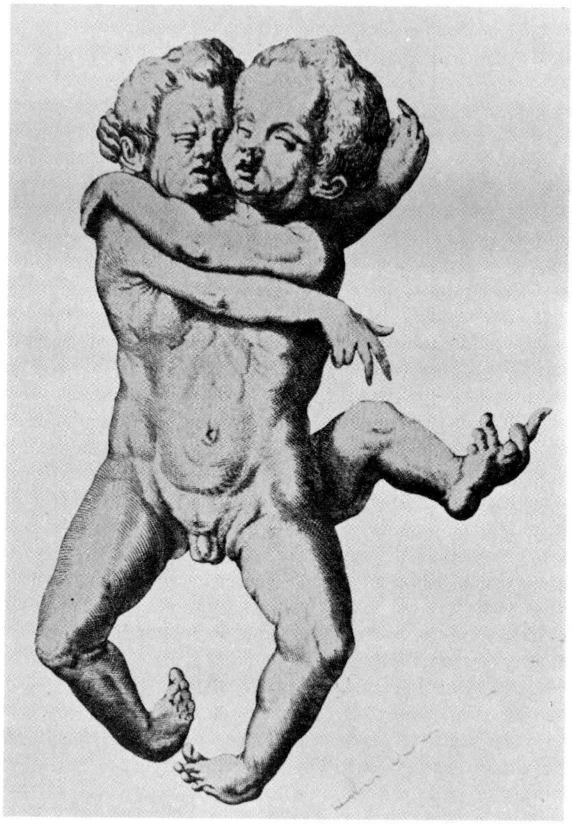

Fig. 70-11.—Conjoined twins, one of whom is affected by complete cleft lip (thoracopagus tetrabrachius tripus), reproduced in a pamphlet of the year 1620. (From E. Holländer: *Wunder, Wundergeburt und Wundergestalt* [Stuttgart: Ferdinand Enke, 1922].)

familial disposition to cleft lip and palate can be discordant in regard to cleft formation.[26,27] In such a case (see Fig. 70-12), the normal twin probably was protected by nongenetic circumstances that interfered with penetrance of the inherited tendency. If we were able to recognize and manage such protective factors, we would have a tool for the prevention of facial clefts. Concordance is more than 40% in monozygotic twins with CL/CP but only 8% in such twins with isolated CP.[10]

Progress has been made in the analysis of genetic factors. It is well known that the CL/CP complex occurs more frequently in boys than in girls (p. 628), but it seems that the genetic prognosis is worse for affected females, as they have a higher incidence of offspring with CL/CP than affected males. In England, Fraser Roberts[28] followed the offspring of 99 males and 52 females with CL/CP. Of the males' offspring, 2% were affected; there was no difference in the incidence of clefts in boys and girls. But among the children of the 52 affected females, 10% of the boys had CL/CP, whereas none of the girls had the malformation. No single-gene explanation seemed applicable, and more complicated explanations seemed likely. The results of Woolf *et al.*[29] in Utah were similar, showing the great risk for male offspring of women with CL/CP and apparent safety for their daughters. These authors thought that many cases have a polygenic mode of inheritance; the threshold number of genes needed for expression of the clefts apparently is lower in males than in females. An affected female will have more of these genes than an affected male, so that the risk for surpassing of the threshold number of genes in her offspring is increased. An increased frequency of the disorder among the siblings of female patients as compared with the siblings of male patients seemed to support this genetic hypothesis,[29] since the parents of an affected female should have more of the predisposing genes than the parents of an affected male. Whatever the explanations, the fact that the children of female CL/CP patients are more endangered than those of male patients requires consideration in genetics counseling.

A possibility of sex-linked cleft palate was considered by Weinstein and Cohen.[30]

There are definite differences in racial groups. In Baltimore, Maryland, the rate of Negro children with clefts was 0.55 per 1,000 live births, whereas it was 1.06 per 1,000 in Caucasians.[2] In Northumberland and Durham,[180] it was 1.4, in Denmark 1.5,[1] in Sweden 1.75, in Birmingham, England 1.76,[31] but in Japan it was 2.7[32] and among Montana Indians 3.6 per 1,000.[33] A low incidence in Negroes was also noted in Pennsylvania, where the rate was 0.25, whereas that of Caucasians was 1.33.[34] It is not certain that such figures can be considered characteristic of "race," since the populations compared differed in environmental conditions also. In Hawaii, for instance, clefts in children of Caucasian mothers were said to occur at a rate of 0.5 per 1,000, whereas in children of Filipino mothers it was 3.5 per 1,000. This seems to indicate a racial difference, but in Hawaii the rate for Caucasians was similar to that of Baltimore Negroes and only about one-third that of northern Europeans. In contrast, in Nairobi, an estimate resulted in a rate of 2.3 per 1,000 in African neonates.[35] Other incidences according to race were tabulated by Greene.[8] No doubt, methods of sampling are of decisive importance too.[36]

Fig. 70-12.—Two short pedigrees showing (probably) inherited clefts, discordant in monozygotic twins. In **A,** one twin had CL/CP; the other twin was normal. The brother of the maternal grandmother had CL/CP.[26] In **B,** one twin had partial CP; the other twin was normal. The father had CP.[27]

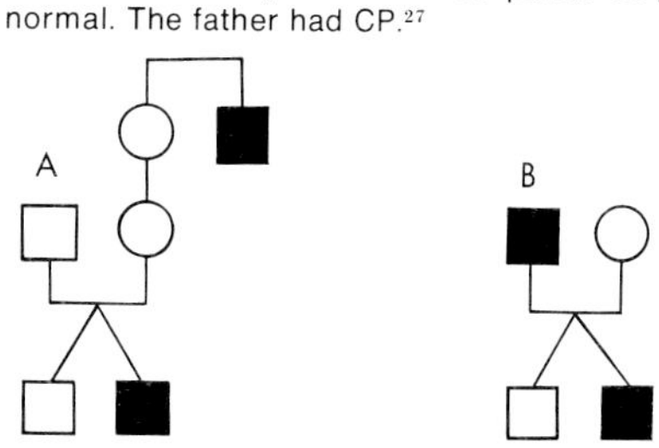

Also, the question of race is intertwined with that of geography.[9]

Assuming that the estimates cited here are correct, one can conclude that the risks for clefts differ in differing populations. But one would err in applying risk figures obtained in a racial group at a certain time and location to all populations considered to be of the same "race." In any population, pockets of high incidences could develop by genetic or environmental constellations, invalidating risk figures obtained in a large over-all survey.

Many genetically determined syndromes have been recognized (p. 650) that include harelip and/or cleft palate but differ in mode of transmission and in penetrance or expressivity of clefts. It is clear that in families in which such specific types of clefts occur, risk figures differ from those of the general population. Even the accepted distinction between the CL/CP complex and isolated CP does not apply to clefts combined with fistulas of the lower lip, in which cleft lip or isolated cleft palate can occur in the same family.[22] Also, the distinction may not hold in certain populations and areas.[37,38]

The CL/CP complex, as well as isolated CP, occurs in infants with *chromosomal anomalies*, particularly trisomy 13-15 (p. 296). A survey in 1966[39] showed that among 40 cases of trisomy 13-15, cleft formations occurred in 30 (75%). In 25 cases, there was CL/CP and in 5 there was isolated CP. In trisomy 18, only 16 of 115 cases had clefts; 13 had CL/CP and 3 had isolated CP. In trisomy 21 (Down syndrome), facial clefts are uncommon, yet they are about ten times more frequent than in the general population. Table 70-1 shows the approximate frequency of clefts in trisomy syndromes.

TABLE 70-1.—Frequency of CL/CP or CP in Trisomy Syndromes

	%
Trisomy 13-15	75
Trisomy 18	15
Trisomy 21	1.5
General neonate population	0.15

Both CL/CP and isolated CP have been described in children with multiple malformations associated with more uncommon chromosomal changes. Only a few examples of such anomalies will be cited. Harelip and cleft palate have been found associated with deletion of the short arms of a B chromosome, probably chromosome 4,[40] with trisomy of the long arm of a C chromosome,[41] with possible trisomy D[42] and in a child with mosaicism involving an isochromosome D and deletion of the short arms of a D chromosome.[43] Isolated cleft palate has been observed in patients with 2/3 translocation,[44] B/C translocation with a trisomy[10] and possible partial trisomy of the C group,[10,45] with ring chromosome 18[46,47] and in sisters with an unidentified extra autosome.[48] A median cleft lip was present in a case of deletion of the short arms of a chromosome 18.[49] One could cite more examples of uncommon chromosomal findings associated with facial clefts but, in many cases, the cytogenetic changes remained ill-defined, being subject to revision.

Turning to anomalies of the sex chromosomes, one commonly finds a high-arched palate in Turner syndrome and occasionally a cleft palate. Haddad and Wilkins[50] mentioned 1 cleft palate in 55 cases of gonadal aplasia. A child with Turner syndrome and cleft palate was seen in the Cincinnati Children's Hospital (Chart No. 93291) before chromosome analyses were possible. A boy with XXXXY karyotype reported by Miller *et al.*[51] had cleft palate among other skeletal malformations. Cleft lip and palate was present in a mongoloid girl with triple-X, trisomy 21 karyotype who also had congenital heart disease and a dystopic left kidney.[161]

In a general population with facial clefts, chromosomal changes probably are rare. From 161 children with clefts, Schutt[10] selected 37 for cytogenetic study because they had associated malformations. No cytogenetic anomalies were found in 17 children who had minor associated defects; in 20 children with major associated defects, 4 had an abnormal chromosome constitution; all 4 patients with chromosomal changes had isolated cleft palate.

The question of localized chromosomal changes in cleft regions was raised by Gropp *et al.*,[52] who reported chromosome counts of 72 and karyotypes with triploidy in cells cultured from palatal mucosa of a boy with CL/CP. But Muramoto *et al.*[53] and Soukup and Warkany[54] failed to find chromosomal anomalies in cells cultured from tissues excised from cleft areas. The genetics of cleft lip and palate was reviewed in 1970 by Fraser.[171]

The role of *environmental or exogenous factors* in the etiology of cleft palate is suggested by numerous experiments in mammals that show that this anomaly can be produced easily by treatment of the mother during gestation with various teratogens (p. 638). Harelip is less readily produced but methods exist to obtain it regularly.[55] Yet, for human beings, not many exogenous causes can be cited. It is certain that the antifolic acid antagonist aminopterin used for abortive purposes can induce harelip[56] and cleft palate,[57,58] but well-documented cases are so rare that one doubts that similar causation is common. Cleft palate was seen in a child whose mother had been treated with busulfan (Myleran) for leukemia.[59] Facial clefts were not conspicuous among the skeletal malformations caused by thalidomide, but Kajii[60] recorded 2 cases of CL/CP in 41 necropsied children damaged by this drug and Fogh-Andersen[22] mentioned 2 cases among a total of approximately 20 thalidomide-damaged children in Denmark. In Germany, facial clefts were not noted in the thalidomide embryopathy. Some antihistamines used as antiemetics during pregnancy were under scrutiny because meclizine in large doses can produce cleft palate in rats.[61] But these drugs taken by pregnant women in moderate doses seem rather innocuous. Lenz found that among 6,124 infants of mothers who had taken meclizine in early pregnancy 12 had cleft lip or palate. This is an incidence of 1.96 per 1,000, which is in line with that in the general population, "thus removing any substance for suspicion of teratogenicity of meclizine."[181] Cortisone, an excellent agent for production of cleft palate in certain strains of mice, is widely used during pregnancy in women. Occasionally, a child is reported who has cleft palate after such maternal treatment,[63,64] but it is difficult to establish a causal relationship because so many embryos of treated mothers are normal. Fogh-Andersen[22] described a child with bilateral cleft lip and palate and absence of the left ear and right thumb whose mother had taken phenmetrazine during the first months of pregnancy. Such single associations do not prove causation by the drug but they deserve recording to alert observers in case of similar occurrences. Meskin[9] found that cigarette smoking by the mother is in some way related to facial clefts, particularly to CP.

Exposure to large doses of x-rays induces cleft palate in rats[65] and mice[66]; it can cause cleft formation in human embryos also.[67,68] Such agents as drugs, chemicals or x-rays probably are not the important nongenetic factors responsible. Disorders within the mother's organism, such as maternal diabetes mellitus, have to be considered,[22,69] but the existence of nongenetic etiologic factors is best illustrated by identical twins discordant in regard to cleft formations (p. 630). These cases suggest local changes of the "microenvironment" affecting one of the twin embryos by factors not yet recognized. Such environmental factors may be of a temporary nature and difficult to ascertain.

Much has been written regarding the role of parental age in cleft lip and palate etiology.[9] McEvitt[70] stated that parental age has no bearing on the incidence of cleft lip and palate, but MacMahon and McKeown[71] found that the incidence of CL/CP increases with maternal age, whereas the incidence of CP was independent of maternal age. Woolf[72] also demonstrated a parental age effect for CL/CP and concluded that the risk of producing a child with this malformation is decreased in younger parents and increased in older ones. Paternal age seemed of etiologic importance. Knox[38] found the mean maternal age higher than in the general population and Fraser and Calnan[73] noted increased paternal age for CL/CP. Hay[74] reported that the incidence of CL/CP and CP of the offspring increased among older parents when the clefts were the only malformation noted. This relationship to parental age did not appear for isolated cleft lip. If cleft formations occurred in conjunction with other congenital malformations, there was a relationship to advanced parental age to all types of clefts. Social class played no role in the etiology of facial clefts in Scotland.[10] Edwards,[75] in Birmingham, England, found the time of highest incidence of cleft lip in March, but others[73,76] denied that seasonal influences play a significant part in the etiology of facial clefts. Cleft lip and palate seem to be independent of birth rank.[71,73]

All these broad epidemiologic investigations shed little light on the causation of facial clefts. More can be learned by consideration of associated malformations. The common CL/CP complex usually occurs in persons who are otherwise free of developmental anomalies, but in approximately 14% of children with clefts associated congenital malformations can be recognized.[71,77] Although associated anomalies can be fortuitous, in many cases they point to a specific and unusual causation. This is particularly true if they constitute a syndrome that in some cases betrays the origin of the cleft. Syndromes that include cleft lip or palate are numerous and only partly recognized at present. In most of these disease pictures, clefts are not obligatory constituents, but their occurrence is too frequent to be considered accidental. This point is best exemplified by the autosomal trisomy syndromes (p. 632). Although these syndromes are well defined by karyotype, and thus recognized as etiologic entities, facial clefts occur in a certain percentage only; even in the trisomy 13–15 syndrome, 25% of the patients escape cleft formation. The situation is similarly variable in many gene-determined syndromes and in some syndromes of exogenous origin. It is of interest in this connection that Meskin[9] noted that children with isolated cleft palate and their siblings have a greater propensity for associated malformations than either of the other two facial cleft groups and their siblings. Since associated malformations and syndromes involving cleft will be discussed later, the reader is referred to the section on associated malformations in which etiologic factors are discussed if they are known (p. 641).

Development of the Face and Palate

In embryos 5 weeks old, an elevation called the frontal process overhangs the stomodeum. Lateral to it, the olfactory placodes, formed during the fourth week, are located in shallow depressions, the olfactory pits. They lie between horseshoe-shaped eminences that are open toward the oral depression. The limbs of the horseshoes are the medial and lateral nasal processes (Fig. 70-13, *B*). Toward the open ends of the "horseshoes" converge the maxillary processes, which are outgrowths of the mandibular arch. The groove separating, on each side, the nasomedial, nasolateral and maxillary processes—termed the "primary palatine groove"—runs from the external nasal opening down to the oral opening. The grooves between the nasolateral and the maxillary processes are best called "naso-optic" grooves. The grooves described, which are recognizable in embryos of approximately 36 days, have disappeared on the forty-fifth day of gestation.[78] According to the modern concept, the molding of the face into processes and grooves is

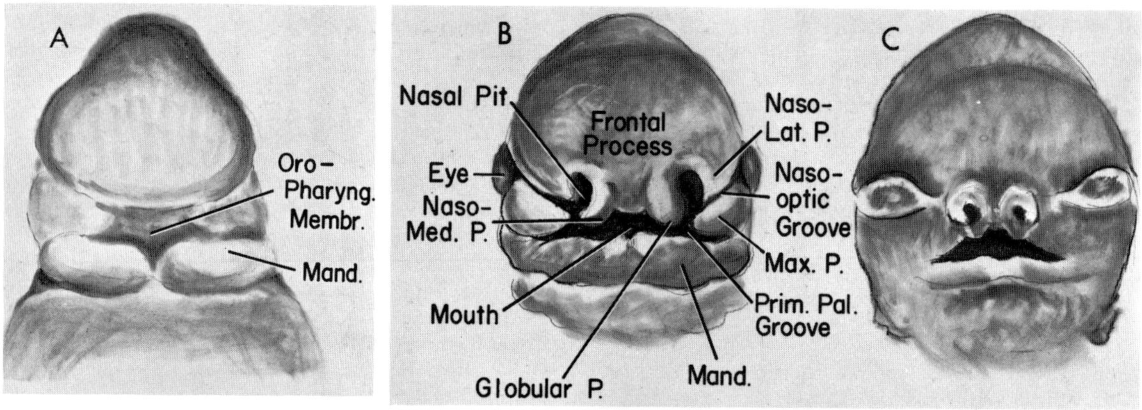

Fig. 70-13. – Diagrammatic presentation of development of the face in an embryo of 2.5 mm. (3 weeks) (**A**), 10 mm. (sixth week) (**B**), to an embryo of 15 mm. (seventh week) (**C**).

due to irregular distribution of mesenchyme that is well developed under the epithelium of the processes but sparse in the grooves where epidermis and epithelium are in close contact. The disappearance of the grooves and processes of the early embryo is due to growth of mesenchyme that invades the areas of the grooves and elevates them to the level of the processes.[78] With the elevation, in the seventh week, of the depressed areas of the primary palatine and the naso-optic grooves and by approximation of the nasomedial processes, the face assumes a more mature appearance. The union of the nasomedial processes with the nasolateral and the maxillary processes and the closer connection of the nasomedial processes with each other lead to formation of the upper lip. The tips of the nasomedial processes remain somewhat prominent as "globular processes" and enclose between them the area of the philtrum. The lower border of the mouth is established by the mandibular arch. By disappearance of the grooves between the maxillary and mandibular arches, the opening of the mouth appears markedly narrowed (Fig. 70-13, *C*).

The morphogenesis of the nasal cavity, which is of importance for an understanding of harelip formation, deserves special consideration. The nasal pockets surrounded–incompletely–by the nasomedial and nasolateral processes become deeper as these processes become more prominent. Posteriorly, in the depth of the nasal pits, the free lower edges of the processes approach each other and grow together, transforming the nasal pits into blind sacs that remain open anteriorly. The concrescence effected by fusion of the epithelial surfaces of the nasal processes (Fig. 70-13, *B*) progresses in posteroanterior direction, narrowing the external nasal aperture. The maxillary processes do not take part in the closure of the nasal cavity. The newly formed floor of the nasal cavity, which becomes a portion of the oral roof, contains a sagittal epithelial fusion line, an "epithelial wall" (Fig. 70-14), which normally is destroyed soon after its formation and replaced by mesenchymal tissue. Posteriorly, a small, purely epithelial area persists, separating the nasal and oral cavities as the "oronasal membrane." This membrane ruptures in the seventh week,[79] and a posterior communication is established between the nasal and oral cavities (primitive choanae). The tissue that at that time separates the nasal pits from the oral cavity has been called the primitive palate. It constitutes a bridge between the frontal process and both maxillary processes for which Peter,[80] who disapproved of the term "primary palate," suggested the names "primitive floor of the nasal cavity" or "anterior palate."

In embryos of 3 weeks (2.5 mm.), on the mandibular arch on either side of the midline there are marked local thickenings brought about by rapid proliferation of mesenchymal tissue (see Fig. 70-13, *A*). Between these elevations there is at first a distinct notch that still can be seen in embryos of 4–5 mm.[81] As the mesenchymal cushions extend to and meet in the midline, the mandibular notch disappears and the arch of the lower jaw is established. The growth of the mandible has a peculiar pattern.[82] At first, the lower jaw is small as compared with the maxillae. Coinciding with the closure of the palatine shelves, it shows a spurt in growth but later the mandible again lags behind the maxillae. Fetuses of 2–3 months still show physiologic micrognathism, which disappears before birth in most fetuses. It is not rare, however, to see in newborn children a receding chin that slowly becomes aligned with the upper jaw without any treatment.

The small triangular shelf that grows from the nasomedial processes into the oral cavity and forms the premaxillary portion of the palate is established early, at a time when there still is a wide posterior communication between the nasal and oral cavities. This shelf is derived from the median palatine or premaxillary processes, which are oral projections of the nasomedial processes. The main portion of the palate is formed later by union of the lateral palatine processes, which are outgrowths of the maxilla. These

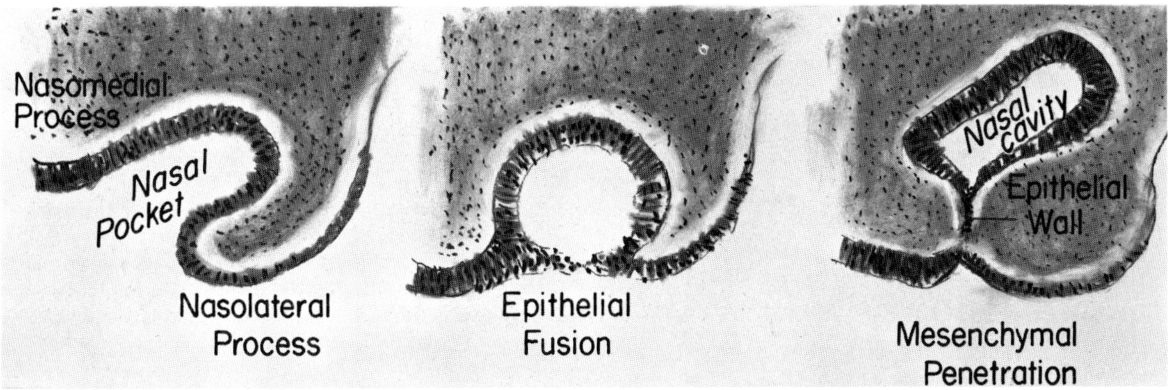

Fig. 70-14. – Diagram showing formation of nasal cavity by epithelial fusion of nasomedial and nasolateral processes and mesenchymal penetration of fusion wall.

processes are directed downward in early stages of development and separated from each other by the tongue. With the growth of the mandible, the tongue grows forward and withdraws from the space between the lateral palatine processes, which then swing upward, approach each other and unite in the midline. In the rostral portion of the mouth, the fused lateral palatine processes contact the premaxillary median palatine processes. Union also is established with the nasal septum, which grows downward to unite with the palate. Thus, two nasal chambers and the definitive oral cavity are established. As remnants of the early communication, the incisive (nasopalatine) canals indicate the place of fusion of the premaxillary (nasomedial) portion of the jaw with the lateral palatine processes. Sometimes these communications are patent in the newborn period but later become covered by mucous membrane, which, in this area, forms the incisive papilla. This somewhat complicated place of union of various primordia can become the site of cyst formations.

The development of the palate had been well described as early as 1869 by Dursy,[83] and in the following 90 years many details were added to his original description. Although some pertinent contributions were made by subsequent authors, many of the discussions were devoted to speculations and semantics rather than to facts. A review of the older literature on the formation of the palate was given by Peter[80] in 1924. Attempts were made to recognize the dynamic processes underlying the closure of the palate from anatomic and histologic material. Since direct observation of these processes was not possible, there was much room for differences of opinion. The intensity of these discussions and the hostility of the various schools to one another are hardly comprehensible at present.

One of the much-discussed questions was how the vertical palatine processes at first are separated by the tongue, move up to a horizontal position and close over the descending tongue. As it was apparent that the union of the lateral palatine processes occurs rather quickly, some authors believed that the tongue was brought down by active muscle contractions and that the rapid upward movement of the palatine shelves was due to their inherent elasticity.[84,85] This opinion was based chiefly on sections of embryos in which, on one side, the tongue appeared depressed and the corresponding palatine process elevated to a horizontal position, whereas on the other side the tongue was still high and the palatine processes vertical. Such sections, resembling to a certain extent Figure 70-15, suggested a quick lowering of the tongue followed by rapid elevation of the lateral palatine processes. The relation between human fetal mouth opening reflexes and closure of the palate was studied and reported by Humphrey.[162]

In contrast to this rapid dynamic picture, Pölzl[86] explained the same processes by a slower mechanism, namely the differing growth of the tongue and the jaws. In young embryos, the upper jaw is much more developed than the tongue and the mandible. The tip of the tongue at first lies behind the posterior border of the premaxilla while its body separates the vertically oriented palatine processes. As the tongue grows, its tip is moved forward under the premaxilla and placed below the upper lip. There also is an absolute and relative increase of the mandible, which grows not only forward but also transversely. Thus, the tongue finds a place between the arch formed by Meckel cartilages, is lowered and removed from its position between the lateral palatine processes. Closure of the secondary palate becomes possible as the tongue grows out of the space between the palatine processes. There is no sudden elevation of the palatine plates, according to Pölzl, but rather a transformation of their form from a vertical fold to a horizontal plate. Schorr[87] explained the elevation of the palatine process by developments in the upper jaw. Condensation of mesenchymal tissue and numerous mitotic figures in this area suggest rapid growth at the time of elevation of the palatine processes. In this way,

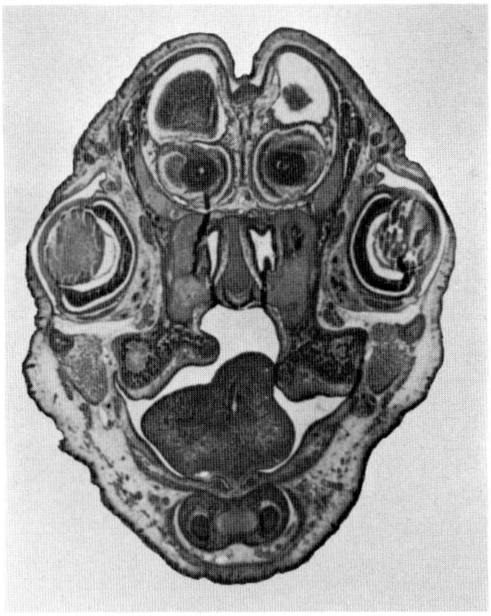

Fig. 70-15.—Frontal section through the head of a newborn rat with cleft palate. On the right side of the animal, the palatine shelf is in the horizontal position but on the left it still is vertical, as if impeded by the tongue in its upward movement (produced by hypervitaminosis A).

the lateral and lower portions of the palatine processes become elongated and elevated as the tongue descends into the mandibular area. The lowering and elongation of the tongue and the tendency of the palate to rise results in a disengagement of the tongue from the "pincers of the palatine processes."

Closure of the palate occurs first just anterior to the middle portion of the hard palate and progresses from there forward and backward. The uvula shows fusion of its lateral primordia relatively late and some separation is still visible even in postnatal life in approximately one-third of all children.[80]

A precise determination of the normal closure of the human palate was made by Fulton,[88] who examined a total of 88 embryos of known age or crown-rump length. It appears that the threshold period of palatal closure lies between 29 and 33 mm. of crown-rump length and between 47 and 49 days of ovulation age, if the embryonic palates are considered "closed" when the maxillary processes are touching at any place along the palatal plane. The palate closes in an X configuration, first at a point somewhat distal to the anterior fourth, continues back through the middle half, then closes through the anterior fourth and, finally, through the posterior fourth. With a single exception, the hard palates were completely closed in all embryos greater than 33 mm. crown-rump length. The soft palate split varied from an opening of 0.3 mm. to a slight notch. All of the embryos below 29 mm. crown-rump length had the maxillary palatal processes in a vertical position, the distance between them averaging 1.5 mm. In these cases, the tongue was found between the vertical processes and extending upward almost to the lower border of the nasal septum.

An excellent study of the development and closure of the secondary palate was made in rodents by Inouye[85] in 1912. More recently, Walker and Fraser[89] studied the closure of the posterior (secondary) palate in several inbred strains of mice. They distinguished seven stages of closure and related the palate stages to the chronologic age and to morphologic criteria of the mouse embryo. They found a better positive correlation between palate stages and the morphologic rating than between palate stage and chronologic age. According to their observations, the secondary palate of the mouse closes by a rapid movement of the palatine shelves from the initial vertical to a final horizontal plane. This movement consists of a bulging of the medial wall and a regression of the ventral (inferior) wall of each shelf, the transformation proceeding in a wave-like motion from the posterior ends of the shelves to their anterior ends. The palatine shelf movement carries the shelf dorsal to the tongue and forces the latter into a more ventral position. Apparently the shelves move by means of an internal elastic force that is sufficiently strong to drive the shelves dorsal to the tongue. Walker and Fraser believed that the elastic force resides in a network of elastic fibers in the connective tissue of the shelves and that an acid mucopolysaccharide may be the substance responsible for shelf movement. It was shown by these investigators that the palate closes at an earlier developmental age in C57B1 than in A/Jax embryos, with time of closure in DBA embryos being intermediate. Autoradiographic studies by Larsson *et al.*[90] showed that ^{35}S-labeled sulfate was incorporated in connective tissue of the palatine shelves of 11–17-day-old mouse embryos; it was assumed that this indicates synthesis of acid mucopolysaccharides in this tissue. The mucopolysaccharide synthesis in the ground substance of the fibroblast zones was considered to be responsible for the internal force that leads to closure of the secondary palate.[91]

Pathogenesis and Experimental Work

Embryologists thought that lateral harelips represent a continuation of the clefts seen in embryos of the sixth week that run down from the nasal aperture to the mouth between the maxillary and nasal processes (see Fig. 70-13, *B*). Failure of fusion of these facial processes in the seventh week was said to result in incomplete development of the upper lip and continuation of the harelip condition, thought to exist in embryonic life. This explanation was based on the supposition that the embryonic facial grooves are actual clefts that penetrate the embryonic tissues completely. Later, Politzer,[92] Veau[93] and others found that the grooves so well described and illustrated by older embryologists were not penetrating clefts but rather thin epithelial layers surrounded by eminences in which epithelial layers were separated by cushions of mesenchymal tissue. The disappearance of facial grooves was not due to healing or true coalescence of processes once separated by clefts but rather to a filling out of the depressed areas by invading mesenchyme. The unification of the processes that form the definitive upper lip is due, therefore, to spread of mesodermal masses from the facial processes into the areas of depression. In the absence of mesodermal penetration, the facial grooves remain thin epithelial areas that break easily and thus establish true clefts in the upper lip.[92,93] Partial mesodermal penetration may result in fleshy connections between the nasal and maxillary processes. Such connections, known as "Simonart bands," occur, according to Veau,[93] in more than 20% of labial clefts.

Careful examination of young embryos with harelip has shown that both the classic theory of "fusion" and the newer theories of "mesodermal penetration" are partially correct. Although the facial grooves generally do not represent true penetrating fissures, a fusion of the nasolateral and nasomedial processes with some sort of epithelial "healing" is necessary before mesodermal connections of these processes can be established. Thus, failure of primary fusion of the nasal processes as well as failure of mesodermal penetration of the fused area can result in harelip. The differences of opinion and the sometimes heated debates of various schools concerning the pathogenesis of harelip may be explained by the fact that this malformation is not uniform and not always of the same origin. Veau[93] distinguished three types of harelip: simple harelip (cheiloschisis), which consists in a cleft limited to the upper lip (36% of the cases); complete harelip (cheilognathoschisis), which involves the lip and the alveolar process reaching from the nasal aperture to the ductus nasopalatinus (42%); and bridged harelip, in which a fleshy connection exists between the two edges of the cleft (22%).

Embryos examined in early stages suggest various modes of abnormal development. Töndury[78] stated that all harelips are due to a disturbance of the development of the nasal cavity. Simple harelip is the result of an early interruption of epithelial fusion of the nasal and maxillary processes. In these cases, the epithelial wall is short and the maxillary and nasomedial processes remain anteriorly separated. The upper lip shows, in a typical place, a cleft of variable size.

Complete harelip, in which the cleft goes through the upper lip and the alveolar process to the ductus nasopalatinus, is due to complete failure of epithelial fusion of the nasal processes. In such cases, the nasolateral process does not grow sufficiently and no epithelial wall is formed. Such complete harelips must be considered *primary* cleft formations. It is possible, however, that some complete harelips may be the result of embryonic cysts formed in the area of the epithelial wall. Rupture of such a cyst would establish a connection between the nasal and oral cavities. In this case, a complete harelip would represent a tear of the embryonic face and a *secondary* cleft formation. However, this process has been observed only in mouse embryos with harelip. A third possibility would be that an epithelial wall is formed that is not penetrated by mesoderm. Subsequently, the wall would be torn by pull of the growing neighboring parts.

Harelips with bridges also can develop in different ways. If the epithelial wall is too short anteriorly and overdeveloped posteriorly, thus reaching to the oronasal membrane, only its middle portion would be reinforced by mesodermal tissue. When the posterior epithelial wall is then dissolved, together with the oronasal membrane, a cleft that is bridged by the reinforced middle portion would result. Or the epithelial wall may persist too long and be replaced only partially by mesoderm. Bridges could also be remnants of the wall of harelip cysts as seen in mouse embryos. Thus, harelips may develop in different ways, and in many cases not represent simple arrest of development.[78]

It is possible to observe the formation of harelips in experimental animals. Occasionally, they occur spontaneously in certain inbred strains of mice. Normally, fusion of the nasal processes progresses in a posteroanterior direction. As in human embryos, an epithelial suture or epithelial wall is formed in the fusion line. It exists for several hours only and soon is penetrated and replaced by mesenchyme. In normal mouse embryos, these developments take place on the tenth and eleventh days of gestation and are finished on the twelfth day.[94] In some embryos of 12 days, one can recognize well-developed harelips in which an epithelial wall was never formed because the nasal processes did not join or fuse.[94,95] In other embryos,[94,96] epithelial walls had been formed but cysts developed in them, which could be seen from the twelfth to the fifteenth day. These harelip cysts were not found in newborn mice and it is believed that they ruptured into the oral and nasal cavities, thus forming complete harelips. It was established that harelip cysts are essentially embryonic formations and that most of them have either ruptured by the time of birth, forming complete labial clefts, or have been filled out by mesodermal tissue if they were small. Sometimes, in newborn animals, bridges within the clefts are found. Such bridges, which are comparable to Simonart bands, are either remnants of embryonic epithelial cysts or imcomplete mesodermal replacements of the epithelial wall. Facial clefts have also been observed in dogs, cats, swine and cattle as hereditary anomalies.[1]

Cleft palate can now be produced by many methods. In the pioneer experiments by Hale,[97] a few of the blind pigs born to vitamin A-deficient sows had harelip and/or cleft palate. However, it is not certain that these facial clefts can be attributed entirely to maternal vitamin A deficiency. Palludan[98] also obtained cleft lip and palate in some young of vitamin A-depleted sows but thought that such oral malformations should not be considered regular components of the deficiency syndrome but rather as occasional malformations. It is obvious that large-scale cleft palate experiments require smaller animals than pigs.

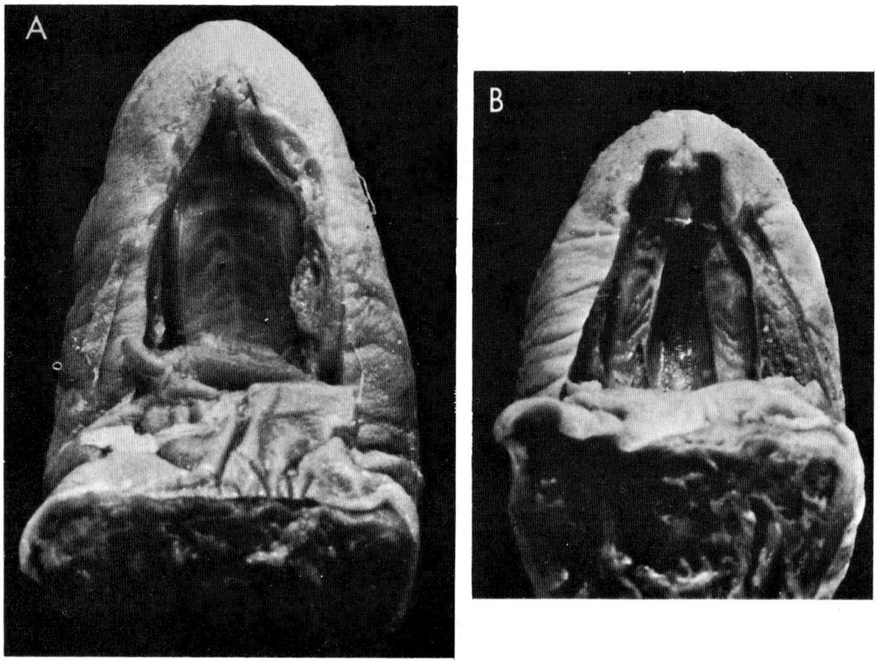

Fig. 70-16. – **A,** palate of a normal newborn rat. **B,** cleft palate produced by maternal riboflavin deficiency.

In rats, vitamin A deficiency results in a variety of malformations but not in facial clefts. Regular experimental production became possible when Warkany *et al.*[20] showed that cleft palate appeared in a syndrome of skeletal defects induced by maternal riboflavin deficiency. Approximately 15% of the young born to riboflavin-deficient rats showed well-developed posterior palate clefts (Fig. 70-16, *B*). Harelip and defects of the anterior palate were seen only in exceptional cases. By a combination of riboflavin deficiency and the use of the antimetabolite galactoflavin, Nelson *et al.*[99] could increase the incidence of cleft palate in rats to 39%. Similar treatment of mice resulted in an almost identical incidence of cleft palate (41%) when the DBA strain was used, but the incidence was much lower in other strains.[100] An acute folic acid deficiency induced with the help of an antimetabolite in rats during days 10–13 of gestation made possible cleft palate induction in 100% of the young. Folic acid deficiency on days 9–11 resulted in 86% cleft palate and 93% cleft lip.[55] This probably is the best method available for producing harelip in rats.

Fraser and Fainstat[101] discovered that large doses of cortisone injected into pregnant females of the inbred A/Jax mouse strain would also cause cleft palate in a large percentage of the offspring. This basic experiment made possible many embryologic and genetic studies. Fraser *et al.*[102] and Kalter[103] noted that cortisone injected from the tenth day of gestation for 4 days resulted in a 100% incidence of cleft palate in the offspring of A/Jax animals but only an 18% incidence in those of strain C57BL. Crosses of these strains were made and the effect of cortisone on the F_1 generation could be studied; it was found that differences in resistance of different strains to the teratogenic action of cortisone was due to a genetically

Fig. 70-17. – A newborn rat with facial clefts produced by salicylate treatment of the mother. The maxillary processes are not united with each other or with the nasomedial and nasolateral processes. The left eye is located between the left maxillary and nasolateral processes.

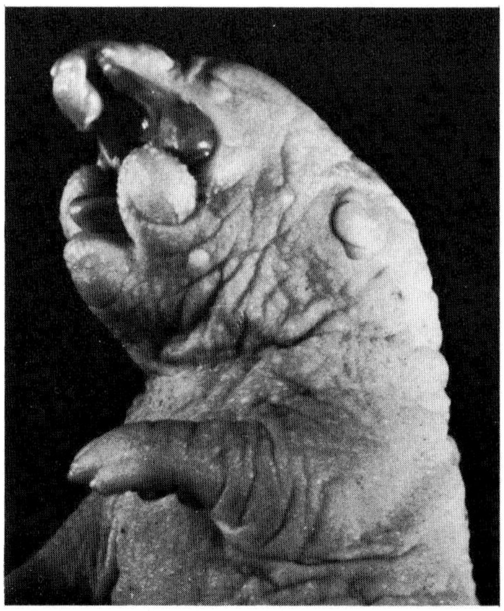

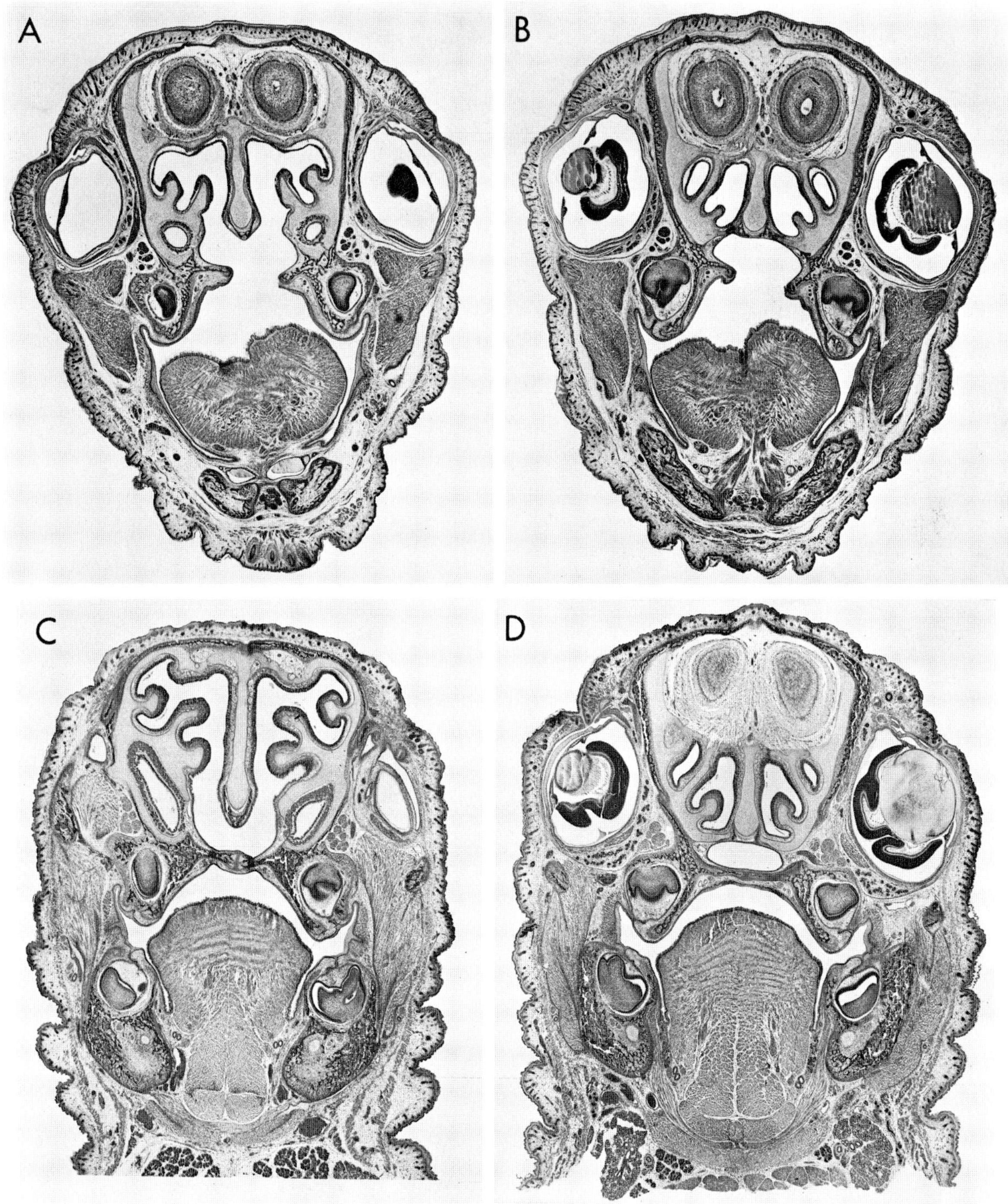

Fig. 70-18. – Frontal sections through the head of a newborn rat with cleft palate produced by maternal riboflavin deficiency. **A,** anterior section shows communication between oral and nasal cavities. **B,** posterior section with communication of oral cavity and nasopharyngeal duct. **C** and **D,** controls.

determined difference in the mothers rather than in the embryos. The fact that, under certain conditions, cleft palate could be induced in approximately 100% of the offspring provided an opportunity for embryologic analysis of the defect.[104,105] It was thought that cortisone treatment causes cleft palate by interfering with the condition within the palatine shelves, which normally forces them to change their alignment from the vertical to the horizontal plane. Delay in shelf movement, apparent inability of the shelves to grow wider without the stimulus of being fused and continued increase in head width result in a palate in which the shelves are too far apart to touch and fuse when they finally become horizontal. The strain difference between C57BL and A/Jax mice in their susceptibility to the teratogenic action of cortisone was found to be due in part to the earlier closing of the palate in C57BL embryos and in part to the lesser inhibition of shelf movement in C57BL embryos as compared with A/Jax embryos. These differences suggested that the C57BL maternal-embryo complex has a more efficient metabolic system for developing palate shelf movement than that of the A/Jax strain. The interplay of many intrinsic and extrinsic factors contributing to these cleft formations could be studied[106] and the role of "shelf force," synthesis of mucopolysaccharides within the shelves, tongue position and movement and mandibular development could be examined.[91,107,108]

Many new methods have been found to produce cleft palate in various mammals. In 1962, Deuschle and Kalter[109] tabulated 30 procedures that result in cleft lip or palate, giving references to original publications. Only a few of these methods have been used for special studies.

Cleft palate can be produced in rats[65] and mice[66] by x-rays, which have been used to study movement of palatine shelves in treated mouse embryos.[110] Hypervitaminosis A is an effective teratogen in rats[111] and mice[112] that was used for analysis of palate development and malformations.[113] It was found that salicylates in toxic doses produce many malformations in rat embryos, including cleft lip and palate.[114] Subsequently, salicylates were found to be teratogenic in mice,[115,116] which made possible studies on the relationship of salicylates to inhibition of mucopolysaccharide synthesis[117] and to cleft lip formation.[116] In addition to vitamin deficiencies and treatment with drugs, chemical compounds or x-rays, amniotic sac puncture,[118] uterine clamping,[119] hypothermia,[120] hypoxia,[121] kidney antisera[122] and other teratogenic procedures resulted in cleft formations.

Many studies could be made of the orofacial complex in rats and mice that had experimentally induced cleft palate[109,123-127,166] and other facial malformations.

Clinical Classifications

Many classifications have been suggested for the various forms of facial clefts. Davis and Ritchie[128] suggested a simple classification that used the alveolar ridge as a line of division between lip and palate anomalies. They distinguished (1) prealveolar, (2) postalveolar and (3) alveolar clefts. Fogh-Andersen[1] proposed (1) clefts of lip (and alveolus) or primary palate clefts, (2) clefts of lip, alveolus and palate or primary and secondary palate clefts, (3) isolated palate clefts or secondary palate clefts and (4) rare, unusual clefts. Stark[129] chose the incisive foramen and not the alveolus as the dividing point and distinguished (1) clefts lying anterior to the incisive foramen, (2) clefts lying posterior to the incisive foramen, clefts due to a failure of fusion of the two palatal processes to form the secondary palate and (3) clefts that combine failure of normal development of both the primary and secondary palate. Such clefts can be unilateral, bilateral or median and total or subtotal.

The rare clefts can be divided[11] into median clefts of the upper lip, oblique facial clefts, transverse facial clefts, clefts of the nose, clefts or defects of the scalp and combinations of these defects with lip and palate clefts. Submucous palate cleft has been defined as an imperfect muscle union across the velum palatinum; the muscle defect often is combined with shortness of the hard palate. Velopharyngeal closure is

Fig. 70-19 (left). – Incomplete cleft lip on left side.
Fig. 70-20 (right). – Complete cleft lip and cleft palate on left side.

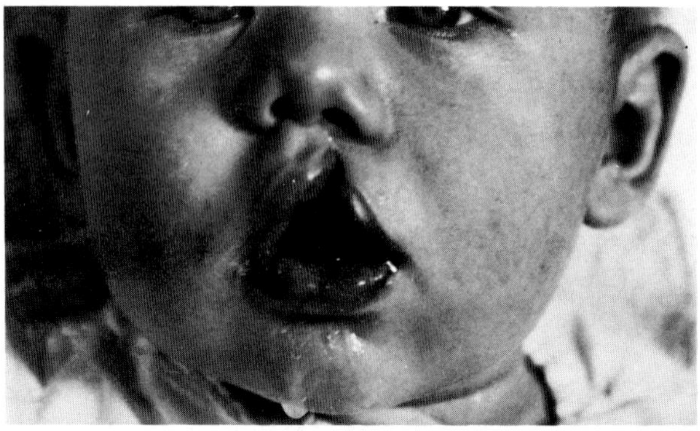

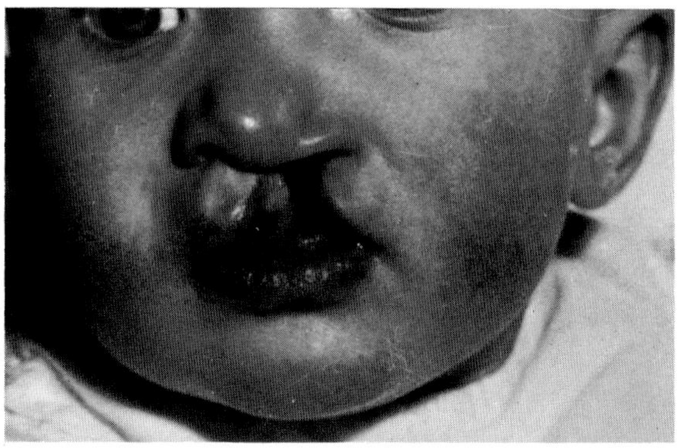

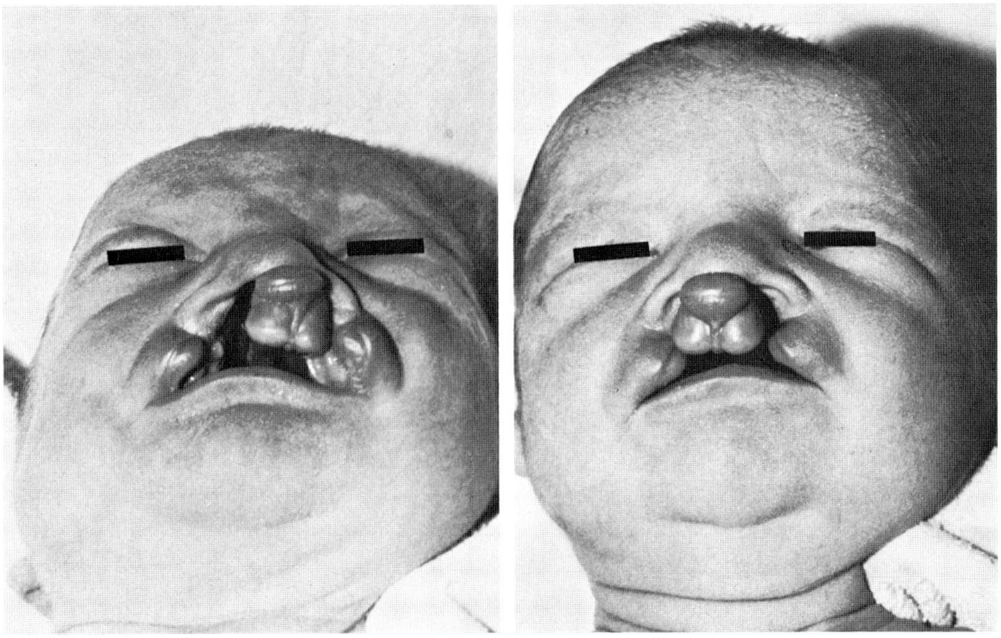

Fig. 70-21. – Bilateral harelip and cleft palate in monozygotic twins.

incomplete, resulting in speech difficulties. The anomaly can be considered a mild form or "forme fruste" of cleft palate. Sometimes submucous palate cleft is found in relatives of persons with cleft lip and overt cleft palate.[130] Submucous palate cleft can be a midline defect in acrocephalosyndactyly, mandibulofacial dysostosis, cleidocranial dysostosis and other syndromes in which it may appear in place of an overt cleft palate.

Fig. 70-22. – Bilateral cleft lip and palate with protruding prolabium.

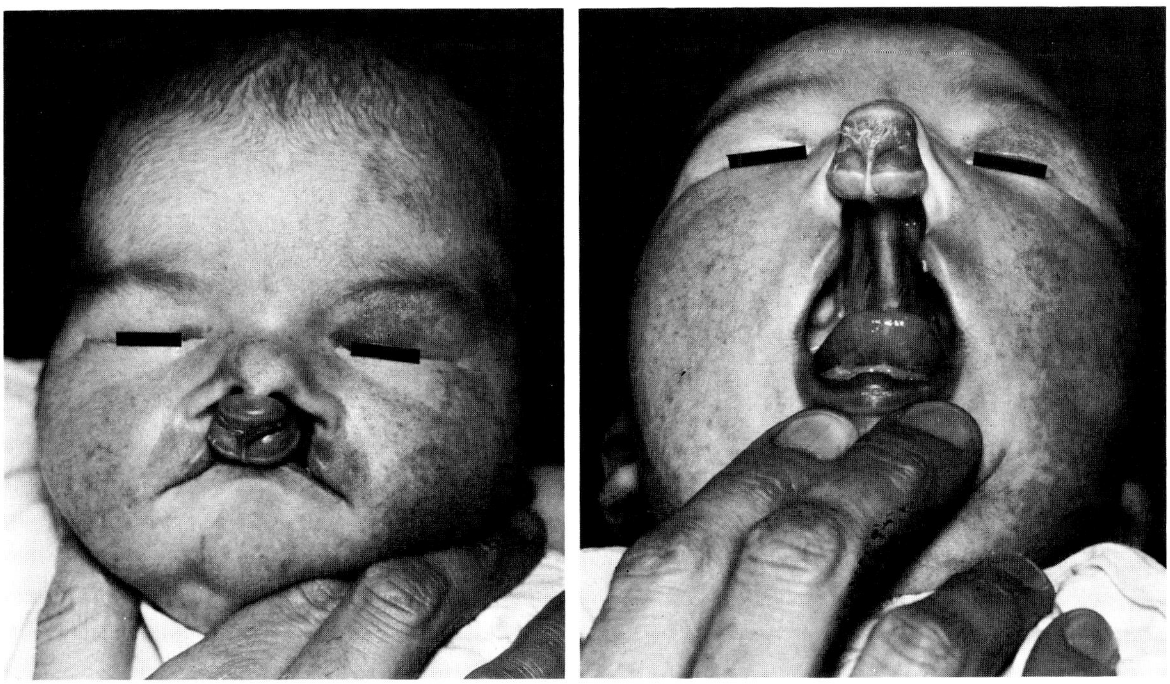

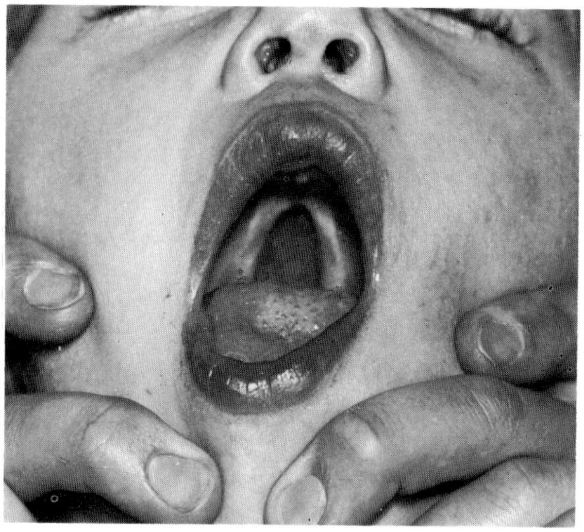

Fig. 70-23. – Posterior palate cleft.

Associated Malformations

It has long been known that patients with facial clefts may have associated malformations. Many combinations and syndromes containing facial clefts have been described in the literature and it is impossible to review all the cases reported. Most of these "interesting cases" represent a selected group, since uncomplicated cases of harelip and/or cleft palate usually are not made the subject of case reports in the medical literature. Thus, rare and complicated cases are overemphasized and a distorted picture is obtained from published reports. It is estimated that not more than 14% of patients with clefts have associated malformations (p. 633).

In 1910, Rischbieth[15] reviewed the literature up to his time and listed most of the associated malformations reported in 122 cases of harelip and cleft palate. In the head region, hydrocephaly, anencephaly, encephalocele, microcephaly and mucous labial sinuses had been observed repeatedly. In four instances, tumors were present in the frontal, lingual, alveolar or nasal area. Among ocular malformations, microphthalmia, coloboma of the lids or of the iris, absence of the eyeballs or eyelids and atresia or asymmetry of the palpebral fissures were noted. The auricles were reported as absent, supernumerary or deformed. The extremities were affected by polydactyly, syndactyly, absence of the radius and other bones or by clubfoot. Congenital heart disease, renal malformations, external and internal genital anomalies, imperforate anus, ventral and diaphragmatic hernias or a single umbilical artery were anomalies mentioned repeatedly in published cases.

In contrast to these selected cases, patients seen by surgeons or in cleft palate clinics generally represent a different picture, as they have a low incidence of associated malformations. From such patients one may get the impression that harelip and cleft palate usually are isolated malformations. This point of view is biased, because infants with severe complicating malformations often are stillborn or they die in the neonatal period without reaching cleft palate centers. An attempt was made by Fogh-Andersen[1] to arrive at correct figures by considering "newborn" material as well as "clinical" material. He came to the conclusion that at birth 10% or more of the children with harelip or cleft palate show severe associated malformations. However, this estimate may be low, because it does not take into account that many internal malformations are not diagnosed in the neonatal period. Of 163 babies, 2 were anencephalic (1 with cystic kidney), 5 had hydrocephaly, 2 had cranioschisis, 1 had exencephaly and an oblique facial cleft, 1 had spina bifida, anal atresia and syndactyly and 1 had diaphragmatic hernia and several malformations of the extremities. In only one of the cases of multiple malformations did the mother also have a malformation (syndactyly). In the "clinical" material, which consisted of survivors, Fogh-Andersen differentiated between "clearly hereditary" and "solitary" cases. It seemed that in hereditary cases associated malformations were rarer than in sporadic cases. Among the latter group there occurred malformations of the extremities or congenital heart disease. The prevalence of facial clefts apparently is somewhat elevated in mentally retarded persons. In Denmark, it was 0.34% in the feeble-minded as compared with 0.1% in the general population. In England, Illingworth[131] observed 8 children with cleft palate among 386 mentally retarded (2%), which is more than ten times the prevalence in the general population. But there are examples of outstanding persons who were born with cleft palate. T. R. Malthus had a cleft palate "inherited from his great-great-grandfather"[132] and the Hungarian prime minister Mihály Károlyi, a member of one of the most powerful families of Hungary, had a harelip and cleft palate.[133] Sir James Berry, surgeon, traveler and scholar, had a clubfoot and cleft palate, "handicaps which he courageously overcame."[134]

Birch-Jensen[135] found 9 cases of harelip and/or cleft palate among 625 patients with severe defects of the upper extremities. If this prevalence of 1.4% is compared with that of 0.1% in the general population, there can be no doubt that cleft formations occur far more often in patients with defects of the upper extremities than in the general population. It has been calculated that 1 of 12,000 persons has both facial clefts and deformities of the extremities. Aplasia of the radius and facial clefts show a significant association.[135] Among children seen by pediatric surgeons because of esophageal atresia, the frequency of harelip and cleft palate was 0.85%; among those with imperforate anus or rectum it was 6.5%.[136] In patients with unilateral renal agenesis or congenital polycystic kidney, facial clefts were observed in 4.5% or 5.7%, respectively.[137] Of 107 children admitted to the Cincinnati Children's Hospital because of cleft palate, 44% had harelip, 7.5% had Pierre Robin syndrome, 4.8% had mental retardation, 3.7% had congenital heart disease and 1.9% had clubfoot. A variety of other congenital malformations, such as absence of the radius and thumb, renal anomalies, microphthalmia, microcephaly, dwarfism and others were listed only once each in these 107 children.

In children born with *gross malformations of the central nervous system*, harelip and/or cleft palate is not rare. It has been mentioned that in Rischbieth's[15] review many cranial anomalies occurred in cases of facial clefts. In anencephalic monsters, harelip and cleft palate have been observed occasionally,[1, 15] but in the majority of anencephalics there is merely a deep depression in the midline extending the length of the hard palate. This depression looks like a palatine cleft on superficial inspection, but it is found to be closed when tested with a probe. A similar high palatine raphe is also seen in acrocephalosyndactyly, but rare patients with this anomaly may have a median cleft of the lip.[138] Facial clefts may also be combined with hydrocephaly,[15] nasal or occipital encephalocele[138, 139] or with arhinencephaly.[138, 140] In some children with facial clefts and severe brain anomalies such as occipital encephalocele, polycystic kidneys were also present. Gruber[138] established a syndrome called "dysencephalia splanchnocystica," which is characterized by encephalocele, facial clefts, polydactyly and polycystic kidneys, liver and pancreas. Some of these cases may have had trisomy 13–15 but others probably had normal karyotypes.[141] In 1822, Meckel (cited by Gruber[138]) reported cleft palate associated with encephalocele, polycystic kidneys and polydactyly in sisters.

Fig. 70-24.—Bilateral harelip and cleft palate in a boy with trisomy 13-15 (D_1).

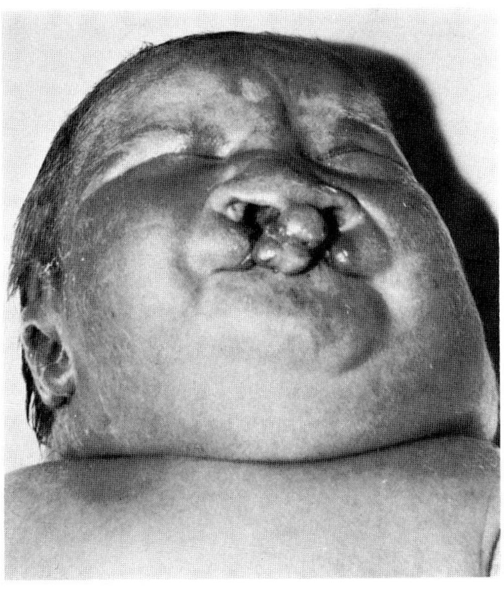

Grebe[140] observed a family in which arhinencephaly and lateral and median CL/CP appeared in combination or alternately.

Lower lip fistulas. The incidence of cleft lip or cleft palate in the syndrome that accompanies congenital lower lip fistulas illustrates the alteration of risk figures for CL/CP or CP in special cases. The rather harmless trait of congenital lip fistulas is due to an autosomal dominant gene (p. 627). Approximately 70% of the patients with lower lip fistulas have lip or palate clefts.[142] Thus, the risk for the offspring of an affected member to have a cleft is about 35% and that of an unaffected member's offspring is zero. These figures are quite different for the over-all risk figures of Fogh-Andersen[1] or Curtis *et al.*[143] The risks of 35% against 0% are influenced by the fact that penetrance of the clefts is not complete, a circumstance that complicates genetic counseling. In affected families, the CL/CP complex and isolated CP can alternate in individual members, which is an exception to the general rule that considers CL/CP and CP different genetic entities.[1, 22] Lower lip fistulas and the syndrome connected with it are quite rare as compared with the common CL/CP or CP malformations. It has been estimated that only one-half of a per cent of CL or CP patients have lower lip fistulas.[144] Some of these patients also have such limb defects as clubfoot, syndactyly or popliteal pterygium.[142]

Popliteal pterygium, genital anomalies and facial clefts combine in a syndrome that has been observed repeatedly in siblings.[13, 142] If the pits of the lower lip are present, differentiation from the foregoing disease picture becomes difficult. The genital anomalies range from minor deviations of the external genitalia to pseudohermaphrodism.[145] The cleft formations also are variable. Expressivity of the syndrome is not constant, and mildly affected patients can have children with serious malformations. Chromosomes are normal; irregular autosomal dominant inheritance has been suggested.[146, 179] This further narrows the gap between this condition and the lower lip fistula syndrome discussed above.

Ectodermal dysplasia combined with facial clefts has been noted in the syndrome described above.[169] A syndrome of anhidrotic ectodermal dysplasia and cleft lip and palate has been described in a mother and 2 of her children as an autosomal dominant trait.[170] Ectodermal dysplasia, ectrodactyly and cleft lip-palate have been associated in a girl reported by Rüdiger *et al.*[172]

Multiple congenital dislocations, clubfoot and vertebral anomalies can occur together with a typical flat face with depressed nasal bridge and hypertelorism.[142, 147] Isolated cleft palate or uvula fissa may be present in this syndrome (Larsen syndrome).

Klippel-Feil syndrome (faulty segmentation of the vertebral column) is not an etiologic entity (p. 909). Patients with this syndrome may have various associated malformations, with cleft palate or bifid uvula among them.[142]

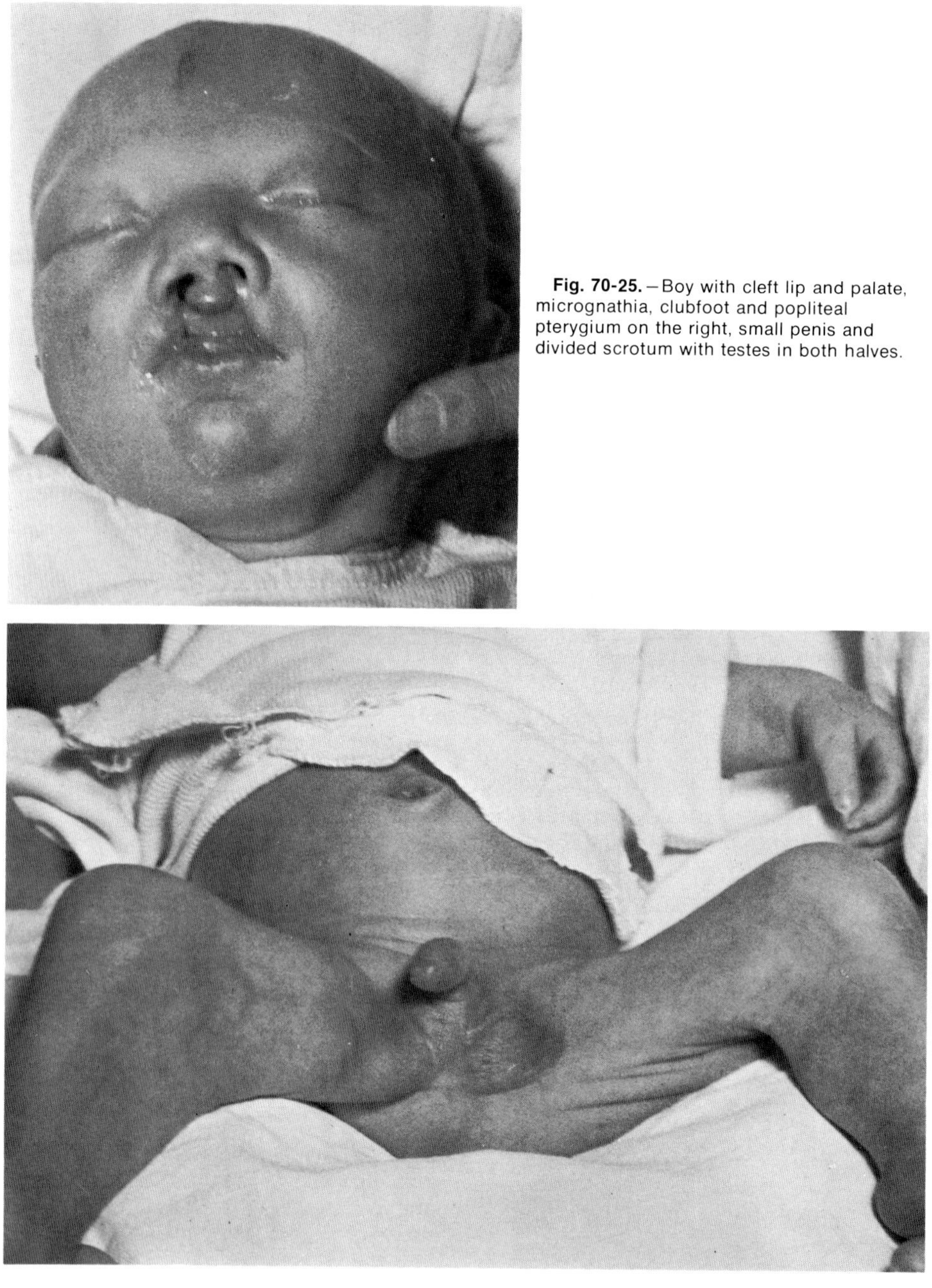

Fig. 70-25.—Boy with cleft lip and palate, micrognathia, clubfoot and popliteal pterygium on the right, small penis and divided scrotum with testes in both halves.

Arthrogryposis sometimes is combined with cleft palate[148,149] (Cincinnati Children's Hospital Chart No. 126420).

The orodigitofacial syndrome (p. 674) is characterized by oral webs that extend to the jaws and are connected to clefts of the lip or palate of unusual types. Partial midline cleft of the upper lip, bilateral hard palate clefts and soft palate clefts occur in this disease picture, which is limited to female members of affected kindreds.[142]

Otopalatodigital syndrome is the name of a disease picture that includes a generalized bone dysplasia, dwarfism, abnormal facial features and deafness. The first digits are spatulate and separated from the second digits; the feet resemble those of "tree frogs" (p. 677).[150,151] Soft palate cleft has been observed in some of the patients.

Microcephaly and cleft palate can be found associated, particularly in infants, with intrauterine growth retardation (p. 137).

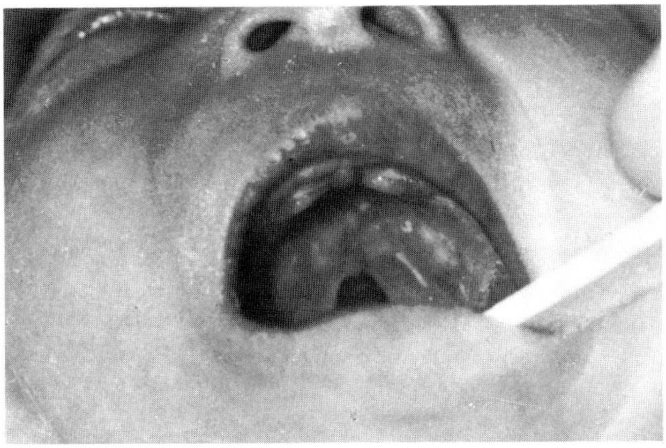

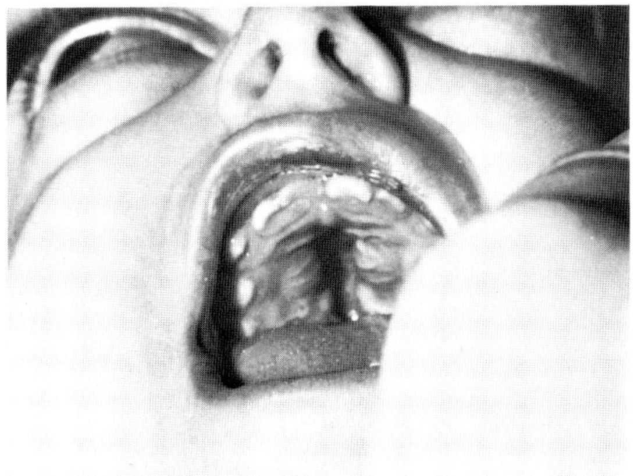

Fig. 70-26 (left). – Posterior palate cleft in a child with severe microcephaly and intrauterine growth retardation.
Fig. 70-27 (right). – High palate in acrocephalosyndactyly.

Craniosynostoses. In acrocephalosyndactyly (p. 899), the hard palate is indented by a narrow median furrow that looks like a palate cleft on superficial inspection. To rule out cleft palate, sometimes one has to make sure with a probe that the oral cavity does not communicate with that of the nose. In some of the patients, the posterior part of the palate or the uvula actually is cleft. The palatal appearance is similar to that of anencephaly (p. 189). *Crouzon disease* (p. 901), a dominantly inherited condition, frequently is complicated by a high-arched palate. Clefts of the hard or soft palate also can occur.[152]

Mandibulofacial dysostosis (p. 650), characterized by antimongoloid slant of the palpebral fissures, colobomas of the lower lids, deformed ears, macrostomia and micrognathia, is a dominant trait that can be transmitted with variable expressivity through many generations. The palate may be high in some affected members of a kindred and cleft in others.[153] Submucous palate cleft can exist in some patients without their knowledge (p. 651), yet overt palate cleft can occur in their children.

Pierre Robin syndrome (glossoptosis and retrognathia) is complicated by cleft palate in the majority of cases (p. 654). Most cases are sporadic, but irregular dominance of the trait has been observed (p. 655). The palate cleft is considered secondary to the retrognathia.[154] Mechanical causative factors have been considered.[155]

Cleidocranial dysostosis is essentially a dysplasia of membrane bones that include the palatine shelves. Cartilage bone is involved to a lesser extent (p. 836). Submucous or complete palate cleft occurs in some patients.[142, 156] The disorder is inherited as a dominant trait.

Arachnodactyly (Marfan syndrome) is transmitted as a dominant trait. High palate is the rule, cleft palate the exception.[142, 157] One patient with Marfan syndrome and cleft palate apparently inherited Marfan syndrome from the father and cleft palate from the mother,[158] which points up the possibility of coincidental association of clefts with syndromes of congenital malformations.

Cleft palate can occur in *diastrophic dwarfism* (p. 801) and clefts have been observed with the *Ellis-van Creveld syndrome* (p. 793). These systemic skeletal disorders are recessively inherited traits.

Associations of facial clefts with malformations of the extremities have been discussed on some of the preceding pages. It remains to mention here some serious *reduction malformations of the extremities* emphasized in a number of publications. Lobster claws have been seen repeatedly in patients with facial clefts.[135, 145, 172-174] Absence of the radius[135, 175] and of other long bones[135, 176] has been observed also. Perodactyly ("amputations"), the most severe appendicular defect, can be combined with cleft lip, ectodermal dysplasia and ear deformities in a recessively inherited syndrome,[178] and tetraphocomelia with cleft lip-palate and hypertrophy of the clitoris in a usually sporadic syndrome.[175] Cleft lip and micromelia of the upper and lower extremities occurred in a fetus exposed to "therapeutic" x-irradiation.[67]

In the *de Lange syndrome*, cleft palate occurs in rare cases.[159]

A strange combination of a hereditary *myelodysplasia* resulting in familial osseous atrophy with harelip and cleft palate has been reported.[160]

Congenital glaucoma and cleft palate were observed in a boy at the Cincinnati Children's Hospital (Chart No. 23812). The father had had buphthalmos attributed to juvenile glaucoma. The patient had an older brother who had cleft palate and reduced vision. Another brother with cleft palate had a daughter with cleft palate and reduced vision. An unrelated patient seen in the Cincinnati Children's Hospital (Chart No. 52881) had cleft lip and palate and bilateral glaucoma. On both sides of the family, cleft lip or/and cleft palate had occurred.

A kindred in which *camptodactyly*, clubfoot and

cleft palate appeared in combination or vicariously in three generations was described by Gordon *et al.*[163] in an African family. Cleft lip and palate were observed in 2 brothers with microcephaly, elbow deformities, hypoplastic thumbs and intrauterine and postnatal growth retardation. Three siblings were also affected by various cranial and digital anomalies. Only one sibling was free of malformations. The parents were normal and there was no known consanguinity.[164] A syndrome of cleft lip, palate and nose combined with hypertelorism, microtia and congenital heart disease was described in sisters by Bixler *et al.*[165]

Association of clefts with *congenital heart disease* is not striking, but with atrial septal defects (p. 480) and tetralogy of Fallot (p. 494) facial clefts are seen with significant frequency.

When a cleft formation can be attributed to a *drug* such as aminopterin (p. 96) or to *x-irradiation*, the risk for recurrence probably is zero if exposure to the teratogenic agent is avoided.

Pituitary dwarfism seldom is combined with cleft lip and palate, but association of the two anomalies has been observed. Many years ago, I saw a girl, considered a pituitary dwarf, who had a congenital scar on the right upper lip that looked like a "healed" or surgically repaired lip. Her maternal uncle and aunt had cleft palate. The question of a hereditary "midline anomaly" causing facial clefts and pituitary deficiency was raised (Cincinnati Children's Hospital Chart No. 42652). In 1966, Francés *et al.*[167] reported a girl with cleft lip and palate and a girl with median cleft lip, both having pituitary dwarfism. Laron *et al.*[168] found growth retardation in 3 of 33 children with cleft lip and palate. In 2 of these children, disturbance in growth hormone secretion was demonstrated. A common embryonic developmental defect was assumed for the skeletal and endocrine anomalies.

REFERENCES

1. Fogh-Andersen, P.: *Inheritance of Harelip and Cleft Palate* (Copenhagen: Arnold Busck, 1942).
2. Davis, J. S.: The incidence of congenital clefts of the lip and palate, Ann. Surg. 80:363, 1924.
3. Erhardt, C. L., and Nelson, F. G.: Reported congenital malformations in New York City, 1958–1959, Am. J. Pub. Health 54:1489, 1964.
4. Davis, W. B.: Congenital deformities of face; types found in series 1,000 cases, Surg., Gynec. & Obst. 61: 201, 1935.
5. McIntosh, R., Merritt, K. K., Richards, M. R., Samuels, M. H., and Bellows, M. T.: The incidence of congenital malformations: A study of 5,964 pregnancies, Pediatrics 14:505, 1954.
6. Fogh-Andersen, P.: Incidence of cleft lip and palate: Constant or increasing?, Acta chir. scandinav. 122:106, 1961.
7. Stevenson, A. C., Johnston, H. A., Stewart, M. I. P., and Golding, D. R.: Congenital malformations. A report of a series of consecutive births in 24 centres, Bull. WHO 34 (supp.):1, 1966.
8. Greene, J. C.: Epidemiology of congenital clefts of the lip and palate, Pub. Health Rep. 78:589, 1963.
9. Meskin, L. H.: An epidemiologic study of factors related to the extent of facial clefts. Thesis, Graduate School, The University of Minnesota, 1966.
10. Drillien, C. M., Ingram, T. T. S., and Wilkinson, E. M.: *The Causes and Natural History of Cleft Lip and Palate* (Baltimore: The Williams & Wilkins Company, 1966).
11. Fogh-Andersen, P.: Rare clefts of the face, Acta chir. scandinav. 129:275, 1965.
12. Moyson, F., and Jeanty, M.: Malformations rares de la face, Arch. franç. pédiat. 21:939, 1964.
13. Rosselli, D., and Gulienetti, R.: *Le Malformazioni Associate* (Torino: Minerva Medica, 1960).
14. Harvey, W. (cited by Ballantyne, J. W.): *Manual of Antenatal Pathology and Hygiene. The Embryo* (Chicago: Chicago Medical Book Company, 1904).
15. Rischbieth, H.: Hare-lip and cleft palate, in Pearson, K. (ed.), *The Treasury of Human Inheritance* (London: Dulau & Company, Ltd., 1910), Vol. I, pt. IV, sec. XIIa.
16. Strean, L. P., and Peer, L. A.: Stress as etiologic factor in development of cleft palate, Plast. & Reconstruct. Surg. 18:1, 1956.
17. Warkany, J., and Kalter, H.: Maternal impressions and congenital malformations, Plast. & Reconstruct. Surg. 30:628, 1962.
18. Fraser, F. C., and Warburton, D.: No association of emotional stress or vitamin supplement during pregnancy to cleft lip or palate in man, Plast. & Reconstruct. Surg. 33:395, 1964.
19. Trew, C. J.: Sistens plura exempla palate deficientis, in *Nova Acta Physico-Medica Academiae Caesareae Leopoldino-Carolinae* (Norimbergae, 1757) (cited by Rischbieth), in Pearson, K. (ed.), *The Treasury of Human Inheritance* (London: Dulau & Company, Ltd., 1910).
20. Warkany, J., Nelson, R. C., and Schraffenberger, E.: Congenital malformations induced in rats by maternal nutritional deficiency. IV. Cleft palate, Am. J. Dis. Child. 65:882, 1943.
21. Hoppe, W.: Lippen-, Kiefer-, Gaumenspalten. Ätiologie, Pathogenese und Therapie, Arch. Kinderh. (supp.) 52:1, 1965.
22. Fogh-Andersen, P.: Genetic and non-genetic factors in the etiology of facial clefts, Scandinav. J. Plast. & Reconstruct. Surg. 1:22, 1967.
23. Sangvichien, S.: A thoracopagus, one with harelip and cleft palate, Anat. Rec. 67:157, 1937.
24. Sinclair, J. G., and McKay, J.: Median harelip, cleft palate and glossal agenesis, Anat. Rec. 91:155, 1945.
25. Robertson, G. S., and McKenzie, J.: Thoracopagous twins with differing first arch defects, Brit. J. Surg. 51: 362, 1964.
26. Verschuer, O.: Die vererbungsbiologische Zwillingsforschung, Ergebn. inn. Med. u. Kinderh. 31:35, 1927.
27. Orgler, A.: Über Erbgleichheit eineiiger Zwillinge, Med. Klin. 31:541, 1935.
28. Fraser Roberts, J. A.: Inherited Diseases, in Burdette, W. J. (ed.), *Methodology in Human Genetics* (San Francisco: Holden-Day, 1962).
29. Woolf, C. M., Woolf, R. M., and Broadbent, T. R.: Cleft lip and heredity, Plast. & Reconstruct. Surg. 34:11, 1964.
30. Weinstein, E. D., and Cohen, M. M.: Sex-linked cleft palate. Report of a family and review of 77 kindred, J. M. Genetics 3:1, 1966.
31. McKeown, T., and Record, R. G.: Malformations in a Population Observed for Five Years after Birth, in Wolstenholme, G. E. W., and O'Connor, C. M. (eds.), *Ciba Foundation Symposium on Congenital Malformations* (London: J. & A. Churchill, Ltd., 1960).
32. Neel, J. V.: A study of major congenital defects in Japanese infants, Am. J. Human Genet. 10:398, 1958.
33. Tretsven, V. E.: Incidence of cleft lip and palate in Montana Indians, J. Speech & Hearing Disorders 28:52, 1963.

34. Ivy, R. H.: The influence of race on the incidence of certain congenital anomalies, notably cleft lip-cleft palate, Plast. & Reconstruct. Surg. 30:581, 1962.
35. Khan, A. A.: Congenital malformations in African neonates, J. Trop. Med. 68:272, 1965.
36. Meskin, L. H., and Pruzansky, S.: Validity of the birth certificate in the epidemiologic assessment of facial clefts, J. Dent. Res. 46:1456, 1967.
37. Rank, B. K., and Thomson, J. A.: Cleft lip and palate in Tasmania, M. J. Australia 2:681, 1960.
38. Knox, G.: Detection of low intensity epidemicity; application to cleft lip and palate, Brit. J. Prev. & Social Med. 17:121, 1963.
39. Warkany, J., Passarge, E., and Smith, L. B.: Congenital malformations in autosomal trisomy syndromes, Am. J. Dis. Child. 112:502, 1966.
40. Wolf, U., and Reinwein, H.: Klinische und cytogenetische Differentialdiagnose der Defizienzen an den kurzen Armen der B-Chromosomen, Ztschr. Kinderh. 98: 234, 1967.
41. de Grouchy, J., Thieffry, S., Aicardi, J., Chevrie, J. J., and Zucker, G.: Trisomie partielle C par translocation t(Cq−; Dp+) et remaniement d'un C(p− q+), Arch. franç. pédiat. 24:859, 1967.
42. Zellweger, H., Mikamo, K., and Abbo, G.: Two cases of multiple malformations with an autosomal chromosomal aberration – partial trisomy D?, Helvet. paediat. acta 17:290, 1962.
43. Therman, E., Patau, K., DeMars, R. I., Smith, D. W., and Inhorn, S. L.: Iso/telo-D_1 mosaicism in a child with an incomplete D_1 trisomy syndrome, Portugal acta biol. 7: 211, 1963.
44. Lee, C. S. N., Bowen, P., Rosenblum, H., and Linsao, L.: Familial chromosome-2, 3 translocation ascertained through an infant with multiple malformations, New England J. Med. 271:12, 1964.
45. Jensen, M. K., and Melchior, J. C.: Possible partial trisomy of a chromosome of group 6-X-12 and familial translocation heterozygosity in a child with congenital abnormalities, Developmental Med. & Child Neurol. 9:313, 1967.
46. Lucas, M., Kemp, N. H., Ellis, J. R., and Marshall, R.: A small autosomal ring chromosome in a female infant with congenital malformations, Ann. Human Genet. 27: 189, 1963.
47. Bernard, R., Stahl, A., Giraud, F., Hartung, M., and Brusquet, Y.: Encéphalopathie avec dysmorphie complexe et chromosome 17-18 en anneau, Semaine hôp. Paris 42: 525, 1966.
48. Gustavson, K-H., Hagberg, B., Finley, S. C., and Finley, W. H.: An apparently identical extra autosome in two severely retarded sisters with multiple malformations, Cytogenetics 1:32, 1962.
49. Pfeiffer, R. A.: Deletion der kurzen Arme des Chromosoms Nr. 18, Humangenetik 2:178, 1966.
50. Haddad, H. M., and Wilkins, L.: Congenital anomalies associated with gonadal aplasia. Review of 55 cases, Pediatrics 23:885, 1959.
51. Miller, O. J., Breg, W. R., Schmickel, R. D., and Tretter, W.: A family with an XXXXY male, a leukaemic male, and two 21-trisomic mongoloid females, Lancet 2:78, 1961.
52. Gropp, A., Jussen, A., and Odunjo, F.: Near-triploid chromosome constitution in epithelial-cell cultures of palatal mucosa from a case of cleft palate, Lancet 1:1167, 1964.
53. Muramoto, J., Aya, T., and Sasaki, M.: A chromosome study of patients with cleft lip and cleft palate based on lesion biopsies in culture, Jap. J. Human Genet. 11:31, 1966.
54. Soukup, S., and Warkany, J.: Chromosomes in cleft-palate tissues, Lancet 1:492, 1966.
55. Nelson, M. M., Wright, H. V., Asling, C. W., and Evans, H. M.: Multiple congenital abnormalities resulting from transitory deficiency of pteroylglutamic acid during gestation in the rat, J. Nutrition 56:349, 1955.
56. Thiersch, J. B.: The control of reproduction in rats with the aid of antimetabolites. Early experiences with antimetabolites as abortifacient agents in man, Acta endocrinol. (supp.) 28:37, 1956.
57. Warkany, J., Beaudry, P. H., and Hornstein, S.: Attempted abortion with 4-amino-pteroylglutamic acid (aminopterin); malformations of the child, A.M.A. J. Dis. Child. 97:274, 1959.
58. Emerson, D. J.: Congenital malformation due to attempted abortion with aminopterin, Am. J. Obst. & Gynec. 84:356, 1962.
59. Diamond, I., Anderson, M. M., and McCreadie, S. R.: Transplacental transmission of busulfan (Myleran) in a mother with leukemia. Production of fetal malformations and cytomegaly, Pediatrics 25:85, 1960.
60. Kajii, T.: Thalidomide experience in Japan, Ann. paediat. 205:341, 1965.
61. King, C. T. G.: Teratogenic effects of meclizine hydrochloride on the rat, Science 141:353, 1963.
62. Lenz, W.: Malformations caused by drugs in pregnancy, Am. J. Dis. Child. 112:99, 1966.
63. Doig, R. K., and Coltman, O. McK.: Cleft palate following cortisone therapy in early pregnancy, Lancet 2:730, 1956.
64. Harris, J. W.S., and Ross, I. P.: Cortisone therapy in early pregnancy: Relation to cleft palate, Lancet 1:1045, 1956.
65. Warkany, J., and Schraffenberger, E.: Congenital malformations induced in rats by roentgen rays, Am. J. Roentgenol. 57:455, 1947.
66. Russell, L. B., and Russell, W. L.: An analysis of the changing radiation response of the developing mouse embryo. J. Cell. & Comp. Physiol. 43 (supp. 1): 130, 1954.
67. Engelhart, E., and Pischinger, A.: Über eine durch Röntgenstrahlen verursachte menschliche Missbildung, München med. Wchnschr. 86:1315, 1939.
68. Kupferberg, H.: Bemerkungen zur gynäkologischen Bestrahlungstechnik, Zentralbl. Gynäk. 48:2031, 1924.
69. Dekaban, A. S.: The outcome of pregnancy in diabetic women. 2. Analysis of clinical abnormalities and pathologic lesions in offspring of diabetic mothers, J. Pediat. 55:767, 1959.
70. McEvitt, W. G.: Cleft lip and palate and parental age, Plast. & Reconstruct. Surg. 10:77, 1952.
71. MacMahon, B., and McKeown, T.: The incidence of harelip and cleft palate related to birth rank and maternal age, Am. J. Human Genet. 5:176, 1953.
72. Woolf, C. M.: Parental age effect for cleft lip and palate, Am. J. Human Genet. 15:389, 1963.
73. Fraser, G. R., and Calnan, J. S.: Cleft lip and palate: Seasonal incidence, birth weight, birth rank, sex, site, associated malformations and parental age; a statistical survey, Arch. Dis. Childhood 36:420, 1961.
74. Hay, S.: Variables in under-reporting of clefts on birth certificates, Pub. Health Rep. 82:985, 1967.
75. Edwards, J. H: Seasonal incidence of congenital disease in Birmingham, Ann. Human Genet. 25:89, 1961.
76. Ingalls, T. H., Taube, I. E., and Klingberg, M. A.: Cleft lip and cleft palate: Epidemiologic considerations, Plast. & Reconstruct. Surg. 34:1, 1964.
77. Smith, D. W., and Bostian, K. E.: Congenital anomalies associated with idiopathic mental retardation, J. Pediat. 65:189, 1964.
78. Töndury, G.: Zum Problem der Gesichtsentwicklung und der Genese der Hasenscharte, Acta anat. 11:300, 1950.
79. Patten, B. M.: *Human Embryology* (New York: Blakiston Division, McGraw-Hill Book Company, 1953).
80. Peter, K.: Die Entwicklung des Säugetiergaumens, Ztschr. Anat. 3:448, 1924.
81. Thoma, K. H.: *Oral Pathology* (3d ed.; St. Louis: The C. V. Mosby Company, 1950).

82. Orban, B.: *Oral Histology and Embryology* (St. Louis: The C. V. Mosby Company, 1957).
83. Dursy, F.: *Zur Entwicklungsgeschichte des Kopfes* (Tübingen: 1869).
84. His, W.: Beobachtungen zur Geschichte der Nasen-und Gaumenbildung beim menschlichen Embryo, Abhandl. math. phys. Kl. Sächs, Gesellsch. Wissensch., Leipzig 27:253, 1901.
85. Inouye, M.: Der Zwischenkiefer, seine Entstehung und der Verlauf der Hasenschartenkieferspalte und der schrägen Gesichtsspalte, Anat. Hefte 45:470, 1912.
86. Pölzl, A.: Entwicklungsgeschichte des menschlichen Gaumens, Anat. Hefte 27:245, 1904.
87. Schorr, G.: Zur Entwicklungsgeschichte des sekundären Gaumens bei einigen Säugetieren und beim Menschen, Anat. Anz., Jena 30:24, 1907.
88. Fulton, J. T.: Closure of the human palate in embryo, Am. J. Obst. & Gynec. 74:179, 1957.
89. Walker, B. E., and Fraser, F. C.: Closure of the secondary palate in three strains of mice, J. Embryol. & Exper. Morphol. 4:176, 1956.
90. Larsson, K. S., Boström, H., and Carlsöö, S.: Studies on the closure of the secondary palate. I. Autoradiographic study in the normal mouse embryo, Exper. Cell Res. 16: 379, 1959.
91. Larsson, K. S.: Closure of the secondary palate and its relation to sulpho-mucopolysaccharides, Acta odont. scandinav. 20:(supp. 31)4, 1962.
92. Politzer, G.: Neue Untersuchungen über die Entstehung der Gesichtsspalten, Monatsschr. Ohrenh. 71:63, 1937.
93. Veau, V.: Hasenscharten menschlicher Keimlinge auf der Stufe 21-23 mm S. St. L., Ztschr. Anat. 108:459, 1938.
94. Steiniger, F.: Neue Beobachtungen an der erblichen Hasenscharte der Maus, Ztschr. menschl. Vererb.-u. Konstitutionslehre 23:427, 1939.
95. Reed, S. C.: An embryological study of harelip in mice, Anat. Rec. 56:101, 1933.
96. Steiniger, F.: Über Hasenschartencysten, Ztschr. menschl. Vererb.-u. Konstitutionslehre 25:1, 1941.
97. Hale, F.: Relation of maternal vitamin A deficiency to microphthalmia in pigs, Texas J. Med. 33:228, 1937.
98. Palludan, B.: *A-Avitaminosis in Swine* (Copenhagen: Munksgaard, 1966).
99. Nelson, M. M., Wright, H. V., Baird, C. D. C., and Evans, H. M.: Effect of 36-hour period of pteroylglutamic acid deficiency on fetal development in rat, Proc. Soc. Exper. Biol. & Med. 92:554, 1956.
100. Kalter, H., and Warkany, J.: Congenital malformations in inbred strains of mice induced by riboflavin-deficient, galactoflavin-containing diets, J. Exper. Zool. 136:531, 1957.
101. Fraser, F. C., and Fainstat, T. D.: Production of congenital defects in the offspring of pregnant mice treated with cortisone, Pediatrics 8:527, 1951.
102. Fraser, F. C., Fainstat, T. D., and Kalter, H.: The experimental production of congenital defects with particular reference to cleft palate, Études néo-natales 2:43, 1953.
103. Kalter, H.: The inheritance of susceptibility to the teratogenic action of cortisone in mice, Genetics 39:185, 1954.
104. Trasler, D. G.: Strain Differences in Susceptibility to Teratogenesis: Survey of Spontaneously Occurring Malformations in Mice, in Wilson, J. G., and Warkany, J. (eds.), *Teratology. Principles and Techniques* (Chicago and London: The University of Chicago Press, 1965).
105. Walker, B. E., and Fraser, F. C.: Embryology of cortisone-induced cleft palate, J. Embryol. & Exper. Morphol. 5:201, 1957.
106. Kalter, H.: Interplay of Intrinsic and Extrinsic Factors, in Wilson, J. G., and Warkany, J. (eds.), *Teratology. Principles and Techniques* (Chicago and London: The University of Chicago Press, 1965).
107. Fraser, F. C.: Cleft lip and cleft palate, Science 158: 1603, 1967.
108. Walker, B. E.: The association of mucopolysaccharides with morphogenesis of the palate and other structures in mouse embryos, J. Embryol. & Exper. Morphol. 9:22, 1961.
109. Deuschle, F. M., and Kalter, H.: Observations on the mandible in association with defects of the lip and palate, J. Dent. Res. 41:1085, 1962.
110. Ross, L. M., and Walker, B. E.: Movement of palatine shelves in untreated and teratogen-treated mouse embryos, Am. J. Anat. 121:509, 1967.
111. Cohlan, S. Q.: Congenital anomalies in the rat produced by excessive intake of vitamin A during pregnancy, Pediatrics 13:556, 1954.
112. Kalter, H., and Warkany, J.: Experimental production of congenital malformations in strains of inbred mice by maternal treatment with hypervitaminosis A, Am. J. Path. 38:1, 1961.
113. Walker, B. E., and Crain, B., Jr.: Effects of hypervitaminosis A on palate development in two strains of mice, Am. J. Anat. 107:49, 1960.
114. Warkany, J., and Takacs, E.: Experimental production of congenital malformations in rats by salicylate poisoning, Am. J. Path. 35:315, 1959.
115. Larsson, K. S., Boström, H., and Ericson, B.: Salicylate-induced malformations in mouse embryos, Acta paediat. scandinav. 52:36, 1963.
116. Trasler, D. G.: Aspirin-induced cleft lip and other malformations in mice, Lancet 1:606, 1965.
117. Larsson, K. S., and Boström, H.: Teratogenic action of salicylates related to the inhibition of mucopolysaccharide synthesis, Acta paediat. scandinav. 54:43, 1965.
118. Trasler, D. G., Walker, B. E., and Fraser, F. C.: Congenital malformations produced by amniotic-sac puncture, Science 124:439, 1956.
119. Field, L. E., Kreshover, S. J., and Lieberman, J. E.: Temporary uterine circulatory arrest as a cause of abnormal fetal development, J. Dent. Res. 39:1240, 1960.
120. Smith, A. U.: The effect on fetal development of freezing pregnant hamsters (Mesocricetus auratus), J. Embryol. & Exper. Morphol. 5:311, 1957.
121. Ingalls, T. H., Curley, F. J., and Prindle, R. A.: Experimental production of congenital anomalies, New England J. Med. 247:758, 1952.
122. Brent, R. L., Averich, E., and Drapiewski, V. A.: Production of congenital malformations using tissue antibodies. I. Kidney antisera, Proc. Soc. Exper. Biol. & Med. 106:523, 1961.
123. Warkany, J., and Deuschle, F. M.: Congenital malformations induced in rats by maternal riboflavin deficiency: Dentofacial changes, J.A.D.A. 51:139, 1955.
124. Deuschle, F. M., and Warkany, J.: Congenital dentofacial malformations in rats induced by maternal nutritional deficiency, J. Dent. Res. 35:674, 1956.
125. Deuschle, F. M., Geiger, J. F., and Warkany, J.: Analysis of an anomalous oculodentofacial pattern in newborn rats produced by maternal hypervitaminosis A, J. Dent. Res. 38:149, 1959.
126. Deuschle, F. M., Takacs, E., and Warkany, J.: Postnatal dentofacial changes induced in rats by prenatal riboflavin deficiency, J. Dent. Res. 40:366, 1961.
127. Kalter, H., and Deuschle, F. M.: Congenital Malformations Experimentally Induced by Hypervitaminosis A, in Kreshover, S. J., and McClure, F. J. (eds.), *Environmental Variables in Oral Disease* (Washington, D.C.: American Association for the Advancement of Science, 1966).
128. Davis, J. S., and Ritchie, H. P.: Classification of congenital clefts of the lip and palate, J.A.M.A. 79:1323, 1922.
129. Stark, R. B.: Embryology, Pathogenesis and Classification of Cleft Lip and Cleft Palate, in Pruzansky, S. (ed.), *Congenital Anomalies of the Face and Associated Structures* (Springfield, Ill.: Charles C Thomas, Publisher, 1961).

130. Calnan, J.: Submucous cleft palate, Brit. J. Plast Surg. 6:264, 1954.
131. Illingworth, R. S.: Congenital anomalies associated with cerebral palsy and mental retardation, Arch. Dis. Childhood 34:269, 1959.
132. Heilbroner, R. L.: *The Worldly Philosophers* (New York: Simon & Schuster, Inc., 1953).
133. Roosevelt, N.: *A Front Row Seat* (Norman, Oklahoma: University of Oklahoma Press, 1953).
134. Keith, A.: *An Autobiography* (New York: Philosophical Library, Inc., 1950).
135. Birch-Jensen, A.: *Congenital Deformities of the Upper Extremities* (Odense, Denmark: Andelsbogtrykkeriet, 1949).
136. Gross, R. E.: *The Surgery of Infancy and Childhood* (Philadelphia: W. B. Saunders Company, 1953).
137. Campbell, M.: *Clinical Pediatric Urology* (Philadelphia: W. B. Saunders Company, 1951).
138. Gruber, G. B.: Über einen akrocephalen Reliefschädel. Ein Beitrag zur Frage der partiellen Chondrodystrophie, Beitr. path. Anat. 97:9, 1936.
139. de Lange, C.: Zum Studium der Encephalocele posterior, Jahrb. Kinderh. 126:253, 1930.
140. Grebe, H.: Zur Ätiologie der Arhinencephalie, Der Erbarzt 12:138, 1944.
141. Marshall, R., Newnham, R. E., Rawstron, J. R., Ellis, J. R., and Stevens, L. J.: Features of 13-15 trisomy syndrome with normal karyotype, Lancet 1:556, 1964.
142. Gorlin, R. J., and Pindborg, J. J.: *Syndromes of the Head and Neck* (New York: McGraw-Hill Book Company, 1964).
143. Curtis, E. J., Fraser, F. C., and Warburton, D.: Congenital cleft lip and palate. Am. J. Dis. Child. 102:853, 1961.
144. Van Der Woude, A.: Fistula labii inferioris congenita and its association with cleft lip and palate, Am. J. Human Genet. 6:244, 1954.
145. Schönenberg, H.: Über die Kombination von Lippen-Kiefer-Gaumen-Spalten mit Extremitätenmissbildungen, Ztschr. Kinderh. 76:79, 1955.
146. Hecht, F., and Jarvinen, J. M.: Heritable dysmorphic syndrome with normal intelligence, J. Pediat. 70:927, 1967.
147. Larsen, L. J., Schottstaedt, E. R., and Bost, F. C.: Multiple congenital dislocations associated with characteristic facial abnormality, J. Pediat. 37:574, 1950.
148. Rossi, E.: Le syndrome arthromyodysplasique congénital, Helvet. paediat. acta 2:82, 1947.
149. James, T.: Multiple congenital articular rigidities, Edinburgh M. J. 58:565, 1951.
150. Dudding, B. A., Gorlin, R. J., and Langer, L. O.: The oto-palato-digital syndrome, Am. J. Dis. Child. 113:214, 1967.
151. Taybi, H.: Generalized skeletal dysplasia with multiple anomalies; note on Pyle's disease, Am. J. Roentgenol. 88:450, 1962.
152. Dodge, H. W., Wood, M. W., and Kennedy, R. L. J.: Craniofacial dysostosis: Crouzon's disease, Pediatrics 23:98, 1959.
153. Weyers, H.: Zur Klinik und Pathologie der Dysostosis mandibulofacialis, Ztschr. Kinderh. 69:207, 1951.
154. Latham, R. A.: The pathogenesis of cleft palate associated with the Pierre Robin syndrome: An analysis of a seventeen-week human foetus, Brit. J. Plast. Surg. 19: 205, 1966.
155. Poswillo, D.: Observations of fetal posture and causal mechanisms of congenital deformity of palate, mandible, and limbs, J. Dent. Res. 45:584, 1966.
156. Avery, H.: Multiple osseous defects, Proc. Roy. Soc. Med. 24:281, 1931.
157. Ross, L. J.: Arachnodactyly. Review of recent literature and report of a case with cleft palate, Am. J. Dis. Child. 78:417, 1949.
158. Wilson, R.: Marfan's syndrome. Description of a family, Am. J. Med. 23:434, 1957.
159. Noé, O.: Amsterdam dwarfs, Clin. Pediat. 3:541, 1964.
160. Reimann, H. A., McKechnie, W. G., and Stanisavljevic, S.: Hereditary sensory radicular neuropathy and other defects in a large family. Reinvestigation after twenty years and report of a necropsy, Am. J. Med. 25:573, 1958.
161. Mirkinson, A. E., and Maitinsky, V.: A triplo-X mongol female with congenital heart disease, cleft palate and hare lip, Bull. St. Francis Hosp. 22:2, 1969.
162. Humphrey, T.: The relation between human fetal mouth opening reflexes and closure of the palate, Am. J. Anat. 125:317, 1969.
163. Gordon, H., Davies, D., and Berman, M.: Camptodactyly, cleft palate, and club foot, J. M. Genetics 6:266, 1969.
164. Juberg, R. C., and Hayward, J. R.: A new familial syndrome of oral, cranial, and digital anomalies, J. Pediat. 74:755, 1969.
165. Bixler, D., Christian, J. C., and Gorlin, R. J.: Hypertelorism, microtia, and facial clefting, Am. J. Dis. Child. 118: 495, 1969.
166. Nanda, R.: *The Normal Palate and Induced Cleft Palate in Rat Embryos* (Nijmegen: Drukkerij Gebr. Janssen N. V., 1969).
167. Francés, J. M., Knorr, D., Martinez, R., and Neuhäuser, G.: Hypophysärer Zwergwuchs bei Lippen-Kiefer-Spalte, Helvet. paediat. acta 21:315, 1966.
168. Laron, Z., Taube, E., and Kaplan, I.: Pituitary growth hormone insufficiency associated with cleft lip and palate, Helvet. paediat. acta 24:576, 1969.
169. Rosselli, D., and Gulienetti, R.: Ectodermal dysplasia, Brit. J. Plast. Surg. 14:190, 1961.
170. Rapp, R. S., and Hodgkin, W. E.: Anhidrotic ectodermal dysplasia: Autosomal dominant inheritance with palate and lip anomalies, J. M. Genetics 5:269, 1968.
171. Fraser, F. C.: The genetics of cleft lip and cleft palate, Am. J. Human Genet. 22:336, 1970.
172. Rüdiger, R. A., Haase, W., and Passarge, E.: Association of ectrodactyly, ectodermal dysplasia, and cleft lip-palate, Am. J. Dis. Child. 120:160, 1970.
173. Walker, J. C., and Clodius, L.: The syndrome of cleft lip, cleft palate and lobster claw deformities of hands and feet, Plast. & Reconstruct. Surg. 32:627, 1963.
174. Jaworska, M., and Popiolek, J.: Genetic counseling in lobster claw anomaly, Clin. Pediat. 7:396, 1968.
175. Appelt, H., Gerken, H., and Lenz, W.: Tetraphokomelie mit Lippen-Kiefer-Gaumenspalte und Clitorishypertrophie – ein Syndrom, Pädiat. und Pädol. 2:119, 1966.
176. Stroer, W. F. H.: Über das Zusammentreffen von Hasenscharte mit ernsten Extremitätenmissbildungen, Der Erbarzt 7:101, 1939.
177. Verschuer, O.: Über das Zusammentreffen von Lippen-Kiefer-Gaumen-spalten mit Missbildungen der Gliedmassen, Der Erbarzt 9:1, 1941.
178. Freire-Maia, N.: A newly recognized genetic syndrome of tetramelic deficiencies, ectodermal dysplasia, deformed ears, and other abnormalities, Am. J. Human Genet. 22:370, 1970.
179. Pfeiffer, R-A, Tünte, W., and Reinken, M.: Das Kniepterygium-Syndrom, Ztschr. Kinderh. 108:103, 1970.
180. Knox, G., and Braithwaite, F.: Cleft lips and palates in Northumberland and Durham, Arch. Dis. Childhood 38:66, 1963.
181. Lenz, W.: How can the teratogenic action of a factor be established in man?, South. M. J. 64(supp. 1):41, 1971.

71

Some Syndromes Involving the Face

Mandibulofacial Dysostosis
(Treacher Collins Syndrome; Franceschetti-Zwahlen Syndrome)

THIS SYNDROME chiefly affects structures formed from the first branchial arch. It is composed of malformations of the eye, the zygoma, the ear and the mandible and is closely related to a syndrome described by McEnery and Brennemann,[1] in which cleft palate was the leading anomaly. Many combinations and transitional forms exist.[2,3] The anomalies may be bilateral or unilateral and the syndrome complete, incomplete or "super-complete." An incomplete form of this syndrome was reported in 1889 by Berry[4] and others by Collins,[5] who recorded the characteristic colobomas of the eyelids associated with hypoplasia of the malar bones. Franceschetti and Klein[2] reviewed the subject thoroughly and extended the syndrome to the following chief symptoms: palpebral fissures sloping downward in antimongoloid direction with coloboma of the lower lid; hypoplasia of the facial bones, especially the malar bones and the mandible; malformations of external and internal ears; macrostomia; high or cleft palate and faulty dentition; fistulas between mouth and ears; and abnormal hair growth on the cheeks. Robbins[6] reviewed 52 cases recorded between 1952 and 1958.

The condition occurs in male and female patients. It has been described in Caucasians, Negroes, Mongols and Indians[7]; it has occurred in one of twins and in a pair of concordant identical twins (see Fig. 71-1, *A*). The trait seems to be relatively common in Kentucky and West Virginia, where several affected kindreds have been observed. Dominant inheritance has been observed repeatedly but the expression may be irregular, some patients showing the entire syndrome and others an incomplete form with only one or two symptoms. A dominant pleiotropic gene is held responsible for all the symptoms. Numerous pedigrees showing transmission through two or three generations have been published.[2,8-10] In the Children's Hospital in Cincinnati a child with the fully developed syndrome (Fig. 71-1, *B*) was observed whose father (Fig. 71-1, *C*) supplied us with a rather reliable family history (Fig. 71-1, *A*) tracing the syndrome through four generations. The name of the family represented as A 1 generation was "S———" and the syndrome was spoken of as the "S – Mark." The family tradition could thus furnish the data on which the pedigree in Figure 71-1, *A* is based. This history is compatible with the hypothesis of dominant inheritance with variable expression of the gene. In the A_1 generation there was a woman who had been considered normal but who transmitted the trait to 2 of her sons. She may have had the anomaly in a mild form, but this was not remembered by our historian. She had 3 sons who were hard of hearing and 1 of them transmitted mandibulofacial dysostosis to 2 of his sons and deafness to another 2. Deafness and frequent middle ear infections apparently can be mild expressions of the anomaly, with the deaf person being capable of transmitting the trait.

But not all cases have a positive family history. There probably are more sporadic cases than those with obvious heritability. An affected child of normal parents could represent a new mutation (Fig. 71-2) or one of the parents could have the disorder in a subclinical form. In both cases, the patient could transmit the condition to some of his children. Another possibility is that some of the cases are not genetically determined but represent phenocopies, produced by environmental interferences with embryonic development. Granrud[11] recorded 5 cases without proof of inheritance but with histories indicating possible maternal disorders during pregnancy. In one instance, maternal rubella occurred in the twelfth week of pregnancy, which is too late to account for most of the symptoms. There was, however, one atypical patient (Case 4) following attempted abortion in the beginning of the second month and again 3–4 weeks later whose malformations could be attributed to embryonic injury. A case showing slight resemblance to the syndrome was caused by aminopterin ingestion by the mother,[12] but in typical cases genetic determination and dominant inheritance should be assumed. The chromosomes appear normal.[7,18]

According to Franceschetti and Klein,[2] an arrest of development toward the end of the second month could explain the micrognathia, the macrostomia and the malposition of the external ears of mandibulofacial dysostosis. In the next stage of development,

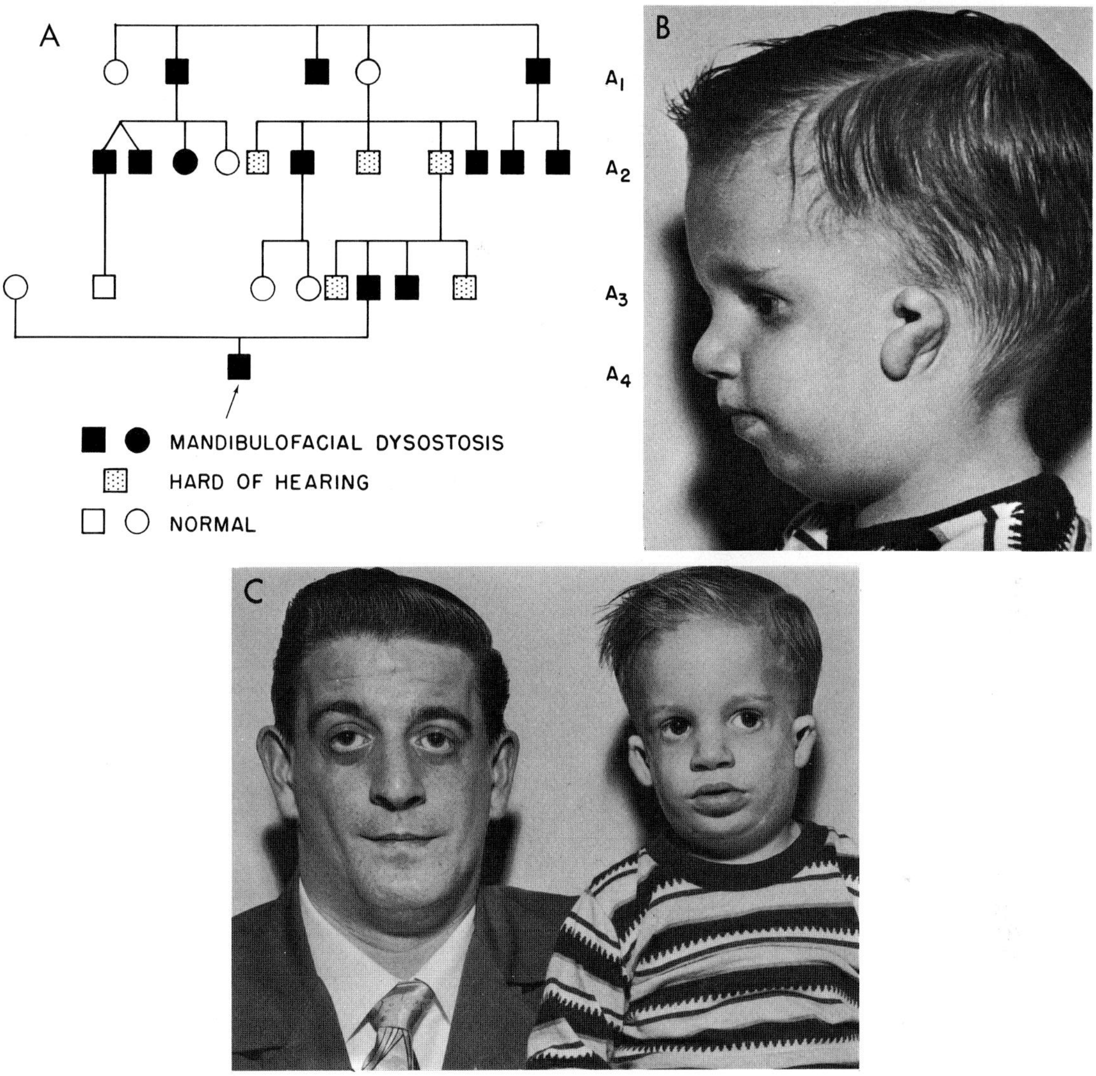

Fig. 71-1. – **A,** pedigree of a kinship in which mandibulofacial dysostosis and related anomálies were inherited as a dominant trait with variable expression. **B,** the propositus, who had posterior cleft palate, anomalies of the external ears, suggestion of coloboma of the lower eyelids and micrognathia. **C,** father and propositus. The father had characteristic shape of eyes and defect in the malar area. He had a high palate with osseous defect in the posterior portion. This defect was completely bridged by soft tissues, which formed a normal uvula. His speech was normal.

formation of the facial bones may be inhibited, with consequent displacement of the bones of the orbit. These skeletal changes are thought to lead to drooping of the lower lids, formation of colobomas and other eye anomalies.

Hövels[13] considered mandibulofacial dysostosis as merely one of the malformations of the first visceral arch and analyzed the entire series of these anomalies from isolated defects to otocephaly. He believed that previous attempts to time the origin of mandibulofacial dysostosis had started from wrong premises arriving at dates that seemed too late to account for the syndrome. He held disturbance of a higher center of organization in the area of the rhombencephalon responsible for the malformations of the first visceral arch.

McKenzie and Craig[14] believed that a defect of the stapedial artery causes maldevelopment not only in its own field of supply but also in the region of the first visceral arch, the vessels of which normally are supported by the stapedial artery during the critical phase between the disappearance of the first aortic arch and the full development of the external carotid artery. McKenzie[15] later differentiated 8 syndromes in

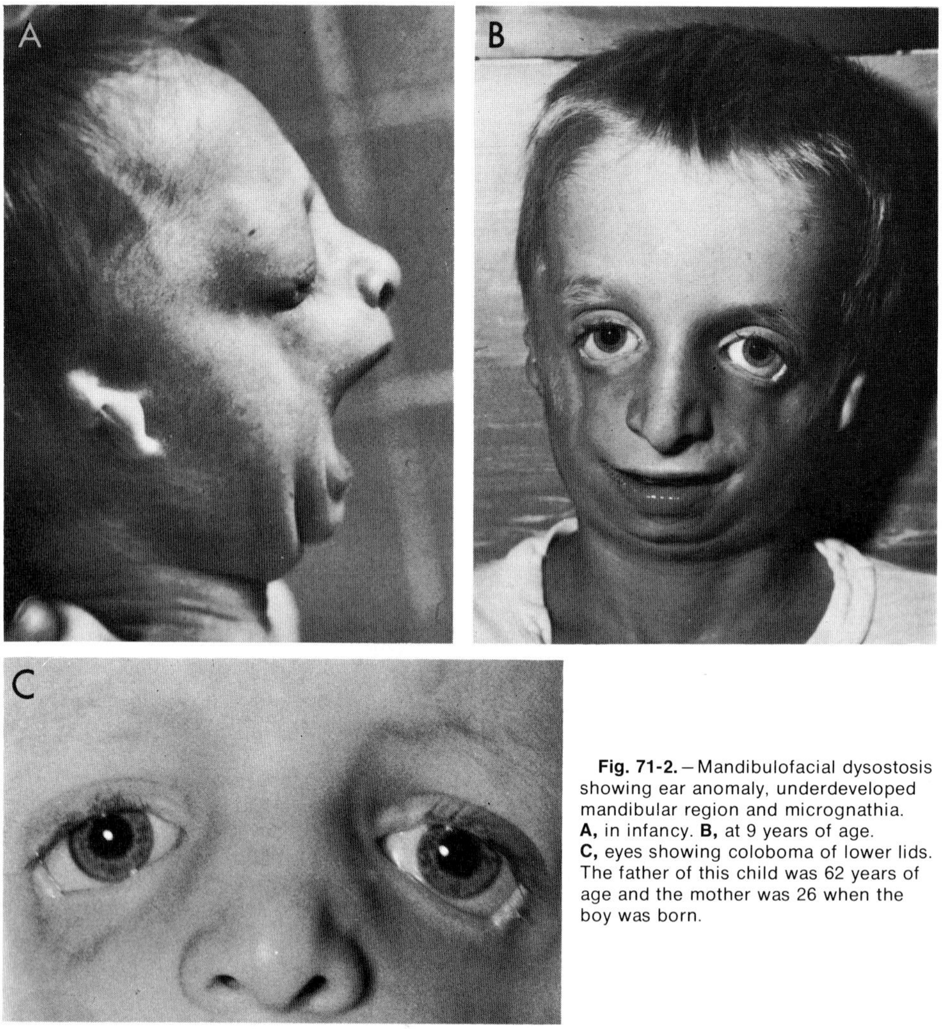

Fig. 71-2. — Mandibulofacial dysostosis showing ear anomaly, underdeveloped mandibular region and micrognathia. **A,** in infancy. **B,** at 9 years of age. **C,** eyes showing coloboma of lower lids. The father of this child was 62 years of age and the mother was 26 when the boy was born.

the "first arch syndrome" and held "a dominant gene or group of dominant genes with variable expressivity and moderate degree of penetrance" responsible for their etiology.

Usually, the skull is normal but it can be asymmetric if the malformations are limited to one side. The width of the face is reduced. The palpebral fissures slope downward in an antimongoloid direction and there are temporal colobomas in the lower lids, which may make the eyes appear "round."[9] Congenital ptosis has been observed and the eyelashes may be absent or growing irregularly in two or three rows. The nasofrontal angle is not developed and the facial bones are hypoplastic. The zygomatic process may be absent and replaced by a depression. In this depressed area, blind fistulas and abnormal hair formation can be found. The external ears may be small, displaced or reduced to "mere nubbins." Sometimes the external auditory canal is obliterated. The middle ear is affected in some of the cases, the tympanic ossicles being absent and the tubes deformed. Hypoplasia of the horizontal semicircular canal and of the cochlea has been observed. Underdevelopment of the mandible and a receding chin are characteristic of the syndrome. The size of the tongue varies. Macrostomia is considered characteristic of the anomaly but microstomia has also been reported.[6] The palate is high; cleft palate complicates the disease picture rather frequently and malposition and malocclusion of the teeth are the rule. Structures surrounding the mouth, such as the parotis and the masseter muscle, may be hypoplastic or absent. In addition to these typical symptoms there often are associated malformations. Absence of the lacrimal glands, atresia of the lacrimal ducts, ectropion and microphthalmia occur, but the anomalies are not always limited to the face. Fusion of cervical vertebrae (Klippel-Feil syndrome) and spina bifida, pectus excavatum, aortic coarctation, ventricular septal defect and anomalies of the extremities have been observed.[2,6] These anomalies may be found in persons with normal mental capacities, but mental retardation was present in some of the patients reported.[6,16]

The syndrome can be recognized at birth. There may be difficulty in breathing and many severely affected children die in the first 6 months of life. A high infant mortality has been noted repeatedly in families with this trait. Respiratory difficulties and their complications are the main reason for early death. Patients who survive the newborn period often are handicapped by harelip, cleft palate, deafness, speech defects and cosmetic problems. Unilateral cases[17] present specific symptoms and problems. In these cases, anomalies of the vertebral column seem to be included in the syndrome.

The respiratory difficulties in the newborn period can be alleviated by putting the infant in a position in which the tongue cannot fall backward and obstruct the respiratory passages. Plastic surgery can improve the appearance of the patients.

REFERENCES

1. McEnery, E. T., and Brennemann, J.: Multiple facial anomalies, J. Pediat. 11:468, 1937.
2. Franceschetti, A., and Klein, D.: *The Mandibulo-facial Dysostosis* (Copenhagen: Ejnar Munksgaard, 1949).
3. Rosselli, D., and Gulienetti, R.: *Le Malformazioni Associate* (Milan: Edizione Minerva Medica, 1960).
4. Berry, G. A.: Note on congenital defect (coloboma) of lower lid, Roy. London Ophth. Hosp. Rep. XII, Part III, 225, 1889.
5. Collins, E. T.: Case(s) with symmetrical congenital notches in the outer part of each lower lid and defective development of the malar bones, Tr. Ophth. Soc. U. Kingdom 20:190, 1900.
6. Robbins, D.: La dysostose mandibulo-faciale, ses associations cliniques et son mode d'hérédité; revue de la littérature récente, J. Génét. Hum. 12:1, 1963.
7. Caldwell, E. E., Anthony, J. A., Brown, H. P., and Crump, E. P.: The Treacher Collins syndrome. Report of studies of an affected Negro infant, and survey of the literature, Clin. Pediat. 6:715, 1967.
8. Debusmann: Familiäre kombinierte Gesichtsmissbildung im Bereich des ersten Viszeralbogens, Arch. Kinderh. 120:133, 1940.
9. Rovin, S., Dachi, S. F., Borenstein, D. B., and Cotter, W. B.: Mandibulofacial dysostosis, a familial study of five generations, J. Pediat. 65:215, 1964.
10. Fazen, L. E., Elmore, J., and Nadler, H. L.: Mandibulofacial dysostosis (Treacher Collins syndrome), Am. J. Dis. Child. 113:405, 1967.
11. Granrud, H.: On the etiology of dysostosis mandibulofacialis, Acta paediat. 42:499, 1953.
12. Warkany, J., Beaudry, P. H., and Hornstein, S.: Attempted abortion with 4-amino-pteroylglutamic acid (aminopterin). Malformations of the child, A.M.A. J. Dis. Child. 97:274, 1959.
13. Hövels, O.: Zur Pathogenese der Missbildungen des 1. Visceralbogens, Ztschr. Kinderh. 73:532, 1953.
14. McKenzie, J., and Craig, J.: Mandibulo-facial dysostosis (Treacher Collins syndrome), Arch. Dis. Childhood 30: 391, 1955.
15. McKenzie, J.: The first arch syndrome, Arch. Dis. Childhood 33:477, 1958.
16. Gibson, R.: Mandibulofacial dysostosis with oligophrenia in siblings, Am. J. Ment. Deficiency 62:504, 1957.
17. Weyers, H.: Zur Klinik und Pathologie der Dysostosis mandibulo-facialis, Ztschr. Kinderh. 69:207, 1951.
18. Moss, M. H., Saphir, R. L., and Gottlieb, M. I.: Mandibulofacial dysostosis; report of two cases with chromosome analysis, Am. J. Dis. Child. 107:304, 1964.

Unilateral Mandibulofacial Dysostosis (Weyers)

UNILATERAL FORMS of mandibulofacial dysostosis, which are rarer than the typical forms,[1,2] were reviewed by Weyers.[3,4] He wrote about "facial scoliosis" with unilateral hypoplasia of the mandible and dental malocclusion. The external ear is low set and rudimentary. On the affected side, the hairline recedes dorsad so that an area free of hair is seen behind the defective ear. The buccal commissure may be enlarged and unilateral macrostomia is formed. Roentgenograms disclose absence of the ramus mandibulae on the affected side and faulty segmentation of the spinal column. In a case described by Weyers,[3] "formes frustes" had occurred in the ancestry. This author distinguished an oculoauricular form from unilateral mandibulofacial dysostosis. Microphthalmia or anophthalmia is included in this syndrome but there is no ocular dermoid as in the Goldenhar syndrome (Chapter 40). As shown in Figure 71-3, anomalies of the hand can be present in a child with unilateral mandibulofacial dysostosis. Transitional forms occur in various combinations.

REFERENCES

1. Franceschetti, A., Brocher, J. E. W., and Klein, D.: Dysostose mandibulo-faciale unilatérale avec déformations multiples du squelette (processus paramastoide, synostose des vertèbres, sacralisation, etc.) et torticolis clonique, Arch. Klaus Stift. Vererbungsforsch. 22:373, 1947.
2. Franceschetti, A., and Klein, D.: The mandibulo-facial dysostosis. A new hereditary syndrome, Acta ophth. 27: 144, 1949.
3. Weyers, H.: Contribution à la sémiotique et à la génétique de la dysostose mandibulo-faciale unilatérale, J. Génét. Hum. 5:89, 1956.
4. Weyers, H., and Thier, C. J.: Malformations mandibulo-faciales et délimitation d'un syndrome oculo-vertébral, J. Génét. Hum. 7:143, 1958.

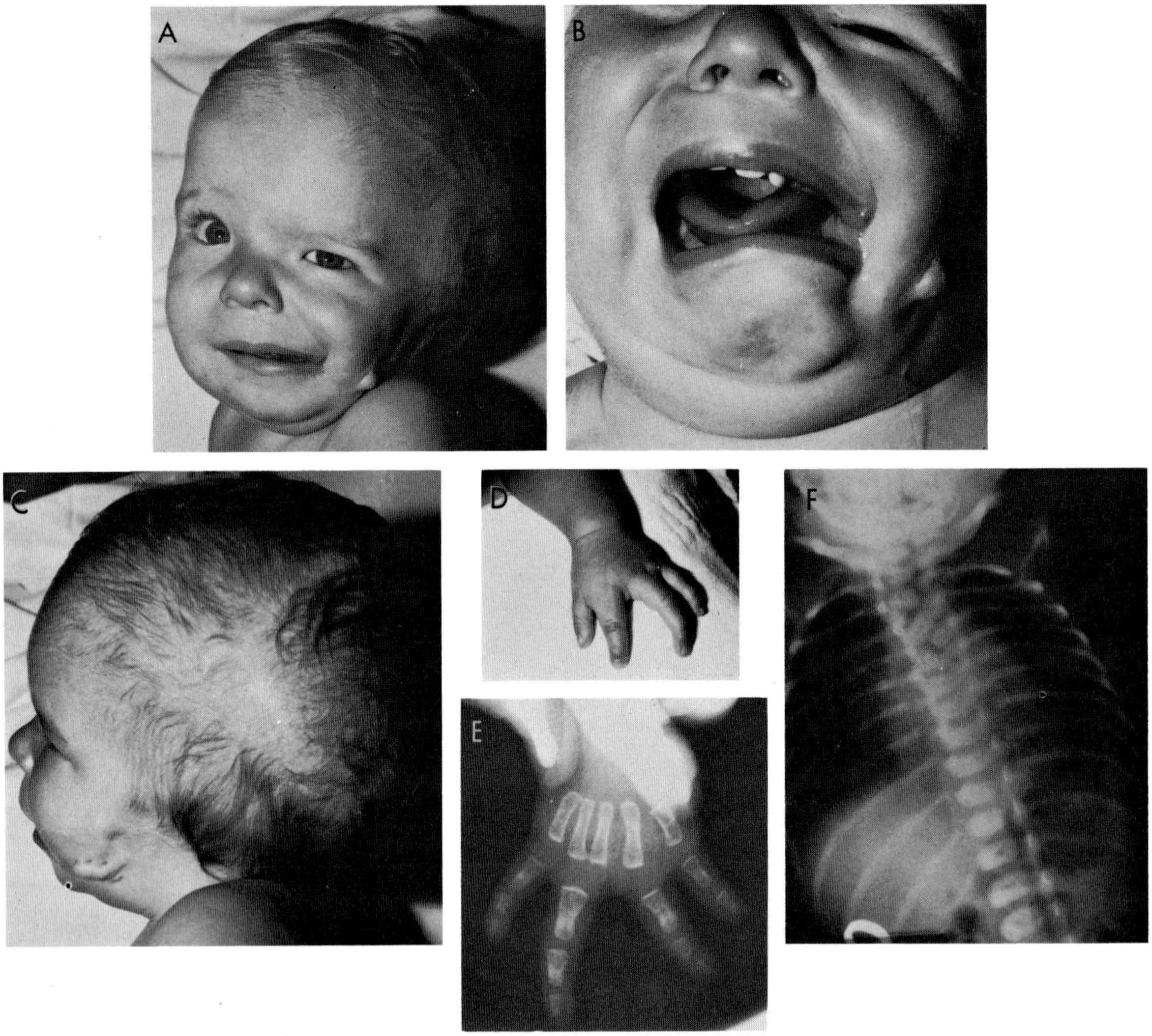

Fig. 71-3.—Unilateral mandibulofacial dysostosis. Family history negative. The patient was the first child of healthy parents. **A** and **B,** macrostomia and ear anomaly are limited to the left side. The upper and lower lips do not meet in the left angle of the mouth. The left palpebral fissure is smaller than the right and has antimongoloid slant. **C,** the skin behind the defective ear is free of hairs. **D** and **E,** there are only 4 fingers on the left hand. **F,** faulty segmentation of upper thoracic vertebrae.

Micrognathia with Glossoptosis
(Pierre Robin Syndrome)

EXTREME FORMS of micrognathia commonly are associated with glossoptosis and narrowing of the respiratory pathway between the tongue and the posterior wall of the pharynx. This leads to a dangerous situation in newborn children, as was recognized by Robin[1-3] and Lenstrup,[4] who pointed out that breathing difficulties arise in such infants through pressure of the base of the tongue on the epiglottis. The breathing difficulties, in turn, lead to retarded physical and mental development. Robin believed that children with this anomaly, if not treated, seldom lived beyond 18 months after birth, but observed that respiration was improved markedly if the mandible could be moved forward. He recommended "orthostatic treatment" for the children during and after feeding. During crying spells, children were to be kept on their stomachs to prevent aspiration of mucus and regurgi-

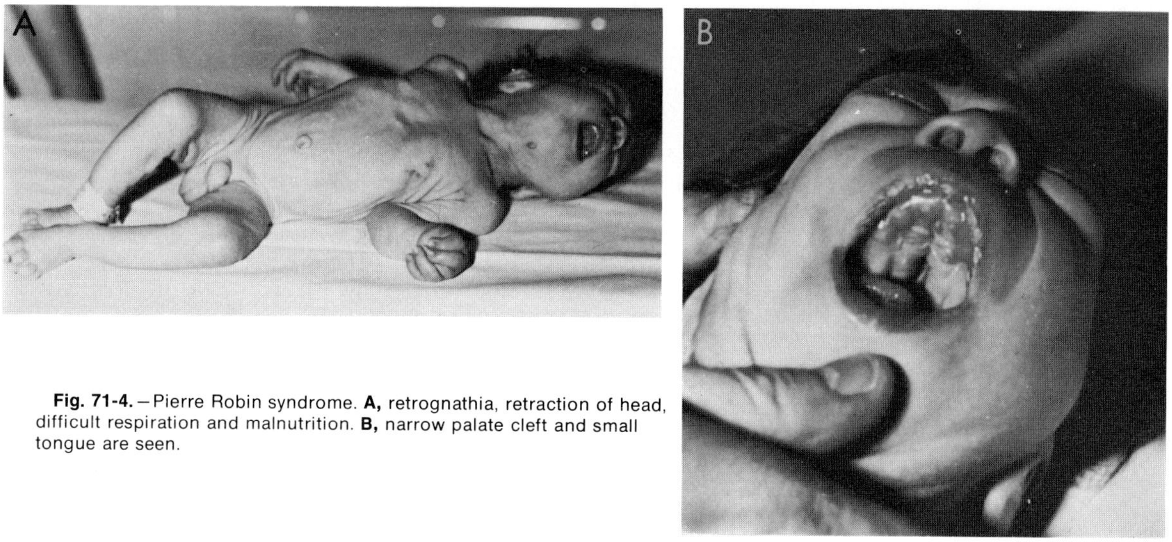

Fig. 71-4. – Pierre Robin syndrome. **A,** retrognathia, retraction of head, difficult respiration and malnutrition. **B,** narrow palate cleft and small tongue are seen.

tated food. Although this complex was clearly recognized, described and treated by earlier authors, it was termed "Pierre Robin syndrome."

Eley and Farber[5] discussed hypoplasia of the mandible as a cause of cyanotic attacks in newborn infants who obviously belong in the same category as those discussed by Robin. Their patients, as those of Lenstrup, also had posterior cleft palate and it is now believed that 60–80% of the infants with micrognathia and glossoptosis have palatal clefts.[6] These authors cited many of the older writers, who discussed this subject in the nineteenth century.

As pointed out before (p. 634), closure of the palatine shelves coincides normally with a growth spurt of the mandible during the second month of embryonic life. If this mandibular growth does not take place, the tongue fails to be carried forward and downward, remaining between the palatine processes, which cannot move up to their horizontal position. They cannot approach each other and form the posterior palate, so that a palatine cleft persists in which the tongue retains its embryonic position.

Although most cases of the Pierre Robin syndrome are sporadic, a genetic origin cannot be excluded. In the Cincinnati Children's Hospital, 2 sisters were affected in one family and in another kinship more distant relatives of the patient with Pierre Robin syndrome were affected by micrognathia or cleft palate (Fig. 71-6). In the Cincinnati Children's Hospital, monozygotic twins were observed, both affected with Pierre Robin syndrome (Chart Nos. 207289 and 207291); a different type of the syndrome and its inheritance are illustrated in Figure 71-5. Smith and Stowe[7] recorded 2 brothers, both with the Pierre Robin syndrome, whose mother stated that the anomaly had occurred in her family for four generations. They also reported a patient with the entire syndrome whose sibling had only a cleft palate.

Associated malformations are not rare. Smith and Stowe[7] stressed ocular anomalies, but aural anomalies, congenital heart disease and malformations of the extremities also were present in their patients with the Pierre Robin syndrome. A combination of Pierre Robin syndrome with atrial septal defect, persistence of the left superior vena cava and talipes equinovarus has been observed and attributed to X-linked recessive inheritance.[15] The combination of marked micrognathia, cleft palate with severe reduction malformations (peromelia) sometimes is called the Hanhart syndrome. There may be ankylosis of the upper and lower jaw, microstomia, hypoplasia of the tongue associated with absence of forearm and lower leg or other defects of the extremities.[16]

Micrognathia and cleft palate have been induced in rats by riboflavin deficiency[8] and other teratogenic methods reviewed by Kalter and Warkany.[9] Such experimental animals can be used for investigation of the relationship of mandibular growth to palatal development and of growth failure to cleft palate formation.[10,11] However, in most of these models, the tongue is large and protrudes over the small mandible, which represents a situation different from that in the Pierre Robin syndrome, in which the tongue usually is held within the oral cavity and is subnormal in size.

Many procedures have been recommended for improvement of the special difficulties of children with marked micrognathia. A review of these treatments was made by Kiskadden and Dietrich.[12] Since Shukowski,[13] in 1911, sutured the tongue to the lip of such a patient, surgical fixation has been used as a remedy, and subsequently Douglas[6] has described in detail surgical fusion of the tongue to the lower lip. All authors stressed that if respiration and feeding can be improved in these infants, the mandible and the pharyngeal space will grow and the children will

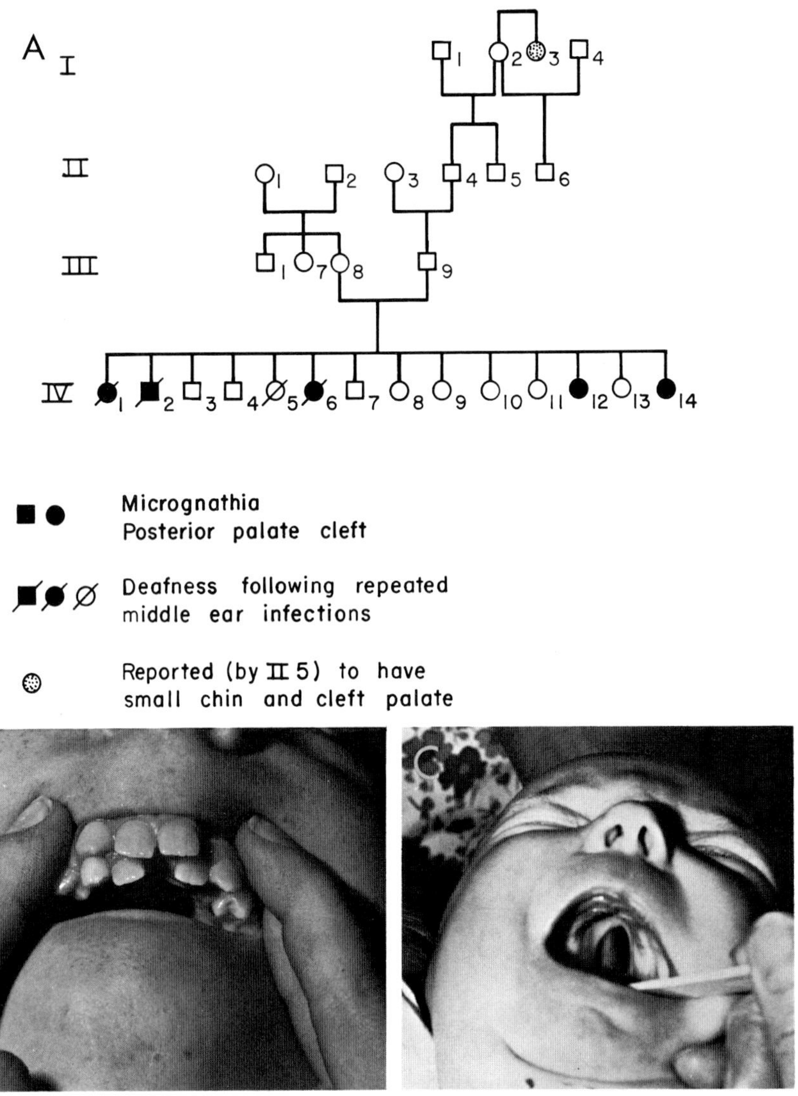

Fig. 71-5. – **A,** pedigree of a family in which 5 of 14 children had Pierre Robin syndrome with posterior palate cleft. Double rows of teeth were present in some of them. **B,** IV_2, showing double row of teeth in upper jaw. **C,** IV_{14}, posterior palate cleft.

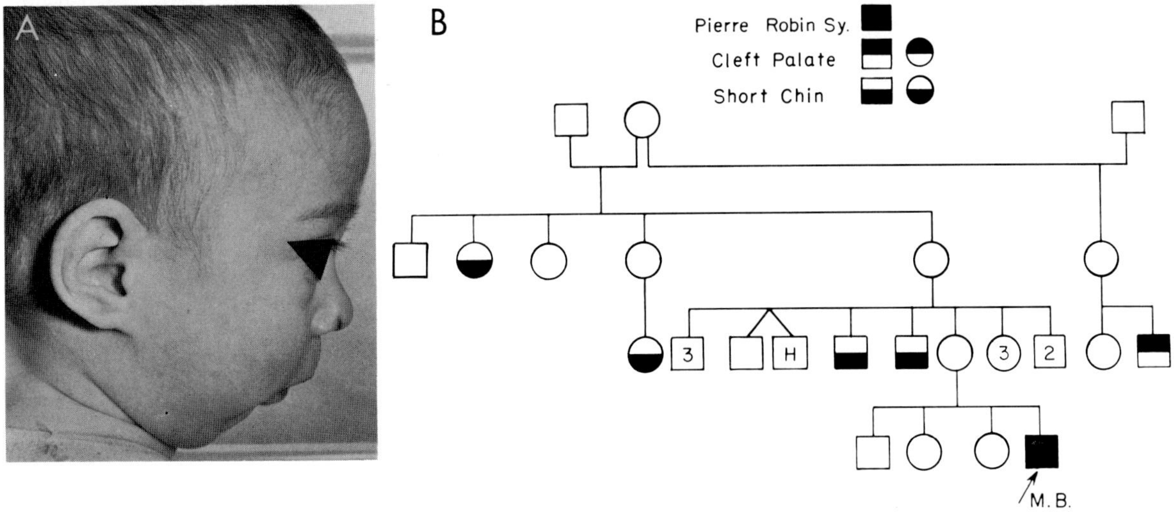

Fig.71-6.—**A,** profile of a child with Pierre Robin syndrome. In this child's kindred, short mandible was present in several members; there also was a relative with cleft palate (**B**). The child had feeding difficulties in early infancy because of cleft palate and extremely short lower jaw. He improved on syringe feeding. Cleft palate was repaired at 3½ years of age.

outgrow their difficulties. Pruzansky and Richmond[14] pointed out that in all instances in which an adequate metabolic situation was provided and the infant gained in weight, mandibular growth during the first 2 months was sufficient to provide for a natural resolution of the symptoms attending the glossoptosis. Lateral cephalometric roentgenograms were found to be a valuable diagnostic aid in assessing the severity of the glossoptosis and obstruction of the airway, since a correlation exists, according to these authors, between the degree of constriction of the airway and the severity of the clinical state. On the basis of these findings, it is possible to recommend either conservative management or tracheotomy in extreme situations.

REFERENCES

1. Robin, P.: La chute de la base de la langue considérée comme une nouvelle cause de gêne dans la respiration naso-pharyngienne, Bull. Acad. méd. Paris 89:37, 1923.
2. Robin, P.: *La glossoptose: Un grave danger pour nos enfants* (Paris: Gaston Doin, 1929).
3. Robin, P.: Glossoptosis due to atresia and hypotrophy of the mandible, Am. J. Dis. Child. 48:541, 1934.
4. Lenstrup, E.: Hypoplasia of mandible as cause of choking fits in infants, Acta paediat. 5:154, 1925.
5. Eley, R. C., and Farber, S.: Hypoplasia of the mandible (micrognathia) as a cause of cyanotic attacks in the newly born infant: Report of 4 cases, Am. J. Dis. Child. 39: 1167, 1930.
6. Douglas, B.: The treatment of micrognathia with obstruction by a plastic operation, Lyon chir. 52:420, 1956.
7. Smith, J. L., and Stowe, F. R.: The Pierre Robin syndrome; a review of 39 cases with emphasis on associated ocular lesions, Pediatrics 27:128, 1961.
8. Warkany, J., and Nelson, R. C.: Skeletal abnormalities in the offspring of rats reared on deficient diets, Anat. Rec. 79:83, 1941.
9. Kalter, H., and Warkany, J.: Experimental production of congenital malformations in mammals by metabolic procedures, Physiol. Rev. 39:69, 1959.
10. Walker, B. E., and Fraser, F. C.: Embryology of cortisone-induced cleft palate, J. Embryol. & Exper. Morphol. 5: 201, 1957.
11. Asling, C. W., Nelson, M. M., Dougherty, H. D., Wright, H. V., and Evans, H. M.: The development of cleft palate resulting from maternal pteroylglutamic (folic) acid deficiency during the latter half of gestation in rats, Surg., Gynec. & Obst. 111:19, 1960.
12. Kiskadden, W. S., and Dietrich, S. R.: Review of the treatment of micrognathia, Plast. & Reconstruct. Surg. 12: 364, 1953.
13. Shukowski, W. P.: Zur Ätiologie des Stridor Inspiratorius Congenitus, Jahrb. Kinderh. 73:459, 1911.
14. Pruzansky, S., and Richmond, J. B.: Growth of mandible in infants with micrognathia, A.M.A. Am. J. Dis. Child. 88:29, 1954.
15. Gorlin, R. J., Cervenka, J., Anderson, R. C., Sauk, J. J., and Bevis, W. D.: Robin's syndrome, Am. J. Dis. Child. 119:176, 1970.
16. Wehinger, H.: Kiefermissbildung und Peromelie, Ztschr. Kinderh. 108:46, 1970.

Cerebro-Costo-Mandibular Syndrome

A SYNDROME of marked micrognathia, palatal changes, vertebral and costal malformations and cerebral hypoplasia has been described in three siblings by McNicholl *et al.*[1] Defects of the elbow, sacrum and coccyx may be present. The inheritance probably is autosomal recessive.

REFERENCE

1. McNicholl, B., Egan-Mitchell, B., Murray, J. P., Doyle, J. F., Kennedy, J. D., and Crome, L.: Cerebro-costo-mandibular syndrome, Arch. Dis. Childhood 45:421, 1970.

PART XI

Malformations of the Oro-gastrointestinal Tract

The Mouth and Pharynx

Fusion of the Gums

CONGENITAL FUSION of the gums associated with fibrous ankylosis of the temporomandibular joint was observed by Snijman and Prinsloo[1] in a newborn Bantu boy. Unilateral fusion of the gums in an infant with facial hemiatrophy was reported by Burket.[2]

Ankyloglossia

Complete inferior ankyloglossia represents a fusion of the tongue to the floor of the mouth. Partial ankyloglossia is due to a short frenum of the tongue that is attached too closely to the tip. Most of these cases do not require any treatment, as the condition corrects itself spontaneously; in rare instances, however, a strong frenum is attached so near the tip that the tongue cannot be protruded over the incisors. When an attempt is made to protrude it, it arches in the middle of the dorsum. This anomaly interferes with free movement and speech. In these cases, simple clipping of the frenum is not sufficient to mobilize the anterior portion, since cicatrization usually pulls the tongue back to its former position. Besides clipping the frenum, a mucosal flap is thrown across the denuded area to prevent immobility.[3,4]

Superior ankyloglossia is rare. Cosack[5] reviewed the literature and described the case of a boy whose tongue tip was attached to the hard palate. In this instance, the premaxilla was rudimentary, the maxilla and upper lip hypoplastic and the incisor teeth were absent. In other cases, the anomaly was combined with cleft palate. Associated malformations of the fingers and of the feet have been observed.

A case of ankyloglossia (superior) combined with amputation of fingers, toes and metatarsals occurred in a premature boy described by Wilson *et al.*[6] The pregnancy had been complicated by hydramnios. The tongue was adherent to the hard palate but could be separated from it by blunt dissection. He survived and was able to walk at the age of 21 months. The family and the chromosomal pattern of the patient were normal. Similar cases of ankyloglossia were associated with cleft palate, the tongue being adherent to the nasal septum.[5] Congenital ankylosis of the tongue and the hard palate, cleft palate, absence of teeth and malformations of the hands and feet have been described as a syndrome.[7]

In mice, lateral ankyloglossia has been induced by hypervitaminosis A. In such specimens, cleft palate due to failure of elevation of the palatine shelves is combined with the anomaly[8] (Fig. 72-1).

Aglossia and Microglossia

Congenital absence of the tongue is extremely rare and only a few cases have been reported in living children. Usually the tongue has been found to be absent in cases of gross underdevelopment of the first visceral arches, especially with congenital agnathia or micrognathia (p. 621). In children who survive, the

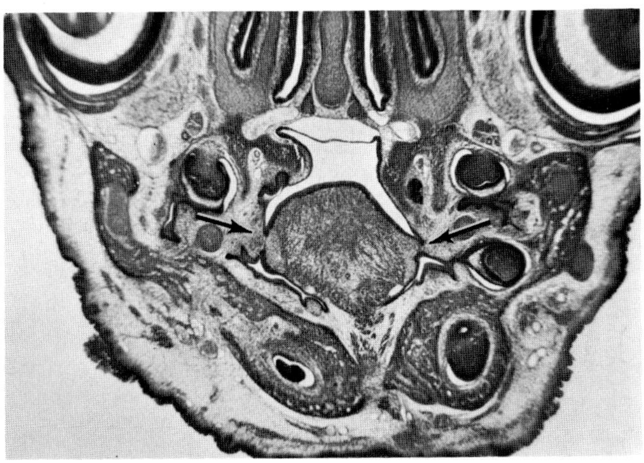

Fig. 72-1.—A newborn mouse with ankyloglossia and cleft palate produced by hypervitaminosis A. (From H. Kalter and J. Warkany[8].) The tongue is bilaterally attached to the gingiva of the upper jaw (**arrows**).

mandible frequently is short and aglossia probably is due to failure of development of the lateral lingual swellings of the mandibular arch, which contribute in large measure to the development of the tongue by fusing with the portions derived from the tuberculum impar and the copula. Historical cases of this anomaly have been reviewed by Rosenthal.[9] The first patient apparently was reported early in the eighteenth century by Jussieu,[10] who described aglossia in a 15-year-old girl who could feed herself with her fingers and could talk. Rosenthal[9] reported a patient of his own who had multiple deformities besides aglossia. In a 3-year-old girl there was retrognathia of the lower jaw, cleft in the lower lip, absence of the lower incisors and absence of the tongue. The tonsils were large and the epiglottis was folded. The speech was not clear but one could understand the patient well. She swallowed with the help of her fingers. There was a tiny rudiment of the anterior portion of the tongue but no evidence of the part normally formed from the tuberculum impar or the copula. This child had associated malformations of both hands and severe anomalies of the right foot. Farrington[11] reported a case of aglossia complicated by a fibrous band extending from the floor of the mouth to the posterior part of the hard palate. After the band was severed, it was noted that the baby did not have a tongue. When the patient was examined at the age of 20 years, he was well developed and appeared normal except for marked retraction in the area of the alveolar processes of the mandible. There was no tongue in the mouth and there was hypertrophy of the submaxillary and sublingual glands. The patient was able to chew normally and to swallow, and his speech was fairly normal. His sense of taste was not impaired. Thoma[3] mentioned a girl in whom absence of the tongue left a large cavity in which the epiglottis could be seen. At birth, the oral membrane was found to be retained, so that breathing was possible only through the nose. Food had to be given through a tube until the membrane was destroyed. Another patient was reported by Fulford,[12] who reviewed 12 previously published cases. He stated that in aglossia the anterior part of the tongue is absent and the posterior part represented by a rudiment. The epiglottis is present in all cases. Among associated malformations there were hypoplasia of the mandible, median harelip (in the upper or lower lip), cleft palate, irregular dentition and remnants of a buccopharyngeal membrane. Deformities of the digits, such as adactyly or syndactyly, are common. Swallowing may improve after the first few months. Pettersson[13] described a case of aglossia congenita with fusion of the jaws by a bony mass between the hard palate and the inside of the mandibular arch. The bone had to be divided before the mouth could be opened. The anomaly was associated with malformations of the hands. On the left thumb there was no nail and the right thumbnail was poorly developed. The second digits of both hands had only two phalanges. Some children with aglossia are not viable. Sinclair and McKay[14] described a case of incomplete median harelip, normal premaxilla, posterior palate cleft, brachydactyly and syndactyly. In this child, who died at the age of 4 weeks, the anterior two-thirds of the tongue were missing.

Microglossia is not so rare. It is seen in cases of micrognathia, particularly with the Pierre Robin syndrome, with mandibulofacial dysostosis and other defects in the facial area. Breathing and ingestion of food usually are difficult. Microglossia is also present in cases of glossopalatine ankylosis (p. 661).

Various forms of aglossia and microglossia combined with dentofacial anomalies in mice were described by Kalter and Deuschle.[15] Such malformations can be produced by maternal hypervitaminosis A (see Fig. 70-4). It is of interest that the micrognathia produced in rats by maternal riboflavin deficiency (see Fig. 4-1, *B*) is regularly associated with a tongue of normal size that protrudes from the mouth.[16]

Macroglossia

Uniform enlargement of the tongue in infancy and in childhood commonly is associated with cretinism, Down syndrome, Hurler syndrome and other types of mental retardation. It is, therefore, an ominous symptom in many cases, yet it must be emphasized that it can occur in otherwise normal children. In cases of thyroid deficiency, the abnormal size of the tongue is due to infiltration with mucoid material that disappears with thyroid treatment, which reduces the size of the tongue. In other mentally retarded children, the tongue merely appears large because of faulty muscular coordination or micrognathia. Tumors such as lipomas, hemangiomas or lymphangiomas (p. 1182) result in enlargement of the tongue. Macroglossia in an otherwise normal child was described in detail by Bronstein *et al.*[17] The tongue was huge and protruding at birth and interfered with nursing. The teeth erupted normally but the tongue pushed the lower dental arch forward so that the lower teeth extended one-half centimeter beyond the upper teeth. The enlargement of the tongue was uniform and the organ was moved freely. Biopsy showed a marked increase in the size of the muscle fibers but no accumulation of glycogen. A slow improvement of the condition was observed.

Bronstein *et al.*[17] distinguished four types of muscular macroglossia: (1) Nodular enlargement is not confined to one-half of the tongue and usually is due to rhabdomyoma. Embryonal muscle cells are present in sections of this lesion, which is seen only rarely in children. (2) Unilateral lingual enlargement associated with localized hypertrophy of the same side of the face or jaw, or with hemihypertrophy of the body. Usually, the anomaly of the tongue constitutes a minor part of the syndrome but sometimes it is the outstanding feature. Occasionally, the entire tongue is enlarged even though the hypertrophy of the other parts of the body is unilateral. (3) The tongue may be uniformly enlarged in certain cases of generalized muscular hypertrophy. This syndrome represents a controversial subject, since it was considered by some authors[18] as a form of hypothyroidism that responds to thyroid treatment, whereas others[19] attributed it to anomalies of the corpus striatum. As a neurologic disorder, it was thought to be refractory to thyroid treatment. An extreme case of this type was reported by Pannullo.[20] The child, born of a mother who had hydramnios, had a huge, protruding tongue that disfigured the nose and face. The protruding portion of the tongue, which measured 6 × 6 × 3 cm., caused marked respiratory difficulty. The child had marked muscular hypertrophy and the "general appearance of a miniature wrestler." The bones were "misshapen" but not achondroplastic and the liver was enlarged. (4) Idiopathic muscular macroglossia like that described by Bronstein *et al.*[17] may be the only malformation of the body or may be associated with other anomalies of the gastrointestinal tract. Enlargement of the fundus of the stomach, malrotation of the intestine and bilateral enlargement of the kidneys have been found associated with this type of macroglossia. In such cases, growth of the tongue may progress slowly or cease after birth. If further enlargement occurs, the growth of the surrounding structures of the mouth and of the jaws eventually leads to a spontaneous correction of the anomaly. It seems that the partial removal of the tongue practiced by some surgeons usually is not necessary.

Macroglossia and exomphalos (p. 171) show a significant association. Irving[74] noted macroglossia in 11.7% of patients admitted for exomphalos to the Liverpool Neo-Natal Surgical Centre. Half of the cases were complicated by hydramnios. Three (of 11) patients were related: 2 were siblings and 1 was their second cousin. Other malformations such as cleft lip and palate, malrotation of the intestine, coarctation of the aorta and congenital Wilms tumor were reported in close relatives. High birth weight was a feature of the syndrome of exomphalos and macroglossia, which also included facial nevus flammeus, indented ear lobes, diaphragmatic anomalies and, less frequently, urogenital deviations. The syndrome is related (if not identical) to visceromegaly (p. 171).

Omphalocele, overgrowth of the kidneys and pancreas and cytomegaly in the adrenal fetal cortex are components of the syndrome, which blends with that of diffuse muscular hypertrophy mentioned above.[21]

Enlargement of the tongue can be a manifestation of neurofibromatosis (p. 1252).

Accessory Tongue

Menzel[22] found an accessory tongue attached to the left tonsil in a boy who also had congenital atresia of the left auditory meatus, microtia and underdevelopment of the left facial nerve. The accessory tongue consisted of muscles covered by glands and papillae characteristic of lingual tissue and was capable of taste perception. In another case, a process arising from the right base of the tongue was associated with absence of the right external ear, tonsil and the right half of the velum palatinum.

Long Tongue

A few instances of extreme length of the tongue have been described. Excessive mobility of the tongue may lead to tongue swallowing and to death from suffocation.[4]

Cleft or Bifid Tongue

In this condition, the anterior part of the tongue is cleft in the midline to a variable degree. This anomaly may be combined with cleft lower lip and cleft mandible. Bifid tongue can be repaired surgically. The so-called clover-leaf tongue is not a malformation but an inherited ability to fold the tongue into a peculiar pattern.[23]

In patients with the orodigitofacial syndrome (p. 674), the tongue may be bifid or cleft in more than two lobes.

Glossitis Rhombica Mediana

This condition is a benign disease of the tongue characterized by the presence of a rhomboid area situated on the dorsum of the tongue just anterior to the foramen cecum. It causes no subjective symptoms and usually is discovered incidentally during examination of the oral cavity. Occasionally, this harmless developmental error is mistaken for an inflammatory lesion or for cancer of the tongue. Martin and Howe[24] believed that the anomaly is due to persistence of the tuberculum impar, which, in the embryo, forms the pharyngeal floor between the first pair of branchial pouches (see Fig. 72-3). Normally, the tuberculum impar is overgrown by the lateral lingual swellings of the mandible and does not appear in the human adult tongue, but in rare instances it is indicated by "glossitis rhombica mediana" – a misleading term, since no inflammation is present in this developmental anomaly.

The typical lesion is a nonulcerated rhomboid plaque that may extend 2–3 cm. anterior to the sulcus terminalis. The surface of the lesion is only slightly raised or it protrudes as much as 5 mm. from the lingual surface. The involved area is distinguished from the normal surface by its color and by absence of the normal papillary pattern of the mucosa. There is no pain or tenderness. For the differential diagnosis, it is important to know that cancer and tuberculous ulcers do not arise in this area of the tongue.[24]

The lesion is limited to the mucous and submucous tissues and does not involve the muscular body of the tongue. Epithelial hypertrophy and lymphocytic infiltration of subepithelial tissue are found on histologic examination. The epithelial growth is always orderly and nonmalignant.

Lingual Thyroid

A comprehensive review on this subject was made by Montgomery[25] in 1936. The thyroid gland develops at the floor of the primitive pharynx, arising from a median bud that grows caudad and becomes bilobed as it develops into the definitive thyroid gland. At first, it is connected with its point of origin by the thyroglossal duct, which, as a rule, disappears in 11-mm. embryos; occasionally, thyroid tissue is left in the area of the foramen cecum, where the thyroid bud arose. In this area, a lingual thyroid may be found as an anomaly. The incidence of thyroid gland elements in the area of the foramen cecum is not known, since only patients who develop symptoms have been recognized and recorded. Montgomery[25] accepted 144 cases as authentic but, since then, others have been observed. Symptom-producing hypertrophies of lingual thyroid have been reported much more frequently in females than in males. According to Goetsch,[26] approximately two-thirds of the persons who had hypertrophy of the lingual thyroid lacked a thyroid gland in the neck. The lingual thyroid may be the size of a pea or as large as a golf ball. Symptoms of thyroid insufficiency arise when special demands are made on the gland by puberty, pregnancy or lactation. Most patients who have a lingual thyroid suffer from such symptoms of pressure and obstruction as dysphagia, dysphonia and dyspnea[26,27] (Chapter 44).

Thyroid insufficiency was reported in approximately 15% of the cases analyzed by Montgomery[25] and in 2 of the patients studied by Goetsch.[26] However, there was no mental retardation. Goetsch pointed out that the abnormal manifestations of these patients are due to thyroid insufficiency; associated developmental anomalies usually are absent. Eighty-five per cent of the tumors arising from lingual thyroid are histologically benign,[25] but carcinoma has been reported in several authentic cases of lingual thyroid.[26,28] Parathyroid tissue in close association with lingual thyroid has been observed.[29]

The lesions usually are median in position immediately posterior to the foramen cecum, sitting on a broad base. Their color is dusky, varying from red to purple. Some are superficial; others penetrate into the deep substance of the tongue. Apnea in the supine position and improvement in the prone position were emphasized as an alerting symptom of a tumor at the base of the tongue in small infants.[30] In the differential diagnosis, adenoma, angioma, salivary tumor and fibroma must be considered. Administration of a tracer dose of radioactive iodine (^{131}I) has been found most helpful in differential diagnosis.[28] In treatment, administration of thyroid may be effective if the lingual thyroid shows compensatory enlargement because of thyroid insufficiency. The effectiveness of treatment with radioactive iodine is doubtful[27] and it may be dangerous in young patients.[28] Surgical removal has been the treatment of choice in most of the cases. Ward *et al.*[28] recommended lateral pharyngotomy as the most satisfactory surgical approach.

Developmental Anomalies of the Thyroid

Complete agenesis of the thyroid is extremely rare. Most cases recorded as athyrosis refer to patients in whom no thyroid was found in its usual location at necropsy. However, one can speak of complete thyroid aplasia only if serial sections of the lingual and cervical areas in which thyroid tissue can occur are found entirely free of it. In a number of cases in the older literature,[31] complete absence of thyroid tissue has been demonstrated; there were more girls than boys among these cases. Before treatment was possible, the life expectancy of such patients was quite limited. The oldest person in whom complete absence of the thyroid was demonstrated was a dwarf woman 28 years of age. Thyroid aplasia shows no geographic concentration and is, therefore, to be distinguished from endemic cretinism, a condition closely related to endemic goiter. As a rule, parathyroids are present in cases of agenesis of the thyroid. In addition, there commonly are accessory parathyroids found at the root of the tongue that consist of epithelial ducts or cysts. Small cystic formations derived from the lingual duct may also be found. Aberrant parathyroid glands in pharyngeal submucosa were described by Herrold *et al.*[32]

Partial Agenesis and Hypoplasia of the Thyroid

Absence of one lobe of the thyroid (hemiaplasia) is uncommon. It has been estimated that it occurs in less than 1 per 1,000 patients operated on for goiter. Hemiaplasia usually is found accidentally at operation or at necropsy. In place of the missing thyroid lobes, small cysts and ducts may be detectable. Absence of the isthmus of the thyroid, which can be considered an exaggerated regression of the thyroglossal duct, occurs more often. It is the rule in birds and occurs in 2–5% of human beings. Sometimes partial agenesis of the thyroid is combined with other congenital defects in the cervical area, such as absence of the parathyroid and irregular formation of the thymus.

In place of an underdeveloped thyroid, mucous glands may be found in the surrounding tissue, and at the root of the tongue heterotopic remnants of thyroid tissue may be detected. In 2 brothers, Rohde (cited by Hückel[31]) found the left thyroid lobe to be underdeveloped; in both cases, the right lobe was goitrous.

Both agenesis and hypoplasia of the thyroid can lead to dwarfism and cretinism.

Fordyce Granules

This is a developmental anomaly involving the mucosa of the lips, cheeks or palate, characterized by discrete yellowish spots that are due to ectopic sebaceous glands. Typically, their site is opposite the molar teeth but they also occur on the inner surface of the lips and in the retromolar regions. Although a developmental disorder, Fordyce granules are rarely seen in children but develop at puberty, when the sebaceous glands reach maximal development; they are more common in males than in females.[3] This anomaly is so frequent among adults that it cannot be considered a disease. It is a harmless condition that does not require treatment.

Leukokeratosis

Leukokeratosis, a whitish discoloration of the buccal mucosa, often simulating *Candida albicans* infection of the mouth, can be inherited as an autosomal dominant trait. Herpetic stomatitis and gingivitis are frequent complicating infections.[33]

Melanin Pigmentation Associated with Intestinal Polyposis (Peutz-Jeghers Syndrome)

In this dominantly inherited syndrome, pigment spots are seen on the face, in the oral cavity and sometimes on the hands and feet. The melanin pigmentations of the lips and oral mucosa usually are present from birth and consist of speckles measuring 1–5 mm. in diameter. In the mouth, the buccal and palatine mucosa, as well as the gingiva, are affected.[34] The tongue is only rarely involved but, externally, pigment spots may be seen around the lips, nostrils and eyes.

Polyps usually are distributed throughout the entire intestine (p. 714), but they manifest themselves clinically chiefly in the small intestine, as many patients suffer from episodes of abdominal pain and signs of minor obstruction that sometimes result in intussusception. The presence of intestinal polyposis is suggested by the oral findings.

Oral Leukoplakias

Leukoplakias are white patches on the oral mucosa that cannot be removed by scraping and cannot be attributed to irritants or any other cause. Some oral leukoplakias undergo malignant epithelial transformation, but conversion from benign epithelium to malignancy cannot be predicted in individual cases.[35] Histochemistry of the epithelial contents has been studied, particularly by glycogen and diastase-resistant periodic acid-Schiff stains.[36] Large doses of vitamin A sometimes cause remissions but, for single lesions, complete surgical removal is the treatment of choice.[35]

Leukoplakia may be a component of a syndrome that is inherited as a recessive trait. Dyskeratosis congenita with pigmentation and nail dystrophy combines with the oral lesions, which can undergo malignant degeneration.[37] In some patients, aplastic anemia develops.[7]

Oral lesions resembling leukoplakia occur as benign hereditary dyskeratoses.[37] *Darier-White disease*, which begins in childhood, manifests itself by crusted patches of the skin and by rough areas or white plaques on the oral mucosa. Irregular autosomal dominance of the trait has been established. *White sponge nevus* (Cannon) results in a thickened, folded mucosa that can be seen in various parts of the mouth and also on the labial, vaginal or oral mucosa. Such lesions can be congenital but they increase in severity until adolescence. Several generations may be affected. The oral lesions of *pachyonychia congenita* resemble those of white sponge nevus, but there are concomitant dystrophic changes in the nails, hyperkeratoses of the palms and soles, hyperhidrosis of the hands and feet and follicular keratosis on the elbows and knees. The disorder is inherited like a dominant autosomal trait.[37]

A congenital and hereditary syndrome of *intra-epithelial dyskeratosis* affecting bulbar conjunctiva and oral mucosa has been reported by Witkop *et al.*[38] The oral lesions, which are present shortly after birth and become more marked with increasing age, may remain symptomless. The mucosal plaques are white, spongy and sometimes folded. On stretching of the mucosa, pinpoint elevations become noticeable. The buccal lesions resemble leukoplakia but they are rather superficial and soft. The eye lesions are more serious than those of the mouth, and may lead to corneal opacities and blindness (p. 367). The disorder is inherited as an autosomal dominant trait with a high degree of penetrance.

Torus Buccalis

This presents a longitudinal fold that starts at the corner of the mouth and extends back as far as the molar teeth. As it often protrudes between the occlusal surfaces of the teeth, it becomes irritated during mastication, causing marked hypertrophy and keratinization, which can be recognized by the light color of the crest. Microscopically, a torus buccalis shows thickening of the epithelium, hyperkeratosis and, in most cases, an inflammatory reaction in the deeper layers.

Torus Palatinus

This is an osseous outgrowth from the midline of the hard palate. It is rare in children and develops slowly, presenting as a broad thickening, as a crest or as a nodular tumor at the roof of the mouth. The anomaly is frequent in Eskimos, Lapps and Chinese but is rare in Negroes. Sometimes it is found in Caucasians as a hereditary trait.[39] Torus palatinus is a benign growth that does not require treatment unless it interferes with speech or the fitting of dentures.[3]

Torus Mandibularis

These benign osseous tumors are found on the inner surface of the mandible in the premolar region. If they are large and multiple, they may interfere with the movement of the tongue and retain food remnants.

Congenital Cysts of the Mouth

Median cysts of the maxilla may occur anteriorly between the roots of the median incisors or posteriorly in the midline of the palate. *Globulo-maxillary cysts* form at the junction of the globular and maxillary processes and are located in the alveolar bone between the roots of the lateral incisors and canines. By expansion, such cysts change the position of the neighboring teeth or protrude on the palate. The anomaly has been observed by Thoma[3] in two generations of a family. *Cysts of the papilla palatina* occur as round swellings expanding the soft tissue beneath the papilla palatina. They are soft and fluctuant, and fluid may exude from the opening of a papilla on pressure. In contrast to these superficial cysts that protrude into the oral cavity, *cysts of the incisive canal* are enclosed in the osseous roof of the mouth and may manifest themselves merely by a salty discharge. These cysts are abnormal remnants of the communications existing in the human fetus between the oral and nasal cavities[3] (p. 635).

Nasoalveolar cysts form at the junction of the nasomedial, nasolateral and maxillary processes. They cause swelling at the attachment of the wing of the nose and bulge into the nostrils and the nasal cavity as they expand. The swelling may also be found in the base of the upper lip, bulge into the vestibule of the oral cavity and cause asymmetry of the face. *Nasopalatine* cysts may be found at the point of fusion of the median palatine process (premaxilla) with the lateral palatine processes. At this point of union, one may find, at the time of birth, the incisive foramen and the incisive canals connecting the oral cavities with the nasal cavities. Later, as mucous membrane covers these communications, the incisive papilla indicates the point of fusion. Cysts of the papilla palatina form from the epithelia. If such a cyst enlarges, it forms a soft swelling covered by mucosa and protrudes into the oral cavity. Incisive canal cysts are enclosed in the bone and therefore at first cause few symptoms but, later, swelling of the papilla may occur. Some patients can suck out fluid with a salty taste from the region of the incisive papilla.

Dermoid cysts of the floor of the mouth originate through faulty placement of epithelial tissue into mesodermal tissue. The walls of such cysts are composed of a stratified epithelial lining that is surrounded by dense connective tissue. The structure of the epithelium is similar to that of normal skin, but sweat glands, sebaceous glands and hair follicles may be included. Such dermoid cysts may be found in the midline behind the chin or to one side below the angle of the jaw. Dermoid cysts are of prenatal origin, but clinical symptoms usually develop late in childhood or in adult life. Then, a slow-growing, smooth and painless mass makes its appearance beneath the chin or within the mouth, where the tongue may be pushed upward. In contrast to ranulae (see below), the color is light yellow. Swallowing and breathing may become impaired when the tumor becomes sizable. Surgical excision is the treatment of choice.

Gingival cysts. A congenital developmental abnormality of the gingiva in the form of visible multiple microcysts appearing in infancy was described by Nichamin and Kaufman.[40] The cysts appear on the gingivae as discrete gray-like nodules along a straight line equidistant from the gingival margin. They can appear in crops, but no general clinical symptoms are evident. Roentgenograms of the mandible and maxilla do not show any anomalies of these structures and the cysts cannot be differentiated roentgenographically from the surrounding tissue. The uninterrupted deciduous teeth are placed normally in the jaws. Eruption of teeth progresses normally and the cysts show spontaneous retrogression.

Ranulae are cysts in the floor of the mouth that usually are considered retention cysts of the sublingual glands. Sometimes they are congenital, and large ranulae that extend downward and backward into the lateral upper neck are thought to be of branchial origin. They are painless, slowly growing, dark red, fluctuating masses located on the floor of the mouth beneath the tongue and behind the incisor teeth. Those extending into the neck can be identified by bulging in the submaxillary region when pressure is exerted on the cystic mass in the floor of the mouth. Treatment consists of surgical dissection of the tumor.[4]

Congenital cysts arising from the base of the tongue may cause respiratory obstruction, inspiratory stridor and attacks of cyanosis. The cysts press on the larynx and may endanger the patient's life. Breast-feeding is impossible and regurgitation occurs after bottle-feeding. The cysts sometimes can be seen with the help of a tongue depressor or by direct laryngoscopy. In the differential diagnosis, lingual thyroids, which are solid tumors, must be considered. The cysts are treated by incision and drainage or by complete excision.

Salivary Glands

Becker[41] discussed the anatomy, embryology and malformations of the parotid gland. A larger lobus superficialis can be distinguished from the smaller lobus profundus. Heterotopic salivary tissues can be found in lymph nodes, in the Rathke pouch or the pituitary and in the middle ear or external meatus. They do not have a duct as accessory glands do but they may be emptied by a fistula in regions quite distant from the mouth. Aplasia, hypoplasia and hyperplasia of the parotid have been observed. They can be unilateral or bilateral. Bilateral absence of the parotid may be associated with dryness of the mouth. Anomalies of the parotid have been found in combination with mal-

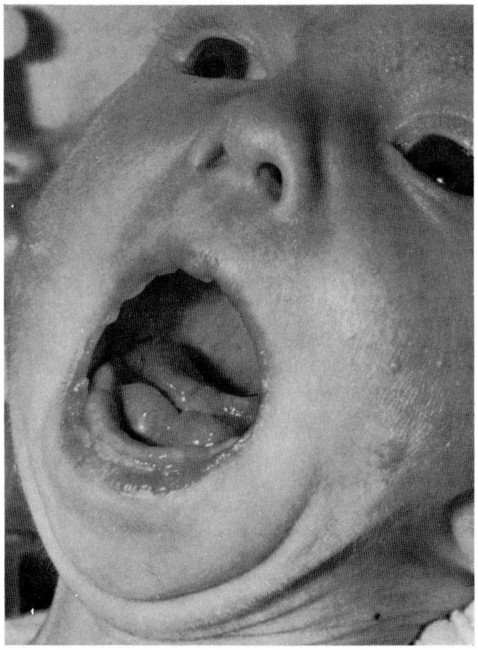

Fig. 72-2.—Enlarged sublingual glands in trisomy 18.

formations of the genitalia.[41] Absence of the parotid gland has been reported in mandibulofacial dysostosis,[42] in hemifacial microsomia[7] and in a stillborn monstrous fetus with cleft face, anophthalmia and many other malformations.[43] Diverticula and ectasias of the parotid duct system are not rare. Becker *et al.*[44] described in detail saccular dilatation of the ducts, resulting in recurrent chronic parotitis. These ectasias, which can occur in children, may be malformations that cause the inflammatory changes.

Hypertrophy of the submaxillary and sublingual glands can be associated with aglossia (p. 661). Enlarged sublingual glands in a child with trisomy 18 are seen in Figure 72-2.

Tumors

Oral tumors of infancy and childhood were discussed by Bhaskar.[45] Many of these tumors are congenital or determined at birth, although they can manifest themselves several years after birth. More than 90% of the tumors are benign. *Hemangiomas* are common; they affect the lip, cheek, tongue or palate. *Lymphangiomas* involve the tongue particularly, but other oral areas may also be affected. Cavernous or simple lymphangiomas may cause macroglossia. Cystic hygromas commonly arise in the neck with extension into the parotid region, cheek, floor of the mouth and tongue. A syndrome of capillary lymphangioma complicated by glossitis was described by Koop and Moschakis.[46] The condition can be associated with cystic hygroma of the neck and with changes in the mandible and dentition. The tongue may become edematous and painful from the eruption of vesicles and hemorrhagic papillary lesions. Enlargement of the tongue usually is present at birth but disturbing symptoms may appear later. *Congenital epulis* is a benign soft tissue tumor that arises from the alveolar ridge and may be sessile or pedunculated. It is much more common in female infants than in males and it originates more often in the maxilla than in the mandible. There are fibrous epulis and giant cell epulis, which differ microscopically, but both are nonmetastasizing tumors that can be treated surgically. Clinically, these tumors may be similar to myoblastomas. *Congenital myoblastomas* represent rare tumors that arise from the anterior alveolar ridges in the region of the future incisors. They occur in the upper or lower jaw and show nodular or polypoid shape. The consistency is rubbery, the epithelium intact or ulcerated. The tumors, which consist of large polygonal cells with small nuclei, also occur on the lips, tongue, larynx or esophagus. Interpretations of the histologic picture vary greatly. Some consider them myomas derived from myoblasts. Others believe that their cells are metabolically disturbed peripheral glia cells.[47] The tumors arising from the alveolar ridges are typically tumors present at birth. They are benign lesions that can be treated successfully by surgical excision.[48] *Hamartomas* and *choristomas* consist of excessive but normal tissues, such as cartilage, bone, glands, muscle, nerve and blood vessels. They are due to developmental errors that may expand in postnatal life. The dorsum of the tongue and the lips are the usual oral sites.[45] Heterotopic gastric mucosa on the tongue was described by Gorlin *et al.*[49] *Neurofibromatosis* can involve the tongue, the oral floor and the cheek (p. 1252). *Tuberous sclerosis* causes oral lesions in more than 10% of the cases.[7]

Many types of tumors of the jaws occur in children. They are divided into odontogenic or nonodontogenic growths. Among the former are the melanoameloblastomas or melanotic progonomas[50] that occur in infancy and are located particularly in the anterior parts of the maxilla. They have been considered "retinal anlage" tumors. Histologically, nests of pigmented cells with large, dark nuclei and scanty cytoplasm are seen. These tumors do not metastasize; they can be removed surgically with little tendency to recurrence. Other odontogenic tumors usually appear in older children. Among the nonodontogenic tumors of the jaws are the *central hemangiomas of bone*, which are considered malformations.[45] The teeth become loose and bleeding occurs in the surrounding tissue. Expansion of the affected region of the jaw results. Sometimes the lesion is associated with hemangiomas of the skin and mental retardation. *Dermoids* at the oropharyngeal border have been observed repeatedly. They may cause respiratory obstruction in the newborn, which can be relieved with little difficulty if the tumor is pedunculated.[51,52] It is thought that they represent inclusion errors in the fusion of the lateral palatine processes. In one child,[53] a dermoid polyp was associated with a cleft lip.

Teratoma of the Tonsil

Baugh and O'Donoghue[54] described a teratoma of the tonsil in a female full-term child showing respiratory difficulties and asphyxia neonatorum. A tumor almost entirely obstructing the pharynx was seen to be protruding from the posterior surface of the left anterior pillar of the tonsil. The tonsil and tumor were removed and on histologic examination showed a disorderly mixture of cartilage, bone, smooth and striated muscle, neuroepithelium and renal, cerebral and adipose tissues.

Teratoid Parasites of the Mouth

These malformations present a striking appearance that has long aroused the interest of teratologists. Schwalbe[55] used them as a basis for the development of his concept of "teratogenetic termination periods" (p. 49). Ehrich[56] pointed out that the term "epignathi" for these anomalies usually is not satisfactory, since many of the parasites are attached to the sphenoid bone, to the lateral wall of the pharynx or to the palate, and only a few oral parasites arise primarily in the jaw. Teratoid parasites of the mouth show all transitions from dermoids through teratomas to incompletely developed twins that sometimes may be affixed to the autosite by an umbilical cord. The parasites may grow into the pharynx and mouth but also into the cranium or in both directions. The intra-oral and intracranial portions of these parasites are connected with each other through the area of the craniopharyngeal canal. Ehrich believed that more highly developed parasites are asymmetric double monsters rather than teratomas due to dislocation of germ tissues, since they show the same axial orientation as their autosites. Hydramnios may be associated with the pregnancy terminating in the birth of such a parasite.

Congenital Atresia of the Oropharynx

In contrast to the relatively frequent congenital atresias of the caudal end of the alimentary canal, those of the cranial end are rare. A case of congenital atresia of the oropharynx, probably representing a persistence of the oral membrane as seen in embryos of 2.5 mm. length in the fourth week, was described by Longacre.[57] The child, when seen at the age of 3 months, had congenital atresia of the fauces, the soft palate being held down tightly across the base of the tongue at the level of the foramen cecum. The only opening into the oral pharynx was a partial cleft of the soft palate measuring 2 cm. in length and 4 mm. in width. Feeding difficulties existed, nursing being followed by severe bouts of choking and coughing. A plastic operation was performed successfully and the child seemed to develop perfectly normally following the operation, although occasional coughing spells persisted. It seemed that the congenital atresia of the fauces was due to persistence of the oral membrane, with only a partial rupture that was represented by the incomplete cleft of the soft palate. A complete imperforation of the oropharynx was reported by Seghers[58] in a newborn child who had deformed ears and costovertebral malformations. It is of interest that the pregnancy was described as normal and hydramnios was not mentioned. An imperforate buccopharyngeal membrane with lateral openings into the oral pharynx was described by Kouyoumdjian and McDonald[59] in a premature child who also showed polydactyly and cataracts. Necropsy showed a metastasizing adrenal neuroblastoma, a hypoplastic kidney and a hydronephrotic kidney, a rudimentary uterus and patent foramen ovale.

The Pharynx

In embryos of approximately 4 weeks, four pairs of pouches become noticeable on the cranial end of the foregut (the pharynx); these grow toward the surface to meet four pairs of corresponding cleft depressions along the sides of the neck. The internal pouches and the external clefts do not contact each other, but remain separated by closing plates consisting of entodermal and ectodermal layers (Fig. 72-3). Between these pouches and clefts the branchial arches become noticeable. The first arch, situated rostral to the first pouch and cleft, is the mandibular arch from which the lower jaw develops. The second branchial arch is the hyoid arch. The branchial arches contain paired arteries, the aortic arches, nerves derived from the hindbrain and cartilages of the visceral skeleton. Meckel cartilage is found in the first mandibular arch, the horns of the hyoid bone in the second and third, the thyroid and cricoid cartilages in the fourth and fifth arches.[60] The first groove is located between the first and second arches. Around the dorsal end of this groove, on the lateral and outer surface of the mandibular and hyoid arches, grow the tubercles from which the auricles are formed. The external auditory canal is a derivative of the first groove.

The mandibular (Fig. 72-3, I) and the hyoid arches (II) grow more rapidly than the caudal branchial arches (III and IV) so that, in embryos of 10 mm., a depression is formed externally caudal to the hyoid arch that later is overgrown by the second arch. In this way, an operculum is formed that covers a depressed area – the cervical sinus. This depression is related to the second, third and fourth pouch. The floor of the cervical sinus is formed by the third branchial arch. The opercular cleft, which represents the opening of the cervical sinus onto the surface, closes by the middle of the second month.[60] The lumen disappears and the cells of the sac normally disintegrate. Failure of regression of these epithelial cells may leave remnants buried and thus give rise to

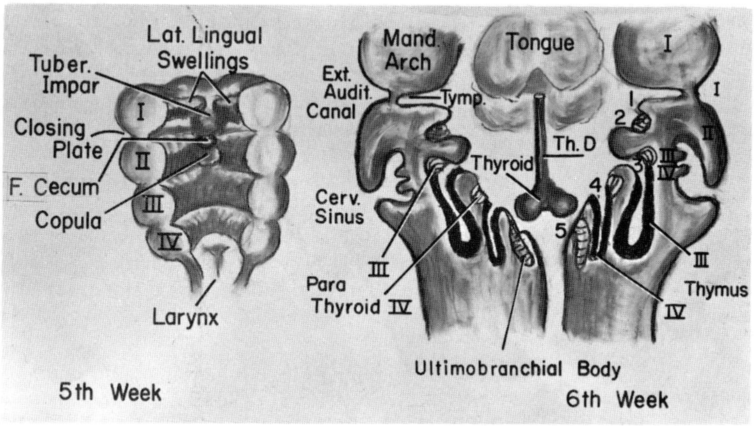

Fig. 72-3. – Diagrams showing branchial arches and pouches with their derivatives. (Th. D = thyroid duct.)

epithelial tumors in the cervical area.[4] Branchial cysts of various types have also been explained by persistence of portions of the cervical sinus.[61]

The thyroid gland appears as the earliest of the pharyngeal derivatives. In embryos 4 weeks old, a median diverticulum becomes noticeable at the floor of the pharynx between the first and second pouches. This thyroid primordium, which is bilobed, soon becomes detached from the floor of the pharynx, but a depression at the base of the tongue – the foramen cecum – remains as a marker of the origin of the thyroid. The thyroid primordium migrates caudad and by the seventh week lies at the level of the laryngeal primordium.[62] The lobes of the thyroid, which are connected by a median isthmus, take their position lateral to the midline. From the endoderm of the grooves or pharyngeal pouches, a number of diverse structures develop. The first pair of pharyngeal pouches located between the first and second branchial arches are directed dorso-laterad. They are converted into the eustachian tubes; their enlarged distal ends form the tympanic cavities of the middle ear. From the second pair of pouches, the tonsils arise. From the walls of the third pouches, diverticula develop that extend down the neck into the thorax, meeting near the midline and forming the thymus (p. 739). A similar but smaller contribution is made to the thymus from the fourth pouch. The lower poles of the thymus follow the pericardium into the thorax, whereas the upper ends lose their connection with the pharynx. From the cranial walls of the third and fourth pouches, nodules are formed that develop into the parathyroids. The ultimobranchial bodies, which develop from a rudimentary fifth pharyngeal pouch, become closely attached to the thyroid but soon lose their identity.

Branchiogenic Fistulas and Cysts

External branchial fistulas or sinuses that open in the lower part of the neck at the anterior border of the sternomastoid muscle represent the most frequent branchial anomaly seen in surgical clinics.[63] In most cases, they are the entrance to incomplete fistulas that take their course upward in the neck, ending blindly. Sections of the tract may be cut off, leaving closed vesicles or cysts along its course. Most of these fistulas are derived from the second branchial cleft. They are bilateral in approximately one-third of the cases, the right side being affected more often than the left. A hereditary tendency has been observed[64] repeatedly, and a single dominant gene is held responsible for the anomaly, which may be associated with preauricular pits.[65] The tracts usually are lined with stratified squamous epithelium but, in the proximal portions, columnar epithelium may be found. The typical cervical fistula is present at birth. In its cephalad course, it parallels the sternomastoid muscle and the carotid artery. Deep or complete fistulas turn inward at the level of the hyoid bone, cross over the hypoglossal nerve and pass between the internal and external carotid arteries to the pharynx.[66] The external opening often is inconspicuous but sometimes it shows signs of irritation by a mucous secretion. Secondary infection is a frequent complication.

Internal branchial fistulas probably are more frequent than one would assume on the basis of the cases that are recognized. They often are symptomless, as they may be closed off by the tonsil or secrete into the pharynx; but they may manifest themselves after tonsillectomy or, if they retain food, by a foul discharge. The tracts derived from the second visceral pouch open posterior to the tonsil or on the posterior palatal arch. Sometimes the opening is located in the lateral pharyngeal wall above the internal laryngeal nerve or in the piriform fossa below that nerve. Such tracts, which are rare and lined by columnar epithelium, have been attributed to remnants of the third or fourth pharyngeal pouch.[66]

Communicating branchial fistulas. If a communication is established between a pharyngeal pouch and a branchial cleft by perforation of a closing plate, which is an abnormal process in man, a perforating pharyngeal fistula is formed. In such instances, the lining of the fistula is in part pharyngeal membrane and in part the skin of the cervical sinus. The whole fistula then includes the pharyngeal pouch, the ruptured closing plate and the open cervical sinus.[60] As a rule, the surface opening of the fistula is found along the opercular line. A perforating fistula of the second pouch will reach the surface along the course of the second cleft, which corresponds in position to the cranial border of the lesser horn of the hyoid bone. Deep fistulas of the second pouch cross cranial to the carotid notch, since the second pharyngeal pouch lies above the third branchial arch, which contains an artery that is transformed into the proximal segment of the internal carotid artery. Fistulas derived from the third pouch run below the notch of the carotid. Fistulas with an open communication between the pharynx and the surface of the neck are rare. They can be demonstrated roentgenographically by injection of a contrast medium into the cervical opening (Fig. 72-4).

Lateral branchial cysts are located in the upper part of the neck at the level of the hyoid bone and anterior to the sternomastoid muscle. They vary considerably in size and usually are unilocular. Most of them are lined with squamous epithelium that may be infiltrated with lymphocytes. Occasionally, the epithelium is ciliated or the lining is skin-like. The cyst content is creamy and bacterial infections are common. These cysts sometimes have pedicles attached to the skin or to the pharyngeal wall. Tumors of branchial cysts are quite rare.[64] Sedgwick and Walsh[67] reviewed the histories of 59 patients with branchial cysts. The cysts became noticeable at various ages from birth to 60 years. Most manifested themselves in the third decade of life. This is in contrast to branchial fistulas, which become noticeable during early childhood. Although most branchial cysts are found anterior to the sternomastoid muscle in the upper third of the neck, other locations in the cervical area are not rare. Although heredity is clearly manifested in some families, it was demonstrable in only 3.5% of the cases reviewed by Sedgwick and Walsh.[67] The patients notice a slowly growing mass that causes pain in some cases. Adenitis and metastatic tumors must be considered in the differential diagnosis. Thyroglossal cysts and dermoids usually are seen in the midline. Treatment consists of enucleation and excision of the cyst.

Fig. 72-4.—Right branchial fistula between surface of neck and pharynx demonstrated by contrast medium.

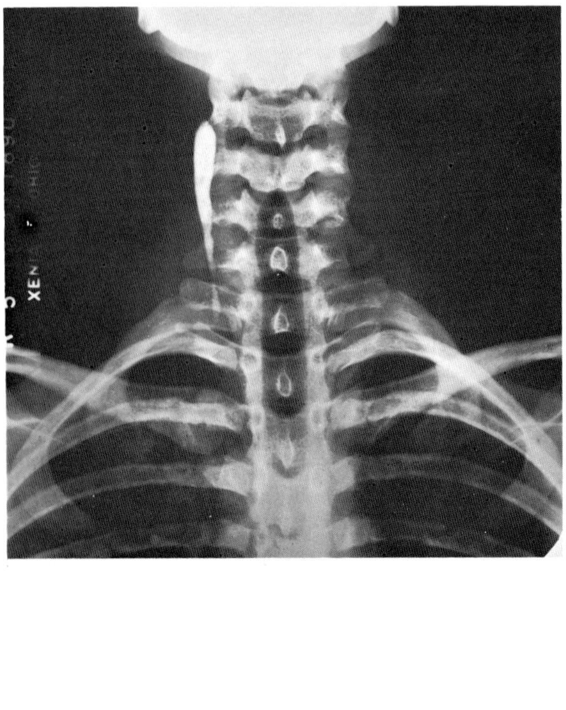

Congenital Pharyngeal Pouches (Diverticula)

Congenital pouches of the pharynx may be found on the lateral or the posterior wall of the pharynx. Lateral pouches are considered remnants of the third or fourth branchial clefts that failed to obliterate during the course of embryonic development. A lateral pharyngeal diverticulum is an open pharyngeal tract with a blind ending, but the morphogenesis of these vestigial structures in the neck and pharynx is not clear and the reader is referred to Raven[68] for a survey of the embryologic and morphologic aspects of these subjects. This author observed three different types of lateral pouches. One, which opened into the pharynx immediately below and lateral to the right tonsillar fossa, was connected by a duct with a cyst that in turn opened on the neck near the anterior border of the right sternomastoid. Raven regarded this vestigial structure as related to the second pharyngeal pouch. A different type was observed in an infant 3 weeks of age who was born with a swelling on the left side of the neck that caused choking attacks during feeding. At necropsy, a pouch was found on the left side of the pharynx opening through a duct into the bottom of the left piriform fossa. This was regarded as a derivative of the third pharyngeal pouch and duct lying in relation to the left piriform fossa. A third specimen showed a pouch on the left lateral aspects of the pharynx, with an opening into the lowest part of the pharynx through the fibers of the inferior constrictor muscle. The neck of the pouch passed behind the termination of the common carotid artery. This pouch was thought to be derived from the fourth embryonic endodermal pouch, the ultimate size being due to repeated distention with food. Kaufman[69] described a lateral pharyngeal diverticulum in a patient 75 years of age who had had difficulty in swallowing for as long as he could remember. A barium study of the pharynx revealed a small pouch arising high on the right lateral wall of the pharynx on the level of the vallecula. It was connected to the pharynx by a narrow aperture that could be seen on endoscopy as a small slit-like groove in the right vallecular wall. A pharyngeal diverticulum discovered by x-ray examination in a woman 65 years of age originated from the posterior lateral aspects of the hypopharynx. The patient also had esophageal diverticula, hiatus hernia of the stomach and chalasia of the esophago-cardiac junction.[70] Zenker diverticula projecting from the posterior hypopharyngeal wall can be variable in size and structure. In adults they consist, as a rule, of mucosal or submucosal tissue, but in infants muscular elements are present in the wall. It is thought that many of the diverticula in older persons are acquired, but congenital forms exist. This can be proved by their existence in infants, in whom they can simulate atresia of the esophagus. Brintnall and Kridelbaugh[71] presented two cases with identical symptoms and roentgenographic findings that suggested atresia of the esophagus; however, in each case the esophagus was entirely normal. Obstructive symptoms were due to the presence of relatively large hypopharyngeal diverticula in the posterior midline that had their openings located above the cricopharyngeus fibers. Such diverticula can be distinguished from atresia of the esophagus by pharyngoscopy. Removal of the diverticula is possible in early life. The congenital nature of Zenker diverticula in adults is made likely by their association with cervical block vertebrae, which prove early malformation in the area of the neck.[72]

Carcinoma has been observed repeatedly as a complication of a pharyngeal pouch.[73]

REFERENCES

1. Snijman, P. C., and Prinsloo, J. G.: Congenital fusion of the gums. Case report, Am. J. Dis. Child. 112:593, 1966.
2. Burket, L. W.: Congenital bony temporomandibular ankylosis with facial hemiatrophy, J.A.M.A. 106:1719, 1936.
3. Thoma, K. H.: *Oral Pathology* (4th ed.; St. Louis: The C. V. Mosby Company, 1954).
4. Padgett, E. C.: *Surgical Diseases of the Mouth and Jaws* (Philadelphia: W. B. Saunders Company, 1938).
5. Cosack, G.: Die angeborene Zungen-Munddach-Verwachsung als Leitmotiv eines Komplexes von multiplen Abartungen, Ztschr. Kinderh. 72:240, 1953.
6. Wilson, R. A., Kliman, M. R., and Hardyment, A. F.: Ankyloglossia superior (palato-glossal adhesion in the newborn infant), Pediatrics 31:1051, 1963.
7. Gorlin, R. J., and Pindborg, J. J.: *Syndromes of the Head and Neck* (New York: McGraw-Hill Book Company, Inc., 1964).
8. Kalter, H., and Warkany, J.: Experimental production of congenital malformations in strains of inbred mice by maternal treatment with hypervitaminosis A, Am. J. Path. 38:1, 1961.
9. Rosenthal, R.: Aglossia congenita, Am. J. Dis. Child. 44: 383, 1932.
10. de Jussieu, M.: Observation sur la manière dont une fille sans langue s'acquitte des fonctions qui dépendent de cet organe, Acad. roy. d. sc., Paris, mém. 6-14, 1718, 1719.
11. Farrington, R. K.: Aglossia congenita: Report of a case without other congenital malformations, North Carolina M. J. 8:24, 1947.
12. Fulford, G. E.: Aglossia congenita, Arch. Dis. Childhood 31:400, 1956.
13. Pettersson, G.: Aglossia congenita with bony fusion of the jaws: Report of one case, Acta chir. scandinav. 122:93, 1961.
14. Sinclair, J. G., and McKay, J.: Median harelip, cleft palate and glossal agenesis, Anat. Rec. 91:155, 1945.
15. Kalter, H., and Deuschle, F. M.: Congenital Malformations Experimentally Induced by Hypervitaminosis A, in Kreshover, S. J., and McClure, F. J. (eds.), *Environmental Variables in Oral Disease* (Washington, D.C.: American Association for the Advancement of Science, 1966), pp. 273-292.
16. Warkany, J., and Nelson, R. C.: Skeletal abnormalities in the offspring of rats reared on deficient diets, Anat. Rec. 79:83, 1941.
17. Bronstein, I. P., Abelson, S. M., Jaffe, R. H., and Bonin, G.: Macroglossia in children; review of the literature, Am. J. Dis. Child. 54:1328, 1937.
18. Debré, R., and Sémelaigne, G.: Syndrome of diffuse muscular hypertrophy in infancy, causing athletic appearance, Am. J. Dis. Child. 50:1351, 1935.
19. de Lange, C.: Congenital hypertrophy of muscles, extrapyramidal motor disturbances, and mental deficiency: Clinical entity, Am. J. Dis. Child. 48:243, 1934.
20. Pannullo, J. N.: Congenital macroglossia, Obst. & Gynec. 7:97, 1956.
21. Goldstein, R.: Congenitale Muskelhypertrophie, Ann. paediat. 189:51, 1957.
22. Menzel, K. M.: Über noch nicht beschriebenes Vorkommen einer Lingua accessoria, zugleich ein Beitrag zur Kenntnis der Atresia auris congenita, Virchows Arch. path. Anat. 288:253, 1933.
23. Whitney, D. D.: Clover-leaf tongues, J. Hered. 41:176, 1950.
24. Martin, H. E., and Howe, M. E.: Glossitis rhombica mediana, Ann. Surg. 107:39, 1938.
25. Montgomery, M. L.: The lingual thyroid. Comprehensive review. West. J. Surg. 43:661, 1935; 44:54, 122, 189, 237, 303, 1936.
26. Goetsch, E.: Lingual goiter, Ann. Surg. 127:291, 1948.
27. Sicher, K.: Lingual thyroid, Brit. M. J. 2:186, 1953.
28. Ward, G. E., Cantrell, J. R., and Allan, W. B.: The surgical treatment of lingual thyroid, Ann. Surg. 139:536, 1954.
29. Asch, R.: Die Zungenstruma, gleichzeitig ein kasuistischer Beitrag zum Myxödem und zur Frage der postoperativen Tetanie, Deutsche Ztschr. Chir. Leipzig 130:593, 1914.
30. Lewison, M. M., and Lim, D. T.: Apnea in the supine position as an alerting symptom of a tumor at the base of the tongue in small infants, J. Pediat. 66:1092, 1965.
31. Hückel, R.: Die Entwicklungsstörungen der Schilddrüse, in Schwalbe, E. (ed.), *Die Morphologie der Missbildungen des Menschen und der Tiere* (Jena: Gustav Fischer, 1932), Vol. 3, pt. 12-15, Chap. 8, p. 600.
32. Herrold, K. M., Rabson, A. S., and Ketcham, A. S.: Aberrant parathyroid gland in pharyngeal submucosa, Arch. Path. 71:60, 1961.
33. Scott, C. R.: Hereditary leukokeratosis; white mouth, J. Pediat. 68:768, 1966.
34. Shafer, W. G., Hine, M. K., and Levy, B. M.: *A Textbook of Oral Pathology* (Philadelphia: W. B. Saunders Company, 1958).
35. Silverman, S., Jr., Renstrup, G., and Pindborg, J. J.: Studies in oral leukoplakias. III. Effects of vitamin A, comparing clinical, histopathologic, cytologic, and hematologic responses, Acta odont. scandinav. 21:271, 1963.
36. Bülow, F. A., and Renstrup, G.: Studies in oral leukoplakias. 10. Periodic acid-Schiff staining of normal and leukoplakic epithelium before and after vitamin A application, Acta path. et microbiol. scandinav. 68:175, 1966.
37. Witkop, C. J., and Gorlin, R. J.: Four hereditary mucosal syndromes, Arch. Dermat. 84:762, 1961.
38. Witkop, C. J., Shankle, C. H., Graham, J. B., Murray, M. R., Rucknagel, D. L., and Byerly, B. H.: Hereditary benign intraepithelial dyskeratosis. II. Oral manifestations and hereditary transmission, Arch. Path. 70:696, 1960.
39. Gates, R. R.: *Human Genetics* (New York: The Macmillan Company, 1946), Vol. 1.
40. Nichamin, S. J., and Kaufman, M.: Gingival microcysts in infancy, Pediatrics 31:412, 1963.
41. Becker, W.: Anatomie, Entwicklungsgeschichte und

Missbildungen der Ohrspeicheldrüse, Fortschr. Kiefer Gesichtschir. 6:194, 1960.
42. McKenzie, J., and Craig, J.: Mandibulo-facial dysostosis (Treacher Collins syndrome), Arch. Dis. Childhood 30: 391, 1955.
43. Ashley, L. M., and Richardson, G. E.: Multiple congenital anomalies in a stillborn infant, Anat. Rec. 86:457, 1943.
44. Becker, W., Matzker, J., and Ruckes, J.: Zur Morphologie der "diffusen, kugelförmigen Gangektasien" in der Glandula Parotis, Ztschr. Laryng. Rhin. Otol. 39:479, 1960.
45. Bhaskar, S. N.: Oral tumors of infancy and childhood; a survey of 293 cases, J. Pediat. 63:195, 1963.
46. Koop, C. E., and Moschakis, E. A.: Capillary lymphangioma of the tongue complicated by glossitis, Pediatrics 27:800, 1961.
47. Hartmann, M. G.: Über sogenannte Myoblastenmyome bei Neugeborenen. (Epulis congenita), Ztschr. Kinderh. 78:613, 1956.
48. Silver, H. K., and Simon, J. L.: Congenital myoblastoma of the newborn, A.M.A. J. Dis. Child. 93:687, 1957.
49. Gorlin, R. J., Kalnins, V., and Izant, R. J.: Occurrence of heterotopic gastric mucosa in the tongue, J. Pediat. 64: 604, 1964.
50. Medenis, R., Slaughter, D. P., and Barber, T. K.: Melanotic progonoma in childhood; report of a case of "Retinal Anlage" tumor of the maxilla in an infant, Pediatrics 29: 600, 1962.
51. Loeb, W. J., and Smith, E. E.: Airway obstruction in a newborn by pedunculated pharyngeal dermoid, Pediatrics 40:20, 1967.
52. Akbay, Y. Z.: Neonatal respiratory distress due to oropharyngeal tumor, J. Pediat. 66:1094, 1965.
53. Wilson, T. G.: Two cases of dermoid polypus of the nasopharynx, J. Laryng. 46:696, 1931.
54. Baugh, C. D., and O'Donoghue, R. F.: Teratoma of the tonsil causing respiratory obstruction in the newborn, Arch. Dis. Childhood 30:396, 1955.
55. Schwalbe, E.: Allgemeine Missbildungslehre, in Schwalbe, E. (ed.), *Die Morphologie der Missbildungen des Menschen und der Tiere* (Jena: Gustav Fischer, 1906), Vol. 1, pt. 1, p. 134.
56. Ehrich, W. E.: Teratoid parasites of mouth (episphenoids, epipalati [epurani], epignathi), Am. J. Orthodontics (Oral Surg. Sect.) 31:650, 1945.
57. Longacre, J. J.: Congenital atresia of the oropharynx, Plast. & Reconstruct. Surg. 8:341, 1951.
58. Seghers, M. J.: Une malformation rare: L'imperforation oropharyngienne, Acta paediat. belg. 20:130, 1966.
59. Kouyoumdjian, A. O., and McDonald, J. J.: Association of congenital adrenal neuroblastoma with multiple anomalies, including an unusual oropharyngeal cavity (imperforate buccopharyngeal membrane?), Cancer 4:784, 1951.
60. Bremer, J. L.: *Congenital Anomalies of the Viscera: Their Embryological Basis* (Cambridge, Mass.: Harvard University Press, 1957).
61. Frazer, J. E.: Disappearance of precervical sinus, J. Anat. 61:132, 1926.
62. Patten, B. M.: *Human Embryology* (2d ed.; New York: Blakiston Division, McGraw-Hill Book Company, Inc., 1953).
63. Gross, P. P.: Epithelioma adenoides cysticum with follicular cysts of maxillae and mandible, J. Oral Surg. 11:160, 1953.
64. Willis, R. A.: *Borderland of Embryology and Pathology* (London: Butterworth & Company, Ltd., 1958).
65. Schull, W. J., and Furuta, M.: Persistent gill slits . . . a dominant trait?, Jap. J. Human Genet. 2:33, 1957.
66. Proctor, B.: Lateral vestigial cysts and fistulas of the neck, Laryngoscope 65:355, 1955.
67. Sedgwick, C. E., and Walsh, J. F.: Branchial cysts and fistulas. A study of 75 cases relative to clinical aspects and treatment, Am. J. Surg. 83:3, 1952.
68. Raven, R. W.: Pouches of pharynx and esophagus, Brit. J. Surg. 21:235, 1933.
69. Kaufman, S. A.: Lateral pharyngeal diverticula, Am. J. Roentgenol. 75:238, 1956.
70. Solis-Cohen, L., Ersner, M., and Friedman, P. S.: Multiple pharyngeal and esophageal diverticula, hiatal hernia of stomach and chalasia of esophageal cardiac junction; case report, Am. J. Roentgenol. 75:242, 1956.
71. Brintnall, E. S., and Kridelbaugh, W. W.: Congenital diverticulum of posterior hypopharynx simulating atresia of esophagus, Ann. Surg. 131:564, 1950.
72. Baeyer, E. V.: Zenker's diverticulum and cervical block vertebra, Am. J. Roentgenol. 84:1037, 1960.
73. Turner, M. J.: Carcinoma as a complication of pharyngeal pouch, Brit. J. Radiol. 36:206, 1963.
74. Irving, I. M.: Exomphalos with macroglossia: A study of eleven cases, J. Pediat. Surg. 2:499, 1967.

73

Some Syndromes Involving Oral and Pharyngeal Anomalies

Craniocarpotarsal Dystrophy (Freeman-Sheldon Syndrome)

A SYNDROME OF microstomia, ulnar deviation of the hands and clubfeet was described in 2 children reported by Freeman and Sheldon.[1] There was thickening of the skin over the forehead, cheeks and hands. The bridge of the nose was flat and hypertelorism was present. The upper lip was elongated, the tongue small and the palate high. Ulnar deviation of the hands and clubfeet indicated inclusion of tissues of the extremities in the disorder. A third case was reported by Otto[2] 15 years later. Rintala[3] added a case report, emphasizing vertical lines on both sides of the chin. Despite the round face and broad nose, the head and chest were flattened laterally. In roentgenograms, the floor of the anterior cerebral fossa ascended steeply. The facial bones, particularly the maxilla and mandible, were hypoplastic and narrow. There was enophthalmia, although the bulbs were of normal size. The mouth was so small that it had to be widened by surgery. Flexion contractures of the fingers resulted in hands resembling those seen in chromosomal disease pictures. Bilateral pes equinovarus was present. Both sexes can be affected and chromosomes are normal.[3] Apparently the syndrome is

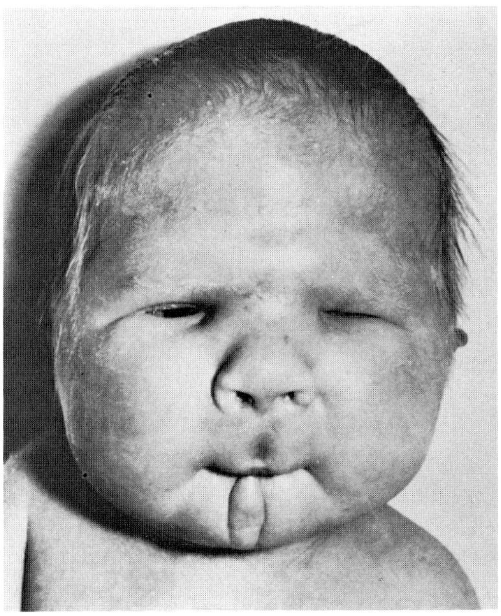

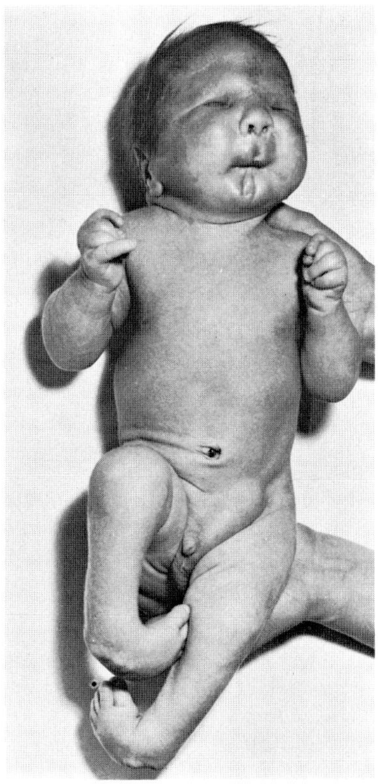

Fig. 73-1.—Child with craniocarpotarsal dystrophy (Freeman-Sheldon syndrome). (From A. E. Rintala.[3])

very rare but it results in a striking appearance. There is a definite resemblance of this disorder to the "whistling face syndrome" suggested by Burian,[4] which is characterized by microstomia with protruding lips, cleft chin and ulnar deviation and contractures of fingers. A case of this type was described by Weinstein and Gorlin,[5] who suggested that the disorder is an autosomal dominant trait. Fraser *et al.*[6] described the syndrome in a father and his son and also suggested autosomal dominant inheritance.

REFERENCES

1. Freeman, E. A., and Sheldon, J. H.: Cranio-carpo-tarsal dystrophy—an undescribed congenital malformation, Arch. Dis. Childhood 13:277, 1938.
2. Otto, F. M.: Die "Cranio-carpo-tarsal dystrophy" (Freeman and Sheldon), Ztschr. Kinderh. 73:240, 1953.
3. Rintala, A. E.: Freeman-Sheldon's syndrome, cranio-carpotarsal dystrophy, Acta paediat. scandinav. 57:553, 1968.
4. Burian, F.: The "whistling face" characteristic in a compound cranio-facio-corporal syndrome, Brit. J. Plast. Surg. 16:140, 1963.
5. Weinstein, S., and Gorlin, R. J.: Cranio-carpo-tarsal dysplasia or the whistling face syndrome, Am. J. Dis. Child. 117: 427, 1969.
6. Fraser, F. C., Pashayan, H., and Kadish, M. E.: Craniocarpo-tarsal dysplasia, J.A.M.A. 211:1374, 1970.

Orodigitofacial Syndrome
(Syndrome of Papillon-Léage and Psaume)

THIS SYNDROME was described in 1954 by Papillon-Léage and Psaume[1] as a hereditary malformation of the buccal mucosa, but additional features have been included in this rare disease picture since. Earlier descriptions were discussed by Stahl and Fuhrmann.[2] It has been estimated that the orodigitofacial syndrome occurs in approximately 1% of cleft lip and palate cases.[3] The face is characterized by short and narrow upper lip, shortened alar nasal cartilages and median notching of the upper lip. Hypertelorism, alopecia and dryness of the skin may be present. There is a true or a submucous cleft palate or a soft palate cleft that may be complete, irregular or asymmetric with ragged edges. Fibrous bands extend from the lower lip to the alveolar processes of the mandible and from the cheek to the alveolar clefts. The tongue is bifid or lobulated and sometimes pedunculated masses or tumors are attached to its dorsal surface. It is fixed to the alveolar ridges of the mandible by fibrous bands and to the floor of the mouth by a thickened frenulum. Similar frenula seem to cleave the jaws. The tumors of the tongue are benign choristomas[4] consisting of aberrant mucus glands, smooth muscle and connective tissue. They are covered by a hyperplastic, keratinized epithelium. There also are small papular lesions on the skin of the face that appear with increasing age. The mandible is hypoplastic and the teeth are irregular. Absence of the lower lateral incisors, malposition of the upper canines and hypoplasia of the mandible result in dental malocclusion. The teeth show enamel defects and early caries.[3] Anomalies of the hands consist of polydactyly of digit I, syndactyly or clinodactyly. Tremor can be observed in some patients and mental retardation in approximately half of them. Hydrocephaly, hydranencephaly and porencephaly are exceptional complications. Speech defects related to the anomalies of the tongue and palate are always present. Doege *et al.*,[4] who described the largest kindred observed to date, considered the typical profile, cleft tongue, cleft or pseudocleft palate and digital anomalies as the most constant signs. Cleft alveolar ridges, cleft lip and abnormally positioned teeth were among the less frequent anomalies. Two postmortem examinations revealed polycystic kidneys in 2 patients and cystic disease of the liver and pancreas in 1 of them. If these findings should be observed more often in patients with the orodigitofacial syndrome, one will have to assume that the external manifestations are only a part of a more generalized "hamartosis" (p. 1251).

The orodigitofacial syndrome is closely related to (if not identical to) the dysostosis acrofacialis described by Weyers in 1953.[5] This syndrome consists of polydactyly, mandibular cleft and oligodontia but goes beyond these malformations. The polydactyly is on the ulnar side and is characterized by fusion of metacarpals V and VI. The two mandibular halves are not fused in the midline and a median dental diastema exists, with the median or all lower incisors missing. In some cases there are frenula from the labial mucosa to the alveolar processes and microforms of palatal clefts, which are also symptoms of the orodigitofacial syndrome.

Not all patients with facial clefts and digital anomalies conform to the orodigitofacial syndrome. Schönenberg[6] described patients who combined cleft lip and palate with polydactyly, syndactyly and split hand without anomalies of the tongue and mucosal bands, but there were defects of the corpus callosum, cysts of the septum pellucidum, tetralogy of Fallot and some form of hermaphrodism. These observations, like those of many other authors cited by Schönenberg, illustrate the great variability of syndromes in which facial clefts occur.

Roentgenographic features of the orodigitofacial syndrome have been described by Schwarz and Fish.[7]

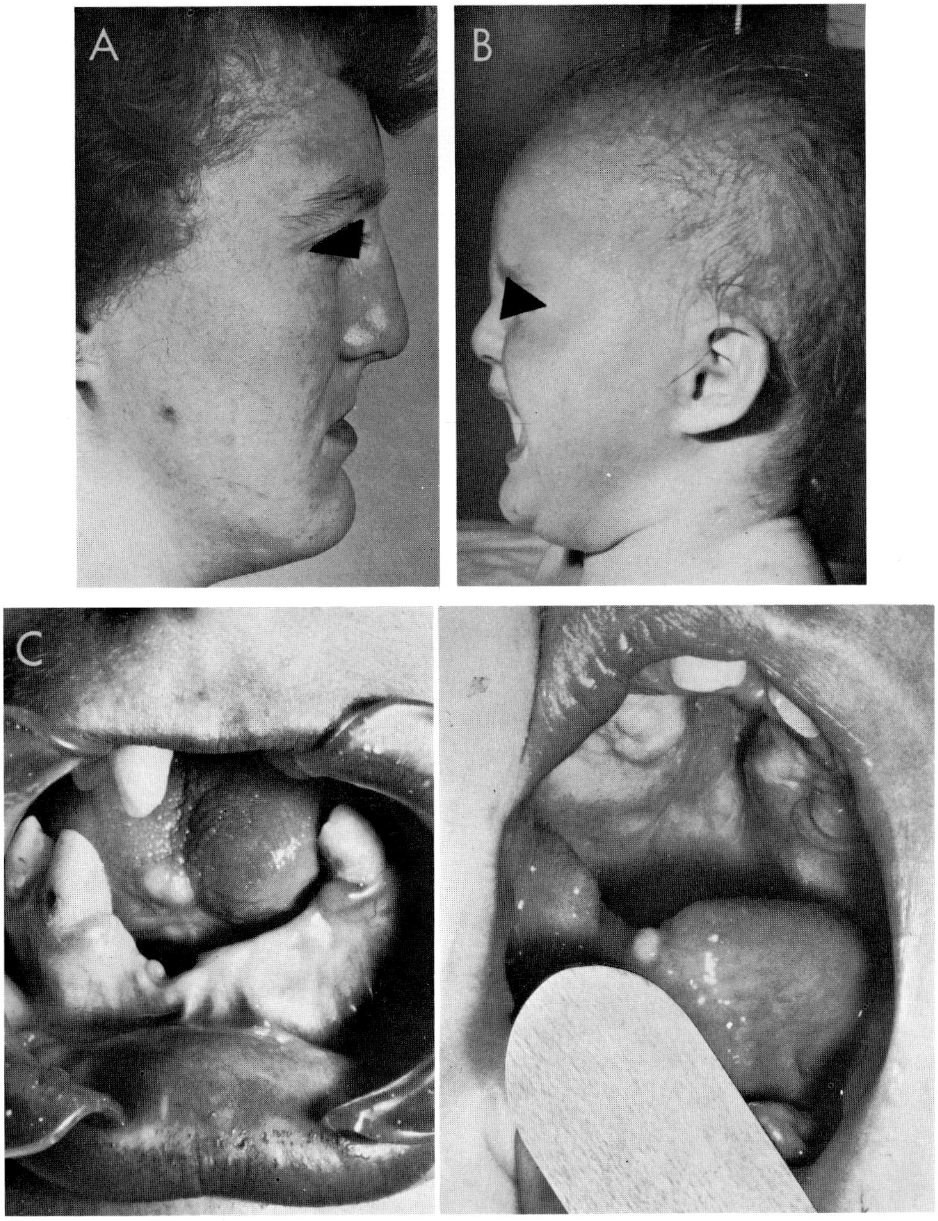

Fig. 73-2.—Orodigitofacial syndrome. An affected mother (**A**) and daughter (**B**) showing short upper lips. **C,** oral cavities with frenula, tongue tumors, pseudocleft palate and cleft tongue. (From T. C. Doege, H. C. Thuline, J. H. Priest, D. E. Norby and J. S. Bryant.[4])

The skull is characterized by a steep anterior fossa and elevation of the lesser wings of the sphenoid and of the cribriform plate. The mandible is small and its rami are shortened. The short tubular bones of the hands and feet are irregularly thickened and the bone structure appears reticular. An association of the syndrome with digital whorls has been suggested.[8]

All patients with the typical orodigitofacial syndrome described so far have been females,[9] but it is possible that a second type exists with manifestations in males,[10] which is now called "Mohr syndrome." Polysyndactyly of the first toe and central alveolar defects in the upper jaw have been mentioned as distinctive features of this syndrome, which can be inherited as an autosomal recessive trait.[18] Doege *et al.*[4] published a pedigree with 15 affected females in four generations with the orodigitofacial syndrome. Dominant inheritance is also suggested by the pedigree published by Gorlin *et al.*,[11] which shows the condition in three generations. This pedigree also illustrates the variable expression of the gene in different members of the same family. A pedigree of 6 affected members in four generations was recorded by Reinwein *et al.*[12] The sex ratio of the progeny was 14 females to 4 males in three generations. Based on the pedigrees available, Doege *et al.*[4] concluded that the syndrome has a dominant mode of inheritance. The absence of affected males in the pedigrees was explained by prenatal lethality of males. At present, either autosomal or sex-linked dominant inheritance – in either case, with lethality in males – must be considered in the etiology. In one family, a chromosomal anomaly was found in an affected mother and her daughter. One of the no. 1 chromosomes had arms that appeared larger than normal and thinned near the centromere. Ruess *et al.*[3] believed that the syndrome is caused by partial trisomy, the extra chromosomal material being inserted into chromosome no. 1 in exceptional cases but being undetectable in others. Doege *et al.*[4] found no chromosomal anomalies in leukocyte cultures of 8 affected females. In a hepatic cell culture of a female patient, an extra chromosome in group G was present, a finding that cannot yet be evaluated. Dodge and Kernohan[13] ascertained normal karyotypes in an affected mother and her 3 affected daughters. Kushnick *et al.*[14] reported a case with findings consistent with the diagnosis of orodigitofacial syndrome in a male infant who had a bilobed tongue with thick frenulum and fixation of the tongue base, pseudocleft of the mid-upper lip, high palate, alopecia, microcephaly, clinodactyly and preaxial polydactyly. The karyotype showed a trisomy probably involving chromosome no. 1. Wahrman *et al.*[15] described a male infant showing all the major features of the orodigitofacial syndrome who had an XXY chromosomal constitution. It was thought that this XXY male was viable because of the normal allele in one X chromosome. Frøland *et al.*[16] observed a boy with pronounced frenula in the upper and lower vestibula and dental anomalies. He had 47 chromosomes with an extra extremely small metacentric. There was only superficial resemblance of the oral symptoms to those of the syndrome discussed here. An orodigitofacial syndrome was described in 2 brothers by Hooft and Jongblaet.[17] Hexadactyly with the extra finger on the ulnar side, microphthalmia and coloboma of the papilla in one case suggest that the syndrome was not identical to that of Papillon-Léage and Psaume.

Treatment of the tongue and palate anomalies is difficult. Surgery and prostheses are utilized, but in the presence of mental retardation the outlook for rehabilitation is poor.[3]

REFERENCES

1. Papillon-Léage, and Psaume, J.: Une malformation héréditaire de la muqueuse buccale, brides et freins anormaux, Rev. stomat. 55:209, 1954.
2. Stahl, A., and Fuhrmann, W.: Oro-facio-digitales syndrom, Deutsche med. Wchnschr. 93:1, 1968.
3. Ruess, A. L., Pruzansky, S., Lis, E. F., and Patau, K.: The oral-facial-digital syndrome: A multiple congenital condition of females with associated chromosomal abnormalities, Pediatrics 29:985, 1962.
4. Doege, T. C., Thuline, H. C., Priest, J. H., Norby, D. E., and Bryant, J. S.: Studies of a family with the oral-facial-digital syndrome, New England J. Med. 271:1073, 1964.
5. Weyers, H.: Hexadactylie, Unterkieferspalt und Oligodontie, ein neuer Symptomenkomplex. Dysostosis acro-facialis, Ann. paediat. 181:45, 1953.
6. Schönenberg, H.: Über die Kombination von Lippen-Kiefer-Gaumen-Spalten mit Extremitätenmissbildungen, Ztschr. Kinderh. 76:79, 1955.
7. Schwarz, E., and Fish, A.: Roentgenographic features of a new congenital dysplasia, Am. J. Roentgenol. 84:511, 1960.
8. Doege, T. C., Campbell, M. M., Bryant, J. S., and Thuline, H. C.: Mental retardation and dermatoglyphics in a family with the oral-facial-digital syndrome, Am. J. Dis. Child. 116:615, 1968.
9. Fuhrmann, W., Stahl, A., and Schroeder, T. M.: Das oro-facio-digitale Syndrom. Zugleich eine Diskussion der Erbgänge mit geschlechtsbegrenztem Letaleffekt, Humangenetik 2:133, 1966.
10. Rimoin, D. L., and Edgerton, M. T.: Genetic and clinical heterogeneity in the oral-facial-digital syndromes, J. Pediat. 71:94, 1967.
11. Gorlin, R. J., Anderson, V. E., and Scott, C. R.: Hypertrophied frenuli, oligophrenia, familial trembling and anomalies of the head. Report of four cases in one family and a forme fruste in another, New England J. Med. 264:486, 1961.
12. Reinwein, H., Schilli, W., Ritter, H., Brehme, H., and Wolf, U.: Untersuchungen an einer Familie mit Oral-Facial-Digital Syndrom, Humangenetik 2:165, 1966.
13. Dodge, J. A., and Kernohan, D. C.: Oral-facial-digital syndrome, Arch. Dis. Childhood 42:214, 1967.
14. Kushnick, T., Massa, T. P., and Baukema, R.: Orofaciodigital syndrome in a male, J. Pediat. 63:1130, 1963.
15. Wahrman, J., Berant, M., Jacobs, J., Aviad, I., and Ben-Hur, N.: The oral-facial-digital syndrome: A male-lethal condition in a boy with 47/XXY chromosomes, Pediatrics 37:812, 1966.
16. Frøland, A., Johnsen, S. G., Andresen, P., Dein, E., Sanger, R., and Race, R. R.: Non-disjunction and XXY men, Lancet 2:1121, 1963.
17. Hooft, C., and Jongblaet, P.: Syndrome oro-digito-facial chez deux frères, Arch. franç. pédiat. 21:729, 1964.
18. Fuhrmann, W., and Stahl, A.: Zur Differentialdiagnose von Papillon-Léage-Psaume-Syndrom und Mohr-Syndrom, Humangenetik 9:54, 1970.

Otopalatodigital Syndrome

A SYNDROME similar in some respects to Pyle disease (p. 870), or "craniometaphyseal dysplasia" was reported by Taybi,[1] but it is now believed that the similarity is superficial. The first patient described had protruding orbital ridges, a flat and broad nasal bridge, long head and digits with markedly enlarged tips. The first toes were extremely short and their nails hypoplastic. Cleft palate, delay of closure of the anterior fontanelle, speech and hearing defects and slow physical and mental development were noted also. Roentgenograms showed increased density of the skeleton, widely open anterior fontanelle and metopic suture, prominent supraorbital ridges, lack of modeling of the long bones, subluxation in the elbow and hip joints and delayed and abnormal ossification, particularly in the hands and feet. An aunt of the mother, who was said to have looked like the patient, had cleft palate and a "soft head." Dudding *et al.*[2] observed a similar disease picture in 3 brothers. There was definite resemblance of the profiles and of the hands and feet of the patients described in the two publications. The feet have been compared to those of a tree frog[2] because of a large cleft between the first and second toes. Posterior palate cleft, loss of hearing and mild mental and physical retardation were also present in these brothers. Skeletal anomalies were similar to those of Taybi's patient but they were generally milder and less distinctive. The name "oto-palato-digital syndrome" suggested by Dudding *et al.*[2] hardly covers the widespread symptomatology of the disorder. The trait is thought to be inherited as a recessive.[3]

REFERENCES

1. Taybi, H.: Generalized skeletal dysplasia with multiple anomalies. A note on Pyle's disease, Am. J. Roentgenol. 88: 450, 1962.
2. Dudding, B. A., Gorlin, R. J., and Langer, L. O.: The oto-palato-digital syndrome. A new symptom-complex consisting of deafness, dwarfism, cleft palate, characteristic facies, and a generalized bone dysplasia, Am. J. Dis. Child. 113:214, 1967.
3. Langer, L. O., Jr.: The roentgenographic features of the oto-palato-digital (OPD) syndrome, Am. J. Roentgenol. 100:63, 1967.

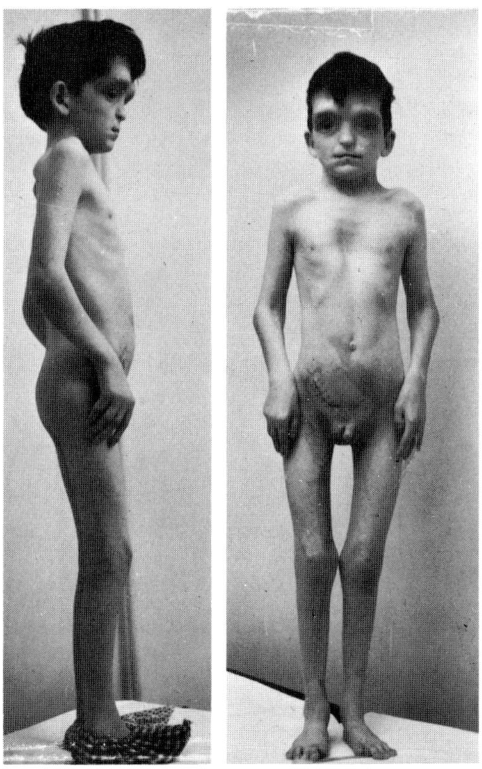

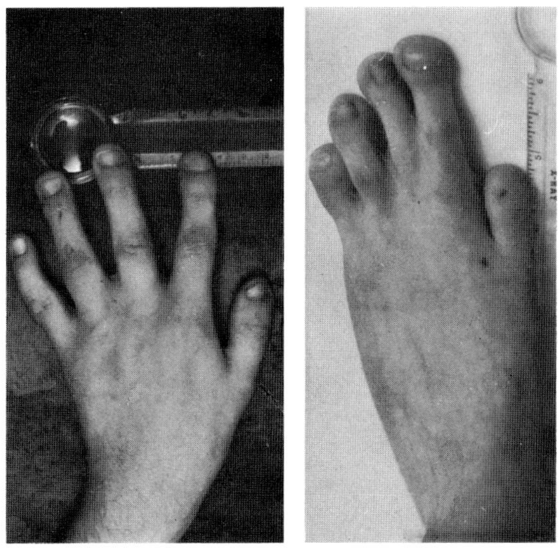

Fig. 73-3.—Boy with a generalized skeletal dysplasia characterized by large distal phalanges, hypoplasia of first digits and nails and cleft palate. (From H. Taybi.[1])

74

The Esophagus

Tracheo-Esophageal Fistula and Esophageal Atresia

HISTORICAL REVIEWS on this subject have been given by Ferguson,[1] Haight[2] and Holder and Ashcraft.[3] Durston,[4] in 1670, generally is credited with having reported the first case of congenital tracheo-esophageal fistula in one of conjoined twins. In 1703, Thomas Gibson[5] described in *The Anatomy of Humane Bodies Epitomized* the clinical and pathologic findings of a patient. The original text, quoted in part by Ferguson[1] and reproduced by Holder and Ashcraft,[3] relates the discovery most vividly:

"About November, 1696, I was sent for to see an infant that could not swallow. The child seem'd very desirous of food and took what was offer'd it in a Spoon with greediness; but when it went to swallow it, it was like to be choaked, and what should have gone down returned by the mouth and nose, and it fell into a strugling convulsive-sort of fit upon it. It was very fleshy and large and was two dayes old when I came to it, but the next day died. The Parents being willing to have it opened. . . . Then we cut open the Thorax. . . . Then we made a slit in the Stomach, and put a pipe into its upper orifice, and blowing, we found the wind had a vent, but not by the top of the Gullet. Then we carefully slit up the backside of the Gullet from the stomach upwards, and when we were gone a little above half way toward the pharynx, we found it hollow no further. Then we begun to slit it open from the pharynx downwards, and it was hollow till within an inch of the other slit, and in the imperforated part it was narrower than in the hollowed. . . . Then searching what way the wind had passed when we blew from the stomach upwards, we found an oval hole (half an inch long) on the fore-side of the gullet opening into the aspera arteria, a little above its first division, just under the lower part of the Isthmus abovementioned."

This excellent description makes it clear that Gibson dissected the most common form of tracheo-esophageal fistula with atresia of the upper portion of the esophagus, as illustrated in Figure 74-1, *C*.

The incidence of esophageal atresia and tracheo-esophageal fistula (TEF) is not known. Belsey and Donnison[6] believed that many cases are overlooked and are diagnosed as atelectasis in case of death without necropsy. They estimated the incidence to be approximately 1 in 800 births. Franklin[7] considered 1 case in 2,500 deliveries, Ingalls and Prindle[8] 1 in 5,000 live births and Holder and Ashcraft[3] 1 in 1,000 births as reasonable estimates. There is no definite sex preponderance. The birth weights of 87 infants with the anomaly were significantly lower than those

Fig. 74-1.—Diagrams representing various esophageal anomalies. **A,** esophageal atresia; there is no communication between the trachea and the esophagus. **B,** the upper esophageal segment communicates with the trachea and the lower segment with the stomach. **C,** the upper esophageal segment ends as a blind pouch and the lower segment communicates with the trachea and the stomach. **D,** both segments communicate with the trachea. **E,** the esophagus is continuous but is connected by a fistula with the trachea. (Modified from R. E. Gross.[9])

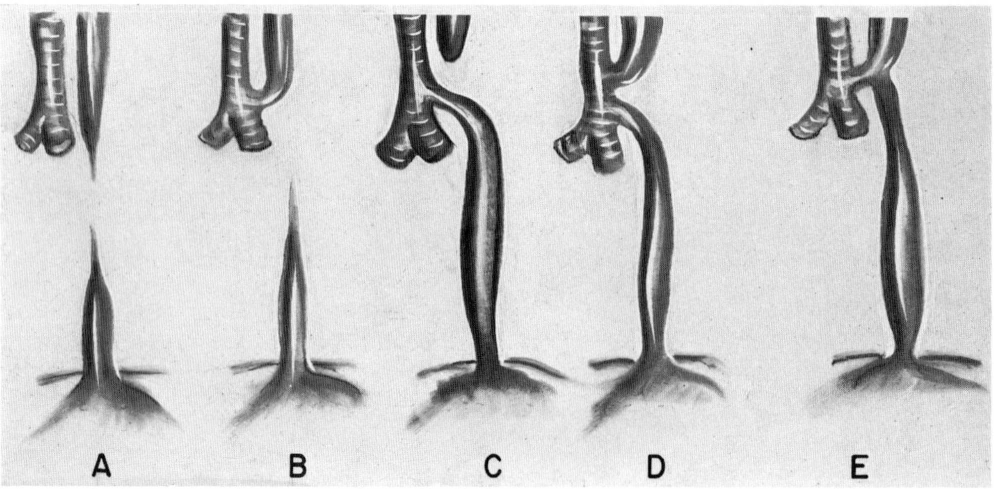

of 1,000 babies of a general lying-in hospital population. Gross[9] believed that there is an unusually high percentage of prematures among babies with esophageal atresia. In a Boston series,[8] the disorder appeared more often than was to be expected by chance among the progeny of older women, although this trend was far less striking than for mongolism. Hydramnios frequently complicates pregnancies resulting in esophageal atresias but is less frequent in those resulting in TEF.[3]

Several types of congenital abnormalities of the esophagus are known and various classifications have been attempted.[9,10] Gross's classification, which is the one usually followed, is shown in Figure 74-1 in modified diagrams. The most common form (87%) of esophageal atresia with tracheo-esophageal fistula is shown in Figure 74-1, *C*, in which the lower segment of the esophagus communicates with the back of the trachea, whereas the upper segment ends as a blind pouch. In Gross's series, more than 90% of all esophageal malformations fell into this group. Figure 74-1, *A* shows an interesting but rare form in which the esophagus is discontinuous and no tracheo-esophageal fistula is formed—"simple esophageal atresia." Another type, Figure 74-1, *E*, shows a tracheo-esophageal fistula without esophageal atresia. This type, although rare and comprising only about 3% of clinical cases, [9,11] is of interest because of its clinical manifestations, which differ somewhat from those of the common tracheo-esophageal fistula with esophageal discontinuity.

Tracheo-esophageal fistula apparently has not been reported as a familial trait in successive generations. If this anomaly were due to a mutation and a dominant gene, it would be understandable that it was not transmitted to subsequent generations, since, until 1939, all children with this anomaly died soon after birth. Instances of tracheo-esophageal fistula in more than one child in a family have been observed repeatedly,[12,13] but it seems that, in general, the incidence in siblings is low, as Haight[2] found, in more than 200 cases, only one family with 2 affected siblings. Mackenzie[14] reported TEF in 3 children fathered by one man but born of different mothers. Hausmann *et al.*[15] noted esophageal atresia in 3 consecutive siblings, the first 2 affected by TEF and the third by an atresia without fistula.

Panse and Gierlich[16] described probably identical twins, both affected by esophageal atresia. One of the twins also had anencephaly, rachischisis and acardia. In a thoracopagus embryo, both sides were affected with TEF.[17] These findings suggest that a genetic factor may be involved in the etiology of TEF, but data are insufficient to attribute the anomaly to a definite mode of inheritance. A considerable number of twins have been described in whom only one of the pair had the anomaly. Some of these twins obviously were dizygotic but others were discordant even though they were monozygotic. In Haight's[2] series of 201 cases of esophageal atresia, the anomaly was discordant in 10 pairs of twins and tracheo-esophageal fistula was discordant in 1 pair. It was believed that at least 6 pairs of the twins were identical, and their discordance suggested to Haight the importance of nongenetic factors in the etiology of the anomaly. Tracheo-esophageal fistula occurs occasionally in children with trisomy 18.[18] Ingalls and Prindle[8] admitted the possibility of a genetic causation of TEF but believed that the syndrome is acquired during early fetal life, with departures from normal development at about the fifth or sixth week. They could, however, find no strong evidence of impairment of maternal health or of abnormalities of the placenta in the majority of cases. Knox[19] noted clustering of TEF and/or esophageal atresia in England, suggesting that the disorders may have an infective origin. Esophageal atresia has been observed in rare cases of thalidomide embryopathy.[20] It seems likely that heterogeneous etiologies can result in esophageal malformations.

It is of interest that tracheo-esophageal fistula has not been produced experimentally with any regularity in teratologic experiments. Warkany, Roth and Wilson,[21] in a large series of embryos adversely influenced by maternal vitamin A deficiency, found only one animal with tracheo-esophageal fistula. Kalter and Warkany[22] found *esophageal atresia* in the young of female mice that received a riboflavin-deficient, galactoflavin-containing diet; there were no tracheo-esophageal fistulas. Such cases (Fig. 74-2) correspond to type A of Gross's classification. Approximately 80% of the young of strains A and DBA showed this esophageal anomaly after such treatment.

The morphogenesis of esophageal atresia must be considered together with the normal separation of the respiratory and upper alimentary tracts. In embryos of 2.5 mm. length (4 weeks), the first indication of the future respiratory organs is seen in a longitudinal laryngotracheal groove that runs in the floor of the gut caudal to the pharyngeal pouches. The endodermal groove is destined to become the larynx and trachea; the more rounded caudal ends represent the primordia of the lungs. Two furrows course longitudinally along the sides of the respiratory primordium and cut inward deeper until they separate it from the esophagus. This separation progresses in a caudocephalic direction, so that the lung bud is the first to become free.[23] Bremer[24] stated that the whole caudal portion of the pharynx below the fourth pair of pouches rapidly grows longer, carrying the lung bud far below the pouches. The lumen of the lengthened portion assumes the shape of a narrow, laterally compressed slit that is divided from below upward into two tubes—the esophagus dorsally and the trachea ventrally. The division is accomplished by the folding in of the lateral walls of the foregut until they meet and fuse, thus turning the slit-like cavity into two parallel channels that are joined only above at the larynx. This method of subdividing can lead to a variety of malformations. If, for instance, the transverse folds do not meet completely at one point of their course, a

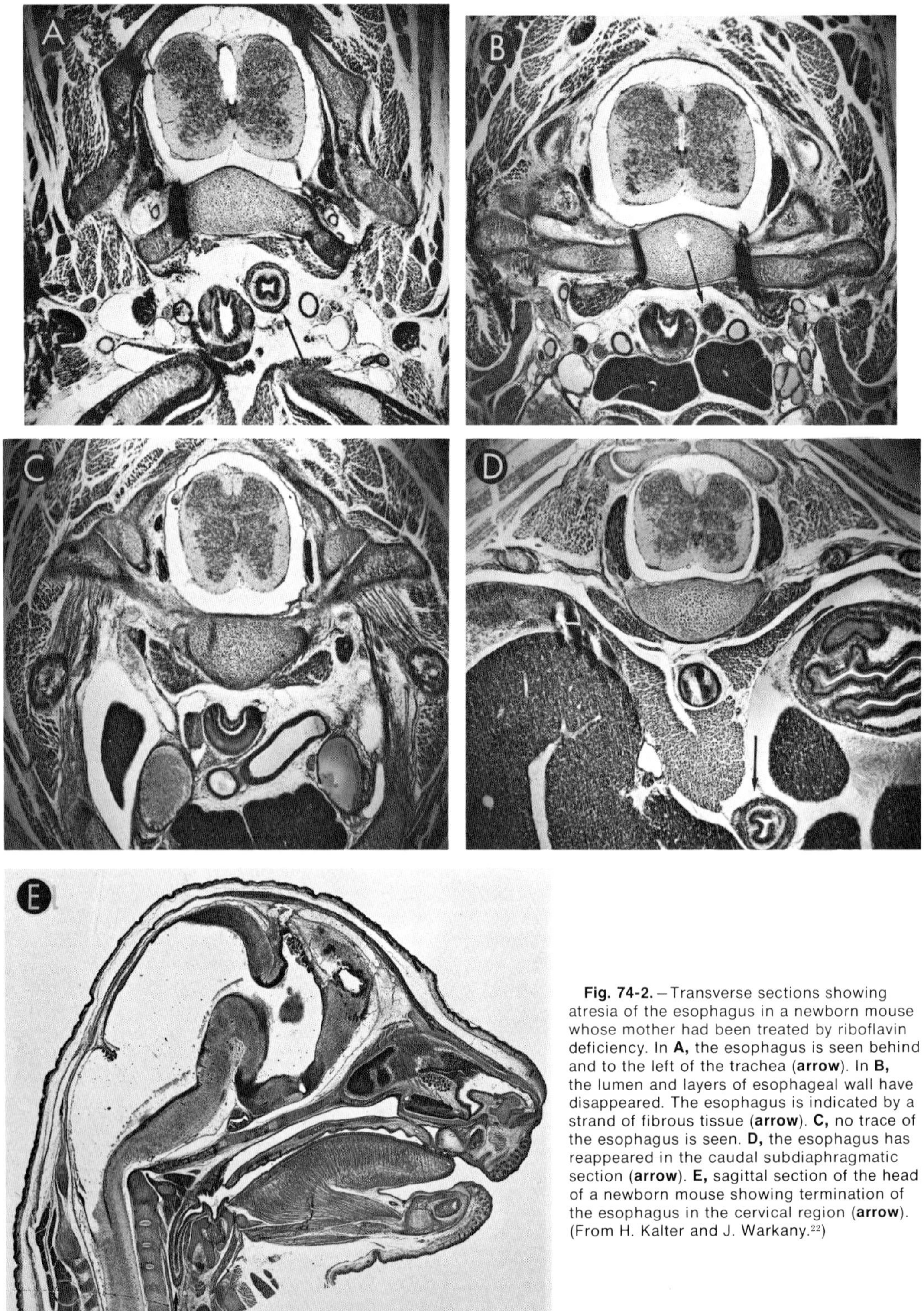

Fig. 74-2. – Transverse sections showing atresia of the esophagus in a newborn mouse whose mother had been treated by riboflavin deficiency. In **A,** the esophagus is seen behind and to the left of the trachea (**arrow**). In **B,** the lumen and layers of esophageal wall have disappeared. The esophagus is indicated by a strand of fibrous tissue (**arrow**). **C,** no trace of the esophagus is seen. **D,** the esophagus has reappeared in the caudal subdiaphragmatic section (**arrow**). **E,** sagittal section of the head of a newborn mouse showing termination of the esophagus in the cervical region (**arrow**). (From H. Kalter and J. Warkany.[22])

fistula would result between the trachea and the esophagus without esophageal atresia (Gross, type E).

It is more difficult to explain the morphogenesis of the more common tracheo-esophageal fistula (type C), which is combined with atresia of the upper segment of the esophagus. Many theories have been advanced; these theories were reviewed by Rosenthal,[25] Ferguson,[1] Smith[26] and Holder and Ashcraft.[3]

Rosenthal[25] did not accept the explanation of arrest of the esophagus at a stage at which the tube had become a solid bar of tissue with no lumen, since the esophagus does not go through any "solid bar" stage as do lower portions of the intestine. He also rejected the various explanations that attribute the anomaly to pressure from a surrounding organ or structure. An aberrant subclavian artery has been observed as an associated defect of tracheo-esophageal fistula in several cases, but it is rather the result than the cause of the esophageal atresia, since the esophageal defect is present before the vascular tree develops. It is also not likely that pressure of the enlarging heart causes tracheo-esophageal fistulas because, if this were the case, the trachea would be compressed also and show atresia like the esophagus. Rosenthal believed that the development of the anomaly is due to early changes of the entodermal cells that give rise to the esophagus and not to concomitant external abnormalities.

Ferguson[1] pointed out that the trachea is developed from the cephalic portion of the primitive foregut. In the 3-mm. stage of the embryo, the normal pulmonary anlage originates from the ventral portion of the primitive foregut just caudal to the pharyngeal pouches, and in the 4-mm. stage this mass of primordial cells has grown caudally so that there are formed, externally along the foregut wall, two lateral longitudinal grooves with corresponding internal elevations, the forerunners of the septum that divides the foregut into the anterior trachea and the posterior esophagus. These changes occur during the second fetal month, so that at the end of 7 or 8 weeks of intrauterine life, the trachea and esophagus have become completely separated. By the time the embryo has reached the 11-mm. stage (the sixth week), either it should have a normal trachea and esophagus or the anomalies under discussion will have been established. In fact, Ysander[17] described a monstrous embryo of 11 mm., a thoracopagus, in which the esophagus and respiratory apparatus were duplicated identically and each half had a typical tracheo-esophageal fistula with associated atresia such as is seen in full-term babies. Gruenwald[27] reported the anomaly in a 9-mm. embryo. He thought that a rapid elongation of the trachea may carry the developing digestive tube caudad so fast that it loses the ability to differentiate into a separate and normal esophagus over the distance that the trachea has grown.

Smith[26] studied the early development of the human trachea and esophagus in relation to atresia of the esophagus and tracheo-esophageal fistula. The tracheo-esophageal abnormalities are well established by the fifth week of embryonic life and probably have their beginning as early as 21 days after fertilization. The defects in question appear to arise from disturbances in the differentiation and growth pattern of the epithelial lining of the foregut. Smith's investigation suggested that both esophageal atresia and tracheo-esophageal fistula may involve hyperplasia of the lateral esophageal ridges. In embryos of about 26 days, a lateral esophageal groove can be seen (Fig. 74-3) that runs caudal and dorsal from the separation point of the trachea and esophagus. Overgrowth of these lateral esophageal grooves with corresponding concrescence of the endothelia could lead to separation of the upper and lower parts of the esophagus and leave a connection between the tra-

Fig. 74-3. – Diagram showing separation of the trachea and the esophagus. **A,** division of pharyngeal area by lateral esophageal groove. **B,** lateral esophageal groove, bv overgrowth, leads to separation of upper and lower segments of the esophagus and to the common (Fig. 74-1, **C**) type of tracheo-esophageal fistula. (After E. I. Smith.[26])

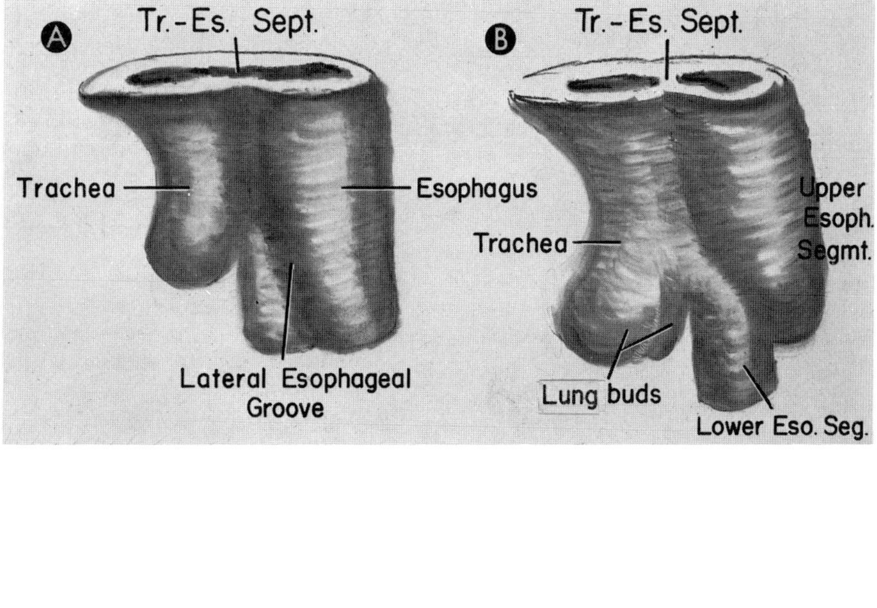

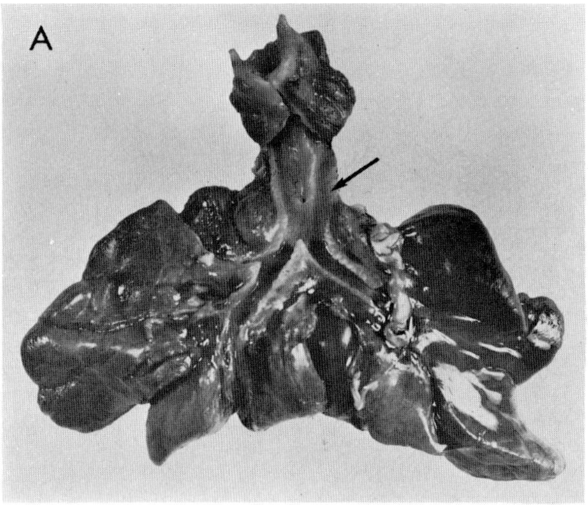

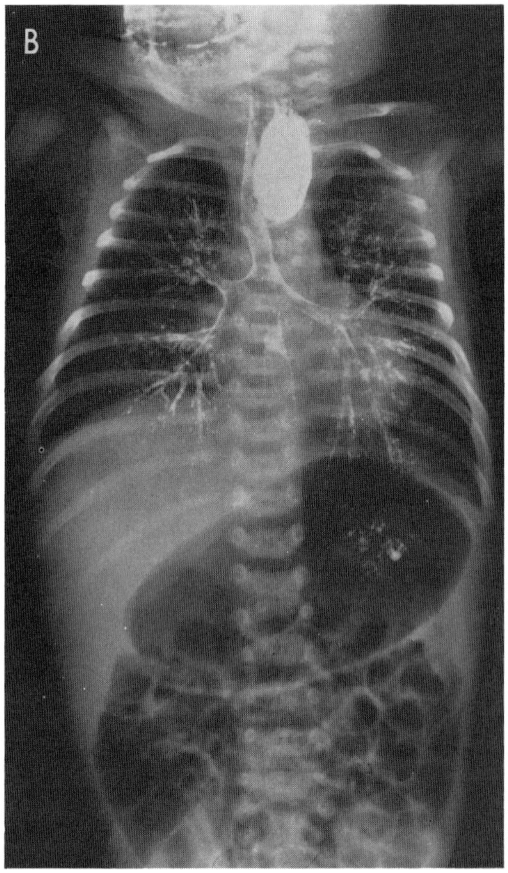

Fig. 74-4. – **A,** tracheo-esophageal fistula (arrow points to opening in midline) in an infant girl. **B,** roentgenogram of the same child. The blind upper segment of the esophagus is filled with contrast medium. Trachea and bronchi are outlined by aspirated contrast medium. Air in the stomach indicates communication of the trachea with the stomach through a fistula and inferior esophageal segment.

chea and the caudal esophageal segment. In this way, the common type (see Fig. 74-1, *C*) of tracheo-esophageal fistula could be formed.[26]

Rosenthal made a study of 8 cases of tracheo-esophageal fistulas and found that the average site of the fistula was 0.5 cm. above the bifurcation of the trachea (Fig. 74-4, *A*), but there are, of course, exceptional cases in which the fistulous tract may extend from a bronchus into the esophagus. In general, the fistula has a crescentic outline and a continuous mucous membrane covers the trachea, esophagus and its communicating tract. The muscle walls frequently blend with each other. The lower portion of the esophagus and the posterior wall of the trachea are closely connected by circular and longitudinal muscle layers, and esophageal glands can be found in the trachea itself. In the posterior tracheal wall, stratified squamous epithelium may extend up as far as the thyroid cartilage, so that some authors considered the posterior tracheal wall as an esophageal structure. Tracheal mucosa can also be found in the lower portion of the esophagus.[25]

Since tracheo-esophageal fistula can now be treated successfully by early surgery, it is important to recognize the symptoms as early as possible. One of the most common findings in Gross's type C is excessive salivation, since the saliva cannot reach the stomach by the normal pathway. The child appears hungry and eager to take the breast or bottle, but attempts to feed are followed by gagging, coughing and respiratory distress. Whenever excess salivation or dysphagia is encountered in a newborn baby, the patency of the esophagus must be investigated by the passing of a catheter, which, in the presence of an atresia of the esophagus, will be stopped by the obstruction. However, in the presence of a tracheo-esophageal fistula without atresia of the esophagus (see Fig. 74-1, *E*), the catheter can pass into the stomach; therefore, the catheter test does not exclude the presence of a tracheo-esophageal fistula. With this anomaly, one finds, in addition to coughing and cyanosis with feeding, abnormal distention of the gastrointestinal tract due to swallowing of air and persistent pneumonitis.[28,29] Excessive salivation will not be a symptom in type E. In both conditions, roentgenographic examinations with introduction of lipidol will contribute to the diagnosis. In the case of esophageal atresia, this procedure shows the end of the blind upper esophageal pouch (Fig. 74-4, *A*). In the case of a fistula without esophageal atresia, the fistula can be demonstrated by the contrast medium if the patient is in the prone position or by a tracheogram that reveals the connection with the esophagus.

Manifestations of esophageal fistulas may be delayed in rare instances. Berman *et al.*[30] described a congenital broncho-esophageal fistula in a Negro woman 40 years of age. A continuous productive cough with hemoptysis, fever, loss of weight and extreme weakness were the presenting symptoms. There was immediate improvement following ligation and removal of the fistulous tract. The authors found reports of congenital tracheo-esophageal or broncho-esophageal fistulas in adults in only 4 proved cases.

Tracheo-esophageal fistula without esophageal atresia is compatible with life and can go unrecognized for many years. Chief manifestations of such fistulas may be chronic bronchopulmonary infections and bronchiectases.[31,32] Congenital broncho-esophageal fistulas are rare; usually they manifest themselves in adult life, when they cause symptoms of bronchiectasis of the lower lobes of the lungs. Cough with swallowing can betray the lesion, which can be demonstrated by esophagography with a contrast medium. Surgical treatment of the fistula or lung resection alleviates the condition.[33] A case of esophageal atresia combined with tracheo-esophageal communication and the right bronchus arising from the esophagus was reported by Higurashi and Shiraki.[34] Duplication of the esophagus accompanied by tracheo-esophageal and tracheo-bronchial fistulas have been observed.[35]

Approximately half the children with congenital esophageal defects have associated anomalies and in half of these the associated anomalies are so serious that survival is not likely.[3] A survey by the Surgical Section of the American Academy of Pediatrics showed that of 1,058 patients reviewed 505 had 848 anomalies. Congenital heart disease was present in 19% of the patients; imperforate anus in 9.4%; other gastrointestinal anomalies in 12.7%; genitourinary anomalies in 10.3%; skeletal and muscular defects in 8.6%; facial anomalies in 5% (of these, 2.6% were facial clefts); central nervous system anomalies in 3.3%; and Down syndrome in 2.6%. The chance for survival after operation was 78% for the infants without associated malformations but only 22% for those with congenital heart disease or those with genitourinary anomalies.

Mellins and Blumenthal[36] noted cardiovascular anomalies in 26% of patients with esophageal atresia. Buchs[37] pointed out that the cardiovascular anomalies associated with stenoses and atresias of the alimentary tract are chiefly derivatives of the distal part of the cardiac tube affecting the bulbus, truncus and the primitive branchial arteries. Septal defects were considered bulbus anomalies. Mehrizi *et al.*[38] emphasized coarctation of the aorta as the most common cardiovascular defect associated with esophageal atresia or TEF. Down syndrome occurs approximately sixteen times more often in infants with esophageal malformation than in the general infant population. A similar relationship exists between facial clefts and esophageal anomalies.

Laryngotracheo-esophageal cleft has been described on page 597. Association of esophageal malformations with chondromalacia of the larynx and upper trachea is of practical importance because of the similarity of the clinical picture of the two conditions.[39] Atresia of the esophagus combined with agenesis of the caudal spinal column and renal agenesis was considered a syndrome by Kučera and Lenz.[40] TEF with limb defects was emphasized by Smith *et al.*,[41] who noted that thumb and radius defects are relatively frequent associations.

The older treatment of multiple-stage repairs for term infants has now been replaced by primary esophageal anastomosis. This operation is performed in one stage by union of the esophageal ends within the mediastinum and by closure of the fistulous connection between the lower esophageal segment and the trachea. But in premature or underweight infants with esophageal anomalies, staged operations are still practiced. Infants with "simple atresia" require special and protracted treatment.[3,9,42,43]

Congenital Esophageal Stenoses

Esophageal stenosis is rarer than esophageal atresia with tracheo-esophageal fistula. Little is known concerning the etiology and morphogenesis of this anomaly, but some cases probably are related to esophageal atresia, since they are, like that anomaly, associated with other malformations of the alimentary tract, such as imperforate anus, duodenal atresia and others.

The symptoms may appear later than those of esophageal atresia. They consist of regurgitation of food and failure to gain weight. Sometimes symptoms do not appear until the child is fed solid food. Dilatation of the esophagus above the level of obstruction may press against the trachea and bronchi and produce wheezing, choking spells, cyanosis and pneumonitis. Most of the segmental lesions that can be demonstrated on x-ray films are located in the middle third of the esophagus.

In most cases, congenital esophageal stenosis can be treated by dilatation, but when nutrition cannot be supplied through the narrow esophagus, gastrostomy is performed.[9]

Congenital esophageal *webs* represent incomplete diaphragms within the esophagus consisting of duplications of mucous membrane. Difficulty in swallowing solids dates back to early life, and impacted foreign bodies may betray the anomaly.[44] Webs of the cervical esophagus may go unrecognized for many decades despite congenital dysphagia.[45]

Congenital Esophageal Ulcer; Esophagitis

The subject of ulcer of the esophagus with melena neonatorum was reviewed in 1926 by Diamantopoulos,[46] who credited Henoch with describing the first child with this lesion. Diamantopoulos reviewed 12 cases published by 1926 that were confirmed by histologic examination and added a case of his own, a 3-day-old infant who was found bleeding from the mouth and was lying in a pool of this blood. The child died on the same day and necropsy revealed an ulcer covered by a large clot of blood in the esophagus above the cardia. Gruenwald and Marsh[47] reviewed the subject of acute esophagitis in infants. Acute esophagitis, usually with ulceration, was found in 1 of every 6 infants in a series of 310 necropsies. This lesion may be an accidental finding or be the principal cause of death. It was suggested that, in many of the cases, esophagitis was a "shock lesion" due to birth trauma including asphyxia. Sullivan *et al.*[48] reported the fatal case of gastrointestinal hemorrhage from a small linear esophageal ulcer just above the gastric cardia in a newborn premature infant. Asphyxia and probably intracranial trauma are thought to be important causal factors in the production of this ulceration.

Spontaneous rupture of the esophagus in the newborn leads to pneumothorax and fluid accumulation in the chest, or subcutaneous and mediastinal emphysema can be noted. Surgical repair has been reported.[49]

Hiatus Hernia, Partial Thoracic Stomach and Short Esophagus

The anatomy and clinical aspects of the gastroesophageal region in infants represent a confused subject. Partial thoracic stomach, hiatus hernia and congenital short esophagus are conditions that are not clearly defined at present and are considered to be of differing clinical importance by different observers.

Gross[9] found only 5 cases of hiatus hernias among 91 cases of congenital hernias of the diaphragm, but Humphreys *et al.*[50] thought that hiatus hernia was approximately equal in number to other congenital defects of the diaphragm. Hernias that appear at the esophageal hiatus always have a sac that limits the upward progression of abdominal viscera so that the sac contains only a portion of the stomach. The gastric fundus or a considerable part of the stomach may be above the level of the diaphragm. Gross[9] distinguished between hiatus hernia with an esophagus of normal length and one in which a portion of the stomach is drawn upward by a congenitally short esophagus, the two conditions to be differentiated roentgenographically. However, Silverman[51] pointed out that the identification of the cardiaesophageal junction is subject to considerable error and that clear differentiation between "chalasia" and partial thoracic stomach is not always possible. It seems that the similarity in manifestations, complications and responses to therapy is such as to suggest that the two conditions may be different stages of the same disturbance. Radiographically demonstrable regurgitation through the cardiaesophageal junction is not rare in children who are vomiting but it can be seen also in normal children.

In 1947, Neuhauser and Berenberg[52] described the mechanism for some cases of persistent vomiting in infancy under the term "cardio-esophageal relaxation or chalasia." The free flow of a barium mixture between the stomach and the persistently dilated esophagus under the influence of position and gravity was attributed to temporary neuromuscular dysfunction involving the diaphragm and the gastroesophageal musculature. This condition was to be differentiated from congenital short esophagus and partial intrathoracic stomach due to diaphragmatic hernia, since prompt and gratifying cessation of symptoms occurred if the infant was maintained in an erect position, which impeded reflux of gastric contents into the esophagus. Within 3–4 weeks, clinical and radiologic recovery was to be expected.

Astley and Carré[53] believed the so-called short esophagus with a small portion of the stomach situated above the diaphragm to be more frequent than "chalasia" as described by Neuhauser and Berenberg.[52] They thought that gastroesophageal incompetence due to a short esophagus and minor degree of partial thoracic stomach is a common cause of vomiting in infancy. In these cases, the vomiting, which usually dates from the neonatal period, often is projectile. Gastric peristalsis is visible, making differentiation from hypertrophic pyloric stenosis difficult. Solid food frequently causes improvement but in a small proportion of cases in which vomiting continues, esophageal stricture develops secondary to reflux esophagitis. These authors believed that the stomach above the diaphragm can be identified radiographically by the change of the esophageal to a gastric mucosal pattern above the diaphragm. Although this concept differs from that of Neuhauser and Berenberg,[52] the positional treatment recommended is essentially the same.

Botha[54] described in detail the anatomy of the gastroesophageal region in infants and criticized some of the prevalent ideas of anomalies in this area. He believed that cardia competence and esophageal fixation are better in normal infants than in adults. A partial thoracic stomach that causes vomiting immediately after birth is, according to this author, a major derangement. In the majority of infants with partial thoracic stomach, symptoms date from birth or the early neonatal period, suggesting a congenital origin. Multiple cases have been seen in some families; the condition has occurred in both of twins and in a mother and daughter. That some of the cases of thoracic stomach are to be considered congenital malformations is suggested by the occurrence of associated malformations.[54,55] In a case reported by Williams,[56] a right-sided aortic arch was associated with congenital short esophagus and partial thoracic stomach. Botha[54] believed that patients with chalasia suffer from mild degrees of partial thoracic stomach and that in such cases the cardia is lying in or just above the hiatus. He also believed that many cases of partial thoracic stomach are due to congenital short esophagus.

In 1959, Carré[57] reviewed the natural history of partial thoracic stomach (hiatus hernia) in children and found that changes of symptoms on weaning to solid food provides a useful guide to a patient's prognosis. Approximately two-thirds of all clinically affected and untreated children recover and are free of symptoms by 2 years of age. But about one-third of the children show no improvement when solid food is given, and vomiting persists up to 4 years of age or longer. Approximately 5% of all patients develop an esophageal stricture; they are responsible for the poor prognosis sometimes given for partial thoracic stomach in retrospective reports from surgical clinics. Humphreys *et al.*[50] reported the treatment and course of 34 patients with esophageal hiatus hernia. Of 16 patients treated without operation 12 had fair results; of 18 treated surgically 15 had good results. The two series are not comparable, since in those treated surgically the diagnosis usually was made too late for effective conservative treatment.

REFERENCES

1. Ferguson, C. F.: Congenital tracheoesophageal fistula not associated with atresia of the esophagus, Laryngoscope 61:718, 1951.
2. Haight, C.: Some observations on esophageal atresias and tracheoesophageal fistulas of congenital origin, J. Thoracic Surg. 34:141, 1957.
3. Holder, T. M., and Ashcraft, K. W.: Esophageal Atresia and Tracheo-Esophageal Fistula, in *Current Problems in Surgery* (Chicago: Year Book Medical Publishers, Inc., August, 1966).
4. Durston, W.: A narrative of a monstrous birth in Plymouth, October 22, 1670, together with the anatomical observations taken thereupon by William Durston, Doctor in Physick, and communicated to Dr. Tim Clerk, Philosophical Transactions Roy. Soc. 5:2096, 1670.
5. Gibson, T.: *The Anatomy of Humane Bodies Epitomized* (6th ed.; London: Awnsham & Churchill, 1703).
6. Belsey, R. H. R., and Donnison, C. P.: Congenital atresia of the oesophagus, Brit. M. J. 2:324, 1950.
7. Franklin, R. H.: Congenital atresia of the oesophagus, Lancet 2:243, 1947.
8. Ingalls, T. H., and Prindle, R. A.: Esophageal atresia with tracheo-esophageal fistula; epidemiologic and teratologic implications, New England J. Med. 240:987, 1949.
9. Gross, R. E.: *Surgery of Infancy and Childhood* (Philadelphia: W. B. Saunders Company, 1953).
10. Vogt, E. C.: Congenital esophageal atresia, Am. J. Roentgenol. 22:463, 1929.
11. Haight, C.: Congenital tracheo-esophageal fistula without esophageal atresia, J. Thoracic Surg. 17:600, 1948.
12. Grieve, J. G., and McDermott, J. G.: Congenital atresia of the esophagus in two brothers, Canad. M.A.J. 41:185, 1939.
13. Lanman, T. H.: Congenital atresia of the esophagus: A study of 32 cases, Arch. Surg. 41:1060, 1940.
14. Mackenzie, M.: *A Manual of Diseases of the Throat and Nose including the Pharynx, Larynx, Trachea, Oesophagus, Nose and Nasopharynx.* Vol. II of *Diseases of the Oesophagus, Nose and Nasopharynx* (New York: Wm. Wood & Company, 1884).
15. Hausmann, P. F., Close, A. S., and Williams, L. P.: Occurrence of tracheoesophageal fistula in three consecutive siblings, Surgery 41:542, 1957.
16. Panse, F., and Gierlich, J.: Zur Pathogenese der Anencephalie, Virchows Arch. path. Anat. 316:135, 1949.
17. Ysander, F.: Zur Frage der Genese der Oesophagusatresien. Human Diploterata, Upsala Läkaref. Förh. 30: 195 and 319, 1925.
18. Warkany, J., Passarge, E., and Smith, L. B.: Congenital malformations in autosomal trisomy syndromes, Am. J. Dis. Child. 112:502, 1966.
19. Knox, G.: Secular pattern of congenital oesophageal atresia, Brit. J. Prev. & Social Med. 13:222, 1959.
20. British Reports on Public Health: Deformities caused by thalidomide. Reports on Public Health and Medical Subjects, no. 112:1–70 (London: Her Majesty's Stationery Office, 1964).
21. Warkany, J., Roth, C. B., and Wilson, J. G.: Multiple congenital malformations: A consideration of etiologic factors, Pediatrics 1:462, 1948.
22. Kalter, H., and Warkany, J.: Congenital malformations in inbred strains of mice induced by riboflavin-deficient, galactoflavin-containing diets, J. Exper. Zool. 136:531, 1957.
23. Arey, L. B.: *Human Histology* (Philadelphia: W. B. Saunders Company, 1957).
24. Bremer, J. L.: *Congenital Anomalies of the Viscera. Their Embryological Basis* (Cambridge, Mass.: Harvard University Press, 1957).
25. Rosenthal, A. H.: Congenital atresia of the esophagus with tracheoesophageal fistula. Report of eight cases, Arch. Path. 12:756, 1931.
26. Smith, E. I.: The early development of the trachea and esophagus in relation to atresia of the esophagus and tracheo-esophageal fistula, Carnegie Institution of Washington Pub. 611, Contrib. Embryol. 36:41, 1957.
27. Gruenwald, P.: Case of atresia of esophagus combined with tracheoesophageal fistula in 9-mm. human embryo and its embryological explanation, Anat. Rec. 78:293, 1940.
28. Ware, G. W., and Cross, L. L.: Congenital tracheoesophageal fistula without atresia of the esophagus, Pediatrics 14:254, 1954.
29. Helmsworth, J. A., and Pryles, C. V.: Congenital tracheoesophageal fistula without esophageal atresia, J. Pediat. 38:610, 1951.
30. Berman, J. K., Test, P. S., and McArt, B. A.: Congenital esophagobronchial fistula in an adult, J. Thoracic Surg. 24:493, 1952.
31. Turpin, R., and Cany, J.: Bronchestasies et malformations congénitales; syndrome d'ectasies broncho-oesophagiennes avec fistule oesophago-trachéale et malformations vertébrocostales, Arch. franç. pédiat. 13:798, 1956.
32. Morton, D. R., Osborn, J. F., and Klassen, K. P.: An apparently congenital bronchoesophageal fistula persistent to adult life, J. Thoracic Surg. 19:811, 1950.
33. Frater, R. W. M., and Dowdle, E. B.: Congenital esophagobronchial fistula, Arch. Surg. 89:949, 1964.
34. Higurashi, M., and Shiraki, K.: An unusual case of congenital esophageal atresia, Paediat. Univ. Tokyo, No. 12, pp. 79–84, June, 1966.
35. Roe, B. B., and Nobis, P. D.: Congenital tracheo-esophageal fistula, Am. J. Dis. Child. 106:489, 1963.
36. Mellins, R. B., and Blumenthal, S.: Cardiovascular anomalies and esophageal atresia, Am. J. Dis. Child. 107:160, 1964.
37. Buchs, S.: Über die Missbildung des Herzens und der Gefässe bei den Stenosen und Atresien des Verdauungstraktes, Ann. paediat. 203:256, 1964.

38. Mehrizi, A., Folger, G. M., Jr., and Rowe, R. D.: Tracheo-esophageal fistula associated with congenital cardiovascular malformations, Bull. Johns Hopkins Hosp. 118:246, 1966.
39. Martin, L. W., and Hogg, S. P.: Esophageal atresia and tracheo-esophageal fistula; association with chondromalacia of the larynx and upper trachea, A.M.A. J. Dis. Child. 99:828, 1960.
40. Kučera, J., and Lenz, W.: Caudale Regression mit Oesophagus-atresie und Nierenagenesie – ein Syndrom, Ztschr. Kinderh. 98:326, 1967.
41. Smith, B., Antunes, C., and Han, C. H.: Thumb points to trachea, Seventh Annual Meeting, Teratology Society, Abst. No. 7, p. 43, 1967.
42. Haight, C., and Towsley, H. A.: Congenital atresia of the esophagus with tracheo-esophageal fistula: Extrapleural ligation of fistula and end-to-end anastomosis of esophageal segments, Surg., Gynec. & Obst. 76:672, 1943.
43. Postlethwait, R. W., and Sealy, W. C.: *Surgery of the Esophagus* (Springfield, Ill.: Charles C Thomas, Publisher, 1961).
44. Greenough, W. G.: Congenital esophageal strictures, Am. J. Roentgenol. 92:994, 1964.
45. Adler, R. H.: Congenital esophageal webs, J. Thoracic & Cardiovas. Surg. 45:175, 1963.
46. Diamantopoulos, S.: Zur Kenntnis der Melaena neonatorum mit Ulcus oesophagi, Ztschr. Kinderh. 42:606, 1926.
47. Gruenwald, P., and Marsh, M. R.: Acute esophagitis in infants, Arch. Path. 49:1, 1950.
48. Sullivan, B. H., Jr., Geppert, L. J., and Ranson, R. F.: Esophageal ulcer in very young infants, A.M.A. Am. J. Dis. Child. 87:49, 1954.
49. Chunn, V. D., and Geppert, L. J.: Spontaneous rupture of the esophagus in the newborn, J. Pediat. 60:404, 1962.
50. Humphreys, G. H., Wiedel, P. D., Baker, D. H. and Berdon, W. E.: Esophageal hiatus hernia in infancy and childhood, Pediatrics 36:351, 1965.
51. Silverman, F. N.: Gastroesophageal incompetence, partial intrathoracic stomach and vomiting in infancy, Radiology 64:664, 1955.
52. Neuhauser, E. B. D., and Berenberg, W.: Cardio-esophageal relaxation as cause of vomiting in infants, Radiology 48:480, 1947.
53. Astley, R., and Carré, I. J.: Gastro-oesophageal incompetence in children with special reference to minor degrees of partial thoracic stomach, Radiology 62:351, 1954.
54. Botha, G. S. M.: The gastro-oesophageal region in infants; observations on the anatomy, with special reference to the closing mechanism and partial thoracic stomach, Arch. Dis. Childhood 33:78, 1958.
55. Radloff, F. F., and King, R. L.: Esophageal hiatus hernia, Gastroenterology 9:249, 1947.
56. Williams, E. R.: A case of right-sided aortic arch associated with congenital short oesophagus and partial thoracic stomach, Brit. J. Radiol. 18:323, 1945.
57. Carré, I. J.: The natural history of the partial thoracic stomach (hiatus hernia) in children, Arch. Dis. Childhood 34:344, 1959.

75

The Stomach

Congenital Gastric Obstruction

THE STOMACH is the least frequent site of congenital obstruction of the alimentary canal. Only 12 cases of complete congenital gastric obstruction were found in the literature by Lafer and Kottmeier.[1] Such obstructions are caused by mucosal diaphragms, gastric atresia, pyloric atresia or pyloric duplication.[43] Intermittent or incomplete gastric obstruction can be due to gastric cysts or ulcers, incomplete mucosal diaphragms, congenital hypertrophic pyloric stenosis and internal herniation.

Complete obstruction results in persistent vomiting of nonbilious material; the stomach is distended in most instances, and there is no air within the distal intestine.

Congenital Prepyloric Gastric Atresia

Whereas hypertrophic pyloric stenosis is a frequent anomaly, intrinsic congenital obstruction of the stomach is extremely rare. In 1940, Touroff and Sussman[2] described a case, then unique, of congenital gastric obstruction due to a complete prepyloric septum of mucous membrane in a premature female infant. The mother was 28 years of age and the pregnancy was complicated by marked polyhydramnios. The presenting symptoms commenced at birth and were those of high obstruction. Roentgenographic examination showed the presence of an obstructive lesion in the distal portion of the stomach or first portion of the duodenum. Operation performed on the fifth day of life consisted of multiple incisions of the prepyloric septum and pyloroplasty. A similar case was reported in 1951 by Benson and Coury.[3] A 4-day-old female infant, weighing 2,724 Gm. and delivered of a hydramniotic mother, vomited all feedings immediately after birth, and developed dehydration and distention. On laparotomy, the entire duodenum and the remaining portion of the gastrointestinal tract were collapsed and free of gas. A gastrotomy was performed and a diaphragm was excised at the prepyloric area. Eventually, an anterior gastroenterostomy had to be performed in the fourth week of life. Anders[4] pointed out that physiologic proliferation of epithelium does not occur in the gastric mucosa, so it cannot be used for explanation of congenital stenosis and atresia of the stomach. Brown and Hertzler[5] reported 2 cases and reviewed the literature up to 1959. Two cases of prepyloric septa were recorded by Rowling.[6]

Hypertrophic Pyloric Stenosis

Hypertrophic pyloric stenosis probably is not a congenital malformation but, rather, a functional anomaly of the pyloric sphincter that is present at or soon after birth. Affected children usually are free of other congenital malformations, but there are interesting familial accumulations in some of the cases. For this reason, this disturbance of the neonatal period is mentioned briefly here.

Hypertrophic pyloric stenosis is a well-known anomaly of infancy. It may be present in some form at birth, but manifestations usually are not noticeable until 2 or 3 weeks after birth. The pylorus shows hypertrophy of its circular musculature, compression of its mucosa and obstruction of its lumen. The mucosa in affected infants under 1 week of age is essentially normal but, later, edema of the mucosa becomes noticeable and its thickening contributes to the obstruction. Gross[7] believed that the secondary reactions of the mucosa explain why infants do not exhibit signs of obstruction until they are 1 or 2 weeks of age, even though the hypertrophied muscle is present at or before birth. Wallgren[8] showed, by routine roentgen examination of 1,000 newborn infants, that babies who later developed pyloric stenosis had a normal roentgenographic pattern immediately after birth. Belding and Kernohan[9] found the number of myenteric ganglion cells and nerve fiber tracts per unit area to be reduced in the pyloric region of affected infants. The majority of myenteric ganglion cells in the pylorus showed degenerative changes resembling those seen after excessive vagus stimulation. Such changes were not seen in the myenteric ganglion cells of the stomach above the pylorus or in the duodenum or in normal individuals. These degenerative changes differed from the congenital absence of myenteric ganglion cells in the affected portion of congenital megacolon. Friesen *et al.*[10] thought that immaturity of ganglion cells rather than paucity was at fault, whereas Zuelzer (cited by Benson[11]) failed to see any significant change in the ganglion cells. Rintoul and Kirkman[12] distinguished type I and type II neurons in the pyloric myenteric plexus of normal children; type I neurons were virtually absent in the pylorus of children with hypertrophic stenosis.

The etiology of pyloric stenosis is a controversial subject. The condition is not analogous to megacolon and there is no reason to believe that it is caused by injury to the central nervous system. There are suggestive facts that point to genetic and other observations that point to nongenetic determinants. Several investigations showed a considerable familial accumulation of the disorder. The incidence varies in different countries and races. It is approximately 3 per 1,000 in England, 4 per 1,000 in Sweden and 1.5 per 1,000 in Scotland. It is 1.26 per 1,000 among white children in Pittsburgh, Pa., but only 0.48 per 1,000 among Negro children in that city.[13] Nielsen[14] ascertained an incidence of 4.2% in the siblings of patients with this disorder, whereas in a comparable control group no siblings were affected. McKeown *et al.*[15] found 5.8% of the siblings born after the propositi affected with pyloric stenosis, whereas the incidence in the general population in Birmingham, England, was 0.3%. Thus, in siblings born after the first affected individual, the incidence was about nineteen times that in the general newborn population. In the same study, the incidence in parents did not seem to be unusually high. But Nielsen,[14] in examining the offspring of individuals who had been treated in infancy for congenital pyloric stenosis, found that 8.6% had the disorder, whereas in a comparable group of control parents only 0.7% of the children were affected. A number of single families have been reported with an unusually high incidence. Gailey[16] saw congenital hypertrophic pyloric stenosis in 4 brothers and, in a family reported by Fenwick,[17] 4 males in two generations were affected. The father of 2 affected boys had manifestations of pyloric stenosis as an adult and in one case the disorder seemed to be transmitted to the son through an unaffected mother. The same author quoted the case of a patient whose father and grandfather both suffered from pyloric stenosis in adult life. Laubscher and Smith[18] reviewed the literature of pyloric stenosis in twins. They noted that when a monovular twin is affected, the other twin probably will be affected also; there were two exceptions to this rule in 13 sets. When a binovular twin is affected, the other twin probably will not be affected; there were two exceptions in 23 sets of binovular twin pairs, and the authors themselves reported an exception of this kind. They stated that twins have approximately the same chance of having pyloric stenosis as infants born singly. These facts do not permit a simple explanation of the etiology of this disorder. Cockayne and Penrose[19] attributed pyloric stenosis to a recessive gene, the manifestation of which is affected by sex and parity, but McKeown *et al.*[20] disagreed with this interpretation. Cockayne and Penrose arrived at their conclusions because they found the proportion of patients with consanguineous parents exceeding expectation and an increased incidence of pyloric stenosis in cousins of affected individuals. The observed incidence of pyloric stenosis in siblings born after an affected child was 1 in 20, an observation that had to be reconciled with the expected incidence of a recessive condition of 1 to 4 by assuming that manifestation is maximal in first-born males but low in later males and in all females. The data of McKeown *et al.*[15] differed from these observations. The proportion of patients with consanguineous parents was not above that in the general population. The observed incidence of pyloric stenosis in cousins was in close agreement with the incidence in the general newborn population. These findings were not considered consistent with the hypothesis that the condition is a Mendelian recessive unless it was attributed to a very common gene of low manifestation that requires an unusual environment. These authors thought that there is a good deal to suggest that the environment is of considerable importance and in 1952[20] they supported their hypothesis by the finding that birth rank plays no role in infants who have manifestations immediately after birth, whereas those with later manifestations show a raised incidence of first births. The onset of symptoms was also earlier in home births than in hospital births. Carter[21] admitted the importance of unknown environmental factors but stressed a predisposing genotype of two components. First, a common dominant gene and, second, a sex-modified multifactorial background. Of great interest are his data concerning the children of patients with pyloric stenosis. Males who survived the disorder had 7% affected boys and 1.5% affected girls. The rare females who had had the disease had 24% affected boys and 4% affected girls. Girls were four times less susceptible than boys but those who were affected had four times as many affected children.[22] MacMahon *et al.*,[23] in a statistical study in Birmingham, England, noted that the incidence of diagnosed cases varied between 3 and 4 per 1,000 live births. Males accounted for 82% of the patients. There was no evidence of increased associated malformations. Knox[24] tested the hypothesis of sex linkage by explaining both the sex ratio of the disorder and the disturbed sex ratio in the parents' siblings, but conclusions derived from the data available were essentially negative.

Occasional mention of pyloric stenosis was made in the older literature on Down syndrome. Association of pyloric stenosis with Hirschsprung disease existed in a male infant with multiple anomalies and an extra chromosome similar in size to no. 16.[25]

It is of interest that there were 7 cases of spastic pyloric hypertrophy among 41 children with internal anomalies attributable to thalidomide damage reported by Kreipe.[26]

Congenital adrenal hypoplasia can manifest itself by symptoms similar to those of pyloric stenosis and, in some cases, the two conditions can occur together (p. 428).

Surgical treatment by the Ramstedt[27] operation generally is practiced with excellent results. Mack[41] published an account of the history of surgical treatment of the condition, and more recent descriptions of the surgical procedures are available.[7, 11]

Congenital Defect of Gastric Musculature and Perforation

Congenital defect of the gastric musculature with spontaneous perforation was described by Braunstein.[28] Rupture of the stomach is rare at birth, and of the cases described only a few were due to congenital defects in the gastric wall. Braunstein observed 5 cases of ruptured stomach in infants. Four of these were encountered in necropsies and 1 was found during surgical exploration. Symptoms consist of respiratory difficulty and cyanosis, abdominal distention, watery discharge from the nose and mouth and regurgitation of gastric contents. Roentgenographic evidence of free air in the peritoneal cavity in the upright position is an important diagnostic feature. Immediate recognition, surgical exploration and repair offer the only chance for survival. Shaw *et al.*[29] doubted that congenital absence of the gastric musculature is the cause of spontaneous perforation of the neonatal stomach. There are potential weak points between interlacing muscle bundles in the gastric wall of the newborn that may lead to rupture with distention strong enough to force apart the muscle bundles in one area of the stomach wall. An alternative explanation is that neonatal asphyxia leading to vascular damage is the cause of the perforation,[11] but a case of prenatal gastric perforation was reported by Sanz *et al.*[30]

Duplication

Goon,[31] in 1953, found only 11 cases of duplication of the stomach in the literature, and in 1957 Kiesewetter[32] noted 28 cases in the English literature. Berg and Marx[33] reported a case of pyloric obstruction secondary to partial duplication of the stomach. The presenting findings were those of high intestinal obstruction with vomiting, marked dehydration and a palpable epigastric mass. Duplications of the stomach may extend into the chest. Duplication of the pylorus has been observed as a rare cause of gastric outlet obstruction.[43] Goon[31] described a boy 2 months of age who had a mass about the size of a tennis ball in the upper quadrant of the abdomen. Roentgenograms revealed a mass below the diaphragm and irregular round masses in the mediastinum coursing behind the heart and displacing the esophagus anteriorly. There also were defective vertebral bodies and hemivertebrae in the lower cervical and upper dorsal regions. Duplication of the stomach and multicystic kidney have been found in an infant with Turner syndrome.[42] Gould and Toffler[34] recorded a case in a 29-year-old man who had been in excellent health until 4 months prior to admission to an Army hospital. Burning epigastric pains were the presenting symptom.

Gastric Diverticula

Ogur and Kolarsick[35] pointed out that few reports on this anomaly deal with the pediatric age group even though true diverticula are considered congenital. They contain all layers of the gastric wall. In adults, the location varies; most diverticula occur either on the posterior wall near the lesser curvature and the cardia or adjacent to the pylorus. Only 6 reports of gastric diverticula were found by Ogur and Kolarsick in children but they added 2 cases of their own. Presenting complaints ranged from signs of intestinal obstruction, hematemesis and passage of blood by bowel to periumbilical pain, but some patients were asymptomatic. In one newborn infant of Ogur and Kolarsick's a diverticulum resulted in intussusception into the stomach, causing gangrene, perforation and peritonitis.

Situs Inversus

In total situs inversus, the stomach is situated on the left side. Almy *et al.*[36] estimated that complete transposition of the viscera occurs once in approximately 6,000–8,000 persons. Partial situs inversus is less frequent.

Isolated situs inversus of the stomach is an extremely rare anomaly. Almy *et al.*[36] described such a case, which was suspected at cholecystectomy and later confirmed by repeated x-ray studies. The affected woman was 56 years of age when the anomaly was found accidentally at operation.

Enterogenous Cysts

Lyall,[37] in 1952, found only 8 cases reported in the literature and added a ninth case—a boy 9 years of age. Recurring vomiting, loss of weight and dehydration were presenting symptoms, so that a provisional diagnosis of intussusception was made. At operation, the distal half of the stomach was found to be replaced by a firm mass thought to be a solid tumor occupying the pyloric half of the stomach. It was found that the pyloric end of the stomach was filled by a mass growing into it from above, and sections revealed that the mass consisted of two cysts that were connected by an opening. The pyloric half of the stomach was reduced to a narrow slit. The wall of the cysts was lined by columnar epithelium.

Teratoma

Tridermal teratoma of the stomach occurring in infancy is extremely rare. The first case probably was described by Selman[38] in a 3-month-old infant who had a nonsymptomatic palpable mass at routine pediatric examination. A second case was described by Large *et al.*[39] in a 7-month-old infant with hematemesis and melena. X-ray studies of the barium-filled stomach showed a large, smooth defect protruding into the gastric lumen. On operation, a cystic tumor confined to the wall of the stomach was found. At first, this tumor was believed to be a reduplication of the stomach. On histologic examination, the tumor was a complex, well-differentiated structure, presenting a disorderly conglomeration of tissues deriving from all three germ layers.

Polyposis

Halsted *et al.*[40] pointed out the possible involvement of the stomach in familial polyposis of the gastrointestinal tract. Usually, patients with this disorder consult a physician because of symptoms originating in the colon, the stomach polyps, as a rule, being symptomless. In one kinship, polyposis involving both the colon and stomach occurred in 2 brothers, an uncle and a son. It has not been decided whether malignant degeneration in the stomach occurs frequently in patients with familial diffuse polyposis.

REFERENCES

1. Lafer, D. J., and Kottmeier, P. K.: Congenital gastric obstruction; case report and subject review, Am. J. Dis. Child. 107:202, 1964.
2. Touroff, A. S. W., and Sussman, R. M.: Congenital prepyloric membranous obstruction in a premature infant, Surgery 8:739, 1940.
3. Benson, C. D., and Coury, J. J.: Congenital intrinsic obstruction of the stomach and duodenum in the newborn, A.M.A. Arch. Surg. 62:856, 1951.
4. Anders, H. E.: Die Missbildungen des Darmkanals und der Verdauungsdrüsen, einschliesslich der Kloakenmissbildungen, in Schwalbe, E. (ed.), *Die Morphologie der Missbildungen des Menschen und der Tiere* (Jena: Gustav Fischer, 1928).
5. Brown, R. P., and Hertzler, J. H.: Congenital prepyloric gastric atresia. A report of two cases, A.M.A. J. Dis. Child. 97:857, 1959.
6. Rowling, J. T.: The prepyloric septum; a rare anomaly, Brit. J. Surg. 47:162, 1959.
7. Gross, R. E.: *The Surgery of Infancy and Childhood* (Philadelphia: W. B. Saunders Company, 1953).
8. Wallgren, A.: Preclinical stage of infantile hypertrophic pyloric stenosis, Am. J. Dis. Child. 72:371, 1946.
9. Belding, H. H., and Kernohan, J. W.: A morphologic study of the myenteric plexus and musculature of the pylorus with special reference to the changes in hypertrophic pyloric stenosis, Surg., Gynec. & Obst. 97:322, 1953.
10. Friesen, S. R., Boley, J. O., and Miller, D. R.: The myenteric plexus of the pylorus: Its early normal development and its changes in hypertrophic pyloric stenosis, Surgery 39:21, 1956.
11. Benson, C. D.: Infantile Hypertrophic Pyloric Stenosis, in Mustard, W. T., Ravitch, M. M., Snyder, W. H., Jr., Welch, K. J., and Benson, C. D. (eds.), *Pediatric Surgery* (2d ed.; Chicago: Year Book Medical Publishers, Inc., 1969), p. 818.
12. Rintoul, J. R., and Kirkman, N. F.: The myenteric plexus in infantile hypertrophic pyloric stenosis, Arch. Dis. Childhood 36:474, 1961.
13. Laron, Z., and Horne, L. M.: The incidence of infantile pyloric stenosis, A.M.A. J. Dis. Child. 94:151, 1957.
14. Nielsen, O. S.: Familial predisposition to congenital pyloric stenosis, Acta paediat. 43:522, 1954.
15. McKeown, T., MacMahon, B., and Record, R. G.: The familial incidence of congenital pyloric stenosis, Ann. Eugenics 16:260, 1951.

16. Gailey, A. A. H.: Congenital hypertrophic pyloric stenosis. Report of 4 cases in brothers, Brit. M. J. 1:100, 1948.
17. Fenwick, T.: Familial hypertrophic pyloric stenosis, Brit. M. J. 2:12, 1953.
18. Laubscher, J. H., and Smith, A. M.: Pyloric stenosis in twins. Review of the literature and report of a case, Am. J. Dis. Child. 73:334, 1947.
19. Cockayne, E. A., and Penrose, L. S.: The genetics of congenital pyloric stenosis, Ohio J. Sc. 43:1, 1943.
20. McKeown, T., MacMahon, B., and Record, R. G.: Evidence of post-natal environmental influence in the aetiology of infantile pyloric stenosis, Arch. Dis. Childhood 27:386, 1952.
21. Carter, C. O.: The inheritance of congenital pyloric stenosis, Brit. M. Bull. 17:251, 1961.
22. Fraser Roberts, J. A.: Inherited Diseases, in Burdette, W. J. (ed.), *Methodology in Human Genetics* (San Francisco: Holden-Day, Inc., 1962).
23. MacMahon, B., Record, R. G., and McKeown, T.: Congenital pyloric stenosis. An investigation of 578 cases, Brit. J. Social Med. 5:185, 1951.
24. Knox, G.: On the nature of the determinants of congenital pyloric stenosis, Brit. J. Prev. & Social Med. 12:188, 1958.
25. Butler, L. J., France, N. E., Russell, A., and Sinclair, L.: A chromosomal aberration associated with multiple congenital anomalies, Lancet 1:1242, 1962.
26. Kreipe, U.: Missbildungen innerer Organe bei Thalidomidembryopathie, Arch. Kinderh. 176:33, 1967.
27. Ramstedt, C.: Zur Operation der angeborenen Pylorusstenose, Med. Klin. 8:1702, 1912.
28. Braunstein, H.: Congenital defect of the gastric musculature with spontaneous perforation, J. Pediat. 44:55, 1954.
29. Shaw, A., Blanc, W. A., Santulli, T. V., and Kaiser, G.: Spontaneous rupture of the stomach in the newborn. A clinical and experimental study, Surgery 58:561, 1965.
30. Sanz, S., Corral, T., Laplana, R., and Tejedor, F. R.: Perforación gástrica neonatal, Bol. Soc. vasco-nav. pediat. 2:41, 1967.
31. Goon, C. D.: Duplication of the stomach with extension into the chest, Am. Surgeon 19:721, 1953.
32. Kiesewetter, W. B.: Duplication of the stomach. A case report, Am. Surgeon 146:990, 1957.
33. Berg, H. F., and Marx, K.: Duplication of the stomach, J. Pediat. 40:334, 1952.
34. Gould, R. J., and Toffler, A. H.: Duplication of the stomach; a case report, Radiology 76:790, 1961.
35. Ogur, G. L., and Kolarsick, A. J.: Gastric diverticula in infancy, J. Pediat. 39:723, 1951.
36. Almy, M. A., Volk, F. H., and Graney, C. M.: Situs inversus of stomach, Radiology 61:376, 1953.
37. Lyall, A.: Enterogenous cyst of the stomach, Brit. J. Surg. 40:286, 1952.
38. Selman, A. N.: Complex tridermal teratoma of stomach (benign); case report, Am. J. Surg. 59:567, 1943.
39. Large, H. L., Jr., Williams, M., and Neel, J. B.: Gastric tridermal teratoma in infancy, J.A.M.A. 149:824, 1952.
40. Halsted, J. A., Harris, E. G., and Bartlett, M. K.: Involvement of the stomach in familial polyposis of the gastrointestinal tract; report of a family, Gastroenterology 15:763, 1950.
41. Mack, H. C.: A history of hypertrophic pyloric stenosis and its treatment, Bull. Hist. Med. 12:465, 595, 666, 1942.
42. Liebert, P. S.: Gastric duplication and multicystic kidney associated with gonadal dysgenesis, Clin. Pediat. 9:60, 1970.
43. Grosfeld, J. L., Boles, E. T., Jr., and Reiner, C.: Duplication of pylorus in the newborn: A rare cause of gastric outlet obstruction, J. Pediat. Surg. 5:365, 1970.

76

The Intestine

Rotation and Malrotation of the Intestine

In embryos of the fourth week, the midgut is in free communication with the yolk sac (Fig. 76-1, *A*), but soon the communication becomes reduced in size to the narrow vitello-intestinal duct within the yolk stalk. At first, the whole midgut is attached closely to the posterior abdominal wall by a short mesentery,[1] but this portion of the gut, from which a large part of the duodenum, jejunum, ileum, cecum, ascending colon and the right and middle thirds of the transverse colon develop, shows a marked growth and rearrangement in position in the second and third month of embryonic life. In a 5-week (10 mm.) embryo, the intestine grows faster than the abdominal cavity, so that a loop formed of the midgut extends into the extra-embryonic coelom of the umbilical cord

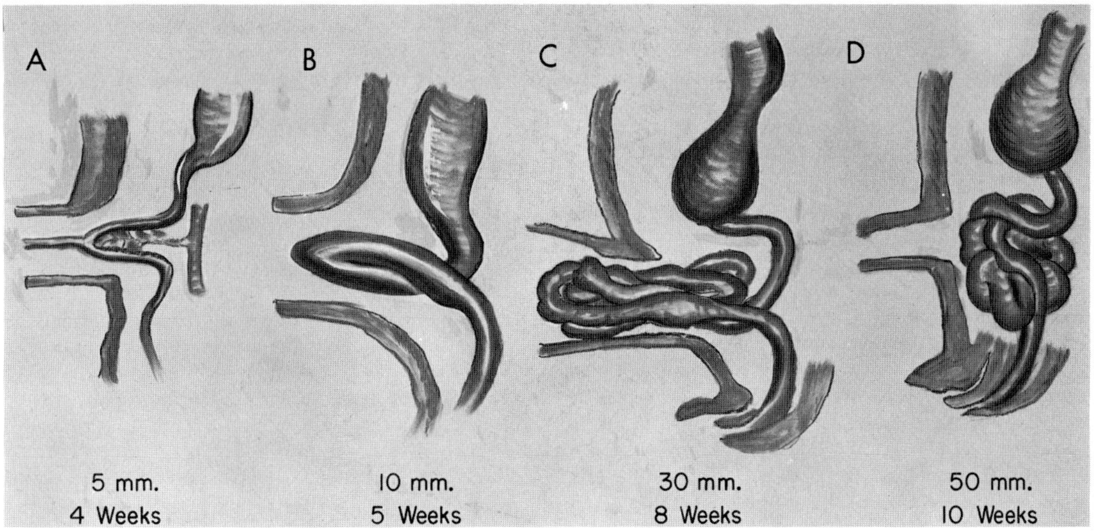

Fig. 76-1. – Diagram showing development of the midgut.

(Fig. 76-1, *B*). At first, this loop has a cranial (proximal) and a caudal (distal) limb, with the yolk stalk at its apex. The corresponding mesentery and the vitelline arteries accompany the extended intestinal loop. Thus, the loop is free and movable, whereas its cephalic and caudal ends are fixed to the posterior abdominal wall, the cranial point of fixation being the duodenum at the level of the papilla and the caudal fixation being a retention band at the colic angle of the upper end of the hindgut. The duodenum and the colic angle are close to each other, so that the two limbs of the midgut loop are attached to two points of the narrow duodenocolic isthmus through which the superior mesenteric artery passes to the distal end of the loop – the vitelline duct.[2]

From the cephalic limb of the umbilical loop between the proximal fixation and the yolk stalk, the jejunum and the greater part of the ileum are formed. The caudal limb between the attachment of the yolk stalk and the point of junction with the hindgut is converted into the terminal portion of the ileum, cecum, appendix, ascending colon and most of the transverse colon. The growth and positioning of the midgut usually are described in three stages of "rotation." The first rotation occurs while the loop lies in the umbilical cord, the second movement during its return into the abdominal cavity at about the tenth embryonic week and the third adjustment from then to well after birth.

In embryos of approximately 7 weeks, the cephalic part of the loop shows distinct enlargement and coiling, the intestinal convolutions occupying mainly the right portion of the extra-embryonic coelomic sac. At about the same time, a counterclockwise (from the observer's point of view) rotation of the loop around its sagittal axis (represented by the superior mesenteric artery) occurs through 90 degrees, so that the cranial limb comes to lie to the (embryo's) right side of the umbilical sac and the caudal limb to its left (first stage of rotation). The intestinal protrusion into the extra-embryonic coelom is at its maximum at 9 weeks and a partial return of the small intestine occurs at 10 weeks. The withdrawal of the intestinal loops into the abdominal cavity in embryos of approximately 45 mm. – in the third lunar month – involves most of the coils of the small intestine with the exception of the caudal loop and the cecum, which enter the abdominal cavity somewhat later. The derivatives of the cranial portion of the intestinal loops occupy the lower and posterior part of the abdominal cavity, whereas the caudal loop and its derivatives normally are situated superior and ventral to the parts developed from the cranial loop. As the cecum returns into the abdomen, it lies at first in the umbilical area but soon it migrates upward and to the right, assuming a position below the right lobe of the liver. This change involves a further rotation by the umbilical loop around the superior mesenteric artery. When this second stage of rotation terminates, the intestinal loop has performed a counterclockwise turn of 270 degrees about the axis of the superior mesenteric artery from the original sagittal position of the midgut loop.[2]

The third stage of "rotation" involves the elongation of the ascending colon in mid-fetal life, leading to descent of the cecum into the right iliac fossa. It also involves fixation of portions of the intestine to the posterior abdominal wall by fusion of their mesenteries with the posterior parietal peritoneum. During this final fixation, the lower part of the duodenum becomes fixed by fusion of its mesentery with the posterior parietal peritoneum. After the descent of the cecum and ascending colon, the greater part of their mesentery disappears by fusing with the peritoneum of the right posterior abdominal wall. The part of the midgut distal to the hepatic flexure and the proximal portion of the hindgut form the transverse colon, which retains its mesentery and stretches across the abdominal cavity. The left end of the transverse colon located at the splenic flexure joins the descending colon, which, as the pelvic colon and rectum, is derived from the hindgut. The mesentery of the descending colon fuses with the peritoneum of the left posterior abdominal wall but the pelvic colon retains its mesentery.

In many cases, this normal pattern has not become established at birth. The cecum may lie in the upper right quadrant or under the ensiform cartilage, or even to the left side. In such cases, the whole colon has lengthened too slowly and the primarily caudal limb of the original midgut loop is composed chiefly of ileum with little colon. The malpositions may persist because of the formation of adhesions or they may be corrected by the continued lengthening of the proximal colon and the shifting of the cecum to a more normal site.

In the formation of the midgut loop and the rapid lengthening of its intestinal portions, a relatively constricted mesenteric base is provided for a large area, and the later rotation of the loop twists this space or pedicle and reduces its linear extent still further. If this situation is accentuated abnormally, there is danger of volvulus, by twisting of a portion of the intestine on itself, with occlusion of the lumen or interference with the blood supply.[3]

Incomplete rotation and fixation of the intestine account for a number of conditions requiring surgical intervention. Snyder and Chaffin[4] established, in a series of abdominal operations performed in infants and children, that the incidence of malrotation accounted for 1%. Gross[5] reported on the treatment of 156 patients with malrotation. Approximately half the children with this anomaly develop symptoms during the neonatal period. The remainder have manifestations later in childhood or during adult life.[6] In some persons, malrotation remains symptomless and the condition is recognized accidentally. Males are affected more often than females. Mobile cecum has been reported in 3 members of a family.[7] Malrotation of the intestine has been reported in patients with Marfan syndrome (p. 850),[8] a condition inherited as a dominant trait. It has been seen repeatedly in children with de Lange syndrome (p. 344). Intestinal malrotation should be suspected in cases of trisomy 18, since it is found in approximately 15% of necropsies of these children.[9] Anomalies of mesenteric attachment also occur in children with trisomy 21 who have congenital duodenal atresia.[10] Gustavson *et al.*[15] described a patient with malrotation of the intestine, anal atresia and other malformations who had a karyotype interpreted as a no. 4 or 5/21 or 22 translocation.

Dott[2] and Gripenberg[11] classified the anomalies of intestinal rotation according to the three stages discussed. If development is arrested in the first stage, with the entire intestinal loop outside the peritoneal cavity, the newborn child has, at the site of the navel, a protrusion covered by a thin membrane from the top of which the umbilical cord arises (omphalocele, p. 758). The protrusion contains intestines that lie in a position corresponding to the first stage of rotation. In addition, it may contain a large abnormal liver and sometimes also the spleen. Dott[2] believed that failure in the first stage occurs in relation to extroversion of the cloaca. Disturbances in the second stage can manifest themselves in a variety of anomalies. Nonrotation of the midgut loop results in abnormal position of the intestinal parts. The small intestine may be found on the right side, the terminal portion of the ileum crossing the midline toward the cecum, which is situated in the left iliac fossa or in the pelvis. The colon ascends on the left side parallel to the distal portions of the colon. These abnormally situated viscera have abnormal fixation and abnormal mesenteries. The cecum usually remains mobile and sometimes the entire midgut loop may remain unaffixed. Dott[2] believed that in such cases an abnormal return into the abdominal cavity has taken place, the colon and cecum preceding the small intestine. A monograph on the anomalies of intestinal rotation and fixation was written by Estrada.[6]

Nonrotation may remain symptomless in postnatal life or lead to clinical manifestations. Failure of intestinal fixation resulting in volvulus is a typical consequence of nonrotation.[2] Volvulus causes obstruction of the alimentary tract by twisting of the intestine around its rudimentary attachment. At the same time, the superior mesenteric vessels may be occluded, leading to infarction of the midgut.

Reversed rotation is a rare anomaly attributable to an error in the second stage of rotation. There, a 90-degree clockwise rotation occurs instead of the normal 270-degree counterclockwise rotation, and, as a result, the prearterial loop becomes situated ventral to the postarterial loop. Some portion between the cecum and the transverse colon lies behind the duodenum. This anomaly may remain symptomless or be complicated by volvulus of the mobile right half of the colon. It may result in a volvulus around the superior mesenteric root and lead to compression of the transverse colon or to obstruction of the duodenojejunal junction. Warthen *et al.*[12] reviewed the cases reported in the literature, adding a case of their own.

The abnormalities of the so-called third stage of malrotation consist of defective or abnormal fixation. Gripenberg[11] distinguished hypofixation and hyperfixation, which predispose to volvulus or to obstruction by abnormal adhesions. Such abnormal fixations are in all probability, and in the majority of cases, consequences of earlier errors of rotation.

Mobile cecum is a minor anomaly that belongs in this chapter. A free cecum in the presence of an attached ascending colon may be normally placed but associated with an unattached mesentery of the proximal portion of the small intestine. A mobile cecum occurs in approximately 10% of all persons without causing pathologic manifestations.[7] However, it may contribute to intussusceptions in infants, which occur with greatest frequency in the ileocolic region. In 17 cases of intussusception Kaufmann[7] found 9 with a mobile cecum and abnormal mesentery. Unusual mobility of the cecum may lead to volvulus. It is of interest that in such cases the congenital anomaly leads to complications in adult life. Patients more than 60 or 70 years of age have been described with cecal volvulus due to mobile cecum. Other complications are repeated and transitory attacks of torsion with colicky pain or chronic inflammatory changes that are attributed to fecal stasis. Inflammation may lead to formation of pericolic membranes and bands that, in turn, can cause obstruction.

Fixation of the cecum apparently is associated with the upright gait of man, since in lower mammals a free cecum occurs normally.[7]

Malrotation often is associated with other malformations, especially those of the urogenital tract.[13] Mesenteric cysts have been observed repeatedly in cases of malrotation.[14] Gross[5] recorded esophageal atresia, pyloric stenosis, duodenal stenosis or atresia, biliary obstruction, annular pancreas and omphalocele as complicating congenital anomalies in 156 patients operated on for malrotation. From the surgeon's point of view, treatment is required in approximately half the children who develop symptoms within the first month of life.[5] In babies, the symptoms usually are those of obstruction demanding immediate surgery. In older children, the symptoms often are intermittent abdominal pain, nausea and vomiting that can lead to a picture of chronic malnutrition and illness. In rare instances, a clinical picture resembling the celiac syndrome may result from malrotation.[5] Because of their irregularity, the symptoms often were considered in older children and adults as psychosomatic or "hysteric."

REFERENCES

1. Hamilton, W. J., Boyd, J. D., and Mossman, H. W.: *Human Embryology* (Baltimore: The Williams & Wilkins Company, 1945).
2. Dott, N. M.: Anomalies of intestinal rotation; their embryology and surgical aspects, Brit. J. Surg. 11:251, 1923.
3. Bremer, J. L.: *Congenital Anomalies of the Viscera–Their Embryologic Basis* (Cambridge, Mass.: Harvard University Press, 1957).
4. Snyder, W. H., Jr., and Chaffin, L.: Embryology and pathology of the intestinal tract: Presentation of 40 cases of malrotation, Ann. Surg. 140:368, 1954.
5. Gross, R. E.: *The Surgery of Infancy and Childhood* (Philadelphia: W. B. Saunders Company, 1953).
6. Estrada, R. L.: *Anomalies of Intestinal Rotation and Fixation* (Springfield, Ill.: Charles C Thomas, Publisher, 1958).
7. Kaufmann, H.: Das Coecum mobile im Kindesalter, Ann. paediat. 179:136, 1952.
8. Ross, L. J.: Arachnodactyly. Review of recent literature and report of a case with cleft palate, Am. J. Dis. Child. 78:417, 1949.
9. Warkany, J., Passarge, E., and Smith, L. B.: Congenital malformations in autosomal trisomy syndromes, Am. J. Dis. Child. 112:502, 1966.
10. Bodian, M., White, L. L. R., Carter, C. O., and Louw, J. H.: Congenital duodenal obstruction and mongolism, Brit. M. J. 1:77, 1952.
11. Gripenberg, L.: On the anomalies of intestinal rotation, Acta chir. scandinav. 104:261, 1952.
12. Warthen, R. O., Lattman, I., and White, C. S.: Reversed rotation of the bowel. Review of the literature and report of an unusual case, A.M.A. Am. J. Dis. Child. 83:487, 1952.
13. Potter, E. L.: *Pathology of the Fetus and the Newborn* (Chicago: Year Book Medical Publishers, Inc., 1952).
14. Bentley, J. F. R., and O'Donnell, M. B.: Mesenteric cysts with malrotated intestine, Brit. M. J. 2:223, 1959.
15. Gustavson, K-H., Finley, S. C., Finley, W. H., and Jalling, B.: A 4-5/21-22 chromosomal translocation associated with multiple congenital anomalies, Acta paediat. 53: 172, 1964.

Underdevelopment of the Intestine

Lack of differentiation or lack of development of large gastrointestinal parts usually is limited to unviable children with severe malformations. Defective intestines have been described in acardii, in conjoined twins and in a sirenomelus.[1,2] Bennington and Haber[3] reported failure of the primitive gut to differentiate into small and large intestines in a child who reached the newborn period. There is a report on an adult male whose small intestine was directly connected with the rectum.[4]

REFERENCES

1. Anders, H. E.: Die Missbildungen des Darmkanals und der Verdauungsdrüsen einschliesslich der Kloakenmissbildungen, in Schwalbe, E. (ed.), *Die Morphologie der Missbildungen des Menschen und der Tiere* (Jena: Gustav Fischer, 1928), Vol. 3, pt. 12–15, Chap. 4, pp. 375–482.
2. Dodek, S. M., and Friedman, J. M.: A sirenomelian monster, J. Internat. Coll. Surgeons 14:226, 1950.
3. Bennington, J., and Haber, S. L.: The embryologic significance of an undifferentiated intestinal tract, J. Pediat. 64: 735, 1964.
4. Morton, J.: Congenital absence of the colon, Brit. M. J. 1: 1118, 1912.

Congenital Atresias of the Intestine

CONGENITAL ATRESIAS of the intestine are serious anomalies that result in early death if unattended. Incidence figures vary greatly according to sampling,[1] but it is known that congenital atresias are more common in the small intestine than in the large. Approximately 15% of all atresias seem to be multiple.[2] More than 50% of Gross's series[3] of 140 patients with intestinal atresia had an ileal obstruction, 23% were duodenal and 13% were jejunal. The remainder were colonic, ileocecal or multiple. Associated anomalies were found in approximately half the patients with duodenal atresia by Moore and Stokes.[4] In Gross's series, 2 of 15 infants who survived operation for duodenal atresia had Down syndrome. The incidence of congenital malformations associated with jejunal or ileal obstruction was 65%, but these complications were rarer in the series of de Lorimier *et al.*[29] Among maternal complications, polyhydramnios is outstanding.[29]

Opinions concerning etiology and pathogenesis vary greatly. Some believe that most intestinal atresias are due to accidental volvulus, intussusception, strangulation of the bowel, peritonitis, meconium ileus or lesions of the mesenteric arteries. Duodenal stenosis and atresia have been observed repeatedly in children damaged by thalidomide.[5] Other observations point to genetic determination. Atresias due to occluding membranes at the ileocecal junction have been observed in identical twins.[6] In another pair of monozygotic twins, one had multiple atresias whereas the other succumbed to a stenosis of the colon and an umbilical hernia.[7] Duodenal atresias have been reported in a brother and sister,[8] and ileal atresias in brothers.[9] "Accidental" atresias in infants with meconium ileus, considered an "acquired" anomaly,[10] can be attributed to fibrocystic disease, a genetically determined disorder. The rare "apple peel" or "Christmas tree" intestinal atresia has been attributed to autosomal recessive inheritance.[30] Duodenal stenosis or atresia in Down syndrome (p. 328) is due to a chromosomal disorder. Since fetal accidents such as volvulus, ileus, and so forth, occur frequently in infants with intestinal malrotation,[4] the cause of the malrotation must be considered an etiologic factor. These facts indicate that unitary explanations of intestinal atresias are bound to be unsatisfactory.

The same is true for pathogenetic theories. In 1900, Tandler[11] showed that the human duodenum passes through a solid stage that is due to epithelial proliferation that begins in the fifth week and lasts to the eighth week; the resulting obliteration of the lumen does not affect the entire duodenum at one time but there is a wave of epithelial overgrowth that passes from below the pylorus to the jejunum.[12] Normally, recanalization of the duodenum occurs by formation of vacuoles that coalesce and re-establish the intestinal lumens. An arrest of development of the duodenum during the solid stage could account for cases of intrinsic duodenal atresias. The observations made by Tandler[11] have been confirmed by many authors,[12] and some of these accepted the theory of the arrested solid stage as an explanation of all congenital duodenal and intestinal occlusions.

Evans[13] doubted that this explanation holds for all types of congenital atresias and believed that some other factors come into play to produce these malformations. It must be pointed out that in the nineteenth century many authors explained the atresias by ischemia of a segment of the fetal bowel, by infarction, volvulus, intussusception, herniations, bands, and so forth,[14] but these explanations were more or less abandoned and supplanted by the theory of arrest during the solid stage. Louw[14] asserted that the theory of vascular insufficiency accounts for all the clinicopathologic features of congenital intestinal atresia. Santulli and Blanc[15] summarized the arguments in favor of heterogeneous pathogenetic factors and pointed out that often meconium, squamous epithelium, lanugo hair or bile droplets are found in the jejunum or ileum distal to the points of atresia. The presence of these elements suggests that occlusion occurred after the eleventh or twelfth week of fetal life, i.e., beyond the time of recanalization, which takes place at the end of the second month. The appearance of the mesenteric defects often seen in association with some of the atresias points to a disturbance of a previously intact bowel and mesentery. Some authors believe that there are two types of atresias, the "true or primary" form attributed to failure of recanalization and the secondary form, which follows fetal accidents befalling a previously normally

Fig. 76-2.—Intestinal loops in a child with meconium ileus. (Courtesy of Dr. L. W. Martin, Cincinnati, Ohio.)

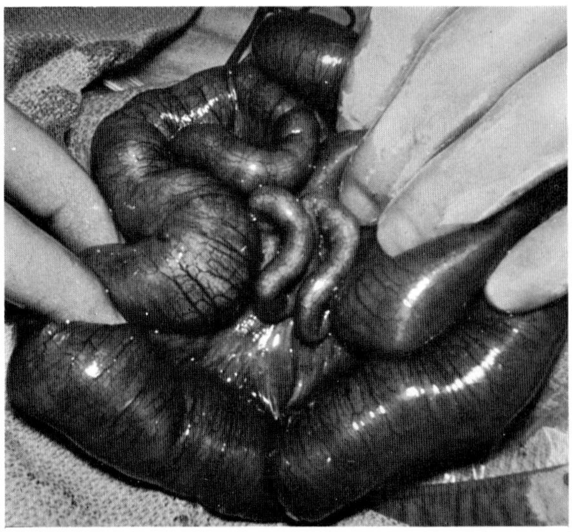

developed intestine. Santulli and Blanc[15] advanced the hypothesis that most, if not all, forms of jejunal and ileal atresia are due to an injury or accident to the fetal intestine. The various forms of atresia seen in newborn infants may be best explained by the differing times of occurrence of the fetal injury. The accidents leading to atresias probably are prepared in many cases by malrotation of the intestine or other anomalies of the gut that often are present in children with jejunal or ileal atresias.[4] Rehbein and Boix-Ochoa[16] attributed duodenal atresias and stenosis to malrotation, volvulus, kinks or annular pancreas in 62% of the cases and to internal stenosis or atresia in 38%. The intrinsic obstructions usually involve the distal duodenum and most of them are due to a diaphragm-like membrane that is either complete or has a narrow central opening. The distal gut is empty or collapsed. Down syndrome, annular pancreas[22] or congenital heart disease suggests that these occlusions are a part of a complicated disease picture. Such membranous atresias are rare in atresias of the jejunum and ileum.[17] Fetal accidents are more likely explanations for these cases. In addition to vascular causation, a number of specific anomalies have been described as sources of such atresias. Strangulation within an umbilical hernia,[17] strangulation of the intestine in the extra-embryonic coelom of the belly stalk,[18] intussusception in utero,[19] secondary occlusion by meconium,[20,21] annular pancreas[22] and others have been described in recent times as pathogenetic factors in intestinal atresia. There usually is complete interruption of the gut, which ends in a blind sac, separated from the following segment or connected with it by a cord or other remnants of previously existing connections. If an obstructing diaphragm is present, it is made up of central connective tissue lined on both sides by the mucosa of the adjacent intestine, but there is no muscularis propria. The blind ends are also lined with mucosa continuous with that of the adjacent gut. Auerbach ganglia are normal in the affected areas.[4] Spencer[28] found that single obstructions are most common in the duodenum, whereas multiple obstructions and those secondary to volvulus and intussusception occur most often in the jejunum and the ileum. He concluded that the higher the obstruction the higher the incidence of prematurity, of multiple malformations, of single, simple obstruction and the higher the mortality rate.

To demonstrate intestinal atresia, meconium is examined by the Farber test, which is negative for cornified epithelial vernix cells in case of occlusion; but, according to Santulli and Blanc,[15] such squamous cells often can be found distal to a secondary jejunal or ileal occlusion, so that finding of such cells does not exclude intestinal atresia.

The chief symptom of congenital intestinal atresia is vomiting beginning on the first day of life. The stools are reduced in amount and abdominal distention develops, particularly if the atresia is at a low level (jejunum or ileum). Roentgenograms often reveal the site of the obstruction as the gas-filled, distended parts proximal to the atresia contrast with the unexpanded distal parts. In a series of 157 infants with neonatal duodenal obstruction, malrotation was found as an associated anomaly in 32%, Down syndrome in 21%, annular pancreas in 20% and congenital heart disease in 18%. Esophageal atresia was noted in 11%, anomalies of the small bowel in 10% and hindgut anomalies in 4%.[27] Marked jaundice occurred in 21% of the children with duodenal obstruction.

Without surgical treatment, infants with intestinal atresia die soon after birth; with treatment, more than 50% survive. Atresias of the ileum tend to postoperative adhesions and complications but, otherwise, the outcome is little influenced by the position of the obstruction.[3]

Congenital atresias of the colon are relatively rare. Gross[3] recorded only 6 cases among 140 intestinal atresias. Wilson *et al.*[23] estimated that they account for 5–10% of the congenital intestinal occlusions. Benson *et al.*[24] stated that of gastrointestinal stenoses or atresias operated on, 10% were located in the colon. The rarity of atresias of the colon is explained by Lynn and Espinas[1] by the fact that plugging of the embryonic colon is rare.

Heckel and Apfelbach[25] reviewed 29 cases of congenital atresia of the colon, i.e., complete occlusion of the lumen resulting from changes in the wall of the large bowel. They also added a case of their own with atresia of the sigmoid portion of the colon. In 7 of the cases, atresia was present in the sigmoid flexure and rectum, in 5, in the ascending colon and in 3, in the transverse portion of the colon. Occlusion of the ileocecal valve, of the splenic flexure and of the descending portion occurred in 2 cases each. In 8 infants, several portions of the colon were continuously occluded. Replacement of a part of the colon by a nonpatent fibrous cord was the rule with the mesocolon present and the cord attached to its free border. In a few instances, the lumen was interrupted only by a membrane of mucosa stretching transversely from wall to wall. In 5 cases there was also occlusion of the small bowel and in 3 there was imperforate anus.

Syndactyly and polydactyly occur occasionally in patients with ano-rectal malformations, and such digital anomalies have been associated with congenital absence of most of the colon.[26] Zaidi[26] also cited cases of partial absence of the large intestine. Atresia of the colon combined with Hirschsprung disease has been reported.[31]

In the past, only a few children with atresia of the colon survived, since treatment often was delayed or was inadequate. But by 1966, 53 successfully treated cases of colonic atresia or stenosis had been reported, and Benson *et al.*[24] added 16 cases to the list. They recommended routine contrast enema in all patients with jejunal or ileal atresia or stenosis to avoid overlooking similar atresias of the colon.

Rectal atresia seems to be rare and must be distinguished from rectal agenesis.[32]

REFERENCES

1. Lynn, H. B., and Espinas, E. E.: Intestinal atresia; an attempt to relate location to embryologic processes, A.M.A. Arch. Surg. 79:357, 1959.
2. Webb, C. H., and Wangensteen, O. H.: Congenital intestinal atresia, Am. J. Dis. Child. 41:262, 1931.
3. Gross, R. E.: *The Surgery of Infancy and Childhood* (Philadelphia: W. B. Saunders Company, 1953).
4. Moore, T. C., and Stokes, G. E.: Congenital stenosis and atresia of the small intestine, Surg., Gynec. & Obst. 97: 719, 1953.
5. Kreipe, U.: Missbildungen innerer Organe bei Thalidomid-embryopathie, Arch. Kinderh. 176:33, 1967.
6. Lewis, F. J.: Intestinal atresia in identical twins, Surgery 33:121, 1953.
7. Denney, E. S., and Sloan, L. H.: Congenital intestinal malformations in identical twins (monozygotic twins with closely related developmental defects. One of extreme rarity), S. Clin. North America 12:227, 1932.
8. Pequet, A. R., and Watson, E H.: Duodenal atresia occurring in siblings, Univ. Michigan M. Bull. 25:363, 1959.
9. Winter, S. T., and Zeltzer, M.: Congenital atresia of the ileum in two brothers, J. Pediat. 49:194, 1956.
10. Bernstein, J., Vawter, G., Harris, G. B. C., Young, V., and Hillman, L. S.: The occurrence of intestinal atresia in newborns with meconium ileus; the pathogenesis of an acquired anomaly, A.M.A. J. Dis. Child. 99:804, 1960.
11. Tandler, J.: Zur Entwicklungsgeschichte des menschlichen Duodenum in frühen Embryonalstadien, Morphol. Jahrb. 29:187, 1900.
12. Boyden, E. A., Cope, J. G., and Bill, A. H., Jr.: Anatomy and embryology of congenital intrinsic obstruction of the duodenum, Am. J. Surg. 114:190, 1967.
13. Evans, C. H.: Atresias of the gastrointestinal tract, Surg., Gynec. & Obst., supp. Internat. Abst. Surg. 92:1, 1951.
14. Louw, J. H.: Congenital intestinal atresia and stenosis in the newborn; observations on its pathogenesis and treatment, Ann. Roy. Coll. Surgeons England 25:209, 1959.
15. Santulli, T. V., and Blanc, W. A.: Congenital atresia of the intestine: Pathogenesis and treatment, Ann. Surg. 154: 939, 1961.
16. Rehbein, F., and Boix-Ochoa, J.: Duodenal stenosis-duodenal atresia, diagnosis and treatment, German M. Monthly 8:466, 1963.
17. Rehbein, F., and Waldmann, I.: Die Dünndarmatresie, Deutsche med. Wchnschr. 89:861, 1964.
18. Okmian, L. G., and Kövamees, A.: Jejunal atresia with intestinal aplasia. Strangulation of the intestine in the extra-embryonic coelom of the belly stalk, Acta paediat. 53:65, 1964.
19. Gherardi, G. J., and Fisher, J. H.: Atresia of the small intestine produced by intussusception in utero, New England J. Med. 264:229, 1961.
20. Carpenter, H. M.: Pathogenesis of congenital jejunal atresia, Arch. Path. 73:390, 1962.
21. Swischuk, L. E.: Meconium plug syndrome: A cause of neonatal intestinal obstruction, Am. J. Roentgenol. 103: 339, 1968.
22. Free, E. A., and Gerald, B.: Duodenal obstruction in the newborn due to annular pancreas, Am. J. Roentgenol. 103:321, 1968.
23. Wilson, B. J., Nelson, A., and Harshbarger, M.: Congenital atresia of the colon, Surg., Gynec. & Obst. 99:34, 1954.
24. Benson, C. D., Lotfi, M. W., and Brough, A. J.: Congenital atresia and stenosis of the colon, J. Pediat. Surg. 3:253, 1968.
25. Heckel, N. J., and Apfelbach, C. W.: Congenital atresia of the colon, Am. J. Dis. Child. 34:1050, 1927.
26. Zaidi, Z. H.: Congenital absence of most of the colon. Anomaly associated with imperforate anus, syndactylism and polydactylism, A.M.A. J. Dis. Child. 98:385, 1959.
27. Young, D. G., and Wilkinson, A. W.: Abnormalities associated with neonatal duodenal obstruction, Surgery 63:832, 1968.
28. Spencer, R.: The various patterns of intestinal atresia, Surgery 64:661, 1968.
29. de Lorimier, A. A., Fonkalsrud, E. W., and Hays, D. M.: Congenital atresia and stenosis of the jejunum and ileum, Surgery 65:819, 1969.
30. Blyth, H., and Dickson, J. A. S.: Apple peel syndrome, J. M. Genetics 6:275, 1969.
31. Hyde, G. A., and de Lorimier, A. A.: Colon atresia and Hirschsprung's disease, Surgery 64:976, 1968.
32. Magnus, R. V.: Rectal atresia as distinguished from rectal agenesis, J. Pediat. Surg. 3:593, 1968.

Duplications of the Alimentary Tract

A VARIETY OF developmental anomalies of the intestine that previously were described as "gastric thoracic cysts, " "enteric cysts," "ileum duplex," "giant diverticula" and so forth are now recognized as duplications of the alimentary tract. They can assume various shapes and they vary in size. Their morphogenesis is also heterogeneous. It seems that males are affected more often than females and that duplications are less frequent in Caucasians than in Negroes.[1]

The majority of duplications encountered by clinicians probably are due to faulty recanalization of the embryonic enteric tract. They can be related to a prenatal condition that is normal at approximately 6 weeks of gestation in embryos 10–12 mm. long. At this time, coincident with the general rapid growth of the intestine, a local multiplication of the epithelial cells occurs in the intestinal lining. Such increase in epithelial tissue leads to formation of cell aggregates that in the narrow embryonic intestine may result in the occlusion of the lumen. In this way, epithelial plugs are formed and a partial and temporary solid stage of the intestine is produced. This solid stage never affects the whole intestinal tract at one time; it is described as a wave of solidification that passes through the intestine. The cell masses secrete a fluid seen in sections as small intercellular droplets, which, by coalescence and arrangement in longitudinal rows, form channels within the intestine. Normally, these intra-intestinal cell masses disappear and the main channel, lined by a single epithelial cell layer, is formed. In pathologic cases, the recanalization is irregular and an accessory row of vacuoles may be retained for a short distance, forming an extra lumen. Intestinal coats may grow between the two channels, which develop their individual submucosal and muscular layers. In most cases, these layers unite the two tubes, but sometimes more independent and separate duplications are formed.[2]

Irregular recanalization of the intestine in embryonic life explains some, but not all, duplications of the enteric tract. Some duplications may date back to adhesions formed in the presomite embryo between the ectodermal and entodermal germ layers, resulting in vertebral anomalies combined with duplications in the posterior mediastinum or within the mesentery.[3] Other duplications, i.e., those of the colon, that are associated with double bladder and urethra[4] have a different embryologic basis. Such anomalies are considered the result of partial twinning of the caudal end of the body. In addition to duplication of the lower urinary tract, double vagina and uterus, double penis or imperforate anus may occur as associated malformations. Duplication of the colon may also be found combined with duplicated vertebral column, spina bifida, omphalocele or exstrophy of the bladder and in parasitic monsters and conjoined twins.[5,6] Kratzer *et al.*[7] described duplication of the colon in a young man 7 years after removal of a parasitic twin attached to the supra-umbilical region. Draining sinuses led to the discovery of a supernumerary bladder and colon, which were remnants of the parasite. A thoracopagus may have duplication of the esophagus and stomach, a single jejunum, duodenum and ileum down to the vitelline duct and from there again a duplication to the anus. A pygopagus may show duplication of the entire small and large intestine with only one anal opening.[6]

Ravitch[5] asserted that it is relatively simple to produce, experimentally, partial twinning in amphibia by constricting ova but that it is impossible so far to produce caudal duplication in this manner. On the other hand, by fusion of two early amphibian embryos, one can produce monsters that are double in some respects and single in others. In mammalian experimental teratology, duplications of the gut have not been described, but Hummel[8] found a variety of duplication phenomena in mice that can be attributed to a gene mutation. A gene called "disorganization gene" (Ds), which disrupts the orderly processes of morphogenesis, results in many anomalies of the skeleton and of visceral structures. The anomalies may occur singly or in various combinations. Among the malformations found in the digestive tract, duplications of the large intestine and rectum were the most frequent. Sometimes the loop had a continuous lumen, but more often one section ended blindly. Two and three cecums were not unusual. Occasionally, one loop of the colon joined the urethra, whereas the other was continuous with a normal rectum and anus. In other cases, the colon entered a cloaca and the rectum and anus were missing. In the same syndrome, a split genital papilla occurred and sometimes doubling of the urinary bladders was present. Gastroschisis and exstrophy of the bladder were not rare. Thus, some animals had changes attributable to the disorganization gene, which showed a striking resemblance to human cases of the extensive duplications reviewed by Ravitch.[5]

Duplications may vary greatly in size, shape, site and epithelial lining. Relatively frequent sites are the esophagus, duodenum, ileum and the ileocecal valve, but they also occur at the base of the tongue, in the stomach, jejunum, cecum, colon, sigmoid or rectum. Some duplications assume the shape of diverticula that can lie within the mesentery or run into distant areas in the abdomen or chest (p. 700). Other duplications take a course parallel to the intestine, with which they are intimately connected. Sometimes ovoid structures arise from some part of the alimentary canal without communication with it. They usually equal the intestine in diameter but they vary in length from a few centimeters to half a meter. The majority of duplications are attached to the main digestive tube and are firmly united with it by common muscular layers. The muscular coat of smooth muscle characterizes duplications and sets them apart from thin-walled mesenteric cysts, which are lymphatic in origin. Mesenteric cysts usually can be peeled off and removed without trauma to the intestine, whereas duplications must be resected together with a portion of the intestine. The lining epithelium resembles that of some part of the alimentary tract but not necessarily the adjacent one. In 20% of the cases, the duplication communicates with the intestinal tract. The blind end, especially that of a long duplication, often is bulbous. The expanded segments may be lined by gastric mucosa, whereas the tubular portion of the duplication shows the mucosa of the parent intestine.[9] The frequent occurrence of ulcers at the communicating opening of a duplication has been explained by juxtaposition of different mucosal types.[2] Duplications may contain clear, hemorrhagic or, if communicating with the intestinal tract, enteric fluid, fecal masses or gas.

Duplications arising in the thorax usually lie alongside the esophagus without communication with this structure. They commonly accumulate fluid, form cysts and manifest themselves by pulmonary compression and respiratory symptoms. Such cysts, which prefer the right side, may fill a large part of the pleural cavity. In many cases, they are lined by gastric mucosa ("gastric thoracic cysts"); the fluid produced by this mucosa can erode the cyst wall and cause inflammatory reaction and adhesions to the esophagus or the adjacent lung. Hemoptysis or hematemesis can occur and fistulas that communicate with the neighboring lung can be established. Gross[9] observed and described duplications arising from the intestine but presenting in the thorax, which can be recognized as diverticula originating from the small intestine, coursing upward through the diaphragm into the thorax, where they may reach the apex of the chest. Such diverticula can compress the heart or lung and produce cardiorespiratory symptoms or they may, like other intrathoracic cysts of intestinal origin, secrete gastric juice, leading to ulceration, hemorrhage, melena and anemia. Fallon *et al.*[10] described enteric cysts in the posterior mediastinum, commonly associated with vertebral anomalies and sometimes with intramesenteric duplications. These authors believed that the muscular wall is characteristic for enteric cysts but that the lining can be ciliated or of any alimentary type. Gastric duplications are discussed on page 688.

Duplication of the entire small intestine, which is rare, poses special problems. Jewett[11] described the case of a 5-month-old boy who had such an anomaly that involved the entire small bowel with the exception of the distal end of the ileum. Melena due to ulceration of the mucosa was the presenting symptom.

Duodenal duplications can be submucous, intramural or retroperitoneal. They can remain symptomless for many years or manifest themselves in infancy. Pyloric stenosis or duodenal atresia has been suspected in many cases; in other instances, symptoms are variable. The subject was reviewed by Schüler and Schüler.[12] Many cases present isolated duodenal duplications. In thoraco-duodenal duplications, the spinal column frequently shows associated anomalies.

Duplication of the colon may be of the simple variety or combined with other duplicated organs. In the majority of cases, there is a normal colon with a diverticulum dorsal to it in the mesentery. The relation between the two—or even three—colons varies from case to case, and from one area in the bowel to another. In some patients, the colons are running parallel and are separated from each other by a septum between the lumina. In other cases, the intestines are separate for a considerable distance and are only slightly connected. The blood supply of the two colons is a common one and, in most cases, there is but a single mesentery.[5] Less frequent types are those combined with double bladder and urethra, which are related to partial twinning (p. 1073).

Symptoms caused by duplications are as variable as their shapes and locations. Gross[9] grouped the manifestations into four categories: (1) A large cyst encroaches on the adjacent intestine and partially obstructs it. (2) A large cyst causes pain by pressure. (3) The duplication presses on the mesenteric blood supply and produces necrosis, sloughing and bleeding of the adjacent intestine. (4) The duplication is lined by gastric mucosa, forms hydrochloric acid and pepsin and leads to ulceration and hemorrhage. Respiratory distress, abdominal pain, a palpable mass, bleeding from the bowel and acute abdomen were listed as clinical manifestations by Mellish and Koop.[1]

Duplications of the colon and rectum gradually compress and partly block the bowel, producing palpable masses. If they are located behind the rectum, they cause compression, constipation and abdominal distention in early infancy. Gross[9] observed 4 patients in whom long segments of the rectum or colon possessed a double loop, each of which contained fecal material. In these patients, imperforate anus, an accessory perineal opening or communication of the secondary colonic tube with the urethra were associated anomalies. Duplications as discovered and treated by the surgeon are chiefly disorders of infancy or childhood. Gross's youngest patient was 1 day of age, the oldest 13 years. In his series,[9] 65% of the cases occurred or manifested themselves in the first year of life, 9% in the second year, 8% in the third year and only a few cases thereafter. Some duplications remain symptomless and others manifest themselves late in life. The patient of van Zwalenburg,[4] who belonged to the complicated type of colon duplication, was 55 years of age when she was treated because of rectal bleeding, and Reilly *et al.*[13] described a 63-year-old woman in whom the anomaly simulated carcinoma of the descending colon.

If duplications cause clinical symptoms, they are treated surgically. Gross[9] stressed that the cystic structure and the adjacent alimentary tube have a common wall and that it is difficult to separate one from the other without injuring the bowel. In addition, arteries and veins of the contiguous portions of the alimentary tract usually course over the surface of the duplication. Consequently, attempts to dissect the supernumerary structure may interrupt these vessels so that there is an impairment of the blood supply. Therefore, in the majority of cases, the treatment of choice is resection of the duplication and its adjacent gut, followed by re-establishment of intestinal or colonic continuity by a primary anastomosis.[9]

Different types of duplication pose different surgical problems. In the case of complete duplication of the small intestine,[11] internal drainage of the duplication into the stomach by creation of a window may be the operation of choice. In this way, the stream of gastric juice produced by the duplication is diverted from the sensitive small intestinal mucosa and the duplication drained to avoid gradual enlargement.

Concerning duplications of the colon, bladder and urethra, van Zwalenburg[4] emphasized that they may be free of clinical symptoms unless there are secondary anomalies such as imperforate anus or a rectovesicular communication. If symptoms are caused by distention of a channel that has an inadequate outlet, drainage of the supernumerary colon into the main channel must be established.[5]

Intestinal Diverticula

Diverticula of the intestine found in children are considered abnormal remnants of a process that occurs regularly in human embryos. In embryos of 20–30 mm. at the end of the second month, development of small buds from the epithelial lining of the gut are observed rather frequently. They grow into the subepithelial connective tissue, chiefly on the antimesenteric surfaces, but they normally disappear as soon as the intestine enlarges. If they persist, they may present as diverticula or as extra-intestinal cysts that have only a mucosal and serosal covering. They may also remain within the intestine, expand within the submucosa, form intra-intestinal cysts and grow to such a size that the lumen of the intestine becomes obstructed.[2] These isolated diverticula of embryonic origin must be distinguished from intestinal diverticulosis of adults (see below). Heredity of such diverticula has not been demonstrated.[14] Gross[9] believed that the outpocketings from the embryonic intestinal tract described by Lewis and Thyng[15] in 1907 may be the source of duplications of the alimentary tract.

A *duodenal diverticulum* causing a valve-like occlusion of the intestine was described by Weyers[16] in a boy 1 year of age. The symptoms were those of pyloric stenosis from birth on, but acute attacks of vomiting occurred after 6 months.

Cecal diverticula may be congenital in origin. They usually are single and occur in somewhat younger age groups than generalized diverticulosis. In one instance, a father and his daughter were affected. In human embryos, an outgrowth from the tip of the cecum has been observed that enlarges during the sixth week of fetal life and atrophies in the seventh week, so that the anomaly could be explained as persistence of an embryonic condition. A cecal diverticulum may manifest itself by abdominal pain that localizes in the right lower quadrant. Occasionally, nausea and vomiting are present, so that, in most cases, appendicitis is diagnosed. A mass may be felt in some cases. In one-third of the cases a fecalith is found. Nissenbaum *et al.*[17] diagnosed a case of cecal diverticulum roentgenographically and suggested that the lesion may be more common than suspected. The operation of choice is excision with inversion as an alternative. Lasher[18] discussed small diverticular duplications of the intestine with peptic ulceration. Such anomalies sometimes are incorrectly considered atypical Meckel diverticula.

Diverticulosis mainly affects the large bowel, particularly the sigmoid flexure of the colon. Symptoms of this anomaly usually are noted in late adult life, but a congenital disposition has been assumed by several authors.[19] In exceptional cases, diverticulosis has been observed in young children. Congenitally weak places in the bowel wall predispose to herniations of the intestinal mucosa and submucosa, which penetrate to the peritoneum. With increasing pressure, the diverticula increase to sac-like pouches, but their connection with the intestinal lumen remains narrow.

The condition is not rare and occurs in approximately 7% of patients examined roentgenographically or at necropsy.[19] Men and women develop diverticulosis in equal numbers. In about 85% of those affected, the anomaly remains symptomless. Diverticulitis (inflammatory manifestations) occurs more often in males than in females.

True *diverticula of the colon* are rare. Morison[20] described giant congenital diverticula of this type with rupture of the bowel opposite one of them. Interestingly, this observation was made in a child with partial hemihypertrophy of the crossed type. There was enlargement of the left side of the brain, cranium and face and the left leg was shorter than the right.

In the past, the literature contained many reports of diverticula, particularly giant diverticula, that now are considered duplications of the alimentary tract (p. 696).

REFERENCES

1. Mellish, R. W. P., and Koop, C. E.: Clinical manifestations of duplication of the bowel, Pediatrics 27:397, 1961.
2. Bremer, J. L.: *Congenital Anomalies of the Viscera—Their Embryological Basis* (Cambridge, Mass.: Harvard University Press, 1957).
3. Beardmore, H. E., and Wiglesworth, F. W.: Vertebral anomalies and alimentary duplications. Clinical and embryological aspects, in Ross, A. (ed.), *Symposium on Recent Clinical Advances*, Pediat. Clin. North America, p. 457, May, 1958.
4. van Zwalenburg, B. R.: Double colon, Am. J. Roentgenol. 68:22, 1952.
5. Ravitch, M. M.: Hindgut duplication—doubling of colon and genital urinary tracts, Ann. Surg. 137:588, 1953.
6. Anders, H. E.: Die Missbildungen des Darmkanals und der Verdauungsdrüsen, einschliesslich der Kloakenmissbildungen, in Schwalbe, E. (ed.), *Die Morphologie der Missbildungen des Menschen und der Tiere* (Jena: Gustav Fischer, 1928), Vol. 3, pt. 12–15, Chap. 4, pp. 375–482.
7. Kratzer, G. L., Dixon, C. F., and Bargen, J. A.: Duplication of the entire colon and terminal part of the ileum associated with parasitic twin, Proc. Staff Meet. Mayo Clin. 26: 15, 1951.
8. Hummel, K. P.: Developmental anomalies in mice resulting from action of the gene, disorganization, a semi-dominant lethal, Pediatrics 23:212, 1959.
9. Gross, R. E.: *The Surgery of Infancy and Childhood* (Philadelphia: W. B. Saunders Company, 1953).
10. Fallon, M., Gordon, A. R. G., and Lendrum, A. C.: Mediastinal cysts of fore-gut origin associated with vertebral abnormalities, Brit. J. Surg. 41:520, 1954.
11. Jewett, T. C.: Duplication of the entire small intestine with massive melena, Ann. Surg. 147:239, 1958.
12. Schüler, H. W., and Schüler, B.: Beitrag zur Klinik der duodenalen Duplikaturen, Ztschr. Kinderh. 100:291, 1967.
13. Reilly, H. F., Weismann, R., and Dyke, J. R.: Duplication of the alimentary tract in an adult simulating carcinoma of the descending colon, Radiology 90:769, 1968.
14. Gutzeit, K., and Lehmann, W.: Erbpathologie des Verdauungsapparates, in Bauer, K. H., Hanhart, E., Lange, J., and Just, G. (eds.), *Handbuch der Erbbiologie des Menschen* (Berlin: Julius Springer, 1940), Vol. 4, pt. 2, pp. 581–673.
15. Lewis, F. T., and Thyng, F. W.: Regular occurrence of intestinal diverticula in embryos of the pig, rabbit and man, Am. J. Anat. 7:505, 1907.
16. Weyers, H.: Duodenaldivertikel mit Ventilverschluss, Arch. Kinderh. 143:179, 1951.
17. Nissenbaum, J., Sparks, A. J., and Ellison, G. R.: Cecal diverticulum; report of a case diagnosed by roentgen ray and surgically proved: Review of the original literature, Am. J. Roentgenol. 73:596, 1955.
18. Lasher, E. P.: Small diverticular duplications of the intestine with peptic ulceration, Am. Surgeon 33:550, 1967.
19. Linde, S. A.: Diverticulosis and diverticulitis, J. Internat. Coll. Surgeons 19:716, 1953.
20. Morison, J. E.: Giant congenital diverticula and neonatal rupture of colon, Arch. Dis. Childhood 19:135, 1944.

Intestinal and Mediastinal Malformations Attributed to Abnormal Neurenteric Connections

A VARIETY of malformations of the intestinal tract have been attributed to abnormal connections between the primitive gut and the notochord or the dorsal ectoderm. Usually, such abnormal connections of primitive entodermal and ectodermal layers are attributed to persistence of the neurenteric canal. However, persistence of this normally short-lived structure, seen in 18-day-old embryos as a communication between the cavities of the yolk sac and amnion,[1] are rare. A case reported by Keen and Coplin[2] may represent an abnormal persistence of the neurenteric canal, since it consisted of a communication between the dorsal wall of the rectum and the dorsal body surface through the skin in the lower sacral region. However, most of the communications between the enteric canal and the structures located dorsal to it probably are due to anomalous endo-ectodermal connections situated cephalad to the neurenteric canal. According to Bremer,[3] the neurenteric canal, an open passage between the enteric cavity and the neural groove, is a minute tube that runs from the yolk sac cavity through the primitive knot (Hensen node) to the amniotic cavity. In presomite human embryos, the primitive knot is a center of cell proliferation that soon becomes unrecognizable because of dispersal of the newly formed cells. In later fetal life, its remnants should be sought at the ends of the spinal cord and the vertebral column. Since the coccygeal tip is the final location of the primitive knot and the former neurenteric canal, any open connection between the intestine and the dorsal surfaces found cranial to the coccyx must be due to an accessory canal or to an abnormal ecto-entodermal connection.

Broad communications between the yolk sac and the dorsal surface of vertebrate embryos have been produced experimentally, and have been called diastematomyelia. They represent models of communications between the intestinal tract and spina bifida. Cases have been described in which broad connections existed between the pharynx, esophagus or intestine with myeloschisis or rachischisis,[4] but such broad connections, found occasionally in stillborn fetuses, are rare in viable children in whom corresponding malformations usually are more limited and more subtle. The roof of the primitive gut may protrude between the separate body halves as a hollow tube or longitudinal ridge, open through the skin of the back, or be obliterated by the meeting of the body halves. If it remains open, the vertebrae and other median structures must grow around it. Such dorsal intestinal fistulas are only rarely patent, but obliterated remnants are found more often. If the fistulous tract disappears soon after its formation, bone may fill the gap, causing merely increased breadth of the vertebral body. If the fistula persists longer, the bodies of one or several vertebrae may grow around the tract so that a hole through the vertebral body is formed. Or a median spur, bony or cartilaginous, may project into a widened spinal canal. In such cases, the two halves of the cord may become separated by the median bony spur, which penetrates between the two contiguous neural leaves. Thus, diastematomyelia is morphogenetically related to dorsal intestinal fistulas and their derivatives (p. 292).

Associations of mediastinal cysts, intestinal duplications and anomalies of the lower cervical and upper thoracic vertebrae have been observed repeatedly. Veeneklaas[5] pointed out that intrathoracic gastrogenic cysts and anomalies of the cervical and thoracic spine commonly occur together. He advanced the theory that adherence of notochord to the foregut persists in such cases. Fallon *et al.*[6] stated that enteric cysts lying in the posterior mediastinum have a well-formed muscular wall and show a lining that can be ciliated or of any alimentary type. They are commonly associated with vertebral abnormalities and sometimes with intramesenteric duplications. Beardmore and Wiglesworth,[7] in discussing mediastinal cysts and spinal anomalies, believed that in the presomite embryo an adhesion between the ectodermal and entodermal germ layers may split or deflect the notochord. This would result in the formation of vertebral anomalies and duplications in the posterior mediastinum that may contain central nervous system tissue. They emphasized a triad consisting of vertebral anomalies in the lower cervical and upper thoracic region, posterior mediastinal cysts and intestinal duplication. Posterior mediastinal masses, if associated with vertebral anomalies, should be recognized as cysts of foregut origin. Cases of Klippel-Feil syndrome or anterior or posterior spina bifida should be screened for the presence of neural or alimentary anomalies.

Nathan[8] also asserted that anomalies such as duplications of the foregut, enterogenous or neurenteric cysts, Klippel-Feil syndrome, anterior spina bifida, posterior spina bifida, diastematomyelia, congenital scoliosis, segmentation defects of vertebrae, enterocystoma of the spinal cord or dorsal intestinal fistula can result from such embryologic errors. Related to these conditions was a gastrocystoma of the spinal cord described by Knight *et al.*[9] in a child 15 months of age. Vertebral anomalies were seen in radiograms extending from the 7th cervical to the 8th thoracic vertebra, with gross enlargement of the neural canal in this region. At operation, the cord was widely expanded with cystic cavities and a red tumor was found occupying the midline of the expanded cord. The cystic tumor showed a lining of gastric and esophageal epithelia thrown into folds and surrounded by smooth muscle with a mass of central nervous tissue at its margins. The tumor was considered a gastrocystoma and explained by the authors by separation of a portion of the endodermal gut from the main portion of the foregut before fusion of the sclerodermss. The ectopic gut growing within the neural canal interfered with the development of the vertebrae at the same level.

REFERENCES

1. Arey, L. B.: *Developmental Anatomy* (6th ed.; Philadelphia: W. B. Saunders Company, 1954).
2. Keen, W. W., and Coplin, W. M. L.: Sacrococcygeal tumor, Surg., Gynec. & Obst. 3:661, 1906.
3. Bremer, J. L.: Dorsal intestinal fistula; accessory neurenteric canal; diastematomyelia, A.M.A. Arch. Path. 54:132, 1952.
4. Lucksch, F.: Über Myeloschisis mit abnormer Darmausmündung, Ztschr. Kinderh. 24:143, 1903.
5. Veeneklaas, G. M. H.: Pathogenesis of intrathoracic gastrogenic cysts, A.M.A. Am. J. Dis. Child. 83:500, 1952.
6. Fallon, M., Gordon, A. R. G., and Lendrum, A. C.: Mediastinal cysts of fore-gut origin associated with vertebral abnormalities, Brit. J. Surg. 41:520, 1954.
7. Beardmore, H. E., and Wiglesworth, F. W.: Vertebral anomalies and alimentary duplications. Clinical and embryological aspects, in Ross, A. (ed.), *Symposium on Recent Clinical Advances,* Pediat. Clin. North America, p. 457, May, 1958.
8. Nathan, M. T.: Cysts and duplications of neurenteric origin, Pediatrics 23:476, 1959.
9. Knight, G., Griffiths, T., and Williams, I.: Gastrocystoma of spinal cord, Brit. J. Surg. 42:635, 1955.

Persistence of the Vitelline Duct and Meckel Diverticulum

THE VITELLINE DUCT normally disappears completely within the peritoneal cavity, but sometimes it can be found as a solid epithelial strand within the umbilical cord. The most frequent case of persistent vitelline duct is Meckel diverticulum, which, in rare cases, is connected with the umbilicus by a thread that contains the vitelline vessels. There exist cysts derived from the vitelline duct or the duct may remain open toward the umbilicus and, after falling off of the umbilical cord, form a fistula through which a thin secretion or intestinal contents exude. It can become the seat of inflammation that may require surgical repair because of its malodorous discharge.[1]

The Meckel anomaly, which arises as a diverticulum from the ileum, is not rare. It is said to occur in approximately 2–3% of all persons.[2] Although described and illustrated long before Meckel, the diverticulum is named after the author who showed that it is a remnant of the vitelline or omphalomesenteric duct.[3] As the intestine returns into the abdominal cavity, it soon becomes detached normally from the yolk stalk, which, in the early embryo, connects the yolk sac with the primitive gut. Various anomalies can arise if the embryonic structure is not completely resolved. The most frequent remnant is a blind diverticulum, 2–5 cm. long, which sits on a broad base on the ileum at a distance, varying with age, of from 25 to 90 cm. from the ileocecal junction. Such an "ileal appendix" usually lies free in the peritoneal cavity,

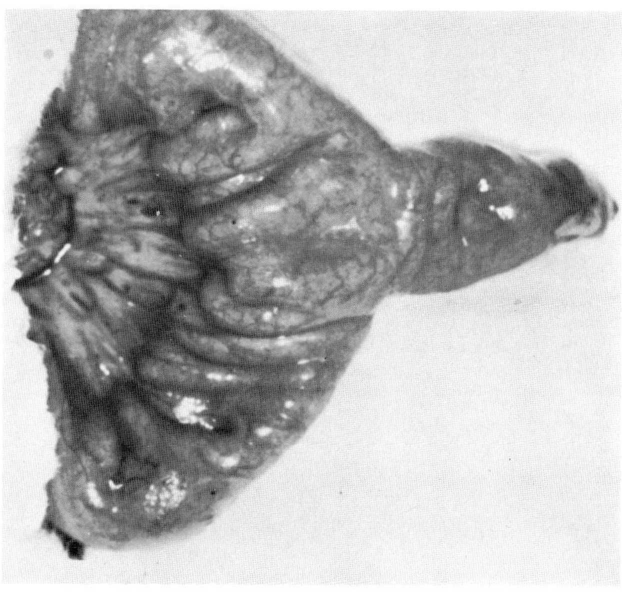

Fig. 76-3.—Resected intestine with Meckel diverticulum. (Courtesy of Dr. L. W. Martin, Cincinnati, Ohio.)

but occasionally it is fixed to the ileum by a mesentery. Variations consist of bifurcation of the diverticulum, narrowness of the base or dilatation of the tip, or its length may be unusual.[4] The diverticulum is lined chiefly by ileal mucosa but in approximately one-third of the cases gastric mucosa is also found in or near the structure. Pancreatic tissue, mucosa characteristic of colon or duodenum or bile ducts may be present also.[5] Rarely, the vitelline duct remains patent in its entire length, forming a fistula between the ileum and the umbilicus through which fecal matter may exude. The distal and proximal patent ends of such a duct may be separated from each other by a fibrotic remnant so that the outer portion forms an umbilical sinus. Partial patency can result in formation of a cyst and the fibrotic band can bring about angulation of the intestine and obstruction.[6] Although Meckel diverticula remain symptomless in the majority of cases, occasionally complications are brought about by these embryologic remnants. Peptic ulceration attributed to heterotopic gastric mucosa probably is the most frequent source of trouble. Such ulcers cause periumbilical pain that is not related to food intake. Hemorrhages and perforation are further complications[1,5] capable of producing fulminant symptoms, since the diverticulum lies free in the peritoneal cavity, which can be infected rapidly by intestinal contents. Massive hemorrhage in small children who have bloody stools without previous warning is rather characteristic of ulceration of such a diverticulum. Chronic pain in the umbilical area sometimes leads to exploration, and relief is obtained by removal of the diverticulum.[1] Inflammation of the structure may simulate acute or chronic appendicitis, the diverticulitis sometimes leading to perforation and peritonitis. A diverticulum may invaginate itself and cause intussusception or it may result in intestinal obstruction by formation of knots, volvulus or herniation.[5] Intestinal obstruction occurs in approximately half of the symptomatic patients.[2] A variety of tumors have been observed in Meckel diverticula. Sarcomas,[7] carcinoma, leiomyomas, lymphomas and polyps have been reported.[5]

There exists a relatively high association between Meckel diverticulum and other congenital malformations. Microcephaly, spina bifida, congenital heart disease, supernumerary spleen, anomalies of the kidneys and ureters, mongolism, umbilical hernia and others have been found in necropsy cases with Meckel diverticulum.[4,5] Such associations are not surprising, since, as already stated, Meckel diverticulum occurs in approximately 2–3% of all persons. But the fact that the diverticulum was found in more than 20% of necropsies of children with trisomy 18 and in approximately 10% of children with trisomy 13-15[8] is significant. Gutzeit and Lehmann[9] cited cases of Meckel diverticulum in siblings, in a mother and her son who had an ileo-umbilical band, in monozygotic twins and in triplets.

Complications usually occur in early life. Perforation of a diverticulum may occur in fetal life, leading to meconium peritonitis.[10,11] In Gross's series[1] approximately half the patients were hospitalized within the first 2 years of life, but complications can occur at any age.

There exists a peculiar predominance of males over females with Meckel diverticulum. In most series, one finds that 75% of the patients are male, [1,4] but there are exceptions to this rule.[12] It seems that the diverticulum is present with equal frequency in males and females but that it causes trouble many more times in boys than in girls.[2,13]

Treatment consists of surgical removal of the diverticulum, but the mortality amounts to 15–20%.[1,12,14]

REFERENCES

1. Gross, R. E.: *Surgery of Infancy and Childhood* (Philadelphia: W. B. Saunders Company, 1953).
2. Jackson, R. H., and Bird, A. R.: Meckel's diverticulum in childhood, Brit. M. J. 2:1399, 1961.
3. Meckel, J. F.: *Handbuch der Pathologischen Anatomie* (Leipzig: C. H. Reclam, 1812).
4. Christie, A.: Meckel's diverticulum; pathologic study of sixty-three cases, Am. J. Dis. Child. 42:544, 1931.
5. Brown, R. G.: Symposium on gastrointestinal diseases; Meckel's curious anomaly, M. Clin. North America 37: 227, 1953.
6. Bremer, J. L.: *Congenital Anomalies of the Viscera – Their Embryological Basis* (Cambridge, Mass.: Harvard University Press, 1957).
7. Moses, W. R.: Meckel's diverticulum, New England J. Med. 237:118, 1947.
8. Warkany, J., Passarge, E., and Smith, L. B.: Congenital malformations in autosomal trisomy syndromes, Am. J. Dis. Child. 112:502, 1966.
9. Gutzeit, K., and Lehmann, W.: Erbpathologie des Verdauungsapparates, in Bauer, K. H., Hanhart, E., Lange, J., and Just, G. (eds.), *Handbuch der Erbbiologie des Menschen* (Berlin: Julius Springer, 1940), Vol. 4, pt. 2, pp. 581–673.
10. Rosza, S., and Gross, R. J.: Intrauterine perforation of Meckel's diverticulum, Am. J. Roentgenol. 69:944, 1953.
11. Gilbert, E. F., and Rainey, J. R., Jr.: Meconium peritonitis caused by a rupture of a Meckel's diverticulum in a newborn infant, J. Pediat. 53:597, 1958.
12. Brooke, W. S.: Meckel's diverticulum, Am. Surgeon 19: 712, 1953.
13. Söderlund, S.: Meckel's diverticulum. A clinical and histologic study, Acta chir. scandinav. (supp. 248) 1:233, 1959.
14. Aitken, J.: Remnants of the vitell-intestinal duct. Clinical analysis of 88 cases, Arch. Dis. Childhood 28:1, 1953.

Malformations of the Appendix

INFLAMMATION of the appendix is attributed to bacterial invasion of the mucosa from infective material accumulated in the lumen. Since such material is present in most appendices, secondary factors must contribute to the etiology of appendicitis. There are a number of reports of families in which appendicitis recurs frequently and appendectomies have to be done in many members of the kindred. Susceptibility to appendicitis may be present in more than one generation.[1-3] The reasons for a familial tendency have not been ascertained. Downs[1] reported a pedigree in which 16 appendectomies were performed in 22 members of three generations. Operation was necessary in early childhood and the susceptibility to inflammation was attributed to a deformity of the appendix consisting of a sharp kink at its base caused by a band of fibrous tissue that bound the appendix to the outer side of the cecum. This deformity was found in every child of this family operated on for appendicitis.

Displacement of the appendix by malrotation can pose a diagnostic problem. Left-sided appendicitis has been reported[4]; it occurs in approximately 1 of 1,000 appendectomies. Incomplete visceral transposition and imperfect fixation of the cecum and ascending colon were the basis of the abnormal situation of the appendix. Nonrotation of the colon or excessive length of the appendix are additional causes of displacement to the left.[5] Inflammation of a Meckel diverticulum can simulate appendicitis.

REFERENCES

1. Downs, T. M.: (Appendix, abnormalities.) Congenital malformations of appendix – familial disease, Ann. Surg. 115: 21, 1942.
2. Flavia, M.: A family pedigree of appendicitis, J. Hered. 31: 113, 1940.
3. Baker, E. G. St.: A family pedigree for appendicitis, J. Hered. 28:187, 1937.
4. Nix, J. T., and Nix, J. T., Jr.: Left-sided appendicitis. A report of three cases, New Orleans M. & S. J. 94:530, 1942.
5. Hembrow, C. H.: Some anomalous forms of appendicitis, M. J. Australia 1:862, 1932.

Congenital Mesenteric Cysts

ALTHOUGH mesenteric cysts are rare, it is said that the Florentine anatomist Benevieni described a case found at necropsy as early as 1507.[1] The origin of these cysts is much debated. They have been attributed to misplaced lymphatic rudiments,[2] to lymphangiomas without active proliferation or to obstruction of lymph vessels.[1] They occur in infants and children but symptoms may be delayed to adult life. Females are affected more often than males.[1] In one instance, a mesenteric cyst was found in a woman 3 months after a large dermoid tumor of an ovary had been removed,[3] but there were no histologic findings to suggest anything but mesenteric cyst. The cysts are found most often in the mesentery of the ileum and of the colon[4]; they also occur in that of the jejunum and sigmoid but are rare near the duodenum. They can be solitary or multilocular. In addition, there exists a (multiple) cystic disease of the mesentery characterized by hundreds of cysts of various sizes that fill the spaces between the mesenteric leaves.[2] The simple cysts arise as small fluid-filled structures that enlarge slowly and sometimes reach remarkable proportions. They may be painless and show shifting dullness and fluid waves. Such cases often have been mistaken for ascites. The cysts may be spheric, dumbbell shaped (bulging out on both sides of the mesentery) or saddle shaped (enveloping the adjacent intestine). More than 1 liter of serous or chylous fluid may be found and aspirated. The composition resembles that of plasma. The walls of these cysts are thin, lined with a flat endothelium and made up of collagen fibers with a few smooth muscle bundles. This is in contrast to enteric cysts (duplications), which are thick-walled, coated with several layers of smooth muscle and lined with mucous membrane. Mesenteric cysts can be found near the intestine or near the root of the mesentery.

As a rule, mesenteric cysts lead to a slow growth of the abdomen that may be painless or be accompanied by brief recurrent attacks of abdominal pain. The chronic stage may be followed by acute intestinal obstruction, which is said to occur in one-third of the cases.[4] Volvulus and infarction of the intestine may complicate the situation. Bentley and O'Donnell[5] described 4 children who had mesenteric cysts with malrotation of the intestine leading to volvulus. It seems possible that such cysts are present in early embryonic life, preventing normal rotation and return. Some mesenteric cysts are associated with anterior spina bifida and tethered to defective vertebral bodies by strands of connective tissue. Excision of mesenteric cysts has been performed successfully in many cases,[2,3] but surgery is not effective in mesenteric cystic disease.[2]

Omental cysts probably are similar in origin to mesenteric cysts. Their structure, growth pattern and symptomatology are also like those of their mesenteric fellows, but they lie anterior to the intestine, a circumstance demonstrable by roentgen studies.

REFERENCES

1. Valcke, J.: Les kystes du mésentère (avec deux cas personnels de kystes lymphatiques), Acta paediat. belg. 6:220, 1952.
2. Gross, R. E.: *The Surgery of Infancy and Childhood* (Philadelphia: W. B. Saunders Company, 1953).
3. Moore, T. C.: Congenital cysts of the mesentery, Quart. Bull. Indiana Univ. M. Center 14:36, 1952.
4. Warfield, J. O.: A study of mesenteric cysts with a report of two recent cases, Ann. Surg. 96:329, 1932.
5. Bentley, J. F. R., and O'Donnell, M. B.: Mesenteric cysts with malrotated intestine, Brit. M. J. 2:223, 1959.

Congenital Megacolon
(Hirschsprung Disease)

In 1887, Hirschsprung[1] described 2 cases of constipation in infancy resulting from dilatation and hypertrophy of the colon. The symptoms in these children dated from birth. Although the abdomen was much enlarged, the children had no pain and vomited only rarely. One child, who died at 11 months of age, had an enormously distended sigmoid and transverse colon at necropsy. The other portions of the colon were dilated also, but the rectum was not enlarged and did not show any constriction. The walls of the enlarged intestines were thickened and their mucous membranes showed erosions and ulcerations. Hirschsprung could not explain these findings and offered no theory concerning their origin; however, he believed that the fundamental anomaly was present in utero and presented either a developmental anomaly or a pathologic fetal process.

Many cases have been observed since Hirschsprung's first description but the incidence of the disorder is still not known. Estimates vary from 1 case in 1,000 to 1 in 20,000 or 30,000 births.[2] Madsen[3] in Denmark and Passarge[4] in Cincinnati, Ohio, arrived at similar incidence figures – 1 in 4,700 and 1 in 5,000. Despite this agreement, incidences could be quite different in other populations and regions. There can be little doubt that the expression of the disorder varies greatly from cases ending in death soon after birth to asymptomatic cases. In the typical patient, difficulty in bowel movements begins in the first weeks or months of life and subsequently the colon becomes enormously distended and filled with gas and fecal material, leading to marked abdominal distention, poor nutrition and respiratory distress (Figs. 76-4 and 76-5).

In general, males are affected more often than females. The sex distribution of published cases is about 4.5 males to 1 female.[3] Familial cases have been observed repeatedly, suggesting genetic determination of the disease. Madsen[3] listed 36 families on record in which more than one member was affected. In his own material of 157 patients there were 6 pairs of affected siblings and in an additional 18 patients there were certain, probable or possible cases in the pedigree. Passarge,[4] reviewing 63 families, noted that in 4, more than one member had certain Hirschsprung disease; in 1 family there was possible, and in another doubtful, familial occurrence. By pooling several studies, one finds that the incidence of the disease in siblings of all index cases is 3.6%. But there is a difference in affected siblings of male and female patients. Whereas only 2.6% siblings of male index cases are affected, there are 7.2% affected siblings of female patients.[4] In the general population, the incidence is thought to be 0.02%. Affected parents have been recorded in several instances,[3] but proved cases are rare. This is understandable, since survival and reproduction was limited before adequate surgical procedures were available. In 1964, Madsen[3] stated that there were 5 pairs of twins on record who were of the same sex and concordant; in some of these, monozygosity had been established.[5] No concordance had been observed in dizygotic twins. The finding in twins and observations of families with repeated cases suggest genetic factors at work in the etiology of Hirschsprung disease. Megacolon occurs

Fig. 76-4. – Hirschsprung disease in a 2½-year-old boy.

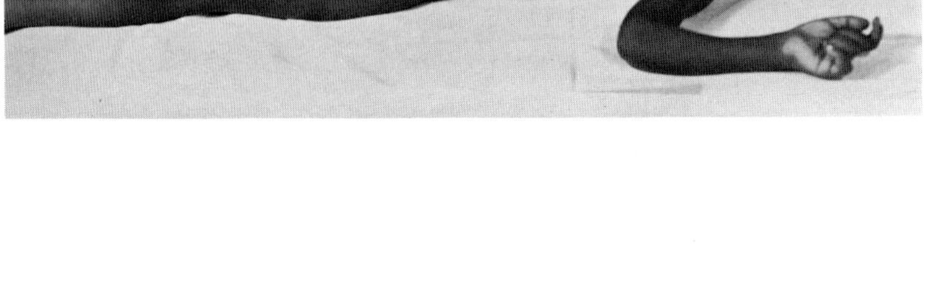

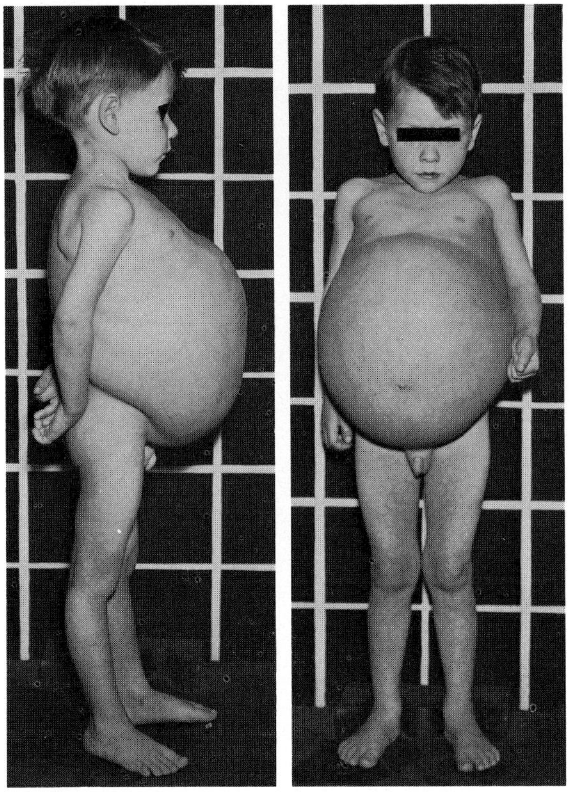

Fig. 76-5.—Hirschsprung disease in a 6-year-old boy.

in 10% of an inbred strain of mice (NZY). The terminal portion is aganglionic and contracted and the remainder of the colon distended. The aganglionic segment is present at birth but manifestations vary according to the length of the segment.[6] Association of megacolon with two recessive spotting genes in the mouse has been reported.[7] But attempts to explain the disease by simple Mendelian inheritance have not been successful. The data available are similar to those ascertained for pyloric stenosis (p. 688) or for cleft lip and palate (p. 631). Such situations, which suggest that the threshold of genes needed for expression of the trait is lower for the male sex than for the female, are attributed to sex-modified multifactorial inheritance[4] (p. 688). The incidence figures in siblings cited above can serve as general risk figures, but it should be kept in mind that they do not imply a unitary etiology of Hirschsprung disease. Bodian and Carter[8] distinguished between "short segment" and "long segment" cases. The over-all sex ratio was 3.6 but for the rarer "long segment" cases it was only 1.5. More important is the fact that Hirschsprung disease can be a constituent of Down syndrome and attributable to trisomy 21. Approximately 2% of patients with aganglionosis have Down syndrome,[4] whereas only 0.17% of the general newborn population are affected by this chromosomal anomaly. A child with XO/XX/XXX mosaicism[9] had Hirschsprung disease and an infant with an extra chromosome similar in size to a chromosome 16 had an aganglionic megacolon, pyloric stenosis and congenital defects.[10]

Ask-Upmark[11] pointed out that associated malformations have been observed in approximately half the children with megacolon. Many of these malformations were limited to the intestinal tract, e.g., anal atresia and underdevelopment of certain portions of the colon, of the small intestine or of the stomach. In addition, deformities of the vertebral column, meningocele, cardiovascular malformations, anomalies of the spleen, limb defects such as syndactyly or clubfoot, iris coloboma and others have been reported. According to Ask-Upmark, mental retardation is present too often to be accidental. Although, in some patients, the mental development could be impaired because of the chronic illness of the child, this would not apply to others, such as those with Down syndrome. Some reports confirmed that patients with Hirschsprung disease have an increased incidence of associated congenital malformations,[4,35] whereas others noted only an elevated incidence of Down syndrome.[8] The relationship of megacolon and megalo-ureter has been accorded special attention. Swenson and Fisher[12] stated that in 50% of their patients the bladder capacity was greater than normal, that defective detrusor contractions could be demonstrated and that in 5% severe bladder dysfunction and dilatation of the upper urinary tract were present. These disturbances were not of a mechanical nature and persisted after successful operation on the intestines. Aganglionic megacolon, pheochromocytoma, megalo-ureter and neurofibroma were found in a patient 18 years of age who had been constipated since birth and presented a rather typical picture of Hirschsprung disease.[13] There was a right hydronephrosis and right megalo-ureter and in the right adrenal gland a tumor was found that showed the signs of a pheochromocytoma. Atresia of the colon can be associated with Hirschsprung disease.[36] The anomaly has been seen in a brother and sister with diastrophic dwarfism[37] (Chapter 85).

Megacolon can be acquired and aganglionosis can be attributed in some instances to malnutrition and to infection with *Trypanosoma cruzi* (Chagas disease) in others. Pseudo-Hirschsprung disease or functional megacolon can be due to hypoplasia of the vegetative nervous system; treatment differs in such cases from that of the congenital form with rectal stenosis.[14] Bentley *et al.*[15] discussed a number of conditions called "pseudo-Hirschsprung's disease" that develop in the presence of normal ganglion cells.

From the time of the description of the striking disease picture by Hirschsprung, many theories have been advanced to explain the disorder.[3] Most of these are now of historical interest only. According to Ask-Upmark,[11] there were three chief hypotheses: (1) the disorder is due to a mechanical obstacle in the intestine; (2) it represents a gross malformation; (3) it is

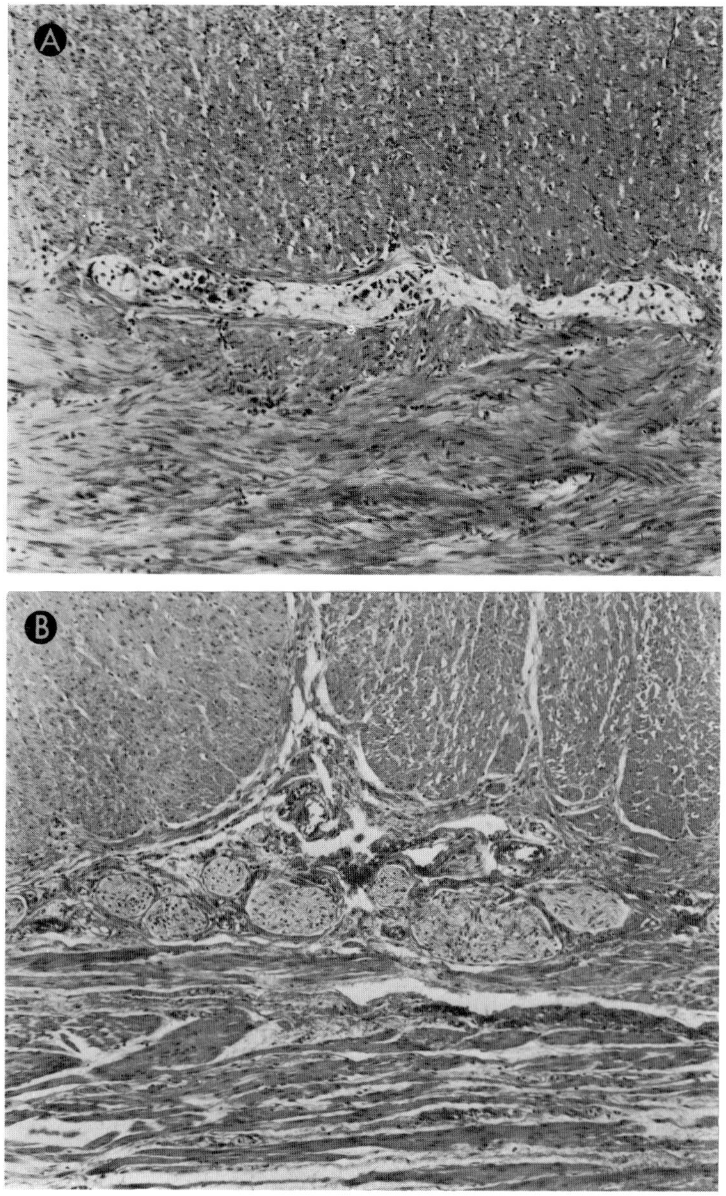

Fig. 76-6.—**A,** myenteric plexus showing ganglion cells. **B,** absence of ganglion cells, hypertrophic nerves in place of myenteric plexus.

due to an abnormal function of the neuromuscular apparatus of the intestine. Since a stenosis or scarring of the wall was not found at any point in the rectum or rectosigmoid, the first hypothesis could not be upheld. The concept of a gross malformation was based on the frequent finding of associated malformations, a finding that has not been generally confirmed. It is now recognized that obstruction is caused by congenital absence of parasympathetic ganglion cells in the rectum, the rectosigmoid or the lower part of the sigmoid itself. Peristaltic waves cannot pass through the rectosigmoid properly because of the neuromuscular deficiency and, consequently, the more proximal portions of the colon are enlarged and thickened by the fecal masses that are not propelled through the end portions of the intestinal tract. This concept, which was proposed by several authors in 1948,[16-18] differed from the old assumption that the enlarged and distended bowel was the abnormal part. In histologic studies of 11 cases of congenital megacolon, Whitehouse and Kernohan[16] found the myenteric (Auerbach) plexus absent in the most distal part of the colon. In a majority of cases, it was also absent in the transitional region, including the lower part of the sigmoid, whereas the upper part of the sigmoid was only rarely affected. In all instances, there were nerves present in place of the myenteric plexus (Fig. 76-6). Zuelzer and Wilson[17] described a series of cases with the clinical picture of acute recurrent (chronic) intestinal obstruction in which no mechanical cause was demonstrable. They thought that the functional disturbance in intestinal motility was related to the congenital absence of nerve cells in the enteric nervous system. The picture of the chronic cases merged with that of idiopathic megacolon. A familial trend was recognized in several instances. Swenson and Bill[18] reported on resection of the rectum and rectosigmoid with preservation of the sphincter for treatment of megacolon and thus prepared the way for the now-accepted surgical procedure for Hirschsprung disease. It is assumed that ganglionic aplasia in Hirschsprung disease extends proximally to the splenic flexure in less than 10% of the cases, but Bowden *et al.*[19] emphasized that in some patients the ganglionic defect may involve the entire large intestine and a portion of the small intestine. Such severe deficits are responsible for acute manifestations in the neonatal period and for early death before megacolon develops.[19] In their series, Bodian and Carter[8] found approximately 20% "long segment" and 80% "short segment" cases. The concepts of the etiology, diagnosis and treatment of congenital megacolon were clearly outlined by Swenson *et al.*[20] in 1949. These authors stated that Hirschsprung disease was due to a functionally abnormal segment of bowel in the sigmoid or rectosigmoid, and that this could be demonstrated by appropriate roentgenologic studies. The bowel dilatation and hypertrophy above this abnormally functioning segment resembled changes commonly found above an area of obstruction. Removal of the functionally abnormal bowel, rectum or rectosigmoid relieved the patient's symptoms. In 1950, Bodian *et al.*[21] examined 28 consecutive cases of Hirschsprung disease and confirmed that there were no intramural ganglion cells in the distal narrow bowel and that there were abnormal nerve bundles in the customary sites of the intramural plexus.

This short note on the search for pathogenesis and treatment of this disorder is not complete. The disease had been described before Hirschsprung and there were many observations suggesting the true situation before 1948.[2,3]

The mechanism leading to the neurologic deficit between the two muscular layers of the rectum has not been elucidated. From the observation of clinical cases, one must assume that the deficit exists in some infants from birth on, although, in other patients, the symptoms do not become manifest before adult life. It is possible that in some late cases the ganglion cells of Auerbach plexus are present at birth and during childhood and that they degenerate with advancing age. But, in most cases of Hirschsprung disease, the aganglionosis probably is congenital. Hüther[22] described the development of intramural ganglia in human embryos. In general, differentiation of the ganglia progresses in a craniocaudal direction but the ganglia of the rectum are formed before those of the more cranial segments of the large intestine. It seems that the intramural ganglia migrate into the intestine during embryonic life, and Hüther[22] assumed that the developmental disturbance leading to rectosigmoid aganglionosis occurs before the eighth week of gestation. It should be emphasized, however, that the ganglion cells of the enteric plexuses have not reached full maturity at birth and that full maturation takes place gradually. If one expects the ganglion cells of the newborn to appear as the large multipolar neurons of adults, the diagnosis of Hirschsprung disease would be made more often than is justified.[34] It has been suggested that the primary defect of aganglionosis is a reduction in the number of neural crest cells or an interference with migration of these cells.[13] The fact that, in certain strains of mice, pigment deficiences and partial aganglionosis of the myenteric plexus are associated is cited as support for the role played by neural crest damage in the pathogenesis of congenital megacolon.[7]

Although the old concept of a gross intestinal malformation as the cause of Hirschsprung disease has been abandoned, the "malformation theory" has been shown to be correct, since congenital absence of myenteric ganglia represents a micro-malformation. At the same time, the advocates of the theory of abnormal function of the neuromuscular intestinal apparatus can also claim to be right. It is not rare that early controversies concerning the pathogenesis or etiology of diseases are reconciled by increased knowledge that shows that both parties were right and wrong.

In typical cases, the colon in its entirety or in parts shows enormous enlargement. The wall of the colon is hypertrophied, thickened and the haustra are not recognizable. The rectum and the rectosigmoid are of normal caliber, whereas the sigmoid and, in many cases, other proximal portions of the colon are greatly distended and hypertrophied. Even the distal parts of the ileum can be distended. In atypical cases, the enlargement of the intestine is not continuous, and in some patients distention of the stomach and esophagus has been observed.[11] In the aganglionic portion of the bowel, ganglion cells are absent in the nerve plexuses, but thick bundles of nonmyelinated nerve fibers are found in their place (see Fig. 76-6). Ulceration of the mucosa as described by Hirschsprung may occur in untreated cases. Perforation of deep-seated ulcers can occur and lead to peritonitis. Enlargement of the bladder frequently is present and megalo-ureter is seen occasionally.[12] Agenesis of peripheral autonomic ganglia characteristic of megacolon is not the cause of coexisting megalo-ureter.[23]

As a rule, Hirschsprung disease makes its appearance soon after birth or in early infancy. There is obstinate constipation and marked enlargement of the abdomen. There may be no bowel movements for many days or even weeks. Distention, fetid odor of breath, anorexia and chronic malnutrition are the outstanding symptoms. The diaphragm may be displaced upward and cause difficulty in respiration and in circulation. Vomiting is not an outstanding symptom in typical cases[24] but in the neonatal period it can be an early manifestation. In the chronic form of megacolon there may be symptom-free periods that alternate with episodes that simulate acute intestinal obstruction. There is no obstruction at the anus and the rectum often is empty. In the neonatal period the clinical picture can differ from that of older children. The presenting symptoms may be failure to pass meconium, constipation from birth, abdominal distention and vomiting, but persistent diarrhea with passing of loose, watery stools and vomiting can also be early manifestations.[19,25] Functional obstruction in the neonatal period leading to perforation and pneumoperitoneum or to fluid and electrolyte imbalance,[26] dehydration, loss of weight and bile-stained or fecal vomiting sometimes also results in a disease picture quite different from that of classic Hirschsprung disease. Swenson and Davidson[27] emphasized the similarity of symptoms in the neonate of aganglionosis and mechanical intestinal obstruction. Rectal biopsy leads to the correct diagnosis. But it has been pointed out that in normal newborn children, particularly in prematures, the enteric plexuses have not yet reached morphologic maturity in the caudal bowels, which could lead to an erroneous diagnosis of Hirschsprung disease.[34] In older children, the clinical picture can also vary greatly. In mild cases, constipation and moderate abdominal distention may be present for years and then improve, so that the patient can grow up, get married and pass on the condition to some of his children. In other patients, the severe disease picture develops (see Figs. 76-4 and 76-5).

Roentgenographic findings are characterized by a rectum and a rectosigmoid that are normal on a barium enema. At the same time, there is tremendous enlargement of the sigmoid and colon. Peristaltic waves coming down the sigmoid terminate abruptly at the rectosigmoid.[20] The urinary tract should be investigated in all persons with Hirschsprung disease, since enlargement of the bladder and megalo-ureter occur in some of the cases.[12]

Conservative medical treatment is possible in some of the patients who can lead a fairly normal life. Diet, cathartics, enemas and parasympathetic stimulants can be employed. Many children must be treated surgically. Gross[24] discussed the results of sympathectomy, cecostomy or colostomy and transabdominal resection. The procedure of choice is now abdominoperineal removal of the rectosigmoid.[18,24] The therapeutic gains have been superior to those that have been attained by other methods. The operation can be done in experienced hands with a low fatality rate, with few postoperative complications and with a promise of curing the patient's complaints in more than 90% of the cases.[24] Alternative surgical procedures have been recommended by Hiatt,[28] State,[29] Duhamel[30] and others.[2,3,31,32] The treatment of infants with congenital megacolon represents a special task that requires cooperation of the pediatrician, radiologist, pathologist and surgeon.[33]

REFERENCES

1. Hirschsprung, H.: Stuhlträgheit Neugeborener in Folge von Dilatation und Hypertrophie des Colons, Jahrb. Kinderh. 27:1, 1887.
2. Pilling, G. P., IV, and Cresson, S. L.: Hirschsprung's Disease, in Mustard, W. T., Ravitch, M. M., Snyder, W. H., Jr., Welch, K. J., and Benson, C. D. (eds.), *Pediatric Surgery* (2d ed.; Chicago: Year Book Medical Publishers, Inc., 1969), p. 961.
3. Madsen, C. M.: *Hirschsprung's Disease. Congenital Intestinal Aganglionosis* (Springfield, Ill.: Charles C Thomas, Publisher, 1964).
4. Passarge, E.: The genetics of Hirschsprung's disease. Evidence of heterogeneous etiology and a study of sixty-three families, New England J. Med. 276:138, 1967.
5. Maltarello, A. A., and Casa, D.: Megacolon idiopatico in madre e due figli gemelli MZ, in Gedda, L., *Novant' anni dell Leggi Mendeliane* (Rome: Instituto Gregorio Mendel, 1955), pp. 472–483.
6. Bielschowsky, M., and Schofield, G. C.: Studies on the inheritance and neurohistology of megacolon in mice, Proc. Univ. Otago M. School 38/2:14, 1960.
7. Lane, P. W.: Association of megacolon with two recessive spotting genes in the mouse, J. Hered. 57:29, 1966.
8. Bodian, M., and Carter, C. O.: A family study of Hirschsprung's disease, Ann. Human Genet. 26:261, 1963.
9. Hayward, M. D., and Cameron, A. H.: Triple mosaicism of the sex chromosomes in Turner's syndrome and Hirschsprung's disease, Lancet 2:623, 1961.
10. Butler, L. J., France, N. E., Russell, A., and Sinclair, L.: A chromosomal aberration associated with multiple congenital anomalies, Lancet 1:1242, 1962.
11. Ask-Upmark, E.: Studien über Megacolon mit besonderer Berücksichtigung der Pathogenese und der Spätresultate, Bruns, Beitr. klin. Chir. 151:267, 1930.
12. Swenson, O., and Fisher, J. H.: The relation of megacolon and megaloureter, New England J. Med. 253:1147, 1955.
13. Shocket, E., and Teloh, H. A.: Aganglionic megacolon, pheochromocytoma, megaloureter, and neurofibroma, A.M.A. J. Dis. Child. 94:185, 1957.
14. Morger, R., and Meier-Ruge, W.: Pseudo-Hirschsprung, Monatsschr. Kinderh. 114:579, 1966.
15. Bentley, J. F. R., Nixon, H. H., Ehrenpreis, Th., and Spencer, B.: Seminar on pseudo-Hirschsprung's disease and related disorders, Arch. Dis. Childhood 41:143, 1966.
16. Whitehouse, F. R., and Kernohan, J. W.: The myenteric plexus in congenital megacolon, Arch. Int. Med. 82:75, 1948.
17. Zuelzer, W. W., and Wilson, J. L.: Functional intestinal obstruction on a congenital neurogenic basis in infancy, Am. J. Dis. Child. 75:40, 1948.
18. Swenson, O., and Bill, A. H., Jr.: Resection of rectum and rectosigmoid with preservation of the sphincter for benign spastic lesions producing megacolon, Surgery 24: 212, 1948.
19. Bowden, D. H., Goodfellow, A. M., and Munn, J. D.: Hirschsprung's disease in the neonatal period. Report of five cases, four of which involved the small intestine, J. Pediat. 50:321, 1957.
20. Swenson, O., Neuhauser, E. B. D., and Pickett, L. K.: New concepts of the etiology, diagnosis and treatment of congenital megacolon (Hirschsprung's disease), Pediatrics 4: 201, 1949.
21. Bodian, M., Stephens, F. D., and Ward, B. C. H.: Hirschsprung's disease, Lancet 1:19, 1950.
22. Hüther, W.: Die Hirschsprungsche Krankheit als Folge

einer Entwicklungsstörung der intramuralen Ganglien, Beitr. path. Anat. 114:161, 1954.
23. Winkelman, J.: Coexistent megacolon and megaureter, Pediatrics 39:258, 1967.
24. Gross, R. E.: *The Surgery of Infancy and Childhood* (Philadelphia: W. B. Saunders Company, 1953).
25. Ehrenpreis, Th.: Hirschsprung's disease in the neonatal period, Arch. Dis. Childhood 30:8, 1955.
26. Donald, J. G., and Donald, J. W.: Unusual manifestations of aganglionic disorder in the newborn, Surgery 56:644, 1964.
27. Swenson, O., and Davidson, F. Z.: Similarities of mechanical intestinal obstruction and aganglionic megacolon in the newborn infant: A review of 64 cases, New England J. Med. 262:64, 1960.
28. Hiatt, R. B.: The surgical treatment of congenital megacolon, Ann. Surg. 133:321, 1951.
29. State, D.: Physiological operation for idiopathic congenital megacolon (Hirschsprung's disease), J.A.M.A. 149: 350, 1952.
30. Duhamel, B.: A new operation for the treatment of Hirschsprung's disease, Arch. Dis. Childhood 35:38, 1960.
31. Rehbein, F., and Zimmermann, H.: Results with abdominal resection in Hirschsprung's disease, Arch. Dis. Childhood 35:29, 1960.
32. Ikeda, K.: New techniques in the surgical treatment of Hirschsprung's disease, Surgery 61:503, 1967.
33. Shim, W. K. T., and Swenson, O.: Treatment of congenital megacolon in 50 infants, Pediatrics 38:185, 1966.
34. Smith, B.: Pre- and postnatal development of the ganglion cells of the rectum and its surgical implications, J. Pediat. Surg. 3:386, 1968.
35. Kilcoyne, R. F., and Taybi, H.: Conditions associated with congenital megacolon, Am. J. Roentgenol. 108:615, 1970.
36. Haffner, J. F. W., and Schistad, G.: Atresia of the colon combined with Hirschsprung's disease, J. Pediat. Surg. 4: 560, 1969.
37. Fauchier, Cl., Régy, J-M., and Combe, P.: Nanisme diastrophique familial avec maladie de Hirschsprung, Ann. pédiat. 16:496, 1969.

Malformations of the Hindgut and Anus

THE PRIMITIVE HINDGUT is first established in early embryos by the ventrad bending of the tailfold, which incorporates a portion of the secondary yolk sac into the embryo. The allantoic diverticulum communicates with the ventral aspect of the early hindgut. In 5-mm. embryos (approximately 32 days), the hindgut is represented by a tube located in the midline that terminates in a dilated blind sac, the primitive cloaca. At about the same stage, a coronal (transverse) mesodermal septum is formed between the allantois and the hindgut that divides the cloaca into the ventral urogenital sinus and the dorsal rectum. This urorectal septum grows toward the cloacal membrane and fuses with it, in embryos 16 mm. in length (seventh week), at the primitive perineum. The portion of the cloacal membrane situated anterior to the point of fusion becomes the urogenital membrane and the posterior portion becomes the anal membrane. From the primitive hindgut are derived the left third of the transverse colon, the descending and pelvic colon, the rectum, the upper part of the anal canal and a portion of the urogenital system.[1] The ecto-endodermal anal membrane becomes surrounded by a mesodermal ring in which the thin membrane appears as a depression (proctodeum). In the third month, the anal membrane ruptures and a communication is established between the rectum and the amniotic cavity.

Bill and Johnson[2] believed that after union of the urorectal septum with the cloacal membrane, the (future) rectal opening is moved backward across the developing perineum by the process of tissue filling in anteriorly until the normal position of the anus is reached. In the meantime, the external sphincter muscles and their nerve supply develop independently at the normal position of the anus. Thus, the rectal opening at first leads into the urogenital sinus until the urorectal septum closes it off. Then the tip of the rectum, its future opening, "migrates" backward to its normal position within the external sphincter muscles until it is finally connected with the outside by disintegration of the cloacal membrane. This migration of the tip of the rectum may stop at any point along its course, whereas the rest of the development of the area of the perineum, including the external anal sphincter,[3] continues normally. In the female, the Müllerian ducts extend downward "at the expense of" the posterior wall of the urogenital sinus, taking over any fistula that already communicates with the rectum. Thus, the vagina receives a fistula to the rectum.[4]

REFERENCES

1. Hamilton, W. J., Boyd, J. D., and Mossman, H. W.: *Human Embryology: Prenatal Development of Form and Function* (2d ed.; Baltimore: The Williams & Wilkins Company, 1952).
2. Bill, A. H., Jr., and Johnson, R. J.: Failure of migration of the rectal opening as the cause for most cases of imperforate anus, Surg., Gynec. & Obst. 106:643, 1958.
3. Bill, A. H., Jr.: Common denominators in rectal anomalies on both sides of the Atlantic, Arch. Dis. Childhood 39:149, 1964.
4. Gross, R. E.: *The Surgery of Infancy and Childhood* (Philadelphia: W. B. Saunders Company, 1953).

Ano-Rectal Malformations

IT IS ESTIMATED that ano-rectal malformations occur once in 5,000 births.[1,2] There seems to be no distinct tendency to prematurity in such births.[3] In some statistics, males and females are affected equally, but some of the males may not appear in hospital statistics, since they often die before they reach a hospital.[1] It seems that males are affected more often by anal (low) lesions and by blindly ending rectum.[4]

That genetic factors play a role in the etiology of ano-rectal malformations is suggested occasionally by their familial occurrence. In one family, a mother who had had imperforate anus with a recto-vaginal fistula had 2 girls with imperforate anus and 3 normal children. One of the girls with imperforate anus had a recto-vaginal fistula and the other had a perineal fistula.[5] Suckling[6] reported congenital abnormalities of the anus and rectum in 3 patients in two generations. Cochran[7] observed imperforate anus in brothers, both having type 3 anomalies (see below). Fuhrmann *et al.*[2] reported 2 brothers with imperforate anus. The older brother also had duplication of the right thumb and probably congenital heart disease. Grebe[8] described necropsy findings in 2 brothers with ano-rectal atresia. One of these children also had exstrophy of the bladder, epispadias and absence of the right kidney and ureter and of the prostate and seminal vesicles. Van Gelder and Kloepfer[9] observed a family in which all 4 children had ano-rectal anomalies. Weinstein[10] reviewed three families with recurrent cases of imperforate anus and noted a distribution suggesting a sex-linked recessive pattern of inheritance in these instances. It is noteworthy that imperforate anus can be an early symptom of the Laurence-Moon-Biedl syndrome (p. 176), particularly if associated with polydactyly. This combination can presage the disorder in an affected child or for subsequently born siblings (p. 179). In a survey of 133 ano-rectal anomalies, Cozzi and Wilkinson[33] found 2 pairs of twins, both affected, and 3 other children who had affected relatives. But Tünte,[34] investigating the case histories of 18 pairs of twins with anal atresia found discordance to be the rule and concluded that genetic factors play only a minor role in the etiology of anal atresia. Imperforate anus occurs occasionally in children with Down syndrome and in children with trisomy 18.[11] Moore and Lawrence[3] listed 2 children with Down syndrome among 120 cases of ano-rectal malformations, an incidence approximately ten times that of Down syndrome in the general newborn population. Zellweger *et al.*[12] recorded the case of a girl with possible partial trisomy D who had multiple congenital malformations, including anal atresia and recto-vaginal fistula, and Gustavson *et al.*[31] described a boy with a 4 or 5/21 or 22 translocation who had anal atresia and other defects. Sparkes *et al.*[32] recorded a boy with a D_2 ring chromosome who was born with imperforate anus and many other malformations. Anal atresia combined with microphthalmia and preauricular skin tags has been described as a syndrome that has been associated repeatedly with an extra small acrocentric chromosome.[35]

Imperforate anus due to extrinsic factors must be considered possible. Among the malformations produced by thalidomide, anal stenosis and imperforate anus have been reported repeatedly. There may be a

Fig. 76-7. – Perineum without anal opening.

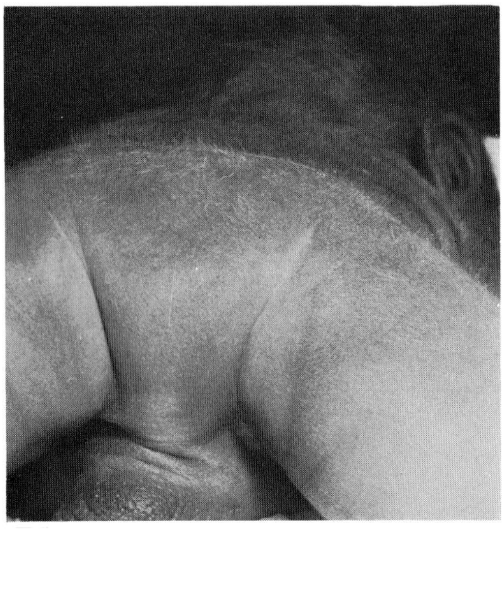

Fig. 76-8. – Imperforate anus in a newborn tailless rat; the mother was treated with trypan blue injections.

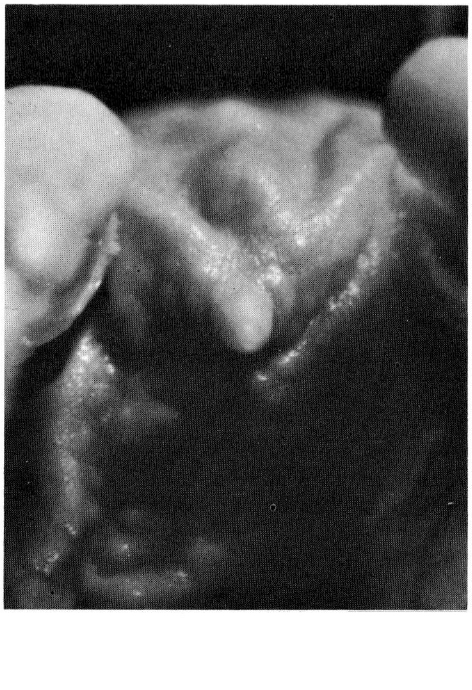

dimple in the skin or a blind pouch several centimeters in length. Sometimes the anal sphincter is missing. Recto-vaginal or recto-urethral fistulas occur.[13,15] In animals, imperforate anus has been produced experimentally, e.g., by trypan blue.[16] Ano-rectal anomalies appeared spontaneously in mice with the "disorganization" mutation,[17] and in mice with the "fused" gene.[18]

Usually, four types of ano-rectal anomalies are described.[19] Type 1 is a stenosis of the anus, type 2 is a membranous obstruction of the anus, type 3 is imperforate anus with a rectal pouch ending some distance above the anus and type 4 is a normal anus with a rectal pouch ending blindly some distance above the anus anterior to the sacrum. Type 3 comprises approximately 80% of the cases.[20] About 70% of the patients with ano-rectal anomalies have fistulas connecting the rectum with the perineum or with the urogenital tract. In males, recto-urethral, recto-vesical and recto-perineal fistulas occur, each type accounting for one-third of the cases. In females, recto-vaginal fistulas make up approximately three-fourths and recto-perineal fistulas one-fourth of the cases; recto-vesical fistulas are rare in females and the recto-urethral form does not occur. In approximately half the patients, the fistulas are large enough to permit evacuation of feces.[19] In the presence of anal or rectal stenosis (type 1), constipation and difficulty in evacuation are observed. With an imperforate membrane (type 2) showing distention, vomiting and absence of meconium, early recognition is the rule. Similar symptoms appear early in infants who have imperforate anus of type 3, if the obstruction is not relieved by a functional fistula. With fistulas, the condition can be tolerated for years. Since in type 4 the anus appears normal, recognition of the anomaly often is delayed for several days until distention, vomiting and dehydration set in. In a monograph, Stephens[4] distinguished anal and rectal deformities in regard to origin and surgical treatment. Rectal anomalies are those with termination of the hindgut at the verumontanum or higher in the male and at corresponding pelvic levels in the female. Anal malformations are those referable to the proctodeal pit and membrane, the perineum and genital folds. The latter group is more common and more accessible to treatment. Snyder[21] reported a series of 42 female patients with some unusual forms of imperforate anus. Reviews have been written by Woolam[22] and Santulli *et al.*[23] and an international classification of the numerous variations has been suggested.[39]

Congenital ano-rectal malformations often are accompanied by anomalies of other organs. Recto-urogenital fistulas usually are not considered associated malformations but rather a part of the rectal anomaly. Estimates of the incidence of associated malformations vary between 22% and 72%,[3] but of children with ano-rectal anomalies who come to necropsy nearly 100% have associated defects. Moore and Lawrence,[3] in reviewing 120 cases, found 72% complicated by associated malformations. In 34%, malformations of the urinary tract were present, with megalo-ureter and hydronephrosis in the lead. This is in agreement with the findings of Garrett and Yurdin,[24] who, finding 45% of their cases complicated by urologic anomalies, emphasized that many children die of urologic lesions years after their ano-rectal malformations have been treated successfully. Some renal malformations of such children (e.g., agenesis) cannot be repaired surgically. Urinary anomalies were present in 57 of 195 patients in a series of ano-rectal anomalies reported by Smith.[36] The urologic problems were more serious with rectal than with anal malformations. Early diagnosis and preventive treatment of these problems were emphasized. Malformations of the spine, particularly those of the sacrococcygeal portion, are also frequent.[1] Atresia of the anus and rectum and malformations of the vertebral column, ribs, radius and tibia have been described as a symptom complex.[38] Stephens[4] pointed out that sacral and coccygeal abnormalities are much more common in rectal defects than in anal defects, and Berdon *et al.*[25] stressed that spinal and urogenital malformations occur much more often in "high" than in "low" types of imperforate anus. Some of these are accompanied by myelomeningocele, but others are not seen externally. Other anomalies of the central nervous system are encountered also. Mongolism associated with ano-rectal malformations[3] has been mentioned (p. 328). Complicating malformations of the gastrointestinal tract are less frequent than those of the urinary tract, but they deserve immediate attention after birth, since some of them, e.g., esophageal or duodenal atresia, are incompatible with life without operation. Congenital heart disease occurred in 15% and malformations of the female genital tract in approximately 20% of the cases reviewed by Moore and Lawrence.[3] Some of these patients have only minor associated malformations, such as deformities of the ears or fingers, whereas others are so deformed that they are classified as monstrosities. Sirenoid monsters usually have ano-rectal malformations. Roentgenologic examinations are important for localization and classification of the ano-rectal anomalies as well as for recognition of associated defects.[25-27] Duplication of the anus and genitourinary system is a rare occurrence; it was reviewed in 1969 by Smith,[37] who found 38 cases reported in the literature and added 2 cases of his own.

Treatment of ano-rectal anomalies and of associated malformations is surgical.[19,20,24,28] Cures are achieved more often in anal than in rectal congenital malformations.[4] Low birth weight and associated malformations contribute greatly to fatal outcome.[29]

The over-all mortality rate for high anomalies (bowel terminating above the pelvic floor) is approximately six times higher than that for low lesions (below the pelvic floor).[30]

REFERENCES

1. Parkkulainen, K. V.: Sacrococcygeal and urological anomalies in connection with congenital malformations of anus and rectum. A preliminary report, Ann. paediat. Fenniae 3:51, 1957.
2. Fuhrmann, W., Rieger, A., and Vogel, F.: Zwei Beobachtungen zur Genetik der Atresia ani, Arch. Kinderh. 158: 264, 1958.
3. Moore, T. C., and Lawrence, E. A.: Congenital malformations of the rectum and anus. Associated anomalies encountered in series of 120 cases, Surg., Gynec. & Obst. 95:281, 1952.
4. Stephens, F. D.: *Congenital Malformations of the Rectum, Anus and Genito-Urinary Tracts* (Edinburgh and London: E. & S. Livingstone, Ltd., 1963).
5. Kaijser, K. A., and Malström-Groth, A.: Ano-rectal abnormalities as a congenital familial incidence, Acta paediat. 46:199, 1957.
6. Suckling, P. V.: Familial incidence of congenital abnormalities of the anus and rectum, Arch. Dis. Childhood 24: 75, 1949.
7. Cochran, J. L.: Imperforate anus in brothers, A.M.A. Am. J. Dis. Child. 89:350, 1955.
8. Grebe, H.: Zur Erblichkeit von Darmmissbildungen, Der Erbarzt 11:104, 1943.
9. Van Gelder, D. W., and Kloepfer, H. W.: Familial anorectal anomalies, Pediatrics 27:334, 1961.
10. Weinstein, E. D.: Sex-linked imperforate anus, Pediatrics 35:715, 1965.
11. Warkany, J., Passarge, E., and Smith, L. B.: Congenital malformations in autosomal trisomy syndromes, Am. J. Dis. Child. 112:502, 1966.
12. Zellweger, H., Mikamo, K., and Abbo, G.: Two cases of multiple malformations with an autosomal chromosomal aberration – partial trisomy D?, Helvet. paediat. acta 17: 290, 1962.
13. Ives, E. J.: Thalidomide and anal abnormalities, Canad. M.A.J. 87:670, 1962.
14. Imdahl, H., Koch, W., and Hermanns, A.: Thalidomid in der Frühschwangerschaft und Enddarmmissbildungen, Bull. Soc. internat. chir. 22:602, 1963.
15. Kreipe, U.: Missbildungen innerer Organe bei Thalidomidembryopathie, Arch. Kinderh. 176:33, 1967.
16. Gillman, J., Gilbert, C., and Gillman, T.: A preliminary report on hydrocephalus, spina bifida and other congenital anomalies in the rat produced by trypan blue, South African J. M. Sc. 13:47, 1948.
17. Hummel, K. P.: Developmental anomalies in mice resulting from action of the gene disorganization, a semi-dominant lethal, Pediatrics 23:212, 1959.
18. Dunn, L. C., and Gluecksohn-Waelsch, S.: A genetical study of the mutation "fused" in the house mouse, with evidence concerning its allelism with a similar mutation "kink," J. Genetics 52:383, 1954.
19. Gross, R. E.: *The Surgery of Infancy and Childhood* (Philadelphia: W. B. Saunders Company, 1953).
20. Orloff, M. J.: Congenital anomalies of the anus and rectum, J. Pediat. 45:316, 1954.
21. Snyder, W. H., Jr.: Some unusual forms of imperforate anus in female infants, Am. J. Surg. 111:319, 1966.
22. Woolam, G. L.: Congenital anomalies of the anus and rectum, Birth Defects Reprint Series, The National Foundation – March of Dimes. Reprinted from Mayo Clin. Proc. 39:866, 1964.
23. Santulli, T. V., Schullinger, J. N., and Amoury, R. A.: Malformations of the anus and rectum, S. Clin. North America 45:1253, 1965.
24. Garrett, R. A., and Yurdin, D.: Urological complications of imperforate anus, J. Urol. 79:514, 1958.
25. Berdon, W. E., Hochberg, B., Baker, D. H., Grossman, H., and Santulli, T. V.: The association of lumbosacral spine and genitourinary anomalies with imperforate anus, Am. J. Roentgenol. 98:181, 1966.
26. Kurlander, G. J.: Roentgenology of imperforate anus, Am. J. Roentgenol. 100:190, 1967.
27. Winslow, O., Litt, R., and Altman, D.: Imperforate anus from a roentgenologic viewpoint, Am. J. Roentgenol. 85: 718, 1961.
28. Browne, D.: Some congenital deformities of the rectum, anus, vagina and urethra, Ann. Roy. Coll. Surgeons England 8:173, 1951.
29. Cozzi, F., and Wilkinson, A. W.: Congenital abnormalities of anus and rectum: Mortality and function, Brit. M. J. 1: 144, 1968.
30. Partridge, J. P., and Gough, M. H.: Congenital abnormalities of the anus and rectum, Brit. J. Surg. 49:37, 1961.
31. Gustavson, K-H., Finley, S. C., Finley, W. H., and Jalling, B.: A 4-5/21-22 chromosomal translocation associated with multiple congenital anomalies, Acta paediat. 53: 172, 1964.
32. Sparkes, R. S., Carrel, R. E., and Wright, S. W.: Absent thumbs with a ring D_2 chromosome: A new deletion syndrome, Am. J. Human Genet. 19:644, 1967.
33. Cozzi, F., and Wilkinson, A. W.: Familial incidence of congenital anorectal anomalies, Surgery 64:669, 1968.
34. Tünte, W.: Analatresie bei Zwillingen, Ztschr. Kinderh. 105:21, 1969.
35. Weber, F. M., Dooley, R. R., and Sparkes, R. S.: Anal atresia, eye anomalies, and an additional small abnormal acrocentric chromosome (47,XX, mar+): Report of a case, J. Pediat. 76:594, 1970.
36. Smith, E. D.: Urinary anomalies and complications in imperforate anus and rectum, J. Pediat. Surg. 3:337, 1968.
37. Smith, E. D.: Duplication of the anus and genitourinary tract, Surgery 66:909, 1969.
38. Schönenberg, H.: Skeletfehlbildungen bei Anal- und Rectumatresie, Monatsschr. Kinderh. 118:149, 1970.
39. Santulli, T. V., Kiesewetter, W. B., and Bill, A. H., Jr.: Anorectal anomalies: A suggested international classification, J. Pediat. Surg. 5:281, 1970.

Exstrophia Splanchnica
(Exstrophy of the Cloaca)

THIS IS A striking malformation for which many expressions have been used in the past. Spencer[1] reviewed the subject in 1965 and suggested the term "exstrophia splanchnica" to indicate that viscera were "turned out" in this condition. Owing to failure of development of the lower parietal mesoderm, the primary cloacal membrane remains a thin entodermal and ectodermal structure. After breakdown of this membrane, the urogenital portion of the endodermal cloaca becomes exposed. In addition, there is failure of development of the uro-rectal septum, so that the dorsal wall of the hindgut is exposed also. The lower ileum, colon and rectum, which, in normal

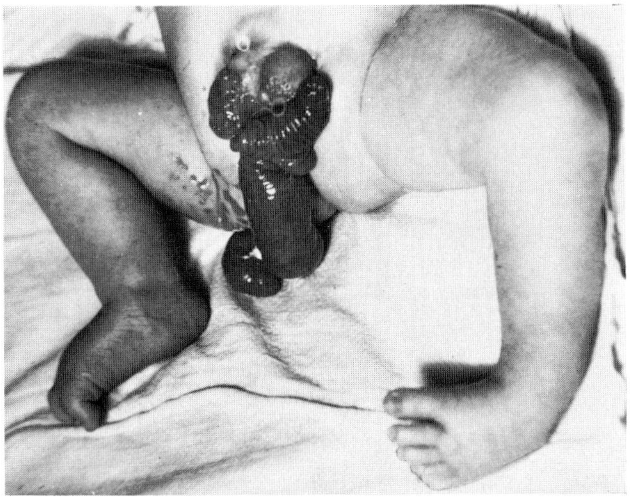

Fig. 76-9. – Exstrophia splanchnica. The upper exposed area represents exstrophy of the bladder. Below it, the prolapsed ileocecal viscus is seen. There are clubfoot deformities.

embryos, are formed from that portion of the hindgut, do not grow properly. The intestine usually terminates with an opening located below the umbilicus between the two halves of the exposed bladder mucosa, but the picture is complicated by prolapse of the viscus, which corresponds to the terminal ileum (Fig. 76-9). Under this prolapse, an opening is found that leads into a short blind colon. The anus is imperforate. One or two appendices may be connected with the exstrophied intestine or the appendix can be absent. Ileocecal exstrophy can be combined with a closed, intra-abdominal bladder, and other variations are possible.[2] Exomphalos occurs as an associated malformation in some of the cases. Ureteral orifices or a vaginal opening may be seen on the bladder mucosa. Associated malformations of the kidneys, genitalia, legs and lower vertebral column, including spina bifida (hydromyelia, p. 292), are common but it

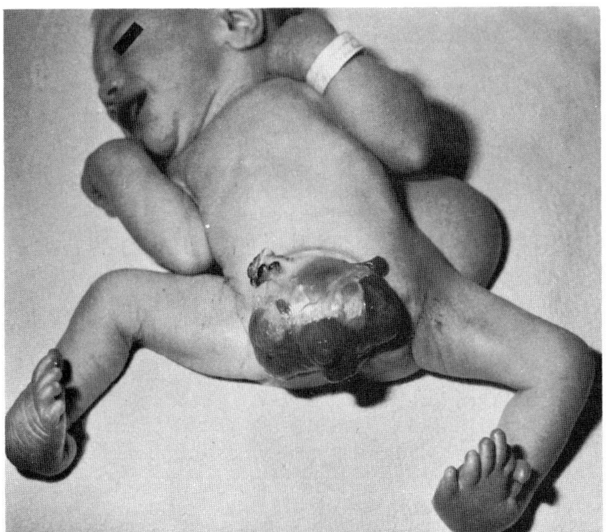

Fig. 76-10. – Exstrophy of the bladder and cloaca. There is a small prolapse of the bowel in the center of the exposed bladder. The child also had spina bifida, clubfeet and polydactyly on the left foot.

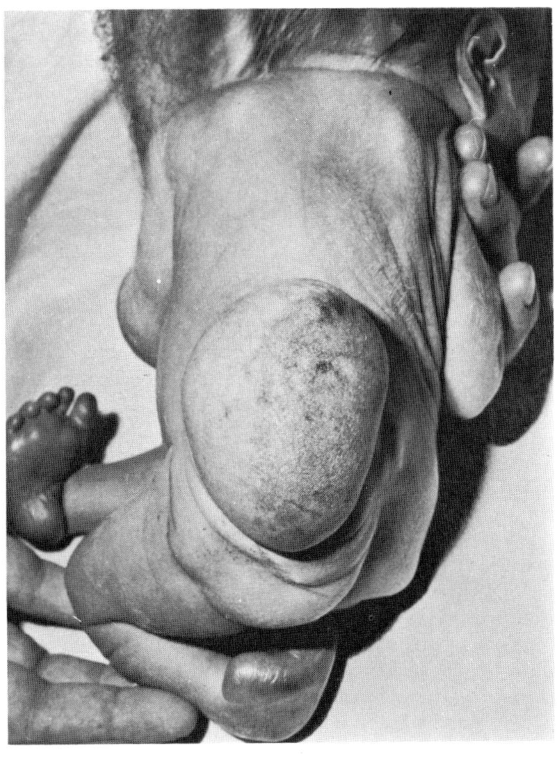

seems that complicating anomalies are limited to the caudal end of the body. It is for this reason that intensive treatment of the urinary and intestinal anomalies is recommended.[1,3]

Because of the variation in the anatomy of the bowel and the observation of prolapse of the bowel between the two halves of the exstrophic bladder, Magnus[4] recommended the descriptive term "vesico-intestinal fistula" for these complicated malformations.

REFERENCES

1. Spencer, R.: Exstrophia splanchnica (exstrophy of the cloaca), Surgery 57:751, 1965.
2. Spencer, R., and Geer, J. C.: Ileocecal exstrophy with bifid intra-abdominal urinary bladder: Incomplete exstrophy of the cloaca, J. Pediat. Surg. 2:69, 1967.
3. Swan, H., and Christensen, S. P.: Exstrophy of the cloaca, Pediatrics 12:645, 1953.
4. Magnus, R. V.: Ectopia cloacae—a misnomer, J. Pediat. Surg. 4:511, 1969.

Polyposes

Gastrointestinal Polyposis with Pigmentation of the Oral Mucosa (Peutz Syndrome)

In 1921, Peutz[1] described the "very remarkable case of familial polyposis of mucous membrane of intestinal tract and nasopharynx accompanied by peculiar pigmentation of skin and mucous membrane." Four years later, van Dijk and Oudendal[2] reported colicky attacks and intussusception of the ileum due to adenomas in siblings who had congenital pigmented spots of the lips. The syndrome of gastrointestinal polyposis and oral pigmentation has since been recognized as a hereditary trait dependent on an autosomal dominant gene with pleiotropic effects. Jeghers *et al.*[3] carefully reviewed the literature and added 10 case reports. Males and females were affected equally and the patients belonged to many ethnic groups. At first it was thought that only persons of dark complexion have the disorder but there are exceptions to this rule.[4,5] The melanin-pigment spots are present at birth or noticeable soon afterward. They occur on the lips and buccal mucosa and consist of brown or black patches usually measuring 1–5 mm. in diameter. The gums, hard palate and tongue are involved less often. In sections, the pigment deposits appear as bands oriented vertically to the surface. The face or the nasal or rectal mucosa sometimes shows similar cutaneous lesions. There also are some pigmented patches on the fingers and toes. The facial spots may fade during adult life but those of the oral mucosa persist.

Observations of these oral pigmentations direct attention to the possibility of polyposis of the intestine. Although polyps can occur in such patients in any portion of the gastrointestinal tract, the typical and prevalent location is in the small intestine. Abdominal pain, vomiting, melena, anemia and intussusception are presenting symptoms and jejunal adenomatous polyps usually are found on examination. Malignant degeneration can set in, but it seems to be rarer than in patients with the more common colonic polyposis.[3] Polyps have been observed also in the stomach, large intestine, bladder and nose. The disorder can be considered a hamartosis.[6] Occasionally, intestinal symptoms appear in children.[7]

Hereditary Polyposis of the Colon

In this uncommon disorder, the colonic mucosa and submucosa form polyps in large numbers, which are scattered throughout the large bowel. The polyps are not detectable at birth but it is estimated that the gene responsible for the development of multiple polyposis is present at birth in 1 of 8,300 newborn children.[8] In exceptional cases, multiple polyps can be found in infancy[9] but, as a rule, polyposis develops between the ages of 15 and 40 years and symptoms appear about 5 years after the development of the growths. Although polyps alone can lead to disturbances, their importance lies in the fact that they have a strong tendency to malignant degeneration, so that their bearers develop early adenocarcinoma of the rectum or colon.[10] Most victims of this disorder die in their forties of carcinoma of the colon. Among the earlier symptoms are rectal bleeding, diarrhea, anemia, weight loss and abdominal cramps, followed by cachexia and death due to carcinoma.

The polyps, which usually appear first in the rectum or sigmoid during adolescence, begin as rather insignificant elevations that later develop into typical sessile or pedunculated adenomatous polyps. Such polyps occur in small numbers in approximately 5% of the general adult population,[11] but in the victims of hereditary polyposis, hundreds or thousands of these growths may cover the colonic lumina. One or several of these undergo malignant degeneration.

In some of the patients, associated connective tissue tumors occur.[10,12,13] Osteomas, fibromas, desmoid tumors, lipomas, leiomyomas and others have been found coexisting with polyposis (Gardner syndrome, p. 1268). It seems that familial polyposis can develop without associated connective tissue tumors,[8] but Smith[14] stressed the occurrence of desmoid tumors, particularly in incisional scars in patients with multiple polyposis, and believed in a general tendency of such patients to mesenchymal cell proliferation.

Multiple polyposis of the colon, as well as Gardner syndrome, can be attributed to an abnormal autosomal dominant gene with high penetrance and variable expression. Many pedigrees supporting this statement have been recorded,[8] the largest one composed of 429 persons, of whom 49 showed, through five generations, evidence of polyposis.[10] In one family mentioned by Gross,[15] 4 children of a mother who had died of polyposis and carcinoma recti at the age of 29 years developed polyposis requiring colectomy during childhood. One of them, a girl 12 years of age, had carcinoma of the rectum. Three maternal uncles had died of carcinoma of the rectum in their twenties and thirties.

Surgical treatment of the disorder has been effected.[10,15]

Benign Lymphoid Polyposis

A syndrome of familial benign lymphoid polyposis associated with facial freckles and café au lait spots was discussed by Louw.[16] Sessile or pedunculated lymphoid polyps were found in the colon or rectum of 4 children belonging to one family. The mother had similar skin lesions but no polyps. Spontaneous regression and possible response to steroids and chemotherapy have been reported.

REFERENCES

1. Peutz, J. L. A.: A very remarkable case of familial polyposis of mucous membrane of intestinal tract and nasopharynx accompanied by peculiar pigmentation of skin and mucous membrane, Nederl. maandschr. geneesk. 10: 134, 1921.
2. van Dijk, J. A., and Oudendal, A. J. F.: Adenoma of small intestine with contribution to knowledge of heredity in tumors, Nederl. tijdschr. geneesk. 69:966, 1925.
3. Jeghers, H., McKusick, V. A., and Katz, K. H.: Generalized intestinal polyposis and melanin spots of oral mucosa, lips and digits; syndrome of diagnostic significance, New England J. Med. 241:993 and 1031, 1949.
4. Young, W. G., Jr.: Jejunal polyps and intussusception associated with abnormal melanin pigmentation, Surgery 34:46, 1953.
5. Crumpacker, E. L.: Intestinal polyposis and pigmentation of the lip; report of a case, New England J. Med. 252:272, 1955.
6. Bartholomew, L. G., Dahlin, D. C., and Waugh, J. M.: Intestinal polyposis associated with muco-cutaneous melanin pigmentation (Peutz-Jeghers syndrome), Gastroenterology 32:434, 1957.
7. Tucker, A. S., and Bolande, R. P.: Duodenal polyposis associated with mucocutaneous melanosis (Peutz-Jeghers syndrome), A.M.A. J. Dis. Child. 99:329, 1960.
8. Reed, T. E., and Neel, J. V.: A genetic study of multiple polyposis of the colon (with appendix deriving a method of estimating relative fitness), Am. J. Human Genet. 7: 236, 1955.
9. LeFevre, H. W., Jr., and Jaques, T. F.: Multiple polyposis in an infant of four months, Am. J. Surg. 81:90, 1951.
10. Kelly, P. B., and McKinnon, D. A.: Familial multiple polyposis of the colon; a review and initial description of a large kindred, McGill M. J. 30:68, 1961.
11. Rider, J. A., Kirsner, J. B., Moeller, H. C., and Palmer, W. L.: Polyps of the colon and rectum. Their incidence and relationship to carcinoma, Am. J. Med. 16:555, 1954.
12. Gardner, E. J., and Richards, R. C.: Multiple cutaneous and subcutaneous lesions occurring simultaneously with hereditary polyposis and osteomatosis, Am. J. Human Genet. 5:139, 1953.
13. Gorlin, R. J., and Chaudhry, A. P.: Multiple osteomatosis, fibromas, lipomas and fibrosarcomas of the skin and mesentery, epidermoid inclusion cysts of the skin, leiomyomas and multiple intestinal polyposis: A heritable disorder of connective tissue, New England J. Med. 263:1151, 1960.
14. Smith, W. G.: Desmoid tumors in familial multiple polyposis, Proc. Staff Meet. Mayo Clin. 34:31, 1959.
15. Gross, R. E.: *The Surgery of Infancy and Childhood* (Philadelphia: W. B. Saunders Company, 1953).
16. Louw, J. H.: Polypoid lesions of the large bowel in children, with particular reference to benign lymphoid polyposis, J. Pediat. Surg. 3:195, 1968.
17. Haggitt, R. C., and Pitcock, J. A.: Familial juvenile polyposis of the colon, Cancer 26:1232, 1970.

77

The Liver

Malformations

THE LIVER makes its appearance in the embryo at the end of the fourth week (3 mm.) as a ventral diverticulum growing from the junction of the foregut with the yolk stalk into the septum transversum. The hepatic diverticulum develops solid cords of cells that grow into the endothelial walls of veins and divide the venous spaces into anastomosing channels or sinusoids. The sinusoids of the liver are derived from the vitelline veins, which take their course from the yolk sac to the sides of the foregut. The liver cords form an anastomosing net that surrounds the sinusoids. The original hepatic diverticulum is drawn out to form the common bile duct (ductus choledochus), the cystic duct and the gallbladder. These ducts, as well as the gallbladder, go through a solid stage that can be seen in embryos of 4–5 weeks (5–7 mm.). By intra-epithelial vacuolization, lumina are formed, first in the ductus choledochus, then in the cysticus and finally in the gallbladder. Failure in luminization and proliferation of the duodenal epithelium can lead to a variety of anomalies, with obstruction and biliary stasis.[1]

The intralobular secretory tubules are formed within the liver cords at about 6 weeks (12 mm.). They take their course toward the center of a lobule, where they contact a branch of the hepatic duct. Normal biliary flow depends on proper contact of the secretory tubules with the hepatic duct system. If contact is not established, the intralobular ducts become distended to intraparenchymal cysts. Normally, bile is secreted at 12 weeks.[2] Comparative embryology and electron microscopy have added new facts to the concepts of the histogenesis of the liver; they have been reviewed by Wilson *et al.*[3]

The liver divides the septum transversum into a thick upper layer, which becomes the fibrous center of the diaphragm; the middle portion, which develops the reticular tissue that supports the cords and the sinusoids; and the lower layer, which forms the capsule of the liver and gallbladder.[4]

The situation of the liver at the junction of the foregut and the yolk stalk is a strategic one, as the veins to the embryo pass through this area. The hepatic sinusoids, which at first run from the yolk sac on either side of the foregut, are changed in their symmetric arrangement as the stomach and the duodenum rotate and the two vitelline veins are replaced by a single vein that gives off the superior mesenteric and the splanchnic veins and then continues as the portal vein. The portal vein supplies the hepatic sinusoids, which send their blood through the hepatic veins to the heart.

The umbilical veins pass from the body stalk into the lateral body wall and reach the sinus venosus. As the lobes of the liver expand, they come into contact with the umbilical veins, which send their blood to the hepatic sinusoids and to the heart. In embryos of 6 mm., the right and the proximal segment of the left umbilical vein atrophy, and in older embryos the enlarged and single distal remainder of the left umbilical vein continues, entering the liver sinusoids and the larger ductus venosus, which join the hepatic veins and the vena cava.[2]

In early embryos, the liver is a single unit but, with increasing size, the organ is divided into two, six and finally thousands of lobules. Each lobule is surrounded by terminal branches of the portal vein and is drained by a single hepatic vessel. In the second month, the right and left lobes of the liver are of equal size, but in the third month the right lobe becomes larger than the left. Early, the caudate lobe appears set off from the mass of the right lobe but, later, the lobus quadratus becomes visible as it bulges between the umbilical vein and the gallbladder.[2]

Absence of the liver – and of the pancreas – occurs in acardiac and other monstrous fetuses that lack the intestinal tract. There is only one case on record, reported in 1836, that showed aplasia of the liver in the presence of an intestinal tract. The umbilical vein received the portal vein and then divided into two branches, one joining the vena cava and one ending blindly in many small vessels.[1]

Abnormal lobation of the liver is rare but, in some instances, the entire left lobe has been absent. Merrill[5] observed complete absence of the left lobe of the liver in 1 of 19,000 necropsies. The elongated right lobe reached down into the right lower quad-

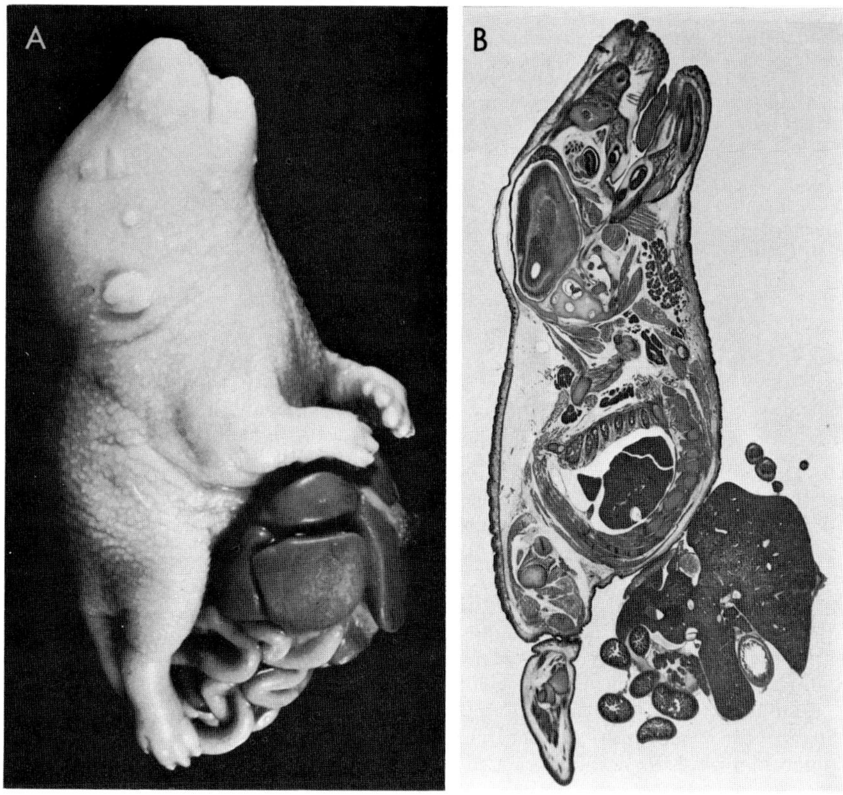

Fig. 77-1. – Exomphalos and iniencephaly produced in a rat by maternal administration of streptonigrin on the ninth day of gestation. Abnormal multiple lobes of the liver are seen in **A**. In the parasagittal section (**B**), the abnormal liver lobes are seen outside the animal.

rant, compensating for the absence of the left lobe. Such an anomalous enlargement of the right lobe could be mistaken for a tumor or hepatomegaly. Abnormal lobation of the liver has been seen repeatedly in necropsies of children with trisomy 18[6] In gastroschisis and in diaphragmatic hernia, the liver often is partially displaced outside the abdominal cavity. In such cases, the liver is always deformed, showing abnormal lobes and constrictions. Accessory livers have been described repeatedly and were attributed to mechanical constrictions of the liver parenchyma.[1] Ectopic liver tissue, detached from the main portion of the organ, can be located in the abdominal cavity,[7] in the thorax[8] or in an omphalocele.[9] Abnormal situation of the lobes of the liver is present in situs inversus.

A small anomalous lobe of the liver protruding through an incomplete diaphragmatic hernia into the pleural space is compatible with good health. Such cases[10] have been discovered in routine roentgenograms; sometimes affected persons have been operated on because of suspected tumor or echinococcus cyst. Awareness of this anomaly should prevent unnecessary operation.

Exaggerated forms of this malformation have been produced experimentally in rats by maternal vitamin A deficiency. In a high percentage of the abnormal young, a large portion of the right hepatic lobe protruded through a diaphragmatic defect into the right pleural cavity. On the left side, this anomaly was rare.[11,12] Much more impressive are gross malformations of the liver in animals in which exomphalos was produced by teratogens such as salicylates, streptonigrin (see Fig. 77-1) and other agents.

REFERENCES

1. Anders, H. E.: Die Missbildungen des Darmkanals und der Verdauungsdrüsen einschliesslich der Kloakenmissbildungen, in Schwalbe, E. (ed.), *Die Morphologie der Missbildungen des Menschen und der Tiere* (Jena: Gustav Fischer, 1928), Vol. 3, pt. 12–15, Chap. 4, pp. 375–482.
2. Arey, L. B.: *Developmental Anatomy. A Textbook and Laboratory Manual of Embryology* (7th ed.; Philadelphia: W. B. Saunders Company, 1965).
3. Wilson, J. W., Groat, C. S., and Leduc, E. H.: Histogenesis of the liver, Ann. New York Acad. Sc. 111:8, 1963.
4. Bremer, J. L.: *Congenital Anomalies of the Viscera–*

Their Embryological Basis (Cambridge, Mass.: Harvard University Press, 1957).
5. Merrill, G. G.: Complete absence of the left lobe of the liver, Arch. Path. 42:232, 1946.
6. Warkany, J., Passarge, E., and Smith, L. B.: Congenital malformations in autosomal trisomy syndromes, Am. J. Dis. Child. 112:502, 1966.
7. Eiserth, P.: Beiträge zur Kenntnis der Nebenleber, Virchows Arch. path. Anat. 307:307, 1941.
8. Kaufman, S. A., and Madoff, I. M.: Intrathoracic accessory lobe of the liver, Ann. Int. Med. 53:403, 1960.
9. Fock, G.: Ectopic liver in omphalocele, Acta paediat. scandinav. 52:288, 1963.
10. Hardisty, N. M., Kearney, E. A., and Brooks, F. P.: Report of a case of an anomalous lobe of the liver, Am. J. Roentgenol. 60:486, 1948.
11. Anderson, D. H.: Incidence of congenital diaphragmatic hernia in the young of rats bred on a diet deficient in vitamin A, Am. J. Dis. Child. 62:888, 1941 (abst.).
12. Warkany, J., Roth, C. B., and Wilson, J. G.: Multiple congenital malformations: A consideration of etiologic factors, Pediatrics 1:462, 1948.

Anomalies of the Bile Ducts

THERE ARE MANY VARIATIONS in the length and course of the bile ducts that are of importance to the surgeon. Hayes and Bishop[1] discussed the developmental basis for bile duct anomalies, pointing out that, in a human embryo 5 weeks of age, the anlage of the gallbladder communicates not only with the cystic duct but also with the primordia of the hepatic ducts and the liver, so that a variety of abnormal connections found in postnatal life can be understood through the pattern of the early embryo. By careful operative exposure of the extrahepatic biliary duct system during operation and by cholangiography, Hayes and Bishop demonstrated that more than 47% of their patients had significant deviations from the conventional picture described in textbooks of anatomy. Accessory ducts, particularly ducts connecting the liver directly with the gallbladder, were found in approximately 18% of the patients, and anomalous length of the common hepatic duct due to its unusually high or low junction with the cystic duct was seen in 26%. Particularly frequent was the low junction of the cystic duct with the common hepatic duct. In addition, there were anomalous insertions of the cystic duct into the common hepatic duct, with occasional winding of the cystic duct around the common hepatic duct. Hayes and Bishop emphasized that knowledge of these variations is necessary for sound surgical practice. They believed that some of the anomalies may play a role in the etiology of chronic cholecystitis.

The most common anomalies of the liver are those of the ducts and of the gallbladder, which, like the intestinal tract, pass through a solid stage before the definitive lumen is formed by the confluence of numerous intracellular vacuoles. This solid stage of the extrahepatic ducts may result in their local atresia or obliteration, or, in the case of double canalization, to duplication of some ducts. Atresia of the cystic duct leads to enlargement of the gallbladder; occurrence of two atretic areas in the common duct may result in the expansion of the duct between the occlusions and formation of a cyst. Such cysts are to be distinguished from idiopathic dilatation of the common bile duct, in which the cyst connects freely with the cystic and hepatic duct (choledochal cysts, p. 721). Another group of congenital cysts is intrahepatic. They are attributed to failure of connection of the bile capillaries with the ducts arising from the hepatic diverticulum. The bile capillaries appear within the solid liver cords at about 6 weeks as lumens filled with secretory droplets. The distal bile capillaries join one another, forming a network of tubules that normally contact the proximal efferent duct system. Intrahepatic cysts located within the liver lobules are explained by failure of junction, stasis and pressure of secretions. Other cysts develop within the connective tissue derived from the hepatic porta, which surrounds the portal veins and bile ducts. Constriction of a bile duct by the invading connective tissue can lead to intraseptal cysts.[2] In polycystic disease of the liver, Moolten[3] found the developmental anomaly primarily in the perilobular ducts, which arise in the hepatic trabeculae in relation to the mesenchyme surrounding the branches of the portal veins. He considered irregular gigantic overgrowth of these ducts and of connective tissue in the periportal areas as characteristic of polycystic disease of the liver (p. 724). There are many authors who do not consider extrahepatic biliary atresias as malformations but rather as the result of a disease or of diseases.[4]

The liver is involved in a number of teratologic syndromes; for instance, in some cases of trisomy 18.[5] Genetically determined syndromes involving anomalies of the liver, kidney, brain and other organs are discussed on page 347.

Congenital Atresia of the Extrahepatic Bile Ducts

The extent of obliteration of extrahepatic bile ducts may vary from a limited stenosis in a single duct to complete atresia of all extrahepatic biliary structures. More than one hundred differing types have been described,[6] although the defect is rare. A good review of these anomalies was given by Moore[7] in 1953, together with a report of 31 cases of his own. It is estimated that extrahepatic atresia occurs once in about 20,000 births.[8,53] Apparently there is no clear sex or race predominance, but in familial cases males predominate.[9] The anomaly has been observed repeatedly in siblings. Sweet[10] reported 3 cases confirmed by necropsy in one family and listed from the literature 6 similar cases with familial occurrence. Krauss[9] recorded 2 brothers with extrahepatic biliary atresia and reviewed other familial cases. It has been estimated that in sibships with 2 affected children the probability of a subsequent recurrence is approximately 20%.[55] But Danks and Bodian[8] were certain that there is no familial tendency in this disorder. Different opinions probably are due to differing terminologies and uncertain criteria of diagnosis.[11] In addition, it is quite likely that the etiology is not uniform. In rare instances, biliary atresia has been seen in cases of trisomy 18.[5,12]

There exist a variety of situations, as the occlusion may be located in different portions of the extrahepatic ducts. Gross[13] attempted a classification and among 145 patients found the following variations: (1) the hepatic and cystic ducts as well as the gallbladder were patent and only the terminal segment of the common duct was occluded (11%); (2) the hepatic duct was patent, the gallbladder normal but other extrahepatic ducts were obliterated (7%); (3) the hepatic duct was open in its upper portion but obliterated below, the common duct was patent and the gallbladder atretic (0.7%). (Types 1, 2 and 3 are operable.) (4) the gallbladder and all ducts were atretic (36%); (5) the gallbladder contained mucoid material but all ducts were obliterated (32%); (6) the hepatic duct was atretic but the gallbladder was connected with the duodenum (13%). (Types 4, 5 and 6 are inoperable.) In Gross's series,[13] they amounted to 81% of the cases, so that only 19% were operable. According to Moore,[7] approximately 25% of the cases are theoretically correctable, but the actual salvage rate is much lower.[15]

In the majority of cases, portal fibrosis with round cell infiltration and bile duct proliferation is well established in children 2 months of age. Evidence of portal hypertension in the form of esophageal varices and splenomegaly also appears early.

Jaundice is a constant finding and may be present at birth or develop within the first 4 weeks. Abdominal enlargement due to hepatomegaly and ascites is not rare, and biliary cirrhosis develops. The children may appear relatively well nourished until the stage of deterioration sets in and signs of malnutrition become evident. The urine is dark and the stools are light and clay colored from birth. Occasionally, they assume a yellowish tint because of excretion of small amounts of pigment through intestinal glands. Bleeding tendency usually is not seen before the patients are 6 months of age. Melena occurs terminally, usually because of a disturbance in the clotting mechanism or through esophageal varices. The icteric index and the serum bilirubin are high. In most of the cases there is a mild anemia but in some instances, especially in the later stages of the illness, the anemia may be severe. The serum protein maintains normal values, but between 6 and 12 months there often occurs a reduction of both albumin and globulin.

Associated malformations occurred in 5 of the 31 patients of Moore.[7] In a larger necropsy material, Stowens[6] noted congenital malformations of differing types and severity in 25% of the patients with biliary atresia, and even higher incidences of associated malformations were listed in other series.[9,15] Anomalies of the cardiovascular and urinary systems were mentioned particularly. Since some of these malformations date back to early embryonic stages, their presence supports the concept of early malformation of the extrahepatic bile ducts. Stowens[6] correlated different types of biliary atresia with various stages of development and times of action of teratogenic agents. The fact that giant cell disease of the liver occurs[6] in approximately 15% of patients with biliary atresia may contribute to the belief that late inflammatory processes have to be considered in the etiology.

In general, the prognosis for extrahepatic atresia of the bile ducts is poor. Although 23% of the cases theoretically appear correctable,[7] only a few patients survive the postoperative period and remain in good health. In Moore's series,[7] only 1 of 31 patients was thought to have a good chance for continued survival and good health. In patients who survive several years, physical and mental retardation may be observed. Osseous abnormalities develop that predispose to traumatic fractures. Roentgenograms show either rachitic changes or an osseous dystrophy with demineralization, ground-glass density, thin cortices, enlarged medullary cavities and undertubulation.[16] A case of congenital bile duct atresia leading to cirrhosis and primary liver cell carcinoma has been observed.[17] The average age at death is approximately 7 months.[7] This poor outlook has been attributed in part to late admission of the patients to medical centers and late operation, but Krovetz[14] pointed out that children in whom only fibrous biliary cords are found at surgical exploration can survive for many years and recommended that in the absence of bile ducts of a size suitable for anastomosis, the patient should be afforded the opportunity to develop the biliary system spontaneously and to clear the jaundice. Hardy[18] reported a patient with congenital stenosis of both the right and left hepatic ducts who, although intermittently jaundiced, reached the age of 14 years before surgical intervention became necessary. The intrahepatic ducts were so dilated that one of them could be joined to the gallbladder, which was anastomosed with a loop of the jejunum. Gross[13] obtained cured jaundice and good health in 8% of his patients. The operation consists in anastomosis of the patent portion of the hepatic duct system with the duodenum. Establishment of an internal hepatic fistula combined with nutritional care resulted in survival of 14 of 72 infants for more than 18 months.[19] Kasai *et al.*[54] found that tiny but patent bile ducts exist in the porta hepatis of nearly all so-called uncorrectable cases and obtained cures in some of them by early hepatic portoenterostomy.

Congenital Atresia of the Intrahepatic Bile Ducts

Congenital absence of the intrahepatic bile ducts is much rarer than congenital absence of the extrahepatic bile ducts. In Gross's series[13] of 146 cases of congenital atresia of the bile ducts, there was only 1 patient with intrahepatic atresia and normal extrahepatic structures. Krovetz[14] reviewed 137 cases of congenital biliary atresia and only 15 of these were of the intrahepatic variety. Among 110 cases of neonatal obstructive jaundice, Danks and Bodian[8] attributed 7 to intrahepatic biliary atresia, 58 to atresia of the major bile ducts and 45 to "neonatal hepatitis." No affected relatives of the patients were ascertained.

Affected infants suffer from obstructive jaundice in the first weeks of life. As they grow older, the jaundice becomes less intense and bile pigment reappears in the feces. In general, patients with intrahepatic bile duct atresia live longer than those whose extrahepatic duct system is occluded. In intrahepatic atresia, one finds enlargement of lymph nodes in the gastrohepatic ligament, with evidence of phagocytosis of bile pigments. This suggests that in these cases the lymphatics may act as accessory channels of bile excretion when the normal pathway is blocked. Since there are no–or only a few–interlobular bile ducts, one sees no distention or duplication of bile ducts and no periductal inflammatory reaction; in short, none of the disorganizing injurious abnormalities typically present in extrahepatic atresia.

It is generally assumed that atresia of the intrahepatic bile ducts is due to a developmental disturbance. If the cases of Sweet[10] are considered as belonging in this group, a familial incidence would be established in at least 2 of them. It is of interest that in Case 2 of Ahrens *et al.*,[20] a sibling had died of intestinal atresia.

The embryologic basis of this anomaly is not clear. It is difficult to understand that intrahepatic bile ducts are absent in the presence of well-developed liver cords. Ahrens *et al.*[20] stated that the presence of fully developed hepatic parenchyma in patients with atresia of bile ducts can be explained only by postulating that biliary epithelium and hepatic cord cells grow independently. Moolten[3] believed that the connective tissue of the portal fields plays the role of an organizer that governs the differentiation of the intrahepatic bile ducts. A functional failure of the connective tissue could result in absence of intrahepatic ducts in the presence of extrahepatic ducts, which are derived directly from the entodermal anlage of the liver. As in the case of extrahepatic bile duct atresia, there are doubts whether intrahepatic biliary atresias are due to malformation or to early destruction of the canaliculi by inflammatory processes. Absence of the cholangioles might be caused by an inflammation of the portal spaces.[21]

Although children with intrahepatic bile duct atresia cannot be helped by surgery, they may survive for several years. Two boys survived to the ages of 10 and 12 years, respectively.[22] Growth usually is retarded; the retardation has been attributed to defective absorption of fatty foods and the ensuing loss of calories. Deficient absorption of vitamin D may lead to rickets.[20]

Xanthomatous cutaneous lesions, usually not seen before the patients are 18 months of age, are characteristic of this anomaly. Pruritus may precede the skin lesions by several months. Elevation of the serum lipids is another feature of the disorder. The serum cholesterol levels usually are very high–well above 500 mg./100 ml. Aside from hyperbilirubinemia and a slightly raised alkaline phosphatase, liver function tests are normal.[22]

Microscopically, the bile ducts are absent from the portal tracts, which show slight infiltration with leukocytes but normal-looking liver cells and normal lobular architecture. Intralobular canaliculi may be present and contain inspissated bile casts. The portal area is prominent because of increase in fibrous tissue.[23]

Other types of neonatal obstructive jaundice differ both clinically and pathologically from the syndrome of congenital absence of the intrahepatic bile ducts. In extrahepatic biliary atresia, jaundice usually persists until the infant dies, but there are exceptions to this rule.[14,18] During the neonatal period, there is marked proliferation of perilobular bile ducts, with gross dilatation of some of the larger bile ducts in the portal tracts. In neonatal hepatitis, the jaundice may persist for a number of weeks to be followed in some cases by recovery. There is a mortality rate of 20% and 10% of the patients develop cirrhosis of the liver.[24] The microscopic picture during the neonatal stage shows marked variation in the size of the liver cells, with distorted multinucleated giant cells scattered throughout the liver substance.[25]

Surgical treatment of patients with absent intrahepatic bile ducts is not possible. Treatment is symptomatic.

Congenital Hepatitis

Congenital biliary atresia can be simulated by hepatitis in the fetal or neonatal period. Craig and Landing[25] reported a group of 20 infants with hepatitis who were admitted to the hospital with severe jaundice, bile in the urine and acholic stools. In 13 of these children, the resemblance to biliary atresia was so pronounced that exploratory operations were performed. In no case was the biliary tree atretic. Histologically active hepatitis was found in all 20 cases. Of 16 patients who could be followed, 12 died and 4 recovered. It seems that serum hepatitis can be transferred through the placenta, and the carrier may be free of jaundice and other symptoms.[26] It was thought that the infection could be carried for several years and transferred by a carrier mother to several children. This would account for the fact that neonatal hepatitis has been reported repeatedly in siblings,[27-30] but Ehrlich and Ratner[29] did not find sufficient evidence to support the theory of viral causation. They thought of a relationship to iso-immunization disease, and Smetana and Johnson[31] thought of failure of development of intercellular bile canaliculi. Hsia *et al.*[32] analyzed 59 families with one or more cases of neonatal hepatitis from the genetic viewpoint. After excluding index cases, there were 11 affected and 50 normal siblings, whereas in a similar survey of 33 families with atresia of the bile ducts no affected siblings were ascertained. An autosomal recessive mode of inheritance appeared possible. Fienberg[33] attributed some familial cases of giant-cell hepatitis to perinatal idiopathic hemochromatosis, and his interpretation was that they were the result of an inborn error of metabolism. Danks and Bodian[8] suggested that a mutant autosomal gene in homozygous form is responsible for "neonatal hepatitis." Twelve of 71 siblings of index cases were affected and there were four consanguineous unions among the parents. In contrast, there was no evidence to show a familial tendency for extrahepatic biliary atresia, which is in disagreement with the findings of other authors (p. 719). As Silverberg *et al.*[11] pointed out, the differential diagnosis between extrahepatic biliary atresia and hepatitis with giant cells is difficult. Subsequently, hepatic lesions in the congenital rubella syndrome were examined by Esterly *et al.*[34] The liver specimens were obtained by necropsy or biopsy in fetuses and children from 26 weeks' gestation to 11 months of age. The histologic lesions observed were identical to those seen in idiopathic neonatal hepatitis, so that an infectious origin for some of the cases of neonatal hepatitis appears established. Whether the histologic picture of giant-cell hepatitis can have a heterogeneous etiology or whether repeated infections can simulate genetic determination of the disorder remains to be seen. Schaffner and Popper[35] considered hepatic giant cells to be a reaction of the liver to a variety of injuries and thought that the use of the term "giant-cell hepatitis" in cases of unknown etiology was not justified.

Congenital Choledochal Cysts

Idiopathic dilatations of the common bile duct are lesions of congenital origin that were considered rare until recently. Now, the number of cases reported in the literature has increased considerably as many more cases are diagnosed clinically and attacked surgically. A number of reviews are available, including those by Zinninger and Cash,[36] Shallow *et al.*,[37] Tsardakas and Robnett[38] and Alonso-Lej *et al.*[39] in 1959, which is based on 419 cases, with an analysis of 94.

The etiology of this condition is puzzling, and many speculations and theories have been advanced as explanations. Alonso-Lej *et al.*[39] enumerated 16 theories that range from infectious causes to "autonomic neurodysplasia." In some of the cases, complete obstruction to bile flow has been found, but in the majority of patients the terminal section of the ductus choledochus is patent, so that no simple explanation can be given. The situation resembles that in hydronephrosis, in which, in some cases, a stenosis of the efferent urinary system can be demonstrated, whereas in the majority of cases no obstruction is found. Similarly, in choledochal cysts, stenosis, angulation or valve-like folding in of the ampulla of Vater can be seen occasionally, whereas, more often, the outlet of the ductus choledochus appears normal or even enlarged. As in idiopathic hydronephrosis (p. 1054), the situation may be clouded by the fact that stenosis or obstruction is present in embryonic or fetal life but has disappeared in postnatal life, leaving a moderate dilatation of the distal portion of the duct system and a weakening of its wall. Normally, the luminization of the bile passages begins near their duodenal termination and progresses toward the liver and the gallbladder. A reversal in the direction of this process would create stasis of secretions distal to the occluded common duct, with dilatation of and damage to the expanded portion. When canalization of the terminal portion finally results, the damage has been done, leaving a weakness in the segment of the common duct that had been dilated in fetal life. The obstruction may be due to a variety of causes, such as abnormal angulation in the lowest part of the common duct, valve-like folds or muscular spasms. As the distention of the cyst increases, torsion, infection or thickening of the wall may add to the obstruction in postnatal life.

A number of associated malformations have been observed that suggest that prenatal factors acting during embryonic life contribute to choledochal cyst formation. Such associated anomalies are double common bile duct, accessory hepatic duct, double gallbladder, absence of the gallbladder and atresia of the bile ducts. In addition, renal agenesis and hypoplastic and polycystic kidneys have been observed.[39] A choledochal cyst has been found in an embryo[40] and in a newborn.[41]

There is a definite predilection for females, who account for more than 80% in some series. The Japanese seem to be particularly affected. Approximately one-third of all the cases reported in the world literature occurred in Japanese people. It is of interest that there is no significant preponderance of the female sex in Asiatic races.[39]

In 92 of the cases analyzed by Alonso-Lej *et al.*,[39] 18% of the patients were less than 1 year of age, 45% less than 10 years and 82% less than 30 years. Thus, choledochal cysts manifest themselves chiefly during childhood or early adulthood. Seven per cent of the cases were detected during pregnancy.

The most common type of congenital choledochal cyst is characterized by a normal intrahepatic tree, moderate dilatation of the biliary ducts above the cyst, sharp demarcation of the cyst against the proximal and distal duct segments and frequent, but not obligatory, narrowing of the terminal common bile duct. As a rule, the cystic dilatation begins below the cystic duct, but in some cases this duct as well as the lower segments of the hepatic ducts are included in the cyst, so that these ducts seem to terminate separately in the cystic portion. In other cases, the cyst is located entirely between two segments of the ductus choledochus.

The dimensions of the cysts vary greatly. Giant cysts containing more than 5 liters of fluid have been reported, but more often the cystic capacity is 1–2 liters. The cyst wall usually is thickened by fibrosis and inflammation. The degree of obstruction influences the quality of the bile contained in the cyst. In cases of complete obstruction with greatly impaired hepatic function, the bile is white. Stones, although uncommon, have been observed in the cyst. Often there is no epithelial lining, but islands of cylindrical or columnar epithelium may be present.[39] The inner surface may be roughened and covered by heavy deposits of inspissated bile pigment or by a purulent exudate.[13] Cirrhosis of the liver, ascites or malignant degeneration of the cyst are rare complications.

Alonso-Lej *et al.*[39] mentioned rare choledochal cysts that may arise from the common bile duct as a diverticulum that is connected merely by a pedicle with the duct. Or a "choledochocele" may develop in the intraduodenal part of the common bile duct and cause symptoms of duodenal obstruction.

Jaundice, epigastric pain and abdominal tumor are the classic symptoms of congenital choledochal cysts. Vomiting, nausea, fever, dark urine and clay-colored stools are other frequent symptoms. Alonso-Lej *et al.*[39] pointed out that, in more recent descriptions, the classic symptoms are not always present because the disease is recognized earlier. In fact, the clinical picture may vary from almost complete absence of symptoms to the terminal picture of bile peritonitis due to rupture of the cyst. Some patients reach a state of anorexia, weakness, hemorrhagic tendencies and malnutrition before the true pathology is recognized, so that adequate treatment may not be possible. There is no complete agreement concerning the treatment. Alonso-Lej *et al.*[39] recommended removal of the cyst with anastomosis of the remaining biliary tree to the duodenum or jejunum as the treatment of choice. They considered choledochal cystojejunostomy an adequate procedure but did not recommend cystoduodenostomy. Gross[13] recommended a primary anastomosis between the biliary system and the intestinal tract, a procedure that may lead to shrinking of the cyst to small dimensions. He considered anastomosis of the cyst directly to the duodenum the best treatment. Spontaneous biliary peritonitis in infancy due to perforation in the common bile duct can occur in infants in the first few weeks of life. A congenital weakness of the duct wall and increasing intraductal pressure caused by inspissated bile have been considered predisposing factors. Similar factors may be responsible for the pathogenesis of choledochal cysts.[42]

Congenital Malformations of the Gallbladder; Absence of the Gallbladder

Reviews on this subject were done by Gross[43] and Stolkind.[44] That the gallbladder may be absent in man was known to Aristotle, who stated that the horse, mule, ass, deer, camel, dolphin and seacalf normally have no gallbladder. Since then, absence of the gallbladder or variations in number have been observed in many species.[44] There is a gallbladder in the mouse but not in the rat. Gross[43] found that, in 1936, more than 400 cases of atresia of the extrahepatic bile passages had been recorded and that approximately one-sixth of these were associated with absence of the gallbladder. In addition to these, 38 cases with normal hepatic and common bile ducts have been reported. The actual incidence is not known, as estimates vary between 0.1 and 0.75 per 1,000 in the general population.[45] In children's hospitals' necropsy material, the incidence may be as high as 3.8 per 1,000,[44] but many of these children died of associated malformations that caused selection of the cases. Combinations with atresia of the hepatic ducts, anencephaly, situs inversus,[46] imperforate anus, hydronephrosis, atresia of the ureter, abnormal lobation of the lungs, two-cusp aortic valves, congenital aneurysm of the circle of Willis, hernias and hydroceles have been observed.[44] Patients in whom absence of the gallbladder is discovered in adult life incidentally or because of symptoms resembling cholecystic disease seem to be free of associated defects.[45,47]

The anomaly is twice as common in females as in males.[47] Heredity has been considered an etiologic factor.[48] Hypoplasia of the gallbladder has been observed in children with trisomy 18.[5] Agenesis of the gallbladder has been seen repeatedly among the malformations caused by thalidomide in children.[49] Stolkind[44] described many cases from London hospitals and reviewed the literature. He reported on 31 patients who had either no gallbladder, a fibrous cord in place of the gallbladder or a rudimentary gallbladder. Absence of the gallbladder may be symptomless and go unrecognized for many years or throughout life. Among the symptoms mentioned in patients who are candidates for operation are pain in the right upper quadrant, nausea, vomiting, chills, fever and jaundice. Some of these symptoms are due to stones in the biliary ducts.[45] Preoperative diagnosis apparently has not been made. Operative cholangiography can demonstrate displaced gallbladder or show its absence.[50]

Treatment deals with complications of the anomaly such as dilatation of the common duct, stones and other findings.[45]

Duplication of the Gallbladder

A double gallbladder seems to occur once in 3,000 or 4,000 persons. Skielboe[51] found 122 cases in the literature. Gross[13] described 28 examples of two sepa-

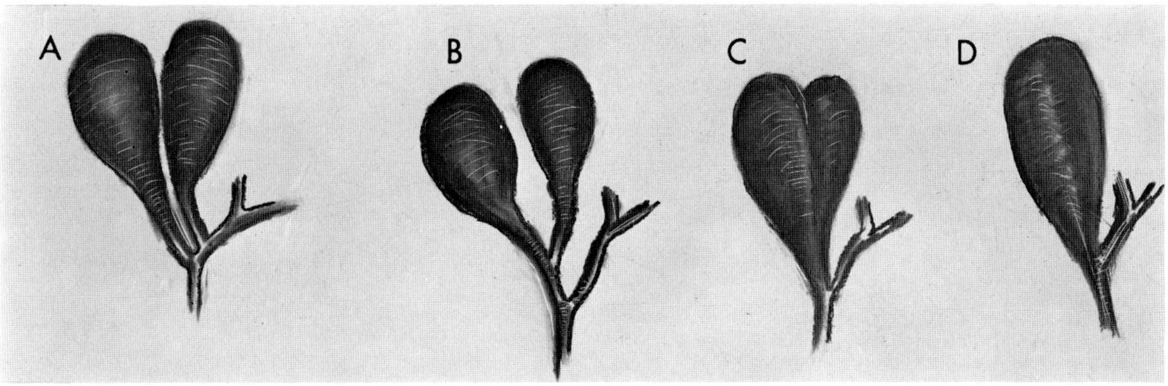

Fig. 77-2.—Anomalies of the gallbladder. **A,** ductular double gallbladder (bladder with separate cystic ducts). **B,** double gallbladder with a Y-shaped cystic duct. **C,** bilobed gallbladder. **D,** septate gallbladder.

rate bladder cavities and two separate cystic ducts. The cystic ducts either joined, forming a Y-shaped structure, or opened separately into the hepatic duct ("ductular type"). The accessory gallbladder may be close to the normal one or be located at some distance—even below the left lobe of the liver.

There are no characteristic clinical signs that suggest duplication of the gallbladder but, in several cases, x-ray studies have revealed two shadows by cholecystography. The accessory gallbladder may be more prone to pathologic changes than the normal.[13] Most double gallbladders are of the ductular type. Parallel double gallbladders with Y-shaped cystic ducts are somewhat rarer.[51]

A case of triple gallbladder has been described in a woman 53 years of age.[51] In this case, all three gallbladders opened with separate cystic ducts into the common hepatic duct. Triple gallbladder has been observed in the cat and the pig.

In bilobed gallbladder, the fundi are duplicated but there is only one bladder neck. In 1958, Skielboe[51] found only 15 case reports of this anomaly in the literature. In some instances, the gallbladder appears single externally, although it is divided into two cavities by an internal septum.[13]

A floating (movable) gallbladder hangs freely suspended from the liver by a peritoneal duplication or mesentery. This variation of gallbladder attachment, which is not too rare, may lead to twisting of the peritoneal fold and to ischemia and infarction. Pain, vomiting, collapse and peritonitis may result.[13]

Abnormal positions of the gallbladder are rare. Some gallbladders are entirely embedded in hepatic tissue and some have been found on the left lobe of the liver. Abnormal position also occurs with situs inversus.

Tracheobiliary Fistula

Tracheobiliary fistula is an extremely rare anomaly that consists of an anastomosis between an accessory bronchus and an accessory outgrowth from the hepatic duct system. Such an aberrant biliary duct can ascend lateral to the esophagus into the lower mediastinum and anastomose with the bronchial system. In this way, the lungs can be flooded with bile.[52]

REFERENCES

1. Hayes, M. A., and Bishop, C. C.: The developmental basis for bile duct anomalies, Surg., Gynec. & Obst. 107:447, 1958.
2. Bremer, J. L.: *Congenital Anomalies of the Viscera—Their Embryological Basis* (Cambridge, Mass.: Harvard University Press, 1957).
3. Moolten, S. E.: Pathogenesis of congenital anomalies of intrahepatic and extrahepatic bile ducts; report of case of polycystic disease of liver and case of atresia of bile ducts, New York J. Med. 43:727, 1943.
4. Gubern-Salisachs, L. G.: La maladie atresiante des voies biliaires extra-hepatiques, Arch. franç. pédiat. 25:415, 1968.
5. Warkany, J., Passarge, E., and Smith, L. B.: Congenital malformations in autosomal trisomy syndromes, Am. J. Dis. Child. 112:502, 1966.
6. Stowens, D.: Congenital biliary atresia, Ann. New York Acad. Sc. 111:337, 1963.
7. Moore, T. C.: Congenital atresia of the extrahepatic bile ducts; report of 31 proved cases, Surg., Gynec. & Obst. 96:215, 1953.
8. Danks, D., and Bodian, M.: A genetic study of neonatal obstructive jaundice, Arch. Dis. Childhood 38:378, 1963.
9. Krauss, A. N.: Familial extrahepatic biliary atresia, J. Pediat. 65:933, 1964.
10. Sweet, L. K.: Congenital malformation of bile ducts: Report of three cases in one family, J. Pediat. 1:496, 1932.
11. Silverberg, M., Graig, J., and Gellis, S. S.: Problems in the diagnosis of biliary atresia, A.M.A. J. Dis. Child. 99:574, 1960.
12. Weichsel, M. E., Jr., and Luzzatti, L.: Trisomy 17-18 syndrome with congenital extrahepatic biliary atresia and congenital amputation of the left foot, J. Pediat. 67:324, 1965.
13. Gross, R. E.: *The Surgery of Infancy and Childhood* (Philadelphia: W. B. Saunders Company, 1953).
14. Krovetz, L. J.: Congenital biliary atresia. Parts I and II, Surgery 47:453 and 468, 1960.
15. Rumler, W.: Über die kongenitale Gallenwegsatresia, zum familiären Vorkommen und zur Genese dieser Fehlbildungen, Arch. Kinderh. 164:238, 1961.
16. Levin, E. J.: Congenital biliary atresia with emphasis on the skeletal abnormalities, Radiology 67:714, 1956.

17. Okuyama, K.: Primary liver cell carcinoma associated with biliary cirrhosis due to congenital bile duct atresia, J. Pediat. 67:89, 1965.
18. Hardy, J. D.: Congenital bile duct stenosis; intrahepatic cholangiochole-cystojejunostomy (Roux Y) with removal of intrahepatic stones, J. Pediat. 59:265, 1961.
19. Sterling, J. A., and Lowenburg, H.: Increased longevity in congenital biliary atresia, Ann. New York Acad. Sc. 111: 483, 1963.
20. Ahrens, E. H., Jr., Harris, R. C., and MacMahon, H. E.: Atresia of the intrahepatic bile ducts, Pediatrics 8:628, 1951.
21. Pilloud, P.: Un cas de syndrome de MacMahon-Thannhauser congénital: Modalité, pathogénique particulière de l'agénésie biliaire intrahépatique, Helvet. paediat. acta 21:327, 1966.
22. Haas, L., and Dobbs, R. H.: Congenital absence of the intrahepatic bile ducts, Arch. Dis. Childhood 33:396, 1958.
23. Rosenthal, I. M., Spellberg, M. A., McGrew, E. A., and Rozenfeld, I. H.: Absence of interlobular bile ducts, Am. J. Dis. Child. 101:228, 1961.
24. Gellis, S. S., Craig, J. M., and Hsia, D. Y-Y.: Prolonged obstructive jaundice in infancy, A.M.A. Am. J. Dis. Child. 88:285, 1954.
25. Craig, J., and Landing, B. H.: Form of hepatitis in neonatal period simulating biliary atresia, A.M.A. Arch. Path. 54:321, 1952.
26. Stokes, J., Jr., Wolman, I. J., Blanchard, M. C., and Farquhar, J. D.: The carrier state in viral hepatitis, J.A.M.A. 154:1059, 1954.
27. Dible, J. H., Hunt, W. E., Pugh, V. W., Steingold, L., and Wood, J. H. F.: Foetal and neonatal hepatitis and its sequelae, J. Path. & Bact. 67:195, 1954.
28. Krainin, P., and Lapan, B.: Neonatal hepatitis in siblings, J.A.M.A. 160:937, 1956.
29. Ehrlich, J. C., and Ratner, I. M.: Congenital cirrhosis of the liver with kernicterus, Am. J. Path. 31:1013, 1955.
30. Cassady, G., Morrison, A. B., and Cohen, M. M.: Familial "giant-cell hepatitis" in infancy, Am. J. Dis. Child. 107: 456, 1964.
31. Smetana, H. F., and Johnson, F. B.: Neonatal jaundice with giant cell transformation of the hepatic parenchyma, Am. J. Path. 31:747, 1955.
32. Hsia, D. Y-Y., Boggs, J. D., Driscoll, S. G., and Gellis, S. S.: Prolonged obstructive jaundice in infancy. V. The genetic components in neonatal hepatitis, Am. J. Dis. Child. 95: 485, 1958.
33. Fienberg, R.: Perinatal idiopathic hemochromatosis: Giant cell hepatitis interpreted as an inborn error of metabolism, Am. J. Clin. Path. 33:480, 1960.
34. Esterly, J. R., Slusser, R. J., and Ruebner, B. H.: Hepatic lesions in the congenital rubella syndrome, J. Pediat. 71: 676, 1967.
35. Schaffner, F., and Popper, H.: Morphologic studies in neonatal cholestasis with emphasis on giant cells, Ann. New York Acad. Sc. 111:358, 1963.
36. Zinninger, M. M., and Cash, J. R.: Congenital cystic dilatation of the common bile duct, Arch. Surg. 24:77, 1932.
37. Shallow, T. A., Eger, S. A., and Wagner, F.: Congenital cystic dilatation of the common bile duct, Ann. Surg. 123: 119, 1946.
38. Tsardakas, E., and Robnett, A. H.: Congenital cystic dilatation of the common bile duct; report of 3 cases, analysis of 57 cases, and review of the literature, Arch. Surg. 72: 311, 1956.
39. Alonso-Lej, F., Rever, W. B., Jr., and Pessagno, D. J.: Collective review. Congenital choledochal cyst, with report of 2, and analysis of 94 cases, Surg., Gynec. & Obst. 108:1, 1959.
40. Heiliger, J.: *Über die congenitale cystenartige Erweiterung des Ductus Choledochus* (Giessen: O. Kindt, 1910).
41. Blummelkamp, R., and Verboon, C. H.: Congenital cyst of the common bile duct in a newborn infant, Arch. chir. neerl. 1:113, 1949.
42. Hammar, B., and Sanders, E.: Spontaneous peritonitis in infancy, J. Pediat. Surg. 3:84, 1968.
43. Gross, R. E.: Congenital anomalies of the gall bladder, Arch. Surg. 32:131, 1936.
44. Stolkind, E.: Congenital abnormalities of the gall-bladder and extra-hepatic ducts. Review of two hundred and forty-five reported cases with reports of thirty-one unpublished cases, Brit. J. Child. Dis. 36:115, 182 and 295, 1939.
45. Vanderpool, D., Klingensmith, W., and Oles, P.: Congenital absence of the gallbladder, Am. Surgeon 30:324, 1964.
46. Anders, H. E.: Die Missbildungen des Darmkanals und der Verdauungsdrüsen, einschliesslich der Kloakenmissbildungen, in Schwalbe, E. (ed.), *Die Morphologie der Missbildungen des Menschen und der Tiere* (Jena: Gustav Fischer, 1928), Vol. 3, pt. 12–15, Chap. 4, pp. 375–482.
47. Mouzas, G., and Wilson, A. K.: Congenital absence of the gallbladder with stone in common bile duct, Lancet 1: 628, 1953.
48. Kobacker, J. L.: Congenital absence of gall bladder; a possible hereditary defect, Ann. Int. Med. 33:1008, 1950.
49. Kreipe, U.: Missbildungen innerer Organe bei Thalidomid-embryopathie, Arch. Kinderh. 176:33, 1967.
50. Navani, S. V., Wilde, W. L., and Kim, R.: Agenesis of the gallbladder, Am. J. Roentgenol. 101:625, 1967.
51. Skielboe, B.: Anomalies of the gallbladder—vesica fellea triplex. Report of a case, Am. J. Clin. Path. 30:252, 1958.
52. Neuhauser, E. B. D., Elkin, M., and Landing, B.: Congenital direct communication between biliary system and respiratory tract, A.M.A. Am. J. Dis. Child. 83:654, 1952.
53. Tünte, W.: Zur Häufigkeit der angeborenen Gallengangsatresie, Ztschr. Kinderh. 102:275, 1968.
54. Kasai, M., Kumura, S., Asakura, Y., Suzuki, H., Taira, Y., and Ohashi, E.: Surgical treatment of biliary atresia, J. Pediat. Surg. 3:665, 1968.
55. Nevin, N. C., Bell, M., Frazer, M. J. L., and Froggatt, P.: Congenital extrahepatic biliary atresia in two brothers, J. M. Genetics 6:379, 1969.

Congenital Polycystic Disease; Congenital Hepatic Fibrosis

POLYCYSTIC DISEASE of the liver represents a part of a syndrome of congenital anomalies that, although hereditary and based on embryologic developmental errors, make their appearance, as a rule, late in life. Polycystic disease of the kidney, of the liver and associated anomalies are best considered a hamartosis with a hereditary tendency to development of multiple tumor-like malformations.[1,2] The disorder can be compared to neurofibromatosis, Hippel-Lindau disease and tuberous sclerosis[1] (p. 1260).

The incidence of polycystic liver is not known. Even in necropsies, estimates vary greatly from 1 in about 700[3] to 1 in 3,400.[4]

The disorder of polycystic kidney, polycystic liver

and associated anomalies as seen in adults is inherited as a dominant trait but the expression of the gene varies greatly. The familial tendency to polycystic liver is less conspicuous than that to polycystic kidney but polycystic liver may occur in siblings. Relatives of patients with this disorder may show cystic manifestations in other organs.[5]

The polycystic renal and hepatic disease seen in infants probably is of different etiology. In such cases, polycystic disease of the kidney dominates the picture, whereas cystic disease of the liver usually has not progressed to severe stages. Therefore, the case reports are concerned chiefly with congenital renal cystic disease. In a number of these cases, several affected children were born to apparently normal parents,[6-8] and a recessive mode of inheritance has to be considered possible for these severe and unviable forms of cystic disease. Infants with this cystic disease sometimes have such associated malformations as meningo-encephalocele, arhinencephaly, polydactyly, facial clefts and others. Some of these anomalies were combined by Gruber[7] into a syndrome and called "dysencephalia splanchnocystica." The orodigitofacial syndrome (p. 674) can include polycystic liver and kidneys.[9,10]

Davis[11] reviewed 499 cases of "nonparasitic" cysts of the liver. Melnick[3] reported on 70 cases of polycystic liver seen in necropsies in Los Angeles and found the disorder rarely manifest in persons under 40 years of age, whereas it was seen relatively often in persons between 40 and 80 years. Cystic liver, although congenital in origin, is recognized rarely in children. In a surgical series, the average age was 53 years.[5] Males and females were affected equally in Melnick's series, but other investigators found a strong preponderance in females.[5,12] Caucasians, Negroes and Mexicans were affected in Melnick's series.

Von Meyenburg[13] emphasized the dual origin of the biliary duct system. Although the larger ducts are derived from elongations of the hepatic diverticulum, the intralobular bile ducts are formed as lumens in the hepatic cords. Normally, the intralobular network joins the larger ducts, but these connections are not established in polycystic livers. Von Meyenburg described conglomerations of small cavities, all connected with one another ("Meyenburg complexes") but not connected with biliary ducts of larger caliber. He recognized the disorder as a developmental disturbance. Many more intrahepatic bile ducts are formed in the embryo than are necessary and normally there is involution of the excess ducts. Meyenburg complexes are groups of these intrahepatic bile ducts that failed to involute, with polycystic liver resulting from their gradual cystic dilatation. Although in most cases of polycystic liver the abundance of atypical bile ducts goes back to embryonic life, new formation of intrahepatic bile ducts from liver cell cords can be seen occasionally in very old people.[3]

The weight of polycystic livers may vary between less than 1,000 Gm. to as much as 4,800 Gm.[3] There is a great variation in the number and size of the cysts, but in typical cases the surface as well as sections of the liver are studded with cysts that vary in diameter from 1 to 10 cm. or more. In some cases, solitary or multilocular cysts are present that may be early manifestations of polycystic liver. The epithelial lining of the cysts usually is cuboidal and rarely flat; sometimes there is no lining. The cysts usually contain a clear fluid but occasionally blood or pus is found within them.

In most cases, there is no evidence of impaired liver function. Symptoms referable to the liver may be absent or abdominal pain, enlargement of the liver or pressure on adjacent viscera may lead to complaints. In rare instances and with increasing age, there may be progressive enlargement of the abdomen, fatigue, dyspnea, epistaxis, ecchymosis, leukopenia and anemia.[4] Polycystic liver disease seldom is fatal but the accompanying renal cystic disease may lead to hypertension, uremia and death. In necropsies, approximately half the cases are combined with polycystic kidneys,[3] whereas polycystic pancreas, spleen, ovary and lung are relatively rare. The incidence of associated congenital anomalies and tumors is higher in these cases than in the general population of comparable age groups.[3] There exists a tendency to diverticulum formation in the esophagus, intestine or in the urinary bladder. Of great interest is the association with aneurysms of the cerebral arteries,[3] an anomaly known to be associated with polycystic kidney (p. 1048).

In most cases, polycystic liver disease of the adult type remains symptomless and requires no therapy but when symptoms become manifest, treatment seldom is satisfactory. Aspiration of the cysts at laparotomy gives temporary relief from symptoms. The anomaly progresses slowly and death usually is due to other causes. Preservation of renal function is the clinical problem in most patients.

Polycystic liver with portal hypertension and bleeding esophageal varices can occur in children or young adults.[14] These juvenile forms may be related to congenital hepatic fibrosis. Lathrop[15] reported a family in which at least 4 and probably 6 of 7 children were affected by cystic disease of the liver and kidney. Two of these patients had portal hypertension and variceal hemorrhages. Campbell *et al.*[16] described 3 siblings with polycystic disease of the liver, portal hypertension and bleeding esophageal varices.

Congenital hepatic fibrosis[17] is considered by some a variant of congenital cystic disease of the liver characterized by fibrous thickening of the portal tracts and an excess of small bile ducts.[18] In contrast to liver cirrhosis, the fibrous tissue of congenital fibrosis is distributed irregularly and is not connected with the lobular structure of the liver. The fibrous tracts contain no inflammatory cells and there is no duplication of bile ducts. The limiting plate of liver cells around the portal tracts is preserved.[19] The hepatomegaly is firm and considerable but the liver function is essentially normal. The anomaly has been described in siblings and in successive generations. It has been attributed to a dominant gene with variable penetrance. The chromosomes are normal.[20] Association with polycystic kidney, cystic pancreas, hydronephrosis, obstruction of the common bile duct, anomalies of the gallbladder and regional adiposity has been reported.[19]

Congenital hepatic fibrosis sometimes is responsible for portal hypertension in children and young adults. Hepatosplenomegaly is present from an early age and gastrointestinal bleeding is a common symptom. General well-being, lack of jaundice and good liver function are the rule, but hepatic failure with ascites can occur. Anemia and recurrent infections were stressed by Thorburn *et al.*[20] Some patients remain symptomless but others have died in childhood or adult life from portal hypertension or renal failure secondary to polycystic disease of the kidneys.[19,21] Portacaval shunt or splenectomy afford relief from portal hypertension and its complications.[22]

REFERENCES

1. Moolten, S. E.: Pathogenesis of congenital anomalies of intrahepatic and extrahepatic bile ducts; report of case of polycystic disease of liver and case of atresia of bile ducts, New York J. Med. 43:727, 1943.
2. Wackerle, L.: Zur Frage der Cystenleber, Virchows Arch. path. Anat. 262:508, 1926.
3. Melnick, P. J.: Polycystic liver, Arch. Path. 59:162, 1955.
4. South, C., Jr., and Haug, W. A.: Congenital polycystic disease of the liver, A.M.A. Arch. Path. 67:650, 1959.
5. Henson, S. W., Gray, H. K., and Dockerty, M. B.: Benign tumors of the liver: IV. Polycystic disease of surgical significance, Surg., Gynec. & Obst. 104:63, 1957.
6. Dunger, R.: Zur Lehre von der Cystenniere mit besonderer Berücksichtigung ihrer Heredität, Beitr. path. Anat. 35:445, 1904.
7. Gruber, G. B.: Beiträge zur Frage "gekoppelter" Missbildungen (Akrocephalo-Syndactylie und Dysencephalia splanchnocystica), Beitr. path. Anat. 93:459, 1934.
8. Potter, E. L.: *Pathology of the Fetus and Infant* (2d ed.; Chicago: Year Book Medical Publishers, Inc., 1961).
9. Doege, T. C., Thuline, H. C., Priest, J. H., Norby, D. E., and Bryant, J. S.: Studies of a family with the oral-facial digital syndrome, New England J. Med. 271:1073, 1964.
10. Tucker, C. C., Finley, S. C., Tucker, E. S., and Finley, W. H.: Oral-facial-digital syndrome with polycystic kidneys and liver: Pathological and cytogenetic studies, J. M. Genetics 3:145, 1966.
11. Davis, C. R.: Liver cysts, non-parasitic, Grace Hosp. Bull., Detroit 20:2, 1936.
12. Clagett, O. T., and Hawkins, W. J.: Cystic disease of the liver, Ann. Surg. 123:111, 1946.
13. von Meyenburg, H.: Über die Cystenleber, Beitr. path. Anat. 64:477, 1918.
14. Sedacca, C. M., Perrin, E., Martin, L., and Schiff, L.: Polycystic liver: An unusual cause of bleeding esophageal varices, Gastroenterology 40:128, 1961.
15. Lathrop, D. B.: Cystic disease of the liver and kidney, Pediatrics 24:215, 1959.
16. Campbell, G. S., Bick, H. D., Paulsen, E. P., Lober, P. H., Watson, C. J., and Varco, R. L.: Bleeding esophageal varices with polycystic liver, New England J. Med. 259:904, 1958.
17. MacMahon, H. E.: Congenital anomalies of the liver, Am. J. Path. 5:499, 1929.
18. Parker, R. G. F.: Fibrosis of the liver as a congenital anomaly, J. Path. & Bact. 71:359, 1956.
19. Hickie, J. B., and Garvan, J. M.: Congenital hepatic fibrosis, Australasian Ann. Med. 11:260, 1962.
20. Thorburn, M. J., Miller, C. G., and Bras, G.: Congenital hepatic fibrosis in Jamaican children, Arch. Dis. Childhood 42:379, 1967.
21. Kerr, D. N. S., Harrison, C. V., Sherlock, S., and Walker, R. M.: Congenital hepatic fibrosis, Quart. J. Med. 30:91, 1961.
22. Hermann, R. E., and Hawk, W. A.: Congenital hepatic fibrosis as a cause of portal hypertension: Report of two cases, Surgery 62:1095, 1967.

Arteriovenous Fistula of the Hepatic Artery and Portal Vein

COMMUNICATIONS BETWEEN the hepatic artery and portal vein are uncommon and clinical recognition and treatment of the anomaly have been achieved only recently. The fistulas can be intrahepatic or extrahepatic. Esophageal or duodenal varices and hemorrhages or abdominal pain may be presenting symptoms. Sometimes a continuous murmur over the abdomen is heard. Such fistulas can be congenital or result from trauma or rupture of a hepatic artery aneurysm. They can be demonstrated by aortography and be resected successfully.[1]

Congenital Absence of the Terminal Portal Vein

Absence of the intrahepatic portal venous system was found in an infant girl who died at the age of 6 months after showing early cyanosis, wheezing and cough. The segment of the portal vein extending from its confluence with the splenic and coronary veins to the point of entry into the liver, as well as its entire intrahepatic distribution, was absent. The usual tributaries of the portal vein drained into a large vessel that took its course behind the liver and joined the hepatic vein to form the inferior vena cava. The subdiaphragmatic portion of the inferior vena cava, formed by the confluence of the iliac veins and joined by the renal veins, passed through the diaphragm to unite with the enlarged azygos vein, which entered the right atrium. Microscopically, the liver showed distortion of the hepatic architecture, irregular hepatic lobules and absence of intrahepatic branches of the portal vein. The left lobe of the liver was larger than the right and the caudate and quadrate lobes were absent. The gallbladder was buried in the liver substance. There was malrotation of the large intestine, multiple prominent hemangiomas of the lip and skin and patent ductus arteriosus. Absence of the intrahepatic portal circulation had the effect of a shunt and contributed to increased cardiac output and hypertrophy. The liver parenchyma was supplied by the hepatic artery. Functionally, this case resembled an Eck fistula, which in itself is not lethal. Embryologically, the case can be explained by interruption of the usual connection of the liver with the vitelline veins and failure of development of the hepatic segment of the inferior vena cava.[2]

REFERENCES

1. Shumacker, H. B, Jr., and Waldhausen, J. A.: Intrahepatic arteriovenous fistula of hepatic artery and portal vein, Surg., Gynec. & Obst. 112:497, 1961.
2. Hellweg, G.: Congenital absence of intrahepatic portal venous system simulating Eck fistula, Arch. Path. 57:425, 1954.

Congenital Tumors

Congenital tumors of the liver have been observed and there are liver tumors that betray a prenatal origin by association with congenital malformations. Reviews of tumors of the liver in infants and children were made by Edmondson[1] and by Cleland[2] but only some of these growths are congenital. In 1940, Wells[3] thought that there were 10 cases of primary carcinoma of the liver on record that suggested prenatal onset of malignancy. Wilbur *et al.*[4] described a 3-day-old boy with congenital hepatoma with extrahepatic metastases. Sawyer[5] reported primary hepatic carcinoma in a girl 2 months of age. In Taiwan, primary carcinoma of the liver accounts for 20% of all the surgically explored abdominal tumors in infancy and childhood. Boys are affected twice as often as girls. Lin *et al.*[6] observed a newborn infant whose enlarged abdomen interfered with delivery. Laparotomy on the third day after birth revealed a hepatoma in the right lobe that extended to the left lobe with nodular metastasis. It was proved by biopsy to be a liver cell carcinoma. The early onset of symptoms in other infants suggests congenital tumors but postnatal origin cannot be excluded. Ishak and Glunz[7] distinguished hepatoblastomas and hepatocarcinomas in infancy and childhood. There were 21 hepatoblastomas but no hepatocarcinomas in infants under 12 months. One of the patients with hepatoblastoma was a premature baby of 34 weeks' gestation and the remainder of them came to medical attention chiefly in the first 2 years of life. Males prevailed, the sex ratio being 2:5. Fraumeni *et al.*[8] made an epidemiologic study of primary carcinoma of the liver in childhood by surveying hospital charts of 76 children with this neoplasm and by studying 282 death certificates for the years 1960-1964. Ten of 282 deaths occurred within 1 month after birth. It appeared that liver cancer often originates in utero, since a large proportion of cases are diagnosed during infancy and there is a sharp decline in mortality in children after 3 years of age. There was some association with hemihypertrophy, Wilms tumor and adrenocortical neoplasm. Association of liver tumor with hemihypertrophy had been reported by Roth[9] in 1938 and several cases have been observed since.[8] Geographic variation in liver cancer mortality was significant in children under 5 years of age, which suggested an environmental influence on the early peak. Okuyama[10] reported primary hepatic carcinoma associated with biliary cirrhosis in a 3-year-old boy. The cirrhosis was due to congenital extrahepatic bile duct atresia. Primary carcinoma of the liver has been reported following giant-cell hepatitis of infancy.[11,12] Fraumeni *et al.*[8] listed 5 children with primary carcinoma of the liver who had antecedent liver diseases such as cirrhosis, neonatal hepatitis, congenital biliary atresia and de Toni-Fanconi syndrome. Familial occurrence of primary hepatocellular carcinoma was reported in 3 adult brothers by Kaplan and Cole,[30] and Hagstrom and Dee Baker[31] described occurrence of such tumors in 3 brothers who died at ages 11, 22 and 31 years. Onset of the disease was not simultaneous. Since the role of environmental factors in primary hepatic cancer has been emphasized in recent years,[32] a search for possible environmental associations was made in these cases but no known hepatic carcinogens were discovered.

Chorioepithelioma

In a newborn male child, malignant tumors were present in the liver and lungs that, on histologic examination, proved to be chorioepitheliomas. There was hyperplasia of the interstitial cells of the testis. The child lived 7 weeks. The mother was in good health during her pregnancy and thereafter.[13]

Hamartomas

Mesenchymal hamartomas of the liver usually are solitary, spherical masses with a tendency to cyst formation. They are congenital and manifest themselves during infancy or early childhood by abdominal enlargement and a palpable mass. Most of the tumors are in the right lobe of the liver or attached by a stalk to it. Surgical removal usually is possible, particularly in those with a pedicle.[14,29] Mixed hamartous adenomas are benign growths of the liver composed of liver cells and bile ducts that show irregular arrangement, the lobular pattern and portal triads being absent. These tumors, which represent developmental anomalies of hepatic segments, vary in size and usually are well circumscribed. Most cases are isolated lesions, but multiple adenomatous nodules have been observed. Occasionally, the lesions are pedunculated and sometimes cystic areas or hemangiomas are included. As congenital anomalies, the tumors have been found repeatedly in infants and young children, but symptoms may be delayed to the fourth decade of life.[15] Abdominal enlargement or pressure symptoms betray the lesion. One case was found incidental to repair of a diaphragmatic hernia.[16] Adenomas of the liver may show malignant tendencies.[17] Hamartoma of the gallbladder developed in a 7-year-old boy who had a diffuse brain sclerosis associated with demyelinization of the white matter (Pelizaeus-Merzbacher disease). Cholecystectomy was performed without complications.[18]

Teratomas

Teratomas of the liver have been observed in infants,[19,20] but they are extremely rare. In at least one case, the teratoma was so large that it made delivery difficult.[21]

Hemangiomas

Congenital hepatic hemangiomas are not rare, but they seldom are diagnosed in the newborn because, if small, they can remain symptomless. Hemangiomas are situated more often in the left than in the right lobe of the liver and they have a predilection for female children.[22] The leading symptom is enlargement of the abdomen; internal hemorrhage may result in anemia and a murmur may be heard over the hepatic tumor. Roentgenograms can be of aid in the diagnosis but needle biopsy is contraindicated. Portal congestion, dilatation of the epigastric veins and enlargement of the spleen may be present in the newborn. Hemangiomatosis of the vena portae in newborn children with thrombopenia and jaundice has been observed.[23,24] Death due to rupture of a hemangioendothelioma of the liver was reported by Caussade *et al.*[25] Korányi *et al.*[22] added a case of liver hemangioma to 8 previously published cases.[26] A giant hemangioma weighing 190 Gm. that had occupied the entire left lobe of the liver was removed successfully.

Multiple hemangiomas of the liver can act as arteriovenous fistulas and shunt a portion of the cardiac output back to the heart, leading to cardiac hypertrophy, dilatation and decompensation. "Benign" hepatic hemangiomas[27] or hemangioendotheliomas[28] may simulate congenital heart disease in infants who have no malformations of the heart or great vessels.

REFERENCES

1. Edmondson, H. A.: Differential diagnosis of tumors and tumor-like lesions of liver in infancy and childhood, A.M.A. Am. J. Dis. Child. 91:168, 1956.
2. Cleland, R. S.: Benign and malignant tumors of the liver, Pediat. Clin. North America 6:427, 1959.
3. Wells, H. G.: Occurrence and significance of congenital malignant neoplasms, Arch. Path. 30:535, 1940.
4. Wilbur, D. L., Wood, D. A., and Willett, F. M.: Primary carcinoma of the liver, Ann. Int. Med. 20:453, 1944.
5. Sawyer, C. D.: Primary hepatoma in infancy, J. Pediat. 36:508, 1950.
6. Lin, T-Y., Chen, C-C., and Liu, W-P.: Primary carcinoma of the liver in infancy and childhood: Report of 21 cases, with resection in 6 cases, Surgery 60:1275, 1966.
7. Ishak, K. G., and Glunz, P. R.: Hepatoblastoma and hepatocarcinoma in infancy and childhood. Report of 47 cases, Cancer 20:396, 1967.
8. Fraumeni, J. F., Jr., Miller, R. W., and Hill, J. A.: Primary carcinoma of the liver in childhood: An epidemiologic study, J. Nat. Cancer Inst. 40:1087, 1968.
9. Roth, F.: Zur Kenntniss und Auffassung der Lebermischgeschwülste und des halbseitigen Riesenwuchses, Frankfurt. Ztschr. Path. 52:163, 1938.
10. Okuyama, K.: Primary liver cell carcinoma associated with biliary cirrhosis due to congenital bile duct atresia, J. Pediat. 67:89, 1965.
11. Roth, D., and Duncan, P. A.: Primary carcinoma of the liver after giant cell hepatitis of infancy, Cancer 8:986, 1955.
12. Fajers, C. M., Falkmer, S., Frisell, E., and Pehrson, M.: Primary carcinoma of the liver and giant cell hepatitis in infancy, Acta paediat. 49:96, 1960.
13. Emery, J. L.: Chorionepithelioma in a newborn male child with hyperplasia of the interstitial cells of the testis, J. Path. & Bact. 64:735, 1952.
14. Sutton, C. A., and Eller, J. L.: Mesenchymal hamartoma of the liver, Cancer 22:29, 1968.
15. Levenson, R. M., and Mason, D. G.: Mixed adenoma (hamartoma) of the liver: Report of a case, Ann. Int. Med. 38:136, 1953.
16. Gross, R. E.: *The Surgery of Infancy and Childhood* (Philadelphia: W. B. Saunders Company, 1953).
17. Packard, G. B., and Stevenson, A. W.: Hepatoma in infancy and childhood, Surgery 15:292, 1944.
18. Brown, R. C., and Brown, R. J.: Hamartoma of the gallbladder in a child, J. Pediat. 52:319, 1958.
19. Hartz, P. H., and van der Sar, A.: Teratoma of the liver in an infant, Am. J. Clin. Path. 15:159, 1945.
20. Yarbrough, S. M.: Report of a case of teratoma of the liver in an infant, Texas J. Med. 40:426, 1944.
21. Froboese, C.: Kindskopfgrosses echtes Teratoma triphyllicum adultum polycysticum congenitum der Leber als absolutes Geburtshindernis, Zentralbl. allg. Path. 89:364, 1952.
22. Korányi, G., Rajk, A., and Róbert, J.: Successfully operated giant hemorrhagic liver hemangioma in a newborn infant, Helvet. paediat. acta 22:201, 1967.
23. Kleint, W.: Ausgedehnte Hämangiomatose im Pfortadergebiet bei einem Neugeborenen, Kinderärztl. Praxis 27: 376, 1959.
24. Haferland, W.: Hämangiomatose im Pfortadergebiet als Kasabach-Merrittsches Syndrom, Ztschr. Kinderh. 85: 125, 1961.
25. Caussade, L., Neimann, N., and Tridon, P.: Hémangioendothéliome du foie chez un nouveau-né mort par rupture du foie, Arch. franç. pédiat. 11:514, 1954.
26. Stone, H. H., and Nielson, I. C.: Hemangioma of the liver in the newborn. Report of a successful outcome following hepatic lobectomy, Arch. Surg. 90:319, 1965.
27. Winters, R. W., Robinson, S. J., and Bates, G.: Hemangioma of liver with heart failure: A case report, Pediatrics 14:117, 1954.
28. Levick, C. B., and Rubie, J.: Haemangio-endothelioma of the liver simulating congenital heart disease in an infant, Arch. Dis. Childhood 28:49, 1953.
29. Sutton, C. A., and Eller, J. L.: Mesenchymal hamartoma of the liver, Cancer 22:29, 1968.
30. Kaplan, L., and Cole, S. L.: Fraternal primary hepatocellular carcinoma in three male adult siblings, Am. J. Med. 39:305, 1965.
31. Hagstrom, R. M., and Dee Baker, T.: Primary hepatocellular carcinoma in three male siblings, Cancer 22:142, 1968.
32. Burdette, W. J.: *Primary Hepatoma* (Salt Lake City: University of Utah Press, 1965).

Familial Intrahepatic Cholestasis

THIS DISORDER, which results in mental and growth retardation, was described by Juberg *et al.*[1] Pruritus, jaundice, light stools, dark urine and abdominal enlargement were noticed in 3 sisters at about 4 months, whereas their brother's symptoms were limited at that age to pruritus and increased abdominal circumference. Three siblings were not affected. Mental development was slow and mild retardation resulted. Physical growth retardation was more marked in height than in weight. Liver biopsies showed bile stasis in the presence of bile ducts. The authors cautiously suggested autosomal recessive inheritance of the disorder.

REFERENCE

1. Juberg, R. C., Holland-Moritz, R. M., Henley, K. S., and Gonzalez, C. F.: Familial intrahepatic cholestasis with mental and growth retardation, Pediatrics 38:819, 1966.

78

The Pancreas

Malformations

IN THE FIFTH WEEK, an embryo of 5 mm. crown-rump length shows two outgrowths from the entodermal lining that represent the earliest rudiments of the pancreas. One of the buds, which arises from the dorsal wall of the intestine near the stomach, is called the dorsal pancreas. The ventral pancreas first appears in the angle between the gut and the ductus choledochus. At about the same time, the epithelial anlage of the respiratory system appears as an outgrowth of the pharyngo-esophageal border area.

In an embryo of 10 mm. (6 weeks fertilization age), the dorsal pancreas is larger than the ventral one and extends backward into the mesentery. The small ventral pancreas has been turned backward by a rearrangement of the lengthened bile duct. Both pancreatic constituents have developed ducts, the dorsal one sending its duct directly into the duodenum, whereas the ventral duct joins the ductus choledochus.

Fusion of the two pancreata to a single organ takes place in 17-mm. embryos (seventh week). The ventral pancreas forms the head and its duct, which remains connected with the common bile duct, becomes the main outlet for the organ. It contacts the duct of the much larger dorsal pancreas and thus develops into the pancreatic duct of Wirsung. The dorsal duct becomes the accessory duct of Santorini. At this stage, the epithelial lining of the duodenum, the esophagus and the rectum grows more vigorously than the intestinal tube, which results in the well-known temporary occlusion of these segments, but such physiologic occlusion of the lumen is not seen in the pancreatic ducts.[1,2]

In embryos of 10 weeks (43 mm.), histologic differentiation has begun. In the pancreas, the acini originate as terminal or lateral buds from the ducts. At first there is a relative preponderance of islands compared to the excretory tissue.[3] The islands are, like the acini, products of differentiation from the ducts. The argyrophilic island cells appear during the eighth week of gestation, followed by the alpha, delta and beta cells during the tenth, eleventh and thirteenth weeks. The first indication of acinar differentiation is an apparent alteration in nucleic acid metabolism, followed by the appearance of zymogen granules, which show no evidence of secretory activity during the fetal period.[4] Meconium is present as far as the ileocolic junction but it does not reach the rectum before the end of the fifth fetal month. Keene and Hewer[5] found pancreatic trypsin in a few human fetuses present at 16 weeks, but in 2 cases it was absent at 22 and 23 weeks. In general, it seems that proteolytic enzymes begin their activity at about the midpoint of gestation. Pancreatic amylase was found at the earliest at 22 weeks, but it may be missing even at term. Pancreatic lipase was present at 32 weeks.

Complete aplasia of the pancreas occurs in monstrous fetuses that lack the portion of the intestine from which the liver and pancreas are derived. It has been seen in acardiacs and anencephalics. A case of agenesis of the exocrine and endocrine pancreas in a female infant with intrauterine growth retardation has been described by Dourov and Buyl-Strouvens.[23] Diabetes mellitus and steatorrhea were present in the neonatal period and death occurred on the nineteenth day. Aplasias of the ventral or dorsal pancreas have been described repeatedly in children. In general, aplasia of the dorsal pancreas has been noted more often than that of the ventral.[6]

Congenital hypoplasia of the exocrine pancreas (lipomatosis of the pancreas). In contrast to cystic fibrosis of the pancreas, which is due to secondary destruction of fetal tissues, congenital hypoplasia of the pancreas is attributed to an embryologic error of development.[7] The clinical pictures of cystic fibrosis and of hypoplasia of the pancreas may be similar to a certain extent, but pathologically and embryologically the two conditions are different. In fibrocystic disease, the pancreas that once was normal is reduced to a small central fibrous core in which are found distended ducts filled with abnormal secretions and a reduced number of islets. In hypoplasia of the exocrine pancreas, the rudimentary duct system, acinar elements and normal islets are scattered throughout the lipomatous tissue and there is no evidence of excessive fibrosis or inflammatory cell infiltration. The larger ducts usually are normally developed but the small ducts are relatively few and branching is imperfect, since there is a lack of differentiation of smaller ducts and acini during the stage of epithelial sprouting. The pancreas may be of normal size and normal shape. The anomaly has been observed in siblings.[7]

Ectopias of the pancreas containing exocrine tissue and islets of Langerhans can be found in the stomach, small and large intestine, Meckel diverticulum, mesentery, gallbladder, lung and spleen.[8,9] Ectopic pancreas has been observed in several cases of trisomy 18.[10] The pancreas can be located outside the abdominal cavity in cases of exomphalos. This has been seen repeatedly in animals in which exomphalos was produced experimentally (Fig. 82-5).

Congenital cystosis of the pancreas may produce a clinical picture simulating fibrocystic disease of the pancreas even though it is not related to it etiologically or pathologically. Some of the cases were associated with polycystic disease of the kidneys and liver and some with malformations of the central nervous system and the eyes. The pancreas may be of normal size, configuration and consistency, but subserous cysts are visible. The alveolar architecture of the pancreas is normal and there is no increase in fibrous stroma except in the vicinity of the cysts. Multiple small cysts containing eosinophilic precipitate and lined by flattened cuboidal epithelium are seen in sections. The duct system is normal, the lumina are patent but not distended. The acinar tissue and the islands of Langerhans are normal in cytology and architecture. There is no inflammatory cell infiltration.[7] This condition probably is not of unitary etiology. It may be part of general cystosis of the liver and kidney or be related in some cases to dysencephalia splanchnocystica[11] and in others to Hippel-Lindau disease (p. 1266).

A *solitary pancreatic cyst* was described by de Lange and Janssen[12] in a premature child who died at 1 week of age. The infant also had polydactyly, dystopia of the anus and enlargement of the cisterna magna, of the fourth ventricle and of the aqueduct of Sylvius. The pancreatic cyst was of grapefruit size and its wall was formed of fibrous connective tissue and lined with cuboidal epithelium. Otherwise, the histologic structure of the pancreas was normal. There were no distended acini or ducts and the connective tissue was not increased. Isolated pancreatic cysts have been seen repeatedly in association with situs inversus and cystic kidneys.[6]

Annular pancreas, once considered a rarity, is now recognized as a relatively common anomaly and as a clinical entity amenable to surgical treatment. Although always congenital, the annular pancreas only rarely leads to serious obstructive symptoms in the newborn, but occasionally it is seen as an incidental necropsy finding. In adults, more often it leads to pathologic manifestations and thus is an example of a congenital malformation that usually manifests itself late in life.

The annular pancreas is an anomaly that can be traced back to the ventral anlage of the pancreas, which appears on the root of the liver diverticulum and accompanies the bile ducts in their dextral migration to the dorsal surface of the duodenum. The ventral pancreatic anlage may be bilobed but the left side normally degenerates very early. If the left bud remains and forms its own lobe, it grows around the left side of the duodenum to join the other parts of the pancreas, thus forming a ring around the intestine.[2] Most pancreatic rings encircle the second part of the duodenum, only a few the first or the third. The ring consists of normal pancreatic tissue, including a duct system and islets. In some instances, the ring around the duodenum is incomplete. In a few newborn children, annular pancreas has caused duodenal obstruction, with vomiting, abdominal distention, small and infrequent stools and characteristic x-ray findings.[13] If the annulus occludes the bile ducts, jaundice may be present. However, in most children, an annular pancreas remains symptomless until supervening disease causes obstruction or pancreatitis, processes that usually do not occur before adult life. Then, pancreatitis may involve the annulus or the body of the organ; the duodenum may be dilated above the ring and gastric or duodenal ulcers may develop subsequently. Such ulcers or gallbladder disease may direct attention to the pancreatic ring. Symptoms appear suddenly or develop slowly; nausea, vomiting, fever or a mass directs attention to the anomaly.[14]

Roentgenograms are characterized by the "double bubble" sign, showing large air bubbles in the stomach and the first part of the duodenum. With barium, the dilatation of the first part of the duodenum, the constricted mid-duodenum and the collapsed third part of the duodenum can be recognized.

As a true malformation, annular pancreas often is associated with other malformations in the intestinal tract, such as duodenal atresia, malrotation, unattached mesentery, tracheo-esophageal fistula or imperforate anus; in addition, facial clefts, congenital heart disease and ectopic kidney have been observed.[6,15,16] Among 10 patients with annular pancreas operated on by Gross,[15] there were 2 with possible mongolism, and there were some with Down syndrome among the cases of annular pancreas cited by Seifert.[6] Of 56 cases of duodenal stenosis with annular pancreas cited by de Wolff,[17] 12 were in patients with Down syndrome. There can be little doubt that the area of the duodenum and of its derivatives – the pancreatic ducts – is adversely affected in many cases of trisomy 21.

Obstructive symptoms in the newborn are treated surgically by duodenojejunostomy, which usually is successful, but associated malformations may dim the prognosis. Direct surgical attack on the ring is not recommended, since the annular tissue and the muscularis of the duodenum often are intermingled.[18]

Congenital tumors. Primary malignant tumors of the pancreas are extremely rare in infants. L'Huillier[19] reported a lymphosarcoma of the pancreas in a 9-day-old girl and Bohn[20] an adenocarcinoma of the head of the pancreas with metastases to the liver and lymph nodes in a 6-month-old infant. Corner[21] described primary carcinoma of the pancreas in an infant 7 months of age. Metastases were present in the liver, pleura and lymph glands. Warthen *et al.*[22] recorded a primary embryonal cancer of the head and body of the pancreas in a 15-month-old boy. Metastases were found in lymph nodes and in the right lung.

REFERENCES

1. Hurwitt, E. S., and Arnheim, E. E.: Meconium ileus associated with stenosis of the pancreatic ducts, Am. J. Dis. Child. 64:443, 1942.
2. Bremer, J. L.: *Congenital Anomalies of the Viscera – Their Embryological Basis* (Cambridge, Mass.: Harvard University Press, 1957).
3. Nakamura, N.: Untersuchungen über das Pankreas bei Foeten, Neugeborenen, Kindern und im Pubertätsalter, Virchows Arch. path. Anat. 253:286, 1924.
4. Conklin, J. L.: Cytogenesis of the human fetal pancreas, Am. J. Anat. 111:181, 1962.
5. Keene, M. F. L., and Hewer, E. E.: Digestive enzymes of human foetus, Lancet 1:767, 1929.
6. Seifert, G.: *Die Pathologie des Kindlichen Pankreas* (Leipzig: Georg Thieme, 1956).
7. Bodian, M.: *Fibrocystic Disease of the Pancreas* (New York: Grune & Stratton, Inc., 1953).
8. Branch, C. D., and Gross, R. E.: Aberrant pancreatic tissue in the gastro-intestinal tract, Arch. Surg. 31:200, 1935.
9. Willis, R. A.: *The Borderland of Embryology and Pathology* (2d ed.; London: Butterworth & Company, Ltd., 1962).
10. Warkany, J., Passarge, E., and Smith, L. B.: Congenital malformations in autosomal trisomy syndromes, Am. J. Dis. Child. 112:502, 1966.
11. Gruber, G. B.: Beiträge zur Frage "gekoppelter" Missbildungen, Beitr. path. Anat. 93:459, 1934.
12. de Lange, C., and Janssen, T. A. E.: Large solitary pancreatic cyst and other developmental errors in a premature infant, Am. J. Dis. Child. 75:587, 1948.
13. Rickham, P. P.: Annular pancreas in the newborn, Arch. Dis. Childhood 29:80, 1954.
14. Dodd, G. D., and Nafis, W. A.: Annular pancreas in the adult, Am. J. Roentgenol. 75:333, 1956.
15. Gross, R. E.: *The Surgery of Infancy and Childhood* (Philadelphia: W. B. Saunders Company, 1953).
16. Shapiro, D. J., Dzurick, F. T., and Gerrish, E. W.: Obstruction of duodenum in the newborn infant due to annular pancreas, Pediatrics 9:764, 1952.
17. de Wolff, E.: Étude clinique de 134 mongoliens, Ann. paediat., vol. 202; supp. 1, 1964.
18. Hyden, W. H.: The true nature of annular pancreas, Ann. Surg. 157:71, 1963.
19. L'Huillier, A.: Über einen Fall von kongenitalem Lymphosarkom des Pankreas, Virchows Arch. path. Anat. 178:507, 1904.
20. Bohn, A.: Krebs der Leber der portalen und retroperitonealen Lymphdrüsen und des Pankreas bei einem halbjährigen Kinde, Jahrb. Kinderh. 23:144, 1885.
21. Corner, B. D.: Primary carcinoma of the pancreas in an infant aged 7 months, Arch. Dis. Childhood 18:106, 1943.
22. Warthen, R. O., Sanford, M. C., and Rice, E. C.: Primary malignant tumor of the pancreas in a fifteen-month-old boy, A.M.A. Am. J. Dis. Child. 83:663, 1952.
23. Dourov, N., and Buyl-Strouvens, M. L.: Agenesie du pancreas, Arch. franç. pédiat. 26:641, 1969.

Congenital Lipomatosis

CONGENITAL LIPOMATOSIS of the pancreas leading to failure to thrive, dwarfism, malabsorption, loose stools and leukopenia has been described as a syndrome.[1] Sweat electrolytes are always normal, thus differentiating the anomaly from cystic fibrosis of the pancreas. On microscopic examination, the acini of the pancreas are almost completely replaced by large, round fat cells and the ducts are absent. The islands of Langerhans are normal.

REFERENCE

1. Goldstein, R.: Congenital lipomatosis of the pancreas, Clin. Pediat. 7:419, 1968.

Cystic Fibrosis of the Pancreas (Mucoviscidosis)

CYSTIC FIBROSIS of the pancreas (CF) is a genetically determined, generalized disorder of many exocrine glands, including the exocrine portion of the pancreas. At first, the anomalies of the pancreas were thought to be the main defect of the disease, but later it was recognized that the sweat glands, mucus-secreting glands and the salivary glands were affected also. In fact, it seems that increased concentration of sodium and chloride in sweat is the most constant feature of the disease, so that the term "cystic fibrosis of the pancreas"[1] now can be considered unjustified. But no term has been suggested that is more appropriate, and it appears of little value to replace the widely accepted name with another that will have to be changed again when the basic metabolic defect is discovered.

The incidence of cystic fibrosis in Caucasian populations is approximately 0.32 per 1,000 or 1 in 3,100 live births.[2,3] Males and females are affected in equal proportions. The disorder is quite rare in Negroes[4] and in Orientals.[5] Parents of the patients are not affected but the incidence in siblings is high. Most authors believe that CF appears in persons homozygous for a recessive autosomal gene[6-8] but there are dissenting opinions.[9,10] Differences of opinion may be due in part to the wide spectrum of manifestations and in part to our ignorance of the basic defect, which is inherited. Manifestation can be present at birth and lead rapidly to death, but survival into the fifth decade is possible.[11] Di Sant'Agnese[4] came to the conclusion that a gene or genes that cause overt disease in homozygotes and partial or no expression of the disorder in heterozygotes may explain the discrepancies found in family investigations. He believed that the most common partial expression recognized so far is an abnormal electrolyte pattern in sweat and that, in some families, heterozygotes have elevated sweat sodium and chloride levels. But the distributions of single values in normal persons and in known heterozygotes overlap in 70–80% of the tests.[13,14] Sproul and Huang[13] performed multiple sweat tests on patients with CF, their parents, siblings and controls. They stated that with a set of four tests, 84% of parents and 83% of the expected number of siblings can be identified as heterozygotes.

Farber[15] attempted experimental production of achylia pancreatica by administration of pilocarpine to kittens over a period of 2–8 weeks to illustrate the effects of overfunction of the parasympathetic system. He observed an increase in the homogeneous material deposited in the ducts of the pancreas that was similar to that of early stages of cystic fibrosis. Attempts to produce cystic fibrosis of the pancreas in young animals also were made by Veghelyi *et al.*[16] They employed deficient diets or toxic compounds for this purpose. Lee *et al.*[17] attempted to produce pancreatic disturbances in the young of female rats by injecting the pregnant animals with ethionine intraperitoneally. By this method, the pancreas of the mother was severely damaged but that of the young remained essentially normal (Fig. 78-1). Neither congenital pancreatic fibrosis nor meconium ileus could be produced in this way.

Cystic fibrosis can begin early in fetal life[10] but the gestation of infants with CF is uneventful and of normal duration.[14] The abortion rate is not increased in affected families.[10] The average birth weight is only slightly reduced,[18] suggesting occasional interference with growth in prenatal life. In general, the disorder is not manifest before birth, and even in cases in which such serious pathologic processes as ileus, volvulus, atresia or intestinal amputation occur, the fetus can continue its intrauterine existence and reach term delivery, since the diseased organs are not essential for prenatal development. This situation exemplifies a failure of the intrauterine screening process owing to maternal protection of the fetus.

Although CF essentially is a disease of postnatal life, some pathologic changes and manifestations are present at birth. These changes and their relationship to congenital malformations will be discussed briefly here.

CF represents an example of anomalies that stand between structural congenital malformations originating in embryonic life and inborn errors of metabolism that, although genetically determined, manifest themselves after birth. In 1938, Andersen[19] distinguished a neonatal group of infants who died before the age of 1 week with intestinal obstruction. A second group was composed of infants who died between the

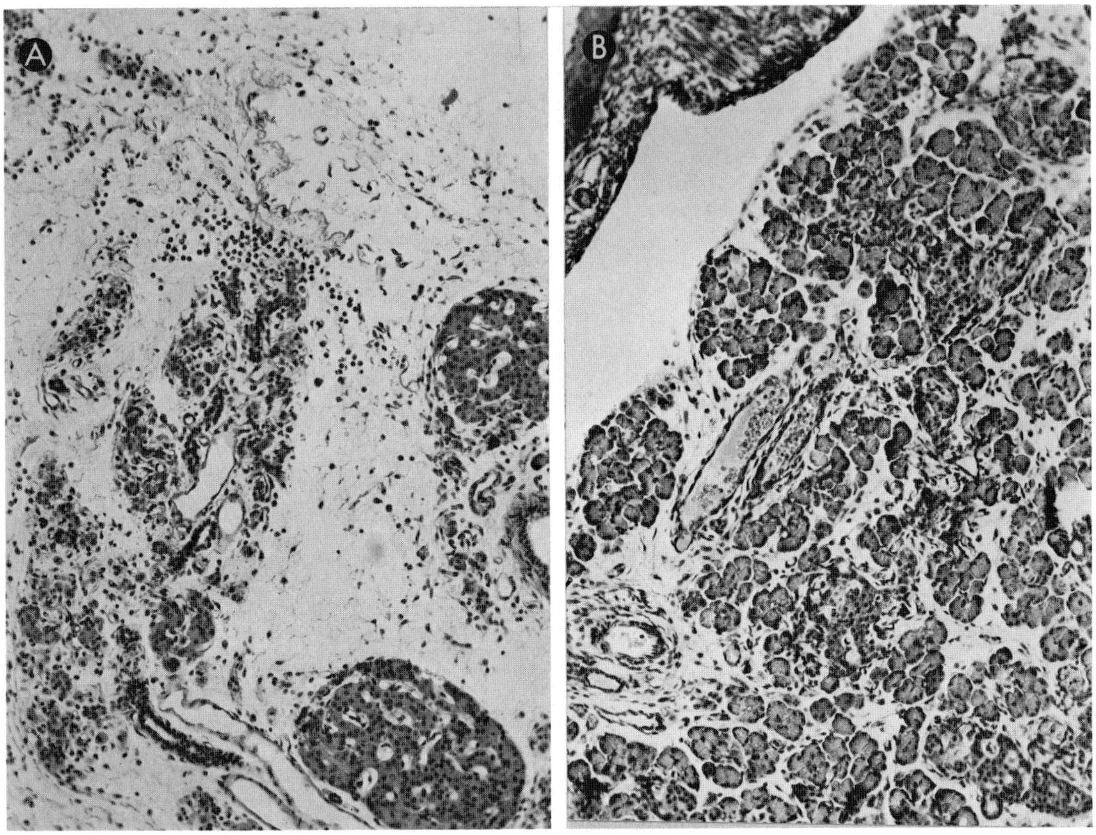

Fig. 78-1.—**A,** section from the pancreas of a pregnant rat treated with a total of 600 mg. of DL-ethionine from the tenth to the twenty-first day of pregnancy, showing almost complete loss of pancreatic exocrine tissue. **B,** section from the pancreas of one of the young of the mother whose pancreas is shown in **A**. The pancreas of the young is essentially normal. (From C. M. Lee, Jr., J. T. Wiseman, S. A. Kaplan and J. Warkany.[17])

ages of 1 week and 6 months. A third group was composed of patients who died between 6 months and adolescence. In the first group of neonates, Andersen encountered infants with meconium ileus and peritonitis, stenosis of the duct of Wirsung, obstructions due to a band of fibrous tissue across the lumen of the terminal portion of the ileum and atresias of the jejunum or of the ileum. In all these cases, the pancreas showed microscopically extensive fibrosis, with formation of cysts. In addition, there were such malformations as Meckel diverticulum, atresia of the cystic duct and ventricular septal defect. The pancreas appeared grossly normal, but Bodian[7] thought that some of these children are born with a pancreatic malformation recognizable on gross examination by loss of the sharp edges of the organ, an oval cross section and a granular surface. In 5 cases of meconium ileus, Baumann[10] found that saccular bronchiectases were already present. He thought that they dated back to fetal life. Oppenheimer and Esterly,[20] reviewing the anomalies of the intestinal tract in children with CF, enumerated volvulus, multiple in-intestinal atresias and stenoses, defective mesenteric attachments, mesenteric cysts and others. Although these structural anomalies must be considered congenital malformations, they represent secondary changes in organs that were primarily normally formed. In this respect, they can be compared with malformations of the central nervous system due to toxoplasmosis or with intrauterine amputations of limbs that at first developed normally and were destroyed later in fetal life. The secondary destruction of the pancreas and other organs affected in fibrocystic disease is due to inability of the organism to produce normal secretions of exocrine glands,[21] particularly normal intestinal mucus and pancreatic secretions. But meconium ileus and its consequences have been observed in patients with minimal microscopic alterations of the pancreas.[14] It is now believed that the abnormal intestinal mucus secreted in fetal life can lead to prenatal meconium ileus, volvulus, atresias, peritoneal bands and intestinal amputations, thus producing secondary, yet congenital, malformations. Associated malformations of the heart or other organ systems are rare and probably fortuitous complications. Defects of other exocrine glands also can be present at birth but they may be less conspicuous than those of the mucus-producing organs. In cases of meconium ileus, elevated sodium and chloride values have been demonstrated in sweat within the first few days of life.[22]

Early changes in the pancreas involve formation of eosinophilic casts in all acini and in some ductules, disorganization of the acini, distention of the ducts and acini with cyst formation, necrosis and infiltration of acinar cells and progressive interlobular and intralobular fibrosis. The cysts can reach a diameter of 2–3 mm. The main pancreatic ducts may be occluded, stenotic or dilated, but usually they are patent. Adipose tissue replaces the shrinking parenchyma. The islands of Langerhans usually are normal in number and appearance, although reduction in number and budding of new islet cells from ductules have been described.[23]

Bodian[7] pointed out that the gradual evolution of the pancreatic lesions differs from other congenital malformations of the pancreas, namely, hypoplasia and cystic disease. In hypoplasia of the pancreas, from birth there is complete or almost complete absence of the acini, but the ducts and islets are normal. As the pancreatic enzymes are absent from the duodenum, some of the clinical symptoms are comparable to those of fibrocystic disease. The symptoms of "cystosis of the pancreas" (p. 730) may also resemble those of cystic fibrosis.

Whether or not *congenital* malformations of the respiratory tract are present in cystic fibrosis is a controversial point. Andersen[23] stated that the lungs appear normal at birth and in most infants who die from congenital intestinal obstruction in the first few weeks of life. The usual findings in infants dying with respiratory symptoms during the first few months are emphysema, chronic bronchitis, lobular pneumonia and atelectasis, changes that cannot be considered congenital malformations. Bodian[7] stated that in children who die from meconium ileus in the first days of life there is invariably an involvement of the mucous glands of the upper and lower respiratory tracts, but most of the gross changes found in the respiratory system seem to be due to postnatal factors. In contrast to these authors, Baumann[10] observed, in 5 cases of meconium ileus that resulted in necropsy within the first days after birth, cylindrical and even saccular bronchiectases. He believed that in such cases of meconium ileus, the mucous membranes of the bronchi are already diseased in fetal life and that bronchiectases are formed before birth.

Fig. 78-2.—Cystic fibrosis of the pancreas, showing distended ducts with laminated concretions. There is increased interstitial connective tissue.

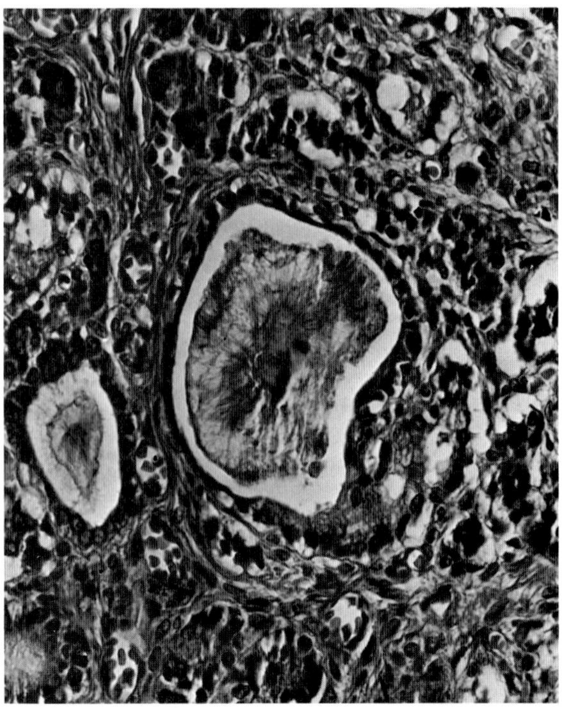

Ten to 15% of infants born with cystic fibrosis of the pancreas have congenital intestinal obstruction due to meconium ileus, and in some series such neonatal complications are even more frequent.[20] In most cases, the site of the obstruction is the terminal ileum. As mentioned before, meconium ileus may lead to volvulus of the largest loop of the ileum, which can perforate before birth, producing meconium peritonitis prenatally or suppurative peritonitis postnatally and, in some instances, volvulus occurs early in fetal life, resulting in secondary atresia of the intestine at the base of the volvulus. Such atresias are not due to faulty luminization but to secondary obstruction of an originally patent intestinal lumen by a fetal disease process. Occasionally, the atresias may lead to hydramnios.[23]

Cirrhotic foci in the liver and fatty infiltration probably are not present at birth, but ductule hyperplasia has been observed in infants with meconium ileus fatal in the first days of life.[7] The number of foci of biliary cirrhosis increases with the age of the patient.[24] With an increasing duration of life in children with CF, the picture of the liver seen at necropsy has changed and hepatic cirrhosis is found with increasing frequency.[25] In approximately one-fourth of the patients, the gallbladder is hypoplastic and the cystic duct is atretic.[7]

Generally, the prognosis of CF was so poor that the trait was considered a lethal one by some authors. Prior to 1945, it was particularly meconium ileus that regularly terminated in early death. Since then, much progress has been made in surgical repair of the condition and subsequent medical treatment or in medical treatment without surgery. Once the obstruction is relieved, the course of the disease is not different from that of CF that begins later in childhood.[26] With antibiotics, vitamin preparations and other measures, the life expectancy of patients with CF has increased considerably.[27]

The disease picture that develops in postnatal life has been described in several monographs.[10,14,19,23,28] Modern treatment has been outlined by Shwachman *et al.*[29]

REFERENCES

1. Fanconi, G., Uehlinger, E., and Knauer, C.: Das Coeliaksyndrom bei angeborener zystischer Pankreasfibromatose und Bronchiektasien, Wien. med. Wchnschr. 86:753, 1936.
2. Pugh, R. J., Pickup, J. D.: Cystic fibrosis in the Leeds region: Incidence and life expectancy, Arch. Dis. Childhood 42:544, 1967.
3. Steinberg, A. G., and Brown, D. C.: On the incidence of cystic fibrosis of the pancreas, Am. J. Human Genet. 12: 416, 1960.
4. Di Sant'Agnese, P. A., Jones, W. O., and Dische, Z.: Cystic fibrosis of the pancreas: Clinical staff conference at the National Institutes of Health, Ann. Int. Med. 54:482, 1961.
5. Kobayashi, Y., Tomisawa, T., Takai, Y., Izumi, R., and Hatakeyama, M.: An autopsied case of fibrocystic disease of the pancreas, Acta paediat. jap. 65:597, 1961.
6. Lowe, C. V., May, C. D., and Reed, S. C.: Fibrosis of the pancreas in infants and children: A statistical study of clinical and hereditary features, Am. J. Dis. Child. 78: 349, 1949.
7. Bodian, M.: *Fibrocystic Disease of the Pancreas* (New York: Grune & Stratton, Inc., 1953).
8. Bulmer, M. G.: Fibrocystic disease of the pancreas: A comment, Ann. Human Genet. 25:163, 1961.
9. Roberts, G. B. S.: Familial incidence of fibrocystic disease of the pancreas, Ann. Human Genet. 24:127, 1960.
10. Baumann, Th.: Die Mucoviscidosis als rezessives und irregulär dominantes Erbleiden. Eine klinische und genetische Studie, Helvet. paediat. acta 13:3, 1958 (supp.).
11. Marks, B. L., and Anderson, C. M.: Fibrocystic disease of the pancreas in a man aged 46, Lancet 1:365, 1960.
12. Di Sant'Agnese, P. A.: Recent observations on pathogenesis of cystic fibrosis of the pancreas, Pediatrics 24:313, 1959.
13. Sproul, A., and Huang, N.: Diagnosis of heterozygosity for cystic fibrosis by discriminatory analysis of sweat chloride distribution, J. Pediat. 69:759, 1966.
14. Lobeck, C. C.: Cystic Fibrosis of the Pancreas, in Stanbury, J. B., Wyngaarden, J. B., and Fredrickson, D. S. (eds.), *The Metabolic Basis of Inherited Disease* (2d ed.; New York: The Blakiston Division, McGraw-Hill Book Company, Inc., 1966).
15. Farber, S.: The experimental production of achylia pancreatica, Am. J. Dis. Child. 64:953, 1942 (abst.).
16. Veghelyi, P. V., Kemeny, T. T., Pozsonyi, J., and Sos, J.: Dietary lesions of the pancreas, Am. J. Dis. Child. 79:658, 1950.
17. Lee, C. M., Jr., Wiseman, J. T., Kaplan, S. A., and Warkany, J.: Effects of ethionine injections on pregnant rats and their offspring, A.M.A. Arch. Path. 59:232, 1955.
18. Boyer, P. H.: Low birth weight in fibrocystic disease of the pancreas, Pediatrics 16:778, 1955.
19. Andersen, D. H.: Cystic fibrosis of the pancreas and its relation to celiac disease; clinical and pathologic study, Am. J. Dis. Child. 56:344, 1938.
20. Oppenheimer, E. H., and Esterly, J. R.: Observations in cystic fibrosis of the pancreas. II. Neonatal intestinal obstruction, Bull. Johns Hopkins Hosp. 3:1, 1962.
21. Di Sant'Agnese, P. A.: Exocrine gland dysfunction in cystic fibrosis of the pancreas, Acta paediat. 46:51, 1957.
22. Elian, E., Shwachman, H., and Hendren, W. H.: Intestinal obstruction of the newborn infant: Usefulness of the sweat electrolyte test in differential diagnosis, New England J. Med. 264:13, 1961.
23. Andersen, D. H.: Cystic fibrosis of the pancreas, J. Chron. Dis. 7:58, 1958.
24. Blanc, W. A., and Di Sant'Agnese, P. A.: Hepatic cirrhosis in cystic fibrosis of the pancreas, Bull. New York Acad. Med. 33:218, 1957.
25. Craig, J. M., Haddad, H., and Shwachman, H.: The pathological changes in the liver in cystic fibrosis of the pancreas, A.M.A. J. Dis. Child. 93:357, 1957.
26. Shwachman, H., Pryles, C. V., and Gross, R. E.: Meconium ileus, A.M.A. Am. J. Dis. Child. 91:223, 1956.
27. Kramm, E. R., Crane, M. M., Sirken, M. G., and Brown, M. L.: A cystic fibrosis pilot survey in three New England states, Am. J. Pub. Health 52:2041, 1962.
28. May, C. D.: *Cystic Fibrosis of the Pancreas in Infants and Children* (Springfield, Ill.: Charles C Thomas, Publisher, 1954).
29. Shwachman, H., Barbero, G. J., Di Sant'Agnese, P. A., Harrison, G. M., Matthews, L. W., and Patterson, P. R.: *Guide to Diagnosis and Management of Cystic Fibrosis* (New York: National Cystic Fibrosis Research Foundation, 1963).

PART XII

Malformations Related to the Oro-gastrointestinal Tract

79

The Thymus

THE HUMAN THYMUS develops at the end of the fourth week of gestation from ventral extensions of the third and fourth pharyngeal pouches, but the connection with the pharynx is lost in the sixth week. At first, the thymic primordia consist of tubules, the lumina of which are soon replaced by solid strands of epithelium. As the primordia enlarge, they extend mediocaudad along the carotid arteries and lateral to the thyroid. For a short time, there occurs an intimate contact of the thymic entoderm with ectoderm, which apparently is of little consequence in man, but in the mole there persists a thymus superficialis that is of ectodermal origin.[1] The primordia grow toward the chest, where the right and left thymic lobes approximate at the level of the aortic arch (without being fused) and then become related to the pericardium. The cranial ends of the thymic primordia become drawn out and thinned until they disappear completely. But many infants have accessory cervical thymic remnants. The mass of the permanent thymus is derived from the third pharyngeal pouches, whereas the contribution of the fourth pouches usually is minimal. If a narrow cervical strand persists, it is called a thymic horn. Its connection with a pharyngeal pouch remnant is called a ductus thymopharyngeus.[1] In the third month of fetal life, the thymic epithelium is transformed into a syncytium that forms the sponge-like framework of the organ. Some of the epidermal cells combine to form round masses (Hassall corpuscles). Their exact mode of formation is not known. Some believe that they begin at the 25-mm. stage as vesicular outgrowths of the epithelial primordia that later become engulfed and distorted by the lobular parenchyma.[2] Others have observed development from one cell, which forms a vacuole at the nuclear-cytoplasmic membrane. Basophilic granules resembling keratohyaline granules of skin appear in the cytoplasm. Other cells join the altered and enlarged cell and undergo similar changes, forming a cluster of epithelial cells with a small cavity within concentric laminations.[3] Toward the end of the third month, cortex and medulla of the thymus become recognizable and lymphocytes begin to fill the reticulum. Whether the lymphocytes are derived from epithelial cells or whether they immigrate into the reticulum is a controversial question.[3] Surrounding mesenchyme forms a capsule and trabeculae that subdivide the organ into thymic lobules.[4,5]

Malformations and maldevelopment of the thymus were considered of little consequence when no function was attributed to the organ. In recent years, the role of the thymus in immune processes has been given much attention, so that congenital variations of the organ deserve increased consideration. It is now thought that the thymus is the central lymphoid tissue with an important function in the maturation of adaptive immunity through its influence on the peripheral lymphoid tissues. Related organs are the tonsils, Peyer plaques of the small intestine and the bursa Fabricii in birds.[6-9] These central lymphoid tissues are considered the source of lymphoid cells responsible for immunologic competence. From the thymus, the peripheral lymphoid tissues are colonized, as assumed by Beard in 1900[10] and demonstrated experimentally in recent years.[11-13] In some disorders, failure of adequate development of the thymus is associated with congenital lymphopenia and in others it is not. But immunologic incompetence of some degree seems to result from complete congenital thymic aplasia.

Agenesis

Congenital absence of the thymus apparently is quite rare; older reports relating frequent agenesis of this organ must be regarded with caution. In most of such studies, morbid involution of the thymus was mistaken for congenital absence. Harington,[14] in 1829, and Clark,[15] in 1896, reported cases of absence of the thymus gland in infants but apparently the neck was not properly searched for thymus tissue. In 20 years, Gruber[1] saw only 1 newborn in whom necropsy and microscopic examination failed to reveal any thymic tissue. The infant was a chondrodystrophic dwarf who also had a small thyroid. In more recent times, additional observations have been made, some of them mentioned in reports of congenital hypoparathyroidism. Since the thymus and parathyroids have common origins in the third and fourth pharyngeal pouches, disturbances in the development of these diverticula can affect both derivatives. Simultaneous malformations of branchiogenic organs, discussed by Rössle[16] in 1932, have been observed repeatedly since, and absence of the thymus and parathyroids has been found to be an important constituent of some broader teratologic syndromes, which have attracted attention because of their effects on immunologic phenomena. In 1959, Lobdell[17] reported the case of an infant who died at the age of 2 months after attacks of tetany. No thymus could be detected in the superior mediastinum or in the cervical region. In addition, the parathyroids and the thyroid isthmus were absent and there was a vascular ring around the trachea and esophagus formed by a double aortic arch and a ductus arteriosus. Subsequently, DiGeorge[18,19] made important contributions to this subject by consideration of the immunologic consequences of the thymo-parathyroid aplasia syndrome, which is called "III and IV pharyngeal pouch syndrome" by some[20] and the "DiGeorge syndrome" by others. But DiGeorge[19] pointed out that the first case of thymic aplasia associated with infantile convulsions already had been described by Harington[14] in 1829, thus preceding recent publications by at least 130 years. Taitz *et al.*[20] observed an infant with progressive lymphopenia who developed tetany, intractable diarrhea and marasmus, although no pathogenic organisms could be isolated from the stools. At necropsy, no thymus or parathyroid could be detected in the neck or mediastinum. The authors believed that, in this and similar cases, absence of the thymus resulted in an immunologic disorder that contributed to the early death of the child. But Huber *et al.*[21] found no signs of immunologic incompetence in a child with congenital aplasia of the thymus and parathyroids. DiGeorge[18,19] noted that the lymphocyte count can be normal in these children, although it declines during the terminal period. He found a negative response to some but not all antigens. Immunoglobulin values were increased slightly. Lymphocyte transfer tests were negative and passive transfer of tuberculin reactivity was not possible. Skin homografts were not rejected. Hart and Schwartz[22] recorded a case of thymic and parathyroid agenesis in an infant boy with mild lymphopenia, low normal levels of immunoglobulins and normal small lymphocytes combined with absence of plasma cells in the gastrointestinal tract. In peripheral lymph nodes, lymphocytes were aggregated cortically and the centers were replaced by hematopoietic tissue and plasma cells. This central deficiency in lymph nodes was not noted in other cases.[21,23]

Thymus and parathyroid agenesis – the "III and IV pharyngeal pouch syndrome" – is not limited to anomalies of these branchiogenic organs. Some of the associated malformations are so serious and domineering that affected fetuses are not viable. Absence of the thymus and parathyroids has been observed in monstrous fetuses with acardia and acephaly.[23] Aortic arch anomalies seem to be common in infants with absent parathyroids and thymus. Patent ductus arteriosus, right aortic arch, anomalous right subclavian artery and transposition of the great vessels have been reported.[17,19,22-24] The heart itself may be involved by ventricular septal defects combined with pulmonary stenosis or atresia.[21-24] Esophageal atresia and tracheo-esophageal fistula can occur together with the branchiogenic anomalies,[19,23] rendering the prognosis dim. But some of the children survive infancy, presenting such rather uncharacteristic external signs as hypertelorism, deformed ears, short philtrum, cleft nose, high-arched palate and micrognathia.[24]

It seems that the syndrome of thymo-parathyroid aplasia occurs only sporadically. In one instance, a sibling of an affected child had anencephaly.[24]

Hypoplasia

It is not always possible to distinguish between primary hypoplasia and secondary involution of the thymus, but if underdevelopment of the thymus is associated with failure of descent into the thorax or with anomalies of other branchiogenic derivatives, a developmental hypoplasia can be assumed. In a premature infant with micrognathia, microstomia and microglossia, Gruber[1] found small, symmetric cervical thymus nodes at the level of the hyoid bone. Böttinger and Wernstedt[25] reported in a child, dead of tetany at the age of 4 months, small cervical thymus lobules on the right side but none on the left and none in the mediastinum. Only one tiny parathyroid rudiment was present under the capsule of the right thyroid lobe. Rössle[16] described a small cervical thymus on the right, combined with a thymus that reached from the left cervical region into the thorax, where it extended over to the right side. Gilmour[26] gave detailed reports of hypoplasia and failure of descent of the left thymus in an anencephalic female and of bilateral hypoplasia and failure of descent of the thymus in an infant 12 weeks of age. Other cases of cervical thymus may also represent hypoplasias, but without necropsy the presence of thoracic thymus tissue cannot be excluded. Thymic hypoplasia combined with thyroid dysfunction has been reported.[58]

Thymic hypoplasia without associated developmental defects can be due to involution secondary to protracted disease. In 1921, Hammar[27] pointed out that descriptions of the thymus gland based on material from diseased or malnourished patients are deceptive. Usually, the parenchyma is reduced and the normal ratio between Hassall corpuscles and lymphoid elements is disturbed. More recently, thymic hypoplasia has become of interest again because of its association with certain immunologic deficiency states. Vestigial thymus has been observed repeatedly in the Swiss type of agammaglobulinemia, an immunologic deficiency accompanied by alymphocytosis or lymphopenia and lack of peripheral lymphoid tissue.[8,28-31] In this disorder, which apparently is transmitted as an autosomal recessive trait, the thymus seen at necropsy consists of epithelial cells only and is devoid of lymphocytes and Hassall bodies and without differentiation of cortex and medulla.[32-34] Sex-linked thymic epithelial hypoplasia in 2 siblings was recorded by Dooren *et al.*[35] The Swiss type of agammaglobulinemia was present and treatment by transplantation with fetal thymus and adult bone marrow was attempted. Thymic epithelial hypoplasia was reported in children who had total absence of white cells[36,37] and it is believed that a spectrum of immune deficiencies may be associated with failure of thymic development.[38] Thymic abnormalities are common in necropsies of children with ataxia telangiectasia (see Chapter 35). The thymuses are small and deficient in lymphocytes and most of the cells found are of an epithelial type. Hassall corpuscles usually are absent. This syndrome is now considered an immunologic deficiency disease, inherited as an autosomal recessive trait. Since children with immunologic disorders suffer from many and protracted infectious diseases, fail to thrive and usually die in a state of emaciation, one could question the specificity of the findings in the thymus, which do not differ greatly from those described by Hammar[27] in malnourished patients dying of prolonged diseases. It seems, however, that thymuses of some children with sex-linked recessive agammaglobulinemia who have died after repeated infections have not been unusual morphologically.[8] Furthermore, hypoplastic thymuses of the type associated with the Swiss type of agammaglobulinemia have been observed in newborn monozygotic twins with total absence of white blood cells.[36] Such thymic hypoplasia in neonates cannot be attributed to prolonged postnatal disease. In fact, a miniscule rudimentary thymus without lymphoctyes and Hassall corpuscles was seen in an aborted 13-week-old embryo who was a sibling of 2 infant boys who had congenital agammaglobulinemia and thymic dysplasia.[39] This observation demonstrates onset of the disease in early fetal life. It seems that there is a need for normal thymic function in fetal life. Observation of XX/XY lymphoid chimerism in immunologic deficiency with thymic alymphoplasia[40] can be interpreted as a developmental disturbance of the immunocompetent system by an early intrauterine graft of maternal cells. Because of failure of thymic differentiation and aplasia of the lymphoreticular system, maternal cells can exist in a male fetus. A normal thymus and immunologically competent lymphoid cells seem to provide a defense against invasion of unwanted similar cells of maternal origin, a property necessary to normal intrauterine development. Thus, there is much evidence that congenital thymic dysplasia precedes the postnatal diseases associated with immunologic deficiencies and is not a sequela of them. One can speak of hereditary, primary and congenital thymic aplasia or dysplasia in cases of the Swiss type of agammaglobulinemia and related disorders, which is clearly different from thymic atrophy characteristic of children who die of protracted infectious diseases and general marasmus.

Abnormal Shape and Position

The shape of the thymus can be modified by spatial conditions within the neck and the thorax and by anomalous descent of the thymic primordium from its cervical position into the chest. Thymus tissue in the cervical area can consist of elongation of thoracic thymus into the neck or of discontinuous cervical lobules in the presence of thoracic thymic tissue or of rudimentary thymus that failed to descend into the chest. In the first two cases, ample thymic tissue may be present, whereas in the third situation hypoplasia is associated with failure of descent. Thymus horns extending from the thyroid down to the thoracic area are due to failure of involution of thymus tissue in its migration from the point of origin to its final position. Such horns usually are unilateral, occurring more often on the left side than on the right. Lewis[41] collected from the medical literature 32 cases of persistence of the thymus in the cervical area and added 2 observations of his own. Thymic remnants in the neck can cause local symptoms of clinical significance. In a 3½-month-old male,[41] a mass in the left side of the neck was noticed when the infant was 2 weeks of age. When removed surgically, the mass proved to consist of normal thymus tissue. Roentgenograms of the chest suggested normal thoracic thymus development. In a second instance, a cystic mass appeared in a 13-year-old boy in the lower third of the left side of the neck. Three thymic cervical remnants were found, one cystic and two solid. Bieger and McAdams[42] described five thymic cysts from the neck; one of these presented as a posterior pharyngeal mass. The epithelial lining had, in part, the appearance of pharyngeal mucosa. Simons *et al.*[43] surveyed 13 cases of cervical thymic cysts reported in the literature. Such cases usually represent (asymptomatic) benign thymus remnants, but some displaced thymic tissues can be life-threatening. Falk[44] reported an infant with a thymic mass in the subglottic space of the trachea that necessitated tracheotomy and finally proved fatal. Ectopic tracheal thymus tissue became malignant in a man 58 years of age.[45] In an 11-year-old child[46] and in a 47-year-old man,[57] thymoma developed in the neck from an undescended thymus. A thymic mass arising from the pharynx and protruding into the mouth like a second tongue has been observed in an infant.[47] In a 35-year-old woman, cervical thymus presenting as a mass attached to the thyroid was associated with myasthenia gravis that subsided after excision of the tumor.[48] A completely different disease picture developed in a man with ectopic thymus tissue. The presenting symptoms were those of pancreatitis and hyperparathyroidism. On surgical exploration of the neck, a mass that consisted of an aggregate of thyroid, parathyroid and thymus tissues was found and excised from the lower pole of the thyroid gland.[49] In a newborn child with a unilateral defect of the left auditory apparatus, a mass of thymus tissue was located in the cavum tympani of the affected side, which shows that thymus anlage occasionally can be displaced or originate above the third pharyngeal pouch. This child, who had normal thymus tissue in the thorax, also had a ventricular septal defect and cryptorchidism.[50]

Normal thymus tissue located in the mediastinum

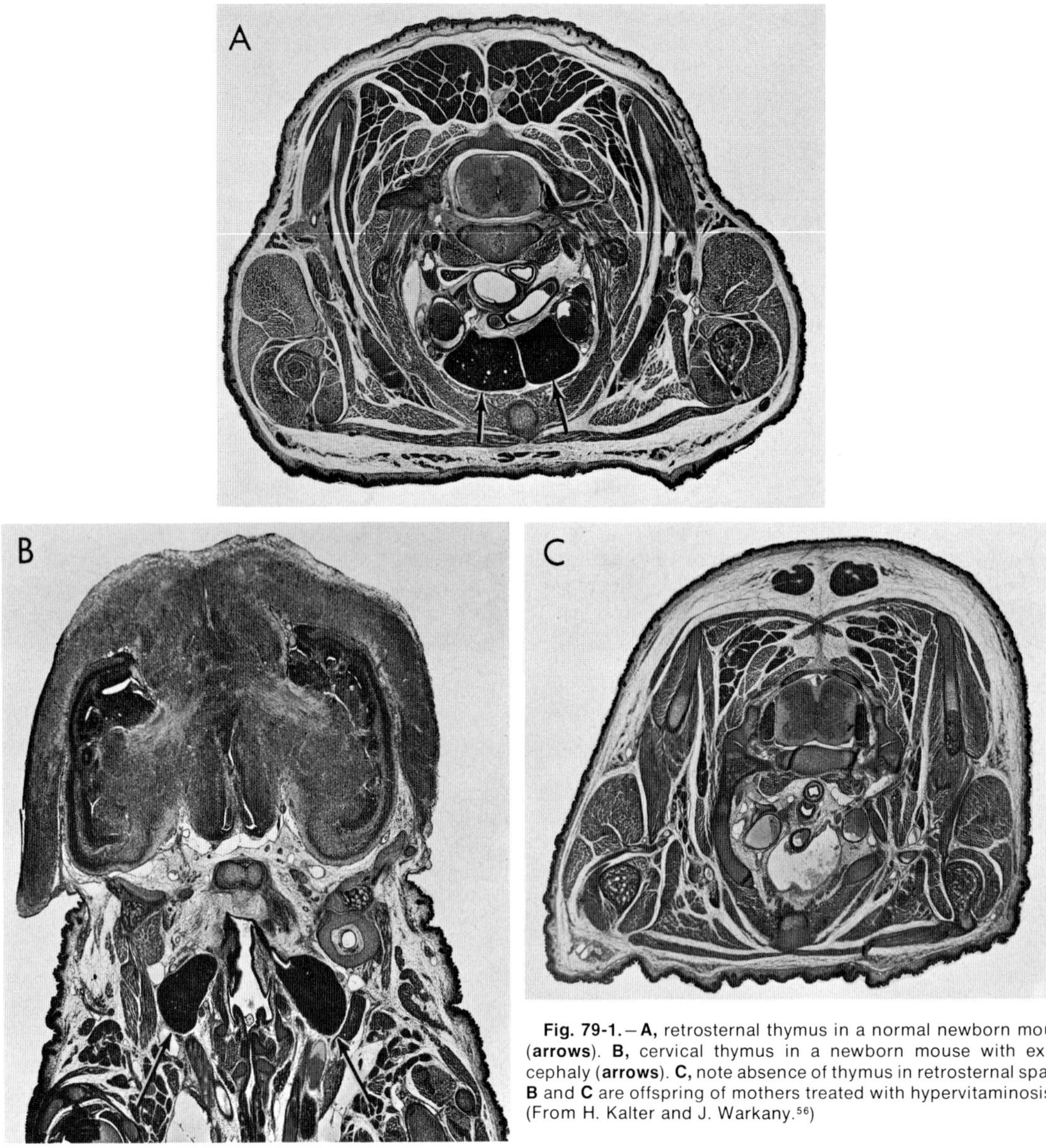

Fig. 79-1.—**A,** retrosternal thymus in a normal newborn mouse (**arrows**). **B,** cervical thymus in a newborn mouse with exencephaly (**arrows**). **C,** note absence of thymus in retrosternal space. **B** and **C** are offspring of mothers treated with hypervitaminosis A. (From H. Kalter and J. Warkany.[56])

sometimes can be displaced laterad and bring about confusing x-ray pictures. Thus, a thymus appearing in the left lung field can be mistaken for a tumor, or a supernumerary thymic lobe can present difficult diagnostic problems.[51] Mediastinal congenital cysts of the thymus may imitate huge cardiac shadows and cause such clinical symptoms as respiratory distress, cough, fever and pain. The cardiac and thymic shadows can be distinguished by angiography. Such cysts are rare; only 40 cases had been reported by 1960.[52] Sometimes mediastinal thymus cysts occur in adults who have few or no symptoms at all. They are discovered in routine roentgenograms of the chest.[53] In one instance, thymus annularis, a ring-shaped gland around the superior vena cava, was considered the cause of chylothorax and chyloabdomen in a 20-month-old girl. The lymph transudate in chest and abdomen disappeared when the superior vena cava was freed of the thymic encirclement.[54]

In guinea pigs and in chickens, the thymus does not descend from the neck into the chest but remains located in the cervical area.[55] In mice and in rats, as well as in man, the thymus is found, at the time of birth, in the upper anterior part of the chest behind the sternum. It is of interest that arrest of development achieved by teratogenic methods can result in cervical thymus glands in mice and rats. In mice, maternal treatment with hypervitaminosis A com-

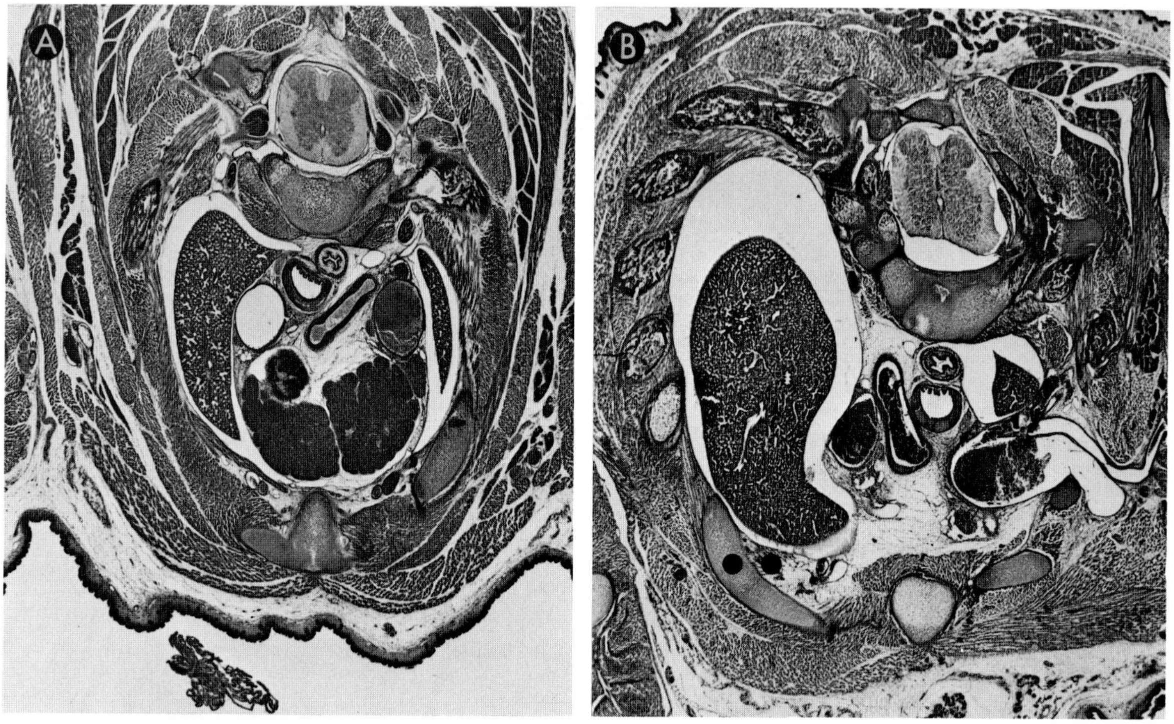

Fig. 79-2.—**A,** retrosternal thymus in a normal control rat fetus (twenty-first day). **B,** absence of the thymus in a rat fetus (twenty-first day) whose mother had been treated with trypan blue injections from the eighth to the tenth day of gestation. Note also situs inversus of aortic arch.

monly produced accessory thymus tissue or various degrees of undescended thymus.[56] The undescended organs ranged in location from a slightly elevated position, just below the thyroid, to a location high in the neck, where they were seen near the pharynx, with which they sometimes were connected by a thymo-pharyngeal duct (Fig. 79-1). In such animals, the superior mediastinum did not contain thymic tissue. Sometimes thymic tissue was also seen in the eustachian tubes.[56] Figure 79-2 shows sections obtained by maternal trypan blue treatment from a rat fetus that had situs inversus. There was no thymus in the upper mediastinum but some thymic tissue could be seen in sections through the neck.

REFERENCES

1. Gruber, G. B.: Die Entwicklungsstörungen der Thymusdrüse, in Schwalbe, E. (ed.), *Die Morphologie der Missbildungen des Menschen und der Tiere* (Jena: Gustav Fischer, 1932), Vol. 3, Chap. 10.
2. Shier, K. J.: The morphology of the epithelial thymus. Observations on lymphocyte-depleted and fetal thymus, Lab. Invest. 12:316, 1963.
3. Siegler, R.: The Morphology of the Thymuses and Their Relation to Leukemia, in Good, R. A., and Gabrielsen, A. E. (eds.), *The Thymus in Immunobiology* (New York: Hoeber Medical Division, Harper & Row, Publishers, 1964).
4. Weller, G. L., Jr.: Development of the thyroid, parathyroid and thymus glands in man, Contrib. Embryol. 24:95, 1933.
5. Arey, L. B.: *Developmental Anatomy* (7th ed.; Philadelphia: W. B. Saunders Company, 1965).
6. Good, R. A., Peterson, R. D., and Gabrielsen, A. E.: The thymus and central lymphoid tissue in immunobiology, Bull. Rheumat. Dis. 15:351, 1964.
7. Good, R. A., Cooper, M. D., Peterson, R. D., Kellum, M. J., Sutherland, D. E., and Gabrielsen, A. E.: The role of the thymus in immune process, Ann. New York Acad. Sc. 135:451, 1966.
8. Good, R. A., and Gabrielsen, A. E. (eds.): *The Thymus in Immunobiology* (New York: Hoeber Medical Division, Harper & Row, Publishers, 1964).
9. Good, R. A., Peterson, R. D., Perey, D. Y., Finstad, J., and Cooper, M. D.: The Immunological Deficiency Diseases of Man: Consideration of Some Questions Asked by These Patients with an Attempt at Classification, in Bergsma, D. (ed.), *Immunological Deficiency Diseases in Man.* Birth Defects Original Article Series, Vol. IV (New York: The National Foundation, 1968).
10. Beard, J.: The source of leucocytes and the true function of the thymus, Anat. Anz. 18:550, 1900.
11. Auerbach, R.: Experimental analysis of the origin of cell types in the development of the mouse thymus, Develop. Biol. 3:336, 1961.
12. Auerbach, R.: Developmental studies of mouse thymus and spleen, National Cancer Institute Monograph No. 11, p. 23, 1963.
13. Miller, J. F.: Immunological function of the thymus, Lancet 2:748, 1961.
14. Harington, H.: Absence of the thymus gland, London M. Gaz. 3:314, 1828–1829.
15. Clark, A.: A case of absence of the thymus gland in an infant, Lancet 2:1077, 1896.
16. Rössle, R.: Über gleichzeitige Missbildungen der branchiogenen Organe und über angeborenen Mangel der Epithel-

körperchen, Virchows Arch. path. Anat. 283:41, 1932.
17. Lobdell, D. H.: Congenital absence of the parathyroid glands, Arch. Path. 67:412, 1959.
18. DiGeorge, A. M.: Discussion of A new concept of the cellular basis of immunity, by Cooper, M. D., Peterson, R. D., and Good, R. A., J. Pediat. 67:907, 1965 (abst.).
19. DiGeorge, A. M.: Congenital Absence of the Thymus and Its Immunologic Consequences: Concurrence with Congenital Hypoparathyroidism, in Bergsma, D. (ed.), *Immunological Deficiency Diseases in Man.* Birth Defects Original Article Series, Vol. IV (New York: The National Foundation, 1968).
20. Taitz, L. S., Zarate-Salvador, C., and Schwartz, E.: Congenital absence of the parathyroid and thymus glands in an infant (III and IV pharyngeal pouch syndrome), Pediatrics 38:412, 1966.
21. Huber, J., Cholnoky, P., and Zoethout, H. E.: Congenital aplasia of parathyroid glands and thymus, Arch. Dis. Childhood 42:190, 1967.
22. Hart, M. N., and Schwartz, D. C.: Thymic agenesis, Arch. Path. 88:437, 1969.
23. Dische, M. R.: Lymphoid tissue and associated congenital malformations in thymic agenesis, Arch. Path. 86:312, 1968.
24. Kretschmer, R., Say, B., Brown, D., and Rosen, F. S.: Congenital aplasia of the thymus gland (DiGeorge's syndrome), New England J. Med. 279:1295, 1968.
25. Böttinger, E., and Wernstedt, W.: Beiträge zur Kenntnis der spasmophilen Diathese, Acta paediat. 6:373, 1927.
26. Gilmour, J. R.: Some developmental abnormalities of the thymus and parathyroids, J. Path. & Bact. 52:213, 1941.
27. Hammar, J. A.: The new views as to the morphology of the thymus gland and their bearing on the problem of the function of the thymus, Endocrinology 5:543, 1921.
28. Glanzmann, E., and Riniker, P.: Essentielle Lymphocytophthise, Ann. paediat. 175:1, 1950.
29. Cottier, H., Bürki, K., Hess, M. W., and Hässig, A.: Pathological Considerations of Immunological Deficiency Diseases in Man, in Bergsma, D. (ed.), *Immunological Deficiency Diseases in Man.* Birth Defects Original Article Series, Vol. IV (New York: The National Foundation, 1968).
30. Hitzig, W. H., Biro, Z., Bosch, H., and Huser, H. J.: Agammaglobulinämie und Alymphozytose mit Schwund des lymphatischen Gewebes, Helvet. paediat. acta 13:551, 1958.
31. Rosen, F. S., Gitlin, D., and Janeway, C. A.: Alymphocytosis, agammaglobulinemia, homografts and delayed hypersensitivity, Lancet 2:380, 1962.
32. Gitlin, D., and Craig, J. M.: The thymus and other lymphoid tissues in congenital agammaglobulinemia. I. Thymic alymphoplasia and lymphocytic hypoplasia and their relation to infection, Pediatrics 32:517, 1963.
33. Gitlin, D., Vawter, G., and Craig, J. M.: Thymic alymphoplasia and congenital aleukocytosis, Pediatrics 33:184, 1964.
34. Delta, B. G., Rothenberg, A. M., Ainsworth, H. D., and Innella, F.: Congenital alymphoplasmacytic agammaglobulinemia with thymic dysplasia, J.A.M.A. 194:507, 1965.
35. Dooren, L. J., de Vries, M. J., van Bekkum, D. W., Cleton, F. J., and de Koning, J.: Sex-linked thymic epithelial hypoplasia in two siblings: Attempt at treatment by transplantation with fetal thymus and adult bone marrow, J. Pediat. 72:51, 1968.
36. deVaal, O. M., and Seynhaeve, V.: Reticular dysgenesia, Lancet 2:1123, 1959.
37. Gitlin, D., Rosen, F. S., and Janeway, C. A.: The thymus and other lymphoid tissues in congenital agammaglobulinemia. II. Delayed hypersensitivity and homograft survival in a child with thymic alymphoplasia, Pediatrics 33:711, 1964.
38. Schaller, J., Davis, S. D., and Wedgwood, R. J.: Failure of development of the thymus, lymphopenia and hypogammaglobulinemia, Am. J. Med. 41:462, 1966.
39. Yakovac, W. C.: Thymic dysplasia in congenital agammaglobulinemia, J. Pediat. 63:699, 1963.
40. Kadowaki, J., Zuelzer, W. W., Brough, A. J., Thompson, R. I., Wooley, P. V., and Gruber, D.: XX/XY lymphoid chimaerism in congenital immunological deficiency syndrome with thymic alymphoplasia, Lancet 2:1152, 1965.
41. Lewis, M. R.: Persistence of the thymus in the cervical area, J. Pediat. 61:887, 1962.
42. Bieger, R. C., and McAdams, A. J.: Thymic cysts, Arch. Path. 82:535, 1966.
43. Simons, J. N., Robinson, D. W., and Masters, F. W.: Cervical thymic cyst, Am. J. Surg. 108:578, 1964.
44. Falk, P.: Über ortsfremde, gutartige Gewebsbildungen, Thymus- und Thyreoidea-gewebe im Kehlkopf, Arch. Ohren- Nasen- u. Kehlkopfh. 141:118, 1936.
45. Wadon, A.: Thymoma intratracheale, Zentralbl. allg. Path. 60:308, 1934.
46. Pirkey, W. P.: Epithelioma of undescended thymus in a child, A.M.A. Arch. Otolaryng. 59:237, 1954.
47. Epstein, H. C., and Loeb, W. S.: Thymic tumor of the pharynx, J. Pediat. 47:105, 1955.
48. Sease, C. I.: Cervical thymoma, Virginia M. Month. 83: 345, 1956.
49. Rankow, R. H., Bruno, M. S., and Ober, W. B.: Congenital pharyngeal pouch formation with hyperparathyroidism, New York J. Med. 64:2568, 1964.
50. Hagens, E. W.: Malformation of the auditory apparatus in the new-born; associated with ectopic thymus, Arch. Otolaryng. 15:671, 1932.
51. Adler, E.: Ein klinischer Beitrag zur Dystopie und Lageanomalie der Thymus, Bruns' Beitr. klin. Chir. 208:233, 1964.
52. Zanca, P., Chuang, T. H., De Avila, R., and Galindo, D. L.: True congenital mediastinal thymic cyst, Pediatrics 36: 615, 1965.
53. Schillhammer, W. R., Jr., and Tyson, M. D.: Mediastinal thymic cysts. Report of three cases and review of the literature, Arch. Surg. 85:410, 1962.
54. Juzbasic, D., and Pasini, M.: Thymus annularis. Contribution to the pathogenesis and treatment of chylothorax and chylo-abdomen, Deutsche med. Wchnschr. 90:1050, 1965.
55. Metcalf, D.: The Thymus and Lymphopoesis, in Good, R. A., and Gabrielsen, A. E. (eds.), *The Thymus in Immunobiology* (New York: Hoeber Medical Division, Harper & Row, Publishers, 1964).
56. Kalter, H., and Warkany, J.: Experimental production of congenital malformations in strains of inbred mice by maternal treatment with hypervitaminosis A, Am. J. Path. 38:1, 1961.
57. Ridenhour, C. E., Henzel, J. H., DeWeese, M. S., and Kerr, S. E.: Thymoma arising from undescended cervical thymus, Surgery 67:614, 1970.
58. Hong, R., Gatti, R., Rathbun, J. C., and Good, R. A.: Thymic hypoplasia and thyroid dysfunction, New England J. Med. 282:470, 1970.

80

The Spleen

IN EMBRYOS of 8–9 mm. length, at the beginning of the sixth week of gestation, a swelling becomes discernible on the left side of the dorsal mesogastrium. This accumulation of mesenchymal cells is located near the fundus of the stomach between the two peritoneal layers. In embryos of 15 mm. length, the swelling has increased and the spleen then consists of three hillocks located on the dorsal body wall between the mesonephric and genital folds. At 25 mm. length, the hillocks are again reduced to two in number and later a single spleen is formed that may show furrows in later fetal life as remnants of previous division.[1] At 3 months, the spleen acquires its characteristic form with a slender connection with the dorsal mesogastrium, which attaches at the hilus as a gastrosplenic ligament. Sinuses, developing as separate cavities within the mesenchyme, are formed by the middle of fetal life. Lymphoid tissue is represented by the splenic corpuscles, which become distinctly recognizable in the sixth month. From the fourth through the eighth month of fetal life, the formation of white blood cells is supplemented by red corpuscles that develop within the splenic mass.[2] The spleen plays a role in the early development of immune bodies of the fetus. Van Furth *et al.*[3] found that the human fetus can synthesize immune globulin C and M from about the twentieth week of gestation on. Whereas synthesis of immunoglobulins could be demonstrated in spleen tissue culture after the nineteenth week, such synthesis was not achieved by thymus tissue.

Agenesis

Congenital absence of the spleen is an impressive anomaly that has long been of interest to anatomists and more recently to clinicians. Early descriptions of the anomaly date back to the seventeenth and eighteenth centuries[4] and it appears that Martin, in 1826,[5] observed it together with cardiovascular and gastric defects. Historical notes and review articles on this subject are available.[6-9]

In 1956, Putschar and Manion[6] listed 19 case reports on agenesis of the spleen without other malformations. Most of these cases concerned adults who died of infectious or other incidental diseases, some of them in the sixth or seventh decade of life. In a case by Riches,[10] a woman 44 years of age developed a round cell sarcoma of the omentum and the mesenteric nodes and died of intestinal obstruction. A 56-year-old man died of a right strangulated inguinal hernia. Gilbert *et al.*[8] culled from the literature 27 instances of asplenia unassociated with intracardiac defects and 16 cases in which no specific mention of the heart was made in the necropsy findings. Among these 43 patients without cardiac involvement there were 8 with partial situs inversus and 5 with multiple congenital malformations. In patients who died of prolonged infectious diseases, destruction of the spleen rather than agenesis may have occurred.

Agenesis of the spleen is of practical importance chiefly because of its frequent association with other congenital malformations. It can be combined with malformations of the heart with or without partial situs inversus or with partial situs inversus but a normal heart.

As stated before, the combination of asplenia with cardiovascular anomalies was recorded by Martin in 1826 and at least 16 other cases of this type had been reported before 1952, when Polhemus and Schafer[11] described atrioventricularis communis, partial situs inversus and splenic agenesis as a syndrome. Ivemark[7] put special emphasis on agenesis and other anomalies of the spleen as related to the pathogenesis of cono-truncal anomalies. Persistent truncus arteriosus (10 cases), pulmonary stenosis or atresia (34 cases) and transposition of the great arteries (14 cases) in various combinations were analyzed as special entities. But attention also was paid to anomalies of the atrioventricular region, septa, pulmonary veins and systemic veins. Abnormal pulmonary return was discussed by Brandt and Liebow.[12]

Putschar and Manion[6] tabulated 49 cases of asplenia combined with congenital heart disease; 20 of these were without situs inversus and 29 were combined with partial situs inversus. The most common anomalies of the heart were atrioventricularis communis (cor biloculare); atresia, stenosis or hypoplasia of the pulmonary artery or ostium; atrial septal defects; cor triloculare biatriatum; transposition of the large arteries; inversion of the chambers of the heart; cor triloculare biventriculare; patent ductus arteriosus; ventricular septal defects; and truncus or pseudotruncus arteriosus. There was considerable overlapping of the anomalies listed. Gilbert *et al.*[8] tabulated 85 cases of splenic agenesis with cardiovascular malformations. Of these, 52 had transposition of the great vessels, 51 common atrioventricular valve, 45 anomalous systemic venous return, 43 anomalous pulmonary venous return, 37 single ventricle, 28 pulmonary atresia, 20 pulmonary stenosis, 12 truncus arteriosus, 7 cor biloculare and 4 cor triloculare. Neimann *et al.*[9] considered malformations associated with asplenia and polysplenia. Of 210 cases, they classified 119 as single ventricle; of 137 cases in which the cardiac situs was mentioned, 59 were listed as dextrocardia and 78 as levocardia.

Partial situs inversus was present in 85 asplenia cases reviewed by Gilbert *et al.*[8] and in 200 of 210 cases of asplenia-polysplenia syndromes listed by Neimann *et al.*[9] Total situs inversus appeared only once in the series of Putschar and Manion[6] and in another instance reported by Terslev.[13] Most cases associated with splenic anomalies represent partial inversions involving an entire organ such as the stomach, liver, duodenum, pancreas, gallbladder, intestine or esophagus; or they affect only parts of an abdominal organ. In addition to situs inversus, abdominal viscera may have other anomalies. Since the spleen develops in the left dorsal mesogastrium, the development of the stomach and the omentum, which are closely related to the dorsal mesogastrium, may be affected also if the spleen is absent. In 6 patients reviewed by Putschar and Manion,[6] the stomach was tubular and without a distinct fundus as in early embryonic life. In 2 cases, rotation had not occurred, so that the stomach retained the midline sagittal position of early embryos. In 2 patients, the stomach was partly intrathoracic, with a short esophagus and a wide esophageal hiatus in the diaphragm. In other cases, the omentum was completely missing or a persistent dorsal mesogastrium and a mobile pancreas were noted. Symmetric lobation of the liver or a larger left than right lobe was seen occasionally. In at least 24 of the asplenic patients there was incomplete rotation of the intestine or anomaly of the mesentery. Supernumerary lobation of the lungs occurred in 47 of 85 cases tabulated by Gilbert *et al.*[8] and symmetric lungs in 114 of the cases of Neimann *et al.*[9] Sometimes bilateral trilobed lungs are combined with bilateral symmetric epiarterial bronchi. The spectrum of associated malformations in the asplenia syndrome may include the central nervous system. Spina bifida cystica,[14-16] hydrocephaly[15,16] and cyclopia[16] have been described. At times, cleft lip, hemivertebrae, complete agenesis of the trachea and lungs,[17] diaphragmatic hernia, anomalous pancreas, agenesis of the gallbladder, horseshoe kidney, absence of one kidney, hydronephrosis, hypospadias, double penis, cryptorchidism, ovarian agenesis, uterus duplex, stenosis and atresia of the rectum, clubfoot and other malformations appear together with splenic anomalies.

In most instances of agenesis of the spleen combined with malformations of the heart (with and without situs inversus), the patients were severely affected by the cardiovascular anomalies and died in infancy or early childhood. The lifetime of 76 of the 85 patients listed by Gilbert *et al.*[8] was less than 1 year. Agenesis of the spleen without associated congenital malformations is, of course, compatible with postnatal life, although a tendency to infectious and thrombotic processes may endanger life at times. Gilbert *et al.*[8] reported the case of a 41-year-old asplenic man who died of multiple thromboses, infarctions and encephalomalacia of the right hemisphere. Ivemark[7] stressed the occurrence of infections, and Hjelt and Hakosalo[18] a tendency to thrombosis. Polycythemia and erythroblastosis observed in some asplenic infants and children probably are responses to congenital cyanotic heart disease. But Heinz-Ehrlich bodies,[19] more closely related to asplenia, can facilitate the clinical diagnosis. Enlargement of lymph nodes was mentioned in many, but not all, patients with asplenia seen at necropsy. Leukemoid reactions to infection have been observed.[20] Of 20 adults with asplenia included in the review by Putschar and Manion,[6] 2 died of lymphosarcoma. Both these patients[10,21] had reached the fifth decade of life. In none of the cases reported in childhood was asplenia associated with lymphosarcoma.

The association of asplenia with other congenital malformations has enticed many authors to find a definite date of the "embryologic timetable" that could explain the various syndromes by arrest of development of the organs involved. Whereas some writers are satisfied to time the morphologic deviations from the normal, others attempted to date and recognize etiologic factors by morphologic considerations – a rather hazardous enterprise.

Ivemark's[7] embryologic studies showed that the early splenic primordia were present in Horizons XV to XVII, when the embryo has, according to Streeter,[22] an estimated ovulation age of 31 – 36 days. Fusion of the atrioventricular canal cushions occurs in the XVIth Horizon, whereas the complete separation of the cono-truncus is accomplished approximately 2 days later in the XVIIth Horizon. Examination of the pathologic material led Ivemark to the view that, in cases of agenesis of the spleen, the anomalies in the atrioventricular region were primary to those of the cono-truncus, so that the syndrome could be attributed to "events" that went into play at the time at which the organ in question was about to be formed, i.e., in embryos with an estimated ovulation age of 31 – 36 days. Gilbert *et al.*[8] arrived at different dates of origin. The most probable explanation for the combination of lesions appeared to be a factor with a wide lethal range operating at about an ovulatory age of 24 days. This factor in its mildest form was thought to cause suppression of the development of the spleen, but in its most severe form to cause also an arrest of development of the primitive heart tube and of the dorsal and ventral mesenteries, so that the structures derived from the gut grow in situ in a symmetric manner instead of the normal asymmetry. Taking into consideration the variability of the syndrome and its severity, Gilbert *et al.*[8] estimated the time of operation of the factor as from 24 to 28 days. They thought that a study of pregnant women 2 weeks after their first missed menstrual period might result in a discovery of the etiologic factor and ultimately lead to preventive measures. Putschar and Manion[6] were less specific about the time of origin of the syndrome and stated that the anomaly seems to originate in approximately the fifth to seventh week of fetal life, which coincides with the teratogenic period of all the associated anomalies of the heart, blood vessels and visceral situs. Polhemus and Schafer[11] thought that early splenic primordia appear at an estimated ovulation age of 31–36 days. It is at this time that fusion of the cushions of the atrioventricular canal occurs, which is followed approximately 2 days later by complete separation of the cono-truncus into two separate channels. At the end of this period, the aortic and pulmonary valves become distinct, but the mitral and tricuspid valves are not yet formed. Polhemus and Schafer believed that in this syndrome something prevents normal development of the systems involved beyond a gestational age of 36 days. These opinions exemplify the difficulties encountered by attempts to ascertain the date of origin of a syndrome of congenital malformations with the help of embryologic timetables (p. 49). There is no agreement on the timetables. In Streeter's horizons, the ages of the embryos were calculated by comparison with macaque embryos of known ovulation age. Textbooks of embryology illustrating developmental stages sometimes mention the length and sometimes the age of the embryo. But, more important, there is no certainty as to the beginning of an organ such as the spleen. Ivemark[7] admitted that the morphologic evidence of the presence of the "first" splenic anlage by definition is subjective and unreliable. It is clear that arrest of development of the branch of a tree may have its cause in a root defect and not necessarily at the bud; it should be equally clear that arrest of development of an embryologic organ may have its cause in a developmental stage that precedes the period in which the organ fails to develop as a visible structure. The disturbing factor *could* interfere with the development of the organ at the time of appearance, but it could also have acted before by damaging an enzyme, an organizer, a chromosome or a gene. The resulting arrest of development would become visible at a much later time. The timing of *the* syndrome is further made impossible by the fact that the disease picture sometimes includes so many heterogeneous malformations that one cannot find an embryologic date at which the organs involved are "about to be formed." To give one example: asplenia can occur together with abnormal lobation of the left lung, but also with complete absence of the trachea and lungs (p. 599). These are quite different malformations, probably with differing times of onset. In addition, it must be remembered that the "asplenia" syndrome occurs not only in patients with absent spleen but also combined with multiple, multilobulated[23] and rudimentary spleens. All one can say is that in the asplenia syndrome and in related disease pictures the disturbing factors generally interfere with early developmental processes; but so do many teratogenic factors that result in completely different syndromes yet permit normal development of the spleen and of the heart. One can agree with Hjelt and Hakosalo,[18] who stated cautiously that the period of influence of the primary disturbing factor and the primary affected area in the embryo varies in different cases of congenital asplenia syndromes and that in many instances the effect obviously was produced before the age of 5 weeks.

There are few leads to explanation of the etiology of the disease pictures involving absence of the spleen.

All reviews show a prevalence of affected males. In one series,[6] 45 patients were male and 29 were female. In the group with situs inversus and malformations of the heart, the sex ratio was 3:1. In another series,[9] 117 of 196 patients were male. The reason for this sex prevalence is not known, but it is of interest that related disorders such as transposition of the great vessels and of splenic gonadal fusion generally show a predilection for males.

There are only isolated observations that suggest genetic determination of the syndromes associated with splenic anomalies. But, in some reports, repetition of some of the symptoms in families is mentioned. Polhemus and Schafer[11] described a girl with transposition of the great vessels, persistent atrioventricularis communis, pulmonary stenosis and atresia, patent ductus arteriosus, incomplete rotation of the intestines, trilobar left lung, "symmetric" and deformed liver and *congenital asplenia*. Her only sibling had died at the age of 11 months with persistent atrioventricularis communis, partial transposition of the abdominal viscera and *multiple accessory spleens*. Schönfeld and Frischman[24] recorded a family of Jews from Iraq in which apparently healthy parents had 5 children, of whom only 1 was free of congenital malformation. The male proband, the third child of the family, died on the ninth day of cyanotic congenital heart disease. At necropsy, atrial and ventricular septal defects, transposition of the great vessels, overriding aorta, "symmetric liver," trilobate left lung and agenesis of the spleen were found. The second pregnancy had resulted in a male child who died of congenital heart disease at the age of 9 months. At necropsy, persistent truncus arteriosus, ventricular septal defect and situs inversus totalis were seen. No mention was made of the spleen. The first-born female child in this family had died an hour after birth. Vaginal atresia, vesicovaginal fistula, bilateral hydronephrosis, polydactyly and clubfeet were present. The fifth child was a girl who was normal except for polydactyly of hands and feet. Apparently, two different and unrelated syndromes of malformation occurred in this family. Two children were affected by severe cardiovascular malformation and situs inversus, and asplenia was present in at least one of them. Interestingly, one of the children had partial and the other total situs inversus. The latter is extremely rare in the asplenia syndrome (p. 746). Two children of the family had polydactyly and one of them had urogenital anomalies, symptoms not characteristic of the asplenia syndrome. Inbreeding was strong in this kindred and the parents were first cousins. In two other cases of the asplenia syndrome, parental consanguinity was mentioned.[9,25]

A variant of the asplenia syndrome was described by Ongley *et al.*[26] Anomalous inferior cava and pulmonary veins, situs inversus and multiple spleens were observed in several cases. The mother of one of these patients had situs inversus of viscera with an apparently normal heart. An interesting case was recorded by Neimann *et al.*[9] The patient had transposition of the great vessels, hypoplasia of one ventricle, abnormal abdominal situs and three small spleens. A sibling had died of congenital heart disease at the age of 6 weeks. The mother was a diabetic. In a few cases, the mother of the affected child reported an infectious episode during pregnancy. A markedly pathologic placenta was found in 3 cases described by Hjelt and Hakosalo.[18] Such observations are valuable but the etiology remains obscure in most cases of asplenia and related syndromes.

Hypoplasia

A tiny spleen was found at necropsy of a 10-month-old girl who had died of an overwhelming infection with *Haemophilus influenzae*.[27] Microscopically, the miniature spleen was normally structured with a congested red pulp but there was a gross deficiency of white pulp. A sister and a brother of this child showed great susceptibility to infection, which also was due to severe splenic hypoplasia. Two siblings in the family were normal. The parents were consanguineous and the hypoplasia of the spleen was attributed to autosomal recessive inheritance.[27]

Accessory Spleens

Accessory spleens are relatively small structures of splenic tissue that develop in addition to a main spleen of approximately normal size. Halpert and Györkey,[28] who made a special search for accessory spleens, observed them in 311 of 3,000 male adult patients (11%). Of 311 persons, 272 had 1, 29 had 2, 7 had 3, 2 had 4 and 1 had 5 accessory spleens. Of these, 208 were located near the splenic hilus, 54 in the tail of the pancreas, 9 along the splenic artery and 1 in the wall of the jejunum. Curtis and Movitz[29] located 54% of accessory spleens at the hilus, 25% in the splenic pedicle, 12% in the great omentum and 6% near the pancreatic tail; others were in rare positions. Various incidence figures were cited by Putschar[30] and Grossman *et al.*[31] Accessory splenic tissue may undergo involution with advancing age. Cahalane and Kiesselbach[55] noted accessory spleens in 10.5% of necropsies in a children's hospital. In more than half of these cases there were congenital malformations of other body systems, with the central nervous and cardiovascular systems predominant. Accessory spleens were present in 9 cases of trisomy 13-15 and ectopic splenic tissue within the pancreas in 2 of 32 cases. In children with trisomy 18, 7% have accessory spleens.[32] Ectopic supradiaphragmatic spleens were present in the thorax of an infant with cyclopia, iniencephaly and many other malformations (Cincinnati Children's Hospital Chart No. C-62-87).

Extra spleens can cause symptoms by torsion of the pedicle, by inducing intestinal obstruction or by preventing proper response to splenectomy in cases of idiopathic thrombocytopenic purpura and hemolytic anemia.[31] But in most cases they remain symptomless.

Moller *et al.*[33] distinguished between accessory spleen and polysplenia in which the bulk of splenic tissue is divided into two and often more nearly equal-sized splenic masses. In a number of patients with such multiple spleens they found a tendency for symmetric development of organs with levo-isomerism or bilateral left-sidedness. Absence of the hepatic segment of the inferior vena cava, absence of the gallbladder, bilobed lungs and malrotation of the bowel were encountered. Cardiac malformations included dextrocardia, bilateral superior venae cavae, anomalous pulmonary venous connection with malposition of the atrial septum and atrial or ventricular septal defects.

Double Spleen

Double spleen is a rare malformation differing from accessory spleens by the nearly equal size and shape of the organs; but, in several cases, both accessory and double spleens were encountered. Double spleen can be associated with situs inversus or with such severe malformations as omphalocele, myeloschisis, craniorachischisis or anencephaly. Occasionally, double spleen is seen at necropsy in persons of advanced age.[30]

Wandering Spleen

When the elongation of the splenic pedicle is sufficient to allow displacement of the spleen to areas outside the left upper abdominal quadrant, one speaks of a wandering or floating spleen. Congenital and acquired forms have been described. Abell[34] reviewed 95 reports of wandering spleen with torsion of the pedicle but only 1 child under 10 years of age was listed among them. Two-thirds of the cases occurred between the ages of 20 and 40 years. In 14% observed before the age of 20 years, congenital factors were thought to be involved.

An interesting case was reported by Simpson and Ashby.[35] A large gangrenous spleen with a long pedicle was removed from a 53-year-old-man whose disease picture of marked laxity of the abdominal musculature, bladder neck obstruction and malrotation of abdominal viscera appears to be identical with "agenesis of abdominal muscles" (p. 1028), with torsion of a wandering spleen as a rare complication.

Perrine[36] described torsion of an accessory splenic pedicle in a 13-year-old girl. Three spleens of various sizes were located in the right lower quadrant of the abdomen. Torsion of an accessory spleen simulating acute appendicitis was reported by Kitchin and Green.[37] An accessory wandering spleen caused symptoms of intestinal obstruction in a 25-year-old pregnant woman. Combination of a prenatal factor with abdominal changes effected by pregnancy led to this complication.[38] Torsion of the spleen associated with congenital absence of the left kidney was recorded by Pearson.[39] A possible association of wandering spleen with partial anomalous venous return was mentioned by Crosett *et al.*[40]

The appearance of a large mass in the abdomen may suggest neoplasm or intestinal complications; wandering spleen should be included in the differential diagnosis.[40]

Cysts and Hemangiomas

Sometimes it is difficult to decide whether cysts of the spleen are of prenatal origin or acquired after birth by trauma or disease. Epithelial cysts – dermoid, epidermoid, entodermal or peritoneal – are rare developmental anomalies. Endothelial cysts are large unilocular or multilocular lymphangiomas or structures in polycystic spleens that may enlarge the organ to tumor size.[30] Fowler[41] reviewed 265 cysts reported in the world literature. Islam[42] encountered four spleens with cysts in 61 splenectomies. He classified nonparasitic cysts as primary and congenital or as secondary and false (acquired). He added developmental "infoliation cysts" to the types enumerated by Putschar.[30] In the process of splenic development from multiple hillocks projecting from the dorsal mesogastrium into the peritoneum, a portion of the peritoneum may be pinched off and form the nidus of a cyst. Among the four splenic cysts observed by Islam,[42] one was thought to be hemagiomatous, one epidermoid and two probably were acquired.

Hemangiomas apparently are the most common benign tumors of the spleen.[43] Giant hemangiomas of the spleen can result – like other large hemangiomas – in thrombocytopenia and fibrinogen deficiency[44,45] by intravascular coagulation and trapping of platelets (Kasabach-Merritt syndrome). Surgical removal of the hemangioma and spleen can lead to marked improvement of the hemorrhagic diathesis.

Splenic-Gonadal Fusion

Abnormal connection between the spleen and the left gonad or derivatives of the left mesonephros was described by Pommer[46] in 1889 and has been observed repeatedly since then. Early reports were reviewed by Putschar and Manion,[47] who distinguished two forms of the anomaly – a continuous fusion in which the spleen and the gonad (or mesonephric derivatives) are connected by a cord-like splenic process and a discontinuous form in which the organs have become separated so that a main spleen and a displaced spleen are found. The anomaly occurs chiefly in males and on the left side. A portion of the spleen attached to the mesonephros descends with the male gonad to the inguinal canal or scrotum. The splenic extension can interfere with normal descent of the testis, which may be located in the iliac fossa, in the inguen, in an inguinal hernia or in the scrotum. In females, descent of the ovary can be inhibited by a splenic process. Splenic-ovarian fusion has been observed in a 44-year-old woman with septate uterus.[48]

In most continuous cases, the cord-shaped splenic elongation arises from the upper pole of the spleen, tapering downward, with a terminal enlargement of splenic tissue at the gonad or ending in a fibrous band that enters the inguinal canal. But sometimes the main spleen is two-lobed and its caudal process arises from the anterior portions of the organ. As a rule, the splenic band crosses ventral to the intestinal loops, where it can cause bowel obstruction in rare cases.[49] Blood from the splenic process may be shunted directly into the vena cava, thus bypassing the liver.[50]

In discontinuous cases, an accessory spleen can be attached to the testis or to the head of the epididymis. Two or even three spleens have been observed in the scrotum or on the spermatic cord.[47] Associated hernias and swelling and pain in the scrotum may be presenting symptoms. An ectopic spleen may be mistaken for a third testis, a testicular tumor or a hydrocele.[51]

Splenic-gonadal fusion has been described repeatedly in association with severe limb defects and with micrognathia. In 37 cases reported by 1961, 8 patients had shown limb defects; some also had micrognathia.[49] One was the case of a child without arms, rudimentary legs, vertebral anomalies, intestinal malrotation and a spleen with a long caudal process reaching down to the left testis. The mother of this child had attempted abortion with quinine during the first 2 weeks of pregnancy.[52]

Putschar and Manion[47] tried to find a common denominator for the anomalies of the spleen, limbs and jaw in the time of critical development of the affected structures. They showed that in a fetus of 17 mm. length the buds of the extremities are differentiating; Meckel cartilage is forming and the spleen is in intimate contact with the mesonephric-gonadal anlage; they thought that a diffuse injury to the fetus at this stage could produce the syndrome of splenic-gonadal fusion, peromelia and micrognathia. Hines and Eggum[49] believed that this set of anomalies results from an insult to the organism at about the eighth week. This period does not tally with that ascertained for limb defects due to thalidomide. Nowack[53] found that severe limb defects followed thalidomide intake between the thirty-eighth and forty-seventh days, i.e., earlier than the eighth week. Actually, in the publication by Putschar and Manion,[47] the illustrations of a 17-mm. embryo show the extremities already fairly well developed and beyond the bud stage, whereas the gonad and spleen are still in close proximity to each other. In addition, it has been found that splenic-gonadal fusion can be combined with a variety of malformations that can be related to differing "critical periods." Sommer[50] and Fritzsche[52] mentioned split vertebrae. In an infant seen in the Cincinnati Children's Hospital, atrial septal defect, hypoplastic larynx and some degree of sexual precocity were noted (Chart No. 118118). In another child, a girl, the spleen adhered to a hypoplastic left ovary. Microcephaly, choanal atresia, pterygia colli, microgastria, anomalies of the bile ducts, hypoplastic kidneys, hydroureter, uterus bicornis, clubfoot and other associated malformations were found. The "critical periods" for all the developmental steps resulting in these malformations probably would encompass the entire organogenic period.

It should be mentioned in this context that reduced spleen size and fragmentation of the spleen occur in a strain of mice with genital hypoplasia and reduction malformations of the limbs. Affected mice also have horseshoe kidney, cystic kidney or absent kidney, with predilection of the renal anomaly for the left side.[54] If such a syndrome appeared in human beings, there would be attempts to find a "critical period" for the deviation of the affected structures from the normal and attempts to search for an "event" that causes the syndrome at the period fitting the embryologic timetable. But the syndrome actually is due to a recessive gene and the malformations occur in animals homozygous for that gene. The event that caused the syndrome did not take place during embryogenesis, when the spleen, the extremities, the kidneys and the gonads went through critical periods, but happened generations before, when a mutation occurred in a male ancestor irradiated with 1,500 R.

REFERENCES

1. Putschar, W.: Die Entwicklungsstörungen der Milz, in Schwalbe, E., and Gruber, G. B. (eds.), *Die Morphologie der Missbildungen des Menschen und der Tiere* (Jena: Gustav Fischer, 1934).
2. Arey, L. B.: *Developmental Anatomy* (Philadephia: W. B. Saunders Company, 1965).
3. Van Furth, R., Schuit, H. R. E., and Hijinans, W.: The immunological development of the human fetus, J. Exper. Med. 122:1173, 1965.
4. Heusinger, C. F.: Die Hemmungsbildungen der Milz, zusammengestellt, Deutsche Arch. Physiol. 6:17, 1820.
5. Martin, G.: Observation d'une déviation organique de l'estomac d'une anomalie dans la situation, dans la configuration du coeur et des vaisseaux qui partent au qui s'y rendent, Bull. Soc. anat. Paris 1:40, 1826.
6. Putschar, W. G. J., and Manion, W. C.: Congenital absence of the spleen and associated anomalies, Am. J. Clin. Path. 26:429, 1956.
7. Ivemark, B. I.: Implications of agenesis of spleen on pathogenesis of cono-truncus anomalies in childhood; analysis of heart malformations in splenic agenesis syndrome, with 14 new cases, Acta paediat. 44:1, 1955.
8. Gilbert, E. F., Nishimura, K., and Wedum, B. G.: Congenital malformations of the heart associated with splenic agenesis, Circulation 17:72, 1958.
9. Neimann, N., Pernot, C., Gentin, G., Vert, P., and Worms, A. M.: Le "syndrome d'Ivemark": Cardiopathie congénitale cyanogène sévère, hétérotaxie thoraco-abdominale complexe et asplénie ou polysplénie, Pédiatrie 21:511, 1966.
10. Riches, R. G.: A case of congenital absence of the spleen, J. Ment. Sc. 60:630, 1914.
11. Polhemus, D. W., and Schafer, W. B.: Congenital absence of the spleen. Syndrome with atrioventricularis and situs inversus, Pediatrics 9:696, 1952.
12. Brandt, H. M., and Liebow, A. A.: Right pulmonary isomerism associated with venous, splenic, and other anomalies, Lab. Invest. 7:469, 1958.
13. Terslev, E.: A case of agenesis of the spleen, congenital heart disease and complete situs inversus, Acta paediat. 47:297, 1958.
14. Breschet, G.: Mémoire sur l'ectopie de l'appareil de la circulation et particulièrement sur celle du coeur, Rép. Gén. Anat. Physiol. Path. 2:1, 1826.
15. Rossman, J. I.: Cor biloculare with transposition of the great cardiac vessels and atresia of the pulmonary artery, Am. J. Clin. Path. 12:534, 1942.
16. Duckett, S.: À propos d'un cas d'agénésie de la rate associée a des malformations abdominales, cardiaques et neurologiques chez l'enfant, Presse méd. 71:2043, 1963.
17. Devi, B., and More, J. R. S.: Total tracheopulmonary agenesis. Associated with asplenia, agenesis of umbilical artery and other anomalies. Acta paediat. scandinav. 55: 107, 1966.
18. Hjelt, L., and Hakosalo, J.: Congenital asplenia. Case reports and a review of the literature, Ann. paediat. Fenniae 5:3, 1959.
19. Gasser, C., and Willi, H.: Spontane Innenkörperbildung bei Milzagenesie, Helvet. paediat. acta 7:369, 1952.
20. Murphy, J. A., and Mitchell, W. A.: Congenital absence of the spleen, Pediatrics 20:253, 1957.
21. Charache, H.: Lymphosarcomatosis and congenital absence of spleen, New York J. Med. 42:1363, 1942.
22. Streeter, G. L.: *Developmental Horizons in Human Embryos* (Washington, D. C.: Carnegie Institution of Washington, 1951).
23. Greenberg, S. D.: Multilobulated spleen in association with congenital heart disease, Arch. Path. 63:333, 1957.
24. Schönfeld, E. A., and Frischman, B.: Syndrome of spleen agenesis, defects of the heart and vessels and situs inversus; report of a case suggesting heredity as an etiological factor, Helvet. paediat. acta 13:636, 1958.
25. Badr-el-Din, M. K.: Syndrome of levocardia, multiple cardiac defects, situs inversus, and absent spleen: A case report, Am. Heart J. 63:115, 1962.
26. Ongley, P. A., Khoury, G. H., and Marshall, H. J.: Anomalous connection of pulmonary veins to right atrium associated with anomalous inferior vena cava, situs inversus and multiple spleen: A developmental complex, Mayo Clin. Proc. 40:609, 1965.
27. Kevy, S. V., Tefft, M., Vawter, G. F., and Rosen, F. S.: Hereditary splenic hypoplasia, Pediatrics 42:752, 1968.
28. Halpert, B., and Györkey, F.: Lesions observed in accessory spleens of 311 patients, Am. J. Clin. Path. 32:165, 1959.
29. Curtis, G. M., and Movitz, D.: The surgical significance of the accessory spleen, Ann. Surg. 123:276, 1946.
30. Putschar, W.: Die Entwicklungsstörungen der Milz, in Schwalbe, E., and Gruber, G. B. (eds.), *Die Morphologie der Missbildungen des Menschen und der Tiere* (Jena: Gustav Fischer, 1934), p. 759.
31. Grossman, S. L.: A case report of ectopic splenic tissue in the scrotum, J. Urol. 81:294, 1959.
32. Warkany, J., Passarge, E., and Smith, L. B.: Congenital

malformations in autosomal trisomy syndromes, Am. J. Dis. Child. 112:502, 1966.
33. Moller, J. H., Nakib, A., Anderson, R. C., and Edwards, J. E.: Congenital cardiac disease associated with polysplenia, a developmental complex of bilateral "left-sideness," Circulation 36:789, 1967.
34. Abell, G.: Wandering spleen with torsion of the pedicle, Ann. Surg. 98:722, 1933.
35. Simpson, A., and Ashby, E. C.: Torsion of wandering spleen, Brit. J. Surg. 52:344, 1965.
36. Perrine, G.: Torsion of the accessory splenic pedicle. A case report, Internat. Surg. 45:164, 1966.
37. Kitchin, R. J., and Green, N. A.: Torsion of an accessory spleen presenting as acute appendicitis, Brit. J. Surg. 50: 232, 1962.
38. Clifford, W. J., and Ilano, A.: Accessory wandering spleen causing intestinal obstruction in pregnancy. A case report, J. Internat. Coll. Surgeons 43:26, 1965.
39. Pearson, J. B.: Torsion of the spleen associated with congenital absence of the left kidney, Brit. J. Surg. 51:393, 1964.
40. Crosett, A. D., Jr., Nestler, W. B., and Cohen, S. J.: Wandering spleen, Johns Hopkins M. J. 124:28, 1969.
41. Fowler, R. H.: Non-parasitic cystic tumours of the spleen, Internat. Abstr. Surg. 96:209, 1953.
42. Islam, N.: Splenic cysts, Postgrad. M. J. 41:139, 1965.
43. Pines, B., and Rubinovitch, J.: Hemangioma of the spleen, Arch. Path. 33:487, 1942.
44. Zervos, N., Vlachos, J., Karpathios, T., and Mantas, J.: Giant hemangioma of the spleen with thrombocytopenia and fibrinogen deficiency, Acta paediat. scandinav. 172: 206, 1967.
45. Thatcher, L. G., Clatanoff, D. V., and Stiehm, E. R.: Splenic hemangioma with thrombocytopenia and afibrinogenemia, J. Pediat. 73:345, 1968.
46. Pommer, G.: Verwachsung des linken kryptorchischen Hodens und Nebenhodens mit der Milz in einer Missgeburt mit zahlreichen Bildungsdefecten, Ber. Naturw. Med. Ver. in Innsbruck, pp. 17, 144, 1887–1889.
47. Putschar, W. G. J., and Manion, W. C.: Splenic-gonadal fusion, Am. J. Path. 32:15, 1956.
48. Almenoff, I. A.: Splenic-gonadal fusion, New York J. Med. 66:1679, 1966.
49. Hines, J. R., and Eggum, P. R.: Splenic-gonadal fusion causing bowel obstruction, Arch. Surg. 83:887, 1961.
50. Sommer, J. R.: Continuous splenic-gonadal fusion with ectromelia: Teratogenesis. A case report, Pediatrics 22: 1183, 1958.
51. Horovitz, L., and Griffel, S.: Aberrant splenic tissue mistaken for hydrococele, Lancet 2:442, 1959.
52. Fritzsche, F.: Lien caudatus mit eigenartiger Implantation des oberen Milzpols in die Leber, Virchows Arch. path. Anat. 329:35, 1956.
53. Nowack, E.: Die sensible Phase bei der Thalidomid-Embryopathie, Humangenetik 1:516, 1965.
54. Freye, H.: Anatomische und entwicklungsgeschichtliche Untersuchungen am Skelett normaler und oligodactyler Mäuse, Wiss. Ztschr. Univ. Halle, Math. Nat. 3:801, 1954.
55. Cahalane, S. F., and Kiesselbach, N.: The significance of the accessory spleen, J. Path. 100:139, 1970.

81

Congenital Diaphragmatic Hernias

THE FIRST SIGN of the diaphragm is seen in human embryos of 3 weeks as a shelf extending dorsad from the ventral body wall between the caudal surface of the heart and the yolk stalk. At first, this septum transversum is located high in the area of the occipital myotomes, separating the thoracic and abdominal cavities ventrally but permitting communication of the cavities in their dorsal aspects through paired pleural canals. As the lung buds develop from the trachea, they protrude into the pleural canals. With growth of the embryo and caudad migration of the heart, the septum transversum also moves steadily caudad so that its position corresponds to the level of the lower thoracic vertebrae in embryos of 6 weeks. The thoraco-abdominal communications are narrowed by two folds that originate bilaterally from the dorsolateral body walls and grow forward toward the mediastinum and septum transversum. The cranial (pleuropericardial) folds develop as shelves supported by the cardinal veins or ducts of Cuvier, establishing contact with the primitive mediastinum and separating the pericardial and pleural cavities. Two caudal mesodermal ridges (pleuroperitoneal folds) develop below the lung buds, narrowing the communications between the pleural and peritoneal cavities. As these folds reach the septum transversum and unite with it, the cavities become separated in the eighth week. The diaphragm formed in this way is composed of the ventral septum transversum, the lateral pleuroperitoneal membranes, a portion of the dorsomedial esophageal mesentery and by ingrowths from the body walls.[1,2,3] The membranous structures are strengthened by striated muscle fibers that accumulate in the sternal, costal and lumbar portions of the diaphragm while the central parts become tendinous. The dorsal component of the diaphragm reaches down to the first lumbar segment. Imperfections of the diaphragm represent possible locations for hernias. Between the sternal and costal portions of the diaphragm is a muscle-free area called Morgagni's trigonum or foramen. Between pars costalis and lumbalis, the trigonum or foramen of Bochdalek represents a weak spot and the area of the passage of the esophagus through the diaphragm is a third location for herniation.

Various etiologic factors must be considered in the etiology. Familial (small) diaphragmatic hernias were reported in 8 adult siblings by Heron.[4] Passarge *et al.*[5] found 4 case reports of diaphragmatic hernia in siblings and described agenesis of the left diaphragm in a sister and her brother. Turpin *et al.*[6] reported diaphragmatic hernia in distant cousins. Thus, in rare instances, recessive inheritance may play a role in the etiology. But in the family recorded by Mertins,[7] in which siblings were affected, the mother had a high and flaccid diaphragm, so that irregular dominant inheritance should be considered also. Absence of the left hemidiaphragm was found in an infant with probable trisomy 18.[40]

Nongenetic factors have been suspected occasionally in man. Thalidomide,[8] quinine[9,10] and phenmetrazine[11] have been mentioned as possible causative agents. There is no doubt that diaphragmatic hernia can be produced experimentally in animals. In rats, it sometimes occurs in severely deformed offspring of mothers treated experimentally with various teratogens. Interesting and curious is the observation that diaphragmatic hernia is present in the young of females subjected to vitamin A deficiency. Andersen[12,13] found, in a certain stock of rats in which diaphragmatic hernia occurred spontaneously with a frequency of 1%, that the anomaly increased to 19% by feeding a vitamin A-deficient diet. Warkany and Roth[14] produced diaphragmatic hernia and other congenital malformations by maternal vitamin A deficiency in various strains of rats in which the anomaly did not occur spontaneously. In many specimens, the right dorsolateral portion of the

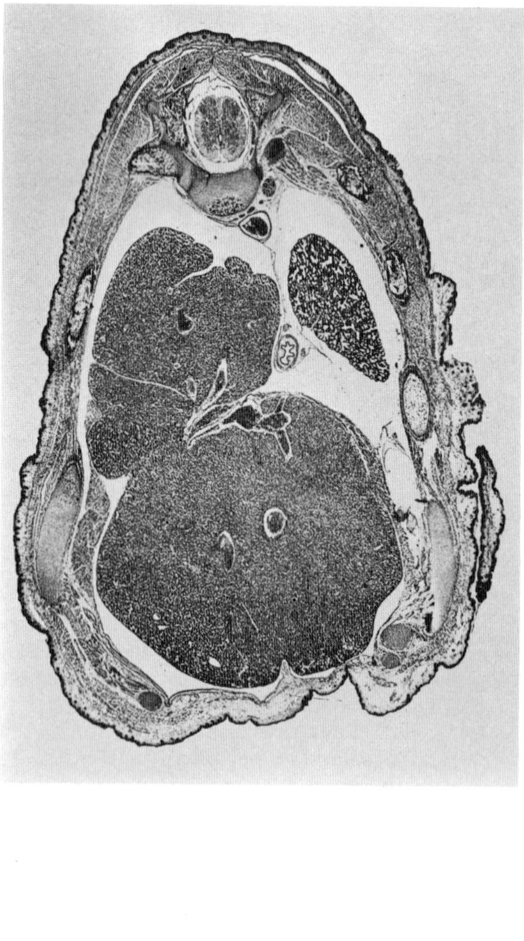

Fig. 81-1 (left). – Congenital diaphragmatic hernia in a newborn rat produced by maternal vitamin A deficiency. Diaphragmatic hernia with liver in right pleural space. Lung is seen in the left pleural space.

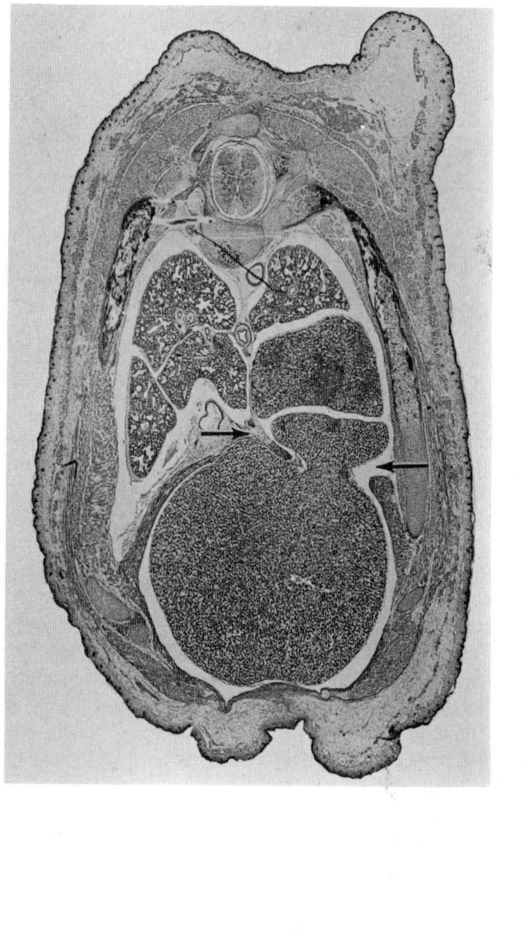

Fig. 81-2 (right). – Congenital diaphragmatic hernia in a newborn rat produced by maternal vitamin A deficiency. Diaphragmatic defect in the left leaf of diaphragm penetrated by liver (**arrows**).

diaphragm was not developed and a lobe of the liver protruded into the pleural space (Fig. 81-1). Rarely, there was a left diaphragmatic defect (Fig. 81-2) and sometimes there was also a defect in the pericardium so that liver and heart were in direct contact (see Fig. 81-6). Supplementing the deficient diet with vitamin A at various days of pregnancy reduced the incidence of diaphragmatic hernia, and the affected animals showed the defect more often on the left side than on the right.[15] The enigmatic role played by vitamin A in the formation of the diaphragm is brought out even more by the fact that diaphragmatic hernia was also caused in pigs by maternal vitamin A deficiency. But the incidence was lower and occurrence more irregular than in rats.[16]

Dorsolateral Hernias

The most frequent and impressive diaphragmatic hernias are found in the dorsolateral portions of the structure, where a circumscribed pleuroperitoneal canal may fail to develop, may fail to close or may remain a weak, membranous spot. In most of the hernias that go through the foramen of Bochdalek there is a complete defect that permits entry of abdominal contents into a pleural cavity. In a minority of cases there is a hernial sac formed by a membranous portion of the dorsolateral diaphragm, which permits protrusion of abdominal viscera into the chest.

The true incidence of the various types of diaphragmatic hernias is not known, since many do not cause symptoms and go unrecognized throughout life. With improved diagnostic measures, recognition of minor defects became possible, resulting in changing incidence figures.

In 1953, Gross,[17] in his surgical material, listed 90% of the diaphragmatic hernias as dorsolateral. Seventy-six per cent were on the left side and 14% on the right. A hernial sac exists in this type in only one-tenth of the cases. Esophageal hiatus hernias and retrosternal hernias together account for only 10%. In 1962, Baffes[18] termed 65% of the congenital hernias as dorsolateral (Bochdalek), 10.4% hiatus hernias, 2.6% retrosternal (Morgagni), 9% short esophagus and 13% eventrations. Eventrations and short esophagus defects increasingly have become known through roentgenographic examinations.

Left Dorsolateral Hernias

This is the well-known type of diaphragmatic hernia that usually causes early clinical symptoms and often a clinical emergency.

The infant may appear normal immediately after birth, but become short of breath and cyanotic when the stomach and intestines fill with gas or food. The symptoms vary with the size of the defect and with the amount of viscera displaced into the pleural cavity. Since the visceral contents may shift between the abdominal and pleural cavities, improvement and aggravation of symptoms can alternate. Labored respiration and cyanosis combined with a sunken abdomen should direct the attention of the examiner to the chest, where dullness to percussion, absence of respiratory sounds, displacement of the heart to the right side and gurgling confirm the suspicion. Roentgenographic examination can demonstrate displaced bowel, stomach or spleen in the left pleural space, with corresponding changes in the heart and lung findings (Fig. 81-4). There often is a defective mesentery and malrotation combined with the defect in the diaphragm that makes possible the extensive movements and dislocations of the bowels. Malrotation is the result and not the cause of the disorder, since normally the intestines return from the cord in 10-week embryos, whereas the diaphragmatic components are joined by 8 weeks. Since the abdominal cavity may be too small for the viscera, the surgeon may encounter difficulties in attempts to adjust the abdominal contents to the limited space available.[17] Herniations with a sac generally are less extensive

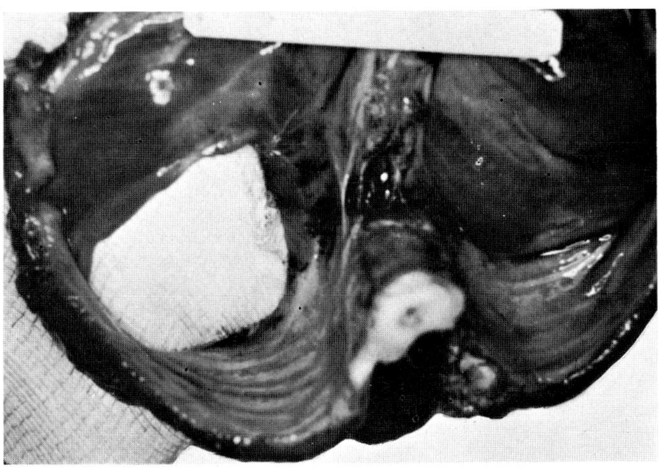

Fig. 81-3. – Left diaphragmatic defect seen from thoracic cavity. (Courtesy of Dr. L. W. Martin, Cincinnati, Ohio.)

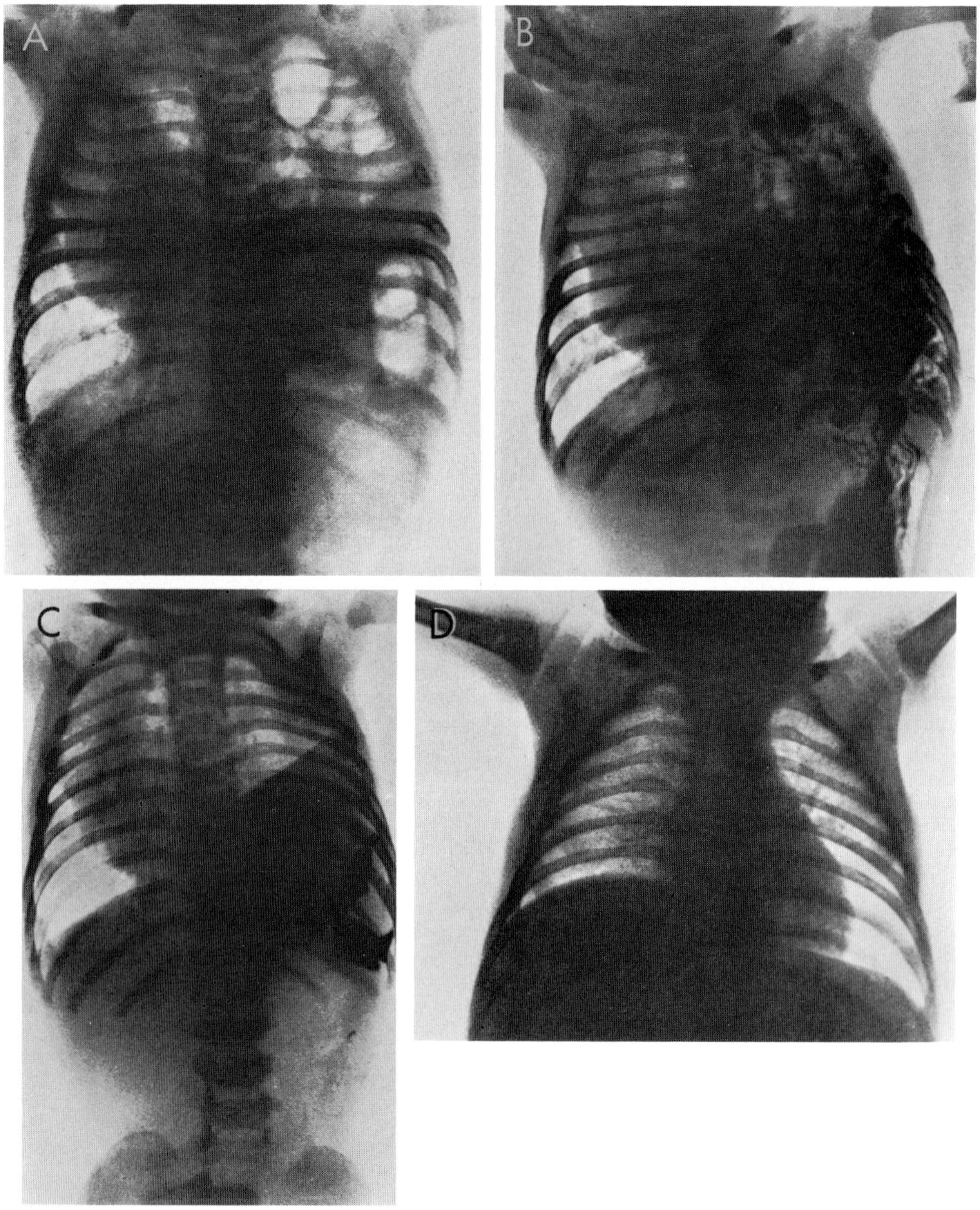

Fig. 81-4.—Congenital diaphragmatic hernia in an infant who appeared well at birth but showed signs of collapse at the age of 2½ months, followed by vomiting, diarrhea, dyspnea and sunken abdomen. **A,** at the age of 3 months, intestinal loops can be seen in the left thoracic cavity; displacement of the heart to the right. **B,** intestinal loops in left thorax shown by contrast medium. **C,** several days later, the picture has changed spontaneously. There are no intestinal loops in the left thoracic cavity. The dense shadow in the left pleural space proved to be spleen at operation. Small intestine, cecum, colon ascendens and transversum and spleen were moved from the left pleural space into the abdominal cavity. The defect in the left leaf of the diaphragm was 3 × 5 cm. Dextroposition of the heart and pneumothorax showed gradual improvement. **D,** 17 days after operation, the position of the heart appeared normal.

than those due to a complete defect of the diaphragm. Without surgical help, extensive herniation into the pleural cavity usually is fatal in infancy. In some cases, however, early symptoms are absent or mild but the disorder becomes manifest during or beyond childhood,[19] when it may present with vomiting, intestinal obstruction, chest or abdominal pain, cough, gastrointestinal bleeding or dyspnea with exertion. Singer and Baue[20] reported Bochdalek hernia and malrotation in a girl whose symptoms were not signif-

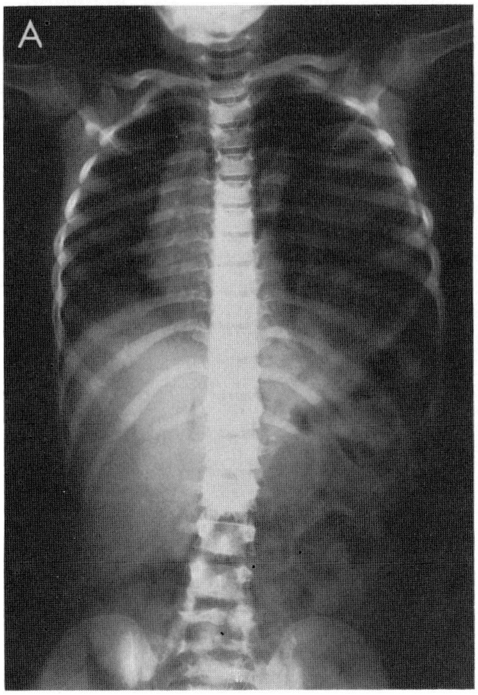

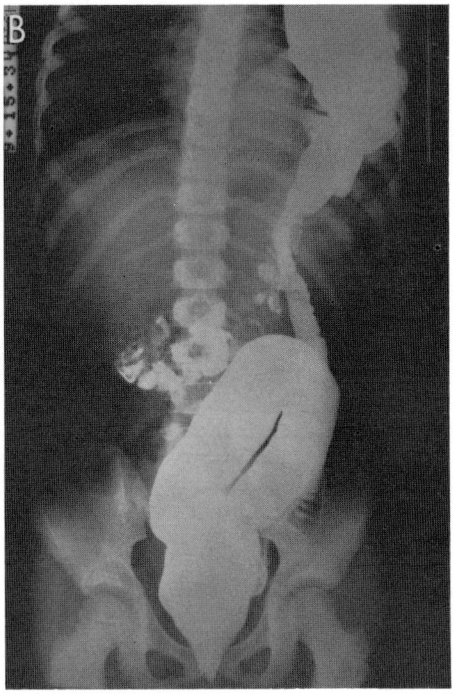

Fig. 81-5.—Diaphragmatic hernia in a child who survived infancy. **A,** a cyst-like structure is shown in the left hemithorax. **B,** large intestine is demonstrated in the left hemithorax by a barium enema.

icant until vomiting and weight loss set in when she was 6½ years of age and duodenal obstruction due to malrotation caused the symptoms. At operation, large and small bowel, spleen and pancreas were found in the pleural space. Intestinal symptoms are more prominent than respiratory signs in children beyond infancy.[21]

In many patients, diaphragmatic hernia is an isolated defect, so that repair can render the child normal. In other cases, diaphragmatic hernia is a component of a syndrome of multiple congenital anomalies that becloud the prognosis. Cleft palate, Klippel-Feil syndrome,[22] spina bifida,[23] ostium atrioventriculare commune,[24] atrial septal defect,[22] coarctation of the aorta,[23] hypoplasia of the left ventricle,[25] aortic atresia,[26] hydronephrosis and hydroureter,[23] malrotation of the intestine,[17,22] horseshoe kidney,[27] omphalocele and situs inversus of thoracic organs[22] have been reported. Diaphragmatic hernia is a rare complication of the asplenia syndrome.[28]

Hernia of the Right Diaphragm

In cases of hernia of the right diaphragm, the liver bulges into the right hemithorax, sometimes covered by a thin membrane or sac that corresponds to the thinned tendinous portion of the diaphragm. According to Gross,[17] the majority of posterolateral herniations have no sac. In man, herniation on the left is about five times more frequent than that on the right.[17,29] Ravitch and Handelsman[30] described cases of attenuation of the central portion of the right diaphragm, which normally is muscular. Through the defect, which may vary greatly in size, a portion of the liver protrudes against the right lung, sometimes displacing the heart to the left. If the diaphragmatic defect is large and a large portion of the liver bulges into the thorax, signs appear in early infancy. Cough may be the only manifestation that leads to x-ray examination and discovery of the anomaly, but sometimes dyspnea and cyanosis are present. Occasionally, the defect remains asymptomatic and is discovered accidentally in roentgenograms.[30] If the defect is very small, symptoms may be delayed to adult life. In one case of this type, strangulation of the protruding portion of the liver occurred in a 47-year-old woman, resulting in epigastric pain, nausea and vomiting.[41] In the differential diagnosis, pneumonia, pulmonary and subdiaphragmatic cysts, pericardial lipoma and mediastinal tumor have been considered. Successful operative treatment has been described.[30]

Retrosternal Hernias

These hernias protrude through the foramen of Morgagni, which, as a rule, does not permit extensive dislocations of abdominal organs. Only 3–6% of diaphragmatic hernias operated on during childhood belong in this group. Approximately half of them have a sac; pericardium and pleural surfaces limit the available thoracic space. Most cases occur on the right side. Small parts of the liver, colon or stomach can be involved.[17, 31] Sometimes such a hernia may be combined with a defect of the pericardium and be much more extensive than a simple Morgagni defect.[32] Thomsen *et al.*[33] reported such a case with displacement of stomach, large and small intestine, liver and spleen into the pericardial space. Tetralogy of Fallot, dextrocardia, septal defect, urinary tract anomalies, spina bifida, Down syndrome and mental retardation can be associated anomalies.[31]

Pericardo-Diaphragmatic Hernia

Reports on this form of diaphragmatic hernia are rare. In 1966, Farriaux *et al.*[32] found only 33 cases reported in the literature, of which 24 were thought to be congenital. Manifestations of the congenital form can occur in infancy or be delayed to the seventh decade. Dyspnea, cyanosis or intestinal disturbances are among the symptoms and enlargement of the heart or abnormal auscultation or visceral displacements are among the signs. Sometimes the anomaly remains silent for months or years to present with serious symptoms later, necessitating prompt surgical treatment.

Fig. 81-6. – Diaphragmatic hernia in a newborn rat produced by maternal vitamin A deficiency (interrupted by vitamin A supplementation on the thirteenth day of gestation). The liver, in close contact with the heart, is in the left pleural space, not separated by pericardium from the heart.

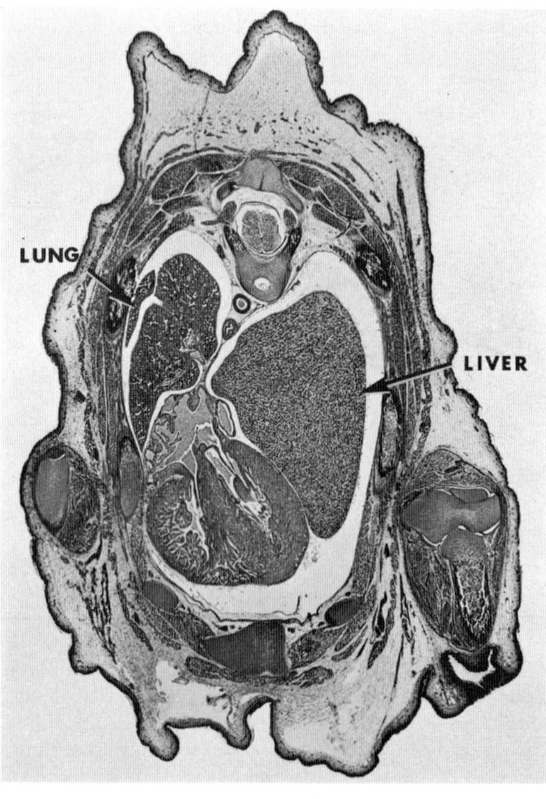

Pericardo-diaphragmatic hernias have been observed in the dog, cat and donkey. Experimental production by vitamin A deficiency has been reported[14] (Fig. 81-6).

Hiatus Hernias

Herniation of all or part of the stomach through an abnormally wide esophageal hiatus is a common disorder in adults, particularly in women. Although a congenital predisposition has been considered in the etiology, the herniation is considered an acquired malady.[34] The disorder is rare in infants and children. Only 5% of the diaphragmatic hernias listed by Gross[17] related to esophageal hiatus, but Engberg *et al.*[35] reported a series of 60 cases diagnosed before the age of 10 years. It is possible that some of these anomalies are not recognized in infancy and that a number of spontaneous cures occur.[35] The disorder manifests itself more often in male than in female children. Familial occurrence has been observed repeatedly.[36, 37] Hiatus hernias have a sac that limits extrusion of viscera into the thoracic cavity. A relatively common type is the sliding hernia with the cardia located above the diaphragm and the contents consisting of the abdominal part of the esophagus and the adjoining part of the stomach. Para-esophageal hernias, which are rarer, consist of herniation of the gastric fundus into the thoracic cavity lateral to the esophagus, leaving the cardia in its normal place. In congenital short esophagus, the segment located above the diaphragm is covered by a layer of gastric mucosa.

Regurgitation of acid secretions, nausea, vomiting and malnutrition may result. The esophageal mucosa can be damaged by regurgitation and develop fibrosis, ulcers or strictures.

Eventration of the Diaphragm

A diaphragm, poor in muscle fibers, may be overstretched and elevated into the pleural space without a break in its continuity. Breathing capacity can be diminished or symptoms are absent. If such eventration is found in an old person, it is likely to be considered acquired, but a case reported by Bulgrin and Holmes[38] casts doubt on this conception. A 65-year-old man died of heart failure, hypertension and uremia. The diaphragm was at the level of the fifth rib posteriorly, with the left kidney immediately beneath. The length of the ureter demonstrated congenital origin of the renal ectopia. These congenital anomalies apparently permitted a normal life to the age of 65 years.

Accessory Diaphragm

This rare anomaly consists of a diaphragmatic leaf that is located in the right chest cavity and separates the lower lobe from the remaining lung. Roentgenographically, the right diaphragm may appear elevated and the oblique fissure thickened. Bronchiectasis of the right lower lobe can be associated with the anomaly.[39]

REFERENCES

1. Patten, B. M.: *Human Embryology* (3d ed.; New York: McGraw-Hill Book Company, Inc., 1968).
2. Wells, L. J.: Development of the human diaphragm and pleural sacs, Contrib. Embryol. 35:107, 1954.
3. Arey, L. B.: *Developmental Anatomy. A Textbook and Laboratory Manual of Embryology* (Philadelphia: W. B. Saunders Company, 1965).
4. Heron, J. C.: Familial diaphragmatic hernia, California Med. 73:497, 1950.
5. Passarge, E., Halsey, H., and German, J.: Unilateral agenesis of the diaphragm, Humangenetik 5:226, 1968.
6. Turpin, R., Petit, P., Chigot, P., Lafourcade, J., and de Parochex, Y.: Hernie diaphragmatique congénitale de type embryonnaire (Fente pleuro-péritonéale gauche). Coincidence chez deux cousins germains de cette malformation isolée, Ann. pédiat. 35:1786, 1959.
7. Mertins, H.: Über eine familiäre Zwerchfellmissbildung, Zentralbl. Gynäk. 74:951, 1952.
8. Hobolth, N.: Drugs and foetal abnormalities, Lancet 2: 1333, 1962.
9. Zolcinski, A., Heimrath, T., and Ujec, M.: Chinina jako przyczyna wad rozwojowych plódu, Ginek. polska 36:935, 1965.
10. Kup, J., von: Zwerchfelldefekt nach Abtreibungsversuch mit Chinin. Kasuistische Beobachtung, München. med. Wchnschr. 109:2582, 1967.
11. Powell, P. D., and Johnstone, J. M.: Phenmetrazine and foetal abnormalities, Brit. M. J. 2:1327, 1962.
12. Andersen, D. H.: Incidence of congenital diaphragmatic hernia in the young of rats bred on a diet deficient in vitamin A, Am. J. Dis. Child. 62:888, 1941.
13. Andersen, D. H.: Effect of diet during pregnancy upon the incidence of congenital hereditary diaphragmatic hernia in the rat, Am. J. Path. 25:163, 1949.
14. Warkany, J., and Roth, C. B.: Congenital malformations induced in rats by maternal vitamin A deficiency, J. Nutrition 35:1, 1948.
15. Wilson, J. G., Roth, C. B., and Warkany, J.: An analysis of the syndrome of malformations induced by maternal vitamin A deficiency. Effects of restoration of vitamin A at various times during gestation, Am. J. Anat. 92:189, 1953.
16. Palludan, B.: *A-Avitaminosis in Swine* (Copenhagen: Ejnar Munksgaard, 1966).
17. Gross, R. E.: *The Surgery of Infancy and Childhood* (Philadelphia: W. B. Saunders Company, 1953).
18. Baffes, T. G.: Diaphragmatic Hernia, in Benson, C. D., Mustard, W. T., Ravitch, M. M., Snyder, W. H., Jr., and Welch, K. J. (eds.), *Pediatric Surgery* (Chicago: Year Book Medical Publishers, Inc., 1962).
19. MacDougall, J. T., Abbott, A. C., and Goodhand, T. K.: Herniation through congenital diaphragmatic defects in adults, Canad. J. Surg. 6:301, 1963.
20. Singer, E. R., and Baue, A. E.: Bochdalek hernia and malrotation beyond infancy, J. Pediat. 66:439, 1965.
21. Hermann, R. E., and Barber, D. H.: Congenital diaphragmatic hernia in the child beyond infancy, Cleveland Clin. Quart. 30:73, 1963.
22. Lester, J., Vesterdal, J., and Winkel Smith, C. C.: Twenty-one cases of anterior and posterior diaphragmatic hernias in children, Acta paediat. 48:175, 1959.
23. Moore, T. C., Battersby, J. S., Roggenkamp, M. W., and Campbell, J. A.: Congenital posterolateral diaphragmatic hernia in the newborn, Surg., Gynec. & Obst. 104:675, 1957.
24. Hambach, R.: Drei Fälle von persistierendem Ostium atrioventriculare commune in einem Fall von grosser Zwerchfellhernie, Ann. paediat. 181:27, 1953.
25. Firestone, F. N., Popper, R. W., Taybi, H., and Leonards, R.: Congenital diaphragmatic hernia and hypoplastic left heart, Pediatrics 40:329, 1967.
26. Peltonen, T.: Diaphragma-Hernie als Ursache der Asphyxie des Neugeborenen, Acta paediat. 41:527, 1952.
27. Lenz, W.: Krankheiten des Urogenitalsystems, in Becker, P. E. (ed.), *Humangenetik* (Stuttgart: Georg Thieme, 1964).
28. Putschar, W. G. J., and Manion, W. C.: Congenital absence of the spleen and associated anomalies, Am. J. Clin. Path. 26:429, 1956.
29. Hedblom, C. A.: Diaphragmatic hernia: A study of 378 cases in which operation was performed, J.A.M.A. 85: 947, 1925.
30. Ravitch, M. M., and Handelsman, J. C.: Defects in right diaphragm of infants and children with herniation of liver, Arch. Surg. 64:794, 1952.
31. Baran, E. M., Houston, H. E., Lynn, H. B., and O'Connell, E. J.: Foramen of Morgagni hernias in children, Surgery 62:1076, 1967.
32. Farriaux, J-P., Ridet, M., Lefebvre, P., Ryckewaert, Ph., and Fontaine, G.: Une curieuse forme de hernie diaphragmatique. La hernie péricardo-diaphragmatique, Ann. pédiat. 42:778, 1966.
33. Thomsen, G., Vesterdal, J., and Smith, C. C. W.: Diaphragmatic hernia into the pericardium, Acta paediat. 43:485, 1954.
34. Edmunds, V.: Hiatus hernia, Quart, J. Med. 26:445, 1957.
35. Engberg, H., Thomsen, G., and Vesterdal, J.: Hiatus hernia in children, Acta paediat. 46:371, 1957.
36. Waterston, D.: Hiatus Hernia, in Benson, C. D., Mustard, W. T., Ravitch, M. M., Snyder, W. H., Jr., and Welch, K. J. (eds.), *Pediatric Surgery* (Chicago: Year Book Medical Publishers, Inc., 1962).
37. Delattre, A., Buisine, A., and Delegrange, P.: Hernie diaphragmatique congénitale de l'estomac chez deux soeurs. (Role probable de l'héredité), J. Sc. M. Lille 69:165, 1951.
38. Bulgrin, J. G., and Holmes, F. H.: Eventration of the diaphragm with high renal ectopia. (A case report), Radiology 64:249, 1955.
39. Nigogosyan, G., and Ozarda, A.: Accessory diaphragm; a case report, Am. J. Roentgenol. 85:309, 1961.
40. Kajii, T., Oikawa, K., Itakura, K., and Ohsawa, T.: A probable 17-18 trisomy syndrome with phocomelia, exomphalos, and agenesis of hemidiaphragm, Arch. Dis. Childhood 39:519, 1964.
41. Wolfson, S. A., and Goldman, A.: Strangulating diaphragmatic hernia of the liver: Report of case with surgical cure, Surgery 24:846, 1948.

82

The Umbilicus

Hernias

THE UMBILICUS is located in the linea alba at the level of the third or fourth lumbar vertebra. At birth, the umbilical ring normally is closed by blood vessels and Wharton's jelly. Incomplete closure of the ring results in defects of various types and sizes that can predispose to herniation. Umbilical hernias are quite common in newborn prematures, particularly in those weighing under 1,500 Gm.[1] They occur in Negro infants about eight times more often than in Caucasians.[2] Cretinism, gargoylism, Down syndrome and conditions that increase intra-abdominal pressure frequently are associated with umbilical hernia. As a rule, infants with umbilical hernia have a tendency to spontaneous healing before the age of 6 years, but large hernias may persist beyond that age. If the fascial defect is greater than 1.5 cm., spontaneous healing is rare.[3] Complications of umbilical hernias are rare, but incarceration and strangulation have been reported. Rupture, ulceration and severe irritation of the covering skin are exceptional aggravations that necessitate surgical intervention.[1] The umbilical protrusion in infants usually is 1–2 cm. in diameter and in older children the hernias can be 3–4 cm. wide. The umbilical swelling becomes larger with crying, coughing and straining. Partial obstruction of intestine entering the hernia can cause cramps, and omentum immobilized in the hernial ring can be painful.

Spontaneous healing of umbilical hernias can be accelerated by reducing the hernia, covering of the umbilicus by longitudinal skin folds and holding the folds in place by adhesive strapping. Large, growing or complicated hernias are treated surgically by umbilical herniorrhaphy.[4]

Fig. 82-1. – Large umbilical hernia in a girl with Hurler syndrome.

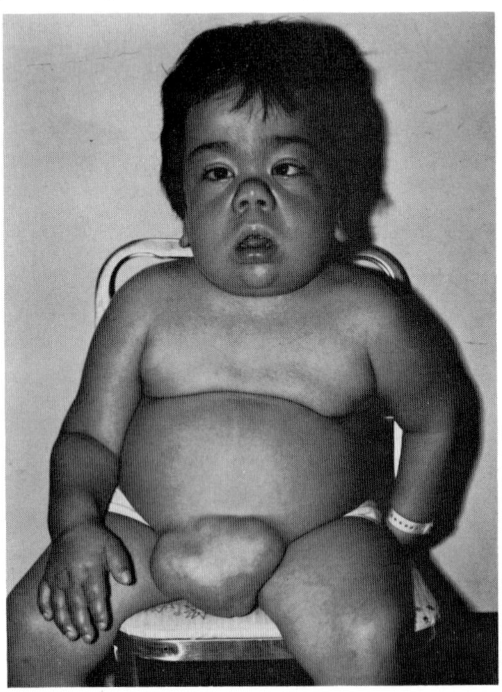

Omphalocele (Exomphalos, Umbilical Eventration)

Omphalocele represents a serious congenital malformation consisting of extrusion of the intestine and of other abdominal contents into the extra-embryonic coelomic cavity. The physiologic herniation of the intestine between the sixth and eleventh weeks of gestation has been described on page 691. Failure to re-enter the abdominal cavity, which normally takes place in about 11-week-old embryos, results in omphalocele. But, as Kermauner[5] pointed out long ago, the stage probably is set for the developmental error much earlier, when growth disturbances occur in the myotomes at the beginning of the third week. Duhamel[6] attributed exomphalos to failure of formation of the lateral folds of the ventral embryonic wall. The prolapse of the intestinal loops into the exomphalos is considered the result and not the cause of the earlier malformation.

Incidence figures of the anomaly vary because of different experiences of the observers. Surgeons often see only liveborn infants with omphalocele who constitute merely half of those actually born. But McKeown *et al.*,[7] who surveyed all infants born in the years 1941–1951 to mothers living in Birmingham, England, ascertained the stillborn and liveborn with exomphalos. Of 69 propositi, 35 were stillborn and 34 liveborn. These authors arrived at an incidence figure of 1 in 3,200. Soper and Green,[8] at the State University of Iowa Hospitals, came to similar figures, namely 1 in 3,800. The samples of omphalocele seen by surgeons probably differ also in severity from those seen by pathologists.

The size of the omphalocele varies according to the contents. The diameter may be from 2 to 15 cm., but the defect of the abdominal wall usually is smaller than the diameter of the sac. Whereas the sac of the omphalocele is translucent and moist immediately after birth, it soon becomes dry and opaque from dehydration and necrosis.[8] As a rule, the thin walls of the sac are well demarcated from the normal skin of the abdominal wall, but sometimes the skin continues over the sac of the hernia.

Small and large omphaloceles should be distinguished because of their different nature and different prognosis.[9] The small omphalocele is a hernia into the umbilical cord; it contains intestine but only rarely liver[10] or other abdominal organs. The umbilical ring is large but normally placed. The umbilical cord arises from the apex of the sac, and its blood vessels continue over the sac to reach the abdominal cavity. In approximately a third of the cases, only one umbilical artery is present.[5] A third type of eventration, "gastroschisis," is discussed below.

In large omphaloceles, the anterior abdominal wall cephalad to the umbilicus is absent, so that the defect extends upward toward the xiphoid process of the sternum. The sac may contain parts of liver, pancreas, spleen or even kidney in addition to intestine. In the most severe forms, which often are lethal, marked scoliosis of the spine, myeloschisis and rib anomalies complicate the disease picture. Anomalies of the cranium and of the extremities have been observed.[5] If the sac ruptures before birth, the eviscerated bowel undergoes degenerative changes and becomes thickened and covered by exudate due to peritoneal changes. Small and large intestine may protrude together with the stomach and other viscera. Prognosis is unfavorable in such cases, but recovery has been reported in some instances.[11, 12]

Recurrence of omphalocele in a sibship is rare but it can occur. Thus, McKeown *et al.*[7] reported 2 siblings in their series. In these children, exomphalos was not associated with other malformations. A first cousin of these siblings also had an uncomplicated omphalocele. There were no consanguineous marriages among the parents of children with exomphalos for which data were available to McKeown *et al.*[7]

It has been recognized relatively recently that some of the children with omphalocele and other congenital malformations may have chromosomal anomalies. Kajii *et al.*[13] reported a child with probable trisomy 18 syndrome that included omphalocele, phocomelia and agenesis of half of the diaphragm. In 13 of 32 necropsies of children with trisomy 13-15, omphalocele or umbilical hernia were mentioned. Gustavson *et al.*[14] recorded a case of a B/G chromosomal translocation manifesting omphalocele, anal atresia, micrognathia and macroglossia. There also was premature synostosis of the sagittal suture, dilatation of the cerebral ventricles and colobomas of the irides. The child had a single umbilical artery. One child with Down syndrome is mentioned in the series of 69 omphaloceles recorded by McKeown *et al.*[7] and another one among 91 patients of O'Leary and Clymer.[15]

Omphalocele as a symptom of visceromegaly was described on page 171. Wiedemann[16] reported a family in which 3 infants were born with omphalocele; 2 of these were boys and 1 was a girl. All were born prematurely and hydramnios was noted in 2. Macroglossia was present in all 3 children and undescended testes in the boys. Diaphragmatic hernia, trilobed liver and adrenal hypoplasia and cysts were also seen. Association of omphalocele and macroglossia has been observed repeatedly (p. 171), and some of these cases may be related to the syndrome of visceromegaly. There was 1 patient with macroglossia among 91 with umbilical hernia recorded by O'Leary and Cly-

Fig. 82-2. – Stillborn fetus with omphalocele or gastroschisis. All viscera are extra-abdominal with the exception of a rudimentary left lobe of the liver and the descending colon. The mother had had infectious hepatitis and secondary syphilis during pregnancy.

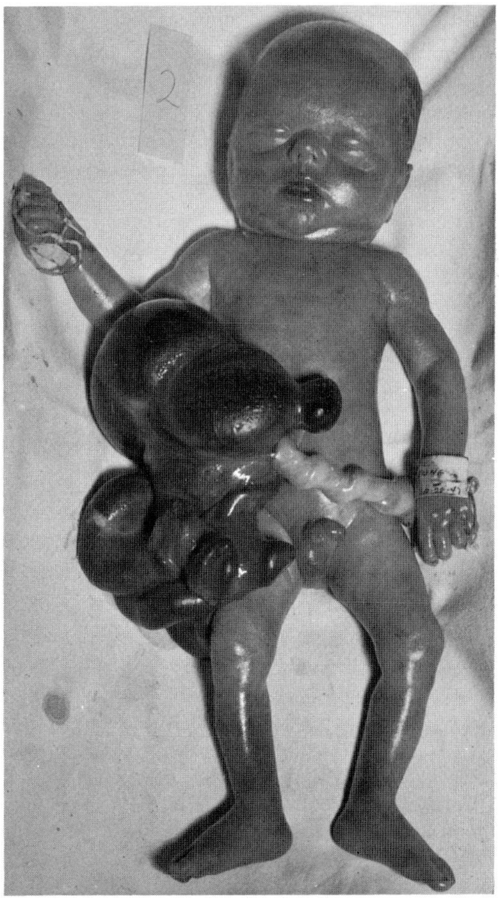

mer.[15] Irving[17] found macroglossia in 11 of 94 children with exomphalos. Three of the children in the series were related, 2 being siblings and 1 their second cousin. The exomphalos-macroglossia combination emerges as a syndrome characterized by a high birth weight, neonatal hypoglycemia, accelerated postnatal growth and ossification, facial nevus flammeus, abnormal pinna, diaphragmatic anomaly, renal enlargement, adrenal cytomegaly and possibly pancreatic islet-cell hyperplasia.[17]

There is little proof that maternal infections play a role in the etiology of omphalocele or eventration. The mother of the child shown in Figure 82-2 had a history of hepatitis and syphilis. Paucot and Gelle[18] reported omphalocele in 3 fetuses from successive pregnancies of a mother with "hereditary syphilis" but there was no proof of syphilis, since the mother's serology was negative and the diagnosis was based merely on reproductive difficulties of the mother.

The prognosis of omphalocele depends on size, preservation of the sac and on associated malformations. Surgical series emphasize complications of the intestinal tract such as malrotation, Meckel diverticulum, volvulus, reduplication and atresias. The various forms and stages of malrotation are discussed on page 691. Extended exstrophies or vesicointestinal fissures consisting of omphalocele, exstrophy of the bladder and colon, ectopic cloaca and anomalies of the genitourinary tract are among the most severe associated malformations. The duodenum usually is normal, but other parts of the intestine may be affected by atresia or stenosis. Imperforate anus associated with exstrophy of the bladder and myelomeningocele were also observed.[7-9] Congenital heart disease,[4, 9] facial clefts and diaphragmatic hernia have been observed repeatedly.[7] Some of these defects are not compatible with postnatal life.[19]

In the series of McKeown *et al.*,[7] the incidence of associated malformations was 52%, in that of Gross[4] 59% and in that of Soper and Green[8] 79%. In Birmingham, England,[7] the association with anencephaly was 20%. It is of interest that in an American series[15] the association with anencephaly was only 2.2% and in other American series anencephaly was not mentioned. The difference between the English and the American series in regard to anencephaly probably is due to the generally high incidence of anencephaly in England; it could also be due to sampling, since anencephalic children only rarely reach a surgical clinic.

We have seen omphalocele in a child with Turner syndrome who also had a bifid uvula and renal malformations (Cincinnati Children's Hospital Chart No. 86328).

The prognosis usually is unfavorable without surgical intervention. Immediate surgical repair is recommended by some, since emptiness of the stomach and intestines facilitates the repair and infection can be avoided.[4, 8] But, in selected cases, conservative treatment can result in surprising spontaneous repair.[9, 20] Sauvage and Bill[21] recommended that those unruptured omphaloceles that can be repaired without producing excessive intra-abdominal pressure should be handled in this way. Those that cannot should have delayed closure. The conservative method is a suitable alternative to primary skin closure of large, irreducible hernias.

Omphalocele can be produced experimentally in mammals. Ingalls *et al.*[22] found the incidence of spontaneous omphalocele in DBA/1 mice to be 1.7%. Exposure of this strain to low oxygen pressure on the ninth day of gestation increased the incidence of the defect to 17.6% and exposure on the fifteenth day to 14%. The malformation varied from a small opening in the abdominal wall from which a sac containing a single loop of gut protruded to an opening of such magnitude that intestines, liver and spleen were almost wholly outside the abdomen. Similar malformations have been induced by folic acid deficiency in rats. Nelson *et al.*,[23] by a combination of folic acid deficiency and administration of x-methyl-folic acid during days 7–9 or 9–11 of gestation, obtained more than 20% young with umbilical hernias or gastroschisis. Most of these animals also had malformations of the central nervous and cardiovascular systems. Omphalocele occasionally is produced in the young of

Fig. 82-3.—Near-term rat fetus whose mother had been treated with 100 mg. of methyl salicylate on the ninth day of pregnancy. Liver, pancreas and intestine protrude through umbilical defect. Note also exencephaly.

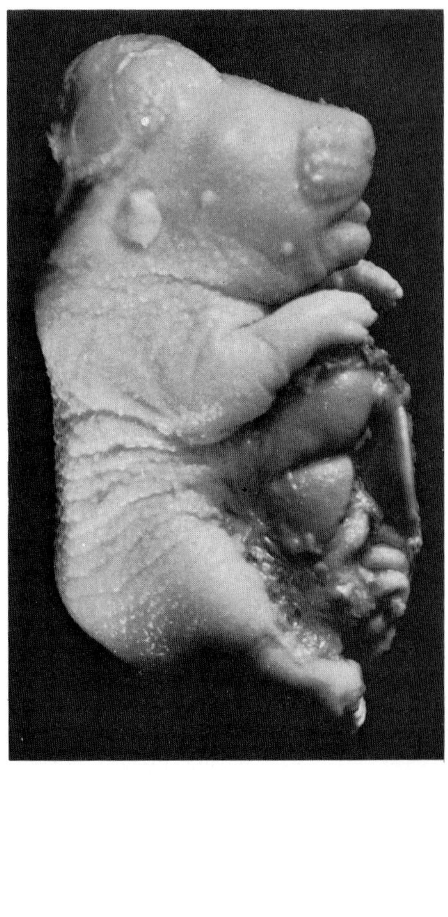

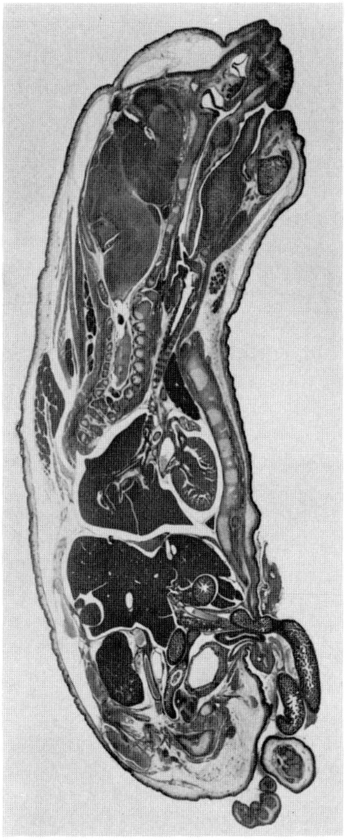

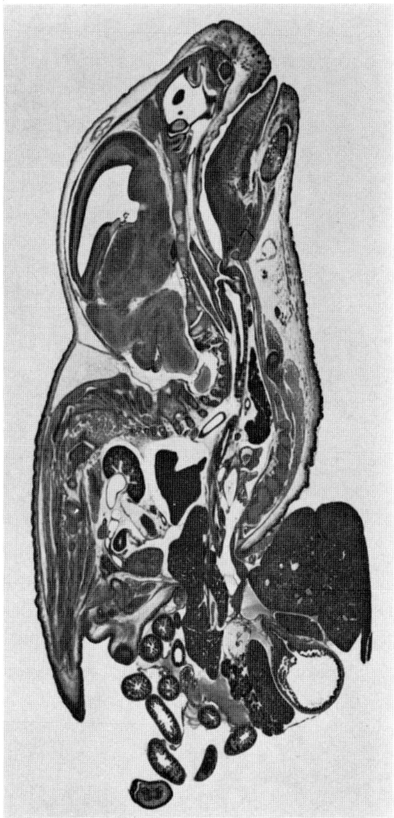

Fig. 82-4 (left). – Sagittal section through a near-term rat fetus whose mother had been treated with streptonigrin on the tenth day. Intestinal loops protrude from the abdominal cavity.

Fig. 82-5 (right). – Sagittal section through a near-term rat fetus whose mother had been treated with streptonigrin on the ninth day. There is a severe deformity of the spinal column and large exomphalos. Lung, liver, pancreas, stomach and intestine are seen outside the body cavities.

female rats injected with trypan blue from the eighth to the tenth day of pregnancy.[24] Association of omphalocele with exencephaly and rachischisis is not rare in the offspring of rats treated with toxic doses of salicylates.[25] Large omphaloceles with extrusion of lung, liver, stomach, pancreas and intestine have been produced in the young of rats treated with streptonigrin.[26] Sometimes it is difficult in such cases to decide whether omphalocele or gastroschisis was produced, since the defects involve large portions of the anterior body wall in some of the specimens.

Gastroschisis

Gastroschisis represents a third and severe type of abdominal wall defect that permits extrusion of abdominal contents without involving the umbilical cord. Often, there is no sac and the protruding viscera are bathed in amniotic fluid, showing rubbery thickening and matting together. True gastroschisis is rare compared with omphalocele, and usually is fatal soon after birth. Sometimes the insertion of the umbilical cord is marginal, so that distinction of exomphalos and gastroschisis is not always clear-cut.

Gastroschisis is an impressive malformation that apparently was first recorded by Lycosthenes in 1557. Many other cases were described by early writers, who attached a variety of names to the anomaly.[27] The term "gastroschisis" is not quite appropriate, since the stomach is not split in these cases, but use has made it acceptable. Pregnancies resulting in children with gastroschisis often are complicated by hydramnios. At birth, the protruding intestines and other abdominal viscera are the presenting parts, which usually are severely injured by the time the child is delivered. Only rarely is a gastroschisis limited to a small defect in the epigastric, mesogastric or hypogastric region, the umbilicus being normal. In most cases, there are large defects in the abdominal wall that can be more pronounced on one side than on the other. Normally, the muscles of the abdominal wall, formed from the somites, grow forward and toward the midline, where they unite to constitute the ventral wall. Disturbance of the early somites may result in partial absence of the abdominal wall with eventration of the viscera.[28] These severe eventrations date back to at least the third week of embryonic life.[5] In the most severe forms, there is no umbilical cord and no umbilicus. The abdominal viscera lie in the extraembryonic coelom in a space limited by amnion and the placenta. The margins of the open abdominal walls usually are continuous with the amnion. The vessels that pass from the placenta to the fetus in the walls of the sac formed by the amnion are short and

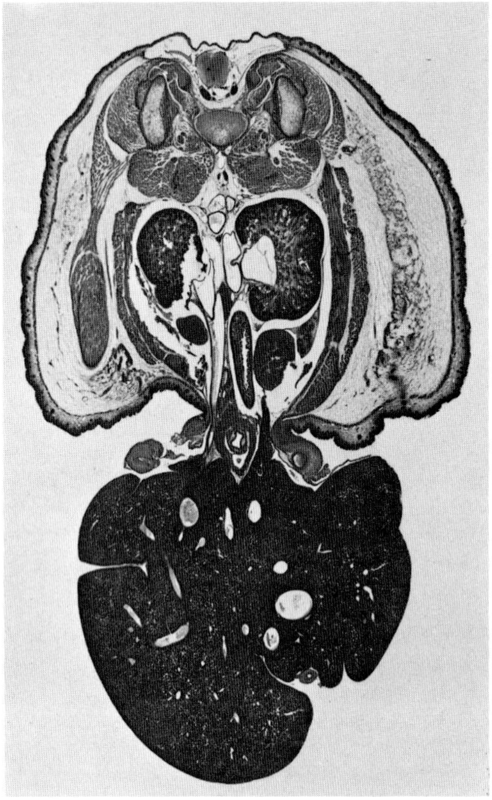

Fig. 82-6.—Transverse section through a near-term rat fetus whose mother had been treated with methyl salicylate on the tenth day. Esophagus and liver are protruding through umbilical opening. On the dorsum, spina bifida occulta is suggested by change of skin to an epithelial layer and absence of posterior vertebral parts.

often there is only one umbilical artery. The placenta is situated nearer to the fetus than is normal. The intestines, the stomach, the liver, the spleen, the kidneys and even the heart and a lung may be extruded.[27] The bladder can be closed and normally located or the abdominal fissure can extend into the hypogastrium and is combined with exstrophy of the bladder. The development of the vessels of the abdomen and pelvis is abnormal. These severe forms of gastroschisis are due to insufficient separation of the embryo from the wall of the blastocyst and defective formation of the body stalk.[29] Concordant gastroschisis has been reported in monozygotic twins.[30]

Infants with this severe anomaly often are affected by associated malformations. There may be varying degrees of defects of the lower bowels such as anal or rectal atresia. The entire large intestine may be missing, the small intestine ending in the wall of the hernial sac or in or near an ectopic bladder (exstrophia splanchnica p. 712). The central nervous system often is involved, as anencephaly, meningocele and spina bifida may accompany visceral ectopia. The scoliotic and lordotic spinal column often is deficient in vertebrae. The spinal retroflexion may be so marked that the back of the head and that of the pelvis can be brought into contact.[27] Iniencephaly and gastroschisis can be combined. Owing to the approach of embryo and placenta, normal position of the extremities may become impossible, so that backward displacement of the lower limbs and abnormal rotation result. The uterus may be bicornuate or duplicated and the genital tubercle divided.

The prognosis for the severe type of gastroschisis is very poor. The large defect of the abdominal wall, premature rupture or absence of the sac and associated malformations contribute to early death of the infant. In recent years, successful surgical treatment of gastroschisis[31, 32] and exstrophia splanchnica has been reported.

A condition that is compatible with life resembles gastroschisis in that it represents an abdominal hernia situated lateral to the umbilicus. Such lateral hernias are seen in the lumbar region, with protrusion of the viscera into a sac covered by normal skin. Survival is possible, since the skin prevents rupture.

Gastroschisis occurs in lower animals as well as in children. It has been observed in calves, pigs, lambs, kittens, reptiles and birds.

Remnants of the Vitelline Duct (Omphalo-Mesenteric Sinus; Omphalo-Enteric Duct)

The retracting intestine may remain attached to the umbilicus by a persistent yolk stalk, a condition described by Meckel in 1812, but apparently known as early as 1598.[33] This connection, or remnants of it, may remain symptomless or cause complications in various ways. The stalk may remain patent, opening to the surface as an umbilical fistula delivering fecal matter; it may be patent at both ends with a fibrous occluding cord between the outer end opening to the surface and secreting to the surface, or it may be closed at both ends, the middle portion forming a cyst. The most common kind of diverticulum is a blind pouch of the ileum 1–3 feet above the cecum, which may be attached to the umbilical scar by a fibrous cord or hang free in the abdominal cavity. Such Meckel diverticula (p. 701) are lined by ileal mucosa, but in approximately 60% of the cases, areas of gastric mucosa are found in the anomalous pouch. There also may be clusters of pancreatic cells.[28] Persistence of the omphalo-enteric duct can result in complication if the umbilical cord is improperly divided or cause difficulties at an exchange transfusion.[42]

Schizosomia Reflexum (Strophosomia)

This anomaly represents the highest degree of ventral body fissure with divergent and reversed growth of the abdominal plates.[5] The condition occurs with relative frequency in cattle, but it has also been observed in the goat, lamb, horse and chick.[34] It presents as a sac that contains all the organs of the thoracic and abdominal cavity as well as the relatively well-formed head, neck and pelvis. The thoracic and abdominal plates, instead of uniting in front of the embryo, fuse posteriorly over its back. There also exists a maximal lordosis, so that head and pelvis are in contact. Kermauner[5] mentioned and illustrated as an example of schizosomia reflexum a human embryo without belly stalk whose back was attached to the chorion, but the condition seems to be extremely rare in man.

Single Umbilical Artery

This anomaly was well known to anatomists of the nineteenth century, but it was considered a curiosity that occurred only in monstrous births. Thus, it was observed that sympodial monsters often had a single median umbilical artery arising directly from the aorta. Omphalocele and acardia[35] are other severe malformations often associated with a single artery in the umbilical cord. As early as 1822, Hermann (cited by Dawson[35]) described 2 cases of congenital umbilical hernia in which there was a single umbilical artery arising from the aorta. Kermauner[5] thought that in about one-third of the infants with omphalocele a second umbilical artery was missing.[35] When it became known that single umbilical artery was also a rather frequent finding in viable infants and that the anomaly could be an early and external sign of internal congenital malformations, the vascular deficiency became of clinical interest. Benirschke and Brown[36] pointed out that in pathologic fetuses there was a high incidence of single umbilical artery, but subsequently it was found[37, 38] that about 1% of all umbilical cords examined routinely have this vascular anomaly. It is true that the results of serial examinations of the cord vary between 0.2% and 3.6%,[39, 40] but the fact remains that the establishment of single umbilical artery at the fetal end of the cord does prove of value by aiding in early detection of internal congenital malformations.[40] The single umbilical artery does not always originate directly from the aorta as seen in sympodia, as it can arise as a branch of a common iliac-hypogastric trunk. Such lateral single umbilical arteries are attributed either to atrophy of the distal portion or to the failure of the primary umbilical root to appear originally. In general, aplasia is associated with more severe fetal malformations than atrophy.[40] A detailed study of the origin of the single umbilical artery in normal and abnormal human fetuses was made by Dawson.[35] Monie[43] thought that single umbilical artery could be due to persistence of the normally transient single umbilical artery of early development in association with degeneration of the truncal portion of either the right or the left umbilical artery. Relatively frequent occurrence of the anomaly in one of monozygotic twins[40] and in fetuses with autosomal trisomies[39] has been emphasized. Absence of one umbilical artery repeatedly has been found associated with thalidomide embryopathies.[40]

The congenital malformations associated with single umbilical artery are heterogeneous in origin and morphology. Cardiovascular, pulmonary, gastrointestinal, cerebrospinal, musculoskeletal, facial and ocular malformations have been observed.[41]

REFERENCES

1. Cresson, S. L.: Lesions about the umbilicus in infants and children, Pediat. Clin. North America 6:1085, 1959.
2. Crump, E. P.: Umbilical hernia, J. Pediat. 40:214, 1952.
3. Walker, S. H.: The natural history of umbilical hernia. A six year follow up of 314 Negro children with this defect, Clin. Pediat. 6:29, 1967.
4. Gross, R. E.: *The Surgery of Infancy and Childhood* (Philadelphia: W. B. Saunders Company, 1953).
5. Kermauner, F.: Die Missbildungen des Rumpfes, in Schwalbe, E. (ed.), *Die Morphologie der Missbildungen des Menschen und der Tiere* (Jena: Gustav Fischer, 1909), Vol. 3, pt. 1, p. 41.
6. Duhamel, B.: Embryology of exomphalos and allied malformations, Arch. Dis. Childhood 38:142, 1963.
7. McKeown, T., MacMahon, B., and Record, R. G.: An investigation of 69 cases of exomphalos, Am. J. Human Genet. 5:169, 1953.
8. Soper, R. T., and Green, E. W.: Omphalocele, Surg., Gynec. & Obst. 113:501, 1961.
9. Smith, W. R., and Leix, F.: Omphalocele, Am. J. Surg. 3: 450, 1966.
10. Fock, G.: Ectopic liver in omphalocele, Acta paediat. 52: 288, 1963.
11. Bell, L. S., and Brown, H. A.: Ruptured omphalocele, J. Pediat. 44:79, 1954.
12. Rickham, P. P.: Rupture of exomphalos and gastroschisis, Arch. Dis. Childhood 38:138, 1963.
13. Kajii, T., Oikawa, K., Itakura, K., and Ohsawa, T.: A probable 17-18 trisomy syndrome with phocomelia, exomphalos, and agenesis of hemidiaphragm, Arch. Dis. Childhood 39:519, 1964.
14. Gustavson, K-H., Finley, S. C., Finley, W. H., and Jalling, B.: A 4-5/21-22 chromosomal translocation associated with multiple congenital anomalies, Acta paediat. 53: 172, 1964.
15. O'Leary, C. M., and Clymer, C. E.: Umbilical hernia, Am. J. Surg. 52:38, 1941.
16. Wiedemann, H-R: Familial malformation complex with umbilical hernia and macroglossia – a "new syndrome?", J. Génét. Hum. 13:223, 1964.
17. Irving, I. M.: Exomphalos with macroglossia: A study of eleven cases, J. Pediat. Surg. 2:499, 1967.
18. Paucot, H., and Gelle, P.: Hernie ombilicale embryonnaire récidivante chez trois foetus successifs, Bull. soc. obst. et gynéc. 25:296, 1936.
19. Aitken, J.: Exomphalos, Arch. Dis. Childhood 38:126, 1963.
20. Grob, M.: Conservative treatment of exomphalos, Arch. Dis. Childhood 38:148, 1963.
21. Sauvage, L. R., and Bill, A. H.: The congenitally malformed. 3. Omphaloceles and gastroschisis defects, Northwest Med. 64:672, 1965.
22. Ingalls, T. H., Avis, F. R., Curley, F. J., and Temin, H. M.: Genetic determinants of hypoxia-induced congenital anomalies, J. Hered. 44:185, 1953.
23. Nelson, M. M., Wright, H. V., Asling, C. W., and Evans, H. M.: Multiple congenital abnormalities resulting from transitory deficiency of pteroylglutamic acid during gestation in the rat, J. Nutrition 56:349, 1955.
24. Gillman, J., Gilbert, C., and Gillman, T.: A preliminary report on hydrocephalus, spina bifida and other congeni-

tal anomalies in the rat produced by trypan blue, South African J. M. Sc. 13:47, 1948.
25. Warkany, J., and Takacs, E.: Experimental production of congenital malformations in rats by salicylate poisoning, Am. J. Path. 35:315, 1959.
26. Warkany, J., and Takacs, E.: Congenital malformations in rats from streptonigrin, Arch. Path. 79:65, 1965.
27. Ballantyne, J. W.: *Manual of Antenatal Pathology and Hygiene. The Embryo* (Edinburgh: W. Green & Sons, 1904).
28. Bremer, J. L.: *Congenital Anomalies of the Viscera. Their Embryological Basis* (Cambridge, Mass.: Harvard University Press, 1957).
29. Potter, E. L.: *Pathology of the Fetus and the Newborn* (Chicago: Year Book Medical Publishers, Inc., 1961).
30. Kikkawa, S., and Matsumoto, K.: A case of abdominal fissure seen in twin babies, Congen. Anom. (Japan) 6:52, 1966.
31. Ament, M. E., and Fonkalsrud, E. W.: Gastroschisis with antenatal intestinal evisceration, J. Pediat. 70:812, 1967.
32. Gilbert, M. G., Mencia, L. F., Brown, W. T., and Linn, B. S.: Staged surgical repair of large omphaloceles and gastroschisis, J. Pediat. Surg. 3:702, 1968.
33. Moses, W. R.: Meckel's diverticulum, New England J. Med. 237:118, 1947.
34. Ancel, P.: *La Chimiotératogenèse*. Réalisation des monstruosités par des substances chimiques chez les vertébrés (Paris: Gaston Doin & Cie, 1950).
35. Dawson, A. B.: The origin and occurrence of the single umbilical artery in normal and abnormal human fetuses, Anat. Rec. 24:321, 1922.
36. Benirschke, K., and Brown, W. H.: A vascular anomaly of the umbilical cord. The absence of one umbilical artery in the umbilical cords of normal and abnormal fetuses, Obst. & Gynec. 6:300, 1955.
37. Little, W. A.: Aplasia of the umbilical artery, Bull. Sloane Hosp. for Women 4:127, 1958.
38. Benirschke, K.: The Number of Vessels in the Umbilical Cord, in Benirschke, K. (ed.), *Comparative Aspects of Reproductive Failure* (New York: Springer-Verlag, 1966).
39. Lenosky, E. F., and Medovy, H.: Single umbilical artery: Incidence, clinical significance and relation to autosomal trisomy, Canad. M.A.J. 87:1229, 1962.
40. Benirschke, K., Sullivan, M. M., and Marin-Padilla, M.: Size and number of umbilical vessels. A study of multiple pregnancy in man and the armadillo, Obst. & Gynec. 24: 819, 1964.
41. Seki, M., and Strauss, L.: Absence of one umbilical artery, Arch. Path. 78:446, 1964.
42. Schellong, G., and Pfeiffer, R. A.: Persistierender Ductus omphaloentericus als Ursache ungewöhnlicher Komplikationen bei der Austauschtransfusion, Arch. Kinderh. 175:204, 1967.
43. Monie, I. W.: Genesis of single umbilical artery, Am. J. Obst. & Gynec. 108:400, 1970.

PART XIII

Systemic Skeletal Malformations

Chondrodystrophies

THERE EXIST a number of types of disproportionate dwarfs in whom the long bones of the extremities seem to be affected more than the bones of the rest of the body. The impressive micromelia of these patients led to the establishment of a disease picture long recognized and recorded in sculptures and paintings, and described by Parrot[1] in the nineteenth century as "achondroplasia." The short-limbed dwarfs with rather normal-sized heads and trunks could be distinguished easily from other dwarfs, so that achondroplasia was considered a well-defined entity for many decades. With increasing interest in systemic skeletal disorders and through investigation of their pathologic, roentgenologic and chemical properties, it evolved that the term "achondroplasia" actually covered many differing entities. Some observers dealt, and are dealing with, micromelic dwarfs who are stillborn or die soon after birth, whereas others describe the survivors. Since the differentiation of the various subgroups was made by different specialists and scientists, the resulting classifications are not uniform. In addition, new subentities are described every year and existing classifications must be revised. It is difficult to deal with this fluctuating situation at present. The differentiation of the numerous types of chondrodystrophy contributes little to the treatment of the patients, but it can aid in prognosis and genetic counseling. There is no doubt that some of the chondrodystrophies are transmitted as autosomal dominant traits, whereas others are recessively inherited. Sex may influence the expression of the gene in some of the disorders. When the mode of inheritance is not revealed by the family history, morphologic distinctive signs sometimes can contribute to the diagnosis and genetic prognosis; in such cases, morphologic classifications may be of great practical importance. But when morphologic details fail to elucidate the etiology or genetic implications, they may be merely of theoretical and temporary interest or at times confuse meaningful classifications.

I have attempted to group the chondrodystrophies mentioned below according to etiology. Achondroplasia and some "atypical chondrodystrophies" attributed to mutant autosomal dominant genes are dealt with in Chapters 83 and 84 and chondrodystrophies considered recessive traits are discussed in Chapter 85. Sex-linked recessive inheritance is mentioned in Chapter 86. This classification is tentative and it must be admitted that we see patients who cannot be diagnosed and classified with certainty, so that their genetic evaluation is not possible. In general, uncertainties of differentiation within the groups with similar inheritance are less disturbing than inconsistencies that make it difficult to arrive at a genetic classification and prognosis.

83

Achondroplasia

ACHONDROPLASIA is a congenital skeletal anomaly that chiefly affects the bones derived from cartilage. It is characterized by slow growth of cartilage, retarded endochondral ossification and almost normal periosteal bone formation. As a result, the tubular bones are short and thick, and affected persons appear dwarfed, having very short extremities and a relatively large head and trunk. This disproportionate dwarfism was recognized as an entity by Parrot[1] in 1878 and was clearly differentiated from other forms of retarded statural growth. Parrot thought that a lack of cartilage formation is at the root of the disorder, which he named "achondroplasia." But Kaufmann[2] pointed out that this name signifies a complete lack of cartilage, thus giving the false impression that no cartilage at all is formed. He introduced, therefore, the term "fetal chondrodystrophy," which indicates an impaired growth of cartilage and characterizes well the essential pathologic feature of this disorder. Unfortunately, a number of other systemic osseous disturbances have been termed "chondrodysplasias," a name that is philologically but not genetically and clinically almost identical with "chondrodystrophy." In order to avoid confusion, it may be better, therefore, to return to the less adequate term "achondroplasia," which has become identified with a well-defined clinical picture recognized by lay persons and physicians alike.

The frequency of births of achondroplastic infants in hospitals has been established in Denmark as well as in Northern Ireland. Mørch,[3] in Copenhagen, found in a hospital, records of 10 achondroplastic births among 94,075 deliveries, i.e., 1 per 9,407, or 0.0106%. Stevenson[4] obtained comparable records in Belfast, where 9 achondroplastics were recognized among 31,753 births, i.e., 0.0283%. Thus, there was a definite difference in the two estimates in northern Europe. Caffey[5] reported that in the Sloane Hospital for Women 4 achondroplastic infants were born in 12,151 deliveries, or 1 in 3,040, an incidence rather close to that of Northern Ireland. There is general agreement about the high mortality of achondroplastic infants. Of the 10 achondroplastic children born in the hospital in Copenhagen, 8 died in the first year of life, and of the 9 born in Belfast, only 1 survived 5 days. Mørch[3] believed that after the first year of life the viability of achondroplastics is normal, but the only survivor in Stevenson's[4] newborn series died at 18 months after a precarious infancy. All 4 achondroplastics in Caffey's[5] series were dead at 6 months.

It is quite likely that the achondroplastics born in hospitals are not representative of the patients as we know them as surviving micromelic dwarfs. Stevenson[4] pointed out that 5 of 9 hospital deliveries resulting in achondroplastic children were complicated by hydramnios and that 2 children diagnosed in the hospital as achondroplastics had cleft palate and polydactyly. It seems that in Belfast, where only about 50% of children are born in a hospital, there is a selection in hospital deliveries for complicated types of the disorder. In general, of the so-called achondroplastics born, approximately 80% die within the first year of life. But recent family studies by Murdoch *et al.*[6] indicate that the outlook for survival of typical achondroplastic infants may be more favorable than previously[3, 4] thought. Affected children who have only one achondroplastic parent (heterozygotes) have a good chance to survive. If both parents are affected, the mortality of their achondroplastic children may be higher, since some of them will be homozygous for the achondroplasia gene.[6]

There are several types of chondrodystrophy that are not compatible with life. One lethal form is characterized by very short ribs and a long, narrow thorax (Figs. 83-1 and 83-2). Infants with this *"thanatophoric" dwarfism*[7] have a large cranial vault with a short base and a depressed nasal root. The vertebral bodies are low and the vertebral interspaces large. The extremities are very short, the humerus and femur are curved and the fibula is shorter than the tibia. There is muscular hypotonia. Cyanosis and respiratory difficulties result from lack of pulmonary ventilation. Death ensues within a few days after birth. A necropsy was reported by Kaufman *et al.*[51] It has been said that these infants usually are male and that there is no familial recurrence. They are considered lethal mutations.[7] Keats *et al.*[8] reported 3 female infants with thanatophoric dwarfism. In another lethal achondroplasia called "achondrogenetic" by Maroteaux and Lamy,[7] the vertebral bodies are not ossified and there is shortness of the trunk. The extremities are very short and the metaphyses wide. A combination of achondroplasia with median cleft lip, cleft palate, hydrocephaly and pulmonary hypoplasia was

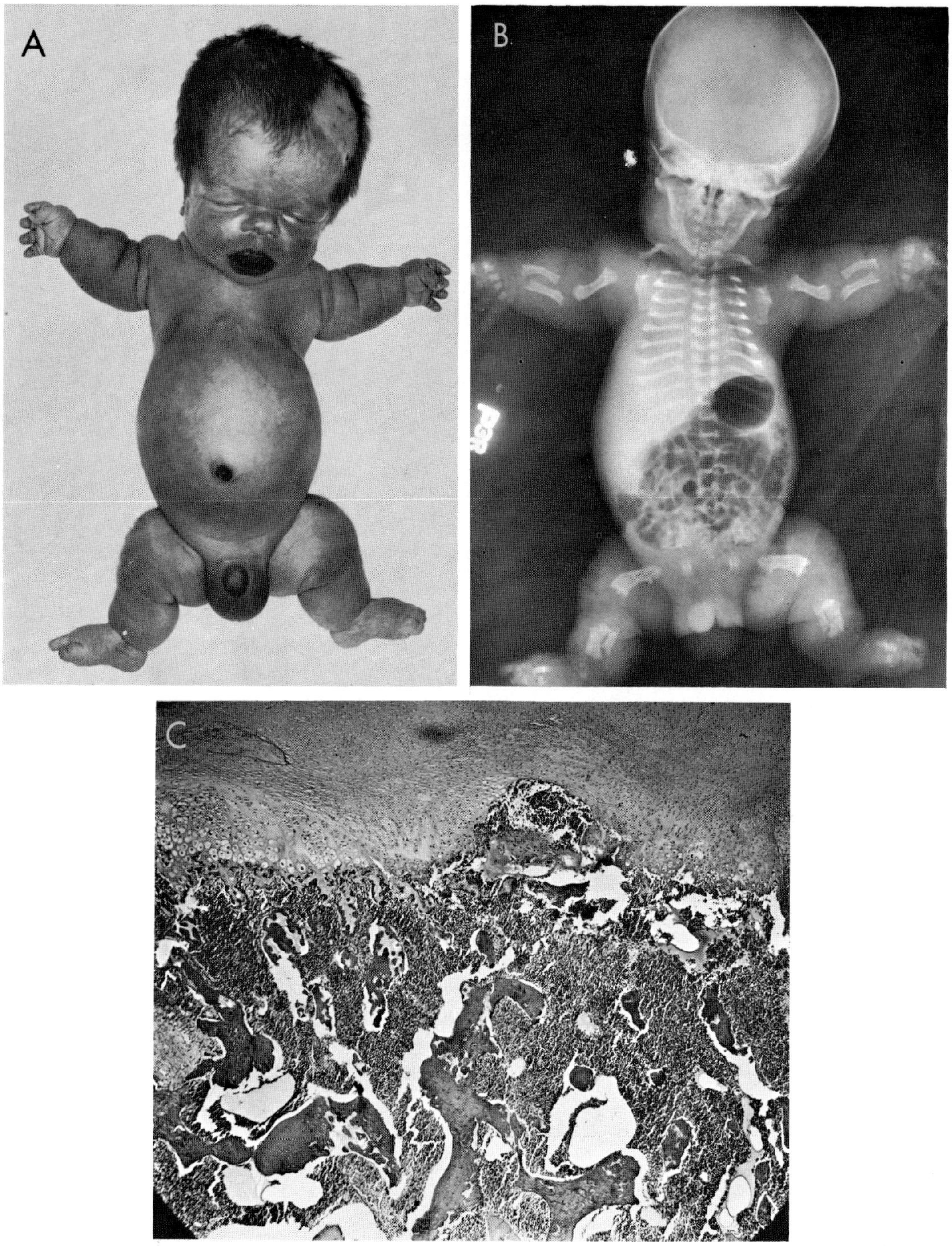

Fig. 83-1. – **A,** achondroplasia in a newborn infant, the child of normal parents. Born after an 8-month pregnancy. The mother had anasarca since the sixth month of pregnancy. Child died on the third day after birth. **B,** roentgenogram of the child showing short tubular bones, short ribs and small pelvis. **C,** section through proximal end of femur. The epidiaphyseal junction is devoid of growing cartilage, with the exception of the left end, which contains a few rows of cartilage. The bone trabeculae are irregular in shape and orientation. This type of achondroplasia corresponds to the hypoplastic form of chondrodystrophy of Kaufmann[2] and to that of "thanatophoric dwarfism."

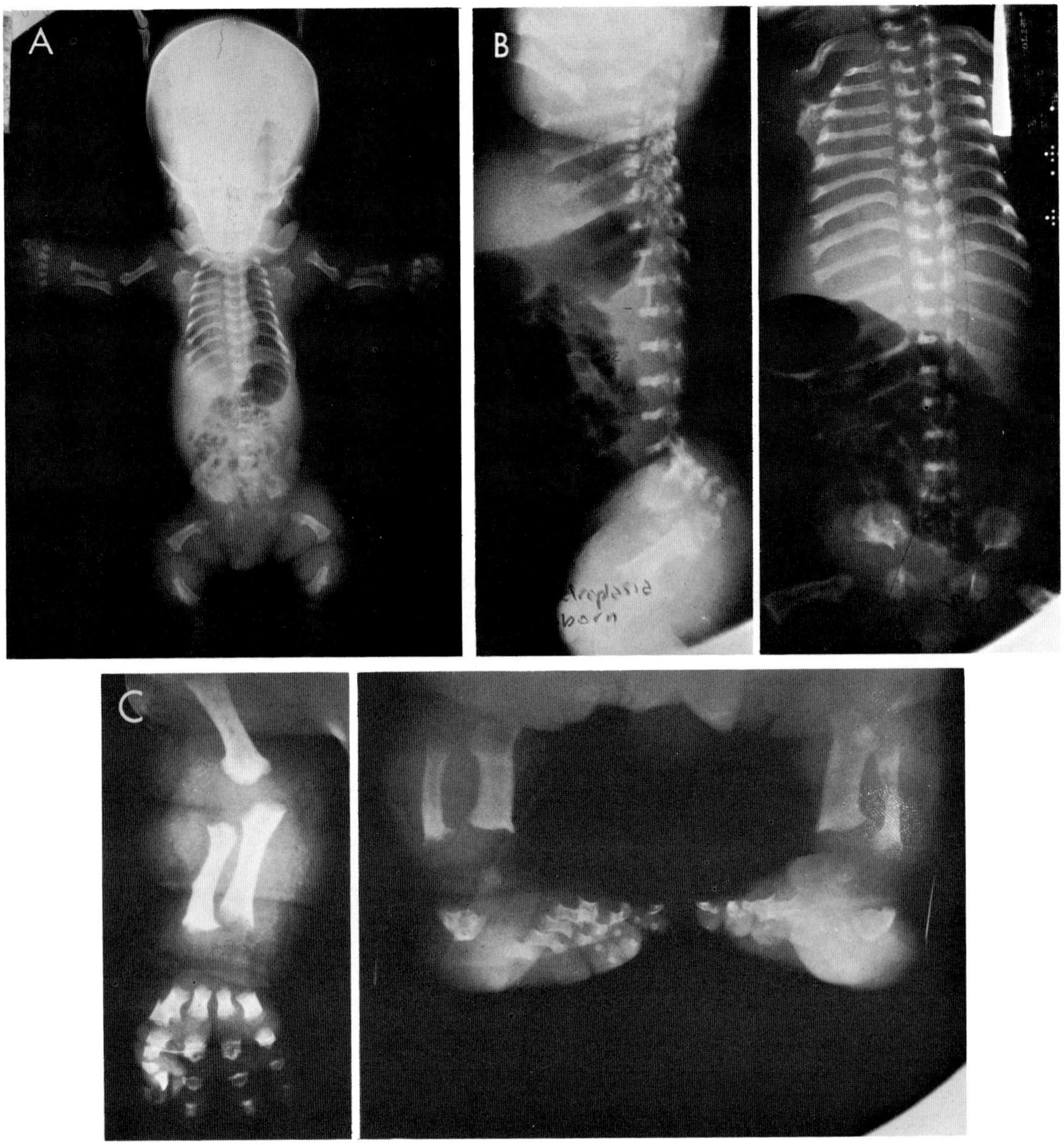

Fig. 83-2.—Lethal ("thanatophoric") achondroplasia. **A,** roentgenogram of a male infant with micromelia. The head is large and there were greatly dilated lateral ventricles found at necropsy done 1 day after birth. **B,** the spine consists of flat vertebral bodies and large intervertebral spaces. There was a well-developed rosary palpable at the costochondral junctions; the distal ends of the ribs are enlarged and cupped. **C,** the tubular bones of the extremities are markedly shortened and relatively thick.

reported by Wallace *et al.*[9] This lethal form, which can recur in a family, is thought to be a recessive hereditary trait. Chondrodystrophy combined with cloverleaf skull ("Kleeblattschädel") is a rare disease picture[10, 11] that can result in stillbirth[12] or early death (Chapter 86).

Other lethal types of micromelic dwarfism may not be achondroplasias but may be mistaken for them. Thus, micromelia with almost complete absence of ossification can be a form of hypophosphatasia (Chapter 92). Diastrophic dwarfism, which accounts for some of the chondrodystrophies with cleft palate, can be lethal before or shortly after birth. Lethal "achondroplasia" with cleft palate and polydactyly[4] probably represents an Ellis-van Creveld syndrome. And lethal cases of osteogenesis imperfecta (p. 827) are micromelic but not achondroplastic.

Data concerning living achondroplastics affected

by milder forms that were gathered in Denmark and Northern Ireland were in good agreement. There were 86 dwarfs of this type in a population of 3,793,000 in Denmark, i.e., the prevalence was 1 in 44,100 persons (0.0023%). In Northern Ireland there were 39 living achondroplastics among a population of 1,387,000, i.e., 1 in 35,560 (0.0028%).

If the prevalence figures of living achondroplastics in northern Europe are considered generally valid, one could estimate that there are about 5,000 dwarfs of this type in the United States and 65,000 on earth. Achondroplastic dwarfs have been reported from all European nations, from India, China, the Philippines and Africa, and the condition has been observed repeatedly in American Negroes and Indians.

Achondroplasia has been described from early times in pictures and sculptures in many races and nationalities. Rischbieth and Barrington[13] have listed and illustrated artistic records of dwarfs of the past, and Mørch[3] has given an account of ancient pictorial recordings that can be interpreted as achondroplastic images. There exists a relief in a temple near Thebes, Egypt, dating back to 1500 B.C. that represents a queen of Punt, Somaliland, and her daughter, of whom Mørch wrote that "after their proportions they were both typical chrondrodystrophics." If this interpretation were correct, this relief would represent an early record of dominantly inherited achondroplasia. Unfortunately, Ruffer[14] doubted that the queen was achondroplastic, and reproductions available[13] are not convincing. The ancient Egyptians apparently were favorably inclined toward achondroplastic dwarfs, as shown by statuettes of benign deities with achondroplastic features. Two of these statuettes are reproduced in Chapter 2. One of them, now in the Hy-Karlsberg Glyptothek in Copenhagen, shows marked shortening of the upper extremities, which do not reach below the umbilicus, short and very muscular bowlegs and a relatively large head and trunk. Ruffer,[14] in his *Studies in the Palaeopathology of Egypt*, pictured a number of achondroplastic dwarfs, records which suggest that the disorder had existed and been recognized 5,000 years ago. A limestone statuette of Chnoum-hotep, who lived in the fifth dynasty, about 2700 B.C., realistically shows a man with a large head and chest out of proportion to the diminutive lower limbs, squat hands and feet, short upper limbs, lordosis and good muscular development. This gentleman apparently was "Chief of the Perfumes" or "Head of the Wardrobe." Other achondroplastic dwarfs in Egypt were in charge of pets or jewelry.[14]

It is believed that Aesop, the Greek teller of fables, and Philetas of Cos, an esteemed poet and grammarian, were dwarfs, possibly achondroplastics. In Rome, emperor Domitian (A.D. 51–96), known for many forms of cruelty, was a great innovator in the realm of circus entertainments and added women and dwarfs to the gladiatorial ranks. He obviously enjoyed the helplessness of small but muscular achondroplastic gladiators (Fig. 83-3) engaged in hopeless combat. Other Roman emperors had achondroplastic court

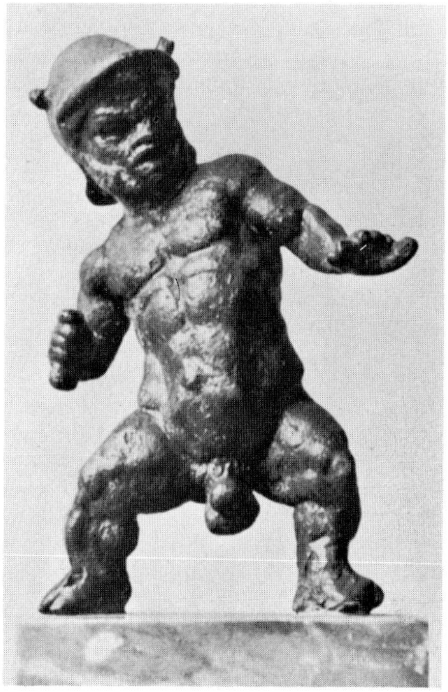

Fig. 83-3.—Achondroplastic gladiator (Coll. Oppenheim). (Reproduced with permission of Bibliothèque Nationale, Paris.)

jesters, a custom that was continued by kings and princes down to the eighteenth century. Good mental development and provocative wit in a person with somewhat grotesque physical features made these dwarfs valuable adjuncts of a princely household. It seems that the demands for achondroplastics was at times greater than the supply, so that increased production was attempted.[3] This was done by dwarf marriages, which usually remained sterile, or by deficient diets imposed on children, which sometimes were effective, probably by producing rachitic dwarfs—substitutes for the achondroplastic. It became customary to have paintings made of successful court dwarfs, and a number of such paintings exist effected by Spanish, French or English painters. It should be pointed out that not all of these paintings represent achondroplastic dwarfs. Thus, a painting by Jacob d'Agar of "Fräulein Else," said to show a typically chondrodystrophic head but a slim figure and fine, narrow hands, should not be considered "an idealization on the part of the painter," as assumed by Mørch, but rather a realistic picture of a hypopituitary dwarf. However, the Roman beggar dwarf, Francesco Ravai, masterfully painted by Jens Juel[3] and the dwarf, Maria Barbola, included in Velasquez' painting "Las Neninas,"[13] were typical achondroplastics. Dwarfs played quite an important role in folklore and literature. The best description of an achondroplastic dwarf was given—before Parrot[1]—in *David Copperfield* by Dickens, who described Miss Mowcher as a waddling dwarf with a very large head with extremely little arms and with legs not worth mentioning although she was "more than full-sized down to where her waist would have been, if she had had any. . . ." Since achondroplasia is now broken down into many disease entities, it can be expected that the micromelic dwarfs presented in sculptures and paintings will be reclassified in the near future. There are some dwarfs who have normal heads and faces that may be considered signs of spondylo-epiphyseal dysplasia (Chapter 84) and there are others who do not agree completely with the classic disease picture.

Achondroplasia, or better chondrodystrophy, is known to occur in animals in many forms. It can affect the entire skeleton or only parts of it. According to Nachtsheim,[15] the Tux-Zillertal cattle and Pekingese and French bulldog are examples of generalized chondrodystrophy, whereas in Niata cattle and Yorkshire swine the anomaly is limited to the head. In some dog races such as the English bulldog and the Boston terrier, head and spine are affected, whereas the extremities are normal. In the dachshund, on the other hand, the extremities are shortened and the head and spine are normal. A short-legged cattle is the English Dexter, which is derived from the normal Kerry cattle raised in Ireland. The Dexter cattle is a small animal with short head, short legs and strong muscles. Crossing of Dexter with the normal Kerry cattle results in 1:1 Kerry and Dexter offspring. Crossing of Dexter and Dexter results also in both types of young but about one-fourth of the offspring are bulldog calves that are born prematurely and unviable. It is assumed that the abnormal factor manifests itself in heterozygotes as Dexter, which are achondroplastic and viable, and in homozygotes as lethal bulldog calves. Yet, the situation may be more complicated, since, in some herds, Dexter crossings give a very high incidence of bulldog calves, whereas in other herds there are none. In the Telemarck breed, chondrodystrophy is inherited as a recessive trait. In dogs, genetic experiments were performed by Stockard[16] and others, resulting in rather complicated phenotypes, particularly when dogs with partial but regionally differing achondroplasias were crossed.[15] Gardner[17] described an achondroplasia in one member of each of four consecutive litters of miniature poodle puppies derived from apparently normal parents. The disorder was semilethal, and inheritance as a simple recessive was assumed. Pearce and Brown[18] studied a recessive form of achondroplasia in purebred Havana rabbits, in which the condition is transmitted by nonachondroplastic heterozygotes, whereas the homozygous achondroplastics are stillborn or die shortly after birth. A different recessive gene inducing achondroplasia was observed by Crary and Sawin[19] in New Zealand white domestic rabbits. The homozygous individual is viable and can be mated. The condition can be recognized early by a small cartilaginous papilla at the base of the external auditory meatus. Achondroplasia has been studied thoroughly in fowl. In the creeper, the disorder is dominantly inherited and creepers are heterozygous for the abnormal gene; the homozygous form is lethal in early embryonic stages.[20] The anomaly, which is due to a single dominant gene, has been observed in many different races. Thus, animals show a great variety of hereditary achondroplasias that are genetically heterogeneous. In addition, there exist "phenocopies" of achondroplastic cattle in the form of "acorn calves,"[21] illustrating that phenotypes resembling achondroplasia can be produced by inadequate nutrition. In rats, disturbance of growth of cartilage has been induced by riboflavin deficiency[22] and other nutritional methods, but the resulting deformities are not those of typical achondroplasia. Achondroplasia occurs as a nonhereditary phenocopy in the fowl, probably as the result of some disturbance in the mother.[23] Although, in animals, crosses can be made experimentally and control of the environment is possible, classification and analysis of chondrodystrophic disease pictures often are difficult.[24] This should caution against oversimplification of the situations encountered in human achondroplasia and other chondrodystrophies. There obviously are many differing forms of chondrodystrophy in human beings that can be distinguished by morphology and course. But more important is recognition of the etiology, since eugenic counseling depends on the understanding of the origin of the disorder and risk of recurrence.

Explanations of the origin of human achondroplasia were given by most authors who described cases of this type. Although most of the older explanations can now be considered baseless, they are still of historical interest. The interested reader can find a detailed account of these early explanations in Mørch's monograph.[3]

Heredity was not considered in scientific reports until Porak[25] described the first hereditary instance, but there can be no doubt that transmission from parent to children was observed before. In the nineteenth century, an increasing tendency to publication of hereditary cases can be noted, and Rischbieth and Barrington[13] reviewed the literature prior to 1912, presenting pedigrees with and without familial recurrence. In 80 pedigrees there were 55 solitary cases of achondroplasia and 25 showing more than one case. Only in 14 (or possibly 17) of the pedigrees were affected members found in two or more generations. In 11 cases, the familial situation was not clear; transmission was either irregular or repetitive cases were reported in families of normal parents. Mørch[3] believed that these 11 pedigrees were not acceptable because some of them did not deal with achondroplasia and others were incomplete. After 1912, many instances of the disorder in two, three and even four generations were published,[3] but such selected reports do not give a true picture of familial occurrence, since there is a tendency to report interesting families with multiple cases and to neglect sporadic ones. The work of Mørch[3] is of outstanding importance because it represents an unbiased collection of all cases of chondrodystrophy detectable in Denmark with their pedigrees. Familial occurrence was rare in Denmark. Among 108 cases, only 18 were familial (distributed in eight families); all repetitive cases were limited to two successive generations. Ninety were solitary incidents in large, otherwise normal families. Seven chondrodystrophics had 1 child, and one had 3 children with the same disorder. Six patients had only normal children. Thus, transmission was directly from parent to children without skipping of generations. More than 1 case in siblings was found only if a parent was affected. Fourteen chondrodystrophics who had offspring had a total of 27 children, of whom 10 were affected and 17 were normal. There were no cousin marriages among the normal parents of chondrodystrophics and there was no chondrodystrophy in distant relatives of the patients. From these observations, Mørch concluded that in the familial cases the disorder was transmitted as a dominant character. The sporadic cases were due to mutation; they were potential initiators of families in which about 50% of the offspring would have been affected. That they did not have families was due to "various, entirely extraneous, social and emotional causes which have nothing to do with the etiology and inheritance of chondrodystrophy." It is true that there were 6 patients who had exclusively normal children, but since they had only small families the possibility existed that subsequent children would have been affected. On the basis of his careful observations—and of a few unproved assumptions—Mørch came to the conclusion that chondrodystrophy arises frequently by mutation, that *all* cases are of genotypic (hereditary) nature and that the condition is transmitted as a dominant character.

Twenty-nine years later, Murdoch *et al.*[6] made a statistical and genetic study of 148 achondroplastic dwarfs in America. Of these, 117 (79%) were sporadic and 31 (21%) were familial, with one or both parents affected. In those attributed to new mutation, paternal age was advanced significantly. There were 57 marriages involving achondroplastic dwarfs and 37 of these were fertile. The 24 affected children who had only one achondroplastic parent all survived; of 16 affected offspring of marriages in which both mates were achondroplastic, 7 died in infancy; it was thought that the majority of these were homozygotes. This relatively favorable survival rate of the offspring of achondroplastic dwarfs suggests that the high mortality rate cited above probably is not that of "regular" achondroplastics but that of various atypical forms with strong lethal tendency (e.g., thanatophorics).

The possibility of recessive forms was denied by Mørch[3] because he did not encounter families in which normal parents had more than 1 affected child and because there were no achondroplastics among distant relatives of the patient. Grebe,[26] discussing recessively inherited achondroplasia, reported rather typical symptoms in 2 distantly related dwarfs from the same village, the offspring of probably consanguineous marriages. The same author also reported 2 achondroplastic stillbirths in a family in which the consanguineous parents were phenotypically normal. Additional families with more than 1 achondroplastic child of apparently healthy consanguineous parents have since been published by Helweg-Larsen and Mørch[27] and by Stevenson.[4] Such cases are suggestive of recessive inheritance. Alternative explanations are reduced expressivity in one of the parents or mutation in a precursor cell of the germ cells (gonadal mosaicism). But it seems advisable to keep in mind the possibility of heterogeneous etiology of the various chondrodystrophies, including achondroplasia. The disorder, once considered a single entity, has now been broken down into many subgroups distinguishable by morphologic, roentgenologic and genetic characteristics.[28-30] The existence of variable origins of achondroplasias in animals (p. 772) should put one on guard against oversimplification of the situations in man.

Concordance has been observed in identical twins and discordance in nonidentical twins.[3,6,31] It is of interest that concordance has been reported in twins of different sex.[31] The occurrence of achondroplasia and mongolism in twin brothers reported by Lapage[32] is remarkable, but interpretation of this single instance is difficult. Achondroplasia and Down syndrome in one and the same individual[33] has also been reported. It is worth mentioning that in two instances of—probably—atypical achondroplasia, the births of the patients were preceded by stillbirths of anencephalic siblings.[34] Chromosome studies in achondroplastic patients have shown normal numbers,[35] but some irregularities were found in some cells of a pair of identical twins.[31]

The results of matings of two achondroplastics are of great interest, but the pregnancies resulting from such matings usually are terminated prematurely. In one instance,[36] abortion was induced in the fourth month and the fetus showed signs of achondroplasia. Potter and Coverstone[37] reported the case of 2 chondrodystrophic parents who had a chondrodystrophic child delivered by cesarean section. Similar cases were listed by Rischbieth and Barrington.[13]

Advanced parental age has been known to be an etiologic factor in achondroplasia since 1912. Bleyer in 1939[38] and Mørch in 1941[3] pointed out that advanced maternal age seemed to play a role in the etiology of this disorder, but Penrose[39] found and Murdoch *et al.*[6] confirmed that paternal age is a major factor in the origin of new mutations for achondroplasia.

The pathologic changes of the skeleton have been explained by the anomalous growth of cartilage, which is followed by abnormal endochondral ossification, but recent biopsies showed that in typical achondroplasia endochondral ossification apparently is regular and well organized. It has been suggested that the basic defect may be a quantitative decrease in the rate of endochondral ossification, which, in conjunction with undisturbed periosteal bone formation, results in the short and thick shapes of tubular bones.[40] But biopsies from ribs and iliac crest may show different pictures from those of long bones.[52] Generalizations should not be made from examinations of one area, since achondroplasia is a disorder of differential growth impairment. Pathologists have described a vascular strip of connective tissue that originates from the periosteum and may be seen in places between the epiphysis and diaphysis. Growth in length is inhibited by such interference, whereas the areas not reached by the strip continue to grow slowly. As a result, the bone bends around the side that contains the periosteal strip and becomes deformed. At points of muscle insertions, osteophytic appositions may be formed.[41]

The process of ossification is rather irregular. In the same skeleton, signs of delayed and precocious ossification have been observed. There may be a delayed appearance of the carpal centers while premature synostoses occur between the phalanges and their epiphyses. In other cases, ossification progresses with normal speed.

Kaufmann[41] emphasized the existence of hypoplastic, hyperplastic and malacic forms. In the hypoplastic, the cartilage is uniformly retarded in all portions of the metaphysis and the epi-metaphyseal junction is smooth. In the hyperplastic type, growth of cartilage may be marked in width, so that mushrooming of the ends of the bones occurs and the epi-metaphyseal junctions are enlarged. Potter[42] and de Groot[34] observed cases of extreme hyperplasia in nonviable fetuses. Attempts are under way to interpret these findings in the light of recent descriptions and classifications of chondrodystrophies.

Slow growth of the cartilage and precocious synostosis of the bones of the base of the skull result in the characteristic shape of the head. Although the base of the skull, which is of cartilaginous origin, remains short, the bones of the calvarium, which develop from membrane bone, grow normally in all directions. As a result, a large vault sits on a small base, and the head becomes pear-shaped. The protrusion of the forehead over the face also leads to depression of the root of the nose and to the "cretinoid" facies of the achondroplastic dwarf. The maxilla is short and broad; the prominence of the mandible is more pronounced in adults than in children. The large head of achondroplastics often suggests hydrocephaly (Fig. 83-4). Although hydrocephaly occurs in some of these patients, it has been pointed out that the enlargement of the brain seen in achondroplastic children can be due to megalencephaly. Dennis *et al.*[43] suggested that megalencephaly could be a part of a general growth disturbance characteristic of achondroplasia. The volume of the posterior fossa is normal for the age of the achondroplastic patient, but is relatively small when compared with the concomitant megalencephaly. In some cases, smallness of the foramen magnum and vertebral canal and eccentric indentation of the foramen magnum by the odontoid process may combine with megalomyelo-encephaly to contribute to neonatal mortality or paraplegia. Cohen *et al.*[44] found that enlargement of the head accompanied by mild dilatation of the ventricles usually is present without increased intracranial pressure. Significant hydrocephaly can occur; it probably is due to obstruction at the level of the foramen magnum and can result in neurologic signs related to cord compression at this level.

Since the trunk is less affected than the extremities, the changes in the axial skeleton have attracted less attention than those of the appendicular skeleton, although in many cases ossification of the vertebrae is irregular. Reduction in height and wedge shape of the vertebral bodies may be seen and abnormal curvatures may be present in the spine. The ribs are broad and their osseous parts are short. The costochondral junctions are enlarged and a "rosary" can be formed.

The chest cavity is small and the heart and lungs may be so compressed that circulatory and respiratory difficulties arise. This is particularly true in achondroplastics who die soon after birth.

The humerus and femur are markedly reduced in length but thick and enlarged at the ends. Bowing is seen in some cases. The bones of the forearm are affected in a similar way; the olecranon usually is overdeveloped, so that extension of the forearm is impaired. In the lower leg, the tibia is shorter than the fibula. The bones of the hands and feet are short, broad and scalloped at their epiphyseal ends. The bones of the basal phalanges often form an angle with the metacarpal bones, so that the fingers assume divergent directions. The pelvis is small and the entrance kidney-shaped; the sacrum is small and in an almost horizontal position; the promontory protrudes into the pelvic entrance. The acetabulum often is flat and underdeveloped, and spontaneous dislocation of the head of the femur may occur.[5] The muscles are well developed and sometimes hypertrophic.

The mean birth weights for males are 3,493 Gm. and for females 3,130 Gm. but if the mother is dwarfed, the birth weights are lower.[6] In the newborn, the head is of normal size but there are frontal and parietal eminences and the root of the nose is depressed. The bones of the skull are of normal hardness and the fontanelles and sutures of normal width. The trunk is of almost normal size but the ribs are flaring and a rosary can be felt at the costochondral junction. The limbs are short, thick and curved. In some patients, the skin appears too large for the size of the bones and it may be folded "like an accordion."

Growth in height is slow after birth and stops early. Achondroplastic dwarfs often can be recognized at a glance by their short extremities, which are attached to a relatively large trunk, and by the large head and typical facial features (Fig. 83-6). The forehead is high and bulging. The root of the nose is broad and depressed and the features are coarse. The mandible

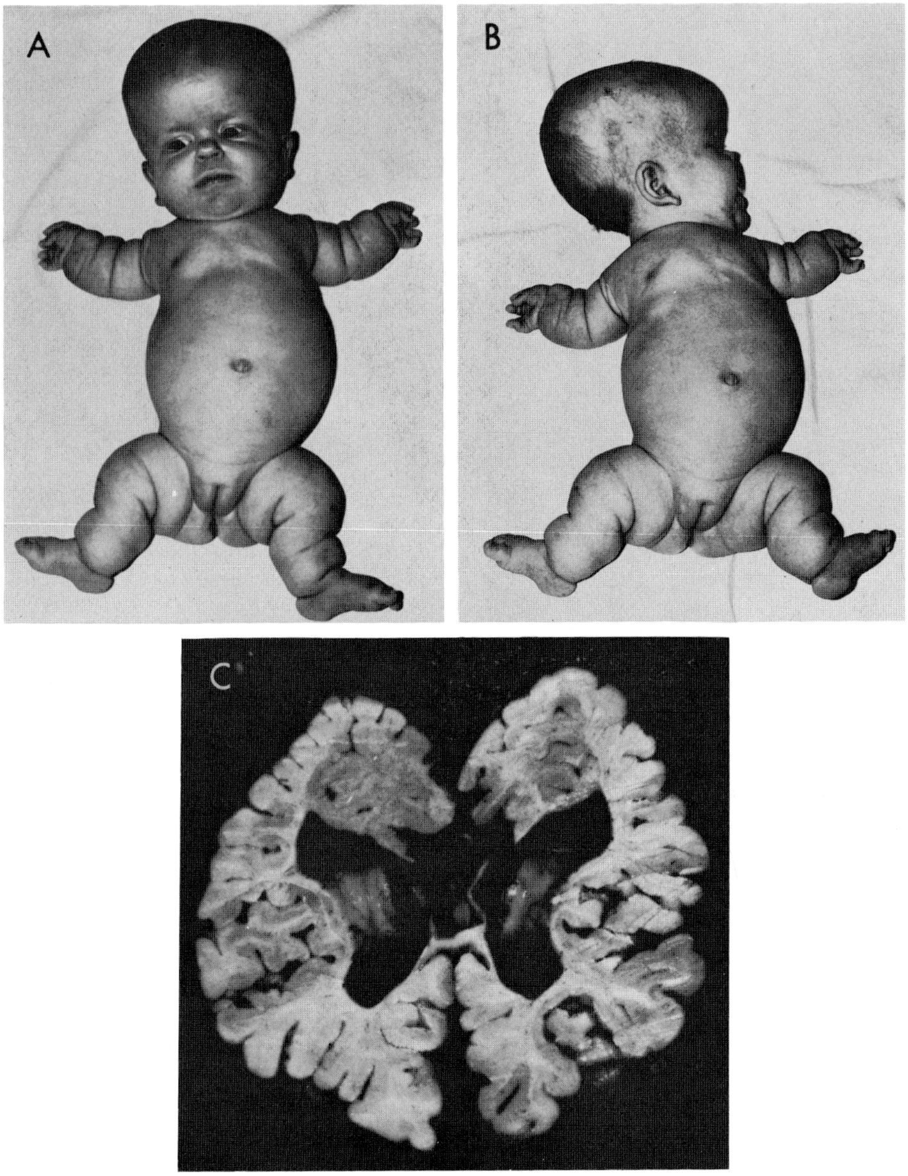

Fig. 83-4.—**A** and **B**, 5-month-old achondroplastic girl with hydrocephaly. Although this child had some roentgenologic signs of "thanatophoric dwarfism," she survived and lived for 8 months. At necropsy, the clinical impression of hydrocephaly was confirmed (**C**).

is disproportionately large and the chin protruding. The palate is high and malposition of the teeth frequently is present. The chest, although of nearly normal length, is contracted in the anteroposterior diameter. A ridge formed by prominent costochondral junctions may be visible. The abdomen is prominent. An exaggerated lumbar lordosis and prominence of the buttocks are characteristic of the disorder. In addition to the well-known lumbar lordosis, some achondroplastics have a localized, low dorsal kyphosis, which is due to wedge-shaped vertebrae. Mørch[3] stressed that the normal cervical and dorsal curvatures frequently are effaced, so that the upper spinal column is straight. Scoliosis is rare. Caffey[5] described characteristic features of the spine seen in roentgenograms of children. The height of the vertebral bodies appears reduced and the intervertebral spaces enlarged (Fig. 83-7). The posterior edges of the vertebrae are concave and the anterior are wedge-shaped in the lumbar area. The lumbar bodies taper in width and with this goes a narrowing of the lumbar spinal canal. In adults, smallness of the spinal canal and

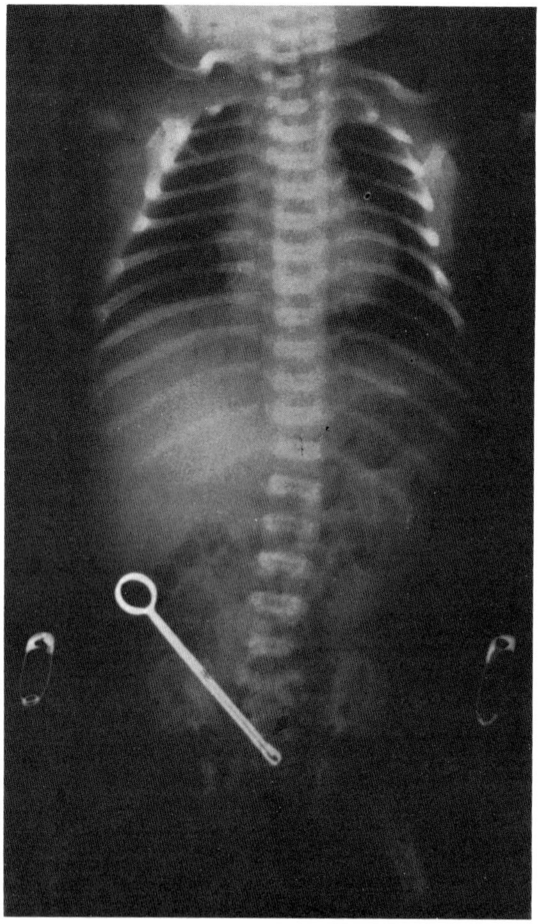

Fig. 83-5.—Roentgenogram of trunk of a newborn achondroplastic. Note the height of vertebral bodies and shape of ribs, which show cupping at the distal ends. Compare these findings with those shown in Figure 83-2, which illustrates a thanatophoric newborn.

herniation of intervertebral disks may lead to neurologic complications. The spinal cord and cauda equina are tightly encased in a narrow vertebral canal and can be compressed easily. Duvoisin and Yahr[45] described adult achondroplastic dwarfs with slowly progressive neurologic deficit; some had long-standing thoracolumbar kyphosis and a mixed picture of spinal cord and cauda equina compression. One who had a straight spine had symptoms of multiple root involvement.

The pelvic changes are of great biologic importance, since they are responsible for the inability of female achondroplastics to deliver without expert help. These changes were described by Porak in 1889[25] and particularly by Breus and Kolisko,[46] who distinguished between a generally reduced ("Grazer") pelvis and the more typical form with kidney-shaped inlet, anteroposterior contraction, reduced ilium, prominent promontorium but almost normal pubic bone. The important defect is the narrowness of the pelvic inlet. Caffey[5] described the characteristic features of the achondroplastic pelvis of children as seen in roentgenograms. He, too, stressed the marked deficiency of the ilium, which is devoid of the portion normally seen below the posteroinferior spine. The greater sciatic notches are reduced to narrow clefts and the acetabular angles are small. The sacrum is narrow. The extremities are short and deformed by various curvatures. With the arms hanging at the sides, the fingertips usually do not reach below the major trochanter of the femur. The shortening is more marked in the proximal than in the distal tubular bones (rhizomelia). The wrists and ankles often are prominent owing to terminal spread of the bones of the forearm and leg. The hands and feet are short and broad. Sometimes there is a divergence of the third and fourth fingers whereby a "trident" hand is formed. Coxa vara frequently is present and the feet are turned inward, which explains the waddling gait so characteristic of achondroplasia. Owing to osseous and cartilaginous deformities, the movements in some joints, particularly the elbow, are impaired; in others, abnormal movements that permit the performance of contortions and stunts are possible. This and the powerful development of their muscles enable some of these dwarfs to act as circus acrobats. Langer *et al.*[47] analyzed roentgenograms of 101 individuals with achondroplasia ranging from newborn to old age and found little variability in the roentgenographic manifestations of this disorder. It is clear that those who establish rules about inclusion and exclusion of cases will find little variations in those

Fig. 83-6.—Achondroplastic boy with large head.

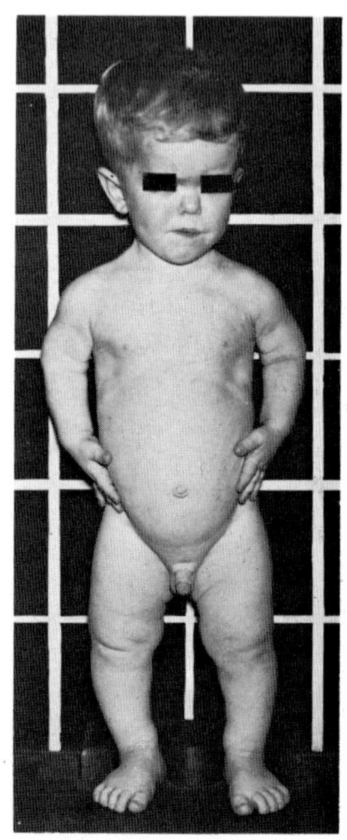

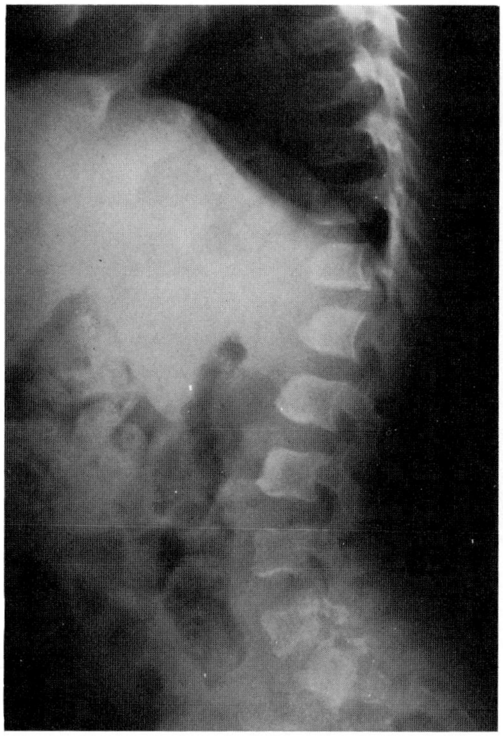

Fig. 83-7 (left).—Spine of an achondroplastic girl, 1½ years of age. Note enlarged intervertebral spaces, concavity of posterior outlines of vertebrae and triangular anterior edges and short pedicles.

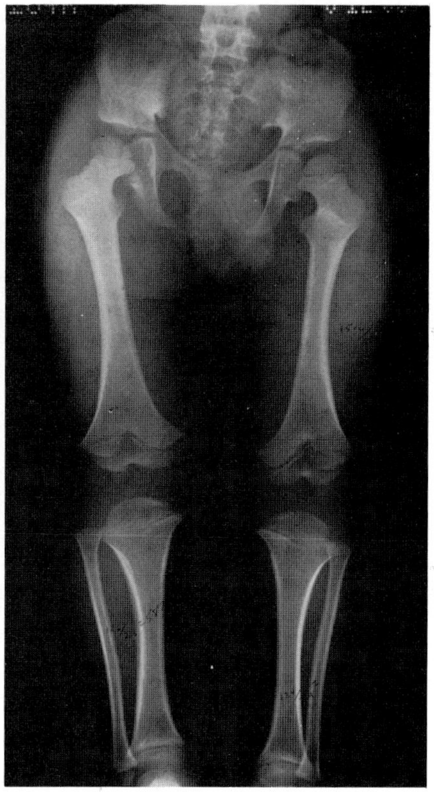

Fig. 83-8 (right).—Pelvis and lower extremities with achondroplastic changes in a boy 5½ years of age.

cases they choose to include in their classification. Since Parrot[1] did not have x-rays at his disposal, one wonders whether all his cases would have been included by Langer *et al.*[47] There seems to be some difference of opinion of the frequency of hydrocephaly in achondroplasia between Parrot[1] and Langer *et al.*[47] The findings of Cohen *et al.*[44] suggest variability of this complication.

The endocrine glands usually are normal, but disturbances have been observed occasionally in achondroplastics. The genitals are normal in function and size, although the male organs sometimes appear relatively large. In Mørch's[3] Danish series, 11 of 30 men were married, but only 1 of 24 women had found a (achondroplastic) husband. Murdoch *et al.*[6] reported on 57 marriages of achondroplastics. Twenty-three of these were married to achondroplastics, whereas the remaining 34 were married to persons with another type of dwarfism or to normal individuals. The 23 couples of which both mates were achondroplastic had a total of 23 children, 7 of whom were normal and 9 were living achondroplastic dwarfs. Seven of the achondroplastic children had died in infancy. Parturition is difficult.[50] The literature reviewed by Guldberg and Mørch[48] showed that of 76 pregnancies, 52 terminated in cesarean section, which was performed in some women repeatedly and usually successfully. In most cases, deliveries per vagina ended with the death of the child and sometimes with the death of the mother. The 76 pregnancies resulted in 78 children, of whom 23 were achondroplastic and 25 normal. Data were not available for the remainder of the children. In the series of Murdoch *et al.*,[6] 8 female achondroplastics had normal mates; of 5 children from these marriages 4 were achondroplastic and 1 was normal.

Delivery in normal women carrying achondroplastic children usually is normal but it can be complicated because of the large head of the child. In Mørch's series,[3] hydramnios was recorded in only 3 of 105 cases, whereas in Stevenson's[4] hospital series, 4 of 9 pregnancies were complicated by hydramnios. Of 3 pregnancies mentioned by Zellweger and Taylor,[31] 2 were associated with hydramnios.

Achondroplasia may occur in association with other congenital anomalies. Microcephaly, highly arched and cleft palate, defective ears, cervical cysts, hypoplastic lungs, spina bifida, clubfeet, umbilical and inguinal hernia, polycystic kidneys and hypospadias have been observed.[13] Hypothyroidism, precocious puberty and obesity may complicate achondroplasia. Some of these associations have been observed re-

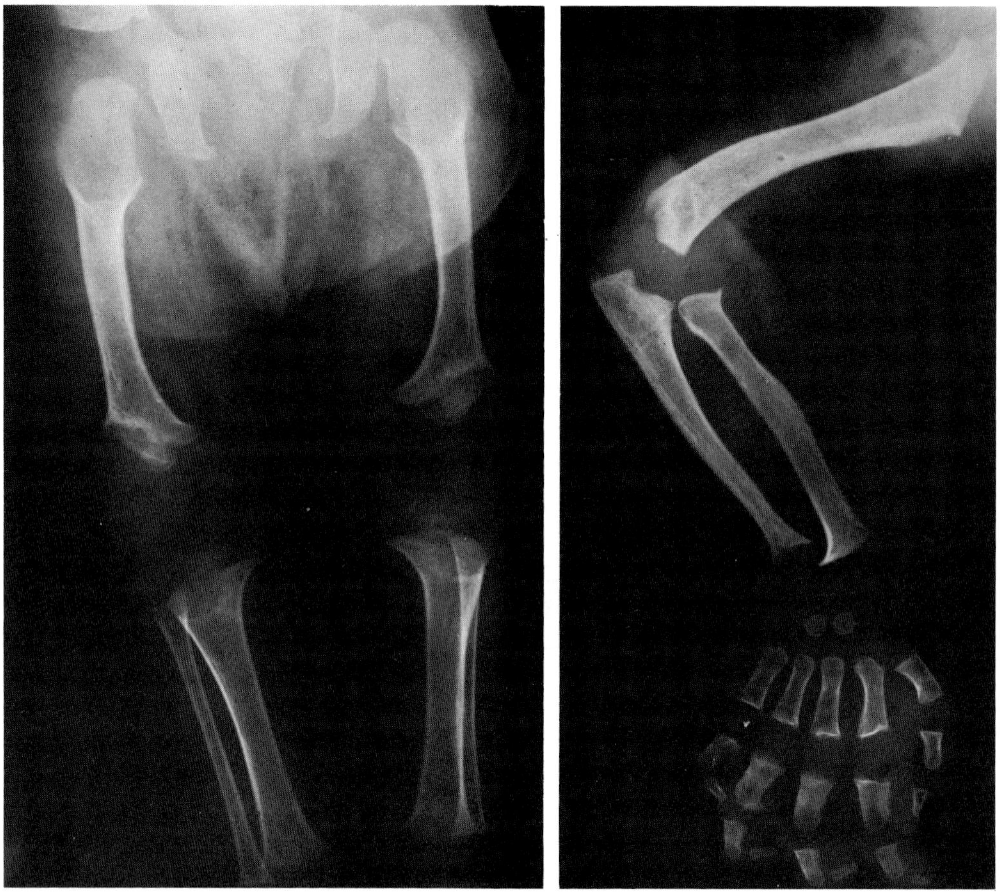

Fig. 83-9.—Roentgenograms of an achondroplastic girl.

peatedly and have become constituents of specific syndromes, e.g., diastrophic dwarfism; others still await classification.

The mentality of achondroplastic dwarfs usually is normal. They have a reputation of being witty and entertaining. In the past, they were in great demand at the courts of Europe and many were employed as court jesters; others were capable of achievement above the average. There also are reports of mentally deficient achondroplastics and of behavioral problems in some cases. In the large Danish series, the mental development of the survivors was essentially normal, their disposition well balanced and their emotional reactions adequate.

Although achondroplastic dwarfs usually can be recognized at a glance, they do not represent as uniform a disease picture as is generally assumed. Mørch,[3] who examined 86 achondroplastics in Denmark, emphasized and illustrated the variability of many symptoms. He found that very severe degrees of shortening of the extremities may be seen in persons with normal heads and facial features. On the other hand, characteristic frontal bossing, retraction of the root of the nose and projection of the lower jaw occurred in patients with moderate shortening of the extremities. The skin was redundant in some achondroplastics and adequate in others. There were variations in the shape of the pelvis and of the spine. The hands sometimes showed slightly shortened fingers or the severely deformed "main en trident." The legs were straight or the patients had bowlegs or knock-knees. There was and is justification and need for establishing valid subgroups, and a number of disease pictures previously confused with achondroplasia already have been separated from the classic form. They are discussed in subsequent pages. Such micromelic dwarfs as those affected by rickets or osteogenesis imperfecta are easily distinguished from achondroplasia, but severe hypophosphatasia (Chapter 92) has been mistaken for achondroplasia in the newborn, since the extremities may be markedly shortened while the head appears large. However, the bones show x-ray changes resembling rickets, the skull bones are not ossified and the phosphatase activity of the serum is very low. Since manifestations of hypophosphatasia may appear in families of apparently normal (heterozygous) parents more than once, it is possible that some pedigrees recorded in the literature showing more than one severe and lethal case of "achondroplasia" in families of normal parents may actually represent pedigrees of hypophosphatasia. Other pedigrees of this type may refer to disorders discussed in Chapters 85 and 86.

Achondroplastic dwarfs who survive the first year often enjoy good general health and their mental development is satisfactory but their growth is slow, and their height rarely exceeds 140 cm. (55 in.). The average height for Danish male achondroplastics was 130 cm. and that of females 124 cm. In the United States, Murdoch *et al.*[6] found a mean adult height of 129 cm. (51.8 in.) for the male and 122 cm. (48.6 in.) for female achondroplastics. Height of the parents did not significantly influence the adult height of the sporadic achondroplastics.

If a eugenic prognosis must be given, it should be based on the assumption that the condition is inherited as a dominant and that the dwarf is heterozygous for the abnormal trait. If he marries a person who is normal, the children will have only a 1:1 chance to be normal. I observed an achondroplastic girl who had normal parents, 4 normal brothers and an otherwise negative pedigree. When she grew up, she married a normal man, but her first child was an achondroplastic (Fig. 83-10). Zellweger and Taylor[31] mentioned an achondroplastic dwarf whose parents, 5 brothers and 3 sisters were normal. Yet, his first child with a normal young woman was an achondroplastic dwarf. Such persons with negative pedigrees can be the first result of a mutation and transmit the disorder to some of their children. The prognosis is further dimmed in achondroplastic women by their inability to deliver children without surgical intervention. In a family in which achondroplasia is inherited dominantly, the members who are normal in appearance and on roentgenogram examination should be considered free of the trait and their eugenic prognosis be favorable. In such cases, a marriage to a normal person should result in normal children, but this prediction must be qualified. Particular caution is advisable for persons who have not been examined by a counselor, since they may have the disorder in a mild form not recognized by the laymen (reduced expressivity). I once met a man short in stature – but not dwarfed – who had peculiar hands with short fingers reminiscent of achondroplasia. I learned later that he had a dwarfed achondroplastic son. Mørch[3] mentioned that the father of an achondroplastic dwarf had multiple cartilaginous exostoses but was otherwise normal. Whether there was a connection between these two dominantly heritable diseases or whether there was a chance association cannot be decided without further observations. For a person with one of the recessively inherited chondrodystrophies, the genetic prognosis should be more favorable, since he should have normal children with a normal mate.

Fig. 83-10. – Beginning of an achondroplastic pedigree, originating with a "sporadic" case. A girl, the only affected member of a healthy family, passed the disorder on to her son.

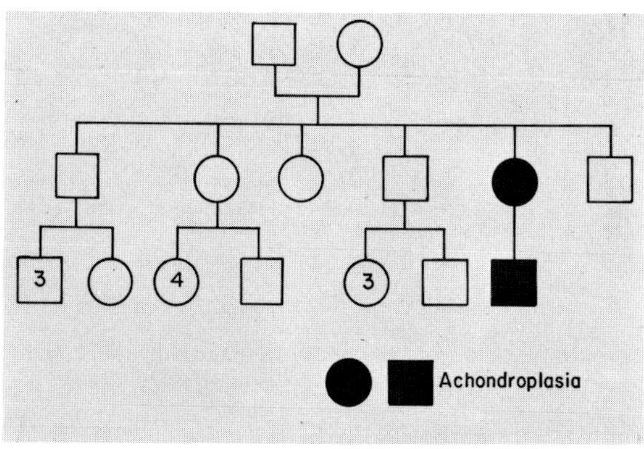

What are the chances for subsequent children in a family into which an achondroplastic is born if the parents, the preceding siblings, the ancestors and collaterals are normal? Such "sporadic" cases usually are considered the result of a new mutation. One may be inclined to assume that the chance for a second mutation of this type is zero and give the normal parents a favorable prognosis for their subsequent children. In most instances, such a prognosis will be correct, but there are families on record[13] in which more than one achondroplastic was born to phenotypically normal parents. The explanation for such repetition is not clear. A recessive gene, or a dominant mutant distributed through a portion of the germinal tissue of one of the parents (gonadal mosaicism), or presence of the disorder in subclinical form in one parent could be held responsible. Whatever the cause, the prognosis cannot be absolutely favorable in such cases.

No specific treatment is known for this disorder. Adequate nutrition, prevention of rickets and early orthopedic corrections of developing deformities can improve the child's appearance to a certain extent. Progressive neurologic deficit and disability can be avoided by early recognition and surgical decompression of encroaching bony structures. Correction of kyphosis of achondroplastic dwarfs who appear to be particularly prone to spinal cord compression syndromes may have prophylactic value.[45]

Human growth hormone given to 2 boys in relatively large doses for 1 or 2 years resulted in an increased growth rate but not in "cure" of the dwarfism.[49] It remains to be seen what the effects of growth hormone will be when it is administered from birth on in large amounts.

Much can be done to develop the abilities of such children, although they are severely handicapped by the shortness and deformity of their extremities. The main aim of their upbringing should be to render them as useful to society as possible. In the past, they often were trained to perform in circuses as acrobats, clowns or athletes, but experience showed that such occupations were not likely to give them emotional

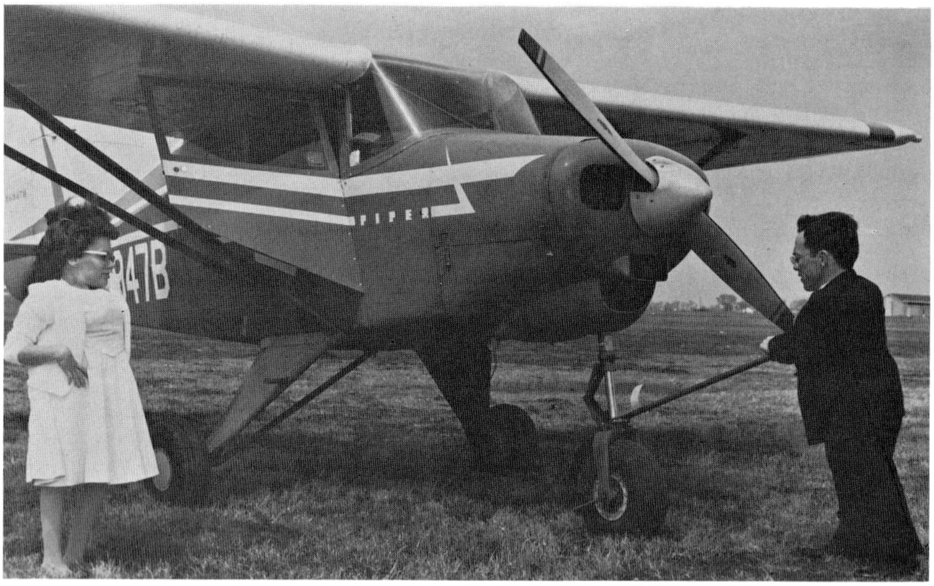

Fig. 83-11. – This picture illustrates better than words the potentials of persons with short stature. Mr. Lee Kitchens, a very successful engineer, is President of Human Growth Foundation, an organization dedicated to research in the processes of growth, and Past President of Little People of America, Inc., an organization devoted to the social development of people of short stature. Both Mr. and Mrs. Kitchens, although chondrodystrophic, pilot their own airplane without difficulty.

stability or permanent satisfaction; alcoholism and suicide were not rare in such circus dwarfs.

In a highly differentiated society such as ours it should be possible to find useful occupations for achondroplastic dwarfs. They are capable of doing many routine tasks in industry and occasionally are superior in certain jobs. Dwarfs have been employed successfully in the manufacture of airplanes, where they are able to work in places inaccessible to taller persons. They have been employed as prompters in theaters, where they can be comfortable in a small prompter box. Mørch's[3] study showed that in Denmark, of 39 men, 28 were usefully employed as artisans, tradesmen or clerks. But of 38 women, only 9 got along fairly well, whereas the majority remained untrained. The mental and artistic faculties of intelligent achondroplastics should be developed. In the past, many of them have made significant contributions as writers, painters, jewelers, linguists and musicians. Today, there exist many more specialties in which the brain rather than the length of the extremities counts. If an achondroplastic dwarf can be made useful or outstanding in his profession, many of his psychologic and emotional difficulties can be relieved.

Fortunately, progress has been made in this respect as the attitude of the general public has been changed through enlightenment about the causes of dwarfism and recognition of the mental abilities of many of the dwarfs. The "little people" themselves have formed organizations such as Little People of America, Inc., and Human Growth Foundation, which help to educate the dwarfs and the general public; they encourage and support each other as well as research in growth and growth retardation. One of the leaders in the movement is an outstanding engineer (Fig. 83-11); others hold posts such as vice-president of a paper company, controller for a food chain, accountants, teachers, businessmen, machinists, television repairmen, and so forth. Unfortunately, there are still many dwarfs who are unemployed or underemployed because of lack of education and training.[53] Education of the dwarfs and education of the general public can and will alleviate this situation.

REFERENCES

1. Parrot, M. J.: Sur la malformation achondroplastique et le dieu Ptah, Bull. Soc. Anthropol. Paris 1:296, 1878.
2. Kaufmann, E.: *Untersuchungen über die sogenannte fötale Rachitis (Chondrodystrophia foetalis)* (Berlin: Reimer, 1892).
3. Mørch, E. T.: *Chondrodystrophic Dwarfs in Denmark* (Copenhagen: Ejnar Munksgaard, 1941).
4. Stevenson, A. C.: Achondroplasia: An account of the condition in Northern Ireland, Am. J. Human Genet. 9:81, 1957.
5. Caffey, J.: Achondroplasia, in Brennemann, J. (ed.), *Practice of Pediatrics* (Hagerstown, Md.: W. F. Prior Company, 1948).
6. Murdoch, J. L., Walker, B. A., Hall, J. G., Abbey, H., Smith, K. K., and McKusick, V. A.: Achondroplasia – a genetic and statistical survey, Ann. Human Genet. 33: 227, 1970.
7. Maroteaux, P., and Lamy, M.: Le diagnostic des nanismes chondrodystrophiques chez les nouveau-nés, Arch. franç. pédiat. 25:241, 1968.
8. Keats, T. E., Riddervold, H. O., and Michaelis, L. L.:

Thanatophoric dwarfism, Am. J. Roentgenol. 108:473, 1970.
9. Wallace, D. C., Exton, L. A., Pritchard, D. A., Leung, Y., and Cooke, R. A.: Severe achondroplasia: Demonstration of probable heterogeneity within this clinical syndrome, J. M. Genetics 7:22, 1970.
10. Meyer, R.: Hydrocephalus chondrodystrophicus mit Bemerkungen über den "Perioststreifen" bei Chondrodystrophie, Virchows Arch. path. Anat. 253:766, 1925.
11. Gruber, G. B.: Über einen akrocephalen Reliefschädel. Ein Beitrag zur Frage der partiellen Chondrodystrophie, Beitr. path. Anat. 97:9, 1936.
12. Welter, H.: Zur Frage des Hydrocephalus chondrodystrophicus congenitus, Beitr. path. Anat. 97:1, 1936.
13. Rischbieth, H., and Barrington, A.: Dwarfism, in *Treasury of Human Inheritance* (London: Dulau & Company, Ltd., 1912) Vol. 1, pts. VII and VIII.
14. Ruffer, M. A.: *Studies in the Palaeopathology of Egypt* (Chicago: University of Chicago Press, 1921).
15. Nachtsheim, H.: Erbpathologie des Stützgewebes der Säugetiere, in Bauer, K. H., Hanhart, E., Lange, J., and Just, G. (eds.), *Handbuch der Erbbiologie des Menschen* (Berlin: Julius Springer, 1940).
16. Stockard, C. R.: Inheritance of localized dwarfism and achondroplasia in dogs, Anat. Rec. 38:29, 1928.
17. Gardner, D. L.: Familial canine chondrodystrophia foetalis (achondroplasia), J. Path. & Bact. 77:243, 1959.
18. Pearce, L., and Brown, W. H.: Hereditary achondroplasia in the rabbit. III. Genetic aspects; general considerations, J. Exper. Med. 82:281, 1945.
19. Crary, D. D., and Sawin, P. B.: A second recessive achondroplasia in the domestic rabbit, J. Hered. 43:255, 1952.
20. Landauer, W.: Studies on the creeper fowl. III. The early development and lethal expression of homozygous creeper embryos, J. Genetics 25:367, 1932.
21. Hart, G. H., Guilbert, H. R., Wagnon, K. A., and Goss, H.: "Acorn calves": A nonhereditary congenital deformity due to maternal nutritional deficiency, Calif. Agric. Exper. Sta. Bull. 699:1, 1947.
22. Warkany, J., and Nelson, R. C.: Skeleton abnormalities induced in rats by maternal nutritional deficiency, Arch. Path. 34:375, 1942.
23. Landauer, W., and Dunn, L. O.: Studies on the creeper fowl. I. Genetics, J. Genetics 23:397, 1930.
24. Crew, F. A. E.: The significance of an achondroplasia-like condition met with in cattle, Proc. Roy. Soc., London 95: 228, 1923.
25. Porak, C.: De l'achondroplasie, Nouv. Arch. Obst. et gynec. 4:551, 1889.
26. Grebe, H.: Gibt es eine recessiv erbliche Chondrodysplasie (Chondrodystrophia foetalis, Achondroplasie)?, Ztschr. Kinderh. 71:473, 1952.
27. Helweg-Larsen, H. F., and Mørch, E. T.: Chondrodistrofi hos to Søskende med Normale Foraeldre, Nord. med. 43: 180, 1950.
28. Lamy, M., and Maroteaux, P.: *Les Chondrodystrophies Génotypiques* (Paris: L'Expansion Scientifique Francaise, 1960).
29. Silverman, F. N.: A differential diagnosis of achondroplasia, Radiol. Clin. North America 6:223, 1968.
30. Kozlowski, K., Maroteaux, P., Silverman, F., Kaufmann, H., and Spranger, J.: Classification des dysplasies osseuses, Ann. radiol. 12:965, 1969.
31. Zellweger, H., and Taylor, B.: Genetic aspects of achondroplasia, Journal-Lancet 85:8, 1965.
32. Lapage, C. P.: Mongolism and achondroplasia in twin brothers, Proc. Roy. Soc. Med. 27:115, 1933.
33. Sommer, A., and Eaton, A. P.: Achondroplasia and Down's syndrome, J. Med. Genetics 7:63, 1970.
34. de Groot, J. W. C.: Two atypical cases of chondrodysplasia, J. Pediat. 39:715, 1951.
35. Ferguson-Smith, M. A.: Chromosomes and Human Disease, in Steinberg, A. G. (ed.), *Progress in Medical Genetics* (New York and London: Grune & Stratton, Inc., 1961).
36. Meyenburg, H.: Über chondrogene Skeletterkrankungen, Schweiz. med. Wchnschr. 68:57, 1938.
37. Potter, E. L., and Coverstone, V. A.: Chondrodystrophy fetalis, Am. J. Obst. & Gynec. 56:790, 1948.
38. Bleyer, A.: Role of advancing maternal age in causing achondroplasia, Am. J. Dis. Child. 58:994, 1939.
39. Penrose, L. S.: Parental age in achondroplasia and mongolism, Am. J. Human Genet. 9:167, 1957.
40. Rimoin, D. L., Hughes, G. N., Kaufman, R. L., Rosenthal, R. E., McAlister, W. H., and Silberberg, R.: Endochondral ossification in achondroplastic dwarfism, New England J. Med. 283:728, 1970.
41. Kaufmann, E.: *Pathology for Students and Practitioners* (Philadelphia: The Blakiston Company, 1929).
42. Potter, E. L.: *Pathology of the Fetus and Newborn* (Chicago: Year Book Medical Publishers, Inc., 1952).
43. Dennis, J. P., Rosenberg, H. S., and Alvord, E. C., Jr.: Megalencephaly, internal hydrocephalus and other neurological aspects of achondroplasia, Brain 84:427, 1961.
44. Cohen, M. E., Rosenthal, A. D., and Matson, D. D.: Neurological abnormalities in achondroplastic children, J. Pediat. 71:367, 1967.
45. Duvoisin, R. C., and Yahr, M. D.: Compressive spinal cord and root syndromes in achondroplastic dwarfs, Neurology 12:202, 1962.
46. Breus, C., and Kolisko, A.: *Die pathologischen Beckenformen* (Wien u. Leipzig: F. Deuticke, 1900).
47. Langer, L. O., Baumann, P. A., and Gorlin, R. J.: Achondroplasia, Am. J. Roentgenol. 100:12, 1967.
48. Guldberg, E., and Mørch, E. T.: Chondrodystrophia foetalis, unter besonderer Berücksichtigung von Geburt und Beckenform, Acta obst. et gynec. scandinav. 21:232, 1941.
49. Escamilla, R. F., Hutchings, J. J., Li, C. H., and Forsham, P.: Achondroplastic dwarfism – effects of treatment with human growth hormone, California Med. 105:104, 1966.
50. Tyson, J. E., Barnes, A. C., McKusick, V. A., Scott, C. I., and Jones, G. S.: Obstetric and gynecologic considerations of dwarfism, Am. J. Obst. & Gynec. 108:688, 1970.
51. Kaufman, R. L., Rimoin, D. L., McAlister, W. H., and Kissane, J. M.: Thanatophoric dwarfism, Am. J. Dis. Child. 120:53, 1970.
52. Ponseti, I. V.: Skeletal growth in achondroplasia, J. Bone & Joint Surg. 52-A: 701, 1970.
53. Kitchens, L.: Personal communication.

84

Atypical Chondrodystrophies I

(Transmitted Like Dominant Hereditary Traits)

IT IS UNDERSTANDABLE that with the discovery of roentgen rays, growth retardations and dwarfism of many types were subjected to renewed analyses, and it was soon discovered that not all dwarfs formerly considered achondroplastic had identical roentgenograms. In addition, it was found that many persons of reduced stature had osseous changes that radiologically resembled in some parts those thought to be characteristic of achondroplasia but differed from them in other parts. Thus, during the past 50 years, a large number of cases have been described by surgeons, orthopedists, pediatricians, internists, pathologists, anthropologists, geneticists and roentgenologists according to the interests of their specialties in a variety of journals and languages with—to put it mildly—confusing results. The names applied to these atypical chondrodystrophies are so numerous that it is almost impossible to mention all of them. They usually have a nucleus made up of "chondro" or "osteo" preceded by prefixes ("a-" or "dys-") and adjectives relating to localization ("epiphyseo-," "metaphyseo-," "diaphyseo-"), distribution ("generalisata," "multiplex," "partial," "systemic"), time of appearance ("congenita," "tarda") or to background ("familial," "hereditary"), terminating finally with various suffixes ("-pathia," "-plasia," "-trophia," "-itis" or "-osis"). It can be seen that by combination and permutation one can arrive at many terms that sound extremely scientific but often are so complicated and devoid of meaning that they hardly can be remembered by anybody except the author. Even *he* may have difficulties at times, as seen by changes suggested by some writers within a few years. The drab picture sometimes is made more colorful by addition of eponyms, which, if melodious, make the disease picture more distinct and alluring. The results of these semantic exercises are, of course, distressing, though understandable. Morphologic examinations and classifications have different results if they are made by inspection, tape measure, roentgen rays or microscope. Etiologic classification, which is needed, is possible only in a limited number of disorders.

Thus, one "familial osseous dystrophy" is now a well-circumscribed disorder known as "Morquio disease" (Chapter 88). A condition once named "dysostosis multiplex," a vague term applicable to any chrondrodystrophy, has become gargoylism (Hurler syndrome) and has been subdivided according to histopathologic changes and chemical findings. Other atypical chondrodystrophies such as the Ellis-van Creveld syndrome or chondrodystrophia calcificans congenita (Chapter 85) have achieved independent status with known hereditary transmission. Unfortunately, familial occurrence—or its absence—does not always reveal etiologic derivation; association with malformations of other organ systems does not always occur. Biochemical differentiation of skeletal disorders is still in the initial stage. The chief confusion still exists in the large group of mild and transitional forms, which do not show characteristic distinguishing signs. Patience will be needed before a satisfactory classification, and terminology will be found for them. In the meantime, it may be advisable to improve descriptions and investigate etiologies but declare a moratorium on fabrication of new names on purely morphologic grounds for disorders of cartilage and bone until a classification based on etiologic and pathogenetic differences becomes possible.

REFERENCES

1. Cocchi, U.: Polytope erbliche enchondrale Dysostosen, Fortschr. Geb. Röntgenstrahlen 72:409, 1950.
2. Hobaek, A.: *Problems of Hereditary Chondrodysplasias* (Oslo: Oslo University Press, 1961).
3. Lamy, M., and Maroteaux, P.: *Les Chondrodystrophies Génotypiques* (Paris: L'Expansion Scientifique Française, 1961).
4. Rubin, P.: *Dynamic Classification of Bone Dysplasias* (Chicago: Year Book Medical Publishers, Inc., 1964).
5. Bergsma, D. (ed.): *Skeletal Dysplasias*, Birth Defects: Original Article Series, Vol. V, Part IV (New York: The National Foundation, 1969).
6. Wiedemann, H-R.: *Dysostosen* (Stuttgart: Gustav Fischer, 1966).

Hypochondroplasia

THERE ARE MILD FORMS of achondroplasia, which have been called "hypochondroplasia." There are no definite changes in the skull and manifestations are mild in the tubular bones and in the pelvis. The disorder usually is not recognized at birth. Although most of the cases described were sporadic,[1] transmission from a mother to 2 of her children has been described.[2] Since it is admitted that transitional and mixed forms exist[1] and since the etiology seems to be the same as that of achondroplasia, hypochondroplasia can hardly be considered an entity of its own. Publications of cases of "semichondroplasia," "sesquichondroplasia," etc., must be expected but they will hardly make great contributions to the field.

REFERENCES

1. Kozlowski, K., and Zychowicz, C.: Hypochondroplasie, Fortschr. Geb. Röntgenstrahlen 100:529, 1964.
2. Kozlowski, K.: Hypochondroplasia, Polish Rev. Radiol. & Nuclear Med. 29:450, 1965.

Peripheral Chondrodysplasia

BRAILSFORD[1] described chondrodystrophic changes limited to the distal portions of the extremities, i.e., the hands and feet. In mild cases, the anomalies can be limited to a few phalanges. Cohen and van Creveld[2] reported the case of a boy who had short and stubby hands with transverse lines in both palms. The feet showed short toes. But the length of the arms and legs appeared normal in relation to the rest of the body. The metacarpals and phalanges were short in roentgenograms but radius, ulna and humerus were of normal length and slender. Movements in the elbow joints were somewhat limited. The situation was similar in the lower extremities, where the bones of the feet were shortened. The boy was "pug-faced" like an achondroplastic with a deep root of the nose and protruding nostrils.

REFERENCES

1. Brailsford, J. F.: *The Radiology of Bones and Joints* (4th ed.; Baltimore: The Williams & Wilkins Company, 1948).
2. Cohen, P., and van Creveld, S.: Peripheral dysostosis, Brit. J. Radiol. 36:761, 1963.

"Pseudoachondroplasia"

(Spondylo-Epiphyseal Dysplasia)

AMONG the newly established subgroups of achondroplasia is one that is characterized by a normal face and delayed manifestation. In 1943, Grebe and Weisswange[1] distinguished between a "pug" and a "dachshund" type of achondroplasia. More recently, it was found that the "dachshund" type with normal facial features at birth appears normal on inspection, as symptoms are not noted until the children are several years of age. Then a waddling gait and growth retardation become noticeable. Roentgenograms reveal irregularities in the epiphyseo-metaphyseal areas with fragmentation of the epiphyseal ossification centers (which is not seen in typical achondroplasia). The ends of the shafts of the tubular bones are flaring. In the pelvis, the sacro-iliac notches are less reduced in size than in the typical form. The spine can be deformed by scoliosis owing to irregularities of the vertebral bodies. The ribs are expanded at the sternal ends. Roentgenograms of the skull are normal. Dominant inheritance has been observed.[2,6]

It is possible that this form of achondroplasia is a clinical and genetic entity, but it is also possible that transitional forms exist and that the delineation from achondroplasia is not sharp. In one case of Ford *et al.*[2] it was noticed that the child was short when she was 7 months of age and another one of their patients showed a "pug" nose. Variations of vertebral anomalies in familial cases are not rare.[3] Thus, it remains to be seen whether the pseudoachondroplastic form can be clearly distinguished from the classic form. Both forms are dominant traits. Association of spondylo-epiphyseal dysplasia with high myopia, retinal detachment, cataracts, buphthalmos and blindness has been described.[5]

The term "spondylo-epiphyseal dysplasia,"[4] now widely accepted by roentgenologists, is unfortunate, since Morquio disease, a recessive trait, has been presented as the prototype of spondylo-epiphyseal dysplasias. In genetic transmission and external appearance, pseudoachondroplasia resembles the typical achondroplasia much more than Morquio disease. Roentgenologically, pseudoachondroplasia may ap-

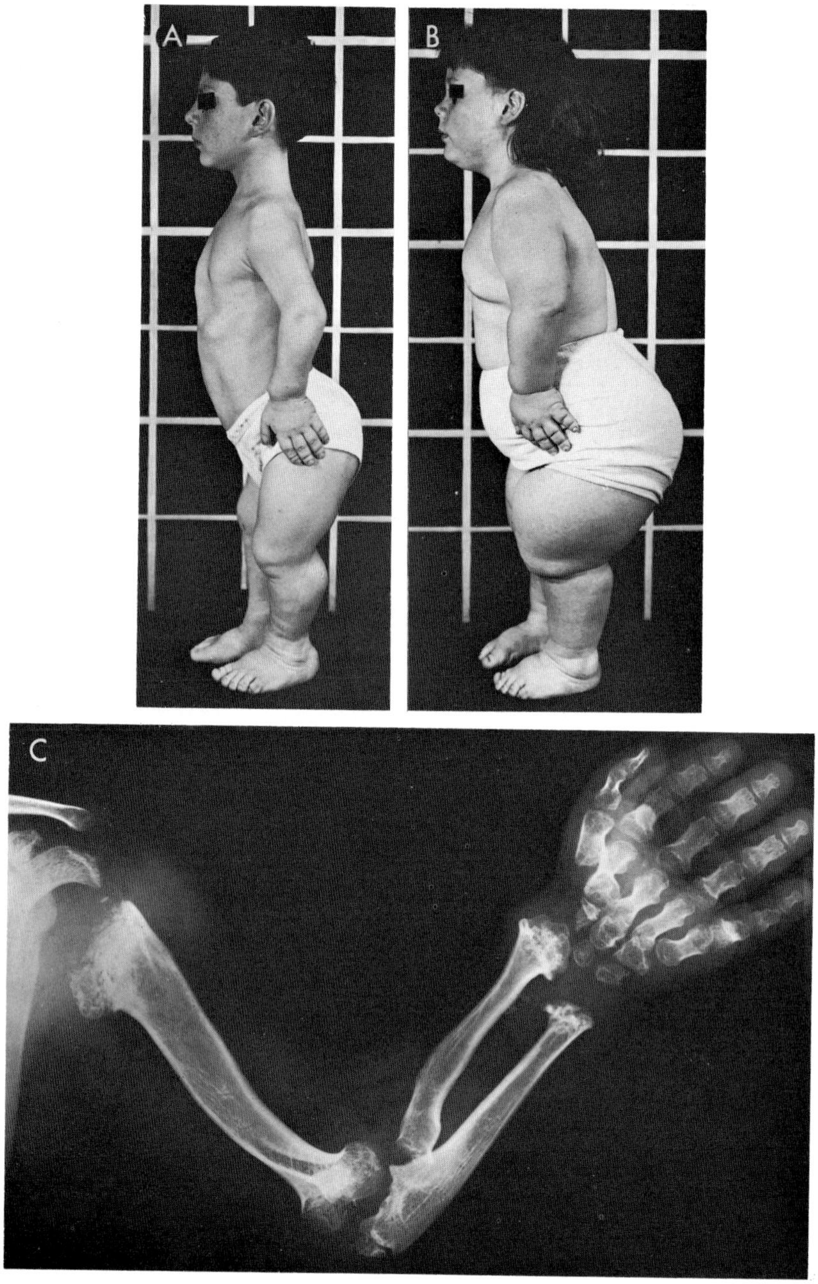

Fig. 84-1. – **A** and **B,** chondrodystrophic siblings, children of a chondrodystrophic father and a normal mother. These children show intrafamilial variability of the disease picture. The brother's face is free of achondroplastic features but the sister's face has some achondroplastic characteristics. This condition is now named spondylo-epiphyseal dysplasia (pseudoachondroplasia).[2] **C,** arm of the male patient showing epiphyseal dysplasia.

pear to be a mild form of Morquio disease,[4] but classification according to genetic behavior seems more advisable. It may be best to speak of an achondroplasia with normal face and late onset and to avoid the term spondylo-epiphyseal dysplasia.

REFERENCES

1. Grebe, H., and Weisswange, W. M. H.: Die Chondrodysplasie (Chondrodystrophia foetalis) und verwandte Systemerkrankungen im Röntgenbild, Fortschr. Geb. Röntgenstrahlen 67:25, 1943.

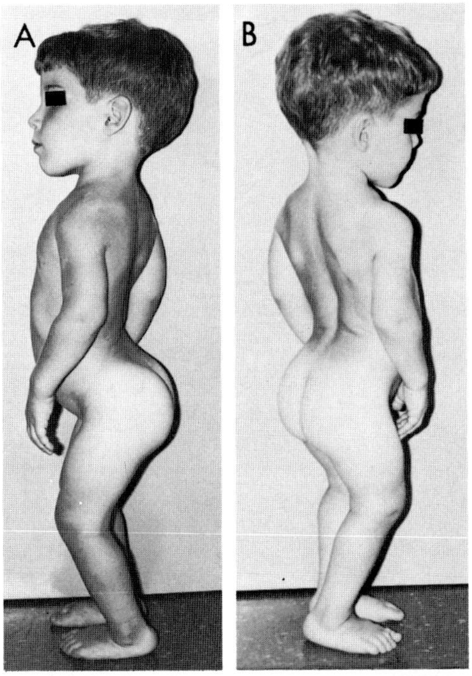

Fig. 84-2. – **A** and **B,** boy, 4 years of age with normal head and chondrodystrophic appearance. His skeletal disorder was not noticed until he was 2 years of age. **C** and **D,** roentgenograms of upper and lower extremities. **E,** spine. At present, the boy is classified as pseudoachondroplastic with spondylo-epiphyseal dysplasia because of his normal facial features and late development of deformities. Yet, the epiphyses seen in **C** and **D** do not show serious epiphyseal changes. The case illustrates that intermediary forms occur that do not conform to present classifications.

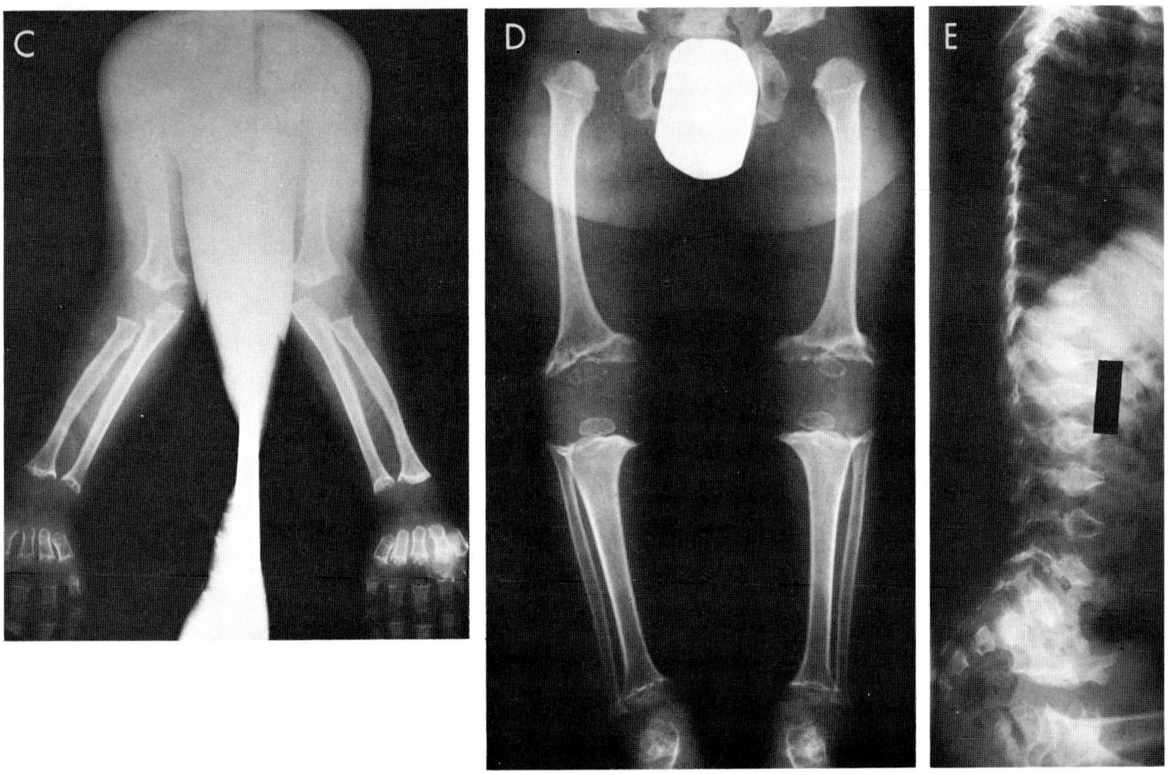

2. Ford, N., Silverman, F. N., and Kozlowski, K.: Spondylo-epiphyseal dysplasia (pseudo-achondroplastic type), Am. J. Roentgenol. 86:462, 1961.
3. Lamy, M., and Maroteaux, P.: *Les Chondrodystrophies Génotypiques* (Paris: L'Expansion Scientifique Française, 1961).
4. Maroteaux, P., and Lamy, M.: Les formes pseudo-achondroplastiques des dysplasies spondylo-epiphysaires, Presse méd. 67:383, 1959.
5. Fraser, G. R., Friedmann, A. I., Maroteaux, P., Glen-Bott, A. M., and Mittwoch, U.: Dysplasia spondyloepiphysaria congenita and related generalized skeletal dysplasias among children with severe visual handicaps, Arch. Dis. Childhood 44:490, 1969.
6. Diamond, L. S.: A family study of spondyloepiphyseal dysplasia, J. Bone & Joint Surg. 52-A: 1587, 1970.

Dysplasia Epiphysealis Multiplex

MØRCH[1] suggested that all cases of achondroplasia are due to a dominant gene that is responsible for all the severe forms of cartilaginous and osseous distortions resulting in the well-known picture of the achondroplastic dwarf. That this unitary theory is not entirely correct has been discussed before (p. 767). It is of interest that much milder forms of chondrodystrophy can also be attributed to dominant inheritance.

A condition that clinically resembles, in some respects, Parrot's achondroplasia and Morquio disease in others sometimes can be observed in two or three generations, transmitted by affected members to some of their offspring. As a rule, this disorder is not noticed at birth but manifests itself during the first few years of childhood and comes to a standstill after adolescence, resulting in variable degrees of reduction in height. In some instances, affected persons have only mild symptoms during childhood and appear externally almost normal as adults. In 1950, Cocchi[2] found in the literature only thirteen families with 42 affected members. Since then, additional families belonging in this category have been recorded under different labels,[3-7] but it seems likely that they represent merely a fraction of the cases attributable to a dominant gene.

To show how early such atypical forms of chondrodystrophy were recognized, the publication by Drysdale and Herringham[8] in 1908 deserves to be mentioned. The authors reported 3 sisters with "an undescribed form of dwarfism associated with a spatulate condition of the hands." The deformities developed late and were too mild to be classified in retrospect as Morquio disease. In 1912, Barrington-Ward[9] described double coxa vara and other mild deformities of late onset in a brother and sister. Dominant inheritance could not be recognized in these early familial cases. In 1912, Schorr[10] wrote about "chondrodystrophia congenita adolescentium sive tarda." It is unfortunate that "chondrodystrophia tarda" was not adopted as a provisional term, which would have been much more fitting for most of these cases of mild skeletal involvement than the complicated names suggested later.

In 1934, we (Warkany and Mitchell[11]) reviewed many cases of atypical chondrodystrophy that could be classified neither as achondroplasia nor Morquio disease and described a case of this type considered a "link" between the two disorders. The patient was a boy 12 years of age of Italian extraction. The father was of small stature. The parents were not consanguineous and none of the 9 children was known to be affected like the patient, who was the fifth child. The child's early development was normal. He could stand at 1 year but at the age of 2 years, when he started to walk, a peculiar waddling gait was noticed, and from that time his physical growth was retarded. From the age of 6 years he complained of pain in the feet and knees, and he was able to run only with considerable difficulty. At the age of 12 years his height was only 127 cm. (Fig. 84-3, *A*). He had a marked lordosis of the spine and the abdomen protruded. The skull appeared large in proportion to the rest of the body. The arms and legs were normal in length but the ends of the shafts were bulging. The hands were large and square and the fingers broad, especially at the terminal phalanges (Fig. 84-3, *B*). The arms could not be lifted above the level of the shoulder and extension and abduction of the thighs were limited. The hips and knee joints were enlarged and there was slight genu valgum. The feet were broad and flat. Roentgenograms revealed vertebral irregularities but there was no platyspondyly (Fig. 84-3, *C*). The epiphyses of the humerus appeared ragged and fragmented. Similar epiphyseal irregularities were seen in the other long bones of the body (Fig. 84-3, *D–G*). The carpal and tarsal ossification centers were small and irregular in outline. The shafts of the bones were affected relatively little but some abnormal bowing was seen in the roentgenograms of the humerus and the radius. Although this case was not included in the later literature under the title "dysplasia epiphysealis multiplex," it clearly belongs in this group of atypical chondrodystrophies as defined by Fairbank,[21] " . . . a rare congenital developmental error characterised by mottling or irregularity in density and outline of several of the developing epiphyses, dwarfism and stubby digits." Onset and course of the disease and (probable) inheritance from the father also agree with the diagnosis.

In the same year (1934), Jansen[12] reported a case of atypical chondrodystrophy that he considered a new osseous growth disturbance, a *metaphyseal* dysosto-

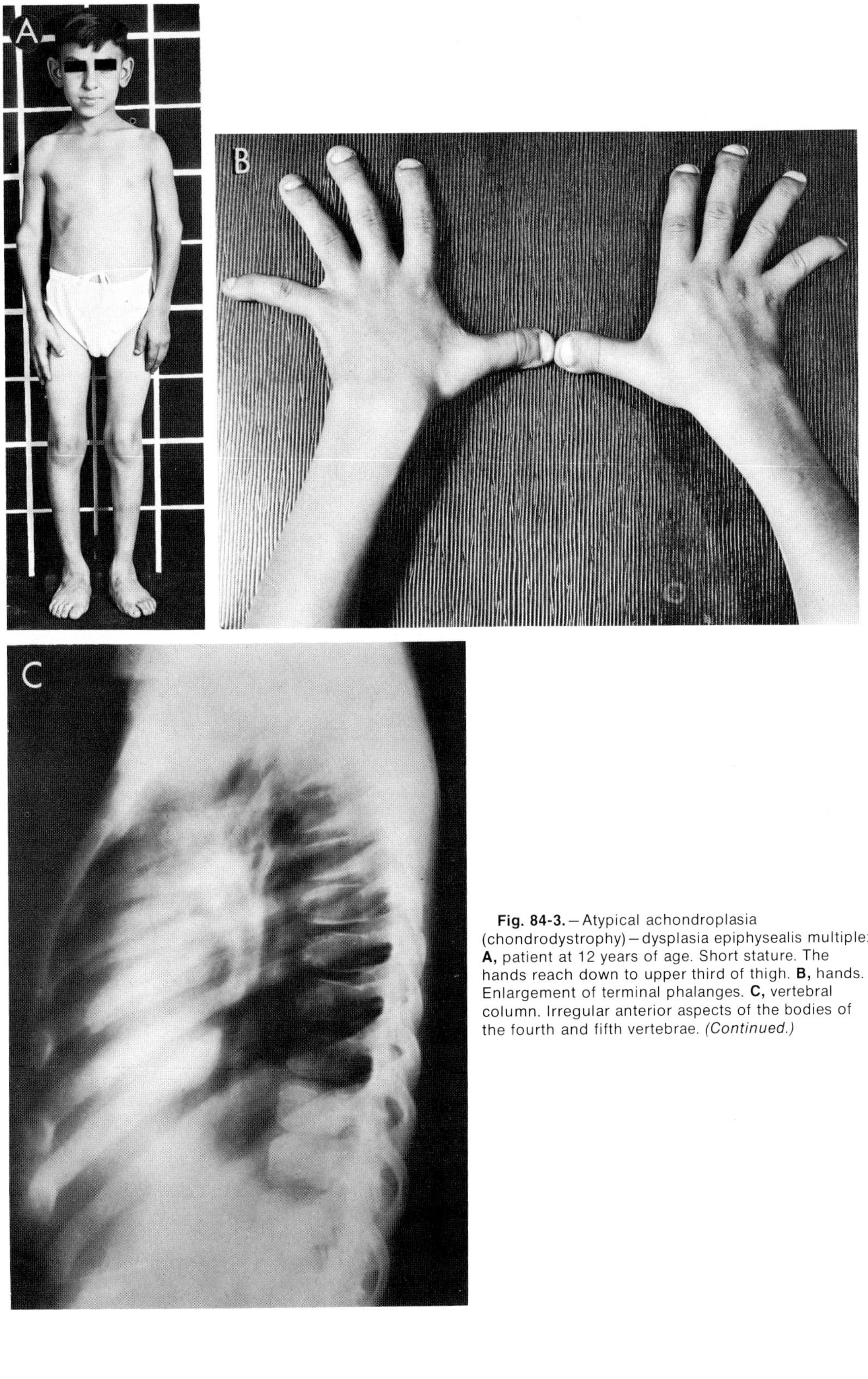

Fig. 84-3.—Atypical achondroplasia (chondrodystrophy)—dysplasia epiphysealis multiplex. **A,** patient at 12 years of age. Short stature. The hands reach down to upper third of thigh. **B,** hands. Enlargement of terminal phalanges. **C,** vertebral column. Irregular anterior aspects of the bodies of the fourth and fifth vertebrae. *(Continued.)*

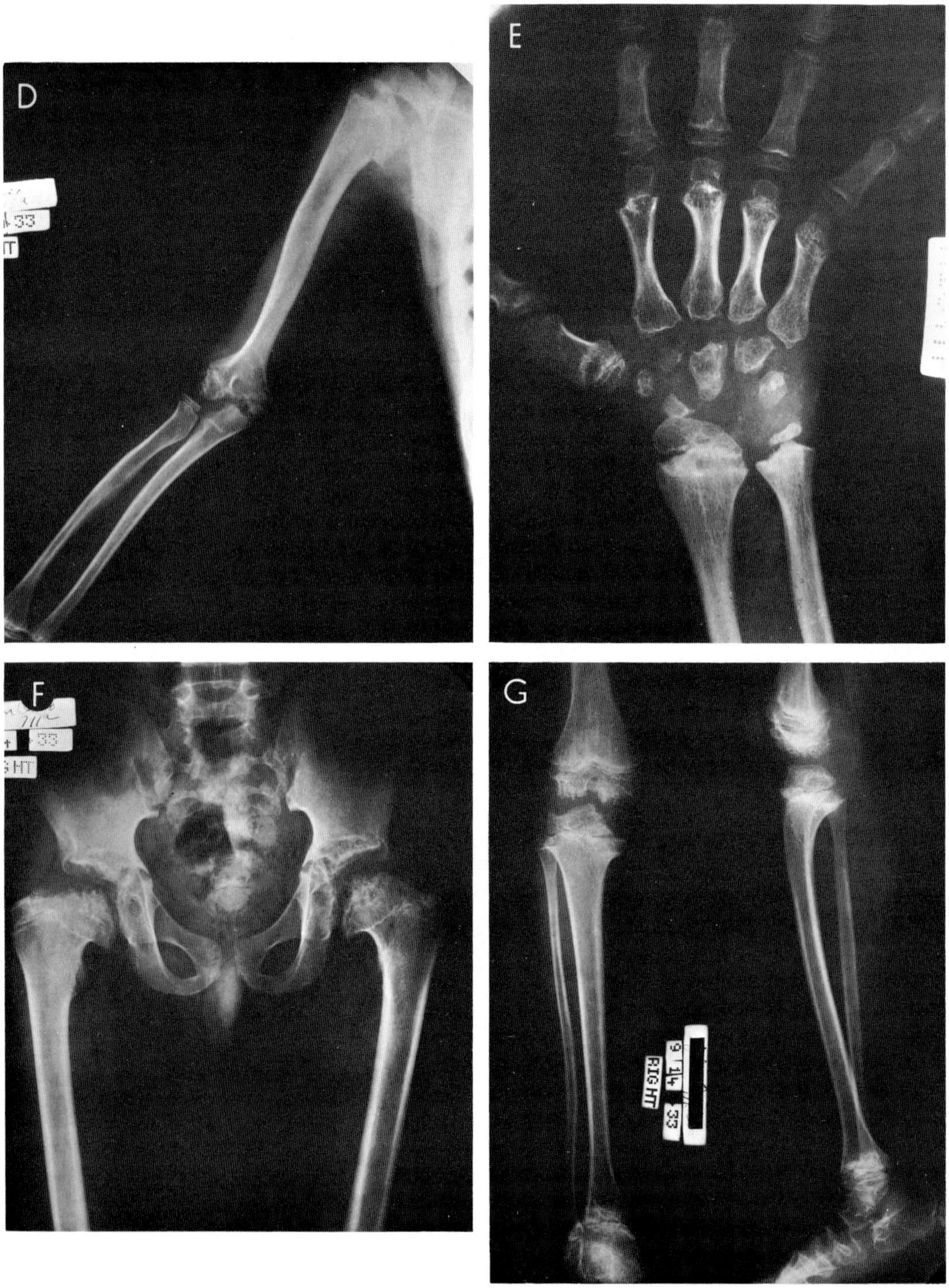

Fig. 84-3 (cont.). – **D,** right upper extremities. Irregular epiphyses of elbow joint. The forearm bones appear long and slender, differing from typical achondroplasia. **E,** right hand. Irregular epiphyses and carpal bones. **F,** the acetabulum is irregular in outline, the epiphysis of the head of the femur is not demonstrable, the outline of the femoral neck is irregular. **G,** right knee and lower leg. The distal epiphysis of the femur appears ragged and the proximal epiphysis of the tibia underdeveloped in its medial aspect. The shafts are long and slender.

sis (see Metaphyseal Dysostosis, p. 791). A case similar to ours was described in 1954 by Cameron *et al.*[13] in a Chinese boy and labeled "metaphyseal dysostosis." In 1937, Hirsch[14] reported the case of an affected mother and her 4 children. Wood and Robertson[15] and Resnick[16] added cases belonging to two generations, and later Fairbank[17] reviewed the literature and established the name "dysplasia epiphysealis multiplex," which has been widely accepted, particularly in the orthopedic and radiologic literatures, where a number of publications of such cases followed, once a label had been found.[18] Barrie *et al.*[6] gave clinical and radiographic descriptions of the disease and attempted a genetic analysis of the cases reported. According to them, all the known examples of the condition, with the exception of those reported by Waugh,[19] can be ascribed to dominant inheritance. Some of the best examples of this – in addition to the cases already mentioned – are a kinship reported by Maudsley[5] with 10 affected members in three generations, and Family A of Barrie *et al.*,[6] in which at least 9 affected persons could be found in three generations. In 1959, Lomas and Boyle[7] published a pedigree in which such an atypical chondrodystrophy occurred in three generations. Of 79 members, 31 were affected, males and females showing manifestations. Interestingly, all grades of the dystrophy were observed, from minor changes involving only the metacarpals, the phalanges or an isolated vertebra to "the florid picture as described by Morquio." The pedigree is a good example of dominant inheritance, although the authors, for unexplained reasons, attribute the disorder to a recessive factor. Concordance as well as discordance has been observed in twins.[14,16]

The disorder occurs in males and in females. The expression of the disease may vary, so that a person with mild manifestations can have severely affected children. This may explain exceptional families[9,19] in which several siblings have the disorder even though the parents appear normal but may have a "forme fruste." It seems probable that some of the so-called sporadic cases also may have a parent with reduced expression of the gene. Other sporadic cases – and there are many of these – could be explained by new mutations. However, such oversimplification may not be heuristic and it should be pointed out that even families showing clear dominant inheritance may exhibit different manifestations and present different entities. Thus, Maudsley[5] described intrafamilial resemblance but interfamilial differences. Barrie *et al.*[6] reported two families in which the disease led to dwarfism and disabling lesions, whereas in a third family the patients had normal height and minimal symptoms. These authors admit the possibility of at least two genetic entities. It would seem that there exists a whole series of dominantly inherited chondrodystrophies with variable manifestations ranging from typical chondrodystrophy (achondroplasia) over spondylo-epiphyseal pseudoachondroplasia[20] to dysplasia epiphysealis multiplex with many intermediate forms. Many show intrafamilial similarity but not necessarily strict identity.

As stated before, dominantly inherited forms of atypical chondrodystrophy show manifestations later than achondroplasia. Vertebral irregularities of ossification with anterior projections and minor wedge formation or biconcave deformity of the vertebral bodies[22] can be seen in roentgenograms. The extremities are characterized by distinct anomalies of the epiphyses, which become visible late in roentgenograms, appearing irregular in outline and ossification. Since the epiphyses show these roentgenographic changes during childhood, when the growth disturbance becomes manifest, they have been made the essential and principal sign of the disease picture by some observers. "Dysplasia epiphysealis multiplex"[17] and similar terms have been adopted, although a glance at roentgenograms shows that the metaphyses and the diaphyses of the affected bones are not spared (see Fig. 84-3, *G*). Thus, Cocchi[2] stated that according to published cases the diaphyses of the tubular bones usually are shortened and bent. Actually, the deformities of the shafts often can be seen in roentgenograms published by authors who stress only epiphyseal changes in the names proposed for the disease.[20,21] Roentgenograms of the usually short and squat hands show involvement of the diaphyses particularly well. The bones of the head and neck are little affected. As a result of these mild changes, the patients remain small but are not dwarfed as adults. There are minor deformities and disabilities but the muscle development and intelligence are normal.

The tibial growth plates of an amputated leg were found to be disorganized, with disordered cartilage cell columns, clefts and areas of degeneration in the matrix. Enchondral ossification was severely disturbed. Urinary mucopolysaccharides are within normal limits.[22]

Osteoarthritis is a frequent complication, beginning as a rule in early adult life. Severe hip involvement may cause difficulty in childbirth.[6]

Physiotherapy was recommended by Barrie *et al.*,[6] who believed that it can prevent disability. Nonweight-bearing exercises are thought to prevent muscular wasting and delay osteoarthritis. Orthopedic treatment and surgery are required in some cases.

REFERENCES

1. Mørch, E. T.: *Chondrodystrophic Dwarfs in Denmark* (Copenhagen: Ejnar Munksgaard, 1941).
2. Cocchi, U.: Polytopic hereditary enchondral dysostoses, Fortschr. Geb. Röntgenstrahlen 72:409, 1950.
3. Turpin, R., and Coste, F.: La polyostéochondrite, Semaine hôp. Paris 34:234, 1958.
4. Jackson, W. P. U., Albright, F., Drewry, G., Hanelin, J., and Rubin, M. I.: Metaphyseal dysplasia, epiphyseal dysplasia, diaphyseal dysplasia, and related conditions. I. Familial metaphyseal dysplasia and craniometaphyseal dysplasia; their relation to leontiasis ossea and osteopetrosis; disorders of bone remodeling, A.M.A. Arch. Int. Med. 94:871, 1954.

5. Maudsley, R. H.: Dysplasia epiphysialis multiplex; report of 14 cases in 3 families, J. Bone & Joint Surg. 37-B:228, 1955.
6. Barrie, H., Carter, C., and Sutcliffe, J.: Multiple epiphysial dysplasia, Brit. M. J. 2:133, 1958.
7. Lomas, J. J. P., and Boyle, A. C.: Osteochondrodystrophy (Morquio's disease) in three generations, Lancet 2:430, 1959.
8. Drysdale, J. H., and Herringham, W. P.: An undescribed form of dwarfism associated with a spatulate condition of the hands, Quart. J. Med. 1:193, 1908.
9. Barrington-Ward, L. E.: Double coxa vara with other deformities occurring in brother and sister, Lancet 1:157, 1912.
10. Schorr, G.: Chondrodystrophie adolescentium s. tarda, Mitt. Grenzgeb. Med. Chir. 25:54, 1912.
11. Warkany, J., and Mitchell, A. G.: Atypical chondrodystrophy, J. Pediat. 4:734, 1934.
12. Jansen, M.: Über atypische Chondrodystrophie (Achondroplasie) und über eine noch nicht beschriebene angeborene Wachstumsstörung des Knochensystems: Metaphysäre Dysostosis, Ztschr. Orthop. Chir. 61:253, 1934.
13. Cameron, J. A. P., Young, W. B., and Sissons, H. A.: Metaphyseal dysostosis: Report of a case, J. Bone & Joint Surg. 36-B:622, 1954.
14. Hirsch, I. S.: Generalized osteochondrodystrophy. The eccentrochondroplastic form, J. Bone & Joint Surg. 19-A: 297, 1937.
15. Wood, B. G., and Robertson, E. G.: Morquio's type of osteo-chondro-dystrophy in father and son, the father also suffering from Parkinson's disease, Roy. Melbourne Hosp. Clin. Rep. 14:78, 1943.
16. Resnick, E.: Epiphyseal dysplasia punctata in mother and identical male twins, J. Bone & Joint Surg. 25-A:461, 1943.
17. Fairbank, T.: Dysplasia epiphysialis multiplex, Brit. J. Surg. 34:225, 1947.
18. Leeds, N. E.: Epiphysial dysplasia multiplex, Am. J. Roentgenol. 84:506, 1960.
19. Waugh, W.: Dysplasia epiphysialis multiplex in 3 sisters, J. Bone & Joint Surg. 34-B:82, 1952.
20. Maroteaux, P., and Lamy, M.: Les formes pseudo-achondroplasiques des dysplasies spondylo-épiphysaires, Presse méd. 67:383, 1959.
21. Fairbank, H. A. T.: *An Atlas of General Affections of the Skeleton* (Edinburgh and London: E. & S. Livingstone, Ltd., 1951).
22. Hunt, D. D., Ponseti, I. V., Pedrini-mille, A., and Pedrini, V.: Multiple epiphyseal dysplasia in two siblings. Histological and biochemical analyses of epiphyseal plate cartilage in one, J. Bone & Joint Surg. 49-A:1611, 1967.

Madelung Deformity and Familial Dyschondrosteosis

MADELUNG,[1] in 1878, described a deformity that presents as a spontaneous volar subluxation of the hand and is due to a growth disturbance of the distal end of the radius. It is likely that the anomaly had been described before by Malgaigne[2] in 1854 and that it is merely a conspicuous part of a generalized skeletal anomaly, later named "dyschondrosteosis" by Léri and Weill.[3] But Madelung is credited with the first clear description and definition of the deformity of the hand and his name has become identified with the anomaly. Externally, there is a bayonet-like volar displacement of the dorsum of the hand against the forearm, which exhibits a dorsal prominence of the styloid process of the ulna and bowing of the radius in the ulnar direction. Abduction of the hand in the radial direction is markedly limited but ulnar abduction is possible. The dislocation of the ulna can be reduced without difficulty but not maintained in proper position. A good review on Madelung deformity was written in 1938 by Anton *et al.*[4]

In roentgenograms, one sees bowing of the radius toward the ulna and bowing of the radius in a dorsovolar plane with a volar concavity. Thus, the distal articular surface of the radius is directed in an ulnar and palmar direction. The radial epiphysis is triangular, with the apex pointing toward the ulnar side, which adds to the curving of the radial distal end. The interosseous space between the radius and ulna is widened. The lunate bone is displaced toward the radius and is crowded between the distal ends of the two forearm bones. The proximal row of carpal bones appears angulated, with the lunate bone at the apex of the angle. On the ulnar border of the radius there often is an area of rarefaction but the ulnar epiphysis shows increased density. The palmar bending of the distal end of the radius leads to a subluxation of the radio-ulnar articulation, so that the distal end of the ulna is seen in lateral views dorsal to the radial end.[5] At the ulnar edge of the radius, a small spur may be noticed projecting into the interosseous space.[5,6]

Madelung deformity is bilateral in 75% of the cases and sometimes is congenital. But pain and weakness are not often disturbing before adolescence, when the anomaly becomes manifest in most cases. There is a predilection of 4:1 for females.[5] The disorder is transmitted like a dominant trait and it has been reported to occur in six generations.[7]

Madelung deformity may occur in the aforementioned more generalized skeletal disorder called "dyschondrosteosis" by Léri and Weill.[3] These authors described a dwarfed woman with proportions of mild achondroplasia or hypochondroplasia. Skull and face appeared normal but the trunk showed a mild scoliosis. The extremities were quite short, the proximal and distal long bones being almost equally shortened. The radius and the carpal bones had the characteristics of Madelung deformity. Kaplan and others[8] reported dyschondrosteosis in a mother and in her daughter. The mother's father, his sister and his father apparently were affected by the same growth disturbance, including Madelung deformity. Herdman *et al.*[9] suggested that Madelung deformity and dyschondrosteosis are manifestations of the same condition. They, as well as Becker,[10] pointed out that in this disorder

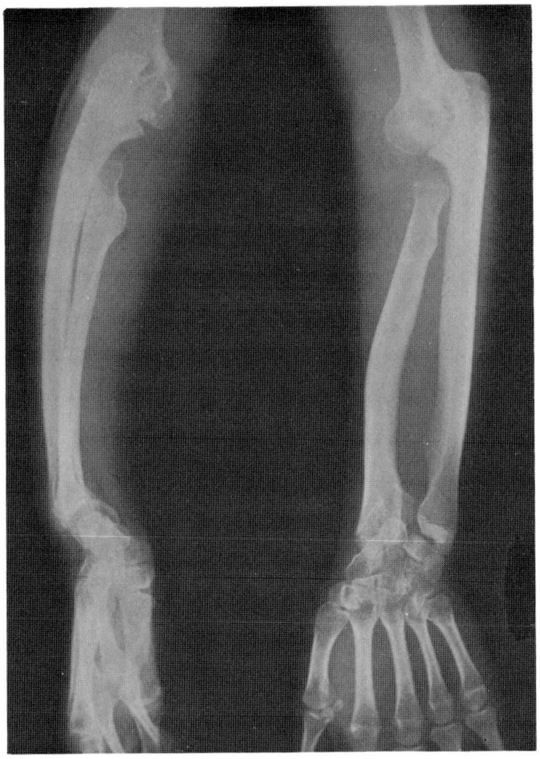

Fig. 84-4.—Dyschondrosteosis (Léri-Weill) with Madelung deformity.

the forearms and the lower legs are more shortened than the upper segments of the extremities, a condition called mesomelia. Thickening of the long bones, metacarpals and phalanges, cubitus valgus and coxa valga, exostoses and scoliosis also occur in such patients. Dyschondrosteosis, like Madelung deformity, is a dominantly inherited trait with variable expressivity. Thus, the wrist deformity may be little developed in some patients and the mesomelic growth retardation not be obvious in others. Such variations can occur in members of the same pedigree.[9] The deformities seem to be less expressed in males than in females.

REFERENCES

1. Madelung: Die spontane Subluxation der Hand nach vorne, Verhandl. deutsch. Gesellach. Chir. 7:259, 1878.
2. Malgaigne: Mémoires sur les luxations de la partie supérieure du radius compliquées de fractures du cubitus, Rev. méd. chir. Paris 15:213, 1854.
3. Léri, A., and Weill, J.: Une affection congénitale et symétrique du développement osseux: La dyschondrostéose, Bull. Soc. méd. hôp. Paris 53:1491, 1929.
4. Anton, J. I., Reitz, G. B., and Spiegel, M. B.: Madelung's deformity, Ann. Surg. 108:411, 1938.
5. Dannenberg, M., Anton, J. I., and Spiegel, M. B.: Madelung's deformity. Consideration of its roentgenological diagnostic criteria, Am. J. Roentgenol. 42:671, 1939.
6. Cocchi, U.: Hereditary Diseases with Bone Changes, in Schinz, H. R., Baensch, W. E., Friedl, E., and Uehlinger, E. (eds.), *Roentgen-Diagnostics* (New York: Grune & Stratton, Inc., 1951).
7. Paus, B.: *Madelung's Deformity* (Oslo: Norske Vid. Akad., 1942).
8. Kaplan, M., Guy, E., and Cantagrel, A.: Dyschondrostéose familiale, Presse méd. 59:1723, 1951.
9. Herdman, R. C., Langer, L. O., and Good, R. A.: Dyschondrosteosis, J. Pediat. 68:432, 1966.
10. Becker, P. E.: Ein weiterer Fall von Dyschondrosteose (Léri-Weill), Humangenetik 1:563, 1965.

Metaphyseal Dysostosis

IN SOME PERSONS of small stature and bowlegs, growth disturbances are noted in roentgenograms in the area of the metaphyses of tubular bones. Changes may be mild and simulate rickets[1] or be severe and deforming. Sometimes, if both epiphyses and metaphyses are abnormal, the disorder is not clearly distinguishable from epiphyseal dysostosis. Thus, the case of Cameron *et al.*[2] showed involvement of the entire ends of the long bones, but was classified as metaphyseal dysostosis. In other cases, the epiphyses were little affected.[3,4] In young children, the metaphyses show cupping, fraying and irregular ossification. Bowing of the ends of the shafts leads to coxa vara, genu varum and other deformities, so that rickets is simulated. Since antirachitic treatment does not give prompt results and transmission through two or more generations may be observed, vitamin D-resistant rickets often is suspected and metabolic studies are made. However, no chemical abnormalities usually associated with rickets and no renal abnormalities have been discovered.[4] Whatever the underlying process, it can be passed on like a dominant hereditary trait. Transmission through four generations has been reported.[3,5] Such hereditary cases may be mild and manifest themselves merely in short stature[6] or bowlegs (Fig. 102-7) or they can be so severe that they result in disproportionate dwarfism.[3] A case published by Jansen[7] in 1934 was re-examined by de Haas *et al.*[8] 34 years later. Normal osseous structures were associated with marked deformity and dwarfism. The joint surfaces remained intact. A syndrome of metaphyseal dysostosis, exocrine pancreatic insufficiency, neutropenia and dwarfism has been described.[9] It was stated that this syndrome, after cystic fibrosis of the pancreas, seems to be the most frequent form of exocrine pancreatic insufficiency in children. Recessive autosomal inheritance has been assumed.[9] There is, of course, no reason why the metaphyses should not be involved by recessively inherited traits. "New metaphyseal dysplasias" that probably are recessively inherited are becoming known.[10, 11]

REFERENCES

1. Schmid, F.: Beitrag zur Dysostosis enchondralis metaphysaria, Monatsschr. Kinderh. 97:393, 1949.
2. Cameron, J. A. P., Young, W. B., and Sissons, H. A.: Metaphyseal dysostosis: Report of a case, J. Bone & Joint Surg. 36-B:622, 1954.
3. Lenk, R.: Hereditary metaphyseal dysostosis, Am. J. Roentgenol. 76:569, 1956.
4. Evans, R., and Caffey, J.: Metaphyseal dysostosis resembling vitamin D-refractory rickets, A.M.A. J. Dis. Child. 95:640, 1958.
5. Stickler, G. B., Maher, F. T., Hunt, J. C., Burke, E. C., and Rosevear, J. W.: Familial bone disease resembling rickets (hereditary metaphysial dysostosis), Pediatrics 29:996, 1962.
6. Kozlowski, K.: Metaphyseal dysostosis; report of five families and two sporadic cases of a mild type, Am. J. Roentgenol. 91:602, 1964.
7. Jansen, M.: Über atypische Chondrodystrophie (Achondroplasie) und über eine noch nicht beschriebene angeborene Wachstumsstörung des Knochensystems Metaphysäre Dysostosis, Ztschr. Orthop. Chir. 61:253, 1934.
8. de Haas, W. H. D., de Boer, W., and Griffioen, F.: Metaphysial dysostosis, J. Bone & Joint Surg. 51-B:290, 1969.
9. Schmerling, D. H., Prader, A., Hitzig, W. H., Giedion, A., Hadorn, B., and Kühni, M.: The syndrome of exocrine pancreatic insufficiency, neutropenia, metaphyseal dysostosis and dwarfism, Helvet. paediat. acta 24:547, 1969.
10. Kozlowski, K., and Sikorska, B.: Dysplasia metaphysaria, Typ Vaandrager-Penna, Ztschr. Kinderh. 108:165, 1970.
11. Wiedemann, H-R., and Spranger, J.: Chondrodysplasia metaphysaria (Dysostosis metaphysaria)–ein neuer Typ[2], Ztschr. Kinderh. 108:171, 1970.

Micromelia with Hypoplasia of Ulna and Fibula

BRAILSFORD[1] described 4 siblings with short arms and legs with hypoplastic ulnae and fibulae. The head was normal. The parents were small but well proportioned. A similar case was reported by Böök.[2] The boy's parents were related members of a kinship in which 21 persons in four generations were small in stature, having short limbs and digits. This moderate reduction in height apparently is transmitted as a dominant trait. In heterozygotes, the condition is harmless and not incapacitating, but in homozygotes dwarfism and micromelia with hypoplastic ulnae and fibulae result. The disorder appears as a "recessive" micromelic dwarfism with hypoplasia of ulna and fibula.[3] Another symmetric distal limb deformity with marked shortening of ulna and fibula in siblings was reported by Blockey and Lawrie.[4] Although radius and tibia were also deformed, they were affected less than their postaxial fellows.

REFERENCES

1. Brailsford, J. F.: Dystrophies of the skeleton, Brit. J. Radiol. 8:533, 1935.
2. Böök, J. A.: A clinical and genetical study of disturbed skeletal growth (chondro-hypoplasia), Hereditas 36:161, 1950.
3. Lenz, W.: Anomalien des Wachstums und der Körperform, in Becker, P. E. (ed.), *Humangenetik* (Stuttgart: Georg Thieme, 1964), Vol. II.
4. Blockey, N. J., and Lawrie, J. H.: An unusual symmetrical distal limb deformity in siblings, J. Bone & Joint Surg. 45-B: 745, 1963.

Dwarfism with Medullary Stenosis of Tubular Bones and Transitory Tetany

CAFFEY[1] described a mother and her son who were affected by proportionate dwarfism and transitory hypocalcemia. The mother had 1 normal son; one pregnancy was terminated during the seventh month by cesarean section, which yielded a dead anencephalic female. In both mother and son there was congenital stenosis of medullary spaces in tubular bones and in the calvaria. The diaphyses were reduced in width. There was no medullary stenosis in the epiphyseal ossification centers, round bones, flat bones of the shoulder girdle and pelvis or in the vertebrae. Hypocalcemic attacks of tetany occurred in both patients. The endocrine relationship of dwarfism, tetany and skeletal changes is not clear.

REFERENCE

1. Caffey, J.: Congenital stenosis of medullary spaces in tubular bones and calvaria in two proportionate dwarfs–mother and son; coupled with transitory hypocalcemic tetany, Am. J. Roentgenol. 100:1, 1967.

Benign Achondroplasias

Robinow *et al.*[1] described 4 cases of a dwarfing syndrome that resembles achondroplasia by brachymelia, depressed nose and bulging forehead present at birth but differs from it by mesomelic dwarfism, normal hands, orbital hypertelorism, widened palpebral fissures, dental malalignment and normal pelvic proportions allowing spontaneous vaginal deliveries by affected female persons. The disorder is not progressive and does not cause ill health. Autosomal dominant inheritance has been established in a kinship in which six generations probably were affected. An epiphyseal dysostosis without dwarfism has been described as a dominantly inherited skeletal disorder.[2]

REFERENCES

1. Robinow, M., Silverman, F. N., and Smith, H. D.: A newly recognized dwarfing syndrome, Am. J. Dis. Child. 117:645, 1969.
2. Rennell, C., and Steinbach, H. L.: Epiphyseal dysostosis without dwarfism, Am. J. Roentgenol. 108:481, 1970.

85

Atypical Chondrodystrophies II

(Transmitted Like Recessive Hereditary Traits)

Chondroectodermal Dysplasia

(Ellis-van Creveld Syndrome)

This syndrome, established by Ellis and van Creveld[1] in 1940, had been described previously by McIntosh[2] in a single case. It is likely that the skeleton reproduced in Figure 85-1 is that of a child with this syndrome. The infant probably had chondrodystrophy and unusually pronounced polydactyly (one foot had nine toes!). This child was found drowned in the river in Amsterdam in 1668 and was dissected and described by the Dutch anatomist Frederic Ruysch.[1] The obligatory constituents of the Ellis-van Creveld syndrome are chondrodystrophy, ectodermal dysplasia and polydactyly. Congenital heart disease and other malformations frequently, but not always, are associated with this triad.

The condition has been observed repeatedly in siblings, children of apparently normal parents.[3-5] Males and females are affected equally. Consanguinity of parents was present in approximately a third of the reported cases. These circumstances strongly suggest inheritance of the disorder as an autosomal recessive. The mother of the child shown in Figure 85-2 had 3 normal children before the patient was born. Subsequently, she had 2 stillborn children and 1 child with polydactyly. The syndrome has been described in many nationalities, with cases occurring in Caucasians as well as in Negroes.[6]

In one case,[7] necropsy showed that the rows of columnar cartilage maintained their parallel arrangement, although there was some disorder of ossification. Mitchell and Waddell[4] found the number of cartilage cells decreased and the columnar arrangement abortive. The epiphyseal line was irregular and showed reduced capillary invasion of the cartilaginous plate. Many types of congenital heart disease have been observed (see below).

In the newborn, the diagnosis can be made by observation of shortening of the extremities, absence or hypoplasia of nails and polydactyly (see Fig. 85-2). Some of the children, particularly those with severe congenital heart disease, succumb soon after birth. Others survive and show good vitality and adequate mental development.

The shortening of the extremities in survivors usu-

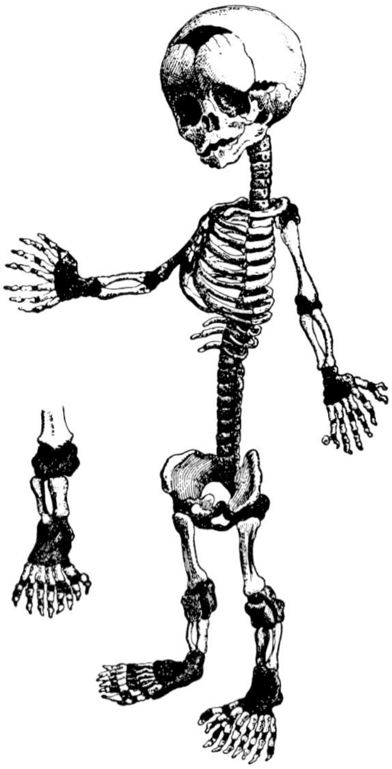

Fig. 85-1.—Skeleton of a polydactylous dwarf found drowned in 1668 in Amsterdam. (From Gould and Pyle, *Anomalies and Curiosities of Medicine*, Philadelphia, 1897. Reproduced with permission of W. B. Saunders Company.)

ally is less pronounced than in typical achondroplasia, the fingertips reaching below the trochanteric region. The extremities show progressive shortening in the proximo-distal direction, which also differs from typical achondroplasia. The head and trunk are of normal size, so that reduction in body length is due to reduction in length of the lower extremities, to genu valgum and to bowing of the bones of the legs. The hands are characterized by polydactyly, sometimes combined with syndactyly, by short and broad fingers and by underdeveloped nails. Seven fingers on the left hand were observed in the patient of Weiss and Crosett.[8] The extra finger is always on the ulnar side. Polydactyly of the feet can occur, but it is rare. The nails often are friable and sometimes distally thickened. The hair may be well developed but alopecia has been observed occasionally.

The shape of the head usually is normal. Strabismus, colobomas of the iris and cataracts have occurred. A pigment ring around the optic disc has been seen in the fundus.[9] The middle portion of the upper lip sometimes is underdeveloped or notched, so that the patients give the impression of a repaired harelip. Harelip and cleft palate have been observed in rare instances.[4,10] A firm attachment of the upper lip to the gum, with loss of the upper vestibular sulcus has been described repeatedly. Teeth can be present at birth or they appear prematurely.[5] They are small, widely spaced and peg-shaped.

The cardiac anomaly, if present, manifests itself by precordial bulging of the chest wall or by murmurs. Various and sometimes severe types of congenital heart disease have been described in more than 50% of the published cases. Ventricular and atrial septal defects, single ventricle, single atrium, atrioventricularis communis, mitral and tricuspid valve defects, transposition of the great vessels, hypoplasia and coarctation of the aorta, patent ductus arteriosus, left superior vena cava and total anomalous venous drainage have been diagnosed by catheterization or necropsy.[6] The frequency of single atrium has been emphasized by Giknis.[11] The anomalies listed above can be found in various combinations. McKusick *et al.*[5] pointed out that, among survivors, congenital heart disease is less prevalent than one would assume from the literature.

The chest is long and narrow and, in this respect, resembles that of asphyxiating thoracic dystrophy (p. 795). Hypoplasia of the lungs and bronchomalacia[12] contribute to respiratory difficulties and early death in some cases.

Fig. 85-2.—This infant had chondrodystrophy, polydactyly and cyanotic congenital heart disease. He died soon after birth.

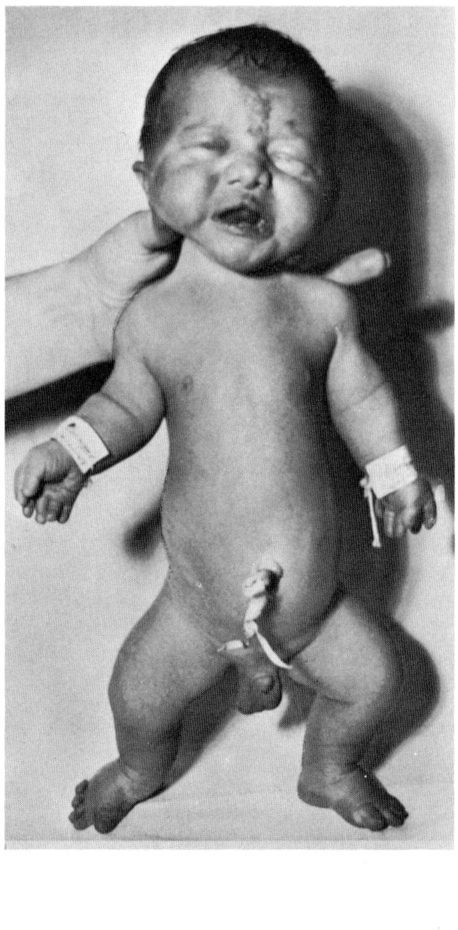

Hepatosplenomegaly has been described in a number of cases.[10] Hypoplastic genitalia, hypospadias and epispadias have been reported.[8] The skin usually is moist and sweat electrolytes are normal.[4]

Mental development of those surviving infancy has been good, with few exceptions. The patient of McIntosh,[2] who has been observed for many years, obtained a college degree[13]; another patient[10] apparently had above-average intelligence.

The radiologic manifestations have been described by Caffey.[13] All of the tubular bones in the extremities are short and thick. In contrast to typical achondroplasia, the shortening of the bones is progressively accentuated from the trunk to the distal phalanges in the Ellis-van Creveld syndrome. The proximal ends of the ulnae and the distal ends of the radii are enlarged, whereas the distal ends of the ulnae and the proximal ends of the radii are small. The proximal tibial metaphysis ends in a paramedian peak, from which a long lateral and a short medial slope descend. Over the short medial slope sits a hypoplastic epiphyseal ossification center. The patellae are normal. Genu valgum is the rule. In contrast to achondroplasia, the tibiae are longer than the fibulae. The hands often have sixth digits, which sit on the ulnar side of forked fifth metacarpals. The capitate and hamate bones are not separated. The acetabular cavities are hypoplastic and irregular in outline.

The outlook for life is poor in cases complicated by cardiac malformations. Survivors with good intelligence are handicapped by their short stature and the deformities of the fingers, which interfere with manual skill. The gait is impaired by changes in the hip joint. There are obvious dental and orthodontic problems.

If a child with chondroectodermal dysplasia is born to apparently healthy parents there is a 25% risk for another child of this type in each subsequent pregnancy. The Ellis-van Creveld syndrome is the most frequent type of dwarfism among the Amish of Lancaster County, Pennsylvania. McKusick *et al.*[5] identified 52 cases in 30 sibships. The incidence was about 5 per 1,000 births and the prevalence 2 per 1,000 living persons. The disorder was a cause of stillbirth and more than a third of the patients died before 2 weeks of age. No case of the syndrome was discovered among the Amish of Ohio or Indiana. It seemed that all the parents of the patients could be traced back to one couple who immigrated to the United States in 1744.

Removal of the sixth finger, orthopedic improvement of the deformities of the legs and dental care with orthodontic corrections are some of the medical measures required by these patients.

REFERENCES

1. Ellis, R. W. B., and van Creveld, S.: A syndrome characterized by ectodermal dysplasia, polydactyly, chondrodysplasia and congenital morbus cordis, Arch. Dis. Childhood 15:65, 1940.
2. McIntosh, R.: Diseases of the Teeth, in Holt, L. E., Jr., and McIntosh, R. (eds.), *Holt's Diseases of Infancy and Childhood* (10th ed.; New York: D. Appleton & Company, 1933), p. 362.
3. Metrakos, J. D., and Fraser, F. C.: Evidence for a hereditary factor in chondroectodermal dysplasia (Ellis-van Creveld syndrome), Am. J. Human Genet. 6:260, 1954.
4. Mitchell, F. N., and Waddell, W. W., Jr.: Ellis-van Creveld syndrome. Report of two cases in siblings, Acta paediat. 47:142, 1958.
5. McKusick, V. A., Egeland, J. A., Eldridge, R., and Krusen, D. E.: Dwarfism in the Amish. I. The Ellis-van Creveld syndrome, Bull. Johns Hopkins Hosp. 115:306, 1964.
6. Lynch, J. I., Perry, L. W., Takakuwa, T., and Scott, L. P.: Congenital heart disease and chondro-ectodermal dysplasia. Report of two cases, one in a Negro, Am. J. Dis. Child. 115:80, 1968.
7. Debré, R., Lamy, M., Minkowski, A., and Grumbach, R.: Syndrome d'Ellis-van Creveld chez un nouveau-né décédé le premier jour, Arch. franç. pédiat. 9:1055, 1952.
8. Weiss, H., and Crosett, A. D., Jr.: Chondroectodermal dysplasia—report of a case and review of the literature, J. Pediat. 46:268, 1955.
9. Rössler, H.: Beitrag zum Ellis-van Creveld-Syndrom, Neue Österr. Ztschr. Kinderh. 3:301, 1958.
10. Walls, W. L., Altman, D. H., and Winslow, O. P.: Chondroectodermal dysplasia (Ellis-van Creveld syndrome), A.M.A. J. Dis. Child. 98:242, 1959.
11. Giknis, F. L.: Single atrium and the Ellis-van Creveld syndrome, J. Pediat. 62:558, 1963.
12. Moore, T. C.: Chondroectodermal dysplasia (Ellis-van Creveld syndrome) with bronchial malformation and neonatal tension lobar emphysema, J. Thoracic & Cardiovas. Surg. 46:1, 1963.
13. Caffey, J.: Chondroectodermal dysplasia, Am. J. Roentgenol. 68:875, 1952.

Asphyxiating Thoracic Dystrophy of the Newborn

JEUNE *et al.*[1] described an atypical form of chondrodystrophy that chiefly involves the thorax and causes serious attacks of cyanosis and asphyxia. These authors observed a brother and sister born with a peculiarly shaped thorax with rib anomalies that interfered with normal respiration. The chest had a cylindrical shape and was narrow in its anteroposterior and transverse diameters but elongated in the craniocaudal direction. Radiograms showed the clavicles high at the level of the 6th cervical vertebra, and taking a horizontal course. The ribs were very short and their osseous parts terminated in the axillary line, rendering the thorax immobile.

Jeune *et al.*[1] believed that they were dealing with a forme fruste of chondrodystrophy. The hands of their patients were short and thick like those of achondroplastics and the sternum was protruding as in Morquio disease. In one case, there was hypotonia and

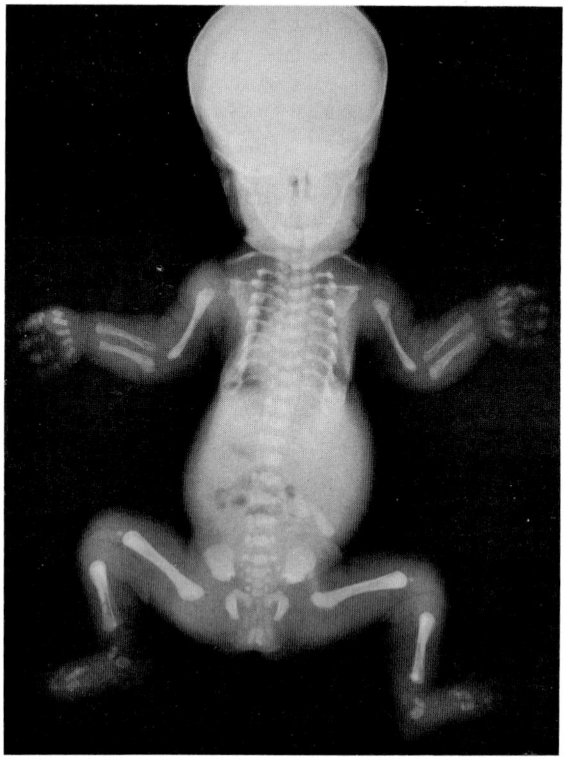

Fig. 85-3. – Roentgenogram of a newborn girl with asphyxiating thoracic dystrophy. Note short ribs, high clavicle and small pelvis with small sciatic notches. Two siblings of this child died in infancy, probably of the same disorder; they also had polydactyly. (Courtesy of Dr. J. C. Willke, Cincinnati, Ohio.)

atrophy of the muscles of the neck. The patients died when they were 13 and 8 months of age, respectively, of infections combined with respiratory difficulty and asphyxia.

The observations by Jeune *et al.*[1] were followed by reports cited by Pirnar and Neuhauser,[2] who observed and described 5 cases. In 1966, Sacrez *et al.*[3] reviewed 23 case reports and added 3 cases to the literature. Hanissian *et al.*[4] reported 4 children with this disorder belonging to two families. Two brothers were Negroes. In 1969, Combe *et al.*[7] reviewed 41 published cases. It seems that in this chondrodystrophy different parts of the fetal skeleton can be affected but the marked thoracic deformity is a constant finding in all the patients. The disturbed ossification in the costochondral junctions of the ribs results in a rosary and in underdeveloped, short, stubby ribs. The head and spine are normal. The extremities may be short and thick but much less so than in achondroplasia. Interestingly, polydactyly has been observed in several patients. The pelvis is very small and in roentgenograms the hypoplastic iliac wings appear square. Deep sciatic notches resemble those of achondroplasia, and ossification around the triradiate cartilages is irregular. Microscopic examination of the costochondral junctions done in one instance showed disorderly enchondral ossification. The proliferating cartilage was hyperplastic and very abundant. The zone of provisional calcification was limited and vessels penetrated it irregularly.

This chondrodystrophy resembles the Ellis-van Creveld syndrome in that it sometimes is associated with polydactyly. Appearance of the pelvis is quite similar in both disorders, but in the Ellis-van Creveld syndrome the involvement of the thorax is less pronounced whereas the long bones are more involved. But some authors consider the thoracic dystrophy a variant of the Ellis-van Creveld syndrome.[4]

Although these patients are prone to develop respiratory difficulties and pneumonia, which often terminate fatally at an early age, some children survive and show improvement of their respiratory functions and chest findings.[2] Some children, despite definite chest deformity, fail to develop respiratory difficulties. For that reason, the term "asphyxiating" thoracic dystrophy has been criticized and the name "infantile thoracic dystrophy" substituted.[4] Hypertension, renal failure and death from uremia have been described in several patients.[6]

Familial recurrence has been frequent. It is possible that in one family 4 siblings were affected.[3,5] The parents are always phenotypically normal. Parental consanguinity has not been recorded so far. Male and female patients have been described. It is quite likely that the trait is inherited as an autosomal recessive.

REFERENCES

1. Jeune, M., Beraud, C., and Carron, R.: Dystrophie thoracique asphyxiante de caractère familiale, Arch. franç. pédiat. 12:886, 1955.
2. Pirnar, T., and Neuhauser, E. B. D.: Asphyxiating thoracic dystrophy of the newborn, Am. J. Roentgenol. 98:358, 1966.
3. Sacrez, T., Levy, J-M., Halb, A., Korn, R., Stoebner (Mme.), Klein, F., and Beauvais, P.: La dystrophie thoracique asphyxiante, Pédiatrie 21:631, 1966.
4. Hanissian, A. S., Riggs, W. W., Jr., and Thomas, D. A.: Infantile thoracic dystrophy – a variant of Ellis-van Creveld syndrome, J. Pediat. 71:855, 1967.
5. Neimann, N., Manciaux, M., Rauber, G., Pernot, C., and Bretagne-de-Kersauson, M. C.: Dystrophie thoracique asphyxiante du nourrisson, Pédiatrie 18:387, 1963.
6. Herdman, R. C., and Langer, L. O.: The thoracic asphyxiant dystrophy and renal disease, Am. J. Dis. Child. 116: 192, 1968.
7. Combe, P., Michel, J., Fauchier, Cl., Régy, J-M., and Casenave, Cl.: La dystrophie thoracique asphyxiante, Ann. pédiat. 16:483, 1969.
8. Jequier, J-C.: La dystrophie thoracique asphyxiante, Arch. franç. pédiat. 27:177, 1970.

Cartilage-Hair Hypoplasia

PATIENTS with this disorder were considered achondroplastics in the past but are now recognized as dwarfs of a specific type. They are characterized by sparse and thin hair, normal cranium and face and normal spine. The tubular bones are short and their metaphyses enlarged. The disorder is transmitted as an autosomal recessive and may account for reports in the literature of achondroplasia with recessive inheritance (p. 773).

Cartilage-hair hypoplasia was discovered as a characteristic form of dwarfism among the Old Order Amish in the United States and Canada by McKusick *et al.*,[1] who ascertained 77 cases and estimated that the incidence was 1–2 per 1,000 live births in that religious group.

The patients are micromelic; the hands are short and the fingers thick, but the fingers can be brought together so that "trident hands" do not occur. In fact, the hands and fingers are overextensible. The elbows are limited in extension. Bowing of the legs is not marked but ankle deformities are common. Adult heights vary from 105 to 145 cm. A rosary at the costochondral junctions resembles that of true achondroplasia, and protrusion of the upper sternal portion can cause chest deformity. The hairs of the scalp, eyebrows and eyelashes are thin, brittle and light in color during childhood.

The radiographic features of children are characteristic. The metaphyses of the tubular bones are broad and scalloped and the ribs show similar changes at the costochondral junctions. The fibula is longer than the tibia but, in contrast to achondroplasia, it is the lower end that shows the elongation clearly and causes ankle deformities. The pelvis does not have the iliac notch characteristic of achondroplasia but its outlet appears compressed in the anteroposterior direction. There is an increased lumbar lordosis owing to marked angulation of the sacrum with the spine.

A tendency to intestinal disorders and reduced resistance to chickenpox have been suspected.[1]

In contrast to the Ellis-van Creveld syndrome that is limited to the Amish of Lancaster County, Pennsylvania, the cartilage-hair hypoplasia is also prevalent among other Amish groups of the United States and Canada. The disorder has been observed in France,[2] in Sweden[3] and in Germany.[4]

REFERENCES

1. McKusick, V. A., Eldridge, R., Hostetler, J. A., Ruangwit, U., and Egeland, J. A.: Dwarfism in the Amish, II. Cartilage-hair hypoplasia, Bull. Johns Hopkins Hosp. 116: 285, 1965.
2. Maroteaux, P., Savart, P., Lefebvre, J., and Royer, P.: Les formes partielles de la dysostose metaphysaire, Presse méd. 71:1523, 1963.
3. Lodin, H., and Sjögren, I.: Chondro-ectodermal dysplasia (Ellis-van Creveld's syndrome), Acta paediat. 53:583, 1964.
4. Wiedemann, H-R., Spranger, J., and Kosenow, W.: Knorpel-Haar-Hypoplasie, Arch. Kinderh. 176:74, 1967.

Chondrodystrophia Calcificans Congenita

(Stippled Epiphyses, Dysplasia Epiphysealis Punctata, Conradi's Disease[1])

INFANTS presenting the fully developed disease picture have bones characteristic of chondrodystrophy and, in addition, stippled epiphyses. Stippling is a striking sign in roentgenograms but it does not represent the most important manifestation. The severe form of the disorder is a generalized anomaly that affects the skeleton very early in embryonic development, as shown by vertebral disorganization, which occurs in some cases.[2] In addition to the effects on the skeleton, there also is involvement of the eyes and of the skin. In the mild forms, stippling of the epiphyses is seen in roentgenograms without pronounced chondrodystrophic changes of the long bones and without involvement of other organ systems. Mild forms are genetically and clinically different disorders.

For the severe and often lethal form, recessive inheritance seems very likely. Fraser and Scriver[3] showed that parental consanguinity is rather frequent, and involvement of more than 1 sibling has been observed sufficiently often to permit the conclusion that autosomal recessive inheritance is responsible for this disorder. A pair of male twins, both affected, has been reported by Raap.[4] In families in which the disorder occurs, there sometimes is a high incidence of stillbirths. Hydramnios has been observed repeatedly in pregnancies resulting in affected children.[5-7]

Whereas chondrodystrophia calcificans congenita can be considered a disease entity, this is doubtful for "stippled epiphyses," which may be a pathologic manifestation of a variety of etiologic factors. Ebel and Keuth[8] mentioned a number of cases in which maternal disease in early pregnancy was reported. In some patients, stippled epiphyses disappear with increasing age, and it is possible that such "cured" persons transmit the disorder to some of their children. Dominant inheritance is difficult to prove in these cases, since the parental disease cannot be demon-

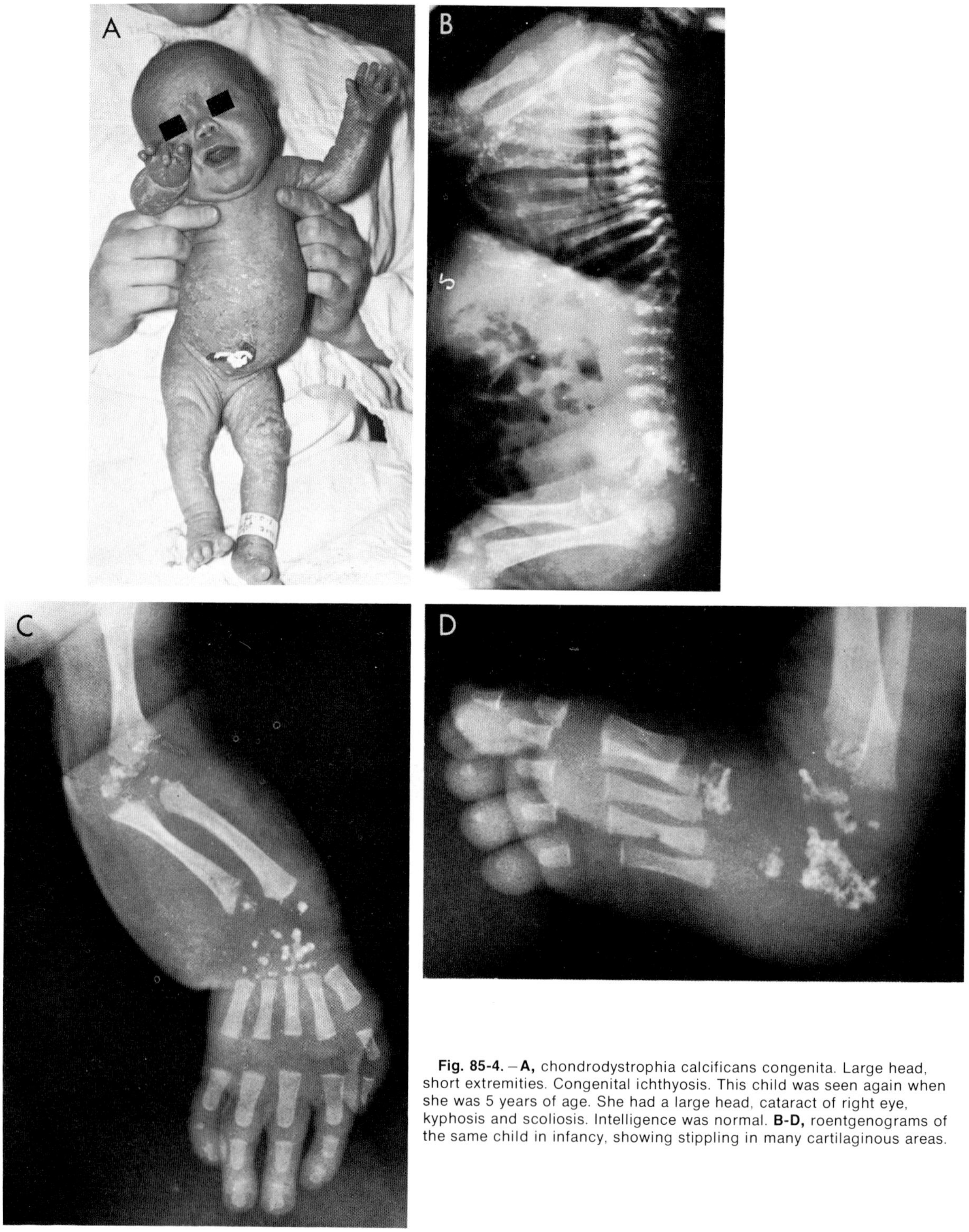

Fig. 85-4. – **A,** chondrodystrophia calcificans congenita. Large head, short extremities. Congenital ichthyosis. This child was seen again when she was 5 years of age. She had a large head, cataract of right eye, kyphosis and scoliosis. Intelligence was normal. **B-D,** roentgenograms of the same child in infancy, showing stippling in many cartilaginous areas.

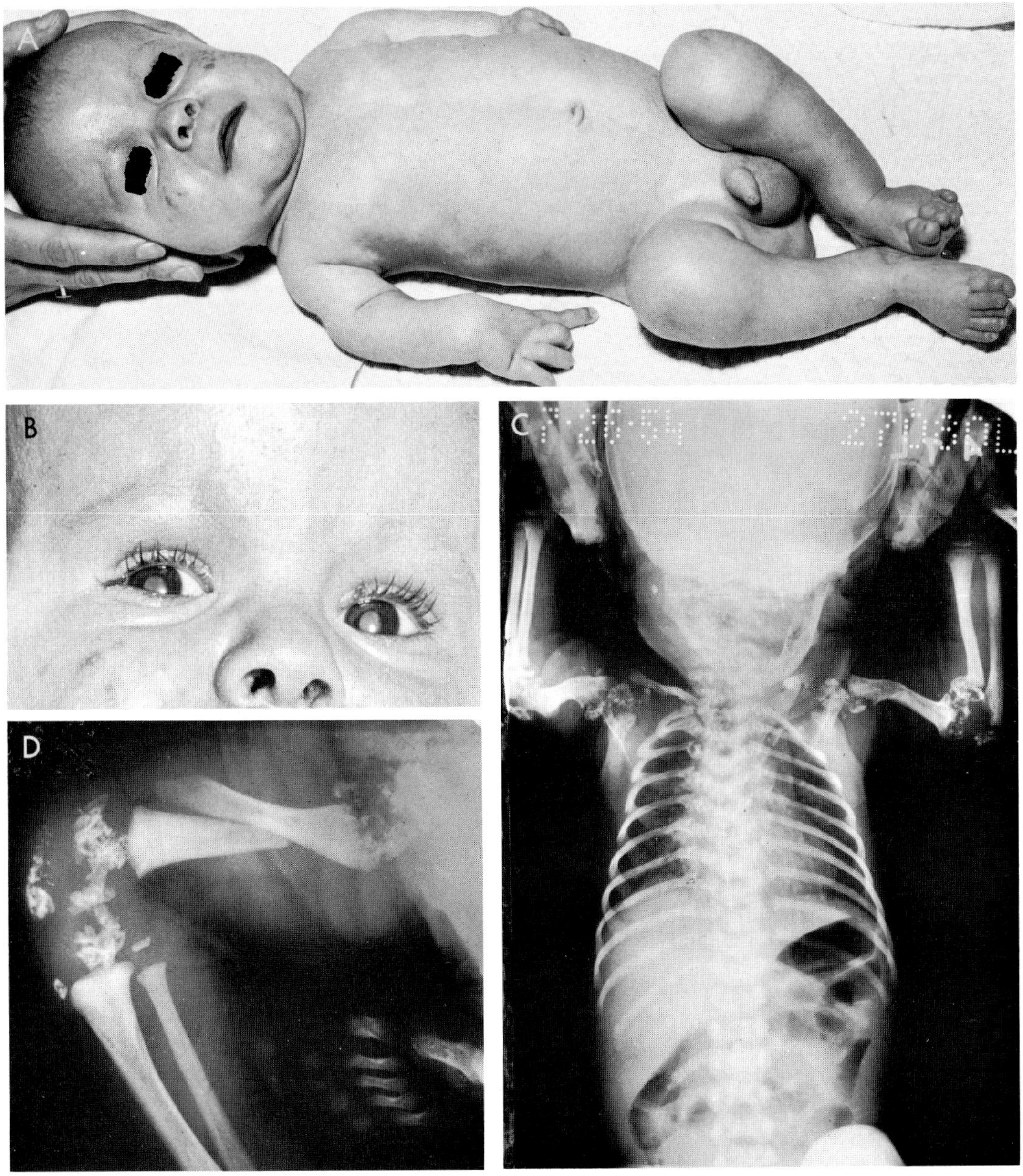

Fig. 85-5. – Chondrodystrophia calcificans congenita in a boy who lived 4 years and died of pneumonia. First child in a family in which no congenital malformations had occurred. **A,** the head is relatively large and the neck short. There were bilateral cataracts and contractures in elbow, knee and wrist joints. Note thickening of metaphyseal areas of wrists. **B,** bilateral cataracts. **C** and **D,** roentgenograms showing large head and stippling about shoulder, elbow and knee joints. Fracture of femur was present at birth.

strated by the time the children are born. At operation or necropsy, calcifications can be recognized macroscopically in cartilage and in connective tissues surrounding joints. Histologic examination shows a reduction of the preparatory zone of calcification and of the columnar cartilage combined with disorganization of the normal cartilage arrangement. In some places, hyaline cartilage may be replaced by fibrous cartilage. The ground substance of cartilage appears swollen, affected by mucoid degeneration and replaced in spots by cysts and calcareous foci that are surrounded by vascular granulation tissue. Similar foci of calcifications can be found in soft tissues and in joint spaces. The belief has been expressed that completely different pathologic processes may effect similar changes in cartilage[9] and result in stippling.

The severe form can be recognized as chondrodystrophy at birth. The head and trunk are relatively large, the extremities short (Fig. 85-4, *A*). As a rule, the proximal tubular bones are more shortened than the distal ones. One extremity may be affected more than the other. The fingers are short and thick in some cases, long and slender in others. Contractures of the joints are the rule in severe cases, and marked limitation of movements in the elbows, hips and knees may be observed. Marked unilateral micromelia has been reported in some cases.[2, 8] Sometimes the hips are dislocated or clubfoot and scoliosis aggravate the disease picture. Calcified foci may be located in connective tissues surrounding the joints. The head sometimes appears normal, sometimes enlarged by accentuated frontal eminences. Saddle nose may be pronounced. The palpebral fissures are narrow. In approximately a third of the cases cataract is present in both eyes (Fig. 85-5, *B*). Congenital heart disease may complicate the situation. The skin often is involved, showing follicular atrophoderma, seborrheic dermatosis, hyperkeratosis, ichthyosis or hair defects. In severe cases, vision is impaired and mental development retarded. Cerebral atrophy and Dandy-Walker malformation have been noted at necropsy.[13] There usually is failure to thrive, general weakness and limited viability, resulting in death within 1 or 2 years. This unfavorable prognosis holds only for fully developed, severe cases and not for all cases of "stippled epiphyses," which often show a remarkable tendency to recovery. In general, the prognosis for life is poor in patients with cataract but survival to adolescence is possible. Comings *et al.*[2] followed a girl with this disorder from birth to age 15 years. The epiphyseal stippling disappeared by the time the child was 6 months of age. The remaining disease picture consisted of severe kyphoscoliosis, marked shortening of the right leg, short stature, cicatricial alopecia, coarse hair, follicular atrophoderma, saddle nose, cataracts, irregular dentition and low normal intelligence. It would be difficult to classify such a case as "chondrodystrophia calcificans" without roentgenograms taken in infancy. The presence of follicular atrophoderma with skeletal changes should raise the question of chondrodystrophia calcificans in the differential diagnosis.[10]

In the mild forms, epiphyseal stippling often is discovered accidentally when x-ray examinations are performed for minor orthopedic anomalies. The disproportioned shortening of the extremities, characteristic of typical chondrodystrophy, usually is absent. Unilateral shortening of an extremity may occur. Children who have the mild type live beyond infancy and show normal mental development. The irregular calcifications of the epiphyses may disappear after the third year of life.

Roentgenograms show in the epiphyses discrete, calcified spots that vary in number. These stippled epiphyseal calcifications sometimes can be seen before the time of normal ossification. They may become less pronounced with time or fuse to form more or less regular ossification centers. The epiphyses of the upper and lower ends of the femur and of the upper ends of the humerus and tibia exhibit the stippling phenomenon most often.[11] However, other epiphyses of long and short bones may be affected, and stippling has been seen at the proximal ends of the ribs, along the vertebrae and in the laryngeal and tracheal cartilages.

In typical cases, the metaphyses show transverse enlargement with irregularities comparable to those of achondroplasia. The shafts are short and thick and their ends are abnormally slanted. The fibula may be longer than the tibia, as is seen in achondroplasia.

No treatment has been found for the basic pathologic process. Orthopedic deformities resulting from this disorder can be corrected to a certain extent in mild cases. The eugenic prognosis is rather serious for families in which a severe case of chondrodystrophia calcificans congenita has occurred, since there exists a risk of repetition in 1 of 4 children.

REFERENCES

1. Conradi, E.: Vorzeitiges Auftreten von Knochen–und eigenartigen Verkalkungskernen bei Chondrodystrophia fötalis hypoplastica: Histologische und Röntgenuntersuchungen, Jahrb. Kinderh. 80:86, 1914.
2. Comings, D. E., Papazian, C., and Schoene, H. R.: Conradi's disease: Chondrodystrophia calcificans congenita, congenital stippled epiphyses, J. Pediat. 72:63, 1968.
3. Fraser, F. C., and Scriver, J. B.: A hereditary factor in chondrodystrophia calcificans congenita, New England J. Med. 250:272, 1954.
4. Raap, G.: Chondrodystrophia calcificans congenita, Am. J. Roentgenol. 49:77, 1943.
5. Haynes, E. R., and Wangner, W. F.: Chondroangiopathia calcarea seu punctata: Review and case report, Radiology 57:547, 1951.
6. Ford, G. D., Schneider, M., and Brandon, J. R.: Congenital stippled epiphyses, Pediatrics 8:380, 1951.
7. Swoboda, W.: Beitrag zur chondrodystrophia calcificans congenita, Ann. paediat. 175:322, 1950.
8. Ebel, D., and Keuth, U.: Extreme Mikromelie bei Chondrodysplasia calcificans congenita. Zugleich ein Beitrag zur Ätiologie, Ztschr. Kinderh. 82:59, 1959.
9. Schönenberg, H., and Schallock, G.: Zur Kenntnis der Chondrodysplasia calcificans congenita und ihrer Beziehungen zur Chondrodysplasia foetalis, Ann. paediat. 180: 129, 1953.
10. Yakovac, W. C.: Calcareous chondropathies in the newborn infant, A.M.A. Arch. Path. 57:62, 1954.
11. Curth, H. O.: Follicular atrophoderma and pseudopelade with chondrodystrophia calcificans congenita, J. Invest. Dermat. 13:233, 1949.
12. Fairbank, T.: *An Atlas of General Affections of the Skeleton* (Edinburgh and London: E. & S. Livingston Ltd., 1951).
13. Tasker, W. G., Mastri, A. R., and Gold, A. P.: Chondrodystrophia calcificans congenita (dysplasia epiphysealis punctata), Am. J. Dis. Child. 119:122, 1970.

Diastrophic Dwarfism

THIS IS an atypical achondroplasia associated with contractures of many joints. The condition was well described and reviewed by Lamy and Maroteaux[1] and named "diastrophic" (i.e., tortuous) dwarfism. A name suggesting chondrodystrophy and joint contractures would have been preferable. Cases were described before and after Lamy and Maroteaux's publication and, by 1967, 40 had been recorded in the literature.[2] In the same year, Monnet *et al*,[3] published 6 new cases and in 1968 Vazquez and Lee[4] added 4.

The disorder can be recognized at birth. Birth weight often is low for gestational age. The extremities are short, flexion contractures at the elbows and knees are present and clubfeet are noticed. The cranium is normal but the facial skeleton is involved, as shown by posterior palate cleft and sometimes by

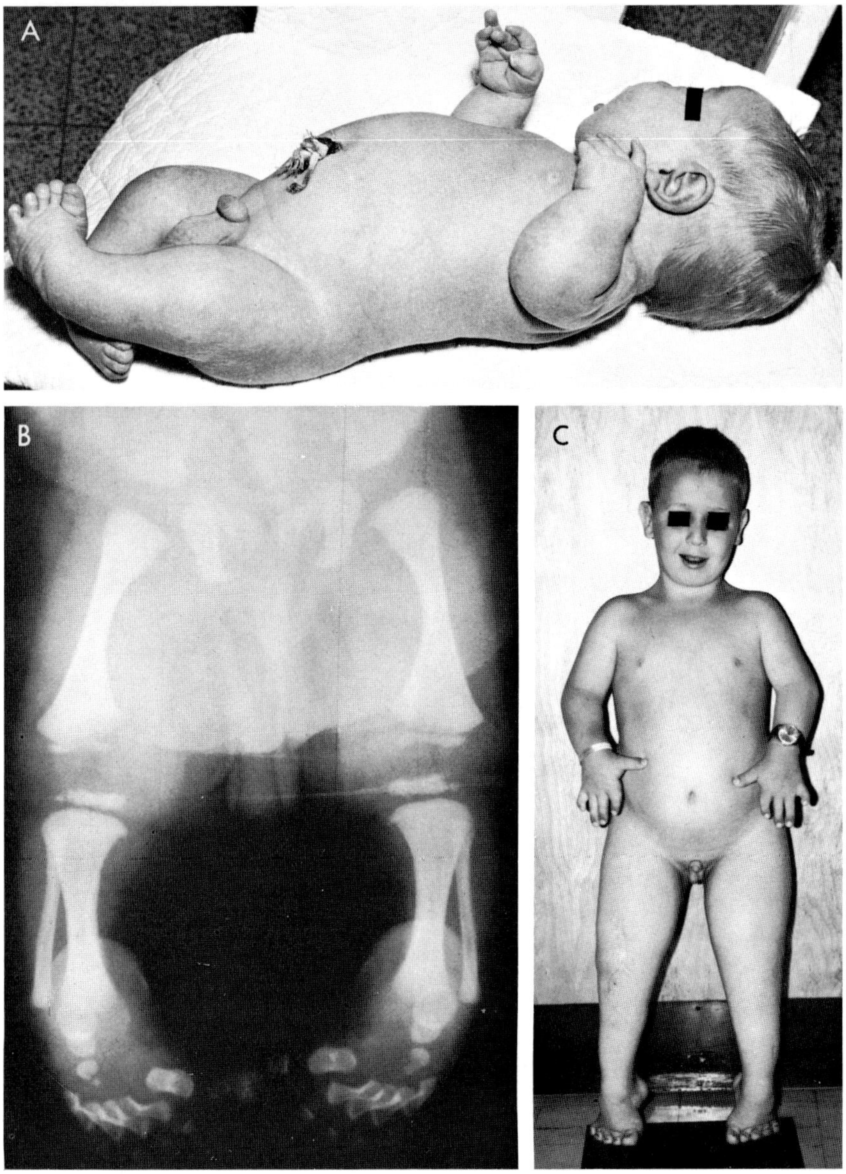

Fig. 85-6.—Chondrodystrophy with contractures of several joints (diastrophic dwarfism). This disorder was present in 2 brothers who were the result of the sixth and seventh pregnancies of an unaffected mother. **A,** chondrodystrophy in an infant with multiple joint contractures. **B,** roentgenogram showing short and thick chondrodystrophic bones with flat, irregular epiphyses. The tibia is longer than the fibula. Severe clubfoot deformity. **C,** the older brother at 11 years of age. Marked growth retardation. The thumbs stand at right angles to the long axis of the hands. Bilateral clubfoot. *(Continued.)*

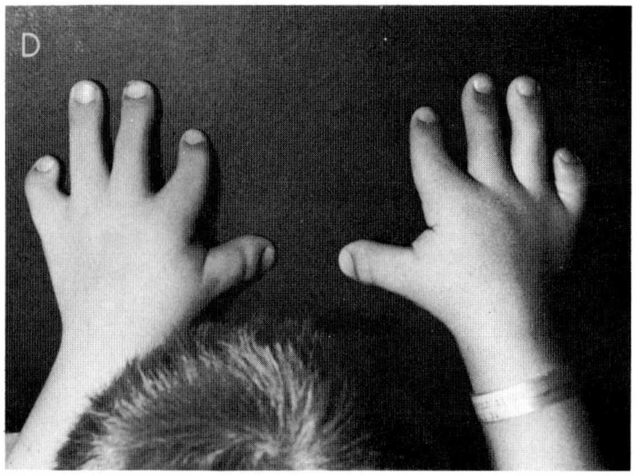

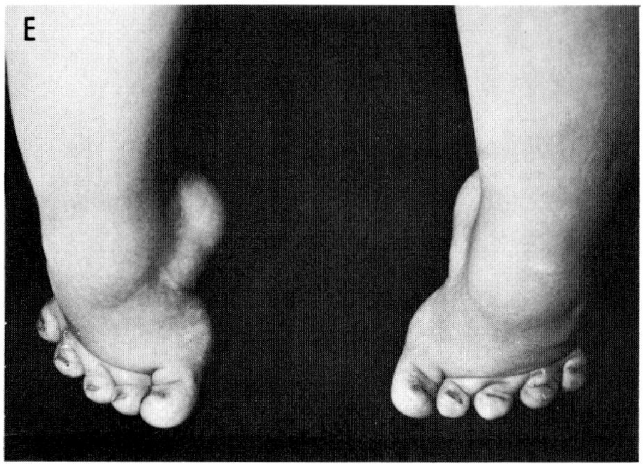

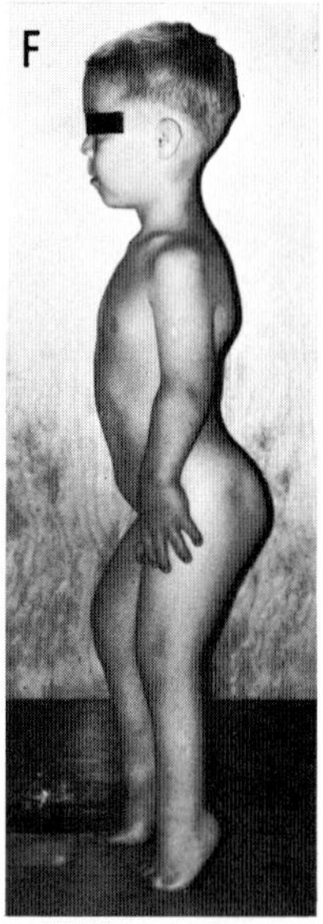

Fig. 85-6 (cont.). – **D** and **E,** hands and feet of patient. **F,** the younger brother, who was born with cleft palate, shows growth retardation, increased lordosis and foot anomaly. **G** and **H,** hands and feet of the same child.

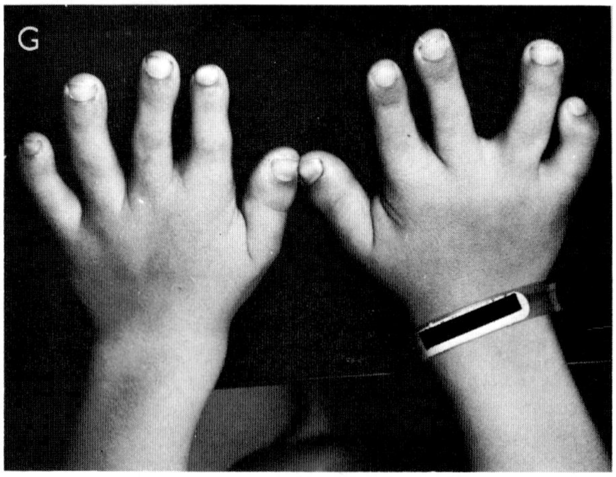

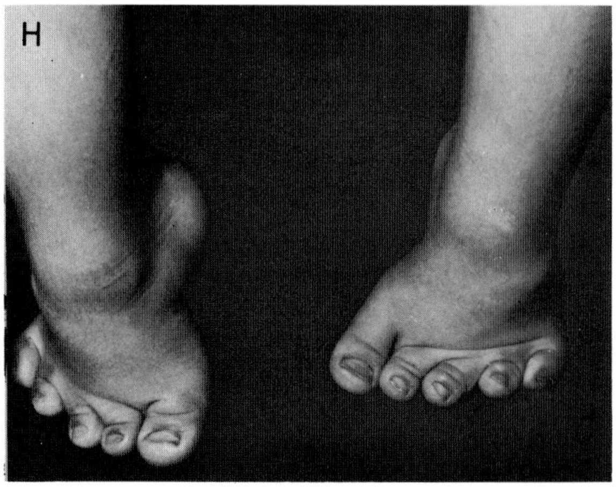

Pierre Robin syndrome.[3] The external ears often are thickened, everted and deformed and the external canals are narrow. The spine may be deformed at birth or become scoliotic later.

General growth and development usually is slow. Dwarfism is severe because of shortness and deformities of the extremities and the spine. Limitation of movement and stiffness of the joints suggest arthrogryposis. There are contractions in the elbow and knee joints. Clubfeet are always present. Hearing and mental development usually are normal.

Roentgenograms show short and thick tubular bones with widely splayed metaphyses and irregular outline. The forearms commonly are more shortened than the upper arms. The ulna is affected more than the radius, which results in radial curving and ulnar deviation of the hands. The wrists and the hands are small, the metacarpals thick and short and their epiphyses are slanting. The thumbs often stand perpendicular to the long axis of the hand. This and the ulnar deviation of the fingers render the appearance of the hand diagnostic. The femoral heads are flat. Genu valgum is pronounced, the lower legs and the patellae may be subluxated and the tibial epiphyses malformed. In contrast to typical achondroplasia, the tibiae are longer than the fibulae. The feet are small, the metatarsal bones incurved and equinus deformity is pronounced. Curvatures of the vertebral column are always present in older children. Flattening of the cervical spine may be caused by anterior dislocation of C3 and C4. There is progressive cephalo-caudal narrowing of the interpedunculate distances of the lumbar vertebrae.[4] Posterior tilt of the sacrum has been observed.[5]

Diastrophic dwarfism is attributed to homozygosity of an autosomal recessive gene. Sex distribution is equal. Siblings have been affected repeatedly (Fig. 85-6). Jackson[6] observed the disorder in 3 children of one family. In a brother and sister the disorder was associated with Hirschsprung disease[9] (Chapter 76). Parental consanguinity was reported in Taybi's[5] cases. Stillbirth[4] or neonatal death[3] eliminates some of the patients early.

REFERENCES

1. Lamy, M., and Maroteaux, P.: Le nanisme diastrophique, Presse méd. 68:1977, 1960.
2. Spranger, J., and Gerken, H.: Diastrophischer Zwergwuchs, Ztschr. Kinderh. 98:227, 1967.
3. Monnet, P., Robert, J-M., Salle, B., and Peytel, J.: Le nanisme diastrophique, Lyon méd. No. 18–30, p. 1306, 1967.
4. Vazquez, A. M., and Lee, F. A.: Diastrophic dwarfism, J. Pediat. 72:234, 1968.
5. Taybi, H.: Diastrophic dwarfism, Radiology 80:1, 1963.
6. Jackson, W. P. U.: Irregular familial chondro-osseous defect with suggestions concerning nomenclature of generalized osseous dystrophies, J. Bone & Joint Surg. 33-B:420, 1951.
7. Amuso, S. J.: Diastrophic dwarfism, J. Bone & Joint Surg. 50-A:113, 1968.
8. Wilson, D. W., Chrispin, A. R., and Carter, C. O.: Diastrophic dwarfism, Arch. Dis. Childhood 44:48, 1969.
9. Fauchier, Cl., Régy, J-M., and Combe, P.: Nanisme diastrophique familial avec maladie de Hirschsprung, Ann. pédiat. 16:496, 1969.

Metatropic Dwarfism

MAROTEAUX *et al.*,[1] in 1966, described as "metatrophic dwarfism" a skeletal systemic malformation in which the proportion of length of trunk to extremities is reversed during childhood. At first, the trunk is too long and the extremities are too short. The length of the children is normal at birth or even above average; the chest is long and narrow and the spinal column kyphoscoliotic. Over the coccygeal area, peculiar longitudinal double folds may be noticed, which reach down into the upper anal fold like a tail. The joints, particularly the knee joints, are enlarged and their mobility is impaired. Abduction is reduced in the hip and shoulder joints and flexion is reduced in the elbow. The fifth digit may be held bent, whereas other fingers can be overextensible. The hands and feet may be slender and the fingers long. Skull and face usually are normal.

In the course of development, there is a change in appearance and proportions. Children fall behind in growth as kyphoscoliosis becomes more marked. Neck, arms and legs are shortened and the hands and feet become plump. The sternum protrudes and a pigeon chest is formed. In infancy, the long trunk and short extremities lead to a mistaken diagnosis of achondroplasia. Later, during childhood, the condition can be mistaken for Morquio disease (p. 819) because of the normal face, short trunk, protruding sternum and deformed spine.

Although the trunk is long in the newborn, roentgenograms show anomalies of the spinal column. There is a retardation of ossification of the vertebral bodies, which appear as narrow, tongue-like, ossified islands lying in front of well-developed pedicles. The centers of ossification are far apart, their distances from each other being two to three times greater than the height of the ossification centers.[3] Thoracic and lumbar vertebrae can be wedge-shaped early and there may be ventral and dorsal ossification centers in lumbar vertebral bodies. In infancy, the chest is very narrow and the ribs are short but respiration is not impaired. With increasing age, the chest becomes reduced in height and enlarged in the anteroposterior direction. At birth, the long bones are short and plump and the metaphyses trumpet-shaped, and separated from the epiphyses by dense calcified zones. The expansion of the metaphyses may become less prominent with increasing age. There is general delay of ossification and the ossification centers are irregular, with alternating denser or lighter areas. Metacarpal bones and phalanges remain short, plump and irregular in outline. The pelvis is low and typically deformed. The iliac crests reach far down and the ventral spines almost touch the upper acetabular margins. The acetabular roofs are horizontally oriented.[4]

Males and females can be affected. Only once did metatropic dwarfism occur in siblings. The parents of patients have not been affected and parental consanguinity has not been observed. Autosomal recessive inheritance has been suggested by Maroteaux *et al.*[1]

The pathogenesis of the disorder is not known. De Groot[2] found, in histologic sections, enchondral ossification lacking. Mucopolysaccharide excretion in the urine seems to be within normal limits.

REFERENCES

1. Maroteaux, P., Spranger, J., and Wiedemann, H-R.: Der metatropische Zwergwuchs, Arch. Kinderh. 173:211, 1966.
2. de Groot, J. W. C.: Two atypical cases of chondrodysplasia, J. Pediat. 39:715, 1951.
3. Gefferth, K.: Beiträge zur Diagnostik des metatropischen Zwergwuchses, Ztschr. Kinderh. 103:325, 1968.
4. Larose, J. H., and Gay, B. B.: Metatropic dwarfism, Am. J. Roentgenol. 106:156, 1969.

Chondrodystrophy with Retinal Detachment and Deafness

Roaf *et al.*[1] described a rare syndrome of bone dysplasia, retinal detachment and deafness. Skeletal changes are present at birth and walking is delayed. The patients are short, have marked lordosis, enlargement of the ends of the long bones and kyphoscoliosis. They resemble achondroplastics and children with spondylo-epiphyseal dysplasia. The facial features are normal. Roentgenograms show splaying of the metaphyseal and epiphyseal regions of the long bones, which have a ground-glass appearance. The pelvis is trefoil shaped and there is coxa vara and genu valgum.

Detached retina develops in the first year or later. Cataract may be congenital and atrophic iritis may be present. Hearing loss develops gradually, with a marked increase in loss in the high frequencies. There is marked mental retardation, which may be due to sensory deprivation.

REFERENCE

1. Roaf, R., Longmore, J. B., and Forrester, R. M.: A childhood syndrome of bone dysplasia, retinal detachment and deafness, Developmental Med. & Child Neurol. 9:464, 1967.

"Achondrogenesis"

The term "achondrogenesis" has been used for different skeletal disorders. A lethal anomaly first described in 1936 as a variant of osteogenesis imperfecta[1] is characterized by lack of ossification of long bones and vertebrae in newborn infants who have large skulls, short limbs and short ribs.

A different disorder that leads to severe dwarfism with extreme shortening of two or four extremities and rudimentary digits can appear repeatedly in a family as a recessive trait. This anomaly has also been termed "achondrogenesis." Grebe[2] reported 2 sisters, children of consanguineous parents, who showed shortening of the upper extremities and severe hypoplasia of the tubular bones of the lower extremities. The digits were rudimentary. The "new type of dwarfism" with bone aplasias and hypoplasias of the extremities reported by Quelce-Salgado[3] resembles these cases to a certain extent. Affected individuals had extremely reduced stature; the short extremities presented variable bone malformations; clubhand was seen frequently; the digits were rudimentary and polydactyly occurred in some cases. Autosomal recessive inheritance seems established.

Since cartilage is formed in patients with either of these conditions, the term "achondrogenesis" probably is unjustified for both disorders.

REFERENCES

1. Parenti, G. C.: La anosteogenesi. Une varieta della osteogenesi imperfecta, Pathologica 28:447, 1936.
2. Grebe, H.: Missbildungen der Gliedmassen, in Becker, P.E. (ed.), *Humangenetik* (Stuttgart: Georg Thieme, 1964), Vol. II.
3. Quelce-Salgado, A.: A new type of dwarfism with various bone aplasias and hypoplasias of the extremities, Acta Genet. 14:63, 1964.

Atypical Chondrodystrophies III (Transmitted Like a Sex-Linked Recessive Trait or of Unknown Etiology)

Hereditary Osteochondrodystrophia Deformans (Jacobsen) (Dysplasia Spondylo-Epiphysealis Tarda)

IN 1939, JACOBSEN[1] reported a kinship in which a disorder resembling Morquio disease to a certain extent affected 20 members in five generations. Gross pathologic changes such as kyphosis, pigeon breast and platyspondyly developed only in males and it seemed that the disorder was transmitted through carrier daughters to approximately half of their sons, so that a sex-linked recessive mode of inheritance can be assumed. Since 2 of the females of this kinship suffered from arthritic changes of the joints, they may have had the disorder with reduced expressivity. It seems that a disorder described in 3 brothers by Nilsonne[2] in 1927 belonged in this group. Lamy and Maroteaux[3] classified it as dysplasia spondylo-epiphysealis tarda and contributed a pedigree that illustrates sex-linked recessive inheritance. The kindred first described by Jacobsen[1] has been followed and restudied by Bannerman.[4]

REFERENCES

1. Jacobsen, A. W.: Hereditary osteochondrodystrophia deformans, J.A.M.A. 113:121, 1939.
2. Nilsonne, H.: Eigentümliche Wirbelkörperveränderungen mit familiärem Auftreten, Acta chir. scandinav. 62:550, 1927.
3. Lamy, M., and Maroteaux, P.: *Les Chondrodystrophies Génotypiques* (Paris: L'Expansion Scientifique Française, 1961).
4. Bannerman, R. M.: X-linked Spondyloepiphyseal Dysplasia Tarda (SDT), in Bergsma, D. (ed.), *The First Conference on The Clinical Delineation of Birth Defects.* Part IV. Skeletal Dysplasias. Birth Defects; Original Article Series (New York: The National Foundation, 1969). Vol. V, No. 4, p. 48.

Chondrodystrophy and Acrocephaly

IN RARE INSTANCES, chondrodystrophy is associated with hydrocephaly and acrocephaly. Meyer[1] reported "hydrocephalus chondrodystrophicus" in a child with moderate shortening of the extremities. The skull appeared subdivided into a frontal and a facio-temporal part. There also was cleft palate and a peculiar occipital encephalocele enclosed in a funnel-shaped canal. There was an upper and a lower skull cavity with a bony shelf within the skull that seemed to separate the two cephalic portions. Hydrocephaly was present. Welter[2] described a chondrodystrophic girl dead half an hour after birth. The tower skull consisted of two parts: an upper high and narrow frontal portion that sat like a second story on the lower temporo-occipital skull. The two parts were separated by a circular furrow that ran from the lateral orbital angles to the posterior fontanelle. Parts of the coronary and sagittal sutures were prematurely obliterated and the skull base was shortened by chondrodystrophic changes. The internal hydrocephaly was explained by narrowing of the jugular foramina. Another newborn with a similar combination of acrocephaly and chondrodystrophy of the skull base was reported by Gruber.[3] This case is interesting because the chondrodystrophy was limited to the skull. These anomalies are related to cloverleaf skulls (Chapter 95).

REFERENCES

1. Meyer, R.: Hydrocephalus chondrodystrophicus mit Bemerkungen über den "Perioststreifen" bei Chondrodystrophie, Virchows Arch. path. Anat. 253:766, 1925.
2. Welter, H.: Zur Frage des Hydrocephalus chondrodystrophicus congenitus, Beitr. path. Anat. 97:1, 1936.
3. Gruber, G. B.: Über einen akrocephalen Reliefschädel. Ein Beitrag zur Frage der partiellen Chondrodystrophie, Beitr. path. Anat. 97:9, 1936.
4. Feingold, M., O'Connor, J. F., Berkman, M., and Darling, D. B.: Kleeblattschädel syndrome, Am. J. Dis. Child. 118: 589, 1969.

87

Epiphyseal Dysgenesis in Cretinism; Kaschin-Beck Disease

Cretinism

THE DANGERS OF CLASSIFYING atypical chondrodystrophies according to roentgenographic similarities is best illustrated by the resemblance of skeletal changes observable in cretins with those of chondrodystrophics of different origin. If in cretins the thyroid deficiency were not betrayed by other symptoms, the skeletal manifestations probably would be classified as "stippled epiphyses," as "dysplasia epiphysealis multiplex" or as "an atypical chondrodystrophy" adorned by an eponym. In cretins, ossification is delayed; after it sets in, epiphyseal dysgenesis (or dysplasia) can be observed in roentgenograms in the form of multiple irregular and fragmented epiphyses. If these centers of ossification are small and numerous, "stippled epiphyses" make their appearance. Fusion of these small centers results in larger centers irregular in shape, size and position that do not differ greatly from those of atypical chondrodystrophies. Wilkins[1] stated that "occasionally chondrodystrophic changes are confined exclusively to the epiphyseal centers and can be distinguished from the abnormality due to thyroid deficiency only by the fact that they are not corrected by thyroid therapy."

Skeletal changes simulating chondrodystrophies can also be seen in *endemic* cretins who show delayed epiphyseal ossification and later irregular, multiple ossification centers.[2] Not only the epiphyses but also the metaphyses and diaphyses can undergo changes simulating atypical chondrodystrophies.[2] The joints, particularly the hip joint and the pelvis, show severe deformities. Many endemic cretins remain dwarfed and "chondrodystrophic." Before the role of the thyroid in the etiology of cretinism was recognized, it often was difficult to differentiate between chondrodystrophic and cretinous dwarfism because of their superficial resemblance. The important point is that the osseous changes characteristic of endemic cretinism resemble to a certain extent "chondrodystrophy" or "epiphyseal dysplasia" of genetic origin. Since more than one endemic cretin can occur in a family, genetic determination could be erroneously assumed for this condition, if it were not for the knowledge that this disorder can be eradicated by simple environmental measures (Chapter 12).

REFERENCES

1. Wilkins, L.: *The Diagnosis and Treatment of Endocrine Disorders in Childhood and Adolescence* (2d ed.; Springfield, Ill.: Charles C Thomas, Publisher, 1957).
2. DeQuervain, F., and Wegelin, C.: *Der endemische Kretinismus* (Berlin and Vienna: Julius Springer, 1936).

Kaschin-Beck Disease

(Osteochondroarthrosis Deformans, Osteoarthritis Endemica, Osteochondral Epiphyseopathy, Urow Disease)

THIS DISEASE, which apparently does not occur in the United States, is mentioned here to illustrate the danger of classification of the osteochondrodystrophies according to morphologic signs only and to emphasize that environmental factors can induce bone changes that simulate hereditary conditions to a great extent. In 1861, Kaschin (cited by Goldstein and Nikiforov[1]) described, in a report on endemic goiter and cretinism in Russia, an osteoarthropathy that was then endemic at the river Urow in Transbaikalia. Although this disease was found in areas in which goiter was endemic, the association between the two anomalies was not a close one. Since the original report, the disease has been seen in different areas of Russia, in Japan, Korea, Manchuria and Italy.[2] It has been attributed to contaminated drinking water and to other toxic factors, to glandular disturbances and to avitaminoses. It is said to be endemic in areas in which drinking water has a very high iron content (0.3–1.0 mg. per liter) and affected persons may have elevated serum iron values and hepatic and pancreatic fibrosis.[3] A hereditary factor may be contributory, but there is general agreement that the disease can be arrested by emigration of the patient to a nonendemic area.

If one looks at pictures of some of the patients with this disease and their roentgenograms[1] without knowledge of the background, a striking resemblance to Morquio disease and other atypical chondrodystrophies cannot be denied. The head appears fairly normal and sits on a dwarfed body. There is shortening of the spine, with increased thoracic kyphosis and lumbar lordosis. The vertebral bodies are flattened and the intervertebral spaces may be reduced or relatively increased. The extremities are shortened to a lesser degree but changes become more noticeable as inspection proceeds in the proximo-distal direction. The shoulder and hip joints are said to be only mildly affected, but flexion contractures can be recognized in some of the illustrations and flattening of the humeral and femoral epiphyses is seen in roentgenograms. Genu valgum occurs in some cases and deformities of the elbow joints have been described.[4] The most marked changes are seen in the hands, which may be deformed at birth. As a rule, however, onset is insidious in postnatal life, beginning at about 5 years and progressing through adolescence to adulthood. The hands are described as broad and short. The epiphyses of the metacarpophalangeal joints are flattened and irregular in outline, the articulations are uneven and movements limited. Similar changes occur in the joints of the foot and in the carpal and tarsal bones. There certainly exists a "dysplasia epiphysealis multiplex." Cartilage changes have been described in embryos of mothers who suffer from the disease[1] and more than one member of a family can be affected. Thus, congenital and hereditary atypical chondrodystrophies can be simulated. It is true that, in contrast to achondroplasia, involvement of soft tissues and of internal organs is possible, but this is also the case in hereditary storage diseases. Although the differentiation from typical achondroplasia and Morquio disease is not difficult, the resemblance to atypical forms may be so great that one wonders whether some of the cases published as examples of Kaschin-Beck disease[1] were not in reality hereditary atypical chondrodystrophies. However, there are so many observations of this disorder on record that its existence should not be doubted or denied.[4-6]

REFERENCES

1. Goldstein, D., and Nikiforov, P. N.: Über die sogenannte Kaschin-Becksche Krankheit, Fortschr. Geb. Röntgenstrahlen 43:321, 1931.
2. Mørch, E. T.: *Chondrodystrophic Dwarfs in Denmark* (Copenhagen: Ejnar Munksgaard, 1941).
3. Stanbury, J. B., Fredrickson, D. S., and Wyngaarden, J. B.: *The Metabolic Basis of Inherited Disease* (New York: McGraw-Hill Book Company, Inc., 1960).
4. Michailow, M.: Das Röntgenbild der Knochenveränderungen bei der Beckschen Krankheit, Fortschr. Geb. Röntgenstrahlen 43:321, 1931.
5. Schipatschoff, W. G.: Die Kaschin-Becksche Krankheit (Osteoarthritis endemica), Deutsches Arch. klin. Med. 170: 133, 1931.
6. Graziansky, W.: Die Kaschin-Beck'sche Krankheit im Röntgenbilde, Fortschr. Geb. Röntgenstrahlen 50:367, 1934.

88

Gargoylism and Other Mucopolysaccharidoses

(Dysostosis Multiplex; Lipochondrodystrophies)

A GROUP OF DWARFING DISORDERS that involve the skeleton and many soft tissues at first were described to separate them from achondroplasia. It evolved that there exist a number of these entities, which can be classified according to clinical, roentgenologic, biochemical or genetic points of view. It is understandable, therefore, that classification is difficult and in flux and that a flexible attitude should be assumed to permit adjustments according to new discoveries.

At present, it is assumed by many writers that the disorders under discussion are due to inborn errors of metabolism that lead to storage of pathologic metabolic products in cells of the affected organs. Although it is likely that mucopolysaccharides are particularly affected by the inborn error of metabolism, it is probable that other chemical constituents of the body, particularly lipids, are also involved. It may be premature to consider the disorders as "mucopolysaccharidoses" and to classify them according to products that appear in the urine in excessive amounts. This is best illustrated by the fact that the Hurler and the Hunter syndromes, which differ clinically and genetically, both show increased urinary excretion of chondroitin sulfate B and heparitin sulfate and by typical cases without amino-aciduria.[65,91] It seems equally premature to select arbitrarily certain clinical or radiologic signs for a rigid classification. Although every branch of medicine and every investigator is entitled to a point of view and classification, nobody can claim as yet to have performed the final analysis in this complex subject. Fortunately, there is much interest in this field and much work is in progress that necessitates frequent revisions of our present conceptions; progress can be hindered by rigid and dogmatic points of view and tubular vision.

In the following pages, various disease pictures will be discussed as they appeared in 1970. Instead of presenting these disorders as final entities in neat and rigid pigeonholes, I shall try to emphasize exceptions and contradictions in our present concepts that require the attention of investigators.

The classic syndrome of gargoylism consists of cloudy corneae, hepatosplenomegaly, mental deficiency and dwarfism combined with typical skeletal changes. Cases of this type were observed and recognized as a disease entity as early as 1900 by Dr. J. Thompson of Edinburgh.[1] Three members of one family showed retarded physical and mental development, dwarfism, short neck, dorsolumbar kyphosis, pigeon breast and stumpy fingers and hands; cloudy corneae and enlargement of the heart, of the liver and of the spleen were present in some but not all of these children. Since there was no name available in the medical literature for this disorder, Thompson called it "Johnny McL-'s disease" after the first child in the afflicted family. In 1917, Hunter[2] published the first description related to this disorder. Although some of the features considered essential for the syndrome, such as cloudy corneae and mental deficiency, were absent in his patients, there were others, such as Sprengel deformity, which were later recognized as part of the disease entity. Hunter observed this "rare disease in two brothers" and thus he, as well as Thompson, early directed attention to the possibility of heredity as an etiologic factor. Absence of some of the cardinal features of the disease is now explained by the assumption that his cases belonged to a special category of the disease with a specific mode of inheritance (p. 816). Three years after Hunter, a more complete description of 2 cases was given by Hurler.[3] In 2 children who appeared normal at birth, dwarfism, kyphosis, deformities of the skull and chest, claw-like hands, cloudy corneae, deafness and mental retardation were recognized as constituents of the syndrome and the differential diagnosis was discussed thoroughly. In 1934, Tuthill[4] recognized the disorder as a storage disease and considered it a form of juvenile amaurotic idiocy. Ellis *et al.*[5] reviewed the cases reported before 1936 and suggested the term "gargoylism." Until 1948, the syndrome generally was considered a lipochondrodystrophy, and subsequently many additional cases were added to the literature. After 1947, thorough studies of the pathologic lesions were reported by Straus *et al.*,[7] Strauss[8] and Lindsay *et al.*[9] These studies confirmed the conception of gargoylism as a storage disease but made it doubtful that the stored material is a lipid substance. In 1952, Brante[10] classified gargoylism as a mucopolysaccharidosis.

There are objections to all of the names suggested for this disorder. Since there were so many "first" authors to recognize the syndrome, it would be difficult to give credit to all of them. The term "dysostosis multiplex" is too broad, being applicable to many other skeletal anomalies; it does not indicate the involvement of soft tissues and, therefore, misses one of the main features of the disease. The name "lipochondrodystrophy" was abandoned because the substance stored in most of the tissues is not a lipid. "Mucopolysaccharidosis" also may not be the ideal term, since other substances may be involved in the faulty metabolism. "Gargoylism" is a useful term, being short and easy to pronounce. Although it has a derogatory implication and the patients do not look like gargoyles, this name appears best suited for the disorders with abnormal facial features until the abnormal substances deposited in the tissues and the metabolic blocks are definitely identified. The subject was reviewed by Ullrich[11] in 1943, by Jervis[12] in 1950 and by McKusick[13] in 1966.

Hurler Syndrome

Both sexes may be affected. The condition is of prenatal origin but few symptoms are present at birth. As a rule, the patients are considered normal for several months, but toward the end of the first year the parents become aware of abnormal traits. If an apparently normal infant is suspected of having gargoylism, as may be the case in a family with a previously affected child, the diagnosis can be made at birth by a combined clinical and roentgenographic examination.[14] Patients have been observed as late as in the third decade of life and even later, but most of those reported were children. The fact that the patients usually are born with a high birth weight indicates that the disorder is compatible with prenatal life. But, after birth or during the first year of life, the children do not develop well; they show little resistance to infections and often they die young. Several children with gargoylism were twins,[15,16] 1 being affected and 1 normal. Craig[17] reported gargoylism in a twin brother and sister. Concordance in identical twins was described by Nonne[18] and Steen.[19] In some of the families with such patients, a tendency to twinning was apparent.[15] Caucasian, Chinese, Indian,[21] Mexican and Negro[22,23] children with this disorder have been observed.

Gargoylism is a genetically determined storage disease, an "inborn error of metabolism" involving mucopolysaccharides. Recessive inheritance of the trait has been considered for some time[24] because of frequent affection of siblings of both sexes, normal parents and increased parental consanguinity. In 1950, Jervis[12] reviewed all the cases then reported in the literature and came to the conclusion that the accumulated data were compatible with the hypothesis that the disorder is determined by a single autosomal recessive gene. Although a prevalence of male over female patients had been observed before, a sex-linked type of gargoylism apparently was considered first by Nja[25] in 1946. A number of families have been reported since in which this mode of transmission seemed to be present (p. 816). Lamy *et al.*[26] reviewed 269 cases of gargoylism and, like others, came to the conclusion that there are two genetic forms of the disease. Autosomal recessive inheritance is more frequent than the sex-linked one. It seems to be characterized by a great frequency of corneal opacities, more marked statural retardation and more rapid progression. The form attributed to sex-linked recessive inheritance and seen exclusively in males, reported first by Hunter,[2] is, according to Lamy *et al.*,[26] free of corneal opacities but affected by a higher percentage of deafness. These authors believed that approximately a third of the male cases are due to sex-linked transmission. McKusick[13] thought that the sex-linked disease having a delayed onset may go unrecognized until the age of 4–8 years, that mental retardation is less pronounced and that the patients live longer than those with the simple recessive form. Despite these differences, in most cases it is difficult to distinguish the two types at an early date, when the distinction would be important for the purpose of genetic counseling. It is also regrettable that heterozygous parents or mothers and carrier sisters of males with the sex-linked form do not betray by clinical or chemical signs their tendency to transmit the disorder.

Gross examination of the skeleton by the pathologist reveals little that cannot be recognized by clinical and roentgenologic examination. The skull is thick, and premature closure of the sagittal and lambdoid sutures may be observed. On the floor of the middle and posterior fossae irregular gyrus-like, osteophytic elevations may be seen. The foramen magnum can be narrowed by such protrusions.[8] The vertebral bodies of the lumbar spine are oval and irregular in outline on sagittal section. "Beaked" vertebrae usually are seen in the dorsolumbar region; they can be recognized by the presistence of cartilage and by lack of ossification in the upper, anterior corner of an affected vertebral body. Sections through the end of the tubular bones show thickening and irregularity of the epiphyseal lines. The articular cartilage is yellow, smooth, gelatinous and, in places, abnormally thick. Histologically, the height of the zone of proliferative cartilage is markedly reduced. In contrast to the normal arrangement, the cells do not form columns but lie in pairs or in irregular small groups between the resting cartilage and the metaphyseal bone. As a result, they form osseous trabeculae that are placed transversely rather than longitudinally under the cartilage. Calcified matrix is almost completely absent in the trabeculae, which consist entirely of bone of osteoblastic origin. The findings explain the slow and irregular growth of the skeleton.[6] Sometimes areas of vascular connective tissue containing large, swollen, vacuolated cells are seen in places where proliferating cartilage cells normally are found. In the thickened periosteum and in the perichondrium, the collagen fibers may be separated by large vacuolated cells. Such changes are found in tubular bones as well as in the flat bones of the skull.[8] Bones of cartilaginous origin as well as membrane bones are affected by the same pathologic process, so that the osseous changes in gargoylism are not completely due to "chondrodystrophy." In some cases, the chondrocytes and osteocytes are swollen, enlarged and vacuolated.[9] In the tendons, the fibroblasts appear round and their cytoplasm is clear and vacuolated.

The liver usually is enlarged and may be twice its normal weight, but the surface remains smooth and normal in appearance. The edges sometimes are rounded and lobulated. The cut surface is soft and the hepatic lobules may be distorted. The cells often are enlarged and foamy or a clear vacuole occupies the center. The vacuole is surrounded by a dense zone of eosinophilic cytoplasm and the nucleus is displaced toward the periphery. The Kupffer cells also may be vacuolated and distended. Enlargement of the spleen is the rule; its weight may be several times the normal and its surface smooth and tense. The endothelial cells lining the sinusoids sometimes are large and vacuolated, whereas malpighian follicles are small and germinal centers are rare.[8,9]

The cloudiness of the cornea has been attributed to islands of clear and vacuolated cells that are located between the anterior epithelium and the substantia propria, thus replacing Bowman's membrane.

Although the brain is subjected to the same pathologic process as other organs, it is, in contrast to the abdominal organs, usually reduced in size and weight. Internal hydrocephaly affecting all parts of the ventricular system and moderate convolutional atrophy have been observed.[27,28] Obstructive hydrocephaly may be due to specific deposits in meningeal cells and to meningeal thickening.[13] Microscopic examination reveals marked changes in the nervous elements. The pyramidal cells are distended, the nuclei displaced to the periphery and the Nissl bodies reduced in number. The neurofibrils are also mostly destroyed or moved to the outer aspects of the cell, whereas the center is occupied by abnormal elements that, according to the solvents used, appear either as vacuoles or as granules. The nerve cells in the subcortical centers show similar changes, but there are wide variations in degree and distribution. The neuroglia and the myelin sheaths are affected less than the nerve cells, but swelling of the glial elements and demyelinated areas can be observed.

Cardiac hypertrophy is present in about two-thirds of the cases and the weight of the heart may be two or even three times normal. Sometimes the epicardium and endocardium are thickened and hypertrophy of the left ventricle is more frequent than that of the right. Valvar lesions occur and, as a rule, the mitral and aortic valves are affected. On the free edges of the valves whitish nodules are noticed and the chordae tendineae are markedly thickened and shortened. The coronary arteries may appear enlarged but their ostia and lumina are narrowed. Yellow streaks and plaques often are seen in the intima of the aorta.[9] Microscopic examination of the myocardium shows infiltration by large and clear polygonal cells, which are found in patches between the muscular elements. The cytoplasm of the muscle fibers remains free of vacuoles.[8] The thickened valves contain large, foamy cells that sometimes are arranged in rows and bands of collagen fibers that are embedded in a homogeneous ground substance. The intima of the aorta and the coronary arteries also show areas of "gargoyle cells." Thickening of dense collagenous tissue with little effect on loose connective tissue has been demonstrated with involvement of the conduction system.[29] It is of interest that the endocardial involvement usually is limited to the left side of the heart and that the marked thickening may simulate endocardial fibrosis. This may occur in patients with severe cardiac symptoms who have gargoylism in an incomplete and atypical form.[30]

The changes in the connective tissue of the lungs, the gastrointestinal tract, the kidneys, the lymph nodes and the glands of internal secretion are essentially the same as those in the heart.

Abnormal granules in leukocytes were first described by Reilly.[31] In 4 of 8 patients with gargoylism, large dark violet granules were found in the cytoplasm of neutrophilic leukocytes and less frequently of lymphocytes stained by the Giemsa-Wright method. Although such cell inclusions are not always present, they have been observed in many cases.[9,32]

There is general agreement concerning the nature of gargoylism as a storage disease due to an inherited metabolic disorder. The typical "gargoyle cells" are found regularly in various organs, but the stored intracellular materials are still under investigation. Whereas some authors based their statements on findings in the brain and considered gargoylism a lipid storage disease, others believed that the accumulated substances are glycoproteins[9] or mucoproteins. In 1952, Brante[10] identified the disorder as a "mucopolysaccharidosis" and his point of view is generally accepted at present. Uzman[33] found in the liver and spleen two stored substances, a complex polysaccharide and a glycolipid. Brown[34] identified the water-soluble stored materials as a group of oligosaccharides, each of which is composed of D-glucosamine and D-glucuronic acid units combined in glycosidic linkage. The histochemical identification is still difficult, but the findings are in agreement with Brante's point of view and it is assumed that the abnormality represents an accumulation of acid mucopolysaccharides in connective tissue and in reticuloendothelial and parenchymal cells of many organs. In different organs, the tissue response may differ and secondary changes be the cause of apparent contradictory findings. Dorfman and Lorincz[35] and Meyer *et al.*[36] discovered increased amounts of mucopolysaccharides in the urine of patients with gargoylism. Chondroitin sulfate B and heparitin can be found in considerable amounts. Kobayashi[37] demonstrated acid mucopolysaccharide granules also in the epithelial cells of the glomeruli. The finding of increased amounts of urinary mucopolysaccharides is, of course, of diagnostic value. Berry and Spinanger[38] developed a diagnostic spot test that is based on the fact that chondroitin sulfuric acid can be detected on paper chromatograms by toluidine blue. From 5 to 25 μl. of urine is placed on separate spots of a piece of filter paper, which then is dipped into a solution of toluidine blue. Urine from children with gargoylism gives a purple spot against a light blue background. A comparison with known amounts of chondroitin sulfate placed on filter paper and treated in the same way permits estimation of the urinary concentration of this substance. It deserves emphasis that the ordinary reactions are positive not only in typical gargoylism but also in some patients who present clinically the symptoms of Morquio disease (p. 819). Chemical analysis of necropsy specimens of patients with gargoylism by Clausen *et al.*[39] showed accumulation of acid mucopolysaccharides in the liver, kidney, spleen and brain. In the liver, spleen and renal cortex there was an accumulation of mono-and di-sialogangliosides and glycolipids. The data suggested a metabolic defect common to the catabolism of both acid mucopolysaccharides and glycolipids in gargoylism. These findings are in agreement with histologic studies, which noted foam cells in viscera as found in Tay-Sachs disease.[40] Wolfe *et al.*[41] made histochemical analyses of 2 patients with mucopolysaccharidoses, 1 with normal mentality and 1 retarded. In the mentally retarded patient, acid mucopolysaccharides and an abnormal glycolipid were accumulated in the central nervous system and viscera; there was only mucopolysaccharide accumulation in the patient with normal intelligence. It was suggested that the acid mucopolysaccharide and glycolipid deposits represent separate but frequently associated abnormalities.

Similarity of gangliosides from the brain of a patient with gargoylism and from a brain of a patient with Tay-Sachs disease[42] was pointed out by Clausen *et al.*,[39] who also cited the case of a family in which 1 child had gargoylism and another Tay-Sachs disease.[43] These reports suggest that gargoylism is not merely a mucopolysaccharidosis and that the metabolic disturbances involved are more complex than is assumed at present.

Fibroblast cultures from skin of patients with Hurler syndrome show metachromatic cytoplasmic granules after staining with toluidine blue.[44] In such cells, dermatan sulfate constituted a larger percentage of the total sulfated glycosaminoglycans than it did in cultured fibroblasts from unaffected individuals.[45]

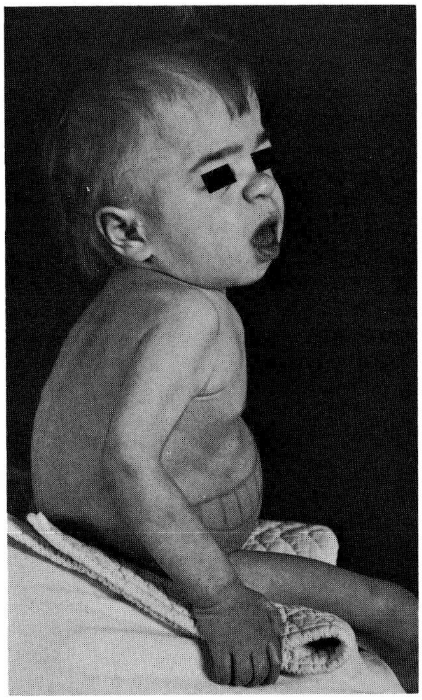

Fig. 88-1. – Girl with gargoylism, showing heavy eyebrows, low-set ears, depressed nasal bridge, kyphosis and outline of enlarged liver. She had corneal opacities and was mentally deficient.

The patients usually are well developed at birth, and in many instances it was stated that they were heavier than their normal siblings. The case of Liebenam[16] is interesting in that of a pair of discordant twin sisters the affected one was heavier at birth than the normal one. Delivery sometimes is difficult because of enlargement or deformity of the head, but, as a rule, the fully developed disease picture is not present before the age of 2 or 3 years. Then, the skull becomes either enlarged or deformed by premature synostosis of sutures. The frontal area protrudes and scaphocephaly, oxycephaly or brachycephaly develops. There may be ridges in place of sutures and protrusions at the base of the skull. The closure of the anterior fontanelle often is delayed. The orbital ridges are prominent and bossing of the temporal region may contribute to the enlargement of the head. The bridge of the nose is depressed and hypertelorism is present. The mandible is described as massive. Dentition is delayed and the erupted teeth are small, spaced and pointed.

The facial features are dull, coarse and grotesque, which has led to the term "gargoylism" for the entire syndrome. The victims also look unhappy, as though they were suffering from discomfort and pain.

The eyes are prominent and there are marked pouches under the palpebral fissures. In approximate-

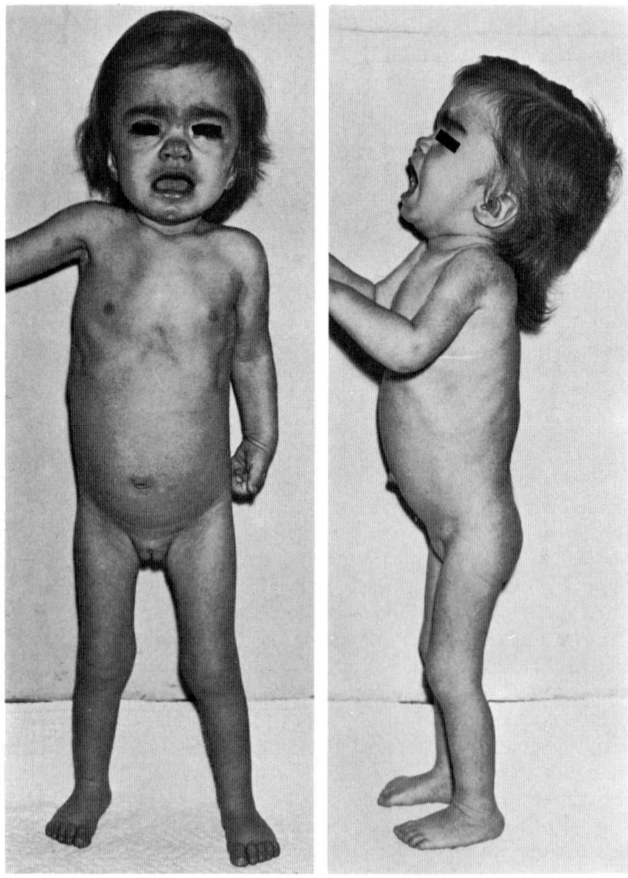

Fig. 88-2.—Child, 2½ years of age, with gargoylism. Note "snub nose" with depressed root, heavy eyebrows and hypertrichosis on shoulder and upper arm.

ly 60% of the cases reported the corneae are cloudy. Cloudiness at birth has been observed in exceptional cases but, as a rule, it develops in later stages of the disease. Even if the corneae appear to be clear, fine punctate dots may be detected with the slit lamp. The cheeks are heavy and the lips thick. The tongue is large, thick, fissured and often protruding. The nose is broad and flat and a profuse nasal discharge is the rule. The ears are broad, "fleshy" and placed low. Many patients are hard of hearing and they have a tendency to infection of the middle ear. The deafness can be attributed to changes in the inner ear.[46]

The neck is short and the head seems to be placed directly on the shoulders. The anteroposterior diameter of the chest is increased and the sternal region bulging or depressed. The heart frequently is enlarged and a systolic murmur can be heard. Dyspnea is noticed on slight exertion and cyanosis is seen in advanced stages. Hemodynamic and angiocardiographic observations in 15 patients with Hurler syndrome were reported by Krovetz *et al.*[47] Sudden death and congestive heart failure terminate many cases of Hurler syndrome (p. 816). Kyphosis in the dorsolumbar region is a characteristic feature of the syndrome. Bilateral congenital elevation of the scapulae (Sprengel deformity) is not always present, but the first cases described by Hunter[2] showed this anomaly, and other authors have since re-emphasized it as a part of the syndrome.[9,20] The abdomen is distended and umbilical and inguinal hernias are noted. Hepatosplenomegaly is found in the majority of cases but, like other symptoms of storage diseases, it may appear late. The liver and spleen are firm and smooth, reaching far below the costal margins. Sexual maturation is slow, but in some patients who survived adolescence good development of the genitalia has been observed.[46] The extremities are limited in movements. Inability to raise the arms above the shoulders and limitation of extension at the elbow and knee are constant features. The upper extremity is short and plump, the appearance of the hand being almost diagnostic. The fingers are short, thick and fleshy and usually held in flexion (Fig. 88-3). The entire hand is broad and claw-like. In the lower extremity, coxa valga and genu valgum occur. The skin is thick and resembles that of myxedema. This thickening is most marked in the face and on the dorsum of the hands and contributes to the resemblance of these patients to cretins. In some patients the skin may be very loose.

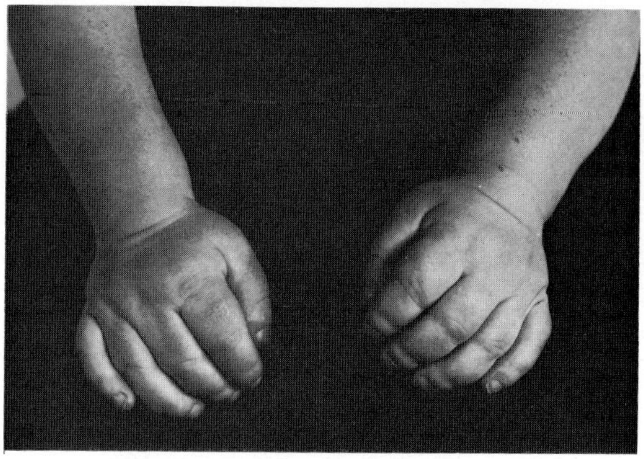

Fig. 88-3.—Hands of a girl with Hurler syndrome.

Symmetrically distributed cutaneous lesions have been observed. They consist of papules or firm nodules of pea size that contain abundant hyaline and collagenous fibers as well as cells characteristic of gargoylism.[48] Localization around the deltoid area seems to be rather characteristic in the beginning but, from there, the specific lesions may spread, forming areas of "Peau d'orange"[49] or "corrugated skin."[50] It is of historic interest that skin lesions now considered typical for gargoylism were present in one of Hunter's cases[2] described in 1917. Hypertrichosis is regularly present. The hair of the scalp sometimes is described as fine and silky and sometimes as coarse and thick. The heavy eyebrows fused over the bridge of the nose represent an almost diagnostic feature.

Dwarfism becomes more pronounced as the patients grow older. The short neck, the kyphosis, the lack of longitudinal growth of the long bones and the semiflexed position of the hip and knee joints account for the small stature of patients with gargoylism.

Neurologic symptoms may develop as the cerebral degeneration proceeds. Convulsions, strabismus, nystagmus, hyperactive tendon reflexes, ankle clonus, positive Babinski signs, spastic paraplegia and ataxic movements have been observed.[28,32]

Mental development is retarded and, in some instances, deterioration below a previously established mental level has been observed. The patients learn to walk and to talk late and acquire only a very limited vocabulary. Many remain incontinent. Mental progress is particularly difficult for patients with impaired hearing. If they are of a friendly disposition, their guidance is not difficult but their ability to learn is very limited. Some of the patients with physical signs of the syndrome are mentally normal and a few were described as definitely intelligent. From these, it was learned what we know about the subjective disturbances of the syndrome. Backaches, headaches, vertigo, dyspnea and inability to use their extremities fully are the complaints proffered. Such intelligent patients usually are shy and retiring. Occasionally, patients with gargoylism survive and reach adulthood. Some of them retain transparent corneae, ability to hear and normal mentality. One patient in whom the diagnosis of gargoylism was confirmed by biopsy had successfully passed through an agricultural and mechanical college; he was in good mental health at the age of 29 years. Many atypical and incomplete cases of gargoylism have been described and designated "formes frustes."[12,51] Many, if not all, of these belong to the milder, sex-linked form (p. 816) or to the Scheie type (p. 817). Sudden and unexpected death is not unusual. Cardiac failure, circulatory collapse, pneumonia or suffocation has been considered the immediate cause of death.

Roentgenograms, although variable, are helpful in the diagnosis of this disorder. In the skull, premature synostosis of sutures may be found. In the majority of cases, the sella turcica is flat and elongated, but the clinoid processes are intact. Encephalograms reveal dilatation of the ventricular system in some of the cases.

The spinal column often is diagnostic, since the vertebral bodies are shortened in the sagittal direction and their anterior and posterior aspects appear concave (Fig. 88-4, *D*) or convex. The spinous processes are directed downward. The first or the second lumbar vertebra is small, wedge shaped and displaced backward, giving rise to the kyphosis typical for this disorder. On the anterior aspect of the reduced vertebra, a hook-like process is seen in many of the cases (Fig. 88-4, *D*). The lower ribs are thin in their proximal parts and become wide and club shaped in their lateral and anterior parts. The tubular bones are irregular in outline and their metaphyseal ends often are grotesquely distorted, their medullary cavities distended and their cortical walls thin. There are great variations in the bone lesions, since the locations of the gargoyle cells in the metaphyses and in the periosteal layers vary. The head of the humerus and the glenoid fossa are flat. The humerus is thickened by irregular swellings and the radius and ulna are expanded and short. The distal ends of the bones of the forearm are flaring or pointed (Fig. 88-4, *B*). The metaphyseal plate of the ulna often is slanted and turned toward the radius. The carpal bones usually are retarded in development and multiform in outline. The metacarpal bones may assume most unusual shapes (Fig. 88-4, *A*), since their shafts are irregularly expanded and their ends are drawn out into thin processes. In Figure 88-4, *A* the "bottle shape" of metacarpals II to IV is well illustrated, and central expansion of the basal phalanges is seen in Figure 88-4, *B*. In such well-developed cases of gargoylism, the roentgenogram of the hand resembles a claw and the diagnosis can be made at a glance (Fig. 88-4, *A*). The acetabulum and the head of the femur are flat and coxa vara or coxa valga may be present. The proximal end of the femur often is bent in a convexity turned laterad, and its width may be markedly reduced.[14] At the knee, the epiphyses sometimes appear small and they assume unusual contours. Figure 88-4,

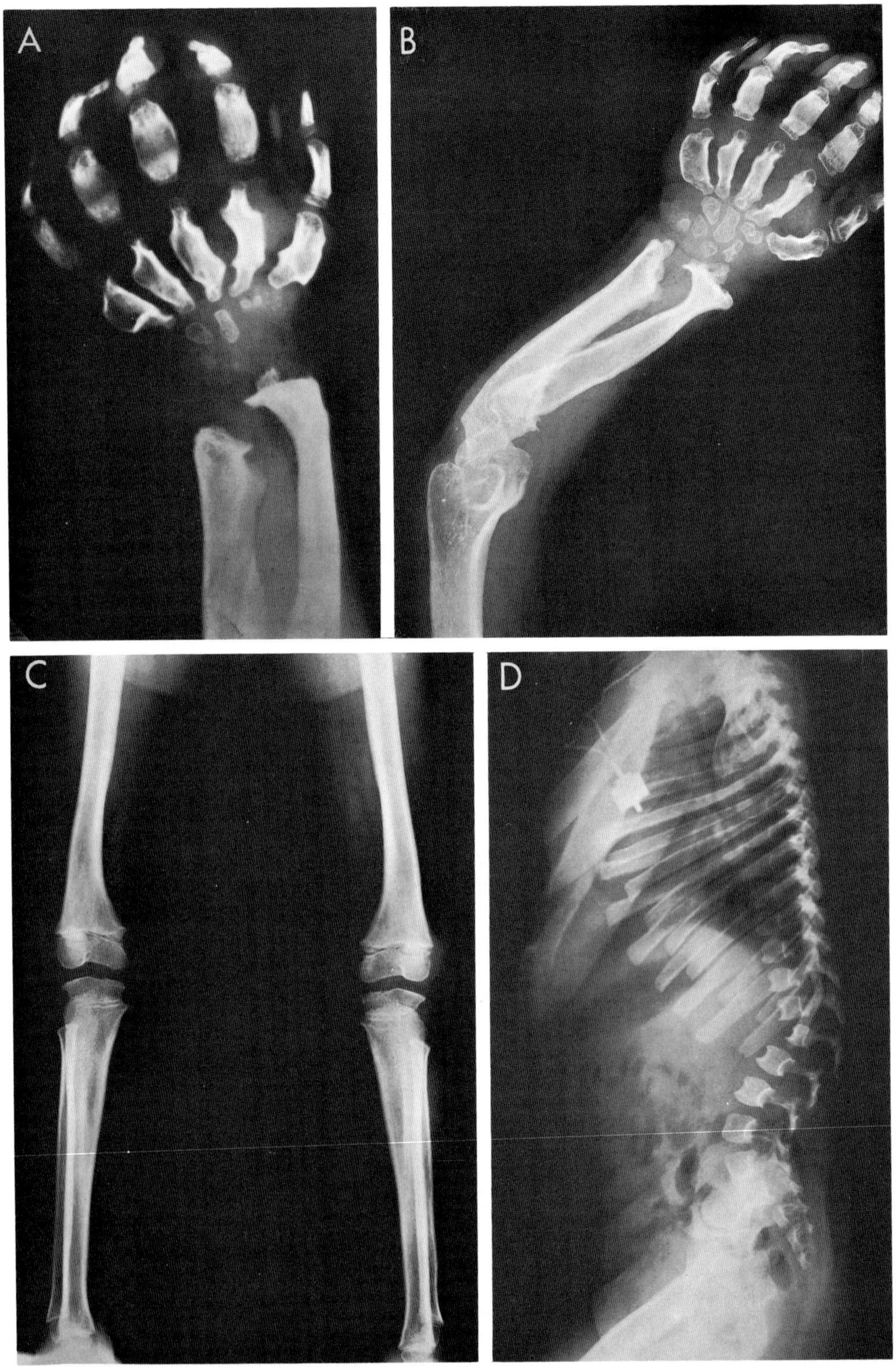

Fig. 88-4. – Hurler syndrome. **A,** roentgenogram of the left hand. Irregularities of metacarpals and phalanges and of metaphyses of radius and ulna. **B,** roentgenogram of the hand of a sister of the girl who also had gargoylism. **C,** lower extremities of a girl with gargoylism, showing irregular epiphyses and markedly shortened fibulae. **D,** roentgenogram of the chest and spine, showing biconcave vertebral bodies and reduction in size and "beaking" of second lumbar vertebra causing kyphosis. Spinous processes are directed downward.

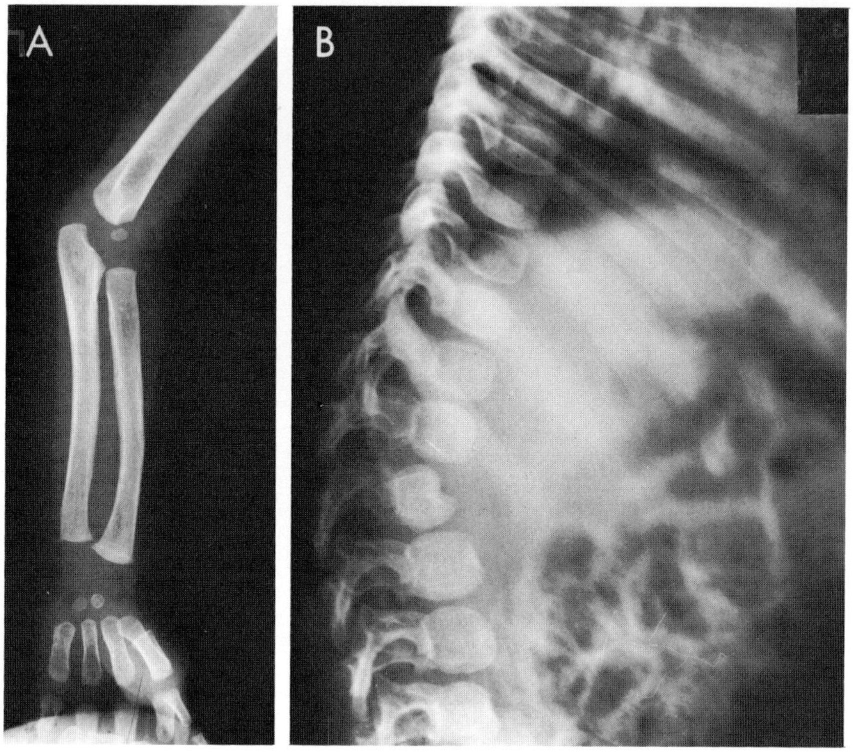

Fig. 88-5.—Roentgenograms of a child with gargoylism and relatively mild skeletal changes. **A,** arm with abnormal curves in radius and ulna. Metacarpal bones show irregularities on both ends. **B,** lateral view of spine. Second lumbar vertebra shows lack of ossification in upper anterior corner, causing kyphosis.

C shows striking shortening of the fibula, which appears reduced in length at both ends. According to Caffey,[14] the earliest bone changes seen immediately after birth are rarefaction, broadening and cupping of the metaphyses of tubular bones, which may appear to be enveloped in cortical cloaks. Differentiation from Morquio disease has been outlined by Langer and Carey.[52]

A typical case of gargoylism can be recognized at a glance on external inspection (see Figs. 88-1 and 88-2) and a roentgenogram of the spine, of the long bones or of the skull will confirm the clinical diagnosis. If, however, the syndrome is incomplete or if the observer is not familiar with the disorder, some other clinical entities will have to be ruled out. In former years, congenital syphilis was brought to mind because of the corneal opacities, the shape of the nose, impaired hearing, mental deficiency and hepatosplenomegaly. Lack of inflammatory signs speaks against keratitis parenchymatosa. The bone changes in the spine, ribs and hands can be distinguished easily from the skeletal changes of syphilis. The external resemblance to cretinism sometimes is striking (see Fig. 4 of Hunter's original publication[2]). Dwarfism, mental retardation, puffiness of the eyelids, thickness of the skin, the shape of the nose, the large tongue, the short neck, the protruding abdomen, umbilical and inguinal hernias, sexual infantilism and limitation of movement of the extremities are common to both conditions. Cloudy corneae, hepatosplenomegaly and the skeletal anomalies are characteristic of gargoylism and distinguish it from hypothyroidism. In Morquio disease, the skull is not severely deformed, the spine shows kyphosis and scoliosis and the vertebrae are flat (platyspondyly). The trunk is very short, the sternum protrudes and the hands and fingers are long but not "claw shaped" and broad. There are no signs of storage disease and the mentality usually is normal. But the differential diagnosis between Morquio disease and gargoylism may be difficult at times and intermediate forms exist (p. 817). Patients have been observed who, during the first years of life, developed skeletal changes compatible with Morquio disease, whereas, in later years, development of cloudy corneae and hepatosplenomegaly established the diagnosis of gargoylism.[32,53,54] The existence of such "late forms" of gargoylism explains the apparent concurrence of these two rare disorders in the same family.[32,55,56] If, in such families, the diagnosis of gargoylism has been established in a child, one is justified in assuming that the child with the syndrome resembling Morquio disease will later also develop signs of gargoylism. Examination of the corneae with the slit lamp helps to show beginning storage disease in the soft tissues (see Morquio-Ullrich syndrome, p. 817). Coffin *et al.*[57] described a syndrome of mental retardation, small stature, coarse facial features, narrow nasopharynx, thick cranium, large fleshy hands, pectus carinatum, tilted radial and ulnar metaphyses, bifid sternum, vertebral anomalies and kyphoscoliosis. These signs suggested an "atypical mucopolysaccharidosis." But many signs of gargoylism were absent, the mothers resembled their children in some respects and urinary mucopolysaccharides were not elevated.

The laboratory contributes to the diagnosis. Reilly[31] described abnormal granules in the leukocytes of children with gargoylism, but the changes are not found in all the patients examined. In the bone marrow, such granules have been seen in macrophages and lymphocytes.[32] The lipids of the blood are normal.[46] In newborn children with gargoylism and rickets-like bone changes, Caffey[14] reported high values of serum alkaline phosphatase. Increased amounts of urinary mucopolysaccharides are very helpful in confirming the diagnosis. Chondroitin sulfate B and heparitin sulfate are excreted in excessive amounts in the urine of patients with Hurler syndrome and in that of patients with Hunter syndrome. Wolfe *et al.*[41] suggested rectal biopsy as a diagnostic and prognostic aid, verifying the presence of Hurler syndrome by acid mucopolysaccharide in foam cells of the colonic wall and predicting the likelihood of normal mental development by absence of lipid storage in the ganglion cells.

Hurler syndrome without abnormal mucopolysacchariduria has been reported.[65,91] Biochemical and ultrastructural studies are being continued.[92]

The outlook for normal development is poor. In the autosomal recessive form, the complete disease picture described above develops during childhood, with all the handicaps of physical and mental retardation. Life expectancy is limited and most patients succumb during the first decade.[58] The sex-linked recessive form often takes a milder course. Impairment of vision and mental deterioration may be absent. Life expectancy is better than in the common form (p. 817). However, in the presence of cardiac lesions, early death is possible even in "incomplete cases," which show little involvement of other organ systems.[30] Deafness is another handicap that contributes to mental impairment of many patients.

The eugenic prognosis depends on the mode of transmission existing in the kinship. If females are among the patients, one is dealing with the autosomal recessive form. After 1 affected child is born in such a family, a risk of recurrence exists for 25% (or 1 in 4) of subsequent children. Some of the phenotypically normal children will be carriers who cannot be identified by clinical or laboratory signs at present.

In the sex-linked recessive type, only males manifest the disease, but it must be emphasized that not all families in which only male patients have been recognized belong in this group. If the disease has occurred in several generations[59,60] in males only who are related through their mothers and if all sisters of the patients are normal, it is quite likely that one is dealing with the sex-linked recessive form. In that case, there is a 50% risk for abnormal male children in subsequent pregnancies, but all female children should be phenotypically normal. Unaffected males in such families are entirely normal but half of the daughters are potential carriers who can transmit the disorder to some of their sons, the risk again being 50% for male children. It is clear that it would be of value for an affected family to know which mode of inheritance is responsible for the disease of their children, but this, for obvious reasons, is not possible in all cases.

There is no satisfactory treatment for gargoylism. The disorder dates back to fetal life, when the deviation from normal development cannot be recognized or suspected and, although many of the pathogenic features develop sometime after birth, as yet there is no way to stop the course of the disease. The finding of chemical anomalies in these patients has raised hopes for alleviation of the symptoms in the future. Prevention of all cases by eugenic advice is hardly possible, since carriers show no signs of their abnormal genotype. Parents who have a child with gargoylism should be informed that the disorder frequently occurs more than once in a family. Orthopedic treatment of the spine or of the extremities may be helpful and advisable, particularly in patients with mild mental retardation.

Hunter Syndrome

In 1917, Hunter[2] described 2 brothers, 10 and 8 years of age, who were dwarfed, had short necks, semiflexed knees, protuberant abdomens, hepatosplenomegaly, coarse facial features, deafness and noisy respiration; in the older brother, cardiomegaly and a diastolic murmur were noted. The corneae were not cloudy, the spine was straight and there was no mental retardation. These patients seem to represent the first description of the sex-linked form of gargoylism, termed the "Hunter" in contrast to the "Hurler" type. In a kinship reported by Beebe and Formel[60] 9 males were affected in four generations.

The disorder is less severe than the autosomal recessive form. Onset of symptoms is delayed, but most cases are more severe than those described by Hunter,[2] since abnormal behavior, feeding problems and mental deterioration become manifest after the boys are 3 years of age. Respiratory difficulties are noted early and hernias develop during the first years.[58] As a rule, cloudy corneae are absent, whereas deafness is pronounced.[26] But there are exceptions and hearing loss is not always severe in the Hunter type.[58] Slit-lamp examination may reveal corneal involvement in older patients. Atypical retinitis pigmentosa, papilledema and optic atrophy have been observed.[13] Growth retardation, stiff joints with contractures, enlargement of the head, coarse features, skin lesions about the shoulders, hepatosplenomegaly and cardiac changes develop at various ages. Death from heart failure occurred repeatedly in late adolescence but some of the patients survived to the fifth or even sixth decade.[13] Although the outlook for good mental development is dim, some of the patients achieve sufficient intelligence to earn their living in menial jobs. In other cases, the management of affected children is so difficult that early institutional care becomes necessary.[58]

Excessive amounts of chondroitin sulfate B and heparitin sulfate are excreted in the urine.

Sanfilippo Syndrome[61] (Polydystrophic Oligophrenia[62, 63])

Patients with this syndrome have severe mental retardation, but skeletal and visceral lesions can be less conspicuous than in the Hurler or Hunter syndrome. Within the first 2 years, slow intellectual and motor development is obvious as deafness and dull facial features become noticeable. There are respiratory and feeding difficulties and drooling is pronounced. The gait is clumsy, coordination is poor and toilet habits are not established. Contractures develop, locomotion becomes difficult and the patients soon are confined to bed.[58]

Cloudy corneae are rare and hepatosplenomegaly is not pronounced. Roentgenograms show only mild changes of the long bones and the vertebrae. Growth in height is fairly adequate.

Parental consanguinity has been recorded. Autosomal recessive inheritance has been established.[63] Excessive amounts of heparitin sulfate are excreted in the urine.[13]

Scheie Syndrome

This syndrome was considered a forme fruste of gargoylism by Scheie *et al.*,[64] since it can be seen in patients with normal intellect and normal stature. But cloudy corneae, retinitis pigmentosa, clawhands and hypertrichosis usually are present. Hepatosplenomegaly and skeletal changes are variable. Aortic valve disease may develop and psychoses have been observed in some of these patients.[13]

Large amounts of chondroitin sulfate B are excreted in the urine.

Polydystrophic Dwarfism

This mucopolysaccharidosis has been described by several authors since 1938[16] and was analyzed by Maroteaux and Lamy in 1965.[62] Lack of growth becomes apparent between the ages of 2 and 3 years. The facial features are reminiscent of Hurler syndrome but they are less pronounced. Trunk and limbs are short. There is lumbar kyphosis, sternal protrusion and genu valgum. Roentgenograms show moderate platyspondyly, wedge-shaped last thoracic and first lumbar vertebrae, obliqueness of the distal ends of the radius and ulna and fragmented epiphyses. Involvement of the corneae and auditory organs varies.

Autosomal recessive inheritance and parental consanguinity have been reported. Excessive amounts of chondroitin sulfate B have been observed but elimination of heparitin sulfate is normal.[62]

Morquio-Ullrich Syndrome (Late Hurler Syndrome)

During the early years of life, some children show characteristic symptoms and signs of Morquio disease limited to the skeleton and later in life develop such signs of Hurler syndrome as cloudy corneae, hepatomegaly or deafness. Such manifestations represent transitions from Morquio to Hurler syndrome. Whether this disorder is a specific entity[66] or a form of Morquio disease[67] is debated.

In 1943, Ullrich[11] reported patients with Morquio disease with normal intelligence, absence of hepatosplenomegaly but with cloudy corneae. Wiedemann[68] added 3 patients, 2 of whom also had hepatosplenomegaly and hearing defects, and by 1960 Noorden *et al.*[69] stated that a total of 15 cases of this type had been recorded. They also described 2 brothers who combined skeletal changes typical of Morquio disease with cloudiness of the corneae demonstrable under the slit lamp as yellowish gray refractile particles distributed throughout the corneal stroma. Both boys also had hearing defects, dental enamel hypoplasia, cardiac murmurs and Reilly granules in about 60% of the polymorphonuclear neutrophils. There was no splenomegaly but the liver was palpable in one case. The urine of the older brother contained "low amounts of mucopolysaccharides." The boys showed a striking external resemblance. Their mental development was slightly retarded. Schenk and Haggerty[56] reported radiologic and morphologic studies in 2 siblings with Morquio disease. A boy died at the age of 12 years, whereas his sister survived and at the age of 17 years developed corneal opacities. It is likely that these patients had Morquio-Ullrich syndrome, and the histologic findings reported in the boy refer to this disorder rather than to Morquio disease. The hyaline cartilage in the boy showed atypical features in all of the matrix components as well as of chondrocytes. In the cartilage matrix, the granular acid mucopolysaccharide component became fibrillar and assumed staining qualities of collagen and reticulin; or the granular acid mucopolysaccharide was absent and increased staining with Bismarck brown of the amorphous material suggested accumulation of keratosulfate. Apparently there was no accumulation of strongly acid mucopolysaccharides such as chondroitin and heparitin sulfate. The chondrocytes were abnormal in shape and size but foam cells contained greater quantities of stainable acid mucopolysaccharides than adjacent chondrocytes. The authors thought that abnormalities of the cartilage matrix were the result of abnormal mucopolysaccharide pro-

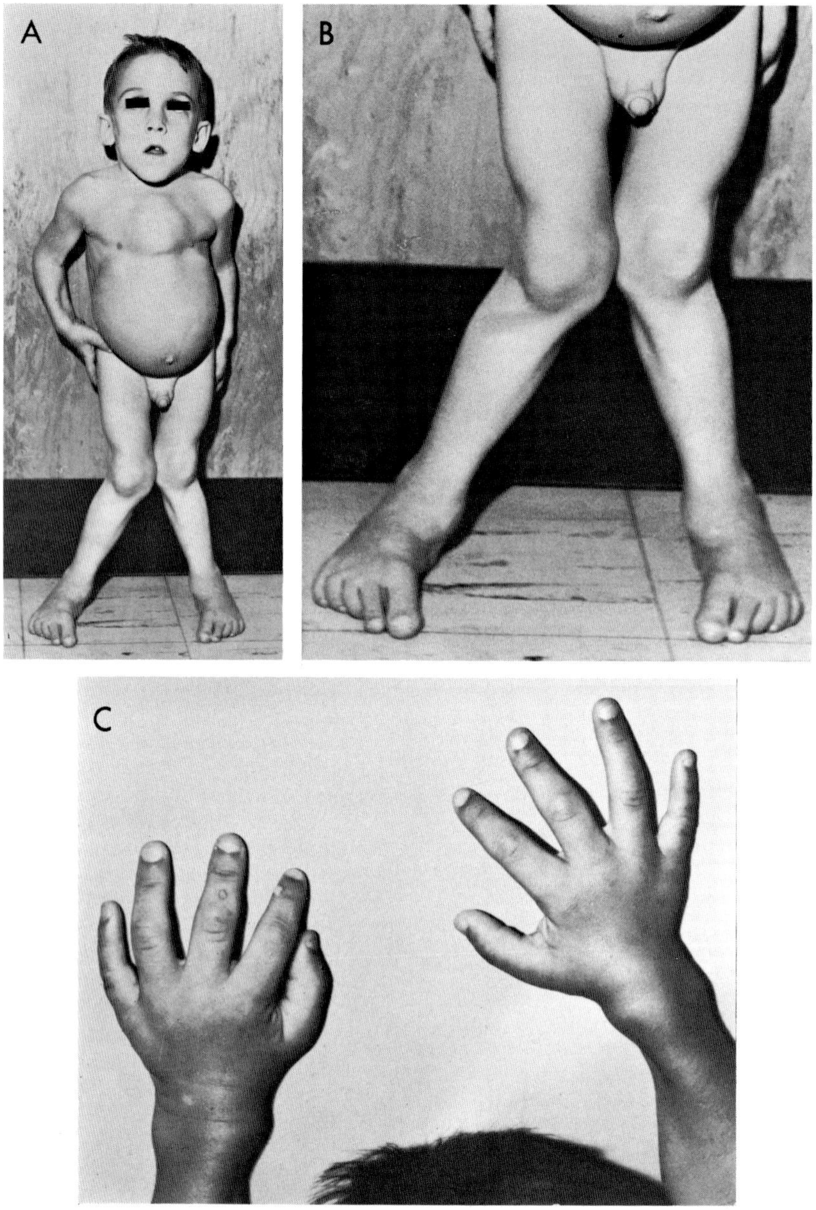

Fig. 88-6.—Boy with Morquio-Ullrich syndrome. Normal facies and skeletal malformations suggesting Morquio disease were present when he was first seen at the age of 2 years. Later, the upper extremities showed changes resembling those of Hurler syndrome. Chondroitin sulfate excretion in the urine was increased and cloudy corneae developed. **A,** at age 6 years. **B,** legs at age 7 years. **C,** hands at age 11 years.

duction by chondrocytes. Although an abnormal accumulation of mucopolysaccharides in foam cells and cartilage matrix was present, no evidence of visceral storage of mucopolysaccharides was found. Robins *et al.*[70] wrote on "Morquio's disease: An abnormality of mucopolysaccharide metabolism." Their findings were in siblings whose roentgenograms were consistent with Morquio disease but who showed corneal opacities, Reilly bodies and excessive mucopolysaccharide excretion. One-third of the excreted mucopolysaccharide in the urine of 1 child was identified as keratosulfate. Goidanich and Lenzi[66] described 3 patients with Morquio-Ullrich disease, including cloudy corneae and hepatomegaly. An increase in total excretion of mucopolysaccharide was found. A large amount of this was keratosulfate, the other fractions being mainly chondroitin sulfate A or chondroitin sulfate C, or both.

We have observed a child of this type who appeared normal at birth but developed pigeon breast with flaring of the ribs when he was 1 year of age. When seen at the age of 2 years he had, in addition, thoracic kyphosis and dislocated hips. He was about 15 cm. below average height for his age. His facial expression was alert and his developmental milestones were within normal limits. The corneae were clear. He presented a rather typical clinical picture of Morquio disease (Fig. 88-6, *A*). The roentgenograms of the spine showing flattening of the vertebrae and increased intervertebral spaces confirmed this diagnosis. But roentgenograms of the hands were characteristic of gargoylism. Reilly bodies were found in the leukocytes in moderate numbers. Mucopolysaccharides were elevated in the urine. A psychologic study was attempted. He did not talk at the examination, but in regard to nonverbal skills he functioned on a level normal for his age.

As he grew older, deafness became more pronounced and his skeletal malformations, particularly genu valgum, became so severe that orthopedic surgery had to be done. The corneae were somewhat clouded but hepatosplenomegaly was hardly noticeable. Mental development was not adequate but the boy could attend special classes. Despite his physical handicaps, he was active in sports and could swim and dive when 10 years of age.

A marked increase in mucopolysaccharide excretion was found, the major part of the uronic acid fraction being chondroitin sulfuric acid A/C.[71]

Morquio Disease (Brailsford Chondro-osteodystrophy; Familial Osseous Dystrophy; Hereditary Osteochondrodystrophy)

This atypical chondrodystrophy has been treated as an entity since 1929, when Morquio[88] reported 4 children of one family with the disorder, and Brailsford[72] described the radiologic features of the disease in 1 patient. The skeletal anomaly had been observed by Drysdale as early as 1908, and between 1910 and 1927 similar cases were reported briefly as atypical chondrodystrophies.[73] Other patients of this type were erroneously thought to have familial and intractable rickets.

A number of patients have been reported in the literature, with more than 1 member of a family affected. Most of these families consisted of apparently normal parents and 2 or more siblings with the disorder. Cocchi[74] collected from the literature 125 families with 184 affected children. Parental consanguinity is found in many instances, as in the original cases of Morquio. Townsend-Coles[75] reported from Khartoum, Sudan, "where consanguineous marriage is the rule rather than the exception," 7 cases occurring in three families. Males and females are affected equally. All these observations suggest that Morquio disease is inherited as an autosomal recessive trait.

Most of the patients described were children of European extraction, but the anomaly also exists in Egyptians,[76] in Sudanese[75] and in Negroes of Bantu and other stock.[77] Among these Negro children, 1 was a dizygotic twin, the other twin and 4 older siblings being normal. Concordance of identical twins with Morquio disease was reported by Neale and Hucknall.[78]

It is quite likely that the changes taking place in patients with this disease are effected by an inherited error of metabolism but, so far, no chemical changes have been demonstrated in typical cases.[79] That in some patients showing the skeletal malformations of Morquio disease, significant amounts of urinary mucopolysaccharides can be found (p. 821) and in others not is somewhat disappointing and it shows how far we are from the understanding of the etiology of deforming inborn errors of metabolism. Even if some chemical deviations are discovered, it is possible that they are the result and not the cause of the disease. Although Morquio disease is presented in recent publications as a mucopolysaccharidosis, this classification is not definitely established. The confusion apparently is due to the fact that some patients with skeletal anomalies resembling those of Morquio disease have a mucopolysaccharidosis with clouding of the cornea and hepatomegaly. Patients with this syndrome (Morquio-Ullrich, p. 817) excrete large amounts of mucopolysaccharides, including keratosulfate. Reports concerning patients with "pure" Morquio disease, who typically have neither corneal opacities, hepatosplenomegaly nor deafness, disagree in regard to increased urinary excretion of keratosulfate.[79,98]

The most striking abnormalities of this disorder are seen in the vertebral column, but information concerning the pathologic processes there is scant. Histologic examination of biopsy material from long bones showed defective ossification and disorderly calcification. In the region of the epiphyses, a paucity of chondrocytes was seen and the interstitial matrix contained foci of vacuolation. The osseous trabeculae were thin and contained cartilaginous masses with an irregularly striated matrix of varied staining intensities.[80] In a case studied at necropsy,[81] the cervical spinal cord was compressed in the anteroposterior diameter and widened in the lateral. Within the spinal cord there was loss of anterior horn cells and glial proliferation. In general, the pathologic process, which must be present at birth, manifests itself clinically only toward the end of the first year and later but, in a number of cases, symptoms have been described that point to early embryonic disturbances. Thus, in some patients, platybasia and abnormal segmentation of cervical vertebrae have been observed. Einhorn *et al.*[81] reported ankylosis of the first five cervical vertebrae and basilar impression of the skull. The boy seen in Figure 88-7 had multiple hemivertebrae, which indicates a relationship to the Klippel-Feil syndrome (p. 909). Congenital clubfeet are seen in some patients and spinal deformities can be recognized at birth occasionally.[82] The necropsy report by Schenk and Haggerty[56] concerns a boy 12 years of age who probably had Morquio-Ullrich syndrome in an early stage.

The clinical manifestation becomes increasingly noticeable during the first year and thereafter. Parents often state that the children were normal at birth, but even then roentgenography may show changes not detectable by inspection of the child. The growth pattern differs in this respect from achondroplasia, which is recognizable at or even before birth. Robinow[83] has shown by measurements gathered from the literature that the growth deficit increases with age. The early changes consist of development of a kyphosis and pigeon breast and enlargement of the osteochondral junctions, whereas knock-knees develop later. It is understandable that such osseous changes appearing during the first and second years of life in the past often led to the erroneous diagnosis of rickets. Antirachitic therapy, however, was of no avail and after several years the fully developed disease picture differed distinctly from vitamin D deficiency rickets. The patients are dwarfed in varying degrees. All cases fall below the lower 5% of the normal range of height.[83] Extreme dwarfing is seen occasionally, as in 1 of the Sudanese patients,[75] a woman who, at age 21 years, had a height of only 86 cm. Since the chief reduction in length is in the spine, the hands reach down to the middle of the thigh. The dwarfism simulates rachitic dwarfism of extreme degree, a condition that is now eradicated in most countries. The head appears rather normal except for its position. It seems sunken into the chest, the chin resting on the protruding sternum. Premature synostosis of the sagittal suture resulting in scaphocephaly has been described.[82] The face usually is well formed and its expression intelligent. Garn and Hurme[84] described in detail dental defects in 3 siblings afflicted with Morquio disease. The deciduous and the permanent teeth were of a dull gray color and lacked luster. The enamel caps were opaque and marked by numerous, irregularly distributed, minute pits. The teeth were small and widely spaced, but were, with the exception of the enamel, of normal structure. The neck is short in all cases, which is due to flattening of the vertebral bodies and sometimes to abnormal segmentation. Changes in the spine, usually observed first by the parents, consist of increasing kyphosis and scoliosis, which as a rule are most marked in the dorsolumbar area. The sternum protrudes almost horizontally in its cranial part and then turns downward at an angle. The costochondral junctions are enlarged and the Harrison groove may be pronounced, as in rickets. The vital capacity is reduced and dyspnea often is marked. The extremities are less reduced in length than the spine but they are not normal. The joints appear swollen; the hands may be normal or short and broad, as in achondroplasia. Owing to abnormal surfaces of articulation, the joints are hyperextensible in some regions and limited in movement in others. Sometimes swelling of the interphalangeal joints and limitation of the movements of the fingers are among the first complaints of patients who develop symptoms relatively late.[85] Such cases have been diagnosed erroneously as rheumatoid arthritis. The lower extremities appear shortened because they are flexed at the hips and knees. Changes in the hip joint are next in frequency to those in the spine. Most patients stand with hips in semiflexion, which accounts in part for their crouching position. Dislocation of the hip, knock-knees and flat feet usually are present. Walking is delayed and the gait slow and difficult. Hair and skin are normal; muscular development is poor and the ligaments are flaccid. If the cervical spinal cord is compressed, paralysis of the extremities, reflex changes and muscular atrophy may develop. Such neurologic complications can occur in patients with hypoplasia or absence of the odontoid process, which can result in atlantoaxial dislocation. Thoracic cord compression can also occur at the level of a thoracic gibbus.[95] Association with aor-

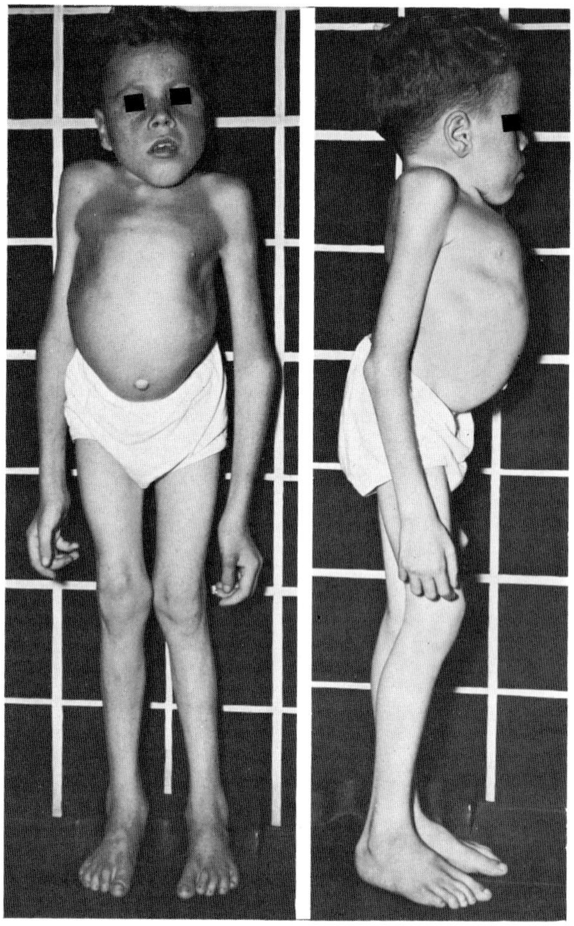

Fig. 88-7.—Morquio disease.

tic stenosis[86] and with patent ductus arteriosus[56] has been observed. Hepatomegaly has been recorded often. Enlargement of the liver suggests Morquio-Ullrich syndrome (p. 817) or gargoylism, but in the absence of splenomegaly, the palpable liver can be due to downward displacement of the organ by the skeletal deformities. The mentality usually is normal, but instances of mental retardation have been reported.[77,87]

In roentgenograms, the skull often is normal and the sella turcica not deformed. Basilar impression (p. 907) has been observed repeatedly. The spine consists of flat and irregularly outlined vertebrae (platyspondyly). The anterior vertebral borders show forward projections or the bodies are wedge shaped. In the cervical region, the atlas may be seen at the level of the foramen magnum, the lordosis be diminished and some of the vertebrae fused. The bodies of the lumbar vertebrae usually are higher than the thoracic but they often are dislocated backward in the upper segments.[83] The epiphyses of the vertebrae as well as those of the bones of the extremities ossify late. They are irregular in shape and fragmented. The metaphyses of the tubular bones are irregularly frayed, expanded in width and sitting obliquely on the shafts. The diaphyses can be long and slender or short and thick, comparable to those of mild achondroplasia. The ulna often is shortened so that the hand shows ulnar deviation. In the hip, the acetabula are large and deep and the femoral heads do not fit into the cavities, particularly if the epiphyses are deformed and fragmented. Coxa valga is present frequently. The proximal ends of the tibiae usually slant downward from the medial to the lateral condyli, with resulting genu valgum. The pelvis may show deficiency of the iliac bones and contraction of the greater sciatic notches.[75,83]

In most cases, the laboratory findings are within normal limits. The hypocalcemia reported by Morquio[88] was not confirmed by subsequent observers. Melkis and Mautner[89] published a case with the typical spine of Morquio disease and severe deformities of the long bones that was associated with marked hypercalcemia and a high basal metabolic rate. In some patients, an elevated serum phosphatase was found.[83] Excretion of large amounts of keratosulfate in the urine has been reported repeatedly,[13,67,98] but this biochemical sign may be characteristic of Morquio-Ullrich syndrome and not of Morquio disease.[79]

In young children, rickets must be excluded in the differential diagnosis; the absence of hypophosphatemia, the normal serum phosphatase, the appearance of the bones in roentgenograms and the resistance to vitamin D treatment support the diagnosis of Morquio disease. In older patients, the changes in the finger joints may suggest rheumatoid arthritis, but the absence of pain speaks against this. In Morquio disease as contrasted to achondroplasia, the trunk is short, the spine and chest are severely deformed and the extremities are relatively long. Differentiation from a well-developed case of gargoylism is not difficult, since in Morquio disease the facial features are normal, whereas the deformities of the spinal column are more pronounced; the shafts of the tubular bones usually are long and the fingers slender; there is absence of cloudy corneae and of hepatosplenomegaly; the mental development usually is normal. The urinary excretion of large amounts of mucopolysaccharides characteristic of gargoylism (p. 816) is absent in Morquio disease.[79] But in atypical cases it may be difficult to differentiate between these two syndromes, as transitional forms exist (p. 817). The same is true for a number of atypical forms of Morquio disease, which are separated with difficulty from the standard type (p. 809). The problem of differential diagnosis is best illustrated by the existence of interfamilial and intrafamilial variations. Robinow[83] has pointed out that the disorder varies greatly in different families in severity as well as in distribution of the anomalies, so that the resulting disease pictures may have little in common clinically.

A thorough discussion of the roentgenographic features of Morquio disease was published by Langer and Carey,[52] who thought that the disease picture of this disorder is well defined and always associated with excretion of keratosulfate in the urine. Since the delineation and differential diagnosis of Morquio disease is still in flux (p. 819), rigid classification according to roentgenographic signs is not recommended at present.

The disease is compatible with life but, with increasing age, there is an increase of complications. Dyspnea is present in many cases and there exists a tendency to respiratory infections that can be fatal. Orthopedic problems vary with the expression of the disease. The disabilities may be minor or they may amount to severe crippling, with inability to stand and walk.[75] Neurologic symptoms and death may be caused by compression of the spinal cord owing to cervical bone changes.

No specific therapy has been found and treatment must be symptomatic. Prevention of spinal cord compression by application of braces during early childhood has been recommended. Surgical intervention is needed when spinal cord damage is recognized.[95] Orthopedic procedures may be helpful but they often are disappointing. The deformities of the hips deserve particular orthopedic attention. Since the mental development usually is good, patients should be trained for occupations compatible with the disease. Ellman[85] reported a patient who successfully studied biochemistry and medicine.

Lipomucopolysaccharidosis

It has been mentioned (p. 810) that both mucopolysaccharide and lipid metabolism may be affected in some patients with gargoylism.[39-43] It is not clear as yet whether the lipid metabolism is abnormal in all patients with gargoylism or whether lipomucopolysaccharidoses are specific storage diseases. Spranger *et al.*[90] recorded a "new" storage disease observed in 2 patients with gargoyle-like features, skeletal malformations, slow cerebral degeneration, vacuolized lymphocytes and granular, metachromatically reacting inclusions in lymphocytes, fibroblasts, bone marrow and liver cells. In the urine there was no excessive excretion of mucopolysaccharides, but in the sediment there was metachromatic material within the cells and outside. The authors thought that this material possibly was a hexosamine-rich unidentified glycoprotein. In the course of the disease, progressive neurologic symptoms developed. Muscular weakness and atrophy, ataxia and tremor were seen in a patient who also had a cherry-red spot in the macula and optic atrophy. Degeneration of peripheral nerve fibers and myelin sheaths occurred with development of metachromatic substances. Similar cases not yet clearly defined were cited by Spranger *et al.*[90]

The area of the mucopolysaccharidoses is under intensive investigation. It is found that some patients do not fit into the established classes and that intermediate forms exist. Classification based on clinical findings may differ from those supported by roentgenologic or biochemical data. Satisfactory classification based on the pattern of mucopolysacchariduria[93,96] may need revision when tissue analyses become available and new cases are recorded. A new mucopolysaccharidosis was reported in 1970 in siblings with multiple soft tissue contractures, normal bones and normal intelligence.[97] One must agree with McKusick,[94] who stated in 1969: "The mucopolysaccharidoses are in a confused state presently" and hope with him that they will be "rectified in the next few years."

REFERENCES

1. Henderson, J. L.: Gargoylism, a review of the principal features with reports of five cases, Arch. Dis. Childhood 15:201, 1940.
2. Hunter, C.: A rare disease in two brothers (elevation of scapula, limitation of movement of joints and other skeletal abnormalities), Proc. Roy. Soc. Med. Vol. X, Sect. Stud. Dis. Child. 104, 1916–1917.
3. Hurler, G.: Über einen Typ multipler Abartungen, vorwiegend am Skelettsystem, Ztschr. Kinderh. 24:220, 1920.
4. Tuthill, C. R.: Juvenile amaurotic idiocy: Marked adventitial growth associated with skeletal malformations and tuberculosis, Arch. Neurol. 32:198, 1934.
5. Ellis, R. W., Sheldon, W., and Capon, N. B.: Gargoylism (chondro-osteo-dystrophy, corneal opacities, hepatosplenomegaly, and mental deficiency), Quart. J. Med. 5:119, 1936.
6. Washington, J. A.: Gargoylism (Hurler's Disease, Dysostosis Multiplex, Lipochondrodystrophy), in Brennemann, J. (ed.), *Practice of Pediatrics* (Hagerstown, Md.: W. F. Prior Company, 1948).
7. Straus, R., Merliss, R., and Reiser, R.: Gargoylism. Review of the literature and report of the sixth autopsied case with chemical studies, Am. J. Clin. Path. 17:671, 1947.
8. Strauss, L.: The pathology of gargoylism. Report of a case and review of the literature. Am. J. Path. 24:855, 1948.
9. Lindsay, S., Reilly, W. A., Gotham, T. J., and Skahen, R.: Gargoylism: A study of pathological lesions and clinical review of 12 cases, Am. J. Dis. Child. 76:239, 1948.
10. Brante, G.: Gargoylism: A mucopolysaccharidosis, Scandinav. J. Clin. & Lab. Invest. 4:43, 1952.
11. Ullrich, O.: Die Pfaundler-Hurler'sche Krankheit. Ein Beitrag zum Problem pleiotroper Genwirkung in der Erbpathologie des Menschen, Ergebn. inn. Med. u. Kinderh. 63:929, 1943.
12. Jervis, G. A.: Gargoylism (lipochondrodystrophy). A study of 10 cases, with emphasis on formes frustes of the disease, Arch. Neurol. 63:681, 1950.
13. McKusick, V. A.: *Heritable Disorders of Connective Tissue* (3d ed.; St. Louis: The C. V. Mosby Company, 1966).
14. Caffey, J.: Gargoylism (Hunter-Hurler disease, dysostosis multiplex, lipochondrodystrophy): Prenatal and neonatal bone lesions and their early postnatal evolution, Bull. Hosp. Joint Dis. 12:38, 1951.
15. Cordes, F. C., and Hogan, M. J.: Dysostosis multiplex (Hurler's disease; lipochondrodysplasia; gargoylism); report of ocular findings in 5 cases, with a review of the literature, Arch. Ophth. 27:637, 1942.
16. Liebenam, L.: Beitrag zur Dysostosis multiplex, Ztschr. Kinderh. 59:91, 1938.
17. Craig, W. S.: Gargoylism in a twin brother and sister. Arch. Dis. Childhood 29:293, 1954.
18. Nonne, M.: Familiäres Vorkommen (3 Geschwister) einer Kombination von imperfekter Chondrodystrophie mit imperfektem Myxoedema infantile, Deutsche Ztschr. Nervenh. 83:263, 1925.
19. Steen, R. E.: Hunter's polydystrophy (gargoylism) with cardiac lesions and some formes frustes, Brit. Heart J. 21:269, 1959.
20. Engel, D.: Dysostosis multiplex: Pfaundler-Hurler syndrome, report of two cases, Arch. Dis. Childhood 14:217, 1939.
21. Mathur, P. S.: Gargoylism, Indian J. Pediat. 24:372, 1957.
22. Lahey, M. E., Lomas, R. D., and Worth, T. C.: Lipochondrodystrophy (gargoylism), J. Pediat. 31:220, 1947.
23. Gilbert, E. F., and Guin, G. H.: Gargoylism, A.M.A. J. Dis. Child. 95:69, 1958.
24. Cockayne, E. A.: Gargoylism (chondro-osteo-dystrophy, hepatosplenomegaly, deafness) in two brothers, Proc. Roy. Soc. Med. 30:104, 1936.
25. Nja, A.: A sex-linked type of gargoylism, Acta paediat. scandinav. 33:267, 1946.
26. Lamy, M., Maroteaux, P., and Bader, J. P.: Étude génétique du gargoylisme, J. Génét. Hum. 6:156, 1957.
27. Jervis, G. A.: Familial mental deficiency akin to amaurotic idiocy, Arch. Neurol. 47:943, 1942.
28. Green, M.: Gargoylism (lipochondrodystrophy), J. Neuropath. 7:399, 1948.
29. Okada, R., Rosenthal, I. M., Scaravelli, G., and Lev, M.: A histopathologic study of the heart in gargoylism, Arch. Path. 84:20, 1967.
30. Vanace, P. W., Friedman, S., and Wagner, B. M.: Mitral stenosis in an atypical case of gargoylism: A case report with pathologic and histochemical studies of the cardiac tissues, Circulation 21:80, 1960.
31. Reilly, W. A.: The granules in the leucocytes in gargoylism Am. J. Dis. Child. 62:489, 1941.
32. Zellweger, H., Giaccai, L., and Firzli, S.: Gargoylism and Morquio's disease, Am. J. Dis. Child. 84:421, 1952.
33. Uzman, L. L.: Chemical nature of the storage substance in gargoylism, Arch. Path. 60:308, 1955.
34. Brown, D. H.: Tissue storage of mucopolysaccharides in Hurler-Pfaundler's disease, Proc. Nat. Acad. Sc. 43:783, 1957.
35. Dorfman, A., and Lorincz, A. E.: Occurrence of urinary acid mucopolysaccharides in the Hurler syndrome, Proc. Nat. Acad. Sc. 43:443, 1957.
36. Meyer, K., Grumbach, M. M., Linker, A., and Hoffman, P.: Excretion of sulfated mucopolysaccharides in gargoylism (Hurler's syndrome), Proc. Soc. Exper. Biol. & Med. 97: 275, 1958.
37. Kobayashi, N.: Acid mucopolysaccharide granules in the glomerular epithelium in gargoylism, Am. J. Path. 35: 591, 1959.

38. Berry, H. K., and Spinanger, J.: A paper spot test useful in study of Hurler's syndrome, J. Lab. & Clin. Med. 55:136, 1960.
39. Clausen, J., Dyggve, H. V., Melchior, J. C., and Lou, H. O.: Chemical studies in gargoylism, Arch. Dis. Childhood 42: 62, 1967.
40. Landing, B. H., Silverman, F. N., Craig, J. M., Jacoby, M. D., Lahey, M. E., and Chadwick, D. L.: Familial neuro-visceral lipidosis. An analysis of eight cases of a syndrome previously reported as "Hurler-variant," "pseudo-Hurler," and "Tay-Sachs" disease with visceral involvement, Am. J. Dis. Child. 108:503, 1964.
41. Wolfe, H. J., Blennerhasset, J. B., Young, G. F., and Cohen, R. B.: Hurler's syndrome, Am. J. Path. 45:1007, 1964.
42. Taghavy, A., Salsman, K., and Ledeen, R.: An abnormal ganglioside pattern from a gargoyle brain, Fed. Proc. 23: 128, 1964.
43. Shanklin, W. M., and Salam, M.: A comparison of the histochemistry of the cerebral cortex from siblings with gargoylism and Tay-Sachs disease, Acta neuroveg. 25:297, 1963.
44. Danes, B. S., and Bearn, A. G.: Hurler's syndrome, a genetic study in cell culture, J. Exper. Med. 123:1, 1966.
45. Schafer, I. A., Sullivan, J. C., Svejcar, J., Kofoed, J., and Robertson, W. van B.: Vitamin C-induced increase of dermatan sulfate in cultured Hurler's fibroblasts, Science 153:1008, 1966.
46. Smith, E. B., Hempelmann, T. C., Moore, S., and Barr, D. P.: Gargoylism (dysostosis multiplex): Two adult cases with one autopsy, Ann. Int. Med. 36:652, 1952.
47. Krovetz, L. J., Lorincz, A. E., and Schiebler, G. L.: Cardiovascular manifestations of the Hurler syndrome, Circulation 31:132, 1965.
48. Andersson, B., and Tandberg, O.: Lipochondrodystrophy (gargoylism, Hurler's syndrome) with specific cutaneous deposits, Acta paediat. scandinav. 41:162, 1952.
49. Cole, H. N., Jr., Irving, R. C., Lund, H. Z., Mercer, R. D., and Schneider, R. W.: Gargoylism with cutaneous manifestations, A.M.A. Arch. Dermat. & Syph. 66:371, 1952.
50. Levin, S.: A specific skin lesion in gargoylism, A.M.A. J. Dis. Child. 99:444, 1960.
51. de Lange, C., Gerlings, P. G., De Kleyn, A., and Lettinga, T. W.: Some remarks on gargoylism, Acta paediat. scandinav. 31:398, 1943.
52. Langer, L. O., Jr., and Carey, L. S.: The roentgenographic features of the KS mucopolysaccharidosis of Morquio (Morquio-Brailsford's disease), Am. J. Roentgenol. 97:1, 1966.
53. Ullrich, O., and Wiedemann, H-R.: Zur Frage der konstitutionellen Granulationsanomalien der Leukocyten in ihrer Beziehung zu enchondralen Dysostosen, Klin. Wchnschr. 31:107, 1953.
54. Wiedemann, H-R.: Zur Spätform der Pfaundler-Hurler'schen Krankheit, Helvet. paediat. acta 4:77, 1949.
55. Böcker, E.: Zur Erblichkeit der Dysostosis multiplex, Ztschr. Kinderh. 63:688, 1943.
56. Schenk, E. A., and Haggerty, J.: Morquio's disease; a radiologic and morphologic study, Pediatrics 34:839, 1964.
57. Coffin, G. S., Siris, E., and Wegienka, L. C.: Mental retardation with osteocartilaginous anomalies, Am. J. Dis. Child. 112:205, 1966.
58. Leroy, J. G., and Crocker, A. C.: Clinical definition of the Hurler-Hunter phenotypes. A review of 50 patients, Am. J. Dis. Child. 112:518, 1966.
59. Millman, C. G., and Whittick, J. W.: A sex-linked variant of gargoylism, J. Neurol., Neurosurg. & Psychiat. 15:253, 1952.
60. Beebe, R. T., and Formel, P. F.: Gargoylism: Sex-linked transmission in 9 males, Tr. Am. Clin. & Climatol. A. 66: 199, 1955.
61. Sanfilippo, S. J., Podosin, R., Langer, L. O., and Good, R. A.: Mental retardation associated with acid mucopolysacchariduria (heparitin sulfate type), J. Pediat. 63:837, 1963.
62. Maroteaux, P., and Lamy, M.: Hurler's disease, Morquio's disease, and related mucopolysaccharidoses, J. Pediat. 67:312, 1965.
63. Maroteaux, P., Frézal, J., Tahbaz-Zadeh, and Lamy, M.: Une observation familiale d'oligophrénie polydystrophique, J. Génét. Hum. 15:93, 1966.
64. Scheie, H. G., Hambrick, G. W., Jr., and Barness, L. A.: A newly recognized forme fruste of Hurler's disease (gargoylism), Am. J. Ophth. 53:753, 1962.
65. Steinbach, H. L., Preger, L., Williams, H. E., and Cohen, P.: The Hurler syndrome without abnormal mucopolysacchariduria, Radiology 90:472, 1968.
66. Goidanich, I. F., and Lenzi, L.: Morquio-Ullrich disease; a new mucopolysaccharidosis, J. Bone & Joint Surg. 46-A: 734, 1964.
67. Maroteaux, P., and Lamy, M.: La maladie de Morquio. Étude clinique, radiologique et biologique, Presse méd. 71:2091, 1963.
68. Wiedemann, H-R.: Ausgedehnte und allgemeine erblich bedingte Bildungs- und Wachstumsfehler des Knochengerüstes, Monatsschr. Kinderh. 102:136, 1954.
69. Noorden, G. K., Zellweger, H., and Ponseti, I. V.: Ocular findings in Morquio-Ullrich's disease; with report of two cases. A.M.A. Arch. Ophth. 64:585, 1960.
70. Robins, M. M., Stevens, H. F., and Linker, A.: Morquio's disease: An abnormality of mucopolysaccharide metabolism, J. Pediat. 62:881, 1963.
71. Dorfman, A.: Heritable Diseases of Connective Tissues: The Hurler Syndrome, in Stanbury, J. B., Wyngaarden, J, B., and Fredrickson, D. S. (eds.), *The Metabolic Basis of Inherited Disease* (2d ed.; New York: McGraw-Hill Book Company, Inc., 1966).
72. Brailsford, J. F.: Chondro-osteo-dystrophy, Am. J. Surg. 7: 404, 1929.
73. Fairbank, H. A. T.: *An Atlas of General Affections of the Skeleton* (Edinburgh: E. & S. Livingstone, Ltd., 1951).
74. Cocchi, U.: Polytope erbliche enchondrale Dysostosen, Fortschr. Geb. Röntgenstrahlen 72:409, 1950.
75. Townsend-Coles, W. F.: A report of seven cases of chondro-osteo-dystrophy (Morquio's disease), Arch. Dis. Childhood 29:7, 1954.
76. Mahmoud, M. E. S.: Chondro-osteo-dystrophy: Report of 3 cases, 2 brothers and 1 sister, J. Egyptian M. A. 37:199, 1954.
77. Feldman, N., and Davenport, M. E.: Osteochondrodystrophia deformans (Morquio-Brailsford disease), Arch. Dis. Childhood 26:279, 1951.
78. Neale, A. V., and Hucknall, R. H.: Chrondrodysplasia in twins, Arch. Dis. Childhood 9:51, 1934.
79. Bitter, T., Muir, H., Mittwoch, U., and Scott, J. D.: A contribution to the differential diagnosis of Hurler's disease and forms of Morquio's syndrome, J. Bone & Joint Surg. 48-B:637, 1966.
80. Shelling, D. H.: Osteochondrodystrophia Deformans (Morquio's Disease), in Brennemann, J. (ed.), *Practice of Pediatrics* (Hagerstown, Md.: W. F. Prior Company, 1948), Vol. IV.
81. Einhorn, N. H., Moore, J. R., and Rowntree, L. G.: Osteochondrodystrophia deformans (Morquio's disease), Am. J. Dis. Child. 72:536, 1946.
82. Whiteside, J. D., and Cholmeley, J. A.: Morquio's disease: Review of the literature with description of 4 cases, Arch. Dis. Childhood 27:487, 1952.
83. Robinow, M.: Morquio's disease, Clin. Orthop. 11:138, 1958.
84. Garn, S. M., and Hurme, V. O.: Dental defects in three siblings afflicted with Morquio's disease, Brit. D. J. 93: 210, 1952.
85. Ellman, P.: Morquio-Brailsford's disease: Simulating the arthritic manifestation of rheumatoid disease, Ann. Rheumat. Dis. 8:267, 1949.
86. Thoenes, W., and Holldack, K.: Aortenstenose bei Morbus Morquio, Monatsschr. Kinderh. 105:26, 1957.
87. Farrell, M. J., Maloney, J. D., and Yakovlev, P. I.: Morquio's disease associated with mental defect, Arch. Neurol. 48:456, 1942.

88. Morquio, L.: Sur une forme de dystrophie osseuse familiale, Bull. Soc. pédiat. Paris 27:145, 1929.
89. Melkis, A., and Mautner, H.: Osteo-chondro-dystrophia hypercalcemica idiopathica. An atypical case of Morquio's disease, Arch. Pediat. 75:285, 1958.
90. Spranger, J., Wiedemann, H-R., Tolksdorf, M., Graucob, E., and Caesar, R.: Lipomucopolysaccharidose. Eine neue Speicherkrankheit, Ztschr. Kinderh. 103:285, 1968.
91. Marchal, C., Grignon, G., Humbel, R., Vidailhet, M., Fall, M., Grignon, M., Pierson, M., and Neimann, N.: Mucopolysaccharidose sans mucopolysaccharidurie, Ann. pédiat. 44:2373, 1968.
92. Loeb, H., Jonniaux, G., Resibois, A., Cremer, N., Dodion, J., Tondeur, M., Gregoire, P. E., Richard, J., and Cieters, P.: Biochemical and ultrastructural studies in Hurler's syndrome, J. Pediat. 73:860, 1968.
93. Kaplan, D.: Classification of the mucopolysaccharidoses based on the pattern of mucopolysacchariduria, Am. J. Med. 47:721, 1969.
94. McKusick, V. A.: The nosology of the mucopolysaccharidoses, Am. J. Med. 47:730, 1969.
95. Blaw, M. E., and Langer, L. O.: Spinal cord compression in Morquio-Brailsford's disease, J. Pediat. 74:593, 1969.
96. Spranger, J. W., and Wiedemann, H-R.: The genetic mucolipidoses, Humangenetik 9:113, 1970.
97. Horton, W. A., and Schimke, R. N.: A new mucopolysaccharidosis, J. Pediat. 77:252, 1970.
98. Linker, A., Evans, L. R., and Langer, L. O.: Morquio's disease and mucopolysaccharide excretion, J. Pediat. 77:1039, 1970.

89

Osteogenesis Imperfecta

(Osteopsathyrosis)

OSTEOGENESIS IMPERFECTA is a disorder of the skeleton characterized by a marked tendency of the bones to fracture on slight provocation. Many patients with this disorder have bluish sclerae and some develop deafness later in life.

In the most severe cases, numerous fractures occur in uterine life and the infants are born with shortened and deformed extremities (micromelia) that resemble those of chondrodystrophy to a certain extent (see Fig. 83-1, *A*). This severe form, *osteogenesis imperfecta gravis* (fetalis, lethalis), has been distinguished from the milder form, *osteogenesis imperfecta tarda* (*osteopsathyrosis*),[1] which results in fractures, usually after birth. Osteogenesis imperfecta gravis and osteogenesis imperfecta tarda originally were described as separate entities, but later many authors considered them manifestations of the same disorder. The merits of these two conceptions will be discussed later.

A few historical remarks may explain and help to dispel the apparent confusion of terminology. A case of multiple congenital fractures was mentioned by Malebranche in 1678 and attributed to shock suffered by the mother while attending the execution of a man whose bones were broken on the wheel, a torture practiced in various countries during the Middle Ages and in Germany as late as 1827.[2] Other cases of osteogenesis imperfecta described in the eighteenth century likewise were related to maternal impressions obtained at executions on the wheel "whereby the child had all its members broken like those of a thief."[3] Intrauterine fractures were reported by Amand in 1714 and anatomically described by Bordenave in 1763. Subsequently, the congenital form was observed repeatedly but usually mistaken for fetal rickets until in 1854 Vrolik,[4] a Dutch anatomist, recognized the disorder as a separate entity, naming it *osteogenesis imperfecta*. The skeleton found in Vrolik's collection and illustrated in his work is that of a newborn child probably representing the severe and lethal form.

The form compatible with extrauterine life, now considered as a dominant hereditary trait, was clearly described in 1788 by Olaus Jacobus Ekman[5] in a doctor's thesis submitted to the faculty of medicine in Uppsala. Although his patients were considered cases of osteomalacia, Ekman's detailed clinical description of a family affected in four generations by fragility of the bones leading to "shocking deformities" represents a factual early report of osteopsathyrosis. Seedorff[6] reprinted this description in its original Latin and added an English translation. The hereditary form of bone fragility was again described by Lobstein[7] in 1833 and named by him *idiopathic osteopsathyrosis*. The distinction of lethal osteogenesis imperfecta gravis and of osteopsathyrosis, a condition compatible with life, is still in use. The term *osteopsathyrosis* seems to me to be preferable to osteogenesis imperfecta tarda,[1] since the viable form may begin early in uterine life or soon after birth, so that the attribute *tarda* can be misleading. Both terms omit the fact that fragility of bones frequently is associated with blue sclerae and deafness. The first recognition of blue sclerae as a related finding is attributed to Spurway.[8] Adair-Dighton[9] first associated deafness and blue sclerae with bone fragility in 1912. A family in which osteopsathyrosis, blue sclerae and osteosclerosis were heritable was reported in 1917 by van der Hoeve and de Kleijn.[10] From a clinical point of view, osteopsathyrosis, whether it manifests itself before or after birth, differs from the most severe forms of osteogenesis imperfecta, which are not compatible with postnatal life. Whether these clinically differing entities are etiologically identical is still undecided. In the following pages, the term "osteopsathyrosis" will be used for the common form of osteogenesis imperfecta, which usually manifests itself in fractures in postnatal life, blue sclerae and late deafness. Occasionally, one or several fractures are present at birth. Familial occurrence can be demonstrated in many cases.

All types of osteogenesis imperfecta are determined before birth by an abnormal development of that part of the mesenchyme that is destined to form the skeleton and the sclerae. According to some authors,[1,11] the nature of the osseous changes is always the same, whether the fractures occur before or after birth. These authors consider osteogenesis imperfecta and osteopsathyrosis, both the severe infantile and the late forms, to be the same disorder. Other students of the disease do not recognize the two as identical entities.[12] The argument between the two factions would be of little interest were it not for the practical problem of eugenic prognosis that depends on it.

There is general agreement that the common form of osteogenesis imperfecta (osteopsathyrosis) is attributable to an autosomal dominant gene. If one parent has the disorder, he may be expected to transmit it to approximately half of his children; members of the family who are free of the abnormal trait should not transmit it to their offspring. But it must be emphasized that the abnormal gene has variable expressivity and only part of the affected members have the complete syndrome—blue sclerae, brittle bones and deafness. The three elements of the syndrome can be found dissociated or in various combinations in different members of the same pedigree.

In his compilation of 60 pedigrees showing the syndrome, Fuss[13] found the abnormal manifestations in 392 affected individuals distributed in the following manner:

Osseous fragility, blue sclerae and deafness	60
Osseous fragility and blue sclerae	148
Osseous fragility and deafness	2
Osseous fragility only	9
Blue sclerae and deafness	20
Blue sclerae only	142
Deafness only	11

Thus, blue sclerae were the most frequent expression of the abnormal gene, since this manifestation was present in 370 of 392 affected persons. This finding must be kept in mind when a eugenic prognosis is made for an apparently healthy member of an osteopsathyrotic family who has no bone fractures but does show blue sclerae. Such a person is capable of passing on the disorder in all its manifestations to some of his children. Or an individual who possesses the abnormal gene may demonstrate no signs that interfere with his health. His bones may be long and slender yet he does not sustain fractures; he may have flaccid joints or slightly blue sclerae without being conscious of these variations; yet he can transmit manifest osteopsathyrosis to half of his children. Complete lack of penetrance with skipping of a generation is very rare if patients are examined thoroughly and x-ray studies are made of the persons who transmit the disorder. But such situations have been observed,[14,15] demonstrating that a clinically normal member of an osteopsathyrotic family can have the abnormal gene and transmit the disorder to some of his offspring. Occasionally, a child with osteopsathyrosis is born with one or several fractures, or suffers fractures soon after birth,[6,16-21] so that osteopsathyrosis does not exclude the possibility of congenital manifestation of the disease.

Many pedigrees showing dominant inheritance of osteopsathyrosis have been reported. Reviews and bibliographies have been published by Bell,[22] Fuss,[13] Kramer,[23] Seedorff,[6] McKusick[24] and others. Hills and McLanahan[25] investigated a family in Maryland in which 27 members of five generations were affected. A large Japanese kindred with a high incidence of blue sclerae but relatively few fractures was recorded by Komai *et al.*[26] But not all cases of osteopsathyrosis have a typical family history. It has been estimated that approximately a third of the cases seen by physicians would be expected to give a family history negative for the disorder.[15] It is possible, of course, that sporadic cases are genetically determined, since they may represent the manifestation of a new mutation of a dominant gene. In that case, the "sporadic" patient may have affected offspring and start a pedigree typical of osteopsathyrosis. Such a pedigree has been published by Herndon.[15] Another genetic explanation of a sporadic case would be that the patient is homozygous for an abnormal recessive gene, his parents being heterozygous and phenotypically normal. Hein[27] observed a newborn child with multiple fractures and blue sclerae whose parents were first cousins. Investigations of 23 relatives were negative for osteopsathyrosis. Kienböck[28] reported the case of a girl who began having fractures of the humeri and femora when she was 9 months of age. The fractures healed rapidly and without deformities. Although blue sclerae were not mentioned, the appearance of the bones spoke for typical osteopsathyrosis. There was no history of bone fractures in the parents and other relatives. The parents were first cousins. Hanhart[29] described hereditary osteopsathyrosis in four kinships. Parental consanguinity of various degrees could be shown in all instances and in no case was a parent affected. All patients had suffered fractures and some had bluish sclerae, but otosclerosis was diagnosed in only 1 of the cases. Simple recessive inheritance was assumed by the author. Other cases with possible recessive inheritance represented more atypical forms of fragilitas ossium. Meyer[30] reported 2 children in one family who had microphthalmia and osteogenesis imperfecta with multiple fractures but did not have blue sclerae. A third sibling had long bones with thin cortex and wormian bones in the skull but had not suffered any fractures. All 3 children, who were mentally retarded, excreted cystine, lysine, arginine and ornithine in amounts characteristic of cystinuria.[31] These siblings probably were the result of incestuous matings. The disorder of the French painter, Henri de Toulouse-Lautrec, whose parents were first cousins, has been considered osteogenesis imperfecta. Toulouse-Lautrec apparently was normal at birth. His childhood pictures[32] show no abnormal facial features or deformities. As an adult he appeared dwarfed because of marked shortness of his legs. The crippling was attributed to falls he had suffered when he was 13 and 14 years of age. He did not have blue sclerae and he was not deaf.[32] The fragility of his bones may have been due to an atypical osteogenesis imperfecta. His parents were free of the disorder and so were other members of his kinship, which can be traced back to A.D. 845.[33] Although this does not prove recessive inheritance, the possibility of a recessively inherited atypical osteogenesis imperfecta exists. In retrospect, Toulouse-Lautrec's case has now been diagnosed as pyknodysostosis[34] (p. 869).

Since the severe and lethal form of osteogenesis imperfecta usually is sporadic, it has been assumed by some authors that its etiology differs from that of osteopsathyrosis. Figure 89-1 shows the roentgenograms of such a newborn child with hundreds of fractures of the long bones and ribs combined with lack of ossification of the cranium. The parents and 3 siblings of this infant were in good health. The relatives in Follis's severe and lethal cases[35,36] also were unaffected. Glanzmann[12] concluded from his and other observations that the severe form is not hereditary. Although this possibility cannot be denied, other explanations can be offered. Such infants could be homozygous for a recessive gene, the heterozygous parents being phenotypically normal. There are some indications that this explanation is correct for some cases. Kaplan and Baldino[37] reported a kindred in which 9 cases of lethal or severe osteogenesis imperfecta occurred. Seven of the 9 patients were derived from consanguineous marriages. There was no osteopsathyrosis in the parents of these children and none of the short-lived patients could transmit the disease. These authors also cited an unpublished case of Perrot, who observed 2 siblings with osteogenesis imperfecta, children of a consanguineous marriage. Rohwedder[38] described a severe congenital form of osteogenesis imperfecta, the result of an incestuous mating. The child died in the fourth week of life. These cases suggest that the most severe forms of osteogenesis imperfecta may be due to recessive inheritance. There are other cases on record that can be explained in this way, although consanguinity of the parents was not known to exist. Schmidt[39] reported a case of unaffected parents who had 5 children with osteogenesis imperfecta. Two of these were stillborn and 2 died in infancy. Goldfarb and Ford[40] reported osteogenesis imperfecta in consecutive siblings born to normal parents and I have seen roentgenograms of 2 siblings with congenital osteogenesis imperfecta, children of unaffected parents. Recently, we have reviewed 2 cases of osteogenesis imperfecta gravis lethalis (Fig. 89-2). Three siblings and the parents were normal clinically and roentgenographically.[41] Although these cases are compatible with the assumption of recessive inheritance, they could also be attributed to the dominant gene responsible for osteopsathyrosis. One of the parents could have the gene that does not manifest itself because of low penetrance. Or a mutation could have occurred in a parental gonad, affecting an immature sex cell from which a cluster of abnormal germ cells was derived, all carrying the mutant dominant gene. The resulting germinal mosaicism could explain that several children of phenotypically normal parents are affected by a disorder attributable to an abnormal dominant gene. Sporadic cases could also be due to a fresh mutation. Since infants with the severe form are not viable, they cannot transmit the disorder to offspring. But if the severe form and osteopsathyrosis are genetically identical, pedigrees should exist in which patients with osteopsathyrosis produce children with the severe, lethal form. Such pedigrees are rare. It is true that congenital fractures have been observed repeatedly in children of osteopsathyrotic patients, but the cases of dominantly inherited osteopsathyrosis with congenital fractures that I could review[16,18,20,42] were not of the most severe type. The fractures resembled in number and healing tendency those seen in postnatal osteopsathyrosis. The child with congenital fractures recorded by Lovett and Nichols[17] died when 10 months old "of an affection not intimately associated with the fractures." In Seedorff's[6] family No. 7, the mother was born (to healthy parents) with fractures of both femora, suffering "innumerable fractures in

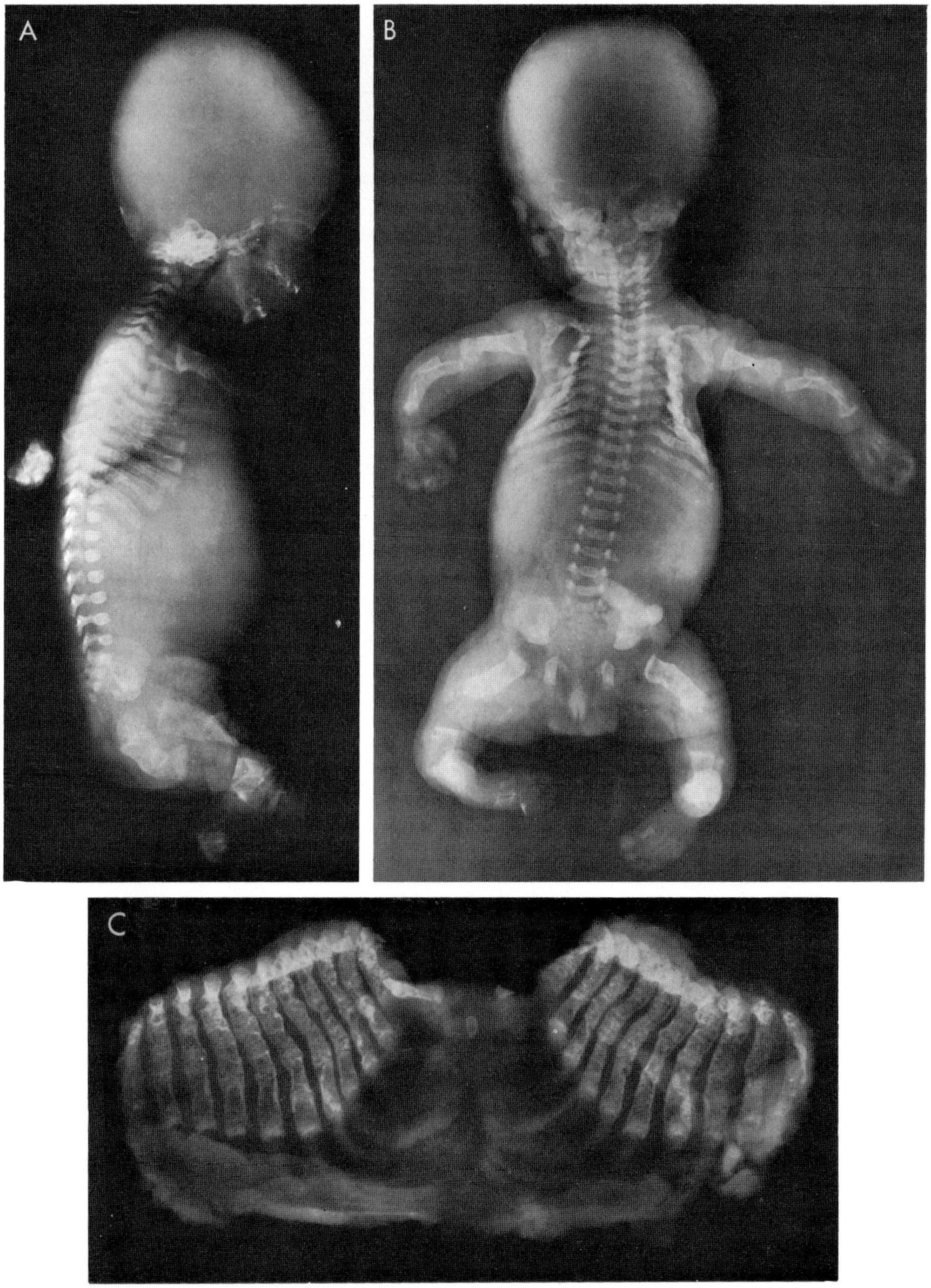

Fig. 89-1.—Sporadic case of osteogenesis imperfecta gravis in a newborn child. Note balloon-like skull, sparsely ossified, misshapen chest and fractured bones of the extremities. **A,** side view. **B,** front view. **C,** roentgenogram of ribs of the child (taken after necropsy), showing innumerable fractures.

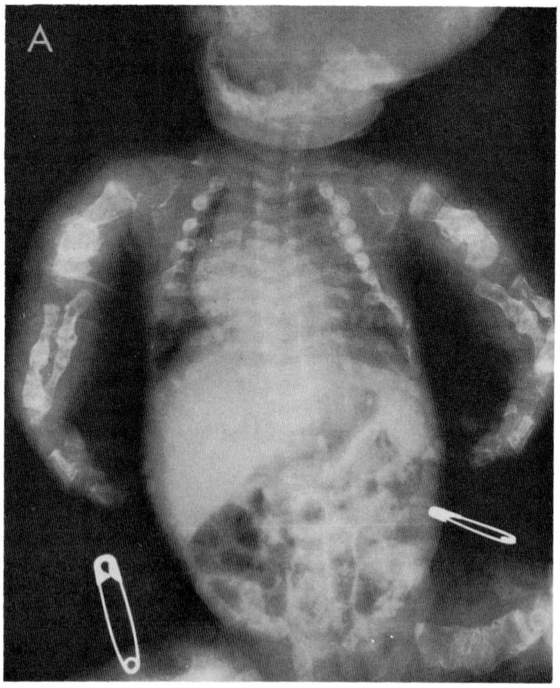

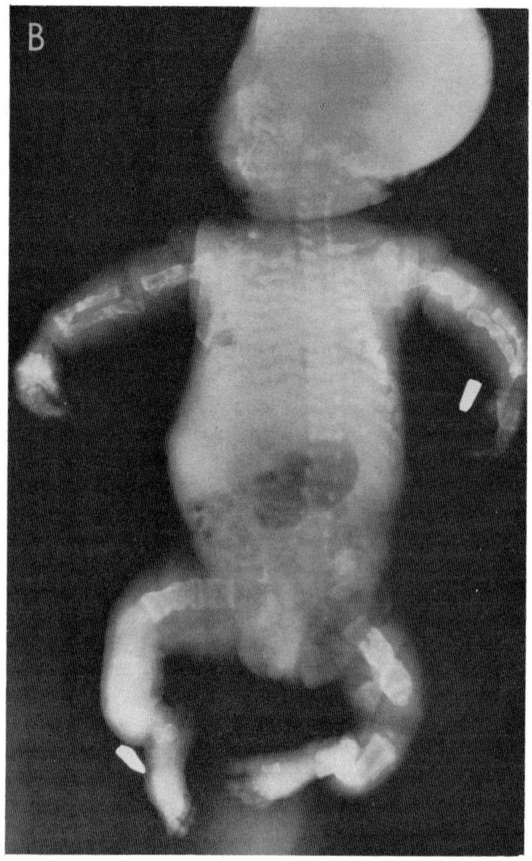

Fig. 89-2.—Severe semilethal osteogenesis imperfecta in sisters whose parents and 3 siblings did not have fractures of blue sclerae. **A,** the first girl in the family died when she was 4 weeks of age. **B,** the fourth girl in the family lived only 30 hours.

the course of her life." At age 22 years, she was delivered by cesarean section of a girl who had numerous fractures at birth. The head presented broad sutures and large fontanelles. She weighed 2,700 Gm. and was 45 cm. long, which does not suggest micromelia. The child died of bronchopneumonia when she was 6 months of age. I do not believe that this child had lethal osteogenesis imperfecta comparable with that illustrated in Figure 89-2. It is of interest that this was the only family in Seedorff's comprehensive Danish study in which osteopsathyrosis and congenital osteogenesis imperfecta occurred in two consecutive generations, which supports the view that most severe and congenital cases occur as "solitary phenomena" and usually are not the offspring of persons who have osteopsathyrosis. But in a pedigree assembled by Heys *et al.*[43] (their Figs. 1–4), a stillborn child with osteogenesis imperfecta gravis was born to a mother with osteopsathyrosis, a member of a kinship with typical manifestation and distribution of this disease. But this case, which proves that the lethal form can appear vicariously with mild forms of osteopsathyrosis, seems to represent an exception rather than the rule.

There is no proof that osteogenesis imperfecta can be induced as a phenocopy by environmental teratogenic factors, but the possibility of such osseous anomalies induced by external factors cannot be excluded. In a case recorded by Hennessy,[44] the mother was treated for "amenorrhea" with quinine and ergot preparations during the first 6 months of pregnancy. The child, delivered at term by cesarean section, had arms and legs that were so flexible that they could almost be tied in knots. The possibility of a toxic injury to the embryo cannot be ignored in this atypical case. We[45] reported an instance of multiple congenital malformations attributable to attempted abortion with aminopterin. The child had almost complete lack of ossification of the skull "reminiscent of the soft skull in the severe type of osteogenesis imperfecta . . . ." The long bones were long and slender but not fractured. I do not wish to present this case as a phenocopy of osteogenesis imperfecta but it is very likely that the defective ossification of the skull can be attributed to an external teratogenic agent. Pregnancy histories deserve recording in cases of severe or atypical osteogenesis imperfecta.

To sum up, it can be stated that osteopsathyrosis, the most frequent form of osteogenesis imperfecta, is a hereditary disorder attributable to an autosomal dominant gene. Reduced penetrance or expressivity and new mutations can explain that some cases of this disorder appear to be sporadic or not clearly transmitted through an affected parent. *Congenital* fractures can be present in patients who have this dominantly inherited form of osteopsathyrosis. Therefore, *congenital* osteogenesis imperfecta does not rule out osteopsathyrosis and not all congenital cases should be considered a specific disease, differing in etiology from "osteogenesis imperfecta tarda" (osteopsathyrosis). On the other hand, it should be emphasized that not all forms of osteogenesis imperfecta or fragilitas ossium need be identical with osteopsathyrosis in symptoms and etiology. Although sporadic cases can be attributed to the autosomal dominant gene of osteopsathyrosis by assuming reduced penetrance, new mutations and so forth, the streamlining tendency of recent authors is not recommended. Pressing all variants of osteogenesis imperfecta into one mold will hinder rather than promote progress in this field. The possibility, in some of the cases, of recessive inheritance or other genetic or nongenetic etiologic mechanisms should not be excluded a priori.

Twin studies have not contributed much to the understanding of osteogenesis imperfecta. Identical twins, both affected with the lethal form, have been reported by Welz and Liebermann[46] and mentally retarded twin sisters, both affected with a milder form of osteogenesis imperfecta, by Faxén.[47] Twins of like sex, discordant in regard to osteopsathyrosis, were encountered by Seedorff[6] and others,[48,49] but there was no proof that they were monozygotic. Discordance in dizygotic twins has been reported also.[50]

Reports concerning pathologic changes in osteogenesis imperfecta are not in complete agreement, since the materials examined were not uniform and different methods of staining were used. Some of the changes described refer to the mild form, others to the severe and some changes are secondary to fractures or to inactivity.

In older studies, the epiphyses and epiphyseal spaces were essentially normal, the pathologic changes being limited to the diaphyses. Although the enchondral ossification was normal and the preparatory calcification adequate, the envelopment of the remnants of calcified cartilage by osseous substance was diminished. Periosteal bone formation also was deficient and no compact cortex was formed. The entire trabecular system lacked the normal coherence and correlation and the marrow assumed a fibrous character.[51] Biopsy specimens from patients with osteopsathyrosis showed irregular lamellae and a reduced compacta. The reduction of the compacta was attributed to numerous large canals in which many osteoblasts were found.[71] The findings of Bauer,[11] who observed abnormalities not only in bones and sclerae but also in cartilage, connective tissue, small arteries, blood-forming organs and lymphatic tissues, have not been confirmed by other authors.[52]

In osteogenesis imperfecta gravis, Follis[35,36] found characteristic changes in several tissues. At the cartilage-shaft junctions, the cartilage appeared normal but osteoblasts and osteoid tissue were absent. The spicules of calcified cartilage did not undergo destruction in the normal fashion and they were fractured in many places. Osteoid tissue, which normally surrounds these spicules, was replaced by a substance that stained intensely red with the periodic acid-Schiff reagents and was interpreted as an immature form of bone matrix, but normal osteoblastic activity could be demonstrated in places in which fractures had occurred. Biophysical examinations revealed that the affected bone matrix consists of immature and short collagen fibers within a ground substance of abnormally staining mucopolysaccharides. This matrix is not replaced by longer collagen fibers arranged in lamellar patterns characteristic of mature bone. It is thought that osteogenesis imperfecta is essentially a disorder of collagen synthesis and maturation.[36,53-55]

The frequent association of osteogenesis imperfecta with an anomaly of the sclerae is not coincidental. Phylogenetically, the sclerae are closely related to, if not a part of, the skeleton.[23] In many fish and amphibia, the sclerae contain cartilage and in those of many reptiles and birds cartilage and ossicles are found. These skeletal characteristics are absent in the sclerae of placental mammals. Nevertheless, the sclerae as well as the skeleton are affected in osteogenesis imperfecta and in osteopsathyrosis, thus indicating that these disorders date back at least to the common precursor of cartilage and bone – to the mesenchymal skeleton.

The sclerae sometimes are reduced in thickness to about one-third of the normal, but in other cases normal thickness and increased transparency have been observed.[23] In a case of the severe and congenital type, Follis[36] found the cornea as well as the sclerae much thinner than normal. The thin fibers in these tissues as well as in the corium of the skin were argyrophilic and metachromatic, and stained red with the periodic acid-Schiff procedure. This behavior was interpreted as a failure of the reticulum to differentiate into mature collagen.

Conceivably, the deafness associated with osteopsathyrosis could be due to osseous changes. Histologic sections of the petrous bone of such a patient showed otosclerotic changes in the anterior part of the cochlea, the footplate of the stapes and the posterior semicircular canal. Both windows were occluded by new sclerotic bone,[56] but there is no complete agreement concerning the pathologic basis of the deafness in osteopsathyrosis. Whereas some authors believe that otosclerosis and osteogenesis imperfecta are due to a common genetic anomaly and that otosclerosis can be a local manifestation of osteogenesis imperfecta,[57] others doubt that the two disturbances have the same basic etiology.[58]

Osteogenesis imperfecta gravis (fetalis) is the most severe form of these disorders. It has been found in fetuses from 7 months to near term. In some cases, the duration of pregnancy is normal, although often the infant is stillborn or dies several hours or days after birth. Frequently, such cases have been made the object of thorough anatomic investigation, so that most necropsy reports refer to the severe type. There is no sharp histologic delineation between this form and milder cases in which the patient may live several years or reach adulthood.

The skull often is soft like a balloon, the bones being only partially ossified, and crackling can be noted on palpation. Infants with entirely membranous skulls usually are not viable. Although the vault may appear completely membranous, some ossification is present at the base of the skull and in lower parts of the frontal and occipital bones (see Fig. 89-1, *A* and *B*). In most cases, the eyes are prominent and the sclerae deep blue. It should be noted, however, that a bluish tint of the sclerae is normal in young infants and not diagnostic of osteogenesis imperfecta. The chest is severely deformed at birth owing to numerous prenatal fractures. The ribs are soft and broken in so many places that it is impossible to count the fractures (see Fig. 89-1, *C*). Often, fractures of the clavicles are present, but in the scapulae and in the pelvic bones they are less frequent. The vertebral column may remain intact, yet the neck usually appears short. The extremities are shortened and deformed (micromelia). The forearms and the lower legs are curved and the hands and feet assume abnormal positions. The extremities can be moved and bent passively in many directions and crepitation may be noted on manipulation. The skin, being too large for the shortened bones, may show transverse folds. The large head and chest, combined with micromelia, simulate achondroplastic proportions to a certain extent, but the fractures, the soft skull and the blue sclerae make possible the correct diagnosis of osteogenesis imperfecta.

Fig. 89-3.—Infant with osteopsathyrosis.

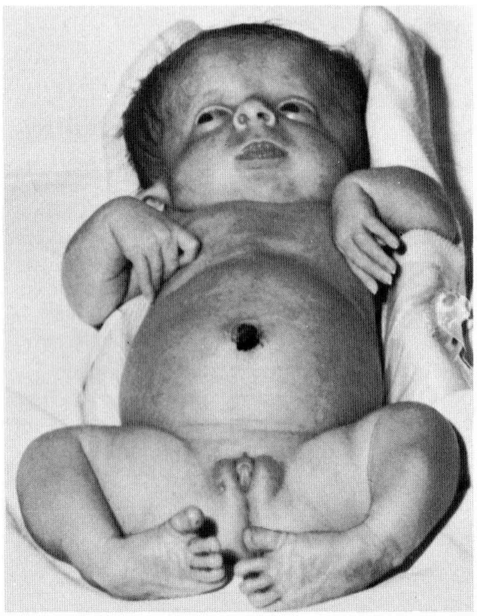

Osteopsathyrosis. As stated before, children born into families in which osteopsathyrosis is transmitted like a dominantly inherited trait may have lack of ossification of the bones of the calvarium and a few fractures at birth. As a rule, such infants are not as severely affected as those described in the preceding paragraphs, although there are exceptions.[43] In those who survive the newborn period, the disorder can continue as a serious handicapping disease or take a more benign course with a tendency to fractures and dislocations, which can be mitigated by avoidance of traumatic situations. In serious forms, fractures continue to occur at slight provocation and the resulting deformities can assume bizarre shapes. The tubular bones become elongated and slender as the child grows or they may become shortened, plump and angulated. Sometimes such patients do not learn to walk and remain bedridden cripples. The skull begins to ossify during the first years and hardens gradually. The ossification proceeds from many centers and numerous wormian bones are visible in roentgenograms for some time. There is marked bulging of the parietal region and the ears are turned downward. The chest and even the spine may be deformed by numerous infractions and abnormal angulations.

There is no treatment available by which this bone fragility may be reduced. Feeding and nursing care are difficult, since any handling of the patient may result in fractures. The fragility is so pronounced in some patients that neither breaks nor deformities can be prevented. In dealing with such patients, one must not blame parental neglect for repeated fractures. Even with the best of care, the outlook is grave, as these exceptional children with serious osteopsathyrosis are unable to stand or walk and their life is endangered by respiratory infections.

The majority of survivors are less affected. They appear normal at birth, although deep blue sclerae may suggest fragility of the bones before breaks occur. The first fractures usually are sustained between the first and second years of life. Only a moderate number of breaks occur and fragility frequently ceases at puberty. The fractures often are not very painful and callus formation is surprisingly good. The healing process, however, is not entirely satisfactory, as endosteal callus formation is insufficient and resorption of the periosteal callus sets in. The apparently healed bone often contains a circular decalcified zone that represents a point of minor resistance at which curvatures, deformities and new fractures are likely to occur. As a rule, fractures caused by minor traumas are not complicated, but after severe accidents, hemorrhages and dislocations may take place. Approximately 70% of the fractures affect the lower extremities, the femur, tibia or fibula being broken most frequently. Fractures of the radius, ulna, humerus or clavicle follow in frequency. In some families, certain

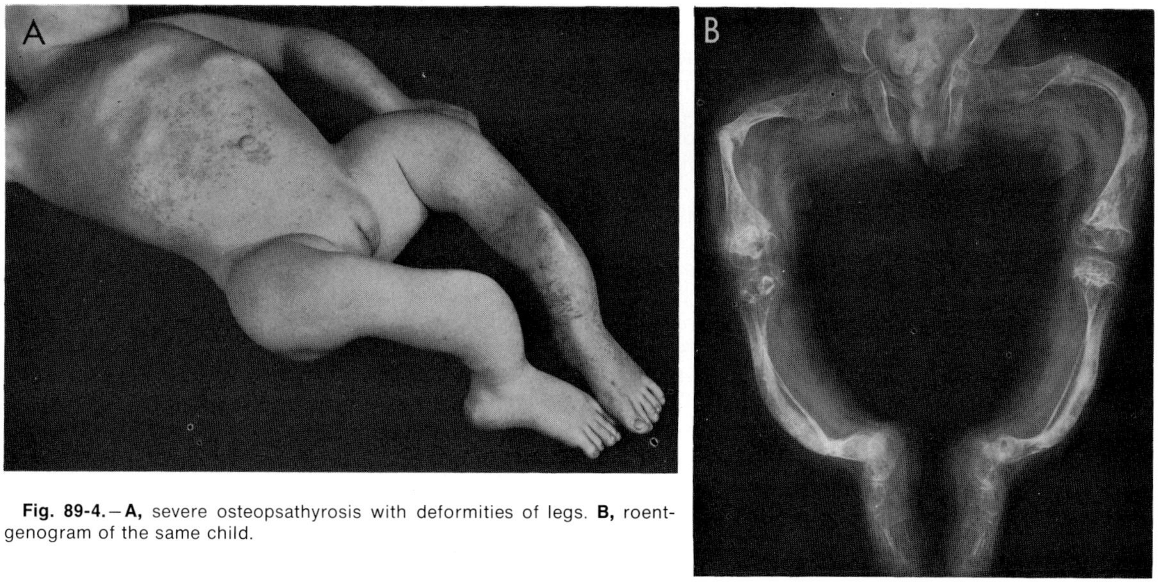

Fig. 89-4.—**A,** severe osteopsathyrosis with deformities of legs. **B,** roentgenogram of the same child.

bones seem to be predisposed and various members suffer breaks in the same location. Marked variations in fragility may be observed at different age periods. In the majority of cases, the years of childhood are most critical, but in rare instances the first fractures occur later. Patients with mild cases may suffer only one or two fractures throughout life and the diagnosis of osteopsathyrosis cannot be made unless the family history or blue sclerae betray the nature of the disorder. In severe cases, more than 100 fractures have occurred in postnatal life. Periods of fragility may alternate with periods of normality during which no breaks are sustained. A patient who suffers his first fracture late in life may transmit the disorder to his offspring before becoming aware of his own anomaly.

Mild osteopsathyrosis does not alter the appearance of the newborn nor does it interfere with early nutrition and growth. The extremities are long and slender and the skull is normally shaped. Later, the head may become flattened in the occipital region and bulging in the parietal region. Blue sclerae in persons with osteopsathyrosis are the rule, but in a few families bone fragility occurs in individuals with normal eyes.[14] Exceptionally, the blue tinge disappears in later life. Eyes with blue sclerae may be otherwise entirely normal, the thinness of the membrane not interfering with ocular function. Arcus senilis and embryotoxon often are seen in older patients with osteopsathyrosis.

As the patients grow older, they may develop curvatures of the spine and of the extremities. The deformities vary according to number, location, healing tendency and treatment of the fractures. Some patients appear almost normal, whereas others develop angulations and distorted curvatures of the legs and arms. Flaccid ligaments and hyperextensible joints are additional symptoms. Consequently, the patients have an increased tendency to sprains and dislocations. Dentition usually is normal but in some families dental changes dominate the disease picture. Heys *et al.*[43] observed five families of this type and eight families in which osteogenesis imperfecta was combined with odontogenesis imperfecta or, better, with *dentinogenesis imperfecta*, the defect being attributed primarily to the mesodermal dentin and not to the ectodermal enamel. The defect is common to both the deciduous and the permanent teeth and is recognizable by discoloration and translucency. The expression of this trait is variable, like that of other constituents of the syndrome.[43,59]

Approximately one-fourth of the patients with osteopsathyrosis develop deafness in the third decade of life or later. Most of these have otosclerosis, but labyrinthine deafness has been diagnosed occasionally. The two types of deafness may be found alternately in the same family.[23]

Many women with mild osteopsathyrosis have had pregnancies without complications and have transmitted their disorder to some of their children. But only a few women with the severe form have given birth to children. Evans[60] reported the remarkable case of such a patient who was so crippled by 65 fractures that she had never walked. She was delivered at 34 weeks' gestation by cesarean section of an apparently normal infant.

Occasionally, osteopsathyrotic patients or families have been known to have associated defects of a different type. Arachnodactyly and osteopsathyrosis have occurred in the same patient[61] but the association may have been accidental. Osteogenesis imperfecta associated with extensive cutaneous pigmentations, precocious puberty and hemihypertrophy has been described.[62] This syndrome represents a transitional complex between osteogenesis imperfecta and polyostotic fibrous dysplasia (p. 878). Combination of osteogenesis imperfecta with Ehlers-Danlos syndrome[63] has also been observed. The simultaneous occurrence of cleft palate, cleft lip, spina bifida, thrombasthenia and various endocrine disturbances probably represents fortuitous association. Congenital heart disease was present in rare cases.[64,65,72] Combination of osteogenesis imperfecta inherited from the father and of another mesenchymal defect from the mother was observed in patients described by Carey *et al.*[73] Calcification of arteries has been emphasized repeatedly.[24]

Osteosarcoma in patients with osteogenesis imperfecta has been reported, and the difficulty of differentiation from hyperplastic callus was pointed out.[66,67] Familial leukemia associated with osteogenesis imperfecta has been observed in siblings.[68]

The calcium and phosphorus values in the serum are within normal limits. The serum phosphatase is found to be normal in the majority of cases. Elevated levels of serum and urinary pyrophosphate have been found in patients with osteogenesis imperfecta, and

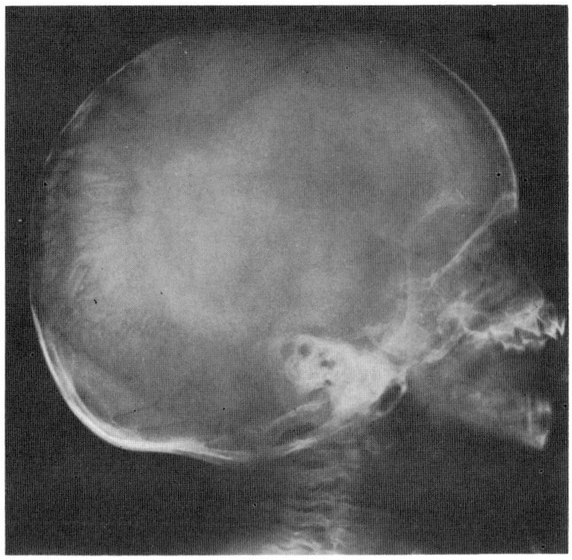

Fig. 89-5.—Skull of infant with osteopsathyrosis.

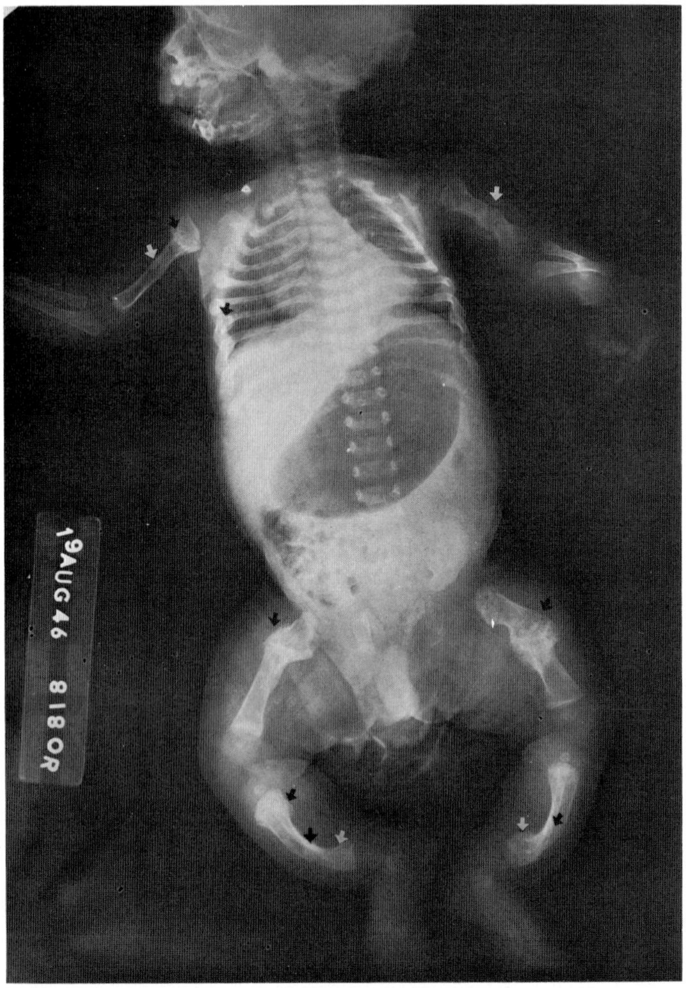

Fig. 89-6.—Congenital osteopsathyrosis in an infant 3 weeks of age. Some of the fractures were present at birth, others occurred after birth. No osteopsathyrosis in parents or other members of kinship.

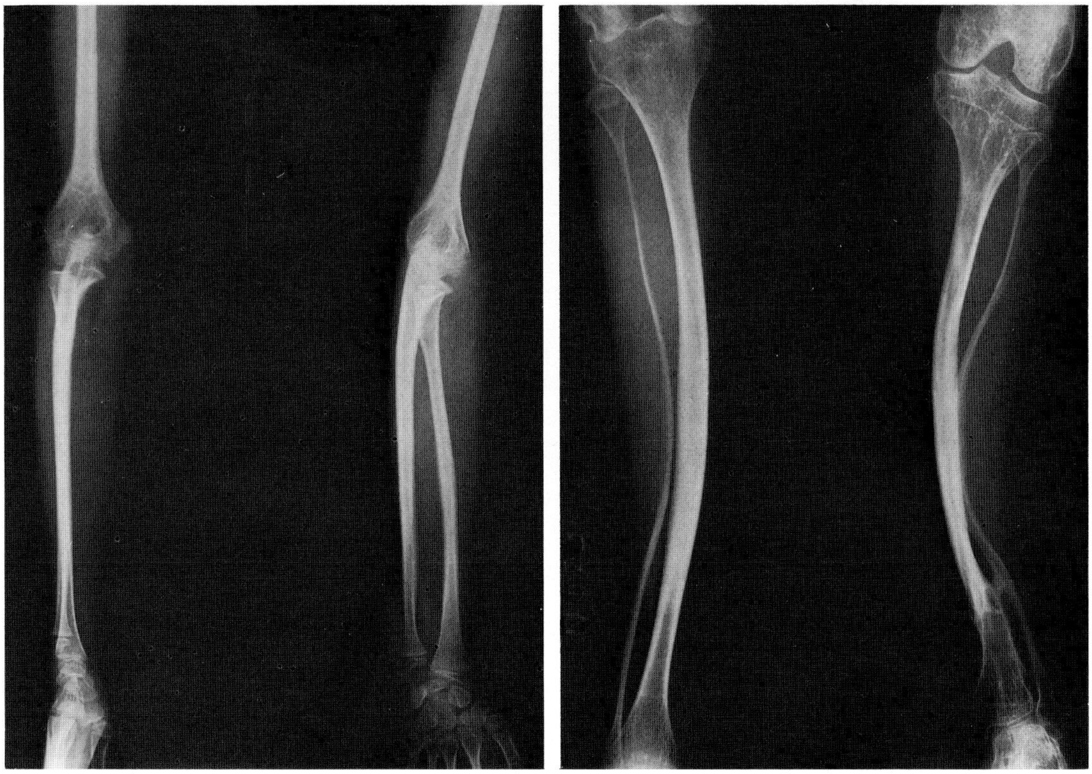

Fig. 89-7.—Roentgenograms of arm and lower leg in osteopsathyrosis. All bones are long and slender. Tibia and fibula show "flaring" of epiphyseal ends and reduction in width of diaphyses. Note bending of these bones caused by numerous fractures.

the possibility of inhibition of calcification by pyrophosphate and treatment with magnesium has been considered.[74] Ash content of the bones is reduced to about one-half of the normal. Estimates of the percentage composition of the minerals in bone vary in each case with the severity, nutritional state and activity of the patient. In osteogenesis imperfecta, the ratio of calcium phosphate to calcium carbonate is relatively high. The phosphatase activity is low in subperiosteal portions of bone but high in areas of callus formation.[69] Mineral balance studies show inadequate retention of calcium and phosphorus, which is accentuated by excessive doses of vitamin D. Favorable effects on mineral retention have been attributed to the administration of sex hormones, but these observations need further confirmation.

Many cases of osteogenesis imperfecta have been diagnosed in utero by roentgenograms. Ossification can be so delayed that the fetal skeleton can hardly be seen in advanced pregnancy; or the lack of ossification is limited to the cranium and fractures are recognized in the long bones and ribs of the fetus.[65]

In the common type of osteopsathyrosis, postnatal roentgenograms of the extremities at first show long slender bones that appear more or less osteoporotic. The diaphyses are thin but the epiphyses and metaphyses are normal. This disproportion creates the impression that the shafts are constricted and the ends enlarged. Considered independently, these x-ray changes are not diagnostic for osteopsathyrosis unless multiple fractures and deformities take place.

The skull bones are thin and osteoporotic and many wormian bones are seen in early life (Fig. 89-5). Later, the sutures between the inlaid bones appear as lines of diminished density, which must not be mistaken for fractures. Diffuse thickening of the calvarium occurs in exceptional cases.[70] The vertebrae sometimes are flat and the intervertebral spaces widened. Repeated fractures of the ribs change the shape of the thoracic cage. The tubular bones may be greatly deformed by repeated fractures and callus formation. Thus, a long, slender bone may become short and thick (Fig. 89-6), showing a pattern of alternating osteoporosis and osteosclerosis. In other instances the diaphyses assume the shape of curved ribbons or threads (Fig. 89-7). Grotesque angulations, pseudarthroses, bowing and malposition of skeletal parts complicate the picture in severe cases. Scoliosis occurs and the pelvis may appear triangular or compressed.

In rare instances, cyst formation and honeycombing are observed in the long bones and excessive callus formation may contribute to the grotesque shapes of the bones.

The outlook for individual patients varies greatly. Some are not troubled by the manifestations of os-

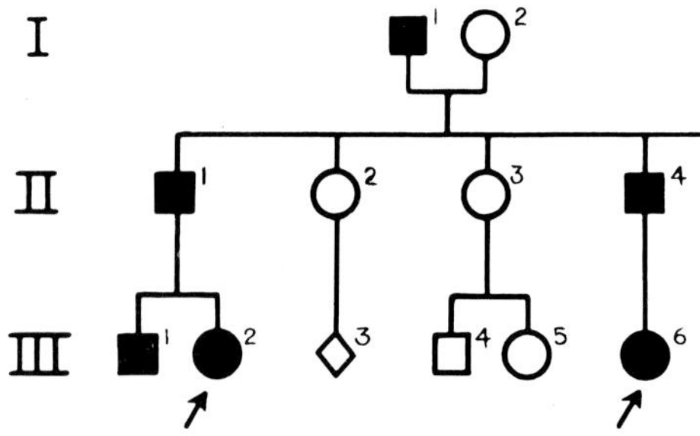

Fig. 89-8.—Pedigree of a kindred with osteopsathyrosis. Persons with blue sclerae are represented by black squares and circles. In addition, II_1 had multiple fractures and was dwarfed. II_4 had multiple dislocations and otosclerosis. III_1 long, gracile bones in roentgenograms. III_2 and III_6 had multiple fractures (personal observation).

teopsathyrosis, which may consist merely of blue sclerae and long and slender bones. Others are more or less handicapped by multiple fractures, dental disorders or otosclerosis. Members of the same sibship may be mildly affected or seriously crippled by the disorder. Some children are born with fractures, others are not affected until later in life.

Because of the variable expression of osteopsathyrosis, a eugenic prognosis is not easy. Persons with a mild form of the disease may have, with a normal mate, children who are severely affected. Affected persons are expected to transmit the trait to approximately half their children. Unaffected members of a family in which the disorder appears established should be free of the trait and the abnormal gene, and should have only normal offspring. But, in rare instances, persons free of symptoms may carry the abnormal gene and have affected children.

Although heredity is less obvious in cases of the severe and lethal form of osteogenesis imperfecta and although most cases of this type remain sporadic, prognosis for subsequent children should be guarded. The possibility of recessive inheritance or of germinal mosaicism must be kept in mind; in either instance, repeated occurrence of severe cases in a family of unaffected parents is possible.

Prevention of fractures is the most important task of the parents or of those who supervise these patients. It is not an easy task, since the children should be brought up as normally as possible yet be excluded from many activities. The child's interest must be diverted to games and toys that do not endanger his fragile bones. Nutrition should be adequate, but vitamins need not be given in excess. Endocrine treatment has been tried with little benefit. Favorable results have been reported following administration of estrogens and androgens,[69] but clinical evaluation of the results is difficult. Many other therapeutic attempts were reviewed by Cattell and Clayton,[55] who tested anabolic steroids in the therapy of severe osteogenesis imperfecta in 8 patients. The treatment was not beneficial and complicatious were severe. Fractures require orthopedic care. Deformities should be prevented by correct application of splints and braces. Surgical treatment of pseudarthroses and deformities has been effective occasionally. The management will be different for each case according to age and the severity of the disease.

REFERENCES

1. Looser, E.: Zur Kenntnis der Osteogenesis imperfecta congenita et tarda, Mitt. Grenzgeb. Med. Chir. 15:161, 1906.
2. *Encyclopedia Britannica*, Vol. 23, p. 566 (14th ed.; New York: Encyclopedia Britannica, Inc., 1953).
3. Griffith, J. P. C.: Idiopathic osteopsathyrosis (fragilitas ossium) in infancy and childhood, Am. J. M. Sc. 113:426, 1897.
4. Vrolik, W.: *Tabulae ad illustrandam embryogenesim hominis et mammalium, tam naturalem quam abnormem* (Leipzig: T. O. Weigel, 1854).
5. Ekman, O. J.: Descriptionem et casus aliquot osteomelaciae sistens, Dissertatio medica (Uppsala, 1788).
6. Seedorff, K. St.: *Osteogenesis Imperfecta* (Copenhagen: Ejnar Munksgaard, 1949).
7. Lobstein, J. G.: *Traité d'Anatomie Pathologique* (Paris: F. G. Levrault, 1833), Vol. 2.

Fig. 89-9.—Pedigree of a kindred with osteopsathyrosis. I_2 was crippled, hard of hearing and had dark blue sclerae. I_4 had dark sclerae and a few fractures. II_2 was crippled after many fractures. II_3 had blue sclerae and a few fractures. II_4 had very dark sclerae, short, twisted arms and dislocations of knees and ankles. II_6 had very dark sclerae, few fractures and a "trick knee." III_1 had many fractures and was crippled. III_3, mother of propositus, had had 9 fractures and dislocations of knee. IV_2 had no fractures but somewhat dark sclerae (history given by III_3).

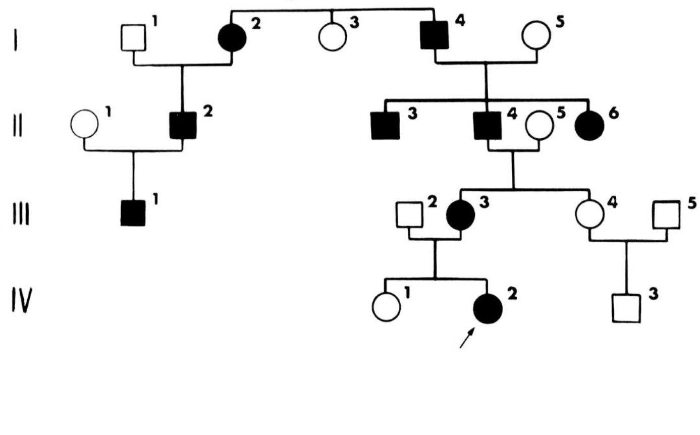

8. Spurway, J.: Hereditary tendency to fracture, Brit. M. J. 2:844, 1896.
9. Adair-Dighton, C. A.: Four generations of blue sclerotics, Ophthalmoscope 10:188, 1912.
10. van der Hoeve, J., and de Kleijn, A.: Blauwe Sclera, Broosheit van het Beemstelsel en Gehoorstornissen, Nederl. tijdschr. geneesk. 1:1003, 1917.
11. Bauer, K. H.: Über Identitaet und Wesen der sogenannten Osteopsathyrosis idiopathica und Osteogenesis imperfecta, Deutsche Ztschr. Chir. 160:289, 1920.
12. Glanzmann, E: Osteogenesis imperfecta (Typus Vrolik) and osteopsathyrosis idiopathica (Typus Lobstein), Schweiz. med. Wchnschr. 66:1122, 1936.
13. Fuss, H.: Die erbliche Osteopsathyrose, Deutsche Ztschr. Chir. 245:279, 1935.
14. Holcomb, D. Y.: A fragile-boned family, J. Hered. 22:105, 1931.
15. Herndon, C. N.: Osteogenesis imperfecta: Some clinical and genetic considerations, Clin. Orthop. 8:132, 1956.
16. Cronental, R.: Über die Osteopsathyrosis hereditaria, Deutsches Arch. klin. Med. 174:228, 1932.
17. Lovett, R. W., and Nichols, H.: Osteogenesis imperfecta, Brit. M. J. 2:915, 1906.
18. Ormerod, E. L.: An account of a case of mollities ossium, Brit. M. J. 2:735, 1859.
19. Puppel, E.: Osteogenesis imperfecta, Monatsschr. Geb. Gynäk. 82:269, 1929.
20. Rosenbaum: Osteogenesis imperfecta familiaris, Klin. Wchnschr. 5:1494, 1926.
21. Simmons, C. C. Osteogenesis imperfecta and idiopathic fragilitas ossium, Ann. Surg. 46:179, 1907.
22. Bell, J.: Blue Sclerotics and Fragility of Bone, in Pearson, K. (ed.), *The Treasury of Human Inheritance* (Cambridge and London: Cambridge University Press, 1928).
23. Kramer, S.: Osteogenesis imperfecta congenita et tarda, Ergebn. inn. Med. u. Kinderh. 56:516, 1939.
24. McKusick, V. A.: *Heritable Disorders of Connective Tissue* (3d ed.; St. Louis: the C. V. Mosby Company, 1966).
25. Hills, R. G., and McLanahan, S.: Brittle bones and blue scleras in 5 generations, Arch. Int. Med. 59:41, 1937.
26. Komai, T., Kunii, H., and Ozaki, Y.: A note on the genetics of van der Hoeve's syndrome, with special reference to a large Japanese kindred, Am. J. Human Genet. 8:110, 1956.
27. Hein, B. J.: Osteogenesis imperfecta with multiple fractures at birth: An investigation with special reference to heredity and blue sclerae, J. Bone & Joint Surg. 10:243, 1928.
28. Kienböck: Über infantile Osteopsathyrose, Fortschr. Geb. Röntgenstrahlen 23:122, 1915.
29. Hanhart, E.: Über eine neue Form von Osteopsathyrosis congenita mit einfachrezessivem Erbgang, sowie 4 neue Sippen mit dominantem Erbgang und die Frage der Vererbung der sogenannten Osteogenesis imperfecta, Arch. Julius Klaus-Stiftung 26:426, 1951.
30. Meyer, H.: Atypical osteogenesis imperfecta; Lobstein's disease, Arch. Pediat. 72:182, 1955.
31. Berry, H. K.: Cystinuria in mentally retarded siblings with atypical osteogenesis imperfecta, A.M.A. J. Dis. Child. 97:196, 1959.
32. Sejournet, G.: La maladie de Toulouse-Lautrec, Presse méd. 63:1866, 1955.
33. Mack, G.: *Toulouse-Lautrec* (New York: Alfred A. Knopf, 1938).
34. Lamy, M.: L'infirmité de Toulouse-Lautrec, Presse méd. 64:249, 1956.
35. Follis, R. H., Jr.: Osteogenesis imperfecta congenita: A connective tissue diathesis, J. Pediat. 41:713, 1952.
36. Follis, R. H., Jr.: Maldevelopment of the corium in the osteogenesis imperfecta syndrome, Bull. Johns Hopkins Hosp. 93:225, 1953.
37. Kaplan, M., and Baldino, C.: Dysplasie périostale paraissant familiale et transmise suivant le mode Mendélien récessif, Arch. franç. pédiat. 10:943, 1953.
38. Rohwedder, H. J.: Ein Beitrag zur Frage des Erbganges der Osteogenesis imperfecta Vrolik, Arch. Kinderh. 147: 256, 1953.
39. Schmidt, O.: *Ein Beitrag zur Kenntnis der sogenannten Osteopsathyrosis idiopathica* (Dissertation, Leipzig, 1901).
40. Goldfarb, A. A., and Ford, D.: Osteogenesis imperfecta in consecutive siblings, J. Pediat. 44:264, 1954.
41. Warkany, J., and Silverman, F. N.: Unpublished material.
42. Zurhelle, E.: Osteogenesis imperfecta bei Mutter und Kind, Ztschr. Geburtsh. u. Gynäk. 74:942, 1913.
43. Heys, P. M., Blattner, R. J., and Robinson, H. B.: Osteogenesis imperfecta and odontogenesis imperfecta: Clinical and genetic aspects in eighteen families, J. Pediat. 56: 234, 1960.
44. Hennessy, J. P.: Osteogenesis imperfecta, Am. J. Obst. & Gynec. 25:590, 1933.
45. Warkany, J., Beaudry, P. H., and Hornstein, S.: Attempted abortion with 4-amino-pteroylglutamic acid (aminopterin); malformations of the child, A.M.A. J. Dis. Child. 97:274, 1959.
46. Welz, W. E., and Liebermann, B. L.: Report of a case of osteogenesis imperfecta in twins, Am. J. Obst. & Gynec. 14:49, 1927.
47. Faxén, N.: A case of twins with osteogenesis imperfecta, Acta paediat. 14:251, 1932.
48. Kusnozoff, J.: Über Osteogenesis imperfecta, Frankfurt. Ztschr. Path. 16:97, 1914.
49. Müller, S.: *Periostale Aplasie mit Osteopsathyrosis unter dem Bilde der sogenannten fötalen Rachitis* (München: J. F. Lehmann, 1893).
50. Levin, E. J.: Intrauterine osteogenesis imperfecta in one of a pair of twins, Am. J. Roentgenol. 93:405, 1965.
51. Kaufmann, E.: *Pathology for Students and Practitioners* (Philadelphia: P. Blakiston's Son & Company, 1929).
52. Friedberg, C. K.: Natur und Wesen des Syndromes: Abnorme Knochenbrüchigkeit, blaue Skleren und Schwerhörigkeit, Ztschr. ges. Anat. (abst. 2) 15:779, 1931.
53. Engfeldt, B., Engström, A., and Zetterström, R.: Biophysical studies of the bone tissue in osteogenesis imperfecta, J. Bone & Joint Surg. 36-B:654, 1954.
54. Spencer, A. T.: Histochemical study of long bones in osteogenesis imperfecta congenita, J. Path. & Bact. 83:423, 1962.
55. Cattell, H. S., and Clayton, B.: Failure of anabolic steroids in the therapy of osteogenesis imperfecta. A clinical, metabolic and biochemical study, J. Bone & Joint Surg. 50-A:123, 1968.
56. Cleminson, F. J.: Otosclerosis associated with blue sclerotics and osteogenesis imperfecta, J. Laryng. 42:168, 1927.
57. Wullstein, H., Ogilvie, R., and Hall, I. S.: Van der Hoeve's syndrome in mother and daughters, J. Laryng. 74:67, 1960.
58. Altmann, F., and Kornfield, M.: Osteogenesis imperfecta and otosclerosis: New investigations, Ann. Otol. 76:89, 1967.
59. Witkop, C. J.: Genetics and dentistry, Eugenics Quart. 5: 15, 1958.
60. Evans, H. D.: Severe osteogenesis imperfecta with pregnancy. Report of a case, Obst. & Gynec. 28:394, 1966.
61. Ross, L. J.: Arachnodactyly. Review of recent literature and report of a case with cleft palate, Am. J. Dis. Child. 78:417, 1949.
62. Fromm, G. A., Parisier, H., Roca, J., and Defilippi Novoa, C. A.: Osteogenesis imperfecta associated with cutaneous pigmentation and other congenital malformations, A.M.A. J. Dis. Child. 96:344, 1958.
63. Riering, A., and Iversen, T.: Osteogenesis imperfecta associated with Ehlers-Danlos syndrome: Addendum. A new syndrome, Acta paediat. scandinav. 45:656, 1956.
64. Voorhoeve, N.: Blue sclerotics in connection with other hereditary or congenital abnormalities, Lancet 2:740, 1918.
65. Navani, S. V., and Sarzin, B.: Intra-uterine osteogenesis imperfecta. Review of the literature and a report of the

radiological and necropsy findings in two cases, Brit. J. Radiol. 40:449, 1967.
66. Jewell, F. C., and Lofstrom, J. E.: Osteogenic sarcoma occurring in fragilitas ossium, Radiology 34:741, 1940.
67. Klenerman, L., Ockenden, B. G., and Townsend, A. C.: Osteosarcoma occurring in osteogenesis imperfecta. Report of two cases, J. Bone & Joint Surg. 49-B:314, 1967.
68. Gilchrist, G. S., and Shore, N. A.: Familial leukemia and osteogenesis imperfecta, J. Pediat. 71:115, 1967.
69. Hansen, A. E.: Osteogenesis Imperfecta, in Brennemann, J. (ed.), *Practice of Pediatrics* (Hagerstown, Md.: W. F. Prior Company, 1948).
70. Keats, T. E.: Diffuse thickening of the calvarium in osteogenesis imperfecta, Radiology 69:408, 1957.
71. Key, J. A.: Brittle bone and blue sclerae. Hereditary hypoplasia of the mesenchyme, Arch. Surg. 13:523, 1926.
72. Heckman, B. A., and Steinberg, I.: Congenital heart disease (mitral regurgitation) in osteogenesis imperfecta, Am. J. Roentgenol. 103:601, 1968.
73. Carey, M. C., Fitzgerald, O., and McKiernan, E.: Osteogenesis imperfecta in twenty-three members of a kindred with heritable features contributed by a non-specific skeletal disorder, Quart. J. Med. 37:437, 1968.
74. Solomons, C. C., and Styner, J.: Osteogenesis imperfecta: Effect of magnesium administration on pyrophosphate metabolism, Calcif. Tissue Res. 3:318, 1969.

90

Other Heritable Skeletal Disorders

Cleidocranial Dysostosis

THIS GENERAL DISORDER of the skeleton is due to retarded ossification of membranous as well as cartilaginous precursors of bone. Its name is derived from the most striking features—congenital absence of the clavicles combined with softness of the calvarium.[1] These main features have been known since the eighteenth century, but with the advent of roentgen rays, abnormalities of many other bones could be demonstrated in severely affected subjects. In milder cases, only the skull may be defective (cranial dysostosis) and in others the clavicles alone show absent or incomplete ossification (cleidal dysostosis). For some time it was thought that only the bones of membranous origin are slow in ossifying, but it is now recognized that cartilage also is affected by retarded and irregular mineralization. Roentgenograms of certain bones resemble those of chondrodystrophies, but the epiphyseal ends do not show overgrowth of cartilage or marked distortions. A tabulation of symptoms in 61 patients was made by Schuch and Fleischer-Peters in 1967.[2]

A number of families have been described in which cleidocranial dysostosis is inherited like an autosomal dominant trait. Estimates of sporadic cases vary between 16% and 50%[2] but such estimates based on reported cases have little meaning, since there is a greater tendency to report familial cases than single ones. There also is the possibility that mild parental forms were overlooked in some reports. Sporadic cases could represent nonhereditary phenocopies or be attributable to recessive inheritance but it is more likely that they are the result of new mutations and that they can be transmitted to the offspring with a 1:1 risk.[3] In some kinships, incomplete manifestations alternate with the fully developed disease picture. Both sexes are affected equally. Monozygotic[4] and dizygotic[5] twins have shown concordance in regard to cleidocranial dysostosis and discordance of twins has been reported also.[6] An interesting pair of probably monozygotic twins has been observed in the Cincinnati Children's Hospital (Fig. 90-1). Both girls had cleidocranial dysostosis but only one had congenital heart disease, a tetralogy of Fallot, successfully operated on when the child was 2 years of age. Concordance in regard to cleidocranial dysostosis and discordance in regard to a malformation of the heart in a pair of monozygotic twins could be explained by genetic causation (mutation) of the former and "environmental" causation of the latter, illustrating possible differences in the environments of identical twins. Chromosome analyses of children with cleidocranial dysostosis showed normal karyotypes.[2]

Patients with cleidocranial dysostosis usually are

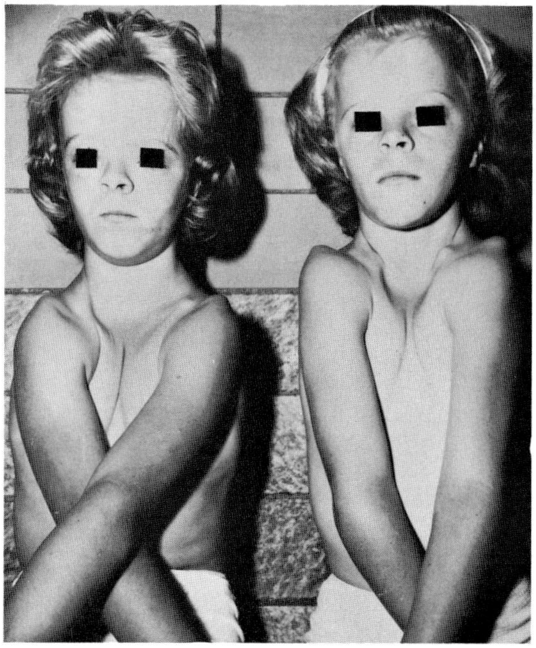

Fig. 90-1.—Twin girls, both affected with cleidocranial dysostosis. The parents were free of the disorder and so were 47 members of the kinship known to the parents. The twins were very similar in most traits, with the exception of tetralogy of Fallot present in one of the girls. The blood groups determined were identical in both girls.

short in stature, although occasionally the anomaly has been observed in tall individuals. The skull is brachycephalic, the frontal and temporal eminences are prominent and the areas of the fontanelles and sutures depressed. The widely spaced eyes are somewhat bulging and the facial skeleton appears underdeveloped. The teeth are irregular in position and form. They wear down prematurely and break easily. Some deciduous teeth may be retained long beyond the usual time and the permanent teeth may not erupt until old age. The enamel of the teeth appears relatively unaffected but the roots are poorly developed. The palate often is highly arched and mandibular prognathism usually is noticeable. The shoulders are sloping. The clavicles cannot be palpated. A characteristic picture is obtained when the shoulders are brought forward passively, since they can be approximated to an unusual extent (see Figs. 90-1–90-3). Slight deformities of the chest and of the spine are attributable to the persistence of cartilage in places in which ossification normally takes place; occasionally, marked scoliosis develops later in life, since traction and pressure can distort the vertebrae. Similar circumstances account for coxa vara and genu valgum, since soft parts of the lower extremities offer insufficient resistance to the weight of the body. The hands and feet show few external anomalies. The thumb and first toes are short, the fingers tapering and slight flaring of the metaphyses may be noticeable.

At birth, palpation of the skull reveals an almost complete absence of the cranial bones. The vault of the skull is as soft as that of newborns with severe

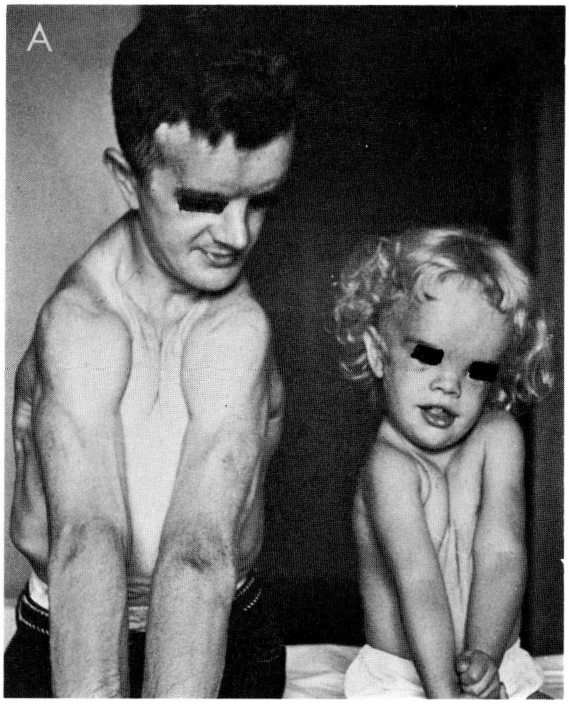

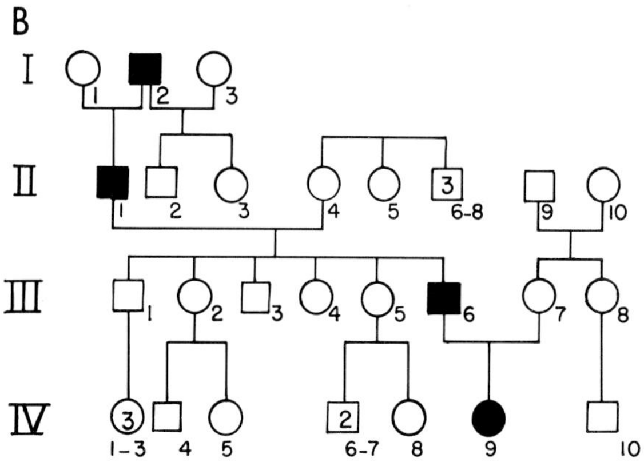

Fig. 90-2.—**A,** cleidocranial dysostosis in a father and his daughter. Disproportion of cranial and facial structures in both. There also is abnormal mobility of shoulders because of absent clavicles. **B,** pedigree of this family, in which at least four generations were affected.

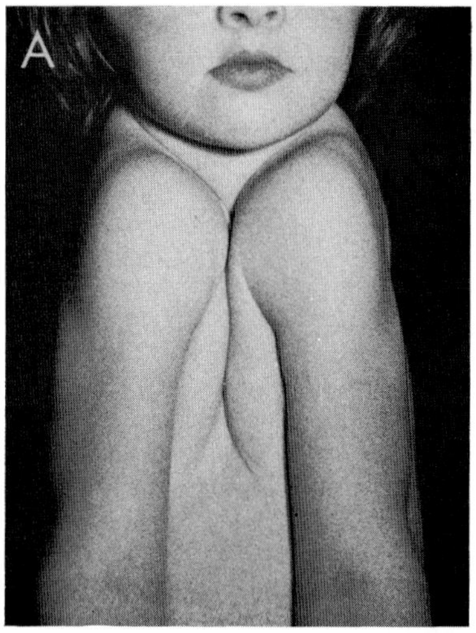

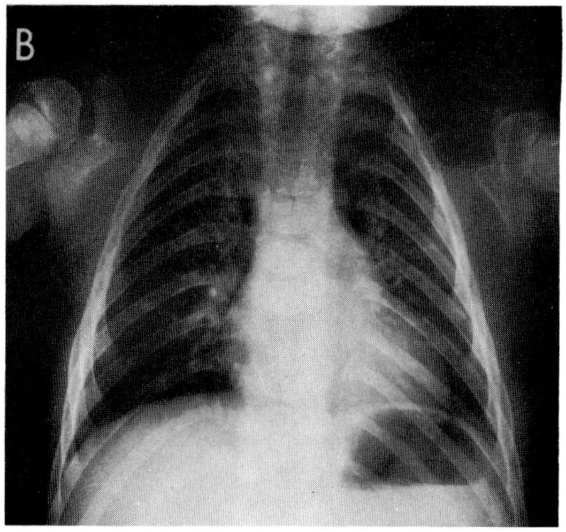

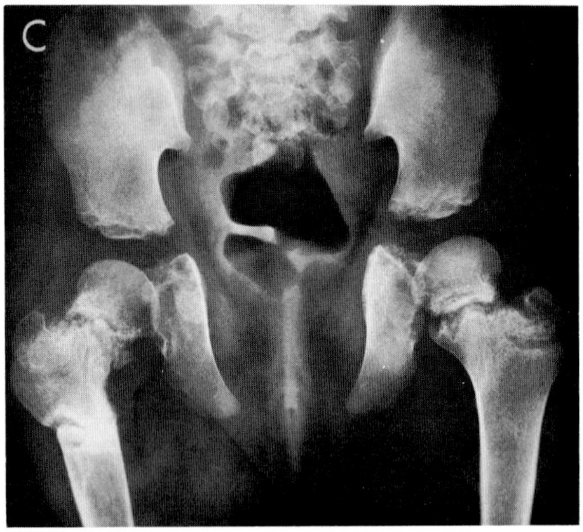

Fig. 90-3.—**A,** absence of clavicle can be demonstrated in this girl, 8 years of age, by approximating the shoulders. **B,** roentgenogram of this child, showing only tiny rudiment of clavicle on left. **C,** pelvis of the same child. Retarded ossification of corpora and rami inferiores of pubic bones.

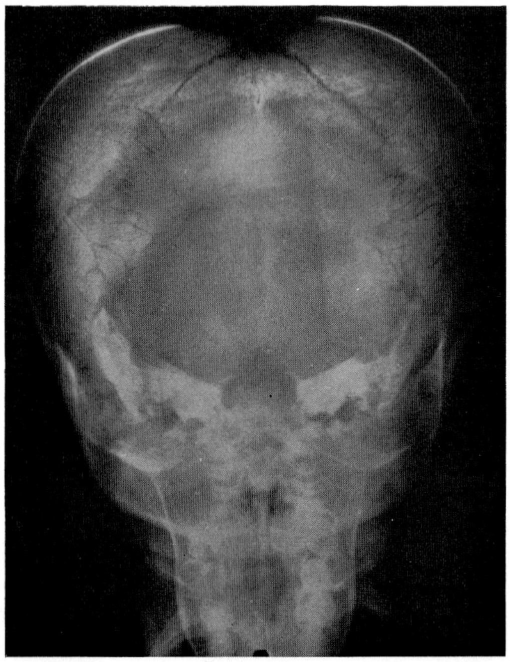

Fig. 90-4.—Roentgenogram of skull of an 8-year-old girl with cleidocranial dysostosis, showing disproportion of cranial and facial skeleton, lack of mineralization of sagittal suture and many sutural bones.

osteogenesis imperfecta. Cyanosis may follow delivery. During the first few years, the sutures—including the metopic—and the fontanelles remain wide open and ossification progresses very slowly (Fig. 90-4).

In the blood, no chemical changes have yet been found. The values of serum calcium, phosphorus and phosphatase are within normal limits. In contrast to osteogenesis imperfecta, there are no fractures present at birth and only rarely later.

As the child grows older, the calvarium slowly becomes mineralized and many irregular foci of mineralization are seen. These foci fuse during childhood but the sutures and fontanelles may remain open until adolescence. Finally, a firm skull is established. A flat skull with deformity of the foramen magnum has been described in a boy who suffered from seizures.[7] The facial bones are underdeveloped and the nasal and zygomatic bones may remain unossified.[2] There is a marked contrast in size of the cranial and facial skeletons (see Fig. 90-4). A chest film reveals absence of the clavicles or rudimentary clavicles (see Fig. 90-3,*B*). If the midportion of the clavicle is not mineralized, a fracture may be simulated even though a fibrous union exists between the clavicular rudiments.

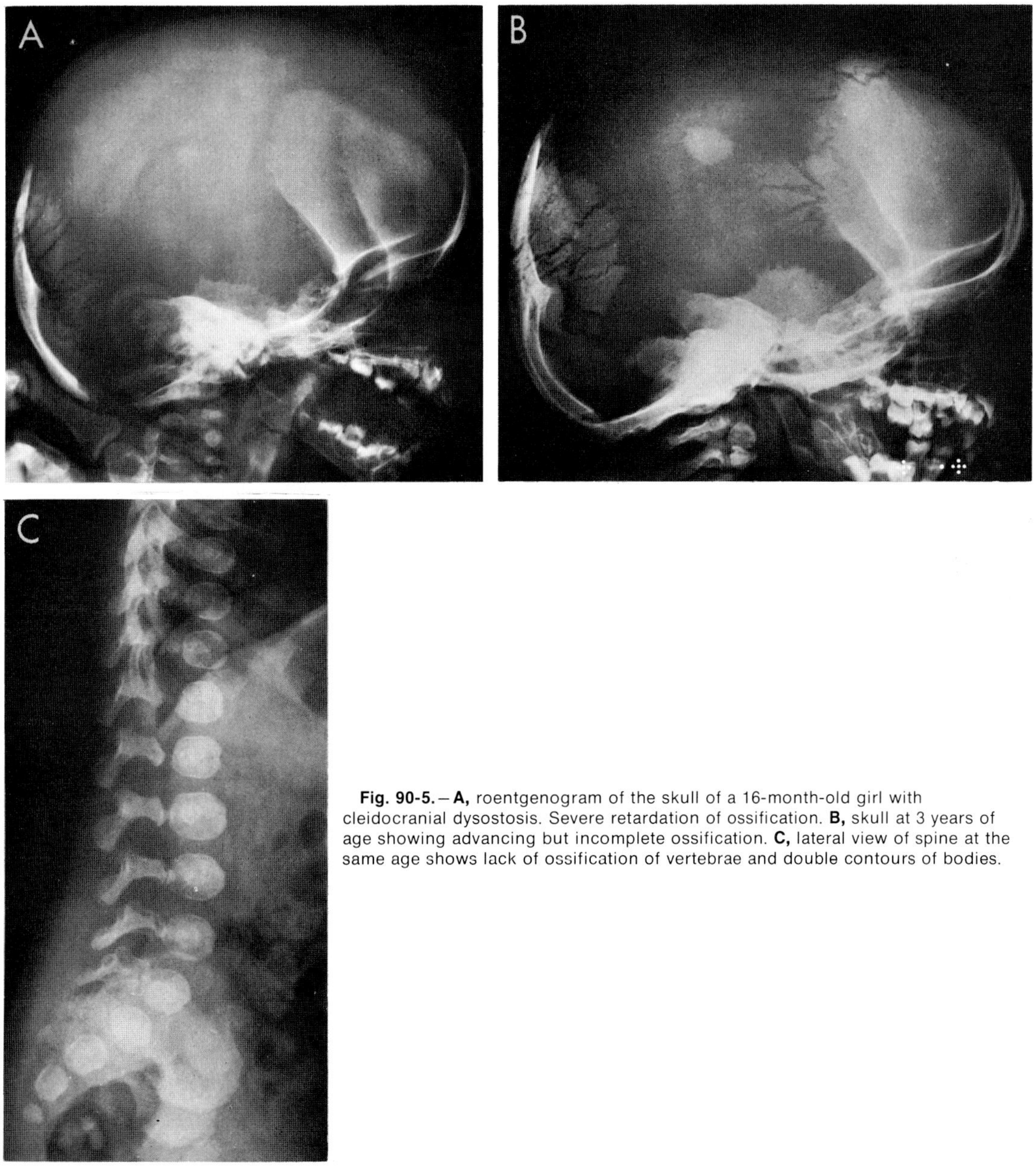

Fig. 90-5.—**A,** roentgenogram of the skull of a 16-month-old girl with cleidocranial dysostosis. Severe retardation of ossification. **B,** skull at 3 years of age showing advancing but incomplete ossification. **C,** lateral view of spine at the same age shows lack of ossification of vertebrae and double contours of bodies.

In many cases, the spine shows irregular ossification and the neural arches of the vertebrae appear open; in lateral views, the vertebral bodies are irregularly outlined and sometimes a center of advanced ossification is seen within a less densely mineralized vertebral body[7] (Fig. 90-5, *C*). Retarded ossification of the symphysis pubis resulting in a wide symphyseal gap is found in roentgenograms of the pelvis (see Fig. 90-3, *C*). Ossification of the proximal ends of the humerus and of the femur is irregular, and pictures reminiscent of metaphyseal dysplasias are seen. Similar irregularities at the distal ends of the radius, ulna, tibia and fibula combined with metaphyseal broadening have been mistaken for signs of rickets. Mineralization of the carpal and tarsal bones is delayed. The metacarpal and metatarsal bones frequently have proximal accessory epiphyseal centers of ossification, which, after final reunion with the shafts, result in their elongation. Irregularities of the phalanges are also seen and the terminal phalanges may appear shortened. There are many variations in the extent of the changes, which range from *cranial dysostosis* (with normal clavicles) to the complete syndrome described above.

Mental development usually is normal and many patients have been described as intelligent. In a number of cases, mental deficiency was present and convulsive disorders have been observed in some instances. In several reported cases, the patients had emotional disturbances. Psychoses were associated with cleidocranial dysostoses in only a few cases. Since these disorders showed dissociation in affected families, the relationship of the two conditions does not appear to be an intimate one.[8] The same seems to be true for occasional associated neurologic disorders.[9] A combination of cleidocranial dysostosis with osteosclerosis and bone fragility has been observed.[10] This disorder has now been recognized as a special entity called pyknodysostosis (p. 869).

As a rule, patients with cleidocranial dysostosis are not seriously handicapped and treatment is limited. Parents who are concerned about the soft skulls of affected infants can be assured of slow but progressive ossification. The prognosis is more favorable in cranial than in cleidocranial dysostosis. In the latter form, rudiments of the clavicle may exert pressure on the brachial plexus, which can be relieved by surgical removal of the rudiments. Dental and orthodontic treatment deserves special attention.[2]

REFERENCES

1. Marie, P., and Sainton, R.: Observation d'hydrocéphalie héréditaire (père et fils), par vice de développement du crâne et du cerveau, Bull. Soc. méd. hôp. Paris 14:706, 1897.
2. Schuch, P., and Fleischer-Peters, A.: Zur Klinik der Dysostosis cleidocranialis, Ztschr. Kinderh. 98:107, 1967.
3. Herndon, C. N.: Cleidocranial dysostosis, Am. J. Human Genet. 3:314, 1951.
4. Liebenam, L.: Zwillingspathologische Untersuchungen aus dem Gebiete der Anomalien der Körperform, Ztschr. menschl. Vererb.-u. Konstitutionslehre 22:373, 1938.
5. Sandler, H. C.: Cleidocranial dysostosis in four siblings, Am. J. Orthodont. 37:584, 1951.
6. Kempfle, B.: Dysostosis cleidocranialis familiaris, Deutsche Zahnärztl. Ztschr. 20:1364, 1965.
7. Keats, T. E.: Cleidocranial dysostosis. Some atypical roentgen manifestations, Am. J. Roentgenol. 100:71, 1967.
8. Kilgore, S., and Lasker, G. W.: Cleidocranial dysostosis with psychosis, Arch. Neurol. & Psychiat. 56:401, 1946.
9. Stewart, R. M.: The nervous system in cleidocranial dysostosis, J. Neurol. & Psychopath. 9:217, 1929.
10. Thomsen, G., and Guttadauro, M.: Cleidocranial dysostosis associated with osteosclerosis and bone fragility, Acta radiol. 37:559, 1952.

Hereditary Multiple Exostoses

(Hereditary Deforming Chondrodysplasia; Diaphyseal Aclasis)

THIS IS A SYSTEMIC DISORDER of the skeleton in which knobby protrusions appear, originating from the metaphyseal areas of the long bones and occasionally from flat bones of cartilaginous origin. The variance in terminology for this rare disease is appalling. One of the earliest reports[1] employed the term "hereditary deforming chondrodysplasia" which, although correct, could also be applied to so many other entities that it would be meaningless. Multiple exostoses have been observed in many races and in such animals as horses, cattle, dogs, cats and lions. A large exostosis has been found on the inner surface of the scapula of a dinosaur.[2]

Hereditary transmission of exostoses is obvious in some families, since the anomaly occurs as an autosomal dominant trait. An affected parent's risk for affected children is 1:1, whereas unaffected members of the family have normal offspring. Occasionally it seems that a generation is "skipped" when a child with exostoses is born to apparently unaffected parents. This may be due to reduced expressivity of the gene; that is, the exostoses may be so small that they are missed by the casual observer as well as by the bearer himself. But such small exostoses sometimes are revealed by roentgenograms of transmitting parents. Expressivity and penetrance seem to be influenced by sex. Exostoses are noticeable more often in males than in females, in whom the abnormal trait can remain latent. It appears – without thorough examination – that 70% of the patients are male,[2] but

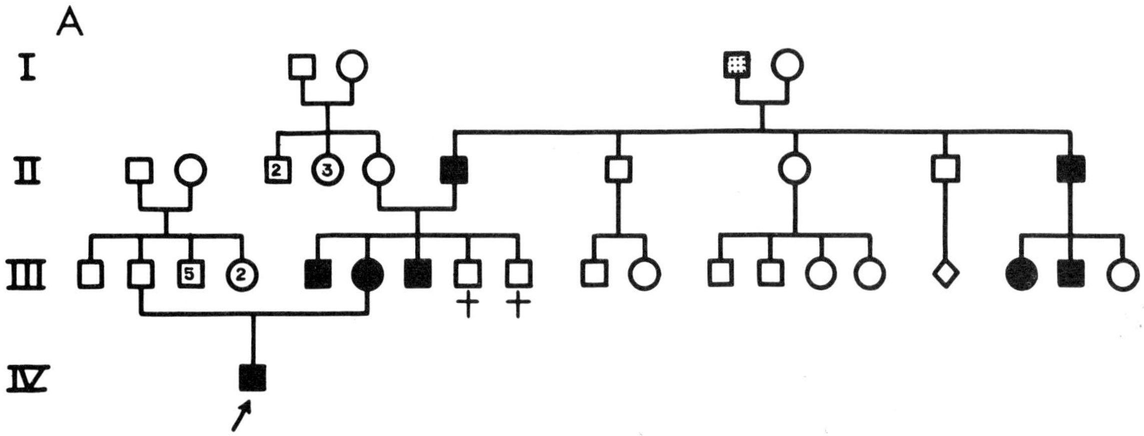

Fig. 90-6.—Multiple exostoses. **A,** pedigree of a kindred showing the anomaly transmitted through three and possibly four generations. The affected male in generation I had a "bone disease" considered tuberculosis (?). **B,** pedigree shows 2 males affected, with an unaffected female apparently transmitting the disorder to her son. However, the "skipping" was only apparent, since the mother showed small exostoses in roentgenograms (reduced expressivity) (personal observations).

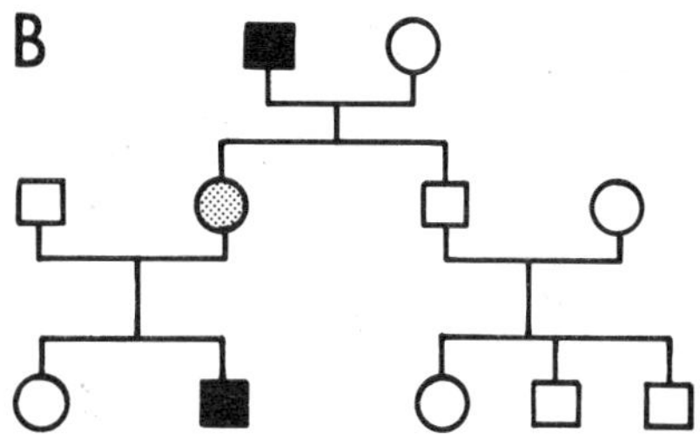

with the help of roentgenograms a more equal sex distribution is found. No satisfactory explanation has yet been given for the difference in expressivity in the two sexes. It is not likely that the male sex hormone is an important factor in the formation of exostoses, since, in males, growth of the exostoses does not coincide with periods of high androgen production. Multiple exostoses usually grow primarily during early childhood, when the hormone production by the testes is low, and they cease growing after adolescence, when the production of sex hormones is high.

Sporadic cases of multiple exostoses are not rare. In a collection of 1,189 cases, Stocks and Barrington,[2] in 1925, found repeated occurrence in 183 families, of which 765 members were affected. In the same series, 424 cases were sporadic. One must not assume that sporadic cases are nonhereditary. A patient either may be the only member of a family who shows clinical expression of the abnormal trait or he may be the first individual who manifests exostoses as the result of a recent mutation. It is not certain that phenocopies exist. If they do, not only the patient's ancestors but also his offspring should be free of the disease. Extensive pedigrees have been pubished by Stocks and Barrington.[2] In a family recorded by Vanzant and Vanzant,[1] a cousin marriage took place. The husband had multiple exostoses and the wife probably had a latent form of the disease. They had 7 children, all of whom had multiple exostoses. In this pedigree, which included five generations, 46% of the members were affected, a percentage close to that expected in the inheritance of a dominant trait. Two females thought to be free of the trait transmitted it to their offspring. In a pair of identical twins with the anomaly,[3] both twins had exostoses but the sites and the number of tumors varied. This suggests that nongenetic factors play a role in the expression of this abnormal hereditary trait.

Exostoses are protuberances that, as a rule, arise from the metaphyses of the bones near attachments of tendons and ligaments. The ends of the affected bones are widened and show a lack of tubulation. Exostoses first appear as small excrescences in the shape of a hook or horn and later assume the form of mushrooms or cauliflower-like outgrowths. They grow away from the epiphyses and toward the shafts (Fig. 90-7, *C* and *E*), but if they become very large they involve and even deform the epiphyses. Bursae often are found between exostoses and overlying muscles. The surface of an exostosis usually is osseous but it may be capped by cartilage and covered by connective tissue to which a tendon is attached. Sometimes masses of calcified cartilage are enclosed within an exostosis. With increasing age, the cartilaginous caps disappear.[4] Exostoses have been explained as derivatives of cartilaginous nests embedded in the periosteum. Both enchondral and perichondral ossification are disturbed, which explains that exostoses can arise in parts of the skeleton that do not have epiphyseal clefts.[5] The epiphyseal centers of ossification develop normally and their fusion with the shafts is not delayed. Multiple exostoses must be clearly differentiated from enchondromatoses (p. 874) and from solitary exostoses, which have different etiologies.

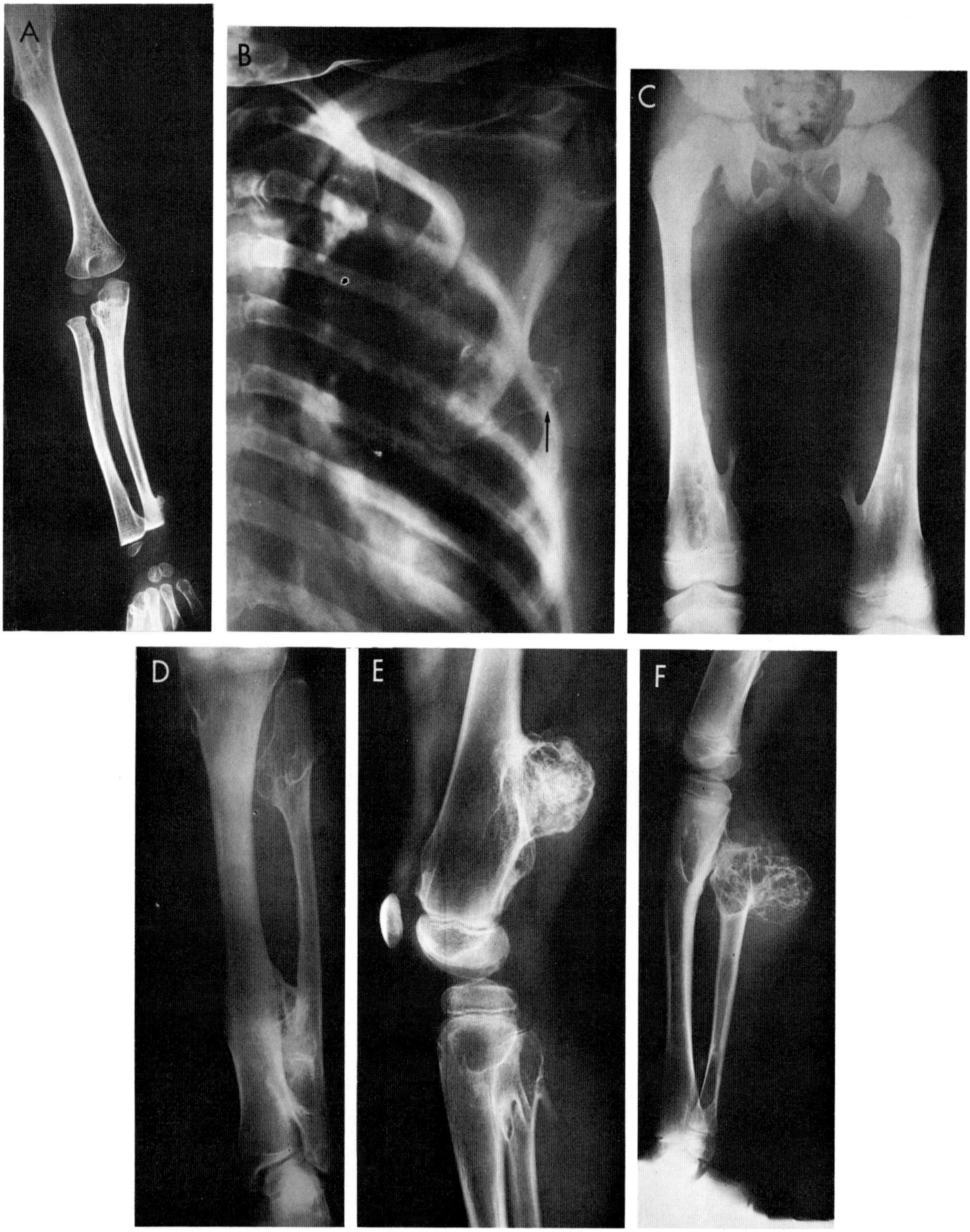

Fig. 90-7.—**A,** knobby exostoses seen best on distal end of ulna and proximal end of humerus. **B,** exostosis of scapula (**arrow**). **C,** exostoses of femora. **D,** exostoses on tibia and fibula with synostosis on distal ends. Note structural changes in the diaphyseal ends of all bones. **E,** large exostosis on distal end of femur. Exostoses of tibia and fibula pointing away from epiphysis. Structural changes clearly seen in the diaphyses of tibia and fibula. **F,** multiple exostoses. The fibula carries a large, deforming osteochondroma, which was removed surgically.

Occasionally, exostoses form large osteochondromas (see Fig. 90-7, *F*), which, in a realtively high percentage of cases, develop into chondrosarcomas. In some cases, the growth of such sarcomas is slow, showing only local invasion of neighboring tissues, but in others, the tumor enters venous channels and metastasizes. Such cases may end fatally within a few months, but most patients with chondrosarcoma developing from exostoses survive for several years. Krooth *et al.*[6] stated that it is estimated that at least 10% of affected persons develop a chondrosarcoma at the site of the tumor during their adult life, but other authors consider malignant degeneration rarer.[5] Hereditary multiple exostoses can be considered as one of the hamartoses that affect only one organ system (p. 1251).

In approximately a third of the cases, exostoses are noticeable at birth, particularly near the knee. In two-thirds of cases, small protrusions appear in various regions of the body during the early years of childhood. They increase in size and number throughout childhood, but after puberty their growth usually stops. When an exostosis resumes growth in later years, the possibility of a malignancy should be considered. Exostoses usually affect both sides of the body, often developing symmetrically. It is of interest that many affected cases are sporadic.[2] They may be etiologically different from hereditary multiple exostoses. Exostoses have a predilection for those parts of the skeleton that show intensive growth. They are most frequent on the bones that form the knee joint. In the arm, the proximal end of the humerus and the distal ends of the radius and ulna are preferred sites. The pelvic bones, phalanges, scapulae, vertebrae, ribs and the base of the skull may be affected, but the cranial vault usually remains free. Size of exostoses ranges from minute to large deforming tumors and their number varies; in some patients, an isolated exostosis may be the only expression of the disorder, whereas in others, as many as 1,000 excrescences have been counted.

Patients with multiple exostoses often are of short stature because of reduced growth of the lower limbs and curvatures of the spine. Deformity of the forearm often is present. The distal end of the ulna shows marked impairment of growth in such cases, whereas the radius is less severely affected. As a result, the head of the radius curves around the distal end of the ulna and the hand is in ulnar deflection. The lower extremities sometimes are unequal in length and genu valgum, talipes valgus and curving of tibia and fibula may be present. Exostoses situated on the lateral border or on the inferior angle of the scapula may be visible and palpable (Fig. 90-8, *A*). The pelvic bones are affected less often, but when large exostoses do occur in that location in female patients, they may complicate parturition. Mobility of the joints can be impaired by abnormal positions of the articular facets or by synostoses formed by coalescent exostoses (see Fig. 90-7, *D*) but hyperextensibility has also been ob-

Fig. 90-8.—**A,** exostosis of left scapula, externally visible in a girl 12 years of age. **B,** deforming exostoses on left lower leg in a boy 10 years of age.

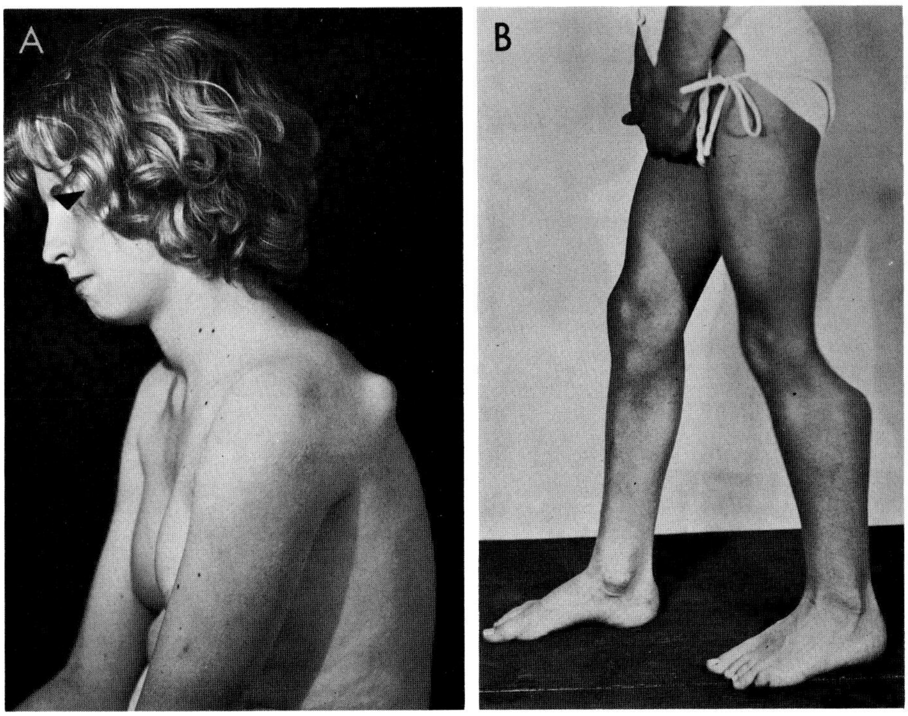

served.[7] Pressure on nerves can give rise to pain, paresthesias, paralysis and even deafness. Pressure on blood vessels sometimes results in dilatation of veins or in arterial aneurysms. Compression of the spinal cord has produced neurologic symptoms. Infection of overlying bursae and necrosis of the skin covering exostoses are occasional complications. The development of chondrosarcoma is rare, as exostoses are benign tumors that interfere little with active life, general health and longevity.

In roentgenograms of the long bones, exostoses appear as hooks or horns that arise on the shaft near its epiphyseal end. If growth continues, mushroom-shaped protuberances develop (see Fig. 90-7, *E*), and, in severe cases, large tumors form, particularly at the proximal end of the fibula. The entire end of the shaft that carries the exostoses undergoes changes that make it appear clumsy and sometimes club-shaped. The interior shows unequal distribution of trabeculae (see Fig. 90-7, *F*) and marrow spaces. Sometimes synostoses between long bones are observed (see Fig. 90-7, *D*). Exostoses of the scapula and changes in the ribs may be seen (see Fig. 90-7, *B*). The outline of the ileum sometimes is irregular owing to exostotic excrescences. The epiphyses appear normal in mild cases, but they can be displaced by bending of the shafts or by formation of large tumors. The prognosis is good in the majority of cases but the development of chondromas impairs the outlook, since they may become malignant.

Surgical removal of exostoses is indicated when pain, limitation of movement, paralysis or deformity requires intervention. It also has been recommended that exostoses be removed early to avoid bowing of tubular bones and deformity.[7] For chondrosarcomatous transformation, amputation beyond the level of the lesion has been recommended.

REFERENCES

1. Vanzant, B. T., and Vanzant, F. R.: Hereditary deforming chondrodysplasia, J.A.M.A. 119:786, 1942.
2. Stocks, P., and Barrington, A.: Hereditary Disorders of Bone Development. Pt. I. Diaphysial Aclasis (Multiple Exostoses), Multiple Enchondromata, Cleido-cranial Dysostosis, in Pearson, K. (ed.), *Treasury of Human Inheritance* (London: Cambridge University Press, 1925), Vol. III, pt. 1.
3. Birkenfeld, W.: Zur Erblichkeit der multiplen kartilaginären Exostosen. (Exostosen bei eineiigen Zwillingen), Deutsche Ztschr. Chir. 226:397, 1930.
4. Jaffe, H. L.: Hereditary multiple exostosis, Arch. Path. 36: 335, 1943.
5. Murken, J-D.: Über multiple kartilaginäre Exostosen, Ztschr. menschl. Vererb.-u. Konstitutionslehre 36:469, 1963.
6. Krooth, R. S., Macklin, M. T., and Hilbish, T. F.: Diaphysial aclasis (multiple exostoses) on Guam, Am. J. Human Genet. 13:340, 1961.
7. Cannon, J. F.: Hereditary multiple exostoses, Am. J. Human Genet. 6:419, 1954.

Osteopathia Hyperostotica Sclerotisans

(Camurati-Engelmann Disease)

THIS DISORDER, described as a bone disease by Engelmann[1] in 1929, and by Cockayne[2] and Camurati[3] before him, apparently has not yet been described in the newborn, and its congenital nature therefore is not certain. It is likely that some cases of diaphyseal hyperostosis are genetically determined. Some cases have been observed in infancy, but most patients were children or adults. It is also possible that some diaphyseal dysplasias represent an osseous reaction to an acquired disease that involves not only the bones but also other organ systems. The condition is rare. In 1956, Griffiths[4] listed 17 certain and 5 probable cases as reported in the literature. The sex incidence seems to be equal and members of several races have been affected. Camurati[3] described the disorder in a child whose father had similar osseous changes and Ortolani and Castagnari[5] reported it in 2 brothers. Clawson and Loop[6] presented a pedigree that shows dominant inheritance with reduced penetrance and variable clinical expression. C. B. Graham[7] observed 8 well-documented cases in four generations, demonstrating dominant inheritance with variable expressivity. "Hereditary, multiple, diaphyseal sclerosis," which was observed by Ribbing[8] in 4 of 6 siblings and by Paul[9] in 2 brothers, may belong in the same category.[15] The roentgenograms of the two disorders are similar and other symptoms are different only in degree. Ribbing diaphyseal sclerosis shows manifestations limited to the skeleton later than Engelmann disease, which probably has its onset in infancy.[10,11]

Pain in the legs, weakness and fatigue, poor appetite, loss of weight and malnutrition accompany Engelmann's osteopathy. Poor muscular development is an integral part of the disease picture.[6] A broad-based, waddling gait, increased lordosis, bowlegs and flat feet often are present. Enlargement of the spleen and lymph nodes is rare. The patients usually are small but have relative elongation of the limbs. Swelling of the long bones may be palpable.[4] A case of an Indian girl was reported by Gulati *et al.*,[12] who described delayed puberty.

Roentgenograms show symmetric, dense, spindle-shaped, cortical expansions of the long bones. The sclerosis is limited to the diaphyses, leaving the metaphyses and epiphyses unaltered. Endosteal and periosteal appositions thicken the cortex. The swelling of bone changes not only the outline of the shaft but also reduces the medullary canal. The long bones of

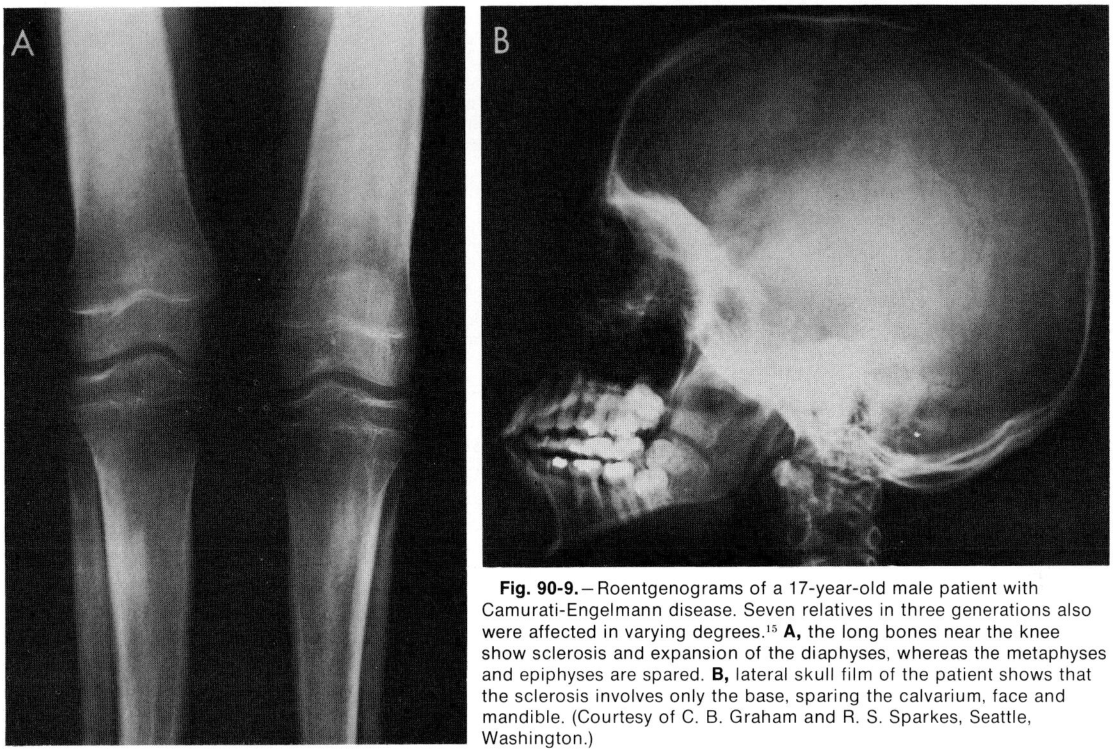

Fig. 90-9.—Roentgenograms of a 17-year-old male patient with Camurati-Engelmann disease. Seven relatives in three generations also were affected in varying degrees.[15] **A,** the long bones near the knee show sclerosis and expansion of the diaphyses, whereas the metaphyses and epiphyses are spared. **B,** lateral skull film of the patient shows that the sclerosis involves only the base, sparing the calvarium, face and mandible. (Courtesy of C. B. Graham and R. S. Sparkes, Seattle, Washington.)

the lower extremity, particularly the femora, are regularly affected and the bones of the upper extremity frequently, although often to a lesser degree. The base of the skull, the frontal bones and the clavicles have been sclerosed in some of the cases.[13]

Biopsies show cortical thickening, regular lamellar structure of bones, abundance of osteoblasts and absence of abnormal cells or tissues.[4]

Progression of sclerosis along the long axis of bone in the distal and proximal directions involving previously normal bone has been observed repeatedly but arrest of the process occurs before the ends of the shafts are affected.

A severe variant of Camurati-Engelmann disease has been described by Joseph *et al.*[14] and named "progressive cranio-diaphyseal dysplasia." It was observed in a boy whose family history was noncontributory. At birth, signs of nasal obstruction were present but the other symptoms developed during early childhood. The nose appeared flat and the palpebral fissures widely separated. Leontiasis ossea developed, with prominence of the malar bones and thickening of the mandible. Vision and hearing became markedly reduced. Hyperostosis was well developed in certain areas of the skeleton at the age of 2 years and progressed as the boy got older. At first, the base of the skull showed increased density in roentgenograms. Thickening of the bones around the orbits and of the maxillae was striking. A year later, the hyperostosis had progressed to the calvarium and the mandible. The changes in the long bones resembled those of Camurati-Engelmann disease: the diaphyses were thickened and the medullary canals reduced in volume, whereas the epiphyses and metaphyses remained unchanged. Hyperostosis also involved the clavicles, ilia and ischia.

At the age of 7 years, the boy, whose intelligence remained normal, showed a very characteristic and bizarre disease picture, with enlargement of the head and flattening of the nose as outstanding external symptoms.

REFERENCES

1. Engelmann, G.: Ein Fall von Osteopathia hyperostotica (sclerotisans) multiplex infantilis, Fortschr. Geb. Röntgenstrahlen 39:1101, 1929.
2. Cockayne, E. A.: Case for diagnosis, Proc. Roy. Soc. Med. 13:132, 1920.
3. Camurati, M.: Di un raro caso di Osteite Simmetrica Ereditaria degli Arti Inferiori, Chir. org. movimento 6:662, 1922.
4. Griffiths, D. L.: Engelmann's disease, J. Bone & Joint Surg. 38-B:312, 1956.
5. Ortolani, M., and Castagnari, G.: L'osteopatia di Camurati-Engelmann, Arch. "Putti" Chir. org. movimento 3:146, 1953.
6. Clawson, D. K., and Loop, J. W.: Progressive diaphyseal dysplasia (Engelmann's disease), J. Bone & Joint Surg. 46-A:143, 1964.
7. Graham, C. B.: Personal communication.
8. Ribbing, S.: Hereditary, multiple, diaphyseal sclerosis, Acta radiol. 31:522, 1949.

9. Paul, L. W.: Hereditary multiple diaphyseal sclerosis (Ribbing), Radiology 60:412, 1953.
10. Cocchi, U.: Hereditary Diseases with Bone Changes, in Schinz, H. R., Baensch, W. E., Friedl, E., and Uehlinger, E. (eds.), *Roentgen-Diagnostics* (New York: Grune & Stratton, Inc., 1951), Vol. I, p. 702.
11. Caffey, J.: *Pediatric X-ray Diagnosis* (5th ed.; Chicago: Year Book Medical Publishers, Inc., 1967).
12. Gulati, P. D., Bhardwaj, O. P., and Vyas, P. B.: Case of Englemann's disease, Brit. M. J. 3:217, 1967.
13. Neuhauser, E. B. D., Shwachman, H., Wittenborg, M. H., and Cohen, J.: Progressive diaphyseal dysplasia, Radiology 51:11, 1948.
14. Joseph, R., Lefèbvre, J., Guy, E., and Job, J. C.: Dysplasia cranio-diaphysaire progressive, Ann. radiol. 1:477, 1958.
15. Graham, C. B., and Sparkes, R. S.: Camurati-Engelmann's disease. (In preparation.)

Osteopoikilosis

(Osteopathia Condensans Disseminata; "Spotted Bones")

THIS SCLEROSING OSTEOPATHY apparently was first described by Stieda[1] in 1905, and by now more than 130 cases have been observed.[2] It is a rare osseous anomaly that is symptomless in most cases and is discovered incidentally on x-ray examinations or in family investigations. Most cases have been described in adults but changes have been seen in children and in a fetus.[2] Although the male sex predominated among reported cases, in family studies, males and females seem to be affected equally. Since Voorhoeve,[3] in 1924, expressed the belief that the condition is hereditary, a number of cases have been found to be transmitted directly from parent to children. Melnick[4] demonstrated the anomaly in four generations. The pedigree published by him is unusual in that it includes a couple, both affected, having 8 children, all showing the anomaly. The condition is transmitted like a dominant trait.

Since the disorder remains clinically symptomless, it is observed chiefly by radiologists. Osteopoikilosis consists of numerous multiform foci of sclerosis varying from a few millimeters to several centimeters in diameter and found in long bones and round bones as well as flat bones. In the diaphyses, condensations may have a striated or linear appearance.[4] The pelvis, femora, carpal and tarsal bones are involved most commonly. Lesions of the skull, ribs and spine are rare, and the sternum seems to be spared.[5] In some cases, striations dominate the picture.[2,3] In histologic sections, the increased densities were found to be due to numerous bone trabeculae of increased thickness.[6]

There is no agreement concerning the course of the anomaly. Some observers believe that the opacities are stationary, whereas others saw them increase with age. Associated anomalies have been found in many patients, but there does not seem to be any definite pattern, with the exception of disseminated lenticular dermatofibrosis, which has been observed repeatedly in patients with the osseous anomaly.[5,7]

Since the condition is asymptomatic and benign, no treatment is required, but it is important to distinguish the areas of increased density from metastatic cancer, tuberculosis, osteomyelitis and osteopetrosis.[5]

Green *et al.*[8] compared osteopoikilosis and melorheostosis. Although these two conditions may show superficial resemblance in roentgenograms, they otherwise have little in common, osteopoikilosis usually being symptomless and melorheostosis painful and disabling. Osteopoikilosis is hereditary and transmitted as a dominant trait; melorheostosis is not.

REFERENCES

1. Stieda, A.: Über umschriebene Knochenverdichtungen im Bereich der Substantia spongiosa im Röntgenbilde, Beitr. klin. Chir. 45:700, 1905.
2. Cocchi, U.: Krankheiten des Skelettsystems, in Becker, P. E. (ed.), *Humangenetik* (Stuttgart: Georg Thieme, 1964).
3. Voorhoeve, N.: L'image radiologique non encore décrite d'une anomalie du squelette, Acta radiol. 3:407, 1924.
4. Melnick, J. C.: Osteopathia condensans disseminata (osteopoikilosis); study of family of 4 generations, Am. J. Roentgenol. 82:229, 1959.
5. Harmston, G. J.: Osteopathia condensans disseminata, Radiology 66:556, 1956.
6. Schmorl, G.: Anatomische Befunde bei einem Falle von Osteopoikilie, Fortschr. Geb. Röntgenstrahlen 44:1, 1931.
7. Windholz, F.: Über familiäre Osteopoikilie und Dermatofibrosis lenticularis disseminata, Fortschr. Geb. Röntgenstrahlen 45:566, 1932.
8. Green, A. E., Jr., Ellswood, W. H., and Collins, J. R.: Melorheostosis and osteopoikilosis; with review of literature, Am. J. Roentgenol. 87:1096, 1962.

Pleonosteosis (Léri)

LÉRI,[1] in 1922, described a rare congenital and hereditary syndrome of the skeleton and the joints that he attributed to precocious and excessive ossification and enlargement of the diaphyses and epiphyses. The manifestations were most pronounced in a father, 35 years of age, clearly recognizable in his 4-year-old daughter and suggestive in a newborn child. Only a few comparable cases have been described since, among them an affected family described by Rukavina *et al.*,[2] who published an excellent review of the subject. It is now known that the anomalous features of this syndrome include the skeleton, the periarticular tissues, the skin and sometimes peripheral nerves. The syndrome probably is due to a pleiotropic dominant autosomal gene with good penetrance but variable expression. Rukavina *et al.* reported a pedigree showing the anomaly in four generations.

In infants, manifestations are rather inconspicuous and noticeable only if an observer acquainted with the anomalies looks for them. Thus, in the families described by Léri[1] and Rukavina *et al.*,[2] deformities of the fingers were noticed in newborn infants who otherwise appeared healthy and normal. Usually the condition is recognized later, when abnormalities of the gait and joints become manifest.

In the fully developed syndrome, short, spade-like hands with broad thumbs and flexion contractures of the interphalangeal joints are present. Comparable changes often are noticed on the feet. Cubitus valgus, genu recurvatum and limitation of motion of many joints supplement the disease picture. The cervical and lumbar lordosis may be reduced, resulting in a stiff, straight and "soldier-like" carriage. The gait is waddling and shuffling. The skin is thick and the palmar skin creases accentuated, so that scleroderma or gargoylism sometimes is suspected. The palms and soles may be hollow because of the cutaneous thickening and the shortening of tendons and fasciae. Contractures and limitations of movements of the fingers impair the proper use of the hands. Sometimes multiple nodules are visible on the deformed fingers. Thickening of the skin probably is responsible for the narrow and somewhat mongoloid palpebral fissures described in these patients. The cutaneous changes are due to marked fibrosis of the corium and widespread hyalinization. Shortness in stature occurs in some affected persons but others reach normal height. Muscular development is good and mental functions usually are normal. Secondary involvement of peripheral nerves has been observed.[3] The patients are handicapped by deformities of their spine and hands, by limitation of movement of the joints and by their abnormal gait. In writing, the pencil sometimes is held between the index and middle fingers. Neurologic symptoms can dominate the clinical picture.[3] Pain, numbness, tingling in the fingers and toes can be very disturbing symptoms.

Watson-Jones[3] believed that the primary pathologic change in pleonosteosis may be in the joint ligaments and that the bone thickening could be due to periosteal traction at their metaphyseal attachments. He also pointed out a certain resemblance to arthrogryposis. Although this is correct, since in both conditions contractures of the joints and small palpebral fissures are present, dominant transmission does not occur in severe, congenital arthrogryposis (p. 1011). In the milder dominant form, the differential diagnosis will be made by the osseous changes characteristic of pleonosteosis.

Laboratory examinations so far have been noncontributory. Roentgenograms reveal skeletal structures that appear massive and strong due to increase of their width. In the cervical spine, the height of the posterior neural arches is increased, whereby the normal cervical lordosis is counteracted. Segmentation of the vertebrae may be incomplete. The vertebral bodies and spinous processes appear enlarged and the lordosis of the lumbar spine diminished. Scoliosis can be present in various parts of the spine. The clavicles and ribs also may manifest osseous overgrowth. The metacarpal and phalangeal bones are characteristically short and broad. In the skull, the clinoid processes appear oversized, so that the outlines of the sella are blurred.

Pain in the hands and feet was relieved in one of Watson-Jones's cases[3] by resection of both anterior carpal ligaments and excision of plantar digital neuroma.

REFERENCES

1. Léri, A.: Dystrophie osseuse généralisée congénitale et héréditaire: La pléonostéose familiale, Presse méd. 30:13, 1922.
2. Rukavina, J. G., Falls, H. F., Holt, J. F., and Block, W. D.: Léri's pleonosteosis. A study of a family with a review of the literature, J. Bone & Joint Surg. 41-A:397, 1959.
3. Watson-Jones, R.: Léri's pleonosteosis, carpal tunnel compression of the median nerves and Morton's metatarsalgia, J. Bone & Joint Surg. 31-B:560, 1949.

Hereditary Hypertrophic Osteoarthropathy

(Familial Idiopathic Osteoarthropathy; Pachydermoperiostosis)

CLUBBING OF THE FINGERS in pulmonary infections, bronchiectasis, neoplasms of the lung and cardiac and hepatic disorders is considered a symptom acquired in postnatal life. Such digital changes often are associated with hypertrophic osteoarthopathy, a condition characterized by periosteal and cortical thickening of the long bones. According to the majority of observers, these two conditions are to be considered closely related, the clubbing of the fingers and toes representing a mild or early osteoarthropathy. In most instances, hypertrophic osteoarthropathy is, like clubbing, secondary to a chronic disease, usually pulmonary or cardiac,[1] and the condition is relatively rare in children. With the use of antibiotics, the secondary form has further decreased in incidence.[2]

Besides the secondary anomalies of the digits and long bones, there are observations that indicate that they sometimes occur primarily in healthy individuals without a preceding disease. Many of these cases are congenital[3] or familial,[4-6] and have been considered essentially different in etiology from those of the secondary type. This "idiopathic" form, which is much rarer than the secondary type, sometimes is associated with pachydermia, thus resulting in a syndrome called "pachydermoperiostosis."[7] The dermal constituent of this syndrome may be represented by cutis verticis gyrata, a congenital malformation of the skin (p. 1192). Here we shall deal only with the congenital forms, but it should be emphasized that idiopathic and secondary osteoarthropathy probably are related, since transitional forms exist and the two types can occur alternately in members of the same family.[8] A person with secondary osteoarthropathy can have children with the idiopathic form[8,9] and a child with an apparently secondary form may have ancestors with "idiopathic" manifestations. In the Cincinnati Children's Hospital, a 4-year-old girl was seen (patient of Dr. Robert H. Kotte) who had cyanotic congenital heart disease and clubbing of the fingers (Fig. 90-10, *A*) and toes. The father, a healthy man engaged in strenuous work when in his thirties, also had clubbing of the fingers (Fig. 90-10, *B*), and his roentgenograms showed long bones with osteophytic changes characteristic of osteoarthropathy (Fig. 90-10, *C*). No acute or chronic disease of the heart or lungs was found on thorough examination. The child's paternal grandfather also had digital clubbing, which had decreased in intensity with increasing age. He stated that his sister had similar clubbing (Fig. 90-10, *D*). This combination of apparently secondary and primary (idiopathic) clubbing of digits in the same family could not be explained and was considered coincidental. However, similar observations have been made by others,[8,9] and it seems likely that such familial clubbing is a manifestation of a hereditary tendency to cutaneous, periosteal and osseous anomalies now labeled "pachydermoperiostosis" or "Touraine-Solente-Golé syndrome."[7] The patients have clubbing of fingers and toes that may be congenital or develop in the second decade of life. Roentgenologically, some of them show periosteal reactions on the long bones of the distal parts of the extremities and swelling of the joints. The skin of these distal parts may be indurated and hyperhidrotic. The complete syndrome, which is rare, includes pachyderma or cutis verticis gyrata. Marked thickening of the skin is most pronounced on the forehead and face. Cutis verticis gyrata (p. 1192) consists of elevated longitudinal skin folds on the scalp reminiscent of convolutions of the brain. This skin anomaly can be congenital or follow inflammatory processes.[10] A relationship to acromegaly and pituitary disease has been considered.[11] Some patients with pachydermia or cutis verticis gyrata also have digital clubbing and osteoarthropathy. Roentgenograms show marked periosteal apposition of bone with widening and irregularities of contour of the affected skeletal parts. The bones have a coarse structure and often narrowed medullary canals. Males apparently are affected much more often than females.[12] Whatever the underlying anomaly, it could be conceived as a dominantly inherited tendency leading to manifestations with or without overt chronic disease of the lungs or the heart. One form of familial idiopathic osteoarthropathy, differing in some respects from the type described, may be due to a recessive hereditary mechanism. Schönenberg[13] described it in brothers who were children of a cousin marriage, both parents being normal. Currarino *et al.*[12] reported a similar disease picture in sisters, children of normal parents. In the sisters, the symptoms present in infancy consisted of widening of the fontanelles and cranial sutures, seborrhoic dermatitis of the scalp, induration of the pretibial skin, hyperhidrosis and subperiosteal new bone formation in the shafts of the long bones. Swelling and tenderness of the knees and ankles developed later during childhood; a younger sister appeared normal at birth but she developed eczema by 1 month of age and the fontanelles and sutures remained large. At the end of the first year, she showed clubbing of the fingers and toes. In all 3 sisters, there was improvement of the disorder with increasing age but small radiolucent areas in the region of the lambdoid sutures persisted into adolescence together with clubbing and joint swelling.[14] The boys described by Schönenberg[13] had symptoms that were noticed later in life. Microscopic examination of the capillaries suggested increased blood flow in the skin examined. This is of interest, since Wilson[15] demonstrated that limited clubbing of

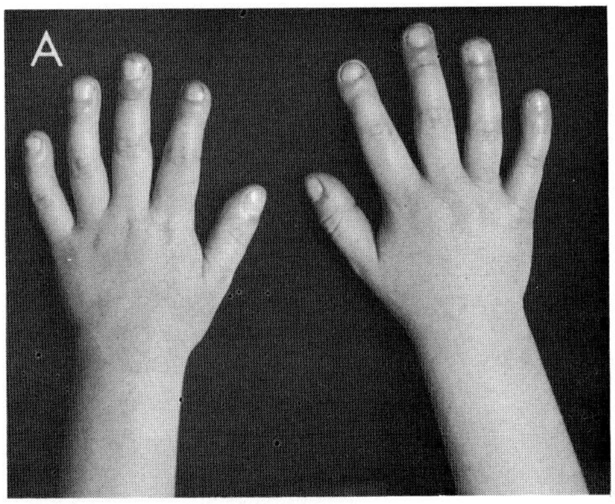

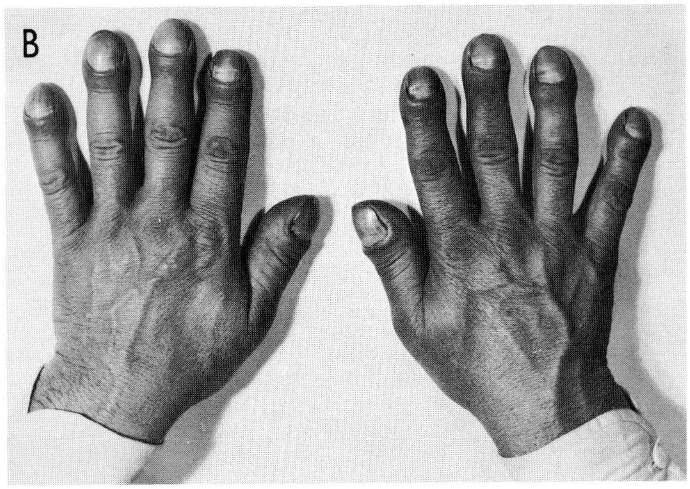

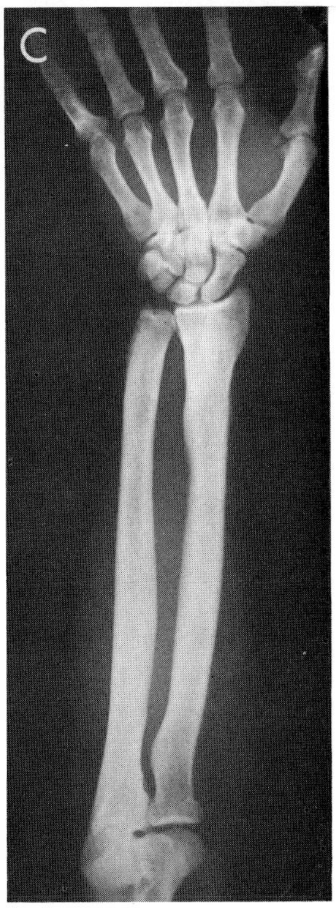

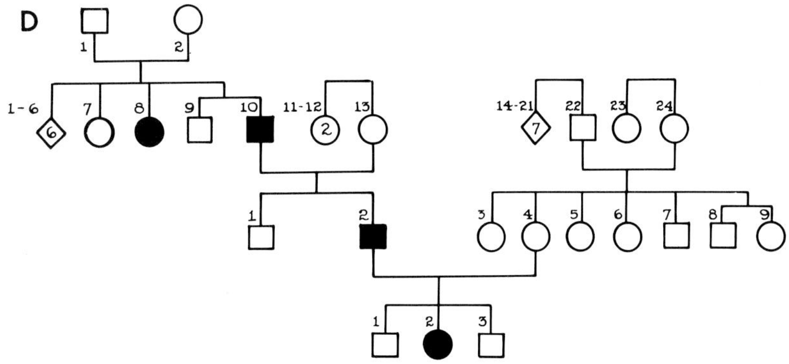

Fig. 90-10. – **A,** hand of child with cyanotic congenital heart disease and clubbing of fingers. **B,** hands of healthy father, showing marked clubbing of fingers. **C,** roentgenogram of hand and forearm of father, showing broad termination of distal phalanges and irregular outlines of radial and ulnar shafts. **D,** pedigree suggesting dominant inheritance of clubbing of fingers transmitted through three generations. Cyanotic congenital heart disease was present in IV_2 only.

the fingers and toes was associated with local and limited circulatory changes (arteriovenous fistulae), and Mendlowitz[1] considered increased peripheral blood flow an important pathogenic factor in secondary clubbing and hypertrophic osteoarthropathy. Schönenberg[13] believed that a disturbance of hypophyseo-diencephalic regulatory mechanisms may play a role in the pathogenesis of osteoarthropathies. In his cases, suprasellar calcifications were seen in the area of the sella turcica, but this was not established in the patients of Currarino *et al.*[12] A hereditary tendency to an unusual allergic reaction seems more likely.

REFERENCES

1. Mendlowitz, M.: Clubbing and hypertrophic osteoarthropathy, Medicine 21:269, 1942.
2. Cavanaugh, J. J. A., and Holman, G. H.: Hypertrophic osteoarthropathy in childhood, J. Pediat. 66:27, 1965.
3. Lewy, E.: Beitrag zur Kenntnis der congenitalen Trommelschlägelfinger, Med. Klin. 17:857, 1921.

4. Ragins, O. B., and Freilich, E. B.: Familial congenital clubbing of fingers and toes; report of case, Ann. Int. Med. 6:946, 1933.
5. Witherspoon, J. T.: Congenital and familial clubbing of fingers and toes with possible inherited tendency, Arch. Int. Med. 57:18, 1936.
6. Weber, F. P. (ed.): A Familial Condition Resembling Clubbed Fingers, in *Further Rare Diseases* (London: Staples Press, 1949).
7. Touraine, A., Solente, O., and Golé, L.: Un syndrome ostéodermopathique: La pachydermie plicaturée avec pachypériostose des extrémités, Presse méd. 43:1820, 1935.
8. de Sèze, S., and Jurmand, S-H.: Pachydermopériostose Hippocratisme digital chez le père atteint de bronchopneumopathie chronique et chez le frère bien portant. Réflexions sur le rôle du facteur héréditaire et familial dans la genèse des hypertrophies des extrémités, Bull. Soc. méd. hôp. Paris 66:860, 1950.
9. Crouzon, E., and Gutmann: Hypertrophie héréditaire des doigts avec ongles en verre de montre sans origine pneumatique chez le descendant, Bull. Soc. méd. hôp. Paris 47:1765, 1931.
10. Ormsby, O. S., and Montgomery, H.: *Diseases of the Skin* (6th ed.; Philadelphia: Lea & Febiger, 1943).
11. Zeisler, E. B., and Wieder, L. M.: Cutis verticis gyrata and acromegaly, Arch. Dermat. 42:1092, 1940.
12. Currarino, G., Tierney, R. C., Giesel, R. G., and Weihl, C.: Familial idiopathic osteoarthropathy, Am. J. Roentgenol. 85:633, 1961.
13. Schönenberg, H.: Zum Krankheitsbild der Osteo-Arthropathie hypertrophiante (Pierre-Bamberger), Ztschr. Kinderh. 74:388, 1954.
14. Chamberlain, D. S., Whitaker, J., and Silverman, F. N.: Idiopathic osteoarthropathy and cranial defects in children (familial idiopathic osteoarthropathy), Am. J. Roentgenol. 93:408, 1965.
15. Wilson, G. M.: Local circulatory changes associated with clubbing of fingers and toes, Quart. J. Med. 21:201, 1952.

91

Arachnodactyly and Homocystinuria

The Arachnodactyly Syndrome

(Marfan Syndrome; Dolichostenomelia)

In 1896, Marfan[1] directed attention to a skeletal anomaly characterized by long and thin tubular bones and contractures in the joints of the fingers, elbows and knees. In the first patient described there also was underdevelopment of the musculature and of the subcutaneous fat. Marfan called this condition "dolichosténomélie" and described the fingers as "spider-like"; the name "arachnodactyly" was created 6 years later by Achard.[2] In the following decades it was realized that patients with arachnodactyly often show a variety of malformations that constitute a syndrome that respects neither the borders of anatomic organs nor those of embryonic germ layers. Rados[3] has reviewed the historical development of this syndrome and the cases reported up to the year 1942, and Ross[4] collected cases published before 1949. In 1966, McKusick[5] believed that at least 400 cases of the Marfan syndrome had been reported in the literature. New facets of this syndrome are still being discovered, particularly in patients beyond childhood, but the syndrome is circumscribed enough already to be of diagnostic and prognostic value. In addition to the skeletal peculiarities noticed by Marfan, ectopia lentis was recognized as a frequent associated anomaly later.[6] Ocular defects occur in approximately 70% of the patients. It should be pointed out that E. Williams,[7] a Cincinnati physician, reported in 1876 —20 years before Marfan—two families in which he observed ectopia lentis, combined with articular changes in one. In one instance, eccentric pupils, luxated lenses and trembling irides were found in a "Frenchwoman, aet. 35," and in her brother, 30 years of age. In the second family, spontaneous bilateral luxation of the lenses, trembling irides and detached retina (in one eye) were present in a woman 28 years of age. Her younger brother also showed trembling irides and both lenses displaced upward. Both patients

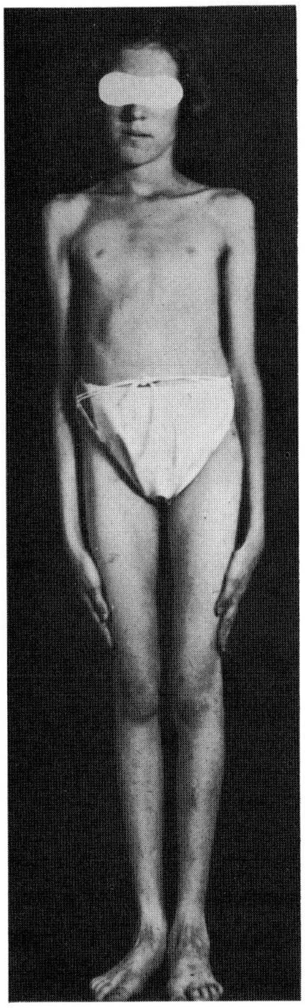

Fig. 91-1.—Arachnodactyly in a girl 10 years of age. Long, slender extremities. Both lenses were dislocated.

were large and *loose-jointed* and the "father's eyes were like theirs." Thus, Williams,[7] in 1876, described not only ectopia lentis in large and loose-jointed patients but also dominant inheritance in one family. He did not give a name to this syndrome and his name was not attached to it. Although in Marfan's case anomalies of the eye were not noticed, the syndrome of arachnodactyly and ectopia lentis has become known as "Marfan syndrome." Since eponymic justice is rare in medicine, there should be no objection to this term. It would be foolish—even for Cincinnati chauvinists—to attempt a change to "Williams syndrome," particularly since pathologic manifestations of other organ systems have been added to the disease picture. The cardiovascular, respiratory, intestinal and other systems may be involved. It has been asserted that Marfan syndrome is a systemic anomaly limited to mesodermal structures. This is not correct, since organs of ectodermal and entodermal origin can be affected also.

The incidence of the arachnodactyly syndrome is hard to evaluate, since many mild cases do not require medical attention and are not diagnosed. This fact has been recognized by many investigators who, on examination of relatives of a patient with a well-developed case, encounter persons with minimal expression of the gene. Incomplete cases and formes frustes often are overlooked. McKusick[5] gave as a minimal figure for prevalence of the Marfan syndrome 1.459 per 100,000 of the population, and for gene frequency 0.729 per 100,000 genes, but I would be inclined to round off the decimals.

Genetic determination can be assumed for most if not all cases. It is true that sporadic cases are seen and reported often, which may give the impression that heredity plays a minor role, but in many of these cases the families were incompletely examined. In addition, some of the cases, probably 15%,[5] may be due to new mutations. They could be the originators of typical pedigrees even though their ancestry is free of the condition.[3] In approximately half of the cases the syndrome is transmitted like a dominant Mendelian trait. Males and females are affected equally and parental consanguinity is rare. Often one member of a kinship shows many of the symptoms that constitute the syndrome, whereas among his relatives the condition may be monosymptomatic. However, as a rule, severe cases tend to be sporadic, whereas milder cases have a positive family history.[8] It is assumed by

Fig. 91-2.—Arachnodactyly in a boy 14 years of age. Bilateral dislocation of the lens was present.

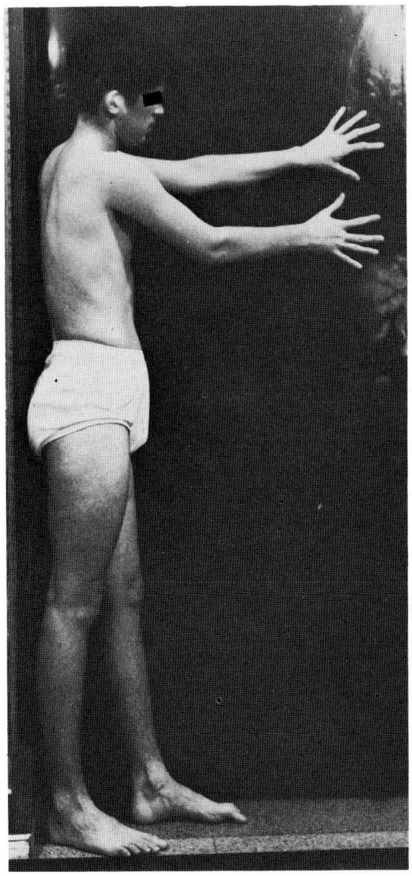

most investigators that the arachnodactyly syndrome is due to a dominant, autosomal and pleiotropic gene. The first report of transmission through two generations apparently was made by Williams[7] in 1876. Achard,[2] in 1902, observed the skeletal peculiarities in 2 girls, their mother and maternal grandfather. Bowers[9] traced the disease through six generations of a kinship with 33 affected persons. To explain the wide phenotypic variations in expression of this gene, modifying influences must be assumed. Modifiers, genetic or environmental, are generally conceded but little is known about them. That the pleiotropic gene responsible for the Marfan syndrome may be influanced by other genes of the affected person, by its genetic milieu, is suggested by observation of patients in whom the skeletal changes appear to be mitigated by the genetic constitution of one small and stocky parent.[5]

It is possible that occasionally a recessive mode of transmission occurs. Apparently normal persons may have more than one affected child,[10] and parental consanguinity has been observed.[11,12] In one instance, the patient was the product of incest between father and daughter.[13] Before recessive inheritance is assumed, the parents of the patients must be examined carefully to exclude the possibility that one of them is affected by a "forme fruste." Another possibility is that patients with homocystinuria (p. 857) simulate the arachnodactyly syndrome.

Marfan syndrome was observed by Steinberg[14] in identical twins, 2 years of age, and reported because of dilatation of the aortic sinuses. Becker[15] encountered identical twins, both affected, in a kinship reported because of ectopia lentis in three generations. Discordance in nonidentical twins was observed by Everberg.[16] An 11-year-old girl with the typical syndrome and a hearing defect had a normal twin brother, and Bowden *et al.*[17] observed an affected infant girl who had a normal twin. Twin observations support the concept of genetic determination of this disorder.

Some reports deal with chromosome anomalies in patients with arachnodactyly. Tjio *et al.*[18] described enlarged satellites in 2 patients with the disorder. In one case, the satellites were on a chromosome of pair no. 18 and in the other on no. 21. Hustinx and van Olphen[19] reported an XYY chromosome pattern in a boy with Marfan syndrome. His sisters, who also had the syndrome, had no chromosome anomalies. We have seen an unusually tall boy with some signs of Marfan syndrome who had an XYY karyotype (p. 1144). In many other patients with Marfan syndrome, normal chromosome number and karyotype were established.[19,20]

The mode of action of the mutant gene is not known at present. Attempts have been made to reduce the kaleidoscopic picture of the syndrome to a concept of alterations of mesoderm or of connective tissue. It is true that mesodermal and connective tissue changes are most obvious in these patients but the lens, which is of ectodermal origin, may be congenitally defective also. An actual defect in the lens substance may be present in some patients rather than changes secondary to deficient zonular fibers.[8] Essentially entodermal structures such as the esophagus and intestine may be involved also. One could attribute such changes to primary defects of connective tissue, which is closely interwoven with the tissues of entodermal origin, but it is difficult to prove this. Another fact that deserves emphasis is that not all mesodermal or connective tissues are affected by the pathologic process. Even elastic tissue—considered by many investigators to be the primary target of the abnormal gene—may not be affected in the skin, trachea, spinal ligaments and intervertebral disks,[21] so that the gene seems to limit its action to certain organs. There also is the possibility that the primary defect involves collagen.[5] It may be better to avoid premature and oversimplified labels for the mechanisms involved in this syndrome.

Only beginnings have been made in chemical investigations of the Marfan syndrome. Sjoerdsma *et al.*[22] found increased amounts of hydroxyproline in the urine of 7 of 10 patients with the syndrome, a finding confirmed by Jones *et al.*[23] and Macek *et al.*[20] Since this amino acid occurs in the body almost entirely in collagen, this finding represented a promising lead. However, Lehmann[24] could not confirm this discovery and found cystinuria instead in 2 members of an affected family. Increased amounts of urinary hydroxyproline are found under conditions of increased growth and are thus not specific for Marfan syndrome. A report on abnormally low levels of serum mucoproteins in affected members of one family[25] remained an isolated observation not confirmed in other studies.[24,26] Large amounts of keratosulfate have been found in cartilage of patients with Marfan syndrome.[27,28]

The production of scoliosis and dissecting aneurysm of the aorta in rats fed with Lathyrus odoratus seeds containing β-glutamylaminopropionitrile[29] is of great interest, since the lesions simulate to a certain extent those of the Marfan syndrome. But the mutant gene may use other methods of achieving its deleterious effects. Phenocopies of other congenital hereditary syndromes have been induced by various methods that do not reveal the mode of action of the mutant gene.

In 1959, Roark[21] found 73 reported necropsies of patients with Marfan syndrome. More than 50 of these contained microscopic studies, mostly of the vascular system, whereas only a few reports included histologic examinations outside the cardiovascular system. The most consistent finding was degeneration in the arterial walls, resembling to a certain extent Erdheim cystic medial necrosis. In the media, necrosis and fragmentation of the elastic fibers, hypertrophy and hyperplasia of smooth muscle and cystic areas rich in mucopolysaccharides can be seen.[30] Microscopic changes are not limited to the aorta but have been found also in other arteries, including the pulmonary. That aneurysmal dilatation usually is limited to the ascending aorta is attributed to continuous expansile pulsation in the arch. Thickening, asymmetry and elongation of valvular cusps are common. Changes in the myocardium, hypertrophy and fibrosis, without other cardiovascular lesions, are rare. When they occur, they can lead to cardiomegaly with relative insufficiency of the mitral and tricuspid valves.[31] Elastic tissue studies of the skin, trachea and lung by Roark[21] failed to demonstrate changes comparable to those found in the cardiovascular tissues. With histologic methods now available, no common denominator has yet been found that could explain the great variety of malformations and anomalies encountered in the arachnodactyly syndrome.

In pronounced cases, the arachnodactyly syndrome can be diagnosed at birth.[73] The birth weight may be low, but usually it is within normal limits; the length can be excessive.[32] Despite a normal birth weight, the infant appears emaciated and the subcutaneous fat reduced, the skin lying in loose folds over the extremities. The head is dolichocephalic and the ears are lowset, large and oblong. Anomalies of the eyes may be suggested by nystagmus or by eccentric pupils. Dislocation of the lens, if present, is only seldom recognized in the newborn period. A high, arched palate is the rule. Cleft palate without harelip has been recorded repeatedly.[4,33-35] It probably is a part of the syndrome, the cleft being an exaggerated expression of the inherited tendency to high palate. But in a report of a patient with arachnodactyly and cleft palate, one of the parents had arachnodactyly and the other cleft palate,[36] so that the combination can be considered coincidental in this case. Micrognathia is not rare. Sometimes asymmetry and deformities of the chest are noticeable at birth and a cardiac murmur may be audible.[37] Winged scapulae are noted often. The extremities are long and thin, but often only the hands and feet show marked elongation. The fingers and toes are strikingly long and slender (spider fingers). The joints may be hyperextensible or contracted, both anomalies sometimes occurring in different joints in the same infant. Arthrogryposis can be combined with Marfan syndrome. We have seen 3 children of this type,[35] and Reeve *et al.*[37] reported 1 case. Congenital dislocation of the clavicle, elbow, hip, femur, patella, tibia and others have been observed. Dislocation of the hips can present the first problem in neonates with Marfan syndrome.[38] Various congenital malformations can be present. In addition to cleft palate and other conditions already mentioned, abnormal segmentation of vertebrae,[4] torticollis, fused and supernumerary ribs,[4,39] microcephaly,[4] turricephaly,[40] abnormal lobation of a lung,[33,41] congenital pulmonary cysts,[5] diaphragmatic defect, short esophagus,[42] malrotation of the colon,[4] clubfoot and many others have been reported. These observations indicate that the mutant gene often exerts its influence in the embryonic period. In former times, the incidence and role of congenital malformations of the heart have been overestimated. Diagnosis often was based on superficial findings, and degenerative, postnatal cardiovascular changes clinically were mistaken for congenital malformations. In recent years, doubt has been expressed that such congenital malformations are a part of Marfan syndrome. But the following congenital cardiovascular malformations have been found in necropsies or were proved by catheterization or angiography: ventricular septal defect,[5,43-46] patent foramen ovale,[6,47-49] large auricular defect,[17,33,34] probable tetralogy of Fallot,[51] stenosis of the aorta,[52] stenosis of the pulmonary artery,[31,45] patent ductus arteriosus,[34,44,53,54] coarctation of the aorta,[24,31,39,55,56] pseudotruncus arteriosus,[45] ventricular septal defect and absence of the pulmonary valve,[57] persistent left superior vena cava,[31] abnormal pulmonary venous return[34] and abnormal numbers of the cusps of the mitral and aortic valves.[5] These observations show that in patients with Marfan syndrome the cardiovascular system may be affected in early embryonic life. It can be assumed safely that congenital structural malformations of the heart are found more often in patients with arachnodactyly than in the general population. One may not accept some of the cases cited above as belonging to the Marfan syndrome because they did not show ectopia lentis and failed to manifest a characteristic familial incidence. But if one deals with a syndrome attributed to a pleiotropic gene, one must expect incomplete cases; and if one deals with a hereditary entity, in which not all carriers of the mutant gene can be discovered and for which de novo mutations are assumed, one cannot hold a negative family history against the diagnosis of the syndrome. It is one of the most interesting properties of the gene responsible for the Marfan syndrome that it already acts adversely in the embryo and that it continues to exert its deleterious influence in postnatal life by "abiotrophic" or "degenerative" processes.

The postnatal development of arachnodactylics sometimes is slower than that of normal children. Weight gain usually is poor and infections of the intestinal or respiratory tract are not rare. Dentition may be normal. Visual defects become manifest sooner or later. As the children begin to sit or stand up, kyphosis or scoliosis develops. Motor activities are impaired by muscular weakness, hypotonia and abnormalities of the joints. The chest deformities present at birth often become more marked during the first years. Cardiac murmurs are heard frequently and cardiovascular changes can be demonstrated by modern cardiologic methods at an early age. Aside from true congenital malformations of the heart, aneurysmal dilatations have been demonstrated very early in some of the cases.[14,58] Marked dilatation of the ascending aorta was found at necropsy in an infant $3\frac{1}{2}$ months of age.[37] In another case,[59] necropsy of a 9-month-old boy revealed an aneurysmal dilatation of the ascending aorta with medial cystic necrosis.

The mitral and tricuspid valves had serrated and thickened borders. Similar valvular changes were observed by Salle[47] in an infant 3½ months of age, so that it is possible that in some cases the degenerative process leading to aneurysmal and valvular changes may be present in intrauterine life or certainly in the first months after birth.[34] Rupture of a dissecting aneurysm into the pericardial sac can occur in early childhood.[58] But in the majority of patients with the arachnodactyly syndrome, cardiac manifestations or even murmurs usually are absent until later in life, when the disease picture is fully developed, or they may never come to the foreground.

Older children or adults with the arachnodactyly syndrome often are unusually tall and the abnormal proportions due to excessive length of their extremities are clearly recognizable. The span of the extended arms exceeds the height by several inches and the lower measurements (pubis to heals) are much greater than the upper (pubis to vertex). The reduction of the sitting height is not only relative and due to the excessive length of the legs but also absolute because of deformities of the spine. The pathologic elongation of the extremities increases in the proximo-distal direction, the fingers and toes presenting the most striking appearance. Some fingers may show more elongation than others. Flexion deformities can affect all fingers, but contracture of the fifth digit occurs more often than that of others. Clawhands are formed by contractures of phalanges in flexion and webbing of fingers is seen occasionally.[4] The feet usually are flat, long and narrow and spurring of the heels contributes to the elongation. The first toes often are excessively long (Fig. 91-3). The ribs are also elongated so that their junctures with the sternum become abnormal. Funnel chest (pectus excavatum) or pigeon breast is the rule. Kyphosis and scoliosis contribute to the deformity of the thorax. Flaccidity of the articular capsules, ligaments and tendons results in hyperextensibility of joints, dislocations, genu recurvatum, pes planus or equinovarus and curvatures of the spine. Muscular hypotonia, seen in many cases, contributes to these anomalies. In infants, muscular underdevelopment may be so striking that systemic muscular atrophies or dystrophies are suspected. Weakness of muscles and their aponeuroses is responsible for the hernias frequently present in these patients. The underdevelopment of the muscles of the lower extremities contributes to the spindly appearance of the legs. Adipose tissue usually is markedly reduced, giving the patients an emaciated appearance.

Of the ocular anomalies, ectopia lentis is considered the cardinal symptom of Marfan syndrome. The lental luxation usually is bilateral and upward. It is due to laxity and fragmentation of the suspensory ligaments. Externally, iridodonesis, (trembling of the iris), heterochromia iridis and pupillary anomalies may be manifest. Megalocornea, buphthalmia and cloudy cornea are rare; blue sclerae have been observed repeatedly. Dilatation of the pupils and visualization of the lental dislocation may be difficult. The lens sometimes is very small[39] and spherical, demonstrating an effect of the gene on an ectodermal struc-

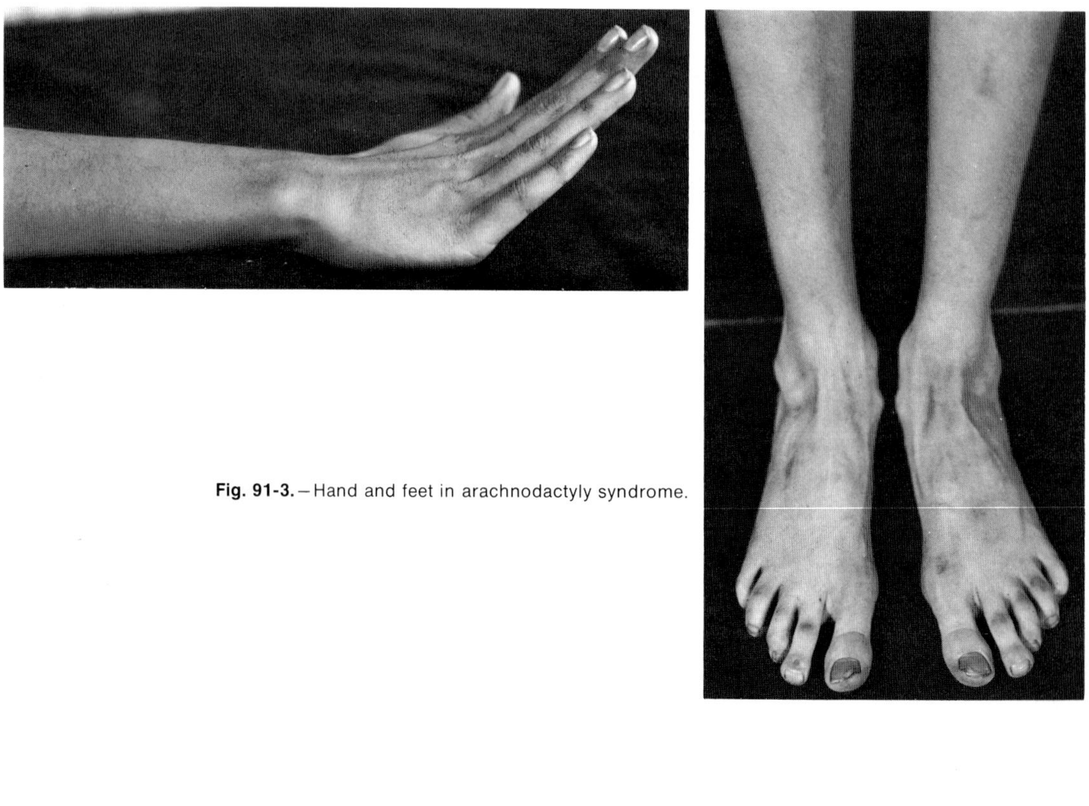

Fig. 91-3.—Hand and feet in arachnodactyly syndrome.

ture. Coloboma of the lens, iris[35,60] or choroid[61] may be seen. Myopia of severe degrees is frequent and detachment of the retina not rare. Iridocyclitis, glaucoma or cataract may complicate the ocular malformations. It has been estimated that ectopia lentis occurs in approximately 70% of the patients with this syndrome. Such estimates depend on the patient material and on the methods of examination. In a department of ophthalmology they will differ from those obtained in an orthopedic department. Whatever the true incidence of ectopia lentis, its absence in a patient showing other manifestations of this pleiotropic gene does not exclude the diagnosis of arachnodactyly or Marfan syndrome. Reduced hearing ability may be due to repeated attacks of otitis media or to nerve deafness.[16]

The cardiovascular anomalies include congenital malformations (p. 853) and pathologic changes that become grossly manifest in postnatal life only. The weakness of the media underlying vascular aneurysmal changes probably is congenital in all cases. The inborn media defect of the aorta and pulmonary artery results in enlargement of the great vessels with continued use and increasing age. Clinical observers have considered this and similar inborn weaknesses to be defects of vitality or growth and termed them "abiotrophic" or "degenerative" disorders. Clinical symptoms based on such areas of decreased resistance can vary in severity and time of appearance. This is true for the changes in the great vessels seen in Marfan syndrome. It has been mentioned that aneurysmal dilatations of the aorta have been observed in infants but it must be stressed that they can be delayed for decades and even to old age. If a dissecting aneurysm occurs in a child or in a young adult, Marfan syndrome frequently is the underlying condition. Early death of patients with Marfan syndrome often is due to cardiovascular anomalies, congenital malformations or dissecting aneurysms usually being responsible. Pathologic dilatation of the aorta begins at the aortic ring, progresses to the valvular cusps and leads to regurgitation. Aortic aneurysms develop as the media is replaced by scar tissue. They usually involve the ascending aorta to the origin of the innominate artery, but in exceptional cases the descending or abdominal aorta, the renal, splenic, carotid and femoral arteries may be involved also.[53,62] Distention of the sinuses of Valsalva occurs which can be recognized roentgenographically.[14] Dissection in young adults has been observed often but it can also occur in children.[58,63] Pregnancy seems to predispose to this complication.[64] Dilatation and rupture of the pulmonary artery have been reported.[54] Noninflammatory valvular changes may lead to insufficiencies and subsequent congestive failure.[30] Subacute bacterial endocarditis can be superimposed on valvular changes.

The respiratory system frequently is affected by infections that sometimes are fatal in young children. Spontaneous pneumothorax has been observed repeatedly.[25,65] Abnormal pulmonary lobation and cyst formation of congenital origin have been reported.[5,50] Diffuse pulmonary emphysema, bullous emphysema[66] with interstitial fibrosis and compression of the left main stem bronchus by a giant left atrium, resulting in atelectasis of the left lung with compensatory emphysema of the right lung are respiratory complications. Intestinal elongation[47] and malrotation[4] occur occasionally. Hiatus hernias may lead to gastrointestinal complications.[60]

Renal cysts and other congenital lesions of the urinary tract have been noted.[34,67] The skin may be affected by a rare disease, Miescher elastoma.[68] Multiple basal cell carcinomas have been recorded in a patient who also developed a bone cyst of the mandible. This patient stated that he had a brother "who looked just like" him, and who also had a tumor of the jaw.[69] Striae distensae occur. This has been cited as evidence of abnormality of the elastic tissue in this disorder.[70]

Involvement of the central nervous system has been observed occasionally and symptoms recalling Friedreich ataxia or syringomyelia have been described.[3] As a rule, the mental development is good and some patients have shown superior mentality. But a relatively large number of children with Marfan syndrome have been described who were mentally retarded.[3,4,71] Homocystinuria must be excluded in patients suspected of Marfan syndrome with mental retardation.

Roentgenograms show long and slender tubular bones, reminiscent of the bones seen in osteopsathyrosis (p. 824), but the bones are not brittle. The abnor-

Fig. 91-4.—Roentgenogram of upper extremity of patient with arachnodactyly and dislocated lenses.

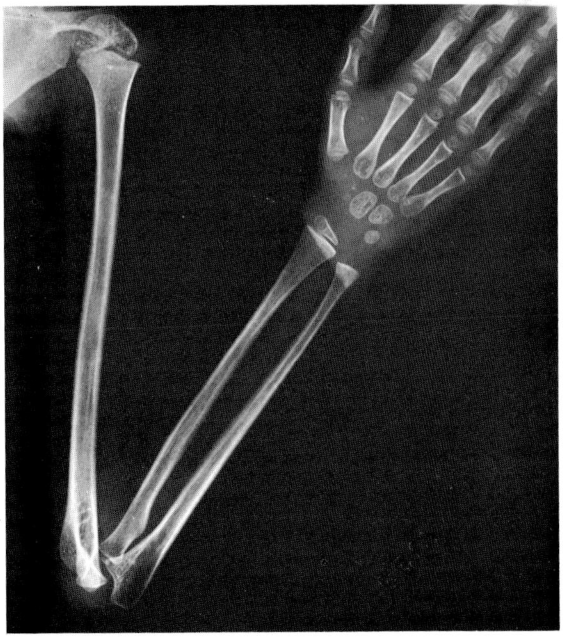

mal elongation increases in the proximo-distal direction, the metacarpals, metatarsals and phalanges being affected most severely. Maturation is normal or even advanced.[3,31] The skull appears dolichocephalic in most cases. Craniostenosis is found occasionally.[4,40] Chest roentgenograms often fail to demonstrate cardiovascular malformations in children.[34] In adults, they often are disappointing also and sometimes misleading, since usually a definite aneurysm is not shown.[72] But angiocardiography, by demonstrating aortic sinus dilatation, may reveal the cardiovascular anomalies of patients with Marfan syndrome.[14,53]

No specific treatment is available, but arachnodactylic patients require many types of symptomatic therapy. This disorder illustrates well the plight of the patient with multiple congenital malformations. To obtain adequate medical treatment, some of these patients need the help of many specialists. They go from the general practitioner or pediatrician to the orthopedic surgeon and to the ophthalmologist. As they grow older, they seek aid from a cardiologist, a lung specialist, a gastroenterologist and possibly an endocrinologist. It surprises no one that they finally consult a psychiatrist, and paranoia[4,51,60] and suicide actually have occurred in several of these unfortunate patients. Other persons with this abnormal gene live a perfectly normal life, reaching old age. Many arachnodactylic patients have proved capable of strenuous work and sports.[55]

Details of the orthopedic treatment cannot be discussed here. Every case needs individual attention. Amelioration of curvatures of the spine, of contractures and of deformities of the feet can be achieved. In some patients, vision can be improved by removal of a dislocated lens or by correction of myopia with glasses. Infections of the lung can be treated by chemotherapy and glandular insufficiency by endocrine preparations. The rare gastrointestinal anomalies of this syndrome sometimes may be amenable to surgery, but the cardiovascular changes are widespread and therefore only in part correctable by the surgeon. Operation for aortic aneurysm has resulted in improvement.[53] A knowledge of the syndrome and the problems created by it will make it possible for the guiding physician to give proper advice and to practice preventive psychiatry.

REFERENCES

1. Marfan, A. B.: Un cas de déformation congénitale des quatres membres plus prononcée aux extremités, charactérisée par l'allongement des os avec un certain degré d'amincissement, Bull. Soc. méd. hôp. Paris 13:220, 1896.
2. Achard, M. C.: Arachnodactylie, Bull. Soc. méd. hôp. Paris 19:834, 1902.
3. Rados, A.: Marfan's syndrome (arachnodactyly coupled with dislocation of the lens), Arch. Ophth. 27:477, 1942.
4. Ross, L. J.: Arachnodactyly. Review of recent literature and report of a case with cleft palate, Am. J. Dis. Child. 78:417, 1949.
5. McKusick, V. A.: *Heritable Disorders of Connective Tissue* (3d ed.; St. Louis: The C. V. Mosby Company, 1966).
6. Börger, F.: Über zwei Falle von Arachnodaktylie, Ztschr. Kinderh. 12:161, 1915.
7. Williams, E.: Rare cases, with practical remarks, Tr. Am. Ophth. Soc., p. 291, 1876.
8. Lutman, F. C., and Neel, J. V.: Inheritance of arachnodactyly, ectopia lentis and other congenital anomalies (Marfan's syndrome) in the E. family, Arch. Ophth. 41: 276, 1949.
9. Bowers, D.: Marfan's syndrome: The S family re-visited, Canad. M.A.J. 89:337, 1963.
10. Lynas, M. A.: Marfan's syndrome in Northern Ireland: An account of thirteen families, Ann. Human Genet. 22:289, 1958.
11. Páez, A. F.: Sobre un caso de aracnodactilia o enfermedad de Marfan, con subluxación de ambos cristalinos y miopia alta, An. argent. oftal. 7:81, 1946.
12. Bortree, L. W. (discussion of Strayhorn, D., and Wells, E. B.): Arachnodactylia with aneurysmal dilatation of the aorta, Tr. Am. Clin. & Climatol. A. 59:205, 1947.
13. Schrader, E.: Ein Beitrag zur Arachnodactylie, Deutsche Ztschr. Chir. 226:423, 1930.
14. Steinberg, I.: Dilatation of the aortic sinuses in the Marfan syndrome: Roentgen findings in five new cases, Am. J. Roentgenol. 83:302, 1960.
15. Becker, F.: Linsenektopie in der I., (II.) und III. Generation, Klin. Monatsbl. Augenh. 94:547, 1935.
16. Everberg, G.: Marfan's syndrome associated with hearing defect. Report of a case in one of a pair of twins, Acta paediat. scandinav. 48:70, 1959.
17. Bowden, D. H., Favara, B. E., and Donahoe, J. L.: Marfan's syndrome, Am. Heart J. 69:96, 1965.
18. Tjio, J. H., Puck, T. T., and Robinson, A.: The human chromosomal satellites in normal persons and in two patients with Marfan's syndrome, Proc. Nat. Acad. Sc. 46: 532, 1960.
19. Hustinx, T. W. J., and van Olphen, A. H. F.: An XYY chromosome pattern in a boy with Marfan's syndrome, Genetica 34:262, 1963.
20. Macek, M., Hurych, J., Chvapil, M., and Kadlecová, V.: Study on fibroblasts in Marfan's syndrome, Humangenetik 3:87, 1966.
21. Roark, J. W.: Marfan's syndrome. Report of one case with autopsy, special histological study and review of the literature, Arch. Int. Med. 103:123, 1959.
22. Sjoerdsma, A., Davidson, J. D., Udenfriend, S., and Mitoma, C.: Increased excretion of hydroxyproline in Marfan's syndrome, Lancet 2:994, 1958.
23. Jones, C. R., Bergman, M. W., Kittner, P. J., and Pigman, W. W.: Urinary hydroxyproline excretion in Marfan's syndrome as compared with age matched controls, Proc. Soc. Exper. Biol. & Med. 116:931, 1964.
24. Lehmann, O.: A family with Marfan's syndrome traced through an affected newborn, including analysis of the mucoproteins in serum and the urinary excretion of amino acids, Acta paediat. scandinav. 49:540, 1960.
25. Bacchus, H.: A quantitative abnormality in serum mucoproteins in the Marfan syndrome, Am. J. Med. 25:744, 1958.
26. Leeming, J. T., and McKusick, V. A.: Serum seromucoid levels in the Marfan syndrome, Bull. Johns Hopkins Hosp. 110:38, 1962.
27. Meyer, K., Hoffman, P., and Linker, A.: Mucopolysaccharides of costal cartilage, Science 128:896, 1958.
28. Dorfman, A.: The biochemistry of connective tissue, J. Chron. Dis. 10:403, 1959.
29. Ponseti, I. V., and Baird, W. A.: Scoliosis and dissecting aneurysm of the aorta in rats with Lathyrus odoratus seeds, Am. J. Path. 28:1059, 1952.
30. Sinclair, R. J. G.: The Marfan syndrome, Bull. Rheumat. Dis. 8:153, 1958.
31. van Buchem, F. S. P.: Arachnodactyly heart, Circulation 20:88, 1959.
32. Kohn, J. L., and Strauss, L.: Marfan's syndrome (arachnodactyly); observation of a patient from birth until death at 18 years, Pediatrics 25:872, 1960.

33. Piper, R. K., and Irvine-Jones, E.: Arachnodactylia and its association with congenital heart disease; report of case and review of literature, Am. J. Dis. Child. 31:832, 1926.
34. Papaioannou, A. C., Agustsson, M. H., and Gasul, B. M.: Early manifestations of the cardiovascular disorders in Marfan syndrome, Pediatrics 27:255, 1961.
35. Warkany, J.: Unpublished data.
36. Wilson, R.: Marfan's syndrome. Description of a family, Am. J. Med. 23:434, 1957.
37. Reeve, R., Silver, H. K., and Ferrier, P.: Marfan's syndrome (arachnodactyly) with arthrogryposis (amyoplasia congenita), A.M.A. J. Dis. Child. 99:101, 1960.
38. Heldrich, F. J., Jr., and Wright, C. E.: Marfan's syndrome. Diagnosis in the neonate, Am. J. Dis. Child. 114:419, 1967.
39. Fischl, A. A., and Ruthberg, J.: Clinical implications of Marfan's syndrome, J.A.M.A. 146:704, 1951.
40. Tung, H. L., and Liebow, A. A.: Marfan's syndrome. Observations at necropsy: With special reference to medionecrosis of the great vessels, Lab. Invest. 3:382, 1952.
41. Bergstrand, C. G.: Beitrag zur pathologischen Anatomie der Arachnodaktylie mit Bericht über einen eigenen Fall, Acta paediat. scandinav. 30:345, 1942.
42. Bronson, E., and Sutherland, G. A.: Ruptured aortic aneurysms in childhood, with the report of a case, Brit. J. Child. Dis. 15:241, 1918.
43. Keith, J. D., Rowe, R. D., and Vlad, P. (eds.): *Heart Disease in Infancy and Childhood* (New York: The Macmillan Company, 1958).
44. Talbert, L. E., and Berchall, R. B.: Marfan's syndrome with interventricular septal defect found at autopsy, Ochsner Clin. Rep. 2:48, 1956.
45. Gottsegen, G., Antony, M., and Szám, I.: Marfan-Syndrom mit Pseudotruncus arteriosus und terminalem Hirnabszess, Wien. klin. Wchnschr. 71:335, 1959.
46. Ross, J. K., and Gerbode, F.: The Marfan syndrome associated with an unusual interventricular septal defect, J. Thoracic & Cardiovas. Surg. 39:746, 1960.
47. Salle, V.: Über eine Fall von angeborener abnormer Grösse der Extermitäten mit einem an Akromegalia erinnernden Symptomenkomplex, Jahrb. Kinderh. 75:540, 1912.
48. Apert, E.: Les formes frustes du syndrome stenomélique de Marfan, Nourrisson 26:1, 1938.
49. Baer, R. W., Taussig, H. B., and Oppenheimer, E. H.: Congenital aneurysmal dilation of the aorta associated with arachnodactyly, Bull. Johns Hopkins Hosp. 72:309, 1943.
50. Oswald, N., and Parkinson, T.: Honeycomb lungs, Quart. J. Med. 18:1, 1949.
51. Lindeboom, G. A., and Westerveld-Brandon, E. R.: Dilatation of the aorta in arachnodactyly, Cardiologia 17:217, 1950.
52. Burry, A. F.: Supra-aortic stenosis associated with Marfan's syndrome, Brit. Heart J. 20:143, 1958.
53. Tuna, N., and Thal, A. P.: Some unusual features of the Marfan syndrome, Circulation 24:1154, 1961.
54. Anderson, M., and Pratt-Thomas, H. R.: Marfan's syndrome, Am. Heart J. 46:911, 1953.
55. Fabre, J., Veyrat, R., and Jeanneret, O.: Syndrome de Marfan avec aneurysme et coarctation de l'aorte; étude anatomo-clinique, Schweiz. med. Wchnschr. 87:49, 1957.
56. Eldridge, R.: Coarctation in the Marfan syndrome, Arch. Int. Med. 113:342, 1964.
57. Childers, R. W., and McCrea, P. C.: Absence of the pulmonary valve; a case occurring in the Marfan syndrome, Circulation 29:(supp.)598, 1964.
58. Wong, F. L., Friedman, S., and Yakovac, W.: Cardiac complications of Marfan's syndrome in a child, Am. J. Dis. Child. 107:404, 1964.
59. Traisman, H. S., and Johnson, F. R.: Marfan's syndrome with aortic aneurysm, A.M.A. Am. J. Dis. Child. 85:706, 1953.
60. Knight, A. M., Jr.: The Marfan syndrome, J. M. A. Georgia 46:413, 1957.
61. Merghoub, S.: Relations entre les colobomes iridochoroïdiens et l'hétérochromie irienne associée ou non à une forme fruste du syndrome de Marfan, J. Génét. Hum. 13: 133, 1964.
62. Langeron, L., Giard, P., Liefooghe, J., and Masson, Ch.: Maladie de Marfan et aneurysme abdominal, Bull. Soc. méd. hôp. Paris 70:374, 1954.
63. Griffith, G. J., Hayhurst, A. P., and Whitehead, R.: Dissecting aneurysm of aorta in mother and child, Brit. Heart J. 13:364, 1951.
64. Husebye, K. O., Wolff, H. J., and Friedman, L. L.: Aortic dissection in pregnancy: A case of Marfan's syndrome, Am. Heart J. 55:662, 1958.
65. Gupta, S. K., and Sharma, V. N.: Chronic pneumothorax in Marfan's syndrome, Brit. J. Tuberc. 51:346, 1957.
66. Bolande, R. P., and Tucker, A. S.: Pulmonary emphysema and other cardiorespiratory lesions as part of the Marfan abiotrophy, Pediatrics 33:356, 1964.
67. Booth, C. C., Loughridge, L. W., and Turner, M. D.: Arachnodactyly with congenital lesions of the urinary tract, Brit. M. J. 2:80, 1957.
68. Haber, H.: Miescher's elastoma (elastoma intrapapillare perforans verruciforme), Brit. J. Dermat. 71:85, 1959.
69. Boyer, B. E., and Martin, M. M.: Marfan's syndrome. Report of a case manifesting a giant bone cyst of the mandible and multiple (110) basal cell carcinomata, Plast. & Reconstruct. Surg. 22:257, 1958.
70. Loveman, A. B., Gordon, A. M., and Fliefelman, M. T.: Marfan's syndrome, Arch. Dermat. 87:428, 1963.
71. Illig, W. P., LoPresti, J. M., and Houck, J. C.: Marfan's syndrome, Clin. Proc. Child. Hosp. (Wash.) 20:73, 1964.
72. Goyette, E. M., and Palmer, P. W.: Cardiovascular lesions in arachnodactyly, Circulation 7:373, 1953.
73. Neimann, N., Rauber, G., Marchal, C., Vidailhet, M., and Fall, M.: Maladie de Marfan chez un nouveau-né avec atteintes polyviscérales, Ann. pédiat. 44:2387, 1968.

Homocystinuria

This inborn metabolic disorder results in anomalies and malformations similar in some respects to those of arachnodactyly or Marfan syndrome, but there is no proof that the malformations of homocystinuria are congenital. Most cases are discovered several years after birth but, as the anomaly becomes better known, defects may be diagnosed earlier.[1-3]

The metabolic disturbance is an autosomal recessive trait, characterized by cystathionine synthetase deficiency.[4] Abnormalities of methionine metabolism have been described.[1,5,6] The defect can recur in families, male and female siblings being affected.

Ocular and skeletal malformations are similar to those of Marfan syndrome, but osteoporosis, thromboembolic phenomena, fatty changes in the liver[7] and mental retardation characterize homocystinuria.

Dislocation of the lens is a leading sign, but keratitis, cataracts, myopia, retinal changes and optic atrophy have been observed also. Glaucoma and hydrophthalmia can complicate the displacement of the lens.[8] Many patients are tall and the lower measurements are much greater than the upper, similar to arachnodactyly. The digits may be elongated, the joints lax or contracted; kyphoscoliosis and pigeon breast develop. Biconcave vertebrae, general osteoporosis and a tendency to fractures are noted in older patients.[3] The central nervous system is more endangered than in Marfan syndrome. Mental retardation is present in approximately half the patients, but this estimate probably is high because many cases were discovered by screening institutionalized persons. There may be mental disturbances simulating schizophrenia. The electroencephalogram often is abnormal and hyperreflexia may be noticed. Convulsions occur in some patients.

A malar flush and blotchy skin can be seen in children, and adults often have intensely red facial skin. Rosy cheeks, fair hair and skin contribute to the facial appearance. As the patients grow older, they develop a tendency to arterial thromboses, which is responsible for many of the cardiovascular symptoms. Death from coronary occlusion can occur at an early age, but aortic aneurysms are not characteristic of this disease.[3]

Some infants show serious complications in early life and die in childhood; other patients reach adulthood and live a rather normal life.

Treatment with a low-methionine and high-cystine diet[9-11] and with pyridoxine[12] supplements are under consideration but clinical effectiveness has not been established.[13,15] It is possible that in homocystinuria two different genetically determined basic defects exist that respond differently to pyridoxine treatment.[14]

REFERENCES

1. Carson, N. A. J., Cusworth, D. C., Dent, C. E., Field, C. M. B., Neill, D. W., and Westall, R. G.: Homocystinuria: A new inborn error of metabolism associated with mental retardation, Arch. Dis. Childhood 38:425, 1963.
2. Gerritsen, T., Vaughn, J. G., and Waisman, H. A.: The identification of homocystine in the urine, Biochem. & Biophys. Res. Commun. 9:493, 1962.
3. McKusick, V. A.: *Heritable Disorders of Connective Tissue* (3d ed.; St. Louis: The C. V. Mosby Company, 1966).
4. Mudd, S. H., Finkelstein, J. D., Irreverre, F., and Laster, L.: Homocystinuria: An enzymatic defect, Science 143: 1443, 1964.
5. Gerritsen, T., and Waisman, H. A.: Homocystinuria, an error in the metabolism of methionine, Pediatrics 33:413, 1964.
6. Brenton, D. P., Cusworth, D. C., and Gaull, G. E.: Homocystinuria: Metabolic studies on 3 patients, J. Pediat. 67: 58, 1965.
7. Carson, N. A. J., Dent, C. E., Field, C. M. B., and Gaull, G. E.: Homocystinuria, J. Pediat. 66:565, 1965.
8. Spaeth, G. L., and Barber, G. W.: Homocystinuria–its ocular manifestations, J. Pediat. Ophth. 3:42, 1966.
9. Komrower, G. M., Lambert, A. M., Cusworth, D. C., and Westall, R. G.: Dietary treatment of homocystinuria, Arch. Dis. Childhood 41:666, 1966.
10. Chase, H. P., Goodman, S. I., and O'Brien, D.: Treatment of homocystinuria, Arch. Dis. Childhood 42:514, 1967.
11. Perry, T. L., Dunn, H. G., Hansen, S., MacDougall, L., and Warrington, P. D.: Early diagnosis and treatment of homocystinuria, Pediatrics 37:502, 1966.
12. Turner, B.: Pyridoxine treatment in homocystinuria, Lancet 2:1151, 1967.
13. Gaudier, B., François, P., Biserte, G., Dautrevaux, M., Nuyts, J-P., and Bombart, E.: L'homocystinurie, Arch. franç. pédiat. 25:541, 1968.
14. Carson, N. A. J., and Carré, I. J.: Treatment of homocystinuria with pyridoxine, Arch. Dis. Childhood 44:387, 1969.
15. Barber, G. W., and Spaeth, G. L.: The successful treatment of homocystinuria with pyridoxine, J. Pediat. 75: 463, 1969.

92

Hypophosphatasia and Hyperphosphatasia

Hypophosphatasia

THIS DISORDER of defective bone formation is associated with a demonstrable enzymatic defect, diminished alkaline phosphatase, and with increased urinary excretion of phosphoethanolamine. It represents a genetically determined error of metabolism that, in its most severe form, manifests itself in congenital malformations. It often is assumed that all hereditary congenital malformations are due to inborn errors of metabolism, but hypophosphatasia is one of the few disorders in which structural congenital deformities can be ascribed to a recognized metabolic defect. But even in this congenital bone disorder it is not certain that the associated inborn error of metabolism, hypophosphatasia, is causative (see below). The condition is rare and the incidence has been estimated to be 1 per 100,000 live births.[1] The disease was considered a "new developmental anomaly" by Rathbun,[2] who, in 1948, first termed it "hypophosphatasia."

The disorder is always congenital, but clinical manifestations may be delayed, appearing in various periods of postnatal life. The most severe type of hypophosphatasia begins in utero, affected infants dying at birth or soon thereafter. Of course, such infants had been seen before 1948, but they probably were mistaken for cases of osteogenesis imperfecta, congenital rickets or achondroplasia. With delayed onset, the disease simulates rickets in many respects, but alkaline phosphatase activity distinguishes the two diseases.

It is very likely that hypophosphatasia is due to an autosomal recessive gene. The heterozygotes seem to be healthy persons who have low serum phosphatase activity, whereas the homozygotes manifest the disease. This has been shown in some families such as that of Case 6 of Currarino *et al.*,[3] in which healthy parents with low serum phosphatase activity had 2 infants with semilethal hypophosphatasia. In addition, 1 daughter, phenotypically normal, had a low phosphatase value. Their Cases 12 and 13 also conform to this concept, since parents with low serum phosphatase activity had 2 children affected by hypophosphatasia and rickets-like symptoms ending in death at age 8 months. The newborn represented by Figure 92-1, *A* and her family also fit the theory very well. In this family, the parents as well as the only surviving brother had low phosphatase values (obtained after the death of the affected infants). The surviving members of the family are heterozygotes, whereas those lost by miscarriage or neonatal death probably were homozygotes. The phosphatase activity—if any—of the lethal cases had not been ascertained. Rathbun *et al.*,[4] studying an affected family, attempted to ascertain the carrier state in 30 relatives in three generations. They concluded that hypophosphatasia is inherited as a recessive characteristic and that the carrier state is represented by adult persons with serum levels below 2 Bodansky units. Parental consanguinity was reported for the case of Bonucci and Agostinelli.[5]

It is doubtful, however, that all cases of hypophosphatasia are inherited in this way. In the case of Sobel *et al.*,[6] only the father's plasma alkaline phosphatase was low, whereas that of the mother was normal. For their patient, whose manifestations were not too severe, one could assume a dominant gene that can manifest itself in heterozygotes. The situation is not clear in Case 1 of Schlesinger *et al.*[7]; this patient's parents had normal phosphatase values. There remains much to be elucidated concerning the etiology of these disturbances. The severity of the disease certainly does not parallel the reduction of alkaline phosphatase activity in the serum. In addition, marked hypophosphatasia can be found in phenotypically normal persons or in persons with renal glycosuria without bone lesions.[1] It must be admitted, therefore, that although low phosphatase activity is closely associated with the hereditary factor, it does not necessarily represent the fundamental expression of the abnormal gene. It is of interest that patients with hypophosphatasia show another metabolic deviation, namely, phosphoethanolaminuria.[8,9] This abnormal urinary metabolite has been attributed to lowered phosphatase activity, which may lead to accumulation of phosphoethanolamine in the body with overflow into the urine.[10] Similarly, hypercalcemia present in many but not in all patients appears to be a secondary effect of a more basic disturbance.

The disorder occurs in both sexes but, so far, more female than male patients have been described. Hypophosphatasia in twins supposed to be monozygotic has been reported.[11] Cases have been observed in many countries. Caucasians and Negroes can be affected. Intrafamilial resemblance of manifestations has been rather striking in cases of repeated occurrence in a pedigree. Chromosome analyses showed normal karyotypes.[11]

Cartilage, osteoid tissue and osteoblasts are abundant in the bones but the zone of provisional calcification is in disorder. Islands of uncalcified cartilage are enclosed in uncalcified bone. Tongues of uncalcified cartilage reach into the marrow of the diaphyses, which are thin and enveloped in subperiosteal osteoid coats. Osteoid is also found in abundance in the uncalcified bones of the calvarium. The disturbance of normal calcification and the presence of excessive amounts of cartilage and osteoid simulate the findings in rickets.[5] The difference is brought out by special stains that demonstrate the absence of alkaline phosphatase in bone. Fraser *et al.*,[9] in in vitro experiments, showed that the serum of a severely affected patient could calcify rachitic rat cartilage, but the patient's costochondral junction did not calcify in the serum of healthy children. Thus, it is believed that the inability to calcify is not humoral but due to an anomaly of the preosseous tissues. Bones of membranous and cartilaginous origin show the defect. The results of the defective osteogenesis and the metaphyseal disorder can be demonstrated in histologic sections as well as in microradiographs.[12]

The renal pathology found in hypophosphatasia probably is secondary to the metabolic disturbance. In the series of Currarino *et al.*,[3] necropsies of newborn patients showed no renal anomalies, but in older children nephritis and scarring were noticeable. Calcific deposits were seen in the tubules and in peritubular tissues. The condition, termed nephrocalcinosis, can be attributed to the hypercalcemia occurring in many of the patients.[1]

Hypophosphatasia has been observed clinically in many forms. In general, the disease picture is the more serious the earlier the manifestations become noticeable. In the most severely affected family observed so far (Fig. 92-1, *B*), miscarriages and premature births with neonatal deaths occurred repeatedly. Pregnancies with affected fetuses may be accompanied by hydramnios, as reported in the X Family and in the case of Malbrain *et al.*[12] In prematurely born infants with hypophosphatasia, the disease is so severe that it is incompatible with life. The lack of ossification is seen in Figure 92-1, *A*. The head is relatively large, but the skull is poorly ossified and soft. The bones, with few exceptions, are not visible in the roentgenogram. There is micromelia and folds are formed by the skin, which is too large for the extremities. Because of micromelia in the presence of a relatively large head and trunk, the child, II_8, as well as two older sisters (II_1 and II_3) were mistaken for achondroplastics. Child II_1 was stillborn after a pregnancy of $6\frac{1}{2}$ months. Infant II_3, born after a pregnancy complicated by hydramnios and lasting $7\frac{1}{2}$ months, lived only 1 hour. The pregnancy resulting in

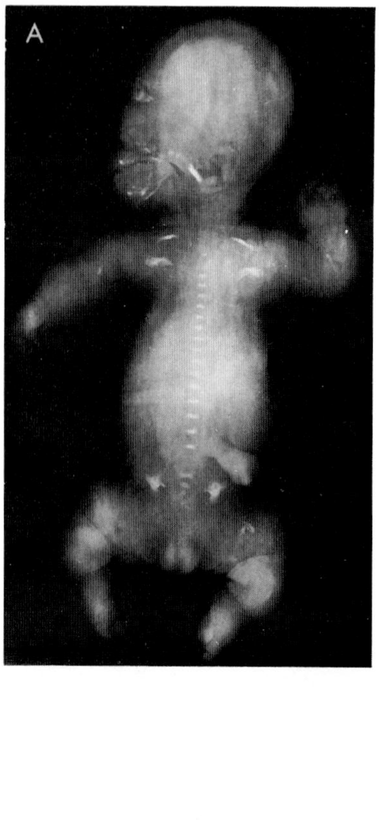

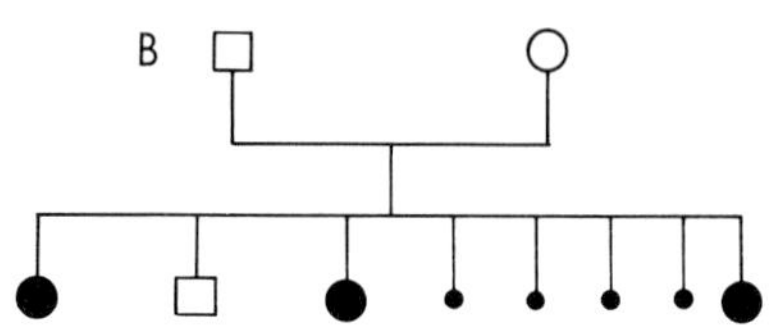

Fig. 92-1.—**A,** roentgenogram of a child with hypophosphatasia. Almost complete lack of ossification. **B,** pedigree of the same child (the X family). Three affected girls died in the neonatal period and there were four miscarriages. Only one phenotypically normal boy survived.

child II_8, whose roentgenogram is shown in Figure 92-1, *A*, was also complicated by hydramnios and lasted 7 months. The infant lived 2 hours. The parents and 1 surviving male child were clinically normal but they all had hypophosphatasia. The serum alkaline phosphatase of the mother was 0.6, that of the father 0.8 and that of their 8-year-old son 3.6 Bodansky units. No blood chemical studies had been made in cases II_3 and II_8. Transitional forms between such lethal cases and children who can survive the first year exist. In newborns described by Currarino *et al.*,[3] the skeleton had many uncalcified parts, some bones showing ossification at their central portions only. The tubular bones were short and thin, the ends—in contrast to osteogenesis imperfecta—being cupped, ragged and frayed. Infractions were common, resulting in angulations and callus deformities. The skull was large and soft because of lack of ossification. The ribs also were only slightly ossified, which made expansion of the thorax and breathing difficult. Exceptionally, the sclerae are blue.[1] Many of these children are dead at birth or die soon after delivery. A few survive for several weeks or months. Congenital bowing of the long bones with skin dimples over the convexities (p. 957) can be an early manifestation. Cupping and fraying of the metaphyses absent at birth can be delayed for several months. If the bowing of the long bones is accompanied by wide cranial sutures and large fontanelles, hypophosphatasia must be considered and confirmed or ruled out biochemically. Partial healing of rickets-like changes can take place spontaneously without changes of phosphatase values.[13]

Other children, although born with the disorder, fail to manifest it for several months. Then, failure to thrive, vomiting, anorexia, fever, irritability, convulsions and cyanosis betray the illness. The cranial sutures and the anterior fontanelle appear enlarged, bulging and tense. The radiolucent bands seen in roentgenograms of the skull are due to abundance of uncalcified osteoid and not to fibrous tissue.[1] Some infants die at this early stage. Others who survive show changes simulating rickets, i.e., a rosary and enlarged ends of the long bones. Growth is slow, and deformities of the spine and of the extremities develop when the children finally begin to walk. Loss of their deciduous teeth soon after their eruption is a characteristic symptom.[6] It can be due to abnormal cementogenesis and be the only overt manifestation of hypophosphatasia.[14] Inadequate growth of alveolar bone and of the dental roots contributes to dental shedding. Another striking feature is development of craniostenosis, leading to an eminence in the area of the anterior fontanelle and increased digital markings of the calvarium.

The childhood form does not manifest itself before the second year, although mild symptoms usually can be traced to infancy. Delayed walking, pain and deformities in the region of the knees, loss of teeth and rickets-like changes are some of the pathologic signs. Spontaneous improvement and healing with deformities is possible. Such cases, erroneously diagnosed as rickets in the past, may flare up again in adult life, leading to arthritic pains, fractures and dental problems.[10]

Laboratory investigations reveal low values for serum alkaline phosphatase. Normally, values between 4 and 15 Bodansky (or 12–20 King-Armstrong) units are found in infants, whereas the corresponding values in hypophosphatasia can be between 0.3 and 3 Bodansky (or 3–5 King-Armstrong) units, respectively. Hypercalcemia is the rule in infants but exceptional in older patients.[3] In the absence of hypercalcemia, urinary calcium excretion can be elevated in infants.[15] Phosphoethanolamine excretion in the urine has been present in most patients but it appears doubtful that this is a specific finding, since it also occurs in other diseases such as scurvy, hypothyroidism and celiac disease. In contrast to rickets, urinary hydroxyproline values are low in hypophosphatasia.[15] Urinary inorganic pyrophosphate excretion is increased.[16]

The newborn form must be distinguished from achondroplasia and osteogenesis imperfecta. The soft and almost boneless skull permits a quick differentiation from achondroplasia. Roentgenograms demonstrate differences from osteogenesis imperfecta, since in hypophosphatasia bone formation is absent in many skeletal parts and the metaphyseal ends of the long bones, if ossified, are frayed and ragged. In infants and children, the disease must be distinguished from rickets. Low alkaline serum phosphatase, high serum calcium and normal inorganic phosphorus values are characteristic for hypophosphatasia.

The prognosis is hopeless for those infants who manifest the most severe form at birth. When symptoms appear several months after birth, death may terminate the disease by cerebral,[17] pulmonary[15] or renal complications. Survivors and children who develop symptoms later show a tendency to slow recovery, but, as a rule, some deformities and shortness of stature remain. Exacerbations may occur in adult life. Neither prednisone nor oral phosphate treatment influences the course of the disease.[15] Delayed union of femoral osteotomies has been reported.[11]

The eugenic prognosis is best based at present on the assumption that the parents are heterozygous for the trait and that there is a risk of one-fourth of the children being affected and one-half being carriers.

REFERENCES

1. Fraser, D.: Hypophosphatasia, Am. J. Med. 22:730, 1957.
2. Rathbun, J. C.: Hypophosphatasia, a new developmental anomaly, Am. J. Dis. Child. 75:822, 1948.
3. Currarino, G., Neuhauser, E. B. D., Reyersbach, G. C., and Sobel, E. H.: Hypophosphatasia, Am. J. Roentgenol. 78: 392, 1957.
4. Rathbun, J. C., Macdonald, J. W., Robinson, H. M. C., and Wanklin, J. M.: Hypophosphatasia: A genetic study, Arch. Dis. Childhood 36:540, 1961.
5. Bonucci, E., and Agostinelli, O.: Radiological and microradiographic features in a case of congenital hypophosphatasia, Radiol. clin. 35:80, 1966.

6. Sobel, E. H., Clark, L. C., Jr., Fox, R. P., and Robinow, M.: Rickets, deficiency of "alkaline" phosphatase activity and premature loss of teeth in childhood, Pediatrics 11:309, 1953.
7. Schlesinger, B., Luder, J., and Bodian, M.: Rickets with alkaline phosphatase deficiency; osteoblastic dysplasia, Arch. Dis. Childhood 30:265, 1955.
8. McCance, R. A., Morrison, A. B., and Dent, C. E.: Excretion of phosphoethanolamine and hypophosphatasia, preliminary communication, Lancet 1:131, 1955.
9. Fraser, D., Yendt, E. R., and Christie, F. H. E.: Metabolic abnormalities in hypophosphatasia, Lancet 1:286, 1955.
10. Bethune, J. E., and Dent, C. E.: Hypophosphatasia in the adult, Am. J. Med. 28:615, 1960.
11. Jacobson, D. P., and McClain, E. J.: Hypophosphatasia in monozygotic twins, J. Bone & Joint Surg. 49-A:377, 1967.
12. Malbrain, H., Ponlot, R., and Denys, P.: L'hypophosphatasie et ses manifestations osseuses, Arch. franç. pédiat. 14:337, 1957.
13. Kellsey, D. C.: Hypophosphatasia and congenital bowing of the long bones, J.A.M.A. 179:187, 1962.
14. Pimstone, B., Eisenberg, E., and Silverman, S.: Hypophosphatasia: Genetic and dental studies, Ann. Int. Med. 65:722, 1966.
15. Teree, T. M., and Klein, L.: Hypophosphatasia: Clinical and metabolic studies, J. Pediat. 72:41, 1968.
16. Russell, R. G. G.: Excretion of inorganic pyrophosphate in hypophosphatasia, Lancet 1:461, 1965.
17. Béthenod, M., Cotte, M. F., Collombel, C., Fréderich, A., and Cotte, J.: Hypophosphatasie à révélation néo-natale. Amélioration osseuse. Encéphalopathie convulsivante fatale, Ann. pédiat. 14:835, 1967.

Hyperphosphatasia

(Familial Osteoectasia with Macrocranium)

Bakwin *et al.*[1] described 2 sisters of Puerto Rican origin with fragilitas ossium that manifested itself early in life but was not associated with blue sclerae and deafness. Bowing of the legs and macrocranium developed. The medullary cavities of the long bones were expanded and the cortices thickened and osteoporotic. The bones of the skull were greatly thickened and round patches of increased density were noticed in roentgenograms. Degenerative changes were present in the retina. Deformities of the pelvis developed. The serum alkaline phosphatase was elevated at times and the serum calcium sometimes was low. The parents of the sisters were first cousins. The mother showed some of the bone changes in a mild degree. Stemmermann[2] made a histologic and histochemical study of a brother and sister of Puerto Rican origin living in Honolulu who had the same disorder. They had large skulls, bowed tubular bones, flared ribs, protruding sterna and marked dwarfism. They suffered many fractures from minor traumas. Roentgenograms showed progressive diaphyseal enlargement of the long bones, thin cortex and active periosteal bone formation. The teeth were carious. Serum alkaline phosphatase levels varied from 40 to 169 Sigma units (high normal, 2.3) and acid phosphatase levels from 1.8 to 3.6 Sigma units (high normal, 0.65). The serum calcium varied from 8.4 to 10.7 mg./100 ml. and the phosphorus level from 4.1 to 6 mg./100 ml.

There were reduced amounts of mature lamellar bone in the diaphyseal cortex and increased membranous osteogenesis with deficient mature bone formation. The conversion of newly formed, coarsely woven bone into mature lamellar bone seemed defective.

Clinical and biochemical data on these children were published by Eyring and Eisenberg,[3] who thought that some cases recorded as osteogenesis imperfecta might be examples of "congenital hyperphosphatasia." Marked elevation of serum alkaline phosphatase, elevated acid phosphatase and elevated leucine amino peptidase are characteristic findings. In the urine, large amounts of hydroxyproline peptide are found. Autosomal recessive inheritance is likely. Gross chromosomal defects cannot be demonstrated. Mabry *et al.*[4] reported a kindred in which 3 siblings and a cousin were affected. The patients had mental retardation, seizures, various neurologic abnormalities and greatly elevated serum alkaline phosphatase. The parents' marriages were consanguineous.

REFERENCES

1. Bakwin, H., Golden, A., and Fox, S.: Familial osteoectasia with macrocranium, Am. J. Roentgenol. 91:609, 1964.
2. Stemmermann, G. N.: An histologic and histochemical study of familial osteoectasia, Am. J. Path. 48:641, 1966.
3. Eyring, E. J., and Eisenberg, E.: Congenital hyperphosphatasia. A clinical, pathological, and biochemical study of two cases, J. Bone & Joint Surg. 50-A:1099, 1968.
4. Mabry, C. C., Bautista, A., Kirk, R. F., Dubilier, L. D., Braunstein, H., and Koepke, J. A.: Familial hyperphosphatasia with mental retardation, seizures, and neurologic deficits, J. Pediat. 77:74, 1970.

Osteopetrosis; Pyknodysostosis; Pyle Disease

Osteopetrosis

(Marble Bones; Albers-Schönberg Disease; Osteosclerosis Fragilis Generalisata)

OSTEOPETROSIS is a rare generalized skeletal disorder that is characterized by increased density of the bones accompanied by loss of their normal structure. Although bones "solid and without marrow" were known at the time of Pliny the Elder, osteopetrosis was not recognized as a clinical entity before the advent of roentgen rays. In 1904, Albers-Schönberg[1] published "Roentgenograms of a rare bone disease" and, for the first time, described the disorder in a living subject. Since then, many instances of osteopetrosis have been reported, and the disease has become established as a pathologic entity. However, it is certain that various types of osteopetrosis exist that differ in etiology, course and prognosis.

In most cases, osteopetrosis is genetically determined. At least two modes of inheritance are known to occur – dominant and recessive – and further subdivisions have been made.[2] As a rule, the severe forms are recessively inherited, whereas asymptomatic mild forms are transmitted as dominant traits. The latter are compatible with life and good health, affected persons having lived into their seventies. In such cases, the slow progress of the disorder can be followed in serial roentgenograms. Members of the same family usually have similar manifestations of osteopetrosis, but there are exceptions to this rule. In a family described by Cocchi,[3] the disorder was transmitted like a dominant trait; the first patient seen was asymptomatic, but other members of the family showed many of the complications of the disease, thus exhibiting intrafamilial variability and a wide range of expressivity. In mild cases, the abnormal gene affects the bones only by increased density, an expression of a disturbed relationship between apposition and resorption of bone. In more severe cases, the osseous anomaly is complicated by fractures, osteomyelitis and optic atrophy. Anemia is attributed to the same gene and is considered a coordinated pleiotropic effect not necessarily dependent on osteosclerosis, since it can occur in patients whose bones are but little affected.[4]

In the severe infantile form, parental consanguinity often can be demonstrated.[2,5,6] The parents are either first cousins or consanguineous in other degrees. Often, children with the infantile form are born in areas of inbreeding; the parents usually appear normal, having 1 or more children with the abnormal trait. It is assumed that this severe infantile form is due to autosomal recessive inheritance; often it is congenital[7] and has been observed and diagnosed in utero.[8] Many fetuses that are severely affected die in utero or in early infancy, but milder cases manifest themselves later at various ages of childhood. Not all recessively inherited forms are severe and lethal.

Hanhart[2] distinguished four types:

1. Simple dominant type limited to osteosclerosis (monophenic) and taking a mild course with good prognosis.
2. Simple dominant type beginning with osteosclerosis but complicated later with severe anemia (polyphenic).[1]
3. Simple recessive type taking a benign course.
4. Simple recessive type with early malignant course involving several organ systems (polyphenic). This form is the most striking and best-known osteopetrosis.

Intrafamilial variability has been observed repeatedly, so that the borderlines between these types are not distinct.[6]

Males and females are affected by osteopetrosis equally. The disease has been observed in Caucasians, Negroes and Japanese. Concordance has been reported in monozygotic twins.[9,10]

A severe hereditary osteopetrosis in rabbits has been discovered and thoroughly studied by Pearce and Brown,[11] who found the anomaly to be congenital and invariably fatal within a few weeks after birth; it is due to a simple recessive factor, affected individuals being homozygous. The condition shows a remarkable resemblance to the severe form that occurs in infants and children.

Although typical cases of osteopetrosis are genetically determined, it should be remembered that a general sclerosis of the bones can be caused by external toxic factors. Therefore, it is necessary to be cautious in the interpretation of sporadic and atypical forms. Chronic fluoride intoxication may result in a generalized density of the bones. Fluoride may be ingested by workers who handle cryolite, which is used in Scandinavia and Canada in the production of aluminum and alum. In the United States, phosphate rock, which contains about 4% fluorine, is incorporated into fertilizers, and bone changes have been found in workers who are in daily contact with these materials.[12] This leads to an increase in bone density without alteration of normal bone structure. The calcifications extend into the ligaments. Fluoride also may be ingested through vegetables and fruits that have been fertilized or sprayed with insecticides containing large amounts of this chemical. Fluoride osteosclerosis from drinking water was reported by Linsman and McMurray[13] in a patient who had lived in areas in which the fluoride content of the water was as high as 4.4 to 12 parts per million. Similar changes have been described in reports from North Africa, India and Argentina. But the use of drinking water containing less than 3 parts per million does not cause sclerosis of the skeleton.[14] Other toxic substances, such as vitamin D in excess,[15] elementary phosphorus, lead and bismuth, may produce increased density of the metaphyseal ends of the long bones. Selye[16] produced increased density in the metaphyses of the long bones and fibrosis of the bone marrow in rats by long-continued administration of large amounts of parathormone. Injections of large doses of estrogen result in overmineralization of the skeleton and in obliteration of the marrow cavities in young rats, in mice and in birds.[17] A transmissible and filterable agent that produces osteopetrosis and lymphoid tumors in chicks has been described, the agent being present in the blood, bone marrow and neoplastic tissue but not in diseased bone.[18]

In osteopetrosis, the cortex and spongiosa of the bones are increased in thickness and density, whereas the bone marrow spaces are reduced in volume. The bones are heavy, hard, not flexible and easily fractured but difficult to cut. The longitudinal growth of the tubular bones usually is retarded. In well-developed cases, the ends of the bones are broad and club shaped, particularly near the distal epiphysis of the femur and the proximal epiphysis of the tibia. If these ends are cut, a transverse striation can be recognized consisting of bands of densely packed trabeculae and bands of decreased density in which bone marrow may be found.[19] The compacta is thickened and the spongiosa is so dense that it looks like compact bone. The Haversian systems are irregularly arranged and small; they are present only in the shaft of the long bones, whereas the structure of the short and small bones is so distorted that the Haversian systems cannot be recognized.[20] A striking anomaly is the persistence of cartilage in areas from which it is removed in the course of normal ossification. Large amounts of cartilaginous ground substance, mostly calcified, can be seen in the metaphyses, but even the diaphyses contain many trabeculae and islands of undestroyed cartilage. Osteoid and bone are found in the form of borders on the cartilaginous ground substance. Osteoblasts occur in normal numbers but osteoclasts are scarce. There is, obviously, faulty resorption of the cartilaginous ground substance and of the primary osseous trabeculae; secondary trabeculae are not formed.[20,21] The endochondral ossification is thus arrested in a primitive state throughout the bone. The marrow spaces are reduced in volume and filled with fibrous tissue or with varying amounts of functioning or even hyperactive marrow. In the newborn with osteopetrosis, the normal bone marrow is replaced by large polygonal cells that have homogeneous protoplasm and large elongated nuclei. These cells have processes that touch one another, so that a reticular tissue is formed.[22]

The trabeculae in the bones of the skull are densely packed but a diploë is not recognizable. The foramina of the cranial nerves and the blood vessels that pass through the skull often are constricted by an overgrowth of bone.

A sagittal section through a vertebra shows, at the anterior and posterior side, large triangular wedges "directed with the points to each other and to the center of the vertebral body."[22] On the superior and inferior surface of the vertebrae, ossification proceeds toward the center of the body but the cartilaginous ground substance persists. The bony lamellae are coarse and thick and the marrow space is reduced in volume. The changes in the vertebrae are also attributed to disturbed endochondral ossification. However important the lack of resorption of cartilage may be in the pathogenesis of osteopetrosis, it cannot be the essential disturbance, since bones of membranous origin are affected also. The transverse bands at the growing ends of the long bones have been interpreted as an indication of an intermittent disease process that is subject to exacerbations and remissions.[21,23] There is a high incidence of rickets among children with osteopetrosis. Although the rachitic process responds to vitamin D, one is left with the impression that osteopetrosis predisposes to rickets. Sometimes rickets develops very early[23] and shows relative refractoriness to antirachitic treatment.[24] Ossification of the epiphyseal centers occurs within normal time limits but, in several cases, closure of the epiphyseal clefts was found to be delayed.

Hydrocephaly or enlargement of the head has been reported, particularly in young children. It can be explained best by the constriction of the foramina, through which the venous blood leaves the skull cavity, and by the resulting increase in venous pressure.[23] In several patients, subdural hematomas were present.

According to Zawisch,[25] manifestations of severe osteopetrosis date back to the "second period" of fetal bone development, which begins at about the fourteenth week of gestation. From that time on, the differentiation of bone is retarded. Resorption is arrested and, as a result, the fetal size and shape of the marrow cavity persist; a thick cortex composed of all embryonic strata and an unusual amount of spongiosa are preserved. The clubbing of the ends of long bones is the result of hyperplasia and persistence of less-differentiated types of bone tissue in the metaphyses. The descriptions of the osseous changes of osteopetrosis refer to severe cases, which usually become the object of histologic examination. One must not assume that in mild cases identical pathologic findings are obtained. Early biopsy specimens may differ greatly from the findings described above.[26]

Hepatosplenomegaly is present in many cases and the lymph nodes may be enlarged. These organs usually show diffuse fibrosis, but signs of extramedullary hemopoiesis have been described. In most cases, the endocrine glands were normal.

The most severe cases of osteopetrosis result in death before or soon after birth. The disorder has been diagnosed roentgenologically in utero by Jenkinson *et al.*[8] Roentgenograms revealed that the bones were dense and had twice the normal thickness. Calcifications were seen in the kidneys. The diagnosis was confirmed when the macerated fetus was delivered after 6 months of gestation. There were radiating spicules in the occipital, parietal and frontal bones. The long bones showed a fine mottling and there was no periosteal thickening.

Osteopetrosis rarely is recognized in the newborn period, but van Creveld and Heybroek[22] described an infant with congenital osteopetrosis who died on the ninth day of life of purulent meningitis. The thorax appeared stiff and immovable; respiration was frequent and of the abdominal type. The face was edematous and cyanotic. The anterior fontanelle was small. The liver could be felt two fingers below the costal margin and the spleen was just palpable. X-ray examination performed because of enlargement of the heart revealed an extraordinary density of the skeleton. Vertebrae, ribs, the proximal end of the clavicle and the pelvis showed a diffuse sclerosis. The base of the skull was very dense but the sella turcica was normal and there was no optic atrophy. The long bones were incompletely sclerosed and the structure of the spongiosa was recognizable. The metaphyseal parts were not broadened and there were no bands of alternating density. On the second day of life, anemia was absent but there was erythroblastosis and thrombopenia; many myelocytes and immature leukocytes were found.

In older infants, in children and in adults, the diagnosis of osteopetrosis usually is made by x-rays, but many of the severe cases described present a clinical picture that suggests the correct diagnosis. The patients are small, of slender body build and underweight. The head is large and frontal and parietal bossae are more or less pronounced (Fig. 93-1). Closure of the anterior fontanelle is delayed. The teeth erupt late and decay early. Sometimes a moderate degree of exophthalmos is present. Blindness may be congenital or develop later, the defective vision being indicated by searching movements of the eyes, nystagmus and sometimes by strabismus. The ophthalmoscope reveals optic atrophy. Deafness develops in some of the patients. Facial palsy and extraocular paralysis occur occasionally. The chest often shows pigeon-breast deformity and respiration may be impaired. In many cases, the liver, spleen and lymph glands are enlarged. The development of secondary sex characteristics is delayed. The extremities appear normal or enlargement of the metaphyseal ends is palpable or visible. Bowing, coxa vara and genu valgum can be attributed to fractures[26] or to rickets. The mentality is not necessarily affected by the disorder.

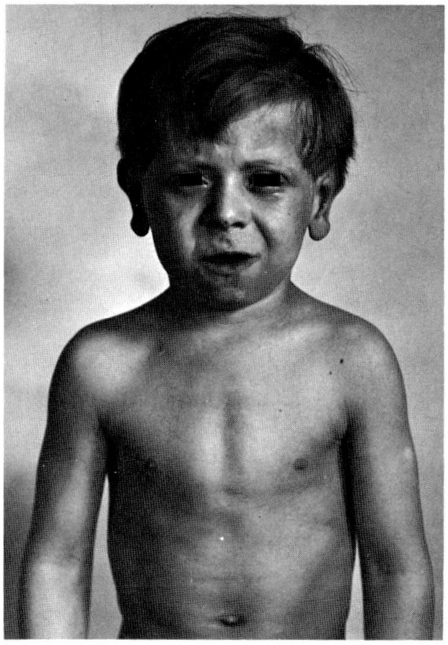

Fig. 93-1.—Osteopetrosis, showing large head and receding mandible (after osteomyelitis).

Anemia frequently is present but its degree is variable and there is no definite correlation between its severity and the sclerosis of the bones. It seems that the anemia is an associated symptom of osteopetrosis but not the result of marrow replacement by bone. The anemia, which may be hypo-, normo- or hyperchromic, reaches severe degrees in the final stage of the disease. Erythroblastosis, anisocytosis and poikilocytosis may be present. Leukocytosis and immature cells of the myeloid series appear in the peripheral blood. Thrombocytopenia and hemorrhagic manifestations occur in advanced cases.[23] Gamsu *et al.*[27] reported hemolytic anemia in 2 siblings with the severe form of the disease. They were surprised by the fact that anemia was absent at birth and suggested that some humoral factor present in the maternal blood had prevented anemia in utero.

The calcium and phosphorus values of the blood are not uniform. Hypercalcemia has been reported in several patients, but it is doubtful that they had true marble bone disease. Metabolic studies have contributed little to the understanding of the pathologic process. It is not surprising that the results have not been uniform, since the patients differed in age, complications and types of the disorder.

Several pathologic conditions have been found associated with osteopetrosis sufficiently often to indicate that they are caused in part by a predisposing factor inherent in marble bones. *Rickets* in a severe form and at an unusually early age was observed repeatedly.[5,23,24,28] It seems that an increased demand for vitamin D exists in these patients, as only intensive antirachitic treatment results in healing. *Subdural hematoma* can occur in children with marble bones. Whether the enlargement of the head is due to such hemorrhages, to rickets or to compression of the veins in the narrowed jugular foramina remains to be decided. Association with port-wine nevus, undescended testes and mental retardation has been reported.[29] Among the complications of osteopetrosis, *fractures* are of importance, since sometimes they are the first manifestation of the disease and roentgenograms taken on their account reveal the general skeletal disorder. In other cases, fractures may go unnoticed and be discovered accidentally after they are healed. Sometimes callus is formed in a satisfactory manner and in great abundance, but occasionally healing is delayed.[26] Complication by osteomyelitis has been observed repeatedly. Before antibiotics were available, osteomyelitis of the mandible was frequent; the maxilla, the scapula and the bones of the extremities also were affected occasionally. Osteogenic *sarcoma* in a femur complicated a case reported by Kerr.[30] The patient was a Negro, 20 years of age, whose father had had an unusually large head. The patient's skull was not only dense in its basal parts but the calvarium was thickened also. There were signs of healed rickets. *Hodgkin disease* in a 41-year-old white male was described by Herscher and Stein.[31] The bones of this patient showed increased density but no transverse bands.

Many cases of osteopetrosis deviate from the syndrome typified by the patient of Albers-Schönberg.[1] Higinbotham and Alexander[32] described a family in which 4 children were affected, and in 3 of them enlargement of the mandible was the main disturbance. The marked prognathism resulted in malocclusion and irregularities of the teeth. The forehead was prominent and there was syndactyly of the fingers and toes. The nails were irregularly formed or entirely missing. The fourth child had similar symptoms but, in addition, had failing vision and hearing. Roentgenograms revealed that in all 4 siblings the entire skeleton was markedly sclerosed. This variant of osteopetrosis associated with syndactyly has been observed in several families in which it probably is inherited as a recessive trait. Absence of nails, atrophy of distal phalanges and thickening of the bones of the head producing a mild degree of leontiasis ossea are characteristic of this syndrome.[33]

A benign type of osteopetrosis sometimes occurs in several generations of a family as a dominantly inherited trait. The cases of Harnapp[28] belong in this group. In a girl, 4½ years of age, roentgenograms showed osteopetrosis of the bones of the chest, vertebral column and skull. The bones of the extremities, however, differed from those seen in the malignant form of osteopetrosis. Sclerosis was found in the proximal parts of the long bones only, the distal ends having normal structure without thickening of the cortex. There was slight broadening of the ends of the humerus and of the femur but transverse bands were absent. The girl's father, a man of athletic body build, appeared entirely normal, with the exception of prominent frontal and occipital bossae and a slight lateral compression of the thorax. Roentgenograms revealed osteosclerosis of the skeleton similar to that of the daughter. The skull showed extreme density, not only of the base but also of the bones of the calvarium. Two brothers and 2 sisters of the patient had similar sclerotic changes of the skeleton, although the intensity of the process varied. None of the affected members of this family was disturbed by the skeletal changes. There were no fractures, no visual impairment and no anemia. Signs of rickets were found in all the children, including those who were free of osteopetrosis. In this family, the roentgenograms had little resemblance to those of patients with the severe form, but in another pedigree with dominant inheritance[34] the roentgenograms of the skeleton resembled those of patients with severe osteopetrosis. Some of the affected individuals showed typical changes of the skull, trunk and long bones. Osseous fragility was marked in some of these patients but all were free of anemia. Osteopetrosis with signs of cleidocranial dysostosis and other distinguishing features has become known as pyknodysostosis (p. 869). Familial occurrence of osteosclerosis, osseous cysts, progressive lipodystrophy and mental deficiency has been reported.[35] An osteopetrosis characterized by a central band-like sclerosis in the vertebral bodies can be inherited as an autosomal dominant trait.[36,37]

Roentgenograms of the bones in typical osteopetrosis show increased density and lack of normal structure. The shadow of the marrow space is reduced or absent. In addition, there are changes in the general shape of the long bones, which have club-like thickening at the metaphyseal ends (Fig. 93-2, *D*). There, transverse bands of varying density are seen that give the bone a characteristic appearance. Curved or circular bands of a similar type occur in the scapula (Fig. 93-2, *B*) and in the pelvic (Fig. 93-2, *C*), carpal and tarsal bones. The base of the skull is markedly thickened and dense (Fig. 93-2, *A*). The pituitary fossa often is reduced in size by the massive development of the posterior clinoid processes, and narrowing of the optic foramina can be demonstrated. The vertebrae show sclerosis near the upper and lower surfaces of the bodies or they are homogeneously dense. The chalky and dense appearance of the ribs found on a routine chest film sometimes betrays the disor-

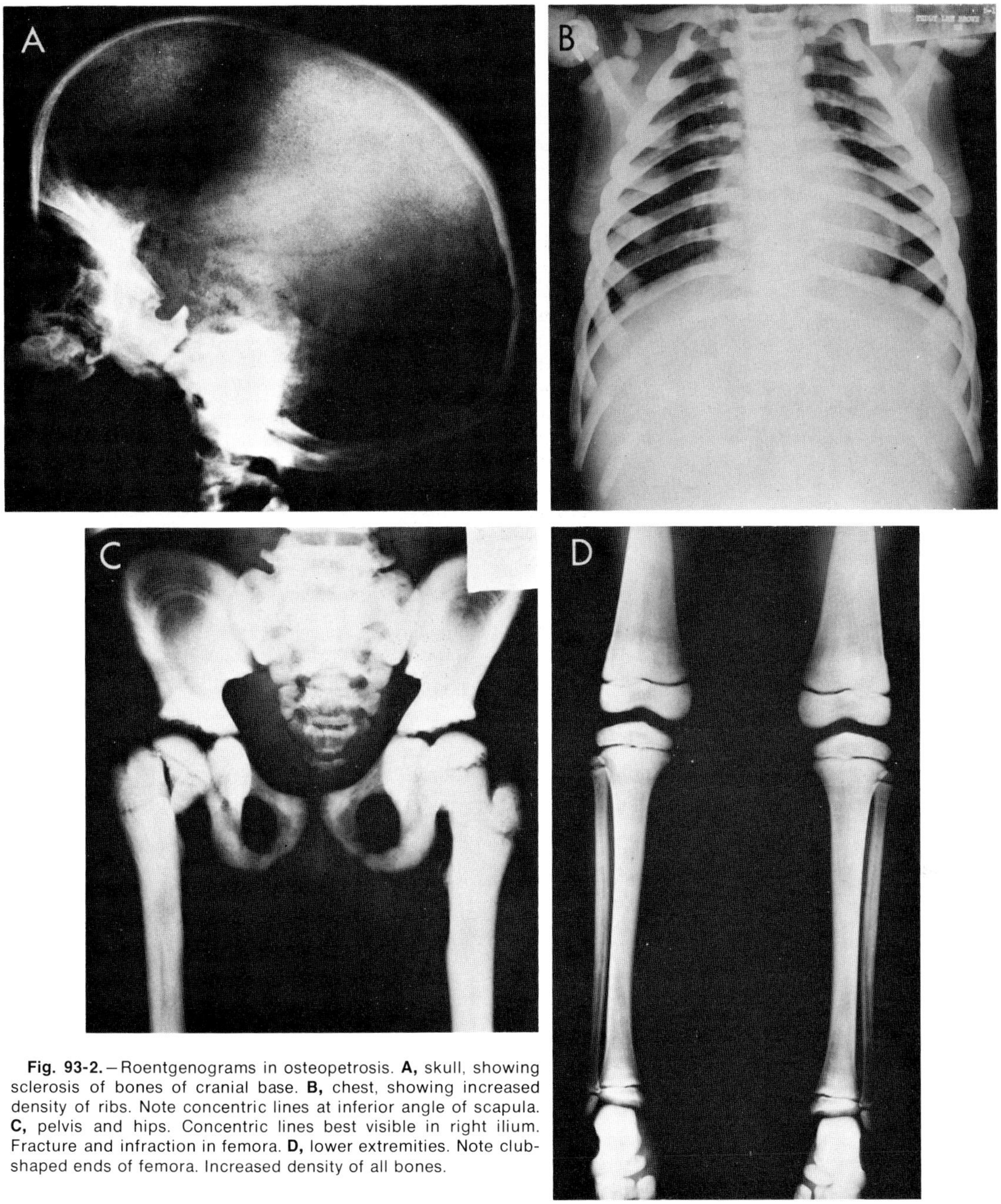

Fig. 93-2.—Roentgenograms in osteopetrosis. **A,** skull, showing sclerosis of bones of cranial base. **B,** chest, showing increased density of ribs. Note concentric lines at inferior angle of scapula. **C,** pelvis and hips. Concentric lines best visible in right ilium. Fracture and infraction in femora. **D,** lower extremities. Note club-shaped ends of femora. Increased density of all bones.

der. Caution should be exercised in the interpretation of general density of the skeleton in the newborn period. The long bones of premature and newborn infants often have a thickened cortex and a more abundant spongiosa, which results in the appearance of osteosclerosis. This osteosclerosis of the newborn is not pathologic and disappears within the first few weeks of postnatal life.[38]

The differential diagnosis of the benign form of osteopetrosis from other osteosclerotic disorders sometimes is difficult. The slowly progressing form, which begins with bands of sclerosis at the ends of the long bones, resembles skeletal changes seen in poisoning with lead, bismuth and phosphorus. In fluorine poisoning, sclerosis is found in all bones but it is most conspicuous in the pelvis, vertebral column, ribs and sternum. In the bones of the extremities, sclerosis develops later and the increased density narrows the marrow space to a certain degree without obliterating it. The cranium is little affected and the clinoid processes are not thickened. In contrast to osteopetrosis, calcification of muscular and ligamentous attachments is found.[39] There are cases reported as "marble bones," which show calcification of soft tissues in addition to increased density of the bones, but they should not be confounded with the well-established syndrome of Albers-Schönberg.[1]

Osteosclerosis of the metaphyseal ends and of the cortex of the long bones and osteosclerosis of the skull occur in a rare syndrome that is characterized by signs of renal insufficiency and hypercalcemia. Dwarfism, mental retardation, craniostenosis and congenital cardiovascular anomalies (p. 578) are additional findings that should permit a clear differentiation from marble bone disease.[40,41] Partial osteosclerosis can occur in cases of infantile myxedema[42] and in chronic renal disease.[43] Pyknodysostosis is discussed on page 869. In Camurati-Engelmann disease (osteopathia hyperostotica sclerotisans) (p. 844), the diaphyses show fusiform enlargement and cortical thickening but the metaphyses and epiphyses are not sclerosed. The localization of the sclerosis, therefore, is very different from that of marble bone disease, which makes differentiation easily possible. In Pyle disease (p. 870), the ends of the shafts are expanded as in osteopetrosis, but they show reduced density rather than sclerosis.

Patients who have generalized osteopetrosis in infancy and early childhood suffer, as a rule, from multiple fractures, blindness, deafness, anemia and osteomyelitis. Their life expectancy is short, since they are endangered by intercurrent infections. Since an early diagnosis is made in such children because of their complications, it is not impossible that osteopetrosis may be present for some time without clinical symptoms, remaining undiagnosed without roentgenography. The patient of Albers-Schönberg,[1] first described when he was 24 years of age, led an active life. He lived to the age of 49 years without impairment of his intellectual capacity but he developed severe anemia and osteomyelitis of the jaw. Osteopetrosis sometimes is lethal before or soon after birth; it sometimes is compatible with life but interferes severely with the well-being of the patient; and, in some cases, manifestations may be absent for several decades. In the same family, patients with frequent fractures and other complications may alternate with affected members who are unaware of their skeletal anomaly.

There is no satisfactory treatment for the severe form of Albers-Schönberg disease. The treatment of manifestations is symptomatic. As a rule, fractures show a good tendency to callus formation and should be treated to restore normal function. Sometimes, however, fractures show little tendency to heal and deformities develop despite adequate treatment. Blood transfusions are helpful in anemia. Antibiotics should be used in combating osteomyelitic complications and other infections. No treatment is available for the blindness and deafness brought about by constriction of the foramina of the base of the skull.

REFERENCES

1. Albers-Schönberg, H. E.: Röntgenbilder einer seltenen Knochenerkrankung, München. med. Wchnschr. 51:365, 1904.
2. Hanhart, E.: Über die Genetik der einfach-rezessiven Formen der Marmorknochenkrankheit und zwei entsprechende Stammbäume aus der Schweiz, Helvet. paediat. acta 3:113, 1948.
3. Cocchi, U.: Hereditary Diseases with Bone Changes, in Schinz, H. R., Baensch, W. E., Friedl, E., and Uehlinger, E. (eds.), *Roentgen-Diagnostics* (1st American ed.; New York: Grune & Stratton, Inc., 1951).
4. Schachenmann, G.: Über die früh-infantile, maligne Form der Marmorknochenkrankheit mit einfach-rezessivem Erbgang, Helvet. paediat. acta 3:126, 1948.
5. Nussey, A. M.: Osteopetrosis, Arch. Dis. Childhood 13: 161, 1938.
6. Cocchi, U.: Krankheiten des Skeletsystems, in Becker, P. E. (ed.), *Humangenetik* (Stuttgart: Georg Thieme, 1964), Vol. II.
7. Ruffenstuhl, G.: Über einen Fall von angeborener Osteosklerose Albers-Schönberg, Beitr. path. Anat. 114:89, 1954.
8. Jenkinson, E. L., Pfisterer, W. H., Latteier, K. K., and Martin, M. E.: Prenatal diagnosis of osteopetrosis, Am. J. Roentgenol. 49:455, 1943.
9. Hesseling: Cited by Cocchi, U.[6]
10. Zetterström, R.: Osteopetrosis (marble bone disease), Ann. paediat. (supp.) 3:488, 1957.
11. Pearce, L., and Brown, W. H.: Hereditary osteopetrosis of the rabbit. I. General factors and course of disease: General aspects, J. Exper. Med. 88:579, 1948.
12. Bishop, P. A.: Bone changes in chronic fluorine intoxication, Am. J. Roentgenol. 35:577, 1936.
13. Linsman, J. F., and McMurray, C. A.: Fluoride osteosclerosis from drinking water, Radiology 40:474, 1943.
14. Hodges, P. C., Fareed, O. J., Ruggy, G., and Chudnoff, J. S.: Skeletal sclerosis in chronic sodium fluoride poisoning, J.A.M.A. 117:1938, 1941.
15. DeWind, L. T.: Hypervitaminosis D with osteosclerosis, Arch. Dis. Childhood 36:373, 1961.
16. Selye, H.: On the stimulation of new bone-formation with parathyroid extract and irradiated ergosterol, Endocrinology 16:547, 1932.
17. Gardner, W. U., and Pfeiffer, C. A.: Inhibition of estrogenic effects on the skeleton by testosterone injections, Proc. Soc. Exper. Biol. & Med. 38:599, 1938.
18. Jungherr, E., and Landauer, W.: Studies on fowl paralysis. III. A condition resembling osteopetrosis (marble bone) in the common fowl, Bull. Connecticut State College 222, February, 1938.
19. Clifton, W. M., and Frank, A.: Osteopetrosis, in Brennemann, J. (ed.), *Practice of Pediatrics* (Hagerstown, Md.: W. F. Prior Company, 1948), Vol. 4, Chap. 23.
20. Laubmann, W.: Über die Knochenstruktur bei Marmorknochenkrankheit, Virchows Arch. path. Anat. 296:343, 1935.
21. Engfeldt, B., Fajers, C-M., Lodin, H., and Pehrson, M.: Studies on osteopetrosis. III. Roentgenological and pathologic-anatomical investigations on some of the bone changes, Acta paediat. 49:391, 1960.
22. van Creveld, S., and Heybroek, N. I.: On Albers-Schönberg's disease (marble bones), Acta paediat. 27:462, 1940.
23. McCune, D. J., and Bradley, C.: Osteopetrosis in an infant, Am. J. Dis. Child. 48:949, 1934.
24. Kramer, B., and Halpert, B.: Marble bones, Am. J. Dis. Child. 57:795, 1939.

25. Zawisch, C.: Marble bone disease; a study of osteogenesis, Arch. Path. 43:55, 1947.
26. Kneal, E., and Sante, L. R.: Osteopetrosis (marble bones); report of a case with special reference to early roentgenologic and pathologic findings, A.M.A. Am. J. Dis. Child. 81:693, 1951.
27. Gamsu, H., Lorber, J., and Rendle-Short, J.: Haemolytic anaemia in osteopetrosis; report of two cases, Arch. Dis. Childhood 36:494, 1961.
28. Harnapp, G. O.: Zum Bilde der Marmorknochenkrankheit, Monatsschr. Kinderh. 69:1, 1937.
29. Wortis, H.: Osteopetrosis (marble bones), Am. J. Dis. Child. 52:1148, 1936.
30. Kerr, H. D.: A case of osteopetrosis (marble bones) complicated by osteogenic sarcoma, Am. J. Roentgenol. 35: 212, 1936.
31. Herscher, H., and Stein, J. J.: Osteopetrosis associated with Hodgkin's disease, Am. J. Roentgenol. 43:74, 1940.
32. Higinbotham, N. L., and Alexander, S. F.: Osteopetrosis; four cases in one family, Am. J. Surg. 53:444, 1941.
33. Truswell, A. S.: Osteopetrosis with syndactyly: A morphological variant of Albers-Schönberg's disease, J. Bone & Joint Surg. 40-B:209, 1958.
34. McPeak, C. N.: Osteopetrosis. Report of 8 cases occurring in 3 generations of one family, Am. J. Roentgenol. 36:816, 1936.
35. van Leeuwen, H. C.: Über familiäres Vorkommen von Lipodystrophia progressiva zusammen mit Otosklerose, Knochenzysten und geistiger Debilität, Ztschr. klin. Med. 123:534, 1933.
36. Sossai, M., and Mignoli, E.: Cited by Cocchi, U.[6]
37. Bonomini, B.: Osteosclerosi generalizzata familiare benigna di tipo nuovo, Radiol. med. 40:273, 1954.
38. Caffey, J.: *Pediatric X-ray Diagnosis* (5th ed.; Chicago: Year Book Medical Publishers, Inc., 1967).
39. Roholm, K.: *Fluorine Intoxication* (London: H. K. Lewis & Company, Ltd., 1937).
40. Fanconi, G., and Girardet, P.: Chronische Hypercalcämie, kombiniert mit Osteosklerose, Hyperazotämie, Minderwuchs und kongenitalen Missbildungen (Zürcher Fall), Helvet. paediat. acta 7:314, 1952.
41. Schlesinger, B., Butler, N., and Black, J.: Chronische Hypercalcämie, kombiniert mit Osteosklerose, Hyperazotämie, Minderwuchs und kongenitalen Missbildungen (Londoner Fall), Helvet. paediat. acta 7:335, 1952.
42. Jeune, M., and Béraud, C.: Ostéopétrose myxoedémateuse, Arch. franç. pédiat. 12:368, 1955.
43. Wolf, H. L., and Denko, J. V.: Osteosclerosis in chronic renal disease, Am. J. M. Sc. 235:33, 1958.

Pyknodysostosis

(Osteopetrosis Acro-osteolytica, etc.)

WHEN THIS FORM of osteopetrosis was named a new disease picture by Andrén *et al.*[1] and Maroteaux and Lamy[2] in 1962, a number of cases already had been recorded under different names. The term "pyknodysostosis," being the most melodious, remained victorious. Patients with this skeletal disorder are characterized by short stature, separated cranial sutures, delayed closure of the fontanelles and hypoplasia of the terminal phalanges. A flattened mandibular angle with receding chin was seen in some patients[2] and prognathism in others.[1] In 1967, Elmore[3] reviewed 33 cases recorded in the medical literature. Sedano *et al.*[4] found 51 families with 73 cases in a review of the literature in 1968.

The disorder sometimes manifests itself by retarded growth, which is due chiefly to shortness of the limbs. The head is relatively large with frontal and occipital bossing. Because of open sutures and fontanelles, hydrocephaly may be suspected.[5] Pneumatization of the sinuses is diminished and the nasal cavities may be small.[1] Parrot-like nose is a frequent finding. Mandibular deformities and malocclusion can be present. The teeth may erupt early, show irregularities and tend to caries. Double rows of teeth in the upper and lower jaws have been observed.[5] Incomplete segmentation of the first and second cervical vertebrae has been noticed. The vertebrae have been described as concave, and "spondylolysis" of the 5th lumbar vertebra has been recorded.[4] The chest is narrow in some of the cases. The extremities are shortened. Faulty articulation and fractures contribute to this feature. The fingers and toes are short and nails spoon shaped and brittle. The joints are hyperextensible.

Roentgenograms show increased density of all bones but, in contrast to typical severe osteopetrosis, the clubbing of the long bones (failure of tubulation) and transverse striations are absent. In the skull, open sutures and fontanelles are seen long after the time of normal closure. The angle between ramus and corpus mandibulae may be obtuse. The metacarpals and metatarsals are short. The same is true of the phalanges, particularly the terminal ones. The clavicles sometimes are underdeveloped and irregular, particularly at their acromial ends.

The course of the disease is more favorable than that of severe osteopetrosis (p. 865). Compression of cranial nerves, anemia and osteomyelitis of the mandible do not develop. But patients have a strong tendency to fractures after minor traumas, chiefly affecting the lower extremities, mandible and clavicle. The bones heal well but deformity and shortening may follow, contributing to reduction in height. Mental retardation was present in approximately a fifth of the patients.[3] Progressive osteolysis of terminal phalanges was demonstrated in roentgenograms by Kajii *et al.*[6]

Both sexes are affected. The disease has been observed repeatedly in siblings and once in monozygotic twin girls.[1] Parental consanguinity was recorded in many cases.[3,4] Autosomal recessive inheritance can be assumed. The parents of these patients usually are normal but some had skeletal anomalies that were interpreted as "microforms in heterozygotes."[7] One chromosome analysis showed a normal karyotype and another a partial deletion in one G-group chromosome.[5] It was thought that the deletion may have permitted the expression of a single autosomal recessive gene located on one of the G-group chromosomes.

It has been asserted that the painter Toulouse-Lautrec suffered from pyknodysostosis.[8,9]

REFERENCES

1. Andrén, L., Dymling, J. F., Hogeman, K. E., and Wendeberg, B.: Osteopetrosis acro-osteolytica, Acta chir. scandinav. 124:496, 1962.
2. Maroteaux, P., and Lamy, M.: La Pycnodysostose, Presse méd. 70:999, 1962.
3. Elmore, S. M.: Pycnodysostosis: A review, J. Bone & Joint Surg. 49-A:153, 1967.
4. Sedano, H. D., Gorlin, R. J., and Anderson, V. E.: Pycnodysostosis. Clinical and genetic considerations, Am. J. Dis. Child. 116:70, 1968.
5. Elmore, S. M., Nance, W. E., McGee, B. J., deMontmollin, M. E., and Engel, E.: Pycnodysostosis, with a familial chromosome anomaly, Am. J. Med. 40:273, 1966.
6. Kajii, T., Homma, T., and Ohsawa, T.: Pycnodysostosis, J. Pediat. 69:131, 1966.
7. Wiedemann, H-R.: Pyknodysostose, Fortschr. Geb. Röntgenstrahlen 103:590, 1965.
8. Maroteaux, P., and Lamy, M.: The malady of Toulouse-Lautrec, J.A.M.A. 191:715, 1965.
9. Lamy, M.: L'infirmité de Toulouse-Lautrec, Presse méd. 64:249, 1956.

Pyle Disease

(Familial Metaphyseal or Craniometaphyseal Dysplasia)

THIS OSSEOUS DYSPLASIA, described in 1931 by Pyle,[1] is rare; only 35 cases had been reported in the literature by 1964.[2] Although skull changes were not stressed in early reports, many patients with this disorder show changes in the cranial skeleton. In contrast to Camurati-Engelmann disease, enlargement of the long bones is seen chiefly at the metaphyseal ends, but it has been pointed out correctly[3] that the changes involving the terminal thirds of the long bones go beyond the metaphyseal zone.

In some instances, siblings, children of normal parents, have been affected and it is thought that recessive inheritance may be responsible for the disease.[4,5] In others, a parent and some of the offspring showed the disease, so that dominant transmission must be considered possible.[2,3,6] Males and females seem to be affected equally. Gorlin *et al.*[10] confirmed that Pyle disease is a recessive trait and emphasized that it is distinguishable from craniometaphyseal dysplasia.

Some persons with typical changes in the long bones have been in good general health. They were tall and slender and had normal sitting height but elongated extremities. The bone changes were not painful, but slight deformities, such as genu valgum, directed medical attention to the underlying disorder. Limitation of extension of the elbows represented a minor handicap. The disease picture is more serious if hyperostosis of the skull is present. There may be enlargement of the head and mandible, hypertelorism, broad, flat nose and cranial nerve anomalies due to narrowing of the cranial foramina. Loss of hearing and vision, peripheral facial paralysis, overflow of tears and dental complications are among the disturbances.[3] In the case of craniometaphyseal dysplasia, the changes in the skull may be so severe that leontiasis ossea dominates the disease picture. Involvement of the skull has occurred in approximately half of the cases.[2]

The laboratory findings are not characteristic.

Roentgenograms of the extremities reveal marked widening of the ends of the shafts resembling the shape of an Erlenmeyer flask but, in contrast to osteopetrosis, the broad ends of the shafts show reduced density and thinning of the cortex. Transverse growth lines are prominent in the broad ends of the shafts. The mid-diaphyseal portion has normal width and structure. The tubular bones are longer than normal. In some cases, osteomalacia is suggested by curvatures of the bones of the lower extremities and by healed fractures.[5] The clavicles and the pelvic bones may be expanded and the vertebral bodies flat and sclerosed.[7] In the skull, hyperostosis is manifested by lack of pneumatization of the paranasal sinuses, the temporal bones and the mastoid processes. In more severe cases, hyperostosis of the cranial vault and base and of the facial bones is revealed in roentgenograms. Thickening of the mandible and encroachment on neural foramina may be visualized also.[3]

Prognosis is good in cases limited to changes in the long bones.[4] If associated with leontiasis ossea, blindness and deafness can complicate the disease picture. Fractures and osteotomy show good tendency to healing.[1,5]

An osseous disorder with roentgen pictures resembling those of Pyle disease was reported by Roy *et al.*[8] in a girl with cutaneous anomalies, progressive neurologic disturbances and mental retardation. The skin lesions ("anetoderma") were seen on the face and neck as round and depressed gray-blue plaques. Unilateral blindness and signs of pyramidal tract disorder remained unexplained.

Another craniometaphyseal disorder was described by Gorlin and Cohen[9] as "frontometaphyseal dysplasia." There is a pronounced osseous supraorbital ridge, agenesis of frontal sinuses, lack of modeling of metaphyses, iliac flare and conductive deafness.

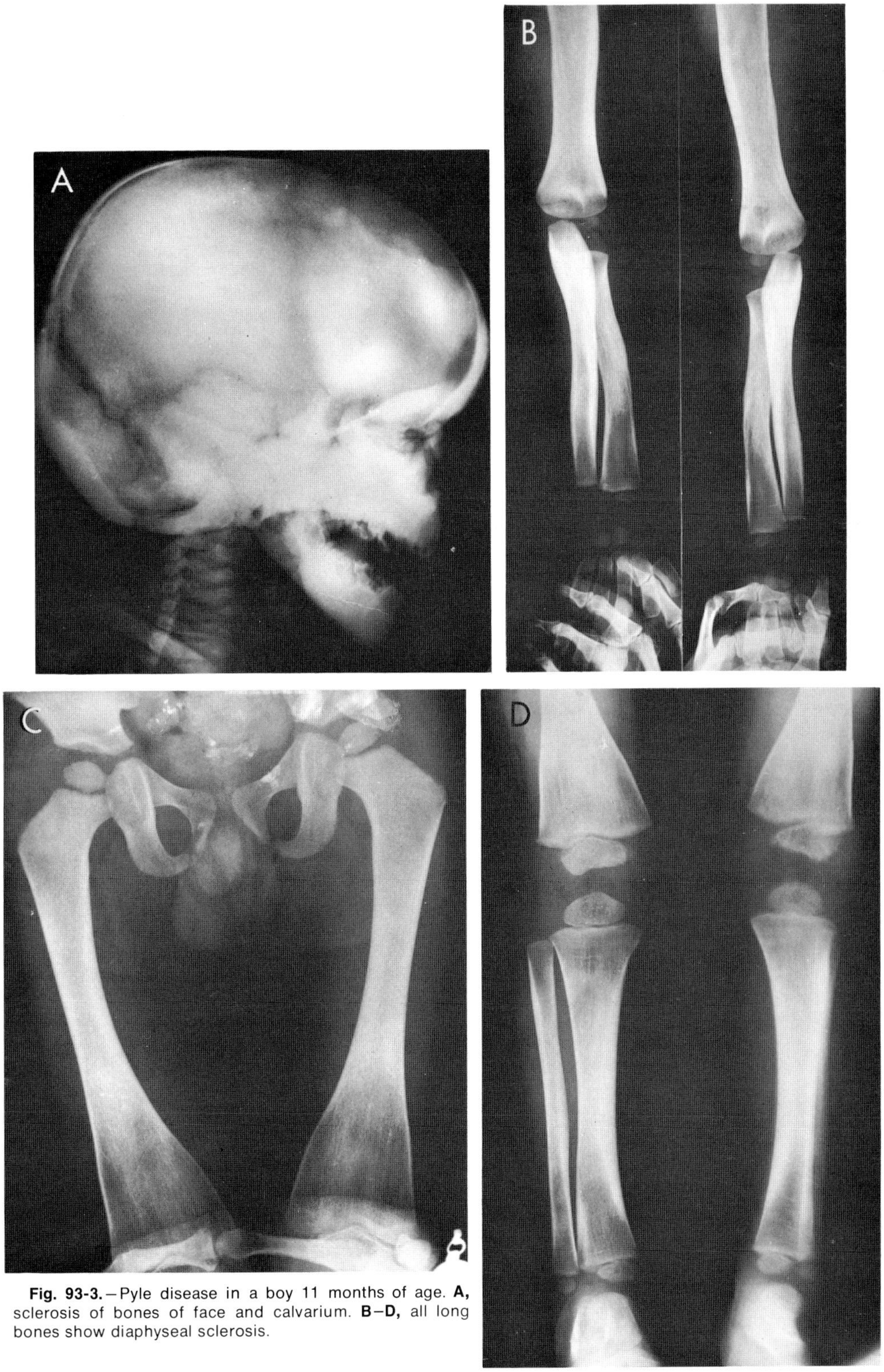

Fig. 93-3.—Pyle disease in a boy 11 months of age. **A,** sclerosis of bones of face and calvarium. **B–D,** all long bones show diaphyseal sclerosis.

REFERENCES

1. Pyle, E.: Case of unusual bone development, J. Bone & Joint Surg. 13:874, 1931.
2. Cocchi, U.: Krankheiten des Skeletsystems, in Becker, P. E. (ed.), *Humangenetik* (Stuttgart: Georg Thieme, 1964), Vol. II.
3. Mori, P. A., and Holt, J. F.: Cranial manifestations of familial metaphyseal dysplasia, Radiology 66:335, 1956.
4. Bakwin, H., and Krida, A.: Familial metaphysial dysplasia, Am. J. Dis. Child. 53:1521, 1937.
5. Hermel, M. B., Gershon-Cohen, J., and Jones, D. T.: Familial metaphyseal dysplasia, Am. J. Roentgenol. 70:413, 1953.
6. Jackson, W. P. U., Albright, F., Drewry, G., Hanelin, J., and Rubin, M. I.: Metaphyseal dysplasia, epiphyseal dysplasia, diaphyseal dysplasia, and related conditions. I. Familial metaphyseal dysplasia and craniometaphyseal dysplasia; their relation to leontiasis ossea and osteopetrosis; disorders of bone remodeling, A.M.A. Arch. Int. Med. 94:871, 1954.
7. Caffey, J.: *Pediatric X-ray Diagnosis* (5th ed.; Chicago: Year Book Medical Publishers, Inc., 1967).
8. Roy, C., Maroteaux, P., Kremp, L., Courtecuisse, V., and Alagille, D.: Un nouveau syndrome osseux avec anomalies cutanées et troubles neurologiques, Arch. franç. pédiat. 25:893, 1968.
9. Gorlin, R. J., and Cohen, M. M., Jr.: Frontometaphyseal dysplasia, Am. J. Dis. Child. 118:487, 1969.
10. Gorlin, R. J., Koszalka, M. F., and Spranger, J.: Pyle's disease (familial metaphyseal dysplasia), J. Bone & Joint Surg. 52-A:347, 1970.

94

Skeletal Disorders of Uncertain Etiology

Ollier Disease

(Dyschondroplasia)

THE DYSCHONDROPLASIA described in 1899 by Ollier[1] is a disorder of the growing areas of bone that is characterized by failure of ossification of cartilage and accumulation of cartilaginous islands in the diaphyseal ends, whereas the middle portions of the shafts remain normal. The disorder usually is unilateral or the lesions predominate strikingly on one side, whereas the other side shows only involvement of small areas. In 1935, Hunter and Wiles[2] reviewed 29 strictly unilateral and 10 almost entirely unilateral cases. They found it impracticable to make a complete list of the bilateral cases because they have been published under widely different names, sometimes as "congenital bone tumors."

There are no indications to permit one to assume that heredity plays a role in this disorder. In contrast to multiple exostoses, in which a dominant mode of inheritance can be demonstrated in the majority of cases, Ollier disease occurs sporadically and, to my knowledge, there is no record of more than 1 proved case in a family. So-called hereditary cases of dyschondroplasia are instances of multiple exostoses that have a vague resemblance to Ollier disease.

Bentzon[3] has pointed out that the fan-like pattern of the affected ends of the bones resembles the pattern seen in bone preparations in which the arteries are made visible by injection of opaque material into the nutrient vessels. He thought that vascular changes caused by a disturbance of the sympathetic nervous system may result in failure of ossification of the type seen in Ollier disease, but experiments to prove this hypothesis have failed.

The fact that several widely separated bones of one half of the body often show similar lesions whereas the bones of the other side are spared or little affected is a striking phenomenon. It has been pointed out that in many cases the entire affected side is smaller than the normal one, so that the reduction in size is not limited strictly to the parts showing dyschondroplasia. Thus, on the affected side the face was described as being smaller than on the normal side in 6 of 29

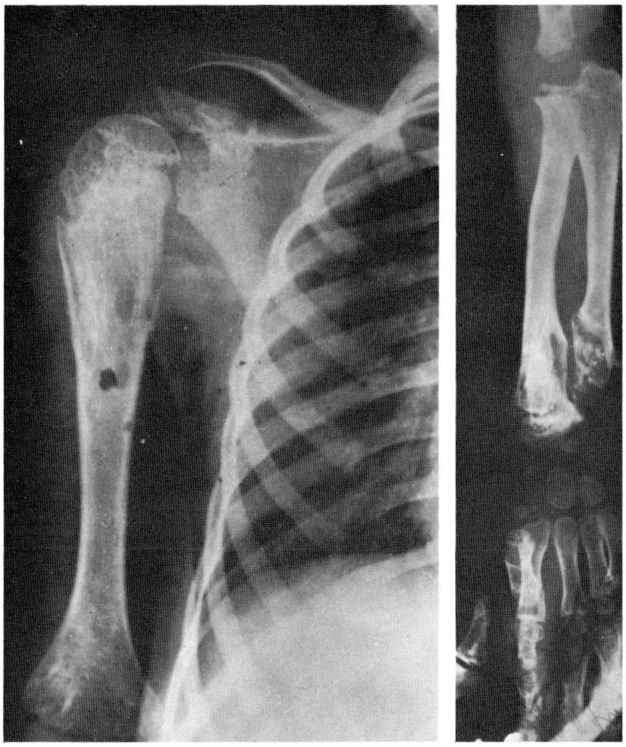

Fig. 94-1.—Ollier disease involving the right humerus, radius and ulna.

cases reviewed by Hunter and Wiles.[2] It seems that Ollier disease is related to hemiatrophy or hemihypertrophy, as shown by a patient recorded by Zellweger and Uehlinger[4] who had a unilateral "dyschondroplasia," nevus ichthyosiformis and growth disturbance. This patient had both Ollier disease and hemiatrophy.

Pathologic changes have been studied in biopsy material, and there is agreement that the rarefied areas seen in roentgenograms consist of hyaline cartilage. The cortex may contain areas of cartilage on which bone is deposited; in other places, cortical cartilage may join directly the fibrous tissue of the periosteum. The periphery of the cartilage is calcified.

Manifestations develop gradually during the early years of childhood. In the second year, it may be noticed that one limb is shorter than the other as a limp becomes apparent when the child begins to walk. By weight-bearing, bowing of an affected leg or enlargement of the diaphyseal ends may become noticeable. In many cases, the upper and lower extremities of one side are affected and the pelvic bones may be involved also. In others, only one bone or one limb is involved. But bilateral changes are compatible with the diagnosis of Ollier disease. At first, the diaphyses only are affected but, after several years, the epiphyses become involved.[2] Affected children do not appear ill and usually remain active and free from pain; occasionally, however, pain is experienced.[5] Limitation of movements of the joints may be caused by malposition of the epiphyses or by the deformities. Sometimes increased mobility is observed. As the children grow older, the difference in size of the extremities increases and scoliosis may develop. Finally, the process becomes stationary and most of the patients reach adult life without serious impairment of their health and activity. In several instances, sarcoma developed in the affected bones.

In the long bones, roentgenograms show changes at both ends, but the ends that grow faster are more affected. The lower end of the femur and the upper end of the tibia usually have an irregular fan-like pattern, the dense striations representing bone and the transparent areas cartilage. Similar striation may be seen in the ileum, whereas the other pelvic bones show round islands of cartilage. In the bones of the upper extremity, in the proximal end of the femur and in the distal end of the tibia more irregular patterns are observed. There may be larger translucent areas enclosed in bone or near the periphery adjoining the periosteum. The ends of the affected bones often assume irregular outlines and, as a result, the roentgenogram may give the impression of a destructive process rather than of a benign malformation. The striations seen in the long bones also may be found in the metacarpals, metatarsals and phalanges, but round enchondromata are observed more often in the short bones. The epiphyses usually are not affected in young children, but in older children irregular calcification and deformity of the epiphyses can be observed. Toward adolescence, the striations may disappear and give way to a mottled pattern that involves the end of the diaphysis and the epiphysis alike.

Roentgenograms make possible the diagnosis of Ollier disease, particularly if the changes are limited to bones of one side and the other side is unaffected. If a single bone is considered, a syphilitic destruction may be suspected or changes seen in leukemia are called to mind. Multiple exostoses (p. 840) are hereditary lesions that affect both sides of the skeleton.

The prognosis is good in most cases. Patients have been seen who had the disease for many years without serious handicaps.[5,6] Others suffered multiple fractures[5] or were disturbed by their deformities. If the fingers are severely involved, the hands can be crippled by chondromata. In rare instances, sarcomas developed in the affected bones.[2]

Orthopedic treatment for the correction of existing malformations and for the prevention of further deformities should be instituted as soon as the disorder is recognized. Fractures through the affected areas show a good tendency to healing. Osteotomy has been performed successfully for the correction of deformities.[2]

REFERENCES

1. Ollier, L.: De la dyschondroplasia, Bull. Soc. Chir. Lyon 3: 22, 1899.
2. Hunter, D., and Wiles, P.: Dyschondroplasia (Ollier's disease) with report of a case, Brit. J. Surg. 22:507, 1935.
3. Bentzon, P. G. K.: Ollier's disease, Acta orthop. scandinav. 19:572, 1950.
4. Zellweger, H., and Uehlinger, E.: Ein Fall von halbseitiger Knochenchondromatose (Ollier) mit Naevus ichthyosiformis, Helvet. paediat. acta 3:153, 1948.
5. Margolis, J.: Ollier's disease, A.M.A. Arch. Int. Med. 103: 279, 1959.
6. Cleveland, M., and Fielding, W.: Chondrodysplasia (Ollier's disease), J. Bone & Joint Surg. 41-A:1341, 1959.

Systemic Chondromatosis
(Enchondroma and Ecchondroma)

THIS SKELETAL ANOMALY probably is related to Ollier disease but the deformities are more severe, particularly in the hands and feet. There are cartilaginous islands within the bones or cartilage tumors develop that expand the bones beyond their normal limits. In contrast to multiple exostoses, which usually are mild in the short bones of the hands and feet, enchondromas are especially well developed in the metacarpal, metatarsal and phalangeal bones.[3] In such cases, one speaks of acroform chondromatosis. Other types have been classified as unilateral, oligotopic or polytopic types, according to extent and localization of the lesions.[1] If the enchondromas are limited to one ray, one speaks of Ollier disease. There is no pronounced tendency to inheritance of these enchondromas but, in rare cases, dominant transmission with reduced penetrance[2] has been reported.[3] In other families, siblings have been affected,[1] so that genetic prognoses should be made with caution.

In acroform chondromatosis, the hands and feet become markedly deformed by the nodes, which protrude from the fingers and toes. The tumors interfere with the use of the fingers and surgical intervention may become necessary. Enchondromas are also found in the long bones, particularly in the marrow spaces, but sometimes the surface is reached also. The vertebrae, ribs, sternum and pelvic bones also can contain cartilaginous masses in polytopic cases. The longitudinal growth of the long bones sometimes is not affected but, in severe cases, shortening of one or several limbs occurs. Fractures through enchondromas are frequent. The cartilaginous islands originate chiefly from the epiphyseal cartilage plate but chondromas may also be formed from the periosteum.

Patients with systemic chondromatosis sometimes show a tendency to formation of other tumors and malformations. The combination of chondromatosis with vascular anomalies represents a syndrome of its own, which, in severe cases, is known as Maffucci syndrome (p. 882).

REFERENCES

1. Cocchi, U.: Krankheiten des Skeletsystems, in Becker, P. E. (ed.), *Humangenetik* (Stuttgart: Georg Thieme, 1964), Vol. II.
2. Rossberg, A.: Zur Erblichkeit der Knochenchondrome, Fortschr. Geb. Röntgenstrahlen 90:138, 1959.
3. Maroteaux, P.: La metachondromatose, Ztschr. Kinderh. 109:246, 1971.

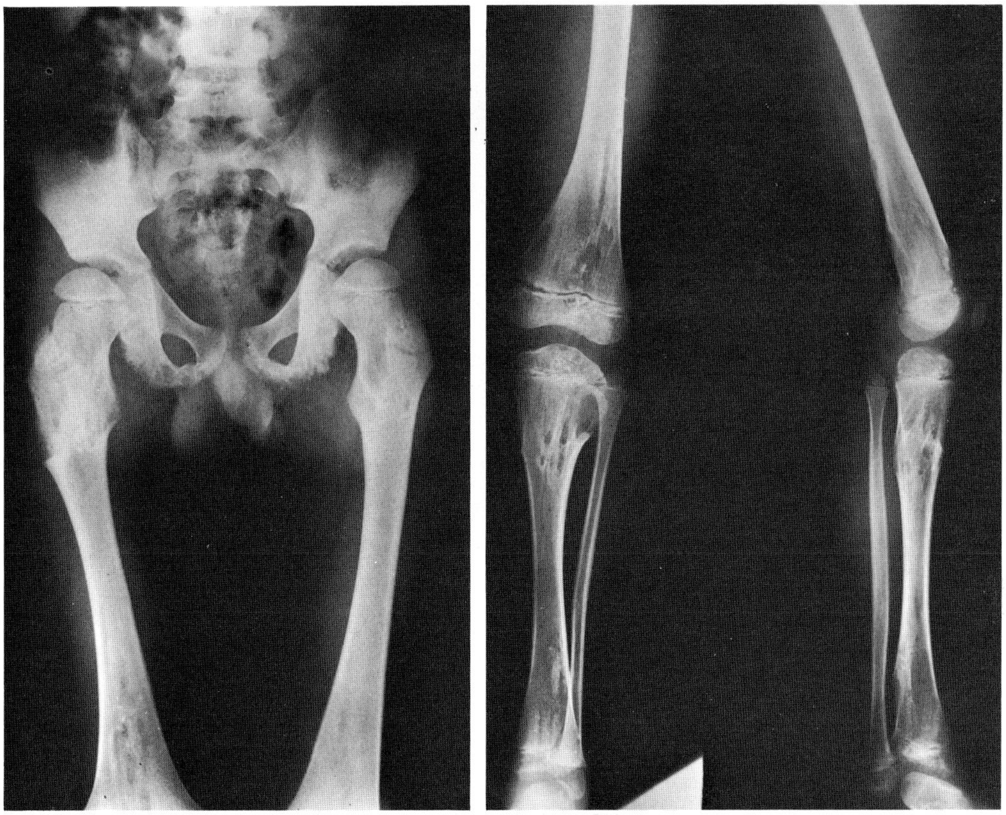

Fig. 94-2.—Generalized chondromatosis as seen in roentgenograms of pelvis and lower extremities.

Fibrous Dysplasia of Bone

Osseous fibrous dysplasia may affect one or many bones of the skeleton; as a rule, the distribution in polyostotic cases tends to be unilateral or, if both sides are involved, one side is definitely more affected than the other. Mild cases probably are not rare; polyostotic cases, which tend to be associated with other anomalies, are described more often in the literature and thus are overemphasized. Lichtenstein and Jaffe,[1] in a survey of 90 cases of fibrous dysplasia, found cutaneous pigmentation in about 35% and manifestations of endocrine disorder in about 22% of the patients. Thus, in the majority of cases, the disorder is limited to the bones.

There is no indication that fibrous dysplasia is hereditary, most of the cases being sporadic. Occasionally, café au lait spots are seen in relatives of these patients, but they probably are of no significance, since a small number of such patches occur frequently in the general population. There is no increased frequency of congenital malformations in patients with fibrous dysplasia.[2] The tendency to develop fibrous dysplasia and associated anomalies probably is due to a congenital developmental defect. Lichtenstein and Jaffe[1] considered the bone lesions as hamartomas, i.e., tumor-like malformations resulting from flaws of development and characterized by defects of tissue combination. They regarded the occurrence of cartilage in the fibrous lesions as significant and emphasized a close relationship to skeletal chondromatosis (p. 874). According to them, these two conditions "may be regarded as first cousins." Transitional cases between fibrous and cartilaginous dysplasia were found by Freund.[3] Some fibrous dysplasias of the jaws do not belong in this chapter. The "cherubism" described by Jones *et al.*[4] and considered a familial fibrous dysplasia of the jaws is inherited like a dominant trait and thus clearly differs from the condition treated in this subchapter. In cherubism, there is absence of a number of permanent teeth, which suggests that the anomaly is a developmental error. Histologically and roentgenographically, the disorder resembles giant cell tumors of the jaw bones.[5] Ossifying fibromas of the facial bones may also differ from fibrous dysplasia, although identity of the two conditions has been considered possible.[6]

The affected areas consist of white or reddish gritty tissue, which is found chiefly in the medullary cavity but may reach the surface of the bone and cause thinning and expansion of the cortex. The cortex is not completely destroyed and the periosteum is not involved at all. Histologically, fibrous connective tissue is found in place of cancellous bone and marrow. The bone surrounding the fibrous areas remains normal and free of generalized osteoporosis. In the fibrous matrix, newly formed immature trabeculae of fiber bone are found. Areas of soft, collagenous tissue or of hyaline cartilage are interspersed within the fibrous tissue and, by focal degeneration, small secondary cysts may be formed. The lesions usually are located in the diaphyses and metaphyses. In exceptional cases only are the epiphyses involved.[7] In some instances, foam cells[8] or lipoid granulomatosis[9] was present in fibrous dysplastic areas, but it is doubtful that such cases belong in this discussion.

In monostotic cases, clinical complaints are rather mild or entirely absent. Occasionally, a lesion is discovered incidentally by roentgenogram. In other cases, a local swelling, a pathologic fracture, pain or functional disturbance may lead to recognition of the disorder. The single bone affected may be a rib, clavicle, maxilla, tibia or femur. If several bones of a limb are affected, clinical complaints are more frequent, pain, dysfunction, bowing or fractures being common manifestations of the disorder. The affected bones may remain normal in contour or become expanded from within by pressure of growing fibrous tissue on the thinned cortex. Flat bones sometimes are distended into tumor-like masses, whereas long bones become curved or shortened, their width increased to several times the original thickness. As a result, affected limbs often appear deformed, particularly when subjected to weight-bearing; coxa vara and genu valgum frequently are present. In the most severe form of the disease, bones of several limbs are involved and the skull, ribs, vertebral column and pelvis show typical changes. In such cases, pigmentation of the skin, endocrine, cerebral or vascular manifestations may complicate the osseous lesions.

The serum calcium and phosphorus often are normal but phosphatase values may be elevated.

In severe cases, the first manifestations occur in childhood and rapid progress is the rule. With the termination of adolescence, the active phase of the disease usually is ended but the patients remain deformed or otherwise injured by the osseous changes. In milder cases, the first clinical signs may appear in adult life or the changes may remain completely asymptomatic.

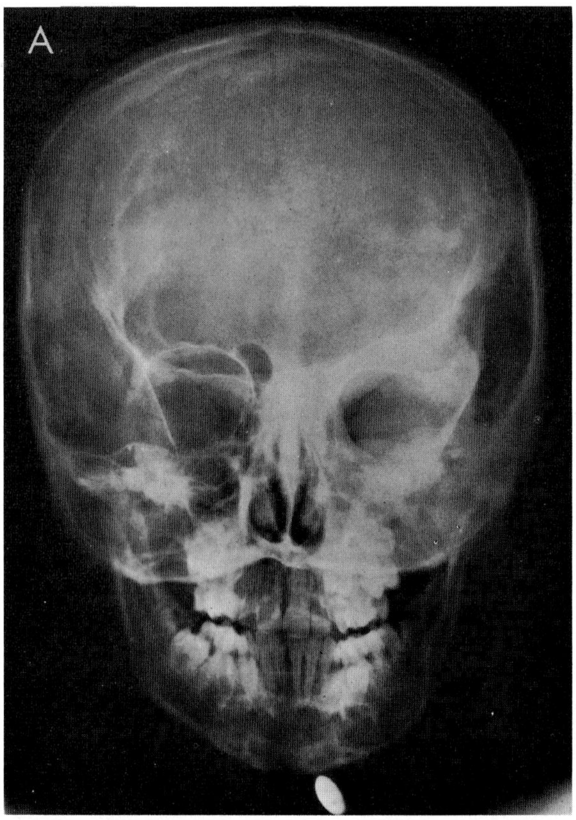

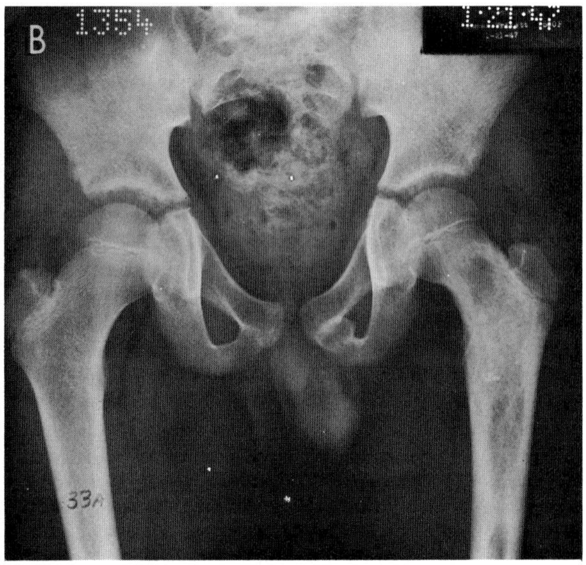

Fig. 94-3.—Fibrous dysplasia in a 13-year-old boy who complained of headaches, showed facial asymmetry and suffered a fracture of the left femur. **A,** sclerosis of bones of the left side of the face and skull. Left orbit diminished in size owing to thickening of bones composing it. The defect in the frontotemporal region is due to surgical intervention undertaken for biopsy. **B,** areas of decreased density and sclerosis in the upper portion of the shaft and neck of the left femur.

The roentgen diagnosis is not difficult in the severe forms but in monostotic cases the lesions seldom are characteristic. A round or oval area of rarefaction can be mistaken for a bone cyst and a mottled and expanded lesion for Ollier disease. If one lesion is found, examination of the entire skeleton is advisable, lest asymptomatic areas be overlooked. The individual lesions that appear as rarefactions represent areas in which bone is replaced by connective tissue. Metaplastic bone trabeculae within the connective tissue cause a mottled, stippled or ground-glass appearance in the rarefied areas.[10] The cortex is thin or entirely missing in some places. There is no periosteal reaction or apposition of bone. Cortical thickening is seen only near healed fractures. Expansion of the outline of bones occurs when the fibrous masses reach the cortex. The resulting deformities, together with those caused by fractures, lead to the grotesque appearance of the bones characteristic of the severe forms. The diaphyses and metaphyses are the usual sites of extended changes. In the differentiation between localized, monostotic fibrous dysplasia and bone cysts, it should be remembered that, in the latter, new bone formation is lacking within the area of decreased density.

Fibrous dysplasia of the skull manifests itself by asymmetry or deformity, by displacement of the eyeball and pressure on the optic nerve or by pathologic fractures of long bones. The frontal bone, sphenoid, ethmoid, maxilla, mandible and zygoma are involved most frequently. Progression takes place during the years of growth. Roentgenography and the difficult differential diagnosis were discussed by Leeds and Seaman.[11] Fibrous dysplasia limited to the face and skull must be differentiated from osteoma, fibro-osteoma, Paget, Recklinghausen and Schüller-Christian disease.[12] Facial fibrous dysplasia may result in a picture resembling leontiasis ossea. In monostotic cases involving the base of the skull exclusively, difficulties may arise in distinguishing the localized fibrous dysplasia from the osseous changes associated with a meningioma. Ocular manifestations are prominent in both disorders; but fibrous dysplasia usually occurs in young people, whereas meningioma appears later in life.[13] Neurologic symptoms may be caused by compression of cranial nerves or by involvement of the brain, which has been observed in some instances. Mental retardation, epilepsy and deafness have been described.[14]

Malignant transformation can occur. The incidence has been estimated to be 1 in 200 cases of fibrous dysplasia. Osteogenic sarcoma is the predominant histologic type and the craniofacial region the most common site.[15]

Treatment is orthopedic and depends on the disturbance caused by the individual lesion. Some solitary asymptomatic lesions are best left alone. If mechanical support is needed, curettage and packing with bone chips are recommended.[1] Good results of surgical treatment of monostotic lesions have been reported.[16] If shortening and deformities of bones have occurred, corrective shoes, braces and corsets are used. It is important to distinguish polyostotic fibrous dysplasia from hyperparathyroidism and to leave the parathyroid glands untouched.

REFERENCES

1. Lichtenstein, L., and Jaffe, H. L.: Fibrous dysplasia of bone; condition affecting one, several or many bones, graver cases of which may present abnormal pigmentation of skin, premature sexual development, hyperthyroidism or still other extraskeletal abnormalities, Arch. Path. 33:777, 1942.
2. Vines, R. H.: Polyostotic fibrous dysplasia, Arch. Dis. Childhood 27:351, 1952.
3. Freund, E.: Osteodystrophia fibrosa unilateralis; report of case, Arch. Surg. 28:849, 1934.
4. Jones, W. A., Gerrie, J., and Pritchard, J.: Cherubism—a familial fibrous dysplasia of the jaws, J. Bone & Joint Surg. 32-B:334, 1950.
5. McDonald, R. E., and Shafer, W. G.: Disseminated juvenile fibrous dysplasia of jaws, A.M.A. Am. J. Dis. Child. 89:354, 1955.
6. Georgiade, N., Masters, F., Horton, C. E., and Pickrell, K.: Ossifying fibromas (fibrous dysplasia) of facial bones in children and adolescents, J. Pediat. 46:36, 1955.
7. Pande, H.: Albright's syndrome in a four-months-old girl, Acta paediat. 48:397, 1959.
8. Denko, J. V., and Perrin, T. L.: Polyostotic fibrous dysplasia of bone, A.M.A. Arch. Path. 59:457, 1955.
9. Harriman, D. G. F., and Millar, J. H. D.: Fibrous dysplasia of bone with skeletal lipoid granulomatosis; report of case with necropsy, J. Bone & Joint Surg. 36-B:95, 1954.
10. Hoboek, A.: Polyostotic fibrous dysplasia of bone, Acta radiol. 36:145, 1951.
11. Leeds, N., and Seaman, W. B.: Fibrous dysplasia of the skull and its differential diagnosis. A clinical and roentgenographic study of 46 cases, Radiology 78:570, 1962.
12. Rosen, H., Lachman, J., and Laufer, A.: Fibrous dysplasia of bone, cranio-facial localisation, Acta oto-laryng. 42: 243, 1952.
13. Feiring, W., Feiring, E. H., and Davidoff, L. M.: Fibrous dysplasia of skull, J. Neurosurg. 8:377, 1951.
14. Wintgens, M., Roland, T., and Evrard, M.: Étude d'un cas de dysplasie fibreuse des os de la face et du crâne associée à un retard mental avec épilepsie et surdité unilatérale, Acta paediat. belg. 22:29, 1968.
15. Schwartz, D. T., and Alpert, M.: The malignant transformation of fibrous dysplasia, Am. J. M. Sc. 247:1, 1964.
16. Stewart, M. J., Gilmer, W. S., and Edmonson, A. S.: Fibrous dysplasia of bone, J. Bone & Joint Surg. 44-B:302, 1962.

Fibrous Dysplasia with Areas of Pigmentation and Endocrine Dysfunction

(Albright Disease)

IN MANY PATIENTS, polyostotic fibrous dysplasia has been found associated with areas of cutaneous pigmentation and manifestations of endocrine disturbance, so that the combination of these disorders has come to be considered a clinical entity since Albright *et al.*[1] directed attention to this syndrome. It is generally assumed that the osseous and cutaneous lesions are independent of each other but that the endocrine lesions may be the result of osseous changes at the base of the skull. In addition to the three manifestations mentioned, other anomalies have been found in association with fibrous dysplasia, so that Albright syndrome may not remain a triad. It seems that Weil,[2] in 1922, first described the syndrome of precocious puberty, pigmentation and spontaneous fractures of the bones in a 9-year-old girl. Then Gaupp,[3] in 1932, recorded 2 cases with precocious puberty and characteristic bone lesions. His second case, in addition, showed abnormal pigmentation, goiter and exophthalmos. In the same year, Freedman[4] described a comparable case, with onset of menstruation at the age of 4 months. Stalmann[5] and Goldhammer[6] made further contributions by pertinent case reports of female children, and McCune and Bruch[7] reviewed the subject, adding an observation of their own. They pointed out that the syndrome need not be limited to girls, since typical polyostotic fibrous dysplasia with pigmentations had been observed in boys before.[8]

The syndrome is not congenital but is most likely somehow determined before birth. In many cases, the pigmentations are present at birth[9] and osseous changes and endocrine symptoms are noticed frequently in infancy.[2,10,11] But cases are on record in which the first symptoms appeared after the fourth decade.[9] The patients reported often are girls who have precocious puberty, whereas those without this symptom remain unrecorded. Precocious puberty is rare in boys with fibrous dysplasia, which may explain why more females than males are included in reviews of the syndrome. Polyostotic fibrous dysplasia with cutaneous pigmentation was observed in a Negro boy by Caplan and Feingold.[12] In two instances, polyostotic fibrous dysplasia has been seen in one of a pair of dizygous twins.[13,14] A case of Caldwell and Broderick[13] is of interest because 7 siblings of the patient – including her twin sister – were normal. In the case of Dockerty *et al.*,[14] the normal twin brother weighed 8 pounds at birth, whereas the affected twin sister weighed only 4 pounds, thus demonstrating intrauterine growth retardation. At first, the patient grew faster in extrauterine life than her twin brother but she stopped growing at the age of 14, attaining a height of 4 ft. 11 in., whereas her brother continued growing to a height of 6 ft. The patient, like others with Albright syndrome, underwent normal pregnancies,[15] and in no case has such a patient born a child with similar symptoms. So far, all cases have been sporadic and there is no suggestion or proof that the syndrome is hereditary, although its multiple manifestations simulate the effects of a pleiotropic gene. Normal chromosomes in cells derived from blood lymphocytes and fibroblasts from pigmented skin have been reported.[16]

It is unlikely that the syndrome can be explained as a result of endocrine changes or of sexual precocity. Fibrous dysplasia and pigmentation are found in female patients without precocious puberty and in males with normal or delayed sex development. It seems, therefore, that one must search for a common cause of the osseous, cutaneous and endocrine changes. It has been thought that an anomaly in the hypothalamus is the central lesion for the syndrome. Although such an anomaly has been found in one case, it has not been demonstrated in others.[17,18] A xanthomatosis such as Schüller-Christian disease could explain the diverse symptoms, but cells typifying that disease are not conspicuous in fibrous dysplasia. The lesions often are unilateral and when both sides are involved there usually is a clear predominance of symptoms on one side. The segmental distribution speaks against a metabolic or hormonal causation of the disorder. In contrast to the lesions of Schüller-Christian disease, those of fibrous dysplasia are not radiosensitive. There are similarities between Albright syndrome, neurofibromatosis and tuberous sclerosis and it has been stated[18] that this suggests similar pathogenic factors in the three diseases. But in both neurofibromatosis and tuberous sclerosis dominant inheritance is well established, which is not the case in the syndromes associated with fibrous dysplasia. There remains then the explanation of an "embryologic defect" of several tissues, more pronounced on one side than on the other.[19] This explanation has much in its favor and groups the fibrous dysplasia syndromes with Ollier disease, Maffucci syndrome, hemihypertrophies and related conditions among the "hemisyndromes" (p. 162). Although this classification does not "explain" the anomalies, it distinguishes them from conditions of different etiology and pathogenesis.

The osseous lesions show replacement of fatty or cellular marrow by fibrous tissue. The cortical bone may be normal in some places and practically absent in others. In the fibrous areas, new bone is laid down by metaplasia and there is formation of fiber bone trabeculae, which are short and closely interwoven but devoid of normal lamination. The trabeculae are surrounded by osteoid zones and there are signs of marked osteoblastic activity. In contrast to hyperparathyroidism, osteoclastic resorption is not conspicuous. The fibers that replace the marrow are coarse and relatively acellular and hyaline zones are seen within the fibrous tissue. Islands of cartilage frequently are found in areas of bone replacement.[20] The changes do not resemble those of lipoid granulomatosis and are distinguishable from those of Recklinghausen neurofibromatosis by the occurrence of cartilage and new bone in fibrous areas.

Pigmented areas of the skin vary in size and location; their outlines are irregular in shape, with many extensions and recesses. The pigmentations are due to melanin deposits in the basal cells of the epidermis. Neurofibromata are absent but pigmented nevi have been observed.

The pathologic basis of the sexual precocity has not been established. In one case there was a diminution in the size of one mamillary body and an accessory nucleus was found in the adjacent tissue.[19] In another case, there was marked hyperplasia of the basophilic cells of the pituitary.[17] Since many of the patients with precocity had thickening of the base of the skull, pressure on the hypothalamus by the underlying bone has been considered a possible cause of precocious puberty and of other endocrine symptoms. The finding of congenital cerebral anomalies in some of the patients[18] makes it appear possible that primary hypothalamic changes may be responsible for the endocrine manifestations. In some instances, diffuse or nodular enlargement of the thyroid gland can be observed. In one patient[17] there was clinical evidence of hyperthyroidism; the gland was hyperplastic and the follicles were of irregular size and shape. Infolding of the epithelium and fetal adenomas were found. In another case,[18] the enlarged thyroid consisted of vesicles extended to an extreme degree and filled with colloid.

In a case with mental retardation with particularly severe involvement of the central nervous system necropsy was performed. There was a severe disorganization of the cerebral cytoarchitecture; giant neurocytes and distorted Purkinje cells were found, suggesting a prenatal deviation of cerebral development.[18] By 1966, 6 necropsies had been reported in cases of fibrous dysplasia. Moldawer and Rabin[21] published a report of a complete necropsy and reconstruction of the skeleton of a man who had polyostotic fibrous dysplasia, a small area of cutaneous pigmentation and thyrotoxicosis.

The clinical symptoms show an insidious onset during the early years of childhood. The osseous changes may progress for some time before deformities or fractures direct the attention of the parents to the disturbance. There is a tendency to limitation of bone changes to one side, or one side may be predominantly affected. Areas of fibrous dysplasia start in the marrow spaces of the diaphyses of the long bones. Roentgenograms reveal areas of rarefaction, and with the formation of fiber bone in the affected regions, the structure of the bone becomes completely altered. The cortex is thinned and the shaft becomes deformed and sometimes expanded. Fractures may be caused by minimal trauma, particularly in the upper end of the femur. Such fractures are not very painful and healing is not unduly delayed. The normal pattern of bone gradually is lost as rarefied areas alternate with patches of increased density. The fractures contribute to the deformities and coxa vara, genu valgum and kyphoscoliosis may develop. As a rule, the affected bones are shortened but in some cases elongation is observed.[15] In the skull and the bones of the face, sclerotic overgrowth predominates, usually on one side, thus making the head and face asymmetric. The nasal sinuses often are obliterated by the sclerosing process and the cranial nerves may be compressed. A picture of leontiasis ossea can result.[20] In roentgenograms, sclerosis is seen of the base of the skull, which can be changed beyond recognition. Patchy sclerotic irregularities are observed in the vault. The spine can be involved and severe changes have been observed in vertebrae, with complete collapse of the bodies.[7] Extra-skeletal symptoms usually occur only in patients with extensive osseous changes.

The pigmentations of the skin may be present at birth or develop in the first years of childhood. They are irregular in outline (in contrast to the smooth borders in neurofibromatosis), light brown, patchy, not elevated and often unilateral. The sacrum, buttocks and upper spine are sites of predilection. If the disorder is limited to one side of the body, the pigmentations usually are on the side of the bony lesions and may extend segmentally along an affected extremity.

As a rule, the blood calcium and phosphorus are normal but the serum phosphatase is elevated.[22] During active phases, the calcium values sometimes are elevated and the inorganic phosphorus depressed.[9]

The developmental changes most often noticed are skeletal and there is sexual precocity. Affected girls usually show advanced development of the centers of ossification and rapid growth. The epiphyses close early and the final stature is below normal. Precocious puberty is most marked in girls. Sometimes menstruation begins in the first year of life and often before the tenth year. Frequently it is preceded by the development of feminine secondary sex characteristics. The ovaries and the adrenals usually show no gross signs of abnormality but ovarian cysts have been observed several times.[9,11,14] Estrogen excretion in the urine may be increased.[7] When women having Albright syndrome become pregnant, gestation may progress normally; several patients of this type have given birth to normal children.[15] The menopausal age is within normal limits. Enlargement of the clitoris was noted only once.[4] Sexual precocity in males occurs occasionally,[20,23,24] but osseous precocity is frequent.[20] In several instances, sexual development was delayed in boys.[8,15,25] In a case observed by us there was marked retardation of growth, ossification and sexual development, so that the diagnosis of pituitary dwarfism had to be considered (Fig. 94-4). Gynecomastia, adiposogenital dystrophy or acromegalic features sometimes are seen in boys with fibrous dysplasia.[15,20] A boy described by Thomas *et al.*[26] is of special interest, since the bone lesions were most pronounced

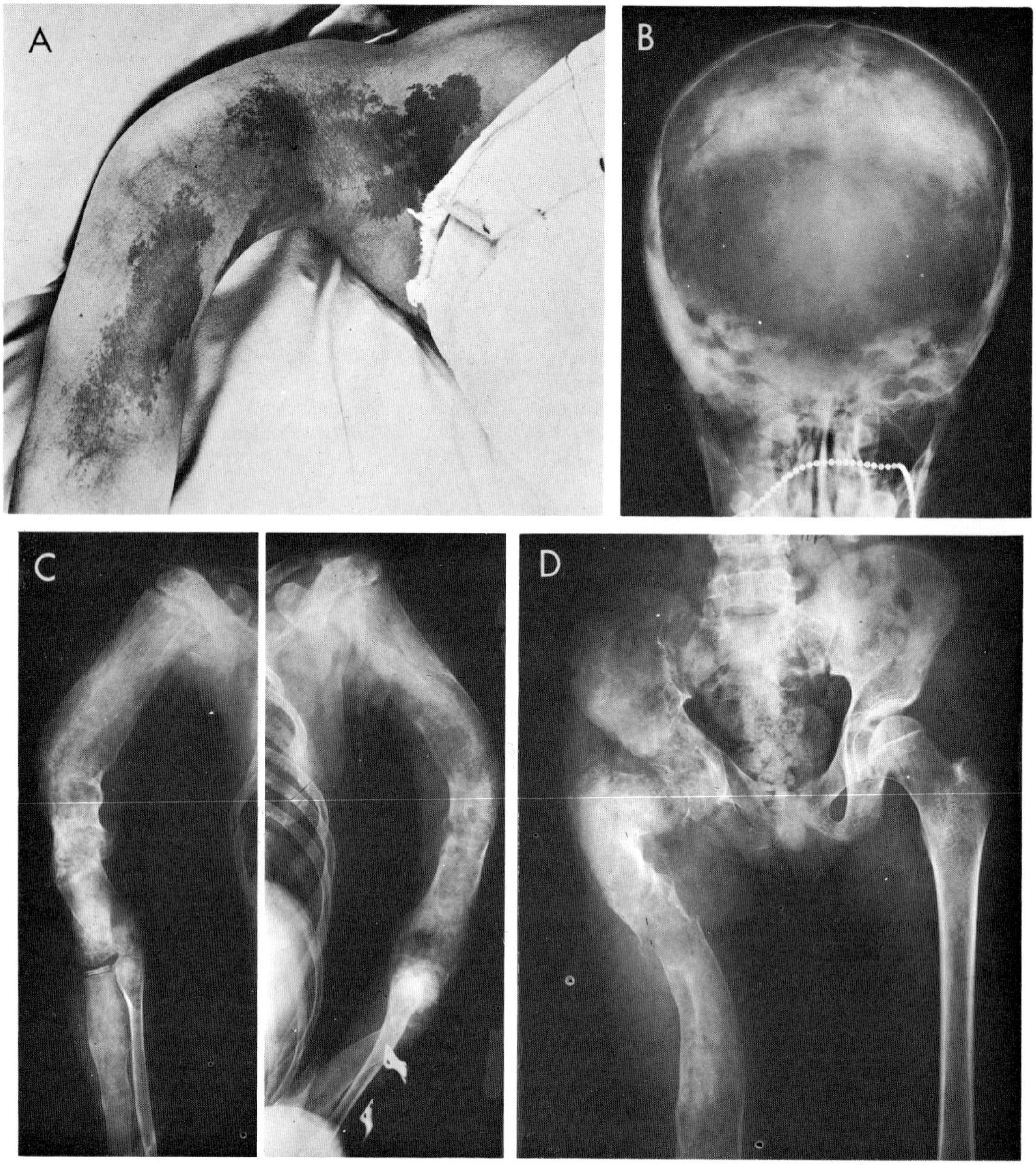

Fig. 94-4. – Polyostotic fibrous dysplasia in a 19-year-old male. His parents and 5 brothers were living and well. He had multiple deformities from previous fractures. Began limping at age 7 years, first fracture age 10. His height (54 in.) and bone development were comparable to those of a boy 10 years of age. His face was child-like and the voice high. The genitalia were infantile. Both testes were descended but small. His mental development was normal. The general impression, aside from the malformations caused by fibrous dysplasia, was that of a pituitary dwarf. **A,** pigmentation in right axilla. There also was pigmentation on right upper arm, chest, on the back and in the sacral region. **B,** roentgenogram of skull, showing thickening of bones on the right side. **C,** roentgenograms of arms, showing bilateral fibrous dysplasia. **D,** roentgenogram of pelvis and femora, showing fibrous dysplasia, predominantly on the right side.

on the right side, whereas marked gynecomastia and testicular enlargement were present on the left. Unilateral enlargement of the testis was also observed in a case of Falconer *et al.*[20] Such unilateral asymmetry cannot be well explained as being by blood-borne hormones.

Enlargement of the thyroid occurs in many patients with polyostotic fibrous dysplasia.[3,9,18,20] This deserves emphasis, since it is a feature that is present – equally unexplained – in some cases with Maffucci syndrome. Hyperthyroidism complicated the disease picture in several instances.[1,9,21,23] McIntosh *et al.*[27] found that polyostotic fibrous dysplasia may be accompanied by high-output cardiac failure. They believed that the osseous lesions of fibrous dysplasia contain functioning A-V fistulas.

Neurologic symptoms may arise through compression of cranial nerves or nerve roots by the osseous destructive processes.[20,23] Mental retardation was present in some of these patients.[13,18] Deafness[9] and visual disturbances[20] complicated some of the cases. Exophthalmos was observed repeatedly.[6,9]

Essentially, this syndrome represents a disorder of childhood and it seems that the underlying process becomes inactive after the epiphyses close. The age at onset is not related to the severity of the disease. Although the prognosis for life is good, there usually is a marked degree of disability caused by deformities and recurrent fractures. Osteogenic sarcoma is rare.[28]

Albright syndrome probably is not limited to osseous, endocrine and cutaneous changes. In a male reported by Stauffer *et al.*,[29] polyostotic fibrous dysplasia, cutaneous pigmentation and congenital arteriovenous aneurysms were combined. Occasionally, additional anomalies such as optic atrophy, hypertelorism, proptosis, deafness, anosmia and changes in sensibility are seen.[20] Whereas such symptoms may be secondary to thickening of the skull, blue sclerae,[28] palpebral coloboma, corneal anomalies,[30] coarctation of the aorta and renal atrophy[25] must be of different origin. Albright syndrome has been observed in a male with situs inversus.[31]

In the differential diagnosis, hyperparathyroidism, Ollier dyschondroplasia and Recklinghausen neurofibromatosis must be considered. In hyperparathyroidism, one finds generalized decalcification of the skeleton without signs of new bone formation; the serum calcium is high, the phosphorus low and the calcium balance is negative. In roentgenograms of the skull, one sees generalized rarefaction. Albright syndrome shows asymmetry of the face and skull combined with dense sclerosis. Hyperparathyroidism is a disorder of adults; Albright syndrome begins and progresses during childhood. In Ollier dyschondroplasia, the skull usually is not involved but facial asymmetry occurs. The pathologic process affects the epiphyses, which usually are not destroyed by fibrous dysplasia. Biopsy specimens in Ollier disease show islands of cartilage in place of bone but lack of marrow fibrosis and new bone formation.

The bone lesions in Recklinghausen neurofibromatosis show a predilection for the lower end of the femur and the upper end of the tibia. The lesions are sharply circumscribed and signs of new bone formation are absent. There usually are multiple cutaneous neurofibromas and the skin pigmentations have smooth margins.[1] Dominant inheritance of neurofibromatosis often is demonstrable.

The osseous changes in Albright syndrome in all probability are identical to those of polyostotic fibrous dysplasia. The differential diagnosis between the two conditions rests on the discovery of cutaneous pigmentation or of signs of endocrine disturbance.

Treatment is not specific. Orthopedic measures are taken as in polyostotic fibrous dysplasia. The osseous lesions are x-ray resistant and irradiation of the pituitary gland has not met with success.

REFERENCES

1. Albright, F., Butler, A. M., Hampton, A. D., and Smith, P.: Syndrome characterized by osteitis fibrosa disseminata, areas of pigmentation and endocrine dysfunction, with precocious puberty in females; report of 5 cases, New England J. Med. 216:727, 1937.
2. Weil: 9-jähriges Mädchen mit Pubertas praecox und Knochenbrüchigheit, Klin. Wchnschr. 1:2114, 1922.
3. Gaupp, V.: Pubertas praecox bei Osteodystrophia fibrosa, Monatsschr. Kinderh. 53:312, 1932.
4. Freedman, H. J.: Disturbances of function of suprarenal glands in children, Am. J. Dis. Child. 44:1285, 1932.
5. Stalmann, A.: Nerven-, Haut- und Knochenveränderungen bei der Neurofibromatosis Recklinghausen und ihre entstehungsgeschichtlichen Zusammenhänge, Virchows Arch. path. Anat. 289:96, 1933.
6. Goldhammer, K.: Osteodystrophia fibrosa unilateralis (kombiniert mit Pubertas praecox und mit gleichseitigen osteosklerotischen Veränderungen des Schädels), Fortschr. Geb. Röntgenstrahlen 49:456, 1934.
7. McCune, D. J., and Bruch, H.: Osteodystrophia fibrosa; report of a case in which condition was combined with precocious puberty, pathologic pigmentation of skin and hyperthyroidism, with review of literature, Am. J. Dis. Child. 54:806, 1937.
8. Priesel, R., and Wagner, R.: Ostitis fibrosa cystica generalisata (osteodystrophia fibrosa), Ztschr. Kinderh. 53:146, 1932.
9. Boenheim, F., and McGavack, T. H.: Polyostotische fibröse Dysplasie, Ergebn. inn. Med. u. Kinderh. 3:157, 1952.
10. Pande, H.: Albright's syndrome in a four-months-old girl, Acta paediat. 48:397, 1959.
11. Peterman, M. G.: Polyostotic fibrous dysplasia (with precocious puberty and pigmentation), J. Pediat. 49:719, 1956.
12. Caplan, D. B., and Feingold, M.: Polyostotic fibrous dysplasia with cutaneous pigmentation. A case in a Negro male, Am. J. Dis. Child. 109:575, 1965.
13. Caldwell, G. A., and Broderick, T. F., Jr.: Polyostotic fibrous dysplasia in one of Negro twin girls, Ann. Int. Med. 27:114, 1947.
14. Dockerty, M. B., Meyerding, H. W., and Wallace, G. T.: Albright's syndrome (fibrous dysplasia of bones with cutaneous pigmentation in both sexes and gonadal dysfunction in females), Proc. Staff Meet. Mayo Clin. 19:81, 1944.
15. Pritchard, J. E.: Fibrous dysplasia of bones, Am. J. M. Sc. 222:313, 1951.
16. Johnston, A. W., Lele, K. P., and Marshall, R.: Chromosomes in Albright's syndrome, Lancet 1:930, 1966.
17. Sternberg, W. H., and Joseph, V.: Osteodystrophia fibrosa combined with precocious puberty and exophthalmic goiter; pathologic report of case, Am. J. Dis. Child. 63:748, 1942.
18. Jervis, G. A., and Schein, H.: Polyostotic fibrous dysplasia (Albright's syndrome); report of case showing central nervous system changes, A.M.A. Arch. Path. 51:640, 1951.
19. Albright, F.: Polyostotic fibrous dysplasia: Defense of entity, J. Clin. Endocrinol. 7:307, 1947.
20. Falconer, M. A., Cope, C. L., and Robb-Smith, A.: Fibrous dysplasia of bone with endocrine disorders and cutaneous pigmentation (Albright's disease), Quart. J. Med. 11:121, 1942.
21. Moldawer, M., and Rabin, E. R.: Polyostotic fibrous dysplasia with thyrotoxicosis. Report of a complete autopsy and skeletal reconstruction, Arch. Int. Med. 118:379, 1966.

22. Vines, R. H.: Polyostotic fibrous dysplasia, Arch. Dis. Childhood 27:351, 1952.
23. Albright, F., Scoville, W. B., and Sulkowitch, H. W.: Syndrome characterized by osteitis fibrosa disseminata, areas of pigmentation and gonadal dysfunction; further observations including report of 2 more cases, Endocrinology 22:411, 1938.
24. Warrick, C. K.: Polyostotic fibrous dysplasia—Albright's syndrome; review of literature and report of 4 male cases, 2 of which were associated with precocious puberty, J. Bone & Joint Surg. 31-B:175, 1949.
25. Coleman, M.: Osteitis fibrosa disseminata; report of case, Brit. J. Surg. 26:705, 1939.
26. Thomas, H. W., Meredith, T. N., and Wunderly, H. L.: Osteodystrophia disseminata; report of case, J. Pediat. 18:638, 1941.
27. McIntosh, H. D., Miller, D. E., Gleason, W. L., and Goldner, J. L.: The circulatory dynamics of polyostotic fibrous dysplasia, Am. J. Med. 32:393, 1962.
28. Coley, B. L., and Stewart, F. W.: Bone sarcoma in polyostotic fibrous dysplasia, Ann. Surg. 121:872, 1945.
29. Stauffer, H. M., Arbuckle, R. K., and Aegerter, E. E.: Polyostotic fibrous dysplasia with cutaneous pigmentation and congenital arteriovenous aneurysms; case report, J. Bone & Joint Surg. 23:323, 1941.
30. Laplane, R., Oehmichen (Mlle.), and Lhermitte, F.: Ostéite pseudo-kystique à prédominance unilatérale avec hémipigmentation cutanée et hémisyndrome sympathique d'origine congénitale, Bull. Soc. méd. hôp. Paris 62: 371, 1946.
31. Verghese, A.: Albright's syndrome in the male with situs inversus, Proc. Roy. Soc. Med. 55:357, 1962.

Maffucci Syndrome

(Dyschondroplasia with Hemangiomatosis)

IN 1881, MAFFUCCI[1] described a woman, 40 years of age, who was of short stature and grossly deformed. In the left scapulohumeral region there was a nodular tumor approximately 50 cm. in circumference, occupying the whole of the acromial end of the clavicle. The left arm was curved and shorter than the right. The hand was replaced by a large nodular mass formed of hard cartilaginous excrescences attached to the phalanges and metacarpals. In the right hand there was a large number of bluish tumors situated on the fingers, which were compressible and tender on pressure. The right leg was greatly deformed by a large, hard tumor in the intercondylar region of the femur and the upper third of the tibia was sharply bent. Bluish tumors were seen on the foot and ankle of the left leg. Because of increasing size of the tumor in the left shoulder, the arm was amputated, but the patient died of pyemia. At necropsy, it was found that the soft tumors were angiomata, many of which contained phleboliths, and the harder tumors attached to the bones were chondromata. The syndrome of bilateral dyschondroplasia with hemangiomata was called Maffucci syndrome by Carleton *et al.*,[2] who reviewed 18 cases from the literature, adding 2 cases of their own. In 1966, Elmore and Cantrell[3] estimated that 75 cases had been recorded.

The etiology of this tissue dysplasia is very puzzling. Although there is a tendency to multiple tissue dysplasia and tumor formation comparable to that of "hamartoses" such as tuberous sclerosis, Hippel-Lindau disease or Recklinghausen neurofibromatosis, there is no evidence of genetic determination and certainly none of dominant inheritance. The condition has not been observed in the ascendants or in the descendants of the patients. In several cases,[1,2] reproduction resulted in normal children. One patient[4] had 9 normal siblings. Parental consanguinity was not recorded and there is no suggestion of recessive inheritance. One patient[5] was a twin and his fraternal twin was normal. Males as well as females can be affected.

The pathogenesis is puzzling also. Although it has been speculated that the vascular anomalies are the primary lesion and the skeletal deformities secondary, there is no proof of this. It seems that the vascular and skeletal anomalies are caused by a common factor. Carleton *et al.*[2] believed that the dysplasia arises in early fetal life, but congenital manifestations are rare. As a rule, the first signs occur between the ages of 1 and 12 years in the form of hard nodules on a finger or toe and other parts of the limbs. Dilated veins or soft bluish tumors appear on the skin of affected parts. Occasionally, the first complaints are in connection with fractures following trivial traumas. A patient described by Bean[5] was plagued by this disease in early life and had suffered 9 fractures when he was 32 years of age. Meckler[6] reported a case of Maffucci syndrome, or one resembling it, which is of interest because there were anomalies present at birth, namely polydactyly and an enlarged right thumb. Later, varices, angiomas and enchondromas developed. The case was unusual in that the patient was tall, having long lower extremities, a feature also present in her father and brother. The deformities are not limited to one side but they are always asymmetric. The two halves of the body may differ in growth. Sometimes there is asymmetry of the face[5] or one side of the body appears dwarfed.[2] Some of the long bones are shortened and bent, with epiphyseal expansion and cartilaginous tumors at the ends. Genu valgum, pes planus and other more bizarre deformities may develop. In severe cases, the hands and feet are transformed into grotesque masses of tumor growth with almost unrecognizable knobby fingers protruding at the periphery.[2] Occasionally, tumors also develop from the vertebrae, ribs, scapulae or pelvic bones. The skull is involved only rarely, but in the severe case reported by Steudel,[7] chondromata were present in the orbita and nasal sinuses. Development of new deformities often ceases in the third decade

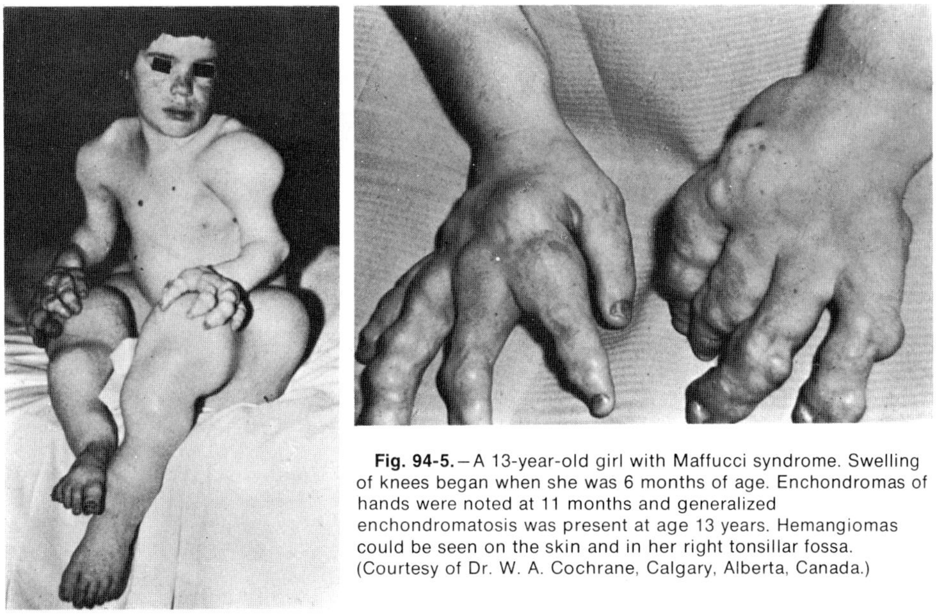

Fig. 94-5.—A 13-year-old girl with Maffucci syndrome. Swelling of knees began when she was 6 months of age. Enchondromas of hands were noted at 11 months and generalized enchondromatosis was present at age 13 years. Hemangiomas could be seen on the skin and in her right tonsillar fossa. (Courtesy of Dr. W. A. Cochrane, Calgary, Alberta, Canada.)

but, after injuries, their growth may be resumed and expanding tumors occur. The growth disturbances result in small stature; in some cases, a partial hemihypertrophy can develop.[5] Vascular anomalies vary and include varicose veins, vascular tumors and hamartomas that may be seen through the skin. Phleboliths can be palpated or visualized in roentgenograms. Vascular tumors have occurred in the lungs, leading to hemoptysis,[5] and in the mesocolon.[2] In general, pain is not one of the outstanding symptoms, but occasionally pressure or hemorrhages result in painful sensations. The central nervous system can be affected by hemorrhages, leading to paralysis,[4,5] or by tumor formation.[2,8] The skin may show, in addition to vascular changes, vitiligo[9] and excessive sweating.[2] Diffuse enlargement of the thyroid has been observed repeatedly. It is illustrated in the patient of Burk[10] and Steudel[7] and was described more recently by Bean.[5] Angiomatous tumors and hemorrhagic cysts seem to be responsible for the thyroid enlargement. In addition to chondromas and angiomas, which are typical of the disease, sarcoma, myxochondrosarcoma,[11] angiosarcoma,[5] pedunculated fibromas[12] and lymphangioma[5] have been observed. In 2 cases, gliomas developed in a temporal lobe[2,13] and in a third[8] an unspecified brain tumor was present. In 1 patient, a teratoid tumor of the ovary was found.[14]

Fig. 94-6.—Patient with Maffucci syndrome reported by Burk[10] and later by Steudel.[7]

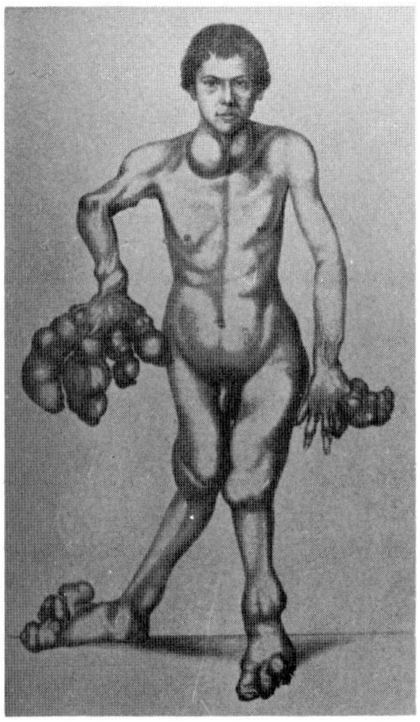

Mild cases probably escape diagnosis, so that the published cases make the prognosis appear very unfavorable. Some patients can live an active and useful life and attain middle and possibly old age. But fractures with poor healing tendency, deformities of limbs requiring amputation and the inclination to malignant tumor formation dim the outlook for a normal life.

Regression of hemangioma after x-ray treatment has been reported.[15] Chromosomes appear to be normal.[3,16]

REFERENCES

1. Maffucci, A.: Di un caso di encondroma ed angioma multiplo. Contribuzione alla genesi embrionale dei tumori, Movimento med. chir. 3:399, 1881.
2. Carleton, A., Elkington, J. St. C., Greenfield, J. G., and Robb-Smith, A. H. T.: Maffucci's syndrome (dyschondroplasia with haemangeiomata), Quart. J. Med. 11:203, 1942.

3. Elmore, S. M., and Cantrell, W. C.: Maffucci's syndrome. Case report with a normal karyotype, J. Bone & Joint Surg. 48-A:1607, 1966.
4. Torri, O.: Angiomi ed encondromi multipli nello stesso individuo, Clin. chir. 10:81, 1902.
5. Bean, W. B.: Dyschondroplasia and hemangiomata (Maffucci's syndrome), Arch. Int. Med. 95:767, 1955.
6. Meckler, L. C.: Dyschondroplasia and hemangiomata, Ohio M. J. 60:672, 1964.
7. Steudel: Multiple Enchondrome der Knochen in Verbindung mit venösen Angiomen der Weichteile, Beitr. klin. Chir. 8:503, 1892.
8. Ashenhurst, E. M.: Dyschondroplasia with hemangioma (Maffucci's syndrome); report of a case complicated by brain tumor, Arch. Neurol. 2:552, 1960.
9. Kast, A., and von Recklinghausen, F. D.: Ein Fall von Enchondrom mit ungewöhnlicher Multiplication, Virchows Arch. path. Anat. 118:1, 1889.
10. Burk, R.: Beitrag zur Lehre vom Enchondrom, Inang. Dissert. Tübingen, 1866.
11. Harbitz, F.: Über das gleichzeitige Auftreten mehrerer selbständig wachsender ("multipler") Geschwülste, Beitr. path. Anat. 62:503, 1916.
12. Casini, A.: Su di un caso di discondroplasia associato ad angiomi e fibromi multipli, Policlinico (seg. chir.) 42:193, 1935.
13. Leu, A.: Zur Frage der systematischen. Enchondromatose des Skelettsystems, Frankfurt. Ztschr. Path. 37:336, 1929.
14. Kuzma, J. F., and King, J. M.: Dyschondroplasia with hemangiomatosis (Maffucci syndrome) and teratoid tumor of ovary, Arch. Path. 46:74, 1948.
15. Umansky, A. L.: Dyschondroplasia with hemangiomata (Maffucci syndrome). Early case with mild osseous manifestations, Bull. Hosp. Joint Dis. 7:59, 1946.
16. Cochrane, W. A.: Personal communication.

Melorheostosis

(Osteosis eburnisans monomelica)

THIS SKELETAL DISORDER is a form of hyperostosis, usually limited to one limb, which manifests itself in infancy or childhood and progresses slowly. There are some indications that in some cases the basic process begins before birth. In other cases, manifestations do not occur before adult life. The hyperostosis "flows" from one bone to another, leaving some bones that are not, in the linear course of progress, free of pathologic changes. Several bones of an upper or a lower extremity may be "vertically" affected, but involvement of more than one extremity is rare. Léri and Joanny[1] termed the disorder melorheostosis because the roentgenographic changes are reminiscent of the flow of molten wax down a candle. Putti[2] suggested the term "osteosis eburnisans monomelica." In biopsy material, formation of new bone is seen around vessels that appear more numerous than normal. Bony lamellae are regularly distributed, but in some areas degenerative changes are found.[2]

The first complaints often are pain and limitation of movement in the affected extremity. Since these manifestations usually occur in older children or in adults, the congenital nature of the disorder can be questioned, but in a number of cases pathologic signs have been observed at birth or in infancy. Léri *et al.*[3] described a patient who had congenital stiffness of the right middle finger. In the case of Widmann and Stecher,[4] the thumb of the left hand assumed an abnormal position from birth on. Zimmer[5] stated that the affected extremity of his patient was longer than the normal one since birth. The observation by Gillespie and Siegling[6] is of interest because it shows that congenital scleroderma and flexion deformity may precede osseous changes, which develop in postnatal life. Thus, it appears that the basic process underlying melorheostosis is present before birth, although marked hyperostosis develops only later. There is no evidence of familial aggregation of cases or of heredity. However, bone changes resembling melorheostosis have been observed in patients with such hereditary conditions as tuberous sclerosis[7] or chondrodystrophy.[8] Melorheostosis has been described in the fibula of an Eskimo buried approximately 1,500 years ago in Alaska.[9] Both sexes can be affected. Little is known concerning the etiology and pathogenesis of the disorder. All theories advanced have been speculative.

In a well-developed case, the patient usually has enlargements and deformities of the fingers or toes. The affected digits are curved and swollen and remind one of macrodactyly. The skin over the enlarged digits is tight and tender and sometimes red and edematous. Scleroderma or trophedema can occur and limit movements. There may be curving and deformity of the proximal bones of the same limb, with limitation of articular movements. As a rule, functional changes and pain increase with age. The disorder usually is monomelic, but bilateral involvement has been described[10,14] and in 1 case both extremities as well as axial bones of the same side were affected.[11] The lower extremity is involved more often than the upper.[12]

Roentgenograms reveal marked hyperostosis of some bones, whereas other bones appear entirely normal. In an affected extremity, the humerus, ulna and the fourth and fifth fingers may show the hyperostotic changes, whereas the radius and digits I–III remain free. Along the long bones, increased wavy cortical densities on one or both sides are characteristic of the disorder. In short bones, dense patchy areas indicate endosteal hyperostosis. Carpal and tarsal bones, the scapulae, pelvic bones and, in rare instances, the skull, spine and ribs may show the disease process.[11] Osseous masses have been found in soft tissues and deposits occur in periarticular areas. Conditions found associated with melorheostosis have been discussed by McGuinness *et al.*[13] These conditions are etiologically so different that one must assume that the osseous manifestations resembled melorheostosis without being identical to the disorder described by Léri and Joanny.[1]

Progress of the osseous changes is slow and sometimes the disease appears stationary.[12] Campbell *et al.*[14] reported 14 cases and pointed out that the disease progresses rapidly in children and slowly in adults. Contracture and deformity were the first findings in childhood, whereas pain and stiffness were the most common complaints in adults. Abnormalities of the soft tissues usually were discovered earlier than hyperostosis.

No satisfactory treatment is known. In 1 case,[8] roentgentherapy was considered effective.

REFERENCES

1. Léri, A., and Joanny: Une affection non-décrite des os: hyperostose "en coulée" sur toute la longeur d'un membre ou mélorhéostose, Bull. Soc. méd. hôp. Paris 46: 1141, 1922.
2. Putti, V.: L'osteosi eburneizzante monomelica, Chir. org. movimento 11:335, 1927.
3. Léri, A., Loiseleur, and Liévre, J. A.: Une nouvelle observation de mélorhéostose. Étude clinique, anatomique et expérimentale, Bull. Soc. méd. hôp. Paris 54:1210, 1930.
4. Widmann, B. P., and Stecher, W. R.: Rhizomonomelorheostosis, Radiology 24:651, 1935.
5. Zimmer, P.: Über einen Fall einer eigenartigen seltenen Knochenerkrankung, Osteopathia hyperostotica-Mélorhéostose, Beitr. klin. Chir. 140:75, 1927.
6. Gillespie, J. B., and Siegling, J. A.: Melorheostosis Léri, Am. J. Dis. Child. 55:1273, 1938.
7. Hall, G. S.: A contribution to the study of melorheostosis: Unusual bone changes associated with tuberose sclerosis, Quart. J. Med. 12:77, 1943.
8. Hilton, G.: Familial chondrodystrophy with rheostosis treated by x-ray therapy, Lancet 1:122, 1934.
9. Lester, C. W.: Melorheostosis in a prehistoric Alaskan skeleton, J. Bone & Joint Surg. 49-A:142, 1967.
10. Carpender, J. W. J., Baker, D. R., Perry, S. P., and Outland, T.: Melorheostosis: Report of a bilateral case, Am. J. Roentgenol. 49:398, 1943.
11. Franklin, E. L., and Matheson, I.: Melorheostosis. Report on a case with a review of the literature, Brit. J. Radiol. 15:185, 1942.
12. Fairbank, H. A. T.: *An Atlas of General Affections of the Skeleton* (Edinburgh and London: E. & S. Livingstone, Ltd., 1951).
13. McGuinness, A. E., Watson, L. C. A., Lindsell, C. K., and Inglis, K.: Melorheostosis: Its relation to associated conditions and a case report, Australasian Ann. Med. 2:84, 1953.
14. Campbell, C. J., Papademetriou, Th., and Bonfiglio, M.: Melorheostosis: A report of the clinical, roentgenographic, and pathological findings in fourteen cases, J. Bone & Joint Surg. 50-A:1281, 1968.

Infantile Cortical Hyperostosis

(Roske-Caffey Disease)

THE BONY CHANGES characteristic of this disease cannot be considered congenital malformations but they are, at least in some cases, congenital anomalies. Infantile cortical hyperostosis has been demonstrated in the fetus in utero[1,2] and immediately after birth.[3,4,13] In the majority of cases, manifestations begin within the first few months of life. Only a few cases had been recorded in the literature before 1945, when Caffey and Silverman[5] described the disease as a new syndrome and gave it the name of "infantile cortical hyperostosis." Before that, Roske[6] had described a typical case with a biopsy report that showed nothing abnormal but "chronic productive periostitis." In recent years, an increasing number of cases have been reported. This may indicate an increase in incidence or a more frequent recognition of the rare disorder for which a label now has been found.

The etiology of infantile cortical hyperostosis presents an interesting and challenging problem. Because of severe and protracted fever and increased sedimentation rate in the patients, infectious agents have been considered repeatedly, but neither syphilis nor tuberculosis or any other pathogenic agent has been demonstrated. No proof of a toxic factor, avitaminosis or endocrine disturbance in mother or child has been established. It is only recently that familial aggregations have been stressed. Van Zeben[7] reported 3 cases occurring in 2 siblings and in a second cousin. Kitchin[8] described a case with manifestations 6 hours after birth, with a history of similar lesions in the mother. Boyes and Demy[3] reported the disease in 2 consecutive cases in one family, affecting a brother and sister. In the latter, swellings were noticed immediately after discharge from the newborn nursery. The mother's maternal grandfather, the mother, her mother and sister had bowing of the legs but it is not possible to diagnose infantile cortical hyperostosis from such a history. Barba and Freriks[1] described a patient born with fusiform swellings of both arms, legs and mandible. A brother of this child had the same condition, swellings being noted at delivery. Sidbury and Sidbury[4] saw the condition in 2 sisters, 1 of them showing swellings of one arm at birth. A remarkable family history was obtained by Van Buskirk *et al.*,[9] who reported 11 cases of infantile cortical hyperostosis in two generations of one family. They believed that their observation lent support to the contention that in some instances this disease is genetically transmitted by males and females but that expressivity varies greatly. Schärer and Szabó[10] wrote on familial infantile cortical hyperostosis with prenatal onset. In a premature infant, severe generalized infantile cortical hyperostosis was observed. The radiologic features were first seen on the flat plate of the mother's abdomen 3 days before birth. Reduced motility and marked osseous deformities were seen until the end of the first year of life. Clinical improvement was thought to be effected by treatment with prednisone. The father of this child presented some residual signs of the same skeletal disorder in the mandible, the styloid process and in the long bones.

An increased amount of citric and aconitic acid was found in the infant's urine. The article gives a good review of familial cases. In some patients, the clinical and roentgenologic manifestations are pronounced, whereas in others they are so mild or atypical that the disease may easily be overlooked. If family histories are taken in all known patients and roentgenographic examinations carried out on both symptomatic and asymptomatic infants in families in which the disease has already been manifest, familial aggregation may be demonstrable more often. There can be little doubt that infantile cortical hyperostosis has been observed repeatedly in familial aggregations, but whether this is due to genetic factors or to familial exposure to a noxious environmental factor has not yet been decided. Reports should not only include pedigrees but also describe the environment, localities in which the parents grew up, their occupations, and so forth. If members of a kinship have the disease despite geographic dispersion, the genetic theory would receive some support.

Infantile cortical hyperostosis occurs in male and female infants. It occurs in cities and rural communities, in all seasons and climates, in various racial strains and social classes.[11]

The symptoms consist of hyperirritability, swellings of the soft tissues and cortical thickening of the underlying bones. The swellings are deeply situated, often tender but not warm or discolored. These swellings can subside and lose their tenderness before the hyperostosis is no longer demonstrable in roentgenograms. Remissions after apparent recovery are not rare. Fever is observed in most of the cases but occasionally patients are afebrile. Increased sedimentation rate of erythrocytes and increased phosphatase activity of the blood serum occur frequently. Serologic tests for both bacterial and viral infections have been consistently negative.[11] Hydroxyproline excretion in the urine has been found greatly increased by Salzer and Schwägerl.[12]

Cortical hyperostosis has been observed in all tubular bones but the phalanges and vertebral bodies remain free. The mandibles, scapulae, ilia, parietals and frontals may show sclerosis and thickening. The mandibles, clavicles and ulnae have been involved most frequently.[11] In long bones and in flat bones, asymmetric distribution is not rare. The lesions of infantile cortical hyperostosis are confined to the middle of the shafts; the metaphyses and epiphyses are not affected.

Clinical and roentgen recovery usually is complete after several weeks or months, but permanent distortion of bones has been reported in some instances.[9,11]

In the differential diagnosis, syphilis probably was considered primarily at times when this disease was prevalent. Now, suppurative infections or tumors occasionally are erroneously diagnosed instead of infantile cortical hyperostosis, and incorrect treatment may be advised.

Since infantile cortical hyperostosis is a self-limited disease with frequent remissions, reports of successful treatment are not convincing. Symptomatic treatment consists of sedation and adequate nursing and nutrition.

REFERENCES

1. Barba, W. P., II, and Freriks, D. J.: Familial occurrence of infantile cortical hyperostosis in utero. J. Pediat. 42:141, 1953.
2. Bennett, H. S., and Nelson, T. R.: Prenatal cortical hyperostosis, Brit. J. Radiol. 26:47, 1953.
3. Boyes, J. G., and Demy, N. G.: Infantile cortical hyperostosis; familial disease?, Am. J. Roentgenol. 65:924, 1951.
4. Sidbury, J. B., Jr., and Sidbury, J. B.: Infantile cortical hyperostosis; inquiry into etiology and pathogenesis, New England J. Med. 250:309, 1954.
5. Caffey, J., and Silverman, W. A.: Infantile cortical hyperostoses: Preliminary report on a new syndrome, Am. J. Roentgenol. 54:1, 1945.
6. Roske, G.: Eine eigenartige Knochenerkrankung im Säuglingsalter, Monatsschr. Kinderh. 47:385, 1930.
7. van Zeben, W.: Infantile cortical hyperostosis, Acta paediat. scandinav. 35:10, 1948.
8. Kitchin, I. D.: Atypical case of infantile cortical hyperostoses, J. Bone & Joint Surg. 33-B:248, 1951.
9. Van Buskirk, F. W., Tampas, J. P., and Peterson, O. S., Jr.: Infantile cortical hyperostosis; an inquiry into its familial aspects, Am. J. Roentgenol. 85:613, 1961.
10. Schärer, K., and Szabó, J.: Familiäre infantile corticale Hyperostose mit pränatalem Beginn, Fortschr. Geb. Röntgenstrahlen 105:154, 1966.
11. Caffey, J.: *Pediatric X-ray Diagnosis* (5th ed.; Chicago: Year Book Medical Publishers, Inc., 1967).
12. Salzer, M., and Schwägerl, W.: Hyperostosis corticalis infantilis (Roske-Caffey-Syndrom), Monatsschr. Kinderh. 115:382, 1967.
13. Kühl, J., Clifton Harris, G. B., Maroteaux, P., and Hansen, H. G.: Ein Beitrag zum Krankheitsbild der infantilen kortikalen Hyperostose, Arch. Kinderh. 179:209, 1969.

PART XIV

Malformations of the Axial and Appendicular Skeleton

95

The Skull

Congenital Defects

CONGENITAL SKULL DEFECTS vary from severe lesions incompatible with life to minor anomalies that are not of practical importance to their carrier. Berry and Berry[1] dealt with minor morphologic variations in adult human skulls and Dedick and Caffey[2] with radiographic findings in the skulls of newborn infants. Head circumference measurements from birth to various ages of childhood and adolescence[3,4] are available and permit comparison with deviations from the normal.

Cranioschisis and Cranium Bifidum

Disturbances of the midline closure of the cranium are called cranioschisis or cranium bifidum. If such cranial defects are very large (*cranioschisis*), affected children are stillborn or they live only a few hours or days. If the squamae of the frontal and temporal bones and the parietal and occipital bones are absent (*holoacrania*), there also may be a complete absence of the brain (*anencephaly*) or the brain may be represented by spongy, vascular remnants (p. 192). A less pronounced cranial defect (*meroacrania*) affects chiefly the sagittal area but does not include defects of the occipital bone. Such severe skull defects usually are associated with severe brain anomalies that, according to their extent, are termed holo- or meroanencephaly. Although children with such severe malformations usually are not viable, their conditions are described (p. 179) because they are relativelv frequent. Defects associated with smaller openings in the skull may be compatible with life. Often they are combined with herniation of the brain or the meninges (*encephalocele* or *cranial meningocele*). The terminology is confusing, since one is dealing with variations of brain defects, skull defects and with differing degrees of secondary brain destruction. *Exencephaly*, for instance, is a congenital exposure of the brain. It is seen often in experimental animals when secondary destruction of the exposed brain is prevented by cesarean section before term. If, however, such animals remain in utero to or beyond term, the exposed brain deteriorates and anencephaly results. Similarly, in human exencephalies, there are only a few cerebral remnants left at birth and anencephaly results (p. 191). The term cranioschisis usually is applied—corresponding to "rachischisis" of the spinal column—to large cranial defects combined with anencephaly. The term cranium bifidum—corresponding to spina bifida—is applied to smaller circumscribed cranial defects. Since transitional forms exist, a clear distinction between cranioschisis-anencephaly and cranium bifidum-encephalocele is not always possible.

Cerebral agenesis or atrophy sometimes is accompanied by *thinning and bulging* of overlying parts of the skull. Childe[5] thought that because of absence of the cushioning effect of normal brain, ventricular fluid exerted localized pressure on the dura and cranium, which gave rise to the cranial changes. But *flattening* of the outer surfaces of the parietal bones with thinning due to diploic dysplasia can be a harmless anomaly that should not be mistaken for a depressed fracture or a tumor. There can be a familial tendency to such diploic dysplasia.[6]

Cranial Dysostosis

Lack of ossification of the calvarium at the time of birth and thereafter represents a striking anomaly

Fig. 95-1.—Cranial dysostosis (lack of ossification) in a newborn child who had clavicles and no associated malformations.

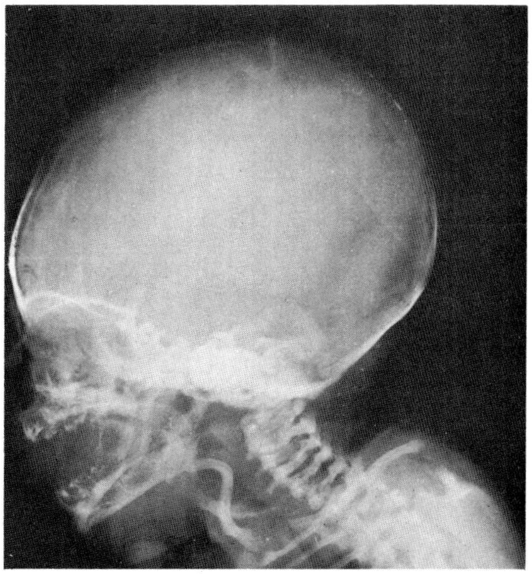

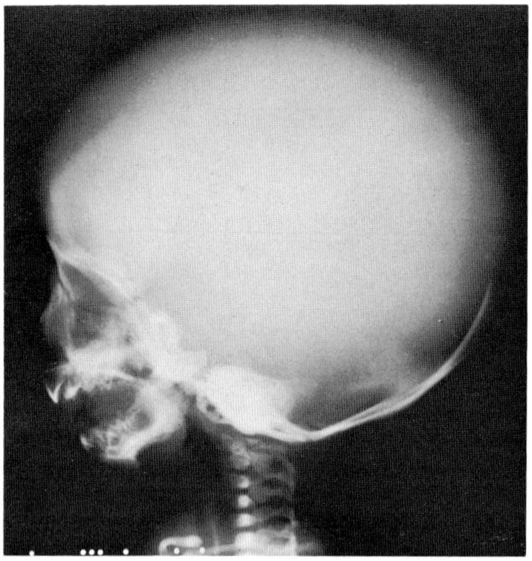

Fig. 95-2.—Cranial dysostosis in a newborn child damaged by aminopterin intake of the mother (p. 97).

that can be associated with systemic skeletal disorders such as osteogenesis imperfecta, hypophosphatasia, cleidocranial dysostosis, pyknodysostosis and others. Cranial dysostosis as an isolated anomaly is rare. In some instances, it is a harmless defect that shows spontaneous repair by delayed ossification. During the existence of the bony defect, the brain can be protected by a hard hat or helmet.

Cranial dysostosis has been observed in infants damaged in utero by aminopterin taken by their mothers in attempted abortions (p. 97). Lesser defects of cranial ossification can be found in various areas and be caused by heterogeneous factors.

Craniolacunia (Lacunar Skull, Lückenschädel)

Craniolacunia is characterized in roentgenograms by round areas of translucency separated by linear shadows formed by strips of bone. As a rule, the defects are due to absence of the inner table and diploë with persistence of the outer table. If the outer table is affected also, fenestration occurs in the skull as bone is replaced by fibrous tissue. The pattern seen in roentgenograms does not correspond to cerebral gyri and sulci. Parietal, frontal and occipital bones are most often the sites of the lacunae. Shopfner *et al.*[7] found craniolacunia in all patients with myelomeningocele if the examination was made before the age of 3 months. There also was a high incidence in infants with encephalocele, but the craniolacunia disappeared within 1–3 months. Hydrocephaly had no influence on the course of the anomaly; in fact, craniolacunia can disappear while hydrocephaly develops. Whereas Shopfner *et al.*[7] denied that craniolacunia persists beyond the fourth month, other authors believed that the anomaly can occur in older children with mental retardation.[8,9] Prenatal diagnosis of craniolacunia has been made by radiography.[10]

Persistent Metopic Fontanelle

This defect occurs in patients with delayed ossification of the cranial bones as seen in cranial or cleidocranial dysostosis, osteogenesis imperfecta, hypophosphatasia and others. It can occur as an isolated ossification defect in the midfrontal region, which is closed by a dense fibrous membrane. The term "congenital cranium bifidum occultum frontale" has been applied to such lesions, which can be inherited as a dominant trait and may be associated with parietal foramina. Spontaneous closure can be expected.[11]

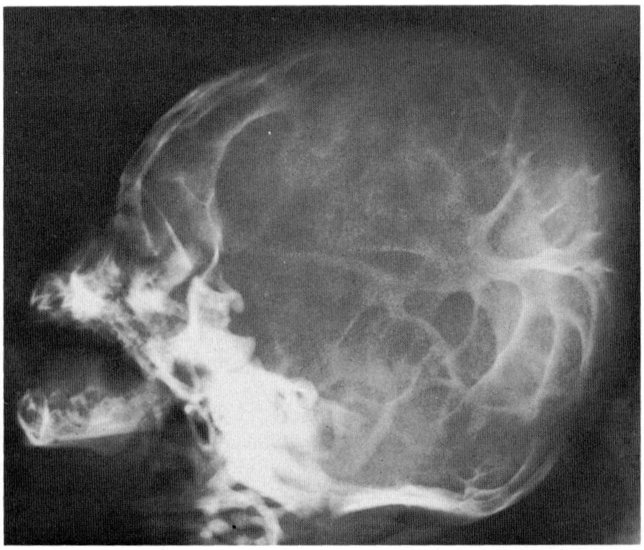

Fig. 95-3.—Lückenschädel in a child with myelomeningocele, Arnold-Chiari malformation and hydrocephaly.

Enlarged Parietal Foramina and Third Fontanelle

Enlarged parietal foramina have been known to anatomists since the eighteenth century, when Lancisi (1707) gave a written account of the anomaly, yet, in 1927, Greig[12] thought the condition to be sufficiently rare to recommend that every example be reported. In the last decades, many more cases have been recognized because roentgenologic examination of the skull can reveal the anomaly in vivo. By 1963, more than 100 cases had been reported.[13]

A parietal foramen is found in approximately 60% of human skulls, more often unilaterally than on both sides. Most foramina do not exceed 1 mm. in diameter, but about 10% are larger, varying in size up to 5 mm. and more. Enlarged foramina have been called foramina parietalia permagna or fenestrae parietales symmetricae. It is believed that they can occur in all races, and the right foramen often is larger than the left.[14] Since some of the defects seen in roentgenograms are filled with fibrous tissue, the term "foramina" may be a misnomer.[13]

The parietal bone ossifies in membrane from an hourglass-shaped center in the area of the parietal eminence at the seventh or eighth week of gestation. In the area of the parietal foramina, ossification toward the median plane is delayed and a diamond-shaped membranous area named the sagittal fontanelle persists for some time. Estimates of the occurrence of a sagittal or third fontanelle in the newborn period vary. The third fontanelle is a deficiency of bone at the suture line approximately 2 cm. rostral to the lambda.[15] The incidence of such a third fontanelle is about 5% in newborn infants, but the soft areas vary in degree. It seems that the incidence is higher in patients with Down syndrome.[16] I often have found a third fontanelle in mongoloid infants but did not compare its incidence with that of normal newborns.

Normally, ossification proceeds from the four sides of the sagittal fontanelle and a cruciform suture is formed. The transverse limbs of the suture become obliterated, whereas the vertical limbs persist as the pars obelica of the sagittal suture. In cases of enlarged parietal foramina, the transverse limb persists and the pars obelica is found obliterated. Large parietal foramina usually begin as one large opening, which is subdivided later.[17,18] In some cases, the enlarged parietal foramina decrease in size with age; in others, they seem to be unchanged after many years.[14]

Enlarged parietal foramina can occur as a dominant hereditary trait. In some families, only a few members are affected, whereas in others the defect is widespread. Thus, in five generations of the Catlin family, described by Goldsmith,[17] 16 of 56 members examined showed the anomaly ("Catlin mark"). Wiedemann[19] reported the anomaly in four genera-

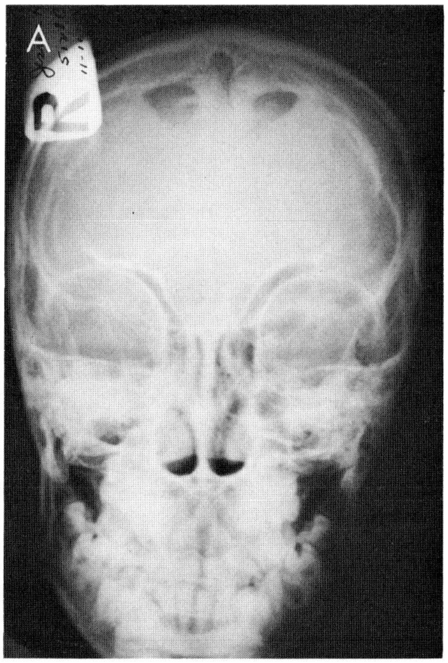

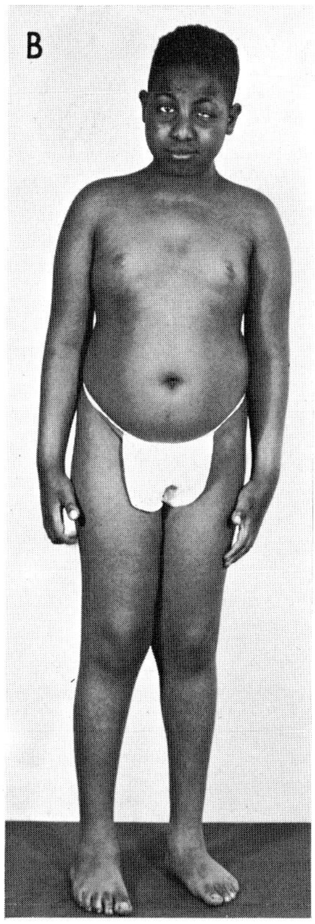

Fig. 95-4. – Boy, 11 years of age, with enlarged parietal foramina (**A**), obesity, microphthalmia, undescended testes and genu valgum (**B**).[20]

tions of a kindred in which an infant of the fifth generation had a large parietal fontanelle considered a forerunner of parietal fenestrae. Hereditary parietal foramina can be associated with clavicular defects.[13]

The statement has been made that enlarged parietal foramina are found in persons or families otherwise perfectly normal. This is only partly true. Various abnormalities of the skull, including microcephaly, hydrocephaly, tower head and cranial asymmetry, have been described in association with large parietal foramina. Abnormalities of the spinal column, funnel chest, coxa valga, syndactyly, polydactyly and supernumerary epiphyses have been observed. Congenital heart disease, ptosis of the eyelid, exophthalmos, microphthalmia, cloudy cornea, nystagmus, strabismus, partial or complete optic atrophy, choked disc, absence of an auricle, atresia of the external auditory canal or deaf-mutism may accompany enlarged parietal foramina. Retardation of growth, ossification and dentition, dwarfism, obesity or cryptorchidism may be found occasionally. Enlarged parietal foramina have been observed in cases of mental retardation and in mongolism. Headaches, choreiform movements and epilepsy occur as neurologic complications.[20]

A variety of etiologically differing conditions may resemble enlarged parietal foramina seen in roentgenograms. Defects in the bones of the skull occur in association with meningo-encephalocele, syphilis, xanthomatosis (Schüller-Christian syndrome), multiple myeloma, multiple malignant metastases, renal and celiac rickets, cleidocranial dysostosis or following trauma or trephining. If one bears in mind the possible occurrence of enlarged parietal foramina, usually symmetrically placed on each side of the posterior third of the sagittal suture and irregularly shaped with well-defined margins, recognition is relatively easy.

Abnormal brains of the cyclopia series, including the arhinencephalies of trisomy 13-15, often are associated with congenital parietal skin defects (p. 1149), and under these skin lesions there may be osseous defects of variable size. Cranial lacunae following trauma in early infancy[21] are irregular in size, shape and location. Such irregular defects are not to be mistaken for craniolacunia or enlarged parietal foramina.

Occipital Foramina

Large foramina are rare in the occipital bone. In the normal occipital bone, an inioendinial canal for the occipital emissary vein may be found or it may be suggested by an internal or external vascular orifice. Of clinical importance are occipital apertures associated with meningo-encephaloceles or dermoid cysts in this area. Such openings usually occur in the midline between the occipital protuberances and the foramen magnum. In rare instances, they have been seen above or at the protuberances.[14,26]

Cranial Defects due to Bone Replacement by Heterologous Tissues

Reticuloendothelioses (eosinophilic granuloma, Schüller-Christian disease, Letterer-Siwe disease) bring about skull lesions in postnatal life but neurofibromatosis, a hamartosis, can cause congenital absence of the superior orbital wall, with pulsating exophthalmos.[22] Similar symptoms can be due to fibrous dysplasia (p. 878), which manifests itself in postnatal life, but in some cases the lesions may be congenital.[23]

Epidermoid cysts are noted as swellings in suture lines. In roentgenograms, they may appear as well-demarcated areas of diminished density surrounded by a well-defined sclerotic border. Osteomas of the calvarium and facial skeleton occur in the hamartosis described by Gardner[24] and others (p. 1268), together with polyposis of the colon and cutaneous tumors. The osseous tumors usually develop at puberty but in at least one case hard projections from the occipital bone were present at birth.[24] A survey of adults showed that the frontal bone, mandible and maxilla were involved most frequently.[25]

REFERENCES

1. Berry, A. C., and Berry, R. J.: Epigenetic variation in the human cranium, J. Anat. 101:361, 1967.
2. Dedick, A. P., and Caffey, J.: Roentgen findings in the skull and chest in 1,030 newborn infants, Radiology 61:13, 1953.
3. Westropp, C. K., and Barber, C. R.: Growth of the skull in young children. Part 1. Standards of head circumference, J. Neurol., Neurosurg. & Psychiat. 19:52, 1956.
4. Nellhaus, G.: Head circumference from birth to eighteen years. Practical composite international and interracial graphs, Pediatrics 41:106, 1968.
5. Childe, A. E.: Localized thinning and enlargement of the cranium with special reference to the middle fossa, Am. J. Roentgenol. 70:1, 1953.
6. Epstein, J. A., and Epstein, B. S.: Deformities of the skull surfaces in infancy and childhood, J. Pediat. 70:636, 1967.
7. Shopfner, C. E., Jabbour, J. T., and Vallion, R. M.: Craniolacunia, Am. J. Roentgenol. 93:343, 1965.
8. Vogt, E. C., and Wyatt, G. M.: Craniolacunia (Lückenschädel), Radiology 36:147, 1941.
9. Pullon, D. H. H.: Craniolacunia and phenylpyruvic oligophrenia, Brit. J. Radiol. 31:634, 1958.
10. Maier, R. J.: Prenatal diagnosis of lacuna skull (Lückenschädel), Radiology 23:615, 1934.
11. Terrafranca, R. J., and Zellis, A.: Congenital hereditary cranium bifidum occultum frontalis, Radiology 61:60, 1953.
12. Greig, D. M.: The skull of the mongolian imbecile, Edinburgh M. J. 34:253, 1927.
13. Eckstein, H. B., and Hoare, R. D.: Congenital parietal "foramina" associated with faulty ossification of the clavicles, Brit. J. Radiol. 36:220, 1963.
14. O'Rahilly, R., and Twohig, N. J.: Foramina parietalia permagna, Am. J. Roentgenol. 67:551, 1952.
15. Carter, C., and MacCarthy, D.: Incidence of mongolism and its diagnosis in newborn, Brit. J. Social Med. 5:83, 1951.
16. Hoyle, C. M., and Franklin, A. W.: Incidence of the third fontanelle. Relation to mongolism, Lancet 1:437, 1954.

17. Goldsmith, W. M.: The Catlin mark; the inheritance of an unusual opening in the parietal bones, J. Hered. 13:69, 1922.
18. Zarfl, M.: Fenestrae parietales symmetricae, Ztschr. Kinderh. 57:54, 1934.
19. Wiedemann, H-R.: Zur Frage der Fenestrae parietales symmetricae, Monatsschr. Kinderh. 105:310, 1957.
20. Warkany, J., and Weaver, T.: Heredofamilial deviations. II. Enlarged parietal foramens combined with obesity, hypogenitalism, microphthalmos and mental retardation, Am. J. Dis. Child. 60:1147, 1940.
21. Charlas, J., Dalloz, J. C., Meyer, B., Paupe, J., and Vialatte, J.: Lacune cranienne secondaire à un traumatisme de la première enfance, Arch. franç. pédiat. 24:1029, 1967.
22. Le Wald, L. T.: Congenital absence of superior orbital wall associated with pulsating exophthalmos. Am. J. Roentgenol. 30: 756, 1933.
23. Wintgens, M., Roland, T., and Evrard, M.: Étude d'un cas de dysplasie fibreuse des os de la face et du crâne associée à un retard mental avec épilepsie et surdité unilatérale, Acta paediat. belg. 22:29, 1968.
24. Gardner, E. J.: Follow-up study of a family group exhibiting dominant inheritance for a syndrome including intestinal polyps, osteomas, fibromas and epidermal cysts, Am. J. Human Genet. 14:376, 1962.
25. Gorlin, R. J., and Chaudhry, A. P.: Multiple osteomatosis, fibromas, lipomas and fibromas of the skin and mesentery, epidermoid inclusion cysts of the skin, leiomyomas and multiple intestinal polyposis: A heritable disorder of connective tissue, New England J. Med. 263:1151, 1960.
26. O'Rahilly, R.: Anomalous occipital apertures, Arch. Path. 53:509, 1952.

Craniostenosis

(Craniosynostosis, Stenocephaly)

CRANIOSTENOSIS, or premature closure of the sutures of the skull, results in deformities of the head and frequently in damage to the brain and eyes. The skull deformities depend on the course of the suture that closes prematurely, since growth is arrested in a direction perpendicular to the affected suture. The most severe abnormalities result when closure precedes birth and when more than one suture is involved.

The deformity is so striking that it was noticed long before the era of modern medicine. Greig[1] gave an illustration of Shou Lao, the Chinese god of long life, which shows an enormous towerhead. The same author explained the term "tête à la Thersite" used by French authors for oxycephaly. It dates back to Homer's description of Thersites in *The Illiad* as "bandylegged, and lame of one foot; and his head was peaked towards the top and thin wooly hair was scattered over it." The combination of tower skull and high palate was known to Hippocrates in the fourth century B.C.[2] Oribasius, anatomist and physician to Julian the Apostate, made reference to the association of a pointed head with palatal and dental defects, deformed ears and headaches.[1] Park and Powers[3] reproduced an engraving from an old, anonymous atlas that shows a child with acrocephaly and symmetric deformities of the hands. In the first half of the nineteenth century, Soemmering as well as Virchow recognized the relation of premature closure of the sutures to the deformities now called craniostenoses. In 1906, Apert[4] established acrocephalosyndactyly as a syndrome and Park and Powers[3] reviewed the subject thoroughly. In 1912, Crouzon[5] described craniofacial dysostosis as a hereditary form of craniostenosis.

According to an analysis by Greig,[1] true oxycephaly, which is present at birth and is due to general craniofacial dysostosis, should be distinguished from delayed and from false oxycephaly. Despite attempts to circumscribe clearly defined disease pictures grouped around the craniostenoses, intermediate forms can be observed that link the entities described and make classification difficult.

Craniostenosis (stenocephaly) signifies any form of skull deformity that is caused by premature closure of one or several cranial sutures. Premature closure of the sagittal suture results in a long, narrow, keel-shaped skull that generally is called *scaphocephalus.* The cephalic index (breadth of skull × length of skull × 100), which normally is between 70 and 80, usually is between 60 and 70 in scaphocephaly. Premature closure of the coronal suture results in the formation of a short, high skull with a cephalic index of 80–95 or more. Patients with this type of craniostenosis have a tendency to premature synostosis of other sutures. According to Greig,[1] the term *oxycephaly* should be applied only to the anomaly that is recognizable at birth as a general craniofacial dysostosis. A premature generalized synostosis of the cranium first manifesting itself during childhood should be differentiated as *delayed oxycephaly.* The term oxycephaly implies a sharp or pointed head and *acrocephaly* is a synonym much more widely used in medical literature. *Tower skull, turricephaly* or the German *Turmschädel* are other expressions used for the same deformity. Since towers are not necessarily pointed, these expressions may be useful for heads that are high, broad and short without coming to a point. If the coronal or lambdoid sutures close prematurely on one side only, an asymmetric craniostenosis called *plagiocephaly* develops. *Hypsicephaly* is a term used by anthropologists for high heads that are neither pathologic nor due to craniostenosis. *Kleeblattschädel* is discussed on page 904. *Microcephaly,* of course, must be distinguished from the craniostenoses, since it is due to a lack of cerebral growth and not to premature synostosis.

Premature closure of cranial sutures probably is due to a variety of causes. In some instances, it is inherited as a dominant trait, whereas in others inheritance cannot be demonstrated. Sometimes the deformity of the head occurs as an isolated anomaly; in other cases, a combination of associated anomalies leads to the formation of syndromes that differ sufficiently to betray various origins. The frequent association of premature synostoses of the skull with other skeletal defects of embryonic origin suggests that the skeleton is adversely affected early in prenatal life. It is likely that the abnormal skeletal development begins in the blastemic stage before chondrification and ossification, since bones of membranous and cartilaginous origin often are affected simultaneously.

Many families have been described in which craniostenosis was inherited through several generations. Crouzon[6] reported craniofacial dysostosis in a mother and son, and in another of his families 2 affected members transmitted the condition to several of their children. Greig[1] cited a number of families in which oxycephaly was observed repeatedly. Ferriman[7] found 188 families with oxycephaly in the literature. Twenty-two of these showed evidence of inheritance; in one family, four generations were affected; the anomaly could be traced through three generations in five instances and in nine families through two generations. In three families, more than 1 child was affected in the same generation. Familial incidence of craniosynostosis was also described and discussed by French and Suechting.[8] Franceschetti and Klein[9] listed 35 pairs of monozygotic twins with oxycephaly; 25 of these were concordant and 10 were discordant. All dizygotic twins known to these authors were discordant. Although inheritance cannot be demonstrated in the majority of the cases, a genetic origin cannot be excluded in all sporadic cases. In order to analyze craniostenosis from an etiologic point of view, cases of various origins must not be pooled but—whenever possible—be separated according to associated symptoms, which may permit a proper classification. Craniostenoses developing in patients with spherocytosis,[10,11] a dominantly transmitted trait, represent a type of their own. Vitamin D-resistant rickets, another disorder of dominant inheritance, may also lead to craniostenosis.[12] In some cases of craniostenosis, recessive inheritance may play a role. Carpenter[13] described 3 children in one family with malformations of the head and extremities showing a certain resemblance to acrocephalosyndactyly without being identical to it. Two of the children probably had congenital heart disease (Carpenter syndrome, p. 901). In two instances mentioned by Franceschetti and Klein,[9] consanguinity of the parents suggested recessive transmission. Craniostenosis in some Ohio Amish sibships probably was due to homozygosity of a recessive gene. In other Amish cases with Crouzon disease, the mode of inheritance was less clear.[68] Hypophosphatasia (p. 859), a condition that often leads to craniostenosis, is considered a recessive trait. In acrocephalosyndactyly there is a striking lack of multiple cases in sibships, only a few instances[14-16] being known in which the condition was observed in two generations.

The occurrence of polyhydramnios, which frequently accompanies pregnancies ending in the delivery of children with acrocephalosyndactyly, is interesting,[17] but at present this association is not understood. Sterility for some years before conception has been observed in mothers who bear children with acrocephalosyndactyly.

How difficult it is to ascertain the role of etiologic factors in craniostenosis may be gathered from studies of this condition in rabbits.[18] Various forms of premature craniosynostosis occur in rabbits and, although they are not identical to those of man, they resemble them sufficiently to permit comparative investigations of pathogenesis and embryology. The cranial deformities are hereditary in the rabbit and experimental test matings can be tried, but the mode of inheritance is not yet established, since many genetic factors seem to be involved. This suggests that the genetics of craniostenosis in man may be more complicated than it appears from some of the statements made in the literature.

High skulls or hypsicephaly occur in twins relatively often. Siemens[19] found such skulls eight times in 86 pairs of twins. In only 1 pair of monozygotic twins did both children show the anomaly, whereas in 4 pairs only 1 twin was affected. It seems possible that in such discordant pairs twinning or the twin pregnancy represents an etiologic factor, but these findings do not permit general conclusions concerning the etiology of craniostenosis, since the twins examined by Siemens had very mild forms of hypsicephaly and premature closure of sutures had not been demonstrated. Older theories that attributed craniostenosis to syphilis or other inflammatory processes, trauma and uterine pressure have been abandoned. That rickets can cause craniostenosis had long been assumed, but this explanation was discarded when prenatal factors were recognized in some cases. But it seems that various types of rickets, deficiency as well as vitamin D-resistant, can be responsible for premature closure of cranial sutures.[20]

Craniostenosis has been observed in many races. It seems that scaphocephaly is relatively frequent in Negroes. Males are affected more often than females. This is particularly true for scaphocephaly, which has a 4:1 predilection for males.[21]

There is little doubt that most craniostenoses are due to premature obliteration of sutures, but the basic mechanisms of premature obliteration of the sutures are not understood. It is true that trauma,[22] inflammation or rickets leads to closure of a suture, but the typical and severe cases of craniostenosis are of different origin. The reasons for premature closure probably will not be understood until we understand why sutures normally remain open for several decades of postnatal life. The entire membranous skull is capable of ossification, except for the small strips that remain fibrous well into the fourth decade of life. What is the intricate mechanism that permits ossification of the peripheral cells of the fibrous strips, while at the same time the central cells remain fibrous and multiply sufficiently to keep the width of the sutures unchanged? It has been suggested that both normal and abnormal sutural fusions are related to tensile forces transmitted to sutural areas by the oriented fiber tracts of the dura mater.[23]

One of the explanations given for premature synostosis is abnormal proximity of the ossification centers of adjacent bones of the cranium in cases of craniostenosis. In both oxycephaly and scaphocephaly, ossification centers are nearer to the obliterated suture than in normal skulls. However, as pointed out by Park and Powers,[3] the displacement of the centers of ossification are not the cause of craniostenosis but only another manifestation of the anomaly. The blastema between the centers is abnormal, permitting the bones to merge. Doerr,[22] after describing 2 cases of cranial deformity attributed to birth trauma, concluded that sutural synostosis in most instances is not the cause but the result of cranial deformities and that brain growth and maturation determine the formation of the cranial vault. Yet, in many cases of acrocephaly, craniectomy prevents or improves damage to the eye and brain, which suggests that the role of craniostenosis must not be underestimated. The differences of opinion concerning the pathognomonic role of craniostenosis and the need for surgical intervention probably result from the fact that premature closure of sutures is not an etiologic entity but a symptom of various disorders.

In the normal newborn infant, the bones of the cranium are still somewhat separated, but soon after birth the definitive sutures are established. In the sutures, the edges of the flat bones are separated by a layer of fibrous tissue, a remnant of the original membranous skull. The bones of the vault grow into this fibrous strip, which, by continuous growth, keeps the sutures open. When this interosseous tissue ceases to grow, the sutures become obliterated. Under normal conditions, only the metopic suture becomes obliterated during childhood, whereas the coronal, sagittal and lambdoid sutures persist into adult life; obliteration does set in before the fourth decade of life.

In the various forms of craniostenosis, obliteration takes place before or soon after birth. The growth of the adjacent bones is inhibited in a direction perpendicular to the course of the obliterated suture. As a result, the diameter of the skull is reduced in this direction but compensatory and abnormal growth takes place in areas and directions in which open fontanelles or open sutures permit it. In oxycephaly, acrocephaly or turricephaly, the coronal suture is chiefly affected, although in many cases the sagittal and

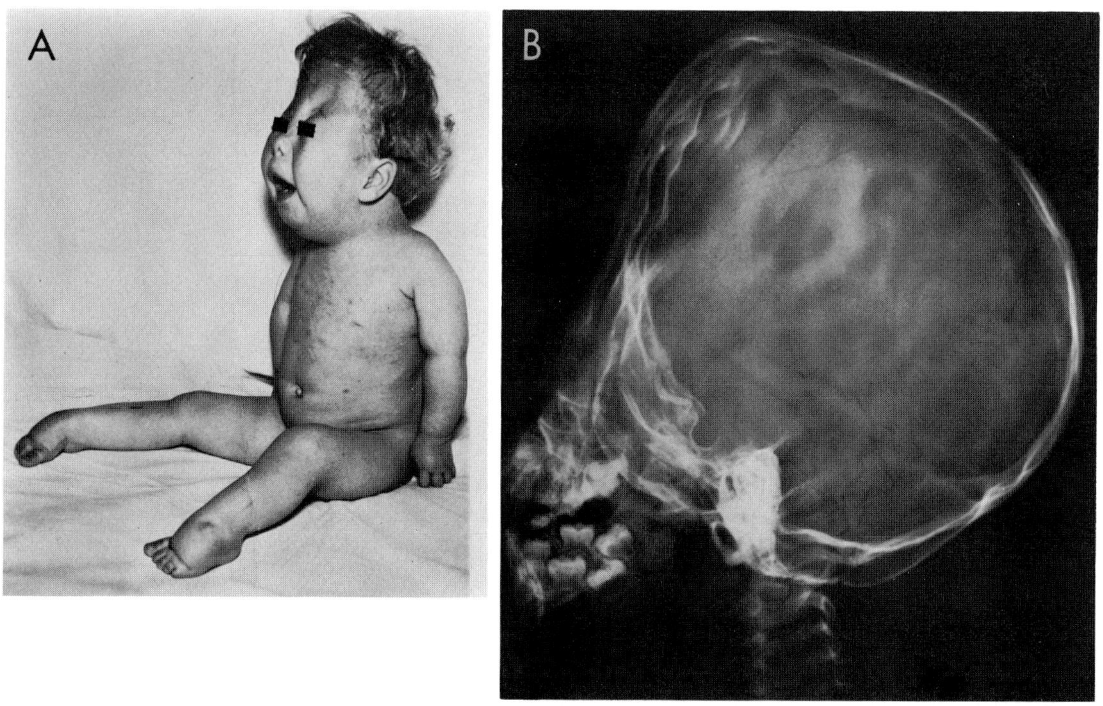

Fig. 95-5. – **A,** acrocephaly, high-arched palate, arthrogryposis, clubfeet, syndactyly of second and third toes. **B,** skull of the child at 28 months of age. The peak of the head is at the bregma. The orbitae are extremely shallow and convolutional markings are pronounced. The sagittal and coronal sutures are obliterated but the lambdoid sutures are clearly visible.

Lower extremities (age 14 months). Right fibula rudimentary, left fibula absent. Extreme varus deformity of both feet shown on page 1003.

lambdoid sutures are also prematurely closed. Sometimes the anterior fontanelle and the metopic suture are widely open and permit limited growth of the skull in abnormal directions. As a result, the frontal, parietal and occipital bones ascend steeply and a high, broad and short skull develops. The highest point is in the region of the anterior fontanelle or the bregma, which is the place in which the last growth is possible. If the sagittal suture is obliterated prematurely, growth in the transverse direction is impaired and a scaphocephalus results. In this condition, the skull is very long and narrow and the parietal protuberances are absent. Owing to brain pressure, the coronal and lambdoid sutures are widened and fronto-occipital elongation takes place. The cephalic index is below 70. Digital impressions and thinning of the bones of the vault are seen in the more severe cases. An osseous crest often develops in place of the obliterated suture.

In oxycephaly or acrocephaly, a bony ridge may be seen or felt along the obliterated coronal suture. The highest point usually is in the place of the anterior fontanelle but it may be near the posterior fontanelle or in an area between the two. The cranial bones are markedly thinned by digital impressions (convolutional atrophy). The internal lamina may be absent and the diploë rarefied. In cases of extreme convolutional atrophy, complete defects are found in the bones of the vault. The frontal and occipital prominences are absent, the circumference of the head is reduced and the cephalic index is above 80 or even over 100. The base of the skull is depressed and the middle and posterior fossae are very deep. The anterior fossa is short in the anteroposterior direction and the sella often enlarged. The vascular foramina sometimes are narrowed, causing venous stasis as manifested by enlargement of the veins of the retina and scalp.

The facial bones often are hypoplastic, particularly in craniofacial dysostosis (Crouzon[5]) (p. 901). The maxilla is small, the palate high and the paranasal sinuses remain undeveloped. The teeth are crowded, deformed and maloccluded. The orbitae are very shallow and their roofs steep. As a rule, the optic foramina are of normal size. The sphenoid bones are widened in the transverse direction and the interorbital distance is increased.

It is understandable that craniostenosis may damage a normal brain. Congenital or early prenatal obliteration of sutures is most injurious. As stressed by Ingraham *et al.*,[24] the brain increases approximately 85% in weight in the first 6 months of life and 135% in the first year. In the following years, growth is slower and after the eighth year little increase occurs. If growth of the brain is inhibited by early craniostenosis, the brain assumes the shape of the deformed skull, the cerebral convolutions are flattened and internal hydrocephaly and optic neuritis and atrophy may develop. The injury to the optic nerve is attributed to traction and distortion of the nerve stem.

However, in some of the cases, brain anomalies can be found that date back to prenatal life. They may not be the result of space limitation but represent associated anomalies caused by the same injurious factors that cause the skeletal anomaly. Aplasia of the corpus callosum or septum pellucidum, meningocele and spina bifida are examples of this type.

Oxycephaly results in very characteristic features. The high, broad and short head has been described. Frontal and parietal bossae and the occipital prominence usually are absent. In infants, membranous regions larger than normal may be palpable in the area of the fontanelles and of those sutures that are not affected by premature synostosis. Owing to the shortness and shallowness of the orbits, exophthalmos is present, sometimes complicated by lagophthalmos and corneal ulcerations. In extreme cases, dislocation of the eyeballs can occur. The palpebral fissures slant outward and downward in an antimongolian fashion. Divergent strabismus is seen frequently and nystagmus sometimes. Vision is defective in the majority of cases. Papilledema or optic atrophy may be seen on ophthalmoscopic examination. The eye ground changes as well as loss of vision progress with age. Headaches are the outstanding subjective signs.

The ears appear to sit low on the head; often they are large and sometimes deformed. Impaired hearing may be observed. The bridge of the nose is broad. The nares are narrow and the septum deviates from the midline. Children thus affected are mouth breathers

Fig. 95-6. – Postural tower head in a boy after immobilization in a cast for congenital dislocation of the hips. There was no craniostenosis demonstrable on x-ray examination.

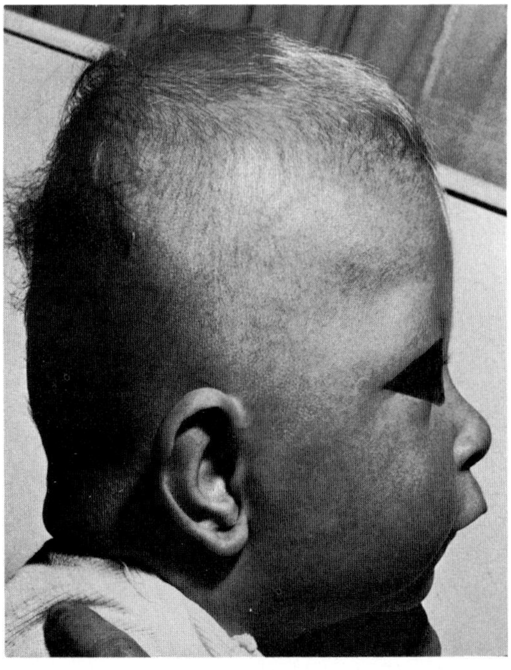

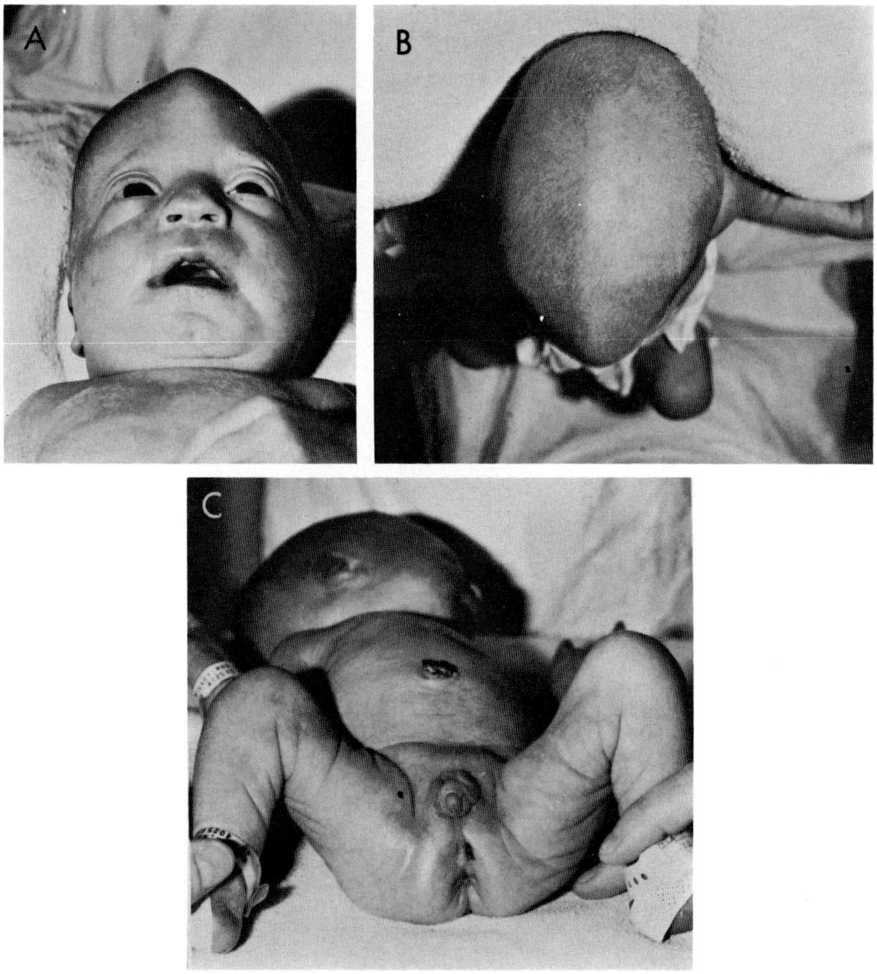

Fig. 95-7. – **A** and **B,** trigonocephaly in a newborn child with ambiguous genitalia (**C**).

and their respiration usually is noisy. The mouth is small, the palate high. Many children with acrocephaly seem to have cleft palate on superficial inspection, since the central part of the hard palate forms a narrow and deep groove. Sometimes it is necessary to insert a sound to prove that the hard palate is closed. The soft palate and the uvula frequently and the hard palate rarely are cleft. The teeth are crowded in malposition, and malocclusion is the rule. The mandible is not characteristically changed; it sometimes is described as micrognathic and sometimes as "protruding." The intracranial pressure may be markedly elevated. It has been estimated that approximately one-fifth of the patients are mentally retarded,[2] but different series differ greatly on this point.[25]

Scaphocephaly is characterized by a long head with marked frontal and occipital protrusion. The head is narrow and the parietal eminences are absent. The obliterated sagittal suture may be indicated by a crest. The bridge of the nose is depressed. Exophthalmos is rare and vision seldom is impaired. Few persons with scaphocephaly develop signs of increased intracranial pressure, but in severe cases of early obliteration, increased intracranial pressure does occur and can be demonstrated by spread of surgically created parasagittal sutures. In some cases, mental retardation occurs concomitantly, but marked scaphocephaly is compatible with superior intelligence.[21]

In oxycephaly, associated malformations are seen frequently. In the skull, enlarged parietal foramina [24,26,27] and platybasia[12] have been observed. Fusion of vertebrae,[26,27] spina bifida[2] and spina bifida occulta[28] can be associated malformations. Occluded choanae occur.[27,29,30] Among cerebral defects, internal hydrocephaly, arhinencephaly[29] and absence of the corpus callosum[31] or of the septum pellucidum[30] have been mentioned. A case of ataxia-telangiectasia presenting with craniostenosis has been described.[32] The extremities participate in syndromes in which syndactyly (p. 899), polydactyly[13,33] clubhands and clubfeet[24,27]

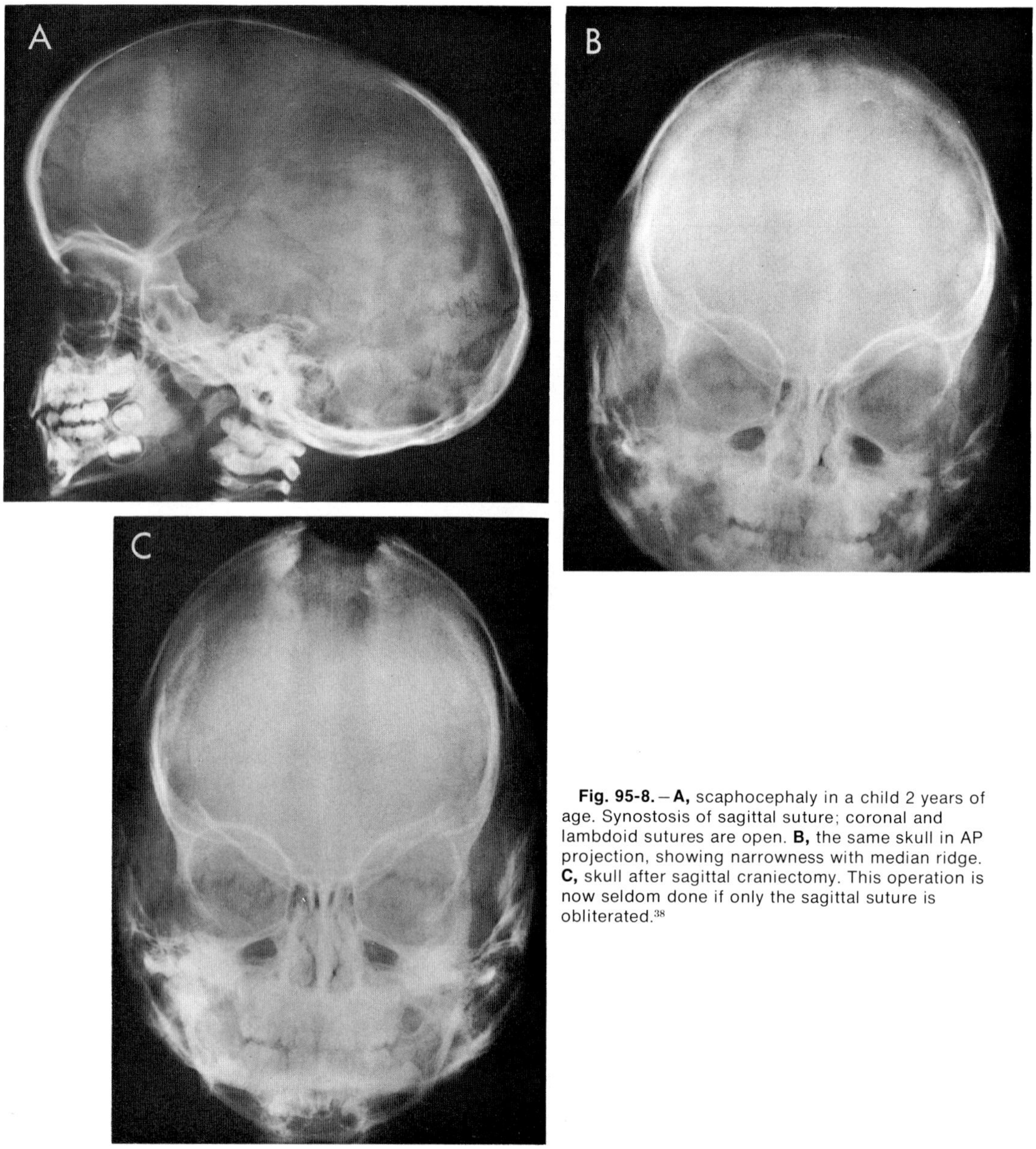

Fig. 95-8. – **A,** scaphocephaly in a child 2 years of age. Synostosis of sagittal suture; coronal and lambdoid sutures are open. **B,** the same skull in AP projection, showing narrowness with median ridge. **C,** skull after sagittal craniectomy. This operation is now seldom done if only the sagittal suture is obliterated.[38]

and ankylosis of the joints of shoulder, elbow, fingers, hip and knees occur.[2] General arthrogryposis was present in 1 of our patients. Congenital heart disease [7,13,30] has been observed repeatedly. Owen[34] described a case in which large ventricular and auricular septal defects and pulmonary stenosis were present. The left innominate vein joined the pulmonary veins and entered the left auricle. There also was congenital hydronephrosis. Cutis frontis gyrata has been observed in monozygotic twins with oxycephaly.[9] In severe and usually lethal cases, exencephaly, arhinencephaly, micromelia, absent fibulae and cystic kidney have been described.[29]

Turricephaly due to craniostenosis can be imitated by deformities of external origin that can occur in the presence of open or even widened cranial sutures. Deformity of the skull can be produced by fixation of the head in postures that mold the cranial bones.[35] There are tower heads produced by tribal customs. For instance, northwest coast American Indians bound the infant's head between two padded boards and the elongated head that resulted was considered a mark of beauty and honor.[36] Although artificial or postural turricephaly can mimic superficially the craniostenotic form, the open sutures can be demonstrated in roentgenograms and craniostenosis ruled out.

Craniostenosis may be found associated with a variety of heterogeneous systemic disorders. It has been observed in patients with chondrodystrophy, Morquio disease, arachnodactyly, osteopetrosis, osteogenesis imperfecta,[12,26] vitamin D-resistant rickets,[12] hypophosphatasia[37] and hemolytic jaundice.[10,11] The association with facial dysostosis is known as Crouzon disease (p. 901) and that with syndactyly as Apert syndrome. In patients with scaphocephaly, associated symptoms occur, but they are rarer and generally of a less serious nature than in those with oxycephaly; mental retardation is also less frequent in scaphocephalics. A long list of anomalies associated with craniostenosis was compiled by Duggan *et al.*[70] The number of combinations probably are unlimited. Association of trigonocephaly (p. 904) and doubtful external genitalia is illustrated in Figure 95-7.

Treatment for craniostenosis causing cerebral or visual disturbances consists of craniectomy. This surgical procedure provides artificial sutures that must remain open during the period of maximum brain growth.[30] Surgical treatment of craniostenosis dates back to the end of the nineteenth century, but success seldom was achieved in such early operations, which often were performed on microcephalic children or with inadequate methods.[38,39] Operative treatment was taken up again in this century to prevent blindness[40] and for the relief of cerebral pressure symptoms; very satisfactory results were obtained in many cases. The operation of choice is linear craniectomy parallel to the suture, which is prematurely fused, with insertion of polyethylene film over the bony margins to delay closure. Operation in early infancy has been advocated to prevent mental retardation and visual impairment and to improve cosmetic appearance. But it must be emphasized that such complications usually fail to develop in cases of scaphocephaly due to isolated premature closure of the sagittal suture and that surgical treatment of such patients seems unwarranted.[38] To obtain good cosmetic results in patients with marked scaphocephaly, deliberate molding of the brain by duraplasty as well as by cranioplasty has been recommended.[21] Surgical treatment has been recommended for all cases with two or more obliterated sutures; whether to operate if only one suture is involved is debatable.[39] In well-defined cases, operation can be performed by the age of 3 months without serious complications.[41]

Acrocephalosyndactyly (Apert Syndrome)

In this syndrome, craniostenosis and syndactyly are the outstanding features. The malformations date back to the mesenchymal stage of development, when incomplete differentiation of localized areas of the skull and of the appendicular skeleton initiates the syndrome. Occasionally, other organs are affected simultaneously; if the heart is involved, the chances of survival are reduced and only a few cases of this type have been observed in older age groups. Articles on this disorder were written by Park and Powers,[3] Ferriman[7] and Grebe.[17] The incidence has been estimated as 1 in 100,000 births[42,43] and the prevalence as 1 in 2,000,000 in the general population.[44]

Only rarely can heredity be demonstrated, since most cases are sporadic. But instances of transmission from a parent to a child have been reported[14,15,44,45] and Pfeiffer[16] observed a "mild form of acrocephalosyndactylism in 3 generations of a kindred in which 8 members were affected." Patients with severe acrocephaly are not likely to reproduce and, therefore, remain "sporadic."

There is a high incidence of hydramnios in pregnancies resulting in this syndrome.[17] Increased paternal age has been cited as a possible etiologic factor.[42-44] Although syndactyly often has been produced experimentally in rodents, craniostenosis—to my knowledge—has not. Acrocephalosyndactyly is not associated with chromosomal anomalies.[46] In one of our cases in which acrocephalosyndactyly was associated with cleft palate, the chromosomal pattern was normal (Cincinnati General Hospital Chart No. 381152). In one instance, enlargement of a chromosome no. 1 has been reported.[47]

The condition can be recognized at birth, since the head as well as the hands and feet show the typical

Fig. 95-9.—Acrocephalosyndactyly and preauricular tab. The palate was high-arched. Pregnancy of mother complicated by hydramnios.

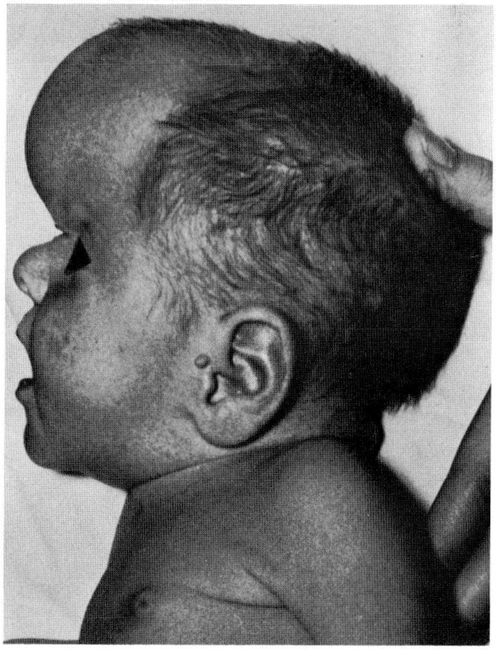

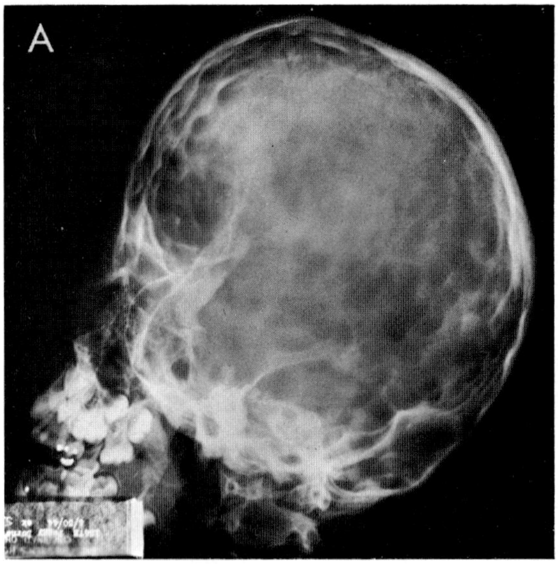

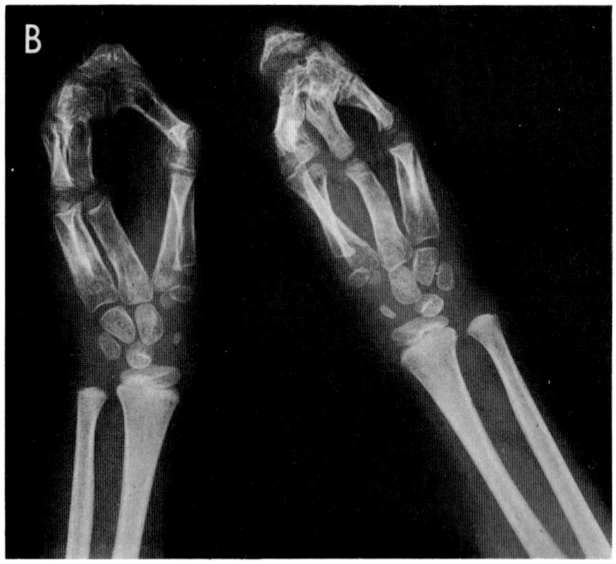

Fig. 95-10. – **A,** acrocephaly in a girl 6 years of age. Steep and high forehead, shallow orbitae, all sutures obliterated. **B,** syndactyly of the hands in the same child. Fusion of fourth and fifth metacarpal bones. The fusion of the phalanges is most marked in the distal parts. The feet showed similar syndactyly.

malformations on first inspection. The sutures of the skull are partly obliterated. The open stretches of the sutures and the open fontanelles yield to the increased intracranial pressure and usually become *larger* than normal. The metopic suture, which separates the two halves of the frontal bone in fetal life, remains open for some time after birth. The veins of the scalp are dilated. As closure of the sutures and fontanelles progresses, a high tower skull develops. The peak of the head is at the bregma, the point of junction of the sagittal and coronal sutures. The forehead is high and ascends steeply. Frontal bossing is seen in many cases but the fronto-occipital diameter usually is reduced. The eyes are far apart, bulging and assume an antimongoloid tilt. Divergent strabismus and visual disturbances may develop. The external ears often are large and sometimes are deformed. Deafness develops in later life. The maxilla is hypoplastic and the nose prominent. The palate is high and may be narrowed to a sagittal cleft in the midline, which often is mistaken for a cleft palate. True cleft palate is rare[42] but the soft palate and the uvula may be split. The nasal cavity is reduced in size; respiration is labored and funnel chest may develop. The mandible is relatively large, so that prognathism becomes apparent. The central part of the face may be depressed between the bulging forehead and the protruding mandible.[28] There is extensive syndactyly of the hands and feet. As a rule, digits II–IV (and sometimes V) appear fused completely into a plate, with distal union of the nails. The shape of the undifferentiated hand has been likened to a spoon. The thumb usually remains separated from the other fingers, but it is short and its terminal phalanx hypoplastic. The toes show similar lack of differentiation and a sixth digit may add to the unusual appearance of the foot.[33,42] The syndactyly, which appears so complete externally, is less complete in roentgenograms. Often the third and fourth phalanges are fused at their distal ends, with irregularities of some of the finger joints. Movements in the elbow, shoulder and hip joints are limited because of deformities of their articular elements. Anomalies in the elbows have been emphasized by Pillay.[42] The ossification centers appear late, the upper ends of the radii are rounded, radii and ulnae are separated and there is subluxation of the proximal radio-ulnar joints. As a rule, the patients are short in stature. Mental development often is subnormal, but deafness and the physical handicaps may contribute more to the mental dullness than cerebral inferiority. Roentgenograms at birth demonstrate the obliteration of the coronal suture, the most important characteristic of the syndrome conducive to treatment. The inner table of the calvarium develops a beaten-silver appearance in untreated cases. In addition, a basilar lordosis, hypoplasia of facial bones with underdeveloped paranasal sinuses and shallow orbital cavities are noticeable in older children. The palate is highly arched and the teeth crowded in the maxilla. Dental malposition is the rule. In the extremities, a few abnormalities may be discovered that are not noticeable externally. Usually, malformations are more pronounced in the upper extremities than in the lower; symmetry of the malformations has been reported in most instances. Transitional forms resembling Crouzon disease (p. 901) exist.[48]

Associated malformations occur. Hydrocephaly, absence of the corpus callosum,[49] congenital heart

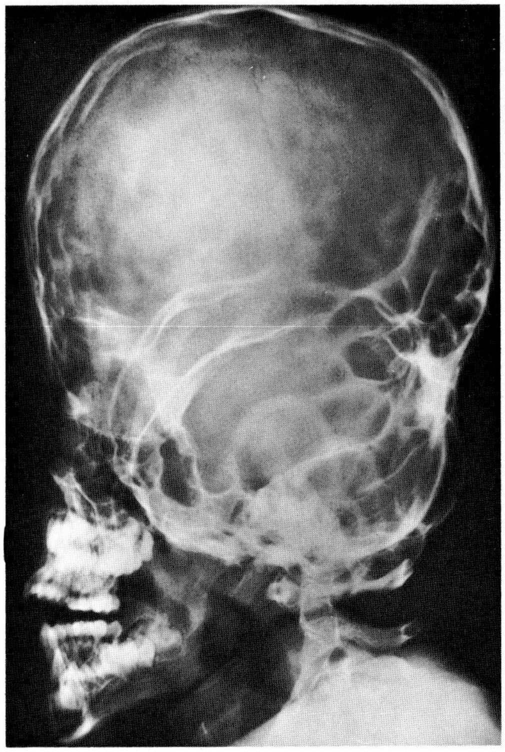

Fig. 95-11.—Tower skull in a girl 2½ years of age. Steep forehead, shallow orbitae, obliteration of all sutures, marked convolutional markings.

disease,[34] hydronephrosis, imperforate anus, polydactyly and others have been recorded.[7] Obesity and acrocephalosyndactyly have been reported by Bravo,[50] and Warkany *et al.*[33] observed the disorder combined with polydactyly, a condition now termed Carpenter syndrome.

To make room for the expanding brain, the prematurely obliterated cranium must be reopened by surgical means.[30] Several operations that allow skull expansion have been recommended, but some of these are only of temporary benefit, since the divided bones have a tendency to heal and to reunite after 4–8 months. For this reason, artificially created sutures or decompression have not proved practical when performed in infancy and before completion of the most intensive brain growth. Spontaneous closure of the opened channels makes secondary operations necessary. Ingraham *et al.*[24] recommended linear craniectomy and prevention of closure by placing polyethylene film over the cut edges of the artificial sutures. For coronal synostosis, a coronal craniectomy is performed, extending from one squamosal suture across the vertex to the other. There should be spreading of the artificial sutures immediately after operation. In well-established cases of craniostenosis, the operation should be performed in early infancy, since damage to the brain and eyes by increased intracranial pressure must be prevented. Yet, it remains to be seen how many persons with premature synostoses require operation. It is likely that many children show some obliteration of cranial sutures in roentgenograms without developing deformities or signs of increased intracranial pressue.[49] The indications for operation in such mild cases are yet to be established.

Carpenter Syndrome

A syndrome standing between acrocephalosyndactyly and the Laurence-Moon-Biedl syndrome was discussed by Temtamy.[51] The author described a patient with acrocephaly, peculiar facies, brachysyndactyly of the fingers, preaxial polydactyly and syndactyly of the toes, hypogenitalism, obesity and mental retardation. There also was coxa valga, genu valgum, pes varus, congenital heart disease and abdominal hernias. It seems that the syndrome has been observed repeatedly in siblings, and autosomal recessive inheritance is suggested. No chromosomal aberrations or biochemical defects were identified. The disorder had been reported before,[13,33] and differentiation from acrocephalosyndactyly is not always easy.[42,67]

Craniofacial Dysostosis (Crouzon)

This syndrome represents craniostenosis of a special type. Although it has many features in common with other forms of oxycephaly, it often can be recognized at a glance by certain external features, and simple dominant inheritance can be proved in many cases. In Crouzon's first description[5] of the syndrome, a mother and her son were affected. Flippen[52] reported the condition in four generations and Dodge *et al.*[48] in three. Pinkerton and Pinkerton[53] illustrated a family in which the mother transmitted the syndrome to 3 of her children, whereas 2 appeared completely free of the trait. This family picture shows well the complete segregation of the trait. Vulliamy and Normandale[54] reported a pedigree with 14 affected members in four generations, demonstrating autosomal dominant inheritance. Disabilities due to the disorder were not pronounced in their kindred, whose affected members developed craniosynostosis after birth. Chromosomes were normal in the cases tested.[66] In some families, mildly affected persons showed only hypertelorism, moderate exophthalmos and prognathism but they transmitted the condition to some of their children, who were severely affected.[55] Thus, intrafamilial variability of expressivity of the gene must be kept in mind by the genetic counselor. Although heredity can be demonstrated in only two-thirds of the cases,[56] the possibility of transmission to the offspring cannot be excluded in a sporadic but otherwise typical case, since it may represent a new mutation. On the other hand, the existence of atypical nonhereditary cases must be considered possible (p. 894).

Well-developed cases are recognizable at birth. The

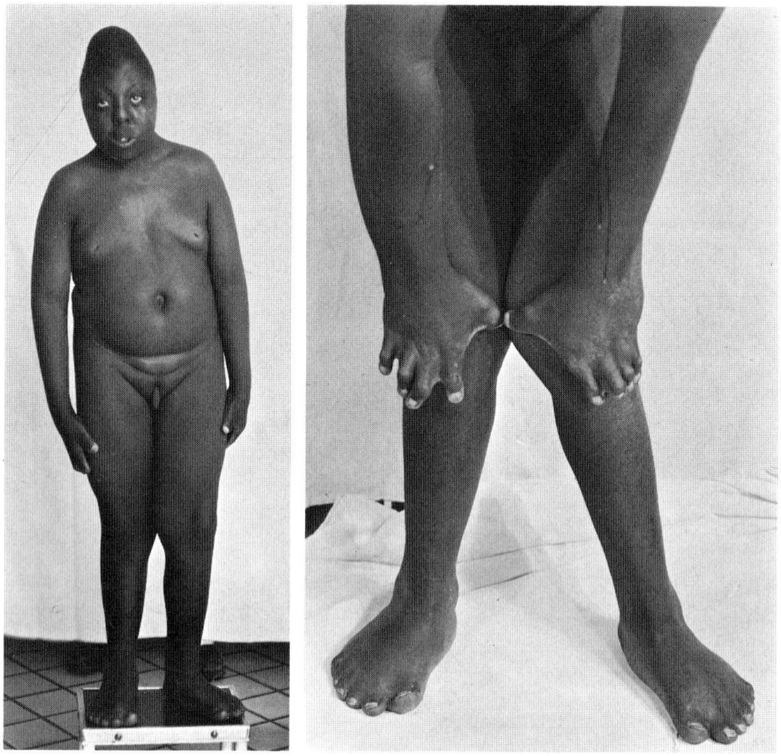

Fig. 95-12.—This patient can be classified as a case of Carpenter syndrome but also as one of acrocephalosyndactyly or Laurence-Moon-Biedl syndrome[33] (hypogenitalism, obesity, polydactyly and mental retardation, Chapter 19).

skull shows a peak at the anterior fontanelle, which is barely open on palpation. The metopic suture may be open but the sagittal and coronal sutures are obliterated and indicated by crests. During the first few years of life, the metopic suture as well as the anterior fontanelle may become permanently fused and replaced by bony eminences. In some patients, premature closure of all sutures can be demonstrated at birth.[55] In such cases, the area of the anterior fontanelle comes to a striking peak and the eyes show hypertelorism, exophthalmos and often strabismus. In later life, vision becomes impaired and optic atrophy may set in. The external ears are set low and sometimes are deformed. Hypoplasia of the maxilla, which is the rule, results in shortness of the upper lip and a high palate. The nose often shows anterior convexity and has been likened to a parrot beak. The nasal cavity and the nasal sinuses are reduced in size. Breathing is loud and labored. The mandible protrudes beyond the alveolar crest of the maxilla. There is poor occlusion of the incisor teeth, since the upper incisors are posterior to the lower ones. In addition to visual disturbances, the patients have headaches and sometimes convulsions. Fifth ventricles demonstrable by pneumoencephalograms have been reported.[48] The mentality is low in many cases, yet some of these patients can lead a full life, marry and pass on their anomaly to some of their children. Syndactyly is not a symptom of Crouzon disease but it can occur, and then the differentiation from acrocephalosyndactyly becomes doubtful.[48] A girl with Crouzon syndrome and congenital heart disease has been observed in the Cincinnati Children's Hospital (Chart No. 162811). She had a normal twin brother and her parents appeared to be normal. A related syndrome occurring in a woman and 2 of her sons included craniosynostosis, hypertelorism, epicanthic folds, commissural lip pits, supernumerary teeth and variations of the oral frenula.[71]

To avoid damage to the brain and to the eyes, early surgical treatment is recommended (p. 901). A warning concerning surgical procedures was expressed by Pinkerton and Pinkerton,[53] and death following operation has been reported. But progressive exophthalmos, optic atrophy or loss of visual acuity, increasing intracranial pressure or signs of mental deterioration are indications for surgical intervention. In severe cases, plastic surgery may be necessary for cosmetic reasons.

Craniofacial Dysostosis with Dental, Cardiac and Genital Anomalies

A syndrome of premature synostosis of the coronal suture, facial hypoplasia (craniofacial dysostosis), patent ductus arteriosus, hypertrichosis, hypoplasia

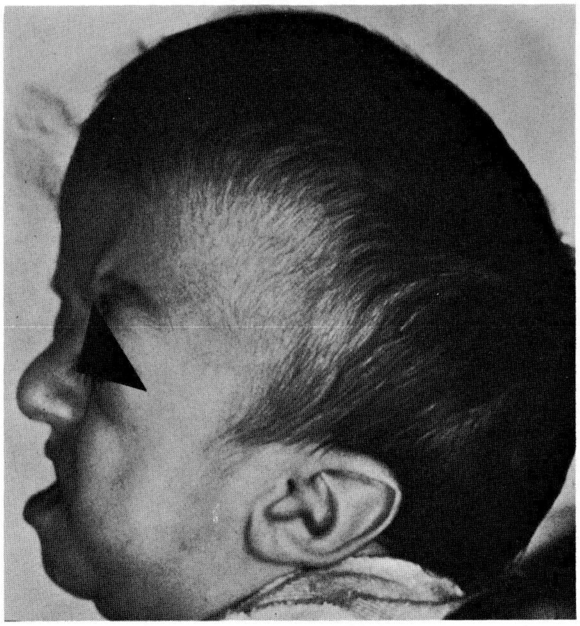

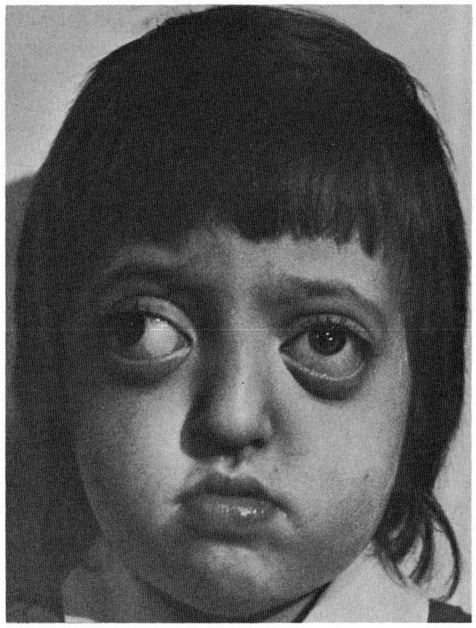

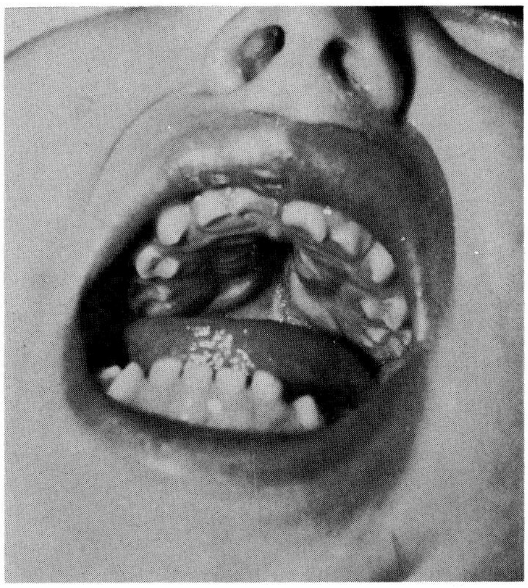

Fig. 95-13 (above left). – Crouzon craniofacial dysostosis in an infant. Sagittal and coronal sutures closed, anterior fontanelle bulging, fingers and toes normal. Negative family history. Child died at 2½ months of age.

Fig. 95-14 (above right). – Girl with Crouzon craniofacial dysostosis. Age 4 years. Cleft of soft palate. Negative family history.

Fig. 95-15 (left). – Palate in a child with Crouzon syndrome. The midline groove in the palate simulates a cleft but there is no connection between the oral and nasal cavities.

of labia majora and dental and ocular anomalies was described in 2 sisters by Gorlin *et al.*[58] The craniofacial profile showed protrusion of the forehead and of the mandible, with concave recession of the facial area. Long and dense hair of the scalp and hypertrichosis of the body added to the peculiar picture. In contrast to severe craniostenosis, the eyes were deep-set and not exophthalmic. The palpebral fissures had an antimongoloid slant and the upper eyelids were notched. Microphthalmia and hyperopia were present. The palate was high-arched and there were many dental anomalies. The syndrome has some features of mandibulofacial dysostosis (p. 650) but it is better classified as a subgroup of the craniostenoses and craniofacial dysostoses.

Sporadic Craniofacial Dysostosis

It has been stated that evidence of heredity can be found in only two-thirds of the reported cases of Crouzon craniofacial dysostosis.[56] The remainder could be explained by assuming that they represent new mutations or that in their ancestors reduced penetrance or expressivity concealed the hereditary aspects of the disorder. It is possible, however, that some sporadic cases showing resemblance to the hereditary type may be of different etiology and possibly be nonhereditary. Dunn[28] described a boy, 5 years of age, with a bird-like facies, wide cleft palate and a large triangular defect in the frontal region, the apex pointing toward the nasion. The ears were low-set and the eyes small and without exophthalmos. The maxillary and mandibular regions were underdeveloped. The skull was scaphoid and there was complete synostosis of the sagittal suture. Hypertelorism, underdeveloped parietal foramina and a V-shaped hypoplastic mandible were additional findings. A spina bifida occulta extending from the tenth thoracic vertebra to the sacrum was seen in roentgenograms. These findings differ from Crouzon syndrome, and Dunn[28] considered the condition nonhereditary.

Craniostenosis with Vitamin D-Resistant Rickets

Craniostenosis due to premature obliteration of the cranial sutures was described by Imerslund[12] in a boy with vitamin D-resistant rickets. His head was long and narrow and the tubera frontalia were prominent. A ridge could be seen in place of the sagittal suture. Roentgenograms of the skull showed increased digital impressions and a prominence in the area of the anterior fontanelle. His mother had a similar skull with a high and narrow head, with platybasia, digital impressions and some prominences over the obliterated sutures. Coleman and Foote[57] pointed out that scaphocephaly had been mentioned previously in the literature on vitamin D-resistant rickets without description of the underlying craniostenosis. They also described a boy with marked scaphocephaly due to premature obliteration of the sagittal suture. In the case of Imerslund,[12] the signs of increased intracranial pressure were sufficiently pronounced to require decompressive craniotomy.

Unilateral Coronostenosis

Premature unilateral coronal synostosis may be betrayed soon after birth by unilateral exophthalmos, asymmetry of the face and flattening of the frontoparietal area. Roentgenograms reveal narrowing of one coronal suture with partial obliteration, deformity of one orbit, shortening of the anterior and deepening of the middle and posterior fossae and depression of the petrous ridge. The nasal septum and the lambda suture are deviating and asymmetric. Hyperopia, astigmatism, optic atrophy and strabismus may be present. Unilateral exophthalmos with flattening of the ipsilateral frontoparietal region is considered pathognomonic for the condition. Mental retardation and associated congenital malformations seem to be rare. Recognition of the condition is of practical importance because it can be relieved by surgical procedures.[59]

Trigonocephaly

This congenital defect of the skull is characterized by a keel-like ridge at the site of the metopic suture. The suture may be closed or open.[60] The head, when seen from above, appears triangular or egg-shaped (oocephaly) (see Fig. 95-7, *B*) and the biparietal diameter is increased. In the presence of a crest over the metopic suture, a vertical bony ridge can be seen or felt in the midline of the forehead and the frontal eminences are absent. Uncomplicated cases can be considered as the mildest form of the cyclopia series (p. 201). In more complex cases, trigonocephaly is associated with arhinencephaly or cyclopia (p. 209). If the rhinencephalon is absent, the lamina cribrosa of the ethmoid bone also may be absent or be imperforate. The frontal ossification centers lie closer together than normal. Currarino and Silverman[61] believed that the metopic suture is always prematurely obliterated in part or completely, the obliteration being demonstrable roentgenographically or post mortem. The orbits are close together (hypotelorism) and their inferior lateral angles sometimes are low-set. Externally, the eyes show mongoloid slanting. The orbital roofs are high in relation to the horizontal plate of the ethmoid, which is reduced in size. The anterior cranial fossa is small.

Whether early obliteration of the metopic suture is the primary defect of trigonocephaly or the result of a defect of the forebrain is a moot point. There probably are different types of this cranial deformity. It can occur in the presence of an entirely normal brain[61] or it can be associated with arhinencephaly and other congenital anomalies such as absence of the falx, corpus callosum, septum pellucidum, premaxilla, nasal septum and philtrum. Microcephaly, lissencephaly (p. 242) and various brain defects of the cyclopia series[61] have been observed. The viability of such severely affected patients is doubtful, but uncomplicated trigonocephaly is compatible with a normal life.

Cloverleaf Head (Kleeblattschädel)

Holtermüller and Wiedemann[62] described a rare congenital malformation of the head characterized by a huge protrusion of the skull and marked broadening of the temporal region and of the face. The protrusion on top of the skull is separated from the facial bulges by a furrow representing the normal dimensions of the face in the plane of the eyes. The result of these changes is a grotesque cloverleaf-shaped head. The external ears, which are situated very low, assume a horizontal position. Corresponding to the externally visible furrow there is within the skull an osseous shelf that separates a frontal vesicle of the brain from two temporal vesicles. The eyeballs protrude because of shortening of the orbital fossa; corneal ulceration and blindness can occur.[63] Antimongoloid palpebral fissures are described in some of the cases. The entire skull base is short owing to premature synostosis of the tribasilare. The foramen magnum and the jugular foramina are narrow. The sagittal, coronal and lambdoid sutures show premature synostosis. The occipital bone is small and protrusion of the brain resembling an occipital exencephalocele may be seen. Cutis verticis gyrata may cover the posterior aspects of the skull (Fig. 95-16, *B*) (Cincinnati Chil-

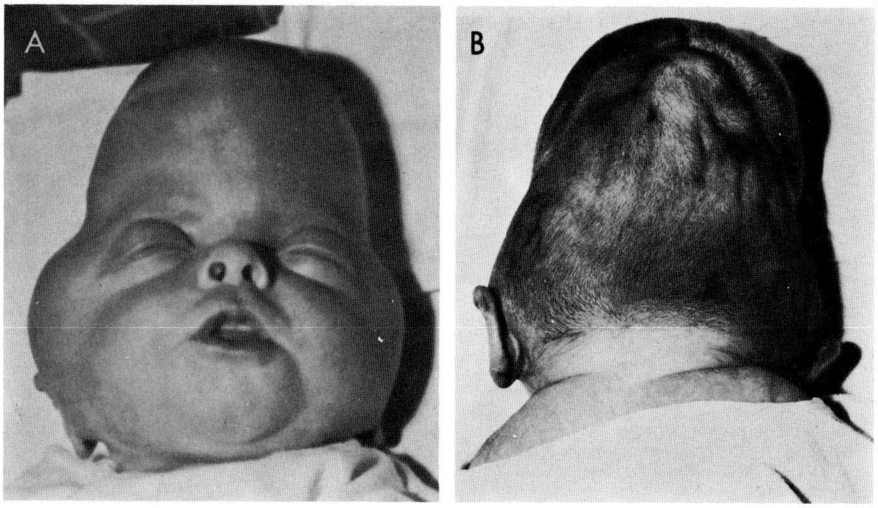

Fig. 95-16. – Cloverleaf head (Kleeblattschädel) in a newborn boy. **A,** front view, showing general shape of head and bulges in the temporal areas. **B,** rear view, showing cutis verticis gyrata and midline protrusion in the occipital area.

dren's Hospital Chart No. 202330). There is marked hydrocephaly. Micromelia with chondrodystrophic changes occurred in some but not in all cases. Cloverleaf head may contribute to the neonatal lethality of chondrodystrophy[69] (Chapter 83). The palate is high but cleft palate is rare. The report by Holtermüller and Wiedemann[62] included a review of 12 cases published previously in the German literature. Comings[64] described a case from Alaska "with almost extraterrestrial appearance." In addition to the features described there was macrostomia, macroglossia and a rudimentary tooth prematurely erupted. Ankylosis of the fingers and joints, syndactyly and contraction of fingers occur. The karyotype appears normal.[63, 64] Survival to 14 years has been observed.[69]

Bathrocephaly

This step-like deformity at the back of the head is due to elevation of the occipital squama over the parietal bones. The anomaly is harmless and occurs in otherwise normal persons.[65]

REFERENCES

1. Greig, D. M.: Oxycephaly, Edinburgh M. J. 33:189, 1926.
2. Günther, H.: Über konstitutionelle Varianten der Schädelform und ihre klinische Bedeutung, Virchows Arch. path. Anat. 278:309, 1930.
3. Park, E. A., and Powers, G. F.: Acrocephaly and scaphocephaly with symmetrically distributed malformations of the extremities, study of so-called "acrocephalosyndactylism," Am. J. Dis. Child. 20:235, 1920.
4. Apert, E.: De l'acrocéphalo-syndactylie, Bull. Soc. méd. hôp. Paris 23:1310, 1906.
5. Crouzon, O.: Dysostose craniofaciale héréditaire, Presse méd. 20:737, 1912.
6. Crouzon, O.: Dysostose cranio-faciale héréditaire, Arch. méd. Enf. 18:529, 1915.
7. Ferriman, D.: The genetics of true oxycephaly and acrocephalosyndactyly, Proc. Internat. Genet. Cong. 7:120, 1941.
8. French, L. A., and Suechting, R. L.: Familial incidence of craniosynostosis, A.M.A. Am. J. Dis. Child. 89:486, 1955.
9. Franceschetti, A., and Klein, D.: Oxycéphalie chez trois paires de jumeaux univitellins, associée dans un des cas à une cutis frontis gyrata, Acta genet. med. 1:48, 1952.
10. Gänsslen, M., Zipperlen, E., and Schüz, E.: Die hämolytische Konstitution, Deutsches Arch. klin. Med. 146:1, 1925.
11. Devine, J.: Familial acholuric jaundice with bone changes, treated by splenectomy, M. J. Australia 1:557, 1947.
12. Imerslund, O.: Craniostenosis and vitamin D-resistant rickets, Acta paediat. 40:449, 1951.
13. Carpenter, G.: Case of acrocephaly with other congenital malformations, Proc. Roy. Soc. Med. Sec. Dis. Child. 2:45, 1908.
14. Weech, A. A.: Combined acrocephaly and syndactylism occurring in mother and daughter, Bull. Johns Hopkins Hosp. 40:73, 1927.
15. Chotzen, F.: Eine eigenartige familiäre Entwicklungsstörung (Akrocephalosyndaktylie, Dysostosis craniofacialis und Hypertelorismus), Monatsschr. Kinderh. 55: 97, 1932.
16. Pfeiffer, R. A.: Dominant erbliche Akrocephalosyndaktylie, Ztschr. Kinderh. 90:301, 1964.
17. Grebe, H.: Die Akrocephalosyndaktylie. Eine klinisch-ätiologische Studie, Ztschr. menschl. Vererb.-u. Konstitutionslehre 28:209, 1944.
18. Greene, H. S. N.: Oxycephaly and allied conditions in man and in the rabbit, J. Exper. Med. 57:967, 1933.
19. Siemens, H. W.: Zur Ätiologie des Turmschädels nebst Mitteilung einer dermatologischen Methode zur Diagnose der Eineiigkeit bei Zwillingen, Virchows Arch. path. Anat. 253:746, 1924.
20. Reilly, B. J., Leeming, J. M., and Fraser, D.: Craniosynostosis in the rachitic spectrum, J. Pediat. 64:396, 1964.
21. Mullan, S.: Late moulding of the scaphocephalic skull, A. M.A. J. Dis. Child. 99:55, 1960.
22. Doerr, W.: Über die geburtstraumatische Nahtsynostose des kindlichen Schädeldaches, Ztschr. Kinderh. 67:96, 1949.
23. Moss, M. L.: Inhibition and stimulation of sutural fusion in the rat calvaria, Anat. Rec. 136:457, 1960.

24. Ingraham, F. D., Matson, D. D., and Alexander, E., Jr.: Experimental observations in treatment of craniosynostosis, Surgery 23:252, 1948.
25. Gordon, H.: Craniostenosis, Brit. M. J. 2:792, 1959.
26. Peter, A. L.: Oxycephaly associated with Klippel-Feil syndrome and other skeletal defects, Am. J. Ophth. 29:685, 1946.
27. Freeman, J. M., and Borkowf, S.: Craniostenosis; review of the literature and report of thirty-four cases, Pediatrics 30:57, 1962.
28. Dunn, F. H.: Nonfamilial and nonhereditary craniofacial dyostosis: A variant of Crouzon's disease, Am. J. Roentgenol. 84:472, 1960.
29. Gruber, G. B.: Beiträge zur Frage "gekoppelter" Missbildungen, Beitr. path. Anat. 93:459, 1934.
30. McLaurin, R. L., and Matson, D. D.: Importance of early surgical treatment of craniosynostosis, Pediatrics 10:637, 1952.
31. Martischnig, E., and Thalhammer, O.: Akrocephalosyndaktylie (Erörterung der Genese vom Gesichtspunkt der Embryopathie), Helvet. paediat. acta 7:257, 1952.
32. Robinson, A.: Ataxia-telangiectasia presenting with craniostenosis, Arch. Dis. Childhood 37:652, 1962.
33. Warkany, J., Frauenberger, G. S., and Mitchell, A. G.: Heredofamilial deviations; 1. The Laurence-Moon-Biedl syndrome, Am. J. Dis. Child. 53:455, 1937.
34. Owen, R. H.: Acrocephalosyndactyly. A case with congenital cardiac abnormalities, Brit. J. Radiol. 25:103, 1952.
35. Pancoast, H. K., Pendergrass, E. P., and Schaeffer, J. P.: *The Head and Neck in Roentgen Diagnosis* (Springfield, Ill.: Charles C Thomas, Publisher, 1940).
36. Josephy, A. M., and Brandon, W.: *The American Heritage Book of Indians* (New York: American Heritage Publishing Company, Inc., 1961).
37. Currarino, G., Neuhauser, E. B. D., Reyersbach, G. C., and Sobel, E.: Hypophosphatasia, Am. J. Roentgenol. 78:392, 1957.
38. Hemple, D. J., Harris, L. E., Svien, H. J., and Holman, C. B.: Craniosynostosis involving the sagittal suture only: Guilt by association?, J. Pediat. 58:342, 1961.
39. Andersson, H., and Gomes, S. P.: Craniosynostosis. Review of the literature and indications for surgery, Acta paediat. scandinav. 57:47, 1968.
40. Faber, H. K., and Towne, E. B.: Early operation in premature cranial synostosis for the prevention of blindness and other sequelae, J. Pediat. 22:286, 1943.
41. Anderson, F. M., and Geiger, L.: Craniosynostosis; a survey of 204 cases, J. Neurosurg. 22:229, 1965.
42. Pillay, V. K.: Acrocephalosyndactyly in Singapore; a study of five Chinese males, J. Bone & Joint Surg. 46-B: 94, 1964.
43. Tünte, W., and Lenz, W.: Zur Häufigkeit und Mutationsrate des Apert-Syndroms, Humangenetik 4:104, 1967.
44. Blank, C. E.: Apert's syndrome (a type of acrocephalosyndactyly)–observations on a British series of thirty-nine cases, Ann. Human Genet. 24:151, 1960.
45. Mohr, O. L.: Dominant acrocephalosyndactyly, Hereditas 25:193, 1939.
46. Ford, C. E.: Human cytogenetics: Its present place and future possibilities, Am. J. Human Genet. 12:104, 1960.
47. Genest, P., Mortezai, M. A., and Tremblay, M.: Le syndrome d'Apert (acrocéphalosyndactylie). Une observation avec un chromosome l abnormal, Arch. franç. pédiat. 23: 887, 1966.
48. Dodge, H. W., Jr., Wood, M. W., and Kennedy, R. L. J.: Craniofacial dysostosis: Crouzon's disease, Pediatrics 23: 98, 1959.
49. Schönenberg, H.: Zur Pathogenese des Turmschädels, der Dysostosis craniofacialis sowie der Acrocephalosyndaktylie, Ztschr. Kinderh. 79:355, 1957.
50. Bravo, T.: Sindrome adiposo-genital con malformaciones congénitas, Rev. neuro-psiquiat. 6:205, 1943.
51. Temtamy, S. A.: Carpenter's syndrome: Acrocephalopolysyndactyly. An autosomal recessive syndrome, J. Pediat. 69:111, 1966.
52. Flippen, J. H., Jr.: Craniofacial dysostosis of Crouzon. Report of a case in which the malformation occurred in four generations, Pediatrics 5:90, 1950.
53. Pinkerton, O. D., and Pinkerton, F. J.: Hereditary craniofacial dysplasia, Am. J. Ophth. 35:500, 1952.
54. Vulliamy, D. G., and Normandale, P. A.: Craniofacial dysostosis in a Dorset family, Arch. Dis. Childhood 41: 375, 1966.
55. Shiller, J. G.: Craniofacial dysostosis of Crouzon. A case report and pedigree with emphasis on heredity, Pediatrics 23:107, 1959.
56. Atkinson, F. R. B.: Hereditary craniofacial dysostosis or Crouzon's disease, M. Press 195:118, 1937.
57. Coleman, E. N., and Foote, J. B.: Craniostenosis with familial vitamin D-resistant rickets, Brit. M. J. 1:561, 1954.
58. Gorlin, R. J., Chaudhry, A. P., and Moss, M. L.: Craniofacial dysostosis, patent ductus arteriosus, hypertrichosis, hypoplasia of labia majora, dental and eye anomalies–a new syndrome?, J. Pediat. 56:778, 1960.
59. Nathan, M. H., Collins, V. P., and Collins, L. C.: Premature unilateral synostosis of the coronal suture, Am. J. Roentgenol. 86:433, 1961.
60. Riemenschneider, P. A.: Trigonocephaly, Radiology 68: 863, 1957.
61. Currarino, G., and Silverman, F. N.: Orbital hypotelorism, arhinencephaly, and trigonocephaly, Radiology 74:206, 1960.
62. Holtermüller, K., and Wiedemann, H-R.: Kleeblattschädel-Syndrom, Med. Monatsschr. 14:439, 1960.
63. Angle, C. R., McIntire, M. S., and Moore, R. C.: Cloverleaf skull: Kleeblattschädel-deformity syndrome, Am. J. Dis. Child. 114:198, 1967.
64. Comings, D. E.: The Kleeblattschädel syndrome–a grotesque form of hydrocephalus, J. Pediat. 67:126, 1965.
65. Epstein, J. A., and Epstein, B. S.: Deformities of the skull surfaces in infancy and childhood, J. Pediat. 70:636, 1967.
66. Alfieri, A., Alù. C., and Ceccarini, M.: Dysostose craniofaciale héréditaire et syndactylie, J. Génét. Hum. 16:1, 1967.
67. Palacios, E., and Schimke, R. N.: Craniosynostosis-syndactylism, Am. J. Roentgenol. 106:144, 1969.
68. Cross, H. E., and Opitz, J. M.: Craniosynostosis in the Amish, J. Pediat. 75:1037, 1969.
69. Feingold, M., O'Connor, J. F., Berkman, M., and Darling, D. B.: Kleeblattschädel syndrome, Am. J. Dis. Child. 118: 589, 1969.
70. Duggan, C. A., Keener, E. B., and Gay, B. B.: Secondary craniosynostosis, Am. J. Roentgenol. 190:277, 1970.
71. Kernohan, D. C., Nevin, N. C., and Dodge, J. A.: Familial craniosynostosis with oral anomalies, Developmental Med. & Child. Neurol. 12:315, 1970.

96

Craniovertebral Anomalies

IN EMBRYOS about 6 weeks old, a cartilaginous plate is formed from the ectomeninx caudal to the hypophysis. Between this basal plate and the first cervical sclerotomes four occipital somites develop that give rise to sclerotomes. By fusion of these occipital sclerotomes, a mass is formed that is interposed between the basal plate and the cervical vertebrae. At the region of the foramen magnum, the mass ("occipital tectum") extends around the neural tube like the neural arch of a vertebra.[1] Subsequently, it is converted by chondrification and ossification into occipital bone. Lateral and dorsal to the chondrocranial portion, additional parts of the occiput develop from membrane bone. In the postcranial axial skeleton, the first cervical sclerotome gives rise to the first cervical vertebra but also to the odontoid process of the second vertebra, so that the odontoid represents developmentally the body of the first cervical vertebra. The most cranial part of the odontoid process may be derived from the most caudal occipital segment.[2] Thus, the connection of the skull to the vertebral column undergoes complicated developmental steps and faulty segmentation can occur in the occipitovertebral area. Occipitalization of the atlas, accessory occipital vertebra, absence or anomaly of the odontoid process combined with one another or with faulty segmentation of the cervical vertebral column are manifestations of error in the development of the occipitovertebral junction. Although such anomalies usually are compatible with prenatal and early postnatal life, they can cause disturbances during adulthood. Since such late manifestations sometimes are correctable by surgery, early diagnosis of the underlying malformations is important. Signs of cranial nerve, root and spinal cord impairment are variable and not specific but roentgenography, including myelography, permits recognition of the skeletal defects.[3–5]

Basilar Impression (Basilar Invagination, Platybasia)

Basilar impression and related malformations of the base of the skull can cause disturbances of the central nervous system that previously were considered incurable but have now become accessible to surgical treatment. A good discussion of these anomalies was given by McGregor[6] in 1948. The structures near the posterior part of the foramen magnum are displaced cranialward, impinging on parts of the central nervous system that rest on the basilar structures. Flattening of the base of the skull or of the basal angle is not necessarily present in basilar impression and not necessarily associated with elevation of the bony structures surrounding the foramen magnum.[7] In fact, Spillane *et al.*,[8] who studied 24 neurologically disabled patients with bony and neural congenital anomalies in the region of the foramen magnum, encountered no case of platybasia. There are two types of basilar impressions: those caused by congenital defects of osseous structures in the cervico-occipital region, which are considered *primary basilar impressions*, and those due to bone disease of the skull, termed *secondary basilar impressions*.

Primary basilar impression leads to upward dislocation of bony structures into the posterior cranial fossa. It is associated with a variety of osseous defects, such as atlanto-occipital fusion, atlantoaxial dislocation, stenosis and deformity of the foramen magnum, failure of fusion of the posterior arch of the atlas, anterior and posterior clefts of the lower cervical vertebrae and fusion of cervical vertebrae (Klippel-Feil syndrome, p. 909). Such generalized osseous disorders as Morquio disease, cleidocranial dysostosis and atypical chondrodystrophies sometimes result in basilar impressions that can be classified as primary.

Secondary basilar impression is attributed to softening of the bones forming the base of the skull. Rickets, osteomalacia, Paget disease, osteitis fibrosa cystica and renal rickets are some of the softening processes considered responsible for such cases.

Basilar impression can cause a variety of clinical symptoms: pain, limitation of movement, shortening of the neck, raised intracranial pressure, hydrocephaly, cerebellar, bulbar or cranial nerve symptoms or degenerative changes in lower cervical segments. Association with spinal arteries and veins in the region of the foramen magnum has been observed. Because of the variety of symptoms produced, basilar impression may be mistaken for tumor of the posterior fossa, syringomyelia, bulbar palsy, amyotrophic lateral sclerosis, transverse myelitis, spinal cord tumor, spastic paraplegia or disseminated sclerosis.[6]

Basilar impression can be diagnosed by roentgenography. In sagittal roentgenograms, a variety of angles can be measured for determination of changes in the cervico-occipital area. The Chamberlain line[9] extends from the dorsal lip of the foramen magnum to the dorsal margin of the hard palate. In the presence of basilar impression, the body of the atlas or the odontoid process is seen above the Chamberlain line. If the posterior lip of the foramen magnum cannot be seen in the roentgenogram, the most caudal point of the occipital curve can be used instead. The resulting line, called the baseline by McGregor,[6] is said to be affected less by basilar impression than the anterior lip of the occipital foramen and therefore is a better index of abnormal position of the odontoid process. There are, however, substantial normal variations of the shortest distance of the tip of the odontoid process from the Chamberlain line, the arithmetical mean position in Europeans being 1 mm. below the baseline, with a standard deviation of 3.6 mm. McGregor[6] measured the same distance in skulls of African Bantu Negroes. He came to the conclusion that when the tip of the odontoid process lies a distance of 4.5 mm. above the baseline, the measurement is on the extreme limit of normality and pathology must be seriously considered. The figure of 4.5 mm. may be taken as the outer limit of normality for both African and European races.[6]

The basal angle of Boogaard can be seen in a lateral roentgenogram of the skull by drawing a line from the nasion to the center of the pituitary fossa, and another line from this point to the anterior lip of the foramen magnum. This basal angle was found to be almost equal in European and African skulls, being 135 degrees, with a minimum of 120 degrees and a maximum of 149. Many authors assumed that an increased basal angle was an indication of basilar impression but, as stated before, it is now believed that estimation of the basal angle is of no value in the diagnosis of basilar impression. Although the basal angle is a poor index of basilar impression, sometimes it may be of clinical significance, since a marked increase in it would cause some elevation of the nasion and an increase in the slope of the foramen magnum. Whether such platybasia would lead to basilar impression remains a matter of speculation.[8]

Primary basilar impression often is associated with other congenital malformations of the cervico-occipital area. It is worth emphasis that such congenital malformations may remain silent until adult life is reached. Then, symptoms closely resembling those of acquired neurologic diseases may develop, and the developmental character of the lesions may not be recognized until operation or necropsy.[8] Isolated basilar impression can be associated with signs of cervical syringomyelia or syringobulbia but the association is not a close one; similar skeletal anomalies may be seen in patients with definite neurologic disorders and in patients without neurologic signs. When basilar impression is combined with other malformations such as occipitalization of the atlas or atlantoaxial dislocation or fusion of vertebrae, the situation is similar, since syringomyelia or spasticity of all four limbs may occur; yet, there also may be little disability despite gross skeletal anomalies.[8] Cerebellar ectopia with herniated flattened tonsils also can be associated with skeletal malformations around the foramen magnum, but in such cases there again is no close relationship between the degree of the skeletal malformations and the degree of neurologic pathology.[8]

Patients with basilar impression and related skeletal malformations, including the Klippel-Feil syndrome, have short necks and, in this respect, sometimes resemble patients with Turner syndrome. The webbing of the neck in the latter disorder is only rarely associated with skeletal malformations such as vertebral fusion or agenesis (p. 909). In the case of skeletal malformation in the atlanto-occipital area, tilting of the head, facial asymmetry, malformation of the ears, abnormal palate, Sprengel deformity, congenital absence of thenar muscles or of digits may be observed as associated malformations. Spontaneous vertical nystagmus, postural loss confined to the upper limbs and mirror movements of the hands may occur. Neurologic symptoms can become aggravated after trauma. Although some of the neurologic symptoms in patients with cervico-occipital skeletal defects cannot be attributed to mechanical impingement on nervous tissue, surgical intervention can arrest, improve or cure some of the neurologic disorders caused by bony abnormalities or dural bands in this area.

Absence of the Odontoid Process

Rowland *et al.*[10] described neurologic syndromes associated with congenital absence of the odontoid process. As with other malformations of this area, pathologic signs can appear late in life, but manifestations during childhood have been observed. The odontoid process develops from three centers of ossification, two lateral and one apical, which unite with one another in the twelfth year. The lateral centers unite with the axis during the third or fourth year.

Cervical pain, torticollis, weakness of the extremities, sensory disturbances, vertigo, seizures or mental deterioration have occurred as neurologic complications. Absence of the odontoid process can be demonstrated roentgenographically. Neurologic symptoms frequently appear after trauma, but slowly progressing myelopathies have been observed also. Compression of the spinal cord or of the vertebral arteries or adhesions around the cord can be the cause of symptoms; in other cases, associated malformations of the central nervous system are responsible for the manifestations.

Occipitalization of the Atlas

Assimilation of the atlas (occipitalization) consists in a bony union between the skull and the atlas, i.e., a continuity between the anterior arch of the atlas and the anterior lip of the foramen magnum. Occipitalization can be complete, the cortex of the anterior arch and the medulla being continuous with the cortex and the medulla of the basiocciput. There also are incomplete cases in which atlanto-occipital joint spaces can be demonstrated. McRae and Barnum[11] presented 25 cases with this bony anomaly but in most of these there were associated malformations in other areas of the cervical skeleton and thoracic spine. The anomaly also was seen in patients who had more serious associated anomalies such as cleft palate, hypoplasia of the jaw, deformities of the external ear, incomplete rotation of the kidney and hypospadias. Associated skeletal malformations included block vertebrae, hemivertebrae, cervical ribs and particularly abnormal size or abnormal position of the odontoid process. In addition to fusion of the anterior arch of the atlas with the occiput, there also were anomalies of the transverse processes of the atlas and abnormal arterial foramina. The posterior arch of the atlas often was rudimentary. The skull, with the exception of assimilation of the atlas, generally was normal. Posterior displacement of the odontoid process of the axis found in 60% of the cases was recognized if the odontoid was seen 4mm. or more posterior to the anterior arch of the atlas. Another pathogenic anomaly associated with occipitalization was a thickened band of dura that constricted the cord. Other complications were cerebellar tonsil herniations, cerebrospinal fluid block and Arnold-Chiari malformations. Although many of the patients showed neurologic signs and symptoms, it was admitted that assimilation of the atlas in itself may not have been responsible for them but rather represented a sign of abnormal development of the entire area.

Important symptoms of cervical cord compression due to soft tissue and bone anomalies associated with occipitalization of the atlas are weakness and ataxia of the lower extremities. Motor disturbances and numbness and pain in the upper extremities occur. Occipital headache may be present. Papilledema, blurring of vision and diplopia could be due to cerebrospinal block of the foramen magnum. Long tract signs in both the upper and lower extremities, ataxia, nystagmus and posterior column signs are seen in some of these patients. McRae and Barnum[11] found that many of their patients had been misdiagnosed because of similarity of symptoms to multiple sclerosis. Foramen magnum decompression can bring about improvement of symptoms.[3]

REFERENCES

1. Hamilton, W. J., Boyd, J. D., and Mossman, H. W.: *Human Embryology* (3d ed.; Baltimore: The Williams & Wilkins Company., 1962).
2. Nicholson, J. T., and Sherk, H. H.: Anomalies of the occipitocervical articulation, J. Bone & Joint Surg. 50-A:295 1968.
3. Bharucha, E. P., and Dastur, H. M.: Craniovertebral anomalies (a report on 40 cases), Brain 87:469, 1964.
4. Michie, M. I., and Clark, M.: Neurological syndromes associated with cervical and craniocervical anomalies, Arch. Neurol. 18:241, 1968.
5. Hohl, M., and Baker, H. R.: The atlanto-axial joint, J. Bone & Joint Surg. 46-A:1739, 1964.
6. McGregor, M.: The significance of certain measurements of the skull in the diagnosis of basilar impression, Brit. J. Radiol. 21:171, 1948.
7. Walsh, M. N., Camp, J. D., and Craig, W.: Basilar invagination of the skull (so-called platybasia). Report of a case with operation, Proc. Staff Meet. Mayo Clin. 16:449, 1941.
8. Spillane, J. D., Pallis, C., and Jones, A. M.: Developmental abnormalities in the region of the foramen magnum, Brain 80:11, 1957.
9. Chamberlain, W. E.: Basilar impression (platybasia). A bizarre developmental anomaly of the occipital bone and upper cervical spine with striking and misleading neurological manifestations, Yale J. Biol. & Med. 11:487, 1939.
10. Rowland, L. P., Shapiro, J. H., and Jacobson, H. G.: Neurological syndromes associated with congenital absence of the odontoid process, Arch. Neurol. 80:286, 1958.
11. McRae, D. L., and Barnum, A. S.: Occipitalization of the atlas, Am. J. Roentgenol. 70:23, 1953.

Klippel-Feil Syndrome

THE KLIPPEL-FEIL SYNDROME is an anomaly of the spine characterized by faulty segmentation of two or more cervical vertebrae. This vertebral anomaly is a representative of many related conditions and it is certain that its etiology is heterogeneous. Klippel and Feil[1] gave a complete description of the clinical course of 1 patient and added a necropsy report, but the condition had been observed before.[2] In patients with cervical "fusion" of the spine, one may detect anomalies in other parts of the spinal column or in other skeletal structures. Neurologic disturbances sometimes are secondary to the skeletal anomalies of the vertebrae or they are due to associated malformations of the central nervous system.

Early theories that attributed the congenital fusion of cervical vertebrae to syphilis or other inflammatory processes in fetal life are of historical interest only. The same is true for explanations by intrauterine pressure and trauma. It can be safely assumed that the vertebral anomalies are not due to "fusion" but to failure of normal segmentation, which can be traced back to the third embryonic week, when segmentation of the mesodermal somites takes place. The factors responsible for the lack of segmentation may vary in different cases. The osseous malformations can be recognized by the seventh week of gestational life but the anomalies date back to earlier mesenchymal stages. Males and females can be affected. The disorder occurs in various races.[3]

Heredity plays a role in many cases.[4,5] Direct transmission from a parent to one or several children has been observed repeatedly. These observations are compatible with the assumption of dominant inheritance. In several families, brothers and sisters were affected, whereas the parents did not show the abnormal trait. This may be interpreted as recessive inheritance or it may be that one of the parents has the anomaly in a subclinical form, whereas one or several of the children show it fully expressed. The observation by Jarcho and Levin[6] bears this out, since in the family described by them a brother and sister were affected, whereas the mother had only minor anomalies such as a defective arch of the 5th cervical vertebra and an accessory nipple on the left side. It is possible, therefore, that in this and similar cases dominant inheritance that is not easily recognized occurs because of reduced expressivity in a parent. Gedda and Iannoccone[7] found that in one-fifth of the cases reported in the literature and in 3 of their own, craniovertebral malformations occurred in some relatives of the patients. In some cases, recessive inheritance seems likely. Einhorn *et al.*[8] described ankylosis of the first five cervical vertebrae and platybasia in a case of Morquio disease. Since Morquio disease is inherited as a recessive trait (p. 819), one can conclude that Klippel-Feil syndrome associated with it is recessively inherited. Gunderson *et al.*[9] investigated the families of 11 patients with cervical fusions. They accepted Feil's[10] classification of these disorders. Type I shows massive fusion of many cervical and upper thoracic vertebrae into bony blocks. In Type II, only one or two interspaces are undeveloped but hemivertebral and atlanto-occipital fusions do not rule out this classification. Patients with cervical and lower thoracic or lumbar fusions were included in Type III. In the study by Gunderson *et al.*, Type II was the most common one, as 7 of the 11 probands' families were assigned to this group and in 6 of them cervical anomalies were found in relatives. Dominant or recessive inheritance seemed to be at work in different families. In the families of probands with Type I, i.e., with the massive involvement, no similarly affected relatives were found, but rachischisis and basilar impression did occur. In one family with Type II, some members apparently had mosaicism of group E and C chromosomes. Occasionally, one sees a combination of Klippel-Feil and Turner syndrome with an XO karyotype, which indicates that fusion of cervical vertebrae can be due to chromosomal abnormality. There was a Klippel-Feil malformation in a case of trisomy 18[11] and in the Cincinnati Children's Hospital (Chart No. 172032) a girl with craniosynostosis and cervical fusions was found to be a mosaic, having 45X/45X + fragment, cells (Fig. 96-1).

Faulty segmentation of the vertebral column owing to environmental factors must be considered possible. There is much experimental evidence for this in lower classes[4] and in mammals, since teratologic experiments frequently result in malformations of the spine. Trypan blue,[12] x-rays,[13] hypoxia,[14] salicylates or streptonigrin[15,16] and other teratogens can lead to severe vertebral malformations that often are associated with abnormalities of the central nervous system.[17] In a case of Type I fusion reported by Gunderson *et al.*,[9] the mother had tried abortion with oral and parenteral agents on three occasions during the first trimester. No other members of this family were affected.

Several or all the cervical vertebrae are fused into a single column. The number of vertebrae may be reduced and, in most cases, the vertebral bodies are flattened. The spinous processes often are small or bifid and the intervertebral foramina smaller than normal. Approximation of the occipital bone to the defect of the spinal column occurs frequently and the atlas and the occiput often are fused. The intervertebral disks are narrow or obliterated and the cervical spine is shortened. Hemivertebrae and other anomalies may be an additional expression of irregular segmentation. Defects of the posterior vertebral arches usually are interpreted as cervical spina bifida. Duplication of the remnants of the notochord, of the spinal cord and of its central canal may be combined with the osseous changes. Feller and Sternberg[18] examined anatomically 5 premature or neonatal infants with severe Klippel-Feil syndrome and spina bifida occulta extending from the upper cervical segments downward to various levels. There also were defects of the occipital bone and displacement of portions of the central nervous system.

The patients with Type I are characterized by a short neck with limited mobility, which gives the impression that the head sits on the shoulders. The hairline is low in the back (Fig. 96-2, *B*). Webbing of the neck (pterygium colli) and webbed armpits may be seen.[19] The mobility of the neck is chiefly reduced in lateral movements. Some of the patients have no further complaints and may remain free of symptoms during their entire lives (Type II). Others are less fortunate and have complications or associated malformations. The vertebrae adjacent to the fused bones show an increased tendency to fracture. Difficulty in breathing and swallowing has been described in children. Scoliosis and kyphoscoliosis of the lower spine frequently are associated with the cervical anomalies (Type III). A variety of neurologic complications have been described. Bimanual synkinesia (mirror movements[20]) are observed frequently and may be present at birth. Every movement of one hand is copied by the other, which may interfere with certain functions. For instance, climbing a ladder may be impossible because of the synchronized movements of the hands. Owing to the narrowness of the foramina, nerve roots may be compressed. Hyperesthesia has been observed in the back of the head and on the neck and chin. In some patients, paralysis of the cranial nerves as well as mental deficiency complicate the disease picture. Attacks of unconsciousness have been observed.[21] Late complications such as spastic paralysis, syringobulbia, syringomyelia and ataxia have been reported.[4,5]

Among associated anomalies, those of the spinal

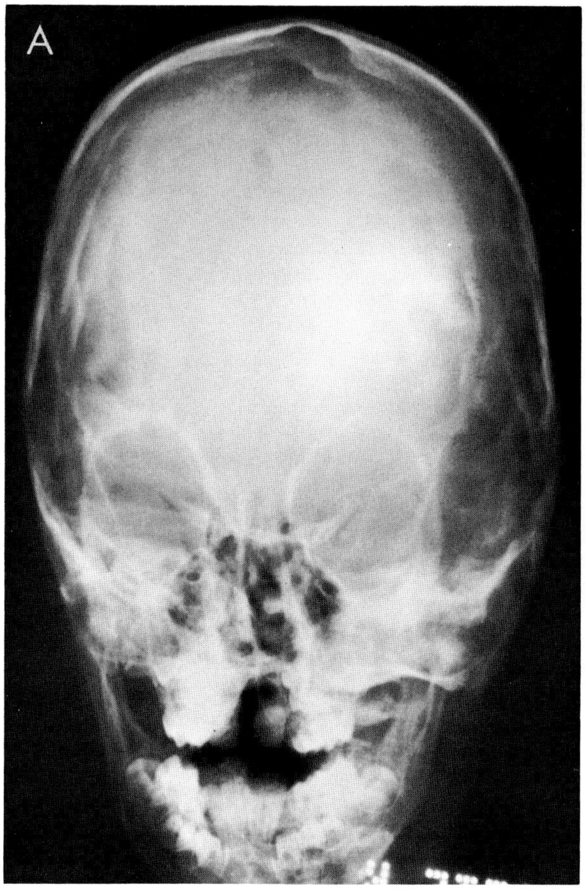

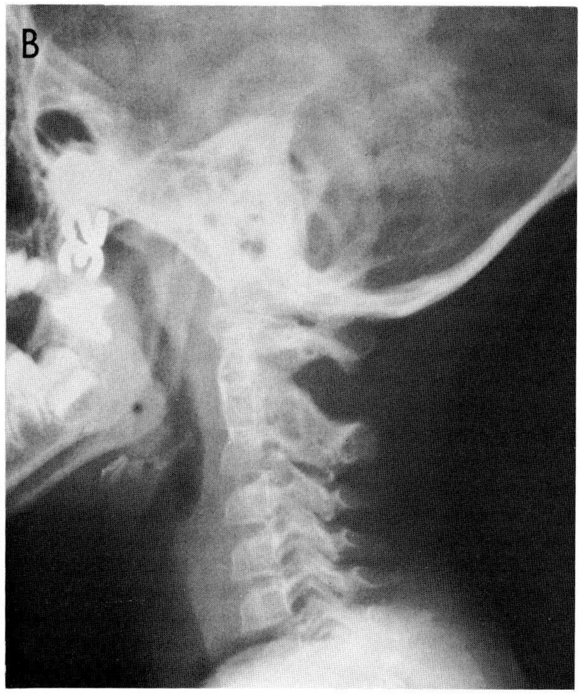

Fig. 96-1.—Roentgenograms of skull and cervical vertebral column of a 6-year-old girl born with intrauterine growth retardation. **A,** skull. Neither the sagittal suture nor the coronal suture appears patent: craniosynostosis. **B,** congenital synostosis of C2 and C3 can be seen. This child is a 45X/45X + fragment, mosaic.

column must be mentioned first. In addition to the cervical vertebrae, other segments of the spinal column often are involved. Abnormal segmentation may reach into the adjacent thoracic spine or it may involve more distant areas. Or the anomaly may be continued cranially and be combined with defects of the occipital bone, platybasia, hydrocephaly and other anomalies of the head. Association with oxycephaly[22] and other forms of craniosynostosis[23] has been observed. Cleft palate, bifid uvula, micrognathia and absence of the external auricular meatus have been seen in combination with the Klippel-Feil syndrome. Osborne[36] wrote a dissertation on the prevalence of anomalies of the upper cervical vertebrae in patients with craniofacial malformations. There, the relationship of cleft lip and palate and the Klippel-Feil syndrome is discussed thoroughly. Deaf-mutism of various types has been described repeatedly.[5] A syndrome of conductive deafness, mitral insufficiency, fusion of cervical vertebrae, fusion of carpal and tarsal bones and short stature was reported by Forney *et al.*[24] Congenital cervical block vertebrae may be combined with Zenker diverticulum, an outpouching of the pharyngeal wall at the junction with the esophagus.[25] Gilmour[26] emphasized the relationship of this condition with iniencephaly, a monstrosity that combines occipital defects with those of the spine (see p. 234).

Extradural hemangiolipoma[27] and a dermoid cyst[28] have been seen as added cervical anomalies. Elevation of the scapula (Sprengel deformity) is associated so often with the Klippel-Feil syndrome that some authors have described it as a part of the disorder (p. 915). Various anomalies of the ribs and low nipple lines have been reported. Klippel-Feil syndrome, elevated scapula and rib anomalies have been observed in association with multiple cysts of the jaws,[29] a disorder related to the syndrome of basal cell nevi (p. 1268). Of other thoracic anomalies, mediastinal cysts deserve to be mentioned. Some of these have been considered bronchogenic[30] but it is more likely that they are of foregut origin.[31] Pulmonary stenosis, patent foramen ovale, ventricular septal defects, dextrocardia, single atrium, single ventricle, aortic arch anomalies and abnormal pulmonary veins have been observed.[5,32] The extremities appear disproportionately long. Malformations of the forearms and of the limbs, clubhand and clubfoot may occur.[5] Some cases of cervical vertebral fusion are manifestations of a general inability to form all joints (arthrodysplasia). Thus, Klippel-Feil syndrome may occur together with

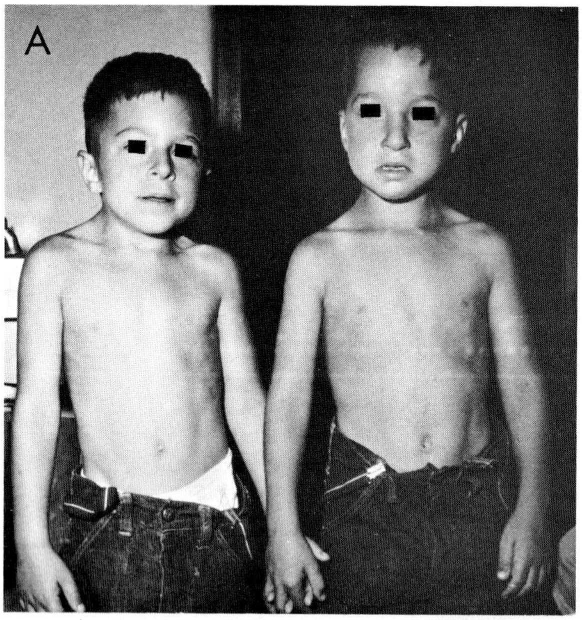

Fig. 96-2.—**A,** brothers with Klippel-Feil syndrome. **B,** rear view of the younger brother, who also has Sprengel deformity. **C,** roentgenogram showing hemivertebrae and block vertebrae of the younger brother's cervical and dorsal spine.

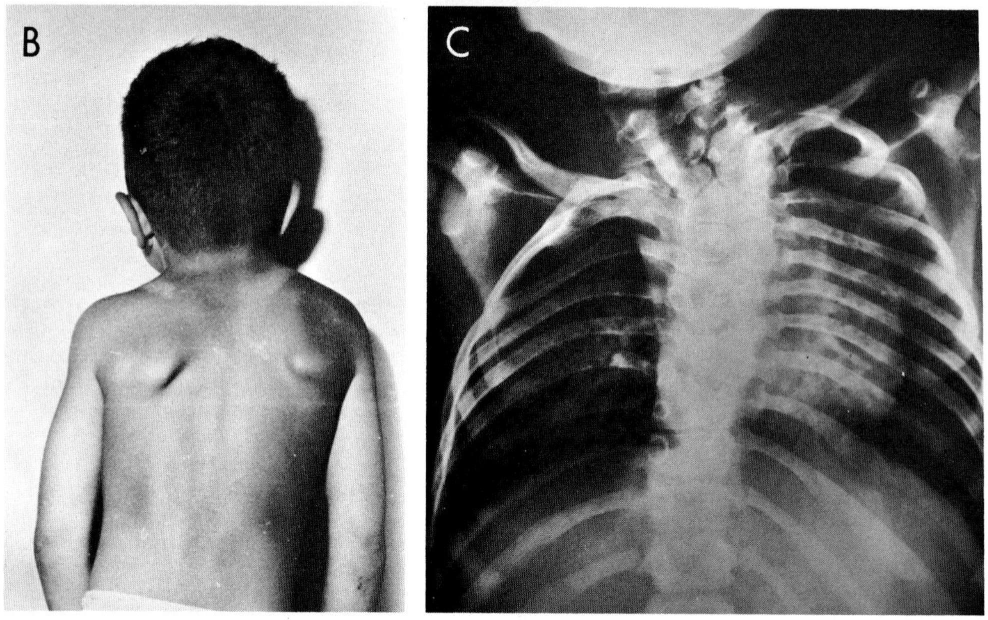

symbrachydactyly (p. 970) or with fusion of carpal and tarsal bones.[24] Congenital malformations of the cervical spine have been observed in patients who develop myositis ossificans progressiva.[33] Pterygium colli in Turner syndrome usually is not associated with vertebral fusion, but in some cases the Klippel-Feil anomaly has been noted in patients with ovarian agenesis.[34,35]

Roentgenograms reveal the synostoses as well as other deformities of the cervical vertebrae. Fusion of transverse processes, spina bifida, hemivertebrae, cervical ribs and other anomalies may be seen. In the differential diagnosis, tuberculosis of the spine, the results of previous fractures and torticollis should be considered because such conditions may be more amenable to treatment than the Klippel-Feil syndrome.

The prognosis varies, since the anomalies of the cervical spine may occur in combination with anomalies of such severity that the affected child is not viable (Type I),[9] or the Klippel-Feil syndrome may be found as an accidental observation at necropsy in aged people who remain asymptomatic throughout life (Type II). In general, the outlook depends on neu-

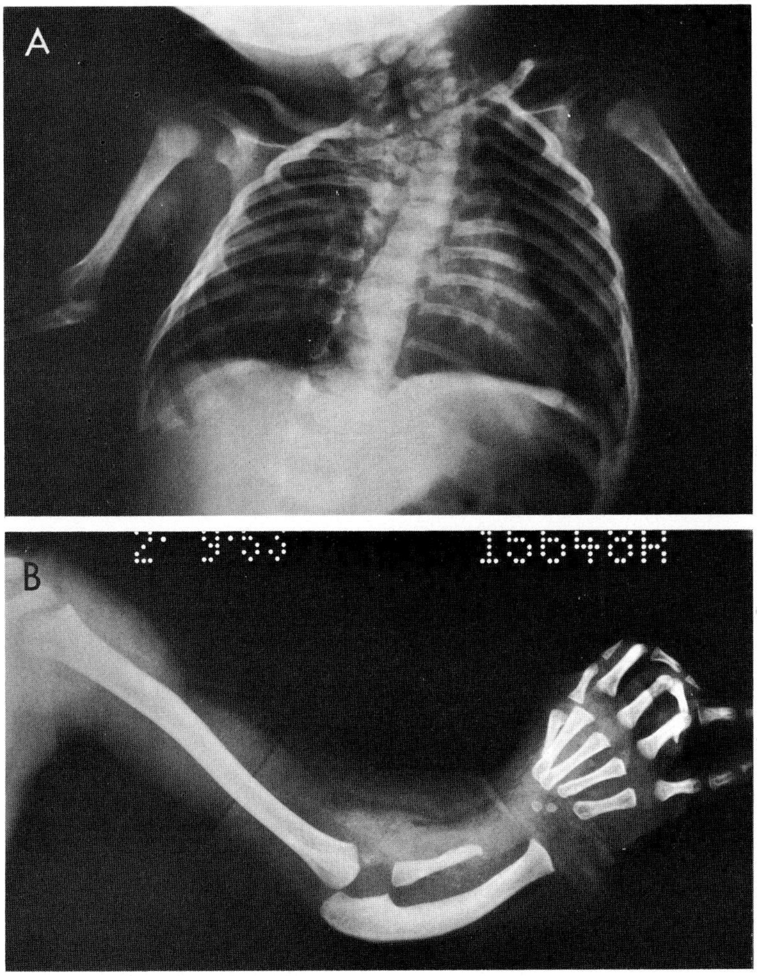

Fig. 96-3.—Roentgenograms of a 2-year-old boy with Klippel-Feil syndrome and other congenital malformations. **A,** abnormal segmentation of cervical vertebrae. Scoliosis. **B,** right arm of the same child. Underdevelopment of radius and ulna; abnormalities of finger joints.

Fig. 96-4.—Roentgenograms of a 6-year-old girl with Klippel-Feil syndrome. **A,** lateral view, showing fusion of the bodies of the 2d and 3d and also fusion of the 4th–6th cervical vertebrae. **B,** roentgenogram in AP projection, showing irregular segmentation and scoliosis of cervical and upper dorsal vertebral column.

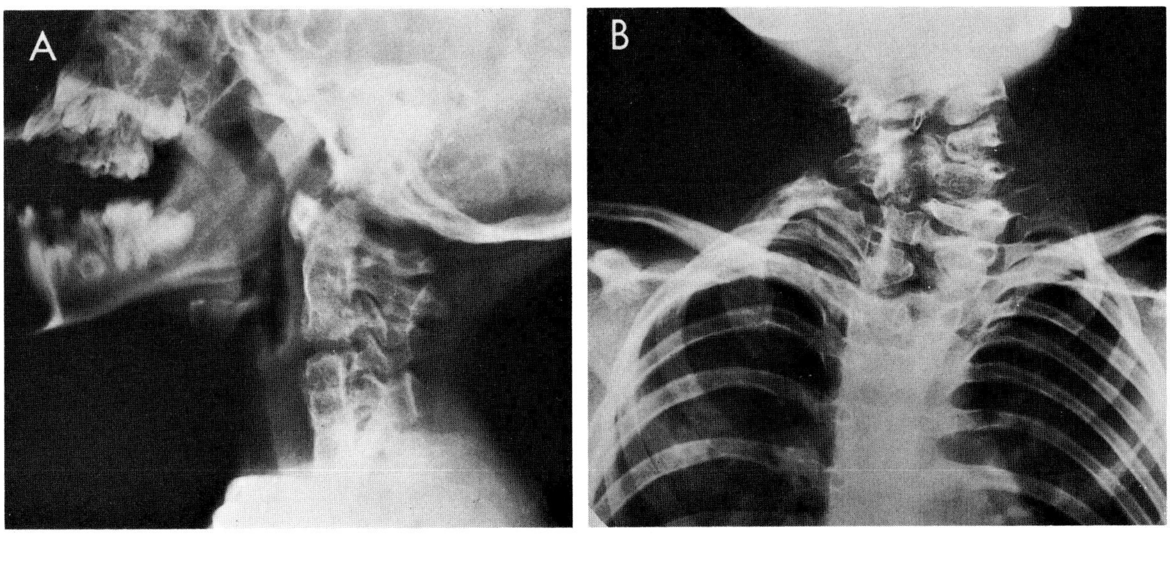

rologic complications and associated malformations. The condition may be stationary and symptomless for many years and then lead to complications. As a rule, death is due to intercurrent disease and not to the Klippel-Feil syndrome itself.

No radical treatment is recommended. The patients should avoid strenuous exercises and athletic performances to prevent fractures in the cervical region. In individual cases, orthopedic measures such as traction, remedial exercises and manipulation have been found useful.

REFERENCES

1. Klippel, M., and Feil, A.: Un cas d'absence des vertèbres cervicales avec cage thoracique remontant jusqu'a la base du crâne (cage thoracique cervicale), Nouv. Icon. Salpêt. 25:223, 1912.
2. Hutchinson, J.: Deformity of shoulder girdle, Brit. M. J. 1: 634, 1894.
3. Jarcho, S.: Anomaly of the vertebral column (Klippel-Feil syndrome) in American aborigines, J.A.M.A. 193:843, 1965.
4. Erskine, C. A.: Analysis of Klippel-Feil syndrome, Arch. Path. 41:269, 1946.
5. Shoul, M. I., and Ritvo, M.: Clinical and roentgenological manifestations of the Klippel-Feil syndrome (congenital fusion of the cervical vertebrae, brevi collis). Report of eight additional cases and review of the literature, Am. J. Roentgenol. 68:369, 1952.
6. Jarcho, S., and Levin, P. M.: Hereditary malformation of vertebral bodies, Bull. Johns Hopkins Hosp. 62:216, 1938.
7. Gedda, L., and Iannaccone, G.: La sindrome di Klippel-Feil nel quadro della schisosinostosi assiale congenita familiare, *Novant' Anni delle Leggi Mendeliane*, Rome, 1956, p. 249.
8. Einhorn, N. H., Moore, J. R., and Rowntree, L. G.: Osteochondrodystrophia deformans (Morquio's disease); observations at autopsy in one case, Am. J. Dis. Child. 72:536, 1946.
9. Gunderson, C. H., Greenspan, R. H., Glaser, G. H., and Lubs, H. A.: The Klippel-Feil syndrome: Genetic and clinical reevaluation of cervical fusion, Medicine 46:491, 1967.
10. Feil, A.: L'absence et la diminution des vertèbres cervicales: Le syndrome de réduction numérique cervicale, Thèse de Paris, 1919.
11. Ozonoff, M. B., Steinbach, H. L., and Mamunes, P.: The trisomy 18 syndrome, Am. J. Roentgenol. 91:618, 1964.
12. Gillman, J., Gilbert, C., and Gillman, T.: A preliminary report on hydrocephalus, spina bifida and other congenital anomalies in the rat produced by trypan blue, South African J. M. Sc. 13:47, 1948.
13. Russell, L. B.: X-ray-induced developmental abnormalities in the mouse and their use in the analysis of embryological patterns, J. Exper. Zool. 131:329, 1956.
14. Ingalls, T. H., Curley, F. J., and Prindle, R. A.: Experimental production of congenital anomalies, New England J. Med. 247:758, 1952.
15. Warkany, J., and Takacs, E.: Experimental production of congenital malformations in rats by salicylate poisoning, Am. J. Path. 35:315, 1959.
16. Warkany, J., and Takacs, E.: Congenital malformations in rats from streptonigrin, Arch. Path. 79:65, 1965.
17. Warkany, J., Wilson, J. G., and Geiger, J. F.: Myeloschisis and myelomeningocele produced experimentally in the rat, J. Comp. Neurol. 109:35, 1958.
18. Feller, A., and Sternberg, H.: Zur Kenntnis der Fehlbildungen der Wirbelsäule, Virchows Arch. path. Anat. 272: 613, 1929.
19. Frawley, J. M.: Congenital webbing, Am. J. Dis. Child. 29: 799, 1925.
20. Baird, P. A., Robinson, G. C., and Buckler, W. S. J.: Klippel-Feil syndrome. A study of mirror movement detected by electromyography, Am. J. Dis. Child. 113:546, 1967.
21. Illingworth, R. S.: Attacks of unconsciousness in association with fused cervical vertebrae, Arch. Dis. Childhood 31:8, 1956.
22. Peter, A. L.: Oxycephaly associated with Klippel-Feil syndrome and other skeletal defects, Am. J. Ophth. 29:685, 1946.
23. Freeman, J. M., and Borkowf, S.: Craniostenosis, Pediatrics 30:57, 1962.
24. Forney, W. R., Robinson, S. J., and Pascoe, D. J.: Congenital heart disease, deafness, and skeletal malformations: A new syndrome?, J. Pediat. 68:14, 1966.
25. Baeyer, E. V.: Zenker's diverticulum and cervical block vertebra, Am. J. Roentgenol. 84:1037, 1960.
26. Gilmour, J. R.: Essential identity of Klippel-Feil syndrome and iniencephaly, J. Path. & Bact. 53:117, 1941.
27. Bucy, P. C., and Ritchey, H.: Klippel-Feil's syndrome associated with compression of spinal cord by extradural hemangiolipoma, J. Neurosurg. 4:476, 1947.
28. Roberts, A. P.: A case of intracranial dermoid cyst associated with the Klippel-Feil deformity and recurrent meningitis, Arch. Dis. Childhood 33:222, 1958.
29. Eisenbud, L., Brooks, H., and Busch, S.: Klippel-Feil syndrome with multiple cysts of jawbones, Oral Surg. 5:659, 1952.
30. Bracher, A. N., and Koontz, A. R.: Mediastinal bronchogenic cyst and Klippel-Feil syndrome; report of case, J.A.M.A. 150:1006, 1952.
31. Fallon, M., Gordon, A. R. G., and Lendrum, A. C.: Mediastinal cysts of fore-gut origin associated with vertebral abnormalities, Brit. J. Surg. 41:2, 1954.
32. Morrison, S. G., Perry, L. W., and Scott, L. P., III: Congenital brevicollis (Klippel-Feil syndrome) and cardiovascular anomalies, Am. J. Dis. Child. 115:614, 1968.
33. Rosborough, D.: Ectopic bone formation associated with multiple congenital anomalies, J. Bone & Joint Surg. 48-B:499, 1966.
34. Cahn, L.: In the Discussion of Eisenbud, L., *et al.*[29]
35. Lenz, W.: *Krankheiten des Urogenitalsystems* (Stuttgart: Georg Thieme, 1964).
36. Osborne, G. S.: The prevalence of anomalies of the upper cervical vertebrae in patients with craniofacial malformations and their effect on osseous nasopharyngeal depth, Thesis for Ph.D. degree, Chicago: Center for Craniofacial Anomalies, University of Illinois Medical Center, 1968.

Sprengel Deformity

IN THIS CONDITION, one or both scapulae are in a congenitally high position, with the lower angle turned toward the spine. These changes usually are associated with other congenital malformations and are closely related to the Klippel-Feil syndrome (see Fig. 96-2 *B*).

Concerning etiology, several theories have been advanced in the past. The anomaly has been attributed, without any proof, to lack of amniotic fluid, to abnormal amniotic bands and to fetal periostitis. There is more truth in the statement that Sprengel deformity is due to an arrest of the scapula in the fetal position. The scapulae and the upper extremities normally are placed higher on the body of the fetus than in older children and there is a gradual descent in prenatal and early postnatal life.[1] In Sprengel deformity, this descent does not take place and there also is retention of the shape of the fetal scapula, which is longer in the transverse diameter than in the vertical. In addition, it has been stressed that the muscles attached to the scapula are abnormal and the lower portion of the trapezius muscle may be absent.[2] It seems likely, however, that both the anomalies of the bones and of the muscles are manifestations of a more generalized developmental anomaly. Heredity can be demonstrated in some of the cases. Neuhof[3] observed a family in which 11 members had either unilateral or bilateral congenital elevation of the scapula. Sometimes the condition was transmitted by members who did not have Sprengel deformity but had other genetically related anomalies such as scoliosis, winged scapula, muscle defects, and so forth. This indicates that the abnormal trait can express itself in various ways in members of a kindred. Dominant inheritance can be assumed in some of the cases,[4,5] but the expression may be so irregular that some investigators assumed recessive inheritance. In general, it is best to remember that in many cases the anomalies of the scapula are only one manifestation of a more fundamental and general disturbance of the shoulder girdle and upper thorax.

"Congenital upward displacement" of the scapula was described by Sprengel[6] in 1891. In addition to upward displacement, the scapula appears removed laterad away from the vertebral column. It also is tilted forward, so that it may appear horizontally oriented. In addition, the scapula is deformed. The change in shape consists of elongation of the transverse diameter and shortening of the vertical. The upper inner angle may be drawn out into a hook. Sometimes there are cartilaginous or fibrous attachments that connect the upper inner angle of the scapula to transverse processes of the cervical spine (omovertebral bone). Often there are anomalies in the vertebral column, particularly in the lower cervical and upper dorsal parts. If fusion of vertebrae is present, one is dealing with a combination of Klippel-Feil syndrome and Sprengel deformity. The clavicles may be short and the ribs deformed. The shoulders slope downward or the concave outline of the neck, which normally is determined by the trapezius muscle, may be deformed by the elevated scapula. The chest is narrow and cylindrical and the ribs slant sharply downward. The muscles frequently are involved. It is particularly the inferior part of the trapezius that is underdeveloped, but the latissimus dorsi, the serratus magnus and the rhomboideus muscles may be involved also. The movements of the shoulder joint are impaired in approximately half the cases, abduction beyond the horizontal being impossible. In order to elevate the arm over the shoulder, it must be swung upward. The scapula moves as soon as abduction begins and becomes almost detached from the chest. However, bilateral undescended scapula associated with omovertebral bones need not interfere with normal function.[7] Snapping of the scapula has been reported by Alvik.[8] Cases complicated by paraplegia or syringomyelia have been observed.[9,10]

Treatment consists of exercises to improve the impaired mobility of the shoulder joint. Surgery should be resorted to only in the most severe cases. It consists of division of the lower portion of the trapezius muscle or of the fibrous bands that are found in its place. Connections with the vertebrae may be severed and the scapula mobilized. Sometimes extensive resection of bone and muscles is necessary to improve mobility.[1]

REFERENCES

1. Steindler, A.: Congenital elevation of the scapula, Pediatrics 5:367, 1924.
2. Fairbank, H. A. T.: Congenital elevation of the scapula, Brit. J. Surg. 1:553, 1914.
3. Neuhof, H.: Congenital elevation of the scapula (Sprengel's deformity) of familial type, Am. J. Dis. Child. 7:357, 1914.
4. Gottesleben, A.: Über den doppelseitigen und einseitigen Schulterblatthochstand, Arch. klin. Chir. 144:723, 1927.
5. Schwarzweller, F.: Der angeborene Schulterblatthochstand und seine Beziehungen zu den Missbildungen der Wirbelsäule, Ztschr. menschl. Vererb.-u. Konstitutionslehre 20:350, 1937.
6. Sprengel, L.: Die angeborene Verschiebung des Schulterblattes nach oben, Arch. klin. Chir. 42:545, 1891.
7. Blair, J. D., and Wells, P. O.: Bilateral undescended scapula associated with omovertebral bone, J. Bone & Joint Surg. 39-A:201, 1957.
8. Alvik, I.: Snapping scapula and Sprengel's deformity, Acta orthop. scandinav. 29:10, 1959.
9. Critchley, M.: Sprengel's deformity with paraplegia, Brit. J. Surg. 14:243, 1926.
10. DuToit, F.: A case of congenital elevation of the scapula (Sprengel's deformity) with defect of the cervical spine associated with syringomyelia, Brain 54:421, 1931.

97

The Spine

THE PRIMITIVE AXIAL SUPPORT of all vertebrates is the notochord, but in mammals a notochordal rod merely represents a transient axial support that is replaced by the vertebrae. The notochord persists only within the nuclei pulposi of the intervertebral disks. The axial skeleton is derived from mesenchyme, most of which traces its origin to the serially arranged pairs of mesodermal somites.[1] During the fourth week (3–4-mm. stage), the ventromesial wall of each somite develops into a mass of mesenchymal cells, the sclerotomes, from which the vertebrae and ribs are formed.

In young embryos, the sclerotomes are separated from one another by the intersegmental arteries, but at the 5-mm. stage (4 weeks) there occurs a rearrangement of the sclerotomes. The caudal half of each sclerotome undergoes proliferation, which results in denser arrangement of cells in these areas. An incomplete and transient sclerotomic fissure separates the looser cranial and the denser caudal halves and, subsequently, each denser (caudal) half joins the looser (cranial) half of the next caudal sclerotome. These recombinations and not the primitive sclerotomes are the primordia of the definitive vertebrae.[1] Thus, a definitive vertebra is not developed from a single somite. A definitive vertebral segment is derived from sclerotomic mesoderm extending longitudinally between two adjacent sclerotomic fissures. The original intersegmental vessels become secondarily intravertebral in position. Each vertebra develops from a sclerotome of secondary origin formed by the union of the caudal sclerotomic half of one segment and the cranial sclerotomic half of the next succeeding segment. The sclerotomic fissure that appears originally within a sclerotome becomes secondarily intersclerotomic and intervertebral in position, marking the limits between two future vertebrae. The intervertebral disk lies caudal to the fissure.[2]

The sclerotomic tissue is derived from the rapidly proliferating lower part of the medial and ventral mesodermal portion of the somite. The mesenchymal tissue grows mesad, surrounds the notochord and forms the primordia of the vertebral bodies. Dorsad proliferation of mesenchymal tissue flanks the neural tube, forming vertebral arches. Ventrolateral outgrowths form the costal processes, the primordia of the ribs. The rearrangement of the sclerotomes establishes intervertebral spaces that are taken over by loose mesenchyme, the substrate of the intervertebral disks in which the notochord persists in the form of nuclei pulposi.[1]

Chondrification of the vertebrae begins at 6 weeks in embryos of 12 mm. length. Centers develop in the vertebral bodies and in each half of the vertebral arches. The four centers unite to a cartilaginous vertebra, but the vertebral arches enclosing the spinal cord do not unite until the third month. At 9 weeks, ossification begins, each lateral half of the arch showing a single center. As a rule, the vertebral body has only one center of ossification, but sometimes two or more separate centers can be distinguished. In embryos of the third month (50 mm.), ossification centers are present only in the thoracic region, but at 4 months, centers are present in all but the sacral and coccygeal vertebrae. Complete union of the centers of ossification is not accomplished until several years after birth.[1]

Late stages of development of the vertebral column were described in detail by Ehrenhaft,[3] who dealt chiefly with chondrification and ossification of the vertebral bodies and with formation of the intervertebral disks. According to this author, not all the developmental defects in the vertebral disk column can be explained on the basis of malformations in the mesenchymal and cartilaginous embryonic state. He believed that many anomalies become understandable if one considers the vascular supply and the changes that occur in the notochord during the different stages. Block and wedge vertebrae, sagittal cleft vertebrae, chordal remnants and congenital weakness of the cartilage plates were interpreted by Ehrenhaft[3] in the light of developmental processes during embryonic and fetal life.

In general, the basic plan of the vertebral column is laid down in early embryonic life. The complex rearrangement of the sclerotomes mentioned above can be disturbed by adverse genetic or environmental factors in the mesenchymal stages of the spinal column. Severe malformations of the spine, therefore, are determined very early in prenatal life. But minor anomalies of the vertebrae and disks could be due to changes in later fetal stages.

Many experimental models exist that can illustrate

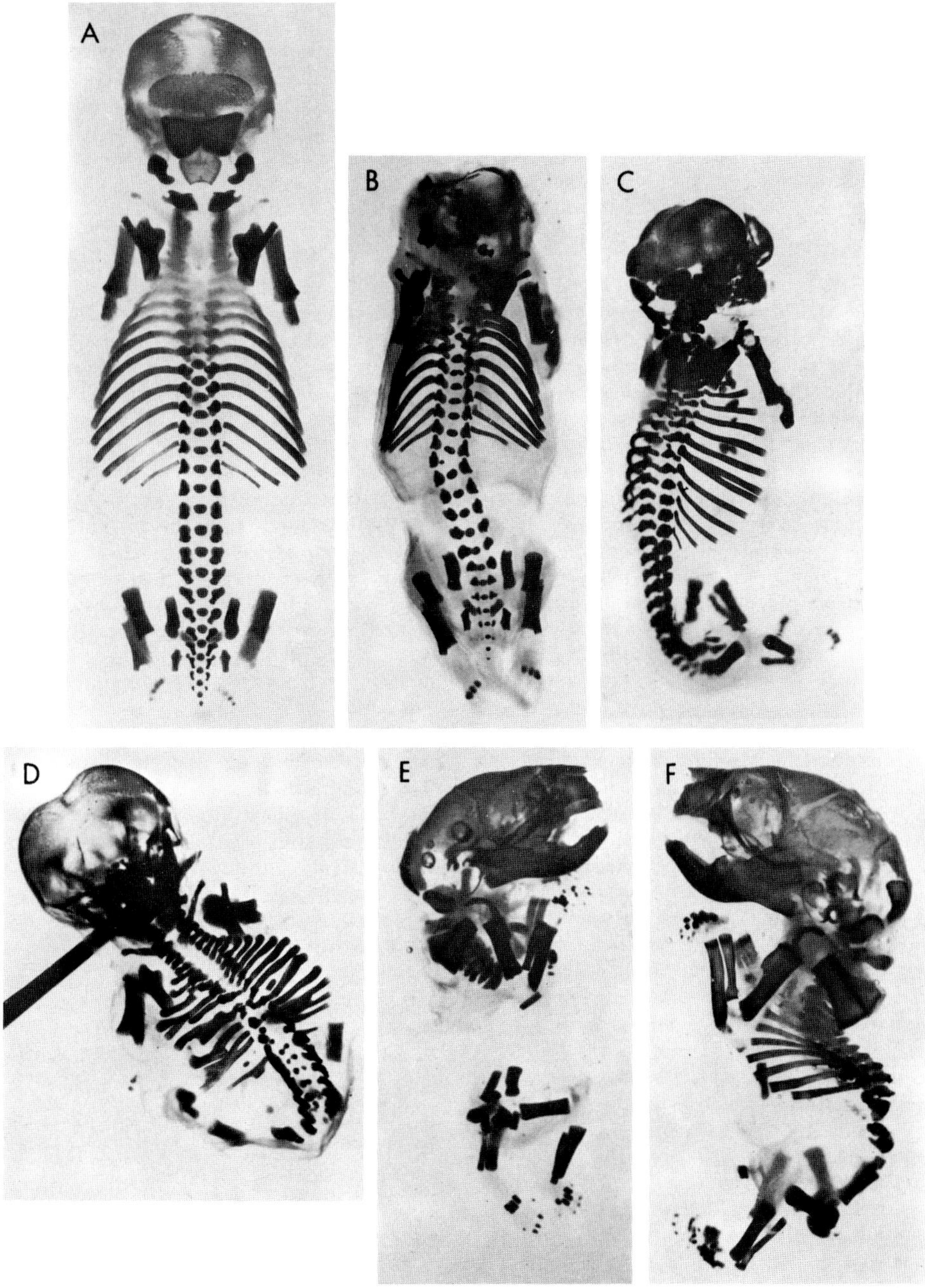

Fig. 97-1. – **A,** cleared specimen of a control rat obtained on the twenty-first day of pregnancy. **B,** 2d lumbar hemivertebra resulting in scoliosis (mother treated with methyl salicylate on the ninth day of gestation). **C,** bifid rib with corresponding vertebral defect (sodium salicylate on the tenth day). **D,** severe disorder of thoracic vertebrae and ribs (methyl salicylate on the eleventh day). **E,** absence of thoracic and lumbar vertebrae (streptonigrin on the tenth day). **F,** block vertebrae in lumbar spine (streptonigrin on the tenth day).

malformation of the spinal column and demonstrate the origins of developmental deviations.

Malformations

Theiler[4] analyzed vertebral malformations by consideration of experimental, genetic and developmental data. The vertebral column develops after formation of the notochord. Experimental evidence in lower animals (Triton) shows that circumscribed defects of the notochord can result in block vertebrae as the intervertebral portions fail to differentiate. The notochord is also important for the development of the vertebral column of mammals, since in some short-tailed mice a failure of the chorda to grow out with the tail bud results in taillessness. This abnormal behavior of the notochord on the tenth day of gestation represents the first manifestation of the abnormal gene. On the same day, which seems to be critical for the axial skeleton of the mouse, environmental disturbances can also produce tail anomalies. There are several abnormal genes that in mice lead to reduction of the tail and to vertebral anomalies, and different mechanisms account for the anomalies. Thus, the recessive gene "tail kinks" (tk) causes severe malformations of the cervical and upper thoracic vertebrae and leaves the lower thoracic and lumbosacral vertebrae intact. Abnormal development can be recognized earlier in "tail kink" embryos than in those of "undulated" as sclerotome differentiation is delayed and irregular. "Bent-tail" (Bn), a sex-linked semidominant gene, manifests itself by a primary reduction in the growth of the tail bud. In brachyury (T/+) and in "taillessness" (T/t^n), the tail shows normal growth at first but the notochord is abnormal in parts of the tail, which is lost secondarily by a constriction that separates the distal portion from the proximal portion. In "vestigial-tail," the tail bud at first appears normal in size in 10-day embryos but 2 days later constrictions begin to separate the tail bud from the rump. In this anomaly, the ventral ectodermal ridge of the tail[5] is reduced in size, which is considered the primary fault of tail development in this strain. In "short-tail" heterozygotes (Sd/+), the tail is reduced in size because of a breakdown of the notochord in parts of the embryonic tail. The Sd/Sd homozygote has imperforate anus, persisting cloaca and renal aplasia. In this syndrome, an abnormality of the ventral ectodermal ridge that is related to the cloacal membrane may be at the root of the tail anomaly. By 1968, approximately 20 genetic factors that influence formation of the spinal column in the mouse were known.[6-8] Studies of these mice showed that the various types of vertebral malformations can be brought about by different mechanisms and that one cannot divine their etiology by morphologic characteristics. Theiler[8] pointed out that changes can be traced back to stages in which somites and notochord develop but vertebrae are not yet formed. He believed that these stages correspond to the fourth week of pregnancy in man. Grüneberg[5] emphasized that the first recognizable changes in the mouse occur at different times of development in different embryonic structures.

To the variety of genetic factors that result in congenital malformations of the spinal column must be added the numerous environmental agents that can produce similar effects. Gillman *et al.*,[9] in 1948, produced many types of vertebral anomalies in rats by trypan blue treatment of the mother and thus devised a simple method for production of axial malformations.[10] Ingalls *et al.*[11] obtained vertebral anomalies in mice whose mothers were exposed to reduced atmospheric pressure and hypoxia during gestation. This method is also effective in rabbits.[12] Exposure to x-rays is also a well-established method for production of spinal malformations.[12,13] Maternal pteroylglutamic acid deficiency together with x-methyl-glutamic acid was used by Nelson *et al.*,[14] which opened up the use of metabolic antagonists in mammalian experimental teratology. Many of these antagonists produce skeletal malformations, including vertebral anomalies. Similar results are obtained by many other teratogenic agents too numerous to be cited here.[15,16] (see Figs. 97-1, 97-4, 97-6 and 97-7).

Genetic influences in the etiology of malformations of the vertebral column are suggested by observations of hemivertebrae in monozygotic twins[17] and by recurrence of the anomaly in certain families. The Klippel-Feil syndrome has been observed repeatedly in more than one member of a family[18] (p. 910) and recurrence has been reported for more widespread vertebral disorders also. Jarcho and Levin[19] described 2 children with hemivertebrae and block vertebrae in the cervical, thoracic and lumbar regions whose mother showed a minor defect of the 5th cervical ver-

Fig. 97-2.—Hemivertebrae, block vertebrae and forking of ribs (**arrow**) in a 6-year-old girl suspected of having Turner syndrome because of a short neck but the chromosomes were normal 46/XX.

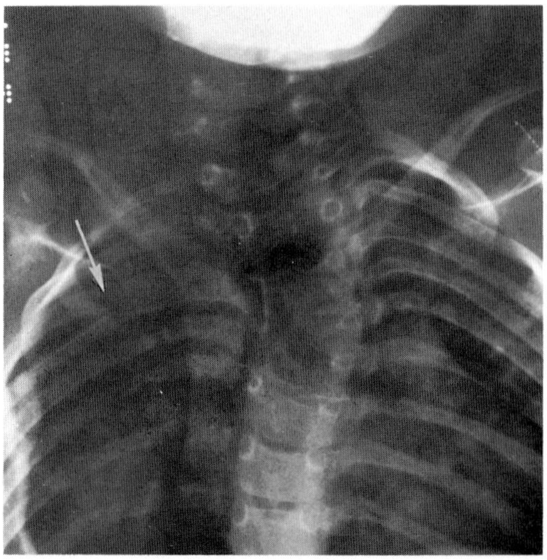

tebra and an accessory nipple. Schwarzweller[20] recorded vertebral malformations transmitted through several generations and Degenhardt[12] published a pedigree that shows structural anomalies of the spine through four generations, but such transmission through several generations is rather rare.

Chromosomal anomalies associated with faulty segmentation of the vertebral column have been described. Turpin *et al.*[21] reported a polyspondyly in a girl with 45 chromosomes and a G/D translocation. Cervical, dorsal and sacral anomalies contributed to the child's growth retardation. In a case of block vertebrae and rib anomalies, a D/D translocation was noted in an affected mother and her child.[22] Fused vertebrae are seen occasionally in trisomy 13-15 (p. 300) and hemivertebrae were described in a patient with a deficiency of part of the long arm of chromosome no. 18.[89] Gunderson *et al.*[18] observed a kindred in which anomalies of segmentation of the cervical spine, kyphoscoliosis and short stature occurred. In some members of the pedigree, a number of cells were found in peripheral blood cultures that were aneuploid. The proband seemed to be a mosaic, showing a small percentage of cells with an extra chromosome 17 or 18. In addition to genetic factors, one must consider the possibility of exogenous influences responsible for spinal malformations[91] (see Fig. 97-1).

As an example of "environmental" factors, one can cite the "caudal dysplasia syndrome" observed in the offspring of diabetic mothers (p. 124). Although the diabetes of these mothers probably is genetically determined, influences of the abnormal genes are indirect, as the children's deformities somehow are due to the changed maternal environment. Gunderson *et al.*[18] mentioned a boy with massive cervical fusion, short neck and cerebrospinal anomalies whose mother had attempted abortion on three occasions during the first trimester of pregnancy.

Since malformations of the axial skeletal system indicate early disturbance of embryonic development, it is understandable that vertebral malformations often are associated with additional skeletal defects or with malformations of other organ systems. In cases of total rachischisis, anencephaly and various monstrous malformations may accompany the defects of the spine (p. 197). Since children with such serious anomalies are not viable, they are better known to pathologists than to pediatricians. In the Cincinnati Children's Hospital, a review of anomalies associated with vertebral defects showed the following malformations: gross brain defects, microcephaly, occipital defect, hypoplastic mandible, cleft palate, microphthalmia, deformed ears, Sprengel deformity, supernumerary nipple, congenital heart disease of many types, agenesis of one lung or abnormal lobation, tracheo-esophageal fistula, malrotation of intestine, imperforate anus, absent or hypoplastic kidney, horseshoe kidney, hydronephrosis, multicystic or malrotated kidney, hypospadias, cryptorchidism, hypoplasia of forearm bones, polydactyly, dislocation of the hip, clubfeet, hemangiomas of the skin and mongolism. Malformations occurring with Klippel-Feil syndrome are mentioned on page 909. Vertebral anomalies as constituents of syndromes are not rare.

Hemivertebrae associated with dwarfism, follicular atrophy of the skin, alopecia of the scalp, unilateral shortening of the tubular bones and mental retardation have been observed repeatedly.[23] In patients with the oculoauriculovertebral (Goldenhar) syndrome, block vertebrae and hemivertebrae can be combined with occipitalization of the atlas (p. 388). Vertebral and costal anomalies sometimes are found in patients with basal cell nevi and odontogenic cysts (p. 1269). Segmentation of the vertebral column may be abnormal in cleidocranial dysostosis. Craniosynostosis can be associated with vertebral anomalies. In patients with brachysyndactyly, abnormal segmentation of the spinal column sometimes appears as a manifestation of irregular joint formation. The same is true for a syndrome of mitral insufficiency, deafness and incomplete differentiation of carpal and tarsal bones (p. 581). An interesting association exists between malformations of the spine and mediastinal cysts of foregut origin.[24] The relationship of these anomalies dates back to the separation of the notochord from the endoderm. Normally, the notochordal cells are completely separated from the primitive alimentary canal by mesodermal cell masses, which later form the vertebral column. If the separation is incomplete and if connections persist between the notochord and the alimentary canal, the formation of vertebrae and disks can be disturbed by the connecting tract and remnants of the endodermal connection can develop into cysts found in postnatal life within the spinal canal or in the mediastinum. Although the connection between the notochord and a mediastinal cyst may have disappeared by the time of birth, an anterior cleft in a vertebral body can remain as testimony to a previous connection.

Rachischisis

Rachischisis is a congenital cleft or fissure of the vertebral column. It can be partial and limited to a few segments (merorachischisis), but the term is applied more often to total rachischisis (holorachischisis), which signifies fissure of the spinal column throughout its length. This form may be combined with anencephaly or exencephaly and cranioschisis. Craniorachischisis, therefore, represents a complete failure of closure of the dorsal osseous covers of the central nervous system. Needless to say, craniorachischisis is not compatible with postnatal life for more than a few hours. Most children with this deformity are stillborn. Sometimes cranioschisis may be combined with a partial rachischisis of the thoracic or lumbosacral area, so that the two clefts of the osseous enclosure of the central nervous system are separated by a normal portion of the spinal column. Rachischisis leaves the underlying portions of the spinal cord exposed to amniotic fluid. This and the inherent abnormalities of the nerve tissue (p. 278) result in partial or total destruction of the exposed neural tissue during fetal life.

In the area of rachischisis, the vertebral bodies are irregularly formed and connected with each other in irregular fashion. Abnormal curvatures of the spine are the rule, since block vertebrae and hemivertebrae are present. The neural arches are incomplete and open dorsally. They also are turned outward, so that they are wider in the transverse direction than normal vertebrae. In holorachischisis, there is a broad, open midline gutter that runs downward from the cranial area to the lumbar area. Ventrally, the bodies of the vertebrae make up the bottom of the gutter, whereas its lateral walls are furnished by the vertebral arches. In fetuses, the gutter is filled out by an open neural plate (p. 197), which usually deteriorates before birth, so that at the time of birth the groove or gutter is covered dorsally by dura mater only. Vestiges of spinal nerves and of ganglia can be found, but there are few remnants of neural plate tissue present at birth (amyelia). The skin defect usually is greater than the osseous cleft and the skin borderline runs outside the rudiments of the arches. A thin epithelium connects the lateral portions of the dura with the borders of the surrounding skin.

Total rachischisis often is combined with cranioschisis and anencephaly. Uranoscopy consists of extreme cervical lordosis and is related to iniencephaly (p. 234). The head is flexed backward so that the occiput touches the open spinal canal in the thoracic or lumbar region. The face is directed upward: uranoscopy. In iniencephaly, the open spinal canal is closed in by the retroflexed head and its skin, which may extend to that of the sacrum. Holorachischisis rarely is associated with omphalocele.

Rachischisis can be limited to the cervical or lumbar region (merorachischisis). In rare instances, anterior clefts of the vertebral bodies constitute ventral rachischisis, resulting in communications between the spinal canal and the thoraco-abdominal cavities, so that the esophagus, stomach, intestine or spleen can appear in the cleft. The extent of the cleft may vary from a limited number of split vertebrae to almost complete anterior cleft of the spinal column. Sometimes the vertebral bodies are cleft but the arches are closed and the spinal cord is normally developed. In such cases, the meninges may form cystic sacs that protrude ventrally. Anterior meningoceles sometimes occur in the sacral region (p. 283).

Meningocele

Incomplete fusion of the neural arch with protrusion of the meninges through vertebral defects may exist under a normal skin or under a thinned epithelial cover. The sac of the meningocele is free of neural tissue and nerve roots but usually there are defects in the vertebrae. In rare instances, a meningocele may be connected with the spinal canal through an intervertebral foramen in the presence of normal vertebrae.

The osseous defects, seen most often in the lumbosacral region, consist of open and spreading pedicles of one or several vertebrae. The affected vertebrae appear broader than normal because of the laterad spreading of the unclosed pedicles. When several segments are affected, a fusiform defect is seen in roentgenograms, with the widest portion at the middle of the lesion. The meningocele does not always correspond to the osseous defect, which, as a rule, is wider than the neck of the sac.[25]

In myeloschisis and spina bifida cystica, the vertebral defects usually are more serious than those of meningocele. Kyphoscoliosis and hemivertebrae are not rare in the spinal column underlying the sac. Vertebral, costal and other skeletal malformations may be present in more distant parts of the body. Diastematomyelia (p. 292) with a bony spur separating two halves of the spinal cord sometimes is associated with these anomalies.[25,26]

Intrathoracic meningoceles occur in neurofibromatosis (p. 1258). Scalloped defects of the posterior portions of the affected vertebral bodies and thinning of the pedicles can be recognized in roentgenograms. The meningocele protrudes through widened intervertebral foramina.[27] Intrathoracic meningoceles also can be combined with developmental vertebral defects. Lateral meningocele with absence of the right halves of the 1st through the 9th thoracic vertebrae and absence of the corresponding ribs was described by Goldman.[28]

Anterior sacral meningocele usually is associated with sacral hemiaplasia (p. 924). An intrapelvic sac containing cerebrospinal fluid protrudes through the osseous defect in such cases. The sac may exert pressure on pelvic structures, causing pain, constipation or urinary difficulties. Roentgenograms show the sacral defect and myelograms demonstrate a meningocele in the pelvis.[29]

Congenital Scoliosis

Congenital deformities of the spine were divided by Putti[30] into five groups: numerical variations, morphologic variations, combinations of numerical and morphologic variations, failure of segmental differentiation and gross unclassifiable changes. This classification is useful for orthopedic surgeons and can be applied to surveys of these anomalies. But sometimes it is difficult to apply in the living infant, since roentgenograms reveal only the ossified parts of the vertebrae and other bony structures may obscure the defects. Kuhns and Hormell,[31] using Putti's classification in 165 patients, found that in half of the cases congenital scoliosis was due to a combination of numerical and morphologic variations and about a third to morphologic variations alone. Failure of differentiation accounted for 13%, numerical variations for 3% and gross unclassifiable changes for 3.6% of the cases.

Numerical variations—decrease or increase in the

number of vertebrae—usually occur in the lumbar region. They cause scoliosis in exceptional cases only, since they need not interfere with normal posture and function. Orthopedic problems arise in children with morphologic vertebral variations, particularly in children in whom such variations are combined with numerical alterations. In the latter type, the changes occur most frequently in the thoracic region, but gross failure of segmental differentiation can occur in all parts of the spine. MacEwen *et al.*[32] described unilateral failure of segmentation of posterolateral vertebral elements of the spine, which results in formation of an osseous bar and severe progressive scoliosis. Fusion of several ribs may be present on the affected side.

Associated extraspinal congenital defects were observed by Kuhns and Hormell[31] in two-thirds of their cases, but the search for concealed malformations was limited and many probably were overlooked. From a list of associated malformations given by these authors, one learns that nearly all parts of the body may be affected and that the etiology of the vertebral malformations is heterogeneous. Shortening of a leg, spasticity or paralysis of muscles, weakness of sphincters or incontinence of urine occurred in 22% of the cases. Many of the patients had a single lateral scoliosis originally, most often in the thoracic region, and in more than one-third multiple scattered anomalies were present at birth. Children with multiple deformities showed a rather slow increase in the progression of the curvature, whereas the most severe curvatures were seen with deformities on one side of the spine, chiefly in the thoracic region. Klippel-Feil syndrome (p. 909), which was included in the series, remained unchanged during the period of growth. Vertebral anomalies on opposite sides of the spine tended to compensate for one another.

It is said that, in general, the prognosis for congenital structural scoliosis is better than for idiopathic forms, since the structural anomalies often counterbalance one another either before birth or later by developing curves in adjacent areas of the spine. But there are exceptions to this rule. Kuhns and Hormell[31] and Shands and Bundens,[33] reporting large series, pointed out that management cannot be uniform. Winter *et al.*[34] thought that most congenital curvatures are progressive, particularly during the preadolescent growth spurt, and that correction and fusion are necessary in many patients. Unilateral thoracic unsegmented bar formation indicates a poor prognosis and requires early operative intervention to prevent a crippling deformity.[32]

Block Vertebrae

Faulty segmentation of the spine manifests itself in many skeletal defects. Lack of differentiation of segmental sclerotomes results in nonseparated, so-called fused, vertebrae, which can form a solid mass. The vertebral bodies, the neural arches and the spinous processes may appear partially or completely fused. The cervical and lumbar vertebrae are affected more often than the thoracic. The intervertebral foramina are smaller than those of neighboring vertebrae. Block vertebrae may correspond in height to that of two normal vertebrae or they may be composed of irregularly formed masses that are asymmetric and joined in an angle. Sometimes block vertebrae are discovered accidentally in roentgenograms, existing without any clinical manifestations. In other cases, they are associated with anomalies of clinical importance.[25] Cervical block vertebrae of differing degrees are present in patients with Klippel-Feil syndrome (p. 909). Block vertebrae in the lower thoracic spine combined with deformities of the appendicular skeleton, advanced ossification, precocious puberty and mental retardation were reported by Meyer.[35]

Transverse (Coronal) Vertebral Clefts

In some fetuses, an anterior and a posterior center of ossification can be recognized in the vertebral bodies. These centers usually fuse after the fourth month, but occasionally fusion is not completed at the time of birth, cartilage still being present between the anterior and posterior halves of the vertebral body. In roentgenograms, such vertebrae seem to have coronal clefts. Fagerberg,[36] in a series of 150 obstetric radiologic investigations, found this anomaly only rarely. If it were seen in a fetus during the last 2 months of pregnancy, it appeared more than 90% probable that the fetus was male. This anomaly in ossification has no pathologic significance in itself, since it disappears during the first year of life, but it may be indicative of more serious associated malformations.[37]

Idiopathic Scoliosis

Idiopathic scoliosis is characterized by lateral spinal curvature without gross congenital malformations attributable to faulty segmentation. Scoliosis develops either in early childhood (infantile idiopathic scoliosis) or during the years of late childhood and adolescence. One cannot speak of congenital scoliosis in most of the cases of idiopathic scoliosis, since they usually develop after birth. But unknown congenital factors may play an imporant role by predisposing to this disorder, which has been observed repeatedly in identical twins.[38–41] In such cases, curvature of the spine may develop after the age of 6 years, showing remarkable similarity in both twins. But concordance has also been noted in dizygotic twins, which suggested to DeGeorge and Fisher[42] that maternal influences predominate. Advanced maternal age was considered a predisposing factor to scoliosis.

James *et al.*[43] distinguished a progressive and a resolving infantile type. Both forms occur more often in males than in females. A few cases can be diagnosed at birth, but most of them make their appearance during the first year of life. There is a definite preponderance of left-sided thoracic curves, which is in contrast to the adolescent form, which shows a preference for right-sided curves.

Ankylosing Spondylitis

This rheumatoid arthritis is not congenital, having its onset in early adult life, but a genetic factor has been considered in its etiology. It is more common among relatives of affected persons than in the general population. Males are affected more often than females.[44]

Cleft Spinous Processes

This is a common and usually inconsequential vertebral anomaly. It consists of lack of fusion of the neural arches and occurs most frequently in the 5th lumbar or 1st sacral segment.[25] Fusion defects also are observed in the lower portion of the sacrum. Such midline defects often are discovered accidentally in roentgenograms of persons who are symptom-free, but sometimes the anomaly is accompanied by low back pain. In such cases, constricting fibrous tissue connected with the dura or the sheaths of nerve roots has been found at operation.[45]

Intervertebral Calcifications

Roentgenograms showing intervertebral calcifications in adults are well known but reports of such changes in children are rarer. Occurrence in newborn children has been reported.[46] Calcifications seen in children may be asymptomatic and found by chance in roentgenograms or they may be associated with a nucleus pulposus hernia or with irritation of nerve roots.

Spondylolisthesis

Junghanns[47] found, in patients with anterior displacement of the spine, bilateral clefts in the interarticular portions of the affected vertebra that he considered congenital even though his patients were of advanced age. Other authors believed that interarticular clefts with or without spondylolisthesis are caused by trauma and are not congenital. Serial examinations of fetuses and neonates failed to demonstrate clefts in the interarticular area comparable to those seen in adults. Spondylolisthesis affects the 5th or 4th lumbar vertebra most often. It is estimated that approximately 4% of the adult population show the abnormality, but the condition is rare in children.[25] In some cases, the congenital nature of the spondylolisthesis is suggested by associated anomalies of the neural arch[48] or by hereditary transmission.[49] Amuso and Mankin[50] reviewed familial cases and published a pedigree in which spondylolisthesis and spina bifida occulta occurred in 5 members of three generations. Wigby and Thomas[51] believed in a

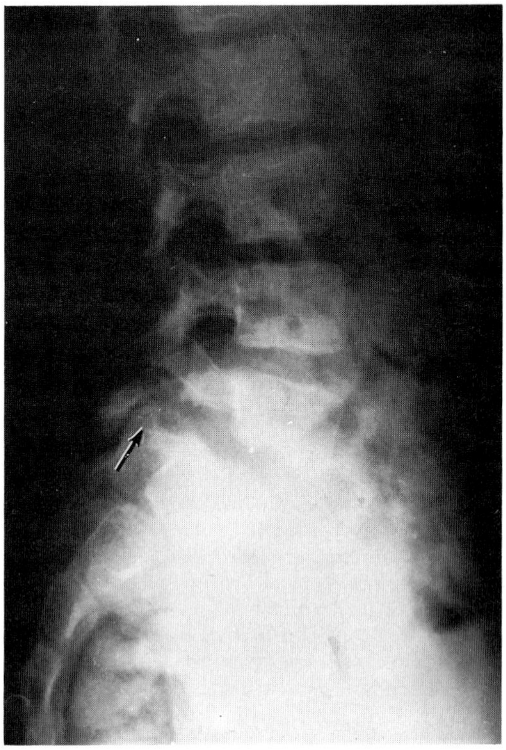

Fig. 97-3.—Spondylolisthesis in an 8-year-old girl. Note separation (**arrow**) of interarticular portion of neural arch, with forward displacement of body of 5th lumbar on the 1st sacral vertebra.

congenital weakness of the vertebral isthmus, with the actual break occurring during childhood.

Malformations of the Caudal Areas of the Body

Severe maldevelopment of the median portions of the caudal body area can result in sirenoid or siren formations. These are, to a certain extent, analogous and comparable to the cyclopian series of the rostral end of the body. Feller and Sternberg[52] pointed out that sirenoid defects must be distinguished from asymmetric monopodia, which, like sirens, have only one extremity; but, in such cases, the defect is limited to one side and there is no "fusion" of the two halves in the midline. In sirens, there is a median, bilateral symmetric defect of the caudal end. The defect can be more pronounced in the dorsal or in the ventral region. In the first case, the legs are not fused but turned backward, approaching each other. This anomaly, called "anchipodia," is associated with aplasia recti. If the ventral area is affected more, the rectum may be formed but the urogenital apparatus is absent. Sympodia are defective in both ventral and dorsal parts. Sirens, which originate very early in embryonic development, show maldevelopment not only in the embryo but also in the body stalk. There are deficiencies of the allantois as well as absence of one umbilical

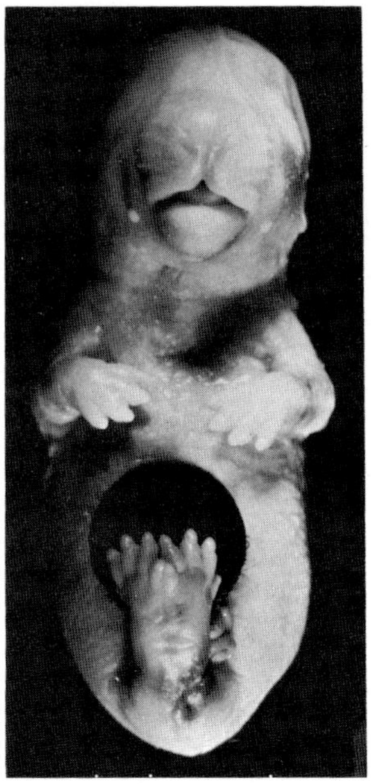

Fig. 97-4. – Sireniform malformation in a 19-day rat fetus produced by treatment of the mother with trypan blue on the ninth and tenth days of gestation.

artery. Sirens are not the result of fusion of previously developed separate skeletal or visceral anlagen but are due to primary lack of median cell masses from which the paired structures normally develop.

Sirens occur occasionally in the offspring of rats treated with trypan blue (Fig. 97-4).

Lumbar Anomalies

Narrow lumbar canal is characteristic of achondroplasia, as the lumbar bodies progressively taper in width in these patients (p. 774). Other disorders due to narrowness of the lumbar canal were discussed by Jones and Thomson.[53] Backache, root pain, paraparesis and intermittent claudication are the symptoms, usually occurring in males. Laminectomy for decompression has been performed with success.

Unilateral absence of lumbar articular facets, although a congenital anomaly, rarely causes trouble during childhood. In adult life, lumbar pain can betray the condition, particularly after trauma.[54]

Agenesis of the Sacrum

According to the medical literature, agenesis of the sacrum is a rather rare anomaly, but its incidence may be higher than is generally believed, since many cases go unreported and others are listed under various names because of more striking associated malformations. Agenesis of the sacrum is an anomaly of segmentation of the spinal column and spinal cord. Often it is the most conspicuous anomaly of the spine, which may show less striking anomalies in its upper part. Agenesis of the caudal end of the spine may vary from the severe forms, with absence of all segments below the 10th or 12th thoracic vertebra, to mild ones with minor coccygeal defects. Freedman[55] tabulated 12 cases according to the lowest vertebra present, from a patient defective from the 10th thoracic vertebra down to one deficient in the lowest coccygeal segments only. These anomalies have been observed in Caucasians, Negroes and Mexicans. Males and females seem to be affected equally.[56] Familial recurrence can be demonstrated only in a minority of cases. Pouzet[57] reported a man with sacral agenesis who had a son with the same malformation. Zeligs[58] described the anomaly in a girl who had a sibling with meningocele. Grand *et al.*[59] observed a patient (Case 2) whose sibling had marked foreshortening of the trunk with a severe kyphoscoliosis, multiple hemivertebrae and rib fusions. In one of our cases with agenesis of the sacrum, Klippel-Feil syndrome, urinary and anal incontinence, undescended testes and bilateral clubfeet, chromosome analysis showed a normal 46/XY constitution (Fig. 97-5).

Fig. 97-5. – Absence of sacrum in a 10-year-old boy. The patient also had Klippel-Feil syndrome, no bladder or bowel control, undescended testes, atrophy of leg muscles and clubfeet. Initially, intelligence was good but later development was retarded as a convulsive disorder developed. There was a normal 46/XY chromosomal pattern. (Cincinnati Children's Hospital Chart No. 121-870.)

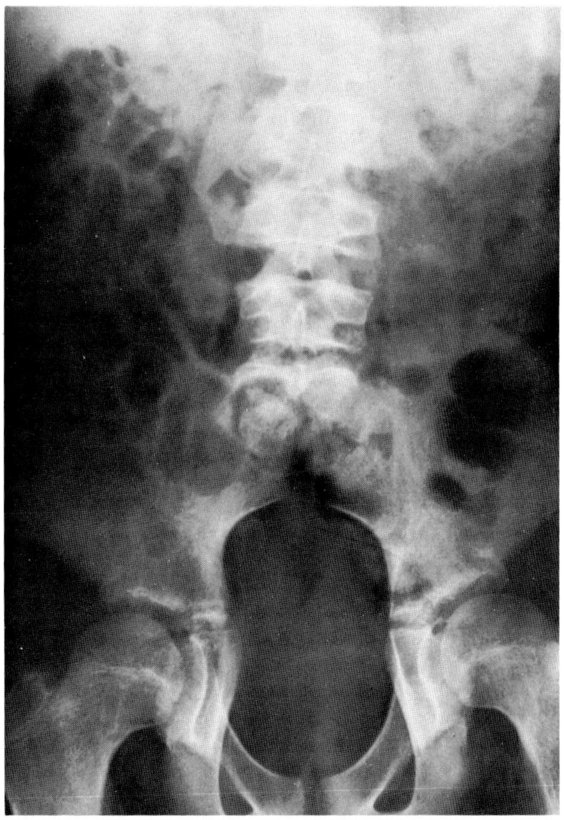

In a tabulation of 50 patients with sacral agenesis, Blumel *et al.*[56] noted that 7 mothers of these patients were diabetic. In Zeligs'[58] Case 2, the mother had not been recognized as diabetic but the deformed baby weighed 5,443 Gm. at birth. Since most babies with sacral agenesis are small at birth, this high birth weight suggests that the mother may have been prediabetic. Absence of the sacrum probably is not an etiologic entity.

In animals, rumpless fowl have been known for several centuries. Landauer[60] produced rumplessness in chickens by mechanical shaking of eggs, but he found that the genetic constitution of the mother played a role in the extent of response. He also induced rumplessness by injection of insulin into eggs of white Leghorn fowl, obtaining an incidence of more than 40% of this malformation. In creeper fowl, the same procedure induced rumplessness in only 17%. Injection of other chemical substances resulted in similar malformations. The role of genetic factors in the "sacral agenesis" syndrome is suggested by observations in mice. Sacrococcygeal agenesis attributed to a recessive mutant gene occurred in a group of Swiss laboratory mice.[61] There is a definite resemblance between the malformations effected by the Sd (short tail) gene in mice and the sacral agenesis syndrome observed in children. In heterozygous mice, there is a shortening of the tail, absence of the 3d and 4th sacral vertebrae and ankylosis of the lower vertebrae. The kidneys may be reduced in size or both kidneys and ureters may be absent, the anomalies being unilateral or bilateral. Some heterozygotes have normal kidneys. In the homozygotes Sd/Sd, which die within 24 hours after birth, the sacral and most of the lumbar vertebrae are missing, the anus is always imperforate and the rectum absent. The colon joins onto the urogenital sinus, the bladder may be absent, the genital papilla reduced and the kidneys usually are absent or dystopic. In both heterozygotes and homozygotes, the syndrome varies in regard to specific malformations, the situation being reminiscent of that of children with sacral agenesis. It is difficult to ascertain how much the morphology of the individual mouse is influenced by nongenetic factors. It is of interest that similar malformations can be produced in genetically "normal" strains of rats by teratogenic agents such as trypan blue,[62] streptonigrin[63] and others. Spina bifida with anomalies of the caudal portion of the spinal column and spinal cord induced in this way have been described.[64,65] An extreme form of agenesis of the spine below the cervical vertebrae is illustrated in Figure 97-6. In mice, various spinal defects, including sacral malformations, can be produced by 6-aminonicotinamide injection.[66]

Approximately 20% of the children with agenesis of the sacrum are delivered in the breech position. It seems that intrauterine growth retardation (p. 134) is not rare. Case 3 of Blumel *et al.*[56] was delivered by breech presentation after a full-term pregnancy, weighing 1,956 Gm. In other patients, intrauterine growth retardation can only be suspected but not proved because either the gestation time or the weight of the baby at birth was not recorded.[56] Some children with the malformation of the sacrum show poor postnatal development (Case 2 of Grand *et al.*[59] was diagnosed as a primordial dwarf because of retarded growth and low weight). A boy observed in the Cincinnati Children's Hospital who weighed only 2,120 Gm. after 37 weeks' gestation did not thrive and weighed 2,270 Gm. when 6 months of age.

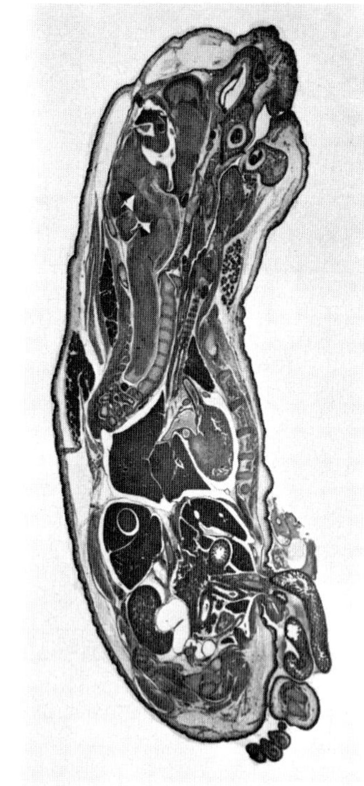

Fig. 97-6. – Absence of vertebral column from upper thoracic segments down. Sagittal section through a 21-day rat fetus whose mother received an injection of streptonigrin on the tenth day of gestation.

There are various degrees of agenesis of the sacrum and various classifications have been suggested. Agenesis of the sacrum can be divided into two subgroups. In incomplete agenesis, the 1st sacral segment is present or the 5th lumbar segment is sacralized, so that a bony ring of the pelvis is formed, resulting in almost normal stance and gait. In complete agenesis, the entire sacrum is missing and the iliac bones meet in the midline posteriorly. This severe form can be recognized by inspection of the patient because the buttocks are flattened, the intergluteal fold is short and there is dimpling over the buttocks. The transverse diameter and the outlet of the pelvis are much reduced, standing and walking may be impossible, the hips are dislocated because of the abnormally vertical position of the pelvic bones and the lower limbs are cone-shaped because of muscular hypoplasia of the lower legs.[55] In the most severe forms, there are serious malformations of the lower limbs, which are functionally useless.[67] Hemisacrum can be total, with absence of all sacral segments on one side and their presence on the other side. In subtotal hemisacrum, all sacral segments are present on one side but on the opposite side development of some bodies and lateral masses is defective.[68]

Manifestations of sacral malformations can be variable. In one case (Case 1 of Blumel *et al.*[56]), there were no clinical complaints and bowel and bladder function was normal. Another (Freedman[55]) patient had thin lower legs and lifelong urinary incontinence but he reached an age of over 61 years. On the other side of the spectrum are cases incompatible with life. In Smith's[68] series, 8 of 26 patients died within the first year. A sireniform, legless, stillborn fetus was described by Brack.[69]

Sometimes sacral agenesis seems merely incidental to a serious syndrome of multiple congenital malformations. Thus, in a child seen in the Cincinnati Children's Hospital (Chart No. 128739), the syndrome consisted of occipital defect, cleft palate, Klippel-Feil syndrome, forked ribs, absence of the left kidney, sacral hypoplasia, imperforate anus and clubfeet. Blumel *et al.*[56] listed a patient (Case 45) with cleft palate, anophthalmia, microcephaly, mandibular ankylosis, congenital heart disease, reduplication of the colon, penis and bladder and imperforate anus.

In typical cases, the patient has urinary and fecal incontinence and often enuresis is the chief complaint. Koontz and Prout[90] reported that in cases of neurogenic bladder dysfunction and serious urologic problems, agenesis of the sacrum should be suspected. Flatness and dimpling of the buttocks, irregularities of the intergluteal fold, a fat pad in place of the sacrum, abnormal posture, dislocation of the hips, marked hypoplasia of the muscles of the lower leg and clubfeet complete the typical picture. Smith[68] compared skeletal with neurologic anomalies. In the majority of his patients, the neurologic deficit paralleled the sacral deficiency, i.e., the sacral nerve supply was absent when the osseous segments had not been formed. In other patients, the neurologic pattern did not conform to the pattern predicted from the bony deficiencies, i.e., function sometimes was better than the skeletal anomalies suggested. It seemed that some sacral roots developed in the absence of vertebral elements.[68]

Associated malformations include skeletal and visceral anomalies. Hemivertebrae and fused vertebrae, Klippel-Feil syndrome, forked ribs, limb deficiencies[69] and Sprengel deformity[70] have been observed. Myelomeningocele (spina bifida) and meningocele frequently are associated with sacral agenesis. Arthrogryposis was listed in 6 of 50 cases of sacral malformations tabulated by Blumel *et al.*[56] In some of these patients, the upper as well as the lower extremities showed the contractures characteristic of arthrogryposis multiplex congenita; in other patients, there were merely "flexion contractures of both hips and knees," i.e., a limited arthrogryposis (p. 1014). The pelvis is contracted in such cases. Imperforate anus and imperforate rectum, partial absence of the genital tract, cryptorchidism, horseshoe kidney, absence or duplication of the kidney, hydronephrosis, agenesis of the lung and other malformations have been observed.[68,71,72] Sacrococcygeal malformations have been observed in approximately a third of the patients who have congenital anorectal anomalies.[73] Mental development may be satisfactory.[71]

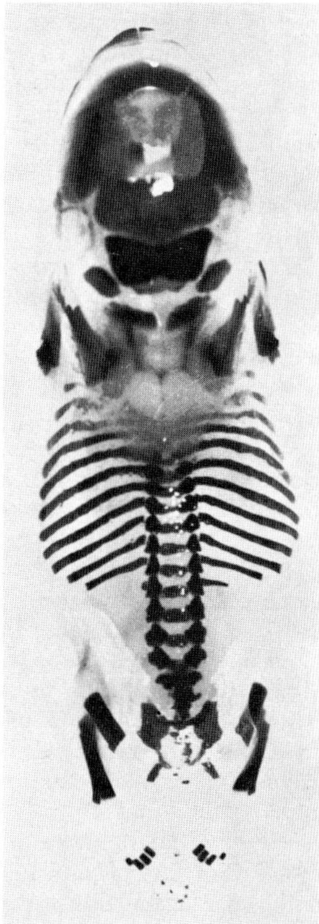

Fig. 97-7.—Abnormal pelvis and defective lower spine in a newborn rat produced by trypan blue injection of the mother on the eighth, ninth and tenth days of gestation.

Roentgenograms show variable sacral defects and often associated skeletal malformations.

Treatment is directed to correction of deformities associated with sacral agenesis. Urinary and rectal anomalies must be alleviated and corrected as far as is possible. In the most severe forms of lumbosacral agenesis with serious involvement of the lower limbs, subtrochanteric amputation and rehabilitation by prosthetic fitting and training has been practiced.[67]

Caudal Appendages (Human Tails)

Legends of tailed men were widespread in the past and tailed races were said to exist in Africa, Asia,

America and Europe. The existence of such tailed tribes has never been confirmed and traditions of their existence must be attributed to observation of people who wore artificial appendages resembling tails or to monkeys mistaken for human beings.

But human individuals with tail-like appendages do exist and old reports concerning such tails of considerable length deserve credence. Gould and Pyle[74] enumerated many cases reported before 1897. Since, in the past, caudal appendages were not removed and since their considerable growth potential has been established, one can believe that the length of such tails could lead to physical discomfort and serious psychologic embarrassment. Human tail-like appendages can arise from various areas of the lower lumbar (Fig. 97-8) or sacrococcygeal midline. They can be straight, segmented or curled. They may be immobile or be "wagged," i.e., moved from side to side.[75] A tail containing vertebrae visible in roentgenograms was reported by Hornitzki.[76]

Harrison[77] reviewed the subject in 1901 and described in great detail a specimen removed from a child 6 months of age. The length of the tail was 4.4 cm. 2 weeks after birth but 7 cm. at the time of removal, thus showing a rapid rate of growth. The child's family was free of congenital malformations; the child itself was well developed, with the exception of hypophalangia of four toes of the right foot. The tail attached in the midline about 1 cm. below the tip of the coccyx was firm but it contained no bone. It was movable and contractile. Hairs were inserted in the skin of the appendage, so that the possibility of hairy tails reported in the past in older persons cannot be excluded. Sections showed normal skin with sweat glands and sebaceous glands. Beneath the skin, the bulk of the tail was made up of areolar tissue containing much fat, with blood vessels, nerves and striated muscle fibers embedded in this mass. There was no

Fig. 97-8.—Tail-like appendage in the lumbar region of a newborn boy.

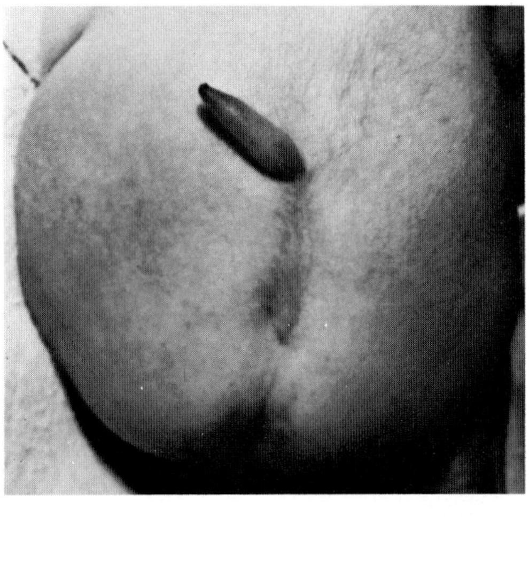

trace of the spinal cord or notochord. Harrison[77] compared his findings with others previously reported. Some of these appendages were similar to the one described by him. In some, there were no muscles and in others there was bone enclosed. Parsons[75] described a soft caudal appendage 4 cm. in length that had its base over the spinous processes of the sacrum in the region of the 3d and 4th vertebrae. This soft structure contained no bone, cartilage or muscle, but near the base there was a capillary hemangioma. Lundberg and Parsons[78] observed a girl born with a firm caudal appendage, 2 cm. long, overlying the tip of the coccyx. This appendage moved from side to side and became elongated when the child cried. On sectioning, longitudinal bundles of muscle fibers were found and at the base of the specimen lay a mass of vascular spaces containing blood, possibly a hemangioendothelioma. In Figure 97-9, a comparable tail-like structure is shown in a newborn boy. The structure was 3.5 cm. in length and sections showed tissues as described by Harrison[77] but no muscle bundles. An unusual tail formation in a newborn Yoruba (Nigeria) girl was reported by Jolly.[79] One end of the tail was attached to the lumbar region and the other to the anterior abdominal wall. There also were ring constrictions on the left leg and malformations of the toes. Giroud *et al.*[80] described a caudal appendage in the lumbar area in a newborn boy who otherwise was entirely normal. They discussed the psychologic impact of this anomaly on the parents and the embryologic basis of the malformation.

Tail-like appendages are now believed to be remnants of structures present in early embryos. Harrison[77] described the caudal structures in human embryos of 14 and 16 mm. length. The embryonic tail, which projects free beyond the cloaca, consists of a portion with and a portion without vertebrae (caudal filament) that contain only notochord and medullary cord. The nonvertebral portion regresses normally. The embryonic tail disappears largely as a result of growth of the extremities and the gluteal region and because of regressive changes in the caudal appendage itself. Many of the anomalous tail-like structures observed in man are due to persistence of the embryonic tail, regression of which may be arrested at various stages of development. The soft and boneless tails are considered remnants of caudal filaments.

It has been suggested that amniotic adhesions could be responsible for persistence of the caudal filament, but this explanation does not hold for the majority of the reported cases.[77] In certain animals, the caudal filament persists normally. Caudal appendages have been found in males and in females of various human races. Associated malformations include meningocele, spina bifida, chondrodystrophy,[81] cleft palate, hemangiomas,[78] syndactyly, hypodactyly[77] and heterotopic anus.[75] But most persons with caudal appendages showed normal general development.

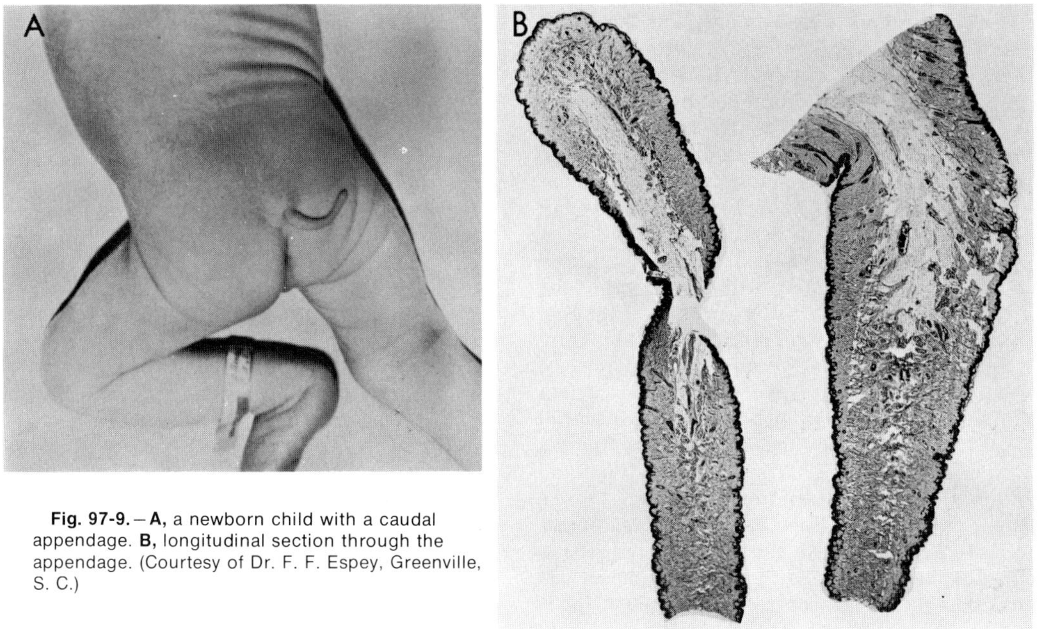

Fig. 97-9. – **A,** a newborn child with a caudal appendage. **B,** longitudinal section through the appendage. (Courtesy of Dr. F. F. Espey, Greenville, S. C.)

Treatment consists of surgical removal of the structure, which usually can be performed without difficulty.

Notochord and Chordoma

The embryonic notochord extends as a continuous rod from the region of the Rathke pouch to the most caudal segments. Around this axial structure the occipital and the vertebral osseous segments are formed. In postnatal life, the notochord is retained by the apical ligament of the dens and within the nucleus pulposus of the intervertebral disks.[82] In a 16-somite human embryo (3 weeks' ovulation age), the notochord is still in contact with the neural tube and is also a component of the mid-dorsal wall of the primitive gut. One week later, the notochord has become separated throughout the cervical and thoracic segments by intervening mesenchyme from both the neural tube and the gut. At the occipital and caudal ends, the notochordal development varies from that of its central portion. In the occipital region, Sensenig[82] found in embryos ranging from 22 to 40 days' gestation age variations of the notochord, such as expansions of its rostral tip, contacts with the pharyngeal epithelium and sacculations. In the caudal region, notochordal elements outside the vertebral anlagen were present frequently and clumps of notochordal cells were left behind following degeneration of the distal caudal segments. There also were adhesions of the notochord with the neural tube in the occipital, cervical and thoracic regions. Such adhesions may become separated from both structures and be left as notochordal remnants at the base of the skull, in vertebral bodies, in the cranial cavity or in the vertebral canal.[83] The remnants may remain harmless and disappear, but they also can be the origin of chordomas, which develop most often in the caudal region (antesacral, retrosacral, central, enteral) or at the cranial end (clivus, hypophyseal, nasopharyngeal, dental). Vertebral chordomas are rare. Two-thirds of the patients with chordoma are male and only one-third female. Manifestations of the tumor usually are delayed to adult life. Antecedent trauma is mentioned often in reports on sacrococcygeal chordomas as a precipitating factor. A few congenital or infantile cases have been recorded.[84] They occurred in the head region, where they may be located in the mouth or retronasally. At the caudal end, they can be found in the hollow of the sacrum and become manifest by pressure on the rectum or by urinary obstruction. They usually are enclosed in a fibrous capsule and show alveolar structure. The tumor cells are arranged in strands that are separated by mucinous secretions. Fibrous trabeculae form an anastomosing network. The cytoplasm of the large and irregular cells is pale and the nuclei are vesicular. After surgical removal, the tumor usually recurs but this can be prevented to a certain extent by irradiation.

Caudal Dysplasia Syndrome (Caudal Regression)

Agenesis of the lower spine was reported in 5 of 920,000 births.[85] Blumel *et al.*[56] reviewed the subject of complete and partial absence of the sacrum with associated malformations. In 7 of 50 cases, the mothers of the affected children were diabetic. Later, Lenz and Maier[86] pointed out that hypoplasia of the femur also was relatively frequent among children of diabetic mothers and it is now assumed that the incidence of the caudal dysplasia syndrome among children of diabetic mothers is 1 per 1,000. By 1966, Passarge and Lenz[87] had collected reports on 43 children with this syndrome associated with diabetes of the mother. Such children have kidney anomalies frequently but anomalies of the upper extremities rarely. Many cases of caudal dysplasia are not related to maternal diabetes, but there is a possibility that exposure of the mother to various chemical substances during pregnancy may be of etiologic significance.[85] Various teratogens used in experimental work produce absence of the lower spine in animals. Streptonigrin is particularly effective in this respect (see Figs. 97-1, *E* and *F*, and 97-6). It has been pointed out that esophageal atresia and renal agenesis combined with caudal dysplasia may represent a syndrome.[85] In the absence of a history of maternal diabetes, prediabetes of the mother must be considered. The caudal regression syndrome has been observed in the child of an 18-year-old mother who showed reduced glucose tolerance.[88] A necropsy revealed hypoplasia and dysplasia of the cord in the region normally occupied by the lumbosacral enlargement, with atrophy of the corresponding spinal roots and defective innervation of the distal musculature in the lower limbs.[92]

REFERENCES

1. Arey, L. B. *Developmental Anatomy* (7th ed.; Philadelphia: W. B. Saunders Company, 1965).
2. Sensenig, E. C.: The early development of the human vertebral column, Contrib. Embryol. 33:21, 1949.
3. Ehrenhaft, J. L.: Development of vertebral column as related to certain congenital and pathological changes, Surg., Gynec. & Obst. 76:282, 1943.
4. Theiler, K.: Beitrag zur Analyse von Wirbelkörperfehlbildungen: Experimente, Genetik und Entwicklung, Ztschr. menschl. Vererb.-u. Konstitutionslehre 31:271, 1953.
5. Grüneberg, H.: Genetical studies on the skeleton of the mouse. XIX. Vestigial-tail, J. Genetics 55:181, 1957.
6. Grüneberg, H.: *The Pathology of Development* (Oxford: Blackwell Scientific Publications, 1963).
7. Kalter, H.: *Teratology of the Central Nervous System* (Chicago: The University of Chicago Press, 1968).
8. Theiler, K.: Das Wirbel-Rippen-Syndrom, Schweiz. med. Wchnschr. 98:907, 1968.
9. Gillman, J., Gilbert, C., and Gillman, T.: A preliminary report on hydrocephalus, spina bifida and other congenital anomalies in the rat produced by trypan blue, South African J. M. Sc. 13:47, 1948.
10. Gillman, J., Gilbert, C., Spence, I., and Gillman, T.: A further report on congenital anomalies in the rat produced by trypan blue, South African J. M. Sc. 16:125, 1951.
11. Ingalls, T. H., Curley, F. J., and Prindle, R. A.: Medical progress: Experimental production of congenital anomalies, New England J. Med. 247:758, 1952.
12. Degenhardt, K. H.: Missbildungen des Kopfes und der Wirbelsäule, in Becker, P. E. (ed.), *Humangenetik* (Stuttgart: Georg Thieme, 1964), Vol. II.
13. Russell, L. B., and Russell, W. L.: An analysis of the changing radiation response of the developing mouse embryo, J. Cell. & Comp. Physiol. 43:103, 1954.
14. Nelson, M. W., Asling, C. W., and Evans, H. M.: Production of multiple congenital abnormalities in young by maternal pteroylglutamic acid deficiency during gestation, J. Nutrition 48:61, 1952.
15. Kalter, H., and Warkany, J.: Experimental production of congenital malformations in mammals by metabolic procedures, Physiol. Rev. 39:69, 1959.
16. Wilson, J. G., and Warkany, J. (eds.): *Teratology: Principles and Techniques* (Chicago and London: The University of Chicago Press, 1965).
17. Haffner, J.: Eineiige Zwillinge mit symmetrischer Wirbelsäulendeformität. Keilwirbel, Acta radiol. 17:529, 1936.
18. Gunderson, C. H., Greenspan, R. H., Glaser, G. H., and Lubs, H. A.: The Klippel-Feil syndrome: Genetic and clinical reevaluation of cervical fusion, Medicine 46:491, 1967.
19. Jarcho, S., and Levin, P. M.: Hereditary malformation of vertebral bodies, Bull. Johns Hopkins Hosp. 62:216, 1938.
20. Schwarzweller, F.: Der angeborene Schulterblatthochstand und seine Beziehungen zu den Missbildungen der Wirbelsäule, Ztschr. menschl. Vererb.-u. Konstitutionslehre 20:350, 1937.
21. Turpin, R., Lejeune, J., Lafourcade, J., and Gautier, M.: Aberrations chromosomiques et maladies humaines. La polydysspondylie à 45 chromosomes, Compt. rend. Acad. Sc. (Paris) 248:3936, 1959.
22. deGrouchy, J., Mlynarski, J. C., Maroteaux, P., Lamy, M., Deshaies, G., Benichou, C., and Salmon, C.: Syndrome polydysspondylique par translocation 14-15 et dyschondrostéose chez un même sujet. Ségrégation familiale, Compt. rend. Acad. Sc. (Paris) 256:1614, 1963.
23. Caffey, J.: *Pediatric X-ray Diagnosis* (5th ed.; Chicago: Year Book Medical Publishers, Inc., 1967).
24. Fallon, M., Gordon, A. R. G., and Lendrum, A. C.: Mediastinal cysts of fore-gut origin associated with vertebral abnormalities, Brit. J. Surg. 41:2, 1954.
25. Epstein, B. S.: *The Spine. A Radiological Text and Atlas* (2d ed.; Philadelphia: Lea & Febiger, 1962).
26. Cameron, A. H.: The Arnold-Chiari and other neuroanatomical malformations associated with spina bifida, J. Path. & Bact. 73:195, 1957.
27. LaVielle, C. J., and Campbell, D. A.: Neurofibromatosis and intrathoracic meningocele, Radiology 70:62, 1958.
28. Goldman, I. R.: Congenital malformation of vertebrae (hemivertebrae) with aplasia of corresponding ribs, associated with lateral meningomyelocele, Arch. Path. 47: 153, 1949.
29. Leigh, T. F., and Rogers, J. V., Jr.: Anterior sacral meningocele, Am. J. Roentgenol. 71:808, 1954.
30. Putti, V.: Die angeborenen Deformitäten der Wirbelsäule, Fortschr. Geb. Röntgenstrahlen 15:65, 1910.
31. Kuhns, J. G., and Hormell, R. S.: Management of congenital scoliosis. Review of one hundred seventy cases, Arch. Surg. 65:250, 1952.
32. MacEwen, G. D., Conway, J. J., and Miller, W. T.: Congenital scoliosis with a unilateral bar, Radiology 90:711, 1968.
33. Shands, A. R., Jr., and Bundens, W. D.: Congenital deformities of the spine, Bull. Hosp. Joint Dis. 17:10, 1956.
34. Winter, R. B., Moe, J. H., and Eilers, V. E.: Congenital scoliosis. A study of 234 patients treated and untreated, J. Bone & Joint Surg. 50-A:1, 1968.
35. Meyer, R.: An unusual form of osseous dysplasia, Am. J. Roentgenol. 73:761, 1955.
36. Fagerberg, S.: Coronal cleft vertebra in foetuses of male sex, Acta obst. et gynec. scandinav. 42:65, 1963.
37. Cohen, J., Currarino, G., and Neuhauser, E. B. D.: Significant variant in ossification centers of vertebral bodies, Am. J. Roentgenol. 76:469, 1956.
38. Weiser, M.: Spiegelbildliche Skoliosen bei Zwillingen, Ztschr. Orthop. 76:264, 1947.
39. Esteve, R.: Idiopathic scoliosis in identical twins, J. Bone & Joint Surg. 40-B:97, 1958.

40. Codorniu, A. H.: "Idiopathic" scoliosis of congenital origin, J. Bone & Joint Surg. 40-B:94, 1958.
41. Murdoch, G.: Scoliosis in twins, J. Bone & Joint Surg. 41-B:736, 1959.
42. DeGeorge, F. V., and Fisher, R. L.: Idiopathic scoliosis: Genetic and environmental aspects, J. M. Genetics 4:251, 1967.
43. James, J. I. P., Lloyd-Roberts, G. C., and Pilcher, M. F.: Infantile idiopathic scoliosis, J. Bone & Joint Surg. 41-B: 719, 1959.
44. Emery, A. E. H., and Lawrence, J. S.: Genetics of ankylosing spondylitis, J. M. Genetics 4:239, 1967.
45. Jelsma, F., and Ploetner, E. J.: Painful spina bifida occulta with review of literature, J. Neurosurg. 10:19, 1953.
46. Lorenz, K., and Berger, G.: Intervertebrale Verkalkungen im Kindesalter, Monatsschr. Kinderh. 114:537, 1966.
47. Junghanns, H.: Über Wirbelabgleiten, Arch. klin. Chir. 159:423, 1930.
48. Roche, M. B., and Bryan, C. S.: Spondylolisthesis; additional variations in anomalies of the pars interarticularis, Arch. Surg. 53:675, 1946.
49. Bailey, W.: Observations on etiology and frequency of spondylolisthesis and its precursors, Radiology 48:107, 1947.
50. Amuso, S. J., and Mankin, H. J.: Hereditary spondylolisthesis and spina bifida. Report of a family in which the lesion is transmitted as an autosomal dominant through three generations, J. Bone & Joint Surg. 49-A:507, 1967.
51. Wigby, P. E., and Thomas, J. R.: Spondylolisthesis. An autopsy study, Radiology 68:94, 1957.
52. Feller, A., and Sternberg, H.: Zur Kenntnis der Fehlbildungen der Wirbelsäule. III. Mitteilung über den vollständigen Mangel der unteren Wirbelsäulenabschnitte und seine Bedeutung für die formale Genese der Defektbildungen des hinteren Körperendes, Virchows Arch. path. Anat. 280:649, 1931.
53. Jones, R. A. C., and Thomson, J. L. G.: The narrow lumbar canal. A clinical and radiological review, J. Bone & Joint Surg. 50-B:595, 1968.
54. Keim, H. A., and Keagy, R. D.: Congenital absence of lumbar articular facets, J. Bone & Joint Surg. 49-A:523, 1967.
55. Freedman, B.: Congenital absence of the sacrum and coccyx, Brit. J. Surg. 37:299, 1950.
56. Blumel, J., Evans, E. B., and Eggers, G. W. N.: Partial and complete agenesis or malformation of the sacrum with associated anomalies, J. Bone & Joint Surg. 41-A:497, 1959.
57. Pouzet, F.: Les anomalies du développement du sacrum, Lyon chir. 35:371, 1938.
58. Zeligs, I. M.: Congenital absence of the sacrum, Arch. Surg. 41:1220, 1940.
59. Grand, M. J. H., Eichenfeld, S., and Jacobson, H. G.: Sacral aplasia (agenesis), Radiology 74:611, 1960.
60. Landauer, W.: Rumplessness of chicken embryos produced by the injection of insulin and other chemicals, J. Exper. Zool. 98:65, 1945.
61. Frye, F. L., McFarland, L. Z., and Enright, J. B.: Sacrococcygeal agenesis in Swiss mice, Cornell Vet. 54:487, 1964.
62. Warkany, J.: Experimental Production of Congenital Malformations of the Central Nervous System, in Bowman, P. W., and Mautner, H. V. (eds.), *Mental Retardation*, Proceedings of First International Conference on Mental Retardation (New York: Grune & Stratton, Inc., 1960).
63. Warkany, J., and Takacs, E.: Congenital malformations in rats from streptonigrin, Arch. Path. 79:65, 1965.
64. Gunberg, D. L.: Spina bifida and the Arnold-Chiari malformation in the progeny of trypan blue injected rats, Anat. Rec. 126:343, 1956.
65. Warkany, J., Wilson, J. G., and Geiger, J. F.: Myeloschisis and myelomeningocele produced experimentally in the rat, J. Comp. Neurol. 109:35, 1958.
66. Nogami, H., and Ingalls, T. H.: Pathogenesis of spinal malformations induced in the embryos of mice, J. Bone & Joint Surg. 49-A:1551, 1967.
67. Frantz, C. H., and Aitken, G. T.: Complete absence of the lumbar spine and sacrum, J. Bone & Joint Surg. 49-A: 1531, 1967.
68. Smith, E. D.: Congenital sacral anomalies in children, Australian & New Zealand J. Surg. 29:165, 1959.
69. Brack, I. E.: Über das Kreuzbein, Virchows Arch. path. Anat. 272:295, 1929.
70. Katz, J. F.: Congenital absence of the sacrum and coccyx, J. Bone & Joint Surg. 35-A:398, 1953.
71. Blumel, J., Butler, M. C., Evans, E. B., and Eggers, G. W. N.: Congenital anomaly of the sacrococcygeal spine, Arch. Surg. 85:982, 1962.
72. Berdon, W. E., Hochberg, B., Baker, D. H., Grossman, H., and Santulli, T. V.: The association of lumbosacral spine and genitourinary anomalies with imperforate anus, Am. J. Roentgenol. 98:181, 1966.
73. Parkkulainen, K. V.: Sacrococcygeal and urological anomalies in connection with congenital malformations of anus and rectum. A preliminary report, Ann. paediat. Fenniae 3:51, 1957.
74. Gould, G. M., and Pyle, W. L.: *Anomalies and Curiosities of Medicine* (Philadelphia: W. B. Saunders Company, 1897).
75. Parsons, R. W.: Human tails, Plast. & Reconstruct. Surg. 25:618, 1960.
76. Hornitzki, P.: Ein Fall des Wirbelschwanzes bei einem Kinde, Zentralbl. Chir. 67:1051, 1940.
77. Harrison, R. G.: On the occurrence of tails in man, with a description of the case reported by Dr. Watson, Bull. Johns Hopkins Hosp. 12:96, 1901.
78. Lundberg, G. D., and Parsons, R. W.: A case of a human tail, Am. J. Dis. Child. 104:72, 1962.
79. Jolly, H.: Baby with a tail, Arch. Dis. Childhood 38:524, 1963.
80. Giroud, A., Salet, J., and Pernet-Robert, J.: L'appendice caudal du nouveau-né, Arch. franç. pédiat. 23:603, 1966.
81. Potter, E. L.: *Pathology of the Fetus and Infant* (2d ed.; Chicago: Year Book Medical Publishers, Inc., 1961).
82. Sensenig, E. C.: Adhesions of notochord and neural tube in the formation of chordomas, Am. J. Anat. 98:357, 1956.
83. Horwitz, T.: Chordal ectopia and its possible relation to chordoma, Arch. Path. 31:354, 1941.
84. Montgomery, A. H., and Wolman, I. J.: Sacrococcygeal chordomas in children, Am. J. Dis. Child. 46:1263, 1933.
85. Kučera, J., and Lenz, W.: Caudale Regression mit Oesophagusatresie und Nierenagenesie – ein Syndrom, Ztschr. Kinderh. 98:326, 1967.
86. Lenz, W., and Maier, W.: Congenital malformations and maternal diabetes, Lancet 2:1124, 1964.
87. Passarge, E., and Lenz, W.: Syndrome of caudal regression in infants of diabetic mothers: Observations of further cases, Pediatrics 37:672, 1966.
88. Thalhammer, O., Lachmann, D., and Scheibenreiter, S.: "Caudale Regression" beim Kind einer 18 jäjrigen Frau mit Prädiabetes, Ztschr. Kinderh. 102:346, 1968.
89. Insley, J.: Syndrome associated with a deficiency of part of the long arm of chromosome no. 18, Arch. Dis. Childhood 42:140, 1967.
90. Koontz, W. W., and Prout, G. R.: Agenesis of the sacrum and the neurogenic bladder, J.A.M.A. 203:481, 1968.
91. Browne, D.: Infantile scoliosis, Clin. Proc. Child. Hosp., Washington 25:157, 1969.
92. Price, D. L., Dooling, E. C., and Richardson, E. P., Jr.: Caudal dysplasia (caudal regression syndrome), Arch. Neurol. 23:212, 1970.

98

The Chest

THE SKELETON OF THE CHEST consists of vertebrae, ribs and sternum. These skeletal elements form a cage that includes and protects the heart and the lungs.

The ribs develop as processes of the primitive mesenchymal anlagen of the vertebrae. In the thoracic area, they grow ventrad, forming bars that follow the body walls. The distal ends of these bars join in lateral sternal bands, forming an early framework for the thoracic organs. In the seventh week, centers of chondrification that are progressively converted into cartilage appear in the dorsal aspects of the ribs. The dorsal costal portions become separated from the vertebrae by joints, and their tubercles articulate with transverse vertebral processes. Ossification begins near the angles of the ribs in the ninth week of gestation. It progresses ventrad but the distal ends remain cartilaginous. In the neck, the rib anlagen remain short, unite with the cervical vertebrae and contribute to the formation of the transverse foramina. In the lumbar area, the ribs are united with the transverse vertebral processes, but in the sacral region they are modified to the lateral masses of the sacrum.[1]

The first condensations of mesoderm, which precede the cartilaginous sternum, appear in the chest wall of embryos 6 weeks old. There are two lateral sternal bands and an anterior median rudiment. The sternal bands at first are widely separated and the heart lies immediately below the skin cover between them. As chondrification sets in, the sternal bands approach each other in their cranial portions and subsequently fuse completely in the midline, including the anterior median rudiment. At 9 weeks, the sternum is preformed in cartilage but unsegmented and solidly united with the ribs.[2] Centers of ossification appear in man in the sixth fetal month, at first in the manubrium and later in the corpus. The center of the xiphoid process ossifies in the third year of postnatal life. Bony union of the four segments of the gladiolus or mesosternum progresses during childhood from below upward, and is completed after puberty. The manubrio-sternal synchondrosis persists in the majority of human beings throughout life, but ossification does occur in approximately 10% of normal persons during postpubertal life.[2] In 90% of children with Down syndrome between the ages of 1 month and 4 years, two and sometimes three ossification centers can be seen in the manubrium sterni, whereas only 20% of control children have two centers in the sternal manubrium.[3]

Experimental teratology shows that rib anomalies can arise in differing manners. Some are associated with disturbances of vertebral segmentation. Owing to absence or malformation of vertebrae, the ribs arise irregularly near the axial skeleton; often they fork as they progress ventrad, as if they tried to "make up" for the central deficiency (Fig. 98-1). Other rib anomalies are seen in their distal parts, their "extremities." They consist of fusions or, better, unions due to failure of differentiation of the distal ends of the costal bars (Fig. 98-2). These distal fusions of ribs were regularly obtained in specimens deformed by riboflavin deficiency.[4] Young with such fused ribs also commonly had sternal anomalies and

Fig. 98-1.—Cleared specimen of a newborn rat with ribs fused at distal ends (produced by maternal riboflavin deficiency). Note reduction malformations of the extremities.

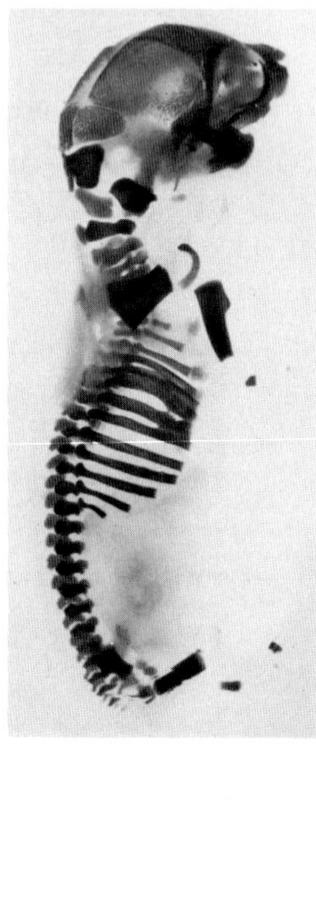

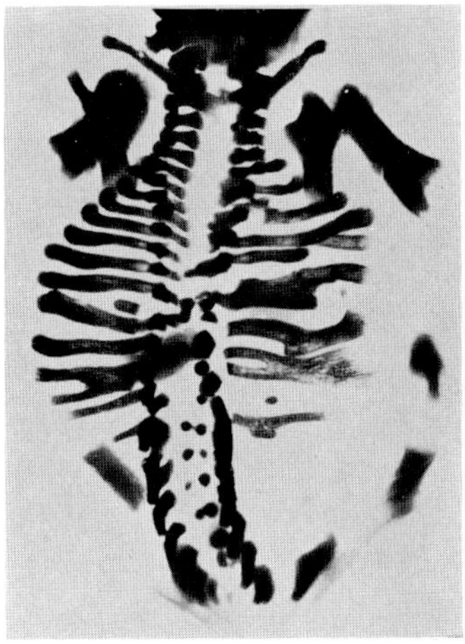

Fig. 98-2.—Disorganization of vertebrae and ribs in a newborn rat, produced by maternal injection of methyl salicylate on the eleventh day of gestation.

malformations of the distal parts of the extremities but the spinal column was normal. Thus, proximal (posterior) and distal (anterior) rib anomalies may have quite different significance in regard to pathogenesis and causation. An interesting observation was made by Smith *et al.*,[5] who described a rib gap as an anomaly in a syndrome of congenital defects. This illustrates another disturbance of development leading to rib anomalies, a disturbance not easily understood with the present knowledge of costal embryology.

Nonsegmentation of the sternum has been found among other effects of a pleiotropic gene in "screw-tail" mice.[6] Faulty segmentation also has been described repeatedly in experimentally induced syndromes of congenital malformations in rats. Warkany and Nelson[4] reported irregular ossification and nonsegmentation of the sternum in the young of female rats fed a riboflavin-deficient diet. Abnormal sternal segmentation also has been induced by thalidomide in rabbits.[7]

Rib Anomalies

Estimates of costal anomalies vary greatly. Steiner[8] found 59 rib anomalies in a series of 38,105 roentgenograms, i.e., approximately 0.15%. Cervical ribs accounted for 32% and lumbar ribs for 29.3% of the abnormalities. Bifurcation of ribs occurred in 5 cases and osseous union between adjoining ribs in 5 cases, with a predilection for males. This is of interest, since cervical and lumbar ribs occur more often in females than in males. Rudimentary first rib was seen in 5 instances. A much higher incidence was noted by Fried[9] in roentgenograms taken for ascertainment of tuberculous lesions. Among more than 50,000 persons, 564, i.e., more than 1%, had rib anomalies. There was male preponderance in this series also. Coury and Delaporte[10] believed that 2% might be a realistic estimate, since most rib anomalies are missed on physical examination and often overlooked in roentgenograms. Another high estimate was made by Martin,[11] who found in roentgenograms of the Cincinnati General Hospital population (Caucasians and Negroes) and of European populations anomalies in 3.4% and 2.7%. Bifid ribs, spurs on ribs and wide or enlarged ribs (BSW) represent a complex that can be distinguished from "fused" ribs, absent ribs and cervical ribs. The BSW type accounted for most rib anomalies. Interesting were the findings in Samoans, who showed an incidence of 10.4%, with BSW anomalies accounting for 9.4%. Half of these anomalies were found in rib IV and one-fourth in rib III. Males were affected twice as often as females. Rib anomalies other than BSW anomalies were not more frequent in the Samoan population. Coury and Delaporte,[10] who made a thorough study of costal anomalies, discussed supernumerary ribs, which were almost exclusively associated with the cervical spine, deficiencies of the first rib and associated anomalies, synostoses, bifid ribs and unusual unclassifiable cases. For details, the reader is referred to this exhaustive article.

Cervical ribs. Cervical ribs usually originate from the costal processes of the 7th cervical vertebrae as bilateral but often asymmetric osseous structures. They may terminate with free ends in the soft tissues or join the first rib or the sternum distally. The relationships of cervical ribs to adjacent anatomic structures have been described in detail.[10,12] Their incidence is seen in roentgenograms of adults in 0.7%.[11]

Cervical ribs occur much more often in females than in males, and symptoms also are noticed more often by females. A genetic background can be demonstrated in some of the cases.[10,13] The anomaly re-

Fig. 98-3.—Infant with congenital heart disease, vertebral anomalies and 10 ribs.

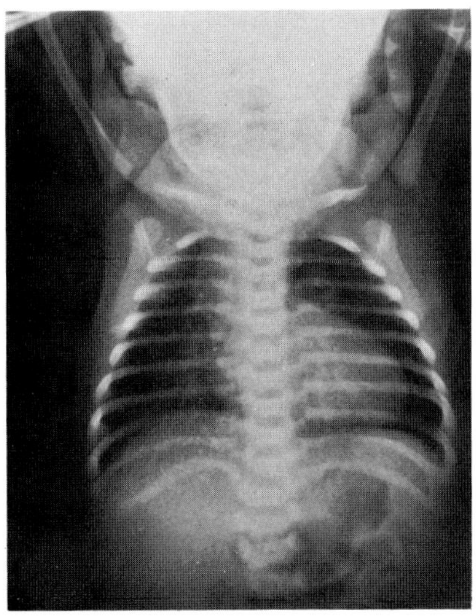

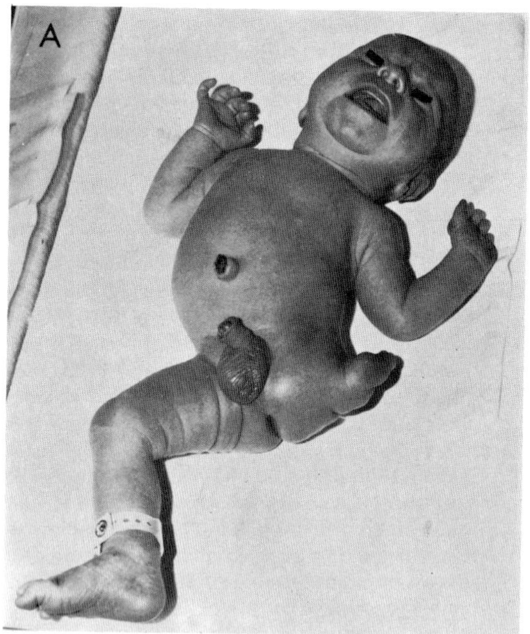

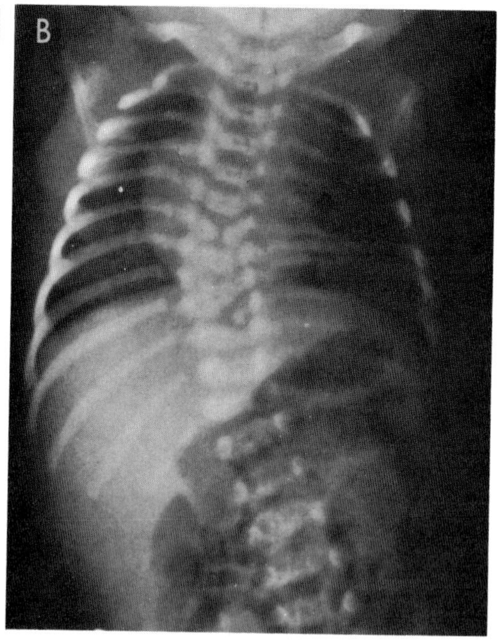

Fig. 98-4. – **A,** boy with reduction malformations of left leg and left undescended testis. **B,** roentgenogram showing vertebral and rib anomalies.

mains without symptoms in approximately 50–75% of the cases.[10] Progressing ossification, physiologic descent of the shoulder, trauma or occupational movements may contribute to the manifestation of symptoms. Disturbances can commence in children, but more often they make their appearance between adolescence and the fifth decade.

Prominence or tumor above the clavicle and a difference in the radial pulse can be signs of the anomaly. If the radial pulse appears normal, it may be obliterated by raising of the arm over the head and turning of the head to the opposite side. Symptoms may be vascular or nervous. Interference with circulation is attributed to compression of the subclavian artery by the cervical rib or by the scalenus anticus muscle. Pressure symptoms referable to the brachial plexus and to fibers reaching the plexus by way of the first thoracic root account for some of the manifestations.[13] Thrombosis of the subclavia or aneurysm formation has been reported.[14] Pain is localized to the back of the neck, shoulder or supraclavicular region. Shooting pain or paresthesia referred to the hand and fingers usually is unilateral. A sensation of coldness may be experienced in the same areas. Muscle weakness and atrophy in the outer portion of the thenar may be present. Objective coldness and blueness of the hands and fingers and redness and numbness of the arm occur in some cases.[13]

Fig. 98-5. – Roentgenogram showing a cervical rib on the left side (**arrows**).

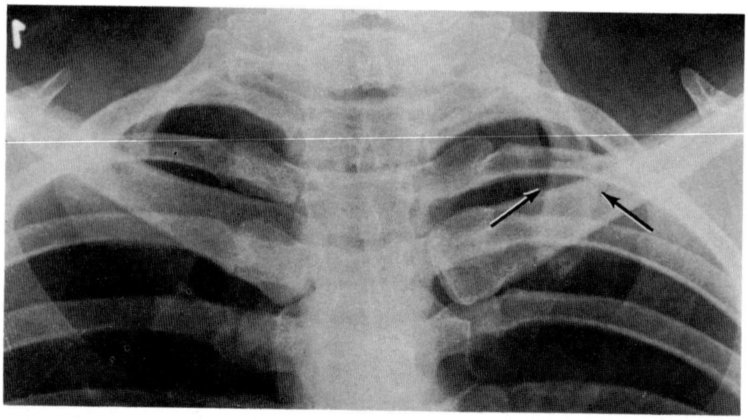

Cervical rib in early life was discussed by Davis and King.[14] As a rule, symptoms caused by the anomaly are delayed to adult life but occasionally they do arise during childhood. Tumor of the neck, edema, "torticollis" or pain may betray the anomaly. If ossification of the abnormal rib is incomplete, roentgenologic demonstration is difficult, but oblique views sometimes can reveal the rib adequately. Davis and King[14] found in 1,000 consecutive roentgenograms of the chest of children 12 cases of cervical ribs, 10 of which were bilateral. In only 3 patients had symptoms been noted. Every patient with cervical rib had a long neck and a hyposthenic thorax. The transverse process of the 7th cervical vertebra was always large so that sometimes it was difficult to differentiate it from the cervical rib. In children under 5 years, the finding of a separate bone adjacent to a transverse process of C7 should be recognized as a costal ossification center and a potential precursor of a cervical rib.[14]

Since most cases of cervical ribs are symptomless, they require no treatment. With mild manifestations, palliative treatment often is successful, but in the presence of neuralgia, muscular atrophy or severe vasomotor symptoms surgical intervention becomes necessary. Section of a band between the cervical and the first rib, removal of the cervical rib and tenotomy of the anterior scalenus muscle are procedures recommended by surgeons.

First ribs. Anomalies of the first ribs are less known than cervical ribs, although they are not rare. Partial agenesis, segmentation and anterior deviation with attachment to the second rib are quite frequent but the majority are symptomless. They may be associated with other skeletal anomalies and rarely with mega-esophagus and bronchiectasis.[10] If upper thoracic ribs are rudimentary or absent, the resulting deformities are noticeable, particularly if there also are muscle deficiencies or malformations.[15] Bilateral synostosis of the seventh rib with the inferior angle of the scapula was reported by Packer *et al.*[16]

Lumbar ribs. Lumbar ribs usually articulate with the transverse processes of the 1st lumbar vertebra. They can vary in length and occur unilaterally or, more often, bilaterally.[8] They are rarer than cervical ribs; they, too, show a predilection for females. Pain and local tenderness in the back or in the area of the affected lumbar vertebra are symptoms of the anomaly.[13]

In addition to the rather orderly costal variations discussed so far, there occur severe malformations of the rib cage with multiple fusions, agenesis and fenestrations combined with disturbances of vertebral segmentation, scoliosis, spina bifida, anencephaly, congenital heart disease or rectal agenesis.[10] Such severe rib anomalies can be produced experimentally by teratogens that disturb vertebral segmentation (p. 931). Figure 98-2 shows such complete disorganization of the vertebrae and ribs produced by methylsalicylate. In children with multiple and severe rib anomalies, respiration may be difficult from birth on. Grislain *et al.*[17] reported such a case in a newborn complicated by bilateral chondromas. Rickham[18] observed lung hernia due to congenital absence of ribs. The ribs are involved in many congenital and systemic skeletal disorders. In achondroplasia, a rosary points to abnormal costochondral junctions; in addition, the ribs are short and the thorax is constricted. Short ribs are characteristic of thanatophoric dwarfism (p. 768) and of asphyxiating thoracic dystrophy (p. 795). Club-shaped ribs typically are seen in Hurler syndrome. In osteogenesis imperfecta gravis, the ribs show deformities due to hundreds of fractures at birth (p. 827). Ossification of the ribs may be quite insufficient in hypophosphatasia, so that respiration may be impeded in the neonate (p. 859). In patients with multiple exostoses (p. 840), bony excrescences can occur on the ribs, usually near their sternal ends. A rib-gap defect was reported as a constituent of a syndrome that includes micrognathia and malformations of tracheal cartilages.[5] The ribs may be involved in thoracic abnormalities produced by neurofibromatosis.[19] Bifid ribs, costal synostoses or partial agenesis combined with vertebral and sternal anomalies have been observed repeatedly in the "basal cell carcinoma syndrome"[20] (p. 1268). Multiple rib anomalies were present in a child with congenital malformations attributed to methotrexate ingestion.[21]

It can be concluded from the foregoing that rib anomalies have differing etiology and pathogenesis. In some of the disorders mentioned, well-defined genetic mechanisms are responsible. That exogenous factors must be considered is shown by numerous teratologic experiments and by the case due to methotrexate exposure.[21] For many patients, the causative factors remain obscure. As a rule, deformities due to absent or irregular ribs do not require treatment, since they may be improved by normal growth. Lester[15] pointed out that fusions of the anterior ends of the ribs need no treatment, whereas fusions of the posterior ends lead to curving of the spine toward the side of the fusion, which requires early orthopedic correction. One of the reasons for the difference in prognosis may be that the posterior rib anomalies often are associated with axial, i.e., vertebral defects, representing, therefore, a more serious developmental disturbance than the anterior ones, which are more related to appendicular defects (p. 939).

Fissure of the Sternum

Sternal fissure, a midline cleft of the anterior chest wall, is a rare deformity. It can be partial or complete. In the mildest form, there is a hole in the center of the sternum. A fissure of the manubrium or continuation of its cleft toward the xiphoid process results in a triangular osseous defect that usually is closed by fibrous tissue and covered by skin. The insertion of the muscles and the position of the viscera may be normal in such cases. In rare instances, ectopia cordis may be present, the heart lying on the body surface connected with the interior of the thorax by the great vessels (p. 475). Greig[22] distinguished between simple cleft sternum and cleft sternum associated with ectopia cordis.

A number of cases of simple cleft were described in the nineteenth century, when the defect afforded examining physicians the opportunity to observe the movements of the heart or of the great vessels. In such cases, the groove formed in place of the absent sternum usually was covered by skin, which bulged during expiration and was drawn in during inspiration. These cases were reviewed by Greig[22] in 1926. Szenes[23] described an 8-year-old boy who was born with a scar-like lesion over the midline of the chest. From the cranial end of the lesion there originated a skin fold that connected the chest with the chin. Below the cutaneous depression, a fissured sternum was present that was laterally limited by cartilaginous bands in which calcified foci were noted roentgenographically. Caudally, the cleft was bridged by a bony lamella that corresponded to the xiphoid process. In contrast to most cases of sternal fissure in which the cleft is closed by firm connective tissue and covered by normal skin, in this case there was a paper-thin scar over the defect.

In the presence of thoracic ectopia cordis, proper formation of the sternum is impossible. In some of these cases, the cranial and central portions of the sternum may be formed in cartilage but the costal cartilages diverge caudad and the heart, without a parietal pericardium, protrudes as a pulsating tumor. Thoracic ectopia cordis may be associated with diaphragmatic defects and with marked diastasis of the recti abdominis. Cardiovascular anomalies usually are present in hearts that protrude through a sternal defect. Atrial and ventricular septal defects and double superior vena cava have been observed repeatedly.[22] In one instance, there was transposition of the great vessels, tricuspid atresia and atrial and ventricular septal defects. The child also had microcephaly and postaxial hexadactyly.[24]

Funnel Chest (Pectus Excavatum)

Funnel chest consists in a depression of the lower parts of the sternum, with the lower costal cartilages running dorsad from their costochondral junctions to their sternal attachments. The tip of the sternum appears depressed and may, in extreme cases, touch the vertebral column. The skeletal changes are associated with abnormal development of the anterior musculature of the diaphragm and shortening of the central tendon, which seems to exert a pull on the sternum and the lower ribs. Many cases of funnel chest are due to muscular and fibrous anomalies, whereas the bones are essentially normal. In other cases, the thoracic malformation is combined with other skeletal deformities representing a part of a serious disease picture. Estimates of the occurrence of pectus excavatum vary between 0.13 and 0.43 per 1,000.[25] Dominant inheritance of the anomaly has been observed repeatedly,[26,27] and there are reports showing that pectus excavatum and pectus carinatum can alternate in families.[28] Narrow and broad types of depression have been described. In the narrow type, there is a thick and dense substernal ligament and a short central attachment of the diaphragm to the lower end of the sternum. In the broad type, the lateral anterior portions of the diaphragm are shortened also. The deformity results in a long and narrow chest, the shoulders are held high and turned forward, the thoracic kyphosis is increased and the abdomen protrudes. The heart usually is displaced to the left. There is retraction with every inspiration.

In some infants, symptoms appear early. Noisy respiration, croup and frequent infections occur. Occasionally, vomiting is a presenting symptom and failure to thrive is noticed. In older children, the symptoms are less striking, but exercise tolerance is decreased and there may be dyspnea on exertion. Spontaneous correction occurs in some children within a few years after birth,[29] but, even in mild cases, symptoms may appear in adult life. The deformity often is a psychologic handicap.

Patients with severe kyphosis, kyphoscoliosis and pectus excavatum eventually may suffer from disturbances of the circulation and respiration and sometimes die of cardiac failure.[30] The lungs of such patients are small and diseased by emphysema, bronchitis, bronchiectasis and pneumonia. Increased resistance in the pulmonary circuit results in hypertrophy and dilatation of the right ventricle and atrium. Be-

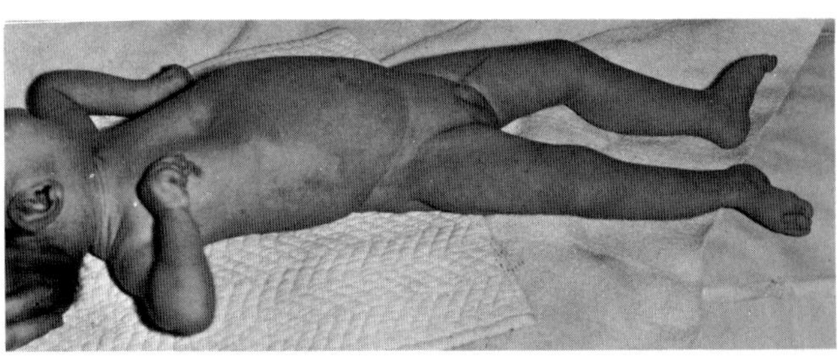

Fig. 98-6.—Funnel chest in an infant.

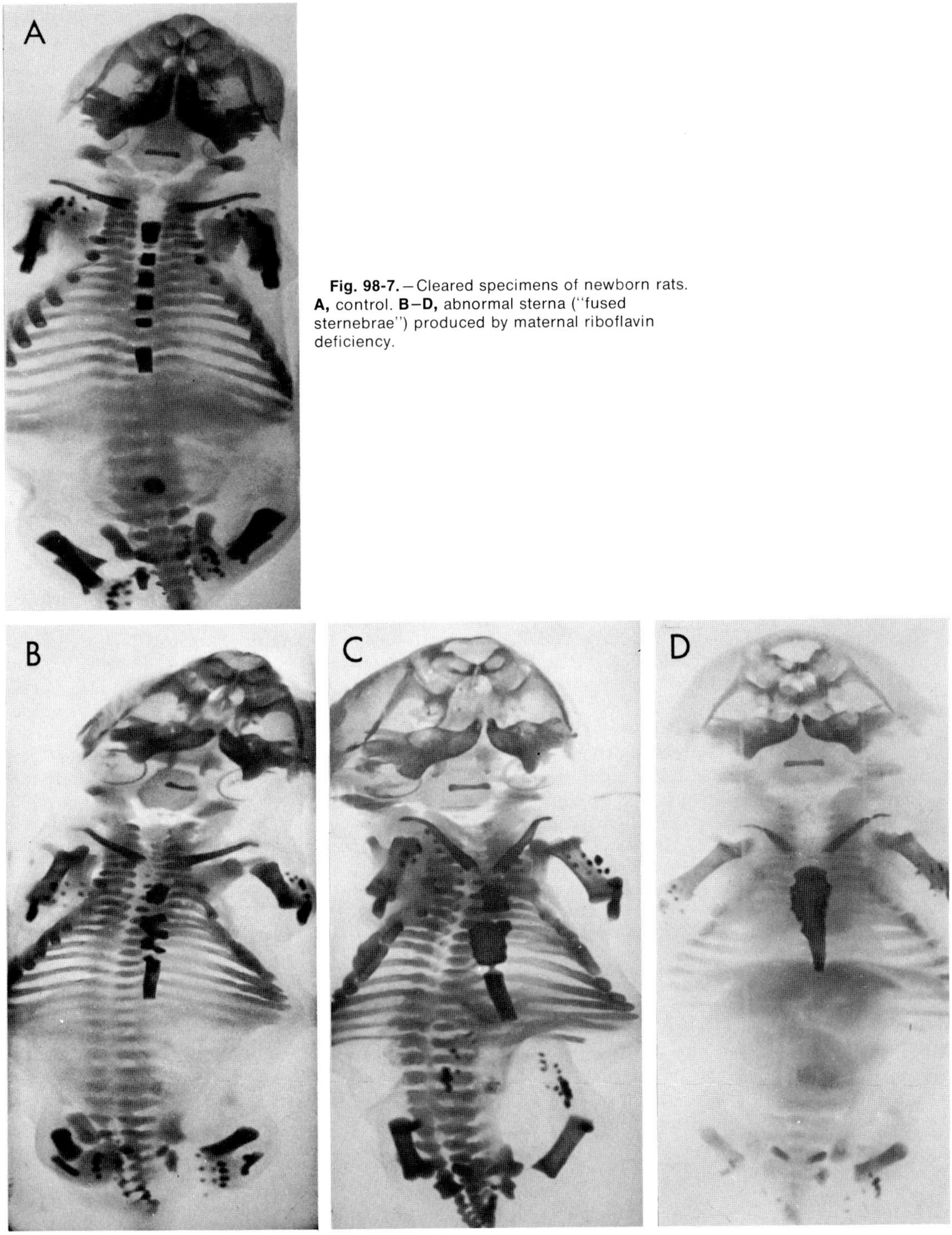

Fig. 98-7. – Cleared specimens of newborn rats. **A,** control. **B–D,** abnormal sterna ("fused sternebrae") produced by maternal riboflavin deficiency.

cause of deformity and rigidity of the deformed thorax, there is no support by negative pressure during inspiration of the flow of venous blood into the right auricle and from the pulmonary capillaries to the left auricle. Dyspnea, often present in such patients, may be due to atelectasis or emphysema. Myocardial insufficiency develops later. Pulmonocardiac symptoms develop in many patients during adolescence or adulthood and dyspnea, cough and palpitation occur. Cyanosis is noticeable in some of the patients but clubbing of the digits is rare. In other patients, pectus excavatum is due to muscle pull and anomalous growth of bone without osseous malformations.[15]

The uncertainty of prognosis explains the differing recommendations for treatment. For infants with severe manifestations, a limited operation is used, which consists of division of the soft tissue attachments of the lower sternum.[31] The tense and thick substernal ligament and the short anterior portion of the central tendon of the diaphragm are divided. In the broad type, the lateral diaphragmatic attachments must be included in the operation also. The limited operation often leads to immediate relief of symptoms in infants, but the deformity may persist and require a complete operation later. The complete operation consists of removal of the lower costal cartilages, which are turned dorsad, and of a wedge-shaped osteotomy across the upper sternum to permit the bone to come forward.[32] This operation has been recommended for children between the ages of 2 and 6 years even in the absence of disturbing symptoms. The reason for this is the fact that some of the cardiopulmonary symptoms appear late, at a time when operation has become difficult. In children, the complete operation is easier and they suffer less pain and disability than do adults.[32] Evaluation of the various approaches to the problem can be found in an article by Lester.[15] Jensen *et al.*[33] discussed the "how, when and why" of surgical correction of pectus excavatum and carinatum. They reviewed the results of surgical treatment in 114 cases.

Pigeon Breast (Congenital Pectus Carinatum)

Protrusion deformities of the chest have been divided into two groups. Midline deformities consist of protrusion of the sternum and the attached cartilages. The second group involves the anterior chest wall lateral to the sternum; the deformity may be limited to one side or, if the costal arches are involved, be bilateral.[15]

Sternal protrusion may be in craniocaudal fashion, with the lowest part being most prominent; or the sternum is arcuate, with the mid-portion most prominent and the lowest portion pointing backward.

In the second group, there can be one ridge or bilateral ridges lateral to the sternum, which remains in a relatively normal position. The protrusions correspond to the costochondral junctions of several consecutive ribs.[15] Such cases often are associated with malformations of ribs, such as forking or irregular fusion of osseous or cartilaginous parts. This situation can be mistaken for funnel chest, but in that condition the distance between xiphoid and vertebral column is decreased and inspiratory retraction occurs. In pigeon breast, the xiphoid moves forward during inspiration, and the distance between xiphoid and vertebrae is normal or increased. Anomalies of ribs and of the diaphragm constitute the basis of these deformities.[15]

Pectus carinatum may be a stationary condition or progress after infancy. There often are no complaints of physical disability. Sometimes dyspnea, chronic bronchitis and fatigability complicate the deformity. The chief complaints concern the cosmetic aspects, and psychologic symptoms may dominate the picture.

Surgical procedures to relieve the protrusion deformities were discussed by Lester.[15]

The arcuate form of pigeon breast has been found associated with faulty segmentation or with premature obliteration of sternal sutures. In such cases, the sternum appears unsegmented in early childhood. In man, it is difficult to decide whether the sternum originated from a single ossification center or whether the various sternal nuclei fused prematurely. The sternum shows a forward angulation in its proximal portion if premature synostosis has taken place. At the same time, the chest wall protrudes and the thorax is enlarged in the sagittal diameter. Nonsegmentation of the sternum usually is found to be associated with various congenital malformations of other parts of the body. Congenital heart disease, facial asymmetry, micrognathia, microphthalmia and other defects can be combined with faulty segmentation of the sternum.[2] Severe pectus carinatum develops in Morquio and Morquio-Ullrich disease (Fig. 98-8) (p. 817).

Fig. 98-8.—Pigeon breast in a boy with Morquio-Ullrich disease (p. 818).

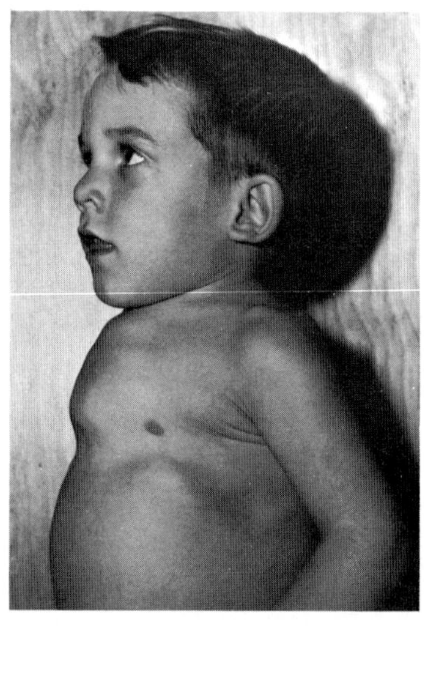

Spondylothoracic Dysplasia

A syndrome of severe spinal and costal malformations leading to early death of affected infants has been described as a recessive hereditary trait.[34] The posterior thorax is shortened, the anteroposterior chest diameter increased and the abdomen protruding. The spinal segmentation is abnormal, resulting in hemivertebrae and block vertebrae; the ribs also show irregularities and radiate fan-like from abnormal vertebrae. The neck is short. Malposition of the extremities occurs. Spina bifida may be limited to neural arches or present as an open myeloschisis.[35,36] Infants with these anomalies who show marked retroflexion of the head are reminiscent of iniencephali (Chapter 27). Many teratogens used in experimental work result in comparable spondylothoracic malformations (see Figs. 97-1 and 98-2).

REFERENCES

1. Arey, L. B.: *Developmental Anatomy* (7th ed.; Philadelphia: W. B. Saunders Company, 1965).
2. Currarino, G., and Silverman, F. N.: Premature obliteration of the sternal sutures and pigeon-breast deformity, Radiology 70:532, 1958.
3. Horns, J. W., and O'Laughlin, B. V.: Multiple manubrial ossification centers in mongolism, Am. J. Roentgenol. 93: 398, 1965.
4. Warkany, J., and Nelson, R. C.: Skeletal abnormalities in the offspring of rats reared on deficient diets, Anat. Rec. 79:83, 1941.
5. Smith, D. W., Theiler, K., and Schachenmann, G.: Rib-gap defect with micrognathia, malformed tracheal cartilages, and redundant skin: A new pattern of defective development, J. Pediat. 69:799, 1966.
6. Bryson, V.: Development of the sternum in screw-tail mice, Anat. Rec. 91:119, 1945.
7. Staples, R. E., and Holtkamp, D. E.: Effects of parental thalidomide treatment on gestation and fetal development, Exper. & Molec. Path. 2:81, 1963.
8. Steiner, H. A.: Rib abnormalities, Radiology 40:175, 1943.
9. Fried, K. H.: Über Rippenanomalien, Deutsches med. J. 7:566, 1956.
10. Coury, C., and Delaporte, J.: Les anomalies congénitales des côtes: Formes anatomo-radiologiques et incidences pratiques; à propos de 288 cas, Semaine hôp. Paris 30:2656, 1963.
11. Martin, E. J.: Incidence of bifidity and related rib abnormalities in Samoans, Am. J. Phys. Anthropol. 18:179, 1960.
12. Adson, A. W., and Coffee, J. R.: Cervical rib, Am. Surgeon 85:839, 1927.
13. Wilson, S. A. K., and Bruce, A. N.: *Neurology* (Baltimore: The Williams & Wilkins Company, 1955), Vol. 2, p. 1203.
14. Davis, D. B., and King, J. C.: Cervical rib in early life, Am. J. Dis. Child. 56:744, 1938.
15. Lester, C. W.: Deformities of the thorax of congenital or developmental origin, J. Pediat. 42:195, 1953.
16. Packer, J. M., Harris, E. J., and Henderson, R. P.: Bilateral synostosis of seventh rib and scapula; a case report, Radiology 74:289, 1960.
17. Grislain, J. R., Mussini, J., de Berranger, P., Mainard, R., and Nomballais, F.: Chondrome costal bilateral du nouveau-né, Ann. pédiat. 44:1789, 1968.
18. Rickham, P. P.: Lung hernia secondary to congenital absence of ribs, Arch. Dis. Childhood 34:14, 1959.
19. Loop, J. S., Akeson, W. H., and Clawson, D. K.: Acquired thoracic abnormalities in neurofibromatosis, Am. J. Roentgenol. 93:416, 1965.
20. Ferrier, P. E., and Hinrichs, W. L.: Basal cell carcinoma syndrome, Am. J. Dis. Child. 113:538, 1967.
21. Milunsky, A., Graef, J. W., and Gaynor, M. F.: Methotrexate-induced congenital malformations, J. Pediat. 72:790, 1968.
22. Greig, D. M.: Cleft sternum and ectopia cordis, Edinburgh M. J. 33:480, 1926.
23. Szenes, A.: Über die fissura sterni und ihre Entstehung, Arch. klin. Chir. 119:116, 1922.
24. Mehrpuyan, T., and Neuhäuser, G.: Totale Sternumspalte kombiniert mit anderen Skeletdeformitäten und seltener Herzmissbildung, Ztschr. Kinderh. 98:86, 1967.
25. Degenhardt, V. K. H.: Missbildungen der Rippen-Brustkorbdeformierungen, in Becker, P. E. (ed.), *Humangenetik* (Stuttgart: Georg Thieme, 1964), Vol. II.
26. Paulsen, I.: Über die Erblichkeit von Thoraxanomalien, Arch. Rassenbiol. 13:1, 1918.
27. Nowak, H.: Die erbliche Trichterbrust, Deutsche med. Wchnschr. 62:2003, 1936.
28. Maneke, M.: Untersuchungen zur Pathogenese der Brustkorbverformungen. (Trichterbrust, Kielbrust, Glockenbrust, Harrisonfurche), Deutsche med. Wchnschr. 84: 504, 1959.
29. Mahoney, E. B., and Emerson, G. L.: Surgical treatment of the congenital funnel-chest deformity, Arch. Surg. 67: 317, 1953.
30. Fischer, J. W., and Dolehide, R. A.: Fatal cardiac failure in persons with thoracic deformities, Arch. Int. Med. 93: 687, 1954.
31. Brown, A. L.: Pectus excavatum (funnel chest), J. Thoracic Surg. 9:164, 1939.
32. Bill, A. H.: Funnel chest; indications for surgery and the time of choice for operation, Pediatrics 2:582, 1953.
33. Jensen, N. K., Schmidt, W. R., Garamella, J. J., and Lynch, M. F.: Pectus excavatum and carinatum: The how, when, and why of surgical correction, J. Pediat. Surg. 5:4, 1970.
34. Lavy, N. W., Palmer, C. G., and Merritt, A. D.: A syndrome of bizarre vertebral anomalies, J. Pediat. 69:1121, 1966.
35. Moseley, J. E., and Bonforte, R. J.: Spondylothoracic dysplasia—a syndrome of congenital anomalies, Am. J. Roentgenol. 106:166, 1969.
36. Eller, J. L., and Morton, J. M.: Bizarre deformities in offspring of user of lysergic acid diethylamide, New England J. Med. 283:395, 1970.

99

The Pelvis

MALFORMATIONS of the female pelvis, congenital and acquired, are of great importance to the birth process and numerous studies have been devoted to this subject by obstetricians and pathologists.[1-3] The problem has been of lesser interest to pediatricians, but in recent years roentgenology has disclosed the diagnostic value of pelvic changes in many systemic disorders.[4,5] In conjoined twins[2,6,7] and in sireniform malformations,[8-10] pelvic configurations have been analyzed by teratologists in great detail.

Aplasia and hypoplasia of the os ilium or os ischii are rarities,[5] whereas agenesis of the sacrum (p. 923) or variations of this bone are well-known anomalies that either can be of little clinical importance or have grave prognostic implications if combined with severe malformations of the cerebrospinal, urogenital or intestinal system. The pelvis often is involved in malformations of the lower extremities,[6,7] particularly in association with defects of the femur (p. 997). Split pelvis commonly is associated with exstrophy of the bladder and sometimes with epispadias. It may be of importance in the management of pregnancy and delivery.[11] Widening of the symphysis pubis has been emphasized as a clue to the presence of anomalies of the urogenital tract.[12]

Involvement of the pelvis has been pointed out in this book in many sections dealing with systemic disorders, but for a thorough review of the subject, including chromosomal aberrations, the reader is referred to the monograph by Kaufmann.[5]

REFERENCES

1. Breus, C., and Kolisko, A.: *Die pathologischen Beckenformen* (Vienna and Leipzig: Deuticke, 1900).
2. Putschar, W.: Spezielle Pathologie des Beckens, in von Lubarsch, O., Henke, F., and Rössle, R. (eds.), *Handbuch der speziellen pathologischen Anatomie und Histologie* (Berlin: Springer-Verlag, 1939).
3. Greenhill, J. P.: *Obstetrics* (13th ed.; Philadelphia: W. B. Saunders Company, 1965).
4. Caffey, J.: *Pediatric X-ray Diagnosis* (5th ed.; Chicago: Year Book Medical Publishers, Inc., 1967).
5. Kaufmann, H. J.: *Röntgenbefunde am kindlichen Becken bei angeborenen Skelettaffektionen und chromosomalen Aberrationen* (Stuttgart: Georg Thieme, 1964).
6. Gruber, G. B., and Eymer, H.: Zur Kenntnis der Dicephalie, Beitr. path Anat. 77:240, 1927.
7. Werthemann, H.: Allgemeine Teratologie mit besonderer Berücksichtigung der Verhältnisse beim Menschen, in Buchner, F., Letterer, E., and Roulet, F. (eds.), *Handbuch d. allgem. Pathologie* (Berlin-Göttingen-Heidelberg: J. Springer, 1955).
8. Feller, A., and Sternberg, L. H.: Über Sirenenbildung, Frankfurt. Ztschr. Path. 47:98, 1934.
9. Frädrich, G.: *Über die menschlichen sireniformen Missbildungen* (Jena: Gustav Fischer, 1938).
10. Töndury, G.: Zur Kenntnis der Fehlbildungen mit Defekten des hinteren Körperendes, Arch. Klaus Stift. Vererbungsforsch. 19:225, 1944.
11. MacKenzie, L. L.: Split pelvis in pregnancy, Am. J. Obst. & Gynec. 29:255, 1935.
12. Muecke, E. C., and Currarino, G.: Congenital widening of the pubic symphysis. Associated clinical disorders and roentgen anatomy of affected bony pelves, Am. J. Roentgenol. 103:179, 1968.

100

The Extremities

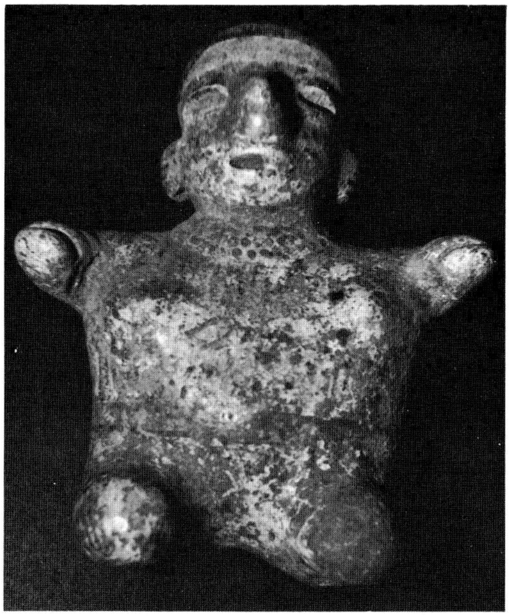

Fig. 100-1.—Reduction malformations of all extremities (Mexican pre-Columbian sculpture). (Courtesy of Dr. A. I. Weisman, from the Weisman Collection of Pre-Columbian Medical Sculpture).

CONGENITAL DEFECTS of the limbs are striking anomalies that did not escape early observation by lay persons or description by early scientists. Terms such as "lobster claw," "crab claw," "seal limbs" and others were used in common language to describe some of these anomalies and "amelia," "phocomelia," "hemimelia," "acheiropodia," "ectrodactyly," "perodactyly," "hypodactyly" and many others adorn and confuse the scientific literature. Adoption of a terminology in this chapter is, to a certain extent, arbitrary and requires explanation. "Amelia" for absence of a limb is an understandable and useful term, but "hemimelia" (absence of half a limb) is not. If "hemimelia" were used only for absence of the forearm and hand (transverse hemimelia) or for absence of one arm and the ipsilateral leg, its use would be justified, but such terms as "radial hemimelia" and "ulnar hemimelia" or "partial hemimelia" make little sense because one cannot call three-quarters of a limb half a limb. The terms "peromelia" (maimed limb) and "ectrodactyly" (aborted fingers) will be used because there is a need for replacing the old concepts of "amputated" limbs and fingers. Peromelia signifies a limb that ends in a stump because the terminal portion had never been formed. Agenesis of the forearm and hand with stump formation would be a more accurate but more awkward term for one of these anomalies. For a hand sitting near the shoulder or a foot attached to the pelvis because of marked underdevelopment of the interposed (intercalary) bones, the term "phocomelia" (seal limb) has long been used. Although it is inaccurate and covers many differing anomalies, it can be retained; it is firmly established and no better name has been suggested. The term has been extended to many single bone aplasias that result in shortening of the limb. There now are proximal (humerofemoral) and distal (forearm and lower leg) phocomelias. Such incomplete phocomelias show little resemblance to the limbs of seals. No doubt seals would consider these human imitations of their flippers to be horrible malformations. "Acheiria" will be used for absence of the hand, "apodia" for absence of the foot and "acheiropodia" for absence of the hand and foot. "Adactyly" for absence and "hypodactyly" for deficiency of fingers are satisfactory terms but, since the medical literature is replete (for the same conditions) with terms such as "ectrodactyly" and "perodactyly," these names cannot be ignored at this time, even though they seem superfluous and inaccurate. "Syndactyly" signifies nonseparation or fusion of fingers or toes, "polydactyly" an excess of fingers or toes. It should be pointed out that the confusion in terminology is due in part to the fact that differing classifications were suggested by different scientific branches. It is understandable that anatomists, pathologists, teratologists and orthopedic and plastic surgeons describe the malformations for different purposes. In recent times, Amputee Centers had a need for classifications useful for prosthetic treatment and they adopted a terminology of their own.[1-3] Their terminology is not the most desirable for other sciences because the terms are unwieldy, not usable as adjectives and not related to pathogenesis or etiology of the anomalies. There is no objection to differing terminologies as long as the authors state what they mean by their terms and use concrete descriptions rather than general expressions.

From the foregoing, it is understandable that specific incidence and prevalence figures are not available for all limb defects. The figures obtained by Birch-Jensen[4] in 1949 refer to congenital deformities of the upper extremities only. The terminology used in Table 100-1 requires various interpretations, but the figures are of permanent value. The frequencies of reduction malformations in the Danish population (then 4,024,000) were as shown in this table.

The incidence of reduction malformations seen in a Child Amputee Center in the United States can be well ascertained from a publication by Frantz and O'Rahilly,[2] who classified their patients as accurately as possible, giving incidences of the various malformations as seen in 300 children. The reader is referred to the original publication for illustrations, details and the authors' terminology. Reference to the data of the Area Child Amputee Center, Grand Rapids, Michigan, will be made with the initials ACAC.

At first, the limb buds of human embryos appear as elevations of the lateral body walls at 4 weeks' fertilization age (5 mm. crown-rump length). The various parts of the limbs develop in proximo-distal sequence, i.e., the proximal structures differentiate in the various stages of development before the distal ones. For instance, the humerus is ahead of the forearm structures and these are ahead of those of the hand in mesenchymal, cartilaginous and osseous development.

The first manifestations of limb development are ridges, which consist of a covering ectoderm and mesoderm of the lateral plate of the embryo. Much has been written about the ectoderm-mesoderm relationship and many of the ruling concepts have been derived from experimental work in chick embryos. Surgical and chemical interventions have been used to elucidate the "ectoderm-mesoderm dialogue,"[5,6] which show the relative importance for limb development of the different tissues in different stages. It has been established that in chicks the thickened ectoderm at the apex of the bud is essential to the formation of the limb,[7] as shown by absence of the ectodermal ridge in chicks with the "wingless syndrome."[8] O'Rahilly *et al.*[9] described in detail the ectodermal thickening and ridge in the limbs of staged human embryos. The mesoderm of the limb buds represents the substrate in which the various skeletal elements are laid down. Such skeletal structures as the humerus, forearm bones, femur, lower leg bones, digits, and so forth differentiate first as mesodermal condensations and become recognizable as such at about 5 weeks. Many important abnormalities of such structures are already present in their mesodermal stage, before chondrification and ossification take place. Chondrification centers appear in embryos 5 weeks old and chondrification progresses during the following week, so that in embryos of the seventh week (15–20 mm.) all skeletal limb structures are clearly recognizable in cartilaginous form.[10] As chondrification and ossification proceed in the proximo-distal direction, the cartilaginous stage of some bones coexists with progressing ossification in others. Ossification of the tubular bones begins with formation of a periosteal collar and vascular invasion of the cartilage by periosteal buds, which establish centers of endochondral ossification in the diaphysis.[10,11] Early signs of ossification can be seen in embryos 7–8 weeks old, but conversion of cartilage into bone continues throughout fetal life and into postnatal stages. If their mesodermal and cartilaginous precursors are abnormal, the bones become deformed by establishment of irregular periosteal collars and irregularly placed ossification centers.

The upper limb bud appears in week 4 and its entire skeleton can be recognized in its mesenchymal stage in week 5. Chondrification begins in the same week, proceeding in the proximo-distal direction, so that the digital phalanges become cartilaginous in week 6 only. The clavicle ossifies early (week 5). Ossification from humerus to terminal phalanges begins between weeks 6 and 7.[10,11]

The lower limb bud can be recognized at 4 weeks and the footplate at 4½ weeks. Mesenchymal and cartilaginous structures appear at about the same time as their homologues in the upper extremity, but there are slight differences that are of theoretical interest and can be ascertained from special publications.[12] Ossification begins a few days later in the lower homologues than in the upper. A roentgenographic study of the human skeleton during early fetal life was made by O'Rahilly and Meyer.[13]

Malformations of the extremities can originate at different stages of development. Formation of an extremity can be suppressed at the time of the earliest appearance of the limb bud. In other cases, adverse factors permit formation of a limb primordium but

TABLE 100-1.—FREQUENCY OF REDUCTION MALFORMATIONS IN THE DANISH POPULATION, 1949*

DEFORMITIES OF REDUCTION (upper extremities)	NUMBER OF PATIENTS	PREVALENCE IN THE POPULATION
Split-hands	36	1 – 111,777
Atypical split-hands	20	1 – 201,200
Ectrodactylism	41	1 – 98,146
Radial defects	73	1 – 55,123
Ulnar defects	19	1 – 211,789
Radio-ulnar defects	44	1 – 91,455
Amputation of upper arm	9	1 – 447,111
Amputation of forearm	161	1 – 24,993
Amputation of hand	54	1 – 74,518
Symbrachydactylism	85	1 – 47,340
Spontaneous amputation	47	1 – 85,617
Exogeneous syndactylism	36	1 – 111,777
TOTAL	625	1 – 6,438

*From A. Birch-Jensen.[4]

interfere with normal differentiation and growth later. As shown in children damaged by thalidomide, absence of a limb and various limb deformities can be present in the same organism. This is true also for limb defects produced in monkeys by a single dose of thalidomide (p. 86). Mutant genes, which result in reduction malformations, can produce defects of very different clinical importance. In the same pedigree, absence of an extremity, phocomelias of varying degree and peromelias can appear vicariously and malformations can vary in extent and character in the extremities of the same individual. A chronic teratogenic procedure, such as riboflavin deficiency, permits development of the limb bud to a certain extent but inhibits adequate differentiation of the mesenchymal skeleton distal to the elbow and knee joints. Other limb defects originate after proper formation of the extremity by secondary destruction in late embryonal or in fetal stages. It is difficult, even in experimental work, to assign times of origin to limb defects but it is possible to speak of termination periods that sometimes permit exclusion of an event as a cause of the deformity. It is clear, for instance, that malformations of excess, such as polydactyly or duplication of the ulna, date back at least to the embryonic period, when they arise as mesodermal structures. Thus, in a 23-mm. (8 week-old) embryo, the digits are well formed and their number is determined. Therefore, a limb defect that includes polydactyly or other anomalies of duplication cannot be blamed on an event or accident that occurred when the embryo was 10 weeks old or older.[14] But the possibility of intrauterine regeneration processes, which can occur at various times of development, should be kept in mind.[54]

Reduction Malformations (Amputations)

Skeletal deficiencies or reduction malformations are characterized by absence or underdevelopment of skeletal elements of the extremities. They can be minor defects of fingers, toes or metacarpals or be serious lesions such as absence of hands, feet or entire limbs. In some instances, children are born with remnants that look like amputation stumps and one finds in the literature the term "intrauterine amputation" applied to many reduction malformations. But absent parts of the appendicular skeleton may never have been formed (aplasia, agenesis), and nonexisting limbs cannot be amputated. It is, therefore, incorrect to call aplastic or hypoplastic limbs "amputations." It is very likely that most reduction malformations are primary defects of development. But, in rare cases, prenatal destruction of limbs, or parts thereof, does occur and such secondary defects can be considered intrauterine amputations. By observation of the end effects, it is not always possible to decide whether a limb reduction is primary or secondary. In the past, primary defects were thought to be genetically determined and, conversely, limb anomalies occurring in families were thought to be primary aplasias. Secondary defects or intrauterine amputations were attributed to outside influences, particularly to mechanical factors, such as amniotic bands, spatial restrictions or traumas. Recent observations in human and animal teratology have shown that these old concepts are not correct. Formation of limbs can be suppressed by genetic or by environmental factors, and amputation can be caused by genetic or environmental mechanisms.

Primary Reduction Malformations (Aplasias or Hypoplasias of Limbs)

As stated before, it is not always possible to recognize primary limb defects by external inspection of the malformation. But intercalary deficiencies, such as phocomelia or absence of one forearm bone, cannot be explained by secondary amputation. It is thought that primary limb defects can be recognized by the presence of distal rudiments on a stump, by good padding of a stump without scar formation or by the near-normal shape of a terminal bone as seen in

Fig. 100-2.—Four children with reduction malformations. **A**, phocomelia with hypoplastic thrombocytopenia. **B**, de Lange syndrome. **C**, Down syndrome. **D**, thalidomide embryopathy.

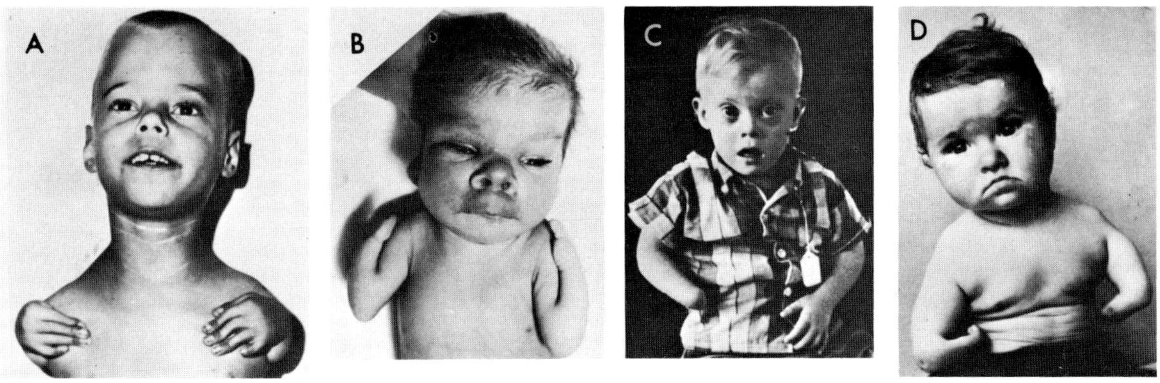

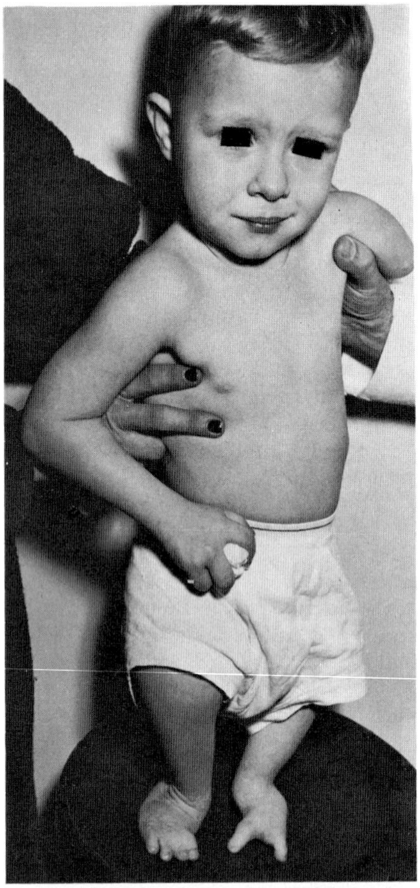

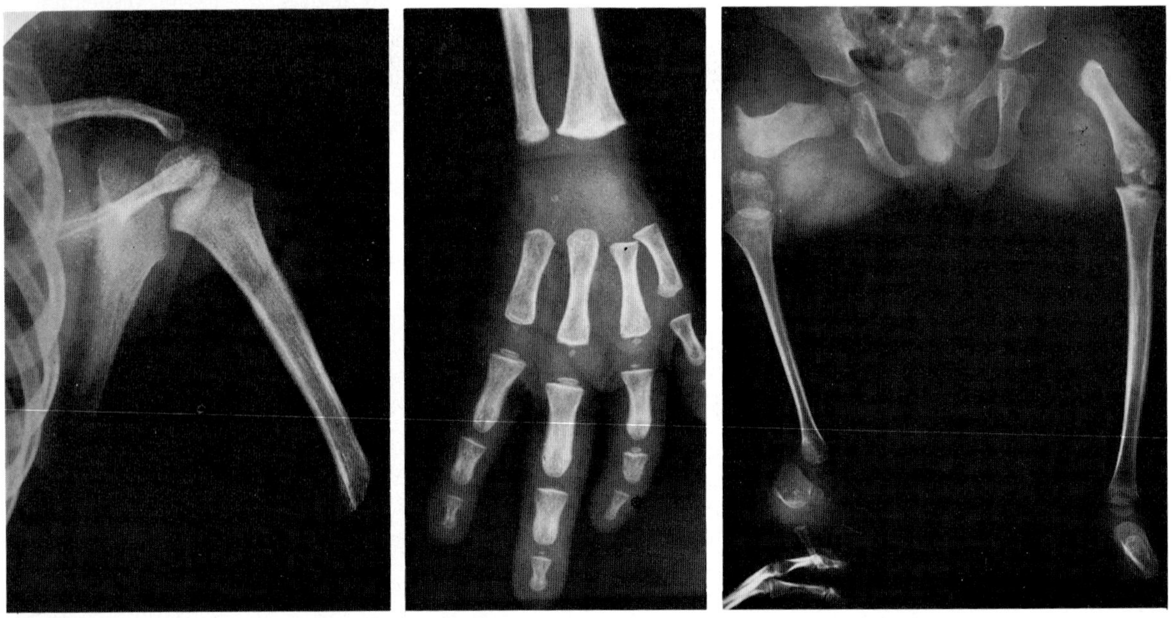

Fig. 100-3.—Reduction malformations of left forearm, femora and fibulae; lobster claw of left foot; absence of fifth finger of right hand. Had the malformation of the left forearm occurred alone, it could have been interpreted as a secondary lesion (amputation) but the other reduction malformations obviously are primary hypoplasias. (The mother had had miscarriages in the early months of pregnancy before and after the birth of the propositus. While pregnant with the propositus, the mother bled for 4 months and did not know that she was pregnant.)

roentgenograms.[4] A distinction can be made better, as a rule, by the presence of associated malformations in the patient, malformations that are clearly due to early arrest of development. Thus, limb defects in an anencephalus will be attributable to faulty differentiation, even when amniotic bands or strands are attached to the abnormal extremity. The same is true for appendicular defects associated with internal developmental errors, such as congenital heart disease, tracheo-esophageal fistula, renal aplasia and the like. Reduction malformations in relatives of the patient do not prove that the limb defects are primary. It will be pointed out later that familial recurrence of secondary destructive processes is possible. But if a patient with a doubtful type of reduction malformation has relatives who have primary developmental defects, it will be reasonable to assume that the patient's malformations are due to the same inhibiting forces that produced the anomalies of arrested development in other family members.

Examples of apparent amputations associated with signs of arrested development can be found in the literature. Schwarzweller[15] reported a Dutch family in which amputation stumps occurred together with reduction malformations that obviously were not due to external amputating forces. In the oldest boy of this family, the right upper arm was represented by a conically reduced stump; the elbow joint, lower arm and hand were missing. This extremity looked like a true or secondary amputation. But the rest of the extremities also were more or less deformed, and these anomalies clearly were due to primary failure of proper development and not to amputation. There were 4 other children in this family of 8 who had malformations of the extremities that showed signs of primary growth disturbance with hypoplastic or missing intercalary bones. A pedigree recorded by Freire-Maia *et al.*[16] contains 4 members with deformed limbs. Two had absence of the left upper extremity resembling true amputations, but they also had osseous malformations that clearly were due to primary defective development. In the other 2 members, all the malformations were hypoplastic and not amputated. Simple recessive heredity was responsible for these malformations, including the lesions that could be mistaken for amputations. Stadler[17] described an infant boy who combined absence of the left upper extremity with hypoplastic anomalies in the other limbs; in addition, he showed mandibular hypoplasia, high palate, abnormal pharynx and atresia of the external auditory canals. Hanhart[18] established a syndrome of peromelia and micrognathia. In one of his cases, the mandibular anomaly was associated with absence of both hands. In the other, the patient, who had a "bird face," was born with three extremities deprived of peripheral parts and one showing hypoplasia of the fingers. The same author also described congenital absence of the right forearm and hand in cousins. Birch-Jensen,[4] in his extensive review of congenital deformities of the upper extremities, attempted a distinction of endogenous and exogenous defects. He considered approximately 13% of the defects as exogenous, since they showed scars or constriction grooves. His findings and a review of the literature suggest that primary reduction malformations are much more frequent than secondary amputations. But distinction between primary arrest of development and secondary destruction of limbs is difficult, since combination of both reducing processes may occur. Sometimes this can be observed directly when portions of extremities showing hypoplastic malformations combined with constricting bands or narrows are progressively destroyed and even amputated in postnatal life.[19,20] If similar complicated deformities arise in prenatal life, inspection of the end effect will not lead to an explanation of the origin and morphogenesis of the malformations of the limb. It is clear that a eugenic prognosis will be very difficult in such cases.

Genetic determination of many primary reduction malformations can be considered established even though most of these deficiencies occur sporadically. Split hand and foot, ectrodactyly, brachydactyly, acheiria and apodia, radial, ulnar and tibial aplasias and even extremely rudimentary limbs sometimes can be shown to be inherited. Reduction malformations of the upper extremities occur in the Holt-Oram syndrome, an autosomal dominant trait, and in Fanconi

Fig. 100-4.—Reduction malformations in a newborn girl whose brother had myelomeningocele. The upper extremities are reduced by deficient growth. The lower extremities probably were impeded in growth also although they look "amputated."

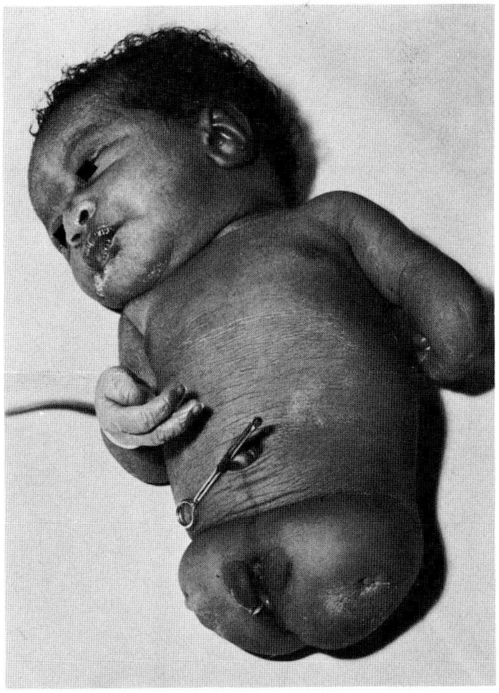

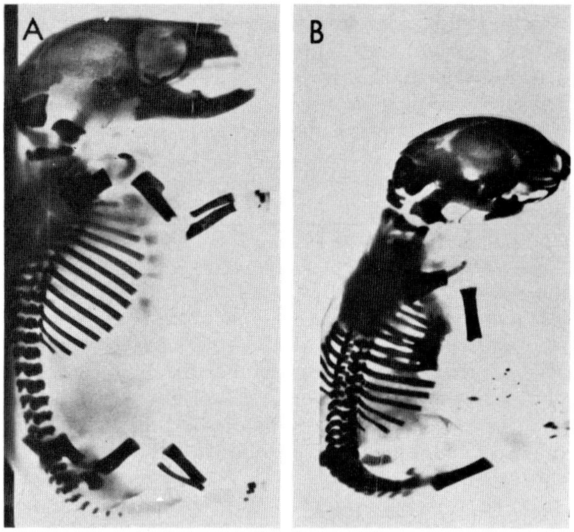

Fig. 100-5.—Cleared specimens of newborn rats. **A,** control. **B,** short mandible and fused ribs are seen. There are no bones visible in the shortened forearms and lower legs. Such anomalies, commonly seen in the offspring of riboflavin-deficient mothers, can be called "distal phocomelia." The humerus shows absence of tuberosity but no shortening.

pancytopenia, an autosomal recessive. But primary limb aplasias can be due to exogenous factors also. The reduction malformations caused by thalidomide are examples of this kind. From many observations in human beings, one can conclude that thalidomide exerts its action during early gestational periods when the extremities are being formed. Although retrospective histories are not entirely reliable (Chapter 7), it seems that the sensitive period lasts from the thirty-fourth to the fiftieth day (postmenstrual) and that after this period thalidomide is not teratogenic.[21,22] More convincing are experiments in Macaca mulatta, which showed that the susceptible period for thalidomide teratogenesis extends from the twenty-fifth through the thirtieth day (after mating), when the limb buds first appear in the monkey embryo.[23] Thalidomide inhibits formation of extremities, thus causing primary reduction malformations. Long before the thalidomide experience, we had found that reduction malformations of the extremities can be produced by maternal riboflavin deficiency. The anomalies were due to limited growth and differentiation and not to secondary destruction of distal parts of the limbs.[24,25] There is a possibility that bacterial toxins can suppress limb formation. Ilberg[26] described a fetus in the third month without any extremities whose mother had a purulent infection of the uterus and pelvic organs. There were no signs of external amputating bands and the author thought that toxins from the maternal endometritis suppressed formation of the limbs. Thus, observations in children and in animal experiments show that primary reduction malformations can be caused by genetic or by environmental mechanisms.

Secondary Reduction Malformations (True Intrauterine Amputations)

True intrauterine amputations can be recognized, as a rule, by the appearance of the stumps, which may show wounds, scarring or osseous projections. The best-proved instances of intrauterine amputations are those of infants born with a stump and the amputated part delivered with or after the deformed child. Occasionally, such cases were described in the nineteenth century and were cited by Ballantyne.[27] One of them dates back to 1825, when Watkinson[28] described such an amputation of the left foot and the editors of the *London Medical and Physical Journal* illustrated the case (Fig. 100-6). The amputated foot was discovered in the mother's vagina and was described as much smaller than the normal attached one. A comparable case was recorded by Hornsby,[29] who delivered a child whose left leg was amputated at the middle of the thigh. The detached portion of the leg and the foot were found also. They were macerated and much smaller than the normal limb, having the size of an extremity of 5 months as compared with the 7½ months of their real gestational age. Streeter[30] illustrated a fetus with amputation of the right foot, which, although smaller than the left, was found as a detached structure. Glessner[31] and Torpin[32] described deliveries of infants born without arms with recovery of the missing extremity. In another fetus, a tiny foot was seen hanging on a thread or band that originated from the stump of the deformed extremity.[33] Such cases represent transitional forms between complete amputations and constriction rings observed more often in recent times. An instructive case was mentioned by Glessner,[31] who illustrated a

Fig. 100-6.—Infant born at the seventh month without a left foot. Foot was found in the mother's vagina after the birth of the child. (Watkinson, London M. & Phys. J. 54:38, 1825 [cited by J. W. Ballantyne, *Manual of Antenatal Pathology and Hygiene,* Vol. 1, p. 152[27]].)

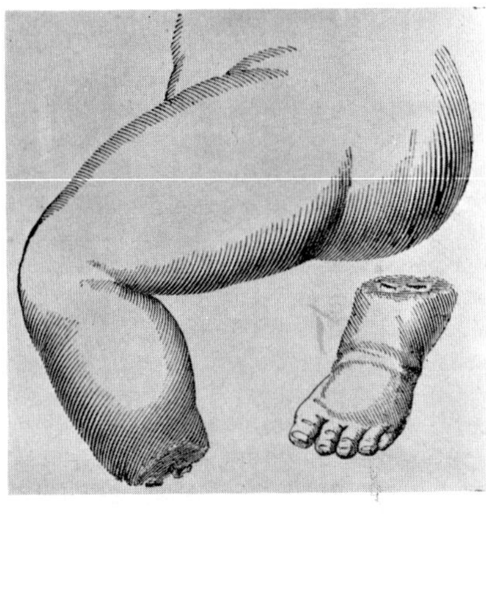

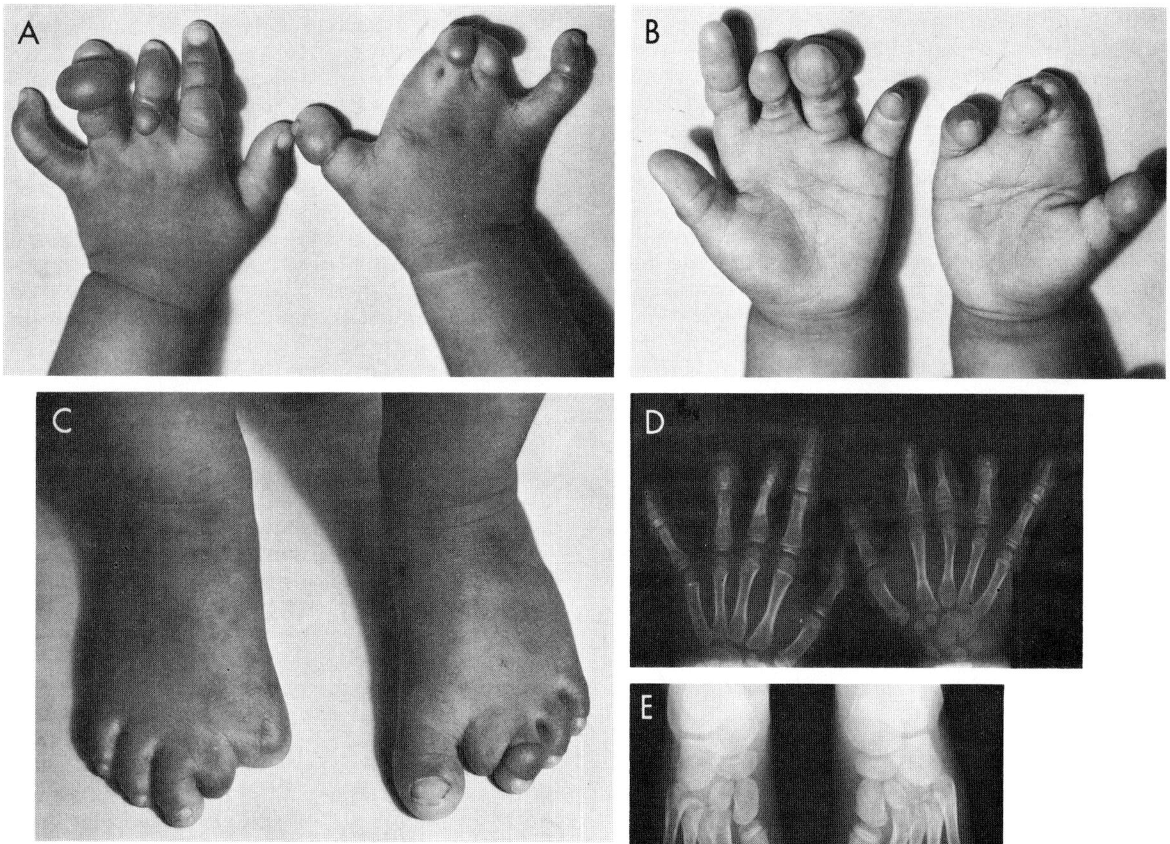

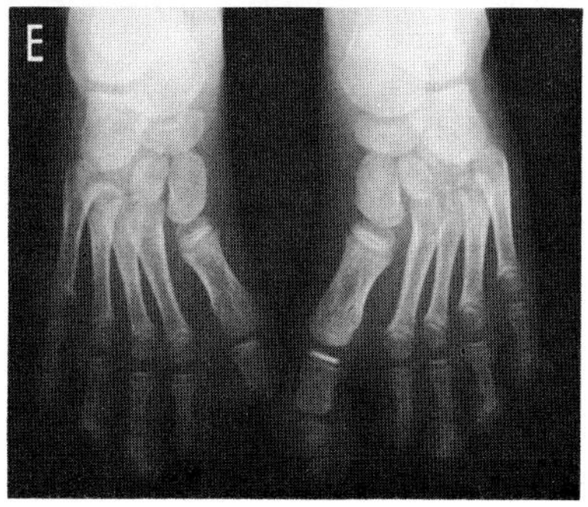

Fig. 100-7.—Hands and feet of a 10-year-old girl with irregular perodactylies that could be interpreted as amputations. The family history was negative for congenital malformations. The mother had had a miscarriage 4 years before the patient's birth. During the pregnancy with the patient, the mother had several bleeding episodes beginning at 3 months. On the right hand there was a congenital band across middle phalanges of second, third and fourth fingers. The thumb and fifth finger also had bands that were less penetrating. On the left hand, the bands involved chiefly the second, third and fourth fingers, with "tumefaction" on the fourth and third (**A**, **B** and **D**). There is partial absence of the distal phalanx on the right first and second toes. On the left there is partial absence of the second toe (**C** and **E**). (Courtesy of Shriner's Hospital, Honolulu, Hawaii.)

patient with absence of the left arm and a deep constricting furrow on the right. The patient apparently shows two stages of the amputating process, an early one on the right and the end result on the left. Sometimes one sees amputations of digits combined with a circular constriction of the leg leading to an hourglass-shaped deformity.[34-36] It seems as if the constricting force was strong enough to amputate fingers and toes but not able to cut through the thicker leg or thigh. In postnatal life, the distal portion of such a limb may become cold, cyanotic,[35] anesthetic[36] or necrotic[31]; it may be affected by trophic disturbances and slough off. But it also can be durable, as shown by a man of 72 years who had been born with constricting bands.[35] Torpin[32] described several infants born with amputated fingers or toes combined with bands and necrotic rings around the remaining extremities. He analyzed 400 cases of ruptured amnion and the consequences of early amnion rupture to the fetus.

Although the occurrence of intrauterine amputations is well established, there are wide differences of opinion concerning their causation. In the older literature, they were attributed to amniotic bands or loops of the umbilical cord,[27] but the latter possibility was later excluded for most cases. It was pointed out that such entanglements would lead to interruption of the blood supply to the fetus and intrauterine death. That this actually can occur was shown by a case of Erlich's,[37] in which the left upper arm and the neck of a fetus were encircled by the umbilical cord. Similar lethal results are attributed to ligation of the umbilical cord by amniotic strands.[32] The theory of amputation by amniotic bands cannot be discarded, since such bands constricting an arm[38,39] with fingers[33,40] have been observed, but Streeter[30] believed that such bands accompany intrauterine amputations but do not sever the limb by mechanical constriction. He stated that the active stages of amputation are to be found in the early weeks of pregnancy, when focal areas of necrosis that lead to an apparent entanglement of fingers or other limb structures appear. Although the enveloping tissue has the appearance of an extraneous mass, it actually consists of degenerated material of the defective parts. Such fibroid material does not increase in size, whereas the adjoining normal tissues grow and surpass the decadent material in extent, so that a *picture* of constricting bands is created. Fibrous appendages connected with constriction rings are surviving remnants of necrotic areas; they have been misinterpreted as amniotic bands. Streeter[30] believed that the real cause of intrauterine amputation is to be found in the subnormal quality or "reduced vitality" of sharply circumscribed areas of limb bud tissue that either become stationary in development or break down and disappear. The subnormal quality of these tissues was primarily determined by the "constitution of the germ plasm."[30] A similar opinion had been expressed before by Ollerenshaw,[41] who thought that congenital defects of long bones are not due to outside interference but due to growth deficiencies of the limb buds during the first few weeks of fetal life.

The occurrence of genetically determined true intrauterine amputations can be demonstrated best by observations in animals. Greene and Saxton,[42] originally working with phenotypically normal rabbits, obtained offspring with reduction malformations of the extremities ranging from shortening of the fingers to complete absence of the paws. The remnants of their digits or legs looked externally very much like so-called exogenous or true amputations. Embryologic studies showed that at first the limbs were normally formed and that they remained normal to about the eighteenth day of gestation (which lasts 32 days in the rabbit), when a dilatation of capillaries became noticeable and areas of red discoloration appeared. Then, cystic lesions developed in these areas and on the twentieth or twenty-first day demarcation lines began to separate normal and abnormal parts. Subsequently, an annular constriction developed and by the twenty-third day the affected portion had sloughed off, with healing achieved in all cases examined after the twenty-fifth day. Genetic studies showed that the abnormalities depended on a simple recessive factor. All animals derived from deformed parents were affected, but the site and extent of the deformity varied greatly in parents and progeny. Histologically, the vascular dilatations and hemorrhages seen in 18-day-old fetuses soon turned into necrotic areas and the necrotic tissues were removed by phagocytosis or by sloughing and sequestration. Thus, it was not the amputations that were hereditary but rather a prenatal disturbance of vascular or nerve tissues.[42] Comparable defects of the extremities and other parts attributable to the hereditary "bleb disease" have been observed in mice.[43]

Reduction deformities in children resembling those observed in the newborn rabbits just described were classified in former years as "exogenous amputations" because it was thought that a once-formed limb could be cut off only by an external structure, such as an amniotic band or an umbilical cord. Observations in rabbits and mice demonstrate that true intrauterine destruction of portions of one or several extremities can be brought about by more subtle mechanisms than mechanical strangulation, mechanisms that can be rightly called "endogenous." There are cases on record of apparently amputated hands or feet that can be attributed to recessive inheritance. The defects of the often published and illustrated Brazilian family,[44] in which 6 of 12 children were born without hands and feet may have arisen in this way. The parents were consanguineous and a recessive mode of inheritance probably was at work. This family has been reinvestigated by Freire-Maia *et al.*,[45] who were able to locate six additional families in Brazil with at least 1 case of acheiria or acheiropodia each. In 1961, Freire-Maia[46] reported his findings in fourteen sibships with 103 members. Of these, 34 were affected and 69 were not. All affected were the offspring of normal parents; all children of the affected persons (married to normal mates) were normal; the frequency of acheiropodia in these sibships agreed with the assumption that the anomaly was due to an autosomal recessive gene; the frequency of consanguineous marriages among the parents of the acheiropodes was 80–90%; perinatal mortality among acheiropodes was significantly higher (37%) than that of their normal siblings (14%), and fertility of affected persons was roughly one-fifth that of their normal siblings.

A different condition, which could be attributed to an inherited amputating disorder, is a familial congenital absence of terminal portions of digits. MacArthur and McCullough[47] reported a kinship in which 15 persons had finger deformities that seemed to be transmitted as a dominant trait. That a teratogenic mechanism different from that of the Brazilian cases was at work was suggested by occasional occurrence of doubling of the thumbs and by the differing mode of inheritance. Such families with more than 1 member affected by such malformations are rare. In general, amputation stumps showing constriction rings, scars and tapering of bones (as seen in roentgenograms) occur sporadically in normal families. Birch-Jensen[4] categorically stated that "exogenous spontaneous amputations" are not hereditary, since they occur sporadically in normal families. But sporadic occurrence does not exclude genetic determination. Streeter,[30] on the other hand, gave no proof that all amputations associated with amniotic bands and constriction rings are determined by the "constitution of the germ plasm." In fact, there exist reports which strongly suggest that uterine disease or spatial limitation occasionally results in destruction of fetal extremities. Ajinkya[34] reported intrauterine amputations, annular constriction rings and amniotic adhesions associated with oligohydramnios in a pregnancy that had been preceded by an abortion, a febrile period and possibly endometrial disease. Hedenstedt[48] described a case of total amelia resulting from a pregnancy that had been preceded by metrorrhagia and curettage. The same author reported another amelus delivered from a uterus narrowed by a myoma the size of a child's head. Barenberg and Greenberg[36] observed a child with congenital amputations of digits whose delivery was associated with presentation of a cyst attached to a pedicle and connected with the limb of the deformed infant. Latta[39] saw stillborn twins, considered identical, one of whom was normal, whereas the other showed various stages of intrauterine amputations from encircling bands to completely severed parts. Although it is not clear what mechanism caused these amputations, it obviously was not a simple genetic one. Torpin[32] believed that in about 1 of 10,000 pregnancies the amnion ruptures without injury to the chorion, whereby the embryo and the amniotic fluid are placed into the chorionic cavity. The amnion may remain as a plaque near the cord-placental insertion or become fragmented into sheets, strands or rope-like bands that can damage the fetus by involving digits, arms or legs and cause amputations. Such explanations are quite convincing when an otherwise normal child has amputations of distal parts, when amputated parts are delivered and recovered or when distal portions of encircled limbs show elephantiasis-like swellings. But when sheets of amnion are attached to an anencephalic head, facial cleft or an exstrophic bladder, it is more likely that the fetal and amniotic anomalies are parallel phenomena due to a common cause.

Nongenetic amputating factors need not be crude mechanical ones. Jost[49] produced amputations experimentally by administration of hypertensive substances to rat fetuses at midpregnancy or thereafter. The amputations produced by posterior pituitary powder, vasopressin or epinephrine resembled those occurring in rabbits and were genetically determined.[42] Jost thought that the abnormal genetic mechanism leading to amputations in rabbits resembles the abnormal physiologic mechanism leading to experimentally induced malformations ("acroblapsies"), an overproduction of vasopressor substances being responsible in both instances. Gruenwald[50] showed that malformations produced in chicken embryos by selenium were due to secondary regression of previously well-formed parts. It could be demonstrated that the wing and leg buds, although normally formed, evidenced necrotic processes in their mesenchyma that resulted in malformations of the limbs. Thus, endocrine, toxic and mechanical forces should be considered as possible causes of secondary destruction of fetal limbs. Streeter[30] probably

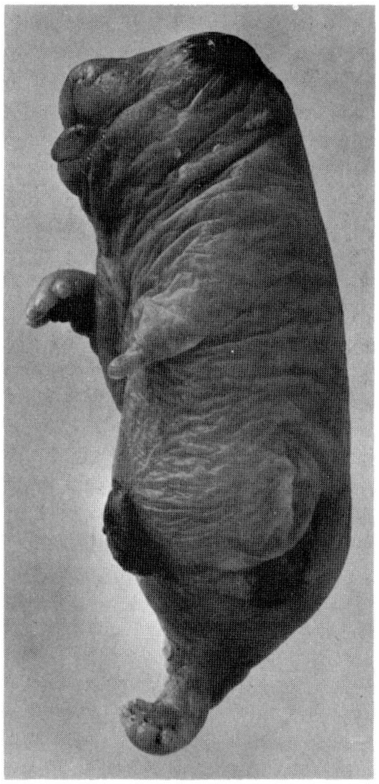

Fig. 100-8.—Malformations in a newborn rat, offspring of a riboflavin-deficient mother. There is an unusually severe reduction malformation of the left upper extremity, which looks like a stump. There is a true amputation of the left lower extremity, indicated by a hemorrhagic scar. Cephalhematoma and umbilical protrusion also are exceptional in this syndrome. This specimen shows primary reduction malformations followed by secondary amputation of the left lower leg.

was correct in pointing out that amniotic bands accompany rather than cause amputations. But the factors causing amputations and bands sometimes may be neither genetic nor gross mechanical. More subtle intrauterine and extrauterine environmental factors should be considered as possible causes of "exogenous spontaneous amputations." There also is the possibility that primary reduction malformations undergo additional secondary destruction. This can be illustrated by occasional specimens with riboflavin-deficiency-induced malformations that show encircling grooves or irregular mutilations (Fig. 100-8). Similar observations were made in reduction malformations due to thalidomide. Knapp and Lenz[51] mentioned that amelia sometimes occurred in such cases by loss of a necrotic rudiment of a limb.

Excess Malformations

In contrast to reduction malformations of the limbs and their parts there exist excess formations that have been given various names and interpretations. Whereas reduction malformations are rather easily understood as failures of development, the mechanisms leading to excess malformations are more puzzling. Whenever a malformation or a syndrome includes overproduction of parts, one is faced with a special phenomenon the etiology and pathogenesis of which arouse uncommon curiosity. Yet, it is known that reduction and excess malformations can occur in the same individual and that both genetic and environmental factors can be responsible for reduplications. Several examples of genetically determined syndromes containing excess anomalies will be cited and thalidomide can be named as an exogenous teratogen that produced reduction malformations as well as extra digits in children. Unequal distribution of primordial tissues accounts for such phenomena. Much experimentation, speculation and writing has been devoted to the phenomena of excess malformations and their coexistence with reduction malformations.[14,52,53] The facts are that the two types of malformation can coexist in one individual or in one hand and that one and the same teratogenic agent can cause both excess and reduction malformations. I do not, therefore, see any good reason to separate the two types of malformations in the following pages.

REFERENCES

1. O'Rahilly, R.: Morphological patterns in limb deficiencies and duplications, Am. J. Anat. 89:135, 1951.
2. Frantz, C. H., and O'Rahilly, R.: Congenital skeletal limb deficiencies, J. Bone & Joint Surg. 43-A:1202, 1961.
3. Hall, C. B., Brooks, M. B., and Dennis, J. F.: Congenital skeletal deficiencies of the extremities. Classification and fundamentals of treatment, J.A.M.A. 181:590, 1962.
4. Birch-Jensen, A.: *Congenital Deformities of the Upper Extremities* (Copenhagen: Ejnar Munksgaard, 1949).
5. Zwilling, E.: Development of fragmented and of dissociated limb bud mesoderm, Develop. Biol. 9:20, 1964.
6. Saunders, J. W.: Control of Growth Patterns in Limb Development, in Frantz, C. H. (ed.), *Normal and Abnormal Embryological Development* (Washington, D. C.: National Research Council, 1967).
7. Saunders, J. W.: The proximo-distal sequence of origin of the parts of the chick wing and the role of the ectoderm, J. Exper. Zool. 108:363, 1948.
8. Zwilling, E.: The role of epithelial components in the developmental origin of the 'wingless' syndrome of chick embryos, J. Exper. Zool. 111:175, 1949.
9. O'Rahilly, R., Gardner, E., and Gray, D. J.: The ectodermal thickening and ridge in the limbs of staged human embryos, J. Embryol. & Exper. Morphol. 4:254, 1956.
10. O'Rahilly, R., Gardner, E., and Gray, D. J.: The skeletal development of the hand, Clin. Orthop. 13:42, 1959.
11. Arey, L. B.: *Developmental Anatomy* (7th ed.; Philadelphia: W. B. Saunders Company, 1965).
12. O'Rahilly, R., Gardner, E., and Gray, D. J.: The skeletal development of the foot, Clin. Orthop. 16:7, 1960.
13. O'Rahilly, R., and Meyer, D. B.: Roentgenographic investigation of human skeleton during early fetal life, Am. J. Roentgenol. 76:455, 1956.
14. O'Rahilly, R.: Normal Development of the Human Embryo, in Frantz, C. H. (ed.), *Normal and Abnormal Embryological Development* (Washington, D. C.: National Research Council, 1967).
15. Schwarzweller, F.: Ein Beitrag fur Genese und Systematik der Gliedmassenmissbildungen, Arch. orthop. Chir. 39:400, 1938.
16. Freire-Maia, N., Quelce-Salgado, A., and Koehler, R. A.: Hereditary bone aplasias and hypoplasias of the upper extremities, Acta Genet. 9:33, 1959.
17. Stadler, J.: Ectromelia and associated developmental defects, J. Pediat. 31:691, 1947.
18. Hanhart, E.: Über die Kombination von Peromelie mit Mikrognathie, ein neues Syndrom beim Menschen, entsprechend der *Akroteriasis congenita* von Wriedt und Mohr beim Rinde, Arch. Klaus Stift. Vererbungsforsch. 25:531, 1950.
19. Kiewe, L.: Zur Frage der Ätiologie der sogenannten "Spontanamputationen," Ztschr. Orthop. Chir. 58:20, 1932.
20. Inglis, K.: The nature of agenesis and deficiency of parts, Am. J. Path. 28:449, 1952.
21. Lenz, W., and Knapp, K.: Die Thalidomid-Embryopathie, Deutsche med. Wchnschr. 87:1232, 1962.
22. Nowack, E.: Die sensible Phase bei der Thalidomid-Embryopathie, Humangenetik 1:516, 1965.
23. Wilson, J. G., and Gavan, J. A.: Congenital malformations in nonhuman primates: Spontaneous and experimentally induced, Anat. Rec. 158:99, 1967.
24. Warkany, J., and Nelson, R. C.: Skeletal abnormalities in the offspring of rats reared on deficient diets, Anat. Rec. 79:83, 1941.
25. Warkany, J., and Nelson, R. C.: Skeletal abnormalities induced in rats by maternal nutritional deficiency, Arch. Path. 34:375, 1942.
26. Ilberg, G.: Fötus ohne Arme und Beine (Amelus); Zusammenstellung von Beobachtungen über Amelie, Ztschr. Geburtsh. u. Gynäk. 114:174, 1937.
27. Ballantyne, J. W.: *Manual of Antenatal Pathology and Hygiene. The Embryo* (Chicago: Chicago Medical Book Company, 1904), p. 152.
28. Watkinson: Case of a foetus in which the left foot was separated from the leg during utero-gestation, London M. & Phys. J. 54:38, 1825.
29. Hornsby, W.: Intrauterine amputation of left leg, Brit. M. J. 1:865, 1926.
30. Streeter, G. L.: The significance of morbid processes in the fetus, Harvey Lect. 1933–1934, p. 204.
31. Glessner, J. R.: Spontaneous intrauterine amputation, J. Bone & Joint Surg. 45-A:351, 1963.
32. Torpin, R.: *Fetal Malformations Caused by Amnion Rupture during Gestation* (Springfield, Ill.: Charles C Thomas, Publisher, 1968).
33. Wolff, J.: Intrauterine Spontan-Amputationen an den oberen Extremitäten bei einem 5 Monate alten Foetus mit vollständiger Erhaltung des die Amputation bedingenden Amnionfadens, Arch. Gynäk. 1:281, 1900.
34. Ajinkya, Y. N.: Intrauterine amputations and annular constrictions in a living infant, now a child of 4, due to amniotic adhesions resulting from oligohydramnios, J. Obst. & Gynaec. Brit. Emp. 45:692, 1938.
35. Johnson, H. M.: Congenital cicatrizing bands, Am. J. Surg. 52:498, 1941.
36. Barenberg, L. H., and Greenberg, B.: Intrauterine amputations and constriction bands, Am. J. Dis. Child. 64:87, 1942.
37. Erlich, N.: Untersuchungen über die congenitalen Defecte und Hemmungsbildungen der Extremitäten, Virchows Arch. path. Anat. 100:109, 1885.
38. Winckel, F.: Ätiologische Untersuchungen über einige sehr seltene fötale Missbildungen, München. med. Wchnschr. 43:389, 1896.
39. Latta, J. S.: Spontaneous intrauterine amputations, Am. J. Obst. & Gynec. 10:640, 1925.
40. Evans, E. L.: Amniotic band, Proc. Roy. Soc. Med. 28:651, 1935.
41. Ollerenshaw, R.: Congenital defects of long bones of lower limb; contribution to study of their causes, effects and treatment, J. Bone & Joint Surg. 7:528, 1925.
42. Greene, H. S. N., and Saxton, J. A.: Hereditary brachydactylia and allied abnormalities in the rabbit, J. Exper. Med. 69:301, 1939.
43. Bagg, H. J., and Little, C. C.: Hereditary structural defects in descendants of mice exposed to roentgen-ray irradiation, Am. J. Anat. 33:119, 1924.

44. Koehler, O.: Die hand-und fusslosen brasilianischen Geschwister, Ztschr. menschl. Vererb.-u. Konstitutionslehre 19:670, 1936.
45. Freire-Maia, A., Freire-Maia, N., and Quelce-Salgado, A.: The achiropody gene. Estimate of the adaptive value of the homozygote; genetic analysis, in search of lethals, of the region where it is located; explanation of the excess of affected men (summary), An. brasil. genet. hum., p. 78, 1959.
46. Freire-Maia, A.: New data on acheiropodia, no. 412, Excerpta Medica, Internat. Cong. Series no. 32, 1961.
47. MacArthur, J. W., and McCullough, E.: Apical dystrophy. An inherited defect of hands and feet, Human Biol. 4: 179, 1932.
48. Hedenstedt, S.: Zwei Fälle von totaler Amelie, Acta obst. et gynec. scandinav. 24:271, 1944.
49. Jost, A.: La dégénerescence des extrémités du foetus de rat sous des actions hormonales (acroblapsie expérimentale) et la théorie des bulles myélencéphaliques de Bonnevie, Arch. franç pédiat. 10:865, 1953.
50. Gruenwald, P.: Malformations caused by necrosis in the embryo, Am. J. Path. 34:77, 1958.
51. Knapp, K., and Lenz, W.: Die Formen der Thalidomid-Embryopathie, Roentgen. Europ. 5:105, 1963.
52. Zwilling, E., and Ames, J. F.: Polydactyly, related defects and axial shifts, Am. Naturalist 92:257, 1958.
53. Carter, T. C.: Genetics of luxate mice. IV. Embryology, J. Genetics 52:1, 1954.
54. Berndorfer, A.: Formalgenetische Diagnostik von Extremitätenmissbildungen in der klinischen Praxis, Ztschr. Orthop. 105:386, 1968.

Amelias

Complete Amelia (Tetra-Amelia)

ABSENCE of upper and lower extremities – total or quadrimembral amelia – is rare. Dresher and Macdonell[1] reviewed the literature and described 2 cases. A total of 13 cases were on record in 1965; 7 of these were stillborn children, 4 died within 8 weeks after birth and 2 lived beyond this period. Dresher and Macdonell described a girl whose mother had had measles during the first trimester of pregnancy. The child was normal except for the limb defects, which were treated with prosthetic devices. In 1969, Aldag[2] listed 19 cases of tetra-amelia recorded in the medical literature without exact specifications and 12 cases with detailed descriptions of the shoulder and pelvic girdles, association malformations and family histories. In this monograph, there also are reviews of published cases of tri-, di- and mono-amelias. A list of 45 amelias encountered in German hospitals and clinics between 1945 and 1967 contained only 1 tetra-amelia.[2] A careful dissection of a child with amelia was made by Lereboullet *et al.*[3] Breech presentation was recorded repeatedly.[2] In some cases, mandibular defects, chest and spine anomalies, congenital heart defects, abnormal lobation of a lung, anal atresia and other associated defects were noted.[1,2] Potter[4] illustrated 1 case of complete amelia combined with hydrocephaly. The ACAC survey by Frantz and O'Rahilly[5] listed 1 case of quadrimembral amelia.

Amelia of arms and legs occurred in rare instances of the thalidomide syndrome.[6-9]

Tri-amelia existed in a girl reported and illustrated

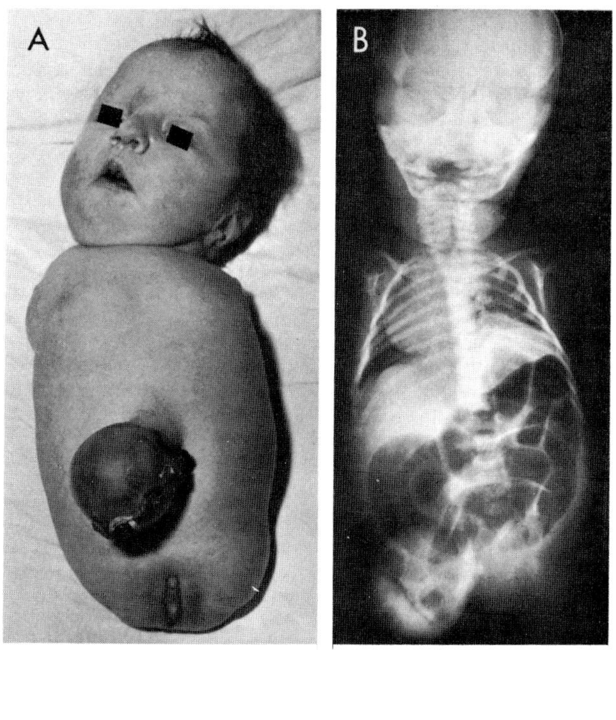

Fig. 100-9. – **A,** infant girl with total amelia, dextrocardia, exomphalos and imperforate anus (Cincinnati Children's Hospital Chart No. 173080). **B,** roentgenogram of the same child.

in several pamphlets of the sixteenth century. Apparently she had only one leg and the arms were missing.[10]

Brachial Amelia

Absence of both arms – bilateral brachial aplasia – was not seen by Birch-Jensen[11] in his Danish survey, but 7 cases were included in the ACAC survey.[5] Harelip, cleft palate, scoliosis and clubfeet were associated malformations. Several bilateral brachial amelias were seen in the Child Amputee Center at Los Angeles and 1 case with prosthetic fitting was described in detail by Hall *et al.*[12] Werthemann[13] described a case of bilateral brachial amelia without complicating malformations and mentioned several case reports from the literature.[3,14,15] The shoulder girdle may be normal or reduced. Associated phocomelia of the lower extremities was mentioned in some of the cases, and 1 child,[14] the product of a consanguineous marriage, had a cleft mandible. Kühne *et al.*,[16] who described a syndrome of defects of the femur and fibula combined with anomalies of the upper extremities, mentioned 9 cases of bilateral brachial amelia among 61 patients with the syndrome.

The mortality of infants with bilateral brachial amelia apparently is high but occasionally such patients survive and some of them have normal mentality and develop great skill in the use of their lower extremities. In the past, such persons sometimes acquired fame because of their skills, and their cases were published in special pamphlets. Thomas Schweicker, born in Halle in 1580, was shown in an engraving at the age of 53 years. He not only could write well but could also paint, carve and bind books. Other talented foot artists without arms were Johannes Wynistarff, who could thread a needle, saw, play cards, write and shoot with his feet. A Swedish woman was able to perform similar acts but she could also serve food and drink, feed her baby at the breast and blow her nose with a handkerchief. In the twentieth century, the painter César Ducornet, born in Lille, France, in 1806, was shown in a lithograph holding his palette with one foot. Gould and Pyle[17] stated that "he was completely deprived of arms, but the rest of the body was well formed with the exception of the feet, of which the second toe was faulty. The deformity of the feet, however, had the happiest results, as the space between the great toe and its neighbor was much larger than ordinary and the toes much more mobile. He became so skillful in his adopted profession that he finally painted a picture eleven feet in height, which was purchased by the Government and given to the city of Lille." The same authors relate that Paré had seen an armless man in Paris who by means of his head and neck could crack a whip or hold an axe. "He ate by means of his feet, dealt and played cards, and threw dice with the same members, exhibiting such dexterity that finally his companions refused to play with him. He was proved to be a thief and a murderer and was finally hanged at Gueldres."

Unilateral absence of one arm was found in 9 patients of the Danish series. An incidence at birth of 1 in 450,000 and a prevalence in the population of 1 in 270,000 were figures cited by Birch-Jensen.[11] The right and the left side were affected equally and 5 of the propositi had congenital deformities of the contralateral arm. It seems that approximately half of the infants with this malformation die soon after birth. In the ACAC survey,[5] 6 cases of unilateral brachial amelia were listed.

Crural Amelia

Absence of both legs seems to be rarer than absence of both arms,[5,12] but it apparently is more frequent than absence of one leg.[12] Pelvic, ulnar and digital defects occur as associated anomalies.[18] A girl with absence of both legs and terminal transverse "hemimelia" of both upper extremities was described by Hall *et al.*[12] Bilateral crural aplasia rarely occurred in the thalidomide syndrome.[19] A pamphlet of 1585 shows a legless girl who possibly was hermaphroditic. She could sing and perform various national dances using her arms and hands.[10]

Absence of one leg (monopodia) was seen in 4 patients in the ACAC survey[5] against 3 with bilateral crural amelia. Werthemann[13] mentioned complete absence of the right leg, right pelvis and right testis in a newborn male with a large exomphalos. The upper extremities and the left leg were essentially normal. In another case, monopodia was combined with segmentation defects of thoracic and lumbar vertebrae, resulting in scoliosis.

Absence of one arm and ipsilateral absence of a leg is very rare. A case was reported by Pires de Lima[20] of a girl with absence of the right arm and right leg; the left foot had four toes. Unilateral left rudimentary extremities, thin and scaly skin on the same side and congenital heart disease were described as a lethal syndrome in sisters by Falek *et al.*[21]

Sympodia

A special kind of monopodia (sympodia) is seen in sireniform monsters that have a median leg. Potter[4] illustrated such a sirenomelus with marked hypoplasia of the fused extremity; there was a single femur but tibiae and fibulae had developed in the lower leg. In other cases, the femora may be separated, whereas the feet are united to a single structure with supernumerary toes. The pelvic bones are not completely differentiated and appear fused. The sacrum is absent and the single acetabulum located on the posterior aspect of the united ilia, as the position of the leg is reversed. Portions of the gastrointestinal tract, kidneys, ureters, bladder and urethra usually are absent but the gonads can be present. A penis-like structure attached to the back of a sirenomelus had corpora cavernosa but no urethra.[4] As a rule, sireniform monsters are male.[22] The case of female identical twins, both with sympodia and absence of kidneys, ureters, bladder, anus and external genital organs, was reported by Roberge.[23] Roentgenograms showed a single femur and a short and pointed tibia; fibulae and feet were absent. Identical twins, discordant in regard to various malformations, were reported by Gruenwald and Mayberger.[24] Both twins had sireniform malformations that differed in degree. Absence of the umbilical cord, exomphalos, cystic kidneys and other malformations were present.

Phocomelia

Seal limbs – phocomelias – are malformations characterized by intercalary deficiency of long bones with relatively good development of hands and feet attached at or near the shoulders or the hips. If the hands or feet sit directly at the shoulder or pelvic girdle, one speaks of complete (or intercalary transverse) phocomelia. If, because of absence of humerus or femur, the forearms and hands or the lower legs and feet are attached to the trunk, one speaks of proximal phocomelia. If the hands or feet contact the upper arms or thighs directly, a distal phocomelia is present.

Complete phocomelia is rare. It occurs, according to Wepler,[25] almost always in combination with such other malformations as distal deficiencies of digits or facial clefts. Phocomelias of various types were frequent manifestations of the thalidomide embryopathy and much has been learned about these malformations since their epidemic occurrence.

Tetraphocomelia of the upper and lower extremities is a rare malformation. Among 93 cases of phocomelia reviewed by Krueger,[26] only 5 involved all extremities. Appelt *et al.*[27] pointed out that only 1 of these cases was free of other malformations. They emphasized that tetraphocomelias usually are combined with facial clefts, lid colobomas and sometimes with hypertrophic clitoris. They described a girl born with marked intrauterine growth retardation and very short, flipper-like extremities who, in addition, had microcephaly, exophthalmos, lid coloboma, antimongoloid palpebral fissures, cleft lip and enlarged clitoris. Occasionally, tetraphocomelia occurs in otherwise normal persons and is compatible with survival to adulthood.[27,28] Most recorded cases of tetraphocomelia were sporadic, but in a family described by O'Brien and Mustard[28] there were 3 affected siblings. In a family reported from Turkey,[29] 2 of 4 children had (proximal) phocomelia. The parents were first cousins. Six cases of complete phocomelia of the upper limbs were listed in the ACAC survey.[5] These patients also had deficient rays of the index to little fingers or syndactyly. The digits present usually were held in flexion. In the same Center, there were 5 cases of complete lower limb phocomelia. When the feet were attached to the trunk walls, the acetabula were absent. Sometimes toes and tarsal bones also were deficient. Proximal phocomelia (absence of the femur) was seen twice. In the absence of the acetabulum, the proximal ends of the tibia and fibula were located close to the external surface of the ilium in an unstable junction. More frequent were distal phocomelias of the upper extremity in 10 patients who had absence or underdevelopment of radius and ulna, resulting in shortening of the arm. The fingers varied in number. Roentgenograms usually showed forking of the distal end of the humerus.

The etiology of phocomelia remains unexplained. In the 5 cases ascertained by Birch-Jensen,[11] there were no affected relatives and one propositus had 3 normal children. The patients seen in the ACAC[5] represented sporadic cases without indications of inheritance. But, in some phocomelias, genetic factors are mani-

Fig. 100-10. – **A,** bilateral distal phocomelia with absence of bones of the forearms and finger anomalies. **B,** there also was shortening of the tibia and absence of the fibula.

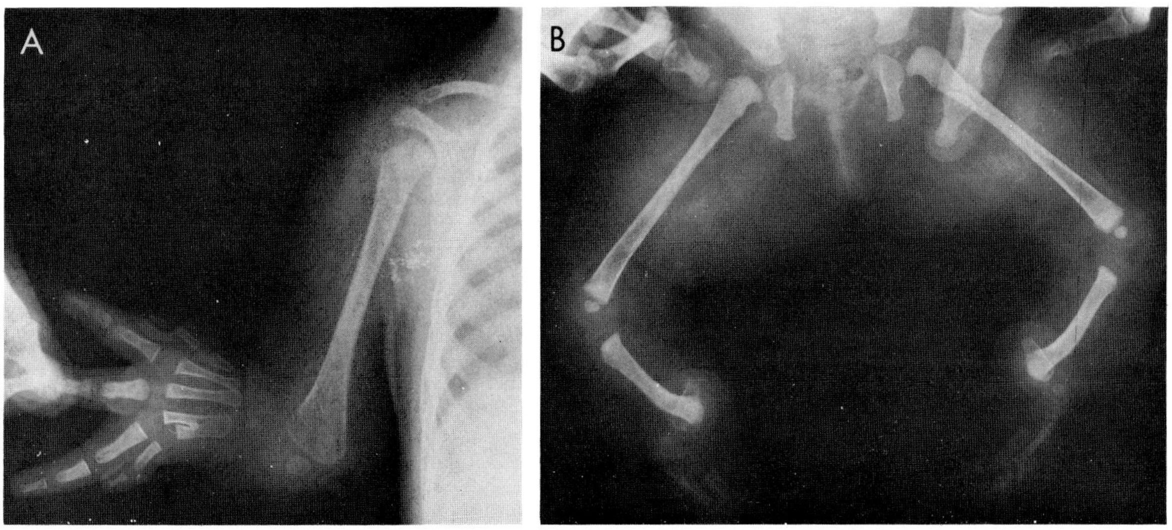

fest. Phocomelia can appear in pedigrees in which malformations of the upper extremities are transmitted as dominant traits. Several kindreds of this type were listed by Grebe.[30] Stiles and Dougan[31] described a father and his 2 sons with phocomelia; minor hand and finger anomalies had been present in their relatives through three generations. A peculiar phocomelia of the lower extremities that is due to short and thick bones of the lower leg[32] has been observed in two successive generations. Some phocomelias appear as constituents of genetically determined syndromes. The Holt-Oram syndrome (p. 571) combines congenital heart disease and such skeletal malformations as reduction of the thumb and of the radius. In some families, the skeletal malformations are more serious and include phocomelia due to shortening of the humerus, radius and ulna. Scapula and clavicle may be reduced in size also.[33,34] Autosomal recessive inheritance of reduction malformations has been documented in many pedigrees. The malformations vary from relatively minor anomalies to very serious limb defects, including phocomelia. Freire-Maia *et al.*[35] recorded a pedigree in which 4 members had severe reduction malformations ranging from aplasia to various degrees of phocomelia. Two of the marriages that gave rise to the patients were consanguineous, and autosomal recessive inheritance can be considered established. O'Brien and Mustard[28] described an adult with phocomelia who had 2 affected and 5 normal siblings. Two sisters reported by Grebe[36] as cases of achondrogenesis, which is considered a recessive trait, had phocomelia of a specific type. The legs were affected more than the arms, and the fingers – tiny soft-tissue buds – radiated in different directions. The appearance of these girls is similar to that of the dwarfs reported by Quelce-Salgado,[37] who had, however, polydactyly as well as manus valga.

Fig. 100-11. – Phocomelia in a boy with congenital hypoplastic thrombocytopenia and myeloid leukemoid reactions. (From P. St. J. Dignan *et al.*[40])

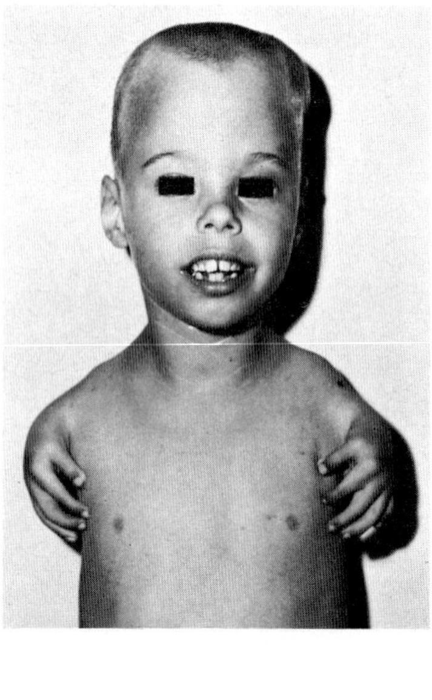

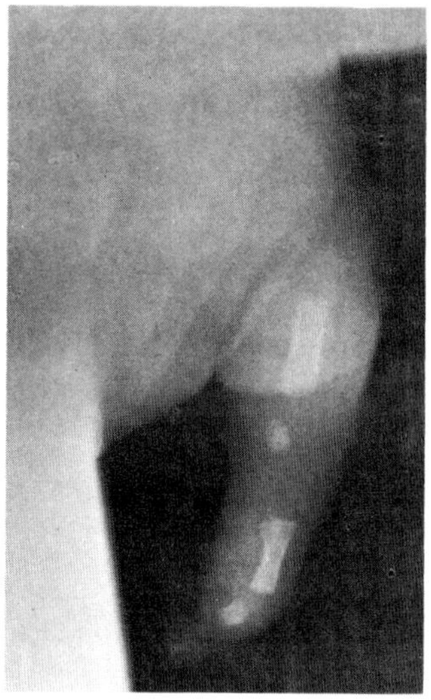

Fig. 100-12. – Phocomelia of left upper extremity with monodactyly.

Phocomelia can occur in syndromes that are recessively inherited. Fanconi pancytopenic anemia often is associated with congenital malformations. Of 68 published cases, 40 had skeletal malformations.[38] Aplasia and hypoplasia of the radius are conspicuous defects and in a few cases absence of the lower arm has been recorded. Less severe anomalies are thumb deformities, deficiencies of metacarpus I and of carpal centers. Such lesser preaxial defects are more common in Fanconi pancytopenia than the major ones mentioned. Autosomal recessive inheritance is held responsible for this disorder and its skeletal malformations. A characteristic bilateral phocomelia of the upper extremities is part of a syndrome that includes thrombocytopenia, megakaryocytopenia, leukemoid reactions and anemia. There are various degrees of shortening of the bones of the upper and lower arms but, as a rule, five rays of the hands are present. Although absence of the radius is the leading symptom, the first ray of the hand usually is present. Ulna and humerus are either hypoplastic or aplastic. In addition, there may be underdevelopment of the scapulae, clavicles and pectoralis muscles. Purpura, gastrointestinal bleeding and thrombocytopenia often are observed in the neonatal period. Later, crises with leukemoid reaction occur without precipitating events. The patient's life sometimes is endangered or terminated by meningeal hemorrhages. Patent ductus arteriosus, auricular septal defect and genital anomalies have been described in some of the cases.[39-41] The disorder has been observed in siblings. McKusick *et al.*[42] found a syndrome of marked unilateral phocomelia of a lower extremity, congenital cataract and progressive scoliosis in an Amish group. In 1 patient, the abnormal limb had a foot with nine toes.

Autosomal recessive inheritance was held responsible for the syndrome. Chromosomal abnormalities have, in rare cases, been associated with phocomelia. Voorhess *et al.*[43] reported absent radius, varus deformity of the hand and rudimentary thumb in a child with trisomy 18. Zellweger *et al.*[44] described a child with malformation and shortening of the left forearm due to absence of the radius, metacarpus I and thumb. There were symptoms and cytogenetic findings typical of trisomy 18. Kajii *et al.*[45] published a case of probable trisomy 18 with bilateral phocomelia.

Some phocomelias participate in syndromes the origin of which is not clarified. In the de Lange syndrome (p. 345), various anomalies of the extremities occur, some of them classifiable as phocomelia. Defects on the ulnar side seem to prevail. In the case of Brachmann,[46] there was symmetric monodactyly with ulna defect, a pattern seen repeatedly in patients with de Lange syndrome recorded later.[47] Hypoplasia of the femora as seen in children of diabetic mothers can result in proximal (femoral) phocomelia. This anomaly is characteristically combined with malformations of the spinal column, particularly agenesis of the sacrum and coccyx. Sometimes the fibula also is underdeveloped and clubfoot results. Dislocation of the hip or absence of the hip joints has been seen repeatedly. In several children, cleft lip and cleft palate were present. Hypoplasia of the femora and proximal phocomelia combined with sacral agenesis and underdevelopment of the fibula also can occur as a syndrome without maternal diabetes.[48] A different type of maternal disease may have contributed to the phocomelia in monozygotic twins reported by Hamilton.[49] In one of the twins, rudimentary hands were set directly onto the shoulders; the feet, which had five toes each, were attached to the lower end of the trunk. In the other twin there were six toes on the right foot and four toes on the left. The twins' mother had a history of infertility and of an enlarged, blocked left uterine tube. Tubal insufflation had been carried out after the last menstrual period and "disestablishment of implantation" was considered a factor in the etiology of the malformations. Hypoplasia of femur and fibula combined with amelia, stump formations of the upper limbs and underdevelopment of the ulna has been established as a syndrome[16] the etiology of which has not been ascertained. In contrast to thalidomide-induced malformations, the syndrome involves preferentially postaxial structures.

The malformations of the extremities produced in children by thalidomide are varied and difficult to classify. This can be seen in an arrangement of pictures by Wiedemann and Aeissen[8] published in 1961 to illustrate the increase in reduction malformations at that time. Some of the children had amelia; others had phocomelias of various degrees or stumps reminiscent of amputations. With the phocomelias went distortions of hands and feet, syndactylies and polydactylies and deficiencies of fingers. Both upper and lower extremities were involved, although the legs were affected less often than the arms[19] and the right side of the upper extremity less than the left.[50] On closer examination, aplastic, rudimentary or triphalangic thumb, thenar hypoplasia and various finger reductions could be seen. In addition to such reduction malformations there occasionally was preaxial polydactyly. Six, seven or eight digits have been observed.[19] Extra first toes were present in approximately 25% of the children but extra thumbs were rare.[50] In general, the preaxial appendicular skeleton was implicated more than the postaxial. Radius and tibia more often were absent or hypoplastic than the ulna and fibula and preaxial rays affected more than the postaxial. In Weicker's[50] series, the radius was absent and the ulna present—although usually reduced in size—in about 60% of the patients with involvement of the upper limb. Absence of the tibia in the presence of a reduced fibula was observed in about 45% of the cases with lower limb anomalies. As a rule, the lower arm was damaged more than the upper. The arms sometimes looked like stumps but there were rudimentary fingers at their ends. The defective tibia—if present—was reduced to a tiny rudiment or represented by a characteristic triangular bone with distal narrowing. Sometimes the fibula was well developed in such cases and sometimes it was hypoplastic. Hypoplasia of the femur was unilateral more often than bilateral. Dislocation or absence of the hip joint occurred frequently.

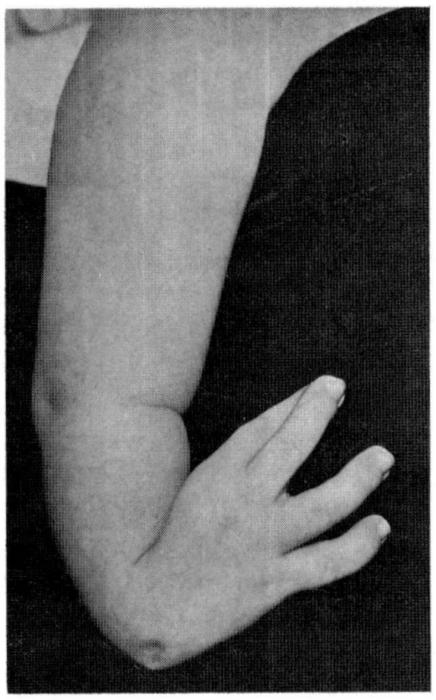

Fig. 100-13.—Congenital absence of right radius and thumb; clubhand. This girl also had abnormal segmentation of upper dorsal vertebrae, dislocation of both hips and clubfeet.

The limb anomalies produced in rats by riboflavin deficiency[51] were distal phocomelias. With relative maintenance of the proximal bones of the upper and lower extremities there typically was reduction of tibia, radius, fibula and ulna (see Fig. 100-5, *B*). Syndactyly and other digital defects were present at the distal ends of the shortened limbs. Very similar reduction malformations were produced in chicks by nitrogen mustard. In milder cases, there was chiefly distal phocomelia; in severe cases, the digits appeared to be inserted directly into the flank of the animal.[52]

Peromelia (Stump Formations; Terminal Transverse Hemimelia)

"Maimed" limbs (peromelia) with stump formation were considered amputations in the past. It is now thought that most of these limbs were never formed completely and were, therefore, not amputated. Since the stumps may represent one-third, one-half or two-thirds of the normal extremity, the term "hemimelia" is misleading and not recommended.

In some instances, all four extremities are reduced to stumps representing the proximal parts of the limbs, whereas distal parts are absent (*tetraperomelia*). Such terminal transverse deficiencies resemble amputations but, in some of the cases, associated micrognathia and other malformations indicate a general peripheral growth retardation rather than severance of distal parts. Werthemann[13] described 2 cases associated with hydromyelia. Stumps of the forearms and lower legs without hands and feet (acheiropodia) were present in 6 siblings of the well-known Brazilian family in which mating between an uncle and a niece had occurred.[53] These and similar cases are attributed to autosomal recessive inheritance.[35] Severe tetramelic deficiencies, deformed auricles, hypotrichosis and abnormal dentition and other congenital anomalies have been observed in another Brazilian family and thought to be due to homozygosity of a rare autosomal recessive gene.[73]

Tetraperomelia has been described in cattle, sheep and pigs. The defects vary in degree and associated malformations. The origin of "amputate" cattle has been traced by Wriedt and Mohr[54] and by Bishop and Cembrowicz[55] and attributed to recessive inheritance. Affected calves may have hydrocephaly, cleft palate, micrognathia and other malformations.

Severe reduction malformations with stump formations of the upper and lower extremities sometimes are associated with splenic-gonadal fusion. Amelia or stumps may alternate in different extremities. Three or all four limbs may be reduced. Micrognathia, hydromyelia, atresia ani or defective coccyx can be associated with this syndrome.[56]

Stumps of both upper arms were present in 3 children of the ACAC and stumps of both thighs in 5 children.[5] There were no persons with bilateral brachial peromelia in the Danish population surveyed by Birch-Jensen.[11] Peromelia on one side can be combined with relatively mild reduction malformations on the other side.[13] Cleft lip and palate, agnathia and congenital heart defects may be associated anomalies.[5]

"Transverse terminal hemimelia," i.e., absence of forearms and hands, was described in a monozygotic twin girl whose co-twin was normal. The defects were symmetric and aplasia rather than amputation of the forearms can be assumed in this case.[57]

Peromelia of one arm was noted in 9 patients of the Danish population by Birch-Jensen.[11] Six were male; the right and left side were affected equally. In 5 of the patients, other malformations occurred on the opposite arms. Approximately 40% of the infants born with these malformations die soon after birth, but survivors of the neonatal period have a good prognosis for life. The families of these patients had no similar defects.

Absence of the distal forearm and hand ("terminal transverse partial hemimelia"), with a stump below the elbow, is one of the more common reduction malformations of the upper extremity, with a prevalence of 1 in 25,000 in the Danish population.[11] It also is a frequent anomaly in Amputee Centers, where it accounts for approximately one-third of the cases.[5,12] The stump of the forearm usually is 4 inches long or less, well padded and without scars. The ulna is fairly well developed in its proximal part but reduced distally; the radius often is somewhat longer than the ulna. Development of the radial head is variable. There usually is a strong biceps and a large tuberosity for its insertion. The elbow flexion power is good.[5] That this anomaly usually is not a true amputation can be gathered from the fact that fingers frequently are present at the distal end of the stump. Roentgenograms also show that the forearm bones are not amputated but hypoplastic and deformed. Occasionally, however, radius and ulna terminate abruptly, so that the possi-

Fig. 100-14. – Peromelia. The rudimentary forearm is fused with the humerus.

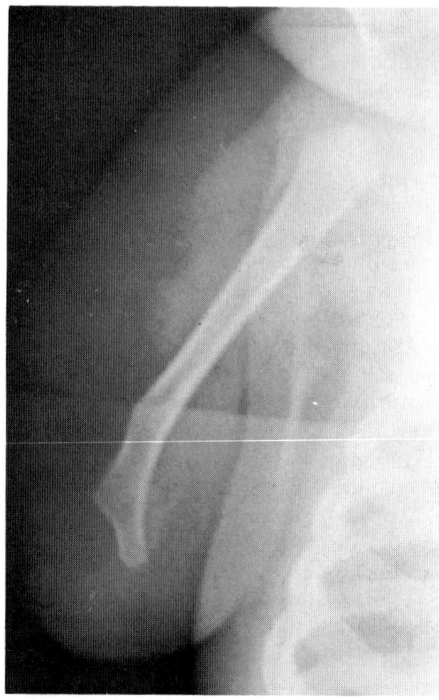

bility of a true amputation cannot be excluded. Absence of forearm and hand is unilateral in the majority and left sided in about two-thirds of the cases.[11] Only 2–3% of the patients have the anomaly on both sides.[12] Predominance of females among these patients has been observed.[5,11] Most of the patients with this anomaly are otherwise normal.[11] Frantz and O'Rahilly[5] mentioned associated skeletal defects in only 9% of their cases. Aglossia and peromelia can occur together.[58] In most families, absence of the distal forearm and hand occurs sporadically. In the Danish series, all 82 children and 10 grandchildren of affected persons were free of the defect. Only once were 2 siblings affected. In two instances, persons with similar reduction malformations married and had normal offspring. But genetic determination could not be excluded in some of the cases, since, in several pedigrees, cousins or more distant relatives showed seemingly related reduction malformations. Grebe[59] reported hypoplasia of the left forearm and hand in a boy in whose kinship brain defects, anencephaly, maxillary anomalies and speech defects had been observed. Absence of one hand with termination of the left forearm at the wrist was observed in one of dizygotic twin girls. The co-twin, although not deformed, died soon after birth. A paternal uncle of the twins' mother had a similar stump of the right forearm. Rudimentary fingers on the girl's stump indicated that aplasia and not amputation was responsible for the defect.[60] A boy with this anomaly and Down syndrome is shown in Figure 100-2, *C*. Risk figures are not available, except that, according to Birch-Jensen,[11] parents who have one child with absent forearm and hand have only about a one-eighth of 1% risk of having another child with this lesion. The Danish survey also showed that the risk for the children of affected persons is slight. The same was suggested in a picture published in 1955 in American newspapers of a Boston mother who had been born without her left forearm. She was shown with her 9 children, all of whom were normal.

Absence of the distal part of the lower leg and the foot with a stump below the knee is much rarer than its counterpart in the upper extremity. It was listed only 12 times as against 112 corresponding arm defects in the ACAC series.[5] Only 1 case was bilateral. Males were affected more often than females. Roentgenograms show a normal proximal epiphysis of the tibia, whereas the distal epiphysis is absent. The distal ends of the tibia and fibula may be pointed. Sometimes the fibula is absent.[5] Below-elbow and below-knee stumps may occur on the same side.[12] A typical stump below the left knee was seen in a girl with trisomy 18 described by Weichsel and Luzzatti.[61] The case was complicated by ventricular septal defect and extrahepatic biliary atresia.

Absence of a hand (acheiria) was seen in 54 persons in the Danish population. Its prevalence was estimated at 1 in 75,000 and its incidence at birth at 1 in 65,000.[11] In Child Amputee Centers, it accounts for about 12% of the cases.[5,12] Acheiria is unilateral in most cases, with a preference for the left side; it was bilateral in 3 of 24 patients in the ACAC series.[5] Bilateral acheiria combined with micrognathia and mental retardation was described by Hanhart.[62] The arm usually terminates at the distal epiphyses of the radius and ulna. Rudimentary digits and skin tabs are seen regularly. Apodia, pectoral agenesis and deformities of the contralateral hands are associated malformations. Most cases are sporadic, but in one pedigree recorded by Birch-Jensen,[11] a woman with acheiria had a great-granddaughter with absence of the hand and distal forearm. Otherwise, all descendants of acheiria patients were normal in that series. Among 192 siblings, 1 had a stump ending at the forearm, another had polydactyly and 2 had cleft lip and palate.

Absence of a foot (apodia) seems to be much rarer than acheiria if one can judge from its appearance in the ACAC.[5] Only 2–3% of their patients have this anomaly. The leg terminates at the ankle with tibial and fibular distal epiphyses. The skin on the plantar surface is cornified. Abnormal tibial torsion may be present.[5] Most cases are unilateral and sporadic. Although the bones of the lower leg at first appear normal, their postnatal growth is retarded in comparison with their contralateral structures.[12]

Absence of hand and foot (acheiropodia) is a rare and very mutilating condition that can affect all four extremities. Freire-Maia[63] reviewed data on 34 persons with this anomaly belonging to fourteen sibships. He found that all those affected were the offspring of phenotypically normal parents and that all children of the affected persons (who had normal mates) were normal. The parents of the acheiropods were consanguineous in more than 80% of the cases. Perinatal mortality of the acheiropods was about 2.5 times that of their normal siblings. The condition is due to homozygosity of a rare autosomal recessive gene. Another kindred in which 6 cases of acheiropodia occurred was reported by Toledo and Saldanha.[72] In the two sibships, the parents were normal and consanguineous; recessive inheritance can be assumed. It is of interest that families with acheiropodia have been reported repeatedly from Brazil.

Hypermelia

Duplication of a limb in a singleton must be distinguished from duplication of limbs in conjoined twins. Duplications in singletons are unilateral and show variable degrees of differentiation. Supernumerary arms attached to fairly normal (left) arms have been observed in otherwise normal children.[64] Stein and Bettman[65] described a rare malformation of a right arm with double humerus, three hands and sixteen fingers. Their patient, a woman 52 years of age, had, on the right, two humeri that joined the scapula in two glenoid fossae. The forearm had two radii and three ulnae ending in diplocheiria. Péterffy and Jona[66] reported a boy who had three upper extremities on the left side and a normal upper extremity on the right.

On the left there was one arm with a normal number of rays and above it brachial duplication with fusion on the ulnar side, resulting in one ulna, two radii and diplocheiria with a digital pattern of I–II–III–IV–IV–III–II–I.

Accessory legs that originate between the pelvic bones have been observed repeatedly.[67-69] In some of the cases, there were duplications of viscera, particularly of the urogenital tract. A different type of accessory leg was reported by Giustra and Podhipleux[70] in a girl born to a family in which twinning had occurred previously. The extra leg was associated with abnormal segmentation of the spinal column, i.e., multiple hemivertebrae. The extra leg originated at the lower part of the back at the level of the upper lumbar vertebrae and terminated with only one metatarsal and toe. Agenesis of the gallbladder, patent ductus arteriosus, persistent superior vena cava on the left, atrial septal defect and bicuspid aortic valve were associated findings. It is not clear what type of stimulus produces hypermelia in man. Supernumerary limbs have been produced in urodela larvae by localized ultraviolet irradiation of the elbow region of the forelimb. Hypermelia in ungulates was discussed thoroughly by Pol.[71]

REFERENCES

1. Dresher, C. S., and Macdonell, J. A.: Total amelia, J. Bone & Joint Surg. 47-A:511, 1965.
2. Aldag, A.: Röntgenologische Differenzierung der Amelie, Inaugural-Dissertation der Rheinischen Friedrich-Wilhelms-Universität zu Bonn (Bonn: R. Schwarzbold, 1969).
3. Lereboullet, P., Hovelacque, A., and Evrard, H.: De l'amélie (à propos de deux observations), Arch. méd. Enf. 40:617, 1937.
4. Potter, E. L.: *Pathology of the Fetus and Infant* (2d ed.; Chicago: Year Book Medical Publishers, Inc., 1961).
5. Frantz, C. H., and O'Rahilly, R.: Congenital skeletal limb deficiencies, J. Bone & Joint Surg. 43-A:1202, 1961.
6. Lenz, W., and Knapp, K.: Die Thalidomid-Embryopathie, Deutsche med. Wchnschr. 87:1232, 1962.
7. Larsen, A., Hole, L. W., and Mackenzie, B.: Congenital deformities associated with the use of thalidomide during pregnancy, British Columbia, 1961–62, Canad. J. Pub. Health 54:505, 1963.
8. Wiedemann, H-R., and Aeissen, K.: Zur Frage der derzeitigen Häufung von Gliedmassen-Fehlbildungen, Med. Monatsschr. 15:816, 1961.
9. Oertel, O.: Amelie bei Zwillingen, Monatsschr. Kinderh. 110:481, 1962.
10. Holländer, E.: *Wunder, Wundergeburt und Wundergestalt* (Stuttgart: Ferdinand Enke, 1922).
11. Birch-Jensen, A.: *Congenital Deformities of the Upper Extremities* (Copenhagen: Ejnar Munksgaard, 1949).
12. Hall, C. B., Brooks, M. B., and Dennis, J. F.: Congenital skeletal deficiencies of the extremities. Classification and fundamentals of treatment, J.A.M.A. 181:590, 1962.
13. Werthemann, A.: Bewegungs-apparatus. V. Teil Die Entwicklungs-Störungen der Extremitäten, in Lubarsch, O., and Henke, F. (eds.), *Handbuch der Speziellen Pathologischen Anatomie und Histologie* (Berlin: Springer-Verlag, 1952).
14. Redenz, E.: Über doppelseitige Aplasie der freien oberen Gliedmasse, Ztschr. Geburtsh. u. Gynäk. 118:442, 1939.
15. Scheer, G.: Ein Fall von Totalmangel der oberen Extremitäten bei einem Neugeborenen, Dissertation, Dusseldorf, 1940.
16. Kühne, D., Lenz, W., Petersen, D., and Schönenberg, H.: Defekt von Femur und Fibula mit Amelie, Peromelie oder ulnaren Strahldefekten der Arme, Humangenetik 3:244, 1967.
17. Gould, G. M., and Pyle, W. L.: *Anomalies and Curiosities of Medicine* (Philadelphia: W. B. Saunders Company, 1897).
18. Rheindt, R.: Amelie der Unterextremitäten, Ztschr. Geburtsh. u. Gynäk. 122:278, 1941.
19. Knapp, K., and Lenz, W.: Die Formen der Thalidomid-Embryopathie, Roentgen. Europ. 5:105, 1963.
20. Pires de Lima, J. A.: À propos d'un nouveau cas d'ectromélie, Ann. anat. path. 10:830, 1933.
21. Falek, A., Heath, C. W., Jr., Ebbin, A. J., and McLean, W. R.: Unilateral limb and skin deformities with congenital heart disease in two siblings. A lethal syndrome, J. Pediat. 73:910, 1968.
22. Kampmeier, O. F.: Sireniform monsters, with consideration of causation and predominance of male sex among them, Anat. Rec. 34:365, 1927.
23. Roberge, J. L.: Sympodia in identical twins, J.A.M.A. 186: 728, 1963.
24. Gruenwald, P., and Mayberger, H. W.: Differences in abnormal development of monozygotic twins, Arch. Path. 70:685, 1960.
25. Wepler, W.: Die sogenannte Phokomelie, Deutsche med. Wchnschr. 63:1302, 1937.
26. Krueger, R.: *Die Phocomelie und ihre Übergänge* (Berlin: August Hirschwald, 1906).
27. Appelt, H., Gerken, H., awd Lenz, W.: Tetraphokomelie mit. Lippen-Kiefer-Gaumenspalte und Clitorishypertrophie–ein Syndrom, Pädiat. und Pädol. 2:119, 1966.
28. O'Brien, H. R., and Mustard, H. S.: An adult living case of phocomelia, J.A.M.A. 77:1964, 1921.
29. Sayli, B. S., Asmaz, A., and Yemisci, B.: Consanguinity, aspirin and phocomelia, Lancet 1:876, 1966.
30. Grebe, H.: Missbildungen der Gliedmassen, in Becker, P. E. (ed.), *Humangenetik* (Stuttgart: Georg Thieme, 1964), Vol. II.
31. Stiles, K. A., and Dougan, P.: A pedigree of malformed upper extremities showing variable dominance, J. Hered. 31:65, 1940.
32. Nievergelt, K.: Positiver Vaterschaftsnachweis auf Grund erblicher Missbildungen der Extremitäten, Dissertation, Zürich, 1944.
33. Pruzanski, W.: Familial-congenital malformations of the heart and upper limbs; a syndrome of Holt-Oram, Cardiologia 45:21, 1964.
34. Lewis, K. B., Bruce, R. A., Baum, D., and Motulsky, A. G.: The upper limb-cardiovascular syndrome, J.A.M.A. 193: 1080, 1965.
35. Freire-Maia, N., Quelce-Salgado, A., and Koehler, R. A.: Hereditary bone aplasias and hypoplasias of the upper extremities, Acta Genet. 9:33, 1959.
36. Grebe, H.: Die Achondrogenesis ein einfach rezessives Erbmerkmal., Folia hered. path. 11:23, 1952.
37. Quelce-Salgado, A.: A new type of dwarfism with various bone aplasias and hypoplasias of the extremities, Acta Genet. 14:63, 1964.
38. Nilsson, L.: Chronic pancytopenia with multiple congenital abnormalities (Fanconi's anaemia), Acta paediat. scandinav. 49:518, 1960.
39. Beaudoing, A., Butin, L-P., Pont, J., Hadjian, A. J., and Bachelot, C.: Un cas de thrombopénie hypoplastique amégacaryocytaire congénitale avec malformations squelettiques et viscérales, Pédiatrie 23:111, 1968.
40. Dignan, P. St. J., Mauer, A. M., and Frantz, C.: Phocomelia with congenital hypoplastic thrombocytopenia and myeloid leukemoid reactions, J. Pediat. 70:561, 1967.
41. Schönenberg, H., and Scheidhauer, E.: Beidseitige radiale Hemimelie mit Megakaryocytopenie. Ein neues Missbildungssyndrom, Ztschr. Kinderh. 97:240, 1966.
42. McKusick, V. A., Weilbaecher, R. G., and Gragg, G. W.: Recessive inheritance of a congenital malformation syndrome, J.A.M.A. 204:113, 1968.

43. Voorhess, M. L., Aspillaga, M. J., and Gardner, L. I.: Trisomy 18 syndrome with absent radius, varus deformity of hand and rudimentary thumb. Report of a case, J. Pediat. 65:130, 1964.
44. Zellweger, H., Huff, D. S., and Abbo, G.: Phocomelia and trisomy E, Acta genet. med. 14:164, 1965.
45. Kajii, T., Oikawa, K., Itakura, K., and Ohsawa, T.: A probable 17-18 trisomy syndrome with phocomelia, exomphalos and agenesis of hemidiaphragm, Arch. Dis. Childhood 39:519, 1964.
46. Brachmann, W.: Ein Fall von symmetrischer Monodactylie durch Ulnadefekt, mit symmetrischer Flughautbildung in den Ellenbeugen, sowie anderen Abnormitäten (Zwerghaftigkeit, Halsrippen, Behaarung), Jahrb. Kinderh. 84:225, 1916.
47. Ptacek, L. J., Opitz, J. M., Smith, D. W., Gerritsen, T., and Waisman, H. A.: The Cornelia de Lange syndrome, J. Pediat. 63:1000, 1963.
48. Kučera, J., Lenz, W., and Maier, W.: Missbildungen der Beine und der kaudalen Wirbelsäule bei Kindern diabetischer Mütter, Deutsche med. Wchnschr. 90:901, 1965.
49. Hamilton, S. G. I.: Congenital phocomelia in monozygotic twins, Brit. M. J. 4:524, 1967.
50. Weicker, H.: 100 children with thalidomide embryopathy, XIth International Congress of Pediatrics, 1965.
51. Warkany, J., and Nelson, R. C.: Skeletal abnormalities in the offspring of rats reared on deficient diets, Anat. Rec. 79:83, 1941.
52. Salzgeber, B.: Production élective de la phocomélie sous l'influence d'ypérite azotée, J. Embryol. & Exper. Morphol. 11:413, 1963.
53. Koehler, O.: Die hand-und fusslosen brasilianischen Geschwister, Ztschr. menschl. Vererb.-u. Konstitutionslehre 19:670, 1936.
54. Wriedt, C., and Mohr, O. L.: Amputated, a recessive lethal in cattle, J. Genetics 20:187, 1938.
55. Bishop, M. W. H., and Cembrowicz, H. J.: A case of amputate, a rare recessive lethal condition of Friesian cattle, Vet. Rec. 76:1049, 1964.
56. Putschar, W. G. J., and Manion, W. C.: Splenic-gonadal fusion, Am. J. Path. 32:15, 1956.
57. Gedda, L., and Torrioli-Riggio, G.: Aplasia subtotale degli arti superiori in coppia gemellare monozigotica discordante, Acta genet. med. 12:228, 1963.
58. Gorlin, R. J., and Pindborg, J. J.: *Syndromes of the Head and Neck* (New York: The Blakiston Division, McGraw-Hill Book Company, Inc., 1964).
59. Grebe, H.: Zur Ätiologie ein-und doppelseitiger Gliedmassenmissbildungen, Ztschr. menschl. Vererb.-u. Konstitutionslehre 32:126, 1954.
60. Kohler, H. G.: Congenital transverse defects of limbs and digits (intrauterine amputation), Arch. Dis. Childhood 37: 263, 1962.
61. Weichsel, M. E., and Luzzatti, L.: Trisomy 17-18 syndrome with congenital extrahepatic biliary atresia and congenital amputation of the left foot, J. Pediat. 67:324, 1965.
62. Hanhart, E.: Über die Kombination von Peromelie mit Mikrognathie, ein neues Syndrom beim Menschen, entsprechend der *Akroteriasis congenita* von Wriedt und Mohr beim Rinde, Arch. Julius Klaus-Stiftung 25:531, 1950.
63. Freire-Maia, A.: New data on acheiropodia, no. 412, Excerpta Medica, Internat. Cong. Series no. 32, 1961.
64. Gruber, G. B.: Hyperdaktylie (Polydaktyly), Diplocheirie und Diplopodie, Hypermelie, Oligodaktylie und Defekte der Röhrenknochen, in Schwalbe, E., and Gruber, G. B. (eds.), *Die Morphologie der Missbildungen des Menschen und der Tiere* (Jena: Gustav Fischer, 1958), Vol. 3, p. 720.
65. Stein, H. C., and Bettman, E. H.: Rare malformation of the arm, double humerus with 3 hands and 16 fingers, Am. J. Surg. 50:336, 1940.
66. Péterffy, P., and Jona, St.: Zwei Fälle von seltener Anomalie der Oberarmentwicklung, Zentralbl. Chir. 21:878, 1942.
67. Deboo, S. N.: A three-legged person, M. Bull. 11:339, 1943.
68. Smillie, I. S., and Murdoch, J. H.: Man with three legs, J. Bone & Joint Surg. 34-B:630, 1952.
69. Norman, W. H.: A child with three lower extremities, J. Bone & Joint Surg. 46-A:1755, 1964.
70. Giustra, F. X., and Podhipleux, P.: Ectopic accessory limb associated with cardiac defects, Am. J. Dis. Child. 112: 467, 1966.
71. Pol, R.: Missbildungen der Extremitaten, in Schwalbe, E., and Gruber, G. B. (eds.), *Die Morphologie der Missbildungen des Menschen und der Tiere* (Jena: Gustav Fischer, 1958), Vol. 3, fasc. 19.
72. Toledo, S. P. A., and Saldanha, P. H.: A radiological and genetic investigation of acheiropody in a kindred including six cases, J. Génét. Hum. 17:81, 1969.
73. Freire-Maia, N.: A newly recognized genetic syndrome of tetramelic deficiencies, ectodermal dysplasia, deformed ears, and other abnormalities, Am. J. Human Genet. 22: 370, 1970.

Prenatal Bowing of Tubular Bones

MANY EARLY OBSERVERS attributed congenital bowing of long bones to uterine pressure. Hippocrates[1] compared the crowded fetus with a tree that "in the earth has not enough space" and believed that crippling results if "in the womb a portion is relatively too narrow for the corresponding part of the infant." Other mechanical theories concerning the origin of congenital malformations have been discussed before (p. 944). The belief in the molding power of the uterine environment still exists in our time and is expressed particularly when prenatal bowing of tubular bones is discussed. A related belief is that fetal posture plays a role in the production of such osseous malformations. Denis Browne[2] stated that even the normal newborn baby shows signs of mechanical compression. The bending of the back, the calcaneus position of the feet and dimples over bony points in contact with the uterine wall were interpreted by him as effects of normal mechanical pressure on a fetus in normal position. Normal pressure in a fetus in abnormal position could bring about talipes equinovarus, malposition of toes, postural torticollis and facial paralysis, but even acrocephalosyndactyly and displaced ears were attributed by this author to fetal malposition. He held normal pressure plus defective development responsible for congenital dislocation of the hip, clubhands and congenital fracture of the tibia (with absence of the fibula). Normal hydraulic pressure, increased mechanical pressure and abnormal position could lead not only to clubfeet but also to spina bifida if the relation between the expanding fetus and its surrounding was disturbed so that the bending of the back was exaggerated, making the sides of the neural groove gape in the lumbar region. Faulty fusion and formation of spina bifida would result. Needless to say, such an explanation of spina bifida leaves unexplained the reasons for the disturbed relation of fetus and surroundings. That this can be due to nonmechanical factors has been discussed elsewhere (p. 273). Chapple and Davidson[3] explained lateral bowing of the femurs by pressure from the wall of the uterus, with the feet opposing the apex of the curvatures acting as fulcra. They found that the child, after birth, enjoyed such a "position of comfort" and established that determination of the position of comfort sometimes led to discovery of unsuspected abnormalities. It should be pointed out that these authors assumed that in their first case the mechanical forces considered acted on "bone softened by syphilis." Caffey[4] reported 3 cases of prenatal bowing and thickening of tubular bones, with multiple cutaneous dimples in the arms and legs. The deformities consisted of symmetric lateral bowing of the femora and symmetric posterior bowing of the humeri, but distal to the knees and elbows the deformities were not symmetric. Serial observations in one of these patients showed regression and disappearance after 2 years. There was no roentgenologic evidence of any osseous dysplasia or disease. The skeletal deformities were explained by the assumption that the fetal arms and legs were packed in attitudes that permitted transmission of deforming uterine pressure from one impacted fetal part to another. The bowing was thought to be due to mechanical forces acting long before birth, possibly at the time when the affected skeletal parts were cartilaginous. Caffey[4] believed that both abnormal fetal position and posture must be assumed as compressing forces applied to the concavities of the affected bones. At birth, one sees in roentgenograms thickening of the cortex on the concave wall of the curve, which was explained as structural adaptation to the forces of compression. The tendency to repair and readjustment in postnatal life added support to the hypothesis of prenatal mechanical molding as the cause of the deformities.

There is a great deal to be said in favor of such mechanical explanations and the postnatal demonstration of the "position of comfort," but it should be remembered that in rickets the deformities of older children could also be "explained" by habitual positions. Thus, bending in the lower third of the tibia and fibula often was due to crossing of the legs and the child's preferred position in bed. Position and posture explained the location of the deformities but there was an underlying softening process—rickets—that made such positional effects possible. It is likely that the situation is similar in cases of prenatal bowing of tubular bones. In some of these cases, the underlying disorder may not be detectable in postnatal life. Yet, rather typical pictures of prenatal bowing have been seen in infants who later developed symptoms of hypophosphatasia (p. 859). Currarino *et al.*[5] pointed out that congenital angulation of long bones with overlying skin dimples was reported in a number of cases of hypophosphatasia. These changes can be the only manifestation of the anomaly at birth; epiphyseal and metaphyseal changes may develop later. Kellsey[6] also reported a case of hypophosphatasia and congenital bowing of the long bones with typical epiphyseal changes developing several months after birth. It seems likely that hypophosphatasia is not the only condition that results in prenatal bowing of tubular bones. Middleton[7] discussed prenatal lesions of striated muscle as a cause of congenital deformities of long bones. In patients of Bound *et al.*[8] and Bain and Barrett,[9] soft palate cleft pointed to early intrauterine disturbance beyond the appendicular skeleton. Bowing of the tibia occurs in the absence of the fibula.[8] Conway[10] described prenatal bowing of the long bones in a brother and sister, one born in the breech and one in the vertex presentation. The mother's uterus was found grossly normal on laparotomy and no mechanical cause was found for the bowing of the bones. All these observations suggest that external pressure and fetal position are merely contributory factors resulting in bowing of skeletal parts if these are abnormal in structure.

In rats, prenatal bowing of tubular bones was induced by feeding the mother a rachitogenic diet.[11] A riboflavin-deficient diet resulted in many skeletal malformations, including angulation of the tibia and radius recognizable in the cartilaginous state.[12] Malformations of the cartilaginous primordia lead to bowing of adjacent bones. There can be little doubt that the intrauterine position of the young conformed to these angulations but the abnormal positions were the result of abnormalities of skeletal parts that had been deformed previously by maternal nutritional deficiencies. Such nutritional deficiencies could not be demonstrated in mothers of children with prenatal bowing. But the experiments suggest that intrauterine pressure and position are teratogenic only if the skeleton is rendered abnormal by other factors in its early stages.

REFERENCES

1. Ballantyne, J. W.: *Manual of Antenatal Pathology and Hygiene. The Embryo* (Chicago: Chicago Medical Book Company, 1904), p. 129.
2. Browne, D.: Congenital deformities of mechanical origin, Proc. Roy. Soc. Med. 29:1409, 1936.
3. Chapple, C. C., and Davidson, D. T.: A study of the relationship between fetal position and certain congenital deformities, J. Pediat. 18:483, 1941.
4. Caffey, J.: Prenatal bowing and thickening of tubular bones, with multiple cutaneous dimples in arms and legs, Am. J. Dis. Child. 74:543, 1947.
5. Currarino, G., Neuhauser, E. B. D., Reyersbach, G. C., and Sobel, E. H.: Hypophosphatasia, Am. J. Roentgenol. 78:392, 1957.

6. Kellsey, D. C.: Hypophosphatasia and congenital bowing of the long bones, J.A.M.A. 179:187, 1962.
7. Middleton, D. S.: Studies on prenatal lesions of striated muscle as cause of congenital deformity; congenital tibial kyphosis; congenital high shoulder; myodystrophia foetalis deformans, Edinburgh M. J. 41:401, 1934.
8. Bound, J. P., Finlay, H. V. L., and Rose, F. C.: Congenital anterior angulation of the tibia, Arch. Dis. Childhood 27:179, 1952.
9. Bain, A. D., and Barrett, H. S.: Congenital bowing of the long bones: Report of a case, Arch. Dis. Childhood 34:516, 1959.
10. Conway, T. J.: Prenatal bowing and angulation of long bones, A.M.A. J. Dis. Child. 95:305, 1958.
11. Warkany, J.: Effect of maternal rachitogenic diet on skeletal development of young rat, Am. J. Dis. Child. 66:511, 1943.
12. Warkany, J., and Nelson, R. C.: Skeletal abnormalities induced in rats by maternal nutritional deficiency, Arch. Path. 34:375, 1942.

101

The Upper Extremities

Hypoplasia of the Shoulder Girdle

LIMITATION of elevation and medial rotation of the humerus was described in a woman and 3 of her children. The glenoid fossa was hypoplastic and brachydactyly and clinodactyly were present.[1]

Malformations of the shoulder girdle were common in children damaged by thalidomide. The scapula was reduced in size in approximately 45% of the cases.[2]

Congenital Hypertrophy of Upper Extremity

Brücke[3] described generalized hypertrophy of the left arm in a newborn premature boy. Bones as well as muscles of the forearm and of the hand were involved. Malposition of the thumb and index finger were noticed. Muscle power was increased and there seemed to be a tendency to progressive hypertrophy after birth. Morrissey[4] reported hypertrophy of the right arm in a boy 9 years of age. The affected arm was stronger and bigger than the left and the muscles were overdeveloped on the same side, giving the impression of the muscles of a wrestler. The hypertrophy also involved the clavicle, scapula, humerus, radius and ulna. The right hand was deformed, showing increased distances between the metacarpal heads. Although his grip was powerful, fine movements were clumsy, the thumb was held in abduction and the index finger in ulnar deviation. This condition has been termed "segmental hypertrophy" or "local acromegaly."

Defects of the Humerus

In his survey of congenital deformities of the upper extremities in Denmark, Birch-Jensen[5] listed only 9 cases of "amputation of the humerus," with an incidence of 1 in 450,000 in the population. Termination at the shoulder joint, in the middle and a few centimeters above the elbow joint occurred. The stumps were conical, rapidly tapering or rounded, carrying a rudimentary hand. Scar foundation may be seen at the site of termination. "Amputation" of the upper arm occurred in some members of the Brazilian family reported by Koehler[6] and the Dutch family recorded by Schwarzweller.[7] As a rule, such humerus defects are combined with hypoplasias and reduction malformations of other parts of the appendicular skeleton. Frantz and O'Rahilly[8] found 13 cases of complete absence of the upper limb (amelia) and 20 cases of absence of the forearm and hand (terminal transverse hemimelia) among 300 patients of the Area Child Amputee Center (ACAC). In addition to associated skeletal defects, cleft lip and palate, agnathia and heart defects were observed in some of these patients. The humerus can be absent or rudimentary in proximal phocomelias with congenital hypoplastic thrombocytopenia[9] or in patients with the Holt-Oram syndrome.[10] In patients with the thalidomide embryopathy, absence or hypoplasia of the humerus often was combined with other skeletal defects.[8] Humeroradial synostosis is a rather rare anomaly that was reviewed by Keutel *et al.*[283] These authors described the anomaly as an autosomal recessive trait but other etiologies should be considered. Humeroradial synostosis was produced experimentally in rats by prenatal x-ray treatment.[27]

Congenital Defects of the Radius

Congenital radial defects (radial hemimelias) are more frequent than ulnar defects. Birch-Jensen[5] estimated that one radial defect occurs in 30,000 births and one ulnar defect in 100,000. Radial defects are unilateral in approximately half of the patients. Many patients die at birth or soon thereafter because of associated defects, so that the prevalence in the (Danish) population was reduced to 1:55,000. Of those who survived, the mortality was still high up to the age of 20 years but patients who reached the twentieth year had a good prognosis as to life. It is of interest that congenital radial defects are relatively seldom combined with defects of the humerus or with defects of the lower extremities. The majority of radial defects occur sporadically. Bilateral complete absence of the radius and thumb has been seen in identical twin boys; three of the hands had four fingers each but one hand had only two fingers.[11] This slight discordance in twins, who otherwise showed striking concordance, illustrates the influence of local prenatal factors. Heredity, dominant or recessive, was suggested by Birch-Jensen[5] for some of his cases of radial defects. Hereditary absence of radius and thumb was described by Dodson,[12] who cited several cases of transmitted radial aplasia. Association with hexadactyly and radial hypoplasia in a family was reported by Schmid.[13] Double thumb has been observed repeatedly as an associated anomaly.[14] Reduction deformities of the radius and the first ray of the hand are included in various syndromes. Such syndromes or other associated malformations sometimes betray the etiology of the forearm defect. Birch-Jensen[5] compiled a list of complicating anomalies from the literature and enumerated congenital defects among his propositi. Congenital heart disease, scoliosis, eye and ear defects, cleft lip and palate, polydactyly, ulnar defects, renal disease, aplastic anemia and mental deficiency were observed. Absence of the radius can occur in patients with laryngeal atresia[15] or with agenesis of a lung.[16] Associations with heart anomalies have been established as syndromes.[132] The Holt-Oram syndrome (p. 572) includes atrial septal defect but ventricular septal defect also can be associated with aplasia or hypoplasia of the radius.[17] The Holt-Oram syndrome, which is a dominant hereditary trait, has been broadened by inclusion of various cardiac and skeletal defects.[10]

In some families, recessive inheritance seems to be responsible for radial aplasia,[18,19] sometimes combined with tower head, ulnar hypoplasia or other skeletal anomalies. Radial reduction malformations and other preaxial defects of the upper limb often are associated with Fanconi pancytopenia,[20] a recessively inherited trait. Bilateral radial defects with megakaryocytopenia[21] probably is related to cases of phocomelia with congenital hypoplastic thrombocytopenia and myeloid leukemoid reactions, in which, despite radial involvement, the hand maintains five fingers. Siblings, children of phenotypically normal parents, have shown this disorder.[9] Rudimentary radius, ulna and thumb may be seen in cases of congenital poikiloderma (Rothmund-Thomson syndrome) (p. 392).

It seems that in the de Lange syndrome postaxial anomalies of the upper extremity prevail,[22] but shortening of the radius and dislocation and angulation of its distal articular surface have been described.[23]

Chromosomal abnormalities can be associated with radial aplasia. Trisomy 18 was present in children with absent radius, varus deformity of the hand and rudimentary thumb.[24,25] In one of these cases, radial agenesis was combined with esophageal atresia, congenital heart disease and thrombocytopenia.[26] Absence of the thumb occurring in such cases differentiates the chromosomal syndrome from the phocomelia-thrombocytopenia syndrome mentioned before, which is characterized by the presence of five fingers.[9] Two cases of bilateral hypoplasia of radial elements, cardiac anomalies and intrauterine growth retardation associated with chromosomal abnormalities were reported by Faed *et al.*[275] In thalidomide phocomelia, absence of the radius was seen in about 70%, reduction in 15% and normal radius in about 15% of the cases with involvement of the upper extremities.[2] The radial defects were commonly associated with defects of the thumb and other preaxial structures. In many instances, aplasia or hypoplasia of the radius and of preaxial structures of the hand was present, whereas the ulna and other postaxial elements were spared. If the ulna and postaxial structures were reduced, the radial structures were affected even more seriously. Such preaxial deficiencies in the upper extremity often were combined with preaxial deficiencies in the leg, i.e., tibial defects and hypoplasia or aplasia of the first and second toes (p. 89).

Most cases of radial reduction are sporadic and their etiology remains obscure. But, as pointed out before, in some of the cases dominant or recessive inheritance, chromosomal aberrations or environmental causes can be identified. The preference of these causes for preaxial structures is puzzling. It is of interest that congenital defects of the radius and of the ulna can be produced experimentally in the rat. By maternal riboflavin deficiency, young can be obtained with a syndrome of skeletal defects in which shortening of both forearm bones is observed. In such animals, the anomaly of the radius is always more pronounced than that of the ulna but, after prenatal x-irradiation, ulnar defects are more frequent and more severe than radial anomalies[27] (Fig. 4-4). Skeletal malformations produced in rabbits by thalidomide also show a predilection for preaxial lesions.

In the presence of aplasia or hypoplasia of the radius, the hand usually is turned radiad because of lack of support by the preaxial bone (manus vara). In most of these cases, the ulna is short, thick and curved. Duplication of the ulna occurs but it is rare. Bilateral absence of the radius and tibia combined with duplication of the ulna and fibula has been reported.[28] In more than 80% of radial aplasia, the scaphoid, trapezium, the first metacarpal and the thumb are absent; the lunate, trapezoid, second metacarpal and index finger occasionally are missing[29] but in some instances the hand is entirely normal.[9] In radial hypoplasia there usually is a proximal rudiment of variable size. It is of interest that idiopathic scoliosis develops in some children with radial and other defects of the upper extremities.[276] Treatment of the clubhand resulting from radial defects was discussed by Bora *et al.*[284]

Duplication of the Radius

Duplication of the radius is a very rare anomaly. Sometimes it is seen in conjoined twins or dicephali, but reports of double radius and single ulna are hard to find.[29]

Congenital Dislocation of the Radius

Unilateral forward displacement of the head of the radius is due to elongation of the radius and hypoplasia of its head. Although the radius can be moved fairly well, it cannot be reduced to normal position. Following an injury, the head of the radius may be felt in the antecubital fossa, a situation that might have gone unnoticed before and the congenital anomaly then be interpreted as the result of trauma. If function is interfered with, the head of the radius can be removed.[30] Bilateral dislocation of the radial head accompanies various anomalies, such as radio-ulnar dysostosis, multiple exostoses and many other systemic disorders.[31] Anterior or posterior dislocation of the radius occurs frequently in a syndrome of small stature and abnormal shape of the external ears, which is transmitted as a dominant trait[31]; bilateral hypoplasia of the capitellum is present in affected persons.

Congenital Defects of the Ulna

Congenital absence of the ulna and other ulnar defects are rare. Incidence at birth was estimated at 1 in 100,000 Danish children and prevalence in the population at 1 in 210,000, which is about one-fourth of the figures given for radial defects.[5] Reviews of ulnar defects were published by O'Rahilly[29] in 1951 and by Lausecker[32] in 1954.

Inheritance of ulnar defects cannot always be demonstrated, but some of the cases occur in families in which there is an accumulation of joint lesions.[5]

A case of ulnar aplasia, including developmental deficiencies of the postaxial carpal and metacarpal bones and fingers, was described by Roberts[33] in 1886. The patient was 73 years of age and 6 feet 4 inches tall. The right extremity was affected more than the left. Heredity played a definite role in that case, since anomalies of the hands or arms were reported in four generations of his kindred. The expressivity of the—probably—dominant gene was variable. Some members of the kinship had merely stiffness of fingers, whereas in others severe reduction malformations occurred. Similar variability of malformations in relatives of persons with ulnar defects was reported by Southwood.[34] Dominantly inherited shortening of the ulna and fibula through four generations was reported by Pfeiffer.[35] The anomaly resulted in shortening and deformity of the forearms and legs in 14 members of a kindred through four generations. Recessive micromelic dwarfism with hypoplasia of the ulna and fibula was reviewed by Lenz.[36] Because of general reduction in height, some of the patients were considered chondrodystrophic. Absence of the ulna usually is combined with ulnar deflection of the hand (manus valga). The radius is curved and the forearm shortened. The radio-humeral joint often is ankylosed or the head of the radius dislocated on the humerus. Any carpal or metacarpal bone may be absent. The pisiform and hamate usually and the triquetrum and capitate often are missing. The metacarpals are absent more often on the ulnar side than on the radial.[29] Although in many cases postaxial structures are deficient, the thumbs also often are abnormal. Failure of joint development has been reported, with synostoses chiefly on the elbows; the distal radio-ulnar joints rarely are affected. Stiffness of fingers due to symphalangism occurs. Aplasia of the fibula, scoliosis and other malformations were mentioned as associated defects by Birch-Jensen.[5] Involvement of the fibula, a homologous structure, has been emphasized by various observers and such ulnar-fibular defects may be combined with sternal, dental, facial and renal anomalies. Weyers[37] used the term "oligodactyly syndrome" for deficiencies of the ulna and other postaxial structures. The radius can be well developed but form a synostosis with the humerus. Only the thumb and the index finger may be present or there is monodactyly. Sometimes postaxial foot anomaly is very mild and consists in shortening of the fifth metatarsal bone, which results in positioning of the low-set fifth over the fourth toe, an anomaly termed "digitus quintus superductus."[37]

Isolated ulnar aplasia was not observed by Weicker[2] among 100 children damaged by thalidomide, but in combination with other osseous defects of the upper extremity the ulna was reduced in size, deformed or absent in 85. It was normal in more than 10% of children who had defects of the upper arm and the hand.

Ulnar Duplication (Ulnar Dimelia)

In ulnar duplication, the forearm contains two ulnar and no radial bones. The ulnae may be of equal size and symmetric. The duplication extends to the carpals, metacarpals and digits. There may be seven or eight fingers. The thumb is always missing and there may be one or two index fingers located near the axis of the extremity. There are two third, fourth and fifth digits symmetrically arranged on both sides of the axis: V, IV, III, II, (II), III, IV, V. All elements are duplicated except the radius, scaphoid trapezium, metacarpal I and digit I.[29] Pintilie *et al.*[38] reviewed the published cases and described a girl with ulnar duplication and eight fingers. They believed that the humerus, scapula and clavicle frequently are abnormal and that the entire arm is deformed in patients with ulnar duplication. Reconstruction of a finger to serve as a thumb is difficult, since not only the radius but its muscles and the thenar muscles are absent. Buettner[39] reported duplication of the ulna and polydactyly in a mother and her child. Bilateral duplication of the ulna and fibula with bilateral absence of the radius and tibia was reported by Laurin *et al.*[28] in a boy born to an otherwise normal family. Polydactyly in the hands was concealed by marked syndactyly, but in each foot approximately ten toes could be identified. Sandrow *et al.*[277] recorded the cases of a man and his daughter, both showing ulnar and fibular dimelia as well as nasal clefts.

Duplication of the ulna has been observed in a syndrome of mice that has been attributed to a "disorganization" gene.[40]

Radio-Ulnar Synostosis

Incomplete differentiation of radius and ulna results in synostosis, which is found most often between the proximal ends of the bones.[41] It does not obliterate the elbow joint but interferes with turning of the forearm, which stays in pronation. Distal radioulnar synostosis is rare. The anomaly often goes unnoticed and is discovered accidentally. It is bilateral more often than unilateral and has a predilection for males. Anomalies of radius and thumb sometimes are associated with the synostosis. Dominant inheritance has been reported in many families. Davenport *et al.*[42] wrote a comprehensive review of this subject and described many different types of radio-ulnar synostosis, with consideration of the phylogenesis and ontogenesis of these bones. Radio-ulnar synostosis and aplasia of the thumb have been observed in patients with mandibulofacial dysostosis.[43] Syndromes of chromosomal abnormalities may include radio-ulnar synostosis. A patient with XXXY karyotype[44] and several patients with XXXXY syndrome[45-47] and with XYY constitution[48] had proximal radio-ulnar union. This anomaly was also observed in 10% of the children whose upper extremity was damaged by thalidomide.[2]

Congenital Ankylosis of the Elbow

This anomaly may occur together with other congenital malformations, such as skeletal anomalies of the hand, synostoses of carpals and metacarpals, absence of the ulna or patella and so forth.[49] The elbow ankylosis may involve a humero-radial, humero-radio-ulnar or a humero-ulnar synostosis. If associated with other malformations, the ankylosis can be unilateral or bilateral. Patients who have congenital ankylosis of the elbow as an isolated anomaly usually show bilateral involvement.[50] Congenital bilateral ankylosis of both elbow joints can be a dominant hereditary trait.[51] Failure of proper formation of the elbow joint in an early mesenchymal stage of development results in connected cell masses—mesenchymal, cartilaginous and, later, osseous. It is understandable that at birth the elbow joint, although fixed at an angle of 90–100 degrees, appears in roentgenograms as a translucent zone between the ankylosed bones but the apparent joint space actually is made up of cartilage, which ossifies within a few months after birth[50] and reveals the existence of a humero-radial bone. Humero-ulnar ankylosis usually occurs in persons who have absence of the radius. Bony ankylosis of the elbow was present in a case of "clover leaf head."[52] Ankylosis of the elbow can be a part of a generalized articular dysplasia (p. 984), which manifests itself in failure of multiple joint formation, such as interphalangeal, intercarpal and intertarsal "fusions." Dominant inheritance of this condition has been reported repeatedly.[53,54]

Both sexes are affected equally by ankylosis of the elbow. Familial occurrence has been observed. In the case described by Card and Strachman,[50] the parents of the patient were first cousins. Humero-radial bones were produced experimentally by Warkany and Schraffenberger[27] in the young of rats x-irradiated on the thirteenth day of gestation (Fig. 4-4). In the newborn rat, a continuous cartilaginous connection between the humerus and the radius is formed (Fig. 4-4).

Hereditary impairment of pronation and supination can be due to flattening of the radial head[55] or to posterior dislocation of the radial head.[56] The latter condition can result also in limitation of flexion and extension.[57] These minor anomalies are of interest because they can be transmitted through several generations.

Contractures of the elbows, short ulna and radius, bilateral corneal opacities, rotational nystagmus, strabismus and mental retardation were anomalies seen in 4 of 6 children of consanguineous parents.[58]

The Hand

The hand, a distal part of the appendicular skeleton, expendable in prenatal life and unnecessary for locomotion, became—together with the human mind—the most important instrument that made man the ruler of the earth. The pentadactylous hands are a continuation of the five-toed paws that were present in early amphibians. The primate hands were improved by their grasping ability, which became essential during life in the trees. The combination of the human brain and hand created the tools and machines that enable man to fly and live under water, to see better and hear better than any animal and to protect him from attacks by other inhabitants of the earth. This combination has achieved an evolutionary step never achieved by any terrestrial organism before without committing man's body to "experimental adaptations in a blind genetic gamble for survival."[59] The hand is used from early infancy to death in functions too numerous to contemplate. Only those who have lost a hand or were born without one can fully appreciate its value. About 1 child in 65,000 is born without a hand,[5] but many more are born with serious deformities of the upper extremity and with impairment of many functions characteristic of human behavior. It is for this reason that numerous studies have been made of congenital malformations of the hand and innumerable efforts aimed at rehabilitation and replacement of hand anomalies.

In 1937, Müller[60] published a monograph on congenital malformations of the human hand. The morphologic deviations from the norm were discussed in great detail in that work and one can find there exact descriptions of abnormalities of the fingers, metacarpals and carpal structures. One section dealt with numerical variations in the number of rays and another section with disturbances of longitudinal differentiation of finger rays. These skeletal anomalies were distinguished from disturbances of the primitive hand plate, which were said to lead to errors in "transverse direction" in syndactylies, ectrodactylies, cleft hand, partial gigantism, and so on. A third section dealt with disturbances of later phases of development and growth and with anomalies that manifest themselves in hands that had originally undergone normal skeletal and soft tissue differentiation. Familial hyperostoses, arachnodactyly, chondrodystrophies, multiple exostoses and other general skeletal disorders affecting the hand were discussed in this group. Hypoplasia of the entire hand occurs in various syndromes, such as Poland syndrome[141,142] or "hand-foot-uterus syndrome."[285] The reader can find in Müller's book most valuable morphologic descriptions of deformities of the hand and many references to case reports in the older literature. Subsequent publications by Werthemann[61] and Gruber[62] devoted much space to changes in the hand in monographs dealing with developmental errors of the extremities. O'Rahilly[29,63] discussed morphologic patterns in limb deficiencies and duplications and surveyed carpal and tarsal anomalies in a special publication. Many hand defects are included in Grebe's[14] monograph on malformations of the extremities. Barsky[64] devoted a book to congenital malformations of the hand and their surgical treatment. This work adds to previous publications the surgical point of view, as remarks concerning treatment and the bibliography refer to plastic surgery and repair of the errors of development. Principles of treatment of congenital anomalies of the hand were also discussed by Kelikian and Doumanian,[65] who pointed out that cosmetic appearance is important, though less important than utility. The hand serves perception by gathering information on the size and shape of objects, their temperature and their position and it reacts to the information by motor actions. Children with congenital malformations of the hand differ from adults who have lost portions of their hand in that they attempt to develop with their remaining parts the same skills and functions shown by their playmates.[66] Surgical treatment depends on the mental abilities of the patient, the condition of the forearm, arm and shoulder and of the musculature. To obtain best function, reconstructive surgery is done as early as feasible—during the preschool age if possible. For details of surgical treatment, the reader is referred to original publications.[64-67]

Split Hands and Split Feet (Lobster Claws; "True Ectrodactyly")

These rather serious deformities represent a type of ectrodactyly that can occur in otherwise entirely normal persons and families. It must be kept in mind that the term "ectrodactyly" is a more comprehensive one than that of split hands and split feet, since not all congenital finger defects conform morphologically and etiologically to the clefts discussed in this section. However, since Geoffroy Saint-Hilaire[68] introduced the term "ectrodactyly" in 1832, it has been used and is being used[69,70] synonymously for split hands and split feet. The terminology is further confused by other authors, who used terms such as "oligodactyly," "perodactyly," "hypodactyly" and "lobster claw" for the same type of malformation. It is possible that the first report on hereditary cleft hand is that by Hartsinck,[71] who described Touvingas or two-fingered Negroes with hands and feet like crayfish claws. An illustration reproduced by Barsky[72] suggests that this tribe had true split hands and split feet. A case published by Martens in 1804[72] was atypical and associated with cleft lip and palate. In 1829, Béchet[73] reported a split-hand family that later was cited by Geoffroy Saint-Hilaire.[68] Many other familial cases have been described since. Dominant Mendelian inheritance was first recognized by Pearson[74] in 1908 but, later, McMullan and Pearson[75] noticed that in their pedigree considerably more than half of the offspring were affected. Since then, many writers have contributed pedigrees demonstrating dominant inheritance.[14,72] Irregularities have been noticed in some of these families, so that Hanhart[76] emphasized irregular dominance, since skipping occurs in one or more generations. Recessive inheritance has been suggested in certain cases, and Popenoe[77] believed that these cleft formations can be transmitted in different modes in different families. Since publications of families with multiple cases usually are selected because of the interest in recurrence of the anomaly, the report by Birch-Jensen[5] on 36 unselected propositi is of great value. These cases represent the patients found in Denmark, where the prevalence of split hands was estimated as 1 per 112,000 in the population and the incidence at birth as 1 per 90,000. The decrease in the number of patients after the early years of life can be attributed to early death of some children who are born with lobster claws in addition to other severe malformations. The limb deformity has been described combined with cyclopia[61] and with congenital heart disease, imperforate anus and hydronephrosis.[78] It is doubtful that such cases of severe and multiple malformations are related to the typical form of lobster claw. "Atypical split hand," which in Denmark has a prevalence of 1 per 200,000, also seems to differ etiologically from the classic type. In the material of Birch-Jensen,[5] there were 21 sporadic and 15 familial cases of typical split hand; but all cases of atypical split hand, which is characterized by unilateral involvement and by irregularities of the digits bordering the cleft, were sporadic without any manifestation in other members of their kinship. Thus, there is justification in Birch-Jensen's distinction of the two types, since the typical and atypical forms differ not only morphologically but also etiologically. Although the majority of propositi with typical split hand were sporadic, the genetic prognosis for their offspring should be guarded, since a sporadic case may represent a new mutation capable of transmission. Even in families with clearly dominant inheritance, the genetic prognosis for the unaffected is made difficult by the possibility of skipping of a generation, which is rare in classic pedigrees[69] but does occur occasionally.[79]

It is of interest that several pedigrees are known in which normal parents had more than 1 affected child who transmitted the trait to some of their offspring,[5,69] so that the new mutation manifested itself in the same generation in several siblings. In one of these cases,[69] a man who had no developmental abnormality by inspection and radiography married twice and had abnormal offspring in both marriages. In another instance,[5] normal parents had 12 children and 6 of these had lobster claws. Four of the affected patients transmitted the condition to their offspring. These observations suggest gonadal mosaicism in one of the parents, resulting in numerous germ cells affected by the mutation. Thus, normality of the parents does not rule out the possibility of recurrence of the deformity in their children.

In 1951, Mackenzie and Penrose[69] published two pedigrees of split hand and split foot with regular transmission in six generations, without skipping but with marked variability of expression. Males and females were affected equally. Of 100 children resulting from matings between one affected and one unaffected parent, 55 manifested the anomaly. Khosrovani[79] confirmed dominant inheritance by recording a pedigree in which 25 members (13 males and 12 females) were affected. In this family, the anomaly was seen most often in the feet. In several pedigrees there was an excess of affected males over females.[80] Stevenson and Jennings[70] re-examined the family first recorded by McMullan and Pearson,[75] in which more than half of the offspring had been affected. They believed that the departure from the expected 1:1 ratio of affected to unaffected could be explained by an excess of affected sons born to affected fathers. This, in turn, was explained by disturbed segregation in the offspring of affected males. It was thought that the sperms at relative advantage in effecting fertilization were those that carried the abnormal gene on an autosome and also carried a Y chromosome. In some families, very irregular dominance has been observed.[76] Concordance and discordance in regard to split hand have been reported in monozygotic twins.[81]

The *typical* split hand (or split foot) is characterized by congenital absence of one or several median digits or rays in the presence of normal rays bordering the cleft. In *atypical* split hand, the remaining rays are also affected by various reduction anomalies. In the typical form, the median portions of the primordial hand or foot plate fail to form the correct mesenchymal condensations that precede chondrification and ossification. A triangular cleft, which narrows proximally, divides the hand or foot into two parts that oppose each other like lobster claws. According to the number of missing rays, various degrees of severity can be distinguished. If the third digit is absent, the third metacarpal bone may be fully developed or be reduced. Rarely, the fourth ray alone is absent. In more severe cases, the second and third rays are affected. Remaining digits on the same side of the cleft can be partially or totally united in syndactyly. The irregular ossification sometimes manifests itself in formation of a cross-bone, which can be interpreted as a proximal phalanx in malposition. In roentgenograms, it usually is seen between the central metacarpals, but many variations are possible, since the cross-bone can be separated from the metacarpals by a joint space or be continuous with one of them; it also varies in length and in position.

In atypical split hand, absence of some of the central rays is combined with reduction of the remaining rays.[5] As a rule, rays II–IV are not developed and rays I and V are reduced, not by amputation but by hypoplasia or aplasia of their middle or proximal phalanx. The extent of the cleft is variable; sometimes the gap is bridged in its proximal portion by a skin fold.

Typical split hands and split feet often occur in the same patient but, according to the Danish study,[5] only half of the patients with the hand deformity also have split foot. Only a few hand deformities were observed in the family described by Khosrovani[79] in which split foot was inherited. Syndactyly is frequent in split hands, with digits I and II and digits IV and V united. Polydactyly is rarer; if it occurs, it usually affects the first digit. The same digit is involved in case of hyperphalangia. Hallux valgus is not rare.[5] Other malformations are not increased in patients with true split hands. Cleft lip and palate have been mentioned repeatedly,[72,80,274] but it is not clear whether typ-

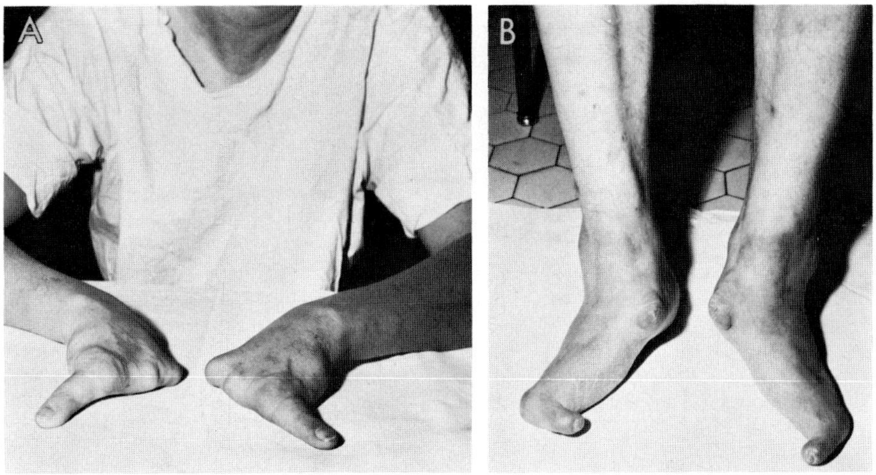

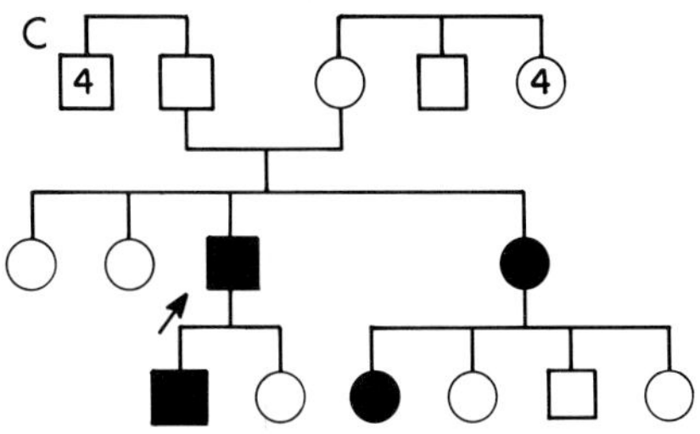

Fig. 101-1.—**A** and **B**, perodactyly (ectrodactyly) in hands and feet of a man whose sister, son and niece had similar malformations. **C,** pedigree of the family. It is possible that in the first generation one of the parents of the patients had gonadal mosaicism (p. 370).

ical or atypical split hands were present.[181] A syndrome of lobster claw deformity and nasolacrimal obstruction[274] has been reported as a dominant autosomal trait.[286] Perceptive deafness in 2 brothers with split hand and split foot was recorded by Wildervanck.[82] Lobster claw has been reported in patients with de Lange syndrome.[83] In lethal or semilethal cases, the clefts of hands and feet are part of a syndrome of multiple malformations (p. 645). Because of the possibility of serious associated malformations, the prognosis for patients with split hand should be guarded in the first years of life when some of them succumb, but after this the prognosis for life is good.[5]

There are many reports that give testimony to the ability of affected persons in acquiring great manual (or pedal) skills with their deformed extremities. Stevenson and Jennings[70] stated that affected and unaffected members of their pedigree showed similar abilities, most doing semi-skilled or unskilled work. All patients were employed, some as mechanics, drivers or packers. Several were outstanding writers and draftsmen. They had problems in obtaining suitable shoes.

In the treatment of split hand, function and usefulness are most essential. "Cosmetic appearance is important, but not as important as utility."[65] Surgical treatment of typical cleft hand was described by Barsky.[72] Atypical forms require various operations or may need no operation at all if adequate function can be obtained by exercise and use. Correction of split foot has been undertaken[84] in order to enlarge the surface of support of the lower extremity but, in many cases, function is satisfactory and surgery can be avoided.

Brachydactyly

Under brachydactyly one understands an abnormal shortness of the fingers and toes. Many types of brachydactyly have been observed and recorded. As a rule, the shortness is due to defects of the phalanges, but sometimes the metacarpal or metatarsal bones are chiefly affected. In the first case, one speaks of brachyphalangy, in the second case of brachymetacarpy or brachymetapody. Brachyphalangy can be subdivided into brachytelephalangy, which is a shortness of the distal phalanx, brachymesophalangy, a shortness of the middle phalanx, and brachybasophalangy, a shortness of the basal phalanx. There may be complete or incomplete absence of a phalanx (hypophalangy) or abnormal segmentation of the phalanges; phalangeal oversegmentation or ankylosis of the interphalangeal joints may contribute to the variability of the anomaly. As a rule, the fingers and toes are both affected and both sides of the body are involved. This is particularly true of the hereditary forms. Brachydactyly may occur as an isolated anomaly or it may be associated with a variety of other congenital malformations and thus be one of the anomalies in a syndrome. The brachydactylies vary

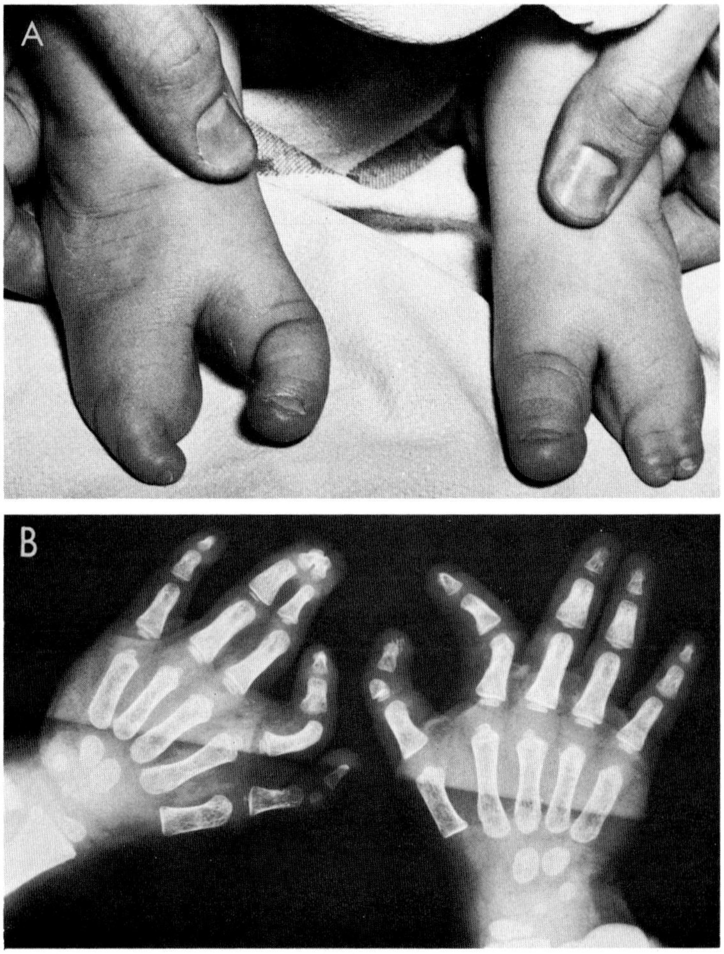

Fig. 101-2. – **A,** "lobster claw" of lower extremity in a boy whose mother, maternal aunt and grandfather had the same anomaly. **B,** hands of the same child, showing syndactyly of digits III and IV on the left and deformities of the index fingers.

greatly in morphology, pathogenesis and etiology. Several extensive reviews have been made of this subject.[14,61,85-88]

Although brachydactyly is not a very frequent anomaly, many cases have been reported. In 1905, Farabee[89] recorded the history of a family in Pennsylvania in which this condition was inherited as a simple dominant trait. This was the first case of Mendelian inheritance demonstrated and recognized as such in man, and many other cases of brachydactyly inherited in a similar fashion have been observed since.[85] As a rule, affected members marry normal persons and approximately half of the offspring show the same anomaly as the affected parent. Pedigrees are known in which the condition is transmitted as an irregular dominant trait. In some pedigrees, brachydactyly is transmitted with surprising uniformity, in others its expression is so variable that one can speak only of inherited irregularities of digital development.[90] Such intrafamilial variability shows that morphologic classifications do not always conform to etiologic entities. Sporadic brachydactyly occurs and it is likely that not all cases are genetically determined. In teratologic experiments, brachydactyly, syndactyly and other finger deformities can be obtained.[27] Brachydactyly can be combined with syndactyly and polydactyly and it can be due to true amputation or symphalangy. The resulting pictures are not easily distinguishable.

Many classifications of brachydactyly have been proposed[61,85,88] but no unitary concept has been developed. Anatomists, roentgenologists, geneticists and surgeons look at the anomalies with different interests. It is not possible to enumerate here all the types that have been recorded, but some of the important groups, their biologic meaning and their role in syndromes will be mentioned.

The hereditary form described by Farabee[89] and Drinkwater[91] represents the more severe type (brachyhypophalangy, major brachydactyly). There are only two phalanges in digits II–V and the proximal phalanx of the thumb is short. The fingers as well as the toes are affected and the metacarpal bones sometimes are reduced in length. Affected persons are of short stature; their hands are broad and short and the palmar skin creases are abnormal. Persons with major brachydactyly cannot play the piano well but may be skillful in many other occupations. The condition is transmitted as a dominant trait in many kindreds.[85]

A milder form, minor brachydactyly, is characterized by short middle phalanges. In roentgenograms, three phalanges can be recognized and there is a joint space between the small middle and the normal terminal phalanx. For details and classification, the reader is referred to Cocchi[88] and Bell.[85] A family belonging in this group[92] is of unusual interest because two consanguineous persons with a mild brachymesodactyly married and produced 8 children, of whom 2 were normal and 1 died young. The parents were second cousins and were of short stature. Two children resembled the parents, having a mild brachydactyly and short stature, but the remaining 3 showed a generalized skeletal defect resembling Morquio disease. It is reasonable to assume that these severely affected children represent the homozygous type of the defect manifested in the parents in its mild and heterozygous form. Absence of middle phalanges, duplicated terminal phalanges of the thumbs—combined with a nail dysplasia transmitted through four generations—was reported by Bass.[93]

Brachytelemesophalangy (apical dystrophy; perodactyly) is a very severe form of brachydactyly. It is characterized by the absence of the entire distal phalanx and nail from each digit of the hands and feet excepting the thumbs and big toes. The middle phalanges of the affected digits may also be absent or very small. The thumbs usually are normal or they are broad and have a bifid terminal phalanx carrying two nails or a single broad nail. Degenhardt and Geipel[94] described a pedigree in which perodactyly was transmitted through four generations. In some of the members there was a tendency to reduplication of the thumbs. But perodactyly can also result from secondary amputation of fingers and sometimes be associated with amniotic constrictions and bands (p. 944).

The carpal and metacarpal bones can be normal in cases of apical dysplasia. The toes are, as a rule, less severely affected than the fingers. In a family reported by Brailsford,[95] a very mild form of brachytelephalangy was associated with bilateral "coxitis" in all the affected members. The condition is transmitted as a dominant trait in some families, with many variations of the anomaly in different members.

Brachydactyly may be limited to a single digit of the hand or foot. Brachydactyly of the first digit (*short thumb, clubbed thumb*) usually occurs in otherwise normal hands and can be limited to one side. It is due to an anomaly of the terminal phalanx, which is short and broad and has a broad shallow nail. The big toes may show the same anomaly but this is not always the case. This brachytelephalangy can be an irregular dominant trait with intrafamilial and interfamilial variation. The short thumb is a cosmetic defect but does not otherwise inconvenience the affected person, except that sewing may be difficult.[86]

Brachydactyly of the second digit is a rare anomaly, but several pedigrees are available in which the inheritance was dominant. Mohr and Wriedt[96] reported a family of this type. The anomaly, which is not incapacitating, was transmitted in the heterozygous form as a dominant trait through six generations. One affected woman married her first cousin, who also had a short index finger. They had 2 daughters; one was normal except for a short index finger and the other was a cripple, with many skeletal anomalies. Her fingers and toes were entirely absent and it was thought that she represented the trait in the homozygous form.

Clinodactyly or incurved little finger is due to a shortening of the middle phalanx of the fifth finger, particularly on its radial side. This anomaly leads to radial deflection of the terminal phalanx. Hersh *et al.*[97] discussed the hereditary forms of clinodactyly and concluded from pedigrees available that the trait depends on an autosomal dominant gene. They divided the hereditary forms into three groups: incomplete ossification, short tendon and fused ossification. Clinodactyly occurred in some members of a kinship described by Vidal,[98] in which hyperphalangy, brachydactyly and other digital anomalies were transmitted by a dominant gene. Hereditary clinodactyly associated with tylosis (tendency to callus formation of the skin) and a tendency to esophageal cancer has been described as a syndrome. A family with tylosis and clinodactyly was investigated by Klintworth and Anderson.[99] Tylosis was transmitted through an autosomal dominant gene with high penetrance, whereas the penetrance of the gene for clinodactyly was low. Myositis ossificans progressiva often is associated with clinodactyly.[88] Clinodactyly without brachymesophalangy is said to occur in approximately 5% of the population, but among schoolchildren even higher prevalence figures have been reported.[92,100] Marked incurving of the little fingers can be due to symmetric bowing of the *terminal* phalanges. This condition, which has been termed "Kirner deformity," can be transmitted as a dominant trait. The curving of the fifth fingers is not congenital but develops during childhood.[101]

Brachydactyly with hyperphalangy (Leboucq type[102]) can be considered a paradoxic brachydactyly, since some of the shortened fingers actually have an excess of phalanges. In a well-developed case, the hand is externally characterized by shortness of the index and middle fingers, elongation of the ring finger and incurving of the little finger. Roentgenograms reveal four instead of the normal three phalanges in the middle and sometimes in the index finger (polyphalangism), shortening of the middle phalanges, elongation of the basal phalanx of the ring finger and clinodactyly of digit V. This anomaly often is combined with muscular hypotonia and overexten-

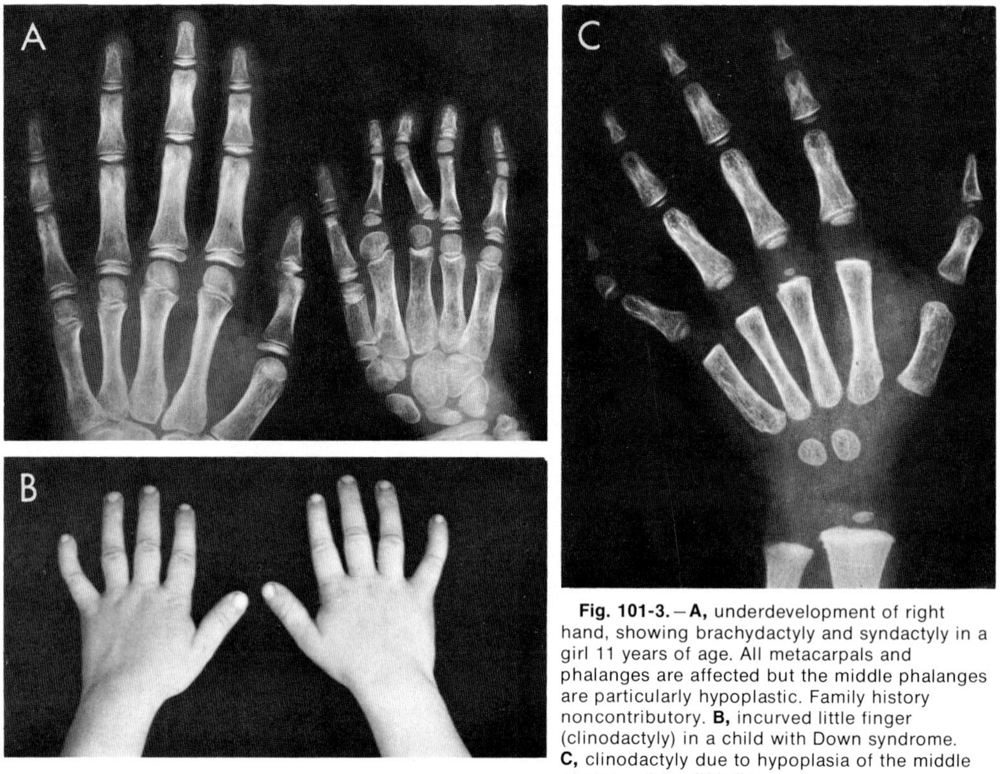

Fig. 101-3. – **A,** underdevelopment of right hand, showing brachydactyly and syndactyly in a girl 11 years of age. All metacarpals and phalanges are affected but the middle phalanges are particularly hypoplastic. Family history noncontributory. **B,** incurved little finger (clinodactyly) in a child with Down syndrome. **C,** clinodactyly due to hypoplasia of the middle phalanx of the fifth finger.

sibility of the joints. Associated malformations such as clubfoot and double-lobed ear have been observed and mental retardation occurs in some of the patients. The supernumerary joint space between the third and fourth phalanges can be mistaken for a fracture line. A hand of this type can be used skillfully for complicated manipulations, but surgical shortening of the elongated ring finger can be done for cosmetic reasons.[103] A different type of hyperphalangy is due to faulty segmentation of several digits. Hyperphalangy and hypophalangy may be combined in such cases. In a foot of this type, the middle and distal phalanges were reported to be absent in the second and third digits, whereas in the fourth and fifth digits four phalanges could be seen. Later, the middle two phalanges in each of the fourth and fifth digits may fuse, so that the number of digits appears normal.[104]

Brachymetacarpy or brachymetapody may be due to shortness of the metacarpal or metatarsal bones. They can be limited to one metacarpal or metatarsal or involve several of these bones in the same hand or foot. They may be bilateral or unilateral. Absence of the first metacarpal in the presence of an unstable but otherwise well-formed thumb represents a problem of plastic surgery.[66] If this anomaly occurs as a dominant hereditary trait, one finds great intrafamilial variation. Sporadic occurrence is more frequent. Short metacarpals may be found along with brachyphalangy of the same or of other rays. They are also associated with certain forms of general developmental retardation, as seen in pseudohypoparathyroidism and related conditions.

Brachydactyly in rabbits has been described by Greene and Saxton.[105] This recessive trait was characterized by secondary destruction of digits, leading to perodactyly and brachydactyly. Brachypodism has been described as a recessive trait in a strain of mice.[106] Warkany and Nelson[107] produced brachydactyly combined with syndactyly experimentally in rats by maternal riboflavin deficiency. In that condition, the anomaly could be traced back to the mesenchymal stage, when the individual digits are differentiated. It is thought that the deficiency interferes with the rapid divisions that take place in mesenchymal cells before they are converted into cartilage or bone. Similar anomalies have been produced since by many teratogenic agents, particularly x-rays.

Brachydactyly occurs in many forms of dwarfism as an expression of general growth retardation. Achondroplasia and various atypical chondrodystrophies exemplify this point. A severe form of symbrachydactyly usually is seen in acrocephalosyndactyly. In the Poland, Laurence-Moon-Biedl and Carpenter syndromes, symbrachydactyly is common (p. 901). Short stature, spherophakia and brachydactyly have been named Marchesani syndrome (p. 395). A skeletal disorder limited to the hands and feet has been described by Sorsby[108] in association with macular dysplasia. There was a tendency to bifurcation of the terminal phalanx of the thumb and of the big toe. There was reduction of the middle phalanx of the little finger and of the terminal phalanges of all digits. The nails of the index finger of each hand and of the big toe of each foot were rudimentary. Brachydactyly, peculiar facies and mental retardation were described as a syndrome by Coffin.[109] This syndrome blends into that of Rubinstein and Taybi[110] as well as into mandibulofacial dysostosis (p. 650). Fuhrmann *et al.*[53] reported a pedigree showing dominantly inherited hypoplasia and aplasia of several phalanges of fingers and toes, hypoplasia and aplasia of interphalangeal joints, synostoses of carpal and tarsal bones and dysplasia of the cubital joints. The anomalies were observed through three generations. The findings were supplemented by dermatoglyphic studies. The otopalatodigital syndrome[111,112] (p. 677) includes brachydactyly and clinodactyly due to shortening of distal and middle phalanges. Shortness of the middle phalanx combined with anomalies of the spine have been described by Pippow.[113] Combination of brachydactyly with "coxitis" has been noted by Brailsford.[95] Dominantly inherited brachydactyly due to disturbance of ossification of the middle phalanges combined with hip disease was reported by Robinson *et al.*[114] Brachydactyly in patients with stenosis of the aorta and pulmonary artery was recorded by Cascos.[115] A syndrome of pear-shaped nose, thin hair and brachydactyly due to epiphyseal disturbances (tricho-rhino-phalangeal syndrome) was described by Giedion.[116] Congenital brachydactyly of the thumbs and great toes is an early manifestation of myositis ossificans.[88] The thumb, the big toe and the little finger usually are affected in this condition, but all fingers may be shortened (p. 976). Keizer[117] recorded a family with hereditary shortness of the thumb and endocrine disorders.

Fig. 101-4. – Bilateral brachymetacarpy in a girl 19 years of age with retarded growth and sex development but no signs of hypoparathyroidism. Note shortness of fourth and fifth metacarpal bones and terminal phalanges of thumbs.

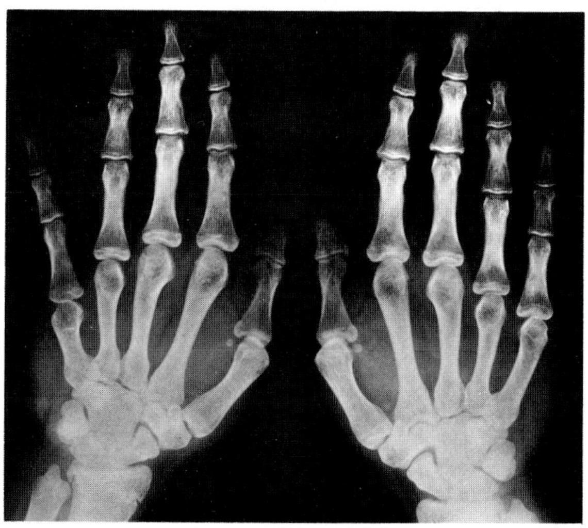

Clinodactyly occurs in more than half of the patients with Down syndrome. There seems to be a positive correlation between mental retardation and marked clinodactyly.[118] Incurved little finger is seen regularly in children with the de Lange (p. 344), Russell and Silver syndromes, which are associated with intrauterine growth retardation (p. 134). It occurs with glossopalatine ankylosis, focal dermal hypoplasia, orodigitofacial[119] and many other syndromes.

Brachymetacarpy typically is found combined with pseudohypoparathyroidism (p. 447). Roentgenograms show shortness of the metacarpal bones with the exception of those of the index finger. There may be metaphyseal spurs, calcifications in soft tissues and stubby distal phalanges. Similar bone changes occur in patients with pseudo-pseudohypoparathyroidism (p. 448). An unusual case of brachyphalangy and brachymetacarpy was recorded by Arkless and Graham,[120] who gave a good discussion of the confusing roentgen pictures of this subject. In Turner syndrome (p. 1128), the fourth metacarpals are short; they do not reach a line drawn between the distal ends of the third and fifth metacarpals.[121] Similar anomalies may be seen in patients with other types of gonadal anomalies.[122]

Symphalangy

The characteristic anomaly of symphalangy is the complete continuity of the middle with the proximal phalanx and immobility of the proximal interphalangeal joint. This anomaly usually is pronounced in the ring and little fingers, whereas in the index and middle fingers the two proximal phalanges may be separated by an incomplete joint space. The distal phalanges and the distal interphalangeal joints are free in all the fingers. The thumb and the big toe are not involved. As a rule, the changes in the toes correspond to those in the fingers but variations are found. Sometimes the middle phalanx of the anomalous fingers is very short. The ends of the fused bones are enlarged at the site of the ankylosis and the fingers appear swollen in this area. The skin creases and folds are normal over the movable joints but absent over the ankylotic joints. All the fingers are movable at the metacarpophalangeal joints; yet, affected persons cannot be made to touch the palm. The affected digits may be shortened.

In 1916, Cushing[123] recorded a pedigree in which symphalangy could be traced through seven generations. The pedigree was brought up to date in 1965 by Strasburger *et al.*,[124] who tabulated ten generations with 684 individuals, of whom 351 were affected. It evolved that anomalies of the ankles and feet caused the affected members more inconvenience than the "stiff fingers" of their hands. Union of the talus and navicular bones was the basis of the foot anomalies but the calcaneus, cuboid and other bones were incompletely separated also. Deafness due to bony union of stapes and the petrous part of the temporal bone appeared in some of the affected persons in the early years of life. The statement made in previous publications that "stiff fingers" are the only trouble of these persons is incorrect; symphalangy in this and other families seems to be a manifestation of a general inability to form all the joints of the body, an articular dysplasia that can be attributed to an autosomal dominant gene. But not all cases of symphalangy can be attributed to the same gene[125] and to the same pathogenesis. In a pedigree from south India, symphalangy was associated with polydactyly and syndactyly.[90] A man with symphalangy was described by Drinkwater[126] in 1917. This man was a direct descendant in the male line from John Talbot, the first Earl of Shrewsbury, who was killed at the battle of Castillon near Bordeaux in the year 1453. His body was brought home and buried at Whitchurch. It was said that when, in 1874, his tomb was repaired and the skeleton removed, the finger bones were found to have ankylosis like those of his descendant and it seemed that symphalangy was inherited in this family through 500 years and fourteen generations.[86] *Se non è vero è ben trovato.* As Fraser Roberts[127] put it: "The chill winds of the higher criticism have recently been blowing around some of the respected and picturesque tales of human genetics" and they brought down some of the leaves so dear to the early geneticists. It seems to be true that in the Talbot family symphalangy is a dominantly inherited trait, but Elkington and Huntsman[128] pointed out that there is little proof that the John Talbot who lived in the fifteenth century had the anomaly. Symphalangy strabismus and hearing loss were described in a mother and daughter.[129] In other pedigrees, hypoplasia and aplasia of digital phalanges and of interphalangeal joints, synostoses of carpal and tarsal bones and dysplasia of cubital joints were transmitted through three generations.[53] Faulty differentiation of cervical vertebrae (Klippel-Feil syndrome) may be included in these syndromes of articular dysplasia, which can be transmitted as dominant traits.[54]

The morphogenesis of symphalangy has been much discussed. If one considers this anomaly as a manifestation of articular dysplasia, one will conceive of it as a failure of joint formation in mesenchymal skeletal primordia during the first 2 embryonic months. As differentiation of the skeleton progresses, the undeveloped joint areas remain fibrous or cartilaginous, i.e., radiolucent, in roentgenograms of young children. In later years, the cartilaginous areas ossify and unite the phalangeal ossification centers. To the roentgenologist, the union will appear as a secondary, postnatal fusion; in reality, failure of joint formation began in early embryonic life.

Dominant inheritance of articular dysplasias including symphalangy is a striking and well-documented phenomenon. It is very likely that some cases of symphalangy have a different etiology. Failure of separation of skeletal elements can be seen in children damaged by thalidomide and failure of joint formation can be observed in teratologic experiments.

Classic symphalangy seems to be rarer than failure of joint formation combined with various digital anomalies. Barsky[64] did not encounter isolated symphalangy among his patients but he saw the anomaly in complicated forms of syndactyly. He pointed out that arthroplasty is not too successful at the middle or distal interphalangeal joint, although it is satisfactory at the metacarpophalangeal joint.

Symbrachydactyly

This malformation of the hand occurred in about 1 per 50,000 of the (Danish) population investigated by Birch-Jensen.[5] It consists of lack of separation and of shortening of fingers. There exist many forms and grades of the anomaly. Hypoplasia affects the central rays more often than the ulnar and radial rays. In mild forms, there may be absence of the middle phalanges and underdevelopment of the distal phalanges of one or more of the central rays. The metacarpals are retained but some reduction can be seen in roentgenograms. Finally, the only remaining digit may be represented by the thumb or all fingers may be reduced to rudiments.[5] Nails usually are well de-

Fig. 101-5. — Symbrachydactyly in a boy.

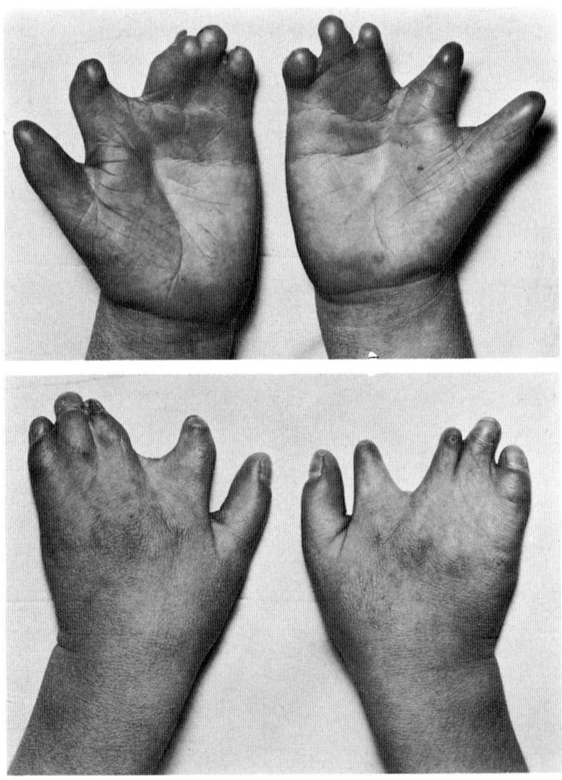

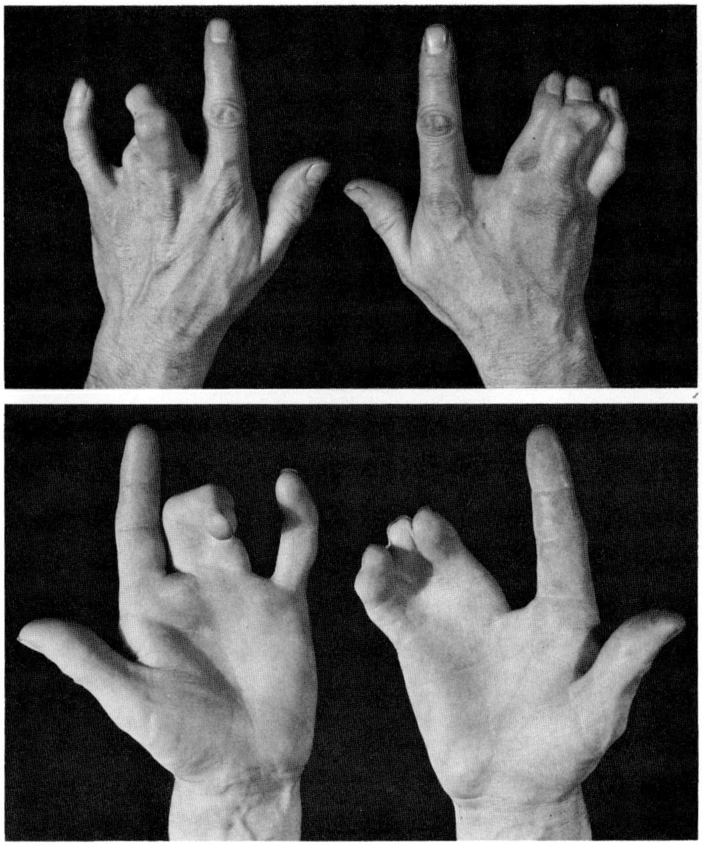

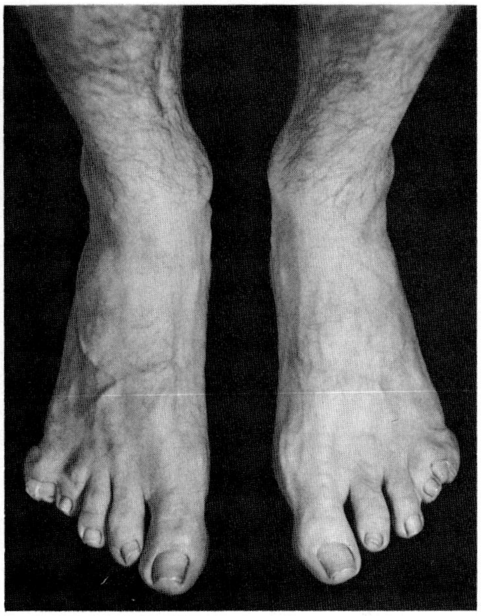

Fig. 101-6.—Symbrachydactyly in a man whose 2 sons had finger deformities of minor degree. One had ulnar polydactyly on the right hand.

veloped. Differentiation from split hand and ectrodactyly sometimes is difficult.

The term "symbrachydactyly" was suggested by Pol[130] and used by Birch-Jensen[5] but other names often are mentioned in the literature. Pol[130] reviewed 33 unilateral cases and more than half of these had defects of the pectoral muscle or chest wall. This suggests that they are related to or identical with Poland syndactyly (p. 973). In the Danish series, the anomaly was bilateral in only 5 of 85 cases; males were affected more often than females. Most cases were sporadic, but in a few families reduction malformations were present in relatives of the propositi, so that inheritance may play a role in some instances. Polydactyly and foot anomalies also occurred in relatives but they may have been coincidental because of their frequency in the population.

Syndactyly

A lack of differentiation between two or more digits is called syndactyly. This condition must be distinguished from symphalangy, which represents a lack of differentiation of two or three phalanges in the proximo-distal direction of a digit. It is customary to speak of fusion of fingers or toes, which would indicate a secondary union of digits. Actually, most cases of syndactyly can be traced back to an early stage of development when the mesenchymal tissue is not differentiated properly into the normal number of digits. The incidence of syndactyly is about 1 in 2,000, with a marked predilection for males.[131] Syndactyly can occur as an isolated defect or in combination with other anomalies of the hand, such as brachydactyly, ectrodactyly, macrodactyly, cleft hand and annular bands. Syndactyly may be cutaneous or osseous, the most common type being a cutaneous connection between digits III and IV.[64] The webbing may be limited to connections between proximal parts of the fingers or involve the entire length of the fingers. If bones, tendons, nerves or nails are joined, the situation is serious from the surgeon's point of view.[64] There are many types and variations, which have been dealt with in monographs.[14,60,134]

Syndactyly is not an etiologic entity but rather a symptom of abnormal differentiation. Dominant inheritance of simple cutaneous syndactyly of digits III and IV was shown in a pedigree published by Schlatter[134] in 1914. It is possible that in that pedigree some of the affected members were homozygous in regard to the anomaly. Yet, the homozygous form did not appear to be more deleterious than the heterozy-

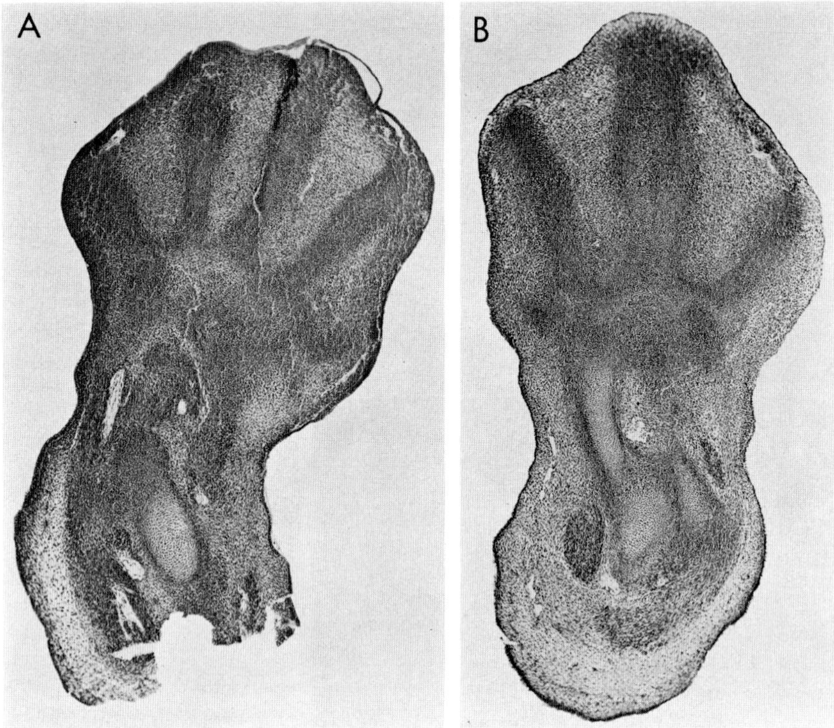

Fig. 101-7. – **A,** forepaw of normal rat embryo, fifteenth day of gestation. **B,** forepaw of rat embryo of mother deficient in riboflavin, fifteenth day of gestation. Syndactyly is clearly recognizable in the precartilaginous state.

gous. Many other pedigrees of dominantly inherited syndactyly have been recorded,[14, 133] including inheritance of more severe syndactylies involving bones and nails.[135] In some kindreds, there is marked intrafamilial variability[136] and in others syndactyly and polydactyly are transmitted.[133] Syndactyly of the ring and little fingers was reported in a pedigree of five generations; it was transmitted as an autosomal dominant trait with incomplete penetrance and variable expression.[137]

The mildest form of syndactyly is *zygodactyly*, a cutaneous webbing between the second and third toes or between the third and fourth fingers. Families have been described in which this mild anomaly is inherited as a dominant trait but sporadic cases are more frequent. This common type of webbing can be found in normal as well as in abnormal children. In an unusual pedigree,[138] webbed toes were recorded in 14 males of four generations; all males of affected sibships had the anomaly but females of affected sibships did not. This pedigree has been interpreted as an example of an abnormal trait located in the Y chromosome, but there exist pedigrees that show zygodactyly in females only and pedigrees in which males and females are affected.[14]

The most severe form of syndactyly, *total syndactyly* or "ladle hand," is rare.[64] In this anomaly, all five digits are joined to a spoon-like structure or the thumb may be separate. This serious condition usually is sporadic and limited to one side. Cenani and Lenz[139] described total syndactyly and distal radioulnar synostosis in 2 brothers; 1 of them also had syndactyly of toes III and IV. Bilateral complete syndactyly with six metacarpals and eight fingernails occurred in a woman and 2 of her children.[140] Total syndactyly with acrocephaly, Apert syndrome or acro-

Fig. 101-8. – Syndactyly of fourth and fifth fingers in a boy whose pedigree contains members with syndactyly through at least five generations. (Cincinnati Children's Hospital Chart No. 162278.)

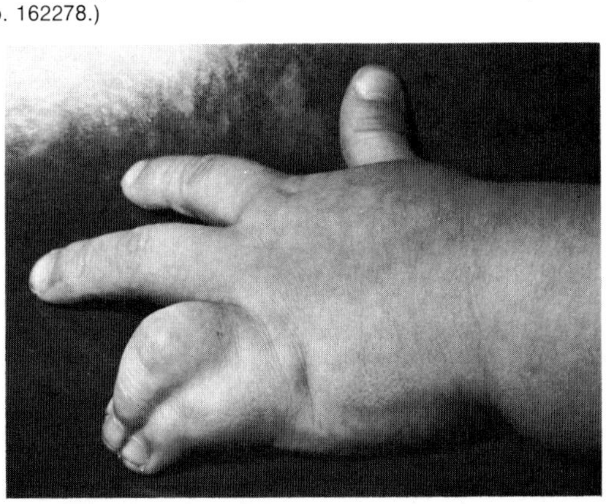

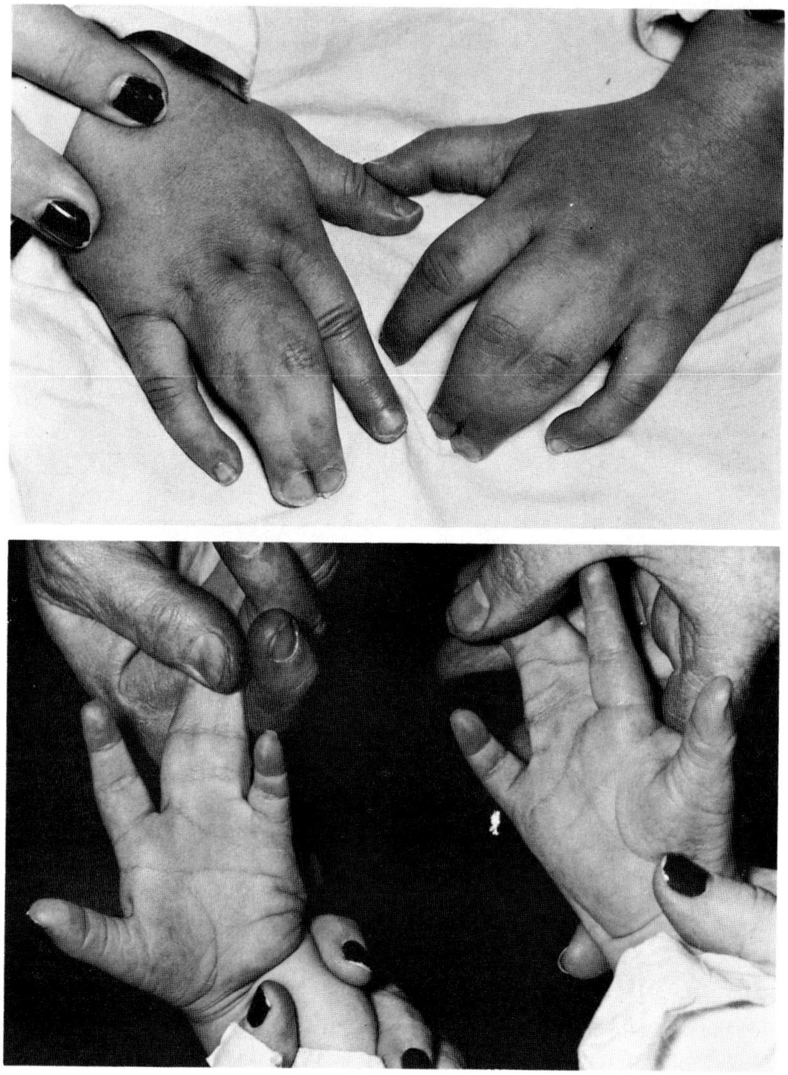

Fig. 101-9.—Bilateral syndactyly of third and fourth fingers in a boy with negative family history.

cephalosyndactyly (p. 899) sometimes is transmitted like a dominant hereditary trait. The hand and Apert syndrome has been described in detail by Hoover *et al.*,[287] who discussed the aspects of surgical treatment.

The heterogeneous etiology of syndactyly is clearly demonstrated by its occurrence in syndromes of differing etiology. In some of these syndromes, syndactyly is an obligatory constituent, in others it participates occasionally.

Poland syndrome, unilateral syndactyly with absence of the sternal head of the pectoralis major muscle of the same side, was named "Poland syndactyly" because the English surgeon Poland described such a case in *Guy's Hospital Reports* of 1841.[141] A review of this condition was published in 1940 by Brown and McDowell.[142] Various and complex forms of syndactyly may be present in such patients and the nipple be absent on the side of the defective muscle.

Syndactyly of the fingers combined with preaxial polydactyly and syndactyly of the toes, acrocephaly, obesity, hypogenitalism and mental retardation has been called Carpenter syndrome (p. 179). Syndactyly sometimes is observed in patients with Laurence-Moon-Biedl syndrome also (p. 178), so that the differentiation from Carpenter syndrome is not always clear-cut. Bilateral syndactyly, polydactyly and adactyly occur together with cutaneous atrophy and linear pigmentation, papillomas of skin and mucous membranes and lip and tooth anomalies in a syndrome

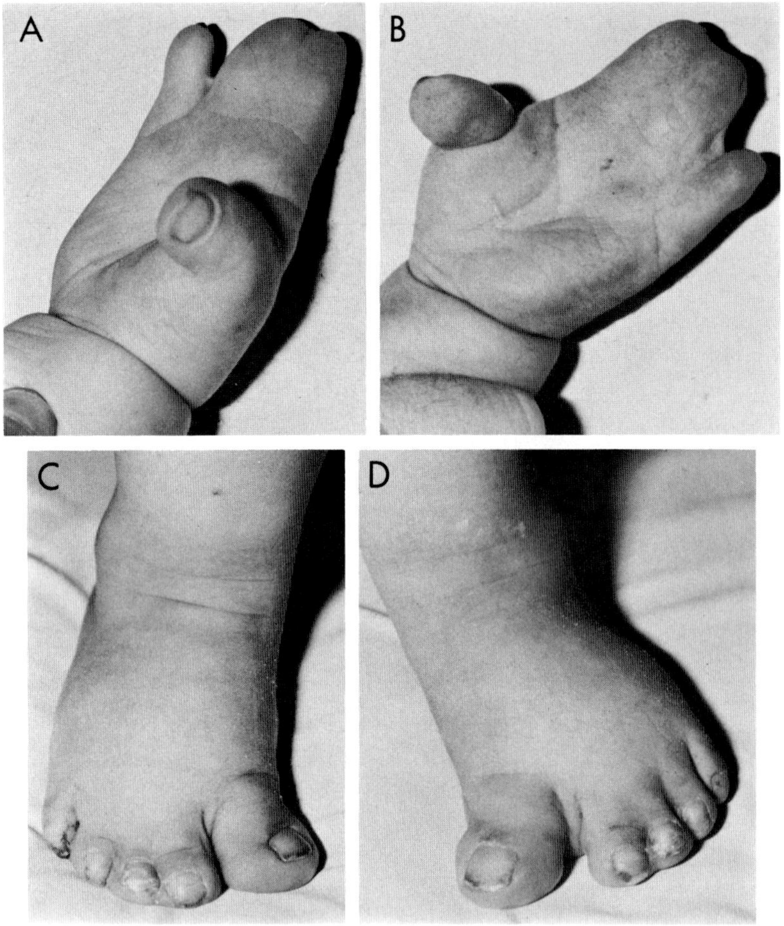

Fig. 101-10. – **A** and **B,** severe forms of syndactyly in a child with acrocephalosyndactyly. Ladle – or spoon – hands. **C** and **D,** syndactyly of toes of the same child is less pronounced.

(Goltz or focal dermal hypoplasia syndrome) that is typically seen in females.[119] Another disease picture limited to females, the orodigitofacial syndrome (p. 674), includes syndactyly and other digital anomalies. In children with intrauterine growth retardation, incomplete separation of digits is not rare. The de Lange (p. 344), Silver (p. 139) and trisomy 18 (p. 303) syndromes frequently include some form of syndactyly. Children with Möbius (p. 397) and with Hallermann-Streiff syndrome (p. 390) have a tendency to syndactyly. Association of aglossia,[143] glossopalatine ankylosis[144] and facial clefts[145,146] with syndactyly has been described. Ectodermal dysplasia and syndactyly[146,147] may be seen in the same patient. Hemihypertrophy (p. 160) and hemifacial hypertrophy[119] sometimes are associated with syndactyly.

Some of the syndromes mentioned are genetically determined; others are of doubtful origin. Exogenous etiologic factors should be considered, since syndactyly can be produced experimentally by unfavorable environmental conditions during the embryonic period. Prenatal riboflavin deficiency, folic acid deficiency, x-ray treatment and others can result in syndactyly.

Adactyly, Oligodactyly, Ectrodactyly, Perodactyly

Congenital underdevelopment of fingers is due to heterogeneous causes and is variable in degree and manifestation. Differing uses of terms complicate the literature. Adactyly, complete absence of fingers, is the most severe digital deficiency, whereas partial lack of fingers can be called oligodactyly. Ectrodactyly, "aborted fingers," is a term used by some authors for irregular digital defects of various types in distinction to split hands and feet[5]; other writers consider split hands a subgroup of ectrodactyly,[64] whereas some equate the two terms.[70] Oligodactyly is a general term used for various types of hands with reduced numbers of digits. Birch-Jensen[5] estimated the prevalence of split hands at about 1 in 112,000, of atypical split hand at 1 in 200,000 and of ectrodactyly at 1 in 98,000. Primary reduction malformations of fingers as well as true amputation of fingers must be considered under these terms.

The distal phalanx, the distal and middle or all three phalanges can be missing (apical deficiencies). Metacarpals may be absent together with their phalanges or they alone may be missing. If central fingers are absent, one speaks of split hand or split foot (p. 963). If radial or ulnar digits are deficient there also may be defects of the radius or ulna. Absence of the radial part of the hand is more frequent than that of the ulnar.[64] Phalangeal absence or hypoplasia occurs in children who develop myositis ossificans. Reduction of digits with preservation of a single ray leads to monodactyly. Systematic reviews of finger anomalies, their variations and combinations are available.[5,14,61,62]

Marginal deficiencies, i.e., radial or ulnar ray defects are more irregular than split hands. Such deficiencies can be clearly hereditary[148,149] or sporadic.[5] If only one finger develops, one speaks of monodactyly. A pedigree with monodactyly was reported in 1908 with only ray V present in 1 male and 4 females belonging to three generations.[150] Monodactyly occurs in children with the thalidomide syndrome[2] and with the de Lange syndrome.[22,151] It was noted, combined with other finger deformities, in a child damaged in utero by methotrexate.[152] A peculiar bilateral monodactyly with absence of both radii was described by Lackey.[153]

Apical deficiencies of fingers can have differing origins. MacArthur and McCullough[154] reported a family with 15 cases in three generations of missing terminal parts of digits II–V. The thumbs were broad and showed a tendency to duplication. Dominant inheritance seemed established. In other instances, heredity cannot be demonstrated in apical deficiencies, and true amputations of previously formed phalanges must be considered possible. Wounds, scars and constricting bands point to secondary destruction of apical structures. Pertinent cases were illustrated by Torpin.[155] As pointed out before (p. 942), such mutilations need not be due to mechanical causes.

Adactyly or oligodactyly occurs in a number of syndromes. Such finger defects are a constituent of the aglossia-adactylia syndrome,[119,156] Möbius syndrome,[157] (ulnar) oligodactyly syndrome,[37] Hanhart micrognathia-peromelia syndrome,[158] focal dermal hypoplasia,[119] spastic paraplegia and mental retardation[159] and the thalidomide embryopathy.[2] Reduction malformations of fingers (perodactyly) in Down syndrome were described by Schönenberg and Pfeiffer.[160] Rudimentary fingers and syndactyly sometimes are seen in patients with Pierre Robin syndrome.[161]

Microdactyly and Progressive Myositis Ossificans

Progressive myositis ossificans usually has its onset in early childhood but it has been congenital in rare instances.[162-165] In 1918, Rosenstirn[163] reviewed 115 published cases, including those reported in the seventeenth and eighteenth centuries. Only about 260 cases were recorded in the medical literature by 1964. In a review, Lutwak[166] discussed mineral, metabolic and radioactive calcium studies of the effect of hormone treatment.

The disorder is characterized by the appearance of bone in fascias, aponeuroses, tendons and muscles, which results in slow immobilization of the joints and the entire body. Since muscle changes are only secondary, the term "myositis" is not quite appropriate and has been replaced by others that are more correct but less popular.[165] Onset usually is blamed on a traumatic episode when a swelling appears in the cervical area, in the back or near a joint of a limb. Subsequently, lumps appear and subside in various locations, but they leave rigidity, ectopic bone formation, calcification or exostoses behind, resulting in progressive disability. In infants, early manifestations may be mistaken for torticollis, but the process slowly involves other areas by ossification of connective tissue and limitation of movement. Complete rigidity "from skull to ankles" may result[167] and lead to death by secondary infections. But some patients survive for many years in a state of immobility and ossification. They may be unable to sit up, stand or walk. Feeding becomes difficult because of ankylosis of the elbow and temporomandibular joints. Episodes of exacerbation may be painful and febrile so that a rheumatic infection can be simulated. This postnatal disease process often is preceded by an unknown prenatal teratogenic process that results in digital or other congenital malformations that presage the process of ossification of later life. Microdactyly, present at birth, has been observed in about two-thirds of the patients who develop myositis ossificans.[163] An association with faulty segmentation of the cervical spine or Klippel-Feil syndrome also seems likely,[168] whereas ectopic testes or hypospadias were observed so seldom that the connection could be fortuitous. Facial asymmetry and sexual infantilism could be the result of the postnatal process.

Microdactyly is the outstanding prenatal anomaly. Patients often are born with symmetric digital malformations. The first toes and the thumbs most often are abnormal but all fingers may be shortened.[169] The disease process affects the phalanges primarily. The proximal phalanges of the first digits may be entirely missing, more often in the toes than in the thumbs. Hallux valgus is observed often. Monophalangic first digits and biphalangic digits II–V have been observed. The terminal phalanges often are pointed and thin. Dysplasia of the middle phalanx of the little finger can result in clinodactyly. Anomaly of the metacarpals is rare but it can occur.[170] In addition, there may be fusion of metatarsals with proximal phalanges and fusion of phalanges with each other, resulting in elimination of joints, bony bridges or exostoses of metatarsal bones and absence of sesamoid

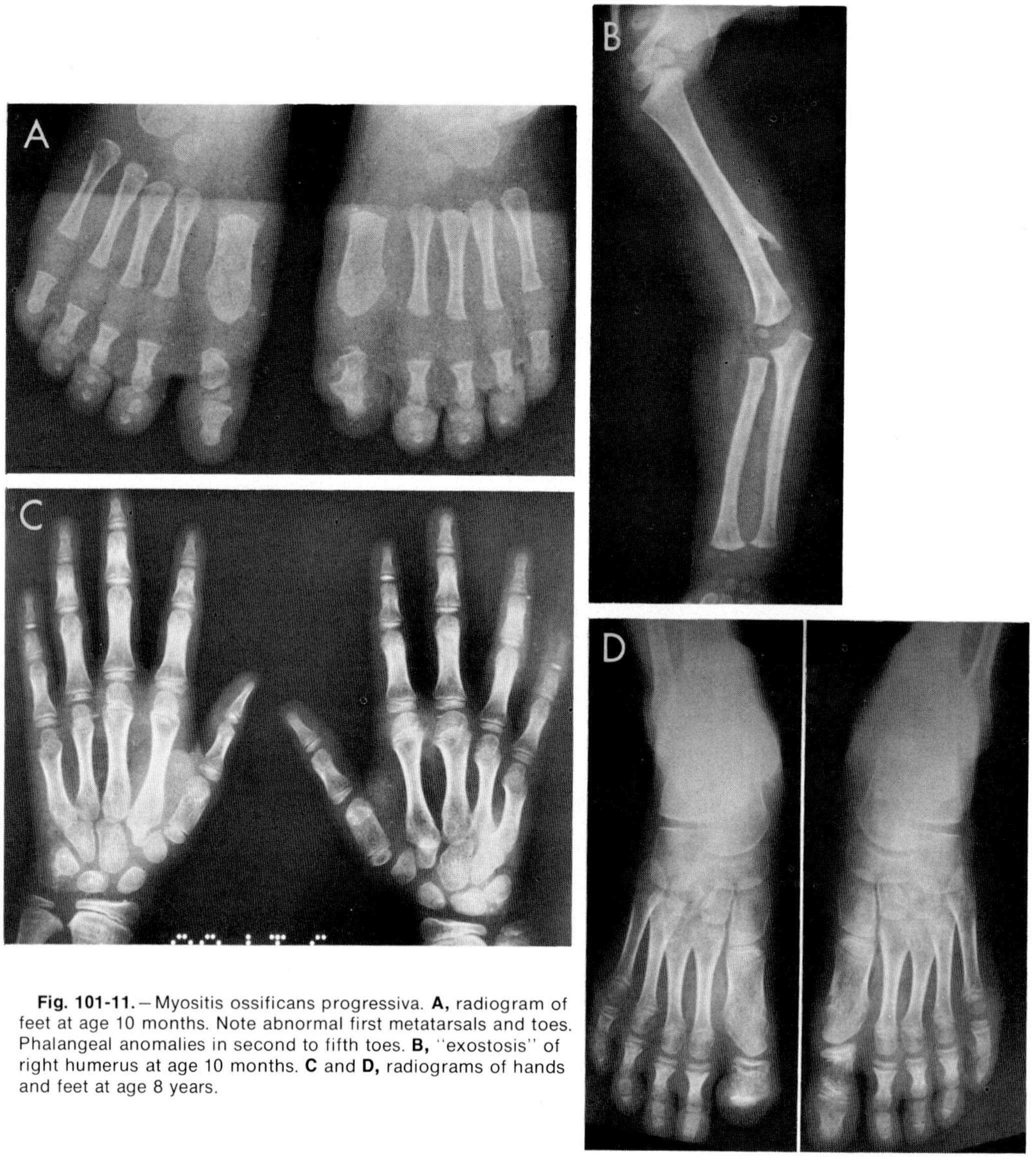

Fig. 101-11.—Myositis ossificans progressiva. **A,** radiogram of feet at age 10 months. Note abnormal first metatarsals and toes. Phalangeal anomalies in second to fifth toes. **B,** "exostosis" of right humerus at age 10 months. **C** and **D,** radiograms of hands and feet at age 8 years.

bones.[165] The big toes may be absent and the thumbs appear mutilated at birth.[166]

The relationship of these congenital digital malformations to the postnatal progressive heterotopic bone development is unexplained. It is of great interest that microdactyly of the type described can be present in a parent and child without myositis ossificans in the parent. There also are a few reports of the generalized disease occurring through more than one generation,[165,166,171] and concordance of progressive myositis ossificans has been reported in homozygotic twins.[172,173] Dominant inheritance is suggested by these observations, but it is important to point out that the expression of the trait can be limited to the digital malformation without development of the disabling generalized ossification. Males are affected more often than females but the ratio was only 138:117 in the cases reviewed by Lutwak[166] and not as significant as in early reports.

Absence of the Thumb

Absence or various anomalies of the thumb often accompany generalized reduction malformations of the extremities and various congenital syndromes.[278] There is a strong association of aplasia and hypoplasia of the radius with similar anomalies of the thumb.[5,14,174] A pedigree of hereditary thumb anomalies without involvement of other skeletal elements and other organs was published by Bilbrey.[175] Absent, vestigial and finger-like thumbs were manifestations of the autosomal dominant gene. It seems that 3 persons in the second generation were affected even though both parents were normal. Gonadal mosaicism in one of the parents could explain this situation similar to that of pedigrees with split hand.[69]

Anomalies of the thumb and other parts of the upper extremity occur in association with congenital heart disease (Holt-Oram syndrome),[176] particularly with atrial and ventricular septal defects. The skeletal defects of this syndrome, which is a dominant trait, vary greatly. Aplasia of the thumb, floating thumb and other skeletal anomalies are illustrated in publications on Holt-Oram syndrome.[177-179] In a child with atrial septal defect recorded by Zetterquist,[180] the thumb was absent on the right and represented by a small triphalangeal finger on the left. Absence of the thumbs or three-phalangeal thumbs, atrial septal defect and a tendency to cardiac arrhythmia sometimes occur together. This syndrome is transmitted as a dominant trait in some families.[180] Absence or anomalies of the thumb were noted in approximately 70% of the patients with Fanconi pancytopenia.[20]

Absence of the thumbs was reported in children with multiple congenital malformations thought to be due to a ring D chromosome.[182-184] Arhinencephaly, trigonocephaly, congenital heart disease and other malformations were seen in these patients. In the thalidomide syndrome, unilateral and bilateral aplasia of the thumb occurred in about 30% of the cases. In other children there was triphalangy of the thumbs. In such cases, the thumbs resembled the index fingers but in roentgenograms showed small middle phalanges. These thumbs, which can be combined with thenar hypoplasia, cannot be opposed. Digital appendages to the index finger were seen in some cases in place of the thumbs.[185]

Floating Thumb ("Pouce Flottant")

This condition is characterized by absence or underdevelopment of metacarpal I in the presence of the phalanges of the thumb. Such a thumb usually is located too far distally and radially for any opposition and function. Surgical improvement is difficult. It seems that transplantation of a metatarsal and of the proximal toe phalanx is required to improve the situation.[64] A floating thumb can be seen in the roentgenogram of the arm of a child with Goldenhar syndrome reported by Gorlin *et al.*[186]

Broad Thumb

Broad thumbs and toes and facial anomalies have been described as a syndrome by Rubinstein and Taybi[110] (p. 1018). There is a short distal phalanx, a short flat nail and radial deviation of the distal phalanx. Hyperextensibility or limitation of opposition of the thumb, broad terminal phalanges of other fingers, webbing, camptodactyly, clinodactyly, sixth toe, absent distal phalanx of the first toe and other anomalies may coexist. Roentgenograms show short and wide terminal phalanges of the thumbs and great toes. Bifid phalanges of the first toes and various kinds of abnormal segmentation of phalanges have been noted.[187] A review of 114 patients with this syndrome[188] showed that mental, motor, language and social retardation, short stature, microcrania, highly arched palate and cryptorchidism in males were common signs in patients with this syndrome, the cause of which is still not known. In one case, a sister of the patient was also mentally retarded and had minor radiologic changes of the first digits.[279] The dermatoglyphics of children with the broad thumb syndrome show distinct characteristics.[280]

Potter's Thumb (Brachymegalodactyly)

The tip of the normal thumb comes nearly to the first interphalangeal joint of the index finger, whereas "hereditary short thumb" as described by Breitenbecher[189] terminates at the junction of the metacarpal and first phalanx of the index finger. The abnormal thumbs are shorter by the length of the first phalanx, are broad and have broad and short nails. In the family recorded by Breitenbecher, the anomaly could be traced as a dominant Mendelian trait through five generations. Hefner,[190] who termed the condition "brachymegalodactylism," pointed out that it can occur on one or both thumbs, with the terminal phalanx as the seat of the anomaly. The thumbs, which have paddle-shaped terminal phalanges, have been called "potter's thumbs" and have been considered by palm readers as "murderers' thumbs."[191] Other fingers of the same hand may be long and slender.

The deformity is present at birth but becomes more marked with adolescence. It is not disabling but it can present a cosmetic problem. In Cleveland,[191] the highest incidence was found in Caucasian women with 0.66% as compared with 0.17% in Caucasian men. In some families, inheritance is irregular, with reduced penetrance in males.

Goodman *et al.*[192] examined the frequency of short thumbs among various ethnic groups in Israel. Approximately 1.6% of Jews and 3% of Arabs had the trait, half of them bilaterally. There was no predilection for one of the sexes. The trait, whether bilateral or unilateral, was autosomal dominant, with a penetrance of about 40%.

Triphalangeal Thumb

Hyperphalangy may occur in digits of normal or excessive length. The best-known cases are those of triphalangeal thumbs and first toes. These digits normally have only two phalanges, a proximal and a terminal one. In hyperphalangism, a middle phalanx is interposed between these two normal phalanges. This phalanx usually is short and wedge shaped and the thumb is therefore inclined toward the center of the hand. This type of hyperphalangia of the thumb sometimes interferes with the normal movements of the hand.[88] The anomaly can be inherited as a dominant familial trait.[193] A different type of hyperphalangy of the thumb is represented by an excess of phalanges of normal length, which leads to a thumb longer than normal. Such a thumb resembles an index finger rather than a normal first digit. A hand with such a long thumb, called a "thumbless hand," has been described as a dominant trait.[88] A third hereditary type combines triphalangeal thumb with polydactyly and syndactyly.[14,194] Triphalangeal thumbs associated with congenital anemia have been reported in brothers, one of whom had also congenital heart disease.[195]

Whether the extra phalanx is a proximal phalanx or a metacarpal is a matter of speculation. There is a theory that in the normal thumb the so-called metacarpal actually is a proximal phalanx, since the epiphysis of this bone is at the proximal end and not at the distal as in other metacarpals. Opinions on this point are divided.[64]

Triphalangy of the thumb became a rather frequent anomaly in Germany during the years 1960–1962 in connection with maternal thalidomide ingestion during early pregnancy. Lenz *et al.*[196] pointed out that some of the hands with this anomaly were so similar to the hereditary type of "double index finger" that one can consider the drug-induced form as a phenocopy. They saw concordance of triphalangeal thumb in a monozygotic and discordance in a dizygotic pair of twins. Lenz *et al.*[196] believed that aplasia of the thumb results from early intake of thalidomide, whereas triphalangy is the result of thalidomide taken toward the end of the susceptible time, i.e., the forty-fifth to fiftieth postmenstrual days.

If in a case of triphalangy of the thumb opposition is impossible, surgery can improve the function of the hand.[64]

Clutched Thumb (Congenital Aplasia of Extensor Tendons of the Thumb and Other Fingers)

This rare deformity of a flexed thumb or thumb-clutched hand is the result of failure of development of the muscles and tendons that extend the thumb and fingers at the metacarpophalangeal joints.[197] Barsky[64] performed a necropsy on a stillborn child with bilateral thumb contracture and found no extensor pollicis brevis; the extensor pollicis longus ended as a fibrous band at the base of the proximal phalanx of the thumb. It is doubtful that such cases are related to arthrogryposis, as no abnormalities are found in the spinal cord.[64] Weckesser *et al.*[198] pointed out that congenital clasped thumb is not a specific entity and that several types can be distinguished. In the most common type, the extensor muscles are either weak or absent but there are no other digital anomalies. Dominant inheritance of such clasped thumbs has been reported.

Restoration of thumb extension has been attempted by various procedures.[197]

Trigger Thumb

With trigger thumb (snapping thumb, stenosing tenovaginitis), the motion from flexion to extension usually is blocked at about 150 degrees, when resistance has to be overcome by pressure to obtain full extension.[199] A thumb persistently locked in this position may be mistaken for a contracture or dislocation of the interphalangeal joint. The correct diagnosis is facilitated by palpation of a hard nodule over the tendon sheath of the flexor pollicis longus at the metacarpophalangeal joint. The locking is due to an enlargement of the tendon, which cannot pass through the sheath. Trigger thumb, which may occur bilaterally or on one side only, is thought to be hereditary in some families. It has been described as a symptom of the trisomy 13–15 (D_1) syndrome.[200]

Polydactyly

Any duplication of one or of several digits is called polydactyly. The term polydactyly usually refers to hexadactyly (six fingers or toes). If the extra finger is on the radial side of the hand, one speaks of preaxial polydactyly; if it is on the ulnar side, it is called postaxial polydactyly. As a rule, either the first or the fifth digit is duplicated but others can be involved also. In the mildest form, the extra finger is only a cutaneous appendage. Such cutaneous appendages may be amputated spontaneously in utero and be recognizable at birth by a residual depression or groove on the previous site of attachment. Polydactyly is a rather frequent anomaly but, because of variation in geographic areas and in races, prevalence and incidence figures cannot be expected to be uniform. In a large population in Germany, a prevalence of about 1 in 2,200 persons was established.[201] In Utah,[281] the incidence of polydactyly with and without associated malformations was about 0.47 in 1,000; polydactyly alone had an incidence of 0.37 in 1,000. But in a New York study, the incidence in Caucasian and Negro infants was 1 in 713.[202] Polydactyly occurred in Boston Caucasian children at a rate of 1 in 1,284 but in Negro children of the District of Columbia it was 1 in 117.[203] In Kampala, Uganda, the incidence of polydactyly in African newborns was 1 in 74.[204] Many extra fingers are tied off or surgically removed soon after birth and there is some decrease in prevalence because of lethality of some syndromes that include polydactyly (p. 213). The mortality of polydactylous fetuses seems to be high before birth. In Japan, the incidence was many times higher in embryos than in infants.[205] These few figures show that any statement concerning incidence and prevalence of polydactyly needs definition of the population sample.

Polydactyly is a striking trait that has been recorded repeatedly since antiquity. In the Bible (II Samuel, 21:20) mention is made of a giant and his 4 sons, 1 of whom had polydactyly: "And there was yet a battle in Gath, where was a man of great stature, that had on every hand six fingers, and on every foot six toes, four and twenty in number; and he also was born to the giant" (see Goliath syndrome, p. 425). The passage is of medical interest, since in modern medicine the combination of gigantism with polydactyly has not been described as a syndrome, yet the association of endocrine symptoms such as obesity and genital underdevelopment with polydactyly and retinitis pigmentosa is well recognized as the Laurence-Moon-Biedl syndrome (p. 176). Polydactyly was known to the Romans, and Pliny mentioned a Roman poet with the surname Sedigitus and also two ladies of a noble Roman family named Sedigitae. Heredity of polydactyly in families, villages and tribes has been recorded. It was said that the Hyabites, an Arab tribe, showed hexadactyly so regularly that a child born with five fingers was considered a product of adultery and was immediately sacrificed.[64] There are reports of hexadactyly in the family of the black sultans of the Ozmani dynasty in southern Arabia, which was continued by marriage of hexadactylous princes to hexadactylous princesses, their cousins. The postaxial polydactyly that was present on hands and feet was considered a rather common and acceptable trait in that area.[62] Hexadactyly was also prevalent in certain groups of Australian aboriginals.[86,206]

In a secluded German village, Lücker[207] observed endemic polydactyly often associated with harelip. De Linares[208] described a village near Madrid with a population of only 150 in which every person was polydactylous. Some had seven fingers that were perfectly formed and could be used like normal fingers. The trait was considered an asset rather than a malformation. Hereditary polydactyly was described before the Mendelian laws were known. Lucas[209] reported a family with dominantly inherited polydactyly in which the expression was variable and harelip and cleft palate occurred as complicating anomalies. Odiorne[210] reported six New England families, all descended from one man who immigrated to New England in the seventeenth century. In this family, postaxial polydactyly was transmitted through ten generations. The anomaly varies in different families. It may be bilateral or unilateral; the hands, the feet or both may be affected or the condition may be com-

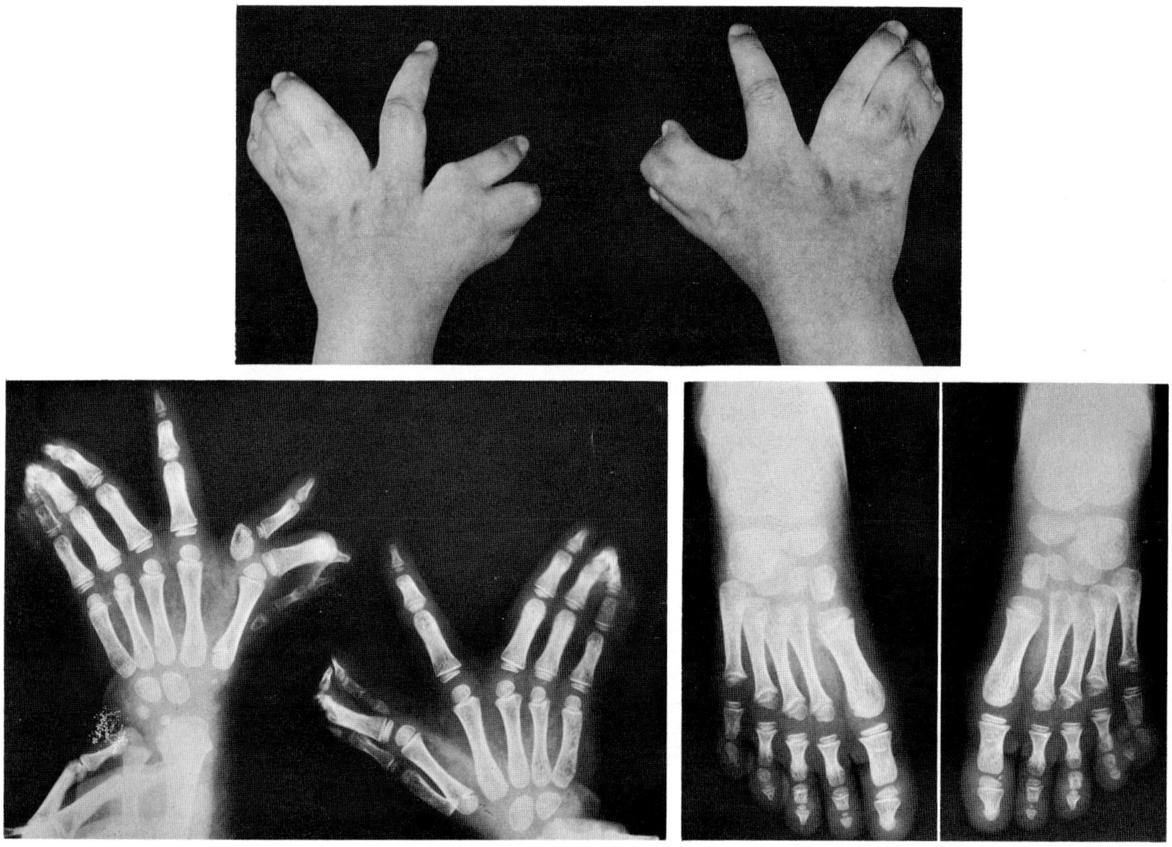

Fig. 101-12. – Polysymbrachydactyly in a girl whose mother, maternal uncle, grandfather and great-grandfather had similar malformations. There are only minor anomalies in the left foot.

pletely or incompletely expressed. Many pedigrees of dominantly inherited polydactyly are recorded in the medical literature.[14,86,211] Although in some pedigrees the polydactyly – for instance double digit V – is transmitted with great regularity, there is great variability in others. A pedigree from south India[90] showed polydactyly, syndactyly, brachydactyly and symphalangy with variable penetrance and expressivity in four generations. When the dominance is very irregular, it may become difficult to decide whether one is dealing with a dominant or a recessive trait, since recessive polydactyly has been established in some cases. Oliver[212] reported a family of Scandinavian ancestry living in Minnesota in which a cousin marriage occurred. Among the children of this consanguineous marriage, 3 were abnormal, showing duplication of the fifth digit, a speech defect and marked mental retardation. Another form of polydactyly inherited in a recessive manner is represented by the Laurence-Moon-Biedl syndrome (p. 176). Sporadic cases of polydactyly, although not rare, usually remain unreported. The sporadic form often occurs in otherwise perfectly normal persons. In a genetic study in Utah,[281] the most common type of polydactyly was partial or complete duplication of the first digit (thumb or large toe); this anomaly with its high incidence in Caucasians was not seen often in relatives of the propositi. Postaxial polydactyly represented by pedunculated postminimus or an extra ulnar or fibular digit showed dominant inheritance in more than one-third of the propositi.

Polydactyly often is associated with syndactyly, brachydactyly, triphalangy of the thumb and other digital anomalies. Facial clefts,[145,207,209] aniridia,[214] iris coloboma,[215] macular coloboma,[108] deafness and dystrophy of the nails,[147] hemihypertrophy (p. 163), acrocephalosyndactyly and other malformations can be combined with polydactyly. Gruber[216] described a disease picture in unviable infants, dysencephalia splanchnocystica, in which polydactyly is associated with encephalocele, microphthalmia and polycystic disease. Polycystic kidneys, hydrocephaly and polydactyly in siblings were reported by Simopoulos *et al.*[217] Unilateral polydactyly and hypertelorism were observed in boys with unilateral cryptorchidism and spermatogenic precocity in the descended testis.[218] Other syndromes that are rather regularly associated with preaxial or with postaxial polydactyly are mentioned below.

Finding of an extra digit may be of diagnostic importance because, when seen in a newborn child, it may point to associated malformations not visible on external inspection or it may point to anomalies that develop later in life. The Laurence-Moon-Biedl syndrome, for instance, is not recognizable at birth. If a sibling of a child with this syndrome is born with polydactyly, the extra finger presages future ocular and endocrine disturbances.

Polydactyly can be associated with tumors. It was present in a premature child with an imperforate buccopharyngeal membrane and metastasizing adrenal neuroblastoma (p. 668). Ganglioneuromas associated with cerebellar hyperplasias and polydactyly have been observed.[219]

The occurrence of polydactyly is not limited to man; it is found also in cattle, horses, dogs, cats, guinea pigs, rats and fowl.[220] This fact makes it possible to breed and study the inheritance of animals showing or carrying the condition. Wright[221] studied polydactyly in guinea pigs, which normally have four toes on the front feet and three on the hind feet. In polydactylous animals, vestigial thumbs were seen on the front feet and an extra big toe and vestigial big toe on the hind feet. Heterozygous animals were well developed but the homozygous generally died in utero. They had short legs and paddle-like feet of double width with seven to twelve digits. They were all microphthalmic and some had nasal clefts and encephalocele. In a strain of rats, polydactyly due to an autosomal recessive gene was associated with partial arhinencephaly, pituitary defects and ocular anomalies.[222] Experimental production of polydactyly resulted from temporary folic acid deficiency of pregnant rats[223] and can be produced by exposure to x-rays in utero.[27] Several strains of mice showed polydactyly[224]; some of them also had hydrocephaly. In one strain, the heterozygotes had slight preaxial polydactyly but homozygotes were unviable, showing high degrees of polydactyly and exencephaly. A highly inbred strain of mice showed only polydactyly and no other anomalies. The first digit was duplicated most often and it is of interest that in such animals the spinal cord showed an excess number of motor neurons innervating the foot on the abnormal side.[225] Polydactyly in fowl usually is due to splitting of the first toe. The condition was studied by Baumann and Landauer,[226] who found in unilateral cases an increased number of anterior horn cells on the side of the extra toe. In fowl, modifications of polydactyly were studied thoroughly. It was shown that polydactyly is linked with multiple spurs and duplex comb and can be suppressed by inhibiting genes.[227] Modification is also possible by environmental factors. Sturkie[228] showed that polydactyly can be suppressed in heterozygous chick embryos by incubation at a temperature below normal. Landauer[229] made a thorough study of the genetic behavior of polydactyly in fowl. He discovered that injection of insulin between 72 and 96 hours of incubation may lead to phenotypic modification of polydactyly. This procedure can result in an increased incidence of heterodactyly or hyperphalangy or in incomplete suppression of polydactyly.

Duplication of Thumb or First Toe

The relative frequency of double thumb and double fifth finger has been discussed in the German and French literature without consensus.[14] In countries with sizable Negro populations, duplication of the fifth finger is definitely more common than that of the

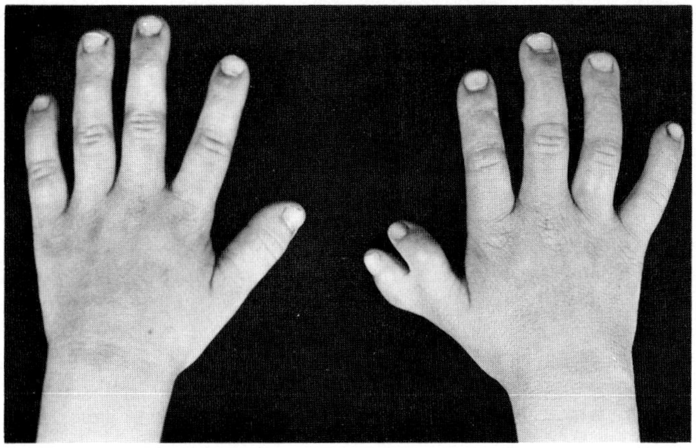

Fig. 101-13.—Bifid thumb of right hand in a mentally retarded girl.

first. Plastic surgeons see double thumb more often than extra little fingers[64]; this is understandable, since the latter often are removed by less specialized physicians or by nurses. Duplications of the first fingers vary in extent and shape from broad thumbs with slight indentation, overforked to completely developed extra thumbs. Gruber[62] and Barsky[64] illustrated the great variability of this anomaly, which needs careful analysis if surgical intervention is considered. Polydactyly can be combined with syndactyly, brachydactyly and triphalangy of the thumb (p. 977). Combination of double thumb with "delta phalanx" was reported by Watson and Boyes.[230] In rare instances, hereditary preaxial and postaxial duplications can occur together[14,233] or an extra little finger in the hands can be combined with duplication of the first toe.[104,231] Pedigrees of dominant inheritance of double thumb through many generations have been published.[14,86,232-235] In some kindreds, penetrance and expressivity are strong and uniform, in others they are variable.

Duplication of the first digits occurs occasionally in syndromes of multiple congenital malformations. Gruber[62] illustrated an acrocephalic infant with cleft lip and palate, bilateral duplication of the fifth finger and unilateral duplication of the right toe. In dominantly inherited acrocephaly, duplication of the terminal phalanges of the thumb was seen in several patients.[236] In a family reported by Sorsby,[108] a mother and 4 of her children had bifurcation of thumbs, clinodactyly and macular colobomas. In the Carpenter[237] syndrome, duplication of the terminal phalanx of the big toe is associated with syndactyly of fingers and acrocephaly. In a kindred with orodigitofacial syndrome, Doege *et al.*[238] described an extra digit, usually occurring at the medial aspect of the first toe. In exceptional cases of the Laurence-Moon-Biedl syndrome, the supernumerary digit may involve the thumb.[239] Extra thumbs were present in sisters with Fanconi anemia.[240] Reber[241] reported a kindred in which 2 cases of heptadactyly occurred in distant relatives. The propositus had seven toes bilaterally, aplasia of the tibiae and "five-finger-hands." His father also had five fingers on both hands and no thumbs. Ectrodactyly occurred in some collaterals. A distant relative had seven fingers on both hands and a rudimentary sixth metatarsal on the right foot. The heptadactyly of the propositus was on the feet and preaxial, that of the relative on the hands and postaxial. It is doubtful that in trisomy 13–15 polydactyly of the first digit occurs in any case. Teller and Pfeiffer[242] showed roentgenograms of the feet of a child with many signs of trisomy 13–15. In the right foot, two terminal phalanges are seen. But there were no chromosome analyses made and the diagnosis is doubtful; in trisomy 13–15, the last digit usually is

Fig. 101-14.—Duplication of basal phalanx of thumb in a boy with Carpenter syndrome (p. 901).

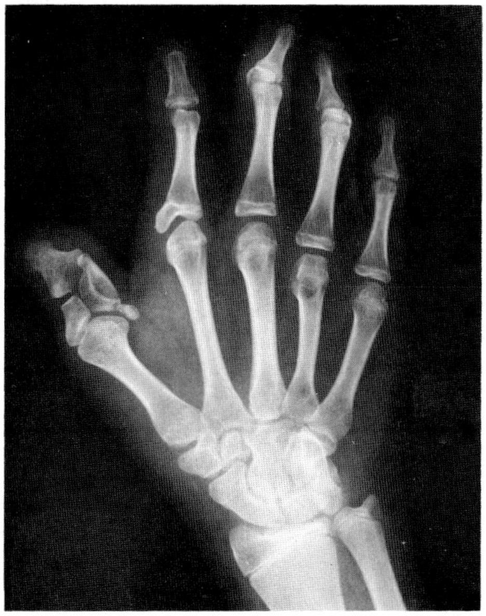

duplicated. Bifid thumb and choanal atresia have been seen in a boy with an abnormal D group chromosome.[288] A syndrome of preaxial polydactyly, imperforate anus and vertebral anomalies has been described.[213]

Duplication of the Fifth Digits

There are many examples of dominantly inherited duplication of fifth fingers and toes,[14,86,211] ranging from rudimentary appendages to well-developed sixth fingers or toes. There are kindreds in which the trait is regularly transmitted and others that show great variance of penetrance and expression. The variations in the expression of a gene causing polydactyly in a Negro family resulted in extra little fingers, extra toes and extra thumbs, i.e., postaxial and preaxial anomalies.[243] In a pair of monozygotic twins, one had duplication of the fifth finger of the left hand and of the fifth toe of the left foot; the other twin had an extra fifth finger on the left hand only; five extremities were normal. This example can be cited to illustrate modification of the trait by nongenetic factors.[244]

Pedunculated "postminimi" were described and discussed by Cummins.[245] They are of interest because of their relation to spontaneous amputations. The postminimi probably represent the most frequent form of polydactyly. Pedunculus minimus is so frequent in Negro children that, if included in comparative tabulations of congenital malformations, higher incidence figures are given for Negroes than for Caucasians; if pedunculus minimus is disregarded, the ratio is reversed.[246] The pedunculated postminimi usually are rotund and the nails are hypoplastic. The skin has no hair follicles or sebaceous glands, but the sweat glands are normal in number and distribution. The dermatoglyphics have recognizable characteristics in some cases, which may aid in ascertainment of postminimi after amputation has occurred. The skeletal framework shows arrested histogenesis and the

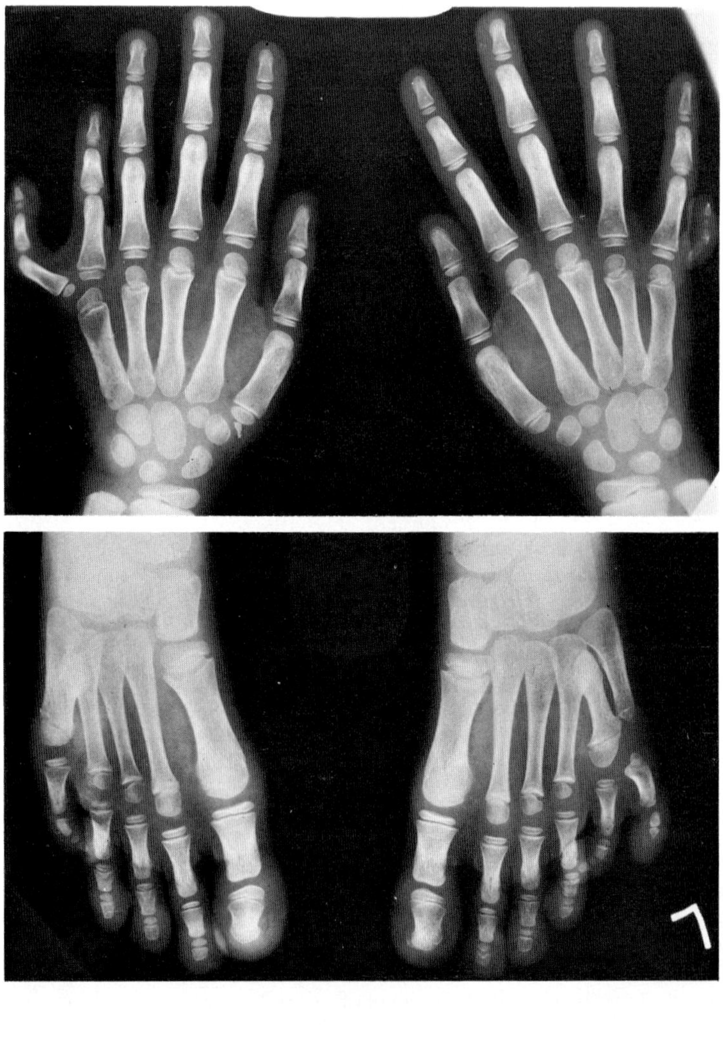

Fig. 101-15. – Various types of duplications of fifth fingers and toes in the same girl.

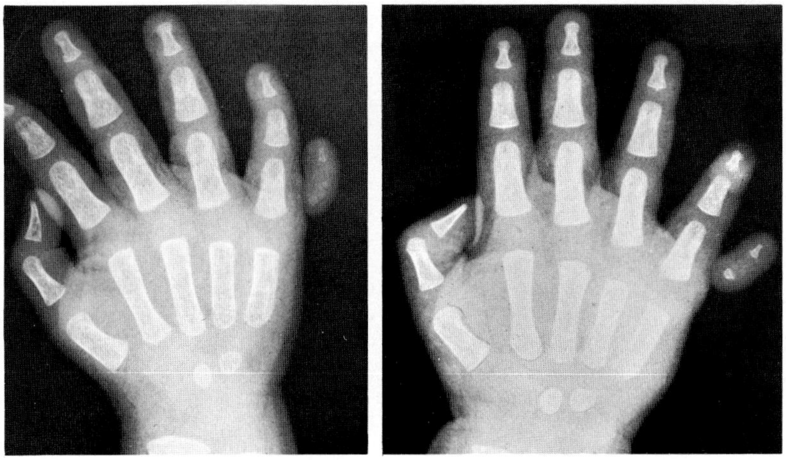

Fig. 101-16.—Hands of identical Negro twin boys, both with bilateral pedunculated postminimi. The toes were normal.

phalanges usually are reduced in size and number. In some instances, no bone can be found even in histologic sections. Polydactyly can be simulated by digital neurofibrosarcomas.[247]

Most syndromes that include polydactyly show a sixth finger or a rudiment on the ulnar side. Trisomy 13–15 typically is seen with postaxial polydactyly. A case showing partial duplication of the first toe and signs of trisomy 21 was not confirmed cytogenetically.[242] It is possible that some of the cases previously published as "typus rostockiensis,"[248] despite their resemblance to trisomy 13–15, were not due to chromosomal anomalies. Postaxial polydactyly is the rule in the following genetically determined syndromes: Ellis-van Creveld, asphyxiating thoracic dystrophy, Laurence-Moon-Biedl, Biemond, total sternal fissure and congenital heart disease,[249] hydrocephaly with polycystic kidneys[217] and others.[289] Occasionally, the extra digit can be in an atypical place in one of these syndromes. Caffey[250] illustrated a case of Ellis-van Creveld syndrome with duplication of sixth fingers and duplication of syndactylous second toes.

Median Duplications

Duplication of a second, third or fourth finger or toe can be called an axial polydactyly. Such duplications often are enclosed in syndactylous hands and combined with synostoses. The second digit is duplicated only rarely[282] but the middle digit is involved relatively frequently.[14] Schatzki[251] dealt with cases of hidden syndactylous polydactyly and triangle formation in the middle hand. Regular duplication of the middle finger in seven generations was reported by Thomsen[233] and many other examples of hereditary duplications of central rays were cited by Grebe.[14] Polydactyly of the second metatarsal with associated defects of the feet is a rare anomaly.[252] A dorsal eminence in the region of the second metatarsal, hallux valgus and overlapping of toes cause pain on weightbearing. The anomaly has been attributed to a dominant gene.

Treatment of polydactyly is complex. Removal of a postminimus usually is very easy but, if the sixth digit is developed to a higher degree, tying off of the finger with a ligature is not recommended. When to leave an extra thumb alone and when to remove it sometimes is not easily decided. It is difficult to decide which digit should be removed, since distribution of nerves, blood vessels and tendons varies.[64]

Polydactylies of High Degrees (Diplocheiria and Diplopodia)

Polydactylies of more than six digits are rare and usually associated with serious—even lethal—malformations. Thus, acrocephalosyndactyly with arhinencephaly, micromelia, cleft lip, choanal atresia or hypoplasia of the tibia may be associated with seven to eight digits.[62,253] But polydactyly of high degrees can be compatible with life. Many years ago, a woman was shown in country fairs in Germany whose legs were so short and deformed that she had to walk on all four extremities. She was named "Lionella" or the "Löwenweib." Her hands showed merely duplication of the thumbs. On the left foot she had eight digits of the formula IV, III, II, I, II, III, IV, V and on the right seven digits with slightly different differentiation, namely, IV, III, II, II, III, IV, V. The symmetric arrangements of rays on each foot suggests incomplete diplopodia on both legs.[62] In a siren, Gruber[62] described almost complete separation of the feet, with each foot showing heptadactyly. The fused legs contained two curved fibulae and very hypoplastic tibiae. Incomplete diplocheiria, indicated by duplication of the digits of the hands, has been observed together with duplication of the ulna and absence of the radius. A roentgenogram showing heptadactyly of a boy of 13 months is illustrated by Gruber.[62] Incomplete diplocheiria and diplopodia with high degrees of polydactyly usually are associated with hypoplasia or absence of the radii and tibiae.

Macrodactyly (Megalodactyly)

Hypertrophy of fingers is a rare anomaly that affects chiefly the second and third digits. True hypertrophy involves enlargement of all the elements of the finger, phalanges, tendons, nerves, vessels, nails and skin but the metacarpals are not affected. Macrodactyly can be unilateral or, rarely, bilateral and be associated with syndactyly. Involvement of a single finger is rarer than multiple digit involvement. Barsky[254] included only those cases in the category of true macrodactyly that show enlargement of all digital elements and he termed digital enlargement by hemangiomas "pseudo-macrodactyly." He distinguished between a congenital (static) and a progressive form. Barsky also reviewed 64 cases of true macrodactyly and thought that this malformation is one of the rarest of the hand. The condition is not familial and chromosome studies done in some of the cases showed no anomalies. Since congenital hypertrophy of digits can occur in neurofibromatosis, this dominant trait should always be considered in the search for a cause of the anomaly.

Camptodactyly

Permanent flexion contracture of a finger in one or more joints is called camptodactyly. There are many variations of this condition and many causes. Anomalies of bones, of their joints or the tendons may result in digital flexures. Sometimes only the little finger is affected but the ring, middle and index fingers may be involved, usually less severely than digit V. Various terms have been used for this anomaly,[86] which appears as a symptom in a variety of pathologic conditions or is inherited through several generations as a specific trait. Murphy[255] reported a pedigree in which 33 members had a flexion deformity of the little finger noticeable at birth. In other cases, the contracture is not observed at birth and remains mild during childhood but becomes worse and progressive during adolescence. There is neither pain nor swelling about the joint[256] and progression may be so gradual that the onset of the contracture is not known. Difficulty in playing an instrument, typing or putting on a glove may direct attention to the anomaly in delayed cases. Camptodactyly is bilateral in two-thirds of the patients. Roentgenograms sometimes show a mild volar subluxation of the proximal end of the second phalanx. The proximal phalanx tapers distally and its capitulum is tilted volarward.[257] Pathologic findings were discussed by Welch and Temtamy.[258] A severe form in which the little finger was so flexed that the first and third phalanges lay parallel was limited to the left hand and to male members of a kindred.[86] In another pedigree, 10 females in three generations had a flexion deformity of the fingers (streblodactyly) and aminoaciduria.[259] Nevin *et al.*[260] reported four families with contracture deformity of the hands characterized by flexion of the fingers at the proximal interphalangeal joints combined with

Fig. 101-17.—Macrodactyly of the second toe. (Courtesy of Dr. H. C. Shirkey.)

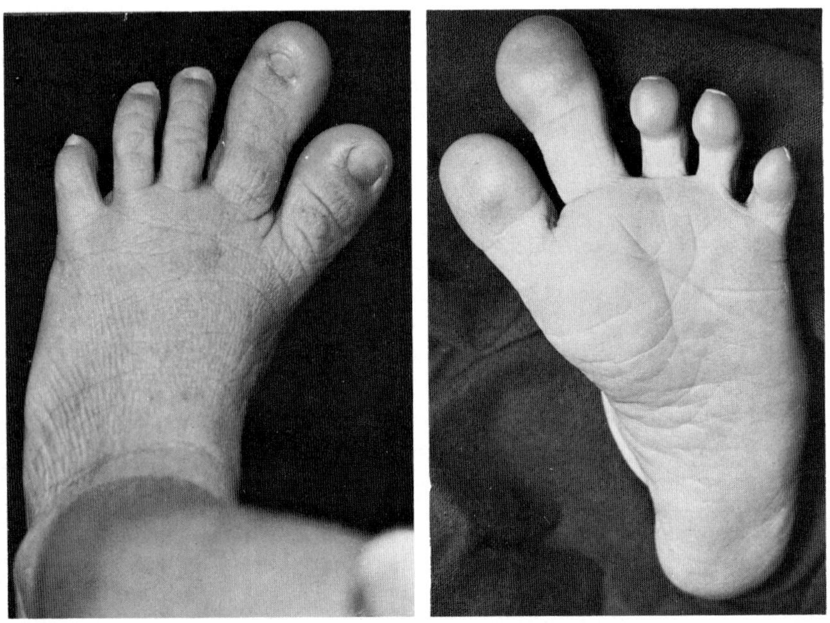

taurinuria. Male and female members were affected and dominant autosomal inheritance seemed likely. A list of other families with hereditary camptodactyly can be found in Grebe's[14] monograph. In Dupuytren contracture, which is hereditary but not congenital, shrinkage of the aponeurosis palmaris superficialis results chiefly in flexion of fingers on the ulnar side of the hand. It usually develops in the fifth decade of life, is more frequent in males than in females and is most common in the ring finger.[256] In some instances, camptodactyly and Dupuytren contracture coexist.[258] Associated anomalies are mentioned in some of the cases. Hammer toes, syndactyly, polydactyly, dislocation of the knee joint, scoliosis, pectus excavatum, arthrogryposis, plenosteosis and others have been observed. Flexion of fingers and elbows is the rule in the syndrome of muscular hypertrophy, extrapyramidal rigidity and mental retardation described by de Lange (p. 1030). Camptodactyly is not rare in combination with severe multiple congenital malformations such as trisomy 13–15, trisomy 18 (with hammer toe) and others.[256,257] It is a constituent of craniocarpotarsaldystrophy[261] and of oculodentodigital dysplasia[262] and occurs frequently in Marfan syndrome. Coexistence of pectus excavatum, scoliosis, ptosis and hypogonadism suggested a syndrome to Welch and Temtamy.[258] Camptodactyly, chondrodystrophia calcificans, glaucoma and cerebral anomalies were reported as a syndrome by Bowen *et al.*[263] Congenital contractures of finger joints, elbows and knees, clubfoot and scoliosis were present in an intelligent man who had 2 children with multiple joint contractures, camptodactyly, hydrocephaly, cleft palate and other malformations.[264] Surgical procedures have been recommended but the results are not uniform.[256,257]

Flexion of hands and fingers has become a highly significant sign of chromosomal anomalies. Although some fingers are maximally flexed in trisomy 18 and 13–15, others can be partially extended and overlie those touching the palm. Sometimes the index finger and the thumb are less contracted than digits III, IV and V but in other cases the thumb and the little finger overlie the central digits. Other anomalies of the nails, thumbs, first toes, hands and feet contribute to the suspicion of chromosomal abnormalities.

Congenital Synostoses

Congenital synostoses are, as a rule, primary aplasias of the joints that form when articulations fail to develop between the skeletal elements of the mesenchymal skeleton of the embryo. Union or nonseparation of skeletal elements often is referred to as "fusion." This term is not correct, since it implies secondary union of parts separated before. Therefore, primary aplasia of joints does not result in fusion but in nonseparation of elements. There exist secondary congenital synostoses in joints that were originally formed. In the spine, for instance, the five sacral vertebrae are at first separated by fibrous disks but later united by ossification of the intervertebral tissues.

The development of joints begins between the fourth and fifth weeks of embryonic life. The future joints become recognizable in the mesenchymal skeleton by condensation of tissue at the base of the skeletal elements of the extremities during the fourth week and they proceed in a distal direction subsequently. The areas of condensation delimit the future bones before the joint spaces are formed. The process of condensation progresses in general in a proximodistal direction. The proximal large joints rarely are affected but intercarpal and interdigital joints are absent more often. Since absence of joints often causes no functional impairment, synostoses frequently remain unrecognized until roentgenograms reveal the defect. At first, synostoses are fibrous and, later, cartilaginous, so that they often are not visible in roentgenograms during early childhood. Later, when the uniting cartilage becomes ossified, synostosis is demonstrable roentgenographically.

Synostoses occur unilaterally or bilaterally. They may be sporadic or be inherited like a dominant trait. They have been transmitted through three or four generations.[265] Such dominant inheritance probably is more frequent than is realized, since synarthroses often do not interfere with the proper use of the extremities.[266] For the same reason, incidence figures are not reliable. Synostosis humero-radialis is considered a rarity, but proximal radio-ulnar synostosis seems to be relatively frequent. According to Cross,[41] about 200 cases had been published in the medical literature by 1939. It is of interest that this peculiar malformation has been observed repeatedly in patients with XXXXY chromosomal constitution.[267,268]

Proximal radio-ulnar synostoses do not affect the elbow joint but interfere with free supination and pronation. In addition to fixation of the joint, there usually is a synostosis between the upper portions of the radial and ulnar shafts to the extent of 1–4 cm. Although fixation occurs in pronation, the use of the upper extremity is little impaired, since compensatory movements can be achieved in the shoulder. A syndrome of corneal opacities, flexion contracture of the elbows, general growth failure and mental retardation was reported by Mietens and Weber.[58] Severe myopia resulting in retinal detachment and blindness combined with premature degenerative joint disease, abnormal vertebral bodies and hearing defect was described as a syndrome transmitted through five generations.[269]

Distal radio-ulnar synostosis seems to be very rare, but union between the radius and the proximal carpal bones has been observed repeatedly. Movements of the hand are little affected by such synostoses. More frequent are synostoses between carpal bones in various combinations and degrees. The most common synostosis occurs between the lunatum and triquetrum; it was observed by O'Rahilly[63] in 0.13% of wrists examined and is said to occur in 6% of West African Negroes. The entire carpus can be united to a single block, which may be attached to the metacarpal bones in synostosis. Hereditary massive synostoses of carpal and tarsal bones have been reported.[270] Synostoses between carpal, tarsal and digital elements are more frequent.[266] Congenital carpal or tarsal "fusions" may occur between almost any two structures. Lunatotriquetral fusion is the most frequent type in the hand.[63] A syndrome of carpal and tarsal fusions with conductive deafness, mitral stenosis and short stature was described by Forney *et al.*[271] Carpal and tarsal fusions and synostosis of the elbow joints combined with brachydactyly (p. 962) can be considered a syndrome of articular dysplasia, which is a dominant hereditary trait.[53,272]

Synostosis between the proximal ends of the tibia and fibula has been observed. Talotibial synostosis is very rare and results in equinus position of the foot. Synostosis talocalcanea interferes with lateral movements of the foot, but compensatory movements can take place between the tibia and the talus. Talonavicular synostosis and union of tarsal and metatarsal bones have been described.[266] "Peroneal spastic flat foot" is due to a talocalcaneal or calcaneonavicular synostosis. Tarsal synostosis is frequent in both tibial and fibular synostoses.[63]

Hereditary transmission of congenital coalition of the calcaneus to the navicular bone has been reported by Wray and Herndon.[273] They observed the anomaly in three generations of a kindred and attributed it to a gene mutation behaving as an autosomal dominant.

REFERENCES

1. Fuhrmann, W., Koch, F., and Rauterberg, K.: Dominant erbliche Hypoplasie und Bewegungseinschränkung beider Schultergelenke, Ztschr. Orthop. 104:584, 1968.
2. Weicker, H.: 100 children with thalidomide embryopathy, XIth International Congress of Pediatrics, 1965.
3. Brücke, H.: Über angeborenen muskulären Riesenwuchs einer oberen Extremität, Virchows Arch. path. Anat. 296:681, 1936.
4. Morrissey, D. M.: Congenital total hypertrophy of the right upper limb, J. Pediat. 42:361, 1953.
5. Birch-Jensen, A.: *Congenital Deformities of the Upper Extremities* (Copenhagen: Ejnar Munksgaard, 1949).
6. Koehler, O.: Die hand-und fusslosen brasilianischen Geschwister, Ztschr. menschl. Vererb.-u. Konstitutionslehre 19:670, 1936.
7. Schwarzweller, F.: Ein Beitrag zur Genese und Systematik der Gliedmassenmissbildungen, Arch. Orthop. Chir. 39:400, 1938.
8. Frantz, C. H., and O'Rahilly, R.: Congenital skeletal limb deficiences, J. Bone & Joint Surg. 43-A:1202, 1961.
9. Dignan, P. St. J., Mauer, A. M., and Frantz, C.: Phocomelia with congenital hypoplastic thrombocytopenia and myeloid leukemoid reactions, J. Pediat. 70:561, 1967.
10. Pruzanski, W.: Familial-congenital malformations of the heart and upper limbs; a syndrome of Holt-Oram, Cardiologia 45:21, 1964.
11. Goldenberg, R. R.: Congenital bilateral complete absence of the radius in identical twins, J. Bone & Joint Surg. 30-A:1001, 1948.
12. Dodson, E. O.: Hereditary absence of radius and thumb, J. Hered. 47:275, 1956.
13. Schmid, O.: Über eine bisher nicht beobachtete Form von partiellem Radiusdefekt, Ztschr. Orthop. Chir. 2:59, 1892.
14. Grebe, H.: Missbildungen der Gliedmassen, in Becker, P. E. (ed.), *Humangenetik* (Stuttgart: Georg Thieme, 1964), Vol. II.
15. Smith, I. I., and Bain, A. D.: Congenital atresia of the larynx. A report of nine cases, Ann. Otol. 74:338, 1965.
16. Booth, J. B., and Berry, C. L.: Unilateral pulmonary agenesis, Arch. Dis. Childhood 42:361, 1967.
17. Harris, L. C., and Osborne, W. P.: Congenital absence or hypoplasia of the radius with ventricular septal defect: Ventriculo-radial dysplasia, J. Pediat. 68:265, 1966.
18. Baller, F.: Radius aplasie und Inzucht, Ztschr. menschl. Vererb.-u. Konstitutionslehre 29:782, 1950.
19. Gerold, M.: Frakturheilung bei einem seltenen Fall kongenitaler Anomalie der oberen Gliedmassen, Zentralbl. Chir. 84:831, 1959.
20. Nilsson, L.: Chronic pancytopenia with multiple congenital abnormalities (Fanconi's anaemia), Acta paediat. scandinav. 49:518, 1960.
21. Schönenberg, H., and Scheidhauer, E.: Beidseitige radiale Hemimelie mit Megakaryocytopenie. Ein neues Missbildungssyndrom, Ztschr. Kinderh. 97:240, 1966.
22. Ptacek, L. J., Opitz, J. M., Smith, D. W., Gerritsen, T., and Waisman, H. A.: The Cornelia de Lange syndrome, J. Pediat. 63:1000, 1963.
23. Gerald, B., and Umansky, R.: The Cornelia de Lange syndrome: Radiographic findings, Radiology 88:96, 1967.
24. Voorhess, M. L., Aspillaga, M. J., and Gardner, L. I.: Trisomy 18 syndrome with absent radius, varus deformity of hand and rudimentary thumb. Report of a case, J. Pediat. 65:130, 1964.
25. Zellweger, H., Huff, D. S., and Abbo, G.: Phocomelia and trisomy E, Acta genet. med. 14:164, 1965.
26. Rabinowitz, J. G., Moseley, J. E., Mitty, H. A., and Hirschhorn, K.: Trisomy 18, esophageal atresia, anomalies of the radius, and congenital hypoplastic thrombocytopenia, Radiology 89:488, 1967.
27. Warkany, J., and Schraffenberger, E.: Congenital malformations induced in rats by roentgen rays, Am. J. Roentgenol. 57:455, 1947.
28. Laurin, C. A., Favreau, J. C., and Labelle, P.: Bilateral absence of the radius and tibia with bilateral reduplication of the ulna and fibula. A case report, J. Bone & Joint Surg. 46-A:137, 1964.
29. O'Rahilly, R.: Morphological patterns in limb deficiencies and duplications, Am. J. Anat. 89:135, 1951.
30. McFarland, B.: Congenital dislocation of the radial head, Brit. J. Surg. 24:41, 1936.
31. Beals, R. K.: Auriculo-osteodysplasia. A syndrome of multiple osseous dysplasia, ear anomaly, and short stature, J. Bone & Joint Surg. 49-A:1541, 1967.
32. Lausecker, H.: Der angeborene Defekt der Ulna, Virchows Arch. path. Anat. 325:211, 1954.
33. Roberts, A. S.: A case of deformity of the fore-arm and hands, with an unusual history of hereditary congenital deficiency, Ann. Surg. 3:135, 1886.
34. Southwood, A. R.: Partial absence of the ulna and associated structures, J. Anat. 61:346, 1927.
35. Pfeiffer, R. A.: Beitrag zur erblichen Verkürzung von Ulna und Fibula, in Wiedemann, H-R. (ed.), *Dysostosen* (Stuttgart: Gustav Fischer, 1966), p. 130.
36. Lenz, W.: Anomalien des Wachstums und der Körperform, in Becker, P. E. (ed.), *Humangenetik* (Stuttgart: Georg Thieme, 1964), Vol. II.
37. Weyers, H.: Das Oligodactylie-Syndrom des Menschen und seine Parallelmutation bei der Hausmaus, Ann. paediat. 189:351, 1957.
38. Pintilie, D., Hatmanu, D., Olaru, I., and Panoza, Gh.: Double ulna with symmetrical polydactyly; case report, J. Bone & Joint Surg 46-B:89, 1964.

39. Buettner, G.: Ulnare Polydactylie bei Ulnarverdoppelung und Radiusdefekt, Ztschr. menschl. Vererb.-u Konstitutionslehre 22:428, 1938.
40. Hummel, K. P.: The inheritance and expression of disorganization, an unusual mutation in the mouse, J. Exper. Zool. 137:389, 1958.
41. Cross, A. R.: Congenital bilateral radio-ulnar synostosis, Am. J. Dis. Child. 58:1259, 1939.
42. Davenport, C. B., Taylor, H. L., and Nelson, L. A.: Radioulnar synostosis, Arch. Surg. 8:705, 1924.
43. Franceschetti, A., and Klein, D.: Mandibulo-facial dysostosis; new hereditary syndrome, Acta ophth. 27:143, 1949.
44. Ferguson-Smith, M. A., Johnston, A. W., and Handmaker, S. D.: Primary amentia and micro-orchidism associated with an XXXY sex-chromosome constitution, Lancet 2:184, 1960.
45. Barr, M. L., Carr, D. H., Pozsonyi, J., Wilson, R. A., Dunn, H. G., Jacobson, T. S., and Miller, J. R.: The XXXXY sex chromosome abnormality, Canad. M.A.J. 87:891, 1962.
46. Atkins, L., and Connelly, J. P.: XXXXY sex-chromosome abnormality, Am. J. Dis. Child. 106:514, 1963.
47. Scherz, R. G., and Roeckel, I. E.: The XXXXY syndrome, J. Pediat. 63:1093, 1963.
48. Cleveland, W. W., Arias, D., and Smith, G. F.: Radioulnar synostosis, behavioral disturbance, and XYY chromosomes, J. Pediat. 74:103, 1969.
49. Romanus, R.: Ein Fall von angeborener Ankylose im Ellbogengelenk, Acta orthop. scandinav. 4:291, 1933.
50. Card, R. Y., and Strachman, J.: Congenital ankylosis of the elbow, J. Pediat. 46:81, 1955.
51. Siwon, P.: Kongenitale, hereditäre, doppelseitige Ankylosen der Ellenbogengelenke, Deutsche Ztschr. Chir. 209:338, 1928.
52. Comings, D. E.: The Kleeblattschädel syndrome—a grotesque form of hydrocephalus, J. Pediat. 67:126, 1965.
53. Fuhrmann, W., Steffens, C., Schwarz, G., and Wagner, A.: Dominant erbliche Brachydaktylie mit Gelenksaplasien, Humangenetik 1:337, 1965.
54. Gaal, S. A., and Larsen, I. J.: Symphalangism, 32d Annual Meeting, Western Orthopedic Association, San Francisco, 1968.
55. Thompson, J. S., McLaughlin, P. R., and Heslin, D. J.: Impaired pronation-supination of the forearm: An inherited condition, J. M. Genetics 5:48, 1968.
56. Gunn, D. R., and Pillary, V. K.: Congenital posterior dislocation of head of radius, Clin. Orthop. 34:108, 1964.
57. Cockshott, W. P., and Omololu, A.: Familial congenital posterior dislocation of both radial heads, J. Bone & Joint Surg. 40-B:483, 1958.
58. Mietens, C., and Weber, H.: A syndrome characterized by corneal opacity, nystagmus, flexion contracture of the elbows, growth failure, and mental retardation, J. Pediat. 69:624, 1966.
59. La Barre, W.: *The Human Animal* (Chicago: University of Chicago Press, 1954).
60. Müller, W.: *Die angeborenen Fehlbildungen der menschlichen Hand* (Leipzig: Georg Thieme, 1937).
61. Werthemann, A.: Bewegungs-apparatus, VI Teil. Die Entwicklungs-Störungen der Extremitäten, in Lubarsch, O., and Henke, F. (eds.), *Handbuch der Speziellen Pathologischen Anatomie und Histologie* (Berlin: Springer-Verlag, 1952).
62. Gruber, G. B.: Hyperdaktylie (Polydaktyly) Diplocheirie und Diplopodie, Hypermelie, Oligodaktylie und Defekte der Röhrenknochen, in Schwalbe, E., and Gruber, G. B. (eds.), *Die Morphologie der Missbildungen des Menschen und der Tiere* (Jena: Gustav Fischer, 1958), Vol. 3, p. 720.
63. O'Rahilly, R.: A survey of carpal and tarsal anomalies, J. Bone & Joint Surg. 35-A:626, 1953.
64. Barsky, A. J.: *Congenital Anomalies of the Hand and Their Surgical Treatment* (Springfield, Ill.: Charles C Thomas, Publisher, 1958).
65. Kelikian, H., and Doumanian, A.: Congenital anomalies of the hand, Parts I and II, J. Bone & Joint Surg. 39-A: 1002, 1249, 1957.
66. Patterson, T. J. S.: Congenital deformities of the hand, Ann. Roy. Coll. Surgeons England 25:306, 1959.
67. Entin, M. A.: Reconstruction of congenital abnormalities of the upper extremities, J. Bone & Joint Surg. 41-A: 681, 1959.
68. Geoffroy Saint-Hilaire, I.: *Histoire générale et particulière des anomalies de l'organisation chez l'homme et les animaux* (Paris: J. B. Baillière et fils, 1832).
69. Mackenzie, H., and Penrose, L. S.: Two pedigrees of ectrodactyly, Ann. Eugenics 16:88, 1951.
70. Stevenson, A. C., and Jennings, L. M.: Ectrodactyly—evidence in favour of a disturbed segregation in the offspring of affected males, Ann. Human Genet. 24:89, 1960.
71. Hartsinck, J. J.: *Beschryving van Guiana, of de wide Kust in Zuid-America* (Amsterdam: Gerrit Tielenburg, 1770), p. 811.
72. Barsky, A. J.: Cleft hand: Classification, incidence, and treatment, J. Bone & Joint Surg. 46-A:1707, 1964.
73. Béchet, J-F.: Essai sur les monstruosités humaines, ou vices congénitaux de conformation (Paris: Didot le Jeune, 1829).
74. Pearson, K.: On inheritance of the deformity known as split-foot or lobster-claw, Biometrika 6:69, 1908.
75. McMullan, G., and Pearson, K.: On the inheritance of the deformity known as split-foot or lobster-claw, Biometrika 9:381, 1913.
76. Hanhart, E.: Stark unregelmässige Dominanz einer Anlage zu Spalthand auf Grund eines schwachen entwicklungslabilen Gens., Arch. Klaus Stift. (supp.) 20: 96, 1945.
77. Popenoe, P.: Split hand, J. Hered. 28:174, 1937.
78. Unterrichter, L.: Beiträge zur Kenntnis der angeborenen Anomalien der Extremitäten, Ztschr. menschl. Vererb.-u. Konstitutionslehre 18:317, 1934.
79. Khosrovani, H.: Malformations des mains et des pieds (ectrodactylie) à travers cinq générations successives dans une grande famille Vaudoise, J. Génét. Hum. 8:1, 1959.
80. Jaworska, M., and Popiolek, J.: Genetic counselling in lobster-claw anomaly. Discussion of variability of genetic influence in different families, Clin. Pediat. 7:396, 1968.
81. Grebe, H.: Spalthand-Spaltfuss, Ectrodactylie, in Schwalbe E., and Gruber, G. B. (eds.), *Die Morphologie der Missbildungen des Menschen und der Tiere* (Jena: Gustav Fischer, 1958), Vol. 3, p. 19.
82. Wildervanck, L. S.: Perceptive deafness associated with split-hand and -foot, a new syndrome?, Acta genet. 13: 161, 1963.
83. Arnand-Battandier, R., and Gillot, F.: Un nouveau cas de typus Amstelodamensis (maladie de Cornelia de Lange), Pédiatrie 8:100, 1953.
84. Meyerding, H. W., and Upshaw, J. E.: Heredofamilial cleft foot deformity (lobster-claw foot or split foot), Am. J. Surg. 74:889, 1947.
85. Bell, J.: On Hereditary Digital Anomalies, I. On Brachydactyly and Symphalangism, in Penrose, L. S. (ed.), *Treasury of Human Inheritance* (London: Cambridge University Press, 1951), Vol. V.
86. Gates, R. R.: *Human Genetics* (New York: The MacMillan Company, 1946).
87. Schinz, H. R.: Erbtypen und Formen bei Brachydaktylie, Arch. Klaus Stift. 18:361, 1943.
88. Cocchi, U.: Hereditary Diseases with Bone Changes, in Schinz, H. R., Baensch, W. E., Friedl, E., and Uehlinger, E. (eds.), *Roentgen-Diagnostics* (New York: Grune & Stratton, Inc., 1951).
89. Farabee, B-C.: Inheritance of digital malformations in man, Papers Peabody Museum, Harvard University, 3: 65, 1905.

90. Savarinathan, G., and Centerwall, W. R.: Symphalangism. A pedigree from south India, J. M. Genetics 3:285, 1966.
91. Drinkwater, H.: A second brachydactylous family, J. Genetics 4:323, 1915.
92. Grebe, H.: Der Nachweis der Heterozygoten bei rezessiven Erbleiden, Der Erbarzt 11:1, 1943.
93. Bass, H. N.: Familial absence of middle phalanges with nail dysplasia, Pediatrics 42:318, 1968.
94. Degenhardt, K. H., and Geipel, G.: Dominant erbliche Perodaktylien in 4 Generationen einer Sippe, Ztschr. menschl. Vererb.-u. Konstitutionslehre 32:277, 1954.
95. Brailsford, J. F.: Familial brachydactyly, Brit. J. Radiol. 18:172, 1945.
96. Mohr. O. L., and Wriedt, C.: A new type of hereditary brachyphalangy in man. Publication of Carnegie Institution No. 295, Washington, D.C., 1919.
97. Hersh, A. H., DeMarinis, F., and Stecher, R. M.: On the inheritance and development of clinodactyly, Am. J. Human Genet. 5:257, 1953.
98. Vidal, E.: Tératologie humaine: Brachydactylie symétrique et autres anomalies osseuses, héréditaires depuis plusieurs génerations, Bull. Acad. méd. Paris 63:632, 1910.
99. Klintworth, G. K., and Anderson, I. F.: Tylosis palmaris et plantaris familiaris associated with clinodactyly, South African M. J. 35:170, 1961.
100. deMarinis, F., and deMarinis, M. R.: Frequency of clinodactyly in children between the ages of 5 and 12, Acta genet. med. 4:192, 1955.
101. Blank, E., and Girdany, B. R.: Symmetric bowing of the terminal phalanges of the fifth fingers in a family (Kirner's deformity), Am. J. Roentgenol. 93:367, 1965.
102. Leboucq, H.: De la brachydactylie et de l'hyperphalangie chez l'homme, Bull. Acad. roy méd. belg. 4:344, 1896.
103. Shoul, M. I., and Rivto, M.: Roentgenologic and clinical aspects of hyperphalangism (polyphalangism) and brachydactylism, New England J. Med. 248:274, 1953.
104. O'Rahilly, R.: Radiological investigation of a case of pedal hyperphalangism and supernumerary phalangeal epiphyses, Brit. J. Radiol. 19:432, 1946.
105. Greene, H. S. N., and Saxton, J. A.: Hereditary brachydactylia and allied abnormalities in the rabbit, J. Exper. Med. 69:301, 1939.
106. Landauer, W.: Brachypodism, J. Hered. 43:293, 1952.
107. Warkany, J., and Nelson, R. C.: Skeletal abnormalities in the offspring of rats reared on deficient diets, Anat. Rec. 79:83, 1941.
108. Sorsby, A.: Congenital coloboma of the macula; together with an account of the familial occurrence of bilateral macular coloboma in association with apical dystrophy of hands and feet, Brit. J. Ophth. 19:65, 1935.
109. Coffin, G. S.: Brachydactyly, peculiar facies and mental retardation, Am. J. Dis. Child. 108:351, 1964.
110. Rubinstein, J. H., and Taybi, H.: Broad thumbs and toes and facial abnormalities; a possible mental retardation syndrome, Am. J. Dis. Child. 105:588, 1963.
111. Taybi, H.: Generalized skeletal dysplasia with multiple anomalies; note on Pyle's disease, Am. J. Roentgenol. 88:450, 1962.
112. Dudding, B. A., Gorlin, R. J., and Langer, L. O.: The oto-palato-digital syndrome. A new symptom-complex consisting of deafness, dwarfism, cleft palate, characteristic facies, and a generalized bone dysplasia, Am. J. Dis. Child. 113:214, 1967.
113. Pippow, G.: Wirbelgelenkaplasien und Brachydaktylie in einer Sippe, Der Erbarzt 10:226, 1942.
114. Robinson, G. C., Wood, B. J., Miller, J. R., and Baillie, J.: Hereditary brachydactyly and hip disease, J. Pediat. 72: 539, 1968.
115. Cascos, A. S.: Brachydactyly and outflow heart tract obstruction. Report of two cases, Cardiologia 50:330, 1967.
116. Giedion, A.: Das tricho-rhino-phalangeale Syndrom, Helvet. paediat. acta 21:475, 1966.
117. Keizer, D. P. R.: A case of brachydactyly (type Brailsford), Brit. J. Radiol. 24:632, 1951.
118. Jürgens, H. W.: Zur Problematik der Klinodaktylie, Ärztl. Jugenkd. 52:341, 1960.
119. Gorlin, R. J., and Pindborg, J. J.: *Syndromes of the Head and Neck* (New York: The Blakiston Division, McGraw-Hill Book Company, Inc., 1964).
120. Arkless, R., and Graham, C. B.: An unusual case of brachydactyly. Peripheral dysostosis?, pseudo-pseudo-hypoparathyroidism?, cone epiphyses?, Am. J. Roentgenol. 99:724, 1967.
121. Archibald, R. M., Finby, N., and DeVito, F.: Endocrine significance of short metacarpals, J. Clin. Endocrinol. 19:1312, 1959.
122. Boczkowski, K., and Fleszar, I.: Radiological studies in patients with gonadal abnormalities, Bull. Polish M. Sc. & Hist. 11:81, 1968.
123. Cushing, H.: Hereditary ankylosis of the proximal phalangeal joints (symphalangism), J. Nerv. & Ment. Dis. 43:445, 1916.
124. Strasburger, A. K., Hawkins, M. R., Eldridge, R., Hargrave, R. L., and McKusick, V. A.: Symphalangism: Genetic and clinical aspects, Bull. Johns Hopkins Hosp. 117:108, 1965.
125. Steinberg, A. G., and Reynolds, E. L.: Further data on symphalangism, J. Hered. 39:23, 1948.
126. Drinkwater, H.: Phalangeal anarthrosis (synostosis, ankylosis) transmitted through fourteen generations, Proc. Roy. Soc. Med. 10:60, 1917.
127. Fraser Roberts, J. A.: *An Introduction to Medical Genetics* (London: Oxford University Press, 1965).
128. Elkington, S. G., and Huntsman, R. G.: The Talbot fingers: A study in symphalangism, Brit. M. J. 1:407, 1967.
129. Vesell, E. S.: Symphalangism, strabismus and hearing loss in mother and daughter, New England J. Med. 263: 839, 1960.
130. Pol, R.: Reduktion der Mittelphalangen in Kombination mit Syndaktylie (Symbrachydaktylie), Arch. path. Anat. 229:447, 1921.
131. MacCollum, D. W.: Webbed fingers, Surg., Gynec. & Obst. 71:782, 1940.
132. Harris, L. C., and Osborne, W. P.: Congenital absence or hypoplasia of the radius with ventricular septal defect: Ventriculo-radial dysplasia, J. Pediat. 68:265, 1966.
133. Stucke, K., and Helbig, D.: Syndaktylie, in Schwalbe, E., and Gruber, G. B. (eds.), *Die Morphologie der Missbildungen des Menschen und der Tiere* (Jena: Gustav Fischer, 1958), pt. 3.
134. Schlatter, C.: Die Mendelschen Vererbungsgesetze beim Menschen an Hand zweier Syndactylie Stammbäume, Cor.-Bl. Schweiz. Ärzter 44:225, 1914.
135. Schade, H.: Zur endogenen Entstehung von Gliedmassendefekten, Ztschr. Morphol. Anthropol. 36:375, 1937.
136. Lucken, K. G.: Über eine Familie mit Syndaktylie, Ztschr. menschl. Vererb.-u. Konstitutionslehre 29:152, 1939.
137. Johnston, O., and Kirby, V. V.: Syndactyly of the ring and little finger, Am. J. Human Genet. 7:80, 1955.
138. Schofield, R.: Inheritance of webbed toes, J. Hered. 12: 400, 1921.
139. Cenani, A., and Lenz, W.: Totale Syndaktylie und totale radioulnare Synostose bei zwei Brüdern, Ztschr. Kinderh. 101:181, 1967.
140. Haas, S. L.: Bilateral complete syndactylism of all fingers, Am. J. Surg. 50:363, 1940.
141. Clarkson, P.: Poland's syndactyly, Guy's Hosp. Rep. 111: 335, 1962.
142. Brown, J. B., and McDowell, F.: Syndactylism with absence of the pectoralis major, Surgery 7:599, 1940.
143. Fulford, G. E.: Aglossia congenita: Cineradiographic findings, Arch. Dis. Childhood 31:400, 1956.
144. Bünnige, M.: Angeborene Zungen-Munddach-Verwach-

sung, Ann. paediat. 195:173, 1960.
145. Schönenberg, H.: Über die Kombination von Lippen-Kiefer-Gaumen-Spalten mit Extremitätenmissbildungen, Ztschr. Kinderh. 76:79, 1955.
146. Rosselli, D., and Gulienetti, R.: *Le Malformazioni Associate* (Turin: Minerva Medica, 1960).
147. Robinson, G. C., Miller, J. R., and Bensimon, J. R.: Familial ectodermal dysplasia with sensori-neural deafness and other anomalies, Pediatrics 30:797, 1962.
148. Stroer, W. F. H.: Familiäres Auftreten von Reihen erblicher Hand-und Fussabweichungen, Der Erbarzt 4:22, 1936.
149. Hofmann, M.: Vererbung von Spalthand und Spaltfuss, Dissertation, Munich, 1936.
150. Looking back: Remarkable case of hereditary monstrosity, Lancet 1:743, 1908.
151. Richter, H.: Drei neue Beobachtungen des Cornelia de Lange Syndrom, Arch. Kinderh. 164:249, 1961.
152. Milunsky, A., Graef, J. W., and Gaynor, M. F.: Methotrexate-induced congenital malformations, J. Pediat. 72:790, 1968.
153. Lackey, W. N.: Unusual congenital deformities of the upper extremities. Absence of the radii with oligodactylia, J.A.M.A. 93:113, 1929.
154. MacArthur, J. W., and McCullough, E.: Apical dystrophy, an inherited defect of hands and feet, Human Biol. 4:179, 1932.
155. Torpin, R.: *Fetal Malformations Caused by Amnion Rupture during Gestation* (Springfield, Ill.: Charles C Thomas, Publisher, 1968).
156. Kelln, E. E., Bennett, C. G., and Klingberg, W. G.: Aglossia-adactylia syndrome, Am. J. Dis. Child. 116:549, 1968.
157. Nisenson, A., Isaacson, A., and Grant, S.: Masklike facies with associated congenital anomalies, J. Pediat. 46: 255, 1955.
158. Hanhart, E.: Über die Kombination von Peromelie mit Mikrognathie, ein neues Syndrom beim Menschen, entsprechend der *Akroteriasis congenita* von Wriedt und Mohr beim Rinde, Arch. Julius Klaus-Stiftung 25:531, 1950.
159. Jancar, J.: Ectrodactyly, spastic paralegia and mental retardation, J. Ment. Defic. Res. 11:207, 1967.
160. Schönenberg, H., and Pfeiffer, R.: Gliedmassenfehlbildungen (Perodaktylie, Symbrachydaktylie) bei 2 Säuglingen mit Down-Syndrom, Ann. paediat. 207:172, 1966.
161. Smith, J. L., and Stowe, F. R.: The Pierre Robin syndrome, Pediatrics 27:128, 1961.
162. Henderson, J. A.: Case of myositis ossificans progressiva in a child, J. Bone & Joint Surg. 5:395, 1923.
163. Rosenstirn, J.: A contribution to the study of myositis ossificans progressiva, Ann. Surg. 68:485, 1918.
164. Mair, W. F.: Myositis ossificans progressiva, Edinburgh M. J. 39:1369, 1932.
165. McKusick, V. A.: *Heritable Disorders of Connective Tissue* (St. Louis: The C. V. Mosby Company, 1966).
166. Lutwak, L.: Myositis ossificans progressiva, Am. J. Med. 37:269, 1964.
167. Maudsley, R. H.: A case of myositis ossificans progressiva, Brit. M. J. 1:954, 1952.
168. Rosborough, D.: Ectopic bone formation associated with multiple congenital anomalies, J. Bone & Joint Surg. 48-B:499, 1966.
169. Fairbank, H. A. T.: *An Atlas of General Affections of the Skeleton* (Baltimore: The Williams & Wilkins Company, 1951).
170. Griffith, G.: Progressive myositis ossificans, Arch. Dis. Childhood 24:71, 1949.
171. Burton-Fanning, F. W.: A case of myositis ossificans, Lancet 2:849, 1901.
172. Vastine, J. H., Vostene, M. F., and Arango, O.: Myositis ossificans progressiva in homozygotic twins, Am. J. Roentgenol. 59:204, 1948.
173. Eaton, W. L., Conkling, W. S., and Daeschner, C. W.: Early myositis ossificans progressiva in homozygotic twins, J. Pediat. 50:591, 1957.
174. Veit, G.: Über familäres Vorkommen von Oligodaktylie, Gleichzeitig ein Beitrag zur genetischen Stellung der Oligodaktylie-innerhalb der Handmissbildungen, Ztschr. menschl. Vererb.-u. Konstitutionslehre 23:620, 1939.
175. Bilbrey, G. L.: Isolated congenital familial thumb deformities, New England J. Med. 274:1057, 1966.
176. Holt, M., and Oram, I.: Familial heart disease with skeletal malformations, Brit. Heart J. 22:236, 1960.
177. Pires de Lima, J. A.: À propos d'un nouveau cas d'ectromélie, Ann. anat. path. 10:830, 1933.
178. Lewis, K. B., Bruce, R. A., Baum, D., and Motulsky, A. G.: The upper limb-cardiovascular syndrome, J.A.M.A. 193:1080, 1965.
179. Holmes, L. B.: Congenital heart disease and upper-extremity deformities. A report of two families, New England J. Med. 272:437, 1965.
180. Zetterquist, P.: The syndrome of familial atrial septal defect, heart arrhythmia and hand malformation (Holt-Oram) in mother and son, Acta paediat. 52:115, 1963.
181. Rüdiger, R. A., Haase, W., and Passarge, E.: Association of ectrodactyly, ectodermal dysplasia and cleft lip-palate, Am. J. Dis. Child. 120:160, 1970.
182. Sparkes, R. S., Carrel, R. E., and Wright, S. W.: Absent thumbs with a ring D2 chromosome: A new deletion syndrome, Am. J. Human Genet. 19:644, 1967.
183. Bain, A. D., and Gould, I. K.: Multiple congenital abnormalities associated with ring chromosome, Lancet 2: 304, 1963.
184. Adams, M. S.: Palm-prints and a ring D chromosome, Lancet 2:494, 1965.
185. Knapp, K., and Lenz, W.: Die Formen der Thalidomid-Embryopathie, Roentgen. Europ. 5:105, 1963.
186. Gorlin, R. J., Jue, K. L., Jacobsen, U., and Goldschmidt, E.: Oculoauriculovertebral dysplasia, J. Pediat. 63:991, 1963.
187. Taybi, H., and Rubinstein, J. H.: Broad thumbs and toes, and unusual facial features. A probable mental retardation syndrome, Am. J. Roentgenol. 93:362, 1965.
188. Rubinstein, J. H.: The Broad Thumbs Syndrome—Progress Report 1968, *Birth Defects: Original Article Series* (New York: The National Foundation, 1969), p. 25.
189. Breitenbecher, J. K.: Hereditary shortness of thumbs, J. Hered. 14:15, 1923.
190. Hefner, R. A.: Inherited abnormalities of the fingers. II. Short thumbs (brachymegalodactylism), J. Hered. 15: 433, 1924.
191. Stecher, R. M.: The physical characteristics and heredity of short thumbs, Acta genet. 7:217, 1957.
192. Goodman, R. M., Adam, A., and Sheba, C.: A genetic study of stub thumbs among various ethnic groups in Israel, J. M. Genetics 2:116, 1965.
193. Roberts, E.: Hereditary hyperphalangism of thumb, J. Hered. 34:291, 1943.
194. Müller, W.: Beiträge zur Kenntnis des dreigliedrigen Daumens, Arch. klin. Chir. 185:377, 1936.
195. Aase, J. M., and Smith, D. W.: Congenital anemia and triphalangeal thumbs: A new syndrome, J. Pediat. 74: 471, 1969.
196. Lenz, W., Theopold, W., and Thomas, J.: Triphalangie des Daumens als Folge von Thalidomidschädigung, München. med. Wchnschr. 106:2033, 1964.
197. Crawford, H. H., Horton, C. E., and Adamson, J. E.: Congenital aplasia or hypoplasia of the thumb and finger extensor tendons, J. Bone & Joint Surg. 48-A:82, 1966.
198. Weckesser, E. C., Reed, J. R., and Heiple, K. G.: Congenital clasped thumb (congenital flexion-adduction deformity of the thumb), J. Bone & Joint Surg. 50-A:1417, 1968.
199. White, J. W., and Jensen, W. E.: Trigger thumb in infants, A.M.A. Am. J. Dis. Child. 85:141, 1953.

200. Patau, K., Therman, E., Smith, D. W., Inhorn, S. L., and Picken, B. F.: Partial trisomy syndromes. I. Sturge-Weber's disease, Am. J. Human Genet. 13:287, 1961.
201. Verschuer, O.: *Genetik des Menschen* (Munich: Urban & Schwarzenberg, 1959).
202. Sesgin, M. Z., and Stark, R. B.: The incidence of congenital defects, Plast. & Reconstruct. Surg. 27:261, 1961.
203. Altemus, L. A., and Ferguson, A. D.: Comparative incidence of birth defects in Negro and white children, Pediatrics 36:56, 1965.
204. Simpkiss, M., and Lowe, A.: Congenital abnormalities in the African newborn, Arch. Dis. Childhood 36:404, 1961.
205. Nishimura, H., Takano, K., Tanimura, T., Yasuda, M., and Uchida, T.: High incidence of several malformations in the early human embryos as compared with infants, Biol. Neonat. 10:93, 1966.
206. Brodsky, I.: Congenital abnormalities, teratology and embryology; some evidence of primitive man's knowledge as expressed in art and lore in Oceania, M. J. Australia 1:417, 1943.
207. Lücker, F. C.: Über Verérbung von Missbildungen, insbesondere Hasenscharte und Polydaktylie, und ihre Beziehungen zur Geburtshilfe, Monatsschr. Geb. Gynäk. 66:327, 1924.
208. de Linares, L. G.: Collective polydactylism in a small town, J.A.M.A. 94:2080, 1930.
209. Lucas, R. G.: On a remarkable instance of hereditary tendency to the production of supernumerary digits, Guy's Hosp. Rep. 25:417, 1881.
210. Odiorne, J. M.: Polydactylism in related New England families, J. Hered. 34:45, 1943.
211. Johnston, O., and Davis, R. W.: On the inheritance of hand and foot anomalies in six families, Am. J. Human Genet. 5:356, 1953.
212. Oliver, C. P.: Recessive polydactylism associated with mental deficiency, J. Hered. 31:365, 1940.
213. Say, B., and Gerald, P. S.: A new polydactyly/imperforate anus/vertebral anomalies syndrome?, Lancet 2:688, 1968.
214. Bornstein, M. B.: Aniridie bilaterale avec polydactylie. Relations des anomalies oculaires du type colobomateux associées à des malformations squelettiques avec les formes atypiques du syndrome de Bardet-Biedl, J. Génét. Hum. 1:211, 1952.
215. Biemond, A.: Het syndroom van Laurence-Biedl en een aanverwant nieuw syndroom, Nederl. tijdschr. geneesk. 78:1801, 1934.
216. Gruber, G. B.: Beiträge zur Frage "gekoppelter" Missbildungen. (Akrocephalo-Syndactylie und Dysencephalia-splanchnocystica), Beitr. path. Anat. 93:459, 1934.
217. Simopoulos, A. P., Brennan, G. G., Alwan, A., and Fidis, N.: Polycystic kidneys, internal hydrocephalus and polydactylism in newborn siblings, Pediatrics 39:931, 1967.
218. Bunge, R. G., and Bradbury, J. T.: Two unilaterally cryptorchid boys with spermatogenic precocity in the descended testis, hypertelorism and polydactyly, J. Clin. Endocrinol. 19:1103, 1959.
219. Ostertag, B.: Die Einzelformen der Verbildungen, in Lubarsch, O., Henke, F., and Rössle, R. (eds.), *Handbuch der Speziellen Pathologischen Anatomie und Histologie* (Berlin: Springer-Verlag, 1956).
220. Pol, R.: Missbildungen der Extremitäten, in Schwalbe, E., and Gruber, G. B. (eds.), *Die Morphologie der Missbildungen des Menschen und der Tiere* (Jena: Gustav Fischer, 1958), Vol. 3, fasc. 19.
221. Wright, S.: A mutation of the guinea pig, tending to restore the pentadactyl foot when heterozygous, producing a monstrosity when homozygous, Genetics 20:84, 1935.
222. Kalter, H.: *Teratology of the Central Nervous System* (Chicago: The University of Chicago Press, 1968).
223. Nelson, M. M., Wright, H. V., Asling, C. W., and Evans, H. M.: Multiple congenital abnormalities resulting from transitory deficiency of pteroylglutamic acid during gestation in the rat, J. Nutrition 56:349, 1955.
224. Grüneberg, H.: *The Genetics of the Mouse* (2nd ed.; The Hague: Martinus Nijhoff, 1952).
225. Tsang, Y-C.: Ventral horn cells and polydactyly in mice, J. Comp. Neurol. 70:1, 1939.
226. Baumann, L., and Landauer, W.: Polydactyly and anterior horn cells in fowl, J. Comp. Neurol. 79:153, 1943.
227. Hutt, F. B., and Mueller, C. D.: The linkage of polydactyly with multiple spurs and duplex comb in the fowl, Am. Naturalist 77:70, 1943.
228. Sturkie, P. D.: Suppression of polydactyly in the domestic fowl by low temperature, J. Exper. Zool. 93:325, 1943.
229. Landauer, W.: The phenotypic modification of hereditary polydactylism of fowl by selection and by insulin, Genetics 33:133, 1948.
230. Watson, H. K., and Boyes, J. H.: Congenital angular deformity of the digits. Delta phalanx, J. Bone & Joint Surg. 49-A:333, 1967.
231. Goodman, R. M.: A family with polysyndactyly and other anomalies, J. Hered. 56:37, 1965.
232. Atwood, E. S., and Pond, C. P.: A polydactylous family, J. Hered. 8:96, 1917.
233. Thomsen, O.: Einige Eigentümlichkeiten der erblichen Poly- und Syndaktylie bei Menschen, Acta med. scandinav. 65:609, 1927.
234. Bell, J.: On Syndactyly and Its Association with Polydactyly, in Penrose, L. S. (ed.), *Treasury of Human Inheritance* (London: Cambridge University Press, 1953), Vol. V, pt. II.
235. Kaul, K. K., and Bhandari, N. R.: Polydactylo-syndactylism in seven generations, Indian J. Pediat. 26:18, 1959.
236. Pfeiffer, R. A.: Dominant erbliche Akrocephalosyndaktylie, Ztschr. Kinderh. 90:301, 1964.
237. Carpenter, G.: Case of acrocephaly with other congenital malformations, Proc. Roy. Soc. Med. II:45, 1909.
238. Doege, T. C., Thuline, H. C., Priest, H. J., Norby, D. E., and Bryant, J. S.: Studies of a family with the oral-facial-digital syndrome, New England J. Med. 271:1073, 1964.
239. Bell, J.: The Laurence-Moon Syndrome, in Penrose, L. S. (ed.), *Treasury of Human Inheritance* (London: Cambridge University Press, 1958), Vol. V.
240. Esparza, A., and Thompson, W. R.: Familial hypoplastic anemia with multiple congenital anomalies (Fanconi's syndrome), Rhode Island M. J. 49:103, 1966.
241. Reber, M.: Un Syndrome osseux peu commun associant une heptadactylie et une aplasie des tibias, J. Génét. Hum. 16:15, 1967–68.
242. Teller, W., and Pfeiffer, R. A.: Die Trisomie D_1 (13-15) als Ursache multipler Abartungen, Ztschr. Kinderh. 89:36, 1964.
243. Callan, R.: Polydactyly in a Negro family, J. Hered. 33:229, 1942.
244. Lehmann, W. E., and Witteler, E. A.: Zwillingsbeobachtung zur Erbpathologie der Polydaktylie, Zentralbl. Chir. 62:2844, 1935.
245. Cummins, H.: Spontaneous amputation of human supernumerary digits: Pedunculated postminimi, Am. J. Anat. 51:381, 1932.
246. Shapiro, R. N., Eddy, W., Fitzgibbon, J., and O'Brien, G.: Incidence of congenital anomalies discovered in neonatal period, Am. J. Surg. 96:396, 1958.
247. Jensen, A. R., Martin, L. W., and Longino, L. A.: Digital neurofibrosarcoma in infancy, J. Pediat. 51:566, 1957.
248. Hövels, O., and Müllereisert, F.: Der "Typus Rostockiensis" als charaktistisches Kombinationsbild multipler Missbildungen (Polydaktylie Hypospadie, Kryptorchismus und Mikrognathie), Ztschr. Kinderh. 77:454, 1955.
249. Mehrpuyan, T., and Neuhäuser, G.: Totale Sternumspalte kombiniert mit anderen Skeletdeformitäten und seltener Herzmissbildung, Ztschr. Kinderh. 98:86, 1967.
250. Caffey, J.: *Pediatric X-ray Diagnosis* (5th ed.; Chicago: Year Book Medical Publishers, Inc., 1967).
251. Schatzki, P.: Über verdeckte syndactyle Polydaktylie und über "Triangelbildung" in der menschlichen Mittelhand,

Arch. Orthop. u. Unfall-Chir. 34:637, 1934.
252. Neel, J. V., and Rusk, M. L.: Polydactyly of the second metatarsal with associated defects of the feet: A new, simply inherited skeletal deformity, Am. J. Human Genet. 15:288, 1963.
253. Davidson, A. J.: A case of congenital deformity of the hands, supernumerary toes and absence of tibiae, Am. J. Roentgenol. 5:434, 1918.
254. Barsky, A. J.: Macrodactyly, J. Bone & Joint Surg. 49-A:1255, 1967.
255. Murphy, D. P.: Familial finger contracture and associated familial knee-joint subluxation, J.A.M.A. 86:395, 1926.
256. Smith, R. J., and Kaplan, E. B.: Camptodactyly and similar atraumatic flexion deformities of the proximal interphalangeal joints of the fingers, J. Bone & Joint Surg. 50-A:1187, 1968.
257. Currarino, G., and Waldman, I.: Camptodactyly, Am. J. Roentgenol. 92:1312, 1964.
258. Welch, J. P., and Temtamy, S. A.: Hereditary contractures of the fingers (camptodactyly), J. M. Genetics 3:77, 1966.
259. Parish, J. G., Horn, D. B., and Thompson, M.: Familial streblodactyly with amino-aciduria, Brit. M. J. 2:1247, 1963.
260. Nevin, N. C., Hurwitz, L. J., and Neill, D. W.: Familial camptodactyly with taurinuria, J. M. Genetics, 3:265, 1966.
261. Freeman, E. A., and Sheldon, J. H.: Cranio-carpo-tarsal dystrophy, Arch. Dis. Childhood 13:277, 1938.
262. Gillespie, F. D.: A hereditary syndrome: "Dysplasia oculodentodigitalis," Arch. Ophth. 71:187, 1964.
263. Bowen, P., Lee, C. S., Zellweger, H., and Linderberg, R.: A familial syndrome of multiple congenital defects, Bull. Johns Hopkins Hosp. 114:402, 1964.
264. Aase, J. M., and Smith, D. W.: Dysmorphogenesis of joints, brain, and palate: A new dominantly inherited syndrome, J. Pediat. 73:606, 1968.
265. Baekh, C. A.: Über congenitale Synostosen zwischen Radius und Ulna, Deutsche Ztschr. Chir. 213:225, 1929.
266. Oeynhausen, R.: Angeborene Synostosen, in Schwalbe, E., and Gruber, G. B. (eds.), *Die Morphologie der Missbildungen des Menschen und der Tiere* (Jena: Gustav Fischer, 1958), p. 893.
267. Fraser, J. H., Boyd, E., Lennox, B., and Dennison, W. M.: A case of XXXXY Klinefelter's syndrome, Lancet 2:1064, 1961.
268. Fraccaro, M., Klinger, H. P., and Schutt, W.: A male with XXXXY sex chromosomes, Cytogenetics 1:53, 1962.
269. Stickler, G. B., and Pugh, D. G.: Hereditary progressive arthro-ophthalmopathy. II. Additional observations on vertebral abnormalities, a hearing defect, and a report of a similar case, Mayo Clin. Proc. 42:495, 1967.
270. Kewesch, E. L.: Über hereditäre Verschmelzung der Hand und Fusswurzelknochen, Fortschr. Geb. Röntgenstrahlen 50:550, 1934.
271. Forney, W. R., Robinson, S. J., and Pascoe, D. J.: Congenital heart disease, deafness, and skeletal malformations: A new syndrome?, J. Pediat. 68:14, 1966.
272. Fuhrmann, W., Steffens, Ch., and Rompe, G.: Dominant erbliche doppelseitige Dysplasie und Synostose des Ellenbogengelenks mit symmetrischer Brachymesophalangie und Brachymetakarpie sowie Synostosen im Finger-, Hand-und Fusswurzelbereich, Humangenetik 3:64, 1966.
273. Wray, J. B., and Herndon, C. N.: Hereditary transmission of congenital coalition of the calcaneus to the navicular, J. Bone & Joint Surg. 45-A:365, 1963.
274. Walker, J. C., and Clodius, L.: The syndrome of cleft lip, cleft palate and lobster claw deformities of hands and feet, Plast. & Reconstruct. Surg. 32:627, 1963.
275. Faed, M., Stewart, A., and Keay, A. J.: Chromosome abnormalities in two cases with bilateral radial element defects, J. M. Genetics 6:342, 1969.
276. Makley, J. T., and Heiple, K. G.: Scoliosis associated with congenital deficiencies of the upper extremity, J. Bone & Joint Surg. 52-A:279, 1970.
277. Sandrow, R. E., Sullivan, P. D., and Steel, H. H.: Hereditary ulnar and fibular dimelia with peculiar facies, J. Bone & Joint Surg. 52-A:367, 1970.
278. Johnson, C. F.: Abnormal thumbs and physical diagnosis, Clin. Pediat. 9:131, 1970.
279. Hayem, F., Boisse, J., Rethore, M. O., Labrune, M., Hambourg, M., and Mozziconacci, P.: Le syndrome de Rubinstein-Taybi, Pédiatrie 25:89, 1970.
280. Giroux, J., and Miller, J. R.: Dermatoglyphics of the broad thumb and great toe syndrome, Am. J. Dis. Child. 113: 207, 1967.
281. Woolf, C. M., and Woolf, R. M.: A genetic study of polydactyly in Utah, Am. J. Human Genet. 22:75, 1970.
282. Wood, V. E.: Duplication of the index finger, J. Bone & Joint Surg. 52-A:569, 1970.
283. Keutel, J., Kindermann, I., and Möckel, H.: Eine wahrscheinlich autosomal recessiv vererbte Skeletmissbildung mit Humeroradialsynostose, Humangenetik 9:43, 1970.
284. Bora, F. W., Nicholson, J. T., and Cheema, H. M.: Radial meromelia. The deformity and its treatment, J. Bone & Joint Surg. 52:966, 1970.
285. Stern, A. M., Gall, J. C., Jr., Perry, B. L., Stimson, C. W., Weitkamp, L. R., and Poznanski, A. K.: The hand-foot-uterus syndrome, J. Pediat. 77:109, 1970.
286. Wiegmann, O. A., and Walker, F. A.: The syndrome of lobster claw deformity and nasolacrimal obstruction, J. Pediat. Ophth. 7:79, 1970.
287. Hoover, G. H., Flatt, A. E., and Weiss, M. W.: The hand and Apert's syndrome, J. Bone & Joint Surg. 52-B:878, 1970.
288. Carter, C. H., Smith, G. F., and Schindeler, J.: Choanal atresia and bifid thumb associated with an abnormal D group chromosome, J. Ment. Defic. Res. 14:221, 1970.
289. Marec, B. L., and Coutel, Y.: La polydactylie. Maladie ou symptome?, Pédiatrie 25:735, 1970.

102

The Lower Extremities

Congenital Dislocation of the Hip (CDH)

IT HAS BEEN SAID that the history of congenital dislocation of the hip is the history of orthopedic surgery and that this disease is the most common of the congenital skeletal deformities.[1] Yet it is very doubtful that the condition usually labeled with that name is a dislocation present at birth in more than 2% of the cases called CDH. The typical and prevalent type, which makes up 98% of the cases of CDH, is represented at birth by a *dysplasia* of the hip consisting of a flat acetabular roof and an underdeveloped proximal end of the femur,[2] i.e., by rather slight anomalies that predispose to *dislocation* after birth. Paradoxically, true congenital dislocation of the hip with bilateral prenatal displacement of the femoral head is also called "atypical" CDH. Because of its association with congenital syndromes or malformations, this form has been called "teratologic" in contrast to the more common "anthropologic" one.[3] The latter name suggests that the disorder is caused by phylogenic "humanization" and is limited to man. This is not correct, since CDH occurs in animals also.[2]

The fact that typical CDH does not exist at birth has important practical consequences. If the dislocation is brought on by faulty handling of infants or by walking and weight bearing, it should be possible to prevent the deforming processes. To do this, children with the predisposing dysplasia of the hip should be recognized as early as possible and prophylactic measures be instituted soon after birth. Thus, modern orthopedics and pediatrics are greatly concerned with the characteristics of congenital dysplasia of the hip and the best procedures for preventing dislocation.

It is said that CDH was well described by Hippocrates, who knew the distortion of the hip, the abnormal gait and the exaggerated lordosis.[2] He also knew that the disorder can occur in utero.[1] Paré pointed out the hereditary tendency and Camper, in the eighteenth century, the predilection for girls and the aggregation in certain localities.[1] Replacement of the femoral head in the socket by traction was attempted in the cadaver by Verduc in 1701, but fixation in the correct position could not be achieved. Pravaz[4] achieved successful reduction preceded by gradual traction and attempted without success to maintain the reduction by a pressure pad. Toward the end of the nineteenth century, open operations were performed in several cases, and about 1895 Lorenz[5] introduced the standard conservative method, with reduction and retention of the femoral head in its normal location. Lorenz also pointed out that dislocation is not present in the newborn period and that only a predisposition exists at birth, but he did not begin treatment in infancy. Several surgeons in the first decade of this century expressed the belief that the tendency to dislocation can be diagnosed during the first weeks of life and that it was possible to prevent serious deformity by abducting the legs in the deflected hip joints; this has now become a widely accepted tenet.[1,2,6,7] The criteria of early diagnosis, however, have not been firmly established and the discussion of this cardinal question continues.[7,8]

CDH is a leading malformation in orthopedic clinics, and some orthopedic surgeons estimate that CDH is about three times as frequent as congenital clubfoot and six times as frequent as congenital torticollis.[2] But in the crippled children's service of the U.S. Children's Bureau (1959), enrollment was due to CDH in only 1.3% of the cases, whereas 6.7% were entered because of clubfoot. Such discrepancies exemplify the need for better prevalence data on orthopedic disorders.

There are numerous statements in the literature about great variations in the incidence and prevalence according to geographic and ethnographic situations. Many reports were based on impressions of orthopedic surgeons and are influenced by the location of the services, interest and reputation of the observers and other variables. It was thought, for instance, that CDH is very rare in China. Such statements should be regarded with caution, since we know that in Japan the incidence increased with interest in the disease,[2] and Plummer,[9] in contrast to earlier statements concerning the rarity of the disease there, found 5 cases among 227 children examined (2.2%) in Hiroshima. In an orthopedic hospital in Honolulu, Stewart[10] listed no case of CDH in Hawaiian patients, although the disorder occurred in other ethnic groups. Among the Lapps, the incidence apparently is particularly high. It is said to be approximately 4% and even considerably higher in certain vil-

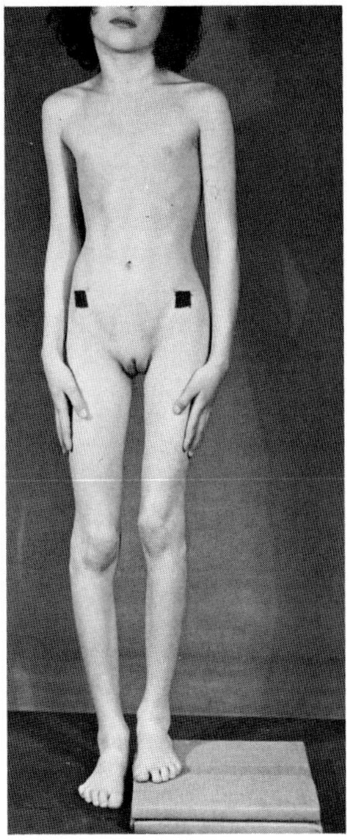

Fig. 102-1.—Dislocation of the left hip in a girl 9 years of age.

lages.[11] In the United States, CDH is rare in Negroes[2] but frequent in Indians.[11] Kraus and Schwartzmann[12] found a minimum of 3% among the Apache Indians and Corrigan and Segal[13] a frequency of 6% among the Indians at Island Lake in Manitoba. In Europe, Bohemia, northern Italy, Tirol, Holland and certain regions of Germany are considered areas of high incidence and many nests of accumulated cases have been described. In France, more cases were observed in the countryside than in Paris.[2] Since attempts are being made to recognize the disorder as early as possible, statistics have been published from Sweden and England that refer to preluxation of the hip joint diagnosed by the click sign and other methods of early diagnosis. In this way, Palmén[1] arrived at an estimate of 0.57% and von Rosen[6] at 0.17%. In Salford, England, Barlow[7] found that about 1 infant in 60 (1.66%) is born with instability of one or both hips but that 88% of these children "recover" in the first 2 months. He believed that 0.16% have congenital dislocations that persist unless treated. Thus, even in recent years, there are great discrepancies in the estimates of the incidences of CDH or preluxation of the hip according to the tests and criteria used by the examiners. In general, an incidence of 1 per 1,000 can be assumed for Caucasian populations.[14] Approximately a third of the children are affected bilaterally and in the remainder the left hip is involved much more often than the right.[15] In stillborn babies and in babies who die soon after birth, congenital hip disease is more frequent than in survivors.[16]

It can be safely assumed that the incidences vary in families,[14] populations and geographic regions. Although epidemiologic observations must be taken into consideration in etiologic studies, their interpretations are not simple or clear, since genetic as well as environmental factors can be held responsible for aggregation of cases in certain populations or localities.

For the *typical and common form* of CDH, heredity has been assumed from early times because of predilection of certain families for the disorder. Beyond such observations, no definite genetic explanations could be given, since the expression of CDH is very irregular in families and kinships. Mendelian ratios are not obvious and in identical twins concordance occurs in less than half of the pairs. But monozygotic twins are ten times more often concordant in regard to CDH than dizygotic twins.[17] This suggests that genetic factors play a role—but not a decisive one—in the etiology of CDH. Years ago, attempts often were made to adjust the facts to Mendelian ratios but the methods were rather tortuous and the results forced. To give an example, it was said that CDH is due to "two recessive, not sex-linked and two dominant sex-linked genes in connection with selective, semilethal genes."[18] Despite the great labor and sagacity employed in such investigations, few adherents of such theories will be found today. The conception advanced by Putti[19] and by Faber[20] seems more attractive. They distinguished between dysplasia, a congenital predisposition to CDH and the overt disease, CDH. Faber[20] examined roentgenologically many members of the pedigrees of patients with CDH and found that dysplasia of the hip was present often in persons who did not have overt dislocation. Dominant inheritance of hip dysplasia could be demonstrated. The female predilection for dysplasia was not as pronounced as that for dislocation. This requires an explanation for the conversion of dysplasia into dislocation and particularly for the tendency to conversion of female dysplasia carriers. Hart[21] accepted the dysplasia concept and stated that classic CDH is secondary to a primary genetic dysplasia of the hip or flat acetabulum, and that dislocation is an incidental phenomenon. In addition to the acetabular changes, dysplasia involves all mesodermal structures of the hip joint. Whether or not a gradual transition occurs from potential to complete dislocation depends on the degree of hypoplasia of the acetabular rim, the sex, the position in utero and the forces of contraction and weight bearing. Dysplasia without dislocation is more frequent than CDH. There is a dominant hip-dysplasia gene with variable expression. In the female, the dysplastic hip can lead much more easily to complete dislocation than in the male, which can be explained by the more perpendicular innominate bone and shallower acetabulum of the female[21] and by a physiologic hormonal joint laxity of girls in early postnatal life.[22] Andrén and Borglin[23] considered a disorder of estrogen metabolism a causal factor in congenital dislocation of the hip. This concept adds to Hart's[21] idea of anatomic dysplasia, laxity of the ligaments, as a pathogenic element.[6] Smith *et al.*[24] thought that acetabular dysplasia is the result rather than the cause of CDH. Record and Edwards[11] questioned the importance of Faber's[20] and Hart's[21] data on statistical grounds. They evaluated various factors, especially environmental influences, related to the etiology of CDH, analyzing data from 167 patients born in Birmingham, England. The sex ratio was 1 male to 6.6 females. Twenty-five per cent of the cases were bilateral, and of the unilateral ones the left hip was involved almost three times as often as the right. The birth weight of affected children was somewhat lower than that of controls but prematurity was not in evidence. The liability of first-born children to dislocation was about double that of second-born and third-born. The influence of maternal age was less marked and maternal fertility was somewhat lowered both before and after the birth of the affected child. As in other series, there was a strong association with breech delivery, particularly in the case of males. The incidence among children born in the winter was double that of children born in the summer (in the series of Woolf *et al.*,[14] infants with the disorder tended to be born during the autumn and early winter months). The risk of the condition occurring in a subsequent child appeared to be 5%. Associated defects were present in 16% of the patients, but this high figure included major and minor malformations. The authors suggested that the stability of the hip joint is determined by multifactorial inheritance and by conditions in the prenatal and postnatal environment, such as attitude and activity of the fetus and of the infant. Breech posture in prenatal life and swaddling after birth are environmental factors that tend to produce CDH.

The *true (atypical, teratologic)* congenital dislocation of the hip is rare and usually is a part of general disorders incorporated into syndromes of multiple congenital malformations. In a series of more than 14,000 infants there were 2 cases of the "teratologic type" against 60 with "dislocatable or common dislocated hips."[15] It is present in utero and at birth and probably affects both sexes equally. Heredity usually is not conspicuous, but genetic factors sometimes can be recognized if the deformity is part of a hereditary syndrome. The fact that congenital hip pathology is more frequent in stillborn infants and babies who die soon after birth[16] points to a high incidence of CDH in children with multiple congenital malformations. In many of these, CDH represents a minor anomaly that is not emphasized. True CDH can be associated with torticollis,[25] spina bifida, agenesis of the sacrum,[26] knee contractures, fibular and femoral hypoplasia, clubfoot and other malformations.[27] It appears in syndromes such as arthrogryposis, arthrochalasia,[2] Ehlers-Danlos syndrome,[28] osteogenesis imperfecta, Morquio disease (Chapter 88), arachnodactyly and others. It has been seen in the syndrome that follows exposure in utero to large doses of x-rays.[27] Limited hip adduction has been noted in approximately 25% of infants with trisomy 18,[29] with a ring 18 chromosome,[30] with a 4/5 translocation[31] and with many other chromosomal abnormalities. Unilateral or bilateral dislocation of the hip was present in 25% of children damaged by thalidomide.[32]

In the newborn, hip joint dysplasia shows few differences from the normal conditions. There exists, according to Hass,[2] hypoplasia of the osseous nuclei, manifested chiefly in the acetabular root of the os ilium, whereas the cartilaginous portions of the joint seem almost intact. In contrast to the dysplastic hip joint, the changes at birth are very pronounced in teratologic dislocation. The osseous nuclei of the ilium, ischium and pubis are closely approximated toward the center. The socket is considerably diminished in size and flattened by accumulation of cartilaginous fatty and connective tissue. The femoral neck is shortened and shows almost no antetorsion.

When dysplasia changes to preluxation, the normal obliquity of the acetabular roof is increased. There is increased anteversion of the head and flatness of the socket, which predisposes the head to dislocation. Ossification of the nucleus of the head of the femur is retarded; the center of ossification always appears later in the affected side than in the normal. A slight lateral upward displacement of the femoral head becomes noticeable, the upper and posterior parts of the capsule protrude and the ligamentum teres is elongated and broader than on the normal side. Yielding of the cartilaginous roof and dilatation of the capsule become manifest. The extensor muscles begin to pull the femoral head from the base of the socket, drawing it upward to subluxation.

In subluxation, the femoral head may protrude more than half-way from the acetabulum but still remain, to some degree, in contact with the original socket. The femoral epiphysis flattens the cartilaginous roof of the socket, which becomes elongated and depressed at the site on which the femoral head rests. The femoral head also is flattened during this process. The roof of the socket passes, without any sharp break, into the lateral surface of the os ilium, so that its resistance to the femoral head disappears. As the femoral head glides farther upward along the inclined plane, the socket is divided into a utilized and an unutilized portion. Subluxation represents an intermediate state in the gradual development of complete luxation from dysplasia.[2] The femoral head moves over the rim of the acetabulum and loses its contact with the original socket. The luxation is always upward but it may be, in addition, anterior, lateral or posterior. As the femoral head moves upward, there is a turn of the cartilaginous limbus toward the center of the socket, so that its free margin is now directed toward the acetabular fossa. Later, the limbus undergoes atrophy or occasionally ossification. The original acetabulum becomes flattened by hypertrophy and chondrification of the fat pad located around the ligamentum teres, the newly formed fibrocartilage fusing with the original hyaline cartilage that lines the socket. A secondary socket is formed opposite the dislocated femoral head. The femoral head is reduced in size with medioposterior flattening. It may assume various shapes and be entirely resorbed in longstanding cases. The femoral neck may be changed in its direction to form a coxa vara or coxa valga deformity. The angle that the femoral neck forms with the transverse axis of the knee joint (anteversion) is, in the normal adult femur, about 10 degrees. In dislocated hips, anteversion may be increased. When the femoral head emerges from the socket, the capsule is drawn out into a tube that shows, at the upper end of the original acetabulum, a narrowing – the so-called isthmus. The upper portion of the capsule forms a hood over the femoral head and undergoes marked hypertrophy. The hood may fuse with the adjoining periosteum of the ilium. The ligamentum teres becomes atrophic and may disappear in some cases. Many anatomicopathologic studies were made by Stanisavljevic.[16]

The present concept of typical "so-called CDH" envisages a congenital dysplasia that is converted into a dislocation during postnatal life. Early signs and symptoms must be distinguished, therefore, from the manifestations of the fully developed disorder. Hass[2] enumerated the following early symptoms: There is a loosening of the hip due to flaccidity of the capsule associated with diminished active and exaggerated passive mobility. The limb shows external rotation and laxity of the skin on the medial aspect of the thigh, where deep transverse folds are visible. Resistance to abduction is an outstanding symptom. If, with flexed hip and knee joints, the knees are bent down toward the examination table and abducted and a slight forward and upward pressure is exerted on the femora, some resistance is felt when 45–60 degrees is reached (in contrast to the normal 90-degree abduction). When this resistance is overcome, a click in the hip joint is perceived as the femoral head slips into the acetabulum and abduction to 90 degrees becomes possible. The method of the "Ortolani click" was considered a very important early diagnostic sign by Palmén,[1] who described the maneuver in great detail. The increased *resistance* to abduction is accompanied by increased *mobility* in adduction and flexion and exaggerated inward and outward rolling movements.[2] Early roentgen diagnosis was based on certain measurements recommended by Hilgenreiner[39] in 1925, particularly on the acetabular angle formed by the Y–Y line and a line drawn through the visible edges of the osseous roof of the acetabulum. In cases of dysplasia, the acetabular angle was thought to be greater than normal, but Plummer[9] found that such early roentgen signs and the clinical outcome show poor correlation. Caffey *et al.*[8] demonstrated that the acetabular angles in the newborn vary to such a degree that the traditional standard of 30 degrees employed as the index of enlargement during infancy appears unacceptable. Difficulties in early roentgen diagnosis of CDH were also encountered and described by Palmén.[1]

Since early and successful treatment depends on early diagnosis of the disorder in its dysplastic stage, early signs assume unusual practical importance but there is no agreement on the symptomatology of neonatal hip dysplasia, i.e., the predislocation stage of the disorder. It seems that the early signs considered characteristic by orthopedic surgeons are not considered characteristic by pediatricians who examine large neonatal populations. It is true that abnormal skin folds, enlarged acetabular angles and limitation of abduction are present in children with CDH, but these symptoms can also be observed in a certain percentage of newborns who do not develop CDH.[8] The click sign described by Froelich[33] and elaborated by Ortolani[34] has been considered diagnostic in recent years, but Hass[2] stated that it is heard most often and most clearly in children in the second and third quarter of the first year of life and that it is not a constant sign of CDH. It remains to be seen whether the modifications of this abduction maneuver by Palmén,[1] von Rosen[6] and Barlow[7] are diagnostic of preluxation and whether they reveal all cases early without giving false positives.

There is less controversy concerning signs of CDH in older children and adults. Externally, prominence of the trochanter, flattening of the gluteal area with changes of the gluteal fold, protrusion of the femoral head, shortening of the leg and increased lumbar lordosis with protrusion of the buttocks are manifestations of CDH. The outstanding symptom of CDH is a limp, which becomes noticeable when the child begins to walk. If the patient is asked to stand on his dislocated leg and to raise his normal leg, the pelvis tilts to the normal side and the trunk is thrown toward the side of the dislocated limb to maintain the equilibrium of the body (Trendelenburg's sign). This shift in weight distribution is necessitated by the functional weakness of the abductors of the dislocated hip joint, the gluteus medius and minimus. The characteristic gait of CDH is a recurring Trendelenburg phenomenon in the standing phase of each step. In addition, there is a vertical gliding movement of the affected limb as the femoral head moves along the lateral pelvic wall. The abnormalities of gait become exaggerated during fatigue and are reduced during dancing or running. Lumbar scoliosis develops, usually toward the sound side, and adduction and flexion contractures of the dislocated hip joint complicate the deformity in advanced cases.[2]

Since typical CDH is not congenital but is present in the preluxation stage at birth, the distressing dislocation of postnatal life should be preventable. If all infants could be screened for dysplasia of the hip and those affected be treated to prevent migration of the femoral head from the socket, the common dislocation of the hip could be eradicated. Because of a tendency to familial recurrence, babies from families with a history of CDH should receive early orthopedic attention and x-ray examination.[35] Palmén[1] examined the hip joints of more than 12,000 newborn children and found 70 with symptoms positive for preluxation. These were treated immediately with fixation in an abduction position and at later re-examination, more than 90% were found to be normal. But Palmén[1] admitted that, left untreated, a number of these cases might have become normal spontaneously. In Malmö, Sweden, almost all children are born in one hospital. Since 1952, routine pediatric examination performed within 2 and again within 7 days after birth included examination of the hip joint, the snapping or clicking phenomenon being considered a symptom of "congenital dislocation." In about 24,000 births, 39 cases of congenital dislocation were discovered and 1 case was missed. Von Rosen[6] believed that the diagnosis could be verified by radiography if the picture was taken with the femoral head dislocated and with the legs fully rotated inward, each abducted 45 degrees. When the affected joint was reduced during the first 2 or 3 days after birth and held reduced for a period not exceeding 3 months, the joint was said to be stabilized and rendered normal. Von Rosen stated that the results were excellent in that the treated children, with the exception of 3, showed normal radiographs in the follow-up studies. Barlow,[7] in Salford, England, reported on more than 9,000 infants born in the Maternity Department. They were examined with a modification of the Ortolani test and with von Rosen's radiographic arrangement. Examination made soon after birth revealed 159 abnormal hips, 81 dislocated and 78 "unstable." But Barlow[7] found before 3½ days more than twice as many abnormal hips than after 3½ days, so that it seemed that about 60% of those diagnosed abnormal "recovered" spontaneously within a few days. Only 12% of those born with instability of the hip were thought to have congenital dislocation. Treatment with a splint begun within the first week resulted in a clinically normal hip and no case of congenital dislocation developed among these children. When one reads about such excellent results, one cannot help asking how they can be considered valid in the absence of well-established criteria of diagnosis and without agreement of the examiners concerning definition of congenital dysplasia and dislocation. It seems very likely that owing to the sensitive diagnostic methods used in such studies many infants receive treatment who would not develop dislocation of the hip. Because of the great responsibility of the examiner who is charged with prevention of CDH, control studies are not feasible, so that we do not know how many false positive diagnoses are made. Yet, if eradication of CDH can be achieved with mass screening and prophylactic methods, it may not be too high a price to treat some children whose tendency to dislocation may be dubious. The good results apparently are due to the great interest of the observers in CDH and continued observation of all patients suspected of having the condition.

Since the end of the nineteenth century, both open surgery and closed reduction have been practiced for fully developed CDH. Closed reduction requires manipulation under anesthesia and fixation of the femur in corrected position in a plaster cast. The child remains in casts for approximately 9 months and receives after-treatment in the form of a posterior shell applied at night for another 6 months. The chances of cure vary, according to severity, laterality, age and definition of cure, between 5 and 70%.[2] Open operative reduction is recommended for teratologic CDH with complete dislocation present at birth and for older children with high degrees of dislocation. For questions of treatment, the reader is referred to textbooks of orthopedic surgery and monographs.[2,15,36-38]

REFERENCES

1. Palmén, K.: Preluxation of the hip joint; diagnosis and treatment in the newborn and the diagnosis of congenital dislocation of the hip joint in Sweden during the years 1948–1960, Acta paediat. 50:(supp. 129)1, 1961.
2. Hass, J.: *Congenital Dislocation of the Hip* (Springfield, Ill.: Charles C Thomas, Publisher, 1951).
3. LeDamany, P.: Die angeborene Hüftgelenkverrenkung, Ztschr. Orthop. Chir. 21:129, 1908.
4. Pravaz, C. A.: Traité théorique et pratique des luxations congénitales du fémur, Paris and Lyon, 1847.
5. Lorenz, A.: Über die unblutige Behandlung der angeborenen Hüftverrenkung, Zentralbl. Chir. 23:1014, 1896.
6. von Rosen, S.: Diagnosis and treatment of congenital dislocation of the hip joint in the newborn, J. Bone & Joint Surg. 44-B:284, 1962.
7. Barlow, T. G.: Early diagnosis and treatment of congenital dislocation of the hip, J. Bone & Joint Surg. 44-B:292, 1962.
8. Caffey, J., Ames, R., Silverman, W. A., Ryder, C. T., and Hough, G.: Contradiction of the congenital dysplasia-predislocation of the hip through a study of the normal variation in acetabular angles at successive periods in infancy, Pediatrics 17:632, 1956.
9. Plummer, G. W.: Congenital dislocation of the hip, Pediatrics 11:28, 1953.
10. Stewart, S. F.: Clubfoot: Its incidence, cause, and treatment; anatomical-physiological study, J. Bone & Joint Surg. 33-A:577, 1951.
11. Record, R. G., and Edwards, J. H.: Environmental influences related to the aetiology of congenital dislocation of the hip, Brit. J. Prev. & Social Med. 12:8, 1958.
12. Kraus, B. S., and Schwartzmann J.: Congenital dislocation of the hip among the Fort Apache Indians, J. Bone & Joint Surg. 39-A:448, 1957.
13. Corrigan, C., and Segal, S.: The incidence of congenital dislocation of the hip at Island Lake, Manitoba, Canad. M.A.J. 62:535, 1950.
14. Woolf, C. M., Koehn, J. H., and Coleman, S. S.: Congenital hip disease in Utah: The influence of genetic and nongenetic factors, Am. J. Human Genet. 20:430, 1968.
15. Finlay, H. V. L., Maudsley, R. H., and Busfield, P. I.: Dislocatable hip and dislocated hip in the newborn infant, Brit. M.J. 4:377, 1967.
16. Stanisavljevic, S.: *Diagnosis and Treatment of Congenital Hip Pathology in the Newborn* (Baltimore: The Williams & Wilkins Company, 1964).
17. Idelberger, K.: *Die Erbpathologie der sogenannten angeborenen Hüftverrenkung* (München and Berlin: Urban & Schwarzenberg, 1951).
18. Isigkeit, E.: Untersuchungen über die Heredität Orthopädischer Leiden, Arch. Orthop. Chir. 26:659, 1928.
19. Putti, V.: Early treatment of congenital dislocation of the

hip, J. Bone & Joint Surg. 15:16, 1933.
20. Faber, A.: Erbbiologische Untersuchungen über die Anlage fur "angeborene" Hüftverrenkung, Ztschr. Orthop. 66:140, 1937.
21. Hart, V. L.: *Congenital Dysplasia of the Hip Joint and Sequelae: In the Newborn and Early Postnatal Life* (Springfield, Ill.: Charles C Thomas, Publisher, 1952).
22. Carter, C. O., and Wilkinson, J. A.: Genetic and environmental factors in the etiology of congenital dislocation of the hip, Clin. Orthop. 33:119, 1964.
23. Andrén, L., and Borglin, N. E.: A disorder of oestrogen metabolism as a causal factor of congenital dislocation of the hip, Acta orthop. scandinav. 30:169, 1960.
24. Smith, W. S., Coleman, C. R., Olix, M. L., and Slager, R. F.: Etiology of congenital dislocation of the hip. An experimental approach to the problem using young dogs, J. Bone & Joint Surg. 45-A:491, 1963.
25. Joachimsthal, G.: Die angeborene Hüftverrenkung als Teilerscheinung anderer angeborener Anomalien, Ztschr. Orthop. Chir. 22:31, 1908.
26. Blumel, J., Evans, E. B., and Eggers, G. W. N.: Partial and complete agenesis or malformation of the sacrum with associated anomalies, J. Bone & Joint Surg. 41-A:497, 1959.
27. Korvin, H.: Über die echte oder teratologische angeborene Hüftverrenkung, Ztschr. Orthop. Chir. 68:33, 1938.
28. Kanof, A.: Ehlers-Danlos syndrome, A.M.A. Am. J. Dis. Child. 83:197, 1952.
29. Warkany, J., Passarge E., and Smith, L. B.: Congenital malformations in autosomal trisomy syndromes, Am. J. Dis. Child. 112:502, 1966.
30. Palmer, C. G., Fareed, N., and Merritt, A. D.: Ring chromosome 18 in a patient with multiple anomalies, J. M. Genetics 4:117, 1967.
31. Shaw, M. W., Cohen, M. M., and Hildebrandt, H. M.: A familial 4/5 reciprocal translocation resulting in partial trisomy B, Am. J. Human Genet. 17:54, 1965.
32. Weicker, H.: 100 children with thalidomide embryopathy, XIth International Congress of Pediatrics, 1965.
33. Froelich, M.: Traitment de la luxation congénitale de la hanche chez le nourisson, Cong. franç. chir. 24:1048, 1911.
34. Ortolani, M.: *Lussazione Congenita Dell' Anca* (Bologna: L. Capelli, 1948).
35. Alldred, A.: Congenital dislocation of the hip, Lancet 2: 608, 1962.
36. Weissman, S. L., and Salama, R.: Treatment of congenital dislocation of the hip in the newborn infant, J. Bone & Joint Surg. 48-A:1319, 1966.
37. Somerville, E. W.: Results of treatment of 100 congenitally dislocated hips, J. Bone & Joint Surg. 49-B:258, 1967.
38. Dickerson, R. C.: Congenital subluxation of the hip, Pediatrics 41:977, 1968.
39. Hilgenreiner, H.: Zur Frühdiagnose und Frühbehandlung der angeborenen Hüftgelenksverrenkung, Med. Klin. 37: 1385 and 1425, 1925.

Other Anomalies Involving the Lower Extremities

Anomalies of the Femur

ABSENCE or marked hypoplasia of the femur is a rare congenital malformation. The isolated form accounted for less than 1% of the cases seen in the ACAC.[1] In 1939, Brussel[2] estimated that only 104 cases of this anomaly had been recorded in almost a century. Reiner[3] distinguished five types: short femur due to delayed development, with coxa vara; upper and lower end developed, with bony nodules in the area of the absent shaft; lower end present and united to the tibia; upper end present, curved and incompletely differentiated; and marked reduction of shaft but hip and knee joints present. Shands and MacEwen,[4] reviewing 19 defects of the femur, found all these types represented except the last. In 12 of these cases, shortening of the femur was associated with other defects, and 7 of these were bilateral. Ring[5] collected 38 examples of the defect, which he considered as the most common of those causing major impairment of limb growth. Half of the cases consisted of simple femoral hypoplasia, with moderate lateral bowing and cortical thickening at the center. Growth was less rapid than that of the contralateral normal femur. Congenital coxa vara with shortening of the femur can be unilateral or bilateral; if combined with marked shortening of the femur, growth of the lower leg is depressed also. Congenital pseudarthrosis is present in some of these cases; usually, the head of the femur is in the acetabulum with the shaft dislocated upward, as head and shaft are not united by bone. Most congenital defects of the femur involve the upper end. So-called complete absence of the femur usually occurs in combination with other limb defects. But, even in these cases, the tibia does not always articulate with the pelvis; the appearance in later childhood of a small ossicle representing the lower femoral end indicates that a rudiment of the femur was present at birth in cartilaginous form. Bilateral femoral defects were rare in Ring's series. A femur with two heads and two necks was described by Lichtblau and Thompson.[6]

Freund[7] pointed out that most of the patients with congenital defect of the femur have other deformities of the same limb. He described 8 cases with the main involvement in the femur but 2 of them were associated with reduction malformations of the upper extremity. In these cases and in those of Ring[5] there was no evidence that heredity played a role and the history of pregnancy failed to yield any clues concerning etiology. Associated skeletal defects were present in 5 of Ring's cases, absent or hypoplastic fibula and scoliosis on a congenital basis being involved. Kühne *et al.*[8] established a syndrome of defects of the femur and fibula combined with amelia, peromelia or ulnar defects of the arms. They collected 55 cases from the literature and described 6 cases. There were no indications that this syndrome was genetically determined. A history of exposure to radiation was given in 2 cases. This is of interest, since Warkany and Schraffenberger,[9] after irradiation of rats in utero

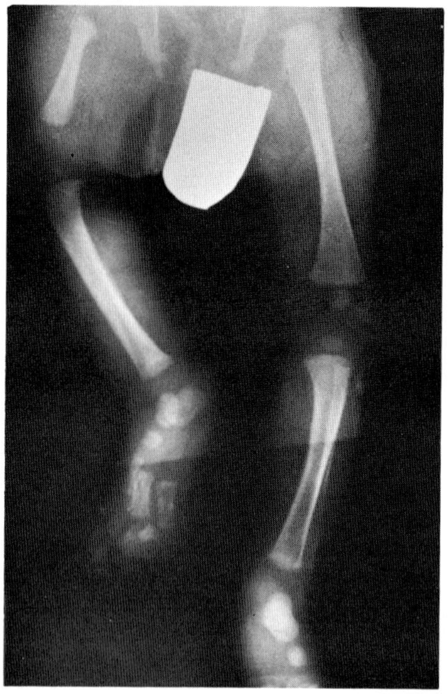

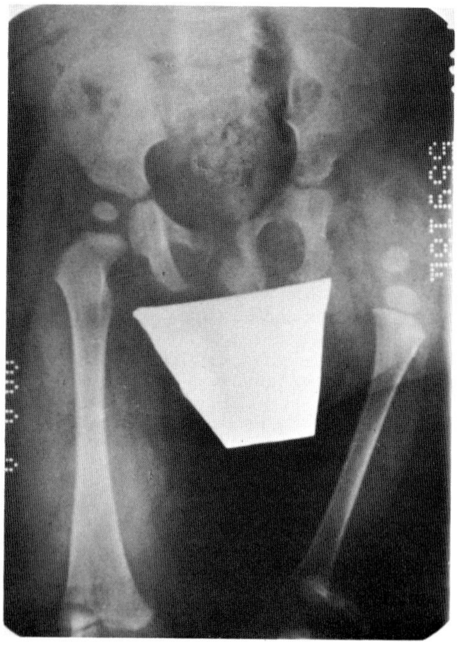

Fig. 102-2 (left).—Shortened femur and hypoplastic fibula of the right extremity.
Fig. 102-3 (right).—The left femur is reduced to a rudiment and the fibula is absent.

on the thirteenth day of gestation, obtained skeletal malformations, including short femur. Distally, there was a predilection for postaxial bones; ulna and fibula were affected more often than radius and ulna. This was in contrast to the syndrome obtained by riboflavin deficiency, which affected preaxial structures more than the postaxial.

The femur is involved in a syndrome observed repeatedly in children of diabetic mothers. In this "caudal dysplasia syndrome" the femur may be absent or hypoplastic. Usually, the sacrum and lower spine are deformed in various ways; deformities of the bones of the lower leg, clubfoot and facial clefts complicate the disease picture in some of the cases.[10]

Aplasia or hypoplasia of the femur was present in many of the children damaged by thalidomide.[11] Often the anomaly was associated with other skeletal defects, particularly tibial aplasia or hypoplasia. But, in a number of patients, the femur was markedly reduced, whereas tibia and fibula were normal (proximal phocomelia).[11]

Inequality in length of the two extremities represents the main problem of adjustment. Treatment varies greatly according to the severity of the shortening. Ring[5] discussed differing methods of alleviation. Guilleminet *et al.*[12] described 13 cases of congenital hypoplasia or aplasia of the femur and recommended prolonged and conservative treatment. In a case of serious femoral deficiency, Shands and MacEwen[4] removed the foot, fused the knee and applied a prosthesis. The result was satisfactory in regard to function and cosmetic improvement.

Congenital tibiofemoral subluxation can occur with or without hyperextension of the knee. The latter type has been observed in siblings.[93] The anomaly may be a component of the Larsen syndrome or of the otopalatodigital syndrome (Chapter 73).

Absence and Hypoplasia of the Patella

Hypoplasia or aplasia of the patella occurs as a constituent of the "nail-patella" syndrome, which is discussed in Chapter 103.

Absence of the patella has been observed in a syndrome that also includes contractures of some finger joints, toe deformities, ear anomalies, hydronephrosis and mental retardation. Three children with this syndrome had chromosomal mosaicism, some cells containing an extra acrocentric[90,91] or submetacentric chromosome.[92]

Defects of the Tibia

Before the thalidomide epidemic, absence of the tibia was much rarer than absence of the fibula and, with the end of that epidemic, tibial defects have again become quite uncommon. In 1932, Aletter[13] collected 120 cases from the literature.

The lower leg is shortened, adducted and flexed. There is pes equinovarus; the plantar surface of the foot is turned medially. The fibula is shortened and may be normal otherwise[14]; it articulates with the femur[41] or is luxated dorsally and proximally.[1] There may be deficiencies of rays[1] or polydactyly.[15] Absence

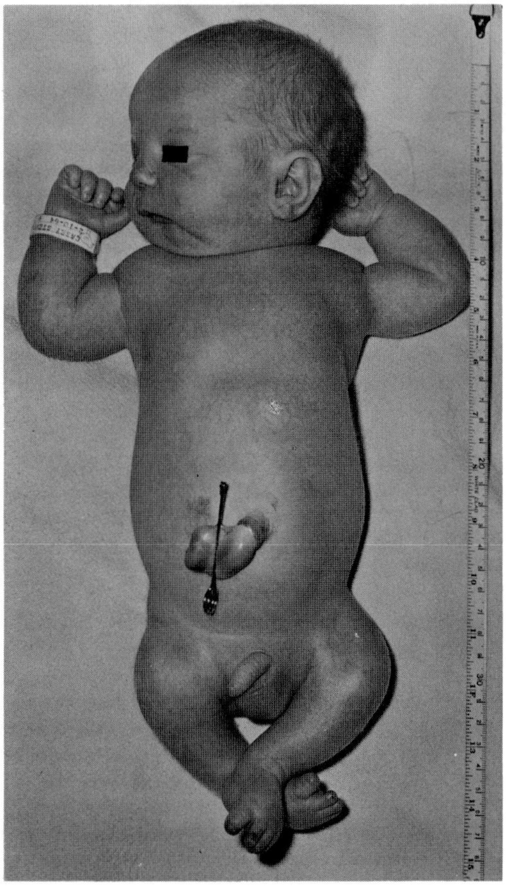

Fig. 102-4.—Shortening of legs with hypoplastic femora in a boy, the child of a diabetic mother. There also was dislocation of the right radius at the elbow. (The case was published by E. Passarge, Lancet 1:324, 1965.)

of the tibia is unilateral more often than bilateral and occurs more often on the right side than on the left[16]; the patella may be present or absent.[41] Partial absence of the tibia differs from complete absence by the existence of a proximal triangular rudiment visible in roentgenograms. The foot is inverted with plantar elevation toward the midline. Since the tibia supports the body, its absence represents a serious malformation that impairs standing and walking.

There is a predilection for the male sex.[16] Among Aletter's 120 cases, heredity had been noted in 3.[13] Heredity plays a role in some kindreds in which polydactyly is an associated anomaly. In one pedigree, clubfoot, polydactyly and tibial defects appeared in three generations.[17] In another family, 2 brothers with tibial aplasia, atrophy of the lower end of the femur and absence of the patella had reduction malformations of the hands and feet.[18] Freund[7] described 2 brothers born with clubfeet whose roentgenograms revealed that each had unilateral hypoplasia of the distal portion of the tibia. The mother had a split-hand and 2 of her cousins had similar deformities. There were no defects of toes in these boys but, in another patient of Freund's, distal deficiency of the tibia was combined with hypoplastic changes of the big toe. Thus, some of these cases are etiologically related to split-hand malformations. Absence of the tibia of the left leg was observed by Ollerenshaw[19] in monozygotic twin girls. These girls, who also had extra toes, were the eleventh and twelfth children of healthy parents; all the preceding children had been normal.

Associated malformations are frequent and strikingly heterogeneous. Davidson[15] described a boy with eight toes on each foot, very short legs with absent tibiae but normal upper legs. He had 5 fingers of equal length but there were no thumbs. This pattern was repeated to a certain extent in a case mentioned by Werthemann.[20] A woman with marked hypoplasia of the tibiae and thickening and bowing of the fibulae had eight toes on the left foot with mirror arrangement V-IV-III-II-II-III-IV-V and absence of the first toe. On the right foot and on both hands she had hexadactyly with duplication of the first digits. Dankmeijer[16] mentioned the following associated malformations recorded in the literature: polydactyly, syndactyly, absence of fibula on the opposite side, defective radius or ulna, hypospadia, hermaphrodism, hernia diaphragmatica, spina bifida and others. A case reported by that author had imperforate anus and mesenterium commune. Absence of the tibia, defective femur, polydactyly, hypertrophy of the penis and anomaly of the anus were described by Ollerenshaw.[19] A syndrome of cleft lip and palate, lip pits, webbing of popliteal fossa and other malformations can include shortening of tibia and fibula. An autosomal dominant gene is responsible for these pleiotropic effects.[21]

Absence of the tibia or hypoplasia played an important role in the thalidomide syndrome. The tibia was more susceptible to thalidomide damage than the fibula. But in a number of cases tibia and fibula were normal, whereas the femur was absent or hypoplastic (proximal phocomelia).[11]

Reduction malformations of the tibia as seen in man have been observed in mice as a hereditary trait. The strains called "souris luxées" or "luxate" have absence of the distal part of the tibia, curved fibula, preaxial polydactyly or oligodactyly, anomalies of the femur, pelvis, kidney and other defects. These mice have been studied in great detail by Carter.[22] Reduction of the tibia combined with preaxial polydactyly, an excess malformation, has led to explanations and controversies.[23] It is of interest, therefore, that complete and partial absence of the tibia can be produced experimentally in rats by riboflavin deficiency in a syndrome that includes oligodactyly but not polydactyly. General embryologic theories should include these experimental results.

Pregnant rats fed riboflavin-deficient diets give birth to young with a syndrome of skeletal malformations (p. 31). Shortness or absence of the tibia is the most frequent anomaly observed.[24] In the short tibiae, the ends remain unossified, whereas the central portion can be seen in cleared specimens as a dot or a curved rod (Fig. 102-6). The unossified ends consist of abnormal cartilage. The fibulae are affected less and the femora are nearly normal. In the upper extremity, the radii are affected more than the ulnae. The paws show syndactyly and brachydactyly. Pregnant rabbits treated with thalidomide give birth to young with skeletal malformations. There may be absence of the tibia or partial absence. In the latter case, the proximal portion of the bone is seen as a wedge with distal tapering. This picture simulates the partial absence of the tibia (incomplete paraxial tibial hemimelia) seen in man. It presents a phenocopy of the hereditary cases described by Freund.[7] In primates, man and macaque, thalidomide causes reduction malformations with particular affinity for the tibia; polydactyly may be associated with bone deficiencies elsewhere.

Treatment depends to a certain degree on the appearance of the fibula, which often is normal or overdeveloped.[14]

Congenital Pseudarthrosis of the Tibia

This term is applied to a condition in which a false joint exists between the two ends of the tibia. There may be local aplasia of cartilage and bone between the ends or there may be a mass of fibrous tissue, which undergoes bending or angulation in early infancy or in utero. In contrast to symmetric bowing of the legs (p. 957), in pseudarthrosis of the tibia there is

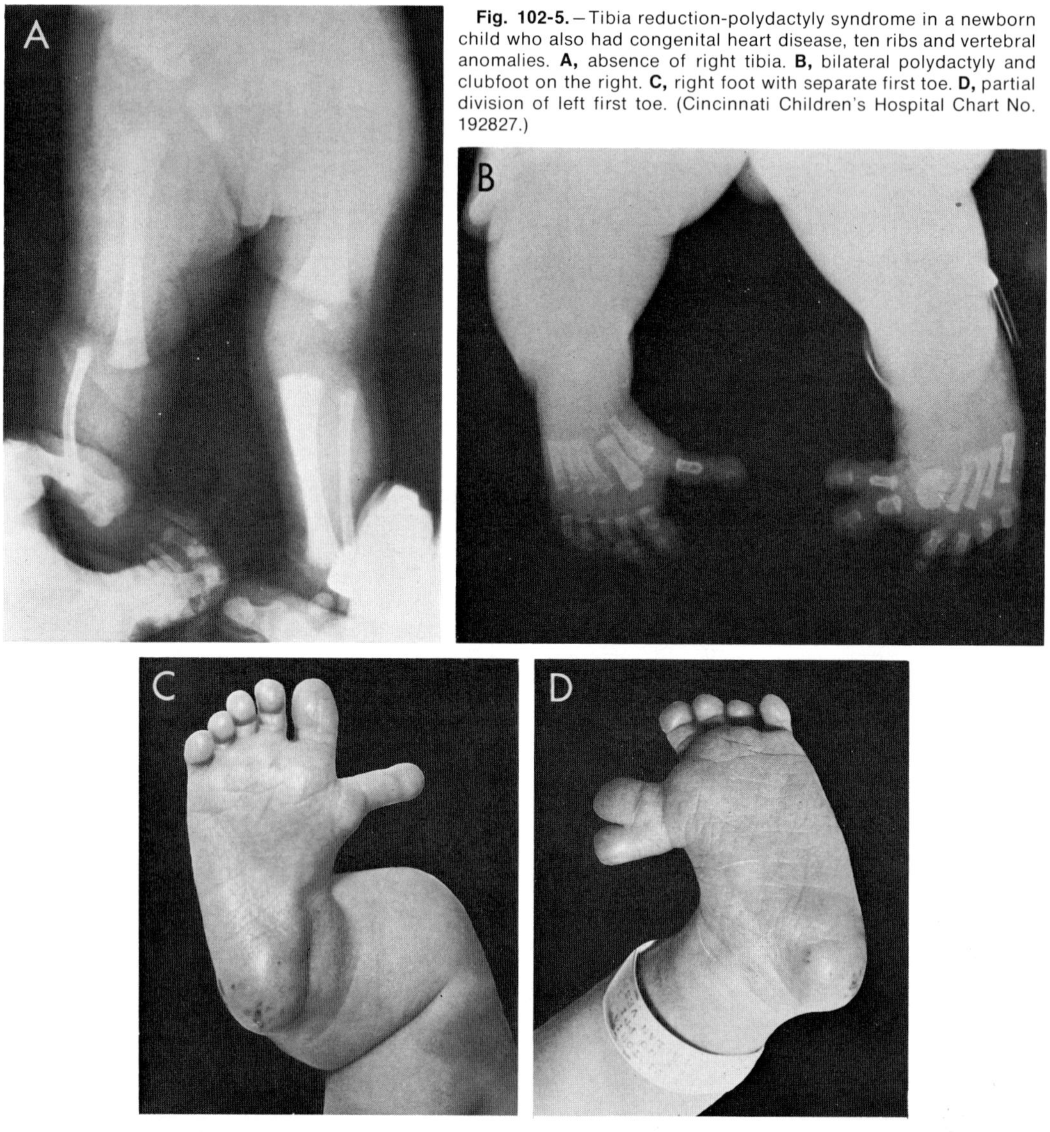

Fig. 102-5. – Tibia reduction-polydactyly syndrome in a newborn child who also had congenital heart disease, ten ribs and vertebral anomalies. **A,** absence of right tibia. **B,** bilateral polydactyly and clubfoot on the right. **C,** right foot with separate first toe. **D,** partial division of left first toe. (Cincinnati Children's Hospital Chart No. 192827.)

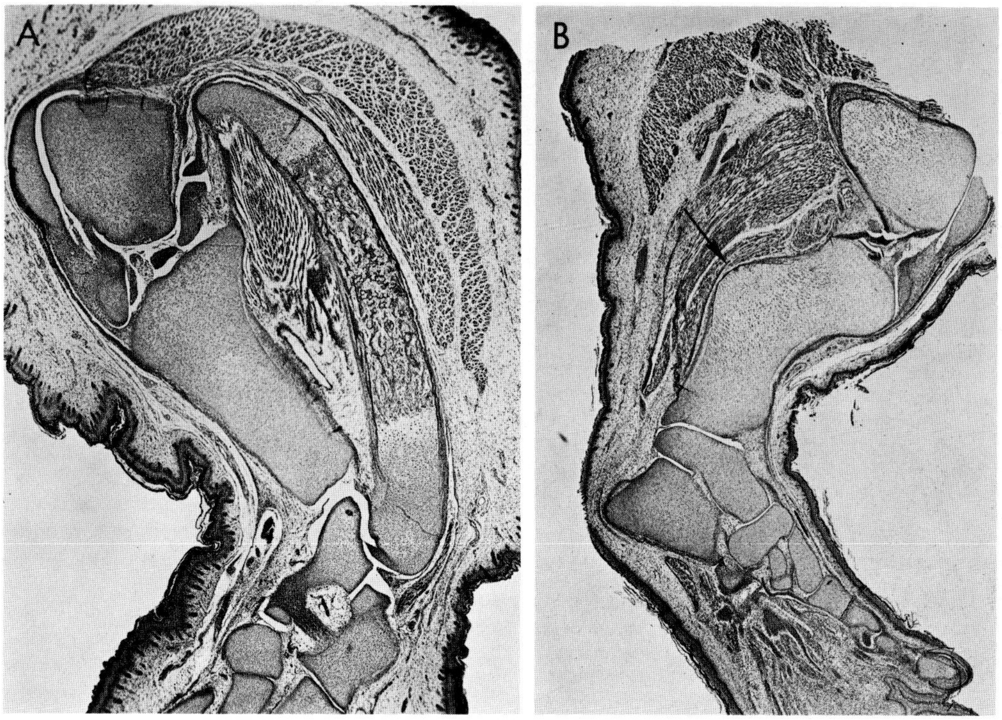

Fig. 102-6.—Longitudinal sections through deformed legs of newborn rats whose mothers had riboflavin deficiency. **A,** the tibia is reduced in length and failed to ossify. The fibula curves around the rudimentary tibia. **B,** the tibia is short and curved. Note that ossification begins in abnormal position on posterior aspect of the bone (**arrow**).

no clubfoot and no dimpling. Fewer than 5% of the cases reported in the literature have been bilateral. The patients often are born with slight bowing of the lower half of the tibia; roentgenograms show a zone of osteoporotic or cystic translucency in the tibia associated with angulation of a thickened fibula. The rarefied area is prone to fractures, which show little tendency to healing and union.

Many theories have been formed concerning the etiology of this condition. An important contribution was made by McCarroll,[26] who related the condition to Recklinghausen neurofibromatosis. Although only a part of the cases can be attributed to this disease, every case should be searched for symptoms of neurofibromatosis. Not only should the patient be examined for café au lait spots and cutaneous nodules but the family pedigree should be investigated also. This is more decisive in the diagnosis than the results of microscopic examination of the pathologic tissue between the tibial ends, since even in cases of overt Recklinghausen disease the tissue of the false joint may not be characteristic of neurofibromatosis. Boyd and Sage[27] found cutaneous manifestations in 9 of 15 patients, but neurofibromata could not be found in the area of the pseudarthrosis. There was only proliferative fibrous tissue with occasional bone trabeculae, poorly formed hyaline cartilage or fibrocartilage and marked thickened periosteum. These authors distinguished two types of congenital pseudarthrosis. In the first, cystic lesions are present in the lower third of the tibia, which is not significantly narrowed. In the second type, there is marked narrowing of the diameter of the tibia, with obliteration of the medullary canal and sclerosis. It is very likely that fibrous dysplasia (p. 875) is a cause of pseudarthrosis in some of the cases.[88] Tibial pseudarthrosis represents a difficult orthopedic problem, and early surgical treatment has been recommended.[88] Multiple operations may be necessary during the growth period.[27] Van Nes[28] reported good results of treatment; of 23 pseudarthroses, 19 had consolidated.

Tibia Vara (Blount Osteochondrosis Deformans Tibiae)

Blount[29] described tibia vara in 28 patients with an osteochondrosis located at the medial side of the proximal tibial epiphysis. The basic disorder may be congenital, but deformities appear after birth. In the infantile form, the varus deformity becomes noticeable when the child begins to walk. The bowing of the legs often was mistaken for rickets. The legs are shortened and the gait waddling.

The changes consist of faulty growth of the epiphyseal cartilage and delayed ossification of the medial portion of the proximal tibial epiphysis. There is a

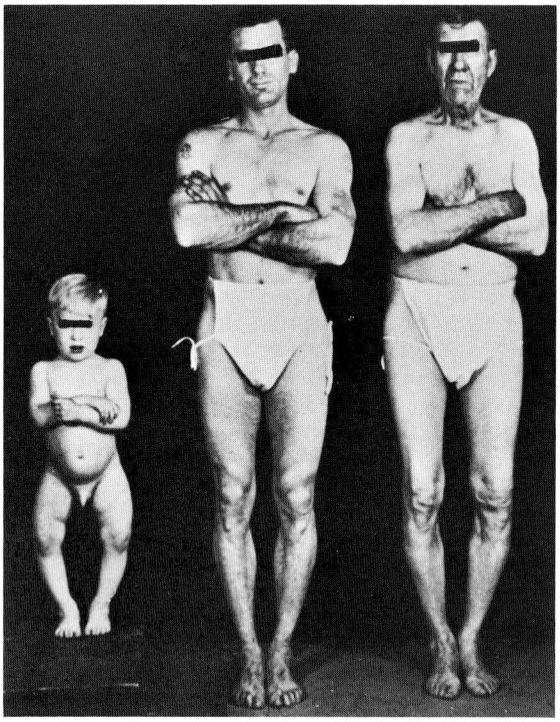

Fig. 102-7.—Genu varum in three generations of one family. The bowing was not corrected with increasing age.

beak-like projection of the tibial metaphysis, with areas of rarefaction visible roentgenographically. These areas consist of islands of hyaline cartilage. The adolescent type usually is unilateral and may be due to trauma or infection.

Bilateral tibia vara develops in young children with hereditary metaphyseal dysostosis. This disorder, the pathogenesis of which is unexplained, shows a tendency to spontaneous improvement.

Congenital Kyphoscoliotic Tibia

This orthopedic disorder is composed of different etiologic entities.[30] Congenitally bent tibia may be found associated with such skeletal deficiencies as hypoplastic fibula, absent fourth and fifth rays of the foot, absence of the foot and ankle and so forth. It may be associated with partial gigantism of fingers or toes and with café au lait spots and other signs of neurofibromatosis (p. 1252). Deformities of the feet often are present and dimpling of the skin at the apex of the curvature is observed frequently. Syndactyly is present occasionally. Pseudarthrosis may develop after birth in patients with bowing of the tibia. There is a mass of dense bone on the concave side of the bent tibia. The trabeculations in the dense area are arranged radially from the apex of the curve.

Prevention of fracture is the basic principle of treatment and no attempts should be made to correct the deformity, since growth from the epiphyseal ends will reduce the deformity. Correction of pes varus or calcaneus is advisable.[30]

Metaphyseal Dysostosis

In some persons of small stature with bowlegs, growth disturbances are noted in roentgenograms in the area of the metaphyses of tubular bones. Changes may be mild and simulate rickets[31] or be severe and deforming. Sometimes, if both epiphyses and metaphyses are abnormal, the disorder is not clearly distinguishable from epiphyseal dysostosis. Thus, the case of Cameron *et al.*[32] showed involvement of the entire ends of the long bones, but was classified as metaphyseal dysostosis. In other cases, the epiphyses were little affected.[33,34] In young children, the metaphyses show cupping, fraying and irregular ossification. Bowing of the ends of the shafts leads to coxa vara, genu varum and other deformities, so that rickets is simulated. Since antirachitic treatment does not give prompt results and transmission through two or more generations may be observed, vitamin D-resistant rickets often is suspected and metabolic studies are made. However, no chemical abnormalities usually associated with rickets and no renal abnormalities have been discovered.[34] Whatever the underlying process, it can be passed on like a dominant hereditary trait. Transmission through four generations has been reported.[33,35] Such hereditary cases may be mild and manifest themselves merely in short stature[36] or bowlegs, or they can be so severe that they result in disproportionate dwarfism.[33] Rosenbloom and Smith[37] described a kindred in which 24 members were affected. Symptomatic and objective improvement began as early as 3 years of age. Only 3 patients had disabilities that required orthopedic surgery.

Absence of the Fibula

This anomaly usually is associated with bowing of the tibia, shortening of the limb and anomalies of the foot. A skin dimple frequently is seen over the convexity of the tibia. The foot is in the equinovalgus position. In the majority of cases, one or several rays of the foot are absent[38] but, in some instances, absence of the fibula occurs in the presence of a normal foot.[1] A gradient exists from patients with partial absence of the fibula, straight tibia and a normal foot to patients with marked shortening of the femur, absent fibula, curved tibia and foot anomalies. From the orthopedic point of view, three types have been distinguished by Coventry and Johnson.[39] Type I includes patients with partial and unilateral absence of the fibula with little bowing of the tibia. This type often remains undiagnosed and makes up 10% of the cases. Type II is characterized by unilateral absence of the fibula, anterior bowing of the tibia with dimpling, foot deformity with absent rays and marked shortening of the limb. This classic form amounted to only 35% in the series of Coventry and Johnson. Type III, the majority of their cases (55%), consisted of bilateral absence of the fibula associated with other congenital deformities. These patients have a poor prognosis in regard to correction and adequate function. In Kruger and Talbott's[40] experience, the classic Type II was prevalent, amounting to 60%.

Complete absence of the fibula is more frequent than partial absence. The fibula—absent as a bone—may be represented by a fibrous band. Unilateral cases are more frequent than bilateral ones; the right side is affected more often than the left.[41] Complete absence of the fibula cannot be diagnosed in infancy by roentgen rays, since a rudimentary fibula may show delayed ossification. Freund[7] recommended delaying the diagnosis of absence of the fibula to the fifth year of life. If this is done, it may be found that partial absence of the fibula is as frequent or even more frequent than complete absence. The proximal or the distal part may be missing or, rarely, the diaphysis may be defective whereas the upper and lower epiphyses are present.

Coventry and Johnson[39] listed associated malformations in other parts of the body in 10 of their 29 cases. The upper extremities were affected in four instances. One patient had one ray missing on the opposite foot. In 3 cases, the femur was deformed. Spina bifida was associated with unilateral defect of the fibula in 2 patients. We observed a child with craniosynostosis, arthrogryposis and defective fibula (Fig. 102-8). A syndrome of defects of fibula, femur and upper extremities was described by Kühne *et al.*[8] (p. 997). A type of micromelic dwarfism is characterized by hypoplasia of the ulna and fibula.[42]

Fig. 102-8.—Roentgenogram of lower extremities of a boy with acrocephalosyndactyly (p. 895), showing hypoplastic fibula on the right side, no fibula on the left and bilateral clubfeet.

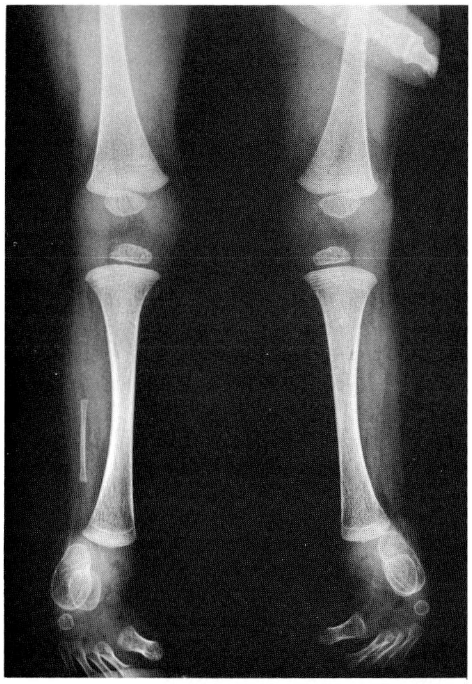

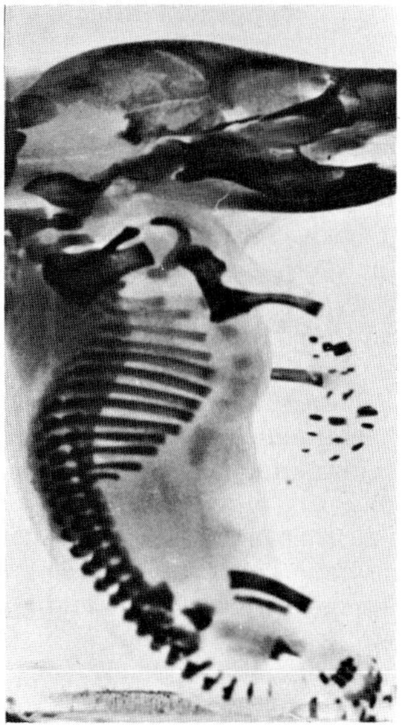

Fig. 102-9.—Cleared specimen of a newborn rat that was irradiated in utero on the thirteenth day of gestation. Note humeroradial bone and absence of the ulna. The fibula is short and hypoplastic.

The fibula is thought to be the most frequent congenitally absent long bone.[7,39] The etiology is not known in most cases. A familial incidence has been recorded in a small percentage of cases.[20] The micromelic dwarfism with marked shortening of the ulna and fibula that was mentioned above is an autosomal recessive trait.[42] But heredity is not manifest in most of the cases. A male patient had a twin brother who was normal.[39] One patient with bilateral hypoplastic femora and unilateral absent fibula had a normal child.[40] The fibula was affected in many children deformed by thalidomide but, as a rule, the tibia was damaged more than the fibula. In mammalian experiments, exposure to x-rays of rat embryos resulted in a greater incidence of fibular than tibial hypoplasia[9] (Fig. 102-9). In contrast, riboflavin deficiency resulted in more tibial than fibular defects[24] (p. 999).

In children, the prognosis for rehabilitation varies. As mentioned above, some patients are affected so mildly that the anomaly escapes recognition. Patients with bilateral involvement may have a more favorable prognosis if length discrepancy of the legs is not marked.[38] Conservative measures include application of casts and braces. Early excision of the tight band replacing the fibula has been recommended.[43] Other operative procedures include plastic repairs, osteotomy of the tibia and amputation.[38-40]

Congenital Dislocation of the Knee

This anomaly, which occurs bilaterally more often than unilaterally, is rare; there is 1 case for about 100 of congenital dislocation of the hip.[44,45] Although mechanical forces, deformity of the distal femoral epiphysis and shortening or fibrosis of the quadriceps muscles have been considered causative, it is much more likely that such anomalies are associated with or caused by the dislocation. The tibia is subluxated and dislocated forward and lateral or rotatory displacement may complicate the picture. The patella is dislocated and often underdeveloped. Abnormal attachments of ligaments and muscles can be present. Dislocation of the knee can be an isolated anomaly but, in the majority of cases, it is associated with other disorders. Dislocation of the hip, deformities of the foot, spina bifida, hydrocephaly, cleft lip and palate, hypoplasia of the fibula, dislocation of the elbow and the anomalies of the nail-patella syndrome may accompany dislocation of the knee.[44,46] In a review of 200 cases, 7 patients had a family history of dislocation of the knee.[47] McFarlane[48] described a family in which a mother and 3 children had genu recurvatum. Small patella can be a dominant hereditary trait that sometimes causes dislocation and flexion contracture of the knee. Congenital lateral dislocation of the patella poses special problems.[49] Lateral dislocation of the patella occurs in the nail-patella syndrome (p. 1016), in which hypoplasia of the patella and of nails is a leading sign. In some families, the knee anomaly goes with general flaccidity of muscles and ligaments[45]; in others, it is associated with muscle contractures. Murphy[50] reported a kindred with subluxation of the knee joint and finger contractures. Genu recurvatum and dislocation of the patella occur in the Ehlers-Danlos syndrome (Chapter 119). Luxation of the knee and of other joints, flat face, cleft palate and clubfoot have been combined in a syndrome[51] that sometimes shows a familial tendency.[52] Recurrent dislocation of the patella and of the shoulder also was seen by Carter and Sweetnam[53] in familial joint laxity.

There are several statements that dislocation of the knee occurs more often in females than in males[45] but this has not been confirmed in some reviews.[47] Breech presentation is more frequent in patients with dislocation of the knee joint than in the general population.

Treatment is conservative in some cases but, in others, associated malformations or general muscular or ligamentous anomalies render the prognosis doubtful.[44,49,54]

Clubfoot (Talipes Equinovarus)

Any foot deformity involving the talus (astragalus, ankle bone) is called talipes. Clubfoot (talipes equinovarus) is a composite deformity. The sole is turned medially so that the lateral margin of the foot touches the ground (varus) and the toes are held lower than the heel (equinus). In addition, the foot is adducted and plantar flexed in the midtarsal joint.[55]

Clubfoot (CF) is one of the most frequent malformations noticeable at birth. Debrunner[56] estimated the incidence of CF in the newborn as 0.6, Müller[57] as 1.3 and Zimmer[58] as 2.0 per 1,000. These incidence figures were obtained in Germany and Switzerland. McIntosh *et al.*,[59] in New York City, found 5.0 per 1,000 of the newborns affected with CF. This figure included live and stillborn infants with and without associated malformations. Eight estimates from various countries[45] averaged 1.8 per 1,000. Incidence differences reported in different parts of the world may be real or be due to variable methods of examination. In the United States, CF is seen more often by orthopedic surgeons in some southern states than in other areas. Stewart[60] noticed great differences among the various ethnic groups of Hawaii, where clubfoot was very frequent among Hawaiians and much rarer among the Japanese. The Hawaiians were also leading in harelip and cleft palate, whereas they apparently were free of congenital dislocation of the hip. Among 240 individuals treated for CF in Honolulu, Stewart[60] found ten families with a history of CF in more than one generation and seven families in which normal parents had more than 1 affected child. Familial CF occurred particularly among Hawaiians. Although this high incidence among Hawaiians probably is best explained by hereditary influences, incidence variations can also be based on differing methods of examination and case-finding. In an obstetric hospital in Zurich, Switzerland, CF was diagnosed in only 0.4 per 1,000 births in 1921–1924, but in 1940–1944, when the newborn infants were more thoroughly examined, the deformity was diagnosed ten times more often, i.e., in 0.4% of the births.[61] The latter figure agrees well with the incidence in New York City ascertained by McIntosh *et al.*,[59] who screened a relatively small number of children thoroughly and repeatedly. In 1969, Ching *et al.*[89] published a genetic and epidemiologic study of clubfoot in Hawaii. They distinguished three types of clubfoot (talipes equinovarus, metatarsus varus and talipes calcaneovalgus). The estimated incidence of talipes equinovarus was 0.57, 1.1 and 6.8 per 1,000 births for unmixed Orientals, Caucasians and Hawaiians, respectively. The incidence of metatarsus varus was 3.2 and for talipes calcaneovalgus 1.2 per 1,000 births for the general population; there was no significance among races in the incidence of metatarsus varus. In Scotland, talipes equinovarus was found in a series of 1,447 institutionalized mentally defectives at a rate of 22.8 per 1,000, which is about ten times that of the general population.[87]

Old explanations of congenital clubfoot relate it to mechanical forces, particularly uterine pressure. Although this explanation usually is attributed to Hippocrates, it is not certain whether "the father of medicine" considered the deforming causes to be within

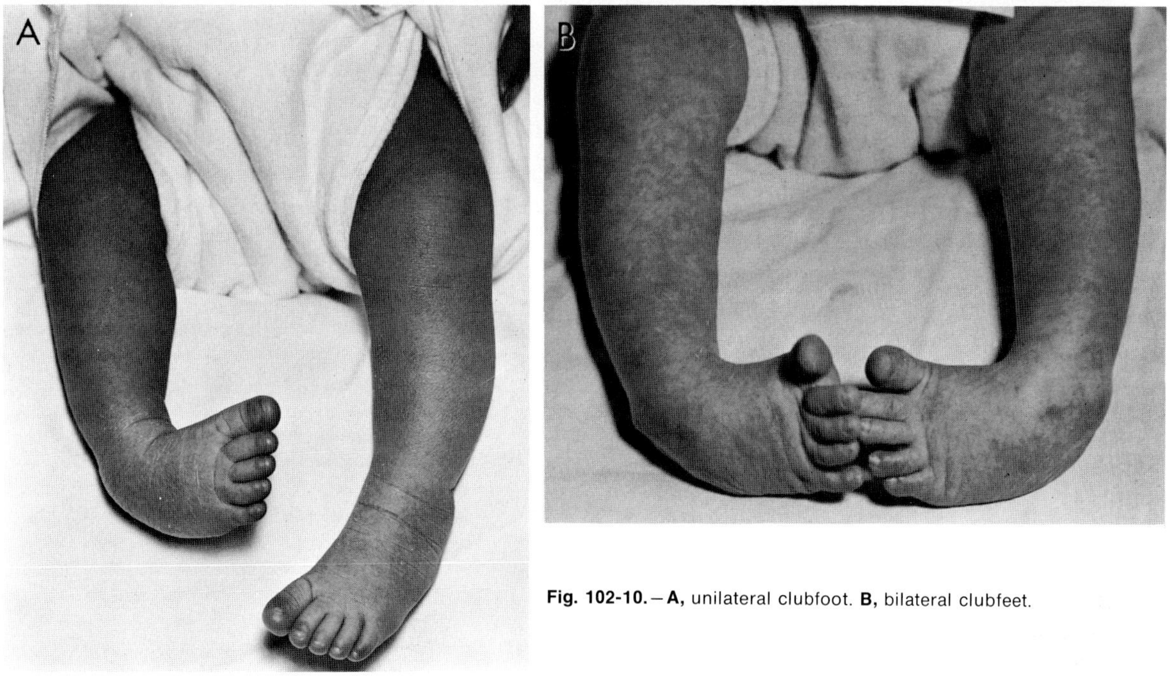

Fig. 102-10. – **A,** unilateral clubfoot. **B,** bilateral clubfeet.

the limb or outside. In fact, he apparently was quite modern, believing in heterogeneous teratogenic factors: "Modus mutilationis non unus est sed plures" (cited by Little[62]). The mechanistic ideas relating to abnormal fetal position in utero or to uterine pressure probably were quite acceptable in the nineteenth century. Boyer, in 1803, believed that congenital varus might be produced by improper intrauterine position of the fetus.[62] Cruveilhier[63] also believed that CF arises from abnormal prenatal positions of the limbs to each other and to the trunk, but did not hold external pressure responsible,[62] since there was no constant association with oligohydramnios or maternal trauma. About 100 years later, some orthopedic surgeons still maintained that the majority of cases of CF are caused by oligohydramnios and limitation of the embryo in utero. Despite early criticism of the pressure theory, Browne, in 1936, continued the idea of congenital deformities of mechanical origin and pointed out that the feet are most likely to be affected by mechanical pressure in utero.[66] Chapple[64] believed that abnormal uterine position forcing bone against bone can cause CF and that reconstruction at the "position of comfort" frequently explains CF. Wiley[65] stated that in CF the primary cause of the deformity is an extrinsic factor maintaining the foot in a deformed position and causing growth deficiencies in the long muscles. Torpin[66] pointed out that conditions that result in oligohydramnios (bilateral renal agenesis, amnion nodosum and extramembranous pregnancy) are correlated with a high incidence of clubfoot in the fetus. Among 400 cases of amnion rupture in gestation, clubfoot was noted in 129 (32%).

Clubfoot as an arrested and continued embryonic position also represents an old and understandable concept. Von Walter, in 1833,[62] stated that "talipes is a natural grade of the development of the foot, and embryos of three or four months very frequently retain one or both feet in this state. . . . The future external margin of the foot is at first drawn downwards; the sole, which is still very concave, presents internally; the future internal margin is directed upwards; and the back of the instep looks outwardly." This theory of arrested development was again advanced 96 years later, when Böhm[67] asserted that a severe CF resembles an embryonic foot at the beginning of the second month of gestation. Since he found the deformity accompanied by underdevelopment of bones and muscles, he assumed it to be due to a primary endogenous disturbance and not to external mechanical forces. But Bechtol and Mossman[68] concluded, after study of 2 fetuses with CF, that the deformity is not just a retained early fetal position and that the skeletal structures of the foot developed normally until displaced by abnormal muscle forces. At an early stage, many abnormal embryonic fibers were found in muscles that normally move the deformed foot. Adams *et al.*[69] confirmed these findings in a premature fetus. The muscle fibers that maintained the foot in the deformed position were of normal size, whereas the opposite muscles, whose action was presumed to be deficient, were reduced in diameter. Attempts to explain the deformity with the help of anatomic studies go back to the nineteenth century, when discussions went on, as today, trying to decide whether abnormal bone formation, muscle defects or anomalies of the central nervous system are primarily at fault. When Little,[62] in 1839, reviewed the literature on "clubfoot and analogous distortions" all these theories already had their champions. Little had a profound interest in this matter: "At an early period of my medical studies," he related, "I devoted much attention to the nature of these distortions, from the circumstance of my being afflicted with Talipes in the left foot. . . . Being particularly desirous of obtaining information respecting the anatomical condition of the limb . . . I obtained only the most discouraging opinions; the affection having invariably been attributed to malformation and ankylosis of the individual bones of the tarsus, the muscular contraction having been regarded as secondary." This conception was a fatalistic one, because it implied that "division of tendo Achillis" would be a useless operation. However, after many inquiries and travels, Little learned that Doctor Stromeyer of Hanover had successfully operated on 2 patients: "I determined on placing myself under the care of Dr. Stromeyer; and to his skill and kindness I am indebted for the restoration of my foot." As "a physician deviating from custom by the performance of a surgical operation," Little had already treated 82 patients when his book appeared in 1839. In his monograph, the history of the theories of clubfoot was related and case reports and good engravings described and illustrated an interesting chapter of orthopedic surgery as practiced about 130 years ago.[62]

Beyond the anomalies of the muscles, peripheral or central nervous lesions have been considered as more

Fig. 102-11.—Clubfeet in a case of spina bifida and other malformations.

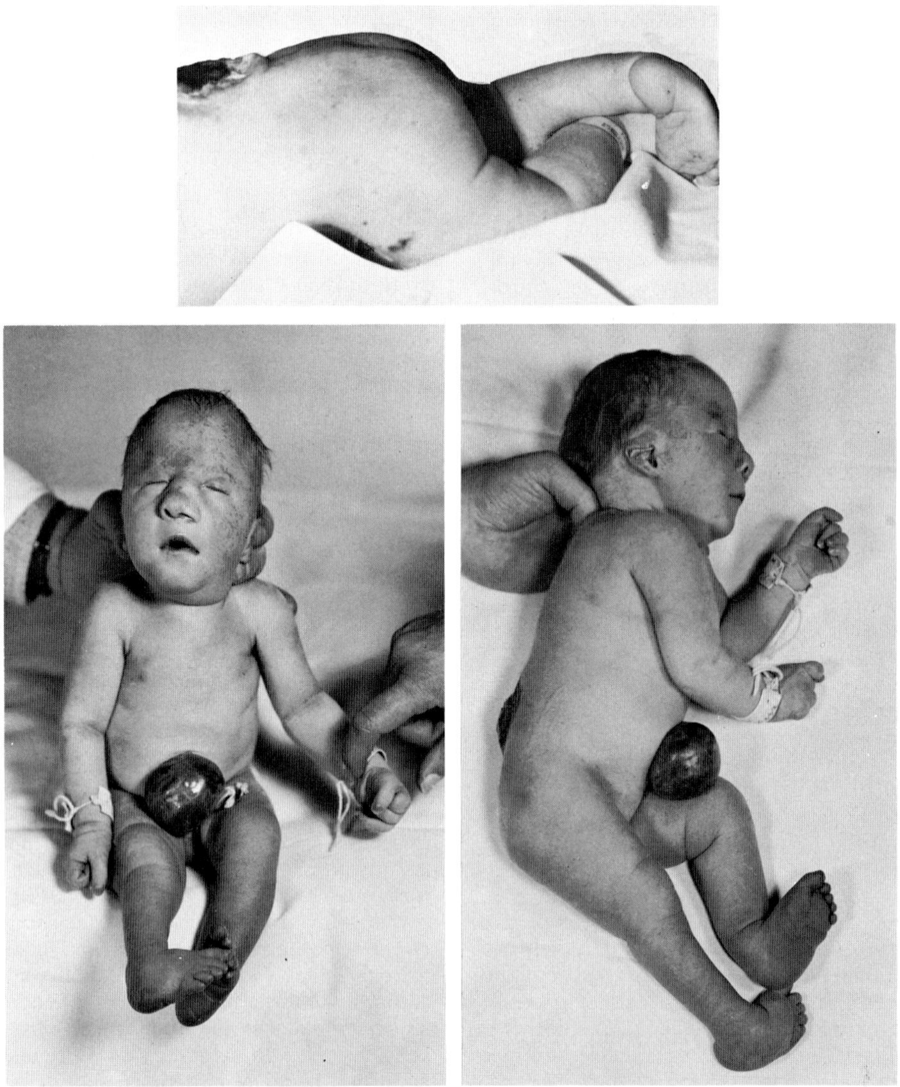

remote causes. Fetuses and infants affected with CF sometimes show simultaneously cyclopia, anencephaly, spina bifida, agenesis of the sacrum, arthrogryposis, Klippel-Feil syndrome, hemivertebrae and other anomalies associated with spinal deficiencies. These findings suggest that the skeleto-muscular imbalance of the leg and foot is due to faulty innervation. This may be true in cases associated with defects of the central nervous system, but since harelip and cleft palate or arachnodactyly sometimes are associated with CF, one is reminded that associated malformations can be merely coordinated and parallel effects of a common cause. In most cases of CF, no primary neurologic abnormality can be demonstrated.[69]

As in other areas of teratology, debates about endogenous versus exogenous causation have lasted for many decades without decisive results. There are many observations and investigations that point to inheritance of CF.[56,70-76] Inheritance is suggested by family histories in approximately 15% of the clinical cases.[74] Some pedigrees recorded in the medical literature indicate direct transmission of CF from parent to child[70,73] but this is rare. Other pedigrees showing skipping of a generation or other irregularities[60,73] have been cited as examples of irregular dominant inheritance, but in most of the cases for which genetic causation is claimed, recessive inheritance is more likely. There are observations of affected siblings, children of unaffected parents.[60,76] Parental consanguinity is relatively high in patients with CF, namely 3.3% as compared with 0.5% in the general population.[74] The fact that CF in Europe is relatively rare in cities and frequent in small and remote communities where consanguineous marriages are frequent has been cited as further proof of recessive inheritance.[74]

A marked preponderance of male CF patients over females, the ratio being 2:1, has been emphasized. This finding, confirmed in many serial investigations, is held against the theories of exogenous causation, especially those that attribute CF to spatial limitation during fetal life. It would be difficult to understand why male embryos are affected more than female by oligohydramnios or uterine anomalies. However, genetic explanations of the sex ratio in CF are also hypothetic and controversial.[74] The sex distribution is equal in unviable children.[58]

There is a marked difference in concordance between monozygotic and dizygotic twins. Concordance is about eleven times higher in monozygotic twins (32%) than in dizygotic twins (3%), a fact that speaks for the role of genetic influences.[74] But the same observations also show discordance in 68% of the monozygotic twins, which can be cited as proof of the importance of nongenetic factors. Such environmental factors, which decide the differences in embryos of identical genetic constitution and similar intrauterine development, usually are rather evasive though of great practical importance. Twinning itself apparently is not a cause of clubfoot. Siblings of probands as well as dizygotic twins of probands with clubfoot have a similar risk figure for clubfoot, namely 3%.[74,77]

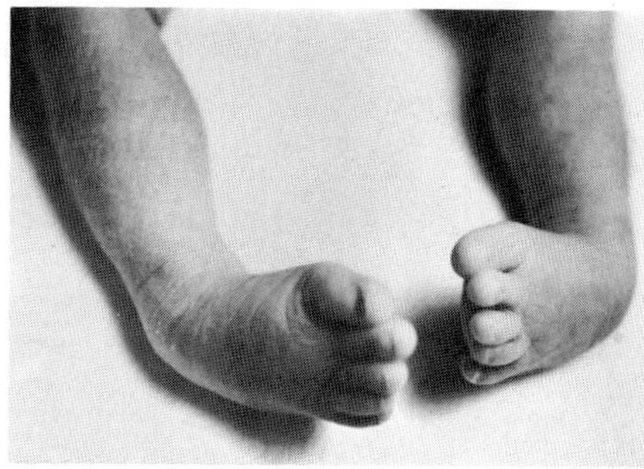

Fig. 102-12.—Clubfeet in a newborn girl with multiple malformations due to aminopterin intake of the mother (p. 96).

Approximately 20% of the infants born with CF are not viable because of severe associated congenital malformations,[59] particularly spina bifida. Estimates of clinical cases complicated by associated malformations vary between 10% and 23%,[56,78] the differences in these estimates being due to differing definitions of the term "malformation." In former times, associated malformations were cited as proof of heredity[56,71] but, since it is known that multiple congenital malformations can be due to environmental factors, exogenous influences must be considered in etiologic studies even if CF is part of a syndrome. Crabbe[78] found an incidence of maternal disease in 21% of his cases but this does not mean that these diseases caused the deformity. In most instances, the cause of CF cannot be ascertained ("idiopathic clubfoot") but, despite our uncertainties, we can safely subscribe to the multifactorial conception of Hippocrates (p. 1004) and state that this malformation may be a symptom of many prenatal disturbances. This can be best illustrated by the fact that clubfoot is a common constituent of such diverse syndromes as arthrogryposis, Möbius syndrome, chondrodystrophia calcificans, diastrophic dwarfism, craniocarpotarsal syndrome, Larsen syndrome, hemihypertrophy, abdominal muscle aplasia, cleft lip with fistulas and others. Clubfoot occurs in at least 15% of the cases of trisomy 18 and less often with trisomy 13–15, cat-cry syndrome (p. 340), deletion of parts of a chromosome 18[79,80] and others. Clubfoot was observed together with other malformations in children damaged by aminopterin, methotrexate or thalidomide. In experimental animals, the deformity can be produced by riboflavin deficiency (Fig. 102-13), by thalidomide (Fig. 102-14) and other teratogens.

To the pediatrician and teratologist, clubfoot as a constituent of syndromes is of greatest interest. The orthopedist usually pays greater attention to the more frequent "idiopathic" and uncomplicated form, but more recent studies by orthopedists included some of the unusual types and arrived at variable risk figures for different groups.[81,82]

The talus and calcaneus show the most marked changes. The talus is thick and heavy and the outer

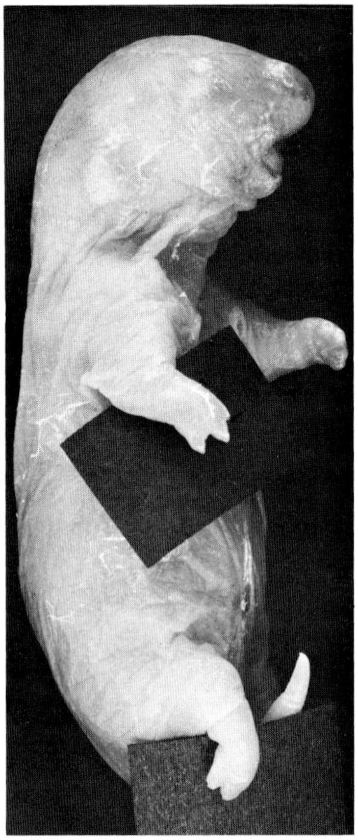

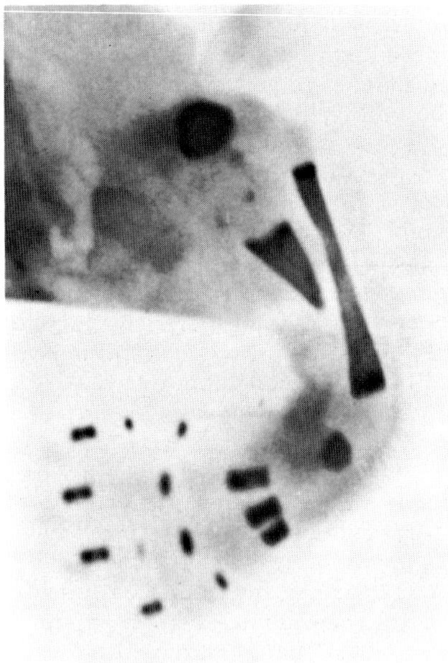

Fig. 102-13 (left).—Clubfoot in a newborn rat whose mother had riboflavin deficiency.
Fig. 102-14 (right).—Clubfoot experimentally produced in a rabbit fetus whose mother was treated with thalidomide. Note typical shortening of the tibia.

side of its body is turned forward. The neck of the bone is elongated and deflected inward and downward. The calcaneus is in a position of plantar flexion with the heel elevated, the anterior process looking downward and inward. The navicular bone is drawn inward and upward so that it approaches the internal malleolus. The cuboid also is displaced medially. The tibia is twisted inward and the fibula lies farther forward then normally.[1] The adductor and flexor muscles are shortened. The opposing muscles, the peronei and the extensors of the toes are elongated. The plantar fascia and the ligaments that bind together the navicular bone, the calcaneus and the internal malleolus are strongly contracted. The calcaneocuboid ligament also is shortened. The deformity may be so severe that the patient walks on the outside of the foot, which is turned directly inward, upward and backward. The muscle mass of the gastrocnemius is reduced and located very high, just below the knee, so that the lower part of the leg appears very thin.

Treatment of CF has been attempted since antiquity, and Hippocrates described bandages that he employed, apparently with great success. He gradually restored the form of the foot by mechanical pressure.[62] The method was modified by introduction of apparatus, stepwise manipulative maneuvers and retention devices. The different components of the deformity were corrected in proper sequence: adduction and inversion, then supination and plantar flexion. Operative treatment began with Stromeyer, who successfully performed tenotomy on W. J. Little.[62] Later, operative methods became more radical, with

Fig. 102-15.—Bilateral clubfeet in a boy with polydactyly of right foot, renal insufficiency and mental retardation.

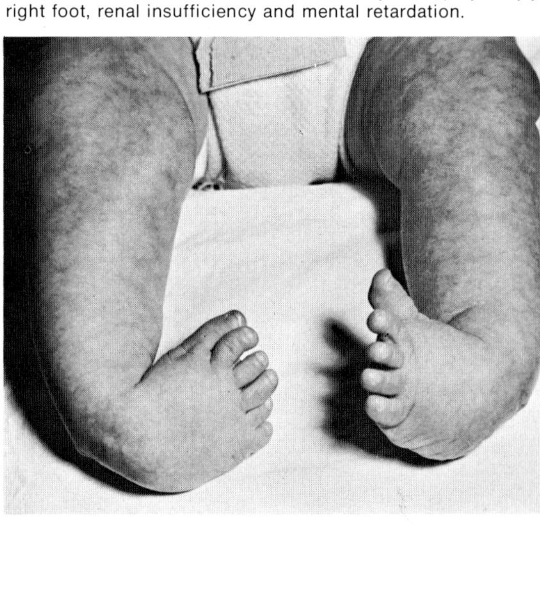

incision of all soft tissues, ligaments and osteotomy.[1]

Modern orthopedic measures attempt correction of CF by conservative means as early as possible. They consist of manipulation and application of plaster dressings. Operative methods are employed only when conservative measures are precluded by the age of the patient or the degree of the deformity. Treatment should begin about 1 week after birth, with gradual manipulation of the foot into proper position. As the foot assumes more normal positions, it must be retained there by casts or splints. Treatments usually are given by orthopedic surgeons at 2-week intervals. Active treatment may last from several months to several years, since CF may have a great tendency to recur. When the child begins to walk, special shoes are prescribed. If treatment is delayed for several months, manipulation becomes more difficult and painful, and anesthesia is required. In neglected or unusual cases, open surgical procedures are employed.

When clubfoot is associated with spina bifida, arthrogryposis or other skeletal defects, treatment is much more difficult and protracted.

The literature concerned with treatment of clubfoot is voluminous. Several monographs have been published in relatively recent years which deal with the practical aspects of diagnosis and treatment of the malformation.[83-86]

REFERENCES

1. Frantz, C. H., and O'Rahilly, R.: Congenital skeletal limb deficiencies, J. Bone & Joint Surg. 43-A:1202, 1961.
2. Brussel, J. A.: Congenital absence of (femur) bones of lower limb (case with psychosis), J.A.M.A. 112:1050, 1939.
3. Reiner, M.: Über den congenitalen Femurdefekt, Ztschr. Orthop. Chir. 9:544, 1901.
4. Shands, A. R., Jr., and MacEwen, G. D.: Congenital abnormalities of the femur, Acta orthop. scandinav. 32:307, 1962.
5. Ring, P. A.: Congenital abnormalities of the femur, Arch. Dis. Childhood 36:410, 1961.
6. Lichtblau, P. O., and Thompson, T. C.: A femur with two heads and necks. A case report, J. Bone & Joint Surg. 36-A:610, 1954.
7. Freund, E.: Congenital defects of femur, fibula and tibia, Arch. Surg. 33:349, 1936.
8. Kühne, D., Lenz, W., Petersen, D., and Schönenberg, H.: Defekt von Femur und Fibula mit Amelie, Peromelie oder ulnaren Strahlendefekten, Humangenetik 3:244, 1967.
9. Warkany, J., and Schraffenberger, E.: Congenital malformations induced in rats by roentgen rays, Am. J. Roentgenol. 57:455, 1947.
10. Kučera, J., Lenz, W., and Maier, W.: Missbildungen der Beine und der kaudalen Wirbelsäule bei Kindern diabetischer Mütter, Deutsche med. Wchnschr. 90:901, 1965.
11. Weicker, H.: 100 children with thalidomide embryopathy, XIth International Congress of Pediatrics, 1965.
12. Guilleminet, M., Michel, L., and Michel, C-R.: Les absences congénitales du femur. (Hypoplasies et aplasies diaphysaires), Rev. chir. orthop. 46:15, 1960.
13. Aletter, C.: Über die angeborenen Defekte der Tibia, Frankfurt. Ztschr. Path. 43:196, 1932.
14. Ferguson, A. D., and Scott, R. B.: Congenital absence of the tibia, A.M.A. Am. J. Dis. Child. 84:84, 1952.
15. Davidson, A. J.: A case of congenital deformity of the hands, supernumerary toes, and absence of tibiae, Am. J. Roentgenol. 5:434, 1918.
16. Dankmeijer, J.: Congenital absence of the tibia, Anat. Rec. 62:179, 1935.
17. Vonnegut, F. A.: Die eugenische Indikation zur Schwangerschaftsunterbrechung, Zentralbl. Gynäk. 48:2197, 1926.
18. Bertaux, M. A.: L'absence congénitale du tibia. Thesis, Paris, 1920.
19. Ollerenshaw, R.: Congenital defects of the long bones of the lower limbs. A contribution to the study of their causes, effects and treatment, J. Bone & Joint Surg. 7:528, 1925.
20. Werthemann, A.: Bewegungsapparatus, in Lubarsch, O., Henke, F., and Rössle, R. (eds.), *Handbuch der Speziellen Pathologischen Anatomie und Histologie* (Berlin: Springer, 1952), Part VI.
21. Hecht, F., and Jarvinen, J. M.: Heritable dysmorphic syndrome with normal intelligence, J. Pediat. 70:927, 1967.
22. Carter, T. C.: The genetics of luxate mice. I. Morphological abnormalities of heterozygotes and homozygotes, J. Genetics 50:277, 1951.
23. Zwilling, E., and Ames, J. F.: Polydactyly, related defects and axial shifts – a critique, Am. Naturalist 92:257, 1958.
24. Warkany, J., and Nelson, R. C.: Skeletal abnormalities in the offspring of rats reared on deficient diets, Anat. Rec. 79:83, 1941.
25. Williams, E. R.: Two congenital deformities of the tibia; congenital angulation and congenital pseudarthrosis, Brit. J. Radiol. 16:371, 1943.
26. McCarroll, H. R.: Clinical manifestations of congenital neurofibromatosis, J. Bone & Joint Surg. 32-A:601, 1950.
27. Boyd, H. B., and Sage, F. P.: Congenital pseudarthrosis of the tibia, J. Bone & Joint Surg. 40-A:1245, 1958.
28. Van Nes, C. P.: Congenital pseudarthrosis of the leg, J. Bone & Joint Surg. 48-A:1467, 1966.
29. Blount, W. R.: Tibia vara; osteochondrosis deformans tibiae, J. Bone & Joint Surg. 19:1, 1937.
30. Badgley, C. E., O'Connor, S. J., and Kudner, D. F.: Congenital kyphoscoliotic tibia, J. Bone & Joint Surg. 34-A: 349, 1952.
31. Schmid, F.: Beitrag zur Dysostosis enchondralis metaphysaria, Monatsschr. Kinderh. 97:393, 1949.
32. Cameron, J. A. P., Young, W. B., and Sissons, H. A.: Metaphyseal dysostosis: Report of a case, J. Bone & Joint Surg. 36-B:622, 1954.
33. Lenk, R.: Hereditary metaphyseal dysostosis, Am. J. Roentgenol. 76:569, 1956.
34. Evans, R., and Caffey, J.: Metaphyseal dysostosis resembling vitamin D-refractory rickets, A.M.A. J. Dis. Child. 95:640, 1958.
35. Stickler, G. B., Maher, F. T., Hunt, J. C., Burke, E. C., and Rosevear, J. W.: Familial bone disease resembling rickets (hereditary metaphysial dysostosis), Pediatrics 29:996, 1962.
36. Kozlowski, K.: Metaphyseal dysostosis; report of five families and two sporadic cases of a mild type, Am. J. Roentgenol. 91:602, 1964.
37. Rosenbloom, A. L., and Smith, D. W.: The natural history of metaphyseal dysostosis, J. Pediat. 66:857, 1965.
38. Arnold, W. D.: Congenital absence of the fibula, Clin. Orthop. 14:20, 1959.
39. Coventry, M. B., and Johnson, E. W., Jr.: Congenital absence of the fibula, J. Bone & Joint Surg. 34-A:941, 1952.
40. Kruger, L. M., and Talbott, R. D.: Amputation and prosthesis as definitive treatment in congenital absence of the fibula, J. Bone & Joint Surg. 43-A:625, 1961.
41. O'Rahilly, R.: Morphological patterns in limb deficiencies and duplications, Am. J. Anat. 89:135, 1951.
42. Lenz, W.: Anomalien des Wachstums und der Körperform, in Becker, P. E. (ed.), *Humangenetik* (Stuttgart: Georg Thieme, 1964), Vol. II.
43. Thompson, T. C., Straub, L. R., and Arnold, W. D.: Congenital absence of the fibula, J. Bone & Joint Surg. 39-A: 1229, 1957.

44. Katz, M. P., Grogono, J. S., and Soper, K. C.: The etiology and treatment of congenital dislocation of the knee, J. Bone & Joint Surg. 49-B:112, 1967.
45. Grebe, H.: Missbildungen der Gliedmassen, in Becker, P. E. (ed.), *Humangenetik* (Stuttgart: Georg Thieme, 1964), Vol. II.
46. Niebauer, J. J., and King, D. E.: Congenital dislocation of the knee, J. Bone & Joint Surg. 42-A:207, 1960.
47. Provenzano, R. W.: Congenital dislocation of the knee, New England J. Med. 236:360, 1947.
48. McFarlane, A. L.: A report on four cases of congenital genu recurvatum occurring in one family, Brit. J. Surg. 34:388, 1947.
49. Green, J. P., Waugh, W., and Wood, J.: Congenital lateral dislocation of the patella, J. Bone & Joint Surg. 50-B: 285, 1968.
50. Murphy, D. P.: Familial finger contracture and associated familial knee-joint subluxation, J.A.M.A. 86:395, 1926.
51. Larsen, L. J.: Multiple congenital dislocations associated with characteristic facial abnormality, J. Pediat. 37:574, 1950.
52. Kaijser, R.: Über kongenitale Kniegelenksluxationen, Acta orthop. scandinav. 6:1, 1935.
53. Carter, C., and Sweetnam, R.: Recurrent dislocation of the patella and of the shoulder; their association with familial joint laxity, J. Bone & Joint Surg. 42-B:721, 1960.
54. Laurence, M.: Genu recurvatum congenitum, J. Bone & Joint Surg. 49-B:121, 1967.
55. Steindler, A.: *Post-Graduate Lectures on Orthopedic Diagnosis and Indications* (Springfield, Ill.: Charles C Thomas, Publisher, 1950).
56. Debrunner, H.: Der Klumpfuss und andere orthopädische Missbildungen als Erbleiden, Schweiz. med. Wchnschr. 75:981, 1945.
57. Müller, R.: Über das Geschlechtsverhältnis beim angeborenen Klumpfussleiden, Ztschr. Orthop. 72:237, 1941.
58. Zimmer, J.: Das Geschlechtsverhältnis beim angeborenen Klumpfuss, Ztschr. Orthop. Chir. 69:126, 1939.
59. McIntosh, R., Merritt, K. K., Richards, M. R., Samuels, M. H., and Bellows, M. T.: The incidence of congenital malformations: A study of 5,964 pregnancies, Pediatrics 14: 505, 1954.
60. Stewart, S. F.: Clubfoot: Its incidence, cause and treatment; anatomical-physiological study, J. Bone & Joint Surg. 33-A:577, 1951.
61. Ehrat, R.: Die Missbildungen der Neugeborenen an der Universitätsfrauenklinik Zürich 1921–1944, Inaugural Dissertation, Zürich, 1948.
62. Little, W. J.: *A Treatise on the Nature of Clubfoot and Analogous Distortions* (London: W. Jeffs, 1839).
63. Cruveilhier, J.: *Anatomie Pathologique du Corps Humain* (Paris: J-B. Baillière, 1830).
64. Chapple, C. C.: Orthopedic Pediatrics, in Nelson, W. E. (ed.), *Textbook of Pediatrics* (Philadelphia: W. B. Saunders Company, 1959).
65. Wiley, A. M.: Clubfoot; an anatomical and experimental study of muscle growth, J. Bone & Joint Surg. 41-B:821, 1959.
66. Torpin, R.: *Fetal Malformations Caused by Amnion Rupture During Gestation* (Springfield, Ill.: Charles C Thomas, Publisher, 1968).
67. Böhm, M.: The embryological origin of clubfoot, J. Bone & Joint Surg. 11:229, 1929.
68. Bechtol, C. O., and Mossman, H. W.: Clubfoot: An embryological study of associated muscle abnormalities, J. Bone & Joint Surg. 32-A:827, 1950.
69. Adams, R. D., Denny-Brown, D., and Pearson, C. M.: *Diseases of Muscle* (New York: Hoeber Medical Division, Harper & Row, Publishers, 1962).
70. Adams, W.: *Clubfoot: Its Causes, Pathology and Treatment* (London: John Churchill and Sons, 1866).
71. Assum, H. W.: Untersuchungen über die Erblichkeit des angeborenen Klumpfussleidens, Ztschr. Orthop. 65:1, 1936.
72. Cavanaugh, C. J.: Clubfoot and congenital hand anomalies, J. Hered. 44:53, 1953.
73. Fetscher, R.: Über die Erblichkeit des angeborenen Klumpfusses, Arch. Rassenbiol. 14:39 and 140, 1922.
74. Idelberger, K.: Der angeborene Klumpfuss, in Schwalbe, E., and Gruber, G. B. (eds.), *Die Morphologie der Missbildungen des Menschen und der Tiere* (Jena: Gustav Fischer, 1958), Part III, No. XIX, Chap. 7, p. 939.
75. Mau, C.: Der Klumpfuss, Ergebn. Chir. Orthop. 20:361, 1927.
76. Schepelmann: Zwei Geschwister mit schwerer kongenitaler Klumpfussbildung, Ztschr. Orthop. Chir. 39:287, 1920.
77. Isigkeit, E.: Untersuchungen über die Heredität orthopädischer Leiden, Arch. Orthop. Chir. 25:535, 1927.
78. Crabbe, W. A.: Aetiology of congenital talipes, Brit. M. J. 2:1060, 1960.
79. Migeon, B. R.: Short arm deletions in group E and chromosomal "deletion" syndromes, J. Pediat. 69:432, 1966.
80. Insley, J.: Syndrome associated with a deficiency of part of the long arm of chromosome no. 18, Arch. Dis. Childhood 42:140, 1967.
81. Palmer, R. M.: The genetics of talipes equinovarus, J. Bone & Joint Surg. 46-A:542, 1964.
82. Wynne-Davies, R.: Family studies and the cause of congenital clubfoot, J. Bone & Joint Surg. 46-B:445, 1964.
83. Kite, J. H.: *The Clubfoot* (New York: Grune & Stratton, Inc., 1964).
84. LeNoir, J. L., III: *Congenital Idiopathic Talipes* (Springfield, Ill.: Charles C Thomas, Publisher, 1966).
85. Hauser, E. D. W.: *Congenital Clubfoot* (Springfield, Ill.: Charles C Thomas, Publisher, 1966).
86. Fripp, A. T., and Shaw, N. E.: *Clubfoot* (Edinburgh and London: E. & S. Livingstone, Ltd., 1967).
87. Primrose, D. A.: Talipes equinovarus in mental defectives, J. Bone & Joint Surg. 51-B:60, 1969.
88. Eyre-Brook, A. L., Baily, R. A. J., and Price, C. H. G.: Infantile pseudarthrosis of the tibia, J. Bone & Joint Surg. 51-B:604, 1969.
89. Ching, G. H. S., Chung, C. S., and Nemechek, R. W.: Genetic and epidemiological studies of clubfoot in Hawaii: Ascertainment and incidence, Am. J. Human Genet. 21: 566, 1969.
90. Warkany, J., Rubinstein, J. H., Soukup, S. W., and Curless, M. C.: Mental retardation, absence of patellae, other malformations with chromosomal mosaicism, J. Pediat. 61:803, 1962.
91. Nakagome, Y., Warkany, J., and Rubinstein, J. H.: Mental retardation, absence of patellae, and other malformations with chromosomal mosaicism, J. Pediat. 72:695, 1968.
92. Riccardi, V. M., Atkins, L., and Holmes, L. B.: Absent patellae, mild mental retardation, skeletal and genitourinary anomalies, and C group autosomal mosaicism, J. Pediat. 77:664, 1970.
93. Curtis, B. H., and Fisher, R. L.: Heritable congenital tibiofemoral subluxation, J. Bone & Joint Surg. 52-A:1104, 1970.

Some Syndromes Involving the Extremities

Arthrogryposis

(Arthrogryposis Multiplex Congenita; Amyoplasia Congenita; Myodystrophia Foetalis Deformans; Multiple Congenital Articular Rigidities)

IN 1923, STERN[1] briefly described arthrogryposis as "a real–though rare–medical entity" of congenital, multiple, incomplete fibrous ankylosis of the joints of the extremities, with complete extension of the arms and legs, not due to muscle or tendon contractures. The terms "arthrogryposis," which signifies "curved joint," has prevailed even though attempts have been made to replace it by possibly more appropriate ones, and doubt can be cast on the statement that it names a real medical entity. Stern[1] described the joint capsules as thickened and the muscles as underdeveloped, but believed that there was no genuine loss of nerve or muscle function, all reflexes and sensations being normal. He emphasized marked limitation of motion in the joints and delay in walking. Mental development also seemed somewhat delayed. The disorder was attributed to intrauterine periarthritis or abnormal intrauterine pressure. Treatment was discussed from the orthopedic point of view.

Long before practical approaches were considered, Otto,[2] in 1841, reported a case in which all the joints of the extremities were in complete flexion, and somewhat later Guérin[3] attributed congenital contractures of the joints to prenatal cerebral or spinal disturbances. Many names suggested for this disorder have been enumerated by James.[4] From the orthopedic point of view, arthrogryposis may appear as a disease entity, but the pathologist and teratologist recognize a variety of entities in children with congenital articular rigidities. Associated anomalies of known etiology often betray the diverse origin of articular anomalies that appear similar clinically.

Arthrogryposis is rare. In 1951, James[4] found 240 cases reported in the medical literature, and Mackenzie[5] based his report on 37 patients seen during 22 years at The Hospital for Sick Children in London. At the Shriners' Hospital for Crippled Children in Chicago, 68 patients were treated for this condition during a period of 31 years.[6]

Many theories have been advanced to explain the origin of congenital articular rigidities but no convincing general explanation has been found. It seems likely that congenital rigidities of the joints can result from a variety of adverse prenatal situations, so that one can possibly ascertain causative factors responsible for some but not for all cases.

Oligohydramnios, hydramnios, increased intrauterine pressure and mechanical compression of the fetus were accused by early authors. Periarthritis and inflammation of muscles in prenatal life have been considered, but pathologists cannot find any evidence for this. Drachman and Coulombre[7] considered temporary immobilization of the embryo a possible cause of congenital ankylosis of the joints, and experiments with chick embryos treated with curare were cited in support of this hypothesis. There is no indication that poliomyelitis is a causative factor. Rubella in early pregnancy occurred in 1 case[6] and exposure of the mother to rubella in 2.[6,8] In some instances, bleeding in early pregnancy has been reported. Fetal movements were weak sometimes[9,10] but not always.[6] Many children with arthrogryposis are born with very low birth weights. Some of them are prematures but others probably have intrauterine growth retardation (p. 134). The child reported by Hanemann and Feye[11] was born at term weighing only 2,100 Gm. Unfortunately, recording of a low birth weight often is not accompanied by an estimate of the gestation time, so that proof of intrauterine growth retardation is difficult. Mackenzie[5] stated that in 10 of his 37 cases the mothers were small during their pregnancy and that fetal movements were weak. Such findings are characteristic for intrauterine growth retardation. In one case,[9] a child with arthrogryposis weighed less than 4 pounds at birth, which was said to have occurred 1 month before term. His intrauterine growth retardation was demonstrated by his normal identical twin brother, who weighed more than 6 pounds at birth.

According to most authors, heredity plays no role in the etiology of arthrogryposis, since most cases appear sporadically in otherwise normal kinships. In the series of Mead *et al.*[6] and that of Mackenzie,[5] who reviewed the histories of 40 and 37 cases respectively, there were no findings suggesting a genetic determination. There are, however, several families on record in which more than 1 child was affected. A most remarkable kindred with 23 cases of arthrogryposis was reported by Lebenthal *et al.*[44] The high consanguinity rate among parents of affected children and the existence of 20 normal offspring of 3 affected males indicated autosomal recessive inheritance. Jacobson *et al.*[12] mentioned that of 13 patients there were 2 who had siblings with similar but milder forms of the disease. Ek,[13] reporting 8 cases of arthrogryposis with cerebral lesions, described 2 siblings whose parents were second cousins and 1 girl whose sister had died previously suffering from articular contractures and cerebral lesions like the patient. Kite[14] mentioned a boy and a girl with arthrogryposis whose healthy parents were first cousins. We observed in the Cincinnati Children's Hospital a girl with typical arthrogryposis whose mother had had another girl with the same disease, and Turpin *et al.*[15] saw the disorder in siblings. But Friedlander *et al.*,[16] who reported on 45 patients and 185 blood relatives, encountered recurrence only once as 2 sisters of one family were affected. Fisher *et al.*,[40] who studied 26 patients with arthrogryposis, found none of the relatives similarly affected. They noted a significantly high birth order of the patients, elevated paternal age and a high incidence of fetal wastage in other pregnancies of the mothers. Other cases with symptoms of arthrogryposis in more than one member of a family showed associated symptoms suggesting etiologic entities differing from the common type. Banker *et al.*[17] reported "arthrogryposis multiplex due to congenital muscular dystrophy" in a boy who was followed by a brother born with hypotonic flaccid weakness without contracture. These cases, which probably represented congenital progressive muscular dystrophy, differed in many respects from those with typical arthrogryposis multiplex congenita. Drachman and Banker[8] believed that these and similar cases of muscular dystrophy are always males showing kyphoscoliosis and a chest deformity. They may or may not have contractures of the extremities, which differs from typical arthrogryposis. The nervous system is not primarily affected in such patients (p. 1032). Sprofkin and Hillman[18] described a boy with Möbius syndrome and arthrogryposis whose sister had arthrogryposis of the upper and lower extremities. A different type of arthrogryposis is now named "diastrophic dwarfism" (p. 801). Kite[14] treated a girl for clubbed hands and extreme flat feet who later had a son with stiff joints, clubbed hands and one clubfoot. Another mother with moderately severe arthrogryposis had a daughter with similar deformities. Kite[14] saw also clubbed hands and clubbed feet transmitted from a father to his son. Although these cases were reported as arthrogryposis, it is not clear whether they can be equated with the severe crippling arthrogryposis described by other authors. In the family reported by Pasma and Wildervanck,[19] in which rigidity of the elbows and knee joints was transmitted through three generations, there were osseous changes showing that the condition was a "pseudo-arthrogryposis" not representative of the disorder under discussion. Contractures of joints were present in children showing such dominant traits as mandibulofacial dysostosis[20] (p. 650) or tuberous sclerosis (p. 1260).[21] Dominant inheritance with variable expressivity was suggested in a case of Aase and Smith,[37] in which a father with joint anomalies had 2 children with arthrogryposis, cleft palate and hydrocephaly. A pair of monozygotic twins concordant in regard to arthrogryposis has been reported.[38] Against this are reports of at least 3 pairs of monozygotic discordant twins,[9,14] so that no conclusions concerning etiology can be drawn from these twin observations. Arthrogryposis was a manifestation in a child with trisomy 18.[22] Environmental intrauterine damage, such as poisoning of the mother with illuminating gas,[23] resulted in atypical arthrogryposis in a child and arthrogryposis has been reported in an infant following treatment of maternal tetanus with the neuromuscular blocking agent tubocurarine.[41] This is of interest because of the previously mentioned joint anomalies produced in chicks by curare. Feeding of lupine and lead to cows produced a "twisted arthrogryposis" in calves.[24] A small epidemic of arthrogryposis, hydranencephaly and blindness in calves was reported by Whittem[25] from Australia, suggesting an environmental causation. The description of arthrogryposis occurring in eight different breeds of cattle closely resembled typical infantile arthrogryposis of neural origin (p. 1013). The joints, the muscles and the spinal cords were very similar to corresponding parts seen in children. Blindness and hydranencephaly, which occur commonly in calves with arthrogryposis, constitute more serious nervous complications than those usually seen in children. Whittem[25] expressed the opinion that absence of ventral horn cells – or a reduction in their number – is the primary lesion and that muscle and joint changes are the result. The disease seems to be degenerative rather than due to failure of formation and differentiation, since it appeared that degenerative changes affect previously normal nerve tissue. There was no evidence pointing to a genetic basis for the disease. Arthrogryposis in sheep seems to be a different condition and may represent the equivalent of congenital muscular dystrophy in man (p. 1032). In lambs examined,[26] there were no changes in the central or peripheral nervous system but the muscles were dystrophic. This condition is genetically determined and is inherited in sheep as an autosomal recessive trait. But locoweeds (*Astragalus* and *Oxytropis*) ingested by pregnant sheep can induce contracted tendons, anterior flexure with hypermobility of the hock joints and flexure of the forelimbs in some of their offspring.[39]

In summary, it can be stated that the etiology of most cases of arthrogryposis remains obscure. There are suggestions of recessive inheritance by involvement of siblings, particularly if they are children of consanguineous marriages.[13,14] There is a possibility that some sporadic cases represent fresh mutations that can be transmitted like a dominant trait,[14] and there are atypical cases (congenital muscular dystrophy) that seem to be due to a sex-linked recessive gene.[17] The situation probably is so confusing because arthrogryposis can be a symptom of many disorders. For genetic counseling, it will be well to remember that most cases are and remain sporadic in families, but in exceptional cases phenotypically normal parents can have more than one affected child and mildly affected persons have transmitted the anomalies to their offspring.

Biopsies and necropsies performed in children showed that the articular rigidities are due to changes in the ligaments, capsules, muscles and primarily the nervous system. There is increased fibrosis around the joints, lack of loose connective tissue under the skin and shortening of the ligaments. Fixation is fibrous and detachment of muscles does not increase articular mobility greatly. The muscles around the affected joints are hypoplastic, pale and soft. In advanced stages of degeneration they are represented by pale, gelatinous tissue strands or they are entirely replaced by fat.[27] Histologically, the muscles show changes of denervation atrophy. Groups of small muscle fibers lie adjacent to normal or large fibers. Interstitial fibrous connective tissue and fatty infiltration are prominent in sections of affected muscles. Drachman and Banker,[8] reviewing 12 cases resulting in necropsies, concluded that typical arthrogryposis multiplex congenita is primarily a disorder of the central nervous system – of the motor neurons of portions of the spinal cord. There is a massive loss of anterior horn cells, reduction of the diameter of the spinal cord, particularly at the cervical and lumbar enlargements, and decrease in thickness of the ventral spinal nerve roots. A moderate increase of glial elements with some signs of neurophagia is seen in the anterior horns. In the case reported by Drachman and Banker,[8] not only the anterior horns of the spinal cord but also the motor nuclei of the trigeminal nerves showed a severe loss of neurons. In other cases,[13,27-29] gross changes in the central nervous system were found. Cortical atrophy, abnormal cortical convolutions, microgyria, enlarged ventricles or myelomeningocele have been observed in some patients with arthrogryposis. The fact that arthrogryposis sometimes is found together with agenesis of the sacrum (p. 923) and related malformations of the spine suggests that the changes in the nervous system in arthrogryposis are due to faulty segmentation or formation of the neural axis and the spine. In the atypical case of Pollak,[23] multiple central canals were found throughout the spinal cord.

The articular immobility due to congenital muscular dystrophy can progress in the presence of a normal central nervous system. Histologically, muscles show striking variation in fiber size within the fascicles, and muscle fibers generally are replaced by fibrous and adipose connective tissue.[17]

Many children with arthrogryposis are born with breech presentation.[10,11,27,30] Of 13 cases collected by Jacobson *et al.*[12] there were four breech presentations; Mead *et al.*[6] recorded breech presentation in 36% and footling presentation in 7.5% of their cases. In one instance, breech presentation was demonstrated in a 7-month fetus[31] and the position remained the same until term. In another case, the affected twin was born in breech position, whereas his normal twin was a vertex presentation.[9] Cyanosis following birth is not rare. Birth fractures occur occasionally.[10,17,30]

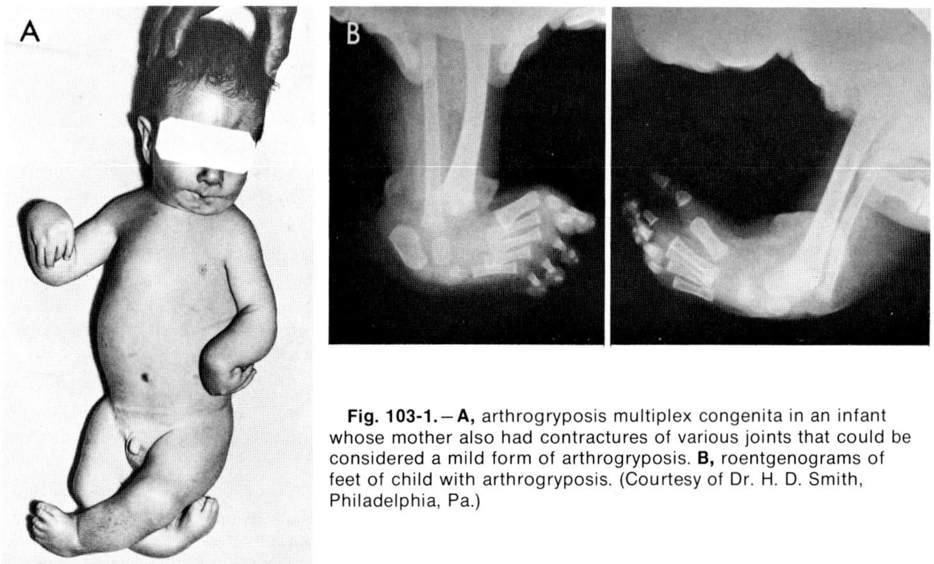

Fig. 103-1. – **A,** arthrogryposis multiplex congenita in an infant whose mother also had contractures of various joints that could be considered a mild form of arthrogryposis. **B,** roentgenograms of feet of child with arthrogryposis. (Courtesy of Dr. H. D. Smith, Philadelphia, Pa.)

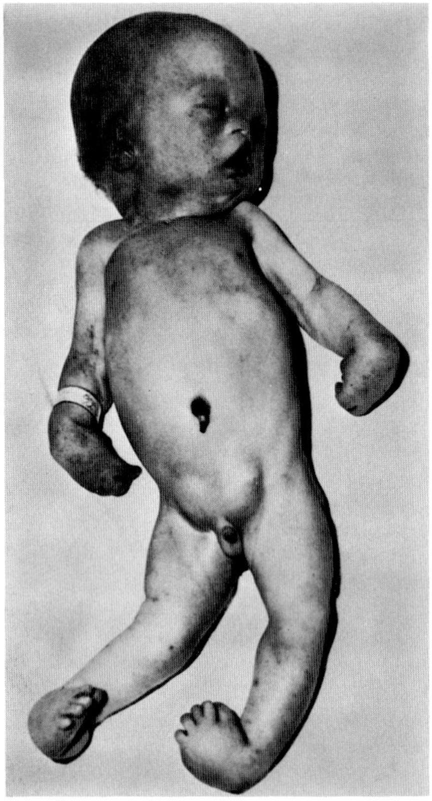

Fig. 103-2.—Child with arthrogryposis, cleft lip and palate, micrognathia, low-set and deformed ears, simian lines, single creases on digit V and bilateral inguinal hernias. The karyotype (skin culture) was 46,XY.

Malformations of the joints are recognized immediately after birth. Fixation of articulations may be present in two or in all four limbs. If only one limb is affected, the diagnosis of arthrogryposis becomes doubtful. Single case reports usually deal with very severe cases, whereas in reports of whole series, mild and doubtful cases are included. This explains some discrepancies in the literature on this subject. According to the terminology of different writers and their definition of arthrogryposis, differing descriptions of the disorder are given. In one-half to two-thirds of the cases, all four extremities are involved. Complete flexion or complete extension of all the joints has been described. Between these two extremes there are reports of all degrees of flexion and extension contractures involving a variable number of joints. As a rule, the anomalies are symmetric. In the series of Mead *et al.*,[6] 39 of 40 patients had deformities of the lower extremities. Flexion deformity and dislocation of the hips, flexion deformity of the knees and talipes equinovarus were the most frequent anomalies but there were fixations in other positions in some of the cases. The upper extremities were affected in 29 of 40 patients. Bilateral shoulder deformities were noticed in 15 patients, extension deformities of the elbows in 11 and flexion deformities in 7. The wrists were abnormal in 23 patients, flexion deformities being the most frequent. As a rule, the joints are rigid, but some active and passive movements are possible. The articular capsules and ligaments are tight and short and the muscles near the joints appear wasted or undeveloped. Subluxation of joints and dislocation of the hips frequently are present. Flexion deformities of the fingers combined with cutaneous syndactyly are seen often. The subcutaneous tissue of the extremities may be thick and doughy, obscuring the normal outlines of the joints, or it may be so reduced that every bone is visible. Mead *et al.*[6] noticed abnormal skin creases in every one of their 40 patients and webbing in about half of them. Dimpling of the skin at the abnormal joints often is noticeable. The bones are involved only indirectly. Owing to rigid fixation of the joints, articular surfaces may be abnormally placed and osteoporosis is marked in bones whose mobility is limited. Absence of the patella is a frequent finding.[32]

Associated malformations are numerous and variable. Hypoplasia of the mandible combined with high or cleft palate is not rare, so that, in addition to arthrogryposis, a disease picture resembling the Pierre Robin syndrome results (p. 654). Craniosynostosis was seen in 2 of our patients and recorded in 1 of Mackenzie's[5] cases. Grossly abnormal brains were observed by Ek,[13] Adams *et al.*,[28] Fowler[27] and others. Mandibulofacial dysostosis associated with arthrogryposis was described by Meier *et al.*[20] Microphthalmia,[4] optic atrophy[27] and cortical blindness[13] are rare complications. Cranial nerve involvement[8,13] or the Möbius syndrome[18,33] may be combined with arthrogryposis. As a rule, the joints of the vertebral column are free, but kyphoscoliosis develops in some cases, particularly when the abdominal muscles are defective.[10,16] Meningocele or myelocele were present in some of the cases.[8] Agenesis of the sacrum and arthrogryposis overlap in some patients.[34] The two disease pictures have much in common; a tendency to breech delivery, intrauterine growth retardation and many associated malformations point to a relationship of the two syndromes (p. 397). Congenital heart disease,[16] renal aplasia,[35] anomalies of the ureters,[8] cryptorchidism and scrotal defects have been reported.[4,20] Mental retardation was present in many published cases,[8,13,30] but in serial observations the incidence was only about 5%.[5,6]

Laboratory studies have so far not contributed to a better understanding of the disease. Routine examinations show no unexpected abnormalities[5] and the changes reported[30] probably are the result of chronic illness, immobilization and muscle degeneration but not indicative of primary pathogenic factors.

Roentgenologically, atrophy of the musculature over affected limbs, contractures of extension or flexion and osteoporosis are clearly evident. Dislocation of the hips, talipes equinovarus and other foot deformities and absence of the patella can be demonstrated in many cases.[12]

The prognosis varies according to the involvement of joints and brain. In severe cases, early death may be due to pneumonia, laryngeal stridor or to sudden respiratory failure. In children who survive infancy, treatment must be adjusted to the individual deformities. In general, the orthopedic treatment of the joint anomalies is less effective in arthrogryposis than in similar lesions of a less general nature.[5] This is not surprising if one considers that the deformities are due not only to changes in the joints but also to muscular and neural degenerative processes. There is no evidence of spontaneous improvement and there is no tendency to postnatal progression. For details of orthopedic and surgical treatment the reader is referred to special orthopedic publications.[5,6,16,36] The need for postoperative care and public health services was emphasized by Swinyard and Mayer.[36]

Kuskokwim Disease

A specific form of arthrogryposis has been observed in Alaskan Eskimos living in the delta of the Kuskokwim River. The disorder is characterized by congenital joint contractures involving particularly the knees and ankles with atrophy or compensatory hypertrophy of associated muscle groups.[42] The knee contractures may be combined with upward migration and hypoplasia of the patella. Elongation of the pedicles of the 5th lumbar vertebra, spondylolisthesis and osteolytic areas in the lateral parts of the clavicle and proximal humerus are additional skeletal anomalies.[43] The disorder, which is attributed to an inherited weakness of connective tissue, probably is transmitted as an autosomal recessive trait. Recurrence in families is common. The patients, although sometimes severely deformed, often are physically very active and usually intellectually unimpaired.[42]

REFERENCES

1. Stern, W. G.: Arthrogryposis multiplex congenita, J.A.M.A. 81:1507, 1923.
2. Otto, A. G.: Monstrorum Sexcentorum Descriptio Anatomica in Vratislaviae Museum, Anatomico-Pathologicum Vratislaviense, 1841.
3. Guérin, J.: Recherches sur les difformités congénitales chez les monstres, le foetus, et l'enfant, Paris, 1880.
4. James, T.: Multiple congenital articular rigidities, Edinburgh M. J. 58:565; 581, 1951.
5. Mackenzie, D. Y.: Arthrogryposis multiplex congenita, Proc. Roy. Soc. Med. 52:1101, 1959.
6. Mead, N. G., Lithgow, W. C., and Sweeney, H. J.: Arthrogryposis multiplex congenita, J. Bone & Joint Surg. 40-A: 1285, 1958.
7. Drachman, D. B., and Coulombre, A. J.: Experimental clubfoot and arthrogryposis multiplex congenita, Lancet 2:523, 1962.
8. Drachman, D. B., and Banker, B. Q.: Arthrogryposis multiplex congenita, Arch. Neurol. 5:77, 1961.
9. Hillman, J. W., and Johnson, J. T.: Arthrogryposis multiplex congenita in twins, J. Bone & Joint Surg. 34-A:211, 1952.
10. Hansen, O. M., and Zachariae, L.: Arthrogryposis multiplex congenita mit sekundärer Skoliose infolge von Bauchmuskelhypoplasie, Ann. paediat. 192:306, 1959.
11. Hanemann, H., and Feye, H.: Beitrag zur Arthrogryposis multiplex congenita, Monatsschr. Kinderh. 101:270, 1953.
12. Jacobson, H. J., Herbert, E. A., and Poppel, M. H.: Arthrogryposis multiplex congenita, Radiology 65:8, 1955.
13. Ek, J. I.: Cerebral lesions in arthrogryposis multiplex congenita, Acta paediat. 47:302, 1958.
14. Kite, J. H.: Arthrogryposis multiplex congenita: Review of 54 cases, South. M. J. 48:1141, 1955.
15. Turpin, R., Cruveiller, J., Lafourcade, J., Bocquet, L., Caille, B., Gorin, R., and Vialettes, M-L.: L'arthrogrypose multiple congénitale, Ann. pédiat. 13:2160, 1966.
16. Friedlander, H. L., Westin, G. W., and Wood, W. L.: Arthrogryposis multiplex congenita, J. Bone & Joint Surg. 50-A: 89, 1968.
17. Banker, B. Q., Victor, M., and Adams, R. D.: Arthrogryposis multiplex due to congenital muscular dystrophy, Brain 80:319, 1957.
18. Sprofkin, B. E., and Hillman, J. W.: Moebius' syndrome: Congenital oculofacial paralysis, Neurology 6:50, 1956.
19. Pasma, A., and Wildervanck, L. S.: Hereditary occurrence of congenital rigidity of the elbows and knees, Arch. chir. neerl. 8:43, 1956.
20. Meier, Z., Poschiavo, and Rothschild, M.: Ein Fall von Arthrogryposis multiplex congenita kombiniert mit Dysostosis mandibulofacialis (Franceschetti-Syndrom), Helvet. paediat. acta 14:213, 1959.
21. Sandbank, U., and Cohen, L.: Arthrogryposis multiplex congenita associated with tuberous sclerosis; a case report, J. Pediat. 64:571, 1964.
22. Pfeiffer, R. A., and Hüther, W.: Trisomie des chromosoms Nr. 18 unter dem Bilde einer Arthrogryposis multiplex congenita, Med. Klin. 58:1110, 1963.
23. Pollak, K.: Kindliche Missbildungen nach Suizidversuch der Mutter während der Schwangerschaft, Zentralbl. Gynäk. 81:1830, 1959.
24. Binns, W., James, L. F., Beeson, K. C., and Holley, R. W.: A congenital deformity experimentally produced in calves by feeding lupine and lead, Proc. Am. Coll. Vet. Toxicologists, p. 29, 1961.
25. Whittem, J. H.: Congenital abnormalities in calves; arthrogryposis and hydranencephaly, J. Path. & Bact. 73: 375, 1957.
26. Middleton, D. S.: Studies on prenatal lesions of striated muscle as cause of congenital deformity, Edinburgh M. J. 34:401, 1934.
27. Fowler, M.: A case of arthrogryposis multiplex congenita with lesions in the nervous system, Arch. Dis. Childhood 34:505, 1959.
28. Adams, R. D., Denny-Brown, D., and Pearson, C. M.: *Diseases of Muscle* (New York: Paul B. Hoeber, Inc., 1953).
29. Rossi, E.: Le syndrome arthromyodysplasique congénital, Helvet. paediat. acta 2:82, 1947.
30. Kanof, A., Aronson, S. M., and Volk, B. A.: Arthrogryposis: A clinical and pathological study of 3 cases, Pediatrics 17:532, 1956.
31. Sheldon, W.: Amyoplasia congenita (multiple congenital articular rigidity; arthrogryposis multiplex congenita), Arch. Dis. Childhood 7:117, 1932.
32. Valentin, B.: Die multiple angeborene Gelenkstarre, in Schwalbe, E., and Gruber, G. B. (eds.), *Die Morphologie der Missbildungen des Menschen und der Tiere* (Jena: Gustav Fischer, 1937), Vol. 3.
33. Rossi, E., and Caflisch, A.: Le syndrome de pterygium, Helvet. paediat. acta 6:119, 1951.
34. Blumel, J., Evans, E. B., and Eggers, G. W. N.: Partial and complete agenesis or malformation of the sacrum with

associated anomalies, J. Bone & Joint Surg. 41-A:497, 1959.
35. Potter, E.: Bilateral absence of ureters and kidneys, Obst. & Gynec. 25:3, 1965.
36. Swinyard, C. A., and Mayer, V.: Multiple congenital contractures, J.A.M.A. 183:23, 1963.
37. Aase, J. M., and Smith, D. W.: Dysmorphogenesis of joints, brain, and palate: A new dominantly inherited syndrome, J. Pediat. 73:606, 1968.
38. Lipton, E. L., and Morgenstern, S. H.: Arthrogryposis multiplex congenita in identical twins, A.M.A. Am. J. Dis. Child. 89:233, 1955.
39. James, L. F., Shupe, J. L., Binns, W., and Keeler, R. F.: Abortive and teratogenic effects of locoweed on sheep and cattle, Am. J. Vet. Res. 28:1379, 1967.
40. Fisher, R. L., Johnstone, W. T., Fisher, W. H., Jr., and Goldkamp, O. G.: Arthrogryposis multiplex congenita: A clinical investigation, J. Pediat. 76:255, 1970.
41. Jago, R. H.: Arthrogryposis following treatment of maternal tetanus with muscle relaxants, Arch. Dis. Childhood 45:277, 1970.
42. Petajan, J. H., Momberger, G. L., Aase, J., and Wright, D. G.: Arthrogryposis syndrome (Kuskokwim disease) in the Eskimo, J.A.M.A. 209:1481, 1969.
43. Wright, D. G.: The Unusual Skeletal Findings of the Kuskokwim Syndrome, in *Birth Defects, Original Article Series* Vol. 6, No. 4: 16 (New York: The National Foundation, 1970).
44. Lebenthal, E., Shochet, S. B., Adam, A., Seelenfreund, M., Fried, A., Najenson, T., Sandbank, U., and Matoth, Y.: Arthrogryposis multiplex congenita: Twenty-three cases in an Arab kindred, Pediatrics 46:891, 1970.

Larsen Syndrome

MULTIPLE congenital dislocations including anterior dislocation of the tibia on the femur, frontal bossing, flat facies, hypertelorism, depressed nasal bridge and clubfeet have been described as a syndrome.[1] The fingers are long and cylindrical and the thumb is spatulate. Cleft palate and abnormal segmentation of vertebrae may occur.[2] Recessive inheritance has been suggested.[2,3]

REFERENCES

1. Larsen, L. J., Schottstaedt, E. R., and Bost, F. C.: Multiple congenital dislocations associated with characteristic facial abnormality, J. Pediat. 37:574, 1950.
2. Gorlin, R. J., and Pindborg, J. J.: *Syndromes of the Head and Neck* (New York: McGraw-Hill Book Company, Inc., 1964), pp. 126–128.
3. McKusick, V. A.: *Mendelian Inheritance in Man. Catalogs of Autosomal Dominant, Autosomal Recessive, and X-Linked Phenotypes* (2d ed.; Baltimore: The Johns Hopkins Press, 1968), pp. 308–309.

Osteo-Onycho Dysplasia
(Nail-Patella Syndrome)

A COMBINATION of rather mild skeletal anomalies of the knee and elbow with dystrophy of the nails has long been known as an occasional familial peculiarity that sometimes is transmitted through many generations. In 1897, Little[1] wrote about congenital absence or delayed development of the patella and mentioned a family in which in four generations 18 persons had no patellae and no thumbnails. In the same year, Mayer[2] described an imbecile man who had congenital absence of the patella associated with broad thumbs showing nails with a central groove; he also had a large head, microphthalmia and other "extraordinary stigmata of degeneration." Changes in the elbow joints were added to the "patella-nail syndrome" by Firth,[3] who reported an affected family in 1911. J. Thompson, in discussing Firth's presentation, mentioned a family in which a mother and 5 of her 9 children had complete absence of both patellae and deformity of the fingernails and toenails. The syndrome was further extended by Turner,[4] who observed ichthyosis, palmar keratosis, hypertrichosis, alopecia, abnormal dentition and mental deficiency in some members of a kinship in which 26 of 39 members were affected by the triad of the patella-elbow-nail dysplasia. Lester[5] re-examined the family presented by Firth and found that some members had, in addition to this triad, scapular and hip deformities and a peculiar anomaly of the iris. Instead of being one color throughout, there was a clear-cut zone of pigment, whereas the darker central part of the iris "was shaped like a clover leaf" (Lester iris sign). Exostoses at the elbow joints[6] or of the frontal bone[7] were noticed before iliac horns were recognized as a part of the syndrome. Kieser[8] described a kinship in which the elbow deformities were so marked that a pterygium formation resulted. Some members of this family also had iliac horns and chronic renal disturbances. Thompson *et al.*[9] emphasized iliac horns as a manifestation of a more complex hereditary syndrome, namely, the patella-elbow-nail triad. Roeckerath[10] coined the term osteo-onycho dysplasia for this triad and associated symptoms. An additional facet of the syndrome was pointed out by Hawkins and Smith,[11] who found renal dysplasia in 4 members of a kinship that had manifestations of osteo-onycho dysplasia in at least five generations. The renal manifestations consisted of albuminuria and urinary casts and red cells. A similar renal dysplasia was present in several members of a large pedigree investigated by

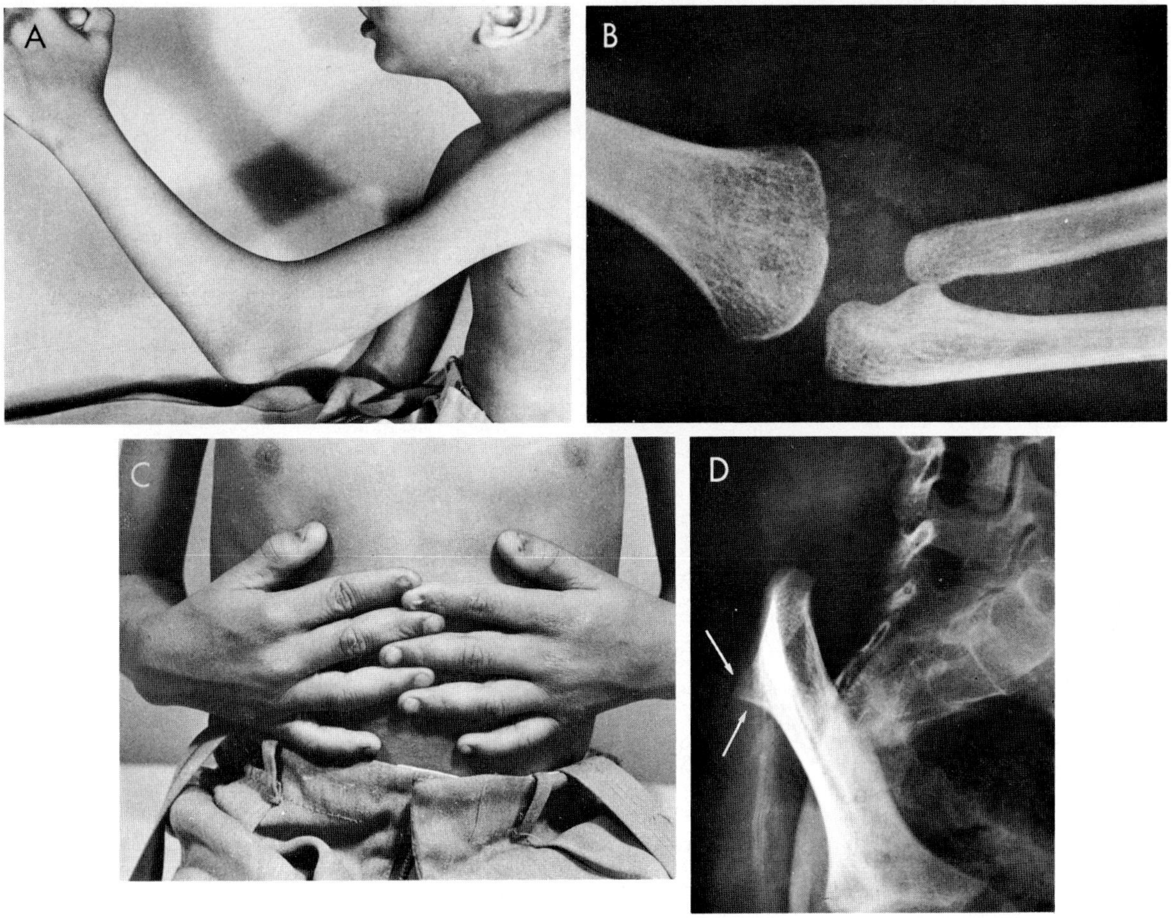

Fig. 103-3.—Nail-patella syndrome. **A,** elbow deformity with mild pterygium formation. **B,** roentgenogram of elbow joint, showing hypoplasia of distal end of humerus and of capitulum radii. **C,** dysplasia of nails seen best on thumb and index finger. **D,** lateral view of pelvic area. Arrows point to iliac horns.

Kieser[8] and Schröder.[12] In this kinship, the deformities of the elbows were very pronounced, whereas the patellar hypoplasia was less marked. Many other reports on familial osteo-onycho dysplasia can be found in reviews by Senturia and Senturia,[13] Mino *et al.*,[7] Schröder[12] and Schleutermann *et al.*[17]

Thus, at present, the syndrome consists of dysplasia of the nails, knees and elbows and of iliac horns. Signs of renal dysplasia appear in some of the affected persons.

Changes in the nails are seen, particularly on the thumbs and index fingers. The nail may be absent in toto or be hemidysplastic, being absent on the outer halves only. In other cases, the nails are thin or grooved. Sometimes they are short and the fleshy end of the finger turns backward, growing over the nail.[11] The toenails are affected only rarely. The patellae may be absent or hypoplastic. There usually are no symptoms connected with this anomaly, but dislocations can occur if the neighboring bones are deformed also. The deformity of the elbows is due to hypoplasia of the radial head and of the capitulum of the humerus. Dislocation, increased carrying angle, limited extension and supination as well as pterygium formation can be observed.

Iliac horns are bilateral, symmetric excrescences on the posterior surfaces of the iliac bones. They can be 1–2 cm. in length and may be palpable or visible through the gluteal musculature. However, the horns usually are missed by the examiner and discovered by the roentgenologist, who sees them best in oblique views. Roentgenograms also show flaring of the iliac bones and elongation of the anterior iliac spines. The iliac horns represent exostoses of a special type and differ from hereditary multiple exostoses (p. 840) in appearance and location. Other exostoses may occur on the os frontale or at the elbow joints.[7] The renal dysplasia manifests itself in the urine like a chronic glomerular nephritis, but there are no acute preceding episodes and blood pressure and ocular fundi are normal; edema and uremia are absent, but some persons with this syndrome die of chronic renal disorder.[12] A necropsy report with special emphasis on skeletal malformations was published by Darlington and Hawkins.[14] In a child with chronic nephropathy, biopsy and necropsy sections of the kidneys showed diffuse hyaline thickening of glomerular basement membranes, progressive fibrosis and tubular atrophy.[15] A nephrosis-like renal disease has been described in a newborn boy with this syndrome belonging to an affected kindred.[19]

The syndrome has been transmitted from generation to generation in many families. It most likely is due to an autosomal dominant gene with pleiotropic effects. It seems that the locus for the nail-patella syndrome and the locus for the ABO blood groups are closely linked[16]; there also is close linkage with the locus for adenylate kinase.[17] But affected persons do not always have the same blood group, as shown in an Indian kindred in which flexion deformities of the hip and hyperextension of the interphalangeal joints of the fingers appeared as additional features.[18] Inter- and intrafamilial variations exist. Iliac horns and renal dysplasia seem to be less constant symptoms than the nail-knee-elbow triad. Rare are other congenital anomalies, such as angiomas,[14] keratosis, cataract, pigeon breast,[14] osseous spina bifida, cervical ribs, polydactyly[11] and cleft palate.[3]

The Ellis-van Creveld syndrome, an autosomal recessive trait (Chapter 85) in which skeletal and nail anomalies occur together, can be distinguished easily from osteo-onycho dysplasia. It consists of dysplasia of nails and teeth, polydactyly, chondrodystrophy and congenital heart disease.

REFERENCES

1. Little, E. M.: Congenital absence or delayed development of the patella, Lancet 2:781, 1897.
2. Mayer, H. N.: Congenital absence or delayed development of the patella, Lancet 2:1384, 1897.
3. Firth, A. C. D.: Congenital absence of patellae and deformity of the nails in a mother and three children, Proc. Roy. Soc. Med., Vol. 5, pt. 1, p. 44, 1911–1912.
4. Turner, J. W.: Hereditary arthrodysplasia associated with hereditary dysplasia of the nails, J.A.M.A. 100:882, 1933.
5. Lester, A. M.: Familial dyschondroplasia associated with anonychia and other deformities, Lancet 2:1519, 1936.
6. Sever, J. W.: Hereditary arthrodysplasia associated with dystrophy of the nails, New England J. Med. 219:87, 1938.
7. Mino, R. A., Mino, V. H., and Livingstone, R. G.: Osseous dysplasia and dystrophy of the nails; review of the literature and report of a case, Am. J. Roentgenol. 60:633, 1948.
8. Kieser, W.: Die sogenannte Flughaut beim Menschen. Ihre Beziehung zum Status dysraphicus und ihre Erblichkeit, Ztschr. menschl. Vererb.-u. Konstitutionslehre 23: 594, 1939.
9. Thompson, E. A., Walker, E. T., and Weens, H. S.: Iliac horns; an osseous manifestation of hereditary arthrodysplasia associated with dystrophy of fingernails, Radiology 53:88, 1949.
10. Roeckerath, W.: Hereditäre Osteo-onycho-dysplasie, Fortschr. Geb. Röntgenstrahlen 75:700, 1951.
11. Hawkins, C. F., and Smith, O. E.: Renal dysplasia in a family with multiple hereditary abnormalities including iliac horns, Lancet 1:808, 1950.
12. Schröder, G.: Osteo-Onycho-Dysplasia hereditaria (albuminurica). Literaturbericht und Einordnung einer Sippe in dieses Missbildungssyndrom, Ztschr. menschl. Vererb.-u. Konstitutionslehre 36:42, 1961.
13. Senturia, H. R., and Senturia, B. D.: Congenital absence of the patellae associated with arthrodysplasia of the elbows and dystrophy of the nails; a hereditary syndrome, Am. J. Roentgenol. 51:352, 1944.
14. Darlington, D., and Hawkins, C. F.: Nail-patella syndrome with iliac horns and hereditary nephropathy, J. Bone & Joint Surg. 49-B:164, 1967.
15. Leahy, M. S.: The hereditary nephropathy of osteo-onychodysplasia; nail-patella syndrome, Am. J. Dis. Child. 112:237, 1966.
16. Renwick, J. H., and Lawler, S. D.: Genetical linkage between the ABO and nail-patella loci, Ann. Human Genet. 19:312, 1955.
17. Schleutermann, D. A., Bias, W. B., Murdoch, J. L., and McKusick, V. A.: Linkage of the loci for the nail-patella syndrome and adenylate kinase, Am. J. Human Genet. 21:606, 1969.
18. Aggarwal, N. D., and Mittal, R. L.: Nail-patella syndrome. Study of an affected family, J. Bone & Joint Surg. 52-B: 29, 1970.
19. Similä, S., Vesa, L., and Wasz-Höckert, O.: Hereditary onycho-osteodysplasia (the nail-patella syndrome) with nephrosis-like renal disease in a newborn boy, Pediatrics 46:61, 1970.

Broad Thumb and Big Toe Syndrome
(Rubinstein-Taybi Syndrome)

A SYNDROME of mental and motor retardation, broad thumbs, broad first toes and facial abnormalities was reported by Rubinstein and Taybi[1] in 1963. By 1965, there were reports on 34 cases that corresponded to the disease picture described. When seen during childhood, the patients usually are small and underweight and the head circumference is reduced. Intelligence quotients range between 17 and 80. Highly arched palate is always present and a beaked nose is seen in the majority of cases. Antimongoloid slant of the palpebral fissures, strabismus, refractive errors, ptosis and epicanthic folds frequently are noted. There is incomplete descent of the testes in the males.

The terminal phalanges of the first digits are broad and sometimes duplicated. Polydactyly and syndactyly occur but they are rare.[2] Brachydactyly was emphasized by Coffin[3] and by Kushnick.[4] Dermatoglyphic studies revealed extensive patterns in the thenar, first interdigital, hypothenar and hallucal areas.[5,6] Simian palmar creases are relatively rare. The bone age commonly is retarded. Vertebral anomalies, including spina bifida, enlarged foramen magnum, sternal and

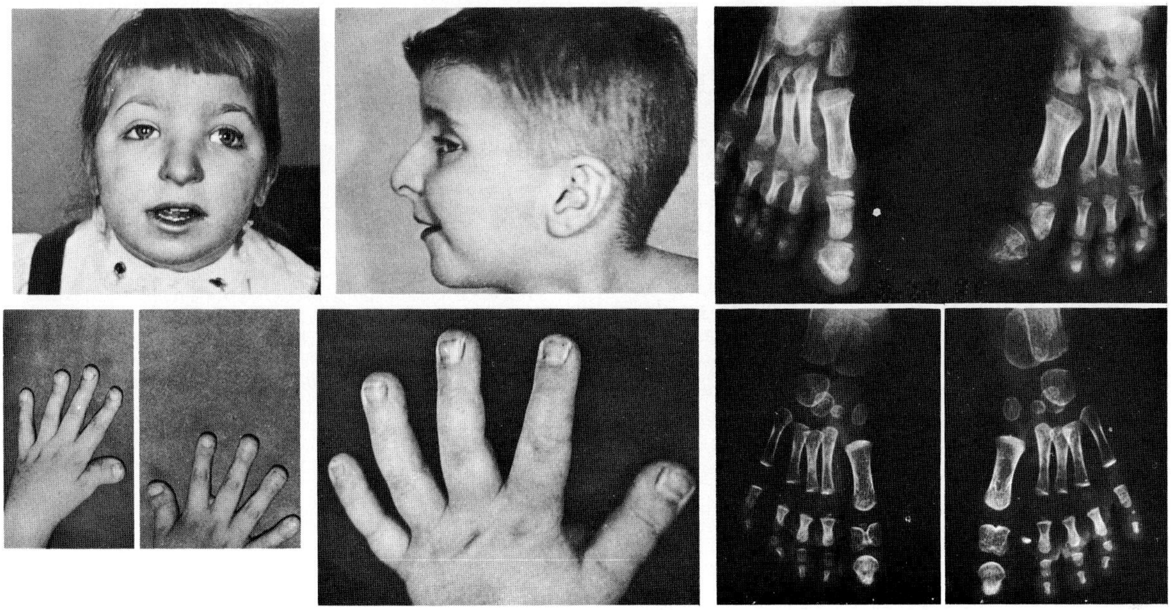

Fig. 103-4.—Broad thumb syndrome (Rubinstein-Taybi). Note typical facies, fingers and toes. (Courtesy of Dr. J. H. Rubinstein, Cincinnati, Ohio.)

rib anomalies, malocclusion, dental anomalies, nevus flammeus on forehead or nape of neck, colobomas and congenital heart and urinary tract defects have been observed in some of the patients.[7,8] Feeding difficulties, recurrent respiratory infections, lack of expressive language[4] and abnormal electroencephalograms without localizing phenomena have been recorded. The syndrome resembles mandibulofacial dysostosis (p. 650) in several respects but does not include the characteristic lid colobomas, malar defects and macrostomia. Dominant inheritance has been observed repeatedly in mandibulofacial dysostosis but not in the Rubinstein-Taybi syndrome. There exist forms of dominantly transmitted thumb anomalies (p. 977) but they are not combined with characteristic facial symptoms. A case resulting from incest has been reported,[10] but parental consanguinity has not been noted in other cases. Sex distribution is equal. In general, family histories are noncontributory. In one instance, siblings appeared to be affected.[7] A pair of twins thought to have de Lange syndrome (Chapter 38) with broad thumbs and toes possibly had the syndrome described by Rubinstein and Taybi.[1] In some cases, relatives of the patients had broad thumbs without other anomalies.[1,7] Chromosome analyses failed to reveal abnormalities.[1,5] The disorder is not rare. In institutions for the mentally retarded, 1 of 400 patients may have this syndrome.[5,10] The condition has been recognized in newborn infants.[11]

Broad thumb and big toe have been observed in a syndrome that also includes frontal bossing, prominent sagittal ridges of the skull and syndactyly. This "frontodigital syndrome," which affects persons with normal intelligence, can be transmitted as a dominant trait.[12]

REFERENCES

1. Rubinstein, J. H., and Taybi, H.: Broad thumbs and toes and facial abnormalities, Am. J. Dis. Child. 105:588, 1963.
2. Rubinstein, J. H.: A syndrome of mental retardation with abnormal facial features and broad thumbs and great toes, International Copenhagen Congress on Scientific Study of Mental Retardation, August 7–14, 1964, p. 812.
3. Coffin, G. S.: Brachydactyly, peculiar facies and mental retardation, Am. J. Dis. Child. 108:351, 1964.
4. Kushnick, T.: Brachydactyly, facial abnormalities, and mental retardation. Rubinstein-Taybi syndrome, Am. J. Dis. Child. 3:96, 1966.
5. Berg, J. M., Smith, G. F., Ridler, M. A. C., Dutton, G., Green, E. A., and Richards, B. W.: On the association of broad thumbs and first toes with other physical peculiarities and mental retardation, J. Ment. Defic. Res. 10:204, 1966.
6. Giroux, J., and Miller, J. R.: Dermatoglyphics of the broad thumb and great toe syndrome, Am. J. Dis. Child. 113: 207, 1967.
7. Johnson, C. F.: Broad thumbs and broad great toes with facial abnormalities and mental retardation, J. Pediat. 68:942, 1966.
8. Taybi, H., and Rubinstein, J. H.: Broad thumbs and toes, and unusual facial features, Am. J. Roentgenol. 93:362, 1965.
9. Kroth, H.: Cornelia de Lange-Syndrom I bei Zwillingen, Arch. Kinderh. 173:273, 1966.
10. Padfield, C. J., Partington, M. W., and Simpson, N. E.: The Rubinstein-Taybi syndrome, Arch. Dis. Childhood 43: 94, 1968.
11. Wilson, M. G.: Rubinstein-Taybi and D_1 trisomy syndromes, J. Pediat. 73:404, 1968.
12. Marshall, R. E., and Smith, D. W.: Frontodigital syndrome: A dominantly inherited disorder with normal intelligence, J. Pediat. 77:129, 1970.

Tricho-Rhino-Phalangeal Syndrome

A SYNDROME of congenital sparseness of the scalp hair, deficiency of the lateral portion of the eyebrows, pear-shaped nose, long philtrum and finger deformities has been described and named by Giedion,[1] who reviewed similar cases previously recorded. The fingers are short, particularly the thumbs, swelling of the middle phalangeal joints develops and axial deviations of the fingers result in deformities of the hands. The nails are thin. Cone-shaped epiphyses and short distal phalanges of the thumbs and large toes are noted in roentgenograms. Multiple exostoses were present in some of the cases.[2] The facial appearance, with frontal baldness, bulbous nose and long upper lip, sometimes is diagnostic. The syndrome has been observed in siblings[3,4] and in a father and his 2 daughters.[5]

REFERENCES

1. Giedion, A.: Das tricho-rhino-phalangeale Syndrom, Helvet. paediat. acta 21:475, 1966.
2. Gorlin, R. J., Cohen, M. M., Jr., and Wolfson, J.: Tricho-rhino-phalangeal syndrome, Am. J. Dis. Child. 118:595, 1969.
3. Klingmüller, G.: Über eigentümliche Konstitutionsanomalien bei zwei Schwestern und ihre Beziehung zu neueren entwicklungspathologischen Befunden, Der Hautarzt 7:105, 1956.
4. Van der Werff ten Bosch, J. J.: The syndrome of brachymetacarpal dwarfism (pseudo-pseudohypoparathyroidism) with and without gonadal dysgenesis, Lancet 1:69, 1959.
5. Fontaine, G., Maroteaux, P., Farriaux, J-P., Richard, J., and Roelens, B.: Le syndrome tricho-rhino-phalangien, Arch. franç. pédiat. 27:635, 1970.

Skeletal Malformations of Patients with Fanconi Anemia

PANCYTOPENIA of the Fanconi type usually is seen in patients with multiple congenital malformations.[1] In addition to skeletal defects, the children may show abnormal pigmentation, stunted growth, microphthalmia, hypogenitalism and mental retardation. The head is small, strabismus often is present and pigmentations are seen mostly on the trunk, in the groin, axillae and around the neck. The skeletal defects are noted often in the upper limbs and rarely in the lower limbs. Distal preaxial structures, particularly the thumbs and the first metacarpals, are affected most often. One or both thumbs may be absent or underdeveloped but duplication of the thumb occurs in some of the cases.[2,3] The entire hand may be small and the fifth finger incurved. The thenar eminence sometimes is hypoplastic and preaxial carpal bones may be missing. The radius often is defective or absent and the hand turned inward. Reduction in size of the humerus and Sprengel deformity have been observed occasionally. Dislocation of the hip, clubfoot and syndactyly of toes are rare signs of the syndrome.[4,5] Cervical rib, fusion of the first two ribs, vertebral anomalies and scoliosis have been noted.[6] The skeletal malformations often are combined with such renal anomalies as horseshoe kidney, aplasia of one kidney, double renal pelvis and ureter, ectopic kidney and hydronephrosis. Ptosis, microphthalmia and retinal detachment have been described.[7] Deafness[2] and atresia of the external auditory canal were present in some of the cases.[7] Heart murmurs are common but congenital cardiac malformations are rare. Patent ductus arteriosus,[3,8] aortic hypoplasia and aortic coarctation[2] have been diagnosed. Cryptorchidism[4] or vaginal atresia with uterus bicornis[6] and delayed puberty[5] have been described. Intrauterine growth retardation occurred in many cases[4] (Chapter 14). In lymphocyte cultures, chromatid-type aberrations are seen frequently, ranging from constrictions to gaps and breaks. Chromatid exchange figures show a variable incidence and endoreduplications sometimes are observed.[9,10] Anemia, thrombocytopenia and pancytopenia develop. Pancytopenia progresses slowly and usually terminates 2–5 years after the appearance of hematologic symptoms, but longer survival has been reported.[6] Severe anemia, hemorrhages and infections are among the causes of death. Cancer[2] and leukemia[11] have been rare complications. A high incidence of leukemia in families of patients with Fanconi syndrome has been reported.[12] In affected families, siblings may show either the hematologic disorder or the malformation syndrome.[13] Most family observations point to autosomal recessive inheritance of the disorder, but other genetic hypotheses have been proposed.[10]

REFERENCES

1. Fanconi, G.: Familiäre infantile perniziosaartige Anämie (perniziöses Blutbild und Konstitution), Jahrb. Kinderh. 117:257, 1927.
2. Esparza, A., and Thompson, W. R.: Familial hypoplastic anemia with multiple congenital anomalies (Fanconi's syndrome)—report of three cases, Rhode Island M. J. 49: 103, 1966.
3. McDonald, R., and Goldschmidt, B.: Pancytopenia with congenital defects (Fanconi's anaemia), Arch. Dis. Childhood 35:367, 1960.
4. Nilsson, L. R.: Chronic pancytopenia with multiple congenital abnormalities (Fanconi's anaemia), Acta paediat. 49:518, 1960.
5. Boivin, P., Bousser, J., Robineaux, R., and Pringuet, C.:

Pancytopénie avec malformations multiples (syndrome de Fanconi). Présentation de 3 nouveaux cas et revue de la littérature, Arch. franç. pédiat. 15:1289, 1958.
6. Dawson, J. P.: Congenital pancytopenia associated with multiple congenital anomalies (Fanconi type). Review of the literature and report of a 20-year-old female with a 10-year follow-up and apparently good response to splenectomy, Pediatrics 15:325, 1955.
7. Levy, W.: Aplastic anemia in siblings with multiple congenital anomalies (Fanconi type), J. Pediat. 40:24, 1952.
8. Zweymüller, E., Stur, O., and Holzner, H.: Beobachtungen an einer konstitutionellen infantilen Panmyelopathie (Fanconi-Anämie), Helvet. paediat. acta 13:97, 1958.
9. Schmid, W.: Familial constitutional panmyelocytopathy, Fanconi's anemia. II. A discussion of the cytogenetic findings in Fanconi's anemia, Seminars Hemat. 4:241, 1967.
10. Hoefnagel, D., Sullivan, M., McIntyre, O. R., Gray, J. A., and Storrs, R. C.: Panmyelopathy with congenital anomalies (Fanconi) in two cousins, Helvet. paediat. acta 21: 230, 1966.
11. Bloom, G. E., Warner, S., Gerald, P. S., and Diamond, L. K.: Chromosome abnormalities in constitutional aplastic anemia, New England J. Med. 274:8, 1966.
12. Garriga, S., and Crosby, W. H.: Incidence of leukemia in families of patients with hypoplasia of marrow, Blood 14: 1008, 1959.
13. Reinhold, J. D., Neumark, E., Lightwood, R., and Carter, C. O.: Familial hypoplastic anemia with congenital abnormalities (Fanconi's syndrome), Blood 7:915, 1952.

PART XV
The Muscular System

104

Malformations of the Muscular System

Congenital Absence of Muscles

CONGENITAL ABSENCE or hypoplasia of muscles has been estimated to occur with a frequency of 1 in 11,000 to 1 in 4,000 persons. This discrepancy indicates a lack of exact knowledge. Observations of muscle defects usually are based on clinical impressions or inspection, palpation and electrical examination. Histories often fail to bring out muscle defects because absence of one or more muscles can go unnoticed if there is no disturbance of function. Most muscle defects are unilateral but there are exceptions. Defects of the abdominal muscles are always bilateral and absence of the pectoral or trapezius muscle sometimes is bilateral. Muscle defects usually are associated with anomalies of the skin and skeleton in the same region of the body, so that one is dealing, in many cases, with syndromes going beyond the muscular system. It often has been asked whether muscle defects are to be considered congenital malformations or, rather, the result of such diseases as progressive muscular dystrophy, atrophy and so forth. This question may be justified in some cases but, in others, combination of muscle defects with skeletal and other malformations indicates embryonic developmental malformation rather than prenatal onset of muscle disease. In some cases, the differentiation may be difficult. Bing[1] pointed out that it happened repeatedly that patients with congenital muscle defects developed progressive muscle atrophy during their later life, so that in such cases the congenital muscle defect must be considered the expression of a general muscle disease. But, as pointed out by Binder,[2] congenital muscle defects are, in contrast to progressive muscle disorders, only rarely hereditary.

Of individual muscle defects, that of the pectoralis has been observed most frequently. In Bing's[1] tabulation, the pectoral muscle was affected five and a half times more often than the trapezius, which was second in frequency. Several hundred cases of pectoralis deficiency have been reported in the literature. Males are affected at least four times more often than females, but there apparently is no preference for the right or left side. Bilateral involvement is very rare. In most cases, there is absence of the sternocostal portion and of the pectoralis minor, whereas the clavicular portion is present. Etiology and pathogenesis are obscure. The family and pregnancy histories usually are not contributory. In exceptional cases, father and son were affected. Sometimes a relative had a skeletal malformation, which could be a different expression of the trait.[2] Liebenam[3] described monozygotic twin girls, one of whom had pectoralis defect, absence of the breast on the same side, vertebral defects and syndactyly. Her twin sister had only minimal skeletal defects and asymmetry of the breasts.

Complicated cases of pectoralis defect are emphasized in the literature, but the majority of patients are well developed except for the muscle aplasia and the abnormal overlying skin. The defect is discovered if the person is made to extend the arms at right angles to the body. It is noted that the anterior axillary fold is absent, whereas the posterior axillary fold stands out as the posterior wall of the axillary space.[4] Absence of the pectoral muscle is compatible with a completely normal life, since functional disturbances usually are mild.

Hypoplasia of the skin attached directly to the underlying ribs is noticeable over the defective muscle; hair and sweat glands may be absent and the mamilla small and poor in pigment. In women, lactation may be wanting on the affected side[4] and sometimes axillary hair is missing also. Associated skeletal anomalies involve chiefly the ribs. The second to the fourth ribs are particularly involved by defects distal to the anterior axillary line or near the costochondral junctions that occasionally lead to herniation of a lung. Cervical ribs or fusion of ribs can occur. The sternum also may be reduced unilaterally and curve toward the normal side. The scapula sometimes is hypoplastic and elevated as in Sprengel deformity (Chapter 96), but in most cases of Sprengel deformity the pectoral muscles are normal. Abnormal curvature of the spine has been observed repeatedly. The ipsilateral upper extremity often is deformed either in its entirety (reduction deformities) or by shortening of the upper or lower arm, syndactyly, brachydactyly, adactyly, radius defect or lobster claw.[1] Absence of the pectoral muscle combined with syndactyly on the same side is called "Poland syndactyly" (p. 973). An

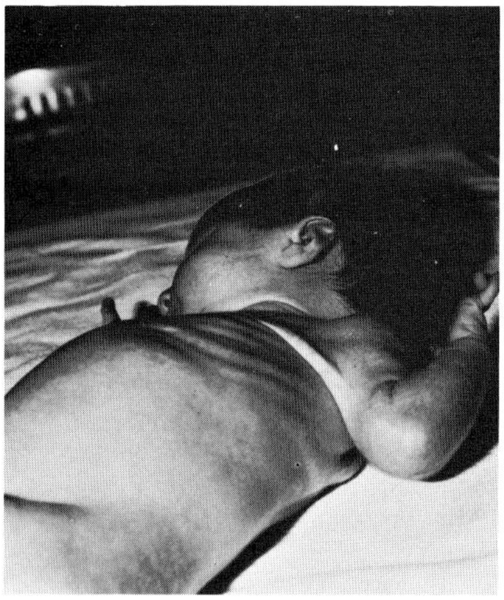

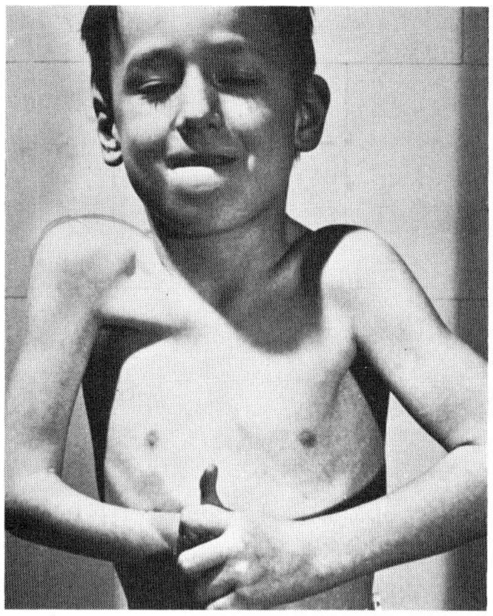

Fig. 104-1 (left).—Absence of the left pectoral muscle in a newborn child with multiple congenital malformations. The axillary pterygium is clearly shown. The infant also had underdevelopment of the left upper extremity, digital syndactyly (Poland syndrome, p. 973) and, in addition, posterior palate cleft, micrognathia and clubfeet.

Fig. 104-2 (right).—Partial absence of the right pectoral muscle in a boy who also had severe finger deformities on the same side. (Courtesy of Dr. R. K. Beals, Portland, Oregon.)

interesting associated anomaly is pterygium or webbing between the thorax and upper arm. It occurs in approximately 15% of the patients with pectoral defects[2] (p. 1025). A fascia or ligament may extend from the sternum to the humerus, impairing normal abduction of the upper arm. Such an anomaly may be noticeable in the newborn and can be removed by operation.[5] Pterygia and muscle aplasias may be present in various syndromes. They are not rare in the Möbius syndrome (Chapter 40), which can include pectoralis defects. They are not rare in a more generalized way in arthrogryposis (p. 1011). Agenesis of one lung associated with ipsilateral pectoralis aplasia has been observed.[6] Web formations, usually combined with muscle aplasias, are discussed on page 1189.

The sternocleidomastoid and the trapezius muscles are developmentally related and sometimes defective in the same person. It seems that isolated defect of the sternocleidomastoid does not occur, but isolated trapezius defects have been observed. Since the trapezius contributes to the outline of the neck-shoulder region, its absence can be recognized by inspection. The defect can be unilateral or bilateral. Position of shoulder and scapula varies. If the sternocleidomastoid is absent, the region between clavicle and mastoid appears empty and the muscle cannot be palpated. The clavicle is more prominent than normal and shows an increased curvature. Function is little impaired, since other muscles of the region can substitute for the missing ones. Defect of the left trapezius has been observed in a father and son.[7]

Defects of the deltoid, supra- and infra-spinatus and the latissimus dorsi are rare and usually associated with other muscle defects, particularly those of the pectoralis. Absence of the serratus anterior major sometimes is combined with defect of the pectoral muscle, but its isolated absence is very rare. Ribs and intercostal spaces are not covered and one can feel the absence by palpation below the scapula, which stands off the thorax and is somewhat approximated to the spine. The scapula moves from the thorax wall if the arms are stretched forward horizontally. The spine is bent toward the side of the defect.

Agenesis of the palmaris longus is common. It is found to be absent in approximately 13% of Americans. Duplication has been observed in 1–3% and triplication occasionally. Dominant inheritance may account for agenesis of the palmaris longus. An accessory palmaris with duplication of the palmaris longus was described by King and O'Rahilly.[8]

Congenital Absence of the Abdominal Muscles

In contrast to congenital absence of the pectoral muscles, absence of the abdominal muscles is a bilateral and symmetric defect associated with visceral anomalies of clinical importance. Most of the patients with congenital absence of the abdominal muscles are male, but the anomaly has been observed exceptionally in females. The condition is rare. When, in 1950, two comprehensive reviews of the literature were published by Silverman and Huang[9] and by Eagle and Barrett,[10] only 45 cases had been recorded. Since then, additional reports have appeared. In a review by Monnet *et al.*[11] in 1959, 83 cases were considered. Only 6 of the patients were females. In the past, many of the patients died in infancy or early childhood of infections or uremia. However, there have been survivors, and lax abdominal muscles have been reported in men 60 or 70 years of age. In recent years, survival was made possible by administration of antibiotics and by surgical repair of bladder obstruction or of intestinal malrotation. Familial recurrence has not been reported and there are no suggestions of genetic determination.

It is thought that Fröhlich,[12] in 1839, wrote the first report on "deficiency of muscles particularly those of the lateral abdominal muscles." Association of abdominal muscle defects with urogenital anomalies apparently was first emphasized in 1895 by Parker.[13]

The abnormal appearance of the abdominal wall usually is fully present at birth or it becomes noticeable in the first weeks of infancy. The abdomen is large and lax, the wall is thin and intestinal loops and their peristalsis can be observed through the thin covers. Palpation of abdominal organs is facilitated. With the child recumbent, the flanks bulge laterally. Skin folds are seen radiating from the umbilicus or as transverse folds. A midline crease from the umbilicus to the symphysis is present in some of the cases.

The order of frequency with which the various abdominal muscles are absent is as follows: (1) transversus abdominis, (2) rectus abdominis below the umbilicus, (3) obliquus internus abdominis, (4) obliquus externus abdominis and (5) the rectus abdominis above the umbilicus.[9] Complete absence of the musculature has been described but, in most instances, the muscles are merely deficient. Often the origins and insertions are present, but the muscles diminish in size and thickness over the bladder. The umbilicus, which usually is in normal position, has been described as a vertical slit-like furrow or as a linear central scar, but it can also be normal. Of great importance are rare communications of the umbilicus with the bladder through a urachus or a urachus cyst.[10] The thorax often is deformed. Flaring of the costal margins or the Harrison groove was noted in about half of the cases. Pigeon breast deformity often narrows the chest in the transverse direction. Enlargement and hypertrophy of the bladder is the rule. It is found attached to the abdominal wall and connected through the urachus to the umbilicus. Greene *et al.*[14] thought that obstruction at the vesical neck, the primary pathologic problem, results in distention of the bladder and residual urine.

Connections of the ureters with the bladder vary. There may be stenosis of the ureterovesical orifice or occlusion. Obstruction may also occur at the ureteropelvic junction. As a rule, the ureters are greatly dilated, sometimes to the size of intestines. But occasionally the enlargement is unilateral or decreasing in the proximo-distal direction. Hydronephrosis, unilateral or bilateral, has been observed repeatedly. In some cases, hydronephrosis was present on one side and a hypoplastic kidney on the other. Renal cysts have been seen also. The urethra usually is patent, but obstructions have been described in several cases. Atresia, folds acting as a valve below the verumontanum, compression by a pouch or diverticulum and hypertrophy of the prostatic urethra have been noted. Hematuria and pyuria reveal the anomalies of the urinary tract in many cases. Cryptorchidism is the rule, the testes being retained in the abdomen and often attached to a ureter. Abnormal fixation of the

Fig. 104-3.—Congenital absence of the abdominal muscles. **A,** transverse folds of abdominal wall in a 19-month-old girl. **B,** lateral bulging of abdominal walls in a 4-day-old boy. (From F. Silverman and N. Huang.[9])

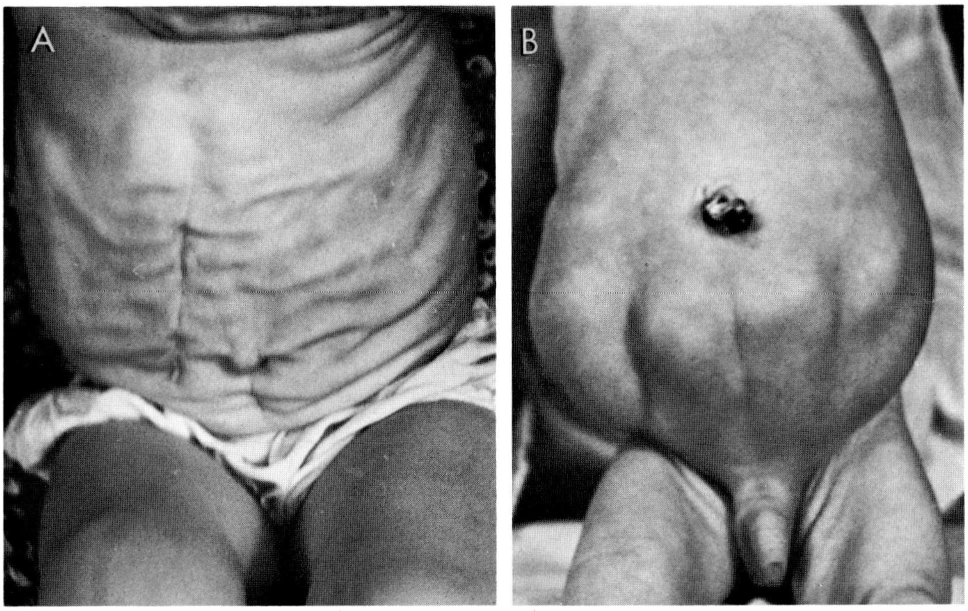

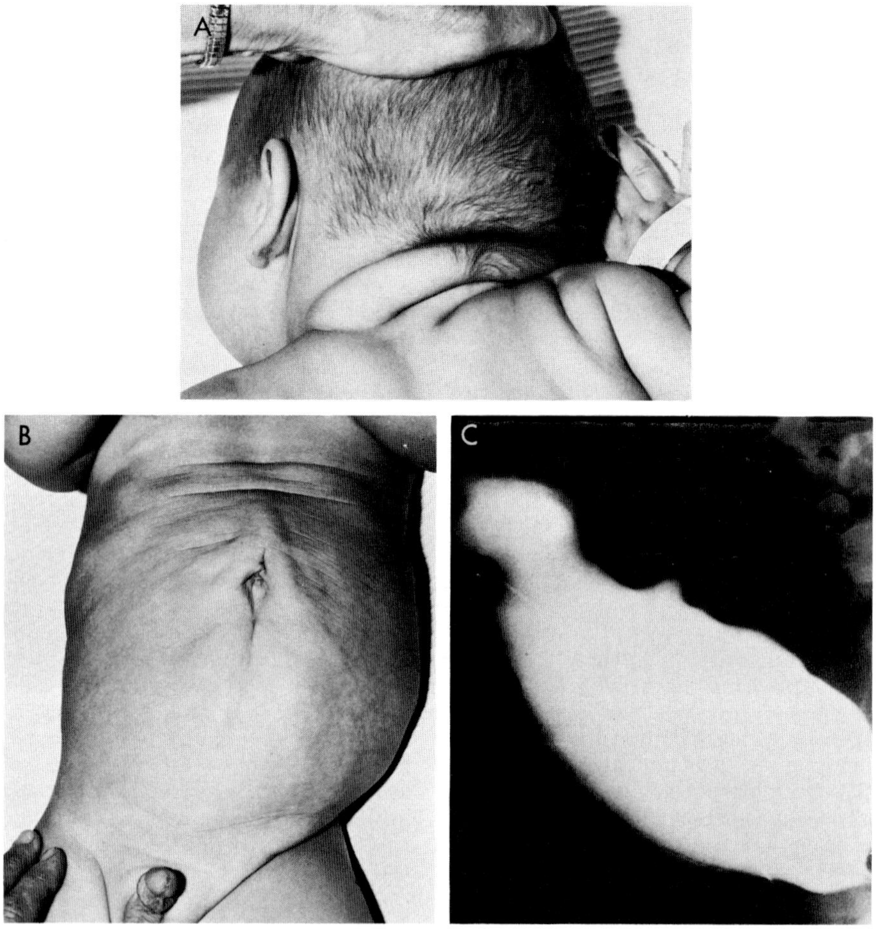

Fig. 104-4.—Boy with loose skin folds of nape (**A**) had hypoplasia of abdominal muscles, midline creases around umbilicus and cryptorchidism (**B**). Roentgenogram (**C**) shows the enlarged bladder extending upward along the abdominal wall toward urachal remnant. (Courtesy of Dr. E. A. Wagner, Cincinnati, Ohio.)

gastrointestinal tract and malrotation with their consequences have been described and emphasized by Silverman and Huang.[9] In an unusual case, abdominal laxity was associated with a wandering spleen and its torsion. Simpson and Ashby[15] reported the case of a 53-year-old mentally subnormal man who was operated on because of torsion of a wandering spleen. The fact that he had been treated before because of renal and vesical calculi with unilateral nephrectomy, cystostomy and bladder neck resection, that he had lax abdominal muscles, scoliosis and limb deformities suggests that the wandering spleen was the result of malrotation, characteristic of the syndrome of agenesis of abdominal muscles.

Explanations of the syndrome have been attempted for many decades. Some writers believed that agenesis of the abdominal muscles is the primary cause of the syndrome, whereas others considered the vesical anomalies as cause of the muscular deficiency. In 1903, Stumme[16] asserted that the bladder becomes obstructed in utero at or distal to the vesical neck after its cranial end has lost its communication with the allantois. Accumulation of urine distends the bladder, the ureter and the renal pelvis. As the bladder enlarges, it causes atrophy of the muscles, either by direct pressure or by interference with their blood supply. Retention of the testes has been attributed to obstruction by a large bladder or to obliteration of the inguinal canals. By the time of birth, the obstruction at the bladder outlet or the urethral obstruction may have been overcome, so that no mechanical obstacle can be demonstrated in postnatal life. There is much to be said for this theory,[10] which is still considered the best explanation by some present-day authors. An alternative theory considers the urinary anomalies as secondary to the abdominal muscular deficiency. With congenital absence of the abdominal muscles, incomplete emptying of the bladder leading to urinary retention and infection is to be expected. Constipation and symptoms of indigestion are possible complications also. Since the abdominal muscles are important for respiration, deformity of the thorax could be explained by their absence. Pros and cons of these alternative theories have been discussed thoroughly by Binder,[2] Silverman and Huang[9] and by Eagle and Barrett.[10] A third possibility is that the muscular deficiency and the urinary anomalies have a common cause that has not yet been elucidated. One has thought of a nervous system defect that could be responsible for early malfunction of abdominal and visceral muscles. Association with spina bifida has been recorded[17] and clubfoot is a fairly common complication. But examination of the spinal cord in some of the cases did not reveal significant alterations.[9]

Malrotation of the intestine, an important complication in some of the cases, has been explained by largeness of the umbilical orifice at the time of withdrawal of the gut into the abdominal cavity. The enlargement could be attributed to absence of the recti muscles. A large umbilical orifice could result in irregular re-entry of the small intestine and cecum and in malrotation of the intestinal tract.[9] But the association with the syndrome of deficient abdominal muscles could have different causes. It must be remembered that some of the patients showed involvement of more distant muscles, such as defects of the latissimus dorsi and quadratus lumborum, and of cardiovascular anomalies, megacolon, imperforate anus, and absence of one leg,[18] clubfoot, genu valgum, dislocation of the hip, torticollis, arthrogryposis and cleft palate.[9,17] Association of aplasia of abdominal muscles with a congenital diverticulum of the anterior urethra was described in detail by Boissonnat and Duhamel[19] as mesodermal defects in midventral regions. Defects of the abdominal musculature have also been reported in a child with Turner syndrome[20] and in a female child with multiple pterygia.[21] In another girl, the syndrome included pinhole urethra, rectum terminating in the bladder, duodenal atresia, two-chambered heart and clubfoot.[18] It is of interest that such complicated disease pictures have been observed in phenotypically female children,[17,20,21] so that one can assume that they represent special syndromes in which defective abdominal muscles are included. In one of these cases,[21] a sibling had malformations of the spine and extremities. This contrasts with the syndrome of congenital absence of the abdominal muscles discussed in this section, which does not tend to familial occurrence of congenital anomalies.

Successful treatment has been reported often. Supportive mechanical and antibiotic measures are important. Early studies and treatment of the urinary and digestive tracts can prevent some of the complications. Greene *et al.*[14] performed resection of the vesical neck, with gratifying results in 4 of 5 cases. But, if there is atresia of the urethra or far-advanced disease of the upper urinary tract, other solutions have to be found. Nephrostomy, pyelostomy, ureteroplasty, ureterovesical reimplantation and other surgical measures have been attempted.[10]

Congenital Muscular Torticollis

Torticollis (wryneck) usually is attributed to injury of the sternocleidomastoid muscle during delivery, and therefore should not be considered a congenital malformation but a birth injury. But the etiology of the anomaly is doubtful and, in many cases, prenatal origin cannot be ruled out. In the presence of anomalies of cervical vertebrae, there is of course no doubt about derangement in early embryonic life, but even muscular torticollis may be present before birth. A comprehensive review of concepts of etiology and pathology was written by Lidge *et al.*,[22] and Jones,[23] in his book on torticollis, expressed the belief that the disorder begins in utero long before birth.

The right and left sides are affected about equally and there is no sex predilection. The incidence is about 0.6 per 1,000.[24] Exceptional cases point to hereditary etiologic factors. There are some pedigrees that include patients in four and even five generations, and there are a number of reports in which a parent and child were affected.[23] This would suggest dominant inheritance in some of the cases. On the other hand, recessive inheritance was considered because of increased parental consanguinity in cases of torticollis. There was concordance in 5 monozygotic pairs of twins and discordance in 1, whereas of 23 dizygotic twin pairs, only 2 were concordant. Although genetic determination or a genetic factor must be suspected in the etiology, the mode of inheritance is obscure. Multifactorial inheritance and environmental influences have been considered in explanations of the anomaly.[24] According to Hulbert,[25] the history of children with congenital torticollis points to obstetric complications in approximately 70% of the cases. About 40% of the patients had breech presentation, 20% were delivered by forceps and 9% were the result of difficult labor.[25] It is understandable that under these conditions a difficult delivery usually is held responsible for the anomaly, but abnormal delivery could be the result and not the cause of it. Jones[23] considered the incidence of obstetric difficulties and traumatic deliveries too low to implicate birth injury as the cause. Explanations by trauma, hemorrhage and hematoma do not seem to be supported by clinical, pathologic or experimental observations.[26] Since the blood supply of the sternomastoid muscle through a branch of the superior thyroid artery, which is an end-artery, is precarious, ischemia of the muscle has been considered as the causative process. This theory has also been doubted, since ligation of an artery does not bring about atrophy and massive fibrosis.[25] For these reasons, forced prenatal malposition has been considered a likely cause of the anomaly and this theory is supported by the fact that torticollis has been observed following extrauterine pregnancy and at cesarean section, with the tumor present at birth.[25]

Chandler and Altenberg[27] reported a case in which roentgenograms taken before birth showed breech presentation, with the fetal head in right lateral flexion. The child was delivered by cesarean section. There was right-sided torticollis, which became increasingly pronounced and a tumor developed after 2 weeks. Such *postural* torticollis can be attributed to intrauterine malposition on the evidence of associated molding of the head with occasional deformity of the ear and facial palsy. However, *muscular* torticollis with an associated sternomastoid tumor is still considered unexplained and some cause, probably acting before birth, is still being sought.[25] Eight theories proposed to explain tumor or fibrosis in the sternomastoid muscle were analyzed by Jones.[23]

In case of torticollis, the muscle fibers of the sternomastoid are replaced by fibrous tissue and the normal elasticity of the muscle is lost. Excised tumors show white glistening tissue interspersed with red muscle fibers. Microscopically, young fibrous tissue is seen but there are no signs of trauma or hematoma.[26]

In most cases, a tumor develops soon after birth and persists for several months. The development of torticollis is delayed for several years and becomes manifest as the neck lengthens. The head is tilted toward the affected side and the chin is turned away from it. Facial and cranial asymmetry develops if the torticollis persists. On the affected side, the frontal eminence is flattened and there is a bulge in the occipital region, whereas on the opposite side the situation is reversed (scoliosis capitis, plagiocephaly). The deformity of the skull and face is decreased after surgical correction of the torticollis. An exostosis of the clavicle may develop on the affected side if there is fibrosis of the clavicular head of the muscle. The auricle on the affected side often is shortened and broadened and a scoliosis of the cervical spine with convexity toward the normal side can develop. Secondary scoliosis must be distinguished from curvatures due to skeletal anomalies. The chest appears pushed upward against the side to the torticollis.[2] The head can be moved with some limitation in all directions and there is no pain. Congenital dislocation of the hip and clubfoot occur as associated anomalies three to four times more often than in the general population.[28] Torticollis can be due to malformations of cervical vertebrae. Such skeletal torticollis differs from the muscular type discussed here in etiology, prognosis and treatment.

In some cases, the condition subsides without treatment. Torticollis noticed soon after birth usually requires no treatment. But in older children the condition is obstinate. In some cases, physiotherapy may be successful. Operative treatment has been practiced since early times, when subcutaneous tenotomy was performed by itinerant practitioners at the fairs of England,[25] but this method is not approved of now because the jugular veins may be endangered. Open tenotomy of the sternal and clavicular heads of the sternomastoid or division of its upper end are followed by overcorrection in a cast or brace.[25]

Muscular Hypertrophy in Hypothyroidism (Kocher-Debré-Sémélaigne Syndrome)

It seems that muscular hypertrophy in hypothyroidism was first mentioned by Kocher[29] in 1892. Debré and Sémélaigne[30] described a syndrome of diffuse muscular hypertrophy in hypothyroid infants with athletic appearance. Najjar and Nachman[31] reviewed the literature and listed 10 reported cases. These children present a characteristic disease picture consisting of typical signs of hypothyroidism combined with enlargement of the skeletal muscles, especially those of the extremities. The gastrocnemius, gluteus, spinalis dorsi, the thenar and hypothenar muscles and the muscles of the forearms are particularly prominent. The tongue also is markedly enlarged. The muscles have a firm consistency but the motor power is reduced. Muscle tone and reflexes are variable. Myotonic reactions, dimpling of the muscle on percussion and slow release of objects have been observed. Histologic changes in the muscles apparently are not uniform. In some cases, the average size of the muscle fibers was normal and in others it was enlarged. Symptoms of hypothyroidism and muscular hypertrophy disappear rapidly after treatment with thyroid. It is not known why the muscular hypertrophy develops in a few children with hypothyroidism but not in the majority of cases.

Congenital Muscular Hypertrophy with Extrapyramidal Motor Disturbances and Mental Deficiency

In 1934, Cornelia de Lange[32] described 3 children with this syndrome and found a fourth case in the literature. In the first patient described by her, the mother noticed immediately after birth the short and broad neck and the massive pectoral muscles. There also was congenital hypertonia and increasing rigidity. At the age of 2 months, the sutures of the skull were closed and marked by elevated ridges. The skin over the cranium was loose and folded and the ears were large and thick. Muscle tonus varied and the tendon reflexes were present. The arms were flexed at the elbows and the fingers rigidly bent. There was marked symmetric hypertrophy of the flexors of the arms but less marked hypertrophy of the pectoralis, deltoid, trapezius and oblique abdominal muscles. The child died and a malformation of the corpus striatum was found. The striatum was underdeveloped, the corpus callosum thin, the fornix hypertrophied and there were many cavities in the brain. It is noteworthy that in the first case described by de Lange a sibling apparently had the same disorder. There were some doubts concerning the specificity of the syndrome, and the opinion was expressed that the affected children had hypothyroidism with muscular hypertrophy. In some of the cases, the protruding tongue contributed to the impression of myxedema. In 1957, Goldstein[33] summarized several cases that seemed to belong to the syndrome of congenital muscle hypertrophy described by de Lange. He reported a patient who had been born with a large omphalocele, operated on immediately after birth. Because of the large tongue, the child was treated with thyroid without effect. The muscles were prominent and the tongue protruding from the mouth. Hypothyroidism and glycogen storage disease could be ruled out, but cerebral hypoplasia with enlargement and deformity of the ventricles could be demonstrated by pneumoencephalography. The author thought that muscular hypertrophy was demonstrated by reduced excretion of creatine in the urine. The combination of omphalocele, macroglossia and muscular hypertrophy suggests that Goldstein's[33] patient may have had visceromegaly. Hyperplasia of the lingual muscles and general overgrowth have been demonstrated in that disorder. A case reported by Pannullo[34] as congenital macroglossia had generalized muscular hypertrophy and probably visceromegaly (see p. 171). Localized muscular hypertrophy limited to the tongue and forearms was observed by Silver and Schroeder.[35] There was an elevated ratio of acid mucopolysaccharide to creatinine in the urine. Mental development was normal. Cocker and Thomson[36] reported multiple smooth muscle hypertrophies in a child dying soon after delivery by a myasthenic mother who had been treated with large doses of neostigmine throughout pregnancy. The authors suggested that the treatment of the mother could have caused the muscle hypertrophies.

REFERENCES

1. Bing, R.: Über angeborene Muskeldefekte, Virchows Arch. path. Anat. 170:175, 1902.
2. Binder, A. W.: Die Missbildungen des Muskelsystems, in Schwalbe, E., and Gruber, G. B. (eds.), *Die Morphologie der Missbildungen des Menschen und der Tiere* (Jena: Gustav Fischer, 1929).
3. Liebenam, L.: Zwillingspathologische Untersuchungen aus dem Gebiet der Anomalien der Körperform. Partieller Riesenwuchs, Angeborener Pektoralisdefekt, Dysostosis cleidocraniofacialis, Ztschr. menschl. Vererb.-u. Konstitutionslehre 22:373, 1939.
4. Hayes, W. M.: Congenital absence of the pectoralis major muscle in whole or in part and the absence of the pectoralis minor muscle (unilateral), South. Surg. 15:417, 1949.
5. Markkula, H., and Korttila, K.: Anomaly of the pectoral muscles; a case report with new observations, Ann. paediat. fenniae 6:203, 1960.
6. Booth, J. B., and Berry, C. L.: Unilateral pulmonary agenesis, Arch. Dis. Childhood 42:361, 1967.
7. Steche, O.: Beitrage zur Kenntnis der kongenitalen Muskeldefecte, Deutsche Ztschr. Nervenh. 28:217, 1905.
8. King, T. S., and O'Rahilly, R.: M. palmaris accessorius and duplication of M. palmaris longus, Acta anat. 10:327, 1950.
9. Silverman, F., and Huang, N.: Congenital absence of abdominal muscles associated with malformation of genitourinary and alimentary tracts; report of cases and review of literature, Am. J. Dis. Child. 80:91, 1950.
10. Eagle, J. F., Jr., and Barrett, G. S.: Congenital deficiency of abdominal musculature with associated genitourinary abnormalities: A syndrome, Pediatrics 6:721, 1950.
11. Monnet, P., Jeune, M., Gauthier, J., and Freycon, F.: Aplasie musculaire congénitale des muscles abdominaux et phénomènes de rétention au niveau des voies urinaires, Semaine hôp. Paris 35:2524, 1959.
12. Fröhlich, F.: *Der Mangel der Muskeln, insbesondere der Seitenbauchmuskeln* (Würzburg: C. A. Zurn, 1839).
13. Parker, R. W.: Case of an infant in whom some of the abdominal muscles were absent, Lancet 1:1252, 1895.
14. Greene, L. F., Emmett, J. L., Culp, O. S., and Kennedy, R. L. J.: Urologic abnormalities associated with congenital absence or deficiency of abdominal musculature, J. Urol. 68:217, 1952.
15. Simpson, A., and Ashby, E. C.: Torsion of wandering spleen, Brit. J. Surg. 52:344, 1965.
16. Stumme, E. G.: Über die symmetrischen kongenitalen Bauchmuskeldefekte und über die Kombination derselben mit anderen Bildungsanomalien des Rumpfes, Mitt. Grenzgeb. Med. Chir. 11:548, 1903.
17. Mathieu, B. J., Goldowsky, S., Chaset, N., and Mathieu, P. L., Jr.: Congenital deficiency of the abdominal muscles (with associated multiple anomalies), J. Pediat. 42:92, 1953.
18. Lattimer, J. K.: Congenital deficiency of the abdominal musculature and associated genitourinary anomalies. A report of 22 cases, Tr. Am. A. Genito-Urin. Surgeons 49: 28, 1957.
19. Boissonnat, P., and Duhamel, B.: Congenital diverticulum of the anterior urethra associated with aplasia of the abdominal muscles in a male infant, Brit. J. Urol. 34:59, 1962.
20. Jeune, M., and Jacquot, F.: Un cas de syndrome d'Ulrich avec aplasie de la musculature abdominale, Pédiatrie 7: 790, 1952.
21. Stanga, E.: Über multiple Abartungen mit Flughautbildung (Pterygium-Syndrom) und kongenitaler Aplasie der Bauchdeckenmuskulatur, Ann. paediat. 187:384, 1956.
22. Lidge, R. T., Bechtol, R. C., and Lambert, C. N.: Congenital muscular torticollis, J. Bone & Joint Surg. 39-A:1165, 1957.
23. Jones, P. G.: *Torticollis in Infancy and Childhood, Sternomastoid Fibrosis and the Sternomastoid "Tumour"* (Springfield, Ill.: Charles C Thomas, Publisher, 1968).
24. Becker, P. E.: Myopathien, in Becker, P. E. (ed.), *Humangenetik* (Stuttgart: Georg Thieme, 1964).
25. Hulbert, K. F.: Congenital torticollis, J. Bone & Joint Surg. 32-B:50, 1950.
26. Garceau, G.: Congenital muscular torticollis. Hematoma, fact or myth, Rhode Island M. J. 45:401, 1962.
27. Chandler, F. A., and Altenberg, A.: "Congenital" muscular torticollis, J.A.M.A. 125:476, 1944.
28. Isigkeit, E.: Untersuchungen über die Heredität orthopädischer Leiden. III. Der angeborene Schiefhals, Arch. orthop. u. Unfall-Chir. 30:459, 1931.
29. Kocher, T.: Zur Verhütung des Cretinismus und cretinoider Zustände nach neuen Forschungen, Deutsche Ztschr. Chir. 34:556, 1892.
30. Debré, R., and Sémélaigne, G.: Syndrome of diffuse muscular hypertrophy in infants causing athletic appearance, Am. J. Dis. Child. 50:1351, 1935.
31. Najjar, S. S., and Nachman, H. S.: The Kocher-Debré-Sémélaigne syndrome, J. Pediat. 66:901, 1965.
32. de Lange, C.: Congenital hypertrophy of the muscles, extrapyramidal motor disturbances and mental deficiency. A clinical entity, Am. J. Dis. Child. 48:243, 1934.
33. Goldstein, R.: Congenitale Muskelhypertrophie, Ann. paediat. 189:51, 1957.
34. Pannullo, J. N.: Congenital macroglossia, Obst. & Gynec. 7:97, 1956.
35. Silver, H. K., and Schroeder, F. A.: Congenital muscular hypertrophy, Am. J. Dis. Child. 108:406, 1964.
36. Cocker, J., and Thomson, R. M.: Multiple smooth muscle hypertrophies in a newborn infant, Arch. Dis. Childhood 41:514, 1966.

Congenital Muscular Dystrophy

IN GENERAL, the progressive muscular dystrophies are disorders of postnatal life and are not dealt with in this book. Congenital muscular dystrophy is a primary myopathy present at birth that is characterized by histologic changes similar to those seen in progressive muscular dystrophy. In infants, the disorder manifests itself either by generalized muscular hypotonia or by arthrogryposis.[1-3] Fetal movements may be weak and delayed and breech presentation is not rare. Muscular hypotonia is combined with poor sucking and sometimes with cyanosis. Muscles near the trunk commonly are weaker than distal ones. Paresis of the muscles of the neck and the face is noticeable. Intercostal and diaphragmatic muscles may be involved. Contractures can be congenital or they develop later. Muscular atrophy often is concealed by fat but pseudohypertrophies are not noticeable. Floppiness in infancy is followed by frequent falling and stumbling later.

Course and prognosis are variable. A severe form (de Lange type[4,5]) can lead to early death or to a stationary disease picture of muscular dystrophy. The benign form (Batten-Turner type[6-8]) consists of hypotonia and weakness of pelvic and neck muscles with a tendency to improvement. Serum enzymes are either normal or slightly elevated. Histologic findings are typical of muscular dystrophy.[9] The disorder occurs in both sexes, and siblings may be affected in the benign and severe forms. Autosomal recessive inheritance has been suggested.[2]

REFERENCES

1. Vasella, F. M., Mumenthaler, M., Rossi, E., Moser, H., and Wiesmann, U.: Die kongenitale Muskeldystrophie, Deutsche Ztschr. Nervenh. 190:349, 1967.
2. Rotthauwe, H. W., Kowalewski, S., and Mumenthaler, M.: Kongenitale Muskeldystrophie, Ztschr. Kinderh. 106:131, 1969.
3. Banker, B. Q., Victor, M., and Adams, R. D.: Arthrogryposis multiplex due to congenital muscular dystrophy, Brain 80: 319, 1957.
4. de Lange, C.: Studien über angeborene Lähmungen bzw. angeborene Hypotonie, Acta paediat. 20: (supp. 3), 1937.
5. Zellweger, H., Afifi, A., McCormick, W. F., and Mergner, W.: Severe congenital muscular dystrophy, Am. J. Dis. Child. 114:591, 1967.
6. Batten, F. E.: Infantile type of myopathy, Brain 26:147, 1903.
7. Turner, J. W. A., and Lee, F.: Congenital myopathy—a fifty year follow-up, Brain 85:733, 1962.
8. Zellweger, H., Afifi, A., McCormick, W. F., and Mergner, W.: Benign congenital muscular dystrophy: A special form of congenital hypotonia, Clin. Pediat. 6:655, 1967.
9. Engel, W. K.: Muscle biopsies in neuromuscular diseases, Pediat. Clin. North America 14:963, 1967.

Dystrophia Myotonica

IN CONTRAST TO congenital myotonia, which is limited to the muscular system, dystrophia myotonica affects many organ systems and there is a possibility that congenital malformations occur with increased frequency in affected kindreds. The fully developed disease seen in adults consists of myotonia, muscular atrophies, ptosis, cataracts, frontal baldness, testicular atrophy, various endocrine disturbances, cardiac anomalies, skeletal changes and mental deterioration. The prevalence among Caucasians is about 3 per 100,000. Males and females are affected and dominant inheritance with variable expressivity seems well established.[1,2] Although the onset of the disease usually is noticed after puberty, there are now many cases on record that prove onset in infancy and childhood.[3-8] Prenatal onset and congenital malformations in patients and their offspring are under consideration.[2,5] Caughey and Myrianthopoulos[2] collected from the literature many cases of congenital malformation occurring in families with dystrophic myotonica. With the exception of congenital clubfoot and ptosis, which were noticed in many cases, there was no pattern of defects that was clearly of prenatal origin. High palate, facial and cranial asymmetries and some other skeletal anomalies could be the result of postnatal factors associated with the disease. Reports on congenital cataracts,[2] oxycephaly and craniosynostosis,[3] cleft lip and palate,[2] congenital heart disease,[2] horseshoe kidney,[8] defects of pectoral muscle,[2] simian crease[8] and radio-ulnar synostosis[3] deserve attention in future examinations, but the association with dystrophia myotonica is not well established at present. There is no doubt that mental retardation is frequent in children with early onset of the disease[7,8] but it is not certain that it is present at the time of birth.

In future studies, congenital malformations occurring in patients with dystrophia myotonica should be listed separately from those occurring in the offspring of affected fathers and of affected mothers and separated from those occurring in the kindred in unaffected persons and their children.

REFERENCES

1. Thomasen, E.: *Myotonia* (Copenhagen: Ejnar Munksgaard, 1948).
2. Caughey, J. E., and Myrianthopoulos, N. C.: *Dystrophia Myotonica and Related Disorders* (Springfield, Ill.: Charles C Thomas, Publisher, 1963).
3. Klein, D.: Manifestations progressives et extensives d'une dystrophie myotonique dans une famille argovienne, Confinia neurol. 14:169, 1954.

4. Vanier, T. M.: Dystrophia myotonica in childhood, Brit. M. J. 2:1284, 1960.
5. Pruzanski, W.: Congenital malformations in myotonic dystrophy, Acta neurol. scandinav. 41:34, 1965.
6. Dodge, P. R., Gamstorp, I., Byers, R. K., and Russell, P.: Myotonic dystrophy in infancy and childhood, Pediatrics 35:3, 1965.
7. Calderon, R.: Myotonic dystrophy: A neglected cause of mental retardation, J. Pediat. 68:423, 1966.
8. Watters, G. V., and Williams, T. W.: Early onset of myotonic dystrophy, Arch. Neurol. 17:137, 1967.

Schwartz-Jampel Syndrome

A DISEASE PICTURE of myotonia, shortness of stature and congenital hip dysplasia has been described.[1,2] The disorder has been observed twice in siblings. In contrast to Thomsen disease, which is inherited as an autosomal dominant, the Schwartz-Jampel syndrome seems to be recessively inherited. It probably is related to "chondrodystrophic myotonia," which is characterized by similar skeletal changes, dwarfism, abnormal posture, narrow palpebral fissures and small chin.[3]

REFERENCES

1. Schwartz, O., and Jampel, R. S.: Congenital blepharophimosis associated with a unique generalized myopathy, Arch. Ophth. 68:52, 1962.
2. Mereu, T. R., Porter, I. H., and Hug, G.: Myotonia, shortness of stature, and hip dysplasia, Am. J. Dis. Child. 117: 470, 1969.
3. Aberfeld, D. C., Namba, T., Vye, M. V., and Grob, D.: Chondrodystrophic myotonia: Report of two cases, Arch. Neurol. 22:455, 1970.

PART XVI

Malformations of the Urogenital System

105

The Kidney

Bilateral Renal Agenesis

THIS IS A LETHAL congenital malformation that is compatible with intrauterine but not postnatal life. Ninety-five per cent of infants born with this anomaly die within the first 24 hours. In rare cases, survival is possible for several days or weeks and in one instance a child lived for 39 days.[1] Reviews on this subject were written by Potter,[2,5] Davidson and Ross,[3] Bain and Scott[4] and Stockhausen.[44]

Incidence figures vary, but it seems that 1 case occurs in about 3,000–4,000 deliveries.[5,6] Davidson and Ross[3] reviewed 232 cases. Approximately 70% of the affected infants are males. As a rule, the siblings of these infants are normal, but Madisson[7] and Baron[8] each reported 2 cases occurring in the same family. Renal agenesis described in sisters by Schmidt *et al.*[9] was found to be a manifestation of a syndrome of renal, genital and middle ear anomalies. In 2 other sisters of that family who survived, unilateral renal agenesis or hypoplasia was demonstrated.[10] Hilson[11] reported a typical case of bilateral renal agenesis in a kindred in which unilateral agenesis, "cystic kidney disease," hypospadias and ear deformities occurred in several members. The anomaly has been observed six times in twins[3] with only one twin being affected. In two instances, the mothers had taken abortive measures in early pregnancy.[12,13] One infant with this anomaly was born to a mother who had pulmonary stenosis[14] and in other cases congenital heart disease was present in siblings of the affected child.[3]

It seems likely that, in some instances, genetic factors play a role in the etiology of this disorder, but the fact that in a pair of identical twins only one twin was affected[3] suggests that nongenetic factors can also be involved. Aside from the cases of admitted use of abortifacients, no disturbances in pregnancy have been found with any regularity. Maternal age and parity do not seem to be significant in the etiology of this disorder. The chromosomes are normal,[15] but in some of the cases apparently male infants have an XX sex chromosome complement.[16]

More than 30% of these children are stillborn. Welch[6] pointed out that the birth weight usually is low for the gestational age of the child and intrauterine growth retardation was well documented by others.[5,17] Sixty per cent of infants with renal agenesis or severe urinary tract dysplasia are delivered in breech presentation and most of them with oligohydramnios. Amniotic fluid is present in rare cases when renal agenesis is combined with anencephaly or iniencephaly.[4] Amnion nodosum is noted in most of the cases and single umbilical artery in some. Children who are born alive have respiratory difficulties to which they succumb.

At necropsy, the kidneys and ureters are absent. If rudimentary ureters are found, there also is rudimentary renal tissue.[5] The renal arteries either are absent or end in the fat surrounding the adrenal glands. The bladder is small, often elongated and sometimes atretic. Other derivatives of the mesonephric and paramesonephric ducts are variable. Sometimes they are present and deformed and sometimes they are absent. As a rule, the gonads are fairly well developed and the testes are located in the scrotum or near the scrotum in the inguinal canal.

Potter[2] established that in most cases bilateral renal agenesis is found in a syndrome that can be recognized on external inspection by the appearance of the face: "The face most characteristically exhibits an increased space between the eyes, a prominent

Fig. 105-1.—This graph shows that most infants with renal agenesis are born with subnormal weights for their gestational age. (From E. L. Potter.[5])

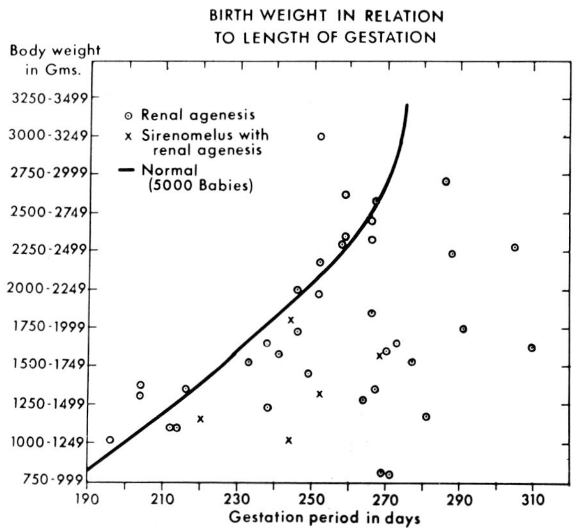

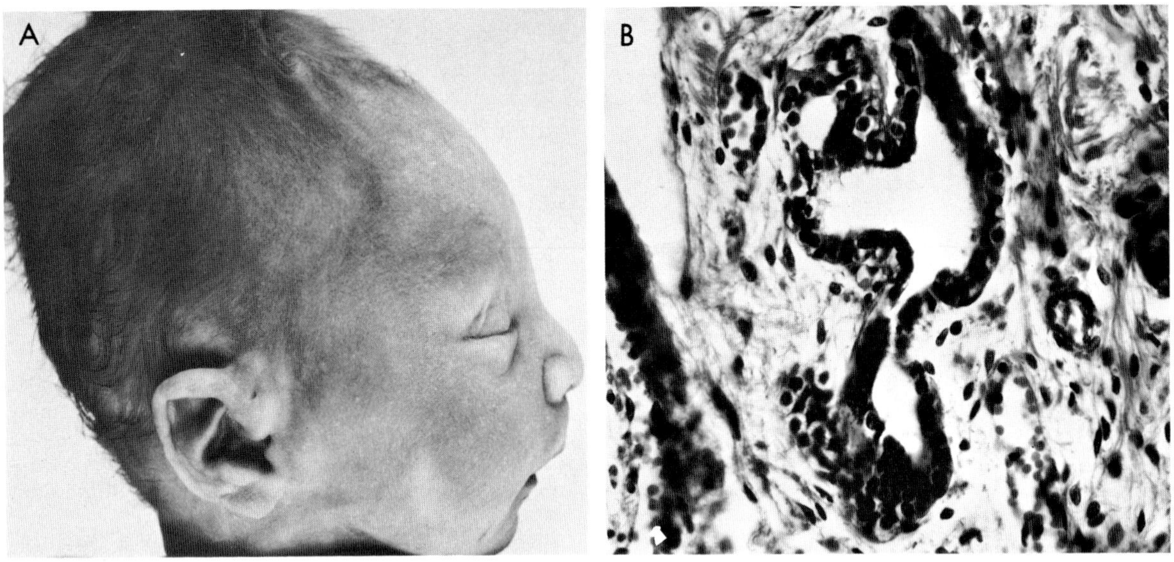

Fig. 105-2. – **A,** head of a child with renal "agenesis."[15] **B,** renal tubular rudiment found near ureter of this child.

fold which arises at the inner canthus and sweeps downward and laterally below the eyes, an unusual flattening of the nose, excessive recession of the chin, and moderate enlargement and decreased chondrification of the ears. The face gives a suggestion of premature senility and is sufficiently characteristic to warrant a diagnosis of coexisting renal aplasia when it is observed." Bilateral agenesis occurs as an isolated malformation in less than 30% of the cases. Hypoplasia of the lungs is present in the majority of cases and may be responsible for early death of the children, who usually have dyspnea and cyanosis before uremia sets in. Congenital heart defects are less common, yet septal defects, patent ductus arteriosus, coarctation of the aorta, truncus arteriosus and transposition of the great vessels have been described.[5,6] Malformations of the ears were emphasized by Hilson.[11]

Talipes is common and sometimes more severe malformations of the lower extremities are present. The lower spine, including the sacrum and coccyx, may be absent.[18] In such cases, the adrenal glands are fused in the midline,[5] but in most infants without kidneys the adrenals are large, flat and oval, assuming some of the space usually occupied by the kidney. Agenesis of the kidneys and Potter syndrome can be

Fig. 105-3. – Typical facies of a newborn child with renal agenesis. (Courtesy of Dr. E. L. Potter, Chicago, Illinois.)

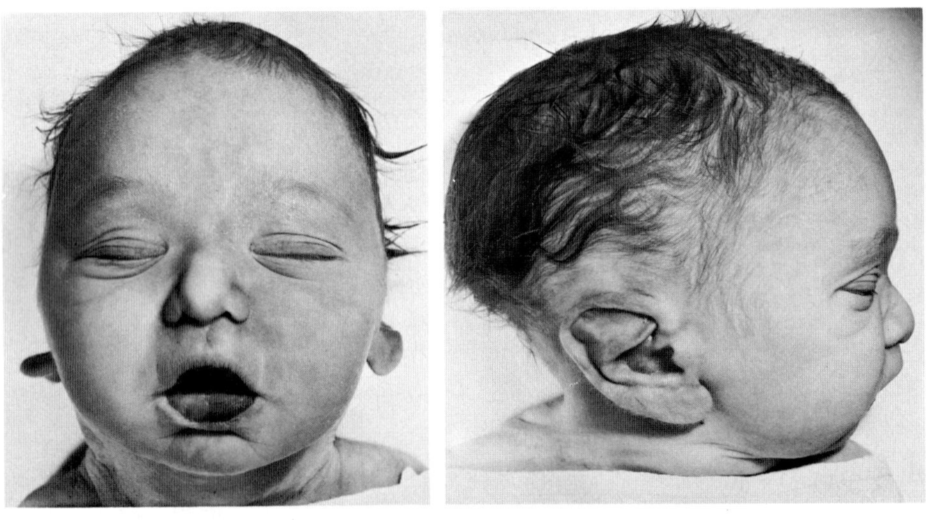

associated with sirenomelia.[5,18,19] In approximately 60% of infants without kidneys the gastrointestinal canal is abnormal; imperforate anus, malrotation of the intestine, Meckel diverticulum and others coexist. Cleft lip or palate is rare; they were noted in only 3 of Potter's[5] 50 cases, but this frequency is about forty times that of the general newborn population. In female fetuses, the external genitalia often are deformed; the vagina and uterus can be absent or rudimentary.[5] A syndrome of absent kidneys associated with esophageal atresia, tracheo-esophageal fistula, small bladder and urethra and contracted lesser pelvis and imperforate anus may represent a specific entity.[45] In rare instances of renal agenesis, infants with male external genitalia have ovaries. In one of these cases of female pseudohermaphrodism,[20] an XX chromosome complement was found.[16]

There is no treatment, and the prognosis is hopeless for infants with bilateral renal agenesis.

Unilateral Renal Agenesis (Congenital Solitary Kidney)

Congenital solitary kidney is a rather frequent anomaly that was known as far back as Aristotle's time.[21] Its incidence is estimated as 1 in 600[22] to 1 in 1,000 necropsies[21]; it is more frequent in necropsies of children than in those of adults.[23] Incidence and prevalence in the population are not known, since no serial examinations have been made in survivors. Doroshow and Abeshouse[24] reviewed all reported cases from 1932 through 1960 and added 37. The world literature at that time contained almost 1,500 cases. Males were affected nearly twice as often as females.[17] Either kidney can be affected. Although unilateral renal agenesis is a congenital anomaly, it is not discovered in two-thirds of the patients until they are 35–45 years of age.[17,21] It has been reported in a boy and in his uncle.[25] In children with Fanconi pancytopenia, solitary kidney has been noted repeatedly. This is an example of the anomaly occurring in a recessively inherited syndrome.[26] Waardenburg[27] observed monozygotic twins, one with a right and the other with a left solitary kidney. In trisomy 18, unilateral renal agenesis or dysplasia was found in 7% of necropsies.[28] A single kidney was present in an infant with partial trisomy B.[29] Several children with renal anomalies possibly due to prenatal rubella have been reported. Menser *et al.*[30] described a male infant with typical rubella syndrome and agenesis of the left kidney. Rubella virus was present in the urine for 10 months. Unilateral renal agenesis has been observed in children damaged by thalidomide.[31-33] The ureter usually is absent on the side of the renal agenesis and rudimentary in some cases. In about half of the patients reported, the functioning kidney was hypertrophic and in some instances it was reduplicated. Although such a kidney can function for a long time, it often is the site of disease and abnormality. It may be malrotated, hydronephrotic, polycystic or ectopic. Crossed renal ectopy with solitary kidney was reviewed by Purpon.[34] Calculi often are found in the renal pelvis. Pyelonephritis with pyuria and hematuria are reported in about one-third of the cases. In the past, when urologic examinations had not yet achieved the perfection of today, such diseased kidneys occasionally were removed, which caused uremic death of the patient.

Congenital solitary kidney often is associated with anomalies of the genitalia. The incidence of associated genital anomalies is about 40% in females and 12% in males.[24] Partial or complete duplication of the uterus is the leading anomaly.[22] Unicornuate, bicornuate, septate, arcuate or double uterus has been observed, and there may be double or absent vagina. Unilateral absence of the ovary has been observed also.[35] In cases of unilateral defect of the genitals, the anomaly usually is on the same side as the renal agenesis. In males, the seminal vesicles, prostate or epididymis may be rudimentary[21] and atrophy of the testes and cryptorchidism occur.[22] Unilateral absence of the adrenal has been described, and absence of the spleen combined with agenesis of the left kidney was reported by Peterman.[36] Among anomalies of the intestinal tract, imperforate anus, esophageal atresia or fistula, malrotation of the intestine and rectovaginal fistula have been observed.[23] In some cases, harelip and cleft palate, patent ductus arteriosus, septal defect, hydrocephaly, anencephaly, meningocele, deformities of the feet, hemivertebrae, polydactyly and syndactyly are associated with solitary kidney. A retroperitoneal cyst arising in a persistent metanephros may be found together with absence of the kidney and ureter.[37] Congenital absence of the right kidney, testis and rectus muscle was described as a "right-sided" syndrome in a male twin who had a normal twin sister.[38]

In many patients, particularly females, anomalies of the genitalia lead to investigation of the urinary tract and to discovery of unilateral renal agenesis. In other patients, manifestation of renal disease leads to urologic investigation. However, congenital solitary kidneys are not discovered often intra vitam but are found as accidental observations at necropsy. The urologic diagnosis is suggested by absence of signs of a kidney in excretory urograms. Enlargement of the shadow of the existing kidney or an ectopic position of that kidney may contribute to the diagnosis. On cystoscopy, the absence of one ureteral opening or hemiatrophy of the trigone will lead to a correct diagnosis.

Congenital solitary kidney is compatible with a long and active life, but since the single kidney present is likely to be diseased, urinary complications are not rare and in about one-quarter of the cases of solitary kidney seen at necropsy renal failure was the cause of death.[23]

Absence of one or both kidneys with absence of ureters and renal vessels occurred in the my/my strain of mice with myelencephalic blebs. By selective breeding of animals with solitary kidneys, the incidence of affected animals could be raised and young with absence of both kidneys occurred. Rarer were mice with one small, polycystic or hydronephrotic kidney.[38] Absence of one or both kidneys and many other urogenital anomalies were also observed in Sd (short-tail) mice.[39,40] Absence of a kidney in an inbred strain of rats was reported by Morgan.[41] About 10% of the animals lacked one kidney. The mode of inheritance was complex.

Unilateral or bilateral renal agenesis was reported by Monie[42] in the young of female rats treated with chlorambucil. We saw unilateral renal agenesis in the offspring of rats treated with methyl salicylate.[43]

REFERENCES

1. Woolf, R. B., and Allen, W. M.: Concomitant malformations; frequent simultaneous occurrence of congenital malformations of reproductive and urinary tracts, Obst. & Gynec. 2:236, 1953.
2. Potter, E. L.: Bilateral renal agenesis, J. Pediat. 29:68, 1946.
3. Davidson, W. M., and Ross, G. I. M.: Bilateral absence of the kidneys and related congenital anomalies, J. Path. & Bact. 68:459, 1954.
4. Bain, A. D., and Scott, J. S.: Renal agenesis and severe urinary tract dysplasia, Brit. M. J. 1:841, 1960.
5. Potter, E. L.: Bilateral absence of ureters and kidneys. A report of 50 cases, Obst. & Gynec. 25:3, 1965.
6. Welch, R. G.: The Potter syndrome of renal agenesis, Brit. M. J. 1:1102, 1958.
7. Madisson, H.: Über das Fehlen beider Nieren (Aplasia renum bilateralis), Zentralbl. allg. Path. 60:1, 1934.
8. Baron, C.: Bilateral agenesis of kidneys in 2 consecutive infants, Am. J. Obst. & Gynec. 67:667, 1954.
9. Schmidt, E. C. H., Hartley, A. A., and Bower, R.: Aplasia in sisters, A. M. A. Arch. Path. 54:403, 1952.
10. Winter, J. S. D., Kohn, G., Mellamn, W. J., and Wagner, S.: A familial syndrome of renal, genital and middle ear anomalies, J. Pediat. 72:88, 1968.
11. Hilson, D.: Malformation of ears as sign of malformation of genito-urinary tract, Brit. M. J. 2:785, 1957.
12. Osmond, R.: Report of 3 cases of bilateral renal agenesis, M. J. Australia 1:42, 1955.
13. Sylvester, P. E., and Hughes, D. R.: Congenital absence of both kidneys; report of 4 cases, Brit. M. J. 1:77, 1954.
14. Peschke, H.: Beitrag zu den Missbildungen am uropoetischen System: (bilaterale Nierenaplasie: Ventilklappenbildung in der Pars prostatica der Urethra mit Hydronephrose), Beitr. path. Anat. 96:528, 1936.
15. Passarge, E., and Sutherland, J. M.: Potter's syndrome, Am. J. Dis. Child. 109:80, 1965.
16. Schlegel, R. J., Aspillaga, M. J., Neu, R. L., Carneiro-Leano, J., and Gardner, L. I.: An XX sex chromosome complement in an infant having male-type external genitals, renal agenesis and other anomalies, J. Pediat. 69: 812, 1966.
17. Ashley, D. J. B., and Mostofi, F. K.: Renal agenesis and dysgenesis, J. Urol. 83:211, 1960.
18. Fritzsche, F.: Dysplasia renofacialis bei Anchipodie, Ztschr. Kinderh. 81:760, 1958.
19. Bearn, J. G.: The association of sirenomelia with Potter's syndrome, Arch. Dis. Childhood 35:254, 1960.
20. Carpentier, P. J., and Potter, E. L.: Nuclear sex and genital malformations in 48 cases of renal agenesis with especial reference to non-specific female pseudohermaphroditism, Am. J. Obst. & Gynec. 76:235, 1959.
21. Longo, V. J., and Thompson, G. J.: Congenital solitary kidney, J. Urol. 68:63, 1952.
22. Thompson, D. P., and Lynn, H. B.: Genital anomalies associated with solitary kidney, Mayo Clin. Proc. 41:538, 1966.
23. Campbell, M.: *Clinical Pediatric Urology* (Philadelphia: W. B. Saunders Company, 1951).
24. Doroshow, L. W., and Abeshouse, B. S.: Congenital unilateral solitary kidney; report of 37 cases and a review of the literature, Urol. Survey 11:219, 1961.
25. Bound, J. P.: Two cases of congenital absence of one kidney in the same family, Brit. M. J. 2:747, 1943.
26. Nilsson, L. R.: Chronic pancytopenia with multiple congenital abnormalities (Fanconi's anaemia), Acta paediat. 49:518, 1960.
27. Waardenburg, P. J.: Einseitige Aplasie der Niere und ihrer Abführwege bei beiden eineiigen Zwillingspaarlingen, Acta genet. med. 1:317, 1952.
28. Warkany, J., Passarge, E., and Smith, L. B.: Congenital malformations in autosomal trisomy syndromes, Am. J. Dis. Child. 112:502, 1966.
29. Shaw, M. W., Cohen, M. M., and Hildebrandt, H. M.: A familial 4/5 reciprocal translocation resulting in partial trisomy B, Am. J. Human Genet. 17:54, 1965.
30. Menser, M. A., Robertson, S. E. J., Dorman, D. C., Gillespie, A. M., and Murphy, A. M.: Renal lesions in congenital rubella, Pediatrics 40:901, 1967.
31. Wiedemann, H-R.: Hinweis auf eine derzeitige Häufung hypo- und aplastischer Fehlbildungen der Gliedmassen, Med. Welt 37:1863, 1961.
32. Weicker, H.: 100 children with thalidomide embryopathy, XIth International Congress of Pediatrics, 1965.
33. Kreipe, U.: Missbildungen innerer Organe bei Thalidomid-embryopathie, Arch. Kinderh. 176:33, 1967.
34. Purpon, I.: Crossed renal ectopy with solitary kidney: A review of the literature, J. Urol. 90:13, 1963.
35. Schumacker, H. B.: Congenital anomalies of the genitalia associated with unilateral renal agenesis, Arch. Surg. 37: 586, 1938.
36. Peterman, M. G.: Congenital absence of spleen and left kidney, J.A.M.A. 99:1252, 1932.
37. Krauss, L. W., and Straus, R.: Retroperitoneal cyst arising in persistent metanephros with congenital absence of right kidney and ureter, J. Urol. 34:97, 1935.
38. Texter, J. H., and Murphy, G. P.: The right-sided syndrome: Congenital absence of the right testis, kidney and rectus. Urologic diagnosis and treatment, Bull. Johns Hopkins Hosp. 122:224, 1968.
39. Grüneberg, H.: *The Genetics of the Mouse* (The Hague: Martinus Nijhoff, 1952).
40. Gluecksohn-Schoenheimer, S.: The morphological manifestation of a dominant mutation in mice affecting tail and urogenital system, Genetics 28:341, 1943.
41. Morgan, W. C.: Inherited congenital kidney, absence in an inbred strain of rats, Anat. Rec. 115:635, 1953.
42. Monie, I. W.: Chlorambucil-induced abnormalities of the urogenital system of rat fetuses, Anat. Rec. 139:145, 1961.
43. Warkany, J., and Takacs, E.: Unpublished data.
44. Stockhausen, H-B.: Beitrag zur Problematik der Dysplasia renofacialis, Ztschr. Kinderh. 105:303, 1969.
45. Currarino, G.: Association of congenitally small pelvic outlet with hypoplasia of bladder and urethra, and absent kidneys, Am. J. Roentgenol. 109:399, 1970.

Renal Hypoplasia and Dysplasia

Renal Hypoplasia

BY DEFINITION, renal hypoplasia refers to kidneys of incomplete development. In the strict sense, "simple hypoplasia" is an underdevelopment that leads to a small kidney with histologically normal parenchyma. Such miniature kidneys exist, but many very small kidneys described in the literature as hypoplastic did not have normal parenchyma and were complicated by dysplastic and cystic processes. If a clear distinction of hypoplastic from small kidneys of other types is difficult for the pathologist, it is almost impossible for clinicians dealing with small kidneys. It is clear, therefore, that clinical statements concerning hypoplastic kidneys do not always refer to the simple miniature type seen by the pathologist. Dysplastic and atrophic kidneys are not easily distinguished from the hypoplastic, and incidence as well as significance of the anomaly are difficult to determine.[1] It seems likely that some generally hypoplastic kidneys have dysplastic areas in some portions. This can result in discussions that lead nowhere and have little significance. Although there exists an extensive literature on this subject, there is little agreement on "what to call hypoplastic kidney."[2] If it were possible to distinguish clinically or etiologically between "normal" miniature kidneys and "abnormal" small kidneys, the differentiation would be important. At present, the situation is so confused[4] that the pathologist's terminology cannot be brought into agreement with that of the clinician, and the following paragraphs will reflect this situation.

Hypoplasia can be unilateral or bilateral. Bilateral hypoplasia, if severe, may lead to neonatal death or growth failure, hypertension and renal failure during childhood. It is suggested by radiography and confirmed by biopsy, which reveals normal parenchyma. It has been suggested that most bilateral hypoplastic kidneys result from retardation of postnatal growth, but they can be associated with developmental abnormalities of other organ systems[1] and with mental retardation.[3] Boissonnat[2] distinguished an upper polar and a bipolar type of hypoplastic kidney and a third type (pseudominiature) characterized by few minor calices that are poorly developed and badly shaped. Since the calices come from the whole external pelvic area, they look, in roentgenograms, like a complete set, although they are reduced in number. The pseudominiature type is less common in unilateral than in bilateral cases.[2] The Ask-Upmark kidney, a special and rare type of renal hypoplasia, is included by pathologists among the true forms of hypoplastic kidneys,[1,4] although it cannot be considered a "miniature kidney." It is a small kidney with a small number of pyramids and a transverse groove on its capsular surface. The groove is separated from a dilated calix by a sclerotic fibrous plate. The anomaly, which can result in hypertension and lithiasis, is attributed to arrest of nephrogenesis in one or several adjacent renal lobules after the formation of juxtamedullary nephrons.[4]

Oligonephronic hypoplasia refers to small kidneys that contain a reduced number of nephrons. The functioning nephrons hypertrophy and, later, interstitial fibrosis and atrophy of nephrons supervene. The condition occurs predominantly in boys who are born with intrauterine growth retardation. Advanced maternal age was noted in about one-third of the cases.[5] Chronic nephritis with inability to concentrate and polydipsia develop, and anemia, growth retardation and renal failure can occur.[1] Bilateral renal hypoplasia with oligonephronia has been described in one of an identical twin pair. Only the affected twin had intrauterine growth retardation.[12] Hypoplasia of the kidney associated with various types of congenital heart disease was emphasized by Bruns.[6]

Clinical observations of patients with hypoplastic kidneys[7,8] probably were derived from small kidneys of various origin and pathology. The symptoms and course of these patients usually cannot be attributed to simple hypoplasia. Unilateral renal hypoplasia can be well tolerated or predispose to nephritis and hypertension. To avoid complications, surgical removal of a hypoplastic kidney has been recommended and segmental hypoplasia with arterial hypertension has been found accessible to surgical treatment.[9]

Renal Dysplasia

The term "dysplasia," indicating malformation, is not used for gross deformities of the kidney but rather for focal histologic malformations found in grossly normal kidneys and attributed to faulty differentiation. Primitive glomeruli, tubules, ductules, ducts and pyramides, metaplastic cartilage and certain cysts are accepted as signs of renal dysplasia but there is disagreement concerning the actual origin of these abnormal structures. It is not certain that all of them result from primary maldevelopment, since it has been shown that some of these faulty tissues are deformed by acquired disease. According to Bernstein and Meyer,[1] only primitive ducts and metaplastic cartilage are signs of congenital maldevelopment. An important factor responsible for renal dysplasia is congenital urinary tract obstruction by anomalies of the ureters, the urethra, the bladder neck or the prostatic utricle.[4]

Unfortunately, the dysplasia defined as focal failure of differentiation in otherwise normally formed kidneys is not the only type of renal dysplasia. Dysplastic areas are found in hypoplastic kidneys; if hypoplasia and dysplasia are extreme, some speak of "aplastic" kidneys, which is to be distinguished from "agenetic" (p. 1037). Aplastic kidney commonly is unilateral; if bilateral and associated with multiple congenital malformations, death in early neonatal life or chronic renal failure results.[1] Since "aplasia," like "agenesis," suggests lack of formation, distinction of the two terms is difficult. The term "renal dysplasia" is also applied to unilateral polycystic and multicystic kidneys, polycystic disease with abundant stroma and segmental and focal defects.[4] The terms used by pathologists so far have little meaning to those interested in etiology, pathogenesis, clinical course and prognosis.

In certain syndromes, dysplasia of the kidneys, liver and pancreas was reported in siblings as a genetically determined disorder.[10] Retinal aplasia in siblings combined with renal dysplasia leading to pyelonephritis and early renal failure has been seen in siblings.[11]

REFERENCES

1. Bernstein, J., and Meyer, R.: Parenchymal Maldevelopment of the Kidney, in Brennemann, J., and Kelley, V. C. (eds.), *Practice of Pediatrics* (Hagerstown, Md.: Hoeber Medical Division, Harper & Row, Publishers, 1967), Vol. III, Chap. 26, p. 1.
2. Boissonnat, P.: What to call hypoplastic kidney?, Arch. Dis. Childhood 37:142, 1962.
3. Roosen-Runge, E. C.: Retardation of postnatal development of kidneys in persons with early cerebral lesions, Am. J. Dis. Child. 77:185, 1949.
4. Kissane, J. M.: Congenital Malformations, in Heptinstall, R. H. (ed.), *Pathology of the Kidney* (Boston: Little, Brown & Company, 1966).
5. Royer, P., Habib, R., Courtecuisse, V., and LeClerc, F.: L'hypoplasie rénale bilatérale avec oligonephronie, Arch. franç. pédiat. 24:249, 1967.
6. Bruns, H. A.: Nierenanomalien bei angeborenen Herzfehlern, Monatsschr. Kinderh. 115:67, 1967.
7. Ekström, T.: Renal hypoplasia: A clinical study of 179 cases, Acta chir. scandinav., Supp. 203, 1955.
8. Campbell, M.: *Clinical Pediatric Urology* (Philadelphia: W. B. Saunders Company, 1951).
9. Mozziconacci, P., Attal, C., Boisse, J., Pham-Huu-Trung, M. T., Guy-Grand, D., and Durand, C.: Hypoplasie segmentaire du rein avec hypertension artérielle, Ann. pédiat. 15:1405, 1968.
10. Ivemark, B. I., Oldfelt, V., and Zetterström, R.: Familial dysplasia of kidneys, liver and pancreas. A probably genetically determined syndrome, Acta paediat. scandinav. 48:1, 1959.
11. Løken, A. C., Hanssen, O., Halvorsen, S., and Jølster, N. J.: Hereditary renal dysplasia and blindness, Acta paediat. 50:177, 1961.
12. Scheinman, J. I., and Abelson, H. T.: Bilateral renal hypoplasia with oligonephronia, J. Pediat. 76:369, 1970.

Congenital Cystic Disease of the Kidney

THIS TERM comprises a variety of cystic renal disorders that are heterogeneous in respect to morphology, pathogenesis and etiology. It seems that the developing kidney responds to many abnormal influences by cyst formation, and neither the gross nor the microscopic appearance of the cysts discloses their causation. Additional data, such as family and pregnancy histories, chromosome findings and listing of associated malformations, sometimes permit a better etiologic understanding. Since, in many reports, the different forms of polycystic kidneys are not distinguished, numerical estimates of incidence, symptoms and prognosis apply to a conglomerate of entities and are therefore of limited value. The disease picture varies in different age groups. Polycystic disease of the kidney occurs in approximately 0.4% of necropsies of children and 0.2% of adult necropsies.[1,2] Age distribution curves uniformly show two definite peaks. The first peak, which represents about 25% of all cases, is made up of infants who are stillborn or who die in neonatal life. It is followed by a sharp decline of manifest cases during the first 2 decades. In the third decade there is an increase of patients, with a second peak reached in the fourth, fifth and sixth decades.[3,4] There is no sex predilection in the adult form,[4,5] but in a series of children's necropsies there were almost twice as many males as females.[1] Congenital polycystic disease usually is bilateral; in unilateral cases, histologic study of the seemingly normal kidney often discloses beginning cyst formation. Several authors[2,3] were of the opinion that infantile and adult polycystic kidneys are pathologically identical, but this applies to some forms only. There is at least one entity, spongy bilateral polycystic giant kidneys, that occurs in infancy only, but other forms affect both infants and adults. There are great variations in degree and it is obvious that a disease process that affects the entire renal parenchyma of a newborn will lead to early death, whereas a similar disorder limited to small portions of the kidney permits not only survival but a marked increase in growth of individual cysts.

The subject of polycystic renal disease has a long history. In 1904, Dunger[6] published a valuable review of 133 articles on cystic kidneys that had appeared up to the twentieth century. He also listed cases of siblings and cases involving two generations. A list of references up to 1941 can be found in an article by Norris and Herman[7] and in a review in 1964 by Osathanondh and Potter.[8] Many of the old controversies appear merely semantic today and conclusions drawn from histologic pictures without consideration of etiology seem outdated and, at best, of historical interest. There is a great need for combination of morphologic and etiologic data that will permit a meaningful classification. In the interim, the morphologic classification of Osathanondh and Potter[8] represents a valuable basis for future investigations concerned with causation. These authors added micro-dissections to the customary gross and histologic examinations of polycystic kidneys and established four types, which clarifies the terminology of the pathologists and helps in the search for etiologic factors. In the following pages, the "types" described and most of the pathologic observations refer to the work and classification of Osathanondh and Potter.[8]

Type 1

This group represents a definite entity seen as bilateral giant kidneys of the newborn, attributed to hyperplasia of interstitial portions of collecting tubules.[8] Other names for this type are "sponge kidney" and "polycystic kidney of the newborn." Type 1 occurs in infants only, since it results in early death, but it is not the only and not the most common type of polycystic kidney encountered in infants. Although many cases of Type 1 have been reported because of their impressive pathologic picture, the incidence seems to be low. In 1961, Potter[9] had found only 2 cases in 100,000 deliveries at the Chicago Lying-in Hospital and these were siblings. Infants with this anomaly usually either are stillborn or they die soon after birth. The most striking cases are characterized by huge kidneys that may weigh many times the normal and present obstacles to normal delivery. The renal anomalies are always accompanied by cystic proliferations of hepatic bile ducts and sometimes by cysts in the lungs, pancreas, spleen and ovaries. If a case appears in a family, there is a definite risk of recurrence; it is likely that the trait is autosomal recessive.

These kidneys are symmetrically enlarged, weigh several hundred grams and expand the entire abdomen. Their surfaces are relatively smooth but minute cysts measuring 1–2 mm. in diameter can be discerned. The "cysts" actually are the ends of long dilated tubules visible on the surface. The renal pelves and calices are enlarged but the ureters and the bladder are normal. On sagittal sections, the kidneys have a spongy appearance because of the grossly enlarged tubular spaces, which run at right angles to the renal surface. Microscopically, the elongated and enlarged tubules are lined by cuboidal cells without signs of flattening or distention. The picture is that of hyperplasia of the tubules and not one of passive expansion. Some of the cylindrical spaces reach the surface, whereas others are separated from it by a zone consisting of more or less normal glomeruli and convoluted tubules. There is no increase in connective tissue or blood vessels between the enlarged spaces. The kidneys are rather normal except for gigantism of the collecting tubules and it seems that only their interstitial but not their terminal portions are affected by the pathologic process.[8]

Micro-dissection shows diverticular cysts in proximal tubules, saccular enlargements in middle tubules and cylindrical cysts in last generation tubules. Most nephrons are normal in number and location, being attached to the last generation collecting tubules.

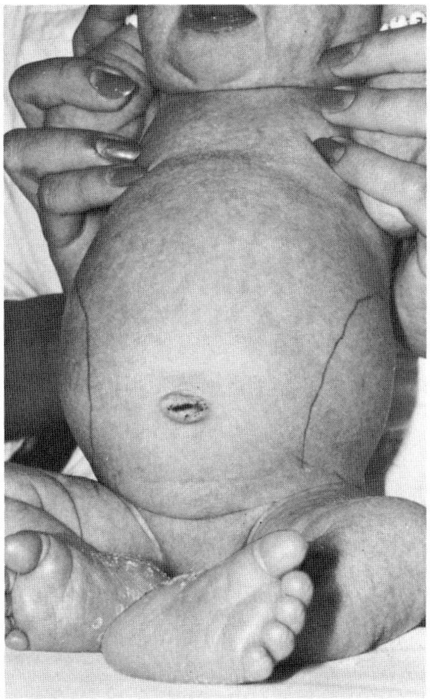

Fig. 105-4.—Newborn girl with enlarged abdomen due to polycystic kidneys. The kidneys (as palpated) are outlined in the picture.

Glomeruli and Bowman capsules are normal. The convoluted tubules sometimes are slightly dilated, and at the angle of the loop of Henle minute cysts can be seen. Norris and Herman[7] traced the enlarged ducts toward the renal surface, where they ended blindly, but Osathanondh and Potter[8] saw no evidence of obstruction or discontinuity in any part. Their findings do not agree with the concept of nonunion of the secretory and collecting renal elements. They asked why children with such kidneys die so soon after birth. Although urine can be excreted through the nephrons and collecting tubules, the life span of infants with such giant kidneys is even shorter than that of children with renal agenesis. The pathologic physiology of these polycystic kidneys remains to be elucidated.

Osathanondh and Potter[8] pointed out that this type of polycystic kidney has never been observed in small fetuses. They believed that the enlargement occurs relatively late, until renal development is well on its way toward completion. This belief is in agreement with the fact that in small rodents, whose gestational period is absolutely and relatively shorter than that of man, no comparable anomalies have been found at birth, although many types of congenital renal anomalies have been produced by a variety of teratogenic procedures. The pleiotropic gene responsible for the cystic enlargements in human kidneys, liver, lungs and other parenchymatous organs may exert its deleterious effects relatively late in fetal life, resulting in

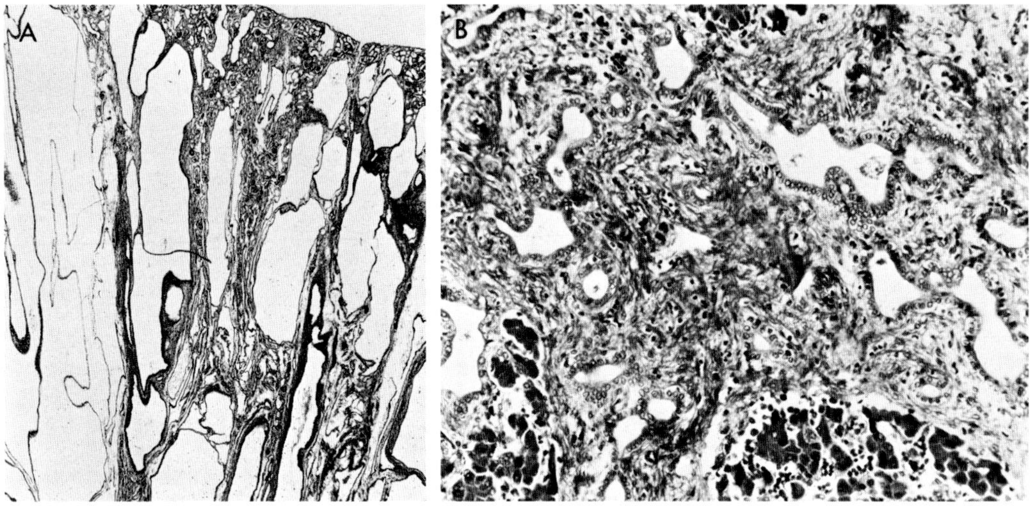

Fig. 105-5. – **A,** polycystic disease of the kidney. Collecting tubules dilated. **B,** cystic hyperplasia of liver of the same child.

a situation compatible with intrauterine but not with postnatal life. Whether this disorder, which undoubtedly goes far beyond the kidneys, should be called a hamartosis[10] depends on the definition of this term. The enlarged kidneys represent "tumors" but it has been pointed out that the kidneys are symmetrically enlarged and that their units are present in normal numbers and in normal arrangement. Only the collecting tubules are increased in volume, which represents a local hyperplasia but not a hamartous alteration. Associated congenital malformations so characteristic of some other types of cystic kidney apparently are not a part of this disorder.[8]

Type 2

These kidneys as well as their cysts are greatly variable in size and shape. The abnormality may be bilateral, unilateral or limited to only a part of a kidney; the portions involved, in contrast to Type 3, do not contain normal renal tissue. The left kidney is involved more often than the right.[11] Kidneys of Type 2 can be enlarged or reduced in size, hypoplastic, aplastic or dysgenetic; they are called multicystic when unilateral and multilocular when limited to a portion of a kidney. If both kidneys are completely involved, the condition is lethal soon after birth, but if only one kidney or a portion of it is affected, symptoms may appear late or not at all. In severe cases, thick-walled cysts forming round elevations under the capsule are embedded in firm connective tissue. Such cysts grow larger in surviving patients as they grow older and distort the shape of the kidney.[8,11]

In histologic sections, oval and round cystic spaces are present in abundance, lined by cuboidal epithelium and surrounded by connective tissue. Nephrons are scarce but collecting tubules are seen in clusters between the cysts. Micro-dissection shows that the collecting tubules are inadequately branched. The number of generations of tubules can be reduced (from the normal 12–20) to 4–12. The tubules are wider than normal, terminating in balloon-like cysts. There always is continuity between the cysts, the collecting tubules and the renal pelvis. Scarce nephrons in various stages of atrophy form islands surrounded by abundant stroma. Hyaline cartilage, calcified areas and even bone may be seen and atresia of the ureter frequently is present.[8,12] The intrarenal blood supply is abnormal. It is believed[8,11] that Type 2, characterized by inadequate branching, is due to inhibition of ampullary activity, resulting in reduction of tubular branching and lack of nephron induction.

It is not yet possible to correlate all clinical cases with the entities established by pathologists. But it seems likely that some of the unilateral polycystic kidneys of the newborn belong to this type and others to Type 3. Some authors assumed that the contralateral kidney always has a tendency to disease in later life, but Weinberg *et al.*[12] believed that unilateral multicystic kidney occurs in children who have one normal kidney and a favorable prognosis if nephrectomy is carried out before inanition supervenes.

The anomaly usually manifests itself as a large palpable unilateral mass. Severe gastrointestinal symptoms such as vomiting, feeding difficulties, dehydration and fever lead to inanition. Roentgen examination discloses evidence of a large mass in the abdomen with nonvisualization of the kidney on the affected side; its mate appears normal.

There is no agreement concerning associated malformations. Whereas Weinberg *et al.*[12] thought that unilateral multicystic kidney occurs in children who are free of other congenital malformations, Osathanondh and Potter[8] showed that microphthalmia, congenital heart disease, diaphragmatic hernia, omphalocele or abnormal sex organs can be associated anomalies. But there are no cystic changes in the liver, pancreas or other parenchymatous organs and familial occurrence is not prominent. The fact that Type 2 and Type 3 can occur in the same patient[8] may explain the difference of opinion concerning association with other malformations. An unusual case of chronic hypoparathyroidism associated with one multicystic kidney has been described by Mitchell.[13] These anomalies were found in the child of a mother who had symptoms of hyperparathyroidism during pregnancy. Polycystic kidneys of Type 2 were found in an unviable child with trisomy C. Flat nasal bridge, epicanthic folds, low-set ears, micrognathia, cleft palate, hyperextensibility and dislocations of joints and hypoplastic lungs were also present.[55]

Weinberg *et al.*[12] thought that surgical removal of a unilateral multicystic kidney results in resolution of symptoms and recovery. It seems that the short-term prognosis is good if nephrectomy is carried out early but that the prognosis must be guarded concerning later developments.

Type 3

Type 3 is characterized by intermingling of normal and abnormal renal elements. As a rule, both kidneys are cystic and enlarged but, at birth, the size of the cysts is variable. Some cysts are only microscopically discernible in grossly normal kidneys, whereas others are big enough to enlarge the entire organ. Thick-walled cysts are located in collecting tubules, thin-walled cysts in nephrons. Minute glomerular cysts located in the outer part of the cortex sometimes are seen in kidneys with pronounced fetal lobulation.[14] Micro-dissection shows the variability of cysts in regard to size and location. There are diffuse or saccular enlargements in the course of tubules with cysts located at their ends. Nephrons, attached irregularly to collecting tubules, sometimes show cystic enlargements at Bowman spaces or at the angles of Henle loops. Cysts are connected to tubules and communicate with the renal pelvis. The anomalies are attributed to irregular division of tubules and failure of formation of calices and papillae. The normal sequence of division of tubules arising from the ureteral bud is disturbed. Proximal tubules may be longer and distal tubules shorter than their normal counterparts. Tubules of any generation may be hyperplastic. Terminal as well as interstitial tubules can be enlarged to cysts, usually surrounded by a dense layer of connective tissue. Nephrons, reduced in number, may be partially dilated and attached to any generation of tubules. There is great variability in the amount of cystic tissue, and the outlook for life varies accordingly. Cystic kidneys of Type 3 can be seen in unviable children and they can be found accidentally in adults who never had experienced any renal symptoms.[8] If the polycystic kidneys in the newborn are very large, the abdomen is markedly distended and the kidneys are palpable. Enlargement of the kidney may interfere with delivery or normal respiration or lead to death by heart failure. In infants who survive birth, discovery of an abdominal tumor, vomiting, failure to thrive, elevation of the urea nitrogen or hypertension may aid in the diagnosis.

Type 3, variable in morphology, extent and prognosis, is even more variable in regard to etiology. Osathanondh and Potter[8] stated that "a family history seems to be often obtainable." If this is the case and adults are affected through several generations, one probably is dealing with polycystic kidneys attributable to an autosomal dominant gene, a disease known to cause symptoms late in life (p. 1046). It is this disease that is responsible for the second peak of the incidence curve of polycystic kidney after the fourth decade of life (p. 1047), which usually is not associated with other congenital malformations,[8] although accompanied by cysts in the liver in about one-quarter of the patients.[15] Type 3 can also be caused by a different autosomal dominant gene, that of tuberous sclerosis. It is likely that polycystic kidneys are also associated with other hamartoses, e.g., Hippel-Lindau disease. Intracranial aneurysms (p. 250) and congenital hepatic fibrosis (p. 724) can be combined with polycystic kidneys.[16] Deformed ears and polycystic kidneys in three generations were reported by Hilson.[17]

Polycystic kidneys in siblings with or without associated anomalies have been reported often.[6] In 1869, Brückner[18] described 2 siblings with polycystic kidneys and exencephaly, short, deformed extremities and polydactyly, and in 1967 Simopoulos *et al.*[19] described 3 male siblings with polycystic kidneys, internal hydrocephaly and polydactyly. Three semilethal cases of neonatal polycystic kidney with brain defects in siblings were reported by Goldston *et al.*[20] In 2 of these infants, Dandy-Walker cysts were present. Stockard[21] mentioned a pair of stillborn identical twins with cystic kidneys, occipital meningoceles and polydactyly. Cortical renal cysts and hepatomegaly with biliary dysgenesis were observed by Smith *et al.*[22] in siblings. Passarge and McAdams[23] reported 5 sisters with cortical renal cysts, hepatomegaly, hypotonia, brain anomalies and certain craniofacial characteristics. Ivemark *et al.*[24] observed familial occurrence of cystic kidneys with hepatic and pancreatic dysplasia. Association of eye anomalies with cystic kidneys is worth mentioning to balance the widespread belief in the prevalence of oto-renal connections.[17] Pierson *et al.*[25] saw 2 sisters with renal microcysts, microcoria, cataracts, retinal hypoplasia and other ocular anomalies. Renal cysts and retinal aplasia were found combined by Reese and Straatsma.[26] Myotonic dystrophy and polycystic disease of the kidney were described in 3 sisters observed by Emery *et al.*[27] Thick-walled renal cysts can be associated with urogenital anomalies in the Laurence-Moon-Biedl syndrome,[28] an autosomal recessive trait (p. 176).

Polycystic kidneys of Type 3 have been found in

infants with trisomy 13-15.[8] The kidneys in such cases show fetal lobulation and glomerular and medullary cysts.[29,30] Cortical renal cysts, microphthalmia and other anomalies were present in a child with 48 chromosomes (trisomy 13-15 and 21-22) reported by Gustavson *et al.*[31] In 10 of 32 necropsies of children with trisomy 13-15, cystic kidneys were noted. In children with trisomy 18, only 8 of 84 had cystic kidneys.[32] The foregoing associations of cystic kidneys with various malformations suggest genetic or chromosomal determination. Other associations still await etiologic clarification. The abundance of concurrence of defects of extrarenal organs is exemplified by the associated malformations collected in 1904 by Dunger[6] from the literature on cystic kidneys: encephalocele, meningocele, hydrocephaly, cleft lip, cleft palate, absence of ductus arteriosus, absence of aortic valve, ventricular septal defect, gastroschisis, horseshoe kidney, absence of renal pelvis, ureter, bladder or urethra, rudimentary penis, hypospadias, uterus bicornis, vagina duplex, absence of tube and ovary, malformations of the limbs and polydactyly of hands and feet were recorded. In 1934, Gruber[33] described in several infants a syndrome termed "dysencephalia splanchnocystica," which consisted of huge cystic kidneys, occipital meningocele, polydactyly, arhinencephaly and microphthalmia. Polycystic disease of the liver and of the pancreas also was present in these cases, some of which may have been related to trisomy 13-15. In 70 children with polycystic kidneys on whom necropsies were performed and who were reported by Campbell,[1] more than half had coexisting anomalies in the urinary tract. Renal reduplication, unilateral agenesis, horseshoe or ectopic kidney and anomalies of the ureter, bladder and urethra were listed. There also were many anomalies in other organs, especially the uterus and vagina. Malformations of the alimentary and cardiovascular systems were encountered repeatedly. Anal atresia, gastroschisis, ectopia cordis and transposition of the great vessels can be striking associated findings. Anomalies of the central nervous system and the skeleton were similar to those listed before.[6,33] There are many opportunities for creation of new syndromes. Unfortunately, it is not possible to ascertain for most of these cases the types of polycystic kidney associated with these anomalies but some undoubtedly were of Type 3.

By taking into consideration family history, character of the disease and associated malformations, at present one can distinguish the following etiologic entities for Type 3: (1) the relatively benign polycystic kidney of adults that produces symptoms late in life and can be transmitted like a dominant trait through several generations, (2) polycystic kidney associated with tuberous sclerosis or other hamartoses that are dominant hereditary traits, (3) a lethal recessive form occurring in several children of the same family that combines polycystic kidneys with various malformations of the urogenital tract, encephalocele, facial clefts, congenital heart disease, clubfoot and polydactyly, (4) various syndromes, recessively inherited, with limited life expectancy, (5) polycystic kidneys associated with microphthalmia, arhinencephaly, facial clefts, congenital heart disease, polydactyly and contracted fingers and attributable to trisomy 13-15 and (6) polycystic kidneys associated with trisomy 18.

In both Type 1 and Type 3, cystic disease of the liver has been observed. Both Type 1 and Type 3 can be lethal in infancy and can appear more than once in a family with phenotypically normal parents.[34] Parental consanguinity has not been conspicuous.[35] Type 2 and Type 3 can occur in the same patient.[8]

Type 4 (Polycystic Kidneys Due to Urethral Obstruction)

Urethral obstruction by membranous folds at the level of the verumontanum can result in renal cyst formation (p. 1228). Cysts are seen under the capsule dilating the terminal ends of collecting tubules, Bowman spaces or Henle loops. The collecting tubules are moderately dilated if obstruction occurs late in fetal life. Obstruction in a young fetus whose collecting tubules are short and straight has more serious effects. The ampullae may be damaged in such cases, resulting in abnormal branching and cystic distention of the early nephrons. Manifestations are variable. If severe damage is present at birth, early death may ensue. In milder cases, removal of the obstruction may lead to repair and normal kidney function.[8]

Simple (Solitary) Cysts in Children

This condition, which is rare in children but more common in adults, has been reviewed by DeWeerd and Simon.[52] Such cysts are unilocular. The cavity of the cyst and the renal pelvis do not communicate and renal elements are not found within the cyst. A localized region of the kidney is involved, leaving the rest of the renal tissue relatively normal and the renal pelvis and ureter patent. Such serous cysts are not always single, yet they are always limited in number. The presenting symptom is an abdominal mass that causes pain in some instances. Roentgenography may permit visualization of the cyst itself or of the effect of the cyst on the configuration of the calices and renal pelvis. The typical picture on pyelography is that of flaring and crescentic deformity of the calices and renal pelvis in the compressed part of the kidney. Displacement of the kidney by the cystic mass may affect its position and later the course of the ureter, a picture not easily differentiated from renal neoplasm. Treatment consists of nephrectomy, excision or incision and drainage of the cyst.

Congenital Polycystic Disease of the Adult Type

This disorder represents an interesting congenital malformation that, as a rule, does not make its clinical appearance before adult life. Although the basic anomaly obviously is present long before birth, manifestations are delayed in the majority of cases. Incidence figures vary, in some hospitals 1 case being reported in 3,500 admissions[5] or 1 in 5,000.[34] There is no predilection for either sex.[4,5]

This form of polycystic disease is considered hereditary and dominant transmission generally is assumed, although transmission from generation to generation cannot be proved in all cases.[2,36] Rall and Odel[4] obtained a positive family history in 34% of their cases. This is understandable, since a person affected by the abnormal trait may have no symptoms for many years or have no symptoms throughout life even though at necropsy the disease is encountered as an accidental finding. Congenital polycystic disease is thus attributed to a gene with low expressivity or penetrance, and apparent skipping of a generation is understandable. Sporadic cases can be explained by the assumption that they represent new mutations, but there is a possibility that some of them are not hereditary at all and merely imitate the dominant form as phenocopies.

In 1925, Cairns[34] described in detail a family in which 8 or probably 10 members were affected by polycystic kidney in three successive generations, and Fuller[36] reported a family with possible transmission through four generations. Werner[35] collected one hundred nine families with 350 affected individuals. Forty families were affected in one generation, 41 in two, 8 in three and 3 in four generations. Reason[37] observed a pair of identical female twins, one of whom transmitted the disease to her son. Although this form of polycystic disease usually occurs in adults, early manifestations of the dominant form have been observed in children.[38,39] This fact explains why some authors believe that the "infantile" and the adult type cannot be clearly distinguished.

Many theories have been advanced concerning the pathogenesis of this disorder. Most of them are merely of historical interest. For a detailed discussion, the reader is referred to the publications of Norris and Herman[7] and of Rall and Odel.[4] When the dual origin of the kidney, namely its derivation from the ureteric bud and from the renal blastema, was recognized, it was logical to assume that failure of union of the two renal primordia results in cyst formation in the excretory elements separated from the collecting ducts. One theory is based on the fact that the early generations of uriniferous tubules and their glomeruli normally are separated from their collecting ducts and in this process normal fetuses pass through a period characterized by the presence of numerous cystic renal tubules that normally degenerate and disappear. This normal transition may be converted into an abnormal condition if such tubules do not give way at the end of their allotted time but continue to grow.[40] Norris and Herman[7] believed that in this case a much greater part of the metanephros than normal is provisional and that growth and anastomoses of cysts derived from uriniferous tubules and collecting ducts during fetal life account for polycystic kidneys. An important part of their findings was that they showed that for a long period in fetal life development of these kidneys appeared normal. Focal cystic dilatations of tubules and of ducts occurred after differentiation of the metanephrogenic anlage and after the union of its elements with collecting ducts, to be followed later by isolation and anastomoses of the cystic spaces. Moolten[41] suggested that the process leading to polycystic disease of the kidney and of the liver is due to faulty organizer action and that this condition should be considered a disseminated hamartosis comparable to tuberous sclerosis and Hippel-Lindau disease.

To test these theories, the use of experimental animals would be valuable if the development of the cysts could be observed directly. Polycystic disease of the kidney occurs in animals spontaneously. In horse fetuses, huge polycystic kidneys resembling those of the infantile form have been observed and in swine, cysts of the adult type can be found.[42] Such kidneys also occur in cattle, goats and sheep but not with sufficient regularity to permit systematic investigation of the pathogenesis of the cysts. In rodents, cystic kidneys are found with greater regularity. Kidney anomalies appeared in the strain of mice derived from animals used in the x-ray experiments of Little and Bagg.[43] In this stock ("my"), the most common anomaly is absence of one kidney. Rarer manifestations are polycystic or hypoplastic kidneys and hydronephrosis with distended ureter.[43] In man, the combination of congenital absence of one kidney with polycystic disease of the kidney present has been observed but it is rare.[44] In another strain of mice studied by Carter,[45] renal cysts were not uncommon but they were found chiefly in adult animals. They were few in number, often single and sometimes so large that they resembled hydronephrosis. Cystic kidneys also were discovered in another strain of mice.[46] They were not seen in newborn and young animals. The polycystic degeneration arose in the cortex of the kidney, and parts of the medulla and of the renal papilla remained unaffected. Degeneration was not due to obstruction as is the case in hydronephrosis, in which the papilla in this strain was affected first, with ensuing complete atrophy of the medulla. Cystic kidneys occur in old mice of the A strain. According to Gorer,[47] the cystic stage is preceded by necrotic lesions on the tip of the renal papilla, which leads to obstruction of urinary flow. Dilatation of the tubules and, later, of the glomerular capsules takes place, resulting in formation of large cysts that resemble, to a certain extent, congenital polycystic kidneys in man. Such a cystic kidney on one side may be accompanied by an atrophic fibrous remnant on the other. It is of interest that this renal disorder may be a local consequence of general amyloidosis, which is, to a certain extent, dependent on the diet of the animals. A high-cystine–low-protein diet reduces both amyloidosis and kidney lesions.[48] Morgan[49] described inherited congenital absence of the kidney in an inbred strain of rats. In a small percentage of these animals, cystic kidneys were found. This seems to be the only known example of hereditary polycystic renal disease with manifestations in the neonatal period in animals. These renal anomalies are not inherited in a simple Mendelian manner. If one considers how complicated the situation is in animals that can be bred, dissected and analyzed systematically, one will understand the confused situation in man and the difficulties of etiologic classification or genetic counseling.

Although it is now possible to produce in animals a variety of anomalies of the urinary system by vitamin deficiencies or by hypervitaminosis A, cystic disorders of the kidneys apparently have not been observed in those abnormal animals who usually were examined in late fetal life or soon after birth. There is a possibility that the renal anomalies produced would eventually lead to cyst formation if the abnormal young could be kept alive but such observations have not been made to the present time. The absence of experimental animals in which cystic kidneys occur or can be produced with regularity explains why the various theories of pathogenesis of polycystic renal disease have not been tested experimentally. In general, the findings in animals seem to point to a confirmation of the concept of Norris and Herman[7] that cystic disease of the kidney has its onset in late fetal life. In exceptional cases, however, cystic changes may be present early, as evidenced by a fetus observed by Potter[9] that was 14 weeks old, weighed 35 Gm. and showed multiple cysts.

Great variability of symptoms exists in patients with the adult type of polycystic disease of the kidney. The average onset of symptoms is approximately 40 years and the average age at death 50 years,[2] but the true average life expectancy may be higher, since only the most severe forms are included in many serial studies. Rall and Odel[4] listed the presenting complaints of their patients at the time of diagnosis as follows: lumbar or abdominal pain, presence of an abdominal mass, elevated blood pressure, difficulties with urination, hematuria and renal failure. In 19% of the cases the presenting complaints were not related to the kidneys. More than 70% of the patients had elevated blood pressure or palpable, enlarged kidneys. In an equal number of patients, changes typical of hypertension were noted in the ocular fundi. Intravenous pyelograms presented a typical appearance, namely, elongation and blunting of the calices and irregularity of outline. Albuminuria, pyuria and hematuria were noted in most and nitrogen retention was demonstrated in more than one-third of the patients. Nephrolithiasis was present occasionally. Causes of death were renal failure with uremia, myocardial infarction, cerebral hemorrhage, cardiac failure and so forth. Unilateral polycystic disease of the kidney was found in 13% of the cases. Associated congenital malformations are rarer in the adult than in the infantile form. However, Oppenheimer[2] found among his patients cystic involvement of the liver in 28.5% and Rall and Odel[4] in 33%. The hepatic involvement usually is symptomless. More than half of the patients show cardiac hypertrophy.

Brown[50] and Bigelow[44] emphasized the association of polycystic kidneys with intracranial aneurysms and other disorders. It is now generally accepted that some intracranial berry aneurysms, especially those in the circle of Willis and its major branches, are due to some developmental defect of the arterial wall. Although it is doubtful that the aneurysmal sac itself is present in early life, the defect in the arterial wall most certainly is. Coarctation of the aorta and polycystic kidneys repeatedly have been found to be associated with such aneurysms. Intracranial hemorrhage occurring in patients with polycystic disease is not rare; in about 6% of cases of congenital intracranial aneurysms, polycystic kidneys have been found. It is of interest that as early as 1904 Dunger[6] recognized a relationship between polycystic kidney of the adult and hereditary type with intracranial arterial aneurysm and hemorrhage.

Multilocular Cysts or Cystadenomas

This type resembles the serous simple cyst, but the space contained in the firm capsule is subdivided, so that a mass of cysts lined by flattened epithelium and containing no renal elements is formed. Hypertension may be present. Differentiation from renal tumors is difficult, and Williams[51] stated that the diagnosis can be made with assurance only from the histology of the specimen. Therefore, nephrectomy must be the treatment of choice.

Cystic Disease of the Renal Medulla

This disorder has been described as an entity characterized clinically by insidious onset of anemia, azotemia and urinary salt wasting. Blood pressure may be normal and albuminuria absent. Osteitis fibrosa has been observed in children and adolescents and parathyroid hyperplasia is the rule. The disease has been seen in siblings and in a pair of identical twins.[53] In one kindred, dominant inheritance and transmission through four generations could be demonstrated.[54]

REFERENCES

1. Campbell, M.: *Clinical Pediatric Urology* (Philadelphia: W. B. Saunders Company, 1951).
2. Oppenheimer, G. D.: Polycystic disease of the kidney, Ann. Surg. 100:1136, 1934.
3. Bell, E. T.: Cystic disease of kidneys, Am. J. Path. 11:373, 1935.
4. Rall, J. E., and Odel, H. M.: Congenital polycystic disease of the kidney: Review of the literature and data on 207 cases, Am. J. M. Sc. 218:399, 1949.
5. Ferguson, J. D.: Observations on familial polycystic disease of the kidney, Proc. Roy. Soc. Med. 42:806, 1949.
6. Dunger, R.: Zur Lehre von der Cystenniere mit besonderer Berücksichtigung ihrer Heredität, Beitr. path. Anat. 35:445, 1904.

7. Norris, R. F., and Herman, L.: The pathogenesis of polycystic kidneys, J. Urol. 46:147, 1941.
8. Osathanondh, V., and Potter, E. L.: Pathogenesis of polycystic kidneys; historical survey, Arch. Path. 77:459, 1964.
9. Potter, E. L.: *Pathology of the Fetus and Infant* (2d. ed.; Chicago: Year Book Medical Publishers, Inc., 1961).
10. Herxheimer, G.: Über Cystenbildungen der Niere und abführenden Harnwege, Virchows Arch. path. Anat. 185: 52, 1906.
11. Vellios, F., and Garrett, R. A.: Congenital unilateral multicystic disease of the kidney; a clinical and anatomic study of seven cases, Am. J. Clin. Path. 35:244, 1961.
12. Weinberg, S. R., O'Connor, W. J., and Senger, F. L.: Unilateral multicystic renal disease of the newborn, A.M.A. Am. J. Dis. Child. 92:576, 1956.
13. Mitchell, R. G.: Chronic hypoparathyroidism associated with a multicystic kidney, Arch. Dis. Childhood 29:349, 1954.
14. Vlachos, J., and Tsakraklidis, V.: Glomerular cysts. An unusual variety of "polycystic kidneys,": Report of two cases, Am. J. Dis. Child. 114:379, 1967.
15. Lathrop, D. B.: Cystic disease of the liver and kidney, Pediatrics 24:215, 1959.
16. Wagenvoort, C. A., Baggenstoss, A. H., and Love, J. G.: Subarachnoid hemorrhage due to cerebellar hemangioma associated with congenital hepatic fibrosis and polycystic kidneys: Report of case, Proc. Staff Meet. Mayo Clin. 37: 301, 1962.
17. Hilson, D.: Malformation of ears as sign of malformation of genitourinary tract, Brit. M. J. 11:785, 1957.
18. Brückner, C.: Zweimalige Entbindung derselben Frau von Missgeburten mit vergrösserten Nieren, Virchows Arch. path. Anat. 46:503, 1869.
19. Simopoulos, A. P., Brennan, G. G., Alwan, A., and Fidis, N.: Polycystic kidneys, internal hydrocephalus and polydactylism in newborn siblings, Pediatrics 39:931, 1967.
20. Goldston, A. S., Burke, E. C., D'Agostino, A., and McCaughey, W. T. E.: Neonatal polycystic kidney with brain defect, Am. J. Dis. Child. 106:484, 1963.
21. Stockard, C. R.: Developmental rate and structural expression: An experimental study of twins, "double monsters" and single deformities, Am. J. Anat. 28:115, 1921.
22. Smith, D. W., Opitz, J. M., and Inhorn, S. L.: A syndrome of multiple developmental defects including polycystic kidneys and intrahepatic biliary dysgenesis in 2 siblings, J. Pediat. 67:617, 1965.
23. Passarge, E., and McAdams, A. J.: Cerebro-hepato-renal syndrome, J. Pediat. 71:691, 1967.
24. Ivemark, B. I., Oldfelt, V., and Zetterström, R.: Familial dysplasia of kidneys, liver and pancreas; a probably genetically determined syndrome, Acta paediat. 48:1, 1959.
25. Pierson, M., Cordier, J., Hervouët, F., and Rauber, G.: Une curieuse association malformative congénitale et familiale atteignant l'oeil et le rein, J. Génét. Hum. 12:184, 1963.
26. Reese, A. B., and Straatsma, B. R.: Retinal dysplasia, Am. J. Ophth. 45:199, 1958.
27. Emery, A. E. H., Oleesky, S., and Williams, R. T.: Myotonic dystrophy and polycystic disease of the kidneys, J. M. Genetics 4:26, 1967.
28. Anderson, N. L.: The Laurence-Moon-Biedl syndrome, J. Clin. Endocrinol. 1:905, 1941.
29. Marin-Padilla, M., Hoefnagel, D., and Benirschke, K.: Anatomic and histopathologic study of two cases of D_1 (13-15) trisomy, Cytogenetics 3:258, 1964.
30. Bartman, J., and Barraclough, C.: Cystic dysplasia of the kidneys studied by microdissection, J. Path. & Bact. 89: 233, 1965.
31. Gustavson, K. H., Ivemark, B. I., Zetterquist, P., and Böök, J. A.: Post-mortem diagnosis of a new double trisomy associated with cardiovascular and other anomalies, Acta paediat. 51:686, 1962.
32. Warkany, J., Passarge, E., and Smith, L. B.: Congenital malformations in autosomal trisomy syndromes, Am. J. Dis. Child. 112:502, 1966.
33. Gruber, G. B.: Beitrage zur Frage "gekoppelter" Missbildungen, Beitr. path. Anat. 93:459, 1934.
34. Cairns, H.: Heredity in polycystic disease of the kidneys, Quart. J. Med. 18:359, 1925.
35. Werner, M.: Erbbiologie und Erbpathologie des Harnapparates, in Bauer, K. H., Hanhart, E., and Just, G. (eds.), *Handbuch der Erbbiologie des Menschen* (Berlin: Julius Springer, 1940), Vol. IV.
36. Fuller, C. J.: Familial polycystic disease of kidneys, Quart. J. Med. 22:567, 1929.
37. Reason, C. H.: Heredity and polycystic disease of the kidneys, Canad. M.A.J. 29:612, 1933.
38. Halbertsma, T.: Über einen klinisch beobachteten Fall erblicher Cystenniere bei einem 10-jährigen Kinde, Ztschr. Kinderh. 52:145, 1932.
39. Kretschmer, H. L.: Renal rickets and polycystic disease of the kidney, J. Urol. 59:773, 1948.
40. Kampmeier, O. F.: A hitherto unrecognized mode of origin of congenital renal cysts, Surg., Gynec. & Obst. 36: 208, 1923.
41. Moolten, S. E.: Pathogenesis of congenital anomalies of the intrahepatic and extrahepatic bile ducts, New York J. Med. 43:727, 1943.
42. Gruber, G. B.: Entwicklungsstörungen der Nieren und Harnleiter, in Henke, F., and Lubarsch, O. (eds.), *Handbuch der Speziellen Anatomie u. Histologie* (Berlin: Julius Springer, 1925).
43. Bagg, H. J.: Hereditary abnormalities of the viscera. I. A morphological study with special reference to the abnormalities of the kidneys in the descendants of x-rayed mice, Am. J. Anat. 36:275, 1925.
44. Bigelow, N. H.: The association of polycystic kidneys with intracranial aneurysms and other related disorders, Am. J. M. Sc. 225:485, 1953.
45. Carter, T. C.: The genetics of luxate mice. III. Horseshoe kidney, hydronephrosis and lumbar reduction, J. Genetics 51:441, 1953.
46. Dunn, L. C., and Gluecksohn-Schoenheimer, S.: A new complex of hereditary abnormalities in the house mouse, J. Exper. Zool. 104:25, 1947.
47. Gorer, P. A.: Renal lesions found in pure lines of mice, J. Path. & Bact. 50:25, 1940.
48. Grüneberg, H.: *The Genetics of the Mouse* (The Hague: Martinus Nijhoff, 1952).
49. Morgan, W. C.: Inherited congenital kidney absence in an inbred strain of rats, Anat. Rec. 115:635, 1953.
50. Brown, P.: Polycystic disease of the kidneys and intracranial aneurysms. The etiology and interrelationship of these conditions, Glasgow M. J. 32:333, 1951.
51. Williams, D.: Urology in Childhood, in *Encyclopedia of Urology* (Berlin, Springer-Verlag, 1958), Vol. XV.
52. DeWeerd, J. H., and Simon, H. B.: Simple renal cysts in children. Review of the literature and report of 5 cases, J. Urol. 75:912, 1956.
53. Strauss, M. B.: Clinical and pathological aspects of cystic disease of the renal medulla, Ann. Int. Med. 57:373, 1962.
54. Goldman, S. H., Walker, S. R., Merigan, T. C., Jr., Gardner, K. D., Jr., and Bull, J. M. C.: Hereditary occurrence of cystic disease of the renal medulla, New England J. Med. 274:984, 1966.
55. Juberg, R. C., Gilbert, E. F., and Salisbury, R. S.: Trisomy C in an infant with polycystic kidneys and other malformations, J. Pediat. 76:598, 1970.

Fused Kidneys
(Horseshoe Kidney)

FUSION OF THE KIDNEYS can result in various shapes, with specific terms for the fused organs. Horseshoe kidney, characterized by fusion of the lower (rarely of the upper) poles, is the most common form, accounting for 90% of the fused kidneys. Such fusion of the kidneys is said to occur in 1 of 400 persons.[1,2] Fusion of both the upper and lower poles results in a disk or doughnut shape, an anomaly that accounts for only 2% of the fused kidneys. Fusion of the lower pole with the upper pole of the contralateral kidney leads to a sigmoid kidney. Extreme fusion, with both kidneys united to one organ, results in formation of lump kidney. Fused kidneys rarely ascend to the normal level and are found, therefore, in the lower lumbar, sacral or pelvic region. They occur about twice as often in males as in females.[1,3]

The portion of the horseshoe kidney that completes the fusion in different degrees is the isthmus. The isthmus may consist of solid, functioning renal tissue, or fusion may be so superficial that only the capsules of the lower poles are connected. The renal pelves point forward and the ureters derived from them cross the isthmus ventrally. Bifurcation of the aorta is behind the isthmus, which usually is situated at the level of the inferior mesenteric artery. The horseshoe formed by the fusion is not always symmetric, the right segment sometimes being smaller than the left.

Various etiologic factors can bring about horseshoe kidneys. Recurrence of horseshoe kidney in families seems to be rare but, in relatives of patients with fused kidneys, alternating anomalies of the urinary tract occur with some frequency.[2,4] Klopstock[5] described 2 brothers with horseshoe kidney and brain malformations of the cyclopia series who were the

Fig. 105-6. – Horseshoe kidney of a girl with trisomy 18.

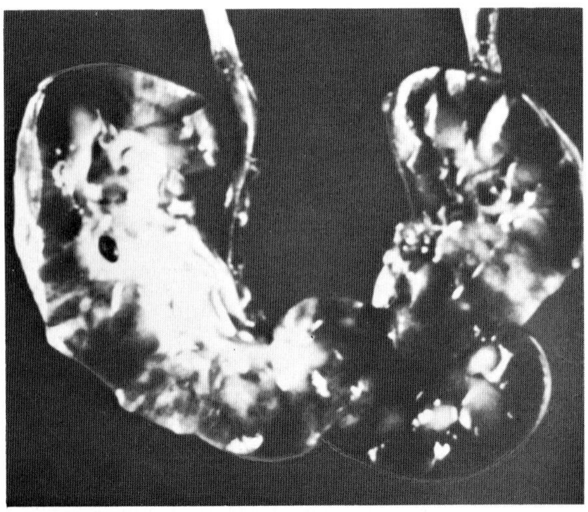

product of a consanguineous marriage. Horseshoe kidney attributable to recessive inheritance has been reported several times in patients with Fanconi pancytopenia.[6] Lump kidneys have been transmitted from parent to child and have recurred in siblings.[7] Concordant horseshoe kidneys have been observed in monozygotic twins.[8,9] Lump kidney has been reported in one pair of monozygotic twins concordantly and discordantly in another.[10]

Chromosomal abnormalities can result in horseshoe kidney, as exemplified by infants with trisomy 18, who show this anomaly in 20% of the cases. Horseshoe kidney also was observed in a mentally retarded boy whose karyotype contained a small mediocentric fragment thought to be a chromosome 18 with deletion.[11] In contrast, horseshoe kidney was not reported in 32 necropsies of the trisomy 13-15 syndrome.[12] It has been seen with Down syndrome[1] but the frequency of this association is not known. Among the urologic malformations occurring with Turner syndrome, horseshoe kidney is quite frequent.[13] It was present in an aborted fetus with 45/XO karyotype[14] and was observed with XO/XX[15] and with XX/XY/XO mosaicism.[16] A puzzling family history was obtained in a child with Turner syndrome seen in the Cincinnati Children's Hospital: a maternal uncle had a horseshoe kidney.

Lump kidneys and horseshoe kidneys have been reported in children damaged by thalidomide.[17-19]

Horseshoe kidneys are formed when the metanephric buds grow upward nearer to the midline than normal. Consequently, the metanephrogenic blastema develops too closely to the midline, so that in the caudal area the kidneys are not separated. Such abnormal course of the ureteric buds can be due to many developmental disturbances.

Horseshoe kidneys are of great biologic interest because of their heterogeneous etiology and because of their relationship to various syndromes of known or unknown origin. They also are examples of congenital malformations that predispose to tumor formation. Development of Wilms tumor in horseshoe kidney has been reported repeatedly. Lathem and Smith[20] described a Wilms tumor in a horseshoe kidney and found 12 cases of this association in the literature. Lattimer *et al.*,[21] reporting 71 cases of Wilms tumor, encountered one in a horseshoe kidney. The combination of these anomalies also evolved in an epidemiologic study by Miller *et al.*,[22] who surveyed abnormalities associated with Wilms tumor. Malignant tubular adenoma in a horseshoe kidney was observed by Ladewig and Eser.[23]

The development of horseshoe kidney can be studied in animals. In a strain of mice (luxate), horseshoe kidney commonly is found associated with a number of congenital defects of the hindlimbs, lumbar vertebrae and abdominal arteries. In this syndrome, studied by Carter,[24,25] various grades of horseshoe kidney occurred. There always were two ureters and the kidney fusion always involved the poste-

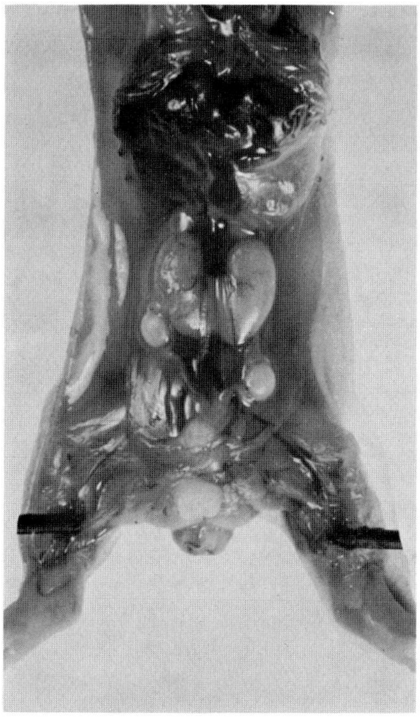

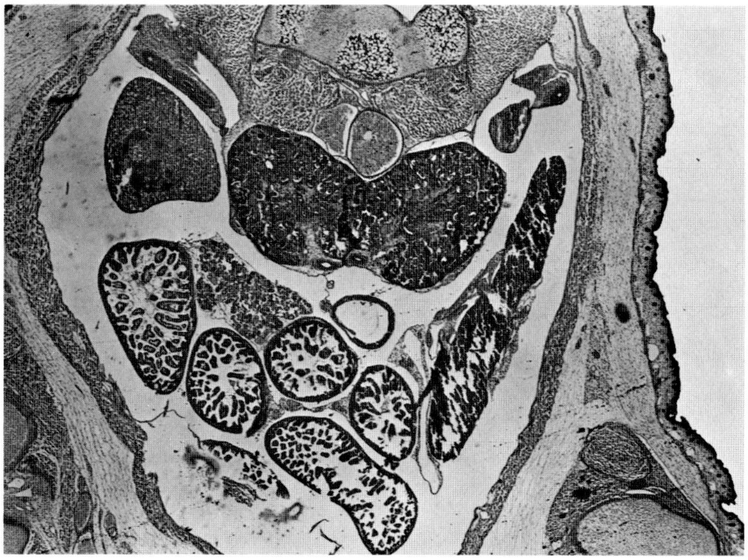

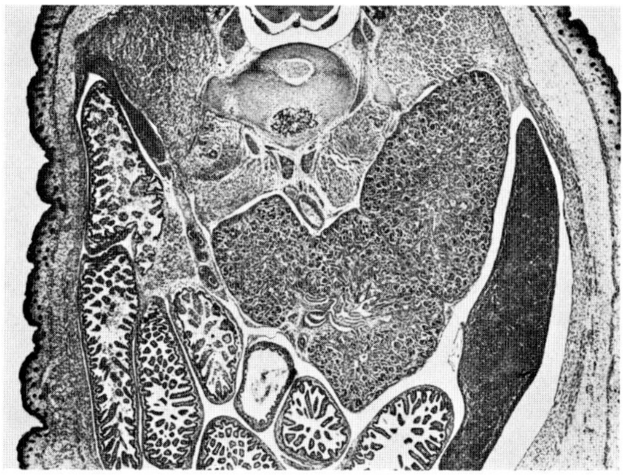

Fig. 105-7 (left).—Horseshoe kidney in a newborn rat produced by maternal vitamin A deficiency. The testes are undescended.

Fig. 105-8. (above).—Transverse section through a rat fetus (twenty-second day) showing fused lower poles of kidneys: horseshoe kidney (produced by maternal vitamin A deficiency).

Fig. 105-9 (below).—Transverse section showing horseshoe kidney in a newborn rat treated with fractionated vitamin A deficiency (p. 1056). Note that the line of fusion of the kidneys is displaced to the left. Both renal components are of equal size but the left portion of the horseshoe appears much bigger than the right.

rior or lower pole. The renal pelves lay on the medioventral or anteroventral margin, the ureters were abnormally close together and the aorta and posterior vena cava lay dorsal to the region of kidney fusion. The inferior mesenteric artery invariably rose anterior to the fused kidney and passed over its ventral surface between the renal pelves and ureters. Thus, these horseshoe kidneys of "luxate" mice resembled the common form of human horseshoe kidney. The reader is referred to the thorough analysis of the syndrome by Carter.[25]

Horseshoe kidneys can be produced experimentally in rats by prenatal vitamin A deficiency (Figs. 105-7–105-9), by x-irradiation and other teratogenic procedures. It is of interest, but remains unexplained, that the syndrome produced by maternal vitamin A deficiency[26] includes horseshoe kidney, whereas the syndrome of folic acid deficiency,[27] which in many respects results in similar urogenital anomalies, does not. The fetuses of vitamin A-deficient mothers studied by Wilson and Warkany[26] showed many renal anomalies. The kidneys usually were closer together than normal, some being almost in contact across the midline. Others were in direct contact or fusion at the caudal poles, forming horseshoe kidneys. Complete fusion of kidneys into a solitary median mass, a lump kidney, occurred in a few instances. Most horseshoe kidneys were found in younger fetuses, whereas older fetuses or mature animals had the anomaly only rarely. This indicated that horseshoe kidney is associated with early fetal death. The majority of the horseshoe kidneys were at a lower than normal level and lump

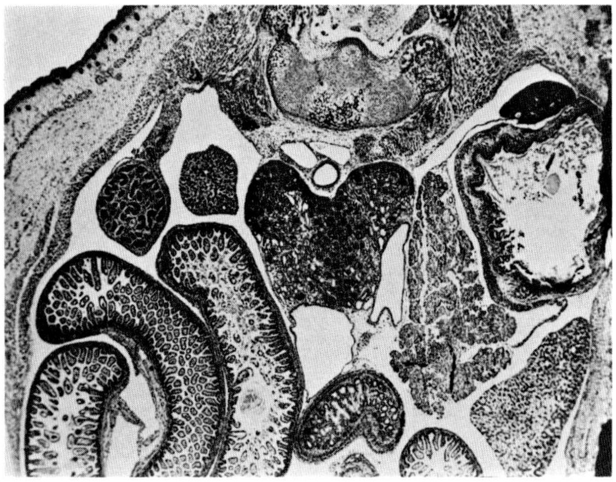

Fig. 105-10. – Lump kidney in a newborn rat produced by x-ray exposure of the mother on the thirteenth day of gestation.

kidneys were always at a low lumbar or sacral level. No obstruction was found to account for the incomplete ascent of the kidneys or for the lack of lateral migration. The pelvis of the abnormal kidneys invariably emerged from the ventromedial or ventral surfaces. These kidneys demonstrated, in their location close to the midline and low in the body, a retardation of development that, in some respects, resembled early embryonic stages.

In man, horseshoe kidney may be asymptomatic during childhood. Because of angulation of the ureters crossing the isthmus, some obstruction occurs, which may lead to stasis, infection, stone formation, hydronephrosis or pain. But many carriers of horseshoe kidney remain asymptomatic for many years.[28] A lump kidney can present as an abdominal tumor or manifest itself by suprapubic protrusion.

Horseshoe kidney often is complicated by hydronephrosis or stricture or duplication of the ureters. Affected kidneys may be polycystic or be deformed by solitary cysts. There may be absence or duplication of the derivatives of the Müllerian ducts. Anomalies of the testes occur occasionally. In rare cases, the adrenals also are fused or one adrenal may be absent. In necropsies, horseshoe kidneys are associated with malformations in other organ systems in approximately 50% of the cases.[3] Understandably, the highest incidence is among stillbirths and infants; it decreases with advancing age. Multiple system involvement is frequent. The skeleton, the central nervous system, the cardiovascular system and the intestinal tract are involved in 24%, 19%, 18% and 17% of the cases, respectively.[3] Those patients with nervous system malformations, particularly spina bifida, die early. The same is true for infants with congenital heart disease and anomalies of the gastrointestinal tract. Tracheo-esophageal and recto-vaginal fistulas, imperforate anus, Meckel diverticulum and other anomalies occur. Malformations of digits are the leading anomalies of the skeletal system. It is of interest that Zondek and Zondek[3] noted associated malformations of the genital system in only 5 of 99 dissected patients. Cretinism was present in 2 cases, cleft palate with or without cleft lip in 6 and exomphalos in 2. Hypoplasia of the lung was seen in 2 cases and fusion of the adrenals in 1. We have seen an achondroplastic boy with a horseshoe kidney (Cincinnati Children's Hospital Chart No. 118261).

Horseshoe kidney does not require any treatment but complications do. In rare cases, the isthmus has been excised. If pain is severe and continuous, division of the two halves of the horseshoe kidney may be helpful.[1]

REFERENCES

1. Campbell, M.: *Clinical Pediatric Urology* (Philadelphia: W. B. Saunders Company, 1951).
2. Lenz, W.: Krankheiten des Urogenitalsystems, in Becker, P. E. (ed.), *Humangenetik* (Stuttgart: George Thieme, 1964), Vol. III.
3. Zondek, L. H., and Zondek, T.: Horseshoe kidney and associated congenital malformations, Urol. Internat. 18:347, 1964.
4. Robertson, P. W.: Horseshoe kidney, renal arterial anomalies, and hypertension: A study of one family, Brit. M. J. 2:793, 1968.
5. Klopstock, A.: Familiäres Vorkommen von Cyklopie und Arrhinencephalie, Monatsschr. Geb. Gynäk. 56:59, 1921.
6. Nilsson, L. R.: Chronic pancytopenia with multiple congenital abnormalities (Fanconi's anaemia), Acta paediat. 49:518, 1960.
7. Rössle, R.: Weitere Beobachtungen über Sektionsbefunde bei Blutsverwandten, Virchows Arch. path. Anat. 308: 495, 1942.
8. Yoshioka, K.: Über Hufeisenniere bei beiden Foeten eineiiger Zwillinge und über die Varietäten der Nierenvenen bei den Zwillingen, cited by Lenz.[2]
9. Bridge, R. A. C.: Horseshoe kidneys in identical twins, Brit. J. Urol. 32:32, 1960.
10. Werner, M.: Erbbiologie und Erbpathologie des Harnapparates, in Bauer, K. H., Hanhart, E., and Just, G. (eds.), *Handbuch der Erbbiologie des Menschen* (Berlin: Springer-Verlag, 1940), Vol. 4/2.
11. Dollman, A., and Jaeger, W.: Überzähliges Chromosomenfragment bei einem oligophrenen Kind mit multiplen Entwicklungsstörungen, Monatsschr. Kinderh. 116:144, 1968.
12. Warkany, J., Passarge, E., and Smith, L. B.: Congenital malformations in autosomal trisomy syndromes, Am. J. Dis. Child. 112:502, 1966.
13. Bishop, P. M. F., Lessof, M. H., and Polani, P. E.: Turner's syndrome and allied conditions, Mem. Soc. Endocrinol. 7: 162, 1960.
14. Singh, R. P., and Carr, D. H.: The anatomy and histology of XO human embryos and fetuses, Anat. Rec. 155:369, 1966.
15. Ferrier, P., Gartler, S. M., Waxman, S. H., and Shepard, T. H., II: Abnormal sexual development associated with sex chromosome mosaicism, Pediatrics 29:703, 1962.
16. Schuster, J., and Motulsky, A. G.: Exceptional sex-chromatin pattern in male pseudohermaphroditism with XX/XY/XO mosaicism, Lancet 1:1074, 1962.
17. Wiedemann, H-R.: Hinweis auf eine derzeitige Häufung hypo- und aplastischer Fehlbildungen der Gliedmassen, Med. Welt 37:1863, 1961.
18. Smithells, R. W.: Thalidomide and malformations in Liverpool, Lancet 1:1270, 1962.
19. Weicker, H.: 100 children with thalidomide embryopathy, XIth International Congress of Pediatrics, 1965.
20. Lathem, J. E., and Smith, K. H.: Wilms tumor in horseshoe kidney: Surviving case, J. Urol. 88:25, 1962.
21. Lattimer, J. K., Melicow, M. M., and Uson, A. C.: Wilms

tumor: A report of 71 cases, J. Urol. 80:401, 1958.
22. Miller, R. W., Fraumeni, J. F., and Manning, M. D.: Association of Wilms' tumor with aniridia, hemihypertrophy and other congenital malformations, New England J. Med. 270:922, 1964.
23. Ladewig, P., and Eser, S.: Malignant tubular adenoma in a horseshoe kidney: Its significance with regard to general cancer pathology, J. Path. & Bact. 57:405, 1945.
24. Carter, T. C.: Genetics of luxate mice; horseshoe kidney, hydronephrosis and lumbar reduction, J. Genetics 51:441, 1953.
25. Carter, T. C.: The genetics of luxate mice. IV. Embryology, J. Genetics 52:1, 1954.
26. Wilson, J. G., and Warkany, J.: Malformations in the genitourinary tract induced by maternal vitamin A deficiency in the rat, Am. J. Anat. 83:357, 1948.
27. Monie, I. W., Nelson, M. M., and Evans, H. M.: Abnormalities of the urinary system of rat embryos resulting from transitory deficiency of pteroylglutamic acid during gestation, Anat. Rec. 127:711, 1957.
28. Glenn, J. F.: Analysis of 51 patients with horseshoe kidney, New England J. Med. 261:684, 1959.

Ectopia and Malrotation

ECTOPIAS OF THE KIDNEY are due to insufficient ascent of the metanephros during embryonic development. According to Patten,[2] the metanephric diverticulum arises opposite the fourth lumbar segment, but toward the end of the third month the center of the kidney lies opposite the 2d or 3d lumbar vertebra and at term it has moved up to the 1st lumbar or the 12th thoracic vertebra. In young embryos, the kidneys lie caudal to the bifurcation of the aorta below the origin of the umbilical arteries. During the seventh week, the kidneys move over the ridges formed by the umbilical arteries and by the ninth week they lie above the aortic fork. During this ascent, a rotation occurs, so that the renal pelves, originally directed forward, become directed toward the midline. The cephalad migration and the rotation of the kidney may be disturbed, so that the caudal position or embryonic anteroposterior orientation is maintained. If the kidney remains in the pelvic or sacro-iliac area, one speaks of pelvic or sacro-iliac kidneys. In rare instances, the kidneys are displaced into the thorax. The length of the ureter depends on the position of the kidney. As a rule, these ectopic organs are deformed and altered in shape, and their vascular supply is abnormal, as they are connected with adjacent blood vessels.[1] The condition occurs about once in 2,000 necropsies.[1] Ectopic kidneys have been found in several infants with trisomy 18.

Ectopia of the kidneys can be bilateral, unilateral, fused or crossed. In unilateral pelvic ectopia, one kidney is located at the level of the promontory or in the pelvic cavity. Such a kidney usually shows malrotation and a blood supply derived from the lower aorta or an iliac artery. A fused pelvic kidney can lie in the sacral region and be drained by two ureters; a solitary pelvic kidney with only one ureter also may be in that position. In malrotation, the ureter passes to the bladder from a greater than normal distance; it may be compressed by overlying blood vessels that produce obstruction and hydronephrosis. Intrathoracic kidney is a rare anomaly that usually is well tolerated and discovered accidentally. Reports on 31 cases were reviewed by Burke et al.,[3] including that of a girl of their own observation. The case is of interest because this anomaly is more common in males than in females. In crossed ectopia, both kidneys are placed on the same side of the body, the crossed organ lying below and medial to the other and usually fused with it. The ureters enter the bladder in the normal position on either side of the trigone after crossing of the midline of one ureter. A crossed renal ectopy with solitary kidney was reported by Purpon,[4] who reviewed the literature on this rare anomaly. Carcinoma in crossed renal ectopia has been reported.[5]

Ectopic kidneys are inclined to disease, such as infection or stone formation, and they can cause pressúre on bowels, nerves or blood vessels. A tumor may betray the ectopia, especially if hydronephrosis is present, as proper drainage is impaired. Pain may be caused by stones or infections.

REFERENCES

1. Campbell, M.: *Clinical Pediatric Urology* (Philadelphia: W. B. Saunders Company, 1951).
2. Patten, B. M.: *Human Embryology* (3d ed.; New York: McGraw-Hill Book Company, Inc., 1968).
3. Burke, E. C., Wenzl, J. E., and Utz, D. C.: The intrathoracic kidney. Report of a case, Am. J. Dis. Child. 113:487, 1967.
4. Purpon, I.: Crossed renal ectopy with solitary kidney: A review of the literature, J. Urol. 90:13, 1963.
5. Langworthy, H. T., and Drexler, L. S.: Carcinoma in crossed renal ectopia, J. Urol. 47:776, 1942.

Supernumerary Kidney

IN CONTRAST TO double kidney, supernumerary kidney is a rare malformation. If there is duplication of the renal pelvis and ureter in one kidney, the term "double kidney" is used, whereas in a supernumerary kidney, the parenchyma is separated from that of the main kidney. As a rule, roentgenography alone does not permit the diagnosis of supernumerary kidney but, in exceptional cases, if the separation of x-ray shadows is so marked that parenchymal connection seems unlikely, supernumerary kidneys sometimes can be recognized by radiography. A woman with six supernumerary kidneys was recorded by Begg,[1] who demonstrated "sextuplicitas renum" by intravenous pyelography.

The few cases on record usually were discovered at necropsy or surgical exploration. Carlson[2] reviewed 51 acceptable cases. In 30,000 necropsies at Boston City Hospital, no supernumerary kidney was found. Burgess[3] encountered a supernumerary kidney incidental to common bile duct exploration; it was mistaken for a lymph node. The patient was a man 77 years of age. But in most cases the extra kidney situated caudal to the normal one is prone to infection; stones, cysts, hydronephrosis and ptosis occur as complications. A clear cell carcinoma in a supernumerary kidney was reported by Exley and Hotchkiss,[4] and Carlson[2] described renal cell carcinoma in normal and supernumerary kidneys on the same side.

REFERENCES

1. Begg, R. C.: Sextuplicitas renum: A case of six functioning kidneys and ureters in an adult female, J. Urol. 70:686, 1953.
2. Carlson, H. E.: Supernumerary kidney: A summary of fifty one reported cases, J. Urol. 64:224, 1950.
3. Burgess, S. B.: Supernumerary kidney; report of a case, A.M.A. Arch. Path. 69:154, 1960.
4. Exley, M., and Hotchkiss, W. S.: Supernumerary kidney with clear cell carcinoma, J. Urol. 51:569, 1944.

Hydronephrosis

HYDRONEPHROSIS consists in dilatation of the renal pelvis usually combined with destruction of renal parenchyma and often with dilatation of the ureters. In many (but not in all) cases of hydronephrosis, an obstruction in the urinary pathways can be demonstrated. This obstruction may be supravesical or infravesical. In a series of Campbell's,[1] 83% of the patients had supravesical and 17% infravesical obstruction. In a series of 41 cases from the Children's Memorial Hospital in Chicago,[2] the obstruction was found at the ureteropelvic junction in 17 patients, in the ureterovesical region in 22 and in the course of the ureter in 1. Only once was no obstruction found. The changes at the ureteropelvic junction have aroused particular interest because of their numerical importance and their operability. Williams[3] stated that the disorder may occur at any age, that it is recognized most often in children who have passed their fifth year and that girls and boys are affected equally. In Campbell's[1] series, the incidence was higher in girls. But Uson *et al.*,[4] who reviewed 130 cases of hydronephrosis in children due to obstruction or dysfunction of the ureteropelvic junction, found it almost twice as often in boys as in girls. As a rule, newborns and infants up to the age of 6 months had the most advanced types. Approximately 40% of the children

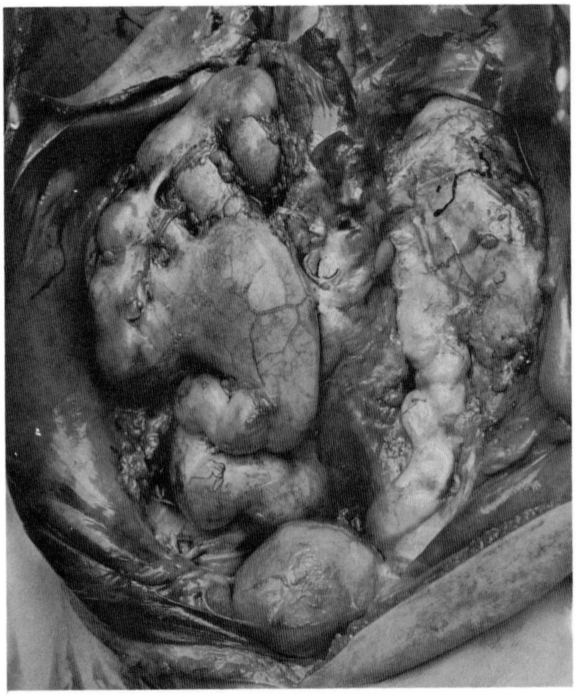

Fig. 105-11 (left).—Bilateral congenital hydronephrosis and hydroureters.

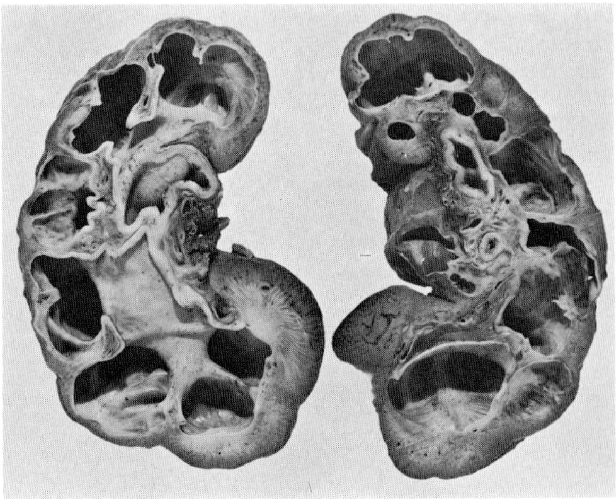

Fig. 105-12 (above).—Congenital hydronephrosis in a girl 8 years of age. Removed by operation.

had another important anomaly of the urogenital tract or elsewhere in the body and about 20% had bilateral hydronephrosis. In two-thirds of the cases, a definite obstructive cause of hydronephrosis was found.

In a family reported by Raffle,[5] the disorder occurred in two generations, all the patients being females. In one generation, 3 of 4 sisters were affected and in the second generation, the daughter of an unaffected brother had congenital hydronephrosis. In this infant, the protuberant abdomen was noticed at birth and, at 4 months of age, large left-sided hydronephrosis was found at operation. Orr[6] observed a woman with hydronephrosis whose brother and 4 children had the same disorder due to ureteropelvic junction obstruction. Campbell[7] saw similar cases of hydronephrosis in a mother, her daughter and her son. Jewell and Buchert[8] reported 4 cases of unilateral hydronephrosis in three consecutive generations. The anomaly has been observed in siblings by Pagliere[9] and by Aaron and Robbins[10] in 2 brothers, aged 12 and 16 years. Hydronephrosis, hydroureter and dilatation of the bladder were present in 2 brothers with congenital nephrogenic diabetes.[27] Mackay[11] described hydronephrosis combined with megaloureter in a most unusual family. Of 7 siblings, 5 had congenital renal lesions, 3 having hydronephrosis with megaloureters and 2 having congenital sarcoma of the kidney. Hydronephrosis has been observed repeatedly in patients with Turner syndrome and it was not rare in children with the thalidomide embryopathy.[12]

The pathogenesis of hydronephrosis due to changes at the ureteropelvic junction has been discussed thoroughly in a monograph by Östling.[13] In normal embryos of 40–50 mm., the uppermost part of the ureter was noticed to be narrower than the lower part and in fetuses of the fourth or fifth month this upper narrowing was more distinct, whereas the lumbar section of the ureter was remarkably wide. In the fetal ureter, there were folds, linear narrows and torsions, and in newborns such normal narrows usually were localized in the upper part of the ureter. Östling could not find mechanical hindrances to the urinary outflow in his fetuses and newborns with dilatations within the upper urinary tract. He thought it improbable that functional disturbances in the ureter and the musculature of the renal pelvis would be significant. The boundary lines between physiologic and pathologic variations in ureters and renal pelves in fetuses are ill defined.

Fixation of the ureter to the renal pelvis is the most common finding in hydronephrosis. In all cases, this fixation is considered to be a congenital malformation as proved by histologic findings. In the majority of cases, muscular hypertrophy and elastic fibrosis were ascertained in the wall of the renal pelvis. Östling[13] believed that an inflammatory swelling of the ureteropelvic junction, a spasm produced by a stone, a temporarily increased diuresis or a pressure at the pelvic outlet may cause a dilatation of the renal pelvis. The adhesion that envelops and fixes the ureter will then be drawn up over the wall of the renal pelvis, pressing the ureter against it. Because of this mechanism, the ureters kink and are subjected to an increased pressure as the dilatation of the hydronephrosis becomes more and more marked. Such changes at the ureteropelvic junction sometimes are combined with renal vessels that cross the ureter and add to the obstruction by pressing the ureter backward, thus accentuating the kink at the ureteropelvic junction. According to Williams,[3] such aberrant renal vessels are found in front of the ureter more often than behind and usually run to the inferior part of the hilum or to the lower pole of the kidney. If the vessel crosses immediately over the ureteropelvic junction, operative separation of the two structures results in emptying of the pelvis, but if the vessel crosses the ureter distal to the junction and binds it down to the surface of the hydronephrotic sac, the urine flow seldom is restored by freeing of the vessel. High insertion of the ureter sometimes is noted in hydronephrosis, particularly in a malrotated, fused or ectopic kidney, which represents a mechanical disadvantage in propelling the urine into the ureter. A narrowing of the ureter immediately below the pelvic ureteric junction has been suspected as the cause of hydronephrosis, but neither fibrotic strictures nor muscular thickening is found in such narrow places. Interruption of the circular element of the musculature also has been claimed to be the primary lesion in hydronephrosis.[3] However, in many cases, no obvious cause of obstruction is found and it is suspected that functional disturbances are at fault.

The complex origin of hydronephrosis is illustrated by observations and experiments in animals. Hydronephrosis has been noticed repeatedly in inbred strains of mice. In no instance does hydronephrosis appear as the only congenital malformation. The abnormal strains show a variety of anomalies of the urogenital system and of other organ complexes. In the strain of "myelencephalic blebs" there exist anomalies of the urinary system in addition to the superficial eye symptoms and foot anomalies. Absence of the kidney, hypoplastic kidneys and unilateral or bilateral hydronephrosis occur in this strain. Bagg[14] attributed the blocking of the urinary flow to occlusion of the ureter just above the vesicoureteral junction. Hydronephrosis also occurs in the strain "luxate" described by Carter[15] in detail. The presence of renal abnormalities was correlated in this case with a reduction in the number of lumbar vertebrae from six to five. Horseshoe kidney and renal cysts were found as well as hydronephrosis. In advanced hydronephrosis, the kidneys sometimes reached an enormous size, distending the abdominal cavity, but the ureter rarely was tortuous and gross examination failed to reveal any obvious blockage. In serial sections it usually was found that the ureter draining a hydropic kidney had one or more kinks close to the

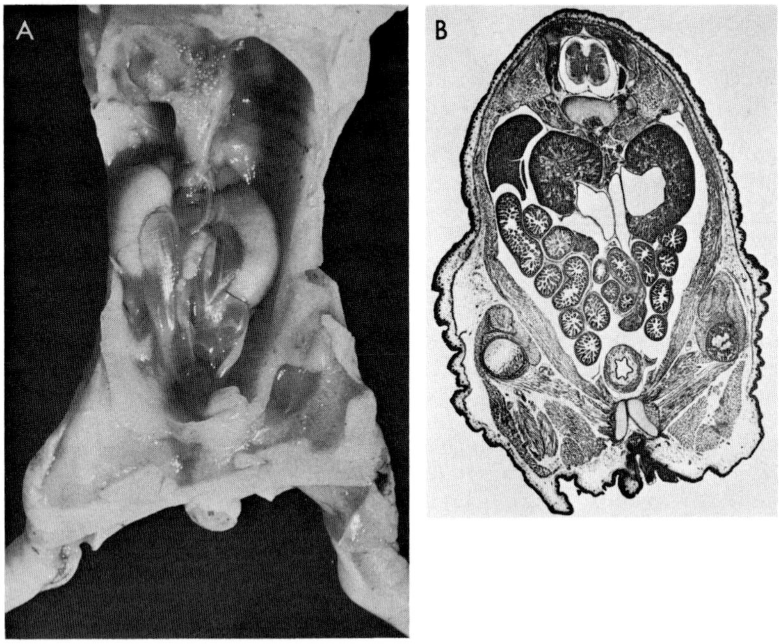

Fig. 105-13.—**A,** bilateral hydronephrosis and hydroureter in a newborn rat. The mother was kept on a vitamin A-deficient diet to the fifteenth day of gestation; the diet then was supplemented by vitamin A. **B,** transverse section showing hydronephrosis.

vesicoureteral opening and within the musculature of the bladder wall. Above this level it was unobstructed. Hydronephrosis was also observed in the complex of hereditary abnormalities in mice homozygous for the gene "U."[16] Association with the short ear gene (Se) was discussed by Wallace and Spickett[17] and compared with the condition in man. Two types of hydronephrosis were found: with and without obvious ureteric constriction. There was a higher incidence of hydronephrosis in males than in females. Hydronephrosis in a substrain of Wistar rats with a predilection for males has been described[18] and a urogenital syndrome has been observed in the golden hamster, with congenital hydronephrosis as one of its manifestations.[19]

Hydronephrosis can be produced in rats by a variety of experimental methods. Vitamin A deficiency of pregnant rats resulted in hypoplasia of the kidneys or in horseshoe kidneys of some of the young, but hydronephrosis was never observed.[20] In these experiments, the depleted rats were kept on vitamin A deficiency throughout pregnancy. In a later experiment,[21] vitamin A was added to the maternal diet at various times during gestation, thus interrupting the vitamin A deficiency. Administration of a single dose of vitamin A before the twelfth day prevented, and administration of vitamin A on days 13, 14 or 15 of gestation reduced, the incidence of renal hypoplasia or horseshoe kidney. But animals that received vitamin A during pregnancy from the eleventh to the fifteenth day had hydronephrotic kidneys, distended by accumulated fluid in the pelvis and calix. These hydronephrotic kidneys apparently were developmentally normal and functionally competent, as evidenced by the fluid accumulated within the pelvis and calix. One could explain the difference in the two experiments by assuming that vitamin A depletion throughout pregnancy resulted in anomalies of the upper and of the lower urinary tract, thus leading to the formation of nonfunctioning hypoplastic kidneys. If, however, vitamin A was given during pregnancy, such a supplement prevented the defects of the kidney but could not repair the anomaly of the lower genital tract. In this case, urinary secretion could take place but the outflow was impeded by the anomalies of the lower urinary tract. This hypothetical explanation was not born out by histologic examination of the lower urinary tract. Renal pelves and ureters were distended in many instances in which the orifices below appeared to be patent. The fluid retention in the ureters and the kidneys was, therefore, not explained by examination of the lower urinary tract as it appeared toward the end of gestation. The hydronephrosis in these cases could be explained by findings of Monie *et al.*[22] These authors pointed out that a temporary closure of the orifices of the ureters normally exists in 16–19-day embryos and that there is a transient narrowing of the urethra in 18–20-day embryos. To achieve normal development of the renal pelvis and ureters, the secretory function of the kidney during intrauterine life must be coordinated with the temporary closure and reopening of the ureteral orifices. If secretion of the kidney proceeds while the orifices are still closed or narrow, distention will take place above the point of

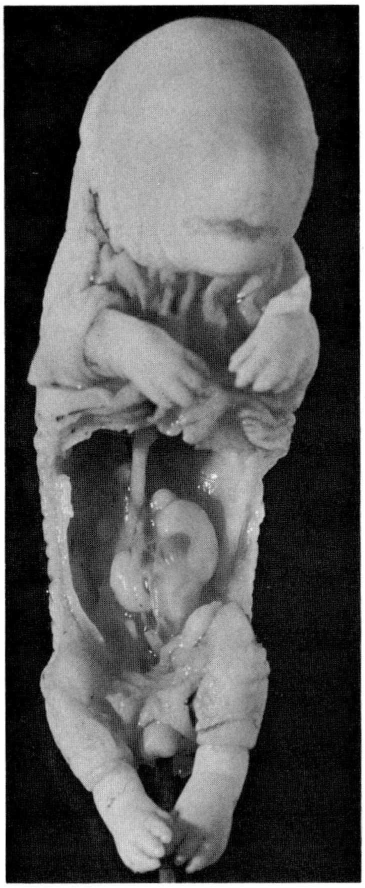

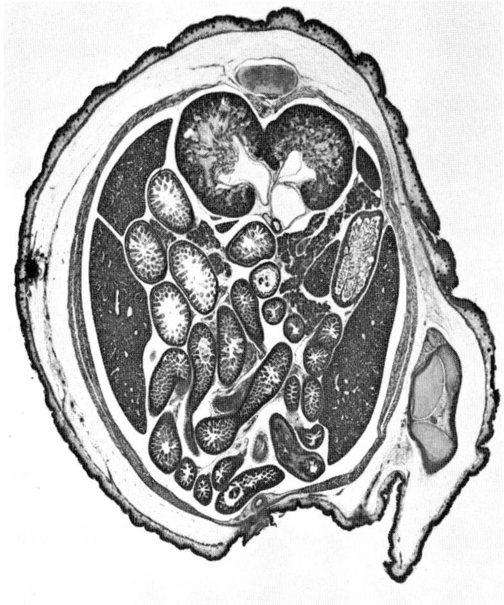

Fig. 105-14 (left). – Abnormal kidneys in a newborn rat whose mother was on a vitamin A-deficient diet that was supplemented with vitamin A on the fifteenth day. The left kidney is enlarged and hydronephrotic. The right kidney is small.

Fig. 105-15 (above). – Transverse section through a rat fetus with horseshoe kidney, hydronephrosis and hydroureter (the mother was injected with streptonigrin on the tenth day of gestation).

temporary obstruction, leading to congenital hydronephrosis and hydroureter. In the case of complete vitamin A deficiency throughout pregnancy, the renal tissue does not develop sufficiently to produce urine, and hydronephrosis cannot develop despite delayed opening of the ureteral orifices or other anomalies of the lower urinary tract. If, however, by vitamin A supplements from the eleventh to the fifteenth day of gestation, development of renal parenchyma is made possible, the urine secreted is held up by the temporary obstruction of the ureter, and hydronephrosis develops.

Hydronephrosis was also observed by Monie *et al.*[22] in the young of rats kept on a folic acid-deficient diet from day 11 of gestation onward and by Roux and Dupuis[23] in the offspring of rats deficient in pantothenic acid. In these animals, the ureteric orifices showed a variable degree of patency. Hydronephrosis was produced by x-irradiation of mouse embryos of 9½ and 10½ days.[24] Giroud *et al.*[25] observed hydroureter and hydronephrosis in embryos whose mothers were treated with large doses of vitamin A (50,000 units) from the eighth to the tenth day of gestation. In these specimens, an obstructive ureteral membrane was found in exceptional cases, but usually epithelial obliteration of the ureter was absent. These authors thought it possible that the membrane existed before birth longer than normally and obstructed elimination of the urine at that time, thus causing dilatation of the pelvis and ureter. They speculated that human hydronephrosis and hydroureter could originate in a similar way in cases in which obstruction of the lower urinary tract is absent. Giroud *et al.*[25] stated that renal function may begin at about 55 days of gestational age and that the ureteral membrane normally is resorbed at the end of the second month. By a prolonged persistence of the obstructive membrane of the ureter, hydronephrosis could be formed in some cases.

According to Williams,[3] congenital ureteropelvic anomalies may cause intermittent acute obstructions or slowly progressive distention of the pelvis and calices. The acute form, which is the most common, is seen chiefly in children over the age of 5 years. During attacks, the children suffer loin pains that last for several hours and may be accompanied by vomiting and pallor. Between attacks, the children are symptom-free. In chronic cases, a more advanced stage of hydronephrosis may be reached, with few symptoms. Sometimes there is some pain in the loin but often the anomaly is discovered by the finding of a large abdominal mass that may vary in size from day to day. Other manifestations, such as hematuria, calculi or infection, sometimes disclose the disorder. Hypertension occurs on rare occasions.

An intravenous pyelogram shows a bulging renal pelvis with no filling of the ureter.[3] The calices have lost their normal cupped appearance and look clubbed and round. As the contrast medium is carried into the ureter in later films, a filling defect may be seen in the ureteropelvic region. In some cases, the intravenous pyelogram shows no secretion in the affected kidney. This may be due to exacerbation of obstruction in a kidney of good function or to advanced destruction of parenchyma. A retrograde pyelogram may demonstrate the anomaly in such cases, or at least show the distorted ureter.

Associated malformations are found in the urogenital tract. Absence or hypoplasia of the contralateral kidney, cystic kidney, hypospadias, cryptorchidism and others are observed. Umbilical hernia, absence of the abdominal muscles, malrotation of the intestine, megacolon, annular pancreas, imperforate anus, congenital heart disease, hemivertebrae and cleft palate and lip have been seen (Cincinnati Children's Hospital) as associated malformations. Hydronephrosis was present soon after birth in 10% of a series of 199 children with myelomeningocele and, after 3 years, 25% had the renal disease.[26] Hydronephrosis has been recognized also in patients with gonadal dysgenesis (p. 1127).

Modern treatment aims not only to relieve the pain and prevent the recurrence of infection but also to preserve and improve the functioning renal tissue. Williams[3] recommended operation in all cases in which obstruction can be demonstrated. Surgical management of 126 infants and children was discussed by Uson *et al.*[4]

REFERENCES

1. Campbell, M.: *Clinical Pediatric Urology* (Philadelphia: W. B. Saunders Company, 1951).
2. Bigler, J. A.: Anomalies of the Urinary Tract, in Brennemann, J. (ed.), *Practice of Pediatrics* (Hagerstown, Md.: W. F. Prior Company, 1959), Vol. 3, Chap. 26.
3. Williams, D.: Urology in Childhood, in *Encyclopedia of Urology* (Berlin: Springer-Verlag, 1958) Vol. XV, p. 353.
4. Uson, A. C., Cox, L. A., and Lattimer, J. K.: Hydronephrosis in infants and children, J.A.M.A. 205:323; 327, 1968.
5. Raffle, R.: Familial hydronephrosis, Brit. M. J. 1:580, 1955.
6. Orr, L. M.: Familial Hydronephrosis, cited by Campbell, M., *Urology* (2d ed.; Philadelphia: W. B. Saunders Company, 1963).
7. Campbell, M.: *Urology* (2d ed.; Philadelphia: W. B. Saunders Company, 1963).
8. Jewell, J. H., and Buchert, W. I.: Unilateral hereditary hydronephrosis: A report of four cases in three consecutive generations, J. Urol. 88:129, 1962.
9. Pagliere, L. E.: Hidronefrosis congénita en dos hermanos, Rev. espec., Buenos Aires 1:938, 1926.
10. Aaron, G., and Robbins, M. A.: Hydronephrosis due to aberrant vessels: Remarkable familial incidence with report of cases, J. Urol. 60:702, 1948.
11. Mackay, H.: Congenital bilateral megalo-ureters with hydronephrosis: A remarkable family history, Proc. Roy. Soc. Med. 38:567, 1945.
12. Lenz, W.: Krankheiten des Urogenitalsystems, in Becker, P. E. (ed.), *Humangenetik* (Stuttgart: Georg Thieme, 1964), Vol. III.
13. Östling, K.: The genesis of hydronephrosis, Acta chir. scandinav. 86 (supp. 72):1–122, 1942.
14. Bagg, H. J.: Hereditary congenital anomalies of the genitourinary organs, Am. J. Surg. 7:211, 1929.
15. Carter, T. C.: The genetics of luxate mice, J. Genetics 51: 441, 1953.
16. Dunn, L. C., and Gluecksohn-Schoenheimer, S.: A new complex of hereditary abnormalities in the house mouse, J. Exper. Zool. 104:25, 1947.
17. Wallace, M. E., and Spickett, S. G.: Hydronephrosis in mouse, rat, and man, J. M. Genetics 4:73, 1967.
18. Astarabadi, I., and Bell, E. T.: Spontaneous hydronephrosis in albino rats, Nature, London 195:392, 1962.
19. Orsini, M. W.: The piebald hamster. A mutation showing growth retardation and urino-genital abnormalities, J. Hered. 43:37, 1952.
20. Wilson, J. G., and Warkany, J.: Malformations in the genitourinary tract induced by maternal vitamin A deficiency in the rat, Am. J. Anat. 83:357, 1948.
21. Wilson, J. G., Roth, C. B., and Warkany, J.: An analysis of the syndrome of malformations induced by maternal vitamin A deficiency. Effects of restoration of Vitamin A at various times during gestation, Am. J. Anat. 92:189, 1953.
22. Monie, I. W., Nelson, M. M., and Evans, H. M.: Abnormalities of the urinary system of rat embryos resulting from transitory deficiency of pteroylglutamic acid during gestation, Anat. Rec. 127:711, 1957.
23. Roux, C., and Dupuis, R.: Urohydronephroses par carence pantothenique, Arch. franç. pédiat. 18:1337, 1961.
24. Russell, L. B.: X-ray induced developmental abnormalities in the mouse and their use in the analysis of embryological patterns. I. External and gross visceral changes, J. Exper. Zool. 114:545, 1950.
25. Giroud, A., Martinet, M., and Roux, C.: Considérations à propos des hydronéphroses par hypervitaminose A chez l'embryon de rat, Arch. Anat. Path. 7:113, 1959.
26. Rose, R. S., and Smith, J. P.: Hydronephrosis in infants with meningomyelocele: Its early recognition, J. Urol. 90: 129, 1963.
27. Bensel, R. W., and Peters, E. R.: Progressive hydronephrosis, hydroureter, and dilatation of the bladder in siblings with congenital nephrogenic diabetes insipidus, J. Pediat. 77:439, 1970.

Hereditary Renal Diseases

It has long been known that in some families renal disorders occur with greater frequency than should be expected by chance alone. Such tendency to renal disorders may manifest itself under such clinical pictures as acute nephritis, chronic nephritis, nephrosclerosis, pyelonephritis or nephrosis. Some pedigrees including many generations go back to times when an exact diagnosis of the renal disease could not be made, and even in modern times classification of hereditary renal disorders is not always possible. In some families, the clinical course of an affected member may be indistinguishable from that of any patient with glomerulonephritis, and progression may be observed from the acute stage, characterized chiefly by hematuria, proteinuria and cylindruria, to the nephrotic stage with massive edema or to the chronic stage with hypertension, azotemia and death from renal failure. Are these familial renal diseases the result of congenital structural anomalies of the kidneys or are they inherited tendencies to abnormal renal or immune reactions after bacterial infections?

An early report dates back to Dickinson[1] in 1875. He observed Bright disease in 12 of 16 members of one kindred.[7] Chronic renal disease through four generations of a family was reported by Pel,[2] Guthrie[3] and Hurst.[4] Alport[5] recognized that the renal disorder frequently was associated with deafness and Sohar[6] described ocular anomalies in some patients. The disease picture has been named "Alport syndrome." It was soon noticed that the disorder was transmitted by females but was far more lethal in males. Robin *et al.*[7] reported a kindred of 200 members, observed in five generations, in which a diagnosis of glomerulonephritis was made in 27 members. Some of the living patients, all males, were in the stage of chronic renal failure and some were nephrotic. Although several females showed abnormal urinary findings, the disorder was not lethal in any of them. In 4 patients, postmortem studies revealed gross and microscopic findings indistinguishable from classic glomerulonephritis. Sixteen of the 27 patients were affected by nerve deafness. Every patient with deafness suffered from nephritis but the converse was not true. In the female, the disease was characterized by proteinuria, hematuria and mild hypertension, and deafness sometimes was present; fecundity was unimpaired and the disease was compatible with longevity. In males, the disease was semilethal and no affected male survived beyond the age of 29. It appeared to these authors that the nephropathy was transmitted as a sex-linked dominant. Only affected members, and no males, transmitted the disease. Hereditary renal disease associated with nerve deafness and ocular lesions was also described by Goldbloom *et al.*[8] They mentioned six kindreds in which hereditary renal disease was connected with nerve deafness, and reported a family in which the mother, who had mild signs of renal disease, had 3 boys, all affected by renal disease. One child died suddenly at the age of 5 years in convulsions. Necropsy showed both kidneys granular and contracted, the picture being that of chronic pyelonephritis. The second child developed hypertension at 7 years followed by signs of chronic glomerulonephritis and bilateral nerve deafness. He died with uremia at the age of 10 years, and again the over-all picture was that of chronic pyelonephritis. The third boy was less affected but at 18 years he showed albuminuria, microscopic hematuria and nerve deafness. He also had an unusual type of bilateral anterior subcapsular cataract. Goldbloom *et al.*[8] believed that nephropathy associated with nerve deafness is due to a dominant gene that may be partially sex-linked, males being affected more severely than females. Auditory and ocular lesions are due to the presence of the same abnormal gene. Hereditary chronic renal disease associated with nerve deafness beginning at age 10 and congenital posterior cortical cataracts were described by Sohar[6] in 4 brothers of a Jewish family from Iraq. Hereditary hematuria, nephropathy and deafness with severe manifestations in the male and mild manifestations in the female were reported by Sturtz and Burke.[9] Perkoff *et al.*[10] studied four generations of a large Mormon family in which 50 members showed evidence of renal disease diagnosed as interstitial pyelonephritis. Fifty members had evidence of renal disorder, males being affected more severely than females. Some of the males also had nerve deafness. In 1958, Perkoff *et al.*[11] reported an extension of their original investigation. They termed the renal disease a chronic nephritis with frequent episodes of bacterial renal infection. The pathologic changes became more severe with advancing age. Foam cells were found in sections from the kidneys of some of the patients, which suggested to the authors a metabolic disturbance leading to increased susceptibility to infection. Sex-linked dominant inheritance seemed the most likely genetic mechanism responsible for the disorder. Other reports on families with Alport syndrome can be found in review articles.[12-16]

Alport syndrome is now characterized by intermittent or permanent hematuria, albuminuria and cylindruria, which appear early in life, sometimes in the newborn period. In some families, urinary tract infections are demonstrable, but in the majority they are not. Deafness apparently is not congenital; it is noticed in children after the age of 8 years and is more pronounced in males. The renal disorder often is fatal in males between 20 and 30 years of age. In females, a milder course is common, although exacerbations occur with infections and pregnancy. Ocular disturbances are frequent in some families and absent in others.[6,16] Pathologico-anatomic examinations show a combination of glomerulonephritis, pyelonephritis and interstitial nephritis with characteristic foam cells in the lower cortex and ringing the corticomedullary junction.[17] In some cases, metabolic disturbances have been described but they are not uniform and seem to be the result rather than the cause of the renal anomalies.[13] Observations have been made in various racial groups. Although transmission from generation to generation indicates dominant inheritance of the disorder, the genetic mechanisms involved are not clear. The increased danger to male patients is unexplained. There is no close association of renal, aural and ocular manifestations. Transmission obviously is irregular. The renal anomaly commonly is transmitted by females, which is not surprising, as males are severely ill by the time they reach maturity; but occasionally the trait is passed on from a father to his son.[11,12] Subtle explanations try to elucidate the confusing genetic situation,[13-15, 18, 19] and speculations concerning the genetic mechanism abound.

Concerning the question of congenital structural anomalies, one can cite that duplication of the renal pelvis and of ureters has been discovered in some members of families with hereditary hematuria and deafness[9] but, since such ureteric variations are found in more than 1% of the population,[20] the significance of such anomalies for the pathogenesis of Alport nephropathy and the etiologically different familial nephrosis[20, 21] is dubious. There also is a possibility that the patients have congenital micro-malformations. Van Buchem and Beetstra[12] did micro-dissection of the kidneys of 3 patients with Alport syndrome and found abnormalities of the distal parts of the nephron. The collecting tubules had few ramifications and there were diverticular protrusions. The proximal tubules were small and only a few glomeruli were found. These authors thought it probable that they were dealing with a developmental disturbance of the kidneys that concerned the ureteral bud as well as the metanephrogenic tissue. Deafness develops during childhood but no congenital substrate has been found. Congenital cataract, spherophakia, lenticonus, retinal detachment, macular pathology or myopia was present in some families; in others, no ocular anomalies were noted.[16] Thus, it is possible that there are congenital roots in Alport familial nephropathy, but in many patients the course is that of a postnatal disease.

Similar considerations apply to other familial renal disorders. Familial nephrosis has been reviewed by Vernier *et al.*,[21] who reported 4 children affected by the nephrotic syndrome. Nephrosis has been observed in twins and in siblings. Such familial nephrosis may begin very early in life and be resistant to all forms of therapy that are known to produce remission in other children with nephrosis. It is likely that such cases of nephrosis are congenital. The spectrum of renal disease may range from transient nephrosis through persistent pure nephrosis, mixed nephrosis and nephritis to chronic glomerulonephritis with nephrotic manifestations. Circulating antibodies to renal tissue in the serum of the mother of the children could not be demonstrated.[21] Braun and Bayer[20] found an association of familial nephrosis with congenital urinary tract anomalies, finger defects and split uvula. The disorder apparently is more common in Finland than in other countries[22]; there, 1 case of congenital nephrosis occurs in 10,000 deliveries. Autosomal recessive inheritance seems to be established. The kidneys show microcystic dilatations of the proximal tubuli and a swan-like neck. Glomerular changes consist of cell proliferation, crescent formation and leukocytic infiltration.[22]

Familial juvenile nephronophthisis is a syndrome that affects several children in one family, leading to early death from renal disease.[23] Polyuria, polydipsia, nycturia and isosthenuria develop, but urine examinations may remain negative and the blood pressure normal. Albuminuria can be absent or mild. The blood phosphorus rises, serum calcium declines and the NPN increases until the children die of uremia. Hackzell and Lundmark[24] observed two families of this type. Necropsies revealed symmetric and diffuse contraction of the kidney with serious injury to the tubules and the glomeruli. Persistent hypokalemia and treatment with potassium chloride were discussed by Mangos *et al.*[25] The disorder occurs in children homozygous for a rare autosomal gene.[25, 26]

Genetically determined tubular nephropathies associated with retinitis pigmentosa present specific problems of heredity.[28-30] Several other renal disorders in which genetic factors play a role are discussed in this chapter.

Comprehensive reviews of hereditary renal diseases, including metabolic disorders, were published by Perkoff in 1967[27] and by Royer *et al.*[31] in 1970.

REFERENCES

1. Dickinson, W. H.: Diseases of the Kidney Characterized by Albuminuria, in Allbut's *A System of Medicine* (New York: The Macmillan Company, 1875), Vol. 4, p. 352.
2. Pel, P. K.: Die Erblichkeit der Chronischen Nephritis, Ztschr. klin. Med. 38:127, 1899.
3. Guthrie, L. G.: Idiopathic or congenital hereditary and family haematuria, Lancet 1:1243, 1902.
4. Hurst, A. F.: Hereditary familial congenital hemorrhagic nephritis, Guys's Hosp. Rep. 73:368, 1923.
5. Alport, A. C.: Hereditary familial congenital hemorrhagic nephritis, Brit. M. J. 1:504, 1927.
6. Sohar, E.: Renal disease, inner ear deafness and ocular changes. A new heredofamilial syndrome, A.M.A. Arch. Int. Med. 97:627, 1956.
7. Robin, E. D., Gardner, F. H., and Levine, S. A.: Hereditary factors in chronic Bright's disease – a study of two affected kindreds, Tr. A. Am. Physicians 70:140, 1957.
8. Goldbloom, R. B., Fraser, F. C., Waugh, D., Aronovitch, M., and Wiglesworth, F. W.: Hereditary renal disease associated with nerve deafness and ocular lesions, Pediatrics 20:241, 1957.
9. Sturtz, G. S., and Burke, E. C.: Hereditary hematuria, nephropathy and deafness. Preliminary report, New England J. Med. 254:1123, 1956.
10. Perkoff, G. T., Stephens, F. E., Dolowitz, D. A., and Tyler, F. H.: Clinical study of hereditary interstitial pyelonephritis, A.M.A. Arch. Int. Med. 88:191, 1951.
11. Perkoff, G. T., Nugent, C. A., Jr., Dolowitz, D. A., Stephens, F. E., Carnes, W. H., and Tyler, F. H.: A follow-up study of hereditary chronic nephritis, A.M.A. Arch. Int. Med. 102:733, 1958.
12. Van Buchem, F. S. P. and Beetstra, A.: Hereditary renal disease associated with deafness; Alport's syndrome, Proc. Kon. Nederl. Acad. Wet. (Series C), p. 350, 1965.
13. Fuhrmann, W.: Das Syndrom der erblichen Nephropathie mit Innenohrschwerhörigkeit, Deutsche med. Wchnschr. 88:525, 1963.
14. Burguet, W., Lefebvre, P., Booz, G., Delwaide, P. J. and van Cauwenberge, H.: Le syndrome d'Alport ou néphropathie héréditaire avec surdité. Nouvelle étude familiale, J. Génét. Hum. 15:7, 1966.
15. Shaw, R. F., and Glover, R. A.: Abnormal segregation in hereditary renal disease with deafness, Am. J. Human Genet. 13:89, 1961.
16. Arenberg, I. K., Dodson, V. N., Falls, H. F., and Stern, S. D.: Alport's syndrome: Reevaluation of the associated ocular abnormalities and report of a family study, J. Pediat. Ophth. 4:21, 1967.
17. Krickstein, H. I., Gloor, F. J., and Balogh, K., Jr.: Renal

pathology in hereditary nephritis with nerve deafness, Arch. Path. 82:506, 1966.
18. Perkoff, G. T., Stephens, F. E., and Tyler, F. H.: Chronic hereditary nephritis and Y-chromosome linkage: Reply to Graham, Am. J. Human Genet. 12:381, 1960.
19. Cohen, M. M., Cassady, G., and Hanna, B. L.: A genetic study of hereditary renal dysfunction with associated nerve deafness, Am. J. Human Genet. 13:379, 1961.
20. Braun, F. C., Jr., and Bayer, J. F.: Familial nephrosis associated with deafness and congenital urinary tract anomalies in siblings, J. Pediat. 60:33, 1962.
21. Vernier, R. L, Brunson, J., and Good, R. A.: Studies on familial nephrosis. 1. Clinical and pathologic study of four cases in a single family, A.M.A. Dis. Child. 93:469, 1957.
22. Hallman, N., Norio, R., and Kouvalainen, K.: Main features of the congenital nephrotic syndrome, Acta paediat. scandinav. 172:75, 1967.
23. Fanconi, G., Hanhart, E., Albertini, A. von, Uhlinger, E., Dolivo, G., and Prader, A.: Die familiäre juvenile Nephronophthise (die idiopathische parenchymatöse Schrumpfniere), Helvet. paediat. acta 6:1, 1951.
24. Hackzell, G., and Lundmark, C.: Familial juvenile nephronophthisis, Acta paediat. 47:428, 1958.
25. Mangos, J. A., Opitz, J. M., Lobeck, C. C., and Cookson, D. U.: Familial juvenile nephronophthisis; an unrecognized renal disease in the United States, Pediatrics 34:337, 1964.
26. Broberger, O., Winberg, J., and Zetterström, R.: Juvenile nephronophthisis. Part 1. A genetically determined nephropathy with hypotonic polyuria and azotaemia, Acta paediat. 49:470, 1960.
27. Perkoff, G. T.: The hereditary renal diseases, New England J. Med. 277:79; 129, 1967.
28. Jackson, W. P. U., and Linder, G. C.: Innate functional defects of the renal tubules, with particular reference to the Fanconi syndrome, Quart. J. Med. 22:133, 1953.
29. Senior, B., Friedman, A. I., and Brando, J. L.: Juvenile familial nephropathy with tapetoretinal degeneration. A new oculo-renal dystrophy, Am. J. Ophth. 52:625, 1961.
30. Bois, E., and Royer, P.: Association de nephropathie tubulo-interstitielle chronique et de degenerescence tapetoretinienne, Arch. franç. pédiat. 27:471, 1970.
31. Royer, P., Frezal, J., Bois, E., and Feingold, J.: Les nephropathies hereditaires, Arch. franç. pédiat. 27:293, 1970.

Wilms Tumor

IT HAS BEEN ASSERTED that 53 names have been applied to this renal tumor of childhood, which is characterized by rapid growth and early metastases. The tumor has no sex preference in children. In adults, there seems to be a predilection for males, but some authors believe that the adult type is not identical to the juvenile. Estimates vary concerning the relative role played by Wilms[1] tumor among the tumors of childhood.[2] Some authors considered it the most common abdominal tumor of childhood,[3] whereas others believed that it ranks second among the cancers of the abdominal region, exceeded only by neuroblastoma.[4] Wilms tumors usually arise within the kidney but occasionally extrarenal location is seen.[5] In 5–10% of the cases, bilateral tumors develop.[6]

Potter[7] pointed out that all the structures found in Wilms tumors are of mesodermal origin and that they are derived from cells of the metanephric blastema that failed to differentiate normally. Metanephric tissue normally ceases to form tubules and glomeruli at about the thirty-fourth week of gestation. Islands of undifferentiated nephroblastic cells that continue to proliferate without undergoing normal differentiation after this period may become Wilms tumors. Such nephroblastic tissue areas can be found in otherwise normal, in polycystic,[7] in horseshoe or hypoplastic

Fig. 105-16. – Wilms tumor of a girl 4 years of age.

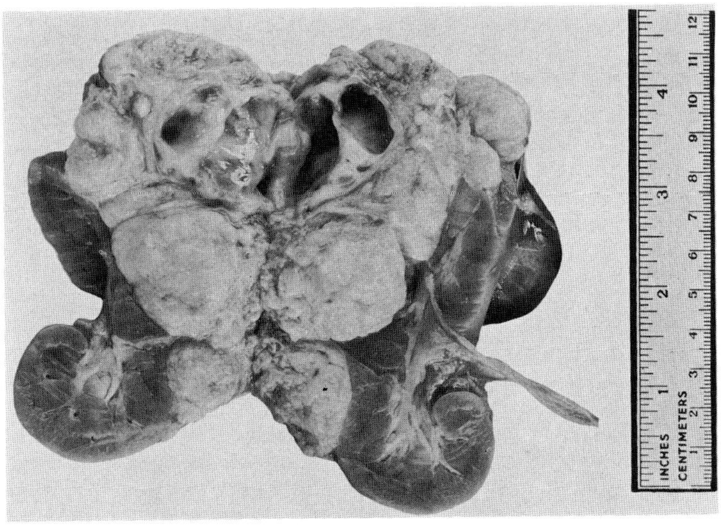

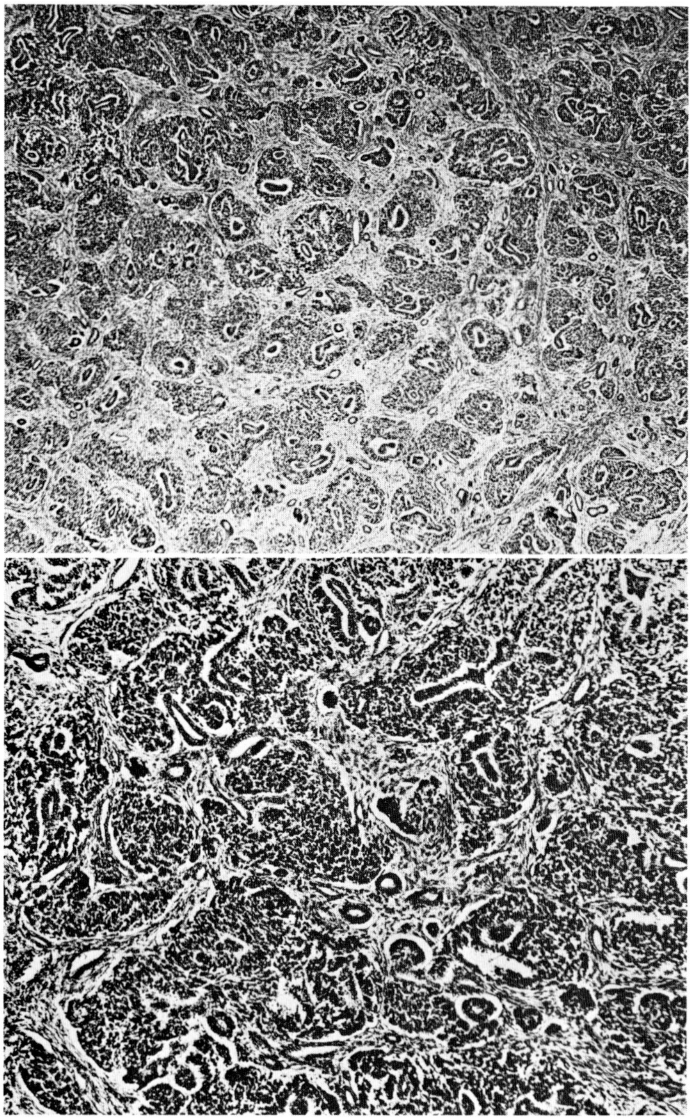

Fig. 105-17. — Sections through Wilms tumor, showing glomeruli-like structures, tubules and undifferentiated and differentiating stroma.

kidneys.[8] Wilms tumors vary in size according to the stage of their discovery. Weights of 5,000 Gm. have been reported,[5] but sometimes they are small and discovered on routine clinical examination or as accidental findings at histologic examination of renal tissue. The cells have large hyperchromatic nuclei but ill-defined boundaries. Structures composed of columnar cells, connective tissue, muscle, cartilage and bone may be seen. Ill-defined tubules and glomeruli are surrounded by immature embryonal mesenchyme. Metastases are most common in the lungs and liver[5] but not in the kidney of the other side.[6] For most cases of Wilms tumor, no association can be demonstrated with other congenital malformations and most renal malformations are not complicated by Wilms tumors. Yet it will be pointed out that many observations suggest a relationship of these tumors with teratogenesis.

Most Wilms tumors are recognized in infancy or early childhood. It seems likely that they are always present at birth in some form and they have been observed repeatedly in fetuses. In 1940, Wells[9] accepted 5 cases recorded in the literature as proved congenital tumors. Presence at birth seemed probable for another 11 cases and there were 2 fetuses among his accepted congenital cases. Since then, Barrett and McCagne[10] reported a case in a 6½-month fetus, and Hon and Holman[11] saw bilateral nephroblastomas in a premature infant who died 13 hours after birth. They considered the transformed kidneys embryonal tumors and malformations. Nicholson[12] described an embryonic tumor of the kidney in a full-term stillborn male fetus. He believed that such tumors are organs malformed before birth and thus developmental congenital malformations in which growth continues but differentiation is aborted. Congenital Wilms tumors have been recorded[13,14] since Wells' publication. Wells[9] pointed out that the definite derivation of these tumors from incompletely developed embryonic structures makes them congenital malignant neoplasms, but it seemed impossible to say in how many the malignant transformation begins before birth. Potter[7] believed that all metanephroblastomas must be congenital, although she found no such tumors in her material of fetuses and newborn children. There were, however, several that contained abnormal metanephric blastema, which "would doubtless have developed into a Wilms tumor." Thus, there apparently is general agreement that these kidney tumors are congenital, at least in the form of abnormal, undifferentiated embryonal tissues that can develop into tumors in postnatal life. The average age of clinical recognition of Wilms tumor is about 3 years, which leads to the question why such undifferentiated embryonal cells usually fail to grow excessively for several years. Wilms tumor in the adult has been observed many times.[15,16] It would be important to understand why such abnormal embryonal tissue remains limited to a small area and then develops into a tumor when its carrier reaches 75 years of age, as in the case of Twinem.[17] It seems that for such cases Cohnheim's theory of oncogenesis (p. 1199) is well applicable, although the delayed growth of the abnormal embryonic tissue remains unexplained. When Wilms tumor occurs in adults, the differential diagnosis from renal cell carcinoma may be difficult.[40] Vice versa, it should be remembered that renal cell carcinoma can occur in children.[41]

The teratologic origin of Wilms tumors suggested by pathologico-anatomic observations is further supported by malformations in patients affected by such tumors. Wilms tumors have been found completely separated from the kidney,[5] thus developing in dystopic renal tissue. They have developed in horseshoe kidneys,[8,18,19] in hypoplastic kidneys and in patients with congenital genitourinary tract anomalies such as hypospadias, cryptorchidism, duplications of the upper urinary tract of the urethra.[4,8,20] They have been observed frequently in patients with extrarenal malformations. In 1876, Weigert[21] reported such a tumor in a male fetus with harelip and cleft palate, malformations seen also in a patient with bilateral nephroblastomas reported by Martin and Kloecker.[22] An association of Wilms tumor with bronchogenic cyst and supernumerary thumb was mentioned by Dargeon.[4] A surprising association of Wilms tumor and congenital aniridia was discovered by Miller *et al.*[8] Wilms tumor with congenital cataract has been observed.[4] By 1967, 26 cases of Wilms tumor had been noted in association with congenital hemihypertrophy.[23] Omphalocele and hemihypertrophy associated with Wilms tumor was recorded by Dargeon.[4] The same author mentioned the combination of Wilms tumor with a "bathing trunk nevus." Bilateral Wilms tumor and polycystic kidneys were described in a 24-day-old male with situs inversus and absent adrenals.[24] Miller *et al.*[8] listed a case of Wilms tumor combined with small penis, cryptorchidism, hypotonia and severe mental retardation in which an extra chromosome in the E group, presumably trisomy 18, was found. Renal blastema nodules apparently are not rare in infants with trisomy 18, but they may be non-neoplastic.[42] A malignant renal tumor in a hermaphroditic child was recorded by Raubitschek[25] in 1912 and bilateral Wilms tumors in a male pseudohermaphrodite in 1954 by Stump and Garret,[26] i.e., at times when karyotypes could not yet be determined. Unilateral nephroblastoma was described by Angström[27] in a patient with ambiguous genitalia and agonadism. Male pseudohermaphrodism combined with Wilms tumor, a nephrotic sydrome in a patient with XX/XY mosaicism, was reported by Denys *et al.*[28] Barr bodies were not noticed in buccal smears but were seen in cells of the testicle, ductus deferens and oviduct. In many cells of the Wilms tumor, multiple Barr bodies were noted. Aneuploidy in cells of nephroblastomas has been reported.[38] Mental development usually is normal in patients with Wilms tumors but retardation sometimes is present.[8,22]

It is estimated that about 8–10% of Wilms tumors occur bilaterally. The mortality in such cases is extremely high and early attention to the contralateral side is recommended in all cases. It is believed that the involvement of the second kidney is due to a separate coexisting malformation and not to metastases. Jagasia *et al.*[6] reported 12 and Martin and Kloecker[22] 3 cases of bilateral nephroblastoma. Before them, Campbell[24] and Hon and Holman[11] had described bilateral and congenital cases. Although the symmetry of these tumors represents an interesting biologic phenomenon, it does not contribute greatly to elucidation of their etiology. Teratogenic factors, whether genetic or environmental, can cause symmetric or unilateral malformations. If there are oncogenic factors that transform the basic developmental error of renal tissue into a malignant tumor, they probably are of a general and nonspecific nature, so that bilateral manifestation can be expected if embryonic cell rests exist in both kidneys. Hemihypertrophy predisposes not only to Wilms tumors but to hepatoblastomas and adrenal neoplasms. There is a patient on record who had a combination of hemihypertrophy with adrenocortical and Wilms tumor.[29]

Not much is known about the etiology of Wilms tumor but there are reports of identical twins, both affected by such tumors.[8,30] Wilms tumors have been observed in siblings of several families.[8,31-33] Association of Wilms tumor with a nephrotic syndrome has been observed in siblings.[34] In two of these families, more than one generation was affected. Strøm[33] described a kindred in which, in the course of three generations, 4 children died and 1 was operated on between the ages of 1 and 3 years, all with a diagnosis of renal or abdominal tumor. In this kindred, the disorder apparently was transmitted through fathers who were not affected. In Fitzgerald and Hardin's[32] cases, a father and 2 of his children were operated on for Wilms tumor. This observation could be interpreted as dominant inheritance made possible through the lifesaving operation on the father. It is possible that many other cases presenting new mutations appear to be sporadic because of the child's early death and failure to produce offspring. Many children with Wilms tumor are now saved by surgical, roentgen and chemotherapeutic measures. Survival is possible for almost half of the treated patients, particularly those recognized before the age of 2 years.[19,35,36] Even metastases are now attacked successfully.[37] It remains to be seen how many successfully treated patients will transmit the disease. Management of bilateral Wilms tumor was discussed by Anderson *et al.*[39]

REFERENCES

1. Wilms, M.: *Die Mischgeschwülste der Niere* (Leipzig: A Georgi, 1899).
2. Deming, C. L.: Renal neoplasms: An enigma and a challenge, J. Urol. 69:1, 1953.
3. Gross, R. E.: *The Surgery of Infancy and Childhood* (Philadelphia: W. B. Saunders Company, 1953).
4. Dargeon, H. W.: *Tumors of Childhood* (New York: Paul B. Hoeber, Inc., Medical Division of Harper & Brothers, 1960).
5. Benzing, W., Jr.: Wilms tumor in infancy and childhood, Radiology 58:674, 1952.
6. Jagasia, K. H., Thurman, W. G., Pickett, E., and Grabstaldt, H.: Bilateral Wilms' tumors in children, J. Pediat. 65:371, 1964.
7. Potter, E. L.: *Pathology of the Fetus and Infant* (2d ed.; Chicago: Year Book Medical Publishers, Inc., 1961).
8. Miller, R. W., Fraumeni, J. F., and Manning, M. D.: Association of Wilms' tumor with aniridia, hemihypertrophy and other congenital malformations, New England J. Med. 270:922, 1964.
9. Wells, H. G.: Occurrence and significance of congenital malignant neoplasms, Arch. Path. 30:535, 1940.
10. Barrett, W. A., and McCagne, E. J.: Histopathology in prognosis of kidney tumors, J. Urol. 71:684, 1954.
11. Hon, L. T., and Holman, R. L.: Bilateral nephroblastoma in a premature infant, J. Path. & Bact. 82:249, 1961.
12. Nicholson, G. W.: An embryonic tumour of the kidney in a foetus, J. Path. & Bact. 34:711, 1931.
13. Silver, H.: Wilms' tumor (embryoma of the kidney), J. Pediat. 31:643, 1947.
14. Hartenstein, H.: Wilms' tumor in a newborn infant, J. Pediat. 35:381, 1949.
15. Culp, O. S., and Hartman, F. W.: Mesoblastic nephroma in adults, J. Urol. 60:552, 1948.
16. Smith, K. H.: Wilms tumor in the adult, Brit. J. Surg. 47: 397, 1960.
17. Twinem, F. P: Wilms' tumor in a 75 year old male; report of a case, J. Urol. 55:246, 1946.
18. Lathem, J. E., and Smith, K. H.: Wilms tumor in horseshoe kidney; surviving case, J. Urol. 88:25, 1962.
19. Lattimer, J. K., Melicow, M. M., and Uson, A. C.: Wilms tumor: A report of 71 cases, J. Urol. 80:401, 1958.
20. Jagasia, K. H., and Thurman, W. G.: Congenital anomalies of the kidney in association with Wilms' tumor, Pediatrics 35:338, 1965.
21. Weigert, C.: Onkologische Beiträge 1. Adenocarcinoma renum congenitum, Virchows Arch. path. Anat. 67:492, 1876.
22. Martin, L. W., and Kloecker, R. J.: Bilateral nephroblastomas, Pediatrics 28:101, 1961.
23. Fraumeni, J. F., Jr., Geiser, C. F., and Manning, M. D.: Wilms tumor and congenital hemihypertrophy: Report of five new cases and review of literature, Pediatrics 40: 886, 1967.
24. Campbell, M. F.: Bilateral embryonal adenosarcoma of kidney (Wilms' tumor), J. Urol. 59:567, 1948.
25. Raubitschek, H.: Über eine bösartige Nierengeschwulst bei einem kindlichen Hermaphroditen, Ztschr. Path. 10: 206, 1912.
26. Stump, T. A., and Garret, R. A.: Bilateral Wilms' tumor in a male pseudohermaphrodite, J. Urol. 72:1146, 1954.
27. Angström, T.: Nephroblastoma in a case of agonadism, Cancer 18:857, 1965.
28. Denys, P., Malvaux, P., Van den Berghe, H., Tanghe, W., and Proesman, W.: Association d'un syndrome anatomopathologique de pseudohermaphrodisme masculin, d'une tumeur de Wilms, d'une nephropathie parenchymateuse et d'un mosaicisme XX/XY, Arch. franç. pédiat. 24:729, 1967.
29. Riedel, H. A.: Adrenogenital syndrome in a male child due to adrenocortical tumor, Pediatrics 10:19, 1952.
30. Gaulin, E.: Simultaneous Wilms tumors in identical twins, J. Urol. 66:547, 1951.
31. Maslow, L. A.: Wilms tumor. Report of three cases and a possible fourth one in the same family, J. Urol. 43:75, 1940.
32. Fitzgerald, W. L., and Hardin, H. C.: Bilateral Wilms tumor in a Wilms tumor family, J. Urol. 73:468, 1955.
33. Strøm, T.: A Wilms tumor family, Acta paediat. 46:601, 1957.
34. Zunin, C., and Soave, F.: Association of nephrotic syndrome and nephroblastoma in siblings, Ann. paediat. 203: 29, 1964.
35. Sukarochana, K. and Kiesewetter, W. B.: Wilms' tumor: Factors influencing long-term survival, J. Pediat. 69:747, 1966.
36. Westra, P., Kieffer, S. A., and Mosser, D. G.: Wilms' tumor. A summary of 25 years of experience before actinomycin-D, Am. J. Roentgenol. 100:214, 1967.
37. Wedemeyer, P. P., White, J. G., Nesbit, M. E., Aust, J. B., Leonard, A. S., D'Angio, G. J., and Krivit, W.: Resection of metastases in Wilms' tumor: A report of three cases cured of pulmonary and hepatic metastases, Pediatrics 41:446, 1968.
38. Cox, D.: Chromosome constitution of nephroblastomas, Cancer 19:1217, 1966.
39. Anderson, E. E., Herlong, J. H., Harper, J. M., Small, M. P., and Atwill, W. H.: Bilateral Wilms' tumor. Diagnosis and management, Clin. Pediat. 7:596, 1968.
40. Olsen, B. S., and Bischoff, A. J.: Wilms' tumor in an adult, Cancer 25:21, 1970.
41. Dehner, L. P., Leestma, J. E., and Price, E. B., Jr.: Renal cell carcinoma in children: A clinicopathologic study of 15 cases and review of the literature, J. Pediat. 76:358, 1970.
42. Bove, K. E., Koffler, H., and McAdams, A. J.: Nodular renal blastema. Definition and possible significance, Cancer 24:323, 1969.

Congenital Mesoblastic Nephromas

IT HAS BEEN RECOMMENDED that congenital mesoblastic nephromas recognized during infancy be clearly distinguished from Wilms tumors. They have received many names, such as congenital fibroma, fibrosarcoma, leiomyoma, leiomyomatous hamartoma and others. In contrast to Wilms tumors, they are free of epithelial and malignant nephroblastic components. Bolande *et al.*[1] described 8 cases discovered in neonates or infants born with palpable abdominal masses. Approximately 10% of the so-called Wilms tumors and 50% of those discovered under 1 year are congenital mesoblastic nephromas, intrarenal tumors without lobulation, necrosis or hemorrhage but containing cartilage and nests of tubules and glomeruli. Although these tumors are hamartomas, they differ from the renal tumors seen in tuberous sclerosis and other generalized hamartoses. Distinction from Wilms tumors is of practical importance, since survival seems to be the rule for children with mesoblastic nephromas after nephrectomy. There is no need for x-ray treatment and chemotherapy. Since treatment with actinomycin can have toxic and even fatal effects, Kay *et al.*[2] recommended that this drug be withheld preoperatively for renal tumors and that it be administered only after growth has been proved to be Wilms tumor at operation.

REFERENCES

1. Bolande, R. P., Brough, A. J., and Izant, R. J., Jr.: Congenital mesoblastic nephroma of infancy, Pediatrics 40:272, 1967.
2. Kay, S., Pratt, C. B., and Salzberg, A. M.: Hamartoma (leiomyomatous type) of the kidney, Cancer 19:1825, 1966.

Renal Lesions in Hamartoses

RENAL CYSTS OR TUMORS can occur as manifestations of generalized hamartoses. In tuberous sclerosis, mixed benign tumors or hamartomas are common. It has been said that tumors of some kind are found in the kidneys of 80% of the patients with tuberous sclerosis. They have been named hypernephromas, liposarcoma, adenosarcoma or angiofibroma, but the common tumors rarely are malignant, invasive or metastasizing. Renal teratomas and polycystic kidneys have been observed also.[1,2] Most of the tumors are small nodules consisting of epithelial cells, smooth muscle and blood vessels located in the renal cortex. Inglis[3] examined the relation of the renal to the cerebral lesions and came to the conclusion that the renal tumors represent a special type that is of neural origin and derived from the neural crest. Most renal tumors are asymptomatic in patients with recognized tuberous sclerosis but in exceptional cases they can be the main lesions. In 1 patient, a renal angiomyolipoma was the first sign of illness[4] and in a woman 62 years of age, renal failure due to massive tumors in the kidney was the cause of death. Although she had cerebral lesions, she was not mentally retarded and had no seizures or skin lesions.[5] Tuberous sclerosis and renal neoplasms were reviewed by Golji.[6]

Roentgenographic findings in the kidneys of patients with tuberous sclerosis were discussed by Crosett.[7] The usefulness of selective renal angiography for differentiation of hamartomas from polycystic kidneys was demonstrated by Viamonte *et al.*[8]

In Hippel-Lindau disease, cystic renal changes and foci of hypernephroma have been seen in some of the patients (p. 1266).

REFERENCES

1. Wilson, S. A. K.: *Neurology* (2d ed.; Baltimore: The Williams & Wilkins Company, 1955), Vol. 2.
2. Crome, L., and Stern, J.: *The Pathology of Mental Retardation* (London: J. & A. Churchill, Ltd., 1967).
3. Inglis, K.: The relation of the renal lesions to the cerebral lesions in the tuberous sclerosis complex, Am. J. Path. 30: 739, 1954.
4. Taylor, J. N., and Genters, K.: Renal angiomyolipoma and tuberous sclerosis, J. Urol. 79:685, 1958.
5. Schnitzer, B.: Tuberous sclerosis complex: Report of a 62 year old patient who died of renal involvement, Arch. Path. 76:626, 1963.
6. Golji, H.: Tuberous sclerosis and renal neoplasms, J. Urol. 85:919, 1961.
7. Crosett, A. D., Jr.: Roentgenographic findings in the renal lesion of tuberous sclerosis, Am. J. Roentgenol. 98:739, 1966.
8. Viamonte, M., Jr., Ravel, R., Politano, V., and Bridges, B.: Angiographic findings in a patient with tuberous sclerosis, Am. J. Roentgenol. 98:723, 1966.

Malformations of Ear and Kidney

MALFORMATION OF THE EARS as a sign of malformation of the urogenital tract has been stressed by Hilson.[1] As mentioned previously, Potter described a typical facies and large, low-set ears with little cartilage in children with renal agenesis (p. 1037). Hilson extended these observations to viable children and believed that malformed ears, particularly if asymmetric, commonly are associated with congenital malformations of the urogenital tract. Such deformed ears may be large and flabby, as were those described by Potter, or they may be folded over with the helix squared across its upper margin, bulbous or small and folded forward. Hilson believed in an association between renal agenesis, unilateral absence of one kidney and other malformations of the urogenital tract with peculiarities in the formation of the ears. In several instances, he could trace malformations of the ears and various anomalies of the kidney through several generations. Double ureters, absence of one kidney, hydronephrosis and polycystic kidneys were found in such families. Hilson thought that a malformed ear in the presence of enuresis, dysuria, abdominal colic or other symptoms referable to the urogenital tract justifies early pyelography. A number of patients with unilateral "bat-ear" deformity were observed in whom the renal tract and the abnormal ear were affected on the same side. Although such an association was stressed by this author, he also emphasized that congenital anomalies of the urogenital tract occur without associated defects of the ears and deformities of the ears without deformities of the urogenital tract. The ear described by Hilson as a sign of renal malformation is only one type of aural deformity seen in patients with anomalies of the kidney. The elongated "gothic" ear in Turner syndrome (Fig. 105-18, *C*) also can be indicative of a renal disorder associated with gonadal aplasia.

To avoid overemphasis of otorenal association, one should remember that anomalies of the kidney also occur in combination with disorders of the eye,[2] (Lowe syndrome, Alport syndrome and so forth), skeleton, heart, lungs, liver, pancreas and particularly the genitalia.

REFERENCES

1. Hilson, D.: Malformation of ears as sign of malformation of genitourinary tract, Brit. M. J. 2:785, 1957.
2. Burguet, W., Lefebvre, P., Booz, G., Delwaide, P. J., and van Cauwenberge, H.: Le syndrome d'Alport ou néphropathie héréditaire avec surdité. Nouvelle étude familiale, J. Génét. Hum. 15:7, 1966.

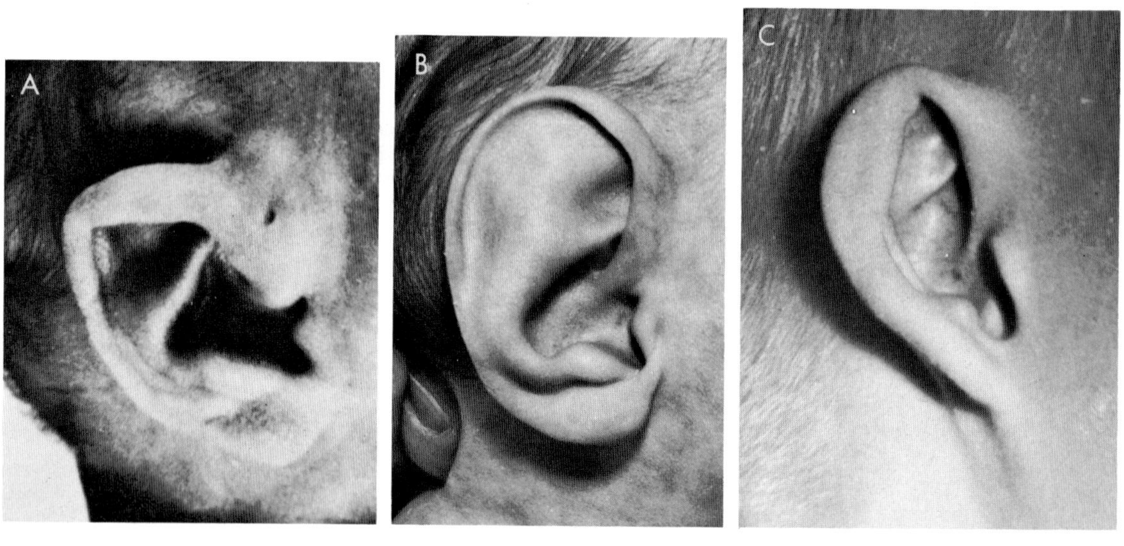

Fig. 105-18. – Ears of children with congenital renal malformations. **A,** renal agenesis. **B,** (familial) hydronephrosis. **C,** male Turner syndrome.

The Ureter

MANY MALFORMATIONS of the kidney observed during childhood or adult life are secondary to obstructive anomalies of the lower urinary tract. They are not congenital but the more distal defects are. Some of the malformations of the ureter, bladder, urethra and meatus are rather inconspicuous; frequently they escaped the pathologist, who was impressed with the striking consequences of the obstruction rather than its imperceptible cause. A few decades ago, many deaths of children were assigned to hydronephrosis, pyelonephritis or cystitis and not to the malformations that caused them. It is clear that early recognition and repair of such injurious congenital defects during infancy and childhood can prevent damage to

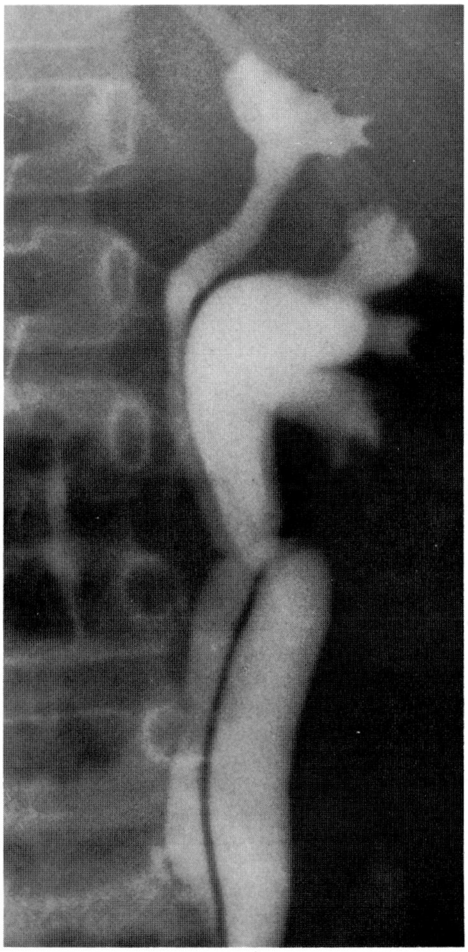

Fig. 106-1 (left). — Duplication of renal pelvis and ureter in a 7-year-old girl. The ureter from the lower pelvis is markedly dilated.

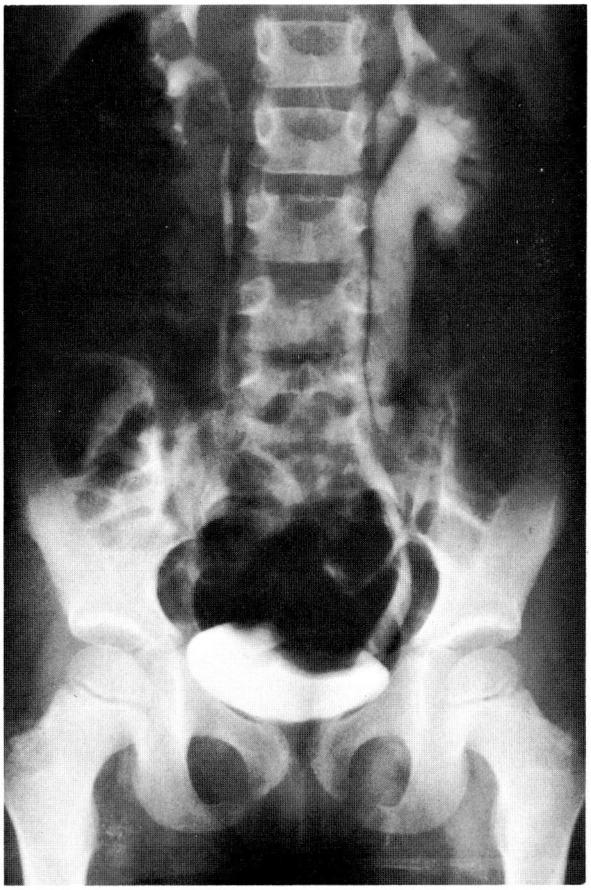

Fig. 106-2 (right). — Pyelogram showing double urinary collecting system with marked dilatation of the lower renal pelvis and ureter.

the kidney and prolong life. Modern urologic and roentgenologic methods make possible early correction of malformations of the lower urinary pathways, which are now recognized as serious disorders of childhood. Several books and monographs deal with these anomalies, their diagnosis and treatment.[2,7,21,23]

Duplication of the Ureter

Ureteral duplication can be complete or incomplete. The incidence of this anomaly is high; it can be found in 1 of 150 necropsies[1] and in 1 of 25 urograms.[2] The higher incidences in urograms are explained by the fact that diagnostic procedures are performed more often in persons who have symptoms of renal disease than in the normal. The condition probably occurs equally often in males and females. Recurrence in families has been observed.[3,4] Three double ureters were noted in 32 necropsies of children with trisomy 13-15 and 14 in 84 necropsies of trisomy 18,[5] i.e., 9% and 17% respectively. Duplication occurs six times more often unilaterally than bilaterally and the right side is affected more often than the left. It is not rare to find complete duplication on one side and a bifid ureter on the other.

Complete duplication arises if two separate ureteric buds develop separately from the Wolffian duct, and incomplete duplication if the accessory bud originates from the ureter. These buds grow cephalad and reach the metanephric blastema, forming separate renal pelves and usually only a single somewhat elongated kidney. As a rule, the upper pelvis and the upper renal portion are smaller than the corresponding lower counterparts. The lower segment has several calices but fewer than a normal kidney. The upper calix usually is single, short and laterally placed. As a rule, the ureter connected with the upper pelvis terminates in the bladder caudal and medial to the ureter from the lower pelvis. This implies that the ureters, after a parallel downward course, cross near the bladder when the upper pelvis ureter passes its companion as it turns toward the midline and to its lower termination.

Incomplete duplication usually is represented by a bifurcated "Y-shaped" structure formed by two ureters uniting in their downward course and terminating with a single orifice in the bladder. The point of union is in the lower third in approximately half of the cases.[2] Other types of incomplete duplication are much rarer, but occasionally an inverted Y-shaped ureter with caudal bifurcation can be found that empties into a single renal pelvis and terminates in two vesical orifices. There also are blind ending duplications that arise if the ureteric bud does not reach nephrogenic blastema. Such ureteric buds usually do not penetrate far in the cranial direction and form structures that resemble vesical diverticula. If separated from the kidney and bladder, incomplete duplications can establish cysts that are not easily recognized as ureteric derivatives. Triplication of the ureter has been observed as a rare anomaly.

Duplication of the ureter need not cause complications and can be found accidentally at necropsy or in urograms, but the anomaly carries increased liability to recurrent infection, pain, hydronephrosis and stone formation, since obstruction occurs in about one-fourth of the cases. Duplication is associated with other malformations in 25% of the cases. Renal agenesis, hypoplasia, ectopy or malrotation, polycystic disease and malformations of the lower urinary tract or of the genital and other systems may be combined with duplicaton of the ureter.[2] Although ectopia of the ureter occurs in but one-half of 1% of the cases of duplication, more than 75% of ureteral ectopias are associated with duplication.[6]

Treatment depends on the type of complication. If only one half of the kidney and one ureter are affected by pathologic processes, uretero-heminephrectomy often is performed successfully.

Ectopic Ureters

Abnormal termination and duplication of the ureter often are combined, and the ureter of the upper renal pelvis usually is the ectopic one. Ectopia of a single ureter often occurs with malrotation, hypoplasia or ectopia of the kidney.[7] An incidence of 1 in 130,000 persons has been suggested,[8] but the anomaly was found by Campbell[2] once in 1,900 necropsies of children. The ectopic ureter almost always is dilated and has a large orifice, and only rarely is a narrowed opening found. The dilatation of the ureter often is attributed to chronic inflammation but it probably is due to prenatal abnormal development and can be present at birth.

In a review of the literature, Burford *et al.*[9] found the ratio of males to females to be 1:3. In males, the anomalous orifice was located in the posterior urethra in 46%, in the seminal vesicle in 24%, in the prostatic utricle in 12%, in the ejaculatory ducts in 7%, in the vas deferens in 5%, in the bladder in 5% and in the rectum in 1% of the cases. In females, the site was in the vestibule in 34%, in the urethra in 32%, in the vagina in 22%, in the bladder in 7%, in the uterus in 3%, in the Gartner duct in 1% and in the rectum in 1% of the cases.

The pathogenesis of ectopic ureter was discussed in great detail by Politzer.[10] Based on the work of Chwalla[11] and other studies of the embryology of the separation of ureter and Wolffian duct, of the relationship of Müllerian and Wolffian ducts[12] and of the formation of the vagina, the various forms of ureteric ectopia can be explained. In embryos of 5–6 mm. length, the Wolffian duct terminates near the cloacal plate but it is still separated from the cloaca by an epithelial layer. In 7-mm. embryos, this layer is already perforated but a portion of the epithelial layer persists as a "terminal bar."[11] At the same time, the termination of the Wolffian duct undergoes a cranial movement and a chamber is formed between the duct and the cloacal plate. When the ureter arises at about this time from the dorsal wall of the Wolffian duct, the two structures at first have this terminal chamber in common. Between the ureter and the Wolffian duct, a tissue spur arises (ureteric spur), which grows caudad toward the terminal bar. When these two structures meet, the terminal chamber is divided and separate end points of ureter and mesonephric ducts are established. Both structures terminate in the ventral portion of the cloaca, which forms the urogenital sinus and the bladder. In this stage, the distal end of the ureter is still closed by an epithelial membrane. Thus, in embryos 13 mm. long, the ureter and the Wolffian duct have separate terminal points but these points lie closely together. Subsequently, differential growth of the ventral cloacal space sets in, which separates the orifices of the two structures, the orifices of the ureters moving craniolaterad, whereas those of the Wolffian ducts remain in a caudal position near the midline. If the ureteric spur formation is insufficient, the ureter and Wolffian duct retain a common terminal duct comparable to that of embryos of less than 7 mm. length. This terminal portion of the mesonephric duct develops into vas deferens, ductus ejaculatorius and seminal vesicle, and consequently the ectopic ureter, not separated from the Wolffian duct, terminates in one of these structures. If the ureter and the Wolffian duct have become properly separated but the craniolateral migration of the ureteric orifice is incomplete, this orifice remains too close to that of the Wolffian duct and the ureter terminates in the urethra or in the bladder caudal to its normal opening.

In the female, incomplete spur formation of the ureter also leads to termination of the ureter in the end portion of the Wolffian duct, which, in such cases, does not retrogress normally but persists in its early embryonic position in the region of the external orifice of the urethra, the hymen or the wall of the vulva between them. The termination of the Wolffian ducts may be placed in the vaginal plate so that a vaginal ectopia is formed. Rare openings of the ureters into the rectum are explained by abnormal growth of the cloacal septum or the cloacal ridges, which brings the ureteric openings into the dorsal portion of the cloaca. This anomaly is combined with severe malformations such as exstrophia vesicae or atresia ani.[2]

Ectopia of the ureter can be induced experimentally in rats. Wilson and Warkany[13] found ureteric ectopia frequently in the young of vitamin A-deficient female rats. Of 42 animals examined histologically, 37 had ureters that emptied in abnormal position. In 15 instances, the ureters retained their primitive juncture with the mesonephric ducts and in 14 fetuses the ureters entered the sinus horns directly. In the rest of the abnormal young, the orifices were found at some point in the upper urogenital sinus between the sinus horns and the base of the bladder or a ureter failed completely to join any part of the lower genitourinary tract due to secondary regression. Monie *et al.*,[14] examining the urinary tract of rat embryos obtained from mothers fed a folic acid-deficient diet from the tenth to the thirteenth days of gestation, found in some fetuses the ureters opening into the vas deferens, the seminal vesicle or the urethra close to the openings of the mesonephric ducts and the paramesonephric ducts. Giroud *et al.*[15] noticed ectopia in some of the ureters of rat fetuses with hydronephrosis experimentally induced by hypervitaminosis A.

In children, presenting symptoms usually are pyuria, fever or incontinence ("enuresis") but, in the female, the ectopia may be symptomless for some time if the ureter opens at the bladder neck or in the upper urethra. In this position, the ectopic ureter does not cause incontinence in the child but infection does occur eventually and recurrent pyuria may be observed.

Symptoms are more serious if the ureter opens in the vicinity of the urethral meatus, in the vestibulum, in the lateral wall of the vagina or in the cervix uteri. Such an ectopic ureter usually is dilated and its kidney is abnormal. Patients with this form of ureteric ectopia often show dribbling, although micturition takes place at normal intervals. In some cases of vestibular ectopia, incontinence is absent because of urinary control by the urethral musculature, and pyuria may be the presenting complaint. In other cases of vestibular ectopia, infection occurs early and the infants fail to thrive. Pus is seen in the vulva and, in the past, gonorrhea often was suspected. If the ectopic ureteric opening is recognized, the course and dilatation of the ureter can be outlined easily by retrograde urography. Surgical removal of the infected organ may result in prompt weight gain and resumption of growth.[16] In infants with vaginal ectopia, sometimes it is possible to recognize the anomaly by a purulent discharge that occurs spontaneously or can be obtained by pressure on the abdomen. Urography can outline the abnormal ureter but the vaginal termination is difficult to localize.

In the male, the ectopic opening usually is above the external sphincter. Incontinence is not an outstanding feature and in the absence of infection the diagnosis often is missed. The ureter may open into the posterior urethra above the level of the verumontanum, in the seminal vesicle and rarely in a vas deferens or epididymis. In such cases, the symptoms may be caused by inflammatory changes in the abnormal ureter. The difficulties in finding ectopic ureteral openings are considerable even if they are suspected.[3,17]

Treatment of ectopic ureter consists of transplantation into the bladder if the kidney and the ureter are sound. If infected, excision of the abnormal ureter and of the renal portion with which it is connected (uretero-heminephrectomy) usually is practiced. Ligation of the ureter can be effective in exceptional cases.[2] Ureteral reimplantation in children was discussed by Hendren.[29]

Ureterocele

Ureterocele is found only once in 3,000 necropsies, according to Campbell,[2] but it is a rather frequent anomaly (1 in 30) in patients with persistent pyuria. Ureterocele is bilateral in approximately 15% of the patients; in unilateral cases, there is no preference as to side. The ureterocele seen in adults may be acquired but the more serious ectopic ureteroceles of childhood are congenital disorders. They occur in females about four times more often than in males, whereas the simple ureteroceles of older age groups show no sex predilection. Concordance of bilateral ureterocele in identical twins has been reported.[19]

A ureterocele is a cystic dilatation of the intravesical ureter that distends the short segment located under the mucosa of the bladder. The wall of the cyst consists of vesical, the lining of ureteral mucosa. As a rule, the orifice of the ureter is very small, the stenosis being attributed to a remnant of the ureteric membrane.[20] The ureter above the stenosis usually is dilated. When the pressure in the bladder is high, the cyst is evaginated into the ureter and presents the picture of a vesical diverticulum. When the bladder is partly filled, the ureterocele protrudes into the bladder. Simple ureterocele usually is a small cystic expansion of a ureter proximal to its opening into the urinary bladder. It is the typical ureterocele of adults but it is relatively rare in children. Ectopic ureterocele is formed when a ureter, usually a supernumerary one, passes submucosally for some distance within the vesical wall before terminating in the urethra blindly or with a small opening. The ureterocele extends behind the vesical neck and has, in contrast to simple ureterocele, no opening into the bladder. The ectopic ureter originates in and communicates with the upper pole of the kidney. The ectopic ureter becomes dilated and bulges into the lumen of the bladder. Ectopic ureteroceles usually are large and often cause obstruction of the other ureters and the vesical neck. They are much more common in girls than in boys and manifest themselves within the first 3 years.[18,21]

Fig. 106-3.—Cystogram in a 2-year-old girl showing filling defect in the opaque bladder lumen.

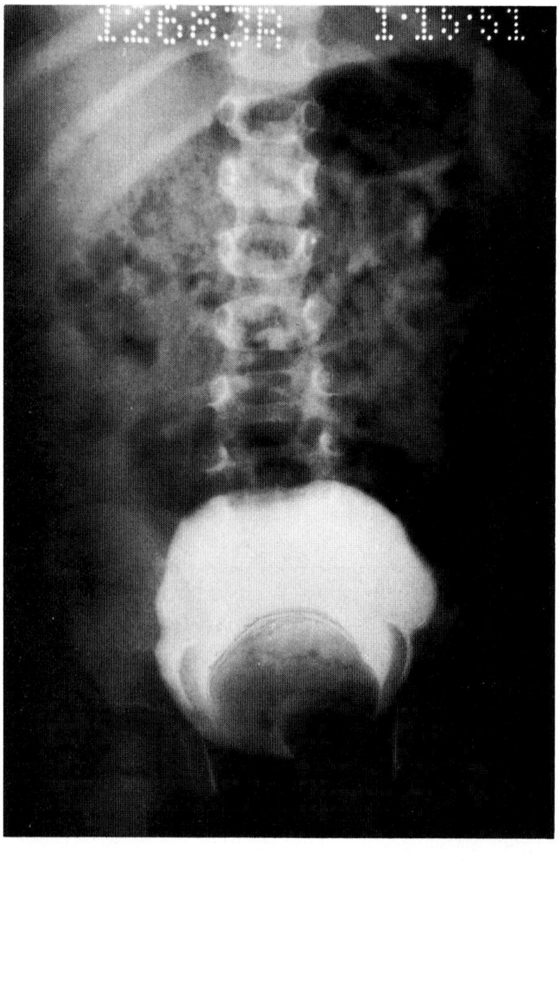

Small ureteroceles can be symptomless but when they cause obstruction they can bring on infection, pain or stone formation. Prolapse into the urethra can occur. Other symptoms are fever, vomiting, urgency and failure to gain weight. Ureteroceles can be observed directly by cystoscopy or be seen in pyelograms as dense, round shadows surrounded by a halo.[7] In approximately half of the cases, ureterocele is associated with other anomalies of the urinary tract,[2] particularly with duplication of the ureter. In such cases, the ureterocele always arises from the orifice of the lower ureter, which drains the upper kidney.

Gross[22] recommended incision of the ureterocele for the majority of cases, a procedure that relieves the obstruction and reduces the attacks of infection. In infants and small children, this is done through a suprapubic opening of the bladder. But in advanced cases of unilateral ureteric dilatation and hydronephrosis, ureteronephrectomy may be required.[7] Details of treatment were discussed by Stephens.[23]

Hydro-ureter and Mega-ureter

In a series of 2,924 necropsies on children, Williams[7] found 103 with ureteric dilatation. Of these, 42 were due to urethral valvular obstructions, and a high percentage could be referred to spinal cord anomalies, obstructive tumors or inflammatory lesions. Only 10 cases belonged in the "mega-ureter group," the type of dilatation for which no explanation can be found. The origin of mega-ureters in the newborn child without obstruction in the lower urinary tract is not well understood. Attempts to elucidate the etiology of mega-ureter go back to the nineteenth century. Vermooten[20] explained certain types of dilated ureters in children by persistence of the ureteric membranes of Chwalla in embryos beyond the stage of normal perforation. If the metanephros begins secretion without perforation of the membrane, fluid cannot escape and hydronephrosis and hydro-ureter will develop. One should expect a return to normal when the membrane eventually breaks, but retrogression of the dilatation may not be possible if the membrane has persisted too long. The findings in experimentally produced congenital hydro-ureter lend support to this theory (p. 1057).

Hydro-ureter due to obstruction of the urethra was found by Williams[7] in 1.4% of children on whom necropsies were performed. In infants, hydro-ureter follows obstruction during fetal life, whereas the renal pelvis dilates only moderately. With the dilatation of the ureter, elongation, kinking and tortuosity develop. At first, an obstructed ureter is hypertrophied but gradual failure follows, so that urinary reflux occurs in advanced stages. That hydro-ureter may be unilateral in the presence of urethral obstruction or neurogenic bladder demonstrates that simple mechanical explanations based on observations after birth probably are not correct in all cases.

Fig. 106-4.—Pyelogram showing right hydronephrosis and hydro-ureter.

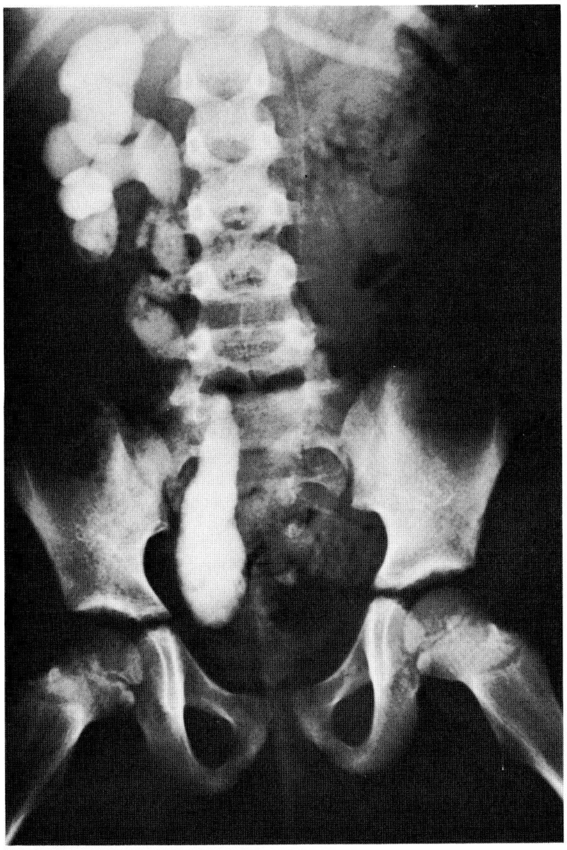

In many patients, hydro-ureter is combined with other malformations of the urinary tract, and, in such cases, the relationship to these anomalies is difficult to establish. Double ureter, ectopic ureter, ureterocele, dysplastic kidney, ureterovesical strictures or solitary kidney often are combined with hydro-ureter, and to these anomalies are added infections, so that an explanation of the origin of the hydro-ureter cannot be found.

Stephens[23] distinguished mega-ureter with from mega-ureter without reflux. The two groups had different clinical patterns and required different treatments. Vesico-ureteric reflux with mega-ureter was concordant in a pair of monozygotic twins and discordant in a pair of dizygotic twins.[23]

Mega-ureter

In simple mega-ureter, the bladder is normal and no anatomic obstruction is found. It has been assumed that a functional abnormality is the basis of this type of ureteric dilatation.[7] Mega-ureter may be unilateral or bilateral. Elongation and kinking usually are present and the lower end of the ureter forms a bulb-like dilatation, whereas the intramural ureter is of normal caliber. Sometimes the narrow is located a short distance above the bladder, so that a supravesical segment of normal caliber can be found. Although, normally, contractions are initiated in the cranial portion of the ureter, it has been observed that in mega-ureters contractions are initiated in the lower segment, in which circular elements of the musculature extend abnormally far down. Another explanation of the dilatation is abnormally long persistence of the ureteric membrane.

Pain, infection, hematuria, stones or renal swelling may be manifestations of mega-ureter. Pyelograms show dilatation of the whole length of the ureter but the lower third usually is affected more than the cranial parts.

Treatment consists of chemotherapy. In the presence of stones and serious infections, unilateral nephro-ureterectomy sometimes is done.[2,7]

Mega-ureter–Megacystis Syndrome

This syndrome is characterized by bilateral mega-ureter with widely gaping ureteric orifices and enlargement of the bladder. The ureters are kinked and have hypertrophied musculature, and the bladder is large with thickened walls. The etiology of this syndrome has been much discussed and it was thought that an obstruction at the bladder neck might be responsible but, as no lower urinary obstructions are found, the etiology remains obscure. One concept assumes that a local giantism and "excess formation" is the basis of the anomaly. Swenson *et al.*[24] likened the syndrome to Hirschsprung disease, as they noted in some patients with megacolon diminution of parasympathetic ganglion cells in the bladder. The mega-ureters would be the result of bladder dysfunction. These authors found that prolonged suprapubic bladder drainage resulted in decrease in size of the mega-ureters and in general improvement of the patient. But in some typical instances of mega-ureter–megacystis syndrome, the ganglion cells were not reduced[25] and in a series of patients operated on because of megacolon no ureteric dilatation was found.[7] In a case of coexistent megacolon and bilateral mega-ureter, colon and rectum were aganglionic but there was normal autonomic innervation of the bladder.[26]

The enlarged bladder and ureter can remain uninfected for many years even though the dilatation is present at birth. Difficult micturition and incontinence are uncommon and signs of renal failure usually appear in adolescence or early adult life. The ureters are capable of powerful contraction but the peristalsis is not always effective and can be retrograde at times. The bladder capacity is large and the urine can be retained in it for long periods. Contraction is powerful but emptying of the bladder is incomplete, probably because of reflux of urine into the large ureters. It is understandable, therefore, that several micturitions are needed to empty the bladder completely. In more severe cases, infections may be recurrent or chronic and lead to renal failure. If infection cannot be brought under control, the ureters and their terminal openings become greatly dilated, so that reflux occurs on micturition. Drug therapy and regular emptying of the urinary tract are recommended for treatment.[7]

Retrocaval Ureter

This is an anomaly of the right ureter that is due to persistence of the ventral limb of the periureteric cardinal venous ring in place of the dorsal limb, which normally forms the inferior vena cava.[27] This anomaly probably occurs in 1 of 1,600 cadaver dissections, but many cases are not recognized during life. Relatively few cases have been reported that were clinically identified and even fewer were diagnosed before operation. Manifestations of the anomaly are rare in children, but the possibility of a retrocaval ureter should be considered in cases of hydronephrosis on the right side, particularly in males, who seem to have a marked predilection for this anomaly. It is of interest that retrocaval ureter has been described in a case of Turner syndrome.[30]

Vascular compression of the ureter can result in dilatation of the upper ureter and renal pelvis. There may be no symptoms or abdominal pain but infection may lead to urologic examination. Urography shows dilatation above the point of obstruction and mesial displacement of the middle portion of the right ureter, which descends over the spine. The anomaly often is associated with a right-sided hydronephrosis. Surgical repair by high ureteral division and placement of the ureter in its normal position can relieve the complaints.[2]

Obstruction of Lower Ureter by Distal Hypogastric Artery

Obstruction of the distal left ureter in an infant with imperforate anus was found to be due to an enlarged, obliterated distal hypogastric (umbilical) artery. Removal of a segment of the vessel in the area of the ureter relieved the obstruction.[28]

The role of vessel obstruction in the pathogenesis of hydronephrosis was discussed by Barnett and Stephens.[23]

REFERENCES

1. Nation, E. F.: Duplication of the kidney and ureter: A statistical study of 230 cases, J. Urol. 51:456, 1944.
2. Campbell, M.: *Clinical Pediatric Urology* (Philadelphia: W. B. Saunders Company, 1951).
3. Frisell, E.: Missbildungen der Harnwege mit familiärem Auftreten von Doppelureter bei Kindern, Acta paediat. 29:418, 1942.
4. Lenz, W.: Krankheiten des Urogenitalsystems, in Becker, P. E. (ed.), *Humangenetik* (Stuttgart: Georg Thieme, 1964), Vol. III.
5. Warkany, J., Passarge, E., and Smith, L. B.: Congenital malformations in autosomal trisomy syndromes, Am. J. Dis. Child. 122:502, 1966.
6. Thompson, I. M., and Amar, A. D.: Clinical importance of ureteral duplication and ectopia, J.A.M.A. 168:881, 1958.
7. Williams, D. I.: Urology in Childhood, in *Encyclopedia of Urology* (Berlin: Springer-Verlag, 1958), Vol. XV.
8. Alldred, A. J., and Higgins, T. T.: The ectopic ureter in childhood, Brit. J. Surg. 38:460, 1951.
9. Burford, C. E., Glenn, J. E., and Burford, E. H.: Ureteral ectopia: A review of the literature on 2 case reports, J. Urol. 62:211, 1949.
10. Politzer, G.: Die dystopische Mündung des Ureters und ihre formale Genese, Ztschr. Path. 64:324, 1953.
11. Chwalla, R.: Über die Entwicklung der Harnblase und der primären Harnröhre des Menschen mit besonderer Berücksichtigung der Art and Weise in der sich die Ureteren von den Urnierengängen trennen, nebst Bemerkungen über die Entwicklung der Müllerschen Gänge und des Mastdarms, Ztschr. ges. Anat. 83:615, 1927.
12. Gruenwald, P., and Surks, S. W.: Pre-ureteric vena cava and its embryological explanation, J. Urol. 49:195, 1943.
13. Wilson, J. G., and Warkany, J.: Malformations in the genitourinary tract induced by maternal vitamin A deficiency in the rat, Am. J. Anat. 83:357, 1948.
14. Monie, I. W., Nelson, M. M., and Evans, H. M.: Abnormalities of the urinary system of rat embryos resulting from transitory deficiency of pteroylglutamic acid during gestation, Anat. Rec. 127:711, 1957.
15. Giroud, A., Martinet, M., and Roux, C.: Urétéro-hydronéphrose expérimentale chez l'embryon par hypervitaminose A, Arch. franç. pédiat. 15:540, 1958.
16. Hryntschak, T.: Ektope Uretermündung und Pyonephrose bei einem sechsmonatlichen Säugling, Wien. klin. Wchnschr. 43:169, 1930.
17. Uson, A. C., and Donovan, J. T.: Ectopic ureteral orifice; a report based on seventeen cases, A.M.A. J. Dis. Child. 98: 153, 1959.
18. Dorst, J. P., Cussen, G. H., and Silverman, F.: Ureteroceles in children with emphasis on the frequency of ectopic ureteroceles, Radiology 74:88, 1960.
19. Riba, L. W.: Ureterocele: With case reports of bilateral ureterocele in identical twins, Brit. J. Urol. 8:119, 1936.
20. Vermooten, J.: New etiology for certain types of dilated ureters in children, J. Urol. 41:455, 1939.
21. Kjellberg, S. R., Ericsson, N. O., and Rudhe, U.: *The Lower Urinary Tract in Childhood* (Chicago: Year Book Medical Publishers, Inc., 1957).

22. Gross, R. E.: *The Surgery of Infancy and Childhood* (Philadelphia: W. B. Saunders Company, 1953).
23. Stephens, F. D.: *Congenital Malformations of the Rectum, Anus and Genito-urinary Tract* (Edinburgh: E. & S. Livingstone, Ltd., 1963).
24. Swenson, O., McMahon, H. E., Jaques, W. E., and Campbell, J. S.: New concept of the etiology of megalo-ureter, New England J. Med. 246:41, 1952.
25. Liebowitz, S., and Bodian, M.: A study of the vesical ganglia in children and the relationship to the megaureter megacystis syndrome and Hirschsprung's disease, J. Clin. Path. 16:342, 1963.
26. Winkelman, J.: Coexistent megacolon and megaureter, Pediatrics 39:258, 1967.
27. Pick, J. W., and Anson, B. J.: Retrocaval ureter: Report of case, with discussion of its clinical significance, J. Urol. 43:672, 1940.
28. Trackler, R. T., and McAlister, W. H.: Obstruction of the lower ureter by the distal hypogastric (umbilical) artery, Am. J. Roentgenol. 98:160, 1966.
29. Hendren, W. H.: Ureteral reimplantation in children, J. Pediat. Surg. 3:649, 1968.
30. Uson, A. C., Braham, S. B., Abrams, C. A., and Berdon, W. E.: Retrocaval ureter in a child with Turner's syndrome, Am. J. Dis. Child. 119:267, 1970.

107

The Bladder

Agenesis; Hypoplasia; Duplication

Agenesis of the Bladder

In complete siren formations, the bladder and the entire urogenital tract are absent, and in monopodal and bipodal sirens, rudiments of the urogenital tract are formed. Agenesis of the bladder is very rare, and Campbell[1] reported 6 cases in 16,000 necropsies of children. In females with this anomaly, the ureters open into the vagina or the uterus and in males into the urethra or the rectum. Most of the infants with the anomaly are stillborn and severely deformed in other parts of the body, but occasionally survival has been reported. Incontinence is the rule and severe infections cause secondary changes, so that it is not always possible to decide whether agenesis or hypoplasia of the bladder was present. Ureters opening into the urethra may act as reservoirs and their orifices can assume sphincter action. In the older literature,[2] some adults were mentioned who had absence of the bladder, the ureters opening into the urethra. Absence of the bladder with ureters opening into the uterus has been observed in twin sisters.[3]

Associated anomalies are sympodia and "dysencephalia splanchnocystica" consisting of polycystic kidneys, meningocele and polydactyly (p. 213). In some stillborn children with absence of both kidneys and ureters, there also is agenesis of the bladder. Agenesis or malformation of the uterus, the vagina or the penis sometimes are associated anomalies.

Hypoplasia of the Bladder

Hypoplasia of the bladder (dwarf bladder) is a rarity that has been seen in stillborn children combined with other anomalies such as horseshoe kidney, absence of the kidneys and ureters and absence of the heart. Survival is possible and the anomaly has been observed in a man who survived to his twenty-first year.[2]

Anomalies of the bladder were observed in short-tail mice (Sd). In homozygotes, the bladder may be absent or underdeveloped. In another strain with the uro-recto-caudal syndrome (ur), absence of the bladder was noted in more than 30% of homozygous newborn mice.[4]

Duplication of the Bladder

Duplication of the bladder can be complete or incomplete. In complete duplication, each bladder receives one or sometimes two ureters and empties into a separate urethra. In such cases, there also may be duplication of the penis, of the uterus and vagina and of the colon or rectum. In incomplete duplication, the bladder appears bilobed but there is only one bladder neck and one urethra. The bladder may be subdivided by a sagittal septum or by a frontal septum. In many cases, it is difficult to distinguish between such incomplete duplications and diverticula. Septation of the bladder may lead to urinary retention and to infection. Burns *et al.*[5] reviewed the older literature and suggested a workable classification.

Duplications of the urinary bladder varying from incomplete to complete separation were observed by Hummel[6] in mice that showed changes due to the disorganization gene. Duplications in other organs also were frequent in such mice.

REFERENCES

1. Campbell, M.: *Clinical Pediatric Urology* (Philadelphia: W. B. Saunders Company, 1951).
2. Gruber, G. B.: Missbildungen der Harnorgane, in Schwalbe, E. (ed.), *Morphologie der Missbildungen des Menschen und der Tiere* (Jena: Gustav Fischer, 1927).
3. Ignatescu, M., Slobozianu, H., and Athanasin-Vergu, E.: Absence de la vessie et abouchement des urèteres, dan l' utérus chez deux jumelles, J. Urol. 45:51, 1938.
4. Grüneberg, H.: *The Genetics of the Mouse* (The Hague: Martinus Nijhoff, 1952).
5. Burns, E., Cummins, H., and Hyman, J.: Incomplete reduplication of the bladder with congenital solitary kidney, J. Urol. 57:257, 1947.
6. Hummel, K. P.: The inheritance and expression of disorganization, an unusual mutation in the mouse, J. Exper. Zool. 137:389, 1958.

Exstrophy of the Bladder and of the Cloaca; Urachal Anomalies

Exstrophy of the Bladder

THIS CONGENITAL MALFORMATION is due to a deficiency of the subumbilical portion of the abdominal wall and of the bladder, which is ventrally open and appears to be everted as its posterior wall protrudes through the defect in the abdomen. The term "ectopia" of the bladder sometimes used is not recommended, since it suggests merely a displacement but not a severe defect of the bladder.

Exstrophy of the bladder can be complete or incomplete. An incomplete form is seen in cases of epispadias combined with slight protrusion of the vesical mucous membrane over the open urethra (inferior vesical fissure). Another incomplete form consists in a defect of the upper part of the bladder with normal union of the pubic skin (superior vesical fissure).[1] The incomplete forms are amenable to surgery and much less detrimental than the complete exstrophy.

The complete form consists in protrusion of the posterior vesical wall, usually combined with epispadias. It may be combined with intestinal fistulas and a cleft perineum, but more often the anus is separated from the open urethra and bladder by a rudimentary penis and a small scrotum. A more serious cleft of the lower anterior wall of the abdomen is exstrophy of the cloaca (p. 712), which sometimes is compatible with life if surgically improved. There are other variations of exstrophies that can be arranged in series according to the extent of the cleft.[2,3] Berndorfer[4] emphasized the forms that seem to have undergone intrauterine healing or "regeneration." In contrast to the clinician, the pathologist sees exstrophy of the bladder in combination with exomphalos, myelocystocele and lordosis of the spine, monstrosities that do not reach urologic services.[2] Occasionally, very complex cases are treated surgically.[5]

The incidence of exstrophy of the bladder was estimated by Campbell[6] as 1 in 40,000–50,000 individuals, but in necropsies of children the incidence was 1 in 936, which indicates that the mortality of affected children is high. Among 72 exstrophies, Uson *et al.*[1] saw 66 complete and 2 incomplete forms and 4 with exstrophy of the cloaca (p. 712) or vesicointestinal fistula. The malformation occurs more often in males than in females, but the ratio has not been established satisfactorily. A ratio of 5:2 is a likely esti-

Fig. 107-1.—Epispadias (exstrophy of the bladder) in a girl 3 months of age.

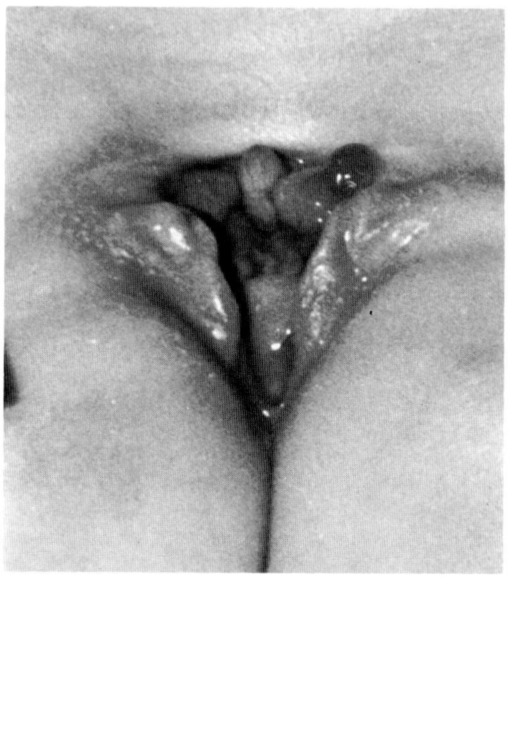

mate.[1,7-9] Exstrophy of the bladder can recur in families. Glaser and Lewis[10] reported it in brothers and Chisholm[11] mentioned that in his series of 90 patients, 4 were siblings. Dr. Mackenzie Smith[12] saw 2 cases in a family. Marshall and Muecke[3] mentioned vesical exstrophy in a twin boy whose twin sister did not have the anomaly. Both had some teratomatous retroperitoneal tissue. Exstrophy of the bladder, epispadias, absence of the right kidney and ureter were associated with atresia recti and imperforate anus in a boy whose brother had rectal and anal atresia.[13] The anomaly has been seen in male identical twins.[14]

Many explanations have been given for the development of this anomaly but they all are based on speculation. Owing to the rarity of the defect, exstrophy of the bladder has not been observed in young embryos. Patten and Barry[15] pointed out that the human embryo does not normally pass through any developmental stage comparable to either exstrophy or epispadias and that, therefore, the concept of developmental arrest cannot be applied to these malformations. Some older investigators believed that the bladder had ruptured after abnormal retention of urine, or they attributed the defect to intrauterine disease. It was noticed early that epispadias frequently is associated with vesical exstrophy, and several investigators saw in this association the clue to the formation of the vesical defect. Patten and Barry[15] reviewed these theories and gave an admittedly hypothetical explanation after discussion of the normal development of the area and the deviations in the pathologic condition. Normally, the paired primordia of the genital tubercle are located lateral to the cephalic border of the cloacal membrane. These paired mounds of mesoderm, noticeable by the fourth week, become higher as they migrate toward the midline along the cephalolateral edge of the cloacal membrane. By the fifth week, they have fused in the midline, forming the genital tubercle situated at the cephalic boundary of the cloacal membrane. Internally, the cloaca is subdivided by the urorectal septum, which, as it reaches the perineal surface, divides the cloacal membrane into the urogenital membrane and the anal plate. When these membranes rupture later, the urogenital orifice is found caudal to the genital tubercle and the anus caudal to the perineum. An accumulation of mesoderm occurs in the infraumbilical portion of the ventral body wall, leading to restriction of the belly stalk and to a marked increase in its distance from the cloacal membrane. According to the theory of Patten and Barry,[15] the exstrophy is initiated by an abnormally caudal origin of the primordia of the genital tubercles and their fusion between the urogenital and the anal orifices. There also is lack of mesodermal tissue between the cloacal plate and the belly stalk, so that the ventral abdominal wall between the cranial end of the cloacal plate and the umbilicus remains without reinforcement. Because of the weakness of the infraumbilical part of the abdominal wall, the rupture of the urogenital membrane could extend farther cephalad than usual and the caudal end of the urogenital sinus as well as the entire ventral wall of the allantois could be split. Owing to the caudal position of the genital tubercle, the urethral groove is formed on its dorsal surface in the position characteristic of epispadias. Many other explanations of the morphogenesis of exstrophy of the bladder have been offered before[2] and after[3] Patten and Barry,[15] but no one has followed its development in human embryos or in animals. To my knowledge, exstrophy of the bladder has not been produced experimentally in mammals. Gruber[2] thought it occurred only very rarely in domestic animals and cited only one report of a horse that urinated from two small papillae located far back on the abdomen. The citation was dated far back in time and was not supported by a detailed description.

In the male, the exstrophic bladder lies on the abdominal wall between the umbilicus and the penis. The umbilicus is situated very low, as the entire suprapubic area is underdeveloped in these patients and often the navel is so defective that it cannot be recognized clearly. An umbilical hernia situated above the exstrophic bladder actually is a hernia through the linea alba that is represented by paper-like, thin tissue, an expression of the mesenchymal deficiency above the open bladder.

The everted bladder is small and covered by a red mucosa that bleeds easily, appears plicated and is

Fig. 107-2.—Exstrophy of the bladder in a female infant who also had myelomeningocele with neurenteric canal remnant. There also was an Arnold-Chiari malformation, hydrocephaly, malformation of the cerebellum, microgyria and hemivertebrae of the lumbar spine.

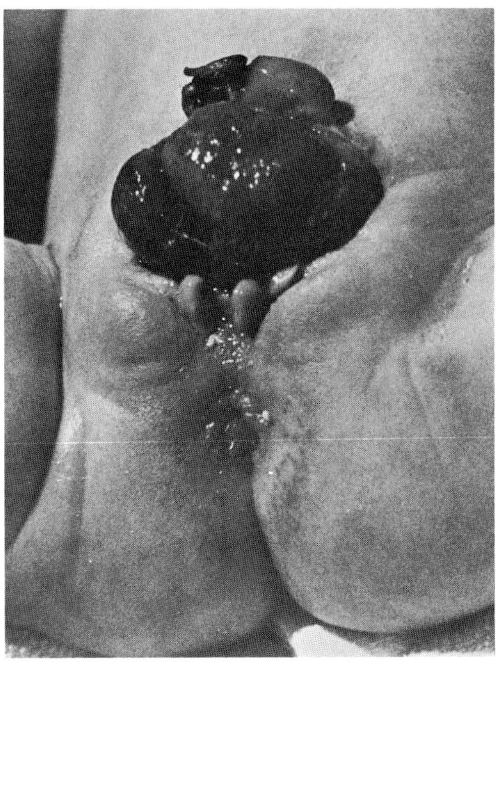

extremely sensitive. The surface is covered by cylindrical as well as squamous epithelium and epithelial strands and glandular structures develop below the surface. Culp[16] studied the histology of exstrophic bladders of patients 2 weeks to 52 years of age and found anomalies in all of them. The submucosa and fibrous tissue growing at the expense of the muscular layers causes protrusion of the bladder over the abdominal skin. The mucosa of the exposed bladder is sharply demarcated from the surrounding skin. The trigone and the openings of the ureters can be recognized, and the open urethra with a well-defined verumontanum is seen over the short and broad penis. The scrotum usually is hypoplastic and the testes are not descended. The anus lies closely behind the scrotum and the rectum tends to prolapse. The pubic bones fail to meet in the midline. They, the acetabula and the femora are rotated outward, which results in a characteristic waddling gait. In the female, the everted bladder ends in a short and open urethral strip. The vaginal opening lies immediately below the urethra and the clitoris is divided into two separate eminences, which are located on both sides of the open urethra.

Severe associated malformations are seen frequently in those infants, who die early in the neonatal period. The abdominal cleft may extend cranially to include the supraumbilical abdominal and the thoracic walls. In such cases, prolapse of the intestines is combined with prolapse of the bladder and the amnion inserts on the edge of the cleft. Omphalocele is present in approximately 4% of children with exstrophy.[1] The ileum may open onto the vesical area, the colon being entirely absent (p. 713). In unviable infants, atresia of the ureter and cystic kidneys,[2] myelomeningocele, clubfoot and cleft lip and palate may be found. In survivors, inguinal hernias, rectal prolapse and fistulas, vaginal anomalies, duplication of the penis, cardiac malformations, cleft palate and Down syndrome have been seen in combination with exstrophy of the bladder.[1]

Aside from complicated cases with exstrophy of the bladder, there are children who have no associated malformations except for those closely connected with the vesical exstrophy. Such children can live for many years but the anomaly causes much distress to the child and to his family. The continuous discharge of urine, the pain caused by ulceration and friction, the maceration of the abdominal skin, the rectal prolapse and the renal infections result in a great deal of suffering. The constant irritation of the exposed mucosa of the bladder may lead to malignant degeneration and formation of adenocarcinomas. These malignancies show little tendency to metastasize. Chronic infection of the ureters and the kidneys occur, but Gross[17] stated that it is quite rare to find marked ureteritis or pyelitis in these patients. Histologic changes of the vesical mucosa may be congenital.[16]

The prognosis for untreated cases cannot be established at this time, since treatment is now given to all patients. It was said in older publications that only about one-third of the patients reach the twentieth year. In the older literature, patients were mentioned who survived their seventieth or eightieth birthday.[2,3] Considering the severity of the malformation and the exposure of the ureteric orifices, this represents a relatively good prognosis. With chemotherapy, the life expectancy of patients not operated on probably would now be longer but the social situation is so serious that surgical intervention is commonly practiced. The resistance of some of these children to secondary diseases is so remarkable that Williams[7] believed that they are far more likely to die from operation than from any other cause. He stated, however, that the improvement in the conditions of life, rather than the prolongation of existence, is the standard by which treatment should be judged.

Some persons with vesical exstrophy have few disturbing symptoms aside from urinary incontinence. Coulter and Sabbagh[18] reported the case of a patient 20 years of age who presented herself complaining of continuous urinary incontinence associated with a "sore" on her lower abdomen since birth. Normal regular menses had started at age 14. Her past history was listed as otherwise noncontributory, although she had a typical and complete exstrophy of the bladder, stenosis of the vaginal orifice and a marked defect of the pubic bones. After excision of the exstrophic bladder, reconstruction of the lower abdominal wall, ureteral transplants into the sigmoid and a plastic vaginal operation, the patient was married, she conceived and delivered at term vaginally a normal living child weighing 2,920 Gm. At the time of the report, the patient was pregnant again. Rubovits and Arnkoff[19] reviewed the literature on pregnancy and exstrophy of the bladder and found that 33 children had been born to 26 women with this anomaly. Vaginal delivery was accomplished in 27 instances and cesarean section performed in 6. Of the infants delivered, 8 were stillborn and 25 were born alive. Epispadic fathers have produced normal offspring. Marshall and Muecke[3] mentioned an epispadic patient who had 5 normal children.

In the newborn child, treatment consists of protection of the open bladder and of the surrounding skin. Erosion of the exposed surfaces can be best treated with a light-cradle, which makes the wearing of diapers unnecessary. Surgical treatment is recommended for most cases. Gross[17] reviewed the history of surgical repair and described in detail the present concepts. He advocated delay of operation until the child is 3 or 4 years of age. Ureterosigmoidostomy with transabdominal exposure and establishment of a long, intramural, submuscular implantation of the ureter was recommended. Removal of the bladder and repair of epispadias can be done 6 months after ureteric transplantation. The results of this surgical treatment have been very satisfactory[6,17] but Williams[7] pointed out that long-term observations give a less encouraging view.

For a discussion of the operative procedures, the reader is referred to the urologic literature.[6,7,9,17,20]

Exstrophy of the Cloaca (Exstrophia Splanchnica)

In this severe defect of the lower abdominal body wall, the exstrophic bladder is divided into a right and a left half between which a field of intestinal mucosa is seen. The ileum opens in this median intestinal field and below this opening additional orifices of the colon or the appendix may be found. The prolapsed ileum hangs like a trunk from the exposed field. In such cases, the colon is short and ends blindly in an imperforate anus. The penis or clitoris consists of two widely separated halves and the vasa deferentia or the Müllerian ducts have openings below the bladder area. Myelocystocele (p. 284), omphalocele and often malrotation of the midgut are present in such cases. In addition to exstrophy of the bladder, the urinary tract may be involved by various anomalies; hydronephrosis, cystic, pelvic or absent kidney, hydro-ureter, atretic or double ureter have been observed.[21] Atypical forms exist. Exstrophy of the bladder and exstrophy of the bowel can be incomplete. Exstrophy of the ileocecal region can be combined with a closed intra-abdominal bladder.[22]

It is clear that repair of these complex malformations is difficult, but some of the patients have survived after surgical intervention.[11,21,23,24]

Urachal Anomalies

Congenital anomalies of the urachus and the bladder can be encountered in patients of various age groups. The bladder, although formed from the ventral cloaca, is continuous with the rudimentary allantois through the urachus, which originally is its cranial apex. Normally, the urachus persists throughout postnatal life as a cord that contains a narrow canal of variable length near its vesical end. The anomalies have been classified by Hinman[25] as completely patent urachus, vesicourachal diverticulum, umbilical cyst and sinus and alternating urachal sinus. In cases of congenital patent urachus, a vesicoumbilical fistula, urine drains from the umbilicus soon after the cord sloughs off. Associated anomalies are hydro-ureter and hydronephrosis, bladder neck obstruction and others. This anomaly, which manifests itself in infancy, must be distinguished from omphalomesenteric duct and omphalitis. Other urachal remnants cause symptoms in adult life. A vesicourachal diverticulum represents a marked enlargement of the narrow canal that normally exists in the middle abdominal ligament. Obstruction at the bladder neck or in the urethra results in dilatation of the canal to a diverticulum that extends about 5 cm. above the apex of the bladder. Calculi may develop in this pocket.[25] If the urachus opens into the umbilicus, a urachal sinus or cyst is formed that tends to infection and gastrointestinal complications. With alternating urachal sinus, umbilical or vesical symptoms can develop either in adults or in children. Treatment of these urachal anomalies was discussed by Hinman.[25]

Fig. 107-3. – Exstrophy of bladder and cloaca in a child who also had myelocystocele, clubfeet and polydactyly (Fig. 76-10). Both ileum and colon open onto the surface.

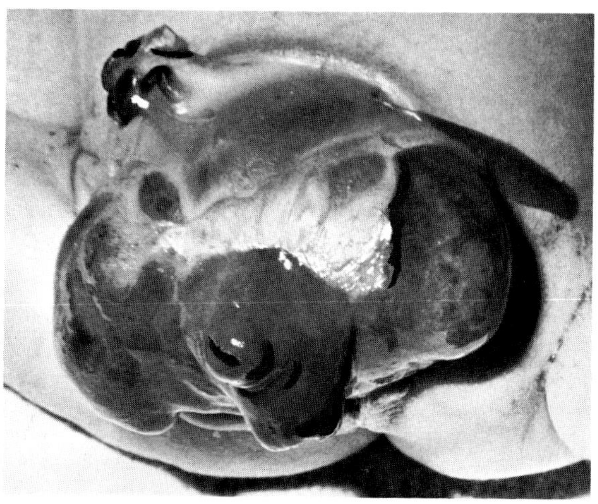

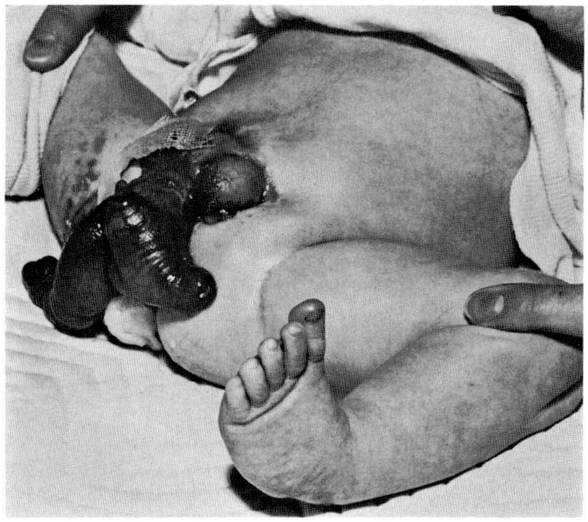

Fig. 107-4. – Exstrophy of the bladder and prolapse of the ileum in a female infant. The child also had myelocystocele, ectopia of the right kidney, bicornuate uterus, hemivertebrae and talipes equinovarus.

REFERENCES

1. Uson, A. C., Lattimer, J. K., and Melicow, M. M.: Types of exstrophy of urinary bladder and concomitant malformations; a report based on 82 cases, Pediatrics 23:927, 1959.
2. Gruber, G. B.: Missbildungen der Harnorgane, in Schwalbe, E. (ed.), *Morphologie der Missbildungen des*

Menschen und der Tiere (Jena: Gustav Fischer, 1927).
3. Marshall, V. F., and Muecke, E. C.: Variations in exstrophy of the bladder, J. Urol. 88:766, 1962.
4. Berndorfer, A.: Die intrauterine Regeneration der Bauch-, Blasen-, Genitalspalten, Paediat. Grenzgeb. 3:174, 1964.
5. Barcat, J., Torre, M. P., Gatelmond, R., Zumer, L., and Mirabel, A.: Un cas tératologique complexe, Arch. franç. pédiat. 17:499, 1960.
6. Campbell, M.: *Clinical Pediatric Urology* (Philadelphia: W. B. Saunders Company, 1951).
7. Williams, D. I.: Urology in Childhood, in *Encyclopedia of Urology* (Berlin: Springer-Verlag, 1958), Vol. XV.
8. Lenz, W.: Krankheiten des Urogenitalsystems, in Becker, P. E. (ed.), *Humangenetik* (Stuttgart: Georg Thieme, 1964).
9. Landau, S. J., and Lattimer, J. K.: Functional closure of bladder exstrophy. A review of fifty cases, Pediatrics 31: 433, 1963.
10. Glaser, L. H., and Lewis, A. P. R.: A case of familial incidence of ectopia vesicae, Brit. M. J. 2:1333, 1961.
11. Chisholm, T. C.: Exstrophy of the Bladder, in Mustard, W. T., Ravitch, M. M., Snyder, W. H., Jr., Welch, K. J., and Benson, C. D. (eds.), *Pediatric Surgery* (2d ed.; Chicago: Year Book Medical Publishers, Inc., 1969).
12. Smith, M.: Personal communication.
13. Grebe, H.: Zur Erblichkeit von Darmmissbildungen, Der Erbarzt 11:104, 1943.
14. Higgins, C. C.: Exstrophy of the bladder in twins, Cleveland Clin. Quart. 10:138, 1943.
15. Patten, B. M., and Barry, A.: The genesis of exstrophy of the bladder and epispadias, Am. J. Anat. 90:35, 1952.
16. Culp, D. A.: The histology of the exstrophied bladder, J. Urol. 91:538, 1964.
17. Gross, R. E.: *The Surgery of Infancy and Childhood* (Philadelphia: W. B. Saunders Company, 1953).
18. Coulter, W. J., and Sabbagh, M. I.: Bladder exstrophy and pregnancy, Obst. & Gynec. 11:104, 1958.
19. Rubovits, F. E., and Arnkoff, M.: Pregnancy associated with exstrophy of the bladder, J. Urol. 62:52, 1949.
20. Boyce, W. H., and Vest, S. A.: New concept concerning treatment of exstrophy of bladder, J. Urol. 67:503, 1952.
21. Spencer, R.: Exstrophia splanchnica (exstrophy of the cloaca), Surgery 57:751, 1965.
22. Spencer, R., and Geer, J. C.: Ileocecal exstrophy with bifid intra-abdominal urinary bladder: Incomplete exstrophy of the cloaca, J. Pediat. Surg. 2:69, 1967.
23. Rickham, P. P.: Vesico-intestinal fissure, Arch. Dis. Childhood 35:97, 1960.
24. Zwiren, G. T., and Patterson, J. H.: Extrophy of the cloaca; report of a case treated surgically, Pediatrics 35:687, 1965.
25. Hinman, F., Jr.: Surgical disorders of the bladder and umbilicus of urachal origin, Surg., Gynec. & Obst. 113: 605, 1961.

Other Bladder Anomalies

Hourglass Bladder

Hourglass bladder is an anomaly formed by horizontal constriction of the bladder so that an upper and a lower compartment are established. Three types can be distinguished. In the first type, extension of the upper portion of the bladder into the urachus results in a cylindrical cavity cranial to the bladder. A second type is characterized by a muscular corpus vesicae above a thin-walled trigonal chamber into which the ureters empty. The third type, which shows a (subtrigonal) constriction under the ureteric orifices, may not be congenital but be acquired in later life.[1] Urinary retention can be a complication of these anomalies.

Vesical Diverticula

The existence of congenital vesical diverticula has been disputed, since most are considered to be due to urinary obstruction in postnatal life. But diverticula have been found in the fetus as well as in the newborn and they constitute approximately 5% of all diverticula. In more than 15,000 necropsies in children there were 9 cases of bladder diverticulum.[2] The sex ratio of congenital diverticula in children is 5 males to 1 female; in adults, it is 10 to 1. According to Campbell,[2] congenital diverticula may have various causes. A patent urachus is held responsible for cases found in the dome of the bladder. Supernumerary ureteric buds, temporary occlusion of the urethra or persistence of the ureteric membrane and other anomalies have been cited as causes of this rare anomaly. Williams[3] pointed out that a diverticulum consists of a herniation of bladder mucosa through a defect in the thickened detrusor coat, so that a local weakness in this coat is responsible for the herniation. In case of a gross defect of muscle, the force of bladder contraction may be sufficient to produce a diverticulum even in the absence of obstruction. The most likely site of the muscle weakness is immediately behind and lateral to the ureteric orifice, but diverticula also occur on the lateral wall of the bladder or near the apex. Recurrent urinary infection and retention with painful bladder distention may be presenting symptoms. The patient, after emptying his bladder, is able after a few seconds to pass additional urine, which may be purulent and fetid (pis en deux).[2] Occasionally, a diverticulum may be palpable in the abdomen as a swelling distinct from the distended bladder. Small diverticula require no special treatment but large diverticula complicated by recurrent urinary infection must be removed.[3]

Congenital "Bladder Neck Obstruction" and Urethral Fibroelastosis

Many urologic conditions leading to urinary obstruction and characterized by a prominent ring at the bladder neck are considered and treated as bladder neck obstructions. Williams[3] pointed out that such findings do not represent an entity and that some bladder neck hypertrophies are not the cause but the result of urinary obstruction. Only when the urethra itself is normal can the bladder neck hypertrophy be regarded as the primary abnormality. In 1957, Bodian[4] demonstrated that severe cases of so-called congenital obstruction of the bladder neck in young males can be due to a fibroelastosis affecting the whole posterior urethra. In such cases, the prostatic tissue is abnormal in structure and the stenosis is distal to the bladder neck. The normal prostate in an infant consists of glandular structures intermingled with smooth muscle fibers. In the abnormal, glands are rare and fibroelastic tissue predominates, particularly below the verumontanum extending to the level of the bulb. It is thought that the fibroelastosis leads to an increased resistance to normal distention, causes obstruction to urine flow and then muscular hypertrophy of the detrusor and bladder neck. Congenital bladder neck obstruction generally occurs more often in boys than in girls.[5] Finkle *et al.*[6] described the condition in male siblings and Wilhelmi[7] reported congenital median bars in the bladder of male identical twins.

The manifestations of this anomaly are similar to those resulting from valves and other types of congenital urethral obstruction. The bladder is distended, there is overflow incontinence and signs of renal failure follow. In older children, a poor urinary stream, recurrent urinary infection, hematuria and abdominal pain may be presenting symptoms. Urethrograms may be normal or the bladder neck hypertrophy produces an unusual indentation in the urethral outline. Residual urine, severe trabeculation of the bladder and ureteric dilatation are characteristic changes, but the ureteric orifices usually are normal. Operation is difficult because the fibroelastosis involves changes in the urethral wall that not only present resistance to normal distention but also interfere with the normal elastic recoil when this resistance has been overcome.[3]

The Urogenital Tract with Absence of the Abdominal Muscles

The syndrome of congenital absence of the abdominal muscles is described on page 1026. The disorder, which usually is seen in males, includes many malformations of the urinary tract. The ureters and the kidneys often are involved and some writers thought that anomalies of the bladder cause the muscle changes (p. 1028). The bladder shows hypertrophy and dilatation with fixation of its apex to the umbilicus. The anomaly of the bladder is considered characteristic for the syndrome by Williams.[3] He found the bladder capacity very large and the detrusor muscle somewhat thickened but trabeculation usually was mild or absent. The trigone is large and there sometimes is a tapering dilatation of the posterior urethra. The ureters usually are long, dilated and tortuous, but in rare instances they are normal or occluded. Imperforate urethra and imperforate anus are rare occurrences.

In some of these children, the upper urinary tract is so severely affected at the time of birth that survival beyond the neonatal period is impossible and death occurs very early. But in other patients with congenital absence of the abdominal muscles, the urinary tract is less severely involved, so that the prognosis is rather favorable.

About one-fourth of the patients have anomalies of the gastrointestinal tract.[8] Cryptorchidism, dislocation of the hip and clubfoot occur in some of the patients. But some of the associated anomalies are above the diaphragm. Pigeon breast, pulmonary hypoplasia and even choanal atresia[9] have been observed.

In the past, many of the children died from uremia in early life, but now treatment of urinary infections and surgical intervention make survival possible in many cases. Some authors assert that obstruction of the bladder neck is the primary cause of the urinary tract anomalies and that removal of this primary obstruction leads to definite improvement.[10] Apparently not all cases respond to such surgical treatment, and Williams[3] emphasized that individual therapy must be applied according to the situation. McGovern and Marshall[8] recommended urinary drainage, preferably by nephrostomy followed by plastic repair of the ureters and vesical outlet.

Tumors

The best-known tumor arising from the bladder, prostate or vagina of infants or young children is a rhabdomyosarcomatous embryonic growth that sometimes is called sarcoma botryoides. The tumor can fill the entire bladder and spread to the ureter and urethra. Eventually it interferes with micturition and leads to pyuria or hematuria. The tumor, which can be congenital, requires radical surgical treatment.[3]

The bladder can be the site of generalized disorders such as neurofibromatosis or polyposis (p. 1256). Neurofibromatosis of the bladder is rare in children but several cases have been recorded.[11-13] Polyposis of the bladder can occur in the syndrome of gastrointestinal polyposis with pigmentation of the mucous membranes (p. 714). Multiple papillomas of the bladder were found in a pair of monozygotic twins who were more than 70 years of age.[14] Cavernous hemangioma of the bladder can be a cause of bleeding in children. Hemangiomas of the skin may betray the nature of the vesical lesion.[3,15] Carcinoma of the bladder was reported by Lowry *et al.*[16]

REFERENCES

1. Gruber, G. B.: Missbildungen der Harnorgane, in Schwalbe, E. (ed.), *Die Morphologie der Missbildungen des Menschen und der Tiere* (Jena: Gustav Fischer, 1927).
2. Campbell, M.: *Clinical Pediatric Urology* (Philadelphia: W. B. Saunders Company, 1951).
3. Williams, D. I.: Urology in Childhood, in *Encyclopedia of Urology* (Berlin: Springer-Verlag, 1958), Vol. V.
4. Bodian, M.: Congenital bladder neck obstruction, Brit. J. Urol. 29:393, 1957.

5. Deakin, R.: Congenital bladder neck obstruction in children, J. Urol. 78:384, 1957.
6. Finkle, A. L., McPhee, V. C., and Van der Reis, L.: Congenital bladder neck contracture in male siblings, California Med. 85:260, 1956.
7. Wilhelmi, O. J.: Congenital median bars occurring in twins, J.A.M.A. 101:847, 1933.
8. McGovern, J. H., and Marshall, V. F.: Congenital deficiency of the abdominal musculature and obstructive uropathy, Surg., Gynec. & Obst. 108:289, 1959.
9. Brierre, J. T., Jr.: Congenital abnormalities of the genitourinary tract: Abdominal muscle dysplasia and choanal atresia, Pediatrics 31:290, 1963.
10. Greene, L. F., Emmett, J. L., Culp, O. S., and Kennedy, R. L. J.: Urologic abnormalities associated with congenital absence or deficiency of abdominal musculature, J. Urol. 68:217, 1952.
11. Kass, J. H.: Neurofibromatosis of the bladder, Am. J. Dis. Child. 44:1040, 1932.
12. Chalkley, T. S., and Bruce, J. W.: Neurofibromatosis of the bladder in a nine-year old boy, J. Pediat. 20:632, 1942.
13. Diekmann, L., Hüther, W., and Pfeiffer, R. A.: Ungewöhnliche Erscheinungsformen der Neurofibromatose (von Recklinghausensche Krankheit) im Kindesalter, Ztschr. Kinderh. 101:191, 1967.
14. Thelen, A., and Schaeuble, J.: Gleichzeitiges Vorkommen von Blasenpapillomen bei eineiigen Zwillingen, Ztschr. Urol. 50:188, 1957.
15. Ballenger, E. G., Elder, O. F., and McDonald, H. P.: Case of cavernous hemangioma of the bladder, Am. J. Surg. 17:409, 1932.
16. Lowry, E. C., Soanes, W. A., and Forbes, K. A.: Carcinoma of the bladder in children: Case report, J. Urol. 73:307, 1955.

108

The Urethra

Congenital Obliteration of the Urethra

This anomaly manifests itself by failure of the child (usually male) to pass urine after birth. If the obliteration is located at the bladder neck, the anomaly is combined not only with dilatation of the bladder but with hydronephrosis or renal hypoplasia. The external genitalia usually are abnormal and such cases end fatally soon after birth. Similarly destructive is occlusion of the membranous urethra unless fistulae through the urachus, the rectum or the vagina permit emptying of the bladder.

Obliteration of the terminal urethra also prevents urination and causes distention of the bladder but, in contrast to more proximal obliteration, the outcome may be favorable if a channel is established soon after birth. The upper urinary tract often is not congenitally distended, so that merely temporary occlusion of the urethra can be assumed. In some cases, urine may escape by an accessory hypospadic meatus.[1]

In 1943, Dourmashkin[2] stated that by then only 50 authentic cases had been reported in living newborn infants, many children with the anomaly being stillborn. The bladder can be so distended that it interferes with delivery of the child. In addition to hydro-uretero-nephrosis, horseshoe kidney, malformations of the genital organs, imperforate anus, spina bifida or cleft lip and palate may be present. Several cases of survival to adulthood have been reported, with urination through the umbilicus via a patent urachus.

Urethral Diaphragms and Strictures

Congenital strictures of the urethra are almost limited to the male sex. Strictures as well as diaphragmatic obstructions, usually located in the prostatic urethra, lead to interference with urinary flow and manifest themselves at birth or in early childhood. They are rarer than urethral valves but can be responsible for death in infancy.[3] There is an abnormal narrow of the canal with dilatation of the proximal urethra. Diaphragms with central perforation occur above or below the verumontanum; they are associated with proximal dilatation of the urethra, detrusor hypertrophy, prominence of the bladder neck, vesical diverticula, hydro-ureter, hydronephrosis or renal hypoplasia. Although a diaphragm can be destroyed easily or a stricture dilated, the outlook is poor because of the renal damage, which usually is advanced when the infant is presented.[1]

Posterior Urethral Valves

Valvular folds of the urethral mucous membrane, although recognized and illustrated by Langenbeck in 1802,[4] are now known as a rather common cause of urinary obstruction in the male. Young and McKay[4] distinguished three main types of posterior urethral valves. In the most common form, type 1, two folds run down from the verumontanum to the urethral wall, forming pockets that prevent flow of urine into the anterior urethra; in type 2, the folds run upward from the verumontanum to the neck of the bladder; in type 3, a transverse iris diaphragm above or below the verumontanum obstructs the urinary flow. As a rule, the folds are symmetric and bilateral but occasionally unilateral obstruction occurs. Type 1, consisting of downward-directed folds, is an exaggerated form of submontanal folds, which are present in the normal male urethra. Watson[5] and Williams[1] observed such ridges as normal prominences in embryos; failure of regression of these ridges in later fetal life may lead to obstruction. It is of interest that congenital malformations in other organ systems usually are absent in patients with such urethral valves but hydronephrosis or renal hypoplasia does occur. The anomaly has been observed in brothers by Hasen and Song.[6] One brother had a type 1 and the other a type 3 valve. The first child died in infancy of complications of the anomaly. The second was thoroughly examined because of his brother's history and could be saved by timely operation. The condition was concordant in a pair of twins.[7] A related anomaly of the urethra combined with hypertrophy of the bladder and cystic kidneys was seen at necropsy in a boy with the Laurence-Moon-Biedl syndrome[8] (p. 179).

Obstruction of urinary flow leads to marked dilatation of the posterior urethra, which acquires thick and muscular walls. The bladder is trabeculated, showing diverticula, detrusor overgrowth and hypertrophy of its neck. The ureters become dilated and tortuous and the kidneys hydronephrotic.

In severe cases, the anomaly can be recognized in the neonatal period by enlargement of the abdomen, failure to thrive, vomiting and signs of uremia. Distention of the bladder is the outstanding symptom, but sometimes the enlarged kidneys become palpable. Ascites may occur in the neonatal period if the bladder is overdistended or ruptured.[9] If such symptoms appear in infancy, the prognosis is poor and early death occurs from renal failure. If the obstruction is less complete, survival for many years is possible. In older children, distention of the bladder, difficulties in micturition and overflow incontinence may reveal the anomaly before the renal damage is too severe. Other manifestations are dwarfism or renal rickets.

Urethrograms show the dilated urethra and a filling defect produced by the hypertrophied bladder neck; urethroscopy reveals the crescentic folds.

Anterior Urethral Valves

This is a rare anomaly consisting of a crescentic, horizontally placed mucosal fold in the region of the penoscrotal junction on the ventral wall of the urethra. During childhood, such folds may cause difficult micturition, distention of the bladder and hydro-ureters. They can be visualized in urethrograms and be removed surgically.[1]

Hypertrophy of the Verumontanum

The verumontanum becomes enlarged as a result of obstructing processes and infections of the urinary tract, so that the question of congenital hypertrophy as a primary cause of obstruction is controversial. Pilcher and Price[10] considered the congenital form a very rare anomaly and thought that in 1940 only 13 cases had been reported. They described a boy, dead at 3 weeks, who showed at necropsy a large and elongated verumontanum projecting into the bladder and acting as an occluding valve. Bugbee and Wollstein[11] observed 7 cases at necropsy and 1 clinical case. Diathermy or resection has been recommended,[1] but Kjellberg *et al.*[12] advocated conservative treatment, since obliteration of the ejaculatory ducts could be caused by operative methods. Polyps of the verumontanum can obstruct the posterior urethra partially and intermittently.[13]

Congenital Urethral Diverticula

In some male fetuses, congenital diverticula of the anterior urethra cause urinary obstruction and renal damage before birth; in others it is possible to correct the anomaly in postnatal life and establish normal urinary flow. Diverticula sometimes occur in the bulb of the urethra, where they open with a narrow orifice. If the diverticulum lies alongside the normal urethra, the latter may be compressed by the filling of the abnormal channel. The anomaly may manifest itself by a swelling on the ventral surface of the penis or remain concealed while causing damage to the proximal urinary pathways.[14] The opening into the urethra can be overlooked easily, but urethrograms show the anomaly and the dilatation of the proximal portion of the urethra. Good results have been reported after excision of the diverticulum.[14,15]

Mega-urethra

Enormous saccular dilatation of the anterior urethra with "monstrous" enlargement of the penis has been described by Nesbitt.[16] There is a great redundance of the skin and tremendous dilatation of the penis on voiding. The corpora cavernosa may be present or absent. The anomaly probably develops secondary to obstruction of the urethral meatus in fetal life. Some of these cases appear to be an exaggerated condition of urethral diverticulum. Surgical repair has been successful.[16] Stephens[13] distinguished a scaphoid and a fusiform mega-urethra. In the first type, the corpus spongiosum only is affected and a sausage-shaped (scaphoid) swelling develops during micturition. The anomaly is a part of a generalized syndrome of dilatations of the prostate, bladder and ureters combined with renal hypoplasia. In the second or fusiform type, the corpus spongiosum and the corpora cavernosa are defective in the pendulous part of the urethra.

Duplication of the Urethra

Duplications of the urethra occur with double bladder or double penis but, in some instances, an isolated accessory urethra is found dorsal to the corpora cavernosa or, rarer, between or ventral to them. A dorsal accessory urethra opens on the dorsum of the penis or on the glans through a broad orifice resembling epispadias. Most accessory urethras do not communicate with the urinary tract and end blindly. In approximately one-sixth of the patients, the accessory tract communicates with the main urethra and in about one-quarter there is a complete accessory urethra that forms a second excretory tract leading from the bladder to some part of the penis. Blind urethral pouches can be infected by gonococci or other organisms. Cases of complete accessory urethra are disturbing because of a double urinary stream or incontinence. Excision can be performed, with cure of the condition.[17] A ventral accessory urethra may cause obstruction of the normal channel or chronic infection.

Duplication of the urethra in the region of its membranous portion can cause urinary retention by constriction of the main urethra and by compression from the dorsally situated blind accessory tract. Such a case was reported by Liban,[18] occurring in a child with polycystic kidneys, cryptorchidism, clubfeet and signs of urinary retention.

Double urethra may occur in the female also and cause urinary incontinence. The accessory urethra usually lies behind the normal opening on or behind the trigone.[1]

Epispadias

Epispadias consists in a lack of closure of the dorsal aspects of the urethra. In males, the epispadic urethra is represented by a broad mucosal strip that lies on the dorsal surface of the corpora cavernosa. The anomaly is associated with exstrophy of the bladder or it occurs as an isolated anomaly. Campbell[19] estimated that the frequency is 1 in 30,000 persons; he observed the anomaly in 1 of 3,570 necropsies of boys. Epispadias can occur in females but it is more frequent in males. Embryologically, the malformation is related to exstrophy of the bladder and can be explained by early malposition of the primordia of the genital tubercle, which do not unite above the cloacal membrane (p. 1074).

In addition to complete epispadias, there are milder forms in which the urethral opening is merely misplaced. If the external urethral orifice is on the dorsum of the glans, one speaks of glandular epispadias. In penile epispadias, the orifice is on the dorsal surface of the penis, usually at its base. A groove that is lined by urethral mucosa is formed on the dorsum. In such cases, the penis usually is small, the corpora are separated and the prepuce is developed only as a skin fold on the ventral surface, leaving the glans uncovered. The urethral groove is covered proximally under a skin fold that conceals the incomplete bladder neck. The pubic bones are not united to a normal symphysis, although they are connected by a strand of fibrous tissue lying in front of the bladder neck. The verumontanum is concealed by the skin fold, under which the urethral groove disappears. In the female, the open urethra is situated between the two rudiments of the clitoris. The urethral slit lies between the mons veneris and the vagina.[1] Only in mild and rare cases is micturition and continence normal. Bladder control usually is disturbed, some children showing incontinence in the standing position.

Surgical repair of the anomaly is possible in many cases. Not only the external deformity is corrected but also the anomaly of the bladder neck.[1] As a rule, the operation is postponed to the third or fourth year, when bladder control can be acquired.

Hypospadias

This congenital defect is characterized by termination of the anterior urethra ventral and proximal to the normal orifice. It occurs in both sexes but males predominate. Hypospadias is, according to Campbell,[19] one of the most common urogenital anomalies, with an incidence estimated from 1 in 1,800 to 1 in 160. In Uppsala, Sweden, it was noted in 1 of 500 newborn boys.[20] It occurred in Campbell's series in 1 of 620 boys on whom necropsy was performed. It may appear repeatedly in families. Kemp,[21] reviewing the older literature, reported that this anomaly has been observed in 2, 3, 4 and even 5 siblings. There also were several observations of dominant transmission of hypospadias from father to son or from father to son and grandson. In two instances, the anomaly was transmitted through five and in one instance through six generations. In some families, one generation may be skipped, so that irregular dominance is assumed. A number of monozygotic twins have been observed with concordant hypospadias. In at least one instance, identical twins were discordant in regard to hypospadias.[21] Hypospadias has been seen repeatedly in boys with chromosomal abnormalities. Several cases of Klinefelter syndrome and 47/XXY karyotype have been reported.[22,23] It also has been associated with trisomy 18,[24] with a ring D_2 chromosome,[25] with deletion on the short arm of a B chromosome[26] and others.

Hypospadias was produced experimentally and described by Wilson and Warkany,[27] who found the anomaly in the young of female rats made vitamin A deficient.

The most common site of the anomaly is at the coronal sulcus, but more serious degrees have penile, penoscrotal and perineal openings. Between the opening of the urethra and the glans, a pink mucosal strip may be visible. The urethra proximal to the meatus can be normal or shortened. A ventral curvature of the penis usually is produced by a fibrous band that connects the area of the orifice to the glans, a condition called "chordee." The glans may be well developed or show a ventral groove corresponding to the open strip of urethral mucosa. Distal to the urethral meatus, one can find blind pits that lead into ducts situated dorsal to the urethra. The prepuce is ventrally incomplete and sits like a hood over the glans.[1]

In perineal hypospadias, the scrotum is bifid and divided by a strip of urethral mucosa. Williams[1] pointed out that the more severe degrees of hypospadias border on the condition of male intersexuality and that there is no well-defined dividing line between the two conditions. The diagnosis may be difficult when the penis is very small, when the testicles are undescended and when a vaginal canal is present. Determination of the sex chromatin and chromosomes is indicated in such cases, since female pseudohermaphrodism could be present.

Difficult micturition and production of a poor urinary stream are the results of coronal hypospadias. In perineal hypospadias, micturition in the sitting position may be necessary. Chordee can cause difficulty in sexual intercourse. According to Williams,[1] there is no treatment required for coronal hypospadias with an adequate orifice and without chordee. When the urethral orifice is placed farther back, operation is indicated to produce a normal urinary stream and permit normal erection. A variety of operations has been recommended for the correction.[1,19] The chordee is eliminated by excision of the fibrous band that unites the glans and the urethral orifice, and the urethral canal is extended to the tip of the penis.

Stenosis of the Urethral Meatus

Such narrows often are seen in children with meatal ulcer and "ammonia dermatitis." It is not always clear whether meatal stenosis is congenital or the result of the inflammatory process. Campbell[19] believed that congenital stenosis of the meatus is a common form of urethral obstruction, particularly in males; the congenital stricture leads to infection, meatal edema, ulceration and formation of rhagades, which in turn result in increasing obstruction. Congenital (pinhole) stenosis of the meatus may be symptomless until the second or third year, although manifestations are present occasionally in the first few weeks of life. Difficult and painful urination, overflow incontinence with distention of the bladder or a purulent urethral discharge may be presenting symptoms. Systemic symptoms result from urinary obstruction, upper urinary tract damage and infections. In female children, meatus stenosis can simulate bladder neck obstruction.[28] Meatotomy and passage of sounds are recommended for treatment.[19]

Malformations of the Urinary Tract Associated with Anal Atresia

In infants with imperforate anus, the division of the cloaca and the urogenital sinus often is imperfect, so that fistulous connections between the terminal bowel and the urogenital tract persist.

In the male, several connections are possible between the rectum and the urethra. The bowel may terminate in a narrow fistula that opens into the urethra below the verumontanum or in the membranous urethra.[1,19] These communications permit entrance of meconium into the urethra and its external orifice or urine can enter the bowel. If such infants are operated on soon after birth for imperforate anus without closure of the fistula, urine may flow from the newly established anal opening. As a result, urinary salts are deposited in the fecal masses or urinary infection occurs. Early separation of the intestinal and urinary tracts should be achieved and the correction followed

Fig. 108-1. – The probe is in the recto-urethral fistula of a boy with imperforate anus and marked distention of the colon. The right kidney was small and cystic.

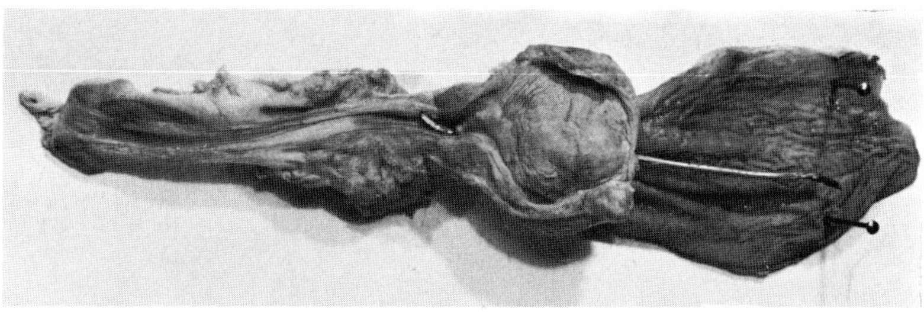

by a "pull-through" of the bowel to form a perineal anus.[1] Sometimes after such operations children show urinary retention or incontinence. There may be anomalies of the posterior urethra that require special surgical attention. Incontinence also may be due to neurologic complications associated with partial agenesis of the sacrum.

A recto-urethral fistula combined with hypospadias results in a common perineal opening for the urethra and the bowel. The bowel also can open independently from the urethra on the ventral surface of the scrotum or the penis.

In rare cases, the rectal fistula opens into the bladder either just above or in the trigone, so that a rectovesical fistula is established. In such cases, associated malformations such as atresia of the urethra, giant bladder, dilatation of the ureters and hypoplasia of the kidney often are present. These anomalies make the outcome of operation doubtful, and death in early infancy occurs frequently.[1]

In the female, anal stenosis may be combined with a bowel opening in the vestibulum or in the perineum. The rectum also may open into the vagina; in such cases, associated malformations occur commonly in the urinary tract. A recto-vaginal fistula may be combined with a vesico-vaginal fistula, so that urine and feces are discharged into a common channel, a persistent cloaca.

Williams[1] pointed out that in all types of imperforate anus, simple or complex upper urinary tract anomalies such as solitary kidney with a unilateral megaureter or ectopic, fused or malrotated kidneys may occur.

REFERENCES

1. Williams, D. I.: Urology in Childhood, in *Encyclopedia of Urology* (Berlin, Springer-Verlag, 1958), Vol. XV.
2. Dourmashkin, R. L.: Complete urethral occlusion in living newborn, J. Urol. 50:747, 1943.
3. Ehrlich, A.: Congenital stenosis of prostatic urethra, A.M.A. Am. J. Dis. Child. 91:625, 1956.
4. Young, H. H., and McKay, R. W.: Congenital valvular obstruction of the prostatic urethra, Surg., Gynec. & Obst. 48:509, 1929.
5. Watson, E. M.: The structure of the verumontanum: A study of the origin and development of its inherent glandular elements, J. Urol. 2:337, 1918.
6. Hasen, H. B., and Song, Y. S.: Congenital valvular obstruction of posterior urethra in 2 brothers, J. Pediat. 47: 207, 1955.
7. Davidsohn, I., and Newberger, C.: Congenital valves of the posterior urethra in twins, Arch. Path. 16:57, 1933.
8. Anderson, N. L.: The Laurence-Moon-Biedl syndrome, J. Clin. Endocrinol. 1:905, 1941.
9. France, N. E., and Back, E. H.: Neonatal ascites associated with urethral obstruction, Arch. Dis. Childhood 29: 565, 1954.
10. Pilcher, F., and Price, H. W.: Congenital hypertrophy of verumontanum, J.A.M.A. 115:2072, 1940.
11. Bugbee, H. G., and Wollstein, M.: Retention of urine due to congenital hypertrophy of the verumontanum, J. Urol. 10:477, 1923.
12. Kjellberg, S. R., Ericsson, N. O., and Rudhe, U.: *The Lower Urinary Tract in Childhood* (Chicago: Year Book Medical Publishers, Inc., 1957).
13. Stephens, F. D.: *Congenital Malformations of the Rectum, Anus and Genitourinary Tract* (Edinburgh: E. & S. Livingstone, Ltd., 1963).
14. Gross, R. E., and Bill, A. H.: Concealed diverticulum of the male urethra as a cause of urinary obstruction, Pediatrics 1:44, 1948.
15. Abeshouse, B. S.: Diverticula of the anterior urethra in the male. A report of four cases and a review of the literature, Urol. & Cutan. Rev. 55:690, 1951.
16. Nesbitt, T. E.: Congenital megalourethra, J. Urol. 73:839, 1955.
17. Gross, R. E., and Moore, J. H.: Urethral reduplication, Arch. Surg. 60:749, 1950.
18. Liban, E.: Rare malformation of urethra as a cause of congenital obstruction of lower urinary tract, A.M.A. Am. J. Dis. Child. 84:340, 1952.
19. Campbell, M.: *Clinical Pediatric Urology* (Philadelphia: W. B. Saunders Company, 1951).
20. Pettersson, F.: Meclozine and congenital malformations, Lancet 1:675, 1964.
21. Kemp, T.: Erbpathologie des männlichen Geschlechtsapparates, in Bauer, K. H., Hanhart, E., Lange, J., and Just, G. (eds.), *Handbuch der Erbbiologie des Menschen* (Berlin: Julius Springer, 1940), Vol. 4, pt. 11.
22. Gray, J.: Hypospadias with 47/XXY karyotype, Lancet 1: 722, 1961.
23. Passarge, E., and Thompson, J. N.: Autoradiography in a boy with XXY karyotype, Am. J. Dis. Child. 108:184, 1964.
24. Townes, P. L., DeHart, G. K., Jr., and Ziegler, N. A.: Trisomy 17-18 – an evaluation of preconceptional parental irradiation as a possible etiologic factor, J. Pediat. 65:870, 1964.
25. Sparkes, R. S., Carrel, R. E., and Wright, S. W.: Absent thumbs with a ring D_2 chromosome: A new deletion syndrome, Am. J. Human Genet. 19:644, 1967.
26. Wolf, U., and Reinwein, H.: Klinische und cytogenetische Differential-diagnose der Defizienzen an den kurzen Armen der B-Chromosomen, Ztschr. Kinderh. 98:235, 1967.
27. Wilson, J. G., and Warkany, J.: Malformations in the genitourinary tract induced by maternal vitamin A deficiency in the rat, Am. J. Anat. 83:357, 1948.
28. Perlmutter, A. D., Colodny, A., Harris, P. D., and Gross, R. E.: Urethral meatal stenosis in female children simulating bladder-neck obstruction, J. Pediat. 69:739, 1966.

Female Genitalia

The Ovaries

Absence of the Ovaries

BILATERAL CONGENITAL ABSENCE of the ovaries in women was generally doubted by older pathologists and reports of such cases encountered "general distrust" until about 40 years ago. Then, several necropsy reports appeared that confirmed the existence of bilateral lack of ovaries.[1-5] In such reports, the genital underdevelopment and small stature of the affected women were described but, otherwise, the external signs now considered diagnostic of ovarian dysgenesis were not mentioned, so that one cannot be sure that these publications concerned patients with Turner syndrome.

Reports of the past require re-evaluation for many reasons. There is confusion in the literature concerning the terms "agenesis" and "dysgenesis," so that some of the old observations dealing with women with streak gonads must be excluded. Some reports were based on surgical findings that, however, cannot establish absence of ovaries with certainty. Without biopsy and serial microscopic sectioning of critical areas, negative results are doubtful. In the past, a patient with external and secondary female sex characteristics was considered a "woman," a concept that cannot be upheld today. Determination of sex chromatin and chromosomes added discrepancies and the finding of cytogenetic mosaics makes it difficult to decide in which cases the existence of an ovary should be expected. Although absence of ovaries is encountered in many patients, it may be doubtful that they can be called "females." For these and other reasons, a definitive chapter on ovarian agenesis (absence of the ovaries) cannot yet be written. A few examples illustrating the confusing situation will be cited here.

Burns *et al*[6] recorded a patient with external genitalia considered male. Surgical exploration did not reveal any internal female genitalia and small masses in the "scrotum" consisted of fat and fibrous tissue. Since the sex chromatin was positive, the patient was considered a female with absent ovaries. Now, men with 46,XX karyotype have been observed repeatedly, so that this paradoxic situation can be considered an established fact. Whether finding of positive sex chromatin and of a 46,XX karyotype proves female genetic sex or whether the genetic sex remains doubtful in such persons because of the possibility of a concealed mosaicism[7] is still under discussion. In 1964, Ferrier *et al.*[8] wrote about nonspecific pseudohermaphrodism as a component of syndromes with multiple congenital malformations. In their article they described an unviable infant with imperforate anus in whom absence of the urethra, vagina and urogenital sinus was noted. An enlarged clitoris was present and, at necropsy, anomalies of the urinary and intestinal tracts were found. Although there was a small uterus and a Fallopian tube on the right, no gonad could be detected on either side. The karyotype was 46,XX.

Other case reports dealing with absence of the ovaries sometimes dealt with male patients or mosaics. In former times, maleness was hard to prove or disprove unless unusual circumstances revealed the presence of ectopic testes. Sellheim[9] described a patient who, on laparotomy, had an "empty" pelvis and no gonad and no duct system. Although raised as a girl, virilization took place after puberty. Burns *et al.*[6] reported a patient raised as a girl because of apparently female external genitalia but absent vagina. On abdominal exploration, no gonads and no internal genitalia were found. There was no evidence of a vas deferens. Sex chromatin was negative, so that male pseudohermaphrodism can be diagnosed.

True agonadism was reviewed by Overzier and Linden,[10] who reported siblings who were considered girls even though they had a phallus with a prepuce and a urethra within the phallus. There was no scrotum and no urogenital sinus. Neither gonads nor sex ducts were present. In former times, the situation could have been described as ovarian agenesis. But, since the sex chromatin was negative, anorchism was diagnosed. Similar cases have been recorded by other authors,[11,12] so that one can assume that some cases of ovarian agenesis described before sex chromatin determinations were possible actually were male.

Ovarian Hypoplasia

Hypoplastic ovaries represent transitions between ovarian agenesis and normal development. Breast development is poor and the uterus small. The ovaries are of bean size and their surface is smooth or gyrate, but sections show merely stroma. Vaginal smears suggest some ovarian function, and corpora fibrosa may be found in sections. There may be primary amenorrhea or a "prepubertal climacterium."[13]

Hypoplastic ovaries have been found repeatedly in patients with atypical Turner syndrome. Such cases with remnants of ovaries were reported occasionally before chromosome analysis was possible.[14-17] Primordial follicles, follicular cysts, developing follicles and even islands of testicular tissue have been found in such cases.[18] In a girl 31 months of age with symptoms of Turner syndrome but positive sex chromatin, Oikawa and Blizzard[19] found, on laparotomy, one normal and one elongated ovary that was similar in appearance to a fibrous streak seen in gonadal agenesis. But both ovaries contained primary follicles. De la Chapelle[18] reported a woman (Case 23) with some symptoms of Turner syndrome and sexual underdevelopment. The karyotype was normal 46,XX. Menstruation was irregular but the patient married and gave birth to a normal boy who was delivered by cesarean section. The ovaries were very small and resembled streak gonads but there was a corpus luteum in the left. Biopsy showed an atrophic ovary with scattered primordial follicles, some of which contained ova. A patient of Bahner *et al.*[20] was short but had no other symptoms of Turner syndrome. The karyotype was 45,XO. Yet, this patient had normal menstruation, breast development and even fertility. Localized mosaicism may be the basis of such paradoxic findings. A patient recorded by Lindsten and Tillinger[21] had some symptoms of Turner syndrome and was seen because of oligomenorrhea. On laparotomy, ovaries with few primordial follicles were found. This patient was a mosaic with cells containing 45,XO chromosomes and cells with 46 and 47 chromosomes. Those with 46 had one normal X and one ring X chromosome and those with 47 one normal X and two ring chromosomes.

Hypoplastic ovaries occur in many other disease pictures of abnormal sex development. Hirschhorn *et al.*[22] reported a newborn child with enlarged phallus and labia majora. The ovaries contained only a few ovarian follicles, much dense fibrous stroma and possibly seminiferous tubes. An XO/XY mosaicism was present. Similar patients with female phenotype except for enlargement of the clitoris were reported by Wilkins[23] as having ovarian dysplasia with medullary elements. The gonadal streaks found in the broad ligaments contained clumps of Leydig cells and some tubular structures. XO/XY and other forms of mosaicism may be the basis of such changes. In a woman seen because of primary amenorrhea, Warren *et al.*[24] found tissue strands in place of normal ovaries that contained no germ cells but hilus-cell hyperplasia in one and a hilus-cell adenoma in the other strand. The karyotype was XO/XX.

Ovarian Deficiencies

Functionally "absent" ovaries occur in many conditions described in this chapter. Women with amenorrhea and other sexual deficiencies may suffer from various clinical disorders and genetic deviations. The background of such disturbances seen in clinical practice was examined by Engel and Forbes,[25] who reviewed cytogenetic and clinical findings in 44 patients with congenitally defective or absent ovaries, elevated urinary gonadotropins, deficient sexual development, primary amenorrhea and low urinary 17-ketosteroids. Chromosomal anomalies were found in 36 (82%) and a normal XX karyotype with 46 chromosomes in only 8 (18%). The classic XO type was found in 16 (36%). Four patients had 46 chromosomes with 2 X chromosomes, but one of the X chromosomes was an isochromosome. Ten patients (23%) showed mosaicism, of which the XO/XX_i (isochromosome) type was the most frequent one with 6 cases. Clinical studies revealed few phenotypic differences between patients with XO constitution and those who had XX_i karyotypes, a finding that agrees with the assumption of genetic inactivity of the abnormal X chromosome. Metabolic studies revealed a high incidence of several metabolic diseases with onset in adult life. Diabetes occurred in 8, clinical or histologic evidence of thyroiditis in 6 and circulating antibody to thyroglobulin in 16 of the patients. Those patients who had normal XX karyotype did not show any of the congenital malformations or anomalies characteristic of Turner syndrome. They did not have a history of congenital lymphedema but 3 out of 4 had adult lymphedema. Genetic determination of infantilism was suggested by Hanhart,[26] who described "universal infantilism" in a girl, the product of incestuous mating. The uterus was absent and the ovaries were hypoplastic. From this and other cases in which incest played a role, Hanhart concluded that recessive inheritance may be responsible for some cases of ovarian dysfunction.

Supernumerary and Accessory Ovaries

A supernumerary ovary is entirely separate in location from the normally placed ovary, whereas an accessory ovary is situated near the normally placed ovary and may be connected with it. Both types contain ovarian follicular tissue. Wharton[27] published 2 cases of supernumerary ovary and 1 case of accessory ovary. He reviewed the literature on this subject and pointed out the great rarity of these anomalies, especially that of supernumerary ovaries. In one of his cases there were four ovaries; the two supernumerary ones were completely separate from the two normally placed ones. One was extraperitoneal and located on the right pelvic wall and the other retroperitoneal in the base of the mesentery of the sigmoid. In a second case, necropsy was performed following chorioepithelioma with cerebral metastases. A supernumerary ovary was "situated to the left of the aorta." Supernumerary ovaries can be mistaken for lymph nodes, but ovarian tissue is seen in histologic sections. Cystic enlargement may occur. In 1 case, absence of the left kidney, ureter and renal artery was found as an associated anomaly; in another case a third, rudimentary, Fallopian tube was present.

Accessory ovaries probably are more frequent than supernumerary ones but proved cases are also rare. Associated congenital malformations have been reported in 5 of 19 accepted cases. Accessory or bifid Fallopian tube, accessory tubal ostium, accessory adrenal gland, lobulated liver and septate uterus have been observed. Lobulated ovaries may be related to accessory ovaries. Uterus bicornis, uterus unicornis and spina bifida have been seen associated with lobulated ovaries.

Pelvic or abdominal but extraovarian tumors such as dermoid cyst, papillary cyst, multilocular cyst, granulosa cell tumor and others have been reported repeatedly as third ovaries. Only in a few of these could ovarian tissue be demonstrated. Yet, it is likely that neoplastic change is much greater in supernumerary and accessory ovaries than in normal ovaries, so that it cannot always be ruled out that abnormal ovaries were the basis of such tumors.

REFERENCES

1. Meyer, R.: Zum Mangel der Geschlechtsdrüsen mit und ohne zwittrige Erscheinungen, Virchows Arch. path. Anat. 255:33, 1925.
2. Olivet, J.: Über den angeborenen Mangel beider Eierstöcke, zugleich ein Beitrag zur Frage der Kastration und Behaarung, Frankfurt. Ztschr. Path. 29:476, 1923.
3. Randerath, E.: Über einen Fall von angeborenem Mangel beider Eierstöcke, Virchows Arch. path. Anat. 254:798, 1925.
4. Schürmann, P.: Über einen Fall von allgemeinem Infantilismus, bedingt durch beiderseitigen Eierstockmangel, Virchows Arch. path. Anat. 263:649, 1927.
5. Rössle, R., and Wallert, J.: Der angeborene Mangel der Eierstöcke und seine grundsätzliche Bedeutung für die Theorie der Geschlechtsbestimmung, Beitr. path. Anat. 84:401, 1930.
6. Burns, E., Segaloff, A., Carrerao, G. M., and Colbert, D. W.: Congenital absence of gonads, J. Urol. 89:450, 1963.
7. Hecht, F., Antonius, J. I., McGuire, P., and Hale, C. G.: XXY cells in a predominantly XX human male: Evidence for cell selection, Pediatrics 38:982, 1966.
8. Ferrier, P., Widgren, S., and Ferrier, S.: Nonspecific pseudohermaphroditism. Report of two cases with cytogenetic investigations, Helvet. paediat. acta 19:1, 1964.
9. Sellheim, H.: Ein Neutrum, Arch. Gynäk. 132:338, 1927.
10. Overzier, C., and Linden, H.: Echter Agonadismus (Anorchismus) bei Geschwistern, Gynaecologia 142:215, 1956.
11. Schoen, E. J., King, A. L., La Mont Baritell, A., and Knigge, W. F.: Pseudohermaphroditism with multiple congenital anomalies, Pediatrics 16:363, 1955.
12. Philipp, E.: Die Fehlbildung der Keimdrüse, Deutsche med. Wchnschr. 81:1298, 1956.
13. Philipp, E.: Die primäre Amenorrhae, Arch. Gynäk. 183: 247, 1953.
14. Atria, A., Sanz, R., and Donoso, S.: Necropsy of a case of Turner's syndrome, J. Clin. Endocrinol. 8:397, 1948.
15. Kerkhof, A. M., and Stolte, L. A. M.: Two cases of "hypoplasia" of ovaries, Acta endocrinol. 21:106, 1956.
16. Hoffenberg, R., Jackson, W. P. U., and Muller, W. H.: Gonadal dysgenesis with menstruation: A report of 2 cases, J. Clin. Endocrinol. 17:902, 1957.
17. Ashley, D. J. B., and Jones, C. H.: Sex reversal: Ovarian tissue with male nuclear sex, Lancet 1:74, 1958.
18. de la Chapelle, A.: Cytogenetical and clinical observations in female gonadal dysgenesis, Acta endocrinol. 40: 1, 1962.
19. Oikawa, K., and Blizzard, R. M.: Chromosomal studies of patients with congenital anomalies simulating those of gonadal aplasia, New England J. Med. 264:1009, 1961.
20. Bahner, F., Schwarz, G., Harnden, D. G., Jacobs, P. A., Hienz, H. A., and Walter, K.: A fertile female with XO sex chromosome constitution, Lancet 2:100, 1960.
21. Lindsten, J., and Tillinger, K-G.: Self-perpetuating ring chromosome in a patient with gonadal dysgenesis, Lancet 1:593, 1962.
22. Hirschhorn, K., Decker, W. H., and Cooper, H. L.: Human intersex with chromosome mosaicism of type XY/XO; report of a case, New England J. Med. 263:1044, 1960.
23. Wilkins, L.: *Diagnosis and Treatment of Endocrine Disorders in Childhood and Adolescence* (3d ed.; Springfield, Ill.: Charles C Thomas, Publisher, 1965).
24. Warren, J. C., Erkman, B., Cheatum, S., and Holman, G.: Hilus-cell adenoma in a dysgenetic gonad with XX/XO mosaicism, Lancet 1:141, 1964.
25. Engel, E., and Forbes, A.P.: Cytogenetic and clinical findings in 48 patients with congenitally defective or absent ovaries, Medicine 44:135, 1965.
26. Hanhart, E.: Zur Phänomenologie und Vererbung des universellen sowie des partiellen Infantilismus, Ztschr. menschl. Vererb.-u. Konstitutionslehre 29:424, 1948.
27. Wharton, L. R.: Two cases of supernumerary ovary and one of accessory ovary, with analysis of previously reported cases, Am. J. Obst. & Gynec. 78:1101, 1959.

The Uterus

INCOMPLETE FUSION of the Müllerian ducts results in various degrees of division of the uterine cavity. Patten[1] arranged abnormal human uteri in a series that closely parallels the organ's evolutionary changes. In uterus septus duplex, two uterine cavities are formed by a complete vertical septum. It may be combined with double vagina. Uterus subseptus unicornis represents a partial division by such a septum, which divides only the fundus so that the duplication is limited to the upper cavity. In uterus bicornis septus, the division is not limited to the cavity but is also seen on the outside in the form of two uterine horns. Uterus bicornis unicollis is a lesser degree of this anomaly. Uterus didelphys (with double vagina) consists of two uteri, each connected with a tube and an ovary. Atresia of the uterus is present at the level of the cervix when the uterus is connected with the vagina by a strand of connective tissue without lumen. Duplications and diverticula of the main Fallopian tubes may occur, and ectopic pregnancies have been reported in such redundant tubes.[2]

Absence of the uterus and many types of rudimentary organs are seen in the various forms of hermaphrodism and pseudohermaphrodism (p. 1105).

As early as 1859, Kussmaul[3] divided uterine malformations into two main groups: (a) deficiencies (agenesis or degeneration) and (b) duplications. Since then, many modifications of his detailed classification have been suggested, but the principal subdivisions still hold in morphologic descriptions. The relationship of these malformations to genic, chromosomal or exogenous teratogenic factors is still not clear in most cases, although some progress has been made in etiologic classification.

Aplasia and Hypoplasia

Complete absence of the genital apparatus does not seem to occur, but aplasia of uterus and vagina in the presence of ovaries and tubes has been observed repeatedly. True agenesis is said to be found only in unviable fetuses such as sirens and those with eventrations and exstrophy of the bladder. Rudimentary uteri can be overlooked and mistaken for agenetic uteri. Adult patients with uterine and vaginal aplasia in the presence of tubes and functioning ovaries have been described, often in conjunction with renal anomalies. A form of uterine hypoplasia consists of uterine rudiments represented by bilateral, noncanalized muscular buds that occur together with absence of the vagina (Rokitansky-Küster-Hauser syndrome, p. 1094). Unilateral absence of uterus and absence of the vagina can be combined with ipsilateral absence of the ovary, tube and kidney, or uterus vaginalis unilateralis can occur even though bilateral ovaries, tubes and round ligaments are present.

Absence of the Uterus

Absence of the uterus is noted in some apparently female patients who have the syndrome of male pseudohermaphrodism with testicular feminization. Such persons are genetic males, have negative sex chromatin and XY karyotype. They do not menstruate and cannot bear children but their external genitalia are normal female and they feminize at puberty, with good breast development. In rare cases, rudimentary tubes and uteri can be present. There are intra-abdominal or inguinal testes with nests of Leydig cells.

The uterus is absent also in the majority of male pseudohermaphrodites with ambiguous genitalia. They may have testes situated intra-abdominally, in the inguinal canal or in the scrotum. The vagina can be of differing size and length, often communicating with a hypospadic urethra. A minority of male pseudohermaphrodites with ambiguous external genitalia have a uterus and tubes. This can be of practical importance if, at laparotomy, gonads at the site of ovaries are seen in a child with tubes, uterus and vagina. Such gonads can be testes.

Bloise *et al.*[4] described a patient with an XO karyotype and intra-abdominal testes who had a rudimentary uterus. Vignetti *et al.*[5] reported a "girl" with a phallus without meatus and a urethral orifice behind it. There was no urogenital sinus. In the "labia," testes were palpable. At operation, no internal female genitalia were found. The chromosomal constitution was XYY. The uterus usually is present in true hermaphrodites, although absence has been reported in exceptional cases.[6]

Uterus Arcuatus

If the uterine fundus remains externally concave due to failure of thickening of the musculature of the roof, one speaks of uterus arcuatus. Uterus arcuatus as seen from the outside can be combined with an internal septum.

Uterus Septus

The Müllerian ducts may join but the uterine cavity can be divided by a septum in two smaller spaces. The septation of the uterovaginal canal can be complete, a condition called uterus septus duplex, or the septation may be limited to cranial portions of the canal–uterus subseptus unicollis. According to the extent and the site of the septa, many variations are possible and their classification is not uniform. The septa usually are sagittally oriented, but occasionally frontal or oblique septa occur and the chambers formed can be unequal in size.

Uterus Bicornis

This anomaly results from separation of the uterine horns in the presence of union of the cervical portion of the Müllerian ducts. Partial cervical and vaginal septation make classification difficult. The uterine horns can be unilaterally or symmetrically underdeveloped. The right horn often is smaller than the left. Various degrees of hypoplasia have been reported. The rudimentary horn may be represented by a thin ligamentous structure or by a round, muscular strand showing cranial egg-shaped enlargement with or without cavitation. Only one horn may be connected with the vagina. The well-developed horn often is elongated (uterus obliquus), whereas the second horn is hardly demonstrable.

Uterus bicornis with symmetric development of the horns may be combined with renal anomalies, duplications of the colon or atresia ani. Inguinal ectopia of the uterine horns and adnexae has been observed repeatedly.[7] Bilateral herniae of the uterus, tubes and ovaries can be combined with absence of the vagina.[8] Asymmetric uterus bicornis is combined in many cases with underdevelopment of the adnexae on the side of the hypoplastic uterine horn. The bladder also may be only unilaterally developed. Uterus bicornis bicollis with left renal and ureteral agenesis was described in detail by Shumacker.[9] The same author reported a case of uterus bicornis unicollis with right renal and ureteral agenesis. An excellent report on concomitant malformations of the reproductive and urinary tracts was written by Woolf and Allen[10] in 1953. A uterus bicornis was present in one of monozy-

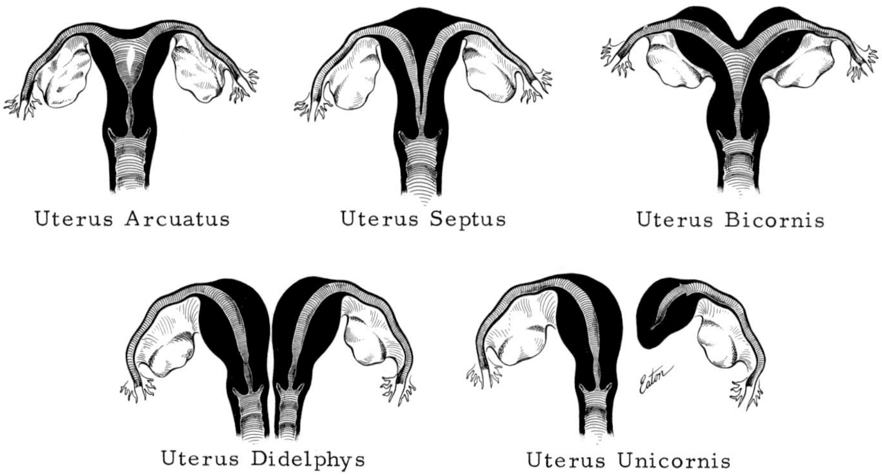

Fig. 109-1. – Diagrams showing various malformations of the uterus.

gous twins with pure gonadal dysgenesis, gonadoblastoma, female external genitalia and 46,XY karyotype. The other twin resembled her "sister" in many respects but the uterine fundus was normal.[11] Hypoplastic uterus bicornis can occur in male pseudohermaphrodites and rarely in true hermaphrodites.[6] Uterus bicornis has been observed in cebocephaly and in several infants with trisomy 13-15.[12,13]

Bicornuate uterus with one cervix and a rudimentary horn may remain symptomless unless a fertilized ovum becomes implanted in the rudimentary horn or if the cavity of the rudimentary horn does not communicate with the main cavity. Menstrual blood that cannot escape from the rudimentary segment can enter the peritoneal cavity through the oviduct. If the oviduct is not open, menstrual blood will accumulate in the rudimentary horn, leading to severe dysmenorrhea, nausea and vomiting with each period. If pregnancy occurs in the main cavity, the periods and the painful attacks stop.[14]

Uterus Didelphys (Uterus Duplex Separatus with Vagina Duplex Separata)

In this anomaly, there is no fusion of the Müllerian ducts, so that the two uteri and two vaginae are formed. This rare condition (presence of a single vagina precludes the term "uterus didelphys") is seen occasionally in unviable fetuses, sometimes combined with omphalocele, double bladder or spina bifida. The rectum is attached anteriorly to the bladder, either directly or through a sagittal rectovesical ligament. This ligament divides the small pelvis into two pockets in which the separate uterine horns lie. One of these horns may be underdeveloped.[7] Ovaries and tubes are present.

Doubling of the vulva, vagina, urethra and bladder have been reported in some of the cases. Absence of the right kidney and ureter has been observed also.[15]

Uterus didelphys can occur in otherwise normal women and may be discovered accidentally or when complicated by pregnancy. Delivery of a normal infant from each uterus has been reported.[16] Of special interest are cases of double pregnancy, such as that described by Brown.[17] Although reported as a case of pseudodidelphys, it could be considered as didelphys, since a vaginal septum was present originally but was destroyed by delivery. In this case, the second infant was delivered 5 minutes after the first. The situation was similar in a case recorded by Vartan.[18] A woman with a double uterus, double cervix and

Fig. 109-2. – Hysterosalpingograph showing a double uterus.[46] (Courtesy of Dr. J. J. Fisher, Jacksonville, Florida, and Am. J. Obst. & Gynec.)

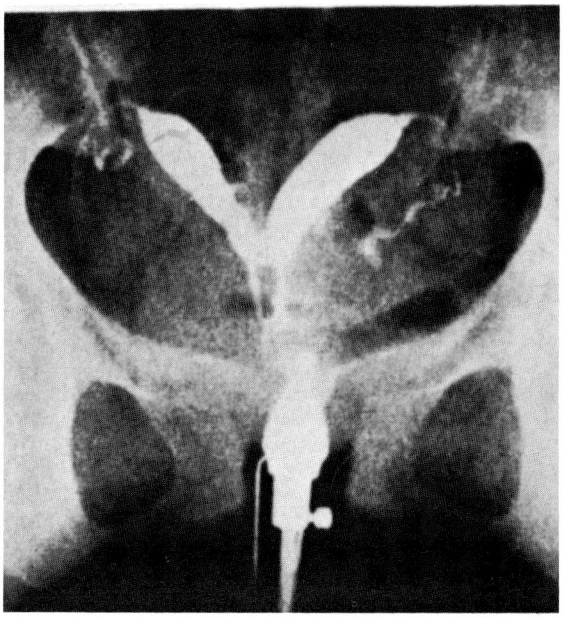

double vagina, pregnant on both sides, delivered at term 2 live girls who weighed 2,400 Gm. and 2,200 Gm., respectively. It is believed that double pregnancies are more frequent in double than in normal uteri. It has been estimated that in double uterus the ratio of double to single pregnancies may be 1 to 16 but this may not be correct, since in single pregnancies duplication of the uterus often is overlooked.

Uterus and vagina duplex has been observed in association with arhinencephaly.[19] A uterus bicornis bicollis with septate vagina was present in an infant girl who had an abnormal chromosome interpreted as an isochromosome.[20] The child also had a ventricular septal defect, patent foramen ovale, absence of gallbladder and left kidney and a pelvic right kidney but normal ovaries. Double vagina and uterus can occur with trisomy 13-15.[21] Double uterus and vagina has been noted in children damaged by thalidomide.[22] A syndrome of duplication of the female genital tract associated with malformations and hypoplasia of the hands and feet and with characteristic dermatoglyphic pattern has been described as a heritable dominant trait.[45]

Uterus Pseudodidelphys (Uterus Bicornis Bicollis; Uterus Duplex Separatus)

This anomaly consists of two uteri but only one vagina. In case of absence of the vagina, distinction between didelphys and pseudodidelphys cannot be made. One uterine horn may be rudimentary. Ovaries and tubes are present but they, too, may show unequal development. According to Brown,[17] duplication of the uterine body and cervix is rare. It was observed 5 times in 50,000 obstetric cases.

The "unusual case of twins" reported by Williams and Cummings[23] probably occurred in a woman with uterus pseudodidelphys. The male infants were born alive 56 days apart. After delivery of the first baby, no lactation set in, but after delivery of the second it was normally established. It was thought that the second placenta, which continued production of estrogen and progesterone, antagonized the action of prolactin. Kennedy[24] recorded a case of double pregnancy and double uterus, the children being born 22 days apart.

The anomaly has been mentioned in combination with anomalies due to thalidomide damage.[22]

Uterus Unicornis

The older literature on this anomaly was reviewed by Shumacker,[9] who reported at the same time a case of left uterus unicornis with right renal and ureteral agenesis and an abnormal umbilical ligament. He tabulated 28 cases, listing the condition of the adnexae and kidneys. The left side was defective in 60% of the cases. In 9 instances, the ovaries and tubes were completely absent on the defective side, in 11 other cases the ovary was ectopic and in 2 cases the ovary was rudimentary. The ovary of the defective side can also be longer and narrower than a normal gonad. The broad ligament commonly is absent on the defective side. The external genitalia are deformed in exceptional cases only. True uterus unicornis is rare,[25] whereas so-called uterus unicornis with a rudimentary second horn (uterus bicornis) is encountered more often.[26] Although these two types were strictly distinguished by older authors, it is known that both kinds frequently are associated with solitary kidney and it seems that they represent related anomalies of differing degrees. Complications such as hematosalpinx, hematometra and pregnancy in the uterine rudimentary horn are, of course, limited to the "so-called" uterus unicornis, which actually is bicornis. In the past, pregnancy in a rudimentary horn often resulted in rupture,[9] as the situation was not recognized in time. Frost [27] reported a case of true uterus unicornis with unilateral renal agenesis and reviewed more recent cases of the anomaly. Uterus unicornis can occur in true hermaphrodism. Gordon *et al.*[28] described a phenotypic boy with hypospadias and a descended testis on the right. With puberty, breasts developed. Chromatin-positive buccal smears were obtained and the karyotype proved to be 46,XX. Laparotomy revealed an ovary, a Fallopian tube and a unicornuate uterus on the left. Another case of true hermaphrodism involved a unicornuate uterus and 46,XX chromosome constitution.[29] In several patients who had a testis on one side and no gonad on the other, unicornuate uterus has been observed.[30] The chromosome constitution is not uniform in such patients, who may be mosaics. In an aborted fetus with 45,XO karyotype, uterus unicornis was observed.[31]

Congenital Prolapse of the Uterus

Congenital prolapse of the uterus has been observed repeatedly in association with spina bifida and clubfoot. Between the labia minora, a mass protrudes with a central opening that represents the uterine cervix. It is thought that defects of sacral nerves result in paralysis of the musculature of the pelvic floor and in prolapse, which sometimes is not congenital but occurs in the first week after birth.[32]

Malformations of the uterus are of practical importance, since menstruation and pregnancy may occur if in such cases ovaries are developed and functioning. Complications are particularly likely if menstrual blood collects in (or if pregnancy occurs in) a hypoplastic horn. If a pregnancy is located in one horn, regular menstruation can continue in the other.[7]

Pregnancy is possible in some of these anomalies if the uterine cavity is connected with the vagina and with a tube. In cases of uterus bicornis, pregnancy can occur in either horn. Sympathetic hypertrophy of the contralateral horn may, in rare cases, interfere with normal pregnancy. There is an increased abortion rate, and premature labor occurs frequently. In many cases, the diagnosis of the uterine anomaly is not made. Uterus unicornis is compatible with a normal pregnancy, but pregnancy in the rudimentary horn of a double uterus can lead to serious complications, particularly if the rudimentary horn does not communicate with the uterine cavity, fertilization having taken place following external migration of spermatozoa.

Pregnancy in uterus didelphys is not uncommon and the anomaly may remain unrecognized even in case of childbearing. In many instances, unusual fertility has been noted, but abortions are relatively common and labor is prolonged because of poor muscular development in the uterus, small cervix and encroaching of the nonpregnant uterus. Pregnancy in bicornuate uterus was discussed by Falls[33,47] and a great number of complications were mentioned. The milder anomalies of incomplete fusion of the Müllerian ducts, uterus bicornis septus, subseptus and arcuatus were said to occur in 1% of pregnant women, but the actual incidence is difficult to ascertain by obstetric observation, since many divided uteri are not diagnosed intra vitam. Other authors[34-36] give much lower incidence figures. Steenstrup[37] arrived at a figure of 0.5% for hospitalized patients. Baker *et al.*[34] analyzed 118 cases of congenital anomalies of the uterus associated with pregnancy and added 9 of their own. They recognized the difficulties of arriving at incidence figures and estimated that 0.3% of all deliveries in their hospital were associated with congenital anomalies of the uterus. The 127 patients reviewed had 275 pregnancies, an average of about 2 pregnancies per patient. The largest number of the women reviewed had either uterus didelphys or uterus bicornis unicollis.

Some affected women are normal except for the uterine anomaly; others have associated malformations, particularly of the genital and urinary tracts. Sterility, abortion, premature labor, fetal asphyxia, breech presentation, oblique and transverse presentation, fetal opisthotonos or placental anomalies may result from uterine malformations, but a large percentage of the women thus affected are delivered spontaneously and without complications. If complications occur, the diagnosis of double uterus often is not made. Steenstrup[37] found that women with uterine deformities usually have normal fertility but that they encounter reproductive difficulties because of a high abortion rate, amounting to 44% of the pregnancies, and because of the low birth weight of the viable children, of whom 34% weighed less than 2,500 Gm. There was an increased number of breech and transverse presentations. The cesarean section rate was 11%. Steenstrup[37] discussed measures to improve the reproductive chances of women with uterine deformities.

Not much is known concerning the babies resulting from these pregnancies. Irregularity of fetal heart tones and possible asphyxia of the fetus were reported by Falls,[33] but he thought that the birth weights and sizes were normal and that the babies were free of malformations. Findley,[15] reviewing 135 cases of double uterus, mentioned the birth of 216 full-term babies, 13 twin pregnancies, 15 premature deliveries, 86 abortions, 13 breech presentations and only 2 malformations of the baby. One of 3 of his own cases was delivered by cesarean section. The child had clubfeet and died within 48 hours. Some authors[38] found no fetal abnormalities in their series, whereas others did.[36] In the 127 patients reviewed by Baker *et al.*,[34] there were 98 viable births and 73 viable term infants. The abortion rate was 19%. In a total of 109 infants, only 3 were noted to be abnormal, 1 developed spastic paralysis, 1 had a clubfoot and 1 had metatarsus varus. A possible connection between maternal uterus bicornis and children with a syndrome of defect of femur and fibula with amelia of the upper extremities was mentioned by Kühne *et al.*[39]

Surgical treatment of double uterus was discussed by Strassmann.[40] Septate uterus, which is rare, can be treated by removal of the septum per vaginam, but if there are partly or completely divided uterine bodies, uterus bicornis unicollis or uterus bicornis bicollis, exposure by laparotomy is followed by plastic unification of the semiuteri.

Tubes

Developmental disturbances of the tubes are rarer than those of the uterus. Absence of the tubes without uterine anomalies apparently does not occur, but aplasia of one tube together with that of a uterine horn is common. Unilateral defect of a tube has been observed in the presence of otherwise normal internal genitalia. Rudimentary tubes occur in hermaphroditic conditions.

Partial absence of a tube has been observed repeatedly; only the fimbriae may be present. The corresponding ovary may be well developed or atretic. Partial atresia of a tube, consisting of connective tissue or muscle fibers, can occur. Despite a normal uterus, the lumen of a tube can be occluded. Diverticula, i.e., epithelial pockets into the tubal musculature, can be congenital but they, as well as partial defects of a tube, can be of postnatal origin. If found in an adult, the origin often is obscure.[41] McNalley[42] demonstrated congenital diverticula in 10 of 12 tubal pregnancies. In 3 of the 10 cases, the malformation was directly responsible for arrest of an ovum. Schoenholz[43] also attributed tubal pregnancies to congenital diverticula or mesh formations in the tube. Inflammatory processes were not considered important as causes of tubal pregnancies by these authors.

A true third tube has been reported only rarely but accessory tubes have been seen repeatedly. They usually appear as small cysts connected by a stalk with the tube. Fimbriae on the cysts identify them as tubal derivatives. Pregnancies in accessory tubes have been described.[44]

REFERENCES

1. Patten, B. M.: *Human Embryology* (Philadelphia: The Blakiston Company, 1946).
2. Bremer, J. L.: *Congenital Anomalies of the Viscera. Their Embryological Basis* (Cambridge, Mass.: Harvard University Press, 1957).
3. Kussmaul, A.: *Von dem Mangel der Verkümmerung und Verdopplung der Gebärmutter* (Würzburg: Stahel, 1859).
4. Bloise, W., DeAssis, L. M., Bottura, C., and Ferrari, I.: Gonadal dysgenesis (Turner's syndrome) with male phenotype and XO chromosomal constitution, Lancet 2:1059, 1960.
5. Vignetti, P., Capotorti, L., and Ferrante, E.: XYY chromosomal constitution with genital abnormality, Lancet 2: 588, 1964.
6. Overzier, C.: True Hermaphroditism, in Overzier, C.: *Intersexuality* (London and New York: Academic Press, 1963).
7. Meyer, R.: Die pathologische Anatomie der Gebärmutter, in Henke, F., and Lubarsch, O. (eds.), *Handbuch der Speziellen Pathologischen Anatomie und Histologie* (Berlin: J. Springer, 1930), Vol. VII.
8. Thomson, G. R.: Complete congenital absence of the vagina associated with bilateral herniae of uterus, tubes and ovaries, Brit. J. Surg. 36:99, 1948.
9. Shumacker, H. B: Congenital anomalies of the genitalia associated with unilateral renal agenesis, Arch. Surg. 37: 586, 1938.
10. Woolf, R. B., and Allen, W. M.: Concomitant malformations. The frequent simultaneous occurrence of congenital malformations of the reproductive and urinary tracts, Obst. & Gynec. 2:236, 1953.
11. Frasier, S. D., Bashore, R. A., and Mosier, H. D.: Gonadoblastoma associated with pure gonadal dysgenesis in monozygous twins, J. Pediat. 64:740, 1964.
12. Smith, D. W., Patau, K., Therman, E., Inhorn, S. L., and DeMars, R. I.: The D_1 trisomy syndrome, J. Pediat. 62: 326, 1963.
13. Teller, W., and Pfeiffer, R. A.: Die Trisomie D_1 (13-15) als Ursache multipler Abartungen, Ztschr. Kinderh. 89:36, 1964.
14. Hall, J. E.: Bicornate unicollic uterus with a rudimentary horn, Brooklyn Hosp. J. 8:25, 1950.
15. Findley, P.: Pregnancy in uterus didelphys, Am. J. Obst. & Gynec. 12:318, 1926.
16. Brown, D. C., and Nelson, R. F.: Uterus didelphys and double vagina with delivery of a normal infant from each uterus, Canad. M.A.J. 96:675, 1967.
17. Brown, D. B.: A case of uterus pseudodidelphis and twin pregnancy, J. Obst. & Gynaec. Brit. Emp. 63:395, 1956.
18. Vartan, C. K.: Uterus didelphys with double pregnancy, J. Obst. & Gynaec. Brit. Emp. 65:120, 1958.
19. Dominok, G. W., and Kirchmair, H.: Familiäre Häufung von Fehlbildungen der Arhinencephaliegruppe, Ztschr. Kinderh. 85:19, 1961.
20. Carr, D. H., Barr, M. L., and Rathbun, J. C.: A probable isochromosome in a child with multiple congenital anomalies, J. Pediat. 62:696, 1963.
21. Marin-Padilla, M., Hoefnagel, D., and Benirschke, K.: Anatomic and histopathologic study of two cases of D_1 (13-15) trisomy, Cytogenetics 3:258, 1964.
22. Kreipe, U.: Missbildungen innerer Organe bei Thalidomidembryopathie, Arch. Kinderh. 176:33, 1967.
23. Williams, B., and Cummings, G.: An unusual case of twins, J. Obst. & Gynaec. Brit. Emp. 60:319, 1953.
24. Kennedy, N.: A case of twin pregnancy in a double uterus, Brit. M. J. 1:486, 1959.
25. Pfleiderer, A.: Über Gebärmuttermissbildungen, Monatsschr. Geb. Gynäk. 82:401, 1929.
26. Eismayer, G.: Über Uterusmissbildung bei kongenitalem Mangel einer Niere, Ztschr. Urol. Chir. 11:191, 1923.
27. Frost, I. F.: Case report of a patient with a true unicornuate uterus with unilateral renal agenesis, Am. J. Obst. & Gynec. 75:210, 1958.
28. Gordon, R. R., O'Gorman, F. J. P., Dewhurst, C. J., and Blank, C. E.: Chromosome count in a hermaphrodite with some features of Klinefelter's syndrome, Lancet 2:736, 1960.
29. Root, A. W., Eberlein, W. R., Briebart, S., Moorhead, P. S., and Mellman, W. J.: Chromosomal analysis of multiple tissues from a true hermaphrodite, J. Clin. Endocrinol. 24:467, 1964.
30. Wilkins, L.: *Diagnosis and Treatment of Endocrine Disorders in Childhood and Adolescence* (Springfield, Ill.: Charles C Thomas, Publisher, 1965).
31. Singh, R. P., and Carr, D. H.: The anatomy and histology of XO human embryos and fetuses, Anat. Rec. 155:369, 1966.
32. Torpin, R.: Prolapsus uteri associated with spina bifida and clubfeet in newborn infants, Am. J. Obst. & Gynec. 43:892, 1942.
33. Falls, F. H.: Study of pregnancy with parturition in primipara with bicornuate uteri, Am. J. Obst. & Gynec. 15:399, 1928.
34. Baker, W. S., Roy, R. L., Bancroft, C. E., McGaughey, H., Dickman, F. N., and Tucker, G. W.: Congenital anomalies of the uterus associated with pregnancy. An analysis of 118 cases from the literature with a report of 9 additional cases, Am. J. Obst. & Gynec. 66:580, 1953.
35. Fenton, A. N., and Singh, B. P.: Pregnancy associated with congenital abnormalities of the female reproductive tract, Am. J. Obst. & Gynec. 63:744, 1952.
36. Smith, F. R.: The significance of incomplete fusion of the Müllerian ducts in pregnancy and parturition, with a report of 35 cases, Am. J. Obst. & Gynec. 22:714, 1931.
37. Steenstrup, O. R.: Congenital uterine anomalies and pregnancy, Acta obst. et gynec. scandinav. 38:143, 1959.
38. Hunter, W.: Pregnancy in the deformed uterus, J. Obst. & Gynaec. Brit. Emp. 64:243, 1957.
39. Kühne, D., Lenz, W., Petersen, D., and Schönenberg, H.: Defekt von Femur und Fibula mit Amelie, Peromelie oder ulnaren Strahldefekten der Arme, Humangenetik 3:244, 1967.
40. Strassmann, E. O.: Strassmann operation for double uterus. A fifty-year experience, Obst. & Gynec. 10:701, 1957.
41. Frankel, O.: Tube, in Henke, F., and Lubarsch, O. (eds.), *Handbuch der Speziellen Pathologischen Anatomie und Histologie* (Berlin: J. Springer, 1930), Vol. VII.
42. McNalley, F. P.: The association of congenital diverticula of the Fallopian tube with tubal pregnancy, Am. J. Obst. & Gynec. 12:303, 1926.
43. Schoenholz, L.: Untersuchungen über die Ursachen der Eileiterschwangerschaft, Arch. Gynäk. 127:609, 1926.
44. Ekler, R.: Gravidität in einer Nebentube, Arch. Gynäk. 113:1920.
45. Stern, A. M., Gall, J. C., Jr., Perry, B. L., Stimson, C. W., Weitkamp, L. R., and Poznanski, A. K.: The hand-foot-uterus syndrome, J. Pediat. 77:109, 1970.
46. Fisher, J. J.: Surgical unification of a double uterus, Am. J. Obst. & Gynec. 81:807, 1961.
47. Falls, F. H.: Pregnancy in the bicornuate uterus, Am. J. Obst. & Gynec. 72:1243, 1956.

Other Anomalies of the Female Genitalia

Duplication of External Genitalia

According to Lister,[1] duplication of the vulva was first recorded in 1552, but 400 years later only 10 cases could be found in the medical literature. Some of these were combined with serious congenital malformations, such as imperforate anus or duplication of the large intestine, so that the infants did not survive. Only 2 of the 10 cases were in adults. Duplication of the genitourinary tract and of the anus was discussed by Smith.[48]

Double vulva with duplication of both lower extremities has been observed[2] and it has occurred together with double vagina and uterus didelphys. Incomplete duplication of female external genitalia with double clitoris was reported by Kurth.[3] There was an accessory papillary structure to the right of apparently normal but obliquely placed, non-midline genitalia. This peculiar anomaly was seen in a child with an incomplete pelvic ring, lumbosacral spina bifida, mild hydrocephaly, probable absence of the right kidney, thoracic hemivertebrae, scoliosis and mental retardation. The sex chromatin was positive.

The case described by Lister[1] was that of an infant who died in the neonatal period owing to cardiac malformations. There were two vulvae, each with labia minora and majora. Only one urethral opening was present on the right side. There were two vaginae. There was a double uterus on the left side and a single uterus on the right. The large bowel was duplicated. Three lumbar vertebrae were cleft. Double vulva with duplication of vagina, uterus and bladder was described by Gemmell and Paterson[4] in a woman 37 years of age who was in labor with her first child.

Double vagina without duplication of the vulva occurs more often than duplication of the external genitalia. It is part of the anomaly known as uterus didelphys, which sometimes is discovered in adults at the time of pregnancy. Double uterus, vagina and rectum may manifest itself earlier because of fecal incontinence and impaction.[5]

Duplication of the clitoris ("diphallus in the female") is of importance because it probably is an epispadias and related to exstrophy of the bladder. The major labia may diverge anteriorly and the pelvis be split.[6]

The fact that partial duplication of the labia minora was described in trisomy 13-15[7] deserves to be mentioned.

Vulvar Fusion

This anomaly is considered of prenatal origin by some[8] and postnatal by others. Nowlin *et al.*,[9] who observed 110 cases within 14 years, stated that the condition was seen only once at birth. The vulva appeared normal at birth in 57 cases in which fusion was diagnosed later during childhood. Inflammatory processes are thought to be responsible for the concrescence of the labia minora, whereas the labia majora are not affected. The clitoris may be covered or there may be a small subclitoric orifice through which urine can be passed. Many cases of this type have been erroneously diagnosed as hermaphrodism or pseudohermaphrodism but when the labia minora are separated, normal female genitalia are found. According to Nowlin *et al.*,[9] the anomaly is not associated with other congenital malformations, but lack of proper urinary drainage leading to infection can result in renal damage. Treatment consists of separation of the labia minora manually or by blunt dissection, but recurrence is not rare.

The Vagina

When the blind ends of the Müllerian ducts make contact with the urogenital sinus, a solid cord of cells – the vaginal bulb – develops. This is a structure of indefinite origin, which was thought to be derived from the Müllerian ducts, the mesonephric ducts or the urogenital sinus. Also, it is not clear whether the solid vaginal bulb forms the entire vagina or only its lower portion. According to Bremer,[10] both comparative embryology and teratology indicate that the entire vagina is derived from the urogenital sinus. Rectovaginal fistulae can best be understood by the assumption that they result from sinu-rectal fistulae representing remnants of the cloaca; otherwise, it would be difficult to explain such fistulae, since the Müllerian ducts reach the urogenital sinus after division of the cloaca. If a fistula met the sinus in the region of the vaginal bulb, it could be carried by its growth onto the vagina and transformed into a rectovaginal fistula. In the same way, an ectopic ureter opening into the vagina could best be explained by considering the vagina as a part of the urogenital sinus into which the ureters normally open.

The vagina remains solid until late in fetal life. Formation of the lumen begins near the fornices and spreads downward, but at the lower end the irregular channel opening forms the hymen. If the channel does not reach the surface in the vulva, an imperforate hymen persists, which results in pathologic conditions such as hydrometrocolpos or hematocolpos.

Congenital Absence of the Vagina

The incidence of this anomaly is not known, as estimates vary greatly.[11] Bryan *et al.*[12] observed 1 case in every 4,000 female patients at the Mayo Clinic and reported on 100 cases. Absence of the vagina can be a symptom of various disorders, which usually are classified according to associated anomalies, endocrine symptoms or etiologic background. No final classification exists at this time, since recent cytogenetic advances have not yet been applied to all cases. Older observations still pertinent in most respects lack laboratory data. In the past, many cases were not recognized or did not come to the attention of physicians. The anomaly is the result of faulty development of the Müllerian ducts or faulty canalization of the vaginal primordia. The external genitalia usually appear normal except for absence of a vaginal introitus. In some cases, a shallow pouch representing the lower portion of the vagina is present. It is understandable that the anomaly, which causes few symptoms, often is overlooked during childhood, since amenorrhea is the presenting symptom. In 1949, Bryan *et al.*[12] thought that the tubes, ovaries or uterus usually are hypoplastic but that some ovarian tissue probably was present in most of the patients, since their secondary sexual characteristics often were normal. On laparotomy, the uterus was found to be bicornuate, unicornuate or absent. In the latter case, the tubes and ovaries could be present. In about one-third of the patients, pelvic kidneys, solitary kidneys, fused kidney, duplication of ureter or renal pelvis and other anomalies were noted. Spina bifida, hemivertebrae and irregularities of the ribs were occasional findings.[11,12] Absence or incomplete development of the uterus often is combined with absence of the vagina. Vaginal aplasia was combined with poorly developed Müllerian derivatives in 12 cases examined by laparotomy by Philipp.[13] The uterine rudiments seen were bilateral horns of the size of a bean without a lumen. Sometimes an immature reduplication of the uterus or only one horn of the uterus was found. The ovaries were normal and secondary sex characteristics were developed. Rarely, absence of the vagina was combined with normal internal genitalia, resulting in blockage of menstrual discharge, hematometra and hematosalpinx. Amenorrhea was considered a manifestation of absence or deficiency of the uterus.

Azoury and Jones[14] examined 12 patients with congenital absence of the vagina cytogenetically. The patients presented themselves because of primary amenorrhea; they had well-developed breasts, normal pubic hair and normal external genitalia. Some had a uterus with anomalous or absent vagina, others had absence of the uterus and vagina and a third group had a combination of these anomalies with other congenital malformations, such as rectovaginal fistula, imperforate anus, renal malrotation and malposition, fusion of cervical vertebrae and others. Of special interest was one woman with webbed neck, deafness, horseshoe kidney situated in the pelvis and a small vaginal pouch. Ovaries and tubes were normal but there was no uterus. All 12 patients had normal 46,XX karyotype! In 1968, Leduc *et al.*[15] reviewed 25 cases seen in a hospital during a 20-year period. Complete physical and laparotomy data were obtained in 14 cases. Of these, 2 were male pseudohermaphrodites and 12 were females with ovaries. There were 2 patients with "pure" vaginal absence and endometriosis. The majority (10) had tubes and uterine rudiments in the form of bilateral, noncanalized, muscular buds or single median buds with normal female sex characteristics, normal endocrine function and 46,XX karyotype. This anomaly, once called "uterus bipartitus solidus rudimentarius cum vagina solida" is now termed, somewhat shorter, the "Rokitansky-Küster-Hauser" syndrome. It can be recognized in the descriptions of other authors[12,13,15] who dealt with vaginal agenesis. The important point is that this syndrome seems to be part of a complex of congenital malformations occurring in females with 46,XX karyotype. Single kidney, bifid ureter, scoliosis, pectus excavatum, syndactyly and situs inversus were associated anomalies among patients of Leduc *et al.*[15] It has long been known that renal anomalies are frequent in women with vaginal agenesis. Pelvic kidney, solitary kidney, horseshoe kidney and ureteric and pelvic duplications had been reported.[16] Phelan *et al.*[11] found significant anomalies of the urinary tract in one-fourth of their patients with vaginal agenesis and Thompson *et al.*[27] in 8 of 17. Miller and Stout[17] recognized single kidney in 8 of 71 patients. Every case of vaginal agenesis should be examined for renal anomalies. Ferrier *et al.*[18] described a child with absent vagina, urethral opening and urogenital sinus; the karyotype was 46,XX. Associated malformations were noted in the face and in the renal and intestinal tracts. The anus was imperforate.

The etiology of these malformations, which occur in patients with 46,XX karyotype, is not known. Only in two instances were sisters involved. Bryan *et al.*[12] obtained negative family histories in 96 cases, but 1 patient had a sister with the same anomaly. Auger *et al.*[19] reported on 3 sisters with a Rokitansky-Küster-Hauser syndrome; no other familial cases are known.[15]

Some female or apparently female patients without vagina can be pseudohermaphrodites or hermaphrodites. Although such cases are numerous in the medical literature, they represent a minority in reports of serial examinations.[14,15]

In female pseudohermaphrodism due to congenital adrenal hyperplasia, the external genitalia can be variously affected. In the first case described by de Crecchio[20] in 1865, the clitoris was markedly enlarged, measuring 6 cm., the urinary meatus was at the base of the penis and the vagina seemed to open into the urethra, measuring 6.5 cm. in length. Jones and Scott[21] based their description of the genitalia of this anomaly on a study of 33 patients. The external urinary meatus was found most often at the base of the phallus but sometimes it extended to its end, where a glans penis and a prepuce were present, as in the male. There was a median perineal raphe, formed by scroto-labial folds in which no gonads could be felt. A vaginal opening was not always found externally but cystoscopy revealed an opening on the floor of the urethra several centimeters from the vesical orifice representing the distal end of the vagina. The vaginal size and length differed. The common urethrovaginal canal opening onto the perineum represented a urogenital sinus. If prenatal virilization was less progressed, there were separate urethral and vaginal openings.[21] Similar external genital changes may exist in female pseudohermaphrodites without adrenal disorders. Uterus, tubes and ovaries are normally formed. The vagina may be absent in female pseudohermaphrodites who are masculinized by a maternal virilizing tumor or by androgens or progestins administered to the mother during pregnancy. The internal genitalia are female in such children and there are no renal anomalies.

Another group of female pseudohermaphrodites cannot be attributed to known etiologic factors. Franks and Northcutt[22] described a girl with absent vagina, underdeveloped labia and clitoral enlargement. At operation, absence of the uterus, normal Fallopian tubes and fibrotic-appearing ovaries were noted. There also was bladder neck obstruction, duplication of the right urinary collecting system and hydro-ureter on the left. The sex chromatin was positive and the karyotype female. Other cases of the same type were reviewed by these authors.

In male pseudohermaphrodites with partial external feminization, absence of the vagina may be a presenting symptom. A case was described by Cooper and Hernits[23] of a patient with XY sex chromosomes and an asymmetry of the no. 1 chromosome pair.

A small vagina and "fetal uterus" can occur in male pseudohermaphrodites. Enlargement of the clitoris but otherwise female external genitalia result in an ambiguous picture. Boczkowski *et al.*[24] reported a patient with 46,XY karyotype who had in place of the ovaries whitish streaks that contained elements of gonadal dysgenesis. Another case of male pseudohermaphrodism was diagnosed in a child with multiple congenital malformations reminiscent of trisomy 13-15.[18] There was a large clitoris, a urogenital sinus and a small vagina and uterus. The gonads located at the normal site of the ovaries were poorly organized testes and the genetic constitution was 46,XY. Similar ambiguous external genitalia with a small vagina can occur in the presence of one testis and an XO karyotype.[25] Among the 14 cases of vaginal agenesis investigated by Leduc *et al.*,[15] there were 2 male pseudohermaphrodites with testes containing Leydig and Sertoli cells but no germinal layers. One patient had female breast development and no axillary or pubic hair; he represented a case of testicular feminization. The second patient was masculinized as evidenced by a hypertrophic clitoris and hirsutism.

Atresia of the vagina can occur with the disease picture of trisomy 18.[26]

Surgical construction of a vagina has been attempted successfully in many cases.[16,27] More recent discussions of surgical techniques were given by Leduc *et al.*,[15] Ulfelder[28] and Cali and Pratt.[29]

Transverse Vaginal Septa

Transverse septa occur at various sites in the vagina. The congenital forms can be explained as remnants of the solid stage that is present in embryos in both components of the vagina, the uterovaginal process and the vaginal plate. Failure of canalization of the vaginal plate or lack of union of the two vaginal primordia – urogenital sinus and Müllerian derivatives – can be considered as possible origins of transverse vaginal septa. Low septa resulting in hematocolpos and hematometra sometimes are taken for imperforate hymens. But in some of the cases the septa are not complete, so that menstruation need not be affected. Septa at more proximal sites result in a short vagina, ending as an apparently blind pouch with the cervix palpable beyond the septum. The external genitalia can be normal. Complications by bicornuate uterus and double cervix[30] or by urethrovaginal fistula[31] have been described.

Congenital Hydrometrocolpos

This anomaly is the result of an obstructive septum of the lower vagina or of an imperforate hymen combined with hypersecretion above the obstructed area. The combination results in cystic dilatation of the vagina and uterus by retained nonsanguineous secretions.[32] The congenital type is rather rare, in contrast to hematocolpos, in which the vaginal obstruction with retained menstrual blood manifests itself after puberty. Uterus duplex may be associated with the anomaly. The cystic enlargement can fill the entire pelvis and the lower abdomen and compression of the ureters may result in hydro-ureters and hydronephrosis.[32]

A low abdominal mass is the most common finding and this often is combined with a bulging mass in the vulva. Urinary retention, with pyuria, diarrhea, constipation and swelling of the vulva or lower extremities are among the symptoms that can be noted within the first weeks or months of life. Roentgenography aids in the diagnosis and cure can be obtained by evacuation of the distended vagina.[33] Mallet *et al.*[34] reported 2 newborn children with hydrocolpos, duplication of the vagina and ipsilateral renal agenesis. Manifestations were delayed several weeks after birth. Vaginography helped in the diagnosis. Hydrometrocolpos with absence of a vaginal opening was reported by Yu *et al.*[35]

In 1962, Spence[49] reviewed the literature on congenital hydrometrocolpos. Only 68 cases had then been reported, including 4 of the author's. The occurrence of familial cases is therefore a noteworthy occurrence. Two sibships each with 2 cases of congenital hydrometrocolpos were observed among Amish people in Pennsylvania and in Ohio. The parents of these siblings could be traced to one ancestral couple born in the eighteenth century. The anomaly was considered by McKusick *et al.*[36] as a simple autosomal recessive trait. It should be stated that hydrometrocolpos was only one striking manifestation of a more complicated hereditary trait. In all patients, the opening of the urethra lay high in the anterior vaginal wall and, in one case, imperforate anus and rectovaginal fistula were associated malformations.

Hematocolpos with Imperforate Hymen

Imperforate hymen can be congenital and due to failure of degeneration of central epithelial cells of the hymenal membrane; some cases may be the result of inflammatory processes before or after birth. If the vagina and the uterus are not distended by estrogen-induced secretions at the time of birth, the imperforate hymen may remain symptomless to the age of puberty, when collection of menstrual material results in enlargement of the vaginal tract, causing pelvic or abdominal pain. It is of historical interest that this condition was known to Aristotle and mentioned in his treatise on the *Generation of Animals:* "We know of instances of women in whom the 'os uteri' was grown together and continued so until the time arrived for the menstrual discharge to begin and pain come on; in some the passage burst open of its own accord, in others, it was separated by physicians; and in some cases, where the opening either was forcibly made or could not be made at all, the patients succumbed."[37]

Approximately two-thirds of the cases become manifest before the age of 15 years. A cystic mass is formed by enlargement of the vagina and uterus that can extend above the symphysis and into the abdominal cavity. Abdominal pain is a regular symptom and urinary difficulties may develop. Examination of the external genitalia reveals a mass protruding between the labia majora. The bulging mass is variable in size, bluish red in color and continuous with the pelvic mass. Constipation results in some of the cases. Following incision of the hymen, thick, darkly colored fluid escapes from the cavities. Infection must be prevented following hymenotomy, since the residual fluid is an excellent culture medium for microorganisms.[38,39]

Double Vagina and Septate Vagina

It seems that double vagina with separate mucosal and muscular layers is a very rare malformation, whereas septate vagina is rather common. But differentiation of the two types is not always easy. In 1966, Samarrae[40] could find only 3 cases in the literature. He added the case of a female girl with double vulva, urethra and bladder. In addition, one can cite a case illustrated by Potter[41] of exstrophy of the bladder with separation of cervix and vagina; and Huffman[42] showed the picture of a double vulva that was associated with uterus didelphys and double vagina. A septate vagina can be complete or partial, i.e., from the cervix down or from the hymen up. It is commonly associated with septate or bicornuate uterus. Brown and Nelson[43] reported on uterus didelphys and double vagina, with delivery of a normal infant from each uterus. Other cases of double vagina were mentioned on page 1089.

Congenital Vaginal Cysts

In the newborn period, vaginal cysts can be located posterior to the urethral meatus at the vaginal introitus arising from the anterior or lateral wall of the vagina and lined by squamous epithelium. Usually they do not cause pathologic manifestation and can rupture spontaneously or they disappear after surgical aspiration and removal of a milky white fluid. Occasionally, the cysts grow large enough to obstruct the urethra, causing urinary retention. Operative removal is indicated in such cases. Cysts in the caudal portion of the vagina probably are derived from the epithelium of the urogenital sinus and formed during the last months of gestation. In younger fetuses, multiple cysts can occur in proximal parts of the vagina. They have been considered derivatives of epithelia of the Müllerian or Wolffian ducts.[44]

Vaginal Fistulae

Rectovaginal fistulae often—but not always—are associated with imperforate anus. They may enter the posterior vaginal wall at any site but they open most often into the fourchette. Urethrovaginal fistulae opening into the anterior wall of the vagina are rare. Fistulous communications between the hindgut and neighboring organs are present in more than half of the patients with imperforate anus. Of 70 such cases reported by Moore and Lawrence,[45] 39 occurred in females and 29 had rectovaginal fistulae. The communications may be small and, in the newborn, plugged by thick meconium; or they can be sufficiently large to permit complete bowel evacuation. The true condition—opening of the bowel into the vagina—may go unnoticed for decades. If recognized, surgical intervention can be delayed for many years until complicating problems arise. Pregnancy represents difficulties, since in such cases vaginal delivery carries risks of postpartum infection and loss of sphincter control. In 1932, Potts[46] reported a case of "atresia ani vaginalis" and reviewed the literature. Several of the patients were unaware of their anomaly until labor occurred. Millar and Black[47] described a primigravida 38 years of age delivered by cesarean section to avoid damage to the pelvic floor muscles, which had provided bowel control.

Urethrovaginal fistulae sometimes are associated with female pseudohermaphrodism. In a case reported by Hightower,[31] the urethra opened into the anterior wall of a vagina that apparently ended in a blind pouch without a cervix. Actually, the vagina was occluded by a transverse septum perforated by a narrow fistula between the uterus and the vagina.

REFERENCES

1. Lister, U. M.: Double vulva, J. Obst. & Gynaec. Brit. Emp. 60:552, 1953.
2. Gould, G. M., and Pyle, W. L.: *Anomalies and Curiosities of Medicine* (Philadelphia: W. B. Saunders Company, 1897).
3. Kurth, M. E.: Incomplete duplication of the female external genitalia or double clitoris, Am. J. Surg. 96:596, 1958.
4. Gemmell, J. E., and Paterson, A. M.: Duplication of bladder, uterus, vagina and vulva, with successive full time pregnancy and labour in each uterus, J. Obst. &. Gynaec. Brit. Emp. 23:25, 1913.
5. Ladd, W. E., and Chisholm, T. C.: Double uterus, vagina and rectum, Am. J. Dis. Child. 66:629, 1943.
6. Jeffcoate, T. N. A.: A case of diphallus in the female, J. Obst. & Gynaec. Brit. Emp. 59:406, 1952.
7. Marin-Padilla, M., Hoefnagel, D., and Benirschke, K.: Anatomic and histopathologic study of two cases of D_1 (13-15) trisomy, Cytogenetics 3:258, 1964.
8. Campbell, M. F.: Vulvar fusion, J.A.M.A. 115:513, 1940.
9. Nowlin, P., Adams, J. R., and Nalle, B. C., Jr.: Vulvar fusion, J. Urol. 62:75, 1949.
10. Bremer, J. L.: *Congenital Anomalies of the Viscera. Their Embryological Basis* (Cambridge, Mass.: Harvard University Press, 1957).
11. Phelan, J. T., Counseller, V. S., and Greene, L. F.: Deformities of the urinary tract with congenital absence of the vagina, Surg., Gynec. & Obst. 97:1, 1953.
12. Bryan, A. L., Nigro, J. A., and Counseller, V. S.: One hundred cases of congenital absence of the vagina, Surg., Gynec. & Obst. 88:79, 1949.
13. Philipp, E.: Die primäre Amenorrhoe, Arch. Gynäk. 183: 247, 1953.
14. Azoury, R. S., and Jones, H. W., Jr.: Cytogenetic finding in patients with congenital absence of the vagina, Am. J. Obst. & Gynec. 94:178, 1966.
15. Leduc, B., van Campenhout, J., and Simard, R.: Congenital absence of the vagina. Observations on 25 cases, Am. J. Obst. & Gynec. 100:512, 1968.
16. Counseller, V. S.: Congenital absence of the vagina, J.A.M.A. 136:861, 1948.
17. Miller, N. F., and Stout, W.: Congenital absence of the vagina, Obst. & Gynec. 9:48, 1957.
18. Ferrier, P., Widgren, S., and Ferrier, S.: Nonspecific pseudohermaphroditism. Report of two cases with cytogenetic investigations, Helvet. paediat. acta 19:1, 1964.
19. Auger, D., Hemet, J., and Ensel, J.: Familial form of Rokitansky-Kuster-Hauser syndrome, Bull. Féd. soc. gynec. et obst. 18:229, 1966.
20. de Crecchio: Cited by Neugebauer, F. L., *Hermaphroditismus beim Menschen* (Leipzig: W. Klinkhardt, 1908).
21. Jones, H. W., and Scott, W. W.: *Hermaphroditism, Genital Anomalies and Related Endocrine Disorders* (Baltimore: The Williams & Wilkins Company, 1958).
22. Franks, R. C., and Northcutt, R.: Female pseudohermaphroditism and renal anomalies, Am. J. Dis. Child. 105: 490, 1963.
23. Cooper, H. L., and Hernits, R.: A familial chromosome variant in a subject with anomalous sex differentiation, Am. J. Human Genet. 15:465, 1963.
24. Boczkowski, K., Philip, J., and Teter, K.: A case of gonadal dysgenesis in a patient with a 46/XY karyotype, phallic enlargement and absence of seminiferous tubules, Acta endocrinol. 47:491, 1964.
25. Atkins, L., and Engel, E.: Absence of the Y chromosome (XO sex-chromosome constitution) in a human intersex with an extra-abdominal testis, Lancet 2:20, 1962.
26. Wolf, U., Reinwein, H., and Schröter, R.: Bericht über vier Trisomien 18 und ein Trisomie-18-Mosaik, Humangenetik 1:232, 1965.
27. Thompson, J. D., Wharton, L. R., and TeLinde, R. W.: Congenital absence of the vagina, Am. J. Obst. & Gynec. 74:397, 1957.
28. Ulfelder, H.: Agenesis of the vagina, Am. J. Obst. & Gynec. 100:745, 1968.
29. Cali, R. W., and Pratt, J. H.: Congenital absence of the vagina. Long-term results of vaginal reconstruction in 175 cases, Am. J. Obst. & Gynec. 100:752, 1968.
30. Bowman, J. A., and Scott, R. B.: Transverse vaginal septum, Obst. & Gynec. 3:441, 1954.
31. Hightower, C. C.: Case of congenital anomaly of the female urethra and vagina, Obst. & Gynec. Surv. 1:135, 1946.
32. Lide, T. N., and Coker, W. G.: Congenital hydrometrocolpos: Review of the literature and report of a case with uterus duplex and incompletely septate vagina, Am. J. Obst. & Gynec. 64:1275, 1952.
33. Klostermyer, L. L., and Thompson, J. J.: Radiographic diagnosis of hydrocolpos in infants, Radiology 58:100, 1952.
34. Mallet, R., Ribierre, M., Labrune, B., and Lozier, E.: Les hydrocolpos du nouveau-né avec duplicité vaginale et agénésie rénale homolatérale, Ann. pédiat. 49:2144, 1966.
35. Yu, S. F., Murugesu, J. J., and Chan, K. Y.: An unusual case of neonatal hydrometrocolpos, Am. J. Roentgenol. 100:186, 1967.
36. McKusick, V. A., Bauer, R. L., Koop, C. E., and Scott, R. B.: Hydrometrocolpos as a simply inherited malformation, J.A.M.A. 189:813, 1964.
37. Aristotle: *Generation of Animals.* English translation by Peck, A. L. (Cambridge, Mass.: Harvard University Press, 1943).
38. Calvin, J. K., and Nichamin, S. J.: Hematocolpos due to imperforate hymen, Am. J. Dis. Child. 51:832, 1936.
39. Warner, R. E., and Mann, R. M.: Hematocolpos with imperforate hymen; report of five cases, Obst. & Gynec. 6: 405, 1955.
40. Samarrae, K.: A case of double vulva, vagina, urethra and bladder, J. Obst. & Gynaec. Brit. Commonwealth 73: 156, 1966.
41. Potter, E. L.: *Pathology of the Fetus and Infant* (2d ed.; Chicago: Year Book Medical Publishers, Inc., 1961).
42. Huffman, J. W.: *The Gynecology of Childhood and Adolescence* (Philadelphia: W. B. Saunders Company, 1968).
43. Brown, D. C., and Nelson, R. F.: Uterus didelphys and double vagina with delivery of a normal infant from each uterus, Canad. M.A.J. 96:675, 1967.
44. Vilas, E.: Cysten in der Scheide von Feten, Arch. Gynäk. 158:1, 1934.
45. Moore, T. C., and Lawrence, E. A.: Congenital malformations of the rectum and anus. Clinical features and surgical management in 120 cases, Surgery 32:352, 1952.
46. Potts, J. E.: Atresia ani vaginalis, Am. J. Obst. & Gynec. 23:892, 1932.
47. Millar, W. G., and Black, W. P.: Pregnancy complicated by imperforate anus with congenital recto-vaginal fistula, J. Obst. & Gynaec. Brit. Emp. 62:441, 1955.
48. Smith, E. D.: Duplication of the anus and genitourinary tract, Surgery 66:909, 1969.
49. Spence, H. M.: Congenital hydrocolpos, J.A.M.A. 180: 1100, 1962.

110

Male Genitalia

The Testes

Absence of the Testes (Congenital Anorchia and Monorchia)

REPORTS ON ANORCHIA are relatively scarce. Sohval and Soffer[1] quoted a case of historical interest, recorded in 1564, of a soldier hanged for rape whose postmortem examination failed to disclose testes in the scrotum or abdomen. Counseller and Walker[2] found 9 acceptable cases in the literature up to 1933 and added 2 of their own. In 1938, Rea[3] collected 29 instances from the literature and added 6 probable cases encountered during operations for apparent cryptorchidism. In more than 10,000 necropsies in boys, Campbell[4] reported bilateral absence of the testes in 26 cases and unilateral absence in 8. In most of the unilateral cases, the testis found was intra-abdominal. Bilateral anorchia also was present in identical twins, dead at 12 hours.

Anorchia may be the only anomaly or there may be, in addition, absence of the epididymis, vas deferens or the entire spermatic tract. Anal atresia, rectourethral and rectovesical fistula, exstrophy of the bladder or absence of the external genitalia may be associated malformations.[1] Campbell[4] mentioned cases combined with horseshoe kidney, Meckel diverticulum, mongolism, congenital heart disease, cleft lip and palate, polydactyly and others. The clinical picture depends on the age of the patient. In young children, hormonal insufficiency is not apparent, but in adults the typical symptoms and signs of eunuchoidism have been described.[1] If no testicle is found at operation, anorchia cannot be considered established, since not all the possible sites can be explored. Williams[5] pointed out that the diagnosis can be made in certain cases when the vas deferens can be traced down into the scrotum, ending in the epididymis without a testicle detectable in the scrotum, the inguinal canal or the pelvis. The karyotype of these patients is XY.[6,7] This and the fact that male ducts are present in most of these patients suggests prenatal destruction of the testes that were formed originally.

A syndrome of anorchia, chest deformities, bronchial anomalies, hypoplasia of muscles and subcutaneous fat and severe mental retardation has been observed in 3 brothers.[52] Anorchia was present in "sisters" described by Overzier and Linden[48] as cases of true agonadism. They reviewed other cases of this type recorded in the literature. Testes could not be found at laparotomy in boys considered male Turner patients by Becker[49] and Heller.[50]

Absence of the testes can be due to the action of an exogenous teratogen, as shown by anorchia observed together with malformations produced by thalidomide.[32]

Undescended Testes (Cryptorchidism)

The testes develop from the genital ridges located on the ventral border of the mesonephros and extending between the diaphragmatic and sacral areas. As the caudal end of the body enlarges, the testes assume a more caudal position until they arrive above the inguinal region at about the fifth month of gestation. The testes are closely connected with mesodermal fibrous strands, the ligamenta or gubernacula testis, which connect them to the ventral body wall. There, the scrotum is first seen in the third month as an eminence that develops later in fetal life into a pouch with peritoneal lining. As the scrotum enlarges, the peritoneal lining becomes the elongated processus vaginalis, which is connected with the peritoneal cavity by a long and thin neck. Toward the end of intrauterine life, the testis descends into the scrotum, where it usually arrives about the time of birth. It develops and remains in an extraperitoneal position, being covered by the visceral layer of the processus vaginalis. With the descent of the testis into the scrotum, the gubernaculum is reduced in length, the cavity of the processus vaginalis is narrowed to a slit and its elongated neck becomes obliterated.

The development and the closure of the processus vaginalis is not always perfectly coordinated with the descent of the testis, so that several types of anomaly can develop. If the neck of the processus vaginalis remains open, inguinal hernias can develop. The closure may be irregular and the remaining spaces expanded to cysts along the course of the spermatic cord. If the processus vaginalis is filled with fluid, a hydrocele is formed. A hydrocele is irreducible if fluid accumulates in a tunica vaginalis that is sealed off.

In the case of an open processus vaginalis, the hydrocele is reducible or shows spontaneous variation in size.

If the testes remain in the pelvic cavity or above the inguinal ring, one speaks of cryptorchidism or undescended testes. Ectopia testis is present if the testis does not reach the scrotum but passes either into the thigh (femoral ectopia), to the penile base, to the perineum or to the contralateral inguinal canal (transverse ectopia). The most frequent aberration is interstitial ectopia, in which the testis lies on the aponeurosis of the external oblique muscle.[4]

At the time of birth, both testes are still undescended in more than 3% of all full-term boys and in 30% of male prematures. In more than 50% of the full-term boys with delayed descent, the testes reach the scrotum during the first month of life.[8] After the end of the first year, about 1% of male children have undescended testes but there is much disagreement concerning the prevalence of cryptorchidism in older children and adults. It is certain and important to know that a very marked reduction in the frequency of undescended testes, unilateral and bilateral, occurs in the age groups of 11 years to 14–17 years.[9] In male adults, approximately 0.3% have cryptorchidism.[4,5,9] Many children with apparently undescended testes have retracting testes that cannot be palpated easily on superficial examination. The frequency of cryptorchidism in necropsies of boys is approximately 3%.[4] This relatively high frequency can be explained by the assumption that in these cases concomitant anomalies caused death, so that in this abnormal material cryptorchidism was relatively frequent. Only about 20% of the cases of undescended testes are bilateral. Right-sided cryptorchidism is found in 50% and left-sided in 30% of the cases. Of 879 cryptorchid testes operated on by Gross,[10] 94% were undescended, 4% absent and 2% perineal.

The mechanisms leading to cryptorchidism are poorly understood. Many mechanical causes, such as absence or smallness of the external inguinal ring, a narrow canal, shortness of the blood vessels of the spermatic cord and others, have been cited. Endocrine factors play a role. It is known that in many patients with endocrine disturbances cryptorchidism is a symptom. Conversely, adolescence, with its hormonal changes, often leads to descent of testes located in a higher position before that period. Retracted testes can be moved into the scrotum by administration of gonadotropic hormones but they return to their former position in many instances.

Many adverse factors can interfere with normal descent of the testes. Hereditary influences sometimes are demonstrated in kindreds in which undescended testes occur in several generations[11,12] or in families with several boys affected by unilateral or bilateral cryptorchidism.[13,14] In over-all surveys, approximately 4% of boys with cryptorchidism have a history of the condition occurring in relatives.[15] A special case is the cryptorchidism of feminizing testes, which is due to an inherited androgen resistance of tissues (p. 1114) and there exists a familial male pseudohermaphrodism that suggests autosomal recessive inheritance.[15]

Cryptorchidism can be concordant or discordant in monozygotic twins. Of 10 pairs, 7 showed concordance, suggesting genetic determination in their cases.[15]

Some cytogenetic entities manifest themselves by cryptorchidism. Whereas this anomaly is rare in XXY Klinefelter patients, it is frequent in more complex karyotypes such as XXXXY and mosaics thereof. Unilateral cryptorchidism can be a manifestation of asymmetric gonadal differentiation (p. 1137). This was the case in a boy observed by us with XXXY/XO constitution,[16] but this syndrome also occurs with different forms of mosaicism such as XO/XY, XO/XY/XX and others.[17] Klein *et al.*[15] reported a patient in whom cryptorchidism was the only physical sign of an XO/XY karyotype. Undescended testes can be associated with the XYY syndrome.[18] Renal agenesis, absence of testicular tissue in the presence of a phallus with centrally placed urethra can occur in infants with XX karyotype.[19] Hypogonadism and cryptorchidism was present in a boy with a presumptive Y/autosome translocation.[20] These examples do not exhaust the many karyotypes of multiple X chromosomes occurring in mosaics of different kinds that result in hypogonadism or cryptorchidism.[21]

Not only in children with abnormal sex chromosomes but also in boys with autosomal anomalies, descent of the testes often is not achieved. In more than 50% of male children with trisomy 13-15, cryptorchidism was mentioned in necropsy reports. The percentage was less impressive, although elevated, in boys with trisomy 18.[22] It has been stated[23] that in about 50% of boys with Down syndrome the testes are not descended at the time of birth; for older children, prevalence figures vary between 5%[24] and 20%.[25] In many other boys with autosomal abnormalities, cryptorchidism is present, as exemplified by cases with a ring D chromosome[26] or with 4/5 translocation.[27]

In a number of syndromes of known or unknown etiology, cryptorchidism is a frequent sign. It is almost always present in patients with abdominal muscular aplasia (p. 1026), with Prader-Willi syndrome (p. 182) and in boys with cleft lip and palate and popliteal pterygium (p. 643), in which it is combined with penile and scrotal anomalies. A syndrome of congenital absence of the right testis, kidney and rectus muscle has been noted in a male dizygotic twin.[28] Cryptorchidism occurs in a substantial number of patients with the male Turner (p. 1132), Lowe (p. 389), Marfan (p. 850), Laurence-Moon-Biedl (p. 176) and Fanconi (p. 1020) syndromes and in many children with intrauterine growth retardation (p. 134). Cryptorchidism and other genital anomalies play an important role in a syndrome of microcephaly, strabismus, short nose, micrognathia, syndactyly, transverse palmar creases, intrauterine growth retardation and failure to thrive.[29,30] Although the appearance of these children suggests a chromosomal abnormality, the karyotypes appear to be normal.

Damage by environmental factors must be considered. In boys with thalidomide embryopathy, cryptorchidism, absence of the scrotum or incomplete testicular descent was among less conspicuous manifestations.[31,32]

Cryptorchidism can be studied in animals but no specific gene has been found for undescended testes in small rodents. Undescended testes have been observed as a secondary symptom of several murine mutations, such as the ichthyotic mouse, the obese mouse and the pigmy mouse.[33] Undescended testes have been induced experimentally in the young of vitamin A-deficient rats.[34] In many male young with urogenital anomalies, the testes were arrested at some point along the course of the descent between their site of formation and the normal neonatal position in the inguinal region. Between the nineteenth and twenty-first days, the testes normally arrive in the pelvis to lie beside the bladder near the inguinal fossa. In the abnormal young, the testes were retained at various levels in the abdominal cavity. About half of them had remained at the site of origin. The urogenital folds persisted as broad connections between the gonads and the dorsal body wall and were not attenuated as the delicate ligaments usually seen in older rat fetuses. Migration of the gonads also was delayed frequently in folic acid-deficient fetuses[35] and in the young of rats treated with various teratogens.

Many boys with cryptorchidism have no disturbing symptoms. They are discovered on routine examination by physicians, or the parents notice that one or both testes are not located in the scrotum. In some cases, pain or development of a hernia leads to discovery of cryptorchidism. In obese boys, puberty often is delayed, the scrotum is poorly developed and the testes are retracted. In most of these children, the testes descend at a later date, together with signs of developing puberty. Cryptorchidism occurs in otherwise normal boys. The testes may be located at the external inguinal ring, at the proximal end of the inguinal canal or in the abdominal cavity.

True cryptorchidism commonly is associated with congenital inguinal hernia. The processus vaginalis remains patent or the inguinal canal is deformed. The epididymis often is elongated or not connected with the testis. Hypospadias, hypogonadism or pseudohermaphrodism may be present. In the last condition, the testes may lie on the ligamentum latum or near the uterus or Fallopian tube or be connected with the lateral pelvic wall by a short pedicle. Retroperitoneal location is possible also. Other conditions occasionally associated with cryptorchidism are hermaphrodism, renal agenesis, agenesis of the abdominal muscles, exstrophy of the bladder and many other severe malformations.[5] Urinary tract anomalies such as double ureters, renal hypoplasia or ectopia, hydronephrosis and others are present in approximately 12% of asymptomatic cryptorchid boys over the age of 2 years.[36]

Uncomplicated cryptorchidism is considered a cosmetic defect that may have adverse psychologic effects on the parents or the child. A testis located in the inguinal canal is more exposed to trauma than a scrotal testis. The concomitant hernia is a complication that may become acutely dangerous by incarceration or strangulation. Pain is attributed to torsion of the testis.[10]

It is assumed by some[37] that undescended testes are never entirely normal, although up to the age of 5 years the histologic appearance of normal and undescended testes does not differ greatly. After this age, retardation of development becomes noticeable in undescended testes. The normal growth of the spermatic tubules and formation of spermatogonia do not take place. Some growth and development of undescended testes occur during puberty but development is not normal. Although interstitial cells appear, many tubules remain immature, devoid of Sertoli cells and germ cells.[5] Moore and Quick[38] demonstrated that the temperature inside the scrotum is lower than the temperature in the peritoneal cavity. They believed that degeneration of seminiferous tubules in cryptorchid testes is due to exposure to a higher temperature in the abdominal cavity. According to these investigators, the scrotum is a thermal regulator for the testes, and normal spermatogenesis depends on a correct temperature. The possibility that undescended testes often have an inherent congenital defect was admitted, but it was thought[37] that by placing the testes in the scrotum, the chances for normal development are improved. But Farrington[51] found that the germinal-cell deficiency of the undescended testis is present from birth and is not significantly influenced by passing of childhood and adolescence. The question of malignant degeneration has led to much controversy. Approximately 11% of all testicular malignancies occur in undescended testes, so that it seems established that undescended testes are more inclined to malignant degeneration than scrotal testes. However, it is not established that this inclination depends on the position of the organ and that operation can avoid malignant degeneration.[37] Cancer may develop in testes after surgical placement in the scrotum.[21,39] A tendency to malignant degeneration seems to be inherent in some undescended testes, but development of cancer is not necessarily the result of their malposition. Testicular descent can be achieved in many cases by administration of gonadotropic hormones. The conventional treatment consists of injections of 500–1,000 units of chorionic gonadotropin twice weekly for 6 weeks. If, after such treatment, the testis appears in the scrotum, it proves that the organ is present, not firmly fixed in the abdomen and capable of descent. This result does not always represent the final status, since the testis may retract again after the treatment is discontinued. It is assumed by some that testes responding to hormonal therapy would descend before or at the time of puberty spontaneously, so that the procedure is not considered a treatment of true cryptorchidism. Injections of gonadotropic hormones can be used as a diagnostic test to demonstrate that a testis is capable of descent and that operation is not indicated. A modification of this test[37] recommended 4,000–5,000 units of gonadotropin for 3 days only, followed by operation if no change occurs within 1 week. It is assumed that the testis does not respond because of an abnormal external ring, absence of the testis or adherence of the fascia outside the external ring. Hormonal treatment of undescended testes is a harmless procedure if not given for a prolonged time. In rare instances, signs of precocious puberty or development of a hernia may complicate the treatment. On the other hand, demonstration of the testis, even though still retractile, can relieve the anxiety of the patient or his parents.

If the testis cannot be demonstrated by palpation or by hormonal treatment, operation usually is performed before puberty. Most surgeons recommend the operation at an age from 9 to 12 years, except in cases of hernias, which require earlier treatment. Orchidopexy treats the inguinal hernia and the undescended testis at the same time. The operation is delayed, if possible, to facilitate elongation of the vas deferens and the spermatic vessels with increasing age. In his large series in 1953, Gross[10] found absence of the testis in only 4% of the patients operated on. If no testes are present, laparotomy may be indicated to search for Müllerian duct derivatives and determination of sex.[5] Gross[10] stated that in about 90% of all patients operated on, a testis of apparently normal size and consistency could be placed into the scrotum. In the rest of the cases, the testis was small and underdeveloped at the time of operation, the organ became atrophied or it retracted after operation. The functional capacity is difficult to evaluate in unilateral, surgically treated cases because the contralateral normal organ is capable of producing spermatozoa and testicular hormones. It was thought that in cases of bilateral cryptorchidism, formation of spermatozoa is better in operated on than in untreated patients,[10] but this is not generally accepted.[40,41] Delay of operation until early puberty does not reduce fertility subsequently. It is obvious that evaluation of surgical results is difficult as long as benign cryptorchidism with a tendency to spontaneous descent is considered together with cases of endocrine and cytogenetic abnormalities. The results will depend on the composition of the sample. Although the surgical placement of a testis into the scrotum has little effect in changing the likelihood of subsequent malignant degeneration, operation is advantageous, since a tumor in the scrotum can be discovered earlier than one developing in the abdomen.[10] As stated before, it has not been proved that surgical placement of the testis into the scrotum reduces malignancy. It seems that testes placed into the scrotum still have an increased risk of becoming malignant.[21,39] It is doubtful that the tendency to malignancy of undescended feminizing testes (p. 1114) or of cryptorchidism due to cytogenetic anomalies[42] can be ascribed to the faulty position of the testis.

Testicular Intratubular Bodies

Unilateral cryptorchidism was described in 2 boys (4 and 6 years of age) whose descended testis showed spermatogenic precocity. Hypertelorism, a large head and polydactyly were present in both. The descended testis contained primary spermatocytes, which normally appear at 12–14 years of age. In the undescended testis, the tubules were small and contained small cells. In each testis, a larger tubule was seen containing a round body with a core, which, in turn, was surrounded by concentric rings of materials varying in density. The nature of this strange structure remained unexplained,[43] but its resemblance to oocytes has been emphasized. Although such bodies have been seen repeatedly in cryptorchid testes and in the testes of pseudohermaphrodites, they apparently are not specific and not indicative of serious disorders.[44]

Supernumerary Testes (Polyorchidism)

A third testicle may manifest itself as a swelling in the scrotum or the groin, where it can be mistaken for a hernia, hydrocele or spermatocele. Anderson[45] reported the case of a 19-year-old man who suddenly developed a painful swelling in the left groin. A strangulated inguinal hernia was diagnosed, but two testes, one of normal size and one small one, were found in the sac. There was no spermatogenesis but proliferation of spermatogonia was noted.

Smith *et al.*[46] described a supernumerary testis in the left scrotum of a man 75 years of age. The testis presented as a painless swelling, and biopsy of two masses found in the left scrotum showed atrophic testicular tissue. Hernias, spermatoceles or ectopic adrenal tissue can be mistaken for supernumerary testes. In cases of splenic-gonadal fusion, a splenic mass may be found attached to the left testis or epididymis. Such a mass must be differentiated from a supernumerary testis (p. 749). Rössler[47] reported a patient with seminoma of a supernumerary abdominal testis in a kindred with hereditary cryptorchidism.

Synorchidism

Fusion of both testes may occur within the scrotum or in the abdomen. Campbell[4] mentioned 2 cases of a solidly fused testicular mass located in the upper pelvis from which two epididymides, vasa deferentia and seminal vesicles originated. Solidly fused lump kidneys were present also. In another case of synorchidism, there was horseshoe kidney, myelomeningocele, scoliosis and fusion of ribs.

REFERENCES

1. Sohval, A. R., and Soffer, L. J.: Congenital familial testicular deficiency, Am. J. Med. 14:328, 1953.
2. Counseller, V. S., and Walker, M. A.: Congenital absence of testes (anorchia), Am. Surgeon 98:104, 1933.
3. Rea, C. E.: Congenital anorchia, with report of 6 probable cases of monorchia, Surgery 4:376, 1938.
4. Campbell, M.: *Clinical Pediatric Urology* (Philadelphia: W. B. Saunders Company, 1951).
5. Williams, D. I.: Urology in Childhood, in *Encyclopedia of Urology* (Berlin: Springer-Verlag, 1958), Vol. XV.
6. Van Wyk, J. J., and Grumbach, M. M.: Disorders of Sex Differentiation, in Williams, R. H. (ed.), *Textbook of Endocrinology* (4th ed.; Philadelphia: W. B. Saunders Company, 1968).
7. Milcou, St. M., Ionescu, B., Strihan, P., Iliescu, I., Augustin, M., and Maximilian, C.: L'anorchidie congénitale, Série d'embryol. 1:89, 1964 (Rev. Roumaine embryol. et cytol.).
8. Scorer, C. G.: The incidence of incomplete descent of the testicle at birth, Arch. Dis. Childhood 31:198, 1956.
9. Ward, B., and Hunter, W. M.: The absent testicle; a report on a survey carried out among schoolboys in Nottingham, Brit. M. J. 1110, 1960.
10. Gross, R. E.: *The Surgery of Infancy and Childhood* (Philadelphia: W. B. Saunders Company, 1953).
11. Wiles, P.: Family tree, showing hereditary undescended right testicle and associated deformities, Proc. Roy. Soc. Med. 28:157, 1934.
12. Lüscher, A.: Über 99 Fälle von Kryptorchism und deren Behandlung an der chirurgischen Abteilung des Kinderspitales Zürich in den Jahren 1928–1937. Thesis, Zürich, 1940.
13. Corbus, B. C., and O'Conor, V. J.: Familial occurrence of undescended testes; report of 6 brothers with testicular anomalies, Surg., Gynec. & Obst. 34:499, 1922.
14. Brimblecombe, S. L.: Bilateral cryptorchidism in three brothers, Brit. M. J. 1:526, 1946.
15. Klein, D., Ferrier, P., and Ammann, F.: La génétique de l'ectopie testiculaire, Path. et biol. 11:1214, 1963.
16. Warkany, J., Chu, E. H. Y., and Kauder, E.: Male pseudohermaphroditism and chromosomal mosaicism, Am. J. Dis. Child. 104:172, 1962.
17. Jeune, M., dePeretti, E., Mollard, P., Hermier, M., Laurent, C., and Couette, Y.: Différenciation testiculaire unilatérale (dysgénésie gonadique mixte), Pédiatrie 21:699, 1966.
18. Sandberg, A. A., Ishihara, T., Crosswhite, L. H., and Kopf, G. F.: XYY genotype. Report of a case in a male, New England J. Med. 268:585, 1963.
19. Schlegel, R. J., Aspillage, M. J., Neu, R. L., Carneiro-Leano, J., and Gardner, L. I.: An XX sex chromosome complement in an infant having male-type external genitals, renal agenesis, and other anomalies, J. Pediat. 69: 812, 1966.
20. Nakagome, Y., Smith, H. D., and Soukup, S. W.: A presumptive Y-autosome translocation in a boy with congenital malformations, Am. J. Dis. Child. 116:205, 1968.
21. Paulsen, C. A.: The Testes, in Williams, R. H. (ed.), *Textbook of Endocrinology* (4th ed.; Philadelphia: W. B. Saunders Company, 1968).
22. Warkany, J., Passarge, E., and Smith, L. B.: Congenital malformations in autosomal trisomy syndromes, Am. J. Dis. Child. 112:502, 1966.
23. Benda, C. E.: *The Child with Mongolism* (New York: Grune & Stratton, Inc., 1960).
24. Hanhart, E.: 800 Fälle von Mongoloidismus (Down-Syndrom) in konstitutioneller Betrachtung, Arch. Klaus Stift Vererbungsforsch. 35:1, 1960.
25. Rosinsky, O. E.: Der Kryptorchismus und seine Behandlung, Med. Klin. 38:843, 1942.
26. Reisman, L. E., Darnell, A., and Murphy, J. W.: Abnormalities with ring chromosome, Lancet 2:445, 1965.
27. Shaw, M. W., Cohen, M. M., and Hildebrandt, H. M.: A familial 4/5 reciprocal translocation resulting in partial trisomy B, Am. J. Human Genet. 17:54, 1965.
28. Texter, J. H., and Murphy, G. P.: The right-sided syndrome: Congenital absence of the right testis, kidney, and rectus. Urologic diagnosis and treatment, Bull. Johns Hopkins Hosp. 122:224, 1968.
29. Smith, D. W., Lemli, L., and Opitz, J. M.: A newly recognized syndrome of multiple congenital anomalies, J. Pediat. 64:210, 1964.
30. Pinsky, L., and DiGeorge, A. M.: A familial syndrome of facial and skeletal anomalies associated with genital abnormality in the male and normal genitals in the female, J. Pediat. 66:1049, 1965.
31. Kajii, T.: Thalidomide experience in Japan, Ann. paediat. 205:341, 1965.
32. Kreipe, U.: Missbildungen innerer Organe bei Thalidomidembryopathie, Arch. Kinderh. 176:33, 1967.
33. Nachtsheim, H.: Erbpathologie der Nagetiere, in *Pathologie der Laboratoriumstiere* (Berlin: Springer-Verlag, 1958).
34. Wilson, J. G., and Warkany, J: Malformations in the genitourinary tract induced by maternal vitamin A deficiency in the rat, Am. J. Anat. 83:357, 1948.
35. Monie, I. W., Nelson, M. M., and Evans, H. M.: Abnormalities of the urinary system of rat embryos resulting from transitory deficiency of pteroylglutamic acid during gestation, Anat. Rec. 127:711, 1957.
36. Grossman, H., and Ririe, D. G.: The incidence of urinary tract anomalies in cryptorchid boys, Am. J. Roentgenol. 103:210, 1968.
37. Robinson, J. N., and Engle, E. T.: Some observations on the cryptorchid testis, J. Urol. 71:726, 1954.
38. Moore, C. R., and Quick, W. J.: The scrotum as a temperature regulator for the testes, Am. J. Physiol. 68:70, 1924.
39. Gilbert, J. B.: Studies in malignant testis tumors: V. Tumors developing after orchidopexy, J. Urol. 46:740, 1941.
40. Charny, C. W., and Wolgen, W.: *Cryptorchidism* (New York: Paul B. Hoeber, Inc., 1957).
41. Charny, C. W.: Spermatogenic potential of undescended testis before and after therapy, J. Urol. 83:697, 1960.
42. Lewis, F. J. W., Mitchell, J. P., and Foss, G. L.: XY/XO mosaicism, Lancet 1:221, 1963.
43. Bunge, R. G., and Bradbury, J. T.: Two unilaterally cryptorchid boys with spermatogenic precocity in the descended testis, hypertelorism and polydactyly, J. Clin. Endocrinol. 19:1103, 1959.
44. Bieger, R. C., Passarge, E., and McAdams, A. J.: Testicular intratubular bodies, J. Clin. Endocrinol. 25:1340, 1965.
45. Anderson, P. St. G.: Case of polyorchidism, Lancet 1:826, 1953.
46. Smith, P. G., Evans, A., and Suder, G.: Polyorchism, J. Urol. 64:515, 1950.
47. Rössler, H. J.: Ein Beitrag zum familiären Vorkommen von Lageanomalien der Hoden und maligner Entartung, Zentralbl. Chir. 85:2160, 1960.
48. Overzier, C., and Linden, H.: Echter Agonadismus (Anorchismus) bei Geschwistern, Gynaecologia 142:215, 1956.
49. Becker, H. W.: Agonadismus mit kongenitalen Missbildungen beim Mann, Med. Welt 10:351, 1957.
50. Heller, R. H.: The Turner phenotype in the male, J. Pediat. 66:48, 1965.
51. Farrington, G. H.: Histologic observations in cryptorchidism: The congenital germinal-cell deficiency of the undescended testis, J. Pediat. Surg. 4:606, 1969.
52. Van Benthem, L. H., Driessen, O., Haneveld, G. T., and Rietema, H. P.: Cryptorchidism, chest deformities, and other congenital anomalies in three brothers, Arch. Dis. Childhood 45:590, 1970.

Other Anomalies of the Male Genitalia

Absence of External Male Genitalia

A VERY UNUSUAL CASE of congenital absence of the external genitalia was reported by Kirshbaum[1] in a monstrous child who had agenesis of the kidneys with characteristic facies (p. 1037), pulmonary hypoplasia with absence of both lower and right middle lobes, a primitive cloaca, imperforate anus, malformation of the vertebral column with spina bifida occulta and clubfeet. Ovaries and Fallopian tubes were present. In place of the external genitalia, a pigmented area was seen. The primitive cloaca with its incomplete division was comparable to that seen in lower mammals or in the human embryo younger than 7 weeks. The child lived only 24 hours.

Congenital Absence of the Penis

Congenital absence of the penis is a very rare malformation attributed to failure of development of the genital tubercle. The scrotum, the testes and the internal urinary tract may be normally developed but the corpora cavernosa are absent or rudimentary. The urethra opens between the two halves of a bifid scrotum, near the anal border, into the rectum or into a cloacal cavity. Survival is possible but the anomaly usually is seen at necropsies or in monsters. It was reported that the anomaly occurs once in 30 million persons[2] and twice in 16,000 necropsies.[3] In a premature child, absence of the penis was combined with absence of the prostate, urethra and anus. The child probably represented a form of sirenomelia.[2] Transposition of a rudimentary penis to the back has been reported in a sirenomelus.[4] In other instances of absence of the penis, associated malformations were anencephaly, accessory lobes of the ears, pigeon breast and clubfeet.[3] In case of survival, the abnormal urethra predisposes to renal infection and hydronephrosis.[3,5]

Micropenis

Micropenis or concealed penis occurs occasionally as an isolated anomaly in the presence of otherwise normal urogenital development. The penis may be concealed in the surrounding fat, the urethra being normal, angulated or stenotic.[3] In such cases, the obstruction must be relieved early to avoid disease of the upper urinary tract. Coitus may be difficult but procreation is possible, as demonstrated in a family in which micropenis occurred in three generations.[5] Micropenis and hypospadias can be combined. In small, obese children, a penis of normal size can appear very small because the organ is concealed by fat.

Congenital absence of the corpora cavernosa and the urethra was observed in a newborn child with imperforate anus, agenesis of the right kidney, hydronephrosis of the left kidney and other malformations. In an infant boy with meatus stenosis and dilatation of the entire anterior urethra, the corpora cavernosa were absent and the corpus spongiosum rudimentary.[6] Absence of portions of the corpora cavernosa can result in diverticula of the urethra (p. 1081).

Torsion of the Penis

Congenital torsion of the penis consists in twisting of the organ on its long axis so that the frenulum faces outward or upward. The torsion is to the left more often than to the right. The anomaly may cause no symptoms and functions may be normal. In some cases, it is associated with hypospadias or epispadias. If stenosis of the external meatus is present, dilatations of the organs of the upper urinary tract develop. In one case, clubfoot was an associated anomaly.[7]

Webbing of the penis commonly is associated with hypospadias or a short urethra. The organ is closely attached to the scrotum, an anomaly that can be corrected, together with the urethral defect, by a plastic operation.

The Prepuce

The prepuce develops by the ingrowth, from the front of the glans backward, of a collar of surface epithelium that is incomplete on the perineal side. The central cells degenerate, whereby a sleeve covering the glans is formed.[8] This splitting of the solid cell lamella is not always complete at birth and congenital preputial adhesions sometimes are present. The prepuce of the newborn infant normally is elongated and redundant. Its orifice appears narrow, which prevents retraction. In the normal course of development, the redundancy is taken up, the orifice widens and the adhesions resolve during the first 6–9 months of life, so that retraction becomes possible and spontaneous freeing of the prepuce occurs in the majority of children.[5]

Congenital absence of the prepuce is seen occasionally; it can be overlooked because it is thought that the child had been circumcised. Several children "born circumcised" were described by James.[9] Aplasia of the prepuce can occur as a dominantly inherited trait in persons who are entirely normal otherwise. However, the condition also has been described together with severe malformation such as congenital absence of one leg.[10] It is of interest that children "born circumcised" were known to the scholars of the Talmud.[9]

Congenital phimosis represents a narrowness of the prepuce, which is rare and difficult to diagnose during the first months of life because preputial adhesions occur normally in the neonatal period. Phimosis is, on rare occasions, responsible for urinary obstruction that is rendered more acute by inflammatory ulceration of the prepuce and sealing off of the orifice by scab formation.[5] There may be back-pressure dilatation and damage to the bladder and upper urinary tract. In rare instances, the prepuce is imperforate.[3]

Cleft of the glans penis usually is vertical and, unless combined with stenosis of the external meatus, represents an anomaly of little clinical concern.[3]

Diphallus

Diphallus (double penis) is a rare anomaly that was observed once by Bokay[11] in 1,000,000 patients of a children's hospital. This author, in a review of published cases, noted that diphallus may be symmetric or there may be a difference in size. Sometimes one penis is located above the other and the degree of division can vary; one penis may contain the urinary and the other the seminal outlet. Vesical duplication is a common association. True diphallus is rare in cases of exstrophy of the bladder but usually there are two halves of one penis because of divided primordia of the genital tubercle. Campbell[3] enumerated many associated malformations. Epispadias, hypospadias, undescended testes, absence of the bladder, ureter or kidney, fused or ectopic kidneys and imperforate anus have been observed. In one instance, the vertebral column was reduplicated. Davis[12] reported a case in which it was uncertain whether two, three or four organs were present. In this viable child, who had a normal penis in normal position over a bifid scrotum, there were three additional appendages between the divergent scrotal halves that imitated penile shapes. One of these supernumerary structures probably was a penis, but another one was thought to be a teratoma or dermoid.

Bifid penis (with duplication of the glans) associated with imperforate anus was described by Cochrane and Saunders.[13] An association with double colon, bladder and urethra was reported by Volpé.[14]

Transposition of the Penis and Scrotum (Prepenile Scrotum)

Only a few cases of this anomaly are on record. Campbell[3] described a patient in whom the penis, with a normal urethra, was located on the perineum behind the bifid scrotum. In this case, the upper urinary tract was normal. In a patient reported by Francis,[15] the anomaly was associated with other severe malformations and the child lived less than 1 hour. The mother had had a tubal pregnancy and a miscarriage before the birth of this child. The child was delivered in the eighth month of gestation and the amniotic fluid was scanty. The scrotum was located above the symphysis and the penis contained no urethra. The anus was present but the colon atretic. The kidneys, ureters, bladder, urachus and the prostate were absent. The testes could be located and their ductus deferentes terminated in the posterior pelvic wall. The abdominal aorta ended as a single umbilical artery.

Campbell[3] was able to divide his patient's scrotum surgically in the midline and to bring the penis forward to normal position. Then the scrotum was closed around the base of the penis, with elimination of the scrotal cleft.

REFERENCES

1. Kirshbaum, J. D.: Congenital absence of the external genitals, J. Pediat. 37:102, 1950.
2. Ruckinstat, G. J., and Hasterlik, R. J.: Congenital absence of the penis, Arch. Path. 27:984, 1939.
3. Campbell, M.: *Clinical Pediatric Urology* (Philadelphia: W. B. Saunders Company, 1951).
4. Potter, E. L.: *Pathology of the Fetus and Infant* (2d ed.; Chicago: Year Book Medical Publishers, Inc., 1961).
5. Williams, D. I.: Urology in Childhood, in *Encyclopedia of Urology* (Berlin: Springer-Verlag, 1958), Vol. XV.
6. Campbell, M. F.: *Urology* (Philadelphia: W. B. Saunders Company, 1963), Vol. 2.
7. Broussard, E. R.: Uncomplicated congenital torsion of the penis, J. Pediat. 46:456, 1955.
8. Bremer, J. L.: *Congenital Anomalies of the Viscera. Their Embryological Basis* (Cambridge, Mass.: Harvard University Press, 1957).
9. James, T.: Aplasia of male prepuce with evidence of hereditary transmission, J. Anat. 85:370, 1951.
10. Goddard, H. S.: Unusual case (congenital absence of leg and foreskin, M. J. Record 133:87, 1931.
11. Bokay, J.: Über Diphallie, Jahrb. Kinderh. 127:127, 1930.
12. Davis, D. M. A case of double, triple or quadruple penis associated with dermoid of the perineum, J. Urol. 61:111, 1949.
13. Cochrane, W. J., and Saunders, R. L.: Rare anomaly of penis associated with imperforate anus, J. Urol. 47:810, 1942.
14. Volpé, M.: Dell'asta doppia, Policlinics 10:46, 1903.
15. Francis, C. C.: A case or prepenial scrotum (marsupial type) associated with absence of urinary system, Anat. Rec. 76:303, 1940.

111

Hermaphrodism

True Hermaphrodism

IN A TRUE HERMAPHRODITE, both ovarian and testicular tissues are present. To verify both types of gonadal tissue, histologic proof usually is required, but there are exceptional patients in whom only ovarian tissue is histologically proved, whereas heterosexual gonadal function is demonstrated by formation of spermatozoa.[1] Menstruation without proof of ovarian tissue is not accepted as proof of hermaphrodism with established testicular tissue.[2]

Gonadal tissues can be distributed in three ways: (1) Bilateral, i.e., testicular and ovarian tissue on both sides. (2) Unilateral, i.e., ovotestis on one side and a testis or ovary on the other. (3) Asymmetric or lateral, i.e., testicular tissue on one side, ovarian tissue on the other side. In 1963, Overzier[2] listed 171 cases of proved hermaphrodism recorded in the medical literature and added a detailed analysis of their anatomic, social and psychologic attributes.

According to the appearance of the external genitalia, five types have been distinguished. Type 1 has completely female external and internal genitalia. On the other side of the series are true hermaphrodites with completely male external and internal sex organs, although ovarian tissue is present in their organism (type 5). Such a case observed by Bregman *et al.*[3] had a 46,XX karyotype. Another patient with entirely male external genitalia and 46,XX chromosomes belonged to the family reported by Rosenberg *et al.*,[4] in which 3 siblings were affected. Yet, in general, this masculine form (type 5) and the feminine form (type 1) are rare. Much more frequent are the intermediate forms (types 2, 3 and 4), all of which have a uterus and an enlarged clitoris or penis with variable development of a urogenital sinus. The derivatives of the Wolffian and Müllerian ducts also show great variations in types 2, 3 and 4. In lateral or alternating hermaphrodism, the duct derivatives may be asymmetrically developed, being male on the side of the testis and female on the side of the ovary. A uterus is present in most cases of true hermaphrodism. Although uterus bicornis and uterus arcuatus have been observed, in the majority of patients the uterus is normal in size and structure. The vagina varies in width and length; it is absent in the rare type 5. Testes and ovotestes may lie in various locations along the path of descent, but in most hermaphrodites the testis is found in the scrotum or in the inguen.[2] Ovaries remain in their normal abdominal position. A descended ovary usually contains some testicular tissue. Histologically, the gonads show various degrees of maturation and differentiation from fully developed ovaries to sperm-producing testes.[2] About two-thirds of true hermaphrodites menstruate. In several cases, both spermatozoa and menstruation have been observed.

The ovaries of hermaphrodites usually are normal in size and appearance. Even in ovotestes, the ovarian portion may show ova, primary follicles, Graafian follicles and corpora lutea. Ovulation can occur and was proved in a patient[5] whose uterus was noncanalized. In general, ovarian tissue is better developed in sex chromatin-positive than in negative cases.[2] The testes of hermaphrodites usually are smaller than normal testes and are underdeveloped. The testicular tissue often is atrophic or rudimentary; living sperm is rare but spermatozoa are found occasionally,[1] and sometimes the testis is well developed. In a hermaphrodite described by Brewer *et al.*,[5] the testes showed seminiferous tubules with spermatogonia, Sertoli cells and well-developed interstitial cells. Despite the presence of spermatic and interstitial cells, female secondary sex characteristics were well developed. There is no difference in the structure of the testes of chromatin-positive and chromatin-negative hermaphrodites. In an ovotestis, the border between male and female gonad may be ill defined or be clearly established by fibrous tissue. Usually, the ovary caps the testicle, but sometimes the testis surrounds ovarian tissue.[2] There also may be islands of ovarian tissue in a testis.[6] Although testicular tissue is present in every true hermaphrodite, female Müllerian duct derivatives persist in the majority of these persons,[7] a fact that throws some doubt on the widely accepted tenet that development of a female duct system depends on the absence of testes.

In infants, a discrepancy in the appearance of the external genitalia will arouse the suspicion of hermaphrodism. Rare cases with completely male or completely female external genitalia can escape recognition before puberty. Gonadal abnormalities may be discovered accidentally during operations or in the presence of herniae. More often, the condition is recognized after puberty or when marriage is contemplated. In exceptional cases, hermaphrodism has been recognized in early infancy[8] or was delayed to old age.[9]

As a rule, true hermaphrodites are regarded as males. Of 138 cases, 94 were registered as males and 44 as females.[2] The phallic structure and the small opening of the orifice of the urogenital sinus suggest that the child is a boy. After puberty, the appearance of the patients is determined by hormonal activities. No definite correlation can be established between the histologic structure of the gonads and the secondary sex characteristics.[10] Biopsy findings of prevalent ovarian or testicular tissue do not mean that the respective secondary sex characteristics will necessarily develop.[7] Thus, the results of early biopsy of the gonads are not necessarily indicative of the trend of development at puberty.

Growth of true hermaphrodites generally is normal; associated malformations are rare but bilateral anophthalmia was present in a patient (46,XX) reported by Root *et al.*[11]

The psychologic orientation varies. The majority of true hermaphrodites live as males according to the sex assigned to them at birth, but there are individual cases that require change of the legal sex. Approximately 15% of the cases reviewed by Overzier[2] were discontented with their legal sex. In most patients, assignment of sex and education decide orientation of the patients.

About 70% of true hermaphrodites are sex chromatin-positive and more than half of the cases reported have 46,XX karyotypes. In a few patients, an XY karyotype was found.[12,13,25] Mosaicism has been reported in several cases. XX/XY,[14,15] XX/XXY, XX/XXY/XXYYY and XX/XXYY[12,13] are mosaicisms in which Y-containing cell lines were recorded but there also were mosaics with XX/XXX[16] and XX/XX+ fragment.[13] The frequent occurrence of true hermaphrodism in persons in whom no Y chromosome can be detected represents an enigma if one believes that testicular tissue cannot be formed without the direction of a Y chromosome. It is not advisable to attribute such cases to an undetected mosaicism. Kladetzky and Rosenbauer[17] found sex chromatin in theca, rete and Leydig cells of an ovotestis, which indicates that testes cells can be XX. A lead to a more plausible explanation of XX karyotype in true hermaphrodites can be obtained through the remarkable family published by Clayton *et al.*[18] and Rosenberg *et al.*,[4] which contained 3 brothers with the condition, all having XX karyotype. These cases show a repetitive mechanism – possibly genetic – that permits formation of testicular tissue in the absence of a Y chromosome. The frequent occurrence of hermaphrodites among Africans in Rhodesia[20] and South African Bantus[21] suggests that racial or unusual environmental factors may be at work. Familial true hermaphrodism was recorded by Milner *et al.*[24] and by Mori and Mizutani.[19] In one of the cases reported by Forbes and Hammar,[20] it seems possible that 2 cases occurred in the same family. True hermaphrodism in patients with XX/XY mosaicism has been explained by double fertilization, i.e., one X-bearing and one Y-bearing sperm forming a chimera.

True lateral (alternating) hermaphrodism has been observed in mice but the condition seems to be rare. The accessory genital organs corresponded to the sex of the neighboring gonad. In one case, an ovotestis was associated with female accessory organs.[22] Palludan[23] saw hermaphrodism in two pigs, the offspring of vitamin A-deficient sows.

REFERENCES

1. McIver, R. B., Seabaugh, D. R., and Mangels, M.: True hermaphroditism: A report of 2 cases, J. Urol. 52:67, 1944.
2. Overzier, C.: True Hermaphroditism, in Overzier, C. (ed.), *Intersexuality* (London and New York: Academic Press, 1963).
3. Bregman, R. U., Bregman, E. T., Cushner, G. B., and Woods, F. M.: Chromosome analysis, nuclear sex, clinical and endocrine studies of a true hermaphrodite, J. Urol. 89:475, 1963.
4. Rosenberg, H. S., Clayton, G. W., and Hsu, T. C.: Familial true hermaphrodism, J. Clin. Endocrinol. 23:203, 1963.
5. Brewer, J. I., Jones, H. O., and Culver, H.: True hermaphroditism, J.A.M.A. 148:431, 1952.
6. Engle, E. T., Yeaw, R. C., and Lattimer, J. K.: True hermaphroditism: A supplementary report of a case, J. Urol. 56:731, 1946.
7. Rosenthal, I. M., Kiefer, J. H., McGrew, E., and Bronstein, I. P.: Unilateral true hermaphroditism. Two cases with sex-chromatin positive cellular pattern, Pediatrics 20: 1006, 1957.
8. Tristan, T. A., Eberlein, W. R., and Hope, J. W.: Roentgenologic investigation of patients with heterosexual development, Am. J. Roentgenol. 76:562, 1956.
9. Armstrong, C. N.: Diversities of sex, Brit. M. J. 1:1173, 1955.
10. Arey, L. B.: Hermaphroditismo Genetico Congenito, in Mussio-Fournier, J. C. (ed.), *Tratodo de Endocrinologia Clinica* (Buenos Aires: Kraft, 1951), Vol. 2.
11. Root, A. W., Eberlein, W. R., Briebart, S., Moorhead, P. S., and Mellman, W. J.: Chromosomal analysis of multiple tissues from a true hermaphrodite, J. Clin. Endocrinol. 24:467, 1964.
12. Van Wyk, J. J., and Grumbach, M. M.: Disorders of Sex Differentiation, in Williams, R. H. (ed.), *Textbook of Endocrinology* (4th ed.; Philadelphia: W. B. Saunders Company, 1968).
13. Miller, O. J.: The sex chromosome anomalies, Am. J. Obst. & Gynec. 90:1078, 1964.
14. Gartler, S. M., Waxman, S. H., and Giblett, E.: An XX/XY human hermaphrodite resulting from double fertilization, Proc. Nat. Acad. Sc. 48:332, 1962.
15. Jasso, N., de Grouchy, J., Auvert, J., Nezelof, C., Jayle, M. F., Moullec, J., Frézal, J., De Casaubon, A., and Lamy, M.: True hermaphroditism with XX/XY mosaicism, probably due to double fertilization of the ovum, J. Clin. Endocrinol. 25:114, 1965.
16. Ferguson-Smith, M. A., Johnston, A. W., and Weinberg, A. N.: The chromosome complement in true hermaphroditism, Lancet 2:126, 1960.
17. Kladetzky, J., and Rosenbauer, K. A.: Sex-Chromatinbe-

stimmung bei Ovotestis, Ztschr. Zellforsch. 70:54, 1966.
18. Clayton, G. W., Smith, D., and Rosenberg, H. S.: Familial true hermaphrodism in pre- and postpuberal genetic females, hormonal and morphologic studies, J. Clin. Endocrinol. 18:1349, 1958.
19. Mori, Y., and Mizutani, S.: Familial true hermaphroditism in genetic females, Jap. J. Urol. 59:857, 1968.
20. Forbes, J. I., and Hammar, B.: Intersex among Africans in Rhodesia, Arch. Dis. Childhood 41:102, 1966.
21. Klempman, S.: The investigation of developmental sexual abnormalities, South African M. J. 38:234, 1964.
22. Grüneberg, H.: *The Genetics of the Mouse* (The Hague: Martinus Nijhoff, 1952).
23. Palludan, B.: *A-Avitaminosis in Swine* (Copenhagen: Ejnar Munksgaard, 1966).
24. Milner, W. A., Garlick, W. B., Fink, A. J., and Stein, A. A.: True hermaphrodite siblings, J. Urol. 79:1103, 1958.
25. Barreiro, E., Peralta, A., Monereo, J., Usandizaga, J. A., Contreras, F., and Swartz, A.: Two new cases of true hermaphroditism, J. M. Genetics 6:426, 1969.

Female Pseudohermaphrodism

Adrenal Female Pseudohermaphrodism (Virilizing Adrenal Hyperplasia)

THIS TYPE OF pseudohermaphrodism usually is described as the "congenital adrenogenital syndrome," since masculinization is due to androgens secreted by the adrenal cortex. Adrenal tumors of a child can cause masculinization after birth but the congenital form is due to adrenal hyperplasia. The patients are females with female sex chromatin, ovaries, uterus and Fallopian tubes. Masculinization is limited to the external genitalia, derivatives of the urogenital sinus and secondary sex characteristics.

This condition has been known since ancient times. It was known in antiquity and Pliny[1] knew that transformation of females into males is not an idle story. In the consulship of Publius Livinius Crassus, a girl at Casinum was changed into a boy and at the order of the augurs was conveyed away to a desert island. Pliny saw in Africa a person who had turned into a male on the day of marriage to a husband.

An early illustrated report of a female pseudohermaphrodite dates back to Regnerus de Graaf in 1678, and Parsons in 1741 cited case histories of persons who in all probability had the adrenogenital syndrome.[2] The association of adrenal tumors with precocious puberty was described by Tilesius in 1803 and by other authors subsequently.[3] But it seems that Marchand, in 1891, gave the first report of adrenocortical hyperplasia with pseudohermaphrodism. Case reports in the early twentieth century were reviewed by Krabbe.[3]

It was estimated that adrenal female pseudohermaphrodism accounts for about 50% of all cases of abnormal sex differentiation,[4] and calculated[5] that 1 case occurred in 67,000 births, but the frequency may vary in different areas.[6] Although the basic anomaly affects both sexes, all series dealing with the adrenogenital syndrome contain more females than males. This deficit of males is attributed to the absence of early signs of abnormal sex development in the males and may, therefore, be apparent rather than real. The anomaly seems to be rare in Negroes.[5] Consanguinity of the parents has been observed repeatedly and siblings often are affected. In a large series,[7] 66 patients had a total of 141 siblings, of whom 34 had the adrenogenital syndrome. Abnormal siblings can alternate with normals. The parents appear normal. Identical twins, concordant in regard to the adrenogenital syndrome, have been recorded.[8,9] In one pair, the genital anomalies were noticed at birth and on the fourth day signs of adrenocortical failure appeared. Adequate treatment stabilized electrolyte balance and made them develop as females.[8] Another pair, although born with enlarged clitoris, went on to progressive virilization until the age of 7½ years. Even that late, some good therapeutic effects could be achieved by treatment with cortisone or prednisone.

Recessive inheritance of this adrenal anomaly was made probable by family studies.[7,10] Childs *et al.*[5] analyzed 46 families with 76 patients who had virilizing adrenal hyperplasia. Comparison of the observed numbers of patients with that expected on the hypothesis of an autosomal recessive gene showed good agreement. There was one consanguineous marriage among the 46 families. Gestation and labor of the mothers of the affected children were normal and there was no evidence of maternal influence on the manifestations of the disease. It is now generally assumed that the virilizing adrenal hyperplasia is a genetically determined inborn error of adrenocortical steroid synthesis. The gene expresses itself in homozygous children, the parents being heterozygous. The risk for affected offspring is 1 in 4. Prenatal diagnosis by amniocentesis has been attempted, but the presence of the disorder could not be predicted during early or midpregnancy.[28]

Congenital malformations of the external genitalia caused by inborn errors of adrenal metabolism are of great practical and theoretical interest. They belong in the small group of structural congenital malformations that can be explained by demonstrable abnormal chemical reactions. It often is asserted that hereditary congenital malformations are due to inborn chemical defects acting in early embryonic development and comparable to those that are now so well investigated in certain types of mental retardation. Actually, there are not many examples to bear out such assertions. It must be assumed that, as a rule, abnormal chemical processes that result in structural congenital malformations cannot be demonstrated in

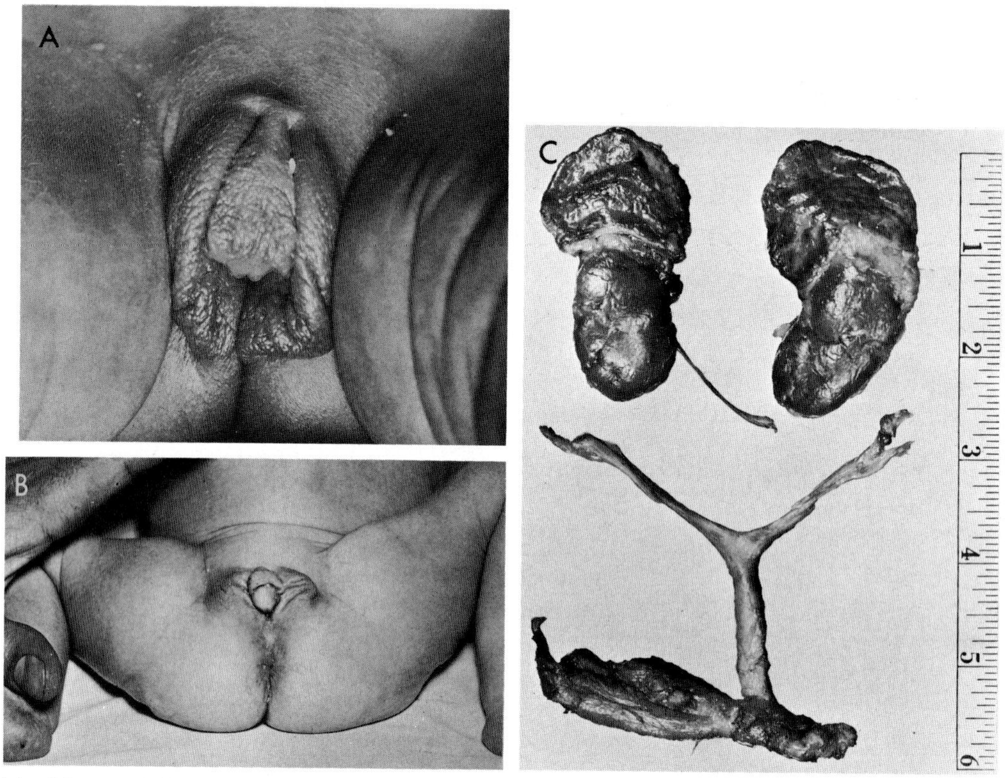

Fig. 111-1.—Adrenogenital syndrome. **A,** external genitalia of infant with female pseudohermaphrodism and bilateral hyperplasia of adrenals. Hypertrophy of clitoris with large labioscrotal folds. Urethra and vagina had separate external orifices. **B,** appearance of external genitalia at age of 2 months. The child died at 13 months of age. **C,** markedly enlarged adrenal glands (combined weight 35 Gm.) over kidneys. Under kidneys: uterus, tubes and rudimentary ovaries. Patient was the eleventh child shown in pedigree, Figure 111-3.

postnatal life, even if they have been present in early embryologic stages. The malformations of the external genitalia associated with or caused by inborn errors of adrenal steroid synthesis are exceptional because they arise relatively late in organogenesis and the abnormal metabolic and teratogenic reactions are still demonstrable at the time of birth and thereafter.

Several types of congenital adrenal hyperplasia can be distinguished according to their basic metabolic defect. They all interfere with cortisol formation, resulting in increased ACTH secretion and hyperplasia of the adrenal cortex. Three defects lead to virilization through prenatal exposure of the female fetus to excessive amounts of adrenal androgens.[11] A partial defect in C-21-hydroxylation results in uncomplicated virilism. Complete C-21-hydroxylase defect blocks C-21-hydroxylation completely, with impairment of aldosterone secretion. Affected infants suffer from salt-losing states, which often prove fatal in early life unless they are adequately treated. Another and rare defect of C-11-hydroxylation[4] results in the adrenogenital syndrome with hypertension. The patients with these metabolic defects have elevated urinary levels of 17-ketosteroids and 3α, 17α, 20α pregnanetriol.

Overproduction of androgens by the adrenals can cause a spectrum of genital changes that vary in newborn girls from slight enlargement of the clitoris with otherwise normal female genitalia to complete virilization of the external organs. Cases of maximal virilization with penile urethra were reviewed by Stolecke.[29] Uterus, tubes and ovaries remain normal. It is assumed that genital development proceeds normally to the twelfth week of intrauterine life, permitting formation of the Müllerian structures and degeneration of the Wolffian ducts and that from about that time on the external genitalia are affected by abnormal adrenal androgens. But the time of onset of virilization is variable. In rare instances, girls with the metabolic defect fail to undergo virilization in prenatal life but develop symptoms after birth, during childhood or adolescence. It also is rare to see complete virilization of the external genitalia with prenatal development of a penis with prepuce, termination of the urethra on the tip of the glans and a scrotum. Prader[12] listed 7 cases of this type and emphasized that such marked virilization usually is paralleled by severe salt-losing symptoms. It is understandable that in the past such girls were mistaken for boys with severe "gastroenteritis" and dehydration until the condition was recognized at necropsy by the finding of female internal genital organs and adrenal hyperplasia. Now positive sex chromatin in buccal

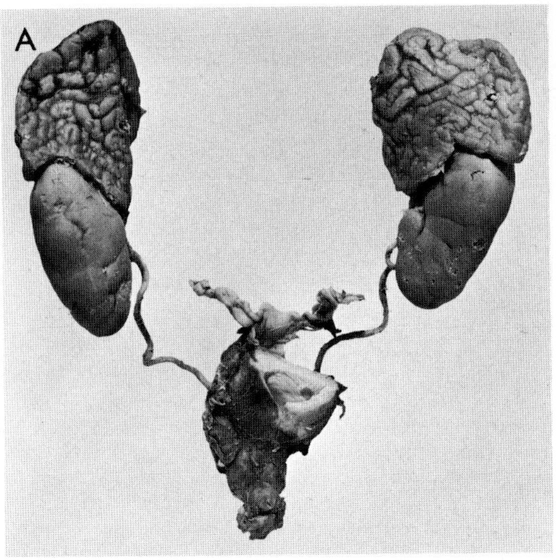

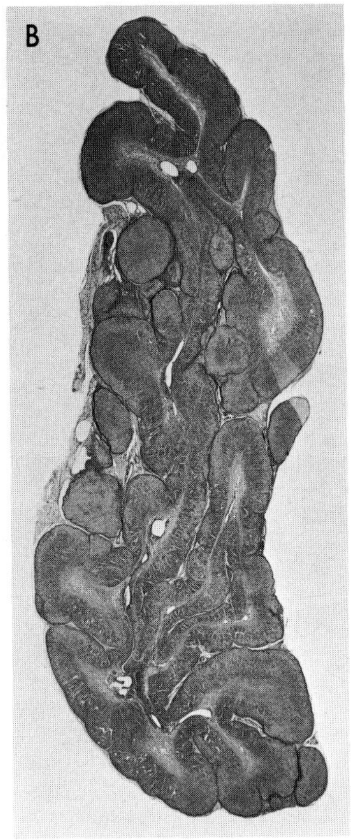

Fig. 111-2. – Adrenogenital syndrome. **A,** adrenocortical hyperplasia in a girl who died at 2 months of age. She had hypertrophy of the clitoris, absence of labia minora and absence of external vaginal opening. A slit-like vagina did not communicate with the urethra, which opened at the base of the clitoris. The adrenals show cortical folds and convolutions. Patient was the sixth child shown in pedigree, Figure 111-3. **B,** histologic section through enlarged and folded adrenal.

smears, normal female karyotype and elevated urinary 17-ketosteroid and pregnanetriol levels can lead to early diagnosis intra vitam. It seems that only 1% or 2% of the girls with the adrenogenital syndrome have complete masculinization. There also are reports of a few cases of such masculinization with hypospadias.[12]

The majority of affected girls show virilization, with varying degrees of fusion of their labial folds. Minor changes consist of formation of a crescent-shaped skin fold across the fourchette and normal vaginal and urethral openings.[4] With more advanced fusion, the urogenital sulcus is partly covered, so that there is a single opening in which both the urethra and the vagina terminate. Further fusion results in a urogenital sinus with a small orifice situated at or near the base of the enlarged clitoris and formation of a "scrotum" by joining of the labial folds. Without treatment, virilization usually progresses during postnatal life. As pubic and axillary hair develop, hypertrophy of the clitoris increases and the voice deepens. Growth and ossification are accelerated. Epiphyseal fusions occur early and the patients end up smaller than average. They have masculine appearance with well-developed musculature, growth of body hair and beards and deep voices. There is no female breast development.

Virilization beginning in postnatal life is rare but a number of cases have been observed, with moderate enlargement of the clitoris developing in later childhood or adolescence. In such cases, the first signs of virilization can occur after secondary female sex characteristics have made their appearance. The clinical pattern usually is consistent within families in which more than one child is affected, but there are variations between families. The anatomic anomalies in affected girls of the same family sometimes are strikingly similar. Thus, in a family reported by Birke *et al.*,[13] there were 3 girls with a phallus with a urethral meatus at the base. But it seems that simple

Fig. 111-3. – Pedigree of a family in which 2 boys and 2 girls had adrenocortical hyperplasia. All 4 died before proper treatment was available, probably in adrenal crises. Necropsy was not performed on the third child, a male, but the ninth had adrenal hyperplasia like his sisters, who had adrenogenital syndrome (Figs. 111-1 and 111-2).

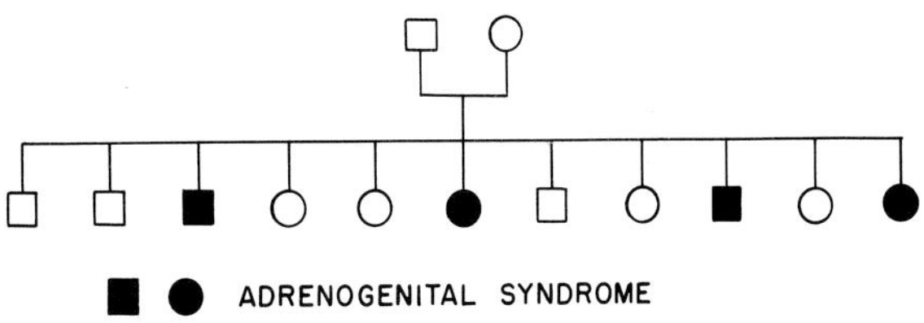

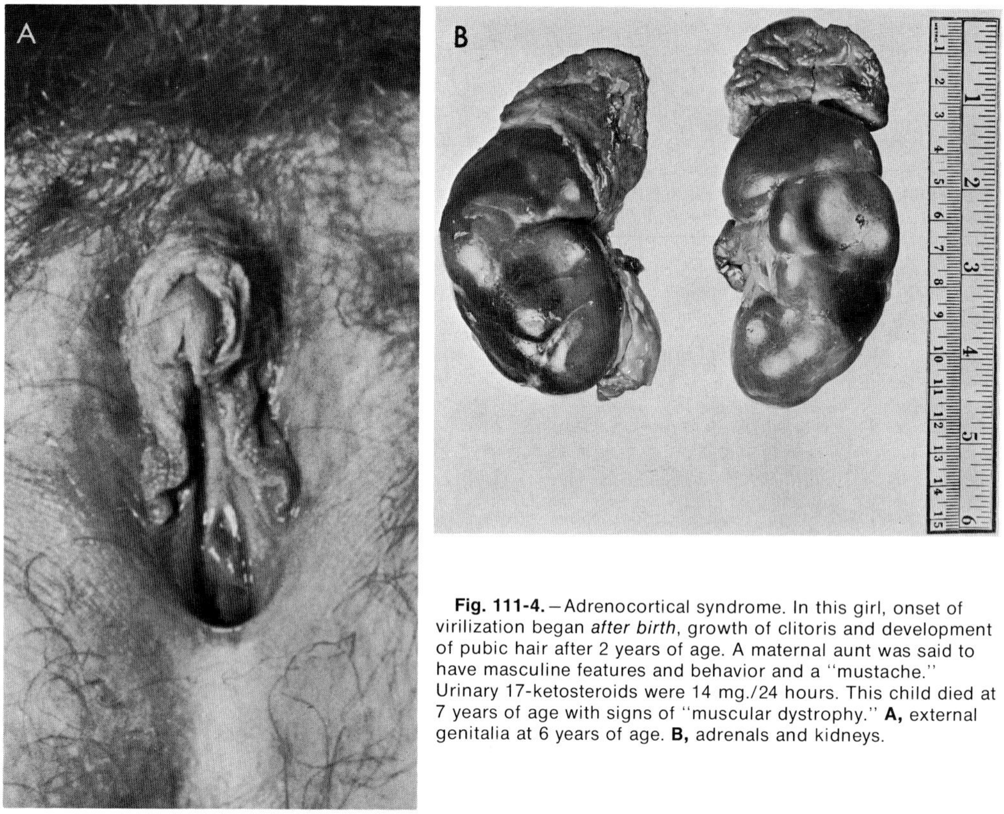

Fig. 111-4. —Adrenocortical syndrome. In this girl, onset of virilization began *after birth*, growth of clitoris and development of pubic hair after 2 years of age. A maternal aunt was said to have masculine features and behavior and a "mustache." Urinary 17-ketosteroids were 14 mg./24 hours. This child died at 7 years of age with signs of "muscular dystrophy." **A,** external genitalia at 6 years of age. **B,** adrenals and kidneys.

virilism and virilism with salt-losing can alternate in the same family.[4,14]

As pointed out before, the genital malformations caused by adrenocortical hyperplasia originate relatively late in fetal life (twelfth week and thereafter), at a time when the "organogenic" period of most organs is terminated. It is not surprising, therefore, that the malformations of the external genitalia characteristic for the adrenogenital syndrome occur in otherwise well-formed children. Associated malformations are rare and probably accidental. Birke *et al.*[13] mentioned stenosis of the pulmonary artery in 1 of 3 sisters with the adrenogenital syndrome. In a case reported by Matheson and Ward,[15] a mucosal valve was found in the posterior urethra below the verumontanum, resulting in vesical hypertrophy and bilateral hydro-ureter.

Treatment with cortisone after birth counteracts virilization and abnormal metabolic processes. The results depend on the degree of virilization and the age at which treatment is begun. Growth and epiphyseal development also are influenced by the treatment and feminization, including menstruation and ovulation, can occur in girls who are at or past the age of adolescence.[4] Malformations of the external genitalia can be corrected surgically. A number of treated females have married and several have gone through normal pregnancy.[16] Successful delivery has been reported in a woman born without distal vagina after combined cortisone and surgical treatment. A normal premature girl was delivered by cesarean section.[17]

In males, the adrenogenital syndrome is manifested by isosexual changes. Neither pseudohermaphrodism nor hermaphrodism results. Virilization in boys with adrenal hyperplasia usually is not present at birth. The external genitalia are normally formed and, according to Wilkins,[4] the testes are always in the scrotum in male patients with the 21-hydroxylase or 11-hydroxylase defect. But patients with the 3-β hydroxysteroid dehydrogenase[18] defect usually have incompletely masculinized genitalia with hypospadias and cleft scrotum. It is thought that in this disorder production of fetal testicular androgens is deficient.

In rare instances, the penis and scrotum can be enlarged at birth and *macrogenitosomia praecox* become evident in early infancy. Such a case was described by Wilkins *et al.*[19] in a patient who had large testes due to aberrant adrenal tissue. In such cases, the enlarged testes are made up of cells resembling cells of the fascicular adrenal zone. Wilkins[4] pointed out that such hyperplastic aberrant adrenocortical tissue can respond to cortisone therapy and shrink like topical hyperplastic adrenals.

Congenital adrenal tumors leading to macrogenitosomia are rare. In a boy with virilizing tumor of the

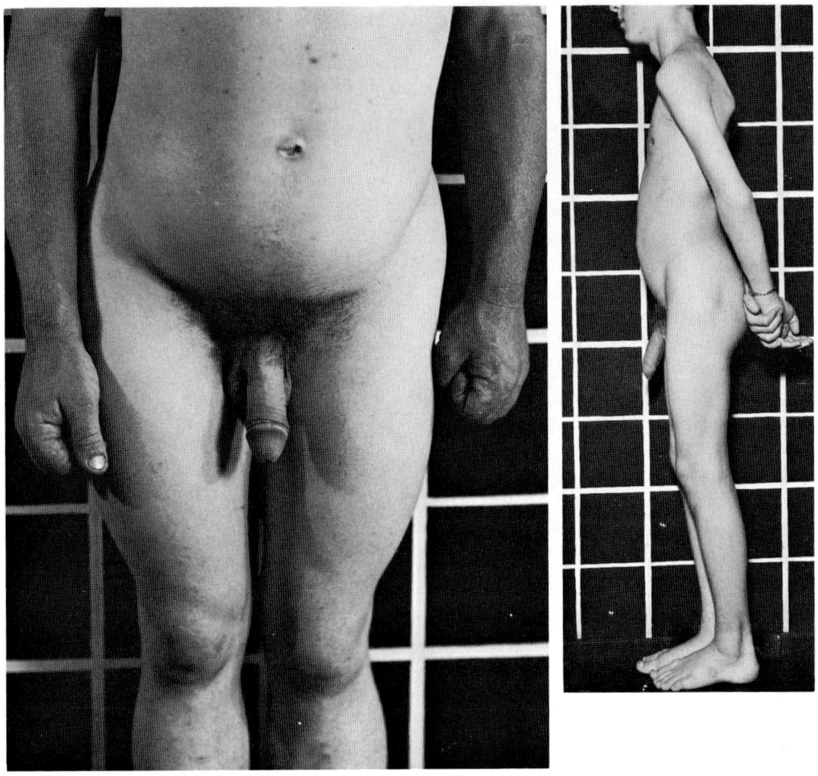

Fig. 111-5. – Macrogenitosomia praecox and adrenogenital syndrome in a boy, 7 years of age. His condition was poor at birth. He was suspected of having pyloric stenosis when he was 1 month of age but there was no obstruction. When he was 7 years of age, he was 21 cm. above average height and about 12 kg. overweight. The penis was much enlarged and the testes of normal size for his age. He had salt craving.

adrenal cortex, gradual enlargement of the abdomen and hirsutism were noticed from birth. At the age of 3 years, a beard, pubic and axillary hair and macrogenitosomia were present. The tumor was removed surgically.[20] A malignant tumor of the adrenal cortex caused virilizing symptoms in a boy 1 year of age. But the growth curve was abnormal from birth on.[21] Lowrey and Brown[22] observed a boy born with enlarged penis who developed pubic hair and acne at 9 months. Operation at 4 years showed an orange-sized carcinoma of the left adrenal cortex.

Nonadrenal Female Pseudohermaphrodism

Compared to the adrenogenital syndrome, nonadrenal female pseudohermaphrodism is rare, as only about 3% of the reported cases with sexual ambiguity belong in this group.[4] Although adrenal and nonadrenal female pseudohermaphrodism show great resemblance externally at the time of birth, it is possible to distinguish the two, since patients with adrenocortical hypertrophy show early endocrine anomalies.

Etiologically, nonadrenal female pseudohermaphrodism is not an entity. Since affected children have signs of prenatal masculinization without showing progressive androgenic changes after birth and since they develop female secondary sex characteristics at the time of puberty, it has been assumed that maternal androgens are responsible for the masculinization. This assumption received support by the finding of female pseudohermaphrodites whose mothers had received androgenic drugs during pregnancy. In other cases, the masculinizing effect could be traced to an arrhenoblastoma of the mother.[23,24] In rare instances, the mother of the affected child showed endocrine anomalies during pregnancy. The occurrence of hirsutism, acne, coarsening of features, deepening of the voice or excessive obesity during pregnancy suggests endocrine disturbances that could be the source of maldevelopment of the external genitalia of a female fetus.[25] But such a simple explanation of androgenic factors at work cannot be applied to all cases of female pseudohermaphrodism. For instance, Perloff *et al.*[26] observed a pair of twins, one a normal female, the other a female pseudohermaphrodite, a situation that cannot be explained by abnormal hormonal conditions of the mother. There also are female pseudohermaphrodites who have, in addition to changes in the external genitalia, malformations of the urinary or intestinal tract. Such cases suggest that the changes in the external genitalia probably are only one manifestation of unknown "pleiotropic" teratogenic factors and demonstrate that pseudohermaphrodism with masculinization can occur as a malformation without the activity of fetal testes (p. 1119).

About 1958, an increase in female pseudohermaphrodites was noticed that was attributed to the extensive use of progesterones and related substances widely used for threatened or habitual abortion. Synthetic steroids such as 17-ethinyl-testosterone and 17α-ethinyl-19-nortestosterone were used under various trade names as oral progesterones in the treatment of threatened abortions. These compounds taken by pregnant women early in pregnancy resulted in virilization of their female fetuses, whereas the mother showed only mild endocrine changes. Such drug-induced female hermaphrodites have various degrees of phallic enlargement and fusion of the labioscrotal folds.[4] If the external genitalia show a high degree of masculinization, the sex may be doubtful, but if there is only a slight enlargement of the clitoris, affected children are reared as girls. The urethra usually opens at the base of the enlarged clitoris but, in some instances, a penile urethra exists. Such children often are mistaken for males until puberty. If the urethra opens at the tip of a micropenis, it sometimes is stenotic and urinary obstruction may occur. In such cases, a minute vaginal opening may be found in the perineum and there may be some communication between the vagina and the urethra.[27] More often, the vagina opens together with the urethra into a urogenital sinus, or the vagina has a separate orifice behind the urethral opening. The cervix and uterus are present; the ovaries are normal, and located in normal position in the abdominal cavity. With beginning puberty, ovulation occurs, corpora lutea are formed, the breasts develop normally and menstruation occurs.

In the differential diagnosis, adrenocortical female pseudohermaphrodism must be excluded. In the nonadrenal form, the urinary metabolites characteristic of adrenal hyperplasia are not elevated, there are no signs of precocious sex development and there is no excessive somatic growth and no precocious ossification. If the sex of patients with enlargement of the clitoris and marked labioscrotal fusion is in doubt, the true situation is ascertained by determination of the sex chromatin, karyotype and biopsy of the gonads.

The correct diagnosis should be established, if possible, in infancy and the children should be reared as girls. Plastic procedures consisting of amputation of the phallus and separation of the labioscrotal folds usually are performed after the age of 2 and before the age of 4 years. Such patients can be married and they have a potential for normal fertility. However, if they had been reared as males for many years, change of sex is not recommended.

REFERENCES

1. Pliny (The Elder): *Natural History.* Translated by Rackham, H. (Cambridge, Mass.: Harvard University Press, 1939), Vol. II.
2. Panos, T. C.: Female pseudohermaphroditism with hypoadrenia, Pediatrics 5:972, 1950.
3. Krabbe, K. H.: The relation between the adrenal cortex and sexual development, New York J. Med. 114:4, 1921.
4. Wilkins, L.: *The Diagnosis and Treatment of Endocrine Disorders in Childhood and Adolescence* (2d ed.; Springfield, Ill.: Charles C Thomas, Publisher, 1965).
5. Childs, B., Grumbach, M. M., and Van Wyk, J. J.: Virilizing adrenal hyperplasia; a genetic and hormonal study, J. Clin. Invest. 35:213, 1956.
6. Prader, A.: Die Häufigkeit der kongenitalen adrenogenitalen Syndrome, Helvet. paediat. acta 13:426, 1958.
7. Iversen, T.: Congenital adrenocortical hyperplasia with disturbed electrolyte regulation. "Dysadrenocorticism," Pediatrics 16:875, 1955.
8. Wolff, S.: Female pseudohermaphroditism with adrenocortical failure in identical twins, Arch. Dis. Childhood 29:132, 1954.
9. Schneeberg, N. G., Steinberg, A., Malen, M.M., Chernoff, B., and Yap, C. L.: Congenital virilizing adrenal hyperplasia in identical twins, J. Clin. Endocrinol. 19:203, 1959.
10. Knudson, A. G., Jr.: Mixed adrenal disease of infancy, J. Pediat. 39:408, 1951.
11. Van Wyk, J. J., and Grumbach, M. M.: Disorders of Sex Differentiation, in Williams, R. H. (ed.), *Textbook of Endocrinology* (4th ed.; Philadelphia: W. B. Saunders Company, 1968).
12. Prader, A.: Vollkommen männliche äussere Genitalentwicklung und Salzverlustsyndrome bei Mädchen mit kongenitalem adrenogenitalem Syndrom, Helvet. paediat. acta 13:5, 1958.
13. Birke, G., Diszfalusy, E., Plantin, L-O., Robbe, H., and Westman, A.: Familial congenital hyperplasia of the adrenal cortex, Acta endocrinol. 29:55, 1958.
14. Rosenbloom, A. L., and Smith, D. W.: Varying expression for salt losing in related patients with congenital adrenal hyperplasia, Pediatrics 38:215, 1966.
15. Matheson, W. J., and Ward, E. M.: Hormonal sex reversal in a female, Arch. Dis. Childhood 29:22, 1954.
16. Wilson, R. B., and Keating, F. R.: Pregnancy following treatment of congenital adrenal hyperplasia with cortisone, Am. J. Obst. & Gynec. 76:388, 1958.
17. Mason, A. S.: Pregnancy in an adrenal pseudohermaphrodite treated with cortisone, Brit. M. J. 1:1003, 1961.
18. Bongiovanni, A. M.: Unusual steroid pattern in congenital adrenal hyperplasia: Deficiency of 3β-hydroxy dehydrogenase, J. Clin. Endocrinol. 21:860, 1961.
19. Wilkins, L., Fleischmann, W., and Howard, J. E.: Macrogenitosomia precox associated with hyperplasia of the androgenic tissue of the adrenal and death from corticoadrenal insufficiency, Endocrinology 26:385, 1940.
20. Weber, E. J., and Menten, M. L.: Histologic studies on virilizing tumor of adrenal cortex, Am. J. Path. 24:293, 1948.
21. Bernheim, M., Wertheimer, P., Guinet, P., François, R., and Sutet, J.: Les syndromes d'hyperfonctionnement cortico-surrénal d'origine tumorale chez l'enfant, Semaine hôp. Paris 41:1, 1954.
22. Lowrey, G. H., and Brown, T. G.: Precocious sexual development, J. Pediat. 38:325, 1951.
23. Bretnall, C. P.: A case of arrhenoblastoma complicating pregnancy, J. Obst. & Gynaec. Brit. Emp. 52:238, 1945.
24. Javert, C. D., and Finn, W. F.: Arrhenoblastoma: The incidence of malignancy and the relation to pregnancy, to sterility and to treatment, Cancer 4:60, 1951.
25. Wilkins, L., and Jones, H. W.: Masculinization of the female fetus, Obst. & Gynec. 11:355, 1958.
26. Perloff, W. H., Conger, K. B., and Levy, L. M.: Female pseudo-hermaphrodism: A description of 2 unusual cases, J. Clin. Endocrinol. 13:783, 1953.
27. Williams, D. I.: Urology in Childhood, in *Encyclopedia of Urology* (Berlin: Springer-Verlag, 1958), Vol. XV.
28. Merkatz, I. R., New, M. I., Peterson, R. E., and Seaman, M. P.: Prenatal diagnosis of adrenogenital syndrome by amniocentesis, J. Pediat. 75:977, 1969.
29. Stolecke, H.: Kongenitale Nebennierenrindenhyperplasie mit maximaler Virilisierung (penile urethra), Ztschr. Kinderh. 107:343, 1970.

Male Pseudo-hermaphrodism

PERSONS with testes and female or ambiguous (external or ductal) genitalia are called male pseudohermaphrodites. There are many types, which can be distinguished according to morphologic characteristics or etiology but classification is not always easy. In some cases, the genital discrepancies are due to chromosomal abnormalities (p. 1118), others have a genetic background (p. 1114), but the most frequent type of male pseudohermaphrodism is of unknown etiology. It affects children with apparently normal 46,XY karyotype who have testes and ambiguous external genitalia. Such patients often are considered girls because of the absence of a penis and scrotum and reared as girls until puberty, when male secondary sex characteristics appear through endocrine activities of the testes.[1] Delayed recognition of such conditions results in confusion, embarrassment and psychiatric complications, which should be avoided by early evaluation of the anomalies. A review of the problems of the "XY female child" as seen in 1970 was made by Dewhurst.[2] There are patients with male pseudohermaphrodism who have normal male external but female internal genital organs.[3]

The accessory genitalia, external and ductal, can assume various shapes in the presence of testes. The penis can be small and hypospadic and labiosacral fusion incomplete; the urethra may open at the base of the phallus; a urogenital sinus, vagina, uterus and tubes may be present. The testes can be in the divided scrotum, which are thought to be major labia, or they are ectopic in the inguen or in the abdomen in various positions, including those of the ovaries. In the last case, they will be mistaken for ovaries unless a biopsy reveals the true nature of the gonad. Such testes can produce masculinizing hormones at puberty. It is not clear, therefore, why they fail to induce male sex characteristics in fetal life. Various alternative endocrine hypotheses have been offered to explain this failure but none has proved satisfactory. It will be advisable to consider nonendocrine teratogenic fac-

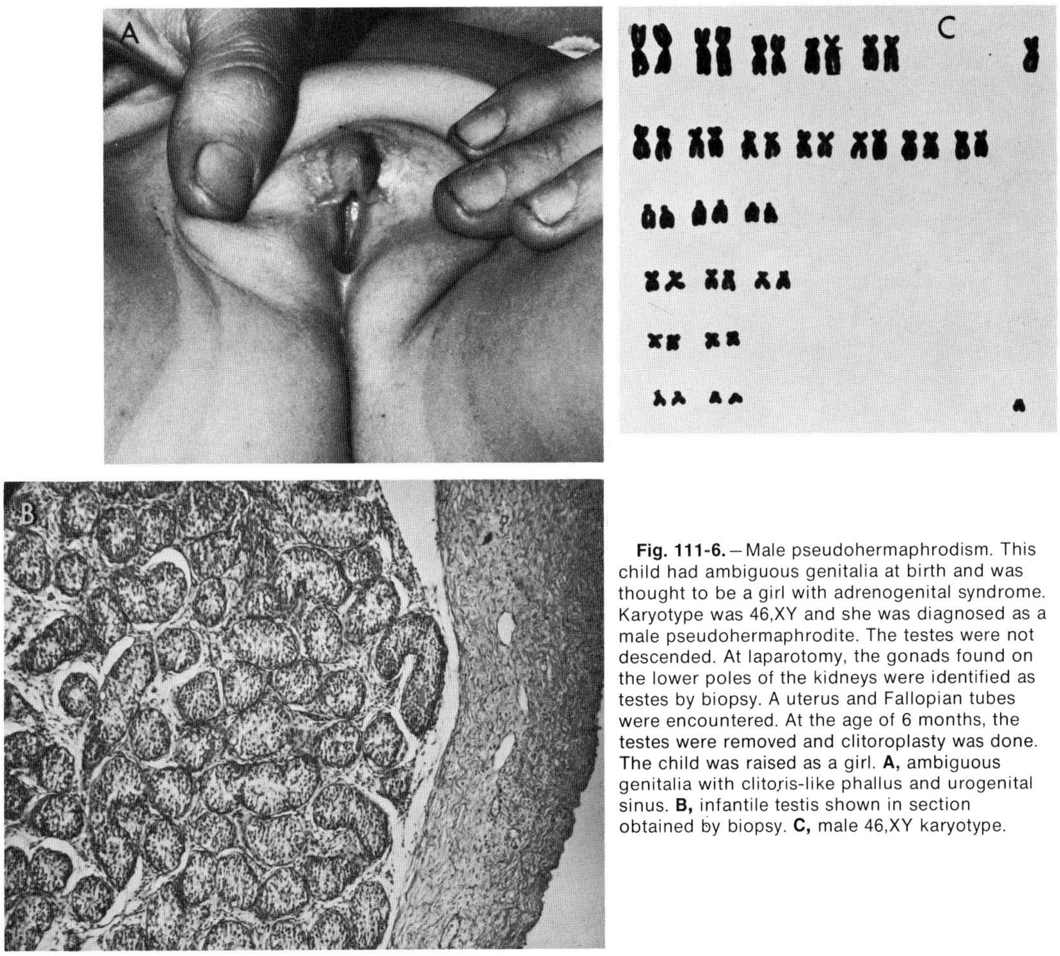

Fig. 111-6. — Male pseudohermaphrodism. This child had ambiguous genitalia at birth and was thought to be a girl with adrenogenital syndrome. Karyotype was 46,XY and she was diagnosed as a male pseudohermaphrodite. The testes were not descended. At laparotomy, the gonads found on the lower poles of the kidneys were identified as testes by biopsy. A uterus and Fallopian tubes were encountered. At the age of 6 months, the testes were removed and clitoroplasty was done. The child was raised as a girl. **A,** ambiguous genitalia with clitoris-like phallus and urogenital sinus. **B,** infantile testis shown in section obtained by biopsy. **C,** male 46,XY karyotype.

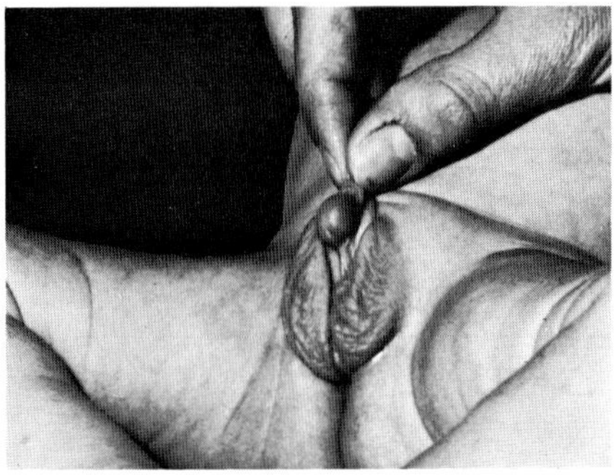

Fig. 111-7. – Ambiguous genitalia of an infant thought to have adrenogenital syndrome. There was a phallus, hypospadias, labioscrotal fusion and urogenital sinus; 17-ketosteroids were normal and the karyotype was 46,XY. Male pseudohermaphrodism was diagnosed but gonads could not be palpated. There were infections of the urinary tract, which were treated, but the child died at age 4½ months of pyelonephritis. The testes were found high in the abdominal cavity, tubules were immature but germinal cells were seen.

tors in the etiology of these cases, since they could deform genital structures as they distort the shapes of other organs (p. 1119).

To avoid complications at the time of puberty, children with ambiguous genitalia should be examined thoroughly soon after birth. The anatomic situation must be evaluated and supplemented by studies of sex chromatin, chromosomes and biopsy of the gonads. Then it can be decided – often with difficulty – how the child should be raised, male or female, without need for changes in later life.

Syndrome of Testicular Feminization

This syndrome represents a form of male pseudohermaphrodism occurring in rather normal-appearing girls or women who have undescended testes. Although such cases had been observed since early

Fig. 111-8. – Ambiguous genitalia of a male pseudohermaphrodite showing small phallus with hypospadias and opening of urogenital sinus; 46,XY karyotype.

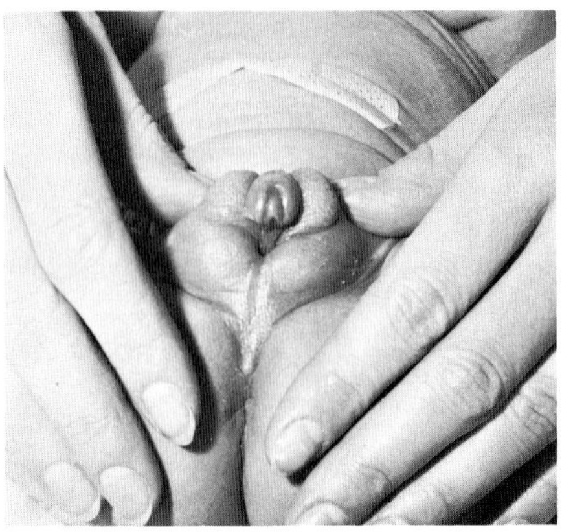

times,[4,20] the syndrome was named and outlined by Morris[5] in 1953, when 80 cases could be collected from the literature. The frequency of the anomaly is about 1 in 50,000.[6] It had been known that certain forms recur in families; it appears now that the syndrome of testicular feminization was present in many familial cases. Before Morris' publication,[5] the disorder usually was discovered by finding gonads in the inguinal canal during herniotomy or at laparotomy performed for abdominal tumors involving the gonads.[4] Now, the condition is suggested by family history, physical signs, sex chromatin and sex chromosomes, which reveal a male genotype.

The disorder is inconspicuous during childhood, when the patients seem to be normal girls. Aside from the sex organs, there are no congenital malformations associated with the syndrome apart from inguinal hernias, which occur in some of the girls.[4] At the time of puberty, some secondary sex characteristics develop. Breasts are formed and often they are well developed, although the nipples may remain juvenile. Pubic and axillary hair is deficient or absent and body hair scanty, whereas scalp hair is developed normally. The external genitalia are female but the labia minora often are underdeveloped; the vagina is short and ends blindly. Primary amenorrhea and sterility may lead to medical consultation if there were no earlier complaints. The growth of these patients is satisfactory but sometimes eunuchoid proportions result. Mental development is good in most of the cases[4,7] and mental retardation is the exception.[4,17] The mental and sexual orientation of these persons is definitely female. Although many are well adjusted to their condition, there is a high incidence of psychosis and suicide, especially when the patients suspect that they are abnormal, which occurs often because of failure to menstruate.[5] Some observations[8] suggest that associated psychopathy is independent of the malformations, since it appears in members of the family who are not intersexes.

In approximately 20% of the patients, a mass appears in the labia majora that can be identified as a testis and in 60% such a mass is located in the inguinal region. The remainder of the patients have abdominal testes.[4] The clitoris is of normal length in most patients. Uterus and Fallopian tubes are absent or very rudimentary.

The intra-abdominal, inguinal or labial testes contain numerous tubules that are filled with undifferentiated cells considered Sertoli cells by some. Specific Sertoli cells and spermatogonia are seen only rarely. Leydig cells abound and tend to form adenomas. Connective tissue around the tubules is thickened and fibrous stroma like that seen in dysgenetic ovaries can be found. Cysts form in the epididymis or in paratesticular structures of many patients.[4]

It seems that the secretory products of the testes of these pseudohermaphrodites do not differ essentially from those of normal males. In young adults, the levels of testosterone in plasma and urine are within the

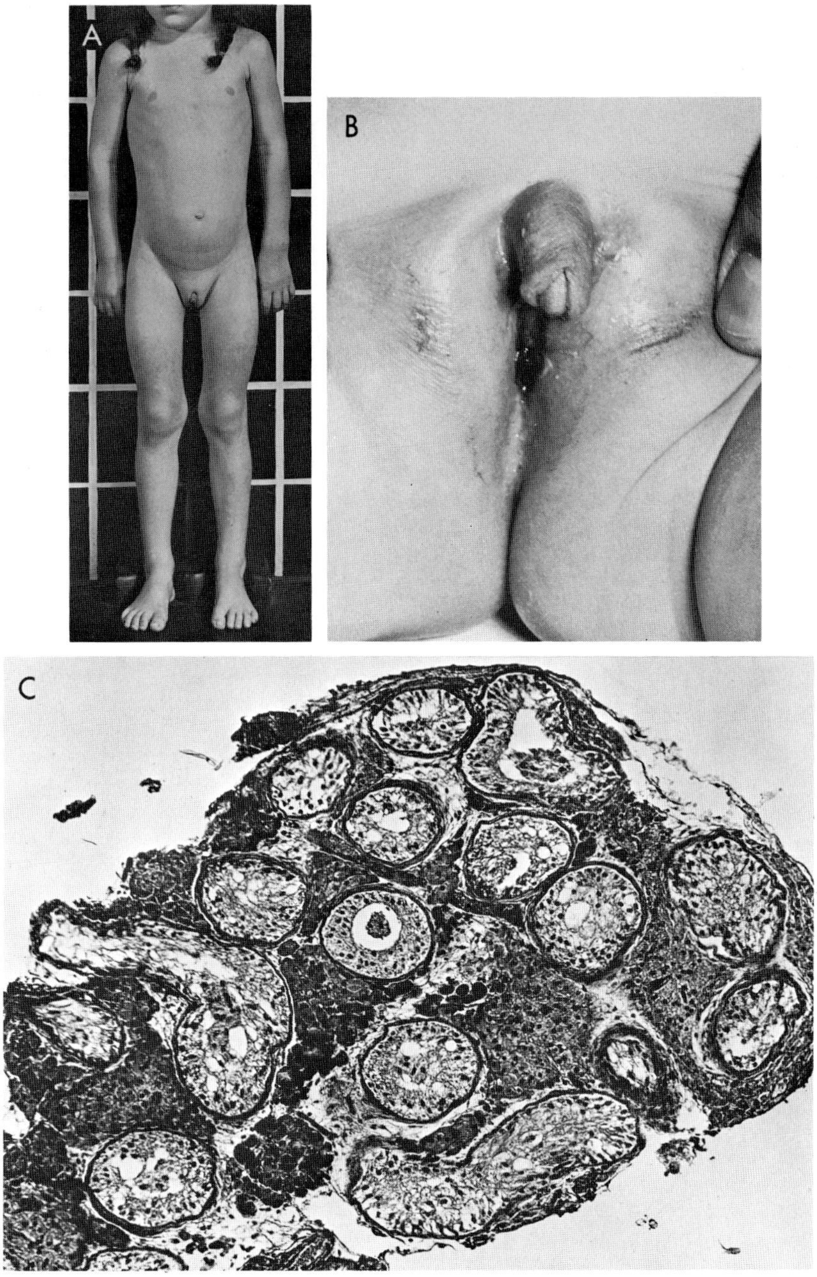

Fig. 111-9. – **A,** male pseudohermaphrodite. The child appeared to be a girl with enlarged clitoris. **B,** at the age of 14 years, virilization occurred. **C,** testes, found in ovarian position, were removed.

range for normal males and higher than in females; the 17-ketosteroid excretion is normal and estrogen levels in plasma and in urine are in the low range of normal females. Following castration, testosterone and estrogen levels fall and gonadotropic hormone levels rise.[9] It is thought that the inherited defect leading to this syndrome is an inability of target tissues to masculinize in utero and to develop secondary sex characteristics at adolescence.[10,11] Administration of large doses of testosterone to women with this syndrome fails to induce masculinization. Feminization is attributed to stimulation by luteinizing hormone of estrogen and testosterone production. Action of testosterone is prevented by a biochemical anomaly at the peripheral cellular level,[9] but the nature of this anomaly is not known. Estrogens

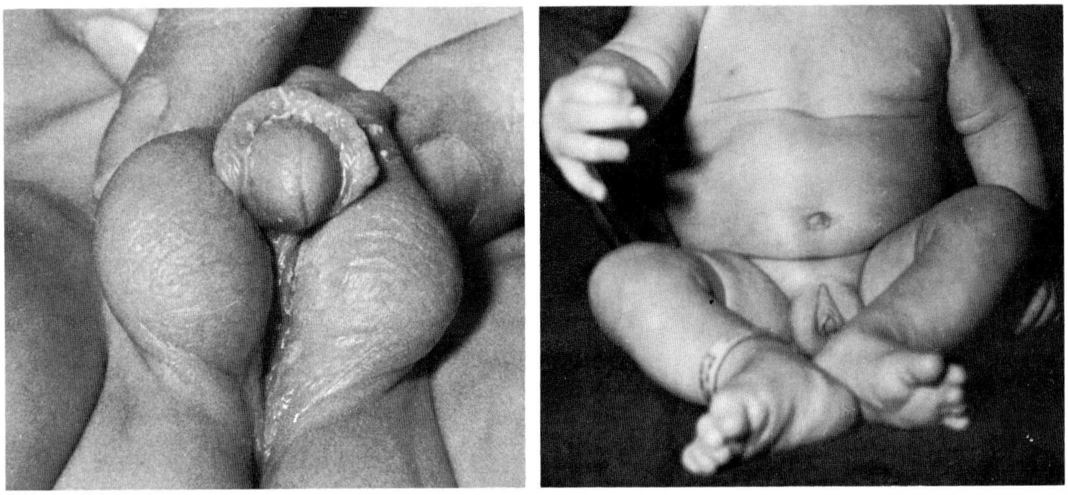

Fig. 111-10. – Ambiguous external genitalia in an infant at first considered to be a girl. The phallus was held down by a chordee, the scrotum was bifid and there was a perineal hypospadias. Gonads found in the inguen were biopsied and identified as testes. Karyotype was 46,XY. Hypospadias was repaired and the child was raised as a boy.

cause growth of breasts but nipples, areolae and gland development often are incomplete. There remains much to be explained in regard to the prenatal and postnatal pathogenesis of this syndrome and it is only fair to state that some investigators consider the testicular anomalies of these patients to be primarily at fault.[4]

There is general agreement that most women with testicular feminization have chromatin-negative cells and XY karyotype. By 1964, there were twenty-one kindreds on record in which the syndrome had occurred in several generations and thirty-one families in which 2 or more siblings were abnormal.[6] In affected kindreds, all the females (XX) are essentially normal in phenotype, whereas half the males (XY) have the disorder and are reared as females. It seems that the facts ascertained are compatible with the assumption of autosomal dominant inheritance with sex limitation and with X-linked recessive inheritance. Some female carriers with XX karyotype are recognizable by sparsity of axillary hair and delayed menarche.[12] Genetic aspects of the syndrome have been discussed by Lenz[6] and Boczkowski.[13]

Although most of the women with testicular feminization have 46,XY karyotype, a number of them have chromosomal abnormalities: XO/XY/XX,[14,15] XO/XY/XXY,[16] XY/XYY/XXY[17] and XXXY[18] mosaicisms have been found in some of the patients. It seems that monozygotic twins with XXY karyotype have been observed.[14] Such exceptional cases cannot be considered accidental; they demonstrate that the genetic origin of the syndrome can be heterogeneous and that genetic counseling must not be oversimplified.

Testicular adenomas are quite frequent in these patients and may amount to 25%. The risk of malignant change is about 5–8%. As more cases are discovered early, the relative tumor incidence decreases.[4]

Fekete[19] described a sexual abnormality in mice that seems comparable to testicular feminization in man. The abnormal animals appeared to be female externally but the vagina ended blindly and no internal female sex organs were found. Undescended testes were located in the abdomen halfway between kidney and bladder. Various degrees of testicular degeneration were observed. These changes were seen in 10 descendants of a pair of mice from an inbred strain that appeared in four generations. In one (possibly two) of these abnormal mice, embryonic carcinoma developed in a testis.

Incomplete Forms of Testicular Feminization

Persons with moderate enlargement of the clitoris, labioscrotal fusion and testes have been described repeatedly. Breast development can occur at adolescence but feminization is incomplete or virilization can take place. This type can recur in families. Lubs *et al.*[21] described 5 male pseudohermaphrodites with labial testes and partial feminization in two generations of a kindred. There was enlargement of the clitoris and sex chromatin was negative. The incomplete and the complete form of testicular feminization can occur in the same family.[9] Two sisters with 46,XY karyotype and incomplete testicular feminization were recorded by Bergman *et al.*[22] One sister noticed that her voice became deep and gruff at the age of 15 years and consulted a speech therapist who referred her to the gynecologic department. Subsequently, she and her sister were recognized as male pseudohermaphrodites.

It is said that the ability of the testes to virilize the

patient at adolescence frequently is a recapitulation of their masculinizing ability in utero. The greater the length of the phallus the greater the tendency to develop secondary sex characteristics, whereas those with feminine appearance tend to remain infantile or to feminize. Unfortunately, there are exceptions to this rule. There are girls with normal vagina and urethra who appear like normal female children except that they have an enlarged clitoris. On laparotomy, a uterus is found and gonads are seen in place of the ovaries; without biopsy, the gonads are taken for ovaries and left in place by the operator. At the time of adolescence, the voice becomes deeper and hair grows on the face and legs. There is no menstruation. When the gonads are removed, they are recognized as testes that lack germinal elements. Signs of masculinization may disappear subsequently and cyclic estrogen therapy can bring about development of secondary sex characteristics. Now, adolescent virilization can be avoided by establishment of negative sex chromatin, 46,XY karyotype, biopsy and removal of the testes during early childhood. Barr *et al.*[23] reported this type of male pseudohermaphrodism in a patient who had a sister with pure gonadal dysgenesis. This observation suggests that the lack of prenatal masculinization in the sister with pure gonadal dysgenesis cannot be attributed to her lack of testes, since her sister, who had testes, also failed to develop a male phenotype.

Reifenstein Syndrome

This form of male pseudohermaphrodism consists of hypospadias, postpubertal atrophy of the testes, azoospermia and gynecomastia. The testes show tubular fibrosis, deficiency of spermatogonia and sometimes Leydig cell hyperplasia. The karyotype is 46,XY and the condition is transmitted to males as a sex-linked recessive or a sex-limited autosomal dominant trait. The patients respond to exogenous androgen administration.[9,24]

Hernia Uteri Inguinalis in the Male (Internal Male Pseudohermaphrodism)

This anomaly occurs in apparently normal males who have, in addition to testes and male ducts, structures derived from Müllerian ducts. The condition can be symptomless or become noticeable by the finding of a uterus or tubes in an inguinal hernia or by inflammation due to retention of secretory uterine products. A rudimentary vagina may terminate in the prostate. Testes can be in the scrotum or ectopic. The patients may be fertile.[25-27] The etiology and pathogenesis are not elucidated. In an unusual case of XO/XXXY mosaicism, a uterus and tube were found in an inguinal canal of a newborn boy who had an inguinal testis on the contralateral side. The child actually had mixed gonadal dysgenesis[28] (p. 1137).

Feminization of Males with Lipoid Adrenal Hyperplasia

Feminization of boys associated with a lipoid hyperplasia of the adrenals was reported by Prader and Siebenmann.[29] Although this rare disease occurs both in boys and girls, the external genitalia are always female. The condition is an ACTH-resistant adrenal insufficiency that can be alleviated through use of cortisone and sodium chloride but survival beyond infancy is rare. Anatomically, the adrenal cortex shows an enormous nodular hyperplasia. With the exception of sparse subcapsular and juxtamedullary areas, the cortical cells are distended with cholesterol and other lipoids. Histochemically detectable ketosteroids are absent. The authors believed that the syndrome is caused by a hereditary enzyme defect in an early stage of steroid synthesis within the adrenal cortex and the Leydig cells. It is possible that these defects involve the transformation of the $\Delta 5$- to $\Delta 4$-steroids. The inhibition of the steroid synthesis leads to both adrenal and testicular insufficiency and the latter occurring in the embryo may explain the female genital development of boys.

Incomplete Masculinization with 3β-Hydroxysteroid Dehydrogenase Deficiency

Male pseudohermaphrodism can occur in patients with adrenal hyperplasia due to 3β-hydroxysteroid dehydrogenase deficiency.[30] In this anomaly, the block is at an early step of steroid synthesis, resulting in failure of the fetal Leydig cells to produce adrenal steroids and testosterone. Masculinization of the external genitalia is incomplete but male genital ducts are present and Müllerian duct derivatives absent. Most of the patients with this anomaly have died in infancy.[9]

Feminizing Adrenal Tumors

Adrenal tumors causing gynecomastia in males occur occasionally in adults but they are very rare in children. Whether prenatal factors are involved in the etiology in any of them is doubtful. In a boy described by Wilkins,[31] breast development was noticed at the age of 6 months and in the case reported by Mosier and Goodwin,[32] signs of virilization in the mother during pregnancy and unilateral cryptorchidism in the patient could be interpreted as symptoms indicative of prenatal onset. In girls, similar tumors bring about isosexual precocity.[10,33] The finding of elevated 17-ketosteroids in the urine leads to recognition of the adrenals as the source of feminization. Adenomas of the adrenal have been found and removed at operation, with alleviation of symptoms.

Pseudohermaphrodism and Wilms Tumor

A syndrome of male pseudohermaphrodism, Wilms tumor, hypertension and degenerative renal disease has been observed in several children.[34]

Male Pseudohermaphrodism with Chromosomal Abnormalities

Most male pseudohermaphrodites have a 46,XY karyotype but some have abnormal chromosomes. Persons with a testis on one side and a dysgenic gonad on the other side are now considered as cases of "mixed gonadal dysgenesis" (p. 1137). In 1961, Shah *et al.*[35] reported a patient reared as a boy despite ambiguous external genitalia, i.e., presence of a phallus and a vagina. At laparotomy, no uterus was found but there were male ducts and testes containing immature seminiferous tubes and Leydig cells. The karyotype established from skin fibroblasts was 46,XX. Despite the karyotype, such a patient with female secondary sex characteristics and testes is phenotypically a male pseudohermaphrodite. Conen and Erkman[36] described an infant who had testes in the position of ovaries, ambiguous genitalia and XX/XO mosaicism. Cooper and Hernits[37] saw a female patient because of amenorrhea and failure of secondary sex development. There was an enlarged clitoris with a urethral opening at its base and bilateral inguinal testes. The karyotype was XY and the chromosomes no. 1 were unequal in size, an anomaly that also was present in a sister and the mother of the patient. An XO/XY/XYY mosaicism and a (familial) translocation were reported by Ferrier *et al.*[38] in a child who had ambiguous genitalia with a uterus, one Fallopian tube, an abnormal abdominal gonad and one scrotal testis. A male pseudohermaphrodite with an XO/XY/XXY mosaicism was also observed by Milcu *et al.*[39] Ambiguous genitalia, hirsutism, lack of breast development and bilateral testes were present in a young "woman" who had an XY/XX/XXY mosaicism.[40] Male pseudohermaphrodism was reported in a patient with XYY karyotype.[41] The clitoris was enlarged, there were separate vaginal and urethral openings and testes in the major labia.

Fig. 111-11.—Bifid scrotum in a newborn boy. The opening of the urethra was at the base of the phallus. Right testis was undescended. Karyotype: XO/XY mosaicism.

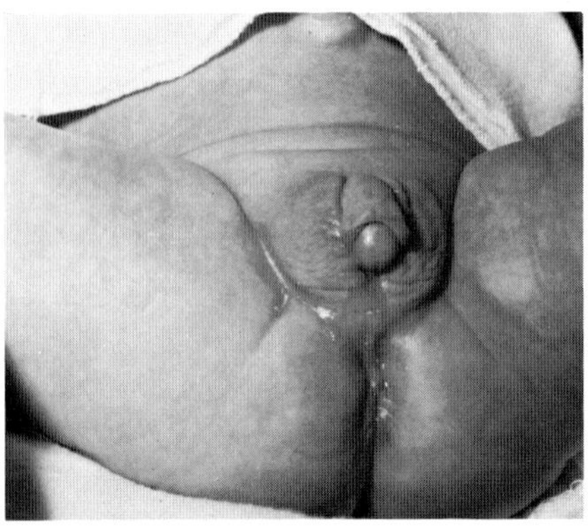

Men with 46,XX Karyotype

A number of men with female XX karyotype have been reported in the literature. De Grouchy *et al.*[42] summarized the reports and added 2 observations. These men are of normal masculine habitus and height and there are no malformations. Intelligence is good in some, below normal in others. Hypoplastic genitalia, reduced sexual activity and azoospermia seem to be the rule. The testes are small, soft and comparable to those of Klinefelter syndrome. Gynecomastia is rare. There are many theories concerning the masculinization of men without a Y chromosome. Hecht *et al.*[43] found a small number of XXY cells in a predominantly "XX man."

REFERENCES

1. Green, O. C., Miller, R. R., Garcia, O., and Hamwi, G. J.: Virilizing male pseudohermaphroditism. Association with abnormal testicular function, J. Clin. Endocrinol. 29:728, 1969.
2. Dewhurst, C. J.: The XY female child, Arch. Dis. Childhood 45:595, 1970.
3. Royer, P., Pellerin, D., Habib, R., Vermeil, G., and Rodriguez-Soriano, J.: Le pseudo-hermaphrodisme masculin interne a organes génitaux externes masculins normaux, Ann. pédiat. 15:143, 1961.
4. Hauser, G. A.: Testicular Feminization, in Overzier, C. (ed.), *Intersexuality* (London and New York: Academic Press, 1963).
5. Morris, J. M.: The syndrome of testicular feminization in male pseudohermaphrodites, Am. J. Obst. & Gynec. 65: 1192, 1953.
6. Lenz, W.: Krankheiten des Urogenitalsystems, in Becker, P. E. (ed.), *Humangenetik* (Stuttgart: Georg Thieme, 1964).
7. Masica, D. N., Money, J., Ehrhardt, A. A., and Lewis, V. G.: IQ, fetal sex hormones and cognitive patterns: Studies in the testicular feminizing syndrome of androgen insensitivity, Johns Hopkins M. J. 124:34, 1969.
8. Burgermaster, J. J.: Contribution a l'étude d'un type familial d'intersexualité, Thèse, Université de Genève Éditions Médecine et Hygiène Genève, 1953.
9. Van Wyk, J. J., and Grumbach, M. M.: Disorders of Sex Differentiation, in Williams, R. H., (ed.), *Textbook of Endocrinology* (4th ed.; Philadelphia: W. B. Saunders Company, 1968).
10. Wilkins, L.: *The Diagnosis and Treatment of Endocrine Disorders in Childhood and Adolescence* (2d ed.; Springfield, Ill.: Charles C Thomas, Publisher, 1957).
11. Prader, A.: Gonadendysgenesie und testikuläre Feminisierung, Schweiz. med. Wchnschr. 87:278, 1957.
12. Puck, T. T., Robinson, A., and Tjio, J. H.: Familial primary amenorrhea due to testicular feminization, Proc. Soc. Exper. Biol. & Med. 103:192, 1960.
13. Boczkowski, K.: Genetical studies in testicular feminization syndrome, J. M. Genetics 5:181, 1968.
14. Miller, O. J.: The sex chromosome anomalies, Am. J. Obst. & Gynec. 90:1078, 1964.
15. Morris, J. M., and Mahesh, V. B.: Further observations on the syndrome, "testicular feminization," Am. J Obst. & Gynec. 87:731, 1963.

16. Uozumi, T., Nozaki, R., Matsumoto, K., Seki, T., and Furuyama, J.: Endocrinological studies of a case of mosaicism (XO/XY/XXY) with clinical appearance of testicular feminization syndrome, Acta endocrinol. 54:193, 1967.
17. Forsberg, J. G., Hall, B., and Rydén, A. B. V.: A case of testicular feminization with chromosome mosaicism, Acta obstet. gynec. scandinav. 44:491, 1965.
18. Botella-Ilusia, J., Clavero-Nunez, J. A., and Nagales, F.: Un caso de feminization testicular con cariotipo XXXY, Acta ginec. 15:389, 1964.
19. Fekete, E.: Sexual abnormalities in an inbred strain of mice, Proc. Soc. Exper. Biol. & Med. 38:59, 1938.
20. Simmer, H., Pion, R. J., and Dignam, W. J.: *Testicular Feminization* (Springfield, Ill.: Charles C Thomas, Publisher, 1965).
21. Lubs, H. A., Jr., Vilar, O., and Bergenstal, D. M.: Familial male pseudohermaphrodism with labial testes and partial feminization: Endocrine studies and genetic aspects, J. Clin. Endocrinol. 19:1110, 1959.
22. Bergman, S., Reitalu, J., and Sundén, B.: Male pseudohermaphroditism in two sisters, Acta obst. et gynec. scandinav. 42:138, 1963.
23. Barr, M. L., Carr, D. H., Plunkett, E. R., Soltan, H. C., and Wiens, R. G.: Male pseudohermaphroditism and pure gonadal dysgenesis in sisters, Am. J. Obst. & Gynec. 99: 1047, 1967.
24. Bowen, P., Lee, C. S., Migeon, C. J., Kaplan, N. M., Whalley, P. J., McKusick, V. A., and Reifenstein, E. C.: Hereditary male pseudohermaphroditism with hypogonadism, hypospadias and gynecomastia: Reifenstein's syndrome, Ann. Int. Med. 62:252, 1965.
25. Nilson, O.: Hernia uteri inguinalis beim Manne, Acta chir. scandinav. 83:231, 1939.
26. Young, D.: Hernia uteri inguinalis in the male, J. Obst. & Gynaec. Brit. Emp. 58:830, 1951.
27. Ashley, D. J. B.: *Human Intersex* (Baltimore: The Williams & Wilkins Company, 1962).
28. Warkany, J., Chu, E. H. Y., and Kauder, E.: Male pseudohermaphroditism and chromosomal mosaicism, Am. J. Dis. Child. 104:172, 1962.
29. Prader, A., and Siebenmann, R. E.: Nebenniereninsuffizienz bei kongenitaler Lipoidhyperplasie der Nebennieren, Helvet. paediat. acta 12:569, 1957.
30. Bongiovanni, A. M.: The adrenogenital syndrome with deficiency of 3β-hydroxysteroid dehydrogenase, J. Clin. Invest. 41:2086, 1964.
31. Wilkins, L.: A feminizing adrenal tumor causing gynecomastia in a boy of 5 years contrasted with a virilizing tumor in a 5 year old girl, J. Clin. Endocrinol. 8:111, 1948.
32. Mosier, H. D., and Goodwin, W. E.: Feminizing adrenal adenoma in a 7-year-old boy, Pediatrics 27:1016, 1961.
33. Snaith, A. H.: A case of feminizing adrenal tumor in a girl, J. Clin. Endocrinol. 18:318, 1958.
34. Drash, A., Sherman, F., Hartmann, W. H., and Blizzard, R. M.: A syndrome of pseudohermaphroditism, Wilms' tumor, hypertension, and degenerative renal disease, J. Pediat. 76:585, 1970.
35. Shah, P. N., Nuik, S. N., Mahagan, D. K., Paymaster, J. C., Dave, M. J., and Tiwari, R.: Male pseudohermaphroditism with female chromosomal complement, J. Clin. Endocrinol. 21:727, 1961.
36. Conen, P. E., and Erkman, B.: Two "new" sex-chromosome mosaics XO/XX;XX/XX (deletion of short arm X) and a further XO/XY mosaic, Lancet 2:1276, 1963.
37. Cooper, H. L., and Hernits, R.: A familial chromosome variant in a subject with anomalous sex differentiation, Am. J. Human Genet. 15:465, 1963.
38. Ferrier, P. E., Ferrier, S. A., Schärer, K. O., Genton, N., Hedinger, C., and Klein, D.: Multiple chromosome aberrations: XO/XY/XYY mosaicism and a translocation in the same family, Helvet. paediat. acta 22:516, 1967.
39. Milcu, S., *et al.*: Pseudohermafroditism masculin cu mozaic cromozomial XO/XY/XYY, Fiziol. Norm. Pat. 10: 145, 1964.
40. Klay, L. J., Sparkes, R. S., and LaGasse, L. D.: Generalized XY/XX/XXY chromosomal mosaicism in a male hermaphrodite, Am. J. Obst. & Gynec. 99:495, 1967.
41. Franks, R. C., Bunting, K. W., and Engel, E.: Male pseudohermaphrodism with XYY sex chromosomes, J. Clin. Endocrinol. 27:1623, 1967.
42. de Grouchy, J., Canivet, J., Canlorbe, P., Mantel, O., Borniche, P., and Poitout, M.: Deux observations d'hommes 46,XX, Ann. Génét. 10:193, 1967.
43. Hecht, F., Antonius, J. I., McGuire, P., and Hale, C. G.: XXY cells in a predominantly XX human male: Evidence for cell selection, Pediatrics 38:982, 1966.
44. Hayata, I., Makina, S., and Sutou, S.: A preliminary note on a phenotypic male with an XX constitution, Proc. Jap. Acad. 45:303, 1969.
45. Ferrier, P. E., Ferrier, S. A., and Kelley, V. C.: Sex chromosome mosaicism in male pseudohermaphrodism, Am. J. Dis. Child. 120:566, 1970.

Pseudohermaphrodism in Syndromes of Congenital Malformations: Ullrich-Feichtiger Syndrome (Typus Rostockiensis); Smith-Lemli-Opitz and Other Syndromes

MANY PSEUDOHERMAPHRODITES, particularly those seen by endocrinologists and gynecologists, are generally well-formed, with the exception of their genital organs. Their manifestations usually can be explained by cytogenetic or endocrine anomalies, although, in some cases, there are discrepancies between their secondary sex characteristics, their karyotype and their gonads. The official tenet that the Y chromosome directs formation of the testes and that the embryonic testes determine the formation of secondary sex characteristics cannot be upheld in all instances. Such irregular cases often are explained by assumptions and hypotheses that have little foundation and cannot be proved or disproved. One point seldom remembered is the fact that external and internal genitalia can be deformed like other organs, such as kidneys, heart, brain, intestines and limbs, by environmental or genetic factors without intervention of gonads or sex chromosomes. In 1950, C. R. Moore,[1] discussing the role of fetal endocrine glands in development, pointed out that modification of embryos and fetuses in utero can be obtained experimentally not only by introduction of chemical hormones into pregnant mothers or direct application to embryos but also by other teratogenic methods such as vitamin A deficiency of the mother. Little attention has been paid to this statement until recently.

Experimental teratology furnishes examples of induced syndromes of congenital malformations that include pseudohermaphrodism. It has been shown in animal experiments that vitamin A deficiency can produce anomalies of the external genitalia and of the Wolffian and Müllerian ducts in the presence of apparently normal gonads. Wilson and Warkany[2] noted that in males there were female ducts, lack of testicular descent, absence or inhibition of bulbo-urethral glands, seminal vesicles, male sex ducts, defective urogenital sinus and hypospadias. In females, male ducts sometimes were found in the absence of Müllerian ducts and of a distal vagina and there was retardation in development of the urogenital sinus. Similar results were obtained by Palludan[3] in pigs damaged by vitamin A deficiency. These modifications of the genital organs were achieved without the use of estrogens and androgens. Newborn rats with anomalies of the genital tract also had malformations of the kidneys, the cardiovascular system, the eyes and the diaphragm. The experiments showed that the external and internal genitalia can be deformed like other organ systems by teratogenic procedures, probably irrespective of the function of the testes and the karyotype. It is likely, therefore, that in some cases lack of testicular function in prenatal life explains feminization, whereas in others masculinization of females and feminization of males is due to interference with normal development of the genital organs by various teratogenic factors, including abnormal genetic constellations. In man, modification of sex characteristics was clearly demonstrated in the syndrome of the thalidomide embryopathy, but genital changes did not get the attention given to limb defects. Absence of uterus and vagina, uterus duplex, bicornis and unicornis and vagina bipartita were observed in females. In males, cryptorchidism, anorchidism, absence of scrotum and hypospadias were noted in some of the cases.[4,5]

Because of the close relationship of genital and urinary organs, it is understandable that malformations of the sex organs often are combined with malformations of the urinary tract. Carpentier and Potter[6] described 3 "male infants" who had ovaries and a positive sex chromatin, although externally there was a phallus, centrally placed urethra and hypoplastic scrotum. These 3 female pseudohermaphrodites were among 48 infants with renal agenesis. Schlegel *et al.*[7] reported the case of a similar newborn infant of assumed male gender who had a small penis, urethral meatus at the tip of the glans, an empty scrotum and gonads that resembled ovaries. There were Fallopian tubes but no uterus. The karyotype was 46,XX. In addition to female pseudohermaphrodism, the infant had an imperforate anus and bilateral renal agenesis. It is difficult to explain the masculinization of these female fetuses by nonexisting fetal testes. It is much more likely that all the malformations in these children have a common cause that is responsible for the malformations of the external genitalia and genital ducts that do not conform to the gonads. Franks and Northcutt[8] reported a case of female pseudohermaphrodism combined with urologic problems in a girl with 46,XX karyotype. They suggested that early examination of the urinary tract of pseudohermaphrodites is of practical importance, since it can reveal renal disease and lead to prompt appropriate treatment. Hypoplastic and cystic kidneys with atretic ureters or hydronephrosis,[9,10] double uterus and unilateral absence of the ovary and of the Fallopian tube may occur. Some renal anomalies combined with genital deformities can be so severe that the infants do not survive the neonatal period. Nonadrenal female pseudohermaphrodism with a cloaca[11] and other intestinal malformations have been recorded.[10] In one case observed in the Children's Hospital at Cincinnati, a diabetic mother who had been treated with progesterone during pregnancy because of threatened and habitual abortion had a child with female pseudohermaphrodism and imperforate anus. Whether such malformations involving the alimentary tract can be attributed to treatment with progestin-like steroids remains to be seen.

Malformations of the genital tract can be associated with defects in many other organs, and various syndromes of congenital malformations have been described that include genital changes. These changes may be limited to the external genitalia or they may be so extensive that pseudohermaphrodism results. Such disease pictures have been considered as "nonspecific" or "teratologic" hermaphrodism by Ferrier *et al.*[12] The latter term would be useful, as it alludes to multiple malformations, which always accompany the genital defects. But, since all types of hermaphrodism are teratologic phenomena, the name is not distinctive enough to be recommended.

Pseudohermaphrodism combined with malformations of the head, including micrognathia and ear anomalies, uvula fissa, atresia ani and polydactyly was reported as early as 1854 and 1862[13] and similar combinations have been described under various headings since. Associated malformations often are lethal or so domineering that affected children fail to reach the endocrinologist or gynecologist. Some of the syndromes involving and deforming the genitalia are of known etiology, others are not. Trisomy 13-15 sometimes results in abnormalities of the penis and cryptorchidism, changes that seldom will lead to a diagnosis of pseudohermaphrodism. But a similar phenotype, called "Ullrich-Feichtiger"[14,15] syndrome or "typus Rostockiensis" (after the town in which Feichtiger's dissertation was published), can include pseudohermaphrodism. Hypospadias, split scrotum, cryptorchidism, uterus septus or bicornis and vagina septa are malformations occurring together with micrognathia, aural and ocular anomalies, polydactyly and other digital defects. Reviews were published by Hövels and Müllereisert[13] and Weber and Schwarz.[16] There is overlapping of this syndrome with "dysencephalia splanchnocystica" (p. 213) and with trisomy 13-15. But infants with such syndromes usually have normal karyotype.

Neither "Ullrich-Feichtiger syndrome" nor "typus Rostockiensis" became popular terms. When Smith *et al.*[17] described as a "newly recognized syndrome" of multiple congenital anomalies cases of 3 unrelated male children with incomplete development of the external genitalia, microcephaly, mental retardation, hypertonicity, peculiar facies and digital anomalies, their publication was followed by many reports on the "Smith-Lemli-Opitz" syndrome. This disease picture is less distinctive than the "typus Rostockiensis," as mild genital changes and syndactyly replaced pseudohermaphrodism and polydactyly of the older entity. But it is clear that the patients recorded as typus Rostockiensis by Hövels and Müllereisert[13] in 1955 and by Weber and Schwarz in 1960[16] had most of the features of the syndrome described by Smith *et al.*[17] in 1964. Polydactyly was present in rudimentary form in Case 2 of Smith *et al.*[17] and in cases observed by Dallaire.[18] The peculiar facial features of the Smith-Lemli-Opitz syndrome, including anteverted nares and micrognathia, can be seen in Figure 2 of the publication by Hövels and Müllereisert.[13] Cleft palate or cleft uvula,[17-20] widened maxillary alveolar ridge, congenital heart defects[18,20] and renal anomalies[17,20-22] seen in some children with Smith-Lemli-Opitz syndrome have been described in the typus Rostockiensis before.[13,16] Intrauterine growth retardation can occur in these syndromes[13,18-21,23] but not all cases are so affected.[17] Autosomal recessive inheritance has been suggested by several authors.[17-19] It must be mentioned that in some familial cases one sibling may show anomalies of the genitalia whereas the other—usually a female—has apparently normal genitalia.

Severe deformities were reported by Ferrier *et al.*,[12] who, in 1964, described a male infant with ambiguous external genitalia, large clitoris, posterior labial fusion opening into a urogenital sinus, vagina and uterus in the presence of small testes at the normal location of ovaries. This male pseudohermaphrodism was combined with microcephaly, arhinencephaly, microphthalmia, micrognathia, anomalous external ears, polydactyly, common mesentery and Meckel diverticulum. The karyotype was 46,XY. The testes of the infant were poorly organized, small and of atypical structure, so that one could "explain" the imperfect masculinization of the child's external and internal genitalia by the deficiency of the embryonic testes. But this probably is as unjustified as blaming the inadequacy of the embryonic testis for the microphthalmia, microcephaly and polydactyly of the child. These anomalies as well as those of the testes probably have a common cause; they are coordinated with the testicular anomalies but are not caused by them. These authors[12] observed another infant with pseudohermaphrodism who had multiple congenital malformations. The external appearance suggested renal agenesis but two (abnormal) kidneys were present. The anus was imperforate and only the upper third of the intestine was present. Bladder and right ureter formed a cystic mass. This child had a clitoris-like organ but no urethra, vagina or urogenital sinus. There was a small uterus, a Fallopian tube on the right and no gonad on either side. The karyotype was 46,XX. Similarity to the typus Rostockiensis was pointed out by the authors.

A syndrome that combines cleft lip and palate, finger deformities, popliteal pterygium and abnormal muscle development, hypospadias, cryptorchidism, absent scrotum, enlarged clitoris and hypoplasia of labia majora[24] may or may not be related to the typus Rostockiensis and its successor syndromes.

Clitoris hypertrophy associated with tetraphocomelia and cleft lip and palate has been considered a syndrome by Appelt *et al.*[25]

The foregoing examples show that malformations of the external genitalia and the sex ducts can be included in various syndromes of multiple congenital defects. The genital malformations may be minor morphologic deviations or they can amount to pseudohermaphroditic changes. The gonads can be involved but it is likely that most of the secondary sex changes are not mediated by endocrine mechanisms but are attributable to abnormal genes, chromosomes or environmental factors that also cause malformations in other organ systems.

REFERENCES

1. Moore, C. R.: The role of the fetal endocrine glands in development, J. Clin. Endocrinol. 10:942, 1950.
2. Wilson, J. G., and Warkany, J.: Malformations in the genitourinary tract induced by maternal vitamin A deficiency in the rat, Am. J. Anat. 83:357, 1948.
3. Palludan, B.: *A-Avitaminosis in Swine* (Copenhagen: Ejnar Munsgaard, 1966).
4. Kreipe, U.: Missbildungen innerer Organe bei Thalidomidembryopathie, Arch. Kinderh. 176:33, 1967.
5. Kajii, T.: Thalidomide experience in Japan, Ann. paediat. 205:341, 1965.
6. Carpentier, P. J., and Potter, E. L.: Nuclear sex and genital malformations in 48 cases of renal agenesis with especial reference to non-specific female pseudohermaphroditism, Am. J. Obst. & Gynec. 76:235, 1959.
7. Schlegel, R. J., Aspillaga, M. J., Neu, R. L., Carneiro-Leano, J., and Gardner, L. I.: An XX sex chromosome complement in an infant having male-type external genitals, renal agenesis, and other anomalies, J. Pediat. 69: 812, 1966.
8. Franks, R. C., and Northcutt, R.: Female pseudohermaphroditism and renal anomalies, Am. J. Dis. Child. 105: 490, 1963.
9. Papadatos, C., and Klein, R.: Nonadrenal female pseudohermaphrodism—report of two patients simulating mixed adrenal disease, J. Pediat. 45:662, 1954.
10. Gross, R. E., and Meeker, I. A., Jr.: Abnormalities of sexual development. Observations from 75 cases, Pediatrics 16:303, 1955.
11. Sieber, W. K., and Klein, R.: Cloaca with non-adrenal female pseudohermaphrodism, Pediatrics 22:472, 1958.
12. Ferrier, P., Widgren, S., and Ferrier, S.: Nonspecific pseu-

dohermaphroditism. Report of two cases with cytogenetic investigations, Helvet. paediat. acta 19:1, 1964.
13. Hövels, O., and Müllereisert, F.: Der "Typus Rostockiensis" als characteristisches Kombinationsbild multipler Missbildungen, Ztschr. Kinderh. 77:454, 1955.
14. Feichtiger, H.: Ein neuer, typischer, vorwiegend die Akren betreffender Fehlbidungskomplex, Inaugural Dissertation, Rostock, 1943.
15. Ullrich, O.: Der Status Bonnevie-Ullrich im Rahmen anderer "Dyscranio-Dysphalangien," Ergebn. inn. Med. u. Kinderh. 2:412, 1951.
16. Weber, J. W., and Schwarz, H.: Der Typus Rostockiensis Ullrich-Feichtiger. Dyskranio-pygo-phalangie, Helvet. paediat. acta 15:163, 1960.
17. Smith, D. W., Lemli, L., and Opitz, J. M.: A newly recognized syndrome of multiple congenital anomalies, J. Pediat. 64:210, 1964.
18. Dallaire, L.: Syndrome of retardation with urogenital and skeletal anomalies (Smith-Lemli-Opitz Syndrome): Clinical features and mode of inheritance, J. M. Genetics 6: 113, 1969.
19. Pinsky, L., and DiGeorge, A. M.: A familial syndrome of facial and skeletal anomalies associated with genital abnormality in the male and normal genitals in the female, J. Pediat. 66:1049, 1965.
20. Park, S. C., Needles, C. F., Dimich, I., and Sussman, L.: Congenital heart disease in an infant with the Smith-Lemli-Opitz syndrome, J. Pediat. 73:896, 1968.
21. Fine, R. N., Gwinn, J. L., and Young, E. F.: Smith-Lemli-Opitz syndrome, Am. J. Dis. Child. 115:483, 1968.
22. Hanissian, A. S., and Summitt, R. L.: Smith-Lemli-Opitz syndrome in a Negro child, J. Pediat. 74:303, 1969.
23. Ruvalcaba, R. H. A., Reichert, A., and Smith, D. W.: Smith-Lemli-Opitz syndrome, Arch. Dis. Childhood 43: 620, 1968.
24. Rosselli, D., and Gulienetti, R.: Ectodermal dysplasia, Brit. J. Plast. Surg. 14:190, 1961.
25. Appelt, H., Gerken, H., and Lenz, W.: Tetraphokomelie mit Lippen-Kiefer-Gaumenspalte und Clitorishypertrophie – ein Syndrom, Pädiat. und Pädol. 2:119, 1966.

112

Sex Chromosomal Anomalies

Turner Syndrome
(Gonadal Dysgenesis)

THERE ARE MANY NAMES for the disorder to be discussed in this section, which indicates that the syndrome is not sharply demarcated and that it has undergone changes according to the knowledge of the times. Endocrinologists place the gonadal dysgenesis and the growth deficit of the patients in the center of the syndrome, but it is clear that many malformations associated with gonadal dysgenesis cannot be explained by endocrine deficiencies and that the patients can be classified according to different points of view and the chief interest of the observers. The syndrome looks entirely different to the pediatrician who sees it in the neonatal period and to the endocrinologist who encounters it at or after the age of adolescence. It looks different to the urologist and different to the cardiologist and the teratologist.

It seems that the first clear description of a patient with gonadal dysgenesis and congenital anomalies often associated with it was given by Funke in 1902.[1] This author observed and described a girl, 15 3/4 years of age, who had pterygium colli, small stature (135 cm.) and high palate. The ears were low-set, large, elongated and standing off. It was reported that she had had swollen feet during her first years. Menstruation had not occurred yet and there was absence of breast development, infantile nipples and lack of axillary and pubic hair. Funke was chiefly interested in the externally recognizable symptoms and explained them by abnormal concrescence of the amnion and epidermis in fetal life. He did not explain the infantilism of his patient, but there can be no doubt that he described an adolescent of the type that later became known as the "Turner syndrome." Baer,[2] in 1927, probably was dealing with a similar patient, a 23-year-old girl of male habitus and sexual infantilism. On laparotomy, no ovaries were found but adrenal tissue was present in place of the ovaries. An 8-year-old girl who belonged in this category was reported by Ullrich in 1930.[3] This child had pterygium colli, ptosis of the eyelids, lack of facial expression, cubitus valgus, irregularities of the nails and rudimentary nip-

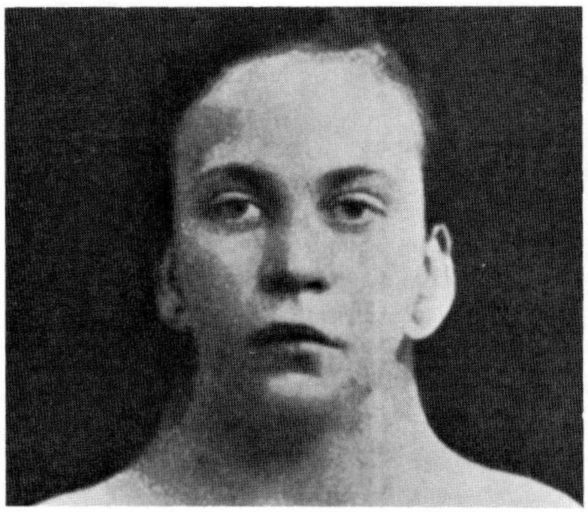

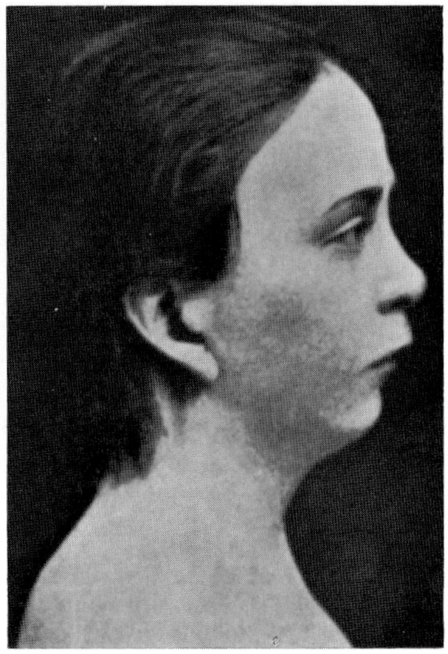

Fig. 112-1.—Patient with pterygium colli, elongated and low-set ears and micrognathia recorded by Funke[1] in 1902. The patient was retarded in growth and sexual maturation. A high-arched palate was emphasized.

ples. The internal organs appeared normal to Ullrich, who, as he was dealing with a child, understandably missed the endocrine nature of the syndrome even though he was faced, in all probability, with a case of gonadal dysgenesis. Since Ullrich was impressed by the anomalies that were recognizable externally, he made these characteristics the center of the syndrome. Unfortunately, he included entities that had little in common with gonadal dysgenesis except some superficial external signs. He strongly advocated an explanation of the pathogenesis based on observations by the embryologist Bonnevie,[4] who had analyzed variable symptoms of a strain of mice derived from the x-rayed mice of Little and Bagg,[5] known to geneticists as "myelencephalic blebs (my)." Bonnevie thought that the anomalies of these mice were the result of overproduction of cerebral spinal fluid, which can leave the myelencephalon to form blebs and migrate under the epidermis. Eyes, feet and other organs located on the surface of the body can be damaged by such blebs. Bonnevie's explanation of the symptoms of mice with blebs is not generally accepted by mouse geneticists, and there certainly is no proof that it applies to human malformations. Most important, the bleb theory cannot explain the numerous internal anomalies found in patients with gonadal dysgenesis. There is, therefore, little justification for maintaining the term "Bonnevie-Ullrich syndrome" and Ullrich himself, in 1949,[6] admitted that the "symmetric form of status Bonnevie-Ullrich" could no longer be reconciled with an unqualified theory of wandering cerebrospinal fluid blebs. In 1931, Meyer[7] reported a patient with sexual infantilism who had follicle-stimulating hormone in the urine despite the absence of secondary sex characteristics. He thus anticipated later investigators, who found increased amounts of gonadotropins in the patients under discussion. In 1938, Turner[8] described a syndrome of infantilism, congenital webbed neck and cubitus valgus in the journal *Endocrinology*. He stressed the combination of the external anomalies with small stature and retardation of sexual and osseus development. Thus, he established and popularized as an endocrine entity the syndrome reported before. Turner did not mention any of the symptoms recognizable at birth, nor did he have knowledge of the anatomy of the gonads, of the increased amounts of gonadotropins excreted in the urine or of the discrepancy between chromatin and external sex of many of these patients. Although Funke,[1] Baer[2] and Meyer[7] had described single cases and given more basic descriptions of gonadal dysgenesis before, Turner[8] established the syndrome as a type by describing several patients. As so often happens when eponymic terms are used for syndromes, the name attached to the syndrome is not identical with the name of the person who described it first. If one is reconciled to the lack of eponymic justice in medicine, one should not object to the use of the term "Turner syndrome," which permits a certain flexibility and is easier to pronounce than other names suggested for this complex of anomalies. In 1942, Varney *et al.*[9] found high urinary gonadotropin titers in a woman of short stature and retarded sexual development. This finding, which already had been established by Meyer,[7] became useful in differentiating gonadal dysgenesis from pituitary dwarfism, but it must be emphasized that this urinary test is not uniformly positive in all patients belonging to this group. Based on biopsy findings of the gonads of some patients, Wilkins and Fleischmann,[10] in 1944, introduced the term "ovarian agenesis." They described the white elongated ridges in the ligamentum latum, which run parallel to the tubes and consist of tissue resembling ovarian stroma without follicles. In 1954, Polani *et al.*[11] and Wilkins *et al.*[12] recognized that many, although not all, patients of this type who externally resembled females had a "male," i.e., negative, chromatin pattern. It seemed then that males and females were affected by this syndrome and that testes or ovaries could be deficient. The name of the disorder was changed to "gonadal dysgenesis."

Although the syndrome of gonadal dysgenesis was very useful in clinical medicine, it blended into many other types of congenital malformations, and a clear definition and demarcation was not possible as long as the etiology was not established. In most recorded cases, the family history was negative, the parents and siblings being normal.

By 1959, it became possible to analyze human chromosomes, and Ford *et al.*[13] reported on a sex chromosome anomaly in a case of gonadal dysgenesis. The patient, a 14-year-old girl, had a chromatin-negative pattern in skin and blood preparations. In cells from bone marrow, only 45 chromosomes were found. In selected cells there were 15 medium-length metacentric chromosomes as compared with the normal female of 16. These observations strongly suggested to the authors that the chromosome constitution of this girl was XO. They emphasized that the patient was a female with abnormal genotype. In the same year, Fraccaro *et al.*[14] reported a similar chromosome complement in gonadal dysgenesis. Numerous confirmations followed and the Turner syndrome with sex chromosome monosomy (XO) is now a fairly well-circumscribed disease picture.

XO (Turner Syndrome)

Whereas a supernumerary X chromosome (XXY) is well tolerated during prenatal life and childhood and does not cause congenital malformations, the lack of an X chromosome (XO) frequently is lethal before birth and usually is associated with congenital anomalies and malformations. There are many girls with XO constitution who go through childhood and adult life without serious (extragenital) handicaps, but they probably are a minority of survivors who escaped the dangers of their chromosomal deficiency. It seems that the most common chromosome abnormality among spontaneous abortions is the XO defect.[15-17] Carr[15] found 12 XO (spontaneous) abortuses among 227, i.e., 1 in 19 (5.3%). It is thought that Turner syndrome occurs in 1 in 5,000 (0.02%) of live-born infants. Carr[15] estimated that only 1 of 40 XO zygotes survives to term. The lack of prenatal viability must be surprising to endocrinologists dealing with adolescent or adult patients with Turner syndrome, since such females often are quite robust despite their endocrine and growth problems. The XO condition is one of the best illustrations of the prenatal and infantile screening process to which abnormal fetuses are subjected. It is not clear why XO embryos and fetuses have such a high mortality. Too few of these unborn have been examined thoroughly so far; in fact, few can be examined, since the conceptuses usually are deteriorated by the time they are obtainable. But cystic hygroma,[17] probably the forerunner of pterygium colli and of edema of the hands and feet seen in the newborn with Turner syndrome, may be the sign of a generalized disease. Anomalies of the kidney, uterus and umbilical artery cannot explain the frequent prenatal deaths. Interestingly, the ovaries were normal in XO fetuses examined by Singh and Carr,[17] pointing to relatively late damage to the gonads. There was no significant difference between the XO and XX gonads up to the third month of intrauterine life. In older fetuses, there was a relative increase in the connective

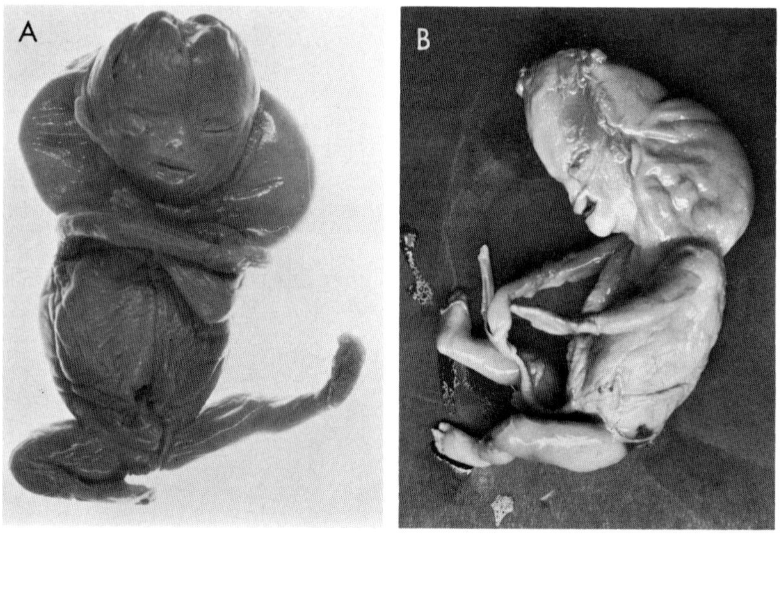

Fig. 112-2.—**A,** phenotypically female fetus, spontaneously aborted, with fluid-filled sac in the nuchal region (cystic hygroma). Tissue cells were chromatin negative. **B,** fetus aborted on 159th day (P.M.), showing bilateral fluid-filled sacs (cystic hygromas), which push the ears forward. The karyotype was 45/XO. (From R. P. Singh and D. H. Carr.[17])

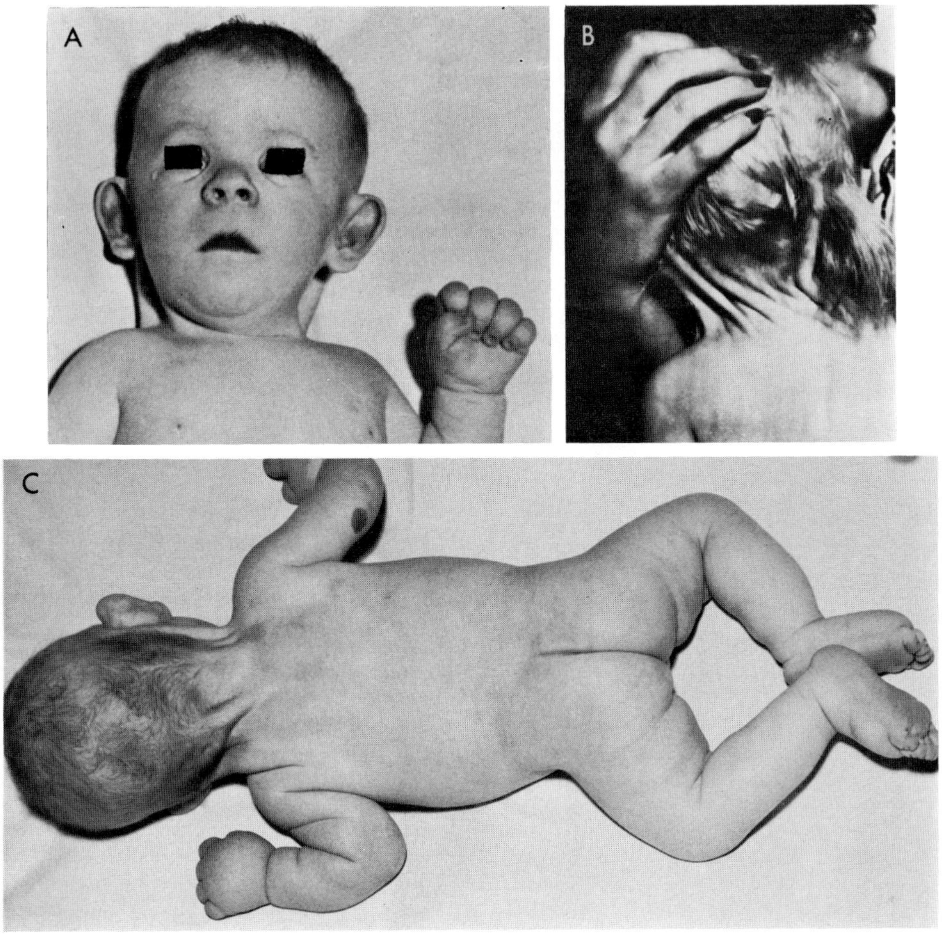

Fig. 112-3.—Children with Turner syndrome. **A,** pterygium colli. **B,** loose skin folds. **C,** loose skin folds, puffy hands and feet.

Fig. 112-4.—Pterygium colli in a girl 10 years of age with 45,XO karyotype.

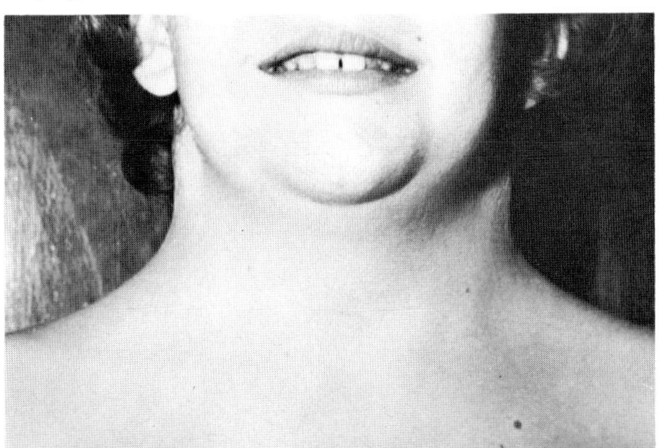

Fig. 112-5.—Feet of newborn girl with 45,XO Turner syndrome, showing loose skin and hypoplastic nails.

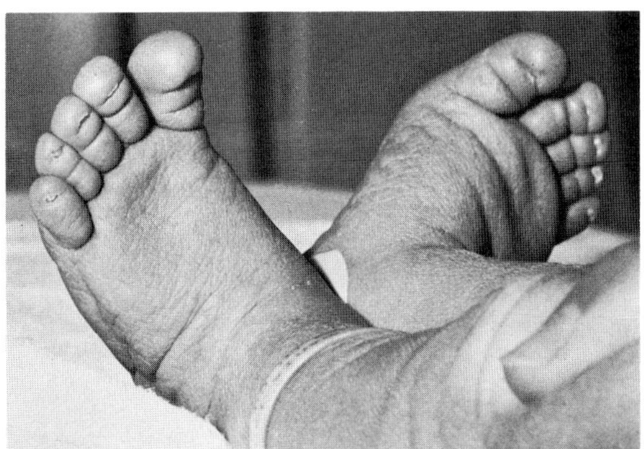

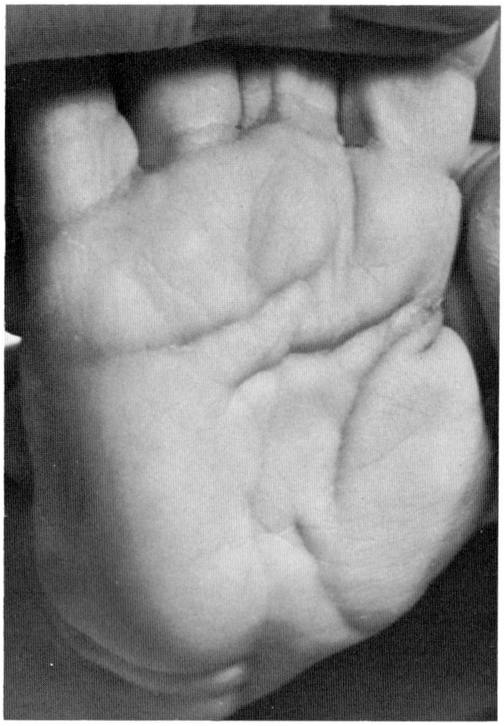

Fig. 112-6.—Thickened skin on palm of right hand of an infant with 45,XO Turner syndrome.

tissue of the XO gonads.[17] There is a great need for further description of XO embryos and fetuses to establish the prenatal phenotype.

Fetuses with marked edema and elephantiasis lymphangiectatica have long been known. Grüenwald and Kornfeld[18] believed that in such cases the spongy structure of the fetal lymphatic system is maintained, that the spongy cavernous structures found in the skin of these fetuses are due to arrested development of the fetal lymphatic system and that larger cysts are formed by confluence of these spaces. There is no proof that those fetuses described before Turner's publication were XO specimens but there is a resemblance to the XO fetuses found by Singh and Carr.[17]

Hypoplasia of the lymphatics and lymphedema, although characteristic of infantile Turner syndrome, can continue into adult life. In some instances, patients develop lymphedema years after birth. In 1957, Hoffenberg and Jackson[19] reported 3 of 27 adolescent patients with gonadal dysgenesis had transient swellings of the limbs or intermittent hydrarthroses. Benson *et al.*[20] demonstrated hypoplasia or aplasia in patients with primary lymphedema using lymphangiography. Examining 32 unselected female patients with primary lymphedema,[21] they found that only 26 had normal karyotypes. Two had XO, 2 had XY, 1 had XO/XX and 1 an X ring/XX karyotype. Males with primary lymphedema had normal karyotypes. It seems that malformations of the lymphatics are an important constituent of Turner syndrome and related sex chromosomal anomalies. Disappearance of lymphedema may be due to establishment of auxiliary lymph channels.[20,21]

Children with Turner syndrome have somewhat lower mean birth weights than normal girls from the same population, but their intrauterine growth retardation is not marked, since the mean duration of pregnancy is also reduced for the patients.[22] Occasionally, the prenatal growth retardation is significant.[23,24] A typical case can be recognized at birth by webbing or loose folds of the short neck, swelling of the dorsa of hands and feet, deep creases on the thickened palms and soles, hypertelorism, epicanthic folds, ptosis of the upper lids, elongated "gothic" ears,

Fig.112-7.—Typical auricles of girls with Turner syndrome. (See also Fig. 112-1.)

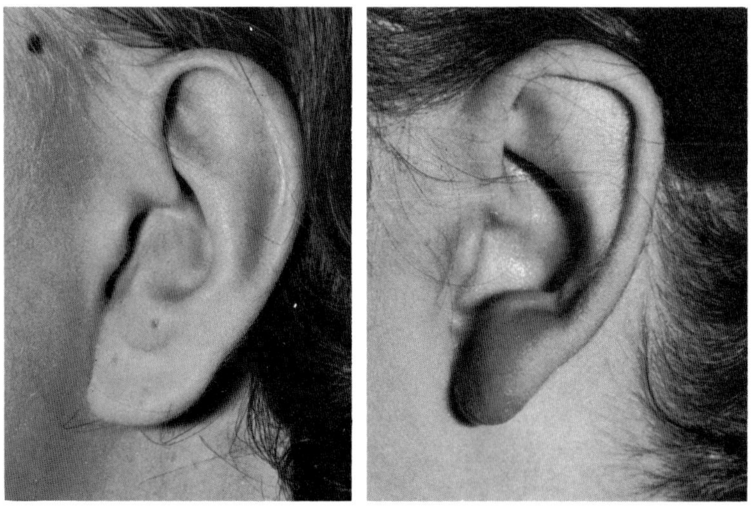

high-arched palate, micrognathia, pinpoint nipples and (sometimes) enlarged clitoris. The fingernails are hypoplastic and appear particularly small if surrounded by lymphedematous skin. Milestones of physical development and teething usually are normal. Growth retardation is noticeable throughout childhood, particularly after the age of 5 or 6 years. The final height reached is about 140 cm. There is no significant difference in the heights of XO, XO/XX mosaicism or isochromosome X patients.[22] Before adolescence, skeletal maturation deviates little from that of normal girls.

Additional ocular manifestations sometimes discovered in later life are refractive errors, color blindness, strabismus, cataract, blue sclerae and, rarely, iris coloboma or glaucoma.[25]

Audiometric analyses reveal hearing impairment of moderate degree. Perceptive and conductive disturbances can be demonstrated but the changes are not noticed by the patients in many instances. Congenital deafness has been observed occasionally.[26]

Taste is partially impaired. Although detection and recognition of salt and sweet are not disturbed, there is impairment in detection of sour and bitter taste. Decrease in olfactory sensitivity has been observed.[27]

Congenital bronchiectases leading to formation of an unusual immune globulin have been reported.[28]

Among patients with Turner syndrome, 25–40% have congenital cardiovascular disease.[29-32] Coarctation of the aorta is the best known anomaly but aortic atresia or stenosis, pulmonary stenosis, ventricular septal defect, tetralogy of Fallot, single ventricle, pseudotruncus, tricuspid stenosis and others have also been observed.[81] Some of these defects cause early death in infancy[31,33] and are not seen by physicians who deal with patients in endocrine clinics. There seems to be a high association of pterygium colli and congenital cardiovascular disease in patients with XO karyotype. Among children with congenital heart disease seen in hospitals, 1–2% have Turner syndrome.[31] Hypertension can develop for various reasons and can occur in the absence of congenital heart disease.

Anomalies of the kidneys, such as horseshoe, cystic and double kidney, were observed in patients of our hospital. Double kidney, hydronephrosis and single kidney have been observed repeatedly.[33,34] The fact that approximately two-thirds of the patients have renal malformations has led to requests to perform routine pyelography.

Gastrointestinal hemorrhages have been reported in many cases.[35-37] Multiple telangiectasias or hemangiomas have been seen in the small bowel, which, through melena, led to anemia.

The chest, which usually is flat in children, remains shield-shaped in later life. The nipples often are small, inverted and widely spaced. Association with Klippel-Feil syndrome (p. 909) occurs.[30,37,38] Spina bifida occulta is not rare. Osteoporosis is found regularly with increasing age[19] and scoliosis develops in some of the patients.[39] Irregularities of the ribs have been noted.[35,39] A highly arched palate was described by Funke[1] and cleft palate has been observed occasionally[37] (Cincinnati Children's Hospital Chart No. 93291). Micrognathia is common.

Fig. 112-8.—Girl, 18 years of age, with 45,XO karyotype. She was only 135 cm. tall and was of stocky build. The neck was webbed and the nipples widely spaced. Cubitus valgus, micrognathia and elongated ears are shown.

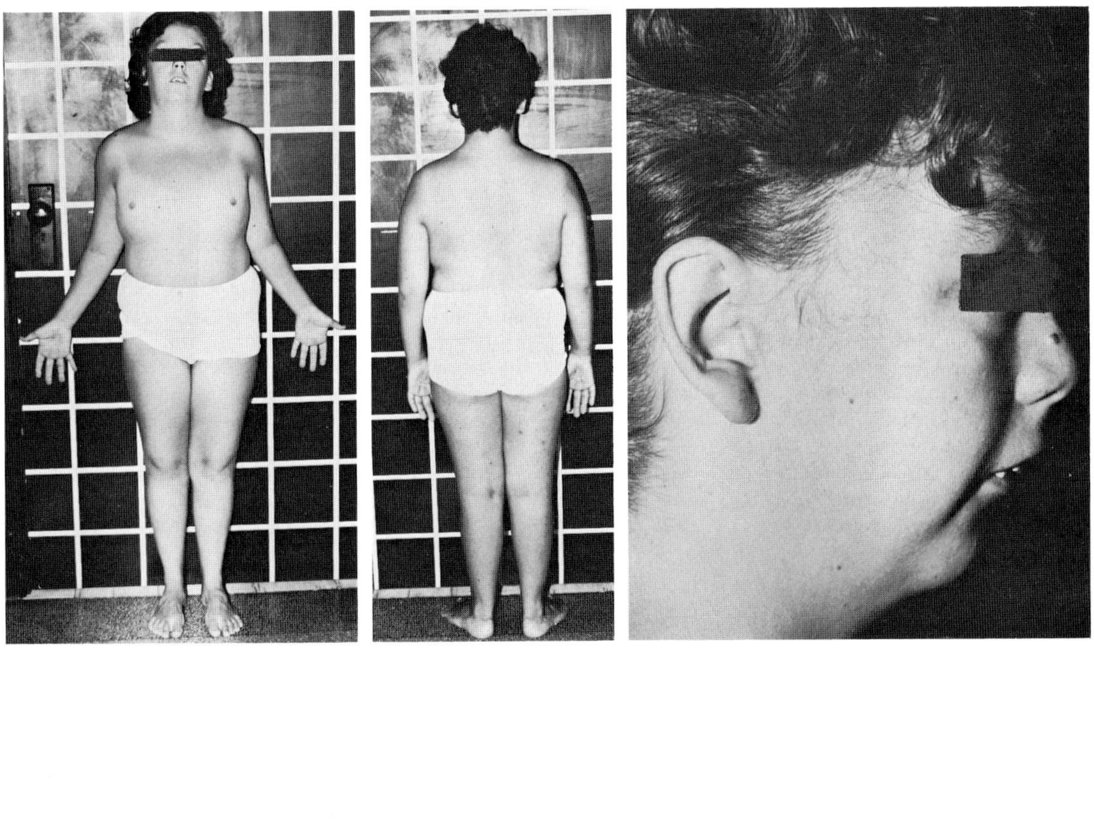

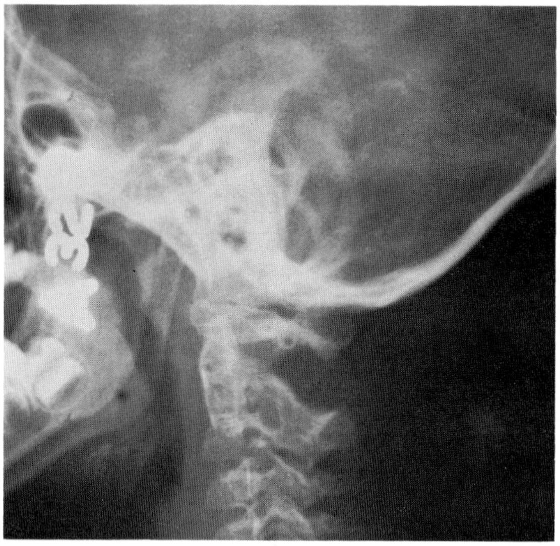

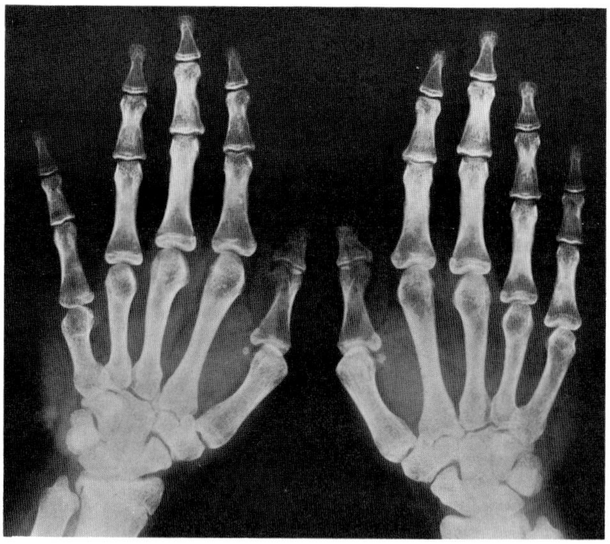

Fig. 112-9 (left). – Klippel-Feil syndrome in a 6-year-old girl with $45,X/46,XX_i$ mosaicism.

Fig. 112-10 (right). – Roentgenogram of hands of a girl with Turner syndrome. She was 135 cm. tall and sexually underdeveloped. Note shortness of fourth and fifth metacarpal bones and of terminal phalanges of thumbs.

Cubitus valgus, a sign emphasized by Turner[8] can be seen in approximately two-thirds of the cases.[32,37] Hoffenberg and Jackson,[19] who saw cubitus valgus in only 1 of their 27 patients, pointed out that abduction of the forearm is normally possible by minor flexion of the elbow joint. Madelung deformity and anomalies of the wrists, shortening of metacarpal, metatarsal and phalangeal bones, clinodactyly, dislocation of the hip and pes planus or pes equinovarus have been reported. The metacarpal sign,[43] shortening of the fourth metacarpal bone relative to the third and fifth, is seen in about 60% of the patients. Many other variations have been pointed out by roentgenologists[39-41] who, however, cannot agree on the question of skeletal maturation in Turner syndrome. Metacarpal defects and stunted growth occur in both gonadal dysgenesis and pseudo-pseudohypoparathyroidism. There is an overlap of these disorders in some patients.[19,42,43]

At the time of expected puberty, sexual infantilism becomes noticeable. There is lack of breast development, pubic hair is scanty and axillary hair absent in most cases. The external genitalia are infantile but the clitoris is enlarged in some cases. The vagina is narrow and the uterus small. The gonads are represented by long, white streaks composed of connective tissue and a few clear hilus cells. Follicles are absent. Estrogen effects are not induced at adolescence and thereafter. There are exceptional cases in which rudimentary ovaries with primordial follicles or follicular cysts develop.[44] In infancy, the ovarian picture is variable. There may be streak ovaries, few ova[15] or almost normal female gonads.[33] In most girls with XO karyotype, germ cells are lost from the ovaries. But there are reports of breast development and other estrogen effects in a girl with Turner syndrome and functioning tissue in one ovary,[45] of girls with regular vaginal bleeding[46,47] and of a case of an XO woman with normal sexual maturation who delivered a normal child. Mosaicism in some tissues[48] cannot be excluded easily.[45]

Ovarian or estrogen deficiency is not the only endocrine disturbance of patients with Turner syndrome. The adrenals may be involved in the syndrome, as is shown in some necropsies. A close connection between the adrenals and the kidneys has been observed, the adrenal glands being embedded within the renal capsule. In addition, adrenal cortex was found in the ligamentum latum near or in the position of the gonad in several cases.[49-51] The role of this ectopic adrenal cortical tissue is still obscure, but Wade *et al*[50] suggested that it plays a role in phallic enlargement of patients with gonadal dysgenesis. As early as 1927, Baer[2] reported finding adrenal tissue in place of the ovaries. A woman with XO Turner syndrome observed in the Cincinnati General Hospital developed an adrenal tumor with signs of Cushing disease. A high incidence of diabetes mellitus in patients with gonadal dysgenesis was pointed out by Forbes and Engel.[52] Patients with XO Turner syndrome and hypothyroidism or Hashimoto thyroiditis have been observed.[26,53,54] Thyroiditis also has been seen in chromatin-positive, x-isochrome Turner patients.[55,56] A woman suffering from Turner syndrome and acromegaly was reported by Willemse.[57] An eosinophilic adenoma of the pituitary was removed when she was 29 years of age. The eosinophilic adenoma did not promote longitudinal growth before operation, although the epiphyseal zones were still open.

Pigmented nevi are numerous and are seen regularly in adolescent or adult patients[19] but they are not

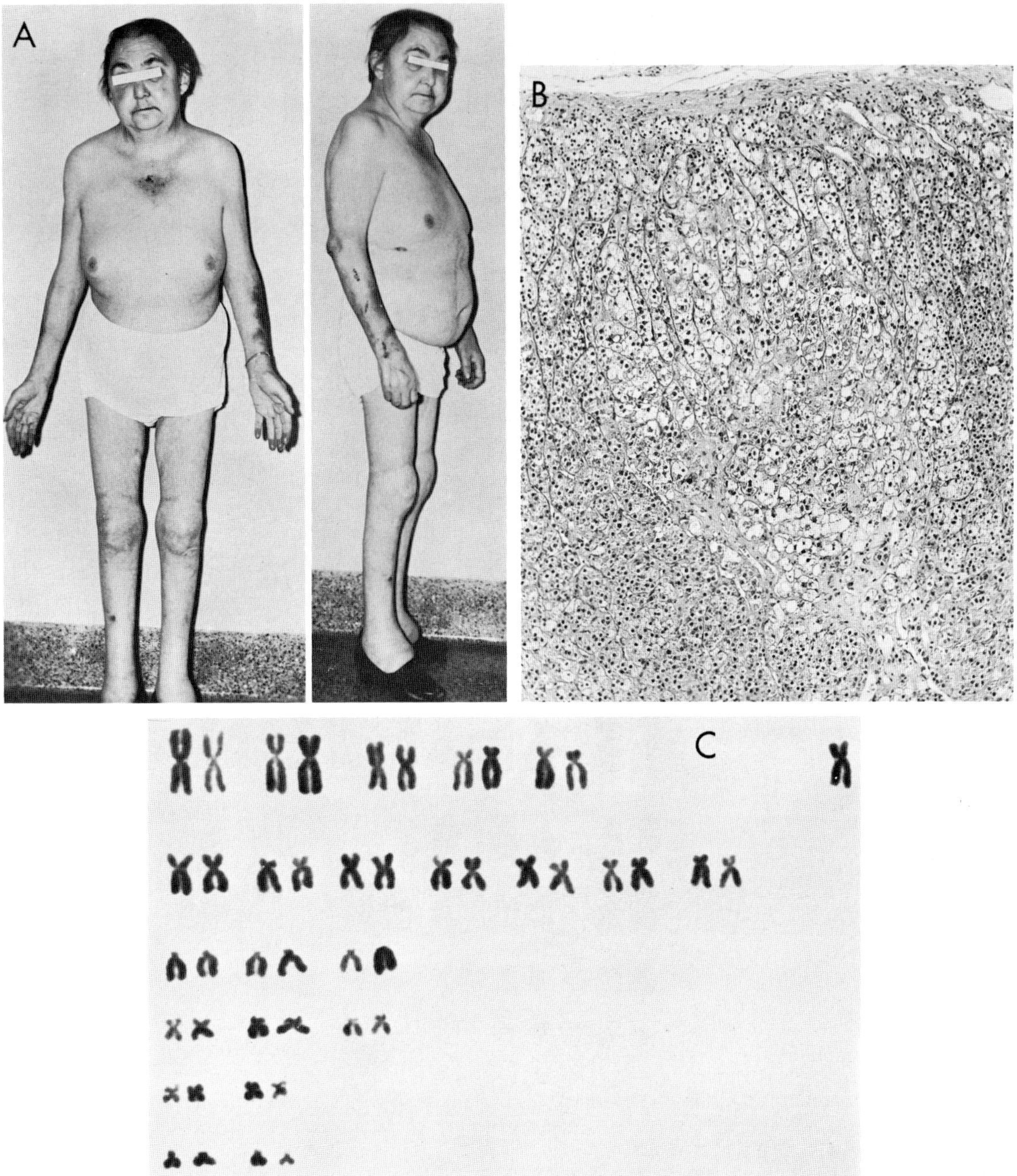

Fig. 112-11. – **A,** Cushing and Turner syndromes in a 48-year-old woman. She developed an adrenal adenoma in the ligamentum latum and died of pulmonary carcinoma. **B,** section through adrenal adenoma. **C,** karyotype 45,XO. (Courtesy of the Metabolism Division, Department of Medicine, University of Cincinnati.)

abundant in young children. Café au lait spots have been observed in several patients and in 2 of 100 patients there were signs of Recklinghausen neurofibromatosis.[30]

The mentality may be normal and Turner[8] pointed out that some of the patients have very good intelligence; but mental retardation is more frequent among them than in the average population. Differences of sampling prevent accurate estimates. Severe retardation occurs in some XO patients[32,37] but the mean I.Q. value for all patients with Turner syndrome is about 100.[22] Women with negative sex chro-

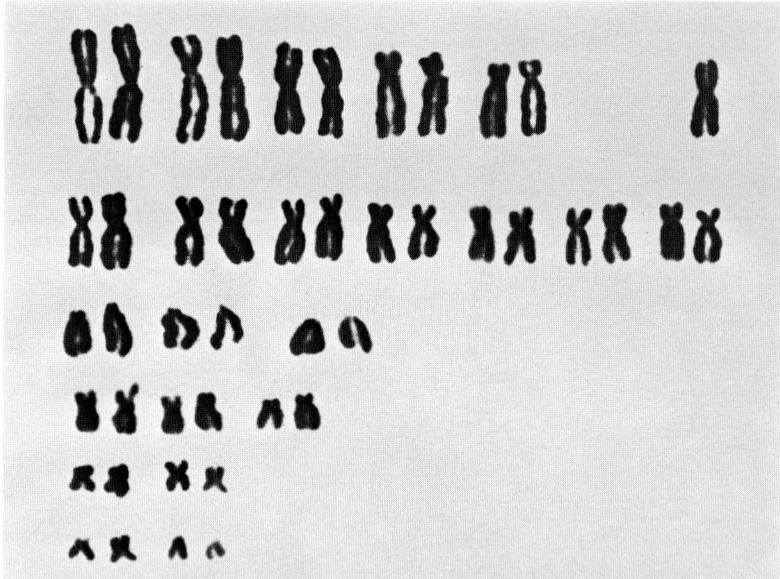

Fig. 112-12.—45,XO karyotype of a girl with Turner syndrome.

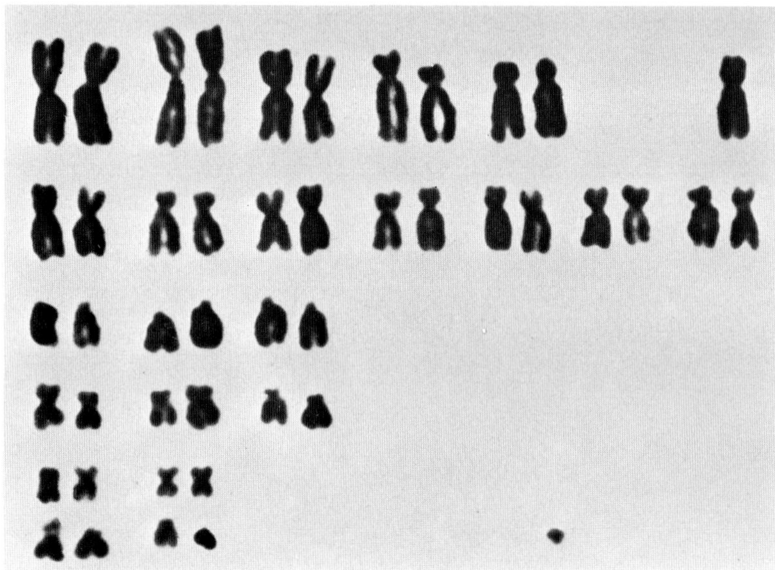

Fig. 112-13.—45,X+ fragment in a girl (who also had 46,XX cells) with some signs of Turner syndrome.

matin are not an important group among patients in mental hospitals.[58]

In approximately 80% of the patients with the Turner phenotype, the sex chromatin pattern is negative and an XO karyotype is present most often. Twenty per cent have positive sex chromatin, and various karyotypes have been ascertained since 1960. Analyses of these karyotypes were described by Court Brown *et al.*[59] and others[60,61,78]; XX, XO/XX, XO/XXX, XX-isochromosome with deletion of short or long arm, mosaics XO with x-isochromosomes, XO/XY, XO/XYY, X with a minute centric fragment, XY and others have been assumed or established.[82,83] Ferguson-Smith[60] listed the relative frequencies of signs and symptoms of fifteen cytogenetic types, attempting an assessment of the correlations between the chromosomal and clinical findings. His conclusion was that monosomy of the short arm of the X chromosome was responsible for short stature and congenital malformations of patients with Turner syndrome. Some patients with Y chromosome defects also show short stature and malformations of the Turner syndrome in addition to testicular defects and ambiguous genitalia. Ferguson-Smith[60] offered a hypothesis that there exists a range of phenotypes from normal male to Turner syndrome and from normal female to Turner syndrome dependent on the degree of sex chromosome deficiency intermediate between

XX and XO and XY and XO complements respectively. An auxiliary hypothesis is that the deficiency involves X- and Y-homologous loci, an assumption that will not be acceptable to all geneticists. Another difficulty encountered in present-day theories is the existence of patients who have testes but no Y chromosomes.[61-65] To assume that such persons have a Y chromosome hidden away in some inaccessible tissue or that they have had a Y chromosome sometime in their embryonic past adds another hypothesis that cannot be proved or disproved. Nars[79] reviewed 43 cases of XO/XY mosaicism and their phenotypes, including symptoms of Turner syndrome. Cyclopia in an infant with trisomy D was reported by Toews and Jones.[80] Although the child had gonadal aplasia, two X chromosomes were present in the karyotype.

The origin of the XO and related constitutions is understandably attributed to cytogenetic errors. They can be explained by nondisjunction or chromosome loss during gametogenesis in a parent. Alternative explanations hold that mitotic errors could be responsible for the XO karyotype by anaphase lag with loss of a sex chromosome or by mitotic nondisjunction with failure of complementary XXX or XYY cell lines to survive.[66]

There are observations pointing to possible origins of gonadal dysgenesis that should be emphasized because they may point to causes of cytogenetic errors or to noncytogenetic etiologies.

Most cases of Turner syndrome and related conditions are sporadic. Reports on familial cases are important but still confusing. Josso *et al.*[67] described a kindred in which two XO Turner syndromes occurred; a maternal aunt and her niece were affected. In another family, a woman with rather typical Turner phenotype and deaf-mutism had a sister with small stature, amenorrhea, gonadal and tubal agenesis and deaf-mutism. These women were products of a consanguineous marriage; their karyotype was normal 46,XX.[67] Migeon and Whitehouse[68] observed 2 brothers with male XY Turner syndrome in one family and a sister and a brother in another, both siblings having apparently normal karyotypes. Elliott *et al.*[69] described 3 sisters with the syndrome and Hauser[70] three families, each comprising 2–4 sisters with gonadal dysgenesis. Bassöe[71] observed a woman with gonadal dysgenesis and her brother, who had hypogonadism resembling Klinefelter syndrome. They belonged to a family in which a form of muscular dystrophy occurred as a hereditary trait. Familial occurrence of the "Turner phenotype" with XX or XY karyotype was also reported by Nora and Sinha.[72] In three kindreds there was direct transmission of Turner phenotypic features from affected women to daughters and sons. All the affected individuals had normal XX or XY constitution in agreement with their sex. A family in which the Turner phenotype was transmitted from a father to his son has been reported.[84] Such cases with normal karyotypes are now distinguished from those with the Turner syndrome and considered as XX or XY Turner phenotype, a genetically determined disorder (see Turner Syndrome in the Male, below).

There are interesting observations of twins with one or both affected by gonadal dysgenesis. Turner[8] described a patient who had a normal twin sister and Turner and Zanartu[73] reported on identical twins with presumptive XO karyotype or possibly XO/XX mosaicism. Another concordant pair of identical twins, both having XO karyotype, was mentioned by Lemli and Smith.[32] Turpin *et al.*[74] observed a pair of monozygotic twins, one of whom was a normal XY boy and the other a girl with typical Turner phenotype and XO karyotype. Mosaicism is suggested in such cases, as was pointed out by Edwards *et al.*,[62] who saw a girl presenting with Turner syndrome and XO karyotype with a small proportion of XY lymphocytes. Her twin brother consistently showed XO lymphocytes and fibroblasts. These authors also described a pair of twins with XO/XX mosaicism. Mikkelsen *et al.*[75] established XO/XX mosaicism in a pair of presumably monozygotic twins, of whom one was phenotypically normal, whereas the other had signs of Turner syndrome and mental retardation. Familial occurrence of the Turner phenotype is of importance but, at present, is unexplained. Rossi and Caflisch,[76] who wrote about the "pterygium syndrome" in 1951, saw it in a father and son. In two of my observations there were malformations often associated with gonadal dysgenesis in otherwise normal relatives. In one case, a brother of the mother had a horseshoe kidney. In a second case, the sister of the mother had a supernumerary kidney and an ectopic ureter. Such family histories deserve recording.

Finally, the possibility of nongenetic, environmental agents as a cause of gonadal dysgenesis should be considered. Diamond *et al.*[77] recorded the case of a girl possibly deformed by Myleran taken by her leukemic mother during pregnancy. There were multiple congenital malformations, including the ovaries, which were identified as two tiny thickenings lying in the broad ligament below the ends of the Fallopian tubes.

Treatment of gonadal dysgenesis is symptomatic. Cardiac, ophthalmologic, orthopedic, renal, surgical, endocrine and psychologic treatment is needed by many of the patients.

Turner Syndrome in the Male

This syndrome suffers from a controversial nomenclature and separatistic tendencies. Since Flavell,[85] in 1943, described "webbing of the neck with Turner's syndrome in the male," many writers have denied the existence of the disorder, others have published additional cases and some have tried to confuse the issue by eponymic zeal. Nobody who has seen cases of Turner syndrome can deny that there are boys who show signs and symptoms very similar to those of their female counterparts. Since we cannot "explain"

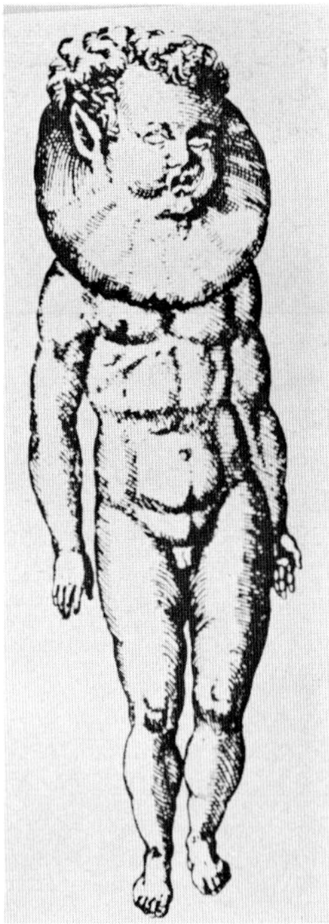

Fig. 112-14.—"Male Turner syndrome" (?) with pterygium colli in a woodcut of 1693 (p. 17). Note elongated ears. (See Figs. 112-1 and 112-7.)

these cases with our present information, we may wish that these patients did not exist, but here they are whether we like the names they are given or not. In 1965, Heller[86] thought that there were 43 cases on record and in 1966, Chaves-Carballo and Hayles[87] counted 86. Since the syndrome varies according to definition and point of view, its limits are not well defined and classifications are diverse. But there *are* boys with short stature, webbed neck, low hairline, cubitus valgus, shield chest and hypoplastic nipples who, at a glance, are reminiscent of Turner syndrome. Many of these patients have congenital heart disease, skeletal anomalies and mental retardation. Two-thirds or more have cryptorchidism or other signs of hypogonadism. The similarity and parallelism of signs to those of XO Turner syndrome are obvious, but the karyotype of the male patients is apparently normal 46,XY. This may be disturbing to those who believe that the Turner syndrome is "explained" by the lack of an X chromosome. Actually, there are many enigmas concerning the female counterpart of the syndrome too. There are such patients with XX karyotype or complex mosaics who demonstrate how incomplete our understanding of the female Turner syndrome is at present.

Webbing of the neck is a striking sign that is not limited to the male Turner syndrome. In 1883, Kobylinski[88] described a man with pterygium colli who apparently was not handicapped by associated anomalies. In 1951, Rossi and Caflisch[76] reviewed the "pterygium syndrome" and distinguished five types of it, gonadal dysgenesis among them. Pterygium colli and a low hairline in the back may be present in the Klippel-Feil syndrome (p. 909), which, however, always shows gross abnormalities of the cervical vertebrae and limitation of motion in the shortened neck. Pterygia around various joints are found in patients with arthrogryposis, absence of the pectoral or other muscles (p. 1025), cleft lip and palate (p. 643) and others. The unilateral disease picture described by Ullrich[89] is characterized by thoraco-brachial hypoplasia with involvement of the pectoral muscles and with shortening of an entire extremity or a part of it. Abnormal hair distribution, malformations of the ears, cranial nerve abnormalities, malformations of the skull, mental retardation and hydrocephaly may be present in this "Ullrich syndrome" as well as in Turner gonadal dysgenesis. All these disease pictures, which include pterygia, can be distinguished easily from the "symmetric" male Turner syndrome.

Some infants with the male Turner syndrome show a loose nuchal skin rather than a well-developed bilateral pterygium. The loose skin as well as a pterygium are remnants of the edematous state of fetuses with Turner syndrome,[17] a condition of great interest that needs explanation (see Fig. 112-2). At birth and for months thereafter, swelling of the dorsa of the hands and feet remains an outstanding sign in many boys with the Turner phenotype. The parents of older children suspected of this disorder should always be asked about these swellings during the child's infancy. With the swelling of the dorsa goes thickening of the skin of the palms and soles, which results in deepening of the skin creases. Together with hypoplastic nails, the symmetric lymphedema is almost diagnostic in these children. There may be swelling around the ears also, with the lobules standing off. Epicanthic folds contribute to the suspicion of male Turner syndrome in the newborn period.

Congenital cardiovascular defects are present in many of these boys; estimates of frequency vary between 35% and 50%.[86,87] In cases discovered in cardiology clinics, the frequency is near 100%; this fact, which is not surprising, explains the distorted point of view of some reports. In many of the older publications, the type of cardiac malformation could not be specified but, with improved diagnostic methods, atrial and ventricular septal defects, aortic and pulmonic stenosis, coarctation of the aorta, truncus arteriosus, patent ductus arteriosus, tetralogy of Fallot and others have been recognized.[72,87,90] Hypertension of differing origins has been noted in several cases.

Skeletal changes include various types of anomalous curvatures of the spine, which are due to reduced height or malformations of vertebrae.[87] When present in the cervical spine, such vertebral defects overlap with the Klippel-Feil syndrome and the differential diagnosis must be made with care. High-arched palate is the rule and micrognathia can be

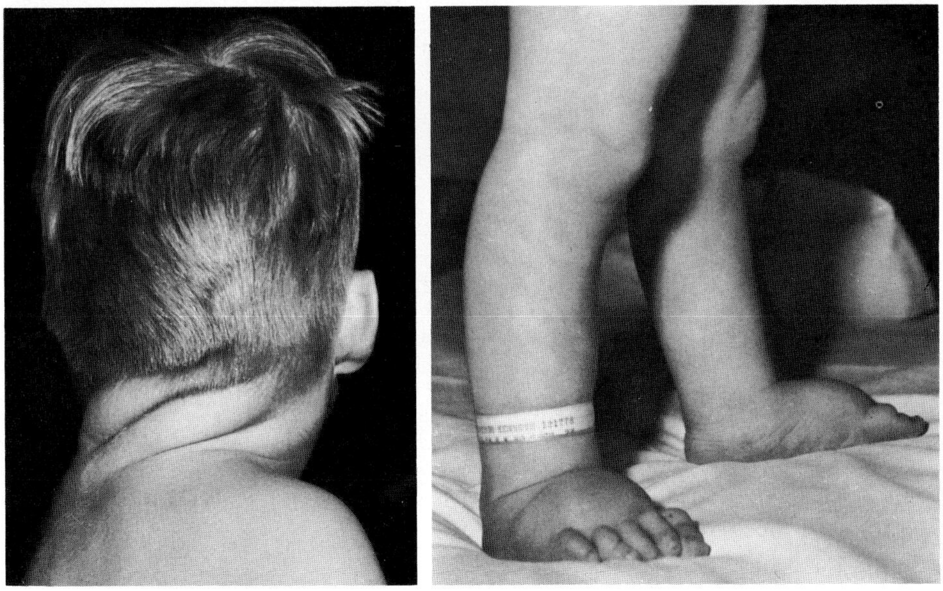

Fig. 112-15. – Loose skin folds and swelling of feet in a boy with male Turner syndrome. He had congenital heart disease (pseudotruncus arteriosus).[94]

present. Shield chest and pectus excavatum, cubitus valgus, simian creases, clinodactyly, bifid thumb and other finger deformities have been observed.[86] Dermatoglyphics have been studied but observations are not sufficient in number to consider a pattern as established.[91]

Growth is stunted in most cases and the height noted is at the 25th percentile or below.

Ocular defects are frequent and varied. There are minor anomalies, such as epicanthic folds, hypertelorism, strabismus, ptosis of lids and slanting palpebral fissures,[86] but such serious complications as hypertensive retinopathy,[92] severe myopia, retinal detachment, cataract and glaucoma have been observed also.[25]

The ears are low-set, elongated in their vertical axis and sometimes deformed. Loss of hearing or deafness has been noted in some of the patients.[86]

The tendency to testicular deficiency represents a challenging problem. Despite the seemingly normal XY karyotype, the patients usually have small, cryptorchid testes.[87] In some cases, there are no testes detectable (anorchia)[93] but the presence of epididymis, vas deferens and gubernaculum suggests that a testis had been present during fetal life. In other patients, the testes were normal.[86] In biopsies, Leydig and Sertoli cells varied in number and in histologic details; germinal hypoplasia is the rule.[86,87]

Renal anomalies have found little attention so far but hypoplasia has been noted[92] and attention should be paid to this aspect of the disorder.

Mental retardation has been recorded in about one-third of the cases[86] but it may be more prevalent, since, in infants, intelligence often is not assessed.

Sex chromatin is negative in most cases and the karyotype appears normal (46,XY) according to present cytogenetic methods.[86,87,94,95] There were some exceptions. XO/XY karotype,[96,97] XO/XY/XYY,[98] XO/XY/XXY[99] and X, iso-X/XX, abnormal Y[100] and others have been recorded. Cases with XO or XXY findings[87] probably were also mosaics that could not be fully investigated. In one instance, a deletion in a chromosome of the C group was assumed[86] and in another a trisomy of a D group chromosome.[101] All these exceptional cases, as well as the apparent nor-

Fig. 112-16. – Small penis and undescended testes in a 13-year-old boy with male Turner syndrome. He had webbed neck, ogival palate, cubitus valgus and congenital heart disease (abnormal venous pulmonary return).

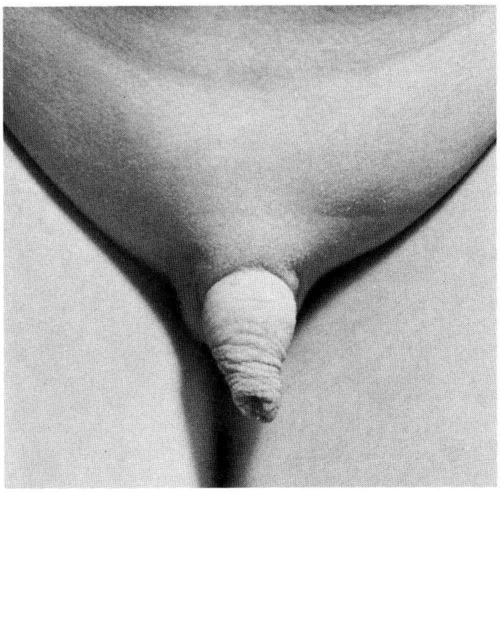

mal XY karyotype, will be studied with more refined cytogenetic methods as they become available.

It is now widely accepted that the male Turner phenotype with XY and the female Turner phenotype with XX karyotype are imitations of the XO Turner syndrome. Cases with the Turner phenotype and apparently normal chromosomes are thought to be gene-determined and hereditary, although the mode of transmission is still uncertain. Families and kindreds with members showing signs of the Turner syndrome have been reported before and after chromosome determinations became possible, so that the karyotypes are not known in all family reports. Rossi and Caflisch[76] pointed out in 1951 that the "pterygium syndrome" can be transmitted through more than one generation. Some of the cases surveyed by them probably were related to the condition now called "male Turner syndrome." Falls and Kertesz[102] described a hereditary syndrome combining pterygium colli with ocular anomalies and disturbances of the lymphatics of the lower extremities. Nora and Sinha[72] reported three families in which women with features of Turner syndrome had male and female offspring with similar features and XY or XX karyotype. Polani *et al.*[104] also observed several families in which fertile women with Turner phenotype and XX karyotype had daughters with similar signs, and Noonan[90] as well as Summitt[105] mentioned an affected mother with affected offspring.

In other families, siblings with Turner phenotype have been seen. Two brothers with male Turner syndrome have been recorded repeatedly[68,103,106] and in one family, 3 brothers were affected.[107] Two sisters with XX Turner phenotype were recorded by Josso *et al.*[67] Abdel-Salam and Temtamy[108] reported 2 brothers and a sister with Turner phenotype who were the offspring of a cousin marriage. Although the mode of inheritance of XY and XX Turner phenotype has not been determined, it is most likely that many of the nonendocrine features seen in XO Turner syndrome can be transmitted in some instances like a genetically determined syndrome with variable expression. Whether all cases of the male Turner syndrome belong in this category remains to be seen. The relationship of point mutations to chromosomal abnormalities resulting in similar phenotypes needs clarification[68] and knowledge that is not available at present. What we do *not* need are new eponyms for old syndromes. "Male Turner syndrome," a term used since 1943,[85] signifies the disease picture of males with XY phenotype, and "XX Turner phenotype" describes its female counterpart. It is not clear why these two conditions should be called "Noonan's syndrome."[105,109] Noonan and Ehmke,[110] reporting briefly in 1963 on noncardiac malformations in children with congenital heart disease, mentioned 6 boys and 3 girls with valvular pulmonic stenosis who had small stature, hypertelorism and mild mental retardation. In some, there also were skeletal malformations, undescended testes and ptosis. Since the karyotypes of these children were not known and since not all patients with XX and XY Turner phenotype have pulmonary stenosis, Noonan and Ehmke[110] did not circumscribe the hereditary Turner phenotype any better than did Kobylinski[88] in 1883. Yet, an editorial[105] that rejected such terms as "male Turner syndrome," "Turner phenotype with normal karyotype," "Ullrich syndrome" and "female pseudo-Turner" found the name "Noonan syndrome" adequate even though only a few of the patients with XX and XY phenotype resemble those mentioned by Noonan and Ehmke.[110] A new label does not shed light on the male Turner syndrome and its female counterpart.

A familial syndrome of short stature associated with facial dysplasia and genital anomalies has been described by Aarskog.[111] It is fully expressed in males only and may be inherited as a sex-linked recessive trait. The sex anomalies consist of undescended testes and a bifid scrotum, with a scrotal skin fold extending ventrad around the base of the penis. The prognosis is good for ultimate height and sexual and mental development.

REFERENCES

1. Funke: Pterygium colli, Deutsche Ztschr. Chir. 63:162, 1902.
2. Baer, W.: Vollkommene angeborene Aplasie beider Ovarien, infantiles Genitale, viriler Habitus, Zentralbl. Gynäk. 51:3241, 1927.
3. Ullrich, O.: Über typische Kombinationsbilder multipler Abartungen, Ztschr. Kinderh. 49:271, 1930.
4. Bonnevie, K.: Embryological analysis of gene manifestation in Little and Bagg's abnormal mouse tribe, J. Exper. Zool. 67:443, 1934.
5. Little, C. C., and Bagg, H. J.: The occurrence of four inheritable morphological variations in mice and their possible relation to treatment with x-rays, J. Exper. Zool. 41:45, 1924.
6. Ullrich, O.: Turner's syndrome and status Bonnevie-Ullrich; synthesis of animal phenogenetics and clinical observations on typical complex of developmental anomalies, Am. J. Human Genet. 1:179, 1949.
7. Meyer, R.: Über gewebliche Anomalien und ihre Beziehung zu einigen Geschwülsten der Ovarien, Arch. Gynäk. 145:2, 1931.
8. Turner, H. H.: A syndrome of infantilism, congenital webbed neck and cubitus valgus, Endocrinology 23:566, 1938.
9. Varney, R. F., Kenyon, A. T., and Koch, F. C.: Association of short stature, retarded sexual development and high urinary gonadotropin titers in women, J. Clin. Endocrinol. 2:137, 1942.
10. Wilkins, L., and Fleischmann, W.: Ovarian agenesis, pathology, associated clinical symptoms and the bearing on the theories of sex differentiation, J. Clin. Endocrinol. 4:357, 1944.
11. Polani, P. E., Hunter, W. F., and Lennox, B.: Chromosomal sex in Turner's syndrome with coarctation of the aorta, Lancet 2:120, 1954.
12. Wilkins, L., Grumbach, M. M., and Van Wyk, J. J.: Chromosomal sex in "ovarian agenesis," J. Clin. Endocrinol. 14:1270, 1954.
13. Ford, C. E., Jones, K. W., Polani, P. E., deAlmeida, J. C., and Briggs, J. H.: A sex-chromosome anomaly in a case of gonadal dysgenesis (Turner's syndrome), Lancet 1: 711, 1959.
14. Fraccaro, M., Kaijser, K., and Lindsten, J.: Chromosome complement in gonadal dysgenesis (Turner's syndrome), Lancet 1:886, 1959.

15. Carr, D. H.: Chromosome anomalies as a cause of spontaneous abortion, Am. J. Obst. & Gynec. 97:283, 1967.
16. Thiede, H. A., and Metcalfe, S.: Chromosomes and human pregnancy wastage, Am. J. Obst. & Gynec. 96: 1132, 1966.
17. Singh, R. P., and Carr, D. H.: The anatomy and histology of XO human embryos and fetuses, Anat. Rec. 155:369, 1966.
18. Grünwald, P., and Kornfeld, W.: Ein Fall von Elephantiasis lymphangiectatica bei einem vier Monate alten menschlichen Fetus, Beitr. path. Anat. 96:341, 1936.
19. Hoffenberg, R., and Jackson, W. P. U.: Gonadal dysgenesis: Modern concepts, Brit. M. J. 2:1457, 1957.
20. Benson, P. F., Gough, M. H., and Polani, P. E.: Lymphangiography and chromosome studies in females with lymphoedema and possible ovarian dysgenesis, Arch. Dis. Childhood 40:27, 1965.
21. Benson, P. F., Taylor, A. I., and Gough, M. H.: Chromosome anomalies in primary lymphoedema, Lancet 1: 461, 1967.
22. Lindsten, J.: *The Nature and Origin of X Chromosome Aberrations in Turner's Syndrome* (Stockholm: Almqvist and Wiksell, 1963).
23. Grumbach, M. M., Judson, J. V. W., and Wilkins, L.: Chromosomal sex in gonadal dysgenesis (ovarian agenesis). Relationship to male pseudohermaphrodism and theories of human sex differentiation, J. Clin. Endocrinol. 15:1161, 1955.
24. Warkany, J., Monroe, B. B., and Sutherland, B. S.: Intrauterine growth retardation, Am. J. Dis. Child. 102: 249, 1961.
25. Khodadust, A., and Paton, D.: Turner's syndrome in a male, Arch. Ophth. 77:630, 1967.
26. Graber, H.: Ein Beitrag zur Frage der Ovarialaplasie unter besonderer Berücksichtigung eines Falles von beiderseitigem Fehlen der Ovarien bei einem Neugeborenen, Virchows Arch. path. Anat. 299:80, 1937.
27. Henkin, R. I.: Abnormalities of taste and olfaction in patients with chromatin negative gonadal dysgenesis, J. Clin. Endocrinol. 27:1436, 1967.
28. Koch, J., and Rossipal, E.: Turnersyndrom mit angeborenen Bronchiektasien und passagerem Auftreten eines ungewöhnlichen Globulins, Arch. Kinderh. 174:342, 1966.
29. Rainier-Pope, C. R., Cunningham, R. D., Nadas, A. S., and Crigler, J. F., Jr.: Cardiovascular malformations in Turner's syndrome, Pediatrics 33:919, 1964.
30. Bishop, P. M. F., Lessof, M. H., and Polani, P. E.: Turner's Syndrome and Allied Conditions, in *Sex Differentiation and Development*, Mem. Soc. Endocrinol. (London: Cambridge University Press, 1960).
31. Damjanova, Zw., Ninova, P., and Damjanova, M.: Herz- und Gefässanomalien beim Turner-syndrom, Arch. Kinderh. 178:86, 1968.
32. Lemli, L., and Smith, D. W.: The XO syndrome: A study of the differentiated phenotype in 25 patients, J. Pediat. 63:577, 1963.
33. Conen, P. E., and Glass, I. H.: 45/XO Turner's syndrome in the newborn: Report of two cases, J. Clin. Endocrinol. 23:1, 1963.
34. Hortling, H.: Congenital kidney anomalies in Turner's syndrome, Acta endocrinol. 18:548, 1955.
35. Lisser, H., Curtis, L. E., Escamilla, R. F., and Goldberg, M.: The syndrome of congenitally aplastic ovaries with sexual infantilism, high urinary gonadotropins, short stature and other congenital abnormalities, J. Clin. Endocrinol. 7:665, 1947.
36. Rosen, K. M., Sirota, D. K., and Marinoff, S. C.: Gastrointestinal bleeding in Turner's syndrome, Ann. Int. Med. 67:145, 1967.
37. Haddad, H. M., and Wilkins, L.: Congenital anomalies associated with gonadal aplasia. Review of 55 cases, Pediatrics 23:885, 1959.
38. Cahn, L. R.: Klippel-Feil syndrome with multiple cysts of the jaw, Oral Surg. 5:659, 1952.
39. Levin, B.: Gonadal dysgenesis; clinical and roentgenologic manifestations, Am. J. Roentgenol. 87:1116, 1962.
40. Kosowicz, J.: The roentgen appearance of the hand and wrist in gonadal dysgenesis, Am. J. Roentgenol. 93:354, 1965.
41. Levin, J., and Kupperman, H. S.: Skeletal abnormalities in gonadal dysgenesis, Arch. Int. Med. 113:730, 1964.
42. van der Werff ten Bosch, J. J.: The syndrome of brachymetacarpal dwarfism ("pseudo-pseudohypoparathyroidism") with and without gonadal dysgenesis, Lancet 1:69, 1959.
43. Archibald, R. M., Finby, N., and deVito, F.: Endocrine significance of short metacarpals, J. Clin. Endocrinol. 19:1312, 1959.
44. de la Chapelle, A.: Cytogenetical and clinical observations in female gonadal dysgenesis, Acta endocrinol. 40 (supp. 65), 1962.
45. MacGillivray, M. H., Cohen, M. M., Aceto, T., Capraro, V. J., and Davidson, R. G.: Spontaneous sexual development in a chromatin negative female with XO blood leucocyte karyotype, Pediatrics 42:825, 1968.
46. Monardo, A.: Gonadal dysgenesis in a woman after seventeen years of regular menses, Am. J. Obst. & Gynec. 91:106, 1965.
47. Kaufman, S.: Vaginal bleeding in gonadal dysgenesis, Pediatrics 37:26, 1966.
48. Bahner, F., Schwarz, G., Harnden, D. G., Jacobs, P. A., Hienz, H. A., and Walter, K.: A fertile female with XO sex chromosome constitution, Lancet 2:100, 1960.
49. Nelson, B. M., and Bailey, B. L.: Gonadal dysgenesis and associated anomalies (Turner's syndrome), A.M.A. Arch. Path. 62:41, 1956.
50. Wade, W. G., Young, R. J., and Creery, R. D. G.: A case of gonadal dysgenesis or the Ullrich-Turner syndrome with androgenic manifestations, Arch. Dis. Childhood 31:354, 1956.
51. Richart, R., and Benirschke, K.: Gonadal dysgenesis in a newborn infant, New England J. Med. 258:974, 1958.
52. Forbes, A. P., and Engel, E.: The high incidence of diabetes mellitus in 41 patients with gonadal dysgenesis, and their close relatives, Metabolism 12:428, 1963.
53. Frey, H. M., and Hoffman, D. L.: Gonadal dysgenesis associated with hypothyroidism, Proc. Staff Meet. Mayo Clin. 34:442, 1959.
54. Hamilton, C. R., Jr., Moldawer, M., and Rosenberg, H. S.: Hashimoto's thyroiditis and Turner's syndrome, Arch. Int. Med. 122:69, 1968.
55. Williams, E. D., Engel, E., and Forbes, A. P.: Thyroiditis and gonadal dysgenesis, New England J. Med. 270:805, 1964.
56. Sparkes, R. S., and Motulsky, A. G.: The Turner syndrome with isochromosome X and Hashimoto's thyroiditis, Ann. Int. Med. 67:132, 1967.
57. Willemse, C. H.: A patient suffering from Turner's syndrome and acromegaly, Acta endocrinol. 39:204, 1962.
58. Maclean, N., Court Brown, W. M., Jacobs, P. A., Mantle, D. J., and Strong, J. A.: A survey of sex chromatin abnormalities in mental hospitals, J. M. Genetics 5:165, 1968.
59. Court Brown, W. M., Harnden, D. G., Jacobs, P. A., Maclean, N., and Mantle, D. J.: Abnormalities of the sex chromosome complement in man, Med. Res. Counc. Spec. Rep. Series No. 305, Her Maj. Staf. Off., p. 239, 1964.
60. Ferguson-Smith, M.A.: Karyotype-phenotype correlations in gonadal dysgenesis and their bearing on the pathogenesis of malformations, J. M. Genetics 2:142, 1965.
61. Miller, O. J.: The sex chromosome anomalies, Am. J. Obst. & Gynec. 90:1078, 1964.
62. Edwards, J. H., Dent, T., and Kahn, J.: Monozygotic twins of different sex, J. M. Genetics 3:117, 1966.
63. Bloise, W., DeAssis, L. M., Bottura, C., and Ferrari, I.: Gonadal dysgenesis (Turner syndrome) with male phen-

otype and XO chromosomal constitution, Lancet 2:1059, 1960.
64. Shah, P. N., Naik, S. N., Mahajan, D. K., Dave, M. J., and Paymaster, J. C.: A new variant of human intersex with discussion on the developmental aspects, Brit. M. J. 2:474, 1961.
65. Conen, P. E., and Erkman, B.: Two "new" sex-chromosome mosaics XO/XX, XX/XX (deletion of short arm X) and a further XO/XY mosaic, Lancet 2:1276, 1963.
66. Van Wyk, J. J., and Grumbach, M. M.: Disorders of Sex Differentiation, in Williams, R. H. (ed.), *Textbook of Endocrinology* (4th ed.; Philadelphia: W. B. Saunders Company, 1968).
67. Josso, N., de Grouchy, J., Frézal, J., and Lamy, M.: Le syndrome de Turner familial. Étude de deux familles avec caryotypes XO et XX, Ann. pédiat. 39:775, 1963.
68. Migeon, B. R., and Whitehouse, D.: Familial occurrence of the somatic phenotype of Turner's syndrome, Johns Hopkins M. J. 120:78, 1967.
69. Elliott, G. A., Sandler, A., and Rabinowitz, D.: Gonadal dysgenesis in three sisters, J. Clin. Endocrinol. 19:995, 1959.
70. Hauser, G. A.: Gonadal Dysgenesis, in Overzier, C.: *Intersexuality* (London and New York: Academic Press, 1963).
71. Bassöe, H. H.: Familial congenital muscular dystrophy with gonadal dysgenesis, Acta endocrinol. (supp. 31): 203, 1957.
72. Nora, J. J., and Sinha, A. K.: Direct familial transmission of the Turner phenotype, Am. J. Dis. Child. 166: 343, 1968.
73. Turner, H. H., and Zanartu, J.: Ovarian dysgenesis in identical twins: Discrepancy between nuclear chromatin pattern in somatic cells and in blood cells, J. Clin. Endocrinol. 22:660, 1962.
74. Turpin, R., Lejeune, J., Lafourcade, J., Chigot, P-L., and Salmon, C.: Présomption de monozygotisme en dépit d'un dimorphisme sexuel: Sujet masculin XY et sujet neutre Haplo X, Compt. rend. séances Acad. Sc. 252: 2945, 1961.
75. Mikkelsen, M., Frøland, A., and Ellebjerg, J.: XO/XX mosaicism in a pair of presumably monozygotic twins with different phenotype, Cytogenetics 2:86, 1963.
76. Rossi, E., and Caflisch, A.: Le syndrome du pterygium, status Bonnevie-Ullrich, dystrophia brevicolli congenita, syndrome de Turner et arthromyodysplasia congenita, Helvet. paediat. acta 6:119, 1951.
77. Diamond, I., Anderson, M. M., and McCreadie, S. R.: Transplacental transmission of busulfan (Myleran) in a mother with leukemia. Production of fetal malformation and cytomegaly, Pediatrics 25:85, 1960.
78. Goldberg, M. B., Scully, A. L., Solomon, I. L., and Steinbach, H. L.: Gonadal dysgenesis in phenotypic female subjects, Am. J. Med. 45:529, 1968.
79. Nars, P. W.: Das XO/XY-Geschlechtschromosomenmosaik, Humangenetik 7:185, 1969.
80. Toews, H. A., and Jones, H. W.: Cyclopia in association with D trisomy and gonadal agenesis, Am. J. Obst. & Gynec. 102:53, 1968.
81. Gunning, J. F., and Oakley, C. M.: Aortic-valve disease in Turner's syndrome, Lancet 1:389, 1970.
82. Finley, W. H., Taylor, P. T., Jr., Rosecrans, C. J., Finley, S. C., Waldrop, E. G., and Pittman, C. S.: Gonadal dysgenesis associated with a deleted X chromosome, Am. J. Ment. Deficiency 74:553, 1970.
83. Weber, F. M., Muller, H., and Sparkes, R. S.: Clinical and cytogenetic variations of gonadal dysgenesis in 3 patients, Am. J. Obst. & Gynec. 107:1092, 1970.
84. Levy, E. P., Pashayan, H., Fraser, F. C., and Pinsky, L.: XX and XY Turner phenotypes in a family, Am. J. Dis. Child. 120:36, 1970.
85. Flavell, G.: Webbing of neck with Turner's syndrome in a male, Brit. J. Surg. 31:150, 1943.
86. Heller, R. H.: The Turner phenotype in the male, J. Pediat. 66:48, 1965.
87. Chaves-Carballo, E., and Hayles, A. B.: Ullrich-Turner syndrome in the male: Review of the literature and report of a case with lymphocytic (Hashimoto's) thyroiditis, Mayo Clin. Proc. 41:843, 1966.
88. Kobylinski, O.: Über eine flughautähnliche Ausbreitung am Halse, Arch. Anthropol. 14:343, 1883.
89. Ullrich, O.: New concepts of mechanism of development of multiple abnormalities and deformities, Klin. Wchnschr. 17:185, 1938.
90. Noonan, J. A.: Hypertelorism with Turner phenotype, Am. J. Dis. Child. 116:373, 1968.
91. Ferrier, P. E., and Ferrier, S. A.: Turner's phenotype in the male, Pediatrics 40:575, 1967.
92. Steiker, D. D., Mellman, W. J., Bongiovanni, A. M., Eberlein, W. R., and Leboeuf, G.: Turner's syndrome in the male, J. Pediat. 58:321, 1961.
93. Becker, H. W.: Agonadismus mit kongenitalen Missbildungen beim Mann (Turnersches Syndrom), Med. Welt 10:351, 1957.
94. Chu, E. H. Y., Warkany, J., and Rosenstein, R. B.: Chromosome complement in a case of the "male Turner syndrome," Lancet 1:786, 1961.
95. Fraccaro, M.: Testicular germinal dysgenesis (male Turner's syndrome), Acta endocrinol. 36:98, 1961.
96. Lambert, A., and Netter, P.: Pseudo-hermaphroditisme male "Turnerien," Semaine hôp. Paris 38:1699, 1962.
97. Ross, G. T., Holland, J. M., Kiser, W. S., and Douglas, G. W.: XO/XY chromosomal mosaicism and extragenital stigmata of Turner's syndrome in a phenotypic male, J. Clin. Endocrinol. 25:141, 1965.
98. Schoen, E. J.: Diminished testicular function in "male Turner's syndrome," J. Clin. Endocrinol. 25:101, 1965.
99. Pelz, L., and Kellner, R.: XO/XY/XXY-Mosaik bei einem Knaben mit Ullrich-Turner-Syndrom, Ztschr. Kinderh. 99:167, 1967.
100. Solomon, I. L., Hamm, C. W., and Green, O. C.: Chromosome studies on testicular tissue cultures and blood leukocytes of a male previously reported to have no Y chromosome, New England J. Med. 271:586, 1964.
101. Milcou, M., Maximilian, C., Stanescu, V., Florea, I., Ionescu, V., and Augustin, M.: Turner's syndrome with male phenotype and trisomy 13-15, Rev. roumaine embryol. & cytol., ser. embryol. 1:1, 1964.
102. Falls, H. F., and Kertesz, E. D.: A new syndrome combining pterygium colli with developmental anomalies of the eyelids and lymphatics of the lower extremities, Tr. Am. Ophth. Soc. 62:248, 1964.
103. Alslev, J., and Reinwein, H.: Über das familiäre Vorkommen des Turner-Ullrich Syndroms und des Kryptorchidism und des Meigs Syndroms bei zwei Brüdern mit kongenitalen Vitien, Deutsche med. Wchnschr. 83:601, 1958.
104. Polani, P. E., Angell, R., and Polani, N.: Ullrich's syndrome, Lancet 2:421, 1967.
105. Summitt, R. L.: Turner's syndrome and Noonan's syndrome, J. Pediat. 74:155, 1969.
106. Kaplan, M. S., Opitz, J. M., and Gosset, F. R.: Noonan's syndrome: A case with elevated serum alkaline phosphatase levels and malignant schwannoma of the left forearm, Am. J. Dis. Child. 116:359, 1968.
107. Simila, S., and Kaski, U.: The Turner phenotype in three brothers with ichthyosis vulgaris, Acta paedit. scandinav. 56 (supp. 177):120, 1967.
108. Abdel-Salam, E., and Temtamy, S. A.: Familial Turner phenotype, J. Pediat. 74:67, 1969.
109. Opitz, J. M., Summitt, R. L., and Sarto, G. E.: Noonan's syndrome in girls: A genocopy of the Ullrich-Turner syndrome, Soc. Pediat. Res. Program and Abstracts, 35th Annual Meeting, Philadelphia, 1965.
110. Noonan, J. A., and Ehmke, D. A.: Associated noncardiac malformations in children with congenital heart disease, J. Pediat. 63:468, 1963.
111. Aarskog, D.: A familial syndrome of short stature associated with facial dysplasia and genital anomalies, J. Pediat. 5:856, 1970.

Mixed Gonadal Dysgenesis

(Asymmetric Gonadal Differentiation)

A GROUP OF PATIENTS who differ from hermaphrodites, pseudohermaphrodites and persons with gonadal dysgenesis has found attention during the past decade because of lateral differences in their gonads.[1,2] They can present as males or females with variable external genitals, gonads and karyotypes. Usually, a streak gonad is present on one side or there may be no gonad. On the other side, there is an ectopic testis or, rarely, a scrotal testis. But the sex chromatin appears to be negative and an XO cell line is found in most cases. On thorough examination, some sex chromatin-positive cells or chromosomal mosaicism is detected in many instances. It was thought at first that XO/XY mosaicism is the basis of the disorder, but it has been learned since that other karyotypes and mosaicisms can result in mixed gonadal dysgenesis.

By 1968, Bitan *et al.*[3] could review 50 cases, 43 of them with cytogenetic analyses. Less than half of the patients had been taken for males. Ambiguous external genitalia were described in almost all patients. In the "girls," the clitoris appears large from birth on or after adolescence; there may be a penile organ with hypospadias and bifid scrotum or a urogenital sinus with a perineal urethra. Cryptorchidism is the rule or a testis is noted in the inguen or, rarely, in the scrotum. In "boys," the penis usually is small and the urethra displaced; chordee or hypospadias sometimes is noted. In the abdomen, one testis may be found in place of an ovary, or the testis is partly descended. In exceptional cases there is a scrotal testis. Histologically, the testis can be normal but more often it is devoid of spermatogonia. In children, it may have the appearance of a normal infantile organ. Sertoli and Leydig cells are variable. The testes have a tendency to tumor formation; seminomas, dysgerminomas, gonadoblastomas or carcinomas[11] have been diagnosed, but in some instances neither the tumor nor the gonad could be clearly identified.

On the contralateral side, a streak gonad is found in the position of the ovary or there is no gonad. In most patients, a uterus is present though hypoplastic and in some there is only one horn developed. A Fallopian tube is seen on the side of the streak gonad but often it is defective on the side of the testis.

In 4 of 43 observations, chromosome analysis revealed an XY karyotype, in 5 XO, in 32 some mosaicism and in 1 a Y/D translocation.[3,4] In the majority of cases, the mosaic was XO/XY, and in some of them a structural anomaly of the Y chromosome seemed likely in the male cell line; or the Y chromosomes were multiple with XO/XYY[5] or XO/XYYY[6]; XO/XY/XX[7] and XY/XX/XXY[8] also have been associated with mixed gonadal dysgenesis. We saw a baby belonging in this category who had rather unusual features. He seemed to be a normal boy with one right undescended testis. The penile shaft was bound to the scrotal skin and the urethra was in the normal position. Aside from these rather inconspicuous signs, inguinal herniae and somewhat deformed ears, the baby appeared strong and healthy. At the age of 2 weeks, a small right inguinal hernia was explored and within it was a structure that proved to be the fundus of a uterus and a Fallopian tube. On the left side, the testis was biopsied and considered infantile but not abnormal. On laparotomy, a large urachal cyst was encountered and in the pelvis of the boy a normal-appearing infantile uterus with a Fallopian tube on each side could be seen. Sex chromatin was essentially negative but approximately 2% of the cells were positive. Cells derived from skin biopsies showed 45,XO karyotype. At the age of 11 months, chromosome analysis from leukocytes showed a mosaicism, 45,XO/48 XXXY, and similar findings were obtained in fibroblasts.[9] The remarkable fact was that the mixed gonadal dysgenesis or combination of Turner and Klinefelter syndromes was present in an apparently healthy boy with normal mentality. Finding of a uterus within a hernia of adult men has been reported before as "hernia uteri inguinalis in the male,"[10] but karyotypes of these patients could not be ascertained in the past. Some of these male pseudohermaphrodites may have had mixed gonadal dysgenesis. They usually have the body build of normal men. But other patients with mixed gonadal dysgenesis sometimes are short of stature and recognizable by external attributes of Turner syndrome.[1,2]

REFERENCES

1. Bergada, C., Cleveland, W. W., and Wilkins, L.: Abnormalities of sex differentiation. Müllerian structures in male pseudohermaphroditism and asymmetric gonadal differentiation, Proc. Soc. Pediat. Res. abstract, p. 62, 1961.
2. Sohval, A. R.: Hermaphroditism with "atypical" or "mixed" gonadal dysgenesis, Am. J. Med. 36:281, 1964.
3. Bitan, A., de Grouchy, J., Jolly, G., and Bach, Ch.: Dysgénésie gonadique mixte (ou différenciation gonadique asymétrique), Sem. Hôp. Paris 44:1, 1968.
4. Federman, D. D., Davidoff, F. M., and Ouellette, E.: Presumptive Y/D translocation in mixed gonadal dysgenesis, J. M. Genetics 4:36, 1967.
5. Ross, G. T., and Tjio, J. H.: Cytogenetics in clinical endocrinology, J.A.M.A. 192:977, 1965.
6. Cox, D., and Berry, C. L.: A patient with 45XO/48XYYY mosaicism, J. M. Genetics 4:132, 1967.
7. Schuster, J., and Motulsky, A. G.: Exceptional sex-chromatin pattern in male pseudohermaphroditism with XX/XY/XO mosaicism, Lancet 1:1074, 1962.
8. Burgio, G. R., Severi, F., and Biscatti, G.: Dysgénésie gonadique mixte a caryotype XY/XX/XXY, Pédiatrie 21:687, 1966.
9. Warkany, J., Chu, E. H. Y., and Kauder, E.: Male pseudohermaphroditism and chromosomal mosaicism, Am. J. Dis. Child. 104:172, 1962.
10. Nilson, O.: Hernia uteri inguinalis beim Manne, Acta chir. scandinav. 83:231, 1939.
11. Pinkerton, J. H. M.: Gonadal dysgenesis complicated by virilizing embryonal carcinoma, J. Reprod. & Fertil. 9:203, 1965.

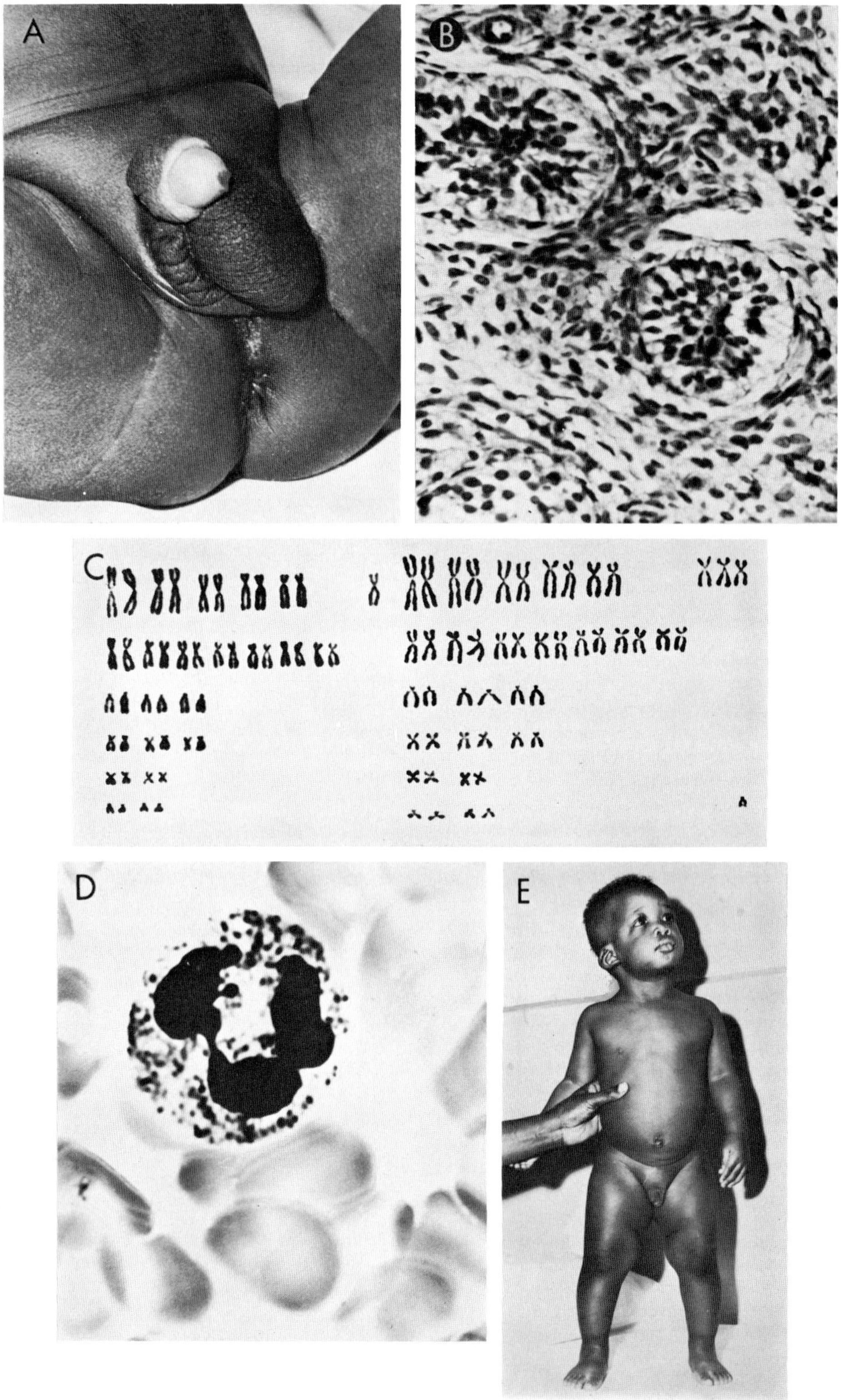

Fig. 112-17.—Mixed gonadal dysgenesis in a boy with XO/XXXY mosaicism.[9] **A,** external genitalia as they appeared at birth. **B,** section through testis found in the left inguinal region. **C,** karyotypes showing mosaicism. **D,** leukocyte showing drumstick. **E,** appearance of the boy at the age of 2½ years.

Pure Gonadal Dysgenesis

THIS TERM is applied to women with gonadal dysgenesis, normal height, eunuchoid body proportions and poorly developed secondary sex characteristics. Although they have streak gonads like patients with Turner syndrome, they are not stunted in growth and do not have congenital malformations characteristic of XO gonadal dysgenesis.[1,2] In 1959, Harnden and Stewart[3] described the chromosomes of a "tall eunuchoid female," 19 years of age, who presented with primary amenorrhea. The secondary sex characteristics were not developed before treatment and urinary excretion of gonadotropins was raised. Sex chromatin was negative and the chromosomes were 46,XY, i.e., like those of a normal male. In 1965, Brøgger and Strand[4] pointed out that congenital malformations commonly found in gonadal dysgenesis (Turner syndrome) can vary between severe disorder and almost normal development and that, therefore, "pure" cases cannot be distinguished sharply from others with characteristic signs. They tabulated 38 cases of pure gonadal dysgenesis, with chromosome analyses in 15. It evolved that the karyotype was not uniform. There were 7 with XY, 2 with XX and 6 with mosaicisms (XY/XX; XY/XO; XY/XO/XYY; 2 XX/XO; deleted-X/XO). Since neither the clinical nor the cytogenetic picture is uniform, the entity is not well circumscribed. In 1968, Boczkowski[5] reviewed 43 cases in which cytogenetic analyses had been done in addition to gynecologic and histologic examinations. The situation remained confused.

The most interesting cases are those that have no signs of male development, female genitalia and XY karyotype. The inability of the Y chromosome to induce formation of testes is remarkable and worth emphasis.

There are families on record in which there are women with pure gonadal dysgenesis and there are oncologic data on such patients that are of interest.

The syndrome has been reported in sisters.[4,6] Frasier *et al.*[7] described gonadal dysgenesis in twin sisters with 46,XY karyotype. Both showed normal female phenotype without signs of Turner syndrome. At the age of 6 years, one of the twins was explored because of lower abdominal pain. A tumor (7 × 7 cm.) could be felt in the right side of her abdomen. On laparotomy, the mass was found attached to a nodule that was connected with the right streak. The left streak also had a nodule at its distal portion. The tumor was considered a solid teratoma containing various tissues and the nodules were gonadoblastomas. The twin sister, who had no symptoms, was explored subsequently and a nodule connected with the right streak gonad also was found to be a gonadoblastoma. Tumors in dysgenetic gonads were reported by Teter and Boczkowski.[8]

Barr *et al.*[9] observed 2 sisters with disturbed sexual development. The older one had pure gonadal dysgenesis with streak ovaries and 46,XY karyotype; the younger was a male pseudohermaphrodite with virilization due to testes in the "ovarian position" and 46,XY karyotype. A nephew of the sisters was a male with hypospadias and a urethral orifice at the base of the penis. Barr *et al.*[9] listed 30 instances of XY gonadal dysgenesis. Only 6 of these had anomalies such as short neck, renal or skeletal changes, whereas 24 could be considered as pure gonadal dysgenesis.

Sternberg *et al.*[10] described XY-pure gonadal dysgenesis in three different sibships in the same kindred and in two generations. Two apparently normal sisters of a patient with pure gonadal dysgenesis transmitted the condition to 2 "XY-daughters."

XY-gonadal dysgenesis was reported in 3 siblings by Chemke *et al.*[11] Two were phenotypic females with pure gonadal dysgenesis and 1 was a phenotypic male with pseudohermaphrodism. The last mentioned sibling had gonads that were found to be nonfunctioning testes. His testosterone was thought to be of adrenal origin.

A review of the problems of the XY female was published by Dewhurst[12] in 1971.

REFERENCES

1. Hoffenberg, R., and Jackson, W. P. U.: Gonadal dysgenesis in normal looking females, Brit. M. J. 1:1281, 1957.
2. Swyer, G. I. M.: Gonadal dysgenesis, Brit. M. J. 1:1421, 1957.
3. Harnden, D. G., and Stewart, J. S. S.: The chromosomes in a case of pure gonadal dysgenesis, Brit. M. J. 2:1285, 1959.
4. Brøgger, A., and Strand, A.: Contribution to the study of the so-called pure gonadal dysgenesis, Acta endocrinol. 48:490, 1965.
5. Boczkowski, K.: The syndrome of pure gonadal dysgenesis, M. Gynaec. Sociol. 3:96, 1968.
6. Cohen, M. M., and Shaw, M. W.: Two XY siblings with gonadal dysgenesis and female phenotype, New England J. Med. 272:1083, 1965.
7. Frasier, S. D., Bashore, R. A., and Mosier, H. D.: Gonadoblastoma associated with pure gonadal dysgenesis in monozygous twins, J. Pediat. 64:740, 1964.
8. Teter, J., and Boczkowski, K.: Occurrence of tumors in dysgenetic gonads, Cancer 20:1301, 1967.
9. Barr, M. L., Carr, D. H., Plunkett, E. R., Soltan, H. C., and Wiens, R. G.: Male pseudohermaphroditism and pure gonadal dysgenesis in sisters, Am. J. Obst. & Gynec. 99: 1047, 1967.
10. Sternberg, W. H., Barclay, D. L., and Kloepfer, H. W.: Familial XY gonadal dysgenesis, New England J. Med. 278:695, 1968.
11. Chemke, J., Carmichael, R., Stewart, J. M., Geer, R. H., and Robinson, A.: Familial XY gonadal dysgenesis, J. M. Genetics 7:105, 1970.
12. Dewhurst, C. J.: The XY female, Am. J. Obst. & Gynec. 109:675, 1971.

Triplo-X, Tetra-X and Penta-X

THE FIRST WOMAN with XXX karyotype reported by Jacobs *et al.*[1] apparently was normal except for sexual underdevelopment and amenorrhea. Triplo-X females can be mentally and physically normal and are capable of reproducing[2] or they can be mentally defective and fertile[3]; or they can have a variety of physical anomalies in addition to mental retardation: mongoloid features, microcephaly, high-arched palate, cleft lip and palate, simian creases, incurved fifth finger and other signs have been observed. Ocular defects, arhinencephaly, congenital heart disease and sporadic cretinism were recorded in single cases[4]; they could be accidental complications. If one considers that the incidence of XXX is approximately 1 in 670 (0.15%) live-born children, and that by 1968 only 65 cases, selected for various reasons, had been described in detail, the finding of heterogeneous anomalies is not surprising, particularly when one looks for them in institutions for the mentally retarded, where they reside with a frequency of 0.42%.[5] Although there is a possibility of an increased tendency to mental retardation in triplo-X females, no increased incidence of congenital malformations has been found in adult and newborn surveys.[5]

Infants with trisomy 18 and triplo-X constitution have the characteristics of their autosomal trisomy.[6] In one case described in detail with necropsy,[7] the ovaries were histologically abnormal.

The fact that a triplo-X woman and one with XX/XXX karyotype each had a son with XXY constitution and "adiposogenital" dystrophy[8] is of great interest and probably of significance. The formation of XXY zygotes can be expected if an XX-containing ovum is fertilized by a normal Y sperm. The women with triplo-X cells had menstrual and reproductive difficulties that required medical treatment. Without knowledge of the karyotypes, one would wonder why women with "hypogonadism" gave birth to boys with genital dystrophy.

Two tetra-X patients were recorded in 1961 by Carr *et al.*[9] They were found through buccal smear examinations of institutionalized defectives. Aside from mental retardation and supernumerary nipples, one girl appeared normal. At the age of 13 years, her reproductive system appeared to be normal for a girl in early adolescence. The second patient also had a reproductive system without unusual features. The degree of mental retardation is variable and physical features are not characteristic.[13] Studies of dermatoglyphics did not give uniform results.[13,14] The few cases on record were reviewed by Telfer *et al.*[15] XXX/XXXX and other mosaics have been observed and reported.[16]

Two penta-X patients had been reported by 1967. Kesaree and Woolley[10] described a 2-year-old girl with somewhat mongoloid features who was retarded in physical and mental development. The child was born 2 months early, weighing 1,800 Gm. A patent ductus was ligated at 10 weeks of age but failure to thrive continued. Her irides were blue, with deeply melanotic sectors. Simian creases and clinodactyly were noted on the hands and overlapping toes on her tiny feet. The external genitalia were female and a small uterus was palpable. A second girl with penta-X karyotype also had patent ductus arteriosus that required surgical treatment.[11] She gained weight following surgery and appeared somewhat mongoloid when photographed at the age of 2 years. Her hands were tiny and there was some clinodactyly. Clubfoot on the right was corrected when she was 2 years of age.

A girl with 48,XXXX/49,XXXXX mosaicism was found who was severely mentally defective and who had various nonspecific congenital anomalies and dermatoglyphic peculiarities.[12]

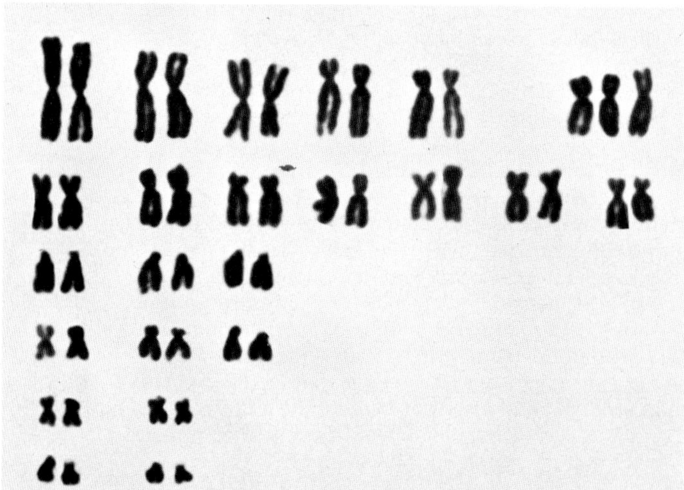

Fig. 112-18.—47,XXX karyotype in a tall 70-year-old woman of normal mentality. She never menstruated and had small breasts, sparse axillary and pubic hair and a hypoplastic uterus. She was married for 25 years but had had no pregnancies.

REFERENCES

1. Jacobs, P. A., Baikie, A. G., Court Brown, W. M., MacGregor, T. N., Maclean, N., and Harnden, D. G.: Evidence for the existence of the human "super female," Lancet 2:423, 1959.
2. Close, H. G.: Two apparently normal triple-X females, Lancet 2:1358, 1963.
3. Stewart, J. S., and Sanderson, A. R.: Fertility and oligophrenia in an apparent triplo-X female, Lancet 2:21, 1960.
4. Pfeiffer, R. A., Palm, D., and Jochmus, J.: Das Erscheinungsbild der Trisomie des X-chromosoms bei Jugendlichen, Monatsschr. Kinderh. 115:9, 1967.
5. Kohn, G., Winter, J. S. D., and Mellman, W. J.: Trisomy X in three children, J. Pediat. 72:248, 1968.
6. Uchida, I. A., and Bowman, J. M.: XXX 18-trisomy, Lancet 2:1094, 1961.
7. Ricci, N., and Borgatti, L.: XXX 18-trisomy, Lancet 2: 1276, 1963.
8. Rosenkranz, W.: Klinefelter Syndrom bei Kindern von Frauen mit Geschlechtschromosomen Anomalien, Helvet. paediat. acta 20:359, 1965.
9. Carr, D. H., Barr, M. L., and Plunkett, E. R.: An XXXX sex chromosome complex in two mentally defective females, Canad. M.A.J. 84:131, 1961.
10. Kesaree, N., and Woolley, P.: A phenotypic female with 49 chromosomes, presumably XXXXX, J. Pediat. 63:1099, 1963.
11. Brody, J., Fitzgerald, M. G., and Spiers, A. S. D.: A female child with five X chromosomes, J. Pediat. 70:105, 1967.
12. Ricci, N., Dallapiccola, B., Ventimiglia, B., Tiepolo, L., and Fraccaro, M.: 48,XXXX/49,XXXXX mosaic: Asynchronies among the late-replicating X chromosomes, Cytogenetics 7:249, 1968.
13. Di Cagno, L., and Franceschini, P.: Feeblemindedness and XXXX karyotype, J. Ment. Defic. Res. 12:226, 1968.
14. Sokolowski, J., Knaus, A., and Kleczkowska, A.: Dermatoglyphics of two cases of X tetrasomy, Am. J. Human Genet. 21:559, 1969.
15. Telfer, M. A., Richardson, C. E., Helmken, J., and Smith, G. F.: Divergent phenotypes among 48,XXXX and 47,XXX females, Am. J. Human Genet. 22:326, 1970.
16. Rerrick, E. G.: Mosaic XXX/XXXX sex chromosome complement. Case report and review of literature, J. Ment. Defic. Res. 14:141, 1970.

XXY to XXXXY
(Klinefelter Syndrome)

THE XXY ORGANISM seems to be well tolerated in prenatal life. By 1966, no case of XXY karyotype had been described among spontaneous abortuses.[1] Furthermore, it is known that most fetuses and newborns with XXY karyotype appear normal and free of malformations at birth. Clinical manifestations such as mental retardation, psychopathic tendencies, behavior problems, small testes, sterility and gynecomastia, which are characteristic of some of the cases, are not recognized in early childhood. It is true that in some patients hypospadias, cryptorchidism[2,4] or bifid scrotum[5,6] was noticed at birth; in others, the XXY state, when combined with trisomy 21,[7] shows congenital anomalies characteristic of Down syndrome. Rohde[8] noted congenital shoulder deformity, brachiomesophalangia, clinodactyly, toe deformities and angiomata in some of his patients with XXY constitution. But such anomalies occur in the general population, too; they will have to be evaluated quantitatively before they can be considered significant. Smallness of the testes is the only sign that is present in all adult patients with Klinefelter syndrome. In 50 patients averaging 38 years, none had cryptorchidism and the length of the penis was judged to be within normal limits in 90%. There were some congenital anomalies but they were heterogeneous and not of any clinical significance.[9] In more than 100 boys with hypospadias, no abnormal karyotypes were found.[6] Mikamo *et al.*[10] noted a reduced number of spermatogonia in testes of chromatin-positive male infants and thought that diminution of germ cells may start in prenatal life.

Fig. 112-19.—Hypospadias in a 4-year-old boy with XXY karyotype.[4]

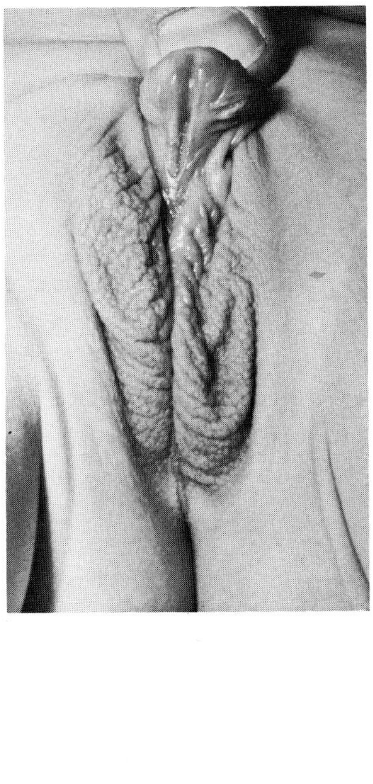

In contrast to the XXY type, the patients with the more complicated karyotypes may have signs of prenatal damage. Uveal coloboma has been observed in a boy with XX/XXY karyotype.[54] In one case of XXXY karyotype, webbing of the neck and bilateral radioulnar synostosis was described[11] and, in another, optic atrophy was seen.[12] A deformed ear has been noted in 1 patient[13] but normal habitus was described in others.[11,14] The serious mental impairment of these patients could be due to prenatal damage but there is

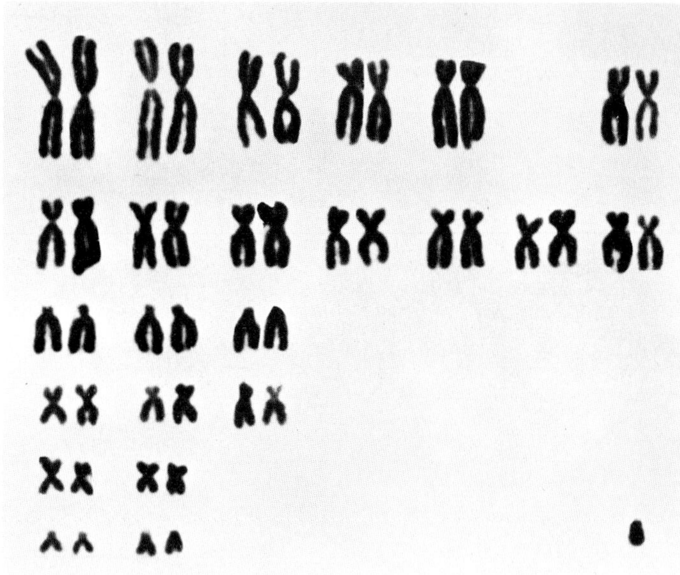

Fig. 112-20.—47,XXY karyotype of a boy with Klinefelter syndrome.

no proof of this. When brain examinations become available, this question may be answered. By 1969, 17 cases had been described and reviewed.[52] Mosaicism can change the clinical picture considerably. We described the case of a boy with XXXY/XO karyotype who appeared externally normal with the exception of unilateral cryptorchidism, a penile chordee and an inguinal hernia; laparotomy revealed the presence of a uterus and of Fallopian tubes but no second gonad was found. The picture was that of male pseudohermaphrodism and hernia uteri inguinalis in the male.[53] The mental development appeared to be normal. With XXXXY karyotype,[15] mental retardation is severe and there also are congenital malformations. Microcephaly, hypertelorism, mongolian slant of palpebral fissures, high-arched or cleft palate, micrognathia, vertebral anomalies, proximal radio-ulnar synostosis, incurved fifth finger and coxa valga have been described in such patients with three "inactive" X chromosomes. The external genitalia usually are abnormal. The penis is small and the scrotum hypoplastic or bifid.[15,16] The genitalia can be so underdeveloped that the sex is doubtful.[17] In a patient with XXXX/XXXXY mosaicism, there was subluxation of the elbow joints, clinodactyly, testes with islands of Leydig cells and few ghost tubules, decreased total ridge counts of fingerprints and severe mental retardation.[55]

Fig. 112-21.—Boy with XXXXY karyotype. He is very small for his age and speech is delayed. At age 6 years he could write a few letters of the alphabet.

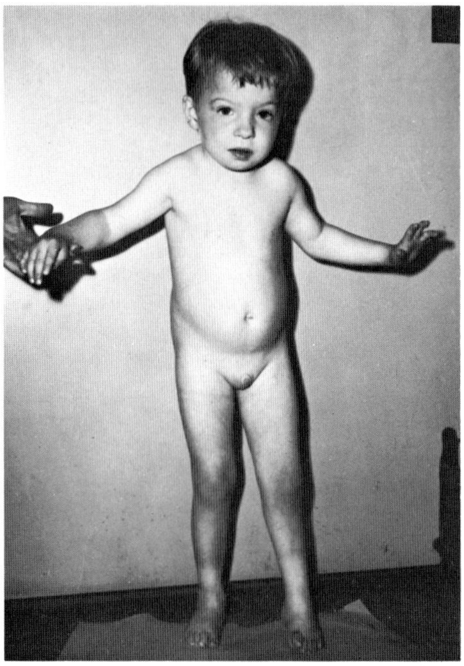

XXYY

Persons with 48 chromosomes and XXYY karyotypes resemble patients with XXY Klinefelter syndrome.[14] Barr *et al.*[18] thought that the addition of a Y chromosome may have a variable and not yet delineated harmful effect, particularly with advancing age. Mental retardation, cryptorchidism, infundibular pulmonary stenosis,[19] clubbing of fingers, incurved little finger[20,21] and other nonspecific signs have been noted. Radio-ulnar synostosis and coxa valga was observed in a boy 7 years of age.[22] Dermatoglyphics have been described and hypothenar patterns were

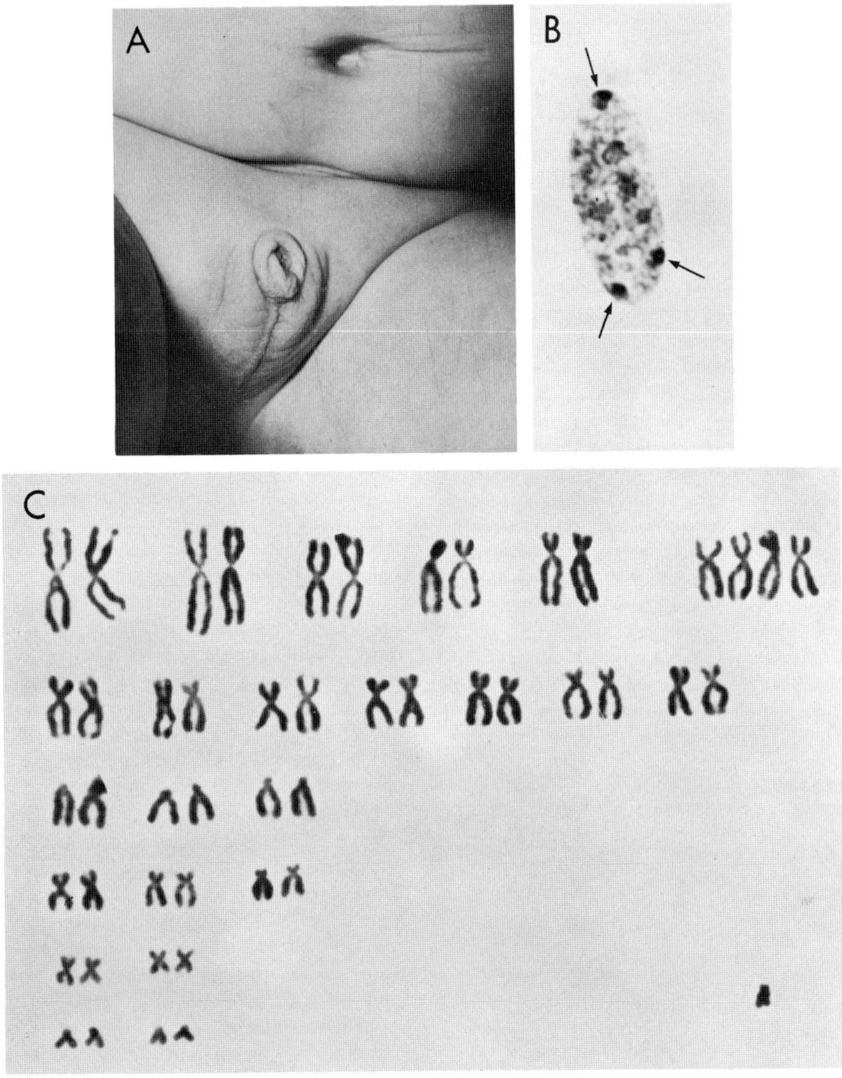

Fig. 112-22.—**A,** genitalia of the boy with XXXXY karyotype shown in Figure 112-21. **B,** cell from buccal smear showing three Barr bodies. **C,** karyotype showing 49 chromosomes with 4 X chromosomes.

thought to be characteristic,[22,23] but this was not confirmed in a more recent case.[21]

The 48,XXYY chromosome pattern seems to be quite rare. Maclean *et al.*[24] found only 1 in 10,725 newborn males with this karyotype, and further studies[25] suggested that the incidence is even lower. Yet, among 942 men in two English special hospitals for dangerous, violent or criminal patients, 7 had an XXYY complement. These 7 males were among 21 who were (singly) sex chromatin positive. The XXYY karyotype also is more frequent among institutionalized mentally retarded than in the general male population.[26] Significantly increased height measurements were ascertained in mentally subnormal patients with XXYY (and XXXYY) constitutions compared with XY and XXY retardates.[27] In maximum security hospitals, the ratio of XXYY to XXY patients was found to be 1 in 3.[25]

By 1967, about 40 cases with XXYY constitution had been reported and 8 were in prepubertal patients.[21] Garcia *et al.*[21] described such a patient who had skeletal anomalies, excessive length of the extremities, abnormal dermatoglyphics, subnormal intelligence and temporary aggressive behavior; they reviewed the cases published by that time.

A patient with 49,XXXYY karyotype had Klinefelter syndrome with mental deficiency. He was 190 cm. tall, had a small penis and small, soft testes that consisted entirely of connective tissue.[28] The palpebral fissures were small and the lower jaw protruding.

XYY and XYYY

In 1961, Sandberg *et al.*[29] reported the case of a man 44 years of age who had an XYY karyotype. He was the father of 8 children from two marriages. A daughter from the first marriage had an apparently normal karyotype, although she had no ovaries and no uterus. A daughter from the second marriage had Down syndrome with trisomy 21. The father, who was obese, had been treated for diaphragmatic and umbilical herniae, peptic ulcer, cystic mandibular lesions and a diffuse neurodermatitis.[30] In 1964, Ricci and Malacarne[31] summarized the findings in several patients with XYY karyotype and stated that no consistent clinical picture is associated with this chromosomal anomaly. It was shown later that some patients with various general disorders had XYY constitution. A patient with Marfan syndrome[32] and another with hypogenitalism, genu varum and valgum and mental retardation had this karyotype.[33] We have seen an extremely tall 13-year-old boy who was suspected of having Marfan syndrome. He had some but not all signs characteristic of that disease picture and was found to have an XYY karyotype. His mental development and behavior were not unusual (Fig. 112-23). Vignetti *et al.*[34] reported a "girl" with a phallus without meatus and a single (urethral) opening in the perineum. The "labia majora" proved to be divided halves of the scrotum containing normal infantile testes. Another "female" child with an enlarged clitoris had separate vaginal and urethral openings and testes in the major labia. Hypertelorism, simian crease and clinodactyly were seen in this XYY case.[35] Severe finger deformities, hypoplastic thenar and hypothenar eminences, short upper lip and prognathism were noted in a boy with XY/XYY constitution.[36] Combination of trisomy 21 and XYY karyotype was discovered in a boy with Down syndrome and rudimentary genitalia with cryptorchidism. Necropsy revealed atrial and ventricular septal defect with transposition of the great vessels.[37] This is of interest, since transposition is rare in patients with "pure" Down syndrome and trisomy 21 (p. 522). Other mosaics containing 47,XYY cell lines have been found.[25]

Fig. 112-23. – A 13-year-old boy with some signs of Marfan syndrome (Chapter 91) and XYY karyotype. Height 204 cm.; span 212 cm. There was a chest deformity and some of the elongated toes had contractures. Mental development and behavior were not unusual.

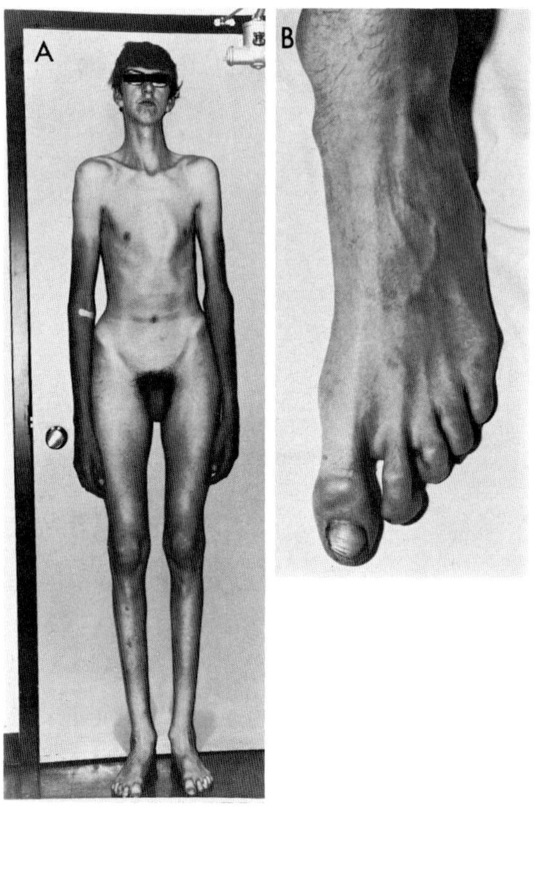

In the majority of persons with 47,XYY, congenital malformations are absent but tall stature and a tendency to delinquency seem to be associated characteristics.[25,38] Casey *et al.*[39] showed that approximately 15% of inmates of maximum security hospitals 183 cm. (6 ft.) or more in height had 47,XYY constitution. Price *et al.*[40] described 9 men with XYY chromosome complement. Eight were mentally retarded, 1 was schizophrenic and all had criminal records. Six of the 9 were more than 181 cm. tall but their physical and sexual features were indistinguishable from those of normal men. In three 47,XYY males, marked elevation of urinary luteinizing hormone (LH) has been noted.[41] The XYY karyotype also may be found in a significant number of mentally subnormal persons[25] and occasionally in boys with multiple congenital malformations that, however, do not conform to a regular disease picture.[42] The "indescribable" behavior of a "tall, handsome, and athletically proportioned boy" with XYY constitution was described by Cowie and Kahn.[43] At the age of 4½ years, he was referred because he was unmanageable, destructive, mischievous and defiant. He was the firstborn, wanted child of a mother aged 23 and a father aged 26 years. Two tall, prepubertal boys with aggressive behavior, mild retardation and radio-ulnar synostosis had an XYY chromosome pattern.[44] A review of the XYY status in children[45] showed a greatly variable phenotype; there were tall as well as undersized patients; psychomotor retardation and genital anomalies were relatively frequent but some of the cases had been selected for chromosome analysis because of the phenotypic changes. The same can be said concerning reports of adults with XYY pattern who often were selected because of tall stature and criminal tendencies. A comparative crimino-biologic study of patients with XYY or Klinefelter syndrome was made by Tsuboi.[56] Before one can make statements about relative frequencies of physical, mental and behavioral features, incidence and prevalence of the XYY karyotype in the general male population have to be ascertained. The incidence at birth has been estimated as 1 per 1,000 males,[25,45] but in one study[46] the XYY condition was in the order of 1 per 250 males. Thus, there is a wide gap between the numbers present in the male population and the small numbers recognized in prisons, hospitals and mental institutions. Interpretation of the XYY constitution will be possible only if those identified at birth will be followed and evaluated subsequently.[25] There may be many persons with XYY karyotype who are normal in size and behavior.

A 5-year-old boy with 48,XYYY karyotype had mild psychomotor retardation, pulmonary valvar stenosis, cryptorchidism, inguinal hernia and simian lines.[47] A male pseudohermaphrodite with hypospadias, a uterus with blindly ending tubes and a single testis on the right side was found to have 48,XYYY/45,XO mosaicism[48] and a "true" hermaphrodite with ambiguous external genitalia and abdominal ovotestis on the left and a primitive testis on the right had a 49,XXYYY/47,XXY/46,XX mosaicism.[49] An XYY/XXY/XY/XO mosaicism in leukocytes was found in an infant with ambiguous external genitalia. No gonads or uterus was found on laparotomy.[50]

A 15-year-old boy with four Y chromosomes was reported by van den Berghe *et al.*[51] He presented a 45,XO/49,XYYYY mosaic. He was mentally defective, had average stature, bilateral cataracts, facial asymmetry, clinodactyly of the fifth finger and general brachymesophalangy. Clinically, he did not show gonadal deficiency but testicular biopsy revealed complete absence of spermatogenesis in tubules that were normal except for Leydig cell hyperplasia.

REFERENCES

1. Kerr, M., and Rashad, M. N.: Chromosome studies on spontaneous abortions, Am. J. Obst. & Gynec. 94:322, 1966.
2. Lamy, M., deGrouchy, J., Frezal, J., Josso, N., and Feintuch, G.: Syndrome de Klinefelter et hypospadias. Présence de deux chromosomes X. Rupture du chromosome Y et translocation de ses fragments, Compt. rend. Acad. Sc. (Paris) 255:581, 1962.
3. Gray, J.: Hypospadias with 47/XXY karyotype, Lancet 1: 722, 1961.
4. Passarge, E., and Thompson, J. N.: Autoradiography in a boy with XXY karyotype, Am. J. Dis. Child. 108:184, 1964.
5. Conen, P. E., Erkman, B., and Jeffs, R. D.: 47/XXY Klinefelter's syndrome in an infant with abnormal genitalia, J. Urol. 91:595, 1964.
6. Frøland, A.: *Klinefelter's Syndrome* (Copenhagen: Costers Bogtrykkeri, 1969).
7. Ford, C. E., Jones, K. W., Miller, O. J., Mittwoch, U., Penrose, L. S., Ridler, M., and Shapiro, A.: The chromosomes in a patient showing both mongolism and the Klinefelter syndrome, Lancet 1:709, 1959.
8. Rohde, R. A.: Chromatin-positive Klinefelter's syndrome: Clinical and cytogenetic studies, J. Chron. Dis. 16:1139, 1963.
9. Becker, K. L., Hoffman, D. L., Albert, A., Underdahl, L. O., and Mason, H. L.: Klinefelter's syndrome. Clinical and laboratory findings in 50 patients, Arch. Int. Med. 118: 314, 1966.
10. Mikamo, K., Aguercif, M., Hazeghi, P., and Martin-Du Pan, R.: Chromatin-positive Klinefelter's syndrome, Fertil. & Steril. 19:731, 1968.
11. Ferguson-Smith, M. A., Johnston, A. W., and Handmaker, S. D.: Primary amentia and micro-orchidism associated with an XXY sex-chromosome constitution, Lancet 2:184, 1960.
12. Makino, S., Takagi, N., and Hikita, M.: Two phenotypic males with XXXXY and XXXY sex chromosomes, Proc. Jap. Acad. 40:427, 1964.
13. Nakagome, Y., Matsui, I., Komiya, K., Momma, K., and Arima, M.: Sex chromosome abnormalities in mentally defective children, Paediat. Univ. Tokyo 11:41, 1965.
14. Carr, D. H., Barr, M. L., Plunkett, E. R., Grumbach, M. M., Morishima, A., and Chu, E. H. Y.: An XXXY sex chromosome complex in Klinefelter subjects with duplicated sex chromatin, J. Clin. Endocrinol. 21:491, 1961.
15. Barr, M. L., Carr, D. H., Poszany, J., Wilson, R. A., Dunn, H. G., Jacobson, T. S., Miller, J. R., Lewis, M., and Chown, B.: The XXXXY sex chromosome anomaly, Canad. M.A.J. 87:891, 1962.
16. Fraccaro, M., Klinger, H. P., and Schutt, W.: A male with XXXXY sex chromosomes, Cytogenetics 1:52, 1962.
17. Turpin, R., Lafourcade, J., Gruveiller, J., Lejeune, J., Bocquet, G., Hoppeler, A., and Cuibert, C.: Dysgénésie gonadosomatique XXXXY. Observation néo-natale, Bull. Soc. méd. hôp. Paris 113:916, 1962.
18. Barr, M. L., Carr, D. H., Soltan, H. C., Wiens, R. G., and Plunkett, E. R.: The XXYY variant of Klinefelter's syndrome, Canad. M.A.J. 90:575, 1964.
19. Schlegel, R. J., Aspillaga, J., Neu, R., and Gardner, L. I.: Studies on a boy with XXYY chromosome constitution, Pediatrics 36:113, 1965.
20. Leisti, J. T., Aula, P. P., and Hjelt, L. H.: Two cases of (prepubertal) Klinefelter's syndrome with XXYY sex chromosomes, Ann. Human Genet. 28:71, 1964.
21. Garcia, H. O., Borgaonkar, D. S., and Richardson, F.: XXYY syndrome in a prepubertal male, Johns Hopkins M. J. 121:31, 1967.
22. Robinson, G. C., Miller, J. R., Dill, F. J., and Kamburoff, T. D.: Klinefelter's syndrome with the XXYY sex chromosome complex, J. Pediat. 65:226, 1964.
23. Uchida, I. A., Miller, J. R., and Soltan, H. C.: Dermatoglyphics associated with the XXYY chromosome complement, Am. J. Human Genet. 161:284, 1964.
24. Maclean, N., Harnden, D. G., Court Brown, W. M., Bond, J., and Mantle, D. J.: Sex chromosome abnormalities in newborn babies, Lancet 1:286, 1964.
25. Court Brown, W. M.: Males with an XYY sex chromosome complement, J. M. Genetics 5:341, 1968.
26. Maclean, N., Mitchell, J. M., Harnden, D. G., Williams, J., Jacobs, P. A., Buckton, K. E., Baikie, A. G., Court Brown, W. M., McBride, J. A., Strong, J. A., Close, H. G., and Jones, D. C.: A survey of sex chromosome abnormalities among 4514 mental defectives, Lancet 1:293, 1962.
27. Hunter, H.: YY chromosomes and Klinefelter's syndrome, Lancet 1:984, 1966.
28. Bray, P., and Sr. Ann Josephine: An XXXYY sex-chromosome anomaly, J.A.M.A. 184:179, 1963.
29. Sandberg, A. A., Koepf, G. H., Ishihara, T., and Hauschka, T. S.: An XYY human male, Lancet 2:488, 1961.
30. Hauschka, T. S., Hasson, J. E., Goldstein, M. N., Koepf, G. F., and Sandberg, A. A.: An XYY man with progeny indicating familial tendency to non-disjunction, Am. J. Human Genet. 14:22, 1962.
31. Ricci, N., and Malacarne, P.: An XYY human male, Lancet 1:721, 1964.
32. Hustinx, T. W. J., and van Olphen, A. H. F.: An XYY chromosome pattern in a boy with Marfan's syndrome, Genetica 34:262, 1963.
33. Thorburn, M. J., Chutkan, W., Richards, R., and Bell, R.:

XYY sex chromosomes in a Jamaican with orthopaedic abnormalities, J. M. Genetics 5:215, 1968.
34. Vignetti, P., Capotorti, L., and Ferrante, E.: XYY chromosomal constitution with genital abnormality, Lancet 2: 588, 1964.
35. Franks, R. C., Bunting, K. W., and Engel, E.: Male pseudohermaphrodism with XYY sex chromosomes, J. Clin. Endocrinol. 27:1623, 1967.
36. Kajii, T., Neu, R. L., and Gardner, L. I.: XY/XYY mosaicism in a prepubertal boy with tall stature, prognathism, and malformations of the hands, Pediatrics 41:984, 1968.
37. Uchida, I. A., Ray, M., and Duncan, B. P.: 21 trisomy with an XYY sex chromosome complement, J. Pediat. 69:295, 1966.
38. Jacobs, P. A., Price, W. H., Brown, W. M. C., Brittain, R. P., and Whatmore, P. B.: Chromosome studies on men in a maximum security hospital, Ann. Human Genet. 31: 339, 1968.
39. Casey, M. D., Blank, C. E., Street, D. R. K., Segall, L. J., McDougall, J. H., McGrath, P. J., and Skinner, J. L.: YY chromosomes and antisocial behavior, Lancet 2:859, 1966.
40. Price, W. H., Strong, J. A., Whatmore, P. B., and McClemont, W. F.: Criminal patients with XYY sex-chromosome complement, Lancet 1:565, 1966.
41. Papanicolaou, A. D., Kirkham, K. E., and Loraine, J. A.: Abnormalities in urinary gonadotrophin excretion in men with a 47,XYY sex chromosome constitution, Lancet 2: 608, 1968.
42. Kosenow, W., and Pfeiffer, R-A.: YY-Syndrom, Monatsschr. Kinderh. 115:24, 1967.
43. Cowie, J., and Kahn, J.: XYY constitution in prepubertal child, Brit. M. J. 1:748, 1968.
44. Cleveland, W. W., Arias, D., and Smith, G. F.: Radioulnar synostosis, behavioral disturbance, and XYY chromosomes, J. Pediat. 74:103, 1969.
45. Keutel, J., and Dauner, I.: XYY-Status bei Kindern, Ztschr. Kinderh. 106:314, 1969.
46. Sergovich, F., Valentine, G. H., Chen, A. T., Kinch, R. A., and Smout, H. S.: Chromosome aberrations in 2159 consecutive newborn babies, New England J. Med. 280:851, 1969.
47. Townes, P. L., Ziegler, N. A., and Lenhard, L. W.: A patient with 48 chromosomes (XYYY), Lancet 1:1041, 1965.
48. Cox, D., and Berry, C. L.: A patient with 45XO/48XYYY mosaicism, J. M. Genetics 4:132, 1967.
49. Fraccaro, M., Taylor, A. I., Bodian, M., and Newns, G. H.: A human intersex ("true hermaphrodite") with XX/XXY/XXYYY sex chromosomes, Cytogenetics 1:104, 1962.
50. Finley, W. H., Finley, S. C., Cocoris, J. G., and Pittman, C. S.: Four stem-line mosaicism (XO/XY/XXY/XYY) in an infant with ambiguous external genitalia, J. Clin. Endocrinol. 28:239, 1968.
51. van den Berghe, H., Verresen, H., and Cassiman, J. J.: A male with 4 Y-chromosomes, J. Clin. Endocrinol. 28:1370, 1968.
52. Zollinger, H.: Das XXXY-Syndrom, Helvet. paediat. acta 24:589, 1969.
53. Warkany, J., Chu, E. H. Y., and Kauder, E.: Male pseudohermaphroditism and chromosomal mosaicism, Am. J. Dis. Child. 104:94, 1962.
54. François, J., Matton-Van Leuven, M. T., and Gombault, P.: Uveal coloboma and true Klinefelter syndrome, J. M. Genetics 7:213, 1970.
55. Rerrick, E. G.: Klinefelter's syndrome variant, XXXX/XXXXY mosaic, J. Maine M. A. 60:90, 1969.
56. Tsuboi, T.: Crimino-biologic study of patients with the XYY syndrome and Klinefelter's syndrome, Humangenetik 10:68, 1970.

PART XVII

Malformations of the Skin

113

Congenital Skin Defects

CONGENITAL DEFECTS of the skin (aplasia cutis congenita) are rare and puzzling anomalies. Such defects usually are seen on the scalp, but they also occur on the extremities, the trunk or the face. At first glance, such defects can be mistaken for birth injuries or for wounds of recent origin, but circumstantial evidence points to an earlier and more fundamental etiology than perinatal trauma. In fact, some children are born with healed skin defects and, in others, a combination of skin defects and scars is seen.[1] In many cases, associated defects of the skull, digits or other parts point to early disturbance of normal development. There is little doubt that congenital skin defects can have differing causes.

The literature before 1960 was reviewed by Gross *et al.*[2] and by Walker *et al.*[3] Of 213 reported cases, 112 had lesions on the scalp and in 21 the scalp and the skull were involved. Without careful palpation and roentgenograms, the osseous defects can be overlooked. The most common form is a single defect in the parietal area near the midsagittal line. The scalp lesions vary in size from pinpoint to 3 inches in diameter, but on the trunk and on the extremities larger areas can be affected. The surface may be represented by raw granulation tissue or by a thin, glistening, parchment-like membrane. Even in relatively mild cases, congenital deformities of fingers and toes have been observed.[3] In more severe cases, several areas can be involved, so that a considerable portion of the skin is missing. In the patients of Gross *et al.*,[2] more than one-fourth of the skin surface was affected. In one case, the skin of the scalp and face and the auricle were absent on the right side.[4] Needless to say, the prognosis is unfavorable in such extensive cases. The shape of the lesion is variable and occasionally an island of normal skin is seen in a large defect. In some patients, vesicles of different sizes accompany the skin defects, so that epidermolysis bullosa must be considered in the differential diagnosis.[5] Epithelialization of the defect, scar formation or ulceration may modify the usual appearance of the skin defects but the skin around the defect that is free of secondary changes shows absence of the sebaceous and sweat glands as well as deficiency of hair papillae. The rete pegs are flattened near the lesion and elastic fibers are lacking around the defective area. Although one sometimes gets the impression that one is dealing with an accidental or traumatic defect, the symmetric arrangement of the lesions, associated malformations and occasional family observations point to a more profound disturbance. Separation of the skin from amniotic bands served as an explanation of congenital skin defects in former times, but such bands are found only in exceptional cases,[6] which probably have little resemblance to the cases discussed here. Hydramnios preceded the birth of some children with congenital skin defects[1,2,4] but this also is not the rule. In some cases, a fetus papyraceus was expelled together with a living co-twin who had congenital skin defects.[2,7] Concordant defects in twins have been recorded.[8,9] Placental infarcts were present repeatedly. Associated defects are frequent and occur in about one-third of the cases.[2] In addition to irregular defects of digits, there are reports of associated syndactyly, polydactyly, clubfeet, harelip, cleft palate, congenital heart disease, horseshoe kidney, iris coloboma, congenital goiter [2] and mongolism.[4] It is clear that some of the older descriptions refer to infants with trisomy 13-15, who commonly have scalp defects (p. 296). They probably account for many cases in which skull and brain defects were noted beneath the skin lesions of the scalp. In other cases, the anomaly can occur in otherwise normal children, who can grow up and transmit the tendency to some of their children. Transmission from a parent to child has been reported.[10,11] In some such cases, the congenital skin defects may be due to epidermolysis bullosa with intrauterine onset. This may have been true for such observations as that by Heinrichsbauer,[5] in which 2 children with congenital bullae and defects of the skin were born to a mother who had a vesicular skin eruption during her first pregnancy. Recessive inheritance may be responsible for some cases.[12] Recessively inherited congenital skin defects have been observed in cattle.[7]

The prognosis is variable. Small lesions heal without great difficulty in utero or in the first few weeks of postnatal life. Other defects require special care and treatment. Plastic surgery is needed, particularly if the scalp and the skull bones are defective, since spontaneous obliteration by normal bone growth does not occur. If scalp, bone and dura are absent, the exposed brain is endangered by trauma and infection. In such cases, a brittle eschar may hide and cover the brain surface, but hemorrhage or infection represents a serious threat to life. For such patients, an early

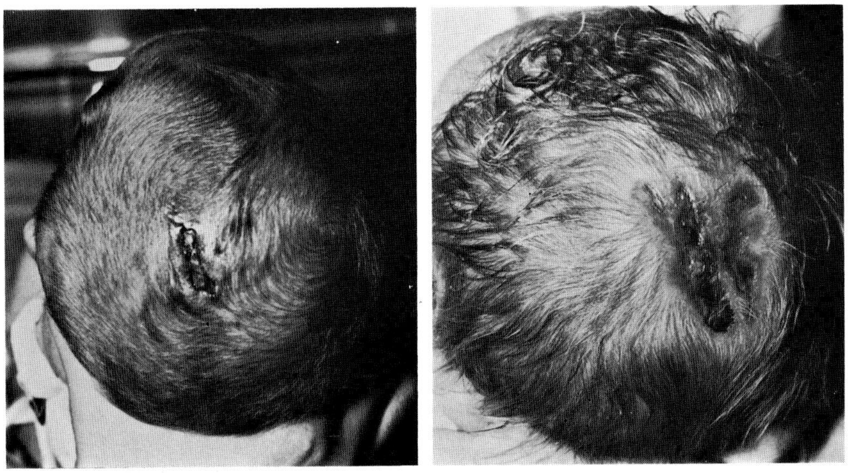

Fig. 113-1.—Congenital skin defects in children with trisomy 13-15.

plastic operation was recommended by Ingraham and Matson.[13] In cases with small defects limited to skin and bone, delay of plastic surgery for several years seems preferable because it permits proper expansion of the skull. For cases of trisomy 13-15, the prognosis is hopeless. It has been estimated that the death rate in infants with congenital defect of the scalp alone amounts to 20%, but if both the skull and scalp are involved, the mortality rate is nearly 60%.[4]

REFERENCES

1. Berndorfer, A.: Ein neugeborenes Kind mit blutenden Wunden und verheilten Narben an der Körperoberfläche, Arch. Kinderh. 168:281, 1963.
2. Gross, H., Lindemayr, W., and Pospisil, G.: Zur Kenntnis der Aplasia cutis, Ztschr. Kinderh. 2:198, 1957.
3. Walker, J. C., Koenig, J. A., Irwin, L., and Meijer, R.: Congenital absence of skin (aplasia cutis congenita), Plast. & Reconstruct. Surg. 26:209, 1960.
4. Conway, H., and Johnson, G.: Congenital absence of the scalp and skull, Ann. Surg. 144:1035, 1956.
5. Heinrichsbauer, F.: Ein weiterer Beitrag zur Frage angeborener Hautdefekte, Arch. Gynäk. 134:673, 1928.
6. Möller, K. O.: Un cas d'acranie et d'hydromicrocéphalie avec une bride amniotique persistante, Acta obst. et gynec. scandinav. 2:380, 1923.
7. Vink, L. P. H. J.: Kongenitaler Hautdefekt bei einem Neugeborenen, Arch. Gynäk. 167:291, 1938.
8. Loewy, E.: Kongenitale Hautdefekte und Keloide bei eineiigen Zwillingen, Dermat. Wchnschr. 79:1660, 1924.
9. Hodgman, J. E., Mathies, A. W., and Levan, N. E.: Congenital scalp defects in twin sisters, Am. J. Dis. Child. 110:293, 1965.
10. Johnsonbaugh, R. E., Light, I. J., and Sutherland, J. M.: Congenital scalp defects in father and son, Am. J. Dis. Child. 110:297, 1965.
11. Cutlip, B. D., Jr., Cryan, D. M., and Vineyard, W. R.: Congenital scalp defects in mother and child, Am. J. Dis. Child. 113:597, 1967.
12. Gedda, L., Muratore, A., and Bernardi, A.: La Gangrena asettica della Teca cranica come Aplasia circoscritta ereditaria del Neonato, Acta genet. med. 12:117, 1963.
13. Ingraham, F. D., and Matson, D. D.: *Neurosurgery of Infancy and Childhood* (Springfield, Ill.: Charles C Thomas Publisher, 1954).

Epidermolysis Bullosa

THIS INHERITED SKIN ANOMALY is characterized by the development of vesicles and bullae on the skin and sometimes on the mucous membranes occurring spontaneously or in response to minimal trauma. Although only the severe forms are congenital, it can be assumed that the basic tendency to epidermolysis bullosa is always determined before birth. Three types of epidermolysis bullosa are distinguished – a simple (or benign) form, a more severe, dystrophic variety and a lethal form. But it should be clear that intermediate forms exist and classification can be difficult.

Although most cases are sporadic, it is likely that all cases are genetically determined. Approximately 20% correspond to the simple or benign form and 10% to the dystrophic form with manifest dominant or recessive inheritance, whereas 70% of the cases are sporadic.[1]

The pathogenesis is not clear. Lack of elastic tissue in the dermis has been observed in some but not in all cases. There also is variability concerning hyperhidrosis. A vascular anomaly seems likely but no histologic proof for it has been found. As early as 1933, Cockayne[1] considered an inborn error of metabolism as the basic hereditary anomaly but until now a metabolic disturbance has not been discovered and only manifestations are known. A relationship to porphyria often has been suspected, since bullous eruptions appear on the skin of patients with that disorder, but elevation of urinary porphyrins has been found only rarely in patients with epidermolysis bullosa.[2] Although both disorders result in bullous skin lesions and both become more pronounced in summer, they differ in that porphyrinuria is adversely influenced by light and epidermolysis bullosa by heat and sweating.

The simple (benign) form of epidermolysis bullosa is inherited as a dominant trait that sometimes skips a generation and is more distinctly expressed in males than in females.[1] Vesicles and bullae appear only rarely in infancy but they develop during childhood, particularly in areas exposed to repeated trauma. The tendency to formation of vesicles is increased in summer by heat and humidity. The lesions often decrease in number at puberty and may disappear in adulthood and old age. The bullae heal rapidly within a few days, usually without scarring. Hyperhidrosis of the palms and soles and dermographism frequently are observed. Mucous membranes, nails and teeth are affected only rarely. General physical and mental development is normal. The bullae form in the epidermis. Elastic tissue deficiency has been observed in some but not in all cases. Noojin *et al.*[3] recorded a pedigree of an Alabama kindred of 283 persons showing transmission of epidermolysis bullosa through eight generations. There were 52 males and 65 females among the affected. Other reports concerning transmission through many generations indicate that incidence of affected members and sex ratio are indicative of autosomal dominant inheritance.[4]

The dystrophic type of epidermolysis bullosa has been subdivided into several varieties.[1] One of the dystrophic forms is inherited as a Mendelian dominant like the simple type. The lesions appear at birth or soon thereafter in otherwise normal children. Minimal trauma can produce lesions that, after healing, leave a thin, atrophic scar containing epidermal cysts or disappear without any scar. The mucous membranes and nails sometimes are involved. Some improvement may be noted at puberty. It is clear from this description that the borderline between the simple and this mild dystrophic form is ill defined.

The recessive dystrophic variety is a serious disorder that occurs in children of apparently healthy parents who are consanguineous in a relatively high percentage of cases. Bullae, which often are present at birth, develop spontaneously or in response to trauma. The lesions often are large and filled with either clear or blood-stained fluid that, at birth, is sterile. On healing, scars, contractures and pigmentations may develop. If the mucous membranes of the respiratory and alimentary tracts are involved, they may heal with scarring and result in stenosis of an affected organ such as the larynx or esophagus or in fusion of the tongue with the roof of the mouth.[1] The conjunctivae can be involved and corneal opacities may develop. Anomalies of the teeth, nails and hair occur. Figure 114-3, *B* and *E* show abnormal shape and spacing of teeth. On the hands or feet, the digits may become tightly fused in contracture and covered with a cutaneous envelope.[5] Roentgenograms reveal overconstriction of the shafts of the long bones, webbing and contractions of fingers, attrition of the teeth or esophageal stenosis.[6] Some of the patients die in childhood but others reach adulthood and then present as small, physically (and sometimes mentally) underdeveloped persons.

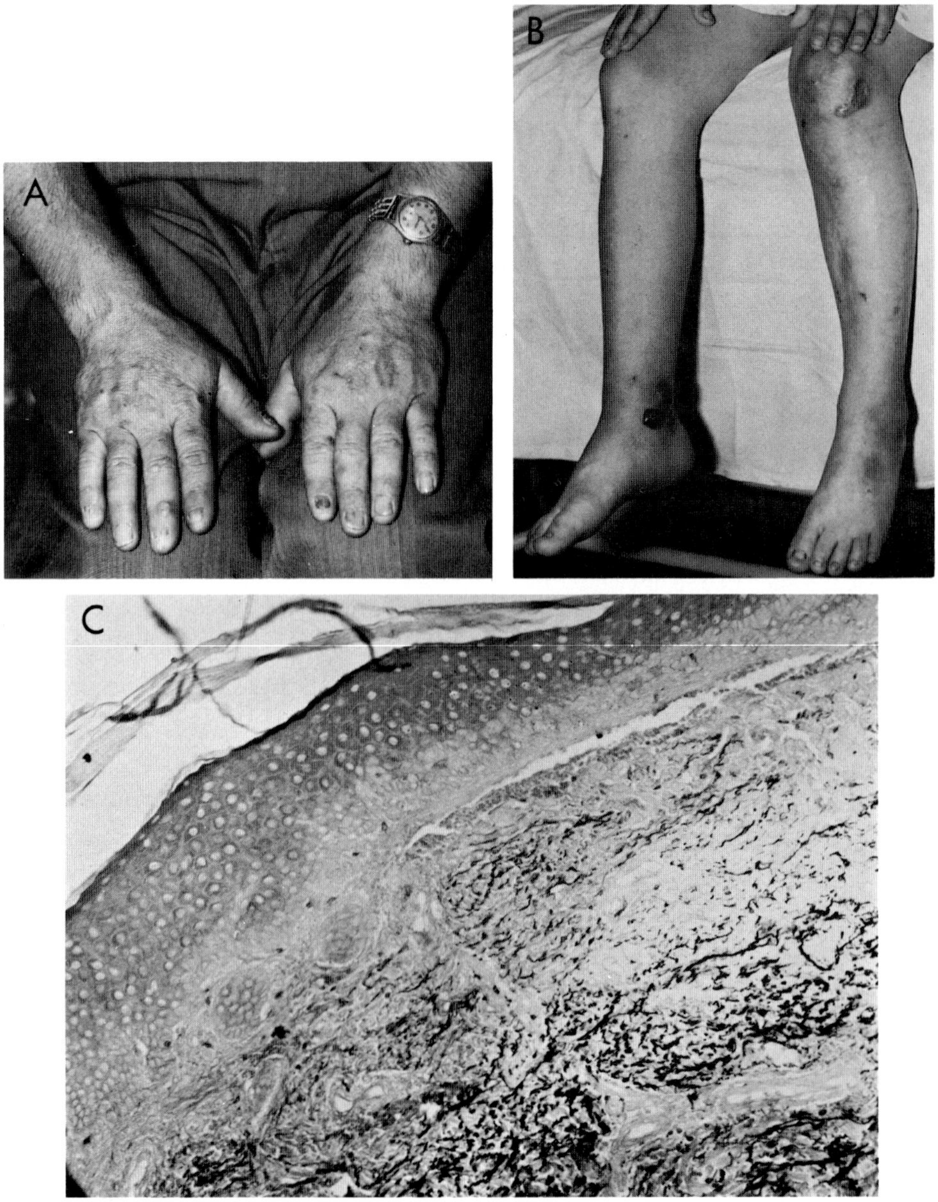

Fig. 114-1. – **A,** epidermolysis bullosa in a man whose daughter, **B,** had the same disorder. The girl's brother was affected also, whereas 2 sisters were normal. **C,** skin of patient shown in **B**. The stratum malpighii is thickened and separating from the underlying dermis. There are no rete pegs or papillae. Only a few elastic (dark) fibers are seen in the upper layers of the corium.

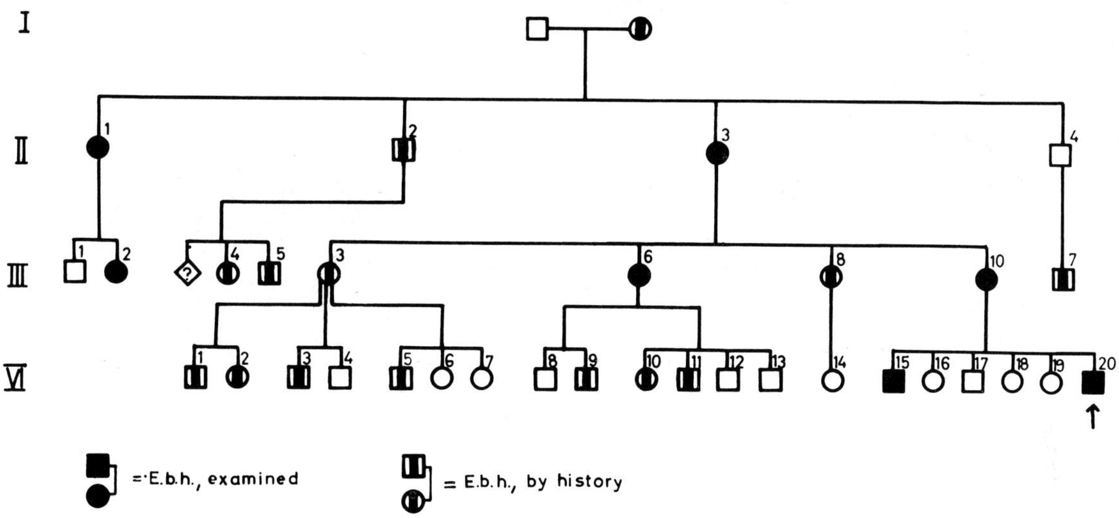

Fig. 114-2.—Pedigree of a kindred with dominantly inherited epidermolysis bullosa hereditaria simplex.[4] (Courtesy of Dr. E. Passarge, Cincinnati, Ohio.)

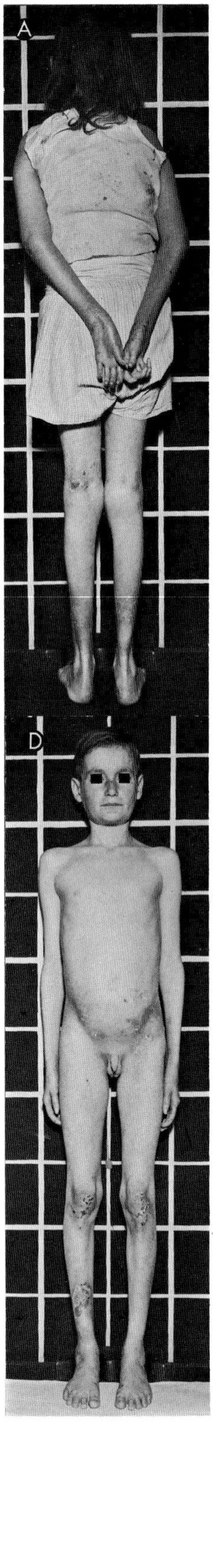

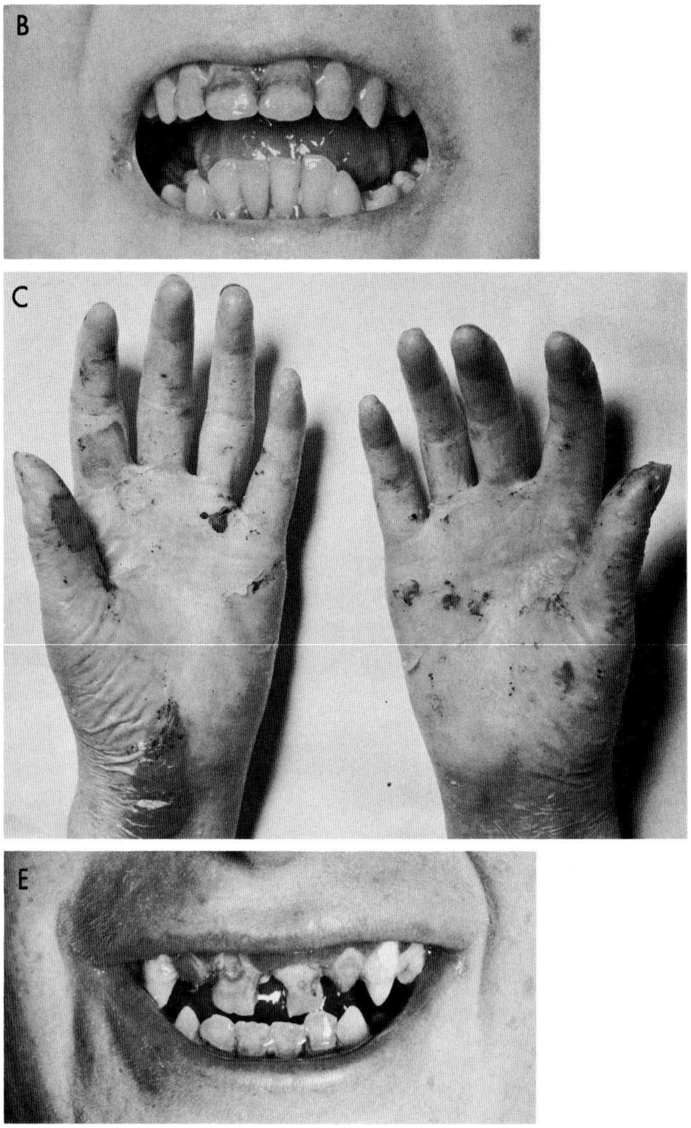

Fig. 114-3.—**A,** epidermolysis bullosa in a girl, 17 years of age. Teeth (**B**) and hands (**C**) of the same girl. **D,** 15-year-old boy with epidermolysis bullosa; brother of the girl shown in **A**. **E,** teeth of the boy. A younger brother of these children also was affected. Three sisters were free of the disease. The father apparently was not affected and 6 of his brothers and 3 sisters were well. But there was a history of "skin disease" in 3 of the father's sisters, who had died young.

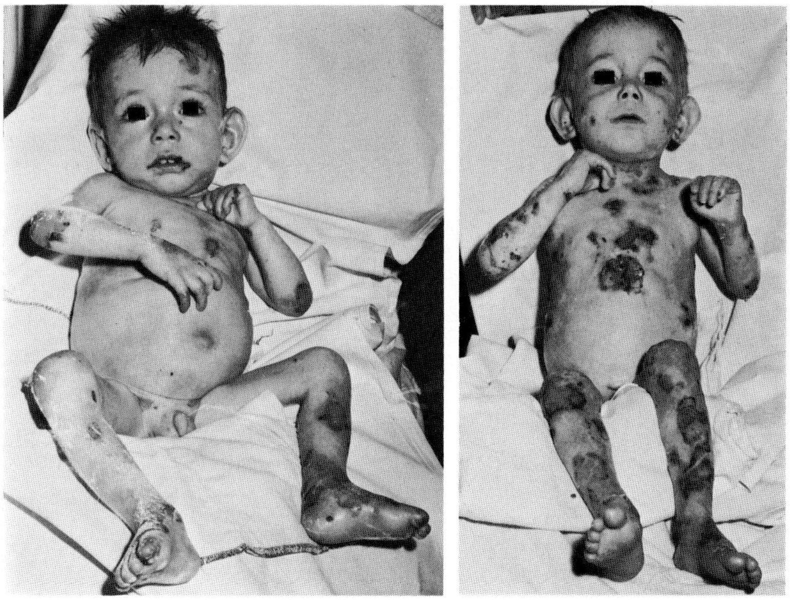

Fig. 114-4. – Severe epidermolysis bullosa in siblings.

The most serious form has been termed *epidermolysis bullosa lethalis*[7]; it was known previously as "hereditary pemphigus."[8] This condition begins in utero or soon after birth and ends fatally within the first year.[9] The fingernails and toenails are markedly deformed. Bullae of the skin and mucous membranes, serous or hemorrhagic, become ulcerated and infected. The denuded skin areas vary in position and extent. Prenatal necrosis is attributed to intrauterine pressure of fetal parts on one another.[10] The fingernails become loose and detached or they can be entirely absent.[9] Vesicles and ulcers can occur on the palate, esophagus and larynx.[9,11,12] Association with renal and cardiovascular anomalies has been reported.[12] It is likely that the most severe prenatal forms end in abortion. Boys and girls can be affected. Recurrence in families has been reported repeatedly[7,9,11,13] and concordance in twins has been observed.[9,10,13] Parental consanguinity was established in several cases[9,11,12] and autosomal recessive inheritance is likely for most of these.[9,11-14] In other instances, incomplete dominant transmission must be considered.[8,10]

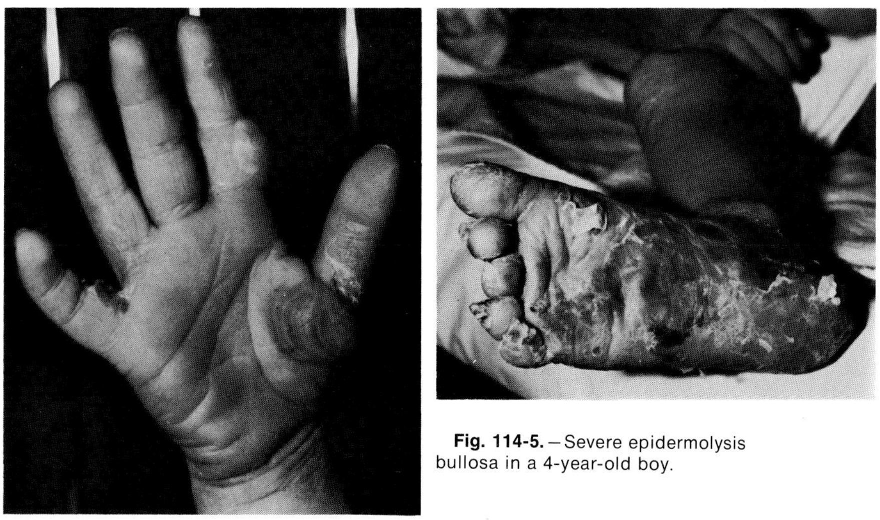

Fig. 114-5. – Severe epidermolysis bullosa in a 4-year-old boy.

The lethal form can alternate in some families with types compatible with life.[5,10] Treatment with ACTH, cortisone and gamma globulin failed to save these children.[12]

REFERENCES

1. Cockayne, E. A.: *Inherited Abnormalities of the Skin and Its Appendages* (New York: Oxford University Press, 1933).
2. Turner, W. J., and Obermayer, M. E.: Studies on porphyria; case of porphyria accompanied with epidermolysis bullosa, hypertrichosis and melanosis, Arch. Dermat. & Syph. 37:549, 1938.
3. Noojin, R. O., Reynolds, J. P., and Croom, W. C.: Genetic study of hereditary type of epidermolysis bullosa simplex, Arch. Dermat. & Syph. 65:477, 1952.
4. Passarge, E.: Epidermolysis bullosa hereditaria simplex, J. Pediat. 67:819, 1965.
5. McDaniel, W. H.: Epidermolysis bullosa, Arch. Dis. Childhood 29:334, 1954.
6. Alpert, M.: Roentgen manifestations of epidermolysis bullosa, Am. J. Roentgenol. 78:66, 1957.
7. Herlitz, G.: Kongenitaler, nicht syphilitscher Pemphigus. Eine Übersicht nebst Beschreibung einer neuen Krankheitsform (Epidermolysis bullosa hereditaria letalis), Acta paediat. 17:315, 1935.
8. Mautner, H.: Über ein familiär auftretendes letales Krankheitsbild mit Blasenbildung (Pemphigus hereditarius), Monatsschr. Kinderh. 22:15, 1922.
9. Jenny, E.: Über eine letal verlaufende Form von Epidermolysis bullosa hereditaria beim Säugling, Ztschr. Kinderh. 43:138, 1927.
10. Walther, T.: Epidermolysis bullosa hereditaria letalis. A review and report of two own cases, Ann. paediat. 180: 382, 1953.
11. Nager: Familiäres Auftreten von Epidermolysis bullosa dystrophica hereditaria, Schweiz. med. Wchnschr. 55: 306, 1925.
12. Gross, H.: Epidermolysis bullosa hereditaria maligna, Neue Österr. Ztschr. Kinderh. 7:225, 1962.
13. Leland, L. S., and Hirschl, D.: Epidermolysis bullosa hereditaria letalis in newborn twins, A.M.A. Am. J. Dis. Child. 87:321, 1954.
14. Cross, H. E., Wells, R. S., and Esterly, J. R.: Inheritance in epidermolysis bullosa letalis, J. M. Genetics 5:189, 1968.

115

Ichthyosis and Keratosis

Ichthyosis Simplex (Vulgaris)

THIS HEREDITARY FORM of ichthyosis usually is not present at birth but develops during infancy and childhood. An association between this condition and infantile eczema and asthma seems to exist.[1] The skin is dry and scaly, particularly at the extensor surfaces of the extremities. Often, the face is spared but the scalp is involved. The hair of the scalp is sparse and the eyebrows are underdeveloped. The palms, soles and nails are dry and the knees and elbows are severely involved. The skin condition improves during the summer months and becomes more severe in winter. Most patients with ichthyosis simplex are in good general health and mentally normal. Some reports mention association with feeble-mindedness, skeletal abnormalities and endocrine disturbances but they seem to be the exception rather than the rule.[2] It is possible that the ichthyosis in such cases is not the simplex form. In patients with Down syndrome, ichthyosis is not present at birth but xerosis (drying of the skin) with scale formation often develops with advancing age.

Histologically, ichthyosis simplex is characterized by hyperkeratosis and thickening of the stratum corneum combined with underdevelopment of the stratum granulosum. The dermis is normal.[3]

Ichthyosis simplex is inherited as a dominant trait, but skipping of one or more generations is common. In some families, the male and in others the female members are affected. This and other genetic variations were discussed by Cockayne.[1] In a male patient 10 months of age who came to the Cincinnati Children's Hospital because of exfoliative dermatitis following vaccination, ichthyosis had been present since birth; the mother, maternal grandmother and great-

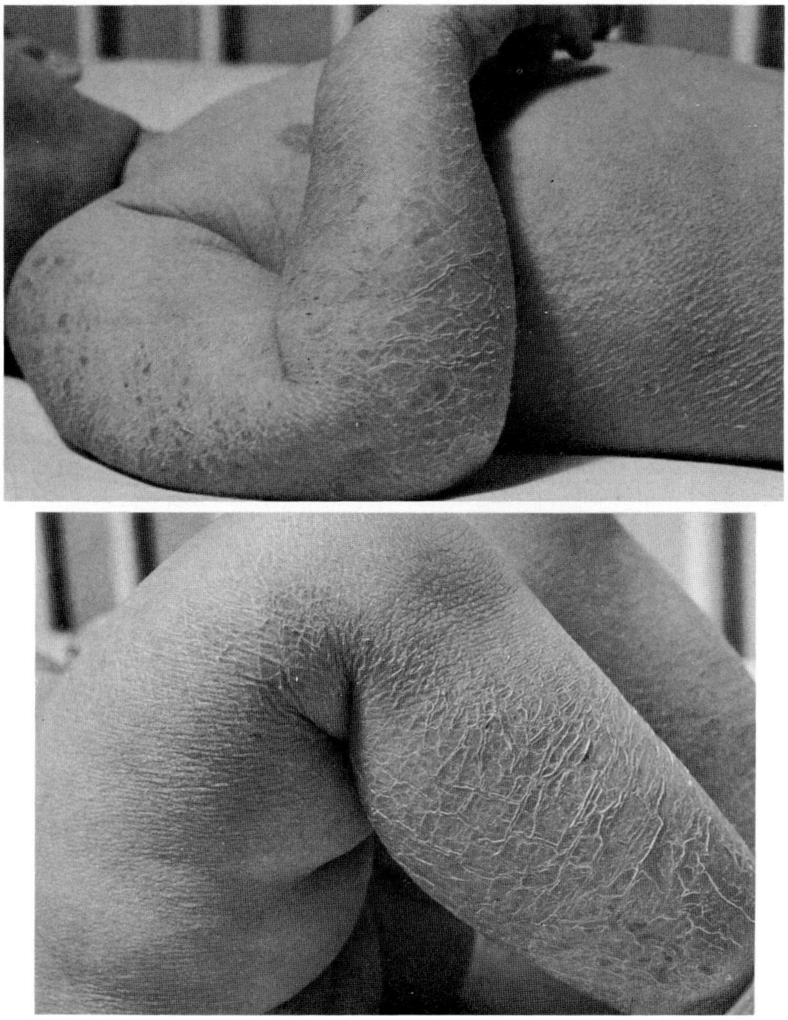

Fig. 115-1.—Ichthyosis simplex in a 1-year-old boy.

grandmother also had ichthyosis (Children's Hospital Chart No. 80270). But in other kinships a dominant gene responsible for faulty keratinization can lead to a variety of clinical entities, such as ichthyosis hystrix, ichthyosis simplex and localized keratoses.[4] There exists a sex-linked recessive form that is clinically rather similar to the autosomal dominant ichthyosis simplex but some differences have been established. It seems that a negative family history of atopy, benefit of warmth as an alleviating factor, absence of scales on the front and sides of the face, presence of scales on the neck, shedding of large scales and failure of improvement with age suggest the sex-linked type.[5] Sex-linked recessive inheritance seems likely for a syndrome of secondary male hypogonadism and congenital ichthyosis reported by Lynch *et al.*[6]

Ichthyosis vulgaris has been observed repeatedly in twins. Concordance in monozygotic twins was reported by Theiss[7] but aside from ichthyosis the twin brothers differed greatly. Whereas one of them was generally sound, the other had cleft lip and palate, cryptorchidism, agenesis of the corpus callosum, epilepsy and severe mental retardation.

Ichthyosis Congenita (Congenital Ichthyosiform Erythroderma)

Under this name a host of congenital entities of ichthyosis may be summarized and it seems that there exist about 20 names for these disorders. The confusion is such that it has been suggested that (in contrast to erythroderma ichthyosiformis fetalis) only those forms be called "congenital" that develop after birth![8] The spectrum of diseases termed ichthyosis congenita includes severe fetal forms on one side and

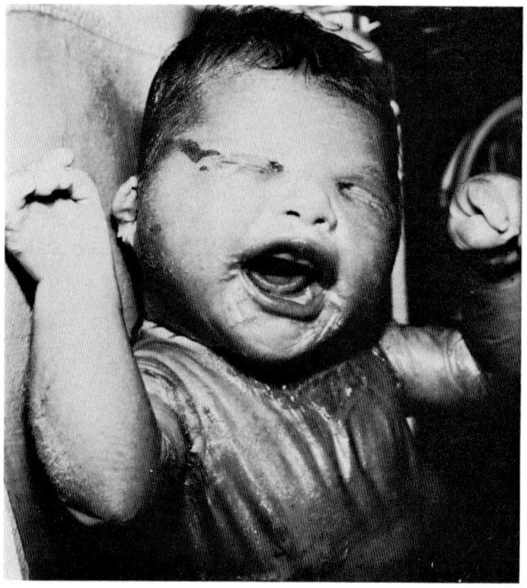

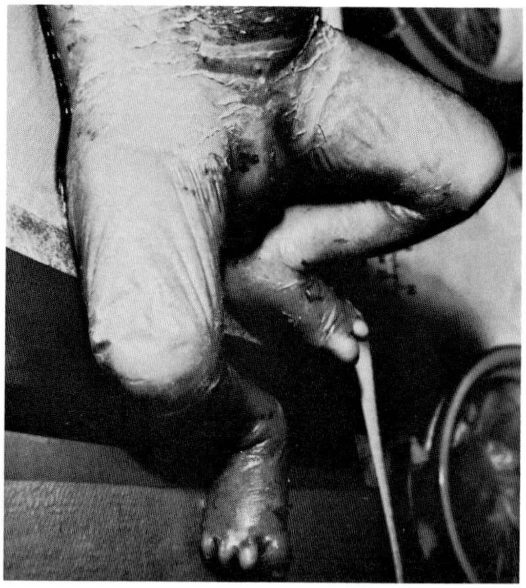

Fig. 115-2. – Congenital ichthyosis in a newborn girl.

mild forms of collodion skin on the other, with many types in between.[9] In some children, the skin is smooth and shiny and red in color, with cracks developing around thickened plates; in others, the skin is loose and involved only in parts of the body. The disease may persist for years, sometimes improving spontaneously. Generally, there is desquamation and reduction of symptoms in summer and return of ichthyosis in winter. Hair and nails may be involved in the process, with complete absence in severe cases. Involvement of the cornea (p. 368) is a serious complication, as opacities and ulcers may interfere with vision. Congenital cataracts may be present.[10] The ears sometimes are deformed or covered by the thickened skin. Sweating is reduced where the epidermis forms thick layers but it occurs between the plates and on the palms and soles, where even hyperhidrosis is present in some cases. Bullae form in some patients and such cases can blend into epidermolysis bullosa[1] (p. 1151). Dominant congenital ichthyosiform erythroderma begins with redness at birth followed by development of hyperkeratosis and bullae. The disorder can be transmitted from a parent to some of the children. A familial exfoliative erythroderma consists of shedding of thin skin flakes followed by reddening of the freed surface and formation of new flakes. Desquamation is present at birth or begins soon thereafter. Small stature and mental dullness of the patients has been reported. The stratum corneum is thin or absent. Autosomal recessive inheritance seems to be established for this form.[1]

There is great variation of general health in patients with ichthyosis congenita.[44] Some cases are not compatible with life, whereas others occur in persons of good general health. A fatal case observed in the Cincinnati Children's Hospital (Chart No. 123736)

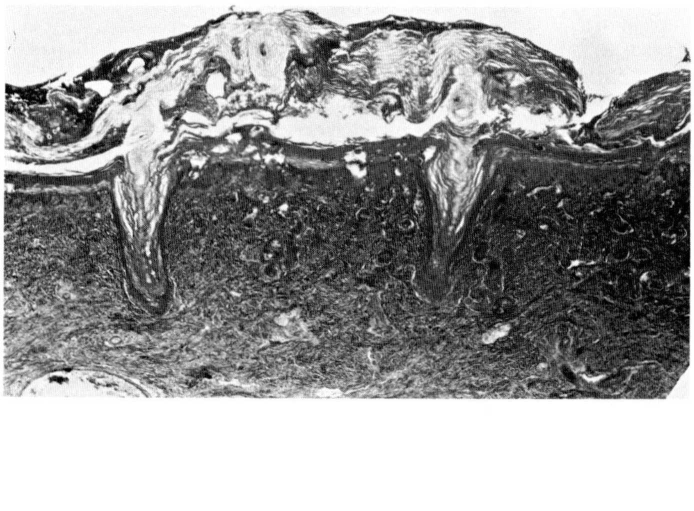

Fig. 115-3. – Ichthyosis congenita. Section shows marked thickening of stratum corneum and stratum lucidum. Hair follicles are dilated and filled with horny material. (Cincinnati Children's Hospital Chart No. 123736.)

was of special interest because of associated congenital malformations. Hydrocephaly with cyst of the fourth ventricle, cleft palate and rudimentary, erupted teeth were present at birth. At first, the skin was erythematous and covered in part by white patches but soon it seemed to thicken, the scales becoming heavier, despite treatment with various ointments. The skin was hyperkeratotic, with a thin stratum germinativum. The sweat glands appared to be normal but their ducts were filled with layers of stratified epithelium. Sebaceous glands were few in number and atrophic (Fig. 115-3).

A syndrome of congenital ichthyosis, mental deficiency and spastic diplegia was described by Sjögren and Larsson[11] (p. 259) as an autosomal recessive trait occurring in an inbred Swedish population. Outside of this endemic area, the condition seems to be rare but isolated cases have been described in the United States[12] and in England.[13] The pathologic findings in skin and brain have been reported.[43] A syndrome of congenital ichthyosis, epilepsy, dwarfism and sexual infantilism was reported by Rud[14] in 1927. Cases fitting this disease picture also may have a variety of other malformations and metabolic deviations, which were reviewed by Ewing.[2] Erythroderma ichthyosiforme congenitum of Brocq, which is one of the many names for the many forms of congenital ichthyosis, can be treated symptomatically and heal within weeks or months.[15] But the same name has been applied to conditions that are resistant to all forms of treatment and show progressive thickening of the skin from birth, reaching a maximum at about the age of 15 years. In a case of this type in which the skin was covered by a black horny layer, treatment with hypnosis resulted in marked improvement.[16] Congenital ichthyosis occurs in children with chondrodystrophia calcificans congenita (p. 797) (Fig. 115-4). Netherton syndrome[17] is a form of congenital ichthyosiform erythroderma combined with an abnormality of the hair shafts (bamboo hair).[18]

Fig. 115-4. – Ichthyosis congenita in a girl with chondrodystrophia calcificans and cataracts.

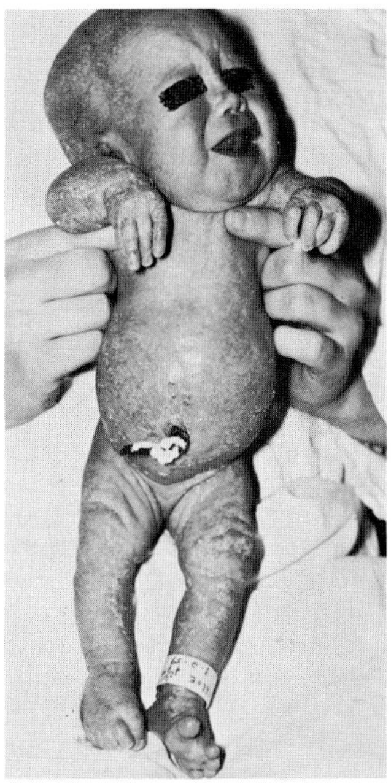

Erythroderma desquamativum, or Leiner disease, which in name resembles the disorder under discussion, is postnatal in origin and considered an allergic disorder. Dermatitis exfoliativa neonatorum, or Ritter disease, is a postnatal infection of the skin that occurred in epidemics in institutions such as foundling houses of the past. The mortality was high. Recent cases responded to antibacterial therapy. Thus, Leiner and Ritter disease are not congenital disorders.

Ichthyosis Fetalis (Harlequin Fetus)

The most severe cases of this disorder are not compatible with life. Affected children usually are born prematurely and alive, but they die within a few hours or days after birth. The skin is formed by thick and hard horny plates of various shapes and between the plates are deep fissures whose corium is exposed and bleeding. On the plates, the epidermis is greatly thickened by hypertrophy of the stratum corneum and stratum lucidum.[45] The hair follicles are dilated and filled with horny material and the hairs are thin. The sebaceous glands may be obliterated but the sweat glands are normal or hypertrophic. The abnormal development of the skin goes back to early fetal life, when unusual thickening and lack of expansion of the skin sets in, resulting in breaks and fissures of the epidermis. The thickest plates are on the back, chest and scalp. The hands and feet are covered either by thinner sheets of epidermis or by smooth, shiny glove-like skin.[19] The eyes and ears have been described as absent by some authors but this is not correct. The red fleshy masses seen between the lids represent swollen conjunctivae exposed by eversion of the eyelids. The external ears may be severely deformed by covering skin plates and the external auditory canals are greatly narrowed or completely covered by deformed skin. The nose is flat and held in the plane of the thick surrounding skin. The nostrils are narrow or plugged by cutaneous debris. The mouth is held open, with the tongue protruding between everted lips. The extremities are held in flexed, "fetal" position. The thyroid gland has been found reduced in size or atrophic and replaced by fibrous tissue. The genitalia and the fingers may be deformed or destroyed by the cutaneous disorder.[19]

According to Cockayne,[1] the difference between ichthyosis fetalis and the milder forms of ichthyosis congenita is one of degree and not of kind. There are transitional forms that cannot be unequivocally classified[46] and in the same sibship a mild and a lethal form can alternate. In a family examined by us, the patient seen in our hospital survived, but a female sibling born several years before her lived only 3 days.

The parents of infants with ichthyosis fetalis usually are free of hyperkeratosis in any form. Repetition of the disorder in sibships has been observed repeatedly and consanguinity of the parents is high, as stressed by Riecke as early as 1900.[20] Males and females are affected. Autosomal recessive inheritance can be assumed.[1,19]

Ichthyosis Lamellaris; Collodion Skin

This rare form of congenital ichthyosis represents a delayed shedding of the fetal epitrichium, which normally disappears at the sixth month of gestation. The embryonic epidermis consists of two layers—a superficial epitrichium composed of large polygonal cells with large nuclei and a deeper layer with cells showing smaller nuclei. In lamellar ichthyosis, the epitrichium is retained until after birth, when it appears as a shining collodion like layer enveloping the infant. Cracks form in this layer soon after birth and desquamation sets in, lasting for weeks or months. Complete recovery is possible.

Although the prognosis generally is favorable, the appearance of the children is at first alarming. The eyelids, the mouth and even the extremities appear fixed and immobile. The face is "dull, pasty and devoid of expression."[21] As desquamation proceeds, the skin acquires a bright copper color until healing sets in. Not all cases clear up completely, as some develop permanent ichthyosis following the shedding of the epitrichium.[22,23] Ichthyosis lamellaris is a rare condition. Most reported cases were sporadic but repetition has occurred in families with normal parents.[1] In one instance,[21] 2 sisters were affected and 1 of them transmitted the disorder to 1 of her daughters.

Ichthyosis Hystrix

Ichthyosis hystrix is a rare but striking malformation of the skin that is of some historical interest. The lesions are wart-like growths with horny tops, brown or black in color, usually limited in distribution. They may be linear and unilateral, chiefly affecting the trunk and sometimes the extremities. The face, the palms and soles usually are not affected. In rare instances, the condition is generalized and results in a picture often compared to the skin covers of animals. Such patients' skin has been described as resembling the pelt of a seal, the hide of an elephant or the quills of a hedgehog.[24] In England, such patients have been on exhibition as "porcupine men."

According to Lever,[3] the condition is histologically not a true ichthyosis but a nevus verrucosus. There is hyperkeratosis, papillomatosis and acanthosis, with elongation of the rete pegs. The lesions are considered epidermal tumors. But Curth and Macklin[4] considered the disorder as related genetically to ichthyosis,

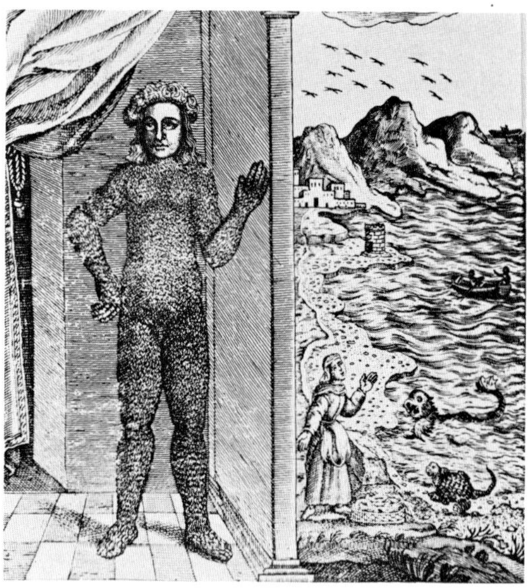

Fig. 115-5.—Ichthyosis hystrix as shown in an Italian broadsheet of 1670. The anomaly was attributed to impressions received by the mother on walks on the beach, where she looked at scaly animals. (From E. Holländer, *Wunder, Wundergeburt und Wundergestalt*, 1922 [Used with permission of Ferdinand Enke, Stuttgart].)

since both conditions occurred in a kinship as manifestations of an inherited tendency to faulty keratinization. There were many skin anomalies with confusing terminology listed in this pedigree. Congenital heart disease, polydactyly and other congenital malformations were recorded also.

In other families, ichthyosis hystrix occurred sporadically as new mutations; in the English kinship mentioned, it was transmitted as a dominant trait through four generations. The history of this family has been cited in many textbooks of genetics as an example of Y chromosome inheritance. It seemed that the unusual skin condition was passed on through several generations from affected males to all their sons and to none of their daughters. But Penrose[24] examined the family records and came to the conclusion that the gene in question arose by mutation in one of the parents of the original "porcupine man," Edward Lambert, in 1716 or 1717 and was transmitted not by a Y chromosome but probably by a dominant autosomal gene. Other cases of ichthyosis hystrix occurred as mutations and were recorded because of their striking appearance before modern dermatology existed. There are several broadsheets in existence dated 1670 and 1688 that tell of the birth of a male, born near Naples, with ichthyosis hystrix. This mutation was attributed to the mother's habit of walking on the beach and looking at scaly animals of the sea.[25] Ichthyosis hystrix can occur in otherwise healthy persons. The members of the English family who were examined by many scientific authorities used their cutaneous malformations to their advantage. They appeared in exhibitions and charged fees for being examined. They married and passed on their anomaly to subsequent generations.

Keratosis Palmarum et Plantarum (Tylosis Palmaris et Plantaris)

This cutaneous anomaly is of interest because, although inherited and to a certain extent congenital, manifestations of hyperkeratosis do not occur until months or years after birth. The anomaly is not brought out in intrauterine life. In some cases, redness of the palms and soles appears soon after birth or a discolored line between ventral and dorsal skin announces early the onset of the disease. In other cases, hyperkeratosis may be delayed for several years. In typical patients, thickening of the skin of the palms and soles develops in the second half of the first year of life and the affected skin is well demarcated from the normal dorsa of the hands and feet. In mild cases, the disorder causes little inconvenience[1] but in others it is a most painful, deforming and crippling disease.[26] The keratosis may involve the fingers and toes as well as the subungual areas. The nails are thickened, discolored and cracked. If the palms are severely involved, the fingers are held in flexion. The skin at the heels may show keratosis several centimeters thick and hyperhidrosis and a rancid odor can be present. The skin condition often improves in warm weather and the horny epidermis is shed in the fall. All layers of the skin are hypertrophic, particularly the epidermis and the stratum corneum. The papillae are increased in depth and the sweat glands and their ducts enlarged. A serious variant of the disease may lead to autoamputation of digits, hands and feet.[27]

Males and females are affected and patients of many races have been observed.[1] Dominant inheritance is the rule and many families have been described showing transmission through several generations.[28] Macauley[29] reported a pedigree involving seven generations with early onset and persistence of the disease throughout life. In another kinship with very early onset of symptoms, the disorder was traced through six generations.[30] Skipping of a generation has been noticed repeatedly and was explained by environmental modifiers. Serum vitamin A has been reduced in a number of cases, whereas carotene was within normal limits.[31] Sporadic cases have been seen often.

There may be families in which the disorder is due to recessive inheritance. This seems to be true particularly for the mal de Meleda, named after a Dalmatian island where intermarriage was frequent and hyperkeratosis endemic. Mal de Meleda was mistaken for leprosy but it actually represents a hyperkeratosis similar to the dominant form described above, yet differing from it in that the backs of the hands and feet, the elbows, knees and forearms may also be involved.[1,32] A syndrome of palmar-plantar hyperkeratosis, premature periodontal destruction of the teeth and calcification of the dura has been reported as a hereditary recessive trait.[33]

Associated anomalies are variable. The keratosis may be present around the mouth and anus[34] or extend into the mouth as leukoplakia of the buccal membranes or as thickening of the gums and tongue.[26] Two families have been described in which the skin disorder was associated with carcinoma of the esophagus.[35] Skeletal malformations such as oxycephaly, clubbed fingers[1] and clinodactyly[31] have been seen in association with the skin disease. Hereditary optic atrophy was reported in a family with keratoderma palmaris and plantaris[36] and a case has been described that was complicated by congenital deafness and total leukonychia.[37] Occasionally, patients with keratosis have been physically or mentally underdeveloped,[1,34] but this is true for a minority of cases only. It has been said that such associated anomalies are more frequent in the recessively inherited than in the common dominant form.[37] Keratosis palmoplantaris hyperhydrotica associated with congenital pachyonychia, follicular keratosis, oral leukokeratosis and granulosis rubra nasi has been described as an entity (*pachyonychia congenita*) by Jadassohn and Lewandowsky.[38] Thickening of the fingernails and toenails can be noticed at birth as a horny brown substance on the undersurface of the nails that turns their edges upward. The changes in the nails seen soon after birth were described and illustrated by Joseph.[39] Various types have been distinguished according to complicating symptoms.[40] In some cases, palmoplantar keratosis develops together with bullae and hyperhidrosis during warm weather. The skin around the larger joints shows follicular elevations with plugging. The hair and skin, with the exception of palms and soles, are dry and the mucosae of the tongue, cheeks and larynx are thickened. An interesting observation is that teeth were erupted at birth in several cases.[41,42] Involvement of the corneae has been reported.[40] Pachyonychia congenita is genetically determined; dominant inheritance has been recorded in several kinships.[39-41]

REFERENCES

1. Cockayne, E. A.: *Inherited Abnormalities of the Skin and Its Appendages* (London: Oxford University Press, 1933).
2. Ewing, J. A.: The association of oligophrenia and dyskeratoses, Am. J. Ment. Deficiency 60:98, 1955; 307, 1955; 575, 1956; and 799, 1956.
3. Lever, W. F.: *Histopathology of the Skin* (4th ed.; Philadelphia: J. B. Lippincott Company, 1967).
4. Curth, H. O., and Macklin, M. T.: The genetic basis of various types of ichthyosis in a family group, Am. J. Human Genet. 6:371, 1954.
5. Merrett, J. D., Wells, R. S., Kerr, C. B., and Barr, A.: Discriminant function analysis of phenotype variates in ichthyosis, Am. J. Human Genet. 19:575, 1967.
6. Lynch, H. T., Ozer, F., McNutt, W., Johnson, J. E., and Jampolsky, N. A.: Secondary male hypogonadism and

congenital ichthyosis: Association of two rare genetic diseases, Am. J. Human Genet. 12:440, 1960.
7. Theiss, B.: Eineiige Zwillinge mit Ichthyosis vulgaris diskordant kombiniert mit multiplen Fehlbildungen, Helvet. paediat. acta 23:429, 1968.
8. Hanak, J., and Raska, B.: Zur Frage der "Ichthyosis" bei Neugeborenen, Ann. paediat. 193:139, 1959.
9. Greither, A.: Zur Klassifikation der Ichthyosis-Gruppe, Dermatologica 128:464, 1964.
10. Rubenstein, R. A., and Eggleston, T. F.: Congenital cataracts associated with congenital ichthyosiform erythroderma, J. Pediat. Ophth. 2:53, 1965.
11. Sjögren, T., and Larsson, T.: Oligophrenia in combination with congenital ichthyosis and spastic disorders, Acta psychiat. et neurol. scandinav. 32:1, 1957.
12. Blumel, J., Watkins, M., and Eggers, G. W. N.: Spastic quadriplegia combined with congenital ichthyosiform erythroderma and oligophrenia, A.M.A. J. Dis. Child. 96: 724, 1958.
13. Richards, B. W.: Congenital ichthyosis, spastic diplegia, and mental deficiency, Brit. M. J. 2:714, 1960.
14. Rud, E.: Case of infantilism with tetany, epilepsy, polyneuritis, ichthyosis, Hosp. København 70:525, 1927.
15. Gross, H.: Erythrodermia ichthyosiformis congenitalis Brocq, Neue Österr. Ztschr. Kinderh. 6:259, 1961.
16. Mason, A. A.: A case of congenital ichthyosiform erythrodermia of Brocq treated by hypnosis, Brit. M. J. 2:422, 1952.
17. Netherton, E. W.: A unique case of trichorrhexia nodosa—bamboo hairs, A.M.A. Arch. Dermat. 78:483, 1958.
18. Porter, P. S., and Starke, J. C.: Netherton's syndrome, Arch. Dis. Childhood 43:319, 1968.
19. Hess, J. H., and Schultz, O. T.: Keratosis diffusa fetalis (ichthyosis congenita), Am. J. Dis. Child. 21:357, 1921.
20. Riecke, E.: Über ichthyosis congenita, Arch. Dermat u. Syph. 54:289, 1900.
21. Dean, C. H.: A case of congenital ichthyosis, J.A.M.A. 77: 465, 1921.
22. Fisher, O. D., and McKee, K. G.: Collodion skin of the newborn, Arch. Dis. Childhood 29:516, 1954.
23. Smith, N. G., and Beach, N.: Lamellar exfoliation of the newborn, or ichthyosis congenita, A.M.A. J. Dis. Child. 98: 249, 1959.
24. Penrose, L. S.: The porcupine man, The Listener, p. 748, May 9, 1957.
25. Holländer, E.: *Wunder, Wundergeburt und Wundergestalt*, in *Einblattdrucken des fünfzehnten bis achtzehnten Jahrhunderts* (Stuttgart: Ferdinand Enke, 1922).
26. Fred, H. L., Gieser, R. G., Berry, W. R., and Eiband, J. M.: Keratosis palmaris et plantaris, Arch. Int. Med. 113:866, 1964.
27. Presley, N. L., and Bonte, F. J.: The roentgen appearance of mutilating palmo-plantar keratosis, Am. J. Roentgenol. 86:944, 1961.
28. Rolleston, J. D.: Hereditary tylosis, Brit. J. Child. Dis. 20: 16, 1923.
29. Macauley, D.: Keratoderma palmaris et plantaris congenitalis, Brit. M. J. 1:334, 1951.
30. Turpin, R., Barochez, Y., and Lejeune, J.: Étude d'une forme familiale de kératodermie palmo-plantaire diffuse (Type Thost-Unna). Recherche d'une liaison factorielle éventuelle, Semaine hôp. Paris 35:1796, 1959.
31. Anderson, I. F., and Klintworth, G. K.: Hypovitaminosis-A in a family with tylosis and clinodactyly, Brit. M. J. 1:1293, 1961.
32. Niles, H. D., and Klumpp, M. M.: Mal de Meleda: Review of the literature and report of four cases, Arch. Dermat. & Syph. 39:409, 1939.
33. Gorlin, R. J., Sedano, H., and Anderson, V. E.: The syndrome of palmar-plantar hyperkeratosis and premature periodontal destruction of the teeth, J. Pediat. 65:895, 1964.
34. Olmsted, H. C.: Keratodermia palmaris et plantaris congenitalis, Am. J. Dis. Child. 33:757, 1927.
35. Howel-Evans, W., McConnell, R. B., Clarke, C. A., and Sheppard, P. M.: Carcinoma of the oesophagus with keratosis palmaris et plantaris (tylosis); a study of two families, Quart. J. Med. 27:413, 1958.
36. Dimsdale, H.: Hereditary optic atrophy in family with keratodermia palmaris et plantaris, Proc. Roy. Soc. Med. 42:796, 1949.
37. Schwann, J.: Keratosis palmaris et plantaris with congenital deafness and total leukonychia, Dermatologica 126:335, 1963.
38. Jadassohn, J., and Lewandowsky, F.: Pachonychia congenita. Ikonograph, Dermatologica 1:29, 1906.
39. Joseph, H. L.: Pachonychia congenita, Arch. Dermat. 90: 594, 1964.
40. Kumer, L., and Loos, H. O.: Über Pachyonychia congenita (Typus Riehl), Wien. klin. Wchnschr. 48:174, 1935.
41. Murray, F. A.: Four cases of hereditary hypertrophy of the nail bed associated with a history of erupted teeth at birth, Brit. J. Dermat. 33:409, 1921.
42. Gorlin, R. J., and Pindborg, J. J.: *Syndromes of the Head and Neck* (New York: McGraw-Hill Book Company, Inc., 1964.
43. Sylvester, P. E.: Pathological findings in Sjögren-Larsson syndrome, J. Ment. Defic. Res. 13:267, 1969.
44. Castanier, J., Hee, P., Lelièvre-Gassin, C., and Gilgenkrantz, S.: Un cas d'erythrodermie ichtyosiforme congénitale associée à diverses malformations, Ann. pédiat. 18:326, 1971.
45. Craig, J. M., Goldsmith, L. A., and Baden, H. P.: An abnormality of keratin in the harlequin fetus, Pediatrics 46:437, 1970.
46. Esterly, N. B., and Solomon, L. M.: Neonatal dermatology. II. Blistering and scaling dermatoses, J. Pediat. 77:1075, 1970.

116

Ectodermal Dysplasias

Mild or Hidrotic Forms

There are many disease pictures that include combinations of defective ectodermal derivatives and which are congenital and hereditary. The combinations vary greatly between families but show rather good intrafamilial resemblance. Yet, even in members of the same kinship or sibship, the expression of the hereditary trait may vary. It is customary to divide the ectodermal dysplasias into a hidrotic and an anhidrotic group, but this classification is not quite satisfactory, since even in the hidrotic type, reduced sweating often is observed.[1] Whereas the classic form of the anhidrotic type usually is transmitted as a sex-linked recessive trait, it can also behave like an irregular dominant. Furthermore, there are great variations in associated symptoms, such as hearing loss, visual disturbances, skeletal defects and cutaneous anomalies. Although it is said that the hidrotic type is more common than the anhidrotic, publications are more numerous on the anhidrotic forms, since they are more interesting medically. It is very difficult to bring order into the kaleidoscopic pictures of which ectodermal dysplasias are a part.

If a mutation occurs in a gene which leads to relatively mild disturbances and is transmitted like a dominant trait, so many persons can be affected that they may outnumber those with the more spectacular recessively inherited disease pictures. A branch of such a kinship was recorded by Jacobsen[2] in 1928, a more inclusive description was given by Clouston[1] of the same kinship in 1929 and the kindred was further studied by Williams and Fraser.[3] Clouston estimated that 6,000 persons with this trait existed in North America; he believed that the mutant gene had been present on this continent prior to 1759 and that it was most widespread among the French Canadians in Quebec Province. The mild ectodermal dysplasia of this kinship is represented chiefly by dystrophy of the nails and hair. Males and females were affected in almost equal numbers and half of the offspring of affected persons manifested the trait, so that it could be attributed to an autosomal dominant gene. Skipping of a generation did not occur: "If a child escapes the defect, he and his heirs are free forever. It never jumps a generation." Skipping, however, was reported by Thompson.[4] In the large kinship reported by Jacobsen[2] and Clouston,[1] dystrophy of the nails was a constant and leading symptom, but the skin, hair, sebaceous glands and "to some extent the sweat glands" were involved also. Thus, this example of the hidrotic type—there were no complaints about lack of

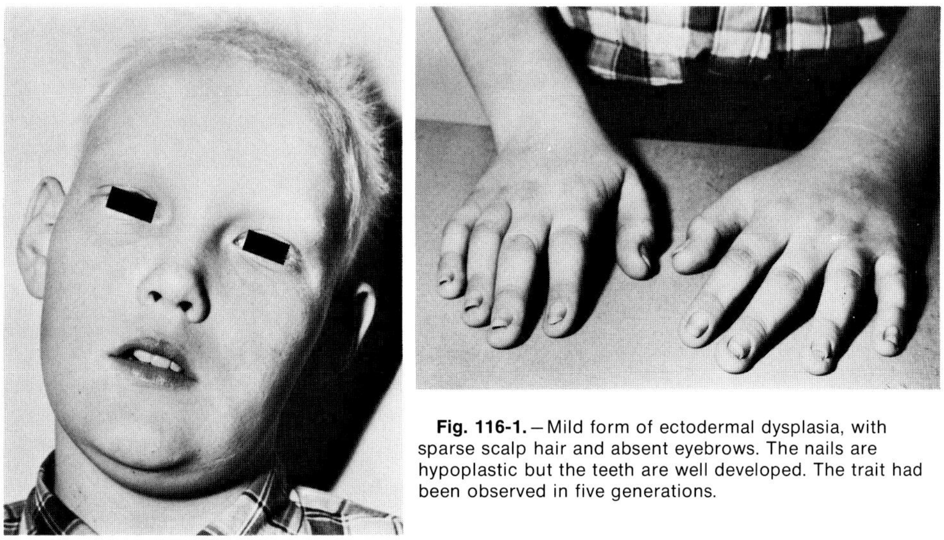

Fig. 116-1.—Mild form of ectodermal dysplasia, with sparse scalp hair and absent eyebrows. The nails are hypoplastic but the teeth are well developed. The trait had been observed in five generations.

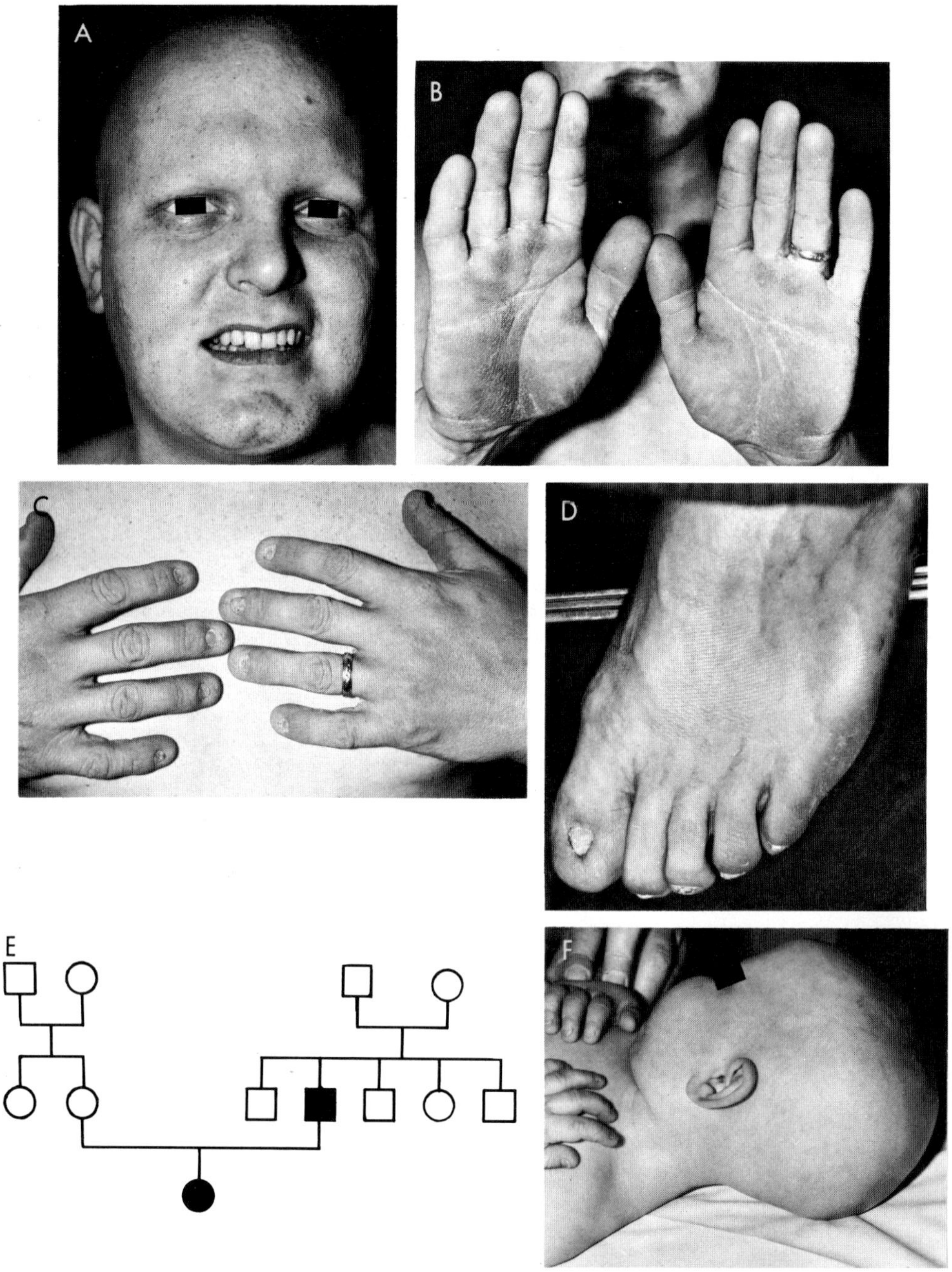

Fig. 116-2. – Ectodermal dysplasia. **A,** a man 27 years of age. He has sparse scalp hair, no eyebrows, no eyelashes but good teeth. **B–D,** the skin of the hands is hyperkeratotic and the nails are dystrophic. **E,** the pedigree shows that the father's condition probably represents a new mutation and that he transmitted the trait to his daughter. **F,** the daughter, 10 months of age, also has ectodermal dysplasia evidenced by sparse hair and absence of eyebrows and eyelashes.

sweat or disturbance of heat regulation – apparently was hypohidrotic to a certain extent. The teeth, the nervous system and the glands of internal secretion also were under suspicion but their involvement was not clearly proved and not noticeable in all patients.

In the mild ectodermal dysplasia, the nails grow slowly and reach the finger tips late or not at all. In some cases, they are merely thickened and discolored but if the disturbance is more severe, the nails split, break or are completely destroyed. Fetid suppuration can be one of the most disturbing manifestations because of the bad odor that emanates from them. The hair grows very slowly and "it does not wear well." It is sparse, thin, fine and "lifeless," particularly in the occipital area. The outer two-thirds of the eyebrows is absent and the eyelashes are underdeveloped or missing. There are many gradations in the nail and hair defects. In some patients, only the nails are defective; in others, there also are abnormal pigmentations or keratosis palmaris and plantaris develops.

The case illustrated in Figure 116-2 is of interest because the disorder affecting the man probably is due to a new mutation. Neither his ancestors nor his siblings had nail or hair anomalies, but his daughter, when seen at the age of 10 months, had no scalp hair and her eyebrows and eyelashes were little developed. The distal nail margins were far from the fingertips. The father's teeth were normal and in the daughter two lower incisors had erupted. The pedigree shown in Figure 116-2, *E* could represent the beginning of a pedigree of autosomal dominant inheritance of a mild ectodermal dysplasia.

Disease pictures reported as "ectodermal dysplasias" vary greatly. Thus, the family group published by Marshall[5] showed somewhat reduced function of sebaceous and sweat glands, underdeveloped teeth and hypoplastic nasal bones, thickening of the outer table of the skull and a characteristic saddle-shaped nasal deformity. They developed early cataract and loss of hearing. The syndrome was inherited like a dominant trait. In contrast to the ectodermal dysplasia reported by Clouston,[1] the patients described by Marshall[5] did not have nail and hair defects, so that the two dominant "ectodermal dysplasias" have little in common.

Another dominant ectodermal dysplasia observed by Robinson *et al.*[6] included nail and tooth defects but the hair was normal. As in the syndrome of Marshall,[5] hearing loss, considered as sensorineural, was one of the leading symptoms, but instead of the nasal deformity, syndactyly or polydactyly was present in some affected persons. Sweating appeared normal but electrolyte concentrations were elevated in sweat.

Another hidrotic ectodermal dysplasia inherited like a dominant trait with variable expression includes nail, hair and skin changes but no tooth anomalies.[7]

Anhidrotic Ectodermal Dysplasia (Hereditary Ectodermal Dysplasia; Congenital Ectodermal Defect)

This severe ectodermal defect is characterized by thin and soft skin, absence of sweat glands, defective growth of hair, defective mucous membranes of the nose, larynx and mouth and abnormal development of the teeth. There also are changes in the skull and fairly characteristic facial features. Heat intolerance is the most serious attribute of the disorder, since it can threaten the life of the patient in infancy.

At birth, scantiness of the hair of the scalp and of the eyebrows, skin lesions, a saddle nose and dry snuffles are noticed. These signs may suggest congenital syphilis. Inability to sweat may lead to fever during infancy and in later life the patients make special adjustments and avoid overheating, vigorous exercise and hot food and drink. Absence or hypoplasia of sebaceous glands is responsible for the dry and sometimes red skin. Papular eruptions on the skin are due to degeneration of sebaceous glands followed by hyperkeratosis. On the trunk and limbs, sebaceous glands are absent and in some patients the lacrimal glands are underdeveloped. Absence of the mammary glands, of the breasts and nipples occurs in rare cases.[8] Alopecia seldom is complete, but the hairs are sparse and thin. Their pigment is deficient and growth is slow. Eyebrows and eyelashes are absent or underdeveloped. Mustaches and beards grow rather well, but hair is lacking on trunk and limbs. As a rule, the nails are normal in the anhidrotic type, although sometimes they are hard and brittle. Atrophy of the nasal mucous membranes leads to atrophic rhinitis, ozena and loss of sense of smell. Atrophy of laryngeal mucous membranes results in a characteristic hoarseness.[29] The teeth are always reduced in number, widely spaced and pointed and they tend to early decay.[9] The incisors have been compared to shark teeth or to teeth of carnivores,[10] whereas the molars often have normal configuration. Deficient dentition can be demonstrated by roentgenograms in the newborn period.[11] The upper lip is short and the mouth resembles that of an old person because of dental deficiencies and underdevelopment of the alveolar processes of the jaws. In many cases, there are prominent supraorbital ridges and a saddle nose attributed to small and flattened nasal bones. The palpebral fissures often are narrow and the skin of the eyelids is thin and wrinkled. The mental development can be entirely normal, but the incidence of inferior intellect is relatively high in patients with anhidrotic ectodermal dysplasia. In 1942, Halperin and Curtis[12] analyzed 66 published cases and recorded 18 as below average in mental development. Although the name of the disorder emphasizes ectodermal deficiencies, involvement of entodermal derivatives, i.e., absence of mucous glands throughout the respiratory tract and esophagus, deserves attention, since recurrent respiratory infections may be due in part to the entodermal anomaly.[11] In infants, unexplained hyperpyrexia can be the leading sign.[13]

Anhidrotic ectodermal dysplasia can be inherited as a typical sex-linked recessive trait.[14] It occurs in males and is transmitted through female carriers. In 1896, Darwin[15] quoted W. Wedderburn's description of a Hindu family with this disorder. It may be cited here as an example of a correct description of inheritance before modern genetic concepts were known in medicine:

". . . ten men, in the course of four generations, were furnished, in both jaws taken together, with only four small and weak incisor teeth and with eight posterior molars. The men thus affected have very little hair on the body, and become bald early in life. They also suffer much during hot weather from excessive dryness of the skin. It is remarkable that no instance has occurred of a daughter thus being affected. . . though the daughters in the above family are never affected, they transmit the tendency to their sons. The affection thus appears only in alternate generations, or after longer intervals."

A later account of this kindred was given by Thadani,[16] who reported on "the toothless man of Sind." Although the female carriers of this disorder appear to be normal, they may have mild manifestations, such as partial anodontia and diminished activity of sweat glands.[17] Whereas sex-linked recessive inheritance is considered the rule, similar disease pictures of anhidrotic ectodermal dysplasia have been observed that are transmitted as autosomal dominant traits. But in such families the females are less severely affected than the males. Dominance sometimes is incomplete, as in a case of Cockayne,[14] who described an affected boy whose mother was phenotypically normal but transmitted the trait, which was well expressed in 2 of her sisters. The genetic situation is further complicated by the fact that autosomal recessive inheritance must be considered also. In the family illustrated in Figure 116-3, there were 3 sisters affected with severe anhidrotic ectodermal dysplasia. A brother had died of "fever" in infancy; 3 sisters and a brother apparently were free of the trait. The father was short in stature and had atrophic rhinitis but none of the other features of the disorder. This family was part of a highly inbred kindred in which three sibships were affected in one generation, with a sex ratio of 1:1 and a 1:4 ratio of affected to unaffected members.[18]

Pure familial congenital anhidrosis, i.e., ectodermal dysplasia limited to the sweat glands, apparently is rare. Mahloudji and Livingston[19] described 3 siblings, 2 boys and 1 girl, who had pure anhidrotic ectodermal dysplasia, i.e., absence of sweat glands without any other congenital anomalies.They were the result of a

Fig. 116-3. – **A–C,** anhidrotic ectodermal dysplasia in 3 sisters, 11, 9 and 7 years of age. A brother and 2 male cousins had the same disorder.[18] Note sparse hair, dental deficiencies and saddle-shaped noses. The youngest sister has an old appearance because of hypoplasia of jaws and teeth. **D,** papular skin eruptions.

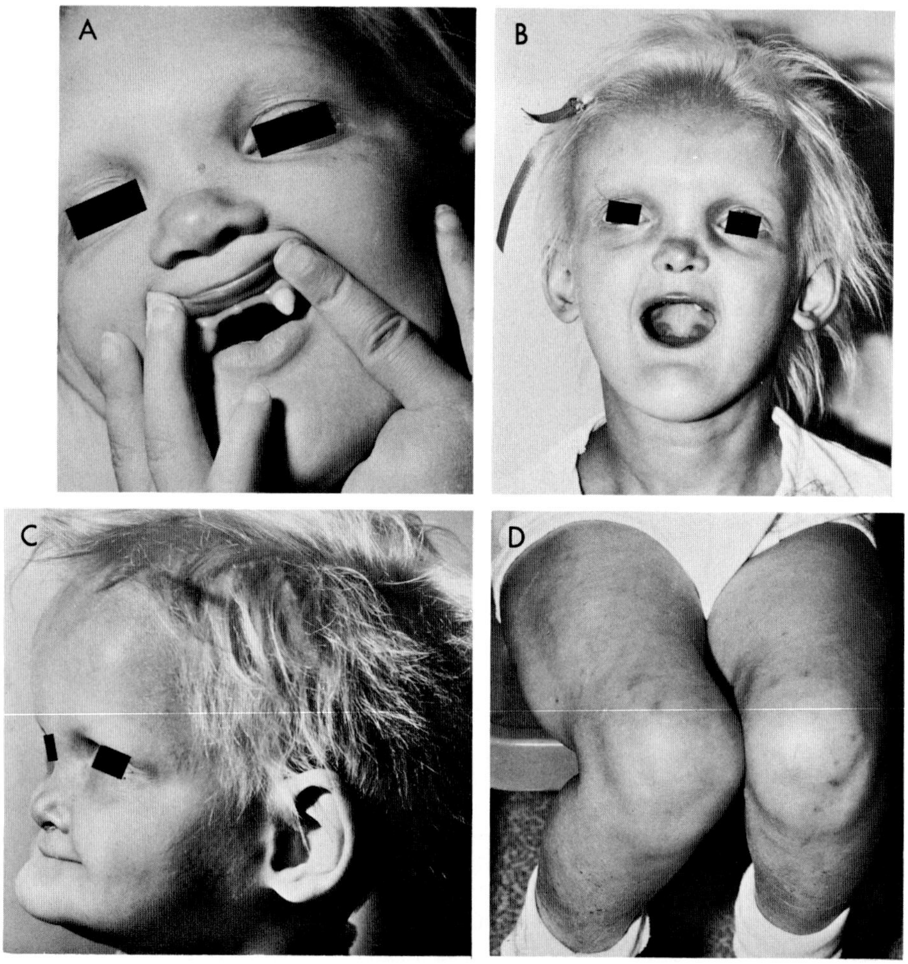

cousin marriage and it is likely that the condition was due to an autosomal recessive gene. These patients were members of a nomadic tribe in Iran. They did well during the periods when the tribe was stationary but complications arose during migration. Their only complaint was their inability to tolerate exposure to heat. They became flushed, uncomfortable, restless and frightened, drinking large quantities of water with only slight relief. Their exercise tolerance was low, especially in hot weather.

Many disease pictures have been described that include symptoms of ectodermal dysplasia but have additional features that often cannot be classified as ectodermal defects. Some of these syndromes are mentioned briefly here.

Chondroectodermal dysplasia, the Ellis-van Creveld syndrome, includes chondrodysplasia, congenital heart defect and polydactyly in addition to hypoplasia of the nails, dental anomalies and scanty hair. Parental consanguinity has been observed repeatedly and autosomal recessive inheritance is the rule (p. 793). In a related disorder, cartilage-hair hypoplasia, the hairs are thin and brittle in patients who have chondrodystrophic manifestations (p. 797).

An ectodermal dysplasia combined with cleft lip and palate, popliteal pterygium, digital anomalies and genital malformations has been described as a syndrome.[20] Rosselli and Gulienetti[21] observed a brother and sister, children of a consanguineous marriage, with a skin dystrophy of "pityriasis type," scanty hair and nails with subungual keratosis, striae and thinned laminae. Both children had harelip and cleft palate, syndactyly and a peculiar pterygial fold over the dorsal aspects of the leg that reached upward to the perineal region. The thumbs were hypoplastic or absent. The genitalia were abnormal in both children. In the boy, the penis was displaced upward and the scrotum was not developed; the labia majora were missing in the girl. Symmetric supernumerary nipples were present in the girl (p. 643).

A boy with hypotrichosis, nail and tooth defects and webbing of fingers and toes had been described before by Hyde[26] and other variations of associated anomalies have been recorded.[20,27]

Ectodermal dysplasia with anomalies of palate and lip was described by Rapp and Hodgkin[28] in a mother and 2 of her children as an autosomal dominant trait.

Ectodermal dysplasia with microphthalmia. Anhidrotic ectodermal dysplasia complicated by microphthalmia, hydrocephaly or absence of nails has been observed as an autosomal dominant trait with variable expressivity.[14]

Ectodermal dysplasia and corneal dysplasia (opacities) in a family were described by Kline *et al.*[22] It appeared that ectodermal dysplasia was transmitted as a dominant trait, expressivity being sex-affected. The corneal dysplasia also was transmitted by a dominant gene that seemed to be neither sex-linked nor sex-affected.

Congenital sensory neuropathy with anhidrosis with recurrent episodes of unexplained fever, self-mutilation and delayed motor and mental development has been described as a possibly recessive hereditary trait.[23,24]

Neurogenic anhidrosis with otherwise normal sweat glands occurs in a syndrome together with pupillary anomalies (Horner syndrome), vasomotor instability, aplasia of dental anomaly, mental retardation and hyporeflexia.[25] Congenital indifference to pain can be recognized. Affected children have shown blond hair and light iris color.

REFERENCES

1. Clouston, H. R.: A hereditary ectodermal dystrophy, Canad. M.A.J. 21:18, 1929.
2. Jacobsen, A. W.: Hereditary dystrophy of the hair and nails, J.A.M.A. 90:686, 1928.
3. Williams, M., and Fraser, F. C.: Hydrotic ectodermal dysplasia—Clouston's family revisited, Canad. M.A.J. 96:36, 1967.
4. Thompson, H. B.: Hereditary dystrophy of the nails, J.A.M.A. 91:1547, 1928.
5. Marshall, D.: Ectodermal dysplasia, Am. J. Ophth. 45: 143, 1958.
6. Robinson, G. C., Miller, J. R., and Bensimon, J. R.: Familial ectodermal dysplasia with sensori-neural deafness and other anomalies, Pediatrics 30:797, 1962.
7. Mallmann-Muhlberger, E., and Helwig, H.: Familiäre ektodermale Dysplasie vom hidrotischen typ, Ann. paediat. 202:358, 1964.
8. Osbourn, R. A.: Congenital ectodermal defect with amastia, J.A.M.A. 148:644, 1952.
9. Weech, A. A.: Hereditary ectodermal dysplasia (congenital ectodermal defect), Am. J. Dis. Child. 37:766, 1929.
10. James, T.: Ectodermal dysplasia, Acta pediat. 41:1, 1952.
11. Capitanio, M. A., Chen, J. T. T., Arey, J. B., and Kirkpatrick, J. A.: Congenital anhidrotic ectodermal dysplasia, Am. J. Roentgenol. 103:168, 1968.
12. Halperin, S. L., and Curtis, G. M.: Anhidrotic ectodermal dysplasia associated with mental deficiency, Am. J. Ment. Deficiency 46:459, 1942.
13. Mills, J.: Anhidrotic ectodermal dysplasia presenting as a pyrexia of undetermined origin in the neonatal period, Postgrad M. J. 44:193, 1968.
14. Cockayne, E. A.: *Inherited Abnormalities of the Skin and Its Appendages* (London: Oxford University Press, 1933).
15. Darwin, C.: *The Variation of Animals and Plants under Domestication* (New York: D. Appleton & Company, 1896), Vol. II.
16. Thadani, K. T.: The toothless man of Sind, J. Hered. 25: 483, 1934.
17. Kerr, C. B., Wells, R. S., and Cooper, K. E.: Gene effect in carriers of anhidrotic ectodermal dysplasia, J. M. Genetics 3:169, 1966.
18. Passarge, E., Nuzum, C. T., and Schubert, W. K.: Anhidrotic ectodermal dysplasia as autosomal recessive trait in an inbred kindred, Humangenetik 3:181, 1966.
19. Mahloudji, M., and Livingston, K. E.: Familial and congenital simple anhidrosis, Am. J. Dis. Child. 113:477, 1967.
20. Gorlin, R. J., and Pindborg, J. J.: *Syndromes of the Head and Neck* (New York: McGraw-Hill Book Company, Inc., 1964).
21. Rosselli, D., and Gulienetti, R.: Ectodermal dysplasia, Brit. J. Plast. Surg. 14:190, 1961.
22. Kline, A. H., Sidbury, J. B., Jr., and Richter, C. P.: The occurrence of ectodermal dysplasia and corneal dysplasia in one family, J. Pediat. 55:355, 1959.

23. Swanson, A. G.: Congenital insensitivity to pain with anhydrosis. A unique syndrome in two male siblings, Arch. Neurol. 8:299, 1963.
24. Vassella, F., Emrich, H. M., Kraus-Ruppert, R., Aufdermaur, F., and Tönz, O.: Congenital sensory neuropathy with anhidrosis, Arch. Dis. Childhood 43:124, 1968.
25. Brown, J. W., and Podosin, R.: A syndrome of the neural crest, Arch. Neurol. 15:294, 1966.
26. Hyde, J. N.: Congenital alopecia as an expression of atavism, J. Cutan. Dis. 27:1, 1909.
27. Cole, H. N., Driver, J. R., Giffen, H. K., Norris, C. B., and Stroud, G., III: Ectodermal and mesodermal dysplasia with osseous involvement, Arch. Dermat. & Syph. 44:773, 1941.
28. Rapp, R. S., and Hodgkin, W. E.: Anhidrodic ectodermal dysplasia: Autosomal dominant inheritance with palate and lip anomalies, J. M. Genetics 5:269, 1968.
29. Beahrs, J. O., Lillington, G. A., Rosan, R. C., Russin, L., Lindgren, J. A., and Rowley, P. T.: Anhidrotic ectodermal dysplasia: Predisposition to bronchial disease, Ann. Int. Med. 74:92, 1971.

117

Pigmented Skin Lesions

Pigmented Nevi

PIGMENTED NEVI consist of nevus cells or melanocytes that are thought to be of neural crest origin. It is said that these cells migrate in early fetal life with the nerves from the neural crest to the epidermis, where they can be identified in the third fetal month. In Negro embryos, the first dendritic melanocytes can be seen within the basal layer of the epidermis by the eleventh week, and 2 weeks later they are seen within the epidermis.[1]

Pigmented nevi may be flat, slightly elevated, papillomatous, dome-shaped or pedunculated. Histologically, one speaks of junction nevi (located in the epidermo-dermal junction), compound nevi (with nevus cell nests within the epidermis and dermis) and intradermal nevi (with nevus cell nests and cords in the dermis), where they are surrounded by collagenous tissue.[1]

Melanocytic nevi are the most common skin lesions; they can be congenital or develop during childhood and adult life. Growth of nevi during childhood seldom leads to malignant change, although pictures resembling those of adult melanomas may be found on histologic examination.[2] As a rule, a period of growth is followed by a stage of stability and finally by atrophy and depigmentation. For discussion of malignancy and treatment, the reader is referred to dermatologic publications.[1–5] It has been said that pedunculated, verrucous and hair-containing nevi do not become malignant.[5] Evenness of pigmentation and sharp definition of the border are reassuring signs.[3] An excellent review of the literature on pigmented nevi and malignant melanoma was published by Beerman *et al.*[6]

Since pigmented nevi occur so commonly that almost any person with light skin shows several of these lesions, it is difficult to establish a hereditary pattern. Yet, families have been reported in which "innumerable" flat pigmented spots of various sizes were seen in members of several generations. In some instances, a few large nevi were seen in the same location in several members of a kinship, inherited like a dominant trait. It was considered possible that families with multiple inherited pigmented nevi are affected by neurofibromatosis (p. 1252) without mollusca fibrosa and neurofibromas.[7] The *café au lait spots* characteristic of neurofibromatosis have smooth borders and are lighter than the common pigmented nevi, but they, too, have increased amounts of melanin and melanocytes in the basal cell layer.[1] They generally are present at or soon after birth but they also may develop during the first or second decade. They do not undergo malignant degeneration. Single café au lait spots occur in 20% of

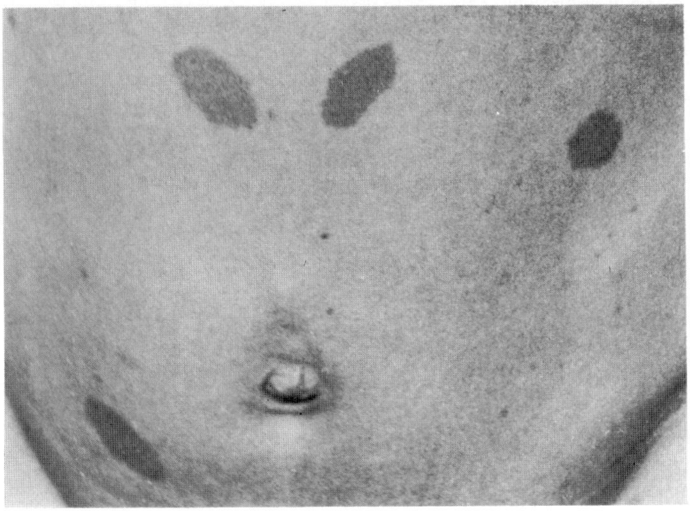

Fig. 117-1.—Café au lait spots in a boy with neurofibromatosis.

normal children under 5 years but fewer than 1% have more than two spots. Multiple café au lait spots are present in 90% of patients with neurofibromatosis.[8,9]

In *fibrous dysplasia (Albright disease)* (p. 878), pigmentations of the skin are irregular in outline, not elevated and often are unilateral, with a preference for the sacrum, buttocks and the spine. If an extremity is affected, the pigmentations and bone lesions usually are on the same side.

Multiple basal cell nevi are constituents of a syndrome that includes odontogenic cysts (p. 1268), bifid ribs, vertebral malformations and many other rather variable anomalies. The syndrome is thought to be inherited as a dominant trait with poor penetrance. The nevi usually are not congenital but some of the associated malformations are. The face, neck, trunk and arms and other parts may be covered by papules that are pigmented or flesh colored. Cysts, milia or keratosis palmaris and plantaris sometimes complicate the cutaneous picture. Some of the nevoid basal-cell epitheliomas appear to bud off from the basal layer of the overlying epithelium, whereas others consist of large masses of basal cells that lie within the corium and show a tendency to cystic degeneration. The lesions may undergo malignant transformation.[10]

The *pigment spots associated with generalized intestinal polyposis* (p. 714) are round or oval, 1–5 mm. in diameter and located chiefly on the oral mucosa, lips and digits. Spots appearing on the skin of the face are grouped around the eyes, nostrils and lips. They are darker than freckles and show a tendency to fade after the age of 25 years. On the fingers and toes, the dorsal and plantar surfaces can be affected. In rare cases, the spots have been observed at birth, but often they are not noticed until later. The pigment consists of melanin deposited in the stratum corneum and to a lesser extent in the cutis. In the epidermis, the melanin deposits are arranged in vertical bands.[11]

A rare but striking neurocutaneous *melanoblastosis* involving the skin, meninges, brain and spinal cord has been described as a syndrome. Pigmented lesions resembling nevi pilosi may be present at birth, with hydrocephaly developing during infancy. The disorder has been considered a congenital systemic disease and has been called a neurocutaneous melanoblastosis.[12] It has been compared to "phakomatoses" or hamartoses such as tuberous sclerosis, Recklinghausen or Hippel-Lindau disease but, in contrast to these conditions, dominant inheritance has not been proved for this melanoblastosis. Since the fully developed disorder commonly is fatal in infancy, it could be due to a new mutation that cannot be transmitted. Only 37 cases had been recorded by 1968.[13]

There are large, partly hairy pigmented nevi on the

Fig. 117-2.—Pigmentations of irregular outline about the axilla as seen in McCune-Albright syndrome.

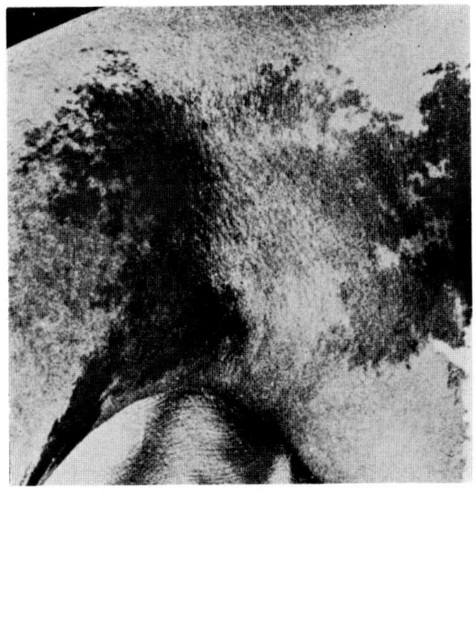

skin, cell proliferations in the leptomeninges with perivascular penetration of the brain substance and melanin storage in perivascular and glial chromatophores of the cerebellum pons and brain stem. Hydrocephaly is attributed to infiltration of the meninges by nevus cells and impairment of cerebrospinal liquor resorption.[12] The disorder has a high malignancy potential, and death in early childhood is the rule.[13,14]

Congenital malignant melanoma can occur in children of mothers with widespread metastases from malignant melanoma. No primary tumor is established in such cases and transplacental transmission can be assumed. In a few children born of normal mothers, cutaneous melanomas present at birth metastasized soon in postnatal life.[15]

Sweet and Connerty[16] reported the case of a male infant who was born with malignant melanomas of the trunk, diaper region, the thighs and other cutaneous parts. The child died when he was 17 days of age and many nodules of tumor tissues were found in the liver, pons and cerebral cortex. Oldhoff and Koudstaal[17] described a boy with a congenital malignant melanoma of the skin of the leg treated by amputation at 3 weeks of age. At the age of 10 years, the boy was in good condition and without evidence of the disease. Malignant melanoma has been observed repeatedly as an autosomal dominant trait,[18] but the lesions are not noted at birth in such cases. Multiple lentigines, hypertelorism, pulmonary stenosis, cardiac conduction defects, genital anomalies, sensorineural deafness and growth retardation have been named the "leopard syndrome."[47] Autosomal dominant inheritance with variable expressivity seems to be established.

Nevus Pilosus (Hairy Mole)

Extended pigmented areas of the skin covered with hair represent serious congenital malformations because of the disfigurement they cause. These sometimes verrucose lesions have a preference for the lower end of the trunk ("bathing-trunk nevi") but they can also involve the face, neck, shoulders and chest, where they are even more disturbing than in the pelvic area.[7] Fortunately, such extended lesions are rare but they present a serious cosmetic problem to those affected. They have been compared to the pelt of animals ("Tierfellnaevus"), with very grave consequences to the parents and the child at times when hybridization of man and animal was consid-

Fig. 117-3. — Extensive nevus pilosus.

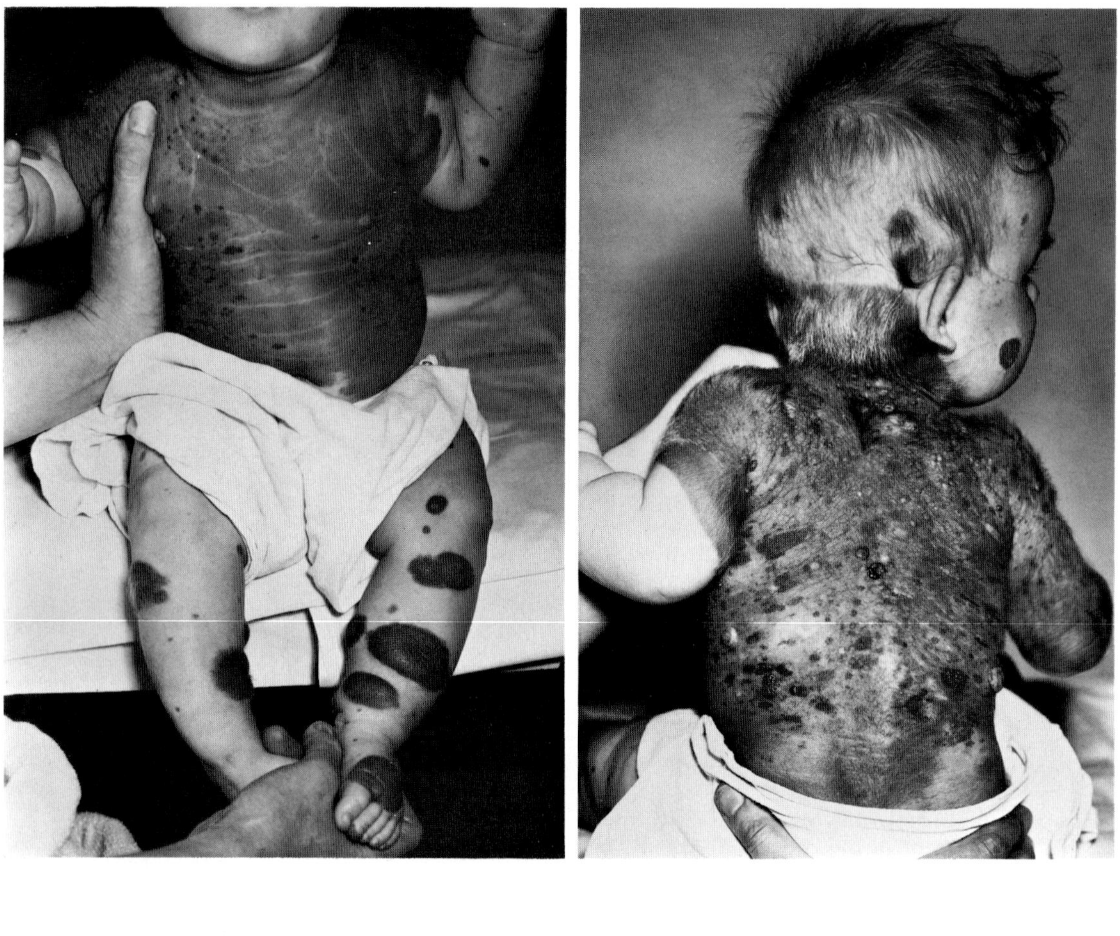

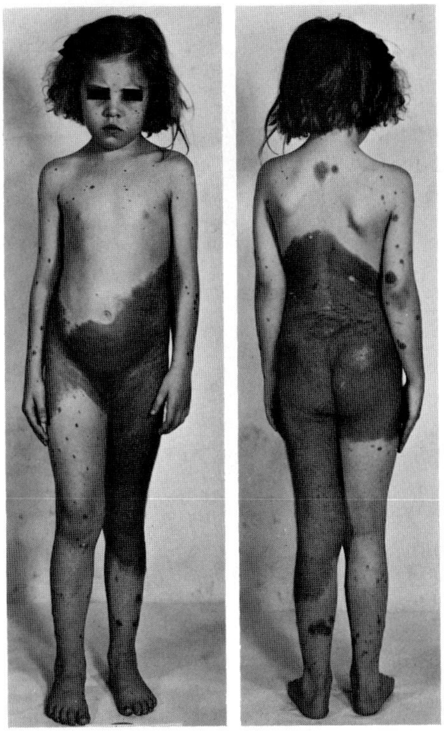

Fig. 117-4.—Nevus pilosus of bathing-trunk type.

ered possible (p. 15). I once saw in Vienna such a child brought to the hospital because of very severe rickets. The parents, living in an Austrian village, had not dared to take the child outdoors, thus depriving him of light and sunshine, which then were the chief antirachitic agents. Unfortunately, treatment of these nevi is difficult and the prognosis unfavorable for cosmetic reconstitution. Nevus pilosus usually appears sporadically, but Gould and Pyle[19] mentioned a Peruvian boy and his sister, both of whom had giant lesions of this type. It is possible that such giant nevi are a manifestation of Recklinghausen neurofibromatosis. They could be due to a new mutation that is not transmitted because it is very disfiguring. A case illustrated by Gould and Pyle[19] showed, in addition to nevus pilosus, several benign tumors (fibroma molluscum), which suggests neurofibromatosis, and the same holds for the child illustrated in Figure 117-3.

Sacral Spot ("Mongolian Blue Spot")

In its typical form, this congenital accumulation of pigment consists of a single patch of bluish color in the lumbosacral region that shows great variability in size, shape and color. Location and distribution of these spots also vary sometimes in different individuals and races.[7] Histologically, they are made up of stellate cells filled with melanin granules and are located chiefly in the midportion of the dermis, where the pigmented cells lie widely scattered or in small groups. The pigment cells give a positive dopa reaction, indicating that they are melanocytes.[1] Sacral blue spots gradually fade during childhood, their duration depending on their intensity. The name "Mongolian spot" is derived from the belief that almost every infant of the Mongolian race has such pigment spots,[7] which, however, also occur in Negroes, American Indians, Polynesians and many other races, including Europeans. Although sacral spots are said to be rare in western Europeans, in Spanish and Portuguese infants their incidence reaches 20%. They are absent in children with blond or red hair. A great deal has been written about the racial distribution of these spots and about their genetics.[7,20] Generally, it can be said that the spots are better developed in individuals and races with more intensive pigmentation and that the visibility of the lumbosacral accumulations is better in Mongolians than in dark Negroes. Much more interesting is the fact that these pigment spots are located in the lumbosacral area, in an area in which spina bifida occulta and aperta appear most often. In this area, the neural crest may have special properties. The cells of the Mongolian spots are regarded as melanocytes, which, in their embryonal migration from the neural crest to the epidermis, failed to reach their goal, becoming arrested in the dermis.[1,4] Why such melanocytes can appear in normal persons in increased amounts in the dermis of an embryologically critical area is not understood at present but is worth investigating.

Blue Nevus

The common blue nevi are small, slate-blue, well-circumscribed, flat or dome-shaped areas that may be present at birth or appear soon thereafter. The pigment-bearing cells are large, spindle-shaped and dendritic, grouped in bundles in the middle and lower strata of the dermis and in the subcutaneous fat. These cells resemble those present in Mongolian spots, but they are more numerous and their granules are so dense that the nucleus cannot be seen. There also occur dopa-negative melanophores in blue nevi. Malignant degeneration of congenital blue nevi is said to be very rare. Blue nevi can be located on the face and in many other regions of the body. Nevus of Ota (ophthalmo-maxillaris) is a blue nevus located in areas of the face supplied by the first and second trigeminal branches. It can be associated with abnormal pigmentation of the conjunctiva, sclera, cornea and iris. Malignant degeneration does not seem to occur in the common blue nevus. But in so-called cellular blue nevi, which form firm, bluish nodules, malignant changes can occur.[1]

Incontinentia Pigmenti (Bloch-Sulzberger Syndrome)

This disorder originally was described as a skin disease but it is now known to involve various additional

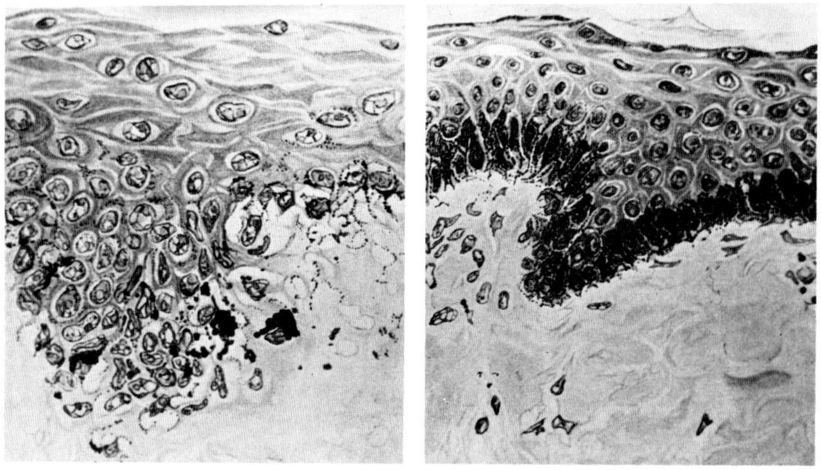

Fig. 117-5.—Incontinentia pigmenti. On the right, normal epidermis is seen and, on the left, changes characteristic of incontinentia pigmenti. (From H. W. Siemens, Arch. Dermat. u. Syph. 157:385, 1929; courtesy of Springer-Verlag, Berlin.)

body systems, particularly the eye, the central nervous system and the teeth. General growth may be impaired also. First described by Bardach[21] in a pair of monozygotic twins, it was named "incontinentia pigmenti" by Bloch[22] and Sulzberger.[23] Skin lesions sometimes are present at birth but, in most cases, they develop soon after birth. Among associated anomalies are some of definite prenatal origin, but some of these could be coincidental and others predisposing to the disorder.

Vesicles, blisters or papules may be present at birth[23-26] or develop within minutes[27] or days after birth.[27-29] In some instances, pigmentation, usually a later development, is also noticeable at birth.[23,24,30] In most cases, vesicular lesions, in linear or patchy arrangement, appear, disappear and recur for many months before the characteristic pigmentation develops. Pigmentations are described as macular, linear, patchy, spattered or spider shaped. The chocolate-brown to slate-gray lesions "do not follow lines of cleavage or distributions of nerves, nor do they respect the limitations of the midline."[27] The legs, pelvic regions and lower trunk are areas of predilection, but other parts can be involved also. The first manifestations usually are nonspecific acute inflammatory reactions with vesiculation. Polymorphonuclear eosinophilic leukocytes may fill the vesicles. Infiltration of papillae and dermis by round cells and polymorphonuclear cells is characteristic of the initial stage. Hyperkeratosis, dyskeratosis and acanthosis follow and then the classic stage of "incontinentia pigmenti" develops, often with reduction of pigment in the basal cell layer of the epidermis and large amounts of melanin within chromatophores in the upper dermis.[27] Basal cells show signs of degeneration and vacuolization. It has been assumed that damage to these cells renders them incapable of holding melanin, but this is not generally accepted.[25,31] Fading of the pigment lesions followed by atrophy of the skin has been observed after the age of 3 years in many but not in all cases. Eosinophilia in skin lesions and in the blood is a sign worth emphasis,[25,32] and which probably holds the key to understanding this disorder.

Associated anomalies and malformations are heterogeneous. Microcephaly, hydrocephaly, spastic paralysis, epilepsy, mental retardation, strabismus, nystagmus, opacities of the cornea and lens, blue sclerae, optic atrophy, retinal changes,[33] pseudoglioma, abnormal dentition, osseous deformities, adrenomedullary aplasia,[30] general growth retardation, alopecia, dystrophy of nails and supernumerary nipple have been described.[27] Micropolygyria, pyramidal hypoplasia and other cerebral changes have been observed.[26] In about one-third of the cases, there are eye lesions and a mass in the posterior chamber has been observed repeatedly.[33] Dentition is delayed and there is a reduction in the number of teeth. Conical crown formation of the incisors, canines and bicuspids is a characteristic symptom.[24]

The etiology of incontinentia pigmenti is under discussion. The condition has been observed in Caucasians, Negroes, Chinese and Japanese and females are almost exclusively affected.[27,32] Lenz,[32] reviewing the literature, found 210 girls among 216 patients and ascertained familial occurrence in 25 observations in which failure of development of dental anlagen was considered a minimal sign of the disorder. The facts available suggested that an X-chromosomal gene, which produces the syndrome in the female and leads to early intrauterine death in the male, could account for the behavior of the disorder. But some investigators considered a virus infection before or after birth as a possible cause.[29,34,35]

Naegeli[36] reported a kinship that showed dominant inheritance of a pigment anomaly with a certain resemblance to incontinentia pigmenti. But this condition probably differed from incontinentia pigmenti by reticular arrangement of pigment, underdeveloped sweat glands with heat intolerance and by mild keratosis palmaris et plantaris.[37] Van Bogaert[38] described in 3 sisters a progressive neurologic disorder that was associated with congenital skin lesions resembling incontinentia pigmenti. The patients' parents were consanguineous and the trait may be an autosomal recessive. It seems that incontinentia pigmenti can be a symptom of various disease pictures.

Acanthosis Nigricans

Hypertrophy of the "prickle-cell layer" of the skin may be a reaction to various stimuli. Acanthosis nigricans may be associated with adenocarcinomas of the stomach, intestine or breast; it may be associated with endocrine disorders such as pituitary hypogonadism, polycystic ovary or adrenal insufficiency; or it may be a benign skin lesion present at birth or developing during childhood.[1] In the last-mentioned form, genetic factors play a role; regular or irregular dominance has been noted.[39] It is possible that there is a connection between the hereditary tendency to acanthosis nigricans and visceral cancer, but this has not been reliably established.[3] The lesions consist of thickened and pigmented skin that has a verrucose, nodular or papillomatous surface. Axilla, neck, genitalia, perianal skin and flexor surfaces of the extremities are areas of predilection. Mucous membranes may show condylomatous lesions and alopecia and dystrophy of nails sometimes are present.[3] In histologic sections, one sees finger-like, pointed papillae projecting toward the surface of the skin. Hyperkeratosis and papillomatosis are distinct but pigmentation is increased only slightly.[1]

Dyskeratosis Congenita

There are large areas of atrophy and reticular pigmentation of the skin with preference for the face, neck and chest. Histologically, the epidermis is thinned, the melanin is increased in amount in the basal layer and melanophores are present in the upper dermis. Hyperhidrosis palmaris et plantaris and acrocyanosis are common. Dystrophy of fingernails and toenails and leukokeratosis of the oral and anal mucous membranes are associated sufficiently often with the cutaneous changes that a clinical syndrome (Zinsser-Cole-Rauschkolb syndrome) seems to be established. The mucous membrane lesions begin as vesicles that change to ulcers and leukoplakia and even carcinoma. Malformation and malposition of teeth have been observed. There is a marked predilection for males, and several sibships have been described in which only brothers were affected. Sex-linked recessive inheritance has been assumed.[1] But some cases were associated with Fanconi pancytopenia,[1] which is an autosomal recessive trait.

Urticaria Pigmentosa

Urticaria pigmentosa was described originally as a skin disease, but it is now known as a systemic disorder that can involve bone marrow, lymph nodes, spleen, liver and other organs. Rarely, it manifests itself at birth[40] as a generalized eruption covering the entire body, with the exception of the hands and feet, with maculopapular lesions, partly surmounted by bullae measuring 1–3 cm. Stroking of the lesions gives rise to urtication. Histologic examination shows an infiltrate below the epidermis consisting of mast cells, the characteristic element of the disease.[1]

The lesions are red in the beginning, turning brown later. Sometimes they are present in infancy and childhood but can appear during adult life also. Affected children gradually improve and are free of symptoms by adolescence or retain lightly pigmented asymptomatic macular lesions. Systemic mast cell involvement is seen chiefly in adult cases.[41] One of the extracutaneous systems most frequently involved is the skeleton, in which thickening of the trabeculae leads to sclerosis of many bones. Such changes usually are manifest in adults only but involvement of a tibia has been described in a 5-year-old girl.[42] Familial occurrence has been observed repeatedly but genetic determination has not been established.[43]

Xeroderma Pigmentosum

The skin lesions of this anomaly are not congenital but develop during early weeks or months of postnatal life (together with photophobia) after exposure to sunlight. Associated defects, i.e., mental retardation, epilepsy, deafness and joint or foot malformations, which have been reported repeatedly, may also be considered as postnatal in origin, but a basic and genetically determined metabolic error must be assumed to be congenital. The first skin reactions to sunlight appear on exposed parts of the body – the face, neck and hands. In these areas, freckles soon make their appearance, followed by larger spots of pigmentation, atrophy and telangiectases. The skin changes have been likened to chronic radiodermatitis.[3] Warty growths and malignant changes – carcinoma, sarcoma or melanoma – develop on the atrophic skin. The eye may be involved by photophobia, leukoma or carcinoma of the cornea, keratitis and ectropion.[44] Two-thirds of the patients die under the age of 15 years.

Jewish, Japanese, Arab and other racial groups have been affected. Parental consanguinity is high and repetition in siblings is frequent. Homozygosity for a single recessive gene seems to be responsible for the disorder. Genetic counseling of an affected family

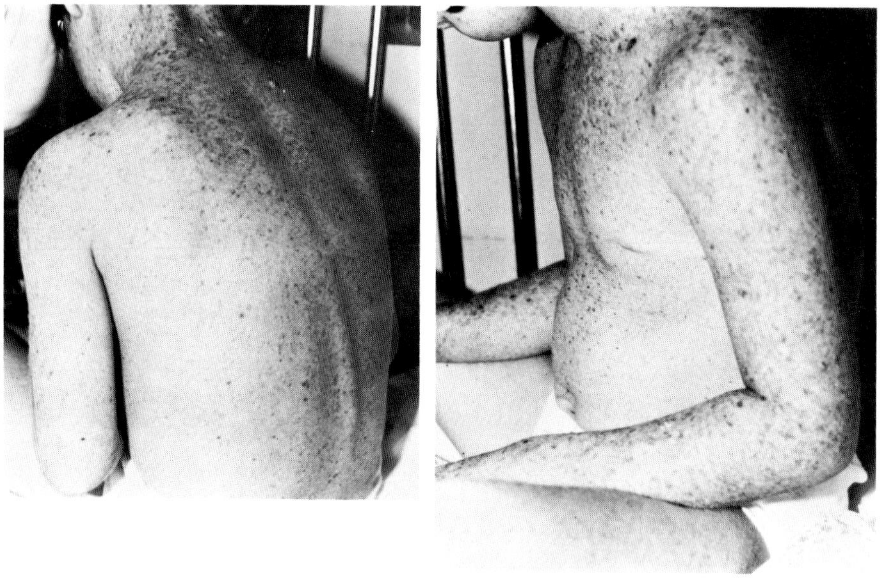

Fig. 117-6. – Xeroderma pigmentosum in a 6-year-old girl.

was discussed in detail by Lynch *et al.*[45] as an example of counseling on cancer. It is possible that freckles or other slight pigment changes of the skin in relatives of the patients are manifestations of the heterozygous state.[7] In one case of xeroderma pigmentosum, "chromosomal asynchrony" has been noted.[46]

REFERENCES

1. Lever, W. F.: *Histopathology of the Skin* (4th ed.; Philadelphia: J. B. Lippincott Company, 1967).
2. Willis, R. A.: *The Pathology of the Tumours of Children* (Springfield, Ill.: Charles C Thomas, Publisher, 1962).
3. Pillsbury, D. M., Shelley, W. B., and Kligman, A. M.: *Dermatology* (Philadelphia: W. B. Saunders Company, 1956).
4. Montgomery, H.: Benign and malignant dermal neoplasma, J.A.M.A. 150:1182, 1952.
5. Lewis, G. M.: Pigmented nevi: Their relationship to malignant melanoma and treatment, New York J. Med. 53: 1654, 1953.
6. Beerman, H., Lane, R. A. G., and Shaffer, B.: Pigmented nevi and malignant melanoma of the skin. A survey of some of the recent literature, Am. J. M. Sc. 229:444, 1955.
7. Cockayne, E. A.: *Inherited Abnormalities of the Skin and Its Appendages* (London: Oxford University Press, 1933).
8. Crowe, F. W., and Schull, W. J.: Diagnostic importance of café-au-lait spot in neurofibromatosis, Arch. Int. Med. 91: 758, 1953.
9. Whitehouse, D.: Diagnostic value of the café-au-lait spot in children, Arch. Dis. Childhood 41:316, 1966.
10. Gorlin, R. J., Vickers, R. A., Kelln, E., and Williamson, J. J.: The multiple basal-cell nevi syndrome. An analysis of a syndrome consisting of multiple nevoid basal-cell carcinoma, jaw cysts, skeletal anomalies, medulloblastoma, and hyporesponsiveness to parathormone, Cancer 18:89, 1965.
11. Jeghers, H., McKusick, V. A., and Katz, K. H.: Generalized intestinal polyposis and melanin spots of oral mucosa, lips and digits; syndrome of diagnostic significance, New England J. Med. 241:993; 1031, 1949.
12. Fanconi, A.: Neurocutane Melanoblastose mit Hydrocephalus communicans bei zwei Säuglingen, Helvet. paediat. acta 2:376, 1956.
13. Battin, J., Vital, C., Alberty, J., Guyonnet-Duperat, J. P., Leger, H., and Fontan, A.: La mélanose neuro-cutanée, Arch. franç. pédiat. 25:277, 1968.
14. Fox, H., Emery, J. L., Goodbody, R. A., and Yates, P. O.: Neurocutaneous melanosis, Arch. Dis. Childhood 39:508, 1964.
15. Skov-Jensen, T., Hastrup, J., and Lambrethsew, E.: Malignant melanoma in children, Cancer 19:620, 1966.
16. Sweet, L. K., and Connerty, H. V.: Congenital melanoma: Report of a case in which antenatal metastasis occurred, Am. J. Dis. Child. 62:1029, 1941.
17. Oldhoff, J., and Koudstaal, J.: Congenital papillomatous malignant melanoma of the skin, Cancer 21:1193, 1968.
18. Anderson, D. E., Smith, J. L., Jr., and McBride, C. M.: Hereditary aspects of malignant melanoma, J.A.M.A. 200:741, 1967.
19. Gould, G. M., and Pyle, W. L.: *Anomalies and Curiosities of Medicine* (Philadelphia: W. B. Saunders Company, 1897).
20. Gates, R. R.: *Human Genetics* (New York : The Macmillan Company, 1946).
21. Bardach, M.: Systematisierte Naevusbildungen bei einem eineiigen Zwillingspaar, Ztschr. Kinderh. 39:542, 1925.
22. Bloch, B.: Eigentümliche bisher nicht beschriebene Pigmentaffektion (incontinentia pigmenti), Schweiz. med. Wchnschr. 56:404, 1926.
23. Sulzberger, M. B.: Über eine bisher nicht beschriebene Pigmentanomalie (incontinentia pigmenti), Arch. Dermat. u. Syph. 154:19, 1928.
24. Gorlin, R. J., and Anderson, J. A.: The characteristic dentition of incontinentia pigmenti, J. Pediat. 57:78, 1960.
25. Oldfelt, V.: Incontinentia pigmenti, J. Pediat. 54:446, 1959.
26. O'Doherty, N. J., and Norman, R. M.: Incontinentia pigmenti (Bloch-Sulzberger syndrome) with cerebral malformation, Developmental Med. & Child Neurol. 10:168, 1968.

27. Carney, R. G.: Incontinentia pigmenti. A report of five cases and review of the literature, Arch. Dermat. & Syph. 64:126, 1951.
28. Loveman, A. B., Fleegelman, M. T., Weedman, A. J., and Rein, C. R.: Incontinentia pigmenti, J. Pediat. 40:442, 1952.
29. Mendelsohn, R. S., Medansky, R. S., and Lazar, M. P.: Incontinentia pigmenti (Bloch-Sulzberger syndrome); a generalized disease, A.M.A. J. Dis. Child. 97:348, 1959.
30. Seidlmayer, H.: Über ein neues Syndrom multipler Abartung. Pigmentanomalie, kongenitale ektodermale Dysplasie, Nebennierenmarkaplasie, Ztschr. Kinderh. 63:451, 1942.
31. Grislain, J. R., Mussini, J., de Berranger, P., Le Bodic, M-F., and Dubigeon, P.: Incontinentia pigmenti (à propos d'une nouvelle observation), Pédiatrie 23:67, 1968.
32. Lenz, W.: Zur Genetik der Incontinentia pigmenti, Ann. paediat. 196:149, 1961.
33. Cole, J. G., and Cole, H. G.: Incontinentia pigmenti associated with changes in the posterior chamber of the eye, Am. J. Ophth. 47:321, 1959.
34. Uebel, H., Ludwig, A., and Karting, G.: Zur Kenntnis der Incontinentia pigmenti (Bloch-Sulzberger), Arch. Dermat. u. Syph. 190:114, 1950.
35. Grüneberg, T.: Zur Frage der Incontinentia pigmenti (Bloch-Sulzberger), Arch. klin. u. exper. Dermat. 201:218, 1955.
36. Naegeli, O.: Cited by Franceschetti and Jadassohn.[37]
37. Franceschetti, A., and Jadassohn, W.: A propos de l' "Incontinentia pigmenti," délimitation de deux syndromes différents figurant sous le même terme, Dermatologica 108:1, 1954.
38. Van Bogaert, L.: D'une atrophie cérébelleuse familiale avec dystrophie maculaire et anomalies congénitales de la pigmentation cutanée du type de l'incontinence pigmenti, Bibl. Ophth. 47:540, 1957.
39. Curth, H. O., and Aschner, B. M.: Genetic studies on acanthosis nigricans, A.M.A. Arch. Dermat. 79:55, 1959.
40. Lipschutz, A., and Shaffer, B.: Urticaria pigmentosa. Report of a case of the bullous variety in a newborn infant, J. Pediat. 39:745, 1951.
41. Caplan, R. M.: The natural course of urticaria pigmentosa, Arch. Dermat. 87:146, 1963.
42. Bendel, W. L., Jr., and Race, G. J.: Urticaria pigmentosa with bone involvement, J. Bone & Joint Surg. 45-A:1043, 1963.
43. Butterworth, T., and Strean, L. P.: *Clinical Genodermatology* (Baltimore: The Williams & Wilkins Company, 1962).
44. Giller, H., and Kaufmann, W. C.: Ocular lesions in xeroderma pigmentosum, A.M.A. Arch. Ophth. 62:130, 1959.
45. Lynch, H. T., Anderson, D. E., Krush, A. J., and Mukerjee, D.: Cancer, heredity and genetic counseling. Xeroderma pigmentosum, Cancer 20:1796, 1967.
46. De Grouchy, J., De Nava, C., Feingold, J., Frézal, J., and Lamy, M.: Asynchronie chromosomique dans un cas de xeroderma pigmentosum, Ann. Génét. 10:224, 1967.
47. Gorlin, R. J.: Multiple lentigenes syndrome, Am. J. Dis. Child. 117:652, 1969.

Nevus Unius Lateralis

NEVUS UNIUS LATERALIS is a striking papillary or verrucose skin lesion limited, or nearly limited, to one side of the body. The lesions are arranged in linear streaks or bands following the long axis of the limbs or extending transversely around the trunk. When Pack and Sunderland[1] reviewed this anomaly in 1941, they found 156 cases reported in the medical literature under (approximately) 40 names. In about half of the cases, the nevus was present at birth or it appeared in the first few months of life. Sensory disturbances may be present. Itching, moisture or fetor are complained of. The distribution of the lesions has been related to the course of cutaneous nerves and to that of blood vessels or of lymph channels.

Marked hyperkeratosis, mild acanthosis, elongation of the papillae and round cell infiltration of the papillary layer and corium have been observed in histologic sections. Many associated malformations have been described. Hypertrophy[2] or underdevelopment of

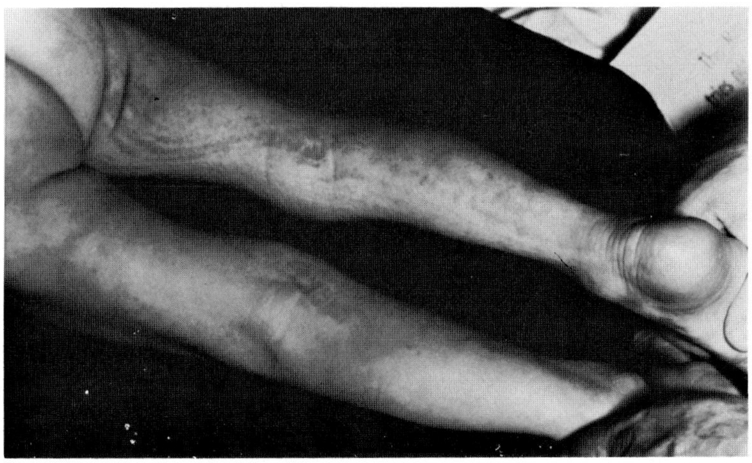

Fig. 117-7.—Linear nevi on the right leg of a boy with left-sided hemihypertrophy. In this case, linear nevi also were present on the left shoulder, back and buttocks (see Fig. 15–2) so that one cannot speak strictly of nevus unius lateralis.

parts[1] has been observed in patients with nevus unius lateralis. Heredity has been suggested by a few cases only.

Growth or retrogression can occur. Malignant transformation has been observed repeatedly, but it is not known in what percentage this occurs.

REFERENCES

1. Pack, G. T., and Sunderland, D. A.: Naevus unius lateris, Arch. Surg. 43:341, 1941.
2. Lenson, N.: Nevus unius lateralis, New England J. Med. 248:757, 1953.

118

Vascular Lesions

Blood Vessels

Nevus Vasculosus (Strawberry Mark and Angioma Vasculosum)

THIS COMMON LESION, occurring at birth or developing soon thereafter, is considered an immature angioma that often shows proliferation for some months, with a subsequent tendency to spontaneous regression. Such nevi (called "superficial cavernous hemangiomas" by Holmdahl[1]) were observed in 12–13% of infants routinely examined, with no significant difference between premature and mature infants. In the areas of proliferation, the endothelial cells are large and lie in several layers around capillary lumina.

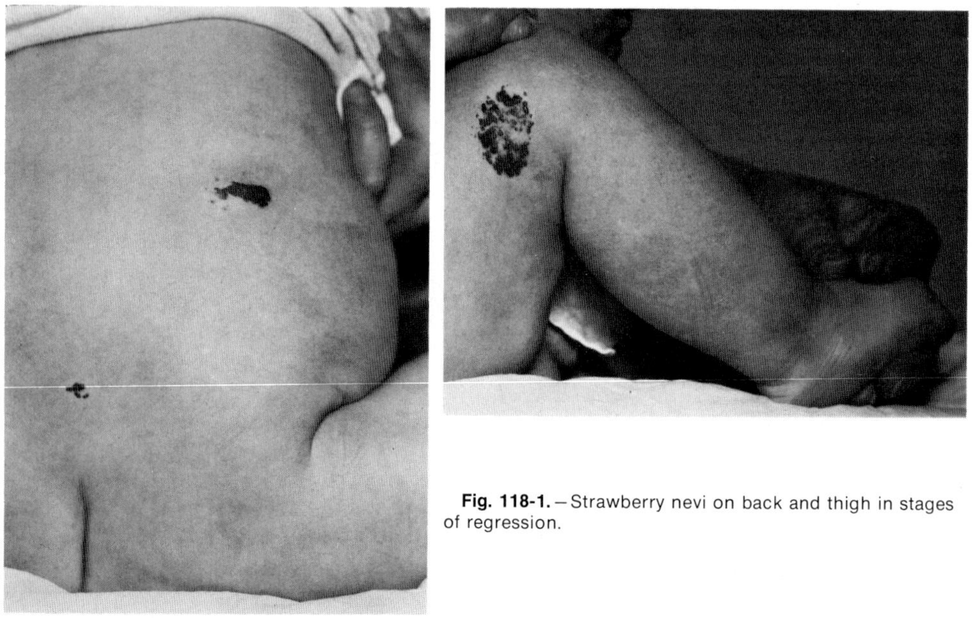

Fig. 118-1. – Strawberry nevi on back and thigh in stages of regression.

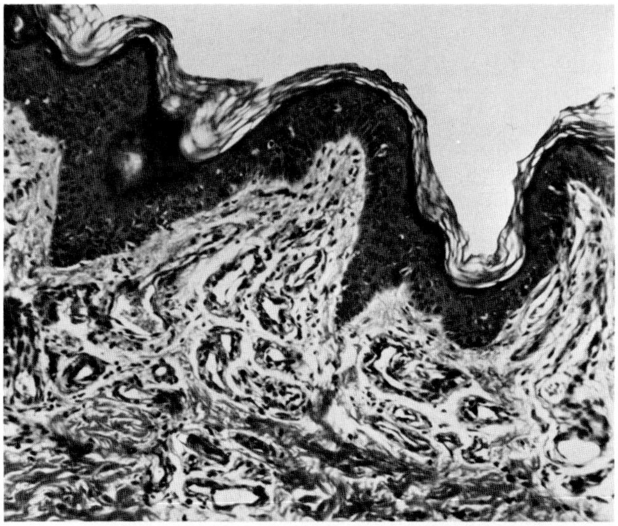

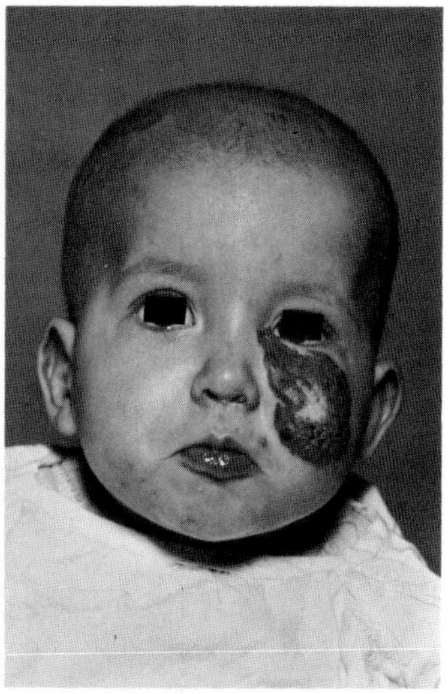

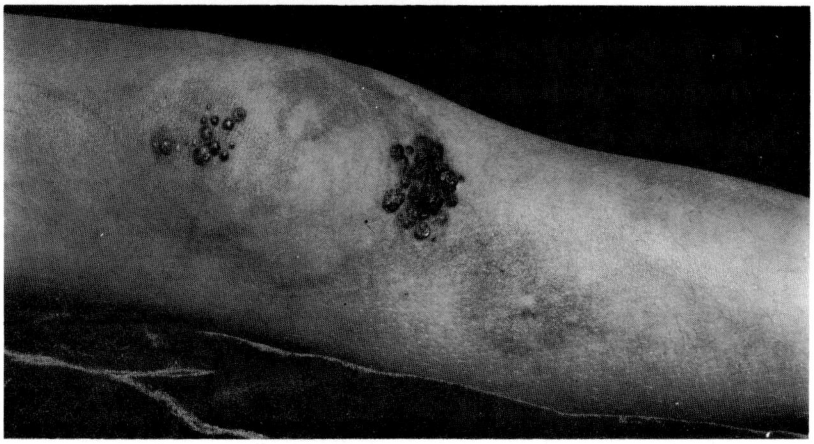

Fig. 118-2 (above left).—Section through superficial capillary hemangioma.
Fig. 118-3 (above right).—Capillary and cavernous hemangioma on left cheek.
Fig. 118-4 (below).—Port-wine hemangioma with hyperkeratotic nodules.

They also can form solid strands and cords without lumina. The microscopic picture can be correlated with clinical phases.[2] Size and color are variable and the nevi can be limited to the skin or reach into the subcutis. Strawberry marks, which eventually regress, may show definite enlargement during the first few months of life, reaching a maximal size in the second half of the first year. Then, a change in color occurs and small white islands of sclerosis appear within the nevus. Involution can lead to disappearance of the lesion or to formation of a skin with minor residual changes. Most strawberry marks occur in the face, but the trunk and the extremities can be affected also. Hemangiomas of the external genitalia are rare. Only 21 cases were found among 2,000 hemangiomas reviewed by Gulienetti[3] and 19 of the 21 were present in females, with localization at the labia majora. Histologically, they were classified chiefly as hemangioma simplex but some were cavernous or phlebectatic. Angioma cavernosum consists of mature blood vessels located in the lower dermis and in the subcutaneous tissue. These blood spaces are lined by a single layer of endothelial cells enveloped by fibrous walls of various thicknesses.[4] There are many arteriovenous shunts and aneurysmal dilatations of the vessels involved. The lesions may be mixed with lymphangiomas, connective tissue and fat.[5] According to Martin,[6] spontaneous regression can be anticipated in many of the cases present at birth but it is less likely when the swelling develops after birth.

Multiple hemangiomas (diffuse neonatal hemangiomatosis) affecting skin, viscera and the central nervous system, deserve special consideration. Hemangiomas consisting of channels ranging from capillary to cavernous size were present in a newborn child described by Cooper and Bolande.[7] Lesions were

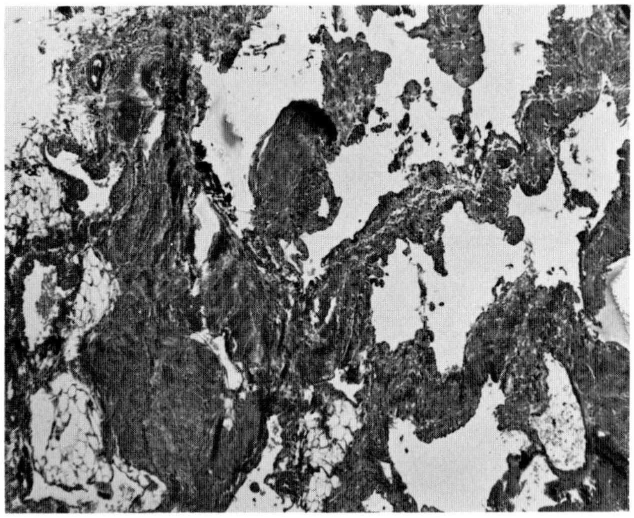

Fig. 118-5.—Section through cavernous hemangioma removed from the back of a child, showing disorganized collection of large vascular spaces with thick walls containing muscle fibers.

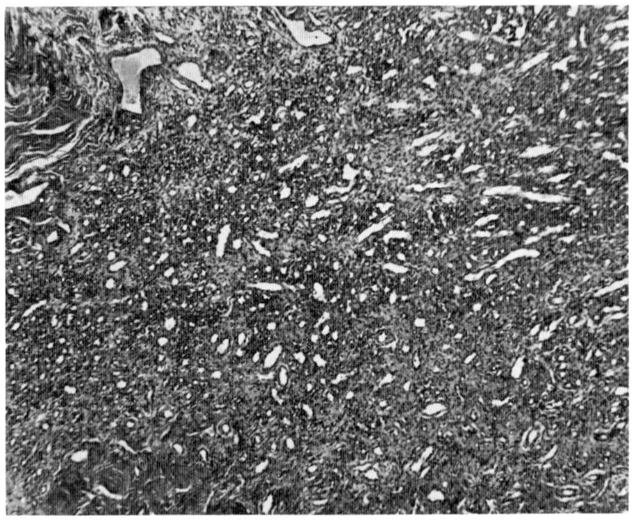

Fig. 118-6.—Section of sclerosing capillary hemangioma of face.

found in the face, mouth, salivary glands, larynx, liver, intestine and leptomeninges. There was enlargement of the heart and congestive heart failure. Postmortem angiograms demonstrated the existence of numerous arteriovenous shunts, which probably were responsible for the cardiac complications. Similar cardiac failure has been observed in infants with hemangioendotheliomas. Burke *et al.*[8] reported disseminated hemangiomatosis in newborn children complicated by central nervous system involvement. Although there was involution of cutaneous lesions in one case, physical and mental development was retarded and hydrocephaly became noticeable. The child died of pneumonia at the age of 2½ years and necropsy revealed multiple tumor masses over the cerebral hemispheres, the cerebellum and within the brain and the pons. A review of diffuse neonatal hemangiomatosis, sites of its lesions, cause of death and malignant potential was published by Holden and Alexander.[29] Another case in which cutaneous hemangiomas were complicated by ocular and intracranial lesions was benign. A generalized type of vascular nevus called "blue rubber-bleb nevus" is described on page 1185.

It is understandable that the waxing and waning of hemangiomas, complicated by the anxiety of parents, have led to much disagreement concerning need for and results of treatment. It is now believed that it is best to leave most vascular nevi to their natural fate, namely spontaneous regression.[5,9] Margileth and Museles[10] observed 210 children with cutaneous hemangiomas (strawberry, cavernous and mixed) and observed that 76% regressed within 7 years. Complications were common in a group that was actively treated. The benign course of the anomaly can be complicated by ulceration or hemorrhage. Ulceration, in turn, may be complicated by infections of various kinds. If bleeding caused by injuries occurs, it usually is easily controlled. Such complications may interfere with spontaneous regression and disappearance of the nevus.[5] Walsh and Tompkins,[2] who believed that there is a correlation between the size of the supplying normal artery and the potential for extensive, rapid growth, recommended immediate treatment because of unusual growth potential of lesions occurring over the head and neck, shoulders, genitalia, thenar eminence and ankles. Other reasons given for initiation of surgical, radiologic or steroid treatment are facial disfigurement, obstruction of a vital orifice or parental pressure. Individualized treatment of angiomas in infants and children was discussed by Martin.[6]

Giant Hemangioma with Thrombocytopenia (Kasabach-Merritt Syndrome)

In 1940, Kasabach and Merritt[11] reported a case of capillary hemangioma with extensive purpura. Since then, many cases of large hemangiomas with thrombocytopenia have been observed and, in 1962, Hill and Longino[12] collected the histories of 43 patients with this syndrome. The majority of the patients had vascular tumors at birth but purpura and petechiae appeared subsequently. The hemangiomas were of different types and locations, single or multiple, superficial and protuberant or deeply penetrating, with involvement of muscles and bones. When the tumor disappeared or was successfully treated, the thrombocytopenia subsided. But not all patients with large hemangiomas have thrombocytopenia.[12] It is now generally assumed that the hemangiomas "collect," utilize and destroy platelets. Masses of platelets have been found on microscopic examination in thrombi within such tumors or platelet counts were higher in blood drawn from the hemangioma than from the peripheral blood. Thrombocytopenia may not be the only hematologic defect of patients with hemangiomas. Leukopenia, leukocytosis and anemia[13] have been observed. Respiratory difficulties can be due to laryngeal and tracheal hemangiomas. Association with arteriovenous fistula, atrial septal defect and anomalous venous return has been reported.[14] A variant of the syndrome was described by Katz and Askin,[28] who saw multiple hemangiomas associated with thrombopenia. Hydronephrosis, renal lithiasis and hepatosplenomegaly also were present in their case. Treatment of the vascular tumor by irradiation[15] or by surgical excision[12] repeatedly resulted in return of the platelet count to normal. Administration of corticosteroids for treatment of hemangiomas with thrombocytopenia must be considered.[28]

Nevus Flammeus

A nevus flammeus (telangiectaticus) consists of one or several dull red or bluish patches that are well defined and not elevated above the level of the skin. It is made up of capillaries within the dermis and often shows segmental distribution (port-wine nevus). Nevus flammeus represents neither a genetic nor a histologic entity.[16] At birth, the color is bright red but with increasing age it becomes dull red or wine red. After the fifth decade of life, there may be tuberous transformation within the lesion. Nevi flammei, which are congenital, grow in proportion with the body as a whole without an abnormal growth tendency. Their distribution may correspond to that of a nerve, particularly the branches of the trigeminus. They often are unilateral and related to the embryonic facial processes and limited by their furrows. Extensive nevi flammei often are merely a part of a more general disorder that can involve soft tissues and bone, tongue, lips and gums. The Sturge-Weber syndrome (p. 349) and the Klippel-Trenaunay syndrome (p. 1180) are combinations for which special terms have been coined.

Schnyder[16] found no dilatation of capillaries in histologic sections of young children. After the tenth year, ectasias appeared with enlarged vascular spaces in the skin. The condition represents a telangiectasia and not a true angioma.

Symmetric or median telangiectatic nevi are very

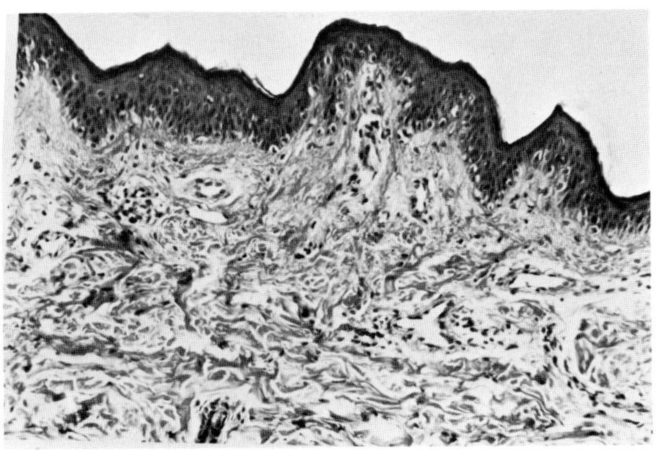

Fig. 118-7. – Section through skin with superficial telangiectasias.

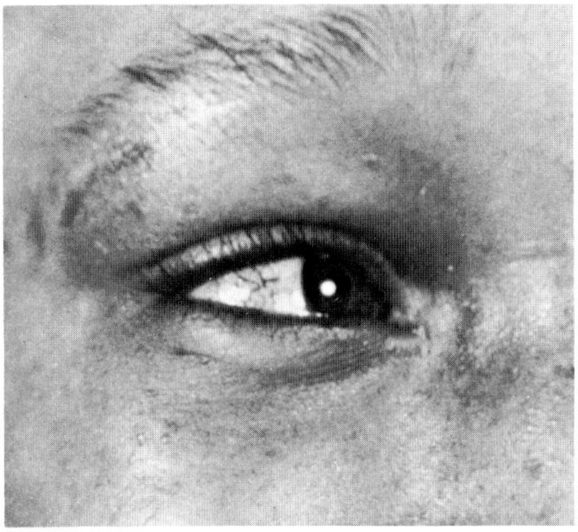

Fig. 118-8.—Telangiectases conjunctivae in a case of ataxia-telangiectasia.

frequent in infancy. They can be found on the nape of the neck in about 50% of all newborn children and they are almost equally frequent on the forehead and the eyelids. The alae nasi and the upper lip are affected in less than 10% of the newborn population. In the area of the neck (nuchal or occipital nevus, nevus Unna), the nevi are rather pale and indistinct. With increasing age, they tend to disappear, but even in the third decade traces can be found in about 20% of the population, twice as often in women as in men.[16]

Nevi flammei at the root of the nose or in the midline of the forehead have a tendency to become pale and to disappear by the third year of life. They often are combined with similar nevi of the upper eyelids and—less frequently—with nevi of the upper lip. These nevi also disappear, as a rule, in early childhood. Nevi flammei in the sacral area are rare.[16]

A different type of telangiectases is an important constituent of the "ataxia-telangiectasia syndrome,"[17] which has been discussed elsewhere (p. 270). The ocular and facial telangiectases are not observed at birth but they appear within the first few years of life of the patients. Characteristically, they are located in the lateral parts of the conjunctiva bulbi, often leaving free the border of the cornea. Telangiectasia progresses to the skin of the face, to the palate, the neck, the antecubital and popliteal areas and to the dorsa of the hands and feet. The telangiectasia is symmetric, predominantly arterial and not visible in infrared photographs. Enlarged veins and venules are found in the meninges and in the cerebellum.[17] Association of these vascular changes with agammaglobulinemia, absence or anomalies of the thymus and with malignancies has been observed.

Dominant inheritance of nuchal nevus flammeus has been reported.[16] The ataxia-telangiectasia syndrome is an autosomal recessive trait. Nevus flammeus occurs in most infants with trisomy 13-15. A tendency to bleeding because of multiple intestinal telangiectases has been observed in patients with Turner syndrome. Hemorrhages from the bowels seem to occur at the time of puberty (p. 1127). There are many reports of well-developed nevi flammei of the forehead, eyelids, nose and lips in children with the thalidomide embryopathy. These examples illustrate the heterogeneous etiology of these vascular lesions.

Nevus Vasculosus or Flammeus with Osteohypertrophy (Klippel-Trenaunay Syndrome)

This syndrome[18] consists of a nevus vasculosus or nevus flammeus combined with enlargement of the affected extremity. Only seldom has the contralateral side been larger than the affected side. The differences in thickness and length of the extremities can amount to several centimeters. The vascular lesion may be present at birth or develop at any time in later life. Spread of the lesion or lesions can occur. In most cases, the vascular nevus involves an extremity, but the neck, the chest or the genitalia can be affected. Vascular lesions also have been observed on the soft and hard palate, on the tongue and gingiva. In such cases, the jaws may be asymmetric and malocclusion can result.[19] Association with hexadactyly on the affected side and syndactyly on the other side has occurred.[20] The skin lesions are considered nevi vasculosi by some authors and nevi flammei by others. Arteriovenous aneurysms and congenital varices have been observed.[21] Hyperhidrosis, moisture and coolness of the abnormal extremity have been reported. Roentgenograms of the bones of the affected side may be normal, but cortical thickening has been described in some cases. Varices and phleboliths have been observed repeatedly. The disorder has been reported more often in males than in females but it is doubtful that the difference is significant.[21] The family history usually is noncontributory, but in several instances there was a tendency to nevus flammeus and cardiovascular anomalies in relatives of the mother.[20,22,23] Chromosome analyses showed normal karyotypes.[20]

Maffucci syndrome (p. 882) is a hemangiomatosis combined with dyschondroplasia. As in Klippel-Trenaunay syndrome, varices, phleboliths and vascular lesions are seen over the skeletal changes. But both the vascular and the skeletal changes differ in the two syndromes and Maffuci syndrome leads to much more serious and bizarre changes than that of Klippel-Trenaunay.

Generalized Congenital Phlebectasia (Cutis Marmorata Telangiectatica Congenita)

This rare congenital skin anomaly appears as mottling of the skin due to interlacing of enlarged superficial veins and formation of venous lakes. Although the disorder looks alarming, it seems to be benign, with a tendency to spontaneous regression.[24] But, in

PART XVIII

Tumors and Malformations

120

Tumors

FROM EARLY TIMES, relationships between congenital malformations and tumors have been explored by pathologists and discussions concerning the common roots of these developmental errors continue to present times. Some of the known facts about their relations and associations will be reviewed in the following pages. Congenital neoplasias will be treated because they, like congenital malformations, date back in origin to prenatal times. Some tumors are congenital malformations. Prenatal factors sometimes are also discernible in tumors that appear many years and even decades after birth, as shown by neoplasias resulting from genic or chromosomal abnormalities; therefore, the discussion will not be limited to congenital tumors. Multiple tumors in individuals and aggregation of neoplasias in families and kindreds will be considered because sometimes they reveal etiologic factors not recognizable in sporadic incidents. In the search for causes of cancers, environmental events were early considered as inciting factors. Chemical oncogens have been suspected since Percival Pott published his "Chirurgical observations relative to the cancer of the scrotum" in 1775.[1] Although other natural and man-made environmental cancerogenic factors became known subsequently, it was not until the second half of the twentieth century that intensive investigations of the role of chemical, actinic and viral carcinogens became possible through animal experimentation, epidemiologic studies, industrial surveillances and tissue culture methods. The possibility that exogenous agents reach the embryo or fetus through the mother must be considered and data concerning transplacental influences will be mentioned.

In the nineteenth century, most pathologists considered postnatal trauma and infection as important oncogenic factors but toward the end of that century attention turned to pathologic-embryologic events and prenatal determinants of tumors. In 1889, Cohnheim[2] rejected the theories of trauma and infection as causes of tumors. He believed that the origins of tumors are to be sought in faults or irregularities of embryonic rudiments and that in early stages of embryonic development more cells are produced than are required for formation of the parts concerned. There remains, according to this concept, an unappropriated quantity of cells—they may be very few in number—that, owing to their embryonic character, are endowed with a marked capacity for proliferation. This opinion was supported by early experiments that showed that fetal tissue introduced into the anterior chamber of the eye or into the abdominal cavity grew there surprisingly well. Cohnheim also based his theory on heredity of certain tumors. He knew of families in which the same kind of tumor appeared in successive generations of a kindred and he knew that certain tumors like enchondromas can be transmitted as systemic entities even though they make their appearance in postnatal life at different sites of the skeleton. It was well established that certain tumors were present at birth: teratomas, angiomas, fibromas, lipomas, enchondromas and many others were known to Cohnheim. True, congenital tumors form but an insignificant minority of all growths, and Cohnheim did not claim that tumors themselves generally are congenital but he believed that their rudiments are. Most newborn infants bring into the world not the tumors but superabundant cell material, and from the latter—if circumstances permit—tumors may develop in later life. Cohnheim thought that the impulse for growth is given when the blood supply becomes adequate, and he cited as an example exostoses, which begin to grow at the time when the general growth of the skeleton is most active, that is, at the period during which blood vessels are formed most abundantly. Dermoid tumors increase chiefly at puberty, when the appearance of the beard points to the occurrence of active developmental processes in the ectoderm. The cystomas of the ovary generally do not commence growing before puberty. It seemed conceivable that oft-repeated arterial congestion, or even inflammatory hyperemias, can stimulate the development of tumor rudiments and in this way theories of traumatic etiology of tumors seemed acceptable. But such exciting factors were recognizable only rarely. For most tumors, physiologic circulation seemed to be sufficient to initiate the development of a rudiment, but many individuals with bodies containing rudiments could complete life without any growth of the tumor anlage. Mechanical irritation did not seem a satisfactory explanation for tumors. Although certain epithelial tumors show a special preference for the orifices of the body, such as the lips, alae nasi, eyelids or rectum, they cannot be attributed entirely to mechanical insults, since the hands and feet, which are exposed to such irritation constantly, do not show the same tendency to development of tumors. The orifices named may be at some embryonic stages the site of developmental complications when some slight irregularity may produce a group of superfluous epithelial cells, that is, rudiments of a tumor. Epithelial pearls in the mouth and in female external genitalia were known at that time as examples of such growths. Cohnheim's theories seemed particularly applicable to heterologous growths, tumors that in structure depart completely from that of the substratum in which they originate; they could be explained by cell rests or embryonic vestiges of heterologous tissue. The theory was best supported by the close resemblance of embryonal tumors with certain types of embryonic tissues. Ribbert[3] expanded and altered the oncogenic theory of embryonal germs by including postnatal separation of cell groups from their natural environment as a cause of blastomatous growth.

Albrecht[4] emphasized organ-like malformations that include various tissues as possible origins of tumors. He considered not only hamartomas and choristomas but also persisting unused cells, postembryonal organ formations, products of regeneration and growths from embryonal clefts. Observations of multiple primary tumors and of systemic tendencies to tumors pointed to developmental origins. The last group, systemic disorders predisposing to oncogenesis, anticipated the concept of hamartoses, which we now recognize as hereditary tendencies to tissue malformations and tumors (Chapters 121–124). Cautious investigators emphasized that one must not consider developmental disturbances as the basis of all tumors (they knew of carcinomas caused by x-irradiation), but they were thought to be on solid ground when they assumed that teratomas, teratoblastomas, choristomas, hamartomas and other "dysontogenetic" tumors had their origin in developmental errors. In 1913, Herxheimer[5] published a critical review on *tissue malformations* in Schwalbe's *Morphologie der Missbildungen des Menschen und der Tiere.* Since most tissue malformations ("Gewebsmissbildungen") discussed by him are microscopic structural anomalies present at birth, they fall within our definition of congenital malformations. Their relations to oncogenesis were, and still are, of great interest to pathologists, oncologists and teratologists. The subject of tissue malformations was new and exciting at Herxheimer's time, and pathologists discussed the fate of abnormal cell aggregations, their transformation, disappearance and growth, including tumor formation. Questions of maturity, maturation, heterotopia and heterochronicity were dealt with in deliberations that are still timely. Relationships of oncology to teratology have been and still are rediscovered through various approaches, particularly by investigators who deal with tumors of children.

Tumors of the fetus, infant and child have certain peculiarities that distinguish them from tumors of adults. Ewing[6] and Andersen[7] thought that most childhood tumors arise as embryonal rests and are, therefore, congenital. This origin seemed particularly evident for mixed tumors, which have a high incidence in children. Ewing,[6] discussing childhood cancers, pointed out that in the first 15 years of life there are many specific neoplastic diseases that are rare in later life. Within the first 7 years, Wilms tumor, retinoblastoma, neuroblastoma and others are relatively frequent occurrences. Then, in the period between 8 and 15 years, there is a sharp decline of malignant tumors. This decrease of cancers was, to Ewing, a "fact of fundamental biologic importance, suggesting that the causative factors of infancy have exhausted themselves and that thereafter new conditions of origin, new types of tumors may be expected. . . ." Ewing also stated that the great majority of tumors of infancy are embryonal in type and that many are of complex teratoid structure, "indicating conditions of origin that fall under the conception of Cohnheim's theory." He believed that the isolation of tissue rests must occur in the embryo before birth and that most of the tumors of infants and children must be regarded as essentially congenital, although they may become manifest later in life. Andersen[7] found it difficult to draw a sharp line between malformations and benign tumors of childhood. Thus, cysts derived from branchial clefts or intestine, epidermoid cysts, hemangiomas and nevi must be considered congenital aberrations. The same is true for many malignant tumors of childhood, according to Andersen.[7] Malignant tumors appearing within the first 5 years show embryonic cells and tissues and many are so different from those of adults that their identification is difficult in terms of adult pathology. She, too, found that after the early years of life, malignant tumors of embryonal origin become rarer. In 1959, Fèvre and Huguenin[8] published a book entitled *Malformations Tumorales et Tumeurs de l'Enfant.* They stated that many tumors of children are at the same time tumors and malformations and emphasized that many transitional forms exist between these developmental anomalies. This book, which combines the view of the pediatric surgeon with that of the oncologist, demonstrates the practical importance and the wide scope of the tumor malformations encountered during childhood. The area is not limited to the interests of pathologists and teratologists; it is an important field of many clinical specialties. Tumors were dealt with in their book according to regions or organ systems with reference to pathogenesis, diagnosis and treatment; etiologic investigations and classifications are still to be made for many of the interesting conditions described by Fèvre and Huguenin.[8]

In Willis'[9] *The Borderland of Embryology and Pathology,* which appeared in 1962, the subject was brought up to date. Detailed chapters were devoted to Developmental Vestiges and Their Pathology, to Developmentally Heterotopic Tissues; to Hamartomas and Hamartomatous Syndromes; and to Embryonic Tumors and Teratomas. In that book and in his *Pathology of Tumors*,[10] Willis dealt with the borderland of malformations and tumors in great detail and exhaustively. Only a few of the subjects treated by him are mentioned in this chapter to illustrate some of the connections of teratology and oncology, to exemplify the relationship of developmental errors to oncogenesis in prenatal and postnatal life and to emphasize the role of malformations in clinical pediatrics. Certain aspects of this borderland of medicine have found special attention in recent years because of rising interests of geneticists and epidemiologists in tumors and malformations. Others still need to be developed. The interactions of genetic tendencies with environmental (prenatal and postnatal) oncogenic factors are under investigation by new methods. Yet, these methods still are not fully established, and sometimes contradictory results are reported.

More than 80 years have passed since Cohnheim[2] formulated his ideas on the etiology of neoplasia and it seems worth while to review some of his thoughts at a time when both oncology and teratology have become fields of intensive research. Although the majority of oncologists now concentrate on investigations of postnatal environmental factors in the search for the causes of cancer, there is room for consideration of prenatal determinants of tumors—genetic or environmental—that may be responsible for or contributory to some oncologic phenomena. It is obvious that tumors of the neonate and the young child are particularly suited for research in prenatal oncogenesis.

Embryonal tumors.—Embryonal tumors are considered both neoplasms and malformations. They are derived from specific organ rudiments, consist of immature tissues and are due to developmental errors during the embryonal and fetal periods. Willis[9] pointed out that certain tissues such as the brain, sympathetic ganglia and kidneys continue differentiating during early postnatal life, so that some of the so-called embryonal tumors may not be truly congenital but develop after birth. They originate from immature tissues but these tissues are already differentiated to a certain extent, demonstrating signs of organ specificity and showing limitation in their ability to form tissues characteristic of other organs. In this respect, they differ from teratomas, which are descended from "regionally undetermined" cells, probably germ cells, capable of much more divergent differentiation.[9] Embryonal tumors such as neuroblastomas, nephroblastomas, rhabdomyomas and others have been seen in fetuses and stillborn infants. Many more have been observed at birth. Others make their appearance in infancy or early childhood and some are delayed until adult life. Thus, there can be no sharp definition of these tumors by the age at which they arise and by the age at which they become manifest.

Although it can be assumed that most tumors of infancy and early childhood originate in fetal life and are congenital, only those neoplasias that have been observed in fetuses and newborn children are proved to be independent of postnatal etiologic factors. If such congenital tumors resemble growths that manifest themselves after birth, their existence supports the view that those discovered later are also prenatal in origin.

Congenital tumors.—Wells[11] pointed out in 1940 that certain types of malignant growth are seen almost exclusively in the very young and some neoplasias develop in the fetus, producing widespread metastases before the brief span of intrauterine existence has been accomplished. These tumors must differ fundamentally from the ordinary adult types of cancer, which require long periods for development, a difference that can throw some light on oncogenesis in general. Wells considered the older literature on congenital cancers, which is unconvincing in many cases, and reviewed the subject thoroughly. He himself had found in about 3,000 necropsies on newborn infants, including many prematures, only four congenital malignant neoplasms; all were neuroblastomas, three in the adrenal and one in the sympathetic nervous system. Of two hundred fifty neoplasms reported by others as malignant and present at birth, he considered only sixty-six as proved. Sarcomas and neuroblastomas were the leading forms of congenital malignancy but there was no convincing proof of congenital carcinomas. Neurogenic malignant tumors derived from the sympathetic nervous system and from the retina were commonly present at birth, but congenital neoplasms of the brain and peripheral nerves were extremely rare. With the exception of retinoblastoma, congenital tumors showed no familial or hereditary influence. Congenital leukemia had not been transmitted from mother to fetus. Since the bulk of human malignant tumors require a large part of the life cycle for development—in contrast to the malignant growths appearing before or soon after birth, which develop within a few months after conception—Wells thought that congenital tumors depend on mechanisms different from those that require years or decades for their formation. It seemed that the tissues that give rise to congenital tumor have metabolic characteristics common to embryos and to tumors.

Since Wells' review in 1940, a great deal of information has been added to the knowledge of congenital tumors. The sarcoma group, which dominated in his survey, probably is still prevalent but it is now broken down into several subgroups. Congenital carcinoma has been reported in the thyroid (p. 1219), in the liver (p. 727) and in connection with various teratomas. Wells[11] had listed 2 cases of congenital glioma reported in the literature. Congenital brain tumors are still not recorded often, but additional intracranial gliomas, teratomas, hemangiomas and others have been observed at birth. It has been recognized that congenital brain tumors may present as hydrocephaly, convulsive disorders and as neurologic or metabolic disturbances. Nasal gliomas (p. 591) usuallly are recognized at birth because of tumors situated at the root of the nose and sacrococcygeal teratomas because of their association with spina bifida. There is little doubt about the congenital nature of most retinoblastomas, although only a limited number are recognized at birth. Neuroblastomas are still a leading form of congenital tumors, as pointed out by Wells,[11] and prenatal metastases have been described repeatedly. Congenital pheochromocytomas apparently have not been reported. Among soft tissue tumors, sarcomas, rhabdomyosarcomas, neurofibromas, fibromatoses, embryonal hepatomas, hemangioendotheliomas of the liver, nephroblastomas (Wilms tumor), mesoblastic nephromas, ovarian cysts, testicular neoplasias and botryoid sarcomas have been observed in the neonate.[9,23] Congenital leukemias are relatively uncommon, yet many instances have been recorded because of their unusual interest. The subject of congenital tumors in animals was reviewed by Misdorp.[12] He observed eight cases of congenital neoplasias in calves: two lymphoid leukemias, two peritoneal mesotheliomas, two nephroblastomas, one lymphangioma on the lower leg and one mixed mesenchymal tumor.

Most congenital neoplasias originate in the fetus. Wells[11] listed only four acceptable instances of malignant growths passed on from mother to fetus. Melanosarcoma, carcinoma and lymphosarcoma were the malignancies transmitted. It is of interest that in the cases of maternal melanosarcoma the children's tumors did not become manifest before 8 months after birth and death occurred at 10 months of age. Similarly, in a case reported later, acute lymphocytic leukemia transmitted from a mother to her fetus was not recognized in the child before the age of 9 months. These observations point to congenital presence of neoplasias that manifest themselves belatedly in infancy or early childhood; they support the view that tumors recognized in infancy or early childhood often are congenital even if disease and death occur only after birth. Thus, distinction between congenital and infantile tumors may be unnecessarily rigorous in many cases. It seems likely today, as pointed out by Ewing[6] in 1940, that many cancers of infancy and childhood have their origin in prenatal life, although their manifestations are delayed; but it seems equally established that some of the embryonal rudiments that form the basis of congenital tumors are capable of maturation or disappearance without trace, as in the case of in situ neuroblastomas or of arrested retinoblastomas (p. 380).

MULTIPLE PRIMARY TUMORS.—Occurrence of multiple primary tumors in patients with cancer and leukemia is of considerable interest to the student of etiology and epidemiology of neoplasia. Sometimes multiplicity of tumors is noted in living patients but, more often, necropsy reveals more than one growth in a person who died of cancer. Early pathologists, who noticed such concurrences, speculated that persons with multiple primary tumors may have a constitutional susceptibility to cancer and other tumors.[13-16] Prenatal factors involved in such constitutional tendencies were suggested by familial incidences[17,18] or by the presence of associated malformations.[19] Much has been written since about multiple primary malignant and benign lesions and there still is no agreement concerning their meaning and interpretation. Multiple primary cancers were found in 3–5% of necropsies[19-21] but, in some studies, multiple primaries were discovered much more often[22,23] and in one necropsy series they amounted to 11%.[24] It is significant that 55% of the second tumors originated in tissues and organs different from the first ones, whereas 45% showed multiplicity in the same organ system.[20] Predisposition to multiple primary tumors seems to be most pronounced in the digestive and respiratory tracts.[19,21,25] Interpretation sometimes is complicated by the fact that some of the tumors are synchronous, whereas others are metachronous in development. In the case of metachronous tumors, i.e., second tumors developing some time after the first, one must consider the possibility that treatment of the original tumor by x-rays or drugs caused the second malignancy.[21] This was best illustrated by a case of thyroid cancer treated by radioactive iodine, when the patient developed pancytopenia soon after treatment and died of acute myelogenous leukemia 2 years later.[26] Malignant neoplasms associated with leukemia have attracted attention. The association exists in many instances but interpretation is difficult.[27] A review by Amromin[28] showed that associated malignant neoplasms are noted most often in patients with chronic lymphatic leukemia, the form that usually is seen in age groups in which malignancy is not rare and in patients who live long enough to allow evolvement of a cancer. X-ray treatment or drug treatment may be causative in some of these cases.[29] In general surveys of multiple primary malignant neoplasms, concurrence of the tumors was thought to be coincidental, since proof for systemic carcinogenic influences or increased susceptibility of affected persons seemed to be lacking.[18] But, in several studies, an excess of blood group A has been found in patients with multiple primary cancers,[25,30] suggesting genetic influences. That multiple tumors, benign or malignant, are not always coincidental is best exemplified by the hamartoses (Chapters 121–123), which frequently are the basis of multiple neoplasia. Genetic influences are obvious in these disorders, which are transmitted like autosomal dominant traits. It is probable that many more hamartoses exist than those recognized and described by now. Multiple tumors also occur in the "multiple endocrine neoplasias," which, like hamartoses, are inherited like autosomal dominant traits. Medullary thyroid carcinoma, pheochromocytoma, tumors of the parathyroid, fibromas and others can occur in "MEN type 2" or pituitary, parathyroid or pancreatic island cell tumors in "MEN type 1" (Chapter 124).

In children with cancer and leukemia, second primary tumors are not frequent but they probably are more significant than those in adults, in whom the general risk for tumors increases with advancing age. Regelson *et al.*[25] found that among 150 children on whom necropsies were performed there were 8 (5.3%) who had two primary tumors; in 2 of these children, sarcomas developed within a radiation portal many years after irradiation treatment of the first tumors, so that the second, metachronous tumors probably were post-therapeutic and postnatal in origin. Salmon *et al.*[31] reported a nephroblastoma in an infant treated surgically and by irradiation, which was followed after 15 months by a sympathoblastoma. A patient who had carcinoma of the colon and neuro-astrocytoma of the right frontal lobe had had a father and a paternal grandfather with neoplasias.[25] A similar kindred with hereditary polyposis and extra-alimentary-tract tumors was reported by Fraumeni *et al.*[32] Other patients in whom glioblastoma multiforme and hepatocarcinoma, retinoblastoma and Hodgkin disease, adrenal neuroblastoma and rhabdomyoma of the heart, neuroastrocytoma and acute lymphocytic leukemia or benign sigmoid polyps and acute myeloblastic leukemia were synchronously linked showed no obvious signs of familial aggregation.

Thus, multiplicity of primary tumors may have different causes. It may be genetically determined and due to hamartoses or to multiple endocrine neoplasia diatheses. Aggregation of such tumors can be striking in certain families or kindreds, although they seem numerically insignificant in general tumor surveys. Environmental carcinogenic factors also could cause multiple and even familial tumors. Viruses and chemical compounds could be suspected in such cases and treatment of a tumor with x-rays or drugs could be responsible for second metachronous tumor.

FAMILIAL TUMORS.—Observations of aggregation of tumors in families and kinships, known to early clinicians and pathologists, have been amplified by many recent investigations. Hamartoses and adenomatoses represent some of the well-established disorders that predispose to benign and malignant tumors (Chapters 121–124). Although dominant autosomal inheritance is clearly suggested for these disorders, the oncogenic factors transmitted are still obscure. Many apparently heterogeneous tumors develop within the framework of these heritable maladies; without knowledge of the familial condition, the tumors may be considered sporadic and accidental. One and the same type of tumor, e.g., glioma, can be a manifestation of neurofibromatosis, tuberous sclerosis or hereditary polyposis; and pheochromocytoma may occur in patients with neurofibromatosis, Hippel-Lindau disease or multiple endocrine neoplasia, type II (Chapters 121–124). Retinoblastomas can be of diverse origin (Chapter 39, p. 380); in some instances, they seem to be transmitted like a dominant hereditary trait; in others, they are associated with a deletion of a chromosome of the 13-15 (D) group; and in many cases, they are sporadic and obscure in etiology. Familial instances of Wilms tumor (p. 1063), hepatoblastoma and other liver cancers (p. 1222), neuroblastoma (p. 1223) and adrenocortical tumors (p. 1226) have been reported.

Although genetic predisposition is strongly suggested in familial cases of tumor, we know nothing about the accessory oncogenic factors that lead to tumor formation in some of the persons who carry the mutant gene, whereas they leave others unaffected. Accessory factors could be genetic or environmental. It should be emphasized that recurrence of tumors in a family must not be attributed to heredity without good proof. To give one example: skin cancer in a father and 2 of his sons could be attributed to dominant inheritance, but if all 3 were chimney sweeps,[1] the familial recurrence could be due to similar exposure to soot and not due to a genetic mechanism. Other environmental oncogens that are more concealed and evasive could cause familial cancers, which should not be glibly attributed to inheritance.

Interaction of genetic and nongenetic factors in the etiology of congenital malformations is demonstrated by observations of monozygotic twins with concordant or discordant tumors. There are reports of concordance of monozygotic twins in regard to leukemia, glioma, retinoblastoma, cardiac rhabdomyoma and neuroblastoma, but there also was discordance in some such twins. Leukemia also has been observed in both members of a pair of dizygotic twins. Such observations demonstrate the complexity of the etiology of neoplasms and the role of accessory and imponderable factors.

ENVIRONMENTAL ONCOGENIC FACTORS.—Carcinogens in the human environment are now under intensive study.[33] Physical, chemical,[34] parasitic agents and particularly viruses[35,36] are known or suspected as oncogenic agents. Some of these agents occur in man's natural environment (ultraviolet radiation, radioactive soil, pollutants of drinking water, *Schistosoma haematobium*), whereas others are man-made. The latter group includes carcinogens that have long been part of the human environment (soot, tobacco, betel nut quids) and, more important, the carcinogens of recent origin that are products of modern industrial development and are under scrutiny by qualified investigators as well as by legislators and the lay public. Some of the carcinogenic factors under consideration are proved contributors to human cancer, others are suspected for various reasons.[33,34] Carcinogenesis by chemicals is of particular importance[37] but actinic[38] and viral causes[36,39] deserve equal attention. Most investigations dealing with environmental carcinogens were and are concerned with postnatal exposures, but it is obvious that prenatal exposure to environmental oncogens must be considered a cause of congenital and postnatal forms of cancer. Studies of prenatal exposure to radiation during obstetric examinations[40,41] illustrate the search for such causes of childhood cancer. It has been suggested that prenatal exposure to x-rays during abdominal radiation or pelvimetry of pregnant women exerts a carcinogenic effect during the first 10 years of postnatal life.[42] On the other hand, there was no significant excess of mortality from leukemia or other cancers in children exposed prenatally in 1945 to the atomic bombs in Hiroshima and Nagasaki.[43]

There is experimental evidence that carcinogenic chemical compounds can reach the fetus transplacentally and bring about tumors in postnatal life. It has been shown that urethan injected into pregnant mice of certain strains enhances the percentage of tumors commonly occurring in such animals,[44-46] but, under appropriate conditions, urethan also can induce de novo neoplasia in a variety of tissues.[47] Carcinogens other than urethan have been shown to initiate neoplasia in utero and in early postnatal life. It seems that susceptible proliferative stages vary in different tissues, so that some tissues respond to carcinogenic stimuli only before birth, whereas others are still responsive in postnatal life.[47] If these experiments have any application to human conditions, they would suggest that neoplasms of infancy and early childhood could be due to perinatal or postnatal environmental events and should caution against the assumption that all tumors of infancy are prenatal in origin.

Transplacental oncogenic experiments have been extended to several species and to many carcinogenic compounds. It was shown that ethylnitrosourea administered to rats in late pregnancy can induce malignant tumors of the brain, spinal cord or peripheral nervous system. Druckrey *et al.*[48] estimated that fetal tissues were at least ten times as sensitive as adult tissues to the carcinogenic action of nitroso-compounds. Reactivity to such chemical oncogens changed with time; the yield of tumors was highest when ethylnitrosourea was given on the last days of pregnancy and zero before the twelfth day.[49] Thus, oncogenesis of this chemical compound seems to begin when teratogenesis declines, although there seems to be intermediate periods when both malformations and tumors can be induced. The relationships between experimental teratogenesis and oncogenesis have been reviewed by DiPaolo and Kotin.[50] Of special interest are experiments by Druckrey *et al.*[49] that showed that rats deformed by injection of ethylnitrosourea developed tumors of the nervous system at the age of 160–165 days. These rats, born with congenital malformations, develop tumors subsequently; in all probability, malformations and tumors are induced in this case by the same chemical substance. The experiment represents a model for a common environmental origin of congenital malformations and tumors. It remains to be seen whether comparable situations occur in man.

CONGENITAL MALFORMATIONS.—Association of neoplasias with congenital malformations give *indirect* evidence of prenatal determination of some tumors, but such associations require analysis, since they may differ in significance. There are malformations that probably are the result and not the cause of the tumor. Large teratomas of the mouth or of the sacrococcygeal region bring about structural anomalies in their surroundings by their size and expansion. Hydrocephaly caused by a brain tumor that obstructs the cerebrospinal fluid circulation is the result of the location of the growth. In other situations, it is difficult to decide whether a tumor or the associated malformations was the primary defect. Nasal gliomas combined with frontal encephaloceles or lipomas in place of an absent corpus callosum exemplify such questionable relationships. Hamartomas and choristomas are malformations as well as tumors. There are congenital malformations that result in tumor formation in a limited number of cases only, so that accessory oncogenic factors must be assumed. Thus, thyroglossal duct cysts, atretic congenital bile ducts and supernumerary, ectopic or horseshoe kidneys predispose to neoplasia.

There are many heritable disorders—hamartoses and multiple endocrine adenomatoses—that result in benign tumors of many kinds and in some patients such benign tumors become the site of malignancies (Chapters 121–124). Multiple exostoses, osteogenesis imperfecta and osteopetrosis have a limited tendency to neoplasias; and xeroderma pigmentosum, epidermolysis bullosa, dyskeratosis congenita and blue rubber-bleb nevus carry a certain risk of malignancy.

Some malformations attributable to chromosomal abnormalities show significant associations with neoplasia. Down syndrome and leukemia or sex anomalies and gonadal tumors exemplify such associations. In the case of sex anomalies, the tendency to tumors is not limited to patients with cytogenetic abnormalities, since testicular feminization—a gene-determined disorder—also has a tendency to gonadal tumor formation. Extragonadal tumors have been observed not only in patients with XO Turner syndrome but also in the male Turner syndrome, which is seen in persons with normal karyotype (p. 1131). There are relationships of tumors to congenital disorders of unknown etiology. Hemihypertrophy and its association with renal, hepatic or adrenocortical tumors will be mentioned in subsequent pages. Through hemihypertrophy, such tumors also are related to a form of aniridia and to visceromegaly. Patients with Maffucci syndrome, a disorder of unknown etiology, have a marked tendency to develop chondromas, angiomas, various types of sarcoma, lymphangiomas and others. Ollier disease and fibrous dysplasia of bone apparently have an increased risk of malignancy (Chapter 94). Thus, there are associations of differing and often unknown causation.

In general epidemiologic reviews, association of congenital malformations and embryonic tumors of childhood may not be obvious. Berry *et al.*[51] examined the records of patients with neuroblastoma, nephroblastoma, hepatoblastoma and teratoma and found no significant association between neoplasia and malformation. An exception were sacrococcygeal teratomas, which showed an increase in frequency of major malformations. But if anomalies attributable to local growth effects of these teratomas were excluded, the over-all incidence of associated malformations was not significantly different from controls. In contrast, a very high incidence of malformations was found by Kobayashi *et al.*[52] in cases of tumors ascertained by the Childhood Cancer Registry of the Tokyo Metropolitan Area. These authors considered major and minor anomalies, including dermatoglyphics, epicanthi and small skin and ear malformations. As controls, they used incidence figures of major and minor anomalies found in patients with nonmalignant disease or without obvious congenital malformations. Congenital anomalies were much more frequent in children with malignancies (41%) than in children with nonmalignant or nondeforming diseases (13%). Major congenital malformations, such as congenital heart disease, facial clefts and other defects requiring surgical intervention, were found associated more often with Wilms tumor and other embryonal and teratomatous tumors than with leukemia and lymphoma. In the latter group, minor congenital anomalies prevailed.

Probably more significant are epidemiologic studies, which revealed associations between specific tumors and specific malformations. An example is the finding of excessive occurrence of aniridia, hemihypertrophy, genitourinary tract anomalies and pigmented nevi and vascular tumors among children with Wilms tumor.[53] Hemihypertrophy also is excessively associated with adrenal and hepatic tumors of childhood.[54,55]

No excessive association was found by Miller *et al.*[56] between neuroblastoma and specific congenital malformations. A lack of association of neuroblastoma and congenital malformations also was noted by other authors.[9,51] But Beckwith and Perrin,[57] who reported on in situ neuroblastomas encountered in necropsies of young infants, observed serious malformations in other organs, particularly in the cardiovascular system in 69% of the cases. Shanklin and Sotelo-Avila[58] described three in situ neuroblastomas and two in situ nephroblastomas, all associated with congenital malformations. Bove *et al.*,[59] in a survey of necropsy records, found multiple, small nodular renal blastemas that were histologically similar to Wilms tumor. The nodules were associated with multiple congenital anomalies in all cases and were detected in serial sections of 5 of 8 cases with the trisomy 18 syndrome. The association of such in situ tumors with congenital malformations must be interpreted with caution; it does not permit application of the findings to such other tumors as neuroblastomas or Wilms tumors of *clinical significance*, since most of the in situ tumors seem to disappear spontaneously without becoming clinically apparent. In addition, the in situ tumors were observed in necropsy material often selected through death resulting from congenital malformations. Through a study of U.S. death certificates, Miller[60] established some relationships between oncogenesis and teratogenesis. In addition to the associations of Wilms tumor with aniridia or renal anomalies and of Down syndrome with leukemia, which had been reported previously, there were associations of leukemia with congenital systemic disorders such as osteogenesis imperfecta, Marfan syndrome, Treacher Collins syndrome and Ollier disease. Concurrences of tetralogy of Fallot and glioma and of cleidocranial dystostosis and medulloblastoma were considered of possible etiologic significance. This study was based on death certificates of 24,457 children who died of cancer, in contrast to 383 children ascertained through hospital records[51] or 371 children registered at a Childhood Cancer Registry.[52] The value of the large death certificate figures is reduced by the fact that, as a rule, congenital defects are greatly underreported in certificates of children who die of cancer. The excess of leukemia in patients with Down syndrome was only 11-fold over the normal, whereas it is found to be 15–20-fold in studies with more complete ascertainment.[51,53,60] Major congenital malformations other than Down syndrome were about twice as numerous among leukemic children as among their matched controls in a national leukemia survey.[62]

Thus, the associations of congenital malformations and tumors are complex in origin, needing further analysis and experimentation. Although well established in certain disorders, they may be coincidental or spurious in others. In the following sections, a variety of neoplasias will be discussed in regard to facts of biologic interest relating to prenatal and postnatal etiology.

REFERENCES

1. Pott, P.: Chirurgical observations relative to the cancer of the scrotum, Nat. Cancer Inst. Monogr. 10:7, 1963.
2. Cohnheim, J.: *Lectures on General Pathology* (London: The New Sydenham Society, 1889), Vol. II.
3. Ribbert, H.: Die Herkunft der Geschwülste, Deutsche med. Wchnschr. 45:1265, 1919.
4. Albrecht, D. P. G.: Hamartomas, Verhandl. deutsch. Gesellsch. Path. 7:153, 1904.
5. Herxheimer, G.: Gewebsmissbildungen, in Schwalbe, E. (ed.), *Die Morphologie der Missbildungen des Menschen und der Tiere* (Jena: Gustav Fischer, 1913), Pt. III, Chap. II.
6. Ewing, J.: A Survey of Cancer in Childhood, in Dargeon, H. W. (ed.), *Cancer in Childhood* (St. Louis: The C. V. Mosby Company, 1940).
7. Andersen, D. H.: Tumors of infancy and children, Cancer 4:890, 1951.
8. Fèvre, M., and Huguenin, R.: *Malformations Tumorales et Tumeurs de l'Enfant* (Paris: Masson & Cie, 1954).
9. Willis, R. A.: *The Borderland of Embryology and Pathology* (Washington, D. C.: Butterworth, 1962).
10. Willis, R. A.: *Pathology of Tumors* (4th ed.; New York: Appleton-Century-Crofts, 1967).
11. Wells, H. G.: Occurrence and significance of congenital malignant neoplasms, Arch. Path. 30:535, 1940.
12. Misdorp, W.: Tumors in newborn animals, Path. Vet. 2:328, 1965.
13. Harbitz, F.: Über das gleichzeitige Auftreten mehrerer selbständig wachsender ("multipler") Geschwülste, Beitr. path. Anat. 62:503, 1916.
14. Rössle, R.: Multiple Tumoren und ihre Bedeutung für die Frage der konstitutionellen Entstehungsbedingungen der Geschwülste, Ztschr. Ang. Anat. 5:126, 1919.

15. Siebke, H.: Über multiple Carcinome, Ztschr. Krebsforsch. 23:66, 1926.
16. Warren, S., and Gates, O.: Multiple primary malignant tumors. A survey of the literature and a statistical study, Am. J. Cancer 16:1358, 1932.
17. Stalker, L. K., Phillips, R. B., and Pemberton, J. de J.: Multiple primary malignant lesions, Surg., Gynec. & Obst. 68:595, 1939.
18. Moertel, C. G., Dockerty, M. B., and Baggenstoss, A. H.: Multiple primary malignant neoplasms. II. Tumors of different tissues or organs, Cancer 14:231, 1961.
19. Hellendahl, H.: Multiple carcinoma. The clinical picture, diagnosis and prognosis, Am. J. Surg. 60:22, 1943.
20. Moertel, C. G., Dockerty, M. B., and Baggenstoss, A. H.: Multiple primary malignant neoplasms. I. Introduction and presentation of data, Cancer 14:221, 1961.
21. Thoma, G. W.: The incidence and significance of multiple primary malignant tumors, Am. J. M. Sc. 247:427, 1964.
22. Warren, S., and Ehrenreich, J.: Multiple primary malignant tumors and susceptibility to cancer, Cancer Res. 4:554, 1944.
23. Lombard, H. L., and Warren, S.: Association of other malignant tumors with cancer of the skin, Am. J. Pub. Health 33:533, 1943.
24. Pickren, J. W.: Cancer often strikes twice, New York J. Med. 63:95, 1963.
25. Regelson, W., Bross, I. D. J., Hananian, J., and Nigogosyan, G.: Incidence of second primary tumors in children with cancer and leukemia, Cancer 18:58, 1965.
26. Delarue, J., Tubiana, M., and Dutreix, J.: Cancer de la thyroide traité par l'iode radioactif: Terminaison par une leucémie aiguë après une amélioration importante, Bull. Assoc. franç. étude cancer 40:263, 1953.
27. Moertel, C. G., and Hagedorn, A. B.: Leukemia or lymphoma and coexistent primary malignant lesions; review of literature and study of 120 cases, Blood 12:788, 1957.
28. Amromin, G. D.: *Pathology of Leukemia* (New York: Hoeber Medical Division, Harper & Row, Publishers, 1968).
29. Faber, M., and Borum, K.: Leukemia and a malignant tumor in the same patient, Brit. J. Haemat. 8:313, 1962.
30. Fadhli, H. A., and Dominquez, R.: ABO blood groups and multiple cancers, J.A.M.A. 185:757, 1963.
31. Salmon, M., Coignet, J., Raybaud, C., Lebreuil, G., and Passeron, P.: Succession d'un sympathoblastome chez un nourrisson, Pédiatrie 25:337, 1970.
32. Fraumeni, J. F., Jr., Vogel, C. L., and Easton, J. M.: Sarcomas and multiple polyposis in a kindred. A genetic variety of hereditary polyposis, Arch. Int. Med. 121:57, 1968.
33. Hueper, W. C.: Carcinogens in the human environment, Arch. Path. 71:237, 1961.
34. Clayson, D. B.: *Chemical Carcinogens* (Boston: Little, Brown & Company, 1962).
35. Gross, L.: *Oncogenic Viruses* (New York: Pergamon Press, 1961).
36. Burdette, W. J.: *Viruses Inducing Cancer* (Salt Lake City: University of Utah Press, 1966).
37. Miller, J. A.: Carcinogenesis by chemicals: An overview. G. H. A. Clowes Memorial Lecture, Cancer Res. 30:559, 1970.
38. Ford, D. D., Paterson, J. C. S., and Treuting, W. L.: Fetal exposure to diagnostic x-rays, and leukemia and other malignant diseases in childhood, J. Nat. Cancer Inst. 22:1093, 1959.
39. Black, P. H.: Recent advances in the study of oncogenic viruses, New England J. Med. 275:377, 1966.
40. Stewart, A., Webb, J., and Hewitt, D.: A survey of childhood malignancies, Brit. M. J. 1:1495, 1958.
41. MacMahon, B.: Prenatal x-ray exposure and childhood cancer, J. Nat. Cancer Inst. 28:1173, 1962.
42. Stewart, A., and Kneale, G. W.: Radiation dose effects in relation to obstetric x-rays and childhood cancers, Lancet 1:1185, 1970.
43. Jablon, S., and Kato, H.: Childhood cancer in relation to prenatal exposure to atomic-bomb radiation, Lancet 2:1000, 1970.
44. Larsen, C. D.: Pulmonary-tumor induction by transplacental exposure to urethane, J. Nat. Cancer Inst. 8:63, 1947.
45. Smith, W. E., and Rous, P.: The neoplastic potentialities of mouse embryo tissues; lung adenomas in baby mice as result of prenatal exposure to urethane, J. Exper. Med. 88:529, 1948.
46. Klein, M.: Influence of age on induction with urethan of hepatomas and other tumors in infant mice, J. Nat. Cancer Inst. 36:1111, 1966.
47. Foulds, L.: *Neoplastic Development* (London: Academic Press, 1969).
48. Druckrey, H., Preussmann, R., Ivankovic, S., and Schmähl, D.: Organotrope carcinogene Wirkungen bei 65 verschiedenen N-Nitroso-Verbindungen an BD-Ratten, Ztschr. Krebsforsch. 69:103, 1967.
49. Druckrey, H., Preussmann, R., and Ivankovic, S.: N-Nitroso compounds in organotropic and transplacental carcinogenesis, Ann. New York Acad. Sc. 163:676, 1969.
50. DiPaolo, J. A., and Kotin, P.: Teratogenesis-oncogenesis: A study of possible relationships, Arch. Path. 81:3, 1966.
51. Berry, C. L., Keeling, J., and Hilton, C.: Coincidence of congenital malformation and embryonic tumours of childhood, Arch. Dis. Childhood 45:229, 1970.
52. Kobayashi, N., Furukawa, T., and Takatsu, T.: Congenital anomalies in children with malignancy, Paediat. Univ. Tokyo No. 16, 31, 1968.
53. Miller, R. W.: Relation between cancer and congenital defects in man, New England J. Med. 275:87, 1966.
54. Parker, D. A., and Skalko, R. G.: Congenital asymmetry: report of 10 cases with associated development abnormalities, Pediatrics 44:584, 1969.
55. Fraumeni, J. F., Jr., and Miller, R. W.: Adrenocortical neoplasms with hemihypertrophy, brain tumors and other disorders, J. Pediat. 70:129, 1967.
56. Miller, R. W.: Relation between cancer and congenital defects: An epidemiologic evaluation, J. Nat. Cancer Inst. 40:1079, 1968.
57. Beckwith, J. B., and Perrin, E. V.: In situ neuroblastomas: A contribution to the natural history of neural crest tumors, Am. J. Path. 43:1089, 1963.
58. Shanklin, D. R., and Sotelo-Avila, C.: In situ tumors in fetuses, newborns and young infants, Biol. Neonat. 14:286, 1969.
59. Bove, K. E., Koffler, H., and McAdams, A. J.: Nodular renal blastema. Definition and possible significance, Cancer 24:323, 1969.
60. Miller, R. W.: Childhood cancer and congenital defects. A study of U.S. death certificates during the period 1960–1966, Pediat. Res. 3:389, 1969.
61. Wald, N., Borges, W. H., Li, C. C., Turner, J. H., and Harnois, M. C.: Leukaemia associated with mongolism, Lancet 1:1228, 1961.
62. Miller, R. W.: Down's syndrome (mongolism), other congenital malformations and cancers among the sibs of leukemic children, New England J. Med. 268:393, 1963.

Leukemias

LEUKEMIAS are the most common of the childhood neoplasias that account for nearly half of all cancer deaths in children.[1] There has been a steady and significant increase of the death rates from leukemias during the past decades,[2] but the rise affected particularly age groups above 55 years[3] and it was doubted that there was any increase in childhood leukemias. Since many leukemias of children show normal or reduced white counts at the time of diagnosis, they often went unrecognized or were misdiagnosed until examination of bone marrow became common practice at about 1940. The inclusion of these "aleukemic leukemias" in present incidence figures may account in part for the apparent rise of children's deaths from leukemia in recent times.[1] In England and Wales, the mortality increase from leukemia in children under 10 years was approximately 4.5% per annum. A peak mortality was present at ages 2–3 years since 1921.[4] In the United States, childhood deaths from acute leukemias also are most common at ages 2–5 years, with a peak at 4 years of age. This peak is due to acute lymphocytic leukemia mortality of white children, whereas nonwhites are spared the early mortality of this leukemia.[5] Ethnic and racial differences, although clearly noticeable, may be spurious, since the racial groups surveyed also differ in socioeconomic conditions, medical attention and other environmental circumstances. The generally observed peaks of acute leukemias at ages 2–5 years possibly could originate in prenatal life, since genetic as well as intrauterine environmental factors could have belated clinical manifestations and result in postnatal leukemia. Between 1960 and 1966, a decrease in leukemia deaths of preschool children has been observed in the United States.[6]

Genetic leukemogenic factors have long been considered. Videbaek[7] compared the families of 209 leukemic patients with the families of 200 normal subjects. Among the relatives of the leukemic patients, 8.1% had leukemia in contrast to only 0.5% in the controls. Relatives of leukemic patients also developed other cancers more frequently than those of the controls. When there was a demonstrable familial tendency, leukemia was more likely to occur at an early age. Simple Mendelian inheritance was not manifest and external factors seemed to play an important role in the etiology of the disease. Similar large-scale family studies by Guasch,[8] Morganti and Cresseri[9] and Steinberg[10] failed to show an excess of leukemia among relatives of leukemic patients. In a study of familial leukemia and lymphoma in Nebraska, 39 families were identified with multiple cases.[11] There are reports of single families or kindreds that show remarkable recurrences of leukemia. Anderson[12] recorded a family in which 5 of 8 siblings developed leukemia between the ages of 5 and 8 years, and Campbell *et al.*[13] described a family in which among 7 siblings 2 had neonatal leukemia and 2 others had blood dyscrasias suggestive of leukemia. There were no chromosomal anomalies in 1 of the leukemic children available for examination and none in the parents. Baikie *et al.*[14] reported a family in which 2 siblings died of leukemia and 1 sibling had a sex chromosome anomaly. A family with 6 cases of acute myelogenous leukemia and 2 cases of reticuloendothelial malignancy was described by Snyder *et al.*[15] In surviving members of this family there was increased susceptibility of skin fibroblasts to in vitro transformation by the oncogenic virus SV40 and in some there were abnormal immunoglobulin levels. Chronic myelocytic leukemia, an uncommon form in childhood, has been observed in 2 sets of infant siblings.[16] A syndrome suggesting chronic or subacute myelogenous leukemia occurred in 9 related children living in various parts of the United States.[17] Lymphocytic leukemia developed in 2 sisters at age 4½ years who had osteogenesis imperfecta.[18] An intensive study was made of a family with chronic lymphocytic leukemia in 3 adult siblings, the progeny of a consanguineous marriage. Two survivors with leukemia and a sibling showed impaired in vitro lymphocyte transformation in response to phytohemagglutinin and selective deficiency of serum immunoglobulin levels. It was thought that a genetically controlled immune mechanism is involved in familial clusters of chronic lymphocytic leukemia.[19] In another family, a man, 53 years of age, died of chronic lymphatic leukemia 27 years after his father, and the father's identical twin had died of the same disease at age 56 years.[20] Concordance in regard to leukemia has been observed repeatedly in identical twins[8,20-22] but occasionally also in nonidentical twins.[8] Discordance has been reported often in identical twins[22]; in England and Wales, for instance, not one pair of identical twins, both affected by leukemia, was discovered in an 8-year period.[1] Yet, the risk of leukemia for an identical twin of a child who developed leukemia before 7 years of age is 1 in 5, the second twin usually falling ill within weeks or months after the first.[5,23]

Chromosomal abnormalities represent a connecting link between certain congenital malformations and some leukemias. Down syndrome is the best known aggregate of malformations with an increased risk of leukemia. In patients with mongolism, the risk of developing leukemia is approximately fifteen to twenty times greater than that of the normal population.[24-28] Myelogenous as well as lymphocytic leukemias can complicate mongolism.[29,30] It seems that Down syndrome is not only more common than usual among leukemic children but also among their siblings.[31] Patients with other autosomal trisomies may have a similar tendency to leukemia but this is not easily demonstrable, since many of them have a limited life span. A case of trisomy 13-15 (D_1) with congenital leukemia[32] suggests that infants with this syndrome have increased risks of developing leukemia. The congenital malformations commonly associated with

Fanconi aplastic anemia may be related to chromosomal breakage observed in cultured blood cells of some of the patients[33] who seem to have an increased risk of leukemia.[34,35] Several constitutional diseases not clearly associated with congenital malformations but with chromosomal instabilities carry an increased risk of leukemia.[36] Thus, it seems that genetic factors play a role in the etiology of some leukemias mediated through inherited mechanisms that are not yet fully understood.

Prenatal environmental damages as causes of postnatal leukemias must also be considered. X-rays, viruses and chemicals have been examined as possible etiologic factors. The peak of childhood leukemia, 3–5 years after birth, could be a late effect of intrauterine exposure to radiation. The mortality from leukemia among survivors of the atomic explosions in Hiroshima and Nagasaki reached a peak 6–7 years after the exposure.[37,38] Similarly, exposure to x-rays in utero could bring about leukemia several years after birth. Several decades ago, embryos and fetuses sometimes were exposed to massive doses of x-rays and children were born with microcephaly, microphthalmia and other signs of actinic damage (Chapter 10). It would be interesting to learn whether any of these children developed leukemia in postnatal life but apparently there are no reports along these lines. There exist suggestive data concerning diagnostic intrauterine x-ray exposures as a cause of leukemia[27,39,40] but interpretations of such data are not uniform.[41,42] One survey of approximately 40,000 children whose mothers had received diagnostic pelvic or abdominal x-ray exposures during pregnancy did not show an increased incidence of leukemia over the expected number.[43] Children exposed in utero to the radiations generated by the atomic bombs in Hiroshima and Nagasaki apparently have not shown an excess of deaths from leukemia.[42,45]

Viruses and drugs as prenatal leukemogenic agents deserve attention but, so far, the evidence for their etiologic role in leukemia of children has not been established.[1,47] Interesting observations have been made of clusters of births with congenital heart disease and of increased prevalence of childhood leukemia. The possibility of an epidemiologic relation between some types of leukemia and some congenital malformations was considered by Heath *et al.*[46] There have been reports of "leukemia houses" and leukemia clusters but, in general, evaluation of these observations provided no solid support for the contention that childhood leukemia aggregates excessively with respect to time and place of birth, diagnosis or death[47] and there was little evidence that aggregates of childhood leukemia represent foci of infection.[48]

Prenatal leukemogenic factors are clearly at work in congenital leukemias. Leukemias present at birth or noticeable soon after birth are rare but, by 1967, more than 50 cases had been recorded.[49] Some of the cases were associated with Down syndrome,[50] trisomy 13-15,[32] Klippel-Feil syndrome or bilateral aplasia of the radius,[51] but in most cases the infants were considered normal with the exception of the blood dyscrasia. Fabia and Drolette[52] pointed out that among 23 mongoloid children with leukemia, 5 died in the neonatal period. In the neonate, granulocytic leukemia is thought to be seven or eight times as frequent as the lymphatic type. The origin of congenital leukemias is obscure. In 1956, Bierman *et al.*,[53] in a review, found that the children born of leukemic mothers were viable and free of the maternal disease, but 2 years later it was reported that a leukemic mother gave birth to a child who developed acute lymphocytic leukemia at the age of 9 months.[54] In a case of acute lymphoblastic leukemia of a neonate, herpesvirus particles were found in the peripheral blood leukocytes of the child and of her mother.[55] Other maternal factors were noted in an investigation of children dying of malignant neoplasms.[56] Mortality from leukemia was associated with both birth order and maternal age. Risk of death was about 50% higher in first than in fifth and later births and about 40% higher in children of women over 40 years of age than in those of women under 20 years of age.

Although it is obvious that prenatal factors play a role in some leukemias and that there exist some suggestive associations between congenital malformations and childhood leukemias, such clues are scarce and must not impede the search for postnatal leukemogenic factors.

REFERENCES

1. Keidan, S. E.: The Leukaemias, in Marsden, H. B., and Steward, J. K. (eds.), *Tumours in Children* (New York: Springer, 1968).
2. Cooke, J. V.: The occurrence of leukemia, Blood 9:340, 1954.
3. Hayhoe, F. G. J.: *Leukaemia Research and Clinical Practice* (Boston: Little, Brown & Company, 1960).
4. Court Brown, W. M., and Doll, R.: Leukemia in childhood and young adult life: Trends in mortality in relation to aetiology, Brit. M. J. 1:981, 1961.
5. Miller, R. W.: Relation between cancer and congenital defects: An epidemiologic evaluation, J. Nat. Cancer Inst. 40:1079, 1968.
6. Miller, R. W.: Decline in U.S. childhood leukaemia mortality, Lancet 2:1189, 1969.
7. Videbaek, A.: *Heredity in Human Leukaemia and Its Relation to Cancer* (London: H. K. Lewis & Company, Ltd., 1947).
8. Guasch, J.: Hérédité des leucémies, Sangre 25:384, 1954.
9. Morganti, G., and Cresseri, A.: Nouvelles recherches génétiques sur les leucémies, Sangre 25:421,1954.
10. Steinberg, A. G.: The genetics of acute leukemia in children, Cancer 13:985, 1960.
11. Rigby, P. G., Pratt, P. T., Rosenlof, R. C., and Lemon, H. M.: Genetic relationships in familial leukemia and lymphoma, Arch. Int. Med. 121:67, 1968.
12. Anderson, R. C.: Familial leukemia, A. M. A. Am. J. Dis. Child. 81:313, 1951.
13. Campbell, W. A. B., Macafee, A. L., and Wade, W. G.: Familial neonatal leukaemia, Arch. Dis. Childhood 37:93, 1962.
14. Baikie, A. G., Court Brown, W. M., Buckton, K. E., and Harnden, D. G.: Two cases of leukaemia and case of sex-chromosome abnormality in same sibship, Lancet 2:1003, 1961.
15. Snyder, A. L., Li, F. P., Henderson, E. S., and Todaro, G.

J.: Possible inherited leukaemogenic factors in familial acute myelogenous leukaemia, Lancet 1:586, 1970.
16. Holton, C. P., and Johnson, W. W.: Chronic myelocytic leukemia in infant siblings, J. Pediat. 72:377, 1968.
17. Randall, D. L., Reiquam, C. W., Githens, J. H., and Robinson, A.: Familial myeloproliferative disease. A new syndrome closely simulating myelogenous leukemia in childhood, Am. J. Dis. Child. 110:479, 1965.
18. Gilchrist, G. S., and Shore, N. A.: Familial leukemia and osteogenesis imperfecta, J. Pediat. 71:115, 1967.
19. Fraumeni, J. F., Jr., Vogel, C. L., and DeVita, V. T.: Familial chronic lymphocytic leukemia, Ann. Int. Med. 71:279, 1969.
20. Gunz, F., and Dameshek, W.: Chronic lymphocytic leukemia in a family, including twin brothers and a son, J.A.M.A. 164:1323, 1957.
21. Anderson, R. C., and Hermann, H. W.: Leukemia in twin children, J.A.M.A. 158:652, 1955.
22. MacMahon, B., and Levy, M. A.: Prenatal origin of childhood leukemia. Evidence from twins, New England Med. J. 270:1082, 1964.
23. Miller, R. W.: Persons with exceptionally high risk of leukemia, Cancer Res. 27:2420, 1967.
24. Krivit, W., and Good, R. A.: The simultaneous occurrence of leukemia and mongolism, A.M.A. Am. J. Dis. Child. 91: 218, 1956.
25. Wald, N., Borges, W. H., Li, C. C., Turner, J. H., and Harnois, M. C.: Leukaemia associated with mongolism, Lancet 1:1228, 1961.
26. Holland, W. W., Doll, R., and Carter, C. O.: The mortality from leukemia and other cancers among patients with Down's syndrome (mongols) and among their parents, Brit. J. Cancer 16:177, 1962.
27. Stewart, A., Webb, J., and Hewitt, D.: A survey of childhood malignancies, Brit. M. J. 1:1495, 1958.
28. Jackson, E. W., Turner, J. H., Klauber, M. R., and Norris, F. D.: Down's syndrome: Variation of leukemia occurrence in institutionalized populations, J. Chron. Dis. 21: 247, 1968.
29. Warkany, J., Schubert, W. K., and Thompson, J.: Chromosome analyses in mongolism (Langdon Down syndrome) associated with leukemia, New England J. Med 268:1, 1963.
30. Miller, R. W.: Childhood cancer and congenital defects. A study of U.S. death certificates during the period 1960–1966, Pediat. Res. 3:389, 1969.
31. Miller, R. W.: Down's syndrome (mongolism), other congenital malformations and cancers among the sibs of leukemic children, New England J. Med. 268:393, 1963.
32. Schade, H., Schoeller, L., and Schultze, K. W.: D-trisomy (Patau-syndrome) with congenital leukemia, Med. Welt 5:2690, 1962.
33. Schmid, W.: Familial constitutional panmyelocytopathy, Fanconi's anemia (F. A.). II. A discussion of the cytogenetic findings in Fanconi's anemia, Seminars Hemat. 4: 241, 1967.
34. Garriga, S., and Crosby, W. H.: Incidence of leukemia in families of patients with hypoplasia of marrow, Blood 14: 1008, 1959.
35. Bloom, G. E., Warner, S., Gerald, P. S., and Diamond, L. K.: Chromosome abnormalities in constitutional aplastic anemia, New England J. Med. 274:8, 1966.
36. Fraumeni, J. F., Jr. : Constitutional disorders of man predisposing to leukemia and lymphoma, Nat. Cancer Inst. Monogr. 32:221, 1969.
37. Moloney, W. C.: Leukaemia in survivors of atomic bombing, New England J. Med. 253:88, 1955.
38. Miller, R. W.: Delayed effects occurring within the first decade after exposure of young individuals to the Hiroshima bomb, Pediatrics 18:1, 1956.
39. MacMahon, B.: Prenatal x-ray exposure and childhood cancer, J. Nat. Cancer Inst. 28:1173, 1962.
40. Graham, S., Levin, M. L., Kilienfeld, A. M., Schuman, L. M., Gibson, R., Down, J. E., and Hempelmann, L.: Preconception, intrauterine, and postnatal irradiation as related to leukemia, Nat. Cancer Inst. Monogr. 19:347, 1966.
41. Burch, P. R. J.: Effects of diagnostic radiation, Lancet 1: 441, 1963.
42. Miller, R. W.: Delayed radiation effects in atomic-bomb survivors, Science 166:569, 1969.
43. Court Brown, W. M., Doll, R., and Hill, A. B.: Incidence of leukaemia after exposure to diagnostic radiation in utero, Brit. M. J. 1539, 1960.
44. Jablon, S., and Kato, H.: Childhood cancer in relation to prenatal exposure to atomic-bomb radiation, Lancet 2: 1000, 1970.
45. Miller, R. W.: Radiation, chromosomes and viruses in the etiology of leukemia, New England J. Med. 271:30, 1964
46. Heath, C. W., Jr., Manning, M. D., and Zelkowitz, L.: Case clusters in the occurrence of leukaemia and congenital malformations, Lancet 2:136, 1964.
47. Miller, R. W., and Fraumeni, J. F., Jr.: Leukemia houses, Ann. Int. Med. 67:675, 1967.
48. Fraumeni, J. F., Jr., and Miller, R. W.: Epidemiology of human leukemia: Recent observations, J. Nat. Cancer Inst. 38:593, 1967.
49. Zussman, W. V., Kahn, A., and Shayesteh, P.: Congenital leukemia, Cancer 20:1227, 1967.
50. Pierce, M. I.: Leukemia in the newborn infant, J. Pediat. 54:691, 1959.
51. Bernhard, W. G., Gore, I., and Kilby, R. A.: Congenital leukemia, Blood 6:990, 1951.
52. Fabia, J., and Drolette, M.: Malformations and leukemia in children with Down's syndrome, Pediatrics 45:60, 1970.
53. Bierman, H. R., Aggeler, P. M., Thelander, H., Kelly, K. H., and Cordes, F. L.: Leukemia in pregnancy, J.A.M.A. 161: 220, 1956.
54. Cramblett, H. G., Freedman, J. L., and Najjar, S.: Leukemia in an infant born of a mother with leukemia, New England J. Med. 259:727, 1958.
55. Carper, J. M., O'Donnell, W. M., and Monroe, J. H.: Neonatal leukemia; detection of herpes virus in the mother and child, Am. J. Dis. Child. 115:61, 1968.
56. MacMahon, B., and Newill, V. A.: Birth characteristics of children dying of malignant neoplasms, J. Nat. Cancer Inst. 28:231, 1962.

Intracranial Tumors

CENTRAL NERVOUS SYSTEM TUMORS occur at all age periods, including fetal life and infancy, but they are rare in early life and increase up to age 7 years, leveling off in succeeding years through adolescence. Approximately 55% of the tumors are infratentorial, in contrast to those of adulthood, which are infratentorial in less than 30%.[1,2] There is an interesting discrepancy between the distribution of brain tumors in childhood and the relative weights of cerebrum and cerebellum. Peller[3] calculated that, considering these weights, there are, per gram substance in the child's cerebellum, about thirty times more primary malignancies than in the cerebrum. It also is noteworthy that, in the past, when tuberculomas were the most frequent intracranial tumors of childhood,[4] they, too, were located more often in the infratentorial than in the supratentorial space. Rich arterial and capillary blood supply, slow capillary circulation and increased venous blood pressure of the cerebellum have been held responsible for the frequency of early cerebellar tumors, since they could favor exposure of the hindbrain to oncogenic agents.[3] In one series of brain tumors[5] it was found that more than 60% of gliomas of childhood arose in the brain stem or vermis even though these structures comprise only 3% of the total mass of the central nervous system. The authors thought that this area contains cells capable of tremendous differentiation during early embryonic development and that the cells could be susceptible, in certain phases, to some carcinogenic influences.

The prevalent brain tumors of childhood have a tendency to midline origin and location; many occur within or near the third or fourth ventricle or they are attached to the brain stem or hypothalamus. It has been stated that displaced cells are seen rather frequently near the midline or raphe of the central nervous system and that they may give rise to tumors. Medulloblastomas, many gliomas and ependymomas exemplify such tumors. Craniopharyngiomas, dermoids, epidermoids and teratomas represent more clearly results of developmental errors. Hamartomas are or develop from congenital tissue malformations consisting of glial cells. Yet, displaced cells near or in the raphe of the spinal cord show little tendency to tumor formation. In addition, displaced cell aggregates generally are much more common than central nervous system tumors, so that accessory oncogenic factors must be sought to explain the formation of tumors. Displaced cells may be the basis or a necessary cause of the tumors but their existence alone does not explain oncogenesis.[3]

Trauma often has been accused as a cause of certain brain tumors but, after thorough review of the subject, Zülch[6] concluded that a traumatic etiology can be accepted for rare cases only. There is no proof that viral or bacterial infections or hypoxia result in brain tumors.[1]

Matson[1] stated that familial incidence of intracranial tumors as seen in the clinic is of no statistical significance. Yet, genetic influences can be recognized in brain tumors that develop in the course of hamartoses. In such cases, there may be no familial recurrence of brain tumors but vicarious manifestations of the hamartosis may be recognizable. Recklinghausen neurofibromatosis (Chapter 121) may lead to neurofibromas, acoustic neurinomas, spongioblastomas, gliomas, ependymomas and meningiomas (p. 1255). There are families in which acoustic neurofibromas occur through several generations,[7] and families in which various types of brain tumors affect members of the pedigree.[6,8] Tuberous sclerosis (Chapter 122) is characterized by nodules or tubers of the cortex, glial nests and ependymal tumors that can obstruct the cerebrospinal fluid circulation. In Hippel-Lindau disease (Chapter 123), cerebellar angioblastomas or Lindau cysts are characteristic intracranial manifestations; angioblastomas of the spine can appear as extracranial lesions of this hamartosis, which sometimes includes retinal, pancreatic and renal tumors. Brain tumors can occur in several generations affected by this disorder. Medulloblastoma has been observed in patients with the "basal cell nevi syndrome" (Chapter 123) and with the "blue rubber-bleb nevus syndrome"[9] (Chapter 118). Gliomas in familial polyposis of the colon[10,11] represent further examples of brain tumors within disease pictures of dominantly inherited hamartoses. Pituitary adenomas can occur within the spectrum of endocrine "adenomatosis-peptic ulcer disorder," which is transmitted like an autosomal dominant trait (MEN type I, p. 1269). These tumors are very rare in children but early signs have been noted in a 16-year-old girl.[12,13] Other brain tumors are rare complications of recessively inherited disorders. In patients with the Laurence-Moon-Biedl syndrome (Chapter 19), tumors have been reported in the hypothalamo-pituitary and in the pineal regions. In another recessively inherited disorder, ataxia-telangiectatica (Chapter 35), frontal-lobe glioma and medulloblastoma have been observed. In the sex-linked recessive Wiskott-Aldrich syndrome, astrocytoma has been recorded.[14]

Familial occurrence of brain tumors has been described repeatedly[6,15-19]; some of the cases probably were associated with the hamartoses mentioned above; others may be connected with similar general disturbances not yet clearly defined. Comparable explanations may apply to multiple primary brain tumors in the same patient.[20] Familial gliomas have been made the subject of genetic studies.[19,21,22] A few monozygotic twins concordant for glioma have been reported[18] but, in most cases, there is discordance in such twins.[18,21,23] Interpretation of the various repetitive tumors is difficult[24] but observations of such cases may lead to discovery of basic oncogenic processes. Most patients with brain tumor are free of congenital malformations but, in some instances, such associations exist and are not incidental. This is particularly true in some teratomas when malignancy develops on the basis of the malformation.[25,26] A hamartoma of the brain in a child with bilateral proboscis and cerebral malformations was described by Gitlin and Behar[27] (Chapter 23). A tumor of the floor of the third ventricle causing precocious puberty, overgrowth and advanced ossification was found in a girl with parieto-occipital meningocele, vertebral malformations and absence of the first rib on the left.[28] Polydactyly and craniofacial and cerebellar hemihypertrophy were noted in patients who developed cerebellar ganglioneuromas.[29] In patients with adrenal malformations, cerebral glioma and brain hypertrophy have been reported.[30]

REFERENCES

1. Matson, D. D.: *Neurosurgery of Infancy and Childhood* (Springfield, Ill.: Charles C Thomas, Publisher, 1969).
2. French, L. A.: Some Aspects of Diagnosis and Treatment of Brain Tumors in Children, in Fields, W. S., and Sharkey, P. C. (eds.), *The Biology and Treatment of Intracranial Tumors* (Springfield, Ill.: Charles C Thomas, Publisher, 1962).
3. Peller, S.: *Cancer in Childhood and Youth* (Baltimore: The Williams & Wilkins Company, 1960).
4. Critchley, M.: Brain tumors in children: Their general symptomatology, Brit. J. Child. Dis. 22:251, 1925.
5. Marsden, H. B., and Steward, J. K.: *Tumours in Children*. Recent Results in Cancer Research No. 13 (New York: Springer-Verlag, 1968).
6. Zülch, K. J.: *Brain Tumors, Their Biology and Pathology* (New York: Springer-Verlag, 1965).
7. Gardner, W. J., and Turner, O.: Bilateral acoustic neurofibromas, Arch. Neurol. 44:76, 1940.
8. Schaltenbrand, G.: Sobre una familia con enfermedad de Recklinghausen, Prensa méd. argent. 20:2011, 1933.
9. Rice, J. S., and Fischer, D. S.: Blue rubber-bleb nevus syndrome, Arch. Dermat. 86:503, 1962.
10. Baughman, F. A., Jr., List, C. F., Williams, J. R., Muldoon, J. P., Segarra, J. M., and Volkel, J. S.: The glioma-polyposis syndrome, New England J. Med. 281:1345, 1969.
11. Turcot, J., Despres, J. P., and St. Pierre, F.: Malignant tumors of central nervous system associated with familial polyposis of the colon: Report of two cases, Dis. Colon & Rectum 2:465, 1959.
12. Wermer, P.: Endocrine adenomatosis and peptic ulcer in a large kindred. Inherited multiple tumors and mosaic pleiotropism in man, Am. J. Med. 35:205, 1963.
13. Steiner, A. L., Goodman, A. D., and Powers, S. R.: Study of a kindred with pheochromocytoma, medullary thyroid carcinoma, hyperparathyroidism and Cushing's disease: Multiple endocrine neoplasis, type 2, Medicine 47:371, 1968.
14. Amiet, A.: Aldrich syndrome, Ann. paediat. 201:315, 1963.
15. Bender, W., and Pause, F.: Familiäres Gliom (Zur Genetik des Glioms), Monatsschr. Psychiat. u. Neurol. 83:253, 1932.
16. Hallervorden, J.: Erbliche Hirntumoren, Nervenarzt 9:1, 1936.
17. Pass, K. E.: Erbpathologische Untersuchungen in Familien von Hirntumorkranken, Ztschr. Neurol. 161:204, 1938.
18. Koch, G.: The genetics of cerebral tumors, Acta neurochir. (supp.) 10:24, 1963.
19. Van der Wiel, H. J.: *Inheritance of Glioma* (Amsterdam: Elsevier Publishing Company, 1960).
20. Austin, G., Barrows, L. J., and Grant, F. C.: Multiple primary brain tumors in opposite hemispheres of the same patient, A.M.A. Arch. Neurol. & Psychiat. 80:170, 1958.
21. Harvald, B., and Hauge, M.: On the heredity of glioblastoma, J. Nat. Cancer Inst. 17:289, 1956.
22. Hauge, M., and Harvald, B.: Genetics of intracranial tumors, Acta Genet. 7:573, 1958.
23. Kuhnen, B.: Beobachtungen an sieben Zwillingspaaren mit Hirntumoren, Acta Genet. 2:407, 1953.
24. Kurland, L. T., Myrianthopoulos, N. C., and Lessell, S.: Epidemiologic and Genetic Considerations of Intracranial Neoplasms, in Fields, W. S., and Sharkey, P. C. (eds.), *The Biology and Treatment of Intracranial Tumors* (Springfield, Ill.: Charles C Thomas, Publisher, 1962).
25. Bruton, O. C., Martz. D. C., and Gerard, E. S.: Precocious puberty due to secreting chorionepithelioma (teratoma) of the brain, J. Pediat. 59:719, 1961.
26. Donnellan, W. A., and Swenson, O.: Benign and malignant sacrococcygeal teratomas, Surgery 64:834, 1968.
27. Gitlin, G., and Behar, A. J.: Meningeal angiomatosis, arhinencephaly, agenesis of the corpus callosum and large hamartoma of the brain, with neoplasia, in an infant having bilateral nasal proboscis, Acta Anat. 41:56, 1960.
28. Bach, C., Bitan, A., Jolly, G., and Grange, G.: Puberté précoce avec tumeur du diencephale. Association à un syndrome de Dandy-Walker et à des anomalies dysraphiques, Ann. pédiat. 45:762, 1969.
29. Ostertag, B.: Die Einzelformen der Verbildungen (einschliesslich Syringomyelie), in Lubarsch, O., Henke, F., and Rössle, R. (eds.), *Handbuch der Speziellen Pathologischen Anatomie und Histologie* (Berlin: Springer-Verlag, 1956), Vol. 13.
30. Miloslavich, E.: Über Bildungsanomalien der Nebenniere, Virchows Arch. path. Anat. 218:131, 1914.

Congenital and Infantile Brain Tumors

Some brain tumors manifest themselves at birth, being responsible for dystocia.[1,2] Others mimic symptoms of hydrocephaly, chronic subdural hematoma or cerebral palsy.[3,4] Because of their rarity, they seldom are recognized clinically, but since some of them are curable, the possibility of such tumors should be considered in the differential diagnosis of the more frequent conditions mentioned above. Wells[5] found 2 published cases of congenital glioma and Arnstein *et al.*[6] 13. Raskind and Beigel[3] added 6 cases in 1964. Although these tumors were listed as occurring in the neonatal period or in early infancy, presence at birth seemed most likely. There were five teratomas among nineteen intracranial tumors. To these can be added the congenital teratomas described by Kimmel *et al.*,[7] Hosoi[8] and Oberman.[9] A congenital pituitary adamantinoma was recorded by Iyer.[10] Other congenital brain tumors were classified as glioma, astrocytoma, papilloma, hemangioma or ependymoma.[2,3] Another report and review on congenital intracranial neoplasm was made in 1964 by Solitare and Krigman.[2] They tabulated twenty-seven definitely congenital, three probably and sixteen possibly congenital intracranial tumors reported in the literature. In addition, they described the necropsy findings of a 32-week-old stillborn fetus with congenital neoplasm of the meninges diagnosed as a mixed hemangiopericytoma and fibroma.

Intracranial tumors encountered during the first 2 years of life include definitely, probably and possibly congenital lesions. They were discussed by Matson,[4] who stressed that many of these tumors are suitable for satisfactory surgical treatment. The medulloblastomas (p. 1213), which represent the largest group of intracranial tumors of infancy, have the least favorable prognosis but the largest of these tumors removed from a 3-month-old infant apparently was checked, as the child survived for at least 7 years. Hamartomas, composed chiefly of glial cells, represent a transition between malformation and neoplasia (glioma). Although they are congenital anomalies, they may remain symptomless for years and decades until they manifest themselves by tumor symptoms. If they are located near hypothalamic midline structures they may cause dwarfism, diencephalic cachexia (Chapter 18) or endocrine disturbances (Chapter 46). Astrocytomas often are benign in infants; in the cerebellar region, they are in part cystic and suitable for surgical removal but benign, slowly growing astrocytomas of the cerebrum involving vital midline structures are critical because of their location.[4] Gliomas of the optic pathways usually are seen in children; Recklinghausen neurofibromatosis, a hamartosis, may be the basic disorder (Chapter 121). Papillomas of the choroid plexus can be congenital or they manifest themselves in early childhood. Most of these lesions are benign and can be removed successfully. Dermoid cysts develop on the basis of congenital dermal sinus tracts in the posterior fossa. They are benign lesions that can be excised if they are treated before repeated infections, meningitis or cerebellar abscesses make the operation difficult. Ependymomas of early infancy occur more often below than above the tentorium. They are benign lesions whose prognosis depends on their location. Congenital ependymomas combined with astrocytoma may be very large and replace half or more of one cerebral hemisphere. Matson[4] emphasized that during the first 2 years of life, intracranial tumors may cause hydrocephaly, increased intracranial pressure, convulsions, spontaneous intracranial hemorrhage, motor weakness, strabismus or other neurologic disturbances. An undiagnosed tumor at the base of the brain was found at necropsy of a 6-week-old boy who, like his brother, had an atypical form of the orodigitofacial syndrome (Chapter 73) with microphthalmia, coloboma of the optic papilla and hexadactyly.[12]

Many brain tumors that have their origin in congenital malformations or errors of prenatal development do not, as a rule, become symptomatic during the first 2 years of life. They include cystic hemangioblastoma, cavernous angioma, craniopharyngioma and colloid cyst of the third ventricle.[4] The relationship of congenital malformation and brain tumor can be illustrated by a pair of monozygotic twins, one of whom died at age 5 years, a microcephalic idiot, whereas the other died of a brain tumor at 6 years of age.[11] It seems unlikely that the two disorders were unrelated.

REFERENCES

1. Wagner, J. A., Douglass, L. H., and Slager, U. T.: Dystocia caused by fetal intracranial teratoma. Report of a case, Obst. & Gynec. 4:647, 1954.
2. Solitare, G. B., and Krigman, M. R.: Congenital intracranial neoplasm. A case report and review of the literature, J. Neuropath. & Exper. Neurol. 23:280, 1964.
3. Raskind, R., and Beigel, F.: Brain tumors in early infancy – probably congenital in origin, J. Pediat. 65:727, 1964.
4. Matson, D. D.: Intracranial tumors of the first two years of life, West. J. Surg. 72:117, 1964.
5. Wells, H. G.: Occurrence and significance of congenital malignant neoplasms, Arch. Path. 30:535, 1940.
6. Arnstein, L. H., Boldrey, E., and Naffziger, H. C.: A case report and survey of brain tumors during the neonatal period, J. Neurosurg. 8:315, 1951.
7. Kimmel, D. L., Moyer, E. K., Peale, A. R., Winborne, L. W., and Gotwals, J. E.: A cerebral tumor containing five human fetuses, Anat. Rec. 106:141, 1950.
8. Hosoi, K.: Teratoma and teratoid tumors of the brain, Arch. Path. 9:1207, 1930.
9. Oberman, B.: Intracranial teratoma replacing brain, Arch. Neurol. 11:423, 1964.
10. Iyer, C. G. S.: Case report of adamantinoma present at birth, J. Neurosurg. 9:221, 1952.
11. Koch, G.: Genetics of microcephaly in man, Acta Genet. 8:75, 1959.
12. Hooft, C., and Jongbloet, P.: Syndrome oro-digito-facial chez deux frères, Arch. franç. pédiat. 21:729, 1964.

Gliomas

Gliomas usually appear sporadically and without intimations concerning their etiology. Yet, some facts have been established that eventually may contribute to the recognition of their etiology in some instances. Classifications of gliomas vary and they may have no relationship with etiologic entities.

Familial recurrence of gliomas has been reported repeatedly.[1-3] A systematic study of hereditary factors in the etiology of gliomas was made by Van der Wiel[4] in the Netherlands. In relatives of tumor patients he found the death rate from glioma to be four times higher than would be expected from that of the general population. Spina bifida, meningocele and anencephaly ("dysraphias") were ascertained more often among relatives of the tumor group than in controls. The fact that café au lait spots were more frequent among relatives of patients than in the control group may explain, in part, familial aggregation, since gliomas are among the tumors that can complicate Recklinghausen neurofibromatosis (Chapter 121). In "central neurofibromatosis," glioblastoma, spongioblastoma, diffuse glioma, ependymoma and ganglioneuroma have been observed. They may alternate with meningioma, neurofibroma and neurinoma.[3,5] Lee and Abbott[6] reported a family with central nervous system neoplasia in three generations. Neurofibromatosis was the basic disorder. Among the tumors, meningioma and neurinoma prevailed. Astrocytoma was found in at least 1 of the cases. Combination of meningioma and glioma in patients with multiple primary brain tumors has been reported repeatedly[7,8] and neurofibromatosis may be the common denominator of such concurrences. The cerebral lesions of tuberous sclerosis (Chapter 122) consist of small nodules as well as of space-consuming brain tumors such as spongioblastoma, astrocytoma, ependymoma and glioblastoma.[8] A hereditary glioma-polyposis syndrome has been described[9,10] that may be related to Gardner syndrome (Chapter 123). Such dominantly inherited hamartoses explain some familial recurrences of gliomas as well as multiple primary brain tumors. Gliomas have been observed concurrent with adrenocortical neoplasms[11] and with adenocarcinoma of the colon, hepatocarcinoma and acute lymphocytic leukemia.[12] Glioma has been seen as a complication of ataxia-telangiectasia[13] (Chapter 35) and of Wiskott-Aldrich syndrome.[14] Concordance in regard to glioma has been observed in monozygotic[15,16] as well as dizygotic twins.[15] Although, in certain cases, genetic factors have been demonstrated in the etiology of gliomas, this is not the case in the majority of the patients.[17]

A great deal of experimental work has been done with mice to elucidate morphogenesis, differentiation and classification of gliomas. It seems that gliogenous tumor cells are incapable of invading blood vessels, which serves as an explanation for the lack of extracranial metastases of these tumors.[18]

REFERENCES

1. Bender, W., and Panse, F.: Familiäres Gliom (zur Genetik des Glioms), Monatsschr. Psychiat. 83:253, 1932.
2. Hallervorden, J.: Erbliche Hirntumoren, Nervenarzt 9:1, 1936.
3. Zülch, K. J.: *Brain Tumors. Their Biology and Pathology* (New York: Springer-Verlag, 1965).
4. Van der Wiel, H. J.: *Inheritance of Glioma* (Amsterdam: Elsevier Publishing Company, 1960).
5. Schaltenbrand, G.: Sobre una familia con enfermedad de Recklinghausen, Prensa méd. argent. 20:2011, 1933.
6. Lee, D. K., and Abbott, M. L.: Familial central nervous system neoplasia. Case report of a family with von Recklinghausen's neurofibromatosis, Arch. Neurol. 20:154, 1969.
7. Austin, G., Barrows, L. J., and Grant, F. C.: Multiple primary brain tumors in opposite hemispheres of the same patient, A.M.A. Arch. Neurol. & Psychiat. 80:173, 1958.
8. Paulson, G. W., and Lyle, C. B.: Tuberous sclerosis, Developmental Med. & Child Neurol. 8:571, 1966.
9. Turcot, J., Despres, J. P., and St. Pierre, F.: Malignant tumors of central nervous system associated with familial polyposis of the colon: Report of two cases, Dis. Colon & Rectum 2:465, 1959.
10. Baughman, F. A., List, C. F., Williams, J. R., Muldoon, J. P., and Volkel, J. S.: The glioma-polyposis syndrome, New England J. Med. 281:1345, 1969.
11. Fraumeni, J. F., Jr., and Miller, R. W.: Adrenocortical neoplasms with hemihypertrophy, brain tumors, and other disorders, J. Pediat. 70:129, 1967.
12. Regelson, W., Bross, I. D. J., Hananian, J., and Nigogosyan, G.: Incidence of second primary tumors in children with cancer and leukemia, Cancer 18:58, 1965.
13. Shuster, J., Hart, Z., Stimson, C. W., Brough, A. J., and Poulik, M. D.: Ataxia-telangiectasia with cerebellar tumor, Pediatrics 37:776, 1966.
14. Amiet, A.: Aldrich syndrome, Ann. paediat. 201:315, 1963.
15. Geyer, H., and Pedersen, P.: Zur Erblichkeit der Neubildungen des Zentralnervensystems und seiner Hüllen, Ztschr. Neurol. u. Psychiat. 165:284, 1939.
16. Koch, G.: Beitrag zur Erblichkeit der Hirngeschwülste, Acta Genet. 3:170, 1954.
17. Koch, G.: The genetics of cerebral tumors, Acta neurochir. (supp.) 10:24, 1963.
18. Zimmerman, H. M.: Experimental Brain Tumors, in Fields, W. S., and Sharkey, P. C. (eds.), *The Biology and Treatment of Intracranial Tumors* (Springfield, Ill.: Charles C Thomas, Publisher, 1962).

Medulloblastomas

THESE NEOPLASIAS, which account for approximately 20% of intracranial tumors in childhood,[1-3] often are cited in support of Cohnheim's theory of the origin of cancer (p. 1199). Medulloblastoma, which has a peak age of 4–6 years[3] at diagnosis, seldom is seen in persons over 20 years. There is a marked sex preponderance, with males affected about three times more often than females.[3,4] Medulloblastomas are midline tumors that probably are derived from abnormal aggregates of cells in the region of the posterior medullary velum. Such cell rests were found in more than 20% of fetuses and infants examined by Raaf and Kernohan.[5] The cells, which are morphologically similar to cells of medulloblastomas, are thought to be remnants of the germinal bud and the external granular layer of the cerebellum, which normally disappear before the end of the first months of extrauterine life.[5] Origin from the posterior medullary velum can be recognized clearly in some medulloblastomas and be assumed in some advanced and widespread ones. More than 80% are in midcerebellar location but supratentorial cases have been reported.[6] French[7] considered a prenatal origin of medulloblastomas because of their site, their occurrence in early life, their occasional presence in newborn children and their occurrence in identical twins.[1,8,9] It is of interest that medulloblastomas developed in children with the basal cell nevi hamartosis (Chapter 123) or in some of their siblings[10] and in a case of blue rubber-bleb nevus (Chapter 118), which probably also represents a hamartosis. Since abnormal cell rests in the posterior medullary velum are quite common in fetuses and infants,[5] it must be assumed that many remain innocuous or disappear as the children grow older.

The medulloblastoma is the most rapidly growing and malignant posterior fossa tumor of childhood and represents "one of the darkest chapters of neurosurgery."[3] Midline location often results in a lack of localizing signs, but there is early obstruction of the cerebrospinal fluid circulation and increased intracranial pressure.[3] Small fragments of the tumor tend to break off, are transported through the cerebrospinal fluid and seeded on the surface of the brain, cerebellum, spinal cord, nerve roots or meninges.[11] Surgical treatment is difficult, since complete removal of the tumor is impossible; the cells are sensitive to deep x-ray therapy, but most patients succumb within the first 2 years after the diagnosis has been made.[3] Prevention would be the only satisfactory answer to this rather hopeless problem. The fact that only a few of the congenital cell rests in the posterior velum become malignant should stimulate searches for secondary oncogenic factors that may act in postnatal life and be preventable.

REFERENCES

1. Cushing, H.: Experiences with the cerebellar medulloblastomas, Acta path. et microbiol. scandinav. 7:1, 1930.
2. Zülch, K. J.: *Brain Tumors, Their Biology and Pathology* (New York: Springer-Verlag, 1965).
3. Matson, D. D.: *Neurosurgery of Infancy and Childhood* (Springfield, Ill.: Charles C Thomas, Publisher, 1969).
4. Marsden, H. B., and Steward, J. K.: *Tumours in Children*. Recent Results in Cancer Research No. 13 (New York: Springer-Verlag, 1968).
5. Raaf, J., and Kernohan, J. W.: Relations of abnormal collections of cells in posterior medullary velum of cerebellum to origin of medulloblastoma, Arch. Neurol. & Psychiat. 52:163, 1944.
6. Bodian, M., and Lawson, D.: The intracranial neoplastic diseases of childhood, Brit. J. Surg. 40:368, 1953.
7. French, L. A.: Some Aspects of Diagnosis and Treatment of Brain Tumors in Children, in Fields, W. S., and Sharkey, P. C. (eds.), *The Biology and Treatment of Intracranial Tumors* (Springfield, Ill.: Charles C Thomas, Publisher, 1962).
8. Leavitt, F. H.: Cerebellar tumors occurring in identical twins, Arch. Neurol. & Psychiat. 19:617, 1928.
9. Wilson, S. A. K., and Wolfsohn, J. M.: Organic nervous disease in identical twins, Arch. Neurol. & Psychiat. 21: 477, 1929.
10. Gorlin, R. J., Vickers, R. A., Kelln, E., and Williamson, J. J.: The multiple basal-cell nevi syndrome. An analysis of a syndrome consisting of multiple nevoid basal-cell carcinoma, jaw cysts, skeletal anomalies, medulloblastoma, and hyporesponsiveness to parathormone, Cancer 18:89, 1965.
11. Kernohan, J. W., and Sayre, G. P.: Tumors of the Central Nervous System, in *Atlas of Tumor Pathology* (Washington, D. C.: Armed Forces Institute of Pathology, 1952).

Craniopharyngiomas and Rathke Pouch Tumors

Craniopharyngiomas and other tumors arising in the critical spot where the notochord, the buccopharyngeal membrane and Rathke pouch meet exemplify growths derived from congenital malformations that may manifest themselves as tumors many years after birth. Of 73 patients with craniopharyngiomas reviewed by Campbell and Hudson,[1] only 21 were operated on in the first decade of life. But in Matson and Crigler's[2] series, 16 of 18 patients were under 12 years of age and Matson[3] stated that the majority of cases were reported in the first 2 decades of life. The peak of incidence occurs between the ages of 13 and 23 years but, in some patients, symptoms developed after the age of 60 years.[4] Among intracranial tumors of childhood, approximately 10% are craniopharyngiomas[3]; they may account for 18% of supratentorial tumors of children.[5] Craniopharyngiomas are said to arise from nests of epithelial cells in the pars tuberalis of the Rathke pouch, the hypophyseo-pharyngeal duct leaving, after incomplete involution, rests of squamous epithelium on the anterior surface of the pituitary near the level of the sellar diaphragm.[6] Derivation from the ectoderm of the primitive stomodeum could explain the adamantinomatous epithelium seen in craniopharyngiomas, but this explanation is not generally accepted because squamous cell nests are found only rarely in pituitary glands from young people. Yet such nests do occur. Goldberg and Eshbaugh[7] noted squamous cells in the pituitaries of 4 newborn infants after a search of 121 glands of premature and full-term newborn infants. Although squamous epithelial cell rests are frequent accidental findings at necropsy of adults, they give rise to tumors in only a few persons. Craniopharyngiomas are tumors and not congenital malformations,[1] although they arise on the basis of developmental errors. The underlying malformation can be demonstrated in some children by early manifestations, such as dwarfism and mental retardation. Other patients appear normal for many years until tumor symptoms become manifest. Some of the manifestations are due to cyst formation or fibrous and glial tissue reaction of surrounding areas. The stroma as well as keratoid substance[4] can undergo calcification, which results in densities so common in roentgenograms of children with this tumor. Craniopharyngiomas grow slowly and do not metastasize. They cause damage by their extension to vital areas. Intrasellar tumors tend to cause pituitary symptoms, whereas suprasellar lesions grow toward the third ventricle and cause obstruction of cerebrospinal fluid pathways. Sometimes, histories suggest the presence of the tumor for as long as 20 years before onset of the signs that lead to hospital admission.[1] Dwarfism, diabetes insipidus,[8,12] obesity, sexual impairment or loss of weight may precede the tumor symptoms. Large *Rathke-cleft cysts* are rarer than craniopharyngiomas but microscopic Rathke-cleft cysts are rather frequent anomalies seen at necropsy[9]; they enlarge only seldom to a size of clinical significance to cause visual difficulties or symptoms of endocrine disturbance. Early retardation of growth is rare but it has been observed[10]; more often, manifestations are delayed for decades after birth. In contrast to craniopharyngiomas, Rathke-cleft cysts are lined by columnar epithelium.[11]

REFERENCES

1. Campbell, J. B., and Hudson, F. M.: Craniobuccal origin, signs, and treatment of craniopharyngiomas, Surg., Gynec. & Obst. 111:183, 1960.
2. Matson, D. D., and Crigler, J. F.: Radical treatment of craniopharyngioma, Ann. Surg. 152:699, 1960.
3. Matson, D. D.: *Neurosurgery of Infancy and Childhood* (Springfield, Ill.: Charles C Thomas, Publisher, 1969).
4. Zülch, K. J.: *Brain Tumors. Their Biology and Pathology* (New York: Springer-Verlag, 1965).
5. Miller, R. H., Craig, W. M., and Kernohan, J. W.: Supratentorial tumors among children, Arch. Neurol. & Psychiat. 68:797, 1952.
6. Erdheim, J.: Über Hypophysengangsgeschwülste und Hirncholesteatome, Sitzungsber. Akad. Wissensch. Math.-naturw. Kl. 113:537, 1904.
7. Goldberg, G. M., and Eshbaugh, D. E.: Squamous cell nests of the pituitary gland as related to the origin of craniopharyngiomas, Arch. Path. 70:293, 1960.
8. Rodeck, H.: Diabetes insipidus und Antidiabetes insipidus als Folge eines Craniopharyngeoms, Monatsschr. Kinderh. 101:417, 1953.
9. Shanklin, W. H.: Incidence and distribution of cilia in the human pituitary with a description of micro-follicular cysts derived from Rathke's cleft, Acta anat. scandinav. 11:361, 1951.
10. Worster-Drought, C., Dickerson, W. E. C., and Archer, B. W. C.: Dyspituitarism of the Lorain type, associated with a pituitary cyst arising from Rathke's cleft and secondary lesions in hypothalamic region and ventricles, Brain 50: 704, 1927.
11. Berry, R. G., and Schlezinger, N. S.: Rathke-cleft cysts, A.M.A. Arch. Neurol. & Psychiat. 1:48, 1959.
12. Warkany, J., and Mitchell, A. G.: Diabetes insipidus in children: A critical review of etiology, diagnosis and treatment, with report of four cases, Am. J. Dis. Child. 57: 603, 1939.

Intracranial Teratomas

THESE INTERESTING GROWTHS are rare; they account for only about 1.5% of intracranial tumors in children and for 3% of teratomas observed in various parts of the body.[1] Among 750 intracranial tumors of children listed by Matson,[2] there were only 11 teratomas. These tumors are always prenatal in origin and some become symptomatic in fetal or neonatal life; others manifest themselves in later childhood or even decades after birth.[3] Although related to epidermoids and dermoids, teratomas differ from these growths, since they contain mesodermal, entodermal and ectodermal tissues. Intracranial teratomas are cystic tumors that cause damage by replacement of or pressure on neural tissues or by interference with cerebrospinal fluid pathways. Almost half of these teratomas are located in the pineal region[4,5]; others are found in the third ventricle, over the sella and in other locations.[2,3,6] Males generally are affected much more often than females, particularly by pineal teratomas,[3,7] but the sex ratio is reversed in newborns with intracranial teratomas.[6] These tumors can lead to congenital hydrocephaly and to dystocia[8-10] or they can replace the brain and occupy the entire cranial cavity.[6,11] Some intracranial teratomas are not limited to the cranium, as they extend to the oral, pharyngeal or orbital region.[6] In the last case, congenital exophthalmia can occur.[12] In 1966, Tamura *et al.*[6] reviewed the publications on intracranial teratomas in fetuses and infants; they found 15 case reports on fetuses and newborns and added 3 cases of their own, including one of a 22-week fetus in which the tumor mass had replaced the brain. They also listed 17 cases observed in infants who had survived birth. Although these teratomas were, of course, congenital also, their manifestations were different from those in patients who died before or soon after birth.[13-16]

In some children, tumor symptoms and signs can be delayed for many years, but the underlying malformation may manifest itself early by hydrocephaly, mental retardation, dwarfism or precocious puberty. Hosoi,[17] who reviewed intracranial teratomas recorded before 1930, described a 27-year-old man who had been hydrocephalic, dwarfed and mentally defective from early childhood. After he died of bronchopneumonia, a teratoma originating from the cerebellum was found. Precocious puberty and rapid weight gain were noted by Bruton *et al.*[18] in a 7-year-old boy. A tumor of the third ventricle was discovered that proved to be malignant teratoma containing many different tissues, such as sarcoma, leiomyosarcoma and epithelial structures resembling glands of the gastrointestinal and respiratory tracts. In addition, there were fields resembling embryonal carcinoma or seminoma of the testis and large areas of choriocarcinoma with malignant syncytial trophoblasts interposed between blood-filled sinuses and sheets of malignant cytotrophoblasts. Chorioepithelial elements also have been noted in pineal tumors leading to precocious puberty (Chapter 47, p. 451). As mentioned before, pineal and juxtapineal teratomas account for about 50% of intracranial teratomas; pineal teratomas constitute about 10% of all the reported pineal tumors.[19] The latter figure could be an underestimate, since many pinealomas may be atypical teratomas.[20] The fact that intracranial teratomas commonly are found in various midline structures has led to the belief that the midline of the developing embryo has potentialities for displacement and subsequent maldevelopment of cells.[5] It also has been suggested that the pineal is a frequent site of teratoma because its anlage is near the surface in intrauterine life and thus susceptible to penetration by foreign tissue elements.[21] Other aspects of pineal tumors, including teratomas, have been discussed in Chapter 46.

Although intracranial teratomas are due to developmental errors, associated malformations are rare in patients with these tumors. An exception was a case reported by Tamura *et al.*,[6] in which the eyeball, the auricles and an external auditory canal were deformed. The orbits also were involved in other cases when an intracranial teratoma extended into that region.[12,22] A pinealoma, possibly a teratoma, was described in a patient with the Laurence-Moon-Biedl syndrome.[23]

REFERENCES

1. Willis, R. A.: *The Pathology of the Tumours of Children* (Springfield, Ill.: Charles C Thomas, Publisher, 1962).
2. Matson, D. D.: *Neurosurgery of Infancy and Childhood* (Springfield, Ill.: Charles C Thomas, Publisher, 1969).
3. Müller, R., and Wohlfart, G.: Intracranial teratomas and teratoid tumors, Acta Psychiat. 22:69, 1947.
4. Zülch, K. J.: *Brain Tumors, Their Biology and Pathology* (New York: Springer-Verlag, 1965).
5. Lichtenstein, B. W.: Teratoma of the pineal body, Arch. Neurol. & Psychiat. 44:153, 1940.
6. Tamura, H., Kury, G., and Suzuki, K.: Intracranial teratomas in fetal life and infancy, Obst. & Gynec. 27:134, 1966.
7. Weber, E.: Die Teratome und Teratoide des Zentralnervensystems, Zentralbl. Neurochir. 4:47, 1939.
8. Baxter, J.: Fetal brain tumor as a cause of dystocia, J. Obst. & Gynaec. Brit. Emp. 54:380, 1947.
9. Wagner, J. A., Douglass, L. H., and Slager, U. T.: Dystocia caused by fetal intracranial teratoma. Report of a case, Obst. & Gynec. 4:647, 1954.
10. Simpson, D. A., Carter, R. F., and Ducrou, W.: Intracranial tumours in infancy, Developmental Med. & Child Neurol. 10:190, 1968.
11. Oberman, B.: Intracranial teratoma replacing brain, Arch. Neurol. 11:423, 1964.
12. Mégevand, A., and Werner, A.: Exophthalmie néo-natale d'origine tumorale, Confinia neurol. 20:125, 1960.
13. Ingraham, F. D., and Bailey, O. T.: Cystic teratomas and teratoid tumors of the central nervous system in infancy and childhood, J. Neurosurg. 3:511, 1946.
14. Arnstein, L. H., Boldrey, E., and Naffziger, H. C.: A case report and survey of brain tumors during the neonatal period, J. Neurosurg. 8:315, 1951.
15. Raskind, R., and Beigel, F.: Brain tumors in early infancy – probably congenital in origin, J. Pediat. 65:727, 1964.
16. Greenhouse, A. H., and Neuberger, K. T.: Intracranial teratoma of the newborn, Arch. Neurol. 3:718, 1960.
17. Hosoi, K.: Teratoma and teratoid tumors of the brain, Arch. Path. 9:1207, 1930.
18. Bruton, O. C., Martz, D. C., and Gerard, E. S.: Precocious puberty due to secreting chorionepithelioma (teratoma) of the brain, J. Pediat. 59:719, 1961.
19. Bochner, S. J., and Scarff, J. R.: Teratoma of the pineal body. Classification of the embryonal tumors of the pineal body. Report of a case of teratoma of the pineal body presenting formed teeth, Arch. Surg. 36:303, 1938.
20. Russel, D. S.: The pinealoma: Its relationship to teratoma, J. Path. & Bact. 56:145, 1944.
21. Krabbe, K. H.: The pineal gland, especially in relation to the problem of its supposed significance in sexual development, Endocrinology 7:379, 1923.
22. Chasan, B.: Eine Missbildung und Mischgeschwulst des Zentralnervensystems, Schweiz. Arch. Neurol. u. Psychiat. 27:64, 1931.
23. Massobrio, E., and Boccuzzi, G.: Tumore (teratoma?) della pineal associato a malformazioni scheletriche come causa di puberta precoce e cindrome iperpituitarica tipo Cushing, Endocrinologia e patologia constituzionale 14:86, 1939.
24. Peyton, W. T., and Baker, A. B.: Epidermoid, dermoid and teratomatous tumors of the central nervous system, Arch. Neurol. & Psychiat. 47:890, 1942.

Epidermoids and Dermoids

THESE TUMORS generally are considered to be the result of embryonic rests. "They are of congenital origin and their foundation is in all probability laid early in intrauterine life."[1] Since such embryonic rests grow very slowly, tumor symptoms are delayed for decades, their peak "incidence" being around the age of 40 years.[2] But dermoid and epidermoid remnants can become symptomatic in children. Some of them develop along congenital dermal sinuses, thus proving their developmental origin.[3,4] The epidermoids produce symptoms somewhat later in life than the dermoids.[1] These tumors account for approximately 1% of intracranial tumors. The predilection for dermoids is around embryonic closure lines, such as the maxillary and frontal processes, and around the pituitary and pons when located within the cranium. Epidermoids occur at the cerebellopontine angle, around the pons or pituitary, in the longitudinal fissure and at other sites.[5,6] The epidermoids show, in their capsule, stratum germinativum, granulosum and corneum and dermoids contain, in addition to epidermal structures, dermal elements such as hair follicles, sebaceous glands and even sweat glands. Epidermoids have a shiny or pearly surface and enclose leafy material arranged in layers like onion skin. Dermoids are covered with a firm capsule that is filled with a greasy mass containing short hairs. Symptoms are caused by cystic growth of the developmental rests and also by inflammatory reactions of surrounding parenchymatous or meningeal tissues.[7] Arachnoiditis, ependymitis and aqueduct stenosis can lead to a variety of signs and symptoms.[2]

REFERENCES

1. Kernohan, J. W., and Sayre, G. P.: Tumors of the Central Nervous System, in *Atlas of Tumor Pathology* (Washington, D. C.: Armed Forces Institute of Pathology, 1952).
2. Zülch, K. J.: *Brain Tumors. Their Biology and Pathology* (New York: Springer-Verlag, 1965).
3. Matson, D. D.: *Neurosurgery of Infancy and Childhood* (Springfield, Ill.: Charles C Thomas, Publisher, 1969).
4. Schwartz, H. G.: Congenital tumors of the spinal cord in infants, Ann. Surg. 136:183, 1952.
5. Peyton, W. T., and Baker, A. B.: Epidermoid, dermoid and teratomatous tumors of the central nervous system, Arch. Neurol. & Psychiat. 47:890, 1942.
6. Price, E. B., Jr., and Mostofi, F. K.: Epidermoid cysts of the testis in children: A report of four cases, J. Pediat. 77:676, 1970.
7. Content, J., Point, G., and Hariga, M.: Kyste dermoïde de la voûte crânienne, Acta paediat. belg. 24:51, 1970.

Congenital Spinal Tumors

TUMORS within the spinal canal are comparatively rare during infancy and childhood[1] and this is particularly true if tumors associated with developmental defects are excluded. In some series, intraspinal tumors were seen frequently in the first few years of life[1] and in others there was no age specificity until a marked rise occurred after the eleventh year.[2] Inclusion of children with tumors associated with congenital anomalies increases the incidence of early tumors. Congenital dermal sinuses, spinal dermoids, teratoids and teratomas represent a continuous series of developmental anomalies.[3] Congenital tumors of the spinal cord commonly are connected with sinus tracts located higher than the typical sinuses seen in the sacrococcygeal region. Dermoids like dermal sinuses are attributed to incomplete separation of neural and cutaneo-epithelial ectoderm. It seems that not only dermoid cysts but also teratoids and teratomas sometimes are connected with the skin by dermal canals,[4] which suggests that both anomalies are due to similar developmental disturbances. Manifestations of congenital spinal cysts and tumors can be delayed for years and be intermittent. Hoefnagel *et al.*[5] made nuclear sex determinations in the tissues of teratomatous cysts found within the vertebral canal and described sex chromatin-positive cells in the tumors of 2 male patients.

It appears that intracranial and intraspinal lipomas like the tumors just discussed show relations to teratoids and teratomas.[6] It has been pointed out[7] that intraspinal lipomas seen in infancy usually are associated with dorsal midline malformations of various types. Intraspinal lipomas found in late childhood and in adults also often are combined with congenital defects that are, however, less obvious than those noted in infants. Slowly progressing neurologic deficits referable to the spinal cord develop in such cases. Swanson and Barnett[7] reported 9 cases of intradural spinal lipomas presenting in childhood or infancy. In all instances, associated congenital defects were present. There is a close relationship of lipomas and lipoblastic tumors of the brain and spine to congenital malformations.[8,9] Spina bifida, including spina bifida occulta,[10] defects or absence of the corpus callosum, hydrocephaly, cataract, harelip and genitourinary anomalies have been listed as associated malformations.

REFERENCES

1. Matson, D. D.: *Neurosurgery of Infancy and Childhood* (Springfield, Ill.: Charles C Thomas, Publisher, 1969).
2. Dodge, H. W., Jr., Keith, H. M., and Campagna, M. J.: Intraspinal tumors in infants and children, J. Internat. Coll. Surgeons 26:199, 1956.
3. Walker, A. E., and Bucy, P. E.: Congenital dermal sinuses: A source of spinal meningeal infection and subdural abscesses, Brain 57:401, 1934.
4. Schwartz, H. G.: Congenital tumors of the spinal cord in infants, Ann. Surg. 136:183, 1952.
5. Hoefnagel, D., Benirschke, K., and Duarte, J.: Teratomatous cysts within the vertebral canal, J. Neurol., Neurosurg. & Psychiat. 25:159, 1962.
6. Vonderahe, A. R., and Niemer, W. T.: Intracranial lipoma. A report of four cases, J. Neuropath. & Exper. Neurol. 3: 344, 1944.
7. Swanson, H. S., and Barnett, J. C., Jr.: Intradural lipomas in children, Pediatrics 29:911, 1962.
8. Caram, P. C., Scorcella, G., and Carton, C. A.: Intradural lipomas of spinal cord; with particular emphasis on "intramedullary" lipomas, J. Neurosurg. 14:28, 1957.
9. Kauffman, S. L., and Stout, A. P.: Lipoblastic tumors of children, Cancer 12:912, 1959.
10. Lassman, L. P., and James, C. C. M.: Lumbosacral lipomas: Critical survey of 26 cases submitted to laminectomy, J. Neurol., Neurosurg. & Psychiat. 30:174, 1967.

Chordomas

THESE TUMORS are thought to arise from vestiges of the notochord or from a nucleus pulposus. They reach tumor size rather late, with a peak incidence in the fifth decade; there is a preponderance in males. In rare cases, chordomas have been observed in the fetus[1] and in children.[2] In one instance, a coccygeal chordoma in a girl was associated with spina bifida occulta.[3] Most often, the site is near either end of the notochord, i.e., at the clivus or at the sacrum or coccyx, but cervical and lumbar vertebrae also can be the origin of these tumors. By 1968, there were 548 chordomas on record, of which 44% were intracranial, 41% sacrococcygeal and 15% vertebral.[4] There are benign chordomas, which usually are discovered accidentally at necropsy. In some such cases, they are associated with other tumors, such as spongioblastoma or rectal carcinoid.[5] Malignant chordomas grow rapidly in exceptional cases but, as a rule, they expand slowly, invading surrounding tissues. Metastases are found in lymph nodes, liver and other organs. Although trauma often is blamed for the development of the tumor, its role is not convincing in all instances.[5]

REFERENCES

1. Henning, L.: Über congenitale echte Sacraltumoren, Beitr. path. Anat. 28:593, 1900.
2. Montgomery, A. H., and Walman, I. J.: Sacrococcygeal chordomas in children, Am. J. Dis. Child. 46:1263, 1933.
3. Willis, R. A.: *The Pathology of the Tumours of Children* (Springfield, Ill.: Charles C Thomas, Publisher, 1962).
4. Wang, C. C., and James, A. E., Jr.: Chordoma: Brief review of the literature and report of a case with widespread metastases, Cancer 22:162, 1968.
5. Congdon, C. C.: Benign and malignant chordomas, Am. J. Path. 28:793, 1952.

Retinoblastoma

RETINOBLASTOMA has been discussed in Chapter 39. It is recognized in 70% of the cases in the first 3 years of life, and in 7% it is sufficiently advanced at birth to manifest itself by the light reflex known as "amaurotic cat eye." Wintersteiner[1] believed that all cases noted in the first year and possibly all those of the second year are congenital. In fact, he assumed that these tumors are always a congenital disease, although the anlage at the time of birth may be so small that it escapes inspection and ophthalmoscopic examination.[2] The development of bilateral retinoblastoma in a premature infant was observed by Hix and Danielson[3] from the time of its first clinical appearance until removal of the eyes. Bilateral involvement occurs in approximately 20% of the cases. The interval between manifestation in the two eyes may be weeks or years. Wells[2] expressed the belief that retinal gliomatous malformations may be frequent but that only a few of them become malignant. This belief is similar to that of Beckwith and Perrin[4] concerning neuroblastoma of the adrenal gland.

Lele *et al.*,[5] examining blood and tissues of a patient with retinoblastoma cytogenetically, noticed in all cells a deletion in the long arm of a large acrocentric chromosome. Five other patients had normal karyotypes. There now are several cases on record in which partial deletion of a D chromosome was noted. In the patient reported by Lele *et al.*,[5] there were no associated malformations. Two patients who developed retinoblastoma had the so-called 13q− deletion syndrome, which is characterized by microcephaly, microphthalmia, protruding upper incisors, micrognathia and other malformations.[6] In a girl with retinoblastoma, cleft palate and transverse palmar creases, deletion of a D chromosome was noted.[7] Retinoblastoma also has been reported in a girl who had an XXX-21 trisomy karyotype.[8] These patients seem to differ in etiology from familial cases that have occurred in several generations and from cases of concordant monozygotic twins.[9] Sporadic cases are more common than familial ones. Eugenic prognosis is difficult for these patients because some of them may have affected children, whereas others have offspring free of the disorder. General risk figures, which are quite tenuous for this anomaly, are discussed in Chapter 39. In some patients who developed retinoblastoma, a familial and individual "tumor diathesis" has been considered. Levene[10] reported a case of congenital retinoblastoma in a patient who later developed vaginal sarcoma botryoides and Bryson and Wolter[11] described a woman who had her left eye removed because of a retinoblastoma at the age of 9 months. She gave birth to 2 children who showed retinoblastoma in infancy and to 1 normal child; she developed choriocarcinoma in her right breast 10 weeks after the birth of her third child.

REFERENCES

1. Wintersteiner, H.: *Das Neuroepithelioma Retinae* (Leipzig: Franz Deuticke, 1897).
2. Wells, H. G.: Occurrence and significance of congenital malignant neoplasms, Arch. Path. 30:535, 1940.
3. Hix, I. E., Jr., and Danielson, R. W.: Bilateral retinoblastoma in a premature infant, Am. J. Ophth. 35:1647, 1952.
4. Beckwith, J. B., and Perrin, E. V.: In situ neuroblastomas: A contribution to the natural history of neural crest tumors, Am. J. Path. 43:1089, 1963.
5. Lele, K. P., Penrose, L. S., and Stallard, H. B.: Chromo-

some deletion in a case of retinoblastoma, Ann. Human Genet. 27:171, 1963.
6. Allerdice, P. W., Davis, J. G., Miller, O. J., Klinger, H. P., Warburton, D., Miller, D. A., Allen, F. H., Jr., Abrams, C. A., and McGilvray, E.: The 13q− deletion syndrome. Am. J. Human Genet. 21:499, 1969.
7. Wilson, M. G., Melnyk, J., and Towner, J. W.: Retinoblastoma and deletion D (14) syndrome, J. M. Genetics 6:322, 1969.
8. Day, R. W., Wright, S. W., Koons, A., and Quigley, M.: XXX-21 trisomy and retinoblastoma, Lancet 2:154, 1963.
9. Klein, D., and Franceschetti, A.: Missbildungen und Krankheiten des Auges, in Becker, P. E. (ed.), *Humangenetik* (Stuttgart: Georg Thieme, 1964), Vol. 4.
10. Levene, M.: Congenital retinoblastoma and sarcoma botryoides of the vagina, Cancer 13:532, 1960.
11. Bryson, J. M., and Wolter, J. R.: Retinoblastoma and choriocarcinoma, J. Pediat. Ophth. 2:41, 1965.

Thyroid Tumors

In 1956, Winship[1] collected from the literature 334 cases of thyroid carcinoma of childhood, a malignancy once considered quite rare before adolescence. He stated that the children were all normal at birth except for 3 with minor developmental anomalies and 12 with congenital thyroid tumors that later proved to be carcinoma. In 1969, the number of reported childhood thyroid cancers had increased to about 900.[2,3] Two-thirds of the patients were female and one-third male. The average age of the children at the time of the diagnosis was 10 years but, in rare instances, thyroid cancer has occurred in infants. The usual manifestation consists of rather painless nodules in the lateral aspects of the neck; carcinoma should be suspected in nodular thyroids of children.[1,4] Local symptoms are rare except in advanced cases. Metastases in the lungs or bones seldom are present when the children are first seen but, in some patients, pulmonary metastases were mistaken for tuberculous lesions.[1] Histologically, papillary, follicular and undifferentiated types can be distinguished but mixed forms are quite frequent. The follicular type has a tendency to bone metastases.

Thyroglossal duct cysts or sinuses give rise to malignant tumors only rarely. Keeling and Ochsner[5] reported 2 cases and collected 5 from the literature. The tumors were carcinomas, two occurring in children. One was located in the tongue, the other appeared as "lumps" in the midline of the neck. In one child, the lump had been present since the age of 2 years, but growth was marked only 1 year before operation, when the child was 9 years of age. The papillary adenocarcinoma of thyroid origin had metastasized to the lymph nodes, lungs and liver. The subject of carcinoma of thyroglossal duct cysts was reviewed again by Bhagavan *et al.*[6] in 1970. Incomplete obliteration of the thyroglossal duct results in an epithelial strand that ends blindly near or in the hyoid bone; dilatation of the tract produces cysts of variable size and variable epithelial lining. Malignant degeneration of thyroglossal duct cysts is rare; only 43 cases had been reported by 1970.[6] The tumors present as masses in or near the midline around the hyoid bone. Adenocarcinoma is more common than follicular carcinoma. It is thought that these tumors are primary carcinomas. The thyroid glands of the patients usually are free of malignant neoplasia and removal of the tumor leads to cure in most cases. Cancers in thyroglossal cysts exemplify malignancy resulting from a developmental error.

Association of thyroid carcinoma with spina bifida occulta, dislocation of the hip, retinal lesions and cerebral calcifications was reported by Langmann and Bruch.[7] A tumor of an accessory thyroid combined with osseous deformities was described by Snapper.[8] In general, there is little evidence that parental thyroid disease or cancer predisposes to thyroid malignancy in the offspring, but there are certain "neoplastic diatheses" with hereditary tendency that involve the thyroid gland. Pendred syndrome (Chapters 41 and 44), which combines nerve deafness with goiter and a tendency to thyroid malignancy, is genetically determined; and heredity plays an important role in a multiple endocrine neoplasia syndrome (Chapter 124) that includes medullary thyroid carcinoma. An unusual case was reported of a mother who died after an operation for thyroid cancer who had had a son and a daughter, both of whom developed thyroid cancer. Interestingly, the son's malignancy proved to be an adenocarcinoma, whereas that of his sister was a medullary carcinoma,[9] which suggests that an inherited etiologic factor can express itself in differing thyroid disease pictures.

It seems that cancer of the thyroid has become more frequent in recent decades. It is thought that these additional cancers are of postnatal origin. There certainly is an increase in the appearance of these tumors with advancing age of children. The incidence of thyroid carcinoma is not increased in areas of endemic goiter and goitrogenic factors such as cobalt medication or soybean diets apparently are not carcinogenic.[2,10] But irradiation of the neck in infancy and early childhood must be accepted as a thyroid carcinogen. Significant numbers of children and adolescents with thyroid cancer have a history of early x-ray treatment for thymic enlargement.[10-12] In 20–40% of children with thyroid cancer, x-irradiation had been given in early childhood for eczema, enlarged tonsils or adenoids, nevi, lymphadenitis or thymic enlargment.[1,3,13] In a controlled study, it was found that the incidence of carcinoma of the thyroid in a group of persons irradiated over the neck, head and chest in infancy and childhood was about one hundred times that expected from morbidity tables; yet, radiation did not appear to be the sole factor responsible for the increased incidence.[14] The nature of the accessory factors has not been recognized and the etiologic role of irradiation is difficult to prove. But a number of careful studies support the belief that childhood irradiation increases the risk of thyroid neoplasia.[15]

The prognosis of thyroid carcinoma in children is relatively good.[16] It is said that differentiated thyroid carcinomas have the best prognosis of all malignant diseases in childhood but the prognosis is poor for undifferentiated tumors.[3] Treatment is outlined and evaluated in a number of publications.[3,16,17]

REFERENCES

1. Winship, T.: Carcinoma of thyroid in childhood, Pediatrics 18:459, 1956.
2. Winship, T.: Management of the patients with cancer of the thyroid, Cancer 20:1815, 1967.
3. Zabransky, S.: Das Schilddrüsenkarzinom beim Kind. Arch. Kinderh. 179:236, 1969.
4. Kennedy, R. L.: Nodular goiter among infants and children, Tr. Am. A. Study of Goiter 322, 1940.
5. Keeling, J. H., and Ochsner, A.: Carcinoma in thyroglossal duct remnants. Review of literature and report of 2 cases, Cancer 12:596, 1959.
6. Bhagavan, B. S., Rao, B-S., and Weinberg, T.: Carcinoma of the thyroglossal duct cyst: Case reports and review of the literature, Surgery 67:281, 1970.
7. Langmann, A. G., and Bruch, H.: Carcinoma of the thyroid gland in children, Am. J. Dis. Child. 56:616, 1938.
8. Snapper, I.: Tumor of accessory thyroid and bone deformities, Nederl. tijdschr. geneesk. 2:4758, 1929.
9. Friedell, G. H., Carey, R. J., and Rosen, H.: Familial thyroid cancer, Cancer 15:241, 1962.
10. Duffy, B. J., and Fitzgerald, P. J.: Thyroid cancer in childhood and adolescence, Cancer 3:1018, 1950.
11. Clark, D. E.: Association of irradiation with cancer of the thyroid in children and adolescents, J.A.M.A. 159:1007, 1955.
12. Simpson, C. L., Hempelman, L. H., and Fuller, L. M.: Neoplasia in children treated with x-rays in infancy for thymic enlargement, Radiology 64:840, 1955.
13. Hiller, H-J., and Bachmann, K. D.: Über das sogenannte Schilddrüsencarcinom im Kindesalter, Monatsschr. Kinderh. 118:157, 1970.
14. Saenger, E. L., Silverman, F. N., Sterling, T. D., and Turner, M. E.: Neoplasia following therapeutic irradiation for benign conditions in childhood, Radiology 74:889, 1960.
15. Janower, M. L., and Miettinen, O. S.: Neoplasms after childhood irradiation of the thymus gland, J.A.M.A. 215: 753, 1971.
16. Horn, R. C., Jr., and Ravdin, I. S.: Carcinoma of thyroid gland in youth, J. Clin. Endocrinol. 11:1166, 1951.
17. Winship, T., and Rosvoll, R. V.: Thyroid carcinoma in childhood: Final report on a 20-year study, Clin. Proc. Child. Hosp., Washington 26:327, 1970.

Cardiac Tumors

CONGENITAL TUMORS OF THE HEART have been discussed in Chapter 65, where their rarity was mentioned. Myxomas, which are the most frequent primary tumors of the heart, have no particular tendency to occurrence in early years. Primary sarcomas of the heart also occur at all ages from infancy to late adult life and not much is known concerning their origin. Rhabdomyomas, however, show a predilection for younger age groups[1]; they have been found in stillborn and newborn babies and it is assumed that many are congenital. One case occurred in a fetus of 6½ months' gestation[2] and many result in early death. It is said that rhabdomyomas are a manifestation of tuberous sclerosis in about half of the cases,[3] but this could be an underestimate, since in patients who die within the first year, tuberous sclerosis may go undiagnosed if rhabdomyoma of the heart is the first manifestation of the disorder. Rhabdomyomas of the heart can simulate pulmonary stenosis[4] or be associated with tetralogy of Fallot.[3] Cardiac rhabdomyomas have been observed in both members of a set of twins.[5] Fibromas, angiomas and pericardial tumors also have been described in infants (Chapter 65). Primary cardiac malignancies in children were reviewed by Arshadi and Watson,[6] who reported a cardiac teratocarcinoma in a 4-year-old girl. Another malignant teratoma of the heart recorded by Solomon[7] was found in a 2-year-old girl.

Successful surgical removal of cardiac tumors[12] has rendered early clinical diagnosis important.[8] Many reports of surgical intervention refer to adult patients[9] but hamartomas have been diagnosed and removed in children. Parks *et al.*[10] excised a large hamartoma of the left ventricular wall in a 2-year-old boy; a sibling of this patient had died at 5 days of age with aortic atresia. May *et al.*[11] reported successful resection of a vascular hamartoma of the right atrium in a 10-year-old boy. The lesion was considered more in the nature of a malformation than a neoplasm.

REFERENCES

1. Longino, L. A., and Meeker, I. A., Jr.: Primary cardiac tumors in infancy, J. Pediat. 43:724, 1953.
2. Bigelow, N. H., Klinger, S., and Wright, A. W.: Primary tumors of the heart in infancy and early childhood, Cancer 7:549, 1954.
3. Golding, R., and Reed, G.: Rhabdomyoma of the heart, New England J. Med. 276:957, 1967.
4. Dupuis, C., Ducoulombier, H., and Nuyts, J. P.: Rhabdomyome du ventricule droit simulant une sténose pulmonaire chez un nourrisson, Pédiatrie 20:585, 1965.
5. Scariano, N.: Rhabdomyoma of the heart in both of a set of twins, Acta Genet. 11:124, 1962.
6. Arshadi, S., and Watson, D. G.: Teratocarcinoma of the heart, Am. J. Dis. Child. 112:87, 1966.

7. Solomon, R. D.: Malignant teratoma of the heart, Arch. Path. 52:561, 1951.
8. Goldberg, H. P., and Steinberg, I.: Primary tumours of the heart, Circulation 11:963, 1955.
9. Abbott, O. A., Warshawski, F. E., and Cobbs, B. W.: Primary tumors and pseudotumors of the heart, Ann. Surg. 155:855, 1962.
10. Parks, F. R., Adams, F., and Sangmire, W. P.: Successful excision of a left ventricular hamartoma, Circulation 26: 1316, 1962.
11. May, I. A., Hardy, K. L., Char, F., and McAdams, J.: Vascular hamartoma of the right atrium with successful resection, Ann. Thoracic Surg. 1:64, 1965.
12. Scannell, J. G., and Grillo, H. C.: Primary tumors of the heart, J. Thoracic Surg. 35:23, 1958.

Tumors of the Respiratory Tract

NASAL GLIOMAS and their relationship to encephaloceles in the nasal area have been discussed (p. 591). In contrast to encephaloceles, gliomas are not connected with the cranial cavity and the brain but there are transitional formations in which the distinction is difficult. The gliomas are congenital; they can be extranasal, intranasal or both. No osseous defect is seen in roentgenograms. In a few cases, growth out of proportion to that of the patient has been reported, but usually they enlarge merely with the rest of the body. Recurrence after surgical removal is exceptional. Males and females can be affected. Associated malformations and familial recurrence have not been reported.[1]

Bronchial hamartomas have been described within the lungs of premature and term infants. Harris and Schattenberg[2] observed 2 newborn infants who survived birth 7 and 5 days, respectively, with tumors that had developed in intrauterine life, replacing entire lobes of the lungs. In one instance, embryonal bronchial budding was perpetuated in a neoplastic mass; in the other, ectodermal and mesodermal derivatives were intermingled. Tumors of mixed germinal layers also were found within bronchi of adult patients and considered embryonal in nature.[2,3] Jones[4] reported the case of a premature baby girl who died 1 hour after birth. A fibrochondromatous hamartoma involved the entire upper lobe of the right lung. Thomas[5] found a hamartoma in the lung of a premature male infant who died 15 minutes after birth. The tumor was interpreted as a malformed accessory lobe in which arrest of maturation had occurred at a stage corresponding to the nineteenth week of fetal life without diminution of the rate of growth. The resulting mass had the appearance of a benign neoplasm. The mother had developed acute hydramnios at the twenty-eighth week of pregnancy, when delivery was induced. The umbilical cord was of average length but twice the average thickness. Goodyear and Shillitoe[6] reported the case of a premature female infant whose right lung was replaced by a hamartomatous lesion.

Endobronchial chondromatous "hamartomas" and similar chondromatous "hamartomas" of the lung are rather common.[7] Willis[8] pointed out that these lesions are metaplastic and not teratologic; they occur in persons of advanced age and not in children.

Primary bronchial carcinoma has occurred in children but it is very rare. The subject was reviewed by Suter,[9] who described the case of a 6-year-old girl. The youngest children observed previously with such tumors were 2 girls, 16 months of age. There is no proof that these tumors arose on the basis of malformations. A case of bronchogenic carcinoma complicating situs inversus totalis was reported by Thompson.[19]

In 1928, an association of tumors and malformations of *the lung* had been suggested by Schwyter,[10] who quoted observations of pulmonary tumors in children and even fetuses. Some of these tumors were benign but carcinomas also were found in tissue malformations, such as congenital pulmonary cysts or bronchiectases. In some cases, associated anomalies were noted in other organs, e.g., polyps in the colon or rectum, intestinal duplication and others. Schwyter[10] considered the possibility of predisposing genetic factors. Today, one would think of tuberous sclerosis,[11,12] polyposis or other hamartoses as disorders predisposing to tumors of the lung. Adenomatous malformations of the lung have been described in newborn infants.[13] Although these lesions are benign, they cause respiratory distress and require surgical intervention. The condition is rare. Only 35 cases had been recorded by 1965[14] and Gillot *et al.*[15] added a case in 1969. The multicystic lesions have been considered hamartomas or congenital pulmonary cysts. Bronchovascular anomalies around the lesion indicate that developmental changes during fetal life are at the root of these anomalies.[16] Anasarca and hydramnios have been noted repeatedly.[15] There is disagreement concerning the nature of hamartomatous lesions found in the lungs of adult patients. They were considered neoplastic rather than developmental in origin, since they are not associated with congenital defects.[17] But mixed tumors of the lung that resemble fetal pulmonary tissue although they manifest themselves in adult life are thought to result from the failure of embryonic bronchial buds to develop into normal structures.[3] They have been considered related to "anlagen" tumors sometimes occurring in newborn children.[2] Chorioepithelioma has been described in the lung of a 7-month-old female infant.[18]

REFERENCES

1. Walker, E. A., Jr., and Resler, D. R.: Nasal glioma, Laryngoscope 73:93, 1963.
2. Harris, W. H., and Schattenberg, H. J.: Anlagen and rest tumors of the lung inclusive of "mixed tumors," Am. J. Path. 18:955, 1942.
3. Womack, N. A., and Graham, E. A.: Mixed tumors of the lung. So-called bronchial or pulmonary adenoma, Arch. Path. 26:165, 1938.
4. Jones, C. J.: Unusual hamartoma of the lung in a newborn infant, Arch. Path. 48:150, 1949.
5. Thomas, M. R.: A cystic hamartoma of the lung in a newborn infant, J. Path. & Bact. 61:599, 1949.
6. Goodyear, J. E., and Shillitoe, A. J.: Adenomatoid hamartoma of the lung in a newborn infant, J. Clin. Path. 12: 172, 1959.
7. Sutherland, T. W., Aylwin, J. A., and Brewin, E. G.: Endobronchial chondromatous hamartoma: A report of two cases, J. Path. & Bact. 65:93, 1953.
8. Willis, R. A.: *The Borderland of Embryology and Pathology* (Washington, D. C.: Butterworth, 1962).
9. Suter, L.: Primäres Bronchialcarcinom im Kindesalter, Ann. Paediat. 179:361, 1952.
10. Schwyter, M.: Über das Zusammentreffen von Tumoren und Missbildungen der Lungen, Frankfurt. Ztschr. Path. 36:146, 1928.
11. Dawson, J.: Pulmonary tuberous sclerosis and its relationship to other forms of the disease, Quart. J. Med. 23: 113, 1954.
12. Milledge, R. D., Gerald, B. E., and Carter, W. J.: Pulmonary manifestations of tuberous sclerosis, Am. J. Roentgenol. 98:734, 1966.
13. Craig, J. M., Kirkpatrick, J., and Neuhauser, E.: Congenital cystic adenomatoid malformation of the lungs in infants, Am. J. Roentgenol. 76:516, 1956.
14. Breckenridge, R. L., Rehermann, R. L., and Gibson, E. T.: Congenital cystic adenomatoid malformation of the lung, J. Pediat. 67:863, 1965.
15. Gillot, F., Bodin, G., Rival, J-M., Nomballais, M. F., Delajartre, A-Y., and Albert, M.: La malformation adénomatöide du poumon chez le nouveau-né, Pédiatrie 24:645, 1969.
16. Herrmann, J. W., Jewett, T. C., Jr., and Galletti, G.: Bronchogenic cysts in infants and children, J. Thoracic Surg. 37:242, 1959.
17. Butler, C., II, and Kleinerman, J.: Pulmonary hamartoma, Arch. Path. 88:584, 1969.
18. Kay, S., and Reed, W. G.: Chorioepithelioma of the lung in a female infant seven months old. Am. J. Path. 29:555, 1953.
19. Thompson, J. R.: Bronchogenic carcinoma complicating situs inversus totalis. Report of a case, Dis. Chest 44:317, 1963.

Hepatic Tumors

Congenital tumors of the liver have been discussed in Chapter 77. Wells[1] listed 10 cases of carcinoma of the liver observed at such an early age as to suggest prenatal malignancy. He also accepted an equal number of hepatic hemangioendotheliomas as congenital. Willis[2,3] distinguished between embryonic hepatomas and mixed hepatoblastomas. Embryonic hepatomas, consisting of immature liver cell parenchyma, manifest themselves in infancy and probably are always congenital. The mixed hepatoblastomas contain not only immature hepatic epithelial tissue but also fibrous tissue, cartilage, osteoid and bone. Rarely, they also show striated muscle fibers. Primary carcinoma of the liver in infancy and childhood was discussed by Bigelow and Wright.[4] Of 21 cases listed, 1 was congenital, showing metastases at 3 days of age, and 10 were under 1 year of age. According to Ishak and Glunz,[5] liver tumors in infants generally are hepatoblastomas and not hepatocarcinomas. Hemangioendotheliomas of the liver are rarities. A case in a newborn child was described by Caussade *et al.*[6] The child, who also showed numerous cutaneous angiomas, died of rupture of the liver at the age of 13 days. Another hepatic hemangioendothelioma simulated congenital heart disease.[7]

After an extensive review of death certificates and hospital charts, Fraumeni *et al.*[8] concluded that liver cancer in children often originates in utero, as indicated by the large proportion of cases diagnosed during infancy and by the sharp decline in national mortality in children after 3 years of age. Among whites, the mortality rates were more than four times higher in children under 5 years than in those 5–14 years of age. In both age groups, a male preponderance was noted. Morbidity, judged by hospital charts, declines sharply in children after 1 year of age.

Owing to the rarity of childhood liver cancer, there are too few observations to ascertain etiologic factors of general significance. Chronic liver diseases have been noted in a number of cases as precursors of hepatic tumors. Thus, a liver cell carcinoma developed in a boy 8 years of age who had de Toni-Fanconi syndrome and liver cirrhosis of several years' duration, and a hepatic mixed tumor was seen in a boy 6 months of age who had a storage disease of uncertain type.[9] Primary cell carcinoma and biliary cirrhosis due to congenital bile duct atresia were reported in a 3-year-old boy.[10] Fraumeni *et al.*[8] established that, in some of their patients, neonatal hepatitis, congenital biliary atresia, cirrhosis, de Toni-Fanconi syndrome or von Gierke disease had preceded formation of the tumor. They cited a number of similar cases from the literature and considered the possibility of a relationship of galactosemia to hepatic neoplasia.[8] These observations show that congenital disorders may be at the root of liver cancer in children who develop the tumor sometime after infancy.

In several instances, hemihypertrophy was an associated anomaly pointing to early prenatal influences. Roth[11] described a huge malignant mixed tumor in the left lobe of the liver in a female infant with complete hemihypertrophy of the left half of the body.

The tumor consisted of epithelial cells resembling liver cells and of cartilage and bone. By 1968, there were 5 cases of liver carcinoma associated with hemihypertrophy on record.[8] The combination of these two rare conditions is of particular interest, since Wilms tumor and adrenocortical tumors also occur in patients with hemihypertrophy. Association of a mixed hepatic tumor with Wilms tumor (without hemihypertrophy) also has been observed, suggesting a relationship of hepatic tumors with the anomalies known to be linked with Wilms tumor (p. 1228). Nephromegaly and other renal anomalies, sexual precocity, hemangiomas, lipoid disorders and demineralization of bone also were recorded in patients with hepatic carcinoma as complicating disorders.[8]

Liver cancer mortality among white children under 5 years of age was significantly higher than average in the North Central areas of the United States.[8] In Taiwan, primary liver cancer accounted for 20.6% of all the abdominal tumors in pediatric patients subjected to laparotomy.[12] Such regional prevalence suggests environmental influences[13] but, as yet, no extrinsic factors have been ascertained.

Familial cases of liver cancer have been reported in adults[8,13] but they must be rare in children.[8] Hepatoblastoma in infant sisters recorded by Fraumeni *et al.*[14] apparently was the first publication on familial occurrence of this neoplasm. No clues to etiology or pathogenesis were found. Hepatic carcinoma and intrahepatic bile duct atresia have occurred as alternate disorders in children of the same family.[15] No conclusions can be drawn from such observations concerning the etiology of the neoplasia, since genetic as well as environmental factors could bring about recurrence of such tumors in families.

In general, it can be stated that the liver responds with tumor formation to various heterogeneous disorders but that there are few leads to explain the hepatic tumors developing in utero or in infancy.

REFERENCES

1. Wells, H. G.: Occurrence and significance of congenital malignant neoplasms, Arch. Path. 30:535, 1940.
2. Willis, R. A.: *The Borderland of Embryology and Pathology* (Washington, D. C.: Butterworth, 1962).
3. Willis, R. A.: *The Pathology of the Tumours of Children* (Springfield, Ill.: Charles C Thomas, Publisher, 1962).
4. Bigelow, N. H., and Wright, A. W.: Primary carcinoma of the liver in infancy and childhood, Cancer 6:170, 1953.
5. Ishak, K. G., and Glunz, P. R.: Hepatoblastoma and hepatocarcinoma in infancy and childhood. Report of 47 cases, Cancer 20:396, 1967.
6. Caussade, L., Neimann, N., and Tridon, P.: Hémangioendotheliome du foie chez un nouveau-né mort par rupture du foie, Arch. franç. pédiat. 11:514, 1954.
7. Levick, C. B., and Rubie, J.: Haemangioendothelioma of the liver simulating congenital heart disease in an infant, Arch. Dis. Childhood 28:49, 1953.
8. Fraumeni, J. F., Jr., Miller, R. W., and Hill, J. A.: Primary carcinoma of the liver in childhood: An epidemiologic study, J. Nat. Cancer Inst. 40:1087, 1968.
9. Cleland, R. S.: Benign and malignant tumors of the liver, Pediat. Clin. North America 6:427, 1959.
10. Okuyama, K.: Primary liver cell carcinoma associated with biliary cirrhosis due to congenital bile duct atresia, J. Pediat. 67:89, 1965.
11. Roth, F.: Zur Kenntniss und Auffassung der Lebermischgeschwülste und des halbseitigen Riesenwuchses, Frankfurt. Ztschr. Path. 52:163, 1938.
12. Lin, T-Y., Chen, C-C., and Lui, W-P.: Primary carcinoma of the liver in infancy and childhood: Report of 21 cases, with resection in 6 cases, Surgery 60:1275, 1966.
13. Hagstrom, R. M., and Dee Baker, T.: Primary hepatocellular carcinoma in three male siblings, Cancer 22:142, 1968.
14. Fraumeni, J. F., Jr., Rosen, P. J., Hull, E. W., Barth, R. F., Shapiro, S. R., and O'Connor, J. F.: Hepatoblastoma in infant sisters, Cancer 24:1086, 1969.
15. Fajers, C. M., Falkner, S., Frisell, E., and Pehrson, M.: Primary carcinoma of the liver and giant cell hepatitis in infancy, Acta paediat. 49:96, 1960.

Neuroblastoma

NEUROBLASTOMA is a collective term used for neoplasms made up of cells of the sympathetic nervous system, which are derived from the neural crest. The term is used for tumors of differing location and differing maturity. In approximately 40% of the cases, the primary site is in an adrenal gland; the remainder originate from the sympathetic nervous system of the chest, abdomen, pelvis or neck. In rare instances, the tumors develop from a kidney or a sacrococcygeal teratoma.[1] Various grades of maturity are distinguished, according to the predominating cells of the tumor. When the most immature cells of the sympathetic system—the sympathogonia—prevail, one speaks of sympathogonioma, and when sympathicoblasts predominate, of sympathicoblastoma. These embryonal and malignant forms usually are summarized under the name of neuroblastoma. When mature sympathetic ganglion cells make up the tumor, one speaks of ganglioneuroma. But there are tumors containing both sympathicoblasts and ganglion cells, so that the pathologic diagnosis often is that of a ganglioneuroblastoma. Since such tumors carry a certain risk of malignancy, they, too, are classified as neuroblastomas. If metastases occur, they are found most frequently in bones, including those of the skull, or in regional lymph nodes, liver, lungs, skin and, rarely, in other locations.[1]

About three-fourths of the cases occur in children under 5 years of age,[1] and one-half in children under 2 years.[2] The mean age in different series was between 2 and 5 years. Patients of higher ages are important exceptions. A man in Willis'[2] series was 51, and a patient mentioned by Vaalasti and Peltokallio[3] was 88 years of age. A good many of these tumors are present at birth; small tissue anomalies, microscopically resembling neuroblastomas, are not rare. Wells[4] stated that neuroblastomas are the most frequent malignant congenital tumors; many produce extensive metastases, especially in the liver, either before or soon after birth. In 1940, Wells[4] tabulated 17 definite, 15 probable and 21 possible congenital cases. Sixteen of these were bilateral. There also were 10 extra-adrenal congenital neuroblastomas on record and several tumors diagnosed as congenital sarcomas that possibly were neuroblastomas. Many congenital neuroblastomas have been reported since; they were noticed at birth or in the neonatal period with a survival rate of about 40%.[5,6] Some of these patients were born with metastases and a third of them were among the long-term survivors.[7] In general, the neuroblastomas are tumors of childhood, whereas ganglioneuromas are tumors of adult life, i.e., they are not discovered before adolescence or later, although they may have been present as silent anomalies during childhood or even earlier. Willis[2] believed that neuroblastomas in adults probably are always the result of growth of tumors that have been clinically dormant since childhood. Neuroblastomas usually are functioning endocrine structures producing catecholamines and their metabolites. Measurements of catecholamines of the urine are important in diagnosis and follow-up care of patients with these tumors. These compounds may betray residual or metastatic tumors that are not evident clinically[8] but they are not specific for the histologic patterns of the growths.

The two sexes are affected equally. Little is known concerning etiologic factors. In one instance, identical twins were concordant, the tumor developing in one twin in the left and in the other twin in the right adrenal.[9] In other twins, there was discordance at the time of the report.[10-12] A few cases of familial neuroblastoma have been observed. There are six kinships on record in which more than 1 member had neuroblastoma and there are some suggestions that a parent may have been affected in two families.[13] A relationship to Recklinghausen neurofibromatosis has been considered in some cases.[7,14,15] Aneuploidy has been observed in tumor cells but the chromosomal abnormalities were not specific.[16]

Congenital malformations may be relatively frequent in children with neuroblastomas, although, in most patients, associated defects are not reported. It is of interest that of 4 cases of congenital neuroblastoma recorded by Wells,[4] 2 were combined with other congenital anomalies. In 1, there was hydrocephaly, spina bifida, partial coarctation of the aorta, absence of the left ureter and a malformation of the second left rib; in the other, there was a thymus cyst and vascular anomalies in the brain. It is noteworthy also that 2 affected infants had intrauterine growth retardation. Mittelbach and Szekely[17] found a neuroblastoma in the left adrenal at the necropsy of a child with cleft lip and palate, micrencephaly and defective corpus callosum. Aase and Smith[18] described an infant with hydrocephaly, absence of the midportion of the cerebellum, deformity of the medulla, cleft palate and flexion deformities of the extremities in whom an early neuroblastoma of the left adrenal gland was found. Patent ductus arteriosus,[15,17] coarctation of the aorta,[4,19] aganglionosis,[13] buccopharyngeal membrane, tracheo-esophageal fistula, patent foramen ovale, rudimentary kidney and uterus, polydactyly,[20] syndactyly,[21] rib anomalies[4,21] and clubfoot[19] have been noted in various combinations. A malformation involving the entire body, hemihypertrophy, was described by Lewis and Geschickter[22] and signs of neurofibromatosis were present in several other patients,[7,13,14,23] suggesting that neuroblastomas can be manifestations of differing general disorders or syndromes of multiple malformations.[21] It is noteworthy in this context that Beckwith and Perrin[24] described 13 cases of minute, incidentally encountered adrenal neuroblastomas in necropsies of young children. Although these tumors were cytologically identical with malignant neuroblastomas, they had not metastasized. The frequency of these "neuroblastomas in situ" found in necropsies was about forty times the expected occurrence of adrenal neuroblastoma. A similar excess of in-situ neuroblastomas over expected frequency of clinical neuroblastomas was noted by Shanklin and Sotelo-Avila.[33] It seemed that only a small proportion of these in-situ neuroblastomas became clinically manifest in survivors, whereas most of them underwent spontaneous resolution. But it must be considered that 9 of the 13 children with in-situ neuroblastomas had various congenital malformations, thus representing a selected group. It is possible, therefore, that there exists in the newborn period a significant association of small neuroblastomas with congenital malformations, an association that is not evident in children who develop clinical signs of neuroblastoma in later life. This would explain why malformations are not noted significantly more often in hospital records of children with neuroblastomas.[25,26] It is somewhat surprising that neuroblastomas are not frequent in children with spina bifida and other defects of closure of the neural tube, since irregularities of the neural crest are a part of these malformations. In fact, one commonly sees abnormal dystopic sympathetic tissue in experimental animals with spinal cord anomalies (Fig. 36-5). Similar misplaced and deformed tissues probably are present in children with dysraphic malformations but apparently they do not give rise to neuroblastomas.

It has long been known that malignant neuroblastoma cells may differentiate with time into mature and nonmalignant cells. It is not known why displaced cell rests can lie quietly for years to become malignant without any noticeable external stimulus and it is not known why neuroblastomas showing all signs of malignancy may become quiescent by maturation of their cells. It seems likely that many neuroblastomas present in infancy disappear without clinical manifestations and there is agreement that neuroblastomatous tumors have the best chance of spontaneous regression or medical cure when they occur in infants or young children.[35] Their behavior suggests the action of a "maturation factor" present in early life that disappears with advancing age. Cushing and Wolbach[27] reported transformation of a malignant paravertebral sympathicoblastoma into a benign ganglioneuroma.[34] It is now believed that about 2–10%[1,28] of neuroblastomatous tumors undergo spontaneous regression. With treatment, cure rates of 40-88% have been reported.[1,28-30] Surgical removal of the tumor, x-ray treatment, chemotherapy and massive vitamin B_{12} injections have been used. The B_{12} treatment was tried with the idea that this vitamin, an essential factor for the normal maturation of hemopoietic cells, might possibly also facilitate maturation of neuroblasts to ganglion cells.[28] Although this attractive hypothesis seemed to be borne out by beneficial therapeutic effects, it was abandoned by its originators because they observed degeneration and disappearance but not maturation of the tumors of their treated patients.[31,32] The results of this treatment and that of other therapeutic measures cannot be evaluated easily, since too many factors enter into such trials to permit judicious analysis. There is general agreement that the outlook is most favorable with treatment during infancy. A remarkable property of neuroblastomas is the possibility of cures despite metastatic spread. Metastases to the liver have responded repeatedly to treatment, whereas metastases to bone and lungs render the prognosis unfavorable. Even congenital subcutaneous and hepatic metastases can undergo spontaneous regression.[7] Maturation of tumor cells and deprivation of blood supply with necrosis and calcification of the malignant tissue have been credited for the cures of neuroblastomas.

REFERENCES

1. Gross, R. E., Farber, S., and Martin, L. W.: Neuroblastoma sympatheticum; a study and report of 217 cases, Pediatrics 23:1179, 1959.
2. Willis, R. A.: *The Borderland of Embryology and Pathology* (Washington, D. C.: Butterworth, 1962).
3. Vaalasti, T., and Peltokallio, P.: A ganglion cell tumour in the neck of a child, Ann. paediat. Fenniae 6:148, 1960.
4. Wells, H. G.: Occurrence and significance of congenital malignant neoplasms, Arch. Path. 30:535, 1940.
5. Schneider, K. M., Becker, J. M., and Krasna, I. H.: Neonatal neuroblastoma, Pediatrics 36:359, 1965.
6. Becker, H.: Sympathikustumoren im Kindesalter, Arch. Kinderh. 176:280, 1967–1968.
7. Griffin, M. E., and Bolande, R. P.: Familial neuroblastoma with regression and maturation to ganglioneurofibroma, Pediatrics 43:377, 1969.
8. Pickett, L. K., and Voorhess, M. L.: Neuroblastoma in childhood, S. Clin. North America 44:1469, 1964.
9. Lee, C. M., Jr.: The surigcal significance of tumors in identical twins: A short review of the literature and a report of sympathicoblastoma occurring in monozygotic twins, Am. Surgeon 19:803, 1953.
10. Brody, H.: Congenital malignant neuroblastoma of the suprarenal gland in one of twin girls, Am. J. Human Genet. 2:371, 1950.
11. Phillips, R.: Neuroblastoma: Hunterian Lecture, Ann. Roy. Coll. Surgeons England 12:29, 1953.
12. Stadler, H. E., and Worley, R. H.: Neuroblastomatosis in one of monozygotic twins, J. Pediat. 47:485, 1955.
13. Chatten, J., and Voorhess, M. L.: Familial neuroblastoma. Report of a kindred with multiple disorders, including neuroblastomas in four siblings, New England J. Med. 277:1230, 1967.
14. Knudsen, A. G., Jr., and Amromin, G. D.: Neuroblastoma and ganglioneuroma in a child with multiple neurofibromatosis: Implications for mutational origin of neuroblastoma, Cancer 19:1032, 1966.
15. Bulmer, J. H.: Scoliosis complicating ganglion cell tumors, Brit. J. Surg. 53:619, 1966.
16. Whang-Peng, J., and Bennett, J. M.: Cytogenic studies in metastatic neuroblastoma, Am. J. Dis. Child. 115:703, 1968.
17. Mittelbach, M., and Szekely, P.: Ein Fall von Neuroblastom des Nebennierenmarkes mit mehreren Missbildungen, Frankfurt. Ztschr. Path. 47:517, 1935.
18. Aase, J. N., and Smith, D. W.: Dysmorphogenesis of joints, brain, and palate: A new dominantly inherited syndrome, J. Pediat. 73:606, 1968.
19. Evans, A. R.: Congenital neuroblastoma, J. Clin. Path. 18:54, 1965.
20. Kouyoumdjian, A. O., and McDonald, J. J.: Association of congenital adrenal neuroblastoma with multiple anomalies including an unusual oropharyngeal cavity (imperforate buccopharyngeal membrane), Cancer 4:784, 1951.
21. Sy, W. M., and Edmonson, J. M.: The developmental defects associated with neuroblastoma; etiologic implications, Cancer 22:234, 1968.
22. Lewis, D., and Geschickter, C. F.: Tumors of the sympathetic nervous system, Arch. Surg. 28:16, 1934.
23. Potter, E. L., and Parrish, J. M.: Neuroblastoma, ganglioneuroma and fibroneuroma in a stillborn fetus, Am. J. Path. 18:141, 1942.
24. Beckwith, J. B., and Perrin, E. V.: In situ neuroblastomas: A contribution to the natural history of neural crest tumors, Am. J. Path. 43:1089, 1963.
25. Miller, R. W.: Relation between cancer and congenital defects in man, New England J. Med. 275:87, 1966.
26. Miller, R. W., Fraumeni, J. F., Jr., and Hill, J. A.: Neuroblastoma: Epidemiologic approach to its origin, Am. J. Dis. Child. 115:253, 1968.
27. Cushing, H., and Wolbach, S. B.: The transformation of a malignant paravertebral sympathicoblastoma into a benign ganglioneuroma, Am. J. Path. 3:203, 1927.
28. Bodian, M.: Neuroblastoma, Pediat. Clin. North America 6:449, 1959.
29. Perez, C. A., Vietti, T. J., Ackerman, L. V., Kulapongs, P., and Powers, W. E.: Treatment of malignant sympathetic tumors in children: Clinicopathological correlation, Pediatrics 41:452, 1968.
30. Gitlow, S. E., Bertani, L. M., Rausen, A., Gribetz, D., and Dziedzic, S. W.: Diagnosis of neuroblastoma by qualitative and quantitative determination of catecholamine metabolites in urine, Cancer 25:1377, 1970.
31. Bodian, M.: Neuroblastoma. An evaluation of its natural history and the effects of therapy, with particular reference to treatment by massive doses of vitamin B_{12}, Arch. Dis. Childhood 38:606, 1963.
32. Sawitsky, A., and Desposito, F.: A survey of American experience with vitamin B_{12} therapy of neuroblastoma, J. Pediat. 67:99, 1965.
33. Shanklin, D. R., and Sotelo-Avila, C.: In situ tumors in fetuses, newborns and young infants, Biol. Neonat. 14: 286, 1969.
34. Fox, F., Davidson, J., and Thomas, L. B.: Maturation of sympathicoblastoma into ganglioneuroma. Report of 2 patients with 20 and 46 year survivals respectively, Cancer 12:108, 1959.
35. Everson, T. C., and Cole, W. H.: Spontaneous Regression of Neuroblastoma, in *Spontaneous Regression of Cancer* (Philadelphia: W. B. Saunders Company, 1966).

Adrenocortical Tumors

ALTHOUGH the adrenal cortex is derived from splanchnic mesoderm, tumors arising from it are termed "adenoma" or "carcinoma." These cortical tumors usually are discussed together, since distinction of benign and malignant tumors is not always possible. Both types can produce hormones or be nonfunctioning. Carcinomas may present with endocrine disorders or as abdominal masses, whereas adenomas usually are discovered because of endocrine syndromes.[1] In a series of 62 cases of adrenocortical tumors reviewed by Fraumeni and Miller,[2] there was marked female predominance. Hemihypertrophy, visceromegaly, astrocytomas of the brain and urinary tract anomalies were associated phenomena in some of the patients. Absence of the contralateral adrenal gland has been noted in some instances. Recurrence of adrenocortical tumors has been observed in several families.[2-4]

Fontaine *et al.*[5] reviewed 34 virilizing and 2 feminizing cases of adrenocortical tumors in boys. A case both virilizing and feminizing has been observed also. Endocrine manifestations consist of precocious puberty, virilization or Cushing syndrome. Feminization in boys can occur but it is rare.[6] Development of an adrenocortical tumor leading to virilism and Cushing syndrome from aberrant adrenal cells located within the liver was reported by Wilkins and Ravitch.[7]

REFERENCES

1. Macfarlane, D. A.: Cancer of the adrenal cortex, Ann. Roy. Coll. Surgeons England 23:155, 1958.
2. Fraumeni, J. F., Jr., and Miller, R. W.: Adrenocortical neoplasms with hemihypertrophy, brain tumors, and other disorders, J. Pediat. 70:129, 1967.
3. Hain, A. M.: Adrenal tumours and pseudohermaphroditism: A hormone study of cases, J. Path. & Bact. 59:267, 1947.
4. Cervino, J. M., Navarro, A., Folle, J. A., Manaro, J. M., Maggiolo, J., De Delfino, E. Z., Muxi, F., and Barges, U. L.: Sindrome de Cushing por carcinoma cortical en una nina de 34 meses, An. Fac. med. Montevideo 44:36, 1959.
5. Fontaine, G., Lacheretz, M., Dupont, A., Fossati, P., Farriaux, J-P., Gnamey, D., and Deparcy, P.: Tumeur de la corticosurrénale avec puberté précoce et gynécomastie chez un garçon de 3 ans 1/2, Ann. pédiat. 17:463, 1970.
6. Mosier, H. D., and Goodwin, W. E.: Feminizing adrenal adenoma in a 7-year-old boy, Pediatrics 27:1016, 1961.
7. Wilkins, L., and Ravitch, M. M.: Adrenocortical tumor arising in the liver of a three year old boy with signs of virilism and Cushing's syndrome, Pediatrics 9:671, 1952.

Pheochromocytoma

THESE TUMORS arise from the chromaffin tissue of the adrenal medulla or the paraspinal ganglia. No congenital pheochromocytomas have been reported and very few have been recognized in early childhood.[1,2] It is thought that fewer than 5% of these tumors occur in children.[1] Although pheochromocytomas and neuroblastomas both are derived from the neural crest and sympathetic tissue, they differ greatly in frequency and age distribution. In a children's registry,[3] neuroblastomas were recorded more than thirty times as often as pheochromocytomas. Most neuroblastomas had their clinical onset during the first 2 years of life, whereas the rare pheochromocytomas occurred late in childhood. By 1963, not more than 100 children's pheochromocytomas had been recorded in the medical literature[1] but additional cases have been described since.[4] Boys are affected twice as often as girls, whereas in adults the sex ratio is reversed. Pheochromocytomas have been reported in Caucasian, Negro, Indian and Chinese children. In 100 cases reviewed by Stackpole *et al.*,[1] more than one tumor was observed in 32 and a single tumor in 68 patients, whereas in adults 86% of pheochromocytomas are single. Extra-adrenal tumors also are more frequent in children than in adults. They can be located in the thorax, bladder wall, preaortic and para-aortic sympathetic chains, in the organ of Zuckerkandl and at the bifurcation of the aorta. Sustained hypertension, episodes of headache, profuse sweating, weight loss and visual disturbances are the most frequent findings in children. Hyperthyroidism, chronic renal disease, essential hypertension, brain tumor, diabetes mellitus,[1] diabetes insipidus,[5] acrodynia or lead poisoning[6] often is suspected before the correct diagnosis is established. Measurements of urinary norepinephrine, epinephrine or VMA (vanillylmandelic acid) aid in the diagnosis of the disease and in evaluation of its course and treatment. Aortography may reveal adrenal or lower retroperitoneal pheochromocytomas.[4]

Although pheochromocytomas appear relatively late in childhood, there are suggestions that prenatal factors play a role in their etiology. Genetic determination is suggested by aggregation of patients in families and kindreds. By 1968, a total of 85 cases appearing in 29 families had been recorded.[7] The tumors occurred in males and females with equal frequency; in several kindreds, autosomal dominant inheritance appeared likely. In familial cases, bilateral adrenal involvement was common but other locations such as the aortic bifurcation and involvement of the organ of Zuckerkandl have been reported.[8] In 20 familial cases, medullary thyroid carcinoma was associated with pheochromocytoma. It evolved that pheochromocytoma may be a manifestation of an "endocrine tumor diathesis" that is transmitted like an autosomal dominant trait; in addition to medullary thyroid carcinoma[9] and pheochromocytoma,[10] the patients may develop hyperparathyroidism, Cushing syndrome[7,11] or multiple neuromatosis[12] (Chapter 124). The tendency to endocrine neoplasia also can lead to nonendocrine manifestations such as cutaneous fibromas and café au lait spots,[13] suggesting a relationship to Recklinghausen neurofibromatosis; but the thyroid-pheochromocytoma "multiple endocrine neoplasia" (MEN, type 2) apparently is genetically different from MEN, type 1, which includes tumors of the pituitary, parathyroids and pancreatic island cells.[7] It is well established, however, that pheochromocytoma can be a manifestation of at least two hamartoses, i.e., Recklinghausen neurofibromatosis and Hippel-Lindau disease[14,15] (Chapters 121 and 123), disorders that have a tendency to autosomal dominant inheritance like the multiple endocrine neoplasias. A connection of the thyroid-pheochromocytoma neoplasia with Wilms tumor is suggested by a unique case recorded by Lynch and Green,[16] who described a woman with bilateral pheochromocytomas of the adrenals, thyroid carcinoma and a mucin-producing breast carcinoma who had a son with congenital heart disease and Wilms tumors. The common denominators of the endocrine neoplasias and their transmission through several generations are still not known and are unexplained, but it is possible that important oncogenic principles may be discovered by analyses of these familial cases.

Despite the emphasis on familial occurrence, sporadic pheochromocytomas are much more frequent than those with familial aggregation.[17] It has been stated that only 6% of the reported pheochromocytomas are familial[18] but this probably is an underestimate, since family investigations of syndromes with late manifestations and variable expressivity are difficult. In addition, there is the possibility that some of the sporadic cases are new mutations and may become "familial" when some of the patients' offspring become affected.

That nongenetic factors may be involved in the development of pheochromocytomas is intimated by development of such tumors in patients with congenital cyanotic heart disease and protracted hypoxemia. Folger *et al.*[19] reported 5 cases of such cyanotic patients that were complicated by pheochromocytomas. Two patients had tetralogy of Fallot, 2 had transposition of the great vessels and 1 had Ebstein deformity. Another child with transposition of the great arteries developed, at the age of 12 years, multiple, malignant extra-adrenal pheochromocytomas.[20] It is thought that chronic hypoxemia may act as a stimulus to growth of chromaffin tissue elements and thus bring about medullary hypoplasia and tumor formation.[19,20] Not only pheochromocytomas but other adrenal, pancreatic or pituitary tumors have been considered as effects of chronic hypoxemia.[21]

REFERENCES

1. Stackpole, R. H., Melicow, M. M., and Uson, A. S.: Pheochromocytoma in children. Report of nine cases and review of the first 100 published cases with follow-up studies, J. Pediat. 63:315, 1963.
2. Neff, F. C., Tice, G., Walker, G. A., and Ockerblad, N.: Adrenal tumor in female infant, J. Clin. Endocrinol. 2: 125, 1942.
3. Marsden, H. B., and Steward, J. K.: *Tumours in Children* (New York: Springer-Verlag, 1968).
4. Weber, A. L., Janower, M. L., and Griscom, N. T.: Radiologic and clinical evaluation of pheochromocytoma in children: Report of 6 cases, Radiology 88:117, 1967.
5. Tevetoğlu, F., and Lee, C-H.: Adrenal pheochromocytoma simulating diabetes insipidus, A.M.A. Am. J. Dis. Child. 91:365, 1956.
6. Insley, J., and Smallwood, W. C.: Phaeochromocytoma in children, Arch. Dis. Childhood 37:606, 1962.
7. Steiner, A. L., Goodman, A. D., and Powers, S. R.: Study of a kindred with pheochromocytoma, medullary thyroid carcinoma, hyperparathyroidism and Cushing's disease: Multiple endocrine neoplasia, type 2, Medicine 47:371, 1968.
8. Cook, J. E., Urich, R. W., Sample, H. G., Jr., and Fawcett, N. W.: Peculiar familial and malignant pheochromocytomas of the organs of Zuckerkandl, Ann. Int. Med. 52: 126, 1960.
9. Sipple, J. H.: The association of pheochromocytoma with carcinoma of the thyroid gland, Am. J. Med. 31:163, 1961.
10. Schimke, R. N., and Hartmann, W. H.: Familial amyloid-producing medullary thyroid carcinoma and pheochromocytoma: Distinct genetic entity, Ann. Int. Med. 63:1027, 1965.
11. Urbanski, F. X.: Medullary thyroid carcinoma, parathyroid adenoma, and bilateral pheochromocytoma, J. Chron. Dis. 20:627, 1967.
12. Schimke, R. N., Hartmann, W. H., Prout, T. E., and Rimoin, D. L.: Syndrome of bilateral pheochromocytoma, medullary thyroid carcinoma and multiple neuromas, New England J. Med. 279:1, 1968.
13. Ljungberg, O., Cederquist, E., and Studnitz, W.: Medullary thyroid carcinoma and phaeochromocytoma: A familial chromaffinomatosis, Brit. M. J. 1:279, 1967.
14. Glushien, A. S., Mansing, M. M., and Littman, D. S.: Pheochromocytoma: Its relationship to neuro-cutaneous syndromes, Am. J. Med. 14:318, 1953.
15. Chapman, R. C., Kemp, V. E., and Taliaferro, I.: Pheochromocytoma associated with multiple neurofibromatosis and intracranial hemangioma, Am. J. Med. 26:883, 1959.
16. Lynch, H. T., and Green, G. S.: Wilms' tumor and congenital heart disease. Report of a case and family, Am. J. Dis. Child. 115:723, 1968.
17. Moorhead, E. L., Brennan, M. J., Caldwell, J. R., and Averill, W. C.: Pheochromocytomata: A familial tumor, Henry Ford Hosp. M. Bull. 13:467, 1965.
18. Hermann, H., and Mornex, R.: *Human Tumours Secreting Catecholamines* (New York: The Macmillan Company, 1964).
19. Folger, G. M., Jr., Roberts, W. C., Mehrizi, A., Shah, K. D., Glancy, D. L., Carpenter, C. C., and Esterly, J. R.: Cyanotic malformations of the heart with pheochromocytoma. A report of five cases, Circulation 29:750, 1964.
20. Reynolds, J. L., and Gilchrist, T. F.: Congenital heart disease and pheochromocytoma, Am. J. Dis. Child. 112:251, 1966.
21. Roberts, W. C., Mason, D. T., and Braunwald, E.: Survival to adulthood in a patient with complete transposition of the great vessels; including a note on the association of endocrine tumors with heart disease, Ann. Int. Med. 57: 834, 1962.

Renal Tumors

As POINTED OUT in Chapter 105, most *Wilms tumors* occur in children who appear generally well formed, i.e., in patients who are free of obvious congenital malformations and associated neoplasms. Yet, in a number of patients with Wilms tumor, the rate of associated malformations and tumors is greater than that expected from incidences ascertained in general children's populations. In most cases, the family history is not contributory, but sometimes siblings or other family members have Wilms tumor or anomalies known to occur in excess in some of the tumor patients. Such observations had been recorded occasionally in the past, and in recent years epidemiologic studies confirmed the significance of earlier case reports. It had been known for some time that Wilms tumors may develop in persons with horseshoe kidneys, hypoplastic kidneys or various extrarenal urogenital tract anomalies. Miller *et al.*,[1] in a review of 440 patients with Wilms tumor, also established an excess of such genitourinary defects, confirming the validity of earlier case reports. The same was found to be true for hemihypertrophy, which had been noted repeatedly in association with Wilms tumor. Among 440 patients with this neoplasm, hemihypertrophy was mentioned three times.[1] That this is an excessive occurrence can be gathered from the report by Parker and Skalko,[2] who found only 10 cases of "total congenital asymmetry" in the records of 860,000 patients admitted to the Cornell Medical Center during 34 years. Through hemihypertrophy, Wilms tumor appears to be linked in etiology with adrenocortical and hepatic neoplasms of childhood[1,2] and with visceromegaly.[2] It should be mentioned here parenthetically that not all kidney anomalies in hemihypertrophic patients are Wilms tumors. Benign enlargement of the kidney, bilateral medullary sponge kidney and deformed renal collecting system[2,3] have been observed in patients with congenital asymmetry, a fact of practical importance, since erroneous diagnosis of Wilms tumor may lead to unnecessary radical and damaging treatment.[4]

Aniridia, sometimes combined with other ocular and cerebral defects, is another malformation associated with Wilms tumor. Miller *et al.*[1] observed aniridia at a rate of 1:73 in their study of 440 Wilms tumor cases. And among 28 children under 4 years of age, hospitalized with congenital aniridia, Wilms tumor developed in 6 and 1 had the neoplasm on admission.[5] Through aniridia, Wilms tumor appears to be related to pseudohermaphrodism and gonadoblastoma.[6] It may be mentioned as a curiosity that a syndrome of horseshoe kidney or renal hypoplasia, aniridia, pseudohermaphrodism and congenital heart disease can be produced in rats by vitamin A deficiency.[7,8] There exists a rare association of Wilms tumor with congenital heart disease,[1,9] and other associated malformations[23] were mentioned in Chapter 105. Nephrogenic rests have been found in infants with trisomy 18, and Wilms tumor has been recorded in a patient with trisomy 18.[1]

Familial occurrence of Wilms tumor has been recorded repeatedly. It has been observed in siblings[10-12] and in identical twins[1,13] and has been reported in successive generations.[11,12] Family histories may lead to the discovery of related syndromes, which can occur in relatives of the Wilms tumor patients.[9,14] Metanephric hamartomas and nephroblastomatosis have been described in siblings.[15] It was suggested that this observation supports the view that abnormal persistence of primitive metanephric tissue into the perinatal period may represent a beginning Wilms tumor.

There exist reports of *carcinoma* developing on the basis of renal malformations, such as crossed renal ectopia[16] and in supernumerary kidneys.[17,18] Renal sarcoma was described in 2 stillborn children of a family in which several cases of hydronephrosis and mega-ureter occurred.[19]

Congenital renal tumors such as *mesoblastic nephromas* (Chapter 105) have been described under many names. They must be distinguished from Wilms tumors,[20] since they should be treated differently. Nephrectomy without chemotherapy and radiotherapy is recommended for these hamartous lesions.[21,22]

REFERENCES

1. Miller, R. W., Fraumeni, J. F., Jr., and Manning, M. D.: Association of Wilms' tumor with aniridia, hemihypertrophy and other congenital malformations, New England J. Med. 270:922, 1964.
2. Parker, D. A., and Skalko, R. G.: Congenital asymmetry: Report of 10 cases with associated developmental abnormalities, Pediatrics 44:584, 1969.
3. Morris, R. C., Yamauchi, H., Palubinskas, A. J., and Howenstine, J.: Medullary sponge kidney, Am. J. Med. 38:883, 1965.
4. Black, W. C., and Ragsdale, E. F.: Wilms' tumor, Am. J. Roentgenol. 103:53, 1968.
5. Fraumeni, J. F., Jr., Geiser, C. F., and Manning, M. D.: Wilms' tumor and congenital hemihypertrophy: Report of five new cases and review of literature, Pediatrics 40: 886, 1967.
6. DiGeorge, A. M., and Harley, R. D.: The association of aniridia, Wilms' tumor, and genital abnormalities, Arch. Ophth. 75:796, 1966.
7. Warkany, J., and Schraffenberger, E.: Congenital malformations induced in rats by maternal vitamin A deficiency. I. Defects of the eye, Arch. Ophth. 35:150, 1946.
8. Warkany, J., Roth, C. B., and Wilson, J. G.: Multiple congenital malformations: A consideration of etiologic factors, Pediatrics 1:462, 1948.
9. Lynch, H. T., and Green, G. S.: Wilms' tumor and congenital heart disease. Report of a case and family, Am. J. Dis. Child. 115:723, 1968.
10. Maslow, L. A.: Wilms' tumor: Report of three cases and possible fourth one in same family, J. Urol. 43:75, 1940.
11. Fitzgerald, W. L., and Hardin, H. C.: Bilateral Wilms tumor in Wilms tumor family: Case report, J. Urol. 73: 468, 1955.
12. Strøm, T.: A Wilms' tumour family, Acta paediat. 46:601, 1957.
13. Gaulin, E.: Simultaneous Wilms tumors in identical twins, J. Urol. 66: 547, 1951.

14. Miller, R. W.: Wilms' tumor, congenital heart defects, pheochromocytomas and thyroid cancer, Am. J. Dis. Child. 116:564, 1968.
15. Liban, E., and Kozenitzky, I. L.: Metanephric hamartomas and nephroblastomatosis in siblings, Cancer 25:885, 1970.
16. Langworthy, H. T., and Drexler, L. S.: Carcinoma in crossed renal ectopia, J. Urol. 47:776, 1942.
17. Exley, M., and Hotchkiss, W. S.: Supernumerary kidney with clear cell carcinoma, J. Urol. 51:569, 1944.
18. Carlson, H. E.: Supernumerary kidney: A summary of 51 reported cases, J. Urol. 64:224, 1950.
19. Mackay, H.: Congenital bilateral megalo-ureters with hydronephrosis, Proc. Roy. Soc. Med. 38:567, 1945.
20. Bolande, R. P., Brough, A. J., and Izant, R. J., Jr.: Congenital mesoblastic nephroma of infancy, Pediatrics 40:272, 1967.
21. Waisman, J., and Cooper, P. H.: Renal neoplasms of the newborn, J. Pediat. Surg. 5:407, 1970.
22. Richmond, H., and Dougall, A. J.: Neonatal renal tumors, J. Pediat. Surg. 5:413, 1970.
23. Haicken, B. N., and Miller, D. R.: Simultaneous occurrence of congenital aniridia, hamartoma, and Wilms' tumor, J. Pediat. 78:497, 1971.

Tumors of the Gonads

Ovary

PREPUBERTAL OVARIAN TUMORS are uncommon; they account for only 1% of all tumors of childhood.[1] Approximately 80% of them are benign and 20% malignant or potentially malignant.[2] Groeber[2] reviewed 263 tumors from 14 reports of serial observations and noted that they are rare in infants but increase in frequency as puberty nears. Benign cystic teratomas accounted for 50% of the cases, being the most frequent type. More primitive solid teratomas were found in 11% and follicular cysts in 16%, whereas cystadenomas, granulosa cell tumors, dysgerminomas, adenocarcinomas and embryonic carcinomas seldom were diagnosed. Bilateral ovarian carcinoma in a 30-week-old fetus was recorded by Ziegler.[3] Although ovarian cysts are rarities in fetuses and in stillborn[4] and premature[5] children, they have been recorded repeatedly. The same is true for ovarian cysts in newborns, which are reported because of their impressive size or symptomatology[6-10]; they sometimes develop to considerable size and may rupture[9] or become twisted.[4] Dermoid cysts account for one-third to one-half of children's ovarian tumors[1,11]; usually they contain sebaceous material, hair and ectodermal tissues. Mixtures of cystic and solid growths occur. Microscopically, ectodermal tissues prevail, mesodermal tissues are common but endodermal elements are rare. More than 80% of dermoid cysts are encountered in patients between 11 and 50 years,[12] but exceptional cases have been reported in patients as young as 2 years.[11,13,14] Only about 2% of dermoid cysts of the ovary are malignant,[12] whereas 15% of solid teratomas show malignant degeneration.[14] Teratomas of the ovary, which contain immature derivatives of all three germ layers, have been seen in a 16-month-old child[15] and in children less than 6 years of age.[14,16] Corpus luteum cysts are rare in children.[14] Ovarian cysts or tumors may occur in hamartoses, such as gastrointestinal polyposis, or with multiple basal cell nevi.[17]

Dysgerminomas, tumors derived from germ cells, can be of heterogeneous origin. They have been described in pseudohermaphrodites[18] and as a dominant hereditary trait[19] in patients with normal karyotype. A case was associated with ataxia-telangiectasia, a recessively inherited disorder.[20] Granulosa cell tumors of the ovary are neoplasms with endocrine functions that may manifest themselves by early breast development, growth of pubic hair and vaginal bleeding in infants or children.[21] Only 5–10% of granulosa-cell tumors occur before adolescence, but bilateral tumors of this type were removed from a child 14 weeks of age[22] and in another patient symptoms began at the age of 16 months.[23] Malignancy is rare in granulosa-cell tumors of childhood but it has been observed in a 19-month-old girl.[16] A virilizing ovarian cell tumor was reported in a 2½-year-old girl.[24] Clitoral enlargement, pubic hair, deepening voice and increased growth were noted. In the right ovary, a tumor was found that was made up of large polygonal cells with eosinophilic cytoplasm. The case is of particular interest because the child developed – 13 months after removal of the ovarian tumor – an undifferentiated sarcoma of the oropharynx that metastasized and led to the child's death at the age of 4 years. In addition to lipoid cell tumors, arrhenoblastoma and gonadoblastoma have been reported as virilizing ovarian tumors in prepubertal children.[24]

Yolk sac tumors of the ovary (Schiller mesonephromas) occur in young individuals but not in infancy.[25]

Tumors developing in dysplastic ovaries are discussed on pages 1232–1234.

Testis

Testicular tumors are rare in infancy and childhood compared to tumors in other organs such as brain, blood, kidneys, and so forth; they also are rare compared to testicular tumors in adults. Campbell,[26] citing J. B. Gilbert, wrote that only 131 of 5,500 testicular tumors reported in the literature occurred in patients under 15 years of age and Young *et al.*[47] stated that only 2–5% of testicular tumors occur in children. Those that occur in children usually make their appearance before the age of 2 years.[27] Julien[28] collected a series of 139 childhood cases and found that twenty-five testicular tumors were present at birth, twenty-five in the first year of life and twenty-five in the second. Dargeon[27] listed 8 patients, only 2 of whom were more than 2 years of age when testicular swelling was noted. The rarity of these tumors was emphasized by Kretschmer,[29] who recorded an embryoma of the testis in a 5-year-old boy as the only testicular tumor in 22,000 hospital admissions of children. Rusche[30] reported 12 cases of testicular tumor occurring in infants and children, four of which were present at birth and, with two exceptions, all were recognized before the children were 3 years of age. Young *et al*,[47] reviewing eighteen embryonal adenocarcinomas in prepubertal testes, listed sixteen as diagnosed at or under 2 years of age.

Classification of testicular tumors was and still is confusing. Mostofi[31] distinguished between "adult teratomas" thought to be derived from early somatic elements of the immature sex cell and embryonal carcinomas, derived from early trophoblastic elements. But there also were tumors of uncertain diagnosis resembling carcinosarcoma though lacking definite malignancy. Rusche[30] classified eight of twelve testicular tumors as teratomas, one as a dermoid cyst and three as embryonal carcinomas. Teratomas of the testes are composed of three germ layers and various combinations of tissues. If they are well differentiated, they are only potentially malignant or of low-grade malignancy.[32] Of Willis'[33] eight specimens of testicular teratoma, six were first noticed in the first year of life and these were all benign. Only 1 childhood case showed malignancy; it developed in an adolescent boy, metastasized and was fatal 19 months after orchidectomy. Other tumors derived from germ cells are diagnosed as embryonal carcinomas, as clear cell carcinomas[32] or as endodermal sinus tumors.[34] The last kind, which occur in ovaries as well as in testes, are considered yolk sac tumors and thought to be derived from embryonal carcinomas by differentiation; they are said to be successfully treatable by surgery before the age of 2 years but rather hopeless after 2 years of age.[35] According to Houser *et al.*,[48] teratomas account for one-fourth of the germinal tumors, whereas the remainder are tumors referred to by a variety of names, some of which were mentioned above. Young *et al.*[47] believed that these names all refer to a single germinal tumor that can be called "embryonal adenocarcinoma of childhood." In 2 cases, these authors saw teratomatous elements in association with embryonal adenocarcinoma in prepubertal testes. There is general agreement that seminomas are very rare in children[26,32,33] but a case has been observed in a boy with Down syndrome. Matsaniotis *et al.*[36] reported this patient with Down syndrome and hypothyroidism who developed, at the age of 2½ years, a tumor in the right testis that was diagnosed as a seminoma. The authors mentioned 2 adult mongoloids who developed testicular tumors, one of which was diagnosed as seminoma.

Interstitial cell tumors or Leydig cell tumors have their onset between the ages of 2 and 9 years. The patients develop macrogenitosomia praecox with a raised excretion of urinary 17-ketosteroids. Signs of sexual precocity are combined with precocious muscular and skeletal development. Gynecomastia, penile erections and aggressive behavior have been reported. The tumor, which usually is nonmalignant and unilateral, may not be obvious initially and virilizing adrenal hyperplasia often is suspected.[37,38] In fact, both adrenocortical hyperplasia and tumors of the testes can occur in the same patient.[39] In contrast to adrenocortical hyperplasia, patients with interstitial cell tumor have a negative family history, normal urinary salt excretion and fail to show effect of steroid therapy on the size of the tumor.[37] A virilizing tumor in one of, probably, monozygotic twins was reported by Martin *et al.*[40] Gonadoblastomas arising in testes are discussed on pages 1232–1234.

Several studies showed that the risk for testicular tumors is ten, twenty or forty times greater in cryptorchidism as in normally situated testes.[41-43] Yet, compared with the frequency of undescended testes, the total incidence of such tumors is low, so that the fear of malignancy should not be the sole indication for operation of cryptorchidism.[26] It is well known that, in children, spontaneous descent is rather frequent. The risk for tumor is higher in abdominal than in inguinal testes. It is very likely that a primary abnormality of the testis is responsible for lack of descent and that such testes have an increased tendency to neoplasia. Sohval[44] believed that the same congenital defect that contributes to lack of descent of a testis may also render it more susceptible to tumor development. This would account, in part, for the increased incidence of testicular neoplasms in undescended testes. This is exemplified by cryptorchidism in phenotypically male patients with XO/XY mosaicism, which may be complicated by development of malignant seminoma[45] or gonadoblastoma.[46] Other examples of testicular neoplasias in the testes of persons with sex anomalies are cited on pages 1232–1234.

REFERENCES

1. Costin, M. E., and Kennedy, R. L. J.: Ovarian tumors in infants and children, Am. J. Dis. Child. 76:129, 1948.
2. Groeber, W. R.: Ovarian tumors during infancy and childhood, Am. J. Obst. & Gynec. 86:1027, 1963.
3. Ziegler, E. E.: Bilateral ovarian carcinoma in a 30 week fetus, Arch. Path. 40:279, 1945.
4. Karrer, F. W., and Swenson, S. A.: Twisted ovarian cyst in a newborn infant, Arch. Surg. 83:921, 1961.
5. Brune, W. H., Pulaski, E. J., and Shucy, H. E.: Giant ovarian cyst: Report of a case in a premature infant, New England J. Med. 257:876, 1957.
6. Bales, E. T., Hardacre, J. M., and Newborn, W. A.: Ovarian tumors and cysts in infants and children, Arch. Surg. 83:580, 1961.
7. Finola, G. C., Quitangon, L., and Pontius, G. V.: Large ovarian cyst in a newborn infant, Am. J. Obst. & Gynec. 73:690, 1957.
8. Kondstaal, J., and Hamming, H. D.: Een nitzonderlijk grote ovariumkyste bij een pasgeborene, Nederl. tijdschr. geneesk. 109:82, 1965.
9. Tietz, K. G., and Davis, J. B.: Ruptured ovarian cyst in a newborn infant, J. Pediat. 51:564, 1957.
10. Tyson, W. T., Kegan, J. M., and Goll, D.: Large ovarian

cyst in a newborn infant, A.M.A. J. Dis. Child. 94:320, 1957.
11. Ein, S. H., Darte, J. M. M., and Stephens, C. A.: Cystic and solid ovarian tumors in children: A 44-year review, J. Pediat. Surg. 5:148, 1970.
12. Marcial-Rojas, R. A., and Medina, R.: Cystic teratomas of the ovary. A clinical and pathological analysis of two hundred sixty-eight tumors, A.M.A. Arch. Path. 66:577, 1958.
13. Obadalek, W.: Stielgedrehte Eierstockcysten im Kindesalter, Monatsschr. Kinderh. 48:419, 1930.
14. Brandesky, G.: Ovarialtumoren im Kindesalter, Monatsschr. Kinderh. 115:434, 1967.
15. Gilman, A., Smith, J., Puziss, I., and Karp, L. M.: Teratoma of the ovary in a sixteen-month-old child, California Med. 75:105, 1951.
16. Einsel, I. H., Bowman, R. E., and Koletsky, S.: Unusual malignant tumor in a young child, A.M.A. Am. J. Dis. Child. 86:568, 1953.
17. Gorlin, R. J., and Pindborg, J. J.: *Syndromes of the Head and Neck* (New York: McGraw-Hill Book Company, Inc., 1964).
18. Goldberg, M. B., and Scully, A. L.: Gonadal malignancy in gonadal dysgenesis: Papillary pseudomucinous cystadenocarcinoma in a patient with Turner's syndrome, J. Clin. Endocrinol. 27:341, 1967.
19. Jackson, S. M.: Ovarian dysgerminoma in three generations?, J. M. Genetics 4:112, 1967.
20. Dunn, H. G., Meuwissen, H., Livingstone, C. S., and Pump, K. K.: Ataxia-telangiectasia, Canad. M.A.J. 91: 1106, 1964.
21. Niswander, K. R., Courey, N. G., and Woodward, T.: Precocious puberty caused by ovarian tumors, Obst. & Gynec. 26:381, 1965.
22. Zemke, E. E., and Herrell, W. E.: Bilateral granulosa cell tumors: Successful removal from a child 14 weeks of age, Am. J. Obst. & Gynec. 41:704, 1941.
23. Cornil, L., and Schachter, M.: On granulosa tumors (folliculomata) of the ovary in children and infants, Med. españ. 6:355, 1941.
24. Ammann, A. J., Kaufman, S., and Gilbert, A.: Virilizing ovarian tumor in a 2½-year-old girl, J. Pediat. 70:782, 1967.
25. Huntington, R. W., Jr., and Bullock, W. K.: Yolk sac tumors of the ovary, Cancer 25:1357, 1970.
26. Campbell, M.: *Urology* (2d ed.; Philadelphia: W. B. Saunders Company, 1963).
27. Dargeon, H. W.: *Tumors of Childhood* (New York: Paul B. Hoeber, Inc., 1960).
28. Julien, R.: Étude des Tumeurs du Testicule chez l'Enfant (Paris, Thèse, 1925) (cited by Campbell[1]).
29. Kretschmer, H. L.: Embryoma of the testicle in a five-year-old child, Am. J. Surg. 76:99, 1948.
30. Rusche, C.: Twelve cases of testicular tumors occurring during infancy and childhood, J. Pediat. 40:192, 1952.
31. Mostofi, F. K.: Infantile testicular tumors, Bull. New York Acad. Med. 28:684, 1952.
32. Michael, P.: *Tumors of Infancy and Childhood* (Philadelphia: J. B. Lippincott Company, 1964).
33. Willis, R. A.: *The Pathology of the Tumours of Children* (Springfield, Ill.: Charles C Thomas, Publisher, 1962).
34. Teilum, G.: Classification of endodermal sinus tumor (mesoblastoma vitellinum) and so-called "embryonal carcinoma" of the ovary, Acta path. et microbiol. scandinav. 64:407, 1965.
35. Pierce, G. B., Bullock, W. K., and Huntington, R. W., Jr.: Yolk sac tumors of the testis, Cancer 25:644, 1970.
36. Matsaniotis, N., Karpouzas, J., and Economou-Mavrou, C.: Hypothyroidism and seminoma in association with Down's syndrome, J. Pediat. 70:810, 1967.
37. Allibone, E. C., Anderson, C. K., and Arthurton, M. W.: Macrogenitosomia praecox due to an interstitial cell tumour of the testis, Arch. Dis. Childhood 44:84, 1969.
38. Johnstone, G.: Prepubertal gynaecomastia in association with an interstitial-cell tumor, Brit. J. Urol. 39:211, 1967.
39. Cohen, H.: Hyperplasia of the adrenal cortex associated with bilateral testicular tumors, Am. J. Path. 22:157, 1946.
40. Martin, M. M., Canary, J. J., and Balsamo, P. A.: Virilizing tumor of the testis in one twin, J. Clin. Endocrinol. 22:345, 1962.
41. Dixon, F. J., and Moore, R. A.: Testicular tumors: A clinicopathological study, Cancer 6:427, 1953.
42. Hinman, F., and Benteen, F. H.: Relationship of cryptorchidism to tumors of testis, J. Urol. 35:378, 1936.
43. Philip, J., and Teter, J.: Significance of chromosomal investigation of somatic cells to determine the genetic origin of gonadoblastoma, Acta path. et microbiol. scandinav. 61:543, 1964.
44. Sohval, A. R.: Testicular dysgenesis in relation to neoplasm of testicle, J. Urol. 75:285, 1956.
45. Lewis, F. J. W., Mitchell, J. P., and Foss, G. L.: XY/XO mosaicism, Lancet 1:221, 1963.
46. Scully, R. E.: Gonadoblastoma. A review of 74 cases, Cancer 25:1340, 1970.
47. Young, P. G., Mount, B. M., Foote, F. W., Jr., and Whitmore, W. F., Jr.: Embryonal adenocarcinoma in the prepubertal testis, Cancer 26:1065, 1970.
48. Houser, R., Izant, R., and Persky, L.: Testicular tumors in children, Am. J. Surg. 110:876, 1965.

Congenital Malformations of the Genital Organs and Tumor Formation

A STRONG ASSOCIATION EXISTS between malformations of the sex organs and development of tumors. It has long been known that persons with somatic sex anomalies have a tendency to develop gonadal neoplasms. As early as 1908, Neugebauer[1] listed 19 cases of benign or malignant genital tumors in "hermaphrodites." In this and many subsequent publications, the diagnoses of the sexual anomalies are doubtful, since the investigations were not complete or modern laboratory methods were not available at the time of observation. But the publications can be trusted in that somatosexual ambiguities were clearly present in the cases described. There also may be doubts concerning the types of tumors reported, since the terminology in this field is not uniform. But there usually is no doubt that a benign or malignant tumor was present in the patients observed. The sex anomalies under consideration range from "undescended testis" to true hermaphrodism.

According to Melicow and Uson,[2] by 1959 there had been 3 cases of dysgerminoma reported in *true hermaphrodites*. Overzier,[3] in 1961, cited 5 cases of malignant gonadal tumors in proved true hermaphrodites. But both reviewers believed that gonadal neoplasms in true hermaphrodites may be more frequent than the reports indicated, since the bivalency of the gonad can be destroyed by the tumor or the diagnosis of true hermaphrodism often cannot be established for various reasons. Cystic degeneration of the gonads is quite common in hermaphrodismus verus.[4]

Gonadal tumors in *female pseudohermaphrodites* were stressed by Meyer,[5] who found that of 46 cases of ovarian tumors resembling seminomas of the testis and named by him "dysgerminomas" 25 were in female pseudohermaphrodites. Many dysgerminomas have been described since in such pseudohermaphrodites, but it is doubtful that the patients observed would be considered female pseudohermaphrodites after examination of their gonads and their chromosomes with present-day methods. Melicow and Uson[2] cited some of them and also described a dysgerminoma in a phenotypic woman who had no contralateral gonad. This patient probably had Turner syndrome (Chapter 112). In another patient considered a female pseudohermaphrodite, a teratocarcinoma developed in one ovary, whereas the other gonad apparently was absent. Claret and Mackintosh[6] observed a benign ovarian teratoma in a 21-year-old female pseudohermaphrodite. Scully[7] described 2 apparently female patients with signs of virilization, each developing a unilateral gonadoblastoma. Neither ovarian nor testicular tissue could be found. In 1961, Perrin and Landing[10] briefly reported bilateral gonadoblastoma in a 14-year-old girl who also had a pituitary stalk oligodendroglioma; she had normal Fallopian tubes, hypoplastic bifid uterus and absence of normal ovarian tissue. A low positive nuclear sex chromatin count was observed, which suggests a mosaicism not recognizable at that time. A hilus cell adenoma was found in a dysgenetic gonad in a woman with XX/XO mosaicism who developed signs of virilization.[8]

Stange[9] stressed the frequent occurrence of neoplasia in underdeveloped gonads, which he explained as reactions to hormonal imbalance. Among 15 patients with underdeveloped gonads and female phenotype, he found 4 who showed tumor formation interpreted as ovarian adenoma, rete-cystoma, epithelial cell nests and Brenner tumor. In 2 patients, surface papillomas were present.

Male pseudohermaphrodites of various types show a marked tendency to tumor development. In 1942, Gilbert[11] reviewed the literature on malignant testicular tumors in pseudohermaphrodites and found 60 cases, to which he added 1 of his own. The tumors most frequently were located in abdominal and sometimes in inguinal but rarely in scrotal testes. Seminomas, teratomas and various malignant types of tumors were diagnosed. By 1954, Taub[12] found that the reports of tumors in male pseudohermaphrodites had risen to 66. He added the description of a remarkable young man who appeared entirely normal with the exception of undescended testes. Laparotomy revealed that the patient was a pseudohermaphrodite with polyorchidism. Choriocarcinoma had developed in the supernumerary testis. The cases of Spielman and Motyloff[13] concern 2 "sisters with hypogenitalism." One of the sisters developed a large pelvic tumor at the age of 40 years. A dysgerminoma was diagnosed in her left gonad, a rudimentary testis and interstitial cell hyperplasia in the right. Melicow and Uson[2] found additional cases in the literature and added 3 of their own. Teter[14] described a gonadoblastoma in a male pseudohermaphrodite with testicular dysgenesis. Of special interest is the case reported by Stump and Garrett,[15] in which *extragonadal* tumors developed. They described a boy recognized as a male pseudohermaphrodite when he was 1 year of age who developed bilateral Wilms tumors at the age of 2 years.

In the older literature, "male pseudohermaphrodism" represented a collective term for several entities. Although classifications of subgroups of these sexual disorders are still changing, certain entities are now well defined and generally accepted.

Patients with *testicular feminization* are phenotypic females with XY chromosomal constitution. They show adequate breast development; the external genitalia are female but the vagina ends as a blind pouch and internal genitalia usually are absent. The gonads are immature testes that can be labial, inguinal or intra-abdominal.[16] In these patients, who are male pseudohermaphrodites (Chapter 111), testicular tubular adenomas are rather common[17,18] and malignant sarcomatous or carcinomatous changes are not rare in the cryptorchid testes. In other cases, seminomas may develop. It is possible that some patients in whom "arrhenoblastomas" were diagnosed belong in this group.[4] In the past, the syndrome of testicular feminization often was not recognized until the displaced testis became enlarged by tumor formation. Such findings led to the recommendation that all patients with testicular feminization syndrome be prophylactically castrated. But new diagnostic methods have shown that the syndrome is more frequent than previously believed and that fewer than 5% of the displaced testes of these patients undergo malignant degeneration; benign adenomas develop in more than 20% of the patients. Taylor *et al.*[16] recommended exploration and removal of the gonad in these patients after completion of their secondary sexual development.

Patients with *pure gonadal dysgenesis* also are phenotypic females with XY karyotype; they differ from patients with testicular feminization by having uteri and Fallopian tubes, by poor development of secondary sex characteristics and by eunuchoid body proportions. Their dysgenetic testes represent a high risk of neoplasia.[43,44] In 26 cases of gonadal dysgenesis without somatic malformations, eight tumors were encountered by Teter and Boczkowski.[19] Dysgerminomas, gonadoblastomas and Brenner tumor were seen. In 5 patients with gonadoblastoma investigated by Philip and Teter,[20] the chromosome pattern was XY. A remarkable incident of gonadoblastoma associated with pure gonadal dysgenesis in monozygotic twins was reported by Frasier *et al.*[21] The (phenotypic) girls, who had no signs of Turner syndrome and had XY sex chromosomes, developed gonadoblastomas of differing sizes near the fibrous gonadal streaks on the posterior aspect of the broad ligament. Associated with one gonadal streak of one twin was a solid teratoma containing smooth muscle, cartilage and glia cells. There also is a report of 2 sisters with pure gonadal dysgenesis and XY karyotype whose streak gonads were replaced by gonadoblastomas.[22] And there were 3 phenotypic females with XY pure gonadal dysgenesis in three different sibships of a kindred reported by Sternberg *et al.*[23] In 1 of these patients, a 14-year-old girl, a sex-cord tumor was present in gonadal streak tissue. The authors thought that the sex anomaly was transmitted in that kindred as an X-linked trait or was carried on an autosome expressed in chromosomal males only. In another family,[24] there were 3 intersexes among 8 siblings. One sibling was considered male and 2 were considered female. All 3 had sex chromosome mosaicism. The abnormal brother was a male pseudohermaphrodite with XYY/XY mosaicism in leukocyte cultures; he had a "potentially malignant testis." His abnormal sisters had XO/XYY/XY mosaicism in varying degree in leukocyte and other tissue cultures. An "ovarian" tumor of unknown type had been removed from 1 of the phenotypic females and a large gonadoblastoma arising from a streak gonad developed in the other. The parents of these siblings were second cousins. Recessive inheritance will have to be considered in such a situation.

Before sex chromatin and chromosomes could be demonstrated, the various forms of hermaphrodism were classified by clinical and anatomic criteria. Since sex has become definable on the cellular level, older classifications are not always applicable. This becomes manifest when one attempts to classify persons with sex anomalies who develop gonadoblastomas, a tumor characteristically occurring in intersexes. In 1970, Scully[25] reviewed 74 such cases. Four-fifths of the patients were phenotypic females, although often they had signs of virilization. Only one-fifth of them were phenotypic male with cryptorchidism, hypospadias and female internal secondary sex organs but almost 90% were chromatin negative, commonly having 46,XY or 45,X/46,XY karyotype. Histologic analyses of these tumors show that they are composed of germ cells and immature cells of Sertoli or granulosa type; cells resembling Leydig and lutein cells usually are present also. Calcification is common and often recognizable in pelvic roentgenograms. Gonadoblastomas can be considered in-situ cancers from which germinomas and occasionally other types of invasive germ cell tumors can develop.[25] That gonadoblastomas in male pseudohermaphrodites can be of microscopic size had been pointed out by Siebenmann[26]; possible early stages of gonadoblastoma have been found in young patients,[21,23,27,46] including an infant with male pseudohermaphrodism and X/XY/XYY mosaicism.[28] Boczkowski *et al.*[29] described a 10-year-old boy with XO/XY karyotype and mixed gonadal dysgenesis who developed a small gonadoblastoma in the undifferentiated gonad. These authors stated that gonadoblastoma is a relatively benign tumor that arises from testicular remnants of dysgenetic testes. In cases in which cytogenetic analysis is performed, a Y chromosome is always present, most often in a normal 46,XY karyotype.[29] Such a Y chromosome[33] can be fragmentary, as shown in a patient reported by Ferenczy *et al.*,[45] who developed a gonadoblastoma having XO/XY fragment gonadal dysgenesis, or it can occur in duplicate.[47]

Turner syndrome complicated by gonadal tumors seems to be rare. Melicow and Uson[2] described a dysgerminoma in the left gonad of an apparently female patient with short stature, cleft palate, absence of parts of the third digit and hypoplastic secondary sex characteristics. The right gonad was not found. Teter and Tarlowski[30] reported the occurrence of a gonadoblastoma developing in the right gonad in a patient with Turner syndrome and clitoromegaly.

Turner syndrome complicated by a teratoblastoma arising from the left gonadal streak of an 18-year-old patient was observed by Tóth and Fehér.[31] The patient was mentally retarded and showed lumbar scoliosis, underdevelopment of a thumb, asymmetric development of the extremities and renal disturbances. The teratoblastoma contained cysts of various sizes, embryonal bone, cartilage, muscle, nerve tissue and epithelial cancer cells as well as sarcomatous tissue. Dysgerminoma of the left gonad in a girl with Turner syndrome was seen by Dominguez and Greenblatt.[32] This chromatin-negative patient had a horseshoe kidney and possibly aortic coarctation. Teter and Boczkowski[19] performed laparotomy in 25 patients with signs of Turner syndrome and found gonadal tumors in 2 cases; one tumor was considered a gonadoblastoma and one an interstitial hilar cell tumor. Both patients had clitoral enlargement and other signs of masculinization. In the patient with gonadoblastoma, a mosaic karyotype, 45,XO/46,XY, was found, so that one cannot consider her a "pure" Turner syndrome. A papillary mucinous cystadenocarcinoma from a 21-year-old patient with Turner syndrome and 45,XO karyotype was reported by Goldberg and Scully.[33] After reviewing the world literature in 1966, these authors listed only 6 cases of Turner syndrome complicated by malignant gonadal tumors. In a review of 289 patients with Turner syndrome by Wertelecki *et al.*,[34] only 1 was found with a gonadal neoplasm, a hilus cell adenoma diagnosed at 19 years of age. Thus, it seems that the gonadal rudiments that usually are present in patients with Turner syndrome have no great tendency to neoplasia; routine prophylactic gonadectomy was not recommended in this disorder except for patients with hypertrophied clitoris or those with XY-mosaic karyotype.[33]

Extragonadal tumors have been observed repeatedly in association with Turner syndrome. In their review of 289 phenotypic females with Turner syndrome, Wertelecki *et al.*[34] found 8 patients with nongonadal neoplasms. There was a preponderance of neurogenic tumors among children and young adults. Adding their cases to others reported in the literature, they listed 25 patients with Turner syndrome complicated by a variety of neoplasms and associated with various hamartomas. Other complications can be caused by endocrine tumors. Willemse[35] observed acromegaly in a patient with Turner syndrome from whom an eosinophilic adenoma of the pituitary was removed at the age of 29 years. Bassøe *et al.*[36] described Cushing disease in a patient with gonadal dysgenesis who had a chromophobe adenoma of the pituitary gland. These authors thought that patients with hypogonadism should be observed for pituitary tumor formation and that adequate substitution therapy in the patients with gonadal dysgenesis may prevent the formation of pituitary tumors. ACTH-like activity in a thymoma associated with Cushing disease and gonadal dysgenesis was reported by Lemon *et al.*[37] An adult patient with 45,XO Turner syndrome observed in the Cincinnati General Hospital (Chart No. 399138) developed signs of Cushing syndrome; she had an adrenal adenoma in the left broad ligament and a pulmonary cylindroma. It is of interest in this context that Stange[9] had pointed out that in hypoplastic gonads adrenocortical tissue is found regularly in the hilus and in the region of the epoophoron. Such adrenal tissue was demonstrated by Richart and Benirschke[38] in a newborn infant with Turner syndrome.

The fact that in a series of 20 patients with *male Turner syndrome* (Chapter 112) and normal karyotype, 1 patient developed a pheochromocytoma and another a ganglioneuroma intimates that the tendency to neoplasia of persons with malformations characteristic of Turner syndrome is independent of the chromosomal anomaly 45,XO. A large number of hamartomas observed in the hospital series of Wertelecki *et al.*[34] could be the basis of neoplasia in some cases of Turner syndrome.

In patients with *mixed gonadal dysgenesis* who have an intra-abdominal dysgenetic testis on one side and a streak gonad on the other, malignant tumors such as seminoma or embryonal carcinoma may develop from the testicular gonad. Such patients may be phenotypic females with XO/XY mosaicism.[16,39]

In patients with *Klinefelter syndrome*, neoplasias have been recorded repeatedly. In 10 men over 50 years, Lubs[40] found 5 cases with neoplasia on record. Leukemias, carcinoma of the testis, reticulum cell sarcoma of the leg and an oat cell carcinoma of the lung were mentioned. Rhode[41] listed angiomas, lipoma and a carcinoma of the lip among 8 cases of chromatin-positive Klinefelter patients and MacSween[42] reported reticulum cell sarcoma in a patient with XY/XXY/XXXY mosaicism. Since the majority of the patients were of advanced age when the neoplasias developed, it is difficult to decide at this time whether Klinefelter syndrome carries an increased risk of neoplasia or whether the reported samples were selected because of unusual features.

REFERENCES

1. Neugebauer, F. L.: *Hermaphroditismus beim Menschen* (Leipzig: Klinkhardt, 1908).
2. Melicow, M. M., and Uson, A. C.: Dysgenetic gonadomas and other gonadal neoplasms in intersexes, Cancer 12: 552, 1959.
3. Overzier, C.: True hermaphroditism, in Overzier, C., *Intersexuality* (New York : Academic Press, 1963).
4. Overzier, C.: *Die Intersexualität* (Stuttgart: Georg Thieme, 1961).
5. Meyer, R.: Über gewebliche Anomalien und ihre Beziehung zu einigen Geschwülsten der Ovarien, Arch. Gynäk. 145:2, 1931.
6. Claret, A. J., and Mackintosh, C. A.: Seudohermafroditismo femenino y tumor mixto de ovario, Rev. argent. urol. 23:137, 1954.
7. Scully, R. E.: Gonadoblastoma, Cancer 6:455, 1953.
8. Warren, J. C., Erkman, B., Cheatum, S., and Holman, G.: Hilus-cell adenoma in a dysgenetic gonad with XX/XO mosaicism, Lancet 1:141, 1964.
9. Stange, H-H.: Über Fehlbildungen der Gonaden und ihre Beziehung zur Geschwulstbildung, Geburtsh. u. Frauenh. 17:63, 1957.
10. Perrin, E. V., and Landing, B. H.: Evidence for a relation between gonadoblastoma and gonadal dysgenesis, Am. J. Dis. Child. 102:575, 1961.
11. Gilbert, J. B.: Studies in malignant testis tumors in pseudohermaphrodites; review of 60 cases and case report, J. Urol. 48:665, 1942.
12. Taub, J.: Malignant testis tumor, cryptorchidism and polyorchidism in pseudohermaphrodite, J. Urol. 71:475, 1954.
13. Spielman, F., and Motyloff, L.: Hermaphroditism and dysgerminoma (neuter cell tumor), New York J. Med. 55: 2168, 1955.
14. Teter, J.: An unusual gonadal tumor (gonadoblastoma) in a male pseudohermaphrodite with testicular dysgenesis, J. Obst. & Gynaec. Brit. Emp. 67:238, 1960.
15. Stump, T. A., and Garrett, R. A.: Bilateral Wilms tumor in a male pseudohermaphrodite, J. Urol. 72:1146, 1954.
16. Taylor, H., Barter, R. H., and Jacobson, C. B.: Neoplasms of dysgenetic gonads, Am. J. Obst. & Gynec. 96:816, 1966.
17. Morris, J. M.: The syndrome of testicular feminization in male pseudohermaphrodites, Am. J. Obst. & Gynec. 65: 1192, 1953.
18. Wachstein, M., and Scorza, A.: Male pseudohermaphroditism; a type showing female habitus, absence of uterus, and male gonads often associated with testicular tubular adenoma. Report of case and review of literature, Am. J. Clin. Path. 21:10, 1951.
19. Teter, J., and Boczkowski, K.: Occurrence of tumors in dysgenetic gonads, Cancer 20:1301, 1967.
20. Philip, J., and Teter, J.: Significance of chromosomal investigation of somatic cells to determine the genetic origin of gonadoblastoma, Acta path. et microbiol. scandinav. 61:543, 1964.
21. Frasier, S. D., Bashore, R. A., and Mosier, H. D.: Gonadoblastoma associated with pure gonadal dysgenesis in monozygous twins, J. Pediat. 64:740, 1964.
22. Cohen, M. M., and Shaw, M. W.: Two XY siblings with gonadal dysgenesis and a female phenotype, New England J. Med. 272:1083, 1965.
23. Sternberg, W. H., Barclay, D. L., and Kloepfer, H. W.: Familial XY gonadal dysgenesis, New England J. Med. 278:695, 1968.
24. Goldstein, A., Hausknecht, R., Hsu, L. Y., Brendler, H., and

Hirschhorn, K.: Sex chromosome mosaicism in 3 sibs, Am. J. Obst. & Gynec. 107:108, 1970.
25. Scully, R. E.: Gonadoblastoma. A review of 74 cases, Cancer 25:1340, 1970.
26. Siebenmann, R. E.: Pseudohermaphroditismus masculinus mit Gonadoblastom, eine besondere Intersexform, Path. et Microbiol. 24:233, 1961.
27. Bergada, C., Cleveland, W. W., Jones, H. W., and Wilkins, L.: Gonadal histology in patients with male pseudohermaphroditism and atypical gonadal dysgenesis: Relation to theories of sex differentiation, Acta endocrinol. 40:493, 1962.
28. Ferrier, P. E., Ferrier, S. A., Scharer, K. O., Genton, N., Hedinger, C., and Klein, D.: Disturbed gonadal differentiation in a child with XO/XY/XYY mosaicism: Relationship with gonadoblastoma, Helvet. paediat. acta 22:479, 1967.
29. Boczkowski, K., Teter, J., Tomaszewska, H., and Philip, J.: Gonadoblastoma (gonocytoma III) in a boy with XO/XY mosaicism. Case report with a survey of literature, Acta path. et microbiol. scandinav. 71:46, 1967.
30. Teter, J., and Tarlowski, R.: Tumors of the gonads in cases of gonadal dysgenesis and male pseudohermaphroditism, Am. J. Obst. & Gynec. 79:321, 1960.
31. Tóth, F., and Fehér, L.: Turner-Syndrom und embryonale Geschwülste, Endokrinologie 43:17, 1962.
32. Dominguez, C. J., and Greenblatt, R. B.: Dysgerminoma of the ovary in a patient with Turner's syndrome, Am. J. Obst. & Gynec. 83:674, 1962.
33. Goldberg, M. B., and Scully, A. L.: Gonadal malignancy in gonadal dysgenesis: Papillary pseudomucinous cystadenocarcinoma in a patient with Turner's syndrome, J. Clin. Endocrinol. 27:341, 1967.
34. Wertelecki, W., Fraumeni, J. F., Jr., and Mulvihill, J. J.: Nongonadal neoplasia in Turner's syndrome, Cancer 26:485, 1970.
35. Willemse, C. H.: A patient suffering from Turner's syndrome and acromegaly, Acta endocrinol. 39:204, 1962.
36. Bassøe, H. H., Godeholt, H., Ronald, K., and Støa, K. F.: Cushing disease in a patient with gonadal dysgenesis and pituitary tumor, Acta endocrinol. 48:72, 1965.
37. Lemon, F. C., Fine, M. B., Grasso, S. G., and Kinsell, L. W.: ACTH-like activity in a thymoma associated with gonadal dysgenesis, J. Clin. Endocrinol. 26:1, 1966.
38. Richart, R., and Benirschke, K.: Gonadal dysgenesis in a newborn infant, New England J. Med. 258:974, 1958.
39. Sohval, A. R.: Hermaphroditism with "atypical" or "mixed" gonadal dysgenesis. Relationship to gonadal neoplasm, Am. J. Med. 36:281, 1964.
40. Lubs, H. A., Jr.: Testicular size in Klinefelter's syndrome in man over fifty. Report of a case with XXY/XY mosaicism, New England J. Med. 267:326, 1962.
41. Rhode, R. A.: Chromatin-positive Klinefelter's syndrome. Clinical and cytogenetic studies, J. Chron. Dis. 16:1139, 1963.
42. MacSween, R. N. M.: Reticulum-cell sarcoma and rheumatoid arthritis in a patient with XY/XXY/XXXY Klinefelter's syndrome and normal intelligence, Lancet 1:460, 1965.
43. Carpentier, P. J., Stolte, L. A. M., and Visschers, G. P.: Gonadal dysgenesis and testicular tumours, Lancet 1:386, 1956.
44. Pinkerton, J. H. M.: Gonadal dysgenesis complicated by virilizing embryonal carcinoma, J. Reprod. & Fertil. 9:203, 1965.
45. Ferenczy, A., Richart, R. M., and Miller, O. J.: Gonadoblastoma occurring in a female with XO/XY fragment gonadal dysgenesis, Am. J. Obst. & Gynec. 109:564, 1971.
46. Taylor, A. I.: Case report. Trisomy of chromosome 16 in a neonate, 47,XY,?16+, J. M. Genetics 8:123, 1971.
47. Suñe, M. V., Centeno, J. V., and Salzano, F. M.: Case report. Gonadoblastoma in a phenotypic female with 45,X/47,XYY mosaicism, J. M. Genetics 7:410, 1970.

Soft Tissue Tumors

THESE ARE NEOPLASMS derived from mesoderm that are situated in connective tissue or fat outside parenchymatous organs.[1-3] Since this definition is not always used in tabulations, exact incidence figures are not obtainable but it can be assumed that 10–20% of children's malignant tumors belong in this category.[3,4] Benign soft tissue tumors are several times more frequent than malignant ones. Many soft tissue tumors can be attributed to embryonal rests and cited in favor of Cohnheim's theory of oncogenesis (p. 1199). Andersen and Perrin[3] pointed out that the prenatal origin of many of these tumors is suggested by the histologic appearance of their cells, which are located in tissues that normally are free of such cell types. Soft tissue tumors behave like many other childhood neoplasms; they consist of two main categories: those that are peculiar to infancy and early childhood and those that are comparable to similar tumors affecting adults. There is a gap of several years between the infantile and the juvenile groups. Both types show definite male prevalence.[6] Infantile fibrous tumors show distinctive features. Despite great cellularity, infiltrative growth and poor differentiation, they do not always imply aggressive clinical behavior. Conversely, growths that appear innocent to the pathologist may recur repeatedly and sometimes even necessitate amputation of an extremity.[6] These tumors' specific behavior raises questions as to their etiology. It is difficult to decide whether they are neoplasms, cellular hypoplasias or congenital tissue malformations. The last possibility is supported by the fact that many of the lesions are present at birth; against their neoplastic nature is the fact that many regress spontaneously.[6] Enzinger,[6] reviewing 98 patients with infantile fibrous tumors, distinguished six separate categories. *Infantile dermal fibromatosis* presents in the form of nodules on the extensor surfaces of the end phalanges of the fingers and toes; it is seen three times as often in males as in females. *Fibrous hamartoma of infancy* also is more prevalent in male infants. The lesions are characteristically located in the axillary or shoulder region. Fibromatosis colli is a subject of its own that has long aroused great interest (Chapter 104). Its frequent association with congenital dislocation of the hip suggests a general prenatal disorder. *Diffuse infantile fibromatosis* histologically resembles fibromatosis colli but the tumors are not limited to any muscle group. The upper extremities, head and neck are the most common sites.[5] *Aggressive infantile fibromatosis* cannot be distinguished easily from fibrosarcoma but the lesions do not metastasize, although they are locally aggressive and have a tendency to recur. The extremities or the trunk can be affected by these rapidly growing tumors. Enzinger[5] separated these lesions from congenital fibrosarcomas and embryonal rhabdomyosarcomas and warned against radical or mutilating surgical procedures as long as growth can be controlled by complete local excision. *Congenital generalized fibromatosis* is a peculiar disorder of prenatal origin that manifests itself by many nodules of apparently fibroblastic mesenchymal tissues located in subcutis, muscle and viscera. The nodules as described by Stout[1] in 2 infants were 2–4 cm. in length, sharply defined and consisting of differentiated fibrous tissue with rare mitoses. In some areas, the picture approached that of differentiated fibrosarcoma. Both infants died in the neonatal period. Shnitka *et al.*[7] reported a third case, giving a detailed history of the mother and her child and a good review of the subject. Their case was that of an infant born with a large tumor mass protruding from the right orbit and displacing the right eye. In addition, multiple tumor nodules were palpable under the skin of the left arm, right chest and back. Death, preceded by irregular respiration and fall of body temperature, occurred unexpectedly 2½ days after delivery. At necropsy, more than 50 grossly identifiable nodules could be dissected from various skeletal muscles, some being located in the musculature of the heart and gastrointestinal tract. The nodules consisted of fibrous tissue composed of spindle cells with infrequent mitoses. Condon and Allen[8] reported the case of an infant[9] with congenital generalized fibromatosis who lived 6 weeks after birth. This case is of special interest because there was involvement of the entire skeletal system with lesions in the ends of the long bones, in the ribs, scapula, vertebrae, pelvis, mandible and skull. There also were multiple nodules in the lungs, heart, liver, intestine and muscles. Deformities of the scapula, clavicle and ribs can be seen in roentgenograms.[10] Occlusion of the pulmonary arteries by fibromatous tissue has been observed.[9] Skeletal lesions could be mistaken for syphilis, reticuloendothelioses, neurofibromatosis, neuroblastoma, fibrous dysplasia, chondromatosis or angiomatosis.

Shnitka *et al.*[7] believed that the lesions arise de novo in interstitial fibrous tissue and not through metastasis. The histologic appearance was much more suggestive of a tissue malformation (hamartoma) than of a neoplasia.

The etiology of this disorder is not known. In 2 of the cases, maternal syphilis treated with large doses of penicillin had preceded the children's birth, but the infants were free of syphilis. Generalized fibromatosis induced in adult guinea pigs by prolonged administration of estrogens[11] simulated the congenital form of fibromatosis in some respects, but there probably is no etiologic relationship between the two conditions. The fact that 4 cases occurred in one family[12] does not elucidate the situation of this mesenchymal dysplasia, which seems to develop during the last months of gestation.[6] Congenital generalized fibromatosis leads to rapid deterioration and early death,[7] but it is possible that sometimes histologically similar lesions are limited to the skin.[6] *Congenital sarcomas and other mesenchymal tumors.* In 1940, Wells[13] listed 29 cases of definite congenital sarcomas found at various sites and 46 cases of possibly congenital sarcomas. He believed that the number of published cases gives a very inadequate idea of the actual incidence. In 1953, Fahey and Bollinger,[14] reviewing the literature, found 35 cases of congenital sarcoma, 17 occurring on the extremities. Other case reports and reviews[15,16] have been published since. Early reports may not be acceptable today, since many conditions have been described in more recent times that resemble fibrosarcomas histologically to a certain degree but differ from them in detail, course and prognosis. The distinction of congenital soft tissue tumors from those appearing in early childhood has lost some importance, as the two groups seem to merge into one that stretches from birth to about 5 years of postnatal life. Prenatal determination of some soft tissue sarcomas that manifest themselves in later childhood sometimes is suggested by their development in patients with congenital malformations, mental retardation[17] or general hamartoses. In a review of 120 congenital mesenchymal tumors, Kauffman and Stout[18] listed fibromatoses as the most common lesions, with 37 cases. There were fifteen congenital rhabdomyosarcomas but only four fibrosarcomas. Mesenchymomas, smooth muscle tumors, hemangiopericytomas and others were among the congenital lesions. Of the one hundred twenty congenital mesenchymal tumors, only six metastasized and seventeen were fatal. Rhabdomyosarcomas, fibrosarcomas and malignant mesenchymomas were the only metastasizing congenital tumors.[18] Rhabdomyosarcomas account for approximately 20% of soft tissue tumors[19] and half of them are of the embryonal type. These embryonal rhabdomyosarcomas can occur at any age, but 75% of the patients develop the tumor within the first decades of life. Li and Fraumeni[33] made an epidemiologic study of rhabdomyosarcoma in children and found a peak mortality before 4 years of age. The neoplasm was present in a number of children before 1 year of age and in some within 1 month of birth. Congenital rhabdomyosarcoma had been observed before.[19,20] Alveolar rhabdomyosarcoma is seen most often in the first 2 decades of life and can occur in infancy.[19]

Congenital rhabdomyomas of the heart are best known as anomalies occurring in tuberous sclerosis (p. 1262) but they also have been seen associated with renal cysts and tumors, with congenital malformations of the pancreas, cleft lip and palate or spina bifida.[22] Congenital or infantile rhabdomyosarcoma of the bladder[20] and of the prostate[23] have been recorded. Rhabdomyomas of the heart in both of a set of probably identical twins have been observed.[34] Botryoid sarcomas of the vagina, urethra, bladder, prostate or in the head region usually occur in children under 5 years of age but only a few are congenital.[24,25]

Various soft tissue tumors occur as manifestations and complications of hamartoses (Chapters 121–123). Although such tumors seldom are congenital, prenatal factors are involved in their origin, since the basic conditions are dominant hereditary traits. In *Recklinghausen neurofibromatosis*, fibroma molluscum, neurofibromas in many forms, hemangiomas, lymphangiomas, lipomas, meningiomas and other tumors appearing at many sites can bring about the variegated disease pictures of this hamartosis. Some of the tumors are present at birth but the majority develop at various periods of postnatal life. Pathologic manifestations of the generally "benign" tumors usually are due to their encroachment on surrounding structures, but malignant degeneration of the lesions, particularly sarcomatous, occurs in some cases. The frequency of malignant complications is not known, as estimates vary between 1.6%[26] and 16%.[27] Overestimates are due to the publication of unusual cases. Through neurofibromatosis, the tumors mentioned above are related etiologically to some gliomas, ependymomas, ganglioneuromas and pheochromocytomas. Although adenoma sebaceum is considered the typical lesion of *tuberous sclerosis*, many other tumors develop in patients with this hamartosis. Fibrous growths such as collagenous plaques, subungual and periungual fibromas, cutaneous tags or polyps, fibrous nodules on the oral mucosa, fibrous hemangiomas, fibrolipomas and lipomyomas appear during the course of the disease.[27] In the heart, congenital rhabdomyomas and myolipomas have been seen. Mixed tumors of the kidneys contain smooth muscles, blood vessels and other tissues (Chapter 122). In *Gardner syndrome* (Chapter 123), soft tissue tumors typically are associated with polyposis of the colon and osteomas. The soft tissue tumors appear in childhood and may be the first sign of this hamartosis. Subcutaneous fibrous tumors develop at many sites and fibrous hyperplasias may be found in retroperitoneal and mesenteric tissues.[27] Fibrosarcomas[28,29] or leiomyomas[29,30] may complicate the disease. In the *basal cell nevi syndrome*, the typical basal cell carcinomas sometimes are combined with fibromas and lipomas (Chapter 123).

A disorder leading to *multiple glomus tumors* can be transmitted like a dominant hereditary trait. These tumors, which have been classified as hamartomas, resemble cavernous hemangiomas but their cavities are lined not only by a single layer of endothelium but by several layers of small polygonal cells with pale cytoplasm and homogeneous round nuclei. Multiple glomus tumors are not encapsulated and may differ in this and other respects from solitary glomus tumors. They can be noticeable soon after birth or make their appearance during childhood or adolescence.[31] It is thought that solitary tumors develop later in life[31,32] but there were six glomus tumors in the series of one hundred twenty congenital mesenchymal tumors reviewed by Kauffman and Stout.[18]

Various neoplasms in siblings and parents of children with rhabdomyosarcoma were recorded by Li and Fraumeni.[33] Some relatives of children with rhabdomyosarcoma developed adrenocortical carcinoma and brain tumors.[33]

In patients with Maffucci syndrome (Chapter 94), sarcomas, myxochondrosarcomas, angiosarcomas, fibromas and lymphangiomas have been observed occasionally in addition to the typical chondromas and angiomas.

REFERENCES

1. Stout, A. P.: Juvenile fibromatoses, Cancer 7:953, 1954.
2. Pack, G. T., and Ariel, I. M.: *Tumors of the Soft Somatic Tissues; A Clinical Treatise* (New York: Paul B. Hoeber, Inc., 1958).
3. Andersen, D. H., and Perrin, E. V.: Soft tissue tumors, Pediat. Clin. North America 6:543, 1959.
4. Marsden, H. B., and Steward, J. K.: *Tumours in Children.* Recent Results in Cancer Research No. 13 (New York: Springer-Verlag, 1968).
5. Enzinger, F. M.: Fibrous Tumors of Infancy, in *Tumors of Bone and Soft Tissue* (Chicago: Year Book Medical Publishers, Inc., 1965).
6. Enzinger, F. M.: Recent Trends in Soft Tissue Pathology, in *Tumors of Bone and Soft Tissue* (Chicago: Year Book Medical Publishers, Inc., 1965).
7. Shnitka, T. K., Asp, D. M., and Horner, R. H.: Congenital generalized fibromatosis, Cancer 11:627, 1958.
8. Condon, V. R., and Allen, R. P.: Congenital generalized fibromatosis. Case report with roentgen manifestations, Radiology 76:444, 1961.
9. Beatty, E. C., Jr.: Congenital generalized fibromatosis in infancy, Am. J. Dis. Child. 103:620, 1962.
10. Levkoff, A. H., Gonzalez, C. G., and Neher, J. L.: Congenital diffuse fibromatosis: A case report, Pediatrics 35:331, 1965.
11. Lipschütz, A., and Vargas, L., Jr.: Structure and origin of uterine and extra-genital fibroids induced experimentally in guinea pig by prolonged administration of estrogens, Cancer Res. 1:236, 1941.
12. Bartlett, R. C., Otis, R. D., and Laakso, A. O.: Multiple congenital neoplasms of soft tissues. Report of 4 cases in one family, Cancer 14:913, 1961.
13. Wells, H. G.: Occurrence and significance of congenital malignant neoplasms, Arch. Path. 30:535, 1940.
14. Fahey, J. J., and Bollinger, J. A.: Congenital sarcoma of foot; case report and review of literature, A.M.A. Am. J. Dis. Child. 86:23, 1953.
15. Reye, R. D. K.: Congenital embryonic mixed leg tumor, Arch. Path. 79:80, 1965.
16. Balsaver, A. M., Butler, J. J., and Martin, R. G.: Congenital fibrosarcoma, Cancer 20:1607, 1967.
17. Sloane, J. A., and Hubbell, M. M.: Soft tissue sarcomas in children associated with congenital anomalies, Cancer 23:175, 1969.
18. Kauffman, S. L., and Stout, A. P.: Congenital mesenchymal tumors, Cancer 18:460, 1965.
19. Albores-Saavedra, J., Butler, J. J., and Martin, R. G.: Rhabdomyosarcoma: Clinicopathologic Considerations and Report of 85 Cases, in *Tumors of Bone and Soft Tissue* (Chicago: Year Book Medical Publishers, Inc., 1965).
20. Houette, C.: Rhabdomyome diverticulaire congénital de la vessie, Ann. anat. path. 6:267, 1929.
21. Golding, R., and Reed, G.: Rhabdomyoma of the heart. Two unusual clinical presentations, New England J. Med. 276:957, 1967.
22. Farber, S.: Congenital rhabdomyoma of heart, Am. J. Path. 7:105, 1931.
23. Grier, E. A., and Phillips, F. L.: Rhabdomyosarcoma of the prostate, J. Urol. 69:695, 1953.

24. Potter, E. L.: *Pathology of the Fetus and Infant* (2d ed.; Chicago: Year Book Medical Publishers, Inc., 1961).
25. Willis, R. A.: *The Borderland of Embryology and Pathology* (Washington, D. C.: Butterworth, 1962).
26. Crowe, F. W., Schull, W. J., and Neel, J. V.: *A Clinical, Pathological and Genetic Study of Multiple Neurofibromatosis* (Springfield, Ill.: Charles C Thomas, Publisher, 1956).
27. Butterworth, T., and Strean, L. P.: *Clinical Genodermatology* (Baltimore: The Williams & Wilkins Company, 1962).
28. Laberge, M. Y., Sauer, W. G., and Mayo, C. W.: Soft tissue tumors associated with familial polyposis, Proc. Staff Meet. Mayo Clin. 32:749, 1957.
29. Collins, D. C.: Frequent association of other body tumors with familial polyposis, Am. J. Gastroenterol. 31:376, 1959.
30. Gumpel, R. C., and Carballo, J. D.: New concept of familial adenomatosis, Ann. Int. Med. 45:1045, 1956.
31. Gorlin, R. J., Fusaro, R. M., and Benton, J. W.: Multiple glomus tumor of the pseudocavernous hemangioma type, Arch. Dermat. 82:776, 1960.
32. Morfit, H. M., Swan, H., and Taylor, E. R.: Carotid body tumors, Arch. Surg. 67:194, 1953.
33. Li, F. P., and Fraumeni, J. F., Jr.: Rhabdomyosarcoma in children: Epidemiologic study and identification of a familial cancer syndrome, J. Nat. Cancer Inst. 43:1365, 1969.
34. Scariano, N.: Rhabdomyoma of the heart in both of a set of twins, Acta Genet. 11:124, 1962.

Osteosarcoma and Other Bone Tumors

Osteosarcomas develop characteristically in the second half of childhood or later. A history of injury often is related but the significance of such incidents often is difficult to assess because of their frequency in that age group. Yet, in some cases, injuries are definite etiologic factors, particularly if the tumor develops in a fracture site. Femur, humerus and tibia are the bones most commonly affected.[1] Despite the relatively late onset of osteosarcomas, prenatal etiologic factors are recognized in some of the cases when the tumor develops in the course of a skeletal disorder that is known to have prenatal determinants.

There are several heritable skeletal anomalies that carry a risk of bone tumor development and there are reports of familial occurrence of bone tumors. The best known osseous disorder with a tendency to tumor formation is that of multiple exostoses, an autosomal dominant trait. Osteochondromas are not rare in this condition and chondrosarcomas are thought to develop in 5–10% of the cases (p. 843). In another dominantly inherited condition—osteogenesis imperfecta—osteosarcoma has been observed in some instances.[2,3] Multiple osteomas are characteristic of Gardner syndrome (Chapter 123), a dominantly inherited hamartosis. Albers-Schönberg osteopetrosis, an autosomal recessive trait, carries a small risk of osteogenic sarcoma (p. 866). Chondrosarcoma[4] and osteogenic sarcoma[5] have developed in siblings of families in which there were no signs of systemic osseous dysplasias. In Ollier disease (p. 874), which seems to be related to hemiatrophy or hemihypertrophy, sarcomas sometimes develop in affected bones.[6] The risk of tumor formation is even greater in Maffucci syndrome (p. 882) but the etiology of that condition is obscure and prenatal etiologic factors have not been established. The same is true for fibrous dysplasias, in which malignant transformation to osteosarcoma can occur.[6,7] Observations of multiple, possibly multicentric, osteogenic sarcomas in adolescents have led to speculations about unknown underlying mesenchymal disturbances in such cases.[8] A correlation of tall stature and osteogenic sarcoma was found by Fraumeni.[9]

Congenital fibrosarcoma of the femur has been reported.[10]

REFERENCES

1. Marsden, H. B., and Steward, J. K.: *Tumours in Children* (New York: Springer-Verlag, 1968).
2. Jewell, F. C., and Lofstrom, J. E.: Osteogenic sarcoma occurring in fragilitas ossium, Radiology 34:741, 1940.
3. Klenerman, L., Ockenden, B. G., and Townsend, A. C.: Osteosarcoma occurring in osteogenesis imperfecta. Report of two cases, J. Bone & Joint Surg. 49-B:314, 1967.
4. Schajowicz, F., and Bessone, J. E.: Chondrosarcoma in three brothers. A pathological and genetic study, J. Bone & Joint Surg. 49-A:129, 1967.
5. Harmon, T. P., and Morton, K. S.: Osteogenic sarcoma in four siblings, J. Bone & Joint Surg. 48-B:493, 1966.
6. Geschickter, C. F.: Mutations and Congenital Abnormalities in Relation to Bone Neoplasms, in *Tumors of Bone and Soft Tissue* (Chicago: Year Book Medical Publishers, Inc., 1965).
7. Schwartz, D. T., and Alpert, M.: The malignant transformation of fibrous dysplasia, Am. J. M. Sc. 247:1, 1964.
8. Amstutz, H. C.: Multiple osteogenic sarcomata—metastatic or multicentric?, Cancer 24:923, 1969.
9. Fraumeni, J. F., Jr.: Stature and malignant tumors of bone in childhood and adolescence, Cancer 20:967, 1967.
10. Drez, D. J., Jr., Akins, W. G., White, P., and King, R. E.: Congenital malignant tumors of the extremities: A report of two cases, Inter-Clinic Information Bull. 9:1, 1970.

Teratomas

OF THE MANY puzzling questions that surround the origin of teratomas, only their etiology and relationship to congenital malformations will be discussed here. The huge and confusing literature on these tumors deals with many interesting problems related to teratology, and teratomas obviously are congenital structural deviations. In fact, some pathologists use the word "teratology" to signify the science of teratomas and refer to factors causing formation of teratomas as "teratogenic." These usages are not to be recommended. The field of teratology is a much larger one than that of teratomas; it is the science of all congenital malformations, whereas teratomas represent merely a specific subgroup of malformations.

Teratomas are tumors consisting of tissues derived from ectoderm, mesoderm and entoderm. Common components of teratomas are skin, central nervous tissue, teeth, glands or respiratory and alimentary mucosa.[1] The relative amounts of these tissues vary greatly and their lack of proper proportions is one of their characteristics. Even in some large ovarian teratomas, skin may be hard to find and in others central nervous tissues are scarce and ectodermal products absent.[2] In teratomas noted at birth, brain tissue makes up a large proportion of the mass, whereas entodermal components are less prominent. Fat, cartilage, bone and muscle are present in all congenitally recognizable teratomas but renal, pulmonary or genital tissues are rare.[3] These formations, which resemble fetuses in that they contain rudimentary organs of many kinds and differ from them by lack of proper organization, have puzzled scientists for centuries. According to Gould and Pyle,[4] the finding of bones, teeth, hairs, fingers, nails and so forth in the abdomen of an unmarried woman was presumptive evidence that she was unchaste. When a fetus in fetu was found in a male or when "a man was pregnant with his sister" one thought of a repetition of the process by which Eve was born of Adam. A report by Gaetano-Nocito, quoted by Gould and Pyle, is of interest because it shows that teratomas were early thought to be related to twinning. From a man of 27 "issued fetal bones and a mass of macerated embryo. His mother had had several double pregnancies. . . ."

In modern times, teratomas were explained as imperfect conjoined twins, parasitic twins or included fetuses (fetus in fetu). There are investigators who believed that gradations exist from normal twins to conjoined twins, parasitic twins, enclosed fetuses and teratomas. Others were strongly opposed to this view and denied that teratomas are related to twins or that they are fetuses. Willis[1] declared that teratomas must be considered tumors; in parasitic twins, one does not see mixtures of embryonic and differentiating tissues, which are present at all stages of growing teratomas. He concluded that the age incidence, sites, structure and mode of growth of teratomas prove that they are tumors derived "from foci of plastic pluripotential embryonic tissue which escaped the influence of the primary organizer during early development." This view is influenced by the work of experimental embryologists who have been able to produce teratoma-like structures in amphibian embryos. Budde,[5] soon after Spemann and Mangold's[6] experiments on induction of embryonal anlagen by implantation of heterologous organizers, explained teratomas by the action of displaced or abnormal organizers. Subsequently, many other writers expressed the belief that organizer phenomena provide the only basis for a modern theory of the origin of teratomas and that these tumors lack the coordinated action of a dominant organizer. Needham[7] attributed teratomas to the liberation of evocators of various grades at times and places where they are not normally released and to persistence of competence to respond to evocators beyond the time at which such competence is normally lost. Since primary evocator is present in most adult tissues of animals in the free state, abnormal competence seemed to be more important for the formation of teratomas than the evocator. Needham[7] concluded that teratomas are formed when either the appropriate evocator has been liberated in a large number of places or when competence has appeared or been retained in a sporadic chaotic way.

Manifestations of teratomas vary with site, age and sex. In Willis's[8] series of one hundred seventy-two teratomas, eighty-one originated in ovaries and thirty-six in testes. There were twenty-two intrathoracic and fourteen sacrococcygeal teratomas, whereas intracranial, retroperitoneal and cervical tumors accounted for only thirteen altogether. These figures, which show that approximately 70% of the teratomas originated in ovaries or testes, demonstrate the predominance of gonadal sites. All types and sites can be observed in children under 16 years; ovarian, testicular and intrathoracic tumors manifest themselves more often in adults than in children. In Willis' series[8] there were no sacrococcygeal, retroperitoneal, cervical or intracranial teratomas in adults. There is an interesting sex distribution. The hosts of epignathous, retroperitoneal and sacrococcygeal teratomas are predominantly female, whereas those of pineal teratomas are male.

Ovarian teratomas have not yet been recognized at birth, but in the second year, several have been diagnosed[8,88] and operated on, usually after torsion, attacks of pain and vomiting. There is a greater tendency of ovarian teratomas to malignancy in children than in adults. Whereas, in adults, malignant degeneration occurs in only 2–3%,[9,87] it develops in about 15% of childhood cases.[10] As in adults, dermoid cysts of children usually are benign, whereas solid or polycystic tumors are potentially malignant. Bilateral ovarian teratomas are rare.[8] Among 75 cases of ovarian cysts and tumors of the ovary in children analyzed by Ein *et al.*,[81] there were thirty-five (47%) considered benign cystic (dermoid) teratomas and three (4%) malignant teratomas. Brandesky[82] encountered in ten ovarian tumors of children five dermoid cysts of which one was a fully developed teratoma. Cells of ovarian teratomas have positive sex chromatin. Normal female 46-chromosome patterns have been described in the cells of benign cystic ovarian teratomas[11] and also in metastatic cells of a malignant ovarian teratoma.[12] But in a malignant ovarian teratoma occurring in a 14-year-old girl, Arias-Bernal and Jones[83] found, in culture of the tumor cells with 47 chromosomes, the extra chromosome similar to one of the A group, probably chromosome 3. The sex chromosome complement was XX like that noted in other ovarian teratomas.

Testicular teratomas are second in frequency and account for approximately 20% of all teratomas. They are more likely to be malignant in adults than in children. They have been recognized repeatedly at birth, and if occurring in children, they usually are detected within the first 2 years. Of thirty-six specimens examined by Willis,[8] eight were found in children under 16 years. Of these eight tumors, six were manifest in the first year of life. One, discovered in a 15-year-old boy, was malignant. There is an association between undescended testis and teratoma in adults, but it is rare in children.[8] There was no testicular teratoma among the tumors of childhood reported by Andersen.[10] Among 12 cases of testicular tumors occurring during infancy and childhood reported by Rusche,[13] there were eight "adult teratomas" and one dermoid cyst. In the first group, two were observed at birth and one of them was mistaken for a hydrocele. In other instances, enlargement of one testis led to the discovery of the teratoma. The sex chromatin of testicular teratomas was found to be positive or negative, an aspect that will be discussed later.

Mediastinal teratomas are recognized most often in the third decade, but about one-fourth of them become manifest during childhood. In Andersen's[10] series, three of twenty-nine teratomas found in children were located in the anterior mediastinum. Even in infants, such tumors can be large enough to cause cyanosis, dyspnea and chest deformity.[14,15] Willis[8] mentioned an intrathoracic teratoma in a stillborn male infant who also had a large occipital encephalocele. Of seven mediastinal teratomas found in children, four were either congenital or manifest within the first few months of life. Hope and Koop[16] stated that such teratomas are the second most common mass lesion found in the anterior mediastinum of infants and children. They can be distinguished from thymic enlargements by their ability to compress the trachea during inspiration and sometimes by dense calcific areas seen within the mass. There apparently is no sex predilection. Another intrathoracic location of teratomas is near the base of the heart, where the tumors can be attached to the great vessels.[8] An intracardial teratoma located in the right ventricle was described by Williams[17] in a male infant who died at the age of 3 weeks and a teratocarcinoma of the heart was recorded by Arshadi and Watson.[18] Schlumberger[19] reported 16 cases of mediastinal teratoma in patients between 18 and 38 years. Six of the tumors were malignant. The author believed that teratomas of the anterior mediastinum arise from tissue dislocations in the anlage of the thymus and not from primordial germ cells.

Sacrococcygeal teratomas are of teratologic interest because most of them can be recognized at birth as congenital malformations. Only rarely are manifestations delayed to later childhood or adulthood.[20] The sex ratio is striking; in the series of Gross *et al.*,[21] 30 of 40, and in that of Gwinn *et al.*,[22] 17 of 18 patients were females. It has been stated that the predilection for the female holds only for benign sacrococcygeal teratomas, whereas the sex ratio is 1:1 in malignant tumors.[23] Yet, in another series of malignant sacrococcygeal teratomas, 17 of 21 patients were female.[84] About one-third of the sacrococcygeal teratomas are malignant.[23] According to Gross *et al.*,[21] other congenital malformations rarely are combined with sacrococcygeal teratomas, but 1 infant in their series had an anomalous development of the thoracic spine and another had an incomplete cleft of the soft palate. Spina bifida combined with teratoma also was mentioned by Ballantyne[24] and Askanazy.[2] Sometimes it may be difficult to distinguish between spina bifida and sacrococcygeal teratoma, even when histologic sections are available. A teratoma associated with duplication of the lower intestinal tract and a communication between one of the "cysts" of enteric origin and the neural canal was described by Esterly and Baghdassarian.[25] There also were duplications of the uterus and vagina and of the left renal pelvis and ureter. Hickey and Layton[26] found reports of associated malformations in eleven of twelve sacrococcygeal teratomas included in their review; anencephaly, spina bifida, meningocele, patent urachus and cleft palate were mentioned. Esophageal and duodenal atresia were present in a case of Ingelrans *et al.*[27] In sacrococcygeal teratomas, one can find cartilage and bone as well as intestinal, pancreatic, respiratory, nervous and ocular rudiments. As a rule, these tissues seem to be mature without signs of malignancy, but occasionally they recur after operation, one of the tissues showing malignant characteristics. The tumors are prenatal in origin and some of their carriers die before birth. The size is variable but large tumors of this type can look like a caudal prolongation of the infant's body, hanging over the posterior aspects of the legs. They adhere to the coccygeal region; a presacral portion sometimes can be palpated on rectal examination. The tumor often is covered by normal skin but cutaneous anomalies such as hemangiomas or ulcers have been observed. Movements within the tumor can be seen or felt in some cases. Roentgenograms show more or less differentiated bones and teeth, but the great mass of the tumor usually is cystic or made up of soft tissues. Some of these tumors grow in proportion to the rest of the body; others grow faster, particularly if they contain malignant tissues. Malignant tumors are primarily intrapelvic. They usually appear after 2 months of age and cause bowel and bladder obstruction, pain and circulatory disturbances.[23] Hunt *et al.*[28] stated that these teratomas, if not treated early, often undergo malignant degeneration. The malignancy rate, which is time-dependent, is 50–60% between age 4 months and 5 years.[28] In addition to malignancy, inflammations and local compression of pelvic organs by presacral tumors must be expected as complications.[29,80]

Retroperitoneal teratomas almost always are recognized in early childhood. In Willis'[8] series, four tumors were seen in children between birth and 9 months, but one came from a girl 13 years of age. Only 1 of the 5 children with retroperitoneal teratomas was a boy. Three children with such tumors observed in the Children's Hospital of Cincinnati were girls. Of the twenty-nine teratomas reported by Andersen,[10] three were from the retroperitoneal region. Such tumors are said to be rather benign, containing highly differentiated tissues. But in Andersen's series, one of three and in Cincinnati two of three were malignant. One of these malignant retroperitoneal teratomas was found in a mongoloid child 4 months of age.

Arnheim[30] reviewed forty-four retroperitoneal teratomas. They commonly were large cystic tumors, arising high in the retroperitoneal space. The malignancy rate was only 6.8% but some teratomas caused death by pressure. More than half of the tumors were detected in the first year of life; more than 60% occurred in females. Abdominal enlargement, a palpable mass and pressure symptoms were among the early manifestations. Later, fever, vomiting, constipation and loss of weight were noted. Teratomas are third in frequency among retroperitoneal tumors of childhood, the two most common being neuroblastoma and Wilms tumor. Roentgenograms often reveal calcified or ossified areas. Arnheim[31] reviewed 15 cases involving combined pelvic and retroperitoneal teratomas that arose in the presacral region and extended upward into retroperitoneal regions. The incidence of malignancy was 38%, with adenocarcinoma developing within the teratoma. Nine of 13 cases were manifest in the first year, usually causing urinary and intestinal obstruction. The mass may appear as an external growth in the sacrococcygeal region or occupy the pelvis and lower abdomen. The prognosis of these tumors is not favorable, the long-term recovery rate being 15% in contrast to 42% for retroperitoneal and 68% for sacrococcygeal teratomas. A sacrococcygeal teratoma in a newborn girl with massive intra-abdominal extension was removed successfully by combined abdominosacral approach.[32]

Cervical teratomas are rare, with only 88 cases on record by 1967. Only four of these had been observed in adults.[33] Approximately half of the reported cases concerned stillborn or newborn children. Males and females were affected equally. Hydramnios complicated pregnancy in a number of cases. A large tumor in a newborn can cause obstruction of the larynx, trachea or esophagus.[34] Cervical teratomas are closely related to the thyroid. Sometimes they replace the thyroid or one of its lobes or they may be enveloped by thyroid tissue.[3,35] Often they are already huge at birth, keeping the head overextended and deflected to one side[36]; or they grow soon after birth,[37] causing dyspnea, cyanosis, stridor and dysphagia. Without operation, large cervical teratomas are rapidly fatal, but surgical removal may result in permanent cure. Newstedt and Shirkey[36] reported a patient operated on at the first day of life; a 7-year follow-up showed normal thyroid function and normal physical and mental development. The tumors found in children usually contain well-differentiated tissues such as neural elements with choroid plexus, cysts lined with squamous or ciliated columnar epithelium, thyroid, cartilage, pancreas and so forth. In the case of Weitzner,[37] two cysts showed epithelial arrangement resembling the trachea and esophagus. Two teratomas of the neck in the newborn were reported by Ruffolo *et al.*[38] By administration of radioiodine, it could be shown that the tumor did not involve the thyroid gland. In adults, only a few cervical teratomas have been observed[33] but, if they occur, they have, in contrast to their counterparts in children, a strong tendency to malignant degeneration.[34] Associated congenital malformations have been mentioned occasionally.[39]

Intracranial teratomas are rare. They account for only about 3% of teratomas in Willis' series,[8] where they were obtained exclusively from children. As intracranial masses, they are discussed with the brain tumors (p. 1215).

Epignathi and other teratoid tumors of the mouth and pharynx were of great interest to pathologists of the nineteenth century, who classified them according to their degree of differentiation and their resemblance to parasitic twins. A more recent review was written by Ehrich,[40] who cited some of the old references. It was thought that teratoid parasites of the mouth show transitions from dermoids (hairy polyps) to incompletely developed twins, sometimes connected to the host or autosite by an umbilical cord. Only a few of these parasites are true epignathi (i.e., attached to a jaw). More often, they are joined to the sphenoid bone or to the palate. Such tumors grow into the pharynx[41] or mouth and sometimes into the cranium (encranii or basicranial teratomas). Kraus[42] and Ehrich[40] described tumors that grew in both directions. The oral and the cranial portions of such growths are connected through the region of the craniopharyngeal canal (p. 421), which seems to be the central point at which, in early embryonic life, the buccopharyngeal membrane, Rathke pouch and the rostral end of the notochord meet. Ehrich[40] believed that the more highly developed epignathous parasites are asymmetric double monsters rather than teratomas. Occlusion of the mouth of the host results in polyhydramnios.[43] Most of the children bearing an epignathous tumor are stillborn and most of them are female. Asphyxia neonatorum due to a nasopharyngeal teratoma was described by Kesson,[44] and similar symptoms are caused by nasopharyngeal dermoids, which occur with a great preference for female children.[41] A teratoma of the face associated with a patent Rathke pouch has been described in a 3-week-old girl.[85]

It is of interest, though not understood, that epignathous and sacrococcygeal teratomas, which are comparable in that they develop near the rostral or near the caudal end of the notochord, show a definite predilection for female hosts.

Only a few cases of *gastric teratomas* have been described.[45] Vomiting, hematemesis, melena or loss of weight are early symptoms in young infants. In one instance, the tumor-bearing portion of the stomach herniated into the thoracic cavity. *Orbital, pulmonary, cardiac,*[17,18] *intrapericardial,*[46] *hepatic and renal teratomas* have been reported as rarities.[8,47] *Paravertebral* teratoids[48] and teratomatous cysts within the *vertebral canal*[49] have been observed.

Are teratomas congenital malformations? We defined congenital malformations as abnormal structures present at birth. Teratomas certainly are abnormal structures, but are they always present at birth? By clinical observation, this question can be answered in the affirmative for many but not all teratomas. One must clearly distinguish between clinical manifestations of teratomas as tumors and their anlage in the organism as abnormal "pluripotential embryonic tissue," which can lie dormant and unrecognized for decades without causing symptoms.

Some teratomas have been seen as tumors in fetuses and many have been seen or felt at birth. Sacrococcygeal, intracranial and epignathous teratomas have been observed in fetuses, and some sacrococcygeal, testicular, retroperitoneal, intrathoracic, cervical, intracranial and epignathous teratomas have been noted at birth. In some cases, renal, gastric or hepatic teratomas became manifest several weeks or months after birth but it can be safely assumed that they, too, were present at birth, escaping recognition because of their concealed location. Examples substantiating early clinical or anatomic verification of such tumors can be found in the comprehensive review by Willis.[8] The most common teratomas, those of the ovary, apparently have not been seen in the newborn and only very rarely in the first year of life. Hertig and Gore[50] stated that ovarian teratomas may "occur" at any age, having been reported in patients from 5 months of age to 78 years. It is certain that several ovarian teratomas have been diagnosed and removed in the second year. It seems justified to assume that those that manifest themselves in early childhood are present at or before birth and that they are not recognized unless a chance torsion of a pedicle leads to their discovery. It is possible that all types of teratomas can be present as small tumors at birth. But manifestations of the majority of teratomas are delayed to adult life. This is true particularly for teratomas of the ovary, testis and anterior mediastinum. But since these growths are very large and of long duration when first discovered, and since congenital teratomas have been observed in these places, there is little doubt that gonadal and mediastinal teratomas also arise at an early period of development. Yet, Andersen[10] and others[19] did not agree with this unitary concept and believed that extragonadal teratomas have a congenital origin whereas teratomas of the ovary and testis have a postnatal, and usually postpubertal, origin.

Schlumberger,[19] who reported on teratomas of the anterior mediastinum, reviewed several theories on the genesis of extragonadal teratomas. For mediastinal teratomas, a close relationship to the thymus can be demonstrated, and Schlumberger[19] believed that teratomas in that region have their origin in faulty embryogenesis of that organ. During embryogenesis of the thymus there is intimate association of ectoderm, entoderm and mesoderm. It is known that there are frequent developmental faults in the branchial cleft area, from where the thymus descends into the anterior mediastinum. Partial degeneration of the cervical vesicle or of Hassal corpuscles could release organizers comparable to those acting in experimental production of testicular teratomas (p. 1243). Schlumberger's[19] explanation of mediastinal teratomas considered faulty embryogenesis as the primary defect, relating them closely to dislocation of tissues and congenital malformations. Sacrococcygeal tumors also are located in a region in which faulty embryogenesis may be facilitated by the presence of an indifferent cell mass, the tail-trunk bud. Holmdahl[51] attributed sacrococcygeal teratomas to pluripotent cells of the tail bud, where organs are formed from undifferentiated cell masses without passing through germ layer stages, and Needham[7] suggested that they could be explained by abnormal gastrulation and compared to partial exogastrulation. Epignathous teratomas also appear in a critical embryologic area in which errors of development are likely to occur (p. 1241).

In contrast to the dual theory of teratoma formation, there is now a tendency to explain all teratomas, gonadal and extragonadal, as derivatives of primordial germ cells. These can be considered as pluripotent cells that, under certain conditions, can form tissues of many types. Genetic as well as environmental factors can influence development of teratomas from primordial germ cells. There is general agreement that germ cells are the original cells from which ovarian and testicular teratomas are formed. But since it is not possible to observe the development of human teratomas from their beginnings to their clinical manifestations, there is much room for speculation and argument. Fortunately, direct observations can be made in mouse strain 129, in which testicular teratomas develop spontaneously in from 1% to 10% of the males. Thus, one knows more about the origin and development of testicular teratomas in mice than about any other teratoma. Stevens[52] studied many facets of the development of testicular teratomas in mice from their beginning in embryos through fetal stages to maturity. After migration from the yolk sac, the germ cells of the male mouse become enclosed in 13-day fetuses by the developing cords of the testes, where they continue to multiply. In the testes of fetal (strain 129) mice, the most primitive teratomas are completely enclosed in testicular tubules, where tumor formation begins. Usually, there are several small tumor foci located within a tubule and it is likely that the foci are derived from a single neoplastic primordial germ cell. The incidence of teratomas is similar in fetuses 15–19 days old to that of older mice, but in 19-day fetuses and newborns, the teratomas are larger and appear older than the tumors in 15–19 day fetuses. Stevens[52] concluded, therefore, that the tumors arise before 19 days of gestation, probably not later than 17 days. Tumors of 15-day fetuses are composed of a small number of cells only, which suggests that they arise during the thirteenth or fourteenth day. Stevens[52] believed that the teratomas originate in these mice during the period from about 13 to 17 days of gestation, i.e., about 1 week before birth. He also gave a description of these tumors during the first 3 weeks of postnatal life.[53]

Before these observations are accepted as a model for all teratomas, some experimental results have to be considered. It has been known for some time that testicular teratomas can be produced experimentally in cocks by zinc chloride injections[54] and it has been shown in subsequent experiments that trauma coupled with administration of hormones can initiate teratoma formation. Bresler[55] induced teratoids in testes of mature mice by injections of testosterone and copper sulfate. It is likely, therefore, that germ cells of mature mice can react to extraordinary external influences by formation of teratomas. If one is permitted to draw conclusions from such observations in cocks and mice, it would appear that most teratomas in man are already present in embryonic and fetal life but that the possibility of postnatal development from a germ cell cannot be completely excluded. Furthermore, it is possible that different kinds of teratomas have different beginnings. There are differences in incidence according to sex, species and location of the tumors; whereas testicular teratomas are relatively frequent in certain strains of mice, ovarian teratomas are very rare in mice.[52] This differing behavior of males and females in teratoma formation may be attributable to the differing behavior of male and female germ cells in fetal life. Male germ cells continue to divide mitotically throughout the life span of the mouse, whereas female germ cells cease to divide mitotically during fetal life. Stevens[52] believed that the prenatal cessation of mitosis in female germ cells prevents the development of ovarian teratomas. How could one then explain the relatively frequent occurrence of ovarian teratomas in the human species? One would have to assume that such teratomas originate before the germ cells have lost the ability to divide mitotically, which is, in the human female, during late fetal life or in the first days of postnatal life.[56]

The origin of extragonadal teratomas also has been attributed to primordial germ cells. The primordial germ cells originate in the entoderm of the yolk sac from where they migrate toward the gonads. On the way, they are widely disseminated throughout the embryo and it seems possible that some of them become lodged in extragonadal sites,[57,58] where they may develop into extragonadal teratomas.[59,60] In the chick embryo, it has been shown that primordial germ cells can be carried long distances in the blood stream before they settle in the gonads.[61] In-vitro experiments suggest that the primordial avian germ cells are attracted to the gonadal germinal epithelium by a specific substance produced by gonadal tissue.[62] Faulty chemotaxis could conduct the primordial germ cells into alien areas, where they could give rise to extragonadal teratomas. That mammalian primordial germ cells also can be carried through embryonic blood channels and be widely distributed to many areas was brought out by observations in twin animals. Ohno *et al.*[63] believed that in cattle some primordial germ cells can be transported from one twin to another through vascular channels. They identified in the testes of newborn chimeric twins abundant XX-mitotic figures. Benirschke and Brownhill[64] found heterosexual cells in testes of chimeric marmoset monkeys. They thought that germ cells could reach through the embryonic vascular bed not only gonads of a co-twin but also other distant extragonadal sites. There they could form teratomas, if such sites provided a favorable location for their survival.

It was hoped that sex determinations in human teratoma cells could shed some light on the origin of these tumors. Sex chromatin and chromosome analyses have been made of teratoma cells to test various theories in existence. Hunter and Lennox[65] found that in ten ovarian teratomas and in two mediastinal teratomas of women the sex chromatin was clearly positive. But, of eight testicular teratomas, four were sex chromatin negative and four sex chromatin positive. Cells of a pineal teratoma also were sex chromatin positive. These findings suggested that teratomas are not ordinary tumors that always have the sex of their host but rather are derived from "separate individuals," since the sex sometimes is independent of the host. Teratomas could arise from the fusion of two gametes, which would always produce an XX zygote in the female but could produce XX, XY or YY zygotes in the male.[65] Tavares,[66] summarizing the results available in 1955, found that 48% of teratomas in males were heterosexual. This ratio did not agree with that to be expected by the hypothesis of Hunter and Lennox,[65] which should be 1 (XX) to 3 (XY + YY) or, if YY cells did not survive, 1 (XX) to 2 (XY). Tavares[66] thought that a 1 to 1 ratio could be explained by parthenogenetic division of haploid cells, followed by chromosome reduplication. This process could account for 100% of XX cells in the female, and 50% of XX and 50% of YY cells in the male. Since nothing was known about the viability of YY cells, this hypothesis was not too attractive. Myers[67] confirmed that teratomas from various sites of female patients were always sex chromatin positive. The cells of thirty-three testicular teratomas were uniformly sex chromatin negative in only thirteen, uniformly positive in ten, mosaic in eight and "abnormal female" in two. Of eight teratomas from other sites of male patients, one from the mediastinum was sex chromatin positive. This author believed that the occurrence of mosaic tumors ruled out parthenogenesis as an explanation of "female" teratomas in males.

Since these reports were made, it has become possible to examine whole sets of chromosomes in teratomas. Corfman and Richart[11] studied epithelial cells from benign ovarian cystic teratomas and found the chromosome number and morphology of such cells to be within normal limits. But, in a malignant ovarian teratoma, karyotype studies revealed 47 chromosomes, with the extra chromosome resembling a normal chromosome A3.[83] Stevens and Bunker[68] found the chromosome number and karyotype of cells of early mouse teratomas indistinguishable from those of cells of normal testes and embryos. They concluded that their findings failed to support theories based on sex chromatin studies of human testicular teratomas, which postulated that these tumors originate from haploid cells, and thought that the simplest explanation is that teratomas arise directly from diploid cells, probably primordial germ cells. Galton *et al.*[69] came to similar conclusions following examination of chromosomes in eight testicular teratomas. Sex chromatin positive stromal, endothelial and epithelial cells were present in five of eight tumors. The modal chromosome numbers ranged from 53 to 111. There was marked karyotypic instability and there was no overall similarity between different tumors. The authors thought that their observations support the idea that teratomas arise from diploid cells, possibly misplaced blastomere or primordial germ cells. Studies of gene segregation in teratomas of human females led to results that were interpreted as evidence that the teratomas were of postmeiotic origin.[86]

If teratomas are congenital malformations comparable to other structural defects present at birth, one should expect a significant incidence of associated malformations in their hosts. Two kinds of associated malformations must be distinguished—malformations in the vicinity of the tumor and more distant and independent malformations. Malformations adjacent to a teratoma may be caused by pressure or by lack of space and cannot be counted as independent associated developmental errors. Thus, absence of a thyroid lobe near a cervical teratoma or absence of coccygeal vertebrae near a sacrococcygeal teratoma or hydrocephaly and precocious puberty with an intracranial tumor cannot be considered independent defects, since they can be explained by expansion and pressure of the tumor on adjoining tissues. But an encephalocele and an intrathoracic teratoma occurring in the same child[8] can be considered independent parallel phenomena that could have a common teratogenic origin. Some combinations such as spina bifida and sacrococcygeal teratoma[2,24,70] are difficult to interpret because of the propinquity of malformation and tumor and because the two lesions sometimes are not distinguishable. But there can be no doubt that in the case of Esterly and Baghdassarian[25] the teratoma and the multiple anomalies of the urogenital tract were separate, associated malformations. By combining the series of Hickey and Layton[26] and that of Gross *et al.*,[21] one arrives at an incidence of about 9 associated malformations per 100 sacrococcygeal teratomas. It seems that the children with sacrococcygeal teratomas have a higher incidence of serious malformations than the general children's population but the difference is not striking. Schmincke,[71] finding a teratoma in place of a left kidney, also observed absence of the left urogenital organs, including the testis. McCurdy[72] described a teratoma in the left lumbar region associated with meningocele, spina bifida, deficiency of the abdominal musculature and hypospadias in a newborn boy. These cases suggested that there may be some connection between the malformations observed and the development of the teratomas, but the number of cases showing such associations is too small to permit definite conclusions.

There are at least 2 reports of multiple teratomas occurring in the same patient. Lovett and Councilman[73] described a newborn child with a testicular teratoma who later developed another teratoma in the parietal region. Goebell[74] reported the combination of a retroperitoneal and an ovarian teratoma in an adult. Tumors in siblings, both possibly teratomas, were reported by Kesson.[44]

Since teratomas have been considered as "twins" by some authors, it is of interest to learn about the tendency to twinning in the families of patients with teratomas. Gross *et al.*,[21] reporting on sacrococcygeal teratomas in infants and children, stated that 3 of their 23 patients were twins and that in at least one of these instances the twins were identical. In addition to these 3, there were twin births in eight of the twenty-three affected families and triplets in one. In a series from the University Hospitals of Cleveland, "A 33% incidence of twinning was found in 18 cases."[75] Hickey and Layton[26] reviewed the histories of one hundred twelve sacrococcygeal teratomas, but there were only 4 twins among their bearers. In 14% of the cases there was a "strong history of twinning."

Fetus in fetu. Although the relationship of teratomas to twinning is a controversial subject, there is general agreement that fetuses in fetu are monozygotic twins of their hosts. The most important characteristic of a fetus in fetu is said to be a vertebral axis sometimes accompanied by appropriate arrangement of other organs or limbs with respect to the axis.[8,76] It is true that tumors with definite axiation resemble fetuses more than tumors without vertebral organization, but a sharp borderline cannot be established under all circumstances, as is well illustrated by the five fetuses found in the brain of a hydrocephalic infant by Kimmel *et al.*[77] Although two of the fetuses had well-defined spinal rudiments, three did not. Thus, according to the definition of Willis,[8] two of the inclusions would be fetuses in fetu, whereas three would not pass as such because they showed no axiation. They probably would be classified as teratomas if it were not for the presence of their fellow quintuplets, who, possessing vertebral axes, betray the fetus in fetu status of their less well-organized fellows. This illustrates the dilemma of those who believe that the presence of an axial skeleton is the decisive criterion in the differentiation between fetus in fetu and teratoma. That this is a rather arbitrary delineation is also illustrated by a case of intracranial teratoma found by Oberman[78] in place of the brain of a stillborn infant. There were no vertebrae in the tumor, but well-formed primitive spinal cord with central canal was seen in every section. Is a spinal cord less representative of "axiation" than a vertebral column?

The five fetuses in fetu recorded by Kimmel *et al.*[77] were found in a hydrocephalic infant who apparently was free of congenital malformations with the exception of those of the brain and skull, which were due to obliteration of the ventricular communications. The intra-abdominal fetuses reviewed by Lord[76] occurred in apparently well-formed children. Of special interest is the fact that one "fetus in fetu" was within a boy who seemed entirely normal except for his abdominal "twin." He lived 15½ years, although he had "been ill with an abdominal tumor since the age of 7."[76] Thus, monozygotic twin fetuses may be enclosed in otherwise normal persons. In contrast to their hosts, the parasitic fetuses always have severe "congenital malformations," ranging from acrania, anencephaly or hydranencephaly to limb defects. In fact, the malformations often are so numerous that the recognizable parts usually are stressed more by the authors than the absent ones.

In summary, one can say that, at present, primordial germ cells are thought to be the pluripotential or totopotential cells from which teratomas arise. Various influences have been recognized as contributory in the formation of teratomas. Genetic influences were discussed by Stevens.[52] Apparently there occur more germinal tumors in white males than in nonwhites.[59] The high incidence of testicular teratomas in one strain of inbred mice indicates that genetic factors are involved in teratoma formation. Chemically induced testicular teratomas are more frequent in white Leghorns than in other varieties of fowl. In different species and in different locations, sex strongly influences the incidence of teratomas. On the other hand, environmental factors also can contribute to the etiology of these tumors. It has been mentioned (p. 1243) that injection of chemical and endocrine compounds into testes can bring about teratomas. In fowl, such experiments are successful only if the treatment is given during the first 3 months of the year. The incidence of teratomas is greatly increased in undescended testes.[79] Age of the host plays an important part in the growth and the time of appearance of the tumors. A maternal influence could be demonstrated in mice of strain 129. The incidence of tumors is lower in the males of first than those of second and later litters.[52] In man, there is a great need for a better knowledge of associated malformations and of twinning in the patients and in their families.

REFERENCES

1. Willis, R. A.: *The Borderland of Embryology and Pathology* (Washington, D. C.: Butterworth, 1962).
2. Askanazy, M.: Die Teratome nach ihrem Bau, ihrem Verlauf, ihrer Genese und im Vergleich zum experimentellen Teratoid, Verhandl. deutsch. Gesellsch. Path. 11:39, 1907.
3. Potter, E. L.: *Pathology of the Fetus and Infant* (2d ed.; Chicago: Year Book Medical Publishers, Inc., 1961).
4. Gould, G. M., and Pyle, W. L.: *Anomalies and Curiosities of Medicine* (Philadelphia: W. B. Saunders Company, 1897).
5. Budde, M.: Über die Genese der Fetalinklusionen, Beitr. path. Anat. 75:357, 1926.
6. Spemann, H., and Mangold, H.: Über Induktion von Embryonalanlagen durch Implantation artfremder Organisatoren, Arch. mikr. Anat. u. Entwicklungsmechanik 100:599, 1924.
7. Needham, J.: *Biochemistry and Morphogenesis* (London: Cambridge University Press, 1942).
8. Willis, R. A.: *Pathology of Tumors* (St. Louis: The C. V. Mosby Company, 1948).
9. Marcial-Rojas, R. A., and Medina, R.: Cystic teratomas of the ovary. A clinical and pathological analysis of two hundred sixty-eight tumors, A.M.A. Arch. Path. 66:577, 1958.
10. Andersen, D. H.: Tumors of infancy and childhood, Cancer 4:890, 1951.
11. Corfman, P. A., and Richart, R. M.: Chromosome number and morphology of benign ovarian cystic teratomas, New England J. Med. 271:1241, 1964.
12. Galton, M., and Benirschke, K.: Forty-six chromosomes in an ovarian teratoma, Lancet 2:761, 1959.
13. Rusche, C.: Twelve cases of testicular tumors during infancy and childhood, J. Pediat. 40:192, 1952.
14. Wilcox, H. B., and Wollstein, M.: Mediastinal teratoma in an infant, Am. J. Dis. Child. 41:89, 1931.
15. Starer, F.: The successful removal of an anterior mediastinal teratoma from an infant, Arch. Dis. Childhood 27: 371, 1952.
16. Hope, J. W., and Koop, C. E.: Differential diagnosis of mediastinal masses, Pediat. Clin. North America 6:379, 1959.
17. Williams, G. E. G.: Teratoma of the heart, J. Path. & Bact. 82:281, 1961.
18. Arshadi, S., and Watson, D. G.: Teratocarcinoma of the heart, Am. J. Dis. Child. 112:87, 1966.
19. Schlumberger, H. G.: Teratoma of the anterior mediastinum in the group of military age, Arch. Path. 41:398, 1946.

20. Marcuse, P. M.: Malignant presacral teratoma in an adult, Cancer 12:889, 1959.
21. Gross, R. E., Clatworthy, H. W., Jr., and Meeker, I. A.: Sacrococcygeal teratomas in infants and children: Report of 40 cases, Surg., Gynec. & Obst. 92:341, 1951.
22. Gwinn, J. L., Doeherty, M. B., and Kennedy, R. L. J.: Presacral teratomas in infancy and childhood, Pediatrics 16: 239, 1955.
23. Donnellan, W. A., and Swenson, O.: Benign and malignant sacrococcygeal teratomas, Surgery 64:834, 1968.
24. Ballantyne, J. W.: *Manual of Antenatal Pathology and Hygiene. The Embryo* (Edinburgh: W. Green & Sons, 1904).
25. Esterly, J. R., and Baghdassarian, O. M.: Presacral neurenteric cyst; an unusual malformation resulting from persistence of the neuroenteric canal, Bull. Johns Hopkins Hosp. 113:202, 1963.
26. Hickey, R. C., and Layton, J. W.: Sacrococcygeal teratoma: Emphasis on biological history and early therapy, Cancer 7:1031, 1954.
27. Ingelrans, P., Lacheretz, M., Debeugny, R., DuBois, R., and Fievez, E.: Les tératomes sacro-coccygiens. À propos de douze observations, Pédiatrie 21:533, 1966.
28. Hunt, P., Van Leeuwen, G., Bingham, H., and Sights, W.: Sacrococcygeal teratomas. A report of three cases and survey of present knowledge, Clin. Pediat. 7:165, 1968.
29. Fèvre, M., and Huguenin, R.: *Malformations Tumorales et Tumeurs de l'Enfant* (Paris: Masson & Cie, 1954).
30. Arnheim, E. E.: Retroperitoneal teratomas in infancy and childhood, Pediatrics 8:309, 1951.
31. Arnheim, E. E.: Combined pelvic and retroperitoneal teratomas in infancy and childhood, Pediatrics 10:198, 1952.
32. Priebe, C. J., Jr.: Sacrococcygeal teratoma in a newborn girl with massive intra-abdominal extension: Combined abdominosacral approach, Surgery 60:1090, 1966.
33. Stone, H. H., Henderson, W. D., and Guidio, F. A.: Teratomas of the neck, Am. J. Dis. Child. 113:222, 1967.
34. Silberman, R., and Mendelson, I. R.: Teratoma of the neck: Report of two cases and review of the literature, Arch. Dis. Childhood 35:159, 1960.
35. Emery, J. L.: Teratomas, Pediat. Clin. North America 6: 573, 1959.
36. Newstedt, J. R., and Shirkey, H. C.: Teratoma of the thyroid region, Am. J. Dis. Child. 107:88, 1964.
37. Weitzner, S.: Benign teratoma of the neck in an infant, Am. J. Dis. Child. 107:84, 1964.
38. Ruffolo, E. H., Dorr, T. W., and Fletcher, J. C.: Teratomas of the neck: Report of two cases, Radiology 84:223, 1965.
39. McGoon, D. C.: Symposium on pediatric surgery; teratomas of the neck, S. Clin. North America 32:1389, 1952.
40. Ehrich, W. E.: Teratoid parasites of the mouth, Am. J. Orthodont. 31:650, 1945.
41. Boeckman, C. R.: Teratoid tumors of the nasopharynx in children, J. Pediat. Surg. 3:735, 1968.
42. Kraus, E. J.: Über ein epignathisches Teratom der Hypophysengegend, Virchows Arch. path. Anat. 271:546, 1929.
43. Raines, D., and Yarington, C. T., Jr.: Adult nasopharyngeal teratoma in the newborn, Ann. Otol. 73:957, 1964.
44. Kesson, C. W.: Asphyxia neonatorum due to a nasopharyngeal teratoma, Arch. Dis. Childhood 29:254, 1954.
45. Cooray, G. H., and Jayaratne, S.: A teratoma arising in the stomach in a young infant, A.M.A. Arch. Path. 67: 383, 1959.
46. Reynolds, J. L., Donahue, J. K., and Pearce, C. W.: Intrapericardial teratoma: A cause of acute pericardial effusion in infancy, Pediatrics 43:71, 1969.
47. Dargeon, H. W.: *Tumors of Childhood* (New York: Paul B. Hoeber, Inc., 1960).
48. Lawson, F. L.: Paravertebral teratoid tumor with scoliosis, J.A.M.A. 151:271, 1952.
49. Hoefnagel, D., Benirschke, K., and Duarte, J.: Teratomatous cysts within the vertebral canal; observations on the occurrence of sex chromatin, J. Neurol., Neurosurg. & Psychiat. 25:159, 1962.
50. Hertig, A. T., and Gore, H.: Tumors of the female sex organs. Part 3. Tumors of the Ovary and Fallopian Tube, in *Atlas of Tumor Pathology* (Washington, D. C.: Armed Forces Institute of Pathology, 1961).
51. Holmdahl, D. E.: Beitrag zur Frage von der Teratomgenese. Die morphogenetische Theorie, Acta path. et microbiol. scandinav. 19:603, 1942.
52. Stevens, L. C.: The biology of teratomas including evidence indicating their origin from primordial germ cells, Ann. Biol. 1:585, 1962.
53. Stevens, L. C.: Embryology of testicular teratomas in strain 129 mice, J. Nat. Cancer Inst. 23:1249, 1959.
54. Michalowsky, I.: Das experimentelle Zinkteratom, Virchows Arch. path. Anat. 274:319, 1929.
55. Bresler, V. M.: Experimental teratoids of white mouse testis induced by testosterone and copper sulphate, Probl. Oncol. 5:24, 1959.
56. Ohno, S., Makino, S., Kaplan, W. D., and Kinosita, R.: Female germ cells of man, Exper. Cell Res. 24:106, 1961.
57. Witschi, E.: Migration of the germ cells of human embryos from the yolk sac to the primitive gonadal folds, Contrib. Embryol. 32:67, 1948.
58. Mintz, B.: Embryological phases of mammalian gametogenesis, J. Cell. & Comp. Physiol. 56:31, 1960.
59. Dixon, F. J., and Moore, R. A.: Tumors of the Male Sex Organs, in *Atlas of Tumor Pathology* (Washington, D. C.: Armed Forces Institute of Pathology, 1952).
60. Friedman, N. B.: Choriocarcinoma of the testis and extragenital choriocarcinoma in men, Ann. New York Acad. Sc. 80:161, 1959.
61. Simon, D.: Contribution à l'étude de la circulation et du transport des gonocytes primoires dans les blastodermes d'oiseau cultivés in vitro, Arch. Anat. Micr. Morphol. et Exper. 49:93, 1960.
62. Dubois, R.: Sur l'attraction des cellules germinales primordiales par la jeune région gonadique chez l'embryon de poulet, Compt. rend. Acad. Sc. (Paris) 258:3904, 1964.
63. Ohno, S., Trujillo, J. M., Stenius, C., Christian, L. C., and Teplitz, R. L.: Possible germ cell chimeras among newborn dizygotic twin calves (Bos taurus), Cytogenetics 1: 258, 1962.
64. Benirschke, K., and Brownhill, L. E.: Heterosexual cells in testes of chimeric marmoset monkeys, Cytogenetics 2: 331, 1963.
65. Hunter, W. F., and Lennox, B.: The sex of teratomata, Lancet 2:633, 1954.
66. Tavares, A. S.: On the sex of cancer and teratoma cells, Lancet 1:948, 1955.
67. Myers, L. M.: Sex chromatin in teratomas, J. Path. & Bact. 78:43, 1959.
68. Stevens, L. C., and Bunker, M. C.: Karyotype and sex of primary testicular teratomas in mice, J. Nat. Cancer Inst. 33:65, 1964.
69. Galton, M., Benirschke, K., Baker, M. C., and Atkin, N. B.: Chromosomes of testicular teratomas, Cytogenetics 5: 261, 1966.
70. Bull, P.: Meningocele vertebrale mit Teratoma kombiniert, München. med. Wchnschr. 54:569, 1907.
71. Schmincke, A.: Beitrag zur Geschwulstpathologie, Beitr. path. Anat. 73:502, 1925.
72. McCurdy, G. A.: Renal neoplasms in childhood, J. Path. & Bact. 39:623, 1934.
73. Lovett, R. W., and Councilman, W. T.: A case of double teratoma, J. Exper. Med. 2:427, 1897.
74. Goebell, R.: Zur Kenntnis der lateral-retroperitonealen Tumoren, Deutsche Ztschr. Chir. 61:1, 1901.
75. Izant, R. J.: Sacrococcygeal Teratoma, in Benson, C. D., Mustard, W. T., Ravitch, M. M., Snyder, W. H., Jr., and Welch, K. J. (eds.), *Pediatric Surgery* (Chicago: Year Book Medical Publishers, Inc., 1962), Vol. 2, p. 849.
76. Lord, J. M.: Intra-abdominal foetus in foetu, J. Path. & Bact. 72:627, 1956.
77. Kimmel, D. L., Moyer, E. K., Peale, A. R., Winborne, L. W., and Gotwals, J. E.: A cerebral tumor containing five human fetuses, Anat. Rec. 106:141, 1950.

78. Oberman, B.: Intracranial teratoma replacing brain, Arch. Neurol. 11:423, 1964.
79. Carmichael, R., and Oldfield, C.: A case of complete pseudohermaphroditism with intra-abdominal teratoma testis, J. Path. & Bact. 39:617, 1934.
80. Dillard, B. M., Mayer, J. H., McAlister, W. H., McGavrin, M., and Strominger, D. B.: Sacrococcygeal teratoma in children, J. Pediat. Surg. 5:53, 1970.
81. Ein, S. H., Darte, J. M. M., and Stephens, C. A.: Cystic and solid ovarian tumors in children: A 44-year review, J. Pediat. Surg. 5:148, 1970.
82. Brandesky, G.: Ovarialtumoren im Kindesalter, Monatsschr. Kinderh. 115:434, 1967.
83. Arias-Bernal, L., and Jones, H. W., Jr.: Chromosomes of a malignant ovarian teratoma, Am. J. Obst. & Gynec. 100: 785, 1968.
84. Chretien, P. B., Milam, J. D., Foote, F. W., and Miller, T. R.: Embryonal adenocarcinomas (a type of malignant teratoma) of the sacrococcygeal region, Cancer 26:522, 1970.
85. Wilson, J. W., and Gehweiler, J. A.: Teratoma of the face associated with a patent canal extending into the cranial cavity (Rathke's pouch) in a three-week-old child, J. Pediat. Surg. 5:349, 1970.
86. Linder, D., and Power, J.: Further evidence for postmeiotic origin of teratomas in the human female, Ann. Human Genet. 34:21, 1970.
87. Caruso, P. A., Marsh, M. R., Minkowitz, S., and Karten, G.: An intense clinicopathologic study of 305 teratomas of the ovary, Cancer 27:343, 1971.
88. Garrett, S. S.: Teratoma of the ovary in an infant twenty months of age, Am. J. Dis. Child. 79:321, 1950.

PART XIX

Hamartoses and Adenomatoses

Hamartoses and Adenomatoses

Hamartomas are tumors formed by tissues of faulty composition. Such tissue malformations appearing in the form of tumors usually are not malignant, but some of them become neoplastic and present as hamartoblastomas.[1] The term "hamartoma" is applied to lesions brought about by a developmental anomaly that is "either an actual malformation with tissue excess already present at birth, or an inborn tissue anomaly which manifests itself by excessive growth during the post-natal maturation of the tissue."[2] These faulty tissue conglomerates (hamartomas) can be single errors of development or they are systemic disorders that appear in various regions of the body. Systemic hamartous disorders may be limited to one organ system, e.g., skeleton, blood vessels or lymphatic vessels, or they affect several body systems. A number of these systemic hamartous disorders show a remarkable inclination to autosomal dominant inheritance. They must be due to specific inherited properties that give rise to tissue malformations and tumors, but the underlying inherited mechanisms are not known at present. A number of these heritable hamartous disease pictures have been recognized and it seems that more come to light as investigations of oncogenesis are extended from single patients to their families and kindreds. In this book, the term "hamartosis" is used for dominantly inherited disorders characterized by formation of multiple hamartomas with or without tendency to neoplasia. Some outstanding examples of hamartoses, such as Recklinghausen neurofibromatosis, tuberous sclerosis, Hippel-Lindau disease and others, are dealt with in this section. Since they affect many organ systems it seemed inappropriate to discuss them in chapters dealing with malformations of specific tissues or organs. The same holds for adenomatoses (multiple endocrine neoplasias) (p. 1269), which involve more than one endocrine gland. Other hamartoses such as multiple exostoses (p. 840), hereditary polyposis of the colon (p. 714), gastrointestinal polyposis (Peutz syndrome) (p. 714), hereditary hemorrhagic telangiectasia (p. 1185), glomus tumors (p. 1185) and the blue rubber-bleb nevus syndrome (p. 1185) have been taken up in preceding chapters, in which anomalies of the respective organ systems were dealt with. Sturge-Weber syndrome (p. 349), Maffucci syndrome (p. 882), fibrous dysplasias (p. 878), melanoblastosis (p. 1169) and others that contain tissue malformations that could be called hamartomas were not considered as hamartoses because there is no proof that they are dominant hereditary traits.

The term "hamartosis" covers a similar, if not identical, concept as the term "phakomatosis." In 1932, van der Hoeve[3] found that tuberous sclerosis, Recklinghausen neurofibromatosis and Hippel-Lindau disease showed retinal and optic disc tumors of lentil shape (phakomas) and recognized that the three disorders, although different, have many points of resemblance and that they belonged to the same group of anomalies, often being congenital and hereditary. Van der Hoeve deserves full credit for recognition of this group of hereditary diseases (phakomatoses), which since has been enlarged by inclusion of other related disorders with a tendency to tumor formation. The reason for using the term "hamartosis" rather than "phakomatosis" is that some of the lesions that constitute these entities are not lentil-shaped spots but quite varied in configuration and hamartous in nature. Another synonym used, "neurocutaneous syndromes," is so nonspecific that it seems meaningless. There are so many syndromes involving skin and nervous system that inclusion of etiologically dissimilar entities is unavoidable and confusing. Time will tell whether these terms, distinctions and classifications are justified but, at this time, it seems that hamartoses and adenomatoses deserve special consideration in their relationships to malformations. The following chapters deal with some of the better-known hamartoses.

REFERENCES

1. Albrecht, D. P. G.: Hamartomas, Verhandl. deutsch. Gesellsch. Path. 7:153, 1904.
2. Willis, R. A.: *The Borderland of Embryology and Pathology* (Washington, D.C.: Butterworth, 1962).
3. van der Hoeve, J.: Eye symptoms in phakomatoses, Tr. Ophth. Soc. U. Kingdom 52:380, 1932.

121

Recklinghausen Neurofibromatosis

THIS DISORDER combines abnormal cutaneous pigmentation, tumors of the central and peripheral nervous system, bone changes and endocrine and growth disturbances, resulting in a great variety of clinical disease pictures.

Although cases of neurofibromatosis had been described before, it was von Recklinghausen[1] who, in 1882, established the entity and correlated the fibromas of the skin to multiple neuromatosis. The disorder, which has become known as "Recklinghausen neurofibromatosis," has been found to go beyond a tendency to formation of neurofibromas, but attempts to find a common denominator for this disease with protean manifestations have failed so far.

Many case reports of multiple neurofibromatosis have been made because of their unusual medical features, and a somewhat distorted picture of the disorder is obtained by the study of such unusual cases. A more balanced impression can be gained by reviews of unselected cases. Such surveys were made by Borberg[2] in Denmark and by Crowe *et al.*[3] in the United States. Neurofibromatosis in childhood was discussed by Fienman and Yakovac.[53]

Multiple neurofibromatosis is attributed to a single dominant gene and has been reported in as many as six generations.[51] Although present in the zygote, the gene has few prenatal manifestations. In general, persons affected by this disorder appear rather normal at birth. But, in many cases, congenital anomalies have been described, café au lait spots being the most frequent manifestation at birth. Neurofibromatosis in infancy was reviewed by Roget *et al.*,[4] who described 3 siblings with manifestations in the neonatal period. Congenital neurofibromas,[5] facial hypertrophy and buphthalmia,[6] glaucoma,[7] glioma of the optic nerve,[8] macroglossia,[9] congenital stridor,[10] vertebral and rib deformities, scoliosis,[11, 12] macrodactyly,[13] hypertrophy of a leg,[7, 12] bowing of the legs, pathologic fractures and pseudarthroses[13-15] are some of the manifestations that have been observed at birth. They are indicative of prenatal existence of the disease, which progresses with variable speed in postnatal life. The disorder apparently is present in some form in the fetus, but most of the manifestations develop in response to physiologic or unphysiologic stimuli after birth. Congenital malformations due to early embryonic maldevelopment such as spina bifida and congenital cardiac or renal deformities were considered coincidental[2] but this may not be the case according to new findings.

Crowe *et al.*[3] collected one hundred seven families in which there occurred one or more cases of neurofibromatosis, with a total of 203 affected persons and 353 normal relatives. In addition, 20 cases were located among 6,873 inmates of three institutions for the mentally deficient (0.23%). Since small and isolated café au lait spots occur rather frequently in persons free of neurofibromatosis, Crowe *et al.*[3] concluded after a survey that persons with more than six café au lait spots that exceed 1.5 cm. in broadest diameter must be presumed to have neurofibromatosis even in the absence of a positive family history and tumors. Borberg[2] studied 84 propositi and their families in Denmark.

Approximately 50% of the cases ascertained by Crowe *et al.*[3] had affected relatives. In all instances of multiple cases within a kindred, the situation was compatible with the hypothesis of dependence on a dominant gene with high penetrance. Inheritance through two, three and four generations has been observed repeatedly.[2] Sporadic cases can and should be considered as new mutations. Such patients can transmit the disease to some of their children with a risk of 50%. Neurofibromatosis limited to a small area or a sector of the body may be attributable to somatic mutation. Patients with this form should be sporadic and not capable of transmitting the disease but it will be difficult to recognize such persons. Mutation probably occurs with a frequency of 10^{-4} per gamete per generation.[3]

The incidence has been estimated as 1 case of multiple neurofibromatosis in 2,500 to 3,300 births.[3]

The disorder occurs in males and females with equal frequency, but certain manifestations show sex predilection. In Borberg's series there were more males than females with central neurofibromatosis and in Crowe's series[3] there were more females than males with palmo-plantar neurofibromata. The incidence of neurofibromatosis apparently is the same in Caucasians and Negroes.[16]

Discordant and concordant monozygotic twins have been described. Discordance as to plexiform neurinoma in face and neck in female monozygotic twins has been observed.[17] Loftis[18] reported Recklinghausen

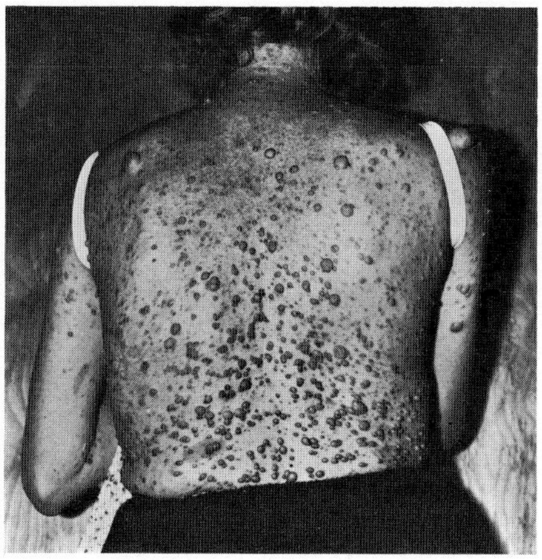
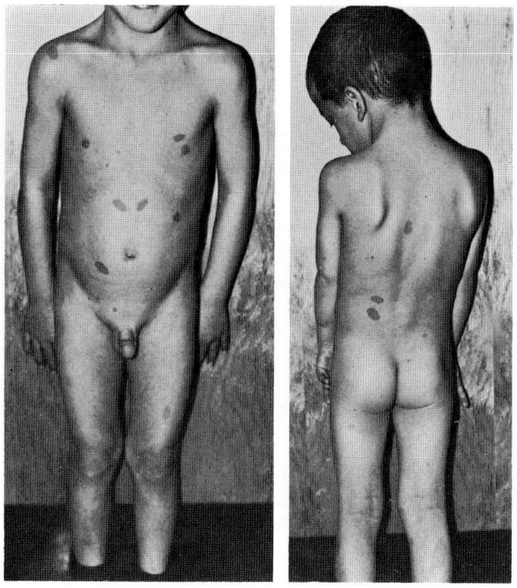

Fig. 121-1.—Cutaneous neurofibromatosis in a woman and her 2 sons.

disease in identical twins, but there were differences in the localization of the lesions. One patient had a tumor on a vocal cord, whereas the twin suffered from deafness. Dresner and Montgomery[19] saw uniovular twins both affected with neurofibromatosis and optic atrophy. Intrafamilial uniformity of the manifestations of neurofibromatosis sometimes is striking. This is particularly true for acoustic neurofibromas. Other examples of similar location of lesions and age of onset were cited by Borberg,[2] but Crowe *et al.*[3] found few examples of intrafamilial uniformity in their series.

Fig. 121-2.—Neurofibromatosis in a young man whose father and paternal uncle had the same disease.

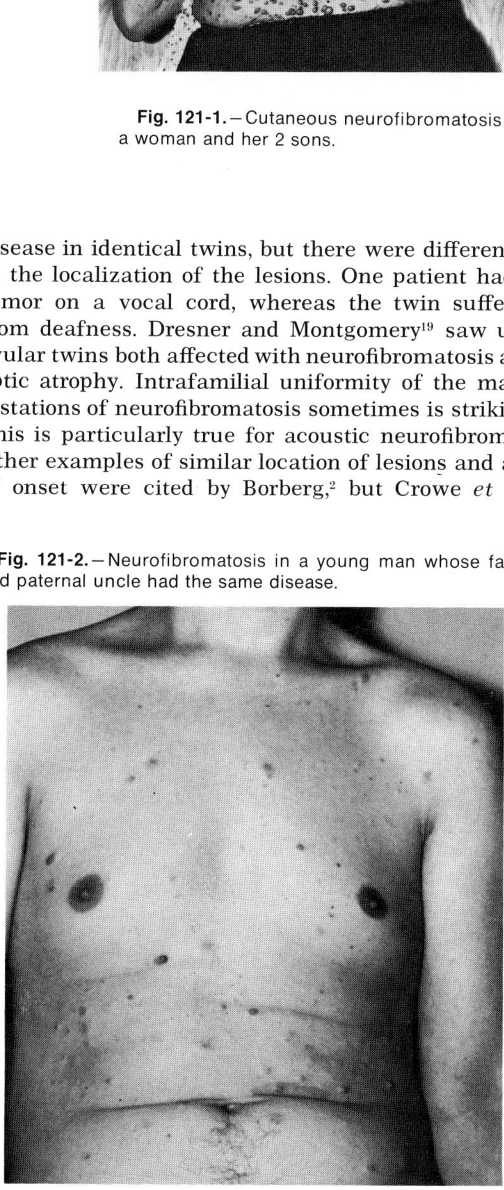

Combination of neurofibromatosis and tuberous sclerosis has been observed, but this may be a chance association.[3] It is worth noting that neurofibromatosis as well as Hippel-Lindau disease (p. 1266), two dominantly inherited hamartoses, can be complicated by formation of pheochromocytomas.[11] Although there is a suspicion that such interrelationships point to some common causative mechanism, it is best to assume at present that these hamartoses are due to different dominant genes. Cutis laxa characteristic of Ehlers-Danlos syndrome (p. 1186) occurs in some patients with neurofibromatosis. Giant nevi of the "bathing trunk" type were observed in 3 of 223 patients with neurofibromatosis.[3] This hardly can be considered a chance association.

Generalized neurofibromatosis as first described by Recklinghausen[1] was considered a disorder of skin manifestations and neurofibromas. Later, it was shown that the entity can involve, in addition to the central and peripheral nervous systems, the eye, the bones and many other organs. Hypertrophy of subcutaneous tissue involving an extremity may simulate elephantiasis, and local gigantism can be seen in one or more digits. Macrodactyly was stressed as a symptom of neurofibromatosis by Moore.[20] Neurofibromas of the stomach, intestine, heart, larynx, kidneys and bladder have been described.[7] Changes in the osseous system have become known through roentgen studies and are recognized as an integral part of the disease.

Café au lait spots are flat, light brown lesions of variable size, melanotic in origin, located on any part of the body, particularly on unexposed sites. The pigment is situated in and around the basal cell layer of the dermis. It was thought that their outline is smooth in contrast to the jagged margins seen in Albright fibrous dysplasia (p. 878), but it seems that the melanotic skin lesions of the two disorders are clinically indistinguishable. Giant pigment granules in Malpighian cells apparently are characteristic for patients with neurofibromatosis[21] but they have to be demonstrated by histologic methods. Café au lait spots often are present at birth, but some develop in the first postnatal decades. Sometimes they are limited to one side of the body (nevus lateralis). Café au lait spots occur in normal persons and their shape is not diagnostic of generalized neurofibromatosis, but there are quantitative differences, especially in children under 5 years.[22] Other skin lesions include lymphangiomas, hemangiomas[13] and vitiligo,[2,7] giant nevi,[2] "bathing trunk" nevi[3] and extensive hairy pigmented nevi.

Cutaneous and subcutaneous tumors may range in diameter from a few millimeters to a meter and be located on almost every part of the epidermis. The number of tumors is variable and increases with advancing age. Infections, puberty, pregnancy and intoxications are held responsible for increases of tumors in size and number. Cutaneous nodules may be only a few or amount to several thousand. They are distributed along the ulnar, radial, orbital, sciatic and crural nerves; the brachial and pelvic plexuses and the cauda equina may be affected severely and involvement of the vagus may cause cardiac symptoms.[14]

Cutaneous tumors (fibroma molluscum) form soft nodules that are cone- or dome-shaped. Early cutaneous tumors have a violaceous color (which can disappear) and a papular shape. They can be invaginated on digital compression. Beneath an epidermis that may be pigmented in its basal layer, a lesion is situated in the dermis, which contains a mixture of connective tissue and nerve fibers. Small whorls and remains of nerve bundles usually occur within the tumors. Subcutaneous tumors can be seen or palpated along the peripheral nerves as hard cord-like structures. They are characterized by an irregular outgrowth of Schwann cells with an increase of reticulin and collagen and penetrated by nerve fibers. Schwannomas, which are encapsulated and rich in reticulin but not in collagen, also can occur in neurofibromatosis.[23] Large granular mast cells may form clusters around small blood vessels of neurofibromas.[3] Cirsoid or plexiform neurofibromas can assume the shape of elephantiasis-like areas or fibroma pendulum. Underlying hemangiomas, lymphangiomas or osseous hypertrophy may be demonstrable. Lipomas, particularly those of hereditary multiple lipomatosis, sometimes simulate neurofibromas in older patients. Neurofibromas can remain latent and painless or cause pain radiating along the nerves.

Crowe *et al.*[3] investigated intrafamilial similarities of tumor location by selecting rare sites for their study. Palmar and plantar and 2d and 8th nerve tumors were selected. In the case of palmar and plantar

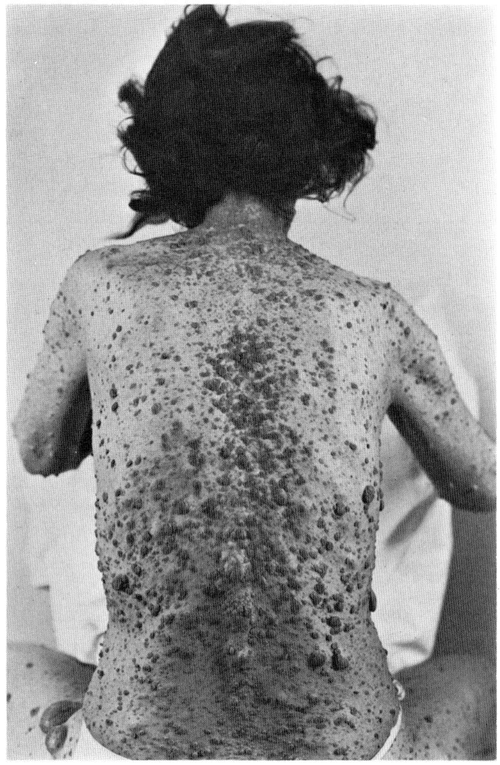

Fig. 121-3. – Recklinghausen neurofibromatosis.

involvement, an intrafamilial site predilection appeared probable, but there was no indication of familial preference for other rare locations. Females seemed more prone than males to develop palmar and plantar tumors. It has been stated that elephantiasis-like deformities, acoustic tumors and sarcomatous degeneration show familial aggregation. Subcutaneous nodules usually appear early in life but some develop after adolescence and their number often increases gradually. Their main site is the trunk, but head, face and limbs can be involved also.

Cranial nerves as well as central parts of the nervous system may undergo pathologic changes. The optic or acoustic nerve is said to be affected most often but, in some necropsy series, neurofibromas of the vagus, trigeminal and hypoglossal nerves were involved more often than the optic or acoustic nerve.[33] Davis[8] reported primary tumors of the optic nerve, gliomas or gliomatoses, in patients with multiple neurofibromatosis. Because of the youth of patients with glioma, he thought the lesions were congenital. Glial tumors of the optic nerve are, according to Davis,[8] in many instances the only manifestation of multiple neurofibromatosis, particularly its abortive form. Plexiform neurofibromatosis can be seen on the upper eyelids, around the orbit and temple and there may be osseous defects. Involvement of the nerves of the choroid, ciliary body and iris often is accompanied by

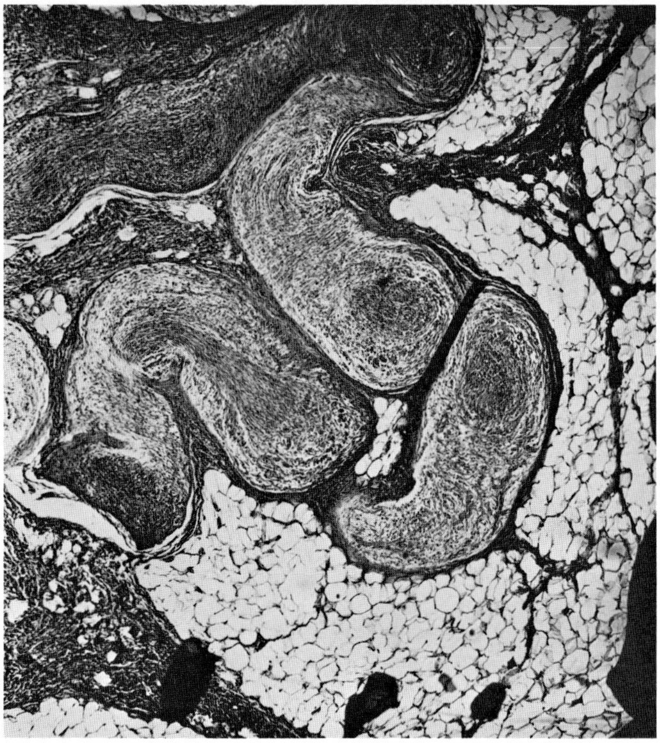

Fig. 121-4. – Section through plexiform neurofibroma.

buphthalmia. Ocular manifestations affecting the globe, optic nerves, the lids and the orbits were tabulated by Marshall,[24] who stated that more than 21% of gliomas of the optic nerve and of the chiasma were associated with neurofibromatosis and that the actual correlation may be even higher. Optic gliomas of this type usually appear in the first or second decade, growing relatively slowly and causing poor vision and exophthalmia. The pedigree of Marshall's case showed dominant inheritance of neurofibromatosis through four generations, but the propositus was the only one affected by optic glioma. Primary optic atrophy with failing vision may be the only symptom and complaint of patients who have few other signs of the disease. A slowly growing prechiasmal tumor of an optic nerve may be present in patients whose cutaneous manifestations can be overlooked. If affecting the chiasma, optic atrophy can be bilateral and if located in the orbit, papilledema may be present.[19] Two sisters with a pigmentary retinopathy and growth retardation simulating Cockayne syndrome (p. 398) had manifestations of neurofibromatosis.[25]

Facial hemihypertrophy and buphthalmia as a manifestation of neurofibromatosis is rare; Turpin *et al.*[6] found only 19 cases on record. They reported a congenital case of unilateral glaucoma and ipsilateral enlargement of one half of the face. Only one café au lait spot was present on the upper lid of the eye but the nature of the disease was betrayed by neurofibromatosis of the mother. Most of the other patients with this syndrome had normal parents and siblings and it must be assumed that they represented new mutations. The buphthalmia can be attributed to neurofibromatosis of the ciliary nerves and the irido-corneal angle.

Bilateral acoustic neurofibromatosis sometimes shows remarkable recurrence in certain kinships. Gardner and Turner,[26] who reviewed this subject, recorded a pedigree in which deafness due to acoustic neurofibromas was transmitted like a dominant trait through six generations, 42 members being affected. Peripheral manifestations may be absent or minimal in such patients. In one case, the acoustic neurofibroma was associated with a psammous meningioma.

Tumors of the meninges, brain and cord, and "central neurofibromatosis"[27] are rarer than peripheral lesions. They seem to have little association with peripheral manifestations, which occur only to a limited degree in central neurofibromatosis.[28] Glioblastoma multiforme, spongioblastoma, Schwannoma and diffuse glioma have been described in the brain and cerebellum. Meningiomas often are multiple and affect both the cranial and spinal areas. They are closely associated with acoustic nerve tumors. Choroid plexus tumors arise in the lateral ventricles.[23] Ependymoma, ganglioneuroma and pheochromocytoma are rarer in neurofibromatosis. Intraspinal neurofibromata represent a substantial part of the spinal cord tumors encountered by neurosurgeons.[29] Ten per cent of the patients of Holt and Wright[15] had intracranial tumors such as meningioma, astrocytoma, spongioblastoma, acoustic neuroma or undifferentiated glioma. In several patients, the intracranial tumors were multiple. Intradural neurofibromas occur occasionally but tumors originating in sheaths of spinal nerve roots are more common. They may be confined to the spinal canal or appear as intrathoracic or intra-abdominal tumors. Sometimes they are dumbbell shaped, emerging on either side of the spinal nerve root canal.[15] As mentioned before, neurofibromatosis may affect the central nervous system with only minimal external manifestations. Crome[27] described a boy born with café au lait spots and a neurofibroma in the right supraclavicular fossa. This patient developed severe mental retardation, deafness, convulsions and possibly diabetes insipidus. When he died at 14 years of age, a necropsy revealed multiple neurofibromata of the vagi, spinal nerve roots and nerves. The brain and spinal cord contained many areas of diffuse and focal gliosis, which resulted in hypertrophy of the hypothalamus, the olfactory bulbs and the medulla oblongata. Sclerotic areas also were found in the cerebellum. The white matter of the cerebral hemispheres showed widespread loss of myelin, with sparing of islands comparable to those found in Pelizaeus-Merzbacher disease. Similar but milder sclerotic changes may be the pathologic basis of mental retardation observed in some patients with multiple neurofibromatosis. Tumors of the central nervous system contribute greatly to the list of fatal complications of neurofibromatosis. Calcifications of the choroid plexus, probably due to meningiomas, may be seen in roentgenograms of the skull.[52] Hydrocephaly was present in 5% of Borberg's[2] patients. Russell[30] recorded hydrocephaly in a girl with neurofibromatosis. The aqueduct was obstructed by two granulations made up of cellular fibrillary neuroglia. Involvement of the septum pellucidum and asymmetry of the lateral ventricles have been reported.[17]

Mental retardation, usually of a moderate degree, is present in some patients with neurofibromatosis. Need for institutionalization is relatively rare, but 20 of the cases of Crowe *et al.*[3] were found in institutions for the mentally retarded. Only 2 of their entire group had completed college and 3 were nurses. Most of the others had failed in their education at early periods and were not successful in holding jobs. In Borberg's[2] series, only 23% of the patients tested had an I.Q. over 90. The reason for intellectual inferiority is not known. Many patients are mentally retarded before clinical manifestations of neurofibromatosis make their appearance. Speech defects and behavior disturbances develop in some.[7] Other neurologic manifestations are proptosis and increased intracranial pressure. Epilepsy can develop in the course of neurofibromatosis, the seizures being focal or generalized and occurring in cycles.[7] Hemiparesis, paraplegia and Brown-Séquard syndrome can be associated with neurofibromatosis.[31] The consequences of basilar impression and syringomyelia[32] can complicate the disease picture.

The intestinal tract can be involved from the lips to the rectum.[33] Macrocheilia, enlargement of the lips due to neurofibromatosis, can be an outstanding symptom. Macroglossia based on neurofibromatosis may be a manifestation of generalized neurofibromatosis or be an isolated lesion. In some patients, it is present at birth, in others it develops within the first few years of life. It takes the form of a unilateral lingual tumor that may be connected with deep structures of the neck and associated with café au lait spots, cutaneous neurofibromas, ipsilateral enlargement of the ear, square head or pilonidal sinus. The anomaly must be distinguished from macroglossia due to lymphangioma, hemangioma and muscular hypertrophy.[9] Neurofibromas as manifestations of generalized neurofibromatosis can be localized also in a maxillary antrum or around the floor and the walls of the oral cavity. The diagnosis can be made by biopsy, which reveals plexiform neuroma with large nerve fibers surrounded by perineurium and containing axon cylinders. Malignant degeneration to neurogenic sarcoma has occurred in some of the cases. Fibromatous tumors in the oral cavity were present in 6% of Borberg's[2] series.

Neurofibromatosis of the stomach, pharynx, larynx,[10,37] small intestine, cecum, colon, mesentery and retroperitoneum has been reported.[32,34-36] Intestinal obstruction has been caused by massive involvement of the colon by neurofibromatosis.[55] Neurofibromatosis of the bladder is rare in children.[38] Pulmonary valvar stenosis and other forms of congenital heart disease sometimes have been combined with neurofibromatosis.[37,39] Hypertension due to neurofibromatosis of a renal artery has been described.[17,40]

Association with endocrine disorders has been seen repeatedly. Although this facet may have been overemphasized because of the interest in such complicated cases, the association is significant but the connection with the basic disorder often remains unexplained. In the series of Crowe *et al.*,[3] 13 of 223 (5.8%) showed sexual and general physical underdevelopment that may have been due to endocrine or other retarding mechanisms. Mental and physical retardation can be the leading symptoms in young patients with neurofibromatosis at a time when cutaneous or tumor symptoms have not yet developed.[41]

Chromaffin tumors of the adrenal have been reported by many observers.[32] Between 5% and 20% of patients with pheochromocytoma show signs of neurofibromatosis, but such tumors occurred in only 1 patient of the series of Crowe *et al.*[3] Glushien *et al.*[11] tabulated 18 cases of multiple neurofibromatosis associated with pheochromocytoma (paraganglioma). Excessive sweating, elevated temperature, high basal metabolic rate, paroxysmal attacks of hypertension, and so forth may be manifestations of pheochromocytoma in patients who also have signs of neurofibromatosis. Epigastric pain, nausea and vomiting, simulating an acute abdominal crisis, also can be presenting symptoms.[42] In the majority of patients with neurofibromatosis and pheochromocytoma, the adrenal tumor was present on the left side. Glushien *et al.*[11] believed that pheochromocytoma also is related to Hippel-Lindau disease (p. 1266). Bilateral pheochromocytoma, medullary thyroid carcinoma and multiple neuromas represent a syndrome that can be transmitted as an autosomal dominant trait and may be related to Recklinghausen neurofibromatosis.[43] There have been observations of acromegaly, myxedema and hypopituitarism[41] in patients with neurofibromatosis.[44] Precocious puberty in patients with fibrous dysplasia and cutaneous pigmentary lesions has been mistaken for neurofibromatosis, but it is now considered a symptom of Albright syndrome (p. 878). Yet, precocious puberty developed in a number of patients with neurofibromatosis.[12,41,45] Pseudoendocrine manifestations can be caused by neurofibromas. Enlargement of the clitoris due to pelvic neurofibromas involving the bladder and uterus was observed in a girl with the generalized disorder by Diekmann *et al.*[17] and neurofibromas simulating a penis and labioscrotal gonads were recorded by Kenny *et al.*[46] A few decades ago, it was thought that neurofibromatosis could be attributed to endocrine disturbances. Now it seems established that neurofibromatosis has many manifestations and that endocrine disorders are among them. On the other hand, it cannot be denied that hormonal factors play an important role in exacerbations of the disease, as manifested by an increase of lesions at the time of puberty or during pregnancy.[2] It deserves to be emphasized that hypertension can occur in neurofibromatosis without the presence of a pheochromocytoma. Stenosis of a renal artery may be responsible for the hypertension.[54]

Osseous changes, as noted clinically or in roentgenograms, include erosions, scoliosis due to structural vertebral defects or inequality of the lower extremities, overdevelopment and underdevelopment of various regions of the skeleton, congenital bowing, pseudarthrosis and intraosseous cysts.[15] None of these changes is diagnostic of neurofibromatosis but their occurrence supports a tentative diagnosis.

Skeletal involvement was recognized in 29% of the patients of Holt and Wright[15] and in more than 50% of those of Hunt and Pugh.[47] Erosions by adjacent neurofibromas have been considered the characteristic osseous lesions of the disorder. "Pits or caves" seen in the bones of the extremities are caused by adjacent neurofibromas. Erosions also can be observed on vertebrae and ribs,[36] where they can bring about notching and a picture similar to that of aortic coarctation. Intrathoracic neurofibromas can result in erosions of thoracic osseous elements. Scoliosis is the most common skeletal anomaly of neurofibromatosis. It shows some predilection for the lower thoracic region, but it can occur in any other area. It has been attributed to asymmetric erosion of vertebrae by periosteal neurofibromatosis or to differences in length of the legs, but pressure from the tumors does not explain all the osseous lesions.[48] Severe angular scoliosis with

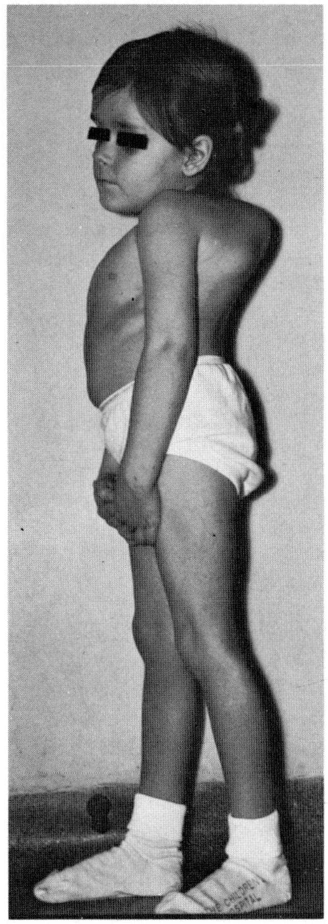

Fig. 121-5.—Kyphoscoliosis in a 6-year-old girl with four café au lait spots on the trunk. Diagnosis of neurofibromatosis was suggested because her brother had ten café au lait spots, kyphoscoliosis and pseudarthrosis on right ulna.

dysplasia of vertebral bodies may lead to cord compression, block of the spinal canal and to serious neurologic complications. In such cases, the ribs may be changed to "twisted ribbons." Congenital vertebral anomalies also have been reported.[11]

Overgrowth of bones usually is associated with cirsoid or plexiform neurofibromas that elevate and invade the periosteum. This infiltrative process results in new bone formation and thickening and lengthening of the affected shaft. Such overgrowth often is associated with elephantiasis neuromatosa. Sometimes the overgrown bones show proportionate enlargement without signs of gross pathology.[12] In other patients, narrowing or shortening of bone may occur.

Congenital bowing and pseudarthrosis of the lower leg have been seen repeatedly in association with neurofibromatosis. Holt and Wright[15] encountered 6 patients with congenital bowing and some signs of neurofibromatosis. McKeown and Frazer[14] reported bowing of the legs, fractures and skin pigmentations in a newborn child. A case of extreme deformity and shortening resulting from congenital pseudarthrosis of the tibia and fibula was illustrated by McCarroll.[13] In such pseudarthroses, neurofibromatous tissue has been found occasionally but in the majority of cases there is just defective bone formation but no tumor.[47] Cystic lesions in bone are thought to arise from neurofibromas of periosteal nerves that erode adjacent bone and subsequently are covered by osseous shells formed by osteogenic elements of the periosteum. There are reports of extensive rarefactions in long bones, ribs and vertebrae in young infants with established congenital neurofibromatosis. Although typical neurofibromas can be found in the skin lesions, the intraosseous lesions are not typical of neurofibromatosis. Spontaneous regression of such osseous defects has been observed.[15]

Congenital absence of the superior orbital wall associated with pulsating exophthalmia was described by LeWald[49] in 1933 and found to be associated with neurofibromatosis in a number of cases. The patients usually also have neurofibromatous tissue within the eyelids or orbital soft tissues. Not only the superior wall but the floor of the orbit may be absent in multiple neurofibromatosis, sometimes without manifestation of ocular symptoms. Defects of the posterosuperior wall of the orbita occurred in more than 6% of the patients of Hunt and Pugh.[47] The resulting gap permits contact of the temporal lobe of the brain with the orbital contents. Pulsating exophthalmia and loss of vision can result. The proptosis may be noticeable in the first months of life. Osseous lesions of various sizes and shapes may be felt[34] or found in roentgenograms of the skull. Radiolucid areas in the left lambdoid suture have been emphasized.[28] Hypertrophy of one half of the facial skull was observed by Borberg[2] in 7% of his patients, particularly in association with plexiform neuroma.

Meningoceles—intrathoracic or lumbar—developed repeatedly in patients with neurofibromatosis. A review of 20 published cases of intrathoracic meningocele with cutaneous neurofibromatosis indicated that the vertebrae had pedicle defects and concave outlines of the posterior aspects of the bodies. Roentgenograms of the chest sometimes show large shadows within a lung field. The herniations of the meninges outside the confines of the vertebral canal and those filling the concavities of the posterior surfaces of the vertebral bodies can be demonstrated by myelograms. A combination of dural weakness with osteomalacia of the vertebrae probably represents points of reduced resistance to spinal fluid pressure, which results in herniation. More than two-thirds of all reported cases of intrathoracic meningocele have been associated with cutaneous neurofibromatosis.[50]

Other changes seen in roentgenograms of the chest have been reported by Levin.[12] A mass in the right upper lung field proved to be an extrapleural neurofibroma. The same author described nodular shadows in the left infraclavicular area of a woman who underwent mastectomy because of a breast tumor. The shadows were not metastases but probably extrapleural neurofibromas that were overlain on the skin by café au lait spots. On the other hand, bronchogenic carcinoma may be present when a mediastinal neurofibroma is suspected.[12] Neurofibromas of the vagus or the sympathetic nerve also occur in the thorax. They may present as large mediastinal masses and erode the anterior walls of vertebral bodies.[47] The kyphoscoliosis of Recklinghausen disease can result in severe impairment of cardiopulmonary function, leading to dyspnea, cyanosis and cardiac failure.[19]

Bone changes resembling melorheostosis have been described by McCarroll[13] in a woman with well-established neurofibromatosis. This is a puzzling finding, since identity of the two disorders is unlikely. Melorheostosis is not hereditary (p. 884), whereas neurofibromatosis is a well-recognized dominant hereditary trait. Cortical thickening and medullary sclerosis[36] probably can simulate melorheostosis. Congenital hypertrophy of digits or limbs was described by McCarroll[13] as overgrowth of soft tissue in which large tortuous nerves are embedded. The nerves proximal to the hamartous enlargement are normal in size and structure. In some tumors, nerve-sheath hypertrophy can be demonstrated; in others the whorls of spindle cells seen in fibrous tissue betray the neurofibromatous origin of the masses. Diffuse increased vascular-

Fig. 121-6.—Cervical glands with neurofibrosarcoma in a girl. Note café au lait spots on her chest. The mother also had Recklinghausen neurofibromatosis.

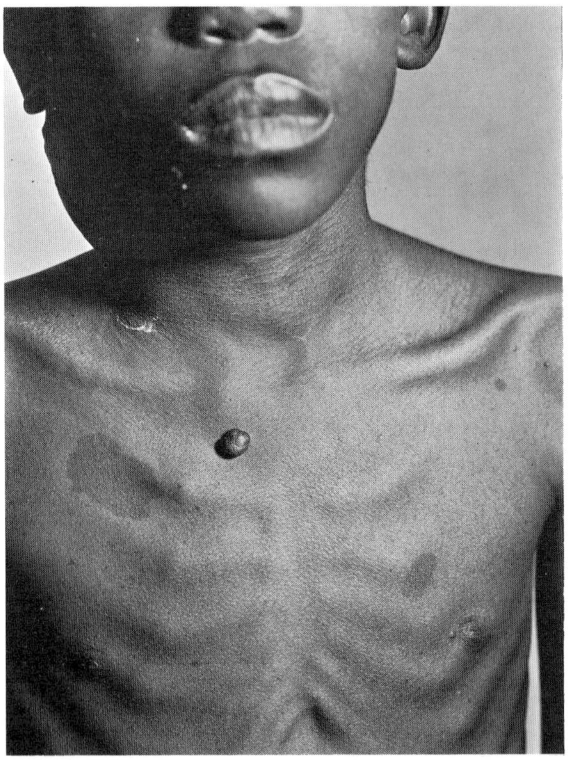

ity is represented by abundant thick-walled veins that are located in the hypertrophic soft tissues. As a rule, the osseous parts of the hypertrophic structures also are enlarged and often sclerosed and generally deformed by osteochondromatous growths.[36]

Neurofibromatosis may undergo malignant degeneration. Estimates of malignancy vary greatly according to selection of the patients. Where serial observations were made, malignant degeneration of lesions occurred in 1.2–2.6% of the patients.[2,3] Sarcoma is the most frequent type of malignancy (Fig. 121-6) but neurilemmomas also may be seen among the tumors. Fibrosarcomas and myxosarcomas can metastasize to the lungs.[32]

REFERENCES

1. Recklinghausen, F.: *Über die multiplen Fibrome der Haut und ihre Beziehung zu den multiplen Neuromen*, Virchow Festschrift (Berlin: A. Hirschwald, 1882).
2. Borberg, A.: Clinical and genetic investigations into tuberous sclerosis and Recklinghausen's neurofibromatosis, Acta psychiat. et neurol. 71:239, 1951.
3. Crowe, F. W., Schull, W. J., and Neel, J. V.: *A Clinical, Pathological and Genetic Study of Multiple Neurofibromatosis* (Springfield, Ill.: Charles C Thomas, Publisher, 1956).
4. Roget, J., Beaudoing, A., Gilbert, Y., and Marchioni, J.: La maladie de Recklinghausen chez le nourrisson. À propos d'une observation familiale, Pédiatrie 19:421, 1964.
5. Scott, B. E., and Cohen, H. J.: Neurofibromatosis in a newborn infant, A.M.A. Am. J. Dis. Child. 82:574, 1951.
6. Turpin, R., Saraux, H., Defranoux, A., Cruveiller, J., Bocquet, H., and Lecoq, F.: L'hémihypertrophie faciale neurofibromateuse avec buphtalmie; à propos d'une nouvelle observation, Ann. pédiat. 36:1921, 1960.
7. Chao, D. H-C.: Congenital neurocutaneous syndromes in childhood. 1. Neurofibromatosis, J. Pediat. 55:189, 1959.
8. Davis, F. A.: Primary tumors of the optic nerve (a phenomenon of Recklinghausen's disease), Arch. Ophth. 23: 735, 1940.
9. Ayres, W. W., Delaney, A. J., and Backer, M. H.: Congenital neurofibromatous macroglossia associated in some cases with von Recklinghausen's disease; case report and review of literature, Cancer 5:721, 1952.
10. Pleasure, J., and Geller, S. A.: Neurofibromatosis in infancy presenting with congenital stridor, Am. J. Dis. Child. 113:390, 1967.
11. Glushien, A. S., Mansuy, M. M., and Littman, D. S.: Pheochromocytoma: Its relationship to the neurocutaneous syndromes, Am. J. Med. 14:318, 1953.
12. Levin, B.: Neurofibromatosis: Clinical and roentgen manifestations, Radiology 71:48, 1958.
13. McCarroll, H. R.: Clinical manifestations of congenital neurofibromatosis, J. Bone & Joint Surg. 32-A:601, 1950.
14. McKeown, F., and Frazer, M. J. L.: Neurofibromatosis with pathological fractures in the newborn, Arch. Dis. Childhood 36:340, 1961.
15. Holt, J. F., and Wright, E. M.: The radiologic features of neurofibromatosis, Radiology 51:647, 1948.
16. Preston, F. W., Walsh, W. S., and Clarke, T. H.: Cutaneous neurofibromatosis (von Recklinghausen's disease), A.M.A. Arch. Surg. 64:813, 1952.
17. Diekmann, L., Hüther, W., and Pfeiffer, R. A.: Ungewöhnliche Erscheinungsformen der Neurofibromatose (von Recklinghausensche Krankheit) im Kindesalter, Ztschr. Kinderh. 101:191, 1967.
18. Loftis, E. L.: Recklinghausen's disease in identical twins, Arch. Dermat. 42:657, 1940.
19. Dresner, E., and Montgomery, D.A.D.: Primary optic atrophy in von Recklinghausen's disease, Quart. J. Med. 18: 93, 1949.
20. Moore, B. H.: Macrodactyly and associated peripheral nerve changes, J. Bone & Joint Surg. 24:617, 1942.
21. Benedict, P. H., Szabo, G., Fitzpatrick, T. B., and Sinesi, S. J.: Melanotic macules in Albright's syndrome and in neurofibromatosis, J.A.M.A. 205:618, 1968.
22. Whitehouse, D.: Diagnostic value of the café-au-lait spot in children, Arch. Dis. Childhood 41:316, 1966.
23. Russell, D. S., and Rubinstein, L. J.: *The Pathology of Tumours of the Nervous System* (London: Edward Arnold, Publishers, Ltd., 1959).
24. Marshall, D.: Glioma of the optic nerve, Am. J. Ophth. 37: 15:1954.
25. Felgenhauser, W. R., and Ammann, F.: Syndrome de Cockayne fruste associé à la neurofibromatose de Recklinghausen, J. Génét. Hum. 16:6, 1967.
26. Gardner, W. J., and Turner, O.: Bilateral acoustic neurofibromas, Arch. Neurol. 44:76, 1940.
27. Crome, L.: A case of central neurofibromatosis, Arch. Dis. Childhood 37:640, 1962.
28. Davidson, K. C.: Cranial and intracranial lesions in neurofibromatosis, Am. J. Roentgenol. 98:550, 1966.
29. Levene, L. J.: Bone changes in neurofibromatosis. Report of a case with coincidental osteitis deformans and review of the literature, A.M.A. Arch. Int. Med. 103:570, 1959.
30. Russell, D. S.: Observations on the pathology of hydrocephalus, Med. Res. Counc. Spec. Rep. No. 265, His Maj. Stat. Off., p. 138, 1949.
31. Hudson, L. H., and Cox, T. R.: Brown-Séquard syndrome with bilateral elephantiasis in neurofibromatosis, J.A.M.A. 161:326, 1956.
32. Willis, R. A.: *The Borderland of Embryology and Pathology* (2d ed.; Washington, D. C.: Butterworth, 1962).
33. Wilson, S. A. K.: *Neurology* (2d ed.; Baltimore: The Williams & Wilkins Company, 1955).
34. Inglis, K.: The influence of intrinsic factors in the causation of disease in man: Illustrated by neurofibromatosis and lesions with which it is sometimes associated, M. J. Australia 1:429, 1956.
35. Luboldt, W., Gregorczyk, K., and Düwell, H. J.: Abdominale Neurofibromatose beim Kind, Ztschr. Kinderh. 100: 35, 1967.
36. Meszaros, W. T., Guzzo, F., and Schorsch, H.: Neurofibromatosis, Am. J. Roentgenol. 98:557, 1966.
37. Pung, S., and Hirsch, E. F.: Plexiform neurofibromatosis of the heart and neck, A.M.A. Arch. Path. 59:341, 1955.
38. Chalkley, T. S., and Bruce, J. W.: Neurofibromatosis of the bladder, J. Pediat. 20:632, 1942.
39. Watson, G. H.: Pulmonary stenosis, café-au-lait spots, and dull intelligence, Arch. Dis. Childhood 42:303, 1967.
40. Cornell, S. H., and Kirkendall, W. M.: Neurofibromatosis of the renal artery. An unusual cause of hypertension, Radiology 88:24, 1967.
41. Ryckewaert, P., Farriaux, J. P., Dubois, O., and Fontaine, G.: La neurofibromatose de von Recklinghausen chez l'enfant, Pédiatrie 22:301, 1967.
42. Healey, F. H., Jr., and Mekelatos, C. J.: Pheochromocytoma and neurofibromatosis. Report of a case, New England J. Med. 258:540, 1958.
43. Schimke, R. N., Hartmann, W. H., Prout, T. E., and Rimoin, D. L.: Syndrome of bilateral pheochromocytoma, medullary thyroid carcinoma and multiple neuromas. A possible regulatory defect in the differentiation of chromaffin tissue, New England J. Med. 279:1, 1968.
44. Sharpe, J. C., and Young, R. H.: Recklinghausen's neurofibromatosis, Arch. Int. Med. 59:299, 1937.
45. Barta, L.: Pubertas praecox bedingt durch Neurofibromatosis generalisata (Recklinghausensche Krankheit), Ann. paediat. 170:15, 1948.
46. Kenny, F. M., Fetterman, G. H., and Preeyasombat, C.: Neurofibromata simulating a penis and labioscrotal gonads in a girl with von Recklinghausen's disease, Pediatrics 37:456, 1966.

47. Hunt, J. C., and Pugh, D. G.: Skeletal lesions in neurofibromatosis, Radiology 76:1, 1961.
48. Loop, J. W., Akeson, W. H., and Clawson, D. K.: Acquired thoracic abnormalities in neurofibromatosis, Am. J. Roentgenol. 93:416, 1965.
49. LeWald, L. T.: Congenital absence of the superior orbital wall associated with pulsating exophthalmos. Report of four cases, Am. J. Roentgenol. 30:756, 1933.
50. LaVielle, C. J., and Campbell, D. A.: Neurofibromatosis and intrathoracic meningocele, Radiology 70:62, 1958.
51. Koch, G.: Phakomatosen, Humangenetik 5:34, 1966.
52. Zatz, L. M.: Atypical choroid plexus calcifications associated with neurofibromatosis, Radiology 91:1135, 1968.
53. Fienman, N. L., and Yakovac, W. C.: Neurofibromatosis in childhood, J. Pediat. 76:339, 1970.
54. Wallis, K., Deutsch, V., and Azizi, E.: Hypertension in a case of von Recklinghausen's neurofibromatosis, Helvet. paediat. acta 25:147, 1970.
55. Raszkowski, H. J., and Hufner, R. F.: Neurofibromatosis of the colon: A unique manifestation of von Recklinghausen's disease, Cancer 27:134, 1971.

122

Tuberous Sclerosis

TUBEROUS SCLEROSIS is a disorder of varied manifestations, observed and described by different investigators from different points of view. The complex disorder was named "tuberous sclerosis" in 1880 by Bourneville[1] and later also became known as "Bourneville disease." There are many other terms in use such as "epiloia," a name not favored at present. Some authors, impressed by the implication of structures derived from the ectoderm, speak of "ectodermosis" or "ectodermal dysplasia." These terms are misleading, since the disease affects not only ectodermal but also mesodermal and endodermal structures. Tuberous sclerosis was named a "phakomatosis"[2] and a "hamartosis" because of the plaque-like or tumor-like malformations occurring in some organs in the course of this disease.[3] Although the descriptive term "tuberous sclerosis" applies chiefly to the brain, it will be used here because it is the best established name in the medical literature.

Tuberous sclerosis is a hereditary and congenital disorder that manifests itself in gross or microscopic malformations from birth on. Although the disease usually is not diagnosed at birth or in early infancy, one can safely assume that histologic or gross changes are present in all cases before birth. It is of interest that the first case on record, published by Recklinghausen in 1862 and showing cardiac tumors and sclerotic plaques in the brain, occurred in an infant who died soon after birth.[4] The connection of such early fatal cases with the neurologic disease occurring in later life was not recognized at first. Whereas some investigators consider tuberous sclerosis a disorder of multiple congenital malformations, it is a neoplastic disease to others. The merits of these differing concepts were discussed thoroughly in the older literature, but the differences of opinion of the past now can be reconciled perhaps by the concept of an inherited and inborn error of metabolism to which the organism responds by formation of abnormal tissues. But no biochemical basis has been found until now for tuberous sclerosis and other hamartoses. Some of the malformations are present at birth (p. 1261) and others develop in postnatal life. In many respects, tuberous sclerosis resembles Recklinghausen neurofibromatosis, to which it may be closely related and with which it overlaps in certain instances. There are families in which tuberous sclerosis and Recklinghausen neurofibromatosis occur alternately, but this does not prove that the two disorders are genetically identical.[5,6] The disorder is attributed to an autosomal dominant gene.[7] This gene is pleiotropic, affects many organs and is variable in expression. It may be very mild and even go undiagnosed in some persons who have no clinical manifestations but show the disease – sometimes after a long life – at necropsy. On the other end of the spectrum are semilethal forms seen in newborn children dying in early infancy and showing rhabdomyomas, renal tumors and sclerotic changes of the brain at necropsy. Between these extremes are the patients, usually encountered by physicians and seen in institutions, who are affected by convulsive disorders in infancy, remain mentally retarded and develop sebaceous adenoma, thus exhibiting the typical picture of tuberous sclerosis. There also are persons with this anomaly who are mentally normal and live outside institutions but who have sebaceous adenoma, possibly occasional convulsions, and sometimes ill-defined psychopathic traits. Such patients and those who have only skeletal or pulmonary manifestations of this gene are considered abortive cases or "formes frustes." As the disease spectrum becomes better known, it is recognized that the disorder can occur in mentally normal persons with a variety of symptoms.[8,9] Such persons can have children with the fully developed disease.[47]

Tuberous sclerosis has been observed in both of identical twins[10] and in one of nonidentical twins.[11,12] It has been transmitted repeatedly in families through several generations. Occurrence in five generations[13] is unusual, but two or three generations are not rarely affected.[5,14] There also are many sporadic cases and some of those must be attributed to new mutations. The severely affected usually do not transmit the disorder to future generations. That this gene can be passed from one generation to another can be explained by the fact that abortive cases exist in which the disorder can be transmitted[14,15] and by a relatively high mutation rate.[7] It is not clear why the same gene manifests itself in mild disturbances in some cases and in severe disease in others. Modifying genes are held responsible for the variability of expression. If environmental factors play a role, they are not known. Order of birth and maternal age are without demonstrable influence and the sexes are affected equally.[7] The incidence of tuberous sclerosis is not known and estimates vary greatly, which is understandable, since the variable expression of the gene makes estimates difficult. Incidence figures vary between 1 in 50,000[12] and 1 in 150,000.[16] In institutions, approximately 0.5% of the inmates have tuberous sclerosis.

In the brain, tuberous sclerosis is characterized by gray or white nodes or nodules with a diameter of from several millimeters to 1–2 centimeters. The nodes, which are hard and have the consistency of cartilage, are located in the cerebral cortex and usually are not sharply demarcated from the more normal brain tissue. In addition, there are small tumors in the walls of the ventricles. Occasionally, large paraventricular tumors develop that can obstruct the cerebrospinal fluid circulation and lead to hydrocephaly. Nodes or tumors in the basal ganglia or the thalamus opticus are rare. Occasionally there are typical changes in the cerebellum, the medulla or the spinal cord.

Histologic examination shows that the demarcation of the white and gray matter is lost and the cytoarchitecture disturbed. Changes are found not only in the sclerotic nodes but in the surrounding cortex. There is a decrease in the number of nerve cells and proliferation of the glia. Some nerve cells are greatly enlarged and contain much tigroid substance, whereas others show signs of regression, sclerosis or loss of staining material. Giant cells with grotesque shapes, abnormal nuclei and cytoplasmic vacuoles are found in nodules as well as in the white matter. Some cells contain much glycogen. The nodes show dense gliosis or nests of large glia cells arranged around blood vessels. The small tumors in the walls of the lateral ventricles show proliferative and degenerative changes, marked gliosis and a tendency to calcification and cyst formation. Paraventricular tumors, sometimes assuming neoplastic proportions, are classified as spongioblastomas.[17,18] The white matter also is affected by demyelination, glial tumors and heterotopias of abnormal nerve cells.[17,19] The phakomas of the eye consist of glial nodes that sometimes are affected by hyaline degeneration or calcification.[12] In the heart, rhabdomyomas form tumors that protrude either onto the outside or into the chambers.[4] They consist of large muscle fibers containing vacuoles and much glycogen. There also may be subendothelial lipomas or fibrolipomas.[19] In some instances, endocardial fibroelastosis has been observed.[18] The tumors of the kidney usually are mixed tumors of embryonic type that have been described under many names (p. 1263). The mixed tumors contain epithelial cells, smooth muscle and blood vessels. The cytoarchitecture of the surrounding renal tissue also is disturbed and the glomeruli and tubules show cellular changes. Tumors found in the kidney have been considered neural in origin.[20] A variety of developmental errors or tumors may be noted in the lung, thyroid, thymus, duodenum, liver, pancreas or spleen.[16,21,22] An early and fundamental error of development, situs inversus, has been observed in several patients.[23] Defects of the corpus callosum and rhinencephalon with atresia of the foramina of Luschka and Magendie in a case of tuberous sclerosis point to early embryonic disturbance.[24]

The tumors in the various organs have been described as hemangiomas, fibromas, lipomyomas or mixed tumors. The sebaceous adenoma of the skin (nevus Pringle) consists chiefly of hypertrophic sebaceous glands embedded in hypertrophic connective tissue and capillaries but there also is an abundance of collagen and fat tissues in such lesions. Heterotopic islands of epithelium and hair follicles are seen in the subcutaneous tissue, and enlargement and cystic changes of the sweat glands can be observed.[19] Fibromata are situated on the forehead or the neck. Subungual fibromas consist of hypertrophic connective tissue located in the corium and the subcutis. The shagreen skin seen chiefly in the area of the iliac crests shows thinning of the epithelium and hypertrophy of

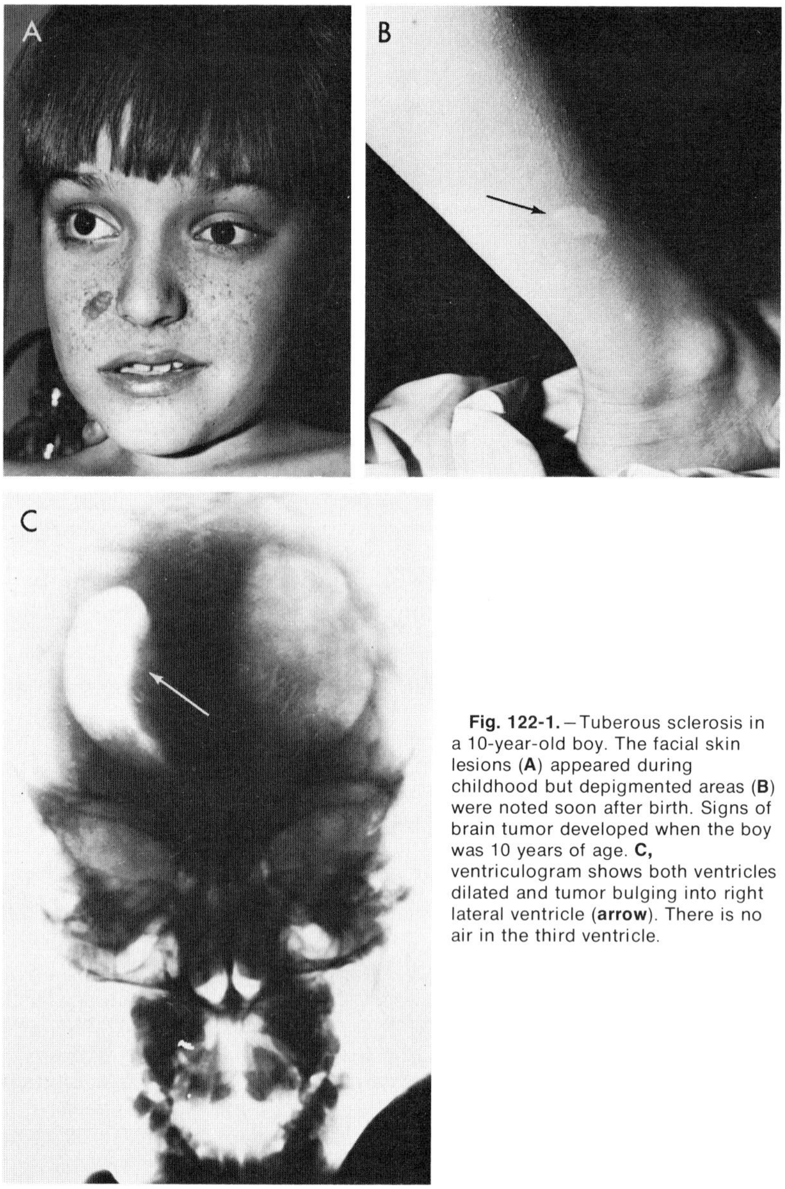

Fig. 122-1.—Tuberous sclerosis in a 10-year-old boy. The facial skin lesions (**A**) appeared during childhood but depigmented areas (**B**) were noted soon after birth. Signs of brain tumor developed when the boy was 10 years of age. **C,** ventriculogram shows both ventricles dilated and tumor bulging into right lateral ventricle (**arrow**). There is no air in the third ventricle.

the connective tissue in the corium. The nerves of the skin are, in contrast to neurofibromatosis, not much affected. The bone is characterized by osteoporosis and "cysts" visible in roentgenograms are attributed to replacement of bone by fibrous tissue.[25]

A typical case of tuberous sclerosis manifests itself by convulsive disorders, by mental retardation and by skin changes. Although the disease is congenital, only 10% of the reported cases described children under 3 years, and most of these were not diagnosed during life but at necropsy. The reason for delay in the diagnosis is that early symptoms such as convulsions and mental retardation are not specific. The cases diagnosed in early infancy were recognized through knowledge of the family history, observation of a parent who had sebaceous adenoma or by the presence of renal tumors in a child with convulsions; but the triad of convulsions, mental retardation and typical skin changes occurred only once in 44 small children with tuberous sclerosis recorded in the literature.[26]

Fatal rhabdomyomas are an outstanding finding in the infantile form of the disease.[26-28] Histologic and histochemical observations have been made in such rhabdomyomas.[29,30] Early recognition of tuberous sclerosis by funduscopic examination is possible.[44] Retinal nodules, conjunctival lesions, cataracts and phthisis bulbi have been observed. Depigmented nevi also have been emphasized as early signs[42,45] and it has been suggested that infantile spasms accompanied by depigmented cutaneous patches suggest tuberous sclerosis.[43] A definite diagnosis can be made by a finding of retinal tumors in such cases.

The development of most children with tuberous sclerosis is retarded from birth on.[31] They are late in sitting up, walking and talking. Many of them have early screaming fits; convulsive disorders occur during the first year in 70% of those who later develop the full disease picture. The convulsive disorders are variable in frequency and type. Some patients have convulsive manifestations daily and others only very rarely. In one instance,[32] a mentally normal person with tuberous sclerosis died suddenly in her first epileptic attack. Head nodding or myoclonus also may be a manifestation of the sclerotic changes. Flexion spasms combined with achromic nevi were emphasized as early manifestations by Aicardi *et al.*[33] In one woman, seizures were due to hypoglycemia brought on by an islet cell tumor of the pancreas.[22] General muscular rigidity, local paralyses or hemiplegias may be present. The mental development is variable, some patients being idiots or imbeciles and others trainable for routine tasks. Some develop psychoses, catatonia and a tendency to mental deterioration. The intracranial pressure can be increased by the growth of the tumors. But, as a more variegated disease picture is recognized, it is found that, at the most, two-thirds of the patients are mentally retarded.[8]

Round gray spots (phakomas) elevated by small tumors can be seen with the ophthalmoscope. Corneal and lens opacities may develop. Coloboma of the choroid is rare; when it occurs, it is a sign of early developmental disturbance (p. 363). Retinal patches that have a rough surface free of blood vessels are only rarely seen in infancy.[26] The most characteristic skin manifestation, the adenoma sebaceum, usually appears about the fourth or fifth year but in the beginning it is rather inconspicuous and consists of small nodules developing in the nasolabial folds. These lesions, brown, yellow or red, are at first pinhead size but they grow larger and spread over the cheeks, assuming a butterfly pattern. There may be fibromata in the face or neck or under the nails, café au lait spots, white patches, vitiligo or pigmented nevi. Shagreen skin usually is seen in the lumbar or iliac area.[34] Cutis verticis gyrata has been observed in several cases.[35] In rare instances, polycystic kidneys and seizures can be early signs of tuberous sclerosis[46] but more often the renal changes go unnoticed during life and renal tumors are rarely palpable. Albuminuria or abnormal pyelograms have been observed in some cases. Renal angiomyolipoma may be the first sign of illness in persons with tuberous sclerosis.[36] In one instance, a 42-year-old woman complaining of abdominal pain was found to have such a tumor. She had given birth to 8 children, 5 of whom were mentally retarded. One of these had the fully developed form of tuberous sclerosis. Crosett[37] described roentgenographic findings in renal lesions. In the course of tuberous sclerosis, tumor masses of an ill-defined but radiotranslucent nature can occur in one or both kidneys associated with pelvocaliceal distortion suggesting polycystic disease. Yet, this picture can be produced by angiomyolipomatous change in the kidney parenchyma. Such anomalies seldom degenerate into malignant lesions, so nephrectomy can be avoided. Pulmonary tuberous sclerosis manifests itself mostly in adults. Cough develops late, but some patients have been observed who suffered from dyspnea, spontaneous pneumothorax and hemoptysis because of involvement of the lungs in the process of tuberous sclerosis.[16] Roentgenograms of the chest are not diagnostic but osseous changes may betray the nature of the pulmonary disease.[38]

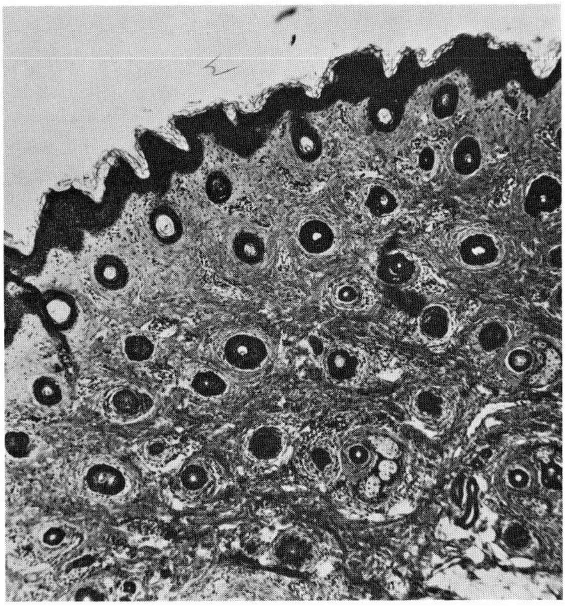

Fig. 122-2.—Section of skin showing adenoma sebaceum.

In many cases, roentgenograms of the skull show calcified foci of variable size. Intracranial calcifications usually are seen as small and discrete shadows representing calcified areas in the basal ganglia or the thalamus. Larger plaques of calcification represent sclerotic changes in the calvarium; they represent bone changes and not cerebral calcifications. Intracranial calcifications or areas of calcifications were noted in roentgenograms of the skull in more than half of the patients with tuberous sclerosis seen at the Mayo Clinic.[39] Encephalograms may reveal brain atrophy, dilatation of the ventricular system or protrusion of subependymal nodules or of tumors into the ventricular spaces. Periosteal thickening and cyst formation may be observed in the long bones. More characteristic are small cysts in the bones of the fingers and toes.[25,38] In some instances, calcification may be demonstrable in renal tumors by x-rays. In the lungs, a fine meshwork or mottling of the parenchy-

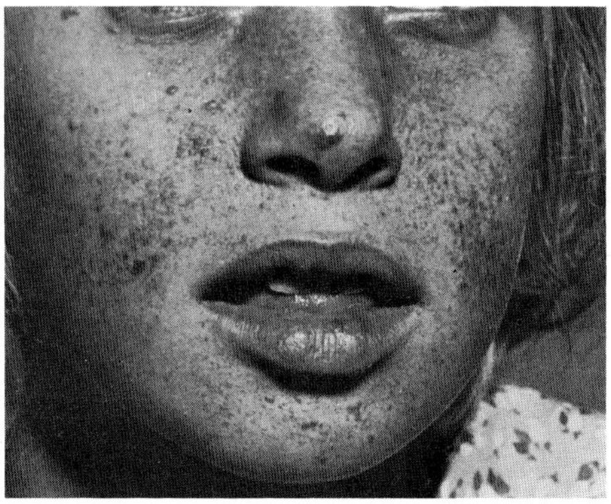

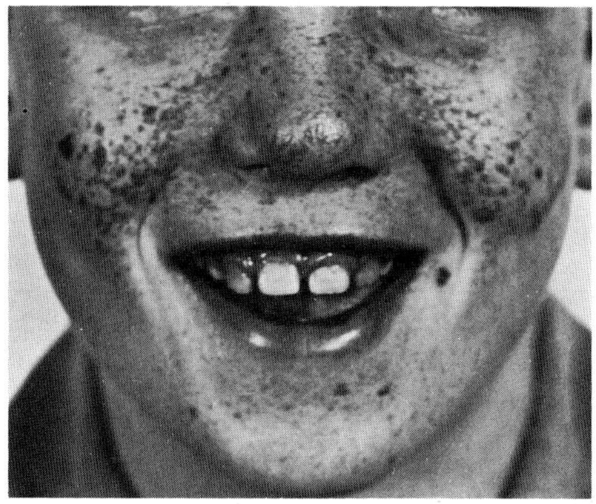

Fig. 122-3. — Tuberous sclerosis in siblings, showing sebaceous adenomas. Convulsions began in both children when they were 4 months of age. Skin lesions began in second and third years, respectively.

ma, cysts or shadows due to adenomas may be observed. Pneumothorax develops in some patients.[16]

A number of authors who look at tuberous sclerosis as a syndrome of multiple congenital malformations have stressed the occurrence of associated congenital defects in these patients. Spina bifida, microcephaly, cleft palate and harelip, pes equinovarus, megacolon, hernias, cataract, keratoconus, dental hypoplasia and intestinal polyposis have been observed.[12,17,19] However, it is undecided whether such differing malformations are a part of the disease process or coincidental findings.

Without a family history and without sebaceous adenoma, the most frequent manifestations of tuberous sclerosis, convulsions and mental retardation, cannot be correctly classified. If calcifications are found in the skull film, toxoplasmosis, Sturge-Weber syndrome, meningiomas and tuberculomas must be considered in the differential diagnosis. Funduscopic findings may aid in the recognition of the disease. Sebaceous adenomas, subungual fibromas and other skin manifestations are very helpful in the differentiation of tuberous sclerosis from other convulsive disorders. As more patients are diagnosed with better knowledge of the disease, it evolves that about one-third of the patients have normal mentality.[8]

Many patients with the fully developed disease picture die before maturity of respiratory diseases or of convulsive disorders and few survive to adult age; but persons with incomplete forms of tuberous sclerosis may live to old age and pass on the disorder to future generations.

Anticonvulsants are employed but are not effective in all cases. Some patients with space-consuming lesions require neurosurgical intervention. The skin manifestations are treated symptomatically. In one case, major and minor seizures in a 10-year-old boy with tuberous sclerosis were controlled by surgical elimination of impulses originating in the basal ganglia.[40] The results of surgery for epilepsy in 7 patients with this disorder were discussed by Perot *et al.*[41]

REFERENCES

1. Bourneville, D.: Scléreuse tubéreuse des circonvolutions cérébrales: Idiotie et epilepsie hémiplégique, Arch. neurol. 1:69; 91; 391, 1880.
2. van der Hoeve, J.: Eye diseases in tuberouse sclerosis and Recklinghausen's disease, Tr. Ophth. Soc. London 43: 534, 1923.
3. Moolten, S. E.: Hamartial nature of tuberous sclerosis complex and its bearing on tumor problem; case with tumor anomaly of kidney and adenoma sebaceum, Arch. Int. Med. 69:589, 1942.
4. Recklinghausen, F.: Ein Herz von einem Neugeborenen, welches mehrere theils nach aussen, theils nach den Höhlen prominierende Tumoren (Myome) trug, Monatsschr. Geburtsk. 20:1, 1862.
5. Borberg, A.: Clinical and genetic investigations into tuberous sclerosis and Recklinghausen's neurofibromatosis, Acta psychiat. et neurol., Supp. 71, 1951.
6. Schull, W. J., and Crowe, F. W.: Neurocutaneous syndromes in the M kindred. A case of simultaneous occurrence of tuberous sclerosis and neurofibromatosis, Neurology 3:904, 1953.
7. Penrose, L. S.: *The Biology of Mental Defect* (2d ed.; New York: Grune & Stratton, Inc., 1954).
8. Lagos, J. C., and Gomez, M. R.: Tuberous sclerosis: Reappraisal of a clinical entity, Mayo Clin. Proc. 42:26, 1967.

9a. Paulson, G. W., and Lyle, C. B.: Tuberous sclerosis, Developmental Med. & Child Neurol. 8:571, 1966.

9b. Paulson, G.: Changing concepts of tuberous sclerosis, Developmental Med. & Child Neurol. 9:493, 1967.

10. Fabing, H.: Tuberous sclerosis with epilepsy in identical twins, Brain 57:227, 1934.
11. Hopwood, A. T.: Tuberous sclerosis: Report of 5 cases, including one case in one of twins, Ohio M. J. 33:277, 1937.
12. Ross, A. T., and Dickerson, W. W.: Tuberous sclerosis, Arch. Neurol. & Psychiat. 50:233, 1943.
13. Fuhs, H.: Über Naevus multiplex Pringle (Adenoma sebaceum), Arch. Dermat. u. Syph. 148:509, 1925.
14. Dickerson, W. W.: Familial occurrence of tuberous sclerosis, A.M.A. Arch. Neurol. & Psychiat. 65:683, 1951.
15. Gupta, S. K.: An unusual case of tuberous sclerosis, Lancet 2:1289, 1956.
16. Dawson, J.: Pulmonary tuberous sclerosis and its relationship to other forms of the disease, Quart. J. Med. 23: 113, 1954.
17. Globus, J. H.: Malformations in the Central Nervous System, in Penfield, W : *Cytology and Cellular Pathology of the Nervous System* (New York: Paul B. Hoeber, Inc., 1932).

18. Crome, L., and Stern, J.: *The Pathology of Mental Retardation* (London: J. & A. Churchill, Ltd., 1967).
19. Hallervorden, J., and Krücke, W.: Die tuberöse Hirnsklerose, in Lubarsch, O., Henke, F., and Rössle, R., (eds.), *Handbuch der Speziellen Pathologischen Anatomie und Histologie* (Berlin: Springer, 1956), Vol. 13, pt. 4.
20. Inglis, K.: The relation of the renal lesions to the cerebral lesions in the tuberous sclerosis complex, Am. J. Path. 30: 739, 1954.
21. Tredgold, A. F.: *A Textbook of Mental Deficiency* (Baltimore: The Williams & Wilkins Company, 1952).
22. Gutman, A., and Lefkowitz, M.: Tuberous sclerosis associated with spontaneous hypoglycemia, Brit. M. J. 2:1065, 1959.
23. Arenillas, L.: Tuberous sclerosis with situs inversus, J. Ment. Defic. Res. 12:108, 1968.
24. Elliott, G. B., and Wollin, D. W.: Defect of the corpus callosum and congenital occlusion of fourth ventricle with tuberous sclerosis, Am. J. Roentgenol. 85:701, 1961.
25. Dickerson, W. W.: Nature of certain osseous lesions in tuberous sclerosis, A.M.A. Arch. Neurol. & Psychiat. 73: 525, 1955.
26. Debré, R., Thieffry, S., Mozziconacci, P., Bargeton, E., and Ramade, J.: La sclérose tubéreuse de Bourneville chez le nourrisson et le petit enfant, Arch. franç. pédiat. 9:342, 1952.
27. Farber, S.: Congenital rhabdomyoma of the heart, Am. J. Path. 7:105, 1931.
28. Simopoulos, A. P., and Breslow, A.: Tuberous sclerosis in the newborn, Am. J. Dis. Child. 3:313, 1966.
29. Elliott, G. B., and McGeachy, W. G.: The monster Purkinje-cell nature of so-called "congenital rhabdomyoma of heart"; a forme fruste of tuberous sclerosis, Am. Heart J. 63:636, 1962.
30. Wolfe, H. J., and Foley, F. D.: Observations on tuberous sclerosis, Arch. Path. 76:197, 1963.
31. Critchley, M., and Earl, C. J. C.: Tuberose sclerosis and allied conditions, Brain 55:311, 1932.
32. Stewart, R. M.: Atypical form of tuberous sclerosis; report of case, Brit. M. J. 2:60, 1935.
33. Aicardi, J., Goutieres, F., Arnaud, M. B., and Thieffry, S.: Sclérose tubéreuse de Bourneville et spasmes en flexion du nourrisson, Ann. pédiat. 42:770, 1966.
34. Butterworth, T., and Wilson, M. C., Jr.: Dermatologic aspects of tuberous sclerosis, Arch. Dermat. & Syph. 43:1, 1941.
35. Akesson, H. O., and Rayner, S.: Epiloia and cutis verticis gyrata, J. Ment. Defic. Res. 12:9, 1968.
36. Taylor, J. N., and Genters, K.: Renal angiomyolipoma and tuberous sclerosis, J. Urol. 79:685, 1958.
37. Crosett, A. D., Jr.: Roentgenographic findings in the renal lesion of tuberous sclerosis, Am. J. Roentgenol. 98:739, 1966.
38. Milledte, R. D., Gerald, B. E., and Carter, W. J.: Pulmonary manifestations of tuberous sclerosis, Am. J. Roentgenol. 98:734, 1966.
39. Lagos, J. C., Holman, C. B., and Gomez, M. R.: Tuberous sclerosis: Neuroroentgenologic observations, Am. J. Roentgenol. 104:171, 1968.
40. Baird, H. W., Wycis, H. T., and Spiegel, E. A.: Convulsions in tuberous sclerosis controlled by elimination of impulses originating in the basal ganglia, J. Pediat. 49:165, 1956.
41. Perot, P., Weir, B., and Rasmussen, T.: Tuberous sclerosis. Surgical therapy for seizures, Arch. Neurol. 15:498, 1966.
42. Gold, A. P., and Freeman, J. M.: Depigmented nevi: The earliest sign of tuberous sclerosis, Pediatrics 35:1003, 1965.
43. Nevin, N. C., and Pearce, W. G.: Diagnostic and genetical aspects of tuberous sclerosis, J. M. Genetics 5:273, 1968.
44. Grover, W. D., and Harley, R. D.: Early recognition of tuberous sclerosis by funduscopic examination, J. Pediat. 75:991, 1969.
45. Hurwitz, S., and Braverman, I. M.: White spots in tuberous sclerosis, J. Pediat. 77:587, 1970.
46. Wenzl, J. E., Lagos, J. C., and Albers, D. D.: Tuberous sclerosis presenting as polycystic kidneys and seizures in an infant, J. Pediat. 77:673, 1970.
47. Bundey, S., Dutton, G., and Wells, R. S.: Tuberose sclerosis without adenoma sebaceum, J. Ment. Defic. Res. 14: 243, 1970.

123

Other Hamartoses

Hippel-Lindau Disease

THIS IS A generalized developmental disorder that is genetically determined and has its origin in early embryonic life. The basic defect that leads to disorganization of mesoderm and entoderm and to the polymorphic clinical syndrome is not known but there is general agreement about the fact that the anlage of the anomalies is congenital. Despite the congenital nature of the syndrome, most pathologic manifestations do not occur, as a rule, before the third or fourth decade of life. The syndrome consists essentially in angiomas (and cysts) of the central nervous system and in angiomatosis of the retina. Cystic changes of the pancreas and of the kidneys and hypernephroma are found frequently at necropsy, sometimes without previous clinical manifestations. The early conception of the syndrome developed by Lindau[1] is expanded when new aspects come to light as more cases are reported. Thus, ependymoma, gliosis of the spinal cord, syringobulbia and syringomyelia, angiomatosis of the liver, ovary and skin, pheochromocytoma, hypernephroma and tumors of the epididymis have been found in patients with cerebellar cysts of the Lindau type. There also are case reports in which one or more of the developmental anomalies were found in patients without angiomatosis of the retina or of the central nervous system. Of special interest to teratologists is a report by Hippel[2] that associates the Hippel-Lindau complex with congenital malformations such as encephalocele, microphthalmia, iris coloboma, cystic liver, kidney and pancreas, cleft palate, polydactyly and other congenital malformations. But it is likely that some of these cases were examples of trisomy 13-15 and not related to the hamartosis.

Approximately 80% of the cases of Lindau disease are sporadic but about 60 families are known in which the disorder was inherited like a dominant abnormal trait.[3] Since the pathologic changes may affect many organs, the clinical manifestations vary and the symptoms can differ in different members of a pedigree but, in general, loss of vision and the symptoms of a brain tumor or of lesions of the spinal cord predominate in the pedigree. Lindau[4] recorded a pedigree with cerebellar hemangioblastomas in 6 members occurring in three generations. König and Schoen[5] reported a patient who had numerous angiomas of the spinal cord with foci of gliosis and syringomyelia. There also were cystic changes in the pancreas and the kidney, which contained foci of hypernephroma. The patient's older brother had a brain tumor that was described as a cyst at necropsy and a sister had died of a brain tumor. These patients' father died after operation for brain tumor and his brother and sister and one of her daughters died of the "family disease" with symptoms suggesting brain tumor. Comparable cases in which angiomatosis retinae and brain tumors occurred in several members of a family were reported by Rochat[6] and by Palin.[7] A South African family with Hippel-Lindau disease was observed by Bird and Krynauw.[8] The father married twice and of 15 offspring of the two marriages, 6 had angioma of the retina and/or cerebellar hemangioblastoma. The cerebellar tumors were removed successfully in some of the patients. One female member of the family had diabetes. At necropsy, her pancreas was found to be entirely replaced by cystic tissue. Diabetes also was a symptom in a member of the interesting family recorded by Rumbaur,[9] which showed marked variation of manifestations. The mother and 3 sons had retinal angioma and a daughter had a brain tumor. Angiomatosis retinae, brain tumor and pancreatic cysts occurred in the mother's sisters. This family was remarkable because it illustrates the pleiotropic effect of the gene and its intrafamilial variability. One daughter had iris coloboma in one eye and microphthalmia in the other, i.e., congenital malformations instead of the more common postnatal disorders. Horseshoe kidney was present in a patient of Glushien *et al.*[10] who had angiomatosis retinae and pheochromocytoma. These findings could be considered coincidental but it is known that in other hamartoses congenital malformations occur in addition to the more conspicuous postnatal manifestations (p. 1257). A kindred in which the disorder was thought to be recessively inherited was recorded by Shokeir.[17] Roentgenologic findings in a family with Lindau disease were described by Isaac *et al.*[11] The various elements of the Lindau complex were recognized at different times. The component first described is the angiomatosis of the retina or Hippel disease.[12] In its typical form, this disorder is characterized ophthalmoscopically by a pair of enlarged vessels, an artery and a vein, that emerge from the disc and run to a small tumor in the periphery. The vessels are of the same color but the vein is larger and the artery often is beaded. If there are several tumors, they are supplied by several paired dilated vessels. It seems that the enlargement of the vessels precedes the formation of the tumor. The tumor is a round red growth that is several times larger than the optic disc. It consists histologically of an angioma that closely resembles those seen in cerebellar Lindau tumors. Like these, the retinal angioma has a tendency to formations of cysts that are, in part, responsible for the secondary changes in the eye, i.e., detachment of the retina, formation of exudates, retinal atrophy, glaucoma and others.[13] In the presence of a cerebellar Lindau tumor, a choked disc may be seen. Secondary changes may conceal the original lesion.[4] Destruction of retinal angiomas by radium and diathermy has been attempted and favorable results have been reported.[9, 14]

Cerebellar hemangioblastomas account for about 2% of all brain tumors.[3, 8] How many cerebellar hemangioblastomas are manifestations of Hippel-Lindau disease is not known; estimates range from 10% to 20%[11, 15] and some authors consider isolated cases of retinal or cerebellar angiomatosis as formes frustes of Hippel-Lindau disease. About one-fourth of the patients with retinal angiomatosis develop cerebellar angiomas or cysts and other complications of Lindau disease but many years may intervene before the other organs are involved.[4, 10] The cerebellar tumors can be solid or cystic; they can be solitary or multiple. In cystic tumors, a mural nodule of hemangioblastoma may be seen. Tumor symptoms such as headaches, papilledema, vomiting and vertigo develop; intensification of symptoms may occur after hemorrhage into the tumor. Polycythemia vera can complicate hemangioblastomas, a fact of theoretical and diagnostic importance.[15]

Hippel-Lindau disease also can manifest itself by angiomas in the medulla and spinal cord. Wyburn-Mason[16] stated that males are affected twice as often as females and that symptoms, as a rule, appear in the fourth decade. Yet, the youngest patient with such a cord lesion was 9 years of age.

The cord tumors lie in the posterior columns or extend from the pia on the dorsal surface into the dorsal columns. They are found most commonly between C3–D1 and D7–L1. The cord usually is compressed into a band around the periphery of the tumor. Microscopically, the tumors are composed of a network of capillary channels opening into thin-walled sinuses and fed by medium-sized vessels that come from the pia-arachnoid. These hemangioblastomas are true neoplasms capable of growth but they do not metastasize and rarely spread along the subarachnoid space. The cord may be damaged by syringomyelic cavitation and be softened as their ascending and descending tracts undergo degeneration. A syringomyelic cavity consists of an irregular, often branching, space in the cord. Syringomyelia was found associated with an intramedullary hemangioblastoma and Lindau disease so often that Wyburn-Mason believed that it is an integral part of the disorder, just as the retinal and visceral tumors are. In many cases of Lindau disease, both the spinal tumor and the syringomyelia produce signs of spinal compression; in others, there are symptoms similar to those of cauda equina tumors. There may be wasting of certain groups of muscles in the upper or lower limbs or signs of spastic paraplegia. Vertebral anomalies, Recklinghausen neurofibromatosis, cerebellar ependymomas and other associated disorders have been observed.

REFERENCES

1. Lindau, A.: Studien über Kleinhirncysten, Acta path. et microbiol. scandinav. (supp.) 1:1, 1926.
2. Hippel, E. V.: Über die Beziehungen von Mikrophthalmus mit Unterlidcyste zu allgemeinen Missbildungen, besonders zum Lindauschen Symptomenkomplex, Arch. Ophth. 132:256, 1934.
3. Koch, G.: Considerations nouvelles sur l'hérédité des maladies de Sturge-Weber et de von Hippel-Lindau, Les Phakomatoses Cérebrales, S.P.E.I.:459, 1963.
4. Lindau, A.: Discussion on vascular tumors of the brain and spinal cord, Proc. Roy. Soc. Med. (Sect. Neurol. and Sect. Ophth.) 24:363, 1931.
5. König, E., and Schoen, H.: Über ausgedehnte Angiomatosis der Medulla oblongata und des Rückenmarks mit zentraler Gliose, Syringomyelie zystisch hypernephroiden Tumoren beider Nieren (Lindausches syndrome), Beitr. klin. Chir. 170:239, 1939.
6. Rochat, G. F.: Familiäre Angiomatosis Retinae und Kleinhirnangiom, Klin. Monatsbl. Augenh. 78:601, 1927.
7. Palin, A.: Lindau-von Hippel's disease, Proc. Roy. Soc. Med. 32:1618, 1939.
8. Bird, A. V., and Krynauw, R. A.: Lindau's disease in a South African family, Brit. J. Surg. 40:1, 1953.
9. Rumbaur, W.: Über angiomatosis retinae, Klin. Monatsbl. Augenh. 106:168, 1941.
10. Glushien, A. S., Mansuy, M. M., and Littman, D. S.: Pheochromocytoma. Its relationship to neurocutaneous syndromes, Am. J. Med. 14:318, 1953.
11. Isaac, F., Schoen, I., and Walker, P.: An unusual case of Lindau's disease. Cystic disease of the kidneys and pancreas with renal and cerebellar tumors, Am. J. Roentgenol. 75:912, 1956.
12. Hippel, E.: Über eine sehr seltene Erkrankung der Netzhaut, Arch. Ophth. 59:83, 1904.
13. Cushing, H., and Bailey, P.: Hemangiomas of cerebellum and retina, Arch. Ophth. 57:447, 1928.
14. Elwyn, H.: *Diseases of the Retina* (Philadelphia: The Blakiston Company, 1946).
15. Cramer, Fr., and Kimsey, W.: The cerebellar hemangioblastomas, A.M.A. Arch. Neurol. & Psychiat. 67:237, 1952.
16. Wyburn-Mason, R.: *The Vascular Abnormalities and Tumors of the Spinal Cord and Its Membranes* (London: Henry Kimpton, 1943).
17. Shokeir, M. H. K.: Von Hippel-Lindau syndrome: A report on three kindreds, J. M. Genetics 7:155, 1970.

Gardner Syndrome

A SYNDROME consisting of intestinal polyps, osteomas, fibromas and epidermal cysts was described by Gardner[1] in a Utah family group. A pattern of inheritance characteristic of a single autosomal dominant gene was established for intestinal polyposis and other manifestations of the syndrome. The most serious aspect from the standpoint of the family was polyposis, which predisposes to carcinoma of the colon and rectum. At the time of the first report, 8 closely related people representing three generations of this kindred had died of carcinoma originating in the lower digestive tract. The osteomas were most noticeable at the mandible, but the maxilla, ethmoid, sphenoid, zygoma and the frontal, temporal and long bones were involved in some of the patients. Impacted supernumerary teeth and other dental irregularities may be present also. Because of the manifestations and the mode of inheritance, this rare syndrome probably is best classified as a hamartosis.[2]

Duncan *et al.*[3] discussed the components of the triad: soft tissue tumors, bone tumors and intestinal polyps. They reported a pedigree that shows skin tumors in members of two generations and the full triad in two subsequent generations. Skin and bone tumors can appear in children as the first manifestations. In such cases, the entire intestine should be searched for potentially malignant polyps and relatives should be examined for similar lesions.

In affected members of the kindred described by Gardner, three kinds of soft tumors were found on or below the skin: epidermal cysts, fibromas and ill-defined masses of connective tissue. The lesions were situated on the face, trunk or extremities. More than one type occurred in the same individuals.[4] Although the tumors usually were noticed in adults, some affected children had the anomalies at birth. One affected girl was born with epidermal cysts, another with a lump on the back considered "diffuse fibromatosis" and a boy with a soft lump on the back and hard projections on the head.[1] As these patients grow older, they develop tumors of various kinds. As stated above, polyps of the colon are the most important manifestations of this hamartosis because they have a tendency to malignancy, but in some of the affected persons, nonmetastasizing fibrosarcoma also has been observed. The clinical manifestations vary greatly within the family.

REFERENCES

1. Gardner, E. J.: Follow-up study of a family group exhibiting dominant inheritance for a syndrome including intestinal polyps, osteomas, fibromas and epidermal cysts, Am. J. Human Genet. 14:376, 1962.
2. Gardner, E. J.: A genetic and clinical study of intestinal polyposis, a predisposing factor for carcinoma of the colon and rectum, Am. J. Human Genet. 3:167, 1951.
3. Duncan, B. R., Dohner, V. A., and Priest, J. H.: The Gardner syndrome: Need for early diagnosis, J. Pediat. 72:497, 1968.
4. Gardner, E. J., and Richards, R. C.: Multiple cutaneous and subcutaneous lesions occurring simultaneously with hereditary polyposis and osteomatosis, Am. J. Human Genet. 5:139, 1953.

Basal Cell Nevi Syndrome

THIS SYNDROME is seen in persons who are born with various vertebral and rib anomalies and develop a peculiar facial and cranial appearance subsequently. There is a broad nasal bridge and increased distance between the inner canthi, with heavy eyebrows meeting in the midline (synophrys). The head is large and brachycephalic and the cranium high. The patients have a tendency to formation of tumors in various organs but most conspicuous are lesions of the skin and the jaws.

Skin lesions may be present in childhood. There are numerous papillary elevations sometimes classified as epithelioma adenoides cysticum and basal cell nevi on face, neck, trunk, abdomen and extremities. Sometimes lipomas and fibromas are present. Multiple nevoid basal cell carcinomas may develop during childhood, becoming more frequent at and after puberty. Dyskeratosis of the palms and soles has been described also.

In the jaws, particularly the mandible, there occur cysts of variable size that are lined by squamous, sometimes keratinized, stratified epithelium. These cysts can become noticeable during childhood but develop more often during adolescence or later, when they may grow so large that the face becomes deformed. Radiographically, the cysts appear as radiolucent areas.

In addition to the craniofacial changes already described, there occur skeletal anomalies that point to early prenatal disturbances. Among these are fused vertebrae, which may be in the cervical spine and present as Klippel-Feil syndrome,[1] and there may be fusion of vertebral bodies in lower regions. With the vertebral malformations go costal anomalies, such as splayed, bifid or fused ribs, and sternal deformities with bulging in the upper and retraction in the lower portions of the bone. Kyphoscoliosis has been described in several cases. Shortened metacarpal bones (brachymetacarpy) have been seen in several patients. A round face, mental retardation and absence of phosphaturic response to parathyroid extract are reminiscent of pseudo-pseudohypoparathyroidism.[2]

Mental deficiency and schizophrenia were observed in several patients. Partial agenesis of the corpus callosum was diagnosed in the patient of Binkley and Johnson.[3] Calcification of the falx cerebri and the tentorium of the cerebellum may be recognized in roentgenograms.[4]

The most important peculiarity of these patients is their strong tendency to formation of various tumors. Of these, basal cell carcinomas as well as lipomas and fibromas have been mentioned. It is of interest that in the basal cell tumors, inability of epidermal cells to keratinize seems to be a basic defect, whereas keratinization of stratified squamous epithelium is conspicuous in the lining of odontogenic cysts. Ovarian fibromas with calcifications may show up in pelvic roentgenograms as calcified areas. Such fibromas, which need not interfere with reproductive ability, are quite frequent in female patients. Lymphatic cysts can occur in the mesentery.[5] Medulloblastomas have developed in several patients or their siblings.[6] Congenital rhabdomyosarcoma has been observed.[8]

The basal cell nevi syndrome apparently is inherited like an autosomal dominant trait, attributable to a single gene with marked penetrance and widely variable expressivity. This genetic behavior also is seen in other hamartoses (p. 1251). Ferrier and Hinrichs[4] published a pedigree in which the disorder occurred in four generations, and other pedigrees were compiled by Witkop.[7]

REFERENCES

1. Eisenbud, L., Brooks, H., and Busch, S.: Klippel-Feil syndrome with multiple cysts of jawbones, Oral Surg. 5:659, 1952.
2. Berlin, N. I., Van Scott, E. J., Clendenning, W. E., Archard, H. O., Block, J. B., Witkop, C. J., and Haynes, H. A.: Basal-cell nevus syndrome. Combined clinical staff conference at the National Institutes of Health, Ann. Int. Med. 64:403, 1966.
3. Binkley, G. W., and Johnson, H. H.: Epithelioma adenoides cysticum: Basal cell nevi, agenesis of the corpus callosum and dental cysts, A.M.A. Arch. Dermat. & Syph. 63:73, 1951.
4. Ferrier, P. E., and Hinrichs, W. L.: Basal cell carcinoma syndrome, Am. J. Dis. Child. 113:538, 1967.
5. Clendenning, W. E., Herdt, J. R., and Black, J. B.: Ovarian fibromas and mesenteric cysts: Their association with hereditary basal cell cancer of the skin, Am. J. Obst. & Gynec. 87:1008, 1963.
6. Gorlin, R. J., Vickers, R. A., Kelln, E., and Williamson, J. J.: The multiple basal-cell nevi syndrome. An analysis of a syndrome consisting of multiple nevoid basal-cell carcinoma, jaw cysts, skeletal anomalies, medulloblastoma, and hyporesponsiveness to parathormone, Cancer 18:89, 1965.
7. Witkop, C. J.: Discussion to Berlin *et al.*[2]
8. Schweisguth, O., Gerard-Marchant, R., and Lemerle, J.: Naevomatose basocellulaire: association à un rhabdomyosarcome congénital, Arch. franç. pédiat. 25:1083, 1968.

124

Adenomatoses
(Multiple Endocrine Neoplasias)

MULTIPLE endocrine adenomatoses or neoplasias resemble, in certain respects, the hamartoses. They occur in families and kindreds and probably are due to an autosomal dominant gene with pleiotropic effects. In contrast to the hamartoses, manifestations usually are delayed until adult life, although symptoms sometimes can be traced back to adolescence and childhood.

Multiple Endocrine Neoplasia, Type 1 and Gastrointestinal Ulcers (MEA or MEN, Type 1)

In this syndrome of multiple endocrine adenomatoses (MEA) the parathyroids, pancreatic islets and the pituitary are involved most often; the adrenals and thyroids are affected less frequently. In more than half of the cases there occur multifocal peptic ulcers, which usually are resistant to the customary treatments.

Association of two or more endocrine tumors in the same patient has been known since Erdheim,[1] in 1903, described a patient with an eosinophilic adenoma of the pituitary who also had four enlarged parathyroid glands. In 1939, Rossier and Dressler[2] reported a family in which 2 sisters manifested pluriglandular disease, whereas the brothers suffered from peptic ulcers. In 1953, Underdahl *et al.*[3] reviewed 14 cases in which pituitary tumor, islet cell adenomas and parathyroid tumors, or a combination of two of these, occurred in the same patient. They added 8 additional cases of this syndrome encountered at the Mayo Clinic. Parathyroid tumors were present in all patients and pituitary tumors in 4 of the 8. Five patients had islet cell tumors and the remaining 3 had attacks of hypoglycemia. Multiplicity of tumors was a striking feature and occurred both in relation to the parathyroids and in relation to the pancreatic islets. All patients described were adults. The syndrome of adenomatosis of endocrine glands was extended by Wermer,[4] who correctly assumed that the disorders of a family thoroughly investigated by him were due to a dominant autosomal gene with a high degree of penetrance. Some patients with this syndrome also had peptic ulcers of the stomach and of the duodenum. In 1963, Wermer[5] extended the pedigree of this family to include four generations. In affected members, most of the tumors were benign, but in exceptional cases malignancy developed in some of the endocrine adenomas. Nineteen of a total of 20 patients suffered from peptic ulceration. The syndrome of peptic ulcer and tumors of the anterior pituitary gland, parathyroid glands and islets of Langerhans sometimes included adenomas of the thyroid and of the adrenal cortex and lipomas in various locations.

In 1964, Ballard *et al.*[6] reviewed the subject monographically. The disorder has been described in both sexes and in all age groups except the first decade. In general, women manifest the disease earlier than men. There were 74 cases on record to which the authors added a Negro kindred with five affected generations. In addition to parathyroid, pituitary and thyroid involvement, benign and malignant tumors of the adrenal cortex, benign and malignant bronchial and intestinal carcinoids, multiple lipomas, giant rugal hypertrophy of the stomach, steatorrhea and intractable diarrhea may be manifestations of the disease. Peptic ulcers occur in more than half of the patients. Many cases of the Zollinger-Ellison syndrome may be variants of the more inclusive multiple endocrine adenomatosis.[6] Since the Zollinger-Ellison syndrome has been seen in children,[7] the adenomatosis may not be limited to adolescence and adulthood as was assumed previously.

Multiple Endocrine Neoplasia, Type 2 (MEN, Type 2)

It seems that this disorder, which is dominated by pheochromocytoma and medullary thyroid carcinoma and includes parathyroid tumors and Cushing syndrome, differs genetically from "MEN, type 1."[8] Both conditions, which are transmitted like autosomal dominant traits, show variable expression in the affected members of the family. It remains to be seen whether "MEN, type 2" represents a link between the endocrine neoplasias and the hamartoses, Recklinghausen and Hippel-Lindau disease, which sometimes encompass sporadic or familial pheochromocytoma. Familial pheochromocytomas become symptomatic, as a rule, in the third or fourth decade of life but they have been recognized in children as early as 3 years.[9] Steiner *et al.*[8] reviewed the subject of "MEN, type 2" and made a study of a kindred with pheochromocytoma, medullary thyroid carcinoma, hyperparathyroidism and Cushing syndrome. In that kindred there were 10 proved and 15 probable cases of pheochromocytoma, 5 of medullary thyroid carcinoma, 2 of parathyroid hyperplasia and 1 of Cushing disease. The pedigree included seven generations; patients were ascertained in four generations. Medullary carcinoma of the thyroid, pheochromocytoma and multiple mucosal neuromas forming "bumpy lips" result in a syndrome belonging in this neoplastic category.[10, 11] The disorder has been observed in a father and his daughter who died at the age of 19 years after an abdominal operation. The neuromas of the lips and tongue may bring about an acromegaloid appearance of the face. In a girl described by Sturtz and Brown,[12] the thickened lips were noted at the age of 3 years and a medullary thyroid carcinoma was removed at the age of 16 years. The face with the "bumpy lip syndrome" was considered typical and it was recommended that patients with the characteristic appearance, which is due to multiple mucosal neuromas, should be examined and followed for the presence of thyroid and adrenal tumors. The chromosomes of these patients appear normal.[13]

REFERENCES

1. Erdheim, J.: Zur normalen und pathologischen Histologie der Glandula thyreoidea, parathyreoidea und Hypophysis, Beitr. path. Anat. 33:158, 1903.
2. Rossier, P. H., and Dressler, M.: Familiäre Erkrankung innersekretorischer Drüsen kombiniert mit Ulcuskrankheit, Schweiz. med. Wchnschr. 20:985, 1939.
3. Underdahl, L. O., Wollner, L. B., and Black, B. M.: Multiple endocrine adenomas. Report of eight cases in which parathyroids, pituitary and pancreatic islets were involved, J. Clin. Endocrinol. 13:20, 1953.
4. Wermer, P.: Genetic aspects of adenomatosis of endocrine glands, Am. J. Med. 16:363, 1954.

5. Wermer, P.: Endocrine adenomatosis and peptic ulcer in a large kindred. Inherited multiple tumors and mosaic pleiotropism in man, Am. J. Med. 35:205, 1963.
6. Ballard, H. S., Frame, B., and Hartsock, R. J.: Familial multiple endocrine adenoma-peptic ulcer complex, Medicine 43:481, 1964.
7. Rosenlund, M. L., Crean, G. P., Johnson, D. G., Holtzapple, P. G., and Brooks, F. P.: The Zollinger-Ellison syndrome in a 10-year-old boy, J. Pediat. 75:443, 1969.
8. Steiner, A. L., Goodman, A. D., and Powers, S. R.: Study of a kindred with pheochromocytoma, medullary thyroid carcinoma, hyperparathyroidism and Cushing's disease: Multiple endocrine neoplasia, type 2, Medicine 47:371, 1968.
9. Greenberg, R. E., and Gardner, L. I.: Pheochromocytoma in father and son: Report of the eighth known affected kindred, J. Clin. Endocrinol. 19:35, 1959.
10. Williams, E. D., and Pollock, D. J.: Multiple mucosal neuromata with endocrine tumors; a syndrome allied to von Recklinghausen's syndrome, J. Path. & Bact. 91:71, 1966.
11. Schimke, R. N., Hartmann, W. H., Prout, T. E., and Rimoin, D. L.: Syndrome of bilateral pheochromocytoma, medullary thyroid carcinoma and multiple neuromas, New England J. Med. 279:1, 1968.
12. Sturtz, G. S., and Brown, R. B.: Medullary carcinoma of the thyroid. Bumpy lip syndrome, Clin. Pediat. 10:81, 1971.
13. Nankin, H., Hydovitz, J., and Sapira, J.: Normal chromosomes in mucosal neuroma. Variant of medullary thyroid carcinoma syndrome, J. M. Genetics 7:374, 1970.

Index

A

ABDOMEN
anomalies, in Down syndrome, 327-328
enlargement
in megacolon, 707
polycystic kidney causing, 1043
muscles
absence, 1026-1028
absence, and urogenital anomalies, 1079
aplasia, undescended testes in, 1099
hypoplasia of, 1029
ABIOTROPHY: in retinitis pigmentosa, 378
ABORTION
aminopterin used, 50
polyploidy and, 59
during second trimester, malformations in, 39
spontaneous, 41
chromosomal anomalies in, 39, 41
chromosomal anomalies in, incidence, 59
threatened, infants surviving, malformations of, 39
toxoplasmosis and, 80
ABSCESS: cerebral, 570
ACANTHOSIS NIGRICANS, 1173
ACARDIA, 473-477
acephalus, 473-474
acormus, 474
amorphus, 474
pathogenesis, 473
ACHEIRIA, 954-955
incidence, 955
unilateral, 955
ACHEIROPODIA, 939, 955
ACHONDROGENESIS, 804
ACHONDROPLASIA, 767, 768-781
(in animals), 772
in antiquity, 9
associated malformations, 777-778
benign, 793
brachydactyly and, 968
characteristics of, 768
diagnosis, differential, 778, 861
growth in, 774-775
growth hormone in, 779
history, 771
hydrocephaly and, 775
hyperplastic, 774
hypoplastic, 774
incidence, 768
inheritance in, 772-773
lethal, 770
malacic, 774
mentality in, 778
nomenclature, 46
ossification in, 774
parental age and, 773
pedigree in, 779
pelvic changes in, 776
prognosis, eugenic, 779
Siamese twins with, 8
skeletal pathology in, 773-774
spine in, 777
ACIDOSIS: metabolic, in Lowe syndrome, 389
ACLASIS, Diaphyseal (*see* Exostoses, multiple, hereditary)
ACOUSTIC NEUROFIBROMATOSIS, 1255
ACROCEPHALOSYNDACTYLY, 899-901, 902, 974
associated malformations, 900-901
clinical characteristics, 900
diagnosis, 899-900
high palate in, 645
hydramnios and, 899
incidence, 899
polyhydramnios and, 894
radiography, 1003
ACROCEPHALY (oxycephaly)
associated malformations, 897-898
cataract and, 375
characteristic features in, 896
chondrodystrophy and, 805-806
definition, 893
delayed, 893
obliterated coronal suture in, 896
radiography, 900
in syndrome of multiple anomalies, 895
true, 893
ACROMEGALY: and hyperpituitarism, 424-425
ACTH: causing cleft palate (in mice), 100
ADACTYLY, 939, 974-976
ADAMANTINOMA (*see* Craniopharyngioma)
ADDISON DISEASE, 432
hypoparathyroidism and, 433
ADENINE, 25
dinucleotide, 32
ADENOHYPOPHYSIS, 419
abnormality due to streptonigrin (in rat), 421
retention in exencephaly, 194
ADENOMA
adrenal, 1129, 1226
sebaceum, 1263, 1264
testicular, in testicular feminization syndrome, 1116
ADENOMATOSIS (*see* Endocrines, neoplasia, multiple)
ADRENAL(s), 427-436
absence, 428
accessory, 429-430
adenoma, 1129, 1226
anatomy, 427
in anencephaly, 430-431
aplasia, 427-428
atrophy, familial, 431-432
carcinoma, 1226
cysts, 431
development, 427
dystopia, 429
ectopic, due to streptonigrin (in rat), 429, 431
fusion, 431
hyperplasia
lipoid, and male feminization, 1117
pedigree in, 1109
virilizing (*see* Pseudohermaphrodism, female)
hypertrophy, 434
hypoplasia, 428-429
pyloric stenosis and, 688
pseudohermaphrodism (*see* Pseudohermaphrodism, female)
tumors
chromaffin, and Recklinghausen neurofibromatosis, 1256-1257
cortex, 1226
feminizing, 1117
hemihypertrophy and, 434-435
visceromegaly and, 435
ADRENOGENITAL SYNDROMES, 26, 1107
AEROCELE, 598
AGANGLIONOSIS, 705
AGE
cystic disease of kidney and, 1042
incidence of anomalies and, 39-40
maternal
in anencephaly, 190
in Down syndrome, 59, 314
in heart disease, 466
parental
in achondroplasia, 773
in clefts, 633
AGENESIS
bladder, 1073
brain, primary and secondary, 256
cerebellum, 268
corpus callosum, 252-254
etiology, 252
gallbladder, 722
kidney (*see* Kidney)
lung (*see* Lung)
nuclear, in Möbius syndrome, 397
palmaris longus muscle, 1026
parathyroid, 740
pulmonary artery, 535-536
rib, and myelomeningocele, 281
sacrum (*see* Sacrum)
spleen, 745-748
thymus, 739-740

AGENESIS (*cont.*)
thyroid, partial, 664
AGLOSSIA, 661-662
clinical characteristics, 662
AGNATHIA, 402, 621
microstomia and, 623
streptonigrin causing (in rat), 622
AGONADISM: true, 1085
AIR ENCEPHALOGRAPHY (*see* Encephalography, air)
ALBERS-SCHÖNBERG DISEASE (*see* Osteopetrosis)
ALBINISM, 370
generalized, 370
ocular, 370
ALBRIGHT DISEASE, 878-882
clinical symptoms, 879
differential diagnosis, 881
osseous changes in, 879
osteodystrophy (*see* Pseudo-pseudohypoparathyroidism)
phosphatase in, 879
pigmentation in, 879
nevi, 1169
sexual precocity and, 879
thyroid in, 880
ALIMENTARY TRACT DUPLICATIONS, 696-699
etiology, 696
surgery, 698
symptoms, 698
ALKALINE PHOSPHATASE
in Down syndrome, 332
in hypophosphatasia, 859, 861
ALKYLATING AGENTS: as teratogens, 35
ALPORT SYNDROME
clinical characteristics, 1059
inheritance in, 1059
AMAUROSIS: congenital, 377
AMELIA, 939, 949-957
brachial, 950
complete, 949-950
crural, 950
thalidomide and, 84, 89
AMELOBLASTOMA (*see* Craniopharyngioma)
AMINO ACID: and genetics, 25
AMNION: rupture, fetal malformations due to, 22
6-AMINONICOTINAMIDE, 35
AMINOPTERIN
attempted abortion with, 50
cleft palate due to, 26
clubfeet due to, 1007
cranial dysostosis due to, 890
ear changes due to, 414
malformations due to, 96-97
as teratogen, 35
p-AMINOSALICYLIC ACID, 127
AMNIOTIC ANOMALIES, 22
AMPUTATIONS
congenital (*see* Extremities, anomalies, reduction)
digits, and ankyloglossia, 661
intrauterine, true (*see* Extremities, anomalies, reduction, secondary)
"postnatal," 295
AMYOPLASIA CONGENITA (*see* Arthrogryposis)
ANASTOMOSIS
esophageal, 683
Potts, 501
ANCHIPODIA, 922
ANDROGEN OVERPRODUCTION: and female pseudohermaphrodism, 1108
ANDROGYNE, 10
laws concerning, 12
ANEMIA
in cytomegalic inclusion disease, 72
Fanconi
clinical characteristics, 1020
differential diagnosis, 94
recessive inheritance of, 144
skeletal malformations in, 1020-1021
undescended testes in, 1099
in osteopetrosis, 865
ANENCEPHALY, 189-200
adrenals in, 430-431
chromosomes and, 190-191
complete, 195
definition, 889
ear in, 410-411
"environmental" factors in, 40
eye in, 361
geographic factors in, 40
holo-anencephaly, 195, 198
hydramnios in, 192
hypervitaminosis A causing (in rat), 359
incidence, 189-190
in autumn and winter, 189-190
malformations in, 195-199
maternal age and, 190
mero-anencephaly, 195, 197
microphthalmia and, 358
morphogenesis, 191-195, 280-281
(in rat), 193-194
origin of, 22
parity in, 190
paternal influences in, 190
pituitary in, 196
postmaturity and, 190
prematurity and, 190
rachischisis and, 920
recurrence, 190
in siblings, 190
spina bifida and, 285
twinning and, 191
ANEUPLOIDY
in Down syndrome, 313
intrauterine growth retardation and, 145
multiple
in Down syndrome, 322
in trisomy 13-15, 298
in trisomy 18, 304-305
ANEURYSM
aortic, 547
coronary artery, 562-563
intracranial
congenital, 250-251
renal cystic disease and, 1048
sinus of Valsalva, 548
ANGIOGRAPHY
in pulmonary arteriovenous fistula, 614
in pulmonary vein connection with inferior vena cava, 566
ANGIOMA
cerebral, 249
CNS, in Hippel-Lindau disease, 1266
elephantiasis and, 1183
lung, 615
skin, in Sturge-Weber syndrome, 349
spine, in Hippel-Lindau disease, 1267
vasculosum, 1176-1179
ANGIOMATOSIS
retina, in Hippel-Lindau disease, 1266
Sturge-Weber syndrome and, 349
ANGIORECTICULOMA, 382
ANHIDROSIS
neurogenic, 1167
pure familial congenital, 1166
sensory neuropathy and, 1167
ANIMALS: teratologic omens in, 10
ANIRIDIA, 369-370
genetic factors in, 369-370
iris coloboma and, 369
partial, differential diagnosis, 362
Wilms tumor and, 1228
ANISOCORIA, 372
in Waardenburg syndrome, 371
ANKYLOGLOSSIA, 661
amputation of digits and, 661
complete inferior, 661
hypervitaminosis A causing (in mice), 661
superior, 661
ANKYLOSIS
elbow, 962
spondylitis and, 922
ANNULAR PANCREAS (*see* Pancreas)
ANOMALIES
(*See also specific sites*)
congenital
definition, 3
differentiated from malformations, 3
Ebstein (*see* Ebstein malformation)
ANOPHTHALMIA, 356-361
methyl salicylate causing (in rat), 360
streptonigrin causing (in rat), 360
in trisomy 13-15, 299
ANORCHIA, 1098
ANOTIA, 401
ANOXIA: research (in mice), 34
ANTIBIOTICS: as teratogens, 35
ANTICONVULSANTS
malformations due to, 98-99
porencephaly and, 248
in sclerosis, tuberous, 1264
ANTIMETABOLITES
cardiovascular malformations due to (in mammals), 471
nutrition research and, 35
ANTIMONGOLISM (Monosomy G), 58, 339
intrauterine growth retardation and, 146
ANTITUBERCULOSIS DRUGS, 99
ANUS
anomalies, 709, 710-712
incidence, 710
inheritance in, 710
polydactyly and, 695
syndactyly and, 695
types, 711
atresia
in Laurence-Moon-Biedl syndrome, 179
urinary tract anomalies associated with, 1083-1084
imperforate
alimentary tract duplication and, 697
amelia and, total, 949
Laurence-Moon-Biedl syndrome and, 710
in syndrome of multiple anomalies, 1084
tracheo-esophageal fistula and, 683
trypan blue causing (in rat), 710
obstruction, 711
prolapse, in antiquity, 10
stenosis, 711
AORTA, 537-548

aneurysm, 547
anomalies, in trisomy 13-15, 298
atresia, 537-538
coarctation (*see* Coarctation of aorta)
enlargement, in tetralogy of Fallot, 497
hypoplasia, and coarctation, 543
right, descending, and left aortic arch, 531
stenosis (*see* Stenosis)
AORTIC ARCH
anomalies, 526-537
incidence, 526
in tetralogy of Fallot, 498
transposition of great vessels and, 522
trypan blue causing (in rat), 471
vitamin A deficiency causing (in rat), 470
development, environmental factors disturbing, 527-528
double, 529-531
esophagography in, 530
left-sided ductus arteriosus and, 530
surgery, 531
surrounding trachea, 530
symptoms, 530-531
fourth
absence, diagram of arterial pattern in, 532
anomalies, 529-534
hypothetic embryonic pattern, diagram of, 527
interruption, 532-533
kinking, 533
left, with right descending aorta, 531
pulmonary, anomalies, 534-536
right, 531-532
clinical characteristics of, 532
mental retardation and facial anomalies, 580
mirror image and, 531
radiography of, 532
right-sided ductus arteriosus and, 531
vitamin A deficiency causing (in rat), 531
sixth, anomalies, 534-536
third, persistence, 528-529
APERT SYNDROME (*see* Acrocephalosyndactyly)
APICAL DYSTROPHY, 967
APLASIA
adrenals, 427-428
cerebellar, 267
cutis congenita, 1149
extensor tendons in hand, 978
extremities, 941-944
femur, 998
kidney, 1041-1042
adrenal fusion and, 431
lung
bilateral agenesis and, 604-605
definition, 604
muscle, 1025
nasal, 587
optic nerve, 379-380
pancreas, complete, 730
pineal, 450
radius
chromosomal anomalies and, 960
inheritance of, 960
retina, 377
thymo-parathyroid, 740
ulna, 961
uterus, 1088
APODIA, 939
clinical characteristics, 955
incidence, 955
APPENDICITIS: familial, 703
APPENDIX
displacement, 703
inflammation, 703
malformations, 703
AQUEDUCT STENOSIS: and myelomeningocele, 285
ARACHNODACTYLY
cardiovascular malformations and, 571
clefts and, 645
heterochromia and, 371
in Marfan syndrome, 377
syndrome (*see* Marfan syndrome)
"ARAPHIA," 294
"AREA CEREBROVASCULOSA," 192
ARHINENCEPHALY, 201-202
cleft of lip and palate in, 208-209
corpus callosum anomaly and, 252
discussion of term, 201
familial, 202
harelip in, median, 207-208
heart disease and, 570
nose in, 587-589
double, 207, 209
in syndrome of multiple anomalies, 213
trigonocephaly and, 209-210
trisomy 13-15 and, 201, 298
ARISTOTLE: on teratology, 17-18
ARNOLD-CHIARI MALFORMATION
craniolacunia and, 890
hydrocephaly and, 220
myelomeningocele and, 286
spina bifida and, 285
in syndrome of multiple anomalies, 1075
ARTERIES
carotid, anomalous left common, 529
cerebral, malformations, 249-250
coronary, 561-563
aneurysm, 562-563
anomalies, 561-562
anomalies, clinical characteristics, 561-562
arising from pulmonary artery, 562
arteriovenous fistula, 563
development, 561
single artery, 562
hepatic, in fistula, 726-727
hypogastric, obstructing ureter, 1072
innominate, anomalous, 529
pulmonary, 548-552
agenesis, 535-536
anomalies, classification, 548-549
anomalies, left pulmonary artery, 535
anomalies, lung sequestration and, 609-610
anomalies, in trisomy 13-15, 298
anomalies, vitamin A deficiency causing (in rat), 605
atresia, 550-551
coronary arteries arising from, 562
fistula (*see* Fistula, arteriovenous, pulmonary)
stenosis (*see* Stenosis)
stapedial, persistent, 405
subclavian, anomalies, 533-534
vitamin A deficiency causing (in rat), 533
umbilical, single, 763
ARTERIOSCLEROSIS: in progeria, 161
ARTERIOVENOUS FISTULA (*see* Fistula)
ARTHROGRYPOSIS, 1011-1016
breech delivery and, 1013
clefts and, 644, 1014
clinical characteristics, 1013
definition, 1011
diagnosis, 1014
etiology, 1011, 1012-1013
history, 1011
incidence, 1011
inheritance in, 1011-1012
intrauterine growth retardation and, 142
karyotype in, 1014
prognosis, 1015
in syndrome of multiple anomalies, 895, 1014
ARTICULAR RIGIDITIES, MULTIPLE CONGENITAL (*see* Arthrogryposis)
ASPHYXIATING THORACIC DYSTROPHY, 795-796
ASPIRIN: causing persistent truncus arteriosus (in rat), 513
ASPLENIA
cardiovascular anomalies and, 745
heart disease and, 745
situs inversus and, partial, 746
syndrome, and supernumerary lung lobation, 608
ASTHMA: and ichthyosis, 1156
ASTROCYTOMA: in diencephalic cachexia, 174
ASYMMETRY (*see* Hemihypertrophy)
ATAXIA
manganese and, 26
in Marinesco-Sjögren syndrome, 392
progressive degenerative, differential diagnosis, 269
-telangiectasia, 270-271, 1180
cerebellum in, 270-271
Purkinje cells in, 270
symptoms, 270
ATELEIOSIS: fetal, 134, 137
ATHYROSIS
cretinism due to, 437
thyroid ectopia and, 438
ATLAS: occipitalization of, 908-909
ATRESIA
anus
in Laurence-Moon-Biedl syndrome, 179
urinary tract anomalies associated with, 1083-1084
aorta, 537-538
bile ducts (*see* Bile ducts)
bronchi, 600
choanal, 594-595
associated malformations, 594-595
bilateral, 594
bilateral complete, treatment, 595
cardiovascular malformations and, 572
familial, 594
nasal development fault and, 588
unilateral, 594
colon, 695
duodenum (*see* Duodenum)
ear, external meatus, 402
microtia and, 401
esophagus (*see* Esophagus)
gut, 51
intestine (*see* Intestine)
larynx, 597
mitral (*see* Mitral valve, atresia)
oropharynx, 668

Atresia (*cont.*)
pulmonary, 550-551
tetralogy of Fallot and, 497
timing of malformation, 51
tricuspid (*see* Tricuspid valve, atresia)
Atrioventricularis Communis, 485
in Down syndrome, 577
Atrium
appendages, juxtaposition of, 489
septum
closure, diagrams showing, 482
defects (*see* Septal defects, atrial)
persistent truncus arteriosus and, 514
Atrophy
adrenal, familial, 431-432
hemiatrophy, 168-169
optic nerve, 380
osseous, familial, 295
prognosis, 295
Auditory (*see* Ear)
Augury: in Roman history, 11
Aural (*see* Ear)
Auriculo-Osteodysplasia, 415
Autoimmune Disease: maternal, and cretinism, 440
Autosomal Recessive Inheritance, 57-58
Autosome Anomalies: and mental retardation, 623-624
Azygos Vein: lobe, 609

B

Babylonia: teratology in, 11
Bardet-Biedl Syndrome, 176
Barr Body, 24
Basal Angle of Boogard: roentgenography, 908
Basal Cell (*see* Nevi, basal cell syndrome)
Basilar Impression, 907-908
clinical symptoms due to, 907
primary, 907
associated malformations, 908
secondary, 907
short neck in, 908
Basilar Invagination (*see* Basilar impression)
Bathing-Trunk Nevi, 1170
Bathrocephaly, 905
Batten-Turner Type: of muscular dystrophy, 1032
Beckwith-Wiedemann Syndrome, 171-172
Best Disease, 379
Biemond Syndrome, 177
Bile Ducts
anomalies, 718-724
atresia, extrahepatic ducts, 718-719
associated malformations, 719
classification by Gross, 719
differential diagnosis, 721
familial, 718-719
jaundice in, 719
prognosis, 719
sex distribution, 718-719
atresia, intrahepatic ducts, 720
case review, 720
embryologic basis, 720
familial, 720
jaundice in, 720
prognosis, 720
xanthoma in, 720
dilatations, idiopathic, 721
polycystic disease and, 725
stenosis, 718
tracheobiliary fistula, 723
Biliary Dysgenesis: in syndrome with multiple anomalies, 44
Biologic Theories: in antiquity, 17-19
Birth
multiple (*see* Multiple birth)
weight
in Down syndrome, 145
low (*see* Low birth weight)
in trisomy 18, 146
Bladder, 1073-1080
agenesis, 1073
diverticula, 1078
double, 697, 1073-1074
dwarf, 1073
enlargement, and muscle absence, 1029
exstrophy, 713, 1074-1077, 1082
associated malformations, 1076
complete, 1074
development of, 1075
in extrophia splanchnica, 1077
familial, 1075
histology, 1076
incidence, 1074-1075
incomplete, 1074
incontinence in, 1076
male, 1075
myelocystocele and, 281
myelomeningocele and, 1075
prognosis, 1076
in syndrome of multiple anomalies, 1077
treatment, 1076-1077
hourglass, 1078
hypoplasia, 1073
megacolon and, 705
neck obstruction, and urethral fibroelastosis, 1078-1079
tumors, 1079
vesico-intestinal fistula, 714
Blalock-Taussig Operation, in Tetralogy of Fallot, 501
"Blastopathies," 61
Blebs, 1190
Blepharophimosis, 355
Bloch-Sulzberger Syndrome (*see* Incontinentia pigmenti)
Block
heart (*see* Heart)
vertebra (*see* Vertebra)
Blood
cells (*see* Leukocytes)
in Down syndrome, 333
pressure elevation, in Cushing syndrome, 434
Bloom Syndrome, 141, 157-159
recessive inheritance of, 144
Blount Osteochondrosis Deformans Tibiae, 1001-1002
Blue
nevi, 1171
rubber-bleb syndrome, 1185
spot, mongolian, 1171
Bochdalek Hernia, 754
Bone
in cretinism, 111
dysplasia (*see* Dysplasia, fibrous, of bone)
facial
in craniostenosis, 896
hypoplasia, and bifid nose, 589
fusion, and cardiovascular malformations, 572
in hemihypertrophy, 165
in Laurence-Moon-Biedl syndrome, 178
marble (*see* Osteopetrosis)
parietal, flattening, 889
in rubella syndrome, 67
spotted, 846
tubular, bowing of, 957-959
tumors, 1238
Bourneville Disease, 1260
Bowel
in diverticulosis, 699
malrotation, in trisomy 13-15, 298
obstruction, and duplications, 698
Bowing: of tubular bones, 957-959
Brachial Amelia, 950
Brachmann-de Lange Syndrome (*see* Cornelia de Lange syndrome)
Brachycephaly: and cretinism, 111
Brachydactyly, 965-969
in achondroplasia, 968
cardiovascular malformations and, 572
classifications, 966
in cretinism, 111
dwarfism and, 968
hyperphalangy and, 967-968
inheritance in, 966
major, 966
in Marchesani syndrome, 395
minor, 967
pedigree in, 24, 25
of second digit, 967
of single digit, 967
syndactyly and, 968
Brachygnathia: (in rat), 31
Brachyhypophalangy, 966
Brachymegalodactyly, 977
Brachymetacarpy, 968-969
bilateral, 969
pseudohypoparathyroidism and, 969
Brachymetapody, 968-969
Brachytelemesophalangy, 967
Brailsford Chondro-Osteodystrophy (*see* Morquio disease)
Brain
agenesis, primary and secondary, 256
anomalies
arteriovenous, 249
in Down syndrome, 324-325
encephalocele and, 215
mental retardation and, 262-263
in porencephaly, 247
arteriovenous malformations, 249
in cytomegalic inclusion disease, 72
damage in craniostenosis, 896
hemihypertrophy, 165
hypertrophy, and adrenal anomalies, 429
injuries, due to mercurial compounds, 27
in sclerosis, tuberous, 1261
in trisomy
13-15, 298
18, 268, 305
tumors, 1211-1212
location, 1210
precocious puberty and, 454
sclerosis and, tuberous, 1262
trauma and, 1210
underdevelopment, and bifid nose, 589

BRANCHIAL
arches and pouches, diagrams, 669
cyst, lateral, 670
fistula (*see* Fistula)
BREAST
in hemihypertrophy, 164
in leprechaunism, 159
pigeon, 936
arcuate form, 936
clinical characteristics, 936
surgery of, 936
BREECH DELIVERY
arthrogryposis and, 1013
sacral agenesis and, 924
BRIGHT DISEASE: inheritance in, 1059
BRONCHI
atresia, 600
eparterial, left, 601
hamartoma, 1221
normal division, 601
pre-eparterial, 601
segmental displacement, 601
segmentation of cartilaginous skeleton, 599
subsegmental displacement, 601
supernumerary apical, 601
tracheal, 600-601
BRONCHIECTASES, 601-602
history, 602
in situs inversus, 186
with nose anomalies, 602-603
BRONCHOBILIARY FISTULA, 603
BRONCHO-ESOPHAGEAL FISTULA, 683
BRONCHOGENIC CYST: of mediastinum, 603
BRONCHOMALACIA, 603
BROWS (*see* Eyebrows)
BRUSHFIELD SPOTS OF IRIS, 371
in Down syndrome, 327
"BUMPY LIP SYNDROME," 1270
BUPHTHALMOS (*see* Hydrophthalmia)
BUSULFAN
intrauterine growth retardation and, 151
malformations due to, 97

C

CACHEXIA: diencephalic, 174-175
CAESAR: and teratology, 11
CAFÉ AU LAIT SPOTS, 1168
age of diagnosis, 39
incidence, 1168-1169
neurofibromatosis and, 1169, 1253-1254
CALCIFICATION
cerebral, and toxoplasmosis, 79
in hypophosphatasia, 860
intervertebral, 922
paraventricular, in cytomegalic inclusion disease, 73
CALCIUM
goiter and, endemic, 107
in osteopetrosis, 865-866
CAMPTODACTYLY, 984
clefts and, 645-646
CAMURATI-ENGELMANN DISEASE (*see* Osteopathia hyperostotica sclerotisans)
CANCER
liver, 1222
familial, 1223
mortality statistics, 1223
multiple tumors and, 1202
CANNON NEVI, 665
CARBON MONOXIDE POISONING: maternal, 128
CARCINOGENS
chemical, 1204
environmental, 1203
CARCINOMA
adrenal, 1226
kidney, 1228
liver, 727, 1222
thyroid, and multiple endocrine neoplasia, 1270
CARDIAESOPHAGEAL JUNCTION: identification, 684
"CARDIO-ESOPHAGEAL RELAXATION," 684
CARDIOMEGALY
aortic stenosis and, subvalvar, 542
familial, 461
CARDIOMYOPATHY: obstructive, 584
CARDIOVASCULAR (*see* Heart, Vessels)
CAROTID ARTERY: anomalous left common, 529
CARPAL: craniocarpotarsal dystrophy, 673-674
CARPENTER SYNDROME, 179, 901, 902
syndactyly in, 973
thumb duplication in, 981
CARTILAGE-HAIR HYPOPLASIA, 797
CATARACT, 372-376
anterior polar, 373
dental disorders and, 376
diffuse, 372
in Down syndrome, 326, 374-375
etiology, 373-374
in galactosemia, 374
genetically determined, 26
in Hallermann-Streiff syndrome, 390
heterochromia and, 370
ichthyosis congenita and, 1159
lamellar, 373
in Lowe syndrome, 389
in Marinesco-Sjögren syndrome, 392
microphthalmia and, 373
posterior polar, 373
in Rothmund-Thomson syndrome, 392-393
in rubella syndrome, 45, 64, 65, 66, 375-376
skeletal disorders and, 375
skin disorders and, 376
suture, 373
total, 372
nuclear, 372-373
toxoplasmosis and, 80
zonular, 373
CAT-CRY SYNDROME, 340-343
ear in, 410
intrauterine growth retardation and, 145
CAUDAL
appendages, 925-927
as embryonic remnants, 926
etiology, 926
history of, 925-926
treatment, 927
areas, malformations, 922-923
dysplasia syndrome, 124-125, 919, 927-928
etiology, 928
femoral anomalies in, 998
maternal diabetes and, 928
regression (*see* dysplasia syndrome *above*)
CAVUM
septi pellucidi, 254-255
veli interpositi, 254-255
vergae, 254-255
CDH (*see* Hip, dislocation)
CEBOCEPHALY, 206-210
discussion of term, 206
nose in, 588
nostril in, 207
single, 588
in trisomy 13-15, 298
CECUM
abnormalities, 692
diverticula, 699
fixation of, 693
mobile, 692-693
incidence, 693
CELLS
basal (*see* Nevi, basal cell syndrome)
blood (*see* Leukocytes)
ganglion, and myenteric plexus, 706
germ, formation of zygote from, diagram, 317
giant, in liver disease, 719
interstitial, tumors, 1230
Leydig (*see* Leydig cell)
Purkinje, in ataxia-telangiectasia, 270-271
subnormal number in intrauterine growth retardation, 152
CENTRAL NERVOUS SYSTEM
adrenocortical atrophy and, 432
angioma, in Hippel-Lindau disease, 1266
changes due to reduced atmospheric pressures (in mice), 34
in Down syndrome, 325
malformations, 187-352
clefts and, 643
in Marfan syndrome, 855
in rubella syndrome, 67
in trisomy
13-15, 298
18, 305
tumors, 1209
CEPHALOCELE, 211-216
occipital, prognosis, 213
parietal, 214-216
CEPHALOSYNDACTYLY: high palate in, 645
CEPHALOTHORACOPAGUS: pituitary duplication in, 420
CEREBELLUM
agenesis, 268
anomalies, 267-271
differential diagnosis, 269
etiology, 267-268
pathology, 268-269
symptoms, 269
in syndrome of multiple anomalies, 1075
in trisomy, 267-268
in trisomy 18, 305
aplasia, 267
in ataxia-telangiectasia, 270-271
clefts, 268
ganglioneuroma, 268
hemangioblastoma, 1267
hyperplasia, 268-269
hypoplasia, 267
prognosis, 269
treatment, 269
CEREBRO-COSTO-MANDIBULAR SYNDROME, 658

CEREBRO-HEPATO-RENAL SYNDROME, 44, 347
CEREBROOCULORENAL SYNDROME (*see* Lowe syndrome)
CEREBROSPINAL FLUID
circulation, blockage of, 219
cysts blocking, 220
hydrocephaly and, 219-220
obstruction, 220
toxoplasmosis and, 79
CEREBRUM
abscess, 570
arteries, malformations, 249-250
arteriovenous fistula, 570
cerebro-hepato-renal syndromes, 347
diplegia, 259
dysplasia, and nasal cleft, 590
gigantism, 173
hypertrophy, and macrencephaly, 244
malformations, 189-271
vascular, 249-251
palsy (*see* Palsy, cerebral)
in rubella syndrome, 67
CERVICAL RIB (*see* Rib)
CERVICAL TERATOMA, 1241
CF (*see* Fibrosis, cystic, pancreas)
CHAGAS DISEASE, 705
"CHALASIA," 684
CHD (*see* Heart disease)
CHEILOGNATHOPALATOSCHISIS, 629
CHEILOGNATHOSCHISIS, 637
CHEILOSCHISIS, 637
CHEMICAL CARCINOGENS, 1204
CHEMICAL MALFORMATIONS, 24, 26
CHERUBISM, 622-623, 875
clinical characteristics, 622
diagnosis, 623
familial, 622
CHEST, 930-937
(See also Thoracic, Thoraco-)
in achondroplasia, 774
development, 930-931
duplications arising in, 697
funnel, 934-936
clinical characteristics, 934
kyphoscoliosis and, 934
kyphosis and, 934
prognosis, 936
symptoms, 934
short, in trisomy 18, 305
wall clefts, 933
CHIMERAS, 59
CHOANAL ATRESIA (*see* Atresia)
CHOLEDOCHAL CYSTS (*see* Cysts)
CHOLEDOCHOCELE, 722
CHOLERA: studies (in swine), 75
CHOLESTASIS: familial intrahepatic, 729
CHONDRIFICATION: of vertebrae, 916
CHONDRODYSPLASIA
(*See also* Ollier disease)
hereditary deforming (*see* Exostoses, multiple, hereditary)
peripheral, 783
CHONDRODYSTROPHY, 767-807
acrocephaly and, 805-806
atypical
discussion of terminology, 782
transmitted like dominant hereditary traits, 782-793
transmitted like recessive hereditary traits, 793-804
transmitted like sex-linked recessive trait, 805-806
calcarea, and cataract, 375
calcificans
congenita, 797-800
ichthyosis congenita and, 1159
in cretinism, endemic, 806
polydactyly and heart disease, 794
retinal detachment and deafness, 804
in siblings, 784
CHONDROECTODERMAL DYSPLASIA (*see* Ellis-van Creveld syndrome)
CHONDROITIN SULFATE: in Morquio-Ullrich syndrome, 818
CHONDROMALACIA: larynx, and esophageal anomalies, 683
CHONDROMATOSIS
acroform, 874
generalized, pelvis and lower extremities in, 875
systemic, 874
types, 874
CHONDRO-OSTEODYSTROPHY, BRAILSFORD (*see* Morquio disease)
CHONDROSARCOMA, 1238
CHORDOMA, 927, 1218
CHORIOEPITHELIOMA: liver, 727
CHORIORETINITIS
optic atrophy after, 380
toxoplasmosis and, 79
CHORISTOMA: mouth, 667
CHOROID: coloboma, 362
CHOROIDEREMIA, 378
CHROMATIN, SEX, 24
in true hermaphrodism, 1106
CHROMOSOMES, 24
aberrations (*see* anomalies *below*)
anencephaly and, 190-191
anomalies, 45
in abortion, spontaneous, 39, 41
in cerebellar malformations, 267-268
in cerebral palsy, 259-260
cleft lip and palate and, 632
etiology, 58-60
fused kidneys and, 1050
in gonadal dysgenesis, mixed, 1137
heart disease and, 462-463, 576-578
in hydrocephaly, 218
incidence, 59
intrauterine growth retardation and, 145-146
leukemia and, 1207-1208
in Marfan syndrome, 852
mental retardation and, 263
in microcephaly, 240
neck webbing and, 1191
omphalocele and, 759
ovarian deficiencies and, 1086
overripe eggs and, 59
pseudohermaphrodism and, male, 1118
radial aplasia and, 960
syndromes of, 296-344
transposition of great vessels and, 516
undescended testes in, 1099
vertebral anomalies and, 919
in Bloom syndrome, 158
clefts and, 630, 632
D, long arm deficiency, 303
deletions, 58-59
18
long arm deficiency, 311
ring, 311
short arm deficiency, 310
5, short arm partial deletion, 340-343
fragments, 59
in hemihypertrophy, 164
mosaicism (*see* Mosaicism)
nondisjunction, environmental factors in, 60
normal complement, 55
ring, 58, 311, 343
intrauterine growth retardation and, 145
1, and microcephalic dwarfism, 343
sex (*see* Sex chromosome)
translocations, 59
trisomy (*see* Trisomy)
X (*see* X chromosome)
Y (*see* Y chromosome)
CHYRURGERY (Paré), 12
CID (*see* Cytomegalic inclusion disease)
CIRCULATION: collateral, and coarctation, 543
CIRRHOSIS
carcinoma and, 727
in cytomegalic inclusion disease, 72
fibrosis and, cystic, of pancreas, 734
CISTRON, 25
CLAVICLE
in cleidocranial dysostosis, 838
in progeria, 160
CLAW, LOBSTER, 963-965
feet, 943, 966
CLEFTS
arachnodactyly and, 645
arthrogryposis and, 644, 1014
camptodactyly and, 645-646
cerebellum, 268
chest wall, 933
chromosome-determined, 630
cleidocranial dysostosis and, 645
clubfoot and, 643
Cornelia de Lange syndrome and, 645
craniosynostosis and, 645
in Crouzon craniofacial dysostosis, 903
dislocations and, 643
dwarfism and
diastrophic, 645
pituitary, 646
ectodermal dysplasia and, 643
Ellis-van Creveld syndrome and, 645
environmental factors causing, 630, 632-633
extremity malformations and, 645
face
oblique, 624-625
oblique, hypervitaminosis A causing (in rat), 625
salicylate causing (in rat), 638
facial development and, 633-636
gene-determined, 630
genital anomalies and, 643
glaucoma and, 645
heart disease and, 646
Klippel-Feil syndrome and, 643
laryngotracheo-esophageal, 597-598, 683
lip
(*See also* Harelip)
in arhinencephaly, 208-209, 588-589
bilateral, of lower lip, 627
cardiovascular malformations and, 573
folic acid deficiency causing (in rat), 35
genetic prognosis in, 630
incomplete, on left side, 640
incomplete, midline, 590
lower, 626, 627
median, in arhinencephaly, 588-589

median, coloboma and, 625
median, of upper lip, 624
nasal development fault and, 588
primary, 637
secondary, 637
lip fistula and, 643
lip and palate, 628-649
associated malformations, 642-646
bilateral, 641
chromosomal anomalies and, 632
classifications, 640-641
complete, on left side, 640
ectodermal dysplasia and, 1167
etiology, 629-633
experimental, 636-640
frequency, 628-629
heredity in, 629
history, 628
pathogenesis, 636-640
popliteal pterygium, and penile, scrotal and testicular abnormalities, 644
mandible, 626
hypervitaminosis A causing (in mice), 626
mandibulofacial dysostosis and, 645
microcephaly and, 644-645
nasal
lateral, 590-591
median, 589-590
midline, incomplete, 590
nostril absence and, 587
orodigitofacial syndrome and, 644
otopalatodigital syndrome and, 644
palatal development and, 633-636
palate
aminopterin and, 26
anoxia and (in mice), 34
in arhinencephaly, 208-209
cardiovascular malformations and, 573
cortisone causing (in mice), 34, 100
diphenylhydantoin causing (in mice), 98
genetic prognosis in, 630
harelip and, 625
hypervitaminosis A causing (in animals), 636, 661
intrauterine growth retardation and, 137
microcephaly and, 240, 241, 348
pedigree in, 366
in Pierre Robin syndrome, 655, 656, 657
posterior, 642
posterior, in syndrome of multiple anomalies, 1026
race and, 40
radiation causing (in rat), 35
riboflavin deficiency causing (in rat), 638, 639
in trisomy 13-15, 18, 298, 301, 306
in twins, 641
parental age and, 633
penis, 1104
Pierre Robin syndrome and, 645
popliteal pterygium and, 643
racial distribution, 631-632
radiation causing, 633
Rathke, cysts, 422-423, 1215
spine, 195, 198, 922
tongue, 663
in orodigitofacial syndrome, 675
tricuspid valve, and atrioventricularis communis, 485
in trisomy, 632
in twins, 630-631
pedigree in, 631
vertebra, 643, 921
CLEIDOCRANIAL DYSOSTOSIS (*see* Dysostosis, cleidocranial)
CLINODACTYLY, 967
Down syndrome and, 968, 969
CLITORIS
duplication, 1093
hypertrophy, in syndrome of multiple anomalies, 1108
in leprechaunism, 159
CLOACA, EXSTROPHY (*see* Exstrophia splanchnica)
CLOVERLEAF HEAD, 904-905
CLUBBING
feet, 1000, 1004-1009
aminopterin causing, 1007
bilateral, 1003, 1005
bilateral, myelomeningocele and, 286
bilateral, in syndrome of multiple anomalies, 1008
clefts and, 643
clinical characteristics, 1004
in craniocarpotarsal dystrophy, 673
etiology, 1004-1005
exstrophia splanchnica and, 713
incidence, 38, 1004
inheritance in, 1007
Möbius syndrome and, 397
myelocystocele and, 281
riboflavin deficiency causing (in rat), 1008
sacral agenesis and, 923
sex distribution, 1007
spina bifida and, 1006
in syndrome of multiple anomalies, 895, 953, 1026, 1077
thalidomide causing (in rabbit), 1008
treatment, 1008-1009
in twins, 1007
unilateral, 1005
uterine prolapse and, 1090
fingers
in osteoarthropathy, hereditary hypertrophic, 848-849
pulmonary arteriovenous fistula and, 614
tetralogy of Fallot and, 499
hand, 953
in trisomy 18, 307
thumb, 967
toes
pulmonary arteriovenous fistula and, 614
tetralogy of Fallot and, 499
CLUTCHED THUMB, 978
CNS (*see* Central nervous system)
COARCTATION OF AORTA, 542-547
abdominal aorta, 546
associated malformations, 545
collateral circulation and, 543
in Cornelia de Lange syndrome, 345
etiology, 543-544
familial, 544
familial heart disease and, 460
incidence, 542
location of, 542-543
pathogenesis, 544-545
in rubella syndrome, 66
severe forms, 546
symptoms, 545
treatment, 545
trisomy and, 544
Turner syndrome and, 544
COCKAYNE SYNDROME, 398
COLLODION SKIN, 1160
COLOBOMA, 355, 361-365
bilateral, 362
cleft lip and, 625
bridge, 362
choroid, 362
heart disease and, 570
history, 362
iris, 361-362
aniridia and, 369
differential diagnosis, 362
optic disc, 379
retina, 362
streptonigrin causing (in rat), 360
in trisomy 13-15, 299
vitamin A deficiency causing (in animals), 33, 363
COLON
anomalies, 1077
atresia, 695
distention, in syndrome of multiple anomalies, 1084
diverticula, 699
duplications, 697
types, 698
in megacolon, 707
polyposis, 714-715
CONGENITAL: definition, 3
CONJUNCTIVA: telangiectasia, 1180
CONRADI'S DISEASE, 797-800
CONSANGUINITY
anomalies and, 40
Laurence-Moon-Biedl syndrome and, 179
CONSCIOUSNESS LOSS: and cardiovascular malformations, 570
CONSTIPATION: in megacolon, 707-708
CONTRACTURES
fingers, 984
joints in diastrophic dwarfism, 801
microcephaly and, 238
CONVULSIONS
cardiovascular malformations and, 570
in sclerosis, tuberous, 1264
in Sturge-Weber syndrome, 350-351
COR
triatriatum, 487
etiology, 487
surgery, 487
symptoms, 487
triloculare biatriatum, 503-504
incidence, 503
mitral atresia and, 510
pathology, 503-504
prognosis, 504
symptoms, 504
transposition and, 504
treatment, 504
triloculare biventriculare, 486
CORD COMPRESSION: cervical, symptoms of, 909
CORECTOPIA, 372
CORNEA
anomalies, 367-368
cloudy, in rubella syndrome, 65
in cutis verticis gyrata, 368
in cystinosis, 368
dermoids, 368
in ectodermal dysplasia, 369, 1167
in epidermolysis bullosa dystrophica, 369

CORNEA (*cont.*)
in gargoylism, 368-369
in Hand-Schüller-Christian disease, 368
in Hurler syndrome, 810
in hydrophthalmia, 366
in ichthyosis, 368
in keratosis palmaris et plantaris, 368-369
in Morquio-Ullrich syndrome, 817, 818
in neurofibromatosis, 368
opacities, 367-368
systemic disorders involving, 368-369
CORNELIA DE LANGE SYNDROME, 344-346
clefts and, 645
clinical characteristics, 344-345
differential diagnosis, 95
extremity anomalies in, 941, 960
familial, 346
history, 344
intestinal malrotation and, 692
intrauterine growth retardation and, 139
CORNELIA DE LANGE TYPE: of muscular dystrophy, 1032
CORONARY ARTERIES (*see* Arteries)
CORPUS CALLOSUM
absence
harelip and, 625
pneumoencephalography of, 254
porencephaly and, 247
trypan blue causing (in rat), 253
agenesis, 252-254
etiology, 252
anomaly in trisomy
13-15, 298
18, 305
hypoplasia, 252-254
arhinencephaly and, 252
CORTISONE
anomalies due to (in mice), 34
cleft palate, 100
in pseudohermaphrodism, female, 1110
CORVISART DISEASE, 495
COUNSELING, GENETIC, 27
COXSACKIE VIRUS: and teratogenesis, 77
CP (*see* Palsy, cerebral)
CRANIOCARPOTARSAL DYSTROPHY, 673-674
CRANIO-DIAPHYSEAL DYSPLASIA: progressive, 845
CRANIOFACIAL DYSOSTOSIS (*see* Dysostosis)
CRANIOLACUNIA, 890
CRANIOMETAPHYSEAL DYSPLASIA, FAMILIAL (*see* Pyle disease)
CRANIOPHARYNGEAL CANAL
persistence, 420-421
streptonigrin causing (in rat), 421
trypan blue causing (in rat), 422
CRANIOPHARYNGIOMA, 423, 1214-1215
case review, 1214
precocious puberty due to, 455
CRANIORACHISCHISIS, 197, 198, 919
methyl salicylate causing (in rat), 194, 195
CRANIOSCHISIS, 195, 889
anoxia and (in mice), 34
rachischisis and, 919, 920
CRANIOSTENOSIS, 893-906
brain damage in, 896
clefts and, 645
definition, 893
ears in, 896
etiology, 893-894
facial bones in, 896
familial, 894
history, 893
racial distribution, 894
rickets and, vitamin D-resistant, 904
systemic disorders associated with, 899
treatment, 899
unilateral, 904
CRANIOSYNOSTOSIS (*see* Craniostenosis)
CRANIOTOMY: in microcephaly, 242-243
CRANIOVERTEBRAL ANOMALIES, 907-915
CRANIUM
aneurysms
congenital, 250-251
renal cystic disease and, 1048
anomalies
bone replacement by heterologous tissue causing, 892-893
in Down syndrome, 374
in Sturge-Weber syndrome, 349
in trisomy 13-15, 299
vascular, 250
bifidum, 889
occultum, hereditary, 216
dermal sinus tracts, 213-214
dysostosis (*see* Dysostosis)
meningocele, 211, 889
location of, 212
in microcephaly, 242
nerves
in Möbius syndrome, 397
in Recklinghausen neurofibromatosis, 1254
teratoma, 1215-1216, 1241
tumors, 1209-1211
diagnosis, differential, 245
incidence, 1210
CRETINISM, 102-124
abnormal iodinated polypeptides in, 442
calcium in, 107
deafness in, 112, 114-115
endemic, 103
(*See also* Goiter, endemic)
chondrodystrophy in, 806
dietary deficiency causing, 23
ear in, 413-414
inheritance of, 108-109
iodine prophylaxis in, 27
mental retardation and, 263
research on, 30-31
thyroid in, 111
environmental factors in, 109
epiphyseal dysgenesis in, 806
etiology, 106-109
fluoride in, 108
incidence, 103-104
iodine deficiency in, 106-107
iodotyrosine coupling failure causing, 441
iodotyrosine deiodination failure causing, 441
life expectancy in, 116
macroglossia in, 662
maternal autoimmune disease and, 440
maternal hyperthyroidism and, 440
maternal hypothyroidism and, 440
mental development in, 115-116
metals in, 107-108
"nervous," 113
neuromuscular deficiencies in, 113
nonendemic goitrous (*see* Goiter, familial)
origin of term, 103
pathogenesis, 109-111
pituitary in, 113
prevention, 116-122
"pseudoheredity" in, 121
sex development in, 116
speech defects in, 114
sporadic, 437-438
hereditary, 439
myxedema, protruding tongue and hernia in, 440
sex distribution, 439
symptomatology, 111-116
thymus in, 113
treatment, 116
vitamin A deficiency in, 108
CRI-DU-CHAT SYNDROME (*see* Cat-cry syndrome)
CROUZON CRANIOFACIAL DYSOSTOSIS (*see* Dysostosis, craniofacial, Crouzon)
CRURAL AMELIA, 950
CRYPTOPHTHALMIA, 361
radiation causing (in rat), 359
CRYPTORCHIDISM (*see* Testes, undescended)
CRYPTOTIA, 401
CSF (*see* Cerebrospinal fluid)
CUBITUS VALGUS: in Turner syndrome, 1127
CUSHING SYNDROME, 433-434
hypothalamus abnormality and, 454
multiple endocrine neoplasia and, 1270
Turner syndrome and, 1129
CUTIS
frontis gyrata, 1193
laxa, 1186-1189
congenital, 1188-1189
marmorata telangiectatica congenita, 1180-1181
verticis gyrata, 905, 1192-1193
clinical characteristics, 1192
cornea in, 368
forms of, 1192-1193
microcephaly and, 1193
CYANOSIS: and toxoplasmosis, 79
CYCLOPHOSPHAMIDE: malformations due to, 97
CYCLOPIA, 201-206
(in animals), 204-205
in antiquity, 10
exomphalos in, 203
eye in, 361
familial, 202-203
head in, 203-204
heart disease and, 570
hydramnios and, 204
incidence, 202
incomplete, 204
iniencephaly and, 204
myelomeningocele and, 204
perfect, 203
proboscis in, 203, 204
(in swine), 15
in trisomy 13-15, 201-202, 298
Veratrum californicum causing (in lamb), 205
"CYEMA," 62

"CYEMOPATHIES," 62
CYST(s)
adrenal, 431
blocking CSF flow, 220
branchial, lateral, 670
choledochal, 721-722
associated malformations, 721
etiology, 721
sex distribution, 721
size of, 722
treatment, 722
dermoid (*see* Dermoids)
enteric, 696
enterogenous, 689
extra-intestinal, 698-699
eye, 361
gastric thoracic, 696, 697
gingival, 666
iris, 371
jaw, 627
kidney (*see* Kidney, cystic disease)
larynx, 597
liver, 725
lymphangiectasis, cystic, 613
maxilla, 666
mediastinum, 700
bronchogenic, 603
mesenteric, 703-704
mouth, 666
nasoalveolar, 666
nasopalatine, 666
omental, 703
orbit, 365
vitamin A causing (in rat), 365
palate, 666
pancreatic, solitary, 730
pathogenesis, 611
pineal, 452
pulmonary, 610-612
ballooning, 610
complications, 612
genetic factors in, 611
incidence, 610
multiple, 610
sex distribution, 611
solitary, 610
solitary, symptoms, 612
Rathke-cleft, 422-423, 1215
spleen, 749
thymus, 742
tongue, 666
vagina, 1096
CYSTADENOMA, 1048
CYSTIC FIBROSIS OF PANCREAS (*see* Fibrosis, cystic, pancreas)
CYSTIC HYGROMA: of Neck, 1182
CYSTINOSIS: cornea in, 368
CYSTOGRAPHY: filling defect in bladder lumen, 1070
CYSTOSIS: of pancreas, 730
"CYTOMEGALIA INFANTUM," 71
CYTOMEGALIC INCLUSION DISEASE, 71-74, 382
brain in, 72
calcification in, paraventricular, 73
cataract and, 376
cells in, 71
intrauterine growth retardation and, 151
microcephaly in, 73, 239
as teratogenic agent, 23
CYTOMEGALOVIRUS: studies (in mice), 75
CYTOMEGALY: and visceromegaly, 171
CYTOPLASM, 25
subnormal amount in intrauterine growth retardation, 152
CYTOSINE, 25

D

D_1 TRISOMY, 296
DARIER-WHITE DISEASE, 665
DARWINIAN TUBERCLE, 404
DEAF-MUTISM, 406
dominantly inherited, 408-409
goiter and, familial, 442
heart disease and, 408
recessively inherited, 407-408
retinitis pigmentosa and, 379, 407
DEAFNESS, 406-409
Bing-Siebenmann type, 406
chondrodystrophy and retinal detachment, 804
classification, 406
in Cockayne syndrome, 398
in cretinism, 112
endemic, 114-115
dominantly inherited, 408-409
drugs causing, 414-415
goiter and, 407
kernicterus and, 414
labyrinthine, and retinitis pigmentosa, 379
Michel type, 406
Mondini type, 408
Mondini-Alexander type, 406
nephritis and, 1059
nerve, 406
in osteogenesis imperfecta, 829
recessively inherited, 407-408
sex-linked, 409
in rubella syndrome, 45, 65, 66
Scheibe type, 406
Siebenmann type, 406
unilateral, 409
DEFINITIONS, 3-5
De Formato Foetu (Fabricius ab Aquapendente), 18
De Generatione Animalium (Harvey), 18
DE LANGE SYNDROME (*see* Cornelia de Lange syndrome)
DELETIONS: of chromosomes, 58-59
DENTAL (*see* Teeth)
DENTINOGENESIS: imperfecta, 831
DEOXYRIBONUCLEIC ACID, 25
DERMATITIS: exfoliativa neonatorum, 1159
DERMATOGLYPHICS
in Down syndrome, 331, 332
palmar, in heart disease, 578
in rubella syndrome, 67
DERMATOMEGALY, 1188-1189
DERMIS
absence of ridges, and milia, 1196
fibromatosis, infantile, 1235
hypoplasia, focal, and associated malformations, 1195-1196
sinus tracts, cranial, 213-214
DERMOIDS, 1216-1217
cornea, 368
epibulbar, and mandibulofacial dysostosis (*see* Goldenhar syndrome)
mouth, 666, 667
nose, 593-594
DEVELOPMENT
disturbances, general, 131-186
pathways of, 56
DEVELOPMENTAL MALFORMATIONS: definition, 5
DEVILS, 15-16
DEXTROCARDIA, 477-480
amelia and, total, 949
etiology, 478
history, 477
isolated, 479
mirror image, 478
pathology, 478-479
situs inversus and, 477-478
trypan blue causing (in rat), 478
twins and, 478
DIABETES
insipidus, 453-454
etiology, 453
hereditary, 453
mellitus, maternal
caudal dysplasia syndrome and, 928
effects of, 124-125
extremity malformations and, 95
femoral anomalies and, 998
femoral hypoplasia and, 999
sacral agenesis and, 924
DIAPHRAGM
accessory diaphragms, 756-757
anomalies due to vitamin A deficiency (in animals), 32
development, 751-752
eventration, 756
hernia (*see* Hernia, diaphragmatic)
urethral, 1080, 1081
DIAPHYSEAL
aclasia (*see* Exostoses, multiple, hereditary)
sclerosis and Pyle disease, 871
DIARRHEA: deaths due to, in infants, 42
DIASTEMATOMYELIA, 291-292, 700
incidence, 292
treatment, 292
DIASTROPHIC DWARFISM, 801-803
clefts and, 645
DICEPHALIC (*see* Siamese twins)
DIENCEPHALIC CACHEXIA, 174-175
DIET DEFICIENCIES (*see* Malnutrition)
DIGEORGE SYNDROME: and thymic agenesis, 740
DIGIT(s)
(*See also* Fingers, Toes)
anomalies, and focal dermal hypoplasia, 1195-1196
fifth, duplication, 982-983
oculodentodigital dysplasia, 388-389
orodigitofacial syndrome (*see* Orodigitofacial syndrome)
otopalatodigital syndrome, 677
clefts and, 644
DIGITALIS: in great vessel transposition, 523
DIHYDROSTREPTOMYCIN, 127
ear changes due to, 414
DIHYDROTACHYSTEROL: in pseudohypoparathyroidism, 447
DILANTIN: cleft palate due to (in mice), 98
DIMELIA: ulnar, 961-962
DIPHALLUS, 697, 1104
DIPHENYLHYDANTOIN: cleft palate due to (in mice), 98

DIPLEGIA
  atonic, differential diagnosis, 269
  cerebral, 259
  facial (*see* Möbius syndrome)
DIPLOCHEIRIA, 983-984
DIPLOIDY, 343
  intrauterine growth retardation and, 134
DIPLOPODIA, 983-984
DISLOCATION
  clefts and, 643
  hip (*see* Hip)
  knee, 1004
  radius, 961, 999
"DISORGANIZATION GENE," 697
DISTICHIASIS, 355
DIVERTICULA
  cecal, 699
  colon, 699
  duodenal, 699
  duplications and, 697
  gastric, 689
  giant, 696
  intestinal, 698-699
    development of, 698-699
  Meckel, 701-702
    anomalies associated with, 702
    complications of, 702
    development of, 702
    incidence, 701
    sex distribution, 702
    treatment, 702
  pharynx, 670-671
  tracheal, 599-600
  urethral, 1081
  vesical, 1078
DIVERTICULOSIS, 699
DL-ETHIONINE: and pancreas (in rat), 733
DNA, 25
DOLICHOCEPHALY: in cerebral gigantism, 173
DOLICHOSTENOMELIA (*see* Marfan syndrome)
DOUBLE-HEADED (*see* Siamese twins)
DOWN SYNDROME, 45, 311-339
  aneuploidies in, multiple, 322
  atrioventricularis communis in, 577
  biochemical data, 331-332
  birth weight in, 145
  blood in, 333
  cardiovascular malformations in, 577
  cataract in, 374-375
  chromosome analysis in, indications for, 322-323
  clefts in, 632
  clinical characteristics, 324-331
  clinodactyly and, 968, 969
  in cretinism, 113
  dermatoglyphics in, 331, 332
  diagnosis, 322-323
    differential, 333-334, 397
  duodenal atresia in, 694
  duodenal stenosis in, 694
  ear in, 409
  etiology, 313-316
    genetic theories, 313
    nongenetic theories, 313
    present theories, 323-324
  extremity reduction anomalies and, 941
  heart disease and, 462, 576-578
  history, 311-312
  incidence, 38, 312-313
  karyotype in, 315, 318-319, 320
    normal, 320-321
  macroglossia in, 662
  maternal age in, 59, 322
    advanced, 314
  maternal, offspring in, 321-322
  megacolon and, 705
  mesenteric attachment anomalies in, 692
  mosaicism, 319-320, 321
  ostium primum in, 577
  partial, 321
  pathologic characteristics, 324-331
  prevention, 334
  prognosis, eugenic, 323
  pyloric stenosis and, 688
  race and, 40
  septal defect in, 577
  teratology and, 21
  thyroid disease and, maternal, 60
  translocation, 316-319
    karyotype, 318-319
    "in tandem," 319
    "in tandem," karyotype, 320
  transposition of great vessels in, 577
  treatment, 334-335
  trisomy 21, prevalence in, 320
  twins and, 314-315
DROPSY: and congenital malformations, 22
DRUGS
  deafness due to, 414-415
  etiology of malformations and, 84-102
  maternal use, causing goiter and hypothyroidism, 442-443
  testing, and experimental teratology, 101-102
DUCTUS ARTERIOSUS, 553-561
  absence, 553-554
    vitamin A deficiency causing (in rat), 554
  anomalies, 534-535
  closure
    intrauterine, 559
    physiologic, 554-556
  coarctation and, 543
  left-sided, and double aortic arch, 530
  patent
    familial, 460, 556
    high altitude and, 465
    persistent (*see below*)
    rubella and, 64, 66, 464, 556
    in siblings, 461
    trisomy and, 306, 556
  patent, persistent, 555-559
    associated malformations, 557, 558
    etiology, 555-557
    familial, 556
    incidence, 555
    murmur of, 557-558
    prognosis, 558-559
    rubella causing, 556
    sex distribution, 557
    symptoms, 557-558
    treatment, 559
    trisomy and, 556
    in twins, 556
  right-sided, and right aortic arch, 531
  stenosis, due to sodium salicylate (in rat), 554
DUODENUM
  atresia
    Down syndrome and, 694
    trisomy 21 and, 692
  diverticular, 699
  duplication, 697
    types, 698
DWARF BLADDER, 1073
DWARFISM, 133-134
  "bird-headed," 137
  brachydactyly and, 968
  in Cockayne syndrome, 398
  in cretinism, 111
  diastrophic, 801-803
    clefts and, 645
  in Hallermann-Streiff syndrome, 390-391
  in Hurler syndrome, 813
  intrauterine growth retardation and, 138, 143
  metatropic, 803-804
    development in, 803
  microcephalic, and ring-1 chromosome, 343
  micromelic, 768, 770
  pituitary, 423-424
    clefts and, 646
    hereditary, 424
  polydystrophic, 817
  Russel intrauterine, 140-141
  senile (*see* Progeria)
  stenosis and tetany, 792
  streptonigrin causing (in rat), 150
  thanatophoric, 768
DYSCEPHALIA MANDIBULO-OCULO-FACIALIS: in Hallermann-Streiff syndrome, 390-392
DYSCHONDROPLASIA (*see* Ollier disease) (*See also* Chondrodysplasia)
DYSCHONDROSTEOSIS: familial, 790-791
DYSENCEPHALIA: splanchnocystica, 725
"DYSENDOCRINISM," 159
DYSGENESIS
  biliary, in syndrome of multiple anomalies, 44
  ectodermal, of eye, 371
  epiphyseal, in cretinism, 806
  gonadal (*see* Gonads, dysgenesis)
  mesodermal, of eye, 371
DYSGERMINOMA, 1229
  in true hermaphrodism, 1231
DYSKERATOSIS, 356, 1173
  intra-epithelial, 665
DYSOSTOSIS, 57
  cleidocranial, 836-840
    clavicle in, 838
    clefts and, 645
    familial, 836
    mental development in, 840
    pedigree in, 837
    skull in, 837-838
    in twins, 836-837
  cranial, 889-890
    aminopterin causing, 890
  craniofacial
    Crouzon (*see below*)
    dental, cardiac and genital anomalies and, 902-903
    in Hallermann-Streiff syndrome, 390-391
    sporadic, 903-904
  Crouzon, craniofacial, 901-902
    associated malformations, 903
    diagnosis, 901-902
    history, 901
    surgery in, 902
  mandibulofacial (*see* Mandibulofacial dysostosis)
  metaphyseal, 786, 789, 791-792, 1002
  multiplex, 808-824

DYSPLASIA
auriculo-osteodysplasia, 415
caudal dysplasia syndrome (*see* Caudal dysplasia syndrome)
cerebral, and nasal cleft, 590
chondroectodermal (*see* Ellis-van Creveld syndrome)
cranio-diaphyseal, progressive, 845
craniometaphyseal, familial (*see* Pyle disease)
ectodermal (*see* Ectodermal dysplasia)
epiphysealis multiplex, 786-790
familial, 789
osteoarthritis in, 789
epiphysealis punctata, 797-800
epiphysealis, spondylo-, 783-786
tarda, 805
fibrous
in Albright disease, 878-882
of bone (*see below*)
pigmented nevi and, 1169
polyostotic, 880
of skull, 877
fibrous, of bone, 875-877
clinical manifestations, 876
inheritance in, 875
malignant transformation in, 877
monostotic, 876
phosphatase in, 876
treatment, 877
frontometaphyseal, 870
hip, 992, 994
jaw (*see* Cherubism)
kidney, 1041-1042
macula, 379
metaphyseal, familial (*see* Pyle disease)
myelodysplasia (*see* Myelodysplasia)
oculodentodigital, 388-389
osteo-onycho, 1016-1018
clinical characteristics, 1016-1017
differential diagnosis, 1018
familial, 1016
radiography, 1017
skeletal, in otopalatodigital syndrome, 677
spondylo-epiphyseal, 783-786
tarda, 805
spondylothoracic, 937
DYSRAPHISM, 268, 294
DYSTOPIA
adrenal, 429
infundibularis, 421
pituitary, 421-422
sodium salicylate causing (in rat), 430
tuberalis, 421
DYSTROPHY
apical, 967
asphyxiating thoracic, 795-796
chondrodystrophy (*see* Chondrodystrophy)
craniocarpotarsal, 673-674
familial osseous (*see* Morquio disease)
hemidystrophy, 167-168
in triploidy, 343
macula, 379
muscular, 1032
Batten-Turner type, 1032
de Lange type, 1032
manifestations, 1032
myotonica, 1032-1033
incidence, 1032
manifestations, 1032
mental retardation in, 1032

E

EAR
in anencephaly, 410-411
anomalies, 399-416
nostril absence and, 587
appendages, 403-404
cardio-auditory syndromes, 581
in cat-cry syndrome, 410
in craniostenosis, 896
in cretinism, 114
endemic, 413-414
Darwinian tubercle, 404
in Down syndrome, 327, 328, 409
external meatus, 402-403
atresia, 402
atresia, and microtia, 401
normal, 403
fistula, 403
in Goldenhar syndrome, 411
in hydrocephaly, 411
inner, 406-407
in kidney disease, 411-412, 1066
lop, 404
in mandibulofacial dysostosis, 411, 652, 654
middle, 404-406
in progeria, 160
pseudohypoparathyroidism and, maternal, 414
in rubella syndrome, 62, 64, 66, 412-413
in syndrome of multiple anomalies, 1014
in thalidomide embryopathy, 89, 94, 413, 414-415
in toxoplasmosis, 413
in trisomy
13-15, 298, 299, 300, 410
18, 305, 306, 409
in Turner syndrome, 410, 1123, 1126
male, 1132, 1133
EBSTEIN MALFORMATION, 507-508
etiology, 507
prognosis, 508
symptoms, 507-508
treatment, 508
ECCHONDROMA, 874
ECHO VIRUS: and teratogenesis, 77
ECTODERMAL DYSGENESIS: of eye, 371
ECTODERMAL DYSPLASIA, 1163-1168
anhidrotic, 1165-1167
clinical characteristics, 1165
inheritance in, 1165-1167
clefts and, 643
lip and palate, 1167
cornea in, 369, 1167
hidrotic, 1163-1165
microphthalmia and, 1167
mild, 1163-1165
inheritance in, 1163-1164
pedigree in, 1164
palatal anomalies and, 1167
ECTODERMOSES: congenital, 351
ECTOPIA
adrenal, due to streptonigrin (in rat), 429
cordis, 475-476
incomplete, 475-476
life expectancy in, 475
streptonigrin causing (in rat), 475
surgery of, 475
thoracic, 934
kidney, 1053
lens (*see* Lens)
pancreas, 730
pupil, 377
thyroid, 438-442
athyrosis and, 438
ureter (*see* Ureter)
ECTRODACTYLY, 939, 974-976
true, 963-965
ECZEMA: and ichthyosis, 1156
EDEMA: and toxoplasmosis, 79
EGG: fertilization of, 55
EHLERS-DANLOS SYNDROME, 1186-1189
clinical characteristics, 1187
inheritance in, 1188
EISENMENGER SYNDROME, 503
ELBOW
ankylosis, 962
in Cornelia de Lange syndrome, 345
in nail-patella syndrome, 1017
in syndrome of multiple anomalies, 1190
ELEPHANTIASIS: congenita angiomatosa, 1183
ELLIS-VAN CREVELD SYNDROME (Chondroectodermal Dysplasia), 793-795, 1167
achondroplasia in, 770
cardiovascular malformations in, 572
clefts and, 645
diagnosis, 793
differential, 1018
familial, 793
heart in, 572, 794
hematosplenomegaly in, 795
septal defects in, 462
EMBRYO
diseases of, 23
exencephalic, 191, 194
EMBRYOLOGIC THEORY: in teratogenesis, 22
EMBRYOLOGIC TIMETABLES: uses and abuses of, 49-52
EMBRYOPATHY, 61
rubella, 62
thalidomide (*see* Thalidomide)
EMPHYSEMA, 612
esophageal rupture and, 684
ENCEPHALITIS: in cytomegalic inclusion disease, 72
ENCEPHALOCELE, 211, 889
brain defect and, 215
etiology, 212
frontal, 216
location of, 212
microcephaly and, 213
microphthalmia and, 358
naso-ethmoidal, 592
nasofrontal, 215, 592, 593
naso-orbital, 592
nose, 215, 591-592
occipital, 212
in syndrome of multiple anomalies, 213
parietal, 214, 215
prenasal, 592
spheno-ethmoidal, 593
surgery of, 216
transethmoidal, 592-593
ENCEPHALOGRAPHY, AIR
in hydrocephaly, 227-228
in porencephaly, 247
ENCEPHALOMENINGOCELE, 211
ENCHONDROMA, 874, 1183
hand, 883
ENCHONDROMATOSIS: and Maffucci syndrome, 883

ENDOCARDITIS: fetal, 459
ENDOCARDIUM
in rubella syndrome, 64
sclerosis, 539
ENDOCRINES
in Albright disease, 878-882
cytomegalic inclusion disease and, 72
in Down syndrome, 328-329
hypothalamic disorders and, 453-456
malformations, 416-456
neoplasia, multiple, 1269-1271
inheritance in, 1269
type 1, 1269-1270
type 1, parathyroid, pancreas and pituitary in, 1269-1270
type 2, 1270
type 2, pheochromocytoma, thyroid carcinoma and Cushing syndrome in, 1270
in neurofibromatosis, Recklinghausen, 1256
ENTERIC CYSTS, 696
ENTERIC-OMPHALO DUCT, 762
ENTERITIS: deaths due to, in infants, 42
ENTEROGENOUS CYSTS, 689
ENVIRONMENTAL CARCINOGENS, 1203
ENVIRONMENTAL FACTORS
in etiology of malformations, 61-62
in intrauterine growth retardation, 146-147
in tumors, 1203-1204
ENZYMES
defect in hypophosphatasia, 859
flavin-dependent, 31
EOSINOPHILIC GRANULOMA, 892
EPENDYMOPATHY: in Down syndrome, 325
EPIBULBAR DERMOIDS AND MANDIBULOFACIAL DYSOSTOSIS (*see* Goldenhar syndrome)
EPICANTHIC FOLDS, 355
in Down syndrome, 374
EPIDEMIOLOGY: and teratology, 26-27
EPIDERMIS: in incontinentia pigmenti, 1172
EPIDERMOIDS, 1216-1217
EPIDERMOLYSIS BULLOSA, 1151-1156
benign form, 1151
dystrophic form, 1151
cornea in, 369
inheritance in, 1151, 1152
lethalis, 1155
pathogenesis, 1151
pedigree in, 1153
simple form, 1151
teeth in, 1154
EPIGNATHI, 1241-1242
EPILOIA, 1260
EPIPHYSEAL-SPONDYLO DYSPLASIA, 783-786
tarda form, 805
EPIPHYSEOPATHY: osteochondral, 807
EPIPHYSIS
dysgenesis in cretinism, 806
dysplasia (*see* Dysplasia epiphysealis)
stippled, 797-800
EPISPADIAS (*see* Bladder exstrophy)
EPONYMIC NOMENCLATURE, 46
EPULIS: mouth, 667
ERYTHEMA: telangiectatic, in Bloom syndrome, 157-159
ERYTHROBLASTEMIA: in cytomegalic inclusion disease, 72
ERYTHRODERMA
desquamativum, 1159
ichthyosiform (*see* Ichthyosis congenita)
ESOPHAGITIS, 684
as shock lesions, 684
ESOPHAGOGRAPHY: in double aortic arch, 530
ESOPHAGUS, 678-686
anastomosis, 683
atresia, 678-683
classification by Gross, 679
diagram of, 678
history, 678
incidence, 678-679
morphogenesis, 679
riboflavin deficiency causing (in mice), 680
stenosis and, 683
in twins, 679
constriction, and double aortic arch, 530
development of, 681
duplication, 697
fistula
broncho-esophageal, 683
tracheo-esophageal (*see* Fistula, tracheo-esophageal)
laryngotracheo-esophageal cleft, 597-598
malformations due to vitamin A deficiency (in rat), 607
rupture, 684
separation from trachea, diagram, 681
short, 684-685
stenosis (*see* Stenosis)
ulcer, 684
varices, and polycystic liver, 725
webs, 683
ESTROGEN
masculinizing, 100
testicular feminization syndrome and, 1115
ETHIONAMIDE, 99, 127
ETHIONINE: causing stunting (in rat), 150
DL-ETHIONINE: and pancreas (in rat), 733
ETHISTERONE: virilizing effects of, 100
ETHMOCEPHALY, 206-210
morphology, 206
nose in, 587-588
ETHNIC FACTORS: and incidence of anomalies, 40
ETIOLOGY, 53-129
chromosomes and, 58-60
drugs and, 84-102
environmental factors in, 61-62
genetic factors in, 57-58
infections and, 62-81
maternal disorders and, 102-129
radiation and, 82-84
EUSTACHIAN TUBE, 406
EUTHYROIDISM, 439
EVENTRATION
diaphragm, 756
umbilical (*see* Omphalocele)
EXENCEPHALIC EMBRYOS, 191, 194
EXENCEPHALY
agnathus and, 621
cervical thymus and (in mice), 742
definition, 889
development during embryogenesis, 194
effect on organs outside CNS, 194
hypervitaminosis A causing (in rat), 625
methyl salicylate causing (in rat), 359
morphogenesis (in rat), 193-194
pituitary in, 196
radiation causing (in rat), 192-193
sodium salicylate causing (in rat), 419
EXOGENOUS FACTORS (*see* Environmental factors)
EXOMPHALOS (*see* Omphalocele)
EXOPHTHALMIA: and Recklinghausen neurofibromatosis, 1258
EXOSTOSES
definition, 841
femur, 842
fibula, 842
humerus, 975
multiple, hereditary, 840-844
inheritance in, 840-841
pedigree in, 841
scapula, 842, 843
tibia, 842
EXPERIMENTAL TERATOGENS: viruses as, 75-76
EXPERIMENTAL TERATOLOGY (*see* Teratology)
EXSTROPHIA SPLANCHNICA (Cloaca Exstrophy), 712-714, 1077
development, 713
myelocystocele and, 287
in syndrome of multiple anomalies, 1077
EXSTROPHY
bladder (*see* Bladder)
cloaca (*see* Exstrophia splanchnica)
EXTRAPYRAMIDAL MOTOR DISTURBANCES: muscular hypertrophy and mental deficiency, 1030-1031
EXTRAUTERINE PREGNANCIES: and congenital malformations, 21
EXTREMITIES, 939-959
anomalies
excess, 947-948
reduction, 939, 941-947
reduction, clefts and, 645
reduction, incidence, 940
reduction, primary, 941-944
reduction, primary, associated malformations, 941
reduction, primary, genetic determination, 942, 944
reduction, primary, riboflavin-deficiency causing (in rat), 944
reduction, secondary, 944-947
reduction, secondary, etiology, 945-946
reduction, secondary, genetic determination, 946
reduction, secondary, stumps in, 944
splenic-gonadal fusion and, 749
terminology, 939
thalidomide causing, 85-93
aplasia, 941-944
development, 940
in Down syndrome, 330-331
hypoplasia, 941-944
lower, 992-1010
accessory, 956
anomalies, and pelvic anomalies, 938
in chondromatosis, 875
length inequality, 998
in osteopsathyrosis, 831
radiation damage (in rat), 1003
in syndrome of multiple anomalies, 932
in osteopsathyrosis, 833

pterygium, 1191
syndromes involving, 1011-1021
upper, 959-991
in Cornelia de Lange syndrome, 960
hypertrophy, 959
lipodystrophy, 1195
in syndrome of multiple anomalies, 1026
EYE
(*See also* Oculo-)
absence, 356
Bartholin's description, 297
albinism, 370
in anencephaly, 361
anomalies, 353-398
cardiovascular anomalies and, 570
dermal hypoplasia and, focal, 1195-1196
salicylate causing (in rat), 638
streptonigrin causing (in rat), 364
in syndrome of multiple anomalies, 213
vitamin A deficiency causing (in animals), 32, 33
changes due to reduced atmospheric pressure (in mice), 34
in cyclopia, 202-206, 361
cystic, 361
in cytomegalic inclusion disease, 72
dislocations in antiquity, 10
in Down syndrome, 326
dyscephalia mandibulo-oculofacialis in Hallermann-Streiff syndrome, 390-392
ectodermal dysgenesis, 371
in Goldenhar syndrome, 388
in hamartosis, 382-383
in hemihypertrophy, 164
in hydrocephaly, 226-227
in Laurence-Moon-Biedl syndrome, 176, 177
mesodermal dysgenesis, 371
in Möbius syndrome, 397
oculocerebrorenal syndrome (*see* Lowe syndrome)
in rubella syndrome, 62, 65
in Russel intrauterine dwarfism, 141
in Silver syndrome, 141
in Sturge-Weber disease, 383
in thalidomide embryopathy, 383
toxoplasmosis of, 381-382
in trisomy
13-15, 299
18, 305
in Turner syndrome, 1127
male, 1133
EYEBROWS
in Cornelia de Lange syndrome, 345
in ectodermal dysplasia, 1163
in Hurler syndrome, 811, 812
EYELASHES: in ectodermal dysplasia, 1164
EYELID, 355

F

FACE
anomalies, 619-657
aortic stenosis and, supravalvar, 578
right-sided aortic arch and mental retardation, 580
in Bloom syndrome, 158
bones
in craniostenosis, 896
hypoplasia, and bifid nose, 589
cardiofacial syndromes, 580-581
clefts (*see* Clefts)
development
clefts and, 633-636
diagrammatic presentation, 634
diplegia (*see* Möbius syndrome)
in Down syndrome, 326-327
dyscephalia mandibulo-oculofacialis in Hallermann-Streiff syndrome, 390-392
in gigantism, cerebral, 173
in Goldenhar syndrome, 388
hemiatrophy, 168
in hemihypertrophy, 164
in leprechaunism, 159
lipodystrophy, bilateral, 1194
mandibulofacial dysostosis (*see* Mandibulofacial dysostosis)
moon, in cat-cry syndrome, 341
nevi of, linear sebaceous, 1194
orodigitofacial syndrome (*see* Orodigitofacial syndrome)
in otocephaly, 621
in renal agenesis, bilateral, 1037-1038
in Rubinstein-Taybi syndrome, 1019
in sclerosis, tuberous, 1262
scoliosis, 653
in thalidomide embryopathy, 92
FALLOPIAN TUBES, 1091
FALLOT TETRALOGY (*see* Tetralogy of Fallot)
FAMILIAL: definition, 4
FANCONI ANEMIA (*see* Anemia)
FARBER TEST: in intestinal atresia, 695
FAT, SUBCUTANEOUS, REDUCTION OF, 1194
in progeria, 161
FEET
absence (*see* Apodia)
clubbing (*see* Clubbing, feet)
in Down syndrome, 331
hand-foot-uterus syndrome, 963
lobster claw, 943, 966
in Marfan syndrome, 854
rocker bottom (*see* Rocker bottom feet)
split, 963-965
pedigree in, 25, 965
in Turner syndrome, 1125
male, 1133
FEMINIZATION, 1226
(*See also* Testicular feminization syndrome)
adrenal tumors and, 1117
in males with lipoid adrenal hyperplasia, 1117
FEMUR
absence, 997
in achondroplasia, 774
anomalies, 997-998
maternal diabetes and, 998
reduction, 943, 998
aplasia, 998
exostoses, 842
hypoplasia, 997
maternal diabetes and, 999
shortened, 998
FERTILIZATION: of ova, 55
FETUS
ateleiosis, 134, 137
effects of maternal malnutrition on, 30
endocarditis, 459
harlequin, 1159-1160
microsomia, 134
FIBROBLASTS: in Hurler syndrome, 811
FIBROELASTOSIS: urethral, and bladder neck obstruction, 1078-1079
FIBROMA: molluscum, 1254
FIBROMATOSIS
aggressive, infantile, 1235-1236
dermal, infantile, 1235
diffused, infantile, 1235
generalized, congenital, 1236
incidence, 1236
FIBROSARCOMA, 1236
FIBROSIS
cystic, pancreas, 732-735
development of, 732
differential diagnosis, 730
incidence, 732
inheritance in, 732
meconium ileus and, 734
prognosis, 734
hamartoma and, infantile, 1235
liver, 724-726
FIBROUS DYSPLASIA (*see* Dysplasia)
FIBULA
absence, 998, 1002-1003
complete, 1003
incidence, 1003
prognosis, 1003
anomalies
reduction, 943
riboflavin deficiency causing (in rat), 1001
exostoses, 842
hypoplasia, 998, 1003
micromelia and, 792
FINGER(S)
(*See also* Digits)
"aborted," 974
amputations, 945
ankyloglossia and, 661
anomalies, 974-976
in hemihypertrophy, 167
mandibulofacial dysostosis and, unilateral, 654
pectoral muscle absence and, 1026
clubbing (*see* Clubbing, fingers)
contractures, 984
in trisomy 13-15, 300
in trisomy 18, 308
in Crouzon craniofacial dysostosis, 903
extensor tendon aplasia, 978
fifth
absence, 943
duplications, 982
syndactyly, 972
flexion in trisomy
13-15, 298, 301
18, 305, 306
fourth, syndactyly, 972, 973
fusion, 900
hypertrophy, 984
median, duplications, 983
third, syndactyly, 973
FINGERNAIL (*see* Nails)
FINGERPRINTS: in heart disease, 578
FISSURES: supernumerary, of lung, 608-609
FISTULA
arteriovenous
cerebral, 570
coronary, 563
hepatic artery, 726-727
portal vein, 726-727
pulmonary, 613-615
pulmonary, developmental defect leading to, 613-614
pulmonary, incidence, 613

FISTULA (*cont.*)
pulmonary, manifestations, 614-615
pulmonary, treatment, 615
branchial
communicating, 669-670
external, 669
internal, 669
right, 670
bronchobiliary, 603
broncho-esophageal, 683
ear, 403
lip, 626-627
clefts and, 643
recto-urethral, 1084
trachea, 600
tracheobiliary, 723
tracheo-esophageal, 678-683
diagram, 678
experimental work, 679
history, 678
incidence, 678-679
inheritance and, 679
morphogenesis, 681
site of fistula, 682
surgery, 683
symptoms, 682-683
vagina, 1096-1097
vesico-intestinal, 714
FLAVIN
adenine dinucleotide, 32
-dependent enzymes, 31
mononucleotide, 32
FLOATING THUMB, 977
FLUORIDE: in endemic goiter, 108
FLUORINE: intoxication, 864
FOLIC ACID DEFICIENCY AND MALFORMATIONS, 35
cardiovascular (in mammals), 471
FONTANELLE
in Crouzon craniofacial dysostosis, 903
persistent metopic, 890
third, 891-892
FOOT (*see* Feet)
FORAMEN
interatrial, prenatal closure, 488
occipital, 892
ovale, 481-482
fenestrae and, 481
parietal, enlarged, 891-892
FORDYCE GRANULES, 664-665
FOREARM: distal, absence, 954-955
FORNIX: absence due to trypan blue (in rat), 253
FRACTURES
in osteopetrosis, 866
in osteopsathyrosis, 829, 832
FRANCESCHETTI
oculo-digital syndrome, and rubella syndrome, 65
-Zwahlen syndrome (*see* Mandibulofacial dysostosis)
FRANÇOIS SYNDROME (*see* Hallermann-Streiff syndrome)
FREEMAN-SHELDON SYNDROME, 673-674
FRONTOMETAPHYSEAL DYSPLASIA, 870
FUCHS SYNDROME: and heterochromia, 370
FUNNEL CHEST (*see* Chest)
FUSION
gums, 661
lung lobes, 608-609

G

GALACTOFLAVIN, 31-32
cardiovascular malformations due to (in mammals), 471
hydrocephaly due to (in mice), 223, 224
GALACTOSEMIA: cataract in, 374
GALLBLADDER
absence of, 722
sex distribution, 722
anomalies, 718, 722-723
bilobed, 723
double, 722-723
ductular, 723
floating, 723
hypoplasia, and trisomy 18, 722
septate, 723
triple, 723
GAMMA GLOBULIN: in rubella immunization, 68
GANGLION CELLS: and myenteric plexus, 706
GANGLIONEUROMA: cerebellar, 268
GARDNER SYNDROME, 714-715, 1268
clinical characteristics, 1268
inheritance in, 1268
tumors and, soft tissue, 1237
GARGOYLISM, 808-824
(*See also* Hurler syndrome)
cardiovascular malformations and, 574-575
clinical characteristics, 808-809
cornea in, 368-369
familial, 808, 809
as genetically determined storage disease, 809
lipid metabolism in, 821
GASTRIC (*see* Stomach)
GASTROSCHISIS, 761-762
in antiquity, 10
associated malformations, 762
history, 761
prognosis, 762
GASTROTOMY: in prepyloric gastric atresia, 687
GENES, 25
clefts and, 630
"disorganization," 697
penetrance, expressivity, 57
GENETIC COUNSELING, 27
GENETICS
(*See also* Inheritance)
etiology of anomalies and, 57-58
intrauterine growth retardation and, 143-146
Laurence-Moon-Biedl syndrome and, 177
molecular, 26
GENITALIA
ambiguous, 1113
trigonocephaly and, 897
anomalies, 1035-1146
abdominal muscle absence and, 1079
cardiovascular malformations and, 574
clefts and, 643
craniofacial dysostosis and, 902-903
microcephaly and, 348
solitary kidney and, 1039
tumors and, 1231-1235
vitamin A deficiency causing (in animals), 32
in Down syndrome, 328-329
female, 1085-1097
external, duplication, 1093
male, 1098-1104
external, absence, 1103
in thalidomide embryopathy, 93
in trisomy
13-15, 300
18, 307
GENOTYPE, 25
GENU
valgum, and parietal foramina enlargement, 891
varum, familial, 1002
GEOGRAPHIC FACTORS: and incidence of anomalies, 40
GERM CELL: formation of zygote from, diagram, 317
GERMAN MEASLES (*see* Rubella)
GIANT CELL: in liver disease, 419
"GIANT TEETH," 164
GIGANTISM, CEREBRAL, 173
familial, 173
GINGIVA
cysts, 666
fusion, 661
GLAUCOMA
clefts and, 645
heterochromia and, 370
infantile (*see* Hydrophthalmia)
oculodentodigital dysplasia and, 388
in rubella syndrome, 65
in Sturge-Weber syndrome, 349
in syndrome of multiple anomalies, 366
GLIOMA, 1212-1213
familial, 1212
nose, 591
optic nerve, 380
GLOBULIN: gamma, in rubella immunization, 68
GLOMERULONEPHRITIS: inheritance in, 1059
GLOMUS TUMORS, 1185-1186
multiple, 1237
GLOSSITIS RHOMBICA MEDIANA, 663-664
GLOSSOPTOSIS AND MICROGNATHIA (*see* Pierre Robin syndrome)
GLUCOSE TOLERANCE: in Down syndrome, 332
GLYCOGEN STORAGE DISEASE: and cardiovascular malformations, 575
GODDESS: double-headed twin, 6-7
GOITER
cretin, endemic, 112
deafness in, 112, 114-115
life expectancy in, 116
mental development in, 115-116
neuromuscular deficiencies in, 113
pathogenesis, 109-111
pituitary in, 113
sexual development in, 116
speech defect in, 114
thymus in, 113
treatment, 116
deafness and, 407
endemic, 102-124
calcium in, 107
effect of iodized salt on, 118
environmental factors in, 109
etiology, 106-109
fluoride in, 108
incidence, 104

inheritance and, 108-109
iodine deficiency in, 106-107
metals in, 107-108
prevention, 116-122
"pseudoheredity" in, 121
research on, 30-31
symptomatology, 111-116
thyroid in, 111
vitamin A deficiency in, 108
familial, 441-442
abnormal iodinated polypeptides in, 442
deaf-mutism and, 442
formation failure in iodine compounds causing, 441
iodide transport failure causing, 442
iodotyrosine coupling failure causing, 441
iodotyrosine deiodination failure causing, 441
iodide during pregnancy causing, 443
maternal drug intake causing, 442-443
maternal, and hypothyroidism, 440
in Mulia, 105
radioactive iodine during pregnancy causing, 443
thiouracil during pregnancy causing, 442-443
veins in, 104
GOLDENHAR SYNDROME, 45, 388
coloboma in, 355
ear in, 411
epibulbar dermoids in, 388
eye in, 388
face in, 388
mandible in, 388
GOLIATH SYNDROME, 425
GONADS
differentiation, asymmetric, 1137-1138
dysgenesis
mixed, 1137-1138
mixed, chromosome anomalies and, 1137
mixed, tumors and, 1234
mixed, XO/XXXY mosaicism in, 1138
pure, 1139
pure, familial, 1139
pure, tumors and, 1232
Turner syndrome (*see* Turner syndrome)
in twins, 1131
fusion with spleen, 749-750
tumors, 1229-1231
hermaphrodism and, true, 1231
pseudohermaphrodism and, female, 1232
pseudohermaphrodism and, male, 1232
Turner syndrome and, 1233
Turner syndrome and, male, 1234
GRANULOMA: eosinophilic, 892
GROWTH
disturbances
general, 131-186
placental insufficiency causing, 136
hormone, in achondroplasia, 779
retardation
in Bloom syndrome, 158
in cretinism, 111
intrauterine (*see* Intrauterine growth retardation)
in Lowe syndrome, 389
in progeria, 160
stunted (*see* Stunting)
GUANINE, 25
GUMS (*see* Gingiva)
GUT: atresia, 51
GYNANDROMORPHISM: (in wasp), 167

H

HAIR
-cartilage hypoplasia, 797
in ectodermal dysplasia, 1163
anhidrotic, 1166
in progeria, 161
over spina bifida occulta, 284
HAIRY MOLE, 1170-1171
HALLERMANN-STREIFF SYNDROME, 390-392
case review, 390
clinical characteristics, 390-392
diagnosis, differential, 161
dwarfism in, 390
heredity in, 391
history, 390
HAMARTOMA
bronchi, 1221
clinical characteristics, 1251
endobronchial, 603
fibrous, infantile, 1235
liver, 727-728
lung, 615
mouth, 667
precocious puberty and, 454-455
HAMARTOSES, 1249-1271
eye in, 382-383
renal lesions in, 1065
vascular, 1185-1186
HAND, 962-965
absence (*see* Acheiria)
clubbing (*see* Clubbing, hand)
in craniocarpotarsal dystrophy, 673
in Down syndrome, 330, 331
in ectodermal dysplasia, 1164
enchondroma of, 883
-foot-uterus syndrome, 963
in Hurler syndrome, 813
ladle, 972, 974
in Maffucci syndrome, 883
in Marfan syndrome, 854
pedunculated postminimi, 982-983
split, 963-965
pedigree in, 965
spoon, 974
in trisomy 18, 308
in Turner syndrome, 1125, 1128
underdevelopment, 968
HAND-SCHÜLLER-CHRISTIAN DISEASE: cornea in, 368
HARELIP, 624
(*See also* Clefts, lip)
bilateral, in twins, 641
bridge, 637
cleft palate and, 625
complete, 637
fusion theory, 637
hypervitaminosis A causing (in rat), 625
incidence, 628
median, in arhinencephaly, 207-208
mesodermal penetration theory, 637
pathogenesis, 636
polydactyly and, endemic, 979
race and, 40
simple, 637
study of, 629-630
in trisomy 13-15, 298
HARLEQUIN FETUS, 1159-1160
HARVEY: on teratology, 18
HEAD
circumferences, normal, during first seven years, 237
cloverleaf, 904-905
in cyclopia, 203-204
in Down syndrome, 324
in hydrocephaly, 226-227
in macrencephaly, 245
monkey (*see* Cebocephaly)
in myelomeningocele, 288
in Pierre Robin syndrome, 655
HEARING: in rubella syndrome, 66
HEART
block, 583-584
associated malformations, 583
familial, 583
cardio-auditory syndromes, 581
cardiofacial syndromes, 580-581
disease (*see* Heart disease *below*)
in Down syndrome, 328, 576-578
failure, congestive
in rubella syndrome, 66
ventricular septal defect and, 492
hypertrophy
asymmetric, 584
in Hurler syndrome, 810
malformations, 457-584
(*See also* Heart disease *below*)
antimetabolites causing (in mammals), 471
asplenia and, 745
associated malformations, 568-569
clefts and, 573, 646
craniofacial dysostosis and, 902-903
deaf-mutism and, 408
in Ellis-van Creveld syndrome, 794
experimental (in mammals), 470-472
extracardiac, 568
gastrointestinal malformations and, 571
genital malformations and, 574
intrauterine growth retardation and, 142
mental complications, 570
metabolic disorders and, 574-576
microphthalmia and, 358
neurologic complications in, 570
ocular complications, 570
skeletal malformations and, 571-573
systemic disorders involving, 568-581
in trisomy 13-15, 299, 300
in trisomy 18, 306
urinary tract malformations and, 574
vitamin A deficiency causing (in animals), 32, 470-471
in Marfan syndrome, 855
myxoma, 1220
parchment, 477
rhabdomyoma, 582, 1236
in rubella syndrome, 62, 64, 65, 66, 459, 464
in situs inversus, 186
(in rat), 185
teratoma, 1242
in thalidomide embryopathy, 92, 465-466
tumors, 582-583, 1220-1221

HEART DISEASE
(*See also* Heart malformations *above*)
chondrodystrophy and polydactyly, 794
chromosomal anomalies and, 462-463
cyanotic, and hereditary hypertrophic osteoarthropathy, 849
dermatoglyphics in, palmar, 578
environmental factors in, 463-466
etiology, 459-470
ontogenic, 459
phylogenic, 459
fingerprints in, 578
hypervitaminosis D and, 466
hypoxia causing, 465
intestinal atresia and, 695
maternal age and, 466
sex distribution, 463
in siblings, 461-462
in succeeding generations, 460-461
in syndrome of multiple anomalies, 1000
tracheo-esophageal fistula and, 683
tumors associated with, 582
in Turner syndrome, 1127
male, 1132
twin studies, 466
vertebral and rib anomalies, 931
HEIGHT: in progeria, 161
HEMANGIOBLASTOMA: cerebellar, 1267
HEMANGIOMA
capillary, 1177
sclerosing, 1178
superficial, 1177
cavernous, 1177, 1178
giant, with thrombocytopenia, 1179
liver, 728
in Maffucci syndrome, 883
mediastinum, 616
meningocele and, pedunculated, 212
mouth, 667
multiple, 1177-1178
port-wine, 1177
in Sturge-Weber syndrome, 350
spleen, 749
subglottic, 596
cry in, 596
incidence, 596
sex distribution, 596
treatment, 596
trachea, 599
in trisomy 13-15, 301
HEMANGIOMATOSIS: in Maffucci syndrome, 882-884
HEMATOCOLPOS: with imperforate hymen, 1096
HEMATOMA, SUBDURAL
differential diagnosis, 227
in osteopetrosis, 866
HEMIAPLASIA: thyroid, 664
HEMIATROPHY, 163, 168-169
face, 168
intrauterine growth retardation and, 168
progressive, 168
HEMICARDIUS, 473
HEMIDYSTROPHY, 167-168
in triploidy, 343
HEMIFACIAL
hyperplasia, 624
hypertrophy, 164
hypoplasia, 624
microsomia, 624
HEMI-HYDRANENCEPHALY, 233
HEMIHYPERTROPHY, 163-167
adrenal tumor and, 434-435
chromosomes in, 164
crossed, 165
etiology, 165
familial, 167
of left, 164, 166-167
liver tumors and, 727
nevus unius lateralis and, 1175
tumors and, 165
Wilms tumor and, 1228
HEMIMELIA, 939
radial, 960
terminal transverse (*see* Peromelia)
HEMIPARESIS: in Sturge-Weber syndrome, 349
HEMIPLEGIA: brain agenesis in, 256
HEMISPHERES: telencephalic, fusion, and harelip, 625
HEMISYNDROMES, 162-170
HEMIVERTEBRA
anoxia and (in mice), 34
associated malformations, 919
in syndrome of multiple anomalies, 1075, 1077
Turner syndrome and, 918
HEMOGLOBIN: in trisomy 13-15, 301
HEMORRHAGE
gastrointestinal, in liver fibrosis, 726
telangiectasia and, 1185
HEPATIC (*see* Liver)
HEPATITIS, 720-721
case review, 720
in cytomegalic inclusion disease, 72
infectious, and congenital anomalies, 60
inheritance in, 721
in rubella syndrome, 65
HEPATOBLASTOMA, 727, 1222
HEPATOCARCINOMA, 727
HEPATOMA, 727, 1222
HEPATOSPLENOMEGALY
in Ellis-van Creveld syndrome, 795
in liver fibrosis, 726
in osteopetrosis, 865
in rubella syndrome, 66
toxoplasmosis and, 79
HEREDITARY: definition, 4
HEREDITY (*see* Inheritance)
HEREDO-RETINOPATHIA CONGENITALIS MONOHYBRIDA RECESSIVA AUTOSOMALIS, 377
HERMAPHRODISM, 1105-1122
as omen in antiquity, 11
true, 1105-1107
dysgerminoma and, 1231
gonadal tissue distribution in, 1105
ovaries in, 1105
psychologic orientation in, 1106
sex chromatin in, 1106
types, 1105
HERNIA
Bochdalek, 754
diaphragmatic, 751-757
in antiquity, 10
etiology, 752-753
familial, 752
-pericardo, 756
right, 755
spina bifida occulta and, 284
vitamin A deficiency causing (in rat), 32, 752, 756
dorsolateral, 753
left, 753-755
left, symptoms, 753-754
hiatus, 684-685, 756
incidence, 684
natural history, 685
inguinal
bilateral, in syndrome of multiple anomalies, 1014
undescended testes and, 1100
retrosternal, 755-756
umbilical, 758
cretinism and, sporadic, 440
in visceromegaly, 172
uteri inguinalis, male, 1117
HERPES, 75
simplex, and teratogenesis, 76
zoster, and teratogenesis, 76
HETEROCHROMIA, 370-371
complicata, 370
history, 370
simplex, 370
sympathetic paralysis and, 370
in Waardenburg syndrome, 371
HETEROZYGOSITY, 25
HEXADACTYLY, 978
HIATUS HERNIA (*see* Hernia)
HINDGUT
development, 709
malformations, 709
HIP
dislocation, 896, 992-997
anomalies predisposing to, 992
atypical, 994-995
diagnosis, 995
history, 992
incidence, 992-993
signs of, 995
surgery of, 996
in syndrome of multiple anomalies, 953
teratologic, 994-995
thalidomide causing, 92
true, 994-995
typical and common forms, 993-994
typical and common forms, inheritance in, 993-994
dysplasia, 992, 994
preluxation and, 994
subluxation and, 994-995
HIPPEL-LINDAU DISEASE, 1266-1267
angioma in
CNS, 1266
spinal, 1267
eye in, 382
familial, 1266
manifestations, 1266
retinal angiomatosis in, 1266
HIROSHIMA STUDY: of Radiation Damage to Fetus, 82
HIRSCHSPRUNG DISEASE (*see* Megacolon)
HIRSUTISM: and Cushing syndrome, 433
Histoire des Monstres (Martin), 14
HODGKIN DISEASE: and osteopetrosis, 866
HOLOACRANIA: definition, 889
HOLO-ANENCEPHALY, 195, 198
"HOLOPROSENCEPHALY," 201, 202
"HOLOSPHERE," 201
"HOLOTELENCEPHALY," 201
HOLT-ORAM SYNDROME
cardiovascular malformations and, 572
diagnosis, differential, 94
familial, 461
thumb absence in, 977
HOMOCYSTINURIA, 857-858
lens dislocation in, 857

HOMOZYGOSITY, 25
HORMONES
growth, in achondroplasia, 779
luteinizing, and testicular feminization syndrome, 1115
maternal imbalance, and triploidy, 59
as teratogens, 34, 35
HORN: iliac, in nail-patella syndrome, 1017-1018
HORNER SYNDROME: heterochromia in, 370
HORSESHOE KIDNEY (*see* Kidney, fused)
HOURGLASS BLADDER, 1078
HUMERUS
in achondroplasia, 774
defects, 959-960
exostosis, 975
in nail-patella syndrome, 1017
in Ollier disease, 873
rudimentary forearm fused to, 954
HUNTER SYNDROME, 816-817
HURLER SYNDROME, 809-816
(*See also* Gargoylism)
cardiac hypertrophy in, 810
cornea in, 810
dwarfism in, 813
eyebrows in, 811, 812
fibroblasts in, 811
hands in, 813
laboratory tests in, 816
late (*see* Morquio-Ullrich syndrome)
leukocytes in, 810
liver in, 810
macroglossia in, 662
mental retardation in, 813
pathology in, 809-810
prognosis, eugenic, 816
sex distribution, 809
spine in, 813
HYBRIDIZATION, 15
HYDRAMNIOS
in acrocephalosyndactyly, 899
in anencephaly, 192
in cyclopia, 204
in iniencephaly, 234
HYDRANENCEPHALY, 231-233
etiology, 233
hemi-hydranencephaly, 233
transillumination in, 232-233
HYDROCEPHALY, 217-231
achondroplasia and, 775
Arnold-Chiari malformation and, 220
cerebrospinal fluid and, 219-220
chondrodystrophicus, 805
chromosomal anomalies and, 218
"communicating," 217
pedigree, 217
craniolacunia and, 890
in cytomegalic inclusion disease, 72
diagnosis, 227-228
differential, 245
ear in, 411
encephalocele and, nasofrontal, 215
encephalography in, air, 227-228
etiology, 217-219
galactoflavin causing (in mice), 223, 224
incidence, 217
internal, and nasal cleft, 590
isosexual precocity and, 455
lumbar puncture in, 228
Macewen sign in, 227
methyl salicylate causing (in rat), 222-223
myelocystocele and, 281
myelomeningocele and, 220-222, 285, 286
natural history of, 228-229
nursing care in, 229
obstructive, 218
optic atrophy and, 380
osteopetrosis and, 864
papilloma of choroid plexus and, 219
parental counseling in, 228
pathogenesis, 219-226
studies (in animals), 222-226
porencephaly and, 247
pseudohydrocephaly, 245-246
riboflavin deficiency causing (in mice), 223-224
spina bifida and, 220
cystica, 284
symptoms, 226-227
in syndrome of multiple anomalies, 1075
syphilis and, 218-219
toxoplasmosis causing, 79, 218, 220
treatment, 228-229
in trisomy
13-15, 298
18, 305
trypan blue causing (in rat), 33, 222-223
twinning and, 218-219
HYDROMETROCOLPOS, 1095-1096
clinical characteristics, 1095
familial, 1095
HYDROMYELIA, 279, 291
(*See also* Myelocystocele)
definition, 272, 273
in Down syndrome, 325
myelocystocele and, 281
pathology, 284
surgery of, 291
symptoms, 291
HYDRONEPHROSIS, 1054-1058
bilateral, and hydroureters, 1054
familial, 1055
ear anomalies and, 1066
kidney fusion complicated by, 1052
pathogenesis, 1055
pyelography, 1071
sex distribution, 1054
streptonigrin causing (in rat), 1057
studies (in animals), 1055-1056
ureter fixed to renal pelvis in, 1055
vitamin A deficiency causing (in rat), 1056
HYDROPHTHALMIA, 365-267
bilateral, 366
cornea in, 366
pedigree in, 366
(in rabbit), 367
rubella causing, 366-367
HYDRO-URETER, 1070-1071
hydronephrosis and, bilateral, 1054
incidence, 1070
pyelography, 1071
streptonigrin causing (in rat), 1057
vitamin A deficiency causing (in rat), 1056
HYDROXYLATION: C-11 and C-21, in female pseudohermaphrodism, 1108
3β-HYDROXYSTEROID DEHYDROGENASE DEFICIENCY: and incomplete masculinization, 1117
HYGROMA, 1181
colli, 1182
cystic, of neck, 1182
HYMEN: imperforate, and hematocolpos, 1096
HYPERAMINOACIDURIA: in Lowe syndrome, 389
HYPERCALCEMIA
aortic stenosis and, supravalvar, 578
in hypophosphatasia, 861
HYPEREXTENSION: in Ehlers-Danlos syndrome, 1187
HYPERMELIA, 955-956
unilateral, 955
HYPEROSTOSIS, INFANTILE CORTICAL, 885-886
bones affected in, 886
differential diagnosis, 886
etiology, 885-886
familial, 885
history, 885
symptoms, 886
HYPERPARATHYROIDISM, 449-450
differential diagnosis, 881
inheritance, 449
maternal, and hypoparathyroidism, 446
HYPERPHALANGY, 977
brachydactyly and, 967-968
HYPERPHOSPHATASIA, 862
HYPERPITUITARISM: and acromegaly, 424-425
HYPERPLASIA
achondroplasia and, 774
adrenal (*see* Adrenals)
cerebellum, 268-269
hemifacial, 624
Leydig cell, and visceromegaly, 171
liver, and renal polycystic disease, 1044
pineal, 451
HYPERTELORISM
in Down syndrome, 374
in gigantism, cerebral, 173
HYPERTENSION, PORTAL
liver fibrosis and, 726
polycystic liver and, 725
HYPERTHYROIDISM
in Down syndrome, 329
maternal, 126
cretinism and, 440
HYPERTROPHY
acquired, classification, 163
adrenal, 434
brain, and adrenal anomalies, 429
cerebral, and macrencephaly, 244
clitoris, in syndrome of multiple anomalies, 1108
congenital, classification, 163
extremities, upper, 959
fingers, 984
heart
asymmetric, 584
in Hurler syndrome, 810
hemifacial, 164
hemihypertrophy (*see* Hemihypertrophy)
in hypothyroidism, 1030
muscle
extrapyramidal motor disturbances and mental deficiency, 1030-1031
in hypothyroidism, 1030
osteoarthropathy and, 848-850
in pyloric stenosis (*see* Stenosis, pyloric, hypertrophic)
ventricle, right, in tetralogy of Fallot, 497

HYPERTROPHY *(cont.)*
verumontanum, 1081
HYPERURICEMIA: in Down syndrome, 332
HYPERVITAMINOSIS A, 35
anencephaly due to (in rat), 359
ankyloglossia due to (in mice), 661
cardiovascular malformations due to (in mammals), 471-472
cervical thymus due to (in mice), 742
clefts due to (in rodent)
exencephaly due to (in rat), 625
face, oblique, 625
mandible, 626
palate, 636, 661
harelip due to (in rat), 625
microstomia due to (in mice), 624
myeloschisis due to (in rat), 280
tongue anomaly due to (in mice), 661
HYPERVITAMINOSIS D: and heart disease, 466
HYPOADRENOCORTICISM: and hypoparathyroidism, 432-433
HYPOCHONDROPLASIA, 783
HYPODACTYLY, 939, 963
HYPOGASTRIC ARTERY: obstructing ureter, 1072
HYPOGENITALISM
in Laurence-Moon-Biedl syndrome, 44
in syndrome of multiple anomalies, 902
HYPOGLYCEMIA: and intrauterine growth retardation, 152
HYPOPARATHYROIDISM, 445-446
Addison's disease and, 433
familial, 445-446
hypoadrenocorticism and, 432-433
maternal hyperparathyroidism and, 446
HYPOPHALANGY, 965
HYPOPHOSPHATASIA, 859-862
alkaline phosphatase in, 859, 861
calcification in, 860
differential diagnosis, 778, 861
forms of, 860-861
hypercalcemia in, 861
inheritance in, 859
kidney in, 860
micromelia and, 770
pedigree in, 860
phosphoethanolamine in, 859
prognosis, 861
sex distribution, 860
HYPOPHYSIODIENCEPHALIC SYNDROME, 174
HYPOPHYSIS, 419
in cachexia, diencephalic, 174
HYPOPLASIA
achondroplasia and, 774
adrenal, 428-429
pyloric stenosis and, 688
aorta, and coarctation, 543
bladder, 1073
cartilage-hair, 797
cerebellar, 267
prognosis, 269
treatment, 269
corpus callosum, 252-254
arhinencephaly and, 252
dermal, focal, and associated malformations, 1195-1196
extremities, 941-944
facial bones, and bifid nose, 589
femur, 997
maternal diabetes and, 999
fibula, 998, 1003
micromelia and, 792
gallbladder, and trisomy 18, 722
hemifacial, 624
kidney, 1041
lung, 606-607
associated malformations, 606-607
definition, 604
scimitar syndrome and, 566
lymphatics, in Turner syndrome, 1126
muscle, 1025
abdominal, 1029
myocardium, due to vitamin A deficiency (in pig), 471
nails, in ectodermal dysplasia, 1163
in trisomy 13-15, 301
in trisomy 18, 308, 722
oligonephronic, 1041
optic nerve, 379-380
ovaries, 1085-1086
in Turner syndrome, 1086
pancreas (*see* Lipomatosis)
patella, 998
pineal, 451
pituitary, 420
shoulder girdle, 959
spleen, 748
thrombocytopenia and (*see* Thrombocytopenia, hypoplastic)
thymus, 740-741
thyroid, 664
tricuspid, 506
ulna, and micromelia, 792
uterus, 1088
HYPOSPADIAS, 1082-1083
in rubella syndrome, 66
XXY karyotype and, 1141
HYPOTELORISM: and oculodentodigital dysplasia, 388
HYPOTHALAMUS
in cachexia, diencephalic, 174
disorders, and endocrine disorders, 453-456
in Laurence-Moon-Biedl syndrome, 176, 177
HYPOTHYROIDISM, 438, 443
discordant, in monozygotic twins, 441
iodide during pregnancy causing, 443
maternal, 126
cretinism and, 440
maternal drug intake causing, 442-443
maternal goiter and, 440
muscular hypertrophy in, 1030
radioactive iodine during pregnancy causing, 443
thiouracil during pregnancy causing, 442-443
HYPOTHYROSIS: causing cretinism, 437
HYPOTONIA: in Lowe syndrome, 389
HYPOTRICHOSIS: in Hallermann-Streiff syndrome, 390-391
HYPOVITAMINOSIS: causing cardiovascular malformations (in mammals), 471-472
HYPOXIA
heart disease due to, 465
intrauterine growth retardation and, 149
malformations due to, 127
HYPSICEPHALY
definition, 893
in twins, 894
HYSTEROSALPINGOGRAPHY: in double uterus, 1089

I

ICHTHYOSIS, 1156-1161
congenita, 1157-1159
chondrodystrophia calcificans and cataracts, 1159
clinical characteristics, 1158
forms of, 1157-1158
cornea in, 368
fetalis, 1159-1160
hystrix, 1160-1161
familial, 1160-1161
histology, 1160
lamellaris, 1160
simplex, 1156-1157
associated malformations, 1156
histology, 1156
inheritance in, 1156-1157
in twins, 1157
vulgaris (*see* simplex *above*)
ILEOCECAL VALVE: duplication, 697
ILEUM
anomalies, 1077
development, 691
duplication, 696, 697
prolapse in syndrome of multiple anomalies, 1077
ILEUS (*see* Meconium ileus)
ILIAC HORNS: in nail-patella syndrome, 1017-1018
IMAGES: in teratology in antiquity, 6-7
IMMUNIZATION, RUBELLA
attenuated live virus, 68
passive, 68
IMPERFORATE ANUS (*see* Anus)
IMPRESSIONS: maternal, 12-15
INCIDENCE: statistical problems concerning, 38-40
INCONTINENCE
bladder exstrophy and, 1076
sacral agenesis and, 925
INCONTINENTIA PIGMENTI, 1171-1173
associated anomalies, 1172
clinical characteristics, 1172
epidermis in, 1172
etiology, 1172
INCUS, 405
INFANTICIDE, 16-17
INFARCTION: placental, 148
INFECTIONS: and etiology of malformations, 61-81
INFERTILITY: in Prader-Willi syndrome, 182
INFLAMMATION: and congenital malformations, 22
INFLUENZA: and teratogenesis, 76-78
INFUNDIBULUM MALFORMATION (in rat) due to
methyl salicylate, 422
streptonigrin, 421
INHERITANCE
(*See also* Genetics)
dominant, 57
recessive, autosomal, 57
sex-linked, 58
INIENCEPHALY, 10, 234-236
cyclopia and, 204
hydramnios in, 234
incidence, 234
pulmonary cyst and, 612
(in rat), 236
spine in, 234
streptonigrin causing (in rat), 717
INNOMINATE ARTERY: anomalous, 529

INTELLIGENCE: in Down syndrome, 326
INTERSTITIAL CELL TUMORS, 1230
INTESTINE, 690-715
absence (history), 10
atresia, 694-696
"apple peel," 694
"Christmas tree," 694
etiology, 694
Farber test in, 695
multiple, incidence, 694
pathogenesis, 694
pathogenesis, theories, 694
symptoms, 695
treatment, 695
vomiting in, 695
development, 690-691
diverticula, 698-699
development, 698-699
duplications, and mediastinal cysts, 700
hemorrhage in liver fibrosis, 726
hyperfixation, 692
hypofixation, 692
irregular recanalization in embryo, 697
malformations
cardiovascular malformations and, 571
megacolon and, 705
neurenteric connection abnormality causing, 700-701
oro-gastrointestinal tract, 659-735
malrotation, 690-693
abdominal muscle absence and, 1028
in Cornelia de Lange syndrome, 345
incidence, 692
symptoms, 692
in meconium ileus, 694
polyposis, 714
melanin pigmentation and, 665, 1169
prolapse (history), 10
rotation, 690-693
reversed, 692
three stages of, 691
in thalidomide embryopathy, 93
in trisomy
13-15, 300
18, 307
ulcer, and multiple endocrine neoplasia, 1269-1270
underdevelopment, 693
vesico-intestinal fistula, 714
INTOXICATION: fluorine, 864
INTRAUTERINE GROWTH RETARDATION, 134-162
alkylating agents and, 151
antimetabolites and, 151
cardiovascular malformations and, 142
cells in, subnormal number, 152
cerebral palsy and, 138
chromosomal aberrations in, 145-146
cleft palate and, 137
cytomegalic inclusion disease and, 73
cytoplasm in, subnormal, 152
de Lange syndrome and, 139
dwarfism and, 143
etiology, 143-147
exogenous factors in, 146-147
genetic factors in, 143-146
hemidystrophy and, 168
hypoglycemia and, 152
hypoxia and, 149
leprechaunism and, 142, 159
macrencephaly and, 138
malnutrition in, 152
Marinesco-Sjögren syndrome and, 138-139
microcephaly and, 136-138
mothers of children with, 147-151
dietary deficiencies of, 147
multiple birth and, 151
pathogenesis, 151-152
pedigree in, 144
placental insufficiency in, 147-149
progeria and, 160
prognosis, 152-153
radiation and, 149
Rothmund-Thomson syndrome and, 142
rubella syndrome and, 63, 66
Russel dwarfism and, 140
Silver syndrome and, 139-140
skull and vertebra after, 911
teratogens in, exogenous, 149-151
treatment, 153-154
in trisomy 18, 305
tumors and, congenital, 142-143
twinning and, 151
vitamin A deficiency (in rat), 149
INTRAUTERINE SCREENING PROCESSES, 41
INTUSSUSCEPTION: and mobile cecum, 693
IODIDE
maternal use, causing goiter and hypothyroidism, 443
transport failure causing familial goiter, 442
IODINE
deficiency, and goiter, 106-107
formation failure causing familial goiter, 441
prophylaxis in endemic cretinism, 27
radioactive, maternal use, causing goiter and hypothyroidism, 443
IODIZED SALT: effect on goiter, 118
IODOTYROSINE CAUSING CRETINISM
coupling failure, 441
deiodination failure, 441
IRIS, 369-371
anatomy, 369
anomalies, color, 370
Brushfield spots of, 371
in Down syndrome, 327
coloboma, 361-362
aniridia and, 369
differential diagnosis, 362
cyst, 371
normal, 369
IRRADIATION (*see* Radiation)
ISONIAZID, 127
ISOSEXUAL PRECOCITY: and hydrocephaly, 455
IUGR (*see* Intrauterine growth retardation)

J

JACOBSEN OSTEOCHONDRODYSTROPHIA DEFORMANS, 805
JAUNDICE
in bile duct atresia, 719, 720
in choledochal cyst, 722
in cytomegalic inclusion disease, 72
toxoplasmosis and, 79
JAW
cyst, 627
development, 635
dysplasia (*see* Cherubism)
shortening due to riboflavin deficiency (in rat), 623
tumors, 667
JEJUNUM: development, 691
JOINTS
contractures in diastrophic dwarfism, 801
in Ehlers-Danlos syndrome, 1187

K

"KANALHYPOPHYSE," 420
KARTAGENER SYNDROME, 602-603
KASABACH-MERRITT SYNDROME, 1179
KASCHIN-BECK DISEASE, 807
KERATOCONUS, 367
KERATOSIS PALMARIS ET PLANTARIS, 1161
cornea in, 368-369
KERNICTERUS: and deafness, 414
KIDNEY, 1037-1066
agenesis, bilateral, 1037-1039
face in, 1037-1038
incidence, 1037
low birth weight in, 1037
talipes and, 1038
agenesis, ear anomalies and, 1066
agenesis, intrauterine growth retardation and, 142
agenesis, unilateral, 1039-1040
genital anomalies and, 1039
history, 1039
incidence, 1039
sex distribution, 1039
aplasia, 1041-1042
adrenal fusion and, 431
carcinoma, 1228
cerebro-hepato-renal syndrome, 44, 347
cerebrooculorenal syndrome (*see* Lowe syndrome)
cystic disease, 1042-1049
adult type, 1046-1048
adult type, inheritance in, 1047
adult type, intracranial aneurysms and, 1048
adult type, pathogenesis, 1047
adult type, symptoms, 1048
age distribution curves in, 1042
history, 1042-1043
inheritance in, 724-725
liver hyperplasia and, 1044
of medulla, 1048
multilocular cysts, 1048
pulmonary cyst and, 612
solitary cyst, 1046
in syndrome of multiple anomalies, 44, 1084
type 1, 1043-1044
type 1, clinical characteristics, 1043
type 2, 1044-1045
type 2, histology, 1044
type 2, manifestations, 1044
type 3, 1045-1056
type 3, clinical characteristics, 1045
type 3, etiology, 1045
type 3, familial, 1045
type 4, 1046
urethral obstruction causing, 1046
in cytomegalic inclusion disease, 72

KIDNEY (*cont.*)
diseases, hereditary, 1058-1061
double, 1053, 1067
dysplasia, 1041-1042
ectopia, 1053
ear anomalies and, 411-412, 1066
in syndrome of multiple anomalies, 1077
fused, 1050-1053
complications, 1052
development (in animals), 1050-1051
etiology, 1050
isthmus in, 1050
streptonigrin causing (in rat), 1057
in trisomy 18, 307, 1050
vitamin A deficiency causing (in rat), 1051
hamartoses and, 1065
horseshoe (*see* fused *above*)
in hypophosphatasia, 860
hypoplasia, 1041
insufficiency, in syndrome of multiple anomalies, 1008
in leprechaunism, 159
malrotation, 1053
overgrowth, and visceromegaly, 171
pelvis
dilatation, pyelography, 1067
duplication, 1067
polycystic (*see* cystic disease *above*)
in rubella syndrome, 66
solitary (*see* agenesis, unilateral *above*)
sponge, 1043
supernumerary, 1053-1054
in syndrome of multiple anomalies, 213
teratoma, 1242
in trisomy 13-15, 300
tumors, 1228-1229
in Turner syndrome, 1127
Wilms tumor and, 1228
KINDRED: definition, 4
KLEEBLATTSCHÄDEL, 893, 904-905
KLINEFELTER SYNDROME, 1141-1146
hypospadias in, 1141
tumors and, 1234
X chromosome duplication in, 58
XXXXY, 1142, 1143
XXY, 1141
47,XXY, 1142
XXYY, 1142-1144
KLIPPEL-FEIL SYNDROME, 909-914
cardiovascular malformations and, 572
clefts and, 643
inheritance in, 909-910
prognosis, 912, 914
sacral agenesis and, 923
scoliosis in, 913
spinal column in, 910-911
Sprengel deformity and, 911, 912
type I, clinical characteristics, 910
type II, clinical characteristics, 910
type III, clinical characteristics, 910
vertebrae in, 912
45,X/46,XX_1 mosaicism in, 1128
KLIPPEL-TRENAUNAY SYNDROME, 1180
KNEE
dislocation, 1004
in Maffucci syndrome, 883
KOCHER-DEBRÉ-SÉMÉLAIGNE SYNDROME, 1030
KUSKOKWIM DISEASE, 1015
KYPHOSCOLIOSIS
funnel chest and, 934
neurofibromatosis and, Recklinghausen, 1257
tibia, 1002
KYPHOSIS: and funnel chest, 934

L

LABIA
fusion in virilization, 1109
majora, in testicular feminization syndrome, 1114
minora, duplication, 1093
LACRIMAL APPARATUS, 355-356
LACUNAR SKULL, 890
LADLE HAND, 972, 974
LARSEN SYNDROME, 1016
LARYNGOCELE, 598
LARYNX, 596-598
atresia, 597
chondromalacia, and esophageal anomaly, 683
cysts, 597
in hemihypertrophy, 167
laryngotracheo-esophageal cleft, 597-598
papilloma, 597
webs, 597
LAURENCE-MOON-BIEDL SYNDROME, 44, 176-181, 902
as autosomal recessive trait, 44
cardiovascular malformations and, 572
deafness in, 407
ectopic pupil and, 372
heart disease and, 462
hypothalamus in, 177
imperforate anus and, 710
inheritance in, 177, 179
male sex characteristics in, 177
obesity in, 177
ocular findings in, 177
pedigree in, 179
polydactyly in, 178-179
retinal aplasia in, 377
symptoms, analysis of, 177
syndactyly in, 973
tumors and, 180
undescended testes in, 1099
urinary tract malformations in, 179
LAWS: concerning androgynes, 12
LEAD POISONING: maternal, 129
LEG (*see* Extremity)
LEINER DISEASE, 1159
LENS, 372-377
dislocation
in homocystinuria, 857
in Marfan syndrome, 851
ectopia, 376-377
lentis and pupillae, 376-377
simple, 376
in rubella syndrome, 64
spherical, in Marchesani syndrome, 395
LEPRECHAUNISM, 159-160
intrauterine growth retardation and, 142
recessive inheritance of, 144, 159
LEPTOMENINGES: in rubella syndrome, 65
LÉRI PLEONOSTEOSIS, 847
LETTERER-SIWE DISEASE, 892
LEUKEMIA, 1207-1209
chromosomal anomalies and, 1207
in Down syndrome, 333
drugs and, 1208
genetic factors in, 1207
mortality statistics, 1207
multiple tumors and, 1202
prenatal environmental damage and, 1208
viruses and, 1208
LEUKEMOID REACTIONS: myeloid, phocomelia and thrombocytopenia, 952
LEUKOCYTES
in Hurler syndrome, 810
in trisomy 13-15, 302
LEUKOKERATOSIS, 665
LEUKOPLAKIA, ORAL, 665
clinical characteristics, 665
familial, 665
treatment, 665
LEVOATRIO-CARDINAL VEIN: anomalies, 564-565
LEVOCARDIA: and situs inversus, 479
LEYDIG CELL
hyperplasia, and visceromegaly, 171
tumors, 1230
LH: and testicular feminization syndrome, 1115
LID (Eyelid), 355
LIMBS (*see* Extremities)
LINDAU DISEASE: eye in, 382
LIP
anomalies, 625-627
mandibulofacial dysostosis and, unilateral, 654
"bumpy lip syndrome," 1270
clefts (*see* Clefts)
double, 626
familial, 626
fistula, 626-627
clefts and, 643
in orodigitofacial syndrome, 675
pits, 626
high palate and, 627
scar, and nasal development fault, 588
upper, short and long, 625-626
LIPID METABOLISM: and gargoylism: 821
LIPOCHONDRODYSTROPHY, 808-824
LIPODYSTROPHY, 1194-1195
case review, 1194
congenital generalized, 174
as autosomal recessive trait, 174
facial, bilateral, 1194
partial, 1195
types, 1194
LIPOID ADRENAL HYPERPLASIA: and male feminization, 1117
LIPOMATOSIS, 732
differential diagnosis, 730
sweat electrolytes in, 732
LIPOMUCOPOLYSACCHARIDOSIS, 821-822
LIVER, 716-729
absence, 716
artery, in fistula, 726-727
cancer (*see* Cancer)
carcinoma, 727, 1222
cells, in rubella syndrome, 65
cerebro-hepato-renal syndrome, 44, 347
cerebrooculorenal syndrome (*see* Lowe syndrome)
chorioepithelioma, 727
cysts, 725
in cytomegalic inclusion disease, 72

development, 716
disease, giant cell, 719
dried, and endemic cretinism, 30
fibrosis, 724-726
hamartoma, 727-728
hemangioma, 728
in Hurler syndrome, 810
hyperplasia, and renal cystic disease, 1044
in leprechaunism, 159
lobation abnormalities, 716-717
malformations, 716-717
polycystic, 724-726
inheritance, 724-725
symptoms, 725
in syndrome of multiple anomalies, 213
weight of, 725
teratoma, 728, 1242
tumors, 727-728, 1222-1223
LOBE(s)
azygos vein, 609
lung, fused, 608-609
Rokitansky, 607-608
LOBSTER CLAW, 963-965
feet, 943, 966
LOP EAR, 404
LOW BIRTH WEIGHT
cerebral palsy and, 258
incidence of congenital malformations in, 39
in renal agenesis, bilateral, 1037-1038
LOWE SYNDROME, 389-390
clinical characteristics, 389
kidney pathology in, 389
pedigree in, 390
sex distribution of, 389
undescended testes in, 1099
LUBCHENKO CHART, 146
LÜCKENSCHÄDEL, 890
LUMBAR
anomalies, 923
puncture, in hydrocephaly, 228
ribs, 933
LUNG, 604-617
(*See also* Pulmonary)
accessory, 607-608
agenesis
bilateral, and aplasia, 604-605
definition, 604
unilateral, 605-606
unilateral, associated malformations, 606
unilateral, diagnosis, 606
unilateral, prognosis, 606
unilateral, treatment, 606
vitamin A deficiency causing (in rat), 605, 607
angioma, 615
anomalies, and tumors, 1221
aplasia (*see* Aplasia)
cyst (*see* Cyst, pulmonary)
fused lobes, 608-609
hamartoma, 615
hypoplasia (*see* Hypoplasia)
in rubella syndrome, 65
sequestration and abnormal pulmonary artery, 609-610
supernumerary, 607-608
supernumerary fissures, 608-609
teratoma, 1242
tumors, 615-616
LUTEINIZING HORMONE: and testicular feminization syndrome, 1115
LYMPH VESSELS, 1181-1184
LYMPHANGIECTASIA, 1183
cystic, 613
LYMPHANGIOMA, 1181-1183
mouth, 667
simplex, 1181
LYMPHATICS: hypoplasia, in Turner syndrome, 1126
LYMPHEDEMA
congenital hereditary, 1183-1184
in Turner syndrome, 1126
LYMPHOID POLYPOSIS: benign, 715

M

MACEWEN SIGN: in hydrocephaly, 227
MACRENCEPHALY, 244-246
cerebral hypertrophy and, 244
differential diagnosis, 228, 245
intrauterine growth retardation and, 138
mild, 245
three varieties of, 245
MACROCRANIA
in gigantism, cerebral, 173
in osteoectasia, familial, 862
MACRODACTYLY, 984
second toe, 985
MACROGENITOSOMIA PRAECOX, 1110-1111
pineal tumors and, 451
MACROGLOSSIA, 662-663
exomphalos and, 663
muscular, types, 662-663
visceromegaly and, 171
MACROGNATHIA, 622
MACROSTOMIA, 623-624
mandibulofacial dysostosis and, unilateral, 654
MACULA
degeneration, hereditary, 379
dysplasia, 379
dystrophy, 379
MADELUNG DEFORMITY, 790-791
MAFFUCCI SYNDROME, 882-884
etiology, 882
hands in, 883
history, 882
knees in, 883
pathogenesis, 882-883
tumors and, 1237
MALADIE DE ROGER, 489
MALFORMATIONS
(*See also specific sites*)
Arnold-Chiari (*see* Arnold-Chiari malformation)
chemical, 24, 26
congenital
bicornuate uterus and, 21
deaths due to, 42
definition, 3
"determination period," 49
differentiated from anomalies, 3
endogenous, 24
exogenous, 24
extrauterine pregnancy and, 21
inherited, 57-58
natural screening and, 40-42
nutritional deficiencies causing, 23
as portents, 7-12
prevention, 27
"termination period," 49
developmental, definition, 5
Ebstein (*see* Ebstein malformation)
synchronisms of, 45
syntropisms of, 45
tumors and, 1197-1247
MALLEUS, 405
MALNUTRITION, MATERNAL
effects on fetus, 30
congenital malformations due to, 23
intrauterine growth retardation and, 147, 152
MALOCCLUSION: in cretinism, 111
MALROTATION
intestine (*see* Intestine)
kidney, 1053
MANDIBLE
absence, 621
cerebro-costo-mandibular syndrome, 658
clefts, 626
hypervitaminosis A causing (in mice), 626
development, 634
in osteopetrosis, 865
in Pierre Robin syndrome, 657
MANDIBULOFACIAL DYSOSTOSIS, 650-654
clefts and, 645
coloboma in, 355
development, 650-651
diagnosis, 652-653
ear in, 411, 652
epibulbar dermoids and (*see* Goldenhar syndrome)
familial, 650
first branchial arch in, 650
mandible in, 652
micrognathia in, 652
nasal development failure and, 587
pedigree in, 651
respiratory difficulties in, 653
sex and racial distribution, 650
skull in, 651-652
unilateral, 624, 653-654
associated malformations, 654
clinical characteristics, 653
scoliosis in, 653
Weyers (*see* unilateral *above*)
MANGANESE: and ataxia, 26
MARBLE BONES (*see* Osteopetrosis)
MARCHESANI SYNDROME, 395
MARFAN SYNDROME, 850-857
arachnodactyly in, 377
cardiovascular malformations and, 571-572, 855
chromosome anomalies in, 852
CNS in, 855
diagnosis, 853
feet in, 854
hands in, 854
heterochromia and, 371
history, 850
incidence, 851
inheritance in, 851-852
intestinal malrotation and, 692
lens in, 377
dislocation, 851
necropsy study, 852-853
respiratory system in, 855
in twins, 852
undescended testes in, 1099
XYY karyotype and, 1144
MARINESCO-SJÖGREN SYNDROME, 392
development in, 392
heredity in, 392
intrauterine growth retardation and, 138-139

MASCULINIZATION
estrogen causing, 100
incomplete, with 3β-hydroxysteroid dehydrogenase deficiency, 1117
progesterone causing, 100
MATERNAL DISORDERS: and etiology, 102-129
MATERNAL IMPRESSIONS, 12-15
MAXILLA
absence, 621
cyst, 666
McCUNE-ALBRIGHT SYNDROME: and pigmentations, 1169
MEASLES
German (*see* Rubella)
teratogenesis and, 77
MECKEL DIVERTICULUM (*see* Diverticula)
MECLIZINE, 99
phocomelia and, 88
MECONIUM ILEUS
cystic fibrosis and, 734
intestinal loops in, 694
MEDIASTINUM
anomalies due to neurenteric connection anomalies, 700-701
cysts, 700
bronchogenic, 603
hemangioma, 616
teratoma, 1240
MEDULLOBLASTOMA, 1212-1213
malignancy of, 1214
sex distribution, 1213
MEGACOLON, 704
associated malformations, 705
constipation in, 707-708
etiology, series, 705-706
familial, 704-705
functional, 705
incidence, 704
sex distribution, 704
surgery, 708
treatment, conservative, 708
MEGACYSTIS SYNDROME, MEGA-URETER, 1071-1072
MEGALENCEPHALY (*see* Macrencephaly)
MEGALOCORNEA, 367
MEGALODACTYLY, 984
second toe, 985
MEGA-URETER, 1070-1072
hydro-ureter and, 1070-1071
incidence, 1070
megacolon and, 705
-megacystis syndrome, 1071-1072
simple, 1071
MEGA-URETHRA, 1081-1082
MELANIN PIGMENTATION: and intestinal polyposis, 665
MELANOCYTIC NEVI, 1168
MELANOMA: congenital malignant, 1170
MELENA
in intestinal duplications, 698
neonatorum, and esophageal ulcer, 684
MELORHEOSTOSIS, 884-885
clinical characteristics, 884
complaints in, 884
history, 884
osseous changes in, 885
MELOTIA: and synotia, 402
MENDEL: on teratology, 19
MENINGOCELE, 920
anterior, 283
clinical characteristics, 920
cranial, 211, 889
location of, 212
definition, 272, 273
intrathoracic, 283
neurofibromatosis and, 920
lumbar, 283
neurofibromatosis and, Recklinghausen, 1258
nose, 590
pedunculated, and hemangioma, 212 (in rat), 213
sacral, 920
symptoms, 286
uncomplicated, surgery of, 289
vertebra in, 920
MENINGOMYELOCELE (*see* Myelomeningocele)
MENTAL COMPLICATIONS: in cardiovascular malformations, 570
MENTAL DEFICIENCY
in basal cell nevi syndrome, 1269
muscular hypertrophy and extrapyramidal motor disturbances, 1030-1031
MENTAL DEVELOPMENT
in cretinism, 115-116
in Down syndrome, 325-326
MENTAL "MODIFICATION": of expectant mothers, 13
MENTAL RETARDATION, 262-266
autosomal abnormalities and, 263-264
aortic stenosis and, supravalvar, 579
bifid thumb and, 981
brain defects in, 262-263
chromosomal aberrations and, 263
deletions, 58
sex chromosome, 264
in Cockayne syndrome, 398
in cretinism, 111
endemic, 263
in cytomegalic inclusion disease, 72
dystrophia myotonica and, 1032
in gigantism, cerebral, 173
heart disease and, 570
in hemihypertrophy, 165
in Hurler syndrome, 813
intrauterine growth retardation and, 138
in Laurence-Moon-Biedl syndrome, 44, 178
in Lowe syndrome, 389
lower extremity anomalies and, 1008
in maternal phenylketonuria, 126
megacolon and, 705
microcephaly and, 240
in microphthalmia, 357
in neurofibromatosis, Recklinghausen, 1256
porencephaly and, 247-248
in Prader-Willi syndrome, 182
pseudoglioma and, 398
in pseudohypoparathyroidism, 447
in pseudo-pseudohypoparathyroidism, 448
radiation damage and, 82
retinitis pigmentosa and, 379
right-sided aortic arch and facial anomalies, 580
in rubella syndrome, 45, 263
in Sturge-Weber syndrome, 349, 351
in syndrome of multiple anomalies, 902
Turner syndrome and, 264
MERCURY
compounds, causing anomalies, 27
methyl, 128
MEROACRANIA: definition, 889
MERO-ANENCEPHALY, 195, 197
MERORACHISCHISIS, 920
MESENCHYME
in osteogenesis imperfecta, 825
tumors, 1236
MESENCHYMOMA, 1236
MESENTERIC ATTACHMENT ANOMALIES, 692
MESENTERIC CYSTS, 703-704
MESENTERIC-OMPHALO SINUS, 762
MESOBLASTIC NEPHROMA, 1065, 1228
MESODERMAL DYSGENESIS: of eye, 371
METABOLISM
disturbances, and cardiovascular malformations, 574-576
inborn errors of, 26
mucopolysaccharidoses and, 808
METACARPAL DWARFISM (*see* Pseudo-pseudohypoparathyroidism)
METACARPALS: fusion, 900
METALS: in endemic goiter, 107-108
METAPHYSEAL DYSOSTOSIS, 786, 789, 791-792, 1002
METAPHYSEAL DYSPLASIA, FAMILIAL (*see* Pyle disease)
METATARSAL AMPUTATION: and ankyloglossia, 661
METATROPIC DWARFISM, 803-804
development in, 803
METHOTREXATE: malformations due to, 97
METHYL MERCURY, 128
METHYL SALICYLATE
anophthalmia due to (in rat), 360
bifid rib due to (in rat), 917
craniorachischisis due to (in rat), 194, 195
exencephaly due to (in rat), 359
hydrocephaly due to (in rat), 222-223
infundibulum abnormality due to (in rat), 422
microphthalmia due to (in rat), 359
omphalocele (exomphalos) due to (in rat), 194, 760
pituitary abnormality due to (in rat), 422
scoliosis due to (in rat), 917
vertebral anomalies due to (in rat), 931
MEYENBURG COMPLEXES, 725
MICRENCEPHALY: in cytomegalic inclusion disease, 72
MICROCEPHALY, 237-244
in cat-cry syndrome, 341
in cephalocele and, 213
cerebral palsy and, 238
chromosome anomalies and, 240, 343
clefts and, 644-645
palate, 240, 241, 348
contractures and, 238
craniotomy in, 242-243
cutis verticis gyrata and, 1193
in cytomegalic inclusion disease, 72, 73, 239
differential diagnosis, 893
dwarfism and ring-1 chromosome, 343
encephalocele and, nasofrontal, 215
etiology, 238-242
familial, 239
genetics of, 26, 239
genital anomalies and, 348
intrauterine growth retardation and, 136-138
mental retardation and, 240
microphthalmia and, 241

olfactory deficiency and, 210
pathology, 242
pedigrees in, 239
petit mal and, 238
phenylketonuria and, 240
radiation causing, 82, 239
(in rat), 241
rubella causing, 239
speech defect and, 240
symptoms, 242-243
toxoplasmosis and, 79, 239
trisomy and, 240
MICROCORNEA, 367
MICRODACTYLY, 976
MICROGLOSSIA, 661-662
MICROGNATHIA, 621-622
clefts and, 644
in Cornelia de Lange syndrome, 345
glossoptosis and (*see* Pierre Robin syndrome)
mandibular, 622
familial, 622
mandibulofacial dysostosis and, 652
maxillary, 621-622
microstomia and, 623
in progeria, 160
splenic-gonadal fusion and, 749
in syndrome of multiple anomalies, 1026
in trisomy 18, 306
Turner syndrome and, 1123, 1127
MICROGYRIA
in cytomegalic inclusion disease, 72
myelocystocele and, 281
in syndrome of multiple anomalies, 1075
MICROMELIA
in dwarfism, 768, 770
hypoplasia of ulna and fibula and, 792
MICROMYELIA: in anencephaly, 196
MICROPENIS, 1103
MICROPHAKIA: in Marchesani syndrome, 395
MICROPHTHALMIA, 356-361
cataract and, 373
ectodermal dysplasia and, 1167
incidence, 357
maternal vitamin A deficiency and, 127
methyl salicylate causing (in rat), 359
microcephaly and, 241
nasal development fault and, 588
oculodentodigital dysplasia and, 388
parietal foramina enlargement and, 891
pedigree, 358
pure, 357
radiation causing (in rat), 359
in rubella syndrome, 64, 65, 66
streptonigrin causing (in rat), 360
thalidomide embryopathy and, 94
toxoplasmosis and, 80
in trisomy 13-15, 298, 301
MICROSOMIA
fetal, 134
hemifacial, 624
MICROSTOMIA, 623
in craniocarpotarsal dystrophy, 673
hypervitaminosis A causing (in mice), 624
MICROTIA
atresia of external meatus and, 401
uncomplicated hereditary, 401
MIDGUT: development, 690-691
MILIA: and dermal ridge absence, 1196
MILROY DISEASE, 1183-1184
MINAMATA DISEASE, 128-129
MIRROR IMAGE
dextrocardia, 478
right aortic arch and, 531
MITOTIC NONDISJUNCTION, 61
MITRAL VALVE
atresia, 510
incidence, 510
pathology, 510
prognosis, 510
duplication, 510-511
malformations, 509-511
stenosis (*see* Stenosis)
MÖBIUS SYNDROME, 397-398
clubfoot and, 397
cranial nerves in, 397
history, 397
intrauterine growth retardation and, 142
MOLE: hairy, 1170-1171
MOLECULAR GENETICS, 26
MONGOLIAN BLUE SPOT, 1171
MONGOLISM (*see* Down syndrome)
MONKEY HEAD (*see* Cebocephaly)
MONODACTYLY: and phocomelia, 952
MONORCHIA, 1098
MONOSOMY G (antimongolism), 58, 339
intrauterine growth retardation and, 146
MONSTER: derivation of word, 12
MONTAIGNE: on monsters, 12
MOON FACE: in cat-cry syndrome, 341
MORBILLI: and teratogenesis, 77
MORQUIO DISEASE, 819-821
clinical manifestations, 820
differential diagnosis, 821
familial, 819
radiography, 821
MORQUIO-ULLRICH SYNDROME, 817-819
chondroitin sulfate in, 818
cornea in, 817, 818
MORTALITY
in leukemia, 1207
in liver cancer, 1223
MOSAICISM, 59
in Down syndrome, 319-320, 321
in triploidy, 343
MOUTH, 661-672
atresia, 668
choristoma, 667
in Cornelia de Lange syndrome, 345
cyst, 666
dermoids, 667
epulis, 667
hamartoma, 667
hemangioma, 667
leukoplakia (*see* Leukoplakia)
lymphangioma, 667
malformations
oro-gastrointestinal tract, 659-735
riboflavin deficiency causing (in rat), 639
syndromes involving, 673-677
mucosal pigmentation and polyposis, 714
myoblastoma, 667
in otocephaly, 621
sclerosis, tuberous, 667
teratoid parasites, 668
in trisomy 18, 305
tumors, 667-668
teratoid, 1241-1242
MUCOIDS, 594
MUCOPOLYSACCHARIDOSES, 808-824
MUCOVISCIDOSIS (*see* Fibrosis, cystic, pancreas)
MULTIPLE BIRTH
incidence of anomalies in, 39
intrauterine growth retardation and, 151
MULTIPLE ENDOCRINE NEOPLASIAS, 1269-1271
MULTIPLE PREGNANCY (*see* Multiple birth)
MUMPS: and teratogenesis, 77
MURMUR: of patent ductus arteriosus, 557-558
MUSCLES, 1023-1033
abdominal (*see* Abdomen, muscles)
absence, 1025-1028
incidence, 1025
anomalies, 1023-1033
aplasia, 1025
in cretinism, endemic, 113
dystrophy (*see* Dystrophy, muscular)
gastric musculature defect, 688
hypertrophy
extrapyramidal motor disturbances and mental deficiency, 1030-1031
in hypothyroidism, 1030
hypoplasia, 1025
palmaris, longus, 1026
pectoralis
absence, 1026
absence, and cutaneous webs, 1190
defects, 1025
stapedius, tendon of, 406
sternocleidomastoid, 1026
torticollis (*see* Torticollis)
trapezius, 1026
MUTAGENESIS, 61
MUTATION, 25
MUTON, 25
MYELOCYSTOCELE, 279
(*See also* Hydromyelia)
cloaca exstrophy and, 287
definition, 272, 273
pathology, 284
in syndrome of multiple anomalies, 281, 1077
MYELODYSPLASIA
discussion of term, 292-293, 294
familial osseous atrophy and, 295
manifestations, 294
in spina bifida, 282
streptonigrin causing (in rat), 293
trypan blue causing (in rat), 293
MYELOMENINGOCELE
aqueduct stenosis and, 285
bladder exstrophy and, 1075
cervical, symptoms, 287-288
craniolacunia and, 890
cyclopia and, 204
definition, 272, 273
head in, 288
hydrocephaly and, 220-222, 285
laterodorsal, and rib agenesis, 281
morphogenesis, 280-281
myeloschisis conversion into, 279
pathology, 283-284
prognosis, 288
sacrolumbar, 593
sagittal section, 280
symptoms, 286-288
in syndrome with multiple anomalies, 286

MYELOMENINGOCELE (*cont.*)
treatment, 288
in trisomy 18, 305
MYELOSCHISIS, 920
conversion to myelomeningocele, 279
in embryos, 39
epithelization and, 285
hypervitaminosis A causing (in rat), 280
pathology, 284
(in rat), 275-276, 280
thoracolumbar, 198
MYENTERIC PLEXUS: and ganglion cells, 706
MYLERAN (*see* Busulfan)
MYOBLASTOMA: mouth, 667
MYOCARDIUM
hypoplasia due to vitamin A deficiency (in pig), 471
in rubella syndrome, 64
MYODYSTROPHIA FOETALIS DEFORMANS (*see* Arthrogryposis)
MYOPIA
pedigree in, 366
in rubella syndrome, 65
MYOSITIS OSSIFICANS PROGRESSIVA, 975, 976
clinical characteristics, 976
MYXEDEMA IN CRETINISM, 112
sporadic, 440
MYXOMA: heart, 1220

N

NAGASAKI STUDY: of radiation damage to fetus, 82
NAIL(s)
hypoplasia, in ectodermal dysplasia, 1163
-patella syndrome (*see* Dysplasia, osteo-onycho)
in trisomies, 301, 308
in Turner syndrome, 1125
NANOSOMIA: fetal, 149
NATURAL SCREENING: and congenital malformations, 40-42
NATURAL SELECTION, 41
NECK
in Cornelia de Lange syndrome, 345
in Down syndrome, 327-328
hygroma, cystic, 1182
short, in basilar impression, 908
thymic remnants in, 741
in trisomy 18, 305
in Turner syndrome, 1127
webbing in male Turner syndrome, 1131-1132
NECROSIS: secondary, 51
NEGROES: polydactyly in, 40
NEOPLASIA (*see* Cancer, Tumors)
endocrine (*see* Endocrines, neoplasia)
NEPHRITIS
deafness and, 1059
inheritance in, 1058
in rubella syndrome, 66
NEPHROBLASTOMA: bilateral, 1062
NEPHROMA: mesoblastic, 1065, 1228
NEPHRONOPHTHISIS: familial juvenile, 1060
NEPHROSCLEROSIS: inheritance in, 1058
NEPHROSIS: inheritance in, 1058
NERVES
cranial
in Möbius syndrome, 397
in Recklinghausen neurofibromatosis, 1254
in cretinism, endemic, 113
deafness and, 406
hypoplasia, 379-380
myelinated fibers in retina, 378
olfactory, absence, and harelip, 625
optic
aplasia, 379-380
atrophy, 380
glioma, 380
NERVOUS SYSTEM (*see* Central nervous system)
NEURENTERIC CANAL: persistence, 700
NEURENTERIC CONNECTIONS: abnormalities causing intestinal and mediastinal malformations, 700-701
NEUROBLASTOMA, 1223-1225
intrauterine growth retardation and, 142
sex distribution, 1224
NEUROCUTANEOUS SYNDROME, 351
NEUROFIBROMATOSIS
acoustic, 1255
café au lait spots and, 1169
"central," 1255-1256
cornea in, 368
cutaneous, 1253
differential diagnosis, 881
eye in, 382
generalized, 1253
meningocele and, intrathoracic, 920
multiple, 1252
plexiform, 1255
Recklinghausen, 1237, 1252-1260
café au lait spots and, 1253-1254
chromaffin adrenal tumors and, 1256-1257
cranial nerves in, 1254
endocrine disorders and, 1256
familial, 1252
incidence, 1252
kyphoscoliosis and, 1257
malignancy of, 1259
meningocele and, 1258
mental retardation in, 1256
sex distribution, 1252
in twins, 1252-1253
ulnar pseudarthrosis and, 1257
NEUROFIBROSARCOMA, 1258
NEUROLOGIC COMPLICATIONS: in cardiovascular malformations, 570
NEUROMUSCULAR (*see* Muscles, Nerves)
NEUROPATHY
mercurial compounds causing, 27
sensory, anhidrosis, 1167
NEVI
basal cell, multiple, 1169
basal cell syndrome, 1268-1269
clinical characteristics, 1268
mental deficiency in, 1269
soft tissue tumors and, 1237
tumor formation in, 1269
bathing-trunk, 1170
blue, 1171
rubber-bleb syndrome, 1185
Cannon, 665
flammeus, 1179-1180
clinical characteristics, 1179
incidence, 1180
inheritance in, 1180
osteohypertrophy and, 1180
in visceromegaly, 172
linear sebaceus, of face, 1194
melanocytic, 1168
pigmented, 1168-1170
clinical characteristics in, 1168
in hemihypertrophy, 163
inheritance in, 1168-1169
in Turner syndrome, 1128-1129
pilosus, 1170-1171
"port-wine," 1177
in Sturge-Weber syndrome, 350
spider, 1181
in thalidomide embryopathy, 92
unis lateralis, 1175-1176
hemihypertrophy and, 1175
vasculosus, 1176-1179
osteohypertrophy and, 1180
white sponge, 665
NICOTENIC ACID: and congenital malformations (in animals), 35
NICOTINAMIDE ANTAGONIST, 35
NIPPLES: in Turner syndrome, 1127
NITROGEN MUSTARD, 33
NONDISJUNCTION
environmental factors in, 60
mitotic, 61
NONNE-MILROY-MEIGE DISEASE, 1183-1184
NORETHISTERONE: virilizing effects of, 100
NORETHYNODREL: virilizing effects of, 100
NORRIE DISEASE, 398
NOSE, 587-596
(*See also* Proboscis)
absence (history), 10
anomalies, bronchiectasis and situs inversus, 602-603
aplasia, 587
in arhinencephaly, 587-589
bifid, 589, 591
in arhinencephaly, 207, 209
cavity
formation, diagram, 635
malformation, riboflavin deficiency causing (in rat), 639
morphogenesis, 634
in cebocephaly, 207
clefts (*see* Clefts, nasal)
cysts, 666
dermoid, 593-594
development failure, 587
microphthalmia and, 588
in Down syndrome, 327
duplication, 589, 591
in arhinencephaly, 207-209
encephalocele, 215-216, 592-593
glioma, 591
meningocele, 590
saddle, 594
in ectodermal dysplasia, anhidrotic, 1166
in trisomy 13-15, 595
NOSOLOGIC THEORY: in teratogenesis, 22
NOSTRIL
absence, 587
in Cornelia de Lange syndrome, 345
NOTOCHORD, 927
NUCLEAR AGENESIS: in Möbius syndrome, 397
NUTRITION
deficiencies (*see* Malnutrition)

teratology and (in animals), 30

O

OBESITY
in Cushing syndrome, 434
in Laurence-Moon-Biedl syndrome, 44, 177
parietal foramina enlargement and, 891
in Prader-Willi syndrome, 182-183
in syndrome of multiple anomalies, 902
OCCIPITAL FORAMINA, 892
OCCIPITALIZATION: of atlas, 908-909
OCULAR (*see* Eye)
OCULOAURICULOVERTEBRAL SYNDROME (*see* Goldenhar syndrome)
OCULOCEREBRORENAL SYNDROME (*see* Lowe syndrome)
OCULODENTODIGITAL DYSPLASIA, 388-389
OCULO-DIGITAL SYNDROME OF FRANCESCHETTI: and rubella syndrome, 65
"OCULOVERTEBRAL" SYNDROME, 358
ODONTOID PROCESS: absence, 908
OLFACTORY DEFICIENCY: and microcephaly, 210
OLIGODACTYLY, 963, 974-976
OLIGONEPHRONIC HYPOPLASIA, 1041
OLIGOPHRENIA: polydystrophic, 817
OLIGURIA, 454
OLLIER DISEASE (dyschondroplasia), 872-874
clinical manifestations, 873
differential diagnosis, 881
history, 872
humerus, radius and ulna in, 873
in Maffucci syndrome, 882-884
pathology in, 873
OMENTAL CYSTS, 703
OMPHALOCELE (EXOMPHALOS), 758-761
amelia and, total, 949
in antiquity, 10
chromosomal anomalies and, 759
clinical characteristics, 758
cyclopia and, 203
exstrophia splanchnica and, 713
incidence, 758-759
intestinal malrotation and, 692
large, 759
macroglossia and, 663
methyl salicylate causing (in rat), 194, 760
prognosis, 760
size of, 759
small, 759
streptonigrin causing (in rat), 717, 761
surgery, 760
visceromegaly and, 171, 759
OMPHALO-ENTERIC DUCT, 762
OMPHALO-MESENTERIC SINUS, 762
ONCOGENIC FACTORS: in tumors, 1203-1204
ONYCHO-OSTEO DYSPLASIA (*see* Dysplasia, osteo-onycho)
OPTIC DISC
coloboma, 379
crescents, 379
OPTIC NERVE (*see* Nerves)
ORAL (*see* Mouth)
ORBIT
absence, and Recklinghausen neurofibromatosis, 1258
cyst, 365
vitamin A causing (in rat), 365
teratoma, 1242
ORODIGITOFACIAL SYNDROME, 674-676
clefts and, 644
clinical characteristics, 674
inheritance, 676
polycystic disease and, 725
radiography, 674-675
sex distribution, 675
treatment, 676
OSSEOUS ATROPHY, familial, 295
prognosis, 295
OSTEOARTHRITIS
in dysplasia epiphysealis multiplex, 789
endemica, 807
OSTEOARTHROPATHY
familial idiopathic (*see* hypertrophic hereditary *below*)
hypertrophic hereditary, 848-850
finger clubbing in, 848-849
heart disease and, cyanotic, 849
pedigree in, 849
OSTEOCHONDRAL EPIPHYSEOPATHY, 807
OSTEOCHONDROARTHROSIS DEFORMANS, 807
OSTEOCHONDRODYSTROPHY
deformans, 805
hereditary (*see* Morquio disease)
OSTEOCHONDROMA, 1238
OSTEOCHONDROSIS: Blount, deformans tibiae, 1001-1002
OSTEODYSTROPHY OF ALBRIGHT (*see* Pseudo-pseudohypoparathyroidism)
OSTEOECTASIA: familial, and macrocranium, 862
OSTEOGENESIS IMPERFECTA, 824-836
(*See also* Osteopsathyrosis)
deafness in, 829
dentinogenesis imperfecta and, 831
differential diagnosis, 861
gravis, 824
sporadic, 827
history, 824
inheritance in, 825
intrauterine growth retardation and, 142
mesenchyme in, 825
osteosarcoma and, 832
pedigrees in, 825-826
sclera in, 825, 829
severe semilethal, in sisters, 828
skull in, 830
tarda, 824
OSTEOHYPERTROPHY: and nevi, 1180
OSTEOMA, 1238
OSTEO-ONYCHO DYSPLASIA (*see* Dysplasia, osteo-onycho)
OSTEOPATHIA
condensans disseminata, 846
hyperostotica sclerotisans, 844-846
biopsies in, 845
sclerosis in, 845
OSTEOPETROSIS, 863-869
acro-osteolytica, 869
anemia in, 865
benign, differential diagnosis, 867-868
calcium in, 865-866
diagnosis, 865
fractures in, 866
hematoma in, subdural, 866
hepatosplenomegaly in, 865
history, 863
Hodgkin disease and, 866
hydrocephaly and, 864
inheritance in, 863
mandible in, 865
phosphorus in, 865-866
(in rabbit), 863
rickets and, 866
sarcoma and, 866
types, 863
vertebra in, 864
OSTEOPOIKILOSIS, 846
OSTEOPSATHYROSIS, 824-826
(*See also* Osteogenesis imperfecta)
extremities in, 833
fractures in, 829, 832
idiopathic, 825
legs in, 831
pedigree in, 834
prognosis, eugenic, 834
skull in, 832
tarda, 825
OSTEOSARCOMA, 1238
fragilis generalisata (*see* Osteopetrosis)
osteogenesis imperfecta and, 832
in osteopetrosis, 863
OSTEOSIS EBURNISANS MONOMELICA (*see* Melorheostosis)
OSTIUM
persistent atrioventriculare commune, 485-486
pathology, 485
symptoms, 485-486
treatment, 486
primum, 483
in Down syndrome, 577
secundum, 482-483
OTOCEPHALY (SYNOTIA), 402
face in, 621
melotia and, 402
mouth in, 621
streptonigrin causing (in rat), 622
OTOPALATODIGITAL SYNDROME, 677
clefts and, 644
OVA
fertilization of, 55
overripeness of, 27, 59
OVARIES, 1085-1087
absence, 1085
accessory, 1086-1087
deficiencies, and chromosomal anomalies, 1086
in hermaphrodism, true, 1105
hypoplasia, 1085-1086
in Turner syndrome, 1086
in leprechaunism, 159
supernumerary, 1086-1087
teratoma, 1229, 1239-1240
tumors, 1229
OVOCYTES: overripeness of, 59
OXYCEPHALY (*see* Acrocephaly)
OXYGEN
consumption in Down syndrome, 332
in transposition of great vessels, 523

P

PACHYDERMOPERIOSTOSIS, 848
PACHYONYCHIA CONGENITA, 665, 1161

Palate
anomalies
ectodermal dysplasia and, 1167
in syndrome of multiple anomalies, 1190
clefts (*see* Clefts)
in Crouzon craniofacial dysostosis, 903
cysts, 666
development, and clefts, 633-636
in gigantism, cerebral, 173
in hemihypertrophy, 164
high
in acrocephalosyndactyly, 645
lip pit and, 627
in syndrome of multiple anomalies, 895
normal closure of, 636
in orodigitofacial syndrome, 675
otopalatodigital syndrome, 677
clefts and, 644
Turner syndrome and, 1123
Palm
in cat-cry syndrome, 341
dermatoglyphics in heart disease, 578
Palmaris Longus Muscle: agenesis, 1026
Palsy, Cerebral, 255-262
associated malformations, 258
chromosomal aberrations and, 259-260
differentiation of prenatal, perinatal and postnatal, 257
diplegia and, 259
etiology, 256-257
heredity in, 259
incidence, 255
intrauterine growth retardation and, 138
low birth weight and, 258
microcephaly and, 238
pathogenesis, 256-257
prematurity in, 256
prenatal factors in, 255-256
Rh incompatibility and, 260
Pancreas, 729-735
absence, 716
annular, 730-731
associated malformations, 731
development, 730-731
intestinal atresia and, 695
surgery, 731
aplasia, complete, 730
cyst, solitary, 730
cystic fibrosis (*see* Fibrosis, cystic, pancreas)
cystosis, 730
development, 729
DL-ethionine and (in rat), 733
ectopia, 730
hypoplasia (*see* Lipomatosis)
in leprechaunism, 159
lipomatosis (*see* Lipomatosis)
malformations, 729-731
in multiple endocrine neoplasia, 1269-1270
overgrowth, and visceromegaly, 171
tumors, 731
Pancytopenia: Fanconi type, 1020
Papilloma
choroid plexus, and hydrocephaly, 219
larynx, 597
Papillon-Léage and Psaume Syndrome (*see* Orodigitofacial syndrome)
Paralysis: sympathetic, and heterochromia, 370
Parathyroid, 445-450
absence, 445-448
agenesis, 740
development, 445
in multiple endocrine neoplasia, 1269-1270
thymo-parathyroid aplasia, 740
Parchment Heart, 477
Parental Counseling, 27
in hydrocephaly, 228
Parietal Bones: flattening, 889
Parietal Foramina: enlarged, 891-892
Parity: in anencephaly, 190
Parotitis: and teratogenesis, 77
Patella
absence, 998
hypoplasia, 998
nail-patella syndrome (*see* Dysplasia, osteo-onycho)
Patent Ductus Arteriosus (*see* Ductus arteriosus)
Pectoralis
absence, 1026
cutaneous webs and, 1190
defects, 1025
Pectus
carinatum (*see* Breast, pigeon)
excavatum (*see* Chest, funnel)
Pedunculated Postminimi, 982-983
Pelvis, 938
changes in achondroplasia, 776
in chondromatosis, 875
in Down syndrome, 329-330
lower extremity malformations and, 938
Pendred Syndrome, 442
deafness in, 407
Penetrance Expressivity: of genes, 57
Penis
absence, 1103
anomalies,
clefts and, 644
XO/XY mosaicism in, 1118
cleft, 1104
double, 697, 1104
torsion, 1103
transposition of penis and scrotum, 1104
in Turner syndrome, male, 1133
Penta-X, 1140-1141
Pentothenic Acid
congenital malformations and, 35
deficiency causing cardiovascular malformations (in mammals), 471
Pericardium: teratoma, 1242
Pericardo-Diaphragmatic Hernia, 756
Perineum: without anal opening, 710
Perodactyly, 939, 945, 963, 974-976
Peromelia, 939, 954-955
forearm absence in, 954-955
hand absence in, 954-955
of one arm, 954
stumps of both upper arms, 954
Pes Equinovarus, 998-999
Petit Mal: and microcephaly, 238
Peutz-Jeghers Syndrome, 665
Peutz Syndrome, 714
Phakoma: and tuberous sclerosis, 1263
Phakomatoses, 351, 1251
Phalangeal-Tricho-Rhino Syndrome, 1020
Phalanx (*see* Finger)
Pharyngeal Pituitary, 421
trypan blue causing (in rat), 422
Pharynx
anomalies, syndromes involving, 673-677
atresia, 668
development, 668-669
diverticula, 670-671
pouches, 670-671
syndrome of (DiGeorge) and thymic agenesis, 740
tumors, teratoid, 1241-1242
Phenocopy, 26
Phenotype, 25
Phenylketonuria, 125-126
microcephaly and, 240
Phenytoin: cleft palate due to (in mice), 98
Pheochromocytoma, 435, 1226-1227
familial, 1227
multiple endocrine neoplasia and, 1270
sex distribution, 1226
Phimosis, 1103-1104
Phlebectasia, 1180-1181
Phocomelia, 939, 951-954
complete, 951
etiology, 951-952
inheritance in, 952
meclizine and, 88
monodactyly and, 952
riboflavin deficiency causing (in rat), 953
thalidomide and, 84
thrombocytopenia and hypoplastic, 941
leukemoid reactions in, 952
Phosphatase
in Albright disease, 879
in fibrous dysplasia of bone, 876
in hypophosphatasia, 859
Phosphoethanolamine: in hypophosphatasia, 859
Phosphorus: in osteopetrosis, 865-866
Pierre Robin Syndrome, 654-657
associated malformations, 655
cardiovascular, 572
clefts and, 645
etiology, 655
familial, 655
pedigree in, 656, 657
Pigeon Breast (*see* Breast, pigeon)
Pigmentation
in Albright disease, 878-882
in McCune-Albright syndrome, 1169
melanin, and intestinal polyposis, 665, 1169
nevi (*see* Nevi)
oral mucosa, and gastrointestinal polyposis, 714
in skin lesions, 1168-1176
Pineal, 450-453
anatomy, 450
aplasia, 450
cyst, 452
development, 450
hyperplasia, 451
hypoplasia, 451
teratoma, 452
tumors, 451-452
sex distribution, 451
Pituitary, 419-426
abnormality due to methyl salicylate (in rat), 422
absence, 419-420

sodium salicylate causing (in rat), 419
anatomy, 419
in anencephaly, 196
in cretinism, endemic, 113
duplication, 420
dwarfism (*see* Dwarfism)
dystopia, 421-422
sodium salicylate causing (in rat), 430
hypoplasia, 420
in leprechaunism, 159
in multiple endocrine neoplasia, 1269-1270
pharyngeal, 421
trypan blue causing (in rat), 422
teratoma, 424
PLACENTA
infarction, 148
insufficiency, causing growth deficiency, 136
intrauterine, 147-149
previa, deformities of conceptuses in, 39
transplacental oncogenic experiments, 1204
PLAGIOCEPHALY: definition, 893
PLATYBASIA (*see* Basilar impression)
PLEIOTROPIC EFFECT: definition, 5
PLEONOSTEOSIS: Léri, 847
PLINY THE ELDER: on teratology, 18
PNEUMOENCEPHALOGRAPHY: of corpus callosum absence, 254
PNEUMONIA
in cytomegalic inclusion disease, 72
in rubella syndrome, 66
toxoplasmosis and, 79
PNEUMONITIS: in rubella syndrome, 64, 66
PNEUMOTHORAX, 684
POIKILODERMA CONGENITALE (*see* Rothmund-Thomson syndrome)
POISONING, MATERNAL
carbon monoxide, 128
lead, 129
POLAND SYNDROME, 963, 1025, 1026
clinical characteristics, 973
POLIOMYELITIS: and teratogenesis, 77
POLYCORIA, 372
POLYCYSTIC DISEASE
kidney (*see* Kidney, cystic disease)
liver (*see* Liver, polycystic)
POLYDACTYLY, 978-980, 1000
age and, 39-40
(in animals), 980
associated malformations, 902, 908, 1008, 1077
ano-rectal, 695
chondrodystrophy and heart disease, 794
imperforate anus, 710
cataract and, 375
in embryos, 39
endemic, and harelip, 979
exstrophia splanchnica and, 713
of high degree, 983-984
history, 979
incidence, 978
inheritance in, 979-980
in Laurence-Moon-Biedl syndrome, 44, 178-179
in Negroes, 40
-tibia reduction syndrome, 1000
in trisomy 13-15, 301
tumors and, 980
POLYDYSTROPHY
in dwarfism, 817
in oligophrenia, 817
POLYHYDRAMNIOS: and acrocephalosyndactyly, 894
POLYORCHIDISM, 1101
POLYPEPTIDES: and genetics, 25
POLYPHALANGISM, 967
POLYPLOIDY, 59
POLYPOSIS, 714-715
colon, 714-715
in Gardner syndrome, 1268
intestinal, 714
melanin pigmentation and, 665, 1169
lymphoid, benign, 715
stomach in, 689
POLYRHINIA, 591
POLYSPLENIA, 748
POLYSYMBRACHYDACTYLY: familial, 979
POMPE DISEASE (glycogen storage disease): and cardiovascular malformations, 575
POPLITEAL PTERYGIUM: and clefts, 643
PORENCEPHALY
air encephalography in, 247
anticonvulsants in, 248
brain defect in, 247
congenital, 246-248
discussion of term, 246, 247
origin of, 247
corpus callosum absence in, 247
hydrocephaly and, 247
mental retardation and, 247-248
(in rat), 248
treatment, 248
PORTAL HYPERTENSION (*see* Hypertension)
PORTAL VEIN (*see* Veins)
PORTENT(S)
derivation of word, 12
malformations as, 7-12
PORT-WINE HEMANGIOMA, 1177
in Sturge-Weber syndrome, 350
POSTENCEPHALITIC CHRONIC DISORDER, 79
POSTMATURITY: and anencephaly, 190
POSTMINIMI: pedunculated, 982-983
"POSTNATAL AMPUTATIONS," 295
POTTER SYNDROME, 1037
POTTER'S THUMB, 977
POTTS ANASTOMOSIS, 501
PRADER-WILLI SYNDROME, 182-183
undescended testes in, 1099
PRECOCIOUS PUBERTY, 454-456
craniopharyngioma causing, 455
etiology, 454
hamartoma and, 454-455
teratoma and, 454
PRECOCITY
isosexual, and hydrocephaly, 455
sexual
Albright disease and, 879
hereditary, 455-456
PREGNANCY
extrauterine, and congenital malformations, 21
multiple (*see* Multiple birth)
tetralogy of Fallot and, 500
toxemia, and intrauterine growth retardation, 147
twin (*see* Twins)
in uterine anomalies, 1090-1091
PRELUXATION: and hip dislocation, 994-995
PREMATURITY
anencephaly and, 190
cerebral palsy and, 256
congenital malformation incidence in, 39
definition, 134-135
incidence, 135
pseudoprematurity, 135
toxoplasmosis and, 80
PREPUCE, 1103-1104
absence, 1103
development, 1103
PROBOSCIS
(*See also* Nose)
bilateral, 589
in cyclopia, 203, 204
double, 589
in arhinencephaly, 207, 209
lateralis, 589
PRODIGY: derivation of word, 12
PROGERIA, 141, 160-162
etiology, 161
familial, 161
as metabolic disturbance, 161
pathogenesis, 161
PROGEROID SYNDROME, 141
PROGESTERONE
masculinizing, 100
pseudohermaphrodism and, female, 1112
as teratogen, 35
PROGNATHISM: in cerebral gigantism, 173
PROTEIN: and genetics, 25
PROTEINURIA: in Lowe syndrome, 389
PSEUDARTHROSIS
tibia, 1000-1001
ulna, and Recklinghausen neurofibromatosis, 1257
PSEUDOACHONDROPLASIA, 783-786
PSEUDOCOLOBOMA, 379
PSEUDOGLIOMA: and mental retardation, 398
"PSEUDOHEREDITY": in cretinism, 121
PSEUDOHERMAPHRODISM
androgen causing (in monkey), 100
female, 1094-1095, 1107-1112
androgen overproduction and, 1108
cortisone in, 1110
gonadal tumors and, 1232
history, 1107
C-11-hydroxylation and, 1108
C-21-hydroxylation and, 1108
incidence, 1107
inheritance in, 1107
nonadrenal, 1111-1112
nonadrenal, differential diagnosis, 1112
nonadrenal, etiology, 1111-1112
nonadrenal, incidence, 1111
progesterone and, 1112
virilization beginning after birth, 1110
male, 1110, 1111, 1113, 1118
chromosomal anomalies and, 1118
gonadal tumors and, 1232
internal, 1117
psychiatric complications in, 1113
46,XY karyotype, 1113
pedigree in, 1109
Smith-Lemli-Opitz syndrome and, 1121

PSEUDOHERMAPHRODISM (*cont.*)
in syndromes of multiple anomalies, 1119-1122
typus Rostockiensis and, 1120-1121
Ullrich-Feichtiger syndrome and, 1120-1121
vitamin A deficiency causing (in animals), 33
Wilms tumor and, 1118
PSEUDO-HIRSCHSPRUNG DISEASE, 705
PSEUDOHYDROCEPHALY, 245-246
PSEUDOHYPOPARATHYROIDISM, 446-448
brachymetacarpy and, 969
dihydrotachysterol in, 447
familial, 447
maternal, and ear of offspring, 414
mental retardation in, 447
symptoms, 447
treatment, 447-448
PSEUDOPREMATURITY, 135
PSEUDO-PSEUDOHYPOPARATHYROIDISM, 448
(*See also* Albright disease)
familial, 448
mental retardation in, 448
PSEUDOXANTHOMA, 382
elasticum, and cardiovascular malformations, 575
PSYCHOSIS: and hemihypertrophy, 165
PTEROYLGLUTAMIC ACID, 35
PTERYGIUM
colli, 1190
clinical characteristics, 1190-1191
history, 17
in syndrome of multiple anomalies, 1123
in Turner syndrome, 1125
in Turner syndrome, male, 1132
extremities, 1191
popliteal, and clefts, 643
syndromes, 1189-1192
review, 1132
PUBERTY (*see* Precocious puberty)
PULMONARY
arteries (*see* Arteries, pulmonary)
stenosis, 549-553
valve, absence, 549
veins (*see* Veins, pulmonary)
PUPIL, 371-372
ectopic, 372, 377
persistent pupillary membrane, 371-372
slit, 372
PUPPET SYNDROME, 349
PURINE, 25
PURKINJE CELLS: in ataxia-telangiectasia, 270-271
PURPURA
thrombocytopenic (*see* Thrombocytopenia)
toxoplasmosis and, 79
PYELOGRAPHY
hydro-ureter and hydronephrosis, 1071
urogenital anomalies, 1067
PYELONEPHRITIS: inheritance in, 1058
PYGOPAGUS: intestinal duplication in, 697
PYKNODYSOSTOSIS, 869-870
clinical manifestations, 869
course of, 869
history, 869
sex distribution, 869-870
PYLE DISEASE, 870-872
clinical characteristics, 870
history, 870
inheritance in, 870
prognosis, 870
PYLORIC STENOSIS (*see* Stenosis)
PYRIMIDINE, 25
PYURIA: in ureterocele, 1070

Q

QUADRIPLEGIA
in carbon monoxide poisoning, 128
in Minimata disease, 128
in rubella syndrome, 67
QUININE CAUSING MALFORMATIONS, 97
ear, 414

R

RACE
clefts and, 631-632
craniostenosis and, 894
Down's syndrome and, 40
harelip-cleft palate complex and, 40
incidence of anomalies and, 40
pyloric stenosis and, hypertrophic, 687
xeroderma pigmentosum and, 1173-1174
RACHISCHISIS, 919-920
clinical characteristics, 919-920
partial, and cranioschisis, 919
spina bifida and, 285
total, 920
vertebrae in, 920
RACHITIC PROCESS, 21
RADIATION
(*See also* X-Ray)
clefts due to, 632
palate (in rat), 35
cryptophthalmia due to (in rat), 359
etiology of malformations and, 82-84
exencephaly due to (in rat), 192-193
intrauterine growth retardation and, 149
lower extremity anomalies due to (in rat), 1003
malformations due to (in rat), 34
microcephaly due to, 239
(in rat), 241
microphthalmia due to (in rat), 359
RADIOIODINE: maternal use, causing goiter and hypothyroidism, 443
RADIO-ULNAR SYNOSTOSIS, 962, 985-986
RADIUS
absence, 953
in Cornelia de Lange syndrome, 345
aplasia
chromosomal anomalies and, 960
inheritance of, 960
defects, 960-961
dislocation, 961, 999
duplication, 961
in Ollier disease, 873
RAMSTED OPERATION: in pyloric stenosis, 688
RANULAE, 666
RATHKE-CLEFT CYST, 422-423, 1215
RATHKE POCKET, 419
RATHKE POUCH TUMORS, 1214-1215
RECKLINGHAUSEN NEUROFIBROMATOSIS (*see* Neurofibromatosis, Recklinghausen)
RECTOSIGMOID: removal in megacolon, 708
RECTO-URETHRAL FISTULA, 1084
RECTUM, MALFORMATIONS, 710-712
incidence, 710
inheritance in, 710
polydactyly and, 695
syndactyly and, 695
types, 711
REIFENSTEIN SYNDROME, 1117
RENAL (*see* Kidney)
RENDU-OSLER-WEBER SYNDROME, 1185
RESPIRATORY
difficulties
in mandibulofacial dysostosis, 653
in Pierre Robin syndrome, 654
distress, and aortic arch interruption, 533
system, in Marfan syndrome, 855
tract
malformations, 585-617
in trisomy 18, 306-307
tumors, 1221-1222
RETARDATION
growth (*see* Growth retardation)
intrauterine (*see* Intrauterine growth retardation)
mental (*see* Mental retardation)
RETICULOENDOTHELIOSES, 892
RETINA, 377-379
angiomatosis, in Hippel-Lindau disease, 1266
aplasia, 377
coloboma, 362
detachment, 377-378
chondrodystrophy and deafness, 804
myelinated nerve fibers in, 378
pigmentation (*see* Retinitis pigmentosa)
RETINITIS PIGMENTOSA, 378-379
in Cockayne syndrome, 398
deafness and, 379, 407
in Laurence-Moon-Biedl syndrome, 44, 177
RETINOBLASTOMA, 380-381, 1218-1219
pedigree in, 380, 381
RETINOSCHISIS: congenital, 378
RETROGNATHIA: in Pierre Robin syndrome, 655
RHABDOMYOMA
heart, 582, 1236
sclerosis and, tuberous, 1262-1263
RHABDOMYOSARCOMA, 1236
RH INCOMPATIBILITY: and cerebral palsy, 260
RHINO-TRICHO-PHALANGEAL SYNDROME, 1020
RIB(s)
agenesis, and myelomeningocele, 281
anomalies, 931-933
etiology, 930-931
heart disease and, 931
incidence, 931
methyl salicylate causing (in rat), 931
in syndrome of multiple anomalies, 932
bifid, due to methyl salicylate (in rat), 917
cervical, 931-933
sex distribution, 931
symptoms, 933
development, 930-931
first, anomalies, 933
forking, and Turner syndrome, 918
fusion
anoxia and (in mice), 34

riboflavin deficiency causing (in rat), 930
lumbar, 933
in syndrome of multiple anomalies, 1000
RIBOFLAVIN
deficiency causing anomalies
cardiovascular (in mammals), 471
cleft lip (in rat), 638
cleft palate (in rat), 639
clubfoot (in rat), 1008
esophageal atresia (in mice), 680
extremity reduction (in rat), 944
fibula (in rat), 1001
hydrocephaly (in mice), 223-224
jaw shortening (in rat), 623
nasal cavity (in rat), 639
oral cavity (in rat), 639
phocomelia (in rat), 953
(in rat), 31, 34
rib fusion (in rat), 930
sternal (in rat), 935
syndactyly (in rat), 972
tibia (in rat), 1001
skeletal defects and, 31
RICKETS
differential diagnosis, 821
in Lowe syndrome, 389
osteopetrosis and, 866
vitamin D-resistant, and craniostenosis, 904
RIEGER DISEASE, 371
RING CHROMOSOMES (*see* Chromosomes)
RITTER DISEASE, 1159
ROCKER BOTTOM FEET IN TRISOMY
13-15, 298
18, 305
ROENTGENOGRAPHY (*see* Radiation)
ROKITANSKY-KÜSTER-HAUSER SYNDROME, 1094
ROKITANSKY LOBES, 607-608
ROSKE-CAFFEY DISEASE (*see* Hyperostosis, infantile cortical)
ROTHMUND-THOMSON SYNDROME, 392-395
cataract in, 392-393
intrauterine growth retardation and, 142
short stature in, 394
skin in, 392-393
RUBELLA, 62-70
clinical manifestations, 65-68
heart disease due to, 459, 464
hydrophthalmia due to, 366-367
immunization
attenuated live virus, 68
passive, 68
intrauterine growth retardation and, 151
mental retardation due to, 263
microcephaly due to, 239
(in monkey), 75
patent ductus arteriosus due to, 464, 556
pathogenesis, 63-65
pathology, 63-65
prevention of, 27, 68-69
prognosis, 68
septal defect due to, 464
stenosis due to, 464
pulmonary, 549
syndrome, 45
cataract in, 45, 64, 65, 66, 375-376
deafness in, 45, 65, 66
ear in, 62, 64, 66, 412-413
as teratogenic agent, 23
tetralogy of Fallot due to, 496
transposition of great vessels due to, 516
virus, 62
RUBEOLA: and teratogenesis, 77
RUBINSTEIN-TAYBI SYNDROME, 1018-1019
clinical characteristics, 1018-1019
facies in, 1019
RUSSEL INTRAUTERINE DWARFISM, 140-141

S

SACROCOCCYGEAL TERATOMA, 1240-1241
SACROLUMBAR MYELOMENINGOCELE, 593
SACRUM
agenesis, 923-925
breech delivery and, 924
classifications, 924-925
incidence, 923
incontinence and, 925
maternal diabetes and, 924
treatment, 925
anomalies, manifestations, 925
meningocele, 920
spot, 1171
SADDLE NOSE, 594
in ectodermal dysplasia, anhidrotic, 1166
SALICYLATE
ear changes due to, 413
eye abnormality due to (in rat), 638
facial cleft due to (in rat), 638
methyl (*see* Methyl salicylate)
sodium (*see* Sodium salicylate)
as teratogen, 35
SALIVARY GLANDS, 666-667
virus disease (*see* Cytomegalic inclusion disease)
SALT, IODIZED
cretinism and, endemic, 30
effect on goiter, 118
SANFILIPPO SYNDROME, 817
SARCOMA, 1236
chondrosarcoma, 1238
osteopetrosis and, 866
osteosarcoma, 1238
osteogenesis imperfecta and, 832
SATAN'S BIRTH OF KRAKOW, 16
SCALP
in progeria, 161
in trisomy 13-15, 298, 301
SCAPHOCEPHALY, 893, 898
clinical characteristics of, 897
SCAPULA
exostosis, 842, 843
in Sprengel deformity, 915
SCHEIE SYNDROME, 817
SCHIZENCEPHALY, 246-248
SCHIZOSOMIA REFLEXUM, 762-763
SCHÜLLER-CHRISTIAN DISEASE, 892
SCHWARTZ-JAMPEL SYNDROME, 1033
SCIMITAR SYNDROME, 567
lung hypoplasia and, 566
SCLERA: in osteogenesis imperfecta, 825, 829
SCLERODERMA: in progeria, 160
SCLEROSIS
(*See also* Tuberous sclerosis)
diaphyseal, in Pyle disease, 871
endocardial, 539
hemangioma and, capillary, 1178
in osteopathia hyperostotica sclerotisans, 845
in osteopetrosis, 863-864
SCOLIOSIS, 920-921
facial, 653
idiopathic, 921-922
clinical characteristics, 921
types, 921
in Klippel-Feil syndrome, 913
methyl salicylate causing (in rat), 917
prognosis, 921
SCREENING
intrauterine processes, 40
natural, and congenital malformations, 40-42
SCROTUM
anomalies, and clefts, 644
bifid, XO/XY mosaicism in, 1118
prepenile, 1104
short, in trisomy 13-15, 298
transposition of penis and scrotum, 1104
SEAL LIMBS (*see* Phocomelia)
SEIZURES: in Sturge-Weber syndrome, 349
SEPTAL DEFECT
atrial, 480-489
anomalous pulmonary venous return and, 567
atrioventricularis communis and, 485
diagrams showing, 483
etiology, 481-483
familial, 460, 481
incidence, 480-481
malformations associated with, 483-484
treatment, 484
in Down syndrome, 577
Ellis-van Creveld syndrome and, 462
in rubella syndrome, 66, 464
in siblings, 461
in trisomy 13-15, 298
ventricular, 489-504
etiology, 490
familial, 460
high, 492
incidence, 489-490
intrauterine growth retardation and, 142
morphogenesis, 490-491
muscular, 492
pathogenesis, 490-491
pathology, 491-492
prognosis, 493
supracristal, 522
symptoms, 492-493
treatment, 493
in trisomy 18, 306
vitamin A deficiency causing (in rat), 470, 491, 607
SEPTUM PELLUCIDUM: anomalies, 254-255
SEX
characteristics, development in male in Laurence-Moon-Biedl syndrome, 177
chromatin, 24
in true hermaphrodism, 1106
chromosomes, 24
anomalies, 1122-1146
in clefts, 632
in heart disease, 463
in mental retardation, 264
-linked inheritance, 58

SEXUAL PRECOCITY (*see* Precocity)
SHOULDER
girdle, hypoplasia of, 959
in syndrome of multiple anomalies, 1190
SIAMESE TWINS
double-headed twin goddess, 6-7
pygopagus type with achondroplasia, 8
SILVER SYNDROME, 139-140
intrauterine growth retardation and, 139-140
SIMIAN LINES: in syndrome of multiple anomalies, 1014
SINUS
tracts, cranial dermal, 213-214
of Valsalva, aneurysm, 548
SIRENIFORM MALFORMATION: due to trypan blue (in rat), 923
SITUS INVERSUS, 183-186
bronchiectasis in, 186
with nose anomalies, 602-603
dextrocardia and, 477-478
etiology, 478
heart (in rat), 185
incidence, 183
levocardia and, 479
partial, and asplenia, 746
pathology, 478-479
recognition of, 186
roentgenogram of, 183
stomach in, 689
(in rat), 185
studies (in animals), 184-185
trypan blue causing (in rat), 184
twinning and, 184
SKELETON
defects, and riboflavin, 31
dysplasia in otopalatodigital syndrome, 677
malformations
axial and appendicular skeleton, 887-1022
cardiovascular malformations and, 571-573
cataract and, 375
in Fanconi anemia, 1020-1021
microphthalmia and, 358
systemic, 765-886
uncertain etiology, 872-886
in trisomy 18, 308
SKIN
anomalies, 1147-1196
case reviews, 1149
cataract and, 376
mandibulofacial dysostosis and, unilateral, 654
prognosis, 1149-1150
vascular, 1176-1186
collodion, 1160
in cretinism, 111
in Ehlers-Danlos syndrome, 1187
in hemihypertrophy, 163-164
lesions, pigmented, 1168-1176
loose, in trisomy 18, 305
neurofibromatosis, 1253
in progeria, 161
in Rothmund-Thomson syndrome, 392-393
in sclerosis, tuberous, 1262
in trisomy 13-15, 1150
in Turner syndrome, 1125
male, 1133
webs, 1189-1192
SKULL, 889-906
bulging, 889
in cleidocranial dysostosis, 837-838
fibrous dysplasia, 877
after intrauterine growth retardation, 911
lacunar, 890
in osteogenesis imperfecta, 830
in osteopsathyrosis, 832
thinning, 889
tower, 893, 901
SMALLPOX: and teratogenesis, 76
SMITH-LEMLI-OPITZ SYNDROME: and pseudohermaphrodism, 1121
SODIUM SALICYLATE
ductus arteriosus stenosis due to (in rat), 554
exencephaly due to (in rat), 419
pituitary absence due to (in rat), 419
pituitary dystopia due to (in rat), 430
SOFT TISSUE TUMORS, 1235-1238
SPEECH
(*See also* Deaf-mutism)
defect
in cretinism, 114
microcephaly and, 240
SPIDER NEVI, 1181
SPINA BIFIDA, 272-291
adrenal fusion and, 431
anencephaly and, 285
anterior, thoracic, 286
aperta (in rat), 276
Arnold-Chiari malformation and, 285
clubfeet and, 1006
cystica, 920
definition, 272
hydrocephaly and, 284
incidence, 272-273
developmental stages of, 275-276
"environmental" factors in, 40
etiology, 273-275
exstrophia splanchnica and, 713
hydrocephaly and, 220
lumbosacral (in rat), 277
nursing care in, 288
occulta
anterior thoracic, symptoms, 286
definition, 272, 273
diastematomyelia and, 292
hair over, with diaphragmatic hernia, 284
incidence, 272
pathology, 282-283
prognosis, 288
prognosis, genetic, 288
streptonigrin causing, (in rat), 293
symptoms, 285-288
optic atrophy and, 380
pathogenesis, 275-282
pathology, 282-285
rachischisis and, 285
(in rat), 224-225
treatment, 288-289
trypan blue causing (in rat), 33, 274, 275, 278, 282
uterine prolapse and, 1090
SPINE, 916-929
in achondroplasia, 777
in anencephaly, 195, 198
angioma, in Hippel-Lindau disease, 1267
anomalies, 918-919
classification, 920
of column, genetic and environmental factors in, 918
of cord, 272-296
trypan blue causing (in rat), 925
cleft, 195, 198
column, anomalies, genetic and environmental factors in, 918
cord
malformations, 272-296
in syringomyelia, 294
development of, 916
in Hurler syndrome, 813
in iniencephaly, 234
in Klippel-Feil syndrome, 910-911
lumbar (*see* Lumbar)
in maternal diabetes, 124
in situs inversus, 186
tumors, 1217
SPINOUS PROCESSES: cleft, 922
SPLEEN, 745-751
absence, 745
etiology, 747
inheritance in, 747
sex distribution, 747
accessory spleens, 748
agenesis, 745-748
cysts, 749
development, 745
double, 748
-gonadal fusion, 749-750
hemangioma, 749
hypoplasia, 748
wandering, 748-749
SPLIT FEET, 963-965
pedigree in, 25, 965
SPLIT HAND, 963-965
pedigree in, 965
SPONDYLITIS: ankylosing, 922
SPONDYLO-EPIPHYSEAL DYSPLASIA, 783-786
tarda form, 805
SPONDYLOLISTHESIS, 922
SPONDYLOTHORACIC DYSPLASIA, 937
SPONGE KIDNEY, 1043
SPOON HAND, 974
SPORADIC: definition, 4
SPOTTED BONES, 846
SPRENGEL DEFORMITY, 915
etiology, 915
Klippel-Feil syndrome and, 911, 912
treatment, 915
STAPEDIAL
arteries, persistent, 405
muscle, tendon of, 406
STAPES, 405
STATISTICS, 38-43
problems with, 38-43
STATUS DYSRAPHICUS, 292-296
discussion of term, 294
heterochromia and, 370
STEIDELE COMPLEX, 532-533
STENOCEPHALY (*see* Craniostenosis)
STENOSIS
anus, 711
aortic, 539-542
associated malformations, 540
classification, 539
etiology, 539-540
familial, 539
prognosis, 540
sex distribution, 540
subvalvar, and cardiomegaly, 542
supravalvar, 541

supravalvar, complex, discussion of, 578-580
supravalvar, facial anomalies and, 578-580
supravalvar, familial, 460
supravalvar, hypercalcemia and, 578-580
symptoms, 540
treatment, 540
aqueduct, and myelomeningocele, 285
bile ducts, 718
cor triatriatum and, 487
in Cornelia de Lange syndrome, 345
craniostenosis (*see* Craniostenosis)
ductus arteriosus, sodium salicylate causing (in rat), 554
duodenum, in Down syndrome, 694
esophagus, 683
symptoms, 683
treatment, 683
medullary, dwarfism and tetany, 792
mitral, 509-510
associated malformations, 510
etiology, 509
incidence, 509
pathology, 509
prognosis, 510
symptoms, 509-510
treatment, 510
pulmonary, 549-553
etiology, 549-550
in rubella syndrome, 66, 464
in siblings, 461
in tetralogy of Fallot, 497
pulmonary, with normal aortic root, 551-553
dome-shaped, 551
incidence, 551
pathogenesis, 551
pathology, 551-552
symptoms, 552
treatment, 552
pyloric, hypertrophic, 687-688
etiology, 687
familial, 687
incidence, 687
manifestations, 687
Ramsted operation in, 688
tenovaginitis, 978
trachea, 599
urethral meatus, 1083
STERNOCLEIDOMASTOID MUSCLE: anomalies, 1026
STERNUM
anomalies (in rat), 31
riboflavin deficiency causing, 935
fissure, 933-934
STILLBIRTH: incidence of anomalies in, 39
STIPPLED EPIPHYSES, 797-800
STOICS: and teratology, 11
STOMACH, 686-690
atresia, prepyloric, 686-687
surgery, 686-687
symptoms, 686
diverticula, 689
duplication, 688
hemorrhage in liver fibrosis, 726
malformations
cardiovascular malformations and, 571
oro-gastrointestinal tract, 659-735
musculature, defect of, 688
obstruction, 686
perforation, 688
polyposis, 689, 714
pyloric stenosis, 687
in situs inversus, 689
(in rat), 185
teratoma, 689, 1242
thoracic cysts, 696, 697
thoracic, partial, 684-685
natural history, 685
in trisomy 18, 307
ulcer, and multiple endocrine neoplasia, 1269-1270
STRABISMUS: in Down syndrome, 326-327
STRAWBERRY MARK, 1176-1179
STREBLODACTYLY, 984
STREPTOCOCCAL INFECTIONS: and congenital anomalies, 60
STREPTOMYCIN, 99, 127
ear changes due to, 414
STREPTONIGRIN, 51
adenohypophysis abnormality due to (in rat), 421
adrenal ectopia due to (in rat), 429, 431
agnathus due to (in rat), 622
anophthalmia due to (in rat), 360
coloboma due to (in rat), 360
craniopharyngeal canal due to (in rat), 421
dwarfism due to (in rat), 150
ectopia cordis due to (in rat), 475
eye abnormality due to (in rat), 364
horseshoe kidney due to (in rat), 1057
hydronephrosis due to (in rat), 1057
hydroureter due to (in rat), 1057
iniencephaly due to (in rat), 717
microphthalmia due to (in rat), 360
myelodysplasia due to (in rat), 293
omphalocele (exomphalos) due to (in rat), 717, 761
otocephaly due to (in rat), 622
spina bifida occulta due to (in rat), 293
undescended testes due to (in rat), 429
vertebral anomalies due to (in rat), 924
absence of vertebrae, 924
STROPHOSOMIA, 762-763
STUMP FORMATIONS (*see* Peromelia)
STUNTING
in Bloom syndrome, 157-159
ethionine causing (in rat), 150
STURGE-WEBER SYNDROME, 349-352
clinical characteristic, 350-351
eye in, 383
SUBCLAVIAN ARTERY (*see* Arteries, subclavian)
SUBDURAL HEMATOMA (*see* Hematoma)
SUBLINGUAL GLAND ENLARGEMENT: in trisomy 18, 667
SUBLUXATION: and hip dislocation, 994-995
SUPRAVALVAR AORTIC STENOSIS, 578
"SYDNEY LINE," 67
SYMBRACHYDACTYLY, 968, 970-971
incidence, 970
inheritance in, 971
SYMPHALANGY, 969-970
clinical characteristics, 969
inheritance in, 970
morphogenesis of, 970
pedigree in, 969
SYMPODIA, 950-951
SYNCHRONISMS: of malformations, 45
SYNDACTYLY, 971-974
in acrocephalosyndactyly, 899-901
ano-rectal malformations and, 695
bilateral, of third and fourth fingers, 973
brachydactyly and, 968
in Carpenter syndrome, 973
cataract and, 375
clinical characteristics, 971
discussion of term, 939
fourth and fifth fingers, 972
high palate in, 645
in Laurence-Moon-Biedl syndrome, 973
lobster claw and, 966
Poland, 963, 1025, 1026
clinical characteristics, 973
radiography, 900
riboflavin deficiency causing (in rat), 972
in syndrome of multiple anomalies, 895, 1026, 1190
total, 972-973
SYNDROMES, 43-48
(*See also specific syndromes*)
classification, 44
by anatomic anomalies, 44
by chemical properties, 44
by embryonic origin of pathology, 44
eponymic nomenclature, 46
by histology, 44
embryologic time tables and, 50-51
hemisyndromes, 162-170
terminologies for, 45
SYNGNATHIA: epithelial, 627
SYNOPHTHALMIA: and agnathus, 621
SYNORCHIDISM, 1101
SYNOSTOSIS, 984-986
in achondroplasia, 774
fibula, 842
radio-ulnar, 962, 985-986
tibia, 842
SYNOTIA (*see* Otocephaly)
SYNTROPISMS: of malformations, 45
SYPHILIS
differential diagnosis, 886
hydrocephaly and, 218-219
SYRINGOMYELIA, 294-295
discussion of term, 293, 294
in Down syndrome, 325
familial, 294
heterochromia and, 370
manifestations, 294
spinal cord in, 294
symptoms, 294
SYRINGOMYELOCELE, 279
definition, 272, 273

T

TAILS (*see* Caudal appendages)
TALIPES
definition, 1004
equinovarus (see Clubbing, feet)
renal agenesis and, bilateral, 1038
TAPETORETINAL DEGENERATIONS, 378-379
TARSAL: craniocarpotarsal dystrophy, 673-674
TASTE: in Turner syndrome, 1127
TEETH
anomalies
cataract and, 376

TEETH *(cont.)*
craniofacial dysostosis and, 902-903
dermal hypoplasia and, focal, 1195-1196
microphthalmia and, 358
in cretinism, 111
in ectodermal dysplasia, anhidrotic, 1166
in epidermolysis bullosa, 1154
"giant," 164
in hemihypertrophy, 164
oculodentodigital dysplasia, 388-389
in Pierre Robin syndrome, 656
in progeria, 160
in rubella syndrome, 64, 67
TELANGIECTASIA
(*See also* Nevi flammeus)
-ataxia (*see* Ataxia-telangiectasia)
conjuctivae, 1180
erythema and Bloom syndrome, 157-159
hemorrhagic, hereditary, 1185
superficial, 1179
TEMPOROMANDIBULAR JOINT: anomalies, 627
TENDON
extensor, of hand, aplasia, 978
of stapedius muscle, 406
TENOVAGINITIS: stenosing, 978
TERATOGEN(S)
definition, 3
exogenous, and intrauterine growth retardation, 149-151
experimental, viruses as, 75-76
hormones as, 34
TERATOGENESIS
critical periods in, 49-52
embryologic theory in, 22
infections and, 76-78
nosologic theory in, 22-23
sensitive periods in, 49-52
TERATOGENIC: definition, 3
TERATOID PARASITES: of mouth, 668
TERATOLOGY
in antiquity, 6-20
Aristotle and, 17-18
in Babylonia, 11
biologic theories in antiquity, 17-19
Caesar and, 11
Down syndrome and, 21
epidemiology and, 26-27
experimental
drug testing and, 101-102
mammalian, 29-37
mammalian, and nutrition, 30
Fabricius ab Aquapendente on, 18
Harvey on, 18
history of, 3
images, 6-7
Mendel and, 19
omens in animals, 10
Pliny the Elder and, 18
present trends, 21-29
Stoics and, 11
TERATOMA, 1239-1247
cervical, 1241
etiology, 1239, 1242-1243
heart, 1242
intracranial, 1215-1216, 1241
intrapericardial, 1242
kidney, 1242
liver, 728, 1242
manifestations, 1239
mediastinum, 1240
multiple, 1244
orbital, 1242
ovaries, 1229, 1239-1240
paravertebral, 1242
pineal, 452
pituitary, 424
precocious puberty and, 454
pulmonary, 1242
retroperitoneal, 1241
sacrococcygeal, 1240-1241
stomach, 689, 1242
testes, 1230, 1240
tonsil, 667
in twins, 1244
TESTES, 1098-1102
absence, 1098
adenoma, in testicular feminization syndrome, 1116
anomalies, and clefts, 644
development, 1098-1099
intratubular bodies, 1101
supernumerary, 1101
teratoma, 1230, 1240
tumors, 1229-1230
classification, 1230
undescended, 1098-1101
(in animals), 1100
chromosomal anomalies in, 1099
incidence, 1099
inguinal hernia and, 1100
inheritance in, 1099
mechanisms leading to, 1099
muscle anomalies and, 1029
parietal foramina enlargement and, 891
in Prader-Willi syndrome, 182
sacral agenesis and, 923
streptonigrin causing (in rat), 429
in syndrome of multiple anomalies, 932, 1099-1100
testicular tumors and, 1230
treatment, 1100-1101
true, 1100
in Turner syndrome, male, 1133
in twins, 1099
uncomplicated, 1100
vitamin A deficiency causing (in rat), 1051
XO/XY mosaicism in, 1118
TESTICULAR FEMINIZATION
incomplete forms, 1116-1117
syndrome, 1114-1116
incidence, 1114
testicular adenoma in, 1116
testosterone, estrogen, and LH in, 1115-1116
XY karyotype, 1116
tumors and, 1232
TESTOSTERONE: and testicular feminization syndrome, 1115
TETANY: dwarfism and medullary stenosis, 792
TETRA-AMELIA, 949
TETRALOGY OF FALLOT, 494-502, 517-518
aortic enlargement in, 497
associated malformations, 499
Blalock-Taussig operation in, 501
clubbing of fingers and toes in, 499
course, 499-500
etiology, 496
incidence, 495-496
history, 494-495
hypertrophic right ventricle in, 497
pathogenesis, 496-497
pathology, 497-499
Peacock's description, 495
Potts anastomosis in, 501
pregnancy and, 500
prognosis, 499-500
radiography, 500
rubella causing, 496
shunt operations in, 501
symptoms, 498-499
treatment, 500-501
Waterston operation in, 501
TETRAPEROMELIA, 954
TETRAPHOCOMELIA, 951
TETRA-X, 1140-1141
THALIDOMIDE, 23, 26, 27, 35, 45, 47, 84-96
embryopathy, 85-95
cardiovascular system in, 92
clubfoot in (in rabbit), 1008
diagnosis, differential, 94
ear in, 89, 94, 413, 414-415
extremity anomalies in, 85-93, 941
eye in, 383
face in, 92
gallbladder agenesis and, 722
genital tract in, 93
heart disease in, 465-466
hip dislocation in, 92
intestinal tract in, 93
microphthalmia in, 94
(in monkey), 86
pyloric hypertrophy and, 688
(in rabbit), 85-86
in twins, 95
urinary tract in, 92-93
THANATOPHORIC DWARFISM, 768
THIOURACIL: maternal use, causing goiter and hypothyroidism, 442-443
THORACIC
(*See also* Chest)
cysts, gastric, 696, 697
dystrophy, asphyxiating, 795-796
stomach, partial, 684-685
natural history, 685
THORACOPAGUS: esophageal and gastric duplication in, 697
THORACOSCHISIS: in antiquity, 10
THROMBOCYTOPENIA
in cytomegalic inclusion disease, 72
hemangioma and, giant, 1179
hypoplastic, and phocomelia, 941
leukemoid reactions in, 952
in rubella syndrome, 65
THUMB
absence, 953, 976-977
bifid, 981
broad, 977
in Rubinstein-Taybi syndrome, 1018-1019
clubbed, 967
clutched, 978
duplication, 980-982
in Carpenter syndrome, 981
floating, 977
Potter's, 977
short, 967
snapping, 978
trigger, 978
triphalangeal, 977-978
in trisomy 13-15, 298
THYMINE, 25
THYMO-PARATHYROID APLASIA, 740
THYMUS, 739-744
absence, 739

trypan blue causing (in rat), 743
agenesis, 739-740
cervical, and hypervitaminosis A (in mice), 742
in cretinism, endemic, 113
cysts, 742
development, 739
horn, 741
hypoplasia, 740-741
in leprechaunism, 159
position abnormalities, 741-743
remnants in neck, 741
retrosternal (in mice), 742
shape abnormalities, 741-743
THYROID, 437-444
agenesis, partial, 664
in Albright syndrome, 880
carcinoma, and multiple endocrine neoplasia, 1270
in cretinism, 111
endemic, 111
development, 437
anomalies of, 664
disease, maternal, 126
Down syndrome and, 60
ectopia, 438-442
athyrosis and, 438
hypoplasia, 664
insufficiency, in lingual thyroid, 664
lingual, 664
clinical characteristics, 664
tumors, 1219-1220
TIBIA
absence, 1000
anomalies, 998-1002
inheritance in, 999
riboflavin deficiency causing (in rat), 1001
sex distribution, 999
exostoses, 842
kyphoscoliosis, 1002
pseudarthrosis, 1000-1001
reduction-polydactyly syndrome, 1000
vara, 1001-1002
TIERFELLNAEVUS, 1170
TOE
(*See also* Digits)
amputations, 945
ankyloglossia and, 661
big (*see* first *below*)
clubbing (*see* Clubbing, toes)
in Cornelia de Lange syndrome, 346
in Crouzon craniofacial dysostosis, 903
in Down syndrome, 330-331
fifth, duplications, 982
first
anomalies, 1000
duplication, 980-982
in Rubinstein-Taybi syndrome, 1018-1019
median, duplications, 983
second, macrodactyly, 985
in trisomy 18, 308
TONGUE
absence, in antiquity, 10
accessory, 663
anomalies due to hypervitaminosis A (in mice), 661
bifid, 663
clefts, 663
in orodigitofacial syndrome, 675
cysts, 666
development, 635
in Down syndrome, 327
in hemihypertrophy, 164
long, 663
in orodigitofacial syndrome, 675
in Pierre Robin syndrome, 655
protruding, and sporadic cretinism, 440
in visceromegaly, 172
TONSIL: teratoma, 667
TORTICOLLIS, 1028-1030
etiology, 1028
incidence, 1028-1029
muscular, 1030
postural, 1030
treatment, 1030
tumor in, 1030
in twins, 1029
TORUS
buccalis, 665
mandibularis, 665-666
palatinus, 665
TOWER SKULL, 893, 901
TOXEMIA: and intrauterine growth retardation, 147
TOXOPLASMOSIS, 78-81
congenital, three stages of, frequencies of, 80
ear in, 413
eye, 381-382
hydrocephaly due to, 218, 220
incidence, 79
macula and, 379
microcephaly due to, 239
optic atrophy after, 380
as teratogenic agent, 23
in twins, 80
TRACHEA
absence, 599
constrictions, 599
development of, 681
diverticula, 599-600
double aortic arch surrounding, 530
fistula, 600
hemangioma, 599
laryngotracheo-esophageal cleft, 597-598
segmentation of cartilaginous skeleton, 599
separation from esophagus, diagram, 681
stenosis, 599
TRACHEAL BRONCHI, 600-601
TRACHEOBILIARY FISTULA, 723
TRACHEO-ESOPHAGEAL FISTULA (*see* Fistula, tracheo-esophageal)
TRANSLOCATIONS OF CHROMOSOMES, 59
intrauterine growth retardation and, 145
TRANSPOSITION
of great vessels, 515-525
associated malformations, 522
chromosome anomalies and, 516
classifications, 515
classifications, by Keith, 521
corrected, 523-524
corrected, life expectancy in, 524
corrected, symptoms, 524
corrected, treatment, 524
definitions, 515
digitalis in, 523
in Down syndrome, 577
etiology, 515
incidence, 515
oxygen and, 523
rubella causing, 516
sex distribution, 516
Spitzer's theory concerning, 518
symptoms, 522-523
trypan blue causing (in rat), 520
types, 517-518
single ventricle and, 504
TRAPEZIUS MUSCLE: anomalies, 1026
TRAUMA: and brain tumors, 1210
TREACHER COLLINS SYNDROME (*see* Mandibulofacial dysostosis)
TRIAZENE: as teratogen, 35
TRICHO-RHINO-PHALANGEAL SYNDROME, 1020
TRICUSPID VALVE
atresia, 505-506
incidence, 505
prognosis, 506
symptoms, 506
treatment, 506
types, 505
cleft, and atrioventricularis communis, 485
duplication, 506-507
hypoplasia, 506
insufficiency, 506
malformations, 505-508
TRIGGER THUMB, 978
TRIGONOCEPHALY, 904
ambiguous genitalia and, 897
arhinencephaly and, 209-210
TRIPLOIDY, 59, 343-344
intrauterine growth retardation and, 145
maternal hormonal imbalance and, 59
TRIPLO-X, 1140-1141
TRISOMY, 58
autosomal, 58
coarctation of aorta and, 544
D_1 syndrome, 58
D_1 (*see* 13-15 *below*)
18, 45, 303-310
birth weights in, 146
brain in, 268
cerebellar malformations in, 267-268
clefts in, 632
clinical characteristics, 305-309
ear in, 409
gallbladder hypoplasia in, 722
heart disease in, 462
history, 303
horseshoe kidney in, 1050
intrauterine growth retardation in, 145
karyotype in, 304
myelomeningocele in, 281
pathologic characteristics, 305-309
sublingual gland enlargement in, 667
triplo-X in, 1140
E syndrome, 58, 303-310
microcephaly and, 240
omphalocele and, 759
patent ductus arteriosus and, 556
13-15, 45, 58, 296-303
arhinencephaly in, 201
cerebellar malformations in, 267-268
chromosomes in, 297
clefts in, 632, 643
corpus callosum hypoplasia and absence in, 252
cyclopia in, 201-202
ear in, 410
heart disease in, 462
history, 296-297

TRISOMY (*cont.*)
incidence, 297
intrauterine growth retardation in, 145
karyotype in, 299
microphthalmia in, 357
nose in, 595
skin anomalies in, 1150
21 (*see* Down syndrome)
ventricular septal defect and, 490
TRUNCUS ARTERIOSUS, PERSISTENT, 512-514
aspirin causing (in rat), 513
associated malformations, 514
incidence, 512
pathology, 512-513
prognosis, 514
sex distribution, 512
symptoms, 513-514
treatment, 514
types, 512
TRYPAN BLUE, 33
aortic arch anomalies due to (in rat), 471
corpus callosum absence due to (in rat), 253
dextrocardia due to (in rat), 478
fornix absence due to (in rat), 253
hydrocephaly due to (in rat), 222-223
imperforate anus due to (in rat), 710
myelodysplasia due to (in rat), 293
pharyngeal pituitary due to (in rat), 422
sireniform malformation due to (in rat), 923
situs inversus due to (in rat), 184
spina bifida due to (in rat), 274, 275, 278, 282
spinal anomalies due to (in rat), 925
thymic absence due to (in rat), 743
transposition of great vessels due to (in rat), 520
TUBERCULOSIS
maternal, 127
pulmonary, inheritance in, 25
TUBEROUS SCLEROSIS, 1260-1265
(*See also* Sclerosis)
anticonvulsants in, 1264
brain in, 1261
convulsions in, 1264
eye in, 382
heart tumors and, 582
histology, 1261
inheritance in, 1260-1261
kidney lesions and, 1065
manifestations, 1262
mouth in, 667
phakoma and, 1263
rhabdomyoma and, 1262-1263
rhabdomyoma and, heart, 1236
in siblings, 1264
skull in, 1263-1264
tumors and, 1237
in twins, 1261
TUBES: fallopian, 1091
TUMORS, 1197-1247
adrenals (*see* Adrenals, tumors)
basal cell nevi syndrome and, 1269
bladder, 1079
bone, 1238
brain (*see* Brain)
CNS, 1209
embryonal, etiology, 1201
as embryonal rests, 1200
environmental oncogenic factors, 1203-1204
etiology, 1200
Anderson on, 1200
Cohnheim on, 1201
Ewing on, 1200
Wells on, 1201
Willis on, 1200-1201
genital anomalies and, 1231-1235
glomus, 1185-1186
multiple, 1237
gonads (*see* Gonads, tumors)
heart, 582-583, 1220-1221
heart disease associated with, 582
hemihypertrophy and, 165
interstitial cell, 1230
intrauterine growth retardation and, 142-143
jaw, 667
kidney, 1228-1229
Laurence-Moon-Biedl syndrome and, 180
Leydig cell, 1230
liver, 727-728, 1222-1223
lung, 615-616
malformations and, 1197-1247
mesenchymal, 1236
mouth, 667-668
teratoid, 1241-1242
multiple primary, 1202-1203
ovaries, 1229
pancreas, 731
pathology, 1199-1200
pharynx, teratoid, 1241-1242
pineal, 451-452
sex distribution, 451
polydactyly and, 980
Rathke pouch, 1214-1215
respiratory tract, 1221-1222
soft tissue, 1235-1238
spine, 1217
testes, 1229-1230
classification, 1230
thyroid, 1219-1220
torticollis and, 1030
Wilms (*see* Wilms tumor)
TURMSCHÄDEL, 893
TURNER SYNDROME, 1122-1136
clefts and, 632
coarctation and, 544
cubitus valgus in, 1128
Cushing syndrome and, 1129
ear in, 410
gonadal tumors and, 1233
hemivertebrae, block vertebrae and rib forking, 918
history, 1122-1123
intrauterine growth retardation and, 146
karyotype in, 1130
male, 1131-1134
ear anomalies and, 1066
familial, 1134
gonadal tumors and, 1234
neck webbing and, 1131-1132
undescended testes in, 1099
mental retardation and, 264
ovaries in, hypoplastic, 1086
X chromosome absence in, 58
XO, 1124-1131
clinical characteristics, 1125-1127
lymphatic hypoplasia and lymphedema in, 1126
TURRICEPHALY, 893
craniostenosis causing, 898-899
TWINS
(*See also* Multiple birth)
anencephaly in, 191
anomalies in, 39
clefts, 630-631
palate, 641
pedigree in, 631
cleidocranial dysostosis in, 836-837
clubfeet in, 1007
dextrocardia in, 478
dizygotic, effects of prenatal rubella, 64
Down syndrome and, 314-315
esophageal atresia and, 679
gonadal dysgenesis in, 1131
harelip in, bilateral, 641
heart disease in, 466
hydrocephaly in, 218-219
hypsicephaly in, 894
ichthyosis simplex in, 1157
intrauterine growth retardation in, 151
Marfan syndrome in, 852
neurofibromatosis in, Recklinghausen, 1252-1253
partial twinning in amphibia, 697
patent ductus arteriosus and, 556
sclerosis in, tuberous, 1261
Siamese (*see* Siamese twins)
situs inversus and, 184
teratoma, 1244
thalidomide embryopathy of, 95
torticollis in, 1029
toxoplasmosis of, 80
undescended testes in, 1099
TYLOSIS: palmaris et plantaris, 1161
TYPUS AMSTELODAMENSIS (*see* Cornelia de Lange syndrome)
TYPUS ROSTOCKIENSIS: and pseudohermaphrodism, 1120-1121

U

ULCER
duplications and, 697
esophagus, 684
gastrointestinal, and multiple endocrine neoplasia, 1269-1270
ULLRICH-FEICHTIGER SYNDROME, 1120-1121
microphthalmia and, 358
ULNA
aplasia, 961
in craniocarpotarsal dystrophy, 673
defects, 961-962
incidence, 961
inheritance in, 961
dimelia, 961-962
duplication, 961-962
hypoplasia, and micromelia, 792
in Ollier disease, 873
pseudarthrosis, and Recklinghausen neurofibromatosis, 1257
radio-ulnar synostosis, 962, 985-986
UMBILICUS, 758-764
artery, single, 763
eventration (*see* Omphalocele)
hernia, 758
in visceromegaly, 172
"UNDERNOURISHED FULL-TERM BABIES," 135-136
URACHAL ANOMALIES, 1077
URETER, 1067-1073

dilation, pyelography, 1067
duplication, 1067, 1068
complete, 1068
incidence, 1068
incomplete, 1068
ectopic, 1068-1070
incidence, 1068
incomplete spur formation, in female, 1069
kidney fusion complicated by, 1052
male, 1069
pathogenesis, 1068-1069
(in rat), 1069
sex distribution, 1068
symptoms, 1069
treatment, 1069-1070
fixed to renal pelvis, in hydronephrosis, 1055
obstruction by hypogastric artery, 1072
retrocaval, 1072
in rubella syndrome, 66
URETEROCELE, 1070
clinical characteristics, 1070
pyuria in, 1070
treatment, 1070
URETHRA, 1080-1084
anomalies, XO/XY mosaicism in, 1118
diaphragms, 1080-1081
diverticula, 1081
double, 697, 1082
fibroelastosis, and bladder neck obstruction, 1078-1079
meatus, stenosis, 1083
obliteration, 1080
obstruction, causing polycystic kidney, 1046
recto-urethral fistula, 1084
strictures, 1080-1081
valves
anterior, 1081
posterior, 1081
URINARY TRACT
anomalies, 1035-1146
abdominal muscle absence and, 1079
anal atresia and, 1083-1084
cardiovascular anomalies and, 574
vitamin A deficiency causing (in animals), 32
in Laurence-Moon-Biedl syndrome, 179
in thalidomide embryopathy, 92-93
in trisomy 18, 307
URINE: double collecting system, pyelography, 1067
UROW DISEASE, 807
URTICARIA PIGMENTOSA, 1173
USHER SYNDROME: deafness in, 407
UTERUS, 1087-1092
absence, 1088
anomalies
classification, 1088
diagrams showing, 1089
aplasia, 1088
arcuatus, 1088
bicornis, 1088-1089
bicollis, 1090
malformations due to, 21
septus, 1087
in syndrome of multiple anomalies, 1077
development, 1087-1088
didelphys, 1087, 1089-1090
hysterosalpingography in, 1089
vagina duplex separata and, 1089-1090
double, 697
growth retardation in (*see* Intrauterine growth retardation)
hand-foot-uterus syndrome, 963
hypoplasia, 1088
prolapse, 1090-1091
pseudodidelphys, 1090
septus, 1088
unicornis, 1090
subseptus, 1087

V

VACCINATION FOR SMALLPOX: and teratogenesis, 76
VAGINA, 1093-1095
absence, 1093-1095
cytogenetics, 1094
etiology, 1094
incidence, 1093
cysts, 1096
development, 1093
double, 697, 1096
uterus didelphys and, 1089-1090
fistula, 1096-1097
septate, 1096
transverse, 1095
VALVES
mitral (*see* Mitral valve)
pulmonary, absence, 549
tricuspid (*see* Tricuspid valve)
urethral (*see* Urethra)
VARICELLA: and teratogenesis, 76
VARICES: esophageal, and polycystic liver, 725
VASCULAR (*see* Vessels)
VEINS
anomalies of venous return, 564-568
pulmonary veins, 565-567
systemic veins, 564-565
arteriovenous fistula (*see* Fistula)
azygos, lobe, 609
cerebral, malformations, 249-250
in goiter, 104
levoatrio-cardinal, anomalies, 564-565
portal
in fistula, 726-727
terminal, absence, 726-727
pulmonary
fistula (*see* Fistula, arteriovenous, pulmonary)
venous connection with inferior vena cava, 566
venous return, partial anomalous, 565-567
pulmonary venous return, total anomalous, 565
malformations associated with, 565
prognosis, 565
surgery, 565
types, 565
VENA CAVA
entering left auricle, 564
inferior
absence, 564
pulmonary vein connection with, 566
superior, persistent left, 564
VENTRICLE
calcification in cytomegalic inclusion disease, 73
cor triloculare biventriculare, 486
in gigantism, cerebral, 173
right, hypertrophy, in tetralogy of Fallot, 497
septum
defect (*see* Septal defect)
persistent truncus arteriosus and, 514
single (*see* Cor triloculare biatriatum)
VENTRICULOGRAPHY: in tuberous sclerosis, 1262
VERATRUM CALCIFORNICUM: causing cyclopia (in lamb), 205
VERTEBRAE
absence due to streptonigrin (in rat), 924
anomalies, 700, 918-919
chromosomal anomalies and, 919
clefts and, 643
craniovertebral, 907-915
genetic influences in, 918-919
heart disease and, 931
mandibulofacial dysostosis and, unilateral, 654
methyl salicylate causing (in rat), 931
streptonigrin causing (in rat), 917
block, 921
clinical characteristics, 921
Turner syndrome and, 918
calcifications, 922
chondrification of, 916
clefts, 921
faulty segmentation of column, 910
fusion, 910
after intrauterine growth retardation, 911
in Klippel-Feil syndrome, 912
megacolon and, 705
in meningocele, 920
in osteopetrosis, 864
in rachischisis, 920
in situs inversus, 186
in syndrome of multiple anomalies, 932, 953, 1000
teratoma, 1242
VERTEBRAL OCULOAURICULO SYNDROME (*see* Goldenhar syndrome)
VERUMONTANUM: hypertrophy, 1081
VESICAL (*see* Bladder)
VESICO-INTESTINAL FISTULA, 714
VESSELS
cerebral, malformations, 249-251
disease, in Turner syndrome, 1127
in Down syndrome, 328, 577
great (*see* Transposition of great vessels)
hamartosis, 1185-1186
intracranial, malformations, 250
malformations, 457-584
antimetabolites causing (in mammals), 471
asplenia and, 745
associated malformations, 568-569
clefts and, 573
cutaneous, 1176-1186
experimental (in mammals), 470-472
gastrointestinal malformations and, 571
genital malformations and, 574
intrauterine growth retardation and, 142
mental complications, 570
metabolic disorders and, 574-576
neurologic complications, 570

VESSELS (*cont.*)
ocular complications, 570
sex distribution, 463
skeletal malformations and, 571-573
systemic disorders involving, 568-581
urinary tract malformations and, 574
vitamin A deficiency causing (in animals), 32, 470-471
in Marfan syndrome, 855
in rubella syndrome, 66
in situs inversus, 186
in thalidomide embryopathy, 92
in trisomy
13-15, 300
18, 306
in Turner syndrome, male, 1132
VESTIBULE: in rubella syndrome, 66
VIRILIZATION, 1226
VIRILIZING ADRENAL HYPERPLASIA (*see* Pseudohermaphrodism, female)
VIRUSES
Coxsackie, and teratogenesis, 77
cytomegaloviruses, studies (in mice), 75
ECHO, and teratogenesis, 77
herpes (*see* Herpes)
leukemia and, 1208
rubella, 63
salivary gland, disease (*see* Cytomegalic inclusion disease)
as teratogens, experimental, 75-76
VISCEROMEGALY, 171-172
adrenal tumor and, 435
omphalocele and, 759
prognosis, 172
VITAMIN A
deficiency
abnormalities due to (in rat), 32
aortic arch anomaly due to (in rat), 470
coloboma due to (in rat), 363
diaphragmatic hernia due to (in rat), 752, 756
esophageal anomaly due to (in rat), 607
eye abnormality due to (in rat), 33
goiter and, 108
horseshoe kidney due to (in rat), 1051
hydronephrosis due to (in rat), 1056
hydroureter due to (in rat), 1056
intrauterine growth retardation and, 149-151
lung agenesis due to (in rat), 605, 607
maternal, 127-128
myocardial hypoplasia due to (in pig), 471
orbital cyst due to (in rat), 365
patent ductus arteriosus due to (in rat), 554
pulmonary artery malformation due to (in rat), 605
right aortic arch due to (in rat), 531
septal defects due to (in rat), 470
septal defects due to, ventricular (in rat), 491, 607
subclavian artery anomaly due to (in rat), 533
(in swine), 30
undescended testes due to (in rat), 1051
resorption, in Down syndrome, 332
as teratogen, 35
VITAMIN D
aortic stenosis and, supravalvar, 579
cretinism and, endemic, 30
deficiency (in swine), 30
-resistant rickets, and craniostenosis, 904
VITAMIN E DEFICIENCY: and congenital malformations, 35
VITELLINE DUCT
persistence, 701-702
remnants, 762
VITREOUS
primary, persistence of, and vitamin A deficiency (in animals), 33
vascular veil in, 378
VOLVULUS, 692
history, 10
mobile cecum and, 693
VOMITING: in intestinal atresia, 695
VON RECKLINGHAUSEN NEUROFIBROMATOSIS (*see* Neurofibromatosis, Recklinghausen)
VULVA
duplication, 1093
fusion, 1093

W

WAARDENBURG SYNDROME, 395-396
anisocoria in, 371
deaf-mutism in, 408
heterochromia in, 371
WATERSTON OPERATION, 501
WEIGHT
birth (*see* Birth weight)
in progeria, 161
WEYERS MANDIBULOFACIAL DYSOSTOSIS (*see* Mandibulofacial dysostosis, unilateral)
WHITE SPONGE NEVUS, 665
WILMS TUMOR, 1061-1064, 1228
bilateral, 1063
etiology, 1063-1064
familial, 1228
mesodermal origin, 1061
pseudohermaphrodism and, 1118
sex distribution, 1061
size, 1062
teratologic origin, 1063
WITCHES, 15-16
WRIST: in syndrome of multiple anomalies, 1190
WRYNECK (*see* Torticollis)

X

X CHROMOSOME, 24
absence in Turner syndrome, 58, 463
duplication and Klinefelter syndrome, 58
penta-X, 1140-1141
tetra-X, 1140-1141
triplo-X, 1140-1141
45/XO karyotype, 1124, 1129, 1130
XO syndrome (*see* Turner syndrome, XO)
XO/XXXY mosaicism, in mixed gonadal dysgenesis, 1138
46,XX karyotype, in male, 1118
XXX, 343
47,XXX karyotype, 1140
45,X/46,XX_1 mosaicism in Klippel-Feil syndrome, 1128
XXXXY
(*See also* Klinefelter syndrome)
intrauterine growth retardation and, 146
XXXY (*see* Klinefelter syndrome)
XXY, 343
(*See also* Klinefelter syndrome)
XY karyotype, in testicular feminization syndrome, 1116
46,XY karyotype, in male, 1113
XANTHOMA: and bile duct atresia, 720
XANTHOMATOSIS: hereditary, and cardiovascular malformations, 575
XANTHURENIC ACID: in Down syndrome, 332
XERODERMA PIGMENTOSUM, 1173-1174
racial distribution, 1173-1174
X-RAY
(*See also* Radiation)
diagnostic
achondroplasia, 769, 776, 778
acrocephalosyndactyly, 900, 1003
Albright syndrome, 880
annular pancreas, 731
arthrogryposis, 1013, 1014-1015
asphyxiating thoracic dystrophy, 796
azygos lobe, 609
basal angle of Boogaard, 908
basilar impression, 907-908
bifid nose, 589
cervical rib, 932
chondrodystrophia calcificans congenita, 800
cleidocranial dysostosis, 838
cretinism, 111
cytomegalic inclusion disease, 72-73
damage to fetus by, 83
diastematomyelia, 291-292
diastrophic dwarfism, 803
Ellis-van Creveld syndrome, 795
exostoses, 842, 843, 844
fibrous dysplasia of bone, 876
gastric atresia, prepyloric, 686
gastric musculature defect, 688
gigantism, cerebral, 173
Hurler syndrome, 813, 814-815
hypophosphatasia, 860
Madelung deformity, 790
Marfan syndrome, 855-856
megacolon, 708
melorheostosis, 884
metatropic dwarfism, 803-804
Morquio disease, 821
myositis ossificans progressiva, 975
nail-patella syndrome, 1017
orodigitofacial syndrome, 674-675
osteoarthropathy, hereditary hypertrophic, 848-849
osteopathia hyperostotica sclerotisans, 844-845
osteopetrosis, 866-867
phocomelia, 951
progeria, 161
pseudohypoparathyroidism, 447
pulmonary arteriovenous fistula, 614
pulmonary cyst, 612
pulmonary venous return, total anomalous, 565
pyknodysostosis, 869
Pyle disease, 870

right aortic arch, 532
sacral agenesis, 923
scaphocephaly, 898
scimitar syndrome and lung hypoplasia, 566
situs inversus, 183
skull and vertebra after intrauterine growth retardation, 911
spondylolisthesis, 922
Sturge-Weber syndrome, 350, 351
tetralogy of Fallot, 500
tower skull, 901
tracheo-esophageal fistula, 682
Turner syndrome, 1128
vertebra in Klippel-Feil syndrome, 912

Y

Y Chromosome, 58
duplication of, 58
46, XY karyotype, in male, 1113
XYY, 343
XYY karyotype in Marfan syndrome, 1144
XYY and XYYY, 1144

Z

Zygodactyly, 972
Zygote, formation, 55
from germ cell, diagram, 317